T025446

KU-160-502

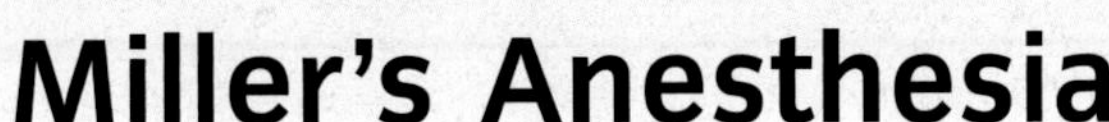

Miller's Anesthesia

Volume 1

Miller's Anesthesia

Seventh Edition

Edited by

Ronald D. Miller, MD

Professor and Chair, Department of
Anesthesia and Perioperative Care
Professor of Cellular and Molecular Pharmacology
University of California, San Francisco, School of Medicine
San Francisco, California

Associate Editors

Lars I. Eriksson, MD, PhD

Professor and Academic Chair
Department of Anaesthesiology and Intensive Care Medicine
Karolinska University Hospital, Solna
Stockholm, Sweden

Lee A. Fleisher, MD

Robert Dunning Dripps Professor and Chair
Department of Anesthesiology and Critical Care
Professor of Medicine
University of Pennsylvania School of Medicine
Philadelphia, Pennsylvania

Jeanine P. Wiener-Kronish, MD

Henry Isaiah Dorr Professor of Research and Teaching in
Anaesthetics and Anaesthesia
Harvard Medical School
Anesthetist-in-Chief
Massachusetts General Hospital
Boston, Massachusetts

William L. Young, MD

James P. Livingston Professor and Vice Chair
Department of Anesthesia and Perioperative Care
Professor of Neurological Surgery and Neurology
Director, UCSF Center for Cerebrovascular Research
University of California, San Francisco, School of Medicine
San Francisco, California

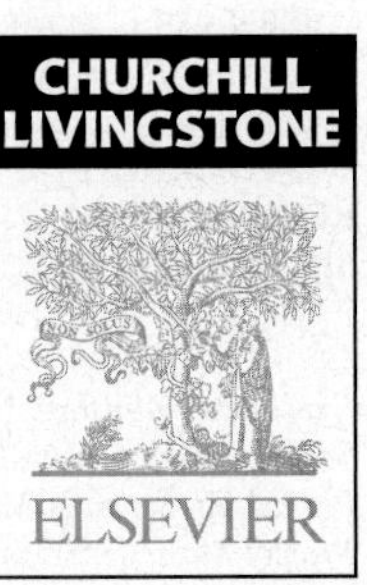

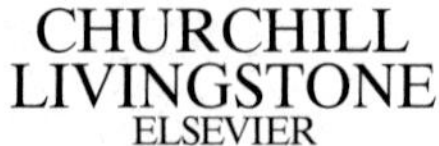

1600 John F. Kennedy Blvd.
Ste 1800
Philadelphia, PA 19103-2899

MILLER'S ANESTHESIA

ISBN: 978-0-443-06959-8
Premium Edition ISBN: 978-1-4160-6624-8
International Edition ISBN: 978-0-8089-2413-5

Notice

Knowledge and best practice in this field are constantly changing. As new research and experience broaden our knowledge, changes in practice, treatment, and drug therapy may become necessary or appropriate. Readers are advised to check the most current information provided (i) on procedures featured or (ii) by the manufacturer of each product to be administered, to verify the recommended dose or formula, the method and duration of administration, and contraindications. It is the responsibility of the practitioner, relying on his or her own experience and knowledge of the patient, to make diagnoses, to determine dosages and the best treatment for each individual patient, and to take all appropriate safety precautions. To the fullest extent of the law, neither the publisher nor the editors assume any liability for any injury and/or damage to persons or property arising out of or related to any use of the material contained in this book.

The Publisher

Note to the Reader

As this edition of *Miller's Anesthesia* was being released to press, a far-reaching fraud involving a researcher in the field of perioperative analgesia came to light, leading to numerous retractions of articles published by several leading anesthesiology journals.[1] Although none of the chapters in this edition cite this research, the readers are advised to continually review the latest literature on the state of knowledge relevant to the practice of anesthesiology.[2]

1. Shafer SL: Tattered threads (editorial). Anesth Analg 108(5), 2009.
2. White PF, Kehlet H, Liu S: Perioperative analgesia: What do we still know? (editorial). Anesth Analg 108(5), 2009.

The Editors

Previous editions copyrighted 2005, 2000, 1994, 1990, 1986, 1981

Library of Congress Cataloging-in-Publication Data
Miller's anesthesia / edited by Ronald D. Miller ; consulting editors,
Lars I. Eriksson … [et al.].—7th ed.
p. ; cm.
Includes bibliographical references and index.
ISBN 978-0-443-06959-8
1. Anesthesia–Atlases. I. Miller, Ronald D. II. Title: Anesthesia.
[DNLM: 1. Anesthesia. 2. Anesthesiology–methods. 3. Anesthetics–therapeutic use.
WO 200 M651 2010]
RD81.M646 2010
617.9′6–dc22

2009010750

Executive Publisher: Natasha Andjelkovic
Senior Developmental Editor: Heather Krehling
Publishing Services Manager: Tina Rebane
Project Manager: Fran Gunning
Design Direction: Steven Stave

Printed in The United States of America

Last digit is the print number: 9 8 7 6 5 4 3 2 1

Contributors

Ted G. Abel, PhD
Professor, Department of Biology, University of Pennsylvania, Philadelphia, Pennsylvania

Olga N. Afonin, MD
Assistant Clinical Professor, Department of Anesthesia and Perioperative Care, University of California, San Francisco, School of Medicine, San Francisco, California

Paul D. Allen, BA, MS(hon), MD, PhD
Professor of Anaesthesia, Harvard Medical School; Senior Anesthesiologist, Brigham and Women's Hospital, Boston, Massachusetts

J. Jeffrey Andrews, MD
Professor and Chair, Department of Anesthesiology, University of Texas Health Sciences Center at San Antonio, San Antonio, Texas

Michael Ang-Lee, MD
Staff Anesthesiologist, Pacific Anesthesia, Bellevue, Washington

Christian C. Apfel, MD, PhD
Associate Professor, Department of Anesthesia and Perioperative Care, University of California, San Francisco, School of Medicine, San Francisco, California

William P. Arnold III, MD
Associate Professor of Anesthesiology, University of Virginia Health System, Charlottesville, Virginia

Solomon Aronson, MD, FACC, FACCP, FAHA, FASE
Professor and Executive Vice Chair, Department of Anesthesiology, Duke University Medical Center, Durham, North Carolina

Angela M. Bader, MD, MPH
Associate Professor of Anaesthesia, Harvard Medical School; Director, Weiner Center for Preoperative Evaluation, Brigham and Women's Hospital; Vice Chair, Department of Anesthesiology, Perioperative and Pain Medicine; Brigham and Women's Hospital, Boston, Massachusetts

David Baker, MPhil, DM, FRCA, FRSM
Consultant Medical Toxicologist, Chemical Hazards and Poisons Division, Health Protection Agency, London, United Kingdom; Consultant Anesthesiologist, SAMU de Paris, Hôpital Necker Enfants Malades, Paris, France

Anis Baraka, MB, BCh, DA, DM, MD, FRCA (Hon)
Professor, Department of Anesthesiology, American University of Beirut, Beirut, Lebanon

Atilio Barbeito, MD
Assistant Professor, Department of Anesthesiology, Duke University Medical Center; Staff Anesthesiologist, Veterans Affairs Medical Center, Durham, North Carolina

Steven J. Barker, MD, PhD
Professor and Chair, Department of Anesthesiology, University of Arizona College of Medicine, Tucson, Arizona

Shahar Bar-Yosef, MD
Assistant Professor, Department of Anesthesiology, Duke University Medical Center; Staff Anesthesiologist, Veterans Affairs Medical Center, Durham, North Carolina

Charles B. Berde, MD, PhD
Professor of Anaesthesia (Pediatrics), Harvard Medical School; Sara Page Mayo Chair in Pediatric Pain Medicine, and Chief, Division of Pain Medicine, Department of Anesthesiology, Perioperative and Pain Medicine, Children's Hospital Boston, Boston, Massachusetts

Darryl H. Berkowitz, MB, BCh
Assistant Professor, Department of Anesthesiology and Critical Care Medicine, University of Pennsylvania School of Medicine; Attending Anesthesiologist, Children's Hospital of Philadelphia, Philadelphia, Pennsylvania

David J. Birnbach, MD, MPH
Professor of Anesthesiology, Obstetrics and Public Health, University of Miami Miller School of Medicine; Vice Provost, University of Miami; Associate Dean and Director, UM-JMH Center for Patient Safety, Miami, Florida

David Bogod, MB, BS, FRCA, LLM
Honorary Senior Lecturer, University of Nottingham; Consultant Anaesthetist, Nottingham University Hospitals NHS Trust, Nottingham, United Kingdom

Russell C. Brockwell, MD
Attending Anesthesiologist, Anesthesia Associates of Naples, Naples, Florida

David L. Brown, MD
Chairman, Institute of Anesthesiology, The Cleveland Clinic, Cleveland, Ohio

Ingrid M. Browne, MB, BCh, MMedSci, FFARCSI
Department of Anesthesiology, National Maternity Hospital; Department of Anesthesiology, St. Vincent's University Hospital, Dublin, Ireland

Michael K. Cahalan, MD
Professor and Chair, Department of Anesthesiology, University of Utah School of Medicine, Salt Lake City, Utah

Enrico M. Camporesi, MD
Professor of Anesthesiology, Surgery, Molecular Pharmacology, and Physiology, University of South Florida, Tampa, Florida

Javier H. Campos, MD
Professor of Anesthesia, University of Iowa College of Medicine; Vice Chair for Clinical Affairs, Medical Director of Operating Rooms, and Director of Cardiothoracic Anesthesia, Department of Anesthesia, University of Iowa Hospitals and Clinics, Iowa City, Iowa

Lydia Cassorla, MD, MBA
Professor, Department of Anesthesia and Perioperative Care, University of California, San Francisco, School of Medicine, San Francisco, California

Charles J. Coté, MD
Professor of Anaesthesia, Harvard Medical School; Director of Clinical Research, Division of Pediatric Anesthesia, Department of Anesthesia and Critical Care, MassGeneral Hospital for Children, Massachusetts General Hospital, Boston, Massachusetts

Bernard J. Dalens, MD, PhD
Associate Professor of Anesthesiology, Laval University; Clinical Professor, Department of Anesthesiology, Centre Hospitalier de l'Université Laval, Quebec City, Quebec, Canada

Clifford S. Deutschman, MS, MD, FCCM
Professor, Department of Anesthesiology and Critical Care, and Director, Stavropoulos Sepsis Research Program, University of Pennsylvania School of Medicine, Philadelphia, Pennsylvania

Peter Dieckmann, PhD
Department of Anaesthesiology and Intensive Care Medicine, University Hospital Tuebingen, Tuebingen, Germany; Researcher, Danish Institute for Medical Simulation, Copenhagen University Hospital Herlev, Herlev, Denmark

Sudhir Diwan, MD, MS, FIPP
Associate Professor of Clinical Anesthesiology, Weill Cornell Medical College; Director, Division of Pain Medicine, New York Presbyterian Hospital, New York, New York

John C. Drummond, MD, FRCPC
Professor of Anesthesiology, University of California, San Diego, School of Medicine; Staff Anesthesiologist, Veterans Affairs Medical Center, San Diego, California

Richard P. Dutton, MD, MBA
Associate Professor of Anesthesiology, University of Maryland School of Medicine; Director, Trauma Anesthesiology, R. Adams Cowley Shock Trauma Center, University of Maryland Medical System, Baltimore, Maryland

David M. Eckmann, PhD, MD
Horatio C. Wood Associate Professor of Anesthesiology and Critical Care and Professor of Bioengineering, University of Pennsylvania, Philadelphia, Pennsylvania

Edmond I. Eger II, MD
Professor, Department of Anesthesia and Perioperative Care, University of California, San Francisco, School of Medicine, San Francisco, California

Christoph Eich, MD, DEAA
Lecturer, Georg-August University School of Medicine; Attending Pediatric Anaesthesiologist, Department of Anaesthesiology, Emergency and Intensive Care Medicine, University Medical Centre Göttingen, Göttingen, Germany

Matthew R. Eng, BS, MD
The University of Texas Southwestern Medical Center, Dallas, Texas

Lars I. Eriksson, MD, PhD
Professor and Academic Chair, Department of Anesthesiology and Intensive Care Medicine, Karolinska University Hospital, Solna, Stockholm, Sweden

Stephen M. Eskaros, MD
Department of Anesthesia and Critical Care, University of California, Los Angeles, Ronald Reagan Medical Center, Los Angeles, California

Neil E. Farber, MD, PhD
Associate Professor of Anesthesiology, Pediatrics, Pharmacology and Toxicology, Medical College of Wisconsin; Director of Pediatric Anesthesia Research, Children's Hospital of Wisconsin, Milwaukee, Wisconsin

Marc Allan Feldman, MD, MHS
Head, Section of Anesthesia, Cole Eye Institute; Director, Cole Eye Institute Operating Rooms, Cleveland Clinic, Cleveland, Ohio

Stephen P. Fischer, BA, MS, MD
Associate Professor, Department of Anesthesia; Medical Director, Anesthesia Preoperative Evaluation Clinic, Stanford University School of Medicine, Stanford, California

Lee A. Fleisher, MD
Robert Dunning Dripps Professor and Chair, Department of Anesthesiology and Critical Care; Professor of Medicine, University of Pennsylvania School of Medicine, Philadelphia, Pennsylvania

Pamela Flood, MD
Associate Professor of Clinical Anesthesiology, Columbia University College of Physicians and Surgeons; Associate Attending Anesthesiologist, New York Presbyterian Hospital, New York, New York

Kazuhiko Fukuda, MD, PhD
Professor, Department of Anesthesiology, Kyoto University Hospital, Kyoto, Japan

David M. Gaba, MD
Professor of Anesthesia and Associate Dean for Immersive and Simulation-Based Learning, Stanford University; Staff Anesthesiologist and Director, Patient Simulation Center of Innovation, VA Palo Alto Health Care System, Palo Alto, California

Michael T. Ganter, MD
Consultant, University Hospital Zurich, Zurich, Switzerland

Adrian W. Gelb, MB, ChB, DA, FRCPC
Professor, Department of Anesthesia and Perioperative Care, University of California, San Francisco, School of Medicine, San Francisco, California

Simon Gelman, MD, PhD, FANZCA
Leroy D. Vandam/Benjamin G. Covino Distinguished Professor of Anaesthesia, Harvard Medical School; Chairman Emeritus, Department of Anesthesiology, Perioperative and Pain Medicine, Brigham and Women's Hospital, Boston, Massachusetts

Peter S. A. Glass, MB, ChB, FFA (SA)
Professor and Chair, Department of Anesthesiology, Stony Brook University Medical Center, Stony Brook, New York

David B. Glick, MD, MBA
Associate Professor, Department of Anesthesiology, University of Chicago; Medical Director, Post-Anesthesia Care Unit, University of Chicago Hospitals, Chicago, Illinois

Lawrence T. Goodnough, MD
Professor of Medicine and Pathology, Stanford University School of Medicine; Director, Transfusion Service, Stanford University Medical Center, Stanford, California

Sumeet Goswami MB, BS
Assistant Professor, Department of Anesthesia and Critical Care, Columbia University College of Physicians and Surgeons, Columbia University Medical Center, New York, New York

Salvatore Grasso, MD
Assistant Professor, Department of Anaesthesia and Intensive Care Medicine, University of Bari, Bari, Italy

Andrew T. Gray, MD, PhD
Professor of Clinical Anesthesia, Department of Anesthesia and Perioperative Care, University of California, San Francisco, School of Medicine; Staff Anesthesiologist, San Francisco General Hospital, San Francisco, California

William J. Greeley, MD, MBA
Chair and Anesthesiologist-in-Chief, Department of Anesthesiology and Critical Care Medicine, The Children's Hospital of Philadelphia; Professor of Anesthesia and Pediatrics, University of Pennsylvania School of Medicine, Philadelphia, Pennsylvania

George A. Gregory, MD
Professor of Anesthesia and Pediatrics, University of California, San Francisco, School of Medicine, San Francisco, California

Alina M. Grigore, MD
Associate Professor of Anesthesiology, Mayo Clinic College of Medicine; Senior Associate Consultant, Mayo Clinic Hospital, Phoenix, Arizona

Thomas E. Grissom, MD, FCCM
Associate Professor, Department of Anesthesiology, University of Maryland School of Medicine, Baltimore, Maryland

Michael A. Gropper, MD, PhD
Professor and Vice Chair, Department of Anesthesia and Perioperative Care, University of California, San Francisco, School of Medicine; Director of Critical Care Medicine, UCSF Medical Center, San Francisco, California

Fouad Salim Haddad, MD, FACA, DABA
Department of Anesthesiology, American University of Beirut, Beirut, Lebanon

C. William Hanson, MD
Professor of Anesthesiology and Critical Care, Surgery and Internal Medicine, University of Pennsylvania School of Medicine, Philadelphia, Pennsylvania

Michael C. Hauser, MD
Associate Professor, Department of Anesthesiology, Cleveland Clinic Lerner College of Medicine, Cleveland, Ohio

Göran Hedenstierna, MD, PhD
Professor of Clinical Physiology, Department of Medical Science, Uppsala University; Head of Nuclear Medicine, Uppsala University Hospital, Uppsala, Sweden

Eugenie S. Heitmiller, MD
Associate Professor, Department of Anesthesiology and Critical Care Medicine and Department of Pediatrics; Vice Chairman for Clinical Affairs, Johns Hopkins University School of Medicine, Baltimore, Maryland

Hugh C. Hemmings Jr., MD, PhD
Professor of Anesthesiology, Vice Chair for Research in Anesthesiology, and Professor of Pharmacology, Weill Cornell Medical College; Attending Anesthesiologist, New York Presbyterian Hospital–Weill Cornell Medical Center, New York, New York

John Henderson, MB, ChB, FRCA
Consultant Anaesthetist, Gartnavel General Hospital, Glasgow, Scotland, United Kingdom

Zak Hillel, PhD, MD
Professor of Clinical Anesthesiology, Columbia University College of Physicians and Surgeons; Director of Cardiac Anesthesia, St. Luke's–Roosevelt Hospital, New York, New York

Christoph K. Hofer, MD, DEAA
Senior Consultant, Institute of Anesthesiology and Intensive Care Medicine, Triemli City Hospital, Zurich, Switzerland

Terese T. Horlocker, MD
Professor of Anesthesiology and Orthopaedics, Mayo Clinic College of Medicine, Rochester, Minnesota

Steven K. Howard, MD
Associate Professor of Anesthesia, Stanford University School of Medicine; Staff Anesthesiologist, VA Palo Alto Health Care System, Palo Alto, California

Yuguang Huang, MD
Professor and Chairman, Department of Anesthesiology, Peking Union Medical College Hospital, Beijing, China

Michael Hüpfl, MD
Department of Anesthesiology and General Intensive Care, Medical University of Vienna; Medical Director, St. John's Ambulance Service, Vienna, Austria

Robert W. Hurley, MD, PhD
Assistant Professor, Department of Anesthesiology and Critical Care, Johns Hopkins University School of Medicine; Medical Director, Blaustein Pain Treatment Center and Center for Neuromodulation at Johns Hopkins University, Baltimore, Maryland

Fumito Ichinose, MD, PhD
Associate Professor of Anaesthesia, Harvard Medical School; Associate Anesthetist, Department of Anesthesia and Critical Care, Massachusetts General Hospital, Boston, Massachusetts

Samuel A. Irefin, MD, FCCM
Associate Professor, Department of General Anesthesia and the Transplant Center, Cleveland Clinic Lerner College of Medicine, Cleveland, Ohio

Ken B. Johnson, MD
Associate Professor, Carter M. Ballinger MD Presidential Chair in Anesthesiology, Department of Anesthesiology, University of Utah School of Medicine, Salt Lake City, Utah

Jean L. Joris, MD, PhD
Professor of Anesthesia, University of Liège; Associate Chief of the Service of Anesthesia and Intensive Care Medicine, CHU de Liège, Liège, Belgium

Alan D. Kaye, MD, PhD, DABPM
Professor and Chairman, Department of Anesthesiology, and Professor of Pharmacology, Louisiana State University Health Sciences Center, New Orleans, Louisiana

Max B. Kelz, MD, PhD
Assistant Professor, Department of Anesthesiology and Critical Care, Mahoney Institute for Neurological Sciences, Center for Sleep and Respiratory Neurobiology, University of Pennsylvania School of Medicine, Philadelphia, Pennsylvania

James D. Kindscher, MD
Professor and Chair, Department of Anesthesiology, Kansas University Medical Center, Kansas City, Kansas

Benjamin A. Kohl, MD
Assistant Professor, Department of Anesthesiology and Critical Care; Director, Critical Care Fellowship, University of Pennsylvania School of Medicine, Philadelphia, Pennsylvania

Andreas Kopf, MD
Instructor, Department of Anesthesiology and Critical Care Medicine, Freie Universität Berlin, Charité Campus Benjamin Franklin, Berlin, Germany

Burkhard Lachmann, MD, PhD
Professor of Anesthesiology, University of Berlin, Berlin, Germany

Arthur M. Lam, MD, FRCPC
Professor of Anesthesiology and Neurological Surgery, University of Washington School of Medicine; Anesthesiologist-in-Chief and Attending Neurointensivist, Harborview Medical Center, Seattle, Washington

Giora Landesberg, MD, DSc, MBA
Associate Professor, Hebrew University Hadassah Medical School; Director of Cardiothoracic and Vascular Anesthesia, Department of Anesthesiology and Critical Care Medicine, Hadassah University Hospital, Jerusalem, Israel

Merlin D. Larson, MD
Professor, Department of Anesthesia and Perioperative Care, University of California, San Francisco, School of Medicine, San Francisco, California

Jae-Woo Lee, MD
Assistant Professor in Residence, Department of Anesthesia and Perioperative Care, University of California, San Francisco, School of Medicine, San Francisco, California

Guillermo Lema, MD
Professor, Department of Anesthesiology, Pontificia Universidad Católica de Chile; Chief of Cardiovascular Anesthesia, Hospital Clinico, Santiago, Chile

Kate Leslie, MBBS, MD, M Epi, FANZCA
Honorary Associate Professor, Department of Pharmacology, University of Melbourne; Staff Anaesthetist, Department of Anaesthesia and Pain Management, Royal Melbourne Hospital, Melbourne, Australia

Cynthia A. Lien, MD
Professor, Department of Anesthesiology, Weill Medical College of Cornell University; Attending Anesthesiologist, New York Presbyterian Hospital, New York, New York

Lawrence Litt, PhD, MD
Professor, Department of Anesthesia and Perioperative Care and Department of Radiology, University of California, San Francisco, School of Medicine; Attending Anesthesiologist, UCSF Hospitals, San Francisco, California

Linda Liu, MD
Associate Professor of Clinical Anesthesia, Department of Anesthesia and Perioperative Care, University of California, San Francisco, School of Medicine, San Francisco, California

David A. Lubarsky, MD, MBA
Emanuel M. Papper Professor and Chair, Department of Anesthesiology, Perioperative Medicine and Pain Management; Senior Associate Dean for Quality, Safety and Risk Prevention, and Assistant Vice-President for Medical Administration, University of Miami Miller School of Medicine; Professor, Department of Management, University of Miami School of Business, Miami, Florida

Michael E. Mahla, MD
Professor of Anesthesiology and Neurosurgery; Associate Chair, Department of Anesthesiology; Assistant Dean for Graduate Medical Education, University of Florida College of Medicine, Gainesville, Florida

Vinod Malhotra, MD
Professor of Clinical Anesthesiology, Weill Medical College of Cornell University; Vice Chair for Clinical Affairs, Department of Anesthesiology and Clinical Director of Operating Rooms, New York Presbyterian Hospital–Weill Cornell Medical Center, New York, New York

Jonathan B. Mark, MD
Professor and Vice Chair, Department of Anesthesiology, Duke University Medical Center; Chief, Anesthesiology Service, Veterans Affairs Medical Center, Durham, North Carolina

Jackie L. Martin, MD
Professor, Department of Anesthesiology and Critical Care Medicine, Johns Hopkins University School of Medicine, Baltimore, Maryland

Elizabeth A. Martinez, MD, MHS
Associate Professor, Department of Anesthesiology and Critical Care Medicine and Department of Surgery, Johns Hopkins University School of Medicine; Medical Director, Adult PACU, Johns Hopkins Hospital, Baltimore, Maryland

Ricardo Martinez-Ruiz, MD
Assistant Professor of Anesthesiology and Surgery, University of Miami Miller School of Medicine; Director, Critical Care Division, and Chief, Surgical Intensive Care Unit, Department of Anesthesiology, Veterans Affairs Medical Center, Miami, Florida

J. A. Jeevendra Martyn, MD, FRCA, FCCM
Professor of Anaesthesia, Harvard Medical School; Anesthetist, Massachusetts General Hospital; Anesthetist-in-Chief, Shriners Burns Hospital; Director, Clinical and Biochemical Pharmacology Laboratory, Massachusetts General Hospital, Boston, Massachusetts

Luciana Mascia, MD, PhD
Assistant Professor, Department of Anesthesiology and Critical Care, Ospedale S. Giovanni Battista, University of Torino, Torino, Italy

George A. Mashour, MD, PhD
Assistant Professor of Anesthesiology, Assistant Professor of Neurosurgery, and Faculty, Neuroscience Graduate Program, University of Michigan Medical School; Director of Neurosurgical Anesthesia, University of Michigan Health System, Ann Arbor, Michigan

Mervyn Maze, FRCA, FRCP, FMedSci, PhD
Professor and Chair, Magill Department of Anaesthetics and Intensive Care, Chelsea and Westminster Hospital, Imperial College, London, United Kingdom

Maureen McCunn, MD, MIPP, FCCM
Associate Professor, Department of Anesthesiology and Critical Care, University of Maryland School of Medicine, Baltimore, Maryland

Matthew D. McEvoy, MD
Assistant Professor of Anesthesiology, Director of Simulation, Associate Dean for Curriculum Reform, College of Medicine, Medical University of South Carolina, Charleston, South Carolina

Brian P. McGlinch, MD
Assistant Professor, Department of Anesthesiology, Mayo Clinic College of Medicine, Rochester, Minnesota

Berend Mets, MB, ChB, PhD, FRCA, FFA(SA)
Eric A. Walker Professor and Chair, Department of Anesthesiology, Pennsylvania State University College of Medicine, Penn State Milton S. Hershey Medical Center, Hershey, Pennsylvania

Ronald D. Miller, MD
Professor and Chair, Department of Anesthesia and Perioperative Care, and Professor of Cellular and Molecular Pharmacology, University of California, San Francisco, School of Medicine, San Francisco, California

Terri G. Monk, MD
Professor, Department of Anesthesiology, Duke University Medical Center, Durham, North Carolina

Richard E. Moon, MD, CM
Professor of Anesthesiology and Medicine, Duke University School of Medicine; Chief, Division of General, Vascular and Transplant Anesthesia; Medical Director, Center for Hyperbaric Medicine and Environmental Physiology, Duke University Medical Center, Durham, North Carolina

Kenjiro Mori, MD, PhD, FRCA
Professor Emeritus, Department of Anesthesia, Kyoto University Hospital, Kyoto, Japan

Jonathan Moss, MD, PhD
Professor, Department of Anesthesia and Critical Care, University of Chicago, Chicago, Illinois

Phillip S. Mushlin, MD, PhD
Associate Professor of Anaesthesia, Harvard Medical School, and Brigham and Women's Hospital, Boston, Massachusetts

Peter Nagele, MD
Assistant Professor, Department of Anesthesiology, Washington University School of Medicine, St. Louis, Missouri; Associate Professor, Department of Anesthesiology and General Critical Care, Medical University of Vienna, Vienna, Austria

Mohamed Naguib, MB BCh, MSc, FFARCSI, MD
Professor, Department of Anesthesiology and Pain Management, The University of Texas MD Anderson Cancer Center, Houston, Texas

Shinichi Nakao, MD, PhD
Associate Professor of Anesthesiology, Kansai Medical University, Moriguchi, Osaka, Japan

Akiyoshi Namiki, MD, PhD
Professor and Chair, Department of Anesthesiology, Sapporo Medical University School of Medicine, Sapporo, Hokkaido, Japan

Aruna T. Nathan, MBBS, FRCA
Attending Anesthesiologist, Department of Anesthesiology and Critical Care Medicine, The Children's Hospital of Philadelphia, Philadelphia, Pennsylvania

Patrick J. Neligan, MA, MB, FFARCSI
Honorary Senior Lecturer in Anaesthesia, University College Galway, National University of Ireland; Consultant in Anaesthesia and Intensive Care Medicine, University College Hospitals, Galway, Ireland

Stanton P. Newman, PhD
Professor of Health Psychology and Director, Centre for Behavioural and Social Sciences in Medicine, Division of Medicine, University College London, London, United Kingdom

Dorre Nicholau, MD, PhD
Clinical Professor, Department of Anesthesia and Perioperative Care, University of California, San Francisco, School of Medicine, San Francisco, California

Claus U. Niemann, MD
Associate Professor of Anesthesia and Surgery, Department of Anesthesia and Perioperative Care, Department of Surgery, Division of Transplantation, University of California, San Francisco, School of Medicine, San Francisco, California

Ervant Nishanian, PhD, MD
Assistant Professor, Department of Anesthesiology and Critical Care, Division of Cardiothoracic Anesthesiology, Columbia University College of Physicians and Surgeons, New York, New York

Edward J. Norris, MD, MBA, FAHA
Associate Professor, Department of Anesthesia and Critical Care, The Johns Hopkins University School of Medicine; Director, Vascular and Endovascular Anesthesia, The Johns Hopkins Hospital and Medical Institutions, Baltimore, Maryland

Florian R. Nuevo, MD
Department of Anesthesiology, University of Santo Tomas Hospital, Manila, Philippines

Nancy A. Nussmeier, MD
Professor and Chair, Department of Anesthesiology, SUNY Upstate Medical University, Syracuse, New York

Christopher J. O'Connor, MD
Professor, Department of Anesthesiology, Rush University Medical Center, Rush Medical College, Chicago, Illinois

Jerome O'Hara, MD
Associate Professor, Cleveland Clinic Lerner College of Medicine; Section Head of Anesthesia, Glickman Urological Institute, Cleveland Clinic, Cleveland, Ohio

Paul S. Pagel, MD, PhD
Professor of Anesthesiology, Medical College of Wisconsin; Staff Anesthesiologist, Clement J. Zablocki Veterans Affairs Medical Center, Milwaukee, Wisconsin

Peter J. Papadakos, MD
Professor of Anesthesiology, Surgery and Neurosurgery, University of Rochester School of Medicine; Director of Critical Care Medicine, University of Rochester Medical Center, Rochester, New York

Anil Patel, MBBS, FRCA
Honorary Senior Lecturer, Institute of Otolaryngology, University College London; Consultant, Royal National Throat, Nose and Ear Hospital and University College Hospital, London, United Kingdom

Piyush M. Patel, MD, FRCPC
Professor of Anesthesiology, University of California, San Diego; Staff Anesthesiologist, Veterans Affairs Medical Center; San Diego, California

Ronald Pauldine, MD
Clinical Associate Professor, Department of Anesthesiology, University of Washington School of Medicine; Attending Anesthesiologist, Veterans Affairs Puget Sound Health Care System, Seattle, Washington

Robert A. Pearce, MD, PhD
Ralph M. Waters, M.D., Distinguished Chair of Anesthesiology and Professor of Anesthesiology, University of Wisconsin School of Medicine and Public Health, Madison, Wisconsin

Misha Perouansky, MD
Professor of Anesthesiology, University of Wisconsin School of Medicine and Public Health, Madison, Wisconsin

Isaac N. Pessah, PhD
Professor, Department of Molecular Biosciences, College of Veterinary Medicine, University of California, Davis; Director, UC Davis Children's Center for Environmental Health and Disease Prevention, Davis, California

Jean-François Pittet, MD
Professor in Residence, Departments of Anesthesia and Surgery; Associate Investigator, Cardiovascular Research Institute, University of California, San Francisco, San Francisco, California

Phillip F. Pratt Jr., PhD
Assistant Professor of Anesthesiology and Pharmacology, Medical College of Wisconsin, Milwaukee, Wisconsin

Peter J. Pronovost, MD, PhD, FCCM
Professor, Departments of Anesthesiology and Critical Care Medicine, Surgery, and Health Policy and Management; Medical Director, Center of Innovations in Quality Patient Care; Director, Quality and Safety Research Group, The Johns Hopkins University School of Medicine, Baltimore, Maryland

Marcus Rall, MD
Director, Center for Patient Safety and Simulation (TuPASS), Department of Anaesthesiology and Intensive Care Medicine, University Hospital Tuebingen, University of Tuebingen Medical School, Tuebingen, Germany

Ira J. Rampil, MS, MD
Professor of Anesthesiology and Neurological Surgery, and Director of Clinical Research, State University of New York at Stony Brook, Stony Brook, New York

V. Marco Ranieri, MD
Professor, Department of Anesthesia and Intensive Care, Ospedale San Giovanni Battista, Torino, Italy

Lars Rasmussen, MD, PhD
Consultant, Department of Anaesthesia, Centre for Head and Orthopaedics, Copenhagen University Hospital, Rigshospitalet, Copenhagen, Denmark

J. G. Reves, MD
Professor, Department of Anesthesia and Perioperative Medicine; Professor, Department of Pharmacology; Dean, College of Medicine; and Vice President for Medical Affairs, Medical University of South Carolina, Charleston, South Carolina

Zaccaria Ricci, MD
Attending Anesthesiologist, Department of Pediatric Cardiac Surgery, Ospedale Bambino Gesù, Rome; Fellow, Ospedale San Bortolo, Vicenza, Italy

James M. Riopelle, MD
Professor, Department of Anesthesiology, Louisiana State University Health Sciences Center, New Orleans, Louisiana

Melissa Rockford, MD
Assistant Professor of Anesthesiology, University of Kansas School of Medicine, Kansas City, Kansas

Michael F. Roizen, MD
Chair, The Wellness Institute, and Chief Wellness Officer, Cleveland Clinic, Cleveland, Ohio

Claudio Ronco, MD
Professor of Medicine and Head, Department of Nephrology, Dialysis and Transplantation, San Bortolo Hospital, Vicenza, Italy

Stanley H. Rosenbaum, MA, MD
Professor of Anesthesiology, Internal Medicine and Surgery, Yale University School of Medicine, New Haven, Connecticut

Steven Roth, MD
Associate Professor of Anesthesia and Critical Care, University of Chicago; Chief of Neuroanesthesia, University of Chicago Medical Center, Chicago, Illinois

David M. Rothenberg, MD, FCCM
The Max S. Sadove Professor of Anesthesiology and Associate Dean, Academic Affiliations of Rush Medical College, Rush University Medical Center, Chicago, Illinois

Marc A. Rozner, PhD, MD
Professor of Anesthesiology and Professor of Cardiology, The University of Texas MD Anderson Cancer Center; Adjunct Assistant Professor of Integrative Biology and Pharmacology, The University of Texas Health Science Center at Houston, Houston, Texas

Muhammad F. Sarwar, MD
Assistant Professor of Anesthesiology, SUNY Upstate Medical University, Syracuse, New York

Rebecca A. Schroeder, MD
Associate Professor, Department of Anesthesiology, Duke University Medical Center; Staff Anesthesiologist, Veterans Affairs Medical Center, Durham, North Carolina

Allan Jay Schwartz, MD, MSEd
Professor of Anesthesiology and Critical Care, University of Pennsylvania School of Medicine; Director of Education and Pediatric Anesthesiology Fellowship Director, Children's Hospital of Philadelphia, Philadelphia, Pennsylvania

Andrew Schwartz, MFA, BA
A. Schwartz Communications, Albany, California

Johanna C. Schwarzenberger, MD
Assistant Professor of Anesthesiology, Columbia University College of Physicians and Surgeons, New York, New York

Debra A. Schwinn, MD
Professor and Chair, Department of Anesthesiology, Adjunct Professor of Pharmacology and Genome Sciences, University of Washington, Seattle, Washington

Bruce E. Searles, BS, CCP
Associate Professor, Department of Cardiovascular Perfusion, College of Health Professions, SUNY Upstate Medical University, Syracuse, New York

Daniel I. Sessler, MD
Professor and Chair, Department of Outcomes Research, The Cleveland Clinic, Cleveland, Ohio

Christoph N. Seubert, MD, PhD
Associate Professor of Anesthesiology and Chief, Division of Neuroanesthesia, University of Florida College of Medicine; Director, Intraoperative Neurophysiologic Monitoring Laboratory, Shands Hospital, Gainesville, Florida

Steven L. Shafer, MD
Professor of Anesthesiology, Columbia University College of Physicians and Surgeons, New York, New York; Adjunct Professor of Anesthesia, Stanford University, Stanford, California; Adjunct Professor of Biopharmaceutical Science, University of California, San Francisco, San Francisco, California

Andrew Shaw, MB, FRCA, FCCM
Associate Professor, Division of Cardiothoracic Anesthesiology, Department of Anesthesiology and Critical Care Medicine, Duke University Medical Center, Durham, North Carolina

Koh Shingu, MD, PhD
Professor and Chair, Department of Anesthesiology, Kansai Medical University, Hirakata Hospital, Hirakata, Osaka, Japan

Frederick E. Sieber, MD
Associate Professor, Department of Anesthesia and Critical Care Medicine, Johns Hopkins University School of Medicine; Clinical Director and Attending Physician, Department of Anesthesia and Critical Care Medicine, Johns Hopkins Bayview Medical Center, Baltimore, Maryland

Sir Peter Simpson, MD, MBBS, FRCA, FRCP, FRCS(Hon), FCARCSI(Hon)
Immediate Past President, Royal College of Anaesthetists; Past President, European Society of Anaesthesiology; Consultant Anaesthetist (Ret.), Frenchay Hospital, Bristol, United Kingdom

Ashish C. Sinha, MD, PhD
Assistant Professor of Anesthesiology and Critical Care, and Assistant Professor of Otorhinolaryngology and Head and Neck Surgery, University of Pennsylvania School of Medicine, Philadelphia, Pennsylvania

Robert N. Sladen, MB, ChB, MRCP(UK), FRCP(C), FCCM
Professor and Vice Chair, Department of Anesthesiology, Columbia University College of Physicians and Surgeons; Director, Cardiothoracic and Surgical Intensive Care Units, Columbia University Medical Center at New York Presbyterian Hospital, New York, New York

Thomas F. Slaughter, MD
Professor, Department of Anesthesiology, Wake Forest University School of Medicine; Head, Section of Cardiothoracic Anesthesiology, Department of Anesthesiology, Wake Forest University Health Sciences, Winston-Salem, North Carolina

Peter D. Slinger, MD, FRCP(C)
Professor, Department of Anaesthesia, University of Toronto; Staff Anesthesiologist, Toronto General Hospital, Toronto, Ontario, Canada

Michael J. Souter, MB, ChB, FRCA
Associate Professor of Anesthesiology and Neurological Surgery, University of Washington School of Medicine; Attending Physician, Anesthesiology and Critical Care, Harborview Medical Center; Medical Co-Director, Neurocritical Care Service, Harborview Medical Center, Seattle, Washington

Mark Stafford-Smith, MD, CM, FRCP(C), FASE
Professor of Anesthesiology, Duke University School of Medicine; Director, Fellowship Education, and Director, Cardiothoracic Anesthesia and Critical Care Fellowship, Duke University Medical Center, Durham, North Carolina

Donald R. Stanski, MD
Emeritus Professor of Anesthesia, Stanford University School of Medicine, Stanford, California; Scientific Advisor to the Director, Center for Drug Evaluation and Research, Food and Drug Administration, Washington, DC

Christoph Stein, MD
Professor and Chair, Department of Anesthesiology and Critical Care Medicine, Freie Universität Berlin, Charité Campus Benjamin Franklin, Berlin, Germany

Paul E. Stensrud, MD
Assistant Professor of Anesthesiology, Mayo Clinic College of Medicine; Consultant in Anesthesiology, Mayo Clinic, Rochester, Minnesota

Gary R. Strichartz, BS, AM (Hon), PhD, FRSM
Professor of Anaesthesia, Pharmacology and Biophysics, Harvard Medical School; Vice-Chairman for Research, Department of Anesthesiology, Perioperative and Pain Medicine, and Director, Pain Research Center, Brigham and Women's Hospital, Boston, Massachusetts

Jan Stygall, MSc
Senior Research Fellow and Health Psychology Unit Research Coordinator, Centre for Behavioural and Social Sciences in Medicine, University College London, London, United Kingdom

Vijayendra Sudheendra, MD
Assistant Professor of Surgery and Anesthesiology, Brown University School of Medicine; Director of Cardiac Anesthesia, Miriam Hospital, Providence, Rhode Island; Medical Director, Southern New England Surgery Center, Attleboro, Massachusetts

Lena S. Sun, MD
Professor of Anesthesiology and Pediatrics, Columbia University College of Physicians and Surgeons; Chief of Pediatric Anesthesia, Columbia University Medical Center, New York, New York

BobbieJean Sweitzer, MD
Associate Professor of Anesthesia and Critical Care, University of Chicago; Director of Anesthesia, Perioperative Medicine Clinic, University of Chicago, Chicago, Illinois

James Szocik, MD
Associate Professor, Department of Anesthesiology, University of Michigan Medical School, Ann Arbor, Michigan

Deepak K. Tempe, MBBS, MD
Professor and Head, Department of Anesthesiology and Intensive Care, G.B. Pant Hospital, University of Delhi, New Delhi, India

Kevin K. Tremper, PhD, MD
Robert B. Sweet Professor of Anesthesiology, University of Michigan Medical School; Chair, Department of Anesthesiology, University of Michigan Medical Center, Ann Arbor, Michigan

Kenneth J. Tuman, MD, FCCM
The Anthony D. Ivankovich Professor of Anesthesiology, Rush Medical College; Chair, Department of Anesthesiology, Rush University Medical Center, Chicago, Illinois

Michael K. Urban, MD, PhD
Associate Professor of Clinical Anesthesia, Weill Medical College of Cornell University; Director, Post-Anesthesia Care Unit, Hospital for Special Surgery, New York, New York

Gail A. Van Norman, MD
Clinical Associate Professor, Department of Anesthesiology, University of Washington; Faculty Associate, Department of Biomedical Ethics, University of Washington, Seattle, Washington

Daniel P. Vezina, MD, MSc, FRCPC
Associate Professor, Department of Anesthesiology, and Associate Professor, Division of Cardiology, Department of Medicine, University of Utah; Director, Echocardiography Laboratory, Department of Anesthesiology, Veterans Administration Hospital, Salt Lake City, Utah

Jørgen Viby-Mogensen, MD, DMSc, FRCA
Professor and Chair, Department of Anesthesia and Intensive Care, Copenhagen University Hospital, Rigshospitalet, Copenhagen, Denmark

David B. Waisel, MD
Associate Professor of Anaesthesia, Harvard Medical School; Senior Associate in Anesthesia, Department of Anesthesiology, Perioperative and Pain Medicine, Children's Hospital Boston, Boston, Massachusetts

David C. Warltier, MD, PhD
Chairman, Department of Anesthesiology, and Professor of Anesthesiology, Pharmacology and Toxicology, Medical College of Wisconsin; Anesthesiologist, Froedtert Memorial Lutheran Hospital; Professor of Biomedical Engineering, Marquette University, Milwaukee, Wisconsin

Denise J. Wedel, MD
Professor, Department of Anesthesiology, Mayo Clinic College of Medicine, Rochester, Minnesota

Charles Weissman, MD
Professor and Chair, Department of Anesthesiology and Critical Care Medicine, Hebrew University Hadassah School of Medicine, Jerusalem, Israel

Paul F. White, PhD, MD, FANZCA
Professor and Holder of the Margaret Milam McDermott Distinguished Chair in Anesthesiology, Department of Anesthesiology and Pain Management, University of Texas Southwestern Medical Center, Dallas, Texas; Visiting Scientist, Department of Anesthesia, Cedars Sinai Medical Center, Los Angeles, California; President, White Mountain Institute, Dallas, Texas

Roger D. White, MD
Assistant Professor, Department of Anesthesiology, Mayo Clinic College of Medicine, Rochester, Minnesota

Jeanine P. Wiener-Kronish, MD
Henry Isaiah Dorr Professor of Research and Teaching in Anaesthetics and Anaesthesia, Harvard Medical School; Anesthetist-in-Chief, Massachusetts General Hospital, Boston, Massachusetts

Christopher L. Wu, MD
Associate Professor, Department of Anesthesia and Critical Care Medicine, The Johns Hopkins University, Baltimore, Maryland

Michiaki Yamakage, MD, PhD
Assistant Professor, Department of Anesthesiology, Sapporo Medical University School of Medicine, Sapporo, Hokkaido, Japan

C. Spencer Yost, MD
Professor, Department of Anesthesia and Perioperative Care, University of California, San Francisco, School of Medicine; Medical Director, Mt. Zion Hospital Intensive Care Unit, San Francisco, California

William L. Young, MD
James P. Livingston Professor and Vice Chair, Department of Anesthesia and Perioperative Care; Professor of Neurological Surgery and Neurology; Director, UCSF Center for Cerebrovascular Research, University of California, San Francisco, School of Medicine, San Francisco, California

Chun-Su Yuan, MD, PhD
Cyrus Tang Professor, Department of Anesthesia and Critical Care, University of Chicago, Pritzker School of Medicine, Chicago, Illinois

Warren M. Zapol, MD
Reginald Jenneg Professor of Anaesthesia, Harvard Medical School; Director, Anesthesia Center for Critical Care Research, Massachusetts General Hospital, Boston, Massachusetts

Jie Zhou, MD, MBA, MS
Instructor in Anaesthesia, Harvard Medical School; Attending Anesthesiologist, Department of Anesthesiology, Perioperative and Pain Medicine, Brigham and Women's Hospital; Consulting Staff, Department of Surgery, Dana-Farber Cancer Institute, Boston, Massachusetts

Maurice S. Zwass, MD
Professor of Anesthesia and Pediatrics, and Associate Director, Pediatric Critical Care Medicine, University of California, San Francisco, School of Medicine, San Francisco, California

Preface to the Seventh Edition

For over 25 years, *Miller's Anesthesia* has been recognized as the most complete and thorough resource on the global scope and practice of contemporary anesthesiology. The seventh edition continues that tradition and represents the most extensive revision we have ever undertaken. These advances include 13 new chapters, more than 30 new authors, and 1500 full-color illustrations. All existing chapters were meticulously revised and updated. The extensive scope of the revision was greatly facilitated by a team of expert and dedicated associate editors: Lee A. Fleisher, MD, Professor and Chair of the Department of Anesthesiology and Critical Care at the University of Pennsylvania; Jeanine P. Wiener-Kronish, MD, Anesthetist-in-Chief, Massachusetts General Hospital and Professor of Anaesthesia at the Harvard Medical School; William L. Young, MD, Professor and Vice Chair of the Department of Anesthesia and Perioperative Care, University of California, San Francisco; and Lars I. Eriksson, MD, PhD, Professor and Academic Chair of Anesthesiology and Intensive Care Medicine at the Karolinska University Hospital in Stockholm.

The 13 new chapters were added in response to an intense analysis of the changes in the scope of anesthesiology. The increasing importance of critical care medicine dictated five separate chapters on nitric oxide, clinical critical care protocols, neurocritical care, renal replacement therapy in the critically ill patient, and prehospital emergency and trauma care, which complements the existing chapter on anesthesia for trauma. The entire state of anesthesia for surgery and other procedures is being examined in more depth in two new chapters on sleep, memory, and consciousness, and perioperative cognitive dysfunction and other long-term implications of anesthetics, the implications being that general anesthesia may have impact long after its administration has been completed. Some rapidly evolving and important subjects in anesthesia are detailed in new chapters on anesthesia for correction of cardiac arrhythmias and anesthesia for bariatric surgery, given that obesity is a major health care issue in many areas of the world, particularly in the United States. The multiple opportunities to interfere with or correct abnormalities in coagulation dictated a separate chapter.

Ultrasound guidance has become a standard of care in the modern practice of regional anesthesia; thus, a dedicated chapter focused on the technique of ultrasound-guided regional anesthesia was clearly warranted. The philosophic question is whether non-ultrasound-guided techniques should continue to be taught, given that many clinicians practice in countries and regions that cannot afford ultrasound technology. Likewise, information technology has become increasingly dominant in medicine as a whole, but especially in anesthesia, necessitating a focused analysis in a dedicated chapter. An ever-growing number of medical centers rely on paperless communication and record keeping, including the anesthetic record. Information technology also allows formation of databases, which can answer important questions related to the institution or individual health care delivery. Chapter 2, entitled Scope of Modern Anesthetic Practice, covers the scope of anesthesia as we know it now with use of modern technology. Lastly, *Miller's Anesthesia* now incorporates the scope and historical development of anesthesia practice in many areas of the world. In Chapter 3, entitled The International Scope and Practice of Anesthesia, the individual contributions from numerous leaders of anesthesia worldwide were compiled into a synopsis of international anesthesia from its origin to the present. Further attesting to the book's global perspective, *Miller's Anesthesia* features contributions from anesthesiologists from all over the world, with 45 contributors to this new edition practicing outside of North America.

Each 2-volume set of the 7th edition of *Miller's Anesthesia* is now accompanied by access to a dedicated *Expert Consult website*, either basic or premium edition. The *basic edition* includes complete, fully searchable online text. The *premium edition* includes all of the above plus additional high-value features such as regular content updates, references linked to Medline abstracts and full-text articles, downloadable image library, drug database, self-assessment questions, and, most importantly, an extensive video library featuring full-length video presentations of anesthesia procedures including airway and ultrasound-guided regional anesthesia techniques.

We wish to acknowledge the long-time participation of Roger A. Johns, MD, and John J. Savarese, MD, who served as consulting editors on the previous edition. We are grateful for the tireless help of Tula Gourdin, who managed all communication with contributors and the publisher, facilitated the flow of manuscripts and page proofs, and checked every detail to make sure the chapters are as accurate and consistent as possible. We also wish to acknowledge our publisher, Elsevier, and the help and dedication of their staff, in particular executive publisher Natasha Andjelkovic, senior developmental editor Heather Krehling, and project manager Fran Gunning.

Ronald D. Miller, MD

Contents

SECTION V ADULT SUBSPECIALTY MANAGEMENT

SECTION IX
ANCILLARY RESPONSIBILITIES AND PROBLEMS

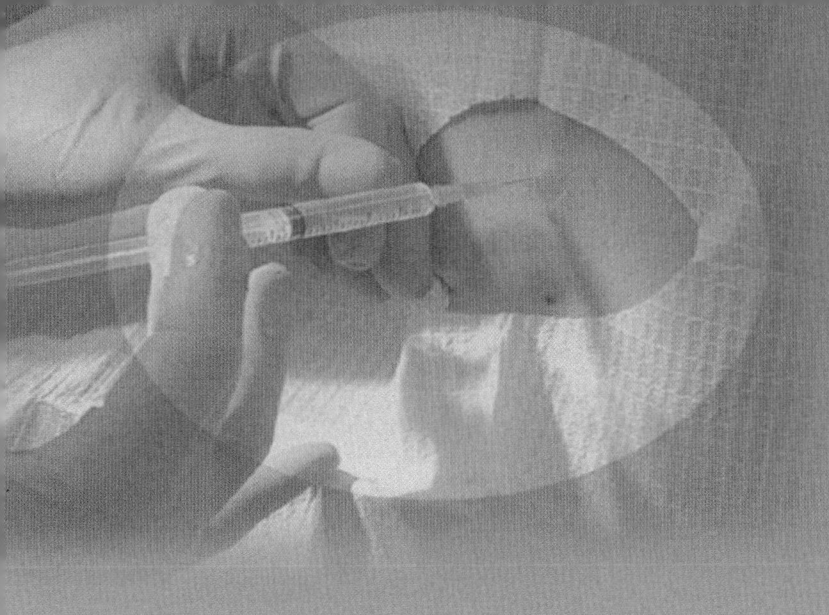

Introduction

Section I

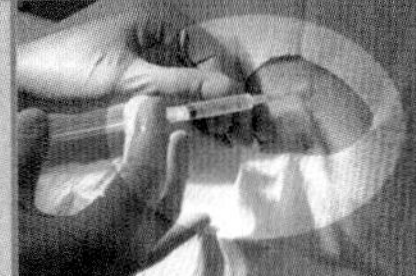

Merlin D. Larson

1 History of Anesthetic Practice

Key Points

1. Methods to safely alleviate severe pain are relatively recent discoveries, as viewed within the time span of human history.
2. The public demonstration of ether anesthesia on October 16, 1846, ranks as one of the most significant events in the history of medicine.
3. No single individual can be said to have discovered anesthesia.
4. The specialty of anesthesia rests on discoveries made from several scientific disciplines.
5. Major discoveries were often made by small groups of curious individuals with diverse backgrounds.
6. Techniques in common use at any one time often seem dangerous to subsequent generations of anesthesiologists.
7. Major innovations were sometimes ignored until their rediscovery several decades later.
8. Developments in anesthesia often arose to meet the needs of patients with severe comorbid conditions that required complex surgical procedures. Consequently, advances within the specialties of surgery and anesthesia are closely integrated.

The first anesthetics were given to ameliorate the pain associated with dental extractions and minor surgery. As the complementary fields of surgery and anesthesiology matured together, new skills were required of the anesthesiologist, including expertise in resuscitation, fluid replacement, airway management, oxygen transport, operative stress reduction, and postoperative pain control. Today, personnel from the anesthesiology department are located throughout the hospital, ranging from the ambulatory care center to the intensive care unit. Organizing a coherent historical document is therefore complicated by the diverse roles of anesthesiologists, in the modern hospital, especially in perioperative medicine.

One approach to the history of anesthesiology is to relate in detail the events surrounding the 1846 public demonstration of ether anesthesia by William T. G. Morton (1819-1868).[1,2] This event represents the starting point from which anesthesiology emerged as a specialty. Although the ether demonstration was dramatic and enacted by interesting personalities, it was just the opening act of the pain control story. Since 1846, there has been enormous progress and change in the specialty of medicine that has become known as anesthesiology, and these changes have often occurred in small, incremental steps that are hardly noteworthy on their own. Most operations in the modern operating room could not have been performed before the great progress in anesthetic practice that took place in the years between 1925 and 1960, but historians often overlook these advances because they were introduced without the drama and spectacle of previous developments.

In addition to examining the advancements of the 20th century, the mid-19th century provided the groundwork laid by inquisitive individuals who sought scientific understanding of cardiopulmonary physiology and pain. These fundamental discoveries provide the physiologic foundation for safe anesthetic practice. A brief survey of these early developments is provided in the opening sections of this chapter. Dentists, priests, musicians, pediatricians, engineers, ophthalmologists, neurophysiologists, pharmacologists, urologists, otolaryngologists, surgeons, ministers, dilettantes, philosophers, physiologists, missionaries, chemists, South American Indians, and anesthesiologists all had a role in shaping the practice of contemporary anesthesiology, one of the most fascinating stories in the history of medicine.

I have attempted to describe and reference the origins of ideas related to modern anesthetic practice, but the issue of priority is vague on some topics and may be open to question by other historians of specific subjects.

Cardiopulmonary Physiology

Respiration

Although volatile anesthetics have changed over the past 150 years, there are two gases that will always be part of anesthetic practice. How oxygen and carbon dioxide are consumed and produced and how they interact with the body have been the subject of intense research over the past 400 years. The ability to manipulate the pressure of these gases in tissues has contributed a great deal to the success of intensive care medicine. Because of the importance that carbon dioxide and oxygen have in the practice of anesthesiology, it is worthwhile to consider how our understanding of respiration came about.

Aristotle (384-322 BC) and Galen (120-200 AD) both thought that the air moving in and out of the lungs served merely to cool the heart, which otherwise became overheated in working to sustain life.[3] In 1678, Robert Hook (1635-1703) attached a bellows to the trachea of a dog with an open chest and demonstrated that the animal could be kept alive by rhythmic and sustained contraction of the bellows. Hook proved that movement of the chest wall was not the essential feature of respiration but instead it was exposure of fresh air to blood circulating through the lungs.[4] Richard Lower (1631-1691), who was the first to transfuse blood from one animal to another, demonstrated in 1669 that blood absorbed a definite chemical substance necessary for life that changed venous blood from dark blue to red and that the process was the chief function of the pulmonary circulation.[5]

Joseph Priestley (1733-1804) (Fig. 1-1A), a complex individual who was a dissenting minister in Leeds, England, and later the "resident intellectual" to the Earl of Shelburne, observed that respiration and combustion had many similarities[6] in that a candle flame would go out and an animal would die if left within a closed space. He thought this effect occurred because the air was putrefied with phlogiston. Priestley discovered photosynthesis by showing that placing plants that imbibed the "phlogistic matter" within the contained space could restore this "bad air." By heating mercuric oxide, he generated a gas that would make flames brighter and keep mice alive longer in a closed space. Priestley called it *dephlogisicated* air, and Carl Scheele[7] (1742-1786) in Sweden, who detected it earlier but failed to publish, called it *feuer luft* ("fire air"). Priestley thought that this process absorbed phlogiston and informed the French chemist Antoine-Laurent Lavoisier (1743-1794) (Fig. 1-1B) of his discovery. Lavoisier then outlined the great facts of respiration: absorption of oxygen through the lungs with liberation of carbon dioxide.

Lavoisier thought that the change from oxygen to carbon dioxide was accomplished in the lungs, but Humphry Davy (1778-1829) (Fig. 1-1C), an English teenager who dropped out of school at the age of 16 years, read the works of Lavoisier and designed his own experiments to study the site of metabolism. Davy heated blood and collected the gases that were produced. By showing that these gases were oxygen and carbon dioxide, he surmised that metabolism takes place in tissues.[8] Davy also estimated rates of oxygen consumption and carbon dioxide production and measured the total and residual volumes

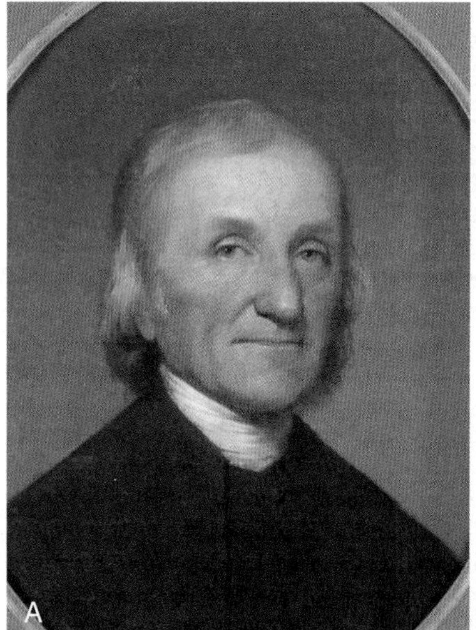

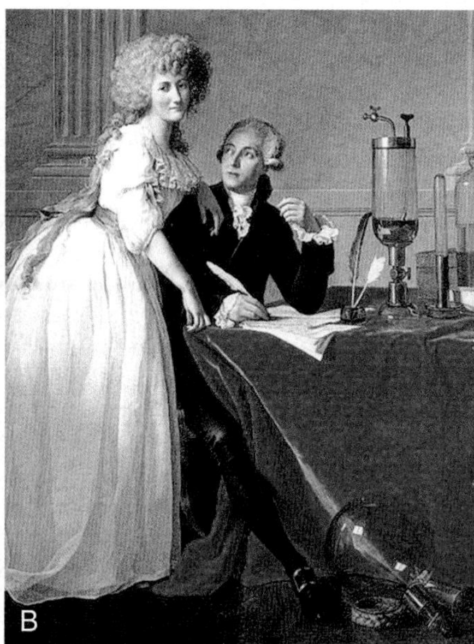

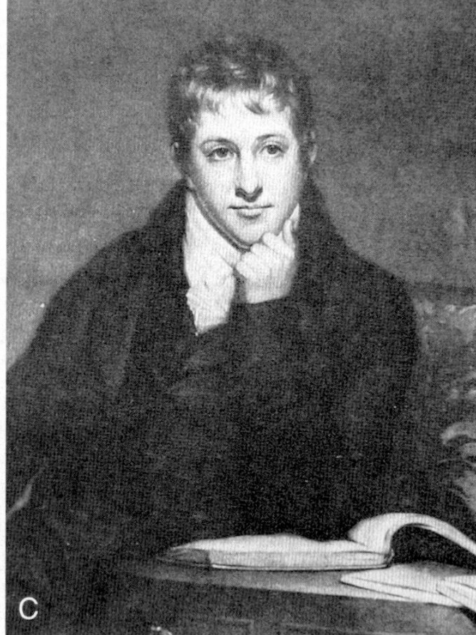

Figure 1-1 A, Joseph Priestley was born in Fieldhead, England, and educated as a minister. His early career was spent as a schoolmaster in Leeds, England. In 1780 he accepted an appointment in Birmingham as minister, where he joined Erasmus Darwin and James Watt in forming the Lunar Society, which met to discuss the new ideas in chemistry and physics emerging at that time. Because of his political views, his chapel and home were vandalized in 1789. Five years later, he joined his sons in Pennsylvania in the United States, where he died in 1804 at the age of 70. **B,** This portrait of Lavoisier and his wife Marie Anne Pierrette Paulz was painted in 1788 by the famous French artist Jacques Louis David. Marie Paulz, who married Lavoisier when she was only 14 years old, was taught to draw by David, and she drew many of the illustrations in Lavoisier's magnum opus *Traite Elementaire de Chimie*. Several experimental devices and gasometers are shown on and below the table. **C,** Humphry Davy was born in Cornwall, England, and became apprenticed to a surgeon, J. B. Borlase of Penzance, at age 17. At 20 years of age he was appointed superintendent of the Beddoe's Pneumatic Institute, where he studied the effects of nitrous oxide inhalation. His later career in chemistry gained him fame and honors. He directed the Royal Institute and was made a baronet in 1818 at the age of 40. *(Courtesy of the Wood Library-Museum of Anesthesiology, Park Ridge, IL.)*

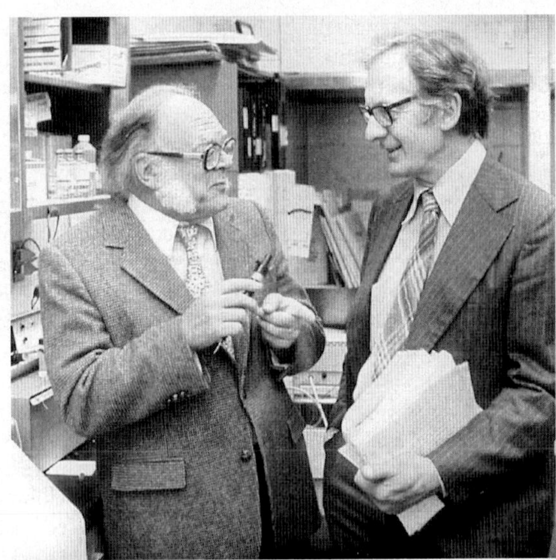

Figure 1-2 This photograph of Leland Clark and John Severinghaus, whose contributions led to modern techniques of blood gas analysis, was taken in Clark's laboratory at the Cincinnati Children's Hospital in 1982. *(From Severinghaus JW, Astrup PB: History of blood gas analysis. Int Anesthesiol Clin 25:1-224, 1987.)*

of the lungs. John S. Haldane (1860-1936) was a pioneer investigator in the study of respiration a century ago. His apparatus for measurement of blood gases was described in 1892.[9] He was the first to promote oxygen therapy for respiratory disease,[10] and in 1905 he discovered that the carbon dioxide tension of blood was the normal stimulus for the respiratory drive.[11] Haldane experimented with self-administration of hypoxic mixtures and coined the ominous phrase that lurks within the inner recesses of the anesthesiologist's mind: "Anoxemia not only stops the machine but wrecks the machinery." He believed until his death, despite experimental evidence, that the lung actively secreted oxygen into the blood from the air. His landmark monograph *Respiration*, published in 1922,[12] summarized his studies on the respiratory system.

At the end of the 19th century it was known that hemoglobin had a vital role in the transport of oxygen to tissues. In 1896, Carl Gustav von Hufner (1840-1908) showed that the presence of hemoglobin in blood greatly enhanced its oxygen-carrying capacity and quantified that 1 g of hemoglobin carried 1.34 mL of oxygen.[13] It was soon observed that delivery of high concentrations of oxygen to patients with advanced pulmonary disease was often inadequate to fully maintain tissue respiration and saturate hemoglobin completely. Gradients for inspired, alveolar, and arterial oxygen partial pressures became apparent after development of the oxygen electrode by Leland C. Clark[14] (1918-) (Fig. 1-2) in 1953. The Clark electrode consisted of a platinum cathode and a silver anode separated from blood by a polyethylene membrane. The platinum was negatively charged to react with any oxygen reaching it through the membrane and was sensitive to the oxygen pressure outside the membrane (i.e., the oxygen tension in blood).

Further understanding of respiratory physiology arose because of the worldwide polio epidemic that occurred roughly between the years of 1930 and 1960. Thousands of afflicted patients were kept alive with mechanical respirators, but the adequacy of ventilation could not be assessed without some measure of carbon dioxide tension (P_{CO_2}) in the blood. Several methods to measure P_{CO_2} indirectly were made by Donald D. Van Slyke[15] (1883-1971) and Paul B. Astrup (1915-2000), but the modern solution rested on development of the carbon dioxide electrode. This problem was solved in 1958, when John W. Severinghaus (1922-) (see Fig. 1-2) improved the accuracy of a prototype carbon dioxide electrode produced by Richard Stow (1916-) that measured the pH of a thin film of electrolyte separated from blood by a Teflon membrane through which carbon dioxide could diffuse and equilibrate. Severinghaus and A. F. Bradley[16] (1932-) constructed the first blood gas apparatus by mounting the carbon dioxide electrode and Clark's oxygen electrode in cuvettes in a bath heated to 37°C. To measure blood P_{O_2} accurately, Severinghaus found it necessary to rapidly stir the blood in contact with Clark's electrode because of its high oxygen consumption rate. A pH electrode was added in 1959. Blood gas analysis made possible rapid assessment of respiratory exchange and acid-base balance. The use of blood gas analysis was rapidly adopted by the anesthesia community and has become one of the most common laboratory tests performed in the modern hospital. The impact of a more in-depth understanding of gas exchange on the practice of anesthesia is summarized by John Nunn in his book *Applied Respiratory Physiology*.[17]

Until the mid-20th century, hemoglobin saturation could be determined only by directly measuring a sample of arterial blood, a technique that required arterial puncture. Oximetry achieves the same measure noninvasively through a finger or ear probe by using optical measures of transmitted light. Glenn Millikan (1906-1947), working in the Johnson Foundation for Medical Physics at the University of Pennsylvania, devised the first ear oximeter in 1942, and it was used to detect hypoxia in pilots, who flew in open cockpits during World War II. Its introduction into anesthesia practice was delayed until the discovery of pulse oximetry by a Japanese engineer, Takuo Aoyagi (1936-).[18] Pulse oximetry added the additional measure of heart rate, and it provided assurance that the signal was actually measuring a biologic parameter. A highly successful commercial product, the Nellcor pulse oximeter was introduced in 1983 and had the unique feature of lowering the pitch of the pulse tone as saturation dropped.

Intravascular Pressures

The first measurement of blood pressure was made by Stephen Hales (1677-1761) (Fig. 1-3A), the curate of Middlesex, England, who occupied himself between sermons with experiments on mechanics of the circulation. He described one of his experiments[19] performed (1733) on an "old mare who was to be killed, as being unfit for service":

> *I fixed a brass pipe to the carotid artery of a mare . . . the blood rose in the tube till it reached to nine feet six inches in height. I then took away the tube from the artery and let out sixty cubic inches of blood, and then replaced the tube to see how high the blood would rise after each evacuation; this was repeated several times until the mare expired. In the three horses, death occurred when the height of the blood in the tube was about two feet.*

Hales also discovered that the resistance of a vascular bed could change by mixing alcohol in the blood, which he observed

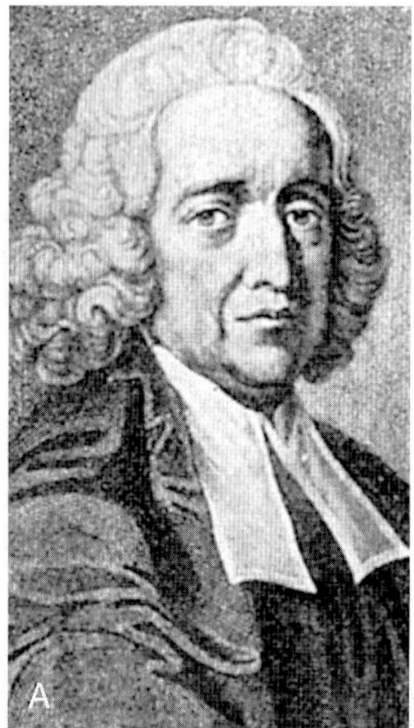

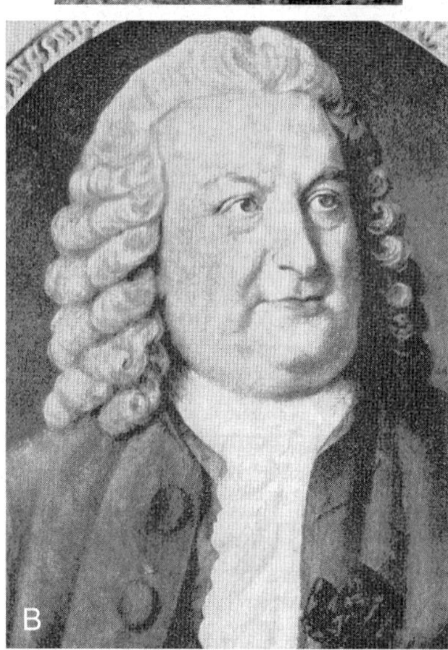

Figure 1-3 Two scientists of the Enlightenment era. **A,** Stephen Hales (1677-1761): detail of an oil painting by T. Hudson, 1759, in the National Portrait Gallery, London. Hales was educated at Cambridge University, England, and ordained as a minister in 1703. He spent his career as minister to the parish of Teddington, England. His rudimentary studies on the gas produced by mixing Walton pyrites (i.e., ferric disulfide) and spirit of nitre (i.e., nitric acid) was the spark that prompted Priestley to pursue his studies on nitric oxide, which led to the discovery of nitrous oxide in 1773. Hales was the first to measure blood pressure and cardiac output. He also developed ventilators that brought fresh air into prisons and granaries. **B,** Albrecht von Haller (1708-1777): detail of an engraving by Ambroise Tardieu. Haller was born in Bern, Switzerland. He served as professor of medicine and surgery at the University of Göttingen, Germany, where he began his encyclopedic work, *Physiological Elements of the Human Body*, published in eight volumes between 1757 and 1766. His demonstration that "irritability" was a property of muscle and "sensitivity" was a property of nerves was derived from nearly 600 experiments on live animals. He returned to Bern in 1753, and while there he published a catalog of the scientific literature containing 52,000 references. *(Portraits courtesy of the National Library of Medicine, Bethesda, MD.)*

could account for changes in blood pressure brought about by diverse ingested agents. In 1828, Jean L. Poiseuille[20] (1799-1869) repeated these experiments and devised a hemomanometer that used mercury instead of the long blood-filled tubes used by Hales. Poiseuille also showed that blood pressure varied with respiration.

In 1854, Karl Vierordt[21] (1818-1884) invented a sphygmograph that acted on the principle that indirect estimation of blood pressure could be accomplished by measuring the counterpressure necessary to obliterate the arterial pulsation. Scipione Riva-Rocci's (1863-1937) sphygmomanometer, described in 1896,[22] involved the same principle but used a rubber cuff that occluded a major arterial vessel and then slowly deflated. In 1905, Nikolai Korotkov[23] (1874-1920) described the sounds produced during auscultation over a distal portion of the artery as the cuff was deflated. These Korotkoff sounds resulted in more accurate determination of systolic and diastolic blood pressure. Oscillometric blood pressure measurement relied on a cuff that sensed changes in arterial pulsations and was described by H. von Recklinghausen in 1931.[24] Automatic blood pressure devices based on the oscillometric method were developed in the 1970s and have become the standard noninvasive measure of arterial pressure in most hospitals.

Venous pressure was of less interest to anesthesiologists until convenient methods for placing cannulas into central vascular structures were described more than 50 years ago by Sven Seldinger.[25] Werner Forssman (1904-1979), a urologist, described methods for central venous access and right heart catheterization in humans in 1929[26]; he originally experimented on himself and was awarded the Nobel Prize in Physiology and Medicine for his work on venous pressure in 1956. The introduction of plastic catheters[27] gradually made it possible to measure central pressure in the clinical setting. Although arm and femoral veins were used initially, subclavian and internal jugular vein cannulation eventually replaced the peripheral sites. Pulmonary artery catheterization with a balloon-tipped, flow-directed catheter was described in 1970[28] and has been used extensively since then by anesthesiologists to measure pulmonary artery pressure and cardiac output via the Fick[29] (Adolf E. Fick—1829-1901) principle. The pulmonary artery catheter also allowed clinicians to use the well-known pressure-volume relationships of the heart described by Ernest H. Starling (1866-1927) in 1918 to maximize cardiac output and oxygen delivery to tissues.

Transesophageal echocardiography (TEE) was described in 1976[30] and used in anesthesia practice a few years later. One of the original probes used during anesthesia was fashioned from an esophageal stethoscope combined with an M-mode echocardiographic probe and was used to calculate cardiac output and ejection fraction in a 65-year-old woman undergoing mitral valve repair.[31] An improved electronic phased-array transducer was initially applied at the University of California, San Francisco, for monitoring regional myocardial function in high-risk surgical patients.[32] Biplane TEE and color flow mapping were introduced in the 1980s and resulted in an explosive growth in TEE applications.[33] With experience and training in TEE, the anesthesiologist can quickly evaluate filling pressures of the heart, as well as obtain measures of myocardial contractility and valvular function. TEE has become a routine monitor for certain surgical procedures.

Autonomic Nervous System and Neurohumoral Transmission

The first hint of involuntary control of glandular and vascular function occurred in the 18th century. In a classic paper written in 1751, Robert Whytt (1714-1766) described the reflex nature of many involuntary activities.[34] Thomas Willis[35] (1621-1675) had described the sympathetic chain as early as 1657. He called it the intercostal nerve because it received segmental branches from the spinal cord at each level.

Pourfour du Petit (1664-1741) observed that there was a corresponding miosis and retraction of the nictitating membrane when this "intercostal" nerve was unilaterally cut in the neck of a cat.[36] Jacob B. Winslow (1669-1760) gave the intercostal nerve the name grand sympathique to stress that this nerve brought the various organs of the body into sympathy,[37] a term that was originally coined by the Greek physician Soranus of Ephesus (98-138) in the first century AD (*sym*, "together," and *pathos*, "feeling"). Claude Bernard (1813-1878) observed vasoconstriction and pupillary dilation after stimulation of the same intercostal (now called the sympathetic) nerve and then described the vasomotor nerves arising between the cervical and lumbar enlargements of the spinal cord.[38]

In 1889, John N. Langley (1852-1925) began his work on sympathetic transmission in autonomic ganglia. He blocked synaptic transmission in the ganglia by painting them with nicotine and then mapped the distribution of the presynaptic and postsynaptic autonomic nerves.[39] He observed a similarity between the effects of injection of adrenal gland extracts and stimulation of the sympathetic nerves.[40] The active principle of adrenal medullary extracts was called epinephrine by John J. Abel[41] (1837-1938) in 1897. Abel was one of the first pharmacologists in the United States, and with his discovery of the hormone epinephrine, he uncovered one of the most commonly used lifesaving agents in the anesthesiologist's pharmacopoeia.

Thomas R. Elliott (1877-1961) postulated that sympathetic nerve impulses release a substance similar to epinephrine and considered this substance to be a chemical step in the process of neurotransmission.[42] George Barger (1878-1939) and Henry H. Dale (1875-1968) then studied the pharmacologic activity of a large series of synthetic amines related to epinephrine and called these drugs sympathomimetic.[43] The different effects on end organs produced by adrenal extracts and sympathetic stimulation were analyzed by Walter B. Cannon (1871-1945) and by Ulf Svante von Euler (1905-1983). In a series of papers, these authors demonstrated that the sympathetic nerves released norepinephrine, whereas the adrenal gland released both epinephrine and norepinephrine.

In 1907, Walter E. Dixon[44] (1871-1931) observed that the alkaloid muscarine had the same effect as stimulation of the vagus nerves on various end organs. He proposed that the nerve liberated a muscarine-like chemical that acted as a chemical mediator. In 1914, Henry H. Dale[45] investigated the pharmacologic properties of acetylcholine and was impressed that its effects reproduced the same effects as stimulation of the craniosacral fine myelinated fibers that Walter H. Gaskell[46] (1847-1914) had called the bulbosacral involuntary nerves and had by then been called parasympathetic by Langley.

The final proof of neurotransmission by acetylcholine was provided through the elegant experiments of Otto Loewi (1873-1961). He stimulated the neural innervation of the frog heart and then allowed the perfusion fluid to come in contact with a second isolated heart preparation.[47] The resulting bradycardia provided evidence that some substance was released from the donor nerves that slowed the heart rate of the second organ.[47] Loewi and Navrail presented evidence that this substance was acetylcholine, as Dale had suggested. Loewi and Dale were jointly awarded the Nobel Prize in 1936 for their work on chemical neurotransmission.

Theodore Tuffier (1857-1929) first demonstrated the relevance of the sympathetic nervous system to the practice of anesthesia in 1900. In a series of experiments on dogs, he demonstrated the sympatholysis that occurs after spinal anesthesia.[48] Further studies on the sympathectomy resulting from neuraxial blockade were performed by G. Smith and W. Porter in 1915.[49] Working with cats, they concluded that the decrease in arterial blood pressure was secondary to sympathetic paralysis of the vasomotor fibers in the splanchnic vessels. Gaston L. Labat[50] (1877-1934) encouraged the use of sympathetic stimulants such as ephedrine to counter the hypotensive effects of spinal anesthesia.

Reversal of neuromuscular blockade rests on a fundamental understanding of two types of cholinergic receptors, muscarinic and nicotinic, originally described in 1914 by Dale.[45] Neostigmine, synthesized in 1931,[51] when given alone during reversal of neuromuscular blockade had produced cardiac arrest in several instances before it was learned that previous administration of an antimuscarinic drug would prevent this complication.[52] Atropine, isolated from the plant *Atropa belladonna* by A. Mein[53] in 1831, blocked peripheral and central nervous system muscarinic receptors. Glycopyrrolate was synthesized in 1960 as an antimuscarinic agent that did not pass the blood-brain barrier.[54] Glycopyrrolate is more titratable, has fewer central nervous system side effects, and has gradually replaced atropine as the preferred anticholinergic during reversal of neuromuscular blockade.

Crucial to the control of arterial blood pressure and heart rate in the perioperative period was the realization that there was more than one type of adrenergic receptor. In 1948, Raymond P. Ahlquist (1914-1983) proposed the designations α- and β-adrenergic receptors,[55] and various subtypes of these two main classes have been characterized since then. Esmolol was introduced in 1985 as a short-acting β-adrenergic antagonist that effectively controls the heart rate during anesthesia. Labetalol, a unique agent introduced in 1976, antagonizes α- and β-adrenergic receptors. α_2-Adrenergic agonists such as clonidine and dexmedetomidine have been shown to be useful agents in certain clinical settings. The α_2-adrenergic agonist effects produce sedation and analgesia through a central effect and, because they do not induce respiratory depression, they may have some advantages over opioids as sedatives in awake subjects.[56]

Manipulation of blood pressure can be achieved rapidly by intravenous nitrates such as nitroglycerin and nitroprusside. These drugs act directly on smooth muscle to allow rapid and more precise control of hemodynamics. Nitroglycerin was synthesized in 1846 by the Italian chemist Ascanio Sobrero (1812-1888) by combining nitric acid and glycerol. The first practical use of the drug was made by Alfred Nobel (1833-1896), who mixed the agent with silica to make dynamite, a highly successful explosive used in building tunnels and canals. A portion of the vast wealth of Nobel was directed by his will to be distributed annually in the form of Nobel Prizes beginning in 1901.[57,58] William Murrell[59] (1853-1912) reported the use of sublingual nitroglycerin in 1879 to treat angina. Intravenous use of the nitrovasodilators during anesthesia was not feasible until the development of continuous arterial monitoring, but for the past 30 years these drugs have been popular for rapid control of hypertensive crises in the operating room.[60] The mechanism of action of nitrates on smooth muscle, through the release of nitric oxide, was demonstrated by Ferid Murad (1936-) in 1986.[61] Nitric oxide, considered a toxic gas by Priestley who discovered it and by Humphry Davy who breathed it, has been shown to be a useful inhaled agent when used in a very low dose of 5 to 10 ppm in cases of life-threatening pulmonary hypertension.[62]

Historical Development of Theories of Pain

An understanding of the mechanism of pain production was not required by the physicians who developed the use of general anesthesia in the second half of the 19th century. Although inhalation of vapors produced a lack of awareness during surgery, anesthesiologists learned that control of perioperative nociception would require a more thorough understanding of pain. Fortunately, by the beginning of the 20th century, there was already a large body of knowledge on pain mechanisms dating from the earliest days of medical inquiry.

In antiquity, pain was thought to be an emotion rather than a sensory modality. Pain control was a function of religious authorities and shamans in primitive cultures, and relief of pain was sought through incantations and prayers. Pain was then often considered to be a punishment for committed sins or a form of religious suffering. The word *pain* is derived from the Greek term *poine* ("penalty"). Aristotle thought that pain was an emotion emanating from the heart, but Galen correctly observed that the brain was required for pain to be manifested in animals. Galen also proposed that sensation was a property of nervous tissue, but his physiologic system was altogether hampered by his idea that an invisible psychic pneuma traveled within hollow nerves.[3]

The 18th and 19th centuries witnessed considerable progress in understanding the mechanisms of pain. Albrecht von Haller[63] (1708-1777) (see Fig. 1-3B) observed that some tissues in the body have a property that he called sensibility: "I call those parts sensible, if the irritation occasions evident signs of pain and disquiet in the animal." Other tissues were insensible, which "if touched occasioned no sign of pain nor convulsion." Some tissues were irritable. "I call that part of the human body irritable, if it becomes shorter upon being touched." von Haller's landmark contribution in 1752[64] concluded that only parts of the body supplied with nerves possess sensibility, whereas irritability is a property of muscular fibers.

The idea of specific neural pathways for painful sensations began with Charles Bell[65] (1774-1842) and François Magendie[66] (1783-1855), who both demonstrated that the dorsal roots transmitted sensory information and that the ventral roots contained the motor nerves. Johannes Müller (1801-1858), in his 1826 paper titled "Of the Peculiar Properties of Individual Nerves," proposed that each sense organ gave rise to its own characteristic sensation and to no other; electrical or mechanical stimulation of the optic nerve, for example, gives rise to only a sensation of light.[67] The evidence that pain was a separate and distinct sense with separate end organs was formulated in 1858 by Moritz S. Schiff (1823-1896).

By the end of the 19th century, the idea was firmly established that acute pain was a distinct sensory modality that was susceptible to interruption through a conduction block initiated with local anesthetics. Pain as a separate sensation that was transmitted through separate neural fiber tracts was supported by clinical observations after neural blockade. Several investigators found, for example, that acute pain could be abolished with cocaine injections, which left some sensory modalities unaffected.[68]

There is evidence that operations undertaken on the battlefield may be associated with less pain than occurs with similar elective operations performed without anesthesia. The amputation of Lord Horatio Nelson's right arm in the battle at Tenerife, Canary Islands, was performed aboard ship after he sustained a musket shot above the elbow that divided the artery and shattered the humerus. Nelson complained only that the knife felt cold and thereafter ordered that all knives on board be heated before entering into conflict because his personal experience had indicated that a warm knife would produce almost no discomfort.[69] Henry Beecher[70] (1904-1976) confirmed during World War II that wounded soldiers had surprisingly little pain.

To further explain some of these central influences on nociception, Ronald Melzack (1929-) and P. D. Wall proposed the gate control theory of pain in 1965.[71] This theory suggested that the nociceptive afferent pain fibers were subjected to the modulating influence of a "gate" at the first synaptic contact in the spinal cord. Whereas large-fiber input tends to close the gate (i.e., inhibit nociceptive transmission), small-fiber input opens it, and descending influences from the cortex and midbrain[72] also profoundly influence the gate. Endogenous opioids, first discovered in 1974 by A. Goldstein[73] and later confirmed by J. Hughes[74] in 1975 and S. H. Snyder and coworkers[75] in 1977, are located at diverse sites in the pain pathway, including the dorsal horn, and they can influence the rostral transmission of pain sensations. Several modalities of pain therapy, such as acupuncture and biofeedback, attempt to activate these endogenous systems to suppress chronic pain syndromes.

The gate theory of pain has had considerable influence on the anesthesiologist's management of pain by focusing attention on the unique pharmacology of the dorsal horn of the spinal cord. By using intrathecal and epidural injections,[76] anesthesiologists have learned to suppress nociceptive transmission at the first synaptic relay in the spinal cord. The technique has implications in acute and chronic pain therapy because neuraxially administered drugs can provide analgesia without some of the systemic side effects of intravenously administered drugs. A typically modern view of perioperative pain is to view it as an impediment to recovery. Aggressive methods are often used to minimize pain and facilitate rapid return to normal functional activity.[77]

Surgical Procedures Before 1846

Greek and Roman surgeons used a variety of surgical instruments that we would recognize today. Drills, saws, syringes, cannulas, probes, and scalpels can all be viewed in the excavations at Her-

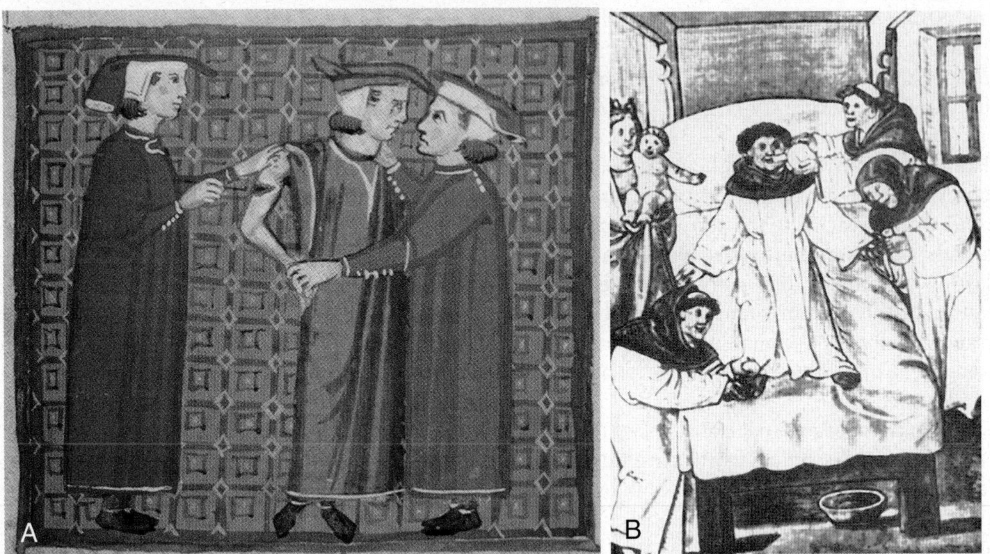

Figure 1-4 **A,** "Operating on the Upper Arm" is taken from the textbook titled *Chirurgia* by Theodoric of Cervia. It is noteworthy because it shows an intense focus by the patient directly into the gaze of an assistant. Although hypnosis is a 19th century term and its use for pain relief during surgery was not widely promoted until then, induction of trances and altered states of being was known to the ancients. Theodoric apparently realized the value of diverting the patient's attention away from the pain of surgery. **B,** Inhalation of the vapor of alcohol was tried in the Middle Ages as a method for pain relief during surgery. The inhaler shown here is remarkably similar to that used by William T. G. Morton on October 16, 1846, which used ether as the volatile agent (compare with Fig. 1-6).

culaneum, Pompeii, and Rheims. Hippocrates (460-377 BC) wrote a treatise on surgery, but it provided little sympathy for the patient. His advice to the patient was "to accommodate the operator . . . and maintain the figure and position of the part operated on . . . and avoid sinking down, and shrinking from or turning away."[78] The most famous Roman surgeon was Pedanius Dioscorides (40-90 AD), a Greek physician who served in the armies of Nero. His *Materia Medica*, written in 77 AD, was the authoritative work on pharmacology for more than 15 centuries. In this book he described the effects of mandragora and wine to produce "anesthesia" in a patient being cut or cauterized. He also described local anesthesia produced by the "stone of Memphis," which "being cut small, and smeared upon the places to be cut or cauterized, produces anesthesia without danger."[3]

During the Middle Ages, attempts were made to use alcohol fumes as an analgesic during surgery (Fig. 1-4B). Another inhaled technique, the soporific sponge, is mentioned in numerous manuscripts written in the Middle Ages. One example[3] from the 9th century comes from a Benedictine monastery at Monte Cassino, near Salerno, Italy:

> *A hypnotic aid, that is a soporific suitable for those who are treated by surgery, so that asleep, they do not feel the pain of cutting. Rx: opium one half ounce, mandragora the juice from the leaves, eight ounces, the juice of fresh hemlock, hyposcyanus three ounces of the juice together with sufficient water so that it forms a liquor, and then absorb in a fresh dry sponge and dry it carefully. And when thou wouldst employ this sponge, dip it in warm water, place it over the nose and cause the patient to breathe deep until he sleeps. And when thou wouldst wake him up, apply to his nose another sponge well soaked with vinegar and thou willst end the sleep.*

The sponge used by Theodoric of Cervia (1205-1296), a member of the Dominican order who practiced in Bologna, contained the same ingredients as the Salernitan sponge.

The effective agents in this sponge were very likely opium and scopolamine.[3] Theodoric was one of the first surgeons to promote methods to ablate pain during surgery (see Fig. 1-4A). One of the great physicians of the Renaissance, Theophrastus Bombastus von Hohenheim, otherwise known as Paracelsus (1493-1541), was familiar with the soporific action of sulfuric ether, a compound that had been synthesized from sulfuric acid and alcohol by the chemist Valerius Cordus (1515-1544). Cordus called the flammable, volatile liquid "sweet vitriol," and in 1740, Frobenius named it ether (from the Greek word for "ignite" or "blaze"). Paracelsus described the effect of ether on chickens and stated that it "quiets all suffering without harm, and relieves all pain." Although he was appointed "surgeon to the Danish army" when they besieged Stockholm in 1518, he had little interest in surgery, and these ideas were not developed clinically.

The suffering associated with surgery is found by examining accounts written by patients who survived major surgical procedures before that time. One comes from Fanny Burney[79] (1752-1840), a novelist and celebrity of the early part of the 19th century. Here is an abbreviated account of her mastectomy for breast cancer by the surgeon Dominique J. Larrey (1766-1842), the celebrated military surgeon in Napoleon's army, on September 30, 1811:

> *I mounted the bed and a cambric handkerchief was placed upon my face. The bed was then surrounded by 7 men and my nurse. Through the cambric I saw the glitter of the polished steel knife. A silence ensued. . . . Oh what a horrible suspension! . . . When the dreadful steel was plunged into the breast, I needed no*

injunctions not to restrain my cries. I began a scream that lasted unintermittently during the whole time of the incision and I almost marvel that it rings not in my ears still, so excruciating was the agony.

Although Fanny Burney lived for another 29 years after this operation, she observed that anything that would recall the surgery to her mind would reactivate the terror of the horrible experience. Apparently, operations performed without anesthesia produced long-lasting emotional and painful side effects. A modern interpretation of this phenomenon could conclude that these patients lacked any form of "preemptive analgesia"[80] and that they therefore experienced lingering side effects after their surgical wounds had healed.

Even though thousands of patients experienced the terror of an operation, countless others suffered with chronic ailments because the risk associated with surgery was too high or because they feared death or severe pain during the operation. For example, even after the introduction of anesthesia in 1846, textbooks on the treatment of hernia continued to have extensive descriptions of hernia belts and trusses.[81]

Introduction of General Anesthesia

Background

Although surgical technique was in development, the patient presented a problem to the surgeon, chiefly because of active physical resistance and because the cries and screams were distracting and often left the patient emotionally and physically exhausted. These factors, combined with the inevitable sepsis, resulted in high mortality rates. No wonder that by the middle of the 19th century there was greater determination by some surgeons to devise ways of improving operating conditions so that these appalling surgical mortality figures could be decreased, which in some reports reached nearly 50%. Bold approaches and risks were required, and these factors came together in Boston, Massachusetts, on October 16, 1846, when William T. G. Morton demonstrated the use of ether inhalation for surgical anesthesia.

Gas Inhalation

As a result of the growing scientific interest in various types of "airs," popular medical treatments involving gas inhalation evolved. Health resorts were popular attractions and financially successful because of their use by prominent members of society. One important "pneumatic" spa was located at Clifton, near Bristol, England, where Thomas Beddoes[82] (1760-1808) furnished airs for therapeutic use and funded research on the manufacture and use of gases. Nitrous oxide, a gas codiscovered by Priestley and Joseph Black, was by then considered to be a dangerous gas after a pronouncement by the influential American physician and U.S. Senator Samuel Latham Mitchill (1764-1831) that the gas was the "principle of contagion" and if breathed would "spread plague." The young scientist Humphry Davy conducted research on nitrous oxide at the Beddoes institute and, undaunted by these pronouncements, made several important observations. He inhaled nitrous oxide and noticed that it provided relief from the pain caused by an erupting wisdom tooth. In 1800 he wrote: "As nitrous oxide in its extensive operation appears capable of destroying physical pain, it may probably be used with advantage during surgical operations in which no great effusion of blood takes place."[83]

Davy was not a surgeon, and clinicians overlooked his suggestion at the time. He resigned his position at the Beddoes Medical Pneumatic Institute in 1801 and moved to London to lecture at the newly founded Royal Institution of Great Britain. Davy was just 20 years old when he performed his studies on nitrous oxide, and his subsequent, highly successful career took him into other areas of scientific study that led to discovery of the elements potassium, sodium, calcium, barium, magnesium, strontium, and chlorine. He was knighted in 1812, became President of the Royal Society in 1820, and never returned to develop his promising early thoughts on nitrous oxide analgesia. Regrettably, he left no students to continue these studies, although his successor at the Royal Institute, Michael Faraday (1791-1867), briefly experimented with ether inhalation and observed that its "effects were similar to those occasioned by nitrous oxide."[84]

The first research specifically directed toward an effective method of providing pain-free surgery was made by a physician working in the village of Ludlow, Shropshire, in northern England. Henry Hill Hickman (1800-1830) was a practicing surgeon who investigated the use of carbon dioxide to induce insensibility in animals. Because of the widespread interest in inhalation therapy at the beginning of the 19th century, it is not surprising that Hickman used an inhaled gas. Unfortunately for him, he used the wrong gas; if he had selected nitrous oxide, which was known to produce analgesia, his results might have achieved further attention. Although he published his work in 1824 in a private letter to T. A. Knight,[85] Hickman failed to find any support from his colleagues in England or France, and he died at an early age without recognition.

Beginning of Inhaled Anesthesia

The story of anesthesia continues with another amateur and itinerant chemist, Gardner Quincy Colton (1814-1898) (Fig. 1-5A). Colton had attended 2 years of medical school at the Crosby Street College of Physicians and Surgeons in New York. While in school, he perfected the manufacture of nitrous oxide by heating ammonium nitrate, and after 2 years of study, he proclaimed himself to be a "Professor of Chemistry" and went on the road to lecture on chemistry and present "scientific exhibitions."

On the night of December 10, 1844, Professor Colton presented his exhibit featuring inhalation of nitrous oxide at Union Hall in Hartford, Connecticut. It was at the Colton exhibit that the dentist Horace Wells (1815-1848) originated an idea that culminated in the first successful demonstration of inhalation anesthesia 22 months later. Wells had experimented with mesmerism to relieve the pain of dental extractions and was aware of the work of Humphry Davy. He attended the Colton demonstration and observed a young man, Samuel A. Cooley, sustain a significant leg injury without pain after nitrous oxide inhalation. Here was the answer to the problem of painful tooth extractions that had occupied his mind. He arranged for Colton to administer nitrous oxide to him on the following day for extraction of one of Wells' own teeth by fellow dentist John M. Riggs. Only a slight tinge of pain was felt, and Wells proceeded to manufacture nitrous

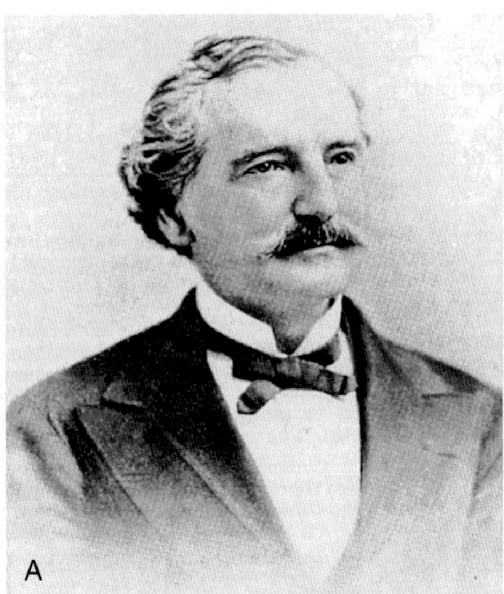

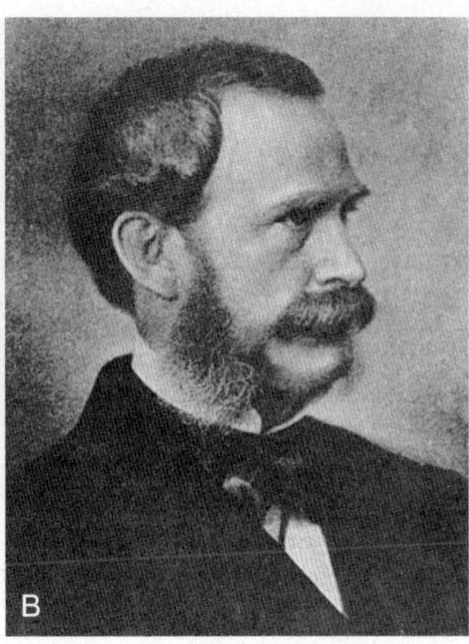

Figure 1-5 A, Gardner Q. Colton was born in Georgia, Vermont, and studied medicine briefly at the College of Physicians and Surgeons in New York City. His demonstrations of nitrous oxide inhalation were the spark that prompted Horace Wells and William T. G. Morton to use gas inhalation for relief of surgical pain. After a long and adventurous career, he died at age 84 in Rotterdam, Holland. **B,** William T. G. Morton was born in 1819 on a farm near Charlton, Massachusetts. After several business failures, he studied at the Baltimore College of Dental Surgery and, in 1842, entered into a partnership in Boston with another dentist, Horace Wells. This partnership was dissolved within a year on amicable terms. During this association, the two dentists had devised a new method for fitting dentures that required removal of all the diseased teeth, a prohibitively painful procedure for most patients. Morton experimented with laudanum and opium without success, and in proceeding with his investigations, he realized that greater knowledge of medicine was essential for further success. He briefly entered Harvard Medical School while continuing a part-time dental practice. During the summer of 1844, Morton, on the advice of Charles T. Jackson, used sulfuric ether for painless tooth extractions, and study of this agent eventually led to his successful demonstration of ether anesthesia at Massachusetts General Hospital on October 16, 1846. The remainder of Morton's life was spent in efforts to patent and receive monetary recognition for the discovery of ether anesthesia. Broken and despondent, he died of a cerebral hemorrhage in New York City in July 1868. *(Images courtesy of the Wood Library-Museum of Anesthesiology, Park Ridge, IL.)*

oxide according to Colton's instructions and use it for extractions of teeth. He recognized the enormous potential of his discovery and used his connections in Boston to arrange a date at the Harvard Medical School to demonstrate the technique of painless surgery.

Wells' appointment was to administer the gas for a leg amputation. The patient scheduled for this procedure refused to proceed with the anesthesia, and a young male student agreed to breathe nitrous oxide for extraction of a wisdom tooth. During the extraction the subject moved and groaned, only later to proclaim that little pain was actually felt. Nevertheless, Wells was discredited and became despondent, eventually withdrawing from further public promotions of his methods.

William T. G. Morton (see Fig. 1-5B), a young dentist from Boston, was acquainted with Wells, having been a former student and colleague of his, and had attended the failed demonstration at Harvard. Morton had lingering thoughts about a more suitable agent, in part arising from his interest in promoting his business of selling dentures. He had invented a new method for fitting dentures, but the process was prohibitively painful, and few patients would submit to the procedure. An adequate analgesic could accelerate his business.

Morton was initially trained as a dentist but had enrolled briefly at Harvard Medical School. Because of financial difficulties, he abandoned these studies and returned to dentistry. In the course of his education he became acquainted with Charles A. Jackson, a professor of chemistry at Harvard Medical School. On Morton's queries, Jackson advised a trial of sulfuric ether as an alternative to nitrous oxide. Later, Jackson was to claim priority in the discovery of anesthesia based on these consultations, but Morton countered that Jackson's role was negligible. Morton obtained the ether and, after performing experiments on himself and his pet animals, administered the agent successfully on September 30, 1846, to Eben Frost for extraction of an upper bicuspid tooth. Prompted by this success, he promoted use of the agent in his dental practice, thereby gaining the attention of another key figure, Henry J. Bigelow (1818-1890), in the unfolding drama. Bigelow, a prominent young surgeon at Massachusetts General Hospital, privately witnessed Morton's success with ether and arranged the time and date for its public demonstration.

The events of October 16, 1846, a complete triumph for Morton, have been recounted several times by others, but certain points are of special interest. The patient, Edward Gilbert Abbott, whom Morton apparently had never met, was to have a vascular tumor of the neck with large tortuous veins excised in the sitting position by 68-year-old Chief Surgeon John Collins Warren (1778-1856). Fearing a difficult airway or air embolism, a modern anesthesiologist might seek special equipment for this case, perhaps a special laryngoscope and central venous catheters. Morton, however, had only a poorly designed inhaler and no intravenous access. Close examination of the circumstances surrounding administration of this anesthetic indicates how dangerous this bold endeavor by Morton actually was and how likely it was to fail miserably. With the inhaler that he used, it seems unlikely that the vapor could be administered during the surgical procedure. Fortunately for Morton, the kinetic properties of ether result in prolonged emergence, and Mr. Abbott responded only briefly at the end of the procedure (Fig. 1-6).

Morton, intending to profit from his discovery, withheld identification of the ether that he used and called it Letheon. He

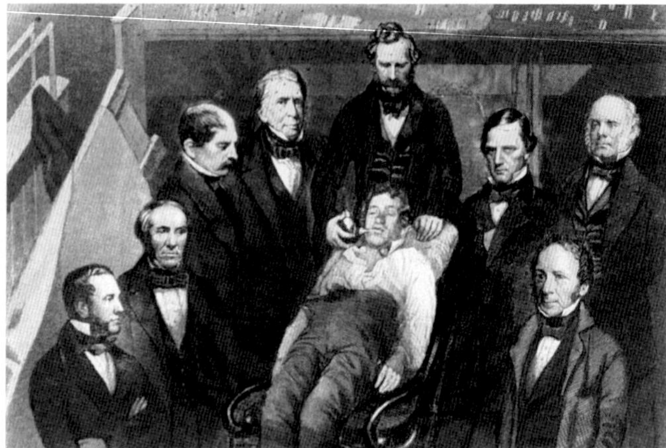

Figure 1-6 Drawing by H. H. Hall in *Rice's Trials of a Public Benefactor* illustrates the first public demonstration of ether anesthesia at Massachusetts General Hospital on October 16, 1846. From the left are Henry J. Bigelow (1818-1890), the earliest advocate and sponsor of William T. G. Morton at the hospital, who also wrote the classic article describing the first experiences with ether anesthesia in the *Boston Medical and Surgical Journal*; Augustus A. Gould, with whom Morton and his wife were boarding and who suggested the design of the first inhaler (Gould also suggested the name Letheon); Jonathan Mason Warren (1811-1867), son of John Collins Warren, who later devised new surgical procedures for nasal deformity and cleft lip (Hall erroneously places him at this event; others [not shown] who were present are George Heywood, house officer, and Eben Frost, who had a tooth pulled by Morton after ether administration on September 30, 1846); John Collins Warren (1778-1856), 68-year-old Chief of Surgery at Massachusetts General Hospital, who performed the operation that day; William T. G. Morton, to whom credit is given for introducing ether anesthesia to the world; Gilbert Abbott, a 28-year-old house painter and printer with a congenital vascular tumor, visible in the drawing as a tumor below the left mandible; and Samuel Parkman, Morton's anatomy instructor at Harvard Medical School; and George Hayward (1791-1863), 53-year-old senior surgeon at Massachusetts General Hospital, who excised an arm mass under ether anesthesia the following day, October 17, 1846. His operation for vesicovaginal fistula is considered to be an original procedure. Also present was Solomon D. Townsend, one of the prominent surgeons at Harvard Medical School. *(Courtesy of the Wood Library-Museum of Anesthesiology, Park Ridge, IL.)*

Insensibility During Surgical Operations Produced by Inhalation

Henry Jacob Bigelow, M.D.
Boston Medical and Surgical Journal
1846

It has long been an important problem in medical science to devise some method of mitigating the pain of surgical operations. An efficient agent for this purpose has at length been discovered. A patient has been rendered completely insensible during an amputation of the thigh, regaining consciousness after a short interval. Other severe operations have been performed without the knowledge of the patients. So remarkable an occurrence will, it is believed, render the following details relating to the history and character of the process, not uninteresting.

Figure 1-7 Title and opening paragraph of Henry J. Bigelow's description of the first ether anesthetics. *(From Bigelow HJ: Insensibility during surgical operations produced by inhalation. Boston Med Surg J 35:309-317, 379-382, 1846.)*

masked the aroma and appearance of ether by adding a colored dye and additional scents. For a fee, he intended to provide instruction on its safe use. The surgeons at Massachusetts General Hospital then denied continued use of the agent until its true nature was identified. After Morton disclosed its chemical nature, further operations were performed with success. Bigelow read his manuscript describing the use of ether for operative surgery on November 3, 1846, before the American Academy of Arts and Sciences and published it (Fig. 1-7) in the November 18, 1846, issue of the *Boston Medical and Surgical Journal*.[86] The name anesthesia (Greek *an*, "without," and *esthesia*, "sensation") was suggested by Oliver Wendell Holmes (1809-1894) in a private letter to Morton dated November 21, 1846. Holmes also considered the words antineurotic, aneuric, neuroleptic, neurolepsia, and neurostasis, but he rejected these as being "too anatomical" because the change induced by ether was physiologic.

Aftermath

It is remarkable that without more explicit instructions or actual demonstration by one of the Boston group, ether anesthesia was adopted so rapidly around the world. Only 63 days after the Morton demonstration, ether was administered in England by James Robinson (1813-1862), a prominent London dentist, for extraction of a deep-seated molar in a 13-year-old girl. Robinson had learned of ether anesthesia through a letter shown to him by a neighboring friend, Francis Boott (1792-1863), who had received the letter from Jacob Bigelow (1786-1879), father of Henry Bigelow, in which the effects of ether inhalation were described. Robinson devised a new inhaler and wrote the first textbook on anesthesia, published in London on March 1, 1847.[87] Two days after Robinson's use of ether, Robert Liston (1794-1847) performed the first operation in England—a leg amputation at University College Hospital, London—with ether as the anesthetic delivered by William Squire. Within a few months, ether anesthesia had spread to the European continent. Nikolai Ivanovitch Pirogoff (1810-1881) used ether in St. Petersburg as early as February 1847, and he wrote a treatise on the subject. Of significant importance for the widespread use of ether was the prestige of the Boston surgeons, who firmly supported its legitimacy.

Many who tried to administer the anesthetic did so without proper preparation, and failures were common. Several questions remained unanswered. Bigelow's article was vague about how it should be administered and simply described a number of cases with the use of Morton's inhaler. How the ether was supposed to be administered after loss of consciousness was not addressed. Nasal breathing or failure to purse the lips around the mouthpiece must have placed a limit on the duration of effective vapor administration. It was another lucky circumstance for Morton that ether was chosen as his agent. Subsequent studies with ether have revealed that it stimulates the sympathetic nervous system at deep levels of anesthesia.[88] This unique property of the drug and its high blood solubility result in a remarkably safe agent that requires only marginal skills to avoid overdose.

Priority for Discovery

Claims of priority for the discovery of ether anesthesia arose quickly. Wells, Morton, and Jackson all claimed to have discovered anesthesia. The issue of priority was further complicated by a report that a surgeon in Jefferson, Georgia, had used ether anesthesia as early as 1842. Crawford Long (1815-1878) published a manuscript in the *Southern Medical and Surgical Journal* in December 1849 describing his use of ether on March 30, 1842, to excise a tumor from the neck of a young man, James M. Venable.[89]

Numerous monuments have been erected to commemorate the man "who discovered anesthesia." At least 15 have been erected for the group of Morton, Wells, and Long. A chair that Charles Jackson sat in while experimenting with ether inhalation is on display in the Pilgrim Memorial Hall in Plymouth, Massachusetts, with the label "Seated in this chair, Dr. Charles T. Jackson discovered etherization February, 1842." In the Public Gardens of Boston, a monument without a name has been erected to those who discovered anesthesia, thus suggesting that the introduction of ether anesthesia was the product of several individuals. Howard R. Raper, in his book *Man Against Pain*, analyzed the controversy about "who discovered anesthesia" and suggested that Crawford Long was the discoverer if only the issue of priority is considered. However, Long continued to use whiskey and other ineffective means after 1842, indicative of his apparent lack of enthusiasm for ether. Wells was the discoverer if the idea of inhalation anesthesia is considered, and Morton was the discoverer if the primary consideration is who introduced inhalation anesthesia to the world. Historians have generally credited the personality who produces the actual change in medical practice, and that individual was William Thomas Green Morton.

Neither honors nor monetary awards were forthcoming during the remaining lives of Wells or Morton. Wells committed suicide in 1848, unaware that the French Academy of Sciences had just named him as the true discoverer of anesthesia. Morton was unsuccessful in his effort to profit from a patent on his discovery or to secure a financial award from the U.S. government and died, broken and despondent, at age 49. Jackson was committed to a hospital for the mentally ill at the age of 68 years, where he died 7 years later. Morton was 27 years old when he demonstrated ether anesthesia. The ages of the other participants at the time of their discoveries were as follows: Wells (1815-1848) was 29; Davy (1778-1829) was 22; Hickman (1800-1830) was 24; Jackson (1804-1880) was 41; Long (1815-1878) was 27; and Colton (1814-1898) was 30 years old.

Development of Inhaled Anesthetics

Chloroform

Within a year after the introduction of ether anesthesia, the search had already begun for other agents that could anesthetize without some of the problems associated with ether. Although ether was a remarkably safe anesthetic, even when administered by untrained hands, there were disadvantages, including flammability, prolonged induction, an unpleasant odor that was persistent, and a high incidence of nausea and vomiting. James Young Simpson (1811-1870), an obstetrician from Edinburgh, Scotland, used ether in 1846 but was determined to find a better anesthetic. As early as January 1847, he began experimenting with a variety of different solvents and volatile liquids.[90]

Marie Jean Flourens (1794-1867) had used chloroform in dogs while studying stages in depression of the central nervous system by chloroform and ether. Simpson and a group of friends learned of the surprising potency of chloroform at a dinner party hosted by Simpson on September 4, 1847. Dinner was followed by the experimental inhalation of volatile drugs, and the use of chloroform was followed by stupor and coma in several participants, including Simpson. Simpson promoted chloroform vigorously, and its use was widely accepted in England. As an obstetrician, he advocated its use during labor and promoted, along with others,[91] the use of analgesics during parturition. Initially, his views conflicted with those of medical authorities, who considered it unsafe during labor, and with those of religious authorities, who opposed it on theologic grounds. Edinburgh had a black history on the issue of pain relief during childbirth. In 1591, a young woman named Euphanie Macalyane was burned alive as punishment for seeking pain relief during labor. Her sentence was on a direct order from the King of Scotland, James VI (1567-1625). Simpson was not a timid man and met the religious controversy with direct quotations from the Bible that appeared to support his views (Genesis 2, 21: "and the Lord God caused a deep sleep to fall upon Adam, and he slept: and he took one of his ribs, and closed up the flesh instead thereof.").

Chloroform was used widely in England, but controversy developed about its safety, particularly in otherwise healthy subjects, those in whom a physician would not anticipate any difficulties. Various commissions and committees were formed, notably the two Hyderabad commissions (1888 and 1890),[92] to investigate the relative safety of chloroform. In the late 19th century, Hyderabad, a city in the middle of the Indian subcontinent, was the capital of the independent state of Hyderabad, ruled by the Nizam Mir Mehboob Ali Khan. The Nizam was persuaded to underwrite an animal investigation into the safety of chloroform anesthesia by Major Edward Lawrie (1846-1915), principal of the Indian Medical School in Hyderabad. Lawrie had a preconceived belief in the safety of chloroform, and the results of his studies understandably concluded that chloroform was entirely safe if given according to his methods. The agent continued in use for several decades, but its slow demise was initiated in 1894, when Leonard G. Guthrie[93] reported several cases of delayed chloroform hepatotoxicity in children. The future use of chloroform anesthesia was doomed after the studies of A. Goodman Levy[94] (1856-1954), who demonstrated that the combination of light chloroform anesthesia and adrenalin produced fatal ventricular fibrillation in experimental animals, thereby explaining the perplexing sudden demise of several healthy subjects who were administered chloroform anesthetics.

Nitrous Oxide

Because of the embarrassing public demonstration by Wells in 1863, revival of nitrous oxide as a surgical anesthetic was delayed until its reintroduction by the same man, Gardner Q. Colton, whose lecture and demonstration Wells had attended in 1844 and from whom he obtained the gas used in his first experiments with inhalation analgesia. Soon after the Wells debacle in 1844, Colton abandoned nitrous oxide demonstrations and joined his brother in California, where he unsuccessfully panned for gold and served briefly as Justice of the Peace for San Francisco. His stay in San Francisco terminated when he was involved in controversial land sales, and he moved to Boston and took a job as a writer for the

Boston Transcript.[95] Colton also resumed his "laughing gas" exhibitions, and in 1863 he joined into a partnership with Joseph H. Smith, a dentist in New Haven, Connecticut, for the "painless extraction of teeth." The business thrived, and between 1864 and 1897, the Colton Dental Association had treated nearly 200,000 patients without a fatality. Colton demonstrated nitrous oxide inhalation in Paris at the First International Congress of Medicine in June 1867, and its wider use in Europe originates from that time. Colton was a unique individual who promoted the continued use of a valuable agent, but he remained ignorant of its true chemical nature. In his writings,[96] he states, for example, the following:

> *The gas is composed of half nitrogen and half oxygen and because oxygen is the life giving principle of the air, a person lives a little faster while under its influence. It acts as an exhilarant, as by supplying an extra supply of oxygen to the lungs, the pulse is increased 15 to 20 beats to the minute.*

Until 1870, nitrous oxide was administered with air, and the livid appearance of many patients raised the question about whether the analgesic properties of the gas were primarily caused by lack of oxygen. The idea of using nitrous oxide with oxygen is usually credited to Edmund Andrews[97] (1824-1904), a Chicago surgeon who was able to provide analgesia without cyanosis, thereby confirming the inherent analgesic properties of nitrous oxide. Andrews noticed that the nitrous oxide provided to dentists in gaseous form was often impure and instead advocated the use of liquid nitrous oxide contained in iron flasks. This pure nitrous oxide, when combined with oxygen, provided satisfactory anesthesia without cyanosis for short procedures. Paul Bert (1833-1886), a French physiologist who contributed significantly to the understanding of blood gas tensions at altered barometric pressures, demonstrated that nitrous oxide and oxygen mixtures produced highly satisfactory surgical anesthesia without hypoxia when delivered at pressures greater than 1 atm. Frederick Hewitt[98] (1857-1916) devised the first anesthesia machine to deliver variable portions of nitrous oxide and oxygen. Johnson demonstrated that the pupillary dilation, lividity, jactitation, and clonic movements of the extremities after the administration of nitrous oxide and air were caused by extreme hypoxia because they could be reproduced exactly by administering nitrogen with only 0.5% oxygen.[99]

These developments led to reintroduction of nitrous oxide into the operating room, where Horace Wells had predicted it would be used with success. Nitrous oxide and oxygen anesthesia was promoted in the United States by Elmer I. McKesson[100] (1881-1935), Paluel J. Flagg (1886-1970), and F. W. Clement (1892-1970). McKesson's method for induction of anesthesia with 100% nitrous oxide did not survive into the latter part of the 20th century. A landmark publication by C. B. Courville described the neuropathologic findings in patients who had sustained hypoxic insults during anesthesia with high concentrations of nitrous oxide.[101] W. D. A. Smith recounts the revival of nitrous oxide after Colton's reintroduction of the agent in an entertaining and informative book on the subject.[102]

Unsatisfactory Inhaled Anesthetics

During the first few decades of the 20th century, practitioners were searching for new and improved anesthetics. An American anesthesia textbook written by James T. Gwathmey (1865-1944) (see Fig. 1-18D) was published in 1914 and briefly discussed more than 600 possible anesthetic agents for the reader to consider. By 1930, all successful anesthetic agents except chloroform and nitrous oxide were explosive. Chloroform by then was thought to be dangerous, and the popularity of nitrous oxide was curtailed by the need for a nearly hypoxic mixture to provide adequate anesthesia. Ethyl chloride was the last agent to be introduced in the 19th century, and like ether, it was flammable. It was a unique agent that was first used as a spray to induce local anesthesia, but if inhaled, it also produced general anesthesia.

In the early 20th century, several unsatisfactory volatile anesthetics were introduced. Ethylene was used clinically in 1923. This agent required high concentrations to achieve anesthesia, had an unpleasant smell, and was explosive. Divinyl ether, developed by Chauncey Leake[103] (1896-1978), had some advantages over ether for induction of anesthesia, but it was also flammable and never widely used. Cyclopropane was introduced in 1934 by Ralph Waters (1884-1979) and was briefly popular, but it was violently explosive. The flammable anesthetics prevented the use of surgical cautery and electronic monitoring. One attempt to produce a nonflammable alternative to ether and cyclopropane was made in 1935, when trichloroethylene was introduced. It was promoted by Christopher L. Hewer[104] (1896-1986) as a nonexplosive agent, but it was eventually withdrawn when it was shown to decompose to the toxic nerve poison dechloroacetylene in the presence of soda lime and to produce phosgene, a severe respiratory irritant, when electrocautery was used. Clearly, new directions were needed.

Fluorinated Anesthetics

In the early 1930s, progress was made in attempts to fluorinate hydrocarbons, and many fluorinated compounds became available commercially, primarily as refrigerants. From a theoretical analysis of hydrocarbon chemistry, it was known that halogenation of the parent hydrocarbon compound would decrease its flammability. One early approach to produce a nonflammable anesthetic was to select a flammable agent and partially fluorinate it. With this in mind, John C. Krantz, Jr., of the University of Maryland, took the flammable anesthetic vinamar, which is ethyl vinyl ether, and produced trifluoroethyl vinyl ether,[105] or fluroxene.

The circumstances surrounding the first anesthesia with fluroxene illustrate the lure of self-experimentation in research related to the advancement of anesthetic practice. Max S. Sadove (1914-1997), an anesthesiologist at the University of Illinois, was a member of the Walter Reed Society, a group of scientists who, following the example of Walter Reed, allowed themselves to be administered the first dose of investigational drugs. Sadove, a close acquaintance of Krantz, insisted that he be given the first fluoride-containing anesthetic, fluroxene, in 1953. Krantz, who had synthesized the drug, was a pharmacologist with no training in anesthesia. Krantz advised Sadove that there was danger that the agent might be administered improperly or might be metabolized to a toxic by-product. Nevertheless, Sadove was insistent, and on April 10, 1953, Krantz administered open-drop fluroxene to Sadove, and recovery was rapid and uneventful.[106]

Fluroxene had marginal success but was eventually withdrawn because of questions about toxicity and the frequent occurrence of postanesthetic nausea and vomiting. Charles Suckling, a chemist at Imperial Chemical Industries, synthesized halothane in 1954 after a theoretical analysis of possible anesthetic halogenated drugs. The pharmacologic properties of halothane were studied by James Raventós[107] (1905-1983), and it was introduced clinically in 1956 by Michael Johnstone.[108] Halothane had definite advantages over ether and cyclopropane because of its more pleasant odor, higher potency, favorable kinetic characteristics, nonflammability, and low toxicity, and it gradually replaced the older agents. Halothane was a highly successful drug that achieved worldwide acceptance, but its unblemished record lasted only a few years before controversy appeared.

In 1958, a case report described a 39-year-old woman who died of fulminant hepatic necrosis 11 days after cholecystectomy with halothane anesthesia.[109] This was followed in 1963 by nine case reports of patients in whom hepatic necrosis developed after halothane anesthesia (also see Chapter 24).[110] The cases were unique in that hepatic failure often followed minor operations in which other causes of hepatic failure were not apparent. Eventually, the term "halothane hepatitis" became a common clinical diagnosis for patients with postoperative liver failure, even when halothane was not used as the anesthetic. A national study formally titled "The National Halothane Study" was established in 1964 and reported that the incidence of liver failure after halothane anesthesia was no more frequent than that reported with other anesthetics.[111] Nevertheless, halothane was extensively metabolized in the body, and in some individuals it seemed that a toxic metabolite might produce liver necrosis. Other halogenated anesthetics were also extensively metabolized, and in the case of methoxyflurane, such metabolism resulted in high levels of fluoride ions. High-output renal failure was an infrequent but potentially morbid side effect of methoxyflurane[112] that was related to increased blood fluoride ion concentrations.

Beginning in 1960, the pharmaceutical industry launched new efforts to synthesize the "ideal anesthetic." Ross C. Terrell at Ohio Medical Products synthesized more than 700 potential anesthetic compounds between 1960 and 1980. During the same period, Edmund I. Eger II (1930-) began a series of studies that significantly enhanced the rational use of inhaled anesthetics. Eger drew on the work of Seymore S. Kety[113] (1915-2000) and Severinghaus,[114] which had previously demonstrated that the end-tidal partial pressure of anesthetic gases at steady state was the same as the brain cerebral partial pressure of those gases. By correlating the end-tidal (alveolar) concentration with the movement response to supramaximal nociceptive stimulation, the concept of minimum alveolar concentration (MAC) was born (also see Chapter 19). By definition, MAC represents the end-tidal concentration of any anesthetic agent at which 50% of patients move in response to a supramaximal stimulus.[115] With this standard measure of potency, new agents could easily be introduced to the anesthesia community. Several further studies by Eger and others on the pharmacokinetics of inhaled anesthetics and factors that alter MAC[116] accelerated an understanding of volatile anesthetic requirements and significantly enhanced the safe use of these drugs.

Two of the anesthetics developed by Ohio Medical Products, enflurane and isoflurane, were introduced about 40 years ago.[117,118] Isofluorane has been highly successful and used extensively since that time. Desflurane was one of the last volatile anesthetics to be synthesized and required a potentially dangerous explosive method of synthesis. Desflurane had a high vapor pressure and the added limitation of requiring more than five times the quantity of vapor to produce anesthesia than needed with isoflurane. Although desflurane was initially overlooked because of these problems, it was studied thoroughly in animals[119] and first used in humans in 1990.[120] Because of its favorable kinetic properties, recovery is more rapid with desflurane than with isoflurane or enflurane.

Sevoflurane was synthesized more than 40 years ago at Travenol Laboratories. Recovery is rapid with this agent, but because the compound is unstable in soda lime, it was not introduced until the late 1980s,[121] first in Japan and then in the United States. The decision to introduce the product was, as with desflurane, spurred by the emphasis on early discharge after anesthesia. Anesthesia has been induced with sevoflurane several million times without apparent complications resulting from the potential by-products arising from contact with carbon dioxide absorbents. Since the introduction of sevoflurane, there have been no additional inhaled anesthetics introduced for clinical use. The inert gas xenon has been under investigation as an anesthetic for several years, but it is expensive and, like nitrous oxide, requires high concentrations to produce anesthesia.

Needles and Syringes

In an attempt to find another parenteral route of drug administration, some physicians raised blisters or excoriated the skin and then deposited drugs on the exposed surface of the wound. Francis Rynd[122] (1801-1861) used a lancet to pierce the skin and devised a syringe to insert medication into the wound by gravity. Alexander Wood[123] (1817-1884) invented a hollow needle that would fit on the end of a piston-style syringe made for him by Daniel Ferguson, an instrument maker from London. Wood used the syringe and needle combination to successfully treat painful neuralgias by local injections of morphine. The syringe and needle combination became a popular item after these reports, and many practitioners used the device to inject morphine subcutaneously for pain relief. The term *hypodermic injection* was coined by Charles Hunter, who argued with Wood that morphine could be injected into the body at any place and achieve the same analgesic effect as that obtained by injection at the site of pain.

The early syringes were inadequate for the work of the developing specialty of regional anesthesia (Fig. 1-8). The rubber or leather plunger cracked or deteriorated after repeated sterilization. During use, the drug contents accumulated proximal to the plunger, or the plunger itself jammed inside the glass barrel. To achieve the fine control required for identification of the epidural space, a more carefully tooled instrument was required. H. Wulfing Luer of Paris introduced the first all-glass syringe in 1896. He sold the patent to partners Maxwell W. Becton and Fairleigh S. Dickinson (Becton, Dickinson and Company) in 1898. The Record syringe was made by Dewitt and Herz of Berlin, Germany, in 1906, and it consisted of an all-metal plunger with a finely ground glass barrel. The fit between the barrel and plunger was precise and sturdy, and Record syringes nearly 100 years old can still be used for identification of the epidural space.

The first hypodermic needles were made of tempered steel, a metal that rusted easily when in contact with water. A small rusted area might not be observed visually, and defective needles sometimes broke below the skin. Meticulous care was taken to

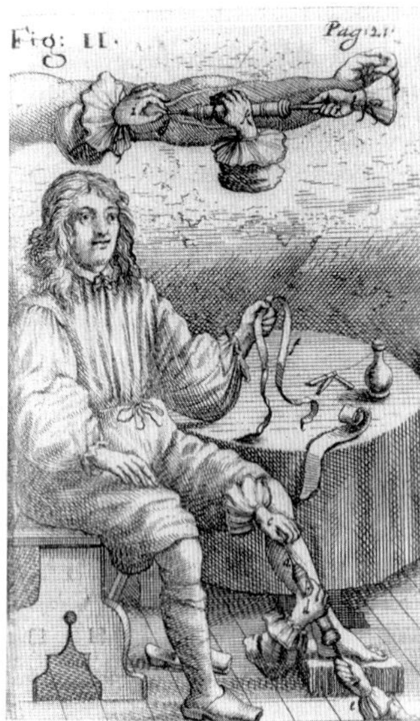

Figure 1-8 Drawing by an unknown artist appearing in *Clysmatica Nova*, a book written by Johan S. Elsholtz (1623-1688) and dated 1667. The artist clearly shows that syringes and rudimentary hollow intravenous tubes were used before the 19th century. Although this book was published in Cologne, Germany, most historians credit the first intravenous injections of pharmaceuticals to Christopher Wren and Timothy Clarck in England. *(Courtesy of the National Library of Medicine, Bethesda, MD.)*

dry each needle after steam sterilization. Specially designed introducers, called rimmers, were used for storage of the needles to prevent rust from developing inside the needle. To avoid the problem with needle breakage, platinum or gold needles were used occasionally. These needles were highly flexible and expensive and never became popular. Stainless steel was produced commercially in 1918 and essentially eliminated the problem with rust. Modern needles are usually disposable stainless steel needles, which has minimized complications resulting from infection and breakage.

The bevel of the needle was a topic of great discussion in the early 20th century. A long bevel produced less trauma to tissues, but it allowed a small portion of the needle to lie in the intrathecal space with the proximal portion of the bevel in the epidural space. To increase the success of spinal anesthesia and minimize side effects, short-beveled needles and pencil-point needles were developed by several regional anesthesia specialists, a process that continues to this day. Fine, 25-gauge spinal needles, designed to produce minimal trauma to the dura, have reduced the incidence of post–dural puncture headache.

Intravenous Fluid Therapy

Awareness of fluid balance had its beginnings in the writings of Claude Bernard, who in his final published work emphasized the importance of extracellular fluid in the support of vital functions.[124] In these writings he stressed that blood and lymph bathe the cells of the body and that these fluids constitute the *milieu interne*, later called the *fluid-matrix* by Walter B. Cannon. These researchers pointed out that an organism's freedom from external disturbances such as hunger, thirst, and cold is brought about by mechanisms that maintain uniformity of body fluids. The concept of the steady state maintained in this internal environment became known as *homeostasis* in the Cannon doctrine. During anesthesia, many of the homeostatic mechanisms are abolished or severely blunted, and the anesthesiologist must assume the role of maintaining a favorable *milieu interne*.

Crystalloids

In the late 19th century, the sodium content of serum was found to be roughly equivalent to an aqueous solution of 0.9% sodium chloride, and this became known as physiologic salt solution. Hartog J. Hamburger (1856-1924) showed a change in the volume of red blood cells at concentrations above and below 0.9% saline.[125] As a result of these experiments, the value of sodium ions in maintenance of osmotic pressure in serum was realized. Ernest H. Starling[126] (1866-1927) extended these observations to explain edema formation on the basis of hydrostatic and colloidal osmotic pressure.

Maintenance of fluid balance was not a priority or even a possibility for those who administered anesthetics during the 19th century. Without intravenous access, there was little that the anesthesia provider could do if the surgeon was recklessly losing blood. The importance of intravenously administered salt to patients with dehydration from cholera was observed in 1831 by William B. O'Shaughnessy[127] (1804-1889). Although there were isolated successful attempts to treat the dehydration of cholera with saline infusions, such treatment did not flourish, and the victory over cholera was finally won only through improved sanitary conditions.

The experimental introduction of saline infusions after surgery was based on work performed by Emil Schwarz[128] (1852-1918), who observed that saline infusions could save the lives of bled rabbits. This work was recognized by Johann J. Bischoff[129] (1841-1892), who reported that a salt infusion saved the life of a woman with severe postpartum hemorrhage. Treatment with salt infusions was generally adopted after surgical hemorrhage, but sepsis and failed attempts to revive the bleeding patient soon became apparent.

Alternative solutions to saline originated with Sydney Ringer[130] (1835-1910), Professor of Medicine at University College, London. Ringer observed that saline prepared from distilled water was not as effective as saline made from pipe water in maintaining contractility of the isolated frog heart. After careful analysis of the pipe water, he learned that it contained calcium and potassium impurities. Adding these cations to the saline made from distilled water proved his hypothesis that these ions played an important role in maintaining normal cardiac function.

In the first decades of the 20th century there were substantial barriers to the successful use of parenteral electrolyte solutions during surgery. Closed sterile administration sets and intravenous cannulas were slow to develop, and alternative methods were therefore used. Most patients received several liters of fluid, usually administered rectally; however, salt was administered, if possible, orally or by subcutaneous injection. With these ineffectual methods, the use of saline in the perioperative period fell into decline. In 1944, a syndrome described as postoperative salt intolerance was caused ostensibly by failure of the kidney to excrete a salt load.[131] These ideas had the support of the influential Francis D. Moore, Chief of Surgery at Peter Bent Brigham Hospital in Boston. When intravenous therapy became more widely available, patients were often administered dextrose and water or dilute sodium-containing solutions. Carl Moyer[132] (1908-1970) presented evidence in 1950 that sodium was avidly retained postoperatively and argued against the use of saline for perioperative fluid maintenance.

The reintroduction of perioperative saline therapy began in 1959, when G. Shires and associates[133] reported the redistribution of extracellular fluid into "third space" compartments during extensive surgical procedures. These reports encouraged preoperative administration of fluid to compensate for the lack of oral intake and intraoperative administration of sodium-containing fluid to replace translocation of extracellular fluid into edematous spaces such as the gut and peritoneum. The increased use of saline reduced the incidence of postoperative renal failure and decreased the requirement for blood transfusions. As a result of these studies, fluid replacement today consists of saline-containing fluids, with the addition of colloid and blood when excessive blood loss occurs. These concepts of fluid management were vigorously promoted by M. T. Jenkins (1917-1994).[134]

Blood Transfusions

The first blood transfusions were not performed as treatment of blood loss. Jean Baptiste Denis (1625-1704) from Montpellier, France, administered lamb's blood[135] to a demented patient with the idea of transferring the attributes of the donating animal to the recipient. Although the first patient survived, a subsequent transfusion resulted in death. Denis was tried for murder, and although he was acquitted, the procedure was condemned and prohibited by the Faculty of Medicine in Paris. Physicians in the 18th and 19th centuries were more prone to remove rather than administer blood.

Successful blood transfusions were performed by James Blundell[136] (1790-1877), who experimented with blood transfusions in animals and rejected the idea of animal-to-human transfusions. Blundell recorded 10 human-to-human transfusions between 1818 and 1828 and recognized that acute blood loss was the primary reason for transfusion. Five of these 10 patients died after the transfusion, possibly as a result of incompatible blood.

In 1900, Karl Landsteiner[137] (1868-1943) described three blood groups: A, B, and O; the fourth blood group (AB) was described by A. V. Decastello[138] 2 years later. George W. Crile (1865-1943) performed the first transfusion of human blood after a preceding compatibility test in 1906. Discovery of the Rh antigens was delayed until 1939.

One hundred years ago, the accepted method of transfusing blood was to surgically anastomose the artery of the donor to the vein of the patient. This method required a long and delicate operation, and there was no way to measure the amount of blood transfused. Blood could not be removed from the body without defibrination, a process that often produced serious reactions and air embolization. In 1914, Albert Hustin[139] (1882-1967) noticed that when sodium citrate was added to blood, it prevented coagulation, and with the addition of dextrose by P. Rous and J. R. Turner in 1916,[140] storage of blood products for up to 21 days became a reality.[141] The familiar drip chamber for estimating infusion rates was devised by R. Laurie in 1909. The effect of these advancements in the use of blood products on the practice of anesthesia is apparent by comparing the American textbook by Gwathmey, dated 1914, in which there is no mention of blood administration, with that of John S. Lundy[142] (1894-1972), dated 1945, which contains an extensive chapter on the subject. Lundy was an early proponent of blood transfusions and opened the first blood bank in the United States at the Mayo Clinic in 1935. The effect of two world wars on the practice of anesthesia in the United States can be appreciated by comparing these two books.

With the increased frequency of contamination of homologous blood by hepatitis virus and human immunodeficiency virus, a new look at an old technique,[143] autologous transfusion, was begun in 1970 (also see Chapter 57). In that year, G. Klebanoff described a disposable autologous transfusion system manufactured by Bentley Laboratories. Klebanoff reported[144] on its use in 53 patients with no deaths if the total volume of blood replaced was less than 3500 mL. Malcolm D. Orr first reported cell-washing techniques in 1975 with the Haemonetics cell-washing system.[145] This system obviated some of the problems when blood was filtered, but not washed after retrieval from the surgical wound. From these early reports it became apparent that washed and concentrated red cells obtained from the surgical site could provide safe alternatives to homologous transfusion. The "cell saver" method of autologous blood transfusion has become an integral part of intraoperative fluid management when large volumes of blood loss are anticipated.

Coagulopathies often develop during large-volume blood transfusions, and their diagnosis and prompt treatment significantly contribute to survival during major surgery. Ronald D. Miller (1939-) and colleagues[146] recognized thrombocytopenia as one of the earliest defects in coagulation after massive blood loss (also see Chapter 55). Advances in specific blood component therapy[147,148] have also contributed to maintenance of normal blood coagulability during large-volume blood loss.

Introduction of Regional Anesthesia

Early Attempts at Local Anesthesia

The first written account of the coca plant being used as a local anesthetic was by the Spanish Jesuit Bernabe Cobo (1582-1657), who chewed the plant to relieve a toothache and wrote about it in 1653.[149] Albert Niemann (1834-1861) of Göttingen, Germany, who isolated the alkaloid from the dried leaves in 1856 (Fig. 1-9B), gave the name *cocaine* to the active drug. Interest in cocaine in Europe and America was directed initially toward the central effects of the drug when taken systemically. Vasili von Anrep[150] (1852-1918) was the first to remark on its local anesthetic properties, and after animal experiments, he suggested its use as a local anesthetic during surgery. This suggestion went unnoticed, and the drug remained a curiosity. A comprehensive pharmacology textbook from 1883 does not mention cocaine or the plant *E. coca*.

Sigmund Freud (1856-1939), a young house officer at the prestigious Allgemeines Krankenhaus in Vienna, had a unique interest in cocaine and tested the drug as a substitute for opioids on a colleague who was addicted to morphine. Although this research met with little success, he had also noticed its ability to

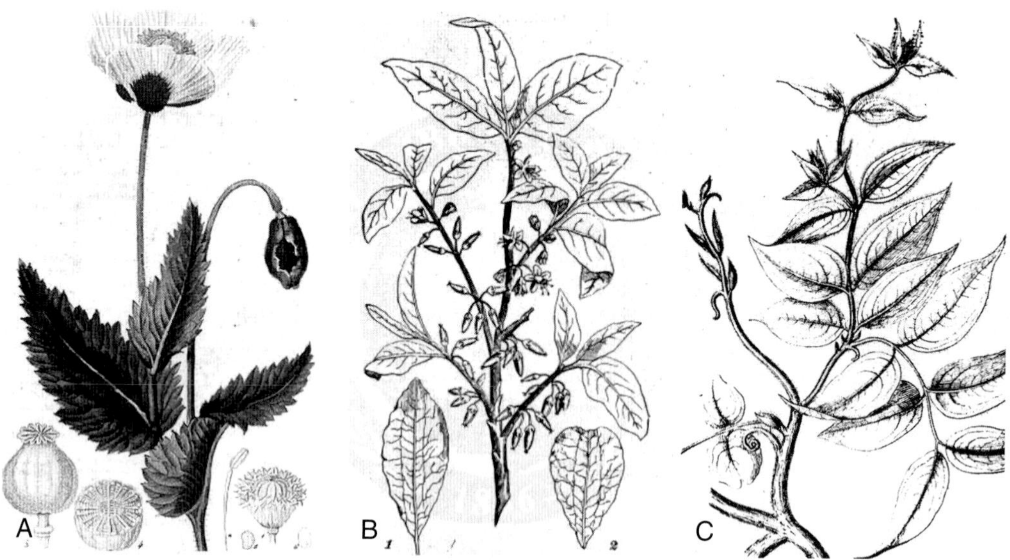

Figure 1-9 Botanical origins of adjuvants used in anesthesiology. **A,** *Papaver somniferum*, from which opium is obtained. The word *opium* is derived from the ancient Greek word for juice because the active alkaloids, which include morphine and codeine, are obtained from juice squeezed from the unripe seed pods. The first undisputed reference to poppy juice is from the writings of Theophrastus (372-287 BC) in the third century BC. **B,** *Erythroxylon coca*, a shrub native to Peru and Bolivia from which cocaine was isolated in 1856. Although the native people of Peru have used the drug for centuries to increase endurance, they may have also used it as a local anesthetic. **C,** *Strychnos toxifera*, a source of curare, as drawn by Robert Schomburgk in 1841. Schomburgk used maps drawn by Waterton to travel into Guiana and obtain several species containing the active drug. Richard Gill's curare was obtained primarily from Ecuador, and the arrow poisons there were made from *Chondodendron tomentosum*. Other botanical drugs that have been used in anesthesia include atropine (*Atropa belladonna*) , scopolamine (*Atropa mandragora*), physostigmine (*Physostigma venenosum*), ether (*Vitus vinifera*), gramine (*Hordeum vulgare*, from which lidocaine was derived), strychnine (*Strychnos toxifera*), ephedrine (*Ephedra sinica*), picrotoxin (*Anamirta cocculus*), theophylline (*Camellia sinensus*), and digitalis (*Digitalis purpurea*). *(Courtesy of the National Library of Medicine, Bethesda, MD.)*

produce numbness of the tongue and provided a small sample to his junior colleague Carl Koller[151] (1858-1944), an intern who was interested in producing local anesthesia for operations on the eye.

Koller had anticipated a career as a scientist in Vienna. He had taken up this question for his research project because the anesthetic methods of the time were highly unsatisfactory for ophthalmic surgery. General anesthetics presented numerous difficulties for the surgeon, and refrigeration anesthesia, although marginally successful for surgery on the extremities, was clearly inappropriate for the eye. Koller observed that after topical application of cocaine he was able to pinch and prick the cornea of dogs without discomfort to the animals. Self-experimentation confirmed complete analgesia of the corneal surface, and he proceeded to use the agent for superficial surgery on the eye.

Koller arranged to demonstrate the use of topical cocaine analgesia at the Ophthalmologic Congress in Heidelberg, Germany, on September 15, 1884. As the time for this presentation approached, he was unable to afford the travel expenses from Vienna, and a colleague from Trieste, Josef Brettauer (1835-1905), presented the three-page manuscript in his absence.[152] The presentation and demonstration were followed by an enthusiastically favorable response. Priority for the discovery was briefly confounded by a report on topical cocaine analgesia at an ophthalmologic meeting in October 1884 by Leopold Koenigstein, who did not mention Koller's previous paper, and by other comments that Sigmund Freud had actually originated the idea of cocaine analgesia. Koenigstein later conceded full credit for the discovery to Koller, and Freud eventually rejected all claims to the idea of topical analgesia with cocaine, although many concede that with his earlier publication on the subject,[153] he was instrumental in reviving interest in a drug that before 1884 was of no interest to pharmacologists.

Koller's career in Vienna seemed secure, but a disagreement arose with another house officer in January 1885. The altercation escalated into a duel with sabers, an activity that was banned in Austria at that time. Koller emerged unscathed from the duel, but the offending party suffered two saber cuts to the face. After this episode, Koller became depressed and ultimately decided to leave Austria. He first immigrated to Holland and then settled in New York City in 1886. There he built a successful private practice while continuing to contribute occasional clinical articles to the ophthalmologic literature. He died in New York City in 1944 after modestly receiving several awards for his seminal role in the development of local and regional anesthesia.[151]

Regional Blocks

It was not obvious that cocaine would produce blockade of sensation if injected directly into peripheral nerves. In 1880, von Anrep had injected cocaine under the skin of his arm and discovered that it produced insensitivity, but this information did not attract attention. At least one Viennese surgeon, Anton Wölfler, first assistant to Theodore Billroth, had attempted hypodermic cocaine injections without producing analgesia and was convinced that it was effective only on the mucous membranes. The idea of injecting cocaine into nerve trunks is credited to William Halsted (1852-1922) and Alfred Hall, who began their injection experiments as early as 8 weeks after the Heidelberg announcement.

Halsted and Hall had studied in Vienna during 1879 and 1880, but it is unlikely that they met Koller during those years because Koller did not finish his medical school training until 1882. During those years Koller was working on a paper about development of the mesoderm and had not developed his interest in cocaine. In 1884, Halsted was occasionally performing operations in the bedroom of his own house in New York City, and it was there that the two surgeons began their work on regional anesthesia. The first report of their success with injection appeared on December 6, 1884, in the *New York Medical Journal* in a letter written by Hall.[154] In this letter, Hall reported that they first injected 4% cocaine (15 mg) into the forearm and concluded that it blocked transmission in the cutaneous nerves because it provided analgesia below but not above the point of injection. They then injected 2 mL (80 mg) into the ulnar nerve at the elbow and produced a block of the entire ulnar distribution distal to the point of injection. Additional blocks were then performed on the brachial plexus and the infraorbital nerves, inferior dental nerves, and the sciatic nerve, all for operative surgery.[155]

With these large doses, it is not surprising that constitutional symptoms developed. Hall described dizziness and nausea. Both Halsted and Hall became addicted to cocaine; Halsted lived with an occult cocaine or morphine addiction the rest of his life. Hall took a position at Columbia University in New York City, but he later moved to Santa Barbara, California, where he died in 1924.

Carl Schleich[156] (1859-1922) introduced infiltration local anesthesia in 1892 as an alternative to direct injection of nerve trunks. His method was to infiltrate cocaine in dilute concentrations (0.01% to 0.2%) directly into subcutaneous tissues. James Leonard Corning[157] (1855-1923), a neurologist from New York, observed that placing a tourniquet on the limb could prolong the analgesic effect of infiltration analgesia, and he reasoned that the tourniquet prevented the blood from removing cocaine from its active site. Heinrich F. Braun[158] (1862-1934) achieved the same prolonged effect of cocaine by adding epinephrine to the solution and producing a "chemical tourniquet." Braun became the pioneer of the new drug procaine, introduced in 1905 as a less toxic drug than cocaine. Braun's textbook,[158] initially published in 1907, was one of the first devoted to regional anesthesia and went through eight editions, with the last one published in 1933.

Although Halsted was the first to block the brachial plexus, he did not use a percutaneous technique. His method in 1884—and that used by George Crile 13 years later—was to surgically expose the roots and then inject each nerve directly. G. Hirschel[159] produced the first percutaneous brachial plexus block in 1911 through an axillary approach (Fig. 1-10A). The axillary brachial plexus block has been modified by several surgeons, including George Pitkin and R. H. de Jong,[160] and remains a popular technique today.

D. Kulenkampff introduced the supraclavicular brachial plexus block[161] a few months after Hirschel described the axillary approach (see Fig. 1-10B). Kulenkampff injected his own plexus with 10 mL of procaine at the midclavicular position, lateral to the subclavian artery, and achieved complete anesthesia of the arm. Early reports indicated a frequent incidence of success with this block, but other practitioners soon reported complications such as pneumothorax and mediastinal emphysema. Several modifications of the supraclavicular block have emerged in an effort to avoid pneumothorax. Infraclavicular approaches to the brachial plexus were described by L. Bazy and V. Pauchet in 1917 and later popularized by P. Raj[162] in 1973 (see also Chapter 52).

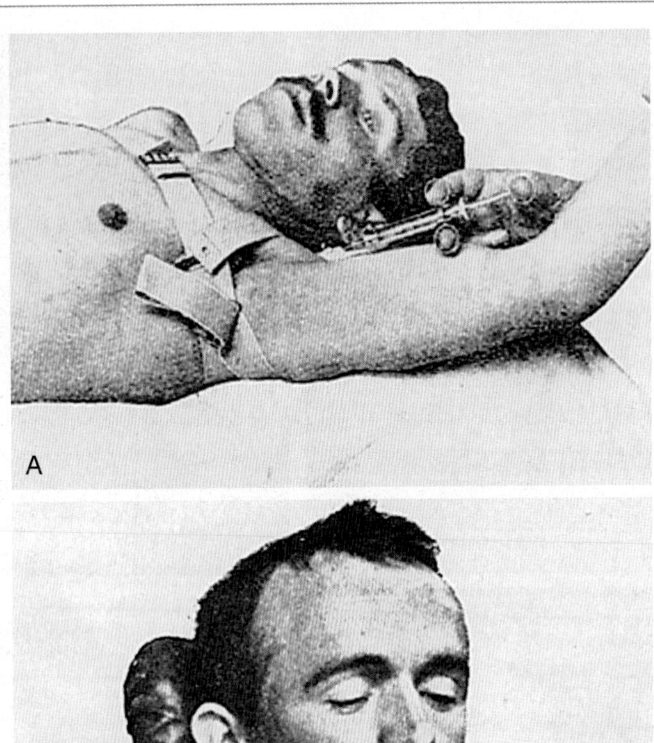

Figure 1-10 **A,** Hirschel performed the first percutaneous axillary block with 20 mL of 2% procaine in 1911. He forced a rubber ball under the pectoral muscles and fixed it with elastic bandages to prevent rapid absorption of anesthetic solution, a maneuver that he later abandoned as unnecessary. **B,** Kulenkampff approached the brachial plexus above the clavicle, just lateral to the subclavian artery. The patients were positioned in the sitting position for the block. An injection of 10 mL of 2% procaine with epinephrine was given only after paresthesia had been achieved. If the first rib was contacted, the injection was directed more medially. *(**A,** From Hirschel G: Die Anasthesierung de Plexus Brachialis fur die Operationen an der oberen Extremitat, Much Med Wochenschr 58:1555-1556, 1911; **B,** from Kulenkampff D: Anesthesia of the brachial plexus. Zentrabl Chr 38:1337-1340, 1911.)*

In an attempt to approach the brachial plexus in the neck and thereby avoid pulmonary complications, M. Kappis[163] in 1912 attempted to perform the block through a posterior paravertebral approach. Because of a high incidence of failures with the posterior approach, several investigators, including J. Etienne, V. Pauchet, and G. Pitkin, used various anterior approaches to the brachial plexus in the neck. In 1970, Alon P. Winnie[164] introduced the interscalene brachial plexus block and emphasized that the scalene muscles are more accurate landmarks to the nerves than the subclavian artery or the midclavicular line is. The block has remained popular for operations on the shoulder and upper part of the arm; the nerves are located by paresthesias or direct nerve

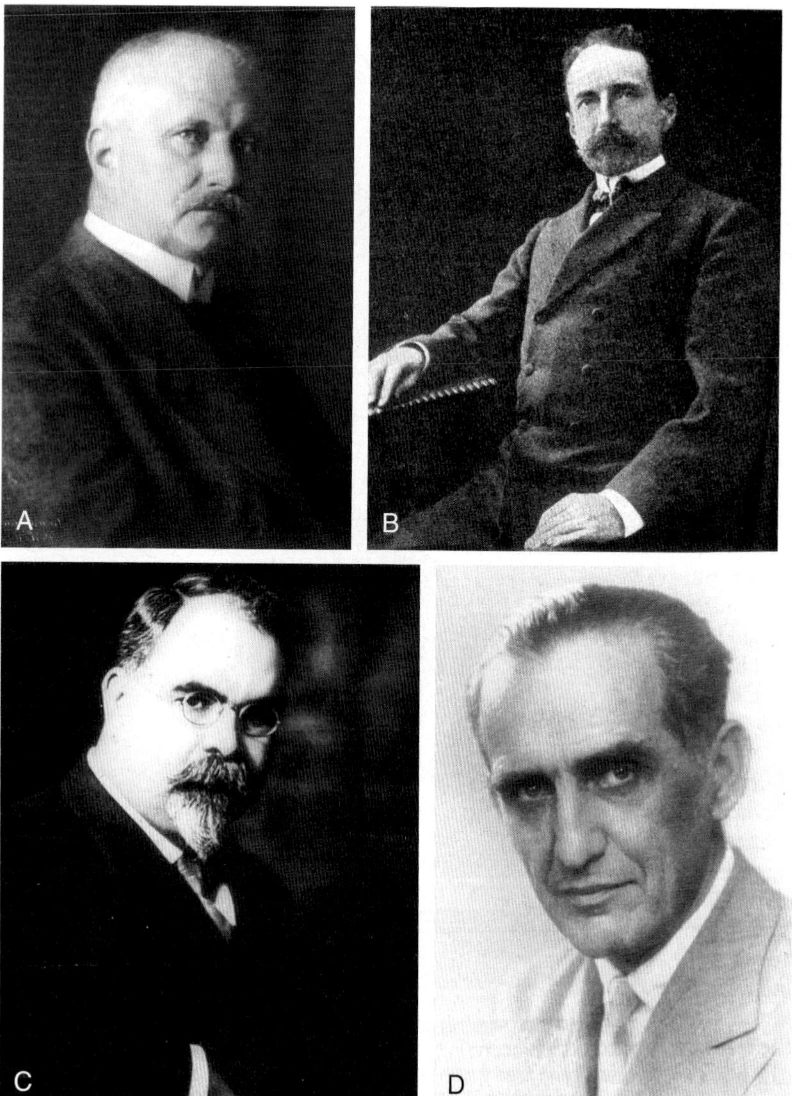

Figure 1-11 Pioneers of the neuraxial block. **A,** August K. G. Bier. **B,** Theodore Tuffier. **C,** Rudolph Matas. **D,** Achille M. Dogliotti. *(Courtesy of the National Library of Medicine, Bethesda, MD.)*

stimulation. Continuous infusion into the roots of the brachial plexus has been introduced and can provide long-lasting analgesia after operations on the arm and shoulder.

A novel method of producing regional analgesia for operations on the extremities was described by August Bier (1861-1949) (Fig. 1-11A) in 1908.[164,165] Bier first exsanguinated the arm with an Esmarch wrap and, after placement of two tourniquets, injected a dilute solution of procaine intravenously. Analgesia was found to develop within minutes and persist until release of the tourniquet. The technique, known now as intravenous regional anesthesia, has been modified with new agents and remains a useful anesthetic technique for surgery on the extremities when a tourniquet is used.

The development of regional anesthesia in the United States was accelerated with the arrival of Gaston Labat at the Mayo Clinic in 1924. Labat had learned regional anesthetic methods from the French authority on injection techniques, Victor Pauchet (1869-1936), and expanded on his work while in Rochester, Minnesota. Labat founded the American Society of Regional Anesthesia and was active during its formative years. John Lundy adopted many of the regional techniques introduced by Labat at the Mayo Clinic and continued their use after Labat relocated to Bellevue Hospital in New York City. Labat's 1922 textbook[50] was one of the first English texts on regional anesthesia and has been followed by several authoritative works on the subject. Labat's influence was also evident in New York City, where Emery A. Rovenstine (1895-1960), his successor as Chairman of the Department of Anesthesiology at Bellevue Hospital, established the first chronic pain clinic. The commitment of anesthesiologists to chronic pain therapy arose as a natural sequel to their emerging expertise in neuraxial and peripheral nerve blocks. Chronic pain clinics today are often modeled after the multidisciplinary clinic established by John J. Bonica (1917-1994) at the University of Washington in Seattle.[166]

The continued success of regional anesthetic techniques can be partially credited to ultrasound techniques for localization of the nerves and also to improved local anesthetics with lower toxicity and longer duration of action. Cocaine was highly toxic, addictive, and of short duration. Procaine was synthesized in 1905 by Alfred Einhorn[167] (1856-1917) and was the most commonly used agent until 1932, when tetracaine, a longer-acting agent, became available. Lidocaine, introduced in 1948 by Torsten

Gordh[168] (1907-), had several advantages, including lower toxicity and intermediate duration of action, and it is still widely used. Other local anesthetics include chloroprocaine (introduced in 1952), mepivacaine (1957), and bupivacaine (1963). Concern about therapy-resistant cardiovascular toxicity with bupivacaine[169] led to introduction of the newer agents ropivacaine (1996) and levobupivacaine.[170] Bupivacaine, ropivacaine, and levobupivacaine are popular agents in low concentration for control of postoperative pain and for obstetric anesthesia because of their long duration of action.

Neuraxial Block and Acute Pain Service

The first neuraxial block was performed 8 months after the demonstration in Heidelberg of the local anesthetic properties of cocaine (see Chapter 87). James Leonard Corning (1855-1923) was a neurologist who had learned of the action of cocaine possibly from observation of Halsted's work in New York City. Corning was interested to know whether the blood could carry cocaine to the spinal cord, similar to what had been demonstrated to occur after the injection of strychnine between the spinous processes. On October 12, 1885, Corning injected a total of 120 mg of cocaine between the T11 and T12 spinous processes in a 45-year-old man and obtained loss of sensation of the legs and perineum. He concluded that this proved cocaine's action on the spinal cord and suggested its use in certain cases of spinal spasticity and for operations on the genitourinary system.

The consensus is that Corning produced an epidural injection of the drug[171] because 120 mg (60 mg initially and then 60 mg 8 minutes later) of intrathecal cocaine would be expected to produce a total spinal anesthetic or a block extending into the cervical dermatomes. It is not surprising that Corning's method of neuraxial blockade was not repeated because the technique of consistently injecting into the epidural space had not yet been described. If any investigators had attempted to repeat the Corning experiment with the dose that he used, it might have ended in disaster and thereby have delayed the development of neuraxial blockade by several years.

Spinal Analgesia (also see Chapter 51)

In Kiel, Germany, during the last decade of the 19th century, preparations were being made for the next major advance in anesthetic practice. At the Kiel University Medical School, Friederich von Esmarch (1823-1908) was the senior surgeon and August Bier one of the junior surgeons. Heinrich I. Quincke (1842-1922) was the leading internist in Kiel and had already contributed several useful clinical observations, among them the Quincke pulse and Quincke edema, to the medical literature. In 1891, Quincke observed that the dural sac, described by Domenico Cotugno (1736-1822) in 1787, could be punctured by inserting a needle between the lumbar spinous processes.[172] This procedure, independently reported by Walter Wynter (1860-1945) of Leeds, England, in the same year, at first was a curiosity without any real purpose. Quincke unsuccessfully attempted to treat hydrocephalus by draining fluid from the dural sac. Microscopic examination of the fluid did have some diagnostic value in cases of inflammation of the central nervous system.

On August 15, 1898, August Bier and his assistant August Hildebrandt (1868-1854) used the Quincke method of entering the intrathecal space and injected between 5 and 15 mg of cocaine to produce spinal anesthesia in six cases for operations on the lower part of the body. They also reported the results of spinal anesthesia given to each other in what has become one of the classic clinical papers in medical literature.[173] Bier thought that it would not replace general anesthesia because of the severity of side effects such as nausea, vomiting, dizziness, and headache. He proposed that these undesirable side effects were caused by escape of cerebrospinal fluid from the dural sac. The method whereby Bier arrived at the correct intrathecal dose of cocaine on the first attempt remains a mystery.

After Bier's report, interest in spinal anesthesia spread rapidly. J. B. Seldowitsch[174] successfully provided spinal anesthesia in St. Petersburg on May 11, 1899; Frederick Dudley Tait (1862-1918) and Guido Caglieri[175] (1871-1951) in San Francisco on October 26, 1899; Theodore Tuffier[176] (see Fig. 1-11B) in Paris on November 9, 1899; and Rudolph Matas[177] (1860-1957) (see Fig. 1-11C) in New Orleans on November 10, 1899. By one report, more than 1000 manuscripts relating to spinal anesthesia had been published within 2 years of the original paper by Bier.

Not all researchers agreed on the technique and indications for spinal anesthesia. Tait and Caglieri suggested the use of cervical intrathecal injections for operating on the upper extremities. A. W. Morton[178] reported success with total spinal anesthesia after lumbar puncture for operations on all parts of the body. Thomas Jonnesco[179] reported no adverse effects from 398 spinal anesthetics administered between vertebrae at the thoracic and lumbar levels with a novocaine and strychnine mixture. Jonnesco called the method general spinal anesthesia. Remarkably, in his series there were 14 operations on the skull, 45 on the face, and 25 on the neck. In 1909, Bier[180] claimed that to be successful with spinal anesthesia, the anesthetist should inject the solution only at body temperature and that tropacocaine was preferable to cocaine.

The early reports of cocaine spinal anesthesia mentioned that after injection, patients frequently became restless and excitable, often exhibiting a significant rise in body temperature. One of the first physicians to specialize in anesthesia, S. Ormond Goldan, maintained accurate anesthesia records from several cases of spinal anesthesia with cocaine.[181] His records reveal a typical increase in heart rate, pupil size, and body temperature after cocaine spinal anesthesia. Matas reasoned that these effects were secondary to an action of cocaine on the central nervous system. He learned that mixing 1.5 mg of morphine with cocaine was useful in mitigating these symptoms. In his 1900 report on spinal anesthesia, he regarded a mixture of cocaine and morphine as his standard agent. This report by Matas appears to be among the first attempts to use spinal opioids to enhance neuraxial analgesia.[177] The Japanese anesthesiologist Otojiro Kitagawa[182] (1864-1922) used intrathecal morphine (10 mg) in the same year to treat the chronic painful conditions of two patients.

It is not surprising that serious complications from the spinal technique were soon observed. F. Gumprecht[183] reported 15 cases of sudden death from lumbar puncture in 1900. Several investigators observed respiratory arrest after high spinal injections. After the introduction of routine blood pressure measurements by Cushing in 1903, it was observed that severe hypotension could occur after spinal anesthesia.

The scientific study of spinal anesthesia began within a few years after its introduction. Investigations were undertaken by Arthur E. Barker[184] (1850-1916) to determine factors involved in spread of the local anesthetic within the subarachnoid space. Barker advised meticulous sterile technique and introduced the use of dextrose to produce hyperbaric solutions. His emphasis on gravity as an essential determinant of local anesthetic spread remains an important facet of the spinal technique today.[185] Several researchers reported the dangers of total spinal anesthesia. Gaston Labat[50] and George P. Pitkin contributed clinical observations that improved the safety of spinal anesthesia.

A widely publicized malpractice trial in 1953 had a negative impact on the use of spinal anesthesia.[186] Albert Woolley and Cecil Roe were healthy subjects who received dibucaine spinal anesthetics on the same day in 1947 at the Chesterfield Royal Hospital in England. Permanent painful spastic paraparesis developed in both patients. Although the cause of the paresis was inconclusive, it was thought that the injuries were caused by contamination of the spinal solution by phenol, in which the dibucaine ampules had been immersed for sterilization. The Wooley and Roe case was followed by other reports of paralysis after spinal anesthesia.[187] However, in 1954, a reassuring study of 10,098 spinal anesthetics with only 71 minor neuropathies, most unrelated to the block itself, was published in a widely circulated medical journal.[188] Spinal anesthesia then re-emerged as a safe anesthetic method, provided that attention was directed to meticulous technique.

Consideration has been given to a syndrome characterized by transient paresthesias after lidocaine spinal anesthesia.[189] However, with the introduction of disposable spinal kits and improved techniques, the spinal route of drug administration is now firmly established. Research is continuing on new drugs and methods of delivery. Reports of cauda equina syndrome after the introduction of lidocaine through spinal microcatheters[190] emphasize the importance of careful clinical observations when new methods of spinal delivery are introduced.

Post–dural puncture headache was an annoying problem for the first practitioners and their patients. The exact cause of this reaction was not agreed on for several years. As late as 1924, Labat had suggested removal of cerebrospinal fluid for the treatment of spinal headache. However, an extensive study by Leroy D. Vandam (1914-2004) and Robert Dripps (1911-1974) confirmed Bier's original suggestion that leakage of cerebrospinal fluid through the dural rent was the causative factor.[191]

The use of small-diameter spinal needles has decreased the incidence of spinal headache after spinal anesthesia. However, inadvertent dural puncture with larger needles can sometimes occur during the placement of epidural catheters. An innovative treatment of headache after dural puncture, the epidural blood patch, was suggested by James B. Gormley[192] in 1960 and further described by Anthony J. DiGiovanni and Burdett S. Dunbar[193] in 1970. The blood patch has been reported to be successful in a high percentage of cases and has withstood the test of time as an effective treatment of this condition.

Epidural Analgesia (also see Chapter 51)

Jean Enthuse Sicard (1872-1929) and Fernand Cathelin (1873-1945) independently introduced cocaine through the sacral hiatus in 1901, thereby becoming the first practitioners of caudal (epidural) anesthesia. Sicard was a neurologist and used the technique to treat sciatica and tabes, but Cathelin used the technique for surgical anesthesia. Arthur Läwen[194] (1876-1958), a pupil of Heinrich Braun (1862-1934) and an early proponent of regional anesthesia, successfully used caudal anesthesia with large volumes of procaine for pelvic surgery. It soon became apparent that caudal anesthesia was sufficient for operations on the perineum, but the drug would have to be deposited into the epidural space at higher levels if the surgeon anticipated operating on the abdomen or thorax. Initial attempts to provide epidural anesthesia through needles placed at higher levels were unsuccessful. B. Heile[195] published an extensive study of the epidural space in 1913, but the focus of his final report was on the treatment of neurologic conditions with epidural injections. His unique approach was to enter the epidural space through the intervertebral foramina (a technique that has recently been revived). Tuffier[196] was aware of the need for entry at higher levels but was unable to perfect a reliable technique for lumbar or thoracic epidural injections.

In 1921, Fidel Pagés[197] (1886-1923), a Spanish military surgeon, devised a technique to introduce epidural procaine at all levels of the neuraxis. His method was to use a blunt needle and then feel and hear entry of the needle through the ligamentum flavum. His report of 43 cases of lumbar and thoracic epidural anesthesia represents a landmark article that went unnoticed because of its publication in an obscure medical journal. Pagés died in an automobile accident soon after his report on epidural analgesia, and no students at the time had learned his technique. Pagés had the idea of producing segmental anesthesia through epidural injections, thereby avoiding some of the side effects of complete neuraxial blockade, which occurred after high subarachnoid administration of local anesthetics. He provided the anesthetics himself and then performed the operations, noting that much time was saved with the epidural technique as compared with general anesthesia. Of the 43 cases, it appears that one subject experienced total spinal anesthesia but survived after assisted ventilation.

Achille Mario Dogliotti[198] (1897-1966) (see Fig. 1-11D) described epidural injections of local anesthetics in 1931, apparently without previous knowledge of the work of Pagés. Dogliotti performed extensive studies to determine the spread of solutions within the epidural and paravertebral space after injection. His work launched one of the most valuable techniques in the modern practice of anesthesiology. An important innovation was Dogliotti's method of identification of the epidural space. His 1939 textbook illustrates the use of continuous pressure on the plunger of a saline-filled syringe as the needle is advanced through the ligamentous structures. In contrast to the methods of Corning and Pagés, the Dogliotti technique was reproducible and easily learned. Dogliotti also observed the extent and duration of analgesia after injection into various spinal interspaces.

Initial acceptance of epidural analgesia was slow to develop in North America, although it gained early acceptance in Europe and South America. A. Gutierrez of Argentina became an enthusiastic advocate for the epidural method and collected valuable data on a large series of successful epidural anesthesia. He also developed the "hanging drop" sign, which is still used by some anesthesiologists to identify the epidural space. Dogliotti's anesthesia textbook was translated into English in 1939 and contained an extensive chapter on epidural analgesia. Textbooks by American authors several years later[142,199] contained only a short description of the technique and considered it a novelty practiced only by those with special expertise. There were some early practitioners of epidural anesthesia in North America. Charles B. Odom of New Orleans published 285 cases of lumbar epidural anesthesia in 1936 and introduced the concept of a test dose to detect intrathecal injection.[200] In Odom's series there was one death attributed to the poor condition of the patient. John R. Harger and coworkers[201] of Cook County Hospital in Chicago reported 1000 cases without a fatality when using single injections of 45 to 50 mL of 2% procaine. Oral Crawford and colleagues[202] reported more than 600 cases of thoracic epidural analgesia for thoracic surgery in 1951, with two deaths.

One major limitation of the neuraxial techniques was the short duration of action of procaine. Bier experimented with the addition of rubber and latex to the spinal anesthetic solution in an attempt to prolong the duration of blockade.[180] These ideas were not expanded on because of complications or lack of effect. To deal with the same problem, William T. Lemmon (1896-1974) used a 17-gauge, malleable, silver needle that was connected through a hole in the operating room table to rubber tubing and a syringe. Injections could then be made at intervals to maintain the spinal block for several hours. Edward B. Tuohy[203] (1908-1959) used a ureteral catheter threaded through a large Huber-tipped spinal needle to provide continuous spinal anesthesia. The Tuohy needle, a simple modification of the Huber needle, was used by him to thread the catheter into the subarachnoid space. Beginning in 1947, Manuel Martinez Curbelo[204] of Havana, Cuba, used the Tuohy needle and a small ureteral catheter to provide continuous lumbar epidural analgesia. He reported 59 successful cases, and in one patient the catheter remained in place for 4 postoperative days with intermittent injections of local anesthetic.

Caudal anesthesia experienced a resurgence in popularity after the report by W. B. Edwards and Robert A. Hingson (1918-1996)[205] in 1942 that analgesia for labor and delivery could be achieved with caudal injections of tetracaine through a malleable needle left in situ within the sacral canal. Their report was widely publicized, and within months the technique was adopted by several hospitals. Although caudal epidural injections had been used for obstetric analgesia for many years, it became apparent that the lumbar approach to the epidural space was more consistent, and it eventually replaced the caudal approach.

Beginning in 1960, coincident with its rising popularity in obstetric anesthesia, the epidural method was taken up by several practitioners in North America. Philip R. Bromage and John J. Bonica performed several studies on epidural dose-response relationships and the hemodynamic changes that followed initiation of the block. Textbooks soon followed that introduced epidural analgesia into the operating room.[206] Although Dogliotti thought that general anesthesia was contraindicated after the initiation of epidural blockade, Massey Dawkins (1905-1975), Philip R. Bromage, and later Michael Cousins[207] discussed the advantages of providing general anesthesia during prolonged surgery while extending epidural analgesia throughout the surgical procedure and into the postoperative period. Although lumbar epidurals were widely used for postoperative pain relief, problems with ambulation and inadequate analgesia led to the current practice of placing epidural catheters between the appropriate interspaces to provide selective antinociception along the surgical incision site.

A report in 1979 by J. Wang and associates[208] demonstrated long-lasting analgesia from the intrathecal administration of morphine in eight patients with cancer pain. This clinical study had firm groundwork from previous basic studies on the spinal effects of opioids in animals. In 1976, Yaksh and Rudy[209] reported that intrathecal morphine produced spinal analgesia in rats. Duggan and North[210] demonstrated evidence of spinal analgesia after iontophoretic application of morphine into the dorsal horn region of the spinal cords of animals. Autoradiographic studies demonstrated a high density of opioid receptors in the substantia gelatinosa of the spinal cord.[211]

The use of spinal opioids spread rapidly after the initial report by Wang and coworkers.[208] Samii and colleagues[212] confirmed that selective opioid spinal analgesia occurs in humans. Cousins and associates[213] noticed that 1 to 2 mg of intrathecal morphine injected into the thoracic intrathecal region relieved the pain of breast or lung cancer for more than 24 hours. Behar and collaborators[214] reported epidural opioid therapy in 1979. The explosive interest in neuraxial opioids that followed these reports was equal to the enthusiasm after the initial report of cocaine spinal anesthesia. The use of epidural catheters to provide long-lasting pain relief after surgery led to the formation of acute pain services.[215] With special attention to drug concentrations and rates of infusion, patients were able to recuperate without pain and ambulate on the first postoperative day, even after extensive thoracic, abdominal, and orthopedic operations. The special advantage of epidural opioids was the synergistic effect that they exhibited with local anesthetics, which allowed a marked decrease in the dose of both drugs to achieve the same level of analgesia.[216]

Intravenous Anesthetics

The development of intravenous anesthetics has been an important component of anesthetic management for more than 70 years (see Chapters 26 and 27). Before the introduction of rapidly acting intravenous agents, induction of general anesthesia necessarily required inhalation of gases or vapors, an unpleasant experience for some patients.

Pierre-Cyprien Oré (1828-1891) performed the first successful attempt at intravenous anesthesia in 1872 by using chloral hydrate to anesthetize a human subject. Although he believed it was superior to chloroform, his contemporaries did not adopt the method. Intravenous paraldehyde was briefly used as an anesthetic during and after World War I. At the same time, the combination of intravenous morphine and scopolamine gained wide popularity, particularly in obstetric anesthesia. The method became known as twilight sleep, but this drug combination was slowly abandoned because of unpredictable side effects when given to some patients. Tribromoethanol (Avertin) was originally promoted as a full anesthetic agent to be administered rectally. Although rectal administration of agents had been promoted by Pirogoff, Gwathmey, and others, the use of rectal tribromoethanol fell into disfavor when rectal ulcerations were reported after use of the agent. Thereafter, tribromoethanol was used briefly as an intravenous agent, but because it had a prolonged duration of action and produced profound respiratory depression and probable hepatotoxicity, other suitable intravenous agents were sought.

Adolf von Baeyer discovered the first barbiturate, barbituric acid, in 1864, but the drug had no sedative properties. It is said that Baeyer celebrated discovery of the compound on Saint Barbara's Day, and he coined the word barbiturate as a combination of Barbara with urea because barbituric acid results from the combination of malonic acid and urea. The first sedative barbiturate was synthesized in 1903 by Emil Fischer (1852-1919) of Berlin, but short-acting intravenous agents such as hexobarbital were not introduced until nearly 30 years later. Helmut Weese[217] (1897-1954), considered by many to be the originator of successful intravenous anesthetic methods, reported several thousand cases of hexobarbital use in 1932. Sodium thiopental followed hexobarbital in 1934, and the first detailed analysis of its use was described by John Lundy of the Mayo Clinic.[218] The use of thiopental was a further refinement of his earlier concept of balanced anesthesia, whereby anesthesia is achieved with the use of multiple agents. According to Lundy, general anesthesia was safer with the use of multiple agents because the dose of any one particular agent was smaller and fewer side effects were observed.

It was soon learned that thiopental could be dangerous to administer in certain circumstances. When the drug was used for induction of anesthesia in injured personnel after the bombing of Pearl Harbor in 1941, the frequent occurrence of sudden death emphasized the profound depressant effect that this drug has on the cardiovascular system.[219] Later analysis of the use of thiopental at Pearl Harbor, however, did not implicate the drug as the cause of the high mortality rate observed at that time.[220] The only other commonly used short-acting barbiturate is methohexital, an oxybarbiturate that has similar depressant effects on the circulation. Because of its unique proconvulsive effect, methohexital is used as an anesthetic for electroshock therapy.

There have been several attempts to replace the barbiturates with shorter-acting drugs that have less cardiovascular depression. Some of these drugs, such as althesin,[221] propanidid, and eltanolone, were withdrawn from clinical use because of unwanted side effects. Etomidate, an intravenous anesthetic introduced in 1973 that was used to induce anesthesia, produces only minimal hemodynamic depression and has found use in patients with hypovolemia and those with significant cardiovascular disease.[222] Etomidate can cause undesirable myoclonic movements during induction in some patients.

The benzodiazepines midazolam, diazepam, and lorazepam are useful intravenous agents that relieve anxiety without the same degree of sedation produced with the barbiturates. Experimental studies on this class of drugs began in 1933 at the University of Cracow in Poland, with the first clinically useful drug, chlordiazepoxide (Librium), introduced in 1960. Diazepam (1963) and midazolam (1978) followed. A specific antagonist can be used to treat overdosage.[223]

Ketamine was synthesized in 1962 as an alternative to phencyclidine, a drug that resulted in severe psychological effects in the postoperative period. Ketamine was one of 200 phencyclidine derivatives that were studied, and it was introduced as an anesthetic in 1966.[224] It was initially used intravenously or intramuscularly as a complete agent by itself, but reports of postoperative hallucinations led to re-evaluation of its use, and it is now typically used only in combination with other sedative agents. Ketamine is a unique agent in the armamentarium of the anesthesiologist because it does not depress the cardiovascular system, even when used in full anesthetic doses.

Propofol, introduced clinically[221,225] in 1977, is an alkylphenol compound that has some advantages over thiopental. It appears to have antiemetic properties and suppresses laryngeal reflexes to a greater extent than thiopental does, thus allowing easy placement of supraglottic airways. It has achieved widespread use since its introduction, partially because of its rapid recovery profile. Propofol is often administered as a continuous infusion for general anesthesia, with or without the addition of inhaled anesthetics. When combined with analgesic agents such as opioids, propofol can provide all the components of satisfactory general anesthesia. This method, often called total intravenous anesthesia (TIVA), can eliminate the need for any gaseous or volatile agents. Propofol is a profound cardiovascular depressant, and it can produce significant pain on injection.

Although intravenous opioids were once considered unsafe in the private rooms of hospitals, a modality of administration called patient-controlled analgesia (PCA) is now routinely used in most hospitals. The rationale is that because pain is a subjective experience, only patients can assess the need for analgesics and balance that with their experience of side effects. Overdose is obviated by lock-out intervals and by the inability to perform the task of drug administration as somnolence ensues. Methods for intravenous PCA therapy in the postoperative setting were developed by anesthesiologists more than 30 years ago,[226] but they are now used by several specialty groups within the hospital.

Muscle Relaxants

Neuromuscular blocking drugs or muscle relaxants are firmly entrenched as an integral part of everyday anesthetic practice (see Chapter 29). Anesthesia providers practiced for nearly 100 years without these drugs, but it would be difficult to provide the same level of anesthetic service today without their use.

Initial Contact with Arrow Poison

Homer (*Odyssey*, I, 260) and Virgil (*Aeneid*, IX, 772) mention poisoned arrows. The word *toxin* is derived from the Greek root *toxon* ("bow"). Medical fascination with the specific arrow poison now called curare began nearly 500 years ago when the first returning explorers from South America told of a poisoned arrow that was used in warfare and to kill game. In 1505, Pietro Martyr d'Anghiera (1457-1525), an Italian monk who visited South America in the early 16th century, wrote the following:

> *This Indian King layd wait for oure men . . . set on them with about seven hundred men armed after theire maner, although they were naked. For only the King and his noblemen were appareled . . . So fiercely assayling oure men with theire venomous arrowes that they slewe of them fortie and seven . . . for that poyson is of such force, that albeit the wounds were not great, yet they dyed thereof immediately.*

Sir Walter Raleigh[227] (1552-1618) was one of the first to report on the wonders of the drug, which his first lieutenant, Laurence Keymis, called ourari, the first English attempt to reproduce the Macusi Indian pronunciation of the poison. Remarkably, the flesh of the poisoned animal was eaten with impunity. The native inhabitants were greatly impressed with gunpowder but noticed that the noise from guns frightened the game, and they

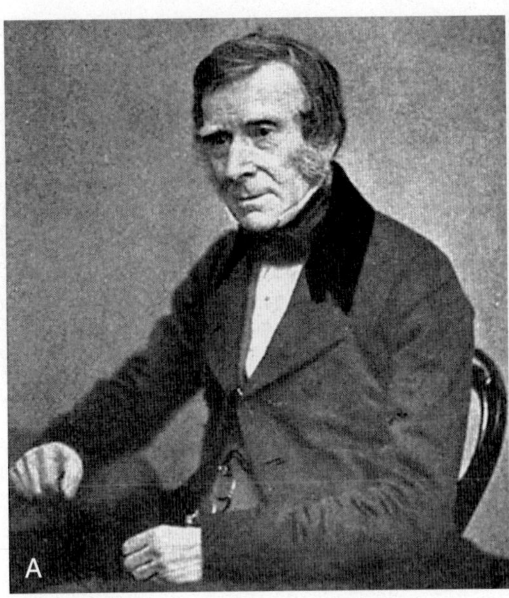

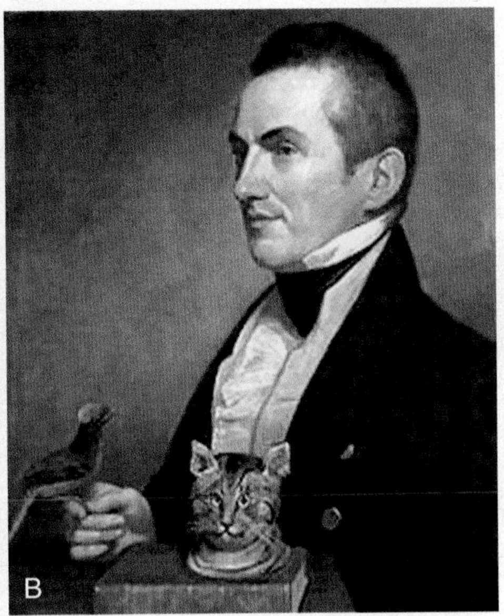

Figure 1-12 Benjamin Brodie (**A**) and Charles Waterton (**B**) collaborated in demonstrating that animals could survive curare poisoning if artificial ventilation was provided. *(Courtesy of the National Library of Medicine, Bethesda, MD.)*

preferred a poison-tipped arrow that was sent quietly from a blowgun. Initial reports indicated that the poison was made from a mixture of rat bones and bark.

Charles-Marie de la Condamine (1701-1774) was the first to bring creditable samples back to Europe. His samples were used by Richard Brocklesby (1722-1797) to demonstrate that the heart of a cat continued to beat for 2 hours after it was apparently dead from curare poisoning. The Florentine Abbot Felix Fontana (1720-1805) injected the drug directly into the exposed sciatic nerve and observed no effect. He concluded that the curare impaired irritability of the muscle.[228]

Mechanism of Action

The collaborative project of Benjamin Brodie (1783-1862) (Fig. 1-12A) and Charles Waterton (1783-1865) (see Fig. 1-12B) initiated our modern understanding of muscle relaxants.[229] Benjamin Brodie was the principal figure of English surgery at that time, and Waterton was the eccentric Squire of Walton Hall, near Wakefield, England. Waterton had traveled extensively, including several expeditions into British Guiana, where he owned property and eventually obtained several samples of the arrow poison.

In 1814, Brodie and Waterton demonstrated that an animal could survive an injection of curare provided that ventilation was continued after injection. For this famous experiment, it seems that Waterton supplied the curare and the animal—a donkey—and Brodie supplied the experimental idea. They injected the donkey with poison in the shoulder, and it was immobilized within 10 minutes.

> *An incision was then made in its windpipe, and through it the lungs were inflated for two hours, with a pair of bellows. The ass held up her head, and looked around, but the inflating being discontinued, she sunk once more in apparent death. The artificial respiration was immediately recommenced and continued without intermission for two hours. This saved the ass from final dissolution: she rose up and walked about; she seemed neither in agitation nor pain.*

Waterton named the donkey Wouralia and nurtured her on his estate, where she died 25 years later. Curiously, in their later correspondence, neither partner mentions the collaboration of the other individual. Waterton's book, titled *Wanderings in South America* and dated 1879, contains an extensive description of the preparation and use of curare, as well as the manner of use of the blowpipe, which he called the "extraordinary tube of death."

The experiment performed by Claude Bernard[230] (1813-1878) demonstrating the action of curare at the junction between the nerve and muscle was deceptively simple (Fig. 1-13). In his studies with curare, Bernard used the drug to open a new area of investigation, the physiology and pharmacology of the junction between the nerve and muscle. Experiments on the specialized apparatus where the action of curare is primarily located, the neuromuscular junction, were begun by one of Bernard's students, Willy Kuhne (1837-1900).

Introduction into Clinical Medicine

Waterton suggested the use of his woraria for the treatment of tetanus and rabies, and the few successful trials of the small samples of curare that were available then were used to treat these conditions.[231] For the next 175 years in Europe and North America, the drug remained a curiosity with no definite purpose. The medical community ignored an early report from 1912 suggesting its use to provide muscular relaxation during closure of the abdomen:

> *Thus far I have used solution of curarine up to 2% by intramuscular injection. With this dose, closure of the abdominal wall was achieved readily. There is not sufficient curare available, so I have not yet been able to ascertain the correct dose for this purpose.*

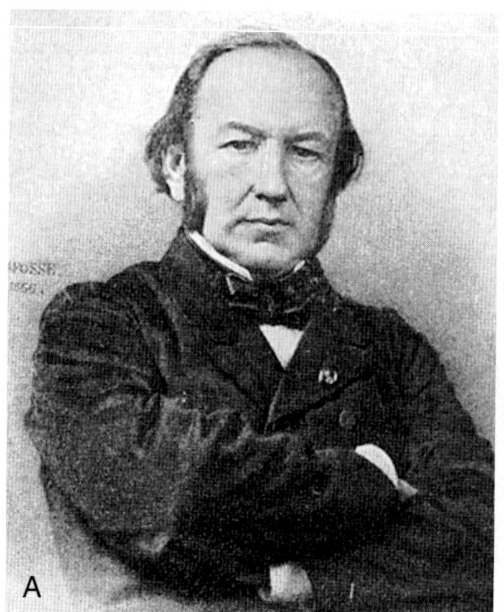

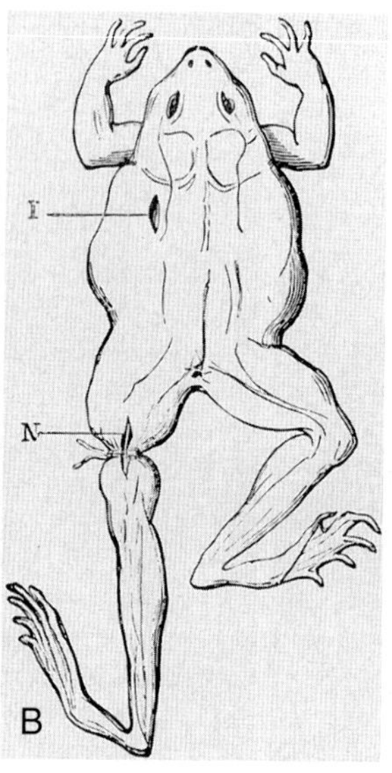

Figure 1-13 **A,** Claude Bernard (1813-1878) was one of the greatest physiologists of all time and made several contributions to the anesthesia literature. Bernard was born in Saint Julien, France, and educated in Paris. After medical training, he became an assistant to François Magendie, the leading physiologist of that era. He never practiced medicine, but his research contributions pervade every field of modern medicine. In 1855, he succeeded Magendie as Professor of Physiology at the College de France. A special Chair of General Physiology was created for him at the Sorbonne. **B,** Experiment by Claude Bernard illustrating the site of action of curare at the junction of the nerve and muscle. A ligature prevented injected curare (I) from reaching the muscle of the frog's hind limb. After systemic injection of curare, Bernard observed that the limb contracted in response to a neural stimulus (N) applied above the ligature. The opposite limb would contract only to direct electric stimulation of the muscle but not to a neural stimulus. He showed that the nerve and muscle were unaffected but that the connection between the nerve and muscle was blocked.[230] *(Courtesy of the National Library of Medicine, Bethesda, MD.)*

The active principle was eventually found in several plant species, primarily *Chondodendron tomentosum* and *Strychnos toxifera* (see Fig. 1-9C). King isolated the active compound from the *Chondodendron* species that he called D-tubocurarine in 1935.

Curare was initiated into clinical practice by several individuals, beginning with Richard C. Gill[232] (1901-1958), whose contributions, like those of Waterton, arose out of a strong sense of wanderlust, combined with an interest in primitive medicine. As a young man growing up in Washington, D.C., Gill was expected to follow his father and older brother into the practice of medicine. Instead, his degree in 1929 from Cornell University was in English, and his career as a teacher was brief. He took a position with a rubber company in Lima, Peru, but with the stock market crash of 1929, he consolidated his savings and, together with his wife Ruth, purchased 750 acres of land in the Ecuadorian jungle. By 1930, Richard and Ruth Gill were the proud owners of a large hacienda on the Eastern slopes of the Andes,[233] where they raised tropical fruits and vegetables and studied the local Indian customs.

While returning to the United States in 1932 for a brief holiday, Gill fell from his horse and a neurologic syndrome, initially thought to be multiple sclerosis, developed and eventually progressed to a painful spastic disorder. His neurologist Walter Freeman (1895-1972) advised him that the arrow poison from South America might help cure his painful spasms, but it was nearly impossible to obtain the drug. Procuring curare and other herbal remedies thereafter became the focus of Gill's life until his death in 1958 at 57 years of age. Gill obtained funding from Sayre Merrill, a wealthy Massachusetts businessman, for an expedition to retrieve indigenous medicinal plants from the Ecuadorian jungle. The primary aim was to retrieve adequate amounts of the crude curare preparation to begin clinical trials with the drug in cases of spasticity. It is noteworthy that Gill was in a unique position to obtain large quantities of curare because the Indian "medicine men," who jealously guarded the secrets of making the poisonous darts, trusted him.

After 4 years of planning, Gill's neurologic condition had improved, and the expedition was launched. In 1938, Richard and Ruth Gill returned with 11 kg of a crude curare mixture and 75 other indigenous medicinal preparations obtained from the Indian shamans. Sadly for the Gills, there was no interest in their jungle remedies. Initially, even the curare failed to generate any interest. Freeman was acquainted with Abram E. Bennett, a psychiatrist at the University of Nebraska who had expressed interest in the drug. Bennett had the crude concoction standardized by the pharmacologist A. R. McIntyre but failed to find any prolonged benefit for it in cases of spasticity (Fig. 1-14A).

Bennett then turned his attention to the use of curare during Metrazol convulsive therapy, which at that time was thought to be therapeutic for depression and mania but was complicated by a high incidence of bone fractures and joint dislocations. By then, E. R. Squibb and Sons had taken the remainder of Gill's curare and was distributing a small quantity of the drug as Intocostrin, an unpurified form of D-tubocurarine. Bennett[234] reported on the successful use of Intocostrin in cases of Metrazol convulsive therapy in 1940. His method was to administer Intocostrin until a head lift was impossible and then give Metrazol. Surprisingly, he reported no respiratory embarrassment and no complications and thought that patients preferred his new method.

E. R. Squibb and Sons, together with their anesthesiologist consultant Lewis H. Wright (1894-1974), were convinced that the true home for curare was with the anesthesiologist, and in 1940, with some urging, Wright convinced Harold R. Griffith (1894-1985) (see Fig. 1-14B) of Montreal, Canada, to use the drug during general anesthesia when muscular relaxation was required by the surgeon. Previous attempts by Wright to generate interest in the drug had failed until Griffith agreed to use Intocostrin during cyclopropane anesthesia. Griffith and his junior colleague Enid Johnson reported the successful use of curare in 43 patients to provide muscular relaxation during surgical anesthesia in 1942.[235] They concluded that the agent provided relaxation without interfering with respiration. This was followed by a study in Iowa by Stuart Cullen[236] (1909-1979), who enthusiastically supported use of the drug to provide muscular relaxation without the need for deep levels of general anesthesia. T. Cecil Gray[237] (1913-) of Liverpool popularized the drug in England and developed an anesthetic technique consisting of profound muscular paralysis and nitrous oxide–oxygen anesthesia. Phyllis Harroun[238,239] used

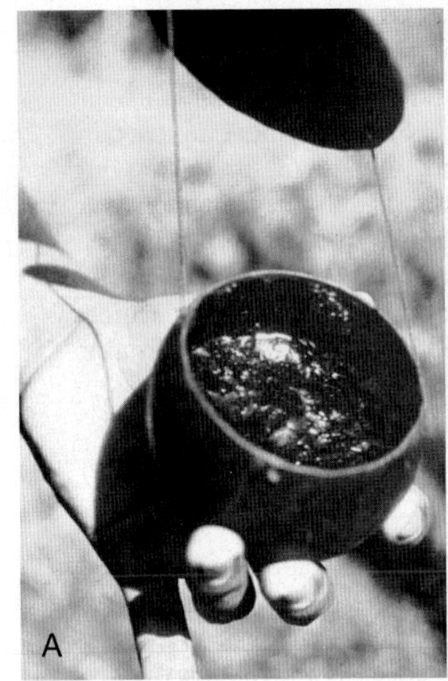

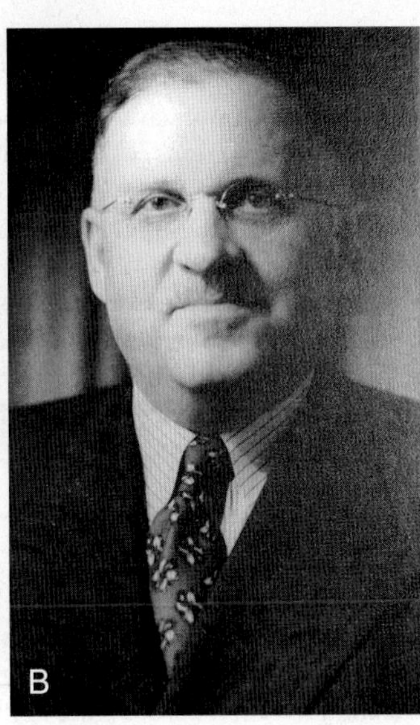

Figure 1-14 A, Richard Gill returned from Ecuador in 1938 with 11 kg of a dark tarlike paste from which Squibb and Sons, Inc., prepared the sterile, injectable solution Intocostrin. **B,** Harold Griffith and Enid Johnson (not shown) used Intocostrin in 43 abdominal surgeries with success in 1942. *(Courtesy of the Guedel Memorial Anesthesia Center, San Francisco, CA.)*

high-dose curare, nitrous oxide, and morphine for thoracic surgery, thereby providing muscular relaxation without the use of flammable agents, a novel technique at the time. In 1947, William Neff used nitrous oxide and oxygen supplemented with meperidine and curare and reported favorable anesthetic conditions. Although Griffith and Cullen had both maintained spontaneous respiration, the technique of Harroun, Gray, and Neff provided profound muscular paralysis with controlled respiration.

In a report from 1954, Henry K. Beecher (1907-1976) and D. P. Todd[240] concluded that the use of curare led to a nearly sixfold increase in postoperative complications and deaths. Similar cautionary articles followed their report but were refuted by others. Churchill-Davidson and Richardson[241] advised in 1952 that a useful technique for monitoring the degree of neuromuscular blockade was to stimulate a peripheral nerve and observe the resulting muscular contraction. Specific devices designed to stimulate the ulnar nerve were promoted in the 1960s.[242,243] Various modifications of the stimulus array to ensure complete return of neuromuscular function before allowing the patient to breathe unassisted have been described since that time.[244]

Since the introduction of curare into anesthesia practice, numerous additional neuromuscular blocking agents have been developed. Gallamine triethiodide was introduced in 1947, but like curare, it had undesirable effects on the autonomic nervous system, which prompted a search for other drugs. Exploration of the structure-activity relationships of plant alkaloids led to development of the methonium compounds. In 1949, the neuromuscular blocking activity of one of this class of drugs, succinylcholine, was recognized,[245] and it was introduced clinically soon thereafter.[246] Daniel Bovet (1907-1992) won the Nobel Prize in 1957, in part related to his discovery of gallamine and succinylcholine. Succinylcholine and other similar agents were shown to depolarize the end plate, thereby preventing additional motor contractions as a result of activity in the motor nerve. Advances in chemistry allowed the synthesis of neuromuscular blocking agents that lacked the autonomic effects of curare. Since the discovery of curare, nearly 50 neuromuscular blocking agents have been introduced, but many of these drugs have been abandoned because of undesirable side effects. Drugs that have maintained favorable safety records are steroid-based synthetic neuromuscular blocking agents such as pancuronium (1966),[247] vecuronium (1980),[248,249] and rocuronium (1991),[250] and they have replaced older drugs such as curare and gallamine in the modern drug armamentarium.

Anesthesia Apparatus

Early Delivery Systems

For the first public demonstration of ether anesthesia, Morton used a specially constructed glass bottle with an attached mouthpiece (see Chapter 25). In England, John Snow developed a new type of ether inhaler and took up the practice of ether anesthesia as a full-time endeavor. His apparatus provided valves to prevent rebreathing, and although he experimented with methods for absorption of carbon dioxide, he did not develop it into a clinically useful technique. John Snow was aware of the difficulties associated with the simple mouthpiece that was used with a noseclip by Wells and Morton. In his book on ether published in 1847, he states the following:

> *For some of the adult patients, after they lost their consciousness, made such strong instinctive efforts to breathe by the nostrils, that the air was forced through the lachrymal ducts, and occasionally they held the breath altogether for a short time, and were getting purple in the face, when the nostrils had to be liberated, for a short time, to allow respiration of the external air, and thus a delay was occasioned.*

Many types of anesthesia machines were developed to provide anesthesia via the insufflation method, whereby a small catheter was placed with its tip near the carina to deliver air and ether or chloroform. These continuous-flow machines did not rely on respiratory movement for oxygenation and were based on the work of Samuel Meltzer (1851-1920) and John Auer (1875-1948), who demonstrated their safe use in animals.[251] It was one solution to the problem of pneumothorax and respiratory decompensation during thoracic surgery. C. A. Elsberg's (1871-1948) continuous-flow machine was described in 1911 and went through several modifications.[252] The popular Shipway model was used by Francis E. Shipway (1875-1968) to provide anesthesia to King George V of England for rib resection and drainage of empyema, a feat for which Shipway was knighted. In retrospect, it is clear that these continuous-flow machines were not capable of eliminating carbon dioxide in all cases,[253] and anesthesia machines eventually were developed that allowed to-and-fro respiration through one large-bore endotracheal tube.

Compressed Gases and Reducing Valves

Of major importance in design of the modern anesthesia machine was compression of gases in metal cylinders. Oxygen and nitrous oxide were available under compression as early as 1885 through the manufacturers S. S. White of Philadelphia and Messrs. Coxeter of London. This allowed the development of compact machines capable of prolonged delivery of anesthetics without the cumbersome feature of low-pressure reservoirs. Frederick Hewitt's first anesthetic gas machine designed for administering oxygen and nitrous oxide mixtures had two nitrous oxide cylinders and one oxygen cylinder; the mixture was fed into a large breathing bag through a double cylinder yoke.[98] Oxygen concentrations could be adjusted at the stopcock near the mask. His preferred oxygen concentrations were 5% to 8%. With the addition of oxygen, he attempted to "dispense with cyanosis, jerky and irregular breathing, deep stertor and clonic movements of the extremities."

Invention of the reducing valve is accredited to Jay Albion Heidbrink (1857-1957), an anesthesiologist from Minneapolis who observed that the opening from high-pressure cylinders often froze closed as the gases were released. He described a valve that reduced the high tank pressures to working pressures and incorporated this device into his Heidbrink Anesthetizer. In Germany, Heinrich Drager (1847-1917) and his son Bernhard Drager (1870-1928) developed reducing valves to control an even, accurate flow of carbon dioxide gas drawn from beer cylinders, and these valves were later used in the early anesthesia machines. Further refinements to the early machines were added by James T. Gwathmey and H. Edmund G. Boyle (1875-1941), chiefly through the addition of bubble-through heated water baths for estimation of gas flow. The Boyle machine passed various amounts of oxygen through ether with a "water-sight" meter. This flow meter estimated the flow through the vaporizer from how many of the holes were generating bubbles. Heidbrink further improved the flow meter by using an inverted float in a tube of varying taper with calibrations marked on the side. Rotating floats, also called rotameters, have slanted grooves cut into the rim that cause them to rotate, and they are more accurate than ball or nonrotating floats. Rotameters were introduced in 1908 by Karl Kuppers and first used in anesthesia in 1910.

Carbon Dioxide Absorption

Anesthesiologists from the first half of the 20th century were not privileged to visit just one hospital during a day's work. Visits to several institutions might take place in a single day, with the practitioners bringing their own delivery systems and drugs with them as they traveled. Understandably, portability and elimination of waste were a priority because these anesthesiologists paid for the agents themselves. One development that conserved gases and vapors was the use of systems that absorbed expired carbon dioxide and allowed rebreathing of expired gases.

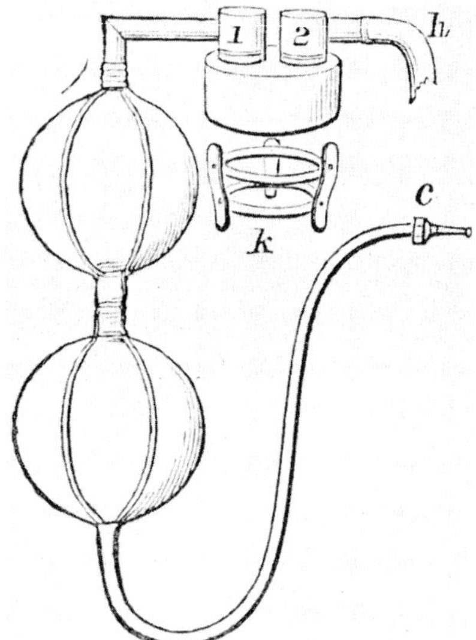

Figure 1-15 Alfred Coleman's economizing device. The anesthetic gases entered the lower bag and passed into the upper bag through a one-way valve. Gases were inhaled and exhaled through the tube (h) and passed over a lime container (1, 2) held in a frame (k) that eliminated carbon dioxide; c, gas inlet. The conserved gas in the upper bag was used during a later anesthetic administration. *(From Coleman A: Mr. Coleman's economizing apparatus for re-inhaling the gas. Br J Dent Sci 12:443, 1869.)*

Several ineffectual attempts were made to introduce carbon dioxide absorption methods in the 19th century. John Snow and Alfred Coleman (1828-1902) were motivated to conserve anesthetic gases that escaped into the atmosphere through nonrebreathing valves. Coleman devised a system of absorbing carbon dioxide by passing the expired gases over slaked quick lime.[254] The recovered gases were then used for subsequent anesthetics (Fig. 1-15). Franz Kuhn (1866-1929) described soda lime absorption of exhaled carbon dioxide in 1905, but the report did not attract attention.

Dennis E. Jackson (1878-1980) demonstrated the use of soda lime absorption to maintain stable levels of anesthesia for several hours in animals with minimal ether consumption.[255] The animals were given additional oxygen to meet metabolic needs, but the anesthetic gases were rebreathed, thereby resulting in economy and improved maintenance of body temperature and airway humidity. In 1923, Ralph Waters (1884-1979) (see Fig. 1-18B), then working as an anesthesia practitioner in Sioux City, Iowa, contacted Jackson and devised a soda lime canister for clinical use.[256] The canister was attached to a breathing hose close to the face, and although it was cumbersome to use, the device was widely distributed. The in-line soda lime canister launched the academic career of Waters, who later became one of the most prominent figures in anesthesiology during the first half of the 20th century. In 1930, Brian C. Sword[257] altered the Waters canister by attaching it to the chassis of a movable cart with two hoses directed to the airway, one for inspired gases and one for exhaled gases.

Controlled Vaporizers

With the introduction of more potent volatile anesthetics such as halothane it became important to control the concentration of inspired vapor carefully. To solve this problem, Lucien Morris[258] invented the copper kettle to vaporize liquid anesthetics. Its advantage rested on the fact that as the agent was vaporized, there was little change in the temperature of the anesthetic liquid. The copper kettle could be used with any agent provided that the practitioner was cognizant of the vapor pressure of the agent and the flow rates of the inspired gases. Without the addition of diluent gases such as nitrous oxide or oxygen, the copper kettle could deliver lethal concentrations of vapor. The vaporizers in common use today use bimetallic strips that bend as the temperature drops and permit more fresh gas to enter the vaporizing chamber. Vaporizers have been designed for all the agents in use today, including halothane, enflurane, isoflurane, desflurane, and sevoflurane. Modern anesthesia machines are also equipped with scavenging systems designed to minimize escape of anesthetic vapors and nitrous oxide into the operating room. Although controversial, some studies have shown that daily exposure to anesthetic vapors in low concentrations can have deleterious side effects.

Ventilators in the Intensive Care Unit

The earliest ventilator, the Fell-O'Dwyer apparatus, was described in 1892.[259] It was used as early as 1896 to provide respiratory support in cases of opium poisoning. Rudolph Matas, a surgeon in New Orleans who contributed significantly to the early development of regional anesthesia in the United States, was one of the first to use the Fell-O'Dwyer ventilator during thoracic surgery.[260] During the polio epidemic, thousands of afflicted patients were kept alive with the Drinker respirator,[261] often referred to as the *iron lung*, a negative-pressure device that surrounded the patient and provided air movement into and out of the lungs. A Swedish ventilator called the Spiropulsator was introduced in 1934 and modified in 1947 by E. Trier Moerch (1908-1995).[262] This ventilator used a piston pump to deliver a fixed volume of gas. Ventilators today are usually an integral part of the anesthesia machine and direct compressed air into a rigid container containing a bellows that inflates the lungs. Bjørn Ibsen[263] (1915-), a Danish anesthesiologist, initiated the concept of intensive care units in the early 1950s to care for polio patients and guided the transition from iron lungs to modern ventilators. Intensive care units have since become an integral part of the modern hospital, with anesthesiologists actively involved in their daily operation.

Stress-Free Anesthesia

Procedures before the discovery of anesthesia were necessarily of short duration. Raper relates that surgical cases lasting longer than 20 minutes would usually result in death of the patient because the stress associated with such intense nociception would exhaust the patient's reserves. Highly stressful procedures such as abdominal surgery were rarely attempted before 1846. Ephraim McDowell[264] (1771-1830), a rural surgeon from Kentucky, performed the first successful intraperitoneal procedure when he excised a 10-kg ovarian cyst from Mrs. Jane Todd Crawford in 1809. McDowell's publication of the case achieved for him a small measure of fame, unusual for a rural practitioner. However, intraperitoneal procedures are among the most highly stressful operations, and McDowell's accomplishment was rarely repeated. The first successful upper abdominal procedure occurred only after the advent of general anesthesia. Theodor Billroth (1829-1894) performed the first gastrectomy with chloroform anesthesia on January 29, 1881.

The idea that reduction of perioperative stress had a beneficial effect on recovery was championed by George W. Crile (1864-1943), chief surgeon at the Cleveland Clinic at the beginning of the 20th century. Crile's operative technique was to infiltrate all tissues with dilute procaine before incision. Patients were lightly anesthetized by mask inhalation of nitrous oxide and oxygen.[265] He describes these concepts of stress-free anesthesia in his book *Anoci-Association*, published in 1914.[266]

An early devotee of Crile's ideas was the prominent neurosurgeon Harvey Cushing[267] (1869-1939), who promoted the use of regional blocks before emergence from ether anesthesia to ensure a smooth postoperative course. Cushing was the first surgeon to use blood pressure measurements on his patients after he learned the Rovi-Rocci method in Italy (Fig. 1-16). Accurate anesthetic records were maintained during Cushing's cases and confirmed his opinion that shock could be prevented by careful attention to avoiding the stresses associated with surgery.

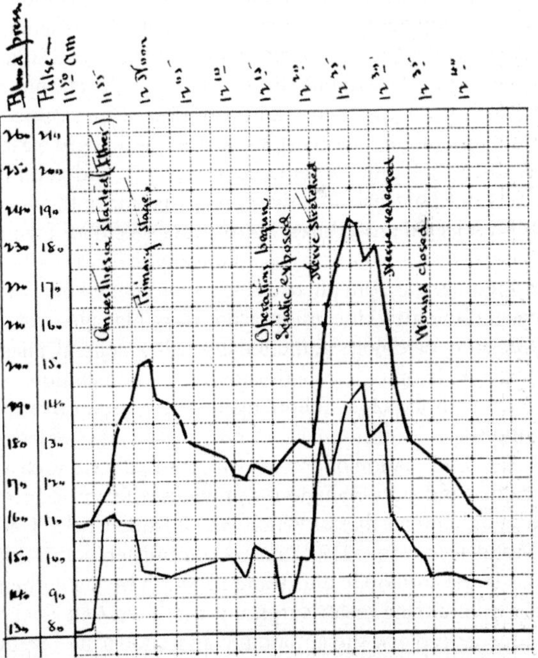

Figure 1-16 One of Harvey Cushing's early anesthesia records shows systolic blood pressure (*top tracing*) and pulse rate (*bottom tracing*). The first rise in blood pressure occurred during the excitement phase of ether induction, and the second rise occurred during the release of adhesions of the sciatic nerve. *Vertical lines* take place 2.5 minutes apart. Systolic blood pressure rose to greater than 230 mm Hg during the operation. Cushing was an early proponent of regional anesthesia, possibly stemming from his observations on blood pressure and heart rate.[267] *(From Cushing H: On routine determination of arterial tension in operating room and clinic. Boston Med Surg J 148:250-256, 1903.)*

Crile's ideas have had a significant impact on how the modern anesthesiologist defines general anesthesia. In 1957, P. Woodbridge[268] defined general anesthesia as consisting of four components: (1) sleep or unconsciousness, (2) blockade of undesirable reflexes, (3) motor blockade, and (4) sensory blockade. These ideas have been discussed and modified by M. Pinsker[269] into three components: (1) paralysis, (2) unconsciousness, and (3) attenuation of the stress response. Lundy's balanced anesthesia is another formulation of the idea that several drugs can be used in combination to produce the state of unconsciousness and analgesia that we define as general anesthesia.

An enduring question during the past century, since Crile's introduction of the concept of stress-free anesthesia, has been how to evaluate the analgesic component of the ideal general anesthetic. Michael Roizen[270] (1947-) observed in 1981 that general anesthetics did not prevent the increase in sympathetic activity in response to a skin incision, even in concentrations that prevented movement. Surgical stimulation often results in intraoperative hypertension and tachycardia, with the corollary that interventions that prevent these hemodynamic reflexes provide "analgesia." Hemodynamic instability was of marginal significance until surgeons began to operate on patients with significant ischemic heart disease. Studies have demonstrated that perioperative β-adrenergic blockade reduces the risk for perioperative myocardial infarction in patients at risk for this complication.[271]

It became apparent that intravenous opioids were highly successful in ablating the hemodynamic markers of stress. Edward Lowenstein and coworkers[272] used large doses of morphine to stabilize the heart rate and blood pressure during cardiac surgery. In 1967, the short-acting opioid fentanyl was introduced to provide intraoperative hemodynamic stability. Theodore H. Stanley and colleagues[273] reported its successful use in large doses for cardiac surgery without the side effect of histamine release that sometimes occurs after administration of morphine. Other short-acting opioids tailored for the anesthesiologist have been added since that time. Alfentanil, sufentanil, and remifentanil have different pharmacokinetic profiles that make them suitable agents for selected procedures. Naloxone, a specific antagonist for this class of drugs, was first used clinically in 1971.[274] Increased understanding of opioid pharmacology has opened up a new role for anesthesiologists, including acute pain management. Rapid detoxification of opioid addiction by using general anesthesia combined with opioid antagonism is a new technique that if combined with judicious follow-up, can be a useful treatment of this condition.[275]

The combination of opioids with tranquilizers such as phenothiazines and butyrophenones provides a form of anesthesia called neuroleptanesthesia, which was introduced by DeCastro and Mundeleer[276] in 1959. Patients administered this form of anesthesia are immobile and tranquil and have stable hemodynamics, even during major surgical procedures. One goal of this technique is to block the autonomic and endocrine response to stress. This unique method of providing anesthesia is another technique for ablating the stress response, but unless other agents such as nitrous oxide or other intravenous agents are administered, there can be a high incidence of awareness. Side effects from dopamine antagonism, such as dysphoria and uncontrolled extrapyramidal motor movements, have limited the widespread use of neuroleptanesthesia.

During the past 30 years, several investigators began a series of studies to measure markers of the stress response during and after surgery. It was learned that during major surgery, patients anesthetized with traditional vapor anesthetics, with or without opioids, displayed increased levels of catabolic hormones postoperatively.[77] Significant elevations in catecholamines and in adrenocorticotropic hormone, cortisol, antidiuretic hormone, and growth hormone were observed. Various methods of preventing postoperative catabolism have been under investigation for several years. The resulting catabolic state is thought by some to delay recovery and, with some operations, can be prevented with the use of neuraxial blockade.[77,277,278] It is apparent from recent reviews on this subject that the formulations of George Crile are still valid 100 years after he promoted them and are likely to be the subject of further studies in the future.

Airway Management and Resuscitation

Masks and Airways

Ventilation during anesthesia was managed without specialized airway devices for more than 50 years after Morton's discovery, and a survey of anesthetic complications during this era attests to the relative safety of inhalation techniques in spontaneously breathing patients (see Chapters 50 and 93). Deaths occurred during this era, and in some reports the anesthetic death rate was alarmingly high, but an obstructed airway was rarely mentioned as the primary cause of death. Friedrich von Esmarch[279] described the jaw thrust (Fig. 1-17) as a lifesaving maneuver in some cases of airway obstruction that resulted from chloroform or asphyxia:

> *Press the lower jaw forwards with both hands by placing the forefingers behind the ascending ramus . . . by this movement the hyoid bone and root of the tongue, and the epiglottis are drawn forwards, and the entrance to the larynx is thus freed from obstruction.*

In 1874 the same maneuver had been previously described, but not popularized by J. Heiberg, a Norwegian surgeon.

Various problems with the Morton inhaler in the United States led to abandonment of inhalers in favor of a simple towel or sponge saturated with ether. In 1850, John Warren,[280] in his

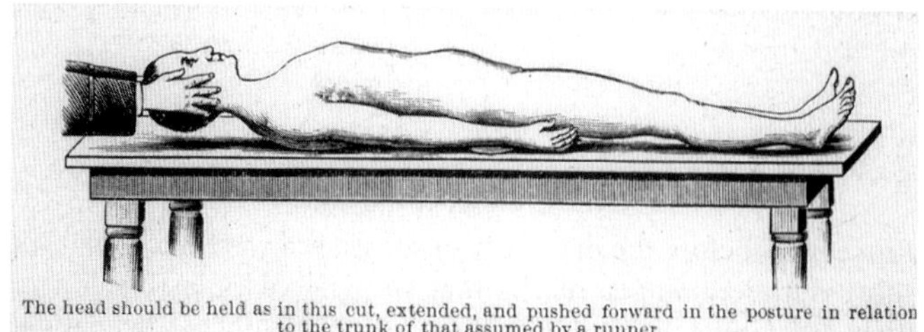

Figure 1-17 Illustration in a treatise by von Esmarch[279] showing the technique of maintaining an open airway in an unconscious patient. *(From von Esmarch F: Handbuch der kriegschirurgischen Technik. Hanover, Carl Rumpler, 1877.)*

address to the American Medical Association, described his preferred technique for administration of ether at the Massachusetts General Hospital: (1) no oral intake for at least 3 hours before surgery, (2) a horizontal position for induction, (3) bleeding the patient before surgery for bloodless operations, (4) pulse and respiration watched carefully by an assistant to the anesthetist, (5) ether applied with a large sponge soaked with ether, and (6) avoidance of cautery.

Several wire frame masks were devised to replace the sponge or folded towel. The popular mask devised by Curl Schimmelbusch (1860-1895) had a trough-shaped rim to prevent liquid chloroform or ether from dropping onto the patient's face. Friederich von Esmarch[279] used a wire mask with a clip that enabled it to be strapped to the patient. The advantages of these masks were low cost, simplicity, and portability. Disadvantages included delivery of vapor throughout the operating room, cooling of the patient, and waste of anesthetic agent.

Development of the modern facemask originated with Francis Sibson[281,282] (1814-1876), who devised a mask made of pliable tinned iron and covered with glove leather. The mask covered the mouth and nose and therefore eliminated the need for noseclips. Snow quickly recognized the superiority of the Sibson mask and incorporated it into his practice.

The first anesthetics were of short duration and rarely required special devices to maintain patency of the airway. With the increasing complexity and duration of surgical procedures, special devices were fashioned to facilitate an open airway. Frederick Hewitt promoted a simple metal tube that projected through the mouth into the hypopharynx. The commonly used Guedel rubber curved airway was described in 1933.[283] At the same time, cuffs were sometimes used on oral airways, a design that has been resurrected in the form of a modern product, the cuffed oral pharyngeal airway (COPA).

Tracheal Tubes

In the 18th century, tubes were passed into the trachea during resuscitation from drowning, but these tubes were passed without direct visualization and were not used for delivery of anesthetic agents. Similarly, the intubations of pediatrician Joseph O'Dwyer (1841-1898) in cases of diphtheria were performed with metal tubes passed blindly.[284] The O'Dwyer metal tube was later attached to a bellows by George Fell (1850-1918) for the treatment of opioid respiratory depression. Placement of tracheal tubes was vigorously opposed by the influential Parisian surgeon Armand Trousseau (1801-1867), who quoted the failures experienced by M. Bouchut in attempting to pass metal tubes for airway obstruction. Bouchut had lost five of seven patients during his procedure, called *le tubage du larynx*, and the other two were rescued only by tracheotomy.[285] Trousseau was the first to perform a tracheotomy in Paris and wrote a treatise promoting its use during airway compromise in 1851.

John Snow had administered chloroform through tracheotomy tubes in animals, and Friedrich Trendelenburg (1844-1924) used the same technique in humans.[286] Sir William Macewen (1848-1924) was the first physician to intubate the trachea orally for the sole purpose of administering anesthesia, and it was done to permit continued administration of chloroform during an operation in the mouth. On July 5, 1878, Macewen[287] performed a blind oral intubation on an awake patient with an ulcerating epithelioma of the tongue. An extensive operation was performed, and the results were excellent. Subsequently, Macewen tracheally intubated three other patients, two for edema of the larynx, and a fourth for another surgical procedure in the mouth. In the fourth case, the pulse was suddenly lost after chloroform was administered, and the patient died on the table.

The use of tracheal intubation was accelerated to meet the needs of surgeons operating on the face and in the thoracic cavity. To operate within the thoracic cavity, some means was required to avoid respiratory compromise, which followed the inevitable pneumothorax when the chest was opened. Ernst Ferdinand Sauerbruch[288] (1875-1951) studied the problem as a young assistant to Johann von Mickulicz-Radecki (1850-1905) in Breslau, Germany, and his solution, the Sauerbruch Box, elevated him into a position of international prominence at a young age. The Sauerbruch Box was a cumbersome solution to the problem of pneumothorax and entailed placing the surgeon and the patient (below the neck) in a negative-pressure chamber while the head of the patient and the anesthetist were outside the box at normal atmospheric pressure. The use of such an awkward construction indicates that surgeons were determined to solve this problem at any cost. The modern solution, endotracheal intubation and controlled ventilation, as it unfolded was relatively simple, but it took several years to become established.

Franz Kuhn (1866-1929) perfected a flexible metal tube and used blind oral or nasal intubation for anesthetic purposes when the surgeon operated in the mouth. Kuhn's first report on tracheal intubation was in 1905 and included an extensive description of a technique using carbon dioxide absorption cartridges. He proposed but did not use inflatable pharyngeal cuffs to prevent air leaks. Insertion of catheters directly into the trachea to insufflate anesthetic agents was begun in the first decades of the 20th century. With this method, gases were introduced under continuous pressure through catheters that allowed exhalation through the space between the catheter and tracheal wall.

The use of to-and-fro respiration through one large-bore endotracheal tube is credited to Ivan W. Magill[289] (1888-1986) (Fig. 1-18A) and Edgar S. Rowbotham[290] (1890-1979) to meet the demands of the maxillofacial surgeon. Their technique of blind nasal intubation was to position patients as if they were "sniffing the morning air." Occasional failures of blind intubation were solved with a special instrument designed by Magill to lift the tube off the posterior wall of the pharynx into the glottic opening. The so-called Magill tubes were formed to fit the airway and were made of red mineralized rubber. The cuffed endotracheal tube was promoted by Arthur Guedel (1883-1956) (Fig. 1-19) and Ralph M. Waters (1883-1979) (see Fig. 1-18B) in 1928,[291] and this refinement allowed the use of intermittent, controlled, positive-pressure ventilation and the potential for one-lung ventilation, introduced by Gale and Waters in 1932.[292] Four years later, Magill introduced the bronchial blocker to confine the secretions of an infected lung to one side. Magill's technique was to pass the blocker before induction of anesthesia with a specially designed bronchoscope.[293] Double-lumen tubes for bronchospirometry were introduced by Carlens in 1949,[294] but the small lumen size made these tubes inconvenient for anesthetized subjects. The commonly used disposable double-lumen tubes in use today are modeled after the Robertshaw tube[295] for the left side and after the Green-Gordon tube[296] for the right side. An opening called the Murphy eye, on the side of the standard endotracheal tube,

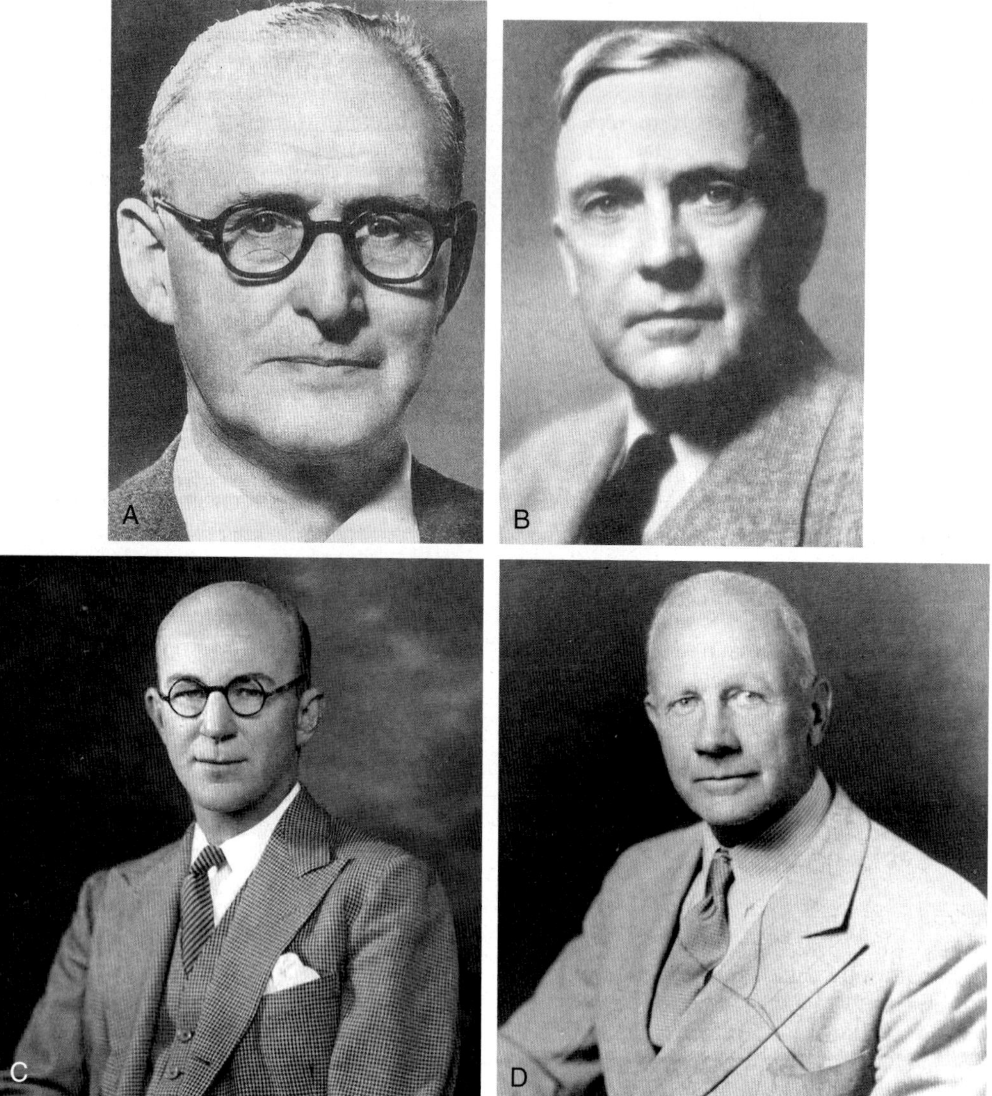

Figure 1-18 Prominent anesthesiologists of the 20th century. **A,** Sir Ivan Whiteside Magill (1888-1986) was born in Larne, Northern Ireland. He obtained a medical degree from Queen's University, Belfast, in 1913. During World War I, he served with the Irish Guards in the Medical Corps. After the war, he and Stanley Rowbotham (1890-1979) pioneered the use of large-bore endotracheal tubes to allow plastic surgeons to operate on the facial injuries of wounded soldiers. He designed many pieces of equipment for the anesthesiologist, some of which are still used today. Before his death at the age of 98 years, he received many awards, including a knighthood awarded personally by the Queen of England in 1960 and the Henry Hill Hickman Award. **B,** Ralph M. Waters was born in North Bloomfield, Ohio, and obtained his medical degree from Western Reserve University in Cleveland. He began his career in general practice in Sioux City, Iowa, and specialized in delivering anesthesia in 1916. Waters established the first academic program of anesthesiology in Madison, Wisconsin, in 1927. His contributions were many and included the carbon dioxide absorption method, endobronchial anesthesia for thoracic surgery, and introduction of cyclopropane. His chief legacy is the many residents he trained who then became leaders within the specialty in the following generation. **C,** Sir Robert R. Macintosh (1897-1989) was born in New Zealand and was a prisoner of war during World War I. He finished medical training in London after the war and began the practice of anesthesia there. In 1937, he was appointed the first Nuffield Professor of Anaesthetics at Oxford University. He was primarily a clinician, and his innovative techniques of airway management were eventually accepted worldwide. He received honorary degrees from universities in several countries and was knighted in 1955. **D,** James T. Gwathmey was born in Roanoke, Virginia, in 1865 and graduated from the Vanderbilt School of Medicine in 1899. In 1903, he limited his practice to the administration of anesthetics, and he is considered one of the first full-time private practice physician-anesthesiologists in the United States. He devised several innovations for the delivery of anesthetic gases and introduced these machines to his European colleagues during World War I. He was an original member of the Long Island Society of Anesthetists, which eventually evolved into the American Society of Anesthesiologists. *(Courtesy of the Wood-Library Museum of Anesthesiology, Park Ridge, IL.)*

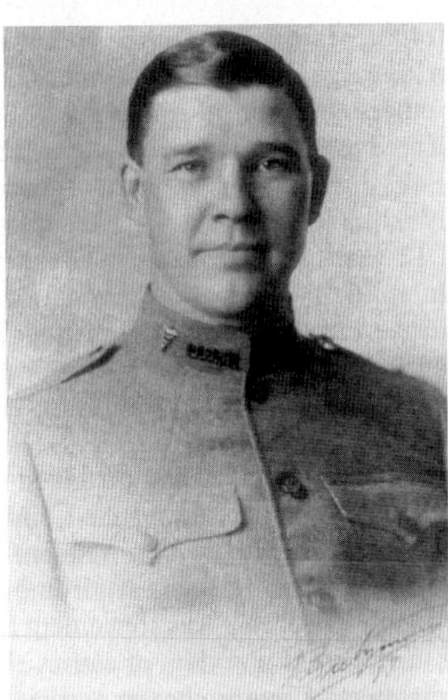

Figure 1-19 Photograph of Arthur Guedel while he was serving in the American Expeditionary Forces in France during World War I. During the war, he was responsible for the safe administration of thousands of anesthetics, often delivered without properly trained personnel. As a guide for teaching nurses and orderlies to administer ether, he devised a wall chart describing the various stages and planes of ether anesthesia that eventually resulted in his classic publication on this topic in 1919. He used a drug sequence of ethyl chloride, chloroform, and ether, which prepared the patient for surgery within 2 minutes.[353] *(Courtesy of the Guedel Memorial Anesthesia Center, San Francisco, CA.)*

was suggested in 1941 as an alternative air passage in the event of distal tip occlusion.[297]

Laryngoscopes

Although blind or tactile tracheal intubation of awake patients could be mastered with extensive practice, an improved technique to accomplish tracheal intubation was developed by Alfred Kirstein[298,299] (1863-1922), Chevalier Jackson[300] (1865-1958), and Gustav Killian (1898-1912), all contributors to the introduction of the hand-held laryngoscope. Before the pioneering efforts of these innovators, the only way to visualize the larynx was by indirect laryngoscopy, a technique introduced by the Spanish singing instructor Manuel Garcia (1805-1868). In 1854, Garcia read a paper before the Royal Society titled "Observations on the Human Voice," wherein he described his use of mirrors to view his student's and his own larynx during vocalization.[301] Alfred Kirstein was charting unknown territory in 1895 when he boldly suggested that the larynx could be directly visualized with instruments similar to the commonly used esophagoscope.[298] Although he abandoned the procedure after 1 year, it was revived 3 years later by Gustav Killian,[302] whose portable laryngoscope was remarkably like the current instrument, but with no light attached.

Direct laryngoscopy did not gain in popularity among anesthesiologists until Chevalier Jackson promoted the use of his hand-held laryngoscope for insertion of tracheal insufflation catheters. Even then, the technique was slow to gain acceptance, but the accelerated use of muscle relaxants eventually required the anesthesiologist to be adept at rapid placement of tubes within the trachea. The first hand-held laryngoscopes, as perfected by Jackson, were U shaped and had no curve at the tip. A light at the end of the blade was a unique contribution by Jackson that has been retained, with the modification that some instruments today use a fiberoptic bundle in the blade.

Anesthesiologists soon began to design their own laryngoscopes that were more suitable for insertion of endotracheal tubes. Robert A. Miller[303] designed a new blade that was remarkably similar to Killian's instrument, except for a slight curve at the distal end. Robert R. Macintosh's (1897-1989) (see Fig. 1-18C) improved laryngoscope featured a short, curved blade that elevated instead of retracted the epiglottis.[304] This promoted a new concept in laryngoscopy specifically designed with the anesthesiologist in mind for timely tracheal intubation. Many intubations were then performed without muscle relaxants, and the Macintosh blade was able to expose the glottis without coming into contact with the sensitive posterior surface of the epiglottis. By this time a detachable joint had been placed between the blade and the handle. The batteries were located in the handle, thereby conveniently avoiding the trailing wires attached to the distal bulb.

Alternatives to the Laryngoscope

Unfortunately, not all patients could be successfully intubated with the hand-held laryngoscope. Several new blades were developed in the 1940s and 1950s to solve the problem of a difficult airway, but none were 100% successful, and it soon became apparent that some airways could not be intubated with any hand-held instrument. In such cases, the few remaining members of the hospital staff who had been trained in blind tactile intubations were called in to secure the airway.

The problem of a difficult or impossible intubation is now solved with a variety of tools, including various modifications of the laryngeal mask airway (LMA) and the flexible laryngoscope, both established tools in the modern anesthesia department. The LMA was developed by A. J. Brain of the Royal Berkshire Hospital, Reading, England, with the commercial product first appearing in 1983.[305] This device is well named, for it is indeed a small mask that covers the glottic opening. The LMA eliminates the need for tracheal intubation in many cases and is useful in managing a difficult airway.

The beginnings of flexible laryngoscopy were rooted in the 19th century. John Tyndall (1820-1893) succeeded the more famous Michael Faraday as Superintendent of the Royal Institution in London in 1867 and published his observation in 1854 that light could follow a curved path through a water tube. In 1930, H. Lamm[306] used this property of light when he introduced the flexible gastroscope, with glass fibers used instead of water. S. Ikeda[307] transferred the same technology to a smaller-diameter instrument and thereby introduced flexible bronchofiberoscopy in 1968. The definitive work followed in 1971.[308]

Resuscitation (see Chapter 97)

Resuscitation from drowning was successfully accomplished by a variety of methods as early as 1792, when James Curry used digital intubation of the trachea and forced air into the lungs with a bellows (see Chapters 93 and 97). J. Leroy criticized the use of positive pressure with bellows as a dangerous procedure in 1827 by showing that it could rupture the alveoli and produce fatal tension pneumothorax. Consequently, several ineffectual techniques developed, such as administration of stimulating vapors, swinging the arms up and down, and pulling the tongue forward in a rhythmic motion, and these futile techniques were slow to dissipate. Largely through the work of O'Dwyer, Tuffier, and Matas, positive-pressure methods were reintroduced in the first few decades of the 20th century. James O. Elam (1918-1995) instinctively demonstrated the efficacy of mouth-to-mouth ventilation in 1946 when ventilators were in short supply during the polio epidemic. Peter Safar (1924-2003) and Elam were influential in converting teaching of the ineffectual arm-lift method to mouth-to-mouth breathing techniques by demonstrating the proficiency of the later technique on volunteer medical students.[309,310]

Rational methods of resuscitation from full cardiac arrest awaited development of the electrocardiogram and its interpretation. Augustus Waller[311] (1856-1922) first produced tracings of the electrical activity of the heart in 1887, but Willem Einthoven[312] (1860-1927) is credited with producing the first modern electrocardiogram by using a string galvanometer in 1903. Tracings compatible with occlusion of the main coronary vessels were demonstrated first in animals and then confirmed in patients by James B. Herrick[313] (1861-1954) of Chicago. John MacWilliam[314] (1857-1937) described ventricular fibrillation in 1887 and provided a case report showing it to be the cause of death in one subject.[315] In 1899, J. L Prevost and F. Battelli[316] showed that small electrical currents passed across the heart could induce ventricular fibrillation and that larger currents could convert fibrillation to a normal rhythm. Claude Beck[317] (1894-1971) performed the first successful use of electric defibrillation in a patient in 1947.

Open cardiac massage was first performed in Norway in 1901[310] and in the following year by Starling,[318] and external massage over the chest was described by W. W. Keen (1837-1932) in 1904.[319] Brief anecdotal reports had been presented on closed chest massage as early as 1883 by Franz Koenig of Göttingen, Germany.[320] William B. Kouwenhoven (1886-1975), Dean of the School of Engineering at Johns Hopkins from 1939 to 1953, began his studies on resuscitation from cardiac arrest in 1929 and 31 years later published the full sequence of external cardiac massage, combined with electric countershock, to restore cardiac rhythm.[321] These methods of resuscitation have been promoted by the American Heart Association and, with some modifications, have become the basis for the widely disseminated educational programs of advanced cardiac life support (ACLS).

Anesthetic Accidents and Complications—Preventive Measures

Anesthetic accidents have occurred since the early days of administration of ether and nitrous oxide. Wells and Morton described patients who required resuscitative measures during anesthesia. Several near deaths were reported after the October 1846 demonstration. Bigelow's first description of ether anesthesia provides a case report of a patient who nearly died after ether administration and was resuscitated by cold effusions, ammonia inhalation, and syringing of the ears.[86] Two other patients "failed to be affected by ether." George Hayward (1791-1863) reported a death occurring after ether inhalation in August 1847. Snow's book on chloroform appeared in 1858 and discusses a number of frightening cases and deaths during administration of anesthesia. The first such tragedy with chloroform struck in 1848, when an anesthetic was given to a 12-year-old girl, Hannah Greener, for a minor surgical procedure. The postmortem examination of this young girl was inconclusive, but the anesthetic was thought to have been administered properly. The controversy surrounding this death has occupied the minds of numerous anesthesiologists for the past 150 years.[322,323]

Most anesthetic deaths were not attributed to the agent or the method of administration but resulted simply from "the patient not taking the anesthetic well." A frequent diagnosis after death during anesthesia was the vague syndrome of "status lymphaticus."[324] Although this phrase was convenient for the anesthesiologist to use, it thwarted a review of causes that might help prevent future disasters. A major change occurred in anesthetic practice with the introduction of morbidity and mortality conferences to examine causes of anesthetic accidents. Originally introduced by Ralph Waters in Madison, Wisconsin, these meetings sought to carefully scrutinize anesthetic complications, thereby shifting the focus of investigation from the patient to the provider and the equipment used to deliver the anesthetic. The postanesthesia care unit, originally designated the recovery room, was promoted for safety reasons by two anesthesiologists from Washington, D.C., in an influential paper in 1951,[325] and these units are now mandated by the accreditation process for all hospitals.

Curtis L. Mendelsohn, an obstetrician from New York City, presented one of the early useful reports of anesthetic complications. In 1945, he reported 66 cases of aspiration of stomach contents during general anesthesia for labor and delivery.[326] He further observed that aspiration of even small volumes of low-pH stomach contents in rabbits would result in fatal pulmonary edema. Since his classic descriptions, the syndrome of acid aspiration is often called the Mendelsohn syndrome.

The cuffed endotracheal tube was one solution to the problem of acid aspiration. Authur Guedel and Ralph Waters were motivated to devise a truly closed system of anesthetic administration with carbon dioxide absorption that would conserve anesthetic gases and body heat. Their 1928 report of the cuffed endotracheal tube[291] achieved these goals with the added benefit of protection of the tracheobronchial tree from aspiration. Others had devised cuffed endotracheal tubes before them,[327] but Guedel and Waters used a novel method to demonstrate and promote the safety features of the cuffed tube. Guedel anesthetized and then intubated his pet dog, appropriately named Airway, with a cuffed endotracheal tube. The dog was submerged in a water tank for several minutes and then removed and awakened unharmed. The demonstration was repeated at several meetings, and this publicity enhanced rapid acceptance of the new endotracheal tube. The cuffed tube is regarded today as an effective measure for preventing acid aspiration.

In 1961, Brian A. Sellick[328] (1918-1996) described rapid-sequence induction for prevention of acid reflux. The method involves the application of firm pressure over the cricoid cartilage to occlude the esophagus during endotracheal intubation. John Hunter[329] had previously described the technique in 1776 for use in resuscitation of individuals "apparently drowned." Rapid-sequence induction remains a popular technique for induction of patients at risk for acid aspiration.

Although few defects in apparatus could occur while applying ether onto a folded towel, the increasing complexity of the anesthetic delivery system brought with it the unfortunate side effect of equipment failure. One of the earliest equipment defects occurred with the simple Morton inhaler. George Hayward reported that a defective intake port led to restricted breathing, lividity, and convulsions in an elderly woman having a leg amputated in January 1847. Wrong gas, wrong agent, wrong concentration, sticky or jammed valves, contaminated agents, and hypoxic mixtures—all of these and others were reported as routes to disaster.

Open discussions of these complications led to adjustments in equipment design.[330] Pin indexing of gas cylinders and hoses eliminated the possibility of introducing air or nitrous oxide into the oxygen lines of the gas machine. In-line oxygen analyzers were placed on the inspiratory limb of the breathing circuit. Fail-safe devices prevented the use of any machine that was not supplied with oxygen. Uniform connectors were adopted, thereby providing rapid assembly of breathing circuits. The American Society of Anesthesiologists (ASA) initiated formation of the Z-79 Committee of the American Standards Institute. This committee recommended safe construction of endotracheal tubes, needles, and connectors. The American Society for Testing and Materials (ASTM), a not-for-profit organization that writes standards for materials and products (through their committee designated F-29), describes the requirements used in the design of safe anesthetic gas machines. The International Standards Organization is also developing global standards for anesthesia equipment.

Further progress in reducing anesthetic-related complications resulted from the formation of professional societies, specialty journals, and certification boards. One of the earliest journals limited exclusively to anesthesiology was *Current Research in Anesthesia and Analgesia*, founded in 1922 largely through the efforts of Francis Hoffer McMechan (1879-1939).[331] McMechan was an anesthesiologist who had retired at an early age for health reasons and devoted the remainder of his career to promoting organizational and political causes of anesthesiologists. An independent American Board of Anesthesiology was formed in 1940 and, through its examination process, continues to elevate standards of anesthetic care. Specialty societies of professional anesthesiologists have formed in most countries practicing modern anesthetic techniques. The ASA was founded as the American Society of Anesthetists in 1936 and currently has approximately 38,000 members. *Anesthesiology*, the official journal of the ASA, began publication in 1940. National anesthesia societies promote safe anesthetic practice through annual meetings, refresher courses, and direct communication with members. Practice guidelines for general anesthesia, obstetric anesthesia, and ambulatory surgery are sent annually to each member of the ASA. Subspecialty societies in cardiac, ambulatory, transplant, pediatric, neurosurgical, and obstetric anesthesia have been formed and strive to improve the anesthetic management of patients within their respective groups.

The Anesthesia Patient Safety Foundation (APSF) was conceived in October 1985, largely through the organizational efforts of Ellison C. Pierce, Jr. This highly successful organization promotes safe anesthesia practice through research grants and periodic mailings to members. As a result of these efforts, anesthesiologists have been recognized as forerunners in promoting agendas that enhance patient safety.[332,333]

Improved monitors have provided the anesthesiologist with methods to fine-tune anesthetic delivery and detect early signs of danger. Auscultation of the chest, an obligatory skill in the current era, had its beginnings in the early 19th century when Rene T. Laennec[334] (1781-1826) used a cylindrical paper tube to listen to the chest. The term *stethoscope* was a combination of the Greek words *stetho* ("chest") and *scope* ("I see") and was used by anesthesia providers as early as 1896 to monitor cardiac and respiratory sounds. The esophageal stethoscope, introduced in 1954 by C. Smith,[335] has been used extensively to detect breathing circuit disconnects, airway obstruction, and bronchospasm in anesthetized patients.

A. E. Codman (1869-1940) of Boston introduced the first anesthetic records in 1894, and the practice was encouraged by Harvey W. Cushing (1869-1939), who promoted recordings of blood pressure, pulse, and respiratory rate on all of his cases.[336] Practice guidelines for minimal monitoring standards were first issued[337] at the nine teaching hospitals of Harvard Medical School, and 2 years later, the ASA issued similar standards that included measures of oxygenation, ventilation, circulation, and body temperature. Electronic monitoring has contributed to the safe practice of anesthesiology significantly. Continuous electrocardiography displays, often with ST-segment analysis, are attached to most anesthesia machines. End-tidal gas analysis using infrared technology developed in the 1940s is in common use. Thermistors offer a continuous measure of core body temperature, thereby providing an early warning of the rare, but potentially lethal syndrome of malignant hyperthermia.[338] Awareness of complications associated with hypothermia in anesthetized patients and the use of methods to prevent its occurrence have contributed significantly to a safer environment for surgical patients.[339,340]

Some complications that may seem trivial to the provider can be highly significant for the patient. Surveys have shown, for example, that postoperative nausea and vomiting are feared complications in a large percentage of patients contemplating surgery.[341] Progress has been made in eliminating this complication through the use of agents with less emetogenic potential. Increased understanding of the neurochemical substrates that regulate the vomiting reflex has resulted in specific therapies to prevent or lessen the gastrointestinal side effects of general anesthetics and opioids.[342] Dopamine antagonists and serotonin 5-HT_3 antagonists have been particularly cost effective.[343]

The increasing use of muscle relaxants by anesthesia providers has led to the terrifying complication of an awake, paralyzed patient who is fully aware of surgical pain. Although early pharmacologic studies of muscle relaxants suggested a central depressant effect of these drugs, this issue was settled when Scott M. Smith[344] (1912-) allowed himself to receive curare without other agents and reported that no sedation or analgesia was present during complete paralysis. R. S. Blacher[345] noticed that complete paralysis with awareness during surgery could sometimes lead to a postoperative traumatic neurotic syndrome characterized by anxiety, irritability, and repetitive nightmares. Various monitors have been used to avoid this rare, but dreaded complication. Tunstall[346] described the isolated arm technique whereby one arm is excluded from the circulation, thereby allowing an awake, paralyzed patient to follow commands by moving that extremity. The electroencephalogram was described in 1929 by Johannes Hans Berger[347] (1873-1941) and first used during administration of anesthesia by Albert Falconer, Jr.[348] (1911-1985). Within the past 30 years, new technologies have been developed that process the electroencephalographic raw signals and provide a number that is indicative of anesthetic depth. The bispectral index (BIS) monitor is a recent commercial product that analyzes the electroencephalographic pattern and provides some assurance that the paralyzed patient is also asleep.[349] Some exceptions have occurred with this device, with paradoxically low BIS numbers being associated with awareness, and solutions to the problem of awake and paralyzed patients continue to evolve.

Allergic reactions to drugs can be life threatening. Anaphylaxis (meaning "without protection") is appropriately named, especially for anesthetized patients, because the symptoms of hypotension and bronchospasm can have many causes and specific treatment can often be delayed. The syndrome was described in 1913 by Charles R. Richet[350] (1850-1935), who was studying the toxicology of various fish poisons and observed the rapid onset of death in dogs that more than 15 days earlier had withstood a much larger dose of the toxin. Richet postulated that an immune response had developed in the interim and produced a fatal reaction to the injection. The role of histamine and vasomotor instability was described in 1932,[351] and this understanding led to the role of vasopressors and antihistamines as treatment.

Even though enormous progress has been achieved toward the goal of zero anesthetic-related morbidity and mortality, no such claim can yet be made at any institution. In part, this is because more extensive procedures are being performed on sicker patients than was the case 100 years ago. In 1914, Gwathmey (see Fig. 1-18D) reported a 0.01% anesthetic-related mortality rate with ether anesthesia, a surprisingly low figure in view of the anesthetic methods in use at the time. However, in 1914 they did not perform extensive procedures such as liver and heart transplantation on patients with life expectancies (without surgical intervention) of only a few weeks. Anesthesiologists have recently focused on postoperative as well as intraoperative pain, and this extension carries with it additional risks to anesthesia providers.

The quest for improving the perianesthetic experience is far from over. A physician has only to ask patients about the experience of having a major surgical procedure to conclude that it is far from pleasant, even in the absence of complications. It is futile to attempt to summarize the current hardships that a surgical patient must undergo in the modern hospital or even attempt possible solutions. Change will occur—that is certain—and if we can learn anything from the past 150 years, there are possibilities for improvement and modalities of practice that we cannot even imagine today. Some methods in use today will appear nonsensical to future practitioners. As portions of the preceding historical survey demonstrate, one barrier to progress is failure by those entrenched in their routines and biases to recognize a breakthrough when it occurs. Perhaps the smarter we are, the more we fail to see our failures. In 1775, while Joseph Priestley[352] was hopelessly lost in the phlogiston theory of combustion, we find these words written in his classic manuscript *Experiments and Observations of Different Kinds of Air*: "The more ingenious a man is, the more effectually he is entangled in his errors; his ingenuity only helping him to deceive himself, by evading the force of truth."

Truth in clinical medicine is perhaps even more difficult to recognize than answers to the questions that chemists were contemplating at the end of the 18th century. However, anesthesiology has made remarkable progress in the more than 150 years since the public demonstration of ether anesthesia, and this progress should continue until safe elimination of all unwanted pain from human experience has been attained.

References

1. Fenster J: Ether Day: The Strange Tale of America's Greatest Medical Discovery and the Haunted Men Who Made It. New York, HarperCollins, 2001.
2. Sykes W: Essays on the One Hundred Years of Anesthesia. Edinburgh, Livingstone, 1960.
3. Major R: A History of Medicine. Springfield, IL, Charles C Thomas, 1954.
4. Hook R: An account of an experiment made by M Hook of preserving animals alive by blowing through their lungs with bellows. Philos Trans R Soc Lond 2:539-540, 1667.
5. Lower R: Tractatus de Corde. London, Redmayne, 1669.
6. Priestley J: Experiments and Observations on Different Kinds of Air. London, Johnson, 1776.
7. Boklund U: Scheele, CW: His Work and Life. Stockholm, Roos Boktrycherier, 1961.
8. Sprigge JS: Sir Humphry Davy: His researches in respiratory physiology and his debt to Antoine Lavoisier. Anaesthesia 57:357-364, 2002.
9. Haldane J: A new form of apparatus for measuring the respiratory exchange of animals. J Physiol 13:419-430, 1892.
10. Haldane J: The therapeutic administration of oxygen. BMJ 1:181-183, 1917.
11. Haldane J, Priestley J: Lung ventilation. J Physiol 32:225-266, 1905.
12. Haldane J: Respiration. New Haven, Yale University Press, 1922.
13. von Hufner CG: Über die Quantitat Sauerstoff welche 1 gramm Hamoglobin zu binden Vermag. Z Physiol Chem 1:317, 1877.
14. Clark LC, Wolf R, Granger D, Taylor Z: Continuous recording of blood oxygen tensions by polarography. J Appl Physiol 6:189-193, 1953.
15. Van Slyke D, Neill J: The determination of gases in blood and other solutions by vacuum extraction and manometric measurement. J Biol Chem 61:523-573, 1924.
16. Severinghaus J, Bradley A: Electrodes for blood Po_2 and Pco_2 determination. J Appl Physiol 13:515-520, 1958.
17. Nunn J: Nunn's Applied Respiratory Physiology, 4th ed. Oxford, Butterworth-Heinemann, 1993.
18. Severinghaus JW, Honda Y: Pulse oximetry. Int Anesthesiol Clin 25:205-214, 1987.
19. Hales S: Statical Essays, Containing Haemastaticks. London, W Innys & R Manby, 1733.
20. Poiseuille J. Recherches sur la Force du Coeur Aortique. Paris, École Polytechnique, 1828.
21. Vierordt K: Die bildliche Darstellung des menschlichen Arterienpulses. Arch Physiol Heilk 13:284-287, 1854.
22. Riva-Rocci S: Un nuovo sfigmomanometro. Gaz Med Torino 47:981-996, 1896.
23. Korotkov N: On methods of studying blood pressure. Izvest Imp Voyenno Med Akad St Petersburg 11:365, 1905.
24. von Recklinghausen H: Neue Wege zur Blutdruckmessung. Berlin, Springer-Verlag, 1931.
25. Seldinger S: Catheter replacement of the needle in percutaneous arteriography. Acta Radiol 39:368-376, 1953.
26. Forssmann W: Die Sondierung des rechten Herzens. Klin Wochenschr 8:2085-2087, 1929.
27. Massa D, Lundy JS, Faulconer A Jr: A plastic needle. Mayo Clin Proc 25:413-415, 1950.
28. Swan HJ, Ganz W, Forrester J, et al: Catheterization of the heart in man with use of a flow-directed balloon-tipped catheter. N Engl J Med 283:447-451, 1970.
29. Fick A: Uber die Messung des Blutquantums in den Herzventrikeln. Sitzber Phys Med Ges Wurzburg July 9, 1870. In Fishman AP, Richards DW (eds): Circulation of the Blood: Men and Ideas. New York, Oxford University Press, 1964.
30. Frazin L, Talano JV, Stephandies L: Esophageal echocardiography. Circulation 54:102-108, 1976.
31. Matsumoto M, Oka Y, Lin YT: Transesophageal echocardiography for assessing ventricular performance. N Y State J Med 79:19-21, 1979.
32. Kremer P, Schwartz L, Cahalan M, et al: Intraoperative monitoring of left ventricular performance by transesophageal M-mode and 2D echocardiography. Am J Cardiol 49:956, 1982.
33. Oka Y: The evolution of intraoperative transesophageal echocardiography. Mt Sinai J Med 69:18-20, 2002.

34. Whytt R: An Essay on the Vital and Other Involuntary Motions of Animals. London, Hamilton, Balfour & Neill, 1751.
35. Willis T: Practice of Physik. London, T Dring, C Harper & J Leigh, 1684.
36. Pourfour Du Petit F: Mémoire dans lequel il est démontré que les nerfs intercostaux fournissent des rameaux que portent des esprits dans les yeux. Hist Acad R Sci 1727, pp 1-19.
37. Winslow J: Exposition Anatomique de la Structure du Corps Humain. Paris, G Desprez, 1732.
38. Bernard C: Influence du grand sympathique sur la sensibilité et sur la calorification. Comptes Rendus Soc Biol 3:163-164, 1852.
39. Langley J, Dickinson W: On the local paralysis of peripheral ganglia, and on the connexion of different classes of nerve fibres with them. Proc R Soc 46:423-431, 1889.
40. Langley J: Observations on the physiological action of extracts of the supra-renal bodies. J Physiol 27:237-256, 1901.
41. Abel J, Crawford A: On the blood-pressure–raising constituent of the suprarenal capsule. Bull Johns Hopkins Hosp 8:151-157, 1897.
42. Elliott TR: On the action of adrenalin. J Physiol 31:xx-xxi, 1904.
43. Barger G, Dale H: Chemical structure and sympathomimetic action of amines. J Physiol 41:19-59, 1910.
44. Dixon W, Hamil P: The mode of action of specific substances with special reference to secretin. J Physiol 38:314-336, 1908-1909.
45. Dale H: The action of certain esters and ethers of choline, and their relation to muscarine. J Pharmacol Exp Ther 6:147-190, 1914.
46. Gaskell W: The involuntary nervous system. Part 1. London, Longmans, Green, 1916.
47. Loewi O: Über humorale Üebertragbarkeit der Herznervenwirkung. Pflüg Arch Ges Physiol 189:239-242, 1921.
48. Tuffier T: Effets circulatoires des injections sousarachnoidiennes de cocaine dans la region lombaire. Soc Biol 18:897-899, 1900.
49. Smith G, Porter W: Spinal anesthesia in the cat. Am J Physiol 38:107-127, 1915.
50. Labat G: Regional Anesthesia: Its Technic and Clinical Application. Philadelphia, WB Saunders, 1922.
51. Aeschlimann J, Reinart MJ: The pharmacological action of some analogues of physostigmine. J Pharmacol 43:413, 1931.
52. MacIntosh R: Death following injection of neostigmine. BMJ 1:852, 1949.
53. Mein A: Ueber die Darstellung des Atropins in weissen Krystallen. Ann Chem Pharm 6:67-72, 1833.
54. Franko B, Lunsford C: Derivatives of 3-pyrrolidinols. III. The chemistry, pharmacology, and toxicology of some *N*-substituted 3-pyrrolidyl alpha-substituted phenylacetates. J Med Pharm Chem 2:523-540, 1960.
55. Ahlquist R: A study of the adrenotropic receptors. Am J Physiol 153:586-600, 1948.
56. Kamibayashi T, Maze M: Clinical uses of alpha2-adrenergic agonists. Anesthesiology 93:1345-1349, 2000.
57. Marsh N, Marsh A: A short history of nitroglycerin and nitric oxide in pharmacology and physiology. Clin Exp Pharmacol Physiol 27:313-319, 2000.
58. Ringertz N: Alfred Nobel—his life and work. Nat Rev Mol Cell Biol 2:925-928, 2001.
59. Murrell W: Nitroglycerin in angina pectoris. Lancet 1:80-81, 1879.
60. Siegel P, Moraca PP, Green JR: Sodium nitroprusside in the surgical treatment of cerebral aneurysms and arteriovenous malformations. Br J Anaesth 43:790-795, 1971.
61. Murad F: Cyclic guanosine monophosphate as a mediator of vasodilation. J Clin Invest 78:1-5, 1986.
62. Frostell C, Fratacci MD, Wain JC, et al: Inhaled nitric oxide: A selective pulmonary vasodilator reversing hypoxic pulmonary vasoconstriction. Circulation 83:2038-2047, 1991.
63. von Haller A: A dissertation on the sensible and irritable parts of animals. London, J Nourse, 1755.
64. von Haller A: De Partibus Corporis Humani Sensibilibus et Irritabilibus. Comment Soc Reg Sci Gottingen 2:114-158, 1752.
65. Bell SC: Idea of a new anatomy of the brain. London, Strahan & Preston, 1811.
66. Magendie F: Expériences sur les fonctions des racines des nerfs rachidiens. J Physiol Exp Pathol 2:276-279, 366-371, 1822.
67. Müller J: Über die phantastischen Gesichtserscheinungen. Leipzig, J Hölscher, 1826.
68. Gasser H, Erlanger J: The role of fiber size in the establishment of a nerve block by pressure or cocaine. Am J Physiol 88:581-591, 1929.
69. Ellis H: Operations That Made History. London, Greenwich Medical Media, 1996.
70. Beecher H: Pain in men wounded in battle. Ann Surg 123:96-105, 1946.
71. Melzack R, Wall P: Pain mechanisms: A new theory. Science 250:971-975, 1965.
72. Reynolds D: Surgery in the rat during electrical analgesia induced by focal brain stimulation. Science 164:444-445, 1969.
73. Goldstein A, Tachibana S, Lowney LI, et al: Dynorphin(1-13), an extraordinarily potent opioid peptide. Proc Natl Acad Sci U S A 76:6666-6670, 1979.
74. Hughes J: Isolation of an endogenous compound from the brain with pharmacological properties similar to morphine. Brain Res 88:295-308, 1975.
75. Simantov R, Childers SR, Snyder SH: Opioid peptides: Differentiation by radioimmunoassay and radioreceptor assay. Brain Res 135:358-367, 1977.
76. Cousins MJ, Mather LE: Intrathecal and epidural administration of opioids. Anesthesiology 61:276-310, 1984.
77. Kehlet H, Brandt MR, Hansen AP, Alberti KG: Effect of epidural analgesia on metabolic profiles during and after surgery. Br J Surg 66:543-546, 1979.
78. Adams F: The Genuine Works of Hippocrates, On Surgery. Baltimore, Williams & Wilkins, 1939.
79. Burney F: A mastectomy, 30 September 1811. In Carey J (ed): Eyewitness to History. Cambridge, Harvard University Press, 1990, pp 272-277.
80. Katz J, Kavanagh BP, Sandler AN, et al: Preemptive analgesia. Clinical evidence of neuroplasticity contributing to postoperative pain. Anesthesiology 77:439-446, 1992.
81. Warren J: A Practical Treatise on Hernia. Boston, Osgood, 1882.
82. Beddoes T, Watts J: Considerations on the Medicinal Use and on the Production of Factitious Airs. Bristol, Bulgin and Rossner, 1795.
83. Davy H: Researches Chemical and Philosophical Chiefly concerning Nitrous Oxide or Dephlogisticated Nitrous Air, and Its Respiration. Bristol, Biggs and Cottle, 1800, pp 1-580.
84. Faraday M: Effects of inhaling the vapors of sulphuric ether. Q J Soc Arts Miscellanea 4:158-159, 1818.
85. Hickman H: A letter on suspended animation containing experiments showing that it may be safely employed on animals, with the view of ascertaining its probable utility in surgical operations on the human subject. Ironbridge, W. Smith, 1824.
86. Bigelow HJ: Insensibility during surgical operations produced by inhalation. Boston Med Surg J 35:309-317, 379-382, 1846.
87. Robinson J: A Treatise on the Inhalation of the Vapour of Ether for the Prevention of pain in Surgical Operations. London, Webster, 1847.
88. Skovsted P, Price HL: Central sympathetic excitation caused by diethyl ether. Anesthesiology 32:202-209, 1970.
89. Long C: An account of the first use of sulphuric ether by inhalation as an anaesthetic in surgical operations. South Med Surg J 5:705-713, 1849.
90. Simpson JY: Discovery of a new anaesthetic agent, more efficient than sulphuric ether. Lond Med Gaz 5:934-937, 1847.
91. Channing W: A Treatise on Etherization in Childbirth. Boston, WD Ticknor, 1848.
92. Hyderabad Chloroform Commission: Report of the first Hyderabad Chloroform Commission. Lancet 1:421-429, 1890.
93. Guthrie LG: On some fatal after-effects of chloroform on children. Lancet 1:193-197, 1894.
94. Levy A: Chloroform Anaesthesia. London, John Bales, Sons & Danielsson, 1922.
95. Smith GB, Hirsch NP: Gardner Quincy Colton: Pioneer of nitrous oxide anaesthesia. Anesth Analg 72:382-391, 1991.
96. Colton G: Anaesthesia. Who Made and Developed This Great Discovery? New York, AG Sherwood, 1886.
97. Andrews E: The oxygen mixture, a new anaesthetic combination. Chicago Med Examiner 9:656, 1868.
98. Hewitt FG: Anaesthetics and Their Administration. London, C Griffin, 1893.
99. Johnson G: On the physiology of asphyxia and on the anaesthetic action of pure nitrogen. Lancet 1:814-815, 1891.
100. McKesson EI: Nitrous oxide-oxygen anaesthesia. With a description of a new apparatus. Surg Gynecol Obstet 13:456-462, 1911.
101. Courville C: Asphyxia as a consequence of nitrous oxide anesthesia. Medicine (Baltimore) 15:129-245, 1936.
102. Smith WD: Under the Influence: A History of Nitrous Oxide and Oxygen. London, Macmillan, 1982.
103. Leake C, Chen M-Y: The anesthetic properties of certain unsaturated ethers. Proc Soc Exp Biol 28:151-154, 1930.
104. Hewer C, Hadfield C: Trichloroethylene as an inhalation anaesthetic. BMJ 1:924-927, 1941.
105. Krantz JC: Anesthesia. XL. The anesthetic action of trifluoroethyl vinyl ether. J Pharmacol 108:488-495, 1953.
106. Krantz J: Historical Medical Classics Involving New Drugs. Baltimore, Williams & Wilkins, 1974.
107. Raventós J: The action of Fluothane—A new volatile anaesthetic. Br J Pharmacol 11:394-410, 1956.
108. Johnstone MW: The human cardiovascular response to Fluothane. Br J Anaesth 28:392-410, 1956.
109. Virtue R, Payne KW: Postoperative death after Fluothane. Anesthesiology 19:562-563, 1958.
110. Lindenbaum J, Leifer E: Hepatic necrosis associated with halothane anesthesia. N Engl J Med 268:525-530, 1963.
111. Bunker JP: Final report of the National Halothane Study. Anesthesiology 29:231-232, 1968.
112. Mazze RI, Shue GL, Jackson SH: Renal dysfunction associated with methoxyflurane anesthesia: A ran-

domized, prospective clinical evaluation. JAMA 216:278-288, 1971.
113. Kety S, Schmidt C: Nitrous oxide method for quantitative determination of cerebral blood flow in man; theory, procedure and normal values. J Clin Invest 27:476-483, 1948.
114. Severinghaus JW: Methods of measurement of blood and gas carbon dioxide during anesthesia. Anesthesiology 21:717-726, 1960.
115. Eger EI 2nd, Saidman LJ, Brandstater B: Minimum alveolar anesthetic concentration: A standard of anesthetic potency. Anesthesiology 26:756-763, 1965.
116. Quasha A, Eger EI, Tinker J: Determination and applications of MAC. Anesthesiology 53:315-334, 1980.
117. Dobkin AB, Heinrich RG, Israel JS, et al: Clinical and laboratory evaluation of a new inhalation agent: Compound 347 (CHF_2-O-CF_2-CHF Cl). Anesthesiology 29:275-287, 1968.
118. Stevens WC, Eger EI, Joas TA, et al: Comparative toxicity of isoflurane, halothane, fluroxene and diethyl ether in human volunteers. Can Anaesth Soc J 20:357-368, 1973.
119. Eger EI 2nd, Johnson BH: Rates of awakening from anesthesia with I-653, halothane, isoflurane, and sevoflurane: A test of the effect of anesthetic concentration and duration in rats. Anesth Analg 66:977-982, 1987.
120. Jones RM, Cashman JN, Eger EI 2nd, et al: Kinetics and potency of desflurance (I-653) in volunteers. Anesth Analg 70:3-7, 1990.
121. Katoh T, Ikeda K: The minimum alveolar concentration (MAC) of sevoflurane in humans. Anesthesiology 66:301-303, 1987.
122. Rynd F: Neuralgia—introduction of fluid to the nerve. Dublin Med Press 13:167-168, 1845.
123. Wood A: Treatment of neuralgic pains by narcotic injections. BMJ 2:721-723, 1858.
124. Bernard C: Leçons sur les Phénoménes de la Vie Communs aux Animaux et aux Végétaux. Paris, Bailliére, 1879.
125. Hamburger H: Osmotischer Druck und Ionenlehre in den Medicinischen Wissenschaften. Wiesbaden, JF Bergman, 1902.
126. Starling E: On the absorption of fluids from the connective tissue spaces. J Physiol 19:312-326, 1896.
127. O'Shaughnessy W: Proposal of a new method of treating the blue epidemic cholera by the injection of highly oxygenized salts into the venous system. Lancet 1:366, 1831-1832.
128. Schwarz E: Ueber den Werth der Infusion alcalischer Kochsalzlosung in das Gefasssystem bei acuter Anamie [dissertation]. Halle, Plotzsche Buchsdruckerei, 1888.
129. Astrup P, Bie P, Engell HC: Salt and Water in Culture and Medicine. Copenhagen, Munksgaard, 1993.
130. Ringer S: Regarding the action of hydrate of soda, hydrate of ammonia, and hydrate of potash on the ventricle of the frog's heart. J Physiol 3:195-202, 1880.
131. Coller F, Campbell K, Vaughan H, et al: Postoperative salt intolerance. Ann Surg 119:533-542, 1944.
132. Moyer CA: Acute temporary changes in renal function associated with major surgical procedures. Surgery 27:198-207, 1950.
133. Shires G, Brown F, Canizaro P, et al: Distributional changes in extracellular fluid during acute hemorrhagic shock. Surg Forum 11:115-117, 1960.
134. Jenkins M: History of Sequestered Edema Associated with Surgical Operations and Trauma: Fluid and Blood Therapy in Anesthesia. Philadelphia, FA Davis, 1982.
135. Denis JB: A letter concerning a new way of curing sundry diseases by transfusion of blood. Philos Trans R Soc Lond 2:489-504, 1667.
136. Blundell J: Experiments on the transfusion of blood by the syringe. Med Chir Trans 9:56-92, 1818.
137. Landsteiner K: Zur Kenntnis der antifermentativen, lyteschen und agglutinierender Wirkungen des Blutserums und der Lymphek. Centralbl Bakteriol Parasit Infekt 27:357-362, 1900.
138. Decastello A, Sturli A: Über die Isoagglutinine im Serum gesunder und kranker Menschen. Munch Med Wochenschr 49:1090-1095, 1902.
139. Hustin A: Note sur une nouvelle méthode de transfusion. Bull Soc R Sci Med Brux 72:104-111, 1914.
140. Rous P, Turner JR: The preservation of living red blood cells in vitro. J Exp Med 23:219-248, 1916.
141. Loutit J, Mollinson P: Advantages of a disodium-citrate glucose mixture as a blood preservative. BMJ 2:744-745, 1943.
142. Lundy J: Clinical Anesthesia. A Manual of Clinical Anesthesiology. Philadelphia, WB Saunders, 1945.
143. Brown A, Debenham M: Autotransfusion. Use of blood from hemothorax. JAMA 96:1223-1225, 1931.
144. Klebanoff G, Rogers W: Clinical experience with autotransfusion. Ann Surg 180:269-304, 1974.
145. Orr M: Autotransfusion: The use of washed red cells as an adjunct to component therapy. Surgery 84:728-732, 1978.
146. Miller RD, Robbins TO, Tong MJ, Barton SL: Coagulation defects associated with massive blood transfusions. Ann Surg 174:794-801, 1971.
147. Blajchman MA, Herst R, Perrault RA: Blood component therapy in anaesthetic practice. Can Anaesth Soc J 30: 382-389, 1983.
148. Robblee JA, Crosby E: Transfusion medicine issues in the practice of anesthesiology. Transfus Med Rev 9:60-78, 1995.
149. Cobo B: Historia del Nuevo Mundo. Manuscrito en Lima, Peru, Libro 5: Capitulo XXIX, 1653.
150. von Anrep V: Über die physiologische Wirkung des Cocain. Pflugers Arch Physiol 21:38-77, 1880.
151. Liljestrand G: Carl Koller and the development of local anesthesia. Acta Physiol Scand Suppl 299:3-29, 1967.
152. Koller C: On the use of cocaine for producing anaesthesia on the eye. Lancet 2:990-994, 1884.
153. Freud S: Über Coca. Centralblatt für die gesamte Therapie 2:289-314, 1884.
154. Hall RJ: Hydrochlorate of cocaine. N Y Med J 40, 1884.
155. Halsted WS: Practical comments on the use and abuse of cocaine; suggested by its invariably successful employment in more than a thousand minor surgical operations. N Y Med J 42:294, 1885.
156. Schleich C: Infiltrationsanästhesie (locale Anästhesie) und ihr Verhältnis zur allgemeinen Narcose (Inhalationsanästhesie), Verhandl D Deutsch Gesellsch F Chir 21:121-127, 1892.
157. Coming JL: On the prolongation of the anaesthetic effect of the hydrochlorate of cocaine, when subcutaneously injected. An experimental study. N Y Med J 42:317-319, 1885.
158. Braun H: Die Lokalanästhesie, ihre wissenschaflichen Grundlagen und praktische Anwendung. Leipzig, Johann Barth, 1907, pp 102-104.
159. Hirschel G: Anesthesia of the brachial plexus for operations on the upper extremity. Med Wochenschr 58:1555-1556, 1911.
160. de Jong R: Axillary block of the brachial plexus. Anesthesiology 22:215-225, 1961.
161. Kulenkampff D: Anesthesia of the brachial plexus. Zentralbl Chir 38:1337-1340, 1911.
162. Raj P, Montgomery S, Nettles D, Jenkins M: Infraclavicular brachial plexus block—a new approach. Anesth Analg 52:897-904, 1973.
163. Kappis M: Conduction anesthesia of the abdomen, breast, arm and neck with paravertebral injection. Med Wochenschr 59:794-796, 1912.
164. Winnie A: Interscalene brachial plexus block. Anesth Analg 49:455-466, 1970.
165. Wulf H: The centennial of spinal anesthesia. Anesthesiology 89:500-506, 1998.
166. Bonica JJ: Basic principles in managing chronic pain. Arch Surg 112:783-788, 1977.
167. Einhorn A: Über die Chemie der lokalen Anästhetica. Munch Med Wochenschr 46:1218-1220, 1254-1256, 1899.
168. Holmdahl M: Xylocaine (lidocaine, lignocaine), its discovery and Gordh's contribution to its clinical use. Acta Anaesthesiol Scand Suppl 113:8-12, 1998.
169. Albright GA: Cardiac arrest following regional anesthesia with etidocaine or bupivacaine. Anesthesiology 51:285-287, 1979.
170. Ruetsch YA, Boni T, Borgeat A: From cocaine to ropivacaine: The history of local anesthetic drugs. Curr Top Med Chem 1:175-182, 2001.
171. Marx GF: The first spinal anesthesia. Who deserves the laurels? Reg Anesth 19:429-430, 1994.
172. Quincke H: Die Lumbalpunktion des Hydrocephalus. Berl Klin Wochenschr 28:929-933, 965-968, 1891.
173. Bier A: Versuche uber Cocainisirung des Ruckenmarkes. Dtsch Z Chir 51:361-369, 1899.
174. Seldowitsch J: Über Kokainisierung des Rückenmarks nach Bier. Centralb Chir 26:1110-1113, 1899.
175. Tait D, Cagliari G: Experimental and clinical notes on the subarachnoid space. Trans Med Soc St Calif 266-271, 1900.
176. Tuffier T: Analgesie chirurgicale par l'injection sousarachnoidienne lombaire de cocaine. Soc Biol 11:882-884, 1899.
177. Matas R: Local and regional anesthesia with cocaine and other analgesic drugs, including the subarachnoid method, as applied in general surgical practice. Phil Med J 6:820-843, 1900.
178. Morton A: The subarachnoid injection of cocaine for operations on all parts of the body. Am Med 3:176-179, 1901.
179. Jonnesco T: Remarks on general spinal analgesia. BMJ 4:1396-1401, 1909.
180. Bier A: Das Zurzeit an der Berliner chirurgischen Universitätsklinik übliche Verfahren der Rückenmarksanästhesie. Dtsch Z Chir 95:373-385, 1909.
181. Goldan SO: Intraspinal cocainization for surgical anesthesia. Phil Med J 6:850-857, 1900.
182. Kitagawa O: On spinal anesthesia with cocaine. J Jpn Soc Surg 3:185-191, 1901.
183. Gumprecht F: Gefahren der Lumbalpunktion; plötzliche Todesfalle danach. Dtsch Med Wochenschr 27:386-389, 1900.
184. Barker A: Clinical experiences with spinal anesthesia in 100 cases. BMJ 23:665-674, 1907.
185. Lee JA: Arthur Edward James Barker 1850-1916. British pioneer of regional analgesia. Anaesthesia 34:885-891, 1979.
186. Cope R: The Wooley and Roe case. Anaesthesia 9:249-270, 1954.
187. Kennedy F, Effron A, Perry G: The grave spinal cord paralysis caused by spinal anesthesia. Surg Gynecol Obstet 91:385-398, 1950.
188. Dripps R, Vandam L: Long term follow-up of patients who received 10,098 spinal anesthetics.

Failure to discover major neurological sequelae. JAMA 156:1486-1491, 1954.
189. Freedman JM, Li DK, Drasner K, et al: Transient neurologic symptoms after spinal anesthesia: An epidemiologic study of 1,863 patients. Anesthesiology 89:633-641, 1998.
190. Rigler ML, Drasner K, Krejcie TC, et al: Cauda equina syndrome after continuous spinal anesthesia. Anesth Analg 72:275-281, 1991.
191. Vandam L, Dripps R: Long term follow-up of patients who received 10,098 anesthetics. JAMA 161:586-591, 1956.
192. Gormley J: Treatment of post-spinal headache. Anesthesiology 21:565-566, 1960.
193. DiGiovanni AJ, Dunbar BS: Epidural injections of autologous blood for postlumbar-puncture headache. Anesth Analg 49:268-271, 1970.
194. Läwen A: Über die Verwertung der Sakralanästhesie fur chirurgische Operationen. Zentralbl Chir 37:708, 1910.
195. Heile B: Der epidurale Raum. Arch Klin Chir 101:845-877, 1913.
196. Tuffier T: Analgesie cocainique par voie extradurale. C R Soc Biol Paris 53:490-492, 1901.
197. Pagés MF: Anestesia metamérica. Rev Sanid Milit 11:351-365, 389-396, 1921.
198. Dogliotti AM: Eine neue Methode der regionären Anästhesie: Die peridurale segmentäre Anästhesie. Zentralbl Chir 58:3141-3145, 1931.
199. Flagg P: The Art of Anaesthesia, 7th ed. Philadelphia, JB Lippincott, 1954.
200. Odom C: Epidural anesthesia. Am J Surg 34:547-558, 1936.
201. Harger J, Christofferson EA, Stokes AJ: Peridural anesthesia: A consideration of 1000 cases. Am J Surg 52:24-31, 1941.
202. Crawford O, Buckingham WW, Ottosen P, Brasher CA: Peridural anesthesia in thoracic surgery: A review of 677 cases. Anesthesiology 12:73-84, 1951.
203. Tuohy E: Continuous spinal anesthesia: Its usefulness and technic involved. Anesthesiology 5:142-148, 1944.
204. Curbelo MM: Continuous peridural segmental anesthesia by means of a ureteral catheter. Anesth Analg 28:13-23, 1949.
205. Edwards WB, Hingson RA: Continuous caudal anesthesia in obstetrics. Am J Surg 57:459-464, 1942.
206. Moore D: Regional Block. Springfield, IL, Charles C Thomas, 1953.
207. Cousins M, Bridenbaugh P: Neural Blockade. Philadelphia, JB Lippincott, 1980.
208. Wang JK, Nauss LA, Thomas JE: Pain relief by intrathecally applied morphine in man. Anesthesiology 50:149-151, 1979.
209. Yaksh TL, Rudy TA: Analgesia mediated by a direct spinal action of narcotics. Science 192:1357-1358, 1976.
210. Duggan AW, North RA: Electrophysiology of opioids. Pharmacol Rev 35:219-281, 1983.
211. Atweh S, Kuhar M: Autoradiographic localization of opiate receptors in rat brain. Brain Res 124:53-67, 1977.
212. Samii K, Chauvin M, Viars P: Postoperative spinal analgesia with morphine. Br J Anaesth 53:817-820, 1981.
213. Cousins MJ, Mather LE, Glynn CJ, et al: Selective spinal analgesia. Lancet 1:1141-1142, 1979.
214. Behar M, Magora F, Olshwang D, Davidson JT: Epidural morphine in treatment of pain. Lancet 1:527-529, 1979.
215. Ready LB, Oden R, Chadwick HS, et al: Development of an anesthesiology-based postoperative pain management service. Anesthesiology 68:100-106, 1988.
216. Wang C, Chakrabarti MK, Whitwam JG: Specific enhancement by fentanyl of the effects of intrathecal bupivacaine on nociceptive afferent but not on sympathetic efferent pathways in dogs. Anesthesiology 79:766-773; discussion 25A, 1993.
217. Weese H, Sscharpff W: Evipan, ein neuartiges Einschlafmittel. Dtsch Med Wochenschr 58:1205-1207, 1932.
218. Lundy J: Intravenous anesthesia: Preliminary report of the use of two new thiobarbiturates. Proc Mayo Clin 10:536-543, 1935.
219. Halford F: A critique of intravenous anesthesia in war surgery. Anesthesiology 4:67-69, 1943.
220. Bennetts FE: Thiopentone anaesthesia at Pearl Harbor. Br J Anaesth 75:366-368, 1995.
221. Kay B, Stephenson DK: ICI 35868 (Diprivan): A new intravenous anaesthetic. A comparison with Althesin. Anaesthesia 35:1182-1187, 1980.
222. Doenicke A, Kugler J, Penzel G, et al: Cerebral function under etomidate, a new non-barbiturate I.V. hypnotic [author's translation]. Anaesthesist 22:357-366, 1973.
223. Hunkeler W, Mohler H, Pieri L, et al: Selective antagonists of benzodiazepines. Nature 290:514-516, 1981.
224. Corssen G, Domino EF: Dissociative anesthesia: Further pharmacologic studies and first clinical experience with the phencyclidine derivative CI-581. Anesth Analg 45:29-40, 1966.
225. Kay B, Rolly G: I.C.I. 35868, a new intravenous induction agent. Acta Anaesthesiol Belg 28:303-316, 1977.
226. White PF: Use of patient-controlled analgesia for management of acute pain. JAMA 259:243-247, 1988.
227. Raleigh W: The Discoererie of the Large, Rich and Beautiful Empire of Guina—Performed in the Year 1595 by Walter Raleigh, Captaine of her Maiests's Guard. London, Robert Robinson, 1596.
228. Betcher A: The civilizing of curare: A history of its development and introduction into anesthesiology. Anesth Analg 56:305-319, 1977.
229. Brodie B: Experiments and observations on the different modes in which death is produced by certain vegetable poisons. Philos Trans R Soc Lond 1:194-195, 1811.
230. Bernard C: Lecons sur les effects des substances toxiques et medicamenteuses. Paris, Bailliere, 1857.
231. Wells T: Three cases of tetanus, in which "woorara" was used. Proc R Med Chir Soc Lond 3:142-157, 1859.
232. Gill R: White Water and Black Magic. New York, Holt, 1940.
233. Gill R: Mrs. Robinson Crusoe in Ecuador. Natl Geog Mag 65:134-150, 1934.
234. Bennett A, McIntyre A, Bennett A: Pharmacologic and clinical investigations with crude curare. JAMA 114:1791, 1940.
235. Griffith H. Johnson G: The use of curare in general anesthesia. Anesthesiology 3:418-420, 1942.
236. Cullen S: The use of curare for improvement of abdominal muscle relaxation during inhalation anesthesia: Report on 131 cases. Surgery 14:261-266, 1943.
237. Gray T, Halton J: A milestone in anaesthesia, D-tubocurarine chloride? Proc R Soc Med 39:400-410, 1946.
238. Harroun P, Beckert F, Hathaway H: Curare and nitrous oxide anesthesia for lengthy operations. Anesthesiology 7:24-28, 1946.
239. Harroun P, Hathaway H: The use of curare in anesthesia for thoracic surgery. Surg Gynecol Obstet 82:229-231, 1946.
240. Beecher HK, Todd DP: A study of the deaths associated with anesthesia and surgery: Based on a study of 599,548 anesthesias in ten institutions 1948-1952. Ann Surg 140:2-34, 1954.
241. Churchill-Davidson H, Richardson AT: Decamethonium iodide (c 10): Some observations on its action using electromyography. Proc R Soc Med 45:179-186, 1952.
242. Cohen AD: A simple inexpensive nerve stimulator. Anaesthesia 18:534-535, 1963.
243. Katz R: A nerve stimulator for the continuous monitoring of muscle relaxant action. Anesthesiology 26:832-833, 1965.
244. Ali HH, Utting JE, Gray T: Quantitative assessment of residual antidepolarizing block (part II). Br J Anaesth 43:478-485, 1971.
245. Bovet D: Proprietá farmacodinamiche di alcuni derivati della succinilcolina dotati di azione curarica. Esteri di trialchiletanolammonio di acidi bicarbossilici alifatici. R C Ist Super Sanita 12:106-137, 1949.
246. Thesleff S, von Dardel O, Holmberg F: Succinylcholine iodide. New muscular relaxant. Br J Anaesth 24:238-244, 1952.
247. Baird WL, Reid AM: The neuromuscular blocking properties of a new steroid compound, pancuronium bromide: A pilot study in man. Br J Anaesth 39:775-780, 1967.
248. Durant NN, Marshall IG, Savage DS, et al: The neuromuscular and autonomic blocking activities of pancuronium, Org NC 45, and other pancuronium analogues, in the cat. J Pharm Pharmacol 31:831-836, 1979.
249. Miller RD: Org Nc 45. Br J Anaesth 52(Suppl 1):71S-72S, 1980.
250. Booij LH, Knape HT: The neuromuscular blocking effect of Org 9426. A new intermediately-acting steroidal nondepolarising muscle relaxant in man. Anaesthesia 46:341-343, 1991.
251. Meltzer S: Continuous respiration without respiratory movements. J Exp Med 11:622-625, 1909.
252. Elsberg C: Anaesthesia by the intratracheal insufflation of air and ether. Ann Surg 53:161-168, 1911.
253. Crafoord C: Pulmonary ventilation and anesthesia in major chest surgery. J Thorac Surg 9:237-253, 1940.
254. Coleman A: Mr. Coleman's economising apparatus for re-inhaling the gas. Br J Dent Sci 12:443, 1869.
255. Jackson D: A new method for the production of general analgesia and anaesthesia with a description of the apparatus used. J Lab Clin Med 1:1-12, 1915.
256. Waters R: Clinical scope and utility of carbon dioxide filtration in inhalation anesthesia. Curr Res Anesth Analg 3:20-22, 1924.
257. Sword B: The closed circle method of administration of gas anesthesia. Curr Res Anesth Analg 9:198-202, 1930.
258. Morris L: A new vaporizer for liquid anesthetic agents. Anesthesiology 13:587, 1952.
259. O'Dwyer J: An improved method of performing artificial forcible respiration with exhibition of instruments. Arch Pediatr 9:30-34, 1892.
260. Matas R: Intralaryngeal insufflation for the relief of acute surgical pneumothorax. Its history and methods with a description of the latest devices for this purpose. JAMA 34:1468-1473, 1900.
261. Drinker P, McKhann C: The use of a new apparatus for the prolonged administration of artificial respiration. I. A fatal case of poliomyelitis. JAMA 92:1658-1660, 1929.

262. Moerch E: Controlled respiration by means of special automatic machines as used in Sweden and Denmark. Proc R Soc Med Lond 40:603-607, 1947.
263. Ibsen B: Anaesthetist's viewpoint on the treatment of respiratory complications in poliomyelitis during the epidemic in Copenhagen, 1952. Proc Roy Soc Med (Lond) 47:72-74, 1954.
264. McDowell E: Three cases of extirpation of diseased ovaria. Med Classics 2:651-653, 1938.
265. Crile G: Nitrous oxide anaesthesia and a note on anoci-association, a new principle in operative surgery. Surg Gynecol Obstet 13:170-173, 1911.
266. Crile G, Lower WE: Anoci-Association. Philadelphia, WB Saunders, 1914.
267. Cushing H: On the avoidance of shock in major amputations by cocainization of large nerve-trunks preliminary to their division. Ann Surg 36:321-345, 1902.
268. Woodbridge P: Changing concepts concerning depth of anesthesia. Anesthesiology 18:536-550, 1957.
269. Pinsker M: Anesthesia: A pragmatic construct. Anesth Analg 65:819-820, 1986.
270. Roizen MF, Horrigan RW, Frazer BM: Anesthetic doses blocking adrenergic (stress) and cardiovascular responses to incision—MAC BAR. Anesthesiology 54:390-398, 1981.
271. Mangano DT, Layug EL, Wallace A, Tateo I: Effect of atenolol on mortality and cardiovascular morbidity after noncardiac surgery. Multicenter Study of Perioperative Ischemia Research Group. N Engl J Med 335:1713-1720, 1996.
272. Lowenstein E, Hallowell P, Levine FH, et al: Cardiovascular response to large doses of intravenous morphine in man. N Engl J Med 281:1389-1393, 1969.
273. Stanley T, Philbin D, Coggins C: Fentanyl oxygen anaesthesia for coronary artery surgery. Cardiovascular and antidiuretic hormone responses. Can Anaesth Soc J 26:168-172, 1979.
274. Clark RB: Transplacental reversal of meperidine depression in the fetus by naloxone. J Ark Med Soc 68:128-130, 1971.
275. Kienbaum P, Thurauf N, Michel MC, et al: Profound increase in epinephrine concentration in plasma and cardiovascular stimulation after mu-opioid receptor blockade in opioid-addicted patients during barbiturate-induced anesthesia for acute detoxification. Anesthesiology 88:1154-1161, 1998.
276. DeCastro J, Mundeleer P: Anesthesie sans sommeil. "La neuroleptanalgesie." Acta Chir Belg 58:689, 1959.
277. Asoh T, Tsuji H, Shirasaka C, Takeuchi Y: Effect of epidural analgesia on metabolic response to major upper abdominal surgery. Acta Anaesthesiol Scand 27:233-237, 1983.
278. Bevan DR: Modification of the metabolic response to trauma under extradural analgesia. Anaesthesia 26:188-191, 1971.
279. von Esmarch F: Handbuch der Kriegschirurgischen Technik. Hannover, Germany, Carl Rumpler, 1877.
280. Warren J: Address before the American Medical Association, Boston, John Wilson, 1850, pp 5-65.
281. Sibson F: On the treatment of facial neuralgia by the inhalation of ether. Lond Med Gaz 4:358-364, 1847.
282. Maltby JR: Francis Sibson, 1814-1876. Pioneer and prophet in anaesthesia. Anaesthesia 32:53-62, 1977.
283. Guedel A: A nontraumatic pharyngeal airway. JAMA 100:1862, 1933.
284. O'Dwyer J: Fifty cases of croup in private practice treated by intubation of the larynx, with a description of the method and of the dangers incident thereto. Med Rec 32:557-561, 1887.
285. Trousseau A: Du tubage de la glotte et de la tracheotomie, par M Bouchut. Bull Acad Med 24:99, 1858.
286. Trendelenburg F: Beiträge zu den Operationen an den Luftwegen. Arch Klin Chir 12:112-133, 1871.
287. Macewan W: Clinical observations on the introduction of tracheal tubes by the mouth instead of performing tracheotomy or laryngotomy. BMJ 2:122-124, 163-165, 1880.
288. Sauerbruch EF: Über die physiologischen and physikalischen Grundlagen bei intrathorakalen Eingriffen in meiner pneumatischen Operationskammer. Verh Dtsch Ges Chir 32:105-115, 1904.
289. Magill I: Endotracheal anesthesia. Proc R Soc Med 22:1-6, 1928.
290. Rowbotham E, Magill I: Anaesthetics in the plastic surgery of the face and jaws. Proc R Soc Med 14:17-27, 1921.
291. Guedel A, Waters, RM: A new intratracheal catheter. Anesth Analg 7:238-239, 1928.
292. Gale J, Waters R: Closed endobronchial anesthesia in thoracic surgery: Preliminary report. Anesth Analg 11:283-287, 1932.
293. Magill I: Anaesthesia in thoracic surgery, with special reference to lobectomy. Proc R Soc Med 29:649-653, 1936.
294. Carlens E: A new flexible double-lumen catheter for bronchospirometry. J Thorac Surg 18:742-746, 1949.
295. Robertshaw F: Low resistance double-lumen endobronchial tubes. Br J Anaesth 34:576-579, 1962.
296. Green R, Gordon W: Right lung anaesthesia. Anaesthesia 12:86-93, 1957.
297. Murphy F: Two improved intratracheal catheters. Anesth Analg 20:102-105, 1941.
298. Kirstein A: Autoskopie des Larynx und der Trachea. Berl Klin Wochenschr 32:476-478, 1895.
299. Hirsch NP, Smith GB, Hirsch PO: Alfred Kirstein: Pioneer of direct laryngoscopy. Anaesthesia 41:42-45, 1986.
300. Jackson C: Tracheobronchoscopy, Esophagoscopy and Gastroscopy. St Louis, CV Mosby, 1907.
301. Garcia M: Observations on the human voice. Proc R Soc Lond 7:399-410, 1854.
302. Killian G: Ueber directe Brochoskopie. Munch Med Wochenschr 45:844-847, 1898.
303. Miller R: A new laryngoscope. Anesthesiology 2:317-320, 1941.
304. Macintosh R: A new laryngoscope. Lancet 1:205, 1943.
305. Brain A: The laryngeal mask: A new concept in airway management. Br J Anaesth 55:801-805, 1983.
306. Lamm H: Biegsame optische Geräte. Z Instrumentenk 50:579-581, 1930.
307. Ikeda S, Yanai N, Ishidawa S: Flexible bronchofiberscope. Keio J Med 17:1-18, 1968.
308. Ikeda S: Atlas of Flexible Bronchofiberoscopy. Baltimore, University Park Press, 1971.
309. Elam J, Greene DG, Brown ES, et al: Oxygen and carbon dioxide exchange and energy cost of expired air resuscitation. JAMA 167:328-334, 1958.
310. Lind B: Recent History of Resuscitation in Norway. Anaesthesia—Essays on Its History. Berlin, Springer-Verlag, 1985.
311. Waller A: A demonstration in man of electromotive changes accompanying the heart's beat. J Physiol 8:229-234, 1887.
312. Einthoven W: The string galvanometer and the human electrocardiogram. Proceedings of the Koninklijke Nederlandse Akademie van Wetenschappen, Amsterdam, Section of Sciences. 6:107-115, 1903.
313. Herrick J: Clinical features of sudden obstruction of the coronary arteries. JAMA 59:2015-2020, 1912.
314. MacWilliam J: Fibrillar contraction of the heart. J Physiol 8:296-310, 1887.
315. MacWilliam J: Cardiac failure and sudden death. BMJ 1:6-8, 1889.
316. Prevost J, Battelli F: La mort par les courants electriques. J Physiol Pathol Gen 1:427, 1899.
317. Beck C, Pritchard W, Feil H: Ventricular fibrillation of long duration abolished by electric shock. JAMA 135:985-986, 1947.
318. Starling E, Lane W: Case report. Lancet 2:1397, 1902.
319. Keen W: A case of total laryngectomy (unsuccessful) and a case of abdominal hysterectomy (successful), in both of which massage of the heart for chloroform collapse was employed, with notes of 25 cases of cardiac massages. Ther Gaz 28:217-230, 1904.
320. Koenig F: Lehrbuch des Allgemeinen. Chirurgie, Göttingen, 1883.
321. Kouwenhoven W, Jude F, Knickerbocker G: Closed chest cardiac massage. JAMA 173:1064-1067, 1960.
322. Beecher H: The first anesthesia death with some remarks suggested by it on the fields of the laboratory and the clinic in the appraisal of new anesthetic agents. Anesthesiology 2:443-449, 1941.
323. Knight PR 3rd, Bacon DR: An unexplained death: Hannah Greener and chloroform. Anesthesiology 96:1250-1253, 2002.
324. Guedel A: Inhalation Anesthesia: A Fundamental Guide. New York, Macmillan, 1937.
325. Lowenthal PJ, Russell A: Recovery room: Life saving and economical. Anesthesiology 12:470-476, 1951.
326. Mendelson C: The aspiration of stomach contents into the lungs during obstetrical anesthesia. Am J Obstet Gynecol 52:191-205, 1945.
327. Dorrance G: On the treatment of traumatic injuries of the lungs and pleura with the presentation of a new intratracheal tube for use in artificial respiration. Surg Gynecol Obstet 11:160-187, 1910.
328. Sellick B: Cricoid pressure to control regurgitation of stomach contents during induction of anaesthesia. Lancet 2:404-406, 1961.
329. Hunter J: Of persons apparently drowned. Philos Trans R Soc Lond 66:415-425, 1776.
330. Rendell-Baker L: Standards for anesthesia: The issues. Contemp Anesth Pract 8:59-88, 1984.
331. Bacon DR: The promise of one great anesthesia society. Anesthesiology 80:929-935, 1994.
332. Gaba DM, Howard SK: Patient safety: Fatigue among clinicians and the safety of patients. N Engl J Med 347:1249-1255, 2002.
333. Cooper JB, Gaba D: No myth: Anesthesia is a model for addressing patient safety. Anesthesiology 97:1335-1337, 2002.
334. Laennec RT: De l'auscultation mediate. Paris, JA Brosson & JS Chaude, 1819.
335. Smith C: An endo-esophageal stethoscope. Anesthesiology 15:566, 1954.
336. Beecher HK: The first anesthesia records. Surg Gynecol Obstet 71:789, 1940.
337. Eichhorn JH, Cooper JB, Cullen DJ, et al: Standards for patient monitoring during anesthesia at Harvard Medical School. JAMA 256:1017-1020, 1986.
338. Denborough M, Lovell R: Anaesthetic deaths in a family. Lancet 2:45, 1960.
339. Sessler DI: Mild perioperative hypothermia. N Engl J Med 336:1730-1737, 1997.
340. Kurz A, Sessler DI, Lenhardt R: Perioperative normothermia to reduce the incidence of surgical-

wound infection and shorten hospitalization. Study of Wound Infection and Temperature Group. N Engl J Med 334:1209-1215, 1996.

341. Orkin F: What do patients want? Preferences for immediate postoperative recovery. Anesth Analg 74:S225, 1992.
342. Watcha M, White P: Postoperative nausea and vomiting—its etiology, treatment, and prevention. Anesthesiology 77:162-184, 1992.
343. Watcha M, Smith I: Cost-effectiveness analysis of antiemetic therapy for ambulatory surgery. J Clin Anesth 6:370-377, 1994.
344. Smith SM, Brown HO, Toman JEP, et al: The lack of cerebral effects of D-tubocurarine. Anesthesiology 8:1-14, 1947.
345. Blacher R: On awakening paralyzed during surgery. A syndrome of traumatic neurosis. JAMA 234:67-68, 1975.
346. Tunstall ME: Detecting wakefulness during general anaesthesia for caesarean section. BMJ 1:1321, 1977.
347. Berger J: Über das Elektroenkephalogramm des Menschen. Arch Psychiatr Nervenkr 87:527-570, 1929.
348. Falconer AJ, Pender JW, Bickford RG: The influence of partial pressure of nitrous oxide on the depth of anesthesia and the electro-encephalogram in man. Anesthesiology 10:601-609, 1949.
349. Glass P, Bloom M, Kearse L, et al: Bispectral analysis measures sedation and memory effects of propofol, midazolam, isoflurane, and alfentanil in healthy volunteers. Anesthesiology 86:836-847, 1997.
350. Richet C: De l'anaphysaxie en general et de l'anaphysoxie par la mytilocongestine en particulier. Ann Inst Pasteur 21:497-524, 1907.
351. Dragstedt C, Gebauer-Fuelnegg E: Studies in anaphylaxis. Am J Physiol 102:512-526, 1932.
352. Priestley J: Observations on different kinds of air. Philos Trans R Soc Lond 62:147-264, 1772.
353. Guedel A: Ethyl Chloride-Chloroform-Ether Anesthesia for Rapid Induction and Minor Surgery in War. In McMechan FH (ed): Year Book of Anesthesia and Analgesia 1917-1918. New York, Surgery Publishing Co.

William L. Young, Jeanine P. Wiener-Kronish, and Lee A. Fleisher

2 Scope of Modern Anesthetic Practice

Key Points

1. With the increase in the elderly population, more of the surgeries performed will be procedures required by elderly patients.
2. Minimally invasive procedures are increasing; anesthesiologists will be performing more anesthetic procedures outside operating rooms. Anesthesia may be the major risk to patients as the surgical procedures become more minimal.
3. The mandates for quality, competency, and uniform process will change the way anesthesia is delivered. More standardization and protocols will be used; this will allow more evaluation and research as to what optimal anesthesia is and what competent anesthesiologists are required to do.
4. The increase in nurses with degrees will change the number of anesthetics delivered by physicians. Team management and relationships between physicians and nurses will become more crucial, and the demand for skills in personnel management will increase.
5. Not enough research is being done by anesthesiologists. Anesthesiologists will need to engage in research to maintain an academic foothold. Opportunities for multidisciplinary research are increasing, and they need to be embraced to increase the number of research-trained anesthesiologists.

Forces That Will Change Anesthetic Practice

Multiple changes are occurring that will affect the role of the anesthesiologist in the United States and perhaps globally. The population of industrialized nations is *aging* so that many more operations are performed on elderly patients; this dictates which operations are being performed. The *cost of medical care* is increasing globally, and perhaps most rapidly in the United States. The increased cost will lead to more scrutiny regarding the need for operations, increased focus on quality and use of care that has documentation by research, changes in Medicare reimbursement, changes in the ability of patients to pay, and a demand for the use of less costly health care providers whenever possible. Technologic advances are leading to less invasive procedures that can be done on patients who heretofore would be denied routine surgical procedures. The mandates for *quality metrics* and *evaluation of processes* will change the way we practice medicine. Changes in *personnel* also will affect the workforce in practices. We can only speculate as to what the practice of anesthesia will be like in the next 10 years, but these forces will likely have a major effect (Fig. 2-1).

Aging of Society

With the aging of the population and improvements in anesthetic and surgical methods, the fraction of the elderly population undergoing surgical procedures is increasing in the United States (see Chapter 71). Use of surgical services in older patients is not unexpectedly higher than in younger patients. In the Centers for Disease Control and Prevention report of inpatient hospitalizations for 2005, there were 45 million procedures performed on inpatients with a similar number of outpatient procedures. From 1995 through 2004, the rate of hip replacements for patients 65 years old and older increased 38%, and the rate of knee replacements increased 70%. There seems to be a direct correlation between age and use of surgical services.[1]

Changes in Location of Care Delivery

Because of the high costs to the insurance industry, the pressure to move less invasive surgical procedures to locations remote from the hospital setting will continue, frequently motivated by changes in reimbursement.[2] Providing anesthesia in ambulatory surgical settings and offices has increased dramatically over the

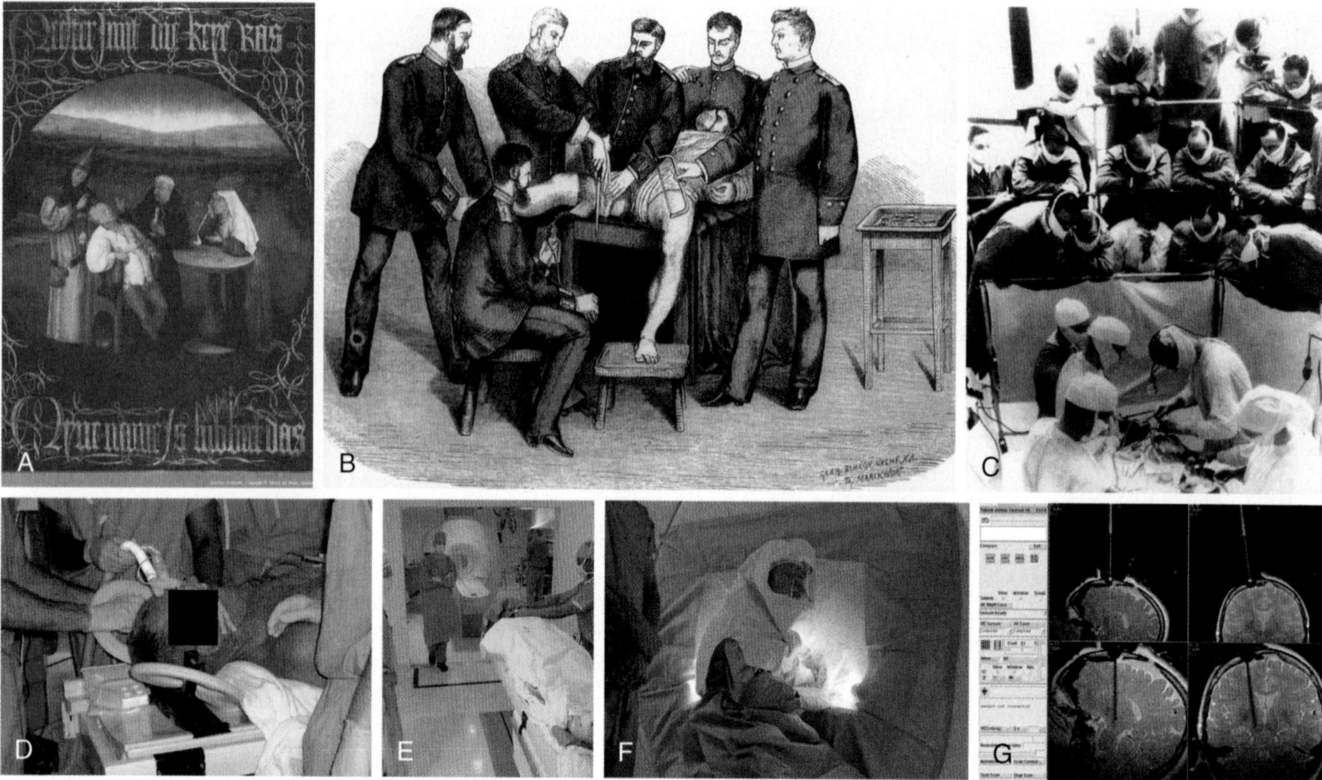

Figure 2-1 Changing scope and settings of anesthesia and perioperative medicine. **A,** *The Cure of Folly,* by Hieronymus Bosch (c. 1450-1516), depicting the removal of stones in the head, thought to be a cure for madness. **B,** Friedrich Esmarch amputating with the use of anesthesia and with antisepsis. Woodcut from Esmarch's *Handbuch der Kriegschirurgischen Technik* (1877). **C,** Harvey Cushing performing an operation, with the Harvey Cushing Society observing, 1932. **D** and **E,** Placement of deep brain stimulator for the treatment of Parkinson's disease using a real-time magnetic resonance imaging technology (MR fluoroscopy). The procedure takes place in the MR suite of the radiology department. The patient is anesthetized (**D**) and moved into the bore of the magnet (**E**). **F** and **G,** A sterile field is created for intracranial instrumentation (**F**), and placement of electrodes is done using real-time guidance (**G**). *(**A,** Courtesy of Museo del Prado, Madrid; **B,** courtesy of Jeremy Norman & Co, Inc; **C,** photograph by Richard Upjohn Light [Boston Medical Library]; **D-G,** courtesy of Paul Larson, MD, UCSF/SF Veterans Administration Medical Center.)*

last several decades (see Chapter 78). As procedures become less invasive than those currently performed in the operating room, they will be performed in procedure units. It will be important to determine the need for anesthesiologists to provide traditional anesthesia and moderate to deep levels of conscious sedation in these settings. Postoperative care has been shifted from the medical setting to the families, which may present difficulties in elderly patients. Anesthesiologists must be involved in determining which patients are appropriate candidates to have different procedures in these different locations of care, and the level of monitoring needed to perform these procedures safely.[3]

Cost of Medical Care

As the cost of health care in the United States approaches 15% of the gross national product, there has been increased interest in determining the factors that are increasing the costs, attempting to find methods to decrease the cost, and obtaining more valuable health care for the money spent. The primary driver of cost in the United States apparently is technical progress, as health care costs are increasing throughout the world, regardless of the insurance system.[4-6] The increase in elderly patients and patients with chronic disease in the population also is increasing health care costs.[7]

The increase in cost has led to a movement to get more value for the money spent. Pay-for-performance programs have been created (i.e., rewarding medical care that is consistent with published evidence and not paying for care that is inconsistent with evidence).[8-10] The concept and reality of pay-for-performance programs has now moved to other countries, including the United Kingdom.[11]

In the nonsurgical arena, the concept of pay-for-performance has been studied for several years.[12,13] In addition to paying for performance, in the United States, there is increasing emphasis on not paying for "never" events, such as decubitus ulcers or urinary tract infections, unless they are present on admission to the hospital. Because of the role of anesthesiologists in the entire continuum of perioperative care, including postoperative intensive care and pain management, we have an opportunity to influence many of the practices that can be associated with poor outcomes and increased cost, but that traditionally have not been considered under our domain of care.

Appropriate and timely administration of antibiotics has a significant impact on surgical site infection, but before the initiation of the Surgical Care Improvement Project, many anesthesiologists were arguing that control of antibiotics was not within their domain (see Chapter 5).[14] Anesthesiologists tend to focus on intraoperative cardiac arrests and other short-term outcomes, such as postoperative nausea and vomiting (see Chapters 33 and 86). Anesthesiologists will need to rethink this approach for other "never" conditions, such as urinary tract infections because they help determine the need for Foley catheters. Anesthesiologists and intensivists also can have a significant impact on the rate of ventilator-associated pneumonia. Some of these proposed measures, particularly the use of ventilator-associated pneumonia as a quality measure, have become quite controversial, however.[15] Pain is considered the fifth vital sign, and the management of postoperative pain is another area in which anesthesiologists can have a significant impact with respect to cost and potential interaction with other members of the hospital team.

Process Assessment and Quality Metrics

Anesthesiology was among the first professions to focus on reducing the risk of complications, and anesthesiologists were among the first groups to develop evidence-based guidelines and standards, as shown by the American Society of Anesthesiologists standards and practice parameters (see Chapter 5).[16] It will be important to continue to be involved in multidisciplinary approaches to surgical care. Examples where anesthesiologists were initially less involved include the Society of Thoracic Surgeons database and the National Surgical Quality Improvement Project.[17,18] More recently, anesthesiologists have become involved in both groups, and the Society of Cardiovascular Anesthesiologists have begun discussions with the Society of Thoracic Surgeons. Anesthesiologists have been involved from an early stage in quality initiatives with the Institute of Healthcare Improvement and the Surgical Care Improvement Project.[19]

Other quality measures that will have an impact on anesthesiologists include the new demand for metrics of competency, to be measured on a focused and an ongoing basis. Defining competency will demand that anesthesiologists adhere to more protocols, and that the concept of safe anesthesia be standardized. Rather than stifling medical innovation, standardization should be viewed as a mechanism for evaluating process and outcomes because comparisons cannot be made without standardization. Anesthesiologists will need to engage in creating quality and competency metrics, or these instruments will be created by others. This is an opportunity to formulate meaningful metrics that can be used in training physicians. Metrics also will be sought for nurse anesthetists and other health care professionals.

Changing processes has become a cottage industry in medical care, with courses being offered on how to change behaviors and processes in medical care. These mandates offer the opportunity for more research as to whether changing processes leads to improved patient outcomes. These mandates also allow anesthesiologists to assume a leadership role in team management. For anesthesiologists to accomplish this role, new skills need to be taught, including leadership training, improved communication skills, and improved relationship training.

One advantage that anesthesiologists have is a long tradition and training in system approaches to care. These date back to the original checklists for the anesthesia machine. It is crucial that this skill set be disseminated beyond the intraoperative setting. Many ambulatory surgery centers are directed by anesthesiologists.

Changes in Personnel

There are approximately 250,000 active physicians, one third of whom are older than 55 years old and likely to retire by 2020.[20] Although in the 1960s enrollment in U.S. medical schools doubled, during the years 1980 through 2005, the enrollment has been flat. There has been zero growth in U.S. medical school graduates. In this same interval, the U.S. population grew by more than 70 million, creating a discrepancy between the supply of medical school graduates and the demand for physician-associated care.

There also has been a significant increase in the number of women in medical schools, so that about 50% of medical students are now women.[21] Women tend not to work as many hours as their male counterparts, even when part-time status is taken into consideration.[22] Also, today's younger physicians choose to work fewer hours than their older counterparts, regardless of gender.[20,23]

There has been a steady use of international medical graduates; 60,000 international medical graduates are used as residents and constitute 25% of all residents in training.[24] There also has been an increase in the number of osteopath schools and schools offering advanced degrees in nursing, including training of nurses to become nurse anesthetists.[20] Given the increase in demand for medical care resulting from the increase in the geriatric population, this need will most likely be met by a combination of physicians and nonphysician personnel.

Research

In terms of creative new investigations, most benchmarks suggest that the specialty of anesthesiology fares poorly compared with other disciplines, especially clinical disciplines. Using data gleaned from publicly available National Institutes of Health (NIH) sources, Reves[25] produced a troubling figure showing that anesthesiology ranked second to the last for many medical disciplines. The exact position on any such figure would undoubtedly change from year to year. The fact that U.S. anesthesiology inhabits the lowest quartile is of concern, however, because the external forces on the practice components are generally applicable to all specialties.

NIH is not the only source of funding that may influence the specialty of anesthesiology; it is not even the largest portion of total research funding in the United States (Fig. 2-2).[26] For all sources, there has been a doubling over the last decade in research expenditures for health and biomedical science research, although compared with biologically based disciplines, health services research is considerably less well funded. In anesthesiology journals, the fraction of non-U.S., original peer-reviewed articles has increased dramatically. This increase does not seem to be attributable directly to research support. Adjusted per capita, research support in Europe is only 10% of that in the United States, even though the proportion of scientists in the population is similar.[27]

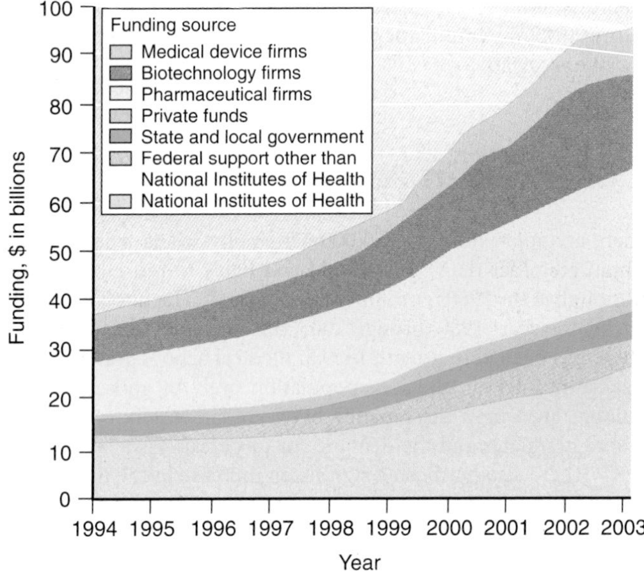

Figure 2-2 Research expenditures in the United States, 1994 to 2003, by funding source (see text).

There is no a priori reason why anesthesiology should differ from any other medical specialty in terms of research output. In our opinion, it should excel. One might argue that practitioners at academic institutions might be better compared in terms of surgical versus medical specialties, but even in that comparison we fare poorly. One line of remedy is to develop clinician-scientist training programs further, such as the NIH T-32 model. This approach is limited, however, by the fact that *selection* of individuals entering the specialty has already occurred.

One of the most exciting and promising developments in this regard has been the initiative by several programs in the United States to construct a special residency track that allows training for scientific independence to occur roughly in parallel with clinical residency training over the course of a 4-year track after internship. Such an approach recognizes that, to change the culture of the specialty, we must build from the ground up. Not all physicians who enter anesthesiology training go on to participate in the research/academic sector. Similar to other highly visible specialties, however, a sufficiently large cadre will be available to replenish those who leave active practice and further build up intellectual capital for future generations.

One of the challenges in training is the inherent and increasingly diverse nature of the disciplines involved in any one-subject area. The term "interdisciplinary research" has become a tautology. Practically all new frontiers lie at the boundaries of established departmental or specialty divisions, which are largely a historical relic of 19th century or early 20th century conceptualizations. A look at any large institution's roster of academic divisions yields a growing number of "centers," "programs," and "institutes," reflecting the ever-increasing interdependency of branches in biomedical knowledge.[28,29] In basic science departments, with conjugate names such as "Physiology and Cellular Biophysics," "Anatomy and Cell Biology," "Biochemistry and Biophysics," and "Cellular and Molecular Pharmacology," it is becoming increasingly difficult to differentiate one faculty research program from another, solely on the basis of the topics and methods of study. Although this differentiation is clearly less complicated for domains that do not involve patient care, the trend is evident. One might cite the example of endovascular surgery as an example in the collision of science, technology, and historical boundaries of medical specialties.[30]

Medical research is at one level original creative work that involves systemic investigation of medical phenomena with the direct or indirect consequence of improving health care. Activity that might be subsumed under "medical research" is scholarly synthesis of available data to generate new insights into phenomena. Scholarship that involves this synthesis is perhaps underappreciated and underemphasized. The most common type of publication in this category is the review article. Although often review articles are written by the individuals performing the original research, this is neither a necessary nor a sufficient precondition for a meaningful review. Especially for clinically oriented reviews, a broad perspective on a particular clinical practice may not only be sufficient, but also desirable.

Ramachandran[31] quotes Medwar: "An imaginative conception of what might be true is the starting point of all great discoveries in science." Ramachandran says that if he would show the reader a talking pig, it is unlikely that he or she would respond: "Ah, but that's just one pig. Show me a few more, and then I might believe you!" In this regard, an unintended consequence of moving toward quantitative indices for impact of biomedical journals has led to the demise of the case report. The case report is just such a Medwarian "imaginative conception of what might be true." It is also an ideal setting in which to perform a synthesis of available knowledge on a particular topic. Well-written and timely case reports can add significantly to the medical literature and provide an "early warning" function before laborious efforts are undertaken to conduct larger scale efforts to characterize a particular complication or phenomenon. Finally, case reports are "entry-level" scholarly activities that students, residents, and junior faculty can use as a stairstep to more complex modes of writing.

An area of potentially increasing contribution of anesthesia and perioperative care is in the realization of clinical trials for efficacy of surgical therapy. It is not unreasonable to assume that reimbursement for delivery of clinical care in the future may be increasingly tied to participation in some form of organized assessment of efficacy, such as a randomized controlled trial (e.g., the case of lung reduction surgery).[32] Such considerations are especially pertinent for procedures that are highly reimbursed, but controversial in terms of efficacy, as in the case of minimally symptomatic cerebrovascular diseases.[30,33] Perverse incentives can drive clinical practice and influence expert opinion. In addition to insights into the delivery of perioperative medical care, anesthesiologists can help provide an "honest broker" function in such settings.

In the clinical and policy research domain, anesthesiologists have an opportunity to study all aspects of surgical care. By joining or leading multidisciplinary teams, they can ask questions relevant to the patient undergoing surgery and not just undergoing anesthesia. Anesthesiologists must take leading roles in helping to define best surgical practice.

Why is it important that anesthesiology maintain the strongest possible profile in research and scholarly contributions to medical knowledge? Besides the intuitive sense that medical specialties must strive for advancing their domains, there is a strategic necessity of significant proactive involvement in scholarly and investigative pursuits. In the modern medical marketplace, physicians are not the only stakeholders in the delivery of health care. Physicians, particularly those in professorial tracks, traditionally conduct the bulk of investigative research, however. The advent of higher-level, doctoral degrees in nursing could significantly change this dynamic. The public that we serve, and the various governmental and institutional bodies that regulate health care delivery, should have a clear vision of our mission and approach.

References

1. National Center for Health Statistics: Health, United States, 2007, with Chartbook on Trends in the Health of Americans. 2007. Available at http://www.ncbi.nlm.nih.gov/books/bv.fcgi?indexed=google&rid=healthus07.chapter.trend-tables.
2. Ruther MM, Black C: Medicare use and cost of short-stay hospital services by enrollees with cataract, 1984. Health Care Financ Rev 9:91-99, 1987.
3. Fleisher LA, Pasternak LR, Herbert R, et al: Inpatient hospital admission and death after outpatient surgery in elderly patients: Importance of patient and system characteristics and location of care. Arch Surg 139:67-72, 2004.
4. Cutler DM: Your Money or Your Life: Strong Medicine for America's Health Care System. New York, Oxford University Press, 2004.
5. Bodenheimer T: High and rising health care costs, part 2: Technologic innovation. Ann Intern Med 142:932-937, 2005.
6. Mongan JJ, Ferris TG, Lee TH: Options for slowing the growth of health care costs. N Engl J Med 358:1509-1514, 2008.
7. Thorpe KE: The rise in health care spending and what to do about it. Health Aff (Millwood) 24:1436-1445, 2005.
8. Rosenthal MB: Nonpayment for performance? Medicare's new reimbursement rule. N Engl J Med 357:1573-1575, 2007.
9. Shortell SM, Rundall TG, Hsu J: Improving patient care by linking evidence-based medicine and evidence-based management. JAMA 298:673-676, 2007.
10. Lee TH: Pay for performance, version 2.0? N Engl J Med 357:531-533, 2007.
11. Campbell S, Reeves D, Kontopantelis E, et al: Quality of primary care in England with the introduction of pay for performance. N Engl J Med 357:181-190, 2007.
12. Lindenauer PK, Remus D, Roman S, et al: Public reporting and pay for performance in hospital quality improvement. N Engl J Med 356:486-496, 2007.
13. Centers for Medicare and Medicaid Services: Medicare Program; Hospital Outpatient Prospective Payment System and CY 2007 Payment Rates; CY 2007 Update to the Ambulatory Surgical Center Covered Procedures List; Medicare Administrative Contractors; and Reporting Hospital Quality Data for FY 2008 Inpatient Prospective Payment System Annual Payment Update Program—HCAHPS Survey, SCIP, and Mortality, Vol 71. Dept of Health and Human Services. Federal Register, 2006.
14. Griffin FA: Reducing surgical complications. Jt Comm J Qual Patient Saf 33:660-665, 2007.
15. Klompas M, Kulldorff M, Platt R: Risk of misleading ventilator-associated pneumonia rates with use of standard clinical and microbiological criteria. Clin Infect Dis 46:1443-1446, 2008.
16. Arens JF: A practice parameters overview. Anesthesiology 78:229-230, 1993.
17. Khuri SF: The NSQIP: A new frontier in surgery. Surgery 138:837-843, 2005.
18. Tong BC, Harpole DH Jr: Audit, quality control, and performance in thoracic surgery: A North American perspective. Thorac Surg Clin 17:379-386, 2007.
19. QualityNet. Available at http://www.qualitynet.org/dcs/ContentServer?pagename=QnetPublic/Page/QnetHomepage.
20. Salsberg E, Grover A: Physician workforce shortages: Implications and issues for academic health centers and policymakers. Acad Med 81:782-787, 2006.
21. AAMC Data Book: U.S. Medical School Women Applicants, Accepted Applicants, and Matriculants. Washington, DC, Association of American Medical Colleges, 2005.
22. Heiligers PJ, Hingstman L: Career preferences and the work-family balance in medicine: Gender differences among medical specialists. Soc Sci Med 50:1235-1246, 2000.
23. Jovic E, Wallace JE, Lemaire J: The generation and gender shifts in medicine: An exploratory survey of internal medicine physicians. BMC Health Serv Res 6:55, 2006.
24. Graduate medical education. JAMA 294:1129-1143, 2005.
25. Reves JG: We are what we make: Transforming research in anesthesiology. Anesthesiology 106:826-835, 2007.
26. Moses H 3rd, Dorsey ER, Matheson DH, et al: Financial anatomy of biomedical research. JAMA 294:1333-1342, 2005.
27. Philipson L: Medical research activities, funding, and creativity in Europe: Comparison with research in the United States. JAMA 294:1394-1398, 2005.
28. Columbia University Medical Center. Academic and Clinical Departments, Centers and Institutions. 2008. Available at http://asp.cumc.columbia.edu/depts/.
29. University of California San Francisco. Department Chairs, ORU Directors, and Assistants. 2008. Available at http://medschool.ucsf.edu/listbuilder/chairs_dirs_assts.htm.
30. Fiehler J, Stapf C: ARUBA—beating natural history in unruptured brain AVMs by intervention. Neuroradiology 50:465-467, 2008.
31. Ramachandran VS, Blakeslee S: Phantoms in the Brain: Probing the Mysteries of the Human Mind. New York, William Morrow, 1998.
32. Centers for Medicare and Medicaid Services. Lung Volume Reduction Surgery (LVRS). 2008. Available at http://www.cms.hhs.gov/MedicareApprovedFacilitie/LVRS/List.asp
33. Mathiesen T: Arguments against the proposed randomised trial (ARUBA). Neuroradiology 50:469-471, 2008.

Ronald D. Miller with Andrew Schwartz, Editors

3 The International Scope and Practice of Anesthesia

Outline

At a recent international anesthesia conference, an American anesthesiologist spoke about the value of using modern electronic monitoring devices in the operating room. Believing that they are essential for improved patient safety, the presenter expressed a hope that hospitals worldwide would adopt and use these devices. During the question and answer session, however, a physician from another country—one whose hospitals have considerably fewer resources than those in the United States—stood to express his frustration with this argument. In his country, he believed, there were other priorities and the sheer cost of monitoring equipment prohibited its widespread adoption. Another physician, also from a country whose hospitals do not have a wealth of resources, disagreed; by understanding what monitoring devices were available, he would pick the most effective monitoring device or devices in accordance with the resources available. A spirited exchange followed. Of course, there is no one right way for hospitals to spend their limited resources. There was, however, enormous value in this exchange among physicians from different countries with different cultures, different resources, and different perspectives. It is through these discussions that the profession can create fully informed baseline standards that foster greater levels of patient safety and improved outcomes worldwide.

Such discussions, which occur with increasing frequency, also inspired this chapter on the global scope and practice of anesthesia. Throughout his career, this book's editor, Ronald D. Miller, has had the privilege and pleasure of speaking and working with leading anesthesiologists from all over the world. His work and discussions with international colleagues spurred a desire to recognize and honor the growth and practice of anesthesia outside North America. He wanted to describe the different ways that anesthesia began from place to place and to follow the regions through time so that we can better understand how the various regions influence each other today.

This chapter is the first step in realizing his hope. Work on this chapter began in earnest when he invited a number of colleagues whom he had met over the years—prominent anesthesiologists in their parts of the world and beyond—to contribute a short summary describing the growth and practice of anesthesia in their country or region. When the contributions arrived, they proved to be a fascinating read: creative, informative, and inspirational. Yet for all their rich content, they also posed an editorial challenge in that the unique cultures, politics, economics, and developments in various regions prompted the contributors to emphasize different ideas, discoveries, or time periods. These differences in emphasis and coverage reflect the freedom that the contributors were given to describe their country or region. In the future we hope to expand on this topic by covering other areas of practice and including world regions not featured in this chapter.

It was in the face of this challenge that Dr. Schwartz was asked to integrate the short individual contributions into a single chapter without compromising their integrity. Dr. Miller and Dr. Schwartz chose to create a chronologic narrative that progresses through three distinct time periods. Each period is broken up by region; each regional narrative draws directly from the work of the international contributors. Our intent was to always acknowledge and document the sources and wherever possible maintain each contributor's individual voice, and we hope that we have achieved that goal.

Dr. Miller is deeply grateful to all the colleagues who contributed to this chapter, for their insightful writing and the time that they devoted to their tasks, and regrets that because of time and space constraints not more contributions of this kind could be included in this edition. He recognizes that the pages you are about to read are only a first step and by no means a comprehensive look at the development of anesthesia around the world. Future editions will deepen and broaden the international focus.

The first section of this chapter is a sprint through a vast stretch of history, from ancient times through the early 20th century. Over these two thousand or so years, with a few notable exceptions, the practice of anesthesia grew independently by region in response to the need for pain relief during medical procedures.

The second section covers the period from the 1920s through the early 1980s. This was a time when modern communications and international travel expanded dramatically, leading to increased cross-pollination of anesthesia techniques. Physicians and researchers began to regularly travel to foreign countries, receive training and education abroad, and hear others speak at conferences. As international journals grew, knowledge about emerging practices in anesthesia spread further.

The third section covers the time from the early 1980s through the present. This has been an exciting period because today nearly all anesthesiologists, no matter where they practice in the world, can gain access to the information necessary to deliver safe anesthesia at the most basic level. Even though significant differences in resource levels still remain, some of which undermine the practice of safe anesthesia, at least all anesthesiologists worldwide today know how to avoid the common complications of anesthesia that can endanger patients' lives. This section details the state of anesthesia in the regions covered—from education, accreditation, professional exchanges, and actual practice to available facilities and equipment.

The chapter concludes by raising questions about what is next in terms of the way various countries and regions practice anesthesia. How integrated should the practice of anesthesia become? What can we do to raise levels of care worldwide? Again, there are no simple answers, but it is a future that anesthesiologists face together.

The Early History of International Anesthesia

Before the early 20th century, those interested in analgesia during surgery rarely had the advantage of being able to learn from what their colleagues around the world were doing. Rather, in response to patient need, physicians from various regions came to different, but often similar conclusions about how to relieve pain. In many, if not most places, herbs, opium, and alcohol were the mainstays of pain relief medication.

Regions were not completely isolated, however. As the narratives herein describe, the traditional ways of spreading culture and information, such as war and trade, enabled at least some sharing of anesthesia techniques. In particular, the first published account of ether used as an anesthetic in 1846 seems to have been anesthesia's "shot heard 'round the world."

India (Deepak K. Tempe)

The history of anesthesia in India dates back to the era of Susruta, the great surgeon of ancient India. During his time, around 600 BC, operations were performed with the use of opium, wine, and Indian hemp (an herb). Surgical science was called "salya-tantra" (*salya*: broken parts of an arrow and other sharp weapons; *tantra*: maneuver).[1]

Much later, in 980 AD, Pandit Ballala mentioned in *Bhoj Prabandh* that Raja (King) Bhoj underwent a cranial operation under the anesthetic influence of a plant called "sammohini." The same plant was applied as healing balm to surgical wounds. A drug called "sanjivan" was administered to revive the Raja and help him regain consciousness.[2]

Nearly 900 years later, after the first widely publicized demonstration of ether anesthesia in the United States in 1846, India quickly followed suit by administering ether anesthesia on March 22, 1847, in Calcutta under the supervision of a surgeon named Dr. O'Shaughnessy.[3] Later, chloroform was also used but fell into disrepute because of the high morbidity associated with it. Despite this—and the fact that the world began to discard chloroform in preference for ether by 1890—India continued to use chloroform until 1928.

Among the several interesting case reports related to anesthetic practice is the emergency appendectomy performed on Mahatma Gandhi on January 12, 1925, at Sassoon Hospital, Pune. During an electricity failure, the mahatma was administered open-drop chloroform anesthesia, with the surgery being completed by the light of a kerosene lamp and battery-operated torch.[4]

The Middle East (Anis Baraka and Fouad Salim Haddad)

With the decline of the Greco-Roman Empire in the fifth century AD, the Middle East witnessed the rise of an Arab/Islamic civilization that within a hundred years (632-732 AD) expanded over a 3000-mile stretch extending from the western borders of India, through north Africa and Sicily, to Andalusia on the Atlantic coast of Spain. This civilization interacted with the ancient Egyptian, Hellenistic, Byzantine, Syrian, Persian, and Indian cultures. Many Arab/Islamic, Christian, and Jewish scholars translated, refined, and augmented the knowledge contained in these cultures. The new civilization that evolved lasted for around 1000 years, carried the torch of knowledge in the Middle Ages, and through its transmission via Spain and Sicily, contributed to the European Renaissance.

In this epoch, some prominent Arab/Islamic, Christian, and Jewish scholars made important contributions in the fields of medicine, philosophy, astronomy, mathematics, and chemistry. A wealth of knowledge was thus inherited by several succeeding ages. Of special interest, the following scholars made contributions to the field of anesthesia: (1) Al-Rhazi (865-925 AD), born in Ray, Persia, described the pupillary reaction to light and the laryngeal branch of the recurrent laryngeal nerve[5]; (2) Avicenna (980-1037 AD), born near Bukhara, Persia, enumerated agents that

A

Et qñqȝ itromittit in gutture cãnula facta de auro aut argento: aut silibus ambobus ad/iuuando ad inspirandũ:

B

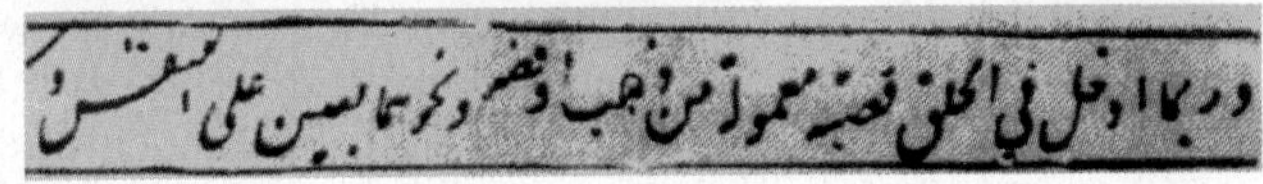

Figure 3-1 **A,** The Latin version of oral intubation: *Et quandoque intromittiture in gutture canula facta de auro aut argento: aut silibus ambobus, adjuvando ad inspirandu.* **B,** The Arabic version of oral intubation: When necessary, a cannula made of gold, silver, or another suitable material is advanced down the throat to support inspiration. *(From Haddad FS: Ibn Sina [Avicenna] advocated orotracheal intubation 1000 years ago: Documentation of Arabic and Latin originals. Middle East J Anesthesiol 17:155-162, 2000.)*

alleviate pain: opium, henbane, and mandrake; in his *Canon of Medicine*, he advocated oral intubation: "When necessary, a cannula of gold, silver, or another suitable material is advanced down the throat to support inspiration" (Fig. 3-1)[6,7]; (3) Ibn Al Nafis (1208-1288 AD), born in Quresh, near Damascus, Syria, criticized in his *Sharh Tashrih Al Qanou* Galen's theory of blood movement, which said that blood from the right ventricle passes into the left ventricle through small invisible pores in the septum (Fig. 3-2A); Ibn Al Nafis asserted that there is no direct pathway between the chambers and the thick septum of the heart is not perforated, and he described the pulmonary circulation as we know it today (see Fig. 3-2B)[8,9]; and (4) Al-Khawarizmi (died 840 AD), born in Balkh, Persia, who was a famed mathematician; the word "algorithm," a mathematical tool, is attributed to him. Algorithm is defined as "a step-by-step problem-solving procedure."[10]

The Use of Spongia Somnifera. In the Middle Ages, the concept of inhalation to induce sedation before surgery with use of the sleeping sponge, or *spongia somnifera*, is attributed to Arab origins.[11,12] With the Arab conquest of Sicily in the ninth century and the Latin translations of Arabic medical books that followed, Arabic medicine, including the soporific sponge, took hold in southern Italy (Salerno, Monte Cassino). From there it spread to other parts of Europe and was used in the Middle Ages.[12] A probability also exists that it was carried from the Andalus of Spain by Michael Scot, who in the 13th century transmitted scientific culture from Toledo to Bologna via the Court of Frederick II Hohenstaufen in Sicily.[13,14]

After the Middle Ages, major political events in the 19th century affected the development of medicine throughout the countries of the Middle East. First, with Napoleon's invasion of Egypt in 1798, the medical awakening of Middle Eastern countries to western medicine can be said to have started. To win the cooperation of the Egyptian people, Napoleon brought with him men of all specialties.[15] After Napoleon's departure from Egypt and the assumption of power by Mohammad Ali in 1805, efforts to propagate knowledge and education continued. Mohammad Ali brought doctors from Europe and France to take care of the health of his army. Of those, the most remarkable was Dr. Antoine Berthelemy Clot (later Clot Bey) (1793-1868), who was brought to Egypt in 1825. In 1835 Bey established a medical school in Kasr Al Aini Hospital in Cairo, the only Arab medical school in the Middle East at the time.[15]

The developing renovation of Egypt then influenced other regions of the Middle East, either through students flocking to

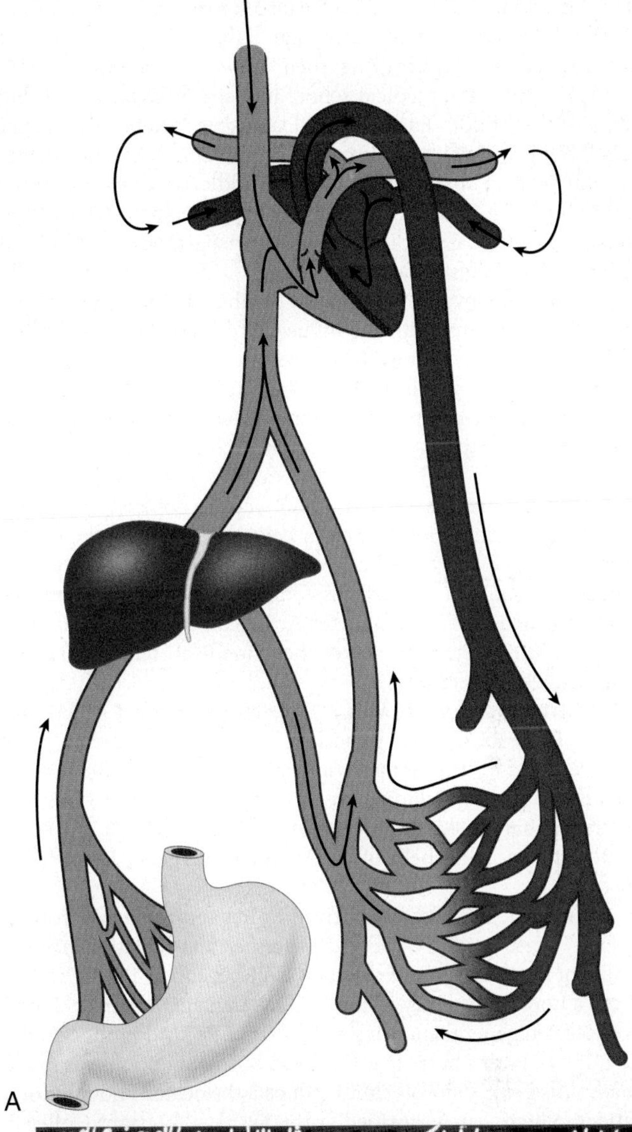

A

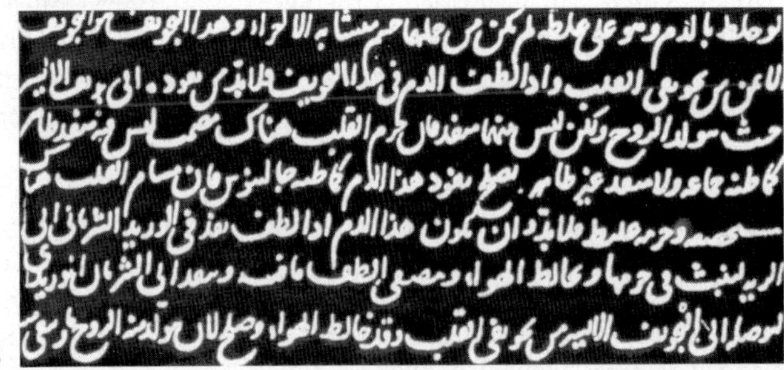

B

Figure 3-2 **A,** Galen's theory of blood movement. According to Galen, blood reached the periphery through the veins (most of it departing from the liver), as well as through the arteries (departing from the heart). Little blood went to the lungs from the right ventricle of the heart. He thought that most of the blood passed from the right to the left ventricle through pores in the intraventricular septum. **B,** Photographic reproduction of the original manuscript of Ibn al-Nafis denying the presence of intraventricular pores and describing the pulmonary circulation as we know it today.

study medicine in Kasr Al Aini Hospital or through the influence of the Egyptian military campaign (Ibrahim Pasha, son of Mohammad Ali) against the then known Syria (1831-1840). Graduates from the medical school in Cairo practiced in all big cities of the Middle East: Beirut, Damascus, Allepo, Jerusalem, Safad, Nablus, Haifa, and Nazareth. It is assumed that the analgesia practiced in major cities of the Middle East was the same technique used in Cairo. Relief of surgical pain in Cairo then consisted of herbal medications and antispasmodics.[15] No kind of inhaled anesthesia was known.

After the invasion of Syria by Ibrahim Pasha from 1831 to 1840, the Egyptians, with the influence of Western missionaries, built two military hospitals—one in Allepo and one in Damascus—and established free medical clinics.[15,16] The presence of Clot Bey in the campaign was instrumental in sending the first five Lebanese students to study medicine at Kasr Al Aini Hospital.[15]

Finally, after massacres in 1860, western powers (American, French, and British) intervened in Lebanon, and with the inflow of missionaries, more medical schools and hospitals were established. In 1866, the Americans founded the Syrian Protestant College, which in 1920 became the American University of Beirut. In 1883, the French founded their medical school (Faculté Française de Médecine).[15]

Introduction of Modern Anesthesia to the Middle East. In 1846, the first published account of the use of ether anesthesia for a surgical operation appeared, and the innovation spread rapidly,[17,18] including to London in December 1846 and Paris in January 1847. Twenty-seven years later, in 1873, it arrived in Beirut[15] with the help of an American surgeon, Dr. George Post.

In 1863, Dr. Post had arrived in Lebanon to assist in missionary work. In 1867, he and others established the medical school of the then Syrian Protestant College, and in 1873, Dr. Post wrote a book on surgery in the Arabic language, which included a chapter on general anesthesia, the first of its kind in the Middle East. It was in this book that for the first time mention was made of administering chloroform to reduce a dislocated shoulder of a patient, which was performed at the Syrian Protestant College's Johanniter Hospital in Beirut. To describe this action, Dr. Post coined the word "kulfera," an Arabization of the word chloroform. Dr. Post rightly deserves the title of the First Pioneer of Modern Anesthesia in Lebanon and the Middle East.[15]

Graduates of the Syrian Protestant College in Lebanon and other graduates of medical schools in the Middle East probably administered open-drop ether or chloroform along with local and spinal anesthesia through the rest of the 19th century and middle of the 20th century. Physicians, students, nurses, nuns, and technicians were most likely also involved.

Russia (Olga N. Afonin)

The history of Russian medicine has its roots in the history of medieval European medicine. Right through the 18th and 19th centuries, much of the information about anesthetic techniques—applying "snow" 15 minutes before surgical procedures and analgesics for the cardiovascular and respiratory systems and wound healing, as well as the use of bellows for lung ventilation—came from various leaders in European medicine. In addition, like their colleagues in the Middle East and India, Russian physicians of course heard of the use of ether on October 16, 1846; that day is still a professional holiday for anesthesiologists in Russia. A brief 4 months later, Dr. F. I. Inozemtzev of Moscow became the first in Russia to use ether for anesthesia during surgery.

Around the same time, the art of local anesthesia was developing rapidly after the publication of an article by the Russian doctor Vassili von Anrep. He described the effects of cocaine as a topical and subcutaneous local anesthetic in 1879. Isolated by the German chemist Friedrich Gaedcke in 1855 and purified by University of Gottingen student Albert Niemann in 1859, cocaine was first given to a patient in 1884. It was the only local anesthetic until 1904, when procaine was synthesized.

von Anrep's ideas of local anesthesia were very popular. Famous physicians of Europe and Russia (Shleich, Lukashevich, Vishnevskiy, Bier) were developing the knowledge of local anesthesia, which gave rise to new methods of preventing pain: local field anesthesia, local infiltration anesthesia, nerve blocks, plexus anesthesia, intravenous anesthesia, and neuraxial anesthesia.

In general anesthesia, the Russian physician Nikolay Pirogov (1810-1881) was a prominent physician and surgeon, well known in Europe. He was the first to describe the negative effects of general anesthesia and the possibility of severe complications. He postulated the necessity of acquiring detailed knowledge of the physiologic and clinical effects of anesthetics and requiring a separate course on anesthesia during medical education. He also described many of the modern methods of anesthesia, including inhaled endotracheal anesthesia, intravenous anesthetics, rectal use of anesthetics, and spinal anesthesia. This had a huge impact on the analgesia provided to wounded soldiers in terms of increasing surgical success and rates of survival.

In 1904, the Russian physicians S. P. Feodorov and N. P. Kravkov described and demonstrated total intravascular anesthesia with the intravenous anesthetic Gedonal. They were also the first to use combined narcosis through induction with Gedonal and maintenance with inhaled chloroform.

Another area in which Russian physicians made advances was in the field of blood transfusions. In 1901, Karl Landsteiner reported his discovery of the possible existence of blood types. In 1909 he expanded his initial discovery by establishing the A, B, AB, and O blood types. He demonstrated that transfusions between individuals with the same blood group do not result in the destruction of new blood cells and that this catastrophe occurs only when a person is transfused with the blood of a person belonging to a different group. In 1930, Landsteiner received the Nobel Prize for his work. In 1907, Russian physician Yanskiy had described four blood types and created the basics of blood transfusion. His work, however, went unnoticed.

Just a few short years later, World War I began, followed by the October Revolution in 1917, which destroyed the monarchy in Russia. Civil war, general poverty, and empowerment of the Communist Party in the early 1920s led to dramatic changes in Russia's political philosophy, economics, and technical and scientific progress, all of which affected the development of medicine. With Joseph Stalin coming to power in the 1920s, communication with other countries in Europe was terminated, exchange of information stopped, and Russian physicians had to continue treating their patients while developing the art of medicine separate from the knowledge and advances in the rest of the world. On the other hand, advances in Russian medicine were not known to the world and, frequently, had to be reinvented.

The Cross-Pollination Period: Approximately 1920-1980

In the late 1970s, the editor took a sabbatical in Holland, during which time he lectured at a local university hospital. Also there at the time was a young anesthesiologist from Ecuador. Over time, the two physicians became friends as they shared ideas about the practice of anesthesiology and its future. This rich exchange about their profession continues to this day. This was the beginning of the editor's understanding of the interesting and varied approaches in different parts of the world to achieve the status of anesthesiology as it now stands.

Their cross-cultural exchange, however, is no aberration. Over the approximately 60 years from the end of World War I through the early 1980s, anesthesiologists from around the world began to meet in a variety of forums facilitated by the advent of air travel and modern communications.

Physicians received training and education abroad. Lecturers from diverse nations spoke frequently outside their home country and brought in new ideas and techniques. Academic and research journals proliferated, as did international congresses and access to textbooks, thereby laying the groundwork for a common understanding about how to practice anesthesia.

India (Deepak K. Tempe)

Up to about 30 years ago, anesthetic equipment in Indian operating rooms often consisted solely of a simple anesthesia machine, a suction unit, and perhaps an electrocardiographic monitor. Even the oxygen supply was mainly via cylinders, with very few hospitals having a centralized medical gas supply. The first medical pipeline system was installed in Vellore in 1954.

Today it is widely accepted that postoperative care is crucial for the success of surgery, but in previous days, many patients were sent back to the ward directly after surgery and only a few would go to the recovery room. In recognition of the fact that surgical patients often need to be observed in a specialized area, India commissioned its first intensive care unit (ICU) in 1963 in an Army hospital in Delhi. Interestingly, that was the same year that an ICU was first established by an anesthesiologist at the University of California, San Francisco.

During this stretch of the 20th century, Indian anesthesiologists also recognized the need for professional societies. The idea of an Indian Society of Anaesthesiologists (ISA) was conceived in 1946; the group was established in 1947. The first ISA meeting was held in 1949 during a surgeons' conference in Mumbai, and the first independent ISA conference was held in Hyderabad in 1965. Professors Macintosh and Gray were the distinguished guests during the conference. The ISA published its first official journal in July 1953 and joined the World Federation of Societies of Anesthesiologists (WFSA) in 1956. The group has grown from 19 members when it began to nearly 12,000 members in 2007.

The Middle East (Anis Baraka and Fouad Salim Haddad)

At the end of World War I, the Middle East was divided by Western powers into small countries that were placed under British and French mandate. The major pattern in the practice of anesthesia was complete dependence on foreign surgeons, who could administer anesthetics, as well as on local and foreign nurses or nonanesthesiologists and technicians, who administered ether or chloroform. This period also witnessed the foundation of faculties of medicine in some countries of the Middle East (Syria, Sudan, and Iraq).[16]

By the end of World War II, the beginning of oil production contributed to an improving economy, which meant more funds available for anesthesia machines, endotracheal tubes, and thiopental, all of which began to appear in many countries of the Middle East. An influx of newly trained surgeons increased the demand for qualified anesthesiologists, thus prompting anesthesia residencies. In addition, in response to a manpower shortage in many countries of the Middle East, nurse and technician training began as well, although this was gradually phased out as locally and internationally trained and certified anesthesiologists began arriving in many countries of the Middle East.

During the second half of the 20th century, all countries of the Middle East were striving to attain state-of-the-art anesthesia. The World Health Organization (WHO) played a great role in encouraging and sponsoring graduate physicians for training in anesthesia at the World Anesthesiology Training Center in Copenhagen.

Raising the Professional Profile of Anesthesia. As in many other places in the world, the status of anesthesia in the Middle East depends partly on the establishment of fully independent departments of anesthesia that have their own structure, staff, residency training, research, and certification by international academic institutions and that offer fellowships in cardiovascular, obstetric, and pediatric anesthesia, as well as pain management. To that end, certain landmark strides were taken during this period.

In 1966, the *Middle East Journal of Anesthesiology* (ISSN 0544-0440) was founded; it continues to thrive to this day. Its main objectives are to act as a forum for education and exchange of opinions and to promote research and publication of Middle Eastern medicine and anesthesia. The journal is accepted for inclusion in the Index Medicus and MEDLARS system.

In addition, in the 1960s and 1970s, many Middle Eastern countries founded their own national societies of anesthesia, which promoted the practice and image of the specialty. In 1990, The Pan Arab Society of Anesthesia and Intensive Care was founded and became a member of the WFSA. Every 2 years, the Pan Arab Society holds The Pan Arab Congress of Anesthesia and Intensive Care in one of the member countries.

Russia (Olga N. Afonin)

In the midst of the economic difficulties and political upheaval after the Russian civil war, medical services underwent dramatic reorganization and expansion, and some positive developments ensued. Campaigns were carried out against diseases and poor hygiene. Thousands of unpaid men and women underwent short courses in nursing. They went all over the country to educate people and treat deadly diseases, often risking their own lives. This remarkable effort was rewarded in just a few years. The epidemics were stopped, and control of many diseases was established. This experience emphasized the importance of preventive measures, including vaccinations, and Soviet physicians began working on preventive medicine.

Meanwhile, in Moscow, Dr. Yurevich was first in the world to begin using citrate for blood conservation. His colleague Dr. Shamov was first to use cadaveric blood for transfusion in 1928, thus giving birth to a new field of medicine—transplantation.

The very first Institute of Blood Transfusion, a scientific center for study and development of the science of blood and blood component use and storage, was formed in 1926 in Moscow by Professor A. A. Bogdanov. Physicians of the institute developed and published the first systematic approach to the treatment of shock, including traumatic, hypovolemic, and "burn related." Another dramatically important innovation of Russian physicians was the introduction of methods of diagnosis and treatment of electrolyte and acid-base imbalances with complex salt solutions, blood substitutes, and total parenteral nutrition solutions.

In 1924, the Russians S. S. Bryuchonenko and S. I. Chechulin constructed and used the very first artificial heart machine in the world, the parent of what is now known to us as a cardiopulmonary bypass machine. Surgical procedures were becoming more complex and required more advanced methods of exposure of the abdominal and thoracic organs. The bellows of Dr. Henry Hickman was transformed into many different machines to provide artificial ventilation, including the famous "iron lung" of Harvard, used first in Boston in 1928.

In 1939, N. L. Gurevich and G. S. Yun'ev developed the physiologic basis and methods of indirect heart massage and electrical defibrillation. These methods were used successfully on patients requiring complicated cardiothoracic surgeries in Russia.

As all these developments grew into complex surgical procedures and as the use of neuromuscular blocking drugs spread, it became necessary in Russia to develop a new kind of subspecialty in medicine: anesthesiology. This would require extensive and detailed knowledge of many disciplines, including physiology, biochemistry, surgery, medicine, neurology, pharmacology, traditional anesthesia, and critical care.

The first Department of Anesthesiology in Russia branched out of the Department of Cardiothoracic Surgery (now the Russian Medical Academy of Physicians Postgraduate Education) in 1959 in Moscow (this is also the same year that the current Department of Anesthesia was formed at the University of California, San Francisco). The first postgraduate courses for physicians to become anesthesiologists lasted 4 months. Later, there were additional courses of anesthesiology that included the basics of intensive care and another couple of months of additional training. The broad variety of topics covered and the complexity of the potential patient care issues meant that the new specialists needed more time to properly prepare for their careers. These careers were in demand as newly formed anesthesiology and intensive care departments required more and more anesthesiologists to teach and take care of patients.

It was in 1969 when the Ministry of Health of the Soviet Union released the "Order of improvement of anesthesiologic and reanimatologic (intensive care) services in the country." That was when anesthesiology finally received the financial and administrative support required at that time for any significant changes to take place.

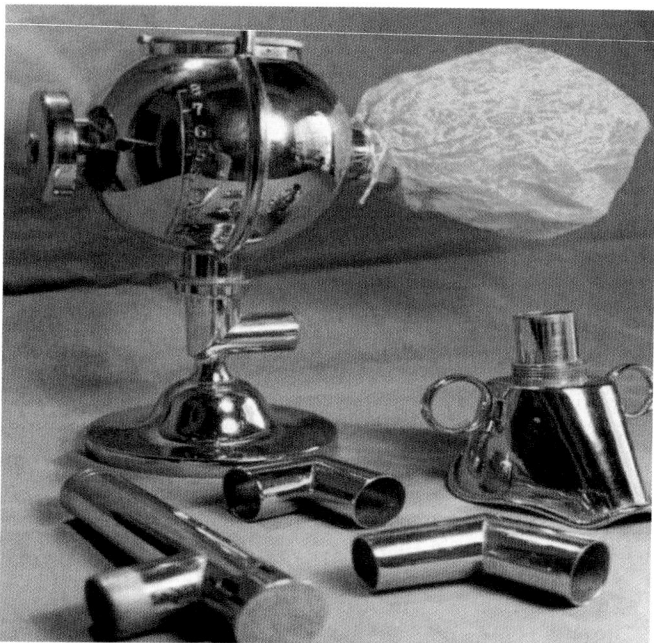

Figure 3-3 The Ombrédanne anesthesia delivery device.

South America (Guillermo Lema)

The main influences on the South American practice of medicine in general, and anesthesia and surgery in particular, come from Europe. For many years and particularly during the first 6 decades of the 20th century, many doctors were trained in different parts of Europe: France, Germany, and Scandinavian countries among others. The European influence was as strong in medicine as it was in other aspects of daily life.

One example of Europe's influence was South Americans' wide use of the Ombredanne (Fig. 3-3). This device, used to deliver anesthesia, was invented in France in 1908 by the surgeon Dr. Louis Ombrédanne (1871-1956). It is believed that South America is the only continent where this particular equipment was clinically acceptable and used widely.

Of course, ether was not the only anesthetic used during this time. Cyclopropane was another, although Chile had a dramatic experience with this gas that eventually caused it to be banned. In 1963 at the Manuel Arriarán Hospital in Santiago, a cyclopropane tank exploded in a pediatric operating room. Two small boys and four physicians—two of them anesthesiologists—died. This remains one of the worst anesthesia-related accidents ever to happen in the world. New standards, including the banning of cyclopropane, were imposed to avoid further accidents.

China (Yuguang Huang)

In the early 20th century, with the introduction of Western medicine into China, modern anesthesia began to be applied in clinics. At that time, anesthesia was implemented mainly by nurses or surgeons. Only a few Western professional anesthesiologists, such as Mr. Yueqing Ma from the Peking Union Medical College, could undertake clinical anesthesia in China.

After the foundation of the People's Republic of China in 1949, some early pioneers—such as Jue Wu and Xingfang Li from Shanghai and Rong Xie, Deyan Shang, and Huiying Tan from Beijing—returned from the United States and Europe to help modern anesthesia take shape in China.

In the 1950s, only simple anesthesia was available in China, such as the ether open-drop method, inhaled tracheal intubation anesthesia, and single procaine spinal anesthesia. Peripheral nerve block and continuous epidural anesthesia were introduced gradually.

From the 1950s to the 1980s, intravenous procaine combined anesthesia and continuous epidural anesthesia were the most common methods in China. When anesthetic drugs and monitoring tools became scarce in the 1960s, Chinese anesthesiologists tried to develop acupuncture anesthesia based on the pain-relieving mechanisms of traditional Chinese acupuncture. In addition, in the 1970s Chinese anesthesiologists investigated the anesthetic effect of Chinese herbal medicine. However, beginning in the late 1970s, because of the success of reform and the government's opening-up policy, many new anesthetic drugs and instruments were introduced into China. At that time, acupuncture anesthesia and herbal anesthesia stepped down from the clinical stage as a result of their unsatisfying anesthetic efficacy and adverse effects.

Raising the Professional Profile of Anesthesia. Chinese anesthesiologists also began raising their profile as early as the 1950s, when they took part in the rescue of critically ill patients via cardiopulmonary resuscitation. For example, in 1959, Professor Yuanchang Wang from Tianjin Medical College shared his experience in the *Chinese Journal of Surgery* by reporting that a woman whose life was in danger during cesarean section was saved by chest compressions. Partly because of the influence of anesthesiologists, since the 1970s ICUs and postanesthesia care units (PACUs) have gradually been established in many domestic hospitals.

China has also participated in numerous international conferences and professional groups (Fig. 3-4). The First National Conference on Anesthesia was held in Nanjing in 1964, during which the development and achievements of Chinese anesthesiology were systematically reviewed. In 1979, the Chinese Society of

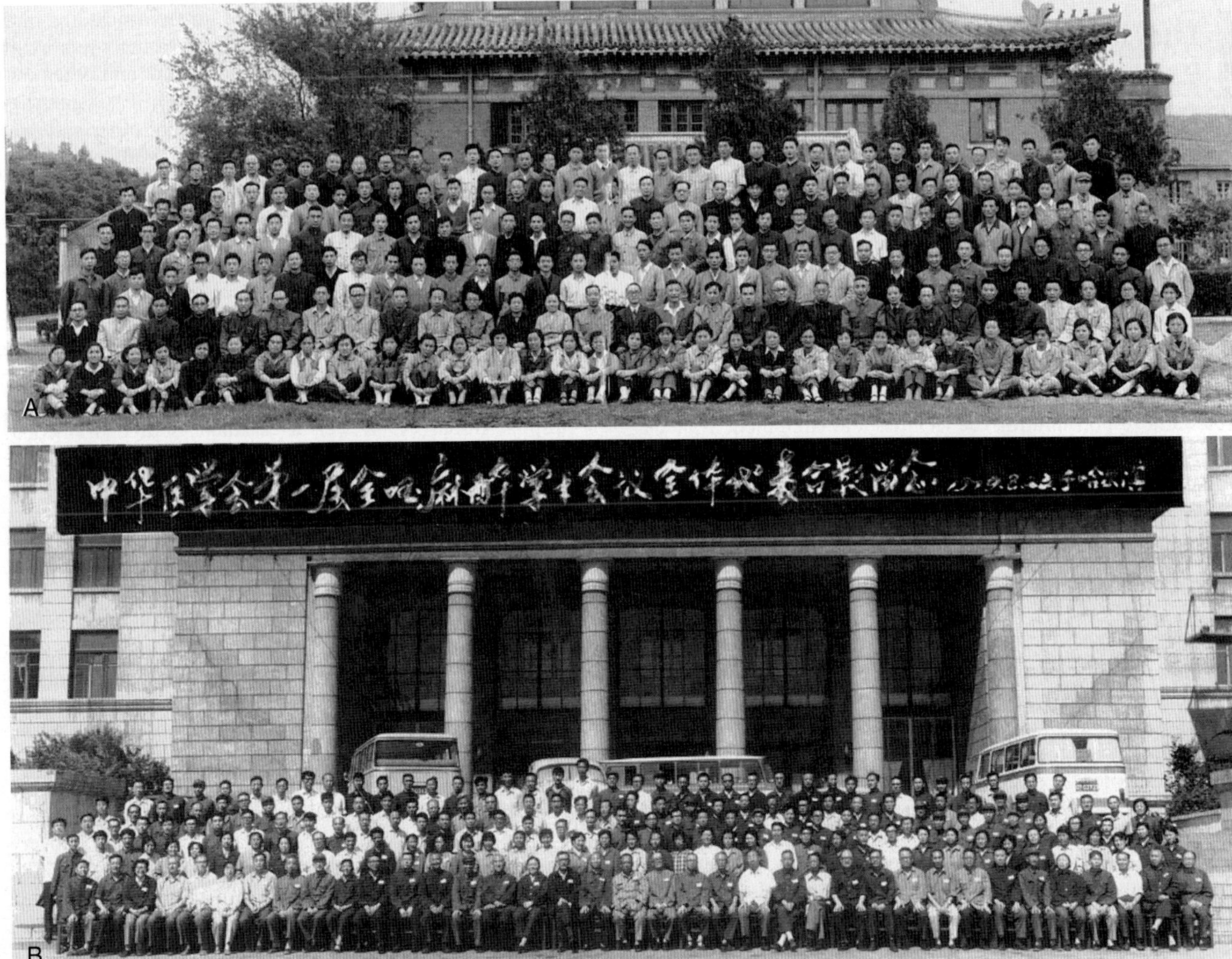

Figure 3-4 A, Participants of the First National Conference on Anesthesia, Nanjing, 1964. **B,** Participants of the Second National Conference on Anesthesia, Harbin, 1979, during which the Chinese Society of Anesthesiology was founded.

Anesthesiology (CSA) was founded during the Second National Conference on Anesthesiology held in Harbin. Professor Deyan Shang was elected as president of the first CSA committee. Since then, national CSA conferences have been held every 3 or 4 years.

During this period there was also a foray into professional publications, most notably Professor Jue Wu, the leader of Chinese anesthesia, who was the lead editor of *Clinical Anesthesiology* in 1954 and *Practical Anesthesiology* in 1976.

Western medicine introduced by the United States also helped promote the development of modern medicine in China. A good example is Peking Union Medical College (PUMC) Hospital, which was founded by the Rockefeller Foundation in 1917. Even today, PUMC Hospital is still regarded as an "ivory tower" of Chinese medicine. Some professors from PUMC Hospital moved to Taiwan in 1949, and some of them changed their specialization from surgery to anesthesiology and became the early practitioners of anesthesiology there. They made important contributions to the foundation and development of modern anesthesiology in Taiwan.

The Modern Period: The Essentials of Modern Anesthesia Around the World

The last 25 years has been an exciting period for anesthesia, largely because the ability to share clinical and research experience has made the practice safer and better than it ever has been.

Today, all anesthesiologists, no matter where they practice in the world, can gain access to the information necessary to deliver safe anesthesia. However, there are still places in the world that do not have access to the equipment or supplies needed to implement that knowledge. This section details the essentials: the roles and responsibilities, the facilities and equipment available, the education and accreditation, the professional societies, and the research conducted by anesthesiologists around the world.

Roles and Responsibilities of Anesthesia Providers

India (Deepak K. Tempe)

In India, anesthesia can be administered only by a qualified anesthesiologist or by a trainee anesthesiologist under the supervision of a qualified anesthesiologist. In some states, such as Delhi, a directive from the government has been issued that states, "Anesthesia must be administered by a qualified anesthesiologist, i.e., an anesthesiologist with a postgraduate qualification and who has been actively working."

The duties and responsibilities of anesthesiologists have been evolving, but they have not yet been clearly defined by the ISA or health care officials (Ministry of Health). Nevertheless, it is now well recognized that an anesthesiologist's work is not limited to the operating room (OR). Typically, anesthesiologists in India are involved in the following types of care: (1) preoperative assessment and preparation of patients; (2) perioperative care of patients; (3) pain relief during the perioperative period; (4) management of critically ill patients; (5) management of acute, chronic, and cancer-related pain; (6) management and teaching of resuscitation skills; (7) provision of outpatient anesthesia services; (8) administrative involvement in setting up and managing health care organizations; (9) disaster management coordinator in the hospital; and (10) teaching and training of the medical and paramedical staff.

In addition to the duties just listed, both natural and man-made disasters have provided an extra challenge for anesthesiologists. By virtue of their ability to administer emergency life support measures, as well as their perioperative management skills, anesthesiologists were at the forefront during the Gujrat earthquake and tsunami disasters and actively participated in setting up operating theaters on site and providing care to victims. Likewise, during the Mumbai and Delhi bomb blasts, anesthesiologists played a leading role in carrying out emergency surgery and perioperative management.

Preoperative Evaluation. Despite preoperative evaluation and preparation of the patient being integral components of safe surgery, there were no dedicated preoperative anesthesia clinics (PACs) in India until recently. That began to change in the early 1980s, and today almost all hospitals have a dedicated PAC in which all patients are screened before surgery (including outpatient day surgery). PACs have become increasingly important because of a growing incidence of cardiovascular and other systemic diseases in patients undergoing surgery. In PACs anesthesiologists review and optimize the treatment of other systemic diseases, as well as detect new diseases and health concerns. In addition to improving patient outcomes, PACs help develop the patient-physician relationship and patient awareness about anesthesia. A few hospitals have started awareness programs wherein a lecture is delivered (with illustrations) on a monthly basis to patients and their relatives to make them familiar with the anesthetic techniques and procedures that they will undergo.

Operating Room. The OR continues to be the mainstay of anesthetic practice, but because ORs are the major consumers of hospital resources, as well as a major source of income for private hospitals, it is imperative that ORs be managed in the most efficient manner. However, there is no consensus on an ideal system to ensure efficiency in this area. The anesthesiologist is actively involved in trying to improve efficiency, especially with triage and scheduling of urgent and emergency cases. Safety is another concern. The professional risks (especially those related to needlestick injuries) of anesthesiologists, as well as other workers in the OR, are well recognized, and preventing such health care hazards has become an important consideration.

Recovery Room and Postoperative Intensive Care Units. Appropriate postoperative care is crucial for the success of surgery. Today in India, depending on the nature of the surgery and the patient's condition, the patient is transferred to either a recovery room or an ICU; some version of an ICU or recovery room exists in almost all major hospitals in India today. The nomenclature of these areas is not uniform, though, so terms that include postoperative ward, recovery room, high-dependence unit, critical care unit, and PACU are often used to describe the same facility. At some hospitals, especially those in which major and complex surgery requiring postoperative ICU management is not performed regularly, there is no demarcation between an

ICU and the recovery room. A single area designated as a recovery room is used for both purposes.

Where there is a distinction, the decision about where a postsurgical patient belongs is governed by the degree of morbidity. If a patient is very sick and requires ventilation and careful hemodynamic monitoring, the patient is transferred to an ICU. If mechanical ventilation and continuous hemodynamic monitoring are not required, the patient is transferred to a recovery room, which is perhaps the equivalent of the PACU. Patients undergoing daycare surgery (if practiced in a given hospital) are also transferred to the recovery room before discharge.

Most recovery rooms are under the charge of an anesthesiologist; in the case of ICUs, sometimes the anesthesiologist is in charge and sometimes not. Practice varies from place to place and is generally governed more by the logistics involved in a particular hospital than by any definite norms.

AMBULATORY CARE AND OTHER AREAS. Although it is recognized and appreciated that ambulatory care is a distinct possibility in a substantial number of patients, it is not practiced as much as it should be. It is difficult to provide exact figures in this matter, but in general, it is the private/corporate hospitals that practice ambulatory care. The number of government hospitals practicing ambulatory care is relatively small, mainly because of logistic reasons. That is likely to change, however, with the increasing availability of short-duration anesthetic drugs and modern surgical facilities (tools for minimally invasive surgery). Saving cost to the patient and the hospital and increasing patient turnover have been the major factors influencing interest in ambulatory care. The safety issues related to ambulatory care are well recognized, but there are no guidelines or recommendations from the ISA or any other regulatory body on this matter.

Anesthesia services are also frequently required in several other areas outside the OR. These areas tend to be less familiar to most anesthesiologists and provide less access to the facilities typically available in an OR. Their proliferation, however, has increased the demands on our profession. Areas where anesthesia is playing an increasingly prominent role include radiology suites (computed tomography, magnetic resonance imaging [MRI], and interventional radiology), the cardiac catheterization laboratory, electrophysiologic laboratories, the endoscopy room, and the electroconvulsive therapy room. In most of these areas patients require sedation, but with some lengthy procedures—such as MRI, electrophysiologic studies, and some interventional procedures—patients tend to get restless and may require general anesthesia. In addition, special considerations such as long breathing circuits or MRI-compatible equipment may be necessary. The anesthesiologist should be familiar with these requirements to maintain safety standards.

CRITICAL CARE MEDICINE. In the beginning, the anesthesiologist's focus on critically ill patients was ventilatory care because anesthesiologists are well versed in cardiorespiratory physiology and ventilatory management. Furthermore, managing a critically ill patient was considered an extension of the job that anesthesiologists performed in the OR. Therefore, the anesthesiologist managed patients receiving controlled ventilation via a ventilator and, ultimately, weaned the patient from mechanical ventilation.

Subsequently, however, it became obvious that respiratory function was only one aspect (albeit a crucial one) of the care of the critically ill. Anesthesiologists therefore became well informed about cardiovascular support, nutrition, infection, and various other diagnostic procedures. However, the interest of anesthesiologists in critical care medicine has been waxing and waning, and other specialists have entered this field. Currently, management of critical care units in India tends to be split: some are managed by physicians not trained in anesthesia, others by anesthesiologists.

There is widespread agreement that a critical care specialist who is devoted full-time to the care of critically ill patients should manage a critical care unit. The consensus includes three key items: (1) a dedicated expert irrespective of the specialty (if not holding a critical care qualification) should be in charge of the critical care unit; (2) each hospital can follow practices according to the availability of trained or experienced personnel with the primary aim of giving the best possible care; and (3) care of critically ill patients is always a team-based process, and the practice of taking the advice of different experts in managing a particular case is encouraged to achieve better outcomes.

Critical care training has long been part of the anesthesia residency program in India, but in 2001 the National Board of Examinations initiated a full-fledged 2-year training program in critical care medicine with 6 seats throughout India; the number has now increased to 25. Anesthesiologists, chest physicians, and general physicians are eligible to seek admission to this program. Clearly, the number of these specialized intensivists is not sufficient to cater to the critical care units that have mushroomed all over the country, so some disparities exist in the personnel involved in the management of critically ill patients.

In summary, critical care medicine has emerged as a new specialty but is still evolving in India. Because the number of persons having a qualification in the critical care area is not sufficient to fill current needs, anesthesiologists and physicians with interest in the specialty continue to practice critical care medicine. Out of a total of around 25 training seats, anesthesiologists account for about half, followed by general physicians (30%) and chest physicians (20%). The fact that all the seats in this program get filled suggests the growing interest in this specialty area.

PAIN MANAGEMENT. Interest in managing pain, both acute and chronic, has been growing over the last 2 decades. Nevertheless, the specialty is in its infancy in India, the number of pain clinics is limited, and there is no formal training program. The focus has largely been on the treatment of chronic pain, including cancer pain. Most anesthesiology departments perform nerve blocks, with a few even practicing acupuncture. There are, however, very few departments that have the facilities to conduct procedures such as radiofrequency ablation, implantation of intrathecal pumps, or spinal cord stimulation. The thrust now is toward treating pain as a disease, especially in patients suffering from nervous disorders or in terminal cancer patients where the only possible form of management is alleviation of pain.

There is also growing awareness of the management of acute pain, including the possibility of providing the patient with a totally pain-free surgical experience. After all, the WHO now recognizes pain as the fifth vital sign, and alleviation of pain is regarded as a basic human right. Various forms of medicine and equipment (patient-controlled analgesia pumps; intrathecal, epidural, and intrapleural techniques) can now offer the possibility of a relatively pain-free course of surgical treatment. Indeed, management of acute pain during the entire perioperative period is a leading concern of all anesthesia departments and is also actively practiced in recovery rooms or PACUs. However, much needs to be done regarding pain management in India. The Indian Society for the Study of Pain was formed in the late 1980s and currently has about 3200 members. The society is working toward improving pain management, but it is facing tough challenges, mainly because of lack of awareness. One looks forward to improving pain relief facilities in the country.

Russia (Olga Afonin)

Until the 1980s, Russia's anesthesia educational system was unified and structured into courses for nurse anesthetists and postgraduate education for physicians that included either a 1-year anesthesiology internship or a 2-year "Orditatura" (analogue of residency). All the programs included intensive care (reanimatology) as an obligatory part of the education. Participants were working in operating rooms and ICUs under the supervision of attending physicians and had a required course of lectures. Self-education was encouraged as well. After completion of training, graduates had to pass an oral qualification examination and were granted a Diploma of a Physician Anesthesiologist-Reanimatologist.

The quality of the education and the amount of experience varied significantly from program to program, and there were no universally accepted standardized examinations. Many conscientious anesthesiologists took additional courses on "qualification improvements" from the Academy of Physicians Postgraduate Education. However, there were also "specialists" whose education was finalized on completion of the courses.

By the end of the 1980s it became clear that the quality of education had to be monitored and the need for standardized examinations was debated to acceptance. Meanwhile, the Iron Curtain had become partially permeable to some of the information about accepted standards of education and care in the other countries. The future promised improvements, but not for long. The "era of stagnation" of the 1980s led to economic imbalance and a gradual decline in political structures. By the end of the 1980s, Communist leaders embarked on major reforms in an effort to revive the country's economics, which led to the collapse of the Soviet Union.

In turn, the continued financial support from the government for the entire medical structure became very thin and eventually disappeared. All the financially unsound programs, such as research, education, and development of new technologies or educational methods, were frozen. The government-funded health care system did not exist any more. Many professionals had to quit their careers for their families to survive. The private sector was in the very beginning of its development, and the great majority of the population could not afford private health care. It was not uncommon for patients to be asked to bring supplies for the medical care that they required, even for surgeries, and it was not uncommon for people to die as a result of the lack of proper medications or proper medical care. This continued until the mid-1990s, when things began to turn around. The damage, however, has not been completely overcome, even now.

As of today, anesthesiology education in Russia still requires revision and improvements. There is a need for structured residency programs that would teach the standards accepted around the world, which are based on decades of experience in the safe practice of anesthesiology. The Academy of Postgraduate Education recently introduced new standardized tests, comparable to internationally accepted graduation examinations, that would permit objective measurement of the knowledge of newly graduated anesthesiologists.

That said, with the exception of very few medical centers, most anesthesiologists have to practice their art of extremely invasive and possibly dangerous science without sufficient monitoring. Pulse oximeters, gas analyzers, and capnographs are still a luxury in many medical centers. Medical science is again government financed, but it is often still subject to the good will of the physicians who carve out time for research from their private lives. Russian anesthesiologists, as well as medics in other specialties, have been raising their concerns to the government. The Ministry of Health recently accepted a new national program for improvement in medical services, but it will take dramatic measures and significant investments in the health of Russian citizens for the country to achieve the goal of a safe and effective health care system in compliance with international standards. Statistics and the experience of multiple countries prove that the huge initial investments are returned as improvements in population health decrease medical and illness-related costs. It would be great to see Russia, the country that contributed so much to the growth and development of medicine and anesthesiology, return to the international scene as a partner in health promotion in all forms of medical science and art.

South America (Guillermo Lema)

For the past 50 years, anesthesiologists have been involved in PACUs and more recently have been responsible for them, including determination of the standards of care for these areas. Pediatric and cardiovascular anesthesia is generally performed by physicians with subspecialty training in these areas. Pain management and critical care reflect important areas where the influence of the anesthesiologist has been important. Anesthesia-trained personnel run most of these units.

Another area of interest is the choice that many physicians, including anesthesiologists, must make between public and private hospitals. For many years, anesthesiologists worked in public hospitals. Private practice came about afterward, in small clinics and in other institutions, with anesthesiologists generally continuing to work in public hospitals in the mornings. Nowadays, anesthesiologists tend to work solely in one hospital, either public or private.

Economic groups own most of the private clinics and run them under strict financial criteria. There are very strict professional duties, and the cost containment issue features heavily. Anesthesiologists, as well as other specialties, have lost control of these institutions, although a few have dedicated their time to administrative duties.

The resources given to public hospitals are increasing, but the benefit of these resources is less than one might expect, probably because of central and nonprofessional administration. Thus, economic restraints and inadequate conditions for anesthesiologists make posts in public practice less attractive than in private institutions.

Southeast Asia (Florian R. Nuevo)

The Association of Southeast Asian Nations (ASEAN) includes Brunei Darussalam, Cambodia, Indonesia, Laos, Malaysia, Myanmar, the Philippines, Singapore, Thailand, and Vietnam. While maintaining their operating room presence, anesthesiologists in this region are beginning to assume duties outside the operating room.

First, having gained the respect of their medical colleagues, anesthesiologists have become an important part of perioperative care and critical care management teams. Many are also moving toward pain management, which has paved the way to the Association of Southeast Asian Pain Societies, with the main goal of promoting further advancement in the study of pain in the region. Some anesthesiologists also practice anesthesia in conjunction with intensive care medicine. Hospice care and palliative medicine are also areas where anesthesiologists are now part of the team. In addition, ASEAN anesthesiologists have emerged as leaders in their national medical organizations and have become essential stakeholders in almost every aspect of medical and surgical care.

However, as we enter areas outside the delivery and operating suites, we must caution ourselves to slow down. ASEAN anesthesiologists must remain focused in our work, within that small space in operating theaters, where we remain the unsung heroes. Physician anesthesiologists should take full responsibility for safeguarding all patients who entrust their whole being to us while undergoing a diagnostic or therapeutic procedure—asleep, immobilized, unable to protect himself from harm—with the hope that as patients regain consciousness, they will not only be healed but comforted as well.

Europe (Lars I. Eriksson and Peter Simpson)

The main areas of work in European anesthesia departments are delivery of operating room anesthesia, postoperative care, critical care medicine, pain medicine, emergency medicine, and prehospital care. In some countries, such as Italy, Germany, Norway, and the United Kingdom, more than 30% of the daily activity of anesthesiologists is devoted to critical care medicine, and in some countries a large proportion of anesthesiologists are also involved in acute and chronic pain medicine.[18]

Delivery of anesthesia in the operating room is most often performed by anesthesiologists and nurse anesthetists, although the number of operating rooms staffed by nurse anesthetists and supervised by a certified anesthesiologist varies between countries. A recent survey has indicated that Greece, Ireland, Italy, Spain, the United Kingdom, Lithuania, Bosnia-Herzegovina, and Israel do not have programs for nurse anesthetists.[18] In all remaining countries, the number of nurse anesthetists per 100,000 population varies largely, from 0.7 in Albania and 4.9 in Turkey to 106.4 in Luxembourg. In most Western European countries (except Luxembourg and Switzerland), nurse anesthetists have undergone formal examination before graduation.

In Western European countries, surveys estimate that more than 70% of an average clinician's time is spent providing operating room anesthesia, with about 20% being spent in critical care medicine, 5% in pain control, and 5% in prehospital care.[18] A similar distribution of working time is found among non–European Union (EU) member countries from all parts of Europe, including the former Eastern Europe. Although most critical care units are staffed by anesthesiologists who have an interest and training in critical care medicine and who are associated with departments of anesthesia, in some countries an increasing number of departments of critical care medicine are staffed by dedicated specialists in critical care medicine.

Facilities and Equipment

India (Deepak K. Tempe)

In India, the journey from open-drop chloroform and ether anesthesia to the present-day high-tech operating theaters with anesthesia workstations and monitors, ICUs, PACUs, pain clinics, and preanesthetic checkup clinics is nearly complete. In fact, the ORs in India have undergone huge change during the last 2 to 3 decades. The present day OR is totally modular in structure with high-tech anesthesia workstations, monitoring systems, and online networking of the various equipment that is used. Such a change has been largely due to the arrival of private investment and management in the health care business. These corporate hospitals have built state-of-the-art ORs that match the best of the ORs in the rest of the world.

One should remember, however, that like many other things in India, diversity is also a hallmark of the health care system. Although corporate and other private hospitals have state-of-the-art ORs, government hospitals—other than those in cities such as Delhi and Mumbai—may not. In general, government hospitals cater to the general population and are overcrowded with long waiting lists. The situation in rural areas in particular is not up to the mark because these places typically have only primary health centers with basic facilities and the ORs are equipped to deal with just minor surgical procedures. Thus, ORs of several varieties can still be seen in India, and one hopes that this diversity gradually changes to uniformity in times to come.

It has been quite a challenging and turbulent journey from the days when Mahatma Gandhi was operated on with the open-drop chloroform technique to today. However, it is satisfying to see that developments in anesthesia have kept pace with time in India. Consider that recently the present Prime Minister Dr. Manmohan Singh underwent prostatectomy at the All India Institute of Medical Sciences (AIIMS). During that procedure, anesthesiologists used a balanced general anesthesia with drugs such as fentanyl, midazolam, sevoflurane, and atracurium and full-fledged monitoring. In addition, they used a patient-controlled analgesia pump for postoperative analgesia.

The Middle East (Anis Baraka)

The anesthetic machinery, monitoring equipment, and anesthetics used match the international standards that are approved by international societies, such as the American Society of Anesthesiologists. Figure 3-5 shows the operating room and illustrates monitoring of a patient undergoing coronary artery bypass grafting at the American University of Beirut Medical Center, which has updated anesthesia equipment.

South America (Guillermo Lema)

In South America, as in other places in the world, the economic resources invested in medicine and anesthesia depend on the economic situation of the country. The huge disparity in economic growth among countries in the region has produced an enormous difference in public resources allocated to health care, which has created diverse conditions for public health management. Moreover, anesthesia has been a relatively low government priority in many countries because governments often perceive anesthesia as having high cost (because of the technology) and little impact on the improvement of health care.

Nevertheless, countries with anesthesia as a mature specialty (Argentina, Brazil, Colombia, Chile, and Uruguay) have modern equipment, advanced monitoring technology, and access to all types of anesthetics and ancillary drugs, comparable to the United States and Europe. Anesthesia techniques vary, and many different types are being practiced. Anesthesia with volatile anesthetics has been used widely for many years and in all of these

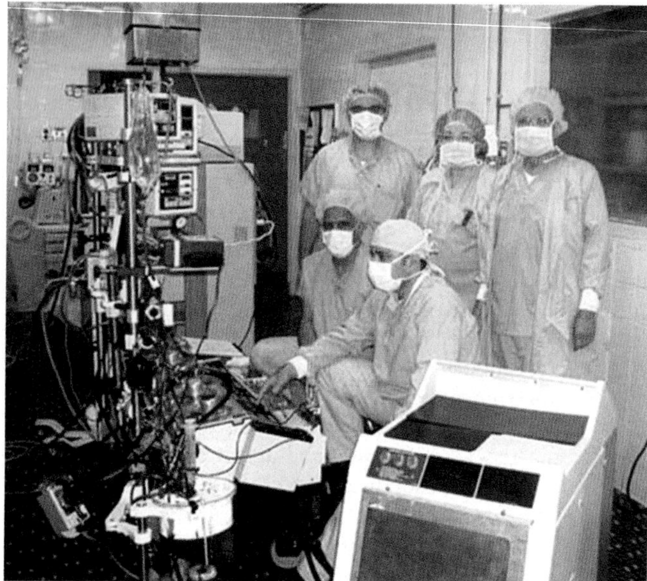

Figure 3-5 The operating room at the American University of Beirut Medical Center, which shows the updated anesthesia equipment and monitoring of a patient undergoing coronary artery bypass grafting.

countries. Total intravenous anesthesia is also common these days, and the use of regional anesthesia has been widespread. Other countries, because of resource constraints, practice a more basic form of anesthesia. Regardless of resources, however, all anesthesiologists in South America need to have a strong focus on cost containment. Indeed, this situation is common globally.

Uganda/Sub-Saharan Africa (D.G. Bogod)

In a 2007 survey of more than a quarter of Uganda's anesthetic practitioners, 23% thought that their facilities met all of the widely accepted minimal standards for the practice of safe, adult anesthesia. Categories surveyed included access to updated information, basic operating room equipment, and the most basic supply of anesthetic drugs. For safe pediatric anesthesia, only 13% thought that their facility met the basic requirements.[19]

For spinal anesthesia techniques, more than half of the anesthesiologists surveyed did not have regular access to the necessary local anesthetics, and others did not have a ready supply of spinal needles. Only 23% could guarantee being able to find a brush to clean their tracheal tube between procedures.[19]

For cesarean sections in women during childbirth, nearly all of the respondents (94%) said that they did not have the facilities to perform this procedure safely. More than three quarters did not have reliable access to magnesium sulfate, and half of them said that they could never get it.[19]

As D. G. Bogod, editor-in-chief of *Anaesthesia*, wrote in the editorial of the issue in which these numbers were published:

> *The figures revealed by this survey show that despite the best efforts of all involved, 27 million Ugandans essentially enter a lottery every time they undergo anaesthesia—a lottery with poor odds of a happy outcome. What the authors cannot tell us is whether this problem is confined to Uganda alone . . . it would be foolish to try to extrapolate from one country to another, but it is unlikely that Uganda data differ wildly from most of sub-Saharan Africa. . . . If the situation in Uganda is bad, it is likely to be far worse in Ethiopia, Somalia, Tanzania and many other neighbouring countries.*[19]

Japan (Michiaki Yamakage)

The following summary of the practice and scope of anesthesia in Japan was excerpted, with permission, from the *Journal of Anesthesia*.[20]

> *In the 1980s, general anesthesia was mainly conducted using halothane or enflurane with nitrous oxide (laughing gas). Fentanyl, an opioid analgesic, was also available, but was rarely used because it was believed to cause delay in awakening. Epidural anesthesia was used more frequently then than it is now. For example, cervical epidural anesthesia was generally used in surgery on upper limbs or for breast cancer. The only intravenous anesthetics available at that time were thiamylal and ketamine, which was administered to asthma patients despite its known secretion-promoting effects. The depolarizing neuromuscular blocking drug (NMBA) succinylcholine was used for induction of anesthesia and the nondepolarizing NMBA pancuronium was the only NMBA available for maintenance of anesthesia. During the 1980s, there was no awareness of the progression of acute renal failure during emergency surgery, and some patients did not awake from anesthesia for a long time after surgery due to the prolonged effect of pancuronium.*
>
> *Since the 1980s, various anesthetic agents have become available in Japan. The availability of a large range of anesthetic agents together with the development of anesthetic monitors has made anesthesia a much safer and more comfortable procedure for patients. However, Japan (maybe due to its unique medical system) lags behind the US and Europe with regard to the use of anesthetic agents other than sevoflurane. The ultrashort-acting opioid analgesic remifentanil has finally been launched in Japan, and the fast-onset nondepolarizing NMBA rocuronium is expected to become available soon. The selective relaxant binding agent sugammadex that is currently being used in phase III clinical trials throughout the world is also expected to be approved for clinical use in the near future.*
>
> *General anesthesia with airway management using a laryngeal mask is increasing in Japan due to the promotion of this device and the widespread use of ProSeal (Laryngeal Mask, Jersey, UK), which has high sealability. The indication for this method of anesthesia depends on the anesthesiologist, although it is generally not used for laparotomy, thoracotomy, or for prolonged general anesthesia. If the device has high sealability and can withstand positive pressure ventilation, anesthetic management is sometimes performed under artificial ventilation with the use of NMBAs. The use of the laryngeal mask is expected to increase further.*
>
> *In the US and Europe, day surgery has become popular due to the high costs of hospitalization. Day surgery in Japan, however, is rare as most patients have national and private medical insurance. However, the duration of hospitalization is expected to become shorter with the introduction of a comprehensive medical system, though it is impossible to predict at present whether this will have an effect on the methods of anesthesia used.*

Methods used for postoperative analgesia differ greatly between countries, and between institutions in Japan. In the US and Europe, patient-controlled analgesia is popular, and intravenous opioids alone are used in about two-thirds of patients. The combination of intravenous opioids with epidural analgesia appears to be used only for patients who have undergone upper abdominal surgery or thoracotomy. In Japan, epidural analgesia with or without intravenous opioids is used for postoperative pain control in almost 50% of patients. When delivery of fentanyl by iontophoresis (Ionsys; Ortho-McNeil, Titusville, NJ, US), which is currently being tested in trials, becomes applicable for clinical use, the methods used for postoperative analgesia might undergo great change.

Finally, . . . the number of surgery cases in specialized hospitals, including university hospitals, is expected to continue to rise in Japan. Due to the increasingly advanced age of patients and an increase in incompatibility complications, the number of cases anesthetically managed by neural block or general anesthesia alone is also growing.

In Japan, with the launch of remifentanil, the anticipated approval of rocuronium, and when sugammadex and the fentanyl iontophoretic transdermal system become available, the methods used for anesthesia will continue to change significantly in the future.

Clinical use in Japan of xenon, an ideal anesthetic, and dexmedetomidine, a respiratory-sparing sedative, is unknown and controversial due to their high cost and prolonged effect/"off label" use, respectively.

Education, Accreditation, and Availability of Practitioners

India (Deepak K. Tempe)

In India, there are mainly two types of postgraduate qualifications that one can obtain in the field of anesthesiology. The first, provided by medical colleges (MD in anesthesiology, a 3-year degree program), is governed by the Medical Council of India (MCI), which oversees the syllabus and other teaching and training standards. The second one is provided by the National Board of Examinations, which awards a degree called Diplomate of National Board (DNB). In addition, the MCI also regulates the "diploma in anaesthesiology (DA)," which is a 2-year training program that is available at medical colleges.

In 1992 it was determined that no new medical college or postgraduate course could be started without the prior approval of the MCI, and the recommendations of the MCI became mandatory for all medical colleges. Thus, it was only after the addition of this section, known as 10a, that teaching and training in the medical field in India were standardized and minimum standards were enforced. The strength of the MCI as a regulatory body was further reinforced in 1998 by a Supreme Court judgment, which ruled that the regulations of the MCI are mandatory and must be applied to all medical colleges in India. As of now, the recognition awarded by the MCI for undergraduate courses must be reviewed every 5 years by an inspection team of the MCI.

However, this is not so for postgraduate courses. Institutions conducting a postgraduate course today can enjoy the benefit of one-time MCI recognition, but the MCI will soon implement a review process every 5 years for postgraduate courses. Thus, teaching and training in anesthesiology in India are standardized through the setting of minimum standards throughout the country in terms of the facilities (space, equipment, manpower, and infrastructure) and the syllabus.

GROWTH OF THE SPECIALTY. The interest of Indian medical students in the specialty of anesthesiology has shown a dramatic increase during the last decade. Candidates for a postgraduate course in anesthesiology used to be admitted on the basis of scores obtained on the MBBS examination. This practice has now changed to conducting a common entrance examination, and admission to a given subject area is decided on the basis of the rank obtained by the student. In a few states such as Delhi, this has been the practice for approximately 20 years.

Table 3-1 shows the top and bottom ranks that were admitted to an MD anesthesiology program between 2002 and 2007 in the states of Maharashtra and Delhi. The table indicates that interest among students to learn and practice anesthesia is increasing. Reasons for the growing interest in anesthesia among students could be related to the increasing scope of anesthesia (as discussed earlier) and better job prospects. It may also be related to resistance to pursuing other fields, such as general surgery and general medicine, which require further subspecialty training. In Delhi, anesthesiology is among the top six specialties preferred by medical students, along with radiology, dermatology, pediatrics, orthopedics, and gynecology. This is in sharp contrast to the situation about 10 to 15 years ago, when anesthesiology was among the last five choices.

There are a total of 269 medical colleges in India with 30,000 undergraduate and 9100 postgraduate seats. Of these, there are 612 seats in MD anesthesia and 528 in DA anesthesia. In addition, the Ministry of Health and Family Welfare of India recognizes the DNB as a qualification in the given field and equates it with the postgraduate degrees awarded by other Indian universities; there are approximately 205 DNB seats in anesthesiology.

One challenge is assigning seats, especially because it remains unclear just how many anesthesiologists India needs. According to one estimate, there are approximately 28,000 anesthesiologists in India and the country requires about 7000

Table 3-1 Overall Rankings of Postgraduate Students Enrolled in Anesthesiology Programs in Maharashtra and Delhi (2002-2007)

	Maharashtra		Delhi	
Year	Top Rank	Bottom Rank	Top Rank	Bottom Rank
2002	228	854	65	98
2004	No exam		53	96
2005	405	642	32	96
2006	160	606	33	99
2007	106	504	61	85

Note: The total number of postgraduate seats in all subjects is 140 in Delhi and 450 in Maharashtra. The students often sit for entrance examinations in several states, which probably explains why the last rank exceeds the number of seats in Maharashtra.

more (data provided by the current president of the ISA at the Uttar Pradesh chapter congress in November 2007).

The Middle East (Anis Baraka)

The departments of anesthesia in the different Middle East countries consist of highly academic staff certified either by the Arab Board or foreign academic bodies, such as the American Board of Anesthesiology of the United States and the Faculty of the Royal College of Anaesthetists of the United Kingdom.

South America (Guillermo Lema)

Training of anesthesiologists is a contentious issue in South America. First, there is a large discrepancy between the views of anesthesia societies and the government with regard to the number of anesthesiologists needed. All countries on the continent have anesthesia training programs of different quality. The governments run a few, but universities conduct most of them.

There is no dispute about the length of time needed for training; regardless of who runs the program, 3 years is required to complete the training. Some countries also have specific scientific organizations run by universities and scientific societies to certify the various places where anesthesia is being taught. There are still places without proper certification that teach residents, but they are gradually being restricted from teaching.

Requirements for anesthesiologists are viewed differently by governments and scientific societies. Governments push for increased numbers of practitioners, whereas universities prefer better trained ones. Despite such difficulties, anesthesiologists and their scientific societies have campaigned for greater influence in the processes of accreditation. To the author's knowledge, only two countries have an anesthesia training program conducted by anesthesia societies; however, in those countries conflict with the government is even greater.

Further training of anesthesiologists is performed abroad, usually in Europe, the United States, or some prominent anesthesia departments in South America: Buenos Aires (Argentina), San Paulo (Brazil), and Santiago (Chile).

China (Yuguang Huang)

In Chinese medical universities, there currently exist 8-year, 7-year, and 5-year options for training in anesthesiology. Specialists in anesthesiology come mostly from undergraduate and postgraduate programs. The system of nurse anesthesiologists is not popular in China. More than 80,000 anesthesia professionals are available in mainland China, based on data from Dr. Shuren Li, Emeritus President of the CSA in 2007.

Southeast Asia (Florian R. Nuevo)

In the Philippines, the certification process for anesthesia includes three phases: a written examination, an oral examination, and practical examinations. Every year, a national anesthesia in-service examination is conducted that gives a percentile assessment of the standing of each trainee. However, even though our medical education has an American flavor, there is no reciprocity with the United States. Everybody must still comply with the licensure requirements or examinations prescribed by the United States to be able to pursue fellowships in anesthesia subspecialties. Thailand, Singapore, Malaysia, and Indonesia have their own framework of certification, one that is more European in context and process.

For basic training on the fundamentals of anesthesiology, many Indonesians prefer to go to the Philippines. In addition, the WFSA supports a regional training center for Southeast Asian countries in Bangkok, Thailand. It is called the Bangkok Anesthesia Regional Training Center and has graduated anesthesiologists from Laos, Myanmar, Cambodia, and Mongolia.

The Anesthesiology Center for the Western Pacific in Manila, Philippines, is a joint activity of the WHO Regional Office for the Western Pacific, the University of the Philippines, the China Medical Board, and the WFSA. It is an 11-month course in anesthesia that was initiated in January 1970. The rationale for this center was to help alleviate the shortage of reliable anesthesiologists in the region and to underscore the importance of administering safe anesthesia. The center does not seek to provide a complete training program, but rather its purpose is to emphasize the basic sciences in anesthesiology. It creates a foundation for students to build on so that they can eventually qualify, through further training, as specialist anesthesiologists. Students come to the center from the Pacific Islands, Southeast Asia, southern Asia, Hong Kong, Taiwan, Korea, Japan, Iraq, Russia, and Sudan. The program has served the region for 16 consecutive years, and many of its graduates have become respected anesthesiologists and contributed to the development of anesthesia programs and safe anesthesia care in their respective countries. If further studies or a fellowship in anesthesia specialties is desired, Singapore and Malaysia are two countries that can offer these particular courses.

At present, only the societies of Malaysia, Singapore, and Philippines have a written monograph on the guidelines for minimum requirements in delivering safe anesthesia practice. The government of Malaysia supports the activity of a national medical audit system and includes respectable physicians from all specialties. Apart from Singapore, most ASEAN anesthesia programs have not developed a quality assurance program. In effect, we have no factual regional database to document and monitor anesthesia-related morbidity and mortality.

Organizations, certification requirements, and recognition of anesthesiologists in Southeast Asian countries are summarized in Table 3-2. Workforce, scope, and type of anesthesiology practice are summarized in Table 3-3.

A shortage of physician anesthesiologists has become a persistent problem in densely populated Southeast Asian countries such as Indonesia, Philippines, and Thailand. The Philippines has the largest number of physician anesthesiologists in this region but is beset by maldistribution of qualified anesthesiologists, with more found in urbanized areas and the majority electing to engage in private (not public) hospital practice.

One strategy to address this personnel shortage is to formally conduct training of nurse anesthesiologists. Unlike the situation in the United States, where nursing programs independently train nurse anesthesiologists, both Indonesia and Thailand have developed formal courses for nurse anesthesiologists. These nurse anesthesiologists are supervised by physician anesthesiologists—and there is a clearly defined demarcation of responsibilities between physician anesthesiologists and nurse anesthesiologists. Hence, through an anesthesia care team composed of physicians and nurses working together, they found the answer to the crying need for anesthesia services in Indonesia and Thailand.

In the Philippines, nurse anesthesia practice is considered illegal. It is not allowed under the Nursing Act of the country. Moreover, the Philippine Society of Anesthesiologists maintains

Table 3-2 Organizations, Certification Requirements, and Recognition of Anesthesiologists in Southeast Asian Countries

	Indonesia	Malaysia	Philippines	Singapore	Thailand
Training	4 years' medicine 1.5 years' internship 3.5 years' residency	Patterned after the British Stringent examination and promotion requirements	Patterned after the United States 3 years' residency	Patterned after the British Stringent examination and promotion requirements	3 years' residency
Certification/certifying organization/continuing medical education	Collegium of Indonesian Anesthesiologist		Philippine Board of Anesthesiology	Singapore Society of Anesthesiologists	Royal College of Anesthesiologists in Thailand
Societies	Indonesian Society of Anesthesiologists & Reanimateurs	Malaysian Society of Anaesthesiologists	Philippine Society of Anesthesiologists	Singapore Society of Anesthesiologists	
Roles outside the operating room			Critical care Pain management	Critical care Pain management	
Recognition by peers/accomplishment	Neuroanesthesia fellowship	National Anesthesia Day		Head of critical care	

that anesthesiology is a practice of medicine and will not allow nurses to deliver anesthesia care.

It is rather sad that the practice of medicine in Philippine government hospitals is not able to provide decent remuneration for the majority of its health care providers, including physician anesthesiologists. Migration of physicians to seek better alternatives in greener pastures is a reality. With the high demand for nurses worldwide, it is also not unusual for some physicians to take a 4-year bachelor's degree in nursing and decide to migrate abroad to work professionally as nurses.

Uganda/Sub-Saharan Africa (D.G. Bogod)

In a survey by Hodges and colleagues, there was only 1 medical anesthesiologist among the 91 anesthesia practitioners who participated in the survey, which means that as is so often the case, many trained physicians in Uganda probably traveled to the West to find a better life for their families. In addition, based on the survey, access to up-to-date textbooks seems iffy at best—fewer than half of those surveyed have access to such texts.[18]

Europe (Lars I. Eriksson and Peter Simpson)

As a geographic area, Europe consists of more than 30 countries, a number of which, during the last decade, have undergone the dynamic process of integration into the EU. Although a core of European countries has had a strong impact for many years on development of the EU, several other countries, many of them belonging to the former Eastern Europe, are still candidates or potential candidates for entry into the EU. Europe is therefore a heterogeneous region and group of countries, which is reflected in the large variation in medical systems, research, and education, as well as language and culture. Over the years, continuous expansion of the number of countries associated with the EU has inevitably affected financial, monetary, labor, and educational systems in the other member states. Inevitably, this has also changed health care systems and provided a new impetus for increased migration of qualified health care workers and academic personnel between member states. Partly because of the large variation in social welfare and financial systems between parts of Eastern Europe and the traditional Western European countries, the net

Table 3-3 Workforce, Scope, and Type of Anesthesiology Practice in Southeast Asian Countries

	Indonesia	Malaysia	Philippines	Singapore	Thailand
Workforce					
Physician anesthesiologist	Yes	Yes	Yes	Yes	Yes
Nurse anesthesiologist	Yes	No	No	None	Yes
Scope of Practice					
Operating room*	Yes	Yes	Yes	Yes	Yes
Intensive care	Yes	Yes	Slowly developing	Yes	Yes
Pain management	Yes	Yes	Yes	Yes	Yes
Type of Practice					
Anesthesia care team (physician, nurse, technician)	Yes (physician has a supervisory role)	No	Limited group practice (consisting of physicians)	No	Yes (physician has a supervisory role)

*Includes anesthesia services for inpatient, ambulatory/office-based, and diagnostic procedures.

migration of health care workers has deprived many low-income countries of their own medical staff. In addition, new working time directives in Western European countries have led to increased demand for physicians, and taken together, these two issues have encouraged emigration from Eastern European countries. In general, the many changes brought about by the integration of new countries into the EU continue to have an impact on the practice of medicine in Europe, and in this context the practice of anesthesiology is no exception.

The average number of anesthesiologists within Western European countries has increased over the last decade from 10.8 to 14.5 per 100,000 population.[18,21] In contrast, among non-EU Eastern European countries, the average number of anesthesiologists is currently 6.1 per 100,000 population.[18] Hence, there is large variation in both the supply and demand of anesthesiologists between parts of Europe.

In most European countries, health care is funded by the government, although local exceptions to this rule exist. Whereas more than 50% of anesthesiologists in some Western European countries (Luxembourg, The Netherlands) are involved in private practice, anesthesiologists within Scandinavia and the United Kingdom rarely (less than 5%) work in private practice.

The European Diploma in Anesthesiology and Intensive Care (EDA). The EDA, introduced in 1984, is a two-part examination intended as a comprehensive test of knowledge of anesthesiology, critical care, and pain management. It provides an international European standard that allows harmonization of training and assessment of knowledge across all European countries and is used by some (Switzerland, Austria, Hungary, and Poland) as part of their internal examination structure. Both parts of the examination take place in designated centers across Europe, depending on demand. Part 1 consists of multilingual, multiple-choice questions available in English, French, German, Italian, Spanish, and Russian. It consists of two multiple-choice sections, one on basic physiology, pharmacology, physics, clinical measurement, and statistics and the other on clinical practice associated with anesthesia and its subspecialty areas. It is intended to be taken after approximately 2 years of anesthesia training. Part 2 consists of four oral examinations, each with two examiners moderating each other. Guidelines for the content of these oral examinations are determined by the examination committee, and each examination is divided again into clinical practice, intensive care medicine, and general anesthesia. Candidates may choose the language in which they wish to be examined within the constraints available at the examination center.

Success in Part 2, which is an end-of-training examination, qualifies the candidate to receive the EDA. Because the EDA is an assessment of anesthetic knowledge, it can in no way substitute for the local assessment of skills and professional attitudes or behavior that takes place in each country according to local systems and is a requirement before an individual can be placed on the specialist register of their country. Because entry onto a person's national specialist register is necessary before award of the EDA, it follows that anyone passing the Part 2 examination also has to provide evidence of specialist registration before receiving the EDA itself. Thus, the EDA examination is a test of knowledge, embedded in and dependent on assessment of clinical skills and attitudes, that is provided by the national training program.

In addition to the examination itself, there is also the option for those wishing to assess their level of knowledge to take the Part 1 EDA as an in-training examination at a much reduced fee. This not only allows personal assessment of one's knowledge but also includes detailed feedback so that candidates can assess their own performance—both in comparison to those in their national peer group and in comparison to candidates in other parts of Europe—in areas as detailed as cardiovascular physiology and other fields.

The ESA/EBA Joint Hospital Visiting and Accreditation Program (HVAP). The HVAP has been in place since January 1996 as a joint permanent committee of the European Society of Anaesthesiology (ESA, formerly the European Academy) and the European Board of Anesthesiology (EBA), its main goal being to encourage and enhance training standards across Europe and to ensure that an academic institution meets the prerequisites of training in anesthesia as set out in the EBA training guidelines (1996). Together with the EDA, the HVAP serves to improve the overall quality of the specialty of anesthesia and to harmonize its activities throughout Europe. The visit consists of a detailed presentation of the staffing and organization of the hospital, the department (or the institute), and the structure of training. This forms the basis for discussion and evaluation of all aspects of the teaching and training process with the staff members involved for the purpose of complementing and building on strengths and encouraging development and change to address areas of weakness. A subsequent comprehensive report of the visit, together with recommendations for improvement or accreditation (or both), is presented by the program committee.

Standardizing the Quality of Patient Care in Anesthesiology and Intensive Care. In recent years the opportunity for accredited specialists in anesthesiology and intensive care to work and move between different European countries has increased considerably. EU legislation allows such free movement of specialists, which in many ways is beneficial to everyone. In such circumstances, it is essential to ensure that the quality and safety of care that patients receive is sustained and enhanced. Training and accreditation programs inevitably vary between member states and even within countries that lack a single national organization. The EBA is uniquely placed to ensure that appropriate standards are set to achieve harmonization in the quality and safety of patient care, and two important areas of standardization are already in place: the joint HVAP and the EDA.

At the present time, although the standards of well-established training and accreditation programs are known and thus acknowledged across many European states, others are not, particularly in some of the countries that have recently joined the EU. As a result, those trained in these countries are potentially unfairly disadvantaged. Their specialists wish to move freely as much as others and should be able to do so. Equally, those appointing them to specialist posts need a uniform quality standard to ensure the delivery of high-quality and safe patient care. Individual countries' specialist qualifications do vary, and an international assessment standard to facilitate free movement of specialists is needed. New proposals for EBA membership and fellowship have been developed and agreed on and build on the initiatives and programs already in place. These proposals are in addition to—but do not replace—national qualifications or competence in discourse or dialogue and allow those who desire to clearly demonstrate their ability to deliver anesthetic care of a uniformly high standard to patients. They are marks of individual excellence in the specialty and can be awarded only after European national accreditation as a medical specialist in anesthesiology is achieved. They will be open to anesthesiologists who are nationals of any country in the world and who are on the specialist anesthesiology register of a European country. They will be strictly awarded to individuals in recognition of their personal achievement and not automatically to all those working in a particular hospital or anesthesiology department. However, they will have no legal standing and do not in themselves confer a right to practice in a country of the EU.

Subspecialization

India (Deepak K. Tempe)

For more than 2 decades, anesthesiologists have recognized the need for dedicated practice in the field of cardiac anesthesia and neuroanesthesia. There are anesthesiologists who are working exclusively in these specialties, but there are no separate departments of cardiac anesthesia and neuroanesthesia. AIIMS is an exception in this respect because it created two such departments in 1986. Postdoctoral courses in these specialties have been started in the country. AIIMS has conducted the courses in both specialties since 2002, whereas the Sri Chitra Tirunal Institute of Medical Sciences, Thiruvananthpuram, has offered a course in cardiac anesthesia since 2003. The number of seats, however, is grossly inadequate, with four seats in cardiac anesthesia and two in neuroanesthesia. The National Board of Examinations started a DNB fellowship program (2 years) in cardiac anesthesia in 2002; it began with four seats, and the number has increased to 18.

South America (Guillermo Lema)

In South America, only Colombia has a specialty law. In all other countries, physicians can perform professional actions without a law to certify the proficiency and quality of care and protect patients. In fact, physicians with a very low level of training have practiced anesthesia for many years; in most of the countries, paramedical personnel have performed anesthesia because of lack of sufficient medical personnel or interest in the specialty. In some countries, surgeons perform both anesthesia and surgery with the help of technical personnel. This practice has been abandoned in most countries, but in a few—Bolivia, Ecuador, Paraguay, Peru, and Venezuela—this situation persists, with government authorization.

Nowadays, the law in most countries specifies that only physicians can provide anesthesia. The problem is a shortage of trained physicians, so some countries are left with inadequately trained ones. Nevertheless, the process of certification of specialties, including anesthesia, is on the way. Most countries have medical organizations and anesthesia societies demanding proper certification methods. In some countries these medical organizations have obtained the support of the government. So even though a law does not exist, there is an intense effort to gain official certification. Medicolegal issues and increased concern from patients have helped. It is interesting that most anesthesiologists are willing to obtain certification; clinics and hospitals are also requiring certification for physicians to work in these institutions.

Professional and Research Activity

India (Deepak K. Tempe)

Since its inception in 1947, the ISA has grown from 19 members in 1947 to nearly 12,000 in 2007. Today, there are also separate Indian associations of cardiothoracic anesthesia and neuroanesthesia. The Indian Association of Cardiovascular and Thoracic Anesthesiologists (IACTA) is 10 years old and holds an annual meeting. IACTA also publishes the journal *Annals of Cardiac Anaesthesia*, which is now in the 10th year of publication and is the first Indian journal in anesthesia to be indexed in the National Library of Medicine and included in the MEDLINE database. In addition, there are societies of critical care medicine (founded in 1992) and for the study of pain.

The Middle East (Anis Baraka)

Most anesthesiologists in the Middle East are in close contact with developments in anesthesia throughout the world through attending congresses and lectures, publications, subscriptions to various international anesthesia journals, and building of worldwide friendships.

Some anesthesiologists in the Middle East, including those who have emigrated abroad, have become leaders in the specialty and have made original contributions in the fields of muscle relaxants,[22-24] semiopen systems, obstetrics,[25] pediatric anesthesia,[26,27] and the pathophysiology of open heart surgery.[28]

South America (Guillermo Lema)

Time, funding, and expertise are the basic requirements for research of sufficient quality to support publications or communications internationally. These requirements are not found widely in South America. Only a few university anesthesia departments have the capability of producing clinical research of high enough quality to be published in esteemed journals such as the Institute for Scientific Information (ISI), most notably in Chile. Some colleagues have argued that research is not important in a continent that has more pressing priorities. I do not agree.

Research is also a tool for learning and it should be encouraged, at least at university-based anesthesia residencies. Unfortunately, research does not generate income, so most of the clinical groups are not willing to dedicate time to this particular activity. Funding is lacking, and although some countries have national research grants to support clinical research, most do not. Support from drug companies is weak and usually depends on the impact that their drugs have in our clinical setting. Because of economic constraints, a large number of generic drugs are used, so major pharmaceutical companies are not willing to support research activities. In short, basic research in anesthesia virtually does not exist in South America.

Anesthesia meetings achieve the goal of educating residents and older generations of anesthesiologists. Anesthesia journals are in existence, and although none of them are ISI, effort is being made to enter the international medical databases.

China (Yuguang Huang)

The CSA was founded in 1979 at the Second National Conference held in Harbin. Professor Deyan Shang was elected president of the first CSA committee. Since then, a national CSA conference has been held every 3 or 4 years. In 1986, the Beijing International Conference on Anesthesia was held successfully. Many famous experts from abroad, including Professor Ronald Miller (this textbook's editor), were invited to join as keynote speakers.

From that point on, Chinese anesthesiologists began to communicate more with international professionals. At the first Sino-Japanese Clinic Anesthesia Symposium held in 1986, the CSA and Japan Society for Clinical Anesthesia agreed to hold a symposium every 2 years. Professor Ailun Luo, after being selected president of CSA in 1997, advocated China's integration into the world anesthesia community. The National Conference on Anesthesia is held annually on the second weekend of every September.

Regarding professional publications, Professor Rong Xie was chief editor of the *Encyclopedia of Chinese Anesthesia Medicine* in 1986. Professor Jun Zhao was the chief editor of *Modern Anesthesiology* in 1987. These books have contributed to the development of clinical and research anesthesiology in China. Two academic journals, *Chinese Journal of Anesthesiology* and *Journal of Clinical Anesthesiology*, were launched in 1981 and 1982 by the Chinese Medical Association. Besides these two journals, the *International Journal of Anesthesiology and Resuscitation* and the *Chinese Journal of Pain Medicine* have formed a good platform for rapid communication among Chinese anesthesiologists.

From the 1990s until today, research in Chinese anesthesiology has moved as fast as the economy of China. The CSA has built good cooperative relationships with many international associations, such as the American Society of Anesthesiologists, the International Anesthesia Research Society, and the Association of Anaesthetists of Great Britain and Ireland, among others. Many well-known journals including, *Anesthesia & Analgesia*, *Anesthesiology*, and *Anaesthesia*, have been published with Chinese editions, which has extended their influence among Chinese professionals. These localized journals will become the window for communication in anesthesiology between China and the world.

Southeast Asia (Florian R. Nuevo)

To lessen the variability in medical practice and anesthesia care—and with the vision of fostering more understanding and cooperation among ASEAN anesthesiologists—two pioneering anesthesiologists (Professor Quintin J. Gomez of the Philippines and Dr. Saywan Lim of Malaysia) conceived of the Confederation of ASEAN Societies of Anesthesiologists (CASA). This took place in Kuala Lumpur in September 1974 during a meeting after the Fourth Asian Australasian Congress of Anaesthesiologists, a regional congress of the WFSA.

The main objective of CASA is to enhance and promote the specialty of anesthesiology in the region by hosting biennial congresses of anesthesia called the ASEAN Congress of Anaesthesiologists. These congresses serve as a venue for ASEAN anesthesiologists to meet experts from the United States and Europe, as well as other international anesthesia leaders, and to learn current practices in anesthesia from them. They also inspire trainees and younger anesthesiologists in Southeast Asia to present their clinical trials and modest research activity and participate in scientific activities as resource speakers or workshop facilitators.

The first such congress was held in December 1979 in Manila, Philippines, under the leadership of Professor Gomez, who was then the incumbent president of the WFSA (1976-1980). More than 400 delegates came from Indonesia, Malaysia, Philippines, Singapore, Thailand, Japan, Taiwan, Hong Kong, and the United States. Professor John Bonica (United States) was the guest of honor and main invited speaker; Professor Bonica would later become president of the WFSA.

Over time, the objectives of CASA have grown. The group has strived to promote closer ties among member societies, to enhance the image of the specialty in the region, and to upgrade the specialty through exchange of information between local and international experts in anesthesia. Indeed, through CASA there has been an information avalanche that has paved the way to further upgrade and develop the practice of anesthesia and anesthesiologists themselves.

Unfortunately, of late, economic depression and terrorism—as well as health threats such as bird flu and severe acute respiratory syndrome (SARS)—have threatened these academic activities. Nevertheless, the ASEAN confederation has persisted in hosting its biennial congress. The five founding members take turns, with much enthusiasm and camaraderie, in hosting these meetings. Attendance has grown from 400 to almost a thousand anesthesiologists coming from ASEAN and non-ASEAN countries, such as Japan, Korea, China, Saudi Arabia, Mongolia, Canada, and the Middle East. The faculty of speakers includes local ASEAN and international anesthesia experts from the United States, Europe, Canada, Australia, and New Zealand, some of whom were supported by the WFSA, by industry, by respective anesthesia societies, and by the faculty themselves.

Currently, each of the CASA member organizations is conducting clinical research activities in anesthesia, but there is much room for improvement. Most research studies involve clinical drug trials funded by pharmaceutical companies, but there is a paucity of published papers in peer-reviewed anesthesiology. What is lacking is translating the research activities into well-written research papers.

The *ASEAN Journal of Anesthesiology* (AJA) is only 8 years old. Thus far it has served as an avenue to publish all of these research endeavors in the region. We encourage all member societies to submit their research papers for publication. The current seat of editorship of the AJA is located in Singapore. Perhaps to encourage more output, future ASEAN Congress of Anaesthesiologists meetings may provide incentives for participation in free papers and poster discussion sessions.

Europe (Lars I. Eriksson and Peter Simpson)

Before formation of the European Academy of Anaesthesiology in 1978 there was no formal representative structure for the specialty within Europe. The five statutory aims of the academy were to (1) raise the scientific level of the discipline; (2) improve the training of anesthetists, their clinical and theoretical education, and their competence at the completion of the training period by holding examinations; (3) hold scientific meetings, conferences, and seminars; (4) facilitate research in anesthesia and its associated disciplines; and (5) promote exchange among anesthetists and discussion of all matters concerning their profession.

The European Academy of Anaesthesiology had a limited number of members and academicians and, as European anesthesiology grew, was perceived by many to be an exclusive organization. In 1992, the ESA was formed and was open to everyone. Its chief aims were to conduct an annual Euroanesthesia meeting to replace the European Congress, which had formerly run on a 4-year cycle alternating with the World Congress, and to support educational and research activities by awarding grants and fellowships. Whereas the ESA was concerned with the practice of clinical anesthesia and supporting its membership, the European Academy of Anaesthesiology had developed formal initiatives such as the EDA, the *European Journal of Anaesthesiology* (EJA), and a system of hospital visiting and accreditation training in conjunction with the Anesthesiology Board and Section of the UEMS (Union Européenne des Médecins Spécialistes or European Union of Medical Specialists).

The fourth organization that existed at that time was the Confederation of European National Societies of Anesthesiology (CENSA), which was effectively the European section of the WFSA.

For some years, the roles of all the various organizations were increasingly complementary, thus making it necessary for an individual anesthesiologist to be a member of more than one body to participate in and benefit from all the variety of activities. As a result, in 1998 a decision was made to amalgamate the former ESA, the European Academy, and CENSA into one organization. A temporary organization, the European Federation of Anaesthesiologists, was established in 2001, under which amalgamation was successfully achieved, and the new European Society of Anaesthesiology, which thus represents every anesthesiologist in Europe, was launched in January 2005 in its interim form before becoming fully established in January 2006. Moreover, because the formal, declared responsibilities of the parent organizations were essentially different and there was very little overlap between them, a strong and comprehensive organization could be established right from the start. Under this new organizational structure, CENSA became the ESA's National Anaesthesiology Societies Committee, now ESA National. Each country has a number of delegates to ESA National, depending on the number of members of its National Society.

The ESA now provides a comprehensive range of activities to support European anesthesiology, primarily aimed at sustaining and enhancing the safety, efficacy, and quality of care of patients. Through publication of the EJA and the Euroanaesthesia organization and other meetings, it supports the interests of its members and facilitates the exchange and dissemination of information related to anesthesiology, critical care, pain, and emergency medicine. It encourages research and scientific progress both by conducting academic meetings and by awarding grants and fellowships and has a key role in raising and harmonizing the standards of anesthesiology. This is achieved by delivering education, training, continuous medical education, and accreditation of anesthetists through educational programs, the EDA, and in-service training examinations, as well as through the HVAP run jointly with UEMS.

UEMS represents national associations of medical specialists in the EU and its associated countries. UEMS provides general and specialist medical advice to ministers. It is also responsible for the European Accreditation Council for Continuing Medical Education. Each specialty has its own board and section, the members of which are drawn from all the EU member states together with Norway and Switzerland. The EBA has two delegates per country, one professional and one academic. UEMS itself is a nonprofit organization concerned with (1) the study, promotion, and harmonization of the highest level of training of medical specialists, medical practice, and health care within the EU; (2) study and promotion of free movement of specialist doctors within the EU; (3) representation, within this framework of medical specialists in the member states of the EU, to EU authorities and to any other authority with similar responsibility; and (4) protection of the professional interests of European medical specialists. UEMS defines a medical specialist as a physician who has satisfactorily completed a specialist training program in a recognized specialty that conforms to the UEMS charter on specialist training.

Thus, European anesthesiologists are represented in several ways. Those in EU member states, together with Norway and Switzerland, are represented nationally through their country's membership in the UEMS Anesthesiology Board and Section. Additionally, anesthesiologists in all European countries are represented nationally as members of their respective national society through that society's delegates to the ESA, through the ESA council via their national elected council member, and individually as active members of ESA.

The *European Journal of Anesthesiology*. The EJA is the official journal of the ESA and is distributed to all ESA members. It is published and owned by the ESA. The EJA is also the official journal of a variety of organizations (EACTA, UEMS, FEEA) and is distributed to all members of these societies. It is published monthly and run by an editorial board that is not directly involved in any editing or editorial work and by a 19-member "group of editors" who are responsible for the content of the journal itself. The EJA has two main functions: to publish peer-reviewed original articles and reviews in the field of anesthesia, pain, emergency medicine, and critical care, together with correspondence pertaining to these articles, and to provide educational material with appropriate methods of self-assessment for ESA members. The ESA also publishes a newsletter four times a year, separately from the EJA, that contains items of interest to ESA members together with information and formal announcements.

Conclusion

As demonstrated in this chapter, anesthesiology as a discipline and a profession has grown dramatically around the world. Differences in the rate of growth and scope of practice exist for a variety of reasons, largely because of disparities in resources and socioeconomic and political factors. Nevertheless, regardless of country of residence, patients can feel much safer today with regard to receiving anesthesia than even 20 or 30 years ago. As noted repeatedly throughout this chapter, some of the most powerful advances are the spread of knowledge, professional integrity, curiosity, and the utmost desire to practice anesthesiology at the highest possible level. This means that anesthesiologists not only can learn of the advances of their colleagues elsewhere but can also better understand and respond to the needs of others.

So where do we go from here? Some authorities suggest that we take advantage of the latest advances to further the interconnectedness of our profession, such as conducting more in-depth comparisons of the effectiveness of various techniques from country to country and engaging in more joint research. Others believe that such comparisons would serve no useful purpose given the disparities in resources and different approaches to care. The editor has dreamed of the day that anesthesiologists worldwide would form global think tanks to ask and answer the most important questions to advance our intellectual foundations and benefit society.

As is noted in the opening paragraph, the purpose of this chapter is not to invite comparisons or highlight differences in the practice of anesthesiology around the world, but rather to encourage and invite anesthesiologists globally to keep talking to each other. The editor was thrilled and honored that his invitation to contribute to this chapter has resulted in so many interesting contributions from leaders of anesthesia worldwide. When viewed together, the journey of anesthesiology has been an amazing story worldwide.

References

1. Agrawal DP: Susruta: The great surgeon of Yore. Available at http://www.infinityfoundation.com.
2. Kothare SN, Pai SA: Sweet slumber. Available at www.histmedindia.org.
3. Divekar VM, Naik LD: Evolution of anaesthesia in India. J Postgrad Med 47:149-152, 2001.
4. Jhaveri VK, Tendulkar DG. Escape from death. *In* Jhaveri VK, Tendulkar DG (eds): Mahatma: Life of Mohandas Karamchand Gandhi, vol 2. The Times of India, 1951, pp 156-166.
5. Baraka A: The contributions of Arabs to medicine. Middle East J Anesthesiol 15:353-359, 2000.
6. Brandt L: The first reported oral intubation of the human trachea. Anesth Analg 66:1198-1199, 1987.
7. Haddad FS: Ibn Sina (Avicenna) advocated orotracheal intubation 1000 years ago: Documentation of arabic and Latin originals. Middle East J Anesthesiol 17:155-162, 2000.
8. Haddad SI, Khairallah AA: A forgotten chapter in the history of the circulation of the blood. Ann Surg 104:1-8, 1936.
9. Takrouri MS, Khalaf M: Ibn al-Nafis contributions to science. Middle East J Anesthesiol 17:163-175, 2003.
10. Baraka A, Salem MR, Joseph NJ: The origin of the "algorithm." Anesthesiology 89:233, 1998.
11. Hunke S: Allah Sonne uber Dem Adenland unser arabisches Erbe. Beirut, Lebanon, Dar Al-Kitab Al-Jadidah, 1982, p 280.
12. Haddad FS: The spongia somnifera. Middle East J Anesthesiol 17:321-327, 2003.
13. Al-Mazrooa AA, Abdel-Halim RE: Anesthesia 1000 years ago. *In* Atkinson RS, Boulton TB (eds): The History of Anaesthesia. London, Royal Society of Medicine Services, Parthenon Publishing Group, 1989, pp 46-48.
14. Science Timeline: Available at http://www.sciencetimeline.net/prehistory.htm.
15. Haddad FS: History of anesthesia in Lebanon 1800-1914. Middle East J Anesthesiol 6:241-280, 1982.
16. Takrouri MSM, Seraj MA: Middle Eastern history of anesthesia. Middle East J Anesthesiol 15:397-413, 2000.
17. Wright AJ: Diffusion of an innovation: The first public demonstration of general anesthesia. Middle East J Anesthesiol 11:93-118, 1991.
18. Egger Halbeis CB, Cvachovec K, Scherpereel P, et al: Anesthesia workforce in Europe. Eur J Anaesthesiol 24:991-1007, 2007.
19. Bogod DG: One day for Africa: Anaesthesia in Uganda and beyond. Anaesthesia 62:1-3, 2007.
20. Yamakage M, Namiki A: Anesthetic practice in Japan: Past, present, and future. J Anesth 21:390-395, 2007.
21. Rolly G, MacRae WR, Blunnie WP, et al: Anaesthesiological manpower in Europe. Eur J Anaesthesiol 13:325-332, 1996.
22. Baraka A: The Influence of carbon dioxide on the neuromuscular block caused by tubocurarine chloride in the human subject. Br J Anaesth 36:272, 1964.
23. Ali HH, Utting JE, Gray C: Stimulus frequency in the detection of neuromuscular block in humans. Br J Anaesth 42:967-978, 1970.
24. Ali HH, Utting JE, Gray C: Quantitative assessment of residual anti depolarizing block (part II). Br J Anaesth 43:478, 1971.
25. Baraka A, Noueihid R, Hajj S: Intrathecal injection of morphine for obstetric analgesia. Anesthesiology 54:136-140, 1981.
26. Naughton P, Mossad E: Retraining the left ventricle after arterial switch operation: Emerging uses for the left ventricular assist device in pediatric cardiac surgery. J Cardiothorac Vasc Anesth 14:454-456, 2000.
27. Verghese ST, Hannallah RS: Postoperative pain management in children. Anesthesiol Clin North Am 23:163-184, 2005.
28. Baraka AS, Baroody MA, Haroun ST, et al: Effect of alpha-stat versus pH-stat strategy on oxyhemoglobin dissociation and whole-body oxygen consumption during hypothermic cardiopulmonary bypass. Anesth Analg 74:32-37, 1992.

C. William Hanson

4 Medical Informatics

Key Points

1. A computer's hardware serves many of the same functions as those of the human nervous system, with a processor acting as the brain and buses acting as conducting pathways, as well as memory and communication devices.
2. The computer's operating system serves as the interface or translator between its hardware and the software programs that run on it, such as the browser, word processor, and e-mail programs.
3. The hospital information system is the network of interfaced subsystems, both hardware and software, that coexist to serve the multiple computing requirements of a hospital or health system, including services such as admissions, discharge, transfer, billing, laboratory, radiology, and others.
4. An electronic health record is a computerized record of patient care.
5. Computerized provider order entry systems are designed to minimize errors, increase patient care efficiency, and provide decision support at the point of entry.
6. Decision support systems can provide providers with best-practice protocols and up-to-date information on diseases or act to automatically intervene in patient care when appropriate.
7. The Health Insurance Portability and Accountability Act is a comprehensive piece of legislation designed in part to enhance the privacy and security of computerized patient information.
8. Providers are increasingly able to care for patients at a distance via the Internet, and telemedicine will continue to grow as the technology improves, reimbursement becomes available, and legislation evolves.

Computer Hardware

Central Processing Unit

The central processing unit (CPU) is the "brain" of a modern computer. It sits on the motherboard, which is the computer's skeleton and nervous system, and communicates with the rest of the computer and the world through a variety of "peripherals." Information travels through the computer on "buses," which are the computer's information highways or "nerves," in the form of "bits." Bits are aggregated into meaningful information in exactly the same way that dots and dashes are used in Morse code. Bits are the building blocks for both the instructions, or programs, and the data, or files, with which the computer works.

Today's CPU is a remarkable piece of engineering, totally comparable in scope and scale to our great bridges and buildings, but so ubiquitous and hidden that most of us are unaware of its miniature magnificence. Chip designers essentially create what can be thought of as a city, complete with transportation, utilities, housing, and a government, every time they create a new CPU. With each new generation of chips, the "cities" grow substantially and yet remain miniaturized to the size of a fingernail.

For the purposes of this text, the CPU can be treated as a black box into which flow two highways: one for data, the other for instructions. Inside that black box, the CPU (Fig. 4-1) uses the instructions to determine what to do with data—for example, how to create this sentence from my interaction with the computer's keyboard. The CPU's internal clock is like a metronome pacing the speed with which the instructions are executed.

Most people think that the clock speed of the CPU, which is measured in megahertz, or millions of instructions per minute, determines the performance speed of the unit. In reality, the performance of a CPU is a function of several factors that should be intuitive to anesthesiologists when an operating room (OR) analogy is used. Let us compare the clock speed to surgical speed, where a fast clock is comparable to a fast surgeon and vice versa. CPUs also have what are called caches, which are holding areas

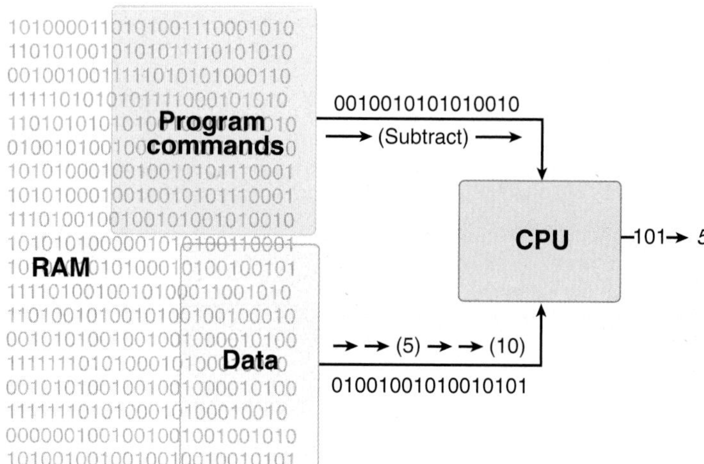

Figure 4-1 Programs and data are stored side by side in memory in the form of single data bits—the program tells the central processing unit (CPU) what to do with the data. RAM, random-access memory.

for data and instructions, quite comparable to preoperative holding areas. Information is moved around in the CPU on buses, which can be likened to the number of ORs. In other words, it is possible to have a CPU that is limited because it has a slow or small cache, in the same way that OR turnover is limited by the lack of preoperative preparation beds or too few ORs for the desired caseload.

The speed of a processor is a function of the width of its internal buses, clock speed, the size and speed of internal caches, and the effectiveness with which it anticipates the future. Although this last concept may seem obscure, an OR analogy would be an algorithm that predicts a procedure's length based on previous operations of the same type by the same surgeon. Without going into detail, modern processors use techniques called *speculation*, *prediction*, and *explicit parallelism* to maximize efficiency of the CPU.

True general-purpose computers are distinct from their predecessor calculating machines in that regardless of whether they are relatively slow and small, as in dedicated devices such as smart phones, or highly streamlined and fast, as in supercomputers, they can perform the same tasks given enough time. This definition was actually formalized by Alan Turing, who is one of the fathers of computing.

Each type of CPU has its own instruction set, which is essentially its language. Families of CPUs, such as Intel's processors, tend to use one common language, albeit with several dialects, depending on the specific chip. Other CPU families use a very different language. A complex–instruction set computer (CISC) has a much more lush vocabulary than a reduced–instruction set computer (RISC), but the latter may have certain efficiencies relative to the former. It is the fact that both types of computer architecture can run exactly the same program (i.e., any windowed operating system) that makes them general-purpose computers.

Memory

Computers have a variety of different kinds of memory ranging from very small, very fast memory in the CPU to much slower, typically much larger memory storage sites that may be fixed (hard disk) or removable (compact disk, flash drive).

Ideally, we would like to have an infinite amount of extremely fast memory immediately available to the CPU, just as we would like to have all of the OR patients for a given day waiting in the holding area ready to roll into the OR as soon as the previous case is completed. Unfortunately, this would be infinitely expensive. The issue of ready data availability is particularly important now, as opposed to a decade ago, because improvements in central processing speed have outpaced gains in memory speed such that the CPU can sit idle for extended periods while it waits for a desired chunk of data from memory.

Computer designers have come up with an approach that ensures a high likelihood that the desired data will be close by. This necessitates the storage of redundant copies of the same data in multiple locations at the same time. For example, the sentence I am currently editing in a document might be stored in very fast memory next to the CPU, whereas a version of the complete document, including an older copy of the same sentence, could be stored in slower, larger-capacity memory (Fig. 4-2). At the conclusion of an editing session, the two versions are reconciled and the newer sentence is inserted into the document.

The very fast memory adjacent to the CPU is referred as cache memory, and it comes in different sizes and speeds. Cache memory is analogous to the preoperative and postoperative holding areas in an OR in that both represent rapidly accessible buffer space. Modern computer architectures have primary and secondary caches that can either be built into the CPU chip or be situated adjacent to it on the motherboard. Cache memory is typically implemented in static random-access memory (SRAM), whereas the larger and slower "main memory" consists of dynamic random-access memory (DRAM) modules. RAM has several characteristics, including the facts that it can be read or written (in contrast with read-only memory), it disappears when the electricity is turned off, and it is much faster than the memory on a disk drive.

To understand the impact of the mismatch in memory access times and CPU speed, consider the following. Today's fastest hard disks have access times measuring about 10 milliseconds (to get a random chunk of information). If a 200-mHz CPU had to wait for 10 milliseconds between each action requiring new data from a hard disk, it would sit idle for 2 *million* clock cycles between each clock cycle used for actual work. Furthermore, it takes 10 times longer for the computer to get data from a compact disk or digital video disk than it does for data from a hard disk.

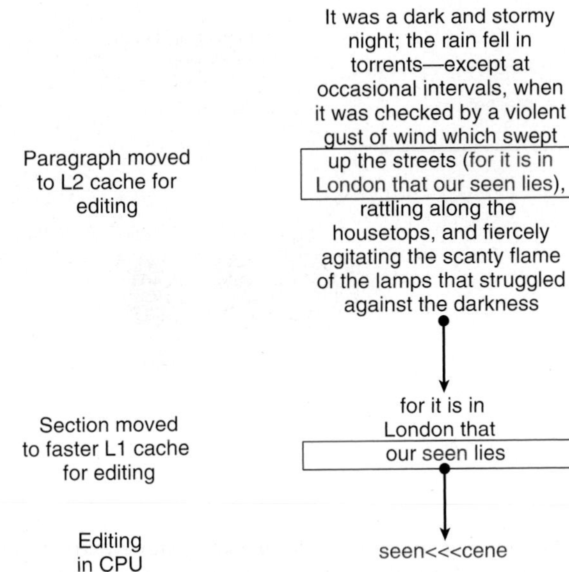

Figure 4-2 Processing of text editing using several "memory" caches in which duplicate copies of the same text may be kept nearby for ready access.

Communications

There are many functionally independent parts of a computer that need to communicate seamlessly and on a timely basis. The keyboard and mouse have to be able to signal their actions, the monitor must be refreshed continuously, and the memory stores have to be read and written correctly. The CPU orchestrates all of this by using various system *buses* as communication and data pathways. Whereas some of the buses are dedicated to specific tasks on newer computers, such as communication with the video processor over a dedicated video bus, others are general-purpose buses.

Buses are analogous to highways traveling between locations in the computer (Fig. 4-3). In most computers, the buses vary in width, with the main bus typically being the widest and other buses narrower and therefore of lower capacity. Data (bits) travel along a bus in parallel, like a rank of soldiers, and at regular intervals determined by the clock speed of the computer. Older computers had main buses 8 bits wide, whereas newer Pentium-class computers use buses as wide as 64 bits.

Input-output buses link "peripherals" such as the mouse, keyboard, removable disk drives, and game controllers to the rest of the computer. These buses have become faster and increasingly standardized. The universal serial bus (USB) is a current widely accepted standard, as is Apple's proprietary Firewire bus. These buses allow "on-the-fly" attachment and removal of peripherals via a standardized plug, and a user can expect that a device plugged into one of these ports will identify itself to the operating system and function without the need for specific configuration. This is a distinct improvement over the previous paradigm, in which a user typically needed to open the housing of the computer to attach a new peripheral and then configure a specific software driver to permit communication between the device and the computer.

In addition to their local computing function, modern personal computers have become our conduits to networks and must therefore act as terminal points on the Internet. As with houses or phones, each computer must have an individual identifier (address, phone number) to receive communications uniquely intended for it. Examples of these kinds of specific addresses are the IP (Internet protocol) address and the MAC (media access control) address. The IP address is temporarily or permanently assigned to a device on the Internet (typically a computer) to uniquely identify it among all of the other devices on the Internet. The MAC address is used to specifically identify the network interface card for the computers that assign IP addresses.

The computer must also have the right kind of hardware to receive and interpret Internet-based communications. Wired and wireless network interface cards are built into all new computers and have largely replaced modems as the hardware typically used

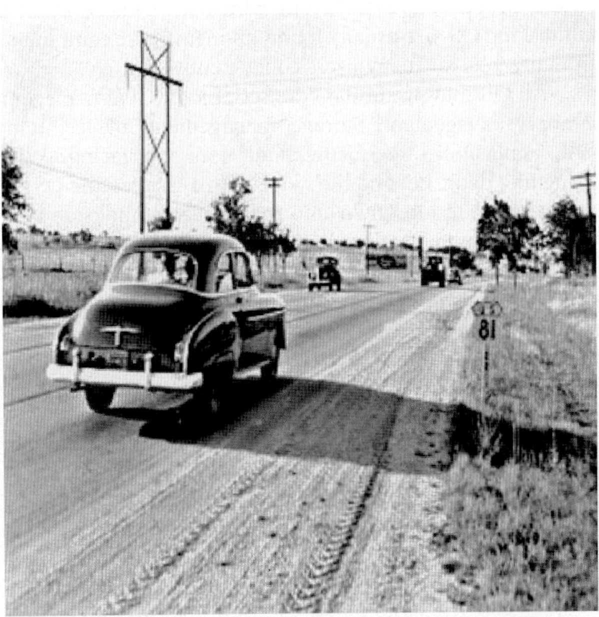

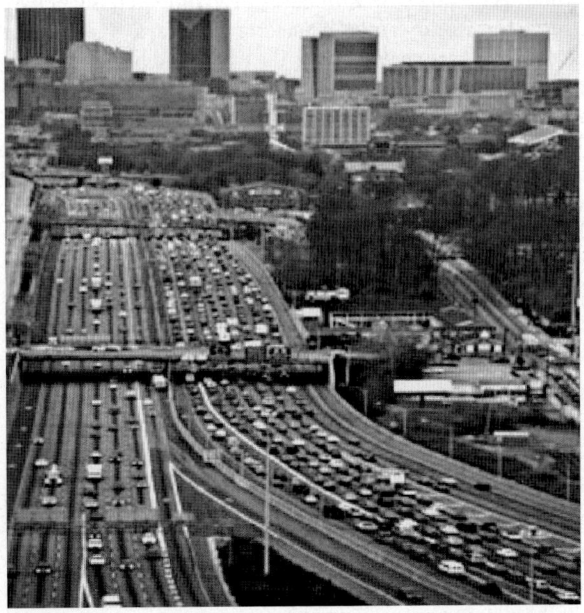

Figure 4-3 Buses are like highways, where the number of available "lanes" relates to bus capacity.

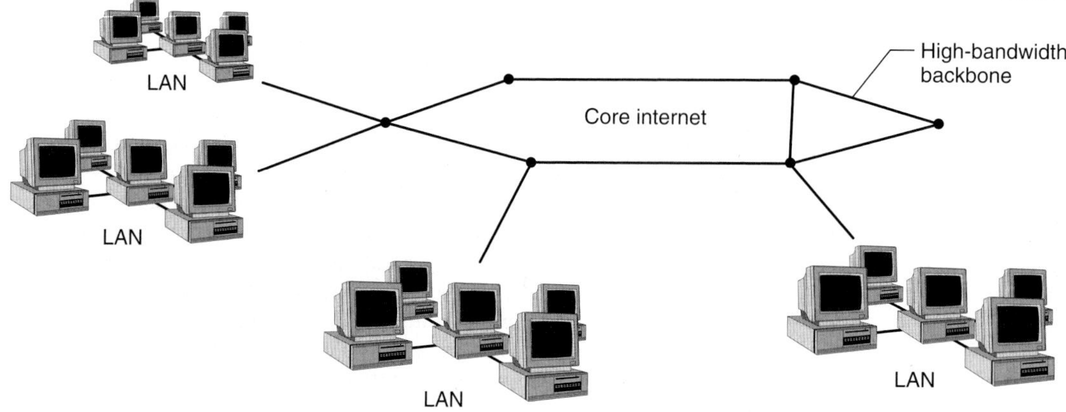

Figure 4-4 Lower-speed networks are attached to high-speed "core" networks that span the globe. LAN, local area network.

for network communications. Whereas a modem communicates over existing phone lines also used for voice communication, network cards communicate over channels specifically intended for computer-to-computer communications and are almost invariably faster than modems.

Although we commonly think of the Internet as being one big network, it is instructive to understand a little bit about the history of computer networking. In the beginning there were office networks and the progenitor Internet. The first office network was designed at the Palo Alto Research Center, which is the Xerox research laboratory where a number of major computer innovations were developed. That office network was called Ethernet and was designed as part of the "office of the future," where word-processing devices and printers were cabled together. Separately, the ARPAnet was the Defense Advanced Research Project Agency's creation and linked mainframe computers at major universities. Over time, the two networks grew toward one another almost organically, and today we have what seems to be a seamless network that links computers all over—and above—the world.

Networking technology has evolved almost as rapidly as computer technology. As with buses in a computer, the networks that serve the world can be likened to highways. Backbone networks (Fig. 4-4) are strung across the world and have tremendous capacity, like interstate highways. Lower-capacity systems feed into the backbones, and traffic is directed by router computers. To facilitate traffic management, before transmission messages are cut up into discrete packets, each of which travels autonomously to its destination, where they are reassembled. Internet packets may travel over hard-wired, optical, or wireless networks en route to their destination.

Computer Software

Operating System and Programming

The operating system (OS) is the government of the computer. As with a municipal government, the OS is responsible for coordinating the actions of disparate components of a computer, including its hardware and various software programs, to ensure that the computer runs smoothly. Specifically, it controls the CPU, memory, interface devices, and all the programs running on the machine at any given time. The OS also needs to provide a consistent set of rules and regulations to which new programs must adhere to participate.

Although most of us think of Apple and Windows synonymously with OSs, there are other OSs that deserve mention. Linux is an open-source, meaning nonproprietary, OS for personal computers that is distributed by several different vendors but continuously maintained by a huge community of passionate programmer devotees who contribute updates and new programs. In addition, every cell phone and smart device has its own OS that performs exactly the same role as for a personal computer OS.

OSs can be categorized into four broad categories (Fig. 4-5). A real-time OS is typically used to run a specific piece of machinery, such as a scientific instrument, and is dedicated solely to that task. A single-user, single-task OS is like that found on a cell phone, where a single user does one job at a time, such as dialing, browsing, or e-mail. Most of today's laptop and desktop computers are equipped with single-user, multitasking OSs, whereby a single user can run several "jobs" *simultaneously*, such as word processing, e-mail, and a browser. Finally, multi-user, multitasking OSs are usually found on mainframe computers and run many jobs for many users concurrently.

All OSs have a similar core set of jobs: CPU management, memory management, storage management, device management, application interfacing, and user interfacing. Without getting into detail beyond the scope of this chapter, the OS breaks a given software job down into manageable chunks and orders them for sequential assignment to the CPU. The OS also coordinates the flow of data among the various internal memory stores, as well as determines where that data will be stored for the long term and keeps track of it from session to session. The OS provides a consistent interface for applications so that the third-party program that you buy at a store will work properly on a given OS. Finally, and of most importance for many of us, the OS manages its interface to you, the user. Typically, today that takes the form of a graphic user interface (GUI).

E-mail

E-mail communication over the Internet antedated the browser-based World Wide Web by decades. In fact, the earliest e-mail

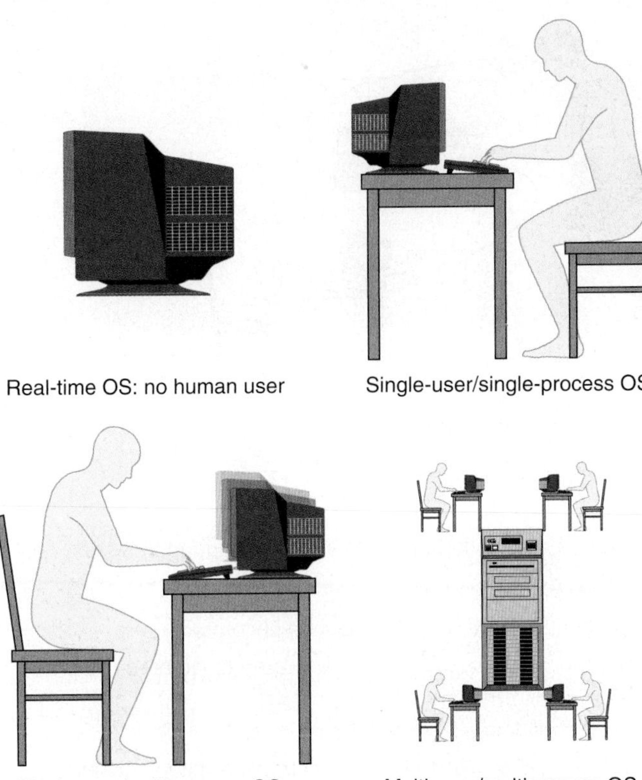

Figure 4-5 Several operating system configurations.

was designed for communication among multiple users in a "time-sharing," multi-user environment on a mainframe computer. E-mail was used for informal and academic communications among the largely university-based user community. Without going into great detail, an e-mail communication protocol was designed so that each message included information about the sender, the addressee, and the body of the message. The protocol is called the Simple Mail Transfer Protocol (SMTP), and the process of message transmission proceeds as follows. The sender composes a message via a software-based messaging program (such as Outlook, Gmail). The sender then applies the recipient's address and dispatches the message. The message travels through a series of mailboxes, much as a regular letter does, and eventually arrives at the addressee's mailbox, where it sits awaiting "pickup."

Although e-mail has had dramatic and largely positive implications for the connectedness of organizations and people, it has also created hitherto unimagined problems, including spam, privacy issues, and the need for new forms of etiquette.

The term *spam* is said to have come from a Monty Python skit. Spam is such a ubiquitous problem that most e-mail crossing the Internet is spam at this point. Spam is essentially bulk e-mail and was never envisioned by the creators of SMTP. Spam is a generic problem with e-mail communications, but the issues of privacy and etiquette are of much greater relevance for medically oriented e-mail.

The American Medical Informatics Association has taken a lead role in defining the issues associated with e-mail in the medical setting. The organization defined patient-provider e-mail as "computer based communication between clinicians and patients within a contractual relationship in which the health care provider has taken on an explicit measure of responsibility for the client's care."[1] A parallel set of issues relates to medically oriented communications between providers.[2-5] Another category of medically oriented communications is that in which a provider offers medical advice in the absence of a "contractual relationship." An egregious example of the latter is the prescription of erectile dysfunction remedies by physicians who review a Web-based form submitted by the "patient" and then prescribe a treatment for a fee.

In theory, e-mail is a perfect way to communicate with patients.[6-9] Because of its asynchronous nature, it allows two parties who may not be available at the same time to communicate efficiently (Fig. 4-6), and it represents the middle road between two other types of asynchronous communication: voice mail and traditional mail. E-mail can also be tailored to brief exchanges, more structured communications, and information broadcasts (such as announcements). As such, a patient could send interval updates (blood pressure, blood sugar) to the physician. Alternatively, the physician could follow up on an office visit by providing educational material about a newly diagnosed condition or planned procedure.

Even though e-mail has many advantages in medicine, there are a variety of risks associated with its use, which has slowed adoption.[10] Some of the problems are generic to any e-mail exchange. Specifically, it is a more informal and often unfiltered form of communication than a letter and often has the immediacy of a conversation but lacks its visual and verbal cues. Emoticons (such as the use of ":)" to indicate that a comment was sent with a "smile") evolved as a remedy for this problem.

E-mail is also permanent in the sense that copies of it remain in mailbox backups even after deletion from local files (Fig. 4-7). Every e-mail should therefore be thought of as discoverable from both a liability and recoverability standpoint. Before dispatch e-mail should be scrutinized for information or content that might be regretted at a later date.

E-mail is also vulnerable to inadvertent or malicious breaches in privacy or disclosure through improper handling of data at any point along the "chain of custody" between the sender and the recipient. Alternatively, a hacker could potentially acquire sensitive medical information from unsecured e-mail or possibly even alter medical advice and test results in an e-mail from physician to patient.

The Healthcare Insurance Portability and Accountability Act (HIPAA) legislation mandates secure electronic communication in correspondence regarding patient care. Three prerequisites for secure communication include authentication (that the

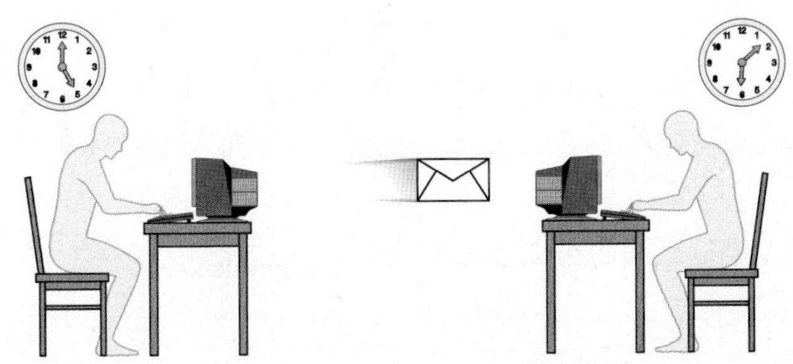

Figure 4-6 E-mail is an effective form of communication between a patient and a physician because it does not require both parties to be present at the same time.

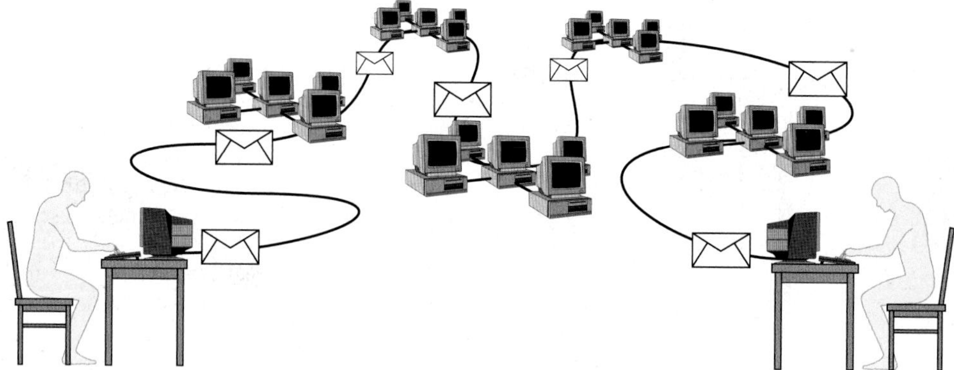

Figure 4-7 E-mail leaves copies of itself as it travels across the Internet.

message sender and recipient are who they say they are), encryption (that the message arrived unread and untampered with), and time/date stamping (that the message was sent at a verifiable time and date), although these techniques are not yet widely deployed in the medical community.

It is beyond the scope of this chapter to go into great detail about the methods used to authenticate, encrypt, and time-stamp e-mail. However, it is possible to ensure that each of these elements by using mathematically linked pairs of numbers (keys), in which an individual's public key is published and freely available through a central registry (like a phone book) whereas a linked private key is kept secret (Fig. 4-8). Public key encryption combined with traditional encryption is used to transmit messages securely across public networks, ensure that messages can be read only by a specific individual, and digitally sign the message.

Although the use of e-mail for medical patient-provider and provider-provider communications is growing, it is not yet universally adopted for several reasons, including physician distrust of the medium, unfamiliarity with software, lack of standards, and lack of clear methods for reimbursement for time spent in e-mail communications. Nevertheless, several professional societies have published consensus recommendations about the management of e-mail in medical practice. Common consensus-based elements are enumerated in (Box 4-1).

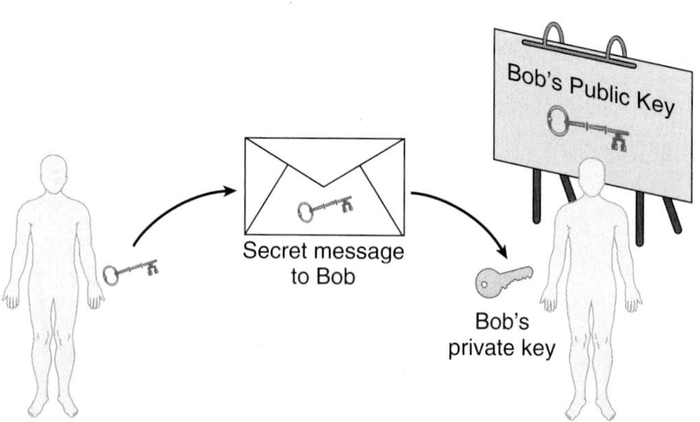

Figure 4-8 Public/private key encryption in which Joe sends a message intended only for Bob by using Bob's public key—the message remains encrypted until Bob decrypts it with his private key.

Box 4-1 Suggested Rules for E-mail Correspondence in a Medical Setting

All patient-provider e-mail should be encrypted.

Correspondents should be authenticated (guarantee you are who you say you are).

Patient confidentiality should be protected.

Unauthorized access to e-mail (electronic or paper) should be prevented.

The patient should provide informed consent regarding the scope and nature of electronic communications.

Electronic communications should (ideally) occur in the context of a preexisting physician-patient relationship.

On-line communications are to be considered a part of the patient's medical record and should be included with the same.

Browser

Many people think of the Internet and the World Wide Web as one and the same. The Internet is the worldwide network, whereas the Web is one of its applications characterized by the browsers with which its users interact. The browser was invented by Tim Berners Lee at the European Organization for Nuclear Research, commonly known as CERN, in 1990. Marc Andreessen wrote the Mosaic browser and subsequently the Netscape browser, which like all subsequent browsers, has a GUI and uses a specific "language" called hypertext markup language (HTML). Microsoft eventually developed its own version of the browser, Internet Explorer, after recognizing the inevitability of the Web.

The browser is a computer program, just like a word-processing or e-mail program, with a GUI. It can be thought of as a radio or television insofar is it serves as an interface to media that do not originate within it. The address of a webpage is analogous to the channel or frequency of a television or radio, and the browser "tunes in" to that address. In actuality, the local browser on your machine communicates with a server somewhere on the Internet (at the address specified in the address line) and uses a communication protocol called HTML as its language. The webpage displayed on your local browser was first constructed on the server and then sent to you.

The original HTML was extremely spare and permitted the construction of very simple webpages. A variety of new "languages" and protocols have subsequently come into existence, such as Java, Javascript, ActiveX, Flash, and others, that allow enhancements to HTML. New browsers support interactivity, security, display of audio and video content, and other functions. Even though the scope of topics that could be covered in discussing browser communications far exceeds that of this chapter, certain issues deserve mention.

"Cookies" is the term used for short lines of text that act like laundry tickets and are used by an Internet server (such as a Google search engine server) to "remember" things about the client computers with which it interacts. Cookies allow the server to keep track, for example, of the items that you have put in your virtual shopping cart as you shop (Fig. 4-9). Although cookies are not inherently risky, there are other risks to the use of a browser.

Like a television, the browser acts like a window on the Internet, and for a long time it was safe to think of that window as being made of one-way glass. Unfortunately, many of the new innovations that allow us to function interactively with websites also have built-in flaws that permit malicious programmers to gain access to your computer. The best way to protect a computer involves timely application of all updates and patches issued by software manufacturers and the use of antivirus software with up-to-date definitions.

Computers and Computing in Medicine

Hospital Information Systems

Modern hospital information systems invariably fall somewhere on the spectrum between a monolithic single comprehensive system design, wherein a single vendor provides all of the components of the system, and a "best-in-breed" model consisting of multiple vendor-specific systems interacting through interfaces or, more typically, an interface "engine."[11-14] The monolithic system has the advantage of smooth interoperability, but some of the component elements may be substantially inferior to those offered by best-in-breed vendors.

Component elements of a hospital information system include administrative, clinical, documentation, billing, and business systems.[15-17] Medical information technology is increasingly subject to governmental regulation, security concerns, and standards. Standards are essential for interoperability among systems and to ensure that systems use uniform terminology.[18]

Health Level 7 (HL7) is an accepted set of rules and protocols for communication among medical devices. Clinical Context Management Specification (also known as CCOW) is a method to enable end users to seamlessly view results from disparate "back-end" clinical systems as though they were integrated. Some of the common medical terminologies or vocabularies include the Systematized Nomenclature of Medicine (SNOMED) and the International Classification of Diseases (the ICD family of classifications).[19]

Modern complicated medical information systems often weave a host of disparate systems at geographically dispersed locations into an extended "intranet." A core hospital, for example, may share an intranet with a geographically remote outpatient practice, or several hospitals in the same health system may coexist within the same intranet. Some of the elements may be physically connected (Fig. 4-10) along a network "backbone," whereas others may use virtual private network (VPN) connections that allow the user to appear to be part of the network while at a remote location.[16]

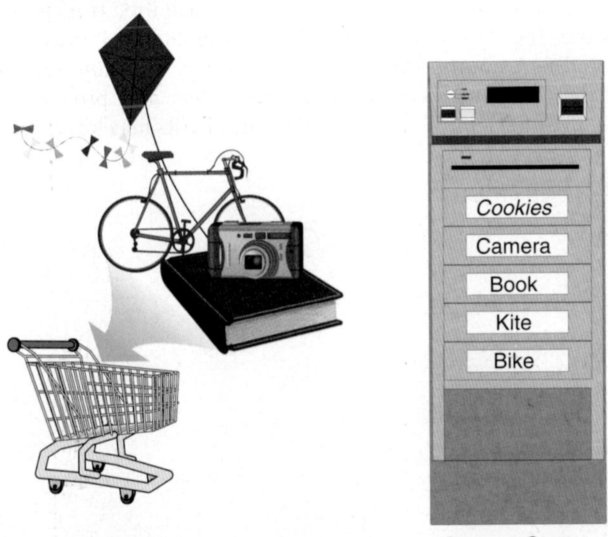

Figure 4-9 Cookies are used by a website, for example, to keep track of the items that a user has put in the "shopping cart."

Electronic Health Record

The electronic record (see Chapter 99) has been described variously as a computerized medical record, computerized patient record, electronic medical record, and electronic health record (EHR).[20-23] It is clear that various settings require radically different EHRs and that EHRs will eventually need to interface seamlessly.[24,25]

The current evolution of software-based EHRs is recapitulating the evolution of hospital information systems as it occurred over the 1980s and 1990s. Best-in-breed commercial systems or "home-grown" site-specific systems are evolving, such as automated anesthesia EHRs[26,27] and intensive care unit (ICU) EHRs (Fig. 4-11). At the same time, large vendors have developed generic inpatient and outpatient EHRs. Health systems will inevitably be faced with the same choices about whether to go with monolithic or best-in-breed EHR software that they have with clinical systems.

The Institute of Medicine issued a recent report characterizing key aspects of an EHR, including an integrated, longitudinal view of patient data; concurrent access to the body of knowledge pertaining both to the patient's condition and to the rules and regulations associated with reimbursement in this age of managed care; order and data entry; and decision support tools that provide current knowledge about diseases, treatments, drug interactions, and risk profiles.

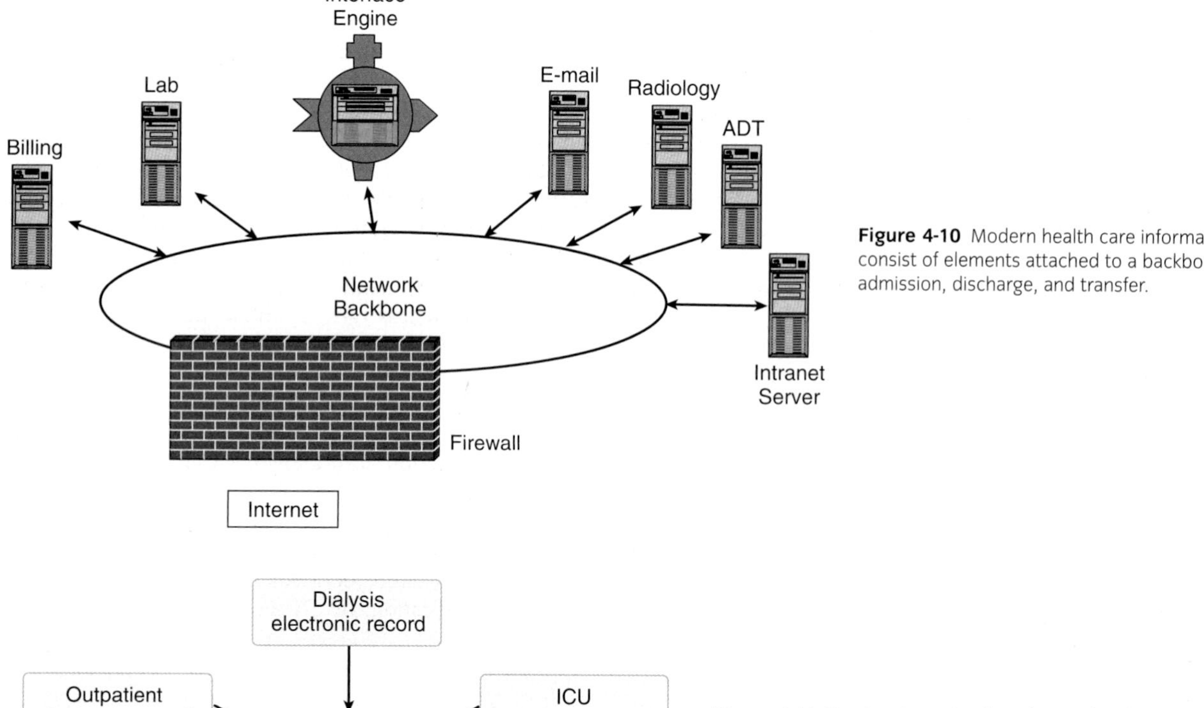

Figure 4-10 Modern health care information systems consist of elements attached to a backbone. ADT, admission, discharge, and transfer.

Figure 4-11 Vendors have developed specialty electronic health records. ED, emergency department; ICU, intensive care unit.

Ideally, the electronic record will provide tools for communication among providers. The EHR should also provide immediate access to population-level information for administrative and research applications.

The Veteran's Health Administration of the United States is an example of a very successful EHR implementation; however, in most hospitals, orders, notes, and reports are still maintained on paper. Additionally, very few small-practice environments have undergone any degree of computerization because the barriers to computerization are formidable.

Technical obstacles to computerization of the medical record are relatively obvious, but there are also organizational, financial, and policy obstacles.[28-30] Adoption of an EHR implies a fundamental reorganization of the way that medicine is practiced in a clinical environment.[31,32] For example, many older physicians have had little occasion to use a computer and are likely to be slowed in their performance of formerly routine tasks, which is a major barrier at a time when demands for efficiency are increasing substantially (Fig. 4-12).

Despite the barriers, governmental and private stakeholders are developing incentives, bonuses, and low-cost capital to encourage use of the EHR. Providers may eventually mandate EHR systems as a condition of participation in certain U.S. insurance plans, such as Medicare.

The EHR is designed to automate the medical record, but once that process occurs, a number of follow-on opportunities become available, such as enhanced patient care delivery, improved efficiency of support processes (e.g., laboratory, radiology, housekeeping, transport), and automated administrative functions (e.g., billing and reimbursement). The EHR can also be used as a vehicle for education, provider regulation, research, public health, and policy support (see Fig. 4-12).

The core functions expected of EHRs fall into eight general categories. The first is management of patient health information and data. Second is presentation of results acquired from patient testing. The third function of EHRs is computerized order entry (CPOE). A fourth key benefit of EHRs is decision support, whereby automatically generated reminders and prompts are used to inform the behavior of clinicians. EHRs may be equipped

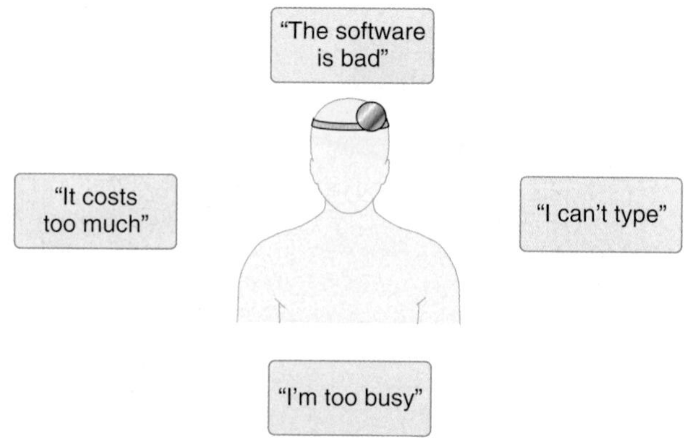

Figure 4-12 Various barriers to adoption of electronic health records.

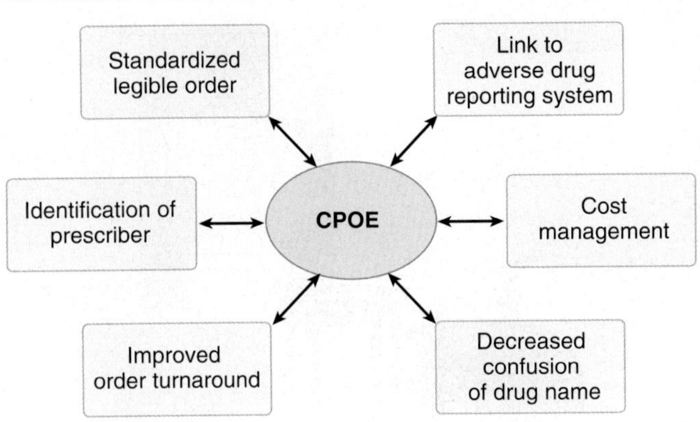

Figure 4-13 Various benefits of a computerized order entry (CPOE).

with communication tools. Patient support tools such as pamphlets describing a disease or discharge directions can be generated automatically. Administrative processes can be integrated into EHRs, including scheduling systems, billing management, and insurance validation. Finally, internal and external reporting requirements can be simplified by using reporting systems built into EHRs.

The concept of a universal medical record deserves specific attention. It has always been desirable for providers in one location to have access to data from a medical record generated at another location, and although there are many models of a universal medical record, such as a record owned and kept by the patient on a piece of hardware such as a flash drive, there are a variety of problems with this approach. A more practical approach is currently being deployed by large vendors such as Microsoft and Google, which now offer patient medical "vaults" that are maintained on line and over which the patient has read-write and access control.

Computerized Order Entry

CPOE systems have begun to gain a foothold in the provision of care at many hospitals, although 50% of American hospitals still lack one. Prescribing errors are the most common source of adverse drug event, and CPOEs, with or without decision support tools, are widely viewed as being integral to reduction in errors and formulary control. CPOEs came into the spotlight after the Institute of Medicine's 1999 report "To Err Is Human: Building a Safer Health System," in which 44,000 to 98,000 deaths per year were attributable to medical errors; however, although CPOE has great potential, poorly designed or deployed systems will either not be adopted or potentially cause errors.

Broadly, the term CPOE is used to refer to computer-based ordering systems designed to automate the ordering process, be it for drugs or for requesting pathologic or radiologic tests. Benefits include the output of standardized, complete, legible orders consistent with the hospital's formulary and automatically sent to the pharmacy (Fig. 4-13). CPOE is also almost invariably associated with a decision support system (DSS), which will be discussed in more detail in the next section.

Successful deployment of CPOE will occur only when the system is deployed as part of a fundamental redesign in the delivery of patient care. The organizational aspects of CPOE deployment have been described by a recent consensus panel from the American Medical Informatics Association in which nine elements of successful systems were highlighted. The first is the development of a clear understanding of all of the institution-specific drivers for implementation of a CPOE system, be they regulatory, regional competition for patients, or internal. A second critical element is sustained internal leadership-level support during implementation of the CPOE system. Third, the CPOE system must be adequately funded in all respects, including training of personnel. A fourth and critical element is prospective understanding of the way in which CPOE will affect workflow at all sites in the organization (Fig. 4-14). A corollary to this element is the fifth, which is ensuring a positive "cost-benefit" ratio for each of the providers who use the system by the creation of time savers such as order sets. The sixth element of successful CPOE systems is the selection of an appropriate deployment strategy, whether it be an all-at-once or a staged approach. The seventh consideration relates to the technical details of CPOE implementation, such as the replacement of legacy systems. Training and support must be comprehensive and is the eighth element. The ninth and final critical aspect is the design of a plan for continuous quality improvement after implementation of the system.

Decision Support Systems/Artificial Intelligence

Decision support tools integrated into the EHR and CPOE can provide immediate access to current medical knowledge, institutional best practices, billing compliance information, and administrative functions and can facilitate cost control. Although there is a wide range of architectures, DSSs fall somewhere on the spectrum between expert systems, in which rules developed by domain experts are used to drive decision support, and autonomous systems that have the ability to "learn" and make observations about large data sets. An example of the latter might be a system that automatically culls through a physician's orders to develop a profile of prescribing patterns.

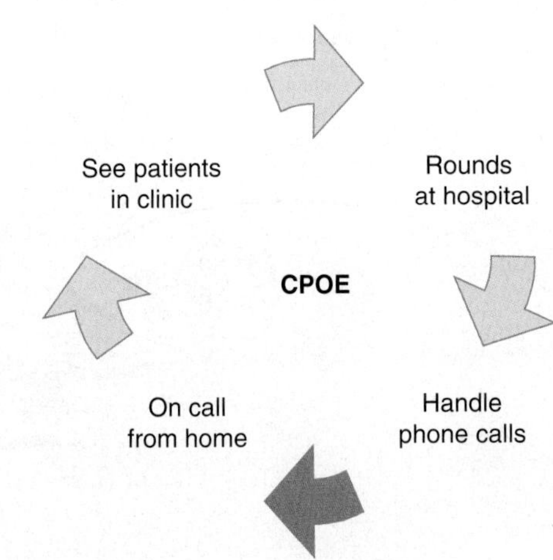

Figure 4-14 Integration of computerized order entry (CPOE) into the workflow of an organization.

A DSS can "act" in one of three ways. It may be a passive system that responds with information when asked. Alternatively, it may be semiactive and provide alerts or alarms only when certain conditions are met. Finally, a system may be active and autonomous and generate an order set or manage a medical process automatically, such as automated weaning of mechanical ventilation according to built-in rules.

Clinicians want certain functions from a DSS, such as access to national consensus guidelines when available, concurrent presentation of relevant patient information when ordering, intelligent alerts, reminders to engage in patient-specific activities (such as immunizations), and the ability to measure their performance versus that of peers in a way that results in continuous improvement in performance.

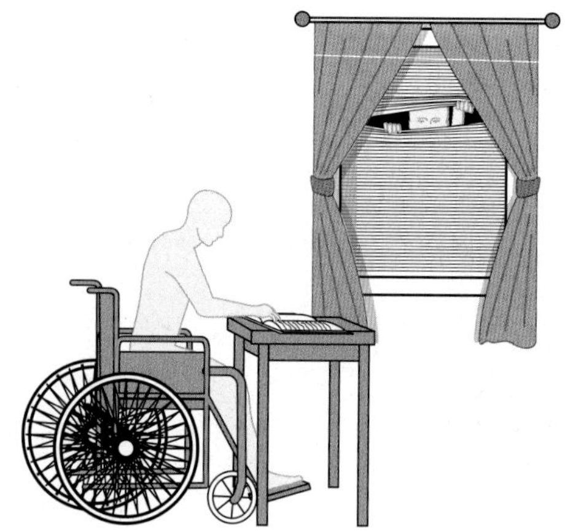

Figure 4-15 Security aspects of the HIPAA legislation relate to the physical aspects protecting unauthorized access to protected health information.

HIPAA and Data Security

Enacted in 1996, the HIPAA was initially designed to protect workers from losing their health insurance (portability) during job transition and to protect the integrity, confidentiality, and availability of their medical information (accountability). HIPAA covers three critical aspects of automated health care information: privacy, universal coding formats, and security.[33-38]

The target of the privacy element is what is known as protected health information, and the bill ensures a patient's right to control the use of that information as it relates to health care, the business of health care, and research. The HIPAA mandates the creation of universal code sets that cover, for example, the classification of diseases and describes both a national provider and national patient identification number. There are a variety of concerns about the latter that have prevented its adoption to date. The security aspect of the legislation relates to the physical and electronic aspects of ensuring the protection of patient health information (Fig. 4-15).

Telemedicine

Telemedicine and telehealth are the application of health care services across space, time, and social and cultural barriers. Telemedicine has been demonstrated in a variety of disciplines, including surgery, emergency medicine, cardiology, dermatology, ophthalmology, neurology, gastroenterology, rehabilitation, and critical care medicine.[26,39-50] However, although telemedicine has already had an enormous impact on the ability of patients to access medical information, there are a variety of barriers to widespread implementation of clinical care at a distance, including licensure, credentialing, malpractice, and reimbursement.

Telemedicine holds great promise as a means of making medical care available to underserved areas, providing access to specialists at remote locations, and allowing patients to receive medical attention in their home when physical contact is not a critical element of an encounter. In addition, new technologies are currently under development, including teleimmersion and telepresence. Teleimmersion permits geographically dispersed people to collaborate in a shared virtual space, whereas telepresence refers to a system in which the human practitioner may have visual and mechanical actuators and sensors permitting them to "see," "feel," and "move" objects in a remote environment (Fig. 4-16).

Telesurgery demonstration projects have been done, for example, with both laparoscopic and robotic instruments to operate at a distance. A number of other demonstration projects are under way in various fields of medicine, and reimbursement agencies are beginning to develop methods of reimbursement for

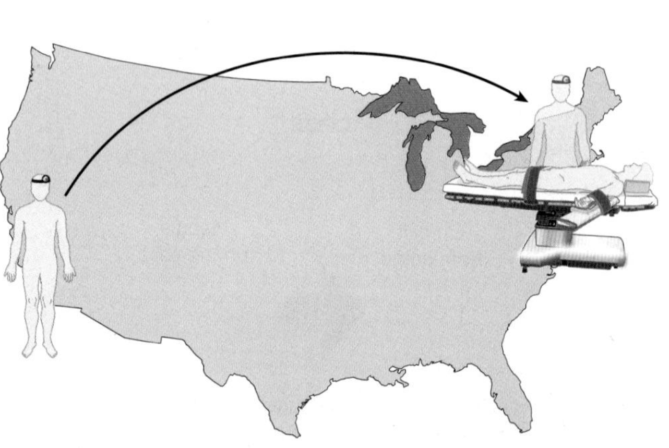

Figure 4-16 Telepresence relates to the ability to be virtually present at a patient's bedside.

telemedicine-based activities. In addition, there are a few commercially available models for delivery of telemedicine, including remote radiographic interpretation, in some cases from appropriately credentialed radiologists interpretation from international locations, and critical care coverage from remote, virtual ICUs.

Telemedicine will eventually change the way that medicine is practiced in many fundamental ways. It is equally certain that the speed of technologic change will outstrip that of regulatory, reimbursement, and legislative change.[51]

References

1. Kane B, Sands DZ: Guidelines for the clinical use of electronic mail with patients. The AMIA Internet Working Group, Task Force on Guidelines for the Use of Clinic-Patient Electronic Mail. JAMIA 5:104-111, 1998.
2. Bones E, Hasvold P, Henriksen E, et al: Risk analysis of information security in a mobile instant messaging and presence system for healthcare. Int J Med Inform 76:677-687, 2007.
3. Car J, Sheikh A: Email consultations in health care: 1—scope and effectiveness. BMJ 329:435-438, 2004.
4. Car J, Sheikh A: Email consultations in health care: 2—acceptability and safe application. BMJ 329:439-442, 2004.
5. Stiles RA, Deppen SA, Figaro MK, et al: Behind-the-scenes of patient-centered care: Content analysis of electronic messaging among primary care clinic providers and staff. Med Care 45:1205-1209, 2007.
6. McGeady D, Kujala J, Ilvonen K, et al: The impact of patient-physician web messaging on healthcare service provision. Int J Med Inform 77:17-23, 2008.
7. Robeznieks A: Don't LOL at virtual visits. Technology is allowing more doctors and patients to consult via e-mail, and insurance companies are reimbursing for it. Mod Healthc 37:6-7, 2007.
8. Stalberg P, Yeh M, Ketteridge G, et al: E-mail access and improved communication between patient and surgeon. Arch Surg 143:164-168, 2008.
9. Stone JH: Communication between physicians and patients in the era of E-medicine. N Engl J Med 356:2451-2454, 2007.
10. Johnson LJ: Patient e-mail perils. Med Econom 84:30, 2007.
11. By the numbers. Information systems. Mod Healthc Suppl 58:16, 18, 20-22, 1960.
12. Lawrence D: Next generation EDIS. The classic "best of breed vs. enterprise" discussion is alive and well among EDIS buyers. Healthc Inform 24:12, 14, 16, 2007.
13. Reichertz PL: Hospital information systems—past, present, future. Int J Med Inform 75:282-299, 2006.
14. Haux R: Health information systems—past, present, future. Int J Med Inform 75:268-281, 2006.
15. Hsieh SL, Lai F, Cheng PH, et al: An integrated healthcare enterprise information portal and healthcare information system framework. *In* Conference Proceedings: Annual International Conference of the IEEE Engineering in Medicine & Biology Society, New York, 2006, pp 4731-4734.
16. Moran EB, Tentori M, Gonzalez VM, et al: Mobility in hospital work: Towards a pervasive computing hospital environment. Int J Electron Healthc 3:72-89, 2007.
17. Raths D: Getting on schedule. Hospitals are dumping manual scheduling for automated systems that tie into other HR software. Healthc Inform 24:22, 24, 2007.
18. Khoumbati K, Themistocleous M, Irani Z, et al: Investigating enterprise application integration benefits and barriers in healthcare organisations: An exploratory case study. Int J Electron Healthc 2:66-78, 2006.
19. Rosenbloom ST, Miller RA, Johnson KB, et al: Interface terminologies: Facilitating direct entry of clinical data into electronic health record systems. J Am Med Inform Assoc 13:277-288, 2006.
20. Mehta NB, Partin MH: Electronic health records: A primer for practicing physicians. Cleve Clin J Med 74:826-830, 2007.
21. Menachemi N, Brooks RG: Reviewing the benefits and costs of electronic health records and associated patient safety technologies. J Med Syst 30:159-168, 2006.
22. Steward M: Electronic medical records. Privacy, confidentiality, liability. J Legal Med 26:491-506, 2005.
23. Stewart WF, Shah NR, Selna MJ, et al: Bridging the inferential gap: The electronic health record and clinical evidence. Health Affairs 26:w181-w191, 2007.
24. Bria WF 2nd, Shabot MM: The electronic medical record, safety, and critical care. Crit Care Clin 21:55-79, 2005.
25. O'Meara E: The effects of electronic documentation in the ambulatory surgery setting. AORN J 86:970-979, 2007.
26. Breslow MJ: Remote ICU care programs: current status. J Crit Care 22:66-76, 2007.
27. Williams JR: Anesthesia information management systems. AANA J 73:178-181, 2005.
28. Agrawal R, Johnson C, Agrawal R, et al: Securing electronic health records without impeding the flow of information. Int J Med Inform 76:471-479, 2007.
29. Bakker AR: The need to know the history of the use of digital patient data, in particular the EHR. Int J Med Inform 76:438-441, 2007.
30. Studer M: The effect of organizational factors on the effectiveness of EMR system implementation—what have we learned? Healthc Q 8:92-98, 2005.
31. Walsh KE, Landrigan CP, Adams WG, et al: Effect of computer order entry on prevention of serious medication errors in hospitalized children. Pediatrics 121:e421-e427, 2008.
32. Walsh SH: The clinician's perspective on electronic health records and how they can affect patient care. BMJ 328:1184-1187, 2004.
33. Califf RM, Muhlbaier LH: Health Insurance Portability and Accountability Act (HIPAA): Must there be a trade-off between privacy and quality of health care, or can we advance both? Circulation 108:915-918, 2003.
34. Hodge JG Jr, Brown EF, O'Connell JP, et al: The HIPAA privacy rule and bioterrorism planning, prevention, and response. Biosecurity Bioterrorism 2:73-80, 2004.
35. Hodge JG Jr: Health information privacy and public health. J Law Med Ethics 31:663-671, 2003.
36. Kulynych J, Korn D: The new HIPAA (Health Insurance Portability and Accountability Act of 1996) Medical Privacy Rule: Help or hindrance for clinical research? Circulation 108:912-914, 2003.
37. Liang BA: Medical information, confidentiality, and privacy. Hematol Oncol Clin North Am 16:1433-1447, 2002.
38. Willerson JT, Kereiakes DJ: Clinical research and future improvement in clinical care: The Health Insurance Portability and Accountability Act (HIPAA) and future difficulties but optimism for the way forward. Circulation 108:919-920, 2003.
39. Anvari M: Remote telepresence surgery: The Canadian experience. Surg Endosc 21:537-541, 2007.
40. Brignell M, Wootton R, Gray L, et al: The application of telemedicine to geriatric medicine. Age Ageing 36:369-374, 2007.
41. Burdick AE: Teledermatology: Extending specialty care beyond borders. Arch Dermatol 143:1581-1582, 2007.
42. Hersh WR, Hickam DH, Severance SM, et al: Telemedicine for the Medicare population: Update. Evidence Report/Technology Assessment1-41, 2006.
43. Jaana M, Paré G: Home telemonitoring of patients with diabetes: A systematic assessment of observed effects. J Eval Clin Pract 13:242-253, 2007.
44. Karunanithi M: Monitoring technology for the elderly patient. Expert Rev Med Devices 4:267-277, 2007.
45. Latifi R, Weinstein RS, Porter JM, et al: Telemedicine and telepresence for trauma and emergency care management. Scand J Surg 96:281-289, 2007.
46. Paré G, Jaana M, Sicotte C, et al: Systematic review of home telemonitoring for chronic diseases: The evidence base. J Am Med Inform Assoc 14:269-277, 2007.
47. Peake SL, Judd N: Supporting rural community-based critical care. Curr Opin Crit Care 13:720-724, 2007.
48. Shore JH, Hilty DM, Yellowlees P, et al: Emergency management guidelines for telepsychiatry. Gen Hosp Psychiatry 29:199-206, 2007.
49. Sood S, Mbarika V, Jugoo, S et al: What is telemedicine? A collection of 104 peer-reviewed perspectives and theoretical underpinnings. Telemed J E-Health 13:573-590, 2007.
50. Thrall JH: Teleradiology. Part I. History and clinical applications. Radiology 243:613-617, 2007.
51. Anderson JG: Social, ethical and legal barriers to e-health. Int J Med Inform 76:480-483, 2007.

Eugenie S. Heitmiller, Elizabeth A. Martinez, and Peter J. Pronovost

5 Quality Improvement

Key Points

1. Quality is a characteristic of the system in which care is delivered, and every system is perfectly designed to achieve the results that it achieves. If we want to improve the quality of care that we provide, we need to reorganize the way that we work.
2. The growing demand for improved quality and safety in health care from patients, providers, insurers, regulators, accreditors, and purchasers calls for anesthesiologists to evaluate the quality of care that they provide.
3. Improving quality of care entails measuring performance. However, health care providers have limited ability to obtain feedback regarding performance in their daily work, in part because of a lack of information systems and lack of agreement on how to measure quality of care.
4. The goal of measurement is to learn and improve. The measurement system must fit into an improvement system; caregivers must have the will to work cooperatively to improve, they must have ideas or hypotheses about changes in the current system of care, and the team must have a model for testing changes and implementing those that result in improvements.
5. Previous efforts to measure performance have focused predominantly on outcome measures, including in-hospital mortality rates. Although important, hospital mortality alone provides an incomplete picture in that it does not provide insight into all domains of quality. A balanced set of structures (how care is organized), processes (what we do), and outcome measures (results we achieve) is needed to obtain a more accurate picture of the quality of care.
6. Future efforts to improve quality of care in the field of anesthesiology should focus on the development of valid, reliable, and practical measures of quality.
7. Developing a quality measure requires several steps: prioritize the clinical area to evaluate; select the type of measure; write definitions and design specifications; develop data collection tools; pilot-test data collection tools and evaluate the validity, reliability, and feasibility of measures; develop scoring and analytic specifications; and collect baseline data.
8. One of the greatest opportunities to improve quality of care and patient outcomes probably will not come from discovering new therapies but from discovering how to better deliver therapies that are known to be effective.
9. Strategies that have been used successfully in the aviation industry to improve performance include interventions to reduce complexity and the creation of redundancies in the system to ensure that critical processes occur. These strategies have not been fully evaluated in the practice of anesthesia.
10. Health care providers can organize their patient safety and quality improvement efforts around three key areas: translating evidence into practice, identifying and mitigating hazards, and improving culture and communication. Although each of these areas requires different tools, they all help health care organizations to evaluate progress in patient safety and quality.

Quality improvement (QI) programs have become a compelling force in virtually all branches of medicine. The Centers for Medicare and Medicaid Services (CMS) and The Joint Commission have put forth regulatory policies to further ensure that patients receive interventions that are evidence based and are broadly accepted as the standard of care. The Agency for Healthcare Research and Quality (AHRQ), the health services research arm of the U.S. Department of Health and Human Services, maintains a website that contains information on clinical practice guidelines and QI initiatives along with data to support their use. These guidelines and initiatives are increasingly being used to maintain accreditation of facilities, achieve optimal reimbursement, and provide quality patient care.

The goal of this chapter is to present a practical framework for developing and implementing QI programs in anesthesiology and critical care medicine that are both scientifically sound and feasible. To accomplish this goal, we review the science of QI, present measures that help evaluate whether QI programs are valid, and offer examples of successful QI efforts.

What Is Quality?

The word *quality* is used to describe the degree or grade of excellence of a trait or characteristic of a system. It is a key word used ubiquitously by many professions and businesses. "Quality is job one" was once the well-known slogan of the Ford Motor Company. It implied that they got it right. However, the recalls on their cars and trucks revealed that such was not always the case. In health care, our "recall" was the 1999 Institute of Medicine (IOM) report *To Err Is Human.*[1] By estimating the number of preventable deaths per year caused by medical errors, the report showed that the need to improve quality in health care was substantial. It still is.

The medical profession has been working for more than a century to improve health care quality. In the early 1900s, Dr. Ernest Codman, a surgeon at Massachusetts General Hospital, began his lifelong pursuit of tracking patient outcomes to serve as a foundation for improving the care of future patients.[2] He went on to lead the founding of the American College of Surgeons and its Hospital Standardization Program, which has become what is known today as The Joint Commission. Over time, quality assurance programs were developed whereby selected indicators were monitored by retrospective chart review to measure compliance with recommended practices. However, we learned that this did not necessarily ensure quality and that it led to fears of punitive action for the health care worker. The intention of monitoring quality of care was, and still is, to learn and improve, not to judge or punish. With this realization, quality assurance became quality improvement. Today, the focus of health care quality is on continuous QI programs.

QI is better facilitated when an interdisciplinary group of health care providers and administrators regularly reviews performance, designs interventions to improve, and creates a team to implement the interventions.[3] It is common to describe "quality improvement" in terms of "patient safety." At times, it is difficult to separate the two. The 2001 IOM report *Crossing the Quality Chasm* classified safety as a component of the broader concept of quality.[4] However, the boundaries between the two remain poorly defined. Among the domains of quality, patient safety generally includes efforts to translate evidence into practice, identify and mitigate hazards, and improve safety culture and communication.

A growing demand continues for improved quality and safety in health care from patients, providers, insurers, regulators, and accreditors. This demand is warranted; evidence suggests that safety and quality of care in hospitals can be improved.[5-7] Improvement is not limited just to programs developed to prevent mistakes of *commission*—things we do to patients—but also includes programs to prevent mistakes of *omission*, whereby patients do not receive the therapies that they should.[8]

Historical Methods of Quality Assessment

Before QI, there was quality assurance. Review of adverse events or defects—peer review, morbidity and mortality conferences, isolated liability claims, and incident reports—has been used historically for quality assurance programs. However, the information provided by these sources is often haphazard and biased. Typically, these adverse events are rare for any given practitioner and are not linked to denominators, thereby limiting the ability to estimate rates and risk, nor do they necessarily reflect quality of care or progress made by QI programs. Moreover, these efforts generally focus on assigning blame (who made the error) rather than on how to reduce the risk for future patients (learning from the mistake).

In an effort to encompass a larger group of adverse events, the American Society of Anesthesiology (ASA) began a Closed Claims Database in 1985.[9] Closed malpractice claims against anesthesiologists provided an enriched environment for collecting information about rare but often catastrophic events. The database provided an opportunity to examine a large set of rare events that might reveal hazards that were common in hospitals and insights that would be otherwise difficult to discern. To be certain, these events represent a biased sample. Most adverse events do not result in claims, and many claims are not the result of preventable adverse events.[10] The information derived from the ASA Closed Claims Database was the impetus for development of QI safety and educational programs with the goal of reducing risk to patients. As an example, a review of adverse respiratory events in the Closed Claims Database, published by Caplan and colleagues in 1990,[11] was followed by organization of an ASA taskforce that established practice guidelines for the difficult airway,[12,13] founding of a Difficult Airway Society in 1995 (http://www.das.uk.com) with its difficult airway guidelines,[14] and development of multidisciplinary difficult airway programs.[15]

Voluntary incident reporting that identifies hazardous systems has been used successfully to improve patient care and foster QI programs.[16] As the potential of voluntary incident reporting is being realized in health care, reporting has become less punitive and more focused on systems rather than individuals. Voluntary incident reporting, when appropriately applied, helps identify hazards to patients, which can then become the focus of QI efforts that seek to mitigate these hazards.[17] Unlike other methods that evaluate harmed patients, voluntary incident reporting provides the potential to also learn from near misses—incidents that did not lead to harm but could have. Although voluntary reporting systems are growing rapidly, most of the effort has been focused on encouraging the actual reporting of events; even more important is the need to focus on learning from these events and reducing risks to patients.

The Intensive Care Unit Safety Reporting System (ICUSRS) project is an example of such an incident reporting system.[18] In the ICUSRS, researchers and caregivers created a web-based, anonymous reporting system that sought to uncover unsafe conditions that could lead to patient harm. They partnered with the Society for Critical Care Medicine to provide expert analysis and feedback to members on lessons learned regarding how to improve patient safety. The ICUSRS has assembled a large community of intensive care units (ICUs) across the United States and is realizing the potential for incident reporting to improve patient care.[19,20] This type of reporting system could be widely applied by anesthesiology to develop QI programs and evidence-based practice.

Measures of Quality Improvement

Key to improving quality in patient care is the ability to measure the progress made. Health care currently has few scientifically sound, feasible measures, and significant effort is necessary to further develop such measures. Health care has borrowed tools from other disciplines (e.g., organizational psychology, sociology, and human-factors engineering) that have developed basic quality and safety-related principles. As Brennan and coworkers noted, other disciplines can be considered the basic science of quality.[21]

At the end of World War II, W. Edwards Deming, an American statistician, introduced the concept of QI in industry, thereby heralding the advent of the modern-day science of improvement. Deming's work helped improve productivity in the United States but made an even bigger impact in Japan, where implementation of his QI methods resulted in Japan becoming renowned for producing innovative, high-quality products.[22] Deming's components for improvement were summarized by Langley and associates[23] as (1) appreciation of a system (people, procedures, equipment), (2) understanding of variation (is a change in outcome a result of a change in practice or simply due to luck?), and (3) theory of knowledge and psychology of change (how people react to change, why they resist, and how to overcome the resistance).

Japan's increased productivity, plus the subsequent adoption of these techniques globally, was a clear measure of the validity of Deming's methods. These methods are rooted in science and depend on robust evaluation. Developing similar measures of quality in health care was (and still is) a challenge. Although patient care cannot necessarily be equated with industry, some similarities exist. Avedis Donabedian was one of the masters of designing measures of health care improvement programs. In the 1980s, Donabedian proposed that we measure the quality of health care by observing its structure (the attributes of the settings where care is delivered), process (whether good medical practices are being followed), and outcome (the impact of the care on health status); this is known as the Donabedian Quality-of-Care Framework.[24,25] This framework may be applied to the clinical setting as follows: First, caregivers must have the will to work cooperatively to improve. Second, the group must have ideas or hypotheses about making changes in the current system of care that are based on scientific fact or expert consensus. Third, the team must have a model for testing changes and implementing those that result in improvement.[23] This ability to measure change in terms of improvement is fundamental to any QI program.[26]

Process and Outcome Measures

As stated earlier, QI measures can be an outcome (morbidity, mortality, length of stay, quality of life, or perceptions of care), a process (β-blockers for patients with coronary artery disease), or a structural measure (ICU physician or nurse staffing ratio).[27,28] Each of these measures has advantages and limitations.[29] Process measures are readily accepted by health care providers because they demonstrate the degree to which caregivers can influence a process, with the intention of improving patient outcomes. Providers generally feel more accountable for the process of care than for its outcomes because outcomes may be affected by many other variables.[29] An obstacle to using process as a measure of quality is sustainability; frequent updating is required as the science of medicine advances.

Process measures that evaluate how care is delivered may be easier to measure and implement and can provide important insight into care.[30] Process measures can provide immediate feedback regarding performance, thereby allowing rapid improvements in care. Additional important advantages of evaluating process measures are (1) that they generally have face validity for providers, which means that providers believe that they can use the data to improve care, and (2) because risk adjustment is less important, broad implementation is feasible. Moreover, joint efforts among providers, professional societies, and external government or payer agencies have made them more feasible.[30]

To be valid, process measures should have causal links to important outcomes; a change in the process should produce a desired change in outcome. One of the greatest opportunities to improve patient outcome may well come from discovering how to deliver therapies (processes) that are known to be effective in producing a desired outcome.[31] For example, prior hand washing and application of chlorhexidine to sterilize the skin site before insertion of a central venous catheter (CVC) are two of five processes known to reduce catheter-related bloodstream infections (CRBSIs).[32] Process measures such as these are indicators of whether patients reliably receive evidence-based interventions known to prevent complications.

When measuring processes, it is essential to remember that patient factors, bias in measurement, and interventions already in place as part of standard practice all play a role in outcomes. The linkage of process to outcomes must be previously demonstrated scientifically or must be widely accepted by peers, although the latter risks being accepted but wrong. In general, a balanced set of process and outcome measures helps to inform improvement efforts and provides evidence that such efforts have made a difference in the lives of patients.

The need for risk adjustment and long-term follow-up is complex. If an outcome occurs infrequently, it will take considerable time before providers can obtain meaningful feedback. For example, evidence of improved rates of CRBSI (an outcome measure) may require 3 months of data (because infections develop in few patients), whereas improved adherence to evidence-based practices to reduce infections (process measures) may be observed within a week (because all patients can be evaluated to determine whether they received the intervention). Nevertheless, consumers and employers are increasingly requesting outcome measures. The relative focus on outcome and process measures will depend on finding the balance between collecting data that are scientifically sound yet feasible.

Analysis of Quality Improvement Data

The QI team must decide how the data will be analyzed and how clinical and statistical significance will be determined. A common feature of a well-run QI project is correlation of several measures over time. The horizontal (x) axis can represent time in days, weeks, or months, and the vertical (y) axis can represent the performance measure (Fig. 5-1). The analyst annotates the plots with the timing of the interventions or other significant events such as, in this example, implementation of an educational program for the appropriate timing of administering antibiotics preoperatively.

Although analysis of rates or proportions is generally clear, analysis of continuous data, such as time, is less clear. There is often uncertainty regarding the unit of analysis when plotting data over time (commonly called a *control chart*). Should the unit of time be days, weeks, months, or years? The unit of analysis should be selected so that learning is optimized; it is influenced by sample-size requirements and by the frequency with which the investigator plans to provide feedback or launch interventions, or both.[33] In general, feedback regarding process measures can be provided more frequently than feedback for outcome measures can. Scales and units of measure should be chosen to optimize learning of the user.[34] Therefore, the user of the information should be involved in deciding which unit of measure to use.

Time series consisting of data from small samples collected continually over time is the standard for QI work. It is less costly to implement than measurements associated with the large, one-time data collection of controlled trials. Study of the patterns of variation in the measures over time determines the performance of the system and its stability. The patterns in time series data contain important information; other methods that rely on averages or other summary statistics can hide this information (e.g., comparing results across the arms of a randomized, controlled trial).

Uncontrolled observational measurement holds higher risk for unrecognized bias and incorrect conclusions about cause and effect than more rigorous designs do. However, unlike these designs, in which measurement ends when the researchers leave, in a health care setting, time series measurement continues to determine whether the perceived improvement is sustainable. This is contingent on having a system to collect, analyze, and report back data. Incorrect claims of improvement that result from faulty inference become apparent in time.

Periodic measurement can be built into daily work and allows the clinical team to continually evaluate performance. Any decline in performance is evident, and a clinical team can quickly respond. If properly planned and coordinated, such local outcomes tracking, when combined with descriptions of evolved systems of care, can enhance learning at both the local and regional level, as well as the national level. This widespread learning and improvement are consistent with the "call for action" issued in 1997 by Lundberg and Wennberg.[35]

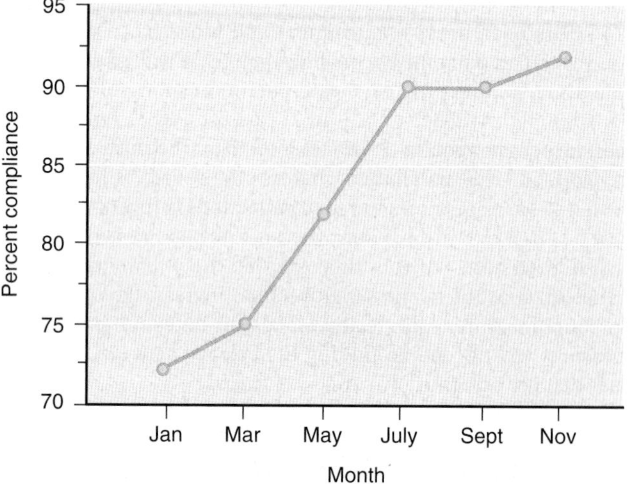

Figure 5-1 Example of a plot of a performance measure over time. The horizontal (x) axis represents time in months, and the vertical (y) axis represents the performance measure—percent compliance with the timing of administration of preoperative antibiotics.

Examples of Quality Improvement Programs and Tools

Voluntary Incident Reporting

Providers who are given a readily available means of reporting incidents can be an excellent source of information for the development of QI programs. However, data from these voluntary reporting systems should not be interpreted as rates or be used to evaluate progress in patient safety. The following is an example of a self-reported medication error and the actions that were taken after a detailed (root cause) analysis of the factors that led to the error.

An ICU patient was administered Zosyn (piperacillin/tazobactam) intravenously despite a documented allergy to penicillin. On cursory review, the physician who wrote the order and the nurse who administered the medication appeared to be at fault because they failed to note the penicillin allergy. An in-depth investigation of this medication error was undertaken, with appropriate scrutiny to identify the system failures that resulted in this error. First, we will review the circumstances that led to the error through the eyes of the caregivers involved.

The patient was exhibiting signs of pneumonia. The physician was interrupted (distracted) while writing the order for Zosyn and failed to review the patient's allergies. The bedside nurse did not realize that Zosyn contained piperacillin and was contraindicated for a patient with an allergy to penicillin. The bedside nurse did know that administering the antibiotic within 1 hour of the diagnosis of pneumonia would dramatically improve the patient's outcome and that the 1-hour rule was a core measure for pneumonia therapy. On further discussion with staff, investigators discovered that the nurse's concern over administering the antibiotic quickly was perpetuated by a broken fax machine and a nonfunctioning pneumatic tube transport system. Orders were normally faxed to the pharmacy, and medications were then dispensed through the pneumatic tube system for a quick turnaround. Because the system for quickly obtaining medications failed, the nurse borrowed the Zosyn from floor stock.

This case is a powerful example of how each step aligned to achieve a catastrophic outcome. By borrowing the antibiotic from floor stock, a crucial safety check of potential medication allergies by the pharmacist was bypassed. The root-cause analysis demonstrated the frontline caregivers' commitment to quality, uncovered several defects that resulted in the event (the drug name Zosyn was unfamiliar and did not indicate that the drug contained piperacillin, the fax machine was broken, the pneumatic tube transport system was broken, and the pharmacy safety check was bypassed), and provided solutions to fix the problem (ongoing preventive maintenance to ensure the functionality of equipment, electronic provider order entry, and possibly hiring staff for transport backup to ensure that medications come from the pharmacy and not floor stock).

It is important to recognize that QI projects often require resources. In this case example, a QI project was undertaken by senior leaders in the organization to intensively evaluate the pneumatic tube used for transport to identify sources of malfunction and reduce defects, develop protocols for handling transport capsules, and determine whether adding staff for transport backup was needed. A plan for electronic order entry was being developed. Each step required measurement and analysis, with the understanding that changes made in a system may introduce new hazards that must be guarded against.

Collaboratives

A collaborative involves the participation of multidisciplinary care providers within a clinical area, across clinical areas, or across multiple health care organizations to improve care. It incorporates a structured program with a shared goal. The team leading the collaborative will (1) determine the evidence-based interventions to be used and, if none are available, generate interventions based on local and broad expert consensus and (2) establish the data collection approach (define measures, collection methods, and feedback mechanisms).

As with all successful QI projects, baseline compliance and change over time are key data points to collect. Collaboratives are successful when they involve a sharing process of interventions and obstacles. Through group discussions (meetings, conference calls), teams can learn about best practices and innovative methods used by other teams to approach a problem. In addition, collaboratives bring a shared momentum that can increase sustainability.[26,36]

Multicentered and single-hospital projects can fail because of inadequate resources, lack of support by leadership, vague expectations and objectives for team members, poor communication, complex study plans, inadequate management of data collection, and wasted effort to "reinvent the wheel" rather than adopting practices proven to be effective. Successful collaboratives require a local culture (the set of values, attitudes, and beliefs of the group) that is ready for change and participants with a shared view of safety, who understand the science of patient quality and safety (i.e., the technical components of how care is organized and delivered). Pronovost and colleagues reported the reproducible success of a collaborative that has adhered to the following steps, which have been validated in several large collaborative efforts.[37,38]

1. Identify evidence-based interventions associated with improved outcome through review of peer-reviewed publications.
2. Select goal-oriented interventions that have the biggest impact on outcomes and transform them into behavior. In selecting behavior, focus on interventions with the strongest treatment effect (lowest number needed to treat) and the lowest barrier to use.
3. Develop and implement measures that evaluate either the interventions (processes) or the outcomes.
4. Measure baseline performance and establish databases to facilitate accurate data management and timely feedback to teams.
5. Ensure that patients receive evidence-based interventions through four basic steps: engagement, education, execution, and evaluation (Table 5-1).

Table 5-1 Four Steps to Ensure That Patients Receive Evidence-Based Interventions through a Collaborative As Illustrated by the Example of Catheter-Related Bloodstream Infections

Step	Action	Example
Engage	Make the problem real	Share information of the local CRBSI rate vs. the national rate
Educate	Develop an educational plan to reach *all* members of the caregiver team	Present evidence-based practices at Grand Rounds and multidisciplinary team meetings Present plans to improve care and measure outcome
Execute	Develop a safety culture Reduce complexity of the processes Introduce redundancy in processes Hold regular team meetings	Develop a culture of intolerance for CRBSI Make certain that all equipment and supplies for sterile CVC insertion are in one place and easily available Use checklists that identify key steps to reduce CRBSI Focus on 1-2 tasks per week and identify team member responsible for the tasks
Evaluate	Measurement and feedback	Develop a data collection plan and database to track progress Give staff real-time feedback; post the progress in a highly visible location Identify causes of defects

CRBSI, catheter-related bloodstream infection; CVC, central venous catheter.

Comprehensive Unit–Based Safety Program: A Strategy To Learn from Mistakes and Improve Culture

The Comprehensive Unit–Based Safety Program (CUSP) is a six-step program that has been tested and successfully used to improve quality and safety in ICUs (Table 5-2).[39,40] It provides a structured approach to improve safety culture and mitigate hazards (i.e., learn from mistakes).[39,41]

Safety culture is assessed in the first step of CUSP and reassessed after 1 year to evaluate the impact of the program. The Safety Attitudes Questionnaire—valid, reliable, and widely recognized—is the survey tool used to assess safety culture.[42,43] The initial measure provides a baseline assessment of staff perceptions of safety culture in their clinical areas and their perceptions of the organization's commitment to patient safety.

Education is a crucial aspect of CUSP; it provides staff with a new set of lenses through which to identify hazards and recommend system changes to improve care. The objectives of

Table 5-2 Six-Step Comprehensive Unit–Based Safety Program

Step	Description
1. Measure safety culture	Assess safety culture by all staff members in each clinical area through the Safety Attitudes Questionnaire
2. Present educational material	Educate staff on the science of safety though lectures and other educational material
3. Complete forms identifying patient safety issues	Ask the following questions: How will the next patient be harmed? How can this harm be prevented? Establish voluntary incident reporting
4. Assign a senior executive responsible for a specific area	The senior executive meets with all staff members of the clinical area to: Help prioritize safety efforts Remove barriers for system changes Provide resources Demonstrate hospital commitment to patient safety Foster relationship between senior leadership and staff
5. Implement projects	Focus on two to three safety issues Keep goals simple: Reduce complexity in the process Create independent redundancies to ensure that critical steps are being accomplished
6. Repeat measure of safety culture	Remeasure safety culture; determine whether scores improve

these educational efforts are to ensure that staff members (1) understand that safety is a system property, (2) learn concepts for reliable health care design, and (3) understand the basics of change management. After an educational lecture on the science of safety, staff members are requested to identify patient safety hazards in their clinical areas and suggest interventions for improvement. For this phase, staff members review incident reports, liability claims, and sentinel events from their unit. In addition, two questions are asked: "How do you think the next patient will be harmed?" and "How can we prevent it from happening?"

After completion of the survey and educational component, a senior leader of the institution (e.g., hospital president, vice-president, director) is partnered with a unit or clinical area and attends monthly rounds on the unit with the staff to help them prioritize safety efforts, ensure that they have the resources to implement improvements, and hold staff accountable for evaluating whether safety has improved. Staff members are asked to learn from one defect per month and implement one tool per quarter that is designed to improve delivery of care, such as a daily goals sheet (see later) to improve communication and teamwork.[44,45]

Our institution pilot-tested CUSP in its ICUs and subsequently implemented it throughout the hospital. In the pilot test, a patient safety team that consisted of staff from the clinical area was responsible for oversight of the program. To be most effective, this team included the ICU director as the ICU physician safety champion, the nurse manager, another ICU physician and nurse, a risk manager or patient safety officer, and a senior executive from the institution. We found that the program worked best if the physician and nurse who led the program dedicated at least 20% of their time to improving patient safety and QI. The first unit was the beta site; subsequent teams from other clinical areas would learn from their successes and failures. The ultimate goal was to have every area in the hospital organizing and managing safety through CUSP.

CUSP has been associated with significant improvements in safety culture. The proportion of staff members reporting a positive safety climate increased from 35% before CUSP to 60% after CUSP.[39,41] In addition, teams identified and mitigated several specific hazards through CUSP. As a result of asking staff how the next patient will be harmed, the ICU created a dedicated ICU transport team, implemented point-of-care pharmacists, put into practice a daily goals sheet, clearly labeled epidural catheters to prevent inadvertent intravenous connection, and standardized the equipment in transvenous pacing kits.[46] Moreover, the use of CUSP was associated with a reduction in patient length of stay and nurse turnover.

In summary, CUSP provides several benefits for improving safety culture and is a primer for compliance of staff in implementing any safety or QI intervention or project. It provides enough structure to convert the often vague goals of improving safety into a focused strategy yet is malleable enough to allow units to work on issues most important to them. CUSP provides a venue to introduce rigorous research methods, acts as a learning laboratory to identify and mitigate hazards, and has the potential to improve patient outcomes.

Quality Improvement Tools

Efforts in QI and patient safety have produced tools with which to reorganize the way that care is delivered. Some of these tools are described briefly in the following sections.

Daily Goals Sheet

The daily goals sheet has been used since July 2001 during multidisciplinary rounds in the ICU at Johns Hopkins to improve communication.[44] A one-page checklist, this tool is completed every morning to establish the care plan, set goals, and review potential safety risks for each patient (Fig. 5-2). The goals sheet stays with the patient, is updated as needed, and is used as an information sheet for all staff involved in the patient's care. It can be modified for use in other nursing units or during operating room sign-out or emergency department rounds.

On initial survey it was found that care team members were unable to answer two simple questions after rounds at each patient's bedside: "Do you understand the patient's goals for the day? and "Do you understand what work needs to be accomplished on this patient today?" The team's inability to answer these questions became the impetus to develop the daily goals sheet. Before implementation of the daily goals sheet, a survey showed that fewer than 10% of the residents and nurses knew the care

	Room Number ____________	Shift: ❒ AM / ❒ PM
Safety	What needs to be done to d/c patient from the ICU?	
	Patient's greatest safety risk? How can we ↓ risk?	
	What events or deviations need to be reported? ICUSRS issues?	
Patient Care	Pain & Sedation Management	Pain goal ____ /10
	Cardiac Review ECGs	HR goal ____ ❒ at goal ❒ ↑ ❒ ↓ beta-blockade
	Volume status Net goal for midnight	Even ❒ Pos ❒ Neg ___ Net ___ (cc) ❒ Patient determined
	Pulmonary: Ventilator, ventilator bundle, HOB ↑, wean	❒ OOB/pulmonary toilet/ambulation
	SIRS/Infection/Sepsis evaluation Temp >38°C or <36°C; HR >90 RR >20 or $Paco_2$ <32 WBC >12000 < 4000 or >10% bands	❒ No current SIRS/sepsis issues ❒ Known/suspected infection ❒ Culture blood ×2/urine/sputum ❒ Antibiotic changes ❒ Discontinue sepsis bundle
	Can catheters/tubes be removed?	Y/N
	GI/Nutrition/Bowel regimen: TPN catheter, ND tube PEG needed?	❒ TPN ❒ NPO/Advance diet
	Is patient receiving DVT/PUD prophylaxis?	Y/N
	Can meds be discontinued, changed to PO, adjusted?	
To Do	Tests/Procedures today	
	Scheduled labs	
	AM labs needed/CXR?	
	Consultations	
Description	Has primary service been updated?	
	Has family been updated? Social issues addressed? Long-term/Palliative care	

Figure 5-2 Example of an intensive care unit (ICU) daily goals sheet. CXR, chest radiograph; d/c, discharge; DVT, deep venous thrombosis; ECG, electrocardiogram; GI, gastrointestinal; HOB, head of bed; HR, heart rate; ICUSRS, ICU self-reporting system; ND, nasoduodenal; NPO, nothing by mouth; OOB, out of bed; PEG, percutaneous endoscopic gastrostomy; PUD, peptic ulcer disease; RR, respiratory rate; SIRS, severe infectious respiratory syndrome; temp, temperature; TPN, total parenteral nutrition; vent, ventilator; WBC, white blood cell count.

plan for the day—a finding that is not surprising because traditional bedside rounds tended to focus on teaching staff about the disease rather than the work that was necessary to treat the patient. Approximately 4 weeks after implementing the daily goals sheet, 95% of the residents and nurses understood the goals for each patient. Moreover, after implementing the daily goals sheet, length of stay in a surgical ICU at Johns Hopkins Hospital decreased from a mean of 2.2 days to just 1.1 days.[44]

Briefings and Debriefings

Similar to the daily goals sheet, briefing and debriefing tools are designed to promote effective interdisciplinary communication and teamwork. Both have been used in the operating room, in sign-out from the ICU nursing staff to the intensivist, and between operating room nursing and anesthesia coordinators.[45,47,48] A briefing is a structured review of the case at hand for all team members before the start of an operative procedure. A debriefing occurs after the procedure; the team reviews what worked well, what failed, and what could be accomplished better in the future (Fig. 5-3).

An example of an operating room briefing includes introduction by name (first and last) and the role of each team member; confirmation of the correct patient, site/side, and procedure ("time-out"); and verbal assurance that all team members agree that they understand the procedure and what is required to ensure its success. A check of all necessary equipment (e.g., electrocautery), medications (e.g., appropriate antibiotic), and blood availability is performed. The question "If something were to go wrong, what would it be?" is asked, and plans to mitigate or respond to the potential hazard are discussed.

Checklists

Checklists have been used in health care and in industry in an effort to ensure that important steps in a process are not forgotten. The Food and Drug Administration recommends that a checklist be used when performing checkout and inspection of an anesthesia machine before use to ensure that the equipment and monitors are functioning properly.[49] As part of a QI project to reduce CRBSI, a checklist was one of several interventions implemented

	Briefing: Before Every Procedure
	Team introductions: First and last names, including roles; write names on board
	Verify: Patient ID band, Informed Consent (read out loud), site marking, OR posting, patient's verbalization of procedure (if patient awake), H&P or clinic note
	Are there any safety, equipment, instrument, implant, or other concerns?
	Have antibiotics been given, if indicated?
	What are the anticipated times of antibiotic redosing?
	Is glucose control or beta-blockade indicated?
	Is the patient positioned to minimize injury?
	Has the prep solution been applied properly, without pooling, and allowed to dry?
	Have the goals and critical steps of the procedure been discussed?
	Is the appropriate amount of blood available?
	Is DVT prophylaxis indicated? If yes, describe.
	Are warmers on the patient?
	Is the time allotted for this procedure an accurate estimate?
	Have the attendings reviewed the latest laboratory and radiology results?
	Debriefing: After Every Procedure
	Could anything have been done to make this case safer or more efficient?
	Has the Surgical Site Infection data collection form been completed?
	Are the patient's name, history number, surgical specimen name, and laterality on the paper work? (must be independently verified by the surgeon)
	Did we have problems with instruments? Were they reported?
	Plan for transition of care to postop unit discussed? ❒ Fluid management? ❒ Blood transfusion paperwork in chart? ❒ Antibiotic dose and interval to be continued postop? ❒ Pain management/PCA plan? ❒ New medications needed immediately postop? ❒ Beta-blockers needed? ❒ Glucose control? ❒ DVT prophylaxis?

Figure 5-3 Example of a checklist for operating room (OR) briefing and debriefing. DVT, deep venous thrombosis; H&P, history and physical examination; ID, identification.

to reduce complexity and introduce a redundant safety check. The checklist, typically completed by a nurse, was attached to the CVC insertion cart to ensure compliance with the best practices for CVC placement. The nurse was empowered to stop the procedure if the checklist was not followed or if sterile technique was compromised. This intervention resulted in a 66% reduction in the overall CRBSI rate, with the median rate reduced from 2.7 per 1000 catheter-days before the intervention to 0 by month 3 and through month 18 of the postintervention period.[50,51] In general, these QI tools seek to standardize communication and technical work.

Sources of Quality Improvement Information

Multiple sources of QI data that span both the clinical and administrative arenas include evidence-based medicine and evidence-based clinical practice guidelines, alerts from accrediting agencies and nonprofit safety organizations, standards and guidelines put forth by medical specialty associations, and administrative (such as those maintained by CMS) and claims databases. U.S. governmental agencies, including AHRQ, CMS, and the National Quality Forum (NQF), promote the development and reporting of health care quality measures.[52]

Peer-reviewed journals have published the results of studies that support evidence-based clinical practice guidelines, as well as individual QI programs, and can be a rich source of ideas to improve clinical decision making and patient care by incorporating the best available evidence with patient values and provider preferences.[53,54] In anesthesiology and critical care medicine, guidelines and protocols have been successful in improving performance in some care processes. Sedation and ventilator weaning protocols in ICUs have been shown to decrease the duration of mechanical ventilation and length of stay in the ICU.[55,56] Moreover, individual QI programs have been used to improve delivery of care and have been shown to have a positive effect on job satisfaction and organizational commitment.[57]

National Programs in Quality Improvement

A growing number of regional and national organizations are developing initiatives that are driving the reporting of specific evidence-based practices and outcomes and determining the local selection of areas for QI (Table 5-3).

The Joint Commission has developed quality measures for several areas (www.jcaho.org). Their ORYX initiative was devel-

Table 5-3 Nonprofit and Government Quality Improvement Organizations Pertinent to Anesthesia

Quality Improvement Organization	Website	Description
Agency for Healthcare Research and Quality (AHRQ)	www.ahrq.gov	Lead federal agency charged with improving the quality, safety, efficiency, and effectiveness of health care
American Health Quality Association (AHQA)	www.ahqa.org	Represents quality improvement organizations and professionals working to improve the quality of health care
Anesthesia Patient Safety Foundation (APSF)	www.apsf.org	Promotes investigations and programs that will provide a better understanding of anesthetic injuries
Centers for Disease Control and Prevention (CDC)	www.cdc.gov	One of the major operating components of the Department of Health and Human Services
Emergency Care Research Institute (ECRI)	www.ecri.org	Uses applied scientific research to discover which medical procedures, devices, drugs, and processes are best
Institute for Healthcare Improvement (IHI)	www.ihi.org	Health care improvement organization based in Cambridge, Massachusetts
Institute for Safe Medication Practices (ISMP)	www.ismp.org	The nation's only 501(c)(3) organization devoted entirely to prevention of medication errors and safe medication use
Medicare Quality Improvement Community (MedQIC)	www.medquic.org	A national knowledge forum for health care and quality improvement professionals
National Quality Forum	www.qualityforum.org	Created to develop and implement a national strategy for health care quality and reporting
National Patient Safety Foundation (NPSF)	www.npsf.org	An independent 501(c)(3) organization, the mission of which is to improve the safety of patients

oped to integrate performance measurement data into the accreditation process and to permit rigorous comparison of the actual results of care across hospitals. In 2004, The Joint Commission partnered with CMS to align measures common to both organizations, called "Hospital Quality Measures." These measures are also endorsed by the NQF.

The NQF is a private, nonprofit membership organization created to develop and implement a national strategy for health care quality measurement and reporting (www.qualityforum.org). One of its functions is to endorse certain quality and safety measures (consensus standards), which are then incorporated into other national quality initiatives. The goal is for NQF-endorsed standards to become the primary standards used to measure the quality of health care in the United States. Anesthesia programs are increasingly focusing on standards that are relevant to them because facilities are being evaluated on their compliance and are required to report their performance regarding these standards to the governing bodies.

The Surgical Care Improvement Project

The Surgical Care Improvement Project (SCIP), a national collaborative of public and private entities that has outlined perioperative QI goals (www.medqic.org) and is in partnership with The Joint Commission and CMS national initiative, was initiated in 2003. This multidisciplinary group uses both process and outcome measures (Box 5-1) to focus on key clinical areas that include preventing surgical-site infections, perioperative myocardial infarctions, venous thromboembolism, and mortality and readmission, as well as increasing the use of fistulas in providing hemodialysis for Medicare beneficiaries with kidney failure.

Private Insurers

Many private insurers now collect data on certain quality elements. The Leapfrog group is one such entity. The Leapfrog Hospital Quality and Safety Survey assesses hospital performance according to four evidence-based safety practices: (1) use of computerized physician order entry, (2) evidence-based hospital referral, (3) ICU physician staffing, and (4) a Leapfrog Safe Practices score, which is based on the level of performance of other NQF-endorsed practices (www.leapfroggroup.org). Leapfrog not only reports the results and rankings of its survey but also uses them as a basis for their selection of hospitals to be covered by the plan for the employees of participating companies.

Pay for Performance

Public and private insurers are demanding increased accountability as a result of rising health care costs and threatened budgets. In response, pay for performance (P4P) has been proposed and implemented as a means of improving quality based on successful examples in business. P4P has been defined as the use of incentives to encourage and reinforce the delivery of evidence-based practices and health care system transformations that promote better outcomes as efficiently as possible. Measures that are incorporated into P4P must be evidence based, consistent with national goals, and based on consensus in the absence of evidence (www.jointcommission.org). Furthermore, it is important that measures be reliable, valid, and feasible and that the programs be voluntary. Although the strategy of P4P is to align quality of care and payment, the impact of P4P on quality of care has thus far been modest.

Box 5-1 Process and Outcome Measures of the Surgical Care Improvement Project

Infection

Prophylactic antibiotics:

- Received within 1 hr before the surgical incision
- Appropriately selected for surgical patients
- Discontinued within 24 hr after the surgical end time (48 hr for cardiac patients)

Cardiac surgery patients with controlled 6 AM postoperative serum glucose

Postoperative wound infection diagnosed during the index hospitalization (***outcome***)

Surgery patients with appropriate hair removal

Colorectal surgery patients with immediate postoperative normothermia

Cardiac

Noncardiac vascular surgery patients with evidence of coronary artery disease who received β-blockers during the perioperative period

Surgery patients who had already received a β-blocker before arrival and then during the perioperative period

Intraoperative or postoperative acute myocardial infarction diagnosed during the index hospitalization and within 30 days of surgery (***outcome***)

Venous Thromboembolism (VTE)

Surgery patients with recommended VTE prophylaxis ordered

Surgery patients who received appropriate VTE prophylaxis within 24 hr before surgery to 24 hr after surgery

Intraoperative or postoperative pulmonary embolism diagnosed during the index hospitalization and within 30 days of surgery (***outcome***)

Intraoperative or postoperative deep venous thrombosis diagnosed during the index hospitalization and within 30 days of surgery (***outcome***)

Respiratory

Number of days ventilated surgery patients had documentation of the head of the bed being elevated from the recovery end date (day 0) through postoperative day 7

Patients in whom postoperative ventilator-associated pneumonia is diagnosed during the index hospitalization (***outcome***)

Number of days ventilated surgery patients had documentation of stress ulcer disease prophylaxis from the recovery end date (day 0) through postoperative day 7

Surgery patients whose medical record contained an order for a ventilator weaning program (***protocol or clinical path***)

Global

Mortality within 30 days of surgery

Readmission within 30 days of surgery

Vascular Access

Proportion of permanent hospital end-stage renal disease vascular access procedures that involve autogenous arterial venous fistulas

The Physician Quality Reporting Initiative is a program in which anesthesiologists can earn a 1.5% bonus from CMS by reporting their compliance with appropriate timing of perioperative antibiotics. Initial steps in this program are payment for participation, with the ultimate goal that successful compliance with the clinical measures will be the basis for bonus payments. The ASA has identified five "quality incentives" or P4P measures to date (www.asahq.org, accessed September 9, 2007):

1. Timely administration of antibiotic prophylaxis
2. Maintenance of normothermia
3. Comprehensive planning for chronic pain management
4. Prevention of ventilator-associated pneumonia
5. Prevention of CRBSIs

All but the chronic pain measure are adaptations of national quality measures. The chronic pain measure was drafted by the ASA Committee on Pain Medicine and subsequently endorsed by five additional specialty organizations representing pain physicians. Additional measures are being evaluated, and the methods by which they will be incorporated into national initiatives or P4P (or both) will continue to evolve.[51,58]

The Future: Research, Education, and Ethics

Much remains to be accomplished in QI research and practice. The opportunity to improve patient care is substantial, and the pressure to improve the quality of perioperative care will continue to increase. Improving quality of care requires the ability to measure and improve performance. Research is needed to develop measures of quality that clinicians believe are valid and to learn how to ensure that all patients reliably receive the recommended interventions. Innovation is needed to develop information systems that can be used by multiple disciplines. Anesthesiologists and professional societies may need to partner with experts in quality measurement to develop and implement quality measures. Future efforts should balance the feasibility and validity of quality measures and develop integrated approaches to improving quality, including strategies to develop care bundles, decrease complexity, and create independent redundancies.

Providers need to be educated in the skills necessary to improve quality. Health care will cross the quality chasm only

Table 5-4 Six Core Competencies of the Accreditation Council of Graduate Medical Education and Six Aims for Improvement of the Institute of Medicine

ACGME Core Competencies	IOM Aims for Improvement
1. Patient Care	Safe
2. Medical Knowledge	Timely
3. Interpersonal and Communication Skills	Effective
4. Professionalism	Efficient
5. System-based Practice	Equitable
6. Practice-based Learning and Improvement	Patient centered

when all view quality and safety as what they do primarily rather than as an added activity and when health care organizations provide the infrastructure to monitor and improve performance. Frontline caregivers must understand the science of quality and safety and evaluate safety risks with lenses that see hazardous systems, not incompetent people.

Anesthesiologists need to train providers in the methodology of improvement. Integral to this goal is the education of our anesthesia resident trainees. Continuous QI has been touted in anesthesia residency training programs for well over a decade.[59] In recent years, residents in training were presented with six core competencies to master, as mandated by the Accreditation Council of Graduate Medical Education (ACGME),[60] and the IOM put forth their six Aims for Improvement[4] (Table 5-4). In an effort to link these two sets of goals and apply them to the clinical setting for training purposes, Bingham and associates developed a framework called a "Healthcare Matrix" that can be used as an educational tool and a research tool for improvement.[61]

With the increasing amount of intellectual focus and health care resources being directed toward QI programs, the ethics of QI have come to light. QI projects have generally been exempt from the rigorous review of human subject research. However, a Hastings Center Report on the ethics of using QI methods to improve health quality and safety suggests that some QI projects may involve risk to patients and should undergo a formal review.[62] This report lists QI initiatives that may trigger the need for a review, such as those with a randomized design, novel treatments, involvement of researchers, or delayed feedback of monitoring or those funded by external sources. Reporting of QI activities should be encouraged, and requiring approval by an internal review board in addition to having a standardized format for reporting the results supports the premise that delivery of quality care is a science as well as an art.

Summary

Health care organizations need a systematic approach to three areas of patient safety: (1) translating evidence into practice, (2) identifying and mitigating hazards, and (3) improving culture and communication. The underlying principle for all of the approaches discussed is that to improve the quality of care that they provide, providers must be able to measure their performance. Health care providers have traditionally had limited ability to obtain feedback regarding performance in their daily work, in part because of a lack of information systems and lack of agreement on how to measure quality of care.[63] As a result, many in health care do not have access to performance data and consequently do not know the results that they achieve (or fail to achieve). As consumers, payers, regulators, and accreditors require evidence regarding quality of care, the demand for quality measures will probably grow. To meet these demands, anesthesiologists must be able to evaluate the quality of care that they provide with valid measures and implement evidence-based best practices in the perioperative care of patients.

References

1. Kohn L, Corrigan J, Donaldson M: To Err Is Human: Building a Safer Health System. Washington, DC, Institute of Medicine, National Academy Press, 1999.
2. Codman EA: The product of a hospital: Surgery. Surg Gynecol Obstet 18:491-496, 1914.
3. Berwick DM: A primer on leading the improvement of systems. BMJ 312:619-622, 1996.
4. Institute of Medicine: Crossing the Quality Chasm: A New Health System for the 21st Century. Washington, DC, National Academy Press, 2001.
5. Chassin MR, Galvin RW: The urgent need to improve health care quality. Institute of Medicine National Roundtable on Health Care Quality. JAMA 280:1000-1005, 1998.
6. President's Advisory Commission on Consumer Protection and Quality in the Health Care Industry: Quality First: Better Health Care for All Americans (Publication No. 5-25-0001). Washington, DC, U.S. Government Printing Office, 1998.
7. Schuster MA, McGlynn EA, Brook RH: How good is the quality of health care in the United States? Milbank Q 76:517-563, 509, 1998.
8. McGlynn EA, Asch SM, Adams J, et al: The quality of health care delivered to adults in the United States. N Engl J Med 348:2635-2645, 2003.
9. Cheney FW, Posner K, Caplan RA, Ward RJ: Standard of care and anesthesia liability. JAMA 261:1599-1603, 1989.
10. Studdert DM, Mello MM, Gawande AA, et al: Disclosure of medical injury to patients: An improbable risk management strategy. Health Aff (Millwood) 26:215-226, 2007.
11. Caplan RA, Posner KL, Ward RJ, Cheney FW: Adverse respiratory events in anesthesia: A closed claims analysis. Anesthesiology 72:828-833, 1990.
12. Practice guidelines for management of the difficult airway. A report by the American Society of Anesthesiologists Task Force on Management of the Difficult Airway. Anesthesiology 78:597-602, 1993.
13. Practice guidelines for management of the difficult airway: An updated report by the American Society of Anesthesiologists Task Force on Management of the Difficult Airway. Anesthesiology 98:1269-1277, 2003.
14. Henderson JJ, Popat MT, Latto IP, Pearce AC: Difficult Airway Society guidelines for management of the unanticipated difficult intubation. Anaesthesia 59:675-694, 2004.
15. Mark L, Akst S, Michaelson J: Difficult airway/intubation implications for anesthesia. *In* Cummings Otolaryngology Head & Neck Surgery, 4th ed. St. Louis, Elsevier Mosby, 2004, pp 232-273.
16. Leape LL: Reporting of adverse events. N Engl J Med 347:1633-1638, 2002.
17. Vincent C: Understanding and responding to adverse events. N Engl J Med 348:1051-1056, 2003.
18. Wu AW, Pronovost P, Morlock L: ICU incident reporting systems. J Crit Care 17:86-94, 2002.
19. Thompson DA, Lubomski L, Holzmueller C, et al: Integrating the intensive care unit safety reporting system with existing incident reporting systems. Jt Comm J Qual Patient Saf 31:585-593, 2005.
20. Vincent C, Taylor-Adams S, Stanhope N: Framework for analysing risk and safety in clinical medicine. BMJ 316:1154-1157, 1998.
21. Brennan TA, Gawande A, Thomas E, Studdert D: Accidental deaths, saved lives, and improved quality. N Engl J Med 353:1405-1409, 2005.
22. Magnier M: The 50 people who most influenced business this century. Los Angeles Times Home, October 10, 1999:U-8.
23. Langley GJ, Nolan KM, Nolan IW, et al: The Improvement Guide: A Practical Approach to Enhancing Organizational Performance. New York, Jossey-Bass, 1996, p 370.
24. Donabedian A: An Introduction to Quality Assurance in Health Care, 44th ed. New York, Oxford University Press, 2003, p 200.

25. Donabedian A: Evaluating the quality of medical care. Milbank Mem Fund Q 44(Suppl)206, 1966.
26. Ovretveit J, Bate P, Cleary P, et al: Quality collaboratives: Lessons from research. Qual Saf Health Care 11:345-351, 2002.
27. Nelson EC, Batalden PB, Mohr JJ, Plume SK: Building a quality future. Front Health Serv Manage 15:3-32, 1998.
28. Nelson EC, Batalden PB, Homa K, et al: Microsystems in health care: Part 2. Creating a rich information environment. Jt Comm J Qual Saf 29:5-15, 2003.
29. Rubin HR, Pronovost P, Diette GB: The advantages and disadvantages of process-based measures of health care quality. Int J Qual Health Care 13:469-474, 2001.
30. Pronovost PJ, Miller MR, Dorman T, et al: Developing and implementing measures of quality of care in the intensive care unit. Curr Opin Crit Care 7:297-303, 2001.
31. Lenfant C: Shattuck lecture—clinical research to clinical practice—lost in translation? N Engl J Med 349:868-874, 2003.
32. O'Grady NP, Alexander M, Dellinger EI, et al: Guidelines for the prevention of intravascular catheter-related infections. Centers for Disease Control and Prevention. MMWR Recomm Rep 51(RR-10):1-29, 2005.
33. Plsek PE: Tutorial: Planning for data collection. Part III—Sample size. Qual Manage Health Care 3:78-92, 1994.
34. Shewhart W: Statistical Method: From the Viewpoint of Quality Control, the Graduate School. Washington, DC, U.S. Department of Agriculture, 1939.
35. Lundberg GD, Wennberg JE: A JAMA theme issue on quality of care. A new proposal and a call to action. JAMA 278:1615-1616, 1997.
36. Mills PD, Weeks WB: Characteristics of successful quality improvement teams: Lessons from five collaborative projects in the VHA. Jt Comm J Qual Saf 30:152-162, 2004.
37. Pronovost PJ, Berenholtz S, Goeschel C: Creating high reliability in healthcare organizations. Health Serv Res 41:1599-1617, 2006.
38. Pronovost P, Needham D, Berenholtz S, et al: An intervention to decrease catheter-related bloodstream infections in the ICU. N Engl J Med 355:2725-2732, 2006.
39. Pronovost PJ, King J, Holzmueller CG, et al: A web-based tool for the Comprehensive Unit-Based Safety Program (CUSP). Jt Comm J Qual Patient Saf 32:119-129, 2006.
40. Pronovost P, Goeschel C: Improving ICU care: It takes a team. Healthcare Exec 20:14-16, 18, 20, 2005.
41. Pronovost P, Weast B, Rosenstein B, et al: Implementing and validating a comprehensive unit-based safety program. J Patient Saf 1:33-40, 2005.
42. Sexton JB, Helmreich RL, Neilands TB, et al: The Safety Attitudes Questionnaire: Psychometric properties, benchmarking data, and emerging research. BMC Health Serv Res 6:44, 2006.
43. Colla JB, Bracken AC, Kinney LM, Weeks WB: Measuring patient safety climate: A review of surveys. Qual Saf Health Care 14:364-366, 2005.
44. Pronovost P, Berenholtz S, Dorman T, et al: Improving communication in the ICU using daily goals. J Crit Care 18:71-75, 2003.
45. Thompson D, Holzmueller C, Hunt D, et al: A morning briefing: Setting the stage for a clinically and operationally good day. Jt Comm J Qual Patient Saf 31:476-479, 2005.
46. Pronovost PJ, Holzmueller CG, Martinez E, et al: A practical tool to learn from defects in patient care. Jt Comm J Qual Patient Saf 32:102-108, 2006.
47. Makary MA, Holzmueller CG, Sexton JB, et al: Operating room debriefings. Jt Comm J Qual Patient Saf 32:407-410, 357, 2006.
48. Makary MA, Holzmueller CG, Thompson D, et al: Operating room briefings: Working on the same page. Jt Comm J Qual Patient Saf 32:351-355, 2006.
49. March MG, Crowley JJ: An evaluation of anesthesiologists' present checkout methods and the validity of the FDA checklist. Anesthesiology 75:724-729, 1991.
50. Berenholtz S, Pronovost PJ, Lipsett PA: Eliminating catheter-related bloodstream infections in the intensive care unit. Crit Care Med 32:2014-2020, 2004.
51. Freund PR, Posner KL: Sustained increases in productivity with maintenance of quality in an academic anesthesia practice. Anesth Analg 96:1104-1108, 2003.
52. Miller T, Leatherman S: The National Quality Forum: A 'me-too' or a breakthrough in quality measurement and reporting? Health Aff (Millwood) 18:233-237, 1999.
53. Sackett DL, Rosenberg WM, Gray JA, et al: Evidence based medicine: What it is and what it isn't. BMJ 312:71-72, 1996.
54. Shojania KG, Duncan BW, McDonald KM, et al: Making health care safer: A critical analysis of patient safety practices. Evid Rep Technol Assess (Summ) i-668, 2001.
55. Brook AD, Ahrens TS, Schaiff R, et al: Effect of a nursing-implemented sedation protocol on the duration of mechanical ventilation. Crit Care Med 27:2609-2615, 1999.
56. Marelich GP, Murin S, Battistella F, et al: Protocol weaning of mechanical ventilation in medical and surgical patients by respiratory care practitioners and nurses: Effect on weaning time and incidence of ventilator-associated pneumonia. Chest 118:459-467, 2000.
57. Wang FL, Lee LC, Lee SH, et al: Performance evaluation of quality improvement team in an anesthesiology department. Acta Anaesthesiol Sin 41:13-19, 2003.
58. Bierstein K: Anesthesiology is in the P4P game. ASA Newsl 70:28-31, 2006.
59. Dubin SA, Jense HG, Yodlowski E, McCranie JM: Continuous quality improvement in an anesthesia residency training program. Int Anesthesiol Clin 30:29-43, 1992.
60. Accreditation Council of Graduate Medical Education (ACGME): The project: Introduction. Available at http://www.acgme.org. Accessed 2001.
61. Bingham JW, Quinn DC, Richardson MG, et al: Using a healthcare matrix to assess patient care in terms of aims for improvement and core competencies. Jt Comm J Qual Patient Saf 31:98-105, 2005.
62. Baily M, Bottrell M, Lynn J, Jennings B: The Ethics of Using QI Methods to Improve Health Care Quality. The Hastings Center Report. 36:S1-S40, 2006.
63. McGlynn EA, Asch SM: Developing a clinical performance measure. Am J Prev Med 14:14-21, 1998.

Marcus Rall, David M. Gaba, Steve K. Howard, and Peter Dieckmann

6 Human Performance and Patient Safety

Key Points

1. Clinical excellence is not achieved by the use of sound medical knowledge alone. Human factors and the interaction of team members, as well as organizational conditions in the system of care, also play major roles. Therefore, the study of human performance and related organizational matters is very important.
2. The health care system in general and clinical institutions in particular must provide appropriate organizational characteristics to allow and foster safe patient care practices (e.g., improve safety culture, integrate effective incident reporting and analysis systems).
3. High-reliability organization theory describes the key features of systems that conduct complex and hazardous work with very low failure rates. Errors do occur in such organizations, but their systems make them more impervious to errors and their sequelae (resilience).
4. In dynamic domains such as anesthesia, continuous decision-making, as described in the cognitive process model, is critical to achieving safe patient care.
5. Several error mechanisms have been demonstrated through human factors research. Understanding these psychological "traps" (for example, "fixation errors") can help anesthetists avoid or mitigate them.
6. The introduction and spread of crisis resource management training, including the application of realistic simulation exercises, is likely to improve patient safety in anesthesia and other acute care domains.
7. Like all human beings, the performance of individual anesthetists can be adversely influenced by "performance-shaping factors," including noise, illness, aging, and especially sleep deprivation and fatigue.
8. A particular technique of human factors research called "task analysis" has been useful in understanding the work of anesthetists.
9. Observation of anesthetists during routine operations or in the handling of adverse events (using realistic patient simulators) has improved our knowledge of critical decision-making and team interactions.
10. Future progress on patient safety in anesthesia will require interdisciplinary research and training, improvements in systems safety and organizational learning, and the involvement of all levels of the health care industry.

Impact of Human Performance on Patient Safety

The most important component of every anesthetic regimen is the human performance of the anesthetist and its relationship to patient safety. More than 70% of accidents are due to "human factors." Because the performance of the anesthetist—embedded in a larger system of care—is such a critical and most determining aspect of patient safety, education and training of health care professionals in this area need improvement. This chapter aims to provide an overview of the importance of human performance and systems safety in anesthesia and to provide start-up knowledge of key safety factors and methods.

Anesthesia is an intrinsically hazardous undertaking, but as hazardous activities go, its track record is indeed a model of patient safety for the rest of health care.[1,2] The Institute of Medicine (IOM) asserts: "Anesthesia is an area in which very impressive improvements in safety have been made."[3,4] However, the theory of organizational safety teaches us that safety is a never-ending process; any patient harmed by an anesthetic is one patient too many (in concert with the "zero vision" statement of the U.S. Anesthesia Patient Safety Foundation [APSF]: "That no patient shall be harmed by anesthesia"). Cooper and Gaba[1] wrote: "Anesthesiologists should remain aware of the hazards they still face, take pride in having been the leaders in patient safety efforts, and stay motivated to continue the pursuit of 'no harm from anesthesia' with the passion it still demands."

Because most of the work on human performance (and also on simulation) has been started and has focused on anesthesiology in the operating room (OR), this chapter deals primarily with aspects of performance and safety in the OR setting. Nevertheless, most of the same principles and issues are relevant to the postanesthesia care unit (PACU), the intensive care unit (ICU), emergency medicine, and to a lesser degree, pain therapy and other domains of importance to anesthesiologists. For readers with a special interest in the ICU, a selection of references is given as a starting point.[5-17]

Safe conduct of anesthesia depends on the appropriate application by skilled anesthetists of knowledge concerning surgical procedures, the physiology of patients during and after anesthesia, the characteristics of anesthetic and adjuvant drugs, and the means of monitoring the patient and the life support equipment throughout the perioperative period. In this chapter the term *anesthetist* refers to any anesthesia professional taking care of a patient, whether a physician, certified registered nurse anesthetist (CRNA), or anesthesia assistant.

Traditionally, an adequately trained anesthetist automatically was assumed to perform appropriately. Deviations from optimal outcomes were understood to be due to imperfections in the art and science of anesthesia, which led to heavy emphasis on the scientific and technical aspect of anesthesia training and care. More rarely, adverse outcomes were ascribed to negligence or incompetence on the part of the anesthetist. Today, there is a more complete understanding that anesthetists themselves, both as a profession and as individuals, have strengths and vulnerabilities pertaining to their work environment. The performance of human beings is incredibly flexible and powerful in some aspects, but is very limited in others. They are vulnerable to distractions, biases, and errors. This chapter surveys some of the human characteristics that define the performance of anesthetists. These characteristics (also termed human factors) are by no means constant; for example, a person may communicate very effectively in one instance and fail to close the loop in the next challenging communication role.

The domain of the anesthetist is very challenging; it is as difficult or more so than other domains that more readily capture the public's imagination, such as aviation. The past 25 years has seen new research on the nature and limitations of professional judgment and decision-making in this dynamic and complex world. Chapter 7, "Patient Simulation," explores developments in the methods of using simulations and simulation technologies that have contributed to this research and that may open new opportunities to prepare anesthetists to handle the challenges that they face in their work.

The literature related to human performance and patient safety is vast (standard reference works are available[18-26]), and this chapter samples only a portion of it as it most closely relates to the work of anesthetists. Moreover, this chapter does not deal to any great extent with human-machine interactions and the physical design of the work environment. These aspects of human factors, or ergonomics, in anesthesia have considerable importance in their own right. The reader is referred to several publications that review these issues in detail.[27-38]

Nature of the Operational Domain of Anesthesiology

The operational domain of anesthesia is a complex, dynamic world that presents a cognitive profile common to many real-world task domains. Analysis of complex dynamic worlds in the last decade has departed sharply from previous conceptions of decision-making.[39] Classic decision-making approaches, such as decision theory and multi-attribute utility theory, are mathematical techniques that were traditionally used as the dominant framework for understanding human performance. They worked well in simplified laboratory experiments on decision-making and action, yet a number of investigators had significant difficulty in applying them to real-world decision and action settings.[39] Orasanu and colleagues[39] identified eight factors that characterize such naturally occurring complex dynamic worlds. They apply to anesthesia as follows:

1. **Ill-structured problems.** Unlike traditional decision experiments, there is not just a single decision to be made. Rather, a variety of interrelated decisions must be made by the anesthetist and surgeon. The patient's physiologic behavior is not an independent random variable but is causally linked to previous decisions and actions.
2. **Uncertain dynamic environment.** Dynamism stems from the frequency of routine and anomalous changes or events, the rapidity with which they evolve, and the unpredictability of the patient's physiology and response to interventions. An anesthetized patient is in a constant state of change during surgery, with many events outside the anesthetist's control. Although preventive measures can reduce the likelihood of some events, others cannot be avoided because they are inevitable side effects of medically necessary procedures (e.g., surgical blood loss). Unpredictable and dynamic occurrences compete with the preplanned aspects of the case and drive the anesthetist's actions. The true state of the patient cannot usually be measured directly. It must be inferred from ambiguous patterns of clinical observations and data from electronic monitors. These data are imperfect because unlike industrial systems that are designed and built with sensors in key areas to measure the most important variables, patients are typically instrumented to measure the variables that are easiest to monitor, predominantly with the use of noninvasive methods. Most physiologic functions are observed indirectly through weak signals available at the body surface and thus are prone to various types of electrical and mechanical interference. Invasive measurements are also vulnerable to artifacts and uncertainties of interpretation. Even if the anesthetist knew the exact state of the patient, the patient's response to interventions would be unpredictable.
3. **Time stress.** Because the OR is a scarce resource, there is an incessant overall time pressure to use it efficiently. There is an even more intense immediate time stress within each case generated by dynamic situations that evolve rapidly and must be dealt with in timely fashion.
4. **Shifting, ill-defined, or competing goals.** Multiple goals of case management (e.g., hemodynamic stability, good operating conditions for the surgeon, rapid emergence from anesthesia) may compete with each other. The surgeon's goals may sometimes compete with those of the anesthetist. All these goals shift as the patient's situation changes dynamically throughout the procedure.
5. **Action/feedback loops.** The time constants of actions and their effects are very short, on the order of seconds to minutes. There is complete intermixing of decision-making and action; these functions are not performed in separate

cycles. Most decisions and actions are implemented and evaluated incrementally, with the effect of one cycle assessed before deciding on further possible actions.

6. **High stakes.** The stakes are high because even for elective surgery in healthy patients, there is an ever-present and very real risk of injury, brain damage, or even death. A catastrophe is often the end result of many pathways that begin with seemingly innocuous triggering events. Each intervention, even if appropriate, is associated with side effects, some of which are themselves serious. Some risks cannot be avoided. Unlike an event such as a commercial flight, which can be delayed or aborted if a problem occurs, during an event in the OR this is not usually possible, and immediate surgery may be necessary to treat a medical problem that is itself life threatening. Analogous to military aviation, balancing the risks of action (anesthesia and surgery) against those of inaction is often extremely difficult.
7. **Multiple players.** Anesthesia domains involve multiple players from different professional backgrounds. Each individual has a set of goals, abilities, and limitations. In some situations, interpersonal interactions, among anesthesia personnel and between them and other OR team members, will dominate the work environment.
8. **Organizational goals and norms.** The anesthetist works within the stated and unstated norms of the OR suite, the anesthesia department, the institution, and the profession as a whole. Decisions are sometimes made to conform to these norms even though they are not wholly subscribed to by the anesthetist.

Although many of these features apply to other domains of medicine, anesthesiology is unique in that all eight factors are prominent. In particular, what sets anesthesia apart from clinic- or ward-based medicine is the intensity of the dynamism, time pressure, and uncertainty, with danger lurking just below the surface.

Safety Culture of the Operating Room and Intensive Care Environment (See Chapters 99-101)

Analyzing the Anesthetist's Domain: The Operational World Versus the Organizational World

Psychologists and cognitive engineers who study real work environments describe each field as a domain. Each domain has specific characteristics that set it apart from others, including the nature of the tasks to be performed, the relationships among the tasks, the time scale over which they must be executed, and the criteria for their successful performance. This chapter deals mainly with the operational domains in which anesthesia care is delivered, primarily the OR, the PACU, and the ICU. However, as pointed out by Reason,[40-43] as well as by Cook, Woods, and McDonald,[44] what goes on in the operational domain is extensively shaped by the organizational and managerial environment in which it is located, even to the point that operational personnel believe themselves to be the "victims" of problematic decisions further back in the system.

In everyday practice, these distinctions are hidden or blurred. The positive and negative contributions of the organizational and management elements are often so embedded in the normal routine that they are difficult to isolate. Interesting information about the system often comes from considering abnormal situations, accidents, or near misses instead of normal events. For example, investigation of the loss of the space shuttle Columbia revealed a variety of latent errors within the procedures and safety culture at the National Aeronautics and Space Administration (NASA):

> *The accident was probably not an anomalous, random event, but rather likely rooted in NASA's history and the space flight program's culture.*[45]

The report placed as much weight on these factors as on the direct technical causes of the accident. Traditionally, one speaks of errors arising in decisions and actions that lead to a mishap. However, the term "error" is increasingly considered an inappropriate way to categorize behavior (being a judgment of attribution and blame) and should be thought of merely as a way to identify behavior at the locus of a critical situation. In this context it must be understood that "errors are not the cause of an accident." Rather, errors are usually the consequence of a combination of several underlying factors. Beyond that, errors must combine with other circumstances to result in an accident or adverse outcome.[46] This concept is illustrated in Figure 6-1. Some errors are actively produced in the operational domain, whereas others are introduced by the organizational environment. James Reason, a psychologist at the University of Manchester, England, described the latter by using the concept of "latent errors"[46]:

Naive view: error causes accidents

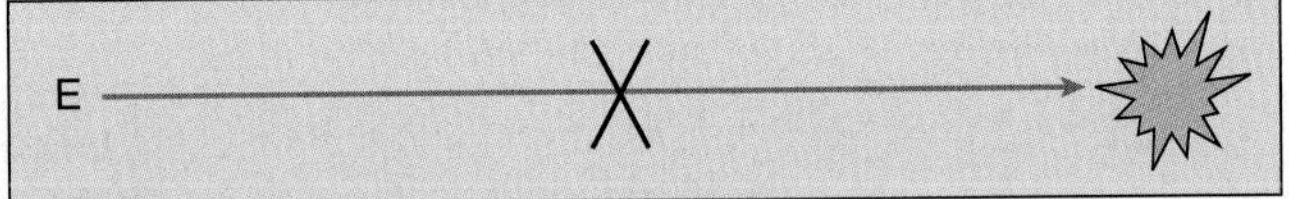

A

Modern view: deeper causes lead to errors that result in accidents

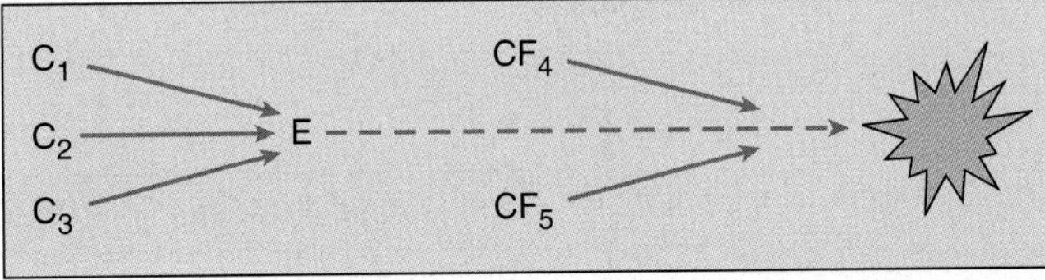

B

Figure 6-1 Relationship between errors (E) and adverse events. **A,** Errors are not the cause of accidents but in rare cases they lead directly to the adverse event. Multiple root causes (C_1, C_2, C_3) lead to the error (**B**). For the most part, additional contributing factors (CF_4, CF_5) are necessary to allow the error to evolve into an adverse event. Incident reporting systems should try to identify as many of the root causes and contributing factors before an accident happens and try to influence these factors in such a way that no accident will happen. *(Adapted from Rall M, Manser T, Guggenberger H, et al: [Patient safety and errors in medicine: Development, prevention and analyses of incidents.] Anästhesiologie, Intensivmedizin, Notfallmedizin, Schmerztherapie 36:321-330, 2001, with permission.)*

... errors whose adverse consequences may lie dormant within the system for a long time, only becoming evident when they combine with other factors to breach the system's defenses. [They are] most likely to be spawned by those whose activities are removed in both time and space from the direct control interface: designers, high-level decision makers, construction workers, managers and maintenance personnel.

Latent errors probably exist in all complex systems, and Reason adopted a medical metaphor to describe them as "resident pathogens." Like microorganisms in the body, the resident pathogens remain under control until sets of local circumstances "combine with these resident pathogens in subtle and often unlikely ways to thwart the system's defenses and bring about its catastrophic breakdown" (Fig. 6-2). This "threat and error model" has also been articulated by the noted aviation-oriented psychologist Robert Helmreich at the University of Texas (Fig. 6-3).[47]

A variety of latent failures can exist in the anesthesia environment. They may include such issues as how surgical cases are booked, how cases are assigned to specific anesthetists, what provisions are made for preoperative evaluation of outpatients, and what relative priority is given to rapid turnover between cases or avoiding cancellation of cases as opposed to avoidance of risk. Latent errors can also result from the design of anesthesia equipment and its user interfaces, which in some cases lead clinicians to err or are unforgiving of errors. Manufacturing defects and routine maintenance failures are also types of latent failure.

Investigation of untoward events must address both latent and active failures and both the organizational and managerial environment and the operational domain. One risk of focusing solely on active failures is that operational personnel may be "victims of the system" in a "Catch-22"–type situation and be pushed to maximize production while admonished to "be safe." Addressing only their actions—and not the latent pressures under which they must work—can make them defensive and uncooperative. Cook, Woods, and McDonald[44] pointed out that if one looks at the chain of events in an accident sequence, one can always find a failure on the part of an operator. If the analysis stops at this point, the operator (i.e., the anesthetist) may be wrongly blamed for a failure, the real roots of which go back to latent failures in the organization. If the underlying latent errors are never identified or never fixed, they remain in the system and

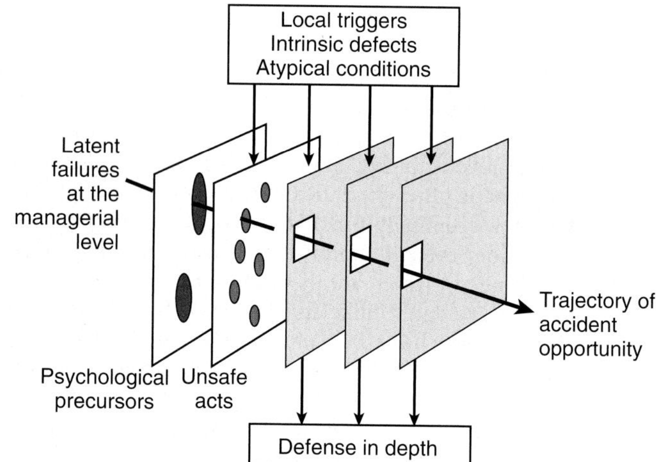

Figure 6-2 James Reason's model of the causation of accidents. Latent failures at the managerial level may combine with psychological precursors and event triggers at the operational level to initiate an accident sequence. Most accident sequences are trapped at one or more layers of the system's defenses. The unforeseen combination of organizational or performance failures with latent errors and triggers may lead to breach of the system's defenses and allow the accident to take place. The diagram should be envisioned as being three-dimensional and dynamic—with "shields" moving around and holes in the defense's opening and closing. *(Redrawn from Reason JT: Human Error. Cambridge, Cambridge University Press, 1990.)*

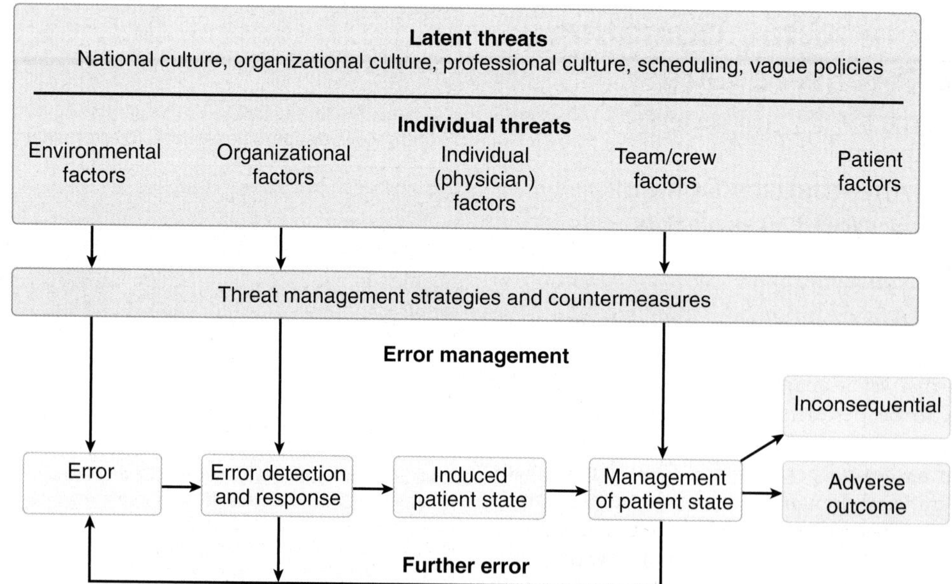

Figure 6-3 University of Texas threat and error model. This model, which illustrates the evolution of errors, is used in the analysis of incidents and accidents (a detailed example is available at http://bmj.bmjjournals.com/misc/bmj.320.7237.781/sld001.htm).

Table 6-1 Asymmetry of Signals of Safety Versus Signals of Production

Production	Safety
Feedback about production is easy to measure reliably and nearly continuously ("revenue,""earnings,"" expenses") and indicates success in a positive fashion	Traditional measures of "safety" are indirect and discontinuous, thus making them noisy and difficult to interpret or even deceptive
Success is indicated "positively" (e.g., increasing earnings), is obviously reinforcing, and has high salience (the bottom line is the "bottom line" for a firm)	Feedback is provided "negatively" (fewer accidents or incidents) and has little reinforcement value in itself. High salience is achieved only after an accident or a scary near miss
The relationship between the application of resources (money, effort, time) and production goals is relatively certain, thus making it easy to use feedback	Even when interpreted correctly, the relationship between application of resources and safety goals is relatively uncertain, thus making it hard to use the feedback

Adapted from Reason JT: Human Error. Cambridge, Cambridge University Press, 1990.

will probably induce another accident chain in the future. This is visualized in Reason's accident trajectory, shown in Figure 6-2.

Asymmetry Between Safety and Production

An additional difficulty in achieving optimal safety is an inherent asymmetry of information and concern about safety versus production (Table 6-1).[46] Investments for production are easy to plan for and measure; feedback about production is easy to obtain and to interpret. Investments for safety are harder to plan for, and the costs are harder to measure. Most importantly, feedback about safety is inherently weak and ambiguous. How can one measure the accidents that could have occurred but did not? Only after a catastrophe takes place do the costs of a safety failure become apparent.

Organizational Safety

Over the last few years there have been many landmark publications and activities concerned with patient safety and the organizational aspects of reducing errors.[3,25,42,48-52] The report of the IOM in 1999, "To Err Is Human,"[3] was a highly publicized awakening in the United States about the problems of patient safety. Summarizing the primary literature, the report stated that "tens of thousands die each year from errors in their care and hundreds of thousands suffer or barely escape from nonfatal injuries that a truly high-quality care system would largely prevent." The most important recommendations of this report, which led to nationwide activities to promote patient safety, are shown in Box 6-1.

The subsequent report of the IOM Committee on Quality of Health Care in America, titled "Crossing the Quality Chasm—A New Health System for the 21st Century,"[48] took a systematic approach to improvement of the entire health care system. It stated that "between the healthcare we have and the care we could have, lies not just a gap, but a chasm" because the health care system today harms too frequently yet routinely fails to deliver its potential benefits. The report concluded: "The current care system cannot do the job. Trying harder will not work. Changing the systems of care will." In the following text we consider the organizational and systems aspects of anesthesia care and patient safety.

There are several schools of thought about organizational safety in highly hazardous activities. Two theories, normal accident theory (NAT) and high-reliability organization theory (HROT), have dominated the discussion of safety in many domains and have been applied individually to health care with increasing frequency over the last 20 years.[43-52,60] NAT was originally promulgated by the sociologist Charles Perrow[57] in the wake of the Three Mile Island nuclear accident and has been applied by him and others to such diverse fields as commercial aviation, maritime transport, and the handling of nuclear weapons. HROT was promulgated initially by a group of researchers at the University of California at Berkeley. It has also been applied to diverse domains, including aircraft carrier flight decks, offshore oil platforms, air traffic control, nuclear power production, and the financial transaction industry (personal communication, Karlene Roberts).

These workers' complementary views of organizational safety are summarized briefly here and in Table 6-2.

Normal Accident Theory (NAT)

NAT focuses primarily on two features of a system: (1) the complexity of interactions among the system's elements and (2) the presence of tight coupling among the system's elements. A system is tightly coupled when a change in one part of the system rapidly alters other parts of the system. For example, some physiologic systems are buffered from changes in others, whereas certain core components, such as oxygen delivery and blood flow, are tightly coupled together and interact strongly. The patient's physiology may become tightly coupled to external systems such as ventilators and infusions of hemodynamically active drugs. When complexity and tight coupling coexist, abnormal sequences of events can sometimes be hidden and have complex or unpredictable consequences. Typically, active errors in the system do not result

Box 6-1 Recommendations of the Institute of Medicine Report "To Err Is Human"

Make patient safety a declared and serious aim.

Provide strong, clear, and visible attention to safety.

Implement nonpunitive systems for reporting and analyzing errors.

Incorporate well-understood safety principles, such as standardizing and simplifying equipment, supplies, and processes.

Establish interdisciplinary programs to improve teamwork and communication by using modalities proven in other industries, including simulation.

Table 6-2 Complementary Views of High-Reliability Organization Theory (HROT) Versus Normal Accidents Theory (NAT)

HROT	NAT
Accidents can be prevented through good organizational design and management	Accidents are inevitable in complex and tightly coupled systems
Safety is the priority organizational objective	Safety is one of a number of competing objectives
Redundancy enhances safety; duplication and overlap can make a reliable system out of unreliable parts	Redundancy often causes accidents because it increases interactive complexity and opaqueness and encourages risk taking by social-shirking and cue-taking behavior
Decentralized decision-making is needed to permit prompt and flexible field-level responses to surprises	Organizational contradiction: decentralization is needed to handle the distributed complexity, but centralization is needed to manage tightly coupled systems
A "culture of reliability" will enhance safety by encouraging uniform and appropriate responses by field-level operators	A military model of intense discipline, socialization, and isolation is incompatible with democratic values
Continuous operations, training, and simulations can create and maintain high-reliability operations	Organizations cannot train for unimagined, highly dangerous, or politically unpalatable operations
Trial-and-error learning from incidents (through effective incident reporting) can be effective and supplemented by anticipation and simulations	Denial of responsibility, faulty reporting, and biased reconstruction of history frequently cripple learning efforts

Modified from Sagan SD: The Limits of Safety. Princeton, NJ, Princeton University Press, 1993.

in an accident because they are trapped at some point by the system's multiple layers of checks and defenses (see Fig. 6-2). Even a minor perturbation can cause normal system behavior to be out of control when there are complex interactions and tight coupling. Perrow called this a "normal accident" because the perturbations are common and arise out of otherwise normal system operations.[57] He suggested that attention should be directed at strengthening the recovery pathways by which small events can be properly handled before they evolve into a serious accident.

Complexity and Tight Coupling: Latent Errors in Anesthesia

Clearly, the anesthesia domain involves complex interactions with tight coupling.[58] The complexity stems to some degree from the variety of devices in use and their interconnections, but these are, in truth, vastly simpler than those found in an oil refinery, a 747 aircraft, or a space shuttle. A more important source of complexity is the "uncertainty complexity" of the patient.[58] The human body is an incredibly complex system containing numerous components, the interactions of which are only vaguely understood. Because many body systems affect each other, the patient is a major site of tight couplings. Furthermore, the anesthetic state tends to ablate the buffers between some of these interconnected systems, thereby strengthening the coupling between them and between the patient and external mechanical supports. Galletly and Mushet[59] studied anesthesia "system errors" and observed tight coupling associated with "the use of neuromuscular blocking drugs, the presence of cardiorespiratory disease, certain types of surgical procedures, and the effect of general anesthetic agents. Looser coupling was observed with the use of high concentrations of oxygen and air mixtures, preoxygenation, and spontaneous breathing techniques."

According to the NAT view, we delude ourselves by believing that we can control our hazardous technologies and forestall disaster; in reality, many of the efforts we make at management and design tend to only increase the opacity and complexity of the system (making more holes in the barriers), thereby increasing the likelihood of accidents. The combination of these factors provides fertile ground for the occurrence of accidents—indeed, according to NAT it makes it inevitable that some of the "normal" everyday faults, slips, and incidents will evolve into tragic accidents. NAT is often considered a "pessimistic" view of the ability of organizations to conduct highly hazardous operations without harmful errors.

The very concept of risk is constructed and negotiated. This was perhaps expressed most clearly by Dianne Vaughan in her powerful analysis of the explosion of the Challenger space shuttle:

> *Risk is not a fixed attribute of some object, but constructed by individuals from past experience and present circumstance and conferred upon the object or situation. Individuals assess risk as they assess everything else—through the filtering lens of individual worldview.*

Vaughan's main thesis is that the Challenger exploded not because "risk-taking" managers "broke the rules" but because the system evolved to make excessive risk a part of "following the rules." This happened because the system had a "culture of production" with ingrained production pressure; it was a regular occurrence that aberrant findings be explained away ("normalization of deviance"), and "structural secrecy" was enforced between departments, between manufacturers and NASA, and between engineers and managers. Sadly, many of these same phenomena occurred yet again and led to the Columbia accident.[45] Unfortunately, each of these system characteristics is also operative in perioperative settings.

High-Reliability Organization Theory

In contrast to these rather pessimistic views of the organizational challenges to safety is the HROT view that although not easy, proper organization of people, technology, and processes can handle complex and hazardous activities at acceptable levels of performance. Even though accidents can never be totally eliminated, high-reliability organizations (HROs) must be judged by the benefits that we derive from their activities and their small absolute risk of failure. This view seems particularly appropriate in anesthesiology because forgoing surgical treatment is not a

Box 6-2 Elements of a Culture of Safety (part of HROT in Box 6-3)

Values

Safety as the most important goal, overriding production or efficiency

Preoccupation with possible "failures" rather than past "successes"

Necessary resources, incentives, and rewards provided for optimal safety, not only for optimal production

Beliefs

Safety must be actively managed

Processes and routines of care are as (or more) important to safety as individual dedication, skill, or effort

Openness about safety and errors is essential; learning from normal and adverse events should be thorough

Norms

Low-ranking personnel raise safety issues and challenge ambiguity regardless of hierarchy or rank

Calling for help is encouraged and occurs frequently, even (or especially) by experienced personnel

Explicit communication is frequent

The hierarchy is flat—leaders listen to juniors; juniors speak up; and calling for help is routine regardless of rank

People are rewarded for rationally erring on the side of safety, even when their credible concerns turn out to be wrong

Adapted from Weick KE: Organizational culture as a source of high reliability. Calif Manage Rev 29:112-127, 1987.

viable option for many patients and challenges to safety must often be met head-on. Although the concepts of HROT have varied over the years, the core characteristics of HROs are shown in Boxes 6-2 and 6-3.

A key aspect of HROT is that of a culture of safety (or "safety culture"). Since publication of the reports from the IOM, health care has begun paying attention to certain elements of "culture." However, most of the attention has been devoted to the "culture of blame" in a system whereby problems are addressed largely in terms of who is to blame rather than what can be done to prevent them. Safety culture goes beyond these issues by dealing with how individuals and groups conduct their work. Culture is made up of values (what is important), beliefs (how things should work), and norms (the way things work). These elements are shown in Box 6-2. It is equally important that the culture is highly uniform throughout the organization and be continually reinforced by peers, more so than by enforcement of rules.

High-Reliability Organization Theory in Anesthesiology

Anesthesiology has traditionally been strong at some elements of an HRO, particularly in redundancy and technical safety measures. There is a growing movement in anesthesia to more fully implement HRO philosophies and techniques.[60] In fact, anesthesiologists have not only been promoters of the patient safety movement in general but have also been leaders at applying HROT principles to health care. In 2003, the APSF began initiatives in high-reliability perioperative health care (see Special

Box 6-3 Key Elements of a High-Reliability Organization (HRO) in Medicine

Established Culture of Safety (see Box 6-2)

Optimal Structures and Procedures

Decision-making rests with those with greatest knowledge or experience about specific issues regardless of rank or job type.

The unit integrates crews from different departments (e.g., cardiac surgery, cardiac anesthesia, OR nursing, perfusion, ICU) into a coherent clinical team. Teamwork and resiliency are emphasized.

There are formal procedures to maximize transfer of information to all team members before a case (e.g., briefings or time-out procedures).

Schedules are designed to keep work hours and duty periods at reasonable levels to avoid undue fatigue. Personnel under excessive stress are supported or replaced as needed.

Standardized procedures, techniques, and equipment are adopted whenever possible so that similar tasks or operations are performed similarly regardless of the personnel involved; conversely, when necessary (in an emergency or adverse event), the team is resilient and responds as needed to the situation without slavish dependence on standard routines.

The use of preplanned algorithms, checklists, and cognitive aids is actively encouraged.

Easy access to current information systems is available at all times and all locations.

Training and Practice in Routine Procedures and Simulations

Debriefings are conducted after each case.

Nonpunitive assessment instruments are used on a regular basis to provide current feedback and identify elements requiring special training.

There is initial and recurrent simulation-based single-discipline and multidisciplinary training in crew resource management (see Chapter 7).

Actual clinical crews and teams conduct periodic drills or simulations of critical situations in the real OR, PACU, and ICU.

Resident training uses a guided curriculum; training goals and the level of responsibility assigned to a resident match the current proficiency level of the trainee with the complexity of the procedure.

Organizational Learning

Robust mechanisms are in regular use for organizational learning, both prospectively (considering in advance how to optimize protocols and procedures, such as failure mode and analysis of effects) and retrospectively (from analyzing reports of adverse events, near misses, or problems such as root cause analysis).

Problems are analyzed primarily to determine what can be improved rather than whom to blame. Altered procedures are assessed and adopted as appropriate. Process changes reflect appropriate analysis.

ICU, intensive care unit; OR, operating room; PACU, postanesthesia care unit.

Issue of APSF Newsletter, Summer 2003, at www.apsf.org). Box 6-3 summarizes key elements of an HRO adapted to health care.

Teams and Communication

Unlike teams in aviation, the military, and police and fire services, the OR team is unusual in that the command structure is ambiguous. Physicians (surgeon and anesthesiologist) are nominally superior to nursing and technical staff, but physicians are coequally responsible for the patient during the immediate perioperative period. Surgeons were historically considered the "captain of the ship," with even a legal doctrine giving them responsibility for the actions of all other OR team members. Although this legal doctrine has formally fallen by the wayside, remnants of it still remain in aspects of the organizational structure and culture of OR environments. Nonetheless, when both an anesthesiologist and surgeon are caring for a patient, they are coequally responsible, which can lead to complex issues of command authority, hierarchy, and control.

Each physician, as well as the nurses and technicians, has a primary territory of knowledge, skill, and responsibility, but there is considerable overlap among them.

Strictly speaking, a team is defined as "a distinguishable set of two or more people who interact, dynamically, interdependently, and adaptively toward a common and valued goal/objective/mission, who have each been assigned specific roles or functions to perform, and who have a limited life-span of membership." A team is distinct from a group in that a group is an ad hoc collection of individuals without a specific mission and without specific roles. In the OR, all team members have the common goal of a good outcome for the patient. However, there can be considerable disagreement about how to achieve this goal and which elements of patient care have the highest priority. These differences are probably traceable to the fact that the OR team is itself made up of several "crews" (i.e., surgery, anesthesiology, nursing, perfusionist, radiology), each of which has its own command hierarchy, its own global properties (professional standing, culture, traditions, and history), and its own set of local goals and objectives for management of the patient. The differences among the crews can be so striking that some investigators refer to them as separate tribes (transcript of Conference on Human Error in Anesthesia, Asilomar, CA, 1991).

Each "crew" has one or more members who must work effectively together, and crews combine to form a team. A critical component of the success of this process is the establishment and maintenance of a shared mental model of the situation. To the degree that this can be accomplished, the different individuals will be able to tailor their efforts toward a common goal. Experience working together as a crew or team will improve the likelihood of generating a shared mental model.

Cooke and Salas[61,62] made some interesting statements on teams and team knowledge (Box 6-4). In their view, "team knowledge" is more than the sum of individual team members' knowledge, and they demonstrate the need for new methods to elicit team knowledge (e.g., a collective holistic approach). In team knowledge they distinguish between "team mental model" and "team situation model." To judge team knowledge, information is also needed on the broader aspect of "team cognition," which involves team knowledge itself, team decision-making, team situation awareness, and team perception. Figure 6-4 reflects these components of team cognition and team knowledge.[61]

Box 6-4 Teamwork Principles

Team leadership matters.

Team members must have clear roles and responsibilities.

Shared understanding of the task, teammates, and objectives goes a long way.

Take time to develop a discipline of prebriefing, performance, and postbriefing.

Teamwork effects matter.

Clinical expertise is necessary but insufficient for patient safety; cooperation, communication, and coordination skills matter.

Teams must have clear and valued visions.

Learning from mistakes, self-correction, and adaptability are the hallmarks of high-performance teams.

From Salas E, Rosen MA, King H: Managing teams managing crises: Principles of teamwork to improve patient safety in the emergency room and beyond. Theoret Issues Ergonomics Sci 8:381-394, 2007.

Status and Hierarchy Effects

Status and hierarchy effects are important in team performance. Especially in crisis situations, the lower-status crew member tends to defer to the higher-status individual, even if that individual is performing poorly. In aviation, some airplane crashes have occurred in which overbearing captains were combined with unassertive subordinates (first officer copilot and flight engineers). The team was not able to respond effectively, even when the subordinates knew that something was wrong.

In aviation, as in academic anesthesia, training is an ongoing activity in the domain. Although the captain is in charge of the flight, the captain and the first officer (who is essentially in training to become a captain) traditionally alternate the roles of "pilot flying" and "pilot not flying" on each leg of a flight. Each of these roles is carefully defined and involves separate but interrelated tasks (the pilot flying handles the flight controls, whereas the pilot not flying handles radio communications and other tasks). In anesthesiology, the roles of the trainee and the faculty member during patient care are rarely made explicit. The trainee is often expected to do all tasks with only occasional assistance from the supervisor (part of a training method known as cognitive scaffolding). The exact responsibility for different tasks in a crisis is not predefined. It is interesting that two factors frequently found to be associated with critical incidents in anesthesia have been "teaching in progress" and "inadequate supervision."[63]

A particular issue of hierarchy is known as "cue giving" and "cue taking," in which people give off "cues" (often without even knowing it) that are taken up by others.[64] Those not at the top are very sensitive to cues emitted by their superiors. The cues sent by high-status personnel can inhibit action or even questions from lower-status people. One effect of this phenomenon is that dyads and teams that expect to have redundancy from "multiple sets of eyes" on a patient may not achieve this goal because the views of a single person dominate the thinking of the group.

<table>
<tr><td rowspan="5">Team cognition</td><td>Team decision-making</td><td colspan="2" rowspan="3">Model and structure of embedded team knowledge in the broader concept of team cognition</td></tr>
<tr><td>Team situation awareness/ vigilance</td></tr>
<tr><td>Team perception</td></tr>
<tr><td rowspan="2">Team knowledge</td><td>Team mental model</td><td>Team situation model</td></tr>
<tr><td>• Long lasting, prior to task
• Through training, experience
• Collective knowledge base, common expectations</td><td>• Fleeting, dynamic
• Through task situation specific
• Interpret situation</td></tr>
</table>

Figure 6-4 Components of team cognition and team knowledge.

Production Pressure

The social and organizational environment may also act as a source of production pressure on anesthetists. Production pressure encompasses the economic and social pressures placed on workers to consider production, not safety, their primary priority.[57] In anesthesiology, this typically means keeping the OR schedule moving speedily, with few cancellations and minimum time between cases. In principle, safety and efficiency can go hand in hand. Many aspects of high reliability, such as standard operating procedures, preprocedure briefings, and flattening the hierarchy, may smooth operation of the system, as well as make it safer. Frequently, however, the pressure for throughput can erode safety.

For example, when anesthetists succumb to these pressures, they may skip appropriate preoperative evaluation and planning or they may fail to perform adequate pre-use checkout of equipment. Even when preoperative evaluation does take place, overt or covert pressure from surgeons (or others) can cause anesthetists to proceed with elective cases despite the existence of serious or uncontrolled medical problems. Production pressure can cause anesthetists to choose techniques that they otherwise believe to be inadvisable.

Gaba and associates[65] reported on a randomized survey of California anesthesiologists concerning their experience with production pressure. They found that 49% of respondents had witnessed a situation in which patient safety was compromised by pressure on the anesthesiologist. Thirty percent reported strong to intense pressure from surgeons to proceed with a case that they wished to cancel. Notably, 20% agreed with the statement that "If I cancel a case, I might jeopardize working with that surgeon at a later date."

Production pressure also leads to haste by the anesthetist, a psychological precursor to the commission of unsafe acts. In the survey, 20% of respondents answered "sometimes" to the statement that "I have altered my normal practices in order to speed the start of surgery," whereas 5% answered "often" to this statement. Twenty percent of respondents rated pressure by surgeons to hasten anesthetic preparation or induction as strong or intense. Repeated exposure to these conflicts can cause the anesthetist to internalize pressures; 38% of survey respondents felt strong to intense internal pressure to "get along" with surgeons, and 48% reported strong internal pressure to avoid delaying cases. Anesthetists may then feel impelled to go ahead with cases against their better judgment, even in the absence of overt pressure.

Investigating these aspects of the work environment is difficult because such relationships are driven by economic considerations, as well as by the complex organizational and interpersonal networks linking the different medical cultures. Changing the environment will be equally challenging.

Assessing Risk Factors in Anesthesia

An innovative attempt was made by a team of engineers and anesthesiologists to apply a technique called "probabilistic risk analysis" (PRA) to model cascading risks and the effects of different types of organizational interventions.[66,67] PRA has been used extensively in nuclear power and other highly hazardous industries (for example, it was used for analysis of the risks to the space shuttle from thermal tile failure). Complete PRA models are very complex and extensive. In the anesthesiology study, a highly simplified PRA model was used to assess the feasibility of applying this technique to health care. The PRA analysis of organizational changes in anesthesia suggested that patient risk could be reduced best by closer supervision of residents, the use of patient simulators for training and periodic recertification, and regular medical examination of anesthetists for fitness for duty. As yet it has not been possible to develop comprehensive PRA models of anesthesia risk because the number of decision and action elements is very large and knowledge of the probability of success or failure for each of the decisions or actions is very limited. The PRA approach might be a useful heuristic to help clinicians lay out critical decision-making and therapy issues, but it may never make any meaningful contribution as a quantitative safety management technique.

There has been growing interest in applying process-oriented systems analysis to patient care flows and processes. For example, a group in Tübingen, Germany, performed a process-oriented systems analysis at a medical university hospital to assess the anesthesia work system's ability to regulate variances and disturbances in the work process.[68] These investigators showed that the internal work process can be regulated well but that the high interdependence of the anesthesia work system with other systems requires extensive coordination activities.

Characteristics of Successful Incident Reporting Systems

Incident Reporting Systems for Learning from Problems

An important strategy for improving patient safety (and a core tenet of HROT) is "organizational learning." Such learning can be both prospective (deliberating in advance of process changes how they might affect safety) and retrospective (learning from events that have already transpired). Most high-hazard and high-reliability industries have made special efforts to create systems for retrospective organizational learning, often concentrating on the reporting, investigation, and analysis of both frank accidents or errors and near-miss events with no negative outcome.[25,46,47,69-72] The details of successful incident reporting systems (IRSs) are covered in a number of publications.[5,7,42,52,73-90]

Historically, investigation of errors in the health care system has been hindered by a "culture of blame"[90-92] in which naming, blaming, and shaming are the main features of event reporting and review rather than analysis by experts and focus on the development of systematic countermeasures. A culture of blame in which it is posited that errors, accidents, and near misses are due primarily to a lack of knowledge, a bad attitude, or a lack of commitment to patients leads to a heavy burden on those involved in adverse events. It may also compound internalized negative feelings over having contributed to patient harm.[92,93]

Anesthesiology as a specialty has played a leading role in the attempt to turn this culture of blame into a safety culture—putting safety first[1,2] and trying to understand how errors, incidents, and adverse events evolve.[5,25,42,60,72,73,75,76,94-103]

Errors Per Se Are Not the Cause of Accidents

Only a minor fraction of errors lead to a negative patient outcome. However, the "harmless" error may well point to a systematic weakness (latent problem) in the system, which if investigated further can lead to a systematic change. Unfortunately, the reverse is often true. The lack of a negative outcome is interpreted as "success" of the system, and the underlying vulnerabilities are ignored. In most cases, errors in complex systems are not the sole causes of accidents and rarely lead inevitably to an adverse event (see Fig. 6-1A). In actuality, first hand there are probably underlying reasons (C_1 to C_3 in Fig. 6-1B) that someone commits an error, and then additional contributing factors (CF_4, CF_5) are "needed" to allow an accident to develop. The main idea of modern IRSs is to identify the factors that make errors more likely to occur, as well as additional factors that allow a negative outcome to ensue. By reporting and analyzing factors C_1 to C_3 and CF_4 and CF_5 in Figure 6-1 regardless of the outcome, it might be possible to eliminate or reduce the probability or the harm potential of the accident long before it ever happens.

"If reporting is safe and provides useful information from expert analysis, it can measurably improve safety."[80]

IRSs, if well structured and operated, can make substantial difference in system safety (Fig. 6-5). The present knowledge about weaknesses and strengths of the health care system that is

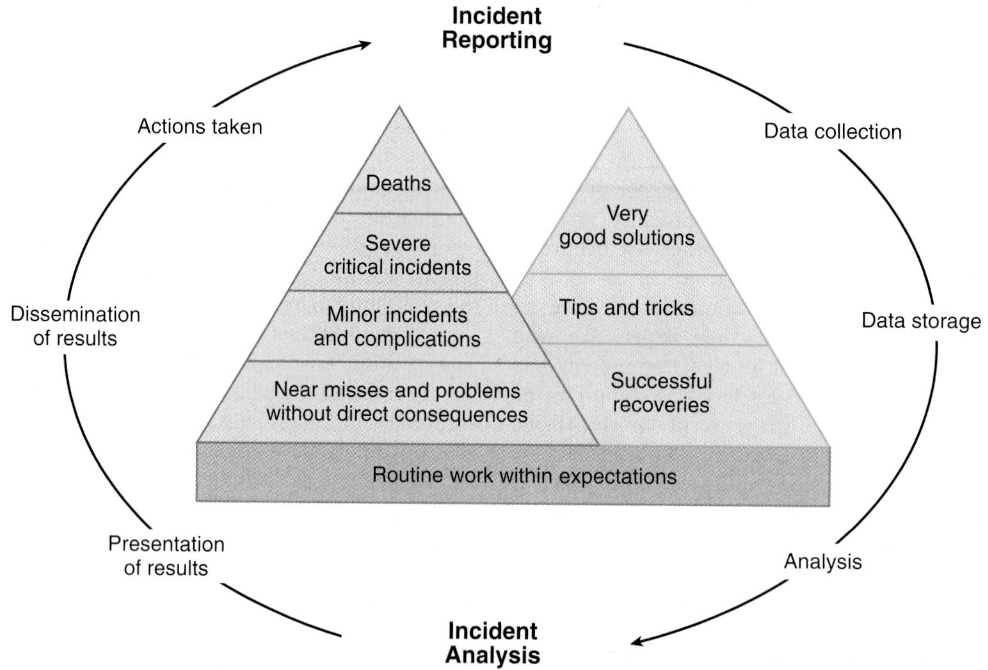

Figure 6-5 Process model of an incident reporting system that is constructed as a complete system. The data need to be collected, saved securely, analyzed independently, and the results need to be visualized in a relevant way, distributed to stakeholders in an applicable way, and result in concrete action by the reporting organization. It should be possible to report all incidents and errors, independent of the outcome. Innovative systems should even include positive reports. (Figure by P. Dieckmann.)

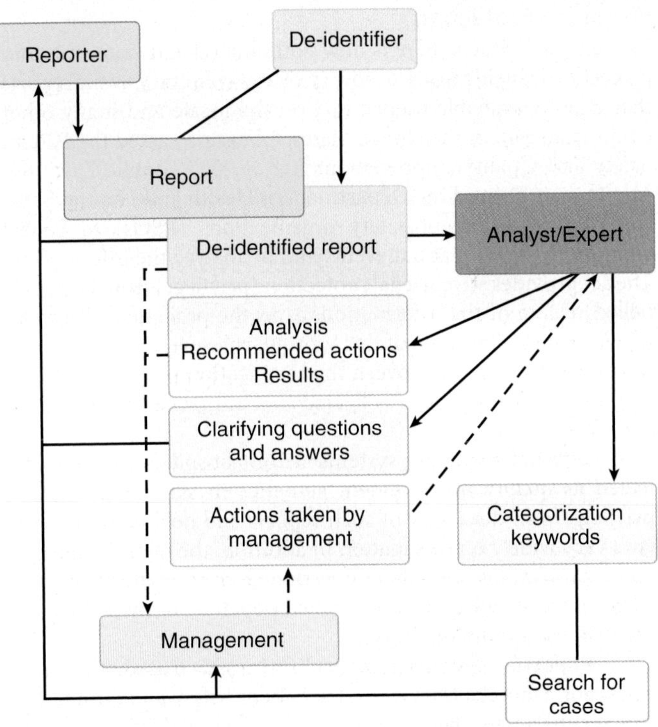

Figure 6-6 Data handling in a modern incident reporting system with de-identification. The incoming reports are first completely de-identified by a trained de-identifier. Only after this step is the report ready to be analyzed. It is important that the reports are analyzed by a multiprofessional team and that recommendations be fed back to the management of the organization from which the report came. The analysis and feedback should be transparent for all stakeholders.

"out there" already can finally be extracted and made available for others. IRSs are often referred to as "learning systems," similar to the National Reporting and Learning System of the National Patient Safety Agency in the National Health Service of the United Kingdom.

Effective IRSs allow insights into the health care system that are otherwise very hard to acquire. In this sense IRSs can open "windows to the system."[94]

Merely having a reporting form or a database of information does not constitute an effective reporting system. They can be effective only when they are constructed, established, and maintained as an entire system (Fig. 6-6; also see Fig. 6-5) and are successfully embedded in the organization or industry. Omission of or faults in any of the requirements in Box 6-5 will limit the success of the system.[88]

What Should Be Reported?

Uncertainty about *what* should be reported is one of the barriers for an IRS.[105] In aviation, it has been necessary to create a reporting system for "incidents" (without negative outcome) that is distinct from systems for reporting or analyzing accidents. Of course, in aviation the occurrence of an accident is usually known immediately, and such events are never "supposed to happen." Yet in health care every human being will get sick and will die; in fact, most people will die in proximity to medical care. Thus, negative outcomes are inherent to the progression of disease, so determining what outcomes are due to "errors" or "accidents" is much harder in health care settings. For this reason many believe that for health care event reporting systems, it should be possible to report all critical incidents, with or without a negative outcome. In fact, the system may also solicit reports of "positive events" in which the outcome was good despite challenging clinical circumstances. In general, the invitation to report should be very broad and cast a "wide net" to find all interesting occurrences.

What Should Report Forms Look Like?

Reporting systems that rely primarily on an array of checkboxes for the reporter to choose from regarding the "causes" of the incident have not proved to be useful. In fact, it is thought in the Aviation Safety Reporting System (ASRS), for example, that "Counting incidents is a waste of time" (quote from Charles

Box 6-5 Important Characteristics of Effective Incident Reporting Systems

- Integration of the incident reporting system into the organization and full support by management
- No negative sanctions for reporters and people involved
- Confidential or anonymous reporting option, with active de-identification (domain expertise required)
- Legal protection and state-of-the-art data security
- Independence of the organizational hierarchy: reports are sent to a trusted subunit outside the hierarchy of the organization or outside the organization (external trust center, e.g., NASA for the ASRS)
- Orientation to a system that enables all stakeholders of patient safety to easily file reports, including physicians, nurses, and technicians
- Easy and fast reporting
- Training of stakeholders to file valuable reports (e.g., focusing on human factors issues, as well as medical-technical aspects)
- Timely feedback about reception of the report, its analysis, and proposed measures to be taken from it
- Analysis of each report by experts (a multiprofessional team that has a background not only in the medical domain but also in issues of human performance and analysis methods)
- Deep analysis of selected cases using root cause analyses or failure modes and effect analyses with the aim of improving systems safety in the future
- Timely implementation of improvements to confirm the "reactivity" of the system and to *make a difference*
- Evaluation of improvements and special care to avoid "improvements for the worse" (quick fixes without improving the underlying latent dangers)
- Organizational support of reporting and analysis of cases, as well as the implementation of improvements
- Supports continuous improvement of the positive proactive safety culture in the department (systems perspective!)

ASRS, Aviation Safety Reporting System; NASA, National Aeronautics and Space Administration.

Data from references 25, 77, 80, 104.

Billings, a founder of the ASRS). In a voluntary reporting system one has no way to estimate the true number of specific problems. Similarly, trend analysis is not feasible because the frequency of events and the frequency of reporting are confounded. A free-text description of the reported incident has been more helpful in identifying what can be learned from the report. This view is also supported by the World Health Organization's Guidelines for Incident Reporting[77]:

> *However, much of what promotes learning in patient safety lacks crisply defined data elements, so most authorities believe it is important for reports to include narrative to convey meaning. Narrative reports provide the opportunity to capture the rich context and storyline that allow the conditions that contributed to the error to be explored and understood.*
>
> *Indeed, some believe that only narrative reports are capable of providing information that provides meaningful insight into the nature of the underlying systems defects that caused the incident (Richard Cook, personal communication).*

Clearly, no reporting system can detect all the problems in a clinical institution, even ones that create a severe vulnerability. For one thing, it is known that between 50% and 96% of critical incidents are not reported[106,107] with current systems, although new thrusts in incident reporting hope to increase the fraction of events that are reported.

Legal Issues of Reporting Systems

Especially in jurisdictions for which medical liability litigation is common, there will be a number of legal issues that affect reporting systems. First, for some kinds of events in some settings there will be legal requirements to report the event to a governmental body. This is true in the United States for certain kind of adverse drug events or for certain failures of medical devices. Moreover, some states have started mandatory reporting programs about so-called never events that are thought should never occur in the absence of a systems failure. In general, voluntary IRSs operate completely in parallel with any other types of reporting systems.

An important question for most reporters is whether the report will be confidential or anonymous and whether the report will confer any immunity to the reporter. Anonymous reporting provides maximum protection for reporters but limits the amount of information that can be acquired about any given event and the cogency of that information. Confidential reporting can allow confidential interaction between analysts and the reporter to acquire all the information and context needed concerning the event, but the linkage between the report and the identity of the reporter exposes a risk even if confidentiality is formally provided. Of note, the ASRS—on which many reporting systems have been modeled—operates as a confidential system but with subsequent de-identification of the reports to make them anonymous. Furthermore, the ASRS was able to offer limited immunity from administrative actions for those who filed a report. This was a major incentive for reporting events. In health care, physicians largely fear malpractice litigation, and it is not possible to offer immunity from litigation to reporters, although offering immunity from administrative action (e.g., an official reprimand) within the hospital itself could be an incentive to report.

Statutory Protection

In the United States there is now both federal and state statutory protection (shield) from discovery of any voluntary event reports that may be available (depending on the locale and many other circumstances). In the United States, Congress passed the Patient Safety and Quality Improvement Act of 2005 (Public Law 109-41). This authorized the Department of Health and Human Services to certify patient safety organizations (PSOs) to collect confidential reports about events and to analyze the information. The act provides strong legal protection (privilege) from any compelled release of the information, as in the process of discovery in a lawsuit. At the time of this writing, rules were in the process of being formulated to govern the certification process for PSOs, so no data have yet been collected that are protected under the act.

Internal reporting systems within hospitals may be protected as quality improvement activities in states that provide privilege from discovery of such reports and deliberations. State laws vary widely on this matter. In addition, the quality improvement protections are often questioned during litigation, and whether the privilege will be applied depends on the ruling of a judge in each individual case.

Reporting systems in other countries have used other strategies. For example, the Center for Patient Safety and Simulation, which runs a national IRS in Germany called PaSOS, has constituted itself as a "press office" (informing the anesthesia public as a journal would); this then brings it under the protection of the "free press act and rights" and makes it almost impossible to use its data in litigation.

De-identification before Information

A common strategy of confidential reporting systems is to quickly convert the data to anonymous status by "de-identification." To do this, it is necessary to edit the reports and delete all information that might be used to identify persons or organizations. Systems vary by what stage of analysis they conduct de-identification and where they set the balance between acquiring needed information versus deleting possibly identifying data. One issue in all reporting systems, especially in health care, is that the key facts of many events might be relatively unique and thereby lead to a high risk of "intrinsic identification" even when all objective identifiers are stripped.

There are now IRSs in many countries with various designs and operational processes (see Appendix 1).[5,7,42,52,73-90] Many systems are installed locally, but more and more national systems, or at least systems with a national common data set, are being installed.[108] Box 6-6 shows some of the features of and lessons learned from the national anesthesia system PaSOS (available at www.pasos-ains.de) in Germany, which is directed by one of this chapter's authors (M.R.).

Human Factors

This part of the chapter deals with human factors in the broadest sense of the meaning. In contrast to the previous part of the chapter, which covered aspects of the health care system and organizational matters, the human factors portion is related to the performance of individuals and teams and to factors influencing their performance and promoting or preventing active or passive errors. Because more than 70% of all errors in medicine can be

Box 6-6 Characteristics of the German National Anesthesia and Intensive Care Incident Reporting System PaSOS (www.pasos-ains.de)

The system is provided by the two German anesthesia societies and run by a professional interdisciplinary group.

Every anesthesia department and ambulatory anesthesia unit in Germany is entitled to take part. The basic functionality, software, server storage, and updates are free of charge (a service by the societies).

The system is Web-based with an anonymous secure login (SSL). No data are stored locally in the hospitals, but users work directly on the central secure server with php technology.

The reports are primarily sent outside one's own institution for de-identification by our independent and interdisciplinary patient safety group (TuPASS), which increases trust of employees in the safety of the system.

All reports undergo a professional four-eye active anonymization and de-identification process by domain experts trained in incident reporting and using checklist protocols to prevent any lapses in de-identification.

After de-identification, most reports can be read in full text by all employees. This is meant to sensitize all by reading all the cases and to stimulate discussion about patient safety in the department and to report your own cases. It also provides very powerful feedback to the reporter, who can read "his" report in the Web.

Every department gets a unique department login that is provided to all employees (physicians, nurses, technicians, etc). This login allows you to separate "your" reports from the national reports. So every department has its own "local" incident reporting system inside the big national system. There are no personal logins because the system is anonymous.

Most reports are readable in the national IRS, open to all anesthesiologists. This should contribute to the national spread of important critical safety information. Of course, on this level, nobody can see where the reports came from. (You can select "your" reports with your department login, but you cannot identify the origin of reports once they are in the national database).

All reports are manually tagged with key words for meaningful search results; they are classified according to the U.K. NHS NPSA contributory factors framework[52,94,95] and also categorized with the CRM key points (see text).[60,109]

A local de-identifier does not exist and can therefore not be interviewed by any legal authorities.

An optional module, "feedback and analysis suggestions," is available on request; it provides expert feedback about every report from the IRS provider team back to the organization's risk management, including systems safety analysis and suggestions for countermeasures.

Several organizational prerequisites need to be fulfilled by departments to take part (organizational embedding before starting to report). For example, all departments have to send their PaSOS representatives to an initial workshop to get briefed about the do's and don'ts of IRS. They also get a set of slides and information material to spread the messages in their local departments (snowball effect).

Departments that do not comply with the minimal requirements, especially prerequisites such as the written "no-blame assurance" to their employees, are not allowed to take part or may even be excluded from the system.

IRS, incident reporting system.
Data from references 60, 104, 108, 110.

attributed to problems with human factors rather than problems with knowledge or practical skills, the impact of human factors cannot be overestimated. On this basis perhaps human factors should take 70% of the whole book! Given that this chapter cannot deal with human factors in a comprehensive way, many topics can be touched on only briefly, and the reader is directed to the available literature. We focus on the most important aspects of human factors that are directly relevant to practicing anesthetists.

Nontechnical Skills in Anesthesia

Over the last 20 years, the health care professions have become more aware of the importance of "nontechnical" skills in the delivery of safe, high-quality medical care. This recognition has brought an increased need for assessment, evaluation, and training of these skills. Patient simulators were perhaps the first opportunity to show and train these skills under realistic stressful conditions.[109,111-113] The introduction of simulators and the associated training concepts accelerated understanding of these human factors by the medical community.[2] Some of the needed "crisis management skills"[20,114] can be trained without the use of simulators, as shown in other domains (aviation, oil platforms, military).[71,115-117] The baseline level of crisis resource management (CRM) performance is somewhat low.[118] Helmreich states that as a first step in establishing error management programs, it is necessary to provide formal training in teamwork, the nature of error, and the limitations of human performance.[47]

There are different ways to group the nontechnical skills that are at the heart of CRM training. One approach is to distinguish between two categories of nontechnical skills: (1) cognitive and mental skills, including decision-making, planning, and situation awareness (Table 6-3), and (2) social and interpersonal skills, including aspects of teamwork, communication, and leadership. Another approach is to split nontechnical skills into five major groups as shown in Figure 6-7.

Crisis Resource Management

What Exactly Is Crisis Resource Management?

Cockpit (later "crew") resource management was introduced in aviation in the mid-1980s and is considered to be successful in

Table 6-3 Nontechnical Skills in Anesthesia: Classification, Markers, and Teaching Points

	Anesthesia Nontechnical Skills (Fletcher et al.[146])		Performance Markers (Gaba et al.[130])	Key Teaching Points in Anesthesia Crisis Resource Management (Gaba et al.[147,148])
Concepts	**Elements**	**Categories**	**Markers**	**Reminders**
Cognitive and mental skills	Planning and preparing	Task management	Orientation to case	Anticipate and plan Know your environment
	Prioritizing		Leadership (also a social and interpersonal skill)	Exercise leadership Set priorities dynamically
	Providing and maintaining standards		Planning	Use cognitive aids
	Identifying and using resources		Workload distribution	Distribute the workload Mobilize all available resources
	Gathering information Recognizing and understanding Anticipating	Situation awareness	Anticipation Vigilance	Use all available information Allocate attention Anticipate and plan
	Identifying options Balancing risks and selecting options Re-evaluating	Decision-making	Preparation Re-evaluation	Prevent and manage fixation errors Re-evaluate repeatedly
Social and interpersonal skills	Coordinating activities with team	Team working	Inquiry/assertion	Communicate effectively Teamwork
	Exchanging information Using authority and assertiveness		Communication feedback Group climate	Communicate effectively Exercise leadership and followership
	Assessing capabilities Supporting others		Followership	Exercise followership
Overall assessment	Not applicable Assessments are made only at the element and category level		Overall nontechnical performance of the primary anesthetist Overall nontechnical performance of the whole team	Teamwork! Concentrate on what is right, not who is right

that industry and other industrial and military settings (although admittedly, there is not what evidence-based medicine would call "level 1 evidence" for this success).[24,25,41,119-122] Crew resource management is now taught systematically to crew members of all major U.S. airlines and at many airlines around the world.[123] A similar program in anesthesiology was first developed by Gaba, Howard, and associates at the Veterans Affairs (VA) Palo Alto Health Care System and Stanford School of Medicine[4,105,109,113,124] originally as anesthesia crisis resource management (ACRM). The ACRM curriculum and its variants have since been adopted by training centers worldwide. A detailed description of the ACRM course is provided.

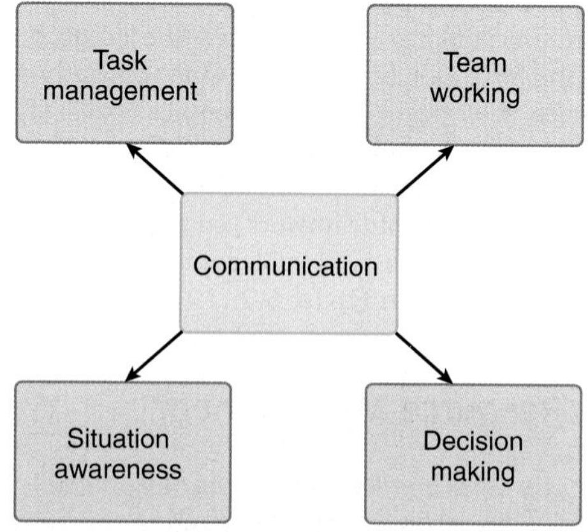

Figure 6-7 Five main groups of nontechnical skills. In this approach, effective communication is like the glue that holds all the other components together.

In overview, CRM means to coordinate, use, and apply all available resources to protect and help the patient as best as possible. Resources include all the personnel involved, along with all their skills, abilities and attitudes—albeit also with their human limitations. Machines, devices, and information sources, including cognitive aids, are also critical resources.

Though termed "crisis management," CRM principles actually also apply before a crisis ensues. CRM includes preventing and intercepting threats and errors and minimizing their negative consequences to the patient.

The key points of CRM as they apply to anesthesia care have been steadily updated and expanded over time (see Box 6-7). Some of the principles might seem obvious or self-evident. However, from our experience in simulation training, it is in fact *not* trivial to actually apply these principles whether during routine work or during crises. More theoretical background on the principles can be found in the textbook on ACRM by Gaba, Fish, and Howard,[125] as well as in related safety literature.[25,41,43,46,47,70,71,72,126-130]

Box 6-7 CRM—Key Points in Healthcare

1. Know the environment.
2. Anticipate and plan.
3. Call for help early.
4. Exercise leadership and followership with assertiveness.
5. Distribute the workload (10-seconds-for-10-minutes principle).
6. Mobilize all available resources.
7. Communicate effectively—speak up.
8. Use all available information.
9. Prevent and manage fixation errors.
10. Crosscheck and double-check (never assume anything).
11. Use cognitive aids.
12. Re-evaluate repeatedly (apply the 10-seconds-for-10-minutes principle).
13. Use good teamwork—coordinate with and support others.
14. Allocate attention wisely.
15. Set priorities dynamically.

Adapted from Rall M, Gaba DM: Human performance and patient safety. *In* Miller RD (ed): Miller's Anesthesia, 6th ed. Philadelphia, Elsevier Churchill Livingstone, 2005.

Like nearly all principles of sound human factors, application of CRM key points to patient care must be supported by top leadership and reinforced in the actual work environment. It is of no worth to study these principles (or even practice them in simulations) only to find that the pressures and culture of the "real OR" make them impossible to implement for real patients. Fully integrating these key points into the structures and processes of clinical practice has proved to be a significant challenge.

Know the environment! (CRM key point 1)

CRM begins before the crisis starts. One of the prerequisites for CRM is to *know the available resources and the details of the specific working environment*. Resources are *personnel*, *equipment* (software, hardware, or cognitive aids), and supplies. It is important to know who can be asked for help, who is available at different times of the day, how to call those helpers quickly, and how long it will take them to arrive. Regarding equipment, it is necessary to not only know *what* is available and *where to find it* but also *how* to operate it. The anesthesiologist is responsible for being well versed in the operation of all relevant equipment and should also use manuals and other cognitive aids to learn to use the gear and as a backup source of information during patient care.

Anticipate and plan (CRM key point 2)

Anticipation is key for goal-oriented behavior. Anesthetists must consider the requirements of a case in advance and plan for the key milestone. They must imagine what could go wrong and plan ahead for each possible difficulty. Savvy anesthetists expect the unexpected, and when it does strike, they then anticipate what could happen next and prepare for the worst. People often talk about "staying ahead of the game" or, conversely, "falling behind" or "being behind the eight ball."

Call for help early (CRM key point 3)

Knowing one's own limitations and calling for help is a sign of a strong character and a competent person. Trying to handle everything alone or toughing out a critical situation is dangerous and unfair for the patient, who should not suffer to protect the anesthetist's pride or ego. In case of an emergency or even a suspected emergency, help should be called early rather than late. Some typical triggers for calling for help that apply to any anesthetist at any level are (1) when there are too many tasks to do, (2) when the situation is already catastrophic (e.g., cardiac arrest, difficulty securing the airway), (3) when serious problems are getting worse or not responding to the usual maneuvers (or both), and (4) when you do not know what is going on. It is important to know in advance who is available and how to call for help and to plan for how best to use the help when it arrives.

Exercise leadership and followership with assertiveness (CRM key point 4)

A team needs a leader. Someone has to take command, distribute tasks, collect information, and make key decisions. Leadership rarely means knowing more than everybody else, doing everything alone, or putting other people down. Leadership is about planning, deciding, and distributing tasks by clear communication. Followership is also an important skill. Followers are key members of the team who listen to what the team leader says and do what is needed. However, it does not mean shutting off their own brains. Followers should be assertive if they think that the team leader is making wrong decisions. It is their responsibility to make sure that the leader is aware of their concerns. Whenever people work together, conflict can ensue; anyone on the team may need to diffuse conflicts to focus the team on care of the patient. Get everyone to concentrate on *what* is right, not on *who* is right.

Distribute the workload "10-seconds-for-10-minutes principle" (CRM key point 5)

One of the main tasks of a team leader is distribution of the workload. Someone is needed to define the necessary tasks and ensure that they are fulfilled properly and that everything fits together. If possible, the team leader should remain free of manual tasks to observe, gather information, and delegate tasks. Team members should also look actively for things that need to be done. It is not a good team if the team leader has to express every idea and nothing is done before it is explicitly ordered.

A corollary is known as the "10-seconds-for-10-minutes principle", which posits that if a team can slow its activities down just a little, it can gain more than enough benefit in rational decision-making and planning to offset the delay. The need to slow down appears to be greatest in critical situations such as the beginning of the diagnosis and treatment planning or when the team "feels stuck" because the usual treatment is not working (Fig. 6-8).

Mobilize all available resources (CRM key point 6)

Everyone and everything that could help deal with the problem at hand should be mobilized, including humans and technology embedded in organizational processes. On the human side, the anesthetist's knowledge and skills (mitigated by knowledge of one's human deficiencies) are the most important resource, com-

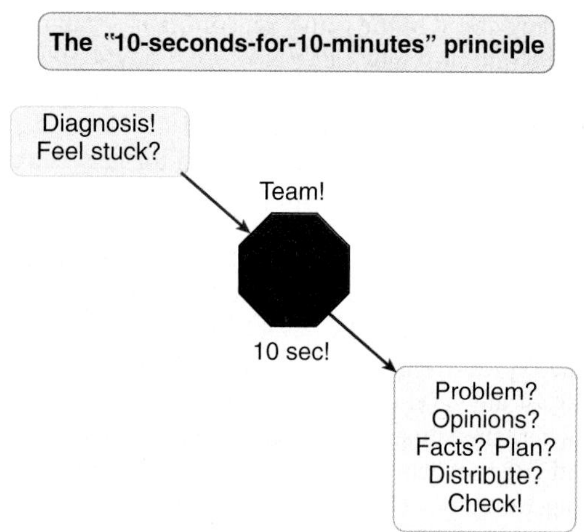

Figure 6-8 The "10-seconds-for-10-minutes principle." When making a *diagnosis* or *feeling stuck*, perform the 10-second team timeout and check to see "what the biggest problem is (the most dangerous aspect right now)" (*Problem*). Clarify this with all available team members (*Opinions*). Gather the information available (*Facts*). *Plan* the treatment, including the desired sequence of actions. *Distribute* the workload by assigning tasks and responsibilities. *Check* with all team members about any further concerns or suggestions.

plemented by the human helpers who can be brought to bear. Equipment and supplies are the means by which knowledge is translated into action. Some equipment will be readily available, but others will need time to be mobilized.

Communicate effectively—speak up (CRM key point 7)

Communication is key in crisis situations. Good team work depends on everybody being on the same page and coordinating their efforts; communication is the glue that holds the disparate members together (see Fig. 6-7). Effective communication is challenging to accomplish. Several aspects make communication difficult sometimes; for example, saying something is meaningful communication only if the messages are received and understood (Fig. 6-9).

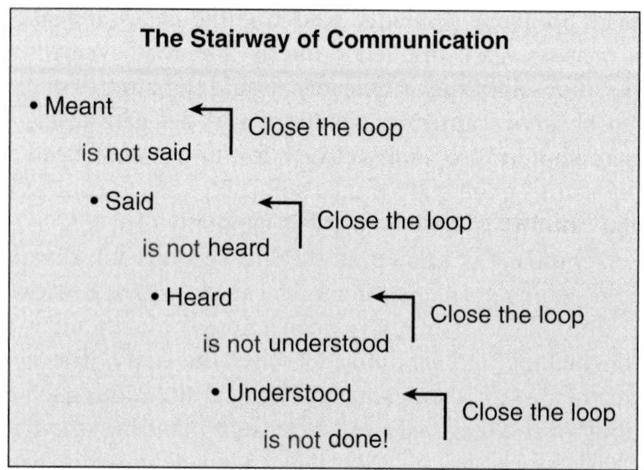

Figure 6-9 Model showing the importance of proper communication. When dealing with complex situations under time pressure, people tend to "mean" a lot but "say" little. It is important to let other team members know what you think (mental model). Not everything that is said is necessarily heard by those who should hear. This is often not the "fault" of the receiving end; acoustic hearing and mental understanding are not the same. It is important for the sender and receiver of a message to close the communication loop. Some tasks need time to be completed and may fail. Let the team know.

Use all available information (CRM key point 8)

Anesthesiology is particularly complex because information must be integrated from many different sources. Every bit of information can assist in understanding a patient's status better and arriving at the correct diagnosis. Information sources include those immediately at hand (the patient, monitors, the anesthesia record), secondary sources such as the patient's chart, and external sources such as cognitive aids (see later) or even the Internet.

Prevent and manage fixation errors (CRM key point 9)

Human actions are based on an instantaneous mental model of the current situation. If the model of the situation is erroneous, the actions will probably be wrong.

The term "fixation error" describes a model that is persistently faulty despite sufficient evidence to correct it. A fixation error is the persistent failure to revise a diagnosis or plan in the face of readily available evidence suggesting that a revision is necessary. This type of error is extremely common in dynamic situations. There are three main types of fixation errors.[131,132]

One type of fixation error is called **"this and only this"**—sometimes also called "cognitive tunnel vision." In this type of error, attention is focused on only one possibility and other (possibly or actually correct) alternatives are not taken into account. Another fixation error is **"everything but this,"** the persistent search for irrelevant information and failure to treat a probable cause with serious consequences.

Perhaps the most insidious fixation error is the persistent claim that **"everything is OK,"** in which all information is attributed to artifact and possible signs of a catastrophic situation are otherwise dismissed. Another form of "everything is OK" is the failure to transition from "routine mode" to "emergency mode" when the situation demands it.

One principle of managing fixation errors is to get a new view—a second opinion—on the situation from someone unaware of the faulty previous assumptions. Although it is appropriate to brief the new person on the situation, it is best to avoid biasing the person with the conclusions already drawn. Even when working alone the anesthetist can deliberately change perspectives (physically or mentally) and look for information not fitting the picture of the situation, as though entering the room for the first time.

The aforementioned 10-for-10 principle (CRM key point 5) might also be helpful in managing fixation errors. More information on fixation error is provided later in the section "Core Process."

Crosscheck and double-check—(never assume anything) (CRM key point 10)

Crosschecking means to correlate information from different sources. There are often three independent sources of information about the patient's heart rate (electrocardiogram [ECG], pulse oximetry, and blood pressure monitor), for example, and two about the rhythm (ECG and pulse oximetry).

Another aspect of crosschecking involves reviewing the status of actions that have been done or are under way. Human memory about actions performed is vulnerable, especially when interruptions have occurred. Moreover, although we often attempt to check things "at a glance," such fleeting observations are prone to error. Checking numbers and settings on equipment by actually touching them and looking carefully may be worth the effort.

ratings, it is possible that the observability or scorability of the desired sets of behavior was greater than in actual simulation scenarios. The scripted scenarios were rather short (4 to 21 minutes), which perhaps made it relatively easy to remember certain aspects of the performance and reduced the likelihood of raters encountering the problem of aggregating a score from fluctuating behavior over time. The window of "accuracy" as "±1 point" on a 4-point scale seems to be rather wide.

On the whole, the ANTS system appears to be a useful tool to further enhance assessment of nontechnical skills in anesthesia and other medical fields, and its careful derivation from a current system of nontechnical assessment in aviation (NOTECHS) may even allow some interdomain comparisons.

Performance-Shaping Factors

With a few exceptions, the foregoing discussion of the performance of skilled anesthetists has assumed that they are normally fit, rested, and acting in a standard working environment. Experience in human performance in the laboratory and other domains suggests that internal and external performance-shaping factors exert profound effects on the ability of even highly trained personnel. The degree to which performance-shaping factors affect the overall performance of anesthetists and the outcome of patients is highly uncertain. In extreme cases, such as profound fatigue, there is no question that these factors can result in severe degradation of the anesthetist's performance or even complete incapacitation. However, these extreme conditions are quite unusual, and it is unclear whether the levels of performance decrement likely to be induced in typical work situations have any significant effect. Although the practice of anesthesia does require an attentive and skilled individual, it does not require peak human performance. It would be unrealistic to expect peak performance for every anesthetic regimen because on the order of 60,000 anesthetic regimens are administered each day in the United States by a total of approximately 40,000 to 60,000 anesthetists. Although it is unrealistic to expect peak performance for every case, society expects anesthesiologists to come to work prepared—not impaired. As stated in the American Society of Anesthesiologists (ASA) guidelines for the ethical practice of anesthesiology, anesthesiologists have ethical responsibilities to themselves. The guideline goes further by stating that "the practice of quality anesthesia care requires that anesthesiologists maintain their physical and mental health and special sensory capabilities. If in doubt about their health, then anesthesiologists should seek medical evaluation and care. During this period of evaluation or treatment, anesthesiologists should modify or cease their practice."

With these caveats in mind, however, there are several performance-shaping factors that are potentially of sufficient magnitude to be of concern. Ambient noise, music, fatigue and sleep deprivation, aging, illness, drug use, and attitudes are discussed later. Several other issues that are not discussed include the level of illumination and environmental temperature. These factors can be shown to have a performance-shaping effect in the laboratory, but it is uncertain how much they affect performance in the OR. Currently, the responsibility for ensuring fitness for duty rests solely with the individual clinician. In HROs, the institution implements measures to mitigate performance-shaping factors.

Ambient Noise and Music in the Operating Room

The OR is a relatively noisy work environment.[153-156] Mean sound levels are considerably higher than in most offices or control rooms (continuous movement of air through an open surgical suction tip is a common source of continuous noise), and peak sound levels can be quite high. Some sources of noise are uncontrollable, such as surgical drills, monitor alarms, and inadvertently dropped instrument pans; other sources are controllable, such as conversation and music (see later). There is evidence in the general literature that noise can adversely affect human performance.[153] Furthermore, studies by Murthy and colleagues[157,158] demonstrated that volume-accurate replay of recordings of OR noise significantly interfered with the speech discrimination ability of anesthesia residents during laboratory testing. The OR noise also caused a significant reduction in residents' performance on psychometric tests of mental efficiency and short-term memory.[157] The potential interference of noise with communication and situation awareness among personnel in the OR is particularly worrisome to those concerned with optimizing teamwork in this complex work environment.

The use of music in the OR is now widespread. Many health care professionals believe that music enlivens the workday and can build team cohesiveness when all team members enjoy the music. A controversial study by two social psychologists, Allen and Blascovich,[159] suggested that surgeon-selected music improved surgeons' performance on a serial subtraction task and reduced their autonomic reactivity (i.e., "relaxed" them) when compared with control conditions consisting of experimenter-selected music or no music at all. The methodology of this study has been criticized.[160]

In response to Allen and Blascovich, several anesthesiologists challenged the notion that the surgeon's preference for the type or volume of music can or should override the needs of other members of the team.[160,161] This issue generated considerable controversy among surgeons and anesthesiologists. In a reply to some of the letters to the editor commenting on their study, Allen and Blascovich[162] stated: "The letters here suggest that not everyone on the surgical team always appreciates the type of music chosen by the surgeon, and anesthesiologists in particular appear to prefer silence in surgery. When we asked the surgeons in our study about this issue, we were told that the environment of surgery does not lend itself to the democratic process, and music was part of the environment in which they felt most comfortable."

Murthy and colleagues studied the effect of OR noise (80 to 85 dB) and music on knot-tying ability in a laparoscopic skill simulator. They found no difference in time or knot quality in the conditions tested and concluded that surgeons can effectively block out noise and music. Invited commentary that accompanied the article brings up important issues: what impact does noise have on other members of the surgical team, how does noise affect communication between team members, does noise affect judgment, and other unanswered questions.

There is no simple answer to the question of the proper role of music in the OR. Clearly, optimal patient care is the primary goal. Some surgical and anesthesia personnel explicitly forbid any type of music in the OR. A more common approach of many OR teams is to allow any team member to veto the

In general it is best to "never *assume* anything"; make sure and double-check important information.

Use cognitive aids (CRM key point 11)

Cognitive aids—such as checklists, handbooks, calculators, and advice hotlines—come in different forms but serve similar functions. They make knowledge "explicit" and "in the world" rather than only being implicit, in someone's brain. Memory and cognitive functioning are vulnerable to error or complete failure, especially in stressful situations. Cognitive aids offload memory and safeguard the recall of critical items. They also help ensure the use of current best practices because during a crisis, people sometimes revert to what they originally learned as the best, not what is the latest recommendation. The use of cognitive aids rather than memory alone is another sign of strength.

Re-evaluate repeatedly (apply the 10-seconds-for-10-minutes principle) (CRM key point 12)

Acute medicine is dynamic. What is correct now might be wrong in the next minute. Some parameters might change slowly over time, and subtle changes can be hard to perceive. Trend monitoring can be helpful to detect slow, but insidious changes.

Furthermore, the dynamic nature of critical events makes it necessary to repeatedly re-evaluate the situation. Box 6-8 shows a set of questions that should be raised repeatedly to check whether one is still treating the most serious problem most effectively.

Implement principles of good teamwork—coordinate with and support others (CRM key point 13)

Teamwork in multidisciplinary teams is at the heart of much patient management in the OR and ICU. Key principles of teamwork in dynamic situations have been delineated, especially in the work of Eduardo Salas and colleagues at University of Central Florida (see Fig. 6-4). Coordination within a team ideally begins before a team gathers. If all members know about the tasks to be done and their roles during these tasks, coordination is easier. Short briefings at the beginning of a task are common in aviation and are worth the time spent. During the acute phase of a crisis situation, it is worth a small amount of time to coordinate the team's activities (see 10-for-10 earlier in CRM key point 5). "Dream teams" support each other continuously, with everybody looking after each other.

Box 6-8 Re-Evaluation Questions—Maintaining Situation Awareness

- Was the initial assessment of the situation or diagnosis correct?
- Did the actions have any effect? (e.g., did the drug reach the patient?)
- Is the problem getting better, or is it getting worse?
- Are there any side effects resulting from previous actions?
- Are there any new problems or other problems that were missed before?
- What further developments can be expected in the (near) future?

Allocate attention wisely (CRM key point 14)

Human attention is very limited and multitasking is very difficult. Attention must be dynamically allocated where it is needed. One can develop rhythms and scan patterns to do this. The "ABC equals airway, breathing, circulation" mnemonic is based on this principle. Other strategies are to alternate between focusing on details and focusing on the big picture and to offload certain responsibilities, tasks, or information streams to other qualified team members, provided that they periodically update the team leader about the situation.

Set priorities dynamically (CRM key point 15)

Dynamic situations demand dynamic measures with decisive, purposeful preliminary decisions and actions that are constantly re-evaluated and modified as new information becomes available or the results of treatment are apparent. What was not a right move at one time may become the right move at another. In addition, having one solution to an obvious problem does not guarantee that it is the best solution to the one problem or that there is only that one problem to deal with. However, one priority is always paramount—ensuring adequate oxygenation and perfusion of critical organs.

How Can CRM Skills Be Learned and Trained

CRM is taught in many different ways. Seminar-based training on human factors and CRM principles has become popular in health care (e.g., programs called "MedTeams," "Medical Team Training," "LifeWings"),[133-140] although the role of such activities versus simulation-based CRM approaches has not yet been fully delineated. Seminars use didactic sessions, group exercises, and sometimes discussion and analysis of "trigger videos." Such training is probably useful for first learning about CRM principles and articulating how they might apply to anesthetists' work environments. Given the experience in the airline industry, it is likely that to completely address CRM skills for both trainees and experienced personnel, a combination of seminars and simulation-based exercises will be needed. We believe that to really practice the execution of CRM skills requires exposure to challenging clinical situations in realistic simulation scenarios, followed by detailed group debriefings (often using video of the simulations) to analyze what transpired. As detailed in Chapter 7, such CRM-oriented simulation training may be available in dedicated simulation centers or as in situ simulation training in actual work environments. Many simulation centers also offer "mobile training," which means that they can bring the simulator and everything else needed (e.g., audio/video equipment) to any facility to train the staff in institutions that do not have a simulator or staff capable of conducting the training.

How Can CRM Skills Contribute to Patient Safety

Although 70% of all errors in anesthesia may be attributable to human factors, interventions to improve this picture have only partially penetrated the fabric of the industry. CRM-oriented training is one component of a comprehensive approach to addressing human factors issues in anesthesia safety, but it is not yet a standard part of clinical training. There is not yet definitive evidence that CRM training in anesthesia improves patient outcomes, and many believe that it may be functionally impossible to acquire such evidence. Nevertheless, CRM training is an integral and accepted part of training in aviation, nuclear power, and other industries in which human errors can lead to catastrophic events. There is no reason to assume that doctors would be less error prone or would benefit less from human factors–based CRM training than the professionals in other high-hazard industries.

Assessing Nontechnical Skills Is More Subjective Than Assessing Technical Skills

A study by Morgan and Cleave-Hogg concluded that "the simulator environment is somehow unique and allows different behaviors to be assessed."[141] As Glavin and Maran stated, "Any scoring system that attempts to address the assessment of clinical competence clearly has to address both technical and non-technical skills"[142]; consequently, there is still a long road ahead in measuring performance.

Two research groups (VA-Stanford and the University of Basel) have studied adaptations of the anchored subjective rating scales developed by the NASA/University of Texas Aerospace Crew Performance Project. The VA-Stanford group published preliminary data reviewing the inter-rater reliability of subjective ratings of behavior on five-point anchored scales.[130,143] Using a fairly stringent test of inter-rater reliability (the topic is quite complex in the statistical literature), they found only moderate reliability when five trained raters used a five-point scale to score 14 anesthesia teams, each managing two different complex critical events in the simulator (malignant hyperthermia and cardiac arrest). Despite some difficulty in agreement on the operational definitions of each type of behavior, the investigators stated that the largest problem in achieving agreement was the high variability of each behavior over the course of a simulation. For example, an anesthesia crew could show evidence of good communication at one instant, only to be shouting ambiguous orders into thin air at the next instant. Aggregating such behavior into a single rating was extremely difficult, even for bounded time segments of the scenario. These data demonstrate the importance of evaluating performance by more than one rater, who no matter how well trained, may produce scores that differ significantly from another single rater. The investigators suggested combining scores from a minimum of a pair of raters inasmuch as it was shown that the mean of scores from two raters had a very low probability of differing from the mean of five raters by more than a single rating point.

The behavioral markers of their score are shown in Table 6-3 and compared with Fletcher's "anesthesia nontechnical skills (ANTS)" score and the ACRM key teaching points (see Box 6-7).

The ANTS System

Fletcher, from the Industrial Psychology Group of Aberdeen (headed by Rhona Flin) and working with clinicians from the Scottish Clinical Simulation Centre (Glavin and Maran), performed an in-depth review of the role of nontechnical skills in anesthesia. Fletcher stated that nontechnical skills have not been explicitly addressed in the traditional education and training of anesthesiologists, even though they have always been demonstrated and used during clinical work. The group analyzed incident reports and observations of real cases, as well as attitude questionnaires and theoretical models.[144] Like others, they recognized that simulation offers the opportunity to identify, develop, measure, and train nontechnical skills in a safe learning environment, so they also included significant observations during realistic simulations.[145]

Incident reports proved very limited because they did "not provide the finer-grained level of information necessary to understand where the skills broke down."[146] They defined nontechnical skills as "attitudes and behaviours not directly related to the use of medical expertise, drugs or equipment." Although nontechnical skills can be seen under the heading of "human factors," it is preferred that they be addressed as "nontechnical skills," which is more specific.

As in the ACRM instructional paradigm,[109,147,148] Fletcher and colleagues identified two categories of nontechnical skills:

- Cognitive and mental skills, including decision-making, planning, and situation awareness
- Social and interpersonal skills, including aspects of team working, communication, and leadership

Fletcher's ANTS scheme is shown in Table 6-4, along with the behavioral markers of Gaba's team and the ACRM key teaching points. A description of the ANTS categories and elements, including examples of good practice and poor practice, is presented in Table 6-4.

The structure of the new ANTS scheme was derived from a system of behavioral markers that had been developed for aviation in an European project called "NOTECHS," which itself was an evolution of the UT-Markers of the University of Texas (Helmreich). A summarized comparison of the aviation systems and explanations about using nontechnical markers for training and evaluation can be found in the downloadable documentation of the "Group Interaction in High Risk Environments" created by an international group of human factors specialists (available at http://www2.hu-berlin.de/gihre/Download/Publications/GIHRE2.pdf). Several comments about the ANTS approach are appropriate.

ANTS' intent is to score only those skills that can be identified unambiguously through observable behavior. Such restriction may enhance the reliability of the scoring but could exclude relevant personal factors such as self-presentation, stress management, and maintaining perspective. ANTS assumes that "communication" is included or "even pervades" all other categories and does not score communication as a separate skill. This approach is in contrast to that of others who believe that communication is a specific skill that should be rated separately.[115,149] The category "task management" of the ANTS includes the element "providing and maintaining standards," which might be a point of discussion if it can be an observable behavior "not directly related to medical expertise" as stated in the definition. In addition, there might be a problem because there are not so many well-accepted standards in medicine (in strong contrast to, e.g., aviation).

Table 6-4 Example of a Description of the Anesthesia Nontechnical Skills System (ANTS System—V1.0)

Task Management—skills for organizing resources and required activities to achieve goals, be they individual case plans or longer-term schedul
It has four skill elements: planning and preparing, prioritizing, providing and maintaining standards, and identifying and using resources.

Planning and preparing—developing primary and contingency strategies in advance for managing tasks, reviewing these tasks, and updating th
required to ensure that goals will be met; making necessary arrangements to ensure that plans can be achieved.

Behavioral Markers for Good Practice	*Behavioral Markers for Poor Practice*
Communicates plan for case to relevant staff	Does not adapt plan in light of new information
Reviews case plan in light of changes	Does not ask for drugs or equipment until the last r
Lays out drugs and equipment needed before starting case that are suitable for the patient	Does not have emergency/alternative drugs availab
Makes postoperative arrangements for patient	Fails to prepare postoperative management plan

Prioritizing—scheduling tasks, activities, issues, information channels, etc., according to importance (e.g., because of time, seriousness, plans); bein
identify key issues and allocate attention to them accordingly; and avoiding being distracted by less important or irrelevant matters

Behavioral Markers for Good Practice	*Behavioral Markers for Poor Practice*
Discusses priority issues in case	Becomes distracted by teaching trainees
Negotiates sequence of cases on list with surgeon	Fails to allocate attention to critical areas
Conveys order of actions in critical situations	Fails to adapt list to changing clinical conditions

Providing and maintaining standards—supporting safety and quality by adhering to accepted principles of anesthesia; following, when possible, co
good practice, treatment protocols or guidelines, and mental checklists

Behavioral Markers for Good Practice	*Behavioral Markers for Poor Practice*
Follows published protocols and guidelines	Does not adhere to emergency protocols or guidelines
Cross-checks drug labels	Does not check blood with patient and notes
Checks machine at beginning of each session	Breaches guidelines such as minimum monitoring standa
Maintains accurate anesthetic records	Fails to confirm patient identity and consent details

From Fletcher GCL, Flin R, Glavin RJ, Maran NJ: Framework for Observing and Rating Anaesthetists' Non-Technical Skills—Anaesthetists' Non-Technical Skills (ANTS) Syst V1.0, 22nd version. Aberdeen, Scotland, University of Aberdeen, 2003.

Flin's group, meanwhile, adapted nontechnical skills scoring systems for several other medical fields, such as for surgeons and ICU care.[25,72,123,128-130,150-152] They have not yet made adaptations that fully describe multidisciplinary crews and teams.

Not all nontechnical skills will be expected to be observed during every scenario or clinical situation. It is important to delineate between "required behaviors" in a given scenario and the generic set of behaviors. If a required behavior is not observed, the rating system advises that one rate that behavior as poor nontechnical skills, whereas the absence of a given nontechnical skill behavior otherwise has no particular meaning and should be rated as "not observed." As in all subjective nontechnical performance systems, training plus calibration of raters is necessary.

Fletcher and coworkers evaluated ANTS by using scripted videotapes taken in a realistic simulator. Fifty consultant anesthetists were given 4 hours of training as raters and then rated eig test scenarios ranging from 4 to 21 minutes each. They rated pe formance at the level of specific elements and also at the broade level of category (see Table 6-3) by using a four-point scale (the could also enter "not observed"). Three investigator anesthetists also rated the scenarios and agreed on a "reference rating" to be used as the benchmark for the study. In questionnaires the ANTS system was evaluated by raters as relatively complete, possibly with superfluous elements. Raters found that nontechnical skills were usually observable, and most thought that it was not difficult to relate observed behavior to ANTS elements. The inter-rater reliability, accuracy, and internal consistency of the ratings were good to acceptable and are presented in Table 6-5.

Although well performed, there are some caveats about these data. Because scripted videos were used as the basis for

Table 6-5 Results of an Evaluation Study of Anesthesia Nontechnical Skills by Fletcher and Colleagues

Measure	Score	Range	Max/Min	Element/Category
Inter-rater agreement	Element level	0.55-0.67	Highest element	Identifying/using resources
			Lowest element	Recognizing/understanding
	Category level	0.56-0.65	Highest category	Task management
				Team working
			Lowest category	Situation awareness
Accuracy relative to the reference rater's score	% within ±1 point	88%-97%	Highest element	Identifying options
			Lowest element	Assessing capabilities
	Mean absolute deviation	0.49-0.84, depending on elements	Highest element	Authority/assertiveness
			Lowest element	Provide standards

From Fletcher R, Flin P, McGeorge R, et al: Anaesthetists' non-technical skills (ANTS): Evaluation of a behavioural marker system. Br J Anaesth 90:580-588, 2003.

choice or volume of music if they believe that it interferes with their work.

Reading in the Operating Room

The observation that some anesthetists were observed to read journals or books casually during patient care led to a vigorous debate of the appropriateness of such activity.[163] Although it is indisputable that reading can distract attention from patient care, there are no data at present to determine the degree to which reading does distract attention, especially if the practice is confined to low-workload portions of a case. Furthermore, many anesthetists pointed out that reading as a distraction is not necessarily any different from many other kinds of activities not related to patient care that are routinely accepted, such as idle conversation among personnel. Many comments about the issue were related not to the actual decrement in vigilance induced by reading but rather to the impact of the negative perception of the practice (and of those who do it) by surgeons and by patients (if they were aware of it).

A noted researcher on human performance in anesthesia, Matt Weinger, was asked to comment on the practice of reading in the OR.[164,165] He pointed out that reading can combat boredom, which can be a significant distractor in its own right. He concluded that in the absence of data specifically on the topic, it is unscientific to condemn the practice outright, but that reading—like all other distractions—should not be allowed to impair vigilance and patient care.

In our training course on ACRM, we teach that the anesthetist is responsible for modulating all controllable distractions—for example, allowing music during routine work (if all agree) but eliminating it when the situation becomes complex or urgent. Similarly, although our own institutions do not have a policy against reading in the OR (or against casual conversation for that matter), we do expect the anesthetist to terminate all incidental activities when necessary and to have a very low threshold for abandoning potential distractions.

Sleep Deprivation and Fatigue*

General Principles

Scientists are discovering the importance of adequate sleep to allow normal human performance. A consensus report[166] by leaders in the field of sleep medicine stated the following:

> *[we] evaluated scientific and technical reports on the distribution throughout the 24-h day of medical incidents (such as heart attack and stroke) and performance failures (such as vehicular accidents and human errors in industrial and technical operations that can affect public safety). We found that these events occur most often at times of day coincident with the temporal pattern of brain processes associated with sleep. It thus appears that the occurrence of a wide range of catastrophic phenomena are influenced by sleep-related processes in ways heretofore not fully appreciated.*

This report goes on to give many examples of catastrophes that have occurred at least in part because of the effects of sleep deprivation and fatigue.

Investigations in other complex industries (aviation, nuclear power, maritime, long-haul trucking) have identified fatigue as the probable cause of or a contributing factor in many accidents. Unlike health care, the transportation industries have a body—the National Transportation Safety Board (NTSB)—that actively evaluates accident causation, including performance-shaping factors such as fatigue and sleep deprivation. By formal analysis, fatigue has been implicated in many famous accidents. For example, fatigue was a contributing factor in the Exxon Valdez grounding, the nuclear disasters at Three Mile Island and Chernobyl, and the decision-making process that led to explosion of the space shuttle Challenger. We have no such mechanism for evaluating fatigue causation in medical error, so what is not looked for will not be found.

Based on these findings, however, it is likely that chronic sleep deprivation, circadian rhythm abnormalities, and fatigue can be blamed for some iatrogenic adverse patient outcomes. As previously mentioned, the IOM report published in 1999 revealed that thousands of patients are harmed each year by preventable error. Some of these errors may have fatigue as a causative factor, and this should be an area of active study. However, it is difficult to determine the degree to which this is true because there is no blood test equivalent for level of impairment secondary to fatigue. Although these factors have long been minimized or ignored by health care professionals, an understanding of them is critical to maximize patient safety, as reflected in recently published reviews.[167,168]

Normal Sleep

Carskadon and coworkers[169] referred to sleep as a reversible behavioral state of perceptual disengagement from and unresponsiveness to the environment that is usually accompanied by postural recumbency, quiescence, closed eyes, and other indicators commonly associated with sleeping. Sleep can be thought of as a physiologic drive state similar to hunger or thirst and is necessary for maintenance of alertness, performance, and overall well-being. The intensity of this drive can be inferred by noting how quickly an individual falls asleep. Just as eating and drinking satiate hunger and thirst states, sleeping reverses the desire to sleep.

The amount of sleep required by any individual is genetically determined and is the amount that allows that individual to be awake and alert throughout the day. The average sleep time for young adults is 7 to 8 hours per 24-hour period, with an approximately 15% inter-individual variation. These sleep requirements do not change with age, and humans can do little to train their physiology to function optimally on less sleep than what is required.

Sleep Debt

If adequate sleep is not obtained for whatever reason, daytime sleepiness and impaired performance ensue. Sleep loss is cumulative and results in what is referred to as sleep debt. An individual who has obtained an optimal amount of sleep is better prepared to perform long periods of sustained work than one who is operating from a sleep debt.

*This section was co-written by Steven K. Howard, M.D., staff anesthesiologist, Veterans Administration Palo Alto Health Care System, and associate professor, Stanford University School of Medicine, Stanford, California.

Because of the additive effects of chronic partial sleep loss, even minor sleep restriction on a nightly basis can insidiously accumulate into a substantial sleep debt.[170] It is important that the only way to pay back a sleep debt is with sleep.

Sleep debts are commonplace in our culture. The National Sleep Foundation's annual survey continues to reveal that Americans chronically undersleep by 60 to 90 minutes each day (website: http://www.sleepfoundation.org/site/c.huIXKjM0IxF/b.3933533/). Shift work, long and irregular work hours, and the demands of family and recreation lead to irregular sleep patterns and prevent restful sleep. This is particularly true for physicians, who often work in shifts, have long duty periods, and must frequently care for patients for long periods.

Circadian Rhythms

Rhythms that fluctuate on a 24-hour time scale are known as circadian rhythms. The biologic clock that is responsible for these rhythms is located in the suprachiasmatic nucleus in the human brain. The best-known circadian rhythms are those of body temperature, hormone secretion, metabolism, and the sleep/wake cycle. The circadian system is synchronized to the 24-hour day by external stimuli referred to as "zeitgebers," the most influential of which is the light/dark cycle of day and night.

The circadian system is biphasic in that it produces a state of increased sleep tendency and decreased performance capacity during two periods throughout the 24-hour day—from 2 AM to 6 AM and from 2 PM to 6 PM. These periods are sometimes referred to as circadian lulls. The circadian clock is very resistant to alterations, and it does not adjust rapidly to changes such as those produced by jet lag or shift work. Disruption of the normal circadian rhythm or incomplete circadian adaptation leads to acute and chronic sleep deprivation, decreased alertness, increased subjective fatigue, and decreased physical and mental performance.[171]

Sleepiness and Alertness

Sleepiness and alertness are at opposite ends of a continuum. Daytime sleepiness is the most obvious effect of failing to obtain adequate sleep. Healthy adults are maximally alert by midmorning. This is sequentially followed by a circadian lull in the early afternoon (causing some cultures to incorporate an afternoon "siesta"), increased alertness in the early evening, and finally increased sleepiness that normally results in falling asleep at night.

The most extreme periods of sleepiness become manifest when one is out of sync with the circadian clock (either staying awake and working when our clock is pressuring sleep or attempting to sleep when our clock is pressuring wakefulness). Data from the U.S. Department of Transportation reveal that the greatest number of single-vehicle accidents takes place during the early morning hours when people are at a circadian lull of alertness. These accidents are thought to be due to inadvertent lapses in driver attention brought about by extremes of sleepiness.[172]

Determinants of Sleepiness

The major factors causing sleepiness are decreased quantity of sleep, poor quality of sleep (sleep fragmentation resulting from multiple awakenings or abnormal progression of sleep states and stages), disrupted circadian rhythms, and the use of certain medications. The amount of sleep obtained is directly related to daytime sleepiness. If sleep is restricted in healthy adults, daytime sleepiness can be demonstrated the following day.[170] If one is allowed to extend sleep beyond the usual sleep time, increased alertness can be demonstrated in the laboratory.[4] Sleep quality is affected by many factors. Sleep fragmentation affects the elderly and patients with sleep disorders such as sleep apnea and periodic limb movements. Sleep fragmentation commonly occurs in physicians who are awakened from sleep to care for patients while in the hospital.

Caffeine[173] and other stronger stimulants are known to reduce nocturnal sleep if ingested close to bedtime, hence decreasing sleep quantity and quality. Potent stimulants such as amphetamines do produce increased alertness and performance, but they have significant side effects and are not an option for health care personnel (e.g., the individual must undergo a substantial amount of recovery sleep ["crash"] after their effect is gone). Newer, nonamphetamine alertness-enhancing drugs (e.g., modafinil) are currently under study and being used in shift workers, including health care workers (see "Fatigue Countermeasures").

Mood

Long work hours, fatigue, and sleep deprivation have also been shown to bring about consistent and dramatic changes in mood and emotions.[174,175] Depression, anxiety, irritability, anger, and depersonalization have all been shown to increase during testing of chronically fatigued house staff. These emotions are an obvious source of stress between anesthetists and their coworkers, patients, and families. The relationship of mood, performance, and patient safety has yet to be determined.

Vigilance

Vigilance, the centerpiece of the ASA logo, is defined as "alert watchfulness." Vigilance is critical, although studies of the performance of anesthesiologists make it clear that vigilance is not the only key characteristic of careful anesthesiologists. Vigilance is a necessary, but not sufficient condition to permit the safe passage of a patient through the perioperative period. If vigilance and other aspects of decision-making are impaired by performance-shaping factors such as sleep deprivation and fatigue, there is a greater likelihood of an adverse patient outcome.

Monitoring of slowly changing stimuli is a classic vigilance task that makes up a significant proportion of the anesthetist's work. This type of task is most sensitive to the degrading effects of sleepiness and fatigue. During the performance of lengthy vigilance tasks, the most common types of decrements include increased reaction time, lapses (transient periods of unawareness), and a reduction in the probability of detecting an alarm. This type of performance impairment has been documented after as little as 30 minutes of time on a task, and the decrement is even more pronounced if the individual is physiologically sleepy at the beginning of the task.

Microsleep Events

The most extreme cause of impaired vigilance is the occurrence of actual sleep episodes (microsleeps) encroaching into periods of wakefulness. Microsleep events typically last a few seconds to a few minutes. They are intermittent in onset, and their impending occurrence is difficult for the individual to predict. Most individuals underestimate their level of sleepiness when they can be objectively shown to be extremely sleepy, thus making this problem even more insidious. In other words, one can fall asleep and not be perceptually aware of it. This has significant meaning in the workplace and when driving home after long work periods. Microsleep episodes are the probable cause of many single-vehicle crashes.

Microsleeps are a sign of extreme sleepiness and are harbingers of the onset of longer sleep periods. Typically, they occur during periods of low workload or stimulation and when an individual is maximally sleepy. In addition, an individual's performance between microsleep episodes is impaired. Frequent and longer microsleeps increase the number of errors of omission.

Driving while drowsy may be less forgiving than practicing medicine while drowsy. It is easy to imagine that if a driver has a microsleep for only seconds while traveling at 60 miles per hour, there is a high likelihood of an accident. Although the anesthetist's work environment does not (usually) evolve as fast as that of the driver, the safety implications of falling asleep while providing care are similarly obvious.[176]

Scientists at the NASA Ames Research Center studied the occurrence of microsleep episodes in pilots during transmeridian flights.[177] These flights involve multiple time zone changes with long, irregular work schedules and resultant disruption of circadian rhythms. This situation causes fatigue, sleepiness, and decreased performance, which are believed to have an impact on flight safety. This particular protocol compared two pilot groups flying equivalent flights: a control (non-nap) group and a nap group. Electroencephalographic monitoring of the pilots was performed to determine the extent of microsleep episodes and also to document whether pilots were actually able to nap if given the opportunity. In brief, the study revealed that (1) crew members were able to nap seated in the cockpit if given the opportunity, (2) the non-nap crew had significantly more microsleep episodes during critical phases of flight than the crew that had napped did, and (3) performance on a standardized test of visual reaction time was worse in the non-nap group than in the group that had napped. This study demonstrated that microsleeps do occur even in a work environment in which sleep is strictly forbidden and in which work hours are tightly regulated. Napping appears to be a reasonable countermeasure to decrease the likelihood of microsleeps and improve performance. Other work on napping supports these conclusions.

Do anesthetists suffer microsleep events? The answer almost certainly is yes. Anecdotal evidence, as well as unpublished reports from our own surveys, suggests that these events do occur from time to time. Microsleeps occurred in a study of anesthesiologists performing work in a simulated environment.[178]

Shift Work

From a practical standpoint, shift work will remain a common method to provide 24-hour care in the hospital setting.[179-181] Workers and managers should learn how circadian factors, sleep-related factors, and social factors affect the lives of workers and their families. Hospital organizations should make it a priority to establish that workers are appropriately rested, just as they try to ensure that workers are not impaired by drugs or alcohol on the job. Given current knowledge concerning shift work and the many factors that affect an individual's ability to cope, there is no single "best" schedule for shift work. Some workers tolerate systems that others find excessively onerous. If given a choice, many workers choose suboptimal shift work rotations when doing so gives them increased pay or more time off work.

Methodologies for Assessing Sleepiness

There are various methods for assessing an individual's level of sleepiness, including behavioral indicators, subjective measures, and physiologic measures. Behavioral indicators of sleepiness include yawning, ptosis, decreased social interaction, and microsleep events. Many of these behaviors are difficult to quantify.

Subjective measures include various types of numeric or visual analog scales that attempt to measure how sleepy the individual feels. These methods are used frequently in studies of sleepiness because they are very easy to implement; however, subjective feelings of fatigue and sleepiness are often underestimated by individuals in comparison to their level of physiologic sleepiness. Both behavioral and subjective sleepiness can be masked by a stimulating environment, even though the individual remains physiologically sleepy. When environmental stimuli wane, physiologic sleepiness manifests itself as an overwhelming propensity to fall asleep. A person who is physiologically alert does not experience sleepiness as environmental stimuli decrease. For example, without physiologic sleepiness, an individual may become bored during a lecture but does not fall asleep.

Physiologic (objective) measures of sleepiness have been used extensively in sleep research and sleep medicine. Carskadon, Dement, and colleagues[182,183] developed the Multiple Sleep Latency Test (MSLT), which is now the standard method for quantifying daytime sleepiness. The MSLT tests the propensity of an individual to fall asleep in a sleep-inducing environment during the daytime. A short sleep latency (i.e., falling asleep quickly) is a sign of increased sleepiness, whereas a long sleep latency is a sign of decreased sleepiness. A normal MSLT score is greater than 10 minutes, whereas pathologic daytime sleepiness is defined as 5 minutes or less. Pathologic levels correspond to the daytime sleepiness typically seen in patients with narcolepsy or sleep apnea or in healthy individuals deprived of sleep for 24 hours.

Evaluation of Physiologic Sleepiness in Anesthesia Residents

Using the MSLT, Howard and colleagues[168,184] evaluated the physiologic daytime sleepiness of anesthesia residents under three different conditions: (1) "baseline" (daytime shift, no on-call duty period in the previous 48 hours), (2) "post-call" (immediately after a 24-hour work and in-house on-call period), and (3) "sleep extended." In the sleep-extended condition, residents were told to maximize sleep and were allowed to arrive for work at 10 AM (3 to 4 hours later than normal) for 4 consecutive days before testing. They were not on call during this time. The sleep-extended condition was included to provide a true control state of maximal rest and optimum alertness.

In this study, anesthesia residents had an MSLT score of 6.7 ± 5.3 minutes in the "baseline" condition and 4.9 ± 4.7 minutes in the "post-call" condition, both scores revealing the nearly pathologic levels of daytime sleepiness seen in patients with narcolepsy or sleep apnea. The "baseline" group slept an average of 7.1 ± 1.5 hours per night, whereas the "post-call" group reported an average of 6.3 ± 1.9 hours of sleep during their night on call. Ironically, although the on-call periods occurred during rotations that often have very busy call nights, only a few subjects were, in fact, awake most of the night. In the "sleep-extended" condition, the subjects extended their sleep to an average of more than 9 hours per night, and MSLT scores were in the normal range (12.0 ± 6.4 minutes). These results clearly demonstrate that medical personnel who have not been on call cannot be assumed to be "rested" when compared with "fatigued" post-call residents. These data also indicate that under "normal" working conditions, the resident physicians studied were physiologically sleepy to nearly pathologic levels. This finding documents a previously unknown level of chronic sleep deprivation in this population. Notably, these data cast substantial doubt on previous studies of the performance of medical personnel that have relied on the assumption that individuals working under "normal" conditions are truly rested.

Evaluation of Subjective Sleepiness

In the previously discussed study, Howard and colleagues also investigated the degree of discrepancy between the residents' subjective sleepiness (how sleepy they felt) and their physiologic sleepiness (how easily they fell asleep). Subjective sleepiness was measured with a validated numeric scale (Stanford Sleepiness Scale); physiologic sleepiness was measured with the MSLT, as described earlier. Subjects' self-reported sleepiness immediately before each sleep opportunity during the MSLT did not, in general, correlate with their MSLT score. As in previous studies, subjective sleepiness correlated better with physiologic sleepiness when subjects were extremely alert or extremely sleepy.

The authors also found that subjects demonstrated little ability to determine whether they had actually fallen asleep during the MSLT sleep opportunities. For example, in 51% of trials in which the electroencephalographic/electro-oculographic measurements showed that the subject had fallen asleep, the subjects thought they had remained awake throughout the test. These results support the contention that medical personnel are physiologically vulnerable to degraded alertness yet are unable to perceive this decrement. Thus, an anesthetist could, in fact, fall asleep during a case, awaken, and be totally unaware of the lapse in vigilance.

Sleep Deprivation and Fatigue in Medical Personnel

Human error represents a significant risk to hospitalized patients,[3] and it has been estimated to play a role in more than 70% of anesthesia mishaps.[185] This is similar to the error rate seen in cognitively similar work environments such as aviation.[186] Clearly, the physiologic capabilities and limitations of the human operator in complex work environments remain central to safe and productive performance. The 24-hour demands of medical care parallel the physiologic challenges present in other operational domains; nevertheless, minimal data are available to quantify the fatigue-related risk to performance and alertness in medical personnel.

Providing quality health care requires physicians to attend to details critical for life, such as monitoring of changing vital signs, administering the correct type and dose of medications, and in general, making crucial decisions to achieve optimal patient care. Physicians, like other workers, are affected by all the physiologic, psychological, and behavioral demands that characterize work environments requiring continuous, around-the-clock operation. However, whereas much of the health care system (e.g., nursing) relies on multiple work shifts to cover the 24-hour day (which is also not a perfect system), physicians more typically work long duty periods and frequently experience sleep loss, circadian disruption, and fatigue. Even minimal levels of sleep loss (for example, obtaining as little as 2 hours less sleep than an individual requires) can lead to lapses in performance, increased physiologic sleepiness during the daytime (including microsleeps), and altered moods.[187] This level of degraded performance and alertness almost certainly contributes to medical error and health care mishaps.[167]

Work Hour Regulations

In July 2003, The Accreditation Council for Graduate Medical Education in the United States instituted common duty hour requirements for all accredited residency training programs. The requirements can be found at www.acgme.org and are as follows:

- Eighty hours per week, averaged over a period of 4 weeks (including all in hospital call)
- One day (continuous 24-hour period) in 7 free of all duties (clinical and educational) averaged over a 4-week period
- In-hospital call occurring no more frequently than every third night averaged over 4 weeks
- In-hospital call not to exceed 24 hours; residents may remain on duty for 6 additional hours to participate in educational activities, transfer care of patients to another team, conduct outpatient clinics, and maintain continuity of care
- No new patients accepted after 24 hours of continuous duty
- Provision of a 10-hour period between all daily duty periods and after in-hospital call
- Moonlighting hours to be included as part of the 80-hour limit
- Exceptions: a residency review committee may grant exceptions for up to a 10% increase in the 80-hour limit to individual programs on a case-by-case basis

Training programs were given little direction on how to accomplish the work hour restrictions, but most anesthesiology training programs have been able to successfully adopt them. Interestingly, there are no work hour restrictions for practitioners or any other care providers beyond residency training. There is no proof that the change has had a positive or negative impact on patient or provider safety, although pundits continue to debate both sides of the issue.[188,189] Recent studies show that the number of hospital-wide adverse drug events remained constant after the limitations[190] and that postoperative outcomes were not affected in the programs studied.[191]

Compliance rates for the common program requirements have been tracked by Landrigan and coworkers.[192] In a survey of interns, they found that more than 80% reported some kind of work hour violation during 1 or more months of the study. Average work duration decreased and sleep time increased when compared with an equivalent time before duty hour limits. Reporting of compliance by individual residents is complicated by many factors, so the true amount of work being performed is not known. Many surgical programs have requested and been given a 10% work hour extension, but it is not known how many of these requests have been turned down.

European and Australian Regulations

Work hours regulations in the European Union and in Australia/New Zealand are much more stringent than they are for trainees in the United States. In 2009, the maximum hours that junior medical staff in the National Health Service (NHS) in the United Kingdom work will be reduced from 58 to 48 under European law. This is a major challenge for the health service and will require new ways of working to be adopted. The NHS National Workforce Projects has been appointed as the lead organization to help support the NHS in finding and implementing solutions to the changes in the work environment (http://www.healthcareworkforce.nhs.uk/). The results of these restrictions on patient and provider safety are still being evaluated, and these findings may have an impact on any further restrictions that may occur in the U.S. system. Empirical studies documenting the effect of the European Union changes are lacking, although there are several argumentative pieces for and against the directive.[193,194]

Harvard Work Hours, Health, and Safety Group Studies

A series of interesting studies has been published recently by a group from the Brigham and Women's Hospital.[195,196] The investigators conducted a randomized study comparing interns working in an ICU on a traditional schedule (every third night on call with shifts longer than 24 hours in duration) and an intervention schedule that reduced work shift duration (to less than 17 hours) and the number of hours worked per week. Interns made 35.9% more serious medical errors and had twice as many attentional failures (microsleeps) during the traditional schedule. Those on the traditional schedule worked more hours per week (85 versus 65 hours) and slept less (5.8 hours), which led the investigators to conclude that elimination of long work shifts reduced errors and decreased manifest sleepiness.

This group also conducted a monthly prospective nationwide survey of interns' first postgraduate year to evaluate the risk for motor vehicle accidents with extended work shifts.[197] They found an increased likelihood of motor vehicle accidents and near-miss accidents after extended work shifts and an increased monthly risk with increasing number of shifts.

Sleep and Performance

Previous studies addressed the effects of sleep deprivation and fatigue on physician performance and well-being. Major reviews of this literature identified little consensus.[198,199] There are several methodologic flaws in the existing literature:

1. The degree of acute sleep deprivation of subjects was poorly defined, and no assessment of chronic fatigue was made. Typically, studies relied on only the previous night's sleep as a level of "fatigue," and subjects could well have been chronically fatigued during baseline (control) trials, which could mask the degree of impairment resulting from the acute fatigue of being on call. This continues to be the greatest weakness in studies of fatigued health care providers.
2. Measuring actual clinical performance is difficult and was not attempted. Most studies had to rely on simple cognitive tasks that probed only short-term memory, immediate recall, and simple reaction time; the validity of using such simple tests to probe complex performance has been challenged because these simple tests do not assess the higher-level cognitive functions most critical to skilled medical care.
3. Most of the performance tests were of very short duration (3 to 5 minutes). Studies have shown that if sufficiently motivated, even fatigued subjects can perform well on short-duration tasks.
4. Practice effects were not adequately accounted for. If subjects have not learned a particular performance test sufficiently to achieve maximum performance, subsequent trials will almost certainly show improvement in performance because of further learning of the task.

Some studies requiring subjects to perform sustained vigilance tasks of long duration have, in fact, shown an impairment in the performance of fatigued physicians. Tasks of this type, which require sustained attention to detail, are highly relevant to the anesthetist's tasks, and they are the most sensitive to the effects of sleep loss and fatigue.

Do Anesthesiologists Perceive Fatigue As a Problem?

The survey by Gaba and associates[200] revealed that more than 50% of respondents believed that they had made an error in clinical management that they thought was related to fatigue. In another survey of anesthesiologists and CRNAs, the majority (61%) of respondents recalled having made an error in the administration of anesthesia that they attributed to fatigue.[201] Data from these surveys and others[202] reveal that issues of sleepiness and fatigue are perceived by anesthesia practitioners as being important causative factors in reducing anesthesia-related patient safety.

Howard and colleagues[178] conducted a study of rested versus sleep-deprived anesthesiology residents using a realistic patient simulator. Multiple measures of performance were collected during this 4-hour experiment (e.g., psychomotor tests, reaction to secondary task probes, response to clinical events). In the rested condition, subjects had 4 consecutive days of sleep extension (showing up at work at 10:00 AM), whereas in the sleep-deprived condition they had remained awake for 25 hours (during a "pseudo"–on-call period) before performing the simulated anesthetic. Subjects in the rested condition were able to increase their total sleep time more than 2 hours from baseline. Psychomotor tests revealed progressive impairment of alertness, mood, and performance over the course of the pseudo–on-call period, as well as on the experimental day, when compared with the well-rested condition. Secondary task probe response times were slower after being sleep deprived, although this reached statistical significance in just one of three probe types. There was no statistical difference in case management between conditions—in fact, subjects in both conditions made significant errors. The behavioral alertness scores in the sleep-deprived condition were different from those of subjects who had increased their sleep time. Even when well rested, the subjects in this experiment did not perform perfectly; however, they did not show any of the behavior indicative of being sleepy (e.g., head nodding, eyes closing). Sleep-deprived subjects cycled (often rapidly) in and out of sleepy behavior, and the most impaired individuals showed such behavior for more than 25% of the experiment (60 minutes).

Fatigue Countermeasures

Studies such as the ones described previously are establishing the true picture of sleepiness and fatigue in medical personnel. From studies of the performance of fatigued individuals in other domains, we know that professionals become increasingly vulnerable to the degrading effects of sleepiness as the sleep debt accumulates. It may be difficult to determine a causal relationship between anesthetist fatigue and patient outcome. However, it is clear that if anesthetists are not awake, they cannot possibly be aware. Such a lapse in vigilance is unacceptable. Furthermore, anesthetists cannot prevent sleep by willpower alone because it is a fundamental physiologic drive. Demands for clinical services must be balanced against the potential for reduced vigilance and error by seriously fatigued practitioners, anesthetists, and surgeons alike.

Because fatigue is such a widespread and insidious problem, it is important to determine ways to counteract its effects. Strategies that institutions or practitioners can use to minimize the negative effects of sleepiness and fatigue on performance, include

- Education
- Improved sleep habits
- Rest breaks at work
- Strategic napping
- Medications
- Light therapy

Education

The first step in addressing sleepiness and fatigue of medical personnel is to educate practitioners and the administrators of health care institutions about the impact of sleep issues on work performance, mood, job satisfaction, and health (see Chapter 8). Education is a relatively simple and inexpensive countermeasure that can be implemented immediately. Educational programs covering sleep deprivation, circadian disruption and fatigue, and countermeasures have been enthusiastically adopted by an increasing fraction of the aviation community.[203,204] Similar programs should be developed for the health care community. Education alone is sufficient for some individuals and institutions to change their work and sleep habits or their organizational and scheduling procedures. However, it is clear at both the individual and organization level that education will not be sufficient to address this issue fully. Other competing forces (e.g., measures of production versus safety) are very powerful and difficult for practitioners to manage.

Improved Sleep Habits

Good sleep habits include the following: regularity of bedtime and wake-up time; sufficient time for sustained and individually adequate sleep; restriction of alcohol, caffeine, and nicotine before bedtime; and use of exercise, nutrition, and environmental factors so that they enhance rather than disturb sleep. A regular sleep schedule is an important part of optimal sleep hygiene, but it is often not possible for medical personnel, given the requirement to cover clinical needs on a 24-hour basis. Medical personnel should make greater effort to maintain as constant a sleep schedule as possible and to maximize sleep opportunities before and after periods of reduced sleep.

Social drug use can have profound effects on sleep. Physicians frequently use caffeine to stay awake during on-call periods, but often its use could be more strategic. Strategic use (i.e., use when its alerting effects are needed) of caffeine requires knowledge about its onset and duration of action. Besides its alerting effects, caffeine produces an increase in awakenings and decreases the total nocturnal sleep time if ingested close to sleep opportunities. Individuals who ingest large amounts of caffeine and who have nocturnal sleep disturbances should limit or cease their intake of caffeine. Chronic use of caffeine, common in our culture, produces tolerance to the alerting effect of the drug, and hence it should be avoided when using it strategically. Nicotine is a stimulant that produces effects similar to those of caffeine. Alcohol is often used successfully to initiate sleep, but its effect on sleep architecture after sleep onset can be devastating. After ingestion of alcohol, frequent awakenings from sleep occur that can be associated with increased sympathetic nervous system activity, often manifested as headache, sweating, and tachycardia. Clearly, use of these substances should be restricted near bedtime.

Physicians often lack good nutritional habits, especially during long duty periods. Meals may be skipped or ingested quickly whenever there is adequate time. If one is hungry before bedtime, it is best to avoid eating or drinking heavily because this, too, can disturb sleep.

The effects of age can make optimum sleep habits difficult to achieve because sleep requirements do not change once reaching adulthood. The number of awakenings per night rises after the age of 45 years and results in decreased sleep efficiency (time in bed versus total sleep time). The ability to initiate sleep at any time during a 24-hour day is diminished after the age of 25 years, and "sleeping in" to make up for lost sleep is more difficult as individuals grow older. Sleep-related disorders such as breathing disruptions (obstructive sleep apnea) and periodic limb movements also become more common with age.

Ideally, the sleep setting should be a dark, quiet room devoid of sources of interruption such as pets, telephones, pagers, and children. The sleeping surface and environmental temperature should be comfortable. Psychological stressors increase baseline physiologic arousal and can impair the quality and quantity of sleep. For example, reviewing the previous day's events or attempting to plan tomorrow's activities while trying to fall asleep is not conducive to sleep. Effort should be made to separate the work of the day with a period of relaxation before attempting to initiate sleep.

Rest Breaks at Work

Although other industries have openly recognized the reality of decrements in vigilance resulting from fatigue and sleepiness, the health care system has not. Rest breaks and rotation of task duties are mandatory for air traffic controllers and are part of naval ship command procedures in an attempt to prevent potential lapses in vigilance. Short breaks have been shown to increase productivity and job satisfaction, and they probably also help alleviate boredom. In anesthesia training programs, residents are frequently given rest breaks during the daytime, but this is often not the case with private practitioners. Private practice anesthesia typically does not provide the mechanisms for rest breaks or task duty rotation, in part because of fiscal issues. An "extra" anesthetist would be necessary to provide these opportunities on a regular basis.

The optimal timing and length of breaks are unknown, but periodic relief from duty should be taken when possible. Cooper and coworkers[205,206] studied the effects of intraoperative exchange of anesthesia personnel. Although in some cases the process of relieving OR personnel caused a problem, it more frequently was associated with the discovery of a preexisting problem. The positive effect of relief of personnel probably depends on the quality of the handover briefing conducted by anesthetists. Studies are currently being performed to address standardized handover of intraoperative care of patients.

If anesthetists are unable to obtain a break during long work periods, there are other measures that they can take to remain alert. They can engage other OR personnel in conversation (although this, too, can be distracting), thereby increasing the level of stimulation in the environment. Walking around and standing up are also techniques that decrease subjective (but not physiologic) sleepiness. If anesthetists are having microsleep events, which may be noticed by other personnel rather than by the anesthetists themselves, fatigue is already very severe, and complete sleep is imminent. In such a situation the practitioner must secure additional assistance in surveillance of the patient and, if necessary, obtain relief to allow time for sleep.

Strategic Napping

If adequate sleep during the night cannot be obtained, naps can be used to decrease sleepiness and improve performance. The optimal nap length for most individuals is about 45 minutes; this duration acutely improves alertness, allows improved performance, and minimizes the possibility of sleep inertia on awakening. Naps as short as 10 minutes have beneficial effects on alertness. A nap of 90 to 120 minutes allows a full sleep cycle and can additionally boost alertness and performance over that of shorter nap periods. Data from NASA studies of flight crews demonstrate that on the whole, napping is a useful countermeasure to fatigue and sleep deprivation.[177]

Smith-Coggins and associates studied the effect of naps during the night shift on health care providers working in a busy suburban university emergency department.[204] Workers were randomized to work a night shift without rest (as was the norm in this facility) or to receive a 40-minute nap opportunity at 3 AM. They found that a nap taken at this time improved performance on some (but not all) measures. The most important result of this study may be the fact that the subjects were able to (1) successfully use this strategy in the real workplace and (2) improve alertness and performance.

Investigators in the Veteran's Hospital at Palo Alto, California, have developed a Strategic Nap Program that has been successfully piloted at two sites within the Veterans' Administration system. This program has been implemented in ICU settings but is equally applicable to other high-risk, dynamic domains such as the OR. Components of the program include a formal educational program, program guidelines for the individual practitioner and the facility, and other guidance for implementation.

There are issues that complicate the appropriate use of naps by medical professionals. Physicians have an individual and cultural tendency to ignore or to minimize the effect of fatigue and sleep deprivation. The culture of medicine views work breaks and naps as signs of weakness. The military has addressed similar attitudes with the concept of "power napping." Troops are strongly encouraged to take naps of 10 minutes to 1 hour when the situation permits to increase their strength and performance. This approach appropriately presents the idea of napping in a positive light as a sign of wisdom and strength rather than one of cowardice and frailty.

Sleep Inertia

Sleep inertia corresponds to the period of reduced ability to function optimally immediately on awakening.[190,207] This phenomenon usually occurs when individuals are awakened out of slow-wave sleep and is manifested as grogginess and impaired performance lasting as long as 15 to 30 minutes after awakening. Sleep inertia can also occur after being awakened from normal sleep and is most common during the early morning circadian trough (2 to 6 AM). Depending on the preexisting level of sleepiness, individuals who take naps longer than 40 minutes are at greater risk for sleep inertia on awakening. Sleep inertia can be important to health care professionals who may be awakened out of deep sleep to provide emergency care to patients (e.g., emergency cesarean section or emergency intubation). If urgent work can be anticipated, the sleeping individual should be awakened with sufficient time (at least 15 minutes) to minimize the fogginess and decrement in performance associated with sleep inertia. If sleep inertia is unavoidable, it would be wise for the affected person to ask for help until the grogginess dissipates.

Medications

A few studies have evaluated the use of sedative-hypnotics for promotion of sleep during nonduty hours by nonmedical personnel (e.g., to assist in daytime sleep after a night shift). Many questions remain unanswered regarding the quality of sleep obtained after using hypnotics, the severity of hangover effects, and the potential risk of abuse. Melatonin, which is a hormone secreted by the pineal gland, may have promise as a nonaddictive daytime sleep-inducing agent, but the results of existing studies are controversial.

Stimulants may have a role in the maintenance of alertness during periods of extreme sleepiness. Modafinil is a nonamphetamine alertness-enhancing drug that has been approved for use in narcolepsy and shift work sleep disorder.[208] The side effect profile of this drug is so promising that it has been studied extensively by the military and shift workers as a nonaddicting adjunct for alertness management. Its use in health care is also being studied but cannot be sanctioned at this point.[209] The use of sedatives and potent stimulants to manipulate sleep is not considered an appropriate option for anesthetists. Caffeine is used frequently to increase alertness temporarily, but there are caveats about its use, as discussed earlier. Caffeine should be used strategically to maximize its effect when needed. Strategic use of caffeine includes (1) knowledge of its onset (15 to 30 minutes) and duration of action (3 to 4 hours) and (2) use when alertness is required and the opportunity to sleep is minimal.

Countermeasures should be studied and implemented in health care. There are major financial incentives to maintain the status quo.[167] If anesthesiologists know that they are impaired (from fatigue or for any other reason), the assistance of a colleague should be enlisted so that patient safety is not negatively affected.

Light Therapy

Timed cycles of bright light and darkness have been used in certain circumstances to facilitate adaptation to shift work. Exposure to bright light (>7000 to 12,000 lux) and darkness at the appropriate points in the circadian cycle has been shown to reset the circadian pacemaker by 12 hours over a period of 2 to 3 days.[210] This important finding demonstrates the ability to make significant changes in the circadian system relatively quickly. However, resetting the circadian timekeeper is critically dependent on the timing, intensity, and duration of exposure to light and to "total" darkness. Being off by only an hour can prevent the desired effect. Adhering to such time-critical schedules for this treatment is probably impractical for anesthetists given the many work-related and social factors that affect their activities. Research on light treatment continues and may eventually result in more practical treatment regimens.

Aging

All individuals understand that their abilities cannot be maintained indefinitely as they age. On average, performance on laboratory tests of discrete sensory-motor and cognitive skills can be shown to decrease with increasing age.[211] However, there are large differences among individuals. Again, except at extreme points of performance failure (e.g., severe impairment of vision or hearing), the contribution of isolated changes in physiologic or cognitive performance is difficult to relate to real work situations.[212] For one thing, the work environment is often rich with redundant cues involving multiple sensory modalities. For another, technologic compensation may be possible, as with the use of hearing aids or glasses. Finally, along with possible physiologic changes of age typically comes greater experience with a variety of situations. For many individuals, the lessons learned from experience more than offset the modest degree of physiologic impairment that they face as they grow older. This compensation has, in fact, been documented for skilled typists, chess players, and bridge players. Middle-aged individuals can use their experience to solve everyday problems better than young individuals can; however, for the elderly (on average), compensation by experience is no longer sufficient to offset cognitive slowing.[212] Age takes a toll on short-term (or "working") memory,[213] and there is evidence that aged workers are more sensitive to the interruptions in attention that are so prevalent in dynamic environments. Nevertheless, few of these deficits have been documented in complex work settings, largely because it is so difficult to measure performance in these domains. The issue of the aging anesthesiologist has raised considerable controversy among anesthesiologists.

What do other industries do about this issue? From 1959 until the end of 2007, U.S. and aviation regulations forced airline pilots to retire at age 60 regardless of their health or competence. When the "Age 60 Rule" was put in force, the rationale was that the "increased speeds and passenger loads of commercial airliners placed greater demands on pilots with respect to their physical fitness and piloting skills." Some may argue that the increasingly challenging nature of anesthesia practice also places greater demands on anesthetists than ever before.

After intense debate and many studies over the last 30 years,[54,214] with partially contradictory studies and little data suggesting that pilots between the ages of 60 and 65 are at greater risk, the Age 60 Rule was modified by law (HR 4343) at the end of 2007. The new rule allows airline pilots to continue flying until age 65, although for captains in international operations, a pilot younger than 60 years must be the copilot.

Federal Aviation Administration (FAA) regulations do require air transport pilots to pass "class I" medical examinations every 6 months. However, the medical examination process appears to be largely aimed at identifying individuals with chronic medical conditions that place them at risk for sudden incapacitation (such as significant coronary heart disease). Pilot incapacitation during high-workload phases of flight has been shown in simulator testing to lead to a significant rate of crashes, even when there is a second pilot at the controls. These physical examinations may weed out pilots with severe cognitive or sensory-motor deficiencies, but they are not designed to assess subtle aspects of changes in performance resulting from age. Of course, there are no requirements whatsoever for medical examination or certification of anesthetists, nor is there any limitation on the practice of anesthesia at any age.

It is likely that age alone does not independently cause a significant decrement in performance, but age correlates with other factors that are likely to affect performance. The concern about aging professionals revolves more around the loss of knowledge and skill as one gets farther from initial training rather than the loss of fundamental mental capacity. Thus, the originally well-trained practitioner who keeps abreast of the changing standard of care and who exercises emergency skills frequently is less likely to be affected by advancing age than is a marginal practitioner whose knowledge and skills were frozen immediately after completion of training and who practices in a low-complexity environment. The FAA regulations deal with this issue for air transport pilots by requiring frequent (every 6 months) evaluation of performance by FAA-certified check pilots. These evaluations are performed during actual flights and in realistic simulators, and they, in essence, check fitness for duty regardless of age. There is currently no similar program in anesthesia to assess the competency of practitioners at any age, except for initial board certification, which is voluntary. Periodic maintenance of certification in anesthesiology is now required by the American Board of Anesthesiology for diplomats attaining certification after the year 2000, but it is not mandatory to be board-certified to practice anesthesia, and the recertification examinations are not as intense, as thorough, or as frequent as those required for air transport pilots. Thus, the issue of age-related effects on anesthetist performance is likely to continue to be raised periodically for the foreseeable future.

Illness and Drug Use

Every anesthetist is vulnerable to transient illnesses, which in some cases probably reduce performance ability (see Chapter 101). All personnel are vulnerable to chronic medical conditions that could directly or indirectly affect their fitness and performance capability. The culture of the caring professions often leads individuals to continue to work with illnesses that would cause other professionals to stay at home or to seek medical advice. The performance-shaping effects of the illness can be exacerbated by the use of either over-the-counter or prescribed medications. The degree to which illness and medications affect anesthetist performance is unknown.

A serious problem for anesthetists is that of drug abuse (see Chapter 101).[55,56,215-218] It is estimated that up to 8% of physicians could be classified as alcoholics. In an anonymous survey of anesthesia personnel from one institution, 75% of respondents reported drinking alcohol on a regular basis. They reported drinking an average of 1.6 drinks per day 2.7 days per week. Just less than 10% of subjects reported having been "hung over" while conducting anesthesia, and 40% reported having given anesthesia within 12 hours of alcohol consumption; 84% stated that alcohol use never adversely affected their clinical performance.

The degree to which small doses of alcohol or hangovers affect the performance of complex, real-world tasks is uncertain. Some studies of general aviation and navy pilots[54,219-221] suggested that hangover effects can degrade performance even when more than 8 hours has elapsed since alcohol consumption and there is no detectable blood alcohol level. Nonetheless, though statistically significant, the changes in performance seen in these studies may not have been functionally significant. These studies[54,219-221] also suggested an interaction among age, workload, and hangover in causing decrements in performance. However, the "aged" cohort was defined as 31 years or older and was compared with a cohort of pilots in their early 20s. Extrapolating these results to the anesthesia domain is difficult.

Nevertheless, the natural history of serious abuse of alcohol, cocaine, sedatives, or narcotics by anesthetists is such that cognitive performance will at some point be seriously compromised. However, addiction specialists frequently report that job performance is one of the last areas of life to become impaired.[222,223] For this reason, the period of time in which an addicted anesthetist's performance in the OR is significantly impaired is a relatively small fraction of the total time during which drugs are abused. Although this in no way excuses the practice of conducting anesthesia while under the influence of drugs, it may account for the fact that reports of addicted anesthesiologists are, unfortunately, common whereas reports of overt patient risk or harm resulting from an addicted physician's errors are unusual.

Anesthesiology has been at the forefront in dealing with impaired medical personnel. Management of those discovered with a drug impairment is fairly standardized,[216,224] but the question of whether to return these individuals to anesthesia practice is increasingly controversial, even when they return under carefully monitored reentry protocols.[216] The main risk appears to be to the addict's own safety, although questions about patient safety can never be eliminated.

Ultimately, in the current medical system the responsibility rests with anesthetists to ensure that their own performance level is sufficient for the work at hand. Pilots use a mnemonic checklist to review the effects of potential performance-shaping factors and are instructed not to fly if they are impaired for any reason. The difficulty in anesthesiology (and to some degree in aviation) is that the real-world organization and incentives of many practice settings do not provide mechanisms for personnel to excuse themselves if they are temporarily impaired. Ironically, there may now be better means to identify and support a practitioner with a serious addiction than there are for the more common occurrences of profound sleep deprivation or impairment by a transient or chronic illness.

The Study of Human Performance

Study of human performance involves research paradigms that are different from those typically used in the science of anesthesia. There are many obstacles to obtaining hard, statistically valid data on human performance. There are no animal models for expert human performance, no "Sprague-Dawley anesthesiologists" to be studied in detail, nor can studies of professional performance be conducted with the psychologist's typical experimental subject, the university undergraduate student. Recruiting expert anesthetists to be the subjects of study is difficult and raises issues of selection bias concerning those who do volunteer. Especially if conducted during actual patient care, investigations of human performance are strongly influenced by concerns about litigation, credentialing, and confidentiality, thus making it difficult to execute optimal studies.

Furthermore, variability among individual anesthetists is quite striking because different anesthetists respond to the same situation in different ways and each individual may act differently on different days or at different times of the same day. The magnitude of this intra-individual variability is often nearly the same as the inter-individual variability.

"Performance" itself is an intuitively meaningful concept that is difficult to define precisely. There are no universal standards for the clinical decisions and actions of anesthetists. They depend heavily on the context of specific situations. In addition, determining how anesthetists perform their jobs, whether successfully or unsuccessfully, means delving into their mental processes. This cannot be measured easily. On the one hand, experimental designs can be used that involve artificial laboratory tasks for which performance can be objectively measured. These tasks will then be far removed from the real world of administering anesthesia. On the other hand, investigating the actual performance of trained practitioners in the real world yields primarily subjective and indirect data. Understanding the anesthetist's performance must be seen as analogous to solving a jigsaw puzzle. Pieces of the puzzle probably come from a variety of sources, none of which by itself captures the entire picture. These pieces include objective data from artificial laboratory tasks, prospective observation of routine patient care, analysis of retrospective reports of near misses or anesthetic mishaps, and prospective observation of the response to simulated events. To achieve the best possible understanding of the situation, it is necessary to accept many data that seem uncomfortably subjective to the physical or biologic scientist. Because the research methodologies may be unfamiliar to anesthetists, some pioneering studies of anesthetist performance are described in detail in this chapter.

Why Study Human Performance in Anesthesia?

How can improved understanding of the human performance of anesthetists help them provide patient care more safely, in a wider variety of clinical situations, with greater efficiency, and with increased satisfaction to both patients and practitioners? The possibilities include the following:

1. Improved operational protocols and enhanced training of anesthetists. The way in which individuals conduct anesthesia is based, in part, on knowing the limits of their performance envelope. Anesthetic techniques and OR practices should draw on anesthetists' abilities and should mitigate their weaknesses. Anesthetists' abilities are strongly affected by training. Understanding the required performance characteristics and inherent human limitations will lead to improved training, which will most fully develop the strengths and counter the existing vulnerabilities of the anesthetist. This process should make patient care safer, less stressful, and more efficient.
2. A more rational view of professional work and legal responsibility (see Chapter 9). Modern medicine, especially in the United States, is strongly influenced by medicolegal concerns. The litigation system has a major selection bias in that every case that comes before it involves an adverse outcome for a patient. The duty of the practitioner is to render care as a "reasonable and prudent" specialist in the area of anesthesia. What is reasonable and prudent? What

type of performance is to be expected from appropriately trained human beings in a complex and dynamic environment? By understanding human performance, it may be possible to generate a more rational view of what is and is not within the standard of care.

3. A more effective work environment. Anesthetists now perform their tasks by using an array of technologies, most of which have not been designed to support the anesthetist's work optimally. By understanding the anesthetist's tasks and performance requirements, the workspace and tools could be improved to better support the most difficult tasks. This, too, can lead to greater safety and to greater efficiency and work satisfaction.
4. A more efficient organizational system (see Chapter 99). Anesthesia is embedded within a larger system of organized medical care that involves interactions among numerous institutions, organizations, and professional domains. Understanding how the anesthetist's work relates to the larger system may enable the development of more rational and efficient flow of information and organizational control.

Although anesthesiologists have been basing analysis of human performance on individual actions, decisions, and mental models and the influence of organizational factors and safety culture for some time (see survey papers[1,2,225]), their importance to health care in general has only recently been appreciated.[3,48]

Box 6-9 Elements of the Core Mental Process

1. Observation
2. Verification
3. Problem recognition
4. Prediction of future states
5. Decision-making
   a. Application of precompiled responses (recognition-primed decision-making)
   b. Decision-making using heuristics and probability
   c. Decision-making including abstract reasoning
6. Action implementation
7. Re-evaluation (avoiding fixation errors)
8. Start again with 1 (loop continues)

Cognitive Process Model of the Anesthetist

The empirical data can best be interpreted in accordance with an explicit model of the cognition involved in an anesthetist's performance. Several investigators[44,58,113,144,226-232] have written about the cognitive elements in anesthesiology.[113,144,226,233-235] The model developed here is explicit, comprehensive, and specific to anesthesia. It is described in detail as a framework for understanding the empirical data and provides a vocabulary for discussing the elements of both successful and unsuccessful performance by anesthetists. This model draws heavily on the work of a number of other investigators[126,235-238] who studied human performance in a variety of complex, dynamic worlds.

Decision-Making Involves Multiple Levels of Mental Activity

The entire model, which is shown in Figure 6-10, depicts the anesthetist as working at five different interacting cognitive levels to implement and control a core process (see Box 6-9) of observation, decision-making, action, and re-evaluation. The core process must then be integrated with the behavior of other team members and with the constraints of the work environment.

The division of mental activities into levels follows the work of Rasmussen and Reason.[237,239,240] Having multiple levels supports parallel processing (performing more than one task at a time) and multitasking (performing only one task at a time but switching very rapidly from one task to another). The anesthesia task analyses[241-245] and the direct observations of anesthetists in Toronto[268] and Tübingen[246-249] have provided clear evidence for the occurrence of parallel processing and multitasking. Table 6-6 gives an overview of the mental activity levels.

At the sensorimotor level, activities involving sensory perception or motor actions take place with minimal conscious control; they are smooth, practiced, and highly integrated patterns of behavior. At the procedural level, the anesthetist performs regular routines in a familiar work situation. These routines have been derived and internalized from training and from previous work episodes. A level of abstract reasoning is used during preoperative planning, and intraoperatively it is used in unfamiliar situations for which no well-practiced expertise or routine is available from previous encounters.

Dynamic Adaptation of the Anesthetist's Thought Processes

Rasmussen's model[237] was extended by the explicit addition of two additional levels of mental activity that provide for dynamic adaptation of the anesthetist's own thought processes. This ability to "think about thinking" in order to control one's own mental activities strategically is called metacognition by psychologists, and it is thought to be an important component of working in complex, dynamic domains. Supervisory control is concerned with dynamically allocating finite attention between routine and nonroutine actions, among multiple problems or themes, and among the five cognitive levels. Resource management deals with the command and control of available resources, including teamwork and communication.

Core Process

An overview of the core process and its elements is given in Box 6-9. The elements are explained in detail in the following sections.

Observation

Management of rapidly changing situations requires the anesthetist to assess a wide variety of information sources, including visual observation of the patient and the surgical field, visual inspection of a multitude of displays from electronic monitors, visual observation of the activities of nurses and the contents of

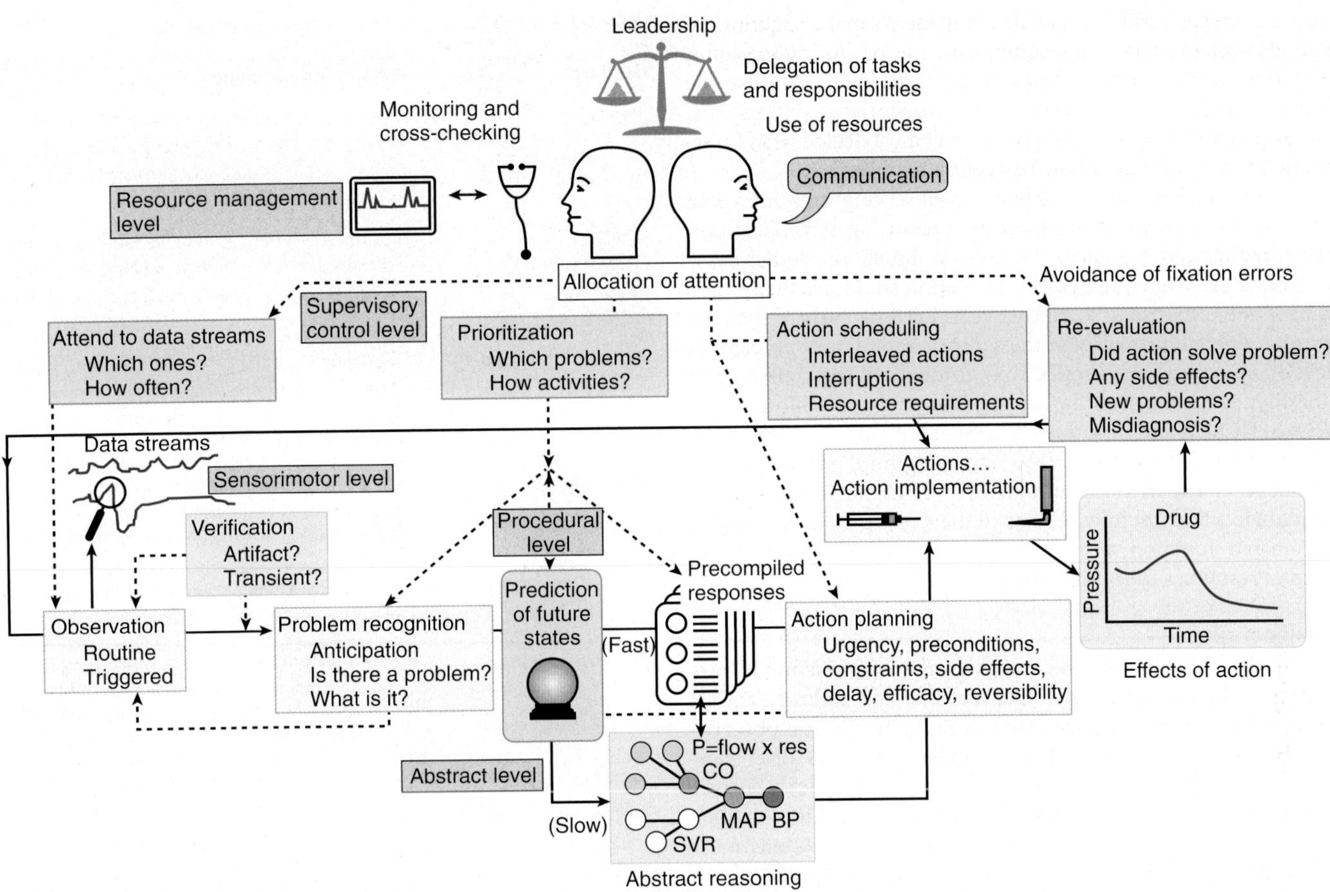

Figure 6-10 Cognitive process model of the anesthetist's real-time problem-solving behavior (see text for a detailed description). Five levels of cognition operate in parallel. The core process involves a main loop (*arrows*) of observation, decision, action, and re-evaluation. The core process is managed by two levels of metacognition that involve supervisory control, allocation of attention, and resource management (above the core process). Each component of the model requires different cognitive skills, and each component is vulnerable to a different set of performance failures or "errors." BP, blood pressure; CO, cardiac output; MAP, mean arterial pressure; SVR, systemic vascular resistance. *(From Gaba DM, Fish KJ, Howard SK: Crisis Management in Anesthesiology. New York, Churchill Livingstone, 1994.)*

Table 6-6 Levels of Mental Activity

Level of Control	Explanation	Comments
Resource management level	Command and control of all resources, including teamwork and communication	Incident analysis shows a huge contribution of lack of resource management and communication skills to the development of incidents and accidents; the importance of these factors is reflected in the ACRM principles and simulation training courses (see Chapter 7)
Supervisory control level	Metacognition: think about thinking	Dynamic adaptation of the thought process, decision-making (e.g., avoiding fixation errors), scheduling, and remembering actions (e.g., prospective memory tasks)
Abstract reasoning level	Use of fundamental medical knowledge, search for high-level analogies, deductive reasoning	Often in parallel with other levels; in emergency situations often too slow and too sensitive to distractions in high-workload situations
Procedural level	Precompiled responses, following algorithms, heuristics, "reflexes"	Recognition-primed decision-making—experts are more often on this level; special errors may occur as a result of not checking for the appropriateness of the "procedure"; less experienced may misuse this level for not-well-considered, unadapted "cookbook medicine"
Sensorimotor level	Use of all senses and manual actions; "feeling, doing, hearing"; sometimes subconscious control of actions	Experts perform smooth action sequences and control their actions by direct feedback from their senses (e.g., action sequences of placing an intravenous line or endotracheal intubation; skill-based errors such as slips and lapses may occur)

ACRM, Anesthesia Crisis Resource Management.

suction canisters and sponges, listening for normal and abnormal sounds from the patient and equipment, interpreting radiographs, and reading the reports of laboratory test results. Because the human mind can attend closely to only one or two items at a time, the anesthetist's supervisory control level must decide what information to attend to and how frequently to observe it.

The multitasking involved in observing multiple data streams was probed by experiments measuring secondary task performance and vigilance. The realistic simulation studies demonstrated the large number of information sources actually used during the response to a critical event. Routine parts of the core process operate primarily at the sensory, motor, and procedural levels and are executed repetitively throughout the course of an anesthetic regimen. Results from the University of California, San Diego (UCSD), and from the Department of Veterans Affairs and Stanford University (UCSD/VA-Stanford group) concerning the vigilance of experienced anesthetists versus novices suggested that novices had not fully developed their core process as a highly automated function and thus were required to devote more mental resources to routine activities.

Verification

In the OR environment, the available information is not always reliable. Most monitoring is noninvasive and indirect and is susceptible to artifacts (false data). Even direct clinical observations such as vision or auscultation can be ambiguous. Brief transients (true data of short duration) can occur that quickly correct themselves. To prevent them from triggering precipitous actions that may have significant side effects, critical observations must be verified before the clinician acts on them. Verification uses a variety of methods, shown in Table 6-7.

It should be noted that if in doubt, it should always be assumed that the patient is at risk and that the parameter in question is real ("rule out the worst case"). The assumption of a technical artifact should be the last step.

Knowing when and how to verify data is a good illustration of strategic knowledge (metacognition). For example, the anesthetist must decide under what conditions it is useful to invest time, attention, and energy in establishing a new information source (e.g., a pulmonary artery catheter) in the middle of a case rather than relying on more indirect information sources that are already in place.

Table 6-7 Methods for Verification of Critical Observations

Method	Explanation, Example
Repeating	The observation or measurement is repeated to rule out a temporary wrong value (e.g., motion artifacts during noninvasive blood pressure measurement)
Checking trend information	The short-term trend is observed for plausibility of the actual value. Trends of physiologic parameters almost always follow curves, not steps
Observing a redundant channel	An existing redundant channel is checked (e.g., invasive arterial pressure and cuff pressure are redundant, or heart rate from an ECG and pulse oximeter)
Correlating	Multiple related (but not redundant) variables are correlated to determine the plausibility of the parameter in question (e.g., if the ECG monitor shows a flat line and "asystole" but the invasive blood pressure curve shows waves)
Activating a new monitoring device	A new monitoring modality is installed (e.g., placing a pulmonary artery catheter). This also adds another parameter for the method of "correlating"
Recalibrating an instrument or testing its function	Checking the quality and reliability of a measurement and testing its function (e.g., if the CO_2 detector shows no values, the anesthetist can exhale through it to see whether the device works). Observation of redundant channels can also help verify a value (see above)
Replacing an instrument	If there is doubt about the function of a device, an entirely new instrument or an alternative backup device may be installed
Asking for help	If the decision on the values remains unclear, help should be sought early to obtain a second opinion from other trained personnel

ECG, electrocardiogram.

Problem Recognition

Anesthetists are taught the importance of scanning their instruments and environment, but they must use these observations to decide whether the patient's course is "on track" or whether a problem is occurring. If a problem is found, a decision must be made regarding its identity and its importance. This process of problem recognition (also known as situation assessment) is a central feature of several theories of cognition in complex, dynamic worlds.[144,250-252]

Problem recognition involves matching sets of environmental cues to patterns that are known to represent specific types of problems. Given the high uncertainty seen in anesthesia, the available information sources cannot always disclose the existence of a problem, and even if they do, they may not specify its identity or origin. Westenskow and colleagues'[253] experiment with the intelligent alarm system mainly probed these parts of problem recognition. In this experiment, subjects were already alerted to the existence of a problem by an alarm, so they could immediately focus their attention specifically on information sources concerning ventilation. In 11 cases, the fault could not be identified, but there was successful compensation for the fault, as described in the next paragraphs.

The supervisory control level mediates the decision when a clear-cut match or "diagnosis" cannot be made. Anesthetists and other dynamic decision-makers use approximation strategies to handle these ambiguous situations; psychologists term such strategies *heuristics*.[254] One heuristic is to categorize what is happening as one of several "generic" problems, each of which encompasses many different underlying conditions. Another is to gamble on a single diagnosis (frequency gambling[239]) by initially choosing the single most frequent candidate event. During preoperative planning, the anesthetist may adjust a mental "index of suspicion" for recognizing certain specific problems anticipated for that particular patient or surgical procedure. The anesthetist must also decide whether a single underlying diagnosis explains all the data or whether these data could be due to multiple causes. This decision is important because excessive attempts to refine the diagnosis can be very costly in terms of allocation of attention. By contrast, a premature diagnosis can lead to inadequate or erroneous treatment.

The use of heuristics is typical of expert anesthetists and often results in considerable time savings in dealing with problems. However, it is a double-edged sword. Both frequency gambling and inappropriate allocation of attention solely to expected problems can seriously undermine problem solving when these gambles do not pay off if the re-evaluation component of the core process does not correct the situation.

Prediction of Future States

Problems must be assessed in terms of their significance for the future states of the patient.[144,250] Problems that are already critical or that can be predicted to evolve into critical incidents receive the highest priority. Prediction of future states also influences action planning by defining the timeframe available for required actions. Cook and colleagues[255] described "going sour" incidents in which the future state of the patient was not adequately taken into account when early manifestations of problems were apparent. It is also known from research in psychology that the human mind is not very well suited to predict future states, especially if things are changing in a nonlinear fashion. Under such circumstances, which are not uncommon for natural systems such as the human body, the rate of change is almost invariably underestimated and the people are surprised at the outcome.[43] Slow but steady and sustained blood loss in a child during surgery may result in few or subtle changes in hemodynamics for some time until rapid decompensation occurs. If the weak signs of the developing problem were not detected, the ensuing catastrophe may seem to have occurred "suddenly."

Decision-making

Having recognized a problem, how does an expert anesthetist respond? The classic paradigm of decision-making posits a careful comparison of the evidence with various causal hypotheses that can explain them.[39] This is then followed by a careful analysis of all possible actions and solutions to the problem. This approach, though powerful, is relatively slow and does not work well with ambiguous or scanty evidence. In complex, dynamic domains such as anesthesia, many problems require "decisions under uncertainty"[233,256] with quick action to prevent a rapid cascade to a catastrophic adverse outcome. For these problems, deriving a solution through formal deductive reasoning from "first principles" is too slow.

Precompiled Responses and Abstract Reasoning

In complex, dynamic domains, the initial responses of experts to the majority of events stem from precompiled rules or response plans for dealing with a recognized event.[239] This method is referred to as recognition-primed decision-making[236,257] because once the event is identified, the response is well known. In the anesthesia domain, these responses are usually acquired through personal experience alone, although there is a growing realization that critical response protocols need to be codified explicitly and taught systematically. Experienced anesthetists have been observed to rearrange, recompile, and rehearse these responses mentally based on the patient's condition, the surgical procedure, and the problems to be expected.[268] Ideally, precompiled responses to common problems are retrieved appropriately and executed rapidly. When the exact nature of the problem is not apparent, a set of generic responses appropriate to the overall situation may be invoked. For example, if a problem with ventilation is detected, the anesthetist may switch to manual ventilation at a higher F_{IO_2} while considering further diagnostic actions.

However, experiments involving screen-only[258] and realistic[109,143,259,260] simulators have demonstrated that even experienced anesthetists show great variability in their use of response procedures to critical situations. This finding led these investigators to target simulator-based training in the systematic training of responses to critical events.[109,226,261-263]

Even the ideal use of precompiled responses is destined to fail when the problem does not have the suspected cause or when it does not respond to the usual actions. Anesthesia cannot be administered purely by precompiled "cookbook" procedures. Abstract reasoning about the problem through the use of fundamental medical knowledge still takes place in parallel with precompiled responses, even when quick action must be taken. This seems to involve a search for high-level analogies[239] or true deductive reasoning using deep medical and technical knowledge and a thorough analysis of all possible solutions. Anesthetists managing simulated crises have linked their precompiled actions to abstract medical concepts.[258] It is unclear whether this represents merely self-justification as opposed to true abstract reasoning, in part because the particular simulated crises they faced did not require novel abstract solutions. At this time, the degree to which abstract reasoning is necessary for optimal intraoperative crisis management is unknown.[113,226,256]

Taking Action

A hallmark of anesthesia practice is that anesthetists do not just write orders in a patient's chart; they are directly involved in implementing the desired actions.

Although such direct involvement has many benefits in timeliness and flexibility of action, it also poses risks. Implementation of action can usurp a large amount of the anesthetist's attention and can be distracting. This is particularly an issue when other tasks have been interrupted or temporarily suspended. The "prospective memory" to complete these tasks can be erased. (For a more detailed explanation of prospective memory, see later.) In addition, anesthetists engaged in a manual procedure are strongly constrained from performing other manual tasks, as demonstrated in several of the mental workload and vigilance studies described earlier.

Errors in executing a task are termed *slips*, as distinguished from errors in deciding what to do, which are termed *mistakes*.[238] Slips are actions that do not occur as planned, such as turning the wrong switch or making a syringe swap. Thus, when critical incident[185,264] and quality assurance studies described "technical errors" in using equipment, they were referring to slips, whereas "judgment errors" referred to mistakes. One particular type of execution error, termed a *mode error*,[238] is becoming more frequent in all domains with the increased use of microprocessor-based instrumentation and devices.[227] In a mode error, actions appropriate for one mode of a device's operation are incorrect for another mode. An example in anesthesiology is the "bag/ventilator" selector valve in the anesthesia breathing circuit, which selects between two modes of ventilation. Failing to activate the ventilator when in the "ventilator mode" can be catastrophic. Mode errors can also occur with monitoring or drug delivery devices if they assign different functions to the same displays or switches depending on the mode of operation selected.

Particularly dangerous slips of execution can be addressed through the use of engineered safety devices[57] that physically prevent incorrect actions. For example, newer anesthesia machines have interlocks that physically prevent the simultaneous administration of more than one volatile anesthetic drug. Other interlocks physically prevent the selection of a gas mixture containing less than 21% O_2.

Certain very complex issues concerning human-machine interactions and the ways in which technology affects behavior in complex patient care environments are beyond the scope of this chapter. Other publications address these issues.[27,29,31-35,37,38,227,265]

Re-evaluation and Situation Awareness

To cope with the rapid changes and profound diagnostic and therapeutic uncertainties seen during anesthesia, the core process must include repetitive re-evaluation of the situation. Thus, the re-evaluation step returns the anesthetist to the observation phase of the core process, but with specific assessments in mind, as shown in Box 6-7 at CRM key point 12, "Re-evaluate repeatedly").

The process of continually updating assessment of the situation and monitoring the efficacy of chosen actions is termed *situation awareness*.[250-252,266,267] Situation awareness is a very interesting and important topic in analyzing performance and reasons for errors.[144,268,269] There has been a review of situation awareness issues in anesthesiology.[144]

Management and Coordination of the Core Process

Empirical studies have clearly demonstrated that attention sharing is needed among cognitive levels, among tasks, and often among problems. The intensive demands on the anesthetist's attention could easily swamp the available mental resources. Therefore, the anesthetist must strike a balance between acting quickly on every small perturbation (which requires a lot of attention) and adopting a more conservative "wait-and-see" attitude. This balance must be constantly shifted between these extremes as the situation changes. However, during simulated crisis situations, some practitioners showed great reluctance to switch from "business as usual" to "emergency mode" even when serious problems were detected. Erring too far in the direction of "wait and see" is an error that can be particularly catastrophic.

In addition to the attentional demands of the anesthetist's core tasks, the OR environment is full of distractions. Routine events, such as turning the OR table or repositioning the patient, distract attention from the main process of conducting the anesthesia. Noise is prevalent, with peak levels exceeding that of a freeway. Practitioners find false auditory alarms from monitors or other equipment to be extremely distracting.[279-281] Other distractions include teaching in progress,[278] incoming telephone calls, background music, and conversation with OR personnel. Expert anesthetists modulate the distractions by eliminating them when the workload is high and allowing them to occur when the workload is low (to improve morale and team building).

Active Management of Workload

One major aspect of strategic control of attention is the active management of workload. Rather than passively dealing with rising or falling workload, the anesthetist actively manages it. Schneider and Detweiler[163] and Gopher (position paper, Conference on Human Error in Anesthesia, Asilomar, CA, 1991) described the theoretical basis for a variety of strategies of workload management. These strategies have been addressed specifically for anesthesiology by several investigators.[226,228] The anesthetist actively manages workload by the following techniques.

Avoiding High-Workload Situations

Experts may choose techniques and plans that reduce the workload (especially when their individual and team resources are limited), even when those plans are marginally inferior from a technical standpoint. For example, a single anesthetist may choose not to use a high-tech, high-workload monitor such as transesophageal echocardiography (TEE) because of the high workload required to use it properly.

Distributing Workload over Time

The anesthetist can prepare for future tasks when the current load is low (preloading) and can delay or shed low-priority tasks when the workload is high (offloading). Resources that require a significant amount of workload to prepare, such as intravenous infusions, are often made ready before the case starts. Multitasking is also a way to distribute work over time. Every task is made up of several subtasks, each of which has a finite duration. Because close attention may not be required during each of these subtasks, they can be interleaved with a fixed amount of attention (multiplexing). Multiplexed tasks must be scheduled and coordinated in real time at the supervisory control level.

Distributing Workload over Personnel

When workload cannot be distributed over time and when additional resources are available, tasks can be distributed to them. Some resources are internal to the individual anesthetist, whereas others require additional personnel. For example, a single anesthetist can simultaneously ventilate the patient by hand, assess cardiac rhythm, and discuss patient care with the surgeon. A single anesthetist cannot simultaneously insert a pulmonary artery catheter and ventilate the patient's lungs by hand. If these tasks are to be performed at the same time, they must be assigned to different individuals.

Changing the Nature of the Task

The nature of a task is not fixed. Surgery and anesthesia can sometimes be postponed or aborted. Tasks can be executed to different standards of performance; as standards are loosened, the workload required to perform them is reduced. For example, during periods of massive blood loss, the anesthetist focuses primarily on administering blood and fluids and on monitoring blood pressure. In such cases, less critical tasks such as writing on the anesthesia record are offloaded to lessen the workload. The acceptable limits of blood pressure will also be widened.

Action Selection and Scheduling

At any time during an anesthetic regimen there may be multiple things to do, each of which is intrinsically appropriate, yet they cannot all be done at once. Simulator experiments have shown that anesthetists sometimes have difficulty selecting, planning, and scheduling actions optimally. The anesthetist must consider the following factors:

1. Preconditions are necessary for carrying out the actions (e.g., it is impossible to measure a thermodilution cardiac output if there is no pulmonary artery catheter in place).
2. Constraints are placed on the proposed actions (some actions are incompatible with other aspects of the situation; e.g., it is impossible to check the diameter of the pupils when the head is fully draped in the surgical field).
3. Side effects of the proposed actions often play a controlling role in choosing among possible drug therapies.
4. The rapidity and ease of implementation of proposed actions are factors; those that are easily and rapidly performed are preferred over those that require more time, attention, and skill.
5. Certainty of success of the actions is often traded off against rapidity and ease of implementation (under some circumstances, the higher certainty of success of a set of actions justifies the investment of time, attention, and resources needed to implement them).
6. Reversibility of the action and the cost of being wrong are considered, with rapidly reversible actions preferred over those that cannot be reversed, especially when potential side effects are significant.
7. Cost of the action in terms of attention, resources, and money is taken into account.

Experts in other complex, dynamic domains (specifically tank commanders and fire chiefs) have been observed[282] to conduct a mental simulation of the actions that they are contemplating to determine whether there are hidden flaws in their plans. Anesthetists have been observed[228] to rehearse a plan mentally in advance of a case, but the degree to which this is done in real time is not known. Because most actions can be executed incrementally, as in titrating a drug in small aliquots, adverse consequences can often be discovered through repetitive re-evaluation.

Resource Management

The ability of the anesthetist to command and control all the resources at hand to execute the anesthetic regimen as planned and to respond to problems that arise is termed *resource management* (another concept first described in aviation that applies equally well to anesthesiology; see the earlier section on CRM key points). Resource management involves translating the knowledge of what needs to be done into effective team activity by taking into account the limitations of the complex and ill-structured OR, PACU, or ICU domain. Resource management explicitly requires teamwork and crew coordination. It is not enough for the anesthetist to know what to do or even to be able to do each task alone. The anesthetist can accomplish only so much in a given time, and there are some tasks that can be performed only by other skilled personnel (e.g., laboratory tests, taking radiographs). When the task load exceeds the resources available, the anesthetist must mobilize help and distribute the tasks among those present. Many issues concerning optimum resource management and crew coordination are not yet well understood and are the focus of active research by cognitive scientists and experts in many complex and dynamic domains.[24,115-117,283-285] Research in aviation has already demonstrated that a large proportion of aircraft accidents are linked to failures on the part of crews with appropriate technical skills to manage the flight deck effectively.[186] The hallmarks of resource management derived from these studies are discussed in detail in the earlier section on CRM key points.

Dynamic Prioritization of Tasks

Complex multiple personnel simulations of anesthetic crises have been used to address the issue of resource management. Although the data from these simulations are still preliminary, it appears that poor supervisory control and resource management were substantial components of suboptimal management of the simulated crises.[260] In other words, like the pilots, anesthetists had the knowledge and technical skill to manage the patient, but they failed to manage their environment properly to achieve success (hence termed CRM skills or nontechnical skills). (In aviation, such situations have often resulted in what is called "controlled flight into terrain.")

Prospective Memory

Prospective memory describes one's ability to remember in the future to perform an action.[270] It is particularly prone to disruption by concurrent tasks or interruptions. Disruption of intentions or on-going tasks is common in everyday life and has also been described in pilots and air traffic controllers.[271-275] In anesthesia, for example, if the anesthetist suspends ventilation temporarily (say to allow a radiograph to be taken), the intention to restart the ventilator depends on prospective memory and can be easily forgotten. Chisholm and associates performed a study in an emergency department and looked for "interruptions" and "breaks in task." They found that during a 3-hour period, the emergency physician was faced with more than 30 interruptions and more than 20 breaks in task. It is likely that similar results would be found in the ICU.[276]

A variety of methods may preserve prospective memory of intentions. Visual or auditory reminders can be used (physiologic monitor alarms often serve this purpose whether intended or not), although the effectiveness of such methods seems to be less than one would expect. Special actions—such as leaving one's finger on the ventilator switch—can be used to indicate that an important intention is pending.

Fixation Errors

Faulty re-evaluation, inadequate adaptation of the plan, or loss of situation awareness can result in a type of human error termed a *fixation error*.[131,132] Fixation errors have been described by all the investigators conducting experimental studies of responses of anesthetists to abnormal situations.[259,260,277] Avoiding fixation errors in the field of anesthesia is CRM key point 9 and is covered in the section on CRM key points.

Hazardous Attitudes

Attitudes are an important component of ability that can affect performance as strongly as physiologic performance-shaping factors can. Psychologists studying judgment in aviators have identified five types of attitude as being particularly hazardous, and they have developed specific antidote thoughts for each hazardous attitude.[195] These attitudes as related to anesthesia are shown in Table 6-8. Aviation psychologists instruct pilots to

Table 6-8 Examples of Hazardous Attitudes and Their Antidote Thoughts

Hazardous Attitude	Antidote Thoughts
Antiauthority: "Don't tell me what to do. The policies are for someone else."	"Follow the rules. They are usually right."
Impulsivity: "Do something quickly—anything!"	"Not so fast. Think first."
Invulnerability: "It won't happen to me. It's just a routine case."	"It *could* happen to me. Serious problems can develop even in routine cases."
Macho: "I'll show you I can do it. I can intubate the trachea of anyone."	"Taking chances is foolish. Plan for failure."
Resignation: "What's the use? It's out of my hands. It's up to the surgeon."	"I'm not helpless. I can make a difference. There is always something else to try that might help."

physically verbalize the antidote thought whenever they find themselves thinking in a hazardous way.

The *invulnerable* and *macho* attitudes are particularly hazardous for anesthetists. They are compounded by production pressures to handle more cases in less time with fewer cancellations and less opportunity for preoperative evaluation. The feeling that a catastrophe "cannot happen to me" and that perfect performance can always be called on to avert a disaster can lead to cavalier behavior and poor planning. It can alter thresholds for believing that abnormal data represent a problem, thereby leading to the fixation error of "everything's OK." In 1984, Cooper[278] wrote the following about studies of critical incidents in anesthesia:

> *Perhaps the most insidious hazard of anesthesia is its relative safety. The individual anesthetist rarely, on average, will be responsible for a serious iatrogenic complication. It is our impression from the process of collecting incidents, that most seemingly minor errors are not taken seriously and that risk management depends almost solely on the anesthetist's ability to react instinctively and flawlessly every time a problem arises.*

Expert human performance is the anesthetist's most powerful tool to safeguard the patient. However, planning to avoid catastrophe is likely to be more successful than battling to avert it.

The Anesthetist's Tasks

Investigation of a complex work environment typically starts with task analysis (reviews of this technique were published in the journal *Human Factors*[286]). One can perform an abstract analysis of the work goals and constraints and then derive the tasks required to achieve the goals. Alternatively, one can observe what skilled practitioners actually do in their work and classify these actions into task elements. Often the techniques are combined. In this section the anesthetist's tasks are examined in the abstract and then the empirical task analysis approach is reviewed. There are two distinct phases of anesthetic care: (1) preoperative evaluation, planning, and preparation and (2) conduct of the anesthetic regimen and immediate postoperative care.

Preoperative Evaluation and Planning

There are few data on how well anesthetists identify important patient conditions through history taking and physical examination (see Chapter 34). A frequent organizational obstacle to the anesthetist's evaluation task is difficulty obtaining the patient's previous medical records. The performance of anesthetists in selecting appropriate laboratory tests has been found to be relatively poor. Roizen and associates[287] state the following:

> *Even when physicians agree to reduce testing by using specific, agreed upon criteria for selectively ordering tests based on history and physical examination, they still make a surprising number of mistakes when ordering tests. Approximately 30% to 40% of patients who should have certain tests … do not get them, and 20% to 40% of patients who should not have tests are subjected to them.*

Roizen has argued for automation of routine patient questioning and selection of laboratory tests and has participated in the development of commercial devices to do so. Whether these devices, in combination with human follow-up for patients with medical problems, will improve the efficiency and accuracy of preoperative evaluation remains to be determined. The performance of anesthetists in interpreting ECGs and chest radiographs also appears to be poor relative to specialists in these fields. The extent to which this factor influences the design of anesthetic plans or patient outcomes is unknown.

Anesthetic Plan

In constructing the plan, the anesthetist uses the preoperative evaluation of the patient to match the technical requirements of the surgical procedure and the physiologic characteristics of the patient to the mental, physical, and technologic resources available. A typical anesthetic plan contains several elements. For example, the plan for general anesthesia includes choices for the means of inducing anesthesia, securing the airway and ensuring proper ventilation, maintaining anesthesia, conducting emergence from anesthesia, and controlling postoperative pain. Skilled planning is as critical as skilled execution in safe patient care. If a significant feature of the situation is missed in formulating the plan, it can leave the patient vulnerable, regardless of how adeptly the plan is implemented.

The technical requirements of most surgical procedures are well known. Most patients do not have medical problems that could significantly alter the anesthetic plan, although Gibby and associates[288] found that 20% of outpatients, most of them with ASA physical status 1 or 2, had conditions identifiable through an anesthetist's history and examination that required changes from a "standard" anesthetic plan. When a procedure is new or challenging, when the patient has significant underlying disease, or when needed resources are not available, creative planning may be needed to identify a set of physiologic goals for the anesthetic regimen. Routine anesthetic plans can be modified or combined to produce a compromise plan that best fits the goals and constraints of the situation.

Although faculty anesthetists routinely critique the anesthetic plans of residents and planning is explicitly probed during the oral examination of the American Board of Anesthesiologists, the process of constructing anesthetic plans has been studied very little. Most of the existing literature on preoperative planning concentrates only on the medical and physiologic aspects of underlying diseases and their anesthetic ramifications.

Pre-use Preparation and Checkout of Equipment

After the plan is established, the anesthetist must prepare the work environment. This involves obtaining the necessary equipment and supplies, assembling infusions, preparing syringes of needed drugs, and conducting pre-use checkouts of life support equipment (see Chapter 38). The performance of anesthetists at these tasks is not optimal. Buffington and coworkers[289] demonstrated that only 3% of anesthetists examining an anesthesia machine could identify all five faults with which it had been rigged; most practitioners found only two of the five. Nearly 30% missed such major faults as complete absence of both unidirectional valve disks in a circle anesthesia breathing system and swap of the nitrous oxide and oxygen cylinders (made possible by a fault in the pin-indexing system).

The Food and Drug Administration (FDA), in cooperation with the ASA, the APSF, and experts from academics and industry, developed a set of recommendations for the checkout of anesthesia apparatus.[290] This checklist was widely disseminated by the ASA and the APSF. However, it was found that use of the checkout procedure was minimal and that the extent of pre-use checkout by practitioners was extremely variable. A newer study[291] was conducted to compare the checkout of anesthesia machines by practitioners with and without use of the FDA checkout procedure. Most of the faults were detected by 50% or fewer participants, regardless of the checkout procedure used. Only for one fault, failure of the oxygen–nitrous oxide ratio protection system, did the FDA checklist offer significant advantages; when using it, the detection rate increased to 65%. Interestingly, 34% of the faults that were not detected were missed by practitioners who had in fact correctly answered three out of three written test questions concerning that fault. This suggests that although some of the performance deficit may be related to lack of knowledge, a substantial proportion are due to the inability to apply abstract knowledge to the practical performance of equipment checkout.

There were many criticisms of the original checklist, particularly its complexity.[292] A streamlined version of the original checklist was published by the FDA in 1994.[293] A study of the new checklist, however, showed no significant benefit from its use and a disturbingly low rate of detection of machine faults (around 50%).[294] In another study, anesthetists using a highly interactive electronic checklist (developed by Blike and Biddle) improved their detection of "easy faults" but still missed a high proportion of difficult faults.[295] A study performed more recently to measure the influence of fatigue on performance in a simulator showed that subjects in both the rested and fatigued conditions left out significant portions of the machine checkout.[178]

Emergency Checklists

One aspect of preparedness is to consider possible emergencies and to mentally rehearse their management. Another approach is the readiness and ability to use critical incident checklists. For example, the Veterans Health Administration has placed a set of emergency checklists on plastic laminated sheets in every OR of 105 hospitals (Fig. 6-11 and Box 6-10 for an example of "anaphylaxis"). Other emergency checklists have been made available electronically.[296,297] Despite these advances, the use of emergency checklists has still not become a regular part of the culture of medical work.

Execution and Adaptation of Plans

Anesthetic plans are dynamic. The anesthetist must monitor the plan as it is executed and must adapt it in response to dynamically changing events. The key features of this task are (1) checking for the achievement of milestones and (2) reactive plan adaptation. These are shown schematically in Figure 6-12. At various points of a procedure there are critical milestones that must be achieved to keep the original plan unaltered. If a milestone is not achieved, the anesthetist must decide whether to delay the next action in the sequence, modify the plan, or suspend or abort the procedure. On some occasions, the milestones are explicitly identified in advance, whereas in others the milestones are implicit.

The anesthetist must also react to a large number of other contingencies, some of which can be predicted in advance based

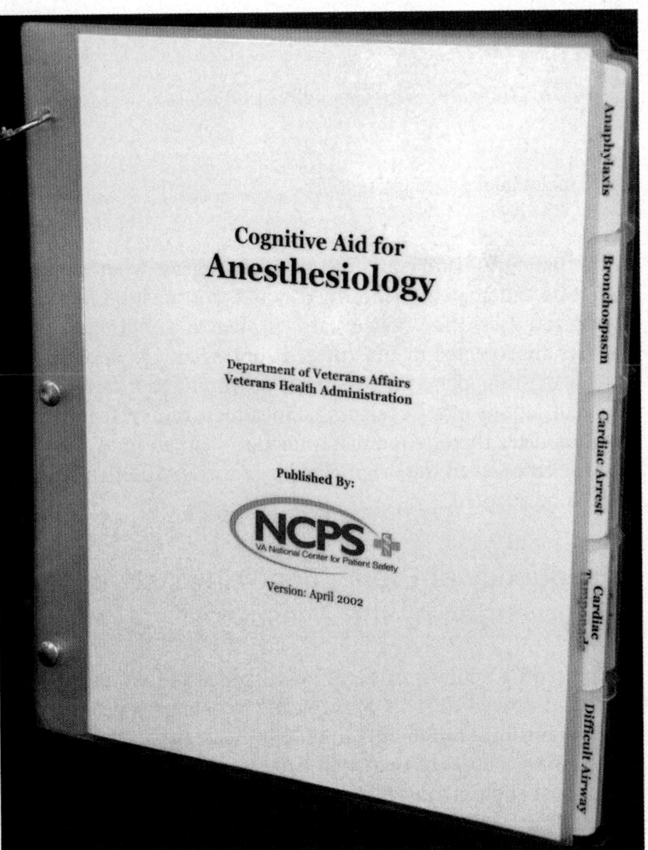

Figure 6-11 Department of Veterans Affairs checklist by NCPS. An example of the cognitive aid is given by Anaphylaxis in Box 6-10.

Box 6-10 VA NCPS Checklist Example (Anaphylaxis)

MANIFESTATIONS

Cardiac

- Hypotension (may be the only sign of anaphylaxis in an anesthetized patient)
- Cardiovascular collapse
- Pulmonary hypertension
- Arrhythmias/tachycardia

Respiratory

- Bronchospasm
- Increased peak inspiratory pressure (high PIP)
- Hypoxemia
- Pulmonary edema
- Stridor, laryngeal edema

Cutaneous

- Rash, flush, hives, angioedema
- In an awake patient, signs and symptoms include
  - Dizziness, decreased level of consciousness, dyspnea and/or chest tightness, pruritus

IMMEDIATE ACTION

- Stop administration of any possible antigen (e.g., antibiotics, muscle relaxants, blood) (transfusion reaction)
- In the absence of any other likely cause, consider *latex allergy*
  - Remove all latex products in contact with the patient
    - Surgical gloves
    - Medications drawn up through a latex stopper
    - Urinary catheter

Maintain the patient's airway and support oxygenation and ventilation
- Increase F_{IO_2} to 100%

Intubate early if the allergic reaction is severe
- The airway and larynx can become very edematous

Inform the surgeons
- Consider terminating the surgical procedure

Expand circulating fluid volume; ensure adequate intravenous access
- Immediate fluid needs may be massive (many liters of crystalloid)

Administer epinephrine intravenously
- Epinephrine is the drug of choice for the treatment of severe anaphylaxis
  - For hypotension or bronchospasm, 10- to 50-μg increments; repeat as necessary with escalating doses
  - For cardiovascular collapse, use ACLS doses, 500- to 1000-μg boluses; repeat as necessary with escalating doses

Treat bronchospasm if present
- Administer inhaled bronchodilators
  - Albuterol: initial dose, 4 to 8 metered puffs
  - Depending on the delivery system, a larger dose of any aerosolized medication may be required when administered via the endotracheal tube

ACLS, advanced cardiac life support.

on the patient's history and the type of surgery, whereas others cannot be anticipated. Incoming data streams must be constantly scrutinized (see the "police cars" in Fig. 6-12) to determine whether an expected or unexpected contingency is occurring. If so, the existing plan may have to be modified. As plans are changed, actions may be taken that invalidate other aspects of the previous plan, thereby requiring further adaptation of the plan. In some cases, even the original goals of the anesthetic plan may need to be adapted.

Frequency of Events Requiring Active Intervention by the Anesthetist

The preceding analysis of Figure 6-12 suggests that anesthetists must be prepared to react dynamically to changing events. How frequent is this requirement? In the Multicenter Study of General Anesthesia,[298] 86% of patients had at least one undesirable outcome. Although most events were minor and caused no injury to the patient, more than 5% of patients had one or more severe events requiring "significant therapy, with or without full recovery." This incidence is probably a lower limit for severe events because the entry criteria of the study precluded the enrollment of critically ill patients or emergency surgeries, for which the likelihood of severe problems requiring intervention would be expected to be high.

In another study by Cooper and associates,[299] impact events, defined as "undesirable, unexpected, and which could cause at least moderate morbidity," occurred in 18% of patients either in the OR or in the PACU, and 3% of all cases involved a "serious" event. These figures are also probably lower limits because for technical reasons the study excluded patients going directly from surgery to an ICU.

Moller and coauthors[300] reported 4439 "impact events" in 10,312 patients either in the OR (2441) or in the PACU (1998). Here again, some patients had several events, whereas others had none. The investigators did not compute the frequency of severe events, but overall, these data appear to be consistent with those from earlier studies.

Model of Event Evolution

The findings just discussed, as well as the larger system issues raised by Reason and Perrow, can be summarized in a model of event evolution (Fig. 6-13).[58,113,226]

Similar models incorporating some of the same features have also been described.[59,301] Underlying aspects of the system can gen-

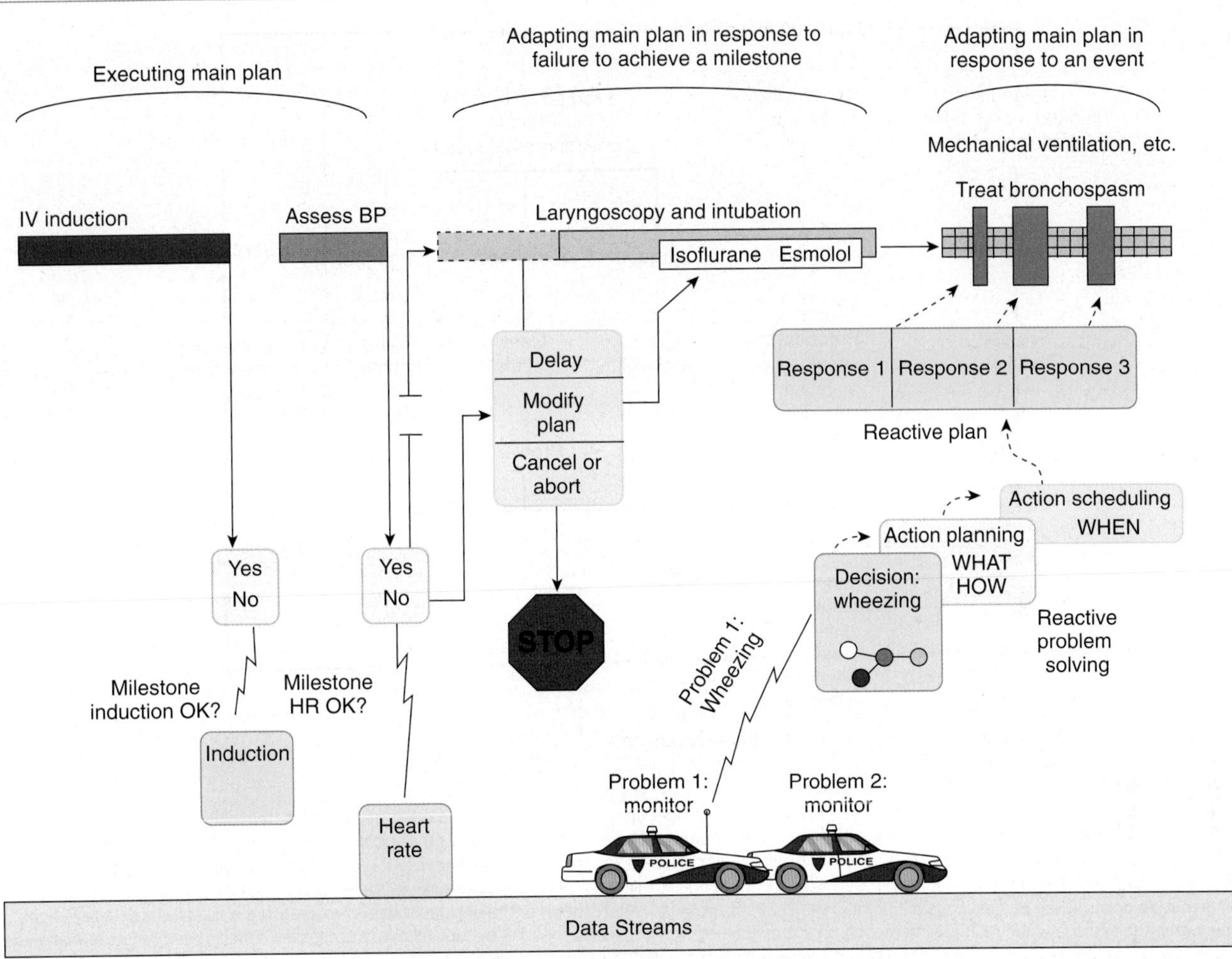

Figure 6-12 Schematic diagram of the dynamic adaptation of preoperative plans. The anesthetist begins with intravenous (IV) induction of anesthesia as planned (*top left*). On achieving the milestone of successful induction of anesthesia, blood pressure (BP) is checked before proceeding with laryngoscopy and intubation (*center*). If BP is not satisfactory, the next step may be delayed and the plan amended to optimize BP. If necessary, the procedure may even be aborted at this stage. Throughout the procedure, the anesthetist is vigilant for the occurrence of new problems ("police cars"). If a problem is detected, a process of reactive problem solving takes place, which may result in new adaptations to the plan (in this case, treatment of bronchospasm). *(From Gaba DM: Human Error in Dynamic Medical Environments. Hillsdale, NJ, Lawrence Erlbaum, 1994, pp 197-224.)*

erate latent failures. Either by random chance or because of interactions between the latent failures, an event may be triggered by one of four components of the operational system in the OR: the anesthetist, the surgeon, the patient, or the equipment. Anesthetists have traditionally been most interested in events that they trigger themselves (such as esophageal intubation), but in fact, most events are initiated by a combination of underlying patient disease and another of the triggering factors. Most problems are not directly harmful to the patient unless they evolve further. Possibilities for evolution of the problem include the following:

1. A single problem worsens and by itself evolves into an adverse outcome.
2. The problem begins to evolve but remains self-limited without any intervention.
3. Multiple small problems combine to trigger a problem that can evolve into an adverse outcome; the original problems by themselves would not have evolved further.
4. A single problem triggers another problem that evolves into an adverse outcome.
5. An evolving problem should be able to be stopped, but the recovery pathway is faulty.
6. Two problems are triggered. Attention focused on one (minor) problem distracts attention from the (serious) evolution of another.

The system has a variety of interruption points at which the occurrence of problems can be prevented (preoperative evaluation of patients and pre-use checkout of equipment). Moreover, although anesthesiology is far more dynamic than many medical domains, it is relatively slow in comparison to many human activities such as sports, driving, and combat flying. Thus, events often evolve slowly enough that the process of accident evolution can be thwarted before an adverse patient outcome actually occurs. The interruption of accident evolution corresponds to the "defense-in-depth" in Reason's "Swiss cheese" model[70] and to recovery from a normal accident in Perrow's paradigm (see Figs. 6-2 and 6-3 and the overview on NAT in Table 6-2).

In the prospective studies of intraoperative events cited earlier, there was a surprisingly high incidence of undesirable situations, whereas the rate of actual patient harm was quite low. The patient's safety was frequently protected only by the skilled intervention of a trained anesthetist. Note that this is a markedly different picture from that in commercial aviation, although the

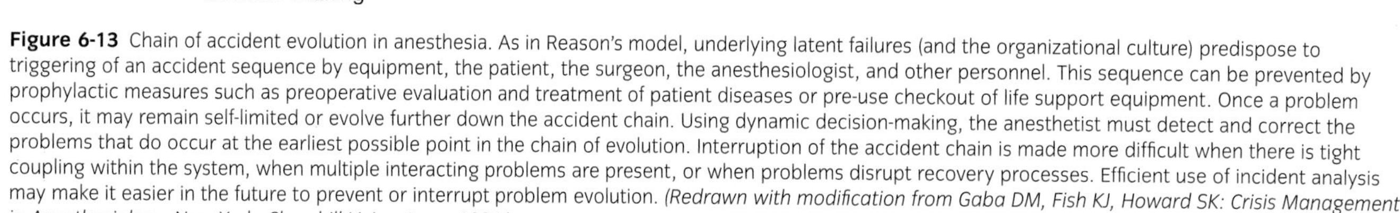

Figure 6-13 Chain of accident evolution in anesthesia. As in Reason's model, underlying latent failures (and the organizational culture) predispose to triggering of an accident sequence by equipment, the patient, the surgeon, the anesthesiologist, and other personnel. This sequence can be prevented by prophylactic measures such as preoperative evaluation and treatment of patient diseases or pre-use checkout of life support equipment. Once a problem occurs, it may remain self-limited or evolve further down the accident chain. Using dynamic decision-making, the anesthetist must detect and correct the problems that do occur at the earliest possible point in the chain of evolution. Interruption of the accident chain is made more difficult when there is tight coupling within the system, when multiple interacting problems are present, or when problems disrupt recovery processes. Efficient use of incident analysis may make it easier in the future to prevent or interrupt problem evolution. *(Redrawn with modification from Gaba DM, Fish KJ, Howard SK: Crisis Management in Anesthesiology. New York, Churchill Livingstone, 1994.)*

accident rate in aviation is very low. About 30,000 airline flights take place each day in the United States, and there are very few serious incidents or accidents, although the exact number is unknown. The total accident rate from all causes (not counting terrorist acts) for major airline flights between 1982 and 2001 was 0.38 per 100,000 departures. Air carrier accidents with one or more fatalities occurred at a rate of 0.045 per 100,000 departures. In 2002 there were no fatalities in U.S. airline or commuter aviation (NTSB website: www.ntsb.gov/aviation/Stats.htm).

The actual number of events in aviation matching the "impact event" criteria given earlier is not known, but it is probably at least 100 times greater than the number of accidents. Even so, this still makes aviation incidents far less frequent than the 3% to 5% rate of "significant" impact events in anesthesia. Based on these data, it is clear that the intraoperative management of abnormal, dynamically changing events remains the critical locus of anesthesia skill.

Empirical Studies of Anesthetists' Tasks

Over the past 20 years there have been a number of studies[31,35-38,40,178,198,235,302-305] of anesthetists' intraoperative activities. In addition, an increasing number of studies have been performed in realistic simulator environments.[2,19,184,306-319]

The earliest studies used time-lapse photography of a handful of anesthetic cases with a frame-by-frame analysis of tasks. One major finding of the first task analysis, by Drui and associates in 1973,[320] was that "the anesthesiologist's attention was often directed away from the patient-surgical field." In subsequent studies,[241-243] it was found that about 40% to 50% of the time the anesthetist's gaze was directed away from the patient or surgical field. McDonald and Dzwonczyk,[242] studying cases from 1981, classified direct patient activity as "one during which the anesthetist had contact with the patient and a view of the surgical field." These investigators explicitly noted "observation of skin color," "palpation of pulse," and "auscultation of heart and breath sounds" as direct patient activities. Observing arterial pressure or the ECG and observing or adjusting the anesthesia machine or intravenous infusions were classified as indirect patient activities. In this study 83% of the anesthetist's time was spent on activities that were not direct patient activities. The same group[243] repeated its study for cases from 1985 and demonstrated a much higher rate of direct patient monitoring than obtained in 1981 (44.8% versus 16.8%). This group attributed the difference to the change from manual ventilation in 1981, which took up much of the anesthetist's visual attention, to the use of mechanical ventilators in 1985, which freed the anesthetist to watch the patient.

It is true that looking at the patient and at the surgical field is a hallmark of an excellent clinician. Opponents of technology decry the degree to which monitors and therapeutic devices distract the anesthetist's gaze from the patient. However, an important distinction has to be made between the anesthetist's attention, which surely must be directed to the patient's needs, and the anesthetist's gaze, which in fact may best serve the patient by being directed elsewhere. Many of the tasks cited in the study by McDonald and Dzwonczyk[243] were highly related to management of the patient, even though they did not involve direct visualization of or contact with the patient. The critical question, which task analysis by itself cannot answer, is when anesthetists gaze at the surgical field, how often are they gathering information, and how often are they just "watching the scenery"? Put more generally, what is the information content of the various observations being made and what is their relationship to action tasks and to the goals of conducting a safe anesthetic regimen?

Intriguingly, Drui and associates[320] had asked physicians who were helping code their films, "What information, if any, do you gain from the direct performance of this activity?" However, these investigators never described what information was available from each activity, although they seem to have assumed that turning the anesthesiologist's gaze away from the patient and surgical field was bad. Boquet and coworkers[241] not only studied the gaze of anesthetists (using a sophisticated eye-tracking system) but also asked consultant anesthetists to grade the importance of different visual targets and manual tasks. "The patient" was assigned the maximal importance on the scale. However, "the surgical field," which occupied 25% of the anesthetist's time, was apparently not listed by the consultants. Perhaps, in their minds, the surgical field was lumped together with the patient.

Another key finding of the study by Drui and coworkers[320] was that 40% of the anesthetist's time was coded as "idle," meaning that no obvious task was seen on that frame of film. In 1988, McDonald and Dzwonczyk[242] stated that this and other "studies showed that the anaesthetist spends most time performing tasks that are either secondary or unrelated to patient care." However, in their original article, Drui and associates[320] correctly recognized that absence of visually apparent activity did not mean that the anesthetist was truly idle; in fact, they hypothesized that this time was used by anesthetists to make the decisions on which the observable tasks were based.

The most detailed task analyses have taken place in a series of studies[198,235,244,245,304,321] carried out by the UCSD/VA-Stanford group. These analyses have used progressively more task categories (11 to 28 to 32) to analyze the activities of novice and experienced anesthetists in day surgery cases and the activities of senior residents during cardiac surgery. The studies have shown that a small number of tasks, repeated frequently, occupy the majority of case time. In one study, four tasks (observing monitors, recording, conversing with attending staff [for novice residents], and adjusting monitors) accounted for 50.1% of the total case time. Specific activities such as airway management (e.g., bag ventilation, laryngoscopy) occurred in brief, but intense clusters (Fig. 6-14). Given the larger number of task categories, the anesthetist was rarely seen to be idle.

Studies by this group have attempted to determine whether there is a difference between the task patterns of novice versus experienced anesthetists. Confirming a priori expectations, the investigators found that novices perform many of the same tasks as experienced personnel do at specific phases of an anesthetic regimen; however, the novices had a longer dwell time, on average, for each task. These studies also showed that experienced providers had lower heterogeneity of tasks and greater efficiency of tasks per unit time.[322]

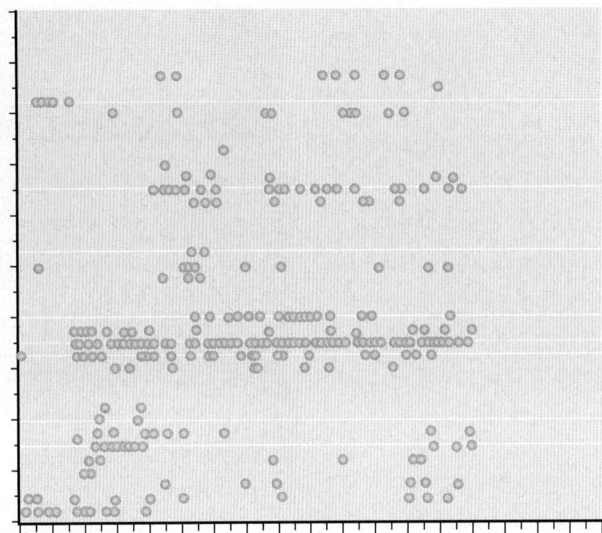

Figure 6-14 Distribution of the anesthetist's tasks during an actual ambulatory surgery procedure. The anesthetist was directly observed by an investigator who recorded a code number for each task as it was performed (there were 28 task codes). Certain tasks, such as bag ventilation, were clustered in specific phases of the case, whereas others, such as observing monitors, were repeated frequently throughout the procedure.

Of note (but also not unexpected), novice residents spent more time speaking to their attending staff (11% of preintubation time) than experienced residents or CRNAs did. Of interest, experienced personnel observed the surgical field more than the novices did. The implications of this finding are not clear. Novices did take longer to complete patient preparation and induction of anesthesia, but it appeared that some of the extra time taken by novices working under supervision was offset by the efficiency of offloading other concurrent tasks to the attending anesthesiologist such that preintubation time was increased by only 6 minutes for novices.[322] This group also reported that as the density of tasks per unit time increased, the dwell time on each task decreased, and vice versa. This finding has important implications for how anesthetists allocate their attention (see "Management and Coordination of the Core Process").

Task Analysis and Action Density

An interdisciplinary research group consisting of the Work and Organisational Psychology Department of the Swiss Federal Institute of Technology in Zurich and the Center for Patient Safety and Simulation of the Department of Anaesthesiology of the University of Tübingen performed several task analysis studies using the Flexible Interface Technique (FIT) system[323] (Fig. 6-15), which facilitates analysis of multiple parallel and overlapping actions.[246] The group produced a set of 41 observation codes—representing a single action (Table 6-9). Because the method allowed true capture of overlapping actions, it was possible to describe a valid task density in the analysis of anesthetists' action sequences.

Figures 6-16 and 6-17 show examples of observations of 24 real OR studies. The observation data contain many short-term fluctuations (dots); the moving average of action density of the previous 5 minutes was charted as well (line). Figure 6-16 shows a complete anesthesia procedure with obvious increases in action

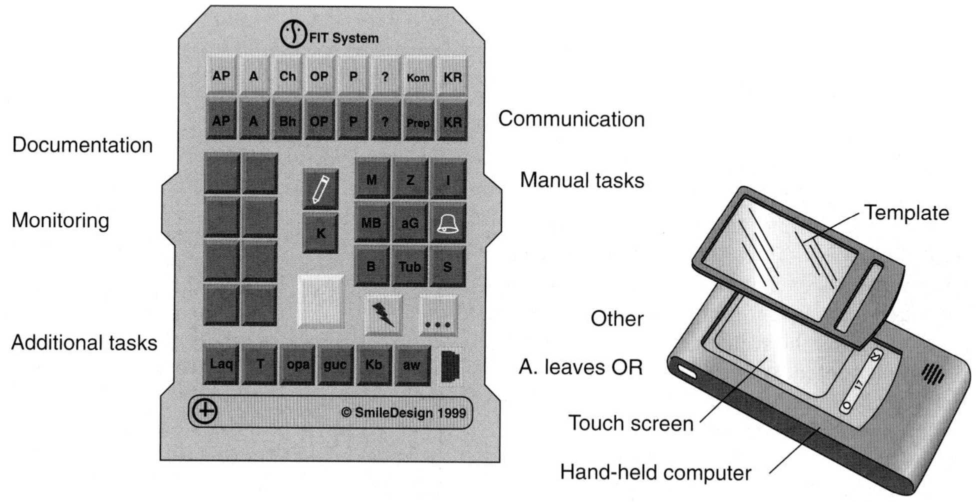

Figure 6-15 Flexible Interface Technique system. The system allows easy reorganization of task analysis items and categories and can properly resolve overlapping actions. OR, operating room.

density during induction and emergence from anesthesia. Figure 6-17 shows two final phases of cardiac cases involving cardiopulmonary bypass. The described task analysis technique was also used successfully by the Tübingen group to study action sequences in a simulator and compare them with findings in the real OR to demonstrate and evaluate the ecologic validity of simulators (see Chapter 7).

Automation

Early task analyses identified repetitive tasks that did not appear to offer substantial information content or therapeutic benefit as candidates for automation. Drui and associates[320] identified filling out anesthesia records, measuring blood pressure, and adjusting intravenous infusions. Kennedy and colleagues[324] identified data display and trend plotting. Many of these tasks have in fact been automated in the past 20 years. Loeb,[325] from University of California, Davis (UCD) showed that anesthesiologists typically observed monitors for about 1 to 2 seconds every 10 to 20 seconds and that it usually took several observing cycles before they detected a subtle cue on the monitor. Gurushanthaiah and coworkers[326] studied the effect of more sophisticated display modalities on detection of signals by anesthesiologists and found that histogram and polygon formats improved response latency in the laboratory setting over formats using raw numbers only. However, the applicability of these laboratory finding to the more complex signal detection that must occur in the midst of patient care is uncertain. Incidentally, the experience in the field of aviation suggests that automation of both monitoring and therapeutic devices produces its own problems in human-machine interactions and may well be a causative or contributing factor in some adverse anesthetic events. Some of the same types of automation-related adverse events seen in aviation are now being observed in anesthesiology.[227]

Table 6-9 Observation Codes Used to Classify Tasks and Actions

Task Group	Actions
Monitoring	Read patient record, observe patient, observe patient monitors, observe anesthesia machine, observe intravenous drip, observe syringe pumps, measurement, scan area
Measures	Placing IV, give drugs, adjust IV, mask ventilation, intubation/extubation, adjust anesthesia machine, use of other equipment, quitting alarms, suctioning
Communication	(1) Active conversation with nurse anesthetist, attending anesthetist, surgeon, OR nurse, patient, others; (2) responsive conversation with nurse anesthetist, attending anesthetist, surgeon, OR nurse, patient, others; and (3) response to pager
Documentation	Patient chart labeling (drugs, drips, laboratory results)
Additional operations	Positioning of patient, patient transfer, tasks of others (circulating nurse, orderly), arrange workplace, conversation with observer ("just looking"), miscellaneous, leaving OR (with possible audiovisual contact with OR)

IV, intravenous line; OR, operating room.

The impact of automation on task distribution is uncertain. The change to mechanical ventilation did affect the analyses of McDonald and Dzwonczyk,[242] as detailed earlier. A study by Allard and coworkers[327] showed no reduction in time spent recording when automated record-keeping devices were used. However, the UCSD/VA-Stanford collaboration published data demonstrating a 20% reduction in the time spent record keeping when automated record keeping was in use during cardiac anesthesia.[322] There was a slight, but not significant increase in time spent on direct patient care activities when electronic record keeping was in use. There is no clear evidence that electronic record keeping will yield a marked enhancement of the anesthetist's ability to perform other patient care tasks, although automated record keeping may yield other benefits. The UCD and UCSD/VA-Stanford groups demonstrated that electronic automated record keeping does not significantly reduce the vigilance of anesthetists.[328,329]

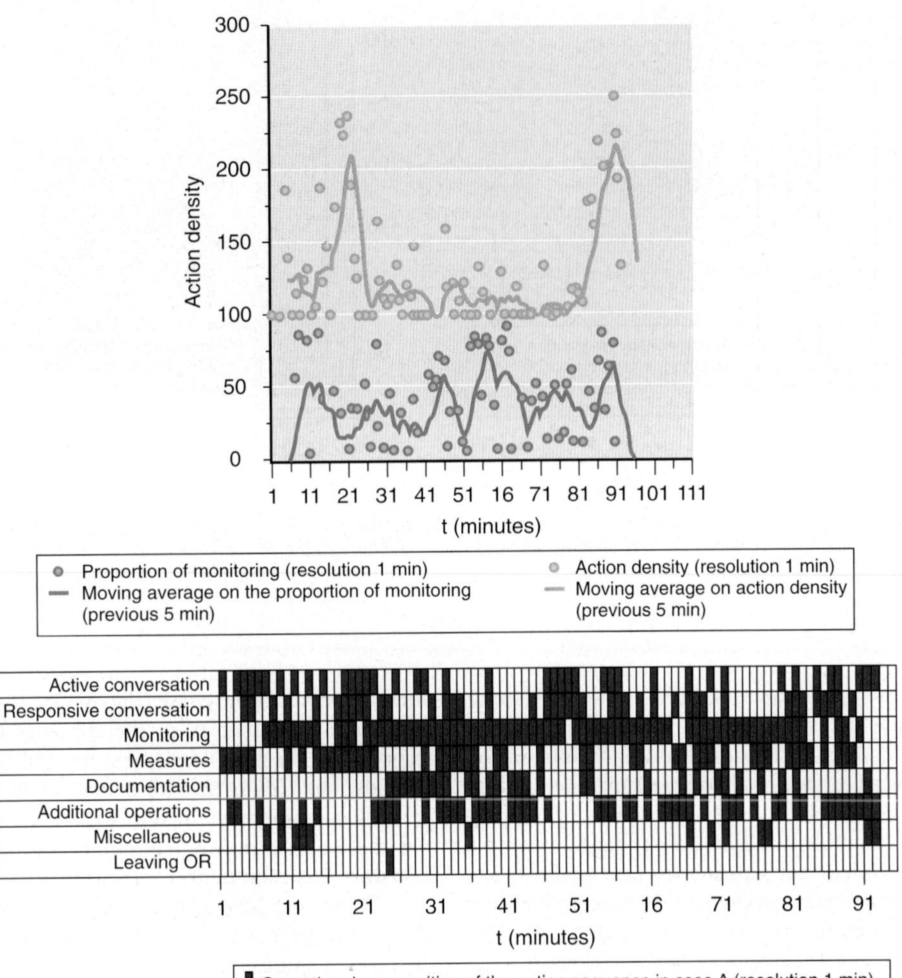

Figure 6-16 Action density diagram illustrating the derived parameter "action density" from induction of anesthesia to emergence in a real anesthetic case. The *top line* in the graph shows the overall action density and the *dots* show the moving average of the density. The *bottom line* shows the contribution of one task group "monitoring" as an example. The table in the lower graph shows the composition of the data for all eight task groups from the same case.

Mental Workload of Administering Anesthesia

The observable tasks do not tell the whole story of what the anesthetist is doing. As Drui and coworkers[320] suggested, mental activity is going on even when the anesthetist appears idle. What, then, is the mental workload of administering anesthesia? Mental workload is another concept that is readily understood but difficult to define precisely. There are various ways to measure workload, none of which are ideal.

Primary Task Performance Measure

The primary task performance measure assesses the subject's performance on standard work tasks as they are made progressively more difficult by increasing the number of tasks, task density, or task complexity. At first the subject is able to keep up with the increasing task load, but at some point the workload exceeds the ability to manage it, and performance on the standard tasks decreases. The disadvantage of the primary task performance measure is that in many complex task domains there is no accepted way to objectively measure the subject's performance on the primary work tasks except by loading to the point of catastrophic performance failure, which is easily detected. In actual high-risk domains, one cannot allow primary task performance to degrade, and one certainly cannot allow it to fail catastrophically. Although experiments of this type are in principle feasible with anesthesia simulators, they have not yet been attempted.

Secondary Task Probing

A more useful technique, secondary task probing, tests the subject with a minimally intrusive secondary task that is added to the primary work tasks. The secondary task is a simple one for which performance can be objectively measured, and the subject is instructed that the primary tasks of patient care take absolute precedence over the secondary task. Therefore, assuming that the secondary task requires some of the same mental resources as the primary task, the performance of the subject on the secondary task is an indirect reflection of the spare capacity available to deal with it; thus, it is an inverse measure of primary task workload (the greater the spare capacity, the lower the primary workload). Secondary tasks such as reaction time (with or without choice), finger tapping, and mental arithmetic have been used for this

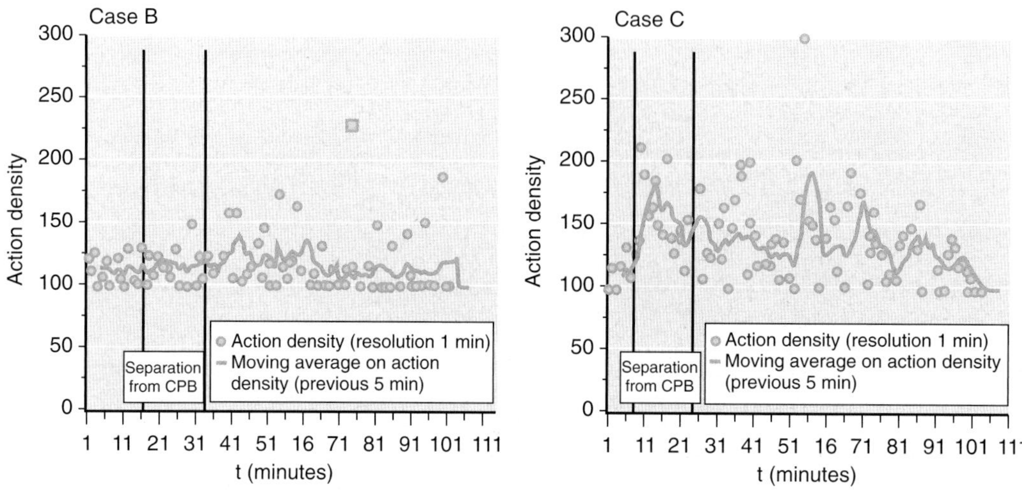

Figure 6-17 Action density during separation from cardiopulmonary bypass (CPB) without and with complications. The graph on the *left* is the density diagram of an uncomplicated case (case B) with a "flat" action density diagram during (between the two *vertical lines*) and after separation from CPB. In contrast, case C, shown in the graph on the *right*, had a complicated weaning from CPB; a very high action density is followed by an elevated density with further peaks after separation.

technique in the psychology laboratory, in high-fidelity simulators, and in some field studies of actual work situations.

Gaba and Lee[330] presented two-digit addition problems on a computer screen placed in the anesthesia workspace at random approximately every 45 seconds. The delay in responding to problems and the number of problems skipped were logged over time and correlated with a concurrent six-category task analysis. The dynamic ebb and flow of mental workload during cases of varying complexity was documented. For example, cardiopulmonary bypass was confirmed as a time of very low workload for the anesthetist, whereas induction of anesthesia was confirmed as a period of high workload. Manual tasks and conversing with the attending physician were correlated with a delayed or absent response to the secondary task.

Subsequent studies by the UCSD/VA-Stanford group[244,245] and the UCD group[325,329,331] used the reaction time to a changing display in or around the clinical monitors as a secondary task to assess mental workload, vigilance, or both. For the UCSD/VA-Stanford group, the display was a red light placed next to the main physiologic monitor. This secondary task was analogous to but totally separate from the standard tasks of clinical work. When the secondary task was embedded in the regular work tasks, it was called an embedded task. The UCD group used a secondary task involving recognition of changes in the alphanumeric display of an unused channel of an actual clinical monitor (a parameter labeled "Vig" on the monitor changed values from "5" to "10"). This task was only partially embedded because although it did involve an actual clinical monitor, it displayed on an otherwise unused channel and was not of clinical significance. The VA-Stanford group has been experimenting with fully embedded secondary tasks during simulator anesthetic cases in which the values of actual clinical variables can be manipulated at will to evaluate the subject's response time to the excursion of data values beyond predefined reporting thresholds.

The mean response time to the red light used by the UCSD/VA-Stanford group was markedly less than 60 seconds for experienced subjects in both the induction and postinduction (maintenance) phases, but it was much higher for novice residents during the induction phase (Fig. 6-18). The probe was not given frequently enough to track the ebb and flow of workload. The response to the UCD task typically (56%) occurred within 60 seconds, but 16% of stimuli overall (27% during the induction period) were not responded to within 5 minutes. The conclusion was that spare capacity may be limited by the workload of the case during certain periods of anesthesia care.

There are several problems with these workload studies. One is interference with the "response channel." If responding to the probe requires manual activity with a mouse or keyboard (as in the studies of Gaba and Lee and the UCD group), it cannot be performed whenever the subject is occupied with a manual task. This is especially true during a sterile procedure. Therefore, it may

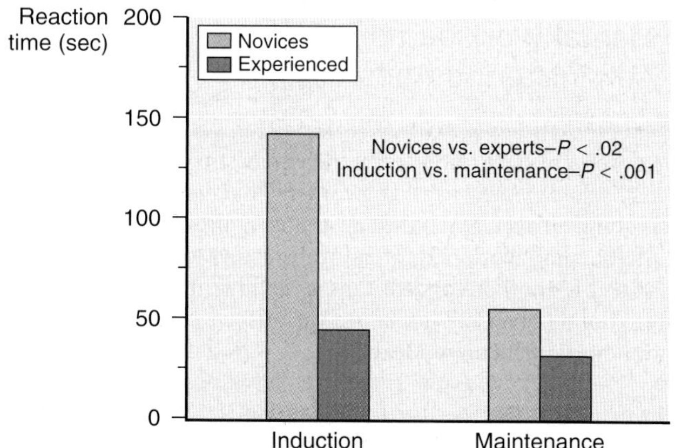

Figure 6-18 A test of the anesthetist's vigilance. Shown is the mean reaction time of novice residents and experienced anesthetists in response to the illumination of a red light placed next to the electrocardiogram monitor display during actual ambulatory surgery procedures. In both groups the reaction was faster in the maintenance phase than during induction of anesthesia. Novices reacted significantly more slowly than experienced anesthetists did. Because the distribution of reaction times was skewed and nongaussian, error bars are not shown and nonparametric statistics were used for hypothesis testing.

be impossible to distinguish between a high primary task load (i.e., no spare capacity to address the secondary task) and a low primary task load that happens to usurp the manual response channel. However, in the Gaba and Lee study,[330] 37% of the problems that were skipped for lack of spare capacity did not occur during a manual task. All of the UCSD/VA-Stanford studies have allowed multiple response channels (manual, voice, and gesture), so there was no response channel interference; however, the potential for interference remains in the UCD studies.

An additional problem with these studies is that even these simple secondary tasks were intrusive when repeated frequently. Thus, there was a tradeoff between temporal resolution of the measurement and its intrusiveness. There is also controversy about whether these probes measure "vigilance" or "workload," although the same techniques probably measure both aspects of performance. When probes occur infrequently, are subtle, have multiple response channels, and are performed with a low level of existing workload, they are more likely to measure vigilance; when they are frequent, readily detectable, require a manual response, and are performed during a high-workload period, they probably are more indicative of spare capacity and workload.

Slagle and colleagues[303] carried out an assessment of an established clinical task analysis methodology regarding intra- and inter-rater reliability. These investigators had one trained observer rating 20 routine anesthesia cases, first rating cases in the OR and then rating the same cases from a videotape, with another observer rating the same videotapes twice. A computerized task analysis program with 38 task categories was used. The results showed good intra-rater reliability and also high concordance between real-time and video analyses. This finding is important because real-time observation is unfeasible in many circumstances. This study had problems in analyzing parallel tasks because the technique of "toggling between the task categories at a rate proportional to the time spent on each task" resulted in big differences in "task duration" and "task occurrences" between the two raters. This problem of recording parallel tasks (two or more) was solved by Manser and colleagues in Tübingen.[246,247,332]

Subjective Measures

A third modality of workload assessment consists of subjective measures in which individuals are asked, either in retrospect or in real time, how much load they were or are under during actual work situations. Subjective measures complement objective measurements because the subjective perceptions of the anesthetist may be an important source of stress and anxiety; conversely, an anesthetist may subjectively underestimate the workload in settings in which objective measurements demonstrate a marked reduction in spare capacity.

Various scales have been proposed to measure dimensions of mental workload that are, in theory, different. However, Gaba and Lee[330] adapted a set of workload scales from those used at NASA and showed that workload ratings on each of the scales were highly correlated. In subsequent studies by the UCSD/VA-Stanford group, a single dimension of overall load was assessed by using an asymmetric numeric scale that minimized biases caused by a tendency to group responses at the middle and extremes of symmetric scales. This group demonstrated that a neutral observer can estimate the subjective workload of the anesthetist in real time with high correlation to the self-rated workload of the subject.[244] Again, as could be expected, subjective workload was highest during induction and emergence from anesthesia, especially for novices.

Physiologic Measures

The final set of techniques for assessing workload consists of physiologic measures. Visual or auditory evoked potentials have been used successfully to assess mental workload, but this technique can be used only in a static laboratory environment. Heart rate is a relatively easily measured variable that may be altered by mental workload. Toung and associates[333] showed that the anesthetist's heart rate increases at the time of intubation and that the amount of increase is inversely related to the amount of overall medical training. Azar and coworkers[334] found that anesthesia faculty members' heart rate and blood pressure increased during induction of anesthesia and that significant ST-segment depression developed in one individual. Bitetti and colleagues[335] confirmed that heart rate changes occurred during anesthesia but did not always correlate with contemporaneous self-recordings of "stress."

Because of the many factors that affect heart rate, the beat-to-beat variability of the heart rate is thought to be a better indicator of mental workload. The frequency components of heart rate variability can be separated by spectral analysis; a component at 0.1 Hz has been linked to mental workload. Although several groups have acquired heart rate data on anesthesiologists, none has reported an analysis of the workload-related frequency components.

Applications of Task Analysis and Workload Methodologies

The results of task analyses and workload measurements have primarily provided objective confirmation of a number of intuitive beliefs about anesthesia practice. The real importance of these studies is that a coherent methodology has been developed that may be useful for studying a variety of interesting questions.[247,336] The question of the impact of electronic automated record-keeping systems was addressed earlier. Another question concerns TEE. This newer monitoring modality has become commonplace during cardiac anesthesia and anesthesia for other patients with cardiovascular disease who undergo complex operations. It is widely recognized that evaluating TEE images and manipulating the TEE probe require substantial visual and mental attention.

The UCSD/VA-Stanford group has published data suggesting that vigilance (as measured by response latency to illumination of a red light) was substantially lower when the anesthesiologist was involved in manipulating, adjusting, or examining the TEE images than when other patient care tasks were being performed (Fig. 6-19).[328] This may be due, in part, to the layout of the workspace. The TEE machine is large and is often placed near the left side of the head of the OR table, whereas the anesthesia machine and attendant monitors, by convention, are typically placed near the right side of the head of the table. Remote displays slaved to the primary monitor are also more likely to be on the patient's right side. This arrangement makes it physically difficult to glance from one modality to another. The degree to which the mental concentration required to use TEE itself detracts from vigilance for other signals remains to be determined explicitly.

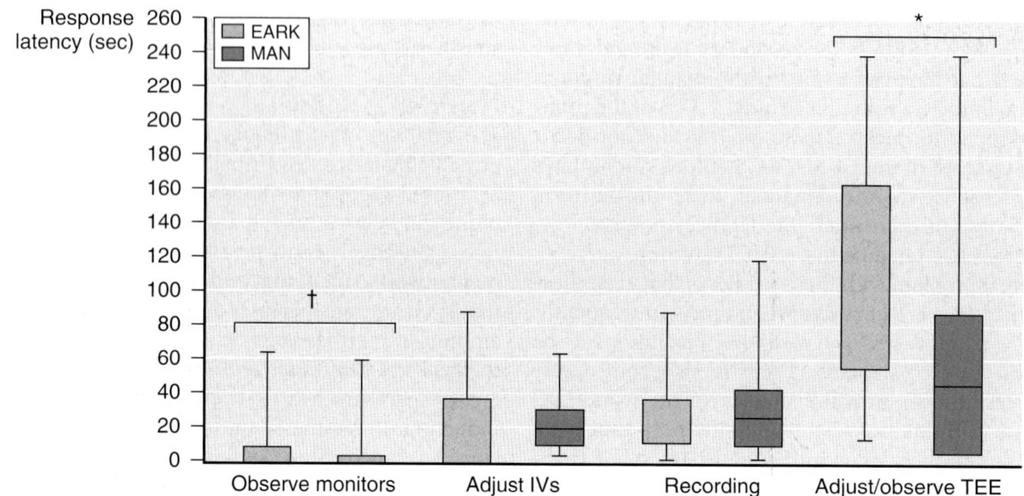

Figure 6-19 Vigilance test data during anesthetic tasks with and without automated record keeping. The range of data is shown for each of four task categories in electronic automated record keeping (EARK) and manual record keeping (MAN). Each box contains 50% of the data for that subgroup (the upper limit of the box is the 75th percentile; the lower limit is the 25th percentile), whereas the maximum and minimum are shown by the upper and lower *horizontal bars*. The response latency during record keeping was not significantly different between EARK and MAN. In both record-keeping groups, subjects had significantly slower responses when observing or adjusting the transesophageal echocardiogram (TEE) than when recording, observing monitors, or adjusting intravenous lines (IVs). Subjects in both groups had faster response latency when observing the monitoring array, which contained a red light, than when performing the other three tasks. $^{*}P < .05$; $^{\dagger}P < .05$. *(From Weinger MB, Herdon OW, Gaba DM: The effect of electronic record keeping and transesophageal echocardiography on task distribution, workload, and vigilance during cardiac anesthesia. Anesthesiology 87:144-145, 1997.)*

It is important to differentiate the various uses of TEE. When it is used to answer specific clinical questions triggered by events or milestones during the procedure, the value of the information may be worth an investment of effort even though there is a reduction in overall vigilance. When it is used as a continuous monitor for myocardial ischemia or when conducting a detailed routine examination, the reduction in vigilance must be considered when evaluating the potential benefits of the technology. Some practitioners describe special ways to handle the attention required for TEE, including tightening alarm thresholds (to provide audio warnings of changed values) and assigning specific patient monitoring functions to another individual while conducting the initial TEE placement and examination.

Many other interesting questions on the performance of anesthetists are still unanswered and can be addressed with the techniques of task analysis and workload and vigilance assessment, including the following:

1. How do task load and task density differ between private practice settings and academic settings?
2. Are there characteristic "patterns" for experts and novices (or should we say for "good" and "bad" anesthesiologists?) in the analysis of tasks and their densities? And if yes,
   a. How do the work patterns of novices change to become those of "experts"? How can the training of novices be focused to support these changes best? Is suboptimal performance of novices detectable through analysis of task distributions and mental workload?
   b. Can work patterns be linked to safe anesthetic practice, or can special patterns be linked to unsafe behavior? Perhaps this could be done by assessing high-workload simulator scenarios. In a proactive safety culture, this would allow us to identify such colleagues and train them individually.
3. How much task load can the average anesthetist handle? How are tasks distributed among personnel (e.g., between resident and faculty, between CRNA and supervisor, and among staff anesthetists) during the high-workload periods of patient care? This question is just beginning to be addressed by applying the task analysis techniques described earlier to videotapes of actual anesthetic cases. With use of these tapes, the task sequences of multiple anesthesia personnel can be elicited separately, as can the communications used to coordinate their activities.

Ability Requirements for Anesthetists

Unlike the situation in military aviation, there are few formal selection criteria for entry into anesthesia practice. Instead, the criteria are decided on by each department's trainee selection committee. Nearly every student who chooses anesthesia as a specialty will be accepted by some training institution. Moreover, few residents are terminated from their anesthesia training—and then usually only because of drug abuse or too persistent or egregious lack of normal or technical skill.

There has been recent work on defining the underlying ability characteristics of a successful anesthetist. Greaves and Grant[21] presented an inventory of 16 characteristics of "good" anesthetic practice—knowledge, skill, perception, confidence, prudence, vigilance, fluency, decisiveness, anticipation, organization, flexibility, responsiveness, good manner, assertiveness, good management, and good communication. This inventory can serve as a basis for discussion of anesthetists' education and training. The authors of the inventory recommended its use for a formalized consultant feedback to trainees, although they pointed out its unproven validity and reliability.

An interdisciplinary group in Germany conducted an evaluation of another list of critical abilities for anesthetists published in German.[337]

Other Studies of "Vigilance" and Decision-Making by Anesthetists

Studies of "Vigilance"

The dominant metaphor for the mental activity of the anesthetist has been that of a vigilance task. "Vigilance" is the motto on the seal of the ASA. What is vigilance and to what degree does it capture the complex nature of the anesthetist's work? "Vigilance, or sustained attention, refers to the ability of observers to maintain their focus of attention and to remain alert to stimuli for prolonged periods of time" (J. Warm, presentation at the Panel on Vigilance, ASA annual meeting, 1992). There is an abundance of literature concerning vigilance. Many laboratory studies have demonstrated decrements in vigilance during prolonged vigilance tasks that are exacerbated or ameliorated by a variety of factors. These studies have generated considerable controversy. Some psychologists believe that the results of laboratory studies of vigilance have little application to complex real-world task domains.[338,339] Certainly, the anesthetist's work involves vigilance as a necessary component because if new stimuli are not perceived, no meaningful work can be accomplished. However, the anesthetist's task is much more complex than just vigilant alertness to stimuli. Therefore, vigilance is a necessary but not sufficient condition for appropriate performance.[58]

Several studies have attempted to quantitate the vigilance of anesthetists to changes in clinically important variables by using low-fidelity simulation. Beatty and associates[340] had anesthetists watch for changes in displays of six vital signs on a video monitor. Denisco and colleagues[341] used videotapes containing abnormal changes in anesthesia flow meter settings and physiologic monitor displays. The raw reaction times were not reported—only the "vigilance scores." Such studies purported to demonstrate a degradation in performance for sleep-deprived and fatigued residents, but there were methodologic flaws. For example, in the study of Denisco and coworkers,[341] the subjects were never told the threshold of change for them to report.

In addition, the work environment of the anesthetist is much more complex than that presented in these low-fidelity simulations. Although it can be argued that complexity will worsen vigilance, such is not necessarily the case. Complexity can combat boredom, which is a distinct possibility in vigilance experiments. In addition, the real work environment often provides redundant data cues on changes, which offers multiple possibilities for their detection.

A study of rested anesthetists[178] using a realistic anesthesia simulator measured detection times (first awareness of a problem) for a variety of intraoperative events embedded within a realistic case situation. Of interest, an event that caused alarms to sound immediately, such as ventricular tachycardia/fibrillation, was detected in 10 seconds or less (thus confirming its veracity, but acting on it took longer in many instances). Another event, occlusion of the intravenous line, was detectable only by visual observation in the direction opposite the anesthesia machine and monitors. This event took several minutes (on average) to detect, but it was corrected quickly after detection. The redundancy of cues in the task domain was confirmed in that six different observational modalities were used by at least 1 of the 19 residents studied to detect endobronchial intubation initially.

Other vigilance studies have focused on detecting the loss of an existing monitoring modality during actual patient care. In one study,[342] the esophageal stethoscope was occluded with a clamp after a staged distraction (conversation or a loud noise). Subjects most commonly detected the occlusion by observing the clamp rather than by noting a loss of sound. Although this study purported to show a difference in vigilance related to the use of automatic blood pressure measurement devices, the artificial distraction could have biased the results; the subjects typically failed to hear the loss of sounds, and there was a significant result for only one group of residents, arbitrarily stratified by length of training. Another study[343] that evaluated reaction time to loss of esophageal stethoscopy more carefully showed that 13% of occlusions were detected after 1 minute. However, this study required a manual response, and the investigators noted that in some instances of delay, the subject was involved in a manual clinical activity such as administering blood or drugs.

Apparent reductions in vigilance could be due either to a reduction in "spare capacity" to attend to the stimuli immediately or to a reduction in the overall alertness of the anesthetist. Enhancements in the display and annunciation of relevant information would be a useful ameliorative strategy in the first case, whereas this strategy would not be useful if the anesthetist's overall alertness were impaired, as by sleep deprivation or illness. The influence and impact of fatigue and possible countermeasures are covered in the earlier section "Performance-Shaping Factors."

Empirical Studies of Complex Decision-Making and Action by Anesthetists

Traditional concepts of decision-making in medicine have concentrated on relatively static, well-structured decisions. For example, should patient A with an elevated blood pressure be treated for hypertension with drug X, or should no treatment be started? Other investigators have looked only at "diagnosis" as an isolated task (specifically, "diagnostic explanation") both in internal medicine[344-346] and in radiology. These approaches to decision-making have not captured the unique aspects of dynamism, time pressure, and uncertainty seen in anesthesiology. Over the past decade, a paradigm has emerged regarding decision-making and action in complex real-world situations.[39,236,250] The cognitive model of dynamic decision-making was described previously. Several teams from inside the anesthesiology profession and from the human performance community have been striving to develop a more comprehensive understanding of the complex performance of anesthetists. Their work has been based on a small number of new experiments (often involving medium- or high-fidelity anesthesia simulators), reinterpretation of previous experiments, direct and indirect observation of the conduct of anesthesia, and extrapolations from other industries to anesthesiology. Each experiment has probed several aspects of decision-making and action, which are described in the following section.

Responding to Simulated Critical Incidents

Using a realistic hands-on anesthesia simulator, Gaba and DeAnda[111,259,347] studied the response of anesthesia trainees and experienced anesthesia faculty and private practitioners to six preplanned critical incidents of differing type and severity:

1. Breathing hoses too short to turn the table 180 degrees, as requested by the surgeon
2. Endobronchial intubation (EI) resulting from surgical manipulation of the tube
3. Occlusion of intravenous tubing
4. Atrial fibrillation (AF) with a rapid ventricular response and hypotension
5. Disconnection between the endotracheal tube and the breathing circuit
6. Ventricular tachycardia/fibrillation

These investigators measured the detection time (as described in the section on vigilance) and the correction time (the time from the event's onset until any one of a predefined set of corrective actions was first taken). They assessed the information sources by which subjects detected the incidents and then confirmed and diagnosed the problem. They asked subjects to "think aloud" to permit subjective analysis of their decision-making strategies. A summary of the data is shown in Figure 6-20. Major findings from this set of studies included the following:

1. Events differed from each other in their inherent ease of solution. Some events (e.g., airway disconnection) were

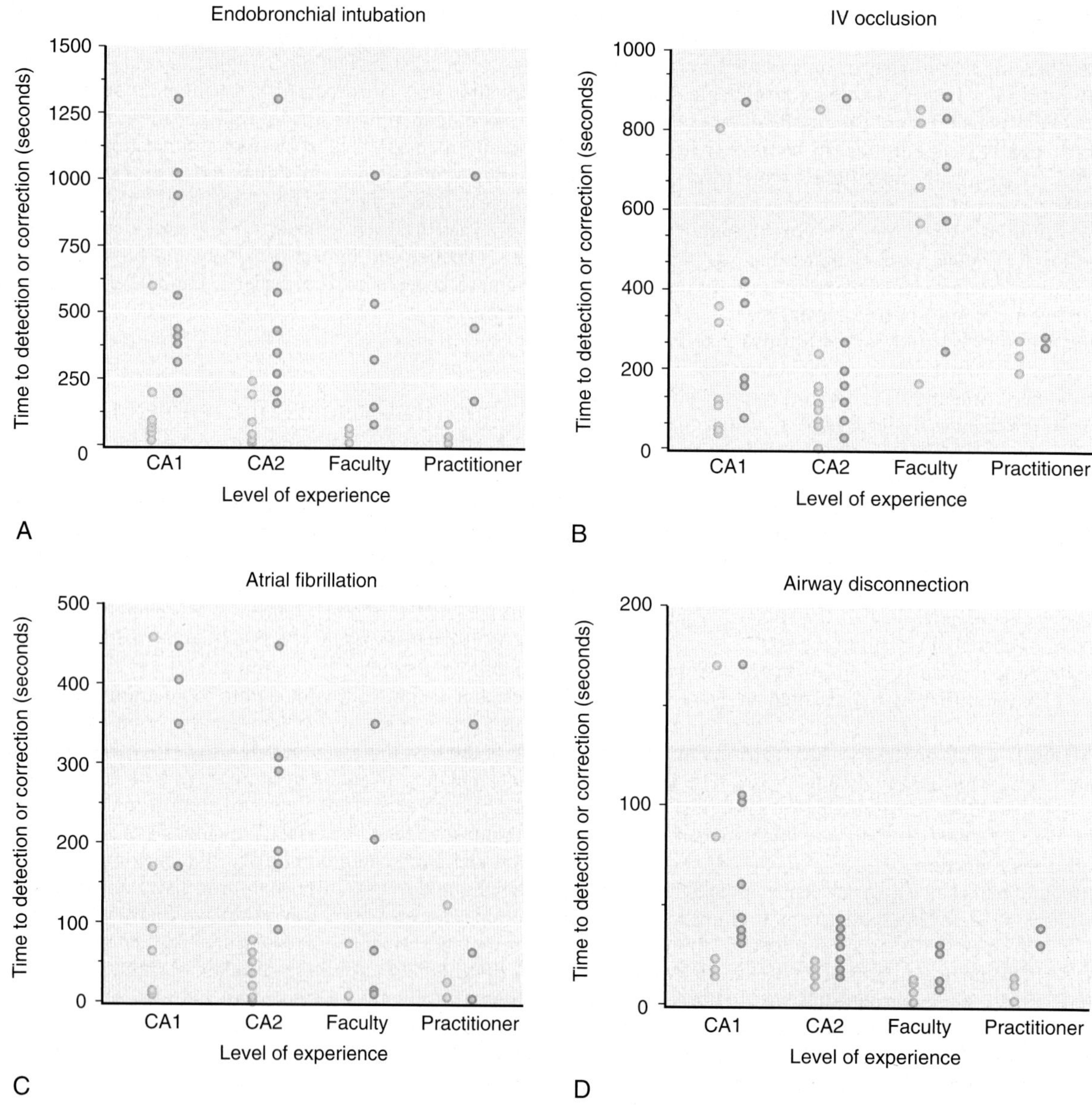

Figure 6-20 Response times of anesthesiologists with different levels of experience to four simulated critical incidents: **A,** endobronchial intubation; **B,** intravenous occlusion (IV); **C,** atrial fibrillation; and **D,** airway disconnection. Detection time is represented by *yellow circles* and correction time by *blue circles* (see text for definitions of these times). Unless there is overlap between response times, each circle represents a single individual. The scale of response times is different for each event. There is substantial variability among incidents and among individuals. Despite a trend to better performance with increased experience, major errors were made by individuals in all groups. *(From DeAnda A, Gaba DM: Role of experience in the response to simulated critical incidents. Anesth Analg 72:308-315, 1991.)*

detected rapidly and corrected. Some problems (e.g., intravenous occlusion) were difficult to detect, but once they were detected, diagnosis and therapy were achieved rapidly. Other problems (EI, AF) were easy to detect by using one of several redundant information sources as the first clue (six for EI, four for AF), but they required additional time (7 to 8 minutes for EI; 1.5 to 4.5 minutes for AF) to confirm the abnormality, establish a diagnosis, and initiate appropriate therapy. Diagnosis and planning and monitoring of therapy used a large number of information sources (11 for EI; 9 for AF).

2. For each incident there was considerable inter-individual variability in detection and correction times, in information sources used, and in the actions taken. In each experience group there were some who required excessive time to solve the problem or who never solved it. In addition, in each experience group at least one individual made major errors that could have had a substantial negative impact on a patient's clinical outcome. For example, one faculty member never used electrical countershock to treat ventricular fibrillation. One private practitioner treated the EI as though it were "bronchospasm" and never assessed the symmetry of ventilation. One resident never found the airway disconnection.
3. The average performance of the anesthetists tended to improve with experience, although this varied by incident. The performance of the experienced groups was not definitively better than that of the second-year residents (who were in their final year of training at that time). Many (but not all) novice residents performed indistinguishably from more experienced subjects.
4. The elements of suboptimal performance were both technical and cognitive. Technical problems included choosing defibrillation energies appropriate for internal paddles when using external paddles, ampule swap, and failure to inflate the endotracheal tube cuff that resulted in a leak. Cognitive problems included failure to allocate attention to the most critical problems and fixation errors.

Schwid and O'Donnell,[258] from the University of Washington, used the Anesthesia Simulator Consultant (ASC) screen-only simulator (Anesoft Corp., Issaquah, WA) (Table 6-10) to perform an experiment similar to those of Gaba and DeAnda with a realistic simulator. This method enabled them to evaluate some elements of anesthetist behavior more carefully, albeit with the limitations imposed by presenting the OR "on the screen." After working on several practice cases without critical incidents, each subject was asked to manage three or four cases involving a total of four serious critical events (esophageal intubation, myocardial ischemia, anaphylaxis, and cardiac arrest). The progression of each event was mediated by the interaction of physiologic and pharmacologic models with the actions taken by the subject. The anesthesiologists studied had varying experience levels. One group was made up of 10 anesthesia residents with at least 1 year of anesthesia training, whereas the other two groups contained 10 anesthesia faculty members and 10 private practitioners, respectively.

Major findings of the study included the following:

1. Significant errors in diagnosis or treatment were made in every experience group. The errors occurred in both diagnosis of problems and in deciding on and implementing appropriate treatment. For example, 60% of subjects did not make the diagnosis of anaphylaxis despite available information on heart rate, blood pressure, wheezing, increased peak inspiratory pressure, and the presence of a rash. In managing myocardial ischemia, there were multiple failures (Table 6-11).
2. Thirty percent of subjects did not compensate for severe abnormalities while considering diagnostic maneuvers.
3. Fixation errors in which initial diagnoses and plans were never revised were frequent, even when they were clearly wrong.

Westenskow and colleagues[253] used a test lung and remotely activated faults in the breathing circuit to test the anesthetist's ability to identify faults related to ventilation and the anesthesia breathing circuit after hearing an alarm. One group of subjects used standard alarms, set to factory defaults, on an anesthesia machine, which included a capnograph. The other group used the same anesthesia machine with the alarms disabled along with a neural network–based intelligent alarm and fault identification system. The mean "human response time," which was the time between sounding of the first alarm and identification of the event, ranged from approximately 15 seconds for airway disconnection to approximately 90 seconds for an endotracheal tube cuff leak. The 10 anesthesiologists tested with the standard alarm setup were unable to identify the fault within 2 minutes on 11 occasions—5 cuff leaks, 3 airway obstructions, and 3 stuck-open expiratory valves. However, in such circumstances they did take appropriate compensatory actions while continuing to search for the cause (e.g., increasing fresh gas flow to compensate for a cuff leak).

The intelligent alarm apparatus used data from three sensors (in-line capnograph, spirometer, and airway pressure). A neural network determined whether any of seven faults was present and, if so, displayed a text message specifying the fault, as well as an animated diagram of the lung, airway, and anesthesia

Table 6-10 Incidence of Totally Correct Diagnosis or Treatment of Simulated Critical Incidents with Use of the Anesthesia Simulator Consultant

Incident	Anesthesia Residents (%)	Anesthesia Attendings (%)	Anesthesiologists in Practice (%)
Diagnosis of esophageal intubation	80	100	100
Treatment of myocardial ischemia	20	40	20
Diagnosis of anaphylaxis	20	60	40
Treatment of cardiac arrest	40	30	20

From Schwid HA, O'Donnell D: Anesthesiologists' management of simulated critical incidents. Anesthesiology 76:495-501, 1992.

Table 6-11 Failure Rate in the Management of Simulated Myocardial Ischemia with the Anesthesia Simulator Consultant

Incident	Anesthesia Residents (%)	Anesthesia Attendings (%)	Anesthesiologists in Practice (%)
Untreated tachycardia	30	50	70
Untreated hypotension	40	60	20
Inappropriate drug	20	10	0
Unable to recall infusion dose	50	20	10
Unable to calculate infusion rate	70	40	40

From Schwid HA, O'Donnell D: Anesthesiologists' management of simulated critical incidents. Anesthesiology 76:495-501, 1992.

breathing circuit with the faulty component highlighted in red. It is interesting that the smart alarm system took slightly longer on average to detect a fault than the conventional alarm system did (25 versus 21 seconds), but the human response time was markedly reduced for three of the seven faults. There were no statistically significant differences between anesthesia residents and faculty members with either alarm system.

The investigators suggested that the more specific alarm messages in their intelligent alarm system could direct the attention of the anesthetist to the occurrence of specific problems and in so doing would decrease workload and reduce the likelihood of fixating on inappropriate information. They stated that such a system's advantages would be even greater in a more realistic clinical environment in which the anesthetist has multiple complex tasks and not just detection and identification of ventilation-related events.

Loeb and Fitch[348] developed and tested an auditory display of six physiologic variables. Encouraged by the popularity of the pulse oximeter's pulse tone,[349-351] they investigated whether the addition of auditory cues would enhance the rate and speed of detection of predefined events. The results showed that the combined display (visual and auditory) lead to faster detection of events, even though the rate for correct identification of the event was slightly higher in the "visual only" display (80% versus 88%). It seems that there is a potential to improve the rate of detection of changes in physiologic variables with more sophisticated display modalities, thereby enhancing the "effective vigilance" of anesthetists.

Complex, Multiple Personnel Simulations of Anesthetic Crises

In the process of evaluating a new type of training for anesthetists involving crisis management, Howard and colleagues[109] collected anecdotal data on the responses of teams of anesthetists, surgeons, and nurses to planned (and unplanned) critical events. These experiments largely confirmed the results of the studies described earlier and extended them to include more complex management issues and team interactions. Howard and colleagues found a substantial incidence of difficulties managing multiple problems simultaneously, applying attention to the most critical needs, acting as team leader, communicating with personnel, and using all available OR resources to best advantage.

Botney and associates[352] analyzed similar videotapes from 18 different simulator training sessions on crisis management. In one event, a volatile anesthetic vaporizer had been left on at 4% and was hidden beneath a printout from the noninvasive blood pressure monitor. Simultaneously, there was a mechanical failure of the capnograph, making it impossible to confirm endotracheal intubation with CO_2 measurements. This event purposefully presented an invitation to become fixated on the endotracheal tube while ignoring other relevant information. Five of 18 subjects never discovered the volatile anesthetic overdose despite catastrophic effects on blood pressure and heart rate and clear evidence that the endotracheal tube was correctly placed. Of those who did detect the vaporizer setting, the average time to detection was nearly 4 minutes, with some subjects taking longer than 12 minutes.

In the second event studied, there was a loss of pipeline O_2 supply while an anesthetist was assuming the care of a critically ill patient who required an FIO_2 of 100% to achieve satisfactory blood oxygenation. The O_2 cylinder on the machine was empty (i.e., it had not been checked by the initial anesthetist, who had left the case after becoming ill). The pipeline failure was quickly detected (19 seconds), but the responses to it were extremely variable and showed a variety of problems. Five of 18 anesthetists closed the anesthesia circuit (which preserves the existing oxygen in the circuit), but all 5 subsequently switched to ventilation with a self-inflating bag using room air or to mouth-to-tube ventilation. Five of 18 could not open the reserve oxygen cylinder because they could not locate the tank wrench attached to the machine (it tended to rest between two gas cylinders). Several teams had trouble mounting a new oxygen tank on the anesthesia machine; problems with the gasket disk were frequent. The individuals did not appear to have a well-formulated plan for managing this event, and they did not optimally coordinate their actions with their assistants or with the other OR personnel.

A study by Byrne and Jones[310] looked at differences in the performance of experienced and less experienced anesthetists. Using a self-developed patient simulator system, they measured time to treatment and deficiencies in patient care in 180 simulations. The results showed significant differences only between the first and second year. As seen in other studies,[319] significant errors occurred at all levels of experience, and most of the anesthetists deviated from established guidelines. These studies underscore the importance of recurrent training for experienced anesthetists and the truism that experience is not a substitute for excellence.

The reader is referred to Chapter 7 for discussion of newer studies with the use of patient simulators and performance assessment as such.[17,20,142,148,312,319,353-357]

Indirect Observation of Anesthetists Involved in Difficult Cases

An unusual approach involving indirect observation of actual cases was used by Cook and colleagues[255] at the Ohio State University. Rather than collecting data on the case itself, these investigators transcribed the discussions of interesting cases occurring at a weekly quality assurance conference. They argued that this approach allowed them to apply a "neutral observer criterion" to the behavior of the anesthetist. The investigators acknowledged the risks of hindsight bias and selection bias with this methodology, but they suggested that their technique provided a unique window on human performance issues.

Fifty-seven cases were analyzed, 21 of which had a full cognitive analysis in the final report. From the presentation and discussion of a case, the investigators classified evolution of the events into one of five categories: acute incident, going-sour incident, inevitable outcome incident, difficult-airway incident, and no-incident incident. For each case, the cognitive analysis was "based on using knowledge about the cognitive demands of the task domain and data about practitioner activities to analyze the practitioner's information-processing strategies and goals, given the resources and constraints of the situation." The investigators postulated a cognitive cycle as a component of data-driven activation of knowledge and knowledge-driven observation and action.

Cook and associates[255] called attention to several issues that surfaced in their cognitive analysis of these cases, including the following:

1. Multiple themes. Many cases involved several lines of concern simultaneously, each of which could have interacted with another (e.g., tight coupling). Each theme had multiple means available to deal with it. Maintaining "situation awareness" was important. The multiple themes sometimes generated competing or conflicting goals. Adaptive planning (as described in the section on abstract task analysis) was sometimes required.
2. Unusual situations. The greatest expertise was seen with infrequent or unusual situations rather than with typical situations.
3. Allocation of attention. Allocation of attention to relevant stimuli or to the most important "theme" was an important issue. The attentional shifts were not always well supported by existing alarm and display technologies.
4. Cognitive workload. Anesthetists attempted to reduce their cognitive workload whenever possible.
5. Team interaction. Cooperative work, team interaction, and communications issues were problems in several cases. These stemmed from both individual and organizational failures to coordinate information and efforts from different organizational components (e.g., ICU and OR, surgeons and anesthesiologists).

Direct Observation of Anesthetists

A team of cognitive scientists and anesthesiologists at the University of Toronto[226] conducted direct observations of anesthesiologists and obtained verbal "think aloud" protocols during actual case management. The group in Tübingen also performed direct observations for their task analysis studies.[247,328] Devitt and coworkers performed a study to assess the validity of performance assessment during simulated scenarios.[19]

Video Analysis of Actual Trauma Resuscitation and Anesthesia

Mackenzie and colleagues[358-362] pioneered in the analysis of actual clinical care of anesthetists captured on videotape, with a focus on trauma resuscitation and anesthesia for trauma patients at the Maryland Shock Trauma Unit. Their sophisticated recording system captures audio, video, and vital signs data and requires only that the clinicians insert a videotape to start the whole system.[363] Analysis of these cases has revealed inadequacies in the availability and arrangement of monitoring equipment, as well as nonexistent or ambiguous communication. Meanwhile, a few groups around the world started to use video for task analysis and assessment of performance for research and training, which is not detailed here.[150,178,270,303,332,364-370]

Problems faced by all investigators are the lack of an accepted standard for objective or subjective evaluation of anesthetist performance and the absence of an agreed-on methodology for analyzing and describing anesthetist performance. Several of the previously mentioned groups are working on methodologies for evaluating technical and behavioral aspects of performance.* Measurement of complex performance is a difficult problem, and it is likely to be some time until there is a well-established metric for assessment of performance.

*See references 20, 79, 81, 142, 143, 198, 235, 244-246, 303, 314, and 357.

References

1. Cooper JB, Gaba D: No myth: Anesthesia is a model for addressing patient safety. Anesthesiology 97:1335-1337, 2002.
2. Gaba DM: Anaesthesiology as a model for patient safety in health care. BMJ 320:785-788, 2000.
3. Kohn LT, Corrigan JM, Donaldson MS: To Err is Human—Building a Safer Health System. Washington, National Academy Press, 1999.
4. Lagasse RS: Anesthesia safety: Model or myth? A review of the published literature and analysis of current original data. Anesthesiology 97:1609-1617, 2002.
5. Beckmann U, Baldwin I, Hart GK, Runciman WB: The Australian Incident Monitoring Study in Intensive Care: AIMS-ICU. An analysis of the first year of reporting. Anaesth Intensive Care 24:320-329, 1996.
6. Bracco D, Favre JB, Bissonnette B, et al: Human errors in a multidisciplinary intensive care unit: A 1-year prospective study. Intensive Care Med 27:137-145, 2001.
7. Buckley TA, Short TG, Rowbottom YM, Oh TE: Critical incident reporting in the intensive care unit. Anaesthesia 52:403-409, 1997.
8. Cullen DJ, Sweitzer BJ, Bates DW, et al: Preventable adverse drug events in hospitalized patients: A comparative study of intensive care and general care units. Crit Care Med 25:1289-1297, 1997.
9. Donchin Y, Gopher D, Olin M, et al: A look into the nature and causes of human errors in the intensive care unit. Crit Care Med 23:294-300, 1995.
10. Frey B, Kehrer B, Losa M, et al: Comprehensive critical incident monitoring in a neonatal-pediatric intensive care unit: Experience with the system approach. Intensive Care Med 26:69-74, 2000.
11. Leape L: Why should we report adverse incidents? J Eval Clin Pract 5:1-4, 1999.
12. Pronovost P, Wu AW, Dorman T, Morlock L: Building safety into ICU care. J Crit Care 17:78-85, 2002.
13. Wu AW, Pronovost P, Morlock L: ICU incident reporting systems. J Crit Care 17:86-94, 2002.
14. Pronovost PJ, Jenckes MW, Dorman T, et al: Organizational characteristics of intensive care

units related to outcomes of abdominal aortic surgery. JAMA 281:1310-1317, 1999.
15. Vande Voorde KM, France AC: Proactive error prevention in the intensive care unit. Crit Care Nurs Clin North Am 14:347-358, 2002.
16. Breslow M: Assessing ICU performance using administrative data. J Crit Care 16:189-195, 2001.
17. Lighthall GK, Barr J, Howard SK, et al: Use of a fully simulated ICU environment for critical event management training for internal medicine residents. Crit Care Med 31:2437-2443, 2003.
18. Colliver JA, Schwartz MH: Assessing clinical performance with standardized patients. JAMA 278:790-791, 1997.
19. Devitt JH, Kurreck MM, Cohen MM, Cleave-Hogg D: The validity of performance assessments using simulation. Anesthesiology 95:36-42, 2001.
20. Gaba DM, Howard SK, Flanagan B, et al: Assessment of clinical performance during simulated crises using both technical and behavioral ratings. Anesthesiology 89:8-18, 1998.
21. Greaves JD, Grant J: Watching anaesthetists work: Using the professional judgement of consultants to assess the developing clinical competence of trainees. Br J Anaesth 84:525-533, 2000.
22. Mackieh A, Cilingir C: Effects of performance shaping factors on human error. Int J Indust Ergonom 22:285-292, 1998.
23. Xiao Y, Hunter W, Mackenzie CF, et al: Task complexity in emergency medical care and its implications for team coordination. Hum Factors 38:636-645, 1996.
24. Salas E, Fowlkes JE, Stout RJ, et al: Does CRM training improve teamwork skills in the cockpit? Two evaluation studies. Hum Factors 41:326-343, 1999.
25. Flin R, O'Connor P, Crichton M: Safety at the Sharp End—A Guide to Non-technical Skills. Aldershot, Ashgate, U.K., 2007.
26. St. Pierre M, Hofinger G, Buerschaper C: Crisis Management in Acute Care Setting: Human Factors and Team Work in a High Stakes Environment. Berlin, Springer-Verlag, 2008.
27. Weinger MB, Smith NT, Ehrenwerth J, Eisenkraft JB: Vigilance, Alarms, and Integrated Monitoring Systems. St Louis, Mosby–Year Book, 1993.
28. Loeb R, Weinger MB, Englund CE, et al: Ergonomics of the Anesthesia Workspace. Malvern, PA, Mosby–Year Book, 1993.
29. Weinger MB, Englund CE: Ergonomic and human factors affecting anesthetic vigilance and monitoring performance in the operating room environment. Anesthesiology 73:995-1021, 1990.
30. Gosbee J: Human factors engineering and patient safety. Qual Saf Health Care 11:352-354, 2002.
31. Fraind DB, Slagle JM, Tubbesing VA, et al: Reengineering intravenous drug and fluid administration processes in the operating room: Step one: Task analysis of existing processes. Anesthesiology 97:139-147, 2002.
32. Held J, Bruesch M, Zollinger A, et al: [Participation-oriented analysis of the anesthesia workplace. A work system for anesthesia in a multidisciplinary operating room.] Anaesthesist 51:110-115, 2002.
33. Schulz-Stubner S, Jungk A, Kunitz O, Rossaint R: [Analysis of the anesthesiologist's vigilance with an eye-tracking device. A pilot study for evaluation of the method under the conditions of a modern operating theatre.] Anaesthesist 51:180-186, 2002.
34. Weinger MB, Pantiskas C, Wiklund ME, Carstensen P: Incorporating human factors into the design of medical devices. JAMA 280:1484, 1998.
35. Weinger MB: Anesthesia equipment and human error. J Clin Monit Comput 15:319-323, 1999.
36. Beuscart-Zephir MC, Anceaux F, Renard JM: Integrating users' activity analysis in the design and assessment of medical software applications: The example of anesthesia. Stud Health Technol Inform 77:234-238, 2000.
37. Berguer R, Loeb RG, Smith WD: Use of the virtual instrumentation laboratory for the assessment of human factors in surgery and anesthesia. Stud Health Technol Inform 39:187-194, 1997.
38. Holst D, Rudolph P, Wendt M: [Practical realization of a patient-accompanying concept in anesthesia and intensive care.] Anasthesiol Intensivmed Notfallmed Schmerzther 35:25-29, 2000.
39. Orasanu J, Connolly T, Klein G, et al: The Reinvention of Decision Making. Norwood, NJ, Ablex, 1993.
40. Reason J: The contribution of latent human failures to the breakdown of complex systems. Philos Trans R Soc Lond B Biol Sci 327:475-484, 1990.
41. Helmreich RL, Merritt AC, Wilhelm JA: The evolution of crew resource management training in commercial aviation. Int J Aviat Psychol 9:19-32, 1999.
42. Secker-Walker J, Taylor-Adams S, Vincent C: Clinical Incident Reporting, Clinical Risk Management—Enhancing Patient Safety. London, BMJ Books, 2001, pp 419-438.
43. Reason JT, Carthey J, de Leval MR: Diagnosing "vulnerable system syndrome": An essential prerequisite to effective risk management. Qual Health Care 10(Suppl 2):ii21-ii25, 2001.
44. Cook RI, Woods DD, McDonald JS: On attributing critical incidents to factors in the environment [letter]. Anesthesiology 71:808, 1989.
45. Columbia Accident Investigation B: Columbia Accident Investigation Board Report, vol 1. Available at http://www.nasa.gov/columbia/home/CAIB_Vol1.html/ Accessed 2003.
46. Reason J: Human Error. Cambridge, UK, Cambridge University Press, 1994.
47. Helmreich RL: On error management: Lessons from aviation. BMJ 320:781-785, 2000.
48. Committee on Quality of Health Care in Anesthesiology, Institute of Medicine: Crossing the Quality Chasm—A New Health System for the 21st Century. Washington, DC, National Academy Press, 2001.
49. Berwick DM, Leape LL: Reducing errors in medicine—it's time to take this more seriously. BMJ 319:136-137, 1999.
50. Gaba DM: Anesthesiology as a model for patient safety in health care. BMJ 320:785-788, 2000.
51. Leape LL, Berwick DM: Safe health care: Are we up to it? [editorial]. BMJ 320:725-726, 2000.
52. Vincent C, Taylor-Adams S, Chapman EJ, et al: How to investigate and analyse clinical incidents: Clinical risk unit and association of litigation and risk management protocol. BMJ 320:777-781, 2000.
53. Hawksworth C, Asbury AJ, Millar K: Music in theatre: Not so harmonious. A survey of attitudes to music played in the operating theatre. Anaesthesia 52:79-83, 1997.
54. Morrow D, Leirer V, Yesavage J, Tinklenberg J: Alcohol, age, and piloting: Judgement, mood, and actual performance. Int J Addict 26:669-683, 1991.
55. Talbott GD: The impaired physician movement. Md Med J 37:216-217, 1988.
56. Talbott GD: The impaired physician: The role of the spouse in recovery. J Med Assoc Ga 76:190-192, 1987.
57. Perrow C: Normal Accidents. New York, Basic Books, 1984.
58. Gaba DM, Maxwell M, DeAnda A: Anesthetic mishaps: Breaking the chain of accident evolution. Anesthesiology 66:670-676, 1987.
59. Galletly DC, Mushet NN: Anaesthesia system errors. Anesth Intensive Care 19:66-73, 1991.
60. Rall M, Dieckmann P: Safety culture and crisis resource management in airway management: General principles to enhance patient safety in critical airway situations. Best Pract Res Clin Anaesthesiol 19:539-557, 2005.
61. Cooke NJ, Salas E, Cannon-Bowers JA, Stout RJ: Measuring team knowledge. Hum Factors 42:151-173, 2000.
62. Cooke NJ, Gorman JC, Duran JL, Taylor AR: Team cognition in experienced command-and-control teams. J Exp Psychol Appl 13:146-157, 2007.
63. Cooper JB, Newbower RS, Kitz RJ: An analysis of major errors and equipment failures in anesthesia management: Considerations for prevention and detection. Anesthesiology 60:34-42, 1984.
64. Sagan S: Toward a political theory of organizational reliability. J Contingencies Crisis Manage 2:228-240, 1994.
65. Gaba DM, Howard SK, Jump B: Production pressure in the work environment. California anesthesiologists' attitudes and experiences. Anesthesiology 81:488-500, 1994.
66. Pate-Cornell ME, Lakats LM, Murphy DM, Gaba DM: Anesthesia patient risk: A quantitative approach to organizational factors and risk management options. Risk Analysis 17:511-523, 1997.
67. Pate-Cornell E: Finding and fixing systems weaknesses: Probabilistic methods and applications of engineering risk analysis. Risk Analysis 22:319-334, 2002.
68. Rall M, Decker K, Manser T: Enhancing patient safety on a system level—results of an interdisciplinary process-oriented analysis of the organisational context in anaesthesia (Erhöhung der Patientensicherheit auf Systemebene—Ergebnisse einer interdisziplinären, prozessorientierten Analyse der organisationalen Unpublished manuscript.
69. Rasmussen J: The role of error in organizing behaviour. Qual Saf Health Care 12:377-383, 2003.
70. Reason J: Human error: Models and management. West J Med 172:393-396, 2000.
71. Helmreich RL: Managing human error in aviation. Sci Am 276:62-67, 1997.
72. Flin R: Safety in health care: Research on safety is happening. BMJ 336:171, 2008.
73. Pronovost PJ, Thompson DA, Holzmueller CG, et al: Toward learning from patient safety reporting systems. J Crit Care 21:305-315, 2006.
74. Thompson DA, Lubomski L, Holzmueller C, et al: Integrating the intensive care unit safety reporting system with existing incident reporting systems. Jt Comm J Qual Patient Saf 31:585-593, 2005.
75. Holzmueller CG, Pronovost PJ, Dickman F, et al: Creating the web-based intensive care unit safety reporting system. J Am Med Inform Assoc 12:130-139, 2005.
76. Leape L: Reporting of adverse events. N Engl J Med 347:1633-1638, 2002.
77. World Health Organization: WHO Draft Guidelines for Adverse Event Reporting and Learning Systems—From Information to Action. Geneva, WHO World Alliance for Patient Safety, 2005, pp 1-72.
78. Runciman WB, Sellen A, Webb RK, et al: The Australian Incident Monitoring Study. Errors, incidents and accidents in anaesthetic practice. Anaesth Intensive Care 21:506-519, 1993.
79. Staender S, Davies J, Helmreich B, et al: The anaesthesia critical incident reporting system: An experience based database. Int J Med Inf 47:87-90, 1997.
80. Leape LL: Reporting of adverse events. N Engl J Med 347:1633-1638, 2002.
81. Morgan C: Incident reporting in anaesthesia. Anaesth Intensive Care 16:98-100, 1988.
82. Williamson J: Critical incident reporting in anaesthesia. Anaesth Intensive Care 16:101-103, 1988.

83. Runciman WB, Webb RK, Lee R, Holland R: The Australian Incident Monitoring Study. System failure: An analysis of 2000 incident reports. Anaesth Intensive Care 21:684-695, 1993.
84. Schwilk B, Muche R, Bothner U, et al: [Quality control in anesthesiology. Results of a prospective study following the recommendations of the German Society of Anesthesiology and Intensive Care.] Anaesthesist 44:242-249, 1995.
85. Short TG, Oregan A, Jayasuriya JP, et al: Improvements in anaesthetic care resulting from a critical incident reporting programme. Anaesthesia 51: 615-621, 1996.
86. O'Leary M, Chappell SL: Confidential incident reporting systems create vital awareness of safety problems. ICAO J 51:11-13, 27, 1996.
87. Vincent C, Stanhope N, Crowley-Murphy M: Reasons for not reporting adverse incidents: An empirical study. J Eval Clin Pract 5:13-21, 1999.
88. Thomas AN, Pilkington CE, Greer R: Critical incident reporting in UK intensive care units: A postal survey. J Eval Clin Pract 9:59-68, 2003.
89. Barach P, Small SD: Reporting and preventing medical mishaps: Lessons from non-medical near miss reporting systems. BMJ 320:759-763, 2000.
90. Rall M, Manser T, Guggenberger H, et al: [Patient safety and errors in medicine: Development, prevention and analyses of incidents.] Patientensicherheit und Fehler in der Medizin. Entstehung, Prävention und Analyse von Zwischenfallen. Anasthesiol Intensivmed Notfallmed Schmerzther 36:321-330, 2001.
91. Hilfiker D: Facing our mistakes. N Engl J Med 310:118-122, 1984.
92. Wu AW: Medical error: The second victim. The doctor who makes the mistake needs help too [editorial]. BMJ 320:726-727, 2000.
93. Dieckmann P, Wehner T, Rall M, Manser T: Prospektive Simulation: Ein Konzept zur methodischen Ergänzung von medizinischen Simulatorsettings. Z Arbeitswissenschaften 59:172-180, 2005.
94. Vincent CA: Analysis of clinical incidents: A window on the system not a search for root causes. Qual Saf Health Care 13:242-243, 2004.
95. Vincent C: Understanding and responding to adverse events. N Engl J Med 348:1051-1056, 2003.
96. Vincent C, Taylor-Adams S: The Investigation and Analysis of Clinical Incidents, Clinical Risk Management—Enhancing Patient Safety. London, BMJ Books, 2001, pp 439-460.
97. Flin R, Burns C, Mearns K, et al: Measuring safety climate in health care. Qual Saf Health Care 15:109-115, 2006.
98. Runciman WB, Merry A: A tragic death: A time to blame or a time to learn? Qual Saf Health Care 12:321-322, 2003.
99. Runciman B, Merry A, Smith AM: Improving patients' safety by gathering information. BMJ 323:298, 2001.
100. Williamson JA, Webb RK, Sellen A, et al: The Australian Incident Monitoring Study. Human failure: An analysis of 2000 incident reports. Anaesth Intensive Care 21:678-683, 1993.
101. Runciman WB: Report from the Australian Patient Safety Foundation: Australasian Incident Monitoring Study. Anaesth Intensive Care 17:107-108, 1989.
102. Pronovost PJ, Martinez EA, Rodriguez-Paz JM: Removing "orange wires": Surfacing and hopefully learning from mistakes. Intensive Care Med 32:1467-1469, 2006.
103. Pronovost PJ, Berenholtz SM, Goeschel CA, et al: Creating high reliability in health care organizations. Health Serv Res 41:1599-1617, 2006.
104. Rall M, Dieckmann P: Characteristics of effective incident reporting systems: To enhance patient safety, to learn from problems, errors and good solutions. *In* Bannister J (ed): Euroanesthesia 2007. Munich, European Society of Anaesthesiology, 2007, pp 179-186.
105. Firth-Cozens J: Barriers to incident reporting. Qual Saf Health Care 11:7, 2002.
106. Leape LL: A systems analysis approach to medical error. J Eval Clin Pract 3:213-222, 1997.
107. Cullen DJ, Bates DW, Small SD, et al: The incident reporting system does not detect adverse drug events: A problem for quality improvement. Jt Comm J Qual Improv 21:541-548, 1995.
108. Rall M, Martin J, Geldner G, et al: Charakteristika effektiver Incident-Reporting-Systeme zur Erhöhung der Patientensicherheit [Characteristics of effective incident reporting systems for the increase of patient safety]. Anaesthesiol Intensivmed 47:9-19, 2006.
109. Howard SK, Gaba DM, Fish KJ, et al: Anesthesia crisis resource management training: Teaching anesthesiologists to handle critical incidents. Aviat Space Environ Med 63:763-770, 1992.
110. Rall M, Dieckmann P, Stricker E: Erhöhung der Patientensicherheit durch effektive Incident Reporting Systeme am Beispiel von PaSIS. *In* Ennker J, Pietrowski D, Kleine P (eds): Risikomanagement in der operativen Medizin. Darmstadt, Germany, Steinkopf, 2007, pp 122-137.
111. DeAnda A, Gaba DM: Unplanned incidents during comprehensive anesthesia simulation. Anesth Analg 71:77-82, 1990.
112. Gaba DM, DeAnda A: A comprehensive anesthesia simulation environment: Re-creating the operating room for research and training. Anesthesiology 69:387-394, 1988.
113. Gaba DM: Human error in anesthetic mishaps. Int Anesthesiol Clin 27:137-147, 1989.
114. Shirely PJ: Reducing error, improving safety. Crew resource management training should be mandatory in anaesthesia. BMJ 321:508-509, 2000.
115. Salas E, Bowers CA, Edens E: Improving Teamwork in Organizations—Applications of Resource Management Training. Mahwah, NJ, Lawrence Erlbaum, 2001.
116. Salas E, Prince C, Bowers CA, et al: A methodology for enhancing crew resource management training. Hum Factors 41:161-172, 1999.
117. Salas E, Rhodenizer L, Bowers CA: The design and delivery of crew resource management training: Exploiting available resources. Hum Factors 42:490-511, 2000.
118. Jacobsen J, Lindekaer AL, Ostergaard HT, et al: Management of anaphylactic shock evaluated using a full-scale anaesthesia simulator. Acta Anaesthesiol Scand 45:315-319, 2001.
119. Helmreich RL, Foushee CH, Benson R, Russini W: Cockpit resource management: Exploring the attitude-performance linkage. Aviat Space Environ Med 57:1198-1200, 1986.
120. Helmreich RL: Does CRM training work? Air Line Pilot 60:17-20, 1991.
121. Federal Aviation Administration: Crew Resource Management Training. Advisory Circular No. 120-51C, 1998.
122. Salas E, Wilson KA, Burke CS, Wightman DC: Does crew resource management training work? An update, an extension, and some critical needs. Hum Factors 48:392-412, 2006.
123. Reader TW, Flin R, Mearns K, Cuthbertson BH: Interdisciplinary communication in the intensive care unit. Br J Anaesth 98:347-352, 2007.
124. Holzman RS, Cooper JB, Gaba DM, et al: Anesthesia crisis resource management: Real-life simulation training in operating room crises. J Clin Anesth 7:675-687, 1995.
125. Gaba DM, Fish KJ, Howard SK: Crisis Management in Anesthesiology. New York, Churchill Livingstone, 1994.
126. Pan E, Cusack C, Hook J, et al: The value of provider-to-provider telehealth. Telemed J E Health 14:446-453, 2008.
127. Thomas EJ, Taggart B, Crandell S, et al: Teaching teamwork during the Neonatal Resuscitation Program: A randomized trial. J Perinatol 27:409-414, 2007.
128. Reader T, Flin R, Lauche K, Cuthbertson BH: Non-technical skills in the intensive care unit. Br J Anaesth 96:551-559, 2006.
129. Yule S, Flin R, Paterson-Brown S, Maran N: Non-technical skills for surgeons in the operating room: A review of the literature. Surgery 139:140-149, 2006.
130. Gaba DM, Howard SK, Flanagan B, et al: Assessment of clinical performance during simulated crises using both technical and behavioral ratings. Anesthesiology 89:8-18, 1998.
131. DeKeyser V, Woods DD, Masson M, Van Daele A: Fixation errors in dynamic and complex systems: Descriptive forms, psychological mechanisms, potential countermeasures. Technical Report for NATO Division of Scientific Affairs, 1988.
132. DeKeyser V, Woods DD, Colombo AG, Bustamante AS: Fixation errors: Failures to revise situation assessment in dynamic and risky systems. *In* Systems Reliability Assessment. Dordrecht, Germany, Kluwer Academic, 1990, p 231.
133. Risser DT, Rice MM, Salisbury ML, et al: The potential for improved teamwork to reduce medical errors in the emergency department. The MedTeams Research Consortium. Ann Emerg Med 34:373-383, 1999.
134. Morey JC, Simon R, Jay GD, et al: Error reduction and performance improvement in the emergency department through formal teamwork training: Evaluation of results of the MedTeams project. Health Serv Res 37:1553-1581, 2002.
135. Rosen MA, Salas E, Wu TS, et al: Promoting teamwork: An event-based approach to simulation-based teamwork training for emergency medicine residents (published online ahead of print July 14, 2008). Acad Emerg Med. 15(11):1190-1198, 2008.
136. Birnbach DJ, Salas E: Can medical simulation and team training reduce errors in labor and delivery? Anesthesiol Clin 26:159-168, viii, 2008.
137. Sundar E, Sundar S, Pawlowski J, et al: Crew resource management and team training. Anesthesiol Clin 25:283-300, 2007.
138. Nielsen PE, Goldman MB, Mann S, et al: Effects of teamwork training on adverse outcomes and process of care in labor and delivery: A randomized controlled trial. Obstet Gynecol 109:48-55, 2007.
139. Marshall DA, Manus DA: A team training program using human factors to enhance patient safety. AORN J 86:994-1011, 2007.
140. Dunn EJ, Mills PD, Neily J, et al: Medical team training: Applying crew resource management in the Veterans Health Administration. Jt Comm J Qual Patient Saf 33:317-325, 2007.
141. Morgan PJ, Cleave-Hogg D: Evaluation of medical students' performance using the anaesthesia simulator. Med Educ 34:42-45, 2000.
142. Glavin RJ, Maran NJ: Development and use of scoring systems for assessment of clinical competence. Br J Anaesth 88:329-330, 2002.

143. Gaba DM, Botney R, Howard SK, et al: Interrater reliability of performance assessment tools for the management of simulated anesthetic crises [abstract]. Anesthesiology 81:A1277, 1994.
144. Gaba DM, Howard SK, Small SD: Situation awareness in anesthesiology. Hum Factors 37:20-31, 1995.
145. Undre S, Sevdalis N, Healey AN, et al: Teamwork in the operating theatre: Cohesion or confusion? J Eval Clin Pract 12:182-189, 2006.
146. Fletcher G, Flin R, McGeorge P, et al: Anaesthetists' Non-Technical Skills (ANTS): evaluation of a behavioural marker system. Br J Anaesth 90(5):580-588, 2003.
147. Howard SK, Gaba DM, Fish KJ, et al: Anesthesia crisis resource management training: Teaching anesthesiologists to handle critical incidents. Aviat Space Environ Med 63:763-770, 1992.
148. Gaba DM, Howard SK, Fish KJ, et al: Simulation-based training in anesthesia crisis resource management (ACRM): A decade of experience. Simulation Gaming 32:175-193, 2001.
149. Roberts KH, Tadmor CT: Lessons learned from non-medical industries: The tragedy of the USS Greeneville. Qual Saf Health Care 11:355-357, 2002.
150. Yule S, Flin R, Maran N, et al: Surgeons' non-technical skills in the operating room: Reliability testing of the NOTSS Behavior Rating System. World J Surg 32:548-556, 2008.
151. Flin R, Yule S, Paterson-Brown S, et al: Teaching surgeons about non-technical skills. Surgeon 5:86-89, 2007.
152. Yule S, Flin R, Paterson-Brown S, et al: Development of a rating system for surgeons' non-technical skills. Med Educ 40:1098-1104, 2006.
153. Koch ME, Kain ZN, Ayoub C, Rosenbaum SH: The sedative and analgesic sparing effect of music. Anesthesiology 89:300-306, 1998.
154. Hawksworth CR, Sivalingam P, Asbury AJ: The effect of music on anaesthetists' psychomotor performance. Anaesthesia 53:195-197, 1998.
155. Morris GN: Reading in the operating theatre. Anaesthesia 50:1089-1090, 1995.
156. Miles C, Auburn TC, Jones DM: Effects of loud noise and signal probability on visual vigilance. Ergonomics 27:855-862, 1984.
157. Murthy VSSN, Malhotra SK, Bala I, Raghunathan M: Detrimental effects of noise on anaesthetists. Can J Anaesth 42:608-611, 1995.
158. Murthy VSSN, Malhotra SK, Bala I, Raghunathan M: Auditory functions in anaesthesia residents during exposure to operating room noise. Indian J Med Res 101:213-216, 1995.
159. Allen K, Blascovich J: Effects of music on cardiovascular reactivity among surgeons. JAMA 272:882-884, 1994.
160. Weinger MB: Cardiovascular reactivity among surgeons: Not music to everyone's ears. JAMA 273:1090-1091, 1995.
161. Stevenson GW, Hall SC: Cardiovascular reactivity among surgeons: Not music to everyone's ears [letter]. JAMA 273:1090, 1995.
162. Allen K, Blascovich J: Cardiovascular reactivity among surgeons: Not music to everyone's ears: In reply [letter]. JAMA 273:1091, 1995.
163. Schneider W, Detweiler M: The role of practice in dual-task performance: Toward workload modeling in a connectionist/control architecture. Hum Factors 30:539-566, 1988.
164. Weinger MB: In my opinion: Lack of outcome data makes reading a personal decision. APSF Newsl 10:13-16, 1995.
165. Weinger MB: OR reading debate continues in my opinion: Lack of outcome data makes reading a personal decision, states OR investigator. J Clin Monit 12:109-110, 1996.
166. Mitler MM, Carskadon MA, Czeisler CA, et al: Catastrophes, sleep, and public policy: Consensus report. Sleep 11:100-109, 1988.
167. Gaba DM, Howard SK: Patient safety: Fatigue among clinicians and the safety of patients. N Engl J Med 347:1249-1255, 2002.
168. Howard SK, Gaba DM, Rosekind MR, Zarcone VP: The risks and implications of excessive daytime sleepiness in resident physicians. Acad Med 77:1019-1025, 2002.
169. Carskadon MA, Dement WC, Kryger MH, Roth T: Normal Human Sleep: An Overview. Philadelphia, WB Saunders, 2000.
170. Carskadon MA, Dement WC: Cumulative effects of sleep restriction on daytime sleepiness. Psychophysiology 18:107-113, 1981.
171. Doran SM, Van Dongen HP, Dinges DF: Sustained attention performance during sleep deprivation: Evidence of state instability. Arch Ital Biol 139:253-267, 2001.
172. Akerstedt T, Kecklund G: Age, gender and early morning highway accidents. J Sleep Res 10:105-110, 2001.
173. Akerstedt T, Ficca G: Alertness-enhancing drugs as a countermeasure to fatigue in irregular work hours. Chronobiol Int 14:145-158, 1997.
174. Engel W, Seime R, Powell V, Doe J: Clinical performance of interns after being on call. South Med J 80:761-763, 1987.
175. Friedman RC, Kornfeld DS, Bigger TJ: Psychosocial problems associated with sleep deprivation in interns. J Med Educ 48:436-441, 1973.
176. Pankratz H: Witness: Doctor Dozed. Denver Post, 1995:1A.
177. Rosekind MR, Gander PH, Miller DL, et al: Fatigue in operational settings: Examples from the aviation environment. Hum Factors 36:327-338, 1994.
178. Howard SK, Gaba DM, Smith BE, et al: Simulation study of rested versus sleep-deprived anesthesiologists. Anesthesiology 98:1345-1355, 2003.
179. Costa G: The problem: Shiftwork. Chronobiol Int 14:89-98, 1997.
180. Harma M: Sleepiness and shiftwork: Individual differences. J Sleep Res 4:57-61, 1995.
181. Roth T, Roehrs T, Zorick F: Sleepiness: Its measurement and determinants. Sleep 5:S128-S134, 1982.
182. Richardson GS, Carskadon MA, Flagg W, et al: Excessive daytime sleepiness in man: Multiple sleep latency measurement in narcoleptic and control subjects. Electroencephalogr Clin Neurophysiol 45:621-627, 1978.
183. Carskadon MA, Dement WC, Mitler MM, et al: Guidelines for the Multiple Sleep Latency Test (MSLT): A standard measure of sleepiness. Sleep 9:519-524, 1986.
184. Howard SK, Rosekind MR, Katz JD, Berry AJ: Fatigue in anesthesia: Implications and strategies for patient and provider safety. Anesthesiology 97:1281-1294, 2002.
185. Cooper JB, Newbower RS, Long CD, McPeek B: Preventable anesthesia mishaps: A study of human factors. Anesthesiology 49:399-406, 1978.
186. Billings CE, Reynard WD: Human factors in aircraft incidents: Results of a 7-year study. Aviat Space Environ Med 55:960-965, 1984.
187. Dinges DF, Pack F, Williams K, et al: Cumulative sleepiness, mood disturbance, and psychomotor vigilance performance decrements during a week of sleep restricted to 4-5 hours per night. Sleep 20:267-277, 1997.
188. Fletcher KE, Davis SQ, Underwood W, et al: Systematic review: Effects of resident work hours on patient safety. Ann Intern Med 141:851-857, 2004.
189. Fletcher KE, Underwood W 3rd, Davis SQ, et al: Effects of work hour reduction on residents' lives: A systematic review. JAMA 294:1088-1100, 2005.
190. Mycyk MB, McDaniel MR, Fotis MA, Regalado J: Hospitalwide adverse drug events before and after limiting weekly work hours of medical residents. Am J Health Syst Pharm 62:1592-1595, 2005.
191. Kaafarani HM, Itani KM, Petersen LA, et al: Does resident hours reduction have an impact on surgical outcomes? J Surg Res 126:167-171, 2005.
192. Landrigan CP, Barger LK, Cade BE, et al: Interns' compliance with Accreditation Council for Graduate Medical Education work-hour limits. JAMA 296:1063-1070, 2006.
193. Costa G, Sartori S, Akerstedt T: Influence of flexibility and variability of working hours on health and well-being. Chronobiol Int 23:1125-1137, 2006.
194. Costa G, Akerstedt T, Nachreiner F, et al: Flexible working hours, health, and well-being in Europe: Some considerations from a SALTSA project. Chronobiol Int 21:831-844, 2004.
195. Lockley SW, Cronin JW, Evans EE, et al: Harvard Work Hours H, and Safety Group: Effect of reducing interns' weekly work hours on sleep and attentional failures. N Engl J Med 351:1829-1837, 2004.
196. Landrigan CP, Rothschild JM, Cronin JW, et al: Effect of reducing interns' work hours on serious medical errors in intensive care units. N Engl J Med 351:1838-1848, 2004.
197. Barger LK, Cade BE, Ayas NT, et al: Harvard Work Hours H, and Safety Group: Extended work shifts and the risk of motor vehicle crashes among interns. N Engl J Med 352:125-134, 2005.
198. Weinger MB, Ancoli-Israel S: Sleep deprivation and clinical performance. JAMA 287:955-957, 2002.
199. Howard SK, Gaba DM: Factors influencing vigilance and performance of anaethetists. Curr Opin Anaesthesiol 11:651-657, 1998.
200. Gaba DM, Howard SK, Jump B: Production pressure in the work environment. California anesthesiologists' attitudes and experiences. Anesthesiology 81:488-500, 1994.
201. Gravenstein JS, Cooper JB, Orkin FK: Work and rest cycles in anesthesia practice. Anesthesiology 72:737-742, 1990.
202. Gander PH, Merry A, Millar MM, Weller J: Hours of work and fatigue-related error: A survey of New Zealand anaesthetists. Anaesth Intensive Care 28:178-183, 2000.
203. Rosekind MR, Neri DF, Gregory KB, et al: A NASA education and training module on alertness management: A survey of implementation and application [abstract]. Sleep 24(Suppl):A415, 2001.
204. Smith-Coggins R, Howard SK, Mac DT, et al: Improving alertness and performance in emergency department physicians and nurses: The use of planned naps. Ann Emerg Med 48:596-604, 2006.
205. Cooper JB, Long CD, Newbower RS, Philip JH: Critical incidents associated with intraoperative exchanges of anesthesia personnel. Anesthesiology 56:456-461, 1982.
206. Cooper JB: Do short breaks increase or decrease anesthetic risk? J Clin Anesth 1:228-231, 1989.
207. Jewett ME, Dijk DJ, Kronauer RE, Dinges DF: Dose-response relationship between sleep duration and human psychomotor vigilance and subjective alertness. Sleep 22:171-179, 1999.
208. Czeisler CA, Cajochen C, Turek FW, et al: Melatonin in the Regulation of Sleep and Circadian Rhythms. Philadelphia, WB Saunders, 2000.

209. Gill M, Haerich P, Westcott K, et al: Cognitive performance following modafinil versus placebo in sleep-deprived emergency physicians: A double-blind randomized crossover study. Acad Emerg Med 13:158-165, 2006.
210. Czeisler CA, Johnson MP, Duffy JF, et al: Exposure to bright light and darkness to treat physiologic maladaptation to night work. N Engl J Med 322:1253-1259, 1990.
211. Rendell PG, Craik FI: Virtual week and actual week: Age-related differences in prospective memory. Appl Cogn Psychol 14:S43-S62, 2000.
212. Denney NW, Poon LW, Rubin DC, Wilson BA: Everyday Problem Solving: Methodological Issues, Research Findings, and a Model. Cambridge, UK, Cambridge University Press, 1989.
213. Leirer VO, Yesavage JA, Morrow DG: Marijuana, aging, and task difficulty effects on pilot performance. Aviat Space Environ Med 60:1145-1152, 1989.
214. Johnson MM: Age differences in decision making: A process methodology for examining strategic information processing. J Gerontol 45(2):P75-P78, 1990.
215. Talbott GD: Treating impaired physicians: Fourteen keys to success. Va Med 113:95-99, 1986.
216. Talbott GD: Alcoholism and other drug addictions: A primary disease entity. J Med Assoc Ga 75:490-494, 1986.
217. Spiegelman WG, Saunders L, Mazze RI: Addiction and anesthesiology. Anesthesiology 60:335-341, 1984.
218. Menk EJ, Baumgarten RK, Kingsley CP, et al: Success of reentry into anesthesiology training programs by residents with a history of substance abuse. JAMA 263:3060-3062, 1990.
219. Yesavage JA, Leirer VO: Hangover effects on aircraft pilots 14 hours after alcohol ingestion: A preliminary report. Am J Psychiatry 143:1546-1550, 1986.
220. Morrow D, Yesavage J, Leirer V, Tinklenberg J: Influence of aging and practice on piloting tasks. Exp Aging Res 19:53-70, 1993.
221. Morrow D, Leirer V, Yesavage J: The influence of alcohol and aging on radio communication during flight. Aviat Space Environ Med 61:12-20, 1990.
222. Spiegel K, Leproult R, Van Cauter E: Impact of sleep debt on metabolic and endocrine function. Lancet 354:1435-1439, 1999.
223. Spiegelman WG, Mazze RI: Addiction and anesthesiology. Anesthesiology 60:335-341, 1984.
224. Talbott GD, Gallegos KV, Wilson PO, Porter TL: The Medical Association of Georgia's Impaired Physicians Program. Review of the first 1000 physicians: Analysis of specialty. JAMA 257:2927-2930, 1987.
225. Pierce EC Jr: Anesthesiologist's leadership in patient safety. Probl Anesth 13:425-429, 2001.
226. Gaba DM, Evans DA, Patel VL: Dynamic Decision-Making in Anesthesiology: Cognitive Models and Training Approaches. Berlin, Springer-Verlag, 1992.
227. Cook RI, Woods DD: Implications of automation surprises in aviation for the future of total intravenous anesthesia (TIVA). J Clin Anesth 8:29s-37s, 1996.
228. Xiao Y, Milgram P, Doyle DJ: Incident evolution and task demands: An analysis and a field study of "going sour" incidents [abstract]. Paper presented at the 36th Annual Meeting of the Human Factors Society, 1992, pp 1279-1283.
229. Gaba DM: Human performance issues in anesthesia patient safety. Probl Anesth 5:329-350, 1991.
230. Cook RI, Woods DD, Howie MB, et al: Unintentional delivery of vasoactive drugs with an electromechanical infusion device. J Cardiothorac Anesth 6:238-244, 1992.
231. Cook RI, Potter SS, Woods DD, McDonald JS: Evaluating the human engineering of microprocessor-controlled operating room devices. J Clin Monit 7:217-226, 1991.
232. Sonenberg EA, Lawrence JA, Zelcer J: Modeling disturbance management in anesthesia: A preliminary report. Artif Intell Med 4:447-461, 1992.
233. Klemola UM, Norros L: Analysis of the clinical behavior of anesthetists: Recognition of uncertainty as a basis for practice. Med Educ 31:449-456, 1997.
234. Mackenzie MD, Horst RL, Mahaffey MA: Group decision-making during trauma patient resuscitation and anesthesia. Paper presented at 37th Annual Meeting of the Human Factors and Ergonomics Society, 1993, pp 372-376.
235. Weinger MB, Slagle J: Human factors research in anesthesia patient safety. Paper presented a symposium of the American Medical Informatics Association, 2001, pp 756-760.
236. Klein GA: Recognition-primed decisions. Adv Man Machine Sys Res 5:47-92, 1989.
237. Rasmussen J: Skills, rules, and knowledge; signals, signs, and symbols, and other distinctions in human performance models. IEEE Trans Systems Man Cybernetics 13:257-266, 1983.
238. Norman DA: Categorization of action slips. Psychol Rev 88:1-15, 1981.
239. Reason J, Rasmussen J, Duncan K, Leplat J: Generic Error-Modeling System (GEMS): A Cognitive Framework for Locating Common Human Error Forms. Chichester, UK, Wiley, 1987.
240. Reason J: Modelling the basic error tendencies of human operators. Reliability Engineering System Saf 20:137-153, 1988.
241. Boquet G, Bushman JA, Davenport HT: The anaesthetic machine, a study of function and design. Br J Anaesth 52:61-67, 1980.
242. McDonald JS, Dzwonczyk RR: A time and motion study of the anaesthetist's intraoperative time. Br J Anaesth 61:738-742, 1988.
243. McDonald JS, Dzwoncyzk R, Gupta B, Dahl M: A second time-motion study of the anesthetist's intraoperative period. Br J Anaesth 64:582-585, 1990.
244. Weinger MB, Herndon OW, Zornow MH, et al: An objective methodology for task analysis and workload assessment in anesthesia providers. Anesthesiology 80:77-92, 1994.
245. Weinger MB, Herdon OW, Gaba DM: The effect of electronic record keeping and transesophageal echocardiography on task distribution, workload, and vigilance during cardiac anesthesia. Anesthesiology 87:144-155, 1997.
246. Manser T, Wehner T: Analysing action sequences: Variations in action density in the administration of anaesthesia. Cognition Tech Work 4:71-81, 2002.
247. Manser T, Dieckmann P, Wehner T, Rall M: Comparison of anaesthetists' activity patterns in the operating room and during simulation. Ergonomics 50:246-260, 2007.
248. Manser T: Dichte als Merkmal komplexer Arbeitshandlungen. *In* Wehner T, Manser T (eds): Komplexes Handeln in der Anästhesie. Lengerich, Germany, Pabst, 2003, pp 100-174.
249. Manser T, Rall M, Schaedle B, et al: Comparison of action density patterns between simulator and clinical settings [Abstract Santander-02-11]. Eur J Anaesthesiol 20:843-844, 2003.
250. Sarter NB, Woods DD: Situation awareness: A critical but ill-defined phenomenon. Int J Aviat Psychol 1:45-57, 1991.
251. Hartman BO, Secrist GE: Situational awareness is more than exceptional vision. Aviat Space Environ Med 62:1084-1089, 1991.
252. Secrist GE, Hartman BO: Situational awareness: The trainability of the near-threshold information acquisition domain. Aviat Space Environ Med 64:885-892, 1993.
253. Westenskow DR, Orr JA, Simon FH, et al: Intelligent alarms reduce anesthesiologist's response time to critical faults. Anesthesiology 77:1074-1079, 1992.
254. Tversky A, Kahneman D: Judgement under uncertainty: Heuristics and biases. Science 185:1124-1131, 1974.
255. Cook RI, Woods DD, McDonald JS: Human Performance in Anesthesia: A Corpus of Cases. Columbus, OH, Cognitive Systems Engineering Laboratory, Department of Industrial and Systems Engineering, Ohio State University, 1991.
256. Hall KH: Reviewing intuitive decision-making and uncertainty: The implications for medical education. Med Educ 36:216-224, 2002.
257. Klein GA, Klein G, Orasanu J, et al: A Recognition-Primed Decision (RPD) Model of Rapid Decision Making. Norwood, NJ, Ablex, 1993.
258. Schwid HA, O'Donnell D: Anesthesiologists' management of simulated critical incidents. Anesthesiology 76:495-501, 1992.
259. DeAnda A, Gaba DM: Role of experience in the response to simulated critical incidents. Anesth Analg 72:308-315, 1991.
260. Botney R, Gaba DM, Howard SK, Jump B: The role of fixation error in preventing the detection and correction of a simulated volatile anesthetic overdose [abstract]. Anesthesiology 79:A1115, 1993.
261. Gaba DM: Improving anesthesiologists' performance by simulating reality [editorial]. Anesthesiology 76:491-494, 1992.
262. Kurrek MM, Fish KJ: Anesthesia crisis resource management training: An intimidating concept, a rewarding experience. Can J Anesth 43:430-434, 1996.
263. Holzman RS, Cooper JB, Gaba DM, et al: Anesthesia crisis resource management: Real-life simulation training in operating room crises. J Clin Anesth 7:675-687, 1995.
264. Cooper JB: Toward prevention of anesthetic mishaps. Int Anesthesiol Clin 22:167-183, 1984.
265. Feigal DW, Gardner SN, McClellan M: Ensuring safe and effective medical devices. N Engl J Med 348:191-192, 2003.
266. Grosjean V, Terrier P: Temporal awareness: Pivotal in performance? Ergonomics 42:1443-1456, 1999.
267. Sloan FA, Whetten-Goldstein K, Stout EM, et al: No-fault system of compensation for obstetric injury: Winners and losers. Obstet Gynecol 91:437-443, 1998.
268. Shrestha LB, Prince C, Baker DP, Salas E: Understanding situation awareness: Concepts, methods, and training. Hum Technol Interact Complex Syst 7:45-83, 1995.
269. McNeese M, Salas E, Engbers FH: New Trends in Cooperative Activities—Understanding System Dynamics in Complex Environments. Santa Monica, CA, Human Factors and Ergonomics Society, 2001.
270. Dieckmann P, Reddersen S, Wehner T, Rall M: Prospective memory failures as an unexplored threat to patient safety: Results from a pilot study using patient simulators to investigate the missed execution of intentions. Ergonomics 49:526-543, 2006.
271. Hazlehurst: The cockpit multiple activity system: A computational model. Int J Aviat Psychol 13:1-22, 2003.

272. Altman EM, Gray WD: Memory for goals: An activation-based model. Cognitive Sci 26:39-83, 2002.
273. Dismukes K: Cockpit interruptions and distractions. ASRS Directline 10:4-9, 1998.
274. Stone M, Dismukes K, Remington R: Prospective memory in dynamic environments: Effects of load, delay, and phonological rehearsal. Memory 9:165-176, 2001.
275. Marsh RL: The demands of an ongoing activity influence the success of evidence-based prospective memory. Psychon Bull Rev 9:604-610, 2002.
276. Chisholm CD, Collison EK, Nelson DR, Cordell WH: Emergency department workplace interruptions: Are emergency physicians "interrupt-driven" and "multitasking"? Acad Emerg Med 7:1239-1243, 2000.
277. Schwid HA, O'Donnell D: Educational computer simulation of malignant hyperthermia. J Clin Monit 8:201-208, 1992.
278. Cooper J: An analysis of major errors and equipment failures in anesthesia management: Considerations for prevention and detection. Anesthesiology 60:34-42, 1984.
279. McIntyre JWR: Ergonomics: Anaesthetists' use of auditory alarms in the operating room. Int J Clin Monit Comput 2:47-55, 1985.
280. Stanford LM, McIntyre JWR, Hogan JT: Audible alarm signals for anaesthesia monitoring equipment. Int J Clin Monit Comput 1:251-256, 1985.
281. Stanford LM, McIntyre JWR, Nelson TM, Hogan JT: Affective responses to commercial and experimental auditory alarm signals for anaesthesia delivery and physiological monitoring equipment. Int J Clin Monit Comput 5:111-118, 1988.
282. Woods DD: Modeling and Predicting Human Error. Boston, Academic Press, 1993, pp 248-274.
283. Paris CR, Salas E, Cannon-Bowers JA: Teamwork in multi-person systems: A review and analysis. Ergonomics 43:1052-1075, 2000.
284. Salas EC, Burke CS, Bowers CA, Wilson KA: Team training in the skies: Does crew resource management (CRM) training work? Hum Factors 43:641-674, 2001.
285. Swezey RW, Owens JM, Bergondy ML, Salas E: Task and training requirements analysis methodology (TTRAM): An analytic methodology for identifying potential training uses of simulator networks in teamwork-intensive task environments. Ergonomics 41:1678-1697, 1998.
286. Cognitive Task Analysis [Special Issue]. Hum Factors 42:1-101, 2000.
287. Roizen MF, Foss JF, Fischer SP, Miller RD: Preoperative Evaluation. New York, Churchill Livingstone, 2000.
288. Gibby GL, Gravenstein JS, Layon AJ, Jackson KI: How often does the preoperative interview change anesthetic management? [abstract]. Anesthesiology 77:A1134, 1992.
289. Buffington CW, Ramanathan S, Turndorf H: Detection of anesthesia machine faults. Anesth Analg 63:79-82, 1984.
290. Anesthesia apparatus checkout recommendations. Fed Reg 52:36-37, 1987.
291. March MG, Crowley JJ: An evaluation of anesthesiologists' present checkout methods and the validity of the FDA checklist. Anesthesiology 75:724-729, 1991.
292. Lees DE: FDA preanesthesia checklist being evaluated, revised. Anesth Patient Saf Found Newsl 6:25-27, 1991.
293. FDA publishes final version of revised apparatus checkout. Anesth Patient Saf Found Newsl 9:35, 1994.
294. Manley R, Cuddeford JD: An assessment of the effectiveness of the revised FDA checklist. AANA J 64:277-282, 1996.
295. Blike G, Biddle C: Preanesthesia detection of equipment faults by anesthesia providers at an academic hospital: Comparison of standard practice and a new electronic checklist. AANA J 68:497-505, 2000.
296. Berkenstadt H, Yusim Y, Ziv A, et al: An assessment of a point-of-care information system for the anesthesia provider in simulated malignant hyperthermia crisis. Anesth Analg 102:530-532, 2006.
297. Berkenstadt H, Yusim Y, Katznelson R, et al: A novel point-of-care information system reduces anaesthesiologists' errors while managing case scenarios. Eur J Anaesthesiol 23:239-250, 2006.
298. Forrest JB, Cahalan MK, Rehder K: Multicenter study of general anesthesia. II. Results. Anesthesiology 72:262-268, 1990.
299. Cooper JB, Cullen DJ, Nemeskal R, et al: Effects of information feedback and pulse oximetry on the incidence of anesthesia complications. Anesthesiology 67:686-694, 1987.
300. Moller JT, Johannessen NW, Espersen K, et al: Randomized evaluation of pulse oximetry in 20,802 patients: II. Perioperative events and postoperative complications. Anesthesiology 78:445-453, 1992.
301. Philip JH, Raemer DB: Selecting the optimal anesthesia monitoring array. Med Instrum 19:122-126, 1985.
302. Weinger MB, Slagle J, Jain S, Ordonez N: Retrospective data collection and analytical techniques for patient safety studies. J Biomed Inform 36:106-119, 2003.
303. Slagle J, Weinger MB, Dinh MT, et al: Assessment of the intrarater and interrater reliability of an established clinical task analysis methodology. Anesthesiology 96:1129-1139, 2002.
304. Weinger MB, Vredenburgh AG, Schumann CM, et al: Quantitative description of the workload associated with airway management procedures. J Clin Anesth 12:273-282, 2000.
305. Weinger MB: Vigilance, boredom, and sleepiness. J Clin Monit Comput 15:549-552, 1999.
306. Devitt JH, Kurrek MM, Cohen MM, et al: Testing internal consistency and construct validity during evaluation of performance in a patient simulator. Anesth Analg 86:1160-1164, 1998.
307. Gaba DM: Simulators in Anesthesiology. Adv Anesth 14:55-94, 1997.
308. Gordon JA: The human patient simulator: Acceptance and efficacy as a teaching tool for students. Acad Med 75:522, 2000.
309. Rosenblatt MAR, Abrams KJ, , et al: The use of a human patient simulator in the evaluation of and development of a remedial prescription for an anesthesiologist with lapsed medical skills. Anesth Analg 94:149-153, 2002.
310. Byrne AJ, Jones JG: Responses to simulated anaesthetic emergencies by anaesthetists with different durations of clinical experience. Br J Anaesth 78:553-556, 1997.
311. Byrne AJ, Greaves JD: Assessment instruments used during anaesthetic simulation: Review of published studies. Br J Anaesth 86:445-450, 2001.
312. Forrest FC, Taylor MA, Postlethwaite K, Aspinall R: Use of a high-fidelity simulator to develop testing of the technical performance of novice anaesthetists. Br J Anaesth 88:338-344, 2002.
313. Gaba DM, Howard SK: Simulated anaesthetic emergencies. Br J Anaesth 79:689-690, 1997.
314. Gaba DM, Howard S, Smith B, Weinger MB: Simulators in anesthesiology education. Anesth Analg 89:805-806, 1999.
315. Halamek LP, Howard SK, Smith BE, et al: Development of a simulated delivery room for the study of human performance during neonatal resuscitation. Pediatrics 100(Suppl):513-524, 1997.
316. Issenberg SB, McGaghie WC, Hart IR, et al: Simulation technology for health care professional skills training and assessment. JAMA 282:861-866, 1999.
317. Morgan PJ, Cleave-Hogg D, McLlory J, Devitt JH: Simulation technology: A comparison of experimental and visual learning for undergraduate medical students. Anesthesiology 96:10-16, 2002.
318. Weller JM, Bloch M, Young S, et al: Evaluation of high fidelity patient simulator in assessment of performance of anaesthetists. Br J Anaesth 90:43-47, 2003.
319. Schwid HA, Rooke GA, Carline J, et al: Evaluation of anesthesia residents using mannequin-based simulation: A multiinstitutional study. Anesthesiology 97:1434-1444, 2002.
320. Drui AB, Behm RJ, Martin WE: Predesign investigation of the anesthesia operational environment. Anesth Analg 52:584-591, 1973.
321. Weinger MB, Herndon OW, Gaba DM: The effect of electronic record keeping and transesophageal echocardiography on task distribution, workload, and vigilance during cardiac anesthesia. Anesthesiology 87:144-155, 1997.
322. Weinger MB, Herndon OW, Paulus MP, et al: Objective task analysis and workload assessment of anesthesia providers. Anesthesiology 80:77-92, 1994.
323. Held J, Krueger H, Landau K: FIT für die Mensch-Maschine-Schnittstelle, Mensch-Maschine-Schnittstellen. Stuttgart, Germany, Institut fuer Arbeits-und Organisation Psychologie, 1998, pp 130-134.
324. Kennedy PJ, Feingold A, Wiener EL, Hosek RS: Analysis of tasks and human factors in anesthesia for coronary artery bypass. Anesth Analg 55:374-377, 1976.
325. Loeb RG: Monitor surveillance and vigilance of anesthesia residents. Anesthesiology 80:527-533, 1994.
326. Gurushanthaiah K, Weinger MB, Englund CE: Visual display format affects the ability of anesthesiologists to detect acute physiologic changes. A laboratory study employing a clinical display simulator. Anesthesiology 83:1184-1193, 1995.
327. Allard J, Dzwonczyk R, Yablock D, et al: Effect of automatic record keeping on vigilance and record keeping time. Br J Anaesth 74:619-626, 1995.
328. Weinger MB, Herndon OW, Gaba DM: The effect of electronic record keeping and transesophageal echocardiography on task distribution, workload, and vigilance during cardiac anesthesia. Anesthesiology 87:144-155, 1997.
329. Loeb RG: Manual record keeping is not necessary for anesthesia vigilance. J Clin Monit 11:9-13, 1995.
330. Gaba DM, Lee T: Measuring the workload of the anesthesiologist. Anesth Analg 71:354-361, 1990.
331. Loeb RG: A measure of intraoperative attention to monitor displays. Anesth Analg 76:337-341, 1993.
332. Manser T, Dieckmann P, Wehner T, Rallf M: Comparison of anaesthetists' activity patterns in the operating room and during simulation. Ergonomics 50:246-260, 2007.
333. Toung TJK, Donham RT, Rogers MC: Effect of previous medical training on the stress of giving anesthesia [abstract]. Anesthesiology 65:A473, 1986.
334. Azar I, Sophie S, Lear E: The cardiovascular response of anesthesiologists during induction of

anesthesia [abstract]. Anesthesiology 63:A76, 1985.
335. Bitetti J, Hartwell P, Chin ML, et al: Stress in the attending anesthesiologist [abstract]. Anesthesiology 73: 1990.
336. Harrison TK, Manser T, Howard SK, Gaba DM: Use of cognitive aids in a simulated anesthetic crisis. Anesth Analg 103:551-556, 2006.
337. Buerschaper C, Harms H, Hofinger G, Rall M: Problemlösefähigkeiten in der Anästhesie. Forum Qualitative Sozialforschung [Forum: Qualitative Social Research] [On-line Journal]. 4, 2003.
338. Mackie RR: Vigilance research—are we ready for countermeasures? Hum Factors 29:707-723, 1987.
339. Adams JA: Criticisms of vigilance research: A discussion. Hum Factors 29:737-740, 1987.
340. Beatty J, Ahern SK, Katz R, Mackie RR: Sleep Deprivation and the Vigilance of Anesthesiologists during Simulated Surgery. New York, Plenum, 1977.
341. Denisco RA, Drummond JN, Gravenstein JS: The effect of fatigue on the performance of a simulated anesthetic monitoring task. J Clin Monit 3:22-24, 1987.
342. Kay J, Neal M: Effect of automatic blood pressure devices on vigilance of anesthesia residents. J Clin Monit 2:148-150, 1986.
343. Cooper JO, Cullen BF: Observer reliability in detecting surreptitious random occlusions of the monaural esophageal stethoscope. J Clin Monit 6:271-275, 1990.
344. Patel VL, Groen GJ, Frederiksen CH: Differences between medical students and doctors in memory for clinical cases. Med Educ 20:3-9, 1986.
345. Patel VL, Evans DA, Kaufman DR: Reasoning strategies and the use of biomedical knowledge by medical students. Med Educ 24:129-136, 1990.
346. Patel VL, Groen GJ, Arocha JF: Medical expertise as a function of task difficulty. Mem Cognit 18:394-406, 1990.
347. Gaba DM, DeAnda A: The response of anesthesia trainees to simulated critical incidents. Anesth Analg 68:444-451, 1989.
348. Loeb RG, Fitch WT: A laboratory evaluation of an auditory display designed to enhance intraoperative monitoring. Anesth Analg 94:362-368, 2002.
349. Runciman WB, Webb RK, Barker L, Currie M: The Australian Incident Monitoring Study. The pulse oximeter: Applications and limitations—an analysis of 2000 incident reports. Anaesth Intensive Care 21:543-550, 1993.
350. Morris RW, Montano SR: Response times to visual and auditory alarms during anaesthesia. Anaesth Intensive Care 24:682-684, 1996.
351. Craven RM, McIndoe AK: Continuous auditory monitoring—how much information do we register? Br J Anaesth 83:747-749, 1999.
352. Botney R, Gaba DM, Howard SK, Jump B: The role of fixation error in preventing the detection and correction of a simulated volatile anesthetic overdose [abstract]. Anesthesiology 79:A1115, 1993.
353. Schwid HA, Rooke GA, Michalowski P, Ross BK: Screen-based anesthesia simulation with debriefing improves performance in a mannequin-based anesthesia simulator. Teach Learn Med 13:92-96, 2001.
354. Schwid HA, Rooke GA, Ross BK, Sivarajan M: Use of a computerized advanced cardiac life support simulator improves retention of advanced cardiac life support guidelines better than a textbook review. Crit Care Med 27:821-824, 1999.
355. Reznek M, Smith-Coggins R, Howard S, et al: Emergency Medicine Crisis Resource Management (EMCRM): Pilot study of a simulation-based crisis management course for emergency medicine. Acad Emerg Med 10:386-389, 2003.
356. Gaba DM: Two examples of how to evaluate the impact of new approaches to teaching [editorial]. Anesthesiology 96:1-2, 2002.
357. Weinger MB, Vora S, Herndon CN, Howard SK, Smith BE, Mazzei WJ, et al: Evaluation of the effects of fatigue and sleepiness on clinical performance of on-call anesthesia residents during actual nighttime cases and in simulated cases. In: Proc Enhanc Patient Safety Reduc Errors Health Care; 1999; Rancho Mirage, CA: National Patient Safety Foundation, 1999, p. 306-310.
358. Mackenzie CF, Hu PF, Horst RL: An audio-video system for automated data acquisition in the clinical environment. LOTAS Group. J Clin Monit 11:335-341, 1995.
359. Mackenzie CF, Martin P, Xiao Y: Video analysis of prolonged uncorrected esophageal intubation. Level One Trauma Anesthesia Simulation Group. Anesthesiology 84:1494-1503, 1996.
360. Xiao Y, Hunter WA, Mackenzie CF, et al: Task complexity in emergency medical care and its implications for team coordination. LOTAS Group. Level One Trauma Anesthesia Simulation. Hum Factors 38:636-645, 1996.
361. Mackenzie CF, Xiao Y, Jaberi M, et al: Strengths and weaknesses of airway teleconsultation. J Clin Monitor 14:526-527, 1998.
362. Xiao Y, MacKenzie C, Orasanu J, et al: Information acquisition from audio-video-data sources: An experimental study on remote diagnosis. The LOTAS Group. Telemed J 5:139-155, 1999.
363. Mackenzie CF, Hu PF, Horst RL: An audio-video system for automated data acquisition in the clinical environment. LOTAS Group. J Clin Monit 11:335-341, 1995.
364. Phipps D, Meakin GH, Beatty PC, et al: Human factors in anaesthetic practice: Insights from a task analysis. Br J Anaesth 100:333-343, 2008.
365. Sanderson PM, Watson MO, Russell WJ, et al: Advanced auditory displays and head-mounted displays: Advantages and disadvantages for monitoring by the distracted anesthesiologist. Anesth Analg 106:1787-1797, 2008.
366. Undre S, Sevdalis N, Healey AN, et al: Observational teamwork assessment for surgery (OTAS): Refinement and application in urological surgery. World J Surg 31:1373-1381, 2007.
367. Salas E, Rosen MA, Burke CS, et al: Markers for enhancing team cognition in complex environments: The power of team performance diagnosis. Aviat Space Environ Med 78:B77-B85, 2007.
368. Friedman Z, Katznelson R, Devito I, et al: Objective assessment of manual skills and proficiency in performing epidural anesthesia—video-assisted validation. Reg Anesth Pain Med 31:304-310, 2006.
369. Guerlain S, Adams RB, Turrentine FB, et al: Assessing team performance in the operating room: Development and use of a "black-box" recorder and other tools for the intraoperative environment. J Am Coll Surg 200:29-37, 2005.
370. Weinger MB, Gonzales DC, Slagle J, Syeed M: Video capture of clinical care to enhance patient safety. Qual Saf Health Care 13:136-144, 2004.

Appendix 1

Links and Useful Resources

Links

Links to Patient Safety and CRM Resources

- http://www.npsf.org/
- www.patientsafety.gov (VA)
- http://www.jcaho.org/
- www.npsa.nhs.uk
- http://anesthesia.stanford.edu/VASimulator
- www.medizin.uni-tuebingen.de/psz

Links to Different Incident Reporting Systems

- www.npsa.nhs.uk/health/reporting
- www.pasis.de
- www.pasos-ains.de
- www.cirrnet.ch
- www.cirsmedical.org
- http://psrs.arc.nasa.gov/
- Pronovost's ICUSRS[75]

Valuable Sources

WHO "World Alliance for Patient Safety"

- "WHO Draft Guidelines for Adverse Event Reporting and Learning Systems—From Information to Action" als pdf
- www.who.int/patientsafety/events/05/Reporting_Guidelines.pdf

U.S. Department of Veterans Affairs Patient Safety Reporting System

- http://www.psrs.arc.nasa.gov
- *U.S. Patient Safety and Quality Improvement Act*
- USA http://www.pso.ahrq.gov/psos/overview.htm

Root-Cause Analysis Tools

- www.va.gov/ncps/rca.html. 2005.
- www.npsa.nhs.uk/health/resources/root_cause_analysis/

Failure Modes and Effects Analysis Tools

- www.va.gov/ncps/HFMEA.html. 2005.

Marcus Rall, David M. Gaba, Peter Dieckmann, and Christoph Eich

7 Patient Simulation

Key Points

1. Simulators and the use of simulation have become an integral part of medical education, training, and research. The pace of developments and applications is very fast, and the results are promising.
2. Different types of simulators can be distinguished: computer-based or screen-based microsimulators versus mannequin-based simulators. The latter can be divided into script-based and model-based simulators.
3. The development of mobile and less expensive simulator models allows for substantial expansion of simulator training to areas where this training could not be applied or afforded previously. The biggest obstacles to providing simulation training are not the simulator hardware but are (1) obtaining access to the learner population for the requisite time and (2) providing appropriately trained and skilled instructors to prepare, conduct, and evaluate the simulation sessions.
4. Realistic simulations are a useful method to show mechanisms of error development (human factors) and to provide their countermeasures. The anesthesia crisis resource management (ACRM) course model with its ACRM key points (see Chapter 6 on Crisis Resource Management) is the de facto world standard for human factor–based simulator training. Curricula should use scenarios that are tailored to the stated teaching goals, rather than focusing solely on achieving maximum "realism."
5. Simulator training is being adapted by many other fields outside anesthesia (e.g., emergency medicine, neonatal care, intensive care, medical and nursing school).
6. Simulators have proved to be very valuable in research to study human behavior and failure modes under conditions of critical incidents and in the development of new treatment concepts (telemedicine) and in support of the biomedical industry (e.g., device beta-testing).
7. Simulators can be used as effective research tools for studying methods of performance assessment.
8. Assessment of nontechnical skills (or behavioral markers) has evolved considerably and can be accomplished with a reliability that likely matches that of many other subjective judgments in patient care. Systems for rating nontechnical skills have been introduced and tested in anesthesia; one in particular (Anaesthetists' Non-Technical Skills [ANTS]) has been studied extensively and has been modified for other fields.
9. The most important part of simulator training that goes beyond specific technical skills is the self-reflective (often video-assisted) debriefing session after the scenario. The debriefing is influenced most strongly by the quality of the instructor, not the fidelity of the simulator.
10. Simulators are just the tools for an effective learning experience. The education and training, commitment, and overall ability of the instructors are of utmost importance.

How can clinicians experience the difficulties of patient care without putting patients at undue risk? How can we assess the abilities of clinicians as individuals and teams when each patient is unique? These are questions that have challenged medicine for years. In recent years, these and related questions have begun to be answered in health care by the application of approaches new to medicine, but borrowed from years of successful service in other industries facing similar problems. These approaches focus on *simulation,* a technique well known in the military, aviation, space flight, and nuclear power industries.

Simulation refers to the artificial replication of sufficient elements of a real-world domain to achieve a stated goal. The goals can include understanding the domain better, training personnel to deal with the domain, or testing the capacity of personnel to work in the domain. The fidelity of a simulation refers to how closely it replicates the domain and is determined by the number of elements that are replicated and the discrepancy between each element and the real world. The fidelity required depends on the stated goals. Some goals can be achieved with minimal fidelity, whereas others require very high fidelity.

Simulation has probably been a part of human activity since prehistoric times. Rehearsal for hunting activities and warfare was most likely an occasion for simulating the behavior of prey or enemy warriors. Technologic simulation probably dates back to the dawn of technology itself. Good and Gravenstein[1] pointed to the medieval quintain as a technologic device that crudely simulated the behavior of an opponent during sword fighting. If the swordsman did not duck at the appropriate time after striking a blow, he would be hit by a component of the quintain. In modern times, preparation for warfare has been an equally powerful spur to the development of simulation technologies, especially for aviation, shipping, and the operation of armored vehicles. These technologies have been adopted by their civilian counterparts, but they have attained their most extensive use in commercial aviation.

Simulation in Aviation

Although some aircraft simulators were built between 1910 and 1927, none of them could provide the proper feel of the aircraft because they could not dynamically reproduce its behavior. In 1930, Link filed a patent for a pneumatically driven aircraft simulator. The Link Trainer was a standard for flight training before World War II, but the war accelerated its use and the further development of flight simulators. In the 1950s, electronic controls replaced pneumatic ones through analog, digital, and hybrid computers. The aircraft simulator achieved its modern form in the late 1960s, but it has been continuously refined. Aviation simulators are so realistic now that pilots with experience flying one aircraft are routinely certified to fly totally new or different aircraft, even if they have never flown the actual aircraft without passengers on board. Similar stories of the development of simulators can be told for numerous other industries.

Uses of Simulators

Although simulators originally were used to provide basic instruction on the operation of aircraft controls, the variety of uses of simulators in general has expanded greatly. Table 7-1 lists possible uses of simulators in all types of complex work situations. Simulation is a powerful generic tool for dealing with human performance issues (e.g., training, testing, and research) (see Chapter 6), for investigating human-machine interactions, and for the design and validation of equipment. As described later in this chapter, each of these uses is potentially relevant to anesthesiology. A few books are devoted solely to the topic of simulation and their use in and outside of anesthesia.[2-4]

Table 7-1 Use of Simulators in Complex Work Environments

Team training, as human factor or CRM training
Training in dynamic plant control
Training in diagnostic skills
Dynamic mockup for design evaluation
Test bed for checking operating instructions
Environment in which task analysis can be conducted (e.g., on diagnostic strategies)
Test bed for new applications (e.g., telemedicine tools such as the "Guardian-Angel-System")
Source of data on human errors relevant to risk and reliability assessment
Vehicle for (compulsory) testing/assessment and recertification of operators

CRM, Crisis resource management.
Adapted from Singleton WT: The Mind at Work. Cambridge, Cambridge University Press, 1989.

Twelve Dimensions of Simulation

Current and future applications of simulation can be categorized by 12 dimensions, each of which represents a different attribute of simulation (Fig. 7-1).[5] Some dimensions have a clear gradient and direction, whereas others have only categorical differences. The total number of unique combinations across all the dimensions is very large (on the order of 4^{12} to 5^{12}—4 million to 48 million). Some combinations overlap strongly with others, and some are inappropriate or irrelevant, so the actual number of meaningful combinations is much lower. Nonetheless, although the demonstrated applications of simulation in health care have been quite diverse, the space of possible applications (a large number, although quite a bit smaller than millions) has by no means been fully examined.

Dimension 1: Purpose and Aims of the Simulation Activity

The most obvious application of simulation is to improve the education and training of clinicians, but other purposes also are important. As used in this chapter, *education* emphasizes conceptual knowledge, basic skills, and an introduction to work practices. *Training* emphasizes the actual tasks and work to be performed. Simulation can be used to *assess performance* and competency of individual clinicians and teams, for low-stakes or formative testing and (to a lesser degree as yet) for high-stakes certification testing.[6,7] Simulation *rehearsals* are now being explored as adjuncts to actual clinical practice; for example, surgeons or an entire operative team can rehearse an unusually complex operation in advance using a simulation of the specific patient.[8-10] Simulators can be powerful tools for research and evaluation, concerning *organizational practices* (patient care protocols) and for the *investigation of human factors* (e.g., of performance-shaping factors, such as fatigue,[11] or of the user interface and operation of medical equipment in high hazard clinical settings[12]). Simulation-based empirical tests of the usability of clinical equipment already have been used in designing equipment that is currently for sale; ultimately, such practices may be required by regulatory agencies before approval of new devices.

Simulation can be a "bottom up" tool for changing the culture of health care concerning patient safety. First, it allows hands-on training of junior and senior clinicians about practices that enact the desired "culture of safety."[13] Simulation also can be a rallying point about culture change and patient safety that can

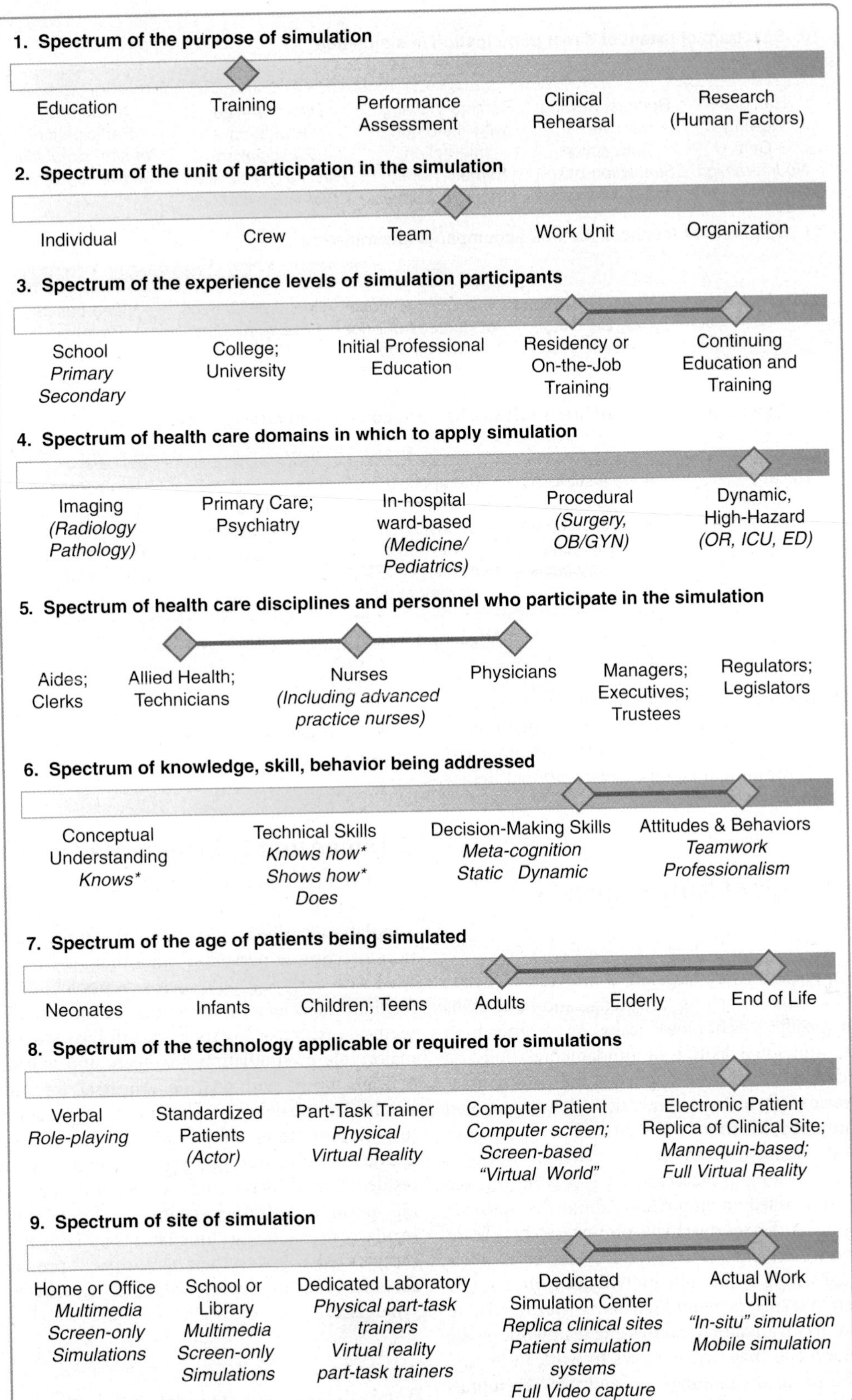

Figure 7-1 The 12 dimensions of simulation applications (10 to 12 shown on next page). Any particular application can be represented as a point or range on each spectrum (shown by *diamonds*). This figure illustrates a specific application—multidisciplinary CRM-oriented decision making and teamwork training for adult intensive care unit personnel. CRM, crises resource management; ED, emergency department; ICU, intensive care unit; OR, operating room. *These terms are used according to Miller's pyramid of learning.

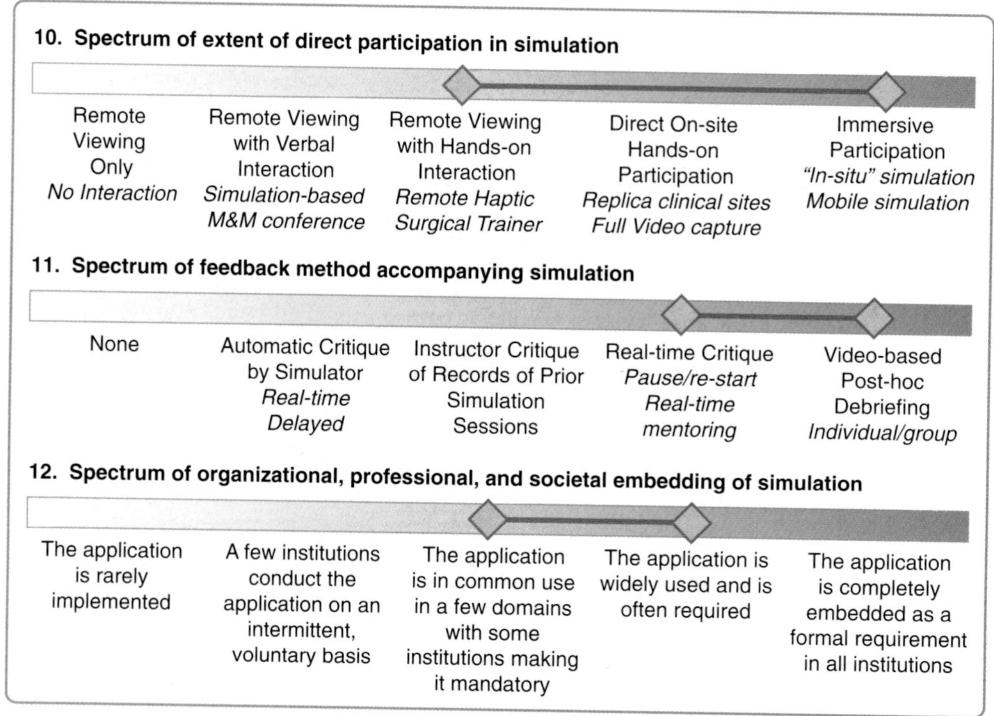

Figure 7-1, cont'd

bring together experienced clinicians from various disciplines and domains (who may be "captured" because the simulations are clinically challenging) along with health care administrators, risk managers, and experts on human factors, organizational behavior, or institutional change.

Dimension 2: Unit of Participation in the Simulation

Many simulation applications are targeted at individuals. These may be especially useful for teaching knowledge and basic skills or for practice on specific psychomotor tasks. As in other high hazard industries, individual skill is a fundamental building block, but a considerable emphasis is applied at higher organizational levels, in various forms of teamwork and interpersonal relations (often summarized under the rubric of *crisis resource management* (CRM) adapted from aviation cockpit resource management) (more on human factors and CRM concepts, see Chapter 6).[14,18] CRM is based on empirical findings that individual performance is not sufficient to achieve optimal safety.[15] Team training may be addressed first to crews (also known as *single discipline teams*), consisting of multiple individuals from a single discipline, and then to teams (or *multidisciplinary teams*).[16] There are advantages and disadvantages to addressing teamwork in the single discipline approach that "trains crews to work in teams" versus the "combined team training" of multiple disciplines together.[21] For maximal benefit, these approaches are used in a complementary fashion.

Teams exist in actual "work units" in an organization (e.g., a specific intensive care unit [ICU]), each of which is its own target for training. There also is growing interest and experience in applying simulation to nonclinical personnel and work units in health care organizations (e.g., to managers or executives)[22] and to organizations as a whole (e.g., entire hospitals or networks).

Dimension 3: Experience Level of Simulation Participants

Simulation can be applied along the entire continuum of education of clinical personnel and the public at large. It can be used with early learners, such as schoolchildren, or lay adults to facilitate bioscience instruction, to interest individuals in biomedical careers, or to explain health care issues and practices. The major role of simulation has been, and will continue to be, to educate, train, and provide rehearsal for individuals actually involved in the delivery of health care. Simulation is relevant from the earliest level of vocational or professional education (students) and during apprenticeship training (interns and residents), and increasingly for experienced personnel undergoing periodic refresher training. Simulation can be applied regularly to practicing clinicians (as individuals, teams, or organizations) regardless of their seniority,[17,18] providing an integrated accumulation of experiences that should have a long-term synergism.

Dimension 4: Health Care Domain in Which the Simulation Is Applied

Simulation techniques can be applied across nearly all health care domains. Although much of the attention on simulation has focused on technical and procedural skills applicable in surgery,[11,20-22] obstetrics,[23,24] invasive cardiology,[25,26] and other related fields, another bastion of simulation has been recreating whole patients for dynamic domains involving high hazard and invasive intervention, such as anesthesia,[27,28] critical care,[29,30] and emergency medicine.[31-34] Immersive techniques can be used in imaging-intensive domains, such as radiology and pathology, and interactive simulations are relevant in the interventional sides of such arenas.[35] In many domains, simulation techniques have been useful for addressing nontechnical skills and professionalism issues, such as communicating with patients and coworkers, or addressing issues such as ethics or end-of-life care.

Dimension 5: Health Care Disciplines of Personnel Participating in the Simulation

Simulation is applicable to all disciplines of health care, not only to physicians. In anesthesiology, simulation has been applied to anesthesiologists, Certified Registered Nurse Anesthetists, and anesthesia technicians. Simulation is not limited to clinical personnel. It also may be directed at managers, executives, hospital trustees, regulators, and legislators. For these groups, simulation can convey the complexities of clinical work, and it can be used to exercise and probe the organizational practices of clinical institutions at multiple levels.

Dimension 6: Type of Knowledge, Skill, Attitudes, or Behavior Addressed in Simulation

Simulations can be used to help learners acquire new knowledge and to understand conceptual relations and dynamics better. Today physiologic simulations allow students to watch cardiovascular and respiratory functions unfold over time and respond to interventions—in essence making textbooks, diagrams, and graphs "come alive." The next step on the spectrum is acquisition of skills to accompany knowledge. Some skills follow immediately from conceptual knowledge (e.g., cardiac auscultation), whereas others involve intricate and complex psychomotor activities (e.g., catheter placement or basic surgical skills). Isolated skills must be assembled into a new layer of clinical practices. An understanding of the concepts of general surgery cannot be combined only with basic techniques of dissecting and suturing or manipulation of instruments to create a capable laparoscopic surgeon. Basic skills must be integrated into actual clinical techniques, a process for which simulation may have considerable power, especially because it can readily provide experience with even uncommon anatomic or clinical presentations. In the current health care system, for most invasive procedures, *novices at a task typically first perform the task on a real patient,* albeit under some degree of supervision. They climb the learning curve, working on patients with varying levels of guidance. Simulation offers the possibility of having novices practice extensively before they begin to work on real patients as supervised "apprentices."

In this way and others, simulation is applicable to clinicians throughout their careers to support lifelong learning. It can be used to refresh skills for procedures that are not performed often. Knowledge, skills, and practices honed as individuals must be linked into effective teamwork in diverse clinical teams, which must operate safely in work units and larger organizations.[36-38] Perpetual rehearsal of responses to challenging events is needed because the team or organization must be practiced in handling them as a coherent unit.

Dimension 7: Age of the Patient Being Simulated

Simulation is applicable to nearly every type and age of patient literally from "cradle to grave." Simulation may be particularly useful for pediatric patients and clinical activities because neonates and infants have smaller physiologic reserves than most adults.[40,41] Fully interactive neonatal and pediatric patient simulators are now available. Simulation also addresses issues of the elderly and end-of-life issues for every age.

Dimension 8: Technology Applicable or Required for Simulations

To accomplish these goals, various technologies (including no technology) are relevant for simulation. Verbal simulations ("what if" discussions), paper and pencil exercises, and experiences with standardized patient actors[41-43] require no technology, but can effectively evoke or recreate challenging clinical situations. Similarly, very low technology—even pieces of fruit or simple dolls—can be used for training in some manual tasks. Certain aspects of complex tasks and experiences can be recreated successfully with little technology. Some education and training on teamwork can be accomplished with role playing, analysis of videos, or drills with simple mannequins.[44]

Ultimately, learning and practicing complex manual skills (e.g., surgery, cardiac catheterization) or practicing the dynamic management of life-threatening clinical situations that include risky or noxious interventions (e.g., intubation or defibrillation) can only be fully accomplished using either animals—which for reasons of cost and issues of animal rights is becoming very difficult—or a technologic means to recreate the patient and the clinical environment. The different types of simulation technologies relevant to anesthesiology are discussed later in this chapter.

Dimension 9: Site of Simulation Participation

Some types of simulation—those that use videos, computer programs, or the Web—can be conducted in the privacy of the learner's home or office using his or her own equipment. More advanced screen-based simulators might need more powerful computer facilities available in a medical library or learning center. Part-task trainers and virtual reality simulators are usually fielded in a dedicated skills laboratory. Mannequin-based simulation also can be used in a skills laboratory, although the more complex recreations of actual clinical tasks require either a dedicated patient simulation center with fully equipped replicas of clinical spaces or the ability to bring the simulator into an actual work setting (in-situ simulation). There are advantages and disadvantages to doing clinical simulations in situ versus in a dedicated center. Using the actual site allows training of the entire unit with all its personnel, procedures, and equipment. There would at best be limited availability of actual clinical sites, and the simulation activity may distract from real patient care work. The dedicated simulation center is a more controlled and available environment, allowing more comprehensive recording of sessions, and imposing no distraction on real activities. For large-scale simulations (e.g., disaster drills), the entire organization becomes the site of training.

Video conferencing and advanced networking may allow even advanced types of simulation to be conducted remotely (see dimension 10). The collaborative use of virtual reality surgical simulators in real time already has been shown, even with locations that are separated by thousands of miles (see later for more on Site of Simulator).

Dimension 10: Extent of Direct Participation in Simulation

Most simulations—even screen-based simulators or part-task trainers—were initially envisioned as highly interactive activities with significant direct "on-site" hands-on participation. Not all learning requires direct participation, however. Some learning can occur merely by viewing a simulation involving others, as one can readily imagine being in the shoes of the participants. A further step is to involve the remote viewers either in the simulation itself or in debriefings about what transpired. Several centers have been using videoconferencing to conduct simulation-based exercises, including morbidity and mortality conferences.[45] Because the simulator can be paused, restarted, or otherwise controlled, the remote audience can readily obtain more information from the on-site participants, debate the proper course of action, and discuss with those in the simulator how best to proceed.

Dimension 11: Feedback Method Accompanying Simulation

Similar to real life, one can learn a great deal just from simulation experiences themselves, without any additional feedback. For many simulations, specific feedback is provided to maximize learning. On screen-based simulators or virtual reality systems, the simulator itself can provide feedback about the participant's actions or decisions,[46] particularly for manual tasks where clear metrics of performance are readily delineated.[47,48] More commonly, human instructors provide feedback. This can be as simple as having the instructor review records of previous sessions that the learner has completed alone. For many target populations and applications, an instructor provides real-time guidance and feedback to participants while the simulation is going on. The ability to start, pause, and restart the simulation can be valuable. For the most complex uses of simulation, especially when training experienced personnel, the typical form of feedback is a detailed post-simulation debriefing session, often using audio-video recordings of the scenario. Waiting until after the scenario is finished allows experienced personnel to apply their collective skills without interruption, and then allows them to see and discuss the advantages and disadvantages of their behaviors, decisions, and actions.

Dimension 12: Organizational, Professional, and Societal Embedding of Simulation

Another important dimension is the degree to which the simulation application is embedded into an organization or industry.[19] Being highly embedded may mean that the simulation is a formal requirement of the institution or is mandated by the governmental regulator. Another aspect of embedding would be that—for early learners—the initial (steep) part of the learning curve would be required to occur in a simulation setting before the learners are allowed to work on real patients under supervision. Also, complete embedding of simulation into the workplace would mean that simulation training is a normal part of the work schedule, rather than being an "add-on" activity attended in the "spare time" of clinicians.

Conceptual Issues about Patient Simulation

"The key is the programme, not the hardware," was a truth about simulation learned early in aviation. Using simulators in a goal-oriented way is equally or more about the conceptual aspects of the technique than it is about the technology of the simulation devices. An understanding of the conceptual and theoretical aspects of the use of simulation techniques can be helpful for determining the right applications of the technique and the important matchups that must be made in the design and conduct of simulation exercises to get the best results. When used most effectively, simulation can be—to borrow a line from the band U2—"even better than the real thing."[20] The concepts discussed in this section concern the nature of "realism" and "reality" as they apply to simulation, and the way that these issues relate to the goals of simulation endeavors to generate a complex social undertaking. The ideas and concepts presented here are largely contributed by Peter Dieckmann and his adaptation of broader psychological concepts to simulation in medicine.

Reality and Realism of Simulation

Unless we are dreaming about it or we are an unrepentant solipsist, a simulation exercise is always "real" (it is actually happening), but it may or may not be a "realistic" replication of the reality that is the target of the exercise. Realism addresses the question of how closely a replication of a situation resembles the target. A key distinction is between a *simulator* (a device) and a *simulation* (the exercise in which the device is used). A simulator could be indistinguishable from a real human being (e.g., a standardized patient actor) and yet be used in an implausible and useless fashion. Conversely, certain kinds of realism (see later) can be evoked by simulation exercises that use very simple simulators or even no simulator at all (as in role-playing when the participants in a sense "become the simulator"). Merely creating a realistic simulation does not guarantee that it would have any meaning or utility (e.g., learning).[21,22] A closely related aspect concerns the question of relevance and the social character of simulation.

Three Distinct Dimensions for Simulation Realism

A lot has been written about simulator and simulation realism using a variety of terms and concepts that are subtly different and often overlapping. These include *physical fidelity* (the device replicates physical aspects of the human body), *environmental fidelity* (the simulation room looks like an operating room), *equipment fidelity* (the clinical equipment works like or is the real thing), and *psychological fidelity*[23] (the simulation evokes behaviors similar to the real situation), and a variety of forms of validity, such as *face validity* ("looks and feels" real to participants), *content validity* (the exercise covers content relevant to the target situation), *construct validity* (the simulation can replicate performance or behavior according to predefined constructs about work in real situations), and *predictive validity* (performance during a simulation exercise predicts performance in an analogous real situation).[24,25]

The results of studies trying to investigate roots and effects of simulation "realism" are not conclusive partly because they may each concentrate on a different aspect of this complex whole. It is simply not true that maximum "realism" is either needed or desired for every type of simulation endeavor. For some applications with some target populations, it can be highly advantageous to reduce the realism to heighten the learning experience.[26]

In 2007, we published an article attempting to clarify some issues about realism, reality, relevance, and the purposes of conducting simulations.[21] We applied the model of thinking about reality by the German psychologist Laucken to the realism of simulation.[21] Laucken described three modes of thinking—physical, semantical, and phenomenal, which have been renamed physical, conceptual, and emotional and experiential modes by colleagues in Boston.[27]

Physical Mode

The *physical mode* concerns aspects of the simulation that can be measured in fundamental physical and chemical terms and dimensions (e.g., centimeters, grams, and seconds). The weight of the mannequin, the force generated during chest compressions, and the duration of a scenario all are physical aspects of the simulation reality. Existing simulator mannequins have many "unrealistic" physical elements despite their roughly human shape: they are made of plastic, not flesh and bone; they may have unusual mechanical noises detectable during auscultation of the chest; the "skin" does not change color. Some physical properties are not readily detectable and can be manipulated. Some clinical equipment used in mannequin-based simulation is fully functional and physically identical to the "real thing," although in some cases functional physical limitations may have been introduced for convenience or for safety.[24] Labeled syringes may contain only water instead of opioids, or a real defibrillator may have been modified so that it does not actually deliver a shock (one manufacturer sells a "Hollywood defibrillator"). That certain physical properties and functions have been altered is not usually apparent to participants, at least without special briefings or labels.

Semantical Mode

The *semantical mode* of thinking concerns concepts and their relationships. Within the semantical mode, a simulation of hemorrhage might be described in conceptual terms as "bleeding" of flow rate *X* beginning at time *Y* occurring at site *Z* and associated with a blood pressure of *B* that is a decrease from the prior value of *A*. In this mode of thinking, it is irrelevant how the information is transmitted or represented. The same pieces of *information* could be represented using a vital signs monitor, a verbal description, or the tactile perception of decreasingly palpable pulses. The semantical *recoding* of physical objects is the cornerstone of simulation. It allows the simulation exercise to represent a real situation, and it allows water-filled syringes to be treated as if they contain a drug.

Phenomenal Mode

The *phenomenal mode* deals with the "experience," including emotions and beliefs triggered by the situation. For many purposes, providing high phenomenal realism is the key goal, and the physical realism and semantic realism are merely means to this end.

Relevance versus Reality

A naive view of simulation would suggest that greater realism in all modes would lead to better achievement of the goals of simulation; this view has been criticized repeatedly.[23,28,29] Simulation is a complex social endeavor, conducted with different target populations for different purposes. The relevance of a simulation exercise concerns the match between the characteristics of the exercise and the reasons for which the exercise is conducted. Different elements of realism are emphasized or sacrificed to maximize the relevance of a simulation exercise. When training on invasive procedures, it is typical to forgo phenomenal realism and emphasize physical and semantic realism so that psychomotor skills can be the focus.

Semantic realism may be sacrificed, especially to help early learners. Situations that might become lethal (e.g., trigger a cardiac arrest) very quickly may be slowed down so that inexperienced clinicians can try to think their way out of the problem. If such a situation were allowed to evolve at its normal speed, it would transition to the management of a cardiac arrest before the participants could deal with the original problem. Other realism-sacrificing strategies for early learners include "cognitive scaffolding," providing various forms of assistance or cues to help them as they struggle with decision making and therapy selection. It is important to select which aspects of the simulation are the most relevant to reach the training goal and should be focused on in terms of optimizing their realism in the different modes.

Setting of the Simulation Exercise

Simulation exercises have a purpose and are generally integrated into a larger training context (often a course or a series of exercises), which influences how they are conducted, how they are perceived by participants, and what kind of effects they might have. This context has been called the *simulation setting*. The typical elements of the simulation setting are discussed next and shown graphically in Figure 7-2.

Setting introduction (SI): The introduction delivers general information on how the exercise will be conducted, logistical information, and some of the known pitfalls of the

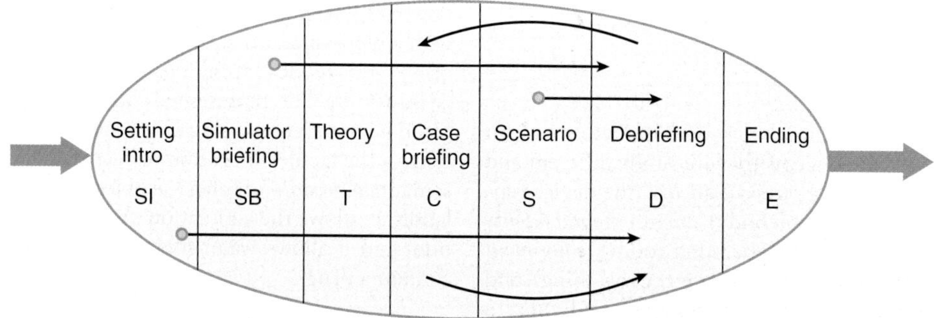

Figure 7-2 The simulator setting. A simulation course consists of different modules or different phases (e.g., setting introduction, simulator familiarization, scenarios, debriefings). This figure shows a typical flow for a course with repeated loops back from debriefing to case briefing for each scenario. The different modules are interrelated, and problems arising in one module can affect other modules (*thin arrows*). For example, it might be difficult to conduct an open, constructive debriefing if the scenario was irrelevant, or the simulator briefing was insufficient, and or the instructor did not succeed in creating an open atmosphere in the beginning of the course. *(Courtesy of Peter Dieckmann.)*

course. Through this introduction and other components of the course, group norms are established explicitly and implicitly.

Simulator briefing (SB) or familiarization: Participants need to be familiar with the simulator and the simulated environment via explanations, demonstrations, and hands-on time. They learn how to use the simulator, what it can and cannot do, what is "normal" (e.g., normal breath sounds), and how they can interact with the environment (e.g., how to call for help, how to request information about the patient that is not directly available in the simulation environment). The familiarization session also is an opportunity for participants to practice the information gathering they must conduct when first entering a new work environment (e.g., for locum tenens practice).

Theory input (T): Most exercises have didactic and theory components on relevant content information. Sometimes this material is made available in advance via readings or online exercises. It may be presented before or after a simulation session. Sometimes there are didactic or group-work modules put in place at different junctures of the course or series.

Breaks (B): For complex courses (e.g., anesthesia crisis resource management [ACRM]), breaks are important for socialization between participants and with instructors. It also is a venue for informal sharing and storytelling.

Case briefing (C): In many simulation scenarios, participants receive a briefing about the upcoming case. Sometimes this is done explicitly before entering the scenario; sometimes it is embedded into a natural "hand-off" of the case from one clinician to another.

Simulation scenario (S): Most simulation exercises involve a scenario that posits a given clinical situation and challenges to be posed for participants to deal with. Commonly, the possible evolutions of the scenario are delineated by instructors in advance, although occasionally an intrinsically challenging situation is started and then allowed to play out naturally depending on how the participants react.

Debriefing (D): Most scenarios are followed by some form of debriefing or feedback. In some courses, there is only minimal feedback, whereas in others there is a dedicated debriefing session (as long or longer than the scenario itself) after each scenario. (See the section on debriefing for more detail.)

Ending (E): Especially for multiple-scenario courses, there may be a separate final session to end the course. This is an opportunity to summarize issues that were covered, to address questions, and to consider how best to apply the principles covered to real patient care.

Components of a course are expected to have a cumulative effect. Similarly, problems in early portions of a course (e.g., inability to create an open learning atmosphere during the introduction) can carry over into later phases. Inadequate familiarization briefings leave participants confused as they try to perform "clinical work" with the patient replaced by a mannequin.

Site of Simulation

Over more than 20 years of experience in simulation, many different variants of simulation have evolved. One particularly rich set of variations is on the site of simulation. The types of "sites" currently in use are described; the advantages and disadvantages of each are summarized in Table 7-2. Many of these variants are not mutually exclusive and can be combined in different hybrids. They are often administratively linked—a simulation group that operates a dedicated center often also conducts in-situ, mobile, and moving patient simulation exercises at various times for different target populations and applications.

Dedicated Simulation Center

One or more simulators are used in a dedicated simulation facility, typically in rooms that can partially or fully replicate, in a relatively generic fashion, various clinical environments (e.g., operating room, ICU, labor and delivery, emergency department). (For more details see the section on Charactistics of Simulation Centers discussed later.)

Table 7-2 Site of Simulation

Site of Simulation	Explanation	Advantages	Disadvantages
Dedicated center	Fixed facility not part of an actual clinical work unit	Equipment permanently installed Facilitates complex audiovisual systems Easy to schedule Personnel not readily "drafted" for clinical work Does not interfere with actual clinical work Multipurpose	Cannot recreate exact work unit, equipment, supplies of diverse target populations May be hard for clinicians to be free to attend training
Temporary in situ	Actual work unit; temporary setup and takedown	Real clinical site Probe or train personnel in their actual work unit, using real equipment and supplies Clinicians can readily attend in proximity to their work	Hard to schedule—may need site for clinical use Interferes with actual clinical work; personnel readily drafted to return to clinical work Great effort of setup and takedown; minimal audiovisual system
Residential in situ	Actual work unit; permanent facility	Same as temporary in situ	Costly to create permanent simulation "bed" in clinical work unit May distract from real clinical work, personnel may be drafted
Patient movement simulations	Transport from site to site is simulated	Transport itself is challenging clinical work Replicates natural flow of patients and handoffs between teams	Requires multiple simulation sites Portable wireless simulators have some technologic limitations
Mobile simulation	Simulation systems and instructor crew travel to client (or neutral) sites	Brings simulation expertise to those who cannot or wish not to invest in it themselves For in-situ use, all advantages thereof	Transport costs can be high (driver, fuel, vehicle) For in-situ use, all disadvantages thereof plus even greater effort for setup and takedown

In-Situ Simulation

In-situ simulation is conducted in an actual clinical workplace; the simulator "replaces" a patient. In-situ simulation is a necessity in the absence of a dedicated center, and can be used in any clinical environment. It is especially useful for unusual workplaces that are difficult to recreate realistically in a simulation center, such as a catheterization laboratory, computed tomography scanner, ambulances, or air rescue aircraft (Figs. 7-3 to 7-9). Most in-situ simulation is performed "mobile" as a temporary setup, but increasingly in-situ simulation is established as "residential simulation," in which a simulator is permanently installed in a clinical workplace (e.g., creating a simulation-specific room in the actual ICU.

Moving Patient Simulation

The advent of completely portable and wireless simulators supports exercises in which the simulated patient can be moved from one clinical site to another. The patient could be brought into the emergency department by ambulance; taken to a computed tomography scanner, interventional radiology, or operating room; and finally transferred to an ICU. Under what circumstances such movements are worth the effort remains to be determined.

Mobile Simulation: "Have Simulator—Will Travel"

Mobile simulation means the simulator and the audiovisual gear are moved (made mobile) outside the originating institution for purposes of the simulation event. In other words, "the simulator comes to the participants." Mobile simulation can be conducted as in-situ simulation in an actual site of a remote client institution, by setting up for simulation in conference rooms or hotel meeting rooms, or by having a simulation facility built into a truck or bus. The built-in mobile facility saves time in setup and takedown, It also is possible to conduct "field exercises" setting up the simulator outside (e.g., in a parking lot or athletic field).

Advantages and Disadvantages of Different Approaches

The advantages and disadvantages of different approaches are summarized in Table 7-2. For sites that lack a dedicated

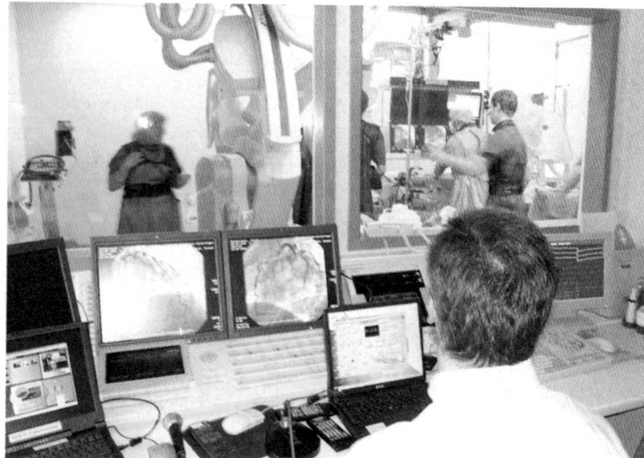

Figure 7-3 In-situ mobile simulation in a catheterization laboratory. The simulator is placed on the catheterization laboratory tables, surrounded by the x-ray machines, complicating the treatment of the patient by limiting space. The vital sign monitor is connected to the real monitors, providing relevant data to the catheterization laboratory team. The simulator is controlled from the catheterization laboratory control room. Multiple mobile cameras and a scan converter for the vital signs provide a live video transmission to a temporary debriefing area for the nonactive part of the training group and allow for CRM-based debriefings. CRM, crisis resource management. *(Picture by team TuPASS, taken at University Hospital, Tübingen, Germany.)*

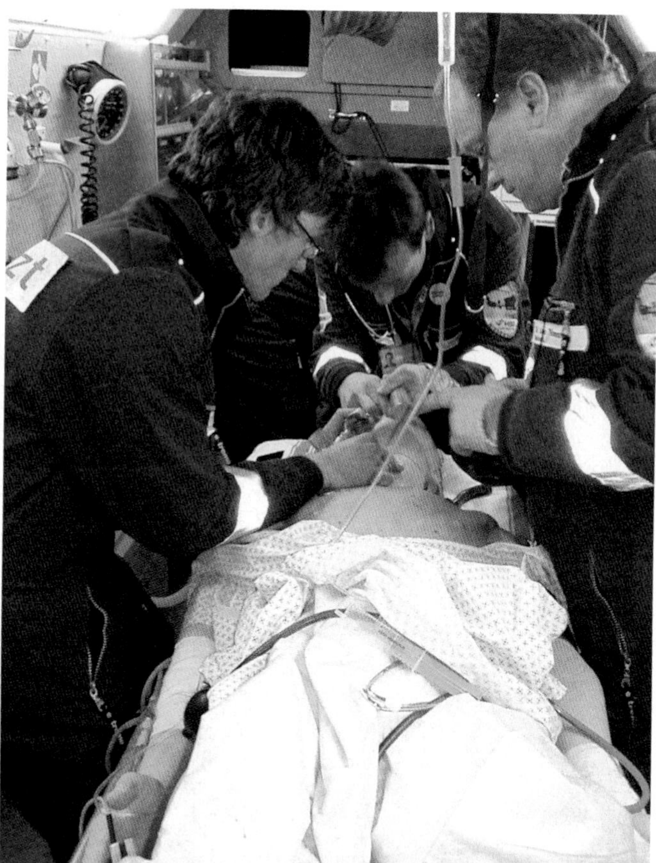

Figure 7-5 In-situ mobile simulation team training in an ambulance. The limitations regarding space to work and move around inside an ambulance are very important. This represents a classic need for in-situ training of prehospital teams (in Germany consisting of three paramedics and a prehospital emergency physician). Also, "take-over scenarios" (e.g., the helicopter team is taking over a patient from the ground-based team) are a challenge for CRM expertise (e.g., information transfer and continuous patient treatment). CRM, crisis resource management. *(Picture by team TuPASS, taken at one of the German Air Rescue centers, Germany.)*

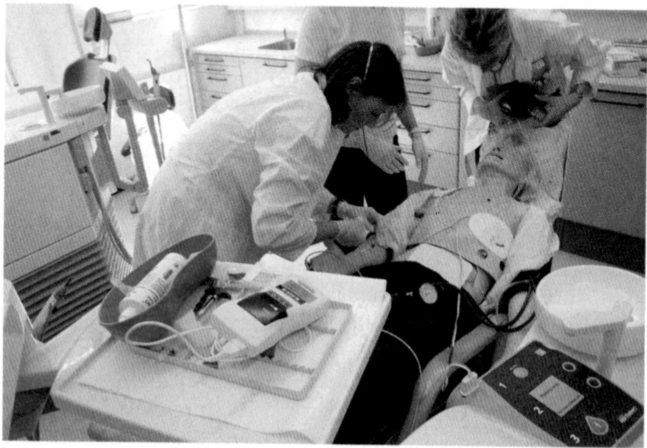

Figure 7-4 In-situ mobile simulation in a dentist chair. The simulator was equipped with artificial teeth gum and a chalk tooth preparation to drill, simulating the dentist's procedures (give anesthetic or drilling). Then emergencies developed, and the team response was trained focusing on CRM key points and important medical aspects, including automated external defibrillator use. CRM, crisis resource management. *(Picture by team TuPASS, taken at University Hospital, Tübingen, Germany.)*

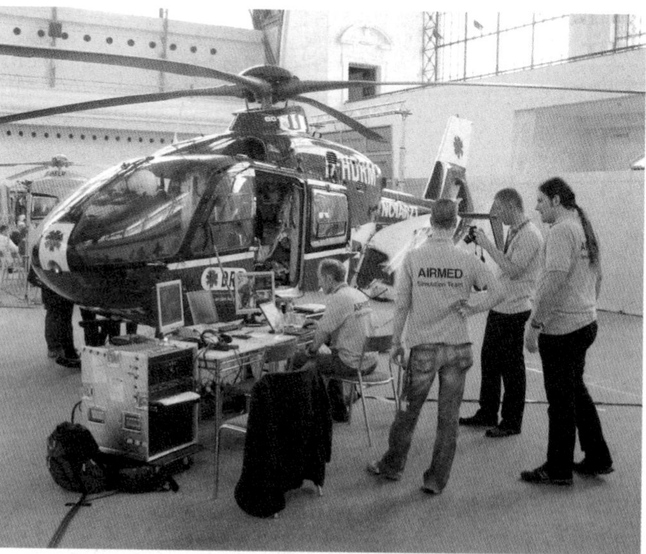

Figure 7-6 In-situ mobile simulation team training in a helicopter. The mobile simulation control room with several cameras and microphones is set up outside the helicopter, also providing a multiperspective view inside to monitor the scenario and react to activities performed. *(Picture by team TuPASS at the German Air Rescue/TuPASS training site at Airmed 2008.)*

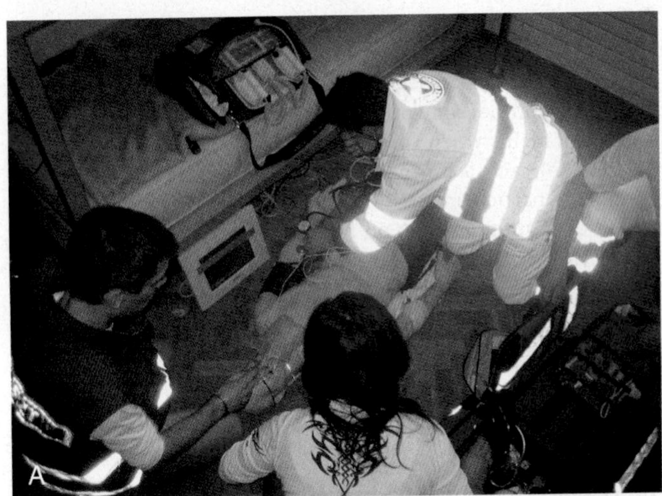

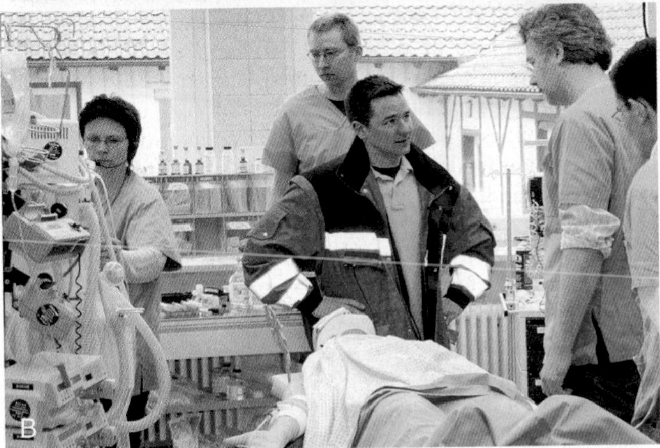

Figure 7-7 **A,** In-situ mobile simulation training in a simulated apartment for prehospital teams. The apartment (living space) scenarios are very common for prehospital teams, requiring adaptation to the local space availability and other circumstances (e.g., bystanders, dogs). **B,** Emergency department simulation with the prehospital team handing over a patient to the hospital staff—always a phase of high-demand and goal-oriented interactions. From a CRM-training perspective, this scenario is a very good opportunity to highlight problems and unsafe practices (in the sense of high reliability), and to show good team performances using video clips of a scenario. CRM, crisis resource management. *(**A,** Picture by team TuPASS at a CRM training session with the South Tyrolian White Cross in Bolzano, Italy. **B,** During an instructor training course at TuPASS, Germany.)*

simulation center, there is no practical alternative to either engage in in-situ simulation or to be a client for mobile simulation. Simulation in the dedicated center facilitates scheduled training and use of complex audiovisual gear. Simulators can be preset, tested, and ready to go. Briefing and debriefing facilities are immediately at hand. In a dedicated center, it is common to use inexpensive discarded, flawed, or outdated clinical equipment and supplies. The major disadvantage to a dedicated center is that regardless of how well equipped it is, it can never replicate the equipment, layout, and clinical processes of actual clinical workplaces. Also, participants know that they are in a simulation center, which may alter their demeanor and reduce the impact of training.

In-situ simulation seems ideal in that it probes and challenges personnel and systems as they actually exist, unmasking real issues of patient care. It is available, in principle, to all sites, even those without a dedicated center, and is conducive to short courses and unannounced mock event drills. In-situ simulation

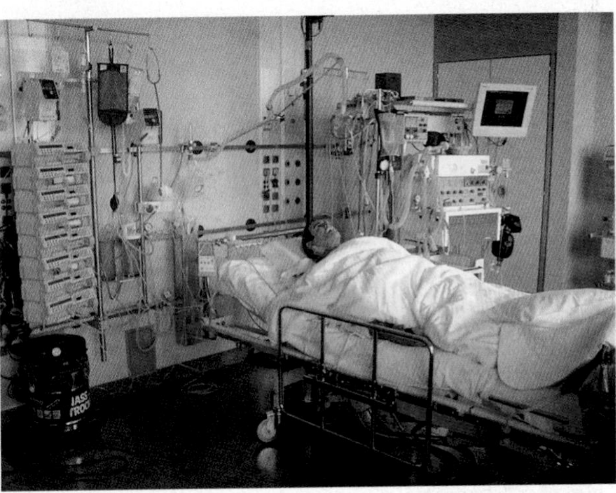

Figure 7-8 In-situ mobile simulation in an intensive care unit (ICU)/ intermediate medical care unit location. The training in actual clinical areas also is especially useful for ICU-like surroundings. CRM-based trainings are very important to highlight the highly complex problems and interactions needed to coordinate high-performing ICU teams. The training also allows for "checking" the local arrangement of equipment and possibilities to react to certain emergencies. There are already a few examples of "residential" in-situ simulation in ICUs (see text). *(Picture by team TuPASS.)*

has disadvantages, however. It is difficult to organize, schedule, and control. The clinical area planned for simulation may not be vacant or may be needed on short notice. The simulations can be distracting to real patient care surrounding them, and the staff engaged in the simulation are prone to being pulled to clinical duty, and there may be constant interruptions of the training sessions. Most clinical supplies must be taken from the stocks of the work unit in order to prevent mix-ups with outdated simulation

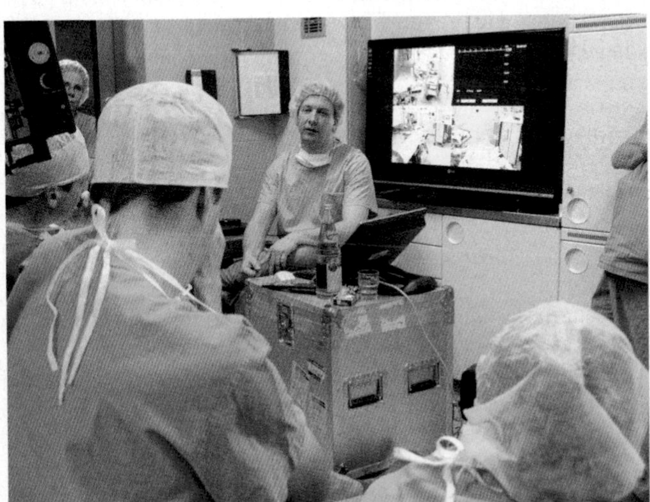

Figure 7-9 In-situ mobile CRM-focused simulation team training inside an actual operating room. The figure shows the debriefing room temporarily set up in an induction room. The use of videos for debriefing (here on a 42-inch flat panel placed over the basin) is highly recommended. Training inside a hospital often includes training actual teams and training a large proportion of employees with the same set-up. These mass training sessions seem to offer a much larger impact and longer lasting effects of the lessons learned, including CRM behaviors (see text on subthreshold training). *(Picture by team TuPASS who performed at a full team training of the Anesthesia department at Steinenberg Medical Center, Reutlingen, Germany.)*

supplies, adding expense. There are major limitations to the audiovisual gear that can be deployed in a real clinical site. A permanent in-situ facility could provide the best of both worlds. Such an arrangement offers unique opportunities, such as the ability to "replay" immediately difficult cases in the simulator "next door," the possibility to use low workload times for spur-of-the-moment simulation sessions, and the ability to conduct long-term simulations (team members responsible for a simulated ICU patient over days or weeks). The major drawback to this approach is that to address diverse clinical domains requires such a site in every domain, and this could be extremely costly.

For dedicated center simulations, single-discipline sessions are simpler logistically because only one discipline needs to be present, rather than scheduling someone from each of the disciplines. In addition, simulations can be applied to some disciplines even in domains where there are not yet credible simulators for the work of each team member. The single-discipline approach may be of particular relevance for trainees who when finished with their training will go on to work in many different settings and with many different kinds of personnel. It also may be of greatest value for individuals who do not work in "fixed" crews or teams and need to acquire generic teamwork skills that can be used with all coworkers.

Team Training, Single Discipline, and Crews

Each discipline in health care can be considered a "crew" containing one or more individuals. Several crews may work together closely as a "team." The operating room team consists of an anesthesia crew, a surgery crew, and a nursing crew (and crews of technicians and support personnel).

Further complementarity exists regarding the homogeneity of the target population in simulations. When the simulation is intended to go beyond specific medical and technical skills for individuals (as in crisis resource management–oriented simulations) and to involve nontechnical skills and teamwork, we distinguish between "single-discipline" approaches ("training crews to work in teams") and true "combined-team" (multidisciplinary) training.

The importance of teamwork and team training is widely accepted,[30-35] although it is still not widely implemented. The prerequisites for effective teamwork (e.g., team leadership, mutual performance monitoring, backup behavior, adaptability and team orientation,[35] and the concept of team cognition) are discussed in Chapter 6.

Single Discipline

Training for single-discipline crews (e.g., anesthesiologists) involves curricula in which all participants are from a single discipline, and other crew members' roles are played either by instructors and confederates or by other simulation participants. This approach allows tailoring simulations to challenge skills, knowledge, and situations specific to the discipline, including material that may be of little relevance to other crews and in the context of a wide variety of types of clinical situations (e.g., cardiac, orthopedic, or general surgery; labor and delivery; intensive care). Single-discipline training can emphasize generic skills of dynamic decision making, resource management, leadership, and teamwork applicable to any challenging clinical situation. In the single-discipline approach, scenarios can be designed that present specific types of personalities and behaviors by other crew or team members, rather than relying on the ad-hoc behavior of real personnel from those disciplines. Even without actual personnel from other disciplines, training crews to work in teams also provides a degree of cross-discipline understanding by allowing participants to discuss other team members' views of the same situation.

Combined Team Training

The complementary approach is to conduct *combined team training*, in which all participants of the team, from crews of several different disciplines (e.g., surgeons, nurses, anesthesiologists), undergo training together. Combined team training allows for more natural team interactions and reinforces understanding across disciplines. There are successful examples of such undertakings in many fields, including obstetrics (combining obstetrics, anesthesia, nursing, neonatology/pediatrics) and intensive care (combining physicians from multiple disciplines with nursing, respiratory therapy, and pharmacy).[32,36-46]

Combined team training may be most effective when a specific group of individuals is to work together clinically as a dedicated team. In dedicated simulation centers, combined team training can be hard to schedule, and it may require instructors from several of the disciplines to conduct the debriefings. Combined team simulations may be easiest to organize when they are conducted as unannounced mock events that activate the actual bedside team (e.g., ward or unit team, rapid response team, or code team). In such situations, the real combined team is mobilized as they would be in real life.

Debriefing for Simulation Training

Debriefing refers to a special time and format for talking about an episode of action in the past; it is the counterpoint to a briefing that occurs before an action or task. The term originally came from the military, for after-action reviews of real missions and simulations. In medicine, the debriefing concept was introduced to simulation training by Gaba and colleagues as part of the whole concept of CRM-based simulation training for anesthesia teams.[16,95] This section focuses on debriefings in the context of simulation team training.

Debriefing—Heart and Soul of Simulation Trainings

In aviation and health care simulations, the debriefing after a simulation team training session is a key element—perhaps the most important element—of simulation training.[47] The debriefing offers an unparalleled instance to reflect and discuss openly and understand other team member's intentions, thoughts, and prob-

Table 7-3 Traditional Teaching versus Facilitation in Simulation Training Courses

Traditional Teaching: "Teacher"	Debriefing Facilitation: "Instructor/Facilitator"
Focus on theoretical knowledge	Focus on human factors and CRM aspects
Focus on what	Focus on why and deeper analysis of why it did (not) work
Teacher is the best (expert)	Instructor just moderates, uses knowledge of participants
Teacher tells participants what to do	Instructor helps participants to find what they could have done and what would be the best way
Teacher knows what is important for participants	Instructor helps to self-reflect and gain realistic self-awareness/consciousness Instructor guides toward interesting areas
Talks most	Stimulates discussion among participants
Domain expert	CRM expert
No teaching training	Extensive instructor training
No video	Use of video of own and others' scenarios
Teacher knows what has been learned (or not)	Instructor might not be aware of all aspects that participants take home

CRM, crisis resource management.

lems. Much of the learning occurs in this self-reflective episode. Eventually, these routines will be applied to clinical medicine (e.g., surgical team timeout).

New Way of Teaching

The debriefing as described in aviation and introduced and refined for medicine by Gaba and others[48,49] requires a complete understanding by instructors of their role in promoting learning (see Chapter 8).[50] The philosophy of teaching and learning in a debriefing of a CRM-based simulation course differs from the traditional clinical teaching style (Table 7-3). The instructor's role is to *facilitate* the learning process, *directing the participants* to the most interesting and important areas for consideration, and *stimulating discussion* among participants to *find the underlying issues* and to seek solutions for future events of similar type.

Facilitation is a new way of teaching and often must be learned anew by instructors, even though they have many years of traditional teaching experience. The use of video for debriefing can advance further the self-reflective component of debriefings, but requires additional expertise to integrate it successfully with self-reflection. Generally, faculty intending to be primary debriefers need special training and practice in this teaching method (see section on Instructor Qualification). Several simulation centers conduct instructor training that emphasizes debriefing skills.

Technique of Debriefing

Although debriefing styles and philosophies differ at centers around the world, a common ground is shared by most centers: A debriefing should *stimulate self-reflection*, and analyze *how* something happened, and what the *underlying concepts* for doing so were, rather than merely finding out *what* happened. Usually the debriefing lasts at least as long as the scenario itself.

Detailed discussions about the different techniques appear in the literature.[47,48,50-54] To prepare a good debriefing, the instructor is challenged during the scenario with performing several tasks in the control room, such as listening to trainees, talking to the instructor team, controlling the simulator, and making notes for the debriefing. Figure 7-10 illustrates the different levels of attendance.

Debriefings by nature have different phases, as shown in Table 7-4. The phases are not meant to be followed in this time sequence and order. Often two or more phases are covered regarding one problem of the scenario—especially clinical problems are often covered while discussing the "how" and "when" they happened (analysis). Then another problem is analyzed and discussed according to different phases. Nevertheless, at the end of a good debriefing, all phases should have been covered according to their respective importance. No debriefing style is associated with a proven better learning outcome, and there may never be defini-

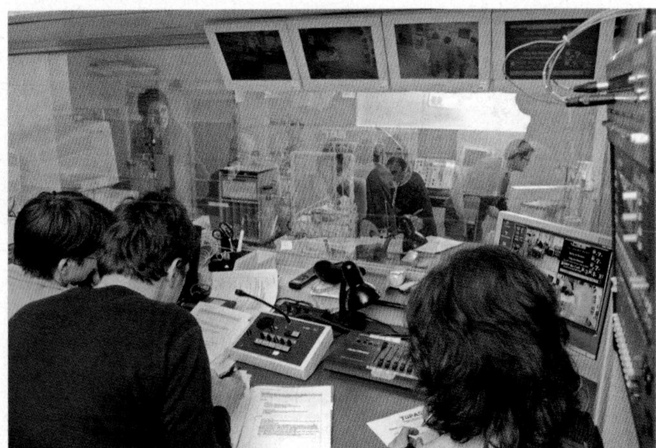

Figure 7-10 The multiple levels of work for CRM-based instructors in the control room. The reflections in the one-way mirror of the control room make the multiple levels of activity transparent. The team of instructors has to control the simulation as such, but also make notes for the CRM-based debriefing. The scenario inside and the audio streams (telephone call) need to be monitored. Also, the instructors have to deal with simulation team role players and instructor trainees inside the control room. These complex tasks need some training and good team organization on the side of the simulation center team. CRM, crisis resource management. *(Picture by B. Schaedle, team TuPASS, taken at a PaedSim training at University Hospital, Tubingen, Germany.)*

Table 7-4 Phases of Debriefings: Issues Relevant to CRM-based Simulation Debriefing

Phase of Debriefing	Explanation
Ending the scenario	When possible, the scenario should not be stopped too early. Participants should be allowed to realize the natural end of the scenario. Ideally, it should not be terminated when participants are in the thick of it
Scenario-to-debriefing transition	Most sites use a "hot" debriefing, in which they enter the debriefing room immediately from the simulation room. This allows the instructor to hear and see participants' direct reactions. Another option is to give the participants a few minutes to discuss the scenario itself while the instructor is planning the debriefing
Emotional venting	All participants who were actively involved are given the opportunity to say how they *felt* during the scenario. This vents pent-up feelings, and may be a time to deal with anomalies in the scenario (e.g., simulator malfunction)
Descriptive phase	Participants describe what happened (or portions of the video are replayed). Different points of view (e.g., hot seat versus first responder versus surgeon confederate) are shared
Self-identification of issues	It can be useful, before anyone else including the instructor is allowed to critique the scenario, to allow active participants to say if they themselves detected any errors or actions that they would do differently. It can be painful and rude to critique participants about something they are aware of themselves
Discussion of clinical content	Any major issues of clinical treatment and related CRM points should be covered. A debriefing should not end without discussing and clarifying any significant clinical errors, and ensuring that participants understand the correct management
Analysis	Debriefings should provide considerable "analysis" of *why* things happened vis-à-vis the intentions of all parties, and alternatives and their pros and cons
Opportunities for systems improvement	Based on the analyses, participants can be asked to suggest how the system can be changed to improve the handling of similar situations in the future
Transfer to the "real world"	Participants can discuss how lessons from the scenario or debriefing can be applied in the real clinical world. They should discuss barriers to improvement and ways to overcome them
Providing a "take-home message" from the scenario and debriefing	A summary of the key points of the debriefing can be useful, either by the instructor or the participants themselves
Terminating the debriefing	Debriefings are rich in content and could extend beyond the time available. Marking the end of the debriefing can be a useful transition to preparing for the next scenario or to the end-of-day activities

CRM, crisis resource management.

tive data on the techniques because of the nature of the topic—reflective practice of high-level cognition.

Use of Video for Debriefings

Although the value is not proven, segments of video recordings to support and deepen the debriefing as a learning and self-awareness experience are frequently used. Anesthesia does not allow for much self-reflection and feedback during routine clinical work. Experienced colleagues typically work alone, and there is often little feedback from other anesthesiologists or from other operating room personnel. This situation is now changing, however, with the use of automatic anesthetic records and information technology (see Chapters 2, 4, 5, and 99).

The lack of feedback leaves a large theoretical gap between the way individuals think they perform and how they do act in reality. Video sequences can correct this gap and provide an awareness of how participants have really acted. Also, one's own video recordings can be compared with the recordings of other participants (either their own course co-participants or "trigger videos" meant to stimulate discussion). "Live transmission" of scenarios to participants not actively involved in the scenario also is useful. When this technique is used, the observers can be given special tasks (e.g., look for CRM key points 10 and 11 in Table 7-8). A study in Tübingen evaluated the use of so-called cooperation scripts in the "passive" phase of watching others perform.

The video should be used in the service of the debriefing, rather than the other way around. The authors believe that if the discussion is active and on-target, it is useless to interrupt it just to show video. Video may have a bigger impact for participants' first simulation experiences. Here they are sometimes struck by what can be revealed on seeing themselves and others work. As they gain more experience with simulation, and when debriefers are experienced, they may not need exposure to the video to hone in on key issues to discuss.

Clinical Application of Debriefing Method

The application of the above-described debriefing techniques to the discussion of real world clinical critical incidents seems very promising. Applying the debriefing technique learned in the simulator after a critical incident in short debriefing circles of the involved clinical team has proven quite valuable.[41,50,55-58]

Scenario Design

The design of scenarios for interactive simulation team trainings is demanding and typically differs from preparing training exercises for traditional curricula, such as "mega codes" in advanced life support. Full simulation scenarios are complex enough that their design is usually an iterative process by which the scenarios are continually improved through experience.

This section can give only an overview of the important aspects of scenario design for realistic simulation team training. The reader is referred to detailed published examples of scenarios in *Simulation in Healthcare*[59] and to more detailed literature about the principles of scenario design.[3,60] The topic also is covered extensively in most of the instructor training curricula that are offered at sites around the world. International and regional simulation meetings often offer workshops on scenario design (IMSH of SSiH, SESAM); the user groups of the major simulator manufacturers also have workshops on the topic. (See section on Simulation Societies discussed later.)

Goal Oriented

Scenarios usually are designed to achieve learning objectives or other goals, such as a formal needs analysis of the relevant target group for training concerning clinical and technical skills or nontechnical CRM skills or both (see Chapter 6). Alternatively, simulation-savvy clinician educators may intuitively know what kinds of scenarios are likely to be valuable for their participant populations, or they may have learned about good examples in their instructor training or in the literature. The cases are not as important as the nature of the underlying challenges that they pose to participants. *Train the causes not the cases.*

Scenarios should be relevant to the trainees. This relevance is more important than realism and depends on many factors, including the trainees' backgrounds and experience, and the method of conducting the scenario and related parts of the simulation course (e.g., familiarization, case briefing, role players).

Constraints and Limitations

It is easy to suggest a scenario on paper but more difficult to translate it into an effective scenario for actual use. There are limitations and constraints to consider, including features and limitations of the simulators available, personnel resources at hand, the props or external systems that would be needed to engage participants, and time available for the proposed scenario. In our experience, most scenarios are first generated with an idea or a "nubbin." The idea is fleshed out by discussion and on paper in an iterative fashion, with limitations addressed either by creative redesign of the proposed situation or by minor technical modifications using the simulator software or simulation environment. The new scenario usually is tested out first by instructors and "simulationists" (the technical staff who operate the simulators and prepare the environment). It can be pilot tested with a volunteer group of participants from the target population. The first one or two sessions typically reveal many problems and flaws in the original scenario layout. After a scenario has been designed and tested, it is advisable to add comments and suggestions for improvement continuously after each training session.

Scenario Templates

Many centers have developed templates for the design of their scenarios. Figure 7-11 is an example of a summary sheet of the template used by TuPASS and taught during their instructor courses. The full version of it is available online (www.tupass.de/scenarioscript.html). Other scenario templates are popular, including the Duke University template (http://simcenter.duhs.duke.edu/SimTemplate1203.doc). The peer-reviewed journal *Simulation in Healthcare* publishes "Simulation Case Reports," which contain detailed scenario descriptions. Some professional societies have created scenario repositories for members; the American Society of Anesthesiologists (ASA) Simulation Committee has a repository for scenarios to be shared between its ASA-endorsed simulation programs.

Instructor Qualification

Teaching with simulation covers a diverse spectrum of applications. In some cases, it is similar to teaching at the bedside, only the patient is a simulator, in which case the skills needed are nearly identical to those used in ordinary clinical supervision and teaching. There are special implications for instructing in courses that involve complex realistic scenarios, with multiple personnel in crews and teams, using video-facilitated debriefings in small groups, and with a focus on human factors and CRM principles and countermeasures. In such courses, the skills needed to be a successful instructor go considerably beyond those typically used by teaching clinicians. Quality of the instructors is *the* key element for any simulation course, captured by the statement "The key is the program, not the hardware."[10] Ensuring instructor competence in using simulation and in debriefing facilitation skills is very important.

Advanced simulation course formats generally reflect very well Kolb's[60a] circle of adult experiential learning: (1) self-experience (participate in the scenario) or vicarious experience (observe scenario live), (2) reflect on experience (debriefing), (3) abstract conceptualization (debriefing, relate to theoretical material), and (4) active experimentation (future scenarios and use of skills in real cases) (Fig. 7-12).

Tasks of Instructors

The tasks of a simulation instructor differ from the tasks of a classic medical educator or a trainer for part-task or skills training. The most prominent differences are the following:

- Need to brief the course participants about an unfamiliar environment
- Creation of relevant, plausible scenarios to reach the intended learning goals
- Theatrical aspects of enacting complex realistic scenarios
- Need for simultaneous control of the simulator, the simulation personnel (instructors, actors, and confederates), and learning objectives during multiperson complex scenarios with built-in problems and challenges and an uncertain flow pathway of action by participants
- Need to provide debriefing and feedback after the scenario, often assisted by replay of video recordings, primarily using a "facilitation style" in small groups; handling group dynamics and individual sensitivities is required

TuPASS Scenario Script Developed by P. Dieckmann & M. Rall, TuPASS, Germany		
Quick reference: Scenario name		
Major problem	Medicine	CRM
Learning goal	Medicine	CRM
Narrative description		
Staffing	Simulator team	Participants
Case briefing	All participants	"Hot seats" only
Simulator setup Mannequin preparation		
Room setup		
Simulator operation		
Scenario lifesavers		
Props needed		

Figure 7-11 The TuPASS Scenario Design Template. The figure shows the summary page of the TuPASS Scenario Design Template, which has more space and details in the full version. The template also includes a script to explain the different fields and their best use. The template is a regular part of the instructor training courses. It can be obtained from the TuPASS webpage (www.tupass.de/scenarioscript.html). *(Template by P. Dieckmann and M. Rall, TuPASS, Germany.)*

- Concentration largely on CRM nontechnical skills of decision making, team management, interpersonal relationships, communication, and professionalism

Instructor Training

For such complex instructor skills, formal training seems warranted. One of the authors (D.G.) pioneered instructor training for CRM-oriented simulation courses in a consortium of the VA–Stanford Simulation Center with the Boston Center for Medical Simulation and the University of Toronto Sunnybrooke Simulation Center. This consortium spread the ideas and format of CRM simulation instructor training around the world. Another author (M.R.) has been running instructor courses in cooperation with a third author (P.D.) for more than 1,000 international participants. Many institutions offer different instructor courses nationally and internationally (ranging from 2 to 6 days in length depending on the course and its scope); the reader is referred to the simulation societies for information about such courses (SSiH, SESAM). The process and impact of instructor training are being evaluated much as the process of simulation training itself is being assessed. Some early evidence is emerging that such courses have value. Also, shorter introductory courses on instructor skills are offered every year at the international health care simulation meetings (e.g., SSH's IMSH conference or the SESAM annual meeting), and there are many workshops at the meeting that cover topics such as debriefing, instructor training, and CRM training.

Table 7-5 presents an example of learning objectives for an instructor training course. For experiences and effects of the instructor course by P. Dieckmann and one of the authors (M.R.), a poster presented at the IMSH 2006 with a short description of the InFacT course and results from a response-shift bias analysis can be downloaded from our website (www.tupass.de/downloads/InFacT.html). The most difficult task for traditional medical teachers is to learn to stop "instructing" and start "facilitating"—guiding participants toward a deep learning experience.

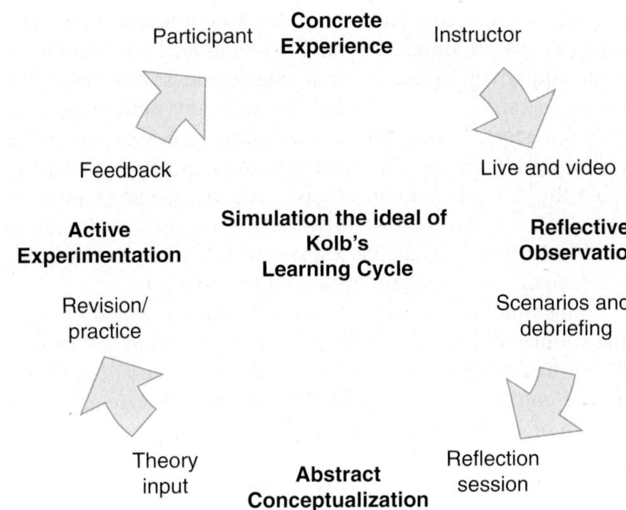

Figure 7-12 Simulation team training with live video transmission as an "ideal" representation of Kolb's learning circle. During the scenario, trainees get a hands-on experience. This is actively reflected in the debriefing. The live video to the nonactive group in the current scenario allows useful reflective observation. During the debriefing, all trainees have a phase of conceptualization, in which the instructor uses generalizations of factors and root causes to show how behavior developed as it did in the scenario (deep learning). During the feedback in the debriefing, but also in the next active scenarios, participants have opportunities to apply and experiment with the newly learned input. *(Figure by P. Dieckmann, modified from Kolb. DA: Experimental learning: Experience as the source of learning and development. Englewood Cliffs, NJ: Prentice Hall, 1984.)*

Certification of Instructors

The original simulation instructors were self-taught in these skills. Should instructors receive documented formal training and certification? CRM-oriented simulation training is probably the most difficult level to achieve. Many institutions have internal systems of levels of training for simulation instructors; they have their own mechanisms for assessing instructor skills and moving instructors up the levels of instructor competency. There is at this time, however, no guideline or agreement regarding criteria for advancement from one level to another.

Table 7-5 Learning Objectives for CRM-oriented Simulation Instructor Courses*

Understand how it feels to be a participant in a simulation scenario, and to be debriefed in a group, seeing oneself on video
Understand the interdependent influence of the different course phases (see Fig. 7-2), and apply this knowledge to a simulation course
Reflect on the changing instructional styles that can be applicable to simulation courses (instruction—facilitation)
Understand basic concepts of human factors, systems theory, and organizational safety
Be able to detect, explain, and discuss CRM key points in the debriefing of scenarios
Use recorded video of scenarios well, selecting the most relevant portions for replay and discussion
Be able to facilitate a debriefing in a nonjudgmental atmosphere with appropriate boundaries
Understand how to manage the individual sensitivities and group dynamics of participants during debriefing
Be able to focus debriefing on the analysis of what happened, why things happened the way they did, and how to apply these lessons to real patient care

*Adapted from the learning objectives of old instructor courses by the authors and P. Dieckmann.

Certification of instructors is just one piece of a larger puzzle of the certification of simulation centers and programs and the certification of specific simulation-based curricula. The ASA in 2008 started a process to endorse (as opposed to accredit or certify) reputable simulation programs capable of delivering high-quality continuing medical education (CME) to ASA members. The Society for Simulation in Healthcare is planning an accreditation program for simulation centers to be accredited in one or more of the areas of assessment, research, training, and patient safety integration. Various other organizations have started or are considering starting similar programs. Specialty and subspecialty societies within anesthesia (including the ASA Simulation Committee) are considering defining one or more uniform curricula to be offered at accredited or approved programs.

It is likely that the skills and certification needed for an instructor would vary greatly with the particular course or curriculum being taught. Competence in conducting a video-based CRM debriefing would not be needed, and would not help, to teach central line placement using part-task trainers for this procedure, and vice versa. Instructor certification probably would be tied to the specific types of courses each individual is capable of conducting. A tiered instructor certification system also would likely provide for advancement from novice instructor to grand master as experience and special training are acquired.

Classification of Patient Simulators

No accepted classification scheme has been devised for the use of patient simulators in anesthesia. Any classification involves some overlapping and gray areas.[19] Cumin and Merry[61] have published a review about available simulators. The following classification and definitions are used in this chapter. In addition to simulators, there are computer-assisted instruction programs and computer-based training devices. Although training devices may replicate certain portions of the clinical domain, they do not attempt to replicate the bulk of the work environment. Some individuals consider the screen-only microsimulator (also known as a screen-based simulator) to be a training device and not a simulator. Computer-assisted instruction programs and training devices are not reviewed in this chapter. This chapter addresses patient simulators in anesthesia that present the overall patient as would be seen by anesthesiologists, intensivists, or others. Devices related purely to emergency medicine (e.g., ResusSim), surgical or procedural simulators that present only the technical work of surgery or invasive manipulations (e.g., bronchoscopy, intravenous access), and partial-task screen-based simulators (e.g., GasMan) are not discussed here.

In this chapter, a *patient simulator* is a system that presents a patient and a clinical work environment of immediate relevance to anesthesiologists (e.g., operating room, postanesthesia care unit, ICU) in one of the following ways:

1. In actual physical reality, defined as a mannequin-based simulator (former and still commonly used synonyms are full-scale simulator, hands-on simulator, realistic simulator, high-fidelity simulator). These simulators can be subdivided in terms of the way that vital signs monitoring is accomplished (interfacing to real clinical monitoring devices or using its own virtual replica of a monitor screen) and in terms of the primary control logic of the simulator (by individual controls and scripts or by using physiologic and pharmacologic modeling).
2. On a computer screen only, defined as a screen-only or screen-based simulator (some prefer the term microsimulator).
3. Using virtual reality, defined as a virtual reality simulator. In such a device, parts or all of the patient and environment are presented to the user by three-dimensional representations with or without "touch" to create a more "immersive" experience. A screen-only simulator could be viewed as a very limited virtual reality simulator.

Components of a Patient Simulator

A patient simulator system contains several components (Fig. 7-13).[19] A set of outputs make up a representation of the patient, the clinical environment, and diagnostic and therapeutic equipment. For screen-only simulators, this representation is generated graphically on the computer screen. For mannequin-based simulators, the representation is generated by using a patient mannequin, plus either actual clinical equipment or virtual replicas of monitor screens, placed (typically) in a recreation of an actual clinical setting. The mannequin and, where appropriate, the clinical equipment are stimulated or actuated by interface hardware. Mannequin-based simulators often use physical stimulation of clinical equipment in addition to electronic stimulation. The mannequin can actually be ventilated with any desired mixture of inspired gases. Carbon dioxide and other gases can be introduced physically by the simulator into the mannequin's lungs to provide the desired elements of gas exchange. A real respiratory gas analyzer can be used to measure the inspired and expired gases. The currently available features of full-scale, mannequin-based patient simulators are presented in Table 7-6.

Any simulator must have control logic by which changes in the simulated patient's condition can be generated, controlled, and sent to the appropriate output of the representation. Originally, the control logic was embedded in the software as a fixed sequence of events, or it consisted largely of continuous input from the instructor working from a script. Some current simulators use upgraded types of manual control logic that allows scripting of combinations of changes in control input. Other current simulators incorporate a more sophisticated technique using mathematical differential equations that model a patient's physiology and pharmacology to provide the bulk of the control logic. These models can be tailored to represent different patients with different pathophysiologic abnormalities.

Not all states or changes in a patient can be modeled by differential equations. Ventricular fibrillation is a totally different state of heart rhythm that does not evolve continuously from normal rhythms. No model can predict exactly when a patient will have a myocardial infarction or when an ischemic heart will begin to fibrillate. A model can only predict factors that increase the likelihood of such events. Most simulators incorporate other modeling techniques in addition to the basic physiologic and pharmacologic mathematical equations, including finite-state

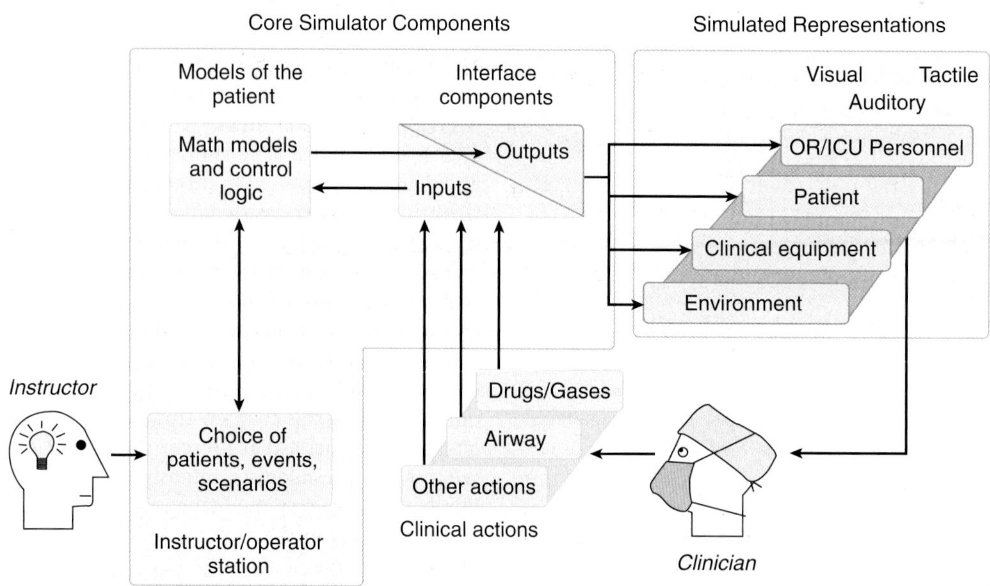

Figure 7-13 Schematic diagram of the generic architecture of patient simulator systems. The simulator generates a representation of the patient and the work environment with appropriate interface hardware, display technologies, or both. The representation is perceived by the anesthesiologist, whose actions are input to the simulator through physical actions or input devices. The behavior of the simulated scenario is manipulated by the instructor or operator through a workstation that allows selection of different patients, abnormal events, and other features of the simulated patient. The control may be manual, script-based, or model-based with manual adaptation to reach optimal learning outcomes. ICU, intensive care unit; OR, operating room. *(Figure by D.M. Gaba, Stanford.)*

Table 7-6 Functionality of Current Mannequin-based Simulator Systems

Clinical Area	Features and Functions	Remarks
Airway	Appropriate pharyngeal and glottic anatomy Placement of facemask, ETT, LMA, LT, Combitube Laryngospasm, tongue and airway swelling, cervical immobility, jaw closure, breakable teeth Cricothyrotomy Transtracheal jet ventilation Bronchial anatomy (to the lobar bronchus level)	Airway often provides acceptable seal for ETT, LMA, Combitube and LT Facemask seal is often difficult as well as placement of ETT
Head	Eyelid movement, pupil dilation, and reaction to light or medications Patient voice and sounds such as coughing and vomiting (through built-in loudspeaker) Palpable carotid pulses Cyanosis by blue light Tearing	Sweating as prototype available The authors prefer "live" voice over prerecorded audio clips, due to higher flexibility in scenarios
Chest	Physiologic and pathophysiologic heart and breath sounds Spontaneous breathing with chest wall movement Bronchospasm Adjustable pulmonary compliance Adjustable airway resistance Pneumothorax Needle thoracotomy and chest tube placement Defibrillation, transthoracic pacing ECG Chest compressions	Breath and heart sounds through loudspeakers; sounds contain artifacts and mechanical noise. Often sound level depends on position of stethoscope relative to loudspeaker
Extremities	Palpable pulses (dependent on arterial pressure) Cuff blood pressure by auscultation, palpation, or oscillometry Modules for fractures and wound modules Intravenous line placement Thumb twitch in response to peripheral nerve stimulation Arm movement Representations of tonic clonic spells	Still very limited movement capabilities at best (as of 2008)
Monitoring (waveforms or numerical readouts)	ECG (including abnormalities in morphology and rhythm) SpO_2 Invasive blood pressure CVP, PAP, PCWP Cardiac output Temperature CO_2 (may be actual CO_2 exhalation) Anesthetic gases (may have actual uptake and distribution of agents) Cardiopulmonary bypass	Simulators interface to actual clinical monitors or provide a simulated virtual vital signs display (or both); may include a virtual heart-lung machine
Automation and sensors	Chest compressions Ventilation rate and volume Defibrillation and pacing (including energy measurement) Gas analyzer (inspired O_2, anesthetics) Drug recognition (drug identification and amount)	Quality of sensors varies greatly from rough ventilation yes/no to almost realistic ventilation loops, etc.

Note: The features listed are each present in some existing simulators, but not all features are present on any single device. Sets of features depend on the device and model.

CVP, central venous pressure; ECG, electrocardiogram; ETT, endotracheal tube; LMA, laryngeal mask airway; LT, larynx tube; PAP, positive airway pressure; PCWP, pulmonary capillary wedge pressure.

Table 7-7 Desirable Features of Future Mannequin-based Simulator Systems

Advanced skin signs such as Change in skin color to cyanotic or pale Diaphoresis Change in skin temperature (e.g., as a result of shock or fever) Rash, hives, or generalized edema
Regurgitation, vomiting, airway bleeding or secretions
Physical coughing (currently only sounds are simulated)
Realistic convulsions
Purposeful movements of extremities
Support for spinal, epidural, or other regional anesthesia procedures
EEG signals (e.g., for BIS, AEP, PSI)
Intracranial pressure
Support for physical central venous and arterial cannulation
Fetal/maternal cardiotocogram

Note: This table shows what features are not currently incorporated (April 2008). Some features may be under development and could be available after publication of this book. In addition, some features are currently available as third-party or homemade add-ons.
AEP, auditory evoked potential; BIS, bispectral index; EEG, electroencephalographic; PSI, patient state index.

models, instructor initiation of abnormal events, and manual modulation of modeled parameters. In finite-state models, different underlying clinical states are defined, each of which has appropriate entry conditions and transition conditions to other states. When an entry or transition condition is met, a new state becomes active, which may directly trigger new observable phenomena (e.g., ventricular fibrillation), or may alter constants in the mathematical models that then evolve in time.[62-64]

The control logic of most simulators is manipulated through an instructor/operator's station that allows the instructor to create specific patients, select and implement abnormal events and faults, and monitor the progress of the simulation session. The system may have a remote-controlled, hand-held instructor/operator's station in addition to the main instructor/operator's station. The instructor/operator's station typically provides logs of physiologic changes and the anesthesiologist's response, and may provide graphics to support the analysis of a simulation run. Some screen-based simulators provide advice and tutorials linked to the management of simulated events. With mannequin-based simulators, especially for applications in which complete work environments are recreated, it is common to obtain detailed records of the simulation and the actions taken from video and audio recording of the personnel working in the replicated clinical environment.

Modern simulators still do not provide many of the desired features listed in Table 7-7. Many different simulator systems are available. No single system is the best choice for all uses, so the decision about the type of simulator required must be based on the objectives and needs of the application. In our experience, the success of a simulator program would not be determined primarily by the type or fidelity of the simulator used, but mostly by the enthusiasm, skill, and creativity of instructors, and the time and effort devoted to preparing and performing credible simulation scenarios.[28]

Virtual Reality Simulators

Virtual reality refers to a set of techniques in which one interacts with a synthetic (*virtual*) environment that exists solely in the computer.[65] In the typical conception of virtual reality, representation of the synthetic environment is fed directly to the eyes (three-dimensional head-mounted displays), the ears, and possibly the hands and limbs (special instrumented "gloves" and sensors). The actions of the user in the environment are translated directly from typical physical activities, not through manipulating a special pointing device. Realization of this ideal is a continuum involving compromises in these input/output modalities. At one end of the continuum, which we call a *complete virtual reality simulation,* the participant is immersed in a virtual world that fully replicates at least three sensory inputs—full three-dimensional vision, hearing, and touch (the last is more technically known as a haptic/kinesthetic system)[65]—and allows complete physical interaction with the world. The "Holodeck" of "Star Trek" would be an example.

At the other extreme of the continuum is a screen-based simulator that generates a limited virtual setting, restricting its output to a screen display, and provides interaction with the virtual world only through a pointing device. Screen-based simulators provide an interface to the human sensory system that is very far from physical reality, whereas a complete virtual reality simulation may be, in its most advanced form, nearly indistinguishable from the real world. A "partial" virtual reality simulator would replicate fewer senses (or less complete replication, such as a three-dimensional visual representation on a two-dimensional screen) or could restrict physical interaction with the world, or both. Finally, one can imagine hybrids of realistic simulators and virtual reality simulators (sometimes called *mixed reality*) in which the virtual reality representation is overlaid onto a real physical environment.

Some surgical and procedural part-task trainers/simulators, such as those used for laparoscopic, endoscopic, or endovascular procedures, might be considered virtual reality because the real procedure is performed only using a two-dimensional television display that can be recreated by the simulator. A comprehensive virtual reality patient simulator would be very complicated, however, because it requires the following:

- Complete computer model of the patient, the environment, and the function of every object in the environment that could be used (e.g., monitoring devices, carts)
- Means of tracking visual, audio, and touch fields of the user to determine what is to be displayed, and to identify what physical actions are being performed
- Appropriate display hardware for every sensory modality and appropriate input hardware for each action pathway (e.g., touch, speech)
- Hardware to compute all the models, to conduct the tracking, and to produce all the output to the display hardware in real time

Immersive virtual reality is a rapidly developing field. It has stimulated intense interest in numerous domains, particularly space flight, the military, and entertainment. Although the potential of this approach is very exciting, virtual reality is still under development. Prototype virtual reality patient simulators in anesthesia or intensive care have been discussed informally, but as of this writing, there is no published experience with any meaningful immersive virtual reality patient simulation system.

A related type of simulation is the virtual environment or virtual world. According to the Wikipedia, a virtual world is a computer-based simulated environment intended for its users to inhabit and interact via "avatars" (users' graphical [often perspective three-dimensional] representation of their "selves"). Such systems typically allow multiple participants each to control simultaneously over a network their own avatar (including speech) and to interact verbally and by virtual physical actions within a commonly perceived virtual environment. This technology currently portrays the virtual world as perspective three-dimensional images on a computer screen plus sound. Virtual worlds have been commonly used for games (the popular "World of Warcraft" game has 9 million monthly subscribers), whereas other virtual worlds encompass online communities (e.g., "Second Life," in which the primary activity is socializing, although commerce and education take place).

In a medical virtual world, the patient may be an automated avatar controlled by the computer, or the patient may be an avatar inhabited by a human participant (an unusual case of a standardized patient actor). Virtual worlds are starting to be used in health care, especially concerning acute care settings such as the ICU, the emergency department, or field resuscitation.

Although virtual reality simulators have many theoretical advantages over screen-based and mannequin-based simulators (e.g., more overall realism in some cases, instantaneous reset of the environment), these advantages are currently offset by the immaturity of the field. Despite considerable hype about virtual reality, such systems are now either very limited in capability or very expensive, and in most cases, they are limited and expensive. A true virtual reality *immersion* experience in a patient care setting comparable to that obtainable with a mannequin-based simulator is not yet on the horizon. Nonetheless, it is likely that virtual reality techniques eventually will eclipse other types of simulators. More than 15 years ago, we (D.G.) predicted this would occur by 2020, but the rate of development of immersive virtual reality has been slower than expected.[66,67]

Development of Patient Simulators

The descriptions given in the following sections are very brief, and the introduction of new or upgraded features in all the simulation systems continues steadily. For up-to-date information about any of the current systems, the reader is advised to contact the manufacturers or authors directly.

The history of the development of patient simulators—particularly the mannequin-based simulators that are in wide use—is well covered in several more recent review articles and book chapters.[5,68-70] The history is of some relevance to anesthesiology because of the dominant role played by anesthesiologists in the early developments in mannequin-based simulation. Anesthesiologists continue to play a major role in this field today, far out of proportion to their numbers relative to other medical domains.

In the late 1960s, a mannequin-based simulator—Sim One—was produced by an aerospace company working with anesthesiologists at the University of Southern California. For that era, it was a technologic marvel and was years ahead of its time.[71] The Sim One project drifted into oblivion, however, largely because the medical professions were not ready to understand the applicability of simulation to key issues of training, research, and assessment, especially regarding the importance of human factors.

Several patient simulators were developed and introduced in the mid to late 1980s. Each was an independent development, and none had any direct connection with the Sim One project. Several factors led to these advances. Most prominent was the new availability of powerful (comparable to advanced minicomputers of a decade earlier) personal computers (PCs) at a relatively cheap price. The popularity of various simulators for PCs (e.g., flight simulators, driving simulators) showed that simulation of complex systems was possible with a PC, and a screen-based simulator could give users some degree of "feel" that they had been in the environment. On the applications side, the public and the anesthesia profession had become more aware of the utility of simulation-based training for military and commercial aviation, space flight, automobile driving, shipping, military command and control, and the operation of nuclear power plants. Media coverage of the space program and corrective responses to the Three Mile Island nuclear power plant accident highlighted the role of simulators. Another pivotal factor was growing interest in anesthesiology in studying the anesthesiologist's performance and the human factors and ergonomics of the anesthesia work environment (see Chapter 6).[72-75]

Screen-Based Simulators (Microsimulators)

Beginning in the mid 1980s, several screen-based simulators were developed by anesthesiologists. These included part-task trainers that simulated isolated aspects of anesthesia, such as the uptake and distribution of anesthetic gases in the body given different physiologic and physical chemistry situations (the well-known GasMan simulator has excelled in this role). Other "full" screen-based simulators represented nearly all aspects of the patient and clinical environment. Originally the control logic was based heavily on mathematical models of physiology and pharmacology, some of the screen-based simulators have converted to control largely from scripts and finite-state models. Originally, the patient was represented by drawings or animations, but increasingly in these systems the representation of the patient is by photos or videos. Vital signs appear on virtual monitors that may mimic real clinical devices. Actions are selected typically using a graphical user interface, pointing and clicking on menus and buttons, and using sliders and numerical entry boxes to allow control of most kinds of interventions that clinicians use on a regular basis.

Experience with Patient Simulators in Anesthesia

Several companies now offer mannequin-based patient simulators with a wide range of capabilities (the term *fidelity* is reserved for the apparent veracity of the simulation; the simulator device has a set of features or capabilities) and with different user interfaces and control logics. The bulk of simulators in use today (coming from several vendors) are considered medium-capability devices. They do approximately 70% as much as a top-of-the-line simulator, but at approximately 15% of the cost of the most expensive simulators. This value proposition has been persuasive to most customers, although for certain applications the high-end simulators still may be required.

The new patient simulators have been in use in anesthesia for more than 20 years, and considerable collective experience with the devices already has been achieved. This section and subsequent sections cover the use of simulators for education, training, evaluation, and research (the last especially in decision making and human factors). The results of simulator studies as regards human performance and patient safety are discussed primarily in Chapter 6.

Simulation for Education and Training of Health Care Personnel

The various available patient simulators offer an unparalleled opportunity for students to experience physiologic and pathophysiologic reactions in a realistic manner. Different objectives are possible for teaching sessions. A study by Morgan and Cleave-Hogg[76] concluded that "the simulator environment is somehow unique and allows different behaviors to be assessed." The objectives of *education* are to provide conceptual understanding and an introduction to skills, whereas the objective of *training* is to implement specific skills and behaviors applicable directly to real-world surroundings. Consistency in objectives is important for evaluating education and training; if we are teaching conceptual understanding, but assessing specific skills, we may obtain misleading results.[77]

A Best Evidence Medical Education (BEME, www.bemecollaboration.org) review by Issenberg and colleagues[25] concluded that high-fidelity medical simulations are educationally effective, but only if the right conditions are met, as follows:

Conditions for the Educational Effectiveness of High-Fidelity Medical Simulations (according to a BEME review by Issenbery[25])

- Educational feedback is provided
- Repetitive practice is used or is allowed
- Simulation is integrated sensibly into the standard curriculum
- The range of task difficulty can be adapted to the level of the learner

Simulation for Education and Training of Medical and Other Health Profession Students

The structured review about simulation effects on simulation-based medical education by Issenberg and colleagues[25] showed that (1) the methodologic quality of educational research is often weak, and (2) in the high-quality studies that were evaluated, there was an effect between hours of simulator practice and learning outcomes equaling a dose-response relationship. Studies by Coates and associates[78] and Gordon and coworkers[79] showed that simulator education for medical students on patient management skills related to dyspnea was superior to problem-based learning.

A variety of curricula exist,[54,77,80-90] including the following:

- Educational sessions and demonstrations concerning basic cardiopulmonary physiology or pharmacology; in some institutions, these sessions replace animal laboratory exercises.[91]
- Introduction to integrated management (i.e., interweaving of diagnosis and treatment) of critically ill patients; this training is offered to immediate preclinical medical students as part of their preparation for clinical medicine courses.
- Anesthesia practicum for clinical students during anesthesia or intensive care clerkships.
- Problem-solving skills training; simulation has been tested as a means of educating and training students in the appropriate response to specific critical events. Morgan and Cleave-Hogg[92] tested simulation versus instructor-facilitated viewing of a videotape for this purpose and found no difference between the two. The generalizability of this finding has been questioned, however.[77]
- Adaptation of curricula originally aimed at experienced trainees or practicing clinicians to students; there is increasing interest in providing early exposure to medical students, and possibly students of nursing or allied health professions, to interdisciplinary team aspects of medical practice. The aim is to inculcate concepts of teamwork and communication at the earliest stages of education and training as a vehicle to implement long-term culture change in the health care system.

A stimulating critical overview of medical education in general was written by Hodges, provocatively titled "Medical education and the maintenance of *incompetence*" (emphasis added).[93] The article points out that any type of education runs a risk of creating or maintaining *incompetence* in certain areas, especially areas that are ignored by the actual educational program. Objective structured clinical examination–style methods in particular are criticized because students may learn to pass the objective structured clinical examination, but still have even gross incompetence in important aspects of real patient care that are not covered by the objective structured clinical examination rating scale. Simulation offers the promise of targeting more thorough integration of different kinds of skills into a better representation of the realities of clinical care. Nonetheless, we recommend that all simulation instructors be especially cognizant of the risks that Hodges articulates.

Anesthesia Crisis Resource Management

In 1989, based on the cognitive process model presented in Chapter 6 and the research results of Cooper and coworkers,[72,94] Howard and associates,[95] and Gaba[73,74] of the VA–Stanford group identified gaps in the training of anesthesiologists regarding several critical aspects of decision making and crisis management that were not systematically taught during standard residency or postgraduate education. These gaps were (1) inadequate learning of precompiled plans for dealing with perioperative events; (2) inadequate skills of metacognition and allocation of attention; and (3) inadequate skill in resource management behavior, including leadership, communication, workload management, monitoring, and cross-checking of all available information. Historically, it had been assumed that anesthesiologists would acquire these plans and skills "by osmosis," solely by experience and by observing role models who had these qualities. As indicated in a previous section, the aviation field had learned that such skills were not acquired unless specifically taught, and CRM training was created to address these issues for flight crews. The VA–Stanford group modeled their ACRM training[95] after CRM, and this approach has been highly influential. ACRM-like curricula are taught at simulation centers around the world, not only in anesthesia, but also in many other domains of health care, including ICU, emergency medicine, labor and delivery, trauma, and field responders.[16,35,38,41,43,44,54,68,96-113] Figure 7-14 shows a typical ACRM team training scenario.

To target the identified gaps in training, approximately 40% of the emphasis of ACRM is on the medical and technical management of specific high-risk perioperative situations, but at least 60% of the emphasis is on generic principles of crisis management that apply to nearly every complex patient care situation. The key teaching points of ACRM are shown in Table 7-8. These points are emphasized during the ACRM simulation course, and their occurrence or omission is highlighted during the video-assisted debriefing sessions (see more on CRM in Chapter 6).

A working group of the original ACRM centers (VA–Stanford, Boston CMS, Toronto Sunnybrooke) has promulgated a set of criteria to be met by a curriculum to be called "ACRM" or "ACRM-like." Table 7-9 presents an excerpt of the criteria. The full set of criteria is available at http://anesthesia.stanford.edu/VASimulator/ACRM_Criteria.htm.

These criteria delineate that special training is needed for instructors in ACRM-like curricula. Experience suggests that the most difficult aspect of ACRM instructing is debriefing, and new instructors require a significant period of experience, preferably under supervision by more senior instructors, before being ready to be fully independent instructors. Several groups working separately or collectively have developed comprehensive training programs on simulation instruction, including substantial modules on debriefing and scenario design.

Table 7-8 Key Points in Anesthesia Crisis Resource Management

1. Know the environment
2. Anticipate and plan
3. Call for help early
4. Exercise leadership and followership with assertiveness
5. Distribute the workload (10 seconds for 10 minutes)
6. Mobilize all available resources
7. Communicate effectively
8. Use all available information
9. Prevent and manage fixation errors
10. Cross and double check (never assume anything)
11. Use cognitive aids
12. Re-evaluate repeatedly (apply the 10 seconds for 10 minutes concept)
13. Use good teamwork
14. Allocate attention wisely
15. Set priorities dynamically

(Detailed explanation of the CRM Key Points are given in Chapter 6.

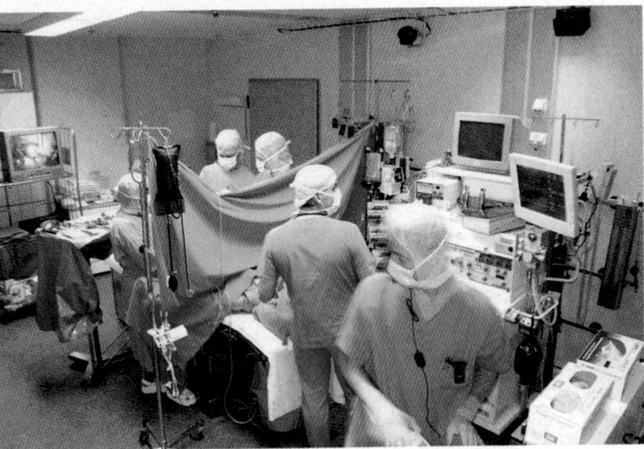

Figure 7-14 Anesthesia crisis resource management team training scenario. A full operating room team (enacted surgeons and nurses) is doing a complicated endoscopic surgery case (replayed on screen). The anesthesia team consisting of the trainee ("hot seat") and the nurse has to solve complex problems. Video cameras (ceiling), microphones, and loudspeakers provide the necessary connectivity and debriefing tools. *(Picture by team TuPASS, taken at Center for Patient Safety and Simulation, University Hospital, Tubingen, Germany.)*

ACRM-like curricula use several teaching modalities to achieve these goals, including the following:

- A comprehensive textbook on anesthesia crisis management (*Crisis Management in Anesthesiology*). This book includes didactic material on ACRM principles and a comprehensive catalog of critical incidents in anesthesia that provides guidelines for preventing, recognizing, and managing 83 perioperative situations in a uniform format. The catalog section of the text is intended to provide study material to increase anesthesiologists' stock of precompiled response plans to common and uncommon situations. This textbook has been translated into Japanese and German (by one of this chapter's authors).
- A brief presentation reviewing the principles of CRM and patient safety.
- Analysis of a videotape of an aviation accident.
- Small group exercises analyzing a videotape of an actual patient care mishap or analyzing written or video presentations about difficult cases.
- Several hours of complex multifaceted realistic simulations in which training participants rotate through different roles, including primary anesthesiologist, first responder (called "cold" with no knowledge of the situation), and scrub nurse. Other personnel play the roles of surgeons, nurses, and technicians as in a real operating room. Each situation is followed by a detailed debriefing with video feedback (see earlier discussion of debriefing).

Several publications have detailed the response of participants with varying levels of experience to ACRM training.[95,109] Participants have been extremely positive about their experience in the ACRM course, and most believe that it contributes to their

Table 7-9 Characteristics of Anesthesia Crisis Resource Management–like Simulator Training

Objectives

Learn generic principles of complex problem solving, decision making, resource management, and teamwork behavior

Improve participants' medical/technical, cognitive, and social skills in the recognition and treatment of realistic, complex medical situations

Enhance capacity for reflection, self-discovery, and teamwork and building a personalized tool kit of attitudes, behaviors, and skills

Aim

Prevent, ameliorate, and resolve critical incidents

Setting Characteristics

Realistic simulation environment replicating a relevant work setting (or an actual patient care setting with in-situ simulation)

Personnel to represent individually those found in the typical work environment of the participant, including nurses, surgeons, and technicians

Bulk of the training course consists of realistic simulations followed by detailed debriefings

Primary participant can request and receive help from other participants

Participants may rotate between different roles during different scenarios to gain different perspectives

Simulation scenarios may be supplemented by additional modalities, including activities such as assigned readings, didactic presentations, analysis of videotapes, role playing, or group discussions

Training involves significant time (>4 hours, typically ≥8 hours) and is conducted with a small group of participants

Content Characteristics

Scenarios require participants to engage in appropriate professional interactions

At least 50% of the emphasis of the course is on crisis resource management behavior (nontechnical skills), rather than medical or technical issues (nontechnical skills are discussed in Chapter 6)

Observation only is not equivalent to actual participation in the course

Faculty Characteristics

Training is intense and entails high level of involvement of faculty with the participants and a low participant-to-faculty ratio

Faculty, especially those leading debriefing, have special training or experience in conducting crisis resource management–oriented training

Debriefing Characteristics

Debriefings are performed with the whole group of participants together and use (as appropriate) audio/video recordings of the simulation sessions

Debriefings emphasize constructive critique and analysis in which the participants are given the greatest opportunity possible to speak and to critique and to learn from each other (debriefing facilitation)

safe practice of anesthesia. Table 7-10 shows the results of one of the earliest studies on that topic.

At VA–Stanford, ACRM has been extended to a multilevel course conducted over several years (i.e., ACRM 1, 2, 3). As the course levels progress, the scenarios become more complex and involve subspecialties of anesthesia. In addition, additional teaching modules cover other important aspects of organizational safety, such as "systems thinking" in morbidity and mortality conference settings or peer review settings, follow-up response to severe adverse perioperative events, and disclosure to the patient or family of "bad news" after an adverse event.

ACRM courses and ACRM-like variants are now being offered worldwide and are often mandatory for trainees (and in some cases for experienced personnel). In Denmark, ACRM-like training courses are a legal requirement for nurse anesthetists (3-day course) and first-year (2-day course) and third-year residents (4-day course), in addition to some other simulator training courses (e.g., difficult airway). Further plans are being made to require simulation training for ICU and recovery room nurses and ICU residents.[114-116] Salas and colleagues[33] published an excellent critical overview about prerequisites for effective CRM training.

Simulation for Training of Anesthesia Residents

Simulation is now a widely used technique in the training of anesthesia residents. It is used in various ways—for technical training on particular procedures or patient care protocols (especially for airway management), for supplementing didactic instruction about anesthesia equipment, and for training about issues of decision making and nontechnical skills as outlined earlier concerning ACRM. Nearly every anesthesia residency program in the United States now offers some cogent simulation training experiences, although the scope, frequency, and target content vary.

Other disciplines and other countries may not have adequate simulation training coverage during residency, as evidenced by a study by Hayes and colleagues[117] about the perception of Canadian internal medicine residents to be qualified for their service on the cardiac arrest team: 49% felt inadequately trained, 50% felt that the provided advanced life support course did not prepare enough to lead the arrest team, and almost none got postevent debriefing or feedback.

Table 7-10 Evaluation of Anesthesia Crisis Resource Management (ACRM) Course in Harvard Anesthesia Simulation Training

		Attending Staff (*n* = 30)		Residents and Fellows (*n* = 34)	
Rating	**Scale**	**Evaluation of Simulator Environment (%)**	**Value of ACRM Course (%)**	**Evaluation of Simulator Environment (%)**	**Value of ACRM Course (%)**
Less favorable	1	13	3	9	1
	2	10	3	6	2
	3	15	15	11	4
	4	10	25	28	28
More favorable	5	33	54	46	75

Modified from Holzman RS, Cooper JB, Gaba DM, et al: Anesthesia crisis resource management: Real-life simulation training in operating room crises. J Clin Anesth 7:675-687, 1995.

Special Considerations in Pediatric Simulation

A sizable body of international experience with simulation in pediatric settings now exists (see Chapter 82).[43,111,118] A study by Overly and coworkers[119] assessing airway management skills in pediatric residents identified many areas of concern about residents' abilities. The authors concluded that high-fidelity simulation can be used to assess residents' airway management, and that the training program was effective to teach these skills.

Many centers use pediatric simulators predominantly for training of the management of critical incidents and medical emergencies, targeting trainees and specialists in anesthesia and pediatric critical care medicine. Because there is frequent organizational and clinical overlap between personnel engaged in pediatric anesthesia, critical care, and emergency medicine, multispecialty (physician crews from different specialties) and multidisciplinary (crews from different professional disciplines), team training can be particularly helpful to prevent failures of cooperation at treatment interfaces (Figs. 7-15 and 7-16). A review by Eppich and colleagues[35] on team training in pediatric acute care settings underlines the impact and effectiveness of team training addressing pediatric teams. The American Academy of Pediatrics now specifically recommends teamwork and communication training for all health care professionals in pediatric emergency settings, and the American Heart Association has included a team concept video and eight elements of team dynamics in its training programs.[120-122]

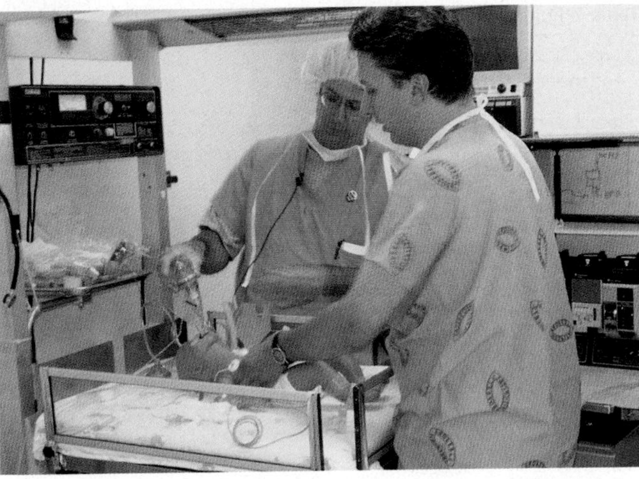

Figure 7-16 Neonatal CRM and resuscitation training at a neonatal emergency workplace. All treatment steps need to be performed in the simulation to show the need to coordinate and delegate. The experienced instructor (on the right side of the infant) is taking part as a team member, while another instructor team is in the control room, presiding over simulation control and debriefing videos. CRM, crisis resource management. *(Picture taken at Stanford Simulation Center.)*

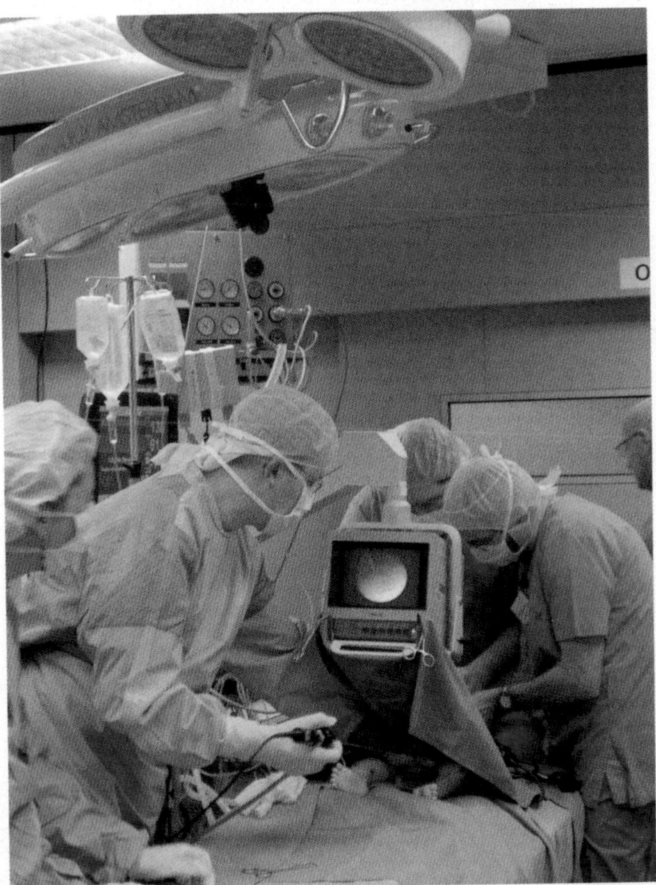

Figure 7-15 Pediatric full team simulation training. The primary trainees (anesthesia) have to solve problems with the infant simulator, while urologic surgical team members perform their procedure. *(Courtesy of C. Eich, University Hospital, Göttingen, Germany.)*

In contrast to adult medicine, the demand in pediatrics for simulation has been largely to address particular points of medical knowledge and technical skill, perhaps because many personnel have little experience with pediatric care, especially for cases involving neonates and infants (Table 7-11).[123] Many simulation courses in pediatric anesthesia or intensive care need extensive involvement by experienced pediatric clinicians. More senior clinical personnel who work regularly in pediatric settings may be comfortable with their pediatric clinical skills, but may be more interested in the generic nontechnical skills that are equally applicable to pediatric and adult care.[120]

There is a positive correlation between the difficulty of pediatric scenarios and the participants' own perception of the learning effect.[123] Scenarios that participants rarely encounter in their clinical practice (e.g., an infant in circulatory shock owing to extensive thermal injury) on the one hand are thought to be threatening, but on the other hand are considered to be particularly beneficial in terms of training effect. A commonplace but interesting aspect inherent in pediatric simulation is the incorporation of role play by family members. Although family members may be present in adult medicine, their presence in pediatrics is nearly ubiquitous.[124] This presence can put further strain and stress on the provider, making it particularly useful to add family role players (either trained actors or instructors or even the participants themselves) to pediatric simulation scenarios.[118]

Continuing Medical Education

Most simulation centers offer CME for experienced practitioners, and nearly all aspects of simulation training for residents (except novice training) can be expanded for this purpose. Several studies

Table 7-11 Unique Aspects of Simulation in Pediatric Anesthesia

Huge discrepancy between high degree of required clinical proficiency and often limited level of expertise
Strong demand for training on medical-technical aspects of management—recommendation to participate in a pediatric advanced life support course before simulation team training course
Need to familiarize with parental presence during pediatric anesthetic care by combination of simulation and role play
The small patient requires an even better organization of the work environment and task responsibilities (in-situ training)
High-impact multidisciplinary team training, including CRM
High level of interest in assessment and certification of trainees and subspecialists for work in pediatric anesthesia

CRM, Crisis resource management.

have shown that experienced anesthesiologists also have deficiencies in the management of critical patient situations and make severe errors comparable to those of anesthesia residents.[64,116,125-129] A study by Jacobsen and associates in Denmark[130] involving 42 specialist anesthesiologists showed major deficiencies in the diagnosis and treatment of anaphylactic shock and in application of the ACRM principles when a score adopted from Gaba and Howard was used.[69,131] Because crisis situations are rare during routine clinical work, these results are not unexpected. In addition, experience in terms of years on the job and hierarchy probably do not correspond to expertise and excellence. It cannot be overemphasized that crisis management training with simulators should be started early in education and training and applied on a recurring basis during practice.

An aspect of CME training in the United States is that it is regulated separately by each of the states, and it is nearly uniformly based only on the number of hours spent in the activity. Reading a short article and answering a handful of questions can generate 1 hour of credit, as can sitting through a lecture. Simulation training is generally much more interactive and much more intensive than other activities. In Australia and Germany, CME requirements are expressed in terms of points to be accrued. Simulation training counts for a large number of points per hour spent, commensurate with its intensity, which might make simulation-based CME financially competitive relative to simpler methods.

The ASA has established a standing Committee on Simulation. The ASA offers an endorsement (analogous to but different from an accreditation) of simulation programs that can show their capability to offer excellent CME curricula to ASA members. The Committee began reviewing applicants for endorsement in 2008.

At the Harvard hospitals, the captive insurer, Harvard Risk Management Foundation, has taken unprecedented steps to link simulation-based CME training to discounts for medical malpractice premium rates for experienced clinicians in anesthesia and in obstetrics (Cooper J: personal communication, 2005). This forward-thinking program is now being adopted by other malpractice carriers. In some jurisdictions, risk managers have chosen to invest directly in simulation activities at their institution, rather than to use the premium discount approach.

Use of Patient Simulation for Training Health Care Personnel outside Anesthesia

Anesthesiology remains a driving force in the use of simulation in health care, but simulation has spread to nearly every discipline and domain. It is proven to be particularly applicable to other areas that share the cognitive profile of anesthesiology—dynamic decision making (played out over seconds, minutes, and hours), with complex teams, wielding highly lethal interventions. ACRM-like training has been performed in settings that include, but are not limited to, intensive care,[113,132] emergency medicine and emergency field responders,[133-138] trauma medicine and surgery, neonatology (neonatal resuscitation and neonatal ICU), labor and delivery (Fig. 7-16),[139,140] cardiac arrest and rapid response teams,[141-143] and radiology. Simulation is such a diverse technique that it is equally applicable—using different modalities of simulation—to nearly all domains. Knudson and colleagues[36] found a significant improvement in overall and teamwork scores in surgical residents when taking care of critically injured simulated trauma patients if they have undergone CRM-like simulation training.

The military and Homeland Security also have been heavy users of simulation in health care, where it has been applied to the initial training of new field medics and to the recurrent training of experienced clinicians and clinical teams.[144] Figure 7-17 shows one room with 10 simulators in a training center for military medics that has more than 100 simulator mannequins altogether.

Simulation is now used more frequently in training for the management of chemical, biologic, or nuclear threats from accidents, weapons of mass destruction, or terrorism. One of our groups in Tübingen, Germany, used their simulator to test the constraints of treating patients in full chemical protection gear (publication of the results is in preparation) to optimize the strategies of the German Ministry of Internal Affairs for dealing with terror attacks or chemical plant disasters (Figs. 7-18 and 7-19) (see Chapter 74). Several investigators have performed multidis-

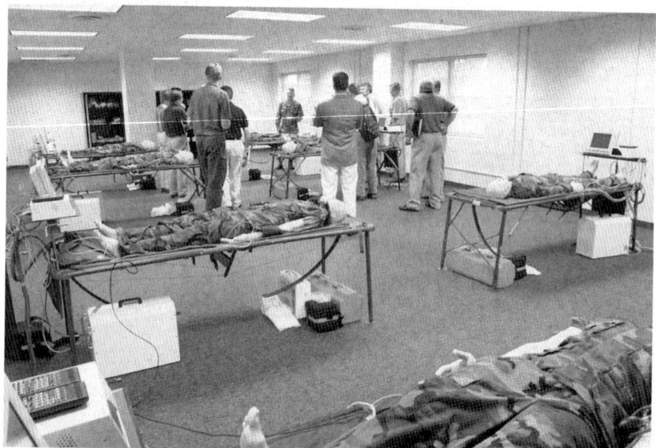

Figure 7-17 Simulation-based training center for military medics. The room is equipped with 10 SimMan training stations. During training sessions, one instructor team is sitting at each foot of each mannequin. Teaching is provided "on scene" during the sessions.

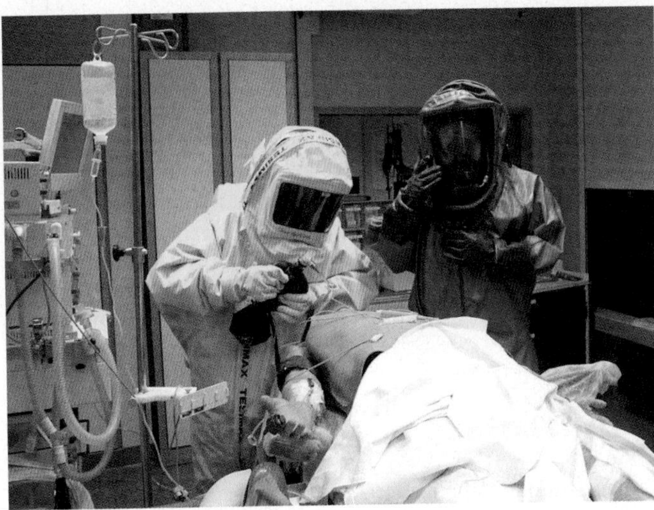

Figure 7-18 Realistic patient simulation as a test bed for studying the performance of medical rescue teams in full chemical protection gear. Teams wore normal uniforms or full protection suits while performing basic resuscitation actions (e.g., placement of intravenous lines, drawing up drugs, intubation). *(Picture taken at the TuPASS Center for Patient Safety and Simulation, Tübingen, Germany.)*

ciplinary studies with combined simulation modalities (script-based, model-based mannequin simulators, and simulated acted patients) to teach the management of victims of an attack with weapons of mass destruction and terrorism.[59,60] The demand for such training is substantial in nations engaged in active military conflicts or with an ongoing need to prepare for war or terrorist attacks (e.g., the United States and Israel).

Use of Patient Simulation for Research

Research in simulation falls into two categories: (1) research *about* simulation—testing or improving the techniques, technologies, and pedagogy of simulation, and (2) research that uses simulation as a tool to study other things, such as human performance, clinical cognition, or clinical care processes (see Chapter 6). Table 7-12 provides a sampling of these latter types of questions. As a research tool, simulation offers some unique features, and it can be thought of as a complementary window on the clinical world relative to other modalities. One can study clinical work using

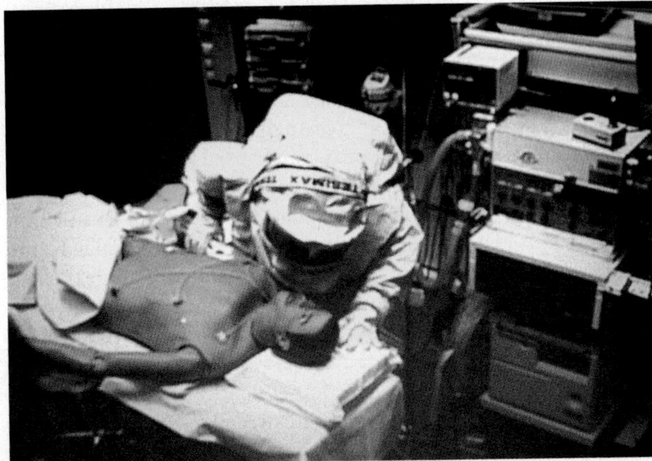

Figure 7-19 In rescue situations with full protective gear, communication within the team and with the patient is difficult. *(Picture taken from a video screen at the TuPASS Center for Patient Safety and Simulation, Tübingen, Germany.)*

Table 7-12 Research Issues That Can Be Addressed by Using Simulation

Cognitive Science of Dynamic Decision Making (see Chapter 6)
What is the interaction of precompiled procedural knowledge versus deep medical knowledge and abstract reasoning?
How does supervisory control of observation relate to vigilance, data overload, and visual scanning patterns?
What is the information content of watching the surgical field?
How are optimal action planning and scheduling implemented?
How does re-evaluation fail and result in fixation errors?
Human-Machine Interactions
What is the distraction penalty for false alarms?
Is there an advantage to integrated monitors and displays versus multiple stand-alone devices and displays?
How easy to use are the controls and displays of existing anesthesia equipment in standard case situations and in crisis situations?
Teaching Anesthesia in the Operating Room
How much teaching can be accomplished in the operating room without sacrificing the anesthesia crew's vigilance?
How well can faculty detect and categorize the performance of anesthesia trainees?
What teaching styles are best integrated with case management in the operating room?
Issues of Teamwork
How does an anesthesia crew (attending anesthesiologist plus resident or Certified Registered Nurse Anesthetist) interact during case and crisis management?
How is workload distributed among individuals?
How do crew members communicate with each other, and how do they communicate with other members of the operating room team?
Effects of Performance-Shaping Factors on Anesthesiologist Performance
How do sleep deprivation, fatigue, aging, and the carryover effects of over-the-counter medications, coffee, or alcohol affect the performance of anesthesiologists?
Intelligent Decision Support
Can smart alarm systems or artificial intelligence provide correct and clinically meaningful decision support in the operating room or intensive care unit?
Development of New Devices and Applications: Research Regarding Technique of Simulation
How well do simulators resemble the operating room and provoke the same actions as use in the operating room (ecologic validity of simulators)?
How much does debriefing add to learning from simulation? Are specific techniques of debriefing (e.g., use of video; participant-centered discussion) of significant utility?
How does the setting of simulation scenarios influence aspects of perceived reality, and how does it influence transfer into the real world?
Does simulation training lead to better clinical practice and improved clinical outcomes?

prospective observation of real cases. This has the benefit of being prospective, but by nature, more cases in most domains would be unremarkable, and one would mostly observe the routine and banal. For some purposes, this study would be more than sufficient. Another source of information is in case reports of challenging cases, whether the challenges were expected or unexpected. These also are real cases, and they are out of the ordinary, but the data obtained from such retrospective reports are usually scanty and biased.

Simulation provides an alternative view of clinical work that can be prospective and about challenging cases, albeit simulated cases. The simulation centers around the world probably have the largest experience by far of observing anesthesiologists managing (simulated) malignant hyperthermia. It is hard to imagine how else one might gather systematic data about how clinicians work while managing this uncommon life-threatening situation.

An important milestone for simulation-based research of both types is the publication by the Society for Simulation in Healthcare since 2007 of a peer-reviewed journal titled *Simulation in Healthcare* (one of the authors, D.G., is the founding editor-in-chief of the journal). In addition, for research that is linked tightly to a specific clinical domain, the traditional medical specialty journals have become more welcoming to articles about simulation or that use simulation as an experimental technique.

Cooperation between simulation directors and instructors with psychologists, human factors engineers, or educators has proved to be helpful in research and training. Such collaborations have helped to delineate the theoretical foundations of simulation-based experiential learning, for improving the understanding of debriefing, and for research on work psychology and human performance in health care.[19,21,22,26,27,145,146] Many institutions have integrated psychologists or educators or both into their simulation center staff.[104] Ways to make such collaborations fruitful and rewarding also have been described.

Use of Patient Simulation in Support of Biomedical Industries

Various simulation activities have involved the pharmaceutical or medical equipment industries. Numerous centers (perhaps the University of Florida at Gainesville was the first) offer training to executives and sales representatives of equipment and pharmaceutical manufacturers. The simulator allows these individuals to gain some understanding of the clinician's task demands during patient care and the situations in which their company's drugs or devices could be useful. At the Boston Center for Medical Simulation, this course is dubbed "Anesthesia for Amateurs." Other industrial uses include training personnel in the use of novel pharmaceuticals. Simulators have been featured in a multifaceted approach to launch the opioid remifentanil. Simulators were used to train the manufacturer's representatives and clinicians in safe use of the drug, and it was possible to train anesthesiologists in the application of remifentanil with the simulator before remifentanil was approved by the U.S. Food and Drug Administration (WB Murray: personal communication, 1998.) Besides offering important educational benefits, the industrial activities are an important source of income for simulation centers to help defray the costs of training students and residents.

Simulators have been used to conduct research on human factors issues in the development of new monitoring and therapeutic devices. The simulator also provides a unique test bed and demonstration modality for preprocurement evaluation of the usability of medical devices from different manufacturers. In our own hospitals (Stanford and Tübingen, Germany), simulators enabled us to conduct evaluations of prototype monitoring systems that were not yet approved for clinical use and could not be evaluated in a preprocurement clinical trial.

Other Uses of Simulators

Other unique applications of simulators have surfaced. Some centers use simulators for conducting outreach programs with high school or college students interested in health care. Simulators have been used to help produce educational videotapes on various patient safety issues. It has been suggested that a "legislator day" could be held in a simulator center to familiarize legislators with the demands of dynamic patient care.

Simulators have been used as adjuncts in medicolegal proceedings.[147] Current patient simulators cannot predict the exact physiologic behavior of a specific patient, but they can be used to illustrate typical perioperative situations and the role of different monitors and therapeutic actions, and provide context for the patient management questions of the litigation.

Effectiveness of Simulation Training

Flanagan and associates[148] provide a thorough review on the literature to date on the efficacy of simulation-based training for learning and assessment. The investigators identified more than 3500 articles, of which 458 were included in the review. The conclusion was that "simulation makes a valuable contribution to learning for students, trainees and clinicians. It enables learning of both routine and non-routine procedures and management of patients."[148] They further concluded that simulation is widely used in teaching and learning, is increasingly being used for formative and low-stakes assessments, and is rarely used (but under growing consideration for) high-stakes summative assessment. Flanagan and associates[148] also observed that the range of simulation modalities used for these activities varies widely. Similar to the BEME review by Issenberg[25], they found that many studies lacked a robust design, and that the level of outcome effectiveness as measured with a modified Kirkpatrick scale rarely exceeded 3 out of 6, with most at the level of 2 or below.

The most important question concerning simulator-based training in anesthesia is its cost-effectiveness. This complicated question has two independent components. The first component is the impact and benefit of the training on the performance abilities of participants, and the second is the cost to achieve that impact. In principle, simulation has many advantages as a training tool, as follows[149]:

- There is no risk to a patient.
- Exercises in routine procedures can be repeated intensively, whereas situations and events involving uncommon, but serious problems can be presented at will.
- Participants can learn to use actual complex devices (with a hands-on simulator).
- The same situation can be presented independently to multiple subjects for evaluating individual or group performance.
- Errors can be allowed to occur that in a clinical setting would require immediate intervention by a supervisor.
- The simulation can be frozen to allow discussion of the situation and its management, and it can be restarted or begun anew to show alternative strategies or techniques.
- Recording, replay, and critique of performance are facilitated because patient safety or confidentiality is not an issue.

The fidelity required of the simulator and the choice between screen-only and realistic simulators depend on the intended goals of the training and the relevant target population. A spectrum of computer-based training is possible. Computer-assisted instruction programs and partial-task trainers can be used to teach basic concepts and technical material, such as the uptake and distribution of inhaled anesthetics or the pharmacokinetics of intravenous drugs. These uses are appropriate for students, novices, advanced residents, and experienced practitioners. Screen-only simulators are inexpensive and easy to use. They allow the presentation of and practice with the concepts and procedures involved in managing normal and abnormal case situations. They also are useful for numerous user populations. Realistic simulators can be used to capture the full complexity of the real task domain, including human-machine interactions and the complications of working with multiple personnel. They are most appropriately used for residents and experienced practitioners. Regardless of the device used, the simulator is only a teaching tool that must be coupled with an effective curriculum for its use.[25]

The evaluations conducted so far suggest that simulator-based training is a powerful technique that novice and experienced anesthesiologists believe to be highly beneficial, and that participants and instructors alike believe may improve clinical performance. As the developers of Sim One 7 pointed out, when simulation provides an opportunity to teach material that cannot be taught in another way, as for the systematic instruction of anesthesiologists in handling severe critical events such as cardiac arrest, anaphylaxis, or malignant hyperthermia, there is nothing with which to compare the simulator. Assessing whether the actual outcome of patients can be affected by this or any other training modality would be extremely difficult and expensive. Individuals investigating simulator-based training do not believe that definitive outcome studies of this type are logistically feasible.[150] Determining the impact of a given type of simulator training on the intermediate variables of "performance" and "ability" is feasible, but it would not be easy. The Leiden group provided data supporting the contention that simulation training improves performance in handling a malignant hyperthermia situation. There is a potential, however, for substantial bias when attempting to measure the impact of simulator training by using performance in the simulator as a criterion. The control procedures used by the Leiden group alleviate this bias, but they cannot eliminate it.[151]

Perhaps of even greater importance, no methodology is currently accepted for measuring the clinical performance of anesthesiologists either in the simulator or in actual practice.[152] Ironically, the simulator itself provides a tool for presenting the same calibrated situation to multiple anesthesiologists and may be a crucial tool in developing such performance measures. Many groups around the world are trying to refine performance measurement tools,[107,140,153-172] but no "gold standard" measurement is yet available to assess a simulation's effectiveness (see the later section on evaluation of performance).[152]

How Simulation Can Be More Effective

Health care has not yet scratched the surface of assessing the impact of simulation-based training. Most simulation is currently targeted at students and trainees (i.e., residents), although programs targeting experienced personnel are growing. The assessment of the impact of simulation to date can be seen using the following analogy to drug development and testing. Suppose we wished to test whether a purported antihypertensive drug actually succeeded in reducing blood pressure in patients, and, more importantly, whether it reduced the occurrence of adverse cardiovascular events, such as myocardial infarction and stroke. Imagine then that we proceeded as follows: Administer a relatively small dose of this drug only a few times per year. Acknowledge variable compliance in taking even these few doses of drug. Immerse all subjects in an environment full of stress and other factors predisposing to cardiovascular events. Use only a few patients, and follow them for a very short time.

Using this methodology, would anyone wonder if no significant effect was found even for a drug otherwise known to be effective? Simulation in health care has so far been tested in this way: very small short-term studies of infrequent (often short) simulation sessions, whose lessons are not fully reinforced in real clinical environments full of production pressure and stress. In truth, the question is not "Does one run through a simulation course make a practitioner better?" To follow the lead of other industries of intrinsic hazard, such as commercial aviation or nuclear power production, the real question is: "What is the impact of health care as an industry adopting a comprehensive integrated strategy of intensive simulation-based training and continued performance assessment of clinical personnel, over a long period of time?" This is the approach in aviation, where no matter how senior and how experienced pilots are, they still undergo training and assessment in simulation every year, for the entirety of their careers.

Even so, industries such as aviation do not have anything resembling level 1A evidence for the benefits of simulation, even though such studies could be grafted onto the existing structure of yearly training and testing. It is unlikely that aviation would ever attempt randomized trials. For one thing, as the saying goes, "Pilots are the first ones at the scene of the accident." It seems unlikely that pilots would forgo simulation training and assessment when their own lives are on the line. For another thing, the public has come to expect that there is a regulatory safety floor imposed by the government to ensure the competency of pilots. The regulator is unlikely to forgo its requirement for mandatory training and testing of pilots. If such requirements continue, there may be only two options: conduct them in real airplanes, with the attendant costs (e.g., fuel) and risks, or conduct them using simulation. With health care heading toward that direction,[37,38,43,46,173-177] we may be able to assess the impact of more effective simulation programs, although we might lose a control group.

Avoiding Subthreshold Training Effects

To date, simulation training has largely been employed in "small doses" given intermittently, not sustained over the long-term, and ignoring many personnel who are crucial in the chain of patient care. When conducted this way, simulation training may not achieve a "critical mass" and may produce a subthreshold effect. It seems likely that a long-term cumulative effect would be achieved only with a long-term comprehensive program of training and performance assessment.

It is possible that it is worth the inherent logistical difficulties and costs to undertake bulk training (>75% of personnel trained in a short time, rather than starting a program of training a few individuals a month and achieving a high penetration rate only in months or years). Where the training is about teamwork and behavioral issues (CRM-focused), this might be especially important so that the lessons taught in the simulator are continuously reinforced by experiences in real patient care. The hope is that creating a critical mass of adherents to CRM principles via simulation would create a self-sustaining reinforcement of safety-oriented behaviors that continues with only occasional refresher sessions of simulation.

An analogy for that effect would be the starting of a fire with wood logs: If you take away the match too early, you do not light the fire, and all you get is a black mark on the wood, but if you keep the match on the wood long enough (similar to activation energy), the fire starts to burn and spread to all logs without any more input—similar to what we would like to see with CRM team behaviors.

Ecologic Validity of Simulators Compared with the Operating Room

The question whether full-scale simulators are an ecologically valid representation of the operating room (i.e., to what extent "the environment experienced by the subjects in a scientific investigation has the properties it is supposed or assumed to have by the experimenter"[178]) has been investigated by an interdisciplinary research group in Tübingen and Zurich.[145] If the actions in the simulator resemble the actions in real operating room environments (*behavioral validity*), it is much more likely that the results of research conducted in a simulator setting or lessons learned in the simulator environment would be transferable to the context of actual patient care. The group developed an improved task analysis method that allows the recording of overlapping activities (41 actions from five categories—monitoring, actions, communication, documentation, and other) to analyze and describe the performance of anesthesia.[179]

This method is described in more detail in Chapter 6. Each of the six anesthesiologists participating in the study was observed during two clinical cases and during three comparable simulator cases (one routine and two involving critical incidents). Analysis of the study showed good comparability of the different action categories (Fig. 7-20). The interpretation of the group is that overall comparability between the operating room and the simulator setting is good, indicating high ecologic validity for simulators in anesthesia. The results of the study also show few, but distinct variations in the task structure of operating room and simulator cases. These variations are mostly due to organizational factors (e.g., fewer "additional tasks" required in the simulator). These studies provide objective confirmation of the favorable sub-

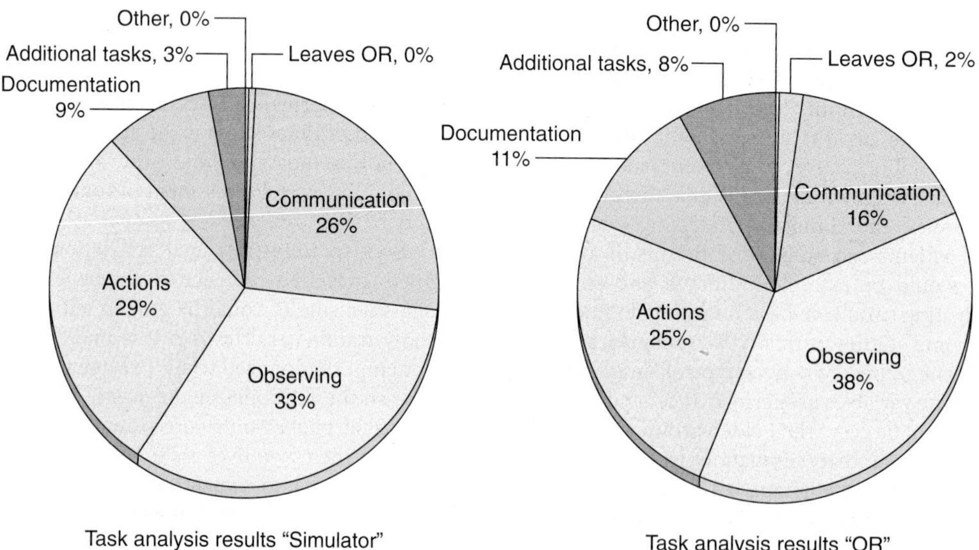

Figure 7-20 Validity of simulator systems versus the operating room (OR). The same anesthesiologists were observed in the OR and the simulator environment with full enactment of the OR personnel, surgical team, and anesthesia nurse. Even though the two settings have some interesting differences, the overall "ecologic validity" of the simulator is good. *(Courtesy of T. Manser, ETH Zurich, and University Hospital, Tübingen, Germany.)*

jective impressions of realistic simulation scenarios by anesthesiologists of varying levels of experience.[126,127,159,161,180-182]

Some differences between simulation and real patient care are inherent to simulation. Subjects realize that they are in a simulator and are likely to be hypervigilant (e.g., many participants neglect documentation in the simulator while waiting for a disaster to happen). In addition, there might be some organizational factors that are usually different in the simulator than in the real operating room (e.g., reflected in fewer "additional tasks" in the simulator compared to the real OR in the study of Manser and Rall). Careful and creative scenario design and introductory briefings may mitigate the hypervigilance and organizational effects.[47,183]

Evaluation of Clinical Performance during Simulation Scenarios

The introduction of patient simulators allowed the study of human performance when responding to critical events (see Chapter 6). Techniques are needed to assess anesthesiologists' performance. Performance can be divided into two components: technical performance, which is the appropriateness and thoroughness of the medical and technical response to the critical event, and behavioral performance, which is the appropriate use of sound crisis management behavior (e.g., leadership, communication, distribution of workload).[184,185] (See Chapter 6 on CRM.) Assessment of medical and technical responses has resulted in "technical scores" suggested by different authors.[151,152,160,161,186-189]

Simulation offers some benefits in assessing performance. Because the nature and cause of the critical incident are known, one can construct in advance a list of essential or appropriate technical activities with relative weights of importance. When assessing technical performance in managing malignant hyperthermia, terminating the trigger agent and administering intravenous dantrolene would be essential items, whereas cooling measures, hyperventilation, and bicarbonate therapy would be among many appropriate (but less critical) technical responses. One also can predict in advance specific technical pitfalls. For malignant hyperthermia, such pitfalls could include diluting dantrolene with the wrong diluent (not sterile water) or an insufficient quantity of diluent. These pitfalls are known to plague clinicians unfamiliar with therapy for malignant hyperthermia.

Can the clinical outcome of the simulator's mathematical physiology predict how a real patient would have fared under that individual's care? This would be possible only where the simulator's control logic used detailed mathematical models of physiology and pharmacology, and not with the script-based control logic. In the latter case, the physiologic state achieved is no different than the checklist of the actions taken that followed the branch points in the script leading to the outcome. The outcome and the actions are essentially the same. Even when mathematical models are used, they are insufficient to predict what would happen to any actual patient after complex sequences of therapy and more subtle patient care judgments. The models have not proven to be robust and have shown a lack of reproducible outcomes even when the same "patient" is given identical perturbations and treatments at exactly the same times.

In extreme cases, the clinical outcome probably does indicate failure or success of performance. A subject who shows totally erroneous decision making (e.g., failure to defibrillate a simulated patient with ventricular fibrillation) unmistakably allows the patient's state to deteriorate quickly. The converse may not be true. Perfect decision making in a resuscitation cannot guarantee that electric countershock would successfully restore a normal cardiac rhythm. We suggest that even with model-driven simulators, the clinical outcome of the simulated patient is at best one datum that can be used to assess the performance of the anesthesiologist on a simulation scenario, but for the foreseeable future, any credible performance measurement technique must involve subjective and semiobjective judgments by clinical experts. In the last few years, there have been many empirical studies attempting to use simulation for different forms of performance assessment in various domains and disciplines.*

Pitfalls of Performance Assessment

Previous trials, experience in other industries, and theoretical analysis suggest that simulation offers substantial opportunities to facilitate performance assessment. Various issues must be resolved, however, to make performance assessment a robust capacity, as follows:

Technical versus nontechnical (CRM) skills. As indicated in previous sections, it is feasible (if difficult) to assess a technical response to specific events and generic nontechnical behaviors (CRM). For which kinds of assessments is it appropriate to measure only technical performance, only nontechnical performance, or some combination of the two?

Number of scenarios. How many different scenarios are needed to achieve robust performance assessment of individuals in all relevant aspects (technical and nontechnical) of patient care? Some emerging results suggest that increasing the number of scenarios is more effective in improving the reliability of ratings than increasing the number of raters is.

Rating individuals versus rating crews or teams. Anesthesiologists work as individuals and in crews and teams with other anesthesiologists and with surgeons, nurses, technicians, and others. Should the performance of individuals working alone be assessed? Should anesthesiologists be able to call for and use help in solving problems? If so, can one still rate the individual when working with a team?

Performance fluctuation. How can performance that fluctuates substantially over time be aggregated into a single rating? This issue was recognized by Gaba and colleagues[185] as a major apparent source of inter-rater disagreement. It is not addressed by the Anaesthetists' Non-Technical Skills (ANTS) system.[162,233] Which techniques would best address this issue, especially as applied to scenarios that represent the actual complexity of clinical practice?

*References 11, 32, 36, 40, 44, 60, 119, 127, 162, 173, 176, 190-215.

Criterion thresholds. What level of performance should be set as criterion thresholds for different purposes? Can benchmarks of performance be established by truly expert clinicians (recognizing that years of experience or hierarchic rank is not a surrogate for expertise or skill)? Similarly, how does the rating system deal with single actions or behaviors that were lethal or harmful in the presence of otherwise good performance? If used for formative assessment, a rating system should indicate the successes of the examinee and the failures. If used for summative or high-stakes assessment, however, it may be critical to ensure that the examinee who risks harming a simulated patient cannot outscore another examinee whose overall performance is less strong, but who at least did not endanger the patient. Not performing chest compressions in a cardiac arrest situation would be such a "knockout" criterion.

Appropriate statistical analysis of validity, inter-rater reliability, and reproducibility of these assessments. Various statistical tests and approaches have been used to evaluate these characteristics. The data on performance show various levels of inter-rater variance and high interindividual (and interteam) variability.[127,151,159-161,180,185,216] As detailed by Gaba and colleagues,[185] some inter-rater reliability statistics are more stringent than others, especially in terms of the nature of the "by chance" benchmark. No firm consensus has been reached regarding which tests are most appropriate to answer key questions about simulation-based performance assessment. Some of the rating systems (including ANTS) have used less stringent tests of inter-rater reliability. Generalizability theory[217,218] offers a set of statistical techniques to sort out the impact of scenario, subject, rater, number of scenarios, and other facets on such assessments. This technique also specifies how comparisons can be made against reference performance levels or as relative comparisons between subjects without a fixed benchmark.

Although simulation should enable performance assessment, a robust set of performance measures of anesthesiologists' skill would be difficult to develop,[219] even if the simulator is used as a tool to present standardized patient scenarios.[220]

Klemola and Norros[221] published a new way of looking at performance that involves anesthesiologists' "habit of actions." These authors distinguish between "reactive habits" (conservative, self-contained, reluctant to construct subjective evaluations) and "interpretative habits" (creative, interactive, continuous integrative reasoning). This article shows that a lot of issues need to be considered when discussing the best method of education and evaluation. Additional issues include defining and assessing professional competence. A more consultant-based method was introduced by Greaves and Grant,[222] who compiled an inventory of characteristics of the anesthesiologist's practice. Epstein and Hundert[223] provide a current review.

Although there are presumed advantages to using simulation as a tool for performance assessment (known scenarios, errors can be allowed to occur and play out, intensive recording and archiving of performance is possible), the anesthesia community should be careful to introduce simulation-based performance evaluation on a slow and measured basis.[224] Performance assessment is expected to be a hot topic for discussion in the simulation and clinical anesthesiology communities in the early 21st century. This controversy should not divert attention from the major application of simulation, which is to improve clinical performance through individual and team training in preventing and managing adverse clinical events.

Can Simulators Be Used for the Evaluation and Testing of Residents or Practitioners?

As discussed previously, patient simulators should be useful tools for evaluating the performance of trainees and others. Scoring or certifying competence by using the simulator is more problematic, however, than using it as a teaching tool.

Anesthesiologists have discussed the possibility of using the simulator as a tool for examinations, either for graduation from a residency or for American Board of Anesthesiologists certification. This use would require independent evaluation of the simulation scenarios and assessment of the predictive power of the subjective judgments made by experts scoring the examinee. An obstacle is the lack of any well-accepted standard for performance evaluation. Another difficulty with using simulation for board certification testing is that the operating room equipment would rarely be the same as that used by the candidate, and the operating room staff's operational protocols could differ from the protocols familiar to the candidate. In the training situation, these difficulties can be overlooked as part of the global suspension of disbelief needed to maximize the benefits of simulator training. In the test situation, these differences potentially could skew the results. This issue could be addressed by allowing candidates preparing to take their examination to undergo sufficient practice sessions to familiarize themselves fully with the standard simulation environment used for the test.

Despite these difficulties, it is likely that if the use of anesthesia simulators does become more widespread, anesthesiologists would become more interested in using them to assist in evaluating performance. The existing system of performance evaluation, which uses a haphazard system of subjective judgment of clinical competency in residency along with written and oral examinations, has itself never been validated. Many believe that the written examination does not correlate well with clinical ability, and the degree to which the oral examination process tests actual clinical skill is unknown. Simulation could offer candidates the opportunity to show their clinical abilities in a controlled clinical domain, while still showing their consulting and language skills through oral examination.

More recently, there have been a few projects on using simulation as a high-stakes test for clinicians.[37,38,96,173,175,197,225,226] Simulation is being used more commonly for "no-jeopardy" formative evaluations of performance in some residencies. This use may then evolve into graded "pass/fail" examinations or demonstrations of skill. Another situation of simulation-based performance assessment would be for the evaluation of residents who have been placed on probation, or for whom dismissal from the residency program is already a distinct possibility. For these residents, the burden of proof is on them to show their skills. The simulator could offer a more controlled environment for them to do so. The same could be true for practitioners who wish to return to clinical work after a hiatus.

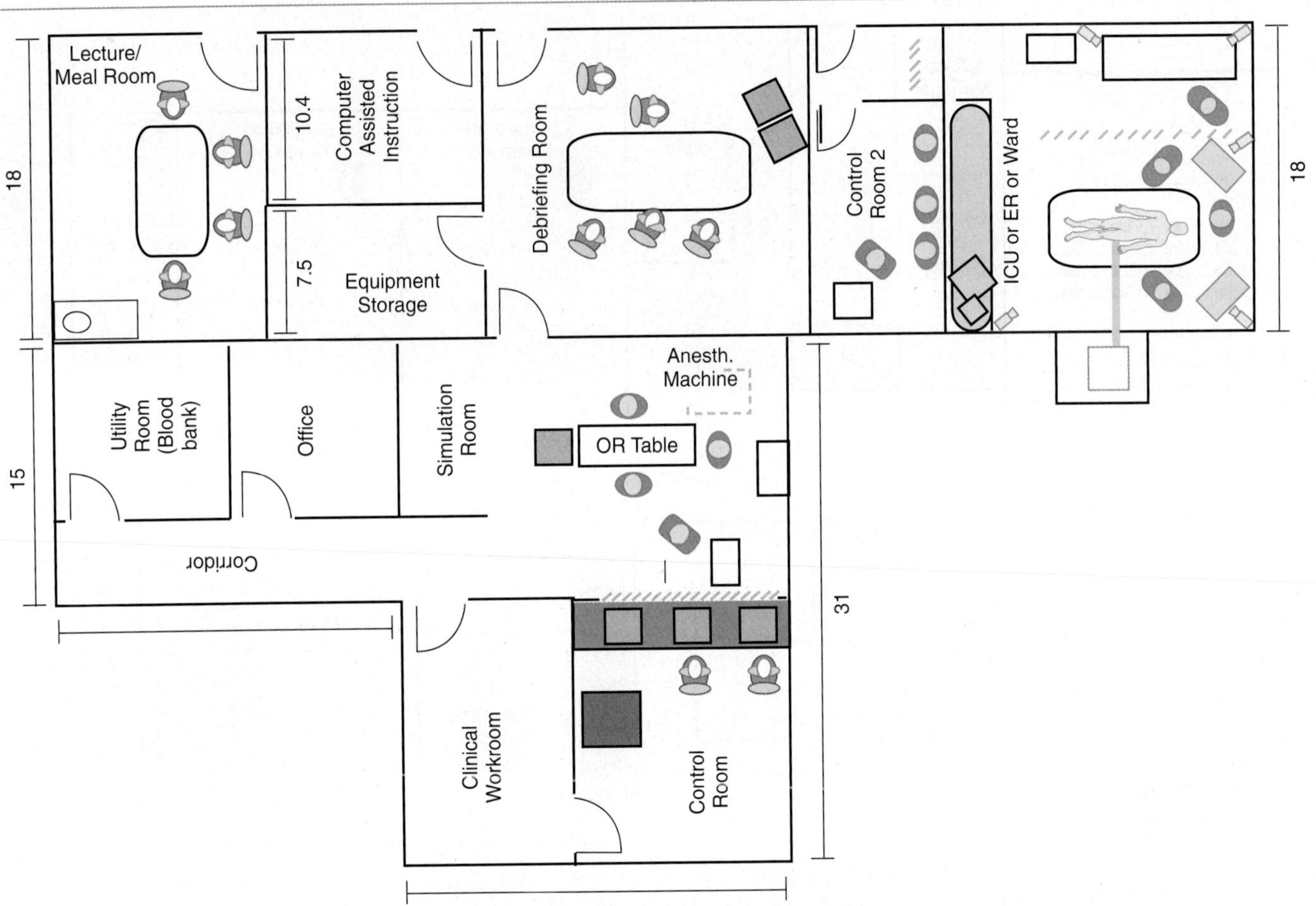

Figure 7-21 Multiroom simulation center at the VA–Palo Alto Health Care System and Stanford University. Two control rooms and two audiovisually interconnected lecture rooms provide the opportunity to run three patient simulators at the same time. ER, emergency room; ICU, intensive care unit; OR, operating room.

In Israel, a simulation examination has become part of the Board certification process. In the United States, the American Board of Anesthesiology has been monitoring the progress of simulation for training and performance assessment. As of 2008, however, there is no prospect of simulation-based board examinations in the United States.

Characteristics of Simulation Centers

Although one can install a simulator in a laboratory or conference room, or conduct only in-situ simulation, many institutions have chosen to construct complete simulation centers. Figures 7-21 and 7-22 show floor plans by the authors (D.G. and M.R.) of medium-sized centers (two to four simulation rooms) for mannequin-based simulation. Figure 7-23 shows the equipment of such a center in more detail. Typically, these centers provide a separate control room to allow complex simulations to be presented without an instructor intruding on the simulated case. The center also provides a debriefing room where videotapes of the simulation session can be reviewed. Some centers have elaborate computer-controlled audio-video systems allowing the recording of multiple views with real-time annotation rapid search to annotated portions of the recording. Figure 7-24 shows the simulator control room with advanced audio-video equipment at the TuPASS Center for Patient Safety and Simulation of one of the authors (M.R.) in Tübingen, Germany.

Universities and hospitals or hospital networks are increasingly constructing very large multidisciplinary and multimodal simulation facilities. Often, these facilities combine all the types of simulation and immersive learning in one large unit, including standardized patient actors (usually in clinic settings), mannequin-based simulation, part-task and surgical/procedural trainers, wet and dry work (e.g., plaster casting or procedures on food products), and different forms of virtual reality. Sometimes these also incorporate facilities for dissection of cadavers or the use of anesthetized animals. Having all forms of simulation together also fosters the hybrid techniques, as when a standardized patient actor is combined with a part-task trainer, or when a surgical simulator is combined with a mannequin-based patient simulator. Large multidisciplinary facilities may have anesthesiologists in leadership positions. Figure 7-25 shows an example of such big centers, the floor plan by one of the authors (D.G.) of the new center for immersive learning at Stanford University, currently under construction (2008).

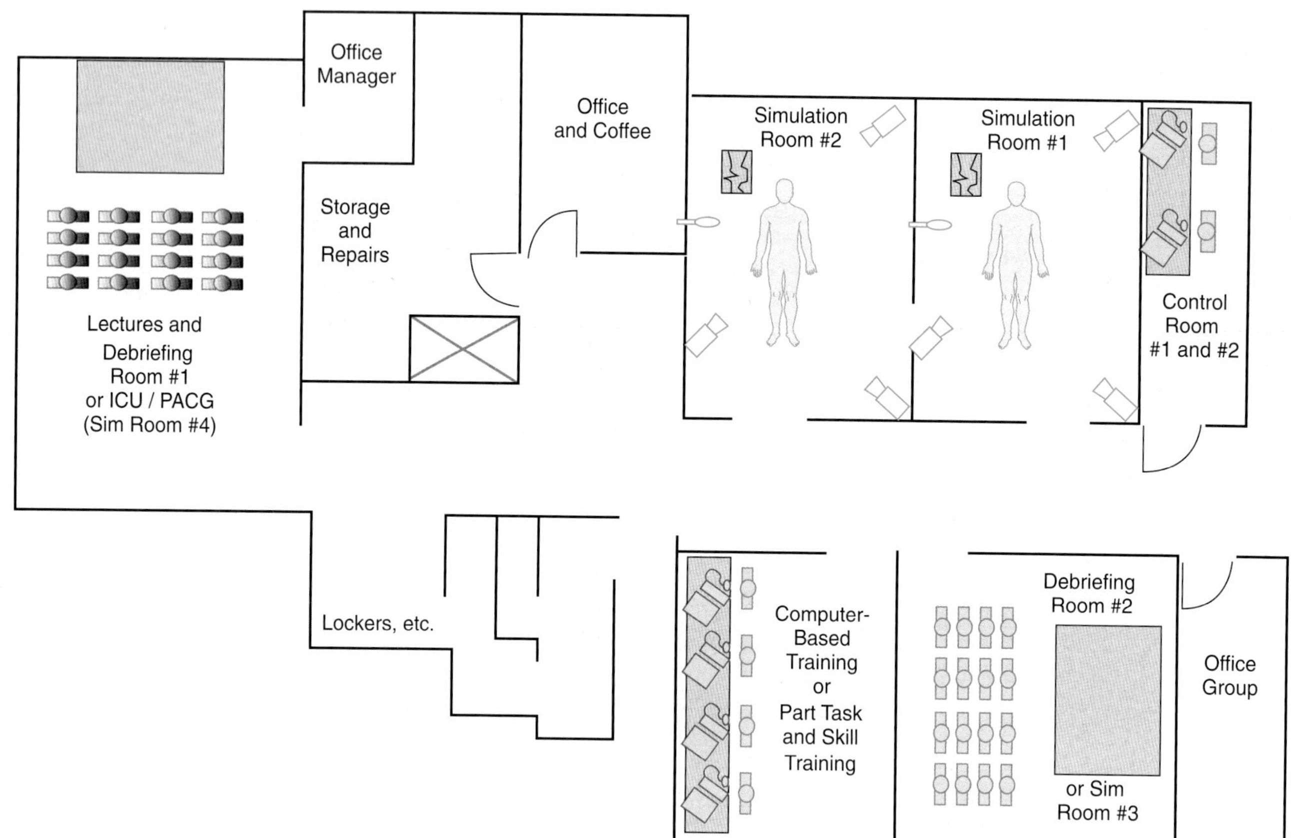

Figure 7-22 An intermediate-sized simulation center with four simulation rooms, a computer-based training room, and several multipurpose rooms, equipped with audio-video patch panels to adjust the room use flexibly to the needs of the different training activities (e.g., the big seminar room also can be used as a big intensive care unit or postanesthesia care unit). *(Picture by E. Stricker from TuPASS Center for Patient Safety and Simulation, Tübingen, Germany.)*

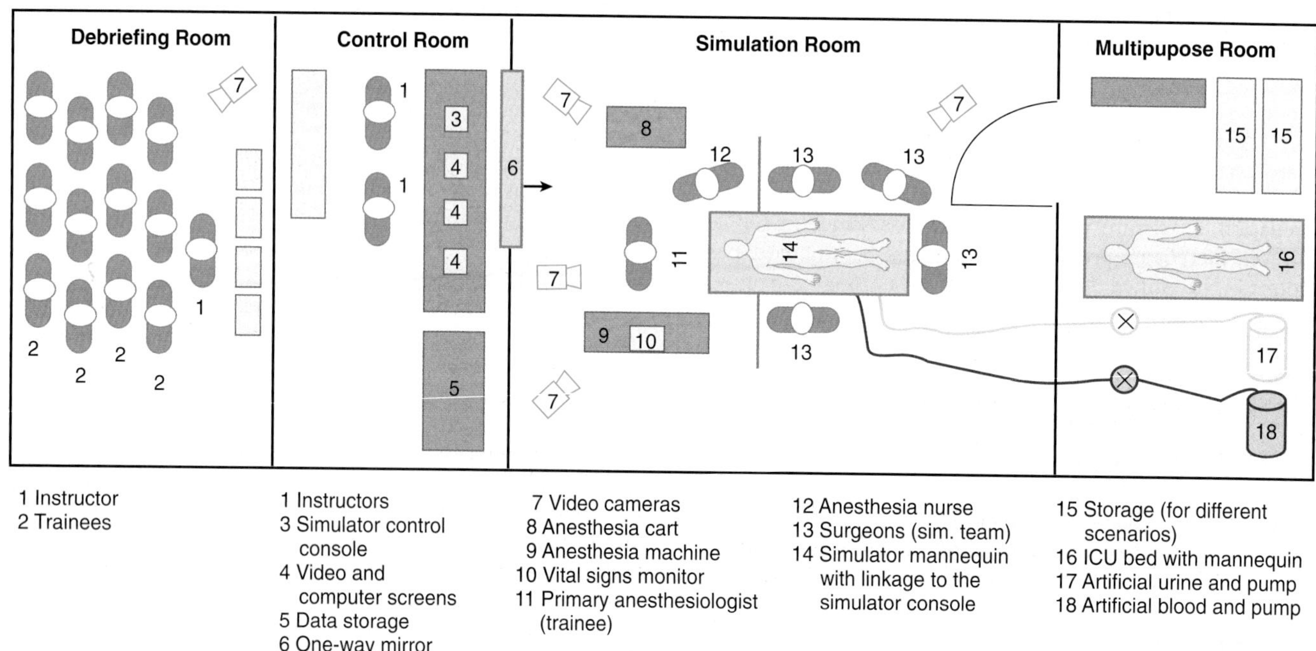

Figure 7-23 Prototypical example of a simulation center (former simulation center at University of Tübingen, Germany). The instructors in the control room look through a one-way mirror into the operating room/intensive care unit (ICU) while they control the "patient" from the simulator workstation and direct the audiovisual recording. Various remote-controllable video cameras, microphones, and loudspeakers in the simulator room provide the best possible view and sound from the "scene." Trainees perform on the simulator mannequin and the vital sign monitors and have to interact with the personnel involved at the same time. Nonactive participants can watch the scenarios live from the adjacent debriefing room, including real-time vital sign transmission, where the video-assisted debriefing session occurs immediately after every scenario. *(From Decker K, Rall M: Simulation in anaesthesia: A step towards improved patient safety. Minim Invasive Ther Allied Technol 9:325-332, 2000.)*

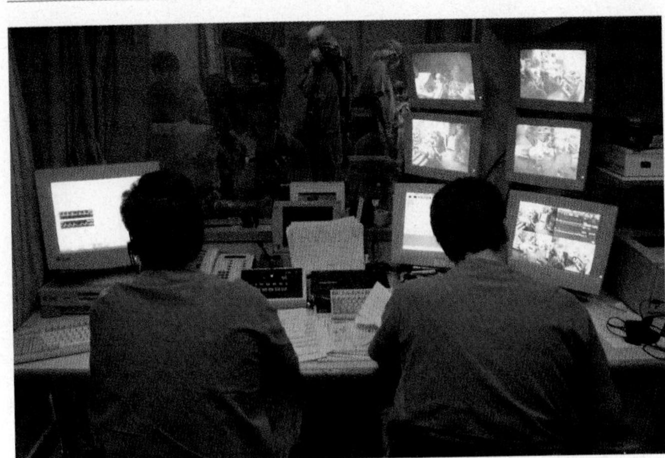

Figure 7-24 Simulator control room. On the left side is the simulator workstation for control of the simulator system itself. In the middle is the audio control desk with integrated control of the simulated patient voice and several wireless headset channels and the remote mixer. On the right are flat screens for selection and control of the multiple views of the video cameras. For anesthesia crisis resource management courses, a multiquad-split view, including the vital sign monitor, is digitally recorded on a hard disk and used for playback. Marks allow jumping to interesting scenes without fast forward or rewind delay. *(Taken at the control room of the TuPASS Center for Patient Safety and Simulation, Tübingen, Germany.)*

The cost structure of a simulation center is a complex issue (see section on Costs). The cost varies greatly depending on the scope of the facility and its programs, the nature of the target populations, and the extent of use by the different possible stakeholder groups. How the costs are allocated to different elements of an institution or consortium is equally complicated and depends highly on local conditions. There is no one formula for success. In some models, the center is wholly responsible for its own costs, but is completely free to generate and retain revenue. At the other extreme is a model whereby the host institution bears all costs of operating a central core facility, but it also collects any and all revenues and may even "tax" components of the institution (e.g., departments) to offset the costs. Perhaps most common are mixed models in which the central authority bears costs of initial construction and outfitting (often funded via philanthropy) and some portion of the ongoing infrastructure (simulation operations personnel, capital refurbishment, utilities), while each user (e.g., department) is responsible for providing instructors and paying for the marginal costs of any specific course or application. To date, few, if any, centers truly generate a profit, but many sites have successfully garnered external funds to offset some of the costs of training their own key target populations.

Costs

What are the costs of simulator-based training? These costs depend on many of the same factors that determine the curriculum, as follows:

Types of training involved, ranging from technology in-service to training in basic anesthesia skills, critical incident management, or CRM

Target populations for the training, whether equipment technicians, medical students, novice residents, experienced residents, nurse anesthetists, teaching faculty, or private practitioners

Organizational and financial characteristics of the institution

The hardware and software costs of the screen-only simulators are quite low (a few hundred dollars), whereas the equivalent cost of a complete hands-on simulator is higher (the prices of commercial simulators range from around $25,000 for intermediate-fidelity simulators to more than $150,000, depending on features; one should contact the manufacturers for detailed information). Cumin and Merry[61] report on available simulators. This cost does not include the necessary clinical equipment (approximately $150,000) and space.[227] Even these large expenditures do not dominate in the cost equation, however, because the capital equipment can be amortized over a relatively long useful life, with appropriate provisions for service and upgrades.

The dominant cost is likely to be the salaries of expert instructors and trainees. An expert must oversee the curriculum, but the type of training and the target population determine the amount of expert instruction required. A single faculty member can review the summaries of exercises performed by residents on a screen-based simulator in a few hours per resident per year. Nonphysician instructors may be suitable for some task training or for drill and practice sessions. A single instructor can use the simulator to show pulmonary or cardiovascular physiology to a whole class of medical students. When training novice residents in basic anesthesia skills, it may be possible to have senior residents or fellows conduct the sessions at a low marginal cost. When training experienced residents and practitioners in complex material, such as the handling of critical events, there is likely to be no substitute for expert instructors. The cost of expert instruction depends on the organizational arrangements of the institution. In a teaching institution where the faculty all have at least some time allocated for teaching or scholarly activities, some of them may choose to fulfill this requirement in simulation-based teaching or scholarship. Where further staffing is needed, payment for clinical release time may be needed.

Another organizational factor that affects the cost has to do with making trainees available for what can be complex, exhausting, and lengthy training sessions. Removing residents from revenue-producing work for training purposes is expensive. If simulator training could allow residents or other anesthesiologists to work more safely and efficiently, the benefit would outweigh the cost. Some residency programs provide protected time for education of residents (e.g., one half day per week). In such cases, residents should be available for educational activities, but faculty time may be even more scarce. Many anesthesia programs have used simulation training as a recruiting tool for residency candidates, although some believe that with the high proportion of programs that already have simulation activities (the scope and quality of which are hard for applicants to judge), the competitive value of simulation has disappeared. Programs that lack such facilities and activities would not be the exception and would likely be seen negatively by applicants.

There is no question that simulation-based training is more costly than exhorting learners to read or putting them in a room with a lecturer. Simulation-based training allows a host of issues to be addressed that cannot be easily tackled in other ways. It is our belief—one that has been borne out by programs "voting with

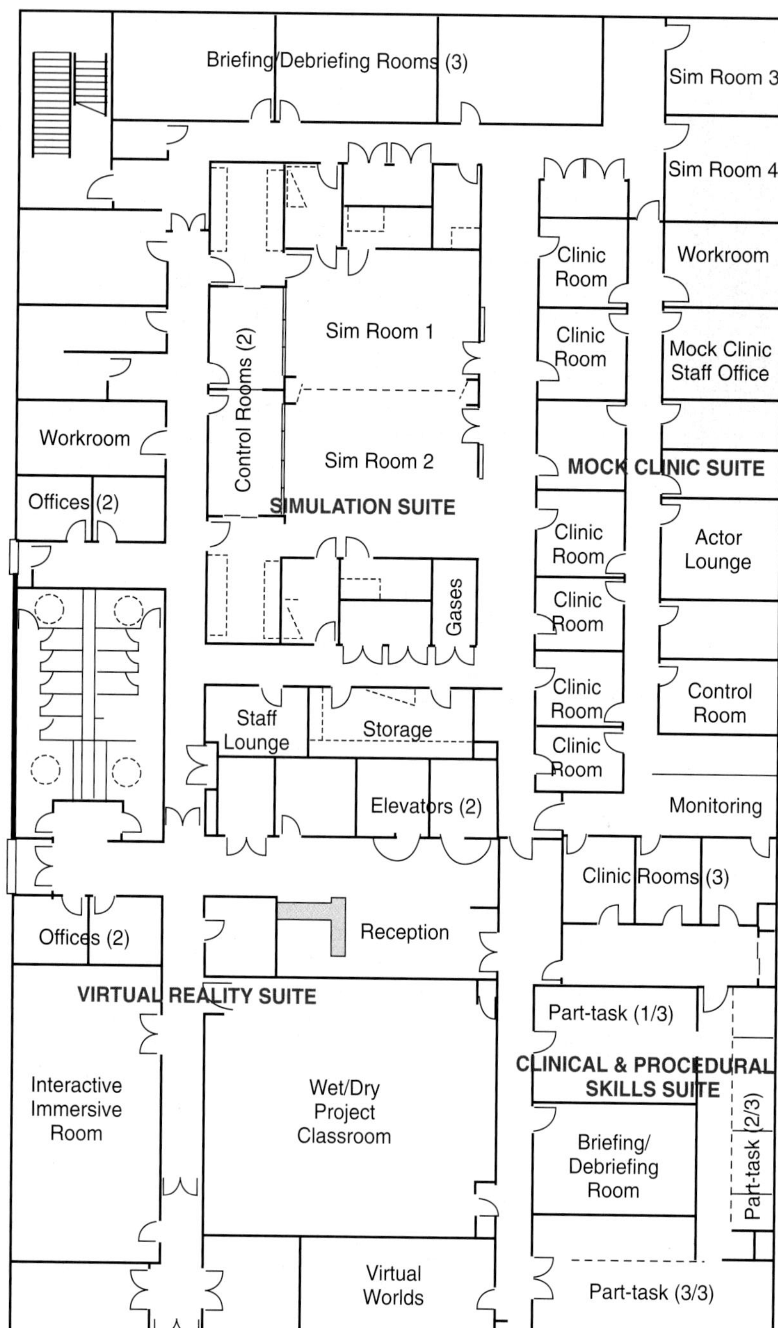

Figure 7-25 Floor plan of a very big interdisciplinary simulation center for multiple domains (anesthesia, surgery, students) with several multipurpose simulation rooms, and skills laboratories. *(Picture by D. M. Gaba, from the Center for Immersive and Simulation-based Learning at Stanford Medical School. Ground floor built as of June 2008.)*

their feet" over the past 15 years—that if simulator-based training is deemed to be desirable, innovative changes in organization would evolve to allow it to occur.

Proliferation of Simulation Centers

Currently, despite the lack of definitive cost-effectiveness data, training with realistic simulators is under way in many sites around the world,[228] with many of them choosing to conduct "high-end" crisis management and critical incident training sessions. Table 7-13 lists useful websites of simulation centers and other resources. These programs have already "voted with their feet" on the issue of cost versus benefit. With so many centers exploring the realities of simulation training, we can expect to see additional data on efficacy and cost within the next few years. A definitive study is in principle possible, but it would require a very large number of subjects evaluated by multiple raters and would be complex and costly.

Still other factors complicate assessment of the effectiveness of simulator-based training. Studying the impact of a single

Table 7-13 Websites of Simulation Centers and Other Useful Resources on Simulation

http://www.ssih.org
Homepage of the Society for Simulation in Healthcare, the largest interdisciplinary society around simulation in Healthcare. Journal Simulation in Healthcare, Elsevier Annual IMSH Meeting (see below).
http://www.hmc.psu.edu/simulation/
Penn State Medical Center, lists of available simulator systems (and links to manufacturers)
www.sesam.ws
Homepage of SESAM (Society in Europe for Simulation Applied to Medicine)
http://www.simulation-users.fsnet.co.uk/
Patient Simulation User's Group, website run by Barts and the London Medical Simulation Centre
http://web.anes.rochester.edu/simulate/simusers.htm
http://web.anes.rochester.edu/simulate/webpages.htm
University of Rochester Medical Center providing lists of and updated links to many simulation centers around the world
http://www.bristol.ac.uk/Depts/BMSC/europe.htm
Bristol Simulation Center, map-based list of simulator sites in Europe and worldwide
http://anesthesia.stanford.edu/VASimulator/simulator.htm
VA–Palo Alto HCS/Stanford University (D. Gaba)
http://www.tupass.de
Center for Patient Safety and Simulation, University of Tübingen (M. Rall)

session of a course that uses a new technology and a new approach to training may underestimate the course's impact when it is used on a regular and repetitive basis. It is widely believed in commercial aviation that CRM training must begin with the initial training of pilots and must be continued throughout their career. Social psychologists Helmreich and Foushee, two of the main architects of CRM training, have written: "Data indicate that even intensive initial CRM training constitutes only an awareness phase and introduction to the concepts, and that continuing reinforcement is essential to produce long-term changes in human factors practice."[229] Similarly, United Airlines states in its CRM manual: "Command/Leadership/Resource management [United's terminology for CRM] cannot be a one-shot approach. It has to be a coordinated long range program. It must therefore be an integral part of the entire training effort: new hire training, transition and upgrade programs, and recurrent training."[230]

Finally, the principles and procedures taught in training must be reinforced within the operational environment. Simulator-based safety training can be totally negated if production pressures or latent failures in the workplace make it impossible to implement its teachings effectively.

It is still too early to make definitive statements about either the benefits or the costs of simulator-based training in anesthesia. To some extent, a "catch 22" is involved. One cannot attempt to determine the true cost-effectiveness until simulation is widespread enough for complex and expensive studies to be undertaken, and until there is more experience on the different organizational aspects of providing the training. Many institutions are likely to shy away from taking the risk until the cost-effectiveness is proven.

Simulation Societies: Society for Simulation in Healthcare and Society in Europe for Simulation Applied to Medicine

One measure of the evolving maturity of simulation in health care is the formation and growth of professional societies focused on this topic. Although anesthesiology was the medical field that initiated work on the fully interactive mannequin-based simulator and that dominated the early developments in the field, simulation is a broad strategy that has now been widely adopted by many different disciplines and domains in health care. For the most part, simulation professional societies have sprung up as explicitly multidisciplinary organizations. Major leadership roles in these societies have been played by anesthesiologists and engineers associated with anesthesiology, however.

The largest simulation organization is the Society for Simulation in Healthcare (SSH; www.ssih.org), which was founded in 2004 as the outgrowth of the group that had operated the International Meeting on Medical Simulation for several years as a satellite to the annual meeting of the Society for Technology in Anesthesia. Under the new auspices of SSH, the meeting was transformed into the International Meeting on Simulation in Healthcare (IMSH), encompassing all health care disciplines and domains, not just medicine. Regular scientific congresses on simulation had been under way since the mid 1990s (the Rochester Conferences on Simulation in Anesthesia). Although they originally had about 100 attendees, Society in Europe for Simulation Applied to Medicine (SESAM) meetings have now around 400 attendees. The IMSH meeting in 2009 is expecting more than 2000 attendees. This puts it in the category of a medium-sized scientific meeting; to put this in the context of anesthesiology, it would rank as the third largest scientific meeting in the United States, falling below only the ASA meeting and the New York Postgraduate Assembly in Anesthesiology (PGA) conference, but ranking ahead of the International Anesthesia Research Society (IARS) annual meeting.

Another sign of the mainstream nature of simulation is that SSH has published a quarterly peer-reviewed journal, *Simulation in Healthcare,* since 2006. It has been integrated in PubMed citations recently (2008). The journal is an official publication of many international professional societies of simulation in health care, including SESAM (www.sesam.ws), the Australian Society for Simulation in Healthcare, and the Association of Standardized Patient Educators. The organizations have become affiliates of the SSH.

Another sign of maturity is the emergence of a trade organization for simulation in health care dedicated to educating and influencing policy makers, primarily concerning federal legislation and health policy. The Advanced Initiatives in Medical Simulation (AIMS) is a 501c6 organization that is allowed to lobby the U.S. government. Supported by universities and industry, AIMS promotes legislation and offers an annual exhibition about simulation in health care on Capitol Hill. What was previously seemingly the province of a few technologically minded anesthesiologists has blossomed into a substantial industry and profession with all the trappings of organizations, meetings, journals, and even lobbyists.

Future of Patient Simulation in Anesthesia

"The future is now—we are it."[231]

Although nearly past 2 decades of consistent development, the field of simulation in health care is still relatively new.[5,16,232] Although there are hundreds to thousands of simulators in use around the world, many targeting anesthesiology and critical care, the fraction of clinicians in these fields who have undergone a meaningful simulation experience is still small.

Simulators have become more sophisticated, and users now can choose from many different models offered by multiple manufacturers. Improvements in simulators depend on the demand for the devices and on the tradeoff between fidelity and cost. Many otherwise desirable improvements may be too costly for the impact that they can be expected to produce. Technologic advances are likely to be targeted at portability and reliability, rather than at supporting increasingly esoteric feature sets. Many users have opted for simpler and cheaper simulators that use direct control, modest scripts, and finite state machines to control the changing state of the simulated patient rather than complex mathematical models. This is partly because the production and use of robust mathematical models has been more difficult than anticipated.

In contrast to aeronautical engineers, physicians do not design and build the system that they wish to model. The fundamental differential equations of fluid mechanics and aerodynamics are firmly established, allowing supercomputers to provide technically meaningful simulations as replacements for many wind tunnel tests. There are still wind tunnel tests, however, and test flights of actual prototype aircraft. Sophisticated instrumentation can be built into test structures to define their behavior accurately. Physicians will never have this type of knowledge about the human body. The advantages and disadvantages of the different types of control logic for different applications is still being sorted out.

There has been growing interest in purely virtual reality simulations, often of a type similar to massive online games or to the popular Second Life system. Participating with others in the same virtual world, linked by the Internet, is appealing for many purposes. Such simulations are only as good as the engines that drive the underlying patients that may be found there, and the quality of the data provided and interventions and choices supported for implementation in these settings. Virtual reality proponents imagine a virtual reality so realistic that it rivals, or is indistinguishable from, the real world. This would approach the Star Trek "Holo-Deck." Although we once predicted that such systems might be in place by 2020, the development of such high-veracity virtual reality has not proceeded as quickly as previously imagined, and it is unclear whether full virtual reality of this nature will be available in the next decade.

Patient simulation has now become a regular part of the initial and recurrent training of most anesthesiologists and many other clinicians in the United States, Australia, and the United Kingdom, and in some European countries. With patient simulation, the human error–based CRM concept was introduced to medicine as ACRM training, revolutionizing the traditional way and content of teaching and learning. The anesthesia community can be proud of its pioneering role in developing patient simulation technology and simulation-based training curricula, and anesthesiologists and others working with them continue to play dominant leadership roles in many settings of simulation, even those devoted to fields outside anesthesia.

References

1. Good ML, Gravenstein JS: Anesthesia simulators and training devices. Int Anesth Clin 27:161-166, 1989.
2. Gallagher CJ, Issenberg SB: Simulation in Anesthesia. Philadelphia, WB Saunders, 2006.
3. Kyle RR, Murray WB: Clinical Simulation—Operations, Engineering and Management. Amsterdam, Academic Press Elsevier, 2008.
4. Smith BE, Gaba DM, Lake C, et al: Simulators. Philadelphia, WB Saunders, 2001.
5. Gaba DM: The future vision of simulation in health care. Qual Saf Health Care 13(Suppl 1):i2-i10, 2004.
6. Sutnick AI, Stillman PL, Norcini JJ, et al: ECFMG assessment of clinical competence of graduates of foreign medical schools. Educational Commission for Foreign Medical Graduates. JAMA 270:1041-1045, 1993.
7. Ziv A, Ben-David MF, Sutnick AI, Gary NE: Lessons learned from six years of international administrations of the ECFMG's SP-based clinical skills assessment. Acad Med 73:84-91, 1998.
8. Stefanich L, Cruz-Neira C: A virtual surgical simulator for the lower limbs. Biomed Sci Instrum 35:141-145, 1999.
9. Krummel TM: Surgical simulation and virtual reality: The coming revolution. Ann Surg 228:635-637, 1998.
10. Meier AH, Rawn CL, Krummel TM: Virtual reality: Surgical application—challenge for the new millennium. J Am Coll Surg 192:372-384, 2001.
11. Howard SK, Gaba DM, Smith BE, et al: Simulation study of rested versus sleep-deprived anesthesiologists. Anesthesiology 98:1345-1355, 2003.
12. Agutter J, Drews F, Syroid N, et al: Evaluation of graphic cardiovascular display in a high-fidelity simulator. Anesth Analg 97:1403-1413, 2003.
13. Singer SJ, Gaba DM, Geppert JJ, et al: The culture of safety: Results of an organization-wide survey in 15 California hospitals. Qual Saf Health Care 12:112-118, 2003.
14. Helmreich RL, Merritt AC, Wilhelm JA: The evolution of Crew Resource Management training in commercial aviation. Int J Aviat Psychol 9:19-32, 1999.
15. Billings CE, Reynard WD: Human factors in aircraft incidents: Results of a 7-year study. Aviat Space Environ Med 55:960-965, 1984.
16. Gaba DM, Howard SK, Fish KJ, et al: Simulation-based training in anesthesia crisis resource management (ACRM): A decade of experience. Simulation and Gaming 32:175-193, 2001.
17. Jensen RS, Biegelski CS: Cockpit Resource Management. Aldershot, U.K. Gower Technical, 1989.
18. Weiner EL, Kanki BG, Helmreich RL: Cockpit Resource Management. San Diego, Academic Press, 1993.
19. Dieckmann P, Rall M: Simulators in anaesthetic training to enhance patient safety. *In* Cashman JN, Grounds RM (eds): Recent Advances in Anaesthesia and Intensive Care. Cambridge, Cambridge University Press, 2007, pp 211-232.
20. Dieckmann P, Wehner T, Rall M, Manser T: Prospektive Simulation: Ein Konzept zur methodischen Ergnzung von medizinischen Simulatorsettings. Zeitschrift Arbeitswissenschaften ZfA 59:172-180, 2005.
21. Dieckmann P, Gaba D, Rall M: Deepening the theoretical foundations of patient simulation as social practice. Simulation in Healthcare 3:183-193, 2007.
22. Dieckmann P, Manser T, Wehner T, Rall M: Reality and fiction cues in medical patient simulation: An interview study with anesthesiologists. Journal of Cognitive Engineering and Decision Making 1:148-168, 2007.
23. Hays RT, Singer MJ: Simulation Fidelity in Training System Design: Bridging the Gap Between Reality and Training. New York, Springer, 1989.
24. Feinstein AH, Cannon HM: Constructs of simulation evaluation. Simulation and Gaming 33:425-440, 2002.

25. Issenberg SB, McGaghie WC, Petrusa ER, et al: Features and uses of high-fidelity medical simulations that lead to effective learning: A BEME systematic review. Med Teach 27:10-28, 2005.
26. Scerbo MW, Dawson S: High fidelity, high performance? Simulation in Healthcare 4:224-230, 2007.
27. Rudolph J, Simon R: Which reality matters? Questions on the path to high engagement in healthcare simulation. Simulation in Healthcare 3:161-163, 2007.
28. Salas E, Bowers CA, Rhodenizer L: It is not how much you have but how you use it: Toward a rational use of simulation to support aviation training. Int J Aviat Psychol 8:197-208, 1998.
29. Salas E, Burke CS: Simulation for training is effective when. Qual Saf Health Care 11:119-120, 2002.
30. Baker DP, Day R, Salas E: Teamwork as an essential component of high-reliability organizations. Health Serv Res 41:1576-1598, 2006.
31. Baker DP, Gustafson S, Beaubien JM, et al: Medical Teamwork and Patient Safety: The Evidence-Based Relation. Literature Review. Rockville, MD, Agency for Healthcare Research and Quality, 2005.
32. Salas E, Rosen MA, Burke CS, et al: Markers for enhancing team cognition in complex environments: The power of team performance diagnosis. Aviat Space Environ Med 78:B77-B85, 2007.
33. Salas E, Wilson KA, Burke CS, Wightman DC: Does crew resource management training work? An update, an extension, and some critical needs. Hum Factors 48:392-412, 2006.
34. Salas E, Bowers CA, Edens E: Improving Teamwork in Organizations—Applications of Resource Management Training. Mahwah, NJ, Lawrence Erlbaum, 2001.
35. Eppich WJ, Adler MD, McGaghie WC: Emergency and critical care pediatrics: Use of medical simulation for training in acute pediatric emergencies. Curr Opin Pediatr 18:266-271, 2006.
36. Knudson MM, Khaw L, Bullard MK, et al: Trauma training in simulation: Translating skills from SIM time to real time. J Trauma 64:255-263; discussion 263-264, 2008.
37. Berkenstadt H, Erez D, Munz Y, et al: Training and assessment of trauma management: The role of simulation-based medical education. Anesthesiol Clin 25:65-74, 2007.
38. Maslovitz S, Barkai G, Lessing JB, et al: Recurrent obstetric management mistakes identified by simulation. Obstet Gynecol 109:1295-1300, 2007.
39. Wallin CJ, Meurling L, Hedman L, et al: Target-focused medical emergency team training using a human patient simulator: Effects on behaviour and attitude. Med Educ 41:173-180, 2007.
40. Rudy SJ, Polomano R, Murray WB, et al: Team management training using crisis resource management results in perceived benefits by healthcare workers. J Contin Educ Nurs 38:219-226, 2007.
41. Dunn EJ, Mills PD, Neily J, et al: Medical team training: Applying crew resource management in the Veterans Health Administration. Jt Comm J Qual Patient Saf 33:317-325, 2007.
42. Gaba D: What does simulation add to teamwork training? AHRQ WebM&M Case Commentary, 2006.
43. Weinstock PH, Kappus LJ, Kleinman ME, et al: Toward a new paradigm in hospital-based pediatric education: The development of an onsite simulator program. Pediatr Crit Care Med 6:635-641, 2005.
44. Shapiro MJ, Morey JC, Small SD, et al: Simulation based teamwork training for emergency department staff: Does it improve clinical team performance when added to an existing didactic teamwork curriculum? Qual Saf Health Care 13:417-421, 2004.
45. Lighthall GK: Toward better outcomes through simulation-based multidisciplinary team training. *In* Dunn WF (ed): Simulators in Critical Care and Beyond. Des Plaines, Society of Critical Care Medicine, 2004, pp 54-60.
46. Ostergaard HT, Ostergaard D, Lippert A: Implementation of team training in medical education in Denmark. Qual Saf Health Care 13(Suppl I):i91-i95, 2004.
47. Rall M, Manser T, Howard S: Key elements of debriefing for simulator training. Eur J Anaesthesiol 17:516-517, 2000.
48. McDonnell LK, Jobe KK, Dismukes RK: Facilitating LOS Debriefings: A Training Manual—Part 1: An Introduction to Facilitation. Moffett Field, Ames Research Center, 1997.
49. Dismukes K, Gaba D, Howard S: So many roads: Facilitated debriefing in healthcare [editorial]. Simulation in Healthcare 1:23-25, 2006.
50. Fanning RM, Gaba DM: The role of debriefing in simulation-based learning. Simulation in Healthcare 2:115-125, 2007.
51. Rudolph JW, Simon R, Rivard P, et al: Debriefing with good judgment: Combining rigorous feedback with genuine inquiry. Anesthesiol Clin 25:361-376, 2007.
52. Savoldelli GL, Naik VN, Park J, et al: Value of debriefing during simulated crisis management: Oral versus video-assisted oral feedback. Anesthesiology 105:279-285, 2006.
53. Rudolph JW, Simon R, Dufresne RL, Raemer DB: There's no such thing as a "nonjudgmental" debriefing: A theory and method for debriefing with good judgment. Simulation in Healthcare 1:49-55, 2006.
54. O'Brien G, Haughton A, Flanagan B: Interns' perceptions of performance and confidence in participating in and managing simulated and real cardiac arrest situations. Med Teach 23:389-395, 2001.
55. Makary MA, Mukherjee A, Sexton JB, et al: Operating room briefings and wrong-site surgery. J Am Coll Surg 204:236-243, 2007.
56. Marshall DA, Manus DA: A team training program using human factors to enhance patient safety. AORN J 86:994-1011, 2007.
57. Makary MA, Holzmueller CG, Sexton JB, et al: Operating room debriefings. Jt Comm J Qual Patient Saf 32:407-410, 2006.
58. Awad SS, Fagan SP, Bellows C, et al: Bridging the communication gap in the operating room with medical team training. Am J Surg 190:770-774, 2005.
59. Kobayashi L, Suner S, Shapiro MJ, et al: Multipatient disaster scenario design using mixed modality medical simulation for the evaluation of civilian prehospital medical response: A "dirty bomb" case study. Simulation in Healthcare 2:72-78, 2006.
60. Kyle RR, Via DK, Lowy J, et al: A multi-disciplinary approach to teach responses to weapons of mass destruction and terrorism using combined simulation modalities. J Clin Anesth 16:(2):152-158, 2004.
60a. Kolb DA. Experiential Learning: Experience as the Source of Learning and Development. Englewood Cliffs, NJ: Prentice Hall, 1984.
61. Cumin D, Merry AF: Simulators for use in anaesthesia. Anaesthesia 62:151-162, 2007.
62. Schwid HA: A flight simulator for general anesthesia training. Comput Biomed Res 20:64-75, 1987.
63. Schwid HA, O'Donnell D: The anesthesia simulator-recorder: A device to train and evaluate anesthesiologists' responses to critical incidents. Anesthesiology 72:191-197, 1990.
64. Schwid HA, O'Donnell D: Anesthesiologists' management of simulated critical incidents. Anesthesiology 76:495-501, 1992.
65. Kalawsky RS: The Science of Virtual Reality and Virtual Environments. Workingham, England, Addison-Wesley Publishing Company, 1993.
66. Gaba DM: Anesthesia simulators—a virtual reality. American Society of Anesthesiologists Newsletter 57:20-23, 1993.
67. Gaba DM: Improving anesthesiologists' performance by simulating reality [editorial; comment]. Anesthesiology 76:491-494, 1992.
68. Cooper JB, Blum RH, Carroll JS, et al: Differences in safety climate among hospital anesthesia departments and the effect of a realistic simulation-based training program. Anesth Analg 106:574-584, 2008.
69. Gaba D, Howard S, Fish K, et al: Simulation-based training in anesthesia crisis resource management (ACRM): A decade of experience. Simulation and Gaming 32:175-193, 2001.
70. Smith B, Gaba D: Simulators. *In* Lake C, Hines R, Blitt C (eds): Clinical Monitoring: Practical Applications for Anesthesia and Critical Care. Philadelphia, WB Saunders, 2001, pp 26-44.
71. Abrahamson S, Denson JS, Wolf RM: Effectiveness of a simulator in training anesthesiology residents. J Med Educ 44:515-519, 1969.
72. Cooper JB, Newborner RS, Kitz RJ: An analysis of major errors and equipment failures in anesthesia management: Considerations for prevention and detection. Anesthesiology 60:34-42, 1984.
73. Gaba DM, Maxwell M, DeAnda A: Anesthetic mishaps: Breaking the chain of accident evolution. Anesthesiology 66:670-676, 1987.
74. Gaba DM: Human error in anesthetic mishaps. Int Anesthesiol Clin 27:137-147, 1989.
75. Weinger MB, Englund CE: Ergonomic and human factors affecting anesthetic vigilance and monitoring performance in the operating room environment. Anesthesiology 73:995-1021, 1990.
76. Morgan PJ, Cleave-Hogg D: A Canadian simulation experience: Faculty and student opinions of a performance evaluation study. Br J Anaesth 85:779-781, 2000.
77. Gaba DM: Two examples of how to evaluate the impact of new approaches to teaching [editorial]. Anesthesiology 96:1-2, 2002.
78. Coates WC, Steadman RH, Huang YM, et al: Full-scale high fidelity human patient simulation vs problem based learning: Comparing two interactive educational modalities. Acad Emerg Med 10:489, 2003.
79. Gordon JA, Shaffer DW, Raemer DB, et al: A randomized controlled trial of simulation-based teaching versus traditional instruction in medicine: A pilot study among clinical medical students. Adv Health Sci Educ Theory Pract 11:33-39, 2006.
80. Gordon JA: The human patient simulator: Acceptance and efficacy as a teaching tool for students. Acad Med 75:522, 2000.
81. Euliano TY: Teaching respiratory physiology: Clinical correlation with a human patient simulator. J Clin Monit Comput 16:465-470, 2000.
82. Gordon J: The human patient simulator: Acceptance and efficacy as a teaching tool for students. Acad Med 75:522, 2000.
83. Gordon JA, Wilkerson WM, Shaffer DW, Armstrong EG: "Practicing" medicine without risk: Students' and educators' responses to high-fidelity patient simulation. Acad Med 76:469-472, 2001.
84. Gordon JA, Pawlowski J: Education on-demand: The development of a simulator-based medical education service. Acad Med 77:751-752, 2002.

85. Gordon JA, Farrell SE, Pawlowski JB, et al: Education "on demand": The development of a simulator-based medical education service. Acad Emerg Med 9:1059, 2002.
86. Gordon JA: The human patient simulator: Acceptance and efficacy as a teaching tool for students. The Medical Readiness Trainer Team. Acad Med 75:522, 2000.
87. Gordon JJ, Saunders NA, Hennrikus D, Sanson-Fisher RW: Interns' performances with simulated patients at the beginning and the end of the intern year. J Gen Intern Med 7:57-62, 1992.
88. Issenberg SB, Gordon DL, Safford RE, Hart IR: Simulation and new learning technologies. Med Teach 23:16-23, 2001.
89. O'Donnell J, Fletcher J, Dixon B, Palmer L: Planning and implementing an anesthesia crisis resource management course for student nurse anesthetists. CRNA 2:50-58, 1998.
90. Rall M, Schaedle B, Zieger J, et al: [Innovative training for enhancing patient safety: Safety culture and integrated concepts]. Unfallchirurg 105:1033-1042, 2002.
91. Ohrn MAK, van Meurs WL, Good ML: Laboratory classes: Replacing animals with a patient simulator [abstract]. Anesthesiology 83:A1028, 1995.
92. Morgan PJ, Cleave-Hogg D: Comparison between medical students' experience, confidence and competence. Med Educ 36:534-539, 2002.
93. Hodges B: Medical education and the maintenance of incompetence. Med Teach 28:690-696, 2006.
94. Cooper JB, Newbower RS, Long CD, McPeek B: Preventable anesthesia mishaps: A study of human factors. Anesthesiology 49:399-406, 1978.
95. Howard SK, Gaba D, Fish KJ, et al: Anesthesia crisis resource management training: Teaching anesthesiologists to handle critical incidents. Aviat Space Environ Med 63:763-770, 1992.
96. Adler MD, Trainor JL, Siddall VJ, McGaghie WC: Development and evaluation of high-fidelity simulation case scenarios for pediatric resident education. Ambul Pediatr 7:182-186, 2007.
97. Murphy JG, Torsher LC, Dunn WF: Simulation medicine in intensive care and coronary care education. J Crit Care 22:51-55, 2007.
98. Ogden PE, Cobbs LS, Howell MR, et al: Clinical simulation: Importance to the internal medicine educational mission. Am J Med 120:820-824, 2007.
99. Thomas EJ, Taggart B, Crandell S, et al: Teaching teamwork during the Neonatal Resuscitation Program: A randomized trial. J Perinatol 27:409-414, 2007.
100. Steadman RH, Coates WC, Huang YM, et al: Simulation-based training is superior to problem-based learning for the acquisition of critical assessment and management skills. Crit Care Med 34:151-157, 2006.
101. Wright SW, Lindsell CJ, Hinckley WR, et al: High fidelity medical simulation in the difficult environment of a helicopter: Feasibility, self-efficacy and cost. BMC Med Educ 6:49, 2006.
102. Pronovost P, Goeschel C: Improving ICU care: It takes a team. Health Exec 20:14-16, 2005.
103. Sundar E, Sundar S, Pawlowski J, et al: Crew resource management and team training. Anesthesiol Clin 25:283-300, 2007.
104. Rall M: Symposium: Simulation in Anaesthesia and Intensive Care Medicine 2000 Annual Meeting of the Society in Europe for Simulation Applied to Medicine (SESAM) [editorial]. Eur J Anaesthesiol 17:515, 2000.
105. Lussi C, Grapengeter M, Schuttler J: [Simulator training in anesthesia: Applications and value]. Anaesthetist 48:433-438, 1999.
106. Lussi C, Grapengeter M, Engl HG, et al: Crisis resource management (CRM) training using a patient simulator: Course evaluation. Anasthesiologie Intensivmedizin 40:729-733, 1999.
107. Schuttler J: [Training in a simulator: Play or indispensable component of the medical learning process?]. Anaesthetist 48:431-432, 1999.
108. Issenberg SB, McGaghie WC, Hart IR, et al: Simulation technology for health care professional skills training and assessment. JAMA 282:861-866, 1999.
109. Kurrek MM, Fish KJ: Anesthesia crisis resource management training: An intimidating concept, a rewarding experience. Can J Anesth 43:430-434, 1996.
110. Yaeger KA, Halamek LP, Coyle M, et al: High-fidelity simulation-based training in neonatal nursing. Adv Neonatal Care 4:326-331, 2004.
111. Halamek LP, Kaegi DM, Gaba DM, et al: Time for a new paradigm in pediatric medical education: Teaching neonatal resuscitation in a simulated delivery room environment. Pediatrics 106:E45, 2000.
112. Smith HM, Jacob AK, Segura LG, et al: Simulation education in anesthesia training: A case report of successful resuscitation of bupivacaine-induced cardiac arrest linked to recent simulation training. Anesth Analg 106:1581-1584, 2008.
113. Lighthall GK, Barr J, Howard SK, et al: Use of a fully simulated ICU environment for critical event management training for internal medicine residents. Crit Care Med 31:2437-2443, 2003.
114. Fellander-Tsai L, Stahre C, Anderberg B, et al: [Simulator training in medicine and health care: A new pedagogic model for good patient safety]. Lakartidningen 98:3772-3776, 2001.
115. Larbuisson R, Pendeville P, Nyssen AS, et al: Use of Anaesthesia Simulator: Initial impressions of its use in two Belgian University Centers. Acta Anaesthesiol Belg 50:87-93, 1999.
116. Lindekaer AL, Jacobsen J, Andersen G, et al: Treatment of ventricular fibrillation during anaesthesia in an anaesthesia simulator. Acta Anaesthesiol Scand 41:1280-1284, 1997.
117. Hayes CW, Rhee A, Detsky ME, et al: Residents feel unprepared and unsupervised as leaders of cardiac arrest teams in teaching hospitals: A survey of internal medicine residents. Crit Care Med 35:1668-1672, 2007.
118. Eich C, Russo SG, Nickel EA, et al: Simulator-based training in paediatric anaesthesia and emergency medicine—thrills, skills and attitudes. Br J Anaesth 98(4):417-419, 2007.
119. Overly FL, Sudikoff SN, Shapiro MJ: High-fidelity medical simulation as an assessment tool for pediatric residents' airway management skills. Pediatr Emerg Care 23:11-15, 2007.
120. Eppich WJ, Brannen M, Hunt EA: Team training: Implications for emergency and critical care pediatrics. Curr Opin Pediatr 2008.
121. Ralston M, Hazinski MF, Zaritsky AL, et al: PALS Course Guide. Dallas, TX, American Heart Association, 2006.
122. Krug SE, Frush K: Patient safety in the pediatric emergency care setting. Pediatrics 120:1367-1375, 2007.
123. Eich C, Russo S, Timmermann A, et al: [New perspectives for simulator-based training in paediatric anaesthesia and emergency medicine]. Anaesthetist 55(2):179-184, 2006.
124. Eppich WJ, Arnold LD: Family member presence in the pediatric emergency department. Curr Opin Pediatr 15:294-298, 2003.
125. Byrne AJ, Jones JG: Responses to simulated anaesthetic emergencies by anaesthetists with different durations of clinical experience. Br J Anaesth 78:553-556, 1997.
126. DeAnda A, Gaba DM: Role of experience in the response to simulated critical incidents. Anesth Analg 72:308-315, 1991.
127. Schwid HA, Rooke GA, Carline J, et al: Evaluation of anesthesia residents using mannequin-based simulation: A multiinstitutional study. Anesthesiology 97:1434-1444, 2002.
128. Gardi T, Christensen UC, Jacobsen J, et al: How do anaesthesiologists treat malignant hyperthermia in a full-scale anaesthesia simulator? Acta Anaesthesiol Scand 45:1032-1035, 2001.
129. Devitt JH, Kurrek MM, Cohen MM, et al: Testing internal consistency and construct validity during evaluation of performance in a patient simulator. Anesth Analg 86:1160-1164, 1998.
130. Jacobsen J, Lindekaer AL, Ostergaard HT, et al: Management of anaphylactic shock evaluated using a full-scale anaesthesia simulator. Acta Anaesthesiol Scand 45:315-319, 2001.
131. Howard SK, Gaba DM, Fish KJ, et al: Anesthesia crisis resource management training: Teaching anesthesiologists to handle critical incidents. Aviat Space Environ Med 63:763-770, 1992.
132. Hammond J, Bermann M, Chen B, Kushins L: Incorporation of a computerized human patient simulator in critical care training: A preliminary report. J Trauma 53:1064-1067, 2002.
133. Ellis C, Hughes G: Use of human patient simulation to teach emergency medicine trainees advanced airway skills. J Accid Emerg Med 16:395-399, 1999.
134. Kaufmann C, Liu A: Trauma training: Virtual reality applications. Stud Health Technol Inform 81:236-241, 2001.
135. Small S, Wuertz R, Simon R, et al: Demonstration of high-fidelity simulation team training for emergency medicine. Acad Emerg Med 6:312-323, 1999.
136. McLaughlin SA, Doezema D, Sklar DP: Human simulation in emergency medicine training: A model curriculum. Acad Emerg Med 9:1310-1318, 2002.
137. Reznek M, Smith-Coggins R, Howard S, et al: Emergency Medicine Crisis Management (EMCM): Pilot investigation of a simulation-based crisis management. Acad Emerg Med 9:430, 2002.
138. Wong SH, Ng KF, Chen PP: The application of clinical simulation in crisis management training. Hong Kong Med J 8:131-135, 2002.
139. Patel RM, Crombleholme WR: Using simulation to train residents in managing critical events. Acad Med 73:593, 1998.
140. Halamek L, Howard S, Smith B, et al: Development of a simulated delivery room for the study of human performance during neonatal resuscitation. Pediatrics 100(Suppl):513-524, 1997.
141. Kurrek MM, Devitt JH, Cohen M: Cardiac arrest in the OR: How are our ACLS skills? Can J Anaesth 45:130-132, 1998.
142. Palmisano J, Akingbola O, Moler F, Custer J: Simulated pediatric cardiopulmonary resuscitation: Initial events and response times of a hospital arrest team. Respir Care 39:725-729, 1994.
143. Christensen UJ, Heffernan D, Andersen SF, Jensen PF: ResusSim 98—a PC advanced life support trainer. Resuscitation 39:81-84, 1998.
144. Hendrickse AD, Ellis AM, Morris RW: Use of simulation technology in Australian Defence Force resuscitation training. J R Army Med Corps 147:173-178, 2001.
145. Manser T, Dieckmann P, Wehner T, Rall M: Comparison of anaesthetists' activity patterns in the

operating room and during simulation. Ergonomics 50:246-260, 2007.
146. Dieckmann P, Reddersen S, Wehner T, Rall M: Prospective memory failures as an unexplored threat to patient safety: Results from a pilot study using patient simulators to investigate the missed execution of intentions. Ergonomics 49:526-543, 2006.
147. Kofke WA, Rie MA, Rosen K: Acute care crisis simulation for jury education. Med Law 20:79-83, 2001.
148. Flanagan B, Clavisi O, Nestel D: Efficacy and effectiveness of simulation based training for learning and assessment in health care (report). Melbourne, 2007, pp 1-90. Available at: http://www.health.vic.gov.au/workforce/research.htm.
149. Gaba D, DeAnda A: A comprehensive anesthesia simulation environment: Re-creating the operating room for research and training. Anesthesiology 69:387-394, 1988.
150. Gaba D: Improving anesthesiologists' performance by simulating reality [editorial]. Anesthesiology 76:491-494, 1992.
151. Chopra V, Gesink B, De Jong J, et al: Does training on an anaesthesia simulator lead to improvement in performance? Br J Anaesth 73:293-297, 1994.
152. Byrne A, Greaves J: Assessment instruments used during anaesthetic simulation: Review of published studies. Br J Anaesth 86:445-450, 2001.
153. Gaba D: The human work environment and anesthesia simulators. *In* Miller R (ed): Anesthesia, 5th ed. New York, Churchill Livingstone, 1999, pp 2613-2668.
154. Howard S, Keshavacharya S, Smith B, et al: Behavioral evidence of fatigue during a simulator experiment. Anesthesiology 89:A1236, 1998.
155. Weinger MB, Herdon OW, Gaba DM: The effect of electronic record keeping and transesophageal echocardiography on task distribution, workload, and vigilance during cardiac anesthesia. Anesthesiology 87:144-155, 1997.
156. Gaba D, Howard S, Small S: Situation awareness in anesthesiology. Hum Factors 37:20-31, 1995.
157. Holzman R, Cooper J, Gaba D, et al: Anesthesia crisis resource management: Real-life simulation training in operating room crises. J Clin Anesth 7:675-687, 1995.
158. Weinger MB, Herndon OW, Zornow MH, et al: An objective methodology for task analysis and workload assessment in anesthesia providers. Anesthesiology 80:77-92, 1994.
159. Howard S, Gaba D, Fish K, et al: Anesthesia crisis resource management training: Teaching anesthesiologists to handle critical incidents. Aviat Space Environ Med 63:763-770, 1992.
160. DeAnda A, Gaba D: The role of experience in the response to simulated critical incidents. Anesth Analg 72:308-315, 1991.
161. Forrest F, Taylor M, Postlehwaite K, Aspinall R: Use of the high-fidelity simulator to develop testing of the technical performance of novice anaesthetists. Br J Anaesth 88:338-344, 2002.
162. Fletcher G, Flin R, McGeorge P, et al: Anaesthetists' Non-Technical Skills (ANTS): Evaluation of a behavioural marker system. Br J Anaesth 90:580-588, 2003.
163. Fletcher GC, McGeorge P, Flin RH, et al: The role of non-technical skills in anaesthesia: A review of current literature. Br J Anaesth 88:418-429, 2002.
164. Glavin RJ, Maran NJ: Development and use of scoring systems for assessment of clinical competence. Br J Anaesth 88:329-330, 2002.
165. Chopra V, Gesink BJ, de Jong J, et al: Does training on an anaesthesia simulator lead to improvement in performance? Br J Anaesth 73:293-297, 1994.
166. Slagle J, Weinger M, Dinh M-T, et al: Assessment of the intrarater and interrater reliability of an established clinical task analysis methodology. Anesthesiology 96:1129-1139, 2002.
167. Weinger MB, Slagle J: Human factors research in anesthesia patient safety. Proc AMIA Symp 756-760, 2001.
168. Devitt J, Kurreck M, Cohen M, Cleave-Hogg D: The validity of performance assessments using simulation. Anesthesiology 95:36-42, 2001.
169. Devitt J, Kurrek M, Cohen M, et al: Testing internal consistency and construct validity during evaluation of performance in a patient simulator. Anesth Analg 86:1160-1164, 1998.
170. Devitt J, Kurrek M, Cohen M, et al: Testing the raters: Interrater reliability of standardized anaesthesia simulator performance. Can J Anaesth 44:924-928, 1997.
171. Byrne A, Hilton P, Lunn J: Basic simulations for anaesthetists. Anaesthesia 49:376-381, 1994.
172. McGaghie WC, Issenberg SB, Gordon DL, Petrusa ER: Assessment instruments used during anaesthetic simulation. Br J Anaesth 87:647-648, 2001.
173. Barsuk D, Ziv A, Lin G, et al: Using advanced simulation for recognition and correction of gaps in airway and breathing management skills in prehospital trauma care. Anesth Analg 100:803-809, 2005.
174. Ziv A, Berkenstadt H: National interdisciplinary, multimodality simulation center: The Israel model and experience. *In* Dunn WF (ed): Simulators in Critical Care and Beyond. Des Plaines, Society of Critical Care Medicine, 2004, pp 67-71.
175. Ziv A, Wolpe PR, Small SD, Glick S: Simulation-based medical education: An ethical imperative. Acad Med 78:783-788, 2003.
176. Rosenstock C, Ostergaard D, Kristensen MS, et al: Residents lack knowledge and practical skills in handling the difficult airway. Acta Anaesthesiol Scand 48:1014-1018, 2004.
177. Ostergaard D: National Medical Simulation training program in Denmark. Crit Care Med 32:S58-S60, 2004.
178. Bronfenbrenner U: The Ecology of Human Development. Cambridge, Harvard University Press, 1979.
179. Manser T, Wehner T: Analysing action sequences: Variations in action density in the administration of anaesthesia. Cognition Tech Work 4:71-81, 2002.
180. Schwid H, O'Donnell D: Anesthesiologists' management of simulated critical incidents. Anesthesiology 76:495-501, 1992.
181. DeAnda A, Gaba D: Unplanned incidents during comprehensive anesthesia simulation. Anesth Analg 71:77-82, 1990.
182. Gaba D, DeAnda A: The response of anesthesia trainees to simulated critical incidents. Anesth Analg 68:444-451, 1989.
183. Dieckmann P, Manser T, Schaedle B, Rall M: How do anesthesiologists experience a simulator setting in comparison with clinical settings? Results from an interview study [Abstract Santander-02-12]. Eur J Anaesthesiol 20:846, 2003.
184. Gaba D, Fish K, Howard S: Crisis Management in Anesthesiology. New York, Churchill Livingstone, 1994.
185. Gaba DM, Howard SK, Flanagan B, et al: Assessment of clinical performance during simulated crises using both technical and behavioral ratings [see comments]. Anesthesiology 89:8-18, 1998.
186. Byrne A, Jones J: Responses to simulated anaesthetic emergencies by anaesthetists with different durations of clinical experience. Br J Anaesth 78:553-556, 1997.
187. Gaba DM, DeAnda A: The response of anesthesia trainees to simulated critical incidents. Anesth Analg 68:444-451, 1989.
188. Gaba DM: Research techniques in human performance using realistic simulation. *In* Henson LC, Lee AC (eds): Simulators in Anesthesiology Education. New York, Plenum Press, 1998, pp 93-102.
189. Weller J, Wilson L, Robinson B: Survey of change in practice following simulation-based training in crisis management. Anaesthesia 58:471-473, 2003.
190. Murray D, Enarson C: Communication and teamwork: Essential to learn but difficult to measure. Anesthesiology 106:895-896, 2007.
191. Jankouskas T, Bush MC, Murray B, et al: Crisis resource management: Evaluating outcomes of multidisciplinary teams. Simulation in Healthcare 2:96-101, 2007.
192. Murray DJ, Boulet JR, Kras JF, et al: A simulation-based acute skills performance assessment for anesthesia training. Anesth Analg 101:1127-1134, 2005.
193. Murray DJ, Boulet JR, Kras JF, et al: Acute care skills in anesthesia practice: A simulation-based resident performance assessment. Anesthesiology 101:1084-1095, 2004.
194. Boulet JR, Murray D, Kras J, et al: Reliability and validity of a simulation-based acute care assessment for medical students and residents. Anesthesiology 99:1270-1280, 2003.
195. Morgan PJ, Pittini R, Regehr G, et al: Evaluating teamwork in a simulated obstetric environment. Anesthesiology 106:907-915, 2007.
196. Nishisaki A, Keren R, Nadkarni V: Does simulation improve patient safety? Self-efficacy, competence, operational performance, and patient safety. Anesthesiol Clin 25:225-236, 2007.
197. Small SD: Simulation applications for human factors and systems evaluation. Anesthesiol Clin 25:237-259, 2007.
198. Ottestad E, Boulet JR, Lighthall GK: Evaluating the management of septic shock using patient simulation. Crit Care Med 35:769-775, 2007.
199. Hunt EA, Heine M, Hohenhaus SM, et al: Simulated pediatric trauma team management: Assessment of an educational intervention. Pediatr Emerg Care 23:796-804, 2007.
200. Harrison TK, Manser T, Howard SK, Gaba DM: Use of cognitive aids in a simulated anesthetic crisis. Anesth Analg 103:551-556, 2006.
201. Savoldelli GL, Naik VN, Joo HS, et al: Evaluation of patient simulator performance as an adjunct to the oral examination for senior anesthesia residents. Anesthesiology 104:475-481, 2006.
202. Scavone BM, Sproviero MT, McCarthy RJ, et al: Development of an objective scoring system for measurement of resident performance on the human patient simulator. Anesthesiology 105:260-266, 2006.
203. Friedman Z, Katznelson R, Devito I, et al: Objective assessment of manual skills and proficiency in performing epidural anesthesia—video-assisted validation. Reg Anesth Pain Med 31:304-310, 2006.
204. Jacobsohn E, Klock PA, Avidan M: Poor inter-rater reliability on mock anesthesia oral examinations. Can J Anaesth 53:659-668, 2006.
205. Reader T, Flin R, Lauche K, Cuthbertson BH: Non-technical skills in the intensive care unit. Br J Anaesth 96:551-559, 2006.
206. Wayne DB, Butter J, Siddall VJ, et al: Mastery learning of advanced cardiac life support skills by internal medicine residents using simulation technology and deliberate practice. J Gen Intern Med 21:251-256, 2006.

207. Kim J, Neilipovitz D, Cardinal P, et al: A pilot study using high-fidelity simulation to formally evaluate performance in the resuscitation of critically ill patients: The University of Ottawa Critical Care Medicine, High-Fidelity Simulation, and Crisis Resource Management I Study. Crit Care Med 34:2167-2174, 2006.

208. Zirkle M, Blum R, Raemer DB, et al: Teaching emergency airway management using medical simulation: A pilot program. Laryngoscope 115:495-500, 2005.

209. Blum RH, Raemer DB, Carroll JS, et al: A method for measuring the effectiveness of simulation-based team training for improving communication skills. Anesth Analg 100:1375-1380, 2005.

210. DeVita MA, Schaefer J, Lutz J, et al: Improving medical emergency team (MET) performance using a novel curriculum and a computerized human patient simulator. Qual Saf Health Care 14:326-331, 2005.

211. Rall M, Gaba DM: Human performance and patient safety. *In* Miller RD (ed): Miller's Anesthesia, 6th ed. Philadelphia, Churchill Livingstone, 2005, pp 3021-3072.

212. Pronovost PJ, Nolan T, Zeger S, et al: How can clinicians measure safety and quality in acute care? Lancet 363:1061-1067, 2004.

213. Gisondi MA, Smith-Coggins R, Harter PM, et al: Assessment of resident professionalism using high-fidelity simulation of ethical dilemmas. Acad Emerg Med 11:931-937, 2004.

214. Shapiro MJ, Kobayashi L, Morchi R: High-fidelity medical simulation and its role in evaluating advanced cardiac life support (ACLS) skills. Acad Emerg Med 10:488, 2003.

215. Weller JM, Bloch M, Young S, et al: Evaluation of high fidelity patient simulator in assessment of performance of anaesthetists. Br J Anaesth 90:43-47, 2003.

216. Weinger M, Herndon O, Zornow M, et al: An objective methodology for task analysis and workload assessment in anesthesia providers. Anesthesiology 77-92, 1994.

217. Brennan RL: Elements of Generalizability Theory. Iowa City, American College Testing Program, 1992.

218. Shavelson R: Generalizability Theory: A Primer. Newbury Park, CA, Sage Publications, 1991.

219. Myerson KR: Can we assess professional behavior in anesthetists? Anesthesia 53:1039-1040, 1998.

220. Kapur P, Steadman R: Patient simulator competency testing: ready for takeoff? Anesth Analg 86:1157-1159, 1998.

221. Klemola UM, Norros L: Practice-based criteria for assessing anaesthetists' habits of action: Outline for a reflexive turn in practice. Med Educ 35:455-464, 2001.

222. Greaves JD, Grant J: Watching anaesthetists work: Using the professional judgement of consultants to assess the developing clinical competence of trainees. Br J Anaesth 84:525-533, 2000.

223. Epstein RM, Hundert EM: Defining and assessing professional competence. JAMA 287:226-235, 2002.

224. Jha AK, Duncan BW, Bates DW: Simulator-based training and patient safety. *In* Shojania KG, Duncan BW, McDonald KM, Wachter RM (eds): Making Health Care Safer: A Critical Analysis of Patient Safety Practices (Evidence Report/Technology Assessment No. 43. AHRQ Publication 01-E058). Rockville, MD, Agency for Healthcare Research and Quality, 2001.

225. Berkenstadt H, Kantor GS, Yusim Y, et al: The feasibility of sharing simulation-based evaluation scenarios in anesthesiology. Anesth Analg 101:1068-1074, 2005.

226. Lamb D: Could simulated emergency procedures practised in a static environment improve the clinical performance of a Critical Care Air Support Team (CCAST)? A literature review. Intensive Crit Care Nurs 23:33-42, 2007.

227. Kurrek M, Devitt J: The cost for construction and maintenance of a simulation centre. Can J Anaesth 44:1191-1195, 1997.

228. Morgan PJ, Cleave-Hogg D: A worldwide survey of the use of simulation in anesthesia. Can J Anaesth 49:659-662, 2002.

229. Wiener E, Kanki B, Helmreich R: Cockpit Resource Management. San Diego, Academic Press, 1993.

230. Orlady H: Airline pilot training today and tomorrow. *In* Wiener E, Kanki B, Helmreich R (eds): Cockpit Resource Management. San Diego, Academic Press, 1993, pp 447-478.

231. Gaba DM: The future vision of simulation in healthcare. Simulation in Healthcare 2:126-135, 2007.

232. Gaba DM: A brief history of mannequin-based simulation and application. *In* Dunn WF (ed): Simulators in Critical Care and Beyond. Des Plaines, Society of Critical Care Medicine, 2004, pp 7-14.

233. Yule S, Flin R, Paterson-Brown S, et al: Development of a rating system for surgeons' non-technical skills. Med Educ 40:1098-1104, 2006.

Alan Jay Schwartz

8 Teaching Anesthesia

Key Points

1. Education is an all-encompassing process (not merely a specific activity) that results in a change in behavior on the part of the student/learner. The focus of education is the learner, not the teacher. It is the student who is educated by interacting with an environment that provides experiences. Education is change in behavior based on experiences.
2. Adult learners learn anesthesiology. Adult learners are those with strong motivation to participate in a set of experiences to learn a specific discipline. The discipline that they want to learn is one that they are interested in or need to know, or both. Adult learners participate in life-centered situational learning in the area or areas in which relevance is most likely.

   Adult learners enter the learning activity with a wealth of previous experience and view the current education in light of their background. Adult learners can capitalize on this previous learning; however, the previous learning may color how the current learning takes place.

   Adult learners are self-directed and initiate their own activities. Adult learning is goal oriented toward relevant life-centered needs. An adult learner tends to pick and choose some, not necessarily all, of the educational activities available.

   Inherent differences among people tend to increase with aging. Adult education must provide for differences in style, time, place, and pace of learning among adult learners. The time factor for learning is especially crucial for adults. Adults perceive that time passes more rapidly; that is, there is less time available to learn—or to do anything for that matter. With time perceived to be in short supply, adult learners tend to be selective in their learning to use what time they have more efficiently.
3. In 2006, there were 4970 resident anesthesiologists in 131 accredited American core anesthesiology residency programs and 360 subspecialty residents in 213 accredited American subspecialty anesthesiology programs.
4. Silber and colleagues,[29] in their study of almost 6000 patients undergoing prostate or gallbladder surgery in multiple hospitals, demonstrated that patient recovery or "rescue" from an adverse event correlated with the proportion of board-certified anesthesiologists in the hospital.
5. The Accreditation Council for Graduate Medical Education has defined six educational areas for which residents and fellows must demonstrate competency. These areas additionally are major components of Maintenance of Certification in Anesthesiology:
   a. Patient Care—Residents must be able to provide patient care that is compassionate, appropriate, and effective for the treatment of health problems and the promotion of health.
   b. Medical Knowledge—Residents must demonstrate knowledge of established and evolving biomedical, clinical, epidemiologic, and social-behavioral sciences, as well as the application of this knowledge to patient care.
   c. Practice-Based Learning and Improvement—Residents must demonstrate the ability to investigate and evaluate their care of patients, to appraise and assimilate scientific evidence, and to continuously improve patient care based on constant self-evaluation and lifelong learning.
   d. Interpersonal and Communication Skills—Residents must demonstrate interpersonal and communication skills that result in the effective exchange of information and collaboration with patients, their families, and health professionals.
   e. Professionalism—Residents must demonstrate a commitment to carrying out professional responsibilities and adherence to ethical principles.
   f. Systems-Based Practice—Residents must demonstrate an awareness of and responsiveness to the larger context and system of health care, as well as the ability to call effectively on other resources in the system to provide optimal health care.*
6. Full-time anesthesiology faculty positions in U.S. medical schools in 2006-2007 numbered 5836.[30] Anesthesiologists represent 5.6% of the clinical teachers and 4.7% of all American medical school teaching faculty.[30] The 5836 anesthesia faculty members in medical schools bear the

major responsibility for teaching some or all of the 69,028 enrolled undergraduate medical students, the 4970 graduate trainees in anesthesiology residency training programs, the 360 graduate trainees in anesthesiology subspecialty fellowship programs, and many of the approximately 104,879 physician house-staff trainees.[12,32]

7. Effective clinical teachers who are able to succeed at the bedside teaching encounter display specific actions noted by their students and themselves.[35] These actions include
   a. Allocating time for teaching
   b. Creating a teaching/learning environment of trust and concern
   c. Demonstrating clinical credibility
   d. An initial orientation
   e. A final evaluation
   f. Learners being able to present a case
   g. Teachers managing the case presentation
   h. Didactic sessions being used to enhance clinical case material
   i. Teaching taking place at the bedside so that students can learn physician-patient relationships
   j. Teachers and students discussing psychosocial issues
   k. Attention being paid to transferring the teaching responsibility

8. Teaching content requires attention to increasingly complex cognitive functions. As described by Bloom,[39] teaching/learning in the cognitive domain for any topic addresses the following:
   a. Knowledge—recall
   b. Comprehension—understanding
   c. Application—use of abstractions
   d. Analysis—break down; seeing the relationship of parts
   e. Synthesis—put together; creating a new entity
   f. Evaluation—judgment of value

9. A systematic methodology to develop a psychomotor skill lesson includes the following steps[54]:
   a. Analyze and separate the skill into its component parts and determine which aspects of the skill are most difficult to perform.
   b. Provide students with a model of the skill, effectively demonstrated in its entirety, that they are expected to perform.
   c. Make provisions for students to practice until the expected behavior is mastered.
   d. Provide adequate supervision and an evaluation of the final performance.

*Adapted from ACGME Outcome Project. Available at www.acgme.org/outcome.

"Pedantic" is a description teachers wish to avoid. In the interest of doing so, I offer a fifth grader's biography of the great teacher Socrates[1]:

Socrates was a man.
Socrates was a Greek.
Socrates went around telling people what to do.
They poisoned him!

This chapter on anesthesia education is not intended in such a manner that I risk Socrates' fate, but rather it is meant to be provocative, to give cause for thought on an important subject not often reflected on. All anesthesia education can be easily considered in the following question (Greenhow DE: personal communication, 1982):

How shall who teach what to whom for what purpose now and in the future?!

Anesthesia education is presented by using this question as the framework for consideration. This chapter provides a philosophy of teaching anesthesia rather than a detailed account of the many aspects of anesthesia education (e.g., operating room anesthesia versus critical care medicine versus cardiopulmonary resuscitation versus chronic pain management). Also, this chapter is exclusively directed toward the teaching organization, regulations, and philosophy of teaching that exist in the United States. See Chapter 3 for perspectives on how other countries are teaching anesthesia and their philosophic approaches that parallel their needs.

Teaching and Education

Teaching, in a narrow sense, the way most of us think about it, is an activity by an individual aimed at causing another person to know some new fact or to know how to accomplish some new task. The focus appears to rest on the teacher and the activity of teaching. It does not take long to realize, however, that this way of looking at the teaching/learning activity has misplaced emphasis. If not with the teaching activity, where does the emphasis belong? The answer to this question lies in understanding the definition of education.

Education is an all-encompassing process (not merely a specific activity) that results in a change in behavior on the part of the student/learner. The focus of education is the learner, not the teacher. It is the student who is educated by interacting with an environment that provides experiences. *Education is change in behavior based on experiences.* The experience most often includes the student interacting with a teacher, but it is almost never limited to that alone. The entire milieu defines the total experience (Fig. 8-1). When the milieu changes, so may the education;

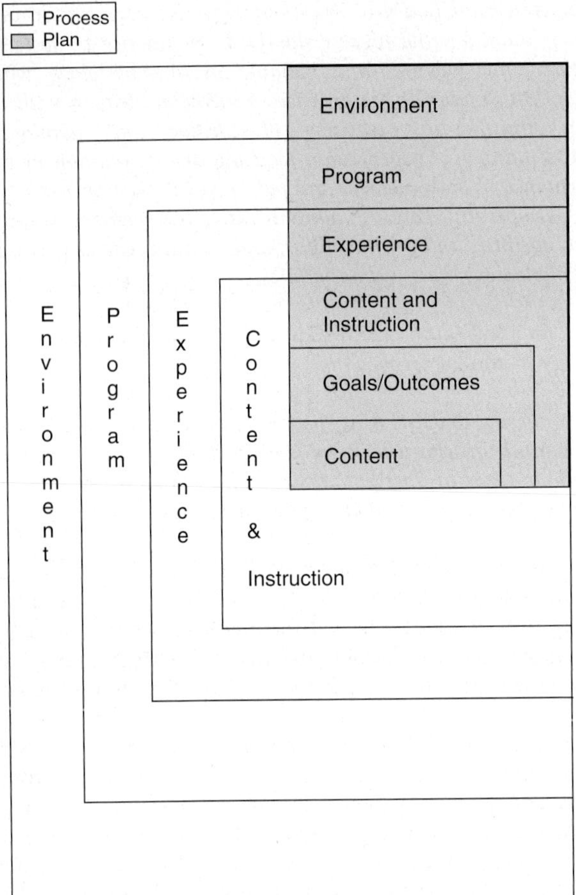

Figure 8-1 Diagrammatic representation of the educational experience. The two major components are the plan for teaching and the process of education that actually occurs. At the core is the content (cognitive, psychomotor, affective, or any combination of the three) to be taught and learned. Growing out of the content are the planned goals of education, the methods and program of instruction, and the environment in which the teaching and learning will occur. In the diagram, each building block of the plan is added to the previous one in an all-encompassing fashion. What is planned as education and what is experienced may or may not be the same. As represented by the diagram, the educational process that actually occurs includes all of the plan and layers on it, both the real environment and the teacher/student interactions that provide the education, that is, the experiences that provide the basis for the ultimate change in student behavior. *(Modified from Atkins E: Curriculum Theorizing as a Scientific Pursuit: A Framework for Analysis [unpublished doctoral dissertation]. University of Pennsylvania, 1982.)*

that is, the change in behavior exhibited by the student may vary dramatically if the milieu is varied.

Picture the educational setting in which an anesthesiology resident is learning how to use epinephrine when weaning a patient from cardiopulmonary bypass. The knowledge and skills that must be learned include application of the pharmacologic principles of catecholamines to the pathophysiology of cardiovascular disease by turning on a mechanical infusion pump to deliver the indicated dose of a medication while technically monitoring for dose response and toxicity. Learning these facts and the skills sufficient to use them is much different when done from a textbook or a preoperative conference with a staff preceptor than when done during the operating room interaction between the surgeon and anesthesiologist, where varied opinions may consider dopamine a more sound physiologic choice or intermittent boluses a better administration technique. The interposition of the concerned surgeon and real-time patient setting between the student and knowledge and skills to be learned changes the learning environment and hence the educational experience for the resident. More is learned than the facts and psychomotor skills. As the attitudes of both the anesthesiologist and the surgeon are displayed during resolution of the question about the "best" drug to use and the "right" way to give it, the resident learns how these two types of practitioners are supposed to relate to one another.

It seems obvious, therefore, that there is more to consider than just teaching. What more is there to the anesthesiologist's responsibility than just teaching those around him or her? The answer is provided by answering the component parts of the question posed at the beginning of this chapter.

Teach to whom?
Why teach?
Who teaches?
What to teach?
How to teach?

Teach to Whom?—The Students

The simplest answer to the question "who learns anesthesiology?" is "those who will provide anesthetic care to patients." Included are the anesthesiologist, nurse anesthetist, and dentist who administers anesthesia for dental procedures.[2] Also to be included are the many varied paramedical personnel who participate in patient care activities related to primary anesthetic care: the anesthesia technician, anesthesia aide, nurse practitioner, postanesthesia recovery room nurse, physician assistant, surgeon assistant, respiratory therapist and aide, intensive care/critical care/emergency room/trauma nurse, perfusionist, emergency medical technician/paramedic, cardiopulmonary technologist, pulmonary function technician, and blood gas laboratory technician.[2] Each of these occupations is intimately related in some way to the body of knowledge that constitutes the practice of anesthesiology.

In a much broader sense, the entire medical community can be considered appropriate learners of anesthesiology. Medical students, for example, are appropriate candidates for learning a core of anesthetic knowledge and skills, specifically those essential for the training of all physicians. Basic central nervous system, cardiovascular, and pulmonary diagnostic monitoring, emergency airway management, and the clinically applied pharmacology of sedative/hypnotic and analgesic medications and local anesthetics are some of these essentials. Medical students, graduate physicians, and paramedical personnel of many types are appropriate learners because all are often faced with the task of educating the lay public about anesthesiology. Who learns anesthesiology, therefore, are those who practice it or perform related duties that require some understanding of the subject.

Another way to address the question of who learns anesthesiology is to answer *adult learners*. What describes an adult learner?[3] How are adult learners unique? Adult learners are those with strong motivation to participate in a set of experiences, such as a curriculum, to learn a specific discipline. The discipline that they want to learn is one that they are interested in, need to know, or both. The resident actively seeks education in anesthesiology. A sixth grader (a child learner), in contrast, does not seek education in arithmetic. Adult learners participate in life-centered situational learning in the area or areas for which relevance is most likely.

Adult learners enter the learning activity with a wealth of previous experience. They view the current educational experience in light of their background. An internist who enters an anesthesiology residency in preparation for a career in intensive care medicine has a rich resource background in medical practice. Adult learners can capitalize on this previous learning. At the same time, however, the previous learning may color how the current learning takes place. The key for the teacher is to acknowledge the adult learner's expertise and build the new education on it rather than downplay it and, in essence, "reject" the adult learner.

Working together in a mutual peer relationship with the teacher, adult learners are self-directed. Whereas child learners need a set of directions that originate from the teacher, adult learners initiate their own activities. Because adult learning is goal oriented toward relevant life-centered needs, an adult learner tends to pick and choose some, not necessarily all, the educational activities available.

Strong commitment and specific intentional attachments uniquely characterize adulthood. Marriage and child rearing are examples of such commitments and attachments. At the same time that adults make commitments, their lives are evolving and they pass through many critical life stages (e.g., assuming financial responsibility, coping with the illness or death of a parent). These strategic choice points in life have an impact on adult learning. The decision by an anesthesiology resident, for example, to extend education an additional year to learn a subspecialty or to participate in research training may be based on the total financial debt incurred for medical education up to the end of residency and the need to repay that debt, weighed against the acuteness of the family's financial needs.

Inherent differences among people tend to increase with aging. Adult education must provide for differences in style, time, place, and pace of learning among adult learners. The time factor for learning is especially crucial for adults. Adults perceive that time passes more rapidly, that is, there is less time available to learn—or to do anything for that matter. With time perceived to be in short supply, adult learners tend to be selective in their learning so that they use what time they have more efficiently. The anesthesiology resident may devote time to learning in the operating room and weekly departmental case conference but may choose to skip the journal club to spend time with the family.

Recognition of the special traits that adult learners possess allows the anesthesiology educator to provide an educational program embraced by the student rather than one that is rejected. Assessing the needs of the adult learner and using these needs as a springboard from which a curriculum is designed are more likely to result in a good educational outcome than to impose on the learner what the teacher alone thinks is right.

Why Teach?—The Reasons

An obvious reason for teaching anesthesiology is that we as a specialty have defined it as part of our identity (see Chapters 1 and 2)[4]:

> *The American Board of Anesthesiology (ABA) exists in order to . . . maintain the highest standards of practice by fostering educational facilities and training in anesthesiology which the ABA defines as the practice of medicine dealing with but not limited to . . . teaching of cardiac and pulmonary resuscitation, . . . supervision, teaching and evaluation of performance of both medical and paramedical personnel involved in perioperative care, . . . administrative involvement in health care facilities and organizations, and medical schools necessary to implement these responsibilities.*[4]

In addition to our own description, others define anesthesiology in similar terms:

> *[An anesthesiologist] May instruct medical students and other personnel in characteristics and methods of administering various types of anesthetics, signs and symptoms of reactions and complications, and emergency measures to employ.*[2]

Teaching anesthesiology is clearly one component of an anesthesiologist's daily activity. In some instances, it means providing the experience needed for physician trainees to achieve consultant anesthesiologist status. In other settings, it means providing the experience needed for other medical and paramedical professionals to achieve a level of expertise appropriate to their required competencies—as examples, for an internist, the ability to understand anesthesiology sufficiently to relate to anesthesiologists and educate patients about anesthesiology; for a postanesthesia recovery room nurse, the ability to understand anesthesiology sufficiently to care appropriately for patients emerging from anesthesia and to be versed in the critical care aspects of the preanesthesia and postanesthesia periods to provide life support if necessary.

A major purpose of teaching anesthesiology is to provide a common set of learning experiences that when mastered by students, will lead to relatively standardized knowledge and behavior. These standards (minimum standards though they may be) become the criteria by which a student candidate can be evaluated (certified) for entry into a specified mastery level.[4-6]

Becoming a consultant anesthesiologist certified by the ABA depends on being able to demonstrate that one possesses a minimum standard of knowledge of, skills in, and attitudes about anesthesiology.[4] Public trust is gained by this process of specialty certification, which ensures that a certified specialist has met the defined standards of anesthesia practice.[4-6] Although specialty certification in anesthesiology culminates in evaluation mechanisms (achieving clinical competence as attested to by the training program and successfully passing written and oral examinations), the certification process is driven by educational activities focused on teaching the resident how to become a consultant anesthesiologist.[4-6] A key part of this process is establishment of the training curriculum or continuum of education in anesthesiology by the ABA.[4]

A resident trainee in anesthesiology voluntarily enrolls in a graduate medical education program and accepts the ABA's approved curriculum and evaluation (testing) protocol. Coupled with the physician candidate *certification* process is the residency education *accreditation* process.[7] Residency program accreditation is a voluntary process whereby an institution applies for recognition of its anesthesiology graduate medical education as meeting a minimum set of teaching standards that will support the curriculum. Such recognition is achieved from the Accreditation Council for Graduate Medical Education (ACGME). The ACGME represents the combined "wisdom" of all specialty residency review committees in its publication dealing with institutional requirements of accredited residencies.[7] More focused training guidelines published as program requirements are defined by the Anesthesiology Residency Review Committee (RRC), a group representing the ABA, the American Society of Anesthesiologists (ASA), and the American Medical Association.[8] These guidelines include program requirements for residency education in (1) anesthesiology (the core program) and fellowship education in its accredited subspecialties, (2) adult cardiothoracic anesthesiology, (3) critical care, (4) pain medicine, (5) pediatric anesthesiology, and (6) undersea and hyperbaric medicine.[8,9]

The teaching responsibilities addressed by the candidate certification and the residency and fellowship education program accreditation processes are clearly articulated by the ABA[4]:

Establish and maintain criteria for the designation of a Board certified anesthesiologist.

Inform the Accreditation Council for Graduate Medical Education (ACGME) concerning the training required of individuals seeking certification as such requirements relate to residency training programs in anesthesiology.

Establish and conduct those processes by which the Board may judge whether a physician who voluntarily applies should be issued a certificate indicating that the required standards for certification or recertification as a diplomate of the American Board of Anesthesiology have been met.

A Board certified anesthesiologist is a physician who provides medical management and consultation during the perioperative period, in pain management and in critical care medicine. A diplomate of the Board must possess knowledge, judgment, adaptability, clinical skills, technical facility and personal characteristics sufficient to carry out the entire scope of anesthesiology practice. An ABA diplomate must logically organize and effectively present rational diagnoses and appropriate treatment protocols to peers, patients, their families, and others involved in the medical community. A diplomate of the Board can serve as an expert in matters related to anesthesiology, deliberate with others, and provide advice and defend opinions in all aspects of the specialty of anesthesiology. A Board certified anesthesiologist is able to function as the leader of the anesthesiology care team.

Because of the nature of anesthesiology, the ABA diplomate must be able to manage emergent life-threatening situations in an independent and timely fashion. The ability to independently acquire and process information in a timely manner is central to assure individual responsibility for all aspects of anesthesiology care. Adequate physical and sensory faculties, such as eyesight, hearing, speech and coordinated function of the extremities, are essential to the independent performance of the Board certified anesthesiologist. Freedom from the influence of or dependency on chemical substances that impair cognitive, physical, sensory or motor function also is an essential characteristic of the Board certified anesthesiologist.

Establish and conduct those processes by which the Board may judge whether a physician who voluntarily applies should be issued a certificate indicating that the required standards for subspecialty certification or recertification in an ABA designated subdiscipline of anesthesiology have been met.[4]

The ABA-ACGME model addresses the purpose of education in anesthesiology and clearly outlines the anesthesiologist's responsibilities in teaching colleagues. Other organizational models similar to the ABA-ACGME example serve the same function for teaching physician anesthesiologists outside the United States.

Meeting the teaching responsibilities for nurse anesthesia is standardized in a fashion similar to that of the ABA-ACGME model. For nurses, the Council on Certification of Nurse Anesthetists and the Council on Accreditation of Nurse Anesthesia Educational Programs serve functions similar to those of the ABA-ACGME model. In 2007, 108 nurse anesthesia educational programs of 24 to 36 months' duration (80% are 27/28 months long) graduated nearly 1200 students educated in approximately 1547 clinical training sites staffed by 8248 certified registered nurse anesthetists (CRNAs) and 4689 anesthesiologists serving as faculty (Council on Accreditation of Nurse Anesthesia Educational Programs: personal communication, 2007). After the first 2 years of certification, CRNAs are required to achieve biennial recertification under the auspices of the Council on Recertification of Nurse Anesthetists.

Education of nonphysician health care professionals is coordinated by 26 agencies that accredit/approve training programs in 71 professions.[10,11] These agencies provide guidelines for education in a standardized fashion so that professionals in 71 allied health occupations can gain certification in their respective disciplines.[10,11] More than 50 professional organizations (including the ASA) serve as experts in their fields and work hand in hand with the 26 agencies to accredit/approve the educational programs for health professions.[10,11] The magnitude of this teaching responsibility becomes clear when one realizes that in 2007-2008, 2468 institutions sponsoring 6873 educational programs educated more than 231,000 students.[10,11]

Occupations related to anesthesiology for which standardized educational programs have been defined by the Accreditation Review Commission on Education for the Physician Assistant (www.arc-pa.org), American Society of Health System–Pharmacists (www.ashp.org), Commission on Accreditation for Health Informatics and Information Management Education (www.cahiim.org), Commission on Accreditation of Allied Health Education Programs (www.caahep.org), and Joint Review Committee on Education in Radiologic Technology (www.jrcert.org) (5 of the 26 accrediting agencies referred to earlier) include anesthesiologist assistant, cardiovascular technologist, electroneurodiagnostic technologist, emergency medical technician-paramedic, health information technician, perfusionist, pharmacy technician, physician assistant, radiation therapist, respiratory therapist (entry level and advanced), specialist in blood bank technology, surgical assistant, and surgical technologist.[10,11] In 2006, these occupations were taught in 1572 accredited or approved programs.[10,11] Students enrolled in these training programs during the 2006 academic year numbered 45,285.[10,11]

In contrast to the teaching responsibility for nonphysician health care professionals, in 2006, 4970 physician resident anesthesiologists (5.6% of all residents in the United States) were educated in 131 accredited American core anesthesiology residency programs and 360 physician subspecialty fellows (2.3% of all subspecialty fellows in the United States) in 213 accredited

American subspecialty anesthesiology programs (30 adult cardiothoracic anesthesiology, 49 critical care medicine, 89 pain medicine, and 45 pediatric anesthesiology programs) (Table 8-1A and B).[12,13] A yearly summary of recruitment of graduating medical students into anesthesiology residencies via the National Resident Matching Program (NRMP) process and how these individuals advance through the residency education years is published in the *ASA Newsletter*.[14,15] Adding the tasks of teaching medical and allied health care students, participating in continuing education for anesthesiologists, and teaching other practicing physicians and allied health care professionals increases the educational responsibilities of anesthesiologists in an exponential fashion.

One fundamental reason that we teach anesthesiology is that we recognize the need to provide uniform educational experiences so that students participating in these activities can reach a goal; that is, they will be acknowledged (certified) as competent in their discipline. So important is this process that it has been incorporated into the very definition that we use to describe ourselves. Now more than ever, competence and physician performance are concepts that are key in the minds of the public consuming medical care, the agencies paying for medical care, and the institutions and individuals providing medical education.[16-18] The United States has a system designed to assess medical competence by defining and ensuring the processes of education, licensing, accreditation, and certification.[16-18]

The American Board of Medical Specialties (ABMS) oversees the certification of physician specialists by 24 medical specialty member boards (including the ABA) in more than 130 specialties (residencies) and subspecialties (fellowships) (Table 8-2).

The primary function of ABMS is to assist its Member Boards in developing and implementing educational and professional standards to evaluate and certify physician specialists.[19]

The ABMS states its mission as being

. . . the organization that establishes standards for physician specialty certification and Maintenance of Certification (MOC), including performance assessment. ABMS communicates information about these standards to support the public's quest for safe, high-quality healthcare.[5,19]

The ABMS has eloquently articulated the goal of MOC by stating that

. . . ultimately, the measure of physician specialists is not merely that they have been certified, but how well they keep current in their specialty. That's why in 2006, ABMS' 24 Member Boards adopted a program of continuous professional development—ABMS Maintenance of Certification—as a formal means of measuring a physician's continued competency in his or her certified specialty and/or subspecialty. By following MOC, physicians demonstrate their commitment to lifelong learning and ongoing self-assessment to advance specialty practice. They live the standards by which medical care is evaluated and demonstrate leadership in the national movement for healthcare quality and patient safety.[19]

In 1989, the ABA established a mechanism (continued demonstration of qualifications [CDQ]) for revalidation of an individual's primary board certificate to address the multitude of questions that had been posed about recredentialing and continued "competence" of physicians initially certified as consultants, especially questions related to public trust.[4,20,21] This program allowed anesthesiologists to demonstrate their continuing qualifications through a *voluntary* recredentialing program.[21] The first implementation of CDQ with its two components—documentation of an anesthesiologist's approved practice credentialing and administration of a secure written examination to assess an anesthesiologist's current knowledge of anesthesia practice—took place in 1993. The CDQ certificate allowed anesthesiologists a means to accomplish recredentialing for needs defined by governmental, health care finance reimbursement, hospital, or other regulatory bodies.

The ABA/ABMS has developed more formal recertification processes since implementation of the voluntary CDQ recredentialing mechanism. In 1994-1995, the ABA adopted time-limited certification; all specialty (anesthesiology) certificates issued by the ABA on or after January 1, 2000, were designated valid for only 10 years from the time of completion of the examination for the initial certification and all subsequent recertifications.[4,22] In 1996, the ABA converted the CDQ mechanism to the recertification process containing the same two components described earlier. Anesthesiologists wishing to remain board certified at the end of the time limit on their certification are required to formally recertify and obtain a new board certificate rather than revalidate the primary certificate.[4,22] Current discussion is focusing on shortening the recertification cycle from 10 years to 5 to 7 years from the time of completion of the examination for the initial certification or subsequent recertifications.

The ABA has also had a certification process for its subspecialties (see Table 8-2).[5] A certification process has existed for critical care medicine since 1985. In 1991, the ABA began certification of pain management subspecialists, and in 2006, the ABA began certification of subspecialists in hospice and palliative medicine. In 1998, time-limited certification for subspecialties in anesthesiology was approved. As of January 2000, all newly issued ABA subspecialty certificates in critical care medicine and pain management were designated valid for only 10 years from the time of completion of the examination for the initial certification. Recertification in critical care medicine, pain management, and hospice and palliative medicine is operative in a fashion similar to that described earlier for recertification in anesthesiology. Similar models for continuing medical education and documentation of physician competence are being developed in other countries as well.[23,24]

Maintenance of Certification in Anesthesiology (MOCA) is the

. . . program [that] enables ABA diplomates holding non–time limited certificates (issued before 2000) to demonstrate continuing qualifications and those with time-limited certificates to maintain their certification. Each MOCA cycle is a 10-year period of ongoing Lifelong Learning and Self-Assessment; continual assessment of Professional Standing; periodic assessments of Practice Performance; and assessment of Cognitive Expertise. MOCA is an opportunity for physicians to document maintenance of their skills in six general competencies, namely, Medical Knowledge; Patient Care; Practice-Based Learning and Improvement; Professionalism; Interpersonal and Communication Skills;

Table 8-1 Number of Anesthesiology Specialty and Subspecialty Graduate Medical Education Programs, Residents, Fellows, and U.S. Medical Students and Full-Time Faculty

A. Core Anesthesiology Residencies and Residents in Graduate Medical Education (GME) Programs in the United States Accredited by the Accreditation Council for Graduate Medical Education (ACGME)

Academic Year	Number of Accredited Core Anesthesiology Residency Programs	Total Number of Core Anesthesiology Residents on Duty	Number (%) of Core Anesthesiology Residents on Duty Who Are U.S. Medical Graduates	Number of Residencies/ Residents on Duty in All ACGME-Accredited and Combined Specialty GME Programs
1990	157	4362	3871 (88.7)	4144/69,798
1995	149	5490	4395 (81.1)	4245/85,732
2000	134	3837	1627 (42.4)	4268/85,460
2005	132	4785	3450 (72.1)	4151/86,975
2006	131	4970	3731 (75.1)	4134/89,269

B. Subspecialty Anesthesiology Fellowships and Fellows in ACGME-Accredited GME Programs in the United States

Academic Year	Number of Accredited Subspecialty Anesthesiology Fellowship Programs	Total Number of Subspecialty Anesthesiology Fellows on Duty	Number (%) of Subspecialty Anesthesiology Fellows on Duty Who Are U.S. Medical Graduates	Number of Subspecialty Programs/Fellows on Duty in All ACGME-Accredited GME Programs
1990	Critical care medicine, 27	7	4 (57.1)	2447/8,006
1995	Critical care medicine, 46	70	52 (74.3)	3264/12,100
	Pain medicine, 55	112	83 (74.1)	
2000	Critical care medicine, 53	59	29 (49.2)	3678/12,529
	Pain medicine, 98	215	100 (46.5)	
	Pediatric anesthesiology, 37	63	33 (52.4)	
2005	Critical care medicine, 47	43	20 (46.5)	4095/14,316
	Pain medicine, 95	190	88 (46.3)	
	Pediatric anesthesiology, 43	91	43 (47.3)	
2006	Adult cardiothoracic, 30	0	0 (0)	4368/15,610
	Critical care medicine, 49	44	22 (50)	
	Pain medicine, 89	206	127 (61.7)	
	Pediatric anesthesiology, 45	110	78 (70.9)	
2007-2008 Projected	Adult cardiothoracic	0		
	Critical care medicine	129		
	Pain medicine	264		
	Pediatric anesthesiology	166		

C. Number of Medical Students and Full-Time Faculty (Total and Anesthesiology Specific) in U.S. Medical Schools

Academic Year	Number of Medical Students in U.S. Medical Schools	Total Number of Full-Time Faculty in U.S. Medical Schools	Number (% of Total Faculty) of Full-Time Anesthesiology Faculty in U.S. Medical Schools
1990	65,081	72,320	3393 (4.7)
1995	67,030	90,016	4535 (5.0)
2000	66,500	102,446	4979 (4.9)
2005	68,280	119,025	5471 (5.7)
2006	69,028	124,725	5836 (4.7)

Data abstracted from the Journal of the American Medical Association, yearly Medical Education editions: 264, 1990; 274, 1995; 284, 2000; 294, 2005; and 298, 2007; and Warner MA: Residency Review Committee for Anesthesiology. ASA Newsl 71:26-27, 2007.

Table 8-2 American Board of Medical Specialties (ABMS) Certificates Issued

	Before 1997	1997-2006	2000-2006
Anesthesiology*	28,515	12,012	7,592
Critical care medicine†		480	267
Pain medicine‡		1,941	1,233
Hospice and palliative medicine§	—	—	—
All specialties	602,578	242,684	167,656
All subspecialties		76,782	51,057

*First ABMS certificate issued in 1938; first time-limited (10 year) certificate issued in 2000.

†First ABMS certificate issued in 1986; first time-limited (10 year) certificate issued in 2000.

‡First ABMS certificate issued in 1993; first time-limited (10 year) certificate issued in 1993.

§First ABMS certificate to be issued in 2008; first time-limited (10 year) certificate to be issued in 2008.

Data abstracted from 2007 Reference Handbook and Certificate Statistics. Evanston, IL, American Board of Medical Specialties, 2007.

and System-Based Practice. There are four requirements for MOCA:

Professional Standing

Diplomates must hold an unrestricted license to practice medicine . . . no medical license . . . can be revoked, suspended or surrendered. . . .

Lifelong Learning and Self-Assessment (LL-SA) Activities

LL-SA is personalized and self-directed professional development, . . . an assessment of . . . current knowledge and practice of anesthesiology . . . [and] continuing medical education (CME) activities and other learning opportunities that meet . . . professional development needs. . . .

Cognitive Examination

The Cognitive Examination is designed to assess core knowledge of the discipline of anesthesiology. It is very clinically oriented, with an emphasis on customary practice. . . .

Practice Performance Assessment and Improvement (PPAI)

The PPAI process consists of the ABA obtaining attestations and evidence of . . . [an anesthesiologist's] clinical activity and ongoing program of practice assessment and performance improvement. The ABA minimum clinical activity requirement is the practice of anesthesiology or a recognized anesthesiology subspecialty, on average, at least one day per week during one of the previous three years. . . . Evidence of PPAI acceptable to the ABA is a prerequisite for the MOCA Cognitive Examination and is a requirement for maintenance of certification in anesthesiology.[25]

The six general competencies for which anesthesiologists need to document maintenance of their skills for the MOCA program are rooted in the graduate medical education process of residency and fellowship education for anesthesiologists. Being concerned that the full range of learning had not been adequately provided for or ensured by an evaluation process, the ACGME developed its Outcome Project in 1999.[26] The ACGME defined six educational areas for which graduate trainees must demonstrate competency (see Appendix 1).[27] The ACGME Outcome Project places the educational responsibility squarely on the shoulders of the residency programs and their faculty to develop innovative curricula and evaluation methods to ensure that trainees graduate with these competencies.[28]

Anesthesiology education for physicians and other health care professionals is, as described earlier, a specific application of assessing medical competence by process evaluation. An equal, and perhaps even more important, question is how to evaluate the outcome of the education rather than the process by which it is achieved.[16,17] The question of why we teach medicine, specifically anesthesiology, is best answered by saying that we want physicians and other health care professionals to perform the activities of anesthesia patient care at a specific level of achievement. Although we are very good at evaluating knowledge, assessment of patient care outcomes is not easily measured. Outcome assessment, that is, evaluation of the practice aspects of anesthesiology, represents the greatest challenge for the future.[16,17]

One such assessment demonstrates the value of the ABA-ACGME model of educating and certifying physician anesthesiologists. Silber and colleagues,[29] in their study of almost 6000 patients undergoing prostate or gallbladder surgery in multiple hospitals, demonstrated that patient recovery or "rescue" from an adverse event correlated with the proportion of board-certified anesthesiologists in the hospital.

Outcome analysis is also becoming a part of the training process for anesthesiologists.[30] An example of this type of approach has been described in an educational setting that makes use of the quality improvement concepts developed in industry.[30] Such an approach is also appearing in post-training practice settings as a form of continuing medical education, as well as a quality assessment tool.[31] We are seeing more of this type of approach as the pressures of health care economics help restructure our clinical practice.

Who Teaches?—The Teachers

Anesthesiology is taught by physician anesthesiologists, the experts in the field, as well as by other expert individuals in related disciplines, examples of whom include pharmacologists, physiologists, biomedical engineers, pediatricians, and neurosurgeons. Full-time anesthesiology faculty positions in U.S. medical schools in 2006 numbered 5836 (see Table 8-1C).[31] Anesthesiologists represent 5.6% of the clinical teachers and 4.7% of all American medical school teaching faculty (see Table 8-1C).[32] The 5836 anesthesia faculty members in medical schools bore the major responsibility for teaching some or all of the 69,028 enrolled undergraduate medical students, the 4970 graduate trainees in accredited anesthesiology residency training programs, the 360 graduate trainees in accredited anesthesiology subspecialty fellowship programs, and many of the other 104,879 physician house staff trainees (see Table 8-1A to C).[12,32]

Clinical care, teaching, research, and administration are major roles assumed by faculty. For anesthesia faculty, clinical care is a prime activity for obvious reasons. The other functions are attended to as time and resources permit. For this reason, teaching is often relegated to a lower level of priority, not always adequately acknowledged in career advancement decisions. Junior faculty members are frequently expected to take on a large part of the teaching load. This expectation, however, could be viewed as a case of reversal of the proper roles for the junior and senior faculty.[33] Junior faculty members have a heavy teaching load during the phase of their career when they lack experience.[33] Senior faculty members, on the other hand, are responsible for departmental, institutional, and specialty roles that limit their availability for teaching, although these same individuals have vast experience and could teach much.[33] The extreme example of this dichotomy is the expectation that house staff teach the more junior of their ranks and medical students. Perhaps the teaching role for house staff would best be accomplished by making the resident a teaching apprentice who not only receives general medical and anesthesiology specialty education but is also educated about education.

Little specific information exists about the teaching credentials or qualities of anesthesiologists, unlike the situation for other physician groups.[34,35] These descriptions can be used to infer what does or could characterize anesthesiology teachers. Physician teachers in general are not trained as educators.[34] They have not had formal training in educational psychology or methodology.[34] Physicians who teach do not use the educational resources available.[34] When faced with a new or difficult educational assignment, physician teachers rarely read medical education journals, nor do they consult educational experts, as they might consult a cardiologist, for example, when treating a patient with a difficult rhythm disturbance.[34] Physician teachers, for the most part, mimic their own teachers, who also had little or no formal training as educators.[34] It seems curious, for example, that at the same time we would not trust a general surgery resident to perform a complicated neurosurgical dissection and achieve a good outcome for the patient without extensive education, we do entrust an anesthesiology trainee to faculty who have limited educational expertise in the hope of achieving a good learning outcome.

What characterizes a good teacher? Effective clinical teachers who are able to succeed at the bedside teaching encounter display specific actions noted by their students and themselves.[35] Table 8-3 presents a schema that was developed by observing internists teaching internal medicine residents and medical students. The similarity of the attending anesthesiologist teaching at the bedside in the intensive care unit or in the operating room is striking.

A teaching responsibility that anesthesiology faculty might consider is how to blend their "expert" status as anesthesiologists with their "novice" status as teachers. As the experts, teachers of anesthesiology can define educational objectives based on the competencies that they believe newly trained anesthesiologists need. Having set the objectives, the teacher can direct the educational process by selecting the appropriate learning activities and then designing tests that assess the learning. As described, the "authoritarian" teacher, the expert, determines the educational ends that must be met, defines the means to these ends, and requires conformity to these ends by the students.

Table 8-3 Traits of Effective Clinical Teachers

Overall instructional effectiveness depends on	1. Allocating time for teaching 2. Creating a teaching/learning environment of trust and concern 3. Demonstrating clinical credibility
A complete educational experience requires	4. An initial orientation 5. A final evaluation
Teaching rounds are facilitated when	6. Learners are able to present a case 7. Teachers manage the case presentation 8. Didactic sessions are used to enhance clinical case material 9. Teaching takes place at the bedside to allow students to learn physician-patient relationships 10. Teachers and students discuss psychosocial issues
Maintained teaching effectiveness occurs when	11. Attention is paid to transferring the teaching responsibility

Adapted from Mattern WD, Weinholtz D, Friedman CP: The attending physician as teacher. N Engl J Med 308:1129, 1983.

Although anesthesiology faculty provide education with this type of curriculum design, few if any know that they are using Tyler's model, nor do they realize that there might be equally good or better alternatives.[36] Dewey's progressive education offers one such alternative.[37] Dewey's philosophy of education elevates students to a level where they can join in a partnership with the teacher. For students of anesthesiology, the adult learners described previously, this type of student-teacher relationship may make very good sense.

An example of these two philosophies put into action clarifies their differences. Let us consider teaching/learning how to manage a patient who is being mechanically ventilated in the operating room. A Tylerian teacher might lecture to residents on how to use the ventilator. It is hoped that the residents will remember what they heard and be able to put what they have learned into action. In contrast, a teacher using Dewey's approach might create a patient simulation exercise in which residents can "experiment" with differing ventilator setups to infer what might occur clinically. A much more meaningful learning environment might be provided by the simulation—coupled with the anesthesiologist faculty member's reactions to and guidance about how the residents "tinkered" with the ventilator—than might be provided by the lecture format. In addition, a teacher using Dewey's philosophy might be more likely to encourage students with previous experience, such as residents who have used different types of ventilators during their internship, to share their know-how with other, less experienced peers.

This chapter is discussing the component parts of the question "How shall who teach what to whom for what purpose now and in the future?" It should be obvious that individually studying the component parts of the question is an artificial separation for teaching purposes. To fully understand the question, its parts must be linked. The consideration "Who teaches anesthesiology?" is an example of how the blending of the individual parts of the total picture of anesthesia education must occur. It is virtually impossible to talk about the teacher without bringing the student and the educational needs into the discussion. This key concept, that is, the importance of knowing not only the component parts of education but also how they interrelate, is essential for understanding and implementing anesthesiology education.

The Curriculum—What to Teach?

The table of contents from any standard anesthesiology textbook provides a broad outline of what to teach in anesthesiology. Similar to a medical school course outline, anesthesiology is a mix of the fundamental basic sciences applied to clinical practice as they relate to specific pathophysiologic disease entities. Patients with these problems are encountered in preoperative, intraoperative, and postoperative settings; therefore, the content is taught as it specifically applies to the time progression of their disease process in these different patient environments. This framework of basic and clinical science is used for teaching anesthesiology to all health professionals, with particular emphasis placed on the areas most pertinent to the particular group being taught (e.g., detailed teaching about the mechanics and clinical application of ventilators is provided to student respiratory therapists).

An accepted uniform content outline exists and has been agreed on for teaching physician anesthesiologists.[38] The major outline headings are listed in Appendix 2. Few teachers would be at a loss to define the content of anesthesiology teaching. Anesthesiology education, however, is not limited to content teaching alone.

The three major areas for teaching/learning all subjects are cognitive, psychomotor, and affective. For anesthesiology, it appears that the cognitive teaching/learning area is well defined. It is the responsibility of the anesthesiology teacher, however, to go further than just listing the content topics. Teaching in the content area requires attention to increasingly complex cognitive functions. Described by Bloom,[39] teaching/learning in the cognitive domain for any topic addresses the following:

1. Knowledge—recall
2. Comprehension—understanding
3. Application—use of abstractions
4. Analysis—break down; seeing the relationship of parts
5. Synthesis—put together; creating a new entity
6. Evaluation—judgment of value

Knowing the facts about pulmonary function is obviously much more basic than being able to apply them to the management of a multiple-trauma patient maintained on a ventilator. Teachers of anesthesiology serve students well by considering the more complex aspects of cognitive learning.

A general taxonomy of psychomotor skill teaching/learning for universal application to all educational settings does not exist because of the great variability among disciplines in this type of domain. A broadly accepted, standardized outline of psychomotor skill learning for anesthesiology also does not exist. There are many psychomotor skills that anesthesiologists and other related health care professionals need to learn. Perhaps a major challenge for teachers of anesthesiology is to codify the fundamental and supplemental psychomotor skills that must be taught and learned. This process is beginning to occur with the introduction of practice parameters or practice guidelines developed by medicine in general and anesthesiology in particular.[40-46]

Affective teaching/learning deals with feelings or emotions. The taxonomy of affective learning addresses the following[47]:

1. Receiving
2. Responding
3. Valuing
4. Organizing
5. Value complexing

Although we actively and consciously teach in the cognitive and psychomotor areas, we are much less aware of our affective teaching. Even though we may not be aware of it, we are nonetheless constantly teaching in the affective arena by the role modeling that we perform. Earlier in this chapter, an example of how affective teaching/learning takes place was described. In the real-life setting, the aggressive, passive-aggressive, or passive posture of the anesthesiology teacher interacting with the surgeon provides a lasting lesson in the affective domain for the resident anesthesiology learner.

Thinking about affective learning results in goals for such learning and permits the development of teaching plans to achieve these goals. Only if we decide how we believe we as anesthesiologists and health care professionals in related fields need to behave in relation to others will we be able to teach professionalism and these psychosocial skills to our students.[48]

Another example of the importance of affective learning concerns our approach to the teaching task. When our students sense our own enthusiasm about and commitment to a particular topic, their attitudes about it follow suit. In similar fashion, if we as teachers are negative about some aspect of learning, we can expect our students to mimic these feelings. The charge that teachers of anesthesiology must accept is that they must be conscious of the emotions that they display and prospectively decide on the values that they wish to teach because affective teaching and learning occur all the time.

Defining the areas of learning (i.e., what to teach) makes it possible for the teacher to devise methods to evaluate the success of the teaching endeavor. For anesthesiology education of physicians, the ABA examination and certification protocol evaluates the three areas of learning. The written examination tests cognitive learning, although perhaps at its simpler levels. Psychomotor and affective learning is evaluated in an ongoing manner by the anesthesiology faculty of residency training programs and is attested to by the faculty granting a "certificate of clinical competence" to successful learners.

> *The Board [ABA] requires every residency training program to file . . . an Evaluation of Clinical Competence in January and July on behalf of each resident who has spent any portion of the prior six months in Clinical Anesthesia training in or under the sponsorship of the residency program and its affiliates. . . . Entry into the examination system is contingent upon the applicant having a Certificate of Clinical Competence on file with the Board attesting to satisfactory clinical competence during the final period of Clinical Anesthesia training in or under the sponsorship of each program. . . . The Board, therefore, will deny entry into the examination system until this requirement is fulfilled.*[4]

The oral examination evaluates cognitive learning, one hopes at its more complex levels. In addition, the oral examination may assess affective learning, although such assessment is accomplished in an unsystematic approach. The goal of the ABA oral examination process is to access the candidate's ability to (1) apply knowledge in the development of a treatment plan, (2) exhibit sound medical judgment in making medical/anesthetic decisions, (3) demonstrate adaptability in handling complications and changing medical situations, and (4) communicate logically and in an organized manner the anesthetic issues and plans for anesthesia patient care.[4]

The Methods—How to Teach

When faculty members talk about education, one of their first considerations is how to teach. Although obviously an important aspect of instruction, it is of relatively minor importance when viewed in the entire context of education. Before one can decide whether a lecture is a better method to teach a specific topic than a group discussion or whether slides, a chalkboard, or computer-assisted instructional software should be used to facilitate making a concept clear, it is essential to understand the student, the student's needs, the purpose of the education, and the content to be taught.

Too often, the instructional methodology, which is easy to consider, receives the major emphasis, whereas the difficult questions about education, such as what is its rationale, are glanced over or never even considered. After the fundamental questions about educational philosophy are answered, selection of a particular instructional technique becomes critical. The specific teaching method selected is intended to be the one best suited to the specific educational goal desired.

The use of simulation games is a good example of how the method satisfies the educational goal. In cardiopulmonary resuscitation training, for example, a simulated cardiac arrest is an exercise during which students play the resuscitator roles and use all the real-life equipment in a real-time setting. The involved students, as well as other students and the teacher or teachers who observe the simulation, review and critique the resuscitation to point out correct knowledge, skills, and attitudes displayed and which of these actions could have been performed better. The goal of the exercise is to teach students to coordinate the entire cardiopulmonary resuscitation effort by bringing together the facts and skills in an atmosphere in which reasonable attitudes are exhibited despite the tense nature of the emergency situation, all without jeopardizing any patient. A lecture, a slide show, or even a small group discussion could not achieve this goal.

Simulation is becoming an integral teaching methodology in anesthesia education.[49,50] Borrowed from flight simulation, which is an essential part of the training and certification of commercial and military pilots, anesthesia patient simulators have been developed and used to educate individuals in the discipline of anesthesiology in two major ways: (1) for specific recognition and management of critical events and (2) in the general comprehensive education about all aspects of anesthesia patient care, such as crew resource management. By coupling a mannequin with a computer and anesthesia patient care equipment, a simulation setting is created that so closely mimics real life that it is a virtual reality. Physiology, pharmacology, pathophysiology, and crisis management are a few of the curricular areas that can be most effectively taught by the anesthesia simulator approach, that is, modeling a real patient scenario for students to manage with zero risk to the simulated patient and no real risk to the student (except for the trainee's self-imposed stress to achieve). Use of this technology is limited only by the ability of the educators and students to create and "live" the scenarios.[49-51] Additional advantages of human patient simulators include their use in teaching all types of students (e.g., medical students, student nurse anesthetists, allied health professionals in a wide variety of disciplines, practitioners in continuing education programs) and the ability to conduct educational research and collect "simulated" patient management outcome data.[49-51]

Scientific evaluation of simulation is being conducted, but there are considerable study design difficulties.[52,53] In addition to the difficulty of designing studies to evaluate simulation, the evidenced-based data that are being collected deal with the performance of providers of simulated care and have yet to effectively answer the question about patient benefit related to simulation-educated physicians.[52,53] Undoubtedly, the field of human simulator education and research will continue to grow exponentially in the next few years.

An in-depth study of individual teaching techniques is appropriate after the links between the questions about educational philosophy and rationale and the methods of teaching have been established. At the teacher's disposal for effective use in the proper situation are lectures; small group discussions; the use of questions; clinical problem solving; psychomotor skill learning at the bedside, in the operating room, or in the classroom; and the use of adjunctive educational media such as slides, chalkboard, videotape, audiotape, overhead projector, computer, and teaching models. Each of these techniques can be used more effectively and efficiently when the method is studied and understood.

Effective use of questioning, for example, occurs when the teacher understands the difference between closed and open questions.[54] Closed questions are used when the teacher is interested in having the student remember facts. Because the range of responses to closed questions is limited, students answer with facts and have limited opportunity to delve into more complex cognitive learning (i.e., problem solving). A teacher uses open questions as a teaching device when desirous of directing the teaching/learning activity toward the application of knowledge to new settings or analysis of information for conceptual learning rather than mere regurgitation of facts. There is a considerable difference in the learning that might occur when a question such as "What might explain postanesthetic stupor in a patient operated on for head trauma?" is asked of a student versus asking a question such as "What are the signs and symptoms of increased intracranial pressure?"

Developing a psychomotor skill lesson is another example of how understanding instructional methodology can lead to effective teaching and learning. The old adage about teaching psychomotor skills in medicine is "see one, do one, teach one." The absurd nature of this approach has been highlighted in the following way: "This is akin to a piano instructor playing 'The Minute Waltz' for a beginner and then saying, 'Now, try it yourself.'"[54] Rather than using the repetitive trial-and-error approach to teaching/learning psychomotor skills, systematic methodology can be used.[54]

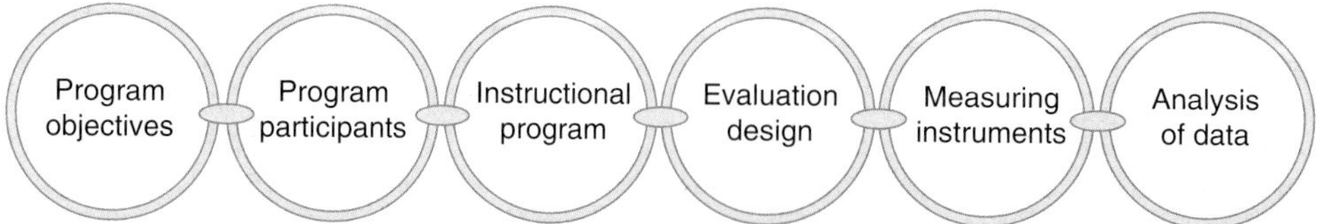

Figure 8-2 Diagrammatic representation of a model to conduct educational outcome analysis. The six components are joined in "chain-link" fashion to signify that the outcome analysis is as strong as its weakest link. Essential to the model, therefore, is sound development and implementation of the educational plan and process. This includes definition of the educational objectives, understanding of both the teaching faculty and student participants, and execution of the instructional activity. Having established the educational experience, its outcome can be assessed by applying an appropriate evaluation design[56] and using the measurement techniques to collect the data for analysis. The final step in the analysis is to apply the results to the program objectives and instructional activities to enhance future desired learner outcomes. *(From Hutchins EB: Unpublished lecture notes: Evaluation Methods in Professional Education. Course ED668, Graduate School of Education. University of Pennsylvania, 1981.)*

1. Analyze and separate the skill into its component parts and determine which aspects of the skill are most difficult to perform.
2. Provide students with a model of the skill, demonstrated effectively in its entirety, that they are expected to perform.
3. Make provisions for students to practice until the expected behavior is mastered.
4. Provide adequate supervision and an evaluation of the final performance.

Anesthesiology instructors need only think of the protocol that they are using to teach, for example, pulmonary artery catheterization by the internal jugular venous route, to assess whether they are expecting their students to perform (learn) with the type of plan just outlined or rather to "learn as they go" on each successive patient as they probe in the neck. The learn-as-you-go method can be quite stressful for both patient and trainee.[55]

A final example of an answer to the question of how to teach comes from review of the effective use of audiovisual aids. Although it is true that "a picture is worth a thousand words," the anesthesiology teacher must be sure that this image is the "text" that the teacher wishes the students to read and absorb. Slides, for example, focus the viewer's attention on an idea or ideas that the lecturer wishes to amplify in some manner. By definition, the entire lecture cannot be put on slides. Only a few important portions of the presentation are conveyed by slides, and these points are emphasized in some specific way by the visual image or images, which add to the verbal presentation. Slides are not the TelePrompTer, although they are often used this way.

Even more basic is the need to understand the proper production formatting of slides so that the message on a 35-mm transparency or a PowerPoint computer image can be seen clearly when projected onto a 12-foot-high screen in a large 800-seat lecture hall. If format is not considered, the slide is not visible and undoubtedly detracts from, rather than enhances, the lecture. Finally, even the best-produced slide is useless if nobody, including the lecturer, knows how to troubleshoot a nonfunctional computer or projector. Surely, the thousands of hours that have been devoted to slide lectures about anesthesiology could have benefitted from teachers taking more responsibility in the preparation of effective visual aids.

Summary

What is the anesthesiologist's responsibility in teaching colleagues and other health care professionals? The answer lies in the answers to the many aspects of the following question:

How shall who teach what to whom for what purpose now and in the future?!

For many, however, this type of review of education is "soft" material that lacks the "hard" research data to prove its validity. Perhaps there is some truth to this. Perhaps by its very nature (i.e., psychosocial) the science of education has its limits. On the other hand, however, enough experimental studies of education may not have been performed. A model to conduct such studies might view the preceding question in terms of educational outcome analysis (Fig. 8-2). Although the educational setting is not a pure, controlled laboratory environment, accepted quasi-experimental design techniques exist for this naturalistic research setting.[56]

What then is the anesthesiologist's responsibility in teaching? It is twofold: to understand all aspects of education and then to scientifically study educational outcome so that future students of anesthesiology will be more effectively taught and better prepared as experts in the field.

Acknowledgment

I wish to thank George E. Miller, M.D., for the insight on Socrates.

Suggested Readings

Barrows HS: Simulated (Standardized) Patients and Other Human Simulations. Chapel Hill, NC, Health Sciences Consortium, 1987.

Bunker JP (ed): Education in Anesthesiology. New York, Columbia University Press, 1967.

Dick W, Reiser RA: Planning Effective Instruction. Englewood Cliffs, NJ, Prentice-Hall, 1989.

Epstein J (ed): Masters: Portraits of Great Teachers. New York, Basic Books, 1981.

Gagné RM, Briggs LJ: Principles of Instructional Design, 2nd ed. New York, Holt, Rinehart & Winston, 1979.

Gawande A: Better: A Surgeon's Notes on Performance. New York, Metropolitan Books, 2007.

Greenberg LW, Jewett LS: Commitment to teaching: Myth or reality? South Med J 76:910, 1983.

Greene NM: Anesthesiology and the University. Philadelphia, JB Lippincott, 1975.

Groopman J: How Doctors Think. New York, Houghton Mifflin, 2007.

Jason H, Westberg J: Instructional Decision-Making Self-Study Modules for Teachers in the Health Professions (Preview Package). Miami, National Center for Faculty Development, University of Miami School of Medicine, 1980.

Joyce B, Weil M: Models of Teaching. Englewood Cliffs, NJ, Prentice-Hall, 1980.

Knowles MS: Andragogy in Action. San Francisco, Jossey-Bass, 1984.

Kohn LT, Corrigan JM, Donaldson MS (Committee on Quality of Health Care in America—Institute of Medicine) (eds): To Err Is Human. Building a Safer Health System. Washington, DC, National Academy Press, 2000.

Lear E (ed): Virtual reality in patient simulators. Am Soc Anesthesiol Newsl 61:October, 1997.

Lyman RA: Disaster in pedagogy. N Engl J Med 257:504, 1957.

McGaghie WC, Frey JJ (eds): Handbook for the Academic Physician. New York, Springer-Verlag, 1986.

McGuire CH, Foley RP, Gorr A, et al: Handbook of Health Professions Education. San Francisco, Jossey-Bass, 1983.

McKeachie WJ: Teaching Tips: A Guidebook for the Beginning College Teacher, 7th ed. Lexington, MA, DC Heath, 1978.

Miller GE: Adventure in pedagogy. JAMA 162:1448, 1956.

Miller GE (ed): Teaching and Learning in Medical School. Cambridge, MA, Harvard University Press, 1961.

Miller GE: Educating Medical Teachers. Cambridge, MA, Harvard University Press, 1980.

Popham WJ, Baker EL: Establishing Instructional Goals. Planning an Instructional Sequence. Englewood Cliffs, NJ, Prentice-Hall, 1970.

Rosenthal MH, Hughes FP: A History of the American Board of Anesthesiology 1938-2003. Raleigh, NC, The American Board of Anesthesiology, 2005.

Schwenk TL, Whitman NA: Residents As Teachers: A Guide to Educational Practice. Salt Lake City, University of Utah, 1984.

Schwenk TL, Whitman NA: The Physician As Teacher. Baltimore, Williams & Wilkins, 1987.

Segall AJ, Vanderschmidt H, Burglass R, et al: Systemic Course Design for the Health Fields. New York, John Wiley & Sons, 1975.

Whitman NA: There Is No Gene for Good Teaching: A Handbook on Lecturing for Medical Teachers. Salt Lake City, University of Utah, 1982.

Whitman NA, Schwenk TL: A Handbook for Group Discussion Leaders: Alternative to Lecturing Medical Students to Death. Salt Lake City, University of Utah, 1983.

Whitman NA, Schwenk TL: Preceptors As Teachers: A Guide to Clinical Teaching. Salt Lake City, University of Utah, 1984.

References

1. Schwartz AJ, Ellison N, Ominsky AJ, et al: Advanced CPR: Student, teacher, administrator, researcher. Anesth Analg 61:629, 1982.
2. Department of Labor: Dictionary of Occupational Titles, 4th ed, Rev 1991. Available at http://www.oalj.dol.gov/PUBLIC/DOT/REFERENCES/DOT01B.HTM U.S. Accessed Nov 18, 2007.
3. Knowles M: The Adult Learner: A Neglected Species. Houston, Gulf Publishing, 1978.
4. Booklet of Information. The American Board of Anesthesiology, Raleigh, NC, March 2007.
5. 2007 Reference Handbook and Certificate Statistics. Evanston, IL, American Board of Medical Specialties, 2007.
6. 2007 Annual Review. Evanston, IL, American Board of Medical Specialties, 2007.
7. ACGME Institutional Review: Available at http://www.acgme.org/acWebsite/navPages/nav_IRC.asp. Accessed Nov 5, 2007.
8. ACGME Anesthesiology Program Requirements: Available at http://www.acgme.org/acWebsite/RRC_040/040_prIndex.asp. Accessed Nov 5, 2007.
9. Rockoff MA, Hall SC: Subspecialty training in pediatric anesthesiology: What does it mean? Anesth Analg 85:1185, 1997.
10. Donini-Lenhoff F (ed): Health Professions Career and Education Directory 2007-2008, 35th ed. Chicago, American Medical Association, 2007.
11. Donini-Lenhoff F (ed): Health Professions Education Data Book 2007-2008. Chicago, American Medical Association, 2007.
12. Brotherton SE, Etzel SI: Graduate Medical Education, 2006-2007. JAMA 298:1081, 2007.
13. Warner MA: Residency Review Committee for Anesthesiology. ASA Newsl 71:26, 2007.
14. Schubert A: National Resident Matching Program Results for 2007: Recruitment maintains all-time high for specialty of anesthesiology. Am Soc Anesthesiol Newsl 71:17, 2007.
15. 2007 Anesthesiology Resident Class Sizes and Graduation Rates: Available at http://www.asahq.org/Newsletters/2007/12-07/schubert1207.html. Accessed Dec 29, 2007.
16. Martini CJM: Evaluating the competence of health professionals. JAMA 260:1057, 1988.
17. Langsley DG: Medical competence and performance assessment: A new era. JAMA 266:977, 1991.
18. Singer I (ed): Physician Competence: Whose Responsibility? Conference Proceedings. Chicago, American Medical Association, 1989.
19. American Board of Medical Specialties: Who we are and what we do. Available at http://www.abms.org/About_ABMS/who_we_are.aspx. Accessed Nov 26, 2007.
20. Epstein RM: The American Board of Anesthesiology: Thoughts on the occasion of its fiftieth anniversary. J Clin Anesth 2:3, 1990.
21. American Board of Anesthesiology: Continued demonstration of qualifications for board-certified anesthesiologists. Anesthesiology 73:770, 1990.
22. Glass DD: Time-limited certification: American Board of Anesthesiology. Anesthesiology 83:413, 1995.
23. Clark AJM: Continuing medical education is as important as patient care [editorial]. Can J Anaesth 39:637, 1992.
24. CMA Policy Summary: Maintenance of competence. Can Med Assoc J 46:264A, 1992.
25. American Board of Anesthesiology: Maintenance of Certification in Anesthesiology. Available at http://www.theaba.org/anesthesiology-maintenance.shtml#components. Accessed Dec 25, 2007.
26. Accreditation Council for Graduate Medical Education: Outcome Project. Available at http://www.acgme.org/Outcome/. Accessed Dec 26, 2007.
27. Accreditation Council for Graduate Medical Education: Common Program Requirements: General Competencies. Available at http://www.acgme.org/outcome/comp/GeneralCompetenciesStandards21307.pdf. Accessed Dec 24, 2007.
28. Schwartz AJ: Innovation in medical education: The Accreditation Council for Graduate Medical Outcome Project. Curr Opin Anaesthesiol 15:659, 2002.
29. Silber JH, Williams SV, Krakauer H, et al: Hospital and patient characteristics associated with death after surgery. Med Care 30:615, 1992.
30. Dubin SA, Jense HG, Yodlowski E, et al: Continuous quality improvement in an anesthesia residency training program. Int Anesthesiol Clin 30:29, 1992.
31. Schisler JQ: Implementing continuous, quality improvement: A private practice's experience. Int Anesthesiol Clin 30:45, 1992
32. Barzansky B, Etzel SI: Medical Schools in the United States 2006-2007. JAMA 298:1071, 2007.
33. Ratzan RM: On teachers. N Engl J Med 306:1420, 1982.
34. Jason H, Westberg J: Teachers and Teaching in U.S. Medical Schools. East Norwalk, CT, Appleton & Lange, 1982.
35. Mattern WD, Weinholtz D, Friedman CP: The attending physician as teacher. N Engl J Med 308:1129, 1983.
36. Tyler RW: Basic Principles of Curriculum and Instruction. Chicago, University of Chicago Press, 1949.
37. Dewey J: Democracy and Education. New York, Macmillan, 1916.
38. American Board of Anesthesiology, American Society of Anesthesiologists: Content Outline. Joint Council on In-Training Examinations. American Board of Anesthesiology Examination Part I. Revised–September 2006. Available at http://www.asahq.org/publicationsAndServices/ContentOutlineREV2006.pdf. Accessed Dec 3, 2007.
39. Bloom BS (ed): Taxonomy of Educational Objectives. Handbook I: Cognitive Domain. New York, David McKay, 1956.

40. Woolf SH: Practice guidelines: A new reality in medicine. I. Recent developments. Arch Intern Med 150:1811, 1990.
41. Woolf SH: Practice guidelines: A new reality in medicine. II. Methods of developing guidelines. Arch Intern Med 152:946, 1992.
42. Arens JF: A practice parameters overview [editorial]. Anesthesiology 78:229, 1993.
43. American Society of Anesthesiologists Task Force on Pulmonary Artery Catheterization: Practice guidelines for pulmonary artery catheterization. Anesthesiology 78:380, 1993.
44. American Society of Anesthesiologists Task Force on Management of the Difficult Airway: Practice guidelines for management of the difficult airway. Anesthesiology 78:597, 1993.
45. American Society of Anesthesiologists Task Force on Pain Management: Practice guidelines for acute pain management in the perioperative setting. Anesthesiology 82:1071, 1995.
46. American Society of Anesthesiologists Task Force on Blood Component Therapy: Practice guidelines for blood component therapy. Anesthesiology 84:732, 1996.
47. Krathwohl DR, Bloom BS, Masia BB: Taxonomy of Educational Objectives. Handbook. II: Affective Domain. New York, David McKay, 1964.
48. Schwartz AJ, Blank LL, Horrow JC, et al: Are anesthesiology residents educated to be professionals? Anesthesiology 87:A950, 1997.
49. Good ML, Gravenstein JS: Training for safety in an anesthesia simulator. Semin Anesth 12:235, 1993.
50. Latif R, Loyd GE, Henson L: Anesthesiology and medical simulation: Past, present and future. AUA Newsletter, Winter 2007. Available at http://www.auahq.org/Winter2007.pdf. Accessed Dec 25, 2007.
51. Euliano T, Good ML: Simulator training in anesthesia growing rapidly. J Clin Monit 13:53, 1997.
52. Murray DJ, Boulet JR, Avidan M, et al: Performance of residents and anesthesiologists in a simulation-based skill assessment. Anesthesiology 107:705, 2007.
53. Weinger MB: Experience ≠ expertise. Can simulation be used to tell the difference? Anesthesiology 107:691, 2007.
54. Foley RP, Smilansky J: Teaching Techniques. A Handbook for Health Professionals. New York, McGraw-Hill, 1980.
55. Gawande A: Complications: A Surgeon's Notes on an Imperfect Science. New York, Metropolitan Books, 2002.
56. Campbell DT, Stanley JC: Experimental and Quasi-experimental Designs for Research. Boston, Houghton Mifflin, 1963.

Appendix 1

Common Program Requirements: General Competencies (Abridged) Approved by the Accreditation Council for the Graduate Medical Education Board on February 13, 2007

The program must integrate the following Accreditation Council for Graduate Medical Education (ACGME) competencies into the curriculum:

- **Patient Care**
  Residents must be able to provide patient care that is compassionate, appropriate, and effective for the treatment of health problems and the promotion of health.
- **Medical Knowledge**
  Residents must demonstrate knowledge of established and evolving biomedical, clinical, epidemiologic, and social-behavioral sciences, as well as application of this knowledge to patient care.
- **Practice-Based Learning and Improvement**
  Residents must demonstrate the ability to investigate and evaluate their care of patients, to appraise and assimilate scientific evidence, and to continuously improve patient care based on constant self-evaluation and lifelong learning. Residents are expected to develop skills and habits to be able to meet the following goals:
  - Identify strengths, deficiencies, and limits in one's knowledge and expertise
  - Set learning and improvement goals
  - Identify and perform appropriate learning activities
  - Systematically analyze practice by using quality improvement methods, and implement changes with the goal of practice improvement
  - Incorporate formative evaluation feedback into daily practice
  - Locate, appraise, and assimilate evidence from scientific studies related to their patients' health problems
  - Use information technology to optimize learning
  - Participate in the education of patients, families, students, residents and other health professionals
- **Interpersonal and Communication Skills**
  Residents must demonstrate interpersonal and communication skills that result in effective exchange of information and collaboration with patients, their families, and health professionals. Residents are expected to
  - Communicate effectively with patients, families, and the public, as appropriate, across a broad range of socioeconomic and cultural backgrounds
  - Communicate effectively with physicians, other health professionals, and health-related agencies
  - Work effectively as a member or leader of a health care team or other professional group
  - Act in a consultative role to other physicians and health professionals
  - Maintain comprehensive, timely, and legible medical records, if applicable
- **Professionalism**
  Residents must demonstrate a commitment to carrying out professional responsibilities and adherence to ethical principles. Residents are expected to demonstrate
  - Compassion, integrity, and respect for others
  - Responsiveness to patient needs that supersedes self-interest
  - Respect for patient privacy and autonomy
  - Accountability to patients, society, and the profession
  - Sensitivity and responsiveness to a diverse patient population, including but not limited to diversity in gender, age, culture, race, religion, disabilities, and sexual orientation
- **Systems-Based Practice**
  Residents must demonstrate awareness of and responsiveness to the larger context and system of health care, as well as the ability to call effectively on other resources in the system to provide optimal health care. Residents are expected to
  - Work effectively in various health care delivery settings and systems relevant to their clinical specialty
  - Coordinate patient care within the health care system relevant to their clinical specialty
  - Incorporate considerations of cost awareness and risk-benefit analysis in patient- or population-based care as appropriate
  - Advocate for quality patient care and optimal patient care systems
  - Work in interprofessional teams to enhance patient safety and improve the quality of patient care
  - Participate in identifying system errors and implementing potential systems solutions

Available from http://www.acgme.org/outcome/comp/GeneralCompetenciesStandards21307.pdf.

Appendix 2

Content Outline—Joint Council on In-Training Examinations

I. Basic Sciences
   A. Anatomy
      1. Topographic anatomy as landmarks
      2. Radiologic anatomy
   B. Physics, monitoring, and anesthesia delivery devices
      1. Mechanics
      2. Flow velocity
      3. Properties of liquids, gases, and vapors
      4. Gas laws
      5. Vaporizers
      6. Uptake and distribution of inhalation agents
      7. Physics of the anesthesia machine/breathing system
      8. Monitoring methods
      9. Instrumentation
      10. Ventilators
      11. Alarms and safety features
      12. Defibrillators
      13. Pacemakers
      14. Electrical, fire, and explosion hazards; basic electronics
      15. Drug delivery devices
   C. Mathematics
      1. Simple mathematics
      2. Statistics
      3. Computer
   D. Pharmacology
      1. General concepts
      2. Anesthetics—gases and vapors
      3. Anesthetics—intravenous
      4. Anesthetics—local
      5. Muscle relaxants

II. Clinical Sciences
   A. Anesthesia procedures, methods, and techniques
      1. Evaluation of the patient and preoperative preparation
      2. Regional anesthesia
      3. General anesthesia
      4. Monitored anesthesia care and sedation
      5. Intravenous fluid therapy during anesthesia
      6. Complications (etiology, prevention, treatment)
      7. Special techniques
      8. Postoperative period

III. Organ-Based Basic and Clinical Sciences (Outline for Sections May Include Physiology, Anatomy, Biochemistry, Pharmacology, Clinical Science)
   A. Respiratory system
   B. Cardiovascular system
   C. Central and peripheral nervous systems
   D. Gastrointestinal/hepatic
   E. Renal/urinary
   F. Endocrine/metabolic
   G. Hematologic
   H. Neuromuscular

IV. Clinical Subspecialties
   A. Painful disease states
   B. Pediatric anesthesia
   C. Obstetric anesthesia
   D. Otolaryngologic anesthesia
   E. Anesthesia for plastic surgery
   F. Anesthesia for laparoscopic surgery
   G. Ophthalmologic anesthesia
   H. Orthopedic anesthesia
   I. Trauma, burn management, mass casualty, biological warfare
   J. Anesthesia for ambulatory surgery
   K. Geriatric anesthesia/aging
   L. Critical care

V. Special Problems or Issues in Anesthesiology
   A. Electroconvulsive therapy
   B. Organ donors
   C. Radiologic procedures
   D. Physician impairment or disability
   E. Ethics, practice management and medicolegal issues

Adapted from American Board of Anesthesiology, American Society of Anesthesiologists Joint Council on In-Training Examinations: American Board of Anesthesiology Examination Part I. Revised—September 2006.[38]

Gail A. Van Norman and Stanley H. Rosenbaum

9 Ethical Aspects of Anesthesia Care

Key Points

1. Anesthesiologists have ethical obligations to promote patients' abilities to make medical decisions, as well as obligations to respect those decisions.
2. Competent patients have the right to refuse medical treatments or tests, even if it appears to be a "bad" decision. Coercing or restraining competent patients is unethical.
3. Children should be involved in medical decision-making to the degree that their abilities allow, and their wishes should usually be respected.
4. Advance directives and decisions by surrogate decision-makers are legally binding.
5. Do-not-attempt-resuscitation orders require reconsideration before anesthesia and surgery and cannot be automatically suspended.
6. Withdrawal or withholding of life-sustaining treatments at the end of life requires specialized training or experience.
7. Anesthesiologists play a pivotal role in caring for both brain-dead and non–heart-beating organ donors and must be familiar with the medical, legal, and ethical issues involved.
8. Human and animal research carries special obligations to protect the subjects from inhumane treatment. Whenever possible, alternatives to human and animal research should be sought.
9. "State-sponsored" activities such as executions (1) are not the practice of medicine, (2) undermine the medical profession, and (3) place the physician on dubious moral grounds.
10. Although physicians have a right to withdraw from some situations in which patient care presents them with personal moral conflicts, this right is limited, and professionally accepted standards and obligations usually prevail (e.g., well-established standards, such as informed consent).

History of Ethics in Medicine and Ethical Theory

Medicine is a respected profession with codes of behavior and definite rules of conduct. In modern times, medical practitioners have tremendous powers, recognized social import, and powerful financial interactions that touch nearly everyone's lives. It is in the context of long-held and highly developed rules and practices that we examine the ethical bases of the practice of medicine and its implications for anesthesiologists.

Ethical Theory

Virtue Ethics, Utilitarianism, and Duty-Driven Ethics

The classic style of medical practice, called "paternalism," is derived from "virtue-based ethics." In this view, the physician is a genuinely virtuous person with inherent qualities of competence, sincerity, confidentiality, and altruism who naturally knows and does what is correct for the patient. The patient, who is not knowledgeable in the art of medicine, should trust the physician to decide what is best. Our society and legal system have changed substantially since paternalism flourished, but some patients and physicians still see this style as a desirable component of medicine.

In utilitarian ethics, actions are judged right or wrong on the balance of their good and bad consequences. A "right" action produces the most good, based on a perspective that gives equal weight to the interests of all affected parties. Although utilitarian theory is compelling (who would not want to do the most good and minimize evil?), it falls short in defining which benefits are most important. Is it the "good" that all reasonable people want or the "good" defined by the individual patient? What if the only way to maximize "good" is to commit an entirely immoral act? Suppose, for example, the only way to win a war is to systematically torture children?

Utilitarian theory may be best when applied to analyzing broad-based policies, in decisions regarding rationing of resources, and when attempting to resolve conflicting ethical obligations.

The premise of Kantian-based ethics (also called "deontological theory") is that there are features of actions other than their consequences that make them right or wrong. Intention is more important than outcome. Furthermore, no person should use another exclusively as a means to an end because each person *is* the end for which we should act. Each person is uniquely valuable and should not be used to further the purposes of other persons without their autonomous consent. Kantian philosophy would, for example, forbid killing one innocent person to save another innocent person.

Deontological and utilitarian theories are both applied to varying degrees in modern medical ethics. Individualism and autonomy are highly valued in Western society, and people tend to turn to Kantian philosophy when ethical questions arise that balance the authority of the physician against the goals and values of individual patients. When broad-based social issues are at stake, such as allocation of scarce medical resources, utilitarian arguments are often used. Some of the toughest ethical questions in medical practice occur when the rights and desires of individual patients are in conflict with social policies. Clashes between deontological and utilitarian principles are common in the intensive care unit (ICU), managed care settings, and the care of poor and elderly patients whose medical management is funded by the government. In each of these settings, the will of the individual patient may be in conflict with the broader principles of minimizing expense, fairly allocating scarce resources, and determining where and how society's health care dollars are best spent.[1]

The American political tradition provides a clear underpinning to individual freedom, hence translation of the Jeffersonian "life, liberty, and the pursuit of happiness" into the contemporary interest in physician beneficence and patient autonomy. It was with the background of this political tradition that contemporary bioethics shifted away from paternalism. At the beginning of the 20th century, the concept of autonomy of patients began to emerge.

Clinical Ethics

Informed Consent

Legal and moral imperatives for informed consent are based on the ethical principle of respect for patient autonomy. "Autonomy" refers to the ability to choose without controlling interference by others and without personal limitations that prevent meaningful choices, such as inadequate information or understanding.[1] Individuals have the right to determine what happens to them to the degree that they are capable of doing so. In the United States, this right is rooted in constitutional guarantees of privacy and noninterference. In 1914, the case of *Schloendorff v Society of New York Hospital* established that it was the right of "every human being of adult years and sound mind to determine what shall happen to his own body."[2] In 1957, the term "informed consent" was first used in the case of *Salgo v Trustees of Leland Stanford Hospital*, which established that it is not sufficient for physicians to simply secure consent; physicians have a duty to inform patients about the risks and alternatives to treatment, in addition to the procedures themselves and their consequences.[3]

Respect for patient autonomy requires physicians to respect decisions made by competent patients and to *promote* autonomy by removing barriers to competent participation in making decisions. Such obstacles range from incomplete or inaccurate information to reversible medical conditions that interfere with a patient's ability to understand the information provided.

Competence or Capacity

Autonomy to make medical decisions cannot exist in the absence of competence. Because "competence" is a legal term, most medical experts prefer the term "capacity" to describe the necessary skills to participate in medical decisions.

Impairment of capacity can be temporary or permanent. Examples include some mental illnesses, dementia, immaturity, anxiety, pain, and effects of medications. The elderly, those suffering from mental impairment, and children are particularly vulnerable to having their participation in medical decisions inappropriately curtailed or even denied because their capacity to participate is frequently underestimated. Hearing loss, dysarthria, and expressive aphasia can create the false impression that capacity is impaired. Many children make medical decisions in ways similar to adults but may be mistakenly excluded from the decision-making process solely because of their age. Language barriers can present significant challenges to communication.

Capacity is both relative and task specific. Patients may be able to understand and make decisions about medical issues while being unable to care for themselves in other ways.

Both prejudice and paternalism permeate physician behavior in the informed consent process. Challenges to patient competence rarely occur unless there is a difference of opinion or values between the patient and physician. Patients are often referred for competency evaluation because they refuse medical advice, although refusal of treatment is not by itself evidence of incompetence.[4] Physicians frequently disagree with patient decisions because they regularly ascribe a lower quality of life to impaired and handicapped patients than the patients themselves do. Doctors are mistaken about patients' preferences regarding life-extending therapies in the majority of cases and underestimate older patients' desire for life-extending therapies in up to 30% of cases.[5] Moreover, surveys indicate that physicians and other health care workers are likely to *act* on personal prejudices regarding handicapped or impaired patients.[6]

Functional capacity for decision-making must be judged separately from the perceived quality of the decision itself. Patients have the right to make "bad" decisions if they are competent and have appropriate information. Otherwise, physicians could merely substitute their own judgment for that of the patient, and autonomy in medical decision-making would be nonexistent.

How do we recognize competence? When assessing a patient for anesthesia care, the anesthesiologist should focus on the following concerns: (1) Can the patient formulate and communicate a decision? (2) Can the patient receive and understand the information relevant to the decision? (3) Can the patient understand potential consequences of the decision, including potential risks and benefits, even if in a very simplified way? (4) Can the patient express a decision and communicate values regarding the medical advice being given?

It is the anesthesiologist's ethical duty to treat reversible conditions that interfere with medical decision-making. Elective surgery may have to be postponed until expert consultation for determination of mental capacity or treatment of reversible conditions can take place. When surgery is urgent or a patient is impaired by an irreversible condition, anesthesiologists may have to rely on a surrogate decision-maker or proceed with their best determination of the patient's interests in mind.

Disclosure

The informed consent process requires honest disclosure of medical information to the patient. U.S. courts currently rely on two standards of disclosure: the reasonable person standard and the subjective standard. A third, "professional standard," in which the physician is obliged to disclose only what other physicians of the same specialty would disclose, was subject to abuse and manipulation and is essentially no longer recognized. In the "reasonable person" standard, the physician must disclose any information that a theoretical "reasonable person" would want to know. This standard does not require an exhaustive recitation of facts and acknowledges that not all information related to the procedure is integral to making a decision about whether to undergo the procedure. The "subjective standard" recognizes that some patients may have special needs for specific information and that when that need is obvious or has been brought to the attention of the physician, the information must be disclosed. For example, a concert violinist may have a specific need to know about the potential for nerve damage from an axillary block. In general, legal and ethical standards now require that (1) the physician accurately discuss the therapy and its potential alternatives—including no therapy—and (2) disclose the common risks (because they are more likely to happen) and the serious risks (because the consequences are severe).

The doctrine of "therapeutic privilege" is sometimes cited to avoid discussing risks under the reasoning that the stress of discussing risks can harm the patient psychologically or physically. Studies of patient stress during the informed consent process *do not* support this concept.[7] Therapeutic privilege is probably invoked in many cases because the physician is uncomfortable with disclosure or wants to curtail discussion. Although it is ethical to forgo or curtail risk discussions at the patient's request, it is not generally ethical for the physician to unilaterally decide to do so.

The physician-patient relationship is an inherently unequal one because of physicians' knowledge and authority and the patient's dependence on them for care. Physicians have ethical obligations to avoid exploiting their influence for the purpose of accomplishing their own ends. Although it is acceptable to offer a rational basis for a medical choice, it is generally unethical to coerce or manipulate patients into decisions by presenting real or implied threats or by omitting or misrepresenting key information.

Legal implications of Informed Consent

The informed consent process does not prevent legal liability when adverse events occur. Flawed informed consent processes have been cited, however, as evidence of a lack of quality of care by the physician. The American Society of Anesthesiologists (ASA) closed claims database reveals that the absence of informed consent is cited in approximately 1% of claims and that cases with inadequate documentation of informed consent are associated with larger monetary awards.[8] Studies repeatedly show that the risk of filing a malpractice claim is directly related to patients' perception of their relationship with the physician.[9] The informed consent process provides one of the few opportunities that anesthesiologists have to establish that relationship, however brief, and should not be underestimated in its medicolegal importance.

Informed Refusal

Informed consent is meaningless if the patient cannot also refuse medical therapy because the consent process is then merely an exercise in patient acquiescence to the physician's will. Examples of informed refusal in anesthesiology include requests to withdraw or withhold life-supporting care in the ICU; do-not-attempt-resuscitation (DNAR) orders in the operating room; cases in which the patient has objections to certain forms of therapy, such as a Jehovah's Witness who refuses blood transfusions; and cases in which a patient refuses preoperative testing, such as human immunodeficiency virus (HIV) or pregnancy testing.

Informed refusal has similar concerns and requirements as informed consent. When patients refuse medical care or insist on what the physician believes is suboptimal care, disclosure of the risks and benefits becomes even more important because these decisions may veer from options that are already widely accepted and for which the risks are believed to be lowest. It is easier to justify agreeing to the unusual preferences of a well-informed patient than to subject a poorly informed patient to unorthodox care.

Despite full information, patients may sometimes request or demand care that is unreasonable, either because it will adversely affect the performance of surgery or because it would be associated with unreasonably high risk. When a patient demands a technique that is inappropriate or outside the realm of reasonable practice, the anesthesiologist is under no ethical obligation to provide that care. No physician can be compelled by a patient to practice negligently.

Special Issues in Informed Consent and Informed Refusal

Jehovah's Witness Patients

The classic example of a patient who refuses therapy in anesthesia practice is that of Jehovah's Witnesses, many of whom believe that accepting a blood transfusion violates a Biblical injunction (also see Chapters 5 and 6). The Jehovah's Witness doctrine has been subject to change over time, which has resulted in inconsistencies in religious practice with regard to which, if any blood components might be acceptable. Individuals interpret religious doctrines in light of their own spiritual contexts, and not all believers hold to the same tenets with equal fervor. Church doctrines, like medical practices, evolve over time, and practices that are acceptable at one time may not be acceptable years later. Anesthesiologists and surgeons have cited individual and doctrinal inconsistencies as justification for ignoring the wishes of Jehovah's Witness patients—but to do so is no more logical than assuming that every hypertensive patient needs or will respond well to identical treatment or that optimal treatments will not evolve over time.[10] Moreover, it is the right of *any* patient to refuse blood transfusion therapy, regardless of whether this desire is founded in a religious preference. Such refusals have become more common in non–Jehovah's Witness patients because blood transfusion therapy was connected to cases of acquired immunodeficiency syndrome (AIDS) in the 1980s and patients began questioning the value and necessity of transfusion therapy in light of its risks.

Because beliefs differ regarding which, if any, blood replacement therapies are acceptable, it is important to have a thorough and detailed discussion of possible therapies with a Jehovah's Witness patient before surgery, and the conclusions should be documented in the patient's chart. If anesthesiologists believe that they cannot comply with an adult patient's desire to forgo transfusion, they have the ethical obligation to find an alternative caregiver whenever possible.[11]

The courts strongly support the rights of adult patients to refuse blood products for themselves but have been inconsistent and have interfered in the cases of some pregnant patients. Transfusion of pediatric Jehovah's Witness patients by court order is common at this time but may become ethically and legally less acceptable as therapy other than blood transfusion to maintain oxygen-carrying capacity evolves, as the Jehovah's Witness church further defines its doctrines with regard to children, and as the capacity of children to consent to or refuse therapy is better understood.

The Pediatric Patient and Other Patients with Impaired Competence

The ethical practice of medicine weighs heavily toward adherence to respect for autonomy in patients who are competent to make medical decisions (also see Chapter 82) or who have executed advance directives when they were competent to do so. Medical care of individuals who have never been autonomous relies on principles such as respect for human dignity, beneficence, avoidance of harm, and adherence to the principle of justice.

Children are an example of persons who may or may not yet be autonomous. Laws in each state define the age at which children become *legally* competent to make medical decisions (usually age 18), but many younger children have the mental and emotional capacity to make medical decisions. Forcing such individuals to undergo treatments that they do not want is unethical and could be illegal as well.

Decision-making capacity in children is variable. Most 2-year-olds are clearly not able to make medical decisions, but there is a wide range of capability present in children as young as 7 or 8, and studies suggest that the average 14-year-old makes medical decisions similar to adults. In one study, children from 6 through 9 years of age invited to participate in influenza vaccine research asked pertinent questions about individual risks and benefits and whether their community and other children would benefit.[12]

Most states recognize "emancipated minor" status whereby a court determines that minors can legally make medical decisions for themselves. Legal exceptions to the age of consent are recognized in most states when treatment is believed to be in the minor's best interest and a requirement for parental consent would interfere with the child's ability to receive medical help. The law recognizes that tragically, some conditions for which a minor seeks therapy may even be the result of parental abuse and that seeking parental permission for treatment may actually further endanger the minor. Thus, minors are allowed in many states to consent to treatment for substance abuse, sexually transmitted disease, mental illness, and medical care affecting pregnancy, including abortion. In situations in which a minor has decision-making capacity but is not "emancipated," a judge may declare the child to be a "mature minor" with decision-making rights.

Ideally, individuals of any age should be involved in medical decisions to the degree that their capacity allows. A minor who possesses the capacity to make decisions should not be coerced or restrained under most circumstances.[13] Determining whether a minor has such capacity may require formal consultation and assessment. The term "assent" rather than "consent" is used to refer to agreement with treatment by children who do not fall into legal categories awarding them adult rights. The American Academy of Pediatrics has stated that physicians who care for children "should give serious consideration to each patient's developing capacities for participating in decision-making, including rationality and autonomy."[14]

When children dissent to undergo medical care, persistent refusals may be ethically binding, particularly in the case of participation in research. Medical personnel should respect the wishes of patients who withhold assent and try to gain a better understanding of their situation or deal with their fears. "A patient's reluctance or refusal to assent should also carry considerable weight when the proposed intervention is not essential to his or her welfare and/or can be deferred without substantial risk."[14,15]

Consent for Laboratory Tests: HIV and Pregnancy Testing

HIV and pregnancy testing has serious ethical considerations (also see Chapters 69 and 101), has limited, if any beneficial impact in the setting of surgery, may create serious social and economic consequences for the patient beyond the operating room, and may require the patient's informed consent.

HIV tests are usually ordered for the purpose of singling out patients for whom "extra universal precautions" could be taken to reduce transmission in the operating room. Most surgeons and anesthesiologists believe that compulsory AIDS testing would reduce their risk of exposure, and many believe that it is the physician's prerogative and can be done without the patient's consent.[16]

However, HIV testing does not necessarily yield safer anesthetic management and is more costly than diligent application of universal precautions.[17] In low-prevalence populations, testing is more likely to give false-negative results that wrongly reassure operating room workers that a patient is not infected. This may paradoxically increase the risk for transmission of HIV if relaxation in vigilance is the result.

Positive HIV tests can result in loss of employment or insurance coverage, or both. Seropositive women often experience marital breakup, abandonment, verbal abuse, and physical violence if their status is disclosed.[18] The threat of compulsory AIDS testing almost certainly would prevent some patients from seeking needed surgical care.[19]

Routine preoperative pregnancy testing has ethical ramifications analogous to HIV testing. Despite pervasive beliefs to the contrary, large, well-designed population studies do not demonstrate that anesthetics lead to early fetal loss or an increased frequency of fetal malformations.[20,21] Studies have also shown that even adolescent girls generally report the possibility of pregnancy accurately when asked privately.[22] Legal ramifications of not routinely testing for pregnancy preoperatively have been virtually nonexistent, and less than a third of U.S. practices require it.[23] A positive pregnancy test may have extremely negative consequences if a vulnerable patient is in a social situation in which pregnancy is not accepted. Abandonment, negative family interactions, and violence to the patient or her fetus (or both) all occur. Adolescent pregnancies are sometimes the result of child abuse or rape, and referral of adolescents who are pregnant to Child Protective Services should be considered.[23] In many states it is illegal to disclose or even insinuate a child's pregnancy status to her parents regardless of her age, thus leaving an anesthesiologist who discovers an adolescent pregnancy with few comfortable or legal options.

Many patients may choose not to undergo elective surgery if they know that they are pregnant. However, coercing a female patient to have a test against her wishes and which she may find insulting explicitly violates patient autonomy. Physician self-interest is not a sufficient justification for disregarding patient autonomy or violating a patient's privacy. It was the joint recommendation of the ASA Task Force on Preoperative Testing and the ASA Committee on Ethics that anesthesiologists offer the *choice* of preoperative pregnancy testing to any female patient who might desire one, explain the potential risks and benefits, and obtain informed consent for the test.[24]

Maternal-Fetal Conflicts

In general, the rights of pregnant women to refuse therapy, even if refusal would be detrimental to their fetuses, are protected under right-to-privacy provisions in the U.S. constitution (also see Chapter 69). These rights are weighed against potential harm to the fetus in a decremental fashion as the fetus approaches and surpasses viable age. When the fetus is of nonviable age, mother's rights prevail. Court decisions have consistently upheld the rights of pregnant women to have abortions, to not be subjected to drug testing, and to forgo transfusions early in pregnancy. Attempts to charge women with child abuse, child endangerment, drug trafficking, murder, and attempted murder for activities deemed dangerous to their fetuses have almost uniformly failed.[25] In general, women do not lose their rights to bodily integrity and informed consent when they become pregnant, and neither fetal "rights" nor state interests supersede a pregnant woman's right as medical decision-maker.

The American Academy of Pediatrics Committee on Ethics has outlined conditions that in their view are necessary to override a mother's refusal of care: (1) the fetus *will* suffer irrevocable harm without the treatment, (2) the treatment is *clearly indicated* and likely to be effective, and (3) the risk to the woman is low.[26] However, the American College of Obstetricians and Gynecologists condemns the use of coercion on pregnant women and advocates counseling the patient carefully about risks, in addition to recommending consultation with an ethics committee.[27]

The Uncooperative Patient—Coercion and Restraint

The use of physical restraint to control medical research subjects was first addressed directly in the Nuremberg Code after the Doctor's Trial in 1947-1949 and is a continuing subject of intense scrutiny (also see Chapter 71).[28] For anesthesiologists, chemical restraints often replace physical ones, but the ethical issues are the same. Anesthesiologists are often asked by medical colleagues to chemically restrain uncooperative patients. Use of restraint is antithetical to promotion of autonomy, and anesthesiologists have both ethical and legal obligations to determine whether such extreme intervention is warranted. Coercing or using physical or chemical means to force competent patients to undergo treatment that they are refusing is both unethical and illegal. Refusal of medical care and angry behavior are not proof of incompetence, intoxication, or inability to make medical decisions.[29]

When faced with an uncooperative adult patient, questions to ask include (1) Is the patient clearly incompetent or merely angry and uncooperative? Is there evidence of neurologic impairment, acute intoxication, or severe mental disability? (2) Is the patient in immediate danger? (3) Does the patient pose a direct threat to staff or other patients? (4) Is there a compelling need to treat life-threatening injuries? In the absence of these considerations, the use of coercion or physical or chemical restraint is neither ethical nor legal. Physicians may be forced in some situations to act within a timeframe that does not permit lengthy evaluation of a patient's competence or a protracted search for a surrogate decision-maker. In such cases, the physician must rely on professional judgment in deciding how to care for uncooperative patients who either cannot speak for themselves or appear incompetent to refuse care at a time when a decision must be made. The standard applied here would be to do what a "reasonable" person would wish. Coercion or restraint (or both) in such situations is not ideal but may be necessary and ethically permissible.

An uncooperative child presents special ethical concerns. When a patient who does not have the capacity to make health care decisions dissents to medical care, the anesthesiologist is ethically required to provide care that is most likely to benefit the patient and prevent harm while preserving the dignity and safety of the patient. Although violation of respect for autonomy is technically not possible in a patient who does not have autonomy, violation of the principles of beneficence, nonmaleficence, and respect for dignity certainly is. Indiscriminate use of physical or chemical restraint is not without physical risk, and the fear and anger provoked by such tactics can lead to future aversion toward medical care and mistrust of health care providers. The American Academy of Pediatrics Committee on Child Abuse and Neglect states that restraint should not be used in pediatric care "unless it is necessary for proper diagnosis and treatment in a sick child, as in the case of a child with a high fever and potential ear infection, or in emergency situations."[30]

Behavioral control in an uncooperative child or incompetent adult should focus on alternatives to physical restraint, such as offering choices on how to go to sleep and use of fantasy or hypnotic suggestion. Although there may be many social, economic, and scheduling pressures to the contrary, delaying or rescheduling surgery on a hysterical patient is better than coercion or force. Delaying elective surgery may reduce stress, allow adequate premedication, and promote safer induction conditions. If medical care is urgent or if delay is unlikely to result in better conditions for the patient, the anesthesiologist should proceed in a manner designed to preserve the patient's dignity and safety.

Advance Directives and Surrogate Decision-Makers

Critical decisions regarding medical care often arise when patients are too ill to formulate or express decisions regarding medical interventions. "Advance directives" were developed after several legal decisions affirmed that patients can refuse even lifesaving medical care and that clear and convincing evidence of the patient's wishes is needed to allow surrogate decision-makers to request withdrawal of life-sustaining therapies.[31] An advance directive is a document executed by patients before incapacity to provide physicians with guidance in medical decision-making when the patients cannot communicate for themselves. Such directives include living wills, which detail which therapies a patient would accept or refuse in the case of terminal incapacity; DNAR orders; and any other information regarding medical care decisions.

A surrogate decision-maker may be someone whom the patient has appointed to make health care decisions for them (a durable power of attorney [POA]) or an individual with other legally recognized authority by virtue of their relationship with the patient.

A durable POA for health care decisions may be given by patients to a specific person whom they designate to make health care decisions for them if they become incapacitated. The authority vested in a POA supersedes most other decision-makers, including family members, except court-appointed guardians.

When the patient has not designated a durable POA, doctors rely on family members to make decisions for the patient. In many states there is no legally defined hierarchy of decision-makers. Usually, the spouse or legally recognized domestic partner is considered the first-line surrogate. Commonly, the surrogate hierarchy after the spouse is the children, if all are in agreement, and then the parents, if both are in agreement, and then the siblings, if all are in agreement. In cases in which there are no advance directives and either a surrogate decision-maker is not available or family members cannot agree, the courts may appoint a guardian ad litem to represent the patient in medical decision-making.

Surrogates explicitly act in "substituted judgment" to provide what the patient would have wanted and, theoretically, are not being asked merely for their own preferences. However, surrogate decision-makers at best only approximate the patient's decisions because their interpretation is subject to their own biases, values, and psychological agendas. Incompetent patients can be emotionally and financially burdensome, and decision-makers may have conflicts of interest that distort their beliefs and testimony about what the patient would have wanted.

Studies demonstrate that patients and their proxies only infrequently discuss issues and values involving life-sustaining technologies. There are often significant discrepancies between patients and proxies in the assessment of patients' emotional health and satisfaction. Neither physicians nor proxies can always accurately predict a patient's preferences for life-sustaining therapy.[32-34] Nevertheless, with all of its imperfections, proxy decision-making may be the only option if a patient has not left specific directives.

Medical Decisions That Cannot Be Made by a Surrogate Decision-Maker

Some medical treatments have intense cultural connotations, may involve limitation on private freedoms such as reproduction, or may have historically been subject to abuse. Decisions regarding such interventions cannot be made by a surrogate decision-maker, even if one is available, and require court review. Examples in some states are sterilization and electroshock therapy.

The anesthesiologist should review the patient record before taking a patient to the operating room and ascertain (1) whether the patient has advance directives, (2) who the patient's surrogate decision-makers are, (3) if the procedure is legally allowed with consent from a surrogate decision-maker, and (4) in special cases, whether an appropriate court order has been obtained.

Special Issues with Advance Directives—Do-Not-Attempt-Resuscitation Orders in the Operating Room

Up to 60% of anesthesiologists incorrectly believe that DNAR orders are automatically suspended during anesthesia and surgery (also see Chapter 97). The ASA,[11] the American College of Surgeons,[35] the Association of Operating Room Nurses,[36] and the Joint Commission on Accreditation of Healthcare Organizations[37] all have published practice guidelines requiring reconsideration, not abandonment, of DNAR orders in the perioperative period.

The DNAR order is, in essence, documentation of the patient's wishes to avoid the medical interventions associated with resuscitation. Because the causes and outcomes expected with cardiac arrest in the operating room are different from what may happen elsewhere and the prognosis is much more favorable, it is very important to reassess the patient's desires when surgery is anticipated.

The ASA has issued guidelines for the management of a patient with DNAR orders and other directives limiting medical care.[11] Although the patient's primary care physician may have introduced the idea of DNAR orders to the patient or surrogate, it is specifically the anesthesiologist's duty to discuss the risks and benefits of resuscitation in the setting of anesthesia and surgery before undertaking the patient's care. The anesthesiologist should include in the discussion the following steps: (1) determine what the patient's goals are regarding surgery and resuscitation; (2) establish exactly what is meant by "resuscitation," in contrast to routine anesthetic care; (3) educate the patient about the risks and benefits of resuscitation in the operating room setting; and (4) document the agreements reached with the patient about which interventions commonly associated with resuscitation are acceptable to the patient. Such interventions might include, but are not limited to, intubation, administration of vasoactive drugs, administration of DC countershock, and institution of chest compressions. Many patients who express reluctance about resuscitation during surgery are fearful of burdensome outcomes, such as permanent neurologic impairment. Education and discussion may reassure them about the favorable outcomes of resuscitation in the operating room and can establish ground rules for discontinuing interventions postoperatively if they do not lead to a chance of meaningful recovery.

Surgery is dependent on the cooperation of many caregivers with differing expertise, each of whom has independent ethical obligations to the patient. It is therefore imperative that resuscitation agreements be discussed with other members of the operating room team. Such a policy prevents crucial disagreements from occurring during a critical event when treatment decisions must be made quickly. It also allows "conscientious objectors" to withdraw from the health care team.

Advance directives are legally and ethically binding. Despite clear, consistent, and forceful legal decisions, many physicians still resist imperatives to respect patient wishes regarding resuscitative care, life-sustaining therapies, or both. Anesthesiologists have ignored DNAR directives under the false assumptions that the legal authority of advance directives and living wills is not binding in the operating room or that the physician has discretion in deciding when to follow or ignore such directives. In response, courts have awarded significant monetary damages for the cost of continued health care and punitive damages for the pain, suffering, and mental anguish of the patients' survivors when DNAR instructions are ignored.[38]

Finally, DNAR orders must never be construed as an excuse to not "care" for the patient. A patient's decision to forgo resuscitation does not imply a wish to avoid other beneficial interventions. Placement of a pulmonary artery catheter, for example, may help ensure optimal management of a frail patient who has a DNAR order by enabling the anesthesiologist to avoid situations in which the patient's DNAR status becomes pivotal.

End-of-Life Decision-Making

A 1996 review by the American Medical Association showed that end-of-life issues of foremost importance to patients were control over the timing and location of death; management of symptoms such as pain, dyspnea, anxiety, and depression; financial management of medical care; and maintenance of therapeutic options, including physician-assisted suicide.[39,40]

Withdrawal/Withholding of Medical Therapy—*Curing* versus *Caring*

More than 80% of deaths in the United States occur in health care facilities, and the majority of deaths in ICUs take place after an explicit decision to withdraw or withhold treatment.[40] Patients and doctors alike recognize that aggressive medical therapy may not be desired or even appropriate in the face of advancing disease. Continued therapy may not be warranted or desired when quality of life is extremely poor, even if the patient is not suffering from terminal disease.

Before the mid-20th century, the concept of "beneficence" in the eyes of physicians was strongly tied to preventing death. Ethical distinctions between acts of omission ("letting die") and acts of commission ("killing") were and remain confusing at best. Worse, physicians faced threats of criminal punishment if patient death resulted from withdrawal of medical treatment. In 1976, the case of Karen Ann Quinlan[41] established that patients have a right to forgo invasive treatment, even if lifesaving, and that surrogate decision-makers could ask for withdrawal of lifesaving therapies if they could show that the patient would not have wanted them. The right to forgo lifesaving treatment was later extended in the cases of Claire Convoy and Nancy Cruzan to include *any* treatment if patients refused or there was clear and convincing evidence that the therapy would have been refused if the patients could speak for themselves.[31] These decisions were revisited and reconfirmed in the tragic case of Theresa Schiavo in 2005.[42]

Arguments that withdrawing or withholding life-sustaining therapy does not violate rules against killing patients are based on ethical differences between killing and letting die and between acts of commission (e.g., lethal injection) and acts of omission (e.g., withdrawal or withholding of ventilator therapy).[43] Because such distinctions are confusing to physicians and patients alike, a "principle of proportionality" is often applied when withholding or withdrawing treatment.[44] In this principle, treatment is "indicated" to the extent that it is likely to present more benefits than burdens to the patient based on the patient's perception of such medical, social, and psychological benefits and burdens. Of course, competent patients still always have the right to refuse therapy, even if the treatment is lifesaving and otherwise indicated.

Two common scenarios in which anesthesiologists may be involved in withdrawal or withholding of life-sustaining interventions are in the ICU or operating room before organ donation after cardiac death. In both cases, the issues and principles of withdrawing/withholding treatment are the same.

Withdrawal of life-sustaining interventions heralds the final phase of end-of-life care. Terminal care requires special physician knowledge and experience. It requires expertise in medically supportive therapy, problematic symptom management, knowledge about physiologic changes in dying patients, support and counseling of patients and families, understanding and respect for patient autonomy and religious and cultural practices and beliefs, ability to work within complex health care teams, ability to communicate well, and empathy.[45] Anyone intimately involved in care of a dying patient should also be intimately familiar with the ethical and legal standards.

Withdrawal of life-sustaining care begins with an assessment of the individual patient's physiology, level of dependence on therapy, degree of consciousness, preferences regarding sedation and analgesia, and preferences regarding privacy and level of involvement of family and other loved ones. All of the patient's treatment orders should be reviewed to meet the new treatment goals. Treatments promoting patient comfort should generally be continued, whereas those directed only at physiologic maintenance might all be withdrawn. Family members and others attending the patient at the end of life should be educated about the physical and mental changes that they can expect to see as treatments are scaled back, including the possibility that death will not occur imminently once support is withdrawn.[46]

Several interventions have ethical implications and deserve special consideration—fluid and nutritional management, administration of sedatives and narcotics that have the potential to hasten death, and administration of neuromuscular blocking agents.

Fluid and nutritional support is controversial. Burdens associated with continuation of fluid and nutritional support include prolongation of the dying process and complications and suffering from placement and maintenance of intravenous or enteral access (or both). However, feeding and hydration may have important connotations for family and members of the health care team in that they allow a sense of nurturing and mitigate feelings that they are "abandoning" the patient.[47] Pain, dyspnea, and depression are all common symptoms that cause suffering in a dying patient. Alleviating the pain and dyspnea carries the risk of hastening death. Medical, legal, and religious authorities have all clearly accepted the principle of "double effect," in which an action intended to produce a benefit for the patient produces not only the expected benefit but also the potential for significant harm. It is entirely ethical and legal to administer high doses of pain medication and sedatives for the intended effect of relieving suffering, even if the treatment has the side effect of hastening death. However, to administer any medication with the explicit intention of hastening death is euthanasia and not medical therapy.[47]

Neuromuscular blocking agents have no anesthetic, analgesic, or sedative properties and have no role in palliative care. Such drugs should not be initiated if withdrawal of ventilatory support is anticipated. When withdrawal of ventilator support is anticipated in a patient already receiving such agents, they should be withheld in all but extraordinary cases. Paralyzing the patient to comfort *the family* so that they see no disturbing movements or respirations as the patient dies is not justifiable. Even worse, it can mask symptoms and signs of distress and prevent relief of suffering during the dying process.[46]

Physician-assisted suicide (PAS) involves the provision of medications or prescriptions to patients by specific request for the purpose of ending their life. PAS requires a patient who is both competent and capable of communicating the request. Euthanasia involves the administration of medication by someone other than the patient for the express purpose of causing death in the belief that this would be best for the patient (but not necessarily at a specific request of the patient). Both practices differ ethically from withdrawing or withholding life-supporting medical treatment. In the former, the primary intent is to cause death, which secondarily ends suffering. In the latter, the primary intention is to discontinue treatments that are causing suffering with an understanding that death may or probably will result.

Currently, euthanasia is legal only in the Netherlands. In the United States, euthanasia remains illegal regardless of circumstance, and PAS is legal in the states of Washington and Oregon at the time of this writing.

Supporters of PAS argue that the right to privacy and respect for autonomy support patients' rights to determine the time, location, and circumstance of their own death. Adequate control of pain, anxiety, dyspnea, and other symptoms at the end of life remains a challenge to the medical profession that has fueled the desire for a means to end life when suffering cannot be controlled. Opponents argue that PAS "medicalizes" death, overly idealizes the physician-patient relationship, and ignores any personal and professional conflicts of interest that might occur. Although many ethicists acknowledge that individual circumstances may make assisted suicide an ethically permissible action, most express concern about potential abuse. Vulnerable members of society, such as the poor, elderly, and handicapped, might be pressed by financial and social factors into a suicide option in preference to palliative care.

An additional argument against PAS or legalized euthanasia is that they might provide simpler and less expensive solutions to the medical, social, and economic problems common to elderly and poor patients than seeking and requiring more difficult, but definitive remedies.

Ethical Issues in Organ Transplantation: Brain Death and Donation after Cardiac Death

Two issues critical to vital organ transplantation that confront anesthesiologists are the concept of brain death and linkage of withdrawal of life-sustaining therapies with organ retrieval and transplantation after cardiac death (donation after cardiac death [DCD]).

Brain Death

Before the 1960s, death was defined as the moment when the heartbeat stopped and respirations ceased. Advances in cardiopulmonary resuscitation and mechanical ventilation then made it possible to postpone death, seemingly indefinitely. In 1968, the Ad Hoc Committee of the Harvard Medical School proposed redefining death as the point at which all cardiorespiratory function had irreversibly ceased *or* all function of the whole brain had irreversibly stopped (brain death).[48] The committee gave two explicit reasons for redefining death. The first was to allow patients to be declared dead and not maintained on machines, thereby limiting expense, reallocating medical resources to other salvageable patients, and allowing the social rituals surrounding death to occur. The second was to allow donation of vital organs before the circulation stopped.

The public has been slow to accept brain death, in part because it requires complete trust in physicians and ignores indicators of death that the public already understands. For nonphysicians, brain-dead donors are superficially indistinguishable in many ways from living persons, and they must therefore rely completely on the physician for both accurate and honest information of a loved one's death.

Diagnosing brain death is relatively straightforward. In the United States it requires demonstration that in the absence of drugs, paralytic agents, hypothermia, and other reversible conditions that mimic loss of brain function, cortical and brainstem function is absent. The diagnosis is usually made either clinically by demonstrating that cortical activity and brainstem reflexes are absent or by radiographic studies demonstrating complete absence of cerebral blood flow.

The definition of brain death is *social* rather than *biologic*. Nevertheless, medical, ethical, theologic, and legal experts generally agree that brain death adequately defines a condition in which a person with ethical and legal rights and moral standing ceases to exist and should no longer be treated as an alive being. Expensive medical interventions can be discontinued without legal ramifications, and vital organs can be donated for transplantation if the patient or surrogate agrees.

Before assuming care of a brain-dead organ donor, the anesthesiologist is obliged to review the chart for documentation of the declaration of brain death, as well as the criteria on which it was based. If there are any questions about the diagnosis, organ donation should be postponed until the anesthesiologist is satisfied that these concerns are addressed.

Donation after Cardiac Death

DCD occurs when a patient desires to have life-sustaining medical therapies withdrawn and also wishes to proceed with donation of vital organs after death. Controlling the time and place of death so that the timing of organ donation can be optimized has obvious medical and ethical advantages. The decision to donate organs is made before death so that discussion and informed consent can take place. Ischemia time can be minimized. The dual decision to withdraw life-sustaining interventions and donate vital organs after death can create ethical conflicts, however. When a dying patient becomes an imminent organ donor, there is a risk that patient interests will be minimized or ignored in favor of the organ recipient.

The Institute of Medicine reviewed DCD in 1997[49] and 2000[50] and found that there were serious ethical questions, such as determining how quickly after asystole organ donation can begin and whether medications can ethically be administered to the donor before death that are solely for the purpose of organ preservation.

Ethical, theologic, and legal principles prohibit us from killing one person to benefit another, but the point at which actual death has occurred in DCD patients is unclear. Although expedient donation is the very purpose of DCD, doctors must never sacrifice any living patient in the process or even take significant risks of doing so—the mistrust that this would engender in the public could place the entire concept of DCD at risk by reducing potential donors and ultimately harming future potential organ recipients.[51-53] Loss of consciousness occurs quickly after asystole, but brain function can continue for some time and irreversible brain injury may not occur for many minutes. Yet many protocols call for organ retrieval to begin only 2 minutes after the circulation has stopped, and in at least one institution, organ donation is allowed to begin within seconds of cardiac arrest.[54] There is both scientific and philosophic uncertainty about when death is complete—this could even lead to accusations of physicians deliberately killing patients to obtain organs for transplantation. Mistakes have occurred in some cases of brain-dead organ donors for which clear clinical criteria exist; DCD is potentially even more prone to error because no such clinical guidelines are universally accepted.[55]

Donation of vital organs after brain death and DCD is both ethical and legal, but the interests of the dying patient must be absolutely protected until death has occurred. Anesthesiologists can play a vital role in the organ donation process by helping hospitals develop reasonable and ethical policies for the management of brain-dead and DCD donors. Every anesthesiologist should be thoroughly familiar with brain death criteria and should review the process of determining brain death before accepting care of a brain-dead donor. Anesthesiologists involved in organ DCD should have appropriate training or expertise in the relevant ethical, legal, and medical issues involved, including end-of-life care.

Research Ethics

Human Subjects Research

The premise that the physician always puts the best interests of the patient first can be jeopardized when research objectives enter the doctor-patient relationship. Human subjects are asked to put aside their own interests to benefit some future, hypothetical group of patients. In extreme cases, the patient becomes a research "object" who will not benefit personally from the experiment at all. Two examples include experiments in healthy subjects and phase I cancer trials in terminally ill patients in which the goal is to determine the toxicity of treatment—not remission, palliation, or cure.

Human subjects research must balance many conflicting interests, such as the needs and rights of the research subject, the hypothetical interests of future patients, and the physician's financial, professional, and personal goals. Academic or corporate advancement, personal prestige, and financial incentives may be disincentives to researchers who are diligently protecting patient interests or remaining objective in designing protocols and analyzing and reporting their findings. Thus, human subjects research is more closely regulated, supervised, and controlled than any other medical endeavor.

Regulation of research began after World War II, with the Nuremburg Code and the Helsinki Declaration outlining the ethical obligations of physicians engaged in human research. The United States was slow to awaken to the parallels between the concentration camp experiments and the sometimes gruesome treatment to which they subjected their own subjects in similar trials.[56] In the years that followed the Doctor's Trial at Nuremburg, Fox[57] and Beecher[58] found that researchers were aware of the standards set at Nuremberg but regularly did not comply with them. In 1974, the National Research Act established the National Commission for the Protection of Human Subjects of Biomedical and Behavioral Research, out of which the modern institutional review board was born.[31]

Ethical conduct of human subjects research follows three principles: (1) respect for autonomy and the obligation to protect subjects with limited autonomy; (2) beneficence, with obligations to minimize risks, maximize benefits, and ensure that the research design is scientifically sound; and (3) justice, the obligation to treat each person with regard to what is morally right and to ensure fair distribution of benefits and burdens.

In addition to comprehensive presentation to research subjects of the risks and benefits of procedures or medications to which they will be subjected, disclosure must include the possibility of commercialization of the results, financial interests of the researchers, and any other actual or perceived conflicts of interest on the part of researchers and their institutions and sponsors. Subjects must be free to refuse or end participation at any time without penalty. "Situational coercion" in which subjects believe that they are not truly free to refuse should be avoided or mitigated. Examples of situational coercion include prisoners whose terms and experiences of incarceration might be affected by their decision to participate or refuse and hospitalized patients who may believe that their care could be compromised if they do not cooperate with researchers.[56]

Monetary or other inducements to participate in research are probably permissible if they do not undermine the freedom of the subject to refuse under reasonable circumstances. Significant monetary awards may have adverse effects on the autonomy of subjects and a negative impact on the scientific quality of the research. If remuneration is high, for example, subjects might conceal factors that would otherwise disqualify them from participating, thereby compromising the research results and exposing themselves to greater risk.

Researchers are obligated to maximize benefit and minimize potential harm, including physical, psychological, social, legal, and financial harm. The research must address a question of sufficient value to justify the level of risk and must follow the approved protocol. Findings must be promptly and accurately reported. The research must be terminated immediately if it is suspected to be harmful to the participants.

Anesthesiology research often involves the treatment or prevention of unpleasant symptoms, such as pain and nausea, for which effective treatments are well established. Such studies should be restricted to comparison of treatments with known efficacy, not placebo-controlled trials, and "escape" analgesics or antiemetics must be provided at the patient's request.[47]

No population group should be unfairly subjected to research without having equal access to its benefits. Finally, in our modern Western research tradition, the interests of the individual subject always prevails over the interests of society.

Children As Research Subjects

Children are particularly vulnerable as research subjects because they may lack the ability to make mature decisions, are subject to the authority of others, may defer to their parents and others in ways that mask underlying dissent, and may have conditions requiring immediate decisions not consistent with informed consent.[59] Children's rights are frequently undervalued, whereas parental authority may be overvalued. Studies show that even children with decision-making capacity are often excluded from the consent process by both parents and physicians.[60]

If a minor child is "able" to assent, assent must usually be obtained in addition to the consent of any legal surrogate decision-makers. In the United States, federal law requires assent of any minor 7 years and older to participate in medical research. Particularly for research in which no substantive individual benefit is expected, many ethicists believe that a child's dissent *must always be honored.*[60,61]

Ethics of Animal Research

The animal rights movement in the United States has gained significant momentum in the last 25 years, following in the wake of the U.S. civil rights movement and paralleling increasing awareness and concern about the human impact on the environment and other animal species. Federal legislation protecting animal welfare began with the Laboratory Animal Welfare Act of 1966. In 1985, the Health Extension Act and amendments to the Animal Welfare Act required the establishment of Institutional Animal Care and Use Committees to oversee conditions of laboratory animals; review and approve animal research protocols; educate and train investigators in ethical issues and aspects of animal handling such as anesthesia, analgesia, and euthanasia; and act as community liaisons.[62]

Some researchers deny that animal experimentation could be subject to any moral reservations and assert that medical advancements have been and continue to be completely dependent on continued animal research. Many animal welfare activists insist on the moral equivalence of animal and human experimentation and accuse researchers of being blind to or, even worse, of being actually unmoved by the suffering of animal subjects. The simplicity of these polarized views does not do justice to the complexity of the issues.

Advancements in the understanding of animal cognition have led most biologists to now believe that many, if not all animals are capable of feeling pleasure, pain, anticipation, and fear and thus experience both enjoyment and suffering. Many bioethicists accept that the higher animals therefore have sufficient awareness to possess moral standing, although how much moral standing is intensely debated.[63,64] Allowing animal suffering as a result of pain, fear, sickness, or poor standards of care is a moral harm that must be avoided, mitigated, and weighed heavily against the benefits that it produces. Many argue that animals should be protected, not only because they have moral standing but also because people who are cruel to animals are more likely to be cruel to other humans.[65]

Researchers have obligations to provide clean and humane conditions and appropriate veterinary care for animal subjects. Researchers should mind the "3 R's"—replacement, reduction, and refinement—that is, use animal subjects only when necessary, minimize any suffering incurred in the study, and seek nonanimate replacements for animal subjects. Mediocre or repetitive research using animal subjects should not be allowed. It is the responsibility of the medical and scientific community to continue to aggressively seek and promote alternatives to the use of animal subjects.[65]

Physician Participation in Executions

U.S. physician professional organizations have consistently stated that physician participation in executions is unethical, yet many physicians admit that they would agree to be involved. The role of physicians in euthanasia and executions is of particular concern to anesthesiologists, who have been identified as ideal candidates for duties that involve killing because of their particular professional skills. Arguments in favor of physician involvement in executions usually cite the principle of beneficence in allowing a humane death.

Historically, however, beneficence arguments have led to "slippery slope" justifications for physicians to be involved in the killing of persons who have never faced an accuser or had a fair hearing—such killings have included persons with physical or mental handicaps and other "social flaws" for the "benefit" of the individual and society as a whole. Once physicians accept a beneficence argument for participating in executions, it is difficult to draw the ethical line at participation in other dubious state-sponsored activities, such as torture, coercion, and "medical incarceration," because these activities are also usually defended as being beneficial to society.[66]

When physicians agree to participate in an execution, they act as agents of the state while appearing to act on behalf of the "patient." This can lead to eventual erosion of public trust and respect. It also at times undoubtedly leads to physician participation in the killing of innocent persons.[67]

Studies clearly demonstrate that to avoid intolerable self-condemnation, virtually all executioners undergo "moral disengagement" in which they dehumanize the convicts and devalue their lives, thereby deflecting moral responsibility for the execution away from themselves by blaming juries, judges, governors, and "the law," rather than accept the responsibility that they share in ending the prisoner's life.[68] It is difficult to reconcile the medical profession's overt ethical imperatives of valuing human life, respecting individuals, and accepting personal moral responsibility with participation in a process that requires rejection of these very values.

Moral Integrity—Can the Physician Be a Conscientious Objector in Medicine?

Anesthesia care of patients can involve ethical controversy, legitimate disagreement, and moral ambiguity. When a physician's personal values run counter to acceptable ethical standards of care, how should the physician resolve such conflicts? Medical professional societies recognize the right to conscientious objection in medical practice. The ASA, the British Medical Association, and the Hastings Center have all issued statements recognizing the physician's right to withdraw from situations in which ethical standards of patient care are in serious conflict with their personal values.[69] The ASA specifically recognizes conscientious withdrawal from patient care in the case of patients with DNAR orders or other directives that limit treatment.[11] However, these rights have limitations. Acceptance of moral objections to certain hotly contentious issues such as abortion or physician-assisted suicide may be reasonable, but objections to well-established standards, such as informed consent, are not. Moral objections of physicians are also likely to carry more weight if they involve concepts that physicians believe supports them as ethical doctors—and not just as ethical persons—because these concepts are more likely to be founded in professionally established standards rather than personal beliefs.[69]

Summary

Anesthesiologists face many ethical challenges, including promotion of patient autonomy, resolution of patient-physician conflicts in medical decision-making, ethical obligations in human subjects and animal research, and ethical conflicts during end-of-life care in the ICU and during organ donation. Knowledge about ethical and professional standards in patient care and research is essential in the specialty of anesthesiology, which is more than just the mere provision of technical service on demand. Anesthesiologists may find that at times accepted values in ethical practice conflict with personal values and goals. This is a common challenge to all physicians, but ethical decisions cannot be left to the individual physician's values, and adherence to ethical principles of the medical profession should prevail.

Suggested Reading

Beauchamp TL, Childress JF: Principles of Biomedical Ethics, 5th ed. Oxford, Oxford University Press, 2001.

References

1. Beauchamp TL, Childress JF: The concept of autonomy. *In* Principles of Biomedical Ethics. Oxford, Oxford University Press, 1994, p 120.
2. Schloendorff v Society of New York Hospital, 311 NY 125, 127, 129; 105 NE 92, 93, 1914.
3. Salgo v Trustees of Leland Stanford Hospital, 154 Col App 2d 560,317 P2d 170 Ct Appl, 1957.
4. Mebane AH, Rauch HB: When do physicians request competency evaluations? Psychosomatics 31:40-46, 1990.
5. Hamel MB, Teno JM, Goldman L, et al: Patient age and decisions to withhold life-sustaining treatments from seriously ill, hospitalized adults. Ann Intern Med 130:116-125, 1999.
6. Madorsky J: Is the slippery slope steeper for people with disabilities? West J Med 166:410-411, 1997.
7. Kain ZN: Perioperative information and parental anxiety: The next generation. Anesth Analg 88:237-239, 1999.
8. Caplan RA, Posner KL: Informed consent in anesthesia liability. ASA Newsl 59:9-12, 1995.
9. Beckman HB, Markakis KM, Suchman AL, Frankel RM: The doctor-patient relationship and malpractice. Lessons from plaintiff depositions. Arch Intern Med 154:1365-1370, 1995.
10. Elder L: Coagulopathy after cardiopulmonary bypass in Jehovah's Witness patients: Management of and for the individual rather than the religious institution. Anesth Analg 104:757-758, 2007.
11. Ethical Guidelines for the Anesthesia Care of Patients with Do-Not-Resuscitate Orders or Other Directives That Limit Treatment. Park Ridge, IL, American Society of Anesthesiologists, 2001.
12. Lewis CE, Lewis MA, Ifekwunigue M: Informed consent by children and participation in an influenza vaccine trial. Am J Public Health 68:1079-1082, 1978.
13. Mutcherson KM: Whose body is it anyway? An updated model of healthcare decision-making rights for adolescents. Cornell J Law Public Policy 14:251-325, 2005.
14. Informed consent, parental permission, and assent in pediatric practice. Committee on Bioethics, American Academy of Pediatrics. Pediatrics 95:314-317, 1995.
15. Komer A, Clayton EW: Informed consent, parental permission and assent in pediatric practice. Pediatrics 95:314-317, 1995.
16. Chapman K, Meadow J, Catalan J, Gassard B: Testing patients for HIV before surgery: The views of doctors performing surgery. AIDS Care 7:125-128, 1995.
17. Lawrence VA, Gafni A, Kroenke K: Preoperative HIV testing: Is it less expensive than universal precautions? J Clin Epidemiol 46:1219-1227, 1993.
18. Lester P, Partridge JC, Cheesny MA, Cooke M: The consequences of a positive prenatal HIV antibody test for women. J Acquir Immune Defic Syndr Hum Retrovirol 10:341-349, 1995.
19. Chapman K, Meadow J, Catalan J, Gassard B: Testing patients for HIV before surgery: The views of doctors performing surgery. AIDS Care 7:125-128, 1995.
20. Mazze RI, Kallen B: Reproductive outcomes after anesthesia and operation during pregnancy: A registry study of 5405 cases. Am J Obstet Gynecol 161:1178-1185, 1989.
21. Reedy MB, Källén, B, Kuehl TJ: Laparoscopy during pregnancy: A study of five fetal outcome parameters with use of the Swedish Health Registry. Am J Obstet Gynecol 177:673-679, 1997.
22. Malviya S, D'errico C, Reynolds P, et al: Should pregnancy testing be routine in adolescent patients prior to surgery? Anesth Analg 83:854-858, 1996.
23. Kempen PM: Preoperative pregnancy testing: A survey of current practice. J Clin Anesth 9:546-550, 1997.
24. Practice Advisory for Preanesthesia Evaluation. ASA Task Force on Preanesthesia Evaluation, Revised. Park Ridge, IL, American Society of Anesthesiologists, 2003.
25. Harris LH, Paltrow L: The status of pregnant women and fetuses in US criminal law. JAMA 289:1697-1699, 2003.
26. Fetal therapy—ethical considerations. American Academy of Pediatrics. Committee on Bioethics. Pediatrics 103:1061-1063, 1999.
27. American College of Obstetricians and Gynecologists: Ethics in Obstetrics and Gynecology, 2nd ed. American College of Obstetrics and Gynecology, Washington, DC, 2004, pp 34-36.
28. Shuster E: Fifty years later: The significance of the Nuremberg Code. N Engl J Med 337:1436-1440, 1997.
29. Clarke JR, Sorenson JH, Hare JE: The limits of paternalism in emergency care. Hastings Center Rep 10(6):20-22, 1980.
30. Krugman RD, Bays J, Chadwick DL, et al: Behavior management of pediatric dental patients [letter]. Pediatrics 90:651-652, 1992.
31. Jonsen A, Beatch R, Walters L: Source Book in Bioethics: A Documentary History. Washington, DC, Georgetown University Press, 1998.
32. Layde P, Beam C, Broste S, et al: Surrogates' predictions of seriously ill patients' resuscitation preferences. Arch Family Med 4:518-523, 1995.
33. Covinsky KE, Fuller JD, Yaffe K, et al: Communication and decision-making in seriously ill patients: Findings of the SUPPORT project. The Study to Understand Prognoses and Preferences for Outcomes and Risks of Treatments. J Am Geriatr Soc 48(5 Suppl):S187-S193, 2000.
34. Hofmann JC, Wenger NS, Davis RB, et al: Patient preferences for communication with physicians about end-of-life decisions. SUPPORT Investigators. Study to Understand Prognoses and Preference for Outcomes and Risks of Treatment. Ann Intern Med 127:1-12, 1997.
35. American College of Surgeons: Statement on advance directives by patients; do not resuscitate in the operating room. ACS Bull 79(9):29, 1994.
36. AORN Position Statement: Perioperative Care of Patients with Do-Not-Resuscitate Orders. Denver, CO, Association of Operating Room Nurses, 1995.
37. Joint Commission on Accreditation of Healthcare Organizations: Patient rights. *In* Manual of the Joint Commission on Accreditation of Health Care Organizations. Chicago, JCAHO, 1994.
38. Osgood v Genesys Regional Medical Center, Mich, No. 94-26731-NH, Circuit Ct for Genesee County.

39. Council on Scientific Affairs, American Medical Association: Good care of the dying patient. JAMA 275:474-478, 1996.
40. Karlawish J: Managing death and dying in the intensive care unit. Am J Respir Crit Care Med 155:1-2, 1997.
41. In the Matter of Karen Quinlan, an Alleged Incompetent, 355 A2d 647, NJ Super Ct Cir 1976.
42. Schiavo v. Schiavo, No. 05-11628, 11th Cir, March 25, 2005.
43. Childress J: Non–heart-beating donors of organs. Are the distinctions between direct and indirect effects and between killing and letting die relevant and helpful? Kennedy Inst Ethics J 3:203-216, 1993.
44. Jonsen A, Siegler M, Winslade W: Clinical Ethics, 3rd ed. New York, McGraw-Hill, 1992.
45. Blank L: Defining and evaluating physician competence in end-of-life patient care: A matter of awareness and emphasis. West J Med 163:297-301, 1995.
46. Cist A, Truog R, Brackett S, Hurford W: Practical guidelines on the withdrawal of life-sustaining therapies. Int Anesthesiol Clin 39:87-102, 2001.
47. Lowenstein E (ed): Medical ethics. Int Anesthesiol Clin 39(3), 2001.
48. A definition of irreversible coma: A report of the ad hoc committee of the Harvard School of Medicine to examine the definition of brain death. JAMA 205:337-340, 1968.
49. Herdman R, Potts J: Non Heart Beating Organ Transplantation: Medical and Ethical Issues in Procurement, a Report of the Institute of Medicine. Washington. DC, National Academy of Sciences, 1997.
50. Cassel C, Allee M, Beasley C, et al: Non–Heart Beating Organ Transplantation: Practice and Protocols, a Report of the Committee on Non–Heart-Beating Transplantation II, Institute of Medicine. Washington, DC, National Academy of Sciences, 2000.
51. Menikoff J: The importance of being dead: Non–heart beating organ donation. Issues Law Med 18:3-20, 2002.
52. DuBois J: Non–heart-beating organ donation: A defense of the required determination of death. J Law Med Ethics 27:126-136, 1999.
53. Youngner S, Arnold R, DeVita M: When is "dead"? Hastings Center Rep 29:14-21, 1999.
54. Stein R: New trend in organ donation raises questions. The Washington Post, March 18, 2007.
55. Van Norman G: A matter of life and death: What every anesthesiologist should know about the medical, legal, and ethical aspects of declaring brain death. Anesthesiology 91:275-287, 1999.
56. Lerner BH: Subjects or objects? Prisoners and human experimentation. N Engl J Med 356:1806-1807, 2007.
57. Final report of the Advisory Committee on Human Radiation Experiments. Washington, DC, Government Printing Office, 1995.
58. Beecher H: Ethics and clinical research. N Engl J Med 74:1354, 1966.
59. Brody JL, Scherer DG, Annett RD, Pearson-Bish M: Voluntary assent in biomedical research with adolescents: A comparison of parent and adolescent views. Ethics Behav 13:79-95, 2003.
60. Olechnowicz JQ, Eder M, Simon C, et al: Assent observed: Children's involvement in leukemia treatment and research discussion. Pediatrics 109:806-814, 2002.
61. Wendler DS: Assent in paediatric research: Theoretical and practical considerations. J Med Ethics 32:229-234, 2006.
62. Shapiro H: Animal rights and biomedical research: No place for complacency. Anesthesiology 64:142-146, 1986.
63. Francione GL: The use of nonhuman animals in biomedical research: Necessity and justification. J Law Med Ethics 35:241-248, 2007.
64. Pluhar EB: Experimentation on humans and nonhumans. Theor Med Bioeth 27:333-355, 2006.
65. Martin J: The rights of man and animal experimentation. J Med Ethics 16:160-161, 1990.
66. Krass ME: How coercive is the medical profession? Can Med Assoc J 119:1340-1344, 1978.
67. Harmon TR, Lofquist WS: Too late for luck: A comparison of post-Furman exonerations and executions of the innocent. Crime Delinquency 51:498-520, 2005.
68. Osofsky MJ, Bandura A, Zimbardo PG: The role of moral disengagement in the execution process. Law Hum Behav 29:371-393, 2005.
69. Wicclair M: Conscientious objection in medicine. Bioethics 14:205-227, 2000.

David B. Waisel

10 Legal Aspects of Anesthesia Care

Key Points

1. The medical malpractice tort system is intended to improve patient care.
2. Medical negligence occurs when a physician's failure to meet the standard of care directly leads to patient injury.
3. A fully informed attorney is the physician's best advocate.
4. Physicians having their medical competence publicly questioned may feel guilt, failure, anger, shame, isolation, depression, fatigue, denial, and physical symptoms.
5. A detailed, legible anesthesia record strengthens the defense against a malpractice suit.
6. More than half the states have laws prohibiting the admission of apology or sympathy as evidence of wrongdoing.
7. The goal of informed consent is to maximize the ability of the patient to make substantially autonomous informed decisions.
8. Evidence of decision-making capacity (the ability to make a particular decision at a specific time) includes the ability to understand medical problems, proposed treatments, alternatives, options to refuse treatment, and the foreseeable consequences of accepting or refusing proposed treatments, as well as the ability to express a preference based on rational, internally consistent reasoning.
9. A reasonable person standard of disclosure requires that the extent of the disclosure be based on what a reasonable person would consider material for choosing whether to undergo the proposed intervention.
10. Anesthesiologists may refuse to provide care when they ethically or morally disagree with the procedure or if they believe that the patient's choice is too inappropriate or likely to result in harm.
11. Competent patients have a virtually unlimited right to refuse life-sustaining medical treatment.
12. Anesthesiologists are responsible for negligent acts made within the scope of defined duties by trainees and certified registered nurse anesthetists.
13. Physicians have been held liable for inadequate pain control.

Statute law, case law, and regulations affect anesthesiologists (Table 10-1).[1-8] Statute law is the body of prescriptive law created by a legislature to achieve a specific purpose. For example, the National Organ Transplant Act is the law that establishes the Organ Procurement and Transplantation Network and authorizes it to maintain a national registry for organ matching. State legislatures subsequently establish state laws governing organ procurement.

When statute laws need interpretation or clash or when there is no definitive statute law, disagreements may be adjudicated by the judicial system. The aggregate of reported cases, known as case law or common law, is used as the basis for future court decisions. The results of these cases are rarely prescriptive and may lead to a collection of confusing, ambiguous, and even contradictory cases that rest on diverse rulings in different jurisdictions. For example, a widow donated the kidney of her deceased husband to a long-time friend. The transplant surgeon, on receiving and examining the kidney, declared it unsuitable because of a renal artery aneurysm. The transplant surgeon then asked for the donor's second kidney. By then, the donor's second kidney had been allocated to another patient. The plaintiff sued, claiming that the organ procurement organization misappropriated the donor's second kidney and alleging in part that under conversion tort, the organ procurement organization interfered with the plaintiff's right of possession of personal property, in this case the kidney. On appeal, the court ruled for the defendant, the organ procurement organization, because the plaintiff had no common law right to the kidney inasmuch as a person cannot have property rights to a dead body.[9]

Regulations often come from administrative authorities such as executive branch agencies or state medical boards. For example, a U.S. Department of Health and Human Services regulation requires hospitals wishing to participate in Medicare to have written polices that an organ procurement organization is notified of potential donors.[10]

Table 10-1 Laws and Regulations That Affect Medical Practice

Law or Regulation	Comment
Health Insurance Portability and Accountability Act (HIPAA)[1]	HIPAA's privacy rules protect individually identifiable health information held or transmitted in any form, whether electronic, paper, or oral. This includes a patient's past, present, or future health or condition, provision of health care, or payment for the provision of health care and either identifies the individual or provides information through which there is a basis to believe that individual may be identifiable. Privacy rules apply to health plans, to health care clearinghouses, and to any health provider who transmits health information. HIPAA is a complex law that includes many other provisions, including making insurance portable from one employer to another.
Emergency in Medical Treatment and Active Labor Act (EMTALA)[2,3]	EMTALA governs when a patient may be refused treatment and when an unstable patient may be transferred from one hospital to another. More commonly stated, the purpose of EMTALA is to prohibit "dumping" of emergency patients onto other hospitals. Hospitals must perform a screening medical examination to determine whether an emergency condition exists, must provide stabilizing treatment if an emergency condition does exist, and may transfer the patient to another hospital only under certain conditions, such as the patient requesting transfer, the patient being stable and transfer will not worsen the patient's condition, and the receiving hospital having treatment abilities unavailable at presenting hospital. The receiving hospital must accept the transfer. Physicians have a central role in this process inasmuch as they must certify that the patient can be safely transferred. EMTALA also requires assigned on-call physicians to respond to emergency situations.
Controlled Substance Act[4]	This act permits the federal government to regulate the manufacture, importation, possession, and distribution of certain drugs to control the traffic of controlled substances. This act permits the federal government to determine whether a drug should be a controlled substance and into what drug schedule it should be placed. This act does not control the medical use of these drugs.
Employment Retirement Income Security Act (ERISA)[5] (A number of amendments to ERISA are relevant to health benefits, including HIPAA)	ERISA established uniform federal standards to protect private employee benefit plans. The U.S. Department of Labor administers and enforces ERISA and federal courts interpret it. The relevance in medicine is that it regulates health benefit plans. Case law interpretation of ERISA affects how, where, and for what indications members may sue health maintenance organizations.[6-8]

Professional Liability

The medical malpractice tort system is intended to "minimize patient injury, maximize patient safety and compensate injured patients." Unfortunately, the malpractice system may not have the desired effects on physician behavior.[11] Physicians are often uninformed about possible standards from malpractice cases.[11] Jury trials of medical malpractice suits do not reliably inform physicians, in part because of inconsistencies in case law and in part because juries tend to correlate liability with severity of harm and not with physician negligence.[12,13] Nonetheless, to improve patient care, anesthesiologists should vigilantly study the medical malpractice tort system.

Medical Malpractice

The most common cause of medical malpractice is medical negligence (Table 10-2). Negligence is breach of a duty that is the proximate cause of a harm.[14] Expanding on that definition, medical negligence occurs when a physician's failure (breach) to meet the standard of care (duty) directly leads (proximate cause) to patient injury (harm). Proximate cause should be tightly coupled and requires proof of "cause-in-fact" and foreseeability. Cause-in-fact, often known as the "but for" test, means that the harm would not have occurred but for the previous negligent act. Foreseeability suggests that injuries must be of the type that would be foreseen by a reasonable practitioner. For example, "but for" the *absence* of an end-tidal carbon dioxide monitor, esophageal intubation would have been recognized because a reasonable practitioner would foresee that this breach of the standard of care may lead to unrecognized esophageal intubation. There must be a harm for which the individual needs to be compensated. Awards

Table 10-2 Causes of Action Most Relevant to Anesthesiologists

Type	Description
Medical negligence	Breech of a duty of a standard of care causing harm
Wrongful death	One that occurs earlier that it would have otherwise. If negligence causes death, survivors may sue for damages
Lack of informed consent	Obligation to provide information material to a reasonable person
Abandonment	Obligation to provide continuity of care once a physician assumes responsibility for the patient
Vicarious liability	Obligation for reasonable oversight of those working for the physician
Loss of chance of recovery or survival	The patient must show that recovery was likely except for the action of the physician
Battery	Touching a person without express or implied consent. There is no need for the plaintiff to prove harm in battery cases
Assault	The attempt to touch another person. There is no need to prove actual harm

From White C, Rosoff AJ, LeBlang TR: Informed consent to medical and surgical treatment. *In* Sanbar AA, Firestone MH, Fiscina S, et al (eds): Legal Medicine, 7th ed. Philadelphia, Mosby Elsevier, 2007, pp 337-343.

may be conferred for noneconomic losses, for the economic costs of repairing the damage, and for loss of income. The amount of time in which a plaintiff can bring an action is governed by state statutes and typically begins on occurrence or discovery of the allegedly negligent act or the harm.

Medical negligence may be adjudged as criminal medical negligence if it deviates greatly from the standard of care, whether unknowingly (criminal negligence) or knowingly (criminal recklessness).[15] Criminal medical negligence is rarely prosecuted, but characteristics of such cases include failure to modify care based on past similar experiences, hiding errors, and practicing in a way that appears to favor financial and personal gains over patient care. For example, an anesthesiologist was prosecuted (but eventually acquitted) for reckless manslaughter when after more than five documented episodes of falling asleep during anesthesia, he fell asleep during a case in which the child died.[16] The anesthesiologist was convicted for criminal medical negligence, although that conviction was eventually overturned because the prosecutors had not brought the criminal medical negligence charge within the legal time limits.[17]

The Process of Being Sued

Some lawsuits may begin "informally" by a request from a potential plaintiff's attorney to review records or to discuss a case. An attorney should be consulted before engaging in these actions to ensure that proper procedure is followed. Lawsuits officially begin with a document called a Summons and Complaint, which is a notification to respond to allegations by the plaintiff.

After initiation of the suit, the process of discovery begins with exchange of documents and a deposition. The purpose of the deposition is for the other side of a legal action to obtain information or clarification otherwise unavailable, particularly about the reasoning underlying actions.[18] At the deposition, oral testimony is taken under oath and transcribed and may be used as evidence at trial. Experts, consultants, clinicians, witnesses to the event, or defendants may be deposed. Some conversations are privileged and may not be discovered by the plaintiff, including discussions with attorneys, risk management personnel, insurance company representatives, personal clinicians (including psychotherapists, clergy, and a spouse). Conversations with close friends are discoverable.

Before the deposition, the physician should inform the attorney about his or her relationship with the plaintiffs and any problems that may have occurred. The physician should educate the attorney about complex medical components of the case and expected weaknesses. A fully informed attorney is the best advocate.

In addition to the defendant, the defendant's attorney, the plaintiff's attorney, and the court reporter, the plaintiff may also be present at the deposition. After the court reporter administers the oath, the plaintiff's attorney will ask standard questions, including education, licensing, and certification. The defendant's attorney will intercede as appropriate. The same questions may be asked several times over. A goal of a plaintiff's attorney is to develop a causal atmosphere to lower the guard of the defendant before asking more relevant questions. A defendant is best served by not speculating about factual matters that may be found in the medical record and answering only the questions asked and asking for clarification if unclear about the meaning of a question.

Malpractice Defense

Physicians having their medical competence publicly questioned may feel guilt, failure, anger, shame, isolation, depression, fatigue, denial, and physical symptoms.[19] It is important to be forthright about these feelings and to manage them, if for no other reason than to be able to participate fully and positively in the legal defense.

Defendants often rebut claims that the standard of care was not met and that the alleged failure to meet the standard of care was a proximate cause of harm. To help support these arguments, expert witnesses, medical texts, journal articles, practice guidelines, and anesthesia records are often used.

Expert witnesses explain the relevant science and offer professional opinions about the standard of care and causation.[20] Although courts commonly accept the expertise of most expert witnesses, courts and juries do use qualifications to modulate the weight that they give the testimony. An expert witness can support the idea that a different explanation or approach, especially one that other physicians would support, may meet a sufficient standard of care. The obligations of expert witnesses include the following: "expert testimony by anesthesiologists should be readily available, objective and unbiased. To limit uninformed and possibly misleading testimony, experts should be qualified for their role and should follow a clear and consistent set of ethical guidelines" (Box 10-1).[21]

Practice guidelines are being used increasingly as evidence of a standard of care.[22] Although authors of practice guidelines routinely state that the guidelines are not intended to set a standard of care, it is highly likely that juries will be strongly influenced by them.[23] Some authors have even proposed that practice guidelines replace expert opinion.[22]

A detailed, legible anesthesia record often strengthens the defense against a malpractice suit. A goal of documentation should be that uninvolved anesthesiologists would be able to recreate the anesthesia care as if they were in the operating room. Uninvolved anesthesiologists should be able to understand interventions, the reasons for interventions, and the outcomes of interventions. Precise documentation and written explanations of thought processes lead to better understanding. For example, when performing regional anesthesia, an anesthesiologist may want to document the length and type of needle used, nerve stimulator type and settings, number of attempts, strength and location of muscle contractions, whether a paresthesia occurred, and how the paresthesia was managed.[24] Alternatively, consider the effect of documentation on the fairly routine event of decreased urine output. Assume that a patient had no urine output over a certain period in a previously functioning bladder catheter. The anesthesiologist treated the decreased urine output with a fluid bolus. The record would ideally indicate a "0" under urine output and indicate a bolus of fluid under fluid administration. Assume, then, that 30 minutes after the fluid bolus there was still no urine output. At this point, it would be reasonable for the anesthesiologist to write a note on the anesthesia record discussing the decreased urine output, the initial interpretation and treatment of the decreased urine output, the results of that

Box 10-1 Guidelines for Expert Witness Qualifications and Testimony

The physician should be board certified in anesthesiology or hold an equivalent specialist qualification. The physician should be familiar with the clinical practice of anesthesiology at the time of the occurrence and should have been actively involved in clinical practice at the time of the event.

The physician's review of the medical facts should be truthful, thorough, and impartial and should not exclude any relevant information to create a view favoring either the plaintiff or the defendant. The ultimate test of accuracy and impartiality is willingness to prepare testimony that could be presented unchanged for use by either the plaintiff or defendant.

The physician's testimony should reflect an evaluation of performance in light of generally accepted standards, as reflected in the relevant literature, neither condemning performance that clearly falls within generally accepted practice standards nor endorsing or condoning performance that clearly falls outside accepted medical practice.

The physician should make a clear distinction between medical malpractice and adverse outcomes not necessarily related to negligent practice.

The physician should make every effort to assess the relationship of the alleged substandard practice to the patient's outcome. Deviation from a practice standard is not always causally related to a poor outcome.

Fees for expert testimony should relate to the time spent and in no circumstances should be contingent on outcome of the claim.

The physician should be willing to submit such testimony for peer review.

From American Society of Anesthesiologists: Guidelines for expert witness qualifications and testimony. Available at http://www.asahq.org/publicationsAndServices/standards/07.pdf. Accessed November 1, 2007.

treatment, and the current interpretation (including differential diagnoses) and planned treatment of the decreased urine output. The anesthesia record should contain certain information (Box 10-2).[25,26]

Countersuits such as abuse of process, malicious prosecution, and defamation have been consistently rejected by the courts.[27] From a public policy perspective, the courts may be concerned that abuse of countersuits may limit the ability of plaintiffs to seek redress.

Box 10-2 Guidelines for Documentation

Preanesthesia Evaluation

Patient interview

Medical history (medication, allergies, family history of anesthesia problems, pertinent review of systems)

Anesthetic history

Medication history

Appropriate physical examination (including pertinent negatives)

Review of objective diagnostic data (e.g., laboratory, electrocardiogram, radiographs)

Assignment of American Society of Anesthesiologists Physical Status

Formulation of the anesthetic plan and discussion and documentation of the risks and benefits of the plan with the patient

If appropriate, explanations of what may be considered atypical choices of the anesthesiologist or the patient

Intraoperative/Procedural Anesthesia (Time-Based Record of Events)

Immediate review before initiation of anesthetic procedures

Patient re-evaluation

Check of equipment, drugs, and gas supply

Monitoring of the patient

Amounts of drugs and agents used and times of administration

Type and amounts of intravenous fluids used, including blood and blood products, and times of administration

Estimated blood loss and urine output

Specifics about the technique or techniques used

Unusual events during the administration of anesthesia, including explanation of recognition of the event, treatment of the event, and outcome of the event

Status of the patient at the conclusion of anesthesia

Postanesthesia Evaluation

Patient evaluation on admission and discharge from the postanesthesia care unit

Time-based record of vital signs and level of consciousness

Time-based record of drugs administered, their dosages, and routes of administration

Type and amounts of intravenous fluids administered, including blood and blood products

Any unusual events, including postanesthesia or postprocedural complications

Medical interventions

Postanesthesia visits

Data from references 23-25.

Apology and Disclosure

Although often inappropriately conflated, an apology, an expression of regret or sorrow, is distinct from disclosure, which is a revelation about what happened. Apologies and disclosures may occur at the same time.

More than half the states have laws prohibiting an admission of apology or sympathy as evidence of wrongdoing.[19] Some recommendations suggest apologizing for the effect on the patient without admitting fault. Sometimes this may make sense, for example, if a previously acceptable antibiotic caused a rash. However, not to take responsibility may seem stilted, such as when an anesthesiologist errantly administers an antibiotic to a patient for whom there is clear documentation of an allergy. In the name of good relationships with patients, apologies should not be limited solely to events that may result in a suit. For example, consider a 6-year-old who on initiation of mask induction starts to scream and cry uncontrollably. After a discussion with the father who is present, a decision is made to, in essence, hold her down and apply the mask. A follow-up discussion with the family may include an apology not only for the induction ("I am sorry that was so unpleasant for Becky and you.") but also to acknowledge that this was not the desired reaction ("That is not our goal for induction. We would like it to be smoother." and "Going without sedation turned out to be a mistake."), as well as a recommendation for the future ("In the future, I would recommend giving oral sedation before going to the operating room."). Although this technically seems to admit wrongdoing, it is simply acknowledging what happened and educating the family for the future.

Although it is my belief that it is better to apologize, there are concerns about apologizing. The action for the physician, particularly if the apology is not readily accepted, may be painful. An apology may also embolden an otherwise unsure plaintiff, and it may be construed as admission of error in court.

It is more complicated whether one should admit fault for something that more likely may be medically negligent. Consider, for example, repeated attempts to place an epidural in a patient who is anesthetized and has previously undergone back surgery. The anesthesiologist tries repeatedly without success and without incorporating other methodologies such as fluoroscopy. The patient awakes with a nerve injury consistent with wayward insertion of an epidural needle. Some would suggest that although it is acceptable to express sympathy for the pain and discomfort ("I am sorry for your discomfort."), it would be legally harmful to acknowledge fault and a desire to do it differently ("I am sorry about your injury. In retrospect, although I am not sure what happened, I suspect that it was due to the needle placement. I should have used direct imaging of the back, such as fluoroscopy."). Others would suggest that the second apology with the disclosure is better because it explains what happened, why it happened, and how it may be prevented in the future. Although this combination of disclosure and apology admits culpability, it discloses only information that would eventually be discovered. I would suggest that the potential advantages gained by a genuine apology outweigh the potential harm of admitting culpability.

Full disclosure is gaining favor. From a wholly practical point of view, the patient will eventually learn what was withheld and will wonder, probably with animosity, why such information was not disclosed. Disclosure may have three components.[28] On realization of the problem, the goal is to give as much information as known, but not to speculate about what is not known, particularly about fault. Physicians should clarify the medical implications of the event, any necessary treatment or follow-up, and who will function as a contact for the patient regarding the event. The next step should be to conduct a thorough investigation with an eye toward minimizing problems in the future. Finally, the patient should be informed about what the investigation found, including the cause of the event and how it will be prevented in the future.

It is not unreasonable to consider responding to patient dissatisfaction by waiving part or all of a bill. This is not generally considered an admission of liability, and it may help satisfy a patient.

Legal Aspects of Informed Consent

Until the 1950s, physicians routinely obtained assent, or general agreement of the patient to have a procedure. The 1957 legal case *Salgo v Trustees of Leland Stanford Hospital* codified the modern concept of informed consent. The judge clarified the difference between informed consent and assent by declaring, "A physician violates his duty to his patient and subjects himself to liability if he withholds any facts which are necessary to form [the] basis of an intelligent consent by the patient to a proposed treatment. . . ."[29]

The goal of informed consent is to maximize the ability of the patient to make substantially autonomous informed decisions. The modifier "substantial" is used because it is unreasonable to expect a patient to be fully informed. The more appropriate goal of substantial informed consent acknowledges that consent may be sufficiently autonomous even if not completely informed. Modern informed consent has seven components.

Components of Informed Consent

Decision-Making Capacity

Decision-making capacity is defined as the ability to make a particular decision at a specific time. Evidence of decision-making capacity includes the ability to understand medical problems, proposed treatments, alternatives, options to refuse treatment, and the foreseeable consequences of accepting or refusing any proposed treatments, as well as the ability to express a preference based on rational, internally consistent reasoning. Decision-making capacity is distinct from the legal concept of competency. Courts determine competency and often make a global determination of competency by declaring that a person is either competent or incompetent for all matters. Adults are presumed to be legally competent unless declared otherwise by a court. On the other hand, anesthesiologists are responsible for assessing decision-making capacity and can make this determination only for specific situations.

Anesthesiologists should permit patients to make decisions to the extent of their ability.[30] For most patients, there are no questions about decision-making capacity. However, anesthesiologists need to actively evaluate the decision-making capacity of patients whose decision-making capacity has been temporarily altered, who do not have legal decision-making authority, or who have preexisting limitations in decision-making capacity. Consider a patient who has received pain medication before giving informed consent. The level of impairment varies depending on the medication, the tolerance of the patient to the medication, and the decision to be made. Indeed, some patients, such as parturients, may have improved decision-making capacity when the pain is decreased. To determine whether a patient has decision-making capacity for a specific decision, anesthesiologists need to balance the medication given and its expected effects with the ability of the patient to show evidence of rational reasoning and understanding. When a patient has temporarily lost decision-making capacity, such as when anesthetized, anesthesiologists should not implement nonemergency care until after the patient regains decision-making capacity and gives consent.

However, in emergencies, anesthesiologists should proceed without obtaining informed consent, based on the presumption that patients want life-sustaining treatment unless they have declared otherwise.[31]

Voluntariness

Physicians should perform procedures only on competent patients who participate willingly. Anesthesiologists compromise voluntariness through manipulation and coercion. Manipulation involves the deliberate distortion or omission of information in an attempt to induce the patient to accept a treatment, such as downplaying or omitting information to influence a patient to make a specific decision. Coercion involves the use of a credible threat to ensure complicity.

Anesthesiologists also hinder voluntariness when they physically restrain or sedate patients who have sufficient decision-making capacity. Competent patients have the legal and moral right to refuse treatment, even in life-threatening emergency situations. It is often hard for physicians to accept that a patient wishes to make what the physician perceives to be a foolish decision. *Shine v Vega* illustrates the complexity of these situations.[32] In 1990, Shine, a competent adult, went to the hospital and received oxygen and an unspecified medication for an asthma attack. Vega, the emergency department attending physician, thought that she was very ill and recommended endotracheal intubation. Shine stated her long-standing refusal of endotracheal intubation (confirmed contemporaneously by her sister and father) and continued to receive oxygen by mask. Later, Shine's sister came into her room in the emergency department and noted that Shine was breathing more easily but was arguing with staff. Shortly thereafter, Shine and her sister attempted to leave but were forcibly detained by a physician and security. Shine was placed in four-point restraints and Vega, choosing to disregard Shine's objection, intubated her trachea. On appeal, the Massachusetts Supreme Court stated that a competent patient has a right to refuse potentially life-sustaining treatment, even if her decision is considered unwise.

Another issue of voluntariness occurs when the interests of a woman and her fetus differ. When a woman refuses a recommended diagnostic or therapeutic procedure, such as cesarean delivery for fetal indications, physicians may choose to respect the patient's autonomy and not proceed, encourage the woman to seek health care elsewhere, or seek judicial involvement. Before seeking judicial involvement, physicians should consider the social, physical, and psychological harm of violating individual liberty and the fallibility and limitations of medical knowledge. Physicians may want to seek judicial involvement only when they are highly confident that the recommended treatment will substantially reduce harm to the fetus, that the risks to the woman are relatively small, and that no comparably effective, less-intrusive option exists.[33] Particularly relevant to anesthesiologists is the American College of Obstetricians and Gynecologists position on forced cesarean section. "Even in the presence of a court order authorizing intervention, the use of physical force against a resistant competent woman is not justified. The use of force will substantially increase the risk to the mother, thereby diminishing the ethical justification of such therapy."[33]

Disclosure

The goal of disclosure is to provide information relevant to the decision-maker and the decision to be made. Skilled disclosure builds trust, helps patients make good decisions, and is a fundamental component of the obligation to respect a patient's autonomy.

Established in 1972, the reasonable person standard requires that the extent of the disclosure be based on what a reasonable person would consider material for choosing whether to undergo the proposed intervention.[34,35] Informed consent discussions should routinely include the specific risks and benefits of reasonable anesthetic options and monitoring techniques, as well as the presence and use of a fallback plan.[31] Anesthesiologists may want to inform patients of common, but less severe risks, such as postoperative nausea and vomiting, and uncommon risks of more long-term significance, such as brain injury and death. If appropriate, the patient should be informed of the quality of the data, such as whether the information has questionable certainty. Anesthesiologists should also inform the patient whether an individual or an anesthesia care team will be providing anesthesia services and, if the latter, the names and specific roles of the team members. It may be appropriate to inform patients if the anesthesiologist is inexperienced in a particular situation.[36] To maintain good relationships with patients, they should be told about other practical matters, such as the probable sequence of events on arrival at the surgical unit, who will be with them at the various stages, what to expect for postoperative pain management, and realistic time estimates.

Exceptions to the obligation to disclose material information include patients who choose not to be informed, emergencies in which a valid informed consent cannot be obtained, and situations of therapeutic privilege. Physicians use therapeutic privilege when they choose to withhold information because they believe that disclosure would cause the patient to become "so ill or emotionally distraught on disclosure as to foreclose a rational decision, or complicate or hinder treatment, or perhaps even pose psychological damage to the patient."[34] Therapeutic privilege has a narrow scope and should be used prudently. Simply because information is undesirable or upsetting to the patient does not mean that such information should be withheld. For example, it may be reasonable to invoke therapeutic privilege when discussing the risk of death with a patient who is having an acute infarction of his myocardium; it would not be reasonable to do the same when discussing the risk of death with the parents of an infant.

Recommendation

Anesthesiologists should offer an opinion about which options are preferable and the advantages and disadvantages of each option. By explaining the value judgments and the quality of data supporting their opinions, anesthesiologists allow the patient not only to receive the benefit of their expertise but also to understand the reasons for the recommendations. Patients can then decide for themselves which choices best fit their priorities.

Understanding

Patients need to understand the risks and benefits of the proposed procedures, the recommendations made, and why those recommendations were made. It is difficult to determine whether a patient fully understands the informed consent discussion, and indeed, many patients may not.[37,38] Pain and distress do not seem to compromise the ability to recall risks, particularly among parturients, and do not preclude obtaining a legally sufficient informed consent.[39-41]

Decision

After considering the information and the anesthesiologist's recommendation, the patient chooses an anesthetic technique. Patients vary in their preferences for participation in decision-making, and anesthesiologists should be sensitive to these preferences. The desire to participate in the decision-making process may be a function of the individual, extent of illness, gender, age, and level of education. Anesthesiologists should attempt to tailor the extent of patient and physician decision-making to the patient and the situation.

When a patient refuses an anesthesiologist's recommendation or requests a technique that the anesthesiologist believes is inappropriate, the focus of conversation moves from informed consent to informed refusal. Informed refusal requirements are similar to informed consent requirements in that the patient should be substantially well versed about the risks, benefits, and alternatives before declining. However, although it may be reasonable to permit a patient agreeing with a recommended or acceptable procedure to refuse extensive information (especially if the likelihood of harm is low), it is more difficult to honor a patient's preference to receive limited information when the patient desires a suboptimal approach.[42] The anesthesiologist may wish to provide additional information about the choice to be sure that the patient has all possible information. If in fact the patient chooses without sufficient information, the anesthesiologist has not fulfilled the obligation of informed refusal. Of course, a patient may still refuse to hear information. In either case, when a patient chooses a technique that the anesthesiologist believes is inappropriate, anesthesiologists are not obligated to provide care in nonemergency situations.

Autonomous Authorization

The informed consent process concludes with the patient intentionally authorizing the anesthesiologist to perform a specific procedure. This authorization is the expression of the patient's self-determination and is the basis of informed consent.

Documentation of Informed Consent

In practice, informed consent for anesthesia may be documented on the surgical consent form, by a handwritten note, or by a separate anesthesia consent form. Use of a surgical consent form is suboptimal because surgeons cannot capably discuss the risks associated with anesthesia and therefore it is unclear what is being documented. Both handwritten notes and anesthesia consent forms may be acceptable. Handwritten notes detail specific discussions with patients. Writing a note for each patient, however, may be impractical and time consuming and may miss key aspects of informed consent. Anesthesia consent forms may act as a prompt for anesthesiologists to discuss key aspects of informed consent. Space for handwritten notes on the consent form will permit additional details to be documented. Having the patient sign the handwritten consent or the consent form gives an indication that some form of communication took place. However, because consent forms by themselves do not fulfill the legal requirement of informed consent, an informed consent discussion must still occur.

Theories of Suit in Informed Consent

Negligence related to the informed consent process may occur if the anesthesiologist provides a disclosure that is insufficient to allow a patient to make an informed decision and an injury subsequently occurs, even if the injury was foreseeable and occured in the absence of a treatment error.[31] To determine whether sufficient information was given, the courts look for materiality and causation. Materiality assesses whether the information given met the standard of care. If the disclosure did not meet the standard of care, it may be considered a breach of duty. Causation then assesses whether sharing the omitted information would have caused the patient to choose a different option.[31] Most jurisdictions use the objective standard, which bases causation on whether a hypothetical reasonable person would have used the additional information to make a different decision. Some jurisdictions use the subjective standard, which is contingent on whether the specific patient involved would have made a different decision. A few jurisdictions combine the two standards by heeding the objective standard while considering factors specific to the patient and situation. Courts also consider how the information was given. The informed consent discussion should occur in a setting conducive to decision-making so that the patient has a chance to ask questions and consider answers.

The disclosure process is not intended to be armor against medical malpractice liability if an adverse event takes place. Informing a patient about a risk does not eliminate liability for its occurrence. Liability is based on negligence theory and depends mainly on whether the standard of care was met and whether failure to meet the standard of care was a proximate cause of the injury.

Refusing to Provide Care

Anesthesiologists may refuse to provide care when they ethically or morally disagree with the procedure or situation, such as elective termination of pregnancy.[43] Although physicians have an obligation to altruistically provide care, this requisite does not always oblige physicians to subjugate their morals. Furthermore, society and medicine have a fundamental interest in preserving the moral fabric of individual physicians. Anesthesiologists should provide care that violates their conscience and possibly weakens their moral constitution only in critical, presumably life-or-death, circumstances. More practically, an anesthesiologist who ethically or morally disagrees with a patient's choice will have difficulty providing the care requested. In a nonemergency situation, such an anesthesiologist should withdraw from or refuse patient care. The anesthesiologist may then be obligated to make a reasonable effort to find a competent and willing replacement.

Physicians may also ethically refuse to provide care if they believe that the patient's choice is too inappropriate or likely to result in harm. Determining that a choice of anesthesia is inappropriate is difficult and should not be invoked lightly or out of convenience. The patient's choice and the resultant risks must be sufficiently extreme that they, say, elicit a similar response from at least several other anesthesiologists. In addition, anesthesiologists may refuse to provide care if they do not feel qualified to provide the needed care.

Legal Aspects of End-of-Life Care

Acknowledgement of patients' rights to refuse life-sustaining treatment began in the mid-20th century with the rise of civil liberties, individual rights, and respect for the importance of self-determination (see Chapters 91 and 98). In 1974, the American Medical Association asserted that "the purpose of cardiopulmonary resuscitation is the prevention of sudden unexpected death. Cardiopulmonary resuscitation is not indicated in cases of terminal irreversible illness where death is not unexpected."[44] Policies acknowledging the need to permit patients to limit resuscitation during terminal illness were prominently published several years later.[45]

Progression of the rights of the individual to refuse potentially life-sustaining care may be seen through case law. The 1976 case of Karen Ann Quinlan first established the right to refuse potentially life-sustaining care. In *Quinlan*, the courts upheld the legality of disconnecting the ventilator from a patient thought to be ventilator dependent and in a permanent vegetative state.[46] The court based this decision on the general constitutional right to privacy. In addition, the court determined that a surrogate had the right to decline medical treatment for an incompetent patient if the surrogate concluded that the patient would have preferred limited care. Quinlan's father thus discontinued his daughter's mechanical ventilation. Quinlan lived for nearly a decade sustained by nasogastric feeding.

The right of a competent person to refuse potentially life-sustaining care was established in the 1984 case of *Bartling v Superior Court*.[47] Bartling was a competent adult patient with an incurable disease who for 6 months received medical therapy against his clear wishes. After pneumothorax from a needle biopsy, Bartling became ventilator dependent. He subsequently received a tracheotomy to facilitate weaning attempts. During this ordeal, Bartling made clear his desire not to receive continued therapy and declared at one point, "While I have no wish to die, I find intolerable the living conditions forced upon me . . . ."[47] Although Bartling died before his case could be adjudicated, the appellate court issued an opinion based on the constitutional right of privacy that supported the right of a competent patient to refuse medical treatment.

The 1990 case of *Cruzan v Director, Missouri Department of Health*, concerned a young woman involved in an automobile accident that left her incapable of expressing a preference.[48] Several years before the accident, Cruzan had expressed to a friend in a somewhat serious conversation a desire not to live in a state of diminished capacity. The Supreme Court of Missouri held that Cruzan's informal statements did not meet Missouri's evidentiary standard of "clear and convincing evidence" of a patient's wish to terminate potentially life-sustaining care and thus mandated continuation of treatment. The case was appealed to the U.S. Supreme Court.[49] Unlike *Quinlan* and *Bartling*, the Supreme Court grounded the right of a competent patient to refuse treatment on the liberty interest of the Fourteenth Amendment, which states, "No State shall make or enforce any law which shall abridge the privileges or immunities of citizens of the United States; nor shall any State deprive any person of life, liberty or property . . . ." The decision also upheld the rights of states to determine standards for the level of certainty required, thereby permitting Missouri to use the "clear and convincing evidence" standard.[48,50]

Competent patients have a virtually unlimited right to refuse life-sustaining medical treatment.[51] For an incompetent patient, three hierarchic levels of judgment direct the decision-making process for end-of-life care. A once-competent patient's previously expressed preferences for end-of-life care should be followed as best as possible. When the patient's declared preferences are not known, substituted judgment, or use of a surrogate's intimate knowledge of the patient's attitudes and beliefs to determine what the patient would have chosen, may be used to direct care. Despite being two distinct categories, both levels require the surrogate to know the patient sufficiently to appropriately choose or interpret the patient's preferences. These standards put significant burdens on decision-makers, who may have legitimate doubts about the appropriateness of their decisions. When a surrogate has to make decisions for a patient who has never been competent, such as a young child or a mentally disabled adult, substituted judgment is impossible, and the surrogate must rely on the best interests standard. The best interests standard requires the surrogate to make decisions based on the surrogate's view of what is best for the patient.

Advanced Care Planning

Advanced care planning permits patients to declare preferences for medical treatment if they become incapacitated. Advance directives are designed to minimize the likelihood of undesired overtreatment and undertreatment. Partially as a result of *Cruzan*, the Patient Self-Determination Act (PSDA) was introduced in 1990 to increase the use of advance directives.[52] The PSDA requires health care institutions, such as hospitals, nursing homes, and hospice programs, to notify individuals about their rights regarding advance directives. Two types of advance directives are living wills and health care proxies (also known as durable power of attorney for health care decisions). Living wills allow patients to declare the extent of desirable interventions, but they may not be able to directly address the subtle differences that characterize clinical situations. The difficulty of applying living wills to clinical situations has led some to prefer the greater flexibility provided by the health care proxy, in which the surrogate decision-maker can consider the specific details when making clinical decisions. Health care proxies permit patients to designate surrogate decision-makers (including non–family members) to make decisions for them should they become unable to make such decisions for themselves. If the patient does not assign surrogacy, most jurisdictions have a hierarchy for assigning surrogacy. Surrogacy is not always effective, particularly for patients who do not make their preferences clearly known to the surrogate before losing their decision-making capacity.[53] Given the strengths and weaknesses of each approach, a combination of the two (a designated proxy with some written form of preferences) may be the best option.

Clinically, advanced care planning should be considered an ongoing process, with the advance directive being used in conjunction with family and friends to help guide the decision-making of patients and surrogates.[54,55] Competent patients may obviously modify their previously declared preferences. Demented patients who previously made an informed choice to limit certain therapy may express an interest in receiving that therapy.[56] If patients have evidence of decision-making capacity, such as being able to provide internally coherent reasoning, their wishes to receive therapy should be honored. However, the process of resolving this situation in a patient without decision-making capacity and with almost no likelihood of regaining decision-making capacity is more complex. In this situation it is better to base judgment on therapy from multiple sources, including significant others, the type of documentation, and the best interests standard.

Refusal of Cardiopulmonary Resuscitation

The right of a patient to reject unwanted therapy in the operating room is now well accepted. Before proceeding to the operating room, preoperative do-not-resuscitate orders should be re-evaluated in light of the surgical procedures, the anesthetic options, and the patient's overall goals. Anesthesiologists are then prepared to clarify and document the desired resuscitation status in the operating room by using either the goal-directed approach or the procedure-directed approach.[57] The process of obtaining and documenting perioperative refusal of resuscitation should comply with hospital policy and jurisdictional law. Written documentation may include the patient's diagnosis and prognosis, the characteristics of perioperative resuscitation, probable outcomes, and the patient's reasoning. If the decision is being made by a surrogate, the record should note the surrogate's relationship to the patient and the basis of the surrogate's decision. It should be signed by the responsible physician.

Refusal of resuscitation in an emergency situation without time to clarify a patient's wishes is inherently different. The traditional bias of providing treatment in the absence of a clear decision not to treat still holds for the anesthesiologist in an emergency situation. The situation can always be clarified later and the patient withdrawn from the ventilator if it is determined that the patient would have preferred not to receive the interventions. In short, the "inconvenience" of a short period of mechanical ventilation is worth the opportunity to correctly ascertain the patient's desires.

The Demand for Life-Sustaining Therapies

Patients or families may demand therapies that clinicians believe are inadvisable because of burden to the patient, cost, or uncertain benefit. When such situations become irreconcilable, the cases may go to court, often not to determine what therapy should be given but to determine who should be the decision-maker for a noncompetent person. For example, an archetypic case involves Helga Wanglie, an 86-year-old patient in a persistent vegetative state who was receiving mechanical ventilation. The medical center believed that further therapy would be futile for Mrs. Wanglie and wanted to withdraw mechanical ventilation. When Mr. Wanglie refused the medical center's request to stop mechanical ventilation, the medical center sought appointment of an independent guardian to supplant Mr. Wanglie as her guardian. The Court declared that Mr. Wanglie was best able to be Mrs. Wanglie's surrogate.[58,59]

In the 1995 case of *Gilgunn*, a jury supported a unilateral refusal of life-sustaining care. Catherine Gilgunn had multiple medical problems, including severe brain damage, and was in a coma.[60] Her daughter Joan, representing the family, requested that everything be done. The Optimum Care Committee of the hospital agreed with the physicians that providing cardiopulmonary resuscitation would be futile in the sense that it was not a genuine therapeutic option. The legal division approved the do-not-resuscitate order because they believed that the physicians were acting in the patient's best interest. Gilgunn was disconnected from ventilator support and died a few days later. The jury supported the actions of the physician and hospital to impose a unilateral do-not-resuscitate order. There was no appeal.

Despite *Gilgunn*, unilateral physician declarations are insufficiently respectful of patient autonomy and may be legally risky. Evidence indicates that negotiation nearly always resolves these problems without the need to resort to unilateral action. However, being able to resolve differences of opinion about applying treatments with a low likelihood of success is important. Policies for resolution based on a procedural approach in which the process for resolving conflict is described are more practical. Good policies are public, reflect the moral values of the community, and include processes for identifying stakeholders, for initiating and conducting the policy, for commencing appellate mechanisms, and for determining relevant information.[61] In a different approach, the Texas Advance Directives Act permits physicians to unilaterally withhold or withdraw treatments that they regard as "futile," provided that they follow guidelines, including obtaining agreement of the hospital ethics committee.[62]

Physician-Assisted Suicide

Physician-assisted suicide is the act of a physician prescribing lethal quantities of medication for self-administration by the patient. In the United states in the cases of *Washington v Glucksberg*[63] and *Vacco v Quill*,[64] the courts held that there was no constitutional right to physician-assisted suicide. It is important to recognize that the courts followed common ethical opinion in drawing a distinction between the positive right to demand an action, such as physician-assisted suicide, and the more powerful negative right to be free of bodily invasion. Although there was no constitutional right to assisted suicide, individual states may choose to legalize or prohibit it.[65] In 1997, Oregon legalized the Oregon Death with Dignity Act, which permitted terminally ill patients to receive prescriptions in lethal quantities for the purpose of self-administration. It does not permit any other forms of physician aid-in-dying, such as another person administering the medication. From 1998 through 2006, 292 patients used 456 prescriptions authorized by this law. The most common diseases in patients choosing to ingest a lethal dose of medication were malignant neoplasms (81% of patients), amyotrophic lateral sclerosis (8% of patients), and chronic lower respiratory tract diseases (4% of patients).[66] In 2006, 40 physicians wrote 65 such prescriptions. Of these 65 patients, 35 used the prescriptions, 19 died of their underlying disease, and 11 lived throughout the year.[66] The financial and educational status of patients did not seem to play a role in the request for physician-assisted suicide.

Other Legal Aspects of Anesthesiology

Care of Jehovah's Witnesses

Jehovah's Witnesses interpret biblical scripture to prohibit taking in blood because it holds the "life force," and anyone who partakes of it shall be "cut off" from eternal life after death (see Chapter 55).[67] Jehovah's Witnesses have different interpretations about the prohibition of blood transfusions, and anesthesiologists must actively clarify what the patient considers acceptable.

Wholly acceptable anesthetic techniques to reduce blood loss include deliberate hypotension, deliberate hypothermia, and hemodilution. Most Jehovah's Witnesses accept synthetic colloid solutions, dextran, erythropoietin, and preoperative iron. Some Jehovah's Witnesses accept autologous banked blood or cell saver blood, and some accept blood removed at the beginning of surgery and returned in a closed loop. Jehovah's Witnesses will colloquially refer to options that are a matter of individual choice as "matters of conscience." Although blood components, autologous blood, and banked blood are generally unacceptable, these specifics must be discussed with the patient. Documenting acceptable interventions crystallizes the patient's desires and provides legal documentation for the anesthesiologist. Anesthesiologists must be certain that they are capable of fulfilling the patient's requests; otherwise, they should not agree to provide anesthesia. Indeed, the anesthesiologist and surgeon should provide non-emergency care to the patient only if all parties can agree on the approach to blood management.

Case law strongly supports the right of an adult patient to refuse blood products. Case law is in flux for pregnant patients, and in such cases the courts are more likely to intervene and mandate transfusion. The ambiguity in legal rulings results from the fact that issues relating to transfusions in Jehovah's Witnesses are based on case law.

Law Regarding Pediatric Patients

For the most part, parents or other surrogate decision-makers of children make health care decisions for minors (in general, children younger than 18 years) (see Chapters 82 and 84). However, the participation of children should increase as they grow older and depends on both the patient's maturity and the consequences involved in the decision. Informed assent acknowledges that although most pediatric patients cannot legally consent to medical care, they should share in decision-making to the extent that their development permits.

Some minors are permitted to consent for themselves.[68] Emancipated minors are patients younger than 18 who have been given the global right to make their own health care decisions. This status varies by state but is generally awarded to patients who are married, parents, in the military, and economically independent and may include patients who are pregnant. The mature minor doctrine holds that minors who have decision-making capacity are legally and ethically capable of giving informed consent in specific situations as determined by a court. Although particulars vary, the mature minor doctrine in general requires patients to be at least 14 years old and tends to permit decisions of lesser risk. The nearer the child is to the age of majority, the more likely the court is to grant the child the ability to consent. The courts will balance the maturity and decision-making capacity of the minor and the risks associated with honoring the minor's wish. As minors near the age of majority, the likelihood increases that the court will support the right of minors to determine therapy. For example, in a case in 2007 that seemed to be on the margin, a judge ruled that a 14-year-old practicing Jehovah's witness would be permitted to refuse transfusion therapy during treatment for a cancer that had a 70% 5-year survival rate. The patient subsequently died.[69]

Even though pediatric patients who are pregnant may be considered emancipated, many states require some form of parental involvement, such as parental consent or notification, before an elective abortion in an adolescent. If a state requires parental involvement, the ability of the minor to circumvent this regulation by seeking relief from a judge, known as judicial bypass, must be available. Requirements and enforcement of statutes vary from state to state. The need for parental involvement in minors having abortions is not always legally straightforward, and it may be best to consult with hospital counsel when determining such issues.[70,71]

Parents and medical personnel may disagree about what is in the best interests of the child. Based on the legal doctrine of *parens patriae*, or the government's obligation to protect the interests of incompetent patients, parents are not permitted to make decisions that are grossly inappropriate overtreatment or undertreatment.[72,73] One way to decide what is in the best interests of the child is to define which choices fall outside the range of acceptable decision-making. The extent to which one intervenes between a patient and the surrogate's decision depends primarily on how harmful the decision is to the patient. Criteria to make this determination include the amount of harm to the child by the intervention or its absence, the likelihood of success, and the overall risk-to-benefit ratio.[74] Charging a parent of not acting in the child's best interests has significant social, fiscal, and familial ramifications. If, however, after exhausting other options the anesthesiologist believes that the parent has chosen unacceptable treatment, the anesthesiologist should report the situation to the proper child welfare authorities for possible legal action.

For anesthesiologists, this is most frequently seen when courts overrule parental wishes and permit transfusion therapy in the children of Jehovah's Witnesses.[75,76] Anesthesiologists caring for a child of a Jehovah's Witness should inform the patient and family that attempts will be made to limit the need for transfusion therapy and abide by their transfusion preferences but that in a life-threatening situation, the anesthesiologist will seek a court order authorizing the administration of life-sustaining blood. In instances in which the likelihood of requiring blood is high or the local judiciary is not that familiar with case law for Jehovah's Witnesses, the anesthesiologist may choose to obtain the court order before the operation. In crisis situations in which no court order exists, anesthesiologists should initiate emergency transfusion therapy before obtaining a court order. As a child becomes older, the courts become less likely to intervene and often grant the emerging adolescent more decision-making latitude. In elective procedures that may be safely delayed, the patient and family may also consider postponing the procedure until the child is of sufficient age and maturity to decide about transfusion therapy.

Supervision and Professional Associations

Attending physicians may be sued because of resident actions. The question of what is considered acceptable resident supervision is affected by local policies and national guidelines, but again, in any individual case, the standard of care is often determined by a jury. Specific guidelines about what trainees are permitted and not permitted to do may provide some protection for the attending physician if the trainee deviates from these guidelines. In addition, residents are being named in lawsuits with increasing frequency. As a general rule, a resident is held to the same standard of care as a practicing attending physician in that specialty.[77]

Under the doctrine of *respondeat superior* and the theory of *vicarious liability*, anesthesiologists are responsible for negligent acts made within the scope of defined duties by certified registered nurse anesthetists.[78] The fundamental issue of vicarious liability is whether the anesthesiologist is controlling the activities of the certified registered nurse anesthetist. Although the question of vicarious liability may depend on who remunerates the certified registered nurse anesthetist, this is likely to be an ineffective defense because anesthesiologists tend to have full authority to medically direct certified registered nurse anesthetists. The scope of defined duties and whether adequate supervision took place may be affected by societal expectations, medical customs, history, practice, manuals, agreements, actions, expert analysis, and written documentation, but it is ultimately determined by a jury in any individual case. For example, in one case, a certified registered nurse anesthetist did not promptly summon the anesthesiologist for help in managing fatal postoperative laryngospasm and bronchospasm.[78] The anesthesiologist was found vicariously liable for negligence, in part because there was a lack of clear understanding between the professional group and certified registered nurse anesthetist about when the anesthesiologist should be called.[79,80]

Many controlling authorities (e.g., state statutes or hospital bylaws) require physicians to participate in certain aspects of anesthesia care when supervising certified registered nurse anesthetists. It is also the responsibility of the professional association to set forth the expectations in a manner that is consistent with law and regulations. Accepting a standard below medically communicated published standards (such as American Society of Anesthesiologists guidelines) risks liability.

Federal regulations for accreditation of hospital and ambulatory surgery facilities require that a certified registered nurse anesthetist be supervised by the physician performing the procedure or an immediately available anesthesiologist.[81,82] State governors may "opt out" of this supervision requirement if they deem doing so to be in the best interests of their citizens. For the opt-out to have practical consequences, however, state laws must also not require supervision. Health care facilities within states that have opted out may still require supervision. To bill for medically directing certified registered nurse anesthetists, anesthesiologists must participate in specific parts of the case.[83]

Anesthesiology professional associations may be held liable if they do not ensure that members are competent and that appropriate policies are followed.[84] Many agreements between professional associations and hospitals require service that complies with governmental and professional standards.[84] Obligations of professional associations may extend to letters of reference. For instance, an anesthesiologist was terminated with cause secondary to abuse of Demerol.[85] When the anesthesiologist went to a locum tenens company, letters of reference from shareholders of the previous professional association did not mention the abuse or that the anesthesiologist was fired with cause. Subsequent negligent care by this anesthesiologist caused severe brain damage to a patient. The court held that the previous professional association was liable for part of the financial award.

Professional associations are responsible for addressing physician impairment. An impaired physician is one who is unable to perform professional or personal responsibilities. Physicians impaired through alcohol and other addictive disorders are considered to have chronic medical illnesses. The Americans with Disabilities Act forbids discrimination against individuals who are in recovery[86] and government agencies from receiving funding if they engage in discrimination. The treatment records of the physician are confidential.

Legal Issues in Pain Management

Inadequate pain management is a health problem, and part of the problem may be due to the tension inherent in unclear regulations, regulatory scrutiny, and criminal investigation and prosecution by state medical boards and drug enforcement agencies (see Chapters 58 and 87).[87,88] For example, the Drug Enforcement Administration's ability to electronically monitor prescriptions for controlled substances gives them access to physicians' prescription histories. Physicians are concerned that knowledge of prescribing practices, divorced from patient-specific context, will lead to misunderstandings and unwarranted investigations. Physicians' concern about being investigated may affect the doses, quantities, number of refills, or even the type of drug used in the care of chronic pain patients.[88] The Drug Enforcement Administration suggests that there should be no effect and has emphasized that only 0.06% of all physicians had investigations initiated, 0.05% of all physicians had actions taken against them, and 0.01% of all physicians were arrested.[89] However, the 0.06% may be fallaciously low because that percentage is out of all practicing physicians. A more relevant percentage would be based on a population of only physicians who prescribe narcotics for pain control and thus are at risk for investigation. A large percentage of the physicians investigated did have actions taken against them.

The *Gonzales v Oregon* decision should comfort physicians because it limits the effects of the Drug Enforcement Administration on physicians.[90] *Gonzales v Oregon* prohibited the U.S. Attorney General from prohibiting physicians in Oregon from prescribing schedule 2 drugs for terminally ill patients to commit suicide.[90] The point of the case is that Congress can set national drug-prescribing rules through the Controlled Substances Act but cannot affect the ability of states to set medical practice standards.[4] The case turns on the Controlled Substances Act. Although there were a number of reasons, the primary reason was that the Controlled Substances Act does not regulate the practice of medicine and, in fact, that the practice of medicine is to be regulated by the state.

Physicians have been held liable for inadequate pain control.[91,92] For example, an 85-year-old man was admitted to a medical center for 5 days in 1998 before his subsequent death several days later.[91] He received inadequate pain control during

Table 10-3 Data Banks

Data Bank	Purpose	Information	Who Can Query
National Practitioner Data Bank (NDPB)[93]	"To restrict the ability of incompetent physicians to move from State to State without disclosure or discovery of the physician's previous damaging or incompetent performance."[93]	Medical malpractice payments Adverse actions: licensing, clinical privileges, professional society, Medicare and Medicaid exclusions, and U.S. Drug Enforcement Administration actions	Hospitals Health care entities with a review process Professional societies State licensing boards Plaintiff attorneys or plaintiffs Self-query
Healthcare Integrity and Protection Data Bank (HIPDB)[94] Established by federal statute	To stop fraud and abuse in health insurance and health care delivery and to promote quality care	Licensing and certification Civil judgments Criminal convictions Exclusions from federal or state health programs	Government agencies Health plans Self-query Researchers
Federation of State Medical Boards (FSMB)[95]	"Continual improvement in the quality, safety and integrity of health care through the development and promotion of high standards for physician licensure and practice."[95]	Records actions by state medical boards against physicians	Medical boards Individuals

his admission. Although a medical malpractice suit was dismissed and the state medical board did not pursue any action against the physician, the family won a civil suit against the physician under the California's Elder Abuse and Adult Civil Protection Act.

Data Banks

Federal databases are designed to improve health care by tracking performance and flagging suspect health care practitioners and entities (Table 10-3).[93-95] By way of context, from 1991 to 2004, the National Practitioner Data Bank recorded 276,274 medical malpractice payments, 8297 of which were related to anesthesia. Over this time, the number of cases with payments has decreased, whereas the median payment has increased.[96]

References

1. Health Insurance Portability and Accountability Act of 1996, Public Law 104-191.
2. 42 USC 1395.
3. 42 CFR 489.24.
4. 21 USC 811.
5. Employee Retirement Income Security Act of 1974, Public Law 93-406.
6. Aetna Health v Davila, 02-1845.
7. Pegram v Herdrich, 530 US 211, 2000.
8. DiFelice v Aetna U.S. Healthcare, No 02-3381, 3d Cir, Oct 15, 2003.
9. Colavito v New York Organ Donor Network, Inc, 860 NE2d 713, NY 2006.
10. U.S. Department of Health and Human Services. 42 CFR 482.
11. Liang BA: Assessing medical malpractice jury verdicts: A case study of an anesthesiology department. Cornell J Law Public Policy 7:121-164, 1997.
12. Brennan TA, Sox CM, Burstin HR: Relation between negligent adverse events and the outcomes of medical-malpractice litigation. N Engl J Med 335:1963-1967, 1996.
13. Cheney FW, Posner K, Caplan RA, Ward RJ: Standard of care and anesthesia liability. JAMA 261:1599-1603, 1989.
14. Sanbar SS, Warner J: Medical malpractice overview. *In* Sanbar AA, Firestone MH, Fiscina S, et al (eds): Legal Medicine, 7th ed. Philadelphia, Mosby Elsevier, 2007, pp 253-264.
15. Filkins JA: Criminalization of medical negligence. *In* Sanbar AA, Firestone MH, Fiscina S, et al (eds): Legal Medicine, 7th ed. Philadelphia, Mosby Elsevier, 2007, pp 507-512.
16. Annas GJ: Medicine, death, and the criminal law. N Engl J Med 333:527-530, 1995.
17. People v. Verbrugge, 998 P2d 43; 1999 Colo App LEXIS 171; 1999 Colo J CAR 3850.
18. Balsamo RR, Brown MD: Risk management. *In* Sanbar AA, Firestone MH, Fiscina S, et al (eds): Legal Medicine, 7th ed. Philadelphia, Mosby Elsevier, 2007, pp 285-303.
19. Mehlman MJ: The shame of medical malpractice. J Leg Med 27:17-32, 2006.
20. Cohen FL: The expert medical witness in legal perspective. J Leg Med 25:185-209, 2004.
21. American Society of Anesthesiologists: Guidelines for expert witness qualifications and testimony. Available at http://www.asahq.org/publicationsAndServices/standards/07.pdf. Accessed November 1, 2007.
22. Moses RE, Feld AD: Legal risks of clinical practice guidelines. Am J Gastroenterol 103:7-11, 2008.
23. Havighurst CC: Practice guidelines as legal standards governing physician liability. Law Contemp Problems 54:87-117, 1991.
24. Liang BA, Ediale KR: Shouldering the evidence burden: Conflicting testimony in a case of interscalene block. J Clin Anesth 17:131-133, 2005.
25. American Society of Anesthesiologists: Documentation of anesthesia care (2003). Available at http://www.asahq.org/publicationsAndServices/standards/21.pdf. Accessed November 1, 2007.
26. Canadian Anesthesiologists' Society: Guidelines to the practice of anesthesia (2007). Available at http://www.cas.ca/members/sign_in/guidelines/practice_of_anesthesia. Accessed January 10, 2007.
27. Lee BH: Countersuits by health care providers. *In* Sanbar AA, Firestone MH, Fiscina S, et al (eds): Legal Medicine, 7th ed. Philadelphia, Mosby Elsevier, 2007, pp 521-526.
28. Wojcieszak D, Saxton JW, Finkelstein MM: Sorry Works! Disclosure, Apology and Relationships Prevent Medical Malpractice Claims. Bloomington, IN, AuthorHouse, 2007.
29. Salgo v Trustees of Leland Stanford Hospital, 154 Col App 2d 560,317 P2d 170 Ct Appl, 1957.
30. Waisel DB, Truog RD: Informed consent. Anesthesiology 87:968-978, 1997.
31. White C, Rosoff AJ, LeBlang TR: Informed consent to medical and surgical treatment. *In* Sanbar AA, Firestone MH, Fiscina S, et al (eds): Legal Medicine, 7th ed. Philadelphia, Mosby Elsevier, 2007, pp 337-343.
32. Shine v Vega, 429 Mass 456,709 NE2d 58, 1999.
33. American College of Obstetricians and Gynecologists Committee on Ethics: Patient choice in the maternal-fetal relationship (2004). Available at http://www.

acog.org/from_home/publications/ethics/ethics034.pdf. Accessed November 1, 2007.
34. Canterbury v Spence, 464 F2d 772, 1972.
35. Cobbs v Grant, 104 Cal Rptr 505,502 P2d 1, 1972.
36. Johnson v Kokemoor, 545 NW2d 495,199 Wis 2d 615, 1996.
37. Byrne J, Napier A, Cuschieri A: How informed is signed consent? BMJ 296:839-840, 1988.
38. Lloyd A, Hayes P, Bell PR, Naylor AR: The role of risk and benefit perception in informed consent for surgery. Med Decis Making 21:141-149, 2001.
39. Affleck PJ, Waisel DB, Cusick JM, Van Decar T: Recall of risks following labor epidural analgesia. J Clin Anesth 10:141-144, 1998.
40. Jackson A, Henry R, Avery N, et al: Informed consent for labour epidurals: What labouring women want to know. Can J Anaesth 47:1068-1073, 2000.
41. Swan HD, Borshoff DC: Informed consent—recall of risk information following epidural analgesia in labour. Anaesth Intensive Care 22:139-144, 1994.
42. Truman v Thomas, 27 Cal, 3d 285,165 Cal Rptr 308, 611 P2d 902, 1980.
43. Annas GJ: Protecting patients from discrimination—the Americans with Disabilities Act and HIV infection. N Engl J Med 339:1255-1259, 1998.
44. Standards for cardiopulmonary resuscitation (CPR) and emergency cardiac care (ECC). JAMA 227(Suppl):833-868, 1974.
45. Rabkin MT, Gillerman G, Rice NR: Orders not to resuscitate. N Engl J Med 295:364-366, 1976.
46. In the Matter of Karen Quinlan, 70 NJ 10,335 A2d 647, cert denied, 429 US 922, 1976.
47. Bartling v Superior Court, 163 Cal App3d 186 [209 Cal Rptr 220], 1984.
48. Cruzan v Director, Missouri Department of Health, 110 SCt 2841, 1990.
49. Bioethicists' statement on the U.S. Supreme Court's Cruzan decision. N Engl J Med 323:686-687, 1990.
50. Emanuel EJ: Securing patients' right to refuse medical care: In praise of the Cruzan decision. Am J Med 92: 307-312, 1992.
51. Council on Ethical and Judicial Affairs, American Medical Association: Decisions near the end of life. JAMA 267:2229-2233, 1992.
52. Patient Self-Determination Act of 1990—Omnibus Budget Reconciliation Act of 1990, Pub. L. No 101-508.
53. Shalowitz DI, Garrett-Mayer E, Wendler D: The accuracy of surrogate decision makers: A systematic review. Arch Intern Med 166:493-497, 2006.
54. Teno JM: Advance directives: Time to move on. Ann Intern Med 141:159-160, 2004.
55. Hammes BJ, Rooney BL: Death and end-of-life planning in one midwestern community. Arch Intern Med 158:383-390, 1998.
56. Woien S: Conflicting preferences and advance directives. Am J Bioeth 7:64-65; discussion W4-W6, 2007.
57. Truog RD, Waisel DB, Burns JP: DNR in the OR: A goal-directed approach. Anesthesiology 90:289-295, 1999.
58. In re the conservatorship of Helga M. Wanglie, No PX-91-283, District Probate Division, 4th Judicial district of the County of Hennepin, State of Minnesota, 1993.
59. Angell M: The case of Helga Wanglie—a new kind of "right to die" case. N Engl J Med 325:511-512, 1991.
60. Gilgunn v Massachusetts General Hospital, SCt Civ Action No 92-4820, Suffolk Co, Mass, verdict April 21, 1995.
61. Consensus statement of the Society of Critical Care Medicine's Ethics Committee regarding futile and other possibly inadvisable treatments. Crit Care Med 25:887-891, 1997.
62. Texas Advance Directive Act. Texas Health & Safety Code Section 166.046.
63. Washington v Glucksberg, 521 US 702, 1997.
64. Vacco v Quill, 521 US 793, 1997.
65. Snyder L, Sulmasy DP: Physician-assisted suicide. Ann Intern Med 135:209-216, 2001.
66. Oregon Department of Human Services: Oregon's Death with Dignity Act. Portland, OR, 2007.
67. Watch Tower Bible and Tract Society of Pennsylvania: How can blood save your life? Brooklyn, NY, Watchtower Bible and Tract Society of New York, 1990.
68. Emancipation of Minors Law. California Family Code, Section 7000-7002.
69. Black C: Boy's death ends battle because of his religion, leukemia patient Dennis Lindberg, 14, didn't want vital transfusions; his biological parents did. A judge sided with the son, who died last night. Seattle Post-Intelligencer, November 29, 2007.
70. Committee on Adolescence, American Academy of Pediatrics: The adolescent's right to confidential care when considering abortion. Pediatrics 97:746-751, 1996.
71. Council on Ethical and Judicial Affairs, American Medical Association: Mandatory parental consent to abortion. JAMA 269:82-86, 1993.
72. Prince v Massachusetts, 321 US 158, 1994.
73. Custody of a Minor, 375 Mass 733,379 NE2d 1053, 1978.
74. Committee on Bioethics, American Academy of Pediatrics: Guidelines on forgoing life-sustaining medical treatment. Pediatrics 93:532-536, 1994.
75. Sampson v. Taylor, 29 NY2d 900, 1972.
76. Wallace v. Labrenz, 104 NE2d 769, 1952.
77. Kachalia A, Studdert DM: Professional liability issues in graduate medical education. JAMA 292:1051-1056, 2004.
78. Coalter JS: The vicarious liability of a physician for the negligence of other medical professionals. Campbell Law Rev 17:375-381, 1995.
79. Doctors Hosp. of Augusta, Inc, v Bonner, 392 SE2d 897, GA App 1990.
80. Liang BA, Hannenberg AA, Johans TG: Negligence in supervision: A case of failed resuscitation. J Clin Anesth 13:44-48, 2001.
81. 42 CFR 482.52.
82. 42 CFR 416.42.
83. 42 CFR 415.110.
84. Liang BA, Katz RL: Professional association liability without personal malpractice: Just who can be liable? J Clin Anesth 16:54-56, 2004.
85. Kadlec Medical Center et al. v Lakeview Anesthesia Associates Interrogatories to the Jury, Civil Action No Civ A 04-0997, Section I/3, ED La, May 19, 2005.
86. 42 USC 126.
87. Quill TE, Meier DE: The big chill—inserting the DEA into end-of-life care. N Engl J Med 354:1-3, 2006.
88. Reddy BS: The epidemic of unrelieved chronic pain. The ethical, societal, and regulatory barriers facing opioid prescribing physicians. J Leg Med 27:427-442, 2006.
89. The myth of the "chilling effect." News release of the Drug Enforcement Administration A, Va, October 30, 2003.
90. Gonzales v Oregon, 126 SCt 904, 2006.
91. Bergman v Wing Chin, MD, and Eden Medical Center, No H205732-1, Cal App Dept Super Ct, 1999.
92. Estate of Henry James v Hillhaven Corp, 89 CVS 64, NC SCt 1991.
93. The Health Care Quality Improvement Act of 1986, as amended in 42 USC Sec 11101.
94. 45 CFR 61.
95. Federation of State Medical Boards: FSMB mission, vision, core values and goals. Available at http://www.fsmb.org/candidates/edusvc_candidates_mission.html. Accessed November 1, 2007.
96. Kain ZN: The National Practitioner Data Bank and anesthesia malpractice payments. Anesth Analg 103:646-649, 2006.

Anesthetic Physiology

Section II

Max B. Kelz, George A. Mashour, Ted G. Abel, and Mervyn Maze

11 Sleep, Memory, and Consciousness

Key Points

1. Sleep is an active process generated in the brain.
2. Structures in the brainstem, diencephalon, and basal forebrain control the sleep-wake cycle and are directly modulated by general anesthetics.
3. Sleep and anesthesia are similar states with distinct traits, with each satisfying neurobiologic features of the other.
4. Distinct memory functions are subserved by distinct neural structures.
5. Limbic system structures such as the hippocampus and amygdala are critical for memory and play a role in anesthetic-induced amnesia.
6. Although brainstem, diencephalon, and basal forebrain structures generate wakefulness, the contents of consciousness are thought to be generated by the cortex.
7. Multiple neural correlates of consciousness are thought to be the targets of general anesthetics.
8. Consciousness and subsequent explicit recall of intraoperative events—known as "awareness during general anesthesia"—occur in 1 to 2 cases per 1000.
9. Monitoring anesthetic depth has evolved to electroencephalographic methods, although limitations still exist.

Within 10 years of Morton's public demonstration of general anesthesia, ether, nitrous oxide, and chloroform were all in widespread use. The existence of three agents with diverse chemical structures led Claude Bernard in 1875 to speculate that the state of general anesthesia must arise through a common mechanism of action. Although decades of research have demonstrated multiple, nonoverlapping molecular targets for individual anesthetics (see Chapters 20 and 26) and appear to refute Bernard's hypothesis, a unitary network theory of anesthetic action remains possible from a systems perspective.

Traditionally, the state of general anesthesia is divided into various behavioral end points, including amnesia, hypnosis (defined as a lack of perceptive awareness to non-noxious stimuli), analgesia, immobility, and blunting of autonomic reflexes. These end points are produced by specific interactions of general anesthetics on discrete neuronal loci. Although volatile anesthetics come closest to being complete and thus capable of producing each of the components of the anesthetized state, the majority of anesthetic drugs fail to satisfy all criteria.

Nonetheless, diverse anesthetics acting at distinct receptor targets might produce common neurophysiologic adaptations in relevant circuits culminating in the behavioral end points that are recognizable as general anesthesia. This chapter considers two distinct anesthetic end points, hypnosis and amnesia. Using sleep as a paradigm to understand the system's neuroscience of control of the arousal state, the first section explores behavioral state transitions, as well as the effects of anesthetics on these circuits. The second section describes the neurophysiology and neurobiology of memory formation and concludes with a discussion of their modulation by anesthetics. Finally, in the last section we address the emerging science of consciousness and discuss how anesthetics reversibly alter its expression.

Neuronal Systems That Regulate Arousal States

Exquisite regulation of the arousal state confers a survival advantage. Predators who fall asleep during the chase may starve, whereas prey caught napping at inopportune times suffer an equally dire fate. Thus, the need to regulate the arousal state seems obvious for all. However, the requirement for sleep in the first place remains mysterious. Prolonged loss of sleep leads to impaired thermoregulation, metabolism, and immune function and, ultimately, to death.[1] Given the tremendous cost of sleep in terms of opportunity—time that might otherwise be spent seeking food or shelter or procreating—one might presume that it offers some as yet unclear selective advantage in an evolutionary sense.[2]

Recent hypotheses about the beneficial effects of sleep include restoration of the neuronal homeostasis essential for synaptic function, consolidation of memories, and initiation and expression of neuronal plasticity (reviewed elsewhere[3-5]).

Whatever its true role, evolution has exerted a selective pressure on organisms to sleep (Table 11-1). Molecular, neuronal, and behavioral conservation of sleep implies that it also carried a survival advantage in ancestral mammals. Hence, it should not be surprising that the neuronal underpinnings for control of arousal lie in subcortical structures deep within the brainstem, thalamus, and hypothalamus in regions where they are conserved across the animal kingdom.

Table 11-1 Sleep Phylogeny—Hours Spent in Each Arousal State

Species	Waking	NREM	REM
Human	16	6	2
Guinea baboon	14.5	8.5	1
Sheep	18.1	5.3	0.6
Horse	20.5	2.5	0.5
Giraffe	19.5	4	0.5
Bottlenose dolphin	14	9.8	<0.2
Platypus	10	6	8
Thick-tailed opossum	6	11.4	6.6
Ferret	9.5	8.5	6
Cat	11	10	3
European hedgehog	13.9	6.6	3.5
Big brown bat	4.3	15.8	3.9
Armadillo	7	14	3
Rat	11	10.5	2.5

NREM, non–rapid eye movement; REM, rapid eye movement.
Data from McGinty DJ, Sterman MB: Sleep suppression after basal forebrain lesions in the cat. Science 160:1253, 1968; and Siegel JM: The REM sleep-memory consolidation hypothesis. Science 294:1058, 2001.

Passive versus Active Theories of Sleep

The discovery on which the neurobiology of control of the arousal state is built belonged to Frederic Bremer (1892-1982). In 1935, Bremer demonstrated that transection of the caudal medulla, although producing paralysis requiring mechanical ventilation, also produced an animal that remained alert, with normal sleep-wake cycles. Conversely, transection through the mesencephalon, immediately caudal to the nucleus of the third cranial nerve, yielded an animal that breathed spontaneously but was unresponsive and displayed a continuous sleep pattern in its electroencephalogram (EEG) (Fig. 11-1). Bremer's discovery formed the foundation for the passive theory of sleep. However, passive notions of sleep predate Bremer. The roots for this idea exist in the surviving sixth century BC writings of the Greek philosopher Alcemaeon and were known to Aristotle, who expounded on them in his treatise *De Somno et Vigilia* ("On Sleep and Waking"). Bremer's experimental evidence lent credence to the ancient Greek idea that sleep is caused by isolation of the brain from the rest of the body. Bremer hypothesized that sleep results anytime that the brain is deprived of its tonic sensory input. Under this passive view, sleep was nothing more than a default state produced by cessation of the active state—waking. A student of Bremer's, Giuseppe Moruzzi (1910-1986), fortified his mentor's hypothesis in collaboration with the physiologist Horace Magoun (1907-1991). Using electrical stimulation of the brainstem reticular formation (which falls in between Bremer's mesencephalic and caudal medullary lesion sites), Moruzzi and Magoun stimulated wakefulness while suppressing sleep and in so doing made the first description of the ascending reticular activating system.[6] Together, they also narrowed the window for inducing a persist-

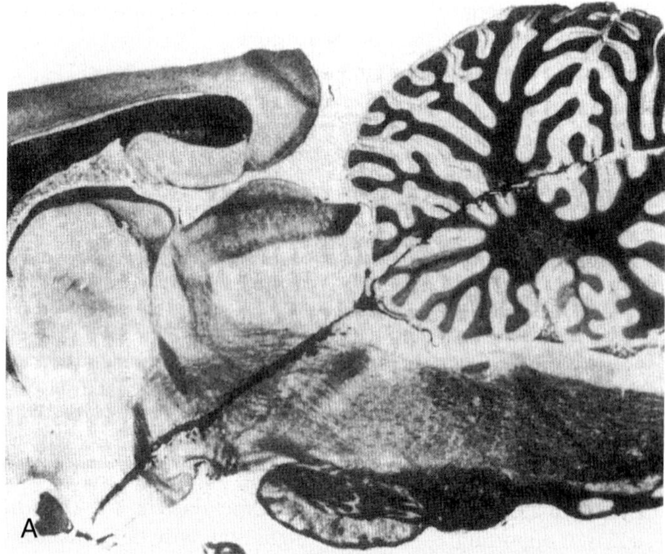

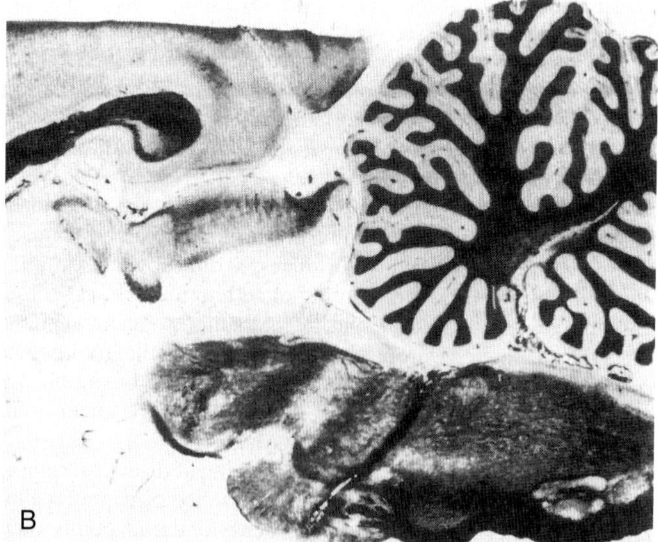

Figure 11-1 Brainstem transections may radically alter the state of arousal. **A,** Bremer's cerveau isole cat in which transection at the collicular level prevents brainstem and hypothalamic arousal-promoting signals from reaching the forebrain, thereby producing a state of deep coma. **B,** This contrasts with the enephale isole cat, in which transection through the caudal medulla disrupts spontaneous ventilation but leaves control of the arousal state intact. *(Modified from Steriade M, Constantinescu E, Apostol V: Correlations between alterations of the cortical transaminase activity and EEG patterns of sleep and wakefulness induced by brain-stem transections. Brain Res 13:177-180, 1969.)*

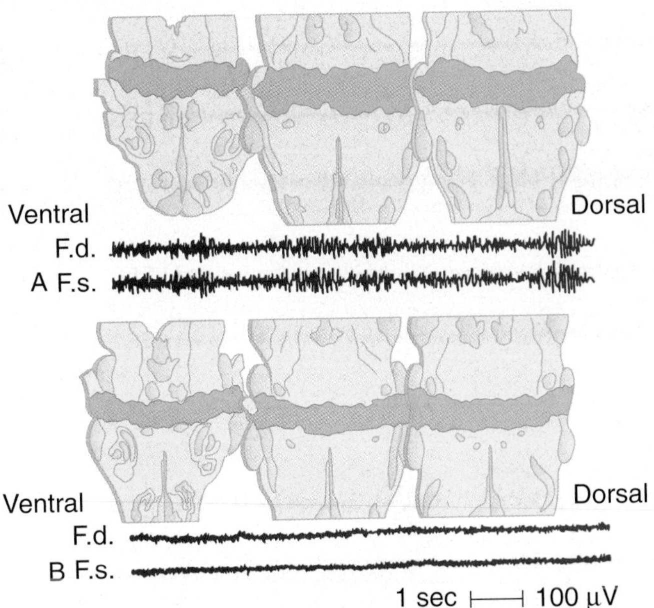

Figure 11-2 Schematic horizontal sections through the cat's brainstem depicting the production of a comatose state resembling continuous sleep in the cat that is immensely similar, if not identical to, the results of barbiturate-induced hypnosis. **A,** Midpontine pretrigeminal lesions that ablate the laterodorsal tegmental (LDT) and pedunculopontine tegmental (PPT) cholinergic neuronal projections to the thalamus and basal forebrain and produce continuous slow-frequency, large-amplitude patterns characteristic of sleep on the electroencephalogram (EEG) in both the right (F.d.) and left (F.s.) frontal EEG leads. **B,** Transections several millimeters more caudad through the rostral pons spare brainstem cholinergic neurons and their projections and lead to preservation of arousal as typified by the fast-frequency low-amplitude patterns on the EEG that characterize normal wakefulness. *(Modified from Batini C, Moruzzi G, Palestini M, et al: Persistent patterns of wakefulness in the pretrigeminal midpontine preparation. Science 128:30-32, 1958.)*

ent state of sleep by demonstrating that lesions through the midpontine pretrigeminal area of the cat did not affect the cyclic nature of control of the arousal state but confirmed that a lesion only a few millimeters more cephalad through the rostral pons at the level of the inferior colliculus produced the identical comatose syndrome as Bremer's (Fig. 11-2).

Nathaniel Kleitman (1895-1999) was another early proponent of the passive theory of sleep genesis. Among his important discoveries was recognition of the paradoxical stage of sleep, termed rapid eye movement (REM) sleep. This state differed dramatically from slow-wave or non-REM (NREM) sleep, as discussed later. For all his careful observations of sleep stages, however, Kleitman pointed out that it was the genesis of wakefulness that required explanation. Before leaving Bremer and the concept of passive sleep, we should return to his studies of the *cerveau isole* cat, in which a mesencephalic lesion deprives the forebrain of all sensory input (save olfactory and visual stimuli, which are carried by cranial nerves I and II). Bremer's insights have direct relevance for anesthetic action. In fact, Bremer's original description of the cerveau isole cat likened the resulting state as being immensely similar, if not identical to barbiturate anesthesia, as well as to natural sleep,[7] a concept to which we shall return in this chapter.

An alternative theory accounting for sleep requires its active genesis. According to the active sleep hypothesis, sleep is generated when specific neuronal systems increase their firing rates and thus inhibit the output of other neuronal structures required for wakefulness. Evidence for an active genesis of sleep has accumulated. During World War I, an outbreak of viral encephalitis reached pandemic proportions. Although many survivors experienced symptoms of profound and prolonged sleepiness (hypersomnolence), a smaller subset of survivors exhibited profound and prolonged insomnia. Based on postmortem neuropathologic observations and correlations with the premortem clinical condition, Baron Constantine von Economo (1876-1931) astutely noticed that the insomniacs had sustained damage within the anterior hypothalamus around the preoptic area, as well as damage to the basal forebrain. Those exhibiting hypersomnolence had sustained posterior hypothalamic damage. von Economo correctly predicted the existence of a sleep-promoting region of brain within the anterior hypothalamus near the optic chiasm, in addition to a wake-promoting region in the posterior hypothalamus.[8] His predictions made more than three quarters of a century ago have withstood the scrutiny of time. Experimental evidence for a hypnogenic center in the preoptic area of the hypothalamus was confirmed in rats and cats inasmuch as insomnia also resulted after lesions to the preoptic area,[9,10] as well as after bilateral microinjection of muscimol, a γ-aminobutyric acid (GABA) agonist, into the preoptic area.[11] Finally, the discovery of a population of inhibitory GABAergic neurons whose activity displays state-dependent firing patterns,[12] with the highest discharge rates occurring during sleep[13] and whose efferent projections inhibit wake-promoting centers (reviewed by Saper and colleagues[14]), fulfills all the criteria for the active generation of sleep.

Although controversy between active and passive mechanisms of the genesis of sleep still remains, these modes need not be mutually exclusive. As we discuss later, the hypnogenic neural substrates that promote sleep antagonize the wake-promoting regions in brain. In the absence of neuropathology, synchronized communication between these sleep- and wake-active neural populations ensures smooth and appropriately timed transitions between arousal states.[15]

Physiologic Patterns of Wakefulness and Sleep

The states of sleep and wakefulness may be characterized physiologically by recording the EEG and electromyogram (EMG). Wakefulness is identified by a fast-frequency, low-amplitude rhythm on the EEG that is "desynchronized," together with the presence of maximal motor activity on the EMG (Fig. 11-3). Broadly speaking, sleep may be subdivided into two distinct patterns, REM sleep and NREM sleep, which is also known as slow-wave sleep. During NREM sleep, the EEG displays large-amplitude, slow frequencies in the δ range of 0.5 to 4 Hz that dominate the power spectrum. Motor tone is lower during NREM sleep than during wakefulness (Fig. 11-3). NREM sleep patterns contrast dramatically with wakefulness, in which the EEG is desynchronized and exhibits low-amplitude, fast frequencies. During REM sleep, the EEG is also desynchronized and is virtually indistinguishable from wakefulness. However, as opposed to wakefulness, EMG activity during REM sleep is minimal to

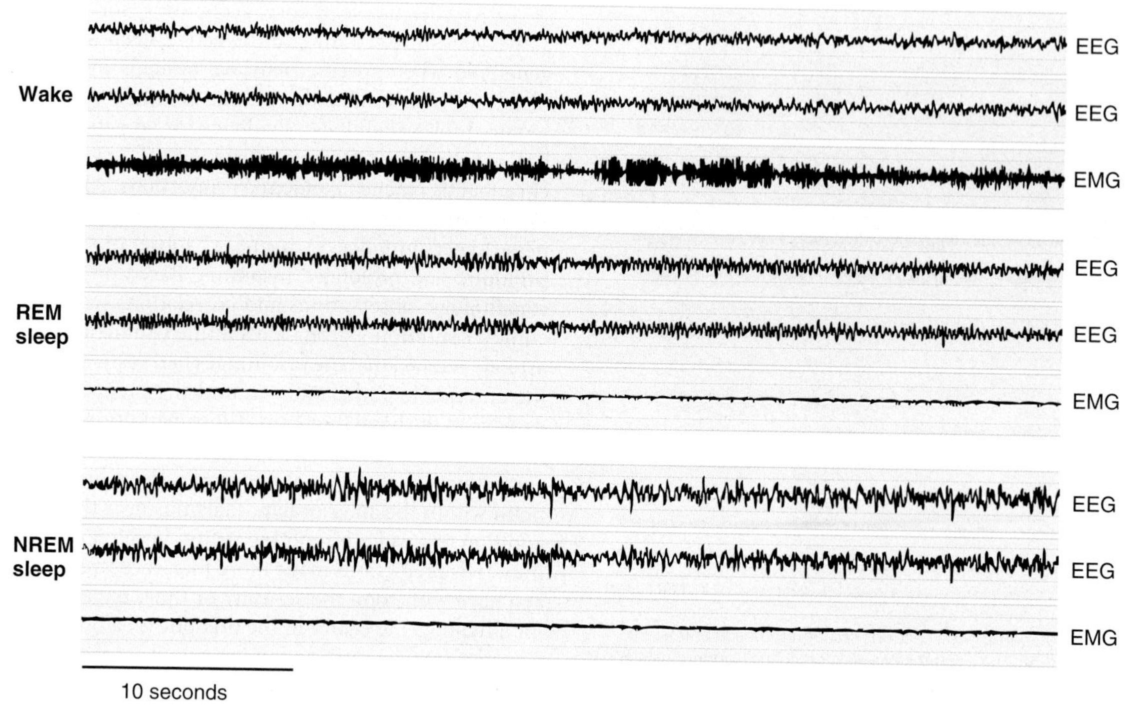

Figure 11-3 Cortical manifestation of wakefulness, rapid eye movement (REM) sleep, and non-REM (NREM) sleep with corresponding muscle tone. Wakefulness is defined by a desynchronized, low-amplitude, fast-frequency electroencephalogram (EEG) with prominent muscle activity. REM sleep shows similar signs of cortical activation with a desynchronized, low-amplitude, fast-frequency EEG in which θ rhythms of 4 to 8 Hz dominate the power spectrum. However, unlike wakefulness, motor activity is minimal in this state. NREM sleep has an EEG appearance that is markedly different from the other two states. During NREM sleep, the EEG displays slow-frequency, large-amplitude oscillations. Motor tone during NREM is dramatically reduced. *(Courtesy of Yihan Chen, University of Pennsylvania, unpublished results.)*

absent. The presence of θ activity (4 to 8 Hz) is also an abundant feature of REM sleep, as is eye movement, which may be recorded with an electro-oculogram (EOG) (for review see Harris[16]).

Wakefulness

Protecting the neural systems responsible for generating wakefulness is so fundamental to survival that evolution has distributed its expression across multiple and partially redundant systems, each contributing in a unique, but nonessential, way to promotion and maintenance of wakefulness. Specific centers in the brain alter their electrical output in proportion to the organism's arousal state. Among these regions, noradrenergic neurons of the locus ceruleus (LC), histaminergic neurons of the tuberomammillary nucleus (TMN), serotonergic neurons of the dorsal and median raphe nuclei (RN), and the newly recognized population of dopaminergic neurons in the ventral periaqueductal gray (vPAG) matter[17] are all monoaminergic centers that display arousal state–dependent firing patterns (Fig. 11-4) (for review see Jones[18]). Their highest discharge rates occur during wakefulness, decrease during NREM sleep, and become virtually quiescent during REM sleep. This pattern contrasts with that of brainstem and basal forebrain cholinergic neurons, which are most active during both wakefulness and REM sleep but decrease their output during NREM sleep, as discussed later. Neurons containing the wake-promoting and wake-sustaining neuropeptide orexin (also known as hypocretin) share similarities with other monoaminergic systems. Although confined to the posterior, lateral, and dorsomedial hypothalamus, orexinergic neurons also innervate the entire neuroaxis of the central nervous system (CNS) from forebrain through the spinal cord. These neurons exhibit maximal activity during wakefulness, reduce their firing during NREM sleep, and become quiescent during REM.[19,20] The orexinergic population positively reinforces wakefulness by stimulating activity in the monoaminergic centers just mentioned. In all mammals studied to date, including humans, impaired orexin signaling causes narcolepsy, a primary disorder affecting the organization of sleep and wakefulness. Although narcoleptics show behavioral state instability and transition to and from sleep at inopportune times, the total amount of sleep and wakefulness remains unchanged. Consistent with this notion, isolated lesion studies in animal models along with pharmacologic and gene knockout experiments have demonstrated that no single monoaminergic, cholinergic, glutamatergic, or orexinergic wake-active center is absolutely required for wakefulness.[21]

Nonetheless, Bremer, Moruzzi, and Magoun demonstrated that complete disruption of the brainstem reticular core, including the laterodorsal tegmentum (LDT) and pedunculopontine tegmentum (PPT), precludes wakefulness. The cholinergic LDT and PPT, the noradrenergic LC, the dopaminergic vPAG, and the serotonergic RN are stimulated by afferent sensory input. Together, these systems ascend through two pathways to stimulate cortical activity and expression of wakefulness (Fig. 11-5). Dorsal fibers synapse in the thalamus, where their input is relayed indirectly to the cortex via glutamatergic thalamocortical afferents. Ventral fibers synapse in the posterior hypothalamus and basal forebrain while communicating with the histaminergic TMN and cholinergic basal forebrain centers on their way to the cortex. Finally, noradrenergic LC and serotonergic RN neurons send afferent input directly to the cortex. Although brainstem and hypothalamic activity modulates wakefulness, the cerebral cortex itself

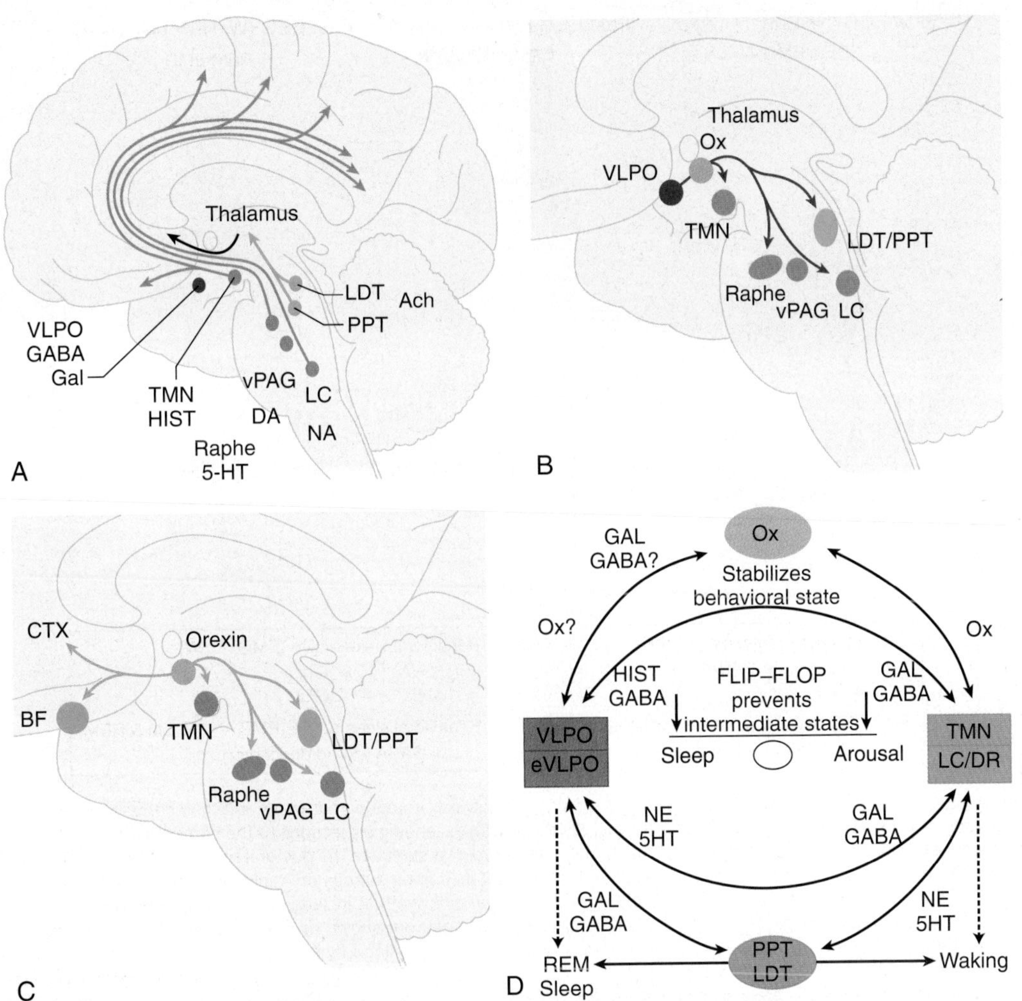

Figure 11-4 Brainstem and hypothalamic regulation of the arousal state. **A,** The ascending arousal system originates in the brainstem and posterior hypothalamus but sends projections throughout the entire central nervous system. Cholinergic neurons of the laterodorsal tegmentum (LDT) and pedunculopontine tegmentum (PPT) project to many forebrain targets, including the thalamus, and are shown in *blue*. Monoaminergic centers (shown in *green*) diffusely project throughout the forebrain and modulate hypothalamic nuclei directly. These wake-active regions include histaminergic neurons of the tuberomammillary nucleus (TMN), serotonergic neurons of the dorsal and median raphe nuclei (Raphe), dopaminergic (DA) neurons of the ventral periaqueductal gray (vPAG) matter, and noradrenergic (NA) neurons of the locus ceruleus (LC). Shown in *red* are the sleep-promoting neurons of the ventrolateral preoptic (VLPO) nucleus, which contain the inhibitory neurotransmitters γ-aminobutyric acid and galanin. **B,** Inhibitory projections from the VLPO antagonize activity in the ascending arousal centers. **C,** Orexinergic (ORX) neurons are confined to the posterior and lateral hypothalamus, yet also communicate with all known arousal centers to promote and reinforce stability of the awake state. **D,** A flip-flop model of control of the arousal state that leads to a bistable circuit in which the individual is predisposed to wakefulness or sleep but should not fluctuate between states of arousal. *(Modified from Saper CB, Chou TC, Scammell TE. The sleep switch: Hypothalamic control of sleep and wakefulness. Trends Neurosci 24:726-731, 2001.)*

contributes to self-awakening through its efferent projections to the thalamus and reticular formation.[22]

NREM Sleep

With a notable exception of the ventrolateral preoptic (VLPO) nucleus, overall electrical activity in most regions of brain is decreased during NREM sleep. This observation correlates with passive notions of sleep in which tonic wake-promoting input dissipates. During NREM sleep, monoaminergic, orexinergic, and cholinergic groups are inhibited by efferent signals emanating from the preoptic anterior hypothalamus, specifically, a cluster of neurons localized to the VLPO nucleus that use the inhibitory neurotransmitters GABA and galanin (see Fig. 11-4). VLPO neurons are sleep active and display increased firing rates and c-Fos immediate early gene expression during sleep.[13,23] Sleep-active VLPO neurons have an antagonistic relationship with wake-active centers such that VLPO activation inhibits firing in wake-active centers. Conversely, rapid firing of wake-active regions inhibits the VLPO nucleus. This network design leads to a bistable behavioral state of arousal favoring either sleep or wakefulness but not rapid transitions between the two. Not surprisingly, destruction of the VLPO nucleus with an excitatory amino acid lesion that destroys cell bodies while leaving fibers of passage intact causes insomnia.[24]

Although preoptic anterior hypothalamic VLPO neurons actively generate NREM sleep, neurons in the thalamus also alter their electrical activity patterns in critical ways during NREM sleep. Thalamic reticular and thalamocortical neurons begin to fire in bursts. This process generates sleep spindles evident on the EEG. Burst firing of thalamocortical neurons transiently causes deafferentation of the cortex by reversibly disconnecting it from sensory stimuli normally conveyed to the cortex from the

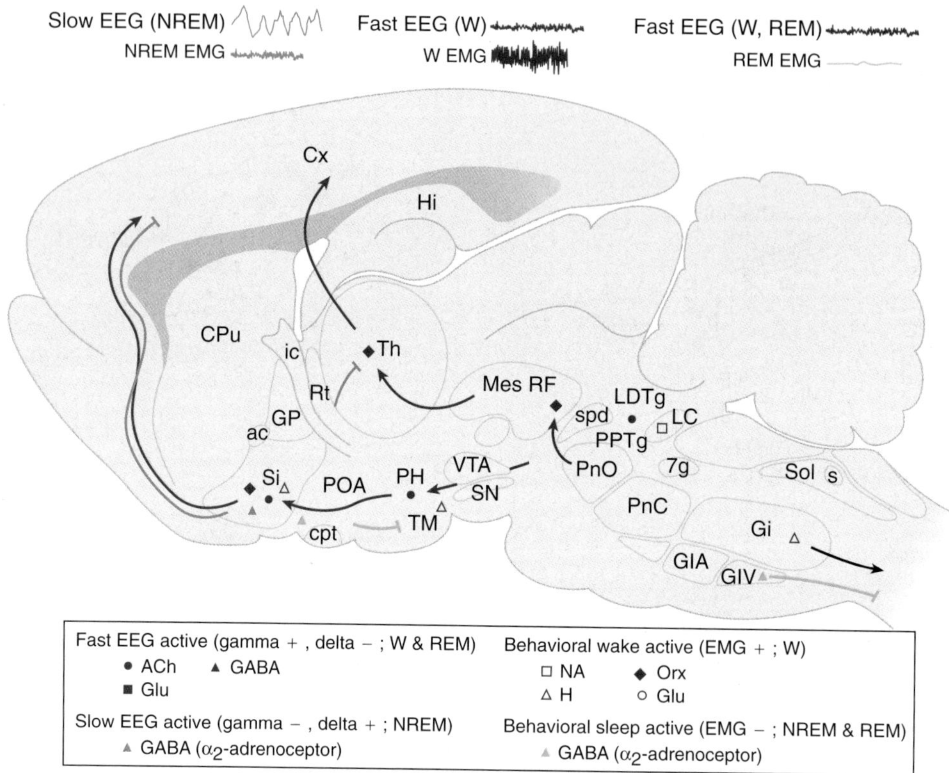

Fast EEG active (gamma + , delta – ; W & REM)	Behavioral wake active (EMG + ; W)
● ACh ▲ GABA	□ NA ◆ Orx
■ Glu	△ H ○ Glu
Slow EEG active (gamma – , delta + ; NREM)	Behavioral sleep active (EMG – ; NREM & REM)
▲ GABA (α_2-adrenoceptor)	▲ GABA (α_2-adrenoceptor)

Figure 11-5 Schematic section through a rat brain depicting conserved sleep- and wake-promoting pathways and their corresponding neurotransmitter signaling systems. Neurons that are active during wakefulness (W) include those with ascending projections to the cortex that stimulate a fast-frequency desynchronized EEG (gamma+), along with descending projections to the spinal cord that stimulate the postural muscle tone required for waking behavior. Wake-active neurons display maximal activity during wakefulness, dramatically slow their firing during non–rapid eye movement (NREM) sleep, and become virtually quiescent during rapid eye movement (REM) sleep. Groups shown with *open pink symbols* include noradrenergic neurons (NA), histaminergic neurons (H), orexinergic neurons (Orx), and glutamatergic (Glu) neurons. Additional wake-active neurons shown by *filled pink symbols* are also active during REM sleep. These largely ascending systems include cholinergic (ACh), glutamatergic (Glu), and some γ-aminobutyric acid (GABA)-containing neurons. Sleep-active neurons (*blue* and *green symbols*) include cells whose cortical ascending projections dampen fast cortical activity and those with descending projections to the spinal cord and brainstem, which diminish behavioral arousal and muscle tone. The sleep-active neurons discharge in association with slow EEG activity (gamma–/delta+) during NREM sleep (*blue triangle*) and include some GABAergic neurons in the basal forebrain and preoptic area (POA) that bear α_2-adrenoceptors and are inhibited by NA. Thalamic GABA-containing neurons of the nucleus reticularis discharge in bursts with sleep spindles and slow waves to inhibit and pace thalamocortical relay neurons. In the basal forebrain and preoptic area, α_2-adrenoreceptor–expressing GABAergic neurons with descending projections increase their firing rates as muscle tone decreases (EMG–) during NREM and REM sleep (*green symbols*). Finally, additional GABAergic (and/or possibly glycinergic) neurons of the medulla descend directly into the spinal cord, where they might inhibit motor neurons during sleep. ac, anterior commissure; CPu, caudate putamen; Cx cortex; EEG, electroencephalogram; EMG, electromyogram; 7g, genu of the 7th nerve; Gi, gigantocellular RF; GiA, gigantocellular, alpha part of the RF; GiV, gigantocellular, ventral part of the RF; GP, globus pallidus; Hi, hippocampus; ic, internal capsule; LDTg, laterodorsal tegmental nucleus; Mes RF, mesencephalic RF; opt, optic tract; PH, posterior hypothalamus; PnC, pontine, caudal part of the RF; PnO, pontine oral part of the RF; POA, preoptic area; PPTg, pedunculopontine tegmental nucleus; RF, reticular formation; Rt, reticularis nucleus of the thalamus; s, solitary tract; scp, superior cerebellar peduncle; SI, substantia innominata; SN, substantia nigra; Sol, solitary tract nucleus; Th, thalamus; TM, tuberomammillary nucleus; VTA, ventral tegmental area. *(Modified from Jones BE: From waking to sleeping: Neuronal and chemical substrates. Trends Pharmacol Sci 26:578, 2005.)*

thalamus.[25] Deafferentation of the cortex by intrinsic thalamic activity is reminiscent of Bremer's lesion studies in which permanent deafferentation of the cortex formed the experimental basis of the passive nature of sleep. Together, VLPO and thalamic activity patterns provide mechanistic neuronal network explanations for the active and passive theories of sleep.

REM Sleep

Control of REM sleep is also regulated in the brain. Although several neuroanatomic centers participate in regulation and coordination of REM onset and offset, the main effector responsible for the generation of REM sleep resides in the pontine reticular formation. Transection studies by Michel Jouvet (1925-) in the cat further localized brainstem REM control within the pons to the nucleus pontis oralis (PnO), which appears to be necessary for REM expression. Direct injection of cholinergic agonists into the PnO (which is slightly rostral and just ventral to the LC) produces a state that mimics natural REM sleep.[26] The endogenous cholinergic tone in the brainstem arises from the LDT and PPT, two nuclei located at the junction between the pons and midbrain. Excitotoxic lesions that ablate the LDT and PPT dramatically impair REM sleep.[27] A subset of LDT and PPT neurons fire selectively during REM sleep, whereas other cholinergic LDT and PPT neurons fire during both REM sleep and wakefulness. Notably, the uniquely REM-active subset increases its firing rates prior to the EEG and behavioral features of REM expression,[28,29] thus suggesting that LDT and PPT cholinergic neuronal activity may initiate REM sleep (REM-on neurons). Neurons of the extended VLPO (eVLPO) nucleus also exhibit preferential activation during REM sleep. Because the eVLPO nucleus communicates directly with brainstem cholinergic LDT neurons along with monoaminergic neurons of the LC and RN and because lesions of the eVLPO nucleus reduce the amount of REM sleep, the eVLPO nucleus appears to play a special role in generation of REM sleep.[30]

The behavioral constellation of REM sleep is dissociable into various components, each with its own specific mechanisms and neuroanatomic controllers. The cardinal signs of REM sleep include rapid eye movement, atonia of all motor groups except for the diaphragm, and activation of a low-voltage, fast-frequency EEG rhythm. Subcortical recordings demonstrate ponto-geniculo-occipital (PGO) waves. This characteristic spiky EEG pattern of REM sleep originates in the pons, is transmitted to the thalamic lateral geniculate, and terminates in the occipital cortex. The REM- and wake-active population of LDT and PPT neurons with rostral projections is important for production of the desynchronized fast-frequency, low-amplitude EEG found in both wakefulness and REM sleep.[26] REM atonia is initiated by a group of pontine reticular neurons that synapse in the bulbar reticular formation before terminating their signal on spinal cord motor neurons. The subset of pontine reticular formation neurons initiating atonia is a non-noradrenergic population of neurons adjacent to the LC, termed either the perilocus ceruleus alpha or subceruleus (SubC) in cats or the sublateral dorsal (SLD) nucleus in rodents.[31,32]

Exit from REM sleep transitions into either NREM sleep or wakefulness and is triggered by "REM-off" groups. The observation that noradrenergic LC neurons decrease their firing rate during NREM sleep and become virtually quiescent during REM sleep, together with pharmacologic and lesion studies, had suggested that inhibition of the LC was a requirement for entry into REM sleep and that LC neurons might serve as REM-off cells. However, genetic studies in noradrenergic-deficient mice have conclusively demonstrated the continued existence of normal, or nearly normal, REM sleep despite the absence of norepinephrine.[33,34] Thus, the adrenergic neurons of the LC cannot be an exclusive REM-off population. Neurons of the ventrolateral periaqueductal gray (vlPAG) matter also serve to terminate REM episodes, as proved by pharmacologic studies during which muscimol inhibition of this region increases REM sleep and also by elegant immunohistochemical mapping combined with vlPAG lesions.[35-37] vlPAG neurons form a mutually antagonistic inhibitory loop with those of the SLD nucleus to efficiently generate or inhibit REM sleep.[35]

Somnogen-Induced Transitions Between Arousal States

Even though cortical EEG and EMG patterns and activity in the sleep- or wake-active centers in the brainstem, hypothalamus, and thalamus are well known during states of sleep or wakefulness, the mechanisms responsible for entry into or exit from a given state remain mysterious. The humoral theory of sleep regulation was independently proposed nearly 100 years ago by French and Japanese neuroscientists. Intrathecal infusion of cerebrospinal fluid (CSF) harvested from sleep-deprived dogs into rested normal dogs caused the recipient dogs to promptly fall asleep.[38,39] This result suggested the existence of an endogenous somnogen, a "hormone" circulating in the CSF whose accumulation could cause the onset of sleep. Over the past century, the list of potential somnogens has grown to include substances as diverse as proteins—δ sleep-inducing peptide (DSIP)[40]; lipids—*cis*-9,10-octadecenoamide[41]; hormones—melatonin; cytokines—interleukin-1; eicosanoids—prostaglandin D_2 (PGD_2); and a nucleoside—adenosine.[42] We shall review data for the latter two putative somnogens, which have been studied most extensively.

Infusion of femtomolar concentrations of PGD_2 into the third ventricle induces both NREM and REM sleep in rats that is indistinguishable from natural sleep.[43] PGD_2 levels fluctuate in the CSF, with circadian frequency paralleling sleep-wake cycles. Sleep deprivation proportionally elevates CSF PGD_2 levels, thus also supporting a role for PGD_2 as an endogenous somnogen. PGD_2 is synthesized by the enzyme prostaglandin D synthetase, which is localized in the arachnoid membrane and choroids plexus (Fig. 11-6), and is secreted directly into CSF, where it is the second most abundant protein. Microdialysis studies confirm a specific sleep-promoting activity of picomolar quantities of PGD_2. However, this somnogenic activity is present only when PGD_2 is infused in the vicinity of the preoptic area of the hypothalamus. The most pronounced activity of PGD_2 is observed when it is

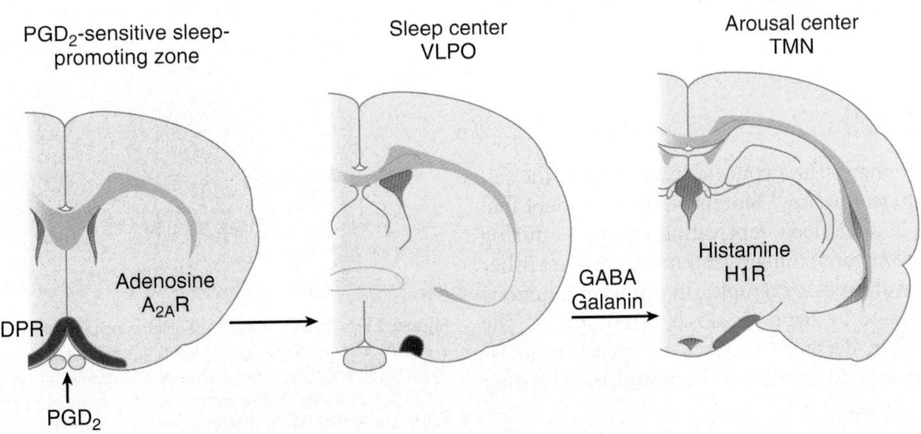

Figure 11-6 Molecular mechanisms of sleep promotion by the endogenous somnogen prostaglandin D_2 (PGD_2). The prostaglandin D_2 receptor (DPR) lines the ventral surface of the basal forebrain and preoptic area (*purple area*). The DPR is thought to transmit the somnogenic PGD_2 signal from cerebrospinal fluid to the ventrolateral preoptic nucleus (VLPO, shown in *red*), with adenosine being used as a signaling molecule. This signal transduction event activates VLPO neurons via the adenosine A_{2A} receptor, which leads to inhibition of wake-active histaminergic groups such as the tuberomammillary nucleus (TMN, shown in *blue*). *(Modified from Hayaishi O, Urade Y: Prostaglandin D_2 in sleep-wake regulation: Recent progress and perspectives. Neuroscientist 8:12, 2002.)*

infused beneath the VLPO nucleus. Infusion of a PGD_2 antagonist into the third ventricle reversibly and dose-dependently inhibits both REM and NREM sleep (for review see Hayaishi and Urade[43]). On binding to the D-type prostanoid receptor (DPR), which is localized to the arachnoid membrane lining the ventral surface of the brain, the somnogenic signal of PGD_2 appears to be transduced indirectly by activation of the VLPO nucleus.[44] The mechanism for VLPO activation after subarachnoid infusion of PGD_2 appears to require adenosine because coadministration of an adenosine receptor A_{2a} antagonist blocks the somnogenic activity of PGD_2. Conversely, administration of an adenosine A_{2a} agonist mimics the somnogenic activity of PGD_2.[45] As adenosine levels accumulate, they activate A_{2a} receptor–expressing neurons to directly or indirectly activate the VLPO nucleus.[46] Hence, it appears that adenosine may function as the neurotransmitter that couples the humoral to the neural mechanisms driving sleep-wake regulation. With this model the homeostatic drive to sleep accumulates proportionally to increases in the endogenous somnogens PGD_2 and adenosine. The existence of such somnogenic substances that accumulate with time argues for active rather than passive generation of sleep.

Anesthesia and Sleep

Anesthesia is a state that shares phenotypic similarities with sleep, and hence the metaphor of "going to sleep" is commonly used to describe induction of general anesthesia in the clinical setting.[47] Not only are anesthesia and sleep similar states, but they also share common neurobiologic traits[48]; indeed, the hypnotic component of anesthesia may result from specific actions of anesthetics on the neural systems that regulate natural sleep. Support for this hypothesis comes from a variety of studies. During sleep and general anesthesia, there is reduced responsiveness to external stimuli. Functional brain imaging during anesthetic-induced unconsciousness has been shown to inhibit thalamic and midbrain reticular formation nuclei.[49] Anesthetic blockade of thalamic information transfer, which disrupts somatosensory input from reaching higher cortical centers, has also been confirmed with more direct microelectrode recordings.[50,51] In both instances, these anesthetic effects on the thalamus resemble the naturally occurring thalamocortical inhibition characteristic of NREM sleep.[25]

Sleep Deprivation

Sleep deprivation potentiates the hypnotic action of anesthetics, including propofol and isoflurane.[52] Moreover, the sleep debt that would otherwise ensue after sleep deprivation dissipates during propofol anesthesia; however, it remains unknown whether other features of sleep deprivation (for example, on immune function) might also be ameliorated by hypnotic doses of propofol.[53] The bispectral index monitor, designed to track the depth of anesthetic-induced hypnosis, also appears to be useful in recording the onset and depth of sleep.[54]

Endogenous Somnogens and Anesthetics

Infusion of adenosine in low doses potentiates the hypnotic actions of intravenous and volatile anesthetics, thereby reducing the amount of anesthetic required to achieve a given depth of anesthesia. This effect is reproduced by 2-chloroadenosine, a potent adenosine analog, and by dipyridamole, an adenosine uptake blocker and adenosine deaminase inhibitor. Conversely, administration of theophylline, an adenosinergic antagonist, produces partial resistance to anesthesia.[55] Mechanistically, these data fit well with an effect of adenosine on activation of the hypothalamic sleep center, the VLPO nucleus (see later discussion). Meanwhile, exposure to anesthetics such as isoflurane affects the levels of endogenous somnogens, with isoflurane altering the balance between prostaglandin E_2, a wake-promoting prostaglandin, and PGD_2, a sleep-inducing prostaglandin, in the hypothalamus.[56]

Effects of Anesthetics on Sleep Circuits

Knowledge of the endogenous arousal systems is an essential prerequisite for any discussion of the mechanisms of action of psychostimulants, sedative-hypnotics, and general anesthetics. Predicted actions of anesthetics based on their known effects at individual cells expressing single recombinant neurotransmitter receptors, including GABAergic, glutamatergic, cholinergic, adrenergic, histaminergic, serotonergic, and orexinergic receptors or voltage-gated calcium, sodium, or potassium channels, allow the generation of testable hypotheses. However, anesthetics distribute throughout the entire brain (Fig. 11-7),[57] and because the majority of sleep- and wake-active nuclei send bidirectional signals that may be either mutually inhibitory, excitatory, or one

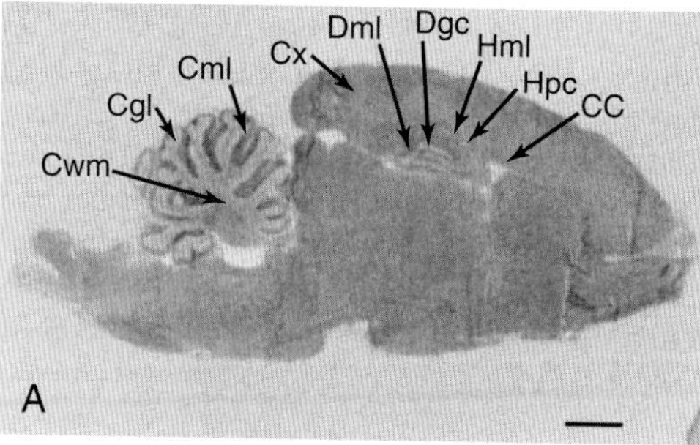

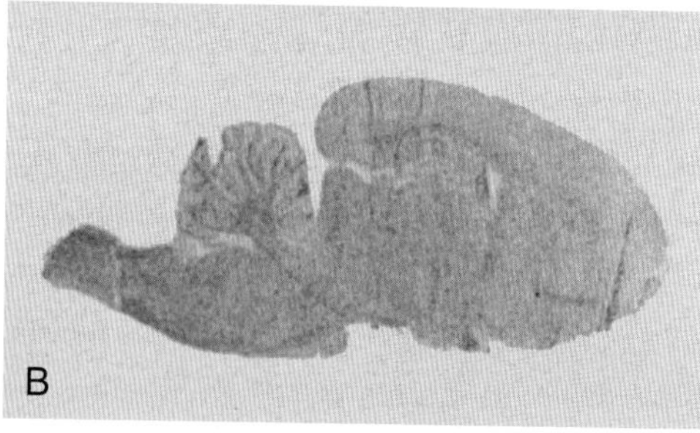

Figure 11-7 Distribution of specific halothane binding throughout the rat brain. **A,** This autoradiogram demonstrates nearly homogeneous binding of the volatile anesthetic halothane at 100 μM by direct photoaffinity labeling with ^{14}C-halothane. Some exceptions to nearly uniform uptake are shown in the cerebellar white matter (Cwm), cerebellar granular layer (Cgl), and subregions of the hippocampus. **B,** Specific binding is competitively inhibited by 2.3 mM nonradioactive halothane. CC, corpus callosum; Cml, cerebellar molecular layer; Cx, cortex; Dgc, dentate granule cell layer; Dml, dentate molecular layer; Hml, hippocampal molecular layer; Hpc, hippocampal pyramidal cell layer. *(Modified from Eckenhoff MF, Eckenhoff RG: Quantitative autoradiography of halothane binding in rat brain. J Pharmacol Exp Ther 285:371, 1998.)*

inhibitory in one direction with an excitatory return, the actual effects of anesthetics on net circuit output must be empirically tested because existing models do not account for all the complexity in the circuits.[58]

Thalamic Sites

The passive theories of sleep set forth by Bremer are similar to many passive concepts of general anesthesia. A central tenet of NREM sleep and anesthesia is that the cortex is deprived of sensory input. Whether by exogenous lesions, as in Bremer's cerveau isole cat, or by endogenous closing of thalamic gates, anesthetics appear to act on NREM sleep circuits, thereby leading to shared mechanisms of action. Within the thalamus, there is a simple architecture of cell types consisting of reticular neurons and thalamocortical neurons that communicate with the cortex while also integrating peripheral input (Fig. 11-8). Activation of the reticular neurons during NREM sleep and anesthesia causes hyperpolarization of thalamocortical relay neurons, which in turn blocks propagation of the action potential through thalamocortical relay neurons. As a result, thalamocortical neurons are prevented from relaying peripheral input to higher cortical centers. This is the mechanism by which the thalamic gates close to transiently, yet reversibly, sever the cortex from the periphery.[25,59,60] Midline thalamic nuclei are thought to play a critical role in generating conscious awareness and appropriately receiving afferent input from most reticular activating arousal-promoting centers.[21] Imaging studies confirm a regionally selective reduction in midline thalamic blood flow, metabolism, and by extension, activity.[49,61] Support for a thalamocortical consciousness switch has recently been strengthened by the finding that microinjection of nicotine into the centromedian nucleus of the thalamus reverses sevoflurane-induced hypnosis (discussed later). These conclusions are mitigated by the fact that administration of nicotine into the centromedian nucleus results in seizures. However, support for the central thalamus as an arousal center that is capable of reversing unconsciousness also comes from literature on the persistent vegetative state. High-frequency stimulation of the central thalamus in the rat has been associated with widespread cortical activation and enhanced cognitive function.[62] Furthermore, deep brain stimulation of the central thalamus has been shown to reverse some of the behavioral deficits in a patient suffering traumatic brain injury.[63]

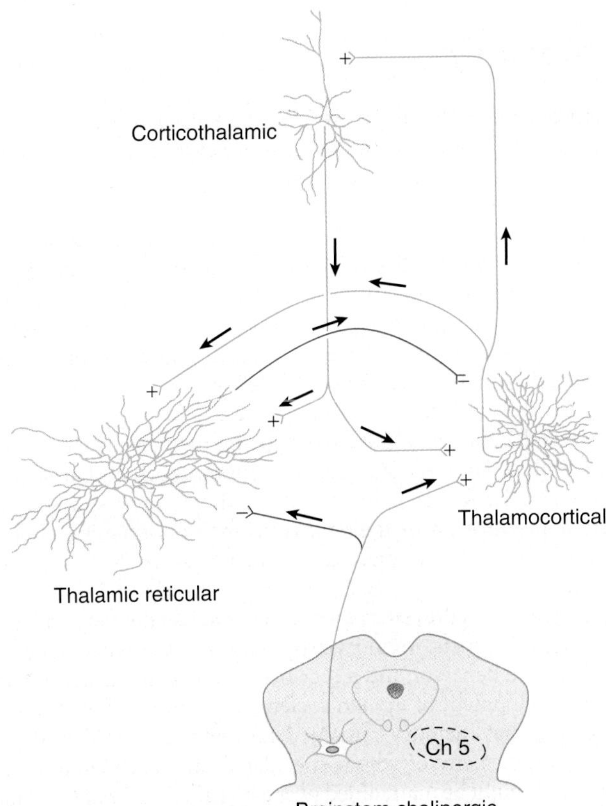

Figure 11-8 The transition from wakefulness to non–rapid eye movement (NREM) sleep is associated with characteristic changes on the electroencephalogram that correlate with underlying changes in the electrical firing patterns of corticothalamic systems. During NREM sleep, thalamocortical neurons are hyperpolarized by thalamic reticular neurons (upper *green* axon). This action prevents incoming peripheral signals from being relayed to corticothalamic neurons in the cortex and transiently, but effectively results in deafferentation of the cortex. Cholinergic input in the brainstem is able to simultaneously hyperpolarize thalamic reticular neurons while depolarizing thalamocortical neurons, thereby returning membrane potential in thalamocortical neurons to baseline and restoring the action potential propagation that transfers peripheral sensory input to corticothalamic neurons. Recent studies suggest that similar changes in the firing properties of corticothalamic loops may also underlie anesthetic-induced hypnosis. Excitatory connections are depicted in *red*, with *plus symbols* at the synapse. Inhibitory connections are displayed in *green*, with *minus signs* at the synapse. *(Modified from Steriade M: The corticothalamic system in sleep. Front Biosci 8:d878, 2003.)*

Because nicotinic acetylcholine receptors are heavily expressed in the thalamus and because many anesthetics inhibit signaling via nicotinic acetylcholine receptors, suppression of the cholinergic arousal system may be one mechanism through which many anesthetics produce unconsciousness.[64] Processed EEG measures of anesthetic depth also reveal an important role for the cholinergic arousal system inasmuch as intracerebroventricular infusions of neostigmine or the muscarinic agonist oxotremorine arouse isoflurane-anesthetized rats.[65]

Hypothalamic Sites

Thalamic nuclei receive input from the ascending brainstem reticular activating system via a dorsal pathway and also receive hypothalamic input from wake-active centers such as histaminergic and orexinergic neurons (see Fig. 11-5). As discussed earlier, the thalamic gates close during NREM sleep and exposure to several anesthetics, and this closure is facilitated by decreased input of monoaminergic, cholinergic, and orexinergic signals during anesthesia. GABAergic anesthetics such as propofol and barbiturates exert their hypnotic effects by inactivating histaminergic neurons of the TMN[66] (see Fig. 11-4). This action may be explained at the molecular level by potentiation of inhibitory GABAergic projection from the sleep center, the VLPO nucleus. Disinhibition of the VLPO nucleus, in turn, shuts down other wake-active groups and further reinforces VLPO activity. This feed-forward mechanism stabilizes the hypnotic state.[14] Blockade of the wake-promoting histaminergic signal is also the mechanism by which the antihistaminergic drug diphenhydramine precipitates sleep. Recovery or emergence from anesthetic hypnosis is facilitated by wake-promoting orexinergic neurons, which are inhibited by volatile anesthetics such as isoflurane and sevoflurane.[67]

Brainstem Sites

One finding that has emerged from studying the hypnotic properties of different anesthetic agents is that there is neither a unitary molecular target nor an invariant neuronal site of action common to all anesthetics. This point is illustrated by dexmedetomidine, an α_2-adrenergic agonist. The behavioral hypnosis of dexmedetomidine results from the drug's ability to inactivate noradrenergic neurons of the LC (Fig. 11-4). This event disinhibits the VLPO nucleus, which subsequently inactivates other arousal centers via the VLPO's GABAergic and galaninergic inhibitory signaling, as discussed earlier.[68] As with propofol and barbiturates acting on the TMN, the common consequence of VLPO disinhibition is stabilization of the hypnotic state. Pharmacologic and lesion experiments that alter both monoaminergic reticular activating function and anesthetic sensitivity can now be reinterpreted in the framework of integrated arousal network activity. Depletion of CNS catecholamines, including norepinephrine, serotonin, dopamine, and histamine, produces hypersensitivity to anesthetics.[69] Conversely, pretreatment with a monamine oxidase inhibitor or acute exposure to amphetamine, both of which increase catecholamine levels in the brain, produces partial resistance to anesthetics.[70] Focusing once again on noradrenergic neurons of the LC, chemical depletion of norepinephrine with 6-hydroxydopamine[71] and electrolytic destruction of LC neurons[72] both produce hypersensitivity to anesthetics, probably by removing an inhibitory signal to the VLPO nucleus.

These pharmacologic treatments affect other monoaminergic systems in addition to the noradrenergic neurons. Moreover, the action of amphetamines or monoamine oxidase inhibitors on serotonergic or dopaminergic systems might also account for a portion of the anesthetic effects. In support of this concept, destruction of serotonergic RN neurons with the toxin 5,6-dihydroxytryptamine or direct electrolytic lesions of serotonergic RN neurons also cause hypersensitivity to anesthetics.[71,72] Once again, as with lesions of the LC, these actions may be interpreted in the light of partial VLPO disinhibition (see Fig. 11-4).

The discovery that pentobarbital and muscimol, a $GABA_A$ agonist, cause behavioral and EEG signs of hypnosis when microinjected into a discrete upper brainstem site, termed the mesopontine tegmentum (MPTA) in rats, has revealed yet another important anesthetic locus.[73] Neuroanatomic tracing studies have shown that MPTA neurons project to thalamic, hypothalamic, and brainstem sites traditionally recognized as part of the ascending reticular activating system. Like other known wake-active systems, MPTA neurons are spontaneously active during wakefulness and are thought to decrease their firing rates during NREM sleep and under anesthesia.[74] MPTA neurons also project to the septohippocampal system, thus providing a link to yet another anesthetic locus (see later).

Limbic System

Strong emotions such as fear, rage, and joy are accompanied by a heightened state of arousal. Hence, it should not be surprising that the limbic system, which responds to emotional content, connects to arousal circuits. Specifically, within the limbic system the medial septum and hippocampus also participate in modulating awareness. This knowledge of neuroanatomy helps explain how inhibition of the medial septum or hippocampus by local injection of muscimol decreases the doses of propofol and pentobarbital needed for hypnosis.[75] The role of limbic system structures such as the hippocampus and amygdala in memory function and anesthetic-mediated amnesia is discussed later.

Summary

Although once considered a passive process in which the cortex loses afferent input, sleep is now recognized as an actively generated state whose genesis depends on the integrated contribution of multiple neuronal input. Increased understanding of the relevant neuronal circuits controlling sleep and wakefulness has opened a series of investigations into anesthetic-induced hypnosis. These studies suggest that anesthetic-induced unconsciousness may arise in part from selective actions of our drugs on these critical nuclei. One basic principle that appears to tie all the neuroanatomic studies together is that inactivation of structures mediating normal arousal appears to enhance the effects of general anesthetic–induced hypnosis. Conversely, activation of these regions appears to produce partial resistance to anesthetic-induced hypnosis.

Memory

In this portion of the chapter we provide a discussion of the major themes in our understanding of memory as it has developed over the past 100 years. Three major themes are clear.[76] First, there are multiple memory systems that are subserved by specific brain regions and neural circuits. Second, there are multiple stages of memory that are mediated by distinct molecular mechanisms. Third, alterations in the strength of connections between neurons—termed *synaptic plasticity*—is a critical component of the way in which memories are stored in neural circuits. After investigating these three major themes of memory research, we describe the molecular mechanisms by which memories are stored and define potential mechanisms by which anesthetics might induce amnesia. Because the hippocampus and amygdala have been the focus of many studies of memory storage and because modulation of their function may underlie anesthetic-induced amnesia, our discussion will focus on these memory systems.

Over the centuries, memory has fascinated poets, philosophers, and scientists. Memory represents an experience-dependent change in behavior, and it is critical to our sense of self, as well as the development of human society and culture. Thus, it is not surprising that memory remained for centuries the domain of philosophers, many of whom speculated on what memory was and how it might be maintained over a lifetime. In *Theatetus*, Plato proposed that thoughts might be stamped into memory the way a signet ring makes an impression in wax. When he discussed a theory of cognition in *Timaeus*, Plato was among the first to suggest that the brain contains the higher, rational soul that controls our actions, but his idea was that this rational soul interacted with a lower, appetitive soul in the gut to form images on the surface of the liver.[77] Experimental work by scientists on memory had its origins in the 19th century when neurologists and psychiatrists such as Jackson, Ribot, and Alzheimer began to identify patients with memory deficits and psychologists such as Hebbinghaus, Müller, and Pilzecker began to define different types and stages of memory.[78] Importantly, the early clinical work on brain-lesioned patients placed memory into the hands of neuroscientists, who defined the importance of the brain in memory, in contrast to earlier proposals by philosophers, in which it was suggested that memory was subserved by other organ systems. As this experimental and clinical work was being carried out on memory, anatomists such as Santiago Ramón y Cajal (1852-1934) were identifying the critical cellular components of the nervous system by using histologic stains to identify distinct classes of neurons and glia within the brain. Cajal's "Neuron Doctorine" led him to postulate that it would be these connections between neurons (later called synapses) that might mediate memory storage.[79] With the work of Ivan Pavlov (1849-1936) on the conditioned reflex, the field of memory began to be a central component of the growing field of psychology.[80]

Distinct Memory Systems Subserve Distinct Types of Memory

The field of memory research was revolutionized in the middle part of the 20th century by study of the patient H.M. by Wilder Graves Penfield (1891-1976), Brenda Milner (1918-), and others. Work in the first half of the 20th century that followed on the work of Pavlov had failed to define specific memory systems, as was suggested by the work of Jackson, Ribot, and Alzheimer and popularized by the phrenologist Joseph Gall. Karl Lashley, working at Harvard, suggested that memories might not be localized to specific brain regions inasmuch as his lesion studies in rodents failed to identify such specific circuits. Rather, Lashley proposed his laws of mass action and "equipotentiality," both based on the ideas that the entire cerebral cortex contributes to memory and that other brain regions can compensate for damage to a certain region of the brain.[81] The study of H.M. thus came in striking contrast to these conclusions of Lashley. At 27 years of age, H.M. underwent surgery to remove portions of his temporal lobe in an effort to treat intractable epilepsy that had developed after a childhood accident. As became clear some 40 years later when H.M.'s brain was studied by magnetic resonance imaging techniques, his neurosurgeon Wilder Penfield had removed the bulk of his hippocampus bilaterally and portions of his amygdala[82] (Fig. 11-9). Thus, it is no surprise that H.M. had severe anterograde memory deficits in the ability to acquire new memories.

Neuropsychological evaluation by Brenda Milner and others revealed two surprising aspects of the amnesia that followed H.M.'s surgery.[76,83] First, he also exhibited retrograde amnesia—that is, certain memories of events before his surgery were lost. As this retrograde amnesia was probed in more detail,

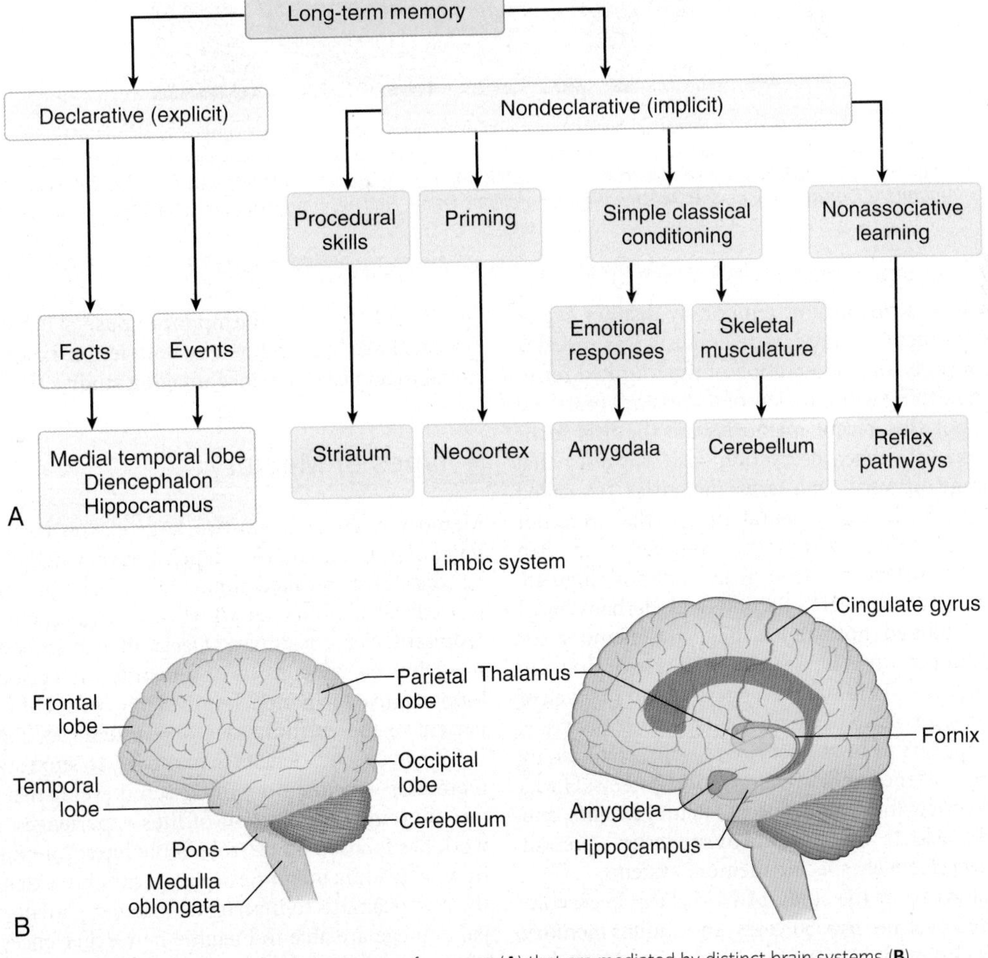

Figure 11-9 There are distinct types of memory (**A**) that are mediated by distinct brain systems (**B**).

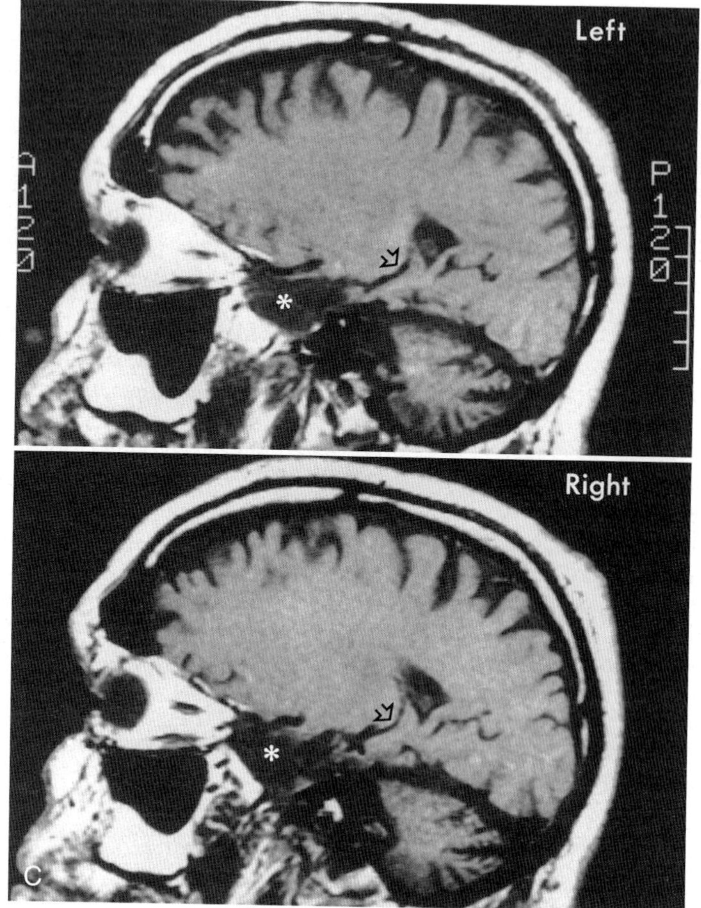

Figure 11-9, cont'd Patient H.M. exhibited selective deficits in declarative memory for facts and events after surgical resection of portions of his medial temporal lobe, including the hippocampus (**C;** the resected portion is marked with an *asterisk*, the remaining portion of the hippocampus is marked with an arrow). *(**A,** Modified from Squire LR, Zola SM: Structure and function of declarative and nondeclarative memory systems. Proc Natl Acad Sci U S A 93:13515, 1996; **C,** from Corkin S, Amaral DG, Gonzalez RG, et al: H. M.'s medial temporal lobe lesion: Findings from magnetic resonance imaging. J Neurosci 17:3964, 1997.)*

it was found that H.M.'s memory of temporally distinct events was intact, and a "gradient" of retrograde amnesia was revealed that decreased with time. This observation of time-limited retrograde amnesia is in keeping with the "law of regression" proposed by Jackson and Ribot that recent memories are the first to be affected by amnesia.[84,85] This observation also suggests that retrieval and storage of very long-term memories (so-called remote memory) are mediated by neural circuits that were not altered by H.M.'s surgery. We now know that these very long-term memories require the cortex—particularly the anterior cingulate cortex, for storage and retrieval.[86] Second and perhaps most important, H.M. exhibited normal learning and memory for certain tasks, a finding that was first shown for a mirror drawing task. This second aspect of H.M.'s amnesia gave rise to the idea of multiple memory systems, each of which mediate particular types of memory. There appears to be at least two reasons why Lashley did not observe the existence of discrete memory systems. H.M.'s lesions were not precisely focused on specific neural circuits, and his behavioral tasks, which were complex maze tasks, were not configured to probe selectively specific memory systems.

The conclusions from the study of H.M. have been confirmed and extended over the past 50 years, and similar memory deficits have been observed in patients with damage limited to specific subregions of the hippocampus.[83,87,88] A variety of memory systems have been defined by both lesion experiments and functional magnetic resonance imaging studies (Fig. 11-9).

Types of Memory

Memory is divided into two large classes termed *declarative* or *nondeclarative* memories, depending on whether the memory can be consciously recalled or not.[89] Nondeclarative memory includes procedural memory, of which bike riding and mirror drawing represent clear examples. Declarative memory, which is consciously recalled, consists of semantic and episodic memory. The hippocampal formation, lesioned in patient H.M., is a major component of the episodic memory system (see Fig. 11-9). Indeed, H.M. had specific deficits in his ability to store and recall episodic memories—the memory of facts and events that provide most of our conscious recollection of life's experiences. Although much work has focused on the role of the hippocampus in the recollection of episodic memories, recent work has extended the study of the hippocampus to investigate whether patients with hippocampal damage are able to imagine new experiences.[90] Patients with hippocampal damage are impaired at imaging new experience, in part because their imagined experiences lack spatial coherence and consist of fragmented images in the absence of configural representation of an environmental setting. Beyond its role in our conscious recollection of our past, the hippocampus also makes a critical contribution to our ability to imagine new experiences.

The existence of multiple memory systems provides a critical analytic tool for the analysis of memory deficits observed in patients. A particularly striking example of such a "double dissociation" between types of memory comes from the work of Damasio and colleagues.[91] They examined a patient with bilateral damage to the amygdala and a patient with bilateral hippocampal damage in classic conditioning tasks. The patient with amygdala damage was unable to acquire conditioning of autonomic responses but did acquire declarative knowledge about the conditioning trials. In contrast, the patient with hippocampal damage learned the conditioned autonomic responses but not the facts. One clinical implication of the existence of multiple memory systems is that appropriate neuropsychological testing combined with structural and functional magnetic resonance imaging can be used to identify the basis of memory deficits in patients.

Memory Consolidation and Different Stages of Memory

In 1900, Georg Elias Müller (1850-1934) and his student Alfons Pilzecker (1865-1949), working at the University of Göttingen, Germany, published a seminal 300-page paper describing 40 experiments on the nature of memory.[92] In this work, Müller and Pilzecker presented clear evidence that memory does not immediately develop after learning but instead takes time to be consolidated and stored. Their primary evidence came from two classes of observations termed perseveration and retroactive inhibition. Using lists of nonsense syllables presented as paired associates, Müller and Pilzecker found a strong tendency for syllable pairs to be maintained in a subject's mind for some minutes after learning. Such "perseveration" was interpreted to reflect the persistence of a memory trace that was necessary to encode the memory. In a set of experiments designed to test this idea, they presented subjects with a second list of words at some time interval after the first list. If this second list followed the first list by 30 seconds, "retroactive interference" was observed—subjects showed less retention of the first word list. If learning of the second list was delayed by 6 minutes, such interference was not seen. Müller and Pilzecker concluded: "After all this, there is no alternative but to assume that after reading a list of syllables, certain physiological processes, which serve to strengthen the associations induced during reading of that list, continue with decreasing intensity for a period of time" (quoted by Lechner and colleagues[92]).

With these pioneering experiments, Müller and Pilzecker laid the groundwork for what today is termed memory consolidation—the idea that memories initially persist in a fragile state and are stabilized over time as they are consolidated into long-term memory.[93] Although it was immediately realized that the work on perseveration and retroactive interference provided an explanation for the temporally graded retrograde amnesia observed in patients by Ribot and Jackson, it took some time for this idea to have an impact on animal studies. It was not until 1949 that two papers reported retroactive interference in rodents with the use of electroconvulsive shock to induce retrograde amnesia.[94,95] In theoretical work at the same time, Hebb and Gerard[95,96] proposed that memory consisted of two "traces" of reverberating neural activity that first gives rise to short-term memory and then to long-term memory (Fig. 11-10). An interesting question that is still actively being explored is whether these short-term and long-term memory traces occur in series or in parallel. Although much work assumes that they are serial, some intriguing experiments suggest that they may form independently in parallel. Despite the fact that much work on memory consolidation has focused on impairing memory after training, memory can also be enhanced during the period of consolidation, as revealed by the work of McGaugh.[93] Thus, the existence of periods of memory consolidation provides an evolutionarily important mechanism to modulate our responses to learned experiences.

The concepts of memory consolidation were critically important for the development of biologically based approaches to memory storage. In particular, postulates that structural

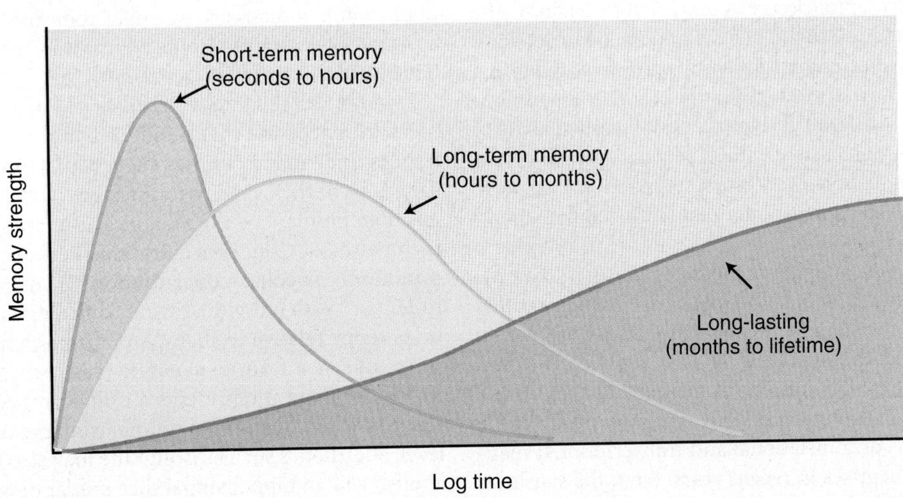

Figure 11-10 Memory consists of distinct phases, including short-term memory, long-term memory, and long-lasting memory. Distinct molecular mechanisms underlie each of these phases. Although these memory phases are shown schematically as though they exist in series, evidence suggests that they may also partially exist in parallel, thus implying that they are mediated by distinct molecular mechanisms acting independently. *(From McGaugh JL: Memory—a century of consolidation. Science 287:248, 2000.)*

changes might underlie memory traces led to development of the idea that proteins might mediate memory storage and then that RNA synthesis was required.[97] With the development of molecular biology, the finding that translation and transcription were critical for memory storage put study of the molecular mechanisms of memory firmly in the realm of the central dogma of molecular biology and led to the use of molecular techniques by many researchers to probe how information is stored in neural circuits. Furthermore, it became clear that it was molecular cascades of signaling molecules, transcription factors, and waves of RNA and protein synthesis that explained the perseveration and retroactive interference observed by experimental psychologists.

Cellular and Molecular Mechanisms of Memory Storage

At the cellular level, the most striking finding about the potential biologic basis of memory came in 1973 when Bliss and Lomo discovered that repeated high-frequency stimulation of input to the hippocampus in vivo resulted in a long-term potentiation (LTP) of synaptic transmission. LTP provides a cellular model of memory.[98,99] Evidence has suggested that processes similar to LTP may mediate memory because induction of LTP impairs ("occludes") subsequent memory formation.[100] LTP is induced after learning.[101] Furthermore, genetic and biochemical manipulations that impair LTP also lead to memory impairment. The development of in vitro slice preparations to study hippocampal LTP and manipulate hippocampal slices pharmacologically and electrophysiologically has been critical for identification of the molecular mechanisms underlying synaptic plasticity and memory.

Like behavioral memory, hippocampal LTP is an experience-dependent process, and extensive evidence suggests that these processes are mediated by similar molecular mechanisms.[98,99] Repeated synaptic stimulation in hippocampal slices, as well as behavioral training, activates the *N*-methyl-D-aspartate (NMDA)-type glutamate receptor, a molecular coincidence detector activated by glutamate and postsynaptic depolarization. When activated, the NMDA receptor becomes permeant to calcium. The resultant influx of calcium into the postsynaptic neuron activates a number of second messenger signaling pathways, including calmodulin kinases (CaMKs), adenylyl cyclase, and mitogen-activated protein kinases (MAPKs)[102] (Fig. 11-11). Synaptic plasticity and behavioral memory are also modulated by neurotransmitters that activate G protein–coupled receptors, such as dopamine and norepinephrine, which in turn also modulate intracellular signaling pathways.

This local synaptic activation mediates plasticity for the first hour or so after induction of LTP. Long-term plasticity, called L-LTP, lasts for many hours and involves the induction of new gene transcription and the synthesis of new proteins.[103] Thus, long-lasting forms of LTP, like long-term memory, are selectively sensitive to inhibition of protein and RNA synthesis. Study of the molecular mechanisms of translational and transcriptional regulation has led to two surprises in recent years. First, the synthesis of new proteins can occur, in part, within the dendrite locally at the synapse, thereby providing a potentially long-lasting synaptic tag to mark synapses that are potentiated.[104] Second, regulation of transcription involves epigenetic mechanisms of chromatin modification, DNA methylation, and chromatin remodeling—mechanisms that were thought to function primarily in a developmental context.[105] It is interesting to suggest that memory may, in part, be stored as epigenetic modifications that alter the expression of select genes.

One important question is how activation of these various signal transduction pathways, changes in gene expression, and epigenetic marks give rise to long-lasting increases in synaptic transmission and memory. The α-amino-3-hydroxy-5-methyl-4-isoxazopropionic acid (AMPA)-type glutamate receptor provides one potential target of these molecular mechanisms. Kinases activated by influx of calcium, such as CaMKII, phosphorylate the GluR1 subunit of the AMPA receptor, which increases its open time and the amount of receptor available on the cell surface at the synapse.[106] Increased levels and activity of the AMPA receptor would increase the depolarization resulting from release of glutamate at the synapse, thereby increasing synaptic strength. Long-lasting forms of LTP activate gene expression and increase transcription of the gene encoding GluR1.[107] Thus, although there are clearly a variety of molecular targets by which synaptic strength can be stably enhanced, the AMPA receptor provides an attractive effector mechanism.

Anesthetic-Induced Amnesia

At larger doses, administration of virtually any anesthetic drug produces loss of consciousness, which in turn results in episodic amnesia. Because monitors capable of assessing memory formation, storage, and retrieval are lacking, one common clinical strategy relies on delivery of hypnotic doses of anesthetics to ensure amnesia. However, anesthetic drugs have the capacity to produce amnesia at subhypnotic doses. The engrams (physical alterations in neural tissue thought to be the substrate for memory) most readily impaired by anesthetic drugs involve episodic memories. Although multiple mechanisms might account for anesthetic-induced amnesia, at subhypnotic doses, benzodiazepines such as midazolam and intravenous anesthetics such as propofol primarily affect either long-term memory storage or its retrieval. At plasma concentrations of 40 ng/mL of midazolam or 0.9 μg/mL of propofol, humans are able to encode and retain memories over a period of 15 to 30 minutes. However, these memories are lost before consolidation.[108]

Even though the circuit-level, neuronal, and molecular mechanisms of anesthetic-induced amnesia remain incompletely understood, animal studies suggest that amnestic doses of anesthetics have the capacity to interfere with memory formation at multiple points. For the volatile anesthetics, memory formation is impaired at drug concentrations between a 25% and 50% the minimum alveolar concentration (MAC) in humans[109] and rodents,[110] with individual agents differing slightly in their amnestic potency relative to their MAC (immobilizing dose).[111]

LTP is a form of synaptic plasticity thought to contribute to memory and it represents a cellular model of memory as discussed earlier. In addition to impairing memory at the behavioral level, anesthetics such as isoflurane may also impair or completely abolish LTP in hippocampal slice preparations.[112] Other anesthetics such as barbiturates, benzodiazepines, and propofol likewise alter the expression of LTP and long-term depression in hippocampal slice preparations, thereby providing cellular correlates of their amnestic properties.[113-115] In these instances, anesthetics are

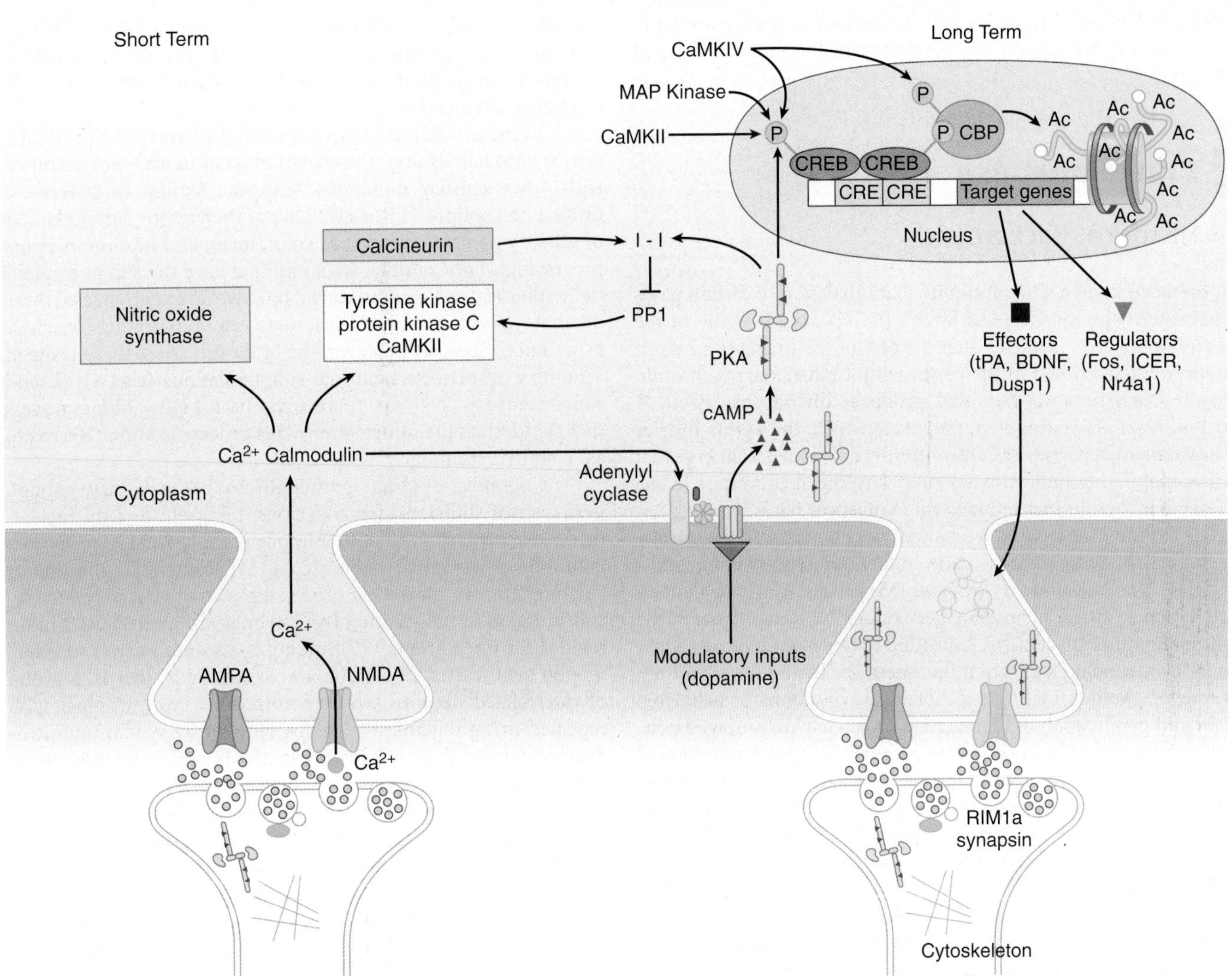

Figure 11-11 Long-term potentiation and long-term memory are mediated by similar molecular mechanisms involving calcium influx through the *N*-methyl-D-aspartate receptor and activation of intracellular signaling pathways that lead to activation of gene expression and synthesis of new proteins. *(Modified from Abel T, Nguyen PV, Barad M, et al: Genetic demonstration of a role for PKA in the late phase of LTP and in hippocampus-based long-term memory. Cell 88:615-626, 1997.)*

thought to impair LTP via GABAergic mechanisms.[112] α_5 Subunit-containing $GABA_A$ receptors are highly sensitive to amnestic concentrations of isoflurane.[116] However, other receptor signaling systems are certainly involved in mediating anesthetic-induced amnesia.[117-119]

Hippocampal θ rhythms (or θ oscillations) are the largest-amplitude synchronous EEG signals that can be recorded from mammalian brain. θ Oscillations have a characteristic frequency in the 5- to 12-Hz range in the behaving rat and dominate the EEG spectrum during NREM sleep (as discussed earlier), as well as during waking behavior essential for survival, such as exploration. Hippocampal θ oscillations are thought to facilitate mnemonic processes in vitro and in vivo. At the circuit level, anesthetics have recently been shown to alter hippocampal θ oscillations, a finding that may underlie anesthetic-induced amnesia.[120]

At the molecular level, propofol inhibits NMDA receptor–mediated activation of one subclass of the MAPK superfamily, extracellular signal–regulated protein kinase 1/2 (ERK1/2), in hippocampal neurons. This results in concurrent inhibition of transcriptional activity inasmuch as interference with MAPKs can uncouple synaptic events from nuclear responses. This finding might provide a molecular mechanism through which an anesthetic impairs transcription-dependent encoding of memory.[117,119] However, whether this mechanism represents a common action of anesthetic-induced amnesia awaits further elucidation.

The hippocampus is not the only limbic system structure thought to be involved in anesthetic-induced amnesia. It has now been established in animal models that the basolateral nucleus of the amygdala is critical for the amnestic effects of general anesthetics. Propofol, benzodiazepines, and sevoflurane lose their amnestic power if the basal nucleus of the amygdala is lesioned.[121,122] These data suggest that the amnestic doses of general anesthetics modulate output of the amygdala in such a way that memory formation is diminished. The role of the amygdala in anesthetic-mediated amnesia may be related to the hippocampus because the two structures are strongly interconnected. Furthermore, the inability of an anesthetic agent to suppress memory has clinical implications for patients who are experiencing intraoperative awareness, a topic to which we turn in the next section.

Consciousness

Historical Background

It has been known since antiquity that inhalation of certain gases may alter consciousness. As Strabo (64 BC-AD 25) wrote of the Delphic oracles: "They say that the seat of the oracle is a cavern hollowed deep down in the earth, with a rather narrow mouth, from which rises a vapor that produces divine possession. A tripod is set above this cleft, mounting which, the Pythia inhales the vapor and prophesies." Only recently did evidence emerge that the general anesthetic ethylene may have been the vapor in the Temple of Apollo that induced these mystical states.[123]

In the modern era, renowned psychologist William James' experiments with nitrous oxide influenced one of his greatest works, *The Varieties of Religious Experience*, and yielded an 1898 article titled "Consciousness under Nitrous Oxide."[124] By the end of the 19th century, James and others regarded consciousness as a fundamental scientific question. In the 20th century, however, the dominating psychological paradigms of behaviorism and psychoanalysis disregarded or actively discouraged consciousness as a subject of serious inquiry. This antipathy toward the scientific study of consciousness persisted until the 1980s. Although Harvard anesthesiologist Henry Beecher promoted general anesthetics as a tool to study consciousness in the mid-20th century,[125] it was not until the 21st century that a true renaissance of interest in consciousness and anesthesia emerged. The current focus on consciousness within the field of anesthesiology is related primarily to anesthetic mechanisms or intraoperative awareness.

Neural Correlates of Consciousness

Whereas philosophers at the time of the Delphic oracles were concerned with the nature of being (ontology), the focus of 18th century thinkers such as Immanuel Kant was the nature and mechanism of knowing (epistemology). In his *Critique of Pure Reason*, Kant argued that our minds affect the ideas that we have about nature. Human experience of reality has two nonintersecting parts: (1) the part accessed by our senses (the phenomenal realm) and (2) the part outside cognition (the noumenal realm). The mind must posses, according to Kant, innate categories to be able to take the information in the phenomenal realm and make inferences about what lies in the noumenal one. Stated another way, he posited that the mind was modular, with discrete faculties that subserved specific cognitive functions. He recognized, however, that for these specific functions to be translated into a unified perceptual experience, there must be a process of integration that is essential.

Consistent with the philosophy of Kant, neuroscientist Giulio Tononi has proposed a 21st-century "information integration" theory of consciousness, as well as a theoretical model that expresses the capacity of neural systems to synthesize information.[126,127] Tononi suggests that consciousness reflects a higher capacity to integrate information processed in functionally specialized modules, which is why, for example, thalamocortical circuits seem to be more relevant to conscious processes than cerebellar circuits do.

In more concrete terms, the neural correlates of particular sensory modalities (e.g., the visual) must ultimately be combined with other sensory modalities (e.g., the tactile) to generate a unified perception. This is also true of the various submodalities of sensory perception (such as color, form, and motion in visual processing). For example, we do not perceive the sun as sequentially spherical, yellow, and warm, but instead experience all these distinct traits at one time. Thus, there is a unity to our conscious experience. Because, however, the brain processes these traits in a number of discrete neuronal subpopulations (e.g., visual and somatosensory cortices), there must be a higher-order process that synthesizes the information. This process is often referred to as "cognitive binding."[128,129]

Cognitive binding is thought to be necessary, though perhaps not sufficient, for consciousness itself. Several mechanisms for integration of neural information have been proposed, including convergence, assembly, and synchrony.[130,131] Binding by convergence is a hierarchic processing strategy characterized by transmission of information from primary to higher-order brain regions for integration.[132-134] Binding by assembly refers to information synthesized in a Hebbian cell assembly, that is, a group of interrelated neurons whose connections grow stronger with repeated firing together.[135] Finally, binding by synchrony introduces a temporal dimension to synthesis and is thought to be associated with neural events at the frequency of 40 Hz.[136-138]

Many of the neural regions or processes that are considered correlates of consciousness are linked to integration of information. Neural correlates may be identified through a number of methods, including clinicopathologic correlation, functional neuroimaging, and neurophysiologic recording. A number of candidates for the neural substrate of consciousness emerged in the 1980s and 1990s, including

- Extended reticular-thalamic activation system[139]
- Intralaminar nucleus in the thalamus[140]
- Reentrant loops in thalamocortical systems[141]
- 40-Hz rhythmic activity in thalamocortical systems[137]
- Neurons in the superior temporal sulcus[142]
- Neural activity in visual area V5/MT[143]
- Neurons in the extrastriate visual cortex projecting to prefrontal areas[144]
- Anterior cingulate system[145]
- Recurrent processing from higher to lower cortical areas[146]

Rees and colleagues discussed the evidence for many of these neural correlates of human consciousness.[147] As we discuss in the following sections, these correlates may serve as the anatomic or neurophysiologic substrates on which general anesthetics act to suppress consciousness.

Effects of Anesthetics on Neural Correlates

General anesthetics may generate unconsciousness by suppressing the activity of the neural correlates at various levels of neural organization, as well as by disrupting processes of information integration. It has become clear that many of the proposed neural correlates of consciousness are modulated by general anesthetics.

Subcortical and Thalamocortical Effects

Functional neuroimaging by positron-emission tomography (PET) during isoflurane or halothane anesthesia demonstrated reduced cerebral glucose metabolism in subcortical structures associated with arousal, including the thalamus and midbrain reticular formation.[49] PET has also revealed suppression of thalamic activity in association with propofol-induced unconsciousness.[61] Other subcortical structures affected include the arousal-promoting TMN in the hypothalamus, which has been associated with anesthetic-induced hypnosis.[66]

Recent data acquired by electrophysiologic techniques in humans have brought into question the role of subcortical structures such as the thalamus. Because PET has poor temporal resolution,[148] Velly and associates compared cortical EEG tracings with recordings from subcortical deep brain electrodes in the human subthalamic nucleus. The authors were able to deduce that their field recordings were actually detecting thalamic rather than subthalamic activity. Loss of consciousness with propofol or sevoflurane was correlated with the cortical EEG, whereas minimal changes in the subcortical recording were identified. As discussed earlier, Alkire and colleagues demonstrated that nicotinic cholinergic agonism in the central medial thalamic nucleus could reverse sevoflurane-induced unconsciousness.[64] Although it would appear that these data contradict the findings of Velly and coworkers, administration of the nicotinic antagonist mecamylamine in the central medial nucleus did not induce anesthesia or even reduce anesthetic requirements. Alkire and associates concluded that the central medial nucleus may be an "on" switch for arousal but not an "off" switch for anesthesia.

The thalamocortical system is thought to be critical for consciousness. The resonance of thalamocortical circuits has been proposed as the "dynamic core" of consciousness[141] and is consistent with cognitive binding by 40-Hz oscillations.[137] Alkire and associates described a "unified theory of narcosis" based on the finding that thalamocortical circuits were disrupted under general anesthesia.[49] It has been demonstrated that isoflurane and halothane disrupt functional connectivity between the thalamus and cortex.[149] Functional connectivity is the causal influence of one brain region on another that occurs beyond a mere anatomic connection.[150] Propofol has also been shown to induce a hyperpolarization block of thalamocortical neurons.[151]

Cortical and Corticocortical Effects

General anesthetics have been demonstrated to affect a number of cortical brain regions. Variable electromagnetic tomographic analysis has demonstrated that multiple general anesthetics induce reversible inhibition of the medial orbital and dorsolateral prefrontal and frontal cortex, anterior cingulate cortex, and paracentral gyrus.[152] The finding of frontal and cingulate cortex inhibition was consistent with previous PET findings of propofol-induced anesthesia.[61] As noted earlier, both the prefrontal and anterior cingulate cortices have been proposed as neural correlates of conscious processing.

It has been demonstrated that general anesthetics of distinct pharmacologic properties affect EEG coherence in a similar way during unconsciousness, an effect that is reversed on the return of consciousness.[152] In 176 cases of human surgical anesthesia using a variety of both inhaled and intravenous anesthetics, there were invariant changes in the electrical uncoupling of brain regions. Multivariate analysis of quantitative EEG recordings showed that γ oscillations (35 to 50 Hz) of the rostral and caudal regions of the brain became uncoupled from one another. These changes were associated with the onset of anesthesia, intensified with increasing depth of anesthesia, and reversed with the termination of anesthesia.

Rostrocaudal dissociation is of particular relevance given the proposed scans of 40-Hz oscillations that sweep from the frontal to the occipital cortex and back again.[137] In addition to this functional rostrocaudal disconnection, the hemispheres themselves became functionally disconnected. The effects of anesthesia on rostrocaudal processing have been studied in animal models as well. It has been demonstrated that processing of visual stimuli during anesthesia can be transmitted from the occipital to the frontal cortex, whereas recurrent processing from the frontal back to the occipital cortex is interrupted.[153] This finding is consistent with the proposed neural correlate of recurrent processing of neural information,[146] that is, transmission of signals from higher-order areas back to primary processing areas.

Other studies in humans have shown functional uncoupling of neural regions in association with general anesthesia. Peltier and colleagues demonstrated loss of functional connectivity in the cerebral cortex during sevoflurane anesthesia.[154] This provides further evidence that anesthetics uncouple the activity of cortical regions that would otherwise influence one another in the waking state.

Information Dissociation and Unconscious States

Based on the effect of anesthetic-mediated interruption of neural information synthesis, a "cognitive unbinding" paradigm of general anesthesia was postulated.[155,156] This framework explicitly stated that anesthetics may function by interrupting various cognitive binding processes from the cellular to the global brain level. This was based, in part, on findings by John and associates[152] that demonstrated functional uncoupling of the hemispheric and rostrocaudal axes of the brain (interruption of synchronous binding). The cognitive unbinding paradigm was also based on interruption of synthetic processes in cortical area MT under isoflurane (interruption of convergent binding).[157]

John and Prichep's "anesthetic cascade" supported the concept of cognitive unbinding while at the same time postulated a specific stepwise process by which anesthetics suppress consciousness.[158] The proposed "cascade" is as follows:

- Depression of the brainstem reduces the influence of the ascending reticular activating system on the thalamus and cortex.
- Depression of mesolimbic-dorsolateral prefrontal cortex interactions leads to blockade of memory storage.
- Further depression of the ascending reticular activating system leads to hyperpolarization of GABAergic neurons in the nucleus reticularis of the thalamus, which results in
- Blockade of thalamocortical reverberations and the associated γ oscillations underlying perception,

Functional uncoupling of parietal-frontal cortical activity, thereby interrupting cognition, and finally
Reduced awareness of and increase in frontal δ- and θ-band activity.

Recent data on the temporal relationship of subcortical anesthetic effects bring into question the first step of the cascade.[148] Furthermore, it is unclear how agents such as ketamine or nitrous oxide, which can lead to EEG activation rather than depression,[159,160] fit within the proposed anesthetic cascade. Nonetheless, the anesthetic cascade is one of the most specific and data-driven theories of anesthetic-induced unconsciousness.

Walling and Hicks supported both cognitive unbinding and the anesthetic cascade based on EEG phase-space analysis of emergence from sevoflurane anesthesia in humans.[161] Return of consciousness was characterized by a higher-dimensional phase space, reflecting a complexity of brain dynamics that could sustain consciousness. The fractal "strange attractors" that were identified on emergence were posited to be the coherence of γ-band frequencies associated with consciousness, in what the authors referred to as "cognitive rebinding."

These frameworks of anesthetic-induced unconsciousness as information dissociation are supported by recent studies of other unconscious states. Studies of brain-injured patients in vegetative states have revealed fragmented cerebral activity[162] and loss of effective cortical connectivity.[163] It has therefore been suggested that vegetative states are "disconnection" syndromes.[164] The neural regions affected in vegetative states include the frontal cortex, cingulate cortex, association cortices, and thalamus,[164] which are also targets for general anesthetics. Like anesthesia, recovery from vegetative states is associated with return of thalamocortical connectivity.[165]

As discussed earlier, sleep is a state with a number of traits similar to general anesthesia.[166] Using transcranial magnetic stimulation and EEG recordings of subjects either asleep or awake, Massimini and coworkers[167] demonstrated that NREM sleep is also characterized by loss of effective cortical connectivity. The loss of cortical connectivity associated with sleep suggests a common feature with anesthetic-induced unconsciousness and vegetative states.

Consciousness in the Operating Room

Although consciousness is emerging as an important scientific problem that is intimately linked to the mechanism of general anesthesia, it can also pose a clinical problem intraoperatively. Awareness during general anesthesia—which denotes both awareness and subsequent explicit recall of intraoperative events—is a complication receiving increased attention by both patients and clinicians. Dreaming is another subjective state that can occur during anesthesia, with an incidence of 22% in patients undergoing elective cases.[168] Although some cases represented "near-miss" experiences of awareness, others were thought to occur during recovery from anesthesia.

Despite recent attention by the medical community and the lay press, the incidence of intraoperative awareness—and hence the magnitude of the problem—remains uncertain. A multicenter study in the United States by Sebel and colleagues[169] estimated an incidence of awareness with explicit recall of approximately 0.13%, a rate consistent with large European studies demonstrating awareness in 1 to 2 per 1000 cases.[170] In contrast, a recent study of awareness in a regional medical system reported a much lower incidence of 1 episode of awareness per 14,560 cases, or 0.0069%.[171] The timing and content of postoperative interviews probably play a role in this discrepancy.

A proportion of patients experiencing awareness may subsequently exhibit serious psychological sequelae, including post-traumatic stress disorder.[172] Earlier studies reported a greater than 50% incidence of post-traumatic stress disorder, whereas more recent studies suggest a much lower rate of occurrence.[173] Because of the profound distress that it can induce in patients, a reliable and practical method of detecting intraoperative consciousness would be an important clinical advance.

Assessing Consciousness Intraoperatively

As early as 1937, Gibbs and coauthors reported that EEG measurements were sensitive to the effects of general anesthetics.[174] However, the use of unprocessed EEG data to assess anesthetic depth in the operating room is impractical for a number of reasons: (1) there is no unique electrical "signature" of an unprocessed EEG that is invariant, (2) the use of standard multiple-channel diagnostic EEG devices is cumbersome in the intraoperative setting, and (3) the use of such diagnostic devices—capable of localizing the source of abnormal signal patterns—generally requires a dedicated interpreter. Because of these limitations, EEG monitors with a minimal number of channels that use processing algorithms have been developed in an attempt to monitor anesthetic depth and detect intraoperative awareness (see Chapter 39).

Fourier transformation of raw EEG data enables the derivation of median power and spectral edge frequencies, and a number of devices available for intraoperative use are based on Fourier-transformed EEG data.[175] The bispectral index (BIS; Aspect Medical Systems, Natick MA) analyzes burst suppression, β-band power, and bispectral coherence of δ and θ waves.[176] The Narcotrend Monitor (MonitorTechnik, Bad Bramstedt, Germany) analyzes stages and substages of anesthesia and was based on a similar developmental process as the BIS (with a distinct algorithm).[177] The Patient State Index (PSI; Physiometrix, Inc., N. Billerica, MA) is derived from quantitative EEG techniques and is based on signal relationships between the frontal and occipital brain regions.[178] Entropy monitors (e.g., S/5, Instrumentarium Corp. [Datex-Ohmeda], Helsinki, Finland) are based on the concept of information entropy posited by Shannon[179] and analyze randomness in frequency and phase relationships with the use of both EEG and frontal EMG.[180] Entropy monitors measure state entropy (response over the range of 0.8 to 32 Hz, reflecting the EEG-dominant spectrum) and response entropy (response over the range of 0.8 to 47 Hz, reflecting both EEG and EMG spectra). Whereas the aforementioned monitors record spontaneous EEG, the stimulus-response technique of auditory evoked potentials has also been used to assess anesthetic depth and can be analyzed in conjunction with other EEG signaling parameters.[181,182] Because the BIS has been extensively studied and is the most frequently used monitor to assess depth of anesthesia, it will be the focus of the remaining sections.

Development and Validation of the BIS Monitor

The BIS monitor was developed empirically by analyzing a high-fidelity database of EEG recordings from approximately 2000 patients who received a variety of commonly used general anesthetics, sedative-hypnotics, and opioids (see Chapter 39).[176] Segments of the EEG were compared with clinical findings of hypnosis; candidate spectral and bispectral features of these segments were computed and tested for their ability to distinguish the clinically described hypnotic states. The best of these features were then combined by multivariate statistical modeling to form a composite index (dimensionless number between 0 and 100, where 0 is isoelectric and 100 is awake), which underwent further prospective testing in a larger database.

In the mid-1990s, a number of studies demonstrated that changes in BIS values were associated with movement in response to noxious stimuli, as well as hemodynamic responses to interventions such as laryngoscopy. A multicentered study using movement as the measured outcome found that BIS values had better response with hypnotic drugs such as isoflurane and propofol than with opiates.[183] Whereas some studies focused on the relationship of BIS to movement in an attempt to validate the BIS in terms of MAC, other studies investigated the relationship of BIS to hypnosis, or MAC-awake. Flaishon and associates[184] used propofol or thiopental to induce anesthesia while continuously monitoring the BIS. BIS values above 60 were highly correlated with the ability of subjects to respond to verbal command. Another multicentered investigation focused on validation of the BIS monitor by comparing BIS values with anesthetic drug concentrations and level of sedation.[185] Other studies confirmed the value of the BIS in measuring hypnotic response to both inhaled and intravenous general anesthetics.[186,187] The BIS has also been validated for assessing the depth of anesthesia in children.[188,189]

One study in a high-risk population showed a significantly decreased incidence of confirmed awareness.[190] When combining both "possible" and "confirmed" awareness events, however, there was no difference between the BIS and control groups. Furthermore, the high number needed to treat (138) and the associated cost ($2200 U.S. dollars) in the high-risk group bring into question use of the BIS to prevent awareness in the general population.

Comparison of the BIS with Other EEG-Based Monitors

Because of validation of the BIS in a number of clinical studies, other emerging technologies have been compared with the BIS for validation. Chen and coworkers[191] demonstrated that the PSI correlated well with the BIS during anesthesia induction, maintenance, and emergence. The PSI and BIS were found to be comparable in a small study of intravenous and inhaled anesthetics, with the PSI reported to have less electrocautery artifact.[192]

The Narcotrend monitor has been shown to correlate well with predicted propofol concentrations in addition to the BIS.[177] The Narcotrend index correlated with the BIS during propofol and remifentanil anesthesia in a small number of patients (n = 26).[193] The BIS and Narcotrend indices were also shown to be comparable in monitoring the depth of isoflurane anesthesia.[177]

State entropy and response entropy show close correlation with the BIS in assessing sevoflurane anesthesia,[194] as well as propofol-remifentanil anesthesia.[195] In a small study evaluating loss of response to verbal command and loss of consciousness during propofol anesthesia, it was suggested that state entropy may be more useful than the BIS.[196] One study also demonstrated comparable performance of the BIS and entropy modules during both intravenous and inhaled anesthesia, with less electrocautery interference by the entropy monitor.[197]

Limitations of the BIS

There are numerous limitations associated with BIS monitoring.[198] One such limitation is that BIS values remain unchanged or even elevated during nitrous oxide anesthesia.[160,199] The intravenous anesthetic ketamine may also elevate BIS levels,[159,200] perhaps reflecting its ability to increase the beta power of the EEG spectrum.[201] It is of interest that both ketamine and nitrous oxide are thought to act primarily through NMDA glutamate receptors.[202] The anesthetic effect of xenon, which also acts on this receptor system, is similarly not reflected with BIS technology.[203] It is of further interest that although spectral entropy values are increased by ketamine in a similar manner to the BIS,[204] the addition of nitrous oxide has been shown to decrease state and response entropy values.[205] Conversely, BIS values are sensitive to nonanesthetic agents routinely administered in the operating room and have been shown to decrease in patients receiving neuromuscular blockers, while fully conscious[206] and while anesthetized.[207] BIS values derived from multiple sensors on the same patient have also been shown to be discordant, suggesting intrapatient variability and poor reproducibility of the index.[208] These and other limitations indicate the need for more sophisticated monitors of anesthetic depth that are linked to the neurophysiologic mechanisms of consciousness.

Conclusion

The oscillating states of sleep and wakefulness are fundamental features of our existence; as such, they have been pondered philosophically since antiquity and explored scientifically in modern times. The field of anesthesiology has much to gain from these investigations and, just as importantly, much to offer in return. Our further understanding of the neuroscientific mechanisms of general anesthesia may provide fundamental insight into the nature of consciousness, unconsciousness, and the memories that bind them together to form a stable sense of self.

References

1. Rechtschaffen A, Bergmann BM, Everson CA, et al: Sleep deprivation in the rat: X. Integration and discussion of the findings. Sleep 25:68, 2002.
2. Rial RV, Nicolau MC, Gamundi A, et al: The trivial function of sleep. Sleep Med Rev 11:311, 2007.
3. Frank MG: The mystery of sleep function: Current perspectives and future directions. Rev Neurosci 17:375, 2006.
4. Gally JA, Edelman GM: Neural reapportionment: An hypothesis to account for the function of sleep. C R Biol 327:721, 2004.
5. Tononi G, Cirelli C: Sleep function and synaptic homeostasis. Sleep Med Rev 10:49, 2006.
6. Moruzzi G, Magoun HW: Brain stem reticular formation and activation of the EEG. Electroencephalogr Clin Neurophysiol 1:455, 1949.
7. Bremer F: Cerveau "isole" et physiologie du sommeil. C R Soc Biol 118:1235, 1935.
8. von Economo C: Sleep as a problem of localization. J Nerv Ment Dis 71:249, 1930.
9. McGinty DJ, Sterman MB: Sleep suppression after basal forebrain lesions in the cat. Science 160:1253, 1968.
10. Nauta W: Hypothalamic regulation of sleep in rats. An experimental study. J Neurophysiol 9:285, 1946.

11. Lin JS, Sakai K, Vanni-Mercier G, et al: A critical role of the posterior hypothalamus in the mechanisms of wakefulness determined by microinjection of muscimol in freely moving cats. Brain Res 479:225, 1989.
12. Sherin JE, Shiromani PJ, McCarley RW, et al: Activation of ventrolateral preoptic neurons during sleep. Science 271:216, 1996.
13. Szymusiak R, Alam N, Steininger TL, et al: Sleep-waking discharge patterns of ventrolateral preoptic/anterior hypothalamic neurons in rats. Brain Res 803:178, 1998.
14. Saper CB, Chou TC, Scammell TE: The sleep switch: Hypothalamic control of sleep and wakefulness. Trends Neurosci 24:726, 2001.
15. Saper CB: Staying awake for dinner: Hypothalamic integration of sleep, feeding, and circadian rhythms. Prog Brain Res 153:243, 2006.
16. Harris CD: Neurophysiology of sleep and wakefulness. Respir Care Clin N Am 11:567, 2005.
17. Lu J, Jhou TC, Saper CB: Identification of wake-active dopaminergic neurons in the ventral periaqueductal gray matter. J Neurosci 26:193, 2006.
18. Jones BE: From waking to sleeping: Neuronal and chemical substrates. Trends Pharmacol Sci 26:578, 2005.
19. Lee MG, Hassani OK, Jones BE: Discharge of identified orexin/hypocretin neurons across the sleep-waking cycle. J Neurosci 25:6716, 2005.
20. Mileykovskiy BY, Kiyashchenko LI, Siegel JM: Behavioral correlates of activity in identified hypocretin/orexin neurons. Neuron 46:787, 2005.
21. Jones BE: Arousal systems. Front Biosci 8:s438, 2003.
22. Steriade M, Timofeev I: Neuronal plasticity in thalamocortical networks during sleep and waking oscillations. Neuron 37:563, 2003.
23. Sherin JE, Elmquist JK, Torrealba F, et al: Innervation of histaminergic tuberomammillary neurons by GABAergic and galaninergic neurons in the ventrolateral preoptic nucleus of the rat. J Neurosci 18:4705, 1998.
24. Lu J, Greco MA, Shiromani P, et al: Effect of lesions of the ventrolateral preoptic nucleus on NREM and REM sleep. J Neurosci 20:3830, 2000.
25. Steriade M: The corticothalamic system in sleep. Front Biosci 8:d878, 2003.
26. McCarley RW: Neurobiology of REM and NREM sleep. Sleep Med 8:302, 2007.
27. Webster HH, Jones BE: Neurotoxic lesions of the dorsolateral pontomesencephalic tegmentum–cholinergic cell area in the cat. II. Effects upon sleep-waking states. Brain Res 458:285, 1988.
28. Kayama Y, Ohta M, Jodo E: Firing of "possibly" cholinergic neurons in the rat laterodorsal tegmental nucleus during sleep and wakefulness. Brain Res 569:210, 1992.
29. Steriade M, Datta S, Pare D, et al: Neuronal activities in brain-stem cholinergic nuclei related to tonic activation processes in thalamocortical systems. J Neurosci 10:2541, 1990.
30. Lu J, Bjorkum AA, Xu M, et al: Selective activation of the extended ventrolateral preoptic nucleus during rapid eye movement sleep. J Neurosci 22:4568, 2002.
31. Jouvet M: What does a cat dream about? Trends Neurosci 2:280, 1979.
32. Sinton CM, McCarley RW: Neurophysiological mechanisms of sleep and wakefulness: A question of balance. Semin Neurol 24:211, 2004.
33. Hunsley MS, Palmiter RD: Norepinephrine-deficient mice exhibit normal sleep-wake states but have shorter sleep latency after mild stress and low doses of amphetamine. Sleep 26:521, 2003.
34. Ouyang M, Hellman K, Abel T, et al: Adrenergic signaling plays a critical role in the maintenance of waking and in the regulation of REM sleep. J Neurophysiol 92:2071, 2004.
35. Lu J, Sherman D, Devor M, et al: A putative flip-flop switch for control of REM sleep. Nature 441:589, 2006.
36. Sastre JP, Buda C, Kitahama K, et al: Importance of the ventrolateral region of the periaqueductal gray and adjacent tegmentum in the control of paradoxical sleep as studied by muscimol microinjections in the cat. Neuroscience 74:415, 1996.
37. Verret L, Fort P, Gervasoni D, et al: Localization of the neurons active during paradoxical (REM) sleep and projecting to the locus coeruleus noradrenergic neurons in the rat. J Comp Neurol 495:573, 2006.
38. Ishimori K: True cause of sleep—a hypnogenic substance as evidenced in the brain of sleep-deprived animals. Tokyo Igakkai Zasshi 23:429, 1909.
39. Legendre R, Pzeron H: Reecherches sur le besoin de sommeil consecutive a une veille prolongee. Z Allg Physiol 14:235, 1913.
40. Schoenenberger GA, Monnier M: Characterization of a delta-electroencephalogram (δ-sleep)-inducing peptide. Proc Natl Acad Sci U S A 74:1282, 1977.
41. Cravatt BF, Prospero-Garcia O, Siuzdak G, et al: Chemical characterization of a family of brain lipids that induce sleep. Science 268:1506, 1995.
42. Hobson JA, Pace-Schott EF: The cognitive neuroscience of sleep: Neuronal systems, consciousness and learning. Nat Rev Neurosci 3:679, 2002.
43. Hayaishi O, Urade Y: Prostaglandin D_2 in sleep-wake regulation: Recent progress and perspectives. Neuroscientist 8:12, 2002.
44. Scammell T, Gerashchenko D, Urade Y, et al: Activation of ventrolateral preoptic neurons by the somnogen prostaglandin D_2. Proc Natl Acad Sci U S A 95:7754, 1998.
45. Satoh S, Matsumura H, Koike N, et al: Region-dependent difference in the sleep-promoting potency of an adenosine A_{2A} receptor agonist. Eur J Neurosci 11:1587, 1999.
46. Morairty S, Rainnie D, McCarley R, et al: Disinhibition of ventrolateral preoptic area sleep-active neurons by adenosine: A new mechanism for sleep promotion. Neuroscience 123:451, 2004.
47. Kopp VJ, Shafer A: Anesthesiologists and perioperative communication. Anesthesiology 93:548, 2000.
48. Lydic R, Biebuyck JF: Sleep neurobiology: Relevance for mechanistic studies of anaesthesia. Br J Anaesth 72:506, 1994.
49. Alkire MT, Haier RJ, Fallon JH: Toward a unified theory of narcosis: Brain imaging evidence for a thalamocortical switch as the neurophysiologic basis of anesthetic-induced unconsciousness. Conscious Cogn 9:370, 2000.
50. Detsch O, Kochs E, Siemers M, et al: Increased responsiveness of cortical neurons in contrast to thalamic neurons during isoflurane-induced EEG bursts in rats. Neurosci Lett 317:9, 2002.
51. Vahle-Hinz C, Detsch O, Siemers M, et al: Local GABA(A) receptor blockade reverses isoflurane's suppressive effects on thalamic neurons in vivo. Anesth Analg 92:1578, 2001.
52. Tung A, Szafran MJ, Bluhm B, et al: Sleep deprivation potentiates the onset and duration of loss of righting reflex induced by propofol and isoflurane. Anesthesiology 97:906, 2002.
53. Tung A, Bergmann BM, Herrera S, et al: Recovery from sleep deprivation occurs during propofol anesthesia. Anesthesiology 100:1419, 2004.
54. Sleigh JW, Andrzejowski J, Steyn-Ross A, et al: The bispectral index: A measure of depth of sleep? Anesth Analg 88:659, 1999.
55. Kaputlu I, Sadan G, Ozdem S: Exogenous adenosine potentiates hypnosis induced by intravenous anaesthetics. Anaesthesia 53:496, 1998.
56. Sato T, Araki I, Kushikata T, et al: Decreased hypothalamic prostaglandin D_2 and prostaglandin E_2 contents during isoflurane anaesthesia in rats. Can J Anaesth 42:1031, 1995.
57. Eckenhoff MF, Eckenhoff RG: Quantitative autoradiography of halothane binding in rat brain. J Pharmacol Exp Ther 285:371, 1998.
58. Dong HL, Fukuda S, Murata E, et al: Excitatory and inhibitory actions of isoflurane on the cholinergic ascending arousal system of the rat. Anesthesiology 104:122, 2006.
59. Alkire MT, Miller J: General anesthesia and the neural correlates of consciousness. Prog Brain Res 150:229, 2005.
60. Steriade M, Amzica F, Contreras D: Cortical and thalamic cellular correlates of electroencephalographic burst-suppression. Electroencephalogr Clin Neurophysiol 90:1, 1994.
61. Fiset P, Paus T, Daloze T, et al: Brain mechanisms of propofol-induced loss of consciousness in humans: A positron emission tomographic study. J Neurosci 19:5506, 1999.
62. Shirvalkar P, Seth M, Schiff ND, et al: Cognitive enhancement with central thalamic electrical stimulation. Proc Natl Acad Sci U S A 103:17007, 2006.
63. Schiff ND, Giacino JT, Kalmar K, et al: Behavioural improvements with thalamic stimulation after severe traumatic brain injury. Nature 448:600, 2007.
64. Alkire MT, McReynolds JR, Hahn EL, et al: Thalamic microinjection of nicotine reverses sevoflurane-induced loss of righting reflex in the rat. Anesthesiology 107:264, 2007.
65. Hudetz AG, Wood JD, Kampine JP: Cholinergic reversal of isoflurane anesthesia in rats as measured by cross-approximate entropy of the electroencephalogram. Anesthesiology 99:1125, 2003.
66. Nelson LE, Guo TZ, Lu J, et al: The sedative component of anesthesia is mediated by GABA(A) receptors in an endogenous sleep pathway. Nat Neurosci 5:979, 2002.
67. Kelz MB, Sun Y, Chen J, et al: An essential role for orexins in emergence from general anesthesia. Proc Natl Acad Sci U S A 105:1309, 2008.
68. Nelson LE, Lu J, Guo T, et al: The alpha2-adrenoceptor agonist dexmedetomidine converges on an endogenous sleep-promoting pathway to exert its sedative effects. Anesthesiology 98:428, 2003.
69. Miller RD, Way WL, Eger EI 2nd: The effects of alpha-methyldopa, reserpine, guanethidine, and iproniazid on minimum alveolar anesthetic requirement (MAC). Anesthesiology 29:1153, 1968.
70. Johnston RR, Way WL, Miller RD: Alteration of anesthetic requirement by amphetamine. Anesthesiology 36:357, 1972.
71. Mueller RA, Smith RD, Spruill WA, et al: Central monaminergic neuronal effects on minimum alveolar concentrations (MAC) of halothane and cyclopropane in rats. Anesthesiology 42:143, 1975.
72. Roizen MF, White PF, Eger EI 2nd, et al: Effects of ablation of serotonin or norepinephrine brain-stem areas on halothane and cyclopropane MACs in rats. Anesthesiology 49:252, 1978.
73. Sukhotinsky I, Hopkins DA, Lu J, et al: Movement suppression during anesthesia: Neural projections from the mesopontine tegmentum to areas involved in motor control. J Comp Neurol 489:425, 2005.
74. Sukhotinsky I, Zalkind V, Lu J, et al: Neural pathways associated with loss of consciousness caused by intracerebral microinjection of GABA(A)-active anesthetics. Eur J Neurosci 25:1417, 2007.

75. Ma J, Shen B, Stewart LS, et al: The septohippocampal system participates in general anesthesia. J Neurosci 22:RC200, 2002.
76. Milner B, Squire LR, Kandel ER: Cognitive neuroscience and the study of memory. Neuron 20:445, 1998.
77. Zalta EN: Stanford Encyclopedia of Philosophy. Available at http://plato.stanford.edu.
78. Squire LR, Kandel ER: Memory: From Mind to Molecules. New York, Owl Books, 2000.
79. Cajal SR: The croonian lecture: La fine structure des centres nerveux. Proc R Soc Lond 5:444-468, 1894.
80. Pavlov IP, Anrep GV II: Conditioned Reflexes; an Investigation of the Physiological Activity of the Cerebral Cortex. London, Oxford University Press, Humphrey Milford, 1927.
81. Lashley KS: Basic neural mechanisms in behavior. Psychol Rev 37:1, 1930.
82. Corkin S, Amaral DG, Gonzalez RG, et al: H.M.'s medial temporal lobe lesion: Findings from magnetic resonance imaging. J Neurosci 17:3964, 1997.
83. Squire LR: Memory and the hippocampus: A synthesis from findings with rats, monkeys, and humans. Psychol Rev 99:195, 1992.
84. Jackson JH: Selected writings of John Hughlings Jackson, vol I and II. London, Hodder, 1931-1932.
85. Ribot T: Diseases of Memory. New York, Appleton, 1882.
86. Frankland PW, Bontempi B: The organization of recent and remote memories. Nat Rev Neurosci 6:119, 2005.
87. Rempel-Clower NL, Zola SM, Squire LR, et al: Three cases of enduring memory impairment after bilateral damage limited to the hippocampal formation. J Neurosci 16:5233, 1996.
88. Squire LR: Memory systems of the brain: A brief history and current perspective. Neurobiol Learn Mem 82:171, 2004.
89. Squire LR, Zola SM: Structure and function of declarative and nondeclarative memory systems. Proc Natl Acad Sci U S A 93:13515, 1996.
90. Hassabis D, Kumaran D, Vann SD, et al: Patients with hippocampal amnesia cannot imagine new experiences. Proc Natl Acad Sci U S A 104:1726, 2007.
91. Bechara A, Tranel D, Damasio H, et al: Double dissociation of conditioning and declarative knowledge relative to the amygdala and hippocampus in humans. Science 269:1115, 1995.
92. Lechner HA, Squire LR, Byrne JH: 100 years of consolidation—remembering Muller and Pilzecker. Learn Mem 6:77, 1999.
93. McGaugh JL: Memory—a century of consolidation. Science 287:248, 2000.
94. Duncan CP: The retroactive effect of electroshock on learning. J Comp Physiol Psychol 42:32, 1949.
95. Gerard RW: Physiology and psychiatry. Am J Psychiatry 106:161, 1949.
96. Hebb DO: The Organization of Behavior. New York, John Wiley & Sons, 1949.
97. Davis HP, Squire LR: Protein synthesis and memory: A review. Psychol Bull 96:518, 1984.
98. Bliss TV, Collingridge GL: A synaptic model of memory: Long-term potentiation in the hippocampus. Nature 361:31, 1993.
99. Martin SJ, Grimwood PD, Morris RG: Synaptic plasticity and memory: An evaluation of the hypothesis. Annu Rev Neurosci 23:649, 2000.
100. Moser EI, Krobert KA, Moser MB, et al: Impaired spatial learning after saturation of long-term potentiation. Science 281:2038, 1998.
101. Whitlock JR, Heynen AJ, Shuler MG, et al: Learning induces long-term potentiation in the hippocampus. Science 313:1093, 2006.
102. Malenka RC, Nicoll RA: Long-term potentiation—a decade of progress? Science 285:1870, 1999.
103. McClung CA, Nestler EJ: Neuroplasticity mediated by altered gene expression. Neuropsychopharmacology 33:3, 2008.
104. ReymannKG, Frey JU: The late maintenance of hippocampal LTP: Requirements, phases, "synaptic tagging," "late-associativity" and implications. Neuropharmacology 52:24, 2007.
105. Levenson JM, Sweatt JD: Epigenetic mechanisms in memory formation. Nat Rev Neurosci 6:108, 2005.
106. Malinow R, Malenka RC: AMPA receptor trafficking and synaptic plasticity. Annu Rev Neurosci 25:103, 2002.
107. Nayak A, Zastrow DJ, Lickteig R, et al: Maintenance of late-phase LTP is accompanied by PKA-dependent increase in AMPA receptor synthesis. Nature 394:680, 1998.
108. Veselis RA: Memory: A guide for anaesthetists. Best Pract Res Clin Anaesthesiol 21:297, 2007.
109. Dwyer R, Bennett HL, Eger EI 2nd, et al: Effects of isoflurane and nitrous oxide in subanesthetic concentrations on memory and responsiveness in volunteers. Anesthesiology 77:888, 1992.
110. Dutton RC, Maurer AJ, Sonner JM, et al: The concentration of isoflurane required to suppress learning depends on the type of learning. Anesthesiology 94:514, 2001.
111. Alkire MT, Gorski LA: Relative amnesic potency of five inhalational anesthetics follows the Meyer-Overton rule. Anesthesiology 101:417, 2004.
112. Simon W, Hapfelmeier G, Kochs E, et al: Isoflurane blocks synaptic plasticity in the mouse hippocampus. Anesthesiology 94:1058, 2001.
113. Akhondzadeh S, Stone TW: Potentiation of muscimol-induced long-term depression by benzodiazepines and prevention or reversal by pregnenolone sulfate. Pharmacol Res 38:441, 1998.
114. Nagashima K, Zorumski CF, Izumi Y: Propofol inhibits long-term potentiation but not long-term depression in rat hippocampal slices. Anesthesiology 103:318, 2005.
115. Takamatsu I, Sekiguchi M, Wada K, et al: Propofol-mediated impairment of CA1 long-term potentiation in mouse hippocampal slices. Neurosci Lett 389:129, 2005.
116. Caraiscos VB, Newell JG, You-Ten KE, et al: Selective enhancement of tonic GABAergic inhibition in murine hippocampal neurons by low concentrations of the volatile anesthetic isoflurane. J Neurosci 24:8454, 2004.
117. Fibuch EE, Wang JQ: Inhibition of the MAPK/ERK cascade: A potential transcription-dependent mechanism for the amnesic effect of anesthetic propofol. Neurosci Bull 23:119, 2007.
118. Gerlai R, McNamara A: Anesthesia induced retrograde amnesia is ameliorated by ephrinA5-IgG in mice: EphA receptor tyrosine kinases are involved in mammalian memory. Behav Brain Res 108:133, 2000.
119. Kozinn J, Mao L, Arora A, et al: Inhibition of glutamatergic activation of extracellular signal–regulated protein kinases in hippocampal neurons by the intravenous anesthetic propofol. Anesthesiology 105:1182, 2006.
120. Perouansky M, Hentschke H, Perkins M, et al: Amnesic concentrations of the nonimmobilizer 1,2-dichlorohexafluorocyclobutane (F6, 2N) and isoflurane alter hippocampal theta oscillations in vivo. Anesthesiology 106:1168, 2007.
121. Alkire MT, Nathan SV: Does the amygdala mediate anesthetic-induced amnesia? Basolateral amygdala lesions block sevoflurane-induced amnesia. Anesthesiology 102:754, 2005.
122. Alkire MT, Vazdarjanova A, Dickinson-Anson H, et al: Lesions of the basolateral amygdala complex block propofol-induced amnesia for inhibitory avoidance learning in rats. Anesthesiology 95:708, 2001.
123. Hale JR, de Boer JZ, Chanton JP, et al: Questioning the Delphic oracle. Sci Am 289:66, 2003.
124. Tymoczko D: The nitrous oxide philosopher. Atlantic Monthly 277, 1996.
125. Beecher HK: Anesthesia's second power: Probing the mind. Science 105:164, 1947.
126. Tononi G: An information integration theory of consciousness. BMC Neurosci 5:42, 2004.
127. Tononi G, Sporns O: Measuring information integration. BMC Neurosci 4:31, 2003.
128. von der Malsburg C: The binding problem of neural networks. *In* Llinas R, Churchland PS (eds): The Mind-Brain Continuum. Cambridge, MA, MIT Press, 1996.
129. von der Malsburg C: The correlation theory of brain function. *In* MPI Biophysical Chemistry, Internal Report. Max Planck Institute for Biophysical Chemistry, Göttingen, 1981, p 81.
130. Singer W: Neuronal synchronization: A solution to the binding problem? *In* Churchland PS (ed): The Mind-Brain Continuum. Cambridge, MA, MIT Press, 1996, p 101.
131. Singer W: Putative functions of temporal correlations in neocortical processing. *In* Koch C, Davis J (eds): Large Scale Neuronal Theories of the Brain. Cambridge, MA, MIT Press, 1994, p 201.
132. Kanwisher N, McDermott J, Chun MM: The fusiform face area: A module in human extrastriate cortex specialized for face perception. J Neurosci 17:4302, 1997.
133. Maunsell JH, Van Essen DC: Functional properties of neurons in middle temporal visual area of the macaque monkey. I. Selectivity for stimulus direction, speed, and orientation. J Neurophysiol 49:1127, 1983.
134. Tanaka K: Neuronal mechanisms of object recognition. Science 262:685, 1993.
135. Hebb DO: The Organization of Behavior: A Neuropsychological Theory. New York, Wiley, 1949.
136. Gray CM: The temporal correlation hypothesis of visual feature integration: Still alive and well. Neuron 24:31, 1999.
137. Joliot M, Ribary U, Llinas R: Human oscillatory brain activity near 40 Hz coexists with cognitive temporal binding. Proc Natl Acad Sci U S A 91:11748, 1994.
138. Rodriguez E, George N, Lachaux JP, et al: Perception's shadow: Long-distance synchronization of human brain activity. Nature 397:430, 1999.
139. Newman J, Baars BJ: A neural attentional model of access to consciousness: A global workspace perspective. Concepts Neurosci 4:255, 1993.
140. Bogen JE: On the neurophysiology of consciousness, parts I and II. Conscious Cogn 4:52 1995.
141. Edelman GM: The Remembered Present: A Biological Theory of Consciousness. New York, Basic Books, 1989.
142. Logothetis NK, Schall JD: Neuronal correlates of subjective visual perception. Science 245:761, 1989.
143. Tootell RB, Reppas JB, Dale AM, et al: Visual motion aftereffect in human cortical area MT revealed by functional magnetic resonance imaging. Nature 375:139, 1995.
144. Crick F, Koch C: Are we aware of neural activity in primary visual cortex? Nature 375:121, 1995.
145. Cotterill R: On the unity of conscious experience. J Consciousness Stud 2:290, 1994.
146. Cauller LJ, Kulics AT: The neural basis of the behaviorally relevant N1 component of the somatosen-

sory-evoked potential in SI cortex of awake monkeys: Evidence that backward cortical projections signal conscious touch sensation. Exp Brain Res 84:607, 1991.
147. Rees G, Kreiman G, Koch C: Neural correlates of consciousness in humans. Nat Rev Neurosci 3:261, 2002.
148. Velly LJ, Rey MF, Bruder NJ, et al: Differential dynamic of action on cortical and subcortical structures of anesthetic agents during induction of anesthesia. Anesthesiology 107:202, 2007.
149. White NS, Alkire MT: Impaired thalamocortical connectivity in humans during general-anesthetic–induced unconsciousness. Neuroimage 19:402, 2003.
150. Friston KJ, Buechel C, Fink GR, et al: Psychophysiological and modulatory interactions in neuroimaging. Neuroimage 6:218, 1997.
151. Ying SW, Abbas SY, Harrison NL, et al: Propofol block of I(h) contributes to the suppression of neuronal excitability and rhythmic burst firing in thalamocortical neurons. Eur J Neurosci 23:465, 2006.
152. John ER, Prichep LS, Kox W, et al: Invariant reversible QEEG effects of anesthetics. Conscious Cogn 10:165, 2001.
153. Imas OA, Ropella KM, Ward BD, et al: Volatile anesthetics disrupt frontal-posterior recurrent information transfer at gamma frequencies in rat. Neurosci Lett 387:145, 2005.
154. Peltier SJ, Kerssens C, Hamann SB, et al: Functional connectivity changes with concentration of sevoflurane anesthesia. Neuroreport 16:285, 2005.
155. Mashour GA: Consciousness unbound: Toward a paradigm of general anesthesia. Anesthesiology 100:428, 2004.
156. Mashour GA: Integrating the science of consciousness and anesthesia. Anesth Analg 103:975, 2006.
157. Pack CC, Berezovskii VK, Born RT: Dynamic properties of neurons in cortical area MT in alert and anaesthetized macaque monkeys. Nature 414:905, 2001.
158. John ER, Prichep LS: The anesthetic cascade: A theory of how anesthesia suppresses consciousness. Anesthesiology 102:447, 2005.
159. Sakai T, Singh H, Mi WD, et al: The effect of ketamine on clinical endpoints of hypnosis and EEG variables during propofol infusion. Acta Anaesthesiol Scand 43:212, 1999.
160. Yamamura T, Fukuda M, Takeya H, et al: Fast oscillatory EEG activity induced by analgesic concentrations of nitrous oxide in man. Anesth Analg 60:283, 1981.
161. Walling PT, Hicks KN: Nonlinear changes in brain dynamics during emergence from sevoflurane anesthesia: Preliminary exploration using new software. Anesthesiology 105:927, 2006.
162. Schiff ND, Ribary U, Moreno DR, et al: Residual cerebral activity and behavioural fragments can remain in the persistently vegetative brain. Brain 125:1210, 2002.
163. Laureys S, Goldman S, Phillips C, et al: Impaired effective cortical connectivity in vegetative state: Preliminary investigation using PET. Neuroimage 9:377, 1999.
164. Laureys S: The neural correlate of (un)awareness: Lessons from the vegetative state. Trends Cogn Sci 9:556, 2005.
165. Laureys S, Faymonville ME, Luxen A, et al: Restoration of thalamocortical connectivity after recovery from persistent vegetative state. Lancet 355:1790, 2000.
166. Lydic R, Baghdoyan HA: Sleep, anesthesiology, and the neurobiology of arousal state control. Anesthesiology 103:1268, 2005.
167. Massimini M, Ferrarelli F, Huber R, et al: Breakdown of cortical effective connectivity during sleep. Science 309:2228, 2005.
168. Leslie K, Skrzypek H, Paech MJ, et al: Dreaming during anesthesia and anesthetic depth in elective surgery patients: A prospective cohort study. Anesthesiology 106:33, 2007.
169. Sebel PS, Bowdle TA, Ghoneim MM, et al: The incidence of awareness during anesthesia: A multicenter United States study. Anesth Analg 99:833, 2004.
170. Sandin RH, Enlund G, Samuelsson P, et al: Awareness during anaesthesia: A prospective case study. Lancet 355:707, 2000.
171. Pollard RJ, Coyle JP, Gilbert RL, et al: Intraoperative awareness in a regional medical system: A review of 3 years' data. Anesthesiology 106:269, 2007.
172. Osterman JE, van der Kolk BA: Awareness during anesthesia and posttraumatic stress disorder. Gen Hosp Psychiatry 20:274, 1998.
173. Samuelsson P, Brudin L, Sandin RH: Late psychological symptoms after awareness among consecutively included surgical patients. Anesthesiology 106:26, 2007.
174. Gibbs FA, Gibbs LE, Lennox WG: Effect on the electroencephalogram of certain drugs which influence nervous activity. Arch Intern Med 60:154, 1937.
175. Rampil IJ: A primer for EEG signal processing in anesthesia. Anesthesiology 89:980, 1998.
176. Rosow C, Manberg PJ: Bispectral index monitoring. Anesthesiol Clin North Am 19:947, 2001.
177. Kreuer S, Bruhn J, Larsen R, et al: Application of Bispectral Index and Narcotrend index to the measurement of the electroencephalographic effects of isoflurane with and without burst suppression. Anesthesiology 101:847, 2004.
178. Dressler O, Schneider G, Stockmanns G, et al: Awareness and the EEG power spectrum: Analysis of frequencies. Br J Anaesth 93:806, 2004.
179. Shannon CE: A mathematical theory of communication. Bell System Technical J 27:379, 623, 1948.
180. Vakkuri A, Yli-Hankala A, Talja P, et al: Time-frequency balanced spectral entropy as a measure of anesthetic drug effect in central nervous system during sevoflurane, propofol, and thiopental anesthesia. Acta Anaesthesiol Scand 48:145, 2004.
181. Scheller B, Schneider G, Daunderer M, et al: High-frequency components of auditory evoked potentials are detected in responsive but not in unconscious patients. Anesthesiology 103:944, 2005.
182. Schneider G, Hollweck R, Ningler M, et al: Detection of consciousness by electroencephalogram and auditory evoked potentials. Anesthesiology 103:934, 2005.
183. Sebel PS, Lang E, Rampil IJ, et al: A multicenter study of bispectral electroencephalogram analysis for monitoring anesthetic effect. Anesth Analg 84:891, 1997.
184. Flaishon R, Windsor A, Sigl J, et al: Recovery of consciousness after thiopental or propofol. Bispectral index and isolated forearm technique. Anesthesiology 86:613, 1997.
185. Glass PS, Bloom M, Kearse L, et al: Bispectral analysis measures sedation and memory effects of propofol, midazolam, isoflurane, and alfentanil in healthy volunteers. Anesthesiology 86:836, 1997.
186. Katoh T, Bito H, Sato S: Influence of age on hypnotic requirement, bispectral index, and 95% spectral edge frequency associated with sedation induced by sevoflurane. Anesthesiology 92:55, 2000.
187. Kearse LA Jr, Rosow C, Zaslavsky A, et al: Bispectral analysis of the electroencephalogram predicts conscious processing of information during propofol sedation and hypnosis. Anesthesiology 88:25, 1998.
188. Denman WT, Swanson EL, Rosow D, et al: Pediatric evaluation of the bispectral index (BIS) monitor and correlation of BIS with end-tidal sevoflurane concentration in infants and children. Anesth Analg 90:872, 2000.
189. Whyte SD, Booker PD: Bispectral index during isoflurane anesthesia in pediatric patients. Anesth Analg 98:1644, 2004.
190. Myles PS, Leslie K, McNeil J, et al: Bispectral index monitoring to prevent awareness during anaesthesia: The B-Aware randomised controlled trial. Lancet 363:1757, 2004.
191. Chen X, Tang J, White PF, et al: A comparison of patient state index and bispectral index values during the perioperative period. Anesth Analg 95:1669, 2002.
192. White PF, Tang J, Ma H, et al: Is the patient state analyzer with the PSArray2 a cost-effective alternative to the bispectral index monitor during the perioperative period? Anesth Analg 99:1429, 2004.
193. Schmidt GN, Bischoff P, Standl T, et al: Comparative evaluation of Narcotrend, Bispectral Index, and classical electroencephalographic variables during induction, maintenance, and emergence of a propofol/remifentanil anesthesia. Anesth Analg 98:1346, 2004.
194. Ellerkmann RK, Liermann VM, Alves TM, et al: Spectral entropy and bispectral index as measures of the electroencephalographic effects of sevoflurane. Anesthesiology 101:1275, 2004.
195. Schmidt GN, Bischoff P, Standl T, et al: Comparative evaluation of the Datex-Ohmeda S/5 Entropy Module and the Bispectral Index monitor during propofol-remifentanil anesthesia. Anesthesiology 101:1283, 2004.
196. Iannuzzi M, Iannuzzi E, Rossi F, et al: Relationship between Bispectral Index, electroencephalographic state entropy and effect-site EC_{50} for propofol at different clinical endpoints. Br J Anaesth 94:492, 2005.
197. White PF, Tang J, Romero GF, et al: A comparison of state and response entropy versus bispectral index values during the perioperative period. Anesth Analg 102:160, 2006.
198. Dahaba AA: Different conditions that could result in the bispectral index indicating an incorrect hypnotic state. Anesth Analg 101:765, 2005.
199. Rampil IJ, Kim JS, Lenhardt R, et al: Bispectral EEG index during nitrous oxide administration. Anesthesiology 89:671, 1998.
200. Vereecke HE, Struys MM, Mortier EP: A comparison of bispectral index and ARX-derived auditory evoked potential index in measuring the clinical interaction between ketamine and propofol anaesthesia. Anaesthesia 58:957, 2003.
201. Hering W, Geisslinger G, Kamp HD, et al: Changes in the EEG power spectrum after midazolam anaesthesia combined with racemic or S- (+) ketamine. Acta Anaesthesiol Scand 38:719, 1994.
202. Sato Y, Kobayashi E, Murayama T, et al: Effect of *N*-methyl-D-aspartate receptor ε1 subunit gene disruption of the action of general anesthetic drugs in mice. Anesthesiology 102:557, 2005.
203. Goto T, Nakata Y, Saito H, et al: Bispectral analysis of the electroencephalogram does not predict responsiveness to verbal command in patients emerging from xenon anaesthesia. Br J Anaesth 85:359, 2000.
204. Hans P, Dewandre PY, Brichant JF, et al: Comparative effects of ketamine on Bispectral Index and

spectral entropy of the electroencephalogram under sevoflurane anaesthesia. Br J Anaesth 94:336, 2005.
205. Hans P, Dewandre PY, Brichant JF, et al: Effects of nitrous oxide on spectral entropy of the EEG during surgery under balanced anaesthesia with sufentanil and sevoflurane. Acta Anaesthesiol Belg 56:37, 2005.
206. Messner M, Beese U, Romstock J, et al: The bispectral index declines during neuromuscular block in fully awake persons. Anesth Analg 97:488, 2003.
207. Liu N, Chazot T, Huybrechts I, et al: The influence of a muscle relaxant bolus on bispectral and Datex-Ohmeda entropy values during propofol-remifentanil induced loss of consciousness. Anesth Analg 101:1713, 2005.
208. Niedhart DJ, Kaiser HA, Jacobsohn E, et al: Intrapatient reproducibility of the BISxp monitor. Anesthesiology 104:242, 2006.

David B. Glick

12 The Autonomic Nervous System

Key Points

1. The autonomic nervous system works in concert with renin, cortisone, and other hormones to respond to internal and external stresses.
2. The hallmark of the sympathetic nervous system is amplification; the hallmark of the parasympathetic nervous system is targeted response.
3. Inhaled and intravenous anesthetics can alter hemodynamics by influencing autonomic function.
4. β-Adrenergic blockade has emerged as important prophylaxis for ischemia and as therapy for hypertension, myocardial infarction, and congestive heart failure.
5. The sympathetic nervous system demonstrates acute and chronic adaptation to stress presynaptically and postsynaptically (e.g., biosynthesis, receptor regulation).
6. Presynaptic α-receptors play an important role in regulating sympathetic release.
7. Many therapies for the treatment of hypertension are based on direct or indirect effects of sympathetic function.
8. The vagus nerve is the superhighway of parasympathetic function; it accommodates 75% of parasympathetic traffic.
9. Aging and many disease states (e.g., diabetes, spinal cord injury) are accompanied by important changes in autonomic function.

The autonomic nervous system (ANS) controls the body's involuntary (i.e., outside of consciousness) activities. It is, at once, the most primitive and among the most essential of the body's systems—primitive in that its characteristics are largely preserved across all mammalian species and essential in that it oversees the body's responses to immediate life-threatening challenges and the body's vital maintenance needs (including cardiovascular, gastrointestinal, and thermal homeostasis). The ANS is divided into two subsystems, the sympathetic nervous system and the parasympathetic nervous system. A third subsystem, the enteric nervous system, has been added to the original characterization of the ANS. Activation of the sympathetic nervous system elicits what is traditionally called the fight-or-flight response, including redistribution of blood flow from the viscera to skeletal muscle, increased cardiac function, sweating, and pupillary dilation. The parasympathetic system governs activities of the body more closely associated with maintenance of function, such as digestive and genitourinary function. A major goal of administration of anesthetics is maintaining optimum homeostasis in patients despite powerful challenges to a sometimes tenuous physiologic balance. Intelligent administration of anesthetic care to patients requires knowledge of ANS pharmacology to achieve desirable interactions of anesthetics with the involuntary control system and to avoid responses or interactions that produce deleterious effects. Disease states may impair ANS function to a significant extent and thereby alter the expected responses to surgery and anesthesia. In addition, possible harmful effects of the human stress response have long been appreciated, and considerable effort has been expended in examining the possibility that modification or ablation of the stress response may actually improve perioperative outcome.

History and Definitions

Initially, nerves were thought to be connected in a giant syncytium. Claude Bernard, a student of Magendie, postulated the theory of transmission via synapses through the release of chemical mediators. Later, Sherrington initiated a systematic study of reflexes and described some characteristics of reflex function. A chemist, J.J. Abel, first synthesized epinephrine in 1899, and his student Langley demonstrated that it caused effects similar to those produced by stimulating postganglionic sympathetic neurons. Furthermore, Langley found that when the nerve was cut and epinephrine was injected, a more profound effect was produced, thus demonstrating denervation supersensitivity. From these observations, the concept of chemical transmission in the ANS developed. Sir Henry Dale isolated choline and studied an ester, acetylcholine, in animals. He demonstrated that it causes a marked decrease in blood pressure and vasodilation.

Nerves are traditionally classified by the chemical transmitters that they contain. Nerves containing acetylcholine are called *cholinergic*, whereas those containing norepinephrine are called *adrenergic*. In addition to classifying nerves, the term cholinergic refers to other structures or functions that relate in some way to acetylcholine. For instance, cholinergic receptors (i.e., cholinoceptors) are proteins in cell membranes that react with acetylcholine and cause the cell to respond in a characteristic way (e.g., muscles contract, glands secrete). Cholinergic agonists are drugs that act like acetylcholine on cholinoceptors to cause the cell to react in its characteristic way. They are sometimes referred to as cholinomimetic drugs. Cholinergic antagonists are drugs that react with cholinoceptors to block access by acetylcholine and thereby prevent its action. These drugs may also be referred to as cholinolytic, cholinergic-blocking, or anticholinergic drugs.

Because muscarine, a chemical isolated from a mushroom, causes effects similar to those produced by activation of the parasympathetic nervous system, it was thought to be the endogenous parasympathetic transmitter. Thus, drugs that mimic the effects of muscarine on parasympathetically innervated structures, including the heart, smooth muscles, and glands, have been called *muscarinic* drugs.

In the early 1900s, nicotine was found to act on ganglionic and skeletal muscle synapses and on nerve membranes and sensory endings. Accordingly, drugs that act on these parts of the cholinergic system are called *nicotinic* drugs. Nicotinic drugs that are more specific in their action have been discovered and are referred to by the name of the system that they affect, such as ganglionic drugs or neuromuscular drugs. Agonists and antagonists exist in each category, with little crossover of effect between drugs acting at the ganglia and those acting at the neuromuscular junction.

For the purposes of this chapter, cholinergic nerves include the following (Fig. 12-1):

1. All the motor nerves that innervate skeletal muscle
2. All postganglionic parasympathetic neurons
3. All preganglionic parasympathetic and sympathetic neurons
4. Some postganglionic sympathetic neurons, such as those that innervate the sweat glands and certain blood vessels
5. Preganglionic sympathetic neurons that arise from the greater splanchnic nerve and innervate the adrenal medulla
6. Central cholinergic neurons

Drugs mimicking the action of norepinephrine are referred to as *sympathomimetic*, whereas drugs inhibiting the effects of norepinephrine are called *sympatholytic*. Adrenergic nerves release norepinephrine at the neuroeffector junction, whereas epinephrine and norepinephrine are released by the adrenal medulla.

Adrenergic receptors have been identified and subdivided into α- and β-receptors and further subdivided into α_1, α_2, β_1, β_2, and other types. α_2-Adrenergic receptors are primarily located on the presynaptic membrane and modulate release of norepinephrine, whereas postsynaptic α_1-adrenergic receptors mediate smooth muscle vasoconstriction (Fig. 12-2). β_1-Adrenergic receptors are found primarily on cardiac tissue, and β_2-adrenergic receptors mediate smooth muscle relaxation in some organs. Adrenergic neurons can be defined as follows (see Fig. 12-1):

1. Postganglionic sympathetic neurons
2. Some interneurons
3. Certain central neurons

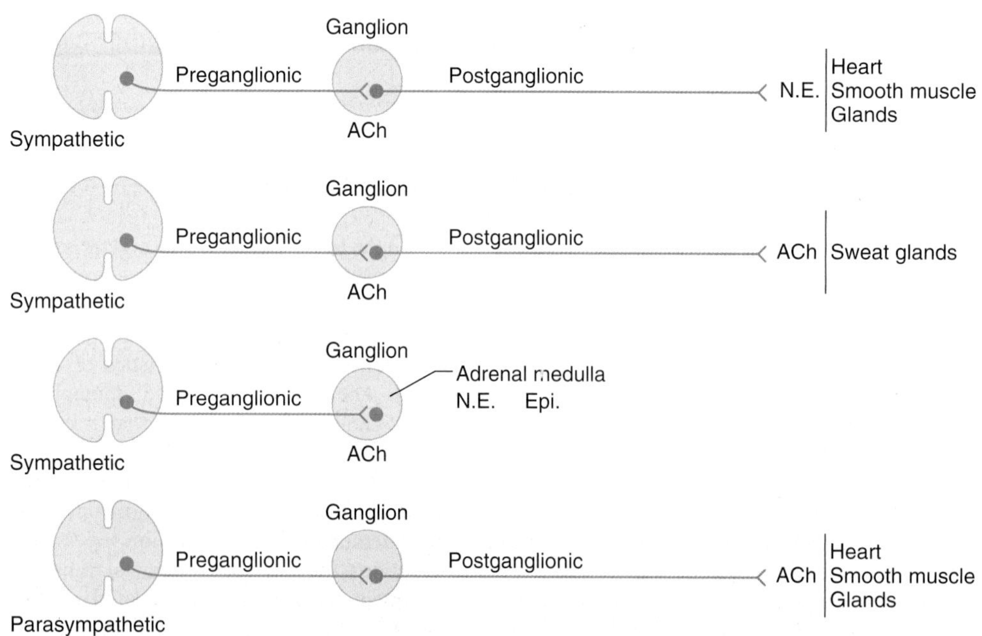

Figure 12-1 Autonomic nervous system neurotransmission. ACh, acetylcholine; Epi, epinephrine; NE, norepinephrine.

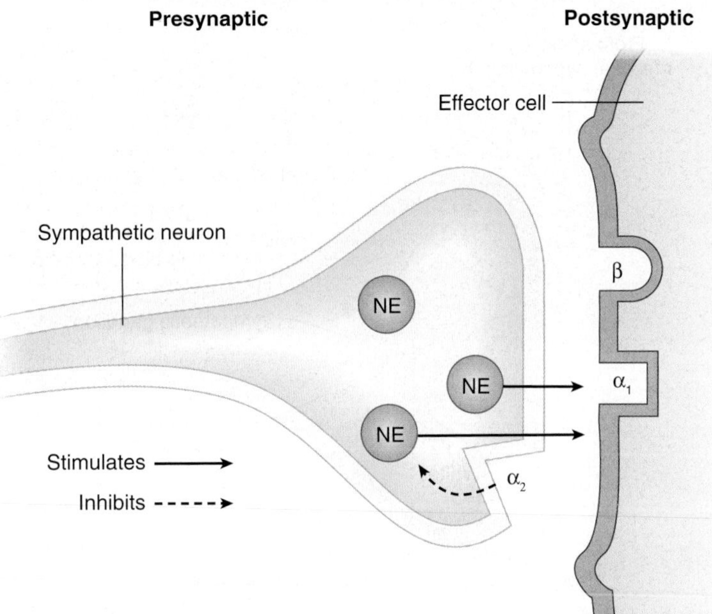

Figure 12-2 Preganglionic and postganglionic α-receptors of the sympathetic nervous system. The α_1-receptor is located postsynaptically on the membrane of the effector cell, whereas the α_2-receptor is located presynaptically on the cell membrane of the sympathetic nerve innervating the effector cell. NE, norepinephrine.

Functional Anatomy

Each branch of the ANS exhibits a different anatomic motif that is recapitulated on a cellular and molecular level. The underlying theme of the sympathetic nervous system is an amplification response, whereas that of the parasympathetic nervous system is a discrete and narrowly targeted response. The enteric nervous system is arranged nontopographically, as would be appropriate for the viscera, and relies on the mechanism of chemical coding to differentiate between nerves serving different functions.

Sympathetic Nervous System

The sympathetic nervous system originates from the spinal cord in the thoracolumbar region, from the first thoracic through the second or third lumbar segment. The preganglionic sympathetic neurons have cell bodies within the horns of the spinal gray matter (i.e., the intermediolateral columns). Nerve fibers from these cell bodies extend to three types of ganglia grouped as paired sympathetic chains, various unpaired distal plexuses, or terminal or collateral ganglia near the target organ.

The 22 paired ganglia lie along either side of the vertebral column. Nerve trunks connect these ganglia to each other, and gray rami communicantes connect the ganglia to the spinal nerves. The preganglionic fibers leave the cord in the anterior nerve roots, join the spinal nerve trunks, and enter the ganglion at their respective level through the white (myelinated) ramus. Leaving the ganglion, postsynaptic fibers reenter the spinal nerve through the gray (unmyelinated) ramus and then innervate the pilomotor and sudomotor (sweat gland) effectors and blood vessels of the skeletal muscle and skin (Fig. 12-3). Sympathetic postganglionic fibers innervate the trunk and limbs via the spinal nerves.

The sympathetic distribution to the head and neck, which enables and mediates vasomotor, pupillodilator, secretory, and pilomotor function, comes from the three ganglia of the cervical sympathetic chain. Preganglionic fibers of these cervical structures originate in the upper thoracic segments. In 80% of people, the stellate ganglion is formed by fusion of the inferior cervical ganglion with the first thoracic ganglion on each side.

The unpaired prevertebral ganglia reside in the abdomen and pelvis anterior to the vertebral column and are the celiac, superior mesenteric, aorticorenal, and inferior mesenteric ganglia. Postganglionic fibers arising from synaptic links of the upper thoracic sympathetic fibers in the vertebral ganglia form the terminal cardiac, esophageal, and pulmonary plexuses. The postganglionic fibers from the celiac, superior and inferior mesenteric plexuses innervate the viscera of the abdomen and pelvis (Fig. 12-4).

Ganglia of the third type, the terminal or collateral ganglia, are small, few in number, and near their target organs (e.g., the adrenal medulla). The adrenal medulla and other chromaffin tissue are homologous to the sympathetic ganglia, and all are derived embryonically from neural crest cells. Unlike sympathetic postganglionic fibers, however, the adrenal medulla releases epinephrine and norepinephrine.

Sympathetic preganglionic fibers are relatively short because sympathetic ganglia are generally close to the central nervous system (CNS), but they are distant from the effector organs; therefore, postganglionic fibers run a long course before innervating effector organs. The distribution is also diffuse and capable of amplification. Preganglionic sympathetic fibers may pass through multiple ganglia before synapsing, and their terminal fibers may contact large numbers of postganglionic neurons. The terminal fibers of preganglionic axons may synapse with more than 20 ganglia, and one cell may be supplied by several preganglionic fibers. Thus, preganglionic sympathetic fibers not only synapse at the ganglion of the level of their origin in the spinal cord but can also course up and down the paired ganglia. Sympathetic response, therefore, is not confined to the segment from which the stimulus originates, thereby allowing an amplified, diffuse discharge.

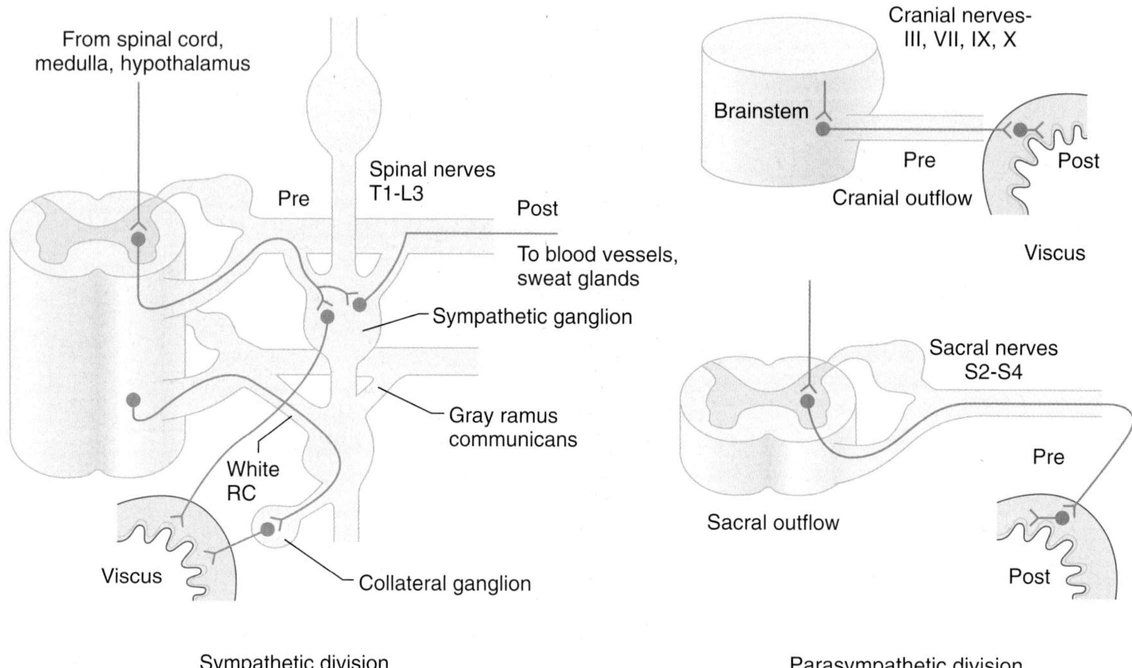

Figure 12-3 Autonomic nervous system. Pre, preganglionic neuron; Post, postganglionic neuron; RC, ramus communicans. *(From Ganong W: The autonomic nervous system.* In *Ganong W [ed]: Review of Medical Physiology, 15th ed. Norwalk, CT, Appleton & Lange, 1991, p 210.)*

Parasympathetic Nervous System

The parasympathetic nervous system arises from cranial nerves III, VII, IX, and X, as well as from sacral segments. Unlike the sympathetic nervous system, ganglia of the parasympathetic nervous system are in close proximity to or within the innervated organ. This location of ganglia makes the parasympathetic nervous system more targeted and less robust than the sympathetic nervous system.

Preganglionic fibers of the parasympathetic nervous system originate in three areas of the CNS: the midbrain, the medulla oblongata, and the sacral part of the spinal cord. Fibers arising in the Edinger-Westphal nucleus of the oculomotor nerve course in the midbrain to synapse in the ciliary ganglion. This pathway innervates the smooth muscle of the iris and the ciliary muscle. In the medulla oblongata lie parasympathetic components of the facial (lacrimatory nucleus), glossopharyngeal, and vagus (dorsal nucleus) nerves. The facial nerve gives off parasympathetic fibers to the chorda tympani, which subsequently synapses in ganglia of the submaxillary or sublingual glands, and to the greater superficial petrosal nerve, which synapses in the sphenopalatine ganglion. The glossopharyngeal nerve synapses in the otic ganglion. These postganglionic fibers innervate the mucous, salivary, and lacrimal glands; they also carry vasodilator fibers.

The vagus is the most important of the parasympathetic nerves and transmits fully three fourths of the traffic of the parasympathetic nervous system. It supplies the heart, tracheobronchial tree, liver, spleen, kidney, and entire gastrointestinal tract except for the distal part of the colon. The preganglionic fibers of the vagus are long, whereas the postganglionic fibers are short. Most vagal fibers do not synapse until they arrive at small ganglia on and about the thoracic and abdominal viscera. Although the parasympathetic nerves may synapse with a 1 : 1 ratio of nerve to effector cells, the vagal innervation of the Auerbach plexus may connect one nerve fiber to 8000 cells.

The second through fourth sacral segments contribute the nervi erigentes, or the pelvic splanchnic nerves. They synapse in terminal ganglia associated with the rectum and genitourinary organs.

Enteric Nervous System

Given the importance of clinical phenomena such as nausea, vomiting, and alterations in bowel and bladder function associated with anesthesia, it is surprising how little is understood about the third branch of the ANS. The enteric nervous system is the network of neurons and their supporting cells found within the walls of the gastrointestinal tract, including neurons within the pancreas and gallbladder. The enteric nervous system contains as many nerve cells as the spinal cord does. It is derived from neuroblasts of the neural crest that migrate to the gastrointestinal tract along the vagus nerve.

One major difference between the enteric nervous system and the sympathetic and parasympathetic branches of the ANS is its extraordinary degree of local autonomy. Digestion and peristalsis occur after spinal cord transection or during spinal anesthesia, although sphincter function may be impaired.

Although functionally discrete, the gut is influenced by sympathetic and parasympathetic activity. The sympathetic preganglionic fibers from T8 through L3 inhibit gut action via the celiac, superior, and inferior mesenteric ganglia; a spinal or epidural anesthetic covering the midthoracic levels removes this inhibition and yields a contracted, small intestine that may afford superior surgical conditions in combination with the profound

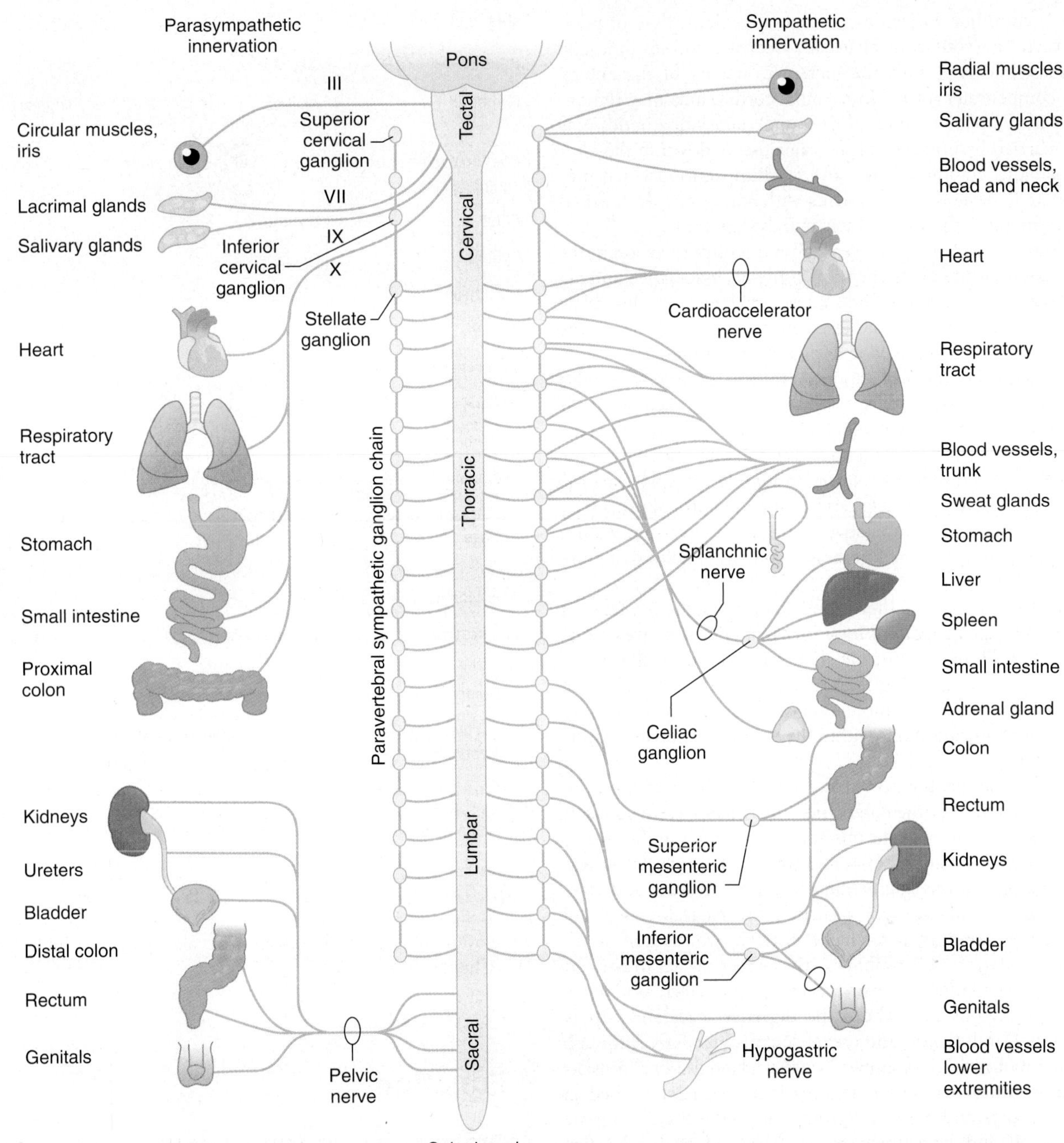

Figure 12-4 Schematic representation of the autonomic nervous system depicting the functional innervation of peripheral effector organs and the anatomic origin of peripheral autonomic nerves from the spinal cord. Although both paravertebral sympathetic ganglia chains are presented, the sympathetic innervation to the peripheral effector organs is shown only on the *right* part of the figure, whereas the parasympathetic innervation of peripheral effector organs is depicted on the *left*. The roman numerals on nerves originating in the tectal region of the brainstem refer to the cranial nerves that provide parasympathetic outflow to effector organs of the head, neck, and trunk. *(From Ruffolo R: Physiology and biochemistry of the peripheral autonomic nervous system. In* Wingard L, Brody T, Larner J, et al [eds]: *Human Pharmacology: Molecular to Clinical. St. Louis, Mosby–Year Book, 1991, p 77.)*

muscle relaxation of a spinal anesthetic. The sphincters are relaxed, and peristalsis is normally active.

Norepinephrine within the gut is the transmitter of postganglionic sympathetic neurons to the gut. For example, if the contents of the upper intestine become overly acidic or hypertonic, an adrenergically mediated enterogastric reflex reduces the rate of gastric emptying. The adrenergic neurons, which run to the myenteric ganglia of the gastrointestinal tract from the thoracic and lumbar spinal segments, are usually inactive in resting individuals. Reflex pathways within and external to the alimentary tract cause discharge of these neurons. When the viscera are handled during abdominal surgery, reflex firing of the adrenergic nerves inhibits motor activity of the intestine for an extended period. This adrenergic inhibition is thought to be the basis of the common condition known as postoperative ileus. Loss of parasympathetic nervous control usually decreases bowel tone and peristalsis, but over time, the increased activity of the enteric plexus compensates for the loss. Spinal cord lesions may remove sacral parasympathetic input, but cranial parasympathetics may still be carried by branches of the vagus nerve down to the end-organ ganglia; colonic dilation and fecal impaction (which may precipitate hypertension in patients with autonomic dysreflexia) occur more often than small intestinal dysfunction.

Enteric neurons can be sensory and monitor tension in the wall of the intestine or its chemical contents, associative and act like interneurons, or motor and contract intestinal muscles, dilate vessels, or transport water and electrolytes. Motor neurons in the enteric nervous system may be excitatory or inhibitory.

Certain plexuses play important roles in the enteric nervous system. The myenteric plexus, also called the Auerbach plexus, is a network of nerve strands and small ganglia lying in the plane between the external longitudinal and circular muscle coats of the intestine. The submucous plexus (Meissner plexus) consists of nerve cell bodies, glial cells, and glial and neuronal processes, but it does not contain connective tissue or blood vessels. Within the ganglia, many neuronal processes contain vesicles that store neurotransmitters.

Unlike the sympathetic and parasympathetic nervous systems, in which geographic location can confer selective action, this is anatomically impossible in the gut, and an alternative pattern of chemical coding for function assumes an important organizational role. The combination of amines and peptides and their relative concentrations within the enteric neuron determine its function.

Acetylcholine, the principal excitatory trigger of the non-sphincteric portion of the enteric nervous system, causes muscle contraction. Cholinergic neurons have several roles in the enteric nervous system, including excitation of external muscle, activation of motor neurons augmenting secretion of water and electrolytes, and stimulation of gastric cells. Neural control of gastrointestinal motility is mediated through two types of motor neurons: excitatory and inhibitory. These neurons act in concert on the circular smooth muscle layer in sphincteric and non-sphincteric regions throughout the digestive tract and supply muscles of the biliary tree and the muscularis mucosae. Although excitatory motor neurons supply the external longitudinal muscle, the role of inhibitory motor neurons is not well established in this muscular layer. Enteric motor neurons to the circular muscle of the small and large intestine are activated by local reflex pathways contained within the wall of the intestine. Distention evokes polarized reflexes, including contraction proximally and relaxation distally, which in synchrony constitute peristalsis. Nicotinic antagonists abolish enteric reflexes, thus suggesting that the sensory neurons or interneurons in the pathway are cholinergic. In cases of cholinergic overload, such as insecticide poisoning or "over-reversal" of muscle relaxants, the gut (in which cholinesterase is inhibited) has a tendency to become hyperreactive.

There are many neuroactive compounds other than norepinephrine and acetylcholine that participate in the autonomic control of intestinal function. The predominant of these nonadrenergic noncholinergic (NANC) neurotransmitters appears to be nitric oxide (NO), a primary intrinsic inhibitor, but other NANC neurotransmitters such as substance P, a variety of opiate peptides, vasoactive intestinal polypeptide (VIP), and a growing population of peptide hormones are also present (Table 12-1) (see Chapter 31).

Table 12-1 Neuropeptides and Their Actions in the Gastrointestinal Tract

Peptide	Action(s)
Bombesin	Multiple stimulatory effects (including gastrin release)
Calcitonin gene–related peptide	Gastric acid secretion, muscle constriction
CCK8	Unknown
Dynorphin	Opiate effects
Endothelin-1	Vasoconstriction
Galanin	Muscle constriction
Leu-enkephalin	Opiate effects
Met-enkephalin	Opiate effects
Neuromedin U	Muscle constriction, vasoconstriction
Neuropeptide Y	Vasoconstriction
Pituitary adenylate cylase	Adenylate cyclase–activating peptide
Peptide histidine methionine	Muscle relaxation, secretion
Somatostatin	Multiple inhibitory effects (including gastrin inhibition)
Substance P	Vasodilation, muscle constriction
Vasoactive intestinal polypeptide	Vasodilation, muscle relaxation, secretion

Modified from Bishop A, Polak J: The gut and the autonomic nervous system. *In* Mathias C, Bannister R (eds): Autonomic Failure: A Textbook of Clinical Disorders of the Autonomic Nervous System, 4th ed. Oxford, Oxford University Press, 1999, p 120.

Function

Organization and Integration

The sympathetic system, in response to internal or external challenges, acts to increase the heart rate, arterial pressure, and cardiac output; dilate the bronchial tree; and shunt blood away from the intestines and other viscera to voluntary muscles. Parasympathetic nervous input acts primarily to conserve energy and maintain organ function and to support vegetative processes.

Most organs of the body exhibit dual innervation, with input from the sympathetic and parasympathetic systems frequently mediating opposing effects (Table 12-2).[1] Stimulation of one system may have an excitatory effect on the end organ, whereas stimulation of the other system may have an inhibitory effect. For example, sympathetic stimulation acts on the heart to increase the rate and vigor of contraction and enhance conduction through the atrioventricular (AV) node, whereas parasympathetic stimulation acts to decrease the heart rate, atrial

Table 12-2 Responses Elicited in Effector Organs by Stimulation of Sympathetic and Parasympathetic Nerves

Effector Organ	Adrenergic Response	Receptor Involved	Cholinergic Response	Dominant Response (A or C)
Heart				
Rate of contraction	Increase	β_1	Decrease	C
Force of contraction	Increase	β_1	Decrease	C
Blood vessels				
Arteries (most)	Vasoconstriction	α_1		A
Skeletal muscle	Vasodilation	β_2		A
Veins	Vasoconstriction	α_2		A
Bronchial tree	Bronchodilation	β_2	Bronchoconstriction	C
Splenic capsule	Contraction	α_1		A
Uterus	Contraction	α_1	Variable	A
Vas deferens	Contraction	α_1		A
Prostatic capsule	Contraction	α_1		A
Gastrointestinal tract	Relaxation	α_2	Contraction	C
Eye				
Radial muscle, iris	Contraction (mydriasis)	α_1		A
Circular muscle, iris			Contraction (miosis)	C
Ciliary muscle	Relaxation	β	Contraction (accommodation)	C
Kidney	Renin secretion	β_1		A
Urinary bladder				
Detrusor	Relaxation	β	Contraction	C
Trigone and sphincter	Contraction	α_1	Relaxation	A, C
Ureter	Contraction	α_1	Relaxation	A
Insulin release from pancreas	Decrease	α_2		A
Fat cells	Lipolysis	β_1		A
Liver glycogenolysis	Increase	α_1		A
Hair follicles, smooth muscle	Contraction (piloerection)	α_1		A
Nasal secretion			Increase	C
Salivary glands	Increase secretion	α_1	Increase secretion	C
Sweat glands	Increase secretion	α_1	Increase secretion	C

A, adrenergic; C, cholinergic.
From Ruffolo R: Physiology and biochemistry of the peripheral autonomic nervous system. *In* Wingard L, Brody T, Larner J, et al (eds): Human Pharmacology: Molecular to Clinical. St. Louis, Mosby–Year Book, 1991, p 77.

contractility, and conduction through the AV node. One of the two systems normally dominates the organ's function and thus provides its "resting tone" (Table 12-3). In a few organs, the sympathetic system alone provides innervation; most blood vessels, the spleen, and piloerector muscles are examples.

To predict the effects of drugs, the interaction of the sympathetic and parasympathetic system in different organs must be understood. Blockade of sympathetic function unmasks preexisting parasympathetic activity, and the converse relationship is also true. For example, administration of atropine blocks the resting muscarinic tone of the parasympathetically dominated heart, and the unopposed sympathetic tone then causes tachycardia. Clinically, cardiac autonomic denervation occurs with cardiac transplantation; it may occur with neuraxial anesthesia, diabetes, and MI; and it can be assessed by changes in the time interval between successive heartbeats (i.e., beat-to-beat or heart rate variability) as a measure of sympathovagal balance.[2]

Adrenergic Function

Overview of the Effects of Sympathetic Mediators

Adrenergic neurons influence and adjust body functions, their effects on circulation and respiration being among the most important (Table 12-4).

The endogenous catecholamines norepinephrine and epinephrine possess α- and β-receptor agonist activity. Norepinephrine has minimal β_2-receptor activity, whereas epine-

Table 12-3 Usual Sympathetic or Parasympathetic Dominance at Specific Effector Sites

Site	Predominant Tone
Ciliary muscle	Parasympathetic
Iris	Parasympathetic
Sinoatrial node	Parasympathetic
Arterioles	Sympathetic
Veins	Sympathetic
Gastrointestinal tract	Parasympathetic
Uterus	Parasympathetic
Urinary bladder	Parasympathetic
Salivary glands	Parasympathetic
Sweat glands	Sympathetic (cholinergic)

phrine stimulates β_1- and β_2-receptors (Table 12-5). α-Receptor–mediated activity is responsible for most of the sympathetically induced smooth muscle contraction throughout the body, including the ciliary muscle of the eye and vascular, bronchial, and ureteral smooth muscle. The gastrointestinal and genitourinary sphincter mechanisms are stimulated by α-adrenergic receptors. α-Receptor agonism also mediates sympathetic nervous system control of pancreatic insulin secretion, with stimulation of α_2-receptors leading to decreased release of insulin from pancreatic beta cells. In the peripheral vasculature, α_1- and α_2-receptors modulate vascular tone in response to humorally borne neurotransmitters and exogenously administered drugs.

β-Receptor agonism is primarily responsible for sympathetic stimulation of the heart, relaxation of vascular and bronchial smooth muscle, stimulation of renin secretion by the kidney,

Table 12-4 Effects of Activation of the Sympathetic Nervous System

Site of Action	Stimulation	Inhibition
Heart	Rate, conduction, contractility	
Blood vessels	Vasoconstriction (skin, gut, liver, heart, kidney)	Vasodilation (skeletal muscle, heart, brain)
Respiration	Respiratory center Bronchodilation	
Gastrointestinal tract	Sphincters	Smooth muscle
Genitourinary tract	Sphincters	Ureteral and uterine muscle
Metabolic and endocrine effects	Glycogenolysis (muscle, liver) Gluconeogenesis Insulin release (β_1) Renin release ADH release	Insulin release (α stimulation or β_1 antagonism) Lipolysis

ADH, antidiuretic hormone or arginine vasopressin.

Table 12-5 Adrenergic Receptor Differentiation

Receptor	Stimulation	Inhibition
Alpha		
Heart		
Blood vessels	Vasoconstriction (skin, gut, kidney, liver, heart)	
Gastrointestinal tract	Sphincters	
Genitourinary tract	Sphincters	
Metabolic and endocrine effects		Insulin release
Beta		
Heart	(1) Rate, conduction contractility	
Blood vessels		(2) Vasodilation (skeletal muscle, heart, brain)
Respiration	(?) Respiratory center (2) Bronchodilation	
Gastrointestinal tract		(2) Smooth muscle
Genitourinary tract		(2) Ureteral and uterine muscle
Metabolic and endocrine effects	(2) Glycogenolysis (muscle, liver) (1) Lipolysis (2) Gluconeogenesis (1) Insulin release (?) Renin release (?) Antidiuretic hormone release	

(1), Mediated by β_1-receptors; (2), mediated by β_2-receptors; (?), controversial.

and several metabolic consequences, including lipolysis and glycogenolysis. The β_1-receptor mechanism is thought to primarily be involved in cardiac effects[3] and release of fatty acids and renin, whereas β_2-receptors are primarily responsible for smooth muscle relaxation and hyperglycemia. In specialized circumstances, however, β_2-receptors may also mediate cardiac activity. Although acute changes in arterial pressure and heart rate can be caused by norepinephrine or epinephrine, chronic hypertension does not appear to be related to circulating levels of these hormones. Eighty-five percent of resting arterial pressure is determined by the level of renin activity (Fig. 12-5). An additional important effect of epinephrine is to increase gap junctions in bone, which causes an increase in circulating blood elements.[4]

Psychological and physical stimuli may evoke different sympathetic compensatory responses. Public speaking activates the adrenal gland with a disproportionate rise in serum epinephrine, whereas physical exercise elicits primarily a marked rise in serum norepinephrine.[5] Thus, the stress response should not be thought of as a uniform response; it can vary in mechanism, intensity, and manifestations.

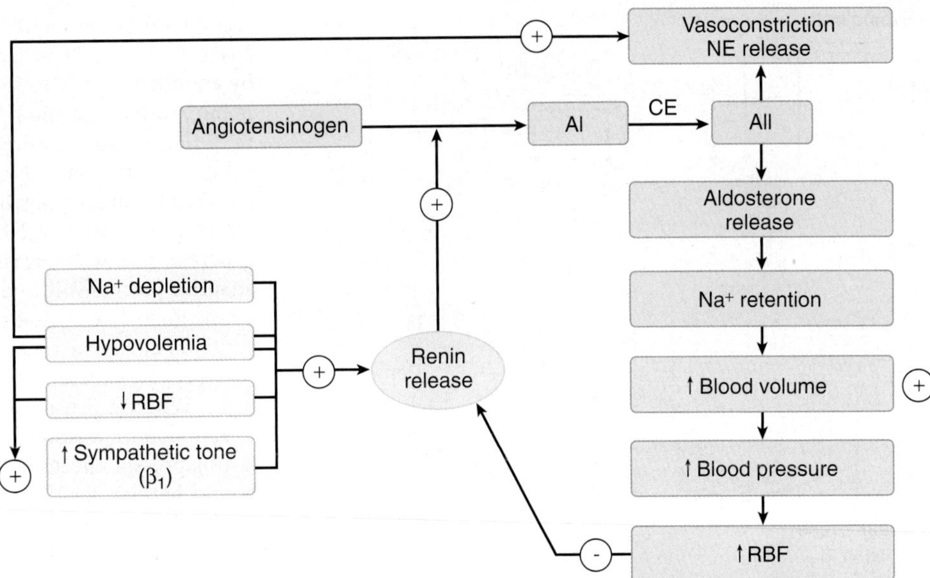

Figure 12-5 Interactions of the renin-angiotensin-aldosterone and sympathetic nervous systems in maintaining blood pressure and volume. AI, angiotensin I; AII, angiotensin II; CE, converting enzyme; NE, norepinephrine; RBF, renal blood flow; +, stimulating effects; –, inhibiting effects.

Blood Glucose

Sympathetic nervous stimulation of β-receptors increases glycogenolysis in liver and muscle and liberates free fatty acids from adipose tissue, thereby ultimately increasing blood glucose levels. In neonates, epinephrine plays an additional role in the exothermic breakdown of brown fat to maintain body temperature (i.e., nonshivering thermogenesis).

Also present in the pancreas are α_2 and β_2 receptors. α_2-Receptor activation suppresses insulin secretion by pancreatic islet cells; blockade of these receptors may increase release of insulin and thus could be associated with significant lowering of blood glucose levels. β_2-Receptor stimulation increases glucagon and insulin secretion and decreases peripheral sensitivity to insulin.[6]

Potassium Shift

Plasma epinephrine also takes part in regulation of the serum potassium concentration. β-Adrenergic activity can initiate transient hyperkalemia as potassium shifts out of hepatic cells with the glucose efflux produced by β_2-adrenergic stimulation. This effect is followed by a more prolonged hypokalemia as β_2-adrenergic stimulation drives potassium into red blood cells and muscle cells. Stimulation of the β_2-receptors of red blood cells by exogenously administered or endogenously released epinephrine activates adenylate cyclase and sodium-potassium adenosine triphosphatase (ATPase) and drives potassium into cells. This leads to a reduction in serum potassium concentration and may contribute to the cardiac arrhythmias accompanying MI and other stresses. β_2-Adrenergic blockade has the theoretical advantage of inhibiting this potassium shift. However, selective and nonselective β-blockers have been shown to be equivalent in protecting the postinfarction heart against arrhythmias.[7-11]

Cholinergic Function

Overview of the Effects of Acetylcholine

In contrast to the diffuse discharge of the sympathetic nervous system that constitutes the fight-or-flight response, the parasympathetic system is anatomically and functionally more localized in its effects. Parasympathetic activation conserves energy and maintains organ function. A massive parasympathetic response would prostrate the organism, leaving it helplessly salivating, weeping, wheezing, vomiting, urinating, defecating, and seizing. Although the sympathetic system is needed for the emergency response to stressful situations, it is not necessary for survival; the parasympathetic system is, however, essential for maintenance of life.

Release of acetylcholine is the hallmark of parasympathetic activation. The actions of acetylcholine are almost diametrically opposed to those of norepinephrine and epinephrine. In general, the muscarinic effects of acetylcholine are qualitatively the same as the effects of vagal stimulation.

Acetylcholine decreases the heart rate, the velocity of conduction in the sinoatrial and AV nodes, and atrial contractility (although this decrease is not as marked as the increase in contractility produced by sympathetic stimulation). In the sinoatrial node, acetylcholine causes membrane hyperpolarization, which delays attainment of the threshold potential and the ability to generate another action potential, thereby slowing the heart rate. In the AV node, acetylcholine decreases conduction velocity and increases the effective refractory period. This decrease in AV nodal conduction accounts for the complete heart block seen when large amounts of cholinergic agonists are given. In the ventricle, acetylcholine decreases automaticity in the Purkinje system, thereby increasing the fibrillation threshold. Cardiac presynaptic and postsynaptic muscarinic receptors are involved in these effects. Acetylcholine inhibits adrenergic stimulation of the heart presynaptically by inhibiting the release of norepinephrine from sympathetic nerve endings and postsynaptically by opposing the effects of catecholamines on the myocardium.

Parasympathetic activation has many effects outside the cardiovascular system. Cholinergic stimulation causes smooth muscle constriction, including that of the bronchial walls. In the gastrointestinal and genitourinary tracts, smooth muscle in the walls constricts, but the sphincter muscles relax, which results in incontinence. Topically administered acetylcholine constricts the smooth muscle of the iris and causes miosis.

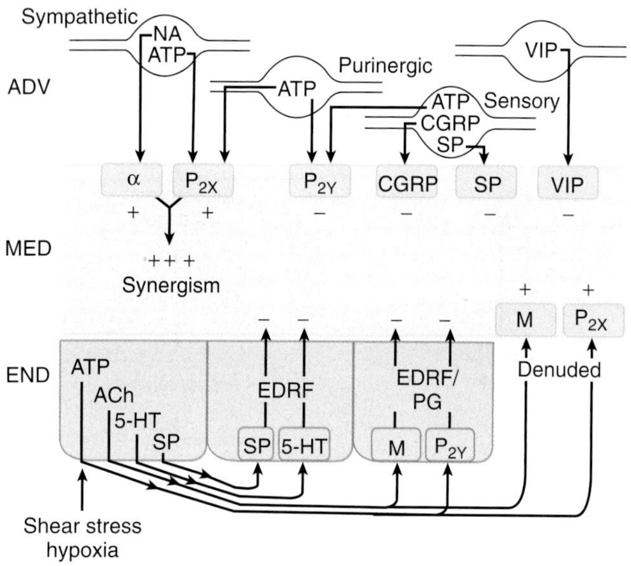

Figure 12-6 Schematic representation of potential modes of regulation of vascular tone by endothelial cell–related mechanisms. Norepinephrine (NA), adenosine triphosphate (ATP), calcitonin gene–related peptide (CGRP), substance P (SP), and vasoactive intestinal polypeptide (VIP) can be released from nerves in the adventitia (ADV) to act on their respective receptors in the media (MED) and cause vasoconstriction or vasodilation. ATP, acetylcholine (ACh), 5-hydroxytryptamine (5-HT), and SP released from endothelial cells (END) by shear stress or hypoxia act on their receptors on endothelial cells to cause release of endothelium-derived relaxing factors (EDRF) or prostaglandins (PG), which act on smooth muscle to cause relaxation. In areas denuded of endothelial cells, opposite effects may be produced by receptors on smooth muscle. α, noradrenaline receptor; M, muscarinic receptor; P_{2X}, P2X purinoceptor; P_{2Y}, P2Y purinoceptor. *(From Lincoln J, Burnstock G: Neural-endothelial interactions in control of local blood flow.* In *Warren J [ed]: The Endothelium: An Introduction to Current Research. New York, Wiley-Liss, 1990, p 21.)*

The signs and symptoms of cholinergic overload reflect all these effects, as well as nausea and vomiting, intestinal cramps, belching, urination, and urgent defecation. All glands innervated by the parasympathetic nervous system are stimulated to produce secretions, including the lacrimal, tracheobronchial, salivary, digestive, and exocrine glands.

Local Control of Vascular Tone

In addition to the pharmacologic effects of acetylcholine that are mediated by the parasympathetic nervous system, blood-borne acetylcholine has a significant effect on blood vessels in that it dilates virtually all vessels in vivo. Endothelial cells respond to acetylcholine stimulation by producing one or more endothelium-derived relaxing factors (EDRFs).[12] It now appears that endothelial cells have receptors for numerous agonists, including serotonin, adenosine, histamine, and catecholamines (Fig. 12-6). The radical NO was the first identified EDRF (see Chapter 31 for details). When the endothelium is damaged, as in atherosclerosis, production of EDRF diminishes and constriction increases. This change explains why patients with damaged or diseased vessels react differently.

An understanding of the biology of NO is fundamental to an appreciation of many vital body functions (see Chaper 31).[13] Endothelial cells play a role in control of the circulation in addition to the production of NO. Endothelial cells metabolize many vasoactive amines, convert angiotensin I to angiotensin II, and secrete prostacyclin and the vasoconstrictive peptide endothelin-1 (ET-1). NO, ET-1, and prostacyclin are local hormones released by endothelial cells to influence their immediate microenvironment. Prostacyclin and NO relax vascular smooth muscle, whereas in the lumen, they act separately or in concert to prevent platelets from clumping onto the endothelium. There is clear synergism between the antiaggregating effect of prostacyclin and subthreshold concentrations of NO. Substances that activate prostacyclin generally stimulate release of NO. Shear stress increases NO as an adaptive mechanism to dilate the circulation actively. NO works by the guanylate cyclase mechanism; prostacyclin works by activation of adenylate cyclase. Thus, although they work in concert, they activate different second messengers.

Whereas prostacyclin and NO are short-lived vasodilators, injection of the vasoconstrictor ET-1 causes a powerful and long-lasting pressor effect. ET-1, which is composed of 21 amino acids bound by two disulfide bonds, is generated enzymatically from the 39–amino acid ET-1 precursor known as big ET-1. The vasoconstrictor action of ET-1 results from activation of endothelin receptors on smooth muscle.[14]

NO, prostacyclin, and ET-1 appear to be operative in local control of the circulation. The prostacyclin system may be a redundant mechanism that reinforces the NO system in the presence of endothelial damage. Acting together, these two dilators are also a strong defense mechanism against intravascular thrombosis. ET-1 can be produced locally in response to trauma, such as wounds to the vessel wall, and it perhaps decreases blood loss. The long-term functions of these local hormones are of considerable interest in the pathophysiology of many disease states, including septic shock, pulmonary hypertension, and renal failure.[15,16] For more information on NO biology, see Chapter 31.

Pharmacology

Adrenergic Pharmacology

Synthesis of Norepinephrine

Norepinephrine is synthesized from tyrosine, which is actively transported into the varicosity of the postganglionic sympathetic nerve ending (Fig. 12-7). Tyrosine is synthesized from phenylalanine. In hypertensive rats, tyrosine may increase central adrenergic transmission, thereby decreasing peripheral sympathetic outflow.[17] In hypotensive (hemorrhaged) rats, tyrosine may increase peripheral synthesis and release of catecholamines. Precursors are taken up in greater amounts in shock and may have beneficial effects on the effort of the sympathetic nervous system to maintain perfusion pressure.

A series of steps results in conversion of tyrosine to norepinephrine and epinephrine (in the adrenal medulla). The first of these steps involves the rate-limiting cytoplasmic enzyme tyrosine hydroxylase (TH). High levels of norepinephrine inhibit TH, and low levels stimulate the enzyme. During stimulation of the sympathetic nervous system, an increased supply of tyrosine also increases the synthesis of norepinephrine. TH activity is modified by phosphorylation. TH depends on a pteridine cofactor and the presence of molecular oxygen. When the quantity of molecular oxygen is reduced, synthesis of norepinephrine may be decreased

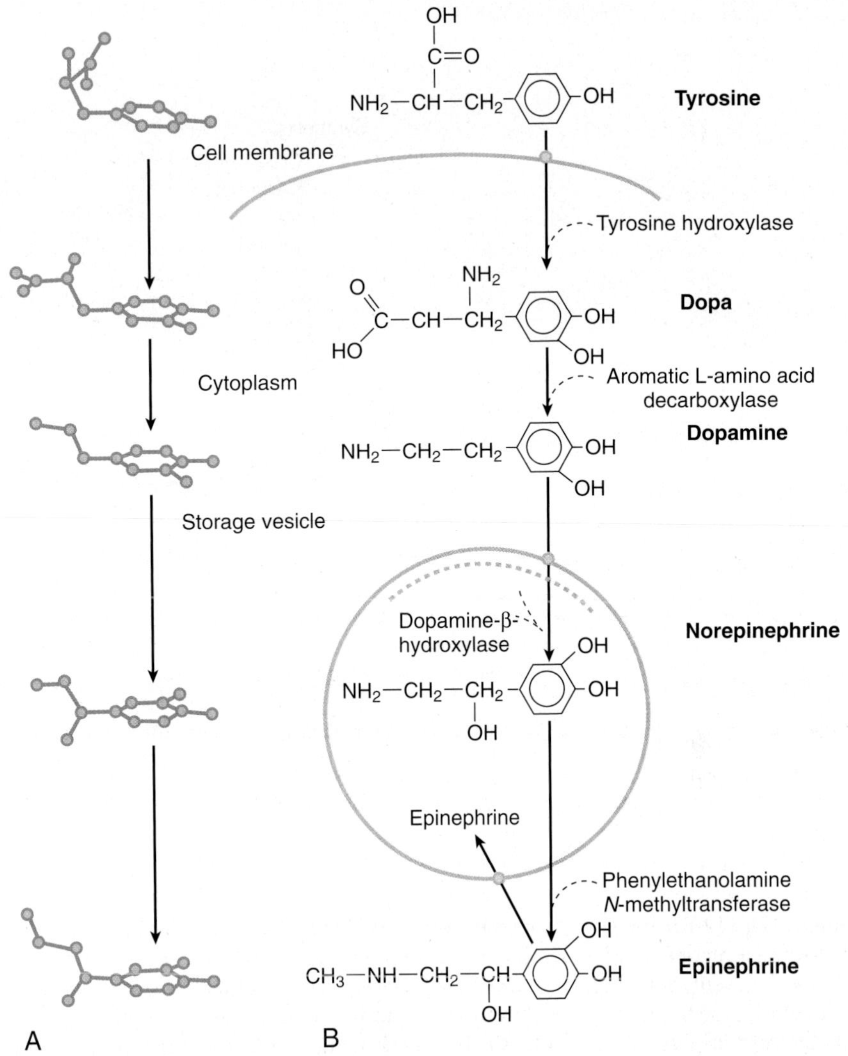

Figure 12-7 Biosynthesis of norepinephrine and epinephrine in sympathetic nerve terminal (and the adrenal medulla). **A,** Perspective view of molecules. **B,** Enzymatic processes. *(From Tollenaeré JP: Atlas of the Three-Dimensional Structure of Drugs. Amsterdam, Elsevier North-Holland, 1979; as modified by Vanhoutte PM: Adrenergic neuroeffector interaction in the blood vessel wall. Fed Proc 37:181, 1978.)*

significantly, which could account for changes in wakefulness. Whereas acute control of TH occurs by altering enzyme activity, chronic stress can elevate TH levels by stimulating the synthesis of new enzyme. Under the influence of TH, tyrosine is converted to dihydroxyphenylalanine (DOPA), which is decarboxylated to dopamine by aromatic amino acid decarboxylase (DOPA decarboxylase), a relatively promiscuous enzyme in its substrate specificity.

Dopamine can and does act as a neurotransmitter in some cells, but most of the dopamine produced is β-hydroxylated within the vesicles to norepinephrine by the enzyme dopamine β-hydroxylase (DβH). In the adrenal medulla and to a limited extent in discrete regions of the brain, another enzyme, phenylethanolamine *N*-methyltransferase (PNMT), methylates about 85% of the norepinephrine to epinephrine. Glucocorticoids from the adrenal cortex pass through the adrenal medulla and can activate the system, and stress-induced steroid release can increase the production of epinephrine. This local circulation amplifies the effects of glucocorticoid release.[18]

Storage of Norepinephrine

Norepinephrine is stored within large, dense-core vesicles. Electron microscopy suggests that the dense cores in these vesicles are filled not only with norepinephrine but also with binding proteins. In addition, the vesicles contain calcium, a variety of peptides, and adenosine 5′-triphosphate (ATP). Depending on the nature and frequency of physiologic stimuli, the ATP can be released selectively for an immediate postsynaptic effect through purinoreceptors. However, norepinephrine is the predominant neurotransmitter at sympathetic nerve endings.

Synaptic vesicles are heterogeneous and exist within functionally defined compartments. An actively recycling population of synaptic vesicles has been defined, together with a reserve population of vesicles that are mobilized only upon extensive stimulation. Functionally, norepinephrine is stored in compartments, 10% of which is readily releasable. In general, 1% of the stored norepinephrine is released with each depolarization, thus implying a significant functional reserve.

Release of Norepinephrine

There are several different processes by which the contents of the vesicle enter the synaptic cleft. The dominant physiologic mechanism of release is exocytosis, during which the vesicle responds to the entry of calcium by initiating vesicular docking, fusion, release of vesicular contents, and ultimately, endocytosis (the process by which the vesicular membrane and proteins are recap-

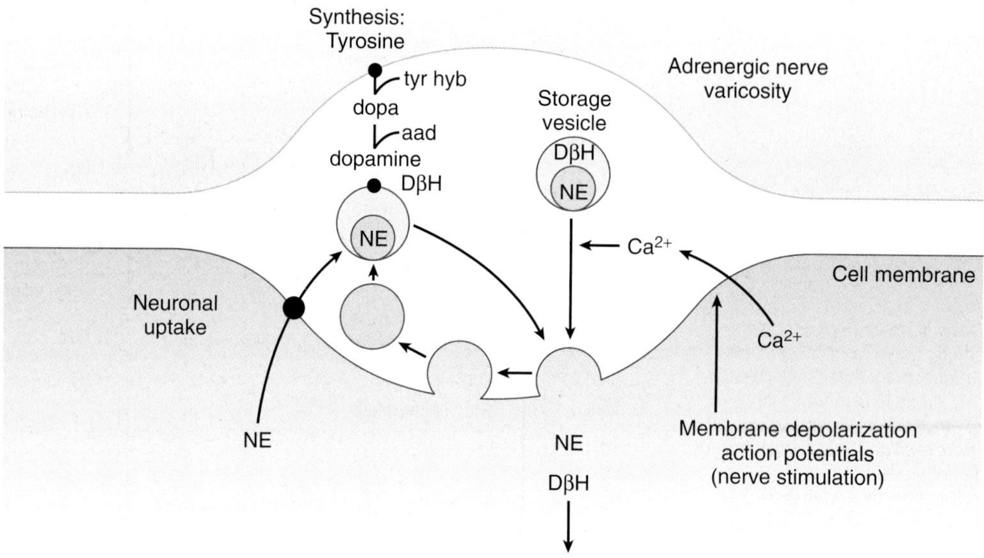

Figure 12-8 Release and reuptake of norepinephrine at sympathetic nerve terminals. aad, aromatic L-amino decarboxylase: DβH, dopamine β-hydroxylase; dopa, L-dihydroxyphenylalanine; NE, norepinephrine; tyr hyd, tyrosine hydroxylase; *solid circle*, active carrier. *(From Vanhoutte PM: Adrenergic neuroeffector interaction in the blood vessel wall. Fed Proc 37:181, 1978; as modified by Shepherd J, Vanhoutte P: Neurohumoral regulation.* In *Shepherd S, Vanhoutte P [eds]: The Human Cardiovascular System: Facts and Concepts. New York, Raven Press, 1979, p 107.)*

tured) (Fig. 12-8). The entire contents of the vesicle are liberated by stimulation of the nerve. The biology of vesicular release is not a random event, but a highly differentiated process. The fact that exocytosis is so highly conserved from species to species indicates its biologic importance. Angiotensin II, prostacyclin, and histamine potentiate release, whereas acetylcholine and prostaglandin E inhibit release.

Further details on neurotransmitter release are discussed in Chapter 23.

Although chromaffin cells in the adrenal medulla synthesize epinephrine and norepinephrine, the two compounds are stored in and secreted from distinct chromaffin cell subtypes. Pharmacologic differences between cells containing norepinephrine and epinephrine have been described, and data suggest that there may be preferential release from one or another form of chromaffin cell contingent on the nature of the stimulus. Nicotinic agonists or depolarizing agents cause the preferential release of norepinephrine, whereas histamine elicits predominantly epinephrine release.[19-21] Protein kinase C plays an important role in regulating secretion of catecholamine from norepinephrine-containing chromaffin cells.[22]

Inactivation

Most of the norepinephrine released is rapidly removed from the synaptic cleft by an amine mechanism (i.e., uptake-1 mechanism) or by non-neuronal tissue (i.e., uptake-2 mechanism). The uptake-1 mechanism represents the first and most important step in the inactivation of released norepinephrine. Most of the norepinephrine released is transported into storage vesicles for reuse. This uptake of neurotransmitter into synaptic vesicles is driven by an electrochemical proton gradient across the synaptic vesicle membrane. The vacuolar proton pump is a large hetero-oligomeric complex that contains eight to nine different subunits. After reuptake, the small amounts of norepinephrine not taken up into the vesicle are deaminated by cytoplasmic monoamine oxidase (MAO). There are several organ-specific forms of this enzyme.

Since its isolation and cloning in 1991, considerable information on the human norepinephrine transporter has accumulated.[23,24] The pharmacologic characteristics of this binding protein identify it as the cocaine binding site, although tricyclic antidepressants (i.e., desipramine and nortriptyline) are also potent antagonists.

Uptake of norepinephrine into the nerve varicosity and its return to the storage vesicle, albeit efficient, are not specific for the neurotransmitter. Some compounds structurally similar to norepinephrine may enter the nerve by the same mechanism and result in depletion of the neurotransmitter. These false transmitters can be of great clinical importance. Moreover, some drugs that block reuptake into the vesicle or into the synaptic ending itself may enhance the response to catecholamines; that is, more norepinephrine is available to receptors. Such drugs include cocaine and tricyclic antidepressants (Table 12-6).

Activity of the uptake-1 system varies greatly among different tissues. Because of anatomic barriers, peripheral blood vessels exhibit almost no reuptake of norepinephrine; consequently, rapid rates of norepinephrine synthesis are needed in peripheral blood vessels to modulate vascular tone. The highest rate of reuptake is found in the heart. Drugs or disease states that alter biosynthesis or storage (e.g., methyldopa decreases storage) have a more profound effect on blood pressure; those

Table 12-6 Comparison of Direct- and Indirect-acting Sympathomimetics

	Response of Effector Organ to	
Pretreatment	**Direct Sympathomimetics (e.g., Epinephrine): Acts at the Receptor**	**Indirect Sympathomimetics (e.g., Tyramine): Causes Release of NE after Its Uptake by Uptake 1**
Denervation Loss of uptake-1 sites Receptor upregulation	Increased	Reduced
Reserpine Blocks vesicular uptake Depletes NE May cause upregulation	Slightly increased	Reduced
Cocaine Blocks uptake 1 Depletes NE	Increased	Reduced

NE, norepinephrine.
Adapted from Moore K: Drugs affecting the sympathetic nervous system. *In* Wingard L, Brody T, Larner J, et al (eds): Human Pharmacology: Molecular to Clinical. St. Louis, Mosby–Year Book, 1991, p 114.

that affect reuptake would be expected to affect cardiac rate and rhythm.

Typically, the lungs remove 25% of the norepinephrine that passes through the pulmonary circulation, whereas epinephrine and dopamine pass through unchanged. Pulmonary uptake of norepinephrine appears to be a sodium-dependent, facilitated transport process in the endothelial cells of precapillary and postcapillary vessels and pulmonary veins. There is no significant uptake by nerve endings. Primary or secondary pulmonary hypertension diminishes uptake of norepinephrine, presumably because of concomitant thickening of the pulmonary vasculature. Although the functional significance of the endothelial uptake mechanism of the pulmonary vascular wall is unknown, uptake of other powerful vasoactive compounds suggests that the pulmonary endothelium functions to protect the left heart.

Defects in the ANS are common in patients with congestive heart failure (CHF). The heart is depleted of catecholamines, and reuptake of norepinephrine is decreased.[25] Sustained sympathoexcitation results in increased neuronal release of norepinephrine.[26] Cardiac norepinephrine spillover rates differ widely, even among patients with end-stage heart failure awaiting cardiac transplantation, but some studies suggest that elevated plasma catecholamine levels portend a poorer prognosis than can be anticipated with traditional cardiovascular indices.[27,28] Because augmentation of catecholamine release is markedly impaired in patients with CHF, compensation for further decreases in systemic vascular resistance requires activation of the renin-angiotensin system. Together, these events result in increased adrenergic drive, desensitization of β-receptors, and depletion of norepinephrine stores, which contribute to insufficient inotropic function.[29,30]

Metabolism

During storage and reuptake, a small amount of norepinephrine escapes uptake into the nerve ending and enters the circulation, where it is metabolized by MAO, catechol *O*-methyltransferase (COMT), or both in the blood, liver, and kidney (Fig. 12-9).

Epinephrine, which is released by the adrenal medulla, is inactivated by the same enzymes. The final metabolic product of inactivation is vanillylmandelic acid (VMA). Because of its rapid clearance, the half-life of norepinephrine (and most biogenic amines) in plasma is short, less than 1 minute. This short half-life necessitates administration of these drugs by infusion. Another consequence of their short half-life is that a more ideal measure of catecholamine production may be metabolic products rather than the catecholamines themselves. For example, screening for a norepinephrine-producing pheochromocytoma is frequently done by measuring the level of urine metanephrine and VMA. Only a small percentage of norepinephrine appears in the urine for assay.

Inhibition of MAO has a large impact on the sympathetic function of a patient. MAO inhibitors (MAOIs) are generally well tolerated, but the stability of the patient belies the fact that amine handling is fundamentally changed. Clinically important, life-threatening drug interactions are discussed later in the section "Drugs and the Autonomic Nervous System."

Other compounds can be metabolized by catabolic enzymes to produce false transmitters. Though not used therapeutically, tyramine is the prototypical drug studied. Tyramine is present in many foods, particularly aged cheese and wine, and it can be synthesized from tyrosine. Tyramine enters the sympathetic nerve terminal through the uptake-1 mechanism and displaces norepinephrine from the vesicles into the cytoplasm. The released norepinephrine leaks out of the cytoplasm and is responsible for the hypertensive effect of tyramine. However, a secondary effect can occur. In the vesicle, tyramine is converted by DβH to octopamine, which is eventually released as a false transmitter in place of norepinephrine, but without the hypertensive effect because it has only 10% of the potency of norepinephrine.

Adrenergic Receptors

Initially, α-adrenergic receptors were distinguished from β-adrenergic receptors by their greater response to epinephrine and norepinephrine than to isoproterenol. The development of α- and β-antagonists further supported the existence of separate α-receptors. Traditionally, adrenergic receptors have been classified as α or β and more recently as α_1, α_2, β_1, or β_2 based on responses to specific drugs. With technologic advances in molecular biology, classification evolved to three major subtypes and nine subtypes (Fig. 12-10).[31] Table 12-7 describes the distribution, response, typical agonists, and antagonists of the α_1-, α_2-, β_1-, and β_2-receptors.

α-Adrenergic Receptors

Functional and binding assays and molecular biologic methods have unequivocally confirmed the classification of α-adrenoceptors into subtypes.[32] Within α_1-adrenergic receptors, $\alpha_{1a/d}$-, α_{1b}-, and α_{1c}-receptors have been characterized. Several α_2-isoreceptors (α_{2a}, α_{2b}, and α_{2c}) have also been described. α_2-Receptors are usually expressed presynaptically or even in nonneuronal tissue. α_2-Receptors are found in the peripheral nervous system, in the CNS, and in a variety of organs, including platelets, liver, pancreas, kidney, and eyes, where specific physiologic functions have been identified.[33] Later, the predominant α_2-receptor of the human spinal cord was identified as the α_{2a}-subtype.[31,34] It appears that mammalian genomes contain two sets of at least three unique genes encoding the α-adrenoceptors. Genes encoding α_2-receptors have been localized to chromosomes 2, 4, and

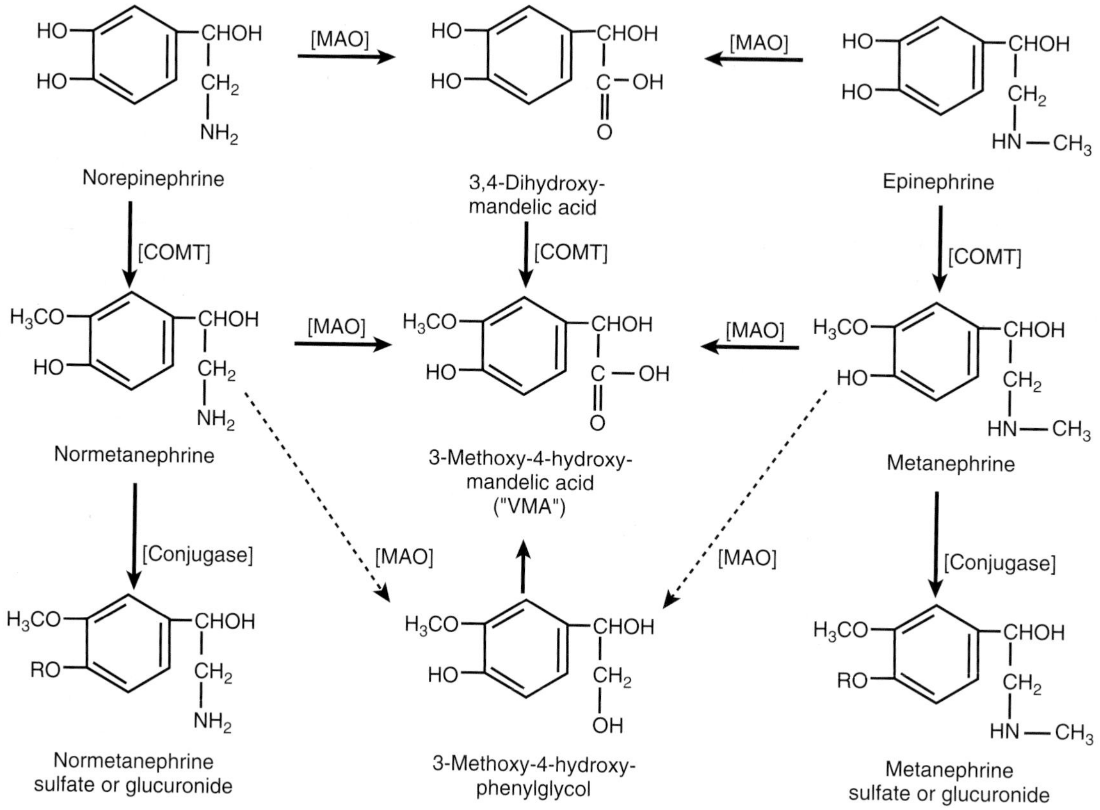

Norepinephrine
[MAO]
3,4-Dihydroxy-mandelic acid
[MAO]
Epinephrine
[COMT]
[COMT]
[COMT]
Normetanephrine
[MAO]
3-Methoxy-4-hydroxy-mandelic acid ("VMA")
[MAO]
Metanephrine
[Conjugase]
[MAO]
[MAO]
[Conjugase]
Normetanephrine sulfate or glucuronide
3-Methoxy-4-hydroxy-phenylglycol
Metanephrine sulfate or glucuronide

Figure 12-9 Metabolism of catecholamines. COMT, catechol *O*-methyltransferase; MAO, monoamine oxidase. *(From Lake CR, Chernow B, Feuerstein G, et al: The sympathetic nervous system in man, its evaluation and the measurement of plasma norepinephrine.* In *Zigler M, Lake C [eds]: Frontiers of Clinical Neuroscience, vol 2. Baltimore, Williams & Wilkins, 1984, p 1.)*

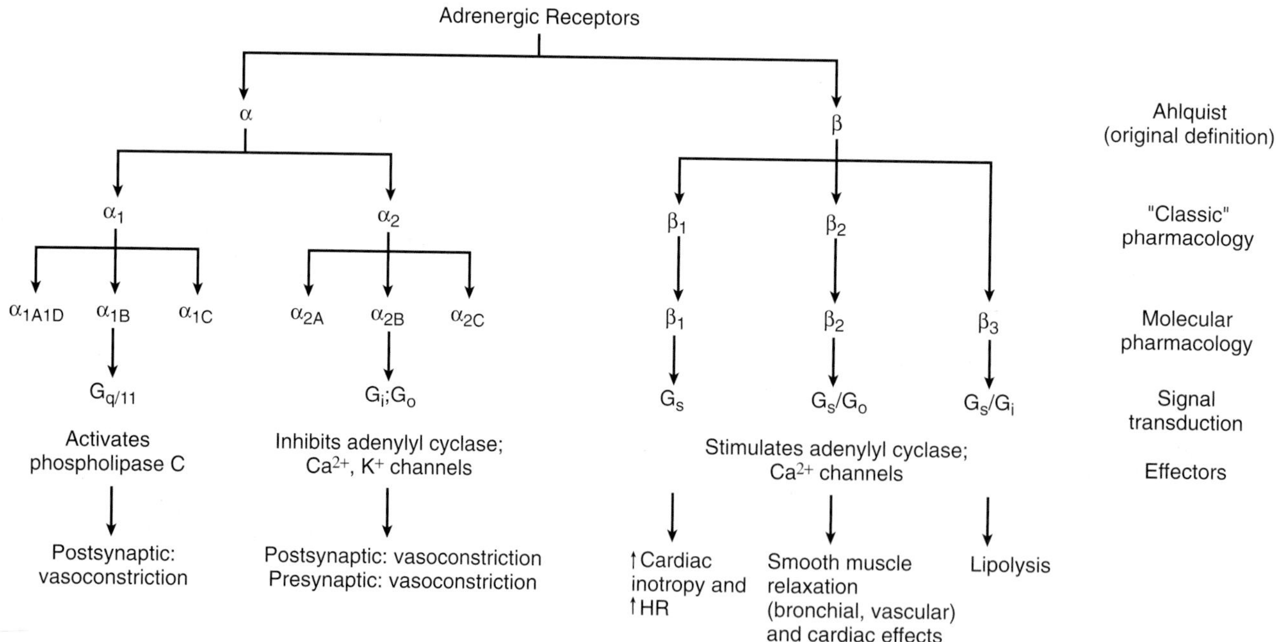

Figure 12-10 Classification of adrenergic receptors. HR, heart rate.

Table 12-7 Distribution of α- and β-Receptors

Receptor	Distribution	Response	Agonist	Antagonist
α_1	Smooth muscle	Constriction	Methoxamine Phenylephrine	Prazosin
α_2	Presynaptic	Inhibits norepinephrine release	Clonidine Dexmedetomidine	Yohimbine
β_1	Heart	Inotropy Chronotropy	Dobutamine	Metoprolol
β_2	Smooth muscle	Dilation Relaxation	Terbutaline	

10. There is more than theoretical relevance in the subclassification of receptors[35] in that mutations that decrease α_{2c} presynaptic function and enhance β_1-receptor linkage cause adrenergic hyperactivity and predispose to CHF.[36]

Amino acid sequence comparisons indicate that α-receptors are members of the seven–transmembrane segment gene superfamily, which uses G protein for signal transduction. A core of 175 amino acids constitutes the seven transmembrane regions and is highly conserved among different family members. The plethora of receptor subtypes remains incompletely explained, although the observation that different signal transduction mechanisms are used suggests finer control and physiologic significance. It may be important that there is considerable variability in α-adrenergic receptor subtypes among species.[37]

Receptors can be presynaptic as well as postsynaptic. Presynaptic receptors may act as heteroreceptors or autoreceptors. An *autoreceptor* is a presynaptic receptor that reacts with the neurotransmitter released from its own nerve terminal to provide feedback regulation. A *heteroreceptor* is a presynaptic receptor that responds to substances other than the neurotransmitter released from that specific nerve terminal. This regulatory scheme is present throughout the nervous system but is particularly important in the sympathetic nervous system.[38]

Although several presynaptic receptors have been identified, the α_2-receptor may have the greatest clinical import. Presynaptic α_2-receptors regulate the release of norepinephrine and ATP through a negative-feedback mechanism.[39] Activation of presynaptic α_2-receptors by norepinephrine inhibits subsequent release of norepinephrine in response to nerve stimulation. A similar inhibitory response is produced by attachment of acetylcholine to presynaptic cholinergic receptors. In the human brain, ligand studies reveal a high density of α_2-receptors, particularly in the cerebral cortex and medulla.[40] This latter distribution may account for the bradycardiac and hypotensive responses to α_2-agonist drugs.

β-Adrenergic Receptors

Like the α-receptor, the β-receptor is one of the superfamily of proteins that have seven helices woven through the cellular membrane. These transmembrane domains are labeled M_1 through M_7; antagonists have specific binding sites, whereas agonists are more diffusely attached to hydrophobic membrane-spanning domains (Fig. 12-11). The extracellular portion of the receptor ends in an amino group. A carboxyl group occupies the intracellular terminal, where phosphorylation occurs. At the cytoplasmic domains, there is interaction with G proteins and kinases, including β-adrenergic receptor kinase. The β-receptor has mechanistic and structural similarities with muscarinic but not nicotinic receptors, primarily in the transmembrane sections.

β-Receptors have been further divided into β_1-, β_2-, and β_3-subtypes, all of which increase cyclic adenosine monophosphate (cAMP) through adenylate cyclase and the mediation of G proteins.[41] Although β_1-receptors were traditionally thought to be isolated to cardiac tissue and β_2-receptors were believed to be restricted to vascular and bronchial smooth muscle, we now know that the β_2-receptor population in human cardiac tissue is substantial and accounts for 15% of β-receptors in the ventricles and 30% to 40% in the atria.[42] β_2-Receptors may help compensate for disease by maintaining response to catecholamine stimulation when β_1-receptors are downregulated during chronic catecholamine stimulation and in CHF.[43] The β_2-population is almost unaffected in end-stage congestive cardiomyopathy.[44] In addition to positive inotropic effects, β_2-receptors in the human atria participate in regulation of the heart rate. Generation of cAMP in the human heart appears to be mediated primarily by β_2-receptors, although this may be an artifact related to the lability of β_1-receptors.[44] Localization of β_3-receptors to fat cells suggests a new therapy for obesity. Polymorphism of this β-receptor subtype is associated with obesity and the potential for the development of diabetes.[45-47] Point mutations in genes encoding β_2-receptors are correlated with decreased downregulation of β-receptors and nocturnal asthma.[48,49]

Dopamine Receptors

Dopamine exists as an intermediate in the biosynthesis of norepinephrine, and in addition, exogenous dopamine exerts α- or β-adrenergic effects (depending on the dose administered). Furthermore, Goldberg and Rajfer[50] demonstrated physiologically distinct dopamine type 1 (DA_1) and dopamine type 2 (DA_2) receptors, and these remain the most important of the five dopamine receptors cloned (Fig. 12-12). DA_1 receptors are postsynaptic and act on renal, mesenteric, splenic, and coronary vascular smooth muscle to mediate vasodilation through stimulation of adenylate cyclase and increased production of cAMP. The vasodilatory effect tends to be strongest in the renal arteries. It is for this action, particularly the redistribution of blood flow to the kidneys, that dopamine is most frequently used. Additional renal DA_1 receptors located in the tubules modulate natriuresis through the sodium-potassium ATPase pump and the sodium-hydrogen exchanger.[50-53] DA_2 receptors are presynaptic; they may inhibit release of norepinephrine and perhaps acetylcholine. There are also central DA_2 receptors that may mediate nausea and vomiting,

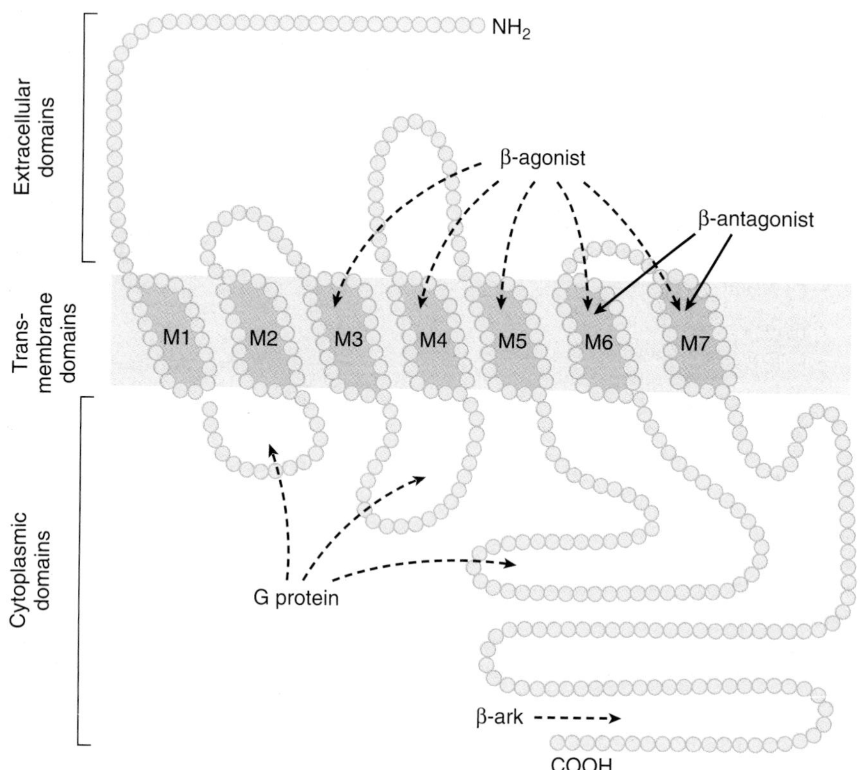

Figure 12-11 Molecular structure of the β-adrenergic receptor. Notice the three domains. The transmembrane domains act as a ligand-binding pocket. Cytoplasmic domains can interact with G proteins and kinases such as β-adrenergic receptor kinase (β-ARK). The latter can phosphorylate and desensitize the receptor. *(From Opie L: Receptors and signal transduction. In Opie LH [ed]: The Heart: Physiology and Metabolism. New York, Raven Press, 1991.)*

which may explain why the antiemetic activity of droperidol is thought to be related to its DA_2 activity.

GTP-Binding Regulatory Proteins (G Proteins)

After adrenergic receptor stimulation, the extracellular signal is transformed into an intracellular signal by a process known as signal transduction in which α_1- and β-receptors are coupled to G proteins. When activated, G proteins can modulate the synthesis or availability of intracellular second messengers (Fig. 12-13). The activated second messenger diffuses through the cytoplasm and stimulates an enzymatic cascade. The sequence of first messenger → receptor → G protein → effector → second messenger → enzymatic cascade is found in a wide variety of cells; the specific entities that fulfill the separate roles vary from cell to cell.[54] G proteins located on the inner surface of the cell membrane can also directly modify the activity of transmembrane ion channels.

G proteins are heterotrimeric compounds composed of three subunits labeled α, β, and γ. The β- and γ-subunits form a stable complex and the α-subunit associates with them in a reversible fashion. The β- and γ-subunits show little variation in their structure. In contrast, 20 different α-subunits have been

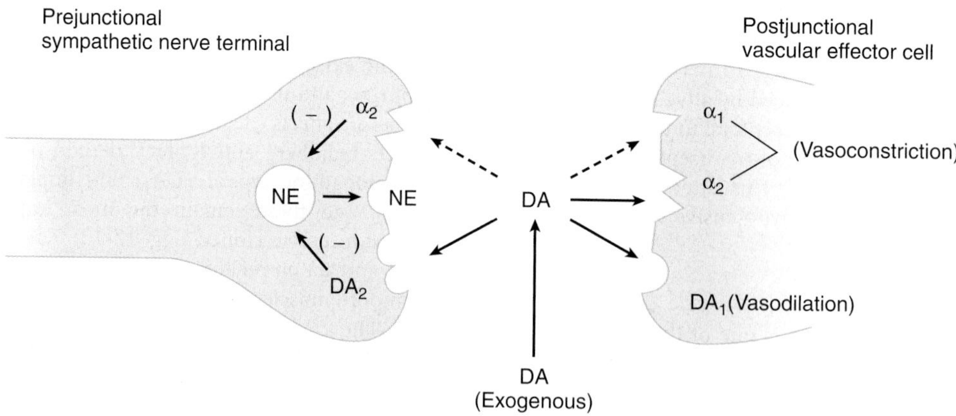

Figure 12-12 Location of dopamine type 1 (DA_1) receptors and α_1- and α_2-adrenoceptors on postganglionic vascular effector cells and DA_2 receptors and α_2-adrenoceptors on the prejunctional sympathetic nerve terminal. When dopamine is administered, activation of DA_1 receptors causes vasodilation, whereas activation of DA_2 receptors causes inhibition (–) of release of norepinephrine (NE) from storage granules. A larger dose of dopamine activates α_1- and α_2-adrenoceptors on the postjunctional effector cells to cause vasoconstriction and α_2-adrenoceptors on the prejunctional sympathetic terminal to inhibit release of NE. NE released from the prejunctional sympathetic terminal also acts on α_1- and α_2-adrenoceptors. *(From Goldberg LI, Rajfer SI: Dopamine receptors: Applications in clinical cardiology. Circulation 72:245, 1985.)*

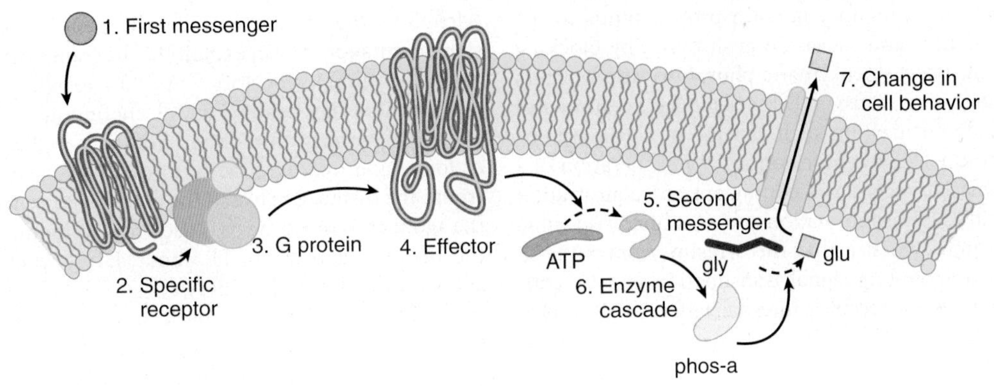

Figure 12-13 Epinephrine-stimulated glycogenolysis in a liver cell demonstrates the role of G proteins in cellular function. The first messenger (epinephrine) binds to its specific receptor and stimulates the G protein (in this case, G_s) to activate the effector adenylyl cyclase. This enzyme converts adenosine triphosphate (ATP) to cyclic adenosine monophosphate, the second messenger, which then triggers a cascade of enzymatic reactions that stimulates the enzyme phosphorylase (phos-a) to convert glycogen into glucose, which the cell extrudes. *(From Linder ME, Gilman AG: G Proteins. Sci Am 267:56, 1992.)*

identified. The structure of the attached α-subunit defines the function of the G protein. Four classes of α-subunits have been defined: α_s, α_i, α_q, and α_{12}. The corresponding G protein complexes formed when these α-subunits bind to the βγ-structure are called G_s, G_i, G_q, and G_o.[55]

Each class of adrenergic receptor couples to a different major subfamily of G proteins, which are linked to different effectors. The major subtypes of α_1-, α_2-, and β-receptors are linked to G_q, G_i, and G_s, respectively, which are linked to activation of phospholipase C (α_1), inhibition of adenylyl cyclase (α_2), or stimulation of adenylyl cyclase (β) (see Fig. 12-10). In its resting state, the G protein is bound to guanosine diphosphate (GDP) and is not in contact with the receptor. When the receptor is activated by the first messenger, it stimulates the G protein to release GDP and bind guanosine triphosphate (GTP) to its α-subunit, thereby activating itself. The bound GTP signals the G protein to split into two parts consisting of the α-GTP structure and the βγ-subunit. The released α-subunit binds to the effector, activates it, and then converts its attached GTP to GDP, thereby returning itself to the resting state. The α-subunit joins with the βγ-unit, and the reconstructed G protein again waits at the inner membrane.

β-Receptor stimulation by G proteins enhances the activity of adenylate cyclase and the formation of cAMP. The briefest encounter of plasma membrane β-adrenergic receptors with epinephrine or norepinephrine results in profound increases (up to 400-fold higher than the basal level within minutes) in intracellular levels of cAMP. Increased cAMP synthesis activates protein kinases, which phosphorylate target proteins to elicit various cellular responses that complete the path between receptor and effect. Stimulation of α_2-receptors results in G_i inhibition of adenylate cyclase. The relative abundance of G proteins results in amplification of receptor agonism at the signal transduction step. The number of G protein molecules greatly exceeds the number of β-adrenergic receptors and adenylate cyclase molecules. It is the receptor concentration and ultimately adenylate cyclase activity that limit the response to catecholamines, which perhaps explains the efficacy of phosphodiesterase inhibitors.[56,57]

Myocardial cells respond to receptor stimulation differently, depending on the identity of the first messenger. Two opposing effects, inhibition and stimulation of contractility, are both produced by the sequence of receptor → G protein → effector → enzymatic cascade. However, the identity of the chemicals in the sequence differs.[58] Norepinephrine causes myocardial cells to contract with more vigor when the α-subunit of the stimulatory protein (G_s) activates adenylate cyclase. The α-subunits of this protein cause potassium channels to open and permit efflux of potassium ion. The force of contraction is diminished when acetylcholine acts as a first messenger and stimulates its receptor to activate the inhibitory protein G_i or G_o. Clinically important, second-to-second changes in heart rate can be explained by the simultaneous activation of G_s and G_o. The current caused by G_o is larger than that caused by G_s, which explains the clinical impression that vagal inhibition of heart rate predominates in the presence of sympathetic stimulation, such as may occur in unpremedicated patients.[58]

Upregulation and Downregulation

β-Adrenergic receptors are not fixed; they change significantly in dynamic response to the amount of norepinephrine present in the synaptic cleft or in plasma. For β-adrenergic receptors, this response is fast; within 30 minutes of denervation or adrenergic blockade, the number of receptors increases. Such upregulation may explain why sudden discontinuation of β-adrenergic receptor blocking drugs causes rebound tachycardia and increases the incidence of MI and ischemia. Many chronic phenomena, such as varicose veins[59] or aging, can decrease adrenergic receptor number or responsiveness systemically.

Clinically and at the cellular level, responses to many hormones and neurotransmitters wane rapidly despite continuous exposure to adrenergic agonists.[60] This phenomenon, called desensitization, has been particularly well studied for the stimulation of cAMP levels by plasma membrane β-adrenergic receptors. Mechanisms postulated for desensitization include uncoupling (e.g., phosphorylation), sequestration, and downregulation. The molecular mechanisms underlying rapid β-adrenergic receptor desensitization do not appear to require internalization of the receptors, but rather an alteration in the functioning of β-receptors themselves that uncouples the receptors from the stimulatory G_s protein. Agonist-induced desensitization involves phosphorylation of G protein–coupled receptors by two classes of serine-threonine kinases. One of these classes initiates receptor-specific or homologous desensitization. The other works through second messenger–dependent kinases and mediates a general cellular hyporesponsiveness called heterologous desensitization. Ultimately, an inhibitory arrestin protein binds to the phosphorylated receptor and causes desensitization by blocking signal transduction. Because enzymatic phosphorylation occurs only in the activated state, transient β-blockade has been used in states of receptor desensitization such as CHF or cardiopulmonary bypass to achieve a "a receptor holiday."[61] Regeneration of a functional β-adrenergic receptor is contingent on sequestration of the receptor, with dephosphorylation and presumed recycling. There has been some evidence that the arrestins contribute to desensitization by uncoupling signal transduction and by contributing to the process of receptor internalization.[62,63] Receptor populations can change rapidly with such sequestration, which does not require protein synthesis.

Downregulation may be distinguished from these rapid mechanisms in that it occurs after hours of exposure to an agonist (as in chronic stress or CHF) and receptors are destroyed. New receptors must be synthesized before return to a baseline state is possible.

Chronic CHF is one of the most important and best-studied pathophysiologic situations in which tolerance or downregulation occurs. It was initially observed that the density of cardiac β-receptors decreases markedly in patients with terminal heart failure in response to the elevated plasma catecholamine levels. This finding explained why administration of exogenous β-agonists was relatively ineffectual in this syndrome. With the demonstration that β_1- and β_2-receptors coexist in human ventricles,[64] Bristow and coworkers, using radioligand techniques, documented that β_1-receptor density decreases without change in the density of β_2-receptors in human ventricles affected by CHF. Consequently, β_2-agonism accounted for 60% of the total inotropic response stimulated by isoproterenol in the failing heart as compared with 40% in a nonfailing heart.[65]

The activity of the thyroid gland influences receptor density, with hyperthyroidism increasing density and hypothyroidism decreasing density. Clinically, β-receptor blockade is important in the acute treatment of hyperthyroidism. There is some evidence that corticosteroids decrease receptor density. Consequently, the reaction of the body to well-characterized sympathetic agonists may be considerably different, depending on the pathologic and environmental circumstances. However, the structural similarity of thyroid hormone and tyrosine suggests that false transmitters may play a role (see Chapter 75).[66]

Cholinergic Pharmacology

Acetylcholine Synthesis

Many of our assumptions about cholinergic pharmacology are drawn from our understanding of cholinergic receptors at the neuromuscular junction. The chemistry of cholinergic synthesis and metabolism is covered in detail in Chapter 14.

Cholinergic Receptors

Traditionally, cholinergic receptors have been organized into two major subdivisions, nicotinic and muscarinic. Muscarinic receptors are present mostly in peripheral visceral organs; nicotinic receptors are found on parasympathetic and sympathetic ganglia (neuronal subtypes) and on the neuromuscular junctions of skeletal muscle (neuronal and muscle subtypes).

Although these two structurally and functionally distinct classes of receptors have significantly different responses to acetylcholine, the chemical itself exhibits no specificity. However, specific antagonists can exploit the difference between muscarinic and nicotinic receptors. As a result, structure-activity relationships have emerged. All cholinergic agonists appear to need a quaternary ammonium group, as well as an atom capable of forming a hydrogen bond through an unshared pair of electrons. The distance between the two sites may determine whether the agonism is nicotinic or muscarinic. With muscarinic agonists, the distance appears to be about 4.4 Å, whereas for nicotinic agonists, the distance is 5.9 Å.

The neuronal and muscle subtypes of nicotinic receptors on ganglia and motor end plates, respectively, differ. Nondepolarizing neuromuscular blocking agents block neuronal nicotinic acetylcholine receptors present in ganglia and at the neuromuscular junction (see Chapter 29),[67] whereas hexamethonium blocks the ganglionic receptors.

Some evidence indicates that ganglionic nicotinic receptors are far more sensitive to anesthetics than receptors in the neuromuscular junction are, but the clinical significance is unclear.[68]

The nicotinic receptors on ganglia and motor end plates are discussed in detail in Chapter 14. In brief, they are pentameric membrane proteins that form nonselective cation channels. There are two α-units (each 40 kd) and one each of the β-, ε-, and δ-units. These five subunits surround each ion channel through which sodium or calcium enters the cell or potassium exits. Each ion has its own separate channel. For the channel to open, acetylcholine must occupy a receptor site on each of the two α-subunits.

In contrast to the ion-gated nicotinic receptors, muscarinic receptors belong to the superfamily of G protein–coupled receptors. Muscarinic receptors therefore have greater homology to α- and β-adrenergic receptors than to nicotinic receptors. Like the other members of the family of receptors with seven helices (i.e., α_2, β_1, β_2, serotonin, rhodopsin, and opsin), muscarinic receptors use G proteins for signal transduction. Five muscarinic receptors (i.e., M_1 through M_5) exist, with the primary structural variability residing in a huge cytoplasmic loop between the fifth and sixth membrane-spanning domains. Although molecular studies have described five forms, four of which are defined pharmacologically (i.e., M_1, M_2, M_3, and M_4), selective muscarinic drugs are not available. The M_2 cholinergic postjunctional receptor predominates in visceral organs. M_2 and M_3 receptors have been identified in the airway smooth muscle of many species. In vitro studies reveal that the M_3 receptor mediates the contractile and secretory response. However, the excess of M_2 receptors could explain the relative ineffectiveness of β-adrenergic agonists in reversing cholinergic bronchoconstriction.[69]

The muscarinic receptors have diverse signal transduction mechanisms. The odd-numbered receptors (i.e., M_1, M_3, and M_5) work predominantly through hydrolysis of polyphosphoinositide, whereas the even-numbered receptors work primarily to regulate adenylate cyclase.[70]

When the M_3 muscarinic receptor is activated, G_q activates phospholipase C, which catalyzes the hydrolysis of phosphatidylinositol bisphosphate into diacylglycerol and inositol triphosphate. Receptors in the muscarinic series are coupled to second messenger systems, such as cyclic nucleotides or phosphoinositides. These are coupled to ion channels. In other cases, influx of a cation is the trigger for cellular response. In some cases, however, the influx of calcium ions acts as a messenger that reacts with and opens other ion channels. In addition to affecting ion channels, the messenger calcium can stimulate various intracellular proteins to alter cell activity. In cardiac atria, activation of muscarinic receptors leads to the efflux of potassium and hyperpolarization of the cell membrane. This hyperpolarization slows conduction and slows or stops atrial pacemakers. In glands, an influx of calcium or sodium, or both, activates intracellular events and causes the cells to secrete. Similarly, influx of these ions into smooth muscle cells causes them to contract.

Muscarinic receptors are found on central and peripheral neurons; a single neuron may have muscarinic receptors with excitatory as well as inhibitory effects. Prejunctional autoreceptors are not as well studied in the parasympathetic nervous system as in the sympathetic nervous system. Presynaptic muscarinic receptors may inhibit the release of acetylcholine from postganglionic parasympathetic neurons; prejunctional nicotinic receptors may increase its release.

Because of the complex coupling, the response of the muscarinic system is sluggish; no response is seen for seconds to minutes after the application of acetylcholine. Similarly, the effect long outlives the presence of the agonist. Even though the transmitter is destroyed rapidly, the train of events that it initiates causes the cellular response to continue for many minutes. Muscarinic receptors are desensitized through agonist-dependent phosphorylation in a mechanism similar to that described earlier for β-adrenergic receptors.

Nonadrenergic, Noncholinergic Neurotransmission in the Autonomic Nervous System

NANC components such as monoamines, purines, amino acids, and polypeptides are part of the ANS. Other transmitter candidates demonstrated in perivascular nerves by histochemical and immunohistochemical techniques include ATP, adenosine, VIP, substance P, 5-hydroxytryptamine (5-HT), neuropeptide Y (NPY), and calcitonin gene–related peptide (CGRP). Immunocytochemical studies show that more than one transmitter or putative transmitter may be colocalized in the same nerve. The most common combinations of transmitters in perivascular nerves are norepinephrine, ATP, and NPY in sympathetic nerves (Fig. 12-14); acetylcholine and VIP in parasympathetic nerves (Fig. 12-15); and substance P, CGRP, and ATP in sensory-motor nerves. Many of these putative transmitters act through cotransmission, which is the synthesis, storage, and release of more than one transmitter by a nerve. Initially, the multiplicity of transmitters released in various combinations appeared random and bewildering, but a pattern is emerging that clarifies the situation. Autonomic nerves exhibit chemical coding—individual neurons serving a specific physiologic function contain distinct combinations of transmitter substances.[71]

The concepts of cotransmission and neuromodulation have become accepted mechanisms in autonomic nervous control. To establish that transmitters coexisting in the same nerves act as cotransmitters, it is necessary to demonstrate that on release, each substance acts postjunctionally on its own specific receptor to produce a response.

For many perivascular sympathetic nerves, there is evidence that norepinephrine and ATP act as cotransmitters and are released from the same nerves but act on α_1-adrenoceptors and P_2-purinoceptors, respectively, to produce vasoconstriction (see Fig. 12-14).[72,73] ATP, once thought to act only as an electrical buffer for the charged norepinephrine, is believed to mediate contraction through P_2 receptors by voltage-dependent calcium channels.[74] The fast component of contraction appears to be mediated by these purinoceptors, whereas norepinephrine sustains contraction of muscle by acting on the α_1-adrenoreceptor through receptor-operated calcium channels. ATP is stored in vesicles along nerve varicosities. It is released into the synaptic cleft via exocytosis and then binds to postsynaptic purinergic receptors. ATP is then broken down to adenosine by membrane-bound ATPases and 5′-nucleotidases. Adenosine is subsequently taken up into the presynaptic neuron, where ATP is resynthesized and incorporated into vesicles for later release.[75]

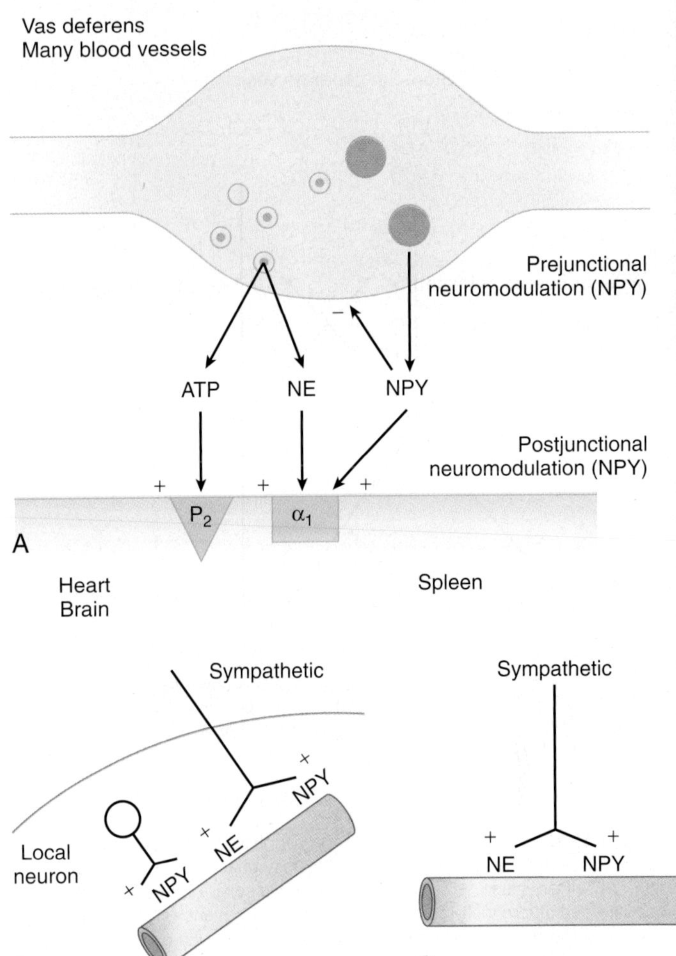

Figure 12-14 Schematic representation of different interactions that occur between neuropeptide Y (NPY) and adenosine triphosphate (ATP) and the norepinephrine (NE) released from single sympathetic nerve varicosities. **A,** Diagram showing what occurs in the vas deferens and many blood vessels, where NE and ATP, probably released from small granular vesicles, act synergistically to contract (+) the smooth muscle through α_1-adrenoceptors and P_2 purinoceptors, respectively. **B** and **C,** Sympathetic neurotransmission in the heart and brain (**B**) and the spleen (**C**). *(From Lincoln J, Burnstock G: Neural-endothelial interactions in control of local blood flow.* In *Warren J [ed]: The Endothelium: An Introduction to Current Research. New York, Wiley-Liss, 1990, p 21.)*

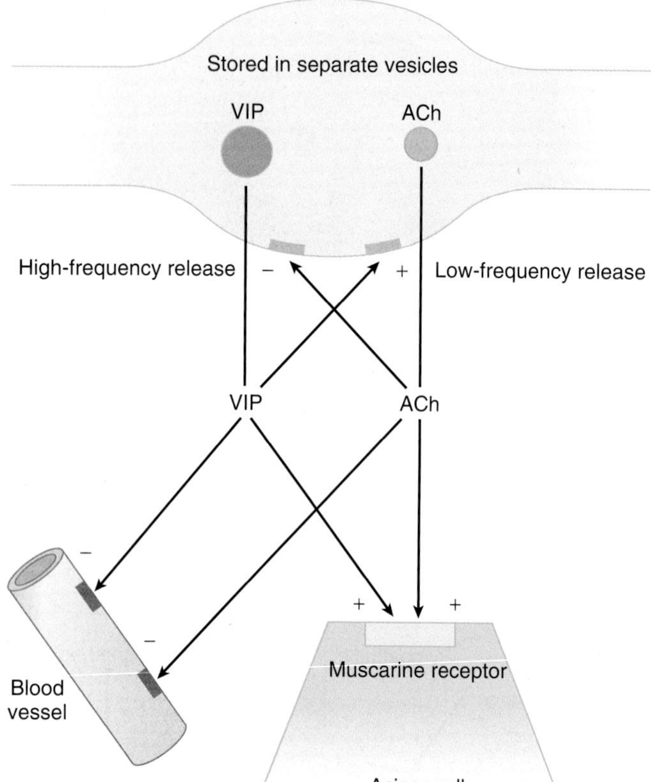

Figure 12-15 The classic transmitter acetylcholine (ACh) coexists with vasoactive intestinal polypeptide (VIP) in parasympathetic nerves supplying the cat salivary gland. ACh and VIP are stored in separate vesicles; they can be released differentially at different stimulation frequencies to act on acinar cells and glandular blood vessels. Cooperation is achieved by the selected release of ACh at low impulse frequencies and VIP at high frequencies. Prejunctional and postjunctional modulation is indicated. *(From Burnstock G: Local mechanisms of blood flow control by perivascular nerves and endothelium. J Hypertens Suppl 8:S95, 1990.)*

Purinergic receptors are categorized as P_1 or P_2 receptors. P_1 receptors bind adenosine, whereas P_2 receptors bind ATP. Four subtypes of P_1 receptors have been identified (A_1, A_{2A}, A_{2B}, and A_3). All the P_1 receptors are coupled to membrane-bound G proteins. There are two subclasses of P_2 receptors (P2X and P2Y). P2X receptors bind ATP and open ligand-gated ion channels. In contrast, P2Y receptors are coupled to G proteins and their associated secondary messenger systems. Seven P2X subtypes ($P2X_{1-7}$) and eight P2Y subtypes ($P2Y_{1,2,4,6,11,12,13,14}$) have been identified. Some P2Y receptors are preferentially activated by adenosine diphosphate rather than ATP, and some can be activated by pyrimidine nucleosides (uridine triphosphate), as well as purinergic agonists.

ATP released at nerve endings in the setting of hypertension leads to marked decreases in arterial pressure. ATP bound to $MgCl_2$ is a potent pulmonary vasodilator used to treat patients with pulmonary hypertension secondary to congenital heart disease. In addition, it is used to treat postischemic renal injury. Purinergic cotransmission is also seen in the gastrointestinal tract, where ATP (and NO) receptor stimulation inhibits peristalsis.

Neuromodulators modify the process of neurotransmission. They may be circulating neurohormones, local agents, or neurotransmitter substances released from the same nerves or from others nearby. Neuromodulation can occur prejunctionally by decreasing or increasing the amount of transmitter released during transmission or postjunctionally by altering the extent or time course of the neurotransmitter's effect. In all known examples in which prejunctional and postjunctional neuromodulation occurs, these substances act in concert to attenuate or augment effective transmission. The rationale for such effects may reflect the variable geometry of the autonomic neuroeffector junction.[76,77] Unlike the neuromuscular junction, the autonomic neuroeffector junction exists in a dynamic state and manifests only modest postjunctional specialization. Biogenic amines often must traverse wide distances. Given the short half-lives of these chemicals, neuromodulation provides a biologic mechanism for augmentation and prolongation of their action.[78]

NPY is also colocalized with norepinephrine and ATP. However, in some vessels, NPY has little or no direct action; instead, it acts as a neuromodulator prejunctionally to inhibit the release of norepinephrine from the nerve or postjunctionally to enhance the action of norepinephrine (see Fig. 12-14A).[79,80] In other vessels, notably those of the spleen, skeletal muscle, and cerebral and coronary vasculature, NPY has direct vasoconstrictor actions. In the heart and brain, local intrinsic (nonsympathetic) neurons use NPY as the principal transmitter (see Fig. 12-14B). In the spleen, NPY appears to act as a genuine cotransmitter with norepinephrine in perivascular sympathetic nerves (see Fig. 12-14C).[81] The frequency of stimulation determines which vesicles are mobilized to release their transmitters.

A classic transmitter such as acetylcholine coexists with VIP in the parasympathetic nerves of many organs, but in this instance, the two transmitters are stored in separate vesicles. They can be released differentially at different stimulation frequencies, depending on where they are located.[82,83] For example, in the salivary gland, they can act independently on acinar cells and glandular blood vessels (see Fig. 12-15).[73] Cooperation is achieved by the selective release of acetylcholine at low frequencies and VIP at high frequencies of stimulation. Elements of prejunctional and postjunctional modulation have also been described. It is becoming increasingly apparent that in many biologic states, including pregnancy,[84] hypertension, and aging, the relationships among cotransmitters may be an important determinant of a compensatory response to allow finer control of important physiologic function. Additionally, the large number of different receptors may provide targets for potential pharmacologic interventions.

Ganglionic Pharmacology

Ganglia serve far more complex functions than simply being a link between the nerve process of one cell and the cell body of its next connection. Integrative and processing functions contribute to the subtlety of response and organization of the ANS. The electrophysiology of ganglionic stimulation is complex, with at least four different types of responses to electrical stimulation (Table 12-8).[85]

The central event at the ganglion is the excitatory postsynaptic potential (EPSP) when acetylcholine interacts with a neuronal-type nicotinic receptor to depolarize the postsynaptic membrane. Depolarization results primarily from the influx of sodium ions through the nicotinic receptor channel, and it is sensitive to nondepolarizing nicotinic blocking drugs such as hexamethonium. The other changes in electrical potential are

Table 12-8 Fast and Slow Responses of Postganglionic Neurons in Sympathetic Ganglia

Potential	Duration	Mediator	Receptor
Fast EPSP	30 msec	Acetylcholine	Nicotinic cholinergic
Slow IPSP	2 sec	Dopamine	D_2
Slow EPSP	30 sec	Acetylcholine	M_1-cholinergic
Late slow EPSP	4 min	GnRH	GnRH

Adapted from Ganong W: The autonomic nervous system. *In* Ganong W (ed): Review of Medical Physiology, 15th ed. Norwalk, CT, Appleton & Lange, 1991, p 210.

D_2, dopamine receptor inhibiting adenylate cyclase through inhibitory G protein; EPSP, excitatory postsynaptic potential; GnRH, gonadotropin-releasing hormone; IPSP, inhibitory postsynaptic potential.

related to secondary or subsidiary pathways that augment or suppress; these pathways are insensitive to classic nicotinic antagonists.

Secondary pathways are indicated by the following changes in potential elicited by electrical stimulation of the ganglia: (1) slow EPSP, (2) late slow EPSP, and (3) inhibitory postsynaptic potential (IPSP).

Autonomic ganglia may be stimulated by two groups of drugs, nicotinic and muscarinic agonists. Nicotinic agonists cause a rapid onset of excitatory effects, mimic the initial EPSP, and are blocked by classic nondepolarizing ganglionic blocking drugs. Muscarinic agonists delay onset of the excitatory effects and are blocked by atropine.

Blockade of ganglionic transmission results primarily from action at the nicotinic receptor to stop or inhibit transmission. Two groups of drugs block ganglionic transmission. The first group is classically represented by nicotine and initially stimulates the receptor but then blocks it. This action is similar to the action of persistent depolarization. The second group does not cause initial stimulation or a change in ganglionic potentials. This group includes the drugs hexamethonium, trimethaphan, and mecamylamine. Trimethaphan acts by competing with acetylcholine at cholinergic receptor sites on the ganglia; hexamethonium blocks the channel when it is open. Either mechanism blocks the initial EPSP and ganglionic transmission.

Muscarinic antagonists or α-agonists are incapable of completely blocking transmission, but they may inhibit normal modulation of the nerve impulse. β-Adrenergic stimulation facilitates nicotinic and muscarinic transmission, whereas α-adrenergic stimulation inhibits it. 5-HT is mostly facilitative, but it can be inhibitory in certain areas. Dopamine may also be inhibitory through stimulation of the IPSP. The adrenal medulla is a specialized ganglionic synapse and is therefore under influences similar to those arising on the autonomic ganglia.

Drugs and the Autonomic Nervous System

The structure and function of the sympathetic and parasympathetic systems are discussed in the preceding sections. Pharmacologic manipulation of autonomic function is the basis of therapy for many acute and chronic illnesses. The complex physiology allows many points for intervention, including enhancement or inhibition of synthesis, storage, or receptor-mediated activity. In the following sections, specific autonomic drugs of interest to anesthesiologists and the mechanisms by which they work are discussed.

Drugs Affecting Adrenergic Transmission

Endogenous Catecholamines

The endogenous sympathetic transmitters norepinephrine, epinephrine, and dopamine are catecholamines, an important subclass of the sympathomimetic drugs (Fig. 12-16). The parent compound of this sympathomimetic group is β-phenylethylamine, the structure of which includes a benzene ring and an ethylamine side chain. Substitution of hydroxyl groups at the 3 and 4 positions of the benzene ring converts benzene to catechol, and these compounds are known as catecholamines. Although synthetic, isoproterenol and dobutamine are likewise catecholamines. Noncatecholamine drugs may also act as sympathomimetics and have a similar structure.

The catecholamines are primarily metabolized by COMT. The loss of either hydroxyl group enhances oral effectiveness and duration of action because the drug is no longer metabolized by COMT. Noncatecholamines are primarily metabolized by MAO. The noncatecholamines that have a substituted α-carbon have a

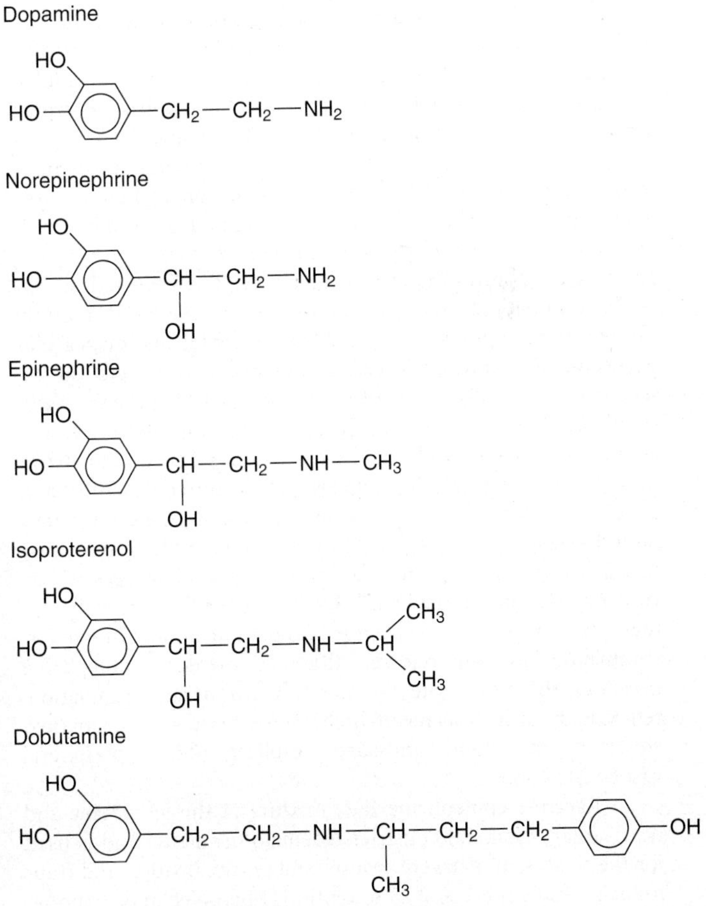

Dopamine

HO, HO–[ring]–CH_2—CH_2—NH_2

Norepinephrine

HO, HO–[ring]–CH(OH)—CH_2—NH_2

Epinephrine

HO, HO–[ring]–CH(OH)—CH_2—NH—CH_3

Isoproterenol

HO, HO–[ring]–CH(OH)—CH_2—NH—CH(CH_3)(CH_3)

Dobutamine

HO, HO–[ring]–CH_2—CH_2—NH—CH(CH_3)—CH_2—CH_2–[ring]–OH

Figure 12-16 Catecholamine structures. A benzene ring with two adjacent hydroxyl groups forms the catechol nucleus.

longer duration of action because they are not metabolized by COMT or MAO.

Epinephrine

Epinephrine is used intravenously in life-threatening circumstances, including the treatment of cardiac arrest, circulatory collapse, and anaphylaxis, but it is also commonly used locally to limit the spread of local anesthetics or to reduce blood loss. The systemic effects of epinephrine are variable and are related to blood levels. The choice of dosing and the route of administration are determined by the indication for use and its urgency.

Epinephrine activates all adrenergic receptors: α_1, α_2, β_1, β_2, and β_3. Potential therapeutic effects of epinephrine include positive inotropy, chronotropy, and enhanced conduction in the heart (β_1); smooth muscle relaxation in the vasculature and bronchial tree (β_2); and vasoconstriction (α_1). With vasoconstriction, aortic diastolic pressure is increased, thereby promoting coronary flow during cardiac arrest, which may be the single most important determinant of survival.[86] Endocrine and metabolic effects of epinephrine include increased levels of glucose, lactate, and free fatty acids.

Epinephrine may be given intravenously as a bolus or by infusion. The usual bolus doses for pressure support begin at 2 to 8 μg given intravenously; 0.02 mg/kg or approximately 1.0 mg is given for cardiovascular collapse, asystole, ventricular fibrillation, electromechanical dissociation, or anaphylactic shock[87] (see also Chapter 97). The larger dose range is recommended in these critical situations to maintain myocardial and cerebral perfusion through peripheral vasoconstriction. High-dose epinephrine (0.1 to 0.2 mg/kg) has been studied in resuscitation from cardiac arrest, but it does not appear to improve rates of survival in adults. In pediatric patients, outcome after asystole and pulseless cardiac arrest is abysmal, and the current recommendation is an initial dose of 0.01 mg/kg repeated every 3 to 5 minutes throughout resuscitative attempts.[41,88] In unusual circumstances, higher doses may be given and doses as large as 0.2 mg/kg may be effective.[89] Patients vary tremendously in their response to epinephrine, and given rates of infusion cannot guarantee the expected serum levels in all patients; the "pressors" should therefore be carefully titrated, and measures to monitor renal, cerebral, and myocardial perfusion are more critical than adherence to a rigid dosing scheme (Table 12-9). A rate of 1 to 2 μg/min, though rarely used, should predominantly activate β_2-receptors, with resulting vascular and bronchial smooth muscle relaxation. A rate of 2 to 10 μg/min (25 to 120 ng/kg/min) increases heart rate, contractility, and conduction through the AV node and decreases the refractory period. Doses in excess of 10 μg/min (100 ng/kg/min) cause marked α-adrenergic stimulation with resultant generalized vasoconstriction. Epinephrine is a potent renal vasoconstrictor that acts directly by α-receptor stimulation and indirectly by stimulation of renin release. Although low-dose epinephrine increases the heart rate by direct β_1-adrenergic stimulation, reflex bradycardia is seen with higher doses because of the marked elevation in blood pressure resulting from peripheral vasoconstriction.

Racemic epinephrine (i.e., mixture of the levorotary and dextrorotary isomers) constricts edematous mucosa and is used for the treatment of severe croup[90] and postextubation and traumatic airway edema. A 2.25% solution (MicroNefrin or Vaponefrin) is diluted with water or saline in a 1:8 ratio and nebulized. Treatments may be given as frequently as every 2 hours, with effects lasting 30 to 60 minutes; the patient should remain under observation for at least 2 hours because initial improvement may be followed by rebound swelling up to 2 hours after administration. Although it is common clinical practice to use the racemic form of epinephrine for these clinical applications, data show that L-epinephrine is 15 to 30 times more potent than the mixture[91] and is equally effective and less expensive for treating these clinical complications.[92]

Bronchospasm may also be treated by subcutaneous administration of epinephrine in doses of 300 μg every 20 minutes with a maximum of three doses. In addition to its direct bronchodilatory effects, epinephrine may decrease antigen-induced release of endogenous bronchospastic substances from mast cells and is particularly useful in anaphylactic reactions.[93] Relative contraindications include advanced age, significant tachycardia, hypertension, and coronary occlusive disease. Absorption of subcutaneous epinephrine is extremely slow because of intense local vasoconstriction, and the effect of a very large subcutaneous dose of 0.5 to 1.5 mg is roughly equivalent to an intravenous infusion of 10 to 30 μg/min. Intravenous injection of epinephrine in a dose appropriate for subcutaneous administration can result in life-threatening ventricular arrhythmias, hypertension, and cerebral hemorrhage. Sus-Phrine, a sustained-release form of epinephrine, may be used in children by subcutaneous injection but should never be given intravenously.

Epinephrine is often applied locally to mucosal surfaces to decrease bleeding in the operative site. It is mixed with local anesthetics for infiltration into tissues or intrathecal injection. The α-mediated vasoconstriction decreases bleeding in the area and slows vascular uptake of local anesthetic, thereby prolonging the duration of effect and decreasing the peak serum level of the

Table 12-9 Dose-Dependent Actions of Inotropes and Chronotropes

Drug* (Proprietary Name)	Receptors	Usual Infusion Rate
Epinephrine (Adrenalin)	β_2 $\beta_1 + \beta_2$ α_1	1-2 μg/min 2-10 μg/min ≥10 μg/min† (bolus: 2-10 μg; 0.5-1.0 mg‡)
Norepinephrine (Levophed)	α_1, β_1, $\gg\beta_2$	4-12 μg/min†
Dopamine (Intropin)	Dopaminergic β α	0-3 μg/kg/min 3-10 μg/kg/min >10 μg/kg/min†
Dobutamine (Dobutrex)	$\beta_1 \gg \beta_2$, α	2.5-10 μg/kg/min†
Isoproterenol (Isuprel)	$\beta_1 > \beta_2$	0.5-10 μg/min
Amrinone (Inocor)	Increase cyclic adenosine monophosphate through inhibition of phosphodiesterase	0.75 mg/kg load over a period of 2-3 min 5- to 10-μg/kg/min infusion

*All agents have elimination half-lives of a few minutes except amrinone ($t_{1/2}$, 3.6 hours; 5.8 hours in congestive heart failure).
†Much higher doses have been used in clinical practice.
‡With anaphylaxis or cardiac arrest.
Data from Hoffman BB, Lefkowitz RJ: Catecholamines and sympathetic drugs. *In* Goodman A, Rall T, Nies A, et al (eds): Goodman and Gilman's the Pharmacological Basis of Therapeutics, 8th ed. New York, Pergamon Press, 1990, p 187.

local anesthetic. Although clinicians express concern about the possible systemic effects of such injections, the increases in plasma levels from vascular uptake are relatively modest and substantially less than levels seen during psychological stress.[94] This conclusion assumes the absence of overt intravenous injection.

Drug interactions with epinephrine are often predictable. Cocaine and other uptake inhibitors enhance the effect and duration of exogenous epinephrine. Preexisting α_1-blockade can cause the paradoxical phenomenon of epinephrine reversal (a hypotensive and tachycardic response) as the β_2-vasodilating effects are unmasked. Patients receiving nonselective β-blockers may demonstrate unopposed α-responses. Cardioselective (β_1) blockade does not have this effect.[95]

Halothane sensitizes the heart to catecholamines, and the potential for troublesome arrhythmias under light inhalational anesthesia has long been appreciated by clinicians. Epinephrine decreases the refractory period, which renders the heart more susceptible to arrhythmias. In adults, the epinephrine dose required to produce three premature ventricular contractions in 50% of patients (ED_{50}) at 1.25 minimum alveolar concentration (MAC) was 2.1 μg/kg for halothane, 6.7 μg/kg for isoflurane, and 10.9 μg/kg for enflurane.[96] Children appear to tolerate higher doses than adults do. It has been suggested that children undergoing halothane anesthesia can receive a maximum of 10 to 15 μg/kg of epinephrine subcutaneously every 10 minutes.[89] Hypocapnia potentiates this drug interaction.

Norepinephrine

Norepinephrine differs structurally from epinephrine only in its lack of a methyl group. Like epinephrine, norepinephrine acts at α- and β-receptors, but it is typically used for its potent α-agonism. It is frequently the pressor of last resort in supporting systemic vascular resistance. Because of its short half-life of 2.5 minutes, continuous infusion is preferred. Whereas less than 2 μg/min (30 ng/kg/min) may uncover the effects of β_1-adrenergic stimulation, the usual infusion rates of greater than 3 μg/min (50 ng/kg/min) elicit peripheral vasoconstriction from α-adrenergic stimulation.

Peripheral vasoconstriction increases blood pressure and may cause reflex bradycardia. Venous return is increased by the powerful venoconstriction. Cardiac output is frequently unchanged or decreased; oxygen consumption is markedly increased. Because pulmonary vascular resistance may be increased, norepinephrine should be used with caution in patients with pulmonary hypertension.[97]

Like epinephrine, norepinephrine is a potent constrictor of the renal and mesenteric vascular beds and can cause renal failure, mesenteric infarction, and peripheral hypoperfusion. The decrease in hepatic flow is of clinical relevance because plasma levels of hepatically metabolized drugs (e.g., lidocaine) are markedly increased. To ameliorate the renal effects, a low-dose dopamine infusion may be added to norepinephrine (see Chapters 92 and 96).[98] Extravasation of norepinephrine can cause tissue necrosis and may be treated by local infiltration of phentolamine. Prolonged infusion has caused gangrene of the digits. The potential for profound vasoconstriction makes careful patient selection and close monitoring mandatory.

Dopamine

Dopamine acts at α-adrenergic, β-adrenergic, and dopaminergic receptors; it also acts to release norepinephrine and therefore has mixed direct and indirect effects. Although dopamine is a precursor of norepinephrine, its most important ANS effect in the periphery may be to cause peripheral vasodilation. Improvement of blood flow through the renal and mesenteric beds in shocklike states is expected through its action at dopamine receptors on the postjunctional membrane. It is rapidly metabolized by MAO and COMT and has a half-life of about 1 minute. Like other endogenous catecholamines, it is given as a continuous intravenous infusion without a loading dose. At low doses (0.5 to 2.0 μg/kg/min), DA_1 receptors are stimulated, and renal and mesenteric vascular beds dilate.[99] In addition to an improvement in renal blood flow, the glomerular filtration rate and sodium excretion increase. With an infusion rate of 2 to 10 μg/kg/min, β_1-receptors are stimulated, and cardiac contractility and output are increased. Rates higher than 5 μg/kg/min stimulate the release of endogenous norepinephrine, which contributes to cardiac stimulation. In larger doses (10 to 20 μg/kg/min), α- and β_1-receptors are stimulated, the α-adrenergic vasoconstrictive effect predominates, and the benefit to renal perfusion may be lost.[100]

In the past, dopamine was frequently used for the treatment of shock (especially in vasodilated states such as sepsis). It was widely believed that infusions of dopamine, by increasing renal blood flow, could protect the kidney and aid in diuresis.[101] However, more recent studies have suggested that dopamine does not have a beneficial effect on renal function in shock states, and its routine use in these patients has therefore been called into question (see Chapters 92 and 96).[102,103]

Dopexamine hydrochloride (Dopacard), an inotropic vasodilator, is a synthetic parenteral dopamine analog (not available in the United States) that may be of use in CHF. Dopexamine is approximately 60 times more potent at β_2-adrenergic receptors than dopamine is, a third as potent at DA_1 receptors, and a seventh as potent at DA_2 receptors.[104,105] Unlike dopamine, it shows no α-adrenergic effects and negligible β_1-adrenergic effects and is consequently devoid of vasoconstrictive activity.[104,106] Dopexamine has a reported half-life of 3 to 7 minutes in healthy patients and approximately 11 minutes in patients with low cardiac output.[107] β_2-Agonism produces systemic vasodilation and indirect inotropic activity (through inhibition of neuronal uptake of norepinephrine).[104-106,108,109] Stimulation of dopaminergic receptors produces selective vasodilation of renal and splanchnic vessels and increases the glomerular filtration rate, diuresis, and natriuresis.[105,110-113]

The use of dopexamine is preferable when vascular resistance is high. Within the dose range of 1 to 6 μg/kg/min, the combined inotropic, vasodilative, diuretic, and natriuretic effects have shown benefit in the management of CHF,[114-117] but an indeterminate outcome in the treatment of septic shock.[116,118-122] Use of this agent has been limited by dose-dependent tachycardia, mainly at doses higher than 4 μg/kg/min.[123,124] The effects of dopexamine on intestinal mucosal and hepatic perfusion remain controversial.[125-130] In general, systemic vasodilation appears more pronounced with dopexamine, and positive inotropic effects appear more marked with dopamine[131] and dobutamine.[132]

Fenoldopam is a selective DA_1 agonist and potent vasodilator (i.e., six to nine times as potent as dopamine) that enhances natriuresis, diuresis, and renal blood flow.[133-137] Because of its poor bioavailability and varied results in clinical trials, fenoldopam is no longer being investigated as a candidate for the treatment of chronic hypertension or CHF. Instead, intravenous fenoldopam, given by infusion at rates of 0.1 to 0.8 μg/kg/min with incremental titration at 0.1 μg/kg/min, has been approved to treat severe hypertension. It is an alternative to sodium nitroprusside, with potentially fewer side effects (i.e., no thiocyanate toxicity, rebound effect, or coronary steal) and improved renal function. Its peak effects occur within 15 minutes.[138,139]

Noncatecholamine Sympathomimetic Amines

The β-agonist isoproterenol and the α-agonists phenylephrine and methoxamine act predominantly at only one type of receptor, but most noncatecholamine sympathomimetic amines act at α- and β-receptors because they have two mechanisms of action: directly at a receptor and indirectly by releasing endogenous norepinephrine.

Mephentermine (Wyamine), ephedrine, and metaraminol (Aramine) are mixed-acting drugs. Ephedrine increases blood pressure and has a positive inotropic effect. Because it does not have detrimental effects on uterine blood flow, ephedrine is widely used as a pressor in hypotensive parturient patients (see Chapter 69). As a result of its β_1-adrenergic–stimulating effects, ephedrine is helpful in treating moderate hypotension, particularly if accompanied by bradycardia. It also has some direct β_2-adrenergic–stimulating effects and has been used orally as a bronchodilator. The usual dose is 2.5 to 25 mg given intravenously or 25 to 50 mg administered intramuscularly. Mephentermine is similar to ephedrine in its effects, whereas metaraminol has relatively stronger direct α_1-adrenergic–stimulating effects and may be associated with reflex bradycardia.

Tachyphylaxis to the indirect effect may develop through depletion of norepinephrine stores. Although all sympathomimetic amines are capable of producing tolerance or tachyphylaxis, the mechanism has been studied best with metaraminol. Metaraminol is taken up into the sympathetic nerve ending, where it displaces norepinephrine and produces its sympathomimetic effect. However, after some time, the drug acts as a false transmitter, and subsequent sympathetic nerve stimulation results in much less effect. Consequently, the drug probably should not be used widely when other, more effective drugs are available. Its indirect action is attenuated in the presence of long-term reserpine or cocaine use, but these drugs may still be efficacious at higher doses. Although indirect-acting drugs are widely used as a first-line therapy for intraoperative hypotension, epidemiologic studies of adverse reactions under anesthesia suggest that dependence on these agents in life-threatening events may contribute to morbidity.[140]

α-Receptor Agonists

Phenylephrine and methoxamine are selective α_1-agonists. These drugs are commonly used when peripheral vasoconstriction is needed and cardiac output is adequate, as in the hypotension that may accompany spinal anesthesia, as well as in patients with coronary artery disease or aortic stenosis to increase coronary perfusion pressure without chronotropic side effects. Phenylephrine (Neo-Synephrine) has a rapid onset and relatively short duration of action (5 to 10 minutes) when given intravenously. It may be given in bolus doses of 40 to 100 μg or by infusion at a starting rate of 10 to 20 μg/min. Larger doses of up to 1 mg are used to slow supraventricular tachycardia through reflex action. Phenylephrine is also used as a mydriatic and nasal decongestant. In anesthetic practice, it is applied topically, alone or mixed with local anesthetic gel, to prepare the nostril for nasotracheal intubation. It is also added to local anesthetic to prolong subarachnoid blockade. In contrast, methoxamine (Vasoxyl) is a much longer-acting drug (30 to 60 minutes).[141] In larger doses, methoxamine possesses some membrane-stabilizing and β-blocking properties.

α_2-Agonists are assuming greater importance as anesthetic adjuvants and analgesics. Their primary effect is sympatholytic. They reduce peripheral norepinephrine release by stimulation of prejunctional inhibitory α_2-adrenoreceptors. They inhibit central neural transmission in the dorsal horn by presynaptic and postsynaptic mechanisms and also have direct sympatholytic effects on spinal preganglionic sympathetic neurons. Traditionally, they have been used as antihypertensive drugs, but applications based on their sedative, anxiolytic, and analgesic properties are being developed.

Clonidine, the prototypical drug of this class, is a selective partial agonist for α_2-adrenoreceptors, with a ratio of approximately 200:1 (α_2 to α_1). Its antihypertensive effects are caused by central and peripheral attenuation of sympathetic outflow and central activation of nonadrenergic imidazoline-preferring receptors.[142-144] The decrease in central sympathetic outflow reduces activity in peripheral sympathetic neurons without affecting baroreceptor reflexes.[145] Arterial blood pressure is thereby decreased without the accompanying orthostatic hypotension produced by many antihypertensive drugs.[146] Because clonidine is lipid soluble, it penetrates the blood-brain barrier to reach the hypothalamus and medulla, and unlike methyldopa, it does not require transformation into another substance.[147] Clonidine withdrawal may precipitate hypertensive crises, so it should be continued throughout the perioperative period (perhaps by patch) or at the least be replaced by close monitoring of blood pressure and ready ability to treat hypertension. The administration of nonselective β-blockers during clonidine withdrawal can worsen hypertension by leaving α_1-receptor–mediated vasoconstriction unopposed. Labetalol has been used to treat this withdrawal syndrome.

Although experience with α_2-agonists as sole anesthetics is limited,[148] these drugs reduce anesthetic requirement and provide a more stable cardiovascular course, presumably because of their sympatholytic effect and the need for lower doses of cardioactive anesthetics.[149,150] Data suggest that oral, intravenous, epidural, and intrathecal administration of clonidine potentiates the anesthetic action of other anesthetics, volatile or injectable, and reduces general and regional anesthetic requirements with correspondingly fewer side effects.[149,151-158] Additionally, a meta-analysis looking at the perioperative use of clonidine and the other α_2-agonists dexmedetomidine and mivazerol indicated a marked decrease in myocardial infarction and perioperative mortality in patients undergoing vascular surgery (see Chapter 62).[159]

Dexmedetomidine has a 1600:1 preference for α_2-receptors relative to α_1-receptors[160]; it was introduced into clinical practice as an adjunct to regional, local, and general anesthetics.[161] Dexmedetomidine has a half-life of 2.3 hours, although its distribution half-life is less than 5 minutes,[162] thus making its clinical effect quite short.

In healthy volunteers, dexmedetomidine increases sedation, analgesia, and amnesia and decreases heart rate, cardiac output, and circulating catecholamines in a dose-dependent fashion.[160] The purported MAC-reducing sedative and analgesic effects demonstrated in preclinical and volunteer studies have largely been borne out in clinical practice. Although dexmedetomidine infusions attenuate the hemodynamic lability of induction, maintenance, and emergence, the dose of other anesthetics must be carefully reduced[163,164] because requirements for other anesthetics may decrease. Another use for this drug is to provide sedation for mechanically ventilated patients during weaning from the ventilator (see Chapter 92).[165]

In addition to their use in the operative setting, α_2-agonists provide effective analgesia for acute and chronic pain, particularly as adjuncts to local anesthetics and opioids. The addition of clonidine increases the duration of analgesia and reduces dose requirements for local and narcotic pain medications.[155,166-180] Epidural clonidine is indicated for the treatment of intractable pain, which is the basis for approval of parenteral clonidine in the United States as an orphan drug.[181] Patients with intractable pain that is unresponsive to maximum doses of oral or epidural opioids benefit from oral, patch, intramuscular, or neuraxial administration of clonidine,[182-185] as do patients with reflex sympathetic dystrophy[186] and neuropathic pain.[187] The intrinsic analgesic effects of α_2-agonists have been demonstrated with large doses of clonidine alone administered intrathecally (as much as 450 µg) or epidurally (1 to 2 µg/kg/hr) to control intraoperative and postoperative pain. Clonidine decreases postoperative oxygen consumption and the adrenergic stress response.[188,189] Although dose-dependent adverse effects such as hypotension and sedation and idiosyncratic adverse effects such as bradycardia do occur, clonidine does not induce profound respiratory depression and only mildly potentiates opiate-induced respiratory depression.[190,191] The relatively minor impact of α_2-induced sedation on respiratory function combined with the short duration of action of dexmedetomidine has led to several reports of the use of dexmedetomidine for awake fiberoptic intubation.[192,193] The authors emphasize the ability to maintain spontaneous ventilation in the context of adequate sedation for the procedure as the reason for selecting the short-acting α_2-agonist for sedation in patients with difficult or at-risk airways. Dexmedetomidine infusions have been used for the perioperative management of obese patients with obstructive sleep apnea to minimize their narcotic needs while providing adequate analgesia.[194]

Aside from its role as an anesthetic adjuvant and antihypertensive agent, clonidine has been used to treat panic disorder[195]; symptoms of opiate, benzodiazepine, and ethanol withdrawal[196]; cigarette craving after smoking cessation[197]; emesis in cancer chemotherapeutic regimens; and diabetic diarrhea. Clonidine may increase blood glucose concentrations by inhibiting release of insulin.[198] Unlike spinal opioids, clonidine does not cause urinary retention and may hasten the time to first micturition after spinal anesthesia.[199,200] Because it has come into wide clinical use only in recent years, the breadth of experience with dexmedetomidine is much less than with clonidine. Nevertheless, infusions of the short-acting intravenous α_2-agonist have been used for sedation during weaning from extubation in the intensive care unit,[201] during neurosurgical cases (to facilitate intraoperative wake-ups and to improve signal quality during neuromonitoring),[202] (see Chapters 46 and 63), and as part of a postoperative pain management regimen.[203] An important characteristic of dexmedetomidine that makes it an attractive choice in these settings is the "rousable" sedation that it creates. Specifically, patients will awaken from apparently deep states of sedation to verbal commands or light tactile stimulation.

β-Receptor Agonists

Nonselective β-Receptor Agonists

DOBUTAMINE. Although at clinical doses it can act at β_2- and α_1-receptors, dobutamine, a synthetic analog of dopamine, has predominantly β_1-adrenergic effects. When compared with isoproterenol, it is reported to affect inotropy more than chronotropy, but it increases conduction velocity through nodal tissue to the same extent. It exerts less of a β_2-type effect than isoproterenol does and less of an α_1-type effect than norepinephrine does. Unlike dopamine, it does not directly release endogenous norepinephrine, nor does it act at dopaminergic receptors.

Dobutamine is particularly useful in CHF and MI complicated by a low-output state, although in cases of severe hypotension, it may not be effective because it lacks a significant α_1-pressor effect. It is relatively safe to use in patients with myocardial ischemia without increasing the size of the infarct or causing arrhythmias. Doses lower than 20 µg/kg/min do not produce tachycardia, but in especially severe CHF, significant tachycardia is the primary adverse effect. Because dobutamine directly stimulates β_1-receptors, it does not rely on norepinephrine stores and may still be effective in catecholamine-depleted states such as chronic CHF. However, in severe chronic CHF, the downregulation of β-adrenergic receptors may hamper its effectiveness.

The β_2-vasodilating effects of dobutamine are almost exactly offset by its α_1-constricting effects, which can be revealed experimentally by administering a nonselective β-blocking drug. Its modest ability to dilate the peripheral vasculature is probably more closely connected with its ability to relieve the high-adrenergic state of decompensated CHF than with specific β_2-mediated vasodilation.[204] Clinical situations that call for distinct afterload reduction may be better served by an agent such as nitroprusside.

Prolonged treatment with dobutamine causes downregulation of β-receptors; tolerance to its hemodynamic effects is significant after 3 days and may be temporarily offset by increasing the rate of infusion.[205] Intermittent infusions of dobutamine have been used in the long-term treatment of heart failure and have improved exercise tolerance[206] but not survival.[207]

ISOPROTERENOL. Isoproterenol (Isuprel) provides relatively pure nonselective β-adrenergic stimulation with no significant effect at α-receptors. Its β_1-adrenergic stimulation is significantly stronger than its β_2 stimulation, but it still causes more β_2-adrenergic activity than dobutamine does. Since the development of other inotropes, its popularity has declined because of its adverse effects of tachycardia and arrhythmias. Isoproterenol was historically used for bradycardia or heart block resistant to atropine, but it is no longer included in the American Heart Association advanced cardiac life support protocol (see Chapter 97). Its primary use at this time is as a chronotropic agent in patients after heart transplantation. These patients are unable to generate an endogenous sympathetic response to challenges because the sympathetic fibers are divided when the native heart is removed. The availability of superior pharmacologic options for most clinical indications has led to removal of isoproterenol from many hospital formularies. Infusion rates start at 0.5 to 5 µg/min for adults. Because it is not taken up into adrenergic nerve endings, its duration of action is slightly longer than that of the natural catecholamines.

Selective β_2-Receptor Agonists

In the past, isoproterenol was used in the treatment of bronchospasm for its β_2-adrenergic–stimulating properties, but unpleasant and dangerous β_1-mediated adverse effects have limited its use. The development of β_2-selective agents has made β-stimulants a cornerstone of the treatment of bronchospasm. However, this β_2-selectivity is only relative, and it may be lost at higher doses; in addition, β_2-receptors in the sinoatrial node may cause tachycardia when stimulated. The structures of these drugs have been modified to slow their metabolism, thereby prolonging their therapeutic benefit and enabling oral administration. In particular, the addition of bulky structures on the catecholamine amino group increases β_2-selectivity, decreases affinity for α-receptors, and protects against metabolism by COMT. These agents are aerosolized and given by inhaler for rapid onset and to minimize systemic drug levels and adverse effects.

An increase in the annual number of deaths from asthma has been well documented, and it has been suggested that this increase may be related to β_2-agonist use.[208-210] Susceptibility to arrhythmia by direct cardiac stimulation or by β_2-induced hypokalemia is a suggested mechanism of these agents. It has also been hypothesized that long-term use of these drugs may increase airway hyperreactivity. Nonetheless, their safe use in many thousands of patients is well documented.

Commonly used drugs include metaproterenol (Alupent, Metaprel), terbutaline (Brethine, Bricanyl), and albuterol (Proventil, Ventolin). Metaproterenol is probably less β_2-selective than albuterol or terbutaline. Terbutaline is the only β_2-selective agent that can be given subcutaneously and may therefore have particular use in status asthmaticus. The normal subcutaneous dose is 0.25 mg, which may be repeated after 15 to 30 minutes.

β_2-Agonists are also used to treat premature labor (see Chapter 69). Ritodrine (Yutopar) has been marketed for this purpose. β_1-Adrenergic adverse effects are common, particularly when the drugs are administered intravenously. The other β_2-selective drugs have also been used as tocolytics, and all have been associated with significant β_1-adrenergic adverse effects and the occasional development of pulmonary edema. As a consequence, their use for the purpose of tocolysis has been questioned.[211]

α-Receptor Antagonists

α_1-Antagonists have long been used clinically as antihypertensives, but they have become less popular over the years. α_1-Blockade vasodilates by blocking the arterial and venous constriction caused by endogenous catecholamines. The effects are potentiated when standing or in the presence of hypovolemia. Reflex tachycardia and fluid retention can ensue.

Phenoxybenzamine (Dibenzyline) is the prototypical α_1-antagonist, although it irreversibly binds to α_1- and α_2-receptors. New receptors must be synthesized before complete offset of its effects occurs. Its half-life after oral administration is unknown, but after an intravenous dose its half-life is about 24 hours. Phenoxybenzamine decreases peripheral resistance and increases cardiac output, and blood flow to the skin and viscera is increased. As expected, its primary adverse effect is orthostatic hypotension; nasal stuffiness may also occur. In addition to receptor blockade, phenoxybenzamine inhibits neuronal and extraneuronal uptake of catecholamines. Phenoxybenzamine is used for the treatment of pheochromocytoma; with extended use, it establishes a "chemical sympathectomy" preoperatively that aids in blood pressure control, permits correction of the contracted plasma volume, and protects against catecholamine-induced cardiac damage. Thus, phenoxybenzamine treatment allows a smoother perioperative course for patients undergoing removal of a pheochromocytoma. When exogenous sympathomimetics are administered after α_1-receptor blockade, their vasoconstrictive effects are inhibited. The effect of phenylephrine is completely blocked, whereas that of norepinephrine is limited to its β_1-adrenergic effect of cardiac stimulation. Epinephrine reversal caused by unopposed β_2-agonism when exogenous epinephrine is given is manifested as severe hypotension and tachycardia. Despite its irreversible binding to the receptor, the recommended treatment of phenoxybenzamine overdosage is norepinephrine infusion because some receptors remain free of the drug.[212]

Phentolamine (Regitine) is a shorter-acting drug that blocks α_1- and α_2-receptors. Historically used to treat pulmonary hypertension, it has largely been supplanted by nitroglycerin and nitroprusside. It is also used to treat the hypertension associated with clonidine withdrawal or with tyramine ingestion during MAOI therapy, but few data have been collected on its efficacy and safety for these indications. Phentolamine has also been infiltrated into affected tissues after extravasation of agents such as norepinephrine in an attempt to relax vasoconstriction; for this purpose, 5 to 10 mg is diluted in 10 mL of saline. Adverse effects of phentolamine include hypotension and gastrointestinal distress; reflex tachycardia and arrhythmias may result from action at α_2-receptors. Coronary artery disease and peptic ulcer disease are relative contraindications to its use. As in phenoxybenzamine overdosage, severe hypotension may require treatment with norepinephrine rather than epinephrine.

Prazosin (Minipress) is a potent selective α_1-adrenergic blocker often used as a prototypical antagonist in pharmacologic experiments. It antagonizes the vasoconstrictor effects of norepinephrine and epinephrine, thereby causing a decline in peripheral vascular resistance and venous return to the heart. Although the heart rate does not normally increase, orthostatic hypotension is a major problem. Unlike other antihypertensive drugs, prazosin improves lipid profiles by lowering low-density lipid levels while raising the level of high-density lipids. It is primarily used to treat hypertension. It has also been used in patients with CHF, but unlike the angiotensin-converting enzyme inhibitors (ACEIs), prazosin does not prolong life. It is metabolized by the liver. Supplied as 1-, 2-, and 5-mg tablets, its starting dose is usually 0.5 to 1 mg given at bedtime because of the orthostatic hypotension. Eventually, it can be taken twice daily.

α_2-Antagonists such as yohimbine increase sympathetic outflow by enhancing release of norepinephrine. These drugs have proved to be of little clinical utility in anesthesia, although they are used in urology.

β-Receptor Antagonists

Pharmacology

β-Adrenergic receptor antagonists (i.e., β-blockers) are among the most commonly prescribed drugs and are frequently taken by patients about to undergo surgery. Current indications for the use of β-blockade include ischemic heart disease, postinfarction management, arrhythmias, hypertrophic cardiomyopathy, hypertension, heart failure, and prophylaxis for migraine headache.

Concern that patients treated with β-blockers would be hemodynamically unstable under anesthesia has proved to be largely unjustified. These drugs are an important part of the armamentarium of the anesthesiologist in the ongoing attempt to limit stress responses perioperatively and to protect the cardiovascular system. A comprehensive analysis by the Agency for Healthcare Research and Quality found that the use of β-blockers perioperatively reduces morbidity and mortality in noncardiac surgery for patients at risk.[213] Several well-known clinical trials[214-218] and the widespread use and safety of these drugs in heart failure[219] have made β-blockade an evolving standard (see Chapter 34).

A wide spectrum of β-adrenergic blockers are available to the clinician. The most important properties to consider when choosing a β-blocker for long-term use are cardioselectivity, intrinsic sympathomimetic activity (ISA), and lipid solubility. In anesthetic practice, cardioselectivity, duration of action, and a formulation suitable for intravenous use are crucial factors (Table 12-10). β-Antagonists resemble isoproterenol in structure and bind competitively to the β-receptor, thereby blocking access by more potent β-agonists (Fig. 12-17). Competitive inhibition at the β-receptor can be overcome by increasing the available concentration of β-agonist. The potency of a β-blocker is often determined by its ability to inhibit induction of tachycardia by isoproterenol. Propranolol is assigned a potency of 1, and the other drugs are evaluated in relation to it.

Nonselective β-adrenergic blockers act at the β_1- and β_2-receptors and include propranolol, nadolol, pindolol, sotalol, oxprenolol, penbutolol, and timolol. Cardioselective β-blockers have stronger affinity for β_1-adrenergic receptors than for β_2-adrenergic receptors, and the predominant effects are therefore cardiac. With β_1-selective blockade, AV conduction velocity, heart rate, and cardiac contractility are decreased, as is release of renin by the juxtaglomerular apparatus and lipolysis at adipocytes. At larger doses, the relative selectivity for β_1-adrenergic receptors is lost and β_2-receptors are also blocked, with the potential for bronchoconstriction, peripheral vasoconstriction, and decreased glycogenolysis.

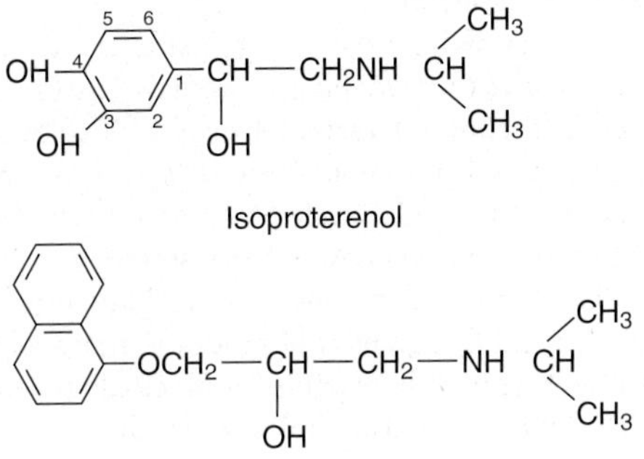

Cardioselective drugs include atenolol, betaxolol, bevantolol, esmolol, and metoprolol. These drugs may be preferable for patients with obstructive pulmonary disease, peripheral vascular disease, Raynaud's phenomenon, and diabetes mellitus. Although previously a matter of controversy, a meta-analysis concluded that cardioselective β-blockers can be given safely to patients with chronic obstructive pulmonary disease.[220] Nevertheless, because the selectivity is only relative and may be lost at conventional clinical doses, extreme care should be taken when administering a β-blocker in the presence of pulmonary disease. Some β-antagonists also have vasodilatory effects, thus making them particularly useful in the treatment of hypertension and

(Catechol) (ethanolamine)

Isoproterenol

Propranolol

Figure 12-17 Structure of isoproterenol and propranolol. *(From Tollenaeré JP: Atlas of the Three-Dimensional Structure of Drugs. Amsterdam, Elsevier North-Holland, 1979.)*

Table 12-10 Pharmacokinetics and Pharmacology of Selected β-Adrenoceptor Blockers

Characteristic	Atenolol	Metoprolol	Propranolol HCl	Labetalol	Esmolol	Carvedilol
Proprietary name	Tenormin	Lopressor	Inderal Ipran	Trandate Normodyne	Brevibloc	Coreg
Relative β sensitivity	+	+	0	0	+	0
Intrinsic sympathetic activity	0	0	0	+	0	0
Membrane-stabilizing activity	0	0	++	0	0	—*
Lipophilicity†	Low	Moderate	High	Low	Low	High
Predominant route of elimination	RE (mostly unchanged)	HM	HM	HM	Hydrolysis by RBC esterase	HM
Drug accumulation in renal disease	Yes	No	No	No	No	No
Elimination half-life (hr)	6 to 9	3 to 4	3 to 4	≈6	9 min	2 to 8
Usual oral maintenance dose	50-100 mg qd	50-100 mg qid	60 mg qid	100-600 mg bid	N/A	25-50 mg bid
Usual intravenous dose (caution)		5 mg q5min × 3	0.1 mg/kg (maximum)	1-2 mg/kg	50 to 300 μg/kg/min infusion	15 mg

*Data not available.
†Determined by the distribution ratio between octanol and water.
HM, hepatic metabolism; N/A, not applicable; RBC, red blood cell; RE, renal excretion; 0, no effect; +, mild effect; ++ moderate effect.

CHF.[221,222] Labetalol vasodilates by blocking α_1-receptors and by direct β_2-receptor agonism.

β-Blockers exerting a partial agonist effect at the receptor while blocking access by more potent agonists possess ISA. Drugs with ISA include acebutolol, carteolol, celiprolol, dilevalol, oxprenolol, penbutolol, and pindolol. These drugs primarily decrease arterial blood pressure and, to a lesser extent, heart rate and left ventricular function. When sympathetic activity is high, such as during exercise, these drugs behave more like conventional β-blockers. The partial β_2-agonism of pindolol induces bronchodilation. ISA may therefore be useful if β-blockade is required in a patient with bradycardia, peripheral vascular disease, or very mild hyperreactive airway disease. Drugs with ISA may not be as effective in controlling symptoms in severe angina or in reducing mortality after MI.[223] ISA may protect against β-blocker withdrawal syndrome.[224]

Propranolol and acebutolol possess membrane-stabilizing activity (MSA), also referred to as the quinidine-like or local anesthetic effect. This effect reduces the rate of rise in cardiac action potential. The MSA of propranolol may explain the decrease in the oxygen affinity of hemoglobin when it is administered. However, MSA is seen only at concentrations 10 times those required for blockade of β-receptors and is probably of little clinical consequence. Overdose with drugs that exhibit MSA is associated with a higher incidence of fatality.[225]

Indications for Use

PERIOPERATIVE β-BLOCKADE. In the late 1990s, two important studies established the value of perioperative β-blockade in patients at risk for coronary ischemia who were undergoing noncardiac operations (see Chapters 34 and 35). Patients are labeled as "at risk" if they fit into one of two categories: they are undergoing high-risk vascular surgery and have no evidence of inducible coronary ischemia, or they are undergoing a nonvascular procedure but have traditional risk factors for coronary artery disease (elderly, high cholesterol, hypertension, cigarette smoking, family history of coronary disease, or diabetes).[226] The Multicenter Study of Perioperative Ischemia Research Group[215] enrolled 200 patients about to undergo surgery who had risk factors for coronary artery disease and randomized them to receive placebo or atenolol before and after surgery. Their results demonstrated that although there was no improvement in in-hospital outcomes (cardiac death or MI) in the atenolol-treated group, the treated group did have a lower incidence of cardiac events at the 6- to 8-month follow-up and a marked decrease in all-cause mortality that persisted at 2-year follow-up (survival rate at 2 years: 68% in the placebo group and 83% in the atenolol-treated group). The second study[216] enrolled patients with known ischemic disease demonstrated on preoperative stress echocardiography. The treatment group in this study was given bisoprolol and the dose was titrated to achieve a heart rate below the patients' ischemic threshold. The results of this study, whose participants were at much higher risk for ischemic events than those of the previous study, demonstrated a 10-fold decrease in perioperative cardiac death and MI (3.4% versus 34%). These powerful demonstrations that β-blockade could decrease perioperative cardiac risk and improve survival out to 2 years led to tremendous political and administrative pressure to increase the use of β-blockers perioperatively.[227] Unfortunately, more recent research has brought the value of routine perioperative β-blockade into question. The POBBLE study[228] results showed no reduction in 30-day cardiovascular morbidity in patients undergoing vascular surgery (one of the "at-risk" groups from previous studies). Similarly, the DIPOM study[229] showed no benefit of β-blockade in diabetics (another "at-risk" group) undergoing major noncardiac operations. Finally, a large retrospective study looking at in-hospital mortality in more than 780,000 patients demonstrated a neutral or even negative effect of perioperative β-blockade in patients without clear-cut coronary artery disease. β-Blockade was associated with a reduced mortality rate in only the 3% of patients who had three or more risk factors (based on the revised Cardiac Risk Index) for coronary ischemia.[230] Thus, until larger studies are completed, the only strong indication for initiating β-blockade preoperatively is for patients undergoing vascular surgery who are at high cardiac risk as a result of the finding of ischemia on preoperative testing.[227]

When perioperative β-blocker therapy is initiated, it should be titrated to a non–ischemia-inducing heart rate (usually 60 to 70 beats per minute) and not given as a standard fixed dose to all patients. β-blockers should be continued in patients who are already taking them as treatment of their angina, symptomatic arrhythmia, or hypertension.

The safety of continuing β-blockade perioperatively is well established, and initial concerns regarding interaction with general anesthesia have not been confirmed. Attempts to discontinue β-blockers increase the risk for rebound tachycardia (with or without atrial fibrillation) and myocardial ischemia in patients with coronary disease. These drugs should be given up to the time of surgery, and intravenous forms in appropriate dosages should be used whenever gastrointestinal absorption may be in question. If β-blockers have been omitted from the preoperative regimen, esmolol or labetalol may be used acutely to blunt tachycardia and hypertension. Cardioselective and nonselective β-blockers appear to be effective in blocking the chronotropic effects of endotracheal intubation and surgical stress.[231]

MYOCARDIAL ISCHEMIA. Propranolol was initially introduced for the treatment of myocardial ischemia more than 3 decades ago, and β-blocking drugs remain an important part of drug therapy for myocardial ischemia (see Chapter 35). This class of drugs reduces oxygen demand by decreasing the heart rate and cardiac contractility. Cardioselective and nonselective β-blockers are effective. Atenolol, metoprolol, nadolol, and propranolol have been approved in the United States for the treatment of angina; metoprolol and atenolol are the only β-blockers approved for intravenous use in patients with acute MI. Although initially there was concern that β_2-receptor blockade could worsen ischemia through unopposed α-mediated vasoconstriction, this phenomenon is rarely seen, even in patients with variant angina. β-Antagonists are used to treat acute MI and on a long-term basis to reduce reinfarction and mortality in patients after infarction.[232-235] Early administration of intravenous β-blocking agents to patients receiving thrombolytic therapy appears to lower the incidence of ischemia and reinfarction[236] and may reduce the incidence of serious ventricular arrhythmias.[237] Long-term use of β-blockers (i.e., timolol, propranolol, metoprolol, and atenolol) has been shown to decrease mortality after MI. In usual clinical practice, the dose is increased until the heart rate is 60 to 80 beats/min at rest and there is no tachycardia with exercise.

CONGESTIVE HEART FAILURE. Over the past 5 to 10 years, β-blockers have become first-line agents for the treatment of CHF of ischemic and nonischemic origin. Clinicians had been disinclined to use β-blockers for heart failure patients because of the drugs' negative inotropic effects. These effects have not turned out to be a significant concern in clinical practice. Early studies demonstrated a significant decrease in all-cause mortality for heart failure patients treated with metoprolol or bisoprolol. Several large studies[238,239] were stopped because the decrease in mortality in treated patients with moderate to severe heart failure was so pronounced. The benefits of β-blockers in patients with heart failure have been attributed to normalization and remodeling of the ventricle, which begin after 1 month of β-blockade[240]; to reduced norepinephrine-related cardiomyocyte apoptosis in the presence of β_1-blockade[241]; to decreased sudden cardiac death because of the β-blockers' antiarrhythmic activity; and most recently, to altered expression of genes in the myocardium that regulate contractility and pathologic hypertrophy.[242] To avoid worsening a patient's heart failure symptoms and to minimize negative inotropic effects, β-blockers are started at very low doses and are titrated to the target dose.[243] The only β-blockers approved for the treatment of CHF by the U.S. Food and Drug Administration are carvedilol and metoprolol, although their efficacy in patients with severe (i.e., New York Heart Association class IV) heart failure is still being studied. If decompensation occurs with the β-blocker, phosphodiesterase inhibitors are the inotropes of choice because their effects are not antagonized by β-blockade.[244]

HYPERTENSION. The mechanisms by which β-antagonists treat hypertension are incompletely understood. Arterial blood pressure is specifically decreased in hypertensive patients because long-term treatment of normotensive individuals does not decrease blood pressure. Reduced cardiac output and renin release have been suggested as mechanisms. In hypertensive patients, β-antagonists without ISA may cause a 15% to 20% reduction in cardiac output and a 60% reduction in renin release. However, pindolol, which has ISA and minimal effect on renin, is also successful in treating hypertension.[245] Maximum renin suppression precedes significant changes in arterial blood pressure.[246] Initially, β-blockade increases peripheral vascular resistance and then over time lowers it.[247] The decrease in cardiac output and eventual lowering of peripheral resistance may account for much of the antihypertensive efficacy of these drugs. However, this too is an incomplete explanation because labetalol is an effective antihypertensive despite its lack of effect on cardiac output. A primary CNS effect is not likely to be a major mechanism because the antihypertensive efficacy of lipophilic and hydrophilic compounds is similar. Generally, β-blockade is ineffective as monotherapy in hypertensive African American patients older than 60 years.

CARDIAC ARRHYTHMIAS. β-Blockers are widely used in the treatment of tachyarrhythmias as class II agents (see Chapters 35, 60, and 61). Two possible mechanisms of action are blockade of catecholamine effects and MSA, although the latter is most likely not clinically significant because antiarrhythmic effects are present in agents without MSA.[248] β-Antagonists slow the rate of depolarization of the sinus node and any ectopic pacemakers, slow conduction through atrial tissue and the AV node, and increase the refractory period of the AV node. These drugs can convert atrial arrhythmias to sinus rhythm,[249] but β-blockade is primarily used to slow the ventricular response. Reentrant tachyarrhythmias and those associated with Wolff-Parkinson-White syndrome, mitral valve prolapse, and a prolonged QT interval may also respond to these drugs. Care should be exercised if AV block is present, as in digitalis toxicity, although these drugs are useful in the treatment of digitalis-associated tachyarrhythmias. Sotalol, a β-blocker with added class III activity, is effective against ventricular tachyarrhythmias; however, in a trial comparing racemic sotalol with D-sotalol in post-MI patients, mortality increased with D-sotalol.[250] The trial was terminated when patients at lowest risk for arrhythmic events after MI had an increased mortality rate with this drug.[251]

TACHYCARDIA. β-Antagonists are frequently used as adjuvants to moderate the reflex tachycardia associated with vasodilators (see Chapter 61). In addition to potentiating a reduction in blood pressure, β-blockade also reduces the velocity of left ventricular ejection (dp/dt) and attenuates the shearing force associated with the increased velocity of ventricular contraction when afterload is reduced with nitroprusside without concomitant β-blockade.[252] Labetalol has been particularly useful in this situation.[253]

THYROTOXICOSIS. Cardiac complications are a primary cause of morbidity in thyrotoxicosis (see Chapter 75). β-Blockade can suppress the tachycardia and rhythm disturbances, although very large doses may be required. β-Antagonists also may be combined with digitalis for their synergistic effect on AV node conduction. Propranolol inhibits conversion of thyroxine to the active form triiodothyronine in the periphery.[254]

MISCELLANEOUS CONDITIONS. Timolol (Timoptic) and betaxolol (Betoptic) are β-blocking drugs used topically in the eye to treat glaucoma. They reduce the production of aqueous humor. Even topical use of these agents has been associated with significant systemic effects of β-blockade. β-Blockers are used in patients with idiopathic hypertrophic subaortic stenosis to reduce the dynamic obstruction to left ventricular outflow. The drugs are also effective in the prophylaxis but not the treatment of migraine headaches and in controlling acute panic symptoms and essential tremor.

Adverse Effects

The adverse effects of most concern are those involving cardiopulmonary function. Severe noncardiopulmonary reactions such as cutaneous reactions or anaphylaxis are rare. Life-threatening bradycardia, even asystole, may occur, and decreased contractility may precipitate CHF in vulnerable individuals. In patients with bronchospastic lung disease, β_2-blockade may be fatal. CNS effects, although an appropriate consideration with long-term therapy, are not a concern with the usual anesthetic use of these agents. Diabetes mellitus is a relative contraindication to the long-term use of β-antagonists because hypoglycemia in the face of sympathetic blockade is not accompanied by warning signs such as tachycardia and tremor and because compensatory glycogenolysis is blunted. However, most non–insulin-dependent diabetic patients can tolerate these drugs, although β-blockade may cause insulin resistance in rare cases. In addition to the potential worsening of peripheral perfusion by β_2-blockade in patients with peripheral vascular disease, Raynaud's phenomenon may be triggered in susceptible patients. Sudden withdrawal of β-blockers may cause myocardial ischemia and possibly infarction, but this is less of a problem with β-blockers that have ISA, such as pindolol.[255] Even though β-antagonists may reduce renal blood flow and the glomerular filtration rate, these agents can be used in renal failure. For such patients, the doses of lipid-insoluble drugs should be reduced. To avoid worsening of hypertension, use in pheochromocytoma should be avoided unless α-receptors have previously been blocked. Nonselective agents may elicit hypertensive responses in cases of high sympathetic stimulation.[256]

Undesirable drug interactions are possible with β-blockers. The rate and contractility effects of verapamil are additive to those of β-blockers,[257,258] and care should be taken when combining these agents, especially the intravenous forms in acute situations such as supraventricular tachycardia. The combination of digoxin and β-blockers can have powerful effects on heart rate and conduction and should be used with special care. Pharmacokinetic interactions are predictable from the degree of lipid solubility of the drug. Cimetidine and hydralazine may reduce hepatic perfusion, thereby increasing plasma levels and half-lives of the lipid-soluble β-antagonists. Barbiturates, phenytoin, rifampin, and smoking may induce hepatic enzymes and enhance metabolism. Propranolol may reduce hepatic clearance of lidocaine and increase the risk for toxicity.

Overdose of β-blocking drugs may be treated with atropine, but isoproterenol, dobutamine, or glucagon infusions (or some combination) may be required along with cardiac pacing to ensure an adequate rate of contraction.

Specific Drugs

The drugs propranolol, metoprolol, labetalol, and esmolol are particularly useful in anesthetic practice because they are widely available in intravenous formulations and have well-characterized effects. If the drug that the patient has taken on a long-term basis is propranolol, metoprolol, or labetalol, it may be continued in intravenous form. In deciding which intravenous β-blocker to substitute in a patient taking a β-blocker on a long-term basis, the need for cardioselectivity is a primary consideration. Cardioselectivity is provided by metoprolol or esmolol. If the long-term agent has ISA, oxprenolol and acebutolol have intravenous forms, but they are not readily available. In many situations, esmolol may be substituted and titrated to effect, with the expectation that its effects will fade relatively rapidly if it is not well tolerated.

Propranolol. Propranolol (Inderal, Ipran), the prototypical β-blocker, is a nonselective β-blocking drug with MSA but no ISA. It readily penetrates the CNS. Because of its high lipid solubility, it is extensively metabolized in the liver, but metabolism varies greatly from patient to patient. Its effective dose is extremely variable: 10 mg to as much as 320 mg may be given orally each day. Clearance of the drug can be affected by liver disease or altered hepatic blood flow. Renal impairment does not require adjustment of dosing. Despite its half-life of 4 hours, its antihypertensive effect persists long enough to permit dosing once or twice daily. Propranolol is available in an intravenous form and was initially given as either a bolus or an infusion. Infusions of propranolol have largely been supplanted by esmolol. For bolus administration, doses of 0.1 mg/kg may be given, although most practitioners initiate therapy with much smaller doses, typically 0.25 to 0.5 mg, and titrate to effect. Propranolol shifts the oxyhemoglobin dissociation curve to the right, which perhaps accounts for its efficacy in vasospastic disorders.[259]

Metoprolol. Metoprolol (Lopressor) is approved for the treatment of angina pectoris and acute MI. It is cardioselective and lacks ISA and MSA. Because it is metabolized in the liver by the monooxygenase system, doses need not be adjusted in the presence of liver failure. The usual oral dose is 100 to 200 mg/day given once or twice daily for hypertension and twice daily for angina pectoris. It may be administered intravenously in doses of 2.5 to 5 mg every 2 to 5 minutes up to 15 mg, with titration to heart rate and blood pressure.

Labetalol. Labetalol (Trandate, Normodyne) is representative of a class of drugs that act as competitive antagonists at the α_1- and β-adrenergic receptors. Labetalol consists of four isomers that block the α_1-, β_1-, and β_2-receptors, inhibit neuronal uptake of norepinephrine (uptake 1), act as a partial agonist at β_2-receptors, and possibly have some direct dilating ability. The potency of the mixture for β-blockade is 5- to 10-fold that for α-blockade. The usual oral dose of labetalol is 200 to 400 mg twice daily, although much larger doses have been used. It is metabolized by the liver, and clearance is affected by hepatic perfusion. The dose need not be adjusted for renal dysfunction. Labetalol may be given intravenously every 5 minutes in 5- to 10-mg doses or up to a 2 mg/min infusion. It significantly blunts cardiovascular responses to tracheal intubation.[260] It can be effective in the treatment of aortic dissection,[252] hypertensive emergencies,[261,262] and postoperative cardiac surgical patients,[263] particularly because vasodilation is not accompanied by tachycardia. It may be used in pregnancy to treat hypertension on a long-term basis and in more urgent situations.[264] Uterine blood flow is not affected, even with a significant reduction in blood pressure (see Chapter 69).[265]

Carvedilol. Carvedilol, a mixed α- and β-antagonist, has been introduced as therapy for mild or moderate hypertension,[266-274] for the management of stable or unstable angina, and after acute MI.[275-279] Clinical trials of carvedilol for the treatment of controlled CHF (New York Heart Association class II to IV) suggest a significant reduction in mortality,[237,238,280,281] especially for patients with diabetes.[282]

Esmolol. Because of its hydrolysis by esterases, esmolol (Brevibloc) has a uniquely short half-life of 9 to 10 minutes, which makes it particularly useful in anesthetic practice. It is administered when β-blockade of short duration is desired or in critically ill patients for whom the adverse effects of bradycardia, heart failure, or hypotension may necessitate rapid withdrawal of the drug. The peak effects of a loading dose are seen within 5 to 10 minutes and diminish rapidly (within 20 to 30 minutes). It is cardioselective and may be given as a bolus of 0.5 mg/kg to blunt cardiovascular responses to tracheal intubation. If used as an infusion for the treatment of supraventricular tachycardia, 500 μg/kg is given over a 1-minute period, followed by an infusion of 50 μg/kg/min for 4 minutes. If the rate is not controlled, a repeat loading dose followed by a 4-minute infusion of 100 μg/kg/min is given, and this sequence is repeated with the infusion increased in 50-μg/kg/min increments up to 200 or 300 μg/kg/min if needed. The effect may persist for 20 to 30 minutes after discontinuation of the infusion. When compared with verapamil, esmolol is more likely to convert atrial fibrillation to sinus rhythm.[248] Esmolol is safe and effective for the treatment of intraoperative and postoperative hypertension and tachycardia.[283-285] If continuous use is required, it may reasonably be replaced by a longer-lasting cardioselective drug such as intravenous metoprolol. It has been used safely even in patients with compromised left ventricular function.[286,287]

Drugs that Inhibit Synthesis, Storage, or Release of Norepinephrine

Some early antihypertensive drugs acted by replacing norepinephrine in the nerve ending with a much less potent false transmitter. Methyldopa (Aldomet) is such a drug and was the most popular nondiuretic antihypertensive used before the development of β-blockers.[213] Like DOPA, methyldopa enters the biosynthetic pathway for norepinephrine (see Fig. 12-7). It is then decarboxylated to α-methylnorepinephrine. Initially, this chemical was thought to act as a false transmitter, but it was found to be almost as potent as norepinephrine. In the CNS, methyldopa may be further metabolized to α-methylepinephrine, and it acts at α_2-receptors to decrease sympathetic outflow, which reduces blood pressure. Because of its sedating qualities, fluid retention, postural hypotension, and occasional reports of hepatic necrosis, methyldopa is now used much less often.

Methylparatyrosine (metyrosine, Demser) is a potent inhibitor of TH, which catalyzes the formation of DOPA from tyrosine (see Fig. 12-7). Because this is the rate-limiting step in the biosynthesis of norepinephrine, the drug significantly decreases levels of endogenous catecholamines and is useful in treating inoperable or malignant pheochromocytomas.

Reserpine affects the uptake of norepinephrine, not at the neuronal membrane but at the vesicular membrane, thereby inhibiting transport and storage of norepinephrine and dopamine. However, this drug is rarely used in modern medicine.

Guanethidine (Ismelin) acts initially by blocking the release of norepinephrine, and then it is taken up into adrenergic nerve endings by the uptake-1 mechanism and depletes norepinephrine stores. It is used to treat hypertension, usually after many other drugs have been tried. Its inability to cross the blood-brain barrier accounts for its lack of sedative effects. Guanadrel (Hylorel) is similar to guanethidine, but it has a faster onset and shorter duration of action.

Bretylium, a class III antiarrhythmic used parenterally to treat life-threatening ventricular tachyarrhythmias, is now largely of historical interest. Like guanethidine, it is taken up into adrenergic nerve terminals, but its mechanism of action is otherwise quite different. Bretylium initially causes release of norepinephrine and subsequently blocks that release by decreasing sympathetic nerve excitability. Unlike guanethidine, bretylium does not deplete norepinephrine stores. The initial catecholamine release may cause marked hypertension and worsen some arrhythmias, such as those associated with digitalis toxicity and myocardial ischemia.[234] As a consequence, bretylium, which had been part of the advanced cardiac life support protocols for treating ventricular arrhythmias, has been dropped from the algorithms.

MAO and COMT are enzymes important in degradation of the catecholamines. MAOIs bind irreversibly to the enzyme and increase the amine concentration within the presynaptic terminal. Chronic MAOI use is associated with antihypertensive, antidepressant, and antinarcoleptic effects. MAOIs are thought to exert their antihypertensive effect through a false transmitter mechanism. Tyramine is usually oxidatively deaminated in the gut by MAO. With administration of an MAOI, tyramine levels rise. When tyramine is taken up into the sympathetic nerve terminal by the uptake-1 mechanism, it enters the varicosities and is transformed by DβH into octopamine. On its subsequent release in place of norepinephrine, octopamine is only weakly reactive at sympathetic receptors, thereby resulting in lowering of blood pressure. The MAOIs are no longer used as antihypertensives because many other drugs with better risk-benefit profiles have been developed.

MAOIs are primarily used in psychiatric practice. The use of MAOIs as antidepressants is based on the theory that depression is caused by decreased amine in the synapses of the CNS. Inhibition of MAO makes more amine available for release. MAOIs available for the treatment of depression include isocarboxazid (Marplan), phenelzine sulfate (Nardil), and tranylcypromine sulfate (Parnate).

Based on substrate specificity, there are at least two forms of MAO. MAO-A acts on 5-HT, epinephrine, norepinephrine, tyramine, and dopamine, whereas MAO-B is specific for tyramine and dopamine. A specific MAO-B inhibitor, selegiline hydrochloride (deprenyl), has been developed for the treatment of Parkinson's disease in the hope that by blocking central dopamine breakdown, more dopamine will be preserved in the affected areas.[288]

Drug and food reactions have been of great concern in patients taking MAOIs. Tyramine-containing foods such as red wine and aged cheese must be avoided by patients taking these drugs. Consumption delivers a huge amount of tyramine to the adrenergic nerve terminal, with a subsequent massive release of norepinephrine. This release is manifested clinically as a hypertensive crisis with the potential for MI, cerebral hemorrhage, and death. Any intake of biogenic amine precursors can be expected to increase catecholamine levels greatly, as seen with the concurrent administration of levodopa with MAOIs. The effects of sympathomimetic amines, particularly the indirectly acting drugs, are enhanced. Narcotics, most notably meperidine, have been associated with hyperpyrexic coma and death in patients treated with MAOIs. The depressant effects of agents such as sedatives, alcohol, and general anesthetics are enhanced in these patients. Interactions between MAOI and tricyclic antidepressants can be disastrous. Anesthetic interactions with deprenyl have not been reported, but experience with this drug is limited. Great concern has been expressed that patients receiving long-term therapy with an MAOI risk life-threatening drug interactions during anesthesia. Emergency surgery in patients given an MAOI can be punctuated by marked hemodynamic instability. Severe reactions to narcotics and indirect-acting sympathomimetics, as well as altered metabolism of endogenous and exogenous catecholamines, make these patients potentially difficult to manage. Because of the possibly dangerous interactions of many drugs with MAOIs, controversy exists about the best way to anesthetize these patients.[289,290] It has been suggested that the level of concern expressed over the years may be excessive. Although prudence and custom dictate discontinuation of MAOIs at least 2 weeks in advance of elective procedures, there appear to be rational anesthetic choices based on pharmacology and risk-benefit considerations for patients when surgery cannot be delayed or no effective alternative psychiatric medications are available.

Drugs Affecting the Renin-Angiotensin System

The renin-angiotensin system maintains blood pressure and fluid balance. The major end product of the system, angiotensin II, is a potent vasoconstrictor that also stimulates release of aldosterone from the adrenal cortex. Aldosterone causes salt and water retention by the kidney. The mechanism by which angiotensin II is produced is as follows. The juxtaglomerular cells of the renal cortex secrete the proteolytic enzyme renin, which cleaves angiotensinogen, a protein synthesized in the liver, and produces the decapeptide angiotensin I. Angiotensin I is converted almost immediately to angiotensin II by angiotensin-converting enzyme (ACE). This converting enzyme is located predominantly in the endothelial tissue of the lung. In addition to its direct vasoconstrictive activity, angiotensin II enhances the prejunctional release of norepinephrine from adrenergic nerve ending and increases efferent sympathetic nerve activity. Angiotensin II also affects sodium and water homeostasis by directly decreasing tubular reabsorption of sodium, increasing antidiuretic and adrenocorticotropic hormone secretion, and stimulating the secretion of aldosterone. ACE is also a kinase that degrades the vasodilator bradykinin. ACE inhibition blocks angiotensin II formation and delays the breakdown of bradykinin, along with effects on associated prostaglandins.[291]

Although only a small percentage of hypertensive patients have high circulating plasma renin levels, 70% of patients will respond to the antihypertensive effects of ACEIs. In patients who have elevated plasma renin levels (e.g., patients with CHF or salt depletion states), ACEI therapy must be initiated at lower doses because these patients are extremely sensitive to the effects of ACEIs and significant hypotension can follow the administration of a standard starting dose of these drugs.[213]

ACEIs have proved to be useful in the treatment of hypertension and CHF and have decreased mortality after MI.[292] Captopril (Capoten) was the first active oral agent available, followed by enalapril (Vasotec) and lisinopril (Prinivil, Zestril). ACEIs affect the renin-angiotensin-aldosterone system by inhibiting ACE activity.[293,294] Enalapril is the only ACEI available as an intravenous preparation at this time. Lisinopril offers once-daily dosing.

All the ACEIs are approved for the treatment of hypertension. Captopril, enalapril, ramipril, and trandolapril all decrease morbidity and mortality in patients with CHF. Captopril is associated with more frequent adverse effects than the other agents are, may have a few more drug interactions, and has a dosing regimen of two or three times daily, in contrast to the other ACEIs, which have a dosing regimen of once or twice daily.

Some adverse effects observed with ACEIs are common to the entire class, such as cough, angioedema, acute renal failure, and hyperkalemia. Angioedema, especially after the first dose, affects the face, extremities, lips, mucous membranes, tongue, glottis, or larynx.[295,296] Some occurrences may be fatal.[291,297] Rash and taste disturbances are more frequent with captopril than with the other ACEIs. Because impairment of renal function with an ACEI is usually reversible after withdrawal of the drug, renal function must be monitored, and because hyperkalemia may result from inhibition of aldosterone secretion, serum potassium levels should be monitored. ACEIs can cause fetal morbidity and mortality in humans. These agents should not be used at all during the second or third trimester of pregnancy.[293] The adverse effect profile of the ACEIs has led to the development of angiotensin II receptor blockers (ARBs). Losartan was the first of this new class of antihypertensive agents, which now includes six other ARBs. Initial trials have not demonstrated ARBs to be superior to ACEIs; however, the addition of these agents during chronic ACEI therapy reduced all-cause mortality and hospitalization in patients with heart failure.[298]

Cholinergic Drugs

Overview of Mechanisms of Action

Cholinergic drugs act by mimicking, amplifying, or inhibiting the effects of acetylcholine. Cholinergic drugs do not behave exactly like acetylcholine; their drug action is more specific, with fewer sites affected than with acetylcholine, and their duration of action is generally longer than that of acetylcholine.

Unlike adrenergic pharmacology, in which the clinician can select from a wide choice of drugs, there is a relative paucity of drugs that influence parasympathetic function. In general, drugs that affect the parasympathetic system act in one of four ways:

1. As an agonist by stimulating cholinergic receptors
2. As an antagonist by blocking or inhibiting the actions mediated by the cholinergic receptor
3. Blocking or stimulating receptors on autonomic ganglia
4. Inhibiting the metabolism of acetylcholine, thereby increasing and prolonging its effect

There are no effective clinically used drugs that act through mechanisms affecting the synthesis of acetylcholine (by inhibiting choline acetyltransferase) or by causing indirect release of acetylcholine. Hemicholinium, which interferes with choline uptake and could deplete acetylcholine stores, is not used clinically. Adenosine may inhibit the release of acetylcholine by decreasing the affinity of binding sites for calcium ions; aminoglycoside antibiotics compete with calcium for membrane calcium channels, as does magnesium. Exocytotic release of acetylcholine is inhibited by botulinum toxin. This toxin is sometimes given by local injection to treat strabismus and blepharospasm and has also been used for trigger point injections in pain clinics and to treat age lines. The popularity of off-label uses of this toxin increases the chance of botulism poisoning. In a full-blown botulism-poisoning syndrome, fatalities may result from muscle weakness and respiratory failure.

Cholinergic Agonists

Cholinergic agonists have limited therapeutic use because of their detrimental effects. As a result of its diffuse, nonselective actions and rapid hydrolysis by acetylcholinesterase and butyrylcholinesterase, acetylcholine has had almost no therapeutic use other than as an intraocular medication for transient constriction of the pupil during ophthalmic surgery.

Cholinergic agonists in clinical use have been derived from acetylcholine, but they resist hydrolysis by cholinesterase, which permits a useful duration of action. The different systemic effects of the cholinergic agonists are more quantitative than qualitative, but some limited organ selectivity is useful therapeutically, as seen with the synthetic choline esters bethanechol and carbachol. Methacholine and bethanechol are primarily muscarinic agonists; carbachol has significant nicotinic and muscarinic effects. Adding a methyl group to the β-position of the choline in acetylcholine produces methacholine, which is almost purely muscarinic and nearly totally resistant to hydrolysis by either of the cholinesterases. An intravenous infusion of methacholine causes hypotension and bradycardia; a small subcutaneous dose causes transient hypotension with a reflex increase in heart rate. The sole current use of methacholine (Provocholine) is as a provocative agent in diagnosing hyperreactive airways, thereby making positive use of the deleterious bronchoconstrictive effect of muscarinic agonists. It is administered only by inhalation; serious adverse effects include gastrointestinal symptoms, chest pain, hypotension, loss of consciousness, and complete heart block when the drug is given orally or parenterally. An excessive bronchoconstrictive response should be treated by an inhaled β-agonist; coexisting β-blockade is considered a contraindication to the use of methacholine.

The carbamate derivative of methacholine, bethanecol (Urecholine), is occasionally used postoperatively to reinstitute peristaltic activity in the gut or to force the extrusion of urine from an atonic bladder. Bethanecol shows preferential activity at intestinal and urinary receptors relative to cardiac sites, so stimulation of the gastrointestinal tract and bladder is achieved with minimal cardiovascular effects. Bethanecol is usually given orally, but if there is inadequate gastrointestinal function to permit absorption of an oral dose, it can be given subcutaneously as well.

Carbachol is used topically or intraocularly to constrict the pupil for the long-term treatment of wide-angle glaucoma. When used topically, it is often better tolerated than the ophthalmic anticholinesterase agents, and it may be effective in patients resistant to pilocarpine and physostigmine. The rapid pupillary constriction is caused by the combination of ganglionic blockade and muscarinic effects. Another natural alkaloid, pilocarpine, was used to treat glaucoma until the advent of more modern drugs.

Muscarinic Antagonists

Muscarinic antagonists are the active ingredients in some common plants used since antiquity for medicinal and poisonous effects. Despite their age, muscarinic antagonists still represent important drugs in anesthesia and critical care.

Muscarinic antagonists compete with neurally released acetylcholine for access to muscarinic cholinoceptors and block its effects. They also antagonize the actions of muscarinic agonists at noninnervated, muscarinic cholinoceptors. Presynaptic muscarinic receptors on the adrenergic nerve terminal may inhibit release of norepinephrine, and muscarinic antagonists may enhance sympathetic activity. With the exception of quaternary ammonium compounds that do not readily cross the blood-brain barrier and have few CNS actions, there is no significant specificity of action among these drugs; they block all muscarinic effects with equal efficacy, although some quantitative differences in effect may be seen (Table 12-11). Research has revealed several subtypes of muscarinic receptors, and agonists and antagonists have been synthesized that bind preferentially to one or another of these subtypes. Pirenzepine preferentially blocks the M_1 receptor, tripitramine shows highest affinity for the M_2 receptor, and darifenacin binds preferentially to the M_3 receptor. The distinctive pharmacology of the various antimuscarinic agents has played a major role in the development of new treatments of overactive bladder disorders. Oxybutynin, tolterodine, darifenacin, solifenacin, and trospium have all been developed to optimize the relief of bladder symptoms while minimizing effects on muscarinic receptors outside the bladder.

Historically, muscarinic antagonists were used for peptic ulcer disease, various forms of spastic bowel syndrome, upper respiratory illness, and asthma. However, with the availability of specific histamine (H_2)-blocking drugs such as cimetidine for peptic ulcer disease, these uses have markedly decreased. Atropine, once used to treat bronchospasm, was displaced with the introduction of β_2-agonist drugs that did not dry secretions or diminish ciliary motility. Topical use of atropine analogs in ophthalmologic practice to dilate the pupil is still common.

The addition of a muscarinic anticholinergic drug to anesthetic premedication for decreasing secretions and preventing harmful vagal reflexes was mandatory in the era of ether anesthesia, but it is less important with modern inhaled agents. Routine preoperative use of these drugs as antisialagogues continues in some pediatric and otorhinolaryngologic cases or when fiberoptic intubation is planned.

Atropine has a tertiary structure that easily crosses the blood-brain barrier (Fig. 12-18). CNS effects have been seen with the relatively large doses (1 to 2 mg) given to block the adverse muscarinic effects of the anticholinesterase drugs that reverse neuromuscular blockade (see Chapter 29). In contrast, one of the synthetic antimuscarinic drugs, glycopyrrolate (Robinul), does not cross the blood-brain barrier because of its quaternary structure and has gained popularity for this use. Glycopyrrolate has a longer duration of action than atropine does.

Scopolamine, which resembles the others of this class in peripheral actions, has pronounced CNS effects. It is the active ingredient in most over-the-counter preparations sold as soporifics, and it is effective in preventing motion sickness. The patch preparation of scopolamine can be used prophylactically for motion sickness and for postoperative nausea and vomiting, but like the oral and parenteral forms, it may be associated with adverse eye, bladder, skin, and psychological effects.[299,300]

Table 12-11 Muscarinic Anticholinergic Drugs

Drug	Duration	Central Nervous System*	Antisialagogue	Heart Rate
Atropine	Short	Stimulation	+	++
Glycopyrrolate	Long	0	++	+
Scopolamine	Short	Sedation	++	0/+

*The effects of atropine are limited with the usual clinical doses, but they can be significant in the elderly.
0, no effect; +, mild effect; ++, moderate effect.

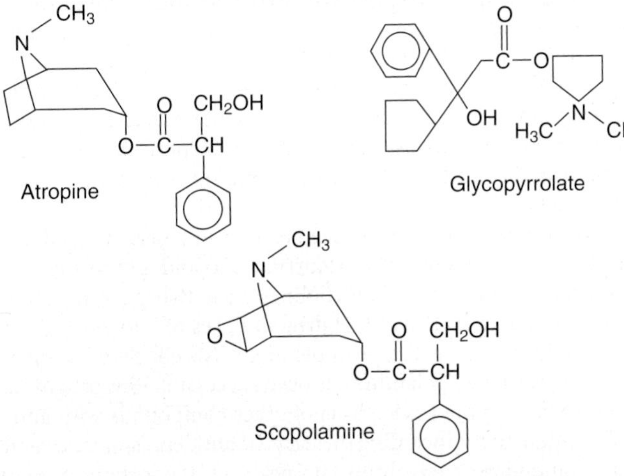

Atropine

Glycopyrrolate

Scopolamine

Figure 12-18 Structural formulas of clinically useful antimuscarinic drugs.

The development of ipratropium (Atrovent) reestablished antimuscarinic drugs for the treatment of asthma and bronchospastic disorders.[301] Although ipratropium is structurally similar to atropine and has essentially the same effects when administered parenterally, an important difference is that ipratropium is a quaternary ammonium compound. It is very poorly absorbed when inhaled and has few extrapulmonary effects, even in extremely large doses by this route. Ninety percent of the inhaled drug is swallowed, but only 1% of the total dose is absorbed systemically.

When administered to normal volunteers, ipratropium provides almost complete protection against bronchospasm induced by a variety of provocative agents. However, in asthmatic patients, results vary. The bronchospastic effects of some agents, such as methacholine or sulfur dioxide, are completely blocked, whereas there is little effect on leukotriene-induced bronchoconstriction. The onset of bronchodilation is slow, and the maximum effect is less than that seen with β-agonists. Unlike atropine, ipratropium has no negative effect on ciliary clearance. In general, the therapeutic effect of antimuscarinics, including ipratropium, is greater in patients with chronic obstructive pulmonary disease than in asthmatic patients.[298] Ipratropium is supplied as a metered-dose inhaler that dispenses 18 μg per puff. Two puffs are taken orally four times each day. Maximum bronchodilation occurs in 30 to 90 minutes and may last 4 hours.

The toxic effects of muscarinic antagonists come from the blockade of muscarinic cholinoceptors in the periphery and the CNS. The peripheral effects (e.g., dry mouth) may be irritating but are not life threatening in healthy adults. However, children depend more than adults on sweating for thermoregulation and can become dangerously hyperthermic when given these agents. Moreover, older individuals may not be able to tolerate the cardiac, ocular, or urinary effects of muscarinic blockade.

CNS effects are the usual cause of death or injury. Increasing doses of atropine or scopolamine cause greater distortions of mentation that progress from thought disorders to hallucinations, delusions, delirium, and severe psychoses. These effects are reversible, but the mental dysfunction can persist for weeks. Left alone, an intoxicated individual will die of starvation, dehydration, or trauma. People who have received more than 500 mg of atropine, which is more than 1000 times the usual dose, and have been disabled for weeks have recovered fully.

Small doses of atropine (0.05 mg) can evoke bradycardia, a finding that has led some clinicians to increase the dose in children. It was thought that a CNS effect of atropine could be responsible, but the time course and the fact that bradycardia occurred in vagotomized animals cast doubt on this explanation. Whether this paradoxical bradycardia is a central or peripheral effect, or both, and the role of muscarinic subtypes are still subjects of debate.[302]

Atropine and scopolamine toxicity has been treated for decades with the naturally occurring alkaloid physostigmine (Antilirium), which is an anticholinesterase that penetrates the blood-brain barrier. Use of this drug in doses of 1 to 2 mg given intravenously to treat the postoperative CNS effects of intravenous atropine or scopolamine has been successful. Physostigmine may also reverse the CNS effects of other compounds with anticholinergic activity, including the tricyclic antidepressants, several major tranquilizers, and antihistamine drugs. Physostigmine may also antagonize the sedative effects of the benzodiazepines, but a specific benzodiazepine antagonist, flumazenil (Romazicon), has supplanted physostigmine for this use.[303] Physostigmine must be administered with care because of its potentially lethal nicotinic effects, which are not prevented by the muscarinic antagonists, and because its half-life rarely matches that of the intoxicant.

Cholinesterase Inhibitors

Anticholinesterase drugs are a common means of producing sustained, systemic cholinergic agonism. These drugs are used to reverse neuromuscular blockade and to treat myasthenia gravis and certain tachyarrhythmias.

Three chemical classes of compounds are used as cholinesterase inhibitors: carbamates, organophosphates, and quaternary ammonium alcohols. Physostigmine, neostigmine, and pyridostigmine are carbamates, whereas edrophonium is a quaternary ammonium alcohol. The cholinesterase enzyme is inhibited as long as the esteratic site is bound to an acetate, carbamate, or phosphate. Carbamate and phosphate bonds are much more resistant to attack by hydroxyl groups than acetate bonds are. The acetylated form lasts for only microseconds, whereas the carbamylated form lasts for 15 to 20 minutes. Organophosphates include diisopropyl fluorophosphate, parathion, malathion, soman, sarin, VX, and a variety of other compounds used as insecticides. Although the toxicity of the organophosphate insecticides is primarily related to their anticholinesterase activity, the mechanism of this effect is different from the clinically used anticholinesterase drugs (see Chapter 74). The organophosphates produce irreversible enzyme inhibition and have CNS effects. Consequently, treatment of organophosphate insecticide poisoning relies on chemical compounds capable of displacing the insecticides from the enzyme to reactivate the cholinesterase activity. The best documented of these chemicals is pralidoxime (2-PAM). Physostigmine and most of the organophosphates are not quaternary ammonium compounds and have major effects on cholinergic functions in the CNS (see Chapter 74).

Because these compounds can increase the effect and duration of neurally released acetylcholine, they are useful in situations in which such release is deficient, such as myasthenia gravis. Anticholinesterase drugs are occasionally used to stimulate intestinal function and are applied topically in the eye as a miotic. An irreversible organophosphate anticholinesterase that is used clinically is echothiophate iodide (Phospholine), which is available as topical drops for the treatment of glaucoma. Its major advantage over other topical agents is its prolonged duration of action. Because this chemical also inactivates plasma cholinesterase, it may prolong the action of succinylcholine. Although prudence dictates discontinuation of echothiophate for 1 week before surgery, there are numerous case reports of successful anesthesia performed without discontinuation of echothiophate under emergency conditions.

Ganglionic Drugs

Ganglionic Agonists

Ganglionic agonists are essential for analyzing the mechanism of ganglionic function, but they have no therapeutic use. Nicotine is the classic ganglionic agonist, and its effects have been well described.

Parasympathetic drugs stimulate ganglia, but this action is usually masked by their other parasympathomimetic effects. Experimentally, relatively large doses of acetylcholine administered intravenously after blockade of muscarinic receptors by atropine cause ganglionic stimulation and release of epinephrine by the adrenal medulla.

Ganglionic Antagonists

Ganglionic antagonists were the first effective therapy for the management of hypertension and were used extensively during the 1950s and 1960s. However, because of interference with transmission through sympathetic and parasympathetic ganglia, their antihypertensive action was accompanied by numerous undesirable effects. Hexamethonium, the prototypical drug of this class, has minimal neuromuscular and muscarinic activity. The systemic effects of ganglionic blockade are determined by the resting tone of a specific body system before the initiation of ganglionic blockade (see Table 12-3). With the disappearance of trimethaphan from clinical use, these drugs are largely of historical interest.

Autonomic Dysfunction

Assessment of Autonomic Function

The increased operative risk of patients with autonomic dysfunction that may occur with aging and diabetes[304] makes the diagnosis of autonomic neuropathy extremely important. A panel of five tests of cardiovascular function has been developed to evaluate autonomic function in diabetic patients (see Chapter 35).[305] The tests include heart rate responses to the Valsalva maneuver, standing up, and deep breathing and blood pressure responses to standing up and sustained handgrip. The tests involving changes in heart rate measure injury to the parasympathetic system, which precedes changes in the measures of blood pressure that reflect sympathetic injury. Early autonomic dysfunction is defined as a single abnormal or two borderline-abnormal results on the tests involving changes in heart rate. Definite involvement is dignosed when the results are abnormal on two of the tests of changes in heart rate. Severe dysfunction is defined as abnormalities in blood pressure assessments. Application of these standards requires that the investigator understand the proper techniques for performing the five tests and the expected results in patients without autonomic neuropathy (Table 12-12). If patients demonstrate an increase in heart rate of more than 20 beats/min with a vigorous handgrip, it can be assumed that they are incompletely β-blocked. The simplicity and effectiveness of this clinical assessment have led to its use in the evaluation of patients with nondiabetic causes of autonomic dysfunction as well.

Table 12-12 Noninvasive Tests for Assessing the Autonomic Nervous System

Clinical Examination	Technique	Normal Value
Parasympathetic		
HR response to a Valsalva maneuver	The seated subject blows into a mouthpiece (while maintaining a pressure of 40 mm Hg) for 15 seconds. The Valsalva ratio is the ratio of the longest R-R interval (which comes shortly after release) to the shortest R-R interval (which occurs during the maneuver)	Ratio of >1.21
HR response to standing	HR is measured as the subject moves from a resting supine position to standing. A normal tachycardic response is maximal around the 15th beat after rising. A relative bradycardia follows that is most marked around the 30th beat after standing. The response to standing is expressed as a 30 : 15 ratio and is the ratio of the longest R-R interval around the 30th beat to the shortest R-R interval around the 15th beat	Ratio of >1.04
HR response to deep breathing	The subject takes six deep breaths in 1 minute. The maximum and minimum heart rates during each cycle are measured, and the mean of the differences (maximum HR – minimum HR) during three successive breathing cycles is taken as the maximum-minimum HR	Mean difference >15 beats/min
Sympathetic		
BP response to standing	The subject moves from resting supine to standing, and standing SBP is subtracted from supine SBP	Difference <10 mm Hg
BP response to sustained handgrip	The subject maintains a handgrip of 30% of the maximum handgrip squeeze for up to 5 minutes. BP is measured every minute, and the initial DBP is subtracted from the DBP just before release	Difference >16 mm Hg

BP, blood pressure; DBP, diastolic blood pressure; HR, heart rate; SBP, systolic blood pressure.

Plasma Catecholamines

Accurate and sensitive techniques for measuring plasma catecholamines have existed for 3 decades, but interpretation of the data that they yield has been controversial. Normal plasma epinephrine and norepinephrine levels are typically in the range of 100 to 400 pg/mL, and they can increase sixfold or more with stress.

Plasma concentrations of epinephrine, which reflect adrenal medullary activity if not overall sympathetic activity, are labile. Significant isolated adrenal medullary secretion results from certain stressful situations, such as public speaking.[5] Moreover, venous samples may reflect epinephrine kinetics in the organ being sampled rather than in the whole body, so arterial samples may be more reliable.

The significance of the norepinephrine concentration in plasma is even more controversial. Even though the adrenal medulla secretes some norepinephrine, levels in plasma generally reflect spillover from sympathetic stimulation that was not taken up again by the nerve terminal. Although reuptake may be tissue specific and markedly influenced by alterations in physiology or diseases, spillover in humans is 10% to 20% of the synthesis rate of norepinephrine at baseline and may be greatly enhanced in periods of sympathetic activation.[306] The most compelling argument for the use of plasma norepinephrine as a marker of sympathetic activity comes from animal studies in which plasma norepinephrine levels directly mirrored nerve stimulation. Many important studies have correlated increases in plasma catecholamines with acute and chronic stress, which has led to the concept of stress-free anesthesia. A striking relationship between mortality rates for patients with CHF and elevated plasma norepinephrine levels resulted in the use of β-adrenergic antagonists to treat ventricular dysfunction.[307,308]

The development of experimental radiotracer techniques to assess the in vivo kinetics of catecholamines has provided additional information that is of clinical importance, particularly in relation to regional kinetics. For example, studies relying only on arterial and venous catecholamines suggested that the hepatomesenteric bed contributes significantly to total-body clearance of catecholamines but only minimally (<8%) to spillover. However, later studies of regional norepinephrine kinetics demonstrated that release of norepinephrine from the gut (≤25% of the total body) was largely obscured by efficient extraction (>80%) in the liver. Similarly, selective elevations in release of norepinephrine from the heart, which may be associated with ischemia, early onset of CHF, and tachyarrhythmias, may not be apparent in measured arterial or venous levels.[309] Observations involving regional spillover led to the realization that although stress may activate a generalized sympathetic response, there may be different patterns contingent on the stimulus. It is possible that the lack of consistency of plasma norepinephrine levels in the presence of clinically significant sympathetic activation may be a function of the measurement technique or the particular stressor.

It is my belief that given the effects of age, posture, and hydration, small changes in plasma catecholamine levels correlate poorly with hemodynamic changes and merit cautious interpretation whereas significant increases (>1000 pg/mL) in levels are good markers of activation of the sympathetic nervous system.

Clinical Syndromes

Surgical Stress Response

Surgical stress, particularly that associated with major operations, results in profound metabolic and endocrine responses. The combination of autonomic, hormonal, and catabolic changes that accompany surgery has been called the surgical stress response.[310] Despite widespread clinical intuition that attenuation of the stress response is beneficial, there has been long-standing debate about whether such a strategy affects outcome. Three separate lines of evidence suggest that attenuation of the surgical stress response can lead to improved outcomes. In a series of studies, interruption of the sympathetic response to surgery markedly reduced surgical stress intraoperatively and postoperatively. The use of continuous thoracic epidural infusions of local anesthetics minimized the rise in plasma catecholamines, cortisol, and glucagon and improved outcomes. Improved outcome was independent of the patient's level of pain because metabolic and endocrine responses to surgery were not similarly reduced in patients receiving other methods of pain relief, including nonsteroidal anti-inflammatory drugs and opioids.[311] Continuation of epidural infusions well into the postoperative period was regarded as essential to improving outcome. Inflammatory and immunologic responses, which are necessary for infection control and wound healing, appear to be unaffected. With the use of similar techniques and other stress-reducing maneuvers, faster and more complete recovery was achieved in elderly patients undergoing colon resection.[312]

A separate line of evidence supporting the hypothesis that long-term attenuation of the stress response alters outcome comes from the pediatric literature. When neonates with complex congenital heart disease underwent cardiac surgery, those who received high-dose sufentanil infusions intraoperatively and for the first 24 hours postoperatively to reduce the stress response had lower β-endorphin, norepinephrine, epinephrine, glucagon, aldosterone, and cortisol levels than controls did.[310] The mortality rate in the opiate group was significantly lower than in the study or historical controls, thus demonstrating that anesthetic techniques can have profound effects on the metabolic and endocrine responses to surgery and that effective management of these reflexes can alter outcomes.

A third line of evidence involves results from the multicenter study of the Perioperative Ischemia Research Group (see "Perioperative β-Blockade").[215] The ability to alter overall survival at 2 years with a perioperative regimen of β-blockade has provided compelling evidence of the benefit of attenuating the stress response[216,217,219] and has altered clinical practice in patients at risk for cardiac morbidity. Similar results have been achieved when perioperative α_2-agonists were given to "at-risk" patients as well.[313] Presumably, the decrease in sympathetic tone that accompanied administration of the β-blocker or the α_2-agonist suppressed the stress response and improved outcomes.

Diabetes Mellitus

Diabetic autonomic neuropathy is the most common form of autonomic neuropathy and the most extensively investigated (see Chapter 35). It occurs in 20% to 40% of all insulin-dependent diabetic patients. The symptoms associated with diabetic autonomic neuropathy confer an increased risk during anesthesia and surgery by direct and secondary mechanisms. Common manifestations of diabetic autonomic neuropathy include impotence, postural hypotension, gastroparesis, diarrhea, and sweating abnormalities. Early small-fiber damage is revealed by loss or impairment of vagally controlled normal heart rate variability, decreased peripheral sympathetic tone with a subsequent increase in blood flow, and diminished sweating. In a diabetic neuropathic foot, the senses of pain and temperature are lost before touch or vibration is affected. With sympathetic denervation, the sympathetic nerves normally found supplying small arterioles are entirely absent or are abnormally distant from their effector sites. When impotence or diarrhea is the sole manifestation, there is little effect on survival; however, with postural hypotension or gastroparesis, 5-year mortality rates are greater than 50%.

Most clinicians recognize that diabetic patients with autonomic neuropathy may be at additional risk during general anesthesia.[314] Gastroparesis is probably caused by vagal degeneration and is of clinical relevance because awake or rapid-sequence intubation may be required. Systemic injury to the vasa vasorum in patients with postural hypotension increases the risk for hemodynamic instability and cardiovascular collapse in the perioperative period. Mechanisms that maintain normal standing blood pressure are altered, and normal precapillary vasoconstriction in the foot on standing may be diminished. Baroreceptors in the carotid sinus and aortic arch are compromised by diabetic neuropathy. Diabetic patients with orthostatic hypotension usually have lower norepinephrine levels.

Even in seemingly minor surgery, diabetic autonomic neuropathy can lead to significant complications.

Diabetics with autonomic neuropathy may have a significantly greater decline in blood pressure with induction and a greater need for vasopressors than diabetic patients without autonomic dysfunction.[314] Page and Watkins[315] reported five cases of unexpected cardiorespiratory arrest in young diabetic patients, all of whom had symptoms of autonomic neuropathy. In a large, prospective study of diabetic autonomic neuropathy involving use of the five evocative clinical tests discussed earlier, parasympathetic dysfunction preceded sympathetic failure in 96% of the patients.[316] This battery of autonomic tests identifies patients with autonomic neuropathy and is highly predictive of mortality and perioperative risk.[304]

Autonomic Changes with Aging

Aging is associated with alterations in vascular reactivity manifested clinically as exaggerated changes in blood pressure—hypertension and orthostatic hypotension (see Chapter 71). Orthostatic hypotension is quite common (about 20%) in the elderly and may result largely from diminished baroreceptor responsiveness. Heart rate responses to changes in blood pressure, the Valsalva maneuver, and the respiratory cycle are blunted with aging.[317]

Resting and exercise-induced norepinephrine levels increase with age in healthy subjects (by about 13% per decade), in part because of decreased clearance.[318] Previously a matter of controversy, it now appears that besides the well-documented reduction in vagal function associated with aging,[319] the primary autonomic defect in aging is an impairment in reuptake of norepinephrine, perhaps as a function of decreased nerve density. Although there is no apparent age-dependent decrement in nerve firing rates from sympathetic efferents in skeletal muscle,[320] kinetic studies reveal selective and dramatic increases in cardiac norepinephrine spillover attributable to the decreased reuptake in elderly patients subjected to mental stress or exercise.[306] This can precipitate clinical complications (i.e., arrhythmogenesis and sudden cardiac death) in patients with cardiac disease. However, end-organ responsiveness is blunted by compensatory downregulation of β_1-adrenoreceptors (i.e., decreased receptor density and affinity) and uncoupling of β_2-adrenoreceptors through decreased G_s activity.[321] Despite increased cardiac spillover, cardiac oxygen consumption is not altered.[322]

Attenuation of presynaptic α_2-adrenoreceptor–mediated inhibition of neuronal norepinephrine release[323-325] also accounts for the increased norepinephrine levels observed with age. Reduced postsynaptic α-adrenoreceptor activity decreases contractile responses and further attenuates vasoconstrictor tone. In a seemingly vicious cycle, the increase in circulating norepinephrine levels is associated with downregulation of platelet α_2-adrenoreceptor density and responsiveness. The loss of adrenergic control through the reduction of α_2- and β-receptor–mediated responses with age causes a decrease in the sympathetic nervous system's ability to maintain cardiovascular homeostasis, thus implying a relationship with or an explanation of the increased incidence of cardiovascular disorders such as CHF in the elderly.

Autonomic Changes in Spinal Cord Transection

The most drastic of all alterations in the ANS that an anesthesiologist may encounter is complete spinal cord transection (see Chapters 46, 63, and 72). Spinal cord transection affects motor and sensory function, and it may also result in profound changes in autonomic activity that can alter anesthetic care. As is obvious from sympathetic and parasympathetic outflow anatomy, spinal cord injuries or transection can cause various degrees of autonomic dysfunction, depending on the site, extent, and timing of the lesion. Many autonomic reflexes are inhibited by the supraspinal feedback that is lost after spinal cord transection. In paraplegic patients, small stimuli can evoke exaggerated sympathetic discharges.

In patients with cervical spinal cord transection, sympathetic and parasympathetic outflow is detached from central control mechanisms. In addition to the expected motor and sensory changes, there are profound abnormalities that alter the cardiovascular, thermoregulatory, gastrointestinal, and urinary systems. The autonomic consequences of transection are not always apparent because the distal portion of the spinal cord may retain some function and thereby result in unanticipated autonomic abnormalities.

There are fundamental differences between the acute and chronic effects of spinal cord transection. Initially, a transient state of decreased excitability occurs. This phenomenon, known as spinal shock, usually takes place immediately after the lesion and may last days to weeks. In these patients, the periphery is generally atonic and the peripheral blood vessels are dilated. In patients with high thoracic lesions who have sustained recent injury, basal supine blood pressure is usually low and accompanied by plasma catecholamine levels that are approximately 35% of normal.[326] Patients with recent low spinal injuries may exhibit compensatory tachycardia from intact parts of the ANS.

Patients with chronic high spinal lesions may fail to respond to hypovolemia with an increased heart rate and may exhibit bradycardia. The only intact efferent component of the baroreflex pathways in quadriplegic patients is the vagus. Bradycardia occurs with changes in position and with Valsalva maneuvers or increased intrathoracic pressure.[327]

One aspect of care that is frequently overlooked is the effect of tracheal suctioning on patients with high spinal transection. Given that many of these patients depend on artificial respiration because of their respiratory muscle paralysis, unopposed vagal stimuli may contribute to profound bradycardia. This vagal response is particularly accentuated during hypoxemia.

Because the sympathetic nervous system may be dysfunctional in these patients, the renin-angiotensin-aldosterone system compensates for the maintenance of blood pressure. Patients with spinal cord transection may be exquisitely sensitive to ACEIs, even with modest changes in intravascular volume or posture. The release of renin may be independent of sympathetic stimulation and may be caused by the renal baroreceptor stimulation that accompanies the decline in renal perfusion pressure.

Although pressure stimuli above the lesion do not usually change blood pressure, the phenomenon of autonomic dysreflexia can occur with stimulation below the lesion. Bladder or bowel distention can elicit the so-called mass reflex. This autonomic reflex includes a dramatic rise in blood pressure, a marked reduction in flow to the periphery, and flushing and sweating in areas above the lesion. In addition, there is often contraction of the bladder and rectum, skeletal muscle spasms, and penile erection.

The patient's heart rate may decline as a reflex. Surprisingly, evidence from microneurography studies indicates that there is only a modest rise in sympathetic nerve activity during activation of the mass reflex,[328] and plasma norepinephrine levels increase only modestly. Speculation has arisen that the exaggerated blood pressure response may be caused by supersensitivity of adrenoreceptors. As anticipated, quadriplegic patients exhibit an increase in sensitivity to exogenously administered pressors.[326] Blood pressure in quadriplegic patients may increase 5- to 10-fold in response to the exogenous administration of angiotensin and to catecholamines. Impairment of the descending inhibitory reflex pathways that are activated during hypertension may contribute to the supersensitivity. This hypothesis is supported by the finding that sensitivity is rarely increased when the lesion is below T5. There is apparently a normal level of adrenoreceptors in these patients with lower spinal lesions, even those with long-standing quadriplegia.

Management of autonomic dysreflexia is of clinical importance. Although the anesthesiologist may be tempted to opt for minimal anesthesia in a patient without sensory or motor function, significant visceral reflexes can be evoked. The anesthesiologist may use spinal anesthesia, general anesthesia, or a vasodilator such as nitroprusside or nitroglycerin to attenuate this reflex, even if pain is not appreciated. There has been some enthusiasm for using clonidine prophylactically to diminish this response.

An additional problem arising from the autonomic denervation of spinal cord transection is thermogenesis. In these patients, hypothermia may result from cutaneous vasodilation and the inability to shiver. Similarly, hyperthermia can occur because the normal sweating mechanism is impaired. It is therefore important to monitor temperature assiduously in these patients during the course of anesthesia.

New Concepts in Autonomic Activity

Genetic Contributors to Autonomic Function and Drug Responsiveness

In the past 5 years there has been an explosion in the knowledge of nonmendelian genetic contributors to human physiologic and pathophysiologic function. The Human Genome Project provided a starting point for the identification of genetic abnormalities. The next logical step is to define the implications of genetic variations on physiologic and pharmacologic responses. Genetic variations as small as a single-nucleotide polymorphism (SNP) to larger genetic insertions or deletions have been identified in the genes coding for essential components of the ANS. SNPs and, to a lesser extent, larger deletion and insertion sequences have been identified in the genes that code for nearly every adrenergic and dopaminergic receptor subtype (all save the α_{1d}-receptor). Genetic coding for the muscarinic receptor subtypes, on the other hand, is remarkably well conserved.[329] In addition to variants in coding for the autonomic receptors, genetic mutations in codes for the proteins responsible for catecholamine synthesis, reuptake, and breakdown have also been identified, as have variants for the receptor-coupled G proteins.[330] Although many potential genetic contributors to autonomic-related disease states (e.g., essential hypertension, lipid and glucose metabolism, and postural tachycardia syndrome[331]) have been identified, no single genetic mutation has completely explained any of the examined autonomic dysfunctions. It is almost certainly true that abnormalities in autonomic function are polygenic in origin and also involve significant environmental input. Thus, future investigations that attempt to explain autonomic diseases will require evaluation of larger genetic sequences (not SNPs or other short-segment variants) that contain multiple associated genetic variants. Once the collection of genetic variants responsible for the majority of the autonomic findings of a given disease are identified, the impact of the combined genetic contribution on responsiveness to a given drug or class of drugs will need to be assessed through directed clinical trials.

References

1. Ruffolo R: Physiology and biochemistry of the peripheral autonomic nervous system. *In* Wingard L, Brody T, Larner J, et al (eds): Human Pharmacology: Molecular-to-Clinical. St. Louis, Mosby–Year Book, 1991, p 77.
2. Fleisher LA, Frank SM, Shir Y, et al: Cardiac sympathovagal balance and peripheral sympathetic vasoconstriction: Epidural versus general anesthesia. Anesth Analg 79:165, 1994.
3. Hoffman B, Lefkowitz R: Adrenergic receptors in the heart. Annu Rev Physiol 44:475, 1982.
4. Radu A, Dahl G, Loewenstein WR: Hormonal regulation of cell junction permeability: Upregulation by catecholamine and prostaglandin E_1. J Membr Biol 70:239, 1982.
5. Dimsdale J, Moss J: Plasma catecholamines in stress and exercise. JAMA 243:340, 1980.
6. Philipson LH: β-Agonists and metabolism. J Allergy Clin Immunol 110:S313, 2001.
7. Kharasch ED, Bowdle T: Hypokalemia before induction of anesthesia and prevention by β_2 adrenoceptor antagonism. Anesth Analg 72:216, 1991.
8. Williams ME, Gervino EV, Rosa RM, et al: Catecholamine modulation of rapid potassium shifts during exercise. N Engl J Med 312:823, 1985.
9. Struthers AD, Reid JL: The role of adrenal medullary catecholamines in potassium homoeostasis. Clin Sci 66:377, 1984.
10. Brown M: Hypokalemia from β_2-receptor stimulation by circulating epinephrine. Am J Cardiol 56:3D, 1985.
11. Vincent HH, ManIn't Veld AJ, Boomsma F, et al: Prevention of epinephrine-induced hypokalemia by nonselective beta blockers. Am J Cardiol 56:10D, 1985.
12. Johns RA: EDRF/nitric oxide: The endogenous nitrovasodilator and a new cellular messenger. Anesthesiology 75:927, 1991.
13. Snyder SH, Bredt DS: Biological roles of nitric oxide. Sci Am 266:68, 1992.
14. Sakurai T, Yanagisawa M, Masaki T: Molecular characterization of endothelin receptors. Trends Pharmacol Sci 13:103, 1992.
15. Nava E, Palmer R, Moncada S: Inhibition of nitric oxide synthesis in septic shock: How much is beneficial? Lancet 338:1555, 1991.
16. Moore K, Wendon J, Frazer M, et al: Plasma endothelin immunoreactivity in liver disease and the hepatorenal syndrome. N Engl J Med 327:1774, 1992.

17. Conlay L, Maher TJ, Wurtman RJ: Tyrosine increases blood pressure in hypotensive rats. Science 212:559, 1981.
18. Nussdorfer GG: Pancrine control of adrenal cortical function by medullary chromaffin cells. Pharmacol Rev 48:495, 1996.
19. Livett BG, Marley PD: Effects of opioid peptides and morphine on histamine-induced catecholamine secretion from cultured, bovine adrenal chromaffin cells. Br J Pharmacol 89:327, 1986.
20. Marley PD, Livett BG: Differences between the mechanism of adrenaline and noradrenaline secretion from isolated, bovine, adrenal chromaffin cells. Neurosci Lett 77:81, 1987.
21. Owen PJ, Plevin R, Boarder MR: Characterization of bradykinin-stimulated release of noradrenaline from cultured bovine adrenal chromaffin cells. J Pharmacol Exp Ther 248:1231, 1989.
22. Cahill A, Perlman RL: Phorbol esters cause preferential secretion of norepinephrine from bovine chromaffin cells. J Neurochem 58:768, 1992.
23. Pacholczyk T, Blakely RD, Amara SG: Expression cloning of a cocaine and antidepressant sensitive human noradrenaline transporter. Nature 350:350, 1991.
24. Eisenhofer G: The role of neuronal and extraneuronal plasma membrane transporters in the inactivation of peripheral catecholamines. Pharmacol Ther 91:35, 2001.
25. Moss J, Lappas D, Slater E: Role of the rennin catecholamine system in hemodynamic performance in man. *In* Usdin E, Kvetnansky R, Kopin IJ (eds): Catecholamines and Stress: Recent Advances in Neurosciences. New York, Elsevier, 1980, p 513.
26. Kaye DM, Lambert GW, Lefkovits J, et al: Neurochemical evidence of cardiac sympathetic activation and increased central nervous system norepinephrine turnover in severe congestive heart failure. J Am Coll Cardiol 23:570, 1994.
27. Cohn J, Levine T, Olivari M, et al: Plasma norepinephrine as a guide to prognosis in patients with chronic congestive heart failure. N Engl J Med 311:819, 1984.
28. Bristow M: The adrenergic nervous system in heart failure [editorial]. N Engl J Med 311:850, 1984.
29. Eisenhofer G, Friberg P, Rundqvist B, et al: Cardiac sympathetic nerve function in congestive heart failure. Circulation 93:1667, 1996.
30. Port JD, Gilbert EM, Larrabee P, et al: Neurotransmitter depletion compromises the ability of indirect-acting amines to provide inotropic support in the failing human heart. Circulation 81:929, 1990.
31. Lawhead R, Blaxall H, Bylund D: α_{2A} is the predominant α_2-adrenergic receptor subtype in human spinal cord. Anesthesiology 77:983, 1992.
32. Bylund DB: Subtypes of α_1 and α_2 adrenergic receptors. FASEB J 6:832, 1992.
33. Szabo B, Hedler L, Starke K: Peripheral presynaptic and central effects of clonidine, yohimbine and rauwolscine on the sympathetic nervous system in rabbits. Naunyn Schmiedebergs Arch Pharmacol 340:648, 1989.
34. Ongioco RR, Richardson CD, Rudner XL, et al: α_2-Adrenergic receptors in human dorsal root ganglia: Predominance of α_{2b} and α_{2c} subtype mRNAs. Anesthesiology 92:968, 2000.
35. Michelotti GA, Price DT, Schwinn DA: α_1-Adrenergic receptor regulation: Basic science and clinical implications. Pharmacol Ther 88:281, 2000.
36. Small KM, Wagoner LE, Levin AM, et al: Synergistic polymorphisms of β_1- and α_{2c}-adrenergic receptors and the risk of congestive heart failure. N Engl J Med 347:1135, 2002.
37. Michel MC, Kenny B, Schwinn DA: Classification of α_1-adrenoceptor subtypes. Naunyn Schmiedebergs Arch Pharmacol 352:1, 1995.
38. Boehm S, Kubista H: Fine tuning of sympathetic transmitter release via ionotropic and metabotropic presynaptic receptors. Pharmacol Rev 54:43, 2002.
39. Szabo B, Schramm A, Starke K: Effect of yohimbine on renal sympathetic nerve activity and renal norepinephrine spillover in anesthetized rabbits. J Pharmacol Exp Ther 260:780, 1992.
40. Limberger N, Singer EA, Starke K: Only activated but not non-activated presynaptic α_2-autoreceptors interfere with neighbouring presynaptic receptor mechanisms. Naunyn Schmiedebergs Arch Pharmacol 338:62, 1988.
41. Raymond J, Hnatowich M, Lefkowitz R, et al: Adrenergic receptors: Models for regulation of signal transduction processes. Hypertension 15:119, 1990.
42. Vanhees L, Aubert A, Fagard R, et al: Influence of β_1- versus β_2-adrenoceptor blockade on left ventricular function in humans. J Cardiovasc Pharmacol 8:1086, 1986.
43. Opie L: Ventricular overload and heart failure. *In* Opie LH (ed): The Heart: Physiology and Metabolism, 2nd ed. New York, Raven Press, 1991, p 386.
44. Brodde O: The functional importance of β_1 and β_2 adrenoceptors in the human heart. Am J Cardiol 62:24C, 1988.
45. Walston J, Silver K, Bogardus C, et al: Time of onset of non–insulin dependent diabetes mellitus and genetic variation in the β_3-adrenergic-receptor gene. N Engl J Med 333:343, 1995.
46. Widen E, Lehto M, Kanninen T, et al: Association of a polymorphism in the β_3-adrenergic receptor gene with features of the insulin resistance syndrome in Finns. N Engl J Med 333:348, 1995.
47. Clement K, Vaisse C, Manning BSF, et al: Genetic variation in the β_3-adrenergic receptor and an increased capacity to gain weight in patients with morbid obesity. N Engl J Med 333:352, 1995.
48. Hall IP, Wheatley A, Wilding P, et al: Association of Glu27 β_2-adrenoceptor polymorphism with lower airway reactivity in asthmatic subjects. Lancet 345:1213, 1995.
49. Turki J, Pak J, Green SA, et al: Genetic polymorphisms of the β_2-adrenergic receptor in nocturnal and non-nocturnal asthma: Evidence that Gly 16 correlates with the nocturnal phenotype. J Clin Invest 95:1635, 1995.
50. Goldberg LI, Rajfer SI: Dopamine receptors: Applications in clinical cardiology. Circulation 72:245, 1985.
51. Bertorello A, Aperia A: Both DA_1 and DA_2 receptor agonists are necessary to inhibit Na^+/K^+ ATPase activity in proximal tubules from the rat kidney. Acta Physiol Scand 132:441, 1988.
52. Bertorello A, Aperia A: Regulation of Na^+/K^+ ATPase activity in kidney proximal tubules: Involvement of GTP binding proteins. Am J Physiol 256:F57, 1989.
53. Gesek FA, Schoolwerth AC: Hormonal interactions with the proximal Na^+/H^+ exchanger. Am J Physiol 258:F514, 1990.
54. Linder ME, Gilman AG: G Proteins. Sci Am 267:56, 1992.
55. Sprang SR: G protein mechanisms: Insights from structural analysis. Annu Rev Biochem 66:639, 1997.
56. Alousi AA, Jasper JR, Insel PA, et al: Stoichiometry of receptor G_s-adenylate cyclase interactions. FASEB J 5:2300, 1991.
57. Post SR, Hilal-Dandan R, Urasawa K, et al: Quantification of signaling components and amplification in the β-adrenergic receptor–adenylate cyclase pathway in isolated adult rat ventricular myocytes. Biochem J 311:75, 1995.
58. Yatani A, Okabe K, Codina J, et al: Heart rate regulation by G proteins acting on the cardiac pacemaker channel. Science 249:1163, 1990.
59. Blochl-Daum B, Schuller-Petrovic S, Wolzt M, et al: Primary defect in α-adrenergic responsiveness in patients with varicose veins. Clin Pharmacol Ther 49:49, 1991.
60. Insel PA: Adrenergic receptors: Evolving concepts and clinical implications. N Engl J Med 334:580, 1996.
61. Bristow MR, Ginsburg R, Minobe W, et al: Decreased catecholamine sensitivity and β-adrenergic receptor density in failing human hearts. N Engl J Med 307:205, 1982.
62. Menard L, Ferguson SS, Zhang J, et al: Synergistic regulation of β_2-adrenergic receptor sequestration: Intracellular complement of β-adrenergic receptor kinase and β-arrestin determine kinetics of internalization. Mol Pharmacol 51:800, 1997.
63. Ferguson SS, Barak LS, Zhang J, et al: G-protein–coupled receptor regulation: Role of G-protein–coupled receptor kinases and arrestins. Can J Physiol Pharmacol 74:1095, 1996.
64. Bristow M, Ginsburg R, Umans V, et al: β_1- and β_2-adrenergic receptor subpopulations in non-failing and failing human ventricular myocardium: Coupling of both receptor subtypes to muscle contraction and selective β_1 receptor downregulation in heart failure. Circ Res 59:297, 1986.
65. Hedberg A, Kemp F Jr, Josephson ME, et al: Coexistence of β_1 and β_2-adrenergic receptors in the human heart: Effects of treatment with receptor antagonists or calcium entry blockers. J Pharmacol Exp Ther 234:561, 1985.
66. Dratman M, Crutchfield F, Axelrod J, et al: Localization of triiodothyronine in nerve ending fractions of rat brain. Proc Natl Acad Sci U S A 73:941, 1976.
67. Jonsson M, Gurley D, Dabrowski M, et al: Distinct pharmacologic properties of neuromuscular blocking agents on human neuronal nicotinic acetylcholine receptors: A possible explanation for the train-of-four fade. Anesthesiology 105:521, 2006.
68. Tassonyi E, Charpantier E, Muller D, et al: The role of nicotinic acetylcholine receptors in the mechanisms of anesthesia. Brain Res Bull 57:133, 2002.
69. Eglen RM, Hedge SS, Watson N: Muscarinic receptor subtypes and smooth muscle function. Pharmacol Rev 48:531, 1996.
70. Hosey MM: Diversity of structure, signaling and regulation within the family of muscarinic cholinergic receptors. FASEB J 12:845, 1992.
71. Bartfai T, Iverfeldt K, Fisone G, et al: Regulation of the release of coexisting neurotransmitters. Annu Rev Pharmacol Toxicol 28:285, 1988.
72. Von Kügelgen I, Starke K: Noradrenaline-ATP cotransmission in the sympathetic nervous system. Trends Pharmacol Sci 12:319, 1991.
73. Burnstock G: Local mechanisms of blood flow control by perivascular nerves and endothelium. J Hypertens Suppl 8:S95, 1990.
74. Ralevic V, Burnstock G: Receptors for purines and pyrimidines. Pharmacol Rev 50:413, 1998.
75. Jacobson KA, Trivedi BK, Churchill PC, et al: Novel therapeutics acting via purine receptors. Biochem Pharmacol 41:1399, 1991.
76. Burnstock G: Overview: Purinergic mechanisms. Ann N Y Acad Sci 603:1, 1990.
77. Goncalves J, Guimaraes S: Influence of neuronal uptake on pre- and postjunctional effects of α-adrenoceptor agonists in tissues with noradrena-

line: ATP cotransmission. Nauryn Schmiedebergs Arch Pharmacol 344:532, 1991.
78. Hirst G, Bramich N, Edwards F, et al: Transmission at autonomic neuroeffector junctions. Trends Neurosci 15:40, 1992.
79. Walker P, Grouzmann E, Burnie M, et al: The role of neuropeptide Y in cardiovascular regulation. Trends Pharmacol Sci 12:111, 1991.
80. Lincoln J, Burnstock G: Neural-endothelial interactions in control of local blood flow. *In* Warren J (ed): The Endothelium: An Introduction to Current Research. New York, Wiley-Liss, 1990, p 21.
81. Lundberg JM, Rudehill A, Sollevi A, et al: Frequency- and reserpine-dependent chemical coding of sympathetic transmission: Differential release of noradrenaline and neuropeptide Y from pig spleen. Neurosci Lett 63:96, 1986.
82. Bloom S, Edwards A: Vasoactive intestinal polypeptide in relation to atropine resistant vasodilatation in the submaxillary gland of the cat. J Physiol 300:41, 1980.
83. Lundberg JM: Evidence for coexistence of vasoactive intestinal polypeptide (VIP) and acetylcholine in neurons of cat exocrine glands: Morphological, biochemical and functional studies. Acta Physiol Scand Suppl 112:1, 1981.
84. Mione M, Cavanagh J, Lincoln J, et al: Pregnancy reduces noradrenaline but not neuropeptide levels in the uterine artery of the guinea-pig. Cell Tissue Res 259:503, 1990.
85. Glusman S: Electrophysiology of ganglionic transmission in the sympathetic nervous system. Int Anesthesiol Clin 27:273, 1989.
86. Paradis NA, Martin GB, Rivers EP, et al: Coronary perfusion pressure and the return of spontaneous circulation in human cardiopulmonary resuscitation. JAMA 263:1106, 1990.
87. Management of cardiac arrest. Circulation 112:IV58, 2005.
88. Pediatric advanced life support. Circulation 112:IV167, 2005.
89. Goetting M, Paradis N: High-dose epinephrine improves outcome from pediatric cardiac arrest. Ann Emerg Med 20:22, 1991.
90. Berry F: Clinical pharmacology of inhalational anesthetic, muscle relaxants, vasoactive agents, and narcotics, and techniques of general anesthesia. *In* Berry F (ed): Anesthetic Management of Difficult and Routine Pediatric Patients, 2nd ed. New York, Churchill Livingstone, 1990, p 64.
91. Waisman Y, Klein BL, Boenning DA, et al: Prospective randomized double-blind study comparing L-epinephrine and racemic epinephrine aerosols in the treatment of laryngotracheitis (croup). Pediatrics 89:302, 1992.
92. Nutman J, Brooks LJ, Deakins KM, et al: Racemic versus L-epinephrine aerosol in the treatment of postextubation laryngeal edema: Results from a prospective, randomized double-blind study. Crit Care Med 22:1591, 1994.
93. Bochner BS, Lichtenstein L: Anaphylaxis. N Engl J Med 324:1785, 1991.
94. Donlon J, Moss J: Plasma catecholamine levels during local anesthesia for cataract operations. Anesthesiology 51:471, 1979.
95. Houben H, Thien T, van't Laar A: Effect of low-dose epinephrine on hemodynamics after selective and nonselective beta-blockade in hypertension. Clin Pharmacol Ther 31:685, 1982.
96. Johnston R, Eger E, Wilson C: A comparative interaction of epinephrine with enflurane, isoflurane, and halothane in man. Anesth Analg 55:709, 1976.
97. O'Neill MJ Jr, Pennock JL, Seaton JF, et al: Regional endogenous plasma catecholamine concentrations in pulmonary hypertension. Surgery 84:140, 1978.
98. Schafer G, Fink M, Parillo J: Norepinephrine alone versus norepinephrine plus low dose dopamine: Enhanced renal blood flow with combination pressor therapy. Crit Care Med 13:492, 1985.
99. Goldberg L: Dopamine: Clinical uses of an endogenous catecholamine. N Engl J Med 291:707, 1974.
100. Goldberg LI, Hsieh Y-Y, Resnekov L: Newer catecholamines for treatment of heart failure and shock: An update on dopamine and a first look at dobutamine. Prog Cardiovasc Dis 19:327, 1977.
101. Maskin C, Oken S, Chadwick B, et al: Comparative systemic and renal effects of dopamine and angiotensin-converting enzyme inhibitor with enalapril in patients with heart failure. Circulation 72:846, 1985
102. Holmes CL, Walley KR: Bad medicine: Low-dose dopamine in the ICU. Chest 123:1266, 2003.
103. Jones D, Bellomo R: Renal-dose dopamine: From hypothesis to paradigm to dogma to myth and finally, superstition? J Int Care Med 20:199, 2005.
104. Brown RA, Dixon J, Farmer JB, et al: Dopexamine: A novel agonist at peripheral dopamine receptors and β_2-adrenoceptors. Br J Pharmacol 85:599, 1985.
105. Foulds RA: Clinical development of dopexamine hydrochloride (Dopacard) and an overview of its hemodynamic effects. Am J Cardiol 62:41C, 1988.
106. Smith GW, O'Connor SE: An introduction to the pharmacologic properties of Dopacard (dopexamine hydrochloride). Am J Cardiol 62:9C, 1988.
107. Fitton A, Benfield P: Dopexamine hydrochloride: A review of its pharmacodynamic and pharmacokinetic properties and therapeutic potential in acute cardiac insuffiency. Drugs 39:308, 1990.
108. Smith GW, Hall JC, Farmer JB, et al: The cardiovascular actions of dopexamine hydrochloride, an agonist at dopamine receptors and β_2 adrenoceptors in the dog. J Pharm Pharmacol 39:636, 1987.
109. Mitchell PD, Smith GW, Wells E, et al: Inhibition of uptake 1 by dopexamine hydrochloride in vitro. Br J Pharmacol 92:265, 1987.
110. Lokhandwala MF: Renal actions of dopexamine hydrochloride. Clin Intensive Care 1:163, 1990.
111. Vyas SJ, Lokhandwala MF: Role of tubular dopamine-1 receptors in the natriuretic and diuretic response to dopexamine. Pharmacologist 31:378, 1989.
112. Bass AS: Contrasting effects of dopexamine hydrochloride on electrolyte excretion in canine kidneys. J Pharmacol Exp Ther 253:798, 1990.
113. Chintala MS, Lokhandwala MF, Jandhyala BS: Protective effects of dopexamine hydrochloride in renal failure after acute hemorrhage in anesthetized dogs. J Auton Pharmacol 10(Suppl):S95, 1990.
114. Leier CV, Binkley PF, Carpenter J, et al: Cardiovascular pharmacology of dopexamine in low output congestive heart failure. Am J Cardiol 62:94, 1988.
115. Baumann G, Felix SB, Filcek SAL: Usefulness of dopexamine hydrochloride versus dobutamine in chronic congestive heart failure and the effects on hemodynamics and urine output. Am J Cardiol 65:748, 1990.
116. Colardyn FC, Vandenbogaerde FE: Use of dopexamine hydrochloride in intensive care patients with low-output left ventricular heart failure. Am J Cardiol 62:68C, 1988.
117. Friedel N, Wenzel R, Matheis G, et al: Haemodynamic effects of different doses of dopexamine hydrochloride in low cardiac output states following cardiac surgery. Eur Heart J 13:1271, 1992.
118. Bredle DL, Cain SM: Systemic and muscle oxygen uptake delivery after dopexamine infusion in endotoxic dogs. Crit Care Med 19:198, 1991.
119. Cain SM, Curtis SE: Systemic and regional oxygen uptake and delivery and lactate flux in endotoxic dogs infused with dopexamine. Crit Care Med 19:1552, 1991.
120. Colardyn FC, Vandenbogaerde JF, Vogelaers DP, et al: Use of dopexamine hydrochloride in patients with septic shock. Crit Care Med 17:999, 1989.
121. Preiser JC, Arminstead C, Le Minh T, et al: Increase in oxygen supply during experimental septic shock: The effects of dobutamine versus dopexamine. J Crit Care 4:40, 1989.
122. Webb AR, Moss RF, Tighe D, et al: The effects of dobutamine, dopexamine and fluid on hepatic histological response to porcine faecal peritonitis. Intensive Care Med 17:487, 1991.
123. Hakim M, Foulds R, Latimer RD, et al: Dopexamine hydrochloride, a β_2-adrenergic and dopaminergic agonist: Haemodynamic effects following cardiac surgery. Eur Heart J 9:853, 1988.
124. Macgregor DA, Butterworth JF IV, Zaloga GP, et al: Hemodynamic and renal effects of dopexamine and dobutamine in patients with reduced cardiac output following coronary artery bypass grafting. Chest 106:835, 1994.
125. Smithies M, Yee TH, Jackson L, et al: Protecting the gut and the liver in the critically ill: Effects of dopexamine. Crit Care Med 22:789, 1994.
126. Lund N, de Asla RJ, Papadakos PJ, et al: Dopexamine hydrochloride in septicemia: Effects on gut, liver and muscle oxygenation [abstract]. Crit Care Med 20(Suppl 4):46, 1992.
127. Trinder TJ, Lavery GG, Fee JPH, et al: Correction of splanchnic oxygen deficit in the intensive care unit: Dopexamine and colloid versus placebo. Anaesth Intensive Care 23:178, 1995.
128. Kuhly P, Oschmann G, Specht M, et al: Dopexamine hydrochloride does not improve gastric and sigmoid mucosal acidosis in patients with sepsis [abstract]. Br J Anesth 74(Suppl 1):121, 1995.
129. Schmidt H, Secchi A, Wellmann R, et al: Dopexamine maintains intestinal villus blood flow during endotoxemia in rats. Crit Care Med 24:1233, 1996.
130. Maynard N, Bihari D, Dalton RN, et al: Increasing splanchnic blood flow in the critically ill. Chest 108:1648, 1995.
131. Jackson NC, Taylor SH, Frais MA: Hemodynamic comparison of dopexamine hydrochloride and dopamine in ischemic left ventricular dysfunction. Am J Cardiol 62:73, 1988.
132. Tan LB, Littler WA, Murray RG: Comparison of the haemodynamic effects of dopexamine and dobutamine in patients with severe congestive heart failure. Int J Cardiol 30:203, 1991.
133. Young JB, Leon CA: Fenoldopam. *In* Messerli FH (ed): Cardiovascular Drug Therapy. Philadelphia, WB Saunders, 1990.
134. Lokhandwala MF: Pre-clinical and clinical studies on the cardiovascular and renal effects of fenoldopam: A DA-1 receptor agonist. Drug Dev Res 10:123, 1987.
135. Goldberg LI: Dopamine and new dopamine analogs: Receptors and clinical applications. J Clin Anesth 1:66, 1988.
136. Aronson S, Goldberg L, Roth S, et al: Preservation of renal blood flow during hypotension induced with fenoldopam in dogs. Can J Anaesth 37:380, 1990.
137. Aronson S, Goldberg LI, Roth S, et al: Effects of fenoldopam on renal blood flow and systemic hemodynamics during isoflurane anesthesia in dogs. J Cardiothorac Vasc Anesth 5:29, 1991.
138. Shusterman NH, Elliott WJ, White WB: Fenoldopam, but not nitroprusside, improves renal function in severely hypertensive patients with impaired renal function. Am J Med 95:161, 1993.
139. Pilmer BL, Green JA, Panacek EA, et al: Fenoldopam mesylate versus sodium nitroprusside in the acute

management of severe system hypertension. J Clin Pharmacol 33:549, 1993.
140. Caplan R, Ward R, Posner K, Cheney F: Unexpected cardiac arrest during spinal anesthesia: A closed claims analysis of predisposing factors. Anesthesiology 68:5, 1988.
141. Shibata S, Seriguchi DG, Iwadare S, et al: The regional and species differences on the activation of myocardial α-adrenoreceptors by phenylephrine and methoxamine. Gen Pharmacol 11:173, 1980.
142. DeVos H, Bricca G, DeKeyser J, et al: Imidazoline receptors, non-adrenergic idazoxan binding sites and α_2-adrenoceptors in the human central nervous system. Neuroscience 59:589, 1994.
143. Hamilton CA: The role of imidazoline receptors in blood pressure regulation. Pharmacol Ther 54:231, 1992.
144. Guyenet PG, Cabot JB: Inhibition of sympathetic preganglionic neurons by catecholamines and clonidine: Mediation by an α-adrenergic receptor. J Neurosci 1:908, 1981.
145. Ruffolo RR Jr: Distribution and function of peripheral α-adrenoceptors on the cardiovascular system. Pharmacol Biochem Behav 22:827, 1985.
146. Muzi M, Goff D, Kampine J, et al: Clonidine reduces sympathetic activity but maintains baroreflex responses in normotensive humans. Anesthesiology 77:864, 1992.
147. Aho M, Erkola O, Korttila K: α_2-Adrenergic agonists in anaesthesia. Curr Opin Anesthesiol 5:481, 1992.
148. Ramsay MA, Luterman DL: Dexmedetomidine as a total intravenous anesthetic. Anesthesiology 101:787, 2004.
149. Flacke J, Bloor BC, Flacke WE, et al: Reduced narcotic requirement by clonidine with improved hemodynamic and adrenergic stability in patients undergoing coronary bypass surgery. Anesthesiology 67:11, 1987.
150. Maze M, Tranguilli W: α_2-Adrenoreceptor agonists: Defining the role in clinical anesthesia. Anesthesiology 74:581, 1991.
151. Ghignone M, Quintin L, Duke P, et al: Effects of clonidine on narcotic requirements and hemodynamic response during induction of fentanyl anesthesia and endotracheal intubation. Anesthesiology 64:36, 1986.
152. Aantaa RE, Kanto JH, Scheinin M: Dexmedetomidine premedication for minor gynecologic surgery. Anesth Analg 70:407, 1990.
153. Richard MJ, Skues MA, Jarvis AP, Prys-Roberts C: Total i.v. anaesthesia with propofol and alfentanil: Dose requirements for propranolol and the effect of premedication with clonidine. Br J Anaesth 65:157, 1990.
154. Murga G, Samso E, Valles J, et al: The effect of clonidine on intra-operative requirements of fentanyl during combined epidural/general anesthesia. Anaesthesia 49:999, 1994.
155. Klimscha W, Chiari A, Drafft P, et al: Hemodynamic and analgesic effects of clonidine added repetitively to continuous epidural and spinal blocks. Anesth Analg 80:322, 1995.
156. Racle JP, Benkhadra A, Poy JY, Bleizal B: Prolongation of isobaric bupivacaine spinal anesthesia with epinephrine and clonidine for hip surgery in the elderly. Anesth Analg 66:442, 1987.
157. Niemi L: Effects of intrathecal clonidine on duration of bupivacaine spinal anaesthesia, haemodynamics, and postoperative analgesia in patients undergoing knee arthroscopy. Acta Anaesthesiol Scand 38:724, 1994.
158. Singelyn FJ, Dangoisse M, Bartholomee S, Gouverneur JM: Adding clonidine to mepivacaine prolongs the duration of anesthesia and analgesia after axillary brachial plexus block. Reg Anesth 17:148, 1992.
159. Wijeysundera D, Naik J, Beattie W: Alpha-2 adrenergic agonists to prevent perioperative cardiovascular complications—a meta-analysis. Am J Med 114:742, 2003.
160. Ebert TJ, Hall JE, Barney JA, et al: The effects of increasing plasma concentrations of dexmedetomidine in humans. Anesthesiology 93:382, 2000.
161. Arain SR, Ebert TJ: The efficacy, side effects, and recovery characteristics of dexmedetomidine versus propofol when used for intraoperative sedation. Anesth Analg 95:461, 2002.
162. Bekker A, Kaufman B, Samir H, Doyle W: The use of dexmedetomidine infusion for awake craniotomy. Anesth Analg 92:1251, 2001.
163. Talke P, Chen R, Thomas B, et al: The hemodynamic and adrenergic effects of perioperative dexmedetomidine infusion after vascular surgery. Anesth Analg 90:834, 2000.
164. Peden CJ, Cloote AH, Stratford N, et al: The effect of intravenous dexmedetomidine premedication on the dose requirement of propofol to induce loss of consciousness in patients receiving alfentanil. Anaesthesia 56:408, 2001.
165. Triltsch AE, Welte M, von Homeyer P, et al: Bispectral index–guided sedation with dexmedetomidine in intensive care: A prospective, randomized, double blind, placebo-controlled phase II study. Crit Care Med 30:1007, 2002.
166. DeKock M, Pichon G, Scholtes JL: Intraoperative clonidine enhances postoperative morphine patient-controlled analgesia. Can J Anaesth 39:537, 1992.
167. Motsh J, Graber E, Ludwig K: Addition of clonidine enhances postoperative analgesia from epidural morphine: A double blind study. Anesthesiology 73:1066, 1990.
168. Bernard JM, Hommeril JL, Passuti N, Pinaud M: Postoperative analgesia by intravenous clonidine. Anesthesiology 75:577, 1991.
169. Carabine UA, Milligan KR, Moore J: Extradural clonidine and bupivacaine for postoperative analgesia. Br J Anaesth 68:132, 1992.
170. Carabine UA, Milligan KR, Mulholland D, Moore J: Extradural clonidine infusions for analgesia after total hip replacement. Br J Anaesth 68:338, 1992.
171. Rostaing S, Bonnet F, Levron JC: Effect of epidural clonidine on analgesia and pharmacokinetics of epidural fentanyl in postoperative patients. Anesthesiology 75:420, 1991.
172. Bonnet F, Boico O, Rostaining S: Clonidine-induced analgesia in postoperative patients: Epidural versus intramuscular administration. Anesthesiology 72:423, 1990.
173. Tryba M, Zenz M, Strumpf M: Clonidine i.v. is equally effective as morphine i.v. for postoperative analgesia—a double blind study [abstract]. Anesthesiology 75:A1085, 1991.
174. DeKock M, Crochet B, Morimont C, Scholtes JL: Intravenous or epidural clonidine for intra- and postoperative analgesia. Anesthesiology 79:525, 1993.
175. Mogensen T, Eliasen K, Ejlersen E, et al: Epidural clonidine enhances postoperative analgesia from a combined low-dose epidural bupivacaine and morphine regimen. Anesth Analg 75:607, 1992.
176. Vercauteren M, Lauwers E, Meert T, et al: Comparison of epidural sufentanil plus clonidine with sufentanil alone for postoperative pain relief. Anaesthesia 45:531, 1990.
177. Rockemann MG, Seeling W, Brinkmann A, et al: Analgesic and hemodynamic effects of epidural clonidine, clonidine/morphine and morphine after pancreatic surgery: A double-blind study. Anesth Analg 80:869, 1995.
178. O'Meara ME, Gin T: Comparison of 0.125% bupivacaine with 0.125% bupivacaine and clonidine as extradural analgesia in the first stage of labour. Br J Anaesth 71:651, 1993.
179. Brichant JF, Bonhomme V, Mikulski M, et al: Admixture of clonidine to epidural bupivacaine for analgesia during labor: Effect of varying clonidine doses [abstract]. Anesthesiology 81:A1136, 1994.
180. Cigarini I, Kaba A, Bonnet F, et al: Epidural clonidine combined with bupivacaine for analgesia in labor: Effects on mother and neonate. Reg Anesth 20:113, 1995.
181. Eisenach JC, DePen S, Dubois M, et al: Epidural Clonidine Study Group: Epidural clonidine anesthesia for intractable cancer pain. Pain 61:391, 1995.
182. Petros AJ, Wright RMB: Epidural and oral clonidine in domiciliary control of deafferentation pain. Lancet 1:1034, 1987.
183. Eisenach JC, Rauck RL, Buzzanell C, Lysak S: Epidural clonidine analgesia for intractable cancer pain: Phase I. Anesthesiology 71:647, 1989.
184. Ferit PA, Aydinli I, Akra S: Management of cancer pain with epidural clonidine [abstract]. Reg Anesth 17(Suppl 3S):173, 1992.
185. Lund C, Hansen O, Kehlet H: Effect of epidural clonidine on somatosensory evoked potentials to dermatomal stimulation. Eur J Anaesth 6:207, 1989.
186. Rauck RL, Eisenach JC, Jackson K, et al: Epidural clonidine treatment for refractory reflex sympathetic dystrophy. Anesthesiology 79:1163, 1993.
187. Zeigler D, Lynch SA, Muir J: Transdermal clonidine versus placebo in painful diabetic neuropathy. Pain 48:403, 1992.
188. Slogoff S: Perioperative ischemia. Semin Anesth 9:107, 1990.
189. Quintin L, Viale JP, Annat G: Oxygen uptake after major abdominal surgery: Effect of clonidine. Anesthesiology 74:236, 1991.
190. Bailey PL, Sperry RJ, Johnson GK, et al: Respiratory effects of clonidine alone and combined with morphine in humans. Anesthesiology 74:43, 1991.
191. Ooi R, Pattison J, Feldman SA: The effects of intravenous clonidine on ventilation. Anaesthesia 46:632, 1991.
192. Bergese S, Khabiri B, Roberts W, et al: Dexmedetomidine for conscious sedation in difficult awake fiberoptic intubation cases. J Clin Anesth 19:141, 2007.
193. Avitsian R, Lin J, Lotto M, Ebrahim Z: Dexmedetomidine and awake fiberoptic intubation for possible cervical spine myelopathy: A case series. J Neurosurg Anesthesiol 17:97, 2005.
194. Ramsay M, Saha D, Hebeler R: Tracheal resection in the morbidly obese patient: The role of dexmedetomidine. J Clin Anesth 18:452, 2006.
195. Uhde TW, Stein MB, Vittone BJ, et al: Behavioral and physiologic effects of short-term and long-term administration of clonidine in panic disorder. Arch Gen Psychiatry 46:170, 1989.
196. Gold MS, Pottash AC, Sweeney DR, Klever HD: Opiate withdrawal using clonidine. A safe, effective, and rapid nonopiate treatment. JAMA 243:343, 1980.
197. Hughes JR: Clonidine, depression, and smoking cessation. JAMA 259:2901, 1988.
198. Metz SA, Halter JB, Robertson RP: Induction of defective insulin secretion and impaired glucose tolerance by clonidine. Selective stimulation of metabolic α-adrenergic pathways. Diabetes 27:554, 1978.
199. Gentili M, Mamelle JC, Le Foll G: Combination of low-dose bupivacaine and clonidine for unilateral

spinal anesthesia in arthroscopic knee surgery. Reg Anesth 20:169, 1995.

200. Kapral S, Kocek S, Krafft P, et al: Intrathecal clonidine delays motor onset of bupivacaine [abstract]. Anesthesiology 81:A935, 1994.
201. Venn R, Hell J, Grounds R: Respiratory effects of dexmedetomidine in the surgical patient requiring intensive care. Crit Care 4:302, 2000.
202. Bekker A, Sturaitis M: Dexmedetomidine for neurological surgery. Neurosurgery 57(Suppl):1, 2005.
203. Wahlander S, Frumento R, Wagener G, et al: A prospective, double-blind, randomized, placebo-controlled study of dexmedetomidine as an adjunct to epidural analgesia after thoracic surgery. J Cardiothorac Vasc Anesth 19:630, 2005.
204. Opie L, Pode-Wilson P: Beta-blocking agents. *In* Opie LH, Gersh B (eds): Drugs for the Heart, 6th ed. Philadelphia, Elsevier Saunders, 2005.
205. Unverferth DV, Blanford M, Kates RE, et al: Tolerance to dobutamine after a 72 hour continuous infusion. Am J Med 69:262, 1980.
206. Leier CV, Huss P, Lewis RP, Unverferth DV: Drug-induced conditioning in congestive heart failure. Circulation 65:1382, 1982.
207. Krell MJ, Kline EM, Bates ER, et al: Intermittent, ambulatory dobutamine infusions in patients with severe congestive heart failure. Am Heart J 112:787, 1986.
208. Spitzer W, Suissa S, Ernst P, et al: The use of β-agonists and the risk of death and near death from asthma. N Engl J Med 326:501, 1992.
209. Robin E, McCauley R: Sudden cardiac death in bronchial asthma, and inhaled with β-adrenergic agonists. Chest 101:1699, 1992.
210. Ziment I: Infrequent cardiac deaths occur in bronchial asthma. Chest 101:1703, 1992.
211. Yaju Y, Nakayama T: Effectiveness and safety of ritodrine hydrochloride for the treatment of preterm labour: A systematic review. Pharmacoepidemiol Drug Saf 15:813, 2006.
212. Westfall T, Westfall D: Adrenergic agonists and antagonists. *In* Brunton L, Lazo J, Parker K (eds): Goodman and Gilman's The Pharmacological Basis of Therapeutics, 11th ed. New York, McGraw-Hill, 2006, p 268.
213. Shojania KG, Duncan BW, McDonald KM, et al: Making health care safer: A critical analysis of patient safety practices. Evidence report/technology assessment No. 43 (Prepared by the University of California at San Francisco–Stanford University Evidence-Based Practice Center under Contract No. 290-97-0013), AHRQ Publication No. 01-E058. Rockville, MD, Agency for Healthcare Research and Quality, July 2001.
214. Stone JG, Foex P, Sear JW, et al: Myocardial ischemia in untreated hypertensive patients: Effect of a single small oral dose of a beta-adrenergic blocking agent. Anesthesiology 68:495, 1988.
215. Mangano DT, Layug EL, Wallace A, et al: Effect of atenolol on mortality and cardiovascular morbidity after noncardiac surgery. Multicenter Study of Perioperative Ischemia Research Group. N Engl J Med 335:1713, 1996.
216. Poldermans D, Boersma E, Bax JJ, et al: The effect of bisoprolol on perioperative mortality and myocardial infarction in high-risk patients undergoing vascular surgery. Dutch Echocardiographic Cardiac Risk Evaluation Applying Stress Echocardiography Study Group. N Engl J Med 341:1789, 1999.
217. Raby KE, Brull SJ, Timimi F, et al: The effect of heart rate control on myocardial ischemia among high-risk patients after vascular surgery. Anesth Analg 88:477, 1999.
218. Urban MK, Markowitz SM, Gordon MA, et al: Postoperative prophylactic administration of beta-adrenergic blockers in patients at risk for myocardial ischemia. Anesth Analg 90:1257, 2000.
219. Stevenson LW: Beta-blockers for stable heart failure. N Engl J Med 346:1346, 2002.
220. Salpeter SS, Ormiston T, Salpeter E, et al: Cardioselective beta-blockers for chronic obstructive pulmonary disease. Cochrane Database Syst Rev 2:CD003566, 2002.
221. MERIT-HF Study Group: Effect of metoprolol CR/XL in chronic heart failure: Metoprolol CR/XL Randomised Intervention Trial in Congestive Heart Failure (MERIT-HF). Lancet 353:2001, 1999.
222. CIBIS-II Investigators and Committees: The Cardiac Insufficiency Bisoprolol Study II (CIBIS-II): A randomised trial. Lancet 353:9, 1999.
223. Furberg C: Secondary prevention trials after myocardial infarction. Am J Cardiol 60:28A, 1987.
224. Rango R, Langlois S: Comparison of withdrawal phenomena after propranolol, metroprolol, and pindolol. Am Heart J 104:437, 1982.
225. Henry J, Cassidy S: Membrane stabilizing activity: A major cause of fatal poisoning. Lancet 1:1414, 1986.
226. London MJ: Con: Beta-blockers are indicated for all adults at increased risk undergoing noncardiac surgery, Anesth Analg 104:11, 2007.
227. Fleisher L, Beckman JA, Brown KA, et al. for the ACC/AHA Task Force on Practice Guidelines: ACC/AHA 2006 guideline update on perioperative cardiovascular evaluation for noncardiac surgery: Focused update on perioperative beta-blocker therapy—a report of the American College of Cardiology/American Heart Association Task Force on Practice Guidelines (Writing Committee to Update the 2002 Guidelines on Perioperative Cardiovascular Evaluation for Noncardiac Surgery). Anesth Analg 104:15, 2007.
228. The POBBLE study (POBBLE Trial Investigators): Perioperative β-blockade (POBBLE) for patients undergoing infrarenal vascular surgery: Results of a randomized double-blind controlled trial. J Vasc Surg 41:602, 2005.
229. Juul AB, Wetterslev J, Gluud C, et al. for the DIPOM Trial Group. Effect of perioperative β blockade in patients with diabetes undergoing major non-cardiac surgry: Randomized placebo controlled blinded multicentre trial. BMJ 332:1482, 2006.
230. Lindenauer PK, Pekow P, Wang K, et al: Perioperative beta-blocker therapy and mortality after major noncardiac surgery. N Engl J Med 353:349, 2005.
231. DeBruijn N, Reves JG, Croughnell N, Knopes K: Comparison of hemodynamic responses to isoproterenol infusion and surgical stress in patients given cardioselective and noncardioselective β-adrenergic antagonists. Anesth Analg 66:637, 1987.
232. Olsson G, Rehnqvist N, Sjogren A, et al: Long-term treatment with metoprolol after myocardial infarction: Effect on 3 year mortality and morbidity. J Am Coll Cardiol 5:1428, 1985.
233. Yusuf S: Interventions that potentially limit myocardial infarct size: Overview of clinical trials. Am J Cardiol 60:11A, 1987.
234. ISIS-1 (First International Study of Infarct Survival) Collaborative Group: Randomised trial of intravenous atenolol among 16,027 cases of suspected acute myocardial infarction: ISIS-1. Lancet 1:57, 1986.
235. Yusuf S, Peto R, Lewis J, et al: Beta blockade during and after myocardial infarction: An overview of the randomized trials. Prog Cardiovasc Dis 27:335, 1985.
236. The TIMI Study Group: Comparison of invasive and conservative strategies after treatment with intravenous tissue plasminogen activator in acute myocardial infarction. N Engl J Med 320:618, 1989.
237. Ryden L, Ariniego R, Arnman K, et al: A double-blind trial of metoprolol in acute myocardial infarction. Effects on ventricular tachyarrhythmias. N Engl J Med 308:614, 1983.
238. Bristow MR, Gilbert EM, Abraham WT, et al: Carvedilol produces dose-related improvements in left ventricular function and survival in subjects with chronic heart failure. MOCHA Investigators. Circulation 94:2807, 1996.
239. Packer M, Colucci WS, Sackner-Bernstein JD, et al: Double-blind, placebo-controlled study of the effects of carvedilol in patients with moderate to severe heart failure. The PRECISE Trial. Prospective Randomized Evaluation of Carvedilol on Symptoms and Exercise. Circulation 94:2793, 1996.
240. Eichhorn EJ, Bristow MR: Medical therapy can improve the biological properties of the chronically failing heart. A new era in the treatment of heart failure. Circulation 94:2285, 1996.
241. Communal C, Singh K, Sawyer D, et al: Opposing effects of β_1- and β_2-adrenergic receptors on cardiac myocyte apoptosis: Role of a pertussis toxin-sensitive G protein. Circulation 100:2210, 1999.
242. Lowes B, Gilbert E, Abraham W, et al.: Myocardial gene expression in dilated cardiomyopathy treated with beta-blocking agents. N Engl J Med 346:1357, 2002.
243. Eichhorn EJ, Bristow MR: Practical guidelines for initiation of beta-adrenergic blockade in patients with chronic heart failure. Am J Cardiol 79:794, 1997.
244. Bristow MR: β-Adrenergic receptor blockade in chronic heart failure. Circulation 101:558, 2000.
245. Frishman W: Pindolol: A new β-adrenoceptor antagonist with partial agonist activity. N Engl J Med 308:940, 1983.
246. Van den Meiracker AH, Man in't Veld AJ, Ritsema van Eck HJ, et al: Hemodynamic and hormonal adaptations to β-adrenoceptor blockade. A 24-hour study of acebutolol, atenolol, pindolol, and propranolol in hypertensive patients. Circulation 78:957, 1988.
247. Man in't Veld AJ, Van den Meiracker AH, Schalekamp MA: Do beta-blockers really increase peripheral vascular resistance? Review of the literature and new observations under basal conditions. Am J Hypertens 1:91, 1988.
248. Shand D: Propanolol. N Engl J Med 293:280, 1975.
249. Platia E, Fitzpatrick P, Wallis D, et al: Esmolol vs verapamil for the treatment of recent-onset atrial afibrillation/flutter. J Am Coll Cardiol 11:170A, 1988.
250. Waldo AL, Camm AJ, deRuyter H, et al: Effect of D-sotalol on mortality in patients with left ventricular dysfunction after recent and remote myocardial infarction. Lancet 348:7, 1996.
251. Doggrell SA, Brown L: D-Sotalol: Death by the SWORD or deserving of further consideration for clinical use? Expert Opin Investig Drugs 9:1625, 2000.
252. DeSanctis RW, Doroghazi RM, Austen WG, Buckley MJ: Aortic dissection. N Engl J Med 317:1060, 1987.
253. Grubb BP, Sirio C, Zelis R: Intravenous labetalol in acute aortic dissection. JAMA 258:78, 1987.
254. Wiersinga WM, Touber JL: The influence of β-adrenergic blocking agents on plasma thyroxine and triiodothyronine. J Clin Endocrinol Metab 45:293, 1977.
255. Psaty B, Koepsell T, Wagner E, et al: The relative risk of incident coronary heart disease associated with recently stopping the use of β-blockers. JAMA 263:1653, 1990.

256. Cleophas T, Kauw F: Pressor responses from non-cardioselective beta-blockers. Angiology 39:587, 1988.
257. Strauss W, Parisi A: Combined use of calcium-channel and β-adrenergic blockers for the treatment of chronic stable angina. Ann Intern Med 109:570, 1988.
258. Wayne VS, Harper RW, Laufer E, et al: Adverse interaction between β-adrenergic blocking drugs and verapamil: Report of three cases. Aust N Z J Med 12:285, 1982.
259. Pendleton RG, Newman DJ, Sherman SS, et al: Effect of propranolol upon the hemoglobin-oxygen dissociation curve. J Pharmacol Exp Ther 180:647, 1972.
260. Bernstein JS, Ebert TJ, Stowe DF, et al: Partial attenuation of hemodynamic responses to rapid sequence induction and intubation with labetalol. J Clin Anesth 1:444, 1989.
261. Huey J, Thomas JP, Hendricks DR, et al: Clinical evaluation of labetalol for the treatment of hypertensive urgency. Am J Hypertens 1:284S, 1988.
262. Gabrielson G, Lingham R, Dimich I, et al: Comparative study of labetalol and hydralazine in the treatment of postoperative hypertension [abstract]. Anesth Analg 66:S63, 1987.
263. Skrobic J, Cruise C, Webster R, et al: Labetalol vs nitroprusside in hypertension post coronary-bypass surgery. Am J Hypertens 2:1295, 1989.
264. Lavies NG, Meiklejohn BH, May AE, et al: Hypertensive and catecholamine response to tracheal intubation in patients with pregnancy-induced hypertension. Br J Anaesth 63:429, 1989.
265. Jouppilla P, Kirkinen P, Koivula A: Labetalol does not alter the placental and fetal blood flow or maternal prostanoids in pre-eclampsia. Br J Obstet Gynaecol 93:543, 1986.
266. Dupont AG, Van der Niepen P, Taeymans Y, et al: Effect of carvedilol on ambulatory blood pressure, renal hemodynamics, and cardiac function in essential hypertension. J Cardiovasc Pharmacol 10(Suppl 1):S130, 1987.
267. Eggertsen R, Sivertsson R, Adren L, et al: Haemodynamic effects of carvedilol, a new β-adrenoceptor blocker and precapillary vasodilator in essential hypertension. J Hypertens 2:529, 1984.
268. Leonetti G, Sempieri L, Cuspidi C, et al: Resting and postexercise hemodynamic effects of carvedilol, a β-adrenergic blocker and precapillary vasodilator in hypertensive patients. J Cardiovasc Pharmacol 10(Suppl 1)1:S94, 1987.
269. Omvik P, Lund-Johansen P: Acute haemodynamic effects of carvedilol in essential hypertension at rest and during exercise. Eur Heart J 12:736, 1991.
270. Cervantes Escarcega JL, Ruiz de Chavez A, Guadalajara Boo J: Double-blind study of the efficacy and tolerability of carvedilol vs nifedipine S.R. in uncomplicated essential hypertension [in spanish]. Invest Med Int 19:142, 1992.
271. Ostergren J, Storstein L, Karlberg BE, et al: Quality of life in hypertensive patients treated with either carvedilol or enalapril. Blood Press 5:41, 1996.
272. Ruilope LM, Group CS: Comparison of a new vasodilating beta blocker, carvedilol, with atenolol in the treatment of mild to moderate essential hypertension. Am J Hypertens 7:129, 1994.
273. Weber K, Bohmeke T, van der Does R, et al: Comparison of the hemodynamic effects of metoprolol and carvedilol in hypertensive patients. Cardiovasc Drug Ther 10:113, 1996.
274. Albergati F, Paterno E, Venuti RP, et al: Comparison of the effects of carvedilol and nifedipine in patients with essential hypertension and non-insulin-dependent diabetes mellitus. J Cardiovasc Pharmacol 19(Suppl 1):S86, 1992.
275. Louis WJ, Krum H, Conway EL: A risk-benefit assessment of carvedilol in the treatment of cardiovascular disorders. Drug Saf 11:86, 1994.
276. van der Does R, Eberhardt R, Derr I, et al: Efficacy and safety of carvedilol in comparison with nifedipine sustained-release in chronic stable angina. J Cardiovasc Pharmacol 19(Suppl 1):S122, 1992.
277. Basu S, Senior R, van der Does R, et al: Carvedilol reduces adverse cardiac events following acute myocardial infarction [abstract]. Circulation 92(Suppl 1):1, 1995.
278. Senior R, Basu S, Lahiri A: Carvedilol prevents remodeling and improves prognosis in patients with left ventricular dysfunction following acute myocardial infarction [abstract]. J Am Coll Cardiol 27(Suppl A):319A, 1996.
279. Zehender M, Faber T, Schnabel P, et al: Benefits and hazards of carvedilol in unstable angina: A double-blind placebo controlled, randomized study [abstract]. Circulation 92(Suppl 1):I, 1995.
280. Cohn JN, Fowler MB, Bristow MA, et al: Effect of carvedilol in severe chronic heart failure [abstract]. J Am Coll Cardiol 27(Suppl A):169A, 1996.
281. Colucci WS, Packer M, Bristow MR, et al: Carvedilol inhibits clinical progression in patients with mild symptoms of heart failure. Circulation 94:2800, 1996.
282. Bristow MR, Gilbert EM, Abraham WT, et al: Effects of carvedilol on LV function and mortality in diabetic versus nondiabetic patients with ischemic or nonischemic dilated cardiomyopathy [abstract]. Circulation 94(Suppl 1):I, 3879, 1996.
283. Gray R, Bateman T, Czer L, et al: Comparison of esmolol and nitroprusside for acute post–cardiac surgical hypertension. Am J Cardiol 59:887, 1987.
284. Reves JG, Croughwell ND, Hawkins E, et al: Esmolol for treatment of intraoperative tachycardia and/or hypertension in patients having cardiac operations, bolus loading technique. J Thorac Cardiovasc Surg 100:221, 1990.
285. Oxorn D, Knox JW, Hill J: Bolus doses of esmolol for the prevention of perioperative hypertension and tachycardia. Can J Anaesth 37:206, 1990.
286. Wallis DE, Littman WJ, Scanlon PJ: Safety and efficacy of esmolol for unstable angina pectoris. Am J Cardiol 62:1033, 1988.
287. Kirshenbaum JM, Kloner RJ, McGowan N, Antman EM: Use of an ultrashort-acting β-receptor blocker (esmolol) in patients with acute myocardial ischemia and relative contraindications to beta-blockade therapy. J Am Coll Cardiol 12:773, 1988.
288. The Parkinson Study Group: Effect of deprenyl on the progression of disability in early Parkinson's disease. N Engl J Med 321:1364, 1989.
289. Roizen MF: Monoamine oxidase inhibitors: Are we condemned to relive history, or is history no longer relevant [letter]? J Clin Anesth 2:293, 1990.
290. Doyle DJ: Ketamine induction and monoamine oxidase inhibitors. J Clin Anesth 2:324, 1990.
291. Materson BJ: Adverse effects of angiotensin-converting enzyme inhibitors in antihypertensive therapy with focus on quinapril. Am J Cardiol 69:46C, 1992.
292. ISIS-4 (Fourth International Study of Infarct Survival) Collaborative Group: A randomised factorial trial assessing early oral captopril, oral mononitrate, and intravenous magnesium sulphate in 58,050 patients with suspected acute myocardial infarction. Lancet 345:669, 1995.
293. Nash DT: Comparative properties of angiotensin-converting enzyme inhibitors: Relations with inhibition of tissue angiotensin-converting enzyme and potential clinical implications. Am J Cardiol 69:26C, 1992.
294. Raia JJ Jr, Barone JA, Byerly WG, Lacy CR: Angiotensin-converting enzyme inhibitors: A comparative review. DICP 24:506, 1990.
295. Weber MA: Safety issues during antihypertensive treatment with angiotensin converting enzyme inhibitors. Am J Med 84(Suppl 4A):16, 1988.
296. Warner JN, Rush JE: Safety profiles of the angiotensin-converting enzyme inhibitors. Drugs 35(Suppl 5):89, 1988.
297. Ferner RE: Adverse effects of angiotensin-converting-enzyme inhibitors. Adverse Drug React Acute Poisoning Rev 141:528, 1990.
298. Jong P, Demers C, McKelvie RS, et al: Angiotensin receptor blockers in heart failure: Meta-analysis of randomized controlled trials. J Am Coll Cardiol 39:463, 2002.
299. Ziskind A: Transdermal scopolamine–induced psychosis. Postgrad Med 84:73, 1988.
300. Wilkinson JA: Side-effects of transdermal scopolamine. J Emerg Med 5:389, 1987.
301. Gross NJ: Ipratropium bromide. N Eng J Med 319:486, 1988.
302. Alcalay M, Izraeli S, Wallach-Kapon R, et al: Paradoxical pharmacodynamic effect of atropine on parasympathetic control: A study by spectral analysis of heart rate fluctuations. Clin Pharmacol Ther 52:518, 1992.
303. Ghoneim MM, Dembo JB, Block RI: Time course of antagonism of sedative and amnesic effects of diazepam by flumazenil. Anesthesiology 70:899, 1989.
304. Charlson ME, MacKenzie CR, Gold JP: Preoperative autonomic function abnormalities in patients with diabetes mellitus and patients with hypertension. J Am Coll Surg 179:1, 1994.
305. Ewing DJ, Martyn CN, Young RJ: The value of cardiovascular autonomic function tests: 10 years experience in diabetes. Diabetes Care 8:491, 1985.
306. Esler M, Thompson J, Kaye D, et al: Effects of aging on the responsiveness of the human cardiac sympathetic nerves to stressors. Circulation 91:351, 1995.
307. Adams K: Current perspectives on β-receptor antagonists in the treatment of symptomatic ventricular dysfunction. Pharmacotherapy 16:69S, 1996.
308. Eichhorn EJ: Do β-blockers have a role in patients with congestive heart failure? Cardiol Clin 12:133, 1994.
309. Rundqvist B, Eisenhofer G, Elam M, Friberg P: Attenuated cardiac sympathetic responsiveness during dynamic exercise in patients with heart failure. Circulation 95:940, 1997.
310. Anand K, Hickey P: Halothane-morphine compared with high dose sufentanil for anesthesia and postoperative analgesia in neonatal cardiac surgery. N Engl J Med 326:1, 1992.
311. Kehlet H: Manipulation of the metabolic response in clinical practice. World J Surg 24:690, 2000.
312. Bardram L, Funch-Jensen P, Jensen P, et al: Recovery after laparoscopic colonic surgery with epidural analgesia, and early oral nutrition and mobilisation. Lancet 345:763, 1995.
313. Wallace A, Galindez D, Salahieh A, et al: Effect of clonidine on cardiovascular morbidity and mortality after non-cardiac surgery. Anesthesiology 101:284, 2004.
314. Burgos LG, Ebert TJ, Asiddao C, et al: Increased intraoperative cardiovascular morbidity in diabetics with autonomic neuropathy. Anesthesiology 70:591, 1989.
315. Page MM, WatKins PJ: Cardiorespiratory arrest and diabetic autonomic neuropathy. Lancet 1:14, 1978.
316. Ewing DJ, Clarke BF: Diagnosis and management of diabetic autonomic neuropathy. BMJ 285:916, 1982.

317. Sato I, Hasegawa Y, Takahashi N, et al: Age-related changes of cardiac control function in man. With special reference to heart rate control at rest and during exercise. J Gerontol 36:564, 1981.
318. Esler MD, Turner AG, Kaye DM, et al: Aging effects on human sympathetic neuronal function. Am J Physiol 268:R278, 1995.
319. Mancia G, Ferrari A, Gregorini L, et al: Blood pressure and heart rate variabilities in normotensive and hypertensive human beings. Circ Res 53:96, 1983.
320. Ng AV, Callister R, Johnson DG, et al: Sympathetic neural reactivity to stress does not increase with age in healthy humans. Am J Physiol 267:H344, 1994.
321. White M, Roden R, Minobe W, et al: Age-related changes in β-adrenergic neuroeffector systems in the human heart. Circulation 90:1225, 1994.
322. Vaz M, Rajkumar C, Wong J, et al: Oxygen consumption in the heart, hepatomesenteric bed, and brain in young and elderly human subjects, and accompanying sympathetic nervous activity. Metabolism 45:1487, 1996.
323. Buchholz J, Duckles SP: Effect of age on prejunctional modulation of norepinephrine release. J Pharmacol Exp Ther 252:159, 1990.
324. Hyland L, Docherty JR: Further examination of the effects of ageing on the adrenoceptor responsiveness of the rat vas deferens. Eur J Pharmacol 110:241, 1985.
325. Fernandes F, Salaices CF, Sanchez-Ferrer JL, et al: Effect of aging and hypertension on [^{3}H]noradrenaline release in rat mesenteric artery. J Hypertens 10(Suppl 4):S65, 1992.
326. Mathias CJ, Christensen NJ, Frankel HL, et al: Cardiovascular control in recently injured tetraplegics in spinal shock. Q J Med 48:273, 1979.
327. Van Lieshout JJ, Imholz BPM, Wesseling KH, et al: Singing-induced hypotension: A complication of high spinal cord lesion. Neth J Med 38:75, 1991.
328. Stjernberg L, Blumberg H, Wallin B: Sympathetic activity in man after spinal cord injury: Outflow to muscle below the lesion. Brain 109:695, 1986.
329. Kirstein S, Insel P: Autonomic nervous system pharmacogenomics: A progress report. Pharmacol Rev 56:31, 2004.
330. Zhu H, Poole J, Lu Y, Harshfield G, et al: Sympathetic nervous system, genes and human essential hypertension. Curr Neurovasc Res 2:303, 2005.
331. Jacob G, Garland E, Costa F, et al: β_2-Adrenoceptor genotype and function affect hemodynamic profile heterogeneity in postural tachycardia syndrome. Hypertension 47:421, 2006.

Piyush M. Patel and John C. Drummond

13 Cerebral Physiology and the Effects of Anesthetic Drugs

Key Points

1. The brain has a high metabolic rate and receives approximately 15% of cardiac output. Under normal circumstances, cerebral blood flow (CBF) is approximately 50 mL/100 g/min. Gray matter receives 80% and white matter receives 20% of this blood flow.
2. Approximately 60% of the brain's energy consumption is used to support electrophysiologic function. The remainder of the energy consumed by the brain is involved in cellular homeostatic activities.
3. CBF is tightly coupled to local cerebral metabolism. When cerebral activity in a particular region of the brain increases, a corresponding increase in blood flow to that region takes place. Conversely, suppression of cerebral metabolism leads to a reduction in blood flow.
4. CBF is autoregulated and held constant over a mean arterial pressure range conservatively estimated at 65 to 150 mm Hg, given normal venous pressure. There is probably appreciable intersubject variability. CBF becomes pressure passive when mean arterial pressure is either below the lower limit or above the upper limit of autoregulation
5. CBF is also under chemical regulation. It varies directly with arterial carbon dioxide tension in the $Pa{CO_2}$ range of 25 to 70 mm Hg. With a reduction in $Pa{O_2}$ to below 60 mm Hg, CBF increases dramatically. Changes in temperature affect CBF primarily by suppression of cerebral metabolism.
6. Systemic vasodilators (nitroglycerin, nitroprusside, hydralazine, calcium channel blockers) vasodilate the cerebral circulation and can, depending on mean arterial pressure, increase CBF. Vasopressors such as phenylephrine, norepinephrine, ephedrine, and dopamine do not have significant direct effects on the cerebral circulation. Their effect on CBF is dependent on their effect on systemic blood pressure. When mean arterial pressure is below the lower limit of autoregulation, vasopressors increase systemic pressure and thereby increase CBF. If systemic pressure is within the limits of autoregulation, vasopressor-induced increases in systemic pressure have little effect on CBF.
7. All modern volatile anesthetics suppress the cerebral metabolic rate (CMR) and, with the exception of halothane, can produce burst suppression of the electroencephalogram. At that level, CMR is reduced by about 60%. Volatile anesthetics have dose-dependent effects on CBF. In doses lower than the minimal alveolar concentration (MAC), CBF is not significantly altered. Beyond doses of 1 MAC, direct cerebral vasodilation results in an increase in CBF and cerebral blood volume.
8. Barbiturates, etomidate, and propofol decrease CMR and can produce burst suppression of the electroencephalogram. At that level, CMR is reduced by about 60%. Flow and metabolism coupling is preserved and therefore CBF is decreased. Opiates and benzodiazepines effect minor decreases in CBF and CMR, whereas ketamine can increase CMR (with a corresponding increase in blood flow) significantly.
9. Brain stores of oxygen and substrates are limited and the brain is exquisitely sensitive to reductions in CBF. Severe reductions in CBF (less than 10 mL/100 g/min) lead to rapid neuronal death. Ischemic injury is characterized by early excitotoxicity and delayed apoptosis.
10. Barbiturates, propofol, ketamine, volatile anesthetics, and xenon have neuroprotective efficacy and can reduce ischemic cerebral injury. Anesthetic neuroprotection is sustained only when the severity of the ischemic insult is mild; with moderate to severe injury, long-term neuroprotection is not achieved. Administration of etomidate is associated with regional reductions in blood flow, and this can exacerbate ischemic brain injury.

This chapter reviews the effects of anesthetic drugs and techniques on cerebral physiology, in particular, their effects on cerebral blood flow (CBF) and metabolism. The final section presents a brief discussion of pathophysiologic states, including cerebral ischemia, as well as discussion of cerebral protection. The chapter gives greatest emphasis to information that is of immediate relevance to the rationale for use of the anesthetic and intensive care management of patients with intracranial pathology. Chapter 63 presents the clinical management of these patients in detail. Neurologic monitoring, including the effects of anesthetics on the electroencephalogram (EEG) and evoked responses, is reviewed in Chapter 46.

Regulation of Cerebral Blood Flow

Anesthetic drugs cause dose-related and reversible alterations in many aspects of cerebral physiology, including CBF, cerebral metabolic rate (CMR), and electrophysiologic function (EEG, evoked responses). The effects of anesthetic drugs and techniques have the potential to adversely affect the diseased brain and conduct of the neurosurgical procedure and are thus of clinical importance in patients with neurosurgical disease. However, in certain instances, the effects of general anesthesia on CBF and CMR can be manipulated to improve both the operative course and the clinical outcome of patients with neurologic disorders.

The adult human brain weighs approximately 1350 g and therefore represents about 2% percent of total-body weight. However, it receives 12% to 15% of cardiac output. This high flow rate is a reflection of the brain's high metabolic rate. At rest, the brain consumes oxygen at an average rate of approximately 3.5 mL of oxygen per 100 g of brain tissue per minute. Whole-brain O_2 consumption (50 mL/min) represents about 20% of total-body oxygen utilization. Normal values for CBF, CMR, and other physiologic variables are provided in Table 13-1.

Approximately 60% of the brain's energy consumption is used to support electrophysiologic function. The depolarization-repolarization activity that occurs and is reflected in the EEG requires expenditure of energy for the maintenance and restoration of ionic gradients and for the synthesis, transport, and reuptake of neurotransmitters. The remainder of the energy consumed by the brain is involved in cellular homeostatic activities. Local CBF and CMR within the brain are very heterogeneous, and both are approximately four times greater in gray matter than in white matter. The cell population of the brain is also heterogeneous in its oxygen requirements. Glial cells make up about half the brain's volume and require less energy than neurons do. Besides providing a physically supportive latticework for the brain, glial cells are important in reuptake of neurotransmitters, in delivery and removal of metabolic substrates and wastes, and in blood-brain barrier (BBB) function.

Table 13-1 Normal Cerebral Physiologic Values

CBF	
Global	45-55 mL/100 g/min
Cortical (mostly gray matter)	75-80 mL/100 g/min
Subcortical (mostly white matter)	≈20 mL/100 g/min
$CMRO_2$	3-3.5 mL/100 g/min
CVR	1.5-2.1 mm Hg/100 g/min/mL
Cerebral venous Po_2	32-44 mm Hg
Cerebral venous So_2	55%-70%
ICP (supine)	8-12 mm Hg

CBF, cerebral blood flow; $CMRO_2$, cerebral metabolic rate of oxygen; CVR, cerebral vascular resistance; ICP, intracranial pressure.

Table 13-2 Factors Influencing Cerebral Blood Flow*

Factor	Comment
Chemical/Metabolic/Humoral	
CMR Anesthetics Temperature Arousal/seizures	CMR influence assumes intact flow-metabolism coupling, the mechanism of which is not fully understood
$Paco_2$	
Pao_2	
Vasoactive drugs Anesthetics Vasodilators Vasopressors	
Myogenic	
Autoregulation/MAP	The autoregulation mechanism is fragile, and in many pathologic states CBF is regionally pressure passive
Rheologic	
Blood viscosity	
Neurogenic	
Extracranial sympathetic and parasympathetic pathways	Contribution and clinical significance poorly defined
Intra-axial pathways	

*See text for discussion.
CBF, cerebral blood flow; CMR, cerebral metabolic rate; MAP, mean arterial pressure.

The brain's substantial demand for substrate must be met by adequate delivery of oxygen and glucose. However, the space constraints imposed by the noncompliant cranium and meninges require that blood flow not be excessive. Not surprisingly, there are elaborate mechanisms for regulation of CBF. These mechanisms, which include chemical, myogenic, and neurogenic factors, are listed in Table 13-2.

Chemical Regulation of Cerebral Blood Flow

Several factors, including changes in CMR, $Paco_2$, and Pao_2, cause alterations in the cerebral biochemical environment that result in adjustments in CBF.

Cerebral Metabolic Rate

Increased neuronal activity results in increased local brain metabolism, and this increase in CMR is associated with a well-matched,

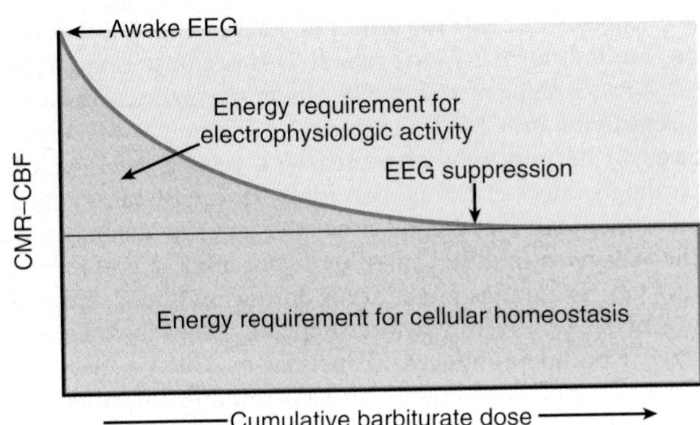

Figure 13-1 Interdependency of cerebral electrophysiologic function and cerebral metabolic rate (CMR). Administration of various anesthetics, including barbiturates, results in a dose-related reduction in the CMR of oxygen ($CMRO_2$) and cerebral blood flow (CBF). The maximum reduction occurs with the dose that results in electrophysiologic silence. At this point, the energy utilization associated with electrophysiologic activity has been reduced to zero, but the energy utilization for cellular homeostasis persists unchanged. Additional barbiturate causes no further decrease in CBF or $CMRO_2$.

proportional change in CBF and is referred to as flow-metabolism coupling. Although the precise mechanisms that mediate flow-metabolism coupling have not been defined, the data available implicate local by-products of metabolism (K^+, H^+, lactate, adenosine, and adenosine triphosphate [ATP]). Glutamate, released with increased neuronal activity, results in the synthesis and release of nitric oxide (NO), a potent cerebral vasodilator that plays an important role in coupling of flow and metabolism. More recent data have highlighted the role of glia in flow-metabolism coupling. Uptake of the glutamate released from neurons by glia triggers increased glial metabolism and lactate production. Glial processes make contact with neurons and capillaries, and hence glia may serve as a conduit for the coupling of increased neuronal activity with increased glucose consumption and regional blood flow. Nerves that innervate cerebral vessels release peptide neurotransmitters such as vasoactive intestinal peptide (VIP), substance P, cholecystokinin, somatostatin, and calcitonin gene–related peptide. These neurotransmitters may also potentially be involved in neurovascular coupling. Flow-metabolism coupling within the brain is a complex physiologic process that is regulated, not by a single mechanism, but by a combination of metabolic, glial, neural, and vascular factors.

CMR is influenced by several phenomena in the neurosurgical environment, including the functional state of the nervous system, anesthetic drugs, and temperature.

Functional State. CMR decreases during sleep and increases during sensory stimulation, mental tasks, or arousal of any cause. During epileptic activity, increases in CMR may be extreme, whereas regionally after brain injury and globally with coma, CMR may be substantially reduced.

Anesthetic Drugs. The effect of individual anesthetic drugs on CMR is presented in greater detail in the second section of this chapter. In general, anesthetic drugs suppress CMR, with ketamine and N_2O being notable exceptions. It appears that the component of CMR on which they act is that associated with electrophysiologic function. With several anesthetics, including barbiturates, isoflurane, sevoflurane, desflurane, propofol, and etomidate, increasing plasma concentrations cause progressive suppression of EEG activity and a concomitant reduction in CMR. However, increasing the plasma level beyond what is required to first achieve suppression of the EEG results in no further depression of CMR. The component of CMR required for maintenance of cellular integrity, the "housekeeping" component, is unaltered by intravenous anesthetic drugs (Fig. 13-1).

The cerebral metabolic rate of oxygen ($CMRO_2$) observed when complete suppression of the EEG is achieved with different anesthetic drugs is very similar. It should be noted, however, that anesthetic-induced EEG suppression is not a single physiologic state and is influenced by the agent that is used to produce suppression. When barbiturates are administered to the point of EEG suppression, a uniform depression in CBF and CMR occurs throughout the brain. When suppression occurs during administration of isoflurane, the relative reductions in CMR and CBF are greater in the neocortex than in other portions of the cerebrum. Electrophysiologic responsiveness also varies. Cortical somatosensory evoked responses to median nerve stimulation can readily be recorded at doses of thiopental far in excess of those required to cause complete suppression of the EEG but are difficult to elicit at concentrations of isoflurane associated with a burst-suppression pattern, such as 1.5 minimum alveolar concentration (MAC) (Fig. 13-2). In addition, the EEG characteristics of the burst-sup-

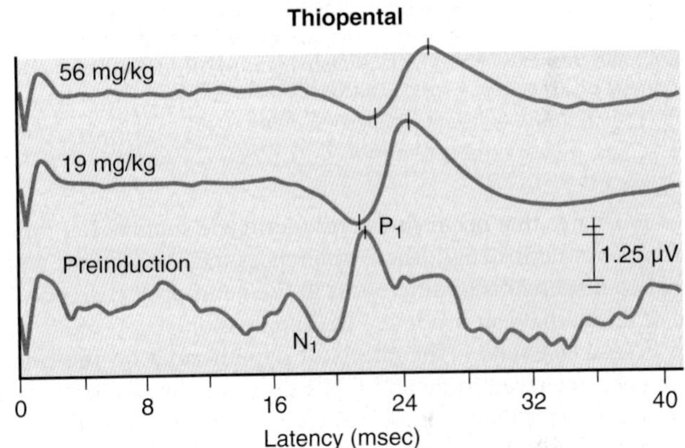

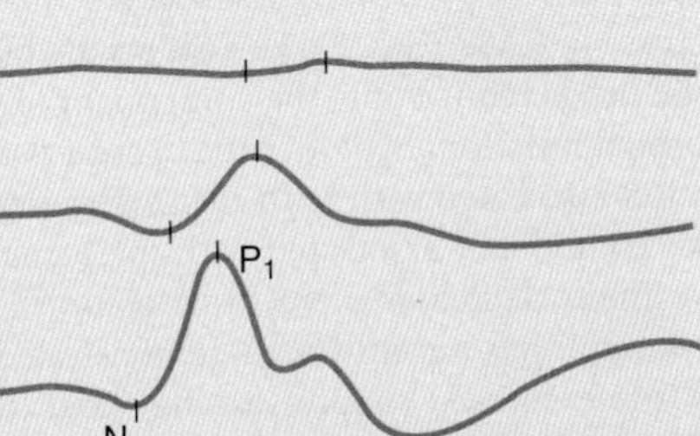
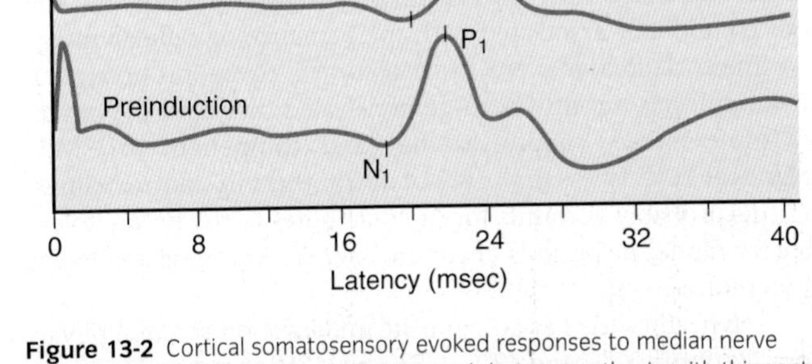

Figure 13-2 Cortical somatosensory evoked responses to median nerve stimulation in humans before induction and during anesthesia with thiopental and isoflurane/N_2O. Despite an equivalent or greater degree of reduction in the cerebral metabolic rate with thiopental, cortical evoked responses are better preserved[1] than during anesthesia with isoflurane.[2] This suggests that the electroencephalographic suppression achieved with different anesthetic drugs should not be assumed to be equivalent electrophysiologic states. The cumulative thiopental doses and expired concentrations of isoflurane and N_2O are indicated in the figure.

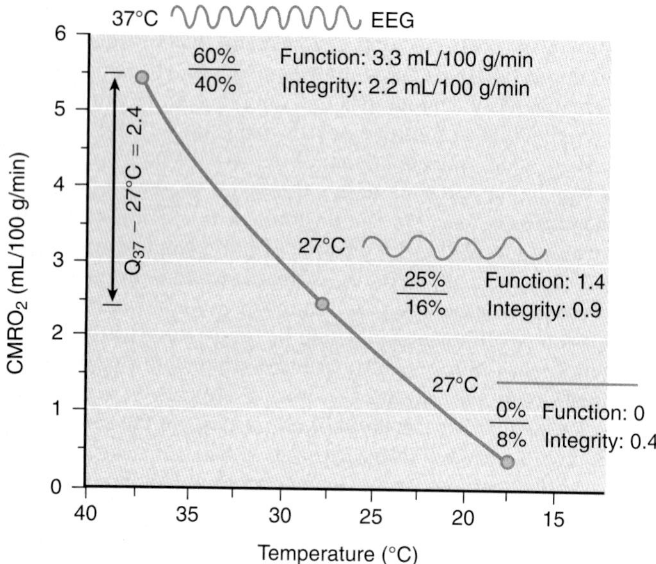

Figure 13-3 Effect of temperature reduction on the cerebral metabolic rate of oxygen ($CMRO_2$). Hypothermia reduces both of the components of cerebral metabolic activity identified in Figure 13-1: that associated with neuronal electrophysiologic activity ("Function") and that associated with maintenance of cellular homeostasis ("Integrity"). This is in contrast to anesthetics that alter only the functional component. The ratio of CMR at 37°C to that at 27°C, the Q_{10} ratio, is shown in the graph. *(Adapted from Michenfelder JD: Anesthesia and the Brain: Clinical, Functional, Metabolic, and Vascular Correlates. New York, Churchill Livingstone, 1988.)*

pression states that occur just before complete suppression differ among anesthetic drugs. These differences may be of some relevance to discussions of differences in the neuroprotective potential of drugs that can produce EEG suppression.

Temperature. The effects of hypothermia on the brain have been reviewed in detail.[3] CMR decreases by 6% to 7% per degree Celsius of temperature reduction. As is the case with some anesthetic drugs, hypothermia can also cause complete suppression of the EEG (at about 18°C to 20°C). However, in contrast with anesthetic drugs, temperature reduction beyond that at which EEG suppression first occurs *does* produce a further decrease in CMR (Fig. 13-3). This occurs because although anesthetic drugs reduce only the component of CMR associated with neuronal function, hypothermia decreases the rate of energy utilization associated with both electrophysiologic function and the basal component associated with maintenance of cellular integrity. These decreases were once assumed to be proportional. However, it has recently been demonstrated that mild hypothermia preferentially suppresses the basal component of CMR. $CMRO_2$ at 18°C is less than 10% of normothermic control values, and this probably accounts for or contributes to the brain's tolerance for moderate periods of circulatory arrest at these and lower temperatures.

Hyperthermia has an opposite influence on cerebral physiology. Between 37°C and 42°C, CBF and CMR increase. However, above 42°C, a dramatic reduction in cerebral oxygen consumption occurs, an indication of a threshold for a toxic effect of hyperthermia that may occur as a result of protein (enzyme) denaturation.

$Paco_2$. CBF varies directly with $Paco_2$ (Fig. 13-4). The effect is greatest within the range of physiologic $Paco_2$ variation. CBF changes 1 to 2 mL/100 g/min for each 1-mm Hg change in $Paco_2$ around normal $Paco_2$ values. This response is attenuated below a $Paco_2$ value of 25 mm Hg. Under normal circumstances, the sensitivity of CBF to changes in $Paco_2$ ($\Delta CBF/\Delta Paco_2$) appears to be positively correlated with resting levels of CBF. Accordingly, anesthetic drugs that alter resting CBF cause changes in the response of the cerebral circulation to CO_2. The magnitude of the reduction in CBF caused by hypocapnia is greater when resting CBF is high (as might occur during anesthesia with volatile agents). Conversely, when resting CBF is low, the magnitude of the hypocapnia-induced reduction in CBF is decreased. However, it should be noted that CO_2 responsiveness has been observed in normal brain during anesthesia with all of the numerous anesthetic drugs that have been studied.

The changes in CBF caused by $Paco_2$ are dependent on pH alterations in the extracellular fluid of the brain. NO, in particular NO of neuronal origin, is an important although not exclusive mediator of CO_2-induced vasodilation. The vasodilatory response to hypercapnia is also mediated in part by prostaglandins. The changes in extracellular pH and CBF occur rapidly after $Paco_2$ adjustments because CO_2 diffuses freely across the cerebrovascular endothelium. Note that in contrast with *respiratory* acidosis, acute systemic *metabolic* acidosis has little immediate effect on CBF because the BBB excludes hydrogen ion (H^+) from the perivascular space. The CBF changes in response to alterations in $Paco_2$ occur rapidly, but they are not sustained. Despite maintenance of an elevated arterial pH, CBF returns to normal over a period of 6 to 8 hours because the pH of cerebrospinal fluid (CSF) gradually normalizes as a result of extrusion of bicarbonate. Consequently, a patient who has had a sustained period of hyperventilation or hypoventilation deserves special consideration. Acute normalization of $Paco_2$ will result in a significant CSF acidosis (after hypocapnia) or alkalosis (after hypercapnia). The former results in increased CBF with a concomitant increase in intracranial pressure (ICP) that depends on the prevailing intracranial compliance. The latter conveys a theoretical risk for ischemia.

Pao_2. Changes in Pao_2 from 60 to greater than 300 mm Hg have little influence on CBF. Below a Pao_2 of 60 mm Hg, CBF

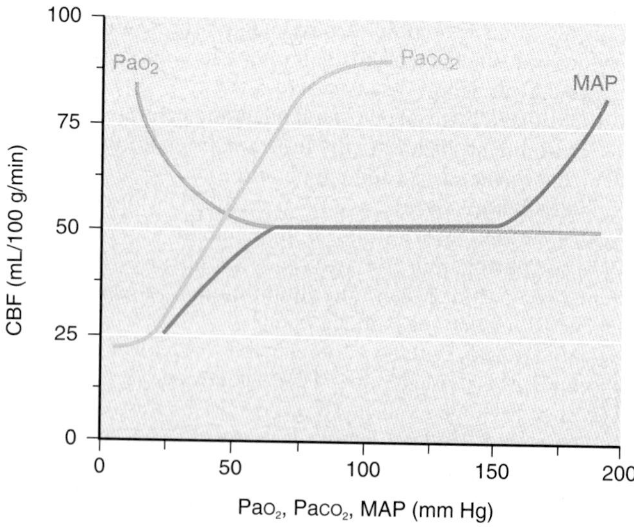

Figure 13-4 Changes in cerebral blood flow (CBF) caused by independent alterations in $Paco_2$, Pao_2, and mean arterial pressure (MAP).

increases rapidly (see Fig. 13-4). The mechanisms mediating cerebral vasodilation during hypoxia are not fully understood but may include neurogenic effects initiated by peripheral and neuraxial chemoreceptors, as well as local humoral influences. At least part of the hyperemic response to hypoxia is mediated by NO of neuronal origin (see Chapter 31). Hypoxia-induced hyperpolarization of vascular smooth muscle by the opening of ATP-dependent K^+ channels also leads to vasodilation. Recent studies have indicated that the rostral ventrolateral medulla (RVM) serves as an oxygen sensor within the brain. Stimulation of the RVM by hypoxia results in an increase in CBF (but not CMR), and lesions of the RVM suppress the magnitude of the CBF response to hypoxia. The response to hypoxia is synergistic with the hyperemia produced by hypercapnia and acidosis. At high $Pa{O_2}$ values, CBF decreases modestly. At 1 atm of oxygen, CBF is reduced by 12%.

Myogenic Regulation (Autoregulation) of Cerebral Blood Flow

Autoregulation refers to the capacity of the cerebral circulation to adjust its resistance to maintain CBF constant over a wide range of mean arterial pressure (MAP). In normal *human* subjects, the best available data—and they are limited—are consistent with the limits of autoregulation occurring at MAP values of approximately 70 and 150 mm Hg (see Fig. 13-4). The lower limit of autoregulation (LLA) has been widely quoted as an MAP of 50 mm Hg. Although this number may be correct for some animal species, the data available argue that the LLA is considerably higher in humans.[4] Note that the units used on the *x* axis of "autoregulation curves" will influence the correct inflection points of the curve. When the *x* axis is "mean arterial pressure", the normal average LLA is not less than 70 mm Hg (with considerable interindividual variation). Because ICP is not usually measured in normal subjects, cerebral perfusion pressure (CPP) (MAP – ICP) is rarely available. Assuming a normal ICP of 5 to 15 mm Hg in a supine subject, an LLA of 70 expressed as MAP corresponds to an LLA of 55 to 60 mm Hg expressed as CPP.

Above and below the autoregulatory plateau, CBF is pressure dependent (pressure passive) and varies linearly with CPP. Autoregulation is influenced by various pathologic processes, as well as the time course over which the changes in CPP occur. Even within the range over which autoregulation normally occurs, a rapid change in arterial pressure will result in a transient (3 to 4 minutes) alteration in CBF.

The "limits of autoregulation" are conceptual constructs for the purpose of analysis. They do not represent physiologic "all-or-none" responses. There is probably a continuum of vascular responsiveness in the knee of the both the lower and upper limits as the ability of the arteriolar bed to dilate or constrict is exhausted. Furthermore, the morphology of the autoregulation is strongly influenced by the background level of vasodilation or vasoconstriction (e.g., $Pa{CO_2}$ or anesthetic conditions).

The precise mechanism by which autoregulation is accomplished and its overlap with flow-metabolism coupling are not known. According to the myogenic hypothesis, changes in CPP lead to direct changes in the tone of vascular smooth muscle; this process appears to be passive. NO may participate in the vasodilation associated with hypotension. Autonomic innervation of cerebral blood vessels may also contribute to autoregulation of blood flow (discussed in the next section).

Neurogenic Regulation of Cerebral Blood Flow

The cerebral vasculature is extensively innervated.[5] The density of innervation declines with vessel size, and the greatest neurogenic influence appears to be exerted on larger cerebral arteries. This innervation includes cholinergic (parasympathetic and nonparasympathetic), adrenergic (sympathetic and nonsympathetic), serotonergic, and VIPergic systems of extra- and intra-axial origin. It is certain that in animals there is an extracranial sympathetic influence via the superior cervical ganglion, as well as parasympathetic innervation via the sphenopalatine ganglion. The intra-axial pathways are less well defined, although there is considerable evidence of innervation arising from several nuclei in animals, including the locus ceruleus, the fastigial nucleus, the dorsal raphe nucleus, and the basal magnocellular nucleus of Meynert. Evidence of the functional significance of neurogenic influences has been derived from studies of CBF autoregulation and ischemic injury. Hemorrhagic shock, a state of high sympathetic tone, results in a lower CBF at a given MAP than occurs when hypotension is produced with sympatholytic drugs, presumably because during shock, a sympathetically mediated vasoconstrictive effect shifts the lower end of the "autoregulatory" plateau (Fig. 13-5) to the right. It is not clear what the relative contributions of humoral and neural mechanisms are to this phe-

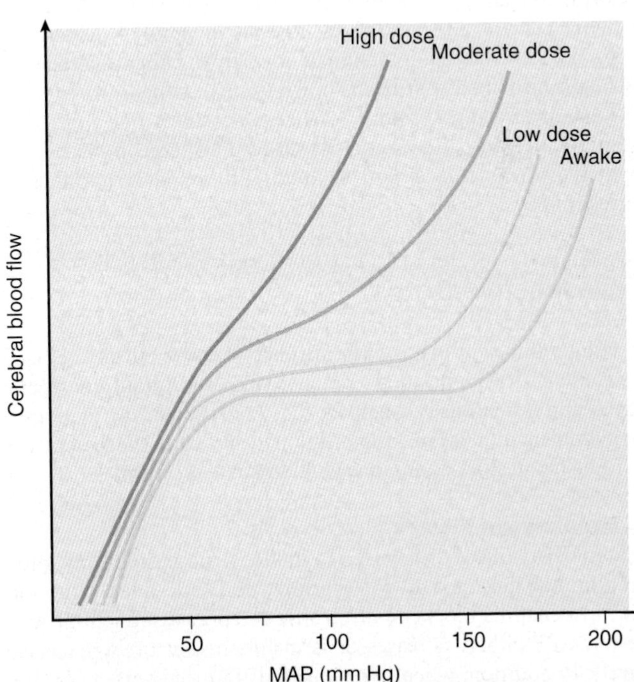

Figure 13-5 Schematic representation of the effect of increasing concentrations of a typical volatile anesthetic drug on autoregulation of cerebral blood flow. Dose-dependent cerebral vasodilation results in attenuation of autoregulatory capacity. Both the upper and lower thresholds are shifted to the left. MAP, mean arterial pressure.

nomenon; however, there is certainly a neurogenic component in some species because sympathetic denervation increases CBF during hemorrhagic shock. Moreover, sympathetic denervation produced by blockade of the stellate ganglion can increase CBF in humans.[6] Activation of cerebral sympathetic innervation also shifts the upper limit of autoregulation to the right and offers some protection against hypertensive breakthrough of the BBB. Experimental interventions that alter these neurogenic control pathways influence outcome after standardized ischemic insults, presumably by influences on vascular tone and therefore CBF. The nature and influence of such pathways in humans are not known, and their manipulation for purposes of clinical management remains to be investigated systematically.

Effects of Blood Viscosity on Cerebral Blood Flow

Blood viscosity can influence CBF. Hematocrit is the single most important determinant of blood viscosity.[7] In healthy subjects, variation of the hematocrit within the normal range (33% to 45%) probably results in only modest alterations in CBF. Beyond this range, changes are more substantial. In anemia, cerebral vascular resistance is reduced and CBF increases. However, this may result not only from a reduction in viscosity but also from reduced oxygen-carrying capacity of blood.[8] The effect of a reduction in viscosity on CBF is more obvious in the setting of focal cerebral ischemia, a condition in which vasodilation in response to impaired oxygen delivery is probably already maximal. In this situation, reducing viscosity by hemodilution results in increases in CBF in the ischemic territory. The best available information suggests that in patients with focal cerebral ischemia, a hematocrit of 30% to 34% will result in optimal delivery of oxygen. However, manipulation of viscosity in patients with acute ischemic stroke has not been shown to be of benefit in reducing the extent of cerebral injury.[9] Hence, viscosity is not a target of manipulation in patients at risk as a result of cerebral ischemia, with the possible exception of those with hematocrit values in excess of 55%.

Vasoactive Drugs

A large number of drugs with intrinsic vascular effects are used in contemporary anesthetic practice, including both anesthetic drugs and numerous vasoactive drugs used specifically for hemodynamic manipulation. This section deals with the latter. The actions of anesthetics are discussed in a later section.

Systemic Vasodilators

The majority of the drugs used to induce hypotension (including sodium nitroprusside, nitroglycerin, hydralazine, adenosine, and calcium channel blockers) also cause cerebral vasodilation. As a result, CBF either increases or is maintained at prehypotensive levels. In addition, when hypotension is induced with a cerebral vasodilator, CBF is maintained at lower MAP values than when induced by either hemorrhage or a noncerebral vasodilator. In contrast to direct vasodilators, the angiotensin-converting enzyme inhibitor enalapril does not have any significant impact on CBF.[10] Anesthetics that vasodilate the cerebral circulation simultaneously cause increases in CBV with the potential to increase ICP. The effects of these anesthetics on ICP are less dramatic when hypotension is induced slowly. This probably reflects the more effective interplay of compensatory mechanisms (shifts in CSF and venous blood) when changes occur more slowly.

Catecholamine Agonists/Antagonists

Numerous drugs with agonist and antagonist activity at catecholamine receptors (α_1, β_2, β, and dopamine) are in common use. The effects of these anesthetics on cerebral physiology are dependent on basal blood pressure, the magnitude of the systemic blood pressure changes that occur as a result of administration of the agent of interest, the status of the autoregulation mechanism, and the status of the BBB. A given agent may have direct effects on cerebral vascular smooth muscle or indirect effects mediated by the cerebral autoregulatory response to changes in systemic blood pressure (or both types of effects). When autoregulation is preserved, increases in systemic pressure would be expected to increase CBF if basal blood pressure is either below or above the lower and upper limits of autoregulation, respectively. When basal pressure is within the normal autoregulation range, an increase in systemic pressure does not affect CBF significantly because the normal autoregulatory response to a rising MAP entails cerebral vasoconstriction (an increase in cerebral vascular resistance) to maintain a constant CBF. When autoregulation is defective, CBF will vary in direct relation to systemic pressure. The information in the following paragraphs and in Table 13-3 emphasizes data obtained from investigations of pressor anesthetics in intact preparations and gives greatest weight to results obtained in humans and higher primates.

Table 13-3 Best Estimates of the Influence of Pure Catecholamine Receptor Agonists and Specific Pressor Substances on Cerebral Blood Flow and Cerebral Metabolic Rate*

Agonist	Cerebral Blood Flow	Cerebral Metabolic Rate
Pure		
α_1	0/–	0
α_2	–	0
β	+	+
β (BBB open)	+++	+++
Dopamine	++	0
Dopamine (high dose)	?–	?0
Fenoldopam	–	?0
Mixed		
Norepinephrine	0/–	0/+
Norepinephrine (BBB open)	+	+
Epinephrine	+	+
Epinephrine (BBB open)	+++	+++

*Where species differences occurred, data from primates were given preference. See text for complete discussion.
BBB, blood-brain barrier; +, increase; –, decrease; 0, no effect; the number of symbols indicates the magnitude of the effect.

α_1-AGONISTS. A frequently encountered clinical concern is that the administration of anesthetics with α_1-agonist effects (phenylephrine, norepinephrine) will lead to a reduction in CBF. Data derived from studies in both humans and nonhuman primates do not support this belief. Intracarotid infusion of norepinephrine in doses that significantly increase MAP result in no change in CBF. Administration of phenylephrine to patients maintained on cardiopulmonary bypass does not decrease CBF.[11] There are, however, some species differences with regard to the CBF response to α-agonists. α_1-Agonists also do not appear to cause cerebral vasoconstriction in rats but do produce modest decreases in CBF in dogs and goats; this reduction in CBF can be blocked by α_1-antagonists.

Increases in CBF have been attributed to norepinephrine. Such increases might occur if autoregulation were defective or its limit exceeded. In some instances the increases may be the result of abnormalities in the BBB. Some data suggest that β-mimetic drugs (norepinephrine has β_1 activity) cause activation of cerebral metabolism[12] with a coupled increase in CBF, and this effect is likely to be most apparent when these drugs can gain greater access to the brain parenchyma via a defective BBB (see the later section on epinephrine).

In summary, it seems likely that circulating α_1-agonists will have little direct influence on CBF in humans with the exception that norepinephrine may cause vasodilation when the BBB is defective.

β-AGONISTS. β-Receptor agonists, in low doses, have little direct effect on the cerebral vasculature. In larger doses and in association with physiologic stress, they can cause an increase in CMR with an accompanying increase in CBF.[13] The β_1-receptor is probably the mediator of these effects. In doses that do not result in substantial changes in MAP, intracarotid epinephrine does not change CBF in unanesthetized humans. However, with larger doses that lead to an increase in MAP, CBF and $CMRO_2$ can increase by about 20%.

There is evidence that a defect in the BBB enhances the effect of β-agonists.[14] Intracarotid norepinephrine, which does not normally affect CBF and CMR, increases CBF and CMR when BBB permeability is increased with hypertonic drugs. Artru and colleagues demonstrated that epinephrine causes an elevation in $CMRO_2$, but only when the BBB was made permeable.[14] These observations beg the interpretation that β-agonists will increase CBF and CMR *only* when the BBB is injured. However, in the human study of King and associates,[15] when epinephrine was given in doses that did not increase MAP significantly, increases in CBF/CMR occurred nonetheless. Accordingly, BBB injury may not be a necessary condition in humans for the occurrence of β-mediated increases in CBF and CMR, although it will probably exaggerate the phenomenon.

β-BLOCKERS. β-Blockers have been variously reported to reduce or to have no effect on CBF and CMR. In two investigations in humans, propranolol, 5 mg intravenously,[16] and labetalol, 0.75 mg/kg intravenously,[17] had no effect on CBF and cerebral blood flow velocity (CBFV), respectively. Modest reductions in CBF occur after the administration of labetalol to craniotomy patients who become hypertensive during emergence from anesthesia. Esmolol has been reported to shorten seizures induced by electroconvulsive therapy (ECT), thus suggesting that it does cross the normal BBB. Catecholamine levels at the time of β-blocker administration or the status of the BBB (or both) may influence the effect of these drugs. The database with respect to these possibilities is incomplete. However, the data suggest that β-blockers are unlikely to have adverse effects on patients with intracranial pathology, other than effects secondary to changes in perfusion pressure.

DOPAMINE. Dopamine is widely used in the treatment of hemodynamic dysfunction. In addition, it is commonly used to augment the function of the normal cardiovascular system when an elevation in MAP is desired as an adjunct to the treatment of focal cerebral ischemia, especially in the setting of vasospasm. Nonetheless, its effects on CBF and CMR have not been defined with certainty. Taken together, the available data[18] suggest that the predominant effect of dopamine in the normal cerebral vasculature, when administered in low doses, is probably slight vasodilation with minimal change in CMR. Increased CMR in discrete regions of the brain, such as the choroid plexus and basal ganglia, has been reported. However, overall cortical blood flow is not influenced.[19] Vasoconstriction of the cerebral circulation is not observed even when dopamine is administered in doses of up to 100 µg/kg/min. In that same investigation, dobutamine was associated with 20% to 30% increases in CBF and CMR.[18] Fenoldopam is a dopamine agonist with activity at the DA_1 receptor and α_2-receptor. Administration of fenoldopam leads to systemic vasodilation and a reduction in systemic blood pressure. In humans, fenoldopam decreased systemic blood pressure to a level that was above the LLA; however, there was a modest (≈15%) reduction in CBF that did not increase to normal levels when systemic blood pressure was supported.[20] This reduction in CBF was attributed to the α_2 activity of fenoldopam. The impact of this reduction in CBF on the injured brain is not known.

α_2-AGONISTS. There is considerable current interest in α_2-agonists because of their analgesic and sedative effects. This class includes dexmedetomidine and clonidine, with the latter being a much less specific and less potent α_2-agonist. Two investigations in human volunteers have confirmed the ability of dexmedetomidine to decrease CBF. Dexmedetomidine dose-dependently decreased middle cerebral artery (MCA) flow velocity, with the maximum reduction being approximately 25%.[21] Dexmedetomidine (1-µg/kg loading dose and infusion at either 0.2 or 0.6 µg/kg/hr) decreased CBF by about 30%[22] in healthy human volunteers. In both these investigations, CMR was not measured and it is not clear whether the reduction in CBF was due to a direct vasoconstrictor activity of dexmedetomidine or to suppression of CMR with a corresponding reduction in CBF. In a more recent study of dexmedetomidine in which both MCA flow velocity and CMR were measured in healthy humans, dexmedetomidine decreased MCA flow velocity in parallel with a reduction in CMR.[23] These data indicate that the effects of dexmedetomidine on CBF are mediated primarily by its ability to suppress CMR. The well-know effect of dexmedetomidine to lower systemic blood pressure merits careful consideration if used in patients who are critically dependent on collateral perfusion pressure, especially in the recovery phase of an anesthetic.

Age

Aging from childhood to late adulthood is associated with a progressive reduction in CBF and $CMRO_2$.[24] This may reflect the progressive neuronal loss that occurs with age.

Effects of Anesthetics on Cerebral Blood Flow and Cerebral Metabolic Rate

This section deals with the effect of anesthetic drugs on CBF and CMR. It includes limited mention of influences on autoregulation, CO_2 responsiveness, and cerebral blood volume (CBV). Effects on CSF dynamics, the BBB, and epileptogenesis are discussed later.

In neuroanesthesia, considerable emphasis is placed on the manner in which anesthetic drugs and techniques influence CBF. The rationale is twofold. First, delivery of energy substrates is dependent on CBF, and in the setting of ischemia, modest alterations in CBF can substantially influence neuronal outcome. Second, control and manipulation of CBF are central to management of ICP because as CBF varies in response to vasoconstrictor-vasodilator influences, CBV varies with it.[25] With respect to ICP, it is CBV that is the more critical variable. In normal brain, CBV is approximately 5 mL/100 g of brain,[26] and over a $Paco_2$ range of approximately 25 to 70 mm Hg, CBV changes by about 0.049 mL/100 g for each 1–mm Hg change in $Paco_2$. In an adult brain weighing about 1400 g, this can amount to a 20-mL change in total CBV for a $Paco_2$ range of 25 to 55 mm Hg. Practically speaking, CBV is much more difficult to measure than CBF, so there is a relatively paucity of data, especially in human subjects.

Although CBV and CBF usually vary in parallel, the magnitude of change in CBV is less than the magnitude of change in CBF (Fig. 13-6); for a given increase in CBF, the increase in CBV is considerably less. In addition, CBV and CBF vary independently under some circumstances. During cerebral ischemia, for example, CBV increases whereas CBF is significantly reduced.[27] Autoregulation normally serves to prevent MAP-related increases in CBV. In fact, as the cerebral circulation constricts to maintain a constant CBF in the face of a rising MAP, CBV actually decreases.[28] When autoregulation is impaired or its upper limit (≈150 mm Hg) is exceeded, CBF and CBV then increase in parallel as arterial pressure rises (see Fig. 13-5). A declining MAP results in a progressive increase in CBV as the cerebral circulation dilates to maintain constant flow, and exaggerated increases in CBV occur as MAP falls below the LLA.[28] In normal subjects, the initial increases in CBV do not result in a significant elevation in ICP because there is latitude for compensatory adjustments by other intracranial compartments (e.g., translocation of venous blood and CSF to extracerebral vessels and the spinal CSF space, respectively). When intracranial compliance* is reduced, an increase in CBV can cause herniation or reduce CPP sufficiently to cause ischemia.

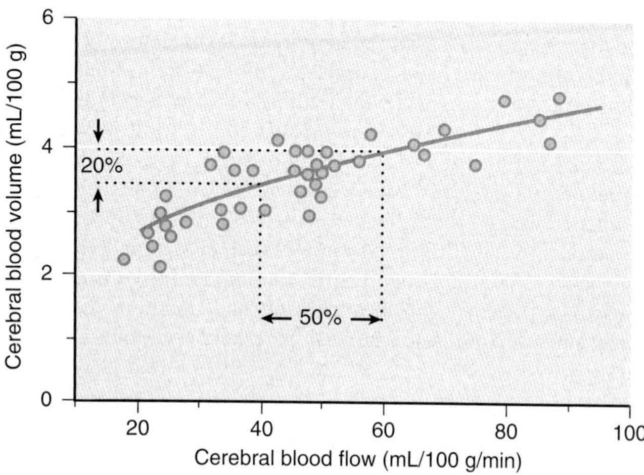

Figure 13-6 Relationship between cerebral blood flow (CBF) and cerebral blood volume (CBV). Note that although there is a linear relationship between CBF and CBV, the magnitude of the change in CBV for a given change in CBF is considerably less. In this figure, an increase in CBF of 50% results in a change in CBV of only 20%.

There have been several investigations of the effects of anesthetics on CBV in normal brain.[30,31] In general, the effects observed confirm a parallel relationship between CBF and CBV. However, the relationship is not consistently 1 : 1,[25,32] and CBF-independent influences on CBV may occur. It is also an unexplored possibility that anesthetic drugs may influence the venous side of the cerebral circulation. Although the intracranial veins are a largely passive compartment, there is evidence that in some species venous caliber is under active control by either neurogenic or humoral mechanisms. At present, there is no evidence that these direct effects have clinical significance. Nonetheless, the importance of blood volume on the venous side of the cerebral circulation should not be overlooked. Passive engorgement of these vessels as a result of the head-down posture, compression of the jugular venous system, or high intrathoracic pressure can have dramatic effects on ICP (see Fig. 63-5).

Intravenous Anesthetic Drugs

The general pattern of the effect of intravenous anesthetics is one of parallel alterations in CMR and CBF. The vast majority of intravenous anesthetics cause a reduction in both. Ketamine, which causes an increase in CMR and CBF, is the exception. The effects of selected intravenous anesthetic drugs on human CBF are compared in Figure 13-7.

It is probable that the changes in CBF induced by intravenous anesthetics are largely the result of effects on CMR with parallel (coupled) changes in CBF. If this were the entire explanation, the CBF/CMR ratio would be the same for all anesthetics. It is not. There are also direct effects on cerebral vascular smooth muscle (e.g., vasoconstriction, vasodilation, alteration of autoregulatory function) that make contributions to the net effect. For instance, although barbiturates are generally thought of as cerebral vasoconstrictors, some barbiturates actually cause relaxation of cerebral vascular smooth muscle in isolated vessel preparations.[45] However, a substantial reduction in CMR occurs in vivo, and the net effect at the point of EEG suppression is vasoconstriction and a substantial decrease in CBF.[46] It appears that in general,

*Note a well-entrenched misuse of terminology.[29] The "compliance" curve that is commonly drawn to describe the intracranial pressure-volume relationship (see Fig. 66-3) actually depicts the relationship $\Delta P/\Delta V$ (elastance) and not $\Delta V/\Delta P$ (compliance). What is here referred to as "reduced compliance" is more correctly described as "increased elastance." However, because the existing literature most commonly uses the "compliance" terminology, we have left the misuse uncorrected herein.

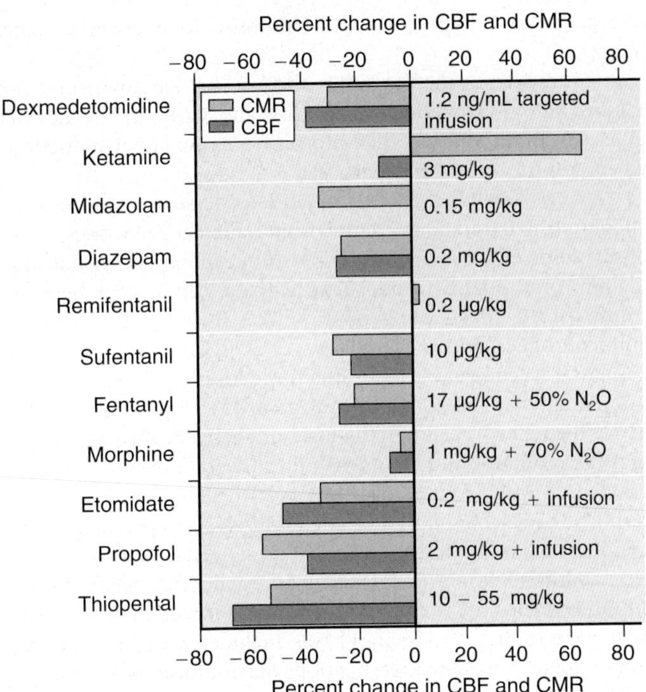

Figure 13-7 Changes in cerebral blood flow (CBF) and the cerebral metabolic rate of oxygen ($CMRO_2$) caused by intravenous anesthetic drugs. The data are derived from human investigations and are presented as percent change from unanesthetized control values. Dexmedetomidine CMR values were determined on a background of 0.5% isoflurane anesthesia. See the text for details. No data for the $CMRO_2$ effects of midazolam in humans are available. *(Data from references 22 and 33-44.)*

autoregulation and CO_2 responsiveness are preserved during administration of intravenous anesthetic drugs.

Barbiturates

A dose-dependent reduction in CBF and CMR occurs with barbiturates. With the onset of anesthesia, CBF and $CMRO_2$ are reduced by about 30%.[47] When large doses of thiopental cause complete EEG suppression, CBF and CMR are reduced by about 50%.[46,48] Further increases in the dose of barbiturate have no additional effect on CMR.[46] These observations suggest that the major effect of nontoxic doses of depressant anesthetics is a reduction in the component of cerebral metabolism that is linked to electrical brain function (e.g., neurophysiologic activity), with only minimal effects on the second component, that related to cellular homeostasis (see Fig. 13-1).

Tolerance to the CBF/CMR effects of barbiturates may develop quickly.[49] In patients with severe head injury in whom "barbiturate coma" was maintained for 72 hours, the blood concentration of thiamylal required to maintain EEG burst suppression was observed to be increased by the end of the first 24 hours and continued to increase over the next 48 hours.[50] During deep pentobarbital anesthesia, autoregulation is maintained up to arterial pressures as low as 60 mm Hg. CO_2 responsiveness also persists.

Propofol

The effects of propofol (2,6-diisopropylphenol) on CBF and CMR appear to be quite similar to those of barbiturates. Investigations in humans have revealed substantial reductions in both CBF and CMR after the administration of propofol.[51] In healthy volunteers, surgical levels of propofol reduced regional CBF by 53% to 79% in comparison with the awake state.[52,53] Alkire and coworkers assessed cerebral glucose metabolism in volunteers by positron emission tomography (PET) before and during infusion of propofol to the point of unresponsiveness.[54] The whole-brain metabolic rate decreased by 48% to 58%, with limited regional heterogeneity observed. When compared with isoflurane-fentanyl or sevoflurane-fentanyl anesthesia, a combination of propofol and fentanyl decreased subdural pressure in patients with intracranial tumors and decreased the arteriovenous oxygen content difference ($AVDo_2$).[55] Collectively, these investigations in human subjects indicate that propofol effects reductions in CMR and secondarily decreases CBF, CBV, and ICP.

Both CO_2 responsiveness and autoregulation appear to be preserved in humans during the administration of propofol,[56,57] even when administered in doses that produce burst suppression of the EEG.[58] The magnitude of the reduction in CBF during hypocapnia is decreased during propofol administration. This effect is probably due to the cerebral vasoconstriction induced by suppression of CMR, which limits further hypocapnia-mediated vasoconstriction.

Etomidate

The effects of etomidate on CBF and CMR are also similar to those of barbiturates. Roughly parallel reductions in CBF and CMR occur in humans,[33,59] and in general they are accompanied by progressive suppression of the EEG. Induction of anesthesia with either thiopental or etomidate resulted in a similar reduction in MCA flow velocity of about 27%.[60] The CBF/CMR changes are substantial. Renou and colleagues[33] gave approximately 0.2 mg/kg of etomidate to adults and observed mean reductions in CBF and CMR of 34% and 45%, respectively. As is the case with barbiturates, no further reduction in CMR occurs when additional drug is administered beyond a dose sufficient to produce EEG suppression. This latter phenomenon has not been demonstrated in humans. However, Bingham and associates[61] observed that etomidate lowered ICP when administered to severely head-injured patients in whom EEG activity was well preserved but was ineffective when there was substantial antecedent EEG suppression. The global CMR suppression attainable with etomidate is slightly less profound than that achieved with isoflurane and barbiturates. This is consistent with the observation that unlike barbiturates, which cause CMR suppression throughout the brain, the CMR suppression caused by etomidate is regionally variable and occurs predominantly in forebrain structures.

Etomidate has been shown to be effective in reducing ICP without causing a reduction in CPP in patients with intracranial tumors[62] and head-injured patients.[63] However, administration of etomidate has been shown to result in an exacerbation of brain tissue hypoxia and acidosis in patients in whom the MCA was temporarily occluded during surgery.[64] Additional concerns regarding the occurrence of adrenocortical suppression and renal injury caused by the propylene glycol vehicle[65] will probably preclude more than episodic use.

Reactivity to CO_2 is preserved in humans during the administration of etomidate.[33,59] Autoregulation has not been evaluated. Myoclonus and epileptogenesis are discussed in a later section.

Narcotics

There are inconsistencies in the information available, but it is likely that narcotics have relatively little effect on CBF and CMR in the normal, unstimulated nervous system. When changes do occur, the general pattern is one of modest reductions in both CBF and CMR. The inconsistencies in the literature probably arise largely because in many studies, the "control" states entailed paralysis and nominal sedation, often with nitrous oxide alone. In these studies, in which substantial reductions in CBF and CMR were frequently observed, the effect of the narcotic was probably a combination of the inherent effect of the drug plus a substantial component attributable to reduction of arousal. Comparable effects related to reduction of arousal may occur and can be clinically important. However, they should be viewed as nonspecific effects of sedation or pain control, or both, rather than specific properties of narcotics. The following discussion emphasizes investigations in which control measurements were unlikely to have been markedly influenced by arousal phenomena.

MORPHINE. When morphine (~1 mg/kg) was administered as the sole drug to humans, Moyer and associates[66] observed no effect on global CBF and a 41% decrease in $CMRO_2$. The latter is a substantial reduction, and the absence of a simultaneous adjustment in CBF is surprising. There have been no other investigations of morphine alone in humans. Jobes and coworkers gave morphine (1 and 3 mg/kg) with 70% N_2O to patients and observed no significant change in CBF or CMR.[34] The N_2O that was used might be expected to have caused a tendency toward increases in CBF and CMR. The relative absence of *net* changes in these variables from awake control measurements suggests a small to moderate depressive effect of morphine on CBF and CMR at this large dose. It should be recalled, however, that morphine can cause substantial release of histamine in individual patients. Histamine is a cerebral vasodilator that will cause an increase in CBV and a CBF effect that will vary depending on the systemic blood pressure response.

Autoregulation was observed to be intact between MAP values of 60 and 120 mm Hg in human volunteers anesthetized with morphine, 2 mg/kg, and 70% N_2O.[67]

FENTANYL. Limited human data are available. Vernhiet and colleagues[35] measured CBF and $CMRO_2$ before and during anesthesia with 12 to 30 (mean, 16) μg/kg of fentanyl and 50% N_2O in patients about to undergo cerebral angiography. Atropine and pancuronium were the only other anesthetics administered. Neither CBF nor $CMRO_2$ changed significantly from awake control values in their group of six subjects. However, one of the patients (an epileptic with normal results on computed tomography [CT]) had dramatic and unexplained increases in both CBF and $CMRO_2$. For the remaining five, CBF and $CMRO_2$ decreased by 21% and 26%, respectively ($P < .05$). The data for fentanyl/N_2O presented in Figure 13-7 are derived from these five patients, who received an average of 17 μg/kg of fentanyl. Murkin and associates measured CBF before and after induction of anesthesia with high-dose fentanyl, 100 μg/kg, and diazepam, 0.4 mg/kg.[68] CBF fell by 25%, although part of this effect may well have been a result of the benzodiazepine (see later) rather than fentanyl. Firestone and coworkers, using PET, observed a heterogeneous CBF response to 1.5 μg/kg of fentanyl in healthy volunteers. Increases occurred in the frontal, temporal, and cerebellar areas simultaneous with decreases in discreet areas associated with pain-related processing.[69] CO_2 responsiveness and autoregulation are unaffected, and the hyperemic CBF response to hypoxia remains intact.

These data, taken together, suggest that fentanyl will cause a moderate global reduction in CBF and CMR in the normal quiescent brain and will, like morphine, cause larger reductions when administered during arousal.

ALFENTANIL. McPherson and associates[70] administered alfentanil, 320 μg/kg, to pentobarbital-anesthetized dogs. They observed no changes in CBF, CMR, CO_2 responsiveness, autoregulation, or the CBF response to hypoxia. There have been no studies of the effects of alfentanil on CMR in humans. Schregel and colleagues administered 25 to 50 μg/kg of alfentanil to patients receiving 60% N_2O after induction of anesthesia with thiopental.[71] CBFV decreased transiently. A Doppler measure of MCA diameter was simultaneously unchanged, thus suggesting that the reduction in CBFV was indicative of a decrease in CBF. Mayberg and coworkers also observed no change in CBFV in response to 25 to 50 μg/kg of alfentanil given to patients during maintenance of anesthesia with isoflurane-N_2O.[72]

Although there are fewer data, the general pattern is similar and the conclusions should be the same as for sufentanil (see the next paragraph).[73-77] Alfentanil was included with fentanyl and sufentanil in two of the investigations of conditions in the surgical field mentioned in connection with sufentanil.[78,79] No adverse effects were noted.

SUFENTANIL. The majority of investigations in both animals[80,81] and humans indicate that sufentanil causes, depending on the dose, either no change or a reduction in CBF and CMR. Stephan and colleagues[36] measured CBF and $CMRO_2$ in patients before and after induction of anesthesia with 10 μg/kg of sufentanil. They observed a 29% reduction in CBF and a 22% reduction in $CMRO_2$. Murkin and coworkers, in a study involving the same dose of sufentanil and a similar design, made essentially identical observations.[82] Mayer and associates gave 0.5 μg/kg of sufentanil to volunteers and observed no change in CBF.[83] Weinstabl and coworkers observed reductions in CBFV when 1.0 and 2.0 μg/kg of sufentanil were given to intensive care unit (ICU) patients with increased ICP.[84] Neither Weinstabl and colleagues[84] nor Mayer and associates,[83] who administered sufentanil to healthy volunteers, observed changes in CBFV after 0.5 μg/kg of sufentanil.

The data from the aforementioned studies led to anticipation of no change or a reduction in ICP as a result of administration of either sufentanil or alfentanil. With respect to sufentanil, the bulk of the data derived in humans[84-88] has revealed no change in ICP after its administration. However, in some investigations in humans, sufentanil was associated with modest increases in intracranial pressure.[73,89] Subsequent investigations appear to indicate that the increases in ICP associated with sufentanil are at least in large part the consequence of a normal autoregulatory response to the sudden reduction in MAP that can occur as a consequence of sufentanil administration.[90] Based on these data, sufentanil (and for that matter fentanyl as well[87]) are best administered in a manner that does not produce sudden reduction of MAP. MAP reduction will clearly reduce CPP and may increase ICP, each of which, in sufficient extreme, may be deleterious. However, it should be noted that the ICP increases attributed to sufentanil have been small. Furthermore, four investigations[78,79,91,92] that compared conditions in the surgical field, including pressure under brain retractors,[78] identified no adverse influences attributable to sufentanil. Accordingly, sufentanil need not be viewed as in any way contraindicated, although it should be used with attention to its effect on MAP.

REMIFENTANIL. Investigations of moderate doses of remifentanil in patients have revealed minimal effects that are very similar to those of the other synthetic narcotics (with the exception of its substantially shorter duration of action). In patients undergoing craniotomy for supratentorial space-occupying lesions, 1 μg/kg of remifentanil caused no change in ICP.[93] In a second investigation in craniotomy patients, approximately 0.35 μg/kg/min of remifentanil resulted in CBF values comparable to those observed with moderately deep anesthesia with either isoflurane/N_2O or fentanyl/N_2O,[94] and CO_2 responsiveness was preserved. Greater doses of remifentanil may have more substantial effects. CBFV in the MCA decreased 30% in response to 5 μg/kg followed by 3 μg/kg/min of remifentanil at a constant MAP in patients being anesthetized for bypass surgery.[37] A lower dose of 2 μg/kg followed by an infusion of 3 μg/kg/min, however, did not affect CBFV. Quantitatively similar observations were made after a large dose of sufentanil in patients undergoing cardiac anesthesia (see earlier).[36]

It should be noted that in the previously mentioned studies, remifentanil was administered with other drugs that might influence cerebral hemodynamics. More recent studies in human volunteers have demonstrated that the infusion of *low* (*sedative*) doses of remifentanil can increase CBF. A PET study in human subjects to whom remifentanil, 0.05 and 0.15 μg/kg/min, was administered revealed increases in CBF in the prefrontal, inferior parietal, and supplementary motor cortices; reductions in CBF were observed in the cerebellum, superior temporal lobe, and midbrain gray matter.[95] The relative increase in CBF was greater with administration of the higher dose of remifentanil. Similar data were obtained by Lorenz and colleagues, who used magnetic resonance imaging for determination of CBF.[96] In a PET investigation in human volunteers, Kofke and coworkers observed remifentanil-induced increases in regional CBF within the limbic system.[97] Although the underlying mechanisms of the increases in CBF are not clear, disinhibition produced by the low-dose remifentanil infusion, or perhaps the sensation of side effects (warmth, comfort, pruritus),[96] may have contributed. It should be noted that when combined with N_2O, CBF and CO_2 reactivity are similar in patients given remifentanil or fentanyl.[98] In aggregate, the available human data indicate that in low sedative doses, administration of remifentanil alone can effect minor increases in CBF. With higher doses or with the concomitant administration of anesthetic adjuvants, CBF is either unaltered or modestly reduced.

Benzodiazepines

Benzodiazepines cause parallel reductions in CBF and CMR in humans. CBF and $CMRO_2$ decreased by 25% when 15 mg of diazepam was given to head-injured patients.[38] The effects of midazolam on CBF (but not CMR) have also been studied in humans. Forster and associates observed a 30% to 34% reduction in CBF[39,99] after the administration of 0.15 mg/kg of midazolam to awake healthy human volunteers. Veselis and coworkers, using PET, observed a global 12% reduction in CBF after a similar dose and noted that the decreases occurred preferentially in the brain regions associated with arousal, attention, and memory.[100] CO_2 responsiveness was preserved.[101]

The foregoing studies indicate that benzodiazepines should cause a moderate reduction in CBF in humans and suggest that the effect may be metabolically coupled. The extent of the maximal CBF/CMR reduction produced by benzodiazepines is probably intermediate between the decreases caused by narcotics (modest) and barbiturates (substantial). It appears that benzodiazepines should be safe to administer to patients with intracranial hypertension, provided that respiratory depression and an associated increase in $Paco_2$ do not occur.

Flumazenil

Flumazenil is a highly specific, competitive benzodiazepine receptor antagonist. It had no effect on CBF when administered to unanesthetized human volunteers.[99,102] However, flumazenil reverses the CBF-, CMR-, and ICP-lowering effects of midazolam. Whereas Knudsen and colleagues[103] observed no change in either CBF or CMR when patients were aroused from midazolam anesthesia with flumazenil at the conclusion of craniotomy for brain tumor resection, Chiolero and coauthors[104] reported severe increases in ICP when flumazenil was given to midazolam-sedated head injury patients in whom ICP was poorly controlled before the administration of flumazenil. These latter observations are consistent with animal investigations in which flumazenil not only reversed the CBF and CMR effects of midazolam but also caused a substantial, though short-lived overshoot above premidazolam levels in both CBF (by 44% to 56%) and ICP (by 180% to 217%). CMR did not rise above control levels, thus indicating that the increase in CBF was not metabolically coupled. The CBF overshoot effect is unexplained, but it may be a neurogenically mediated arousal phenomenon. Flumazenil should be used very cautiously to reverse benzodiazepine sedation in patients with impaired intracranial compliance.

Droperidol

There have been no human investigations of the CBF/CMR effects of droperidol in isolation. However, the information available from animal investigations and combination drug administration in humans,[105,106] taken together, suggests that droperidol is not a cerebral vasodilator and probably has little effect on CBF and CMR in humans. The occasional increases in ICP that have been observed[105] probably reflect normal autoregulation-mediated vasodilation in response to an abrupt fall in MAP.

Ketamine

Among the intravenous anesthetics, ketamine is unique in its ability to cause increases in both CBF and CMR.[107] Animal studies indicate that the changes in CMR are regionally variable. In rats, substantial increases occur in limbic system structures with modest changes or small decreases in cortical structures.[108] PET studies in humans have demonstrated that subanesthetic doses of ketamine (0.2 to 0.3 mg/kg) can increase global CMR by about 25%.[109] The greatest increase in CMR occurred in the frontal and anterior cingulated cortex. A relative reduction in CMR in the cerebellum was also observed. Commercially available formulations of ketamine contain both the (*S*)- and (*R*)-ketamine enantiomers. The (*S*)-ketamine enantiomer increases CMR substantially, whereas the (*R*) enantiomer tends to decrease CMR, particularly in the temporomedial cortex and in the cerebellum.[110] These changes in CMR are accompanied by corresponding changes in CBF.[111] Increases in global (as well as regional) CBF in humans that were not accompanied by similar increases in $CMRO_2$ after the administration of (*S*)-ketamine have been observed. However, the majority of investigations indicate that autoregulation is maintained during ketamine anesthesia[112]; the observed effects of ketamine on cerebral hemodynamics indicate that ketamine increases CMR and secondarily increases CBF. CO_2 responsiveness is preserved.

The anticipated ICP correlate of the increase in CBF has been confirmed to occur in humans. However, anesthetic drugs (diazepam, midazolam, isoflurane/N_2O, propofol) have been shown to blunt or eliminate the increases in ICP or CBF associated with ketamine.[113-115] In fact, decreases in ICP have been reported in response to relatively large doses of ketamine (1.5 to 5 mg/kg) administered to propofol-sedated head-injured patients.[116] Accordingly, although ketamine is probably best avoided as the sole anesthetic agent in patients with impaired intracranial compliance, it may be reasonable to use it cautiously in patients who are simultaneously receiving the other drugs mentioned earlier.

Lidocaine

Lidocaine produces a dose-related reduction in $CMRO_2$ in experimental animals.[117] In dogs, 3 mg/kg lowered $CMRO_2$ by 10% and 15 mg/kg reduced it by 27%. When very large doses (160 mg/kg) were given to dogs maintained on cardiopulmonary bypass, the reduction in $CMRO_2$ was apparently greater than that seen with high-dose barbiturates.[118] This may occur because the membrane-stabilizing effect of lidocaine also reduces the energy required for maintenance of membrane integrity. In unanesthetized human volunteers, Lam and colleagues observed reductions in CBF and CMR of 24% and 20%, respectively, after the administration of 5 mg/kg of lidocaine over a 30-minute period, followed by infusion of 45 µg/kg/min.[119]

Bedford and coworkers[120] compared the effectiveness of bolus doses of thiopental, 3 mg/kg, and lidocaine, 1.5 mg/kg, in controlling the acute increase in ICP that occurred after the application of a pin head holder or skin incision in craniotomy patients. The two regimens were equally effective in causing a reduction in ICP. However, the decrease in MAP was greater with thiopental. Accordingly, a bolus dose of lidocaine is a reasonable adjunct to the prevention or treatment of acute elevations in ICP and has been recommended for preventing increases in ICP associated with endotracheal suctioning. Note that large doses of lidocaine can produce seizures in humans and some experimental animals. Lidocaine-induced seizures have not been reported in anesthetized humans. Nonetheless, it seems appropriate to restrict lidocaine doses to amounts that achieve serum levels less than the seizure threshold (>5 to 10 µg/mL) in awake humans. After a 2-mg/kg bolus, peak serum concentrations of 6.6 to 8.5 µg/mL are below this seizure threshold. Bolus doses of 1.5 to 2.0 mg/kg therefore seem appropriate.

Inhaled Anesthetics

Volatile Anesthetics

The pattern of volatile anesthetic effects on cerebral physiology is a striking departure from that observed with the intravenous anesthetics, which generally cause parallel reductions in CMR and CBF. All volatile anesthetics, similar to intravenous sedative-hypnotic drugs, suppress cerebral metabolism in a dose-related manner.[121-125] Volatile anesthetics also possess intrinsic cerebral vasodilatory activity as a result of direct effects on vascular smooth muscle. The net effect of volatile anesthetics on CBF is therefore a balance between a reduction in CBF caused by CMR suppression and augmentation of CBF caused by the direct cerebral vasodilation. When administered at a dose of 0.5 MAC, CMR suppression–induced reduction in CBF predominates, and net CBF decreases in comparison to the awake state. At 1.0 MAC, CBF remains unchanged; at this dose, CMR suppression and vasodilatory effects are in balance. Beyond 1.0 MAC, the vasodilatory activity predominates, and CBF increases significantly even though CMR is substantially reduced.

The increase in CBF produced by volatile anesthetics at doses greater than 1.0 MAC has been interpreted as evidence of uncoupling of flow and metabolism. However, there is considerable evidence that coupling (CBF adjustments paralleling changes in CMR) persists during anesthesia with volatile agents.[126-129] Accordingly, it is probably more accurate to say that the CBF/CMR ratio is altered (increased) by volatile anesthetics. This alteration is dose related, and under steady-state conditions there is a positive correlation between MAC multiples and the CBF/$CMRO_2$ ratio[123,130]; that is, higher MAC levels cause greater "luxury" perfusion.

The important clinical consequences of administration of volatile anesthetics are derived from the increases in CBF and CBV—and consequently ICP—that can occur. Of the commonly used volatile anesthetics, the order of vasodilating potency is approximately halothane >> enflurane > desflurane ≈ isoflurane > sevoflurane.

Effects on Cerebral Blood Flow. Volatile anesthetics possess intrinsic vasodilatory activity, and they not only modify cerebral autoregulation but also produce dose-dependent reductions in systemic blood pressure. Hence, their effects on CBF and CMR are best evaluated when arterial pressure is supported to a common level. In addition, the cerebrovascular effects of volatile anesthetics are modulated by the simultaneous administration of other central nervous system (CNS)-active drugs. It is therefore important to understand the control state (awake, sedated, or anesthetized) against which the CBF and CMR effects of volatile anesthetics are compared. The best information about the cerebrovascular effects of volatile anesthetics is obtained in studies in which a nonanesthetized awake control state is used.

Data on the cerebrovascular effects of halothane and enflurane are limited. Initial studies in humans demonstrated that administration of 1 MAC halothane significantly increases CBF, even when systemic blood pressure is substantially reduced, in comparison to preanesthetic CBF.[131] The same investigators subsequently showed that in humans, when MAP is maintained at 80 mm Hg, 1.1 MAC levels of halothane increase CBF by as much as 191% and decrease CMR by about 10% (Fig. 13-8).[131,132] When compared with awake values, 1.2 MAC enflurane also increase CBF and decrease CMR by 45% and 15%, respectively.[136] The dramatic increases in CBF with a simultaneous modest reduction in CMR attest to the cerebral vasodilatory properties of halothane and enflurane. Isoflurane, by contrast, does not increase CBF as much as halothane or enflurane does. Human studies have shown that at doses of 1.1 MAC, isoflurane increases CBF by about 19% when systemic pressure is maintained within the normal range. CMR is reduced by about 45%.[129]

More recent investigations have shown that both sevoflurane and desflurane can significantly reduce CBF in humans

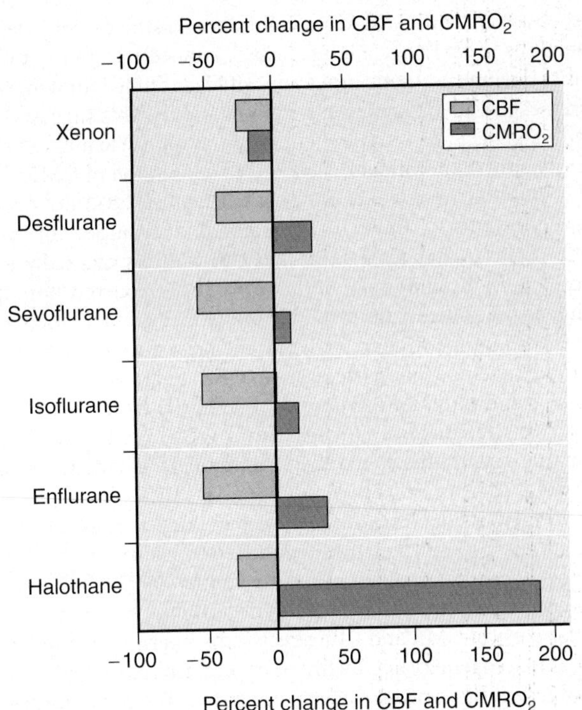

Figure 13-8 Estimated changes in cerebral blood flow (CBF) and the cerebral metabolic rate of oxygen ($CMRO_2$) caused by volatile anesthetics. The CBF data for halothane, enflurane, and isoflurane were obtained during anesthesia (with blood pressure support) at 1.1 minimum alveolar concentration (MAC) in humans[132] and are expressed as percent change from awake control values. The $CMRO_2$ data for halothane, enflurane, and isoflurane were obtained in the cat[123,133] and are expressed as percent change from N_2O-sedated control values. The data for sevoflurane were obtained during 1.1 MAC anesthesia in the rabbit and are expressed as percent change from a morphine/N_2O-anesthetized control state.[125] CBF values were obtained in patients who received 1 MAC sevoflurane anesthesia.[134] Desflurane data were obtained in patients to whom 1 MAC desflurane was administered.[135]

when compared with CBF in awake, nonanesthetized patients. At 1.0 MAC concentrations, sevoflurane[134] and desflurane[136] decreased CBF by 38% and 22% and CMR by 39% and 35%, respectively. These results, which suggest that the cerebral vasodilation produced by isoflurane is greater than that produced by sevoflurane and desflurane, were obtained with CBF measured by the inert gas technique. This technique measures CBF primarily within the cortex and therefore may have substantially underestimated global CBF. PET studies in healthy humans have shown that sevoflurane dose-dependently suppresses $CMRO_2$ and CBF; at 1 MAC levels, the reduction in CBF and $CMRO_2$ is approximately 50% and 50% to 60%, respectively.[52,53] In addition, other investigations in humans, most using measurement of MCA flow velocity by transcranial Doppler, indicate that differences in the effects of isoflurane, desflurane (Fig. 13-9), and sevoflurane are, at best, modest.[137,138,151] It should be noted that a strictly quantitative comparison between these volatile anesthetics is not possible given the variations in blood pressure among study group patients. In addition, there is some discrepancy among studies in the literature regarding the magnitude of the effects of volatile anesthetics on CBF. Much of this may occur as a result of the interaction of regionally selective CBF methods with the heterogeneity within the cerebrum of the CBF effects of volatile anesthetics. See the later section "Distribution of Changes in Cerebral Blood Flow/Cerebral Metabolic Rate."

There is considerable interest in use of the inert gas xenon in the modern practice of anesthesia. The anesthetic properties of xenon were recognized several decades ago, but it is only now that the agent is being evaluated for possible use in patients. The MAC

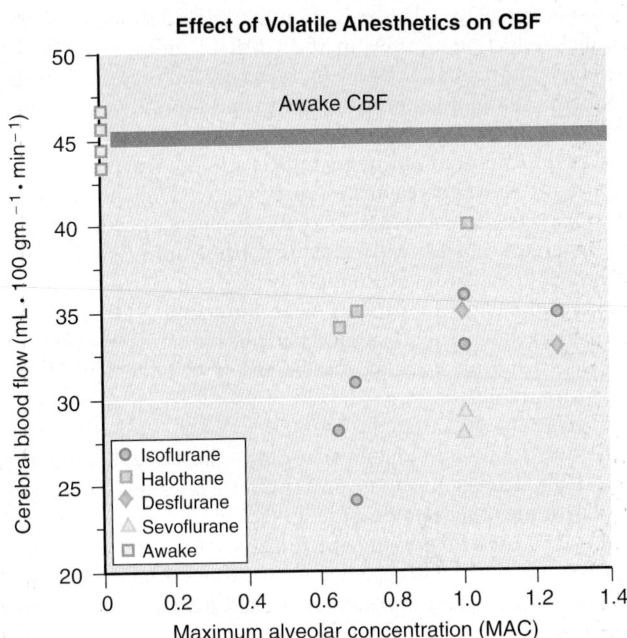

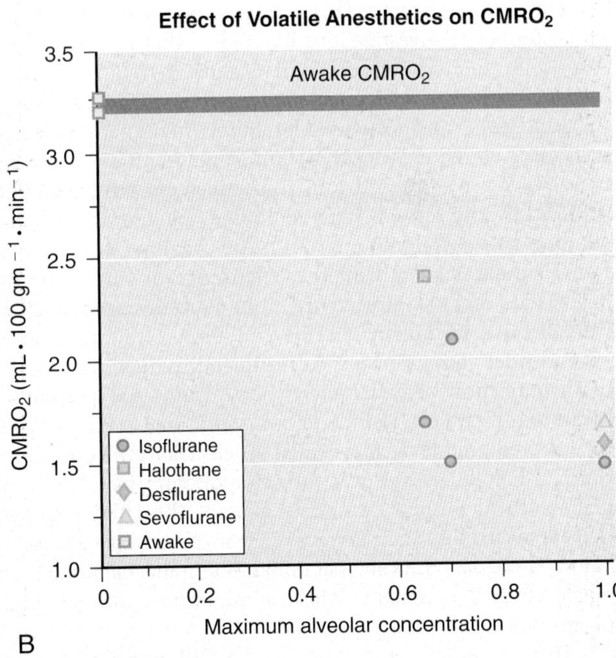

Figure 13-9 Effect of volatile anesthetics on cerebral blood flow (CBF) (**A**) and the cerebral metabolic rate of oxygen ($CMRO_2$) (**B**) in humans. The results are a composite of CBF and $CMRO_2$ values obtained from a number of separate investigations.[54,96,134,135,138-150] In these studies, $Paco_2$ was maintained in the normocapnic range (~35 to 40 mm Hg) and mean arterial pressure was supported. In most of the investigations, CBF was measured by the inert gas technique. This technique measures primarily cortical CBF and, as such, might underestimate global CBF.

of xenon has been estimated to be 63% to 71%, with females having significantly lower MAC values (51%).[152] Xenon is thought to exert its anesthetic effect primarily via noncompetitive antagonism of the N-methyl-D-aspartate (NMDA) receptor,[153] although activation of the TREK two-pore K^+ channel might also play a role.[154] In healthy humans, administration of 1 MAC xenon resulted in a reduction in CBF by approximately 15% in the cortex and by 35% in the cerebellum; interestingly, CBF in white matter increased by 22%.[155] This reduction in CBF is accompanied by a parallel reduction of 26% in the CMR of glucose (CMRg).[156] Cerebral autoregulation and CO_2 reactivity are preserved during xenon anesthesia in animals.[157] Under background pentobarbital anesthesia in an experimental model of increased ICP, administration of xenon did not increase ICP, and the response to both hypocapnia and hypercapnia was preserved.[158] Diffusion of xenon into air-containing spaces such as the bowel does occur, although the magnitude of air expansion is considerably less than that with N_2O.[159] Accordingly, caution will have to be exercised with the use of xenon in patients with intracranial air. Although the use of xenon in neurosurgical patients has not been evaluated, the data available suggest that it has a favorable profile for neuroanesthesia.

Effects on Cerebral Metabolic Rate. All of the volatile anesthetics cause reductions in CMR. The degree of reduction in $CMRO_2$ that occurs at a given MAC level is less with halothane than with the other four anesthetics (see Fig. 19-8). Sevoflurane's effect on $CMRO_2$ is very similar to that of isoflurane. The available information, derived in separate investigations, suggests that desflurane causes slightly less suppression of $CMRO_2$ than isoflurane does, especially at concentrations above 1.0 MAC.[124] Although a direct comparison of the $CMRO_2$ effects of all of the volatile anesthetics has not been performed in humans, collation of data from a number of investigations has shown that at doses of 1.0 MAC, isoflurane, sevoflurane, and desflurane reduce $CMRO_2$ ($AVDO_2$ in arterial and jugular bulb blood samples) by 25%,[139] 38%,[134] and 22%,[160] respectively. PET studies in humans have also shown that halothane (0.9 MAC) and isoflurane (0.5 MAC) can decrease CMRg by 40% and 46%, respectively.[54,140] The reduction in $CMRO_2$ is dose related. With isoflurane (and almost certainly desflurane and sevoflurane as well), the maximal reduction is attained simultaneously with the occurrence of EEG suppression.[124] This occurs at clinically relevant concentrations, such as 1.5 to 2.0 MAC in humans. In dogs, additional isoflurane up to 6.0% end-tidal volume results in no further reduction in CMR and no indication of metabolic toxicity. Halothane presents a contrast to this pattern. Halothane concentrations in excess of 4.0 MAC are required to achieve EEG isoelectricity in dogs, and additional halothane causes a further reduction in $CMRO_2$ in concert with alterations in energy charge. The latter changes, which are reversible, suggest interference with oxidative phosphorylation. These data indicate that unlike isoflurane, halothane can produce reversible toxicity when administered in very high concentrations.

There is some nonlinearity in the CBF and CMR dose-response relationships for volatile anesthetics. The initial appearance of an EEG pattern associated with the onset of anesthesia with halothane, enflurane, and isoflurane is accompanied by a precipitous decline in $CMRO_2$.[47] Thereafter, $CMRO_2$ declines in a slower dose-dependent manner. Such an effect has also been demonstrated for sevoflurane. In a dose escalation study in humans, the greatest reduction in entropy (a measure of anesthetic depth) was observed with 1 MAC sevoflurane anesthesia, with lesser reductions occurring at increasing concentrations.[161] Other studies during anesthetic induction with halothane found marked increases in CBF before any alteration in CMR. This suggests that the direct effect of a volatile agent on smooth muscle may develop more rapidly than influences related to depression of CMR.

Distribution of Changes in Cerebral Blood Flow/Cerebral Metabolic Rate. The regional distribution of anesthetic-induced changes in CBF and CMR differs markedly with halothane and isoflurane. Halothane produces relatively homogeneous changes throughout the brain. CBF is globally increased and CMR is globally depressed. The changes caused by isoflurane are more heterogeneous. Increases in CBF are greater in subcortical areas and hindbrain structures than in the neocortex.[128,162,163] For CMR the converse is true, with a greater reduction in the neocortex than in the subcortex.[164] In humans, 1.0 MAC sevoflurane (Fig. 13-10) results in a reduction in CBF within the cortex and an increase in CBF within the cerebellum.[141] These effects of sevoflurane are similar to those produced by isoflurane.[141,163] Desflurane has not been submitted to similar local CBF studies. However, given the similarity of its effects on the EEG (suggesting similar cortical CMR and CBF effects), the interim assumption of similar heterogeneity in CBF distribution seems reasonable. These distribution differences may explain certain apparent contradictions in reported CBF effects in the existing literature for isoflurane. Methods that assess global hemodynamic effects reveal greater changes than those that emphasize the cortical compartment. For instance, Eintrei and coworkers found no increase in CBF by surface Xe washout when isoflurane was administered to patients undergoing craniotomy,[165] yet others[166-168] have reported that administration of isoflurane to normocapnic subjects with intracranial pathology can result in increases in CSF pressure.

Cerebral Vasodilation by Volatile Anesthetics—Clinical Implications. Isoflurane, desflurane, and sevoflurane may have a modest cerebral vasodilating effect in the human cortex when administered at doses of 1 MAC or less. In fact, administration of volatile anesthetics can effect net decreases in CBF (see Fig. 13-9). These data, however, should be interpreted with considerable caution because the critical variable that is of interest in the clinical sphere is CBV. Although there is a direct correlation between CBF and CBV, as noted earlier, the relationship is not strictly 1 : 1. The magnitude of the changes in CBV is significantly less than the magnitude of the changes in CBF, and modest reduction in CBF may not necessarily be accompanied by reductions in CBV. This is exemplified by clinical investigations in which a significant increase in ICP (and by extension, CBV) was observed in patients to whom isoflurane was administered at doses that would be expected to effect a reduction in CBF.[166,168] Although induction of hypocapnia mitigated the increase in ICP in these studies, other investigations have revealed that hyperventilation may not be effective in blunting isoflurane-induced increases in ICP in patients with intracranial tumors.[167] In experimental investigations of cerebral injury, volatile anesthetics increased ICP significantly, and this rise in ICP was not ameliorated by hypocapnia.[169] Collectively, these data suggest that volatile anesthetics will have minimal effects on cerebral hemodynamics in patients with normal intracranial compliance. However, in patients with abnormal intracranial compliance, the potential for volatile agent–induced increases in CBV and ICP exists. Accordingly, there should be discretion in the use of volatile anesthetics in the setting of large or rapidly expanding mass lesions, unstable

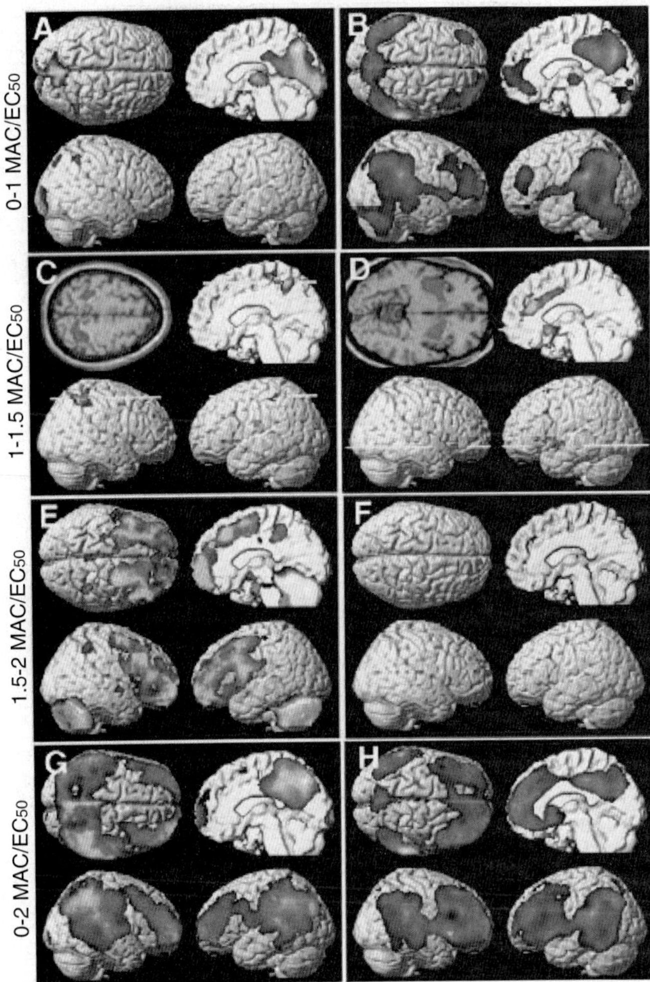

Figure 13-10 Dose-dependent redistribution of cerebral blood flow (CBF) in humans. **A** to **H**, Positron emission tomography (PET) scans demonstrate a dose-dependent reduction in CBF in both sevoflurane-anesthetized (*left*) and propofol-anesthetized (*right*) subjects. During sevoflurane anesthesia, an increase in concentration from 1.5 to 2.0 minimum alveolar concentration (MAC) leads to an increase in CBF within the subcortex, particularly in the cerebellum. There was a gradual reduction in mean arterial pressure (MAP) with increasing concentrations of sevoflurane, and MAP was not supported. The CBF values would be expected to be considerably greater had blood pressure been maintained within the normal range. Therefore, the CBF values represented in the figure probably *underestimate* true CBF during sevoflurane anesthesia. In propofol-anesthetized subjects, CBF was uniformly decreased and redistribution of CBF was not observed. *(Data from Kaisti K, Metsahonkala L, Teras M, et al: Effects of surgical levels of propofol and sevoflurane anesthesia on cerebral blood flow in healthy subjects studied with positron emission tomography. Anesthesiology 96:1358-1370, 2002.)*

Situations in which there has been substantial antecedent lowering of CMR by drug administration or disease processes should also justify caution in the use of volatile anesthetics. If a volatile agent has a substantial direct vasodilating effect on the cerebral vasculature that is normally offset by an opposing metabolically mediated vasoconstricting influence, it might be surmised that when near-maximal reduction of CMR has occurred, introduction of the volatile agent will have a predominantly vasodilating effect.[58,127] There are data to support this prediction. Maekawa and colleagues[164] measured CBF and local CMRg in rats both awake and during anesthesia with increasing concentrations of isoflurane. One MAC isoflurane resulted in an average decrease in CMRg of 54% of the awake control value in five cortical areas and no change in average CBF. An additional 1.0 MAC (i.e., a total of 2.0 MAC) caused a further reduction in CMRg of only 20% of the control value, and CBF simultaneously increased by 70% (Fig. 13-11). These data together suggest that isoflurane is a significant cerebral vasodilator when administered in concentrations at and above those associated with near-maximal CMR suppression or, perhaps, when administered in situations in which the component of CMR that is associated with electrophysiologic function is already suppressed by other drugs[58,127] or pathologic processes, such as traumatic brain injury.

The net vasodilating effect of equi-MAC concentrations of isoflurane, desflurane, and sevoflurane is less in humans than that of halothane, and the former are probably therefore preferable if a volatile agent is to be used in the setting of impaired intracranial compliance. That is not to say that halothane is contraindicated in these circumstances. It has been clearly demonstrated that when hypocapnia is established before the introduction of halothane, the increases in ICP that might otherwise occur in a nor-

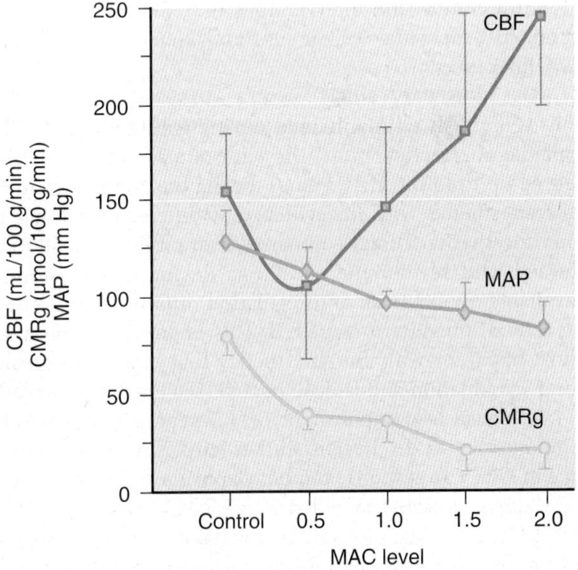

Figure 13-11 Relationship between changes in the cerebral metabolic rate of glucose (CMRg) and cerebral blood flow (CBF) in the motor-sensory cortex in rats during isoflurane anesthesia. The majority of the suppression in CMR caused by isoflurane has occurred by 1.0 minimum alveolar concentration (MAC), and in this concentration range CBF is not increased. Thereafter, additional isoflurane causes little further reduction in CMR, and cerebral vasodilation occurs. These data (±SD), from Maekawa and colleagues,[164] suggest the importance of metabolic coupling in determining the effects of isoflurane on CBF. MAP, mean arterial pressure.

ICP, or other significant derangements of cerebral physiology in which CO_2 responsiveness and flow-metabolism coupling may be impaired. When they occur (a somnolent, vomiting patient with papilledema, a large mass, and compressed basal cisterns), the clinician may well be advised to use a predominantly intravenous technique until such time as the cranium and dura are open and the effect of the anesthetic technique can be assessed directly. Such circumstances will be relatively rare in elective neurosurgery.

mocapnic patient with poor intracranial compliance can be prevented or greatly attenuated. Nonetheless, most clinicians will prefer isoflurane, desflurane, or sevoflurane because the margin for error is probably wider than with halothane.

Time Dependence of Cerebral Blood Flow Effects. The effect of volatile anesthetic drugs on CBF has been shown to be time dependent in animal investigations. After an initial increase, CBF falls substantially and reaches a steady state near pre–volatile agent levels between 2½ and 5 hours after exposure.[162,170,171] The mechanism of this effect is not understood, and the phenomenon was not evident in humans studied during 3- or 6-hour exposure to halothane, isoflurane, desflurane, or sevoflurane.[151,172]

Cerebral Blood Volume. The extensive investigation of the influence of volatile anesthetics on CBF has been based primarily on the concern that the cerebral vasodilation produced by volatile anesthetics might increase ICP. It should be noted, however, that it is CBV and not CBF per se that influences ICP. The vast majority of intracranial blood is within the cerebral venous circulation, and although there is a reasonable correlation between vasodilation-induced increases in CBF and CBV, the magnitude of changes in CBF is considerably greater than that in CBV (see Fig. 13-6). Hence, changes in CBF do not reliably predict changes in CBV and, by extension, in ICP. Nonetheless, the available data do indicate that CBV is considerably greater during isoflurane anesthesia than during propofol or pentobarbital anesthesia.[25] In human volunteers, 1 MAC sevoflurane reduced regional CBF but not regional CBV; by contrast, propofol reduced both regional CBF and regional CBV (Fig. 13-12).[53] In addition, CBV responds to changes in $Paco_2$ by a reduction in CBV with hypocapnia and an increase in CBV with hypercapnia. The magnitude of the change in CBV is, however, less than the change in CBF. In aggregate, these data indicate clearly that although the effect of anesthetics and interventions on CBF may parallel the effect on CBV, there may well be substantial qualitative and quantitative differences.

CO_2 Responsiveness and Autoregulation. CO_2 responsiveness is well maintained during anesthesia with all of the volatile anesthetics.[142,173,174] As with all vasodilators, CBF is preserved up to lower MAP values during the administration of volatile anesthetics with no evidence of differences among the various anesthetics. Direct comparisons of CBF with isoflurane, desflurane, and sevoflurane anesthesia during hypotension are not available. By contrast, autoregulation of CBF in response to rising arterial pressure is impaired. This impairment appears to be most apparent with the anesthetics that cause the greatest cerebral vasodilation and is dose related (see Fig. 13-5). Sevoflurane may cause less impairment of autoregulation than other volatile anesthetics do. Recent studies surprisingly reported no change in CBFV in response to phenylephrine-induced increases in MAP during anesthesia with 1.2 to 1.5 MAC sevoflurane[175,176] or in CBF during hemorrhagic hypotension.[177] The autoregulatory response to rising pressure may be pertinent during acute episodes of hypertension, such as during laryngoscopy or mismatch of surgical stimulation to anesthetic depth. There may be some relevance to hyperemic states after carotid endarterectomy or resection of arteriovenous malformations (see Chapter 63).

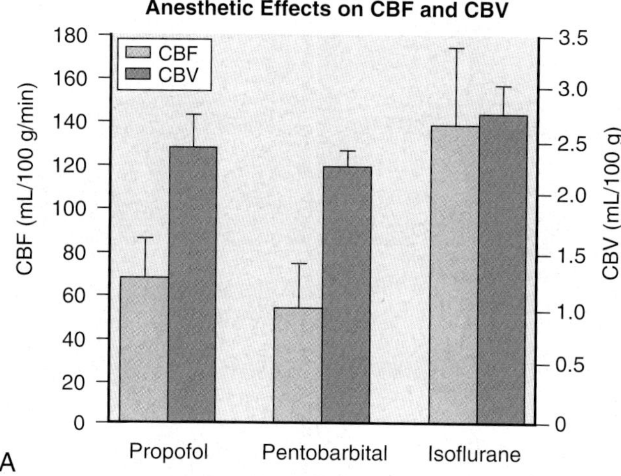

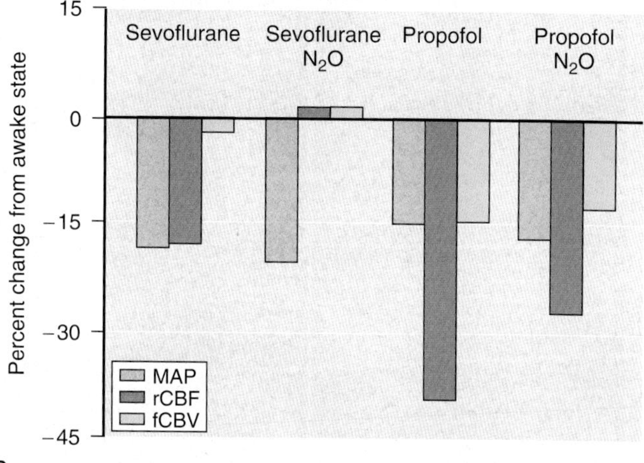

Figure 13-12 Effect of anesthetic drugs on cerebral blood flow (CBF) and cerebral blood volume (CBV). **A,** When compared with isoflurane, propofol and pentobarbital effected substantial reductions in CBF. However, reductions in CBV were more modest.[156] **B,** Although sevoflurane effected a significant reduction in regional CBF (rCBF), regional CBV (rCBV) was unchanged; had blood pressure been supported to normal levels, rCBV may have been greater than the awake state. By contrast, propofol effected a significant reduction in both rCBF and rCBV. These data indicate that the magnitude of the effect of anesthetics on rCBF is substantially greater than on rCBV. Hence, a reduction in rCBF may not lead to equivalent reductions in rCBV. MAP, mean arterial pressure.

Nitrous Oxide

The available data indicate that N_2O can cause increases in CBF, CMR, and ICP. At least a portion of the increases in CBF and CMR may be the result of a sympathoadrenal-stimulating effect of N_2O. The magnitude of the effect varies considerably according to the presence or absence of other anesthetic drugs (Fig. 13-13). When N_2O is administered alone, very substantial increases in CBF and ICP can occur. In sharp contrast, when N_2O is administered in combination with intravenous drugs, including barbiturates, benzodiazepines, narcotics, and propofol, its cerebral-vasodilating effect is attenuated or even completely inhibited. The addition of N_2O to anesthesia established with a volatile agent will result in moderate increases in CBF.

N_2O Administered Alone. The most dramatic reported increases in ICP or CBF in humans[181] and experimental animals[182] have occurred when N_2O was administered alone or with minimal background anesthesia. For instance, Henriksen and Jorgensen[181] recorded ICP before and during spontaneous breathing of 66% N_2O by patients with intracranial tumors. Mean ICP rose from

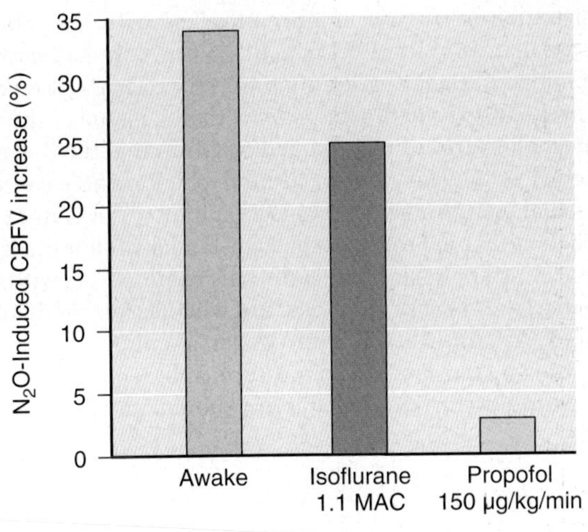

Figure 13-13 Mean percent increases in cerebral blood flow velocity (CBFV) in the middle cerebral artery of normocapnic subjects exposed to 60% N_2O after control recording in three conditions: awake[178]; 1.1 minimum alveolar concentration (MAC) of isoflurane[179]; and propofol, 150 µg/kg/min.[180]

13 to 40 mm Hg. The increases in CBF observed in humans are more modest than those observed in animals but are still substantial.[178] Whether these substantial increases represent the effects of N_2O per se or whether they reflect the nonspecific effects of a "second-stage" arousal phenomenon is not known.

N_2O Administered with Intravenous Anesthetics. When N_2O is administered in conjunction with certain intravenous anesthetics, its CBF effect may be considerably attenuated. Phirman and Shapiro[183] observed that a reproducible increase in ICP that had occurred in response to administration of 70% N_2O to a comatose patient was prevented by the previous administration of a combination of thiopental and diazepam despite no change in baseline ICP. In an investigation of patients with intracranial tumors and poor intracranial compliance (mean preinduction ICP, 27 mm Hg),[184] 50% N_2O introduced during barbiturate anesthesia and after the induction of hypocapnia had a negligible effect on ICP. Jung and associates compared lumbar CSF pressure in patients with brain tumors during administration of 0.7% isoflurane or 70% N_2O after induction of anesthesia with a barbiturate. Lumbar CSF pressure was modestly but significantly greater with N_2O.[185] That the increase was less dramatic than those cited earlier for N_2O alone may reflect the presence of residual barbiturate. Benzodiazepines administered alone have been shown to blunt the CBF response to N_2O in both animals and humans.[96] Narcotics appear to have a similar effect. Jobes and coauthors[34] reported that anesthesia with 1 mg/kg of morphine plus 70% N_2O resulted in no change in CBF from awake control values. Because of the very minor effect of morphine on CBF, these data suggest that N_2O did not cause substantial cerebral vasodilation. Although the addition of N_2O to propofol anesthesia in children increased MCA flow velocity,[186] such increases have not been demonstrated by other investigators.[180]

N_2O Administered with Volatile Anesthetics. In the majority of investigations, including several in humans, in which N_2O has been added to an anesthetic of 1.0 MAC or greater, substantial increases in CBF have been recorded.[179-187-190] Algotsson and associates[143] examined the effect of an approximately equi-MAC substitution of N_2O for isoflurane. They compared CBF in patients anesthetized with 1.5 MAC isoflurane and 0.75 MAC isoflurane with 65% N_2O. They observed 43% greater CBF with the latter, again consistent with a substantial vasodilating effect of N_2O in the presence of a volatile agent. Similar observations were made by Lam, Strebel, and their colleagues.[179,190] Several investigations have confirmed that CBF will be less with 1.0 MAC isoflurane than with a 1.0 MAC combination achieved with 50% to 65% N_2O and isoflurane.[143,144,191]

The result of an investigation in humans indicates that this vasodilating effect of N_2O may be positively correlated with the concentration of inhaled drug[190] and suggests that in general, the increase in CBF caused by N_2O is exaggerated at higher concentrations of both halothane and isoflurane. Of importance, however, is the observation of Reinstrup and coworkers, who demonstrated that administration of 50% N_2O to healthy volunteers did not significantly alter CBV.[192] In support of this observation, Kaisti and colleagues did not observe any effect of N_2O on CBV when added to a background of 1 MAC sevoflurane anesthesia.[53] These data indicate that although N_2O can increase CBF, its effect on CBV is modest at best.

Effects of N_2O on Cerebral Metabolic Rate. There is no uniform agreement about the effect of N_2O on CMR. Parallel changes in CBF and CMR,[182] increases in CBF without alteration of CMR,[193] and CMR alteration occurring without changes in CBF[194] have all been reported. This is doubtless the product of differences in species, methods, depth of background anesthesia, and interactions with simultaneously administered anesthetics. In a recent investigation in humans, administration of 70% N_2O on a background of either sevoflurane or propofol anesthesia resulted in modest increases in $CMRO_2$, thus indicating that N_2O does indeed increase cerebral metabolism.[53]

The CBF response to CO_2 is preserved during administration of N_2O.[195]

Clinical Implications. Despite the inconsistencies that are evident, data indicate that the vasodilatory action of N_2O can be clinically significant in neurosurgical patients with reduced intracranial compliance. However, it appears that N_2O-induced cerebral vasodilation can be considerably blunted by the simultaneous administration of intravenous anesthetics, although not all anesthetics have been evaluated and the dose-response relationships are not well defined. By contrast, addition of N_2O to a volatile drug–based anesthetic can increase cerebral metabolism and blood flow modestly. N_2O has been widely used in neurosurgery, and banishing it is inconsistent with the experience accumulated. Nonetheless, in circumstances wherein ICP is persistently elevated or the surgical field is persistently "tight," N_2O should be viewed as a potential contributing factor. Because N_2O rapidly enters a closed gas space, it should be avoided or omitted when a closed intracranial gas space may exist or intravascular air is a concern.

Muscle Relaxants

Nondepolarizing Relaxants

The only recognized effect of nondepolarizing relaxants on the cerebral vasculature occurs via the release of histamine (see Chapter 29). Histamine can result in a reduction in CPP because of the simultaneous increase in ICP (caused by cerebral vasodilation) and decrease in MAP.[196] It is not entirely clear, when the BBB is intact, whether histamine directly causes cerebral vasodilation or whether it is a secondary (autoregulatory) response to a reduction in MAP. D-Tubocurarine is the most potent histamine releaser among available muscle relaxants. Metocurine, atracurium, and mivacurium also release histamine in lesser quantities. This effect is likely to be clinically inconsequential unless these anesthetics are administered in the large doses necessary to achieve intubating conditions rapidly. Of this group of drugs, cisatracurium has the least histamine-releasing effect. No evidence of histamine release was seen after the administration of 0.15 mg/kg (three times the ED_{95} for twitch depression) of cisatracurium to neurosurgical ICU patients.[197]

Vecuronium, in relatively large doses of 0.1 to 0.14 mg/kg, had no significant effect on cerebral physiology in patients with brain tumors.[198] Pipecuronium and rocuronium have not been studied but should similarly be without direct effect, and no adverse events have been reported.

The indirect actions of relaxants may also have effects on cerebral physiology. Pancuronium given as a large bolus dose can cause an abrupt increase in arterial pressure. This might elevate ICP in patients with impaired intracranial compliance and defective autoregulation; however, no significant clinical event has ever been reported. Muscle relaxation may reduce ICP because coughing and straining are prevented, and this results in lowering of central venous pressure with a concomitant reduction in cerebral venous outflow impedance.

A metabolite of atracurium, laudanosine, may be epileptogenic. However, although large doses of atracurium caused an EEG arousal pattern in dogs, CBF, CMR, and ICP were unaltered.[199] In rabbits, administration of laudanosine did not increase the severity of the epileptoid activity caused by direct application of a cephalosporin to the cortical surface.[200] It appears highly unlikely that epileptogenesis will occur in humans with atracurium.[201]

In summary, vecuronium, pipecuronium, rocuronium, atracurium, mivacurium, cisatracurium, metocurine, and pancuronium (if acute MAP increases are prevented with the latter) are all reasonable muscle relaxants for use in patients with or at risk for intracranial hypertension. Doses of metocurine, atracurium, and mivacurium should be limited to ranges not associated with hypotension.

Succinylcholine

Succinylcholine can produce modest increases (~5 mm Hg) in ICP in lightly anesthetized humans. This effect appears to be the result of cerebral activation (as evidenced by EEG changes and increases in CBF) caused by afferent activity from the muscle spindle apparatus.[202] Note, however, that there is poor correlation between the occurrence of visible muscle fasciculations and an increase in ICP. As might be expected with what appears to be an arousal phenomenon, deep anesthesia has been observed to prevent succinylcholine-induced increases in ICP in the dog. In humans, the increase in ICP is also blocked by paralysis with vecuronium and by "defasciculation" with metocurine, 0.03 mg/kg.[198] The efficacy of other defasciculating anesthetics has not been examined in humans.

Although succinylcholine *can* produce increases in ICP, it need not be viewed as contraindicated in circumstances in which its use for rapid attainment of paralysis is otherwise seen as appropriate. Kovarik and coauthors observed no change in ICP after the administration of succinylcholine, 1 mg/kg, to 10 nonparalyzed, ventilated neurosurgical ICU patients, 6 of whom had sustained a head injury.[203] Their observations are very relevant because it is in precisely this population of patients that the issue of the use of succinylcholine arises most frequently. Given that the ICP effects of succinylcholine may be an arousal phenomenon caused by increased afferent traffic from muscle spindles,[202] it is not unreasonable that disease processes that substantially blunt the level of consciousness might similarly blunt this response. As with many anesthetics, the concern should be not whether it is used but how it is used. If administered with proper attention to control of carbon dioxide tension, blood pressure, and depth of anesthesia and after defasciculation, little hazard should attend its use.

Other Effects of Anesthetics on Cerebral Physiology

Cerebrospinal Fluid Dynamics

There is approximately 150 mL of CSF in the adult human, half within the cranium and half in the spinal CSF space. CSF, which is formed in the choroid plexuses and to a lesser extent in the brain's interstitium with transependymal diffusion into the ventricular system, is replaced about three to four times per day. It functions both as a cushion for the CNS and as an excretory pathway. Anesthetics have been shown to influence both the rate of formation and the rate of reabsorption of CSF. Table 13-3 provides nonquantitative information about the direction of the influences of common anesthetic drugs. All the information has been derived from animals,[30,204-209] and these processes have not been examined in humans. Of the volatile anesthetics, halothane decreases secretion of CSF, isoflurane has no effect, and enflurane and desflurane increase secretion. Absorption of CSF is reduced by halothane and enflurane, unchanged by desflurane, and increased by isoflurane. Though probably of minimal relevance to clinical practice, a theoretical concern might be in the setting of a prolonged closed-cranium procedure in a patient with poor intracranial compliance. The most deleterious potential combination of effects in a patient with poor intracranial compliance is increased CSF production and decreased reabsorption. In the dog this pattern occurs with enflurane, which is perhaps another reason (in addition to the potential for epileptogenesis in the presence of cerebral injury and hypocapnia) for omission of enflurane in this circumstance.

Blood-Brain Barrier

In the majority of the body's capillary beds, there are fenestrations approximately 65 Å in diameter between endothelial cells. In the brain, with the exception of the choroid plexus, the pituitary, and the area postrema, tight junctions reduce this pore size to approximately 8 Å. As a result, large molecules and most ions are prevented from entering the brain's interstitium. There is little evidence that anesthetics alter the function of this "blood-brain barrier" in most circumstances. However, acute hypertension can breach the barrier, and certain anesthetics facilitate this phenomenon.[210] Forster and colleagues[211] observed that extravasation of Evan blue into rabbit brain was greater when acute hypertension occurred during anesthesia with halothane than with thiopental. It is likely that the effect is a nonspecific result of cerebral vasodilation rather than a specific effect of halothane. These results were obtained in the setting of extreme, abrupt hypertension in animals with an initially normal BBB. To our knowledge, no peer-reviewed investigation has attempted a comparison of anesthetic effects on BBB function during anesthesia in normotensive humans.

Epileptogenesis

An extensive review of the convulsant and anticonvulsant effects of anesthetics and adjuvants is available.[212,213] Several commonly used anesthetics have some epileptogenic potential, particularly in predisposed individuals. A concern is that seizure activity may go unrecognized in an anesthetized and paralyzed patient and result in neuronal injury if substrate demand (CMR) exceeds supply for a prolonged period.[214] A second concern is that the epileptogenic effect will persist in the postanesthesia period when seizures may occur in less well controlled circumstances than exist in the operating room. In practice, it appears that spontaneous seizures during or after anesthesia have been extremely rare events. Nonetheless, in patients with processes that might predispose to seizures, it seems prudent to avoid the use of potentially epileptogenic drugs in situations in which there are reasonable alternatives.

Volatile Anesthetics

Enflurane is potentially epileptogenic in the clinical setting. Of particular relevance to neuroanesthesia is the observation that hypocapnia potentiates seizure-type discharges during enflurane anesthesia.[215] A 50% decrease in $CMRO_2$ was noted in human volunteers anesthetized with 3% enflurane, but with the onset of seizure activity, $CMRO_2$ returned to normal,[216] thus indicating preservation of flow-metabolism coupling. Note that there is no evidence that this type of EEG activity is deleterious when oxygen delivery is maintained during the event. However, because seizure activity can elevate brain metabolism by as much as 400%, the use of enflurane, especially at high doses and with hypocapnia, should probably be avoided in patients predisposed to seizures or with occlusive cerebrovascular disease.

The EEG-activating property of enflurane has been used intraoperatively to activate and identify seizure foci that are to be surgically resected, and in this situation spike activity not present preoperatively has been observed to persist after surgery.[217] There have also been two reports of seizures in the immediate postoperative period after enflurane anesthesia in both predisposed[218] and non-predisposed individuals.[219] No permanent sequelae appeared to occur as a result of these events, and in fact, this association is not a rigorously proven one. At worst, such occurrences are extremely uncommon.

Isoflurane can cause EEG spiking and myoclonus, but in the experimental setting it has not been associated with the frank epileptoid activity induced by enflurane. The clinical experience with isoflurane is very large, and unexplained "seizure-like activity" has been reported in only two patients. One occurrence was intraoperative[220] and the other immediately postoperative.[221] It therefore appears that epileptogenesis is not a clinical concern with isoflurane. In fact, isoflurane has been successfully used to control EEG seizure activity in refractory status epilepticus.[222]

Seizures occur during induction of anesthesia with high concentrations of sevoflurane in children, including those without a recognized seizure diathesis.[223] In two healthy human subjects, EEG burst suppression with 2 MAC sevoflurane was accompanied by epileptiform discharges that were observed during EEG monitoring.[224] These discharges were associated with a significant increase in CBF, thus demonstrating that flow-metabolism coupling was preserved. In patients with temporal lobe epilepsy, administration of 1.5 MAC sevoflurane elicited widespread paroxysmal interictal EEG activity. Of note was the observation that paroxysmal activity was not restricted to the ictal focus and that the administration of sevoflurane was not of any assistance in localization of the epileptogenic region of the brain.[225] The development of tonic-clonic movements indicative of seizure activity has also been reported in otherwise healthy patients on emergence from sevoflurane anesthesia.[226,227] In all of the reported cases of seizure activity attributable to sevoflurane anesthesia, untoward sequelae have not been documented. These reports highlight sevoflurane's ability, albeit small, to evoke epileptiform activity, and accordingly, the use of sevoflurane in patients with epilepsy should be undertaken with appropriate caution.

Methohexital

Myoclonic activity is sometimes observed with methohexital, and this agent has been used to activate seizure foci during cortical mapping.[224,228] In neurosurgical patients to whom larger doses of methohexital were administered to produce burst suppression of the EEG, refractory seizures have occurred.[229] Accordingly, it appears that patients with seizures of temporal lobe origin, typically of the psychomotor variety, or those to whom high doses are administered are at risk for seizure activation by methohexital. However, it should be noted that prolonged seizure activity after single-dose methohexital administration has not been reported in patients who undergo ECT.

Ketamine

Ketamine can elicit seizures in patients with an epileptic diathesis.[230] Depth electrode recordings in epileptic patients have revealed the occurrence of isolated subcortical seizure activity originating in the limbic and thalamic areas during ketamine anesthesia and demonstrated that this subcortical activation may not be reflected in surface EEG recordings.[231] Seizures have also been reported to occur after ketamine anesthesia in neurologically normal subjects on only two occasions,[232,233] and in one of these instances seizure thresholds may have been lowered by aminophylline.

Etomidate

Etomidate frequently produces myoclonus that is not associated with epileptiform activity on the EEG.[234] A single instance of severe, sustained myoclonus immediately after anesthesia with etomidate by infusion has been reported.[235] Etomidate has also been shown to precipitate generalized epileptic EEG activity in epileptic patients,[236] and its use in this population should probably be avoided. However, it has been used electively, in low doses, to activate seizure foci for the purposes of intraoperative EEG localization.[237] In our experience (unpublished), selective activation of a quiescent focus can be achieved with 0.1 mg/kg. Larger doses are more likely to lead to generalized activation.

Etomidate is also associated with longer seizures in response to ECT than occur after methohexital or propofol. Remarkably, etomidate, in the dose range of 0.15 to 0.3 mg/kg, does not cause dose-related seizure inhibition during ECT as is readily demonstrated with the other two drugs.

The preceding information not withstanding, there are no convincing reports to indicate epileptogenesis in normal subjects, and use of etomidate need not be restricted on this basis. In fact, it has been used to control refractory status epilepticus.

Propofol

Seizures and opisthotonos have been reported to occur after propofol anesthesia. However, systematic studies in both humans[238] and animals,[239] though identifying the occurrence of occasional dystonic and choreiform movements, have failed to confirm the notion that propofol is proconvulsant. In fact, propofol appears to be anticonvulsant in mice.[239] Furthermore, ECT seizures were shorter after induction with propofol than after induction with methohexital,[240] which is more consistent with an *anticonvulsant* effect. In addition, propofol sedation has been widely used during "awake" resection of seizure foci and other intracranial lesions. Although pronounced high-amplitude β-frequency activity in the EEG has been observed,[241] there has not been an unexpected incidence of seizures.

Narcotics

Seizures or limbic system hypermetabolism (or both) can be readily elicited in some animal species with narcotics. Although an increase in CBF in deep brain structures associated with pain processing has been observed in human volunteers,[69] humans do not have a clinically apparent correlate of the hypermetabolism effect seen in animals. Several anecdotal accounts, unaccompanied by EEG recordings, have reported the occurrence of grand mal convulsions in patients who received both high and low doses of fentanyl. However, systematic investigations of EEG changes during the administration of relatively large doses of fentanyl, sufentanil, and alfentanil in humans have *not* documented neuroexcitatory activity,[242-244] and the "seizures" may have been an exaggerated rigidity phenomenon. There are exceptions. Tempelhoff and coauthors reported on induction of anesthesia with fentanyl for secondary craniotomy and anterior temporal lobectomy in patients with partial complex seizures. Eight of the nine patients displayed electrical seizure activity at a range of clinically relevant fentanyl doses (mean, 26 μg/kg).[245] Another study found that alfentanil, 50 μg/kg, augmented temporal lobe spike activity in patients with temporal lobe epilepsy.[246] Note that untreated rigidity may itself also have important CNS consequences. ICP elevation can occur during narcotic-induced rigidity, probably as a consequence of cerebral venous congestion.

Atracurium

See discussion regarding the atracurium metabolite laudanosine in the section on nondepolarizing muscle relaxants.

Neonatal Anesthetic Neurotoxicity

This subject is covered in detail in Chapter 82.

Cerebral Physiology in Pathologic States

Cerebral Ischemia—Pathophysiology

Critical Cerebral Blood Flow Thresholds

The brain has a high rate of energy utilization and very limited energy storage capacity. It is therefore extremely vulnerable in the event of interruption of substrate (oxygen, glucose) supply. Under normal circumstances, global CBF is maintained at approximately 50 mL/100 g/min. In the face of a declining CBF and therefore oxygen supply, neuronal function deteriorates progressively rather than in an all-or-none fashion (Fig. 13-14). There is a substantial reserve below normal CBF levels, and it is not until CBF has fallen to approximately 20 mL/100 g/min that EEG evidence of ischemia begins to appear. At a CBF level of approximately 15 mL/100 g/min, the cortical EEG is isoelectric. However, only when CBF is reduced to about 6 mL/100 g/min are indications of potentially irreversible membrane failure (elevated extracellular potassium[247] and loss of the direct cortical response) rapidly evident. As CBF decreases in the flow range between 15 and 10 mL/100 g/min, a progressive deterioration in energy supply occurs and eventually leads, with a time course that may last hours rather than minutes, to membrane failure and neuronal death. The brain regions falling within this CBF range (6 to 15 mL/100 g/min) encompass brain tissue in which neuronal dysfunction is temporarily reversible but within which neuronal death will occur if flow is not restored; such regions are referred to as the ischemic penumbra.[247,251] Studies defining progression to cerebral infarction within the penumbra have been performed principally in the cerebral cortex of primates, and the actual CBF levels at which the various decrements in function occur may vary with both anesthetic[250] and species. However, in humans anesthetized with halothane and

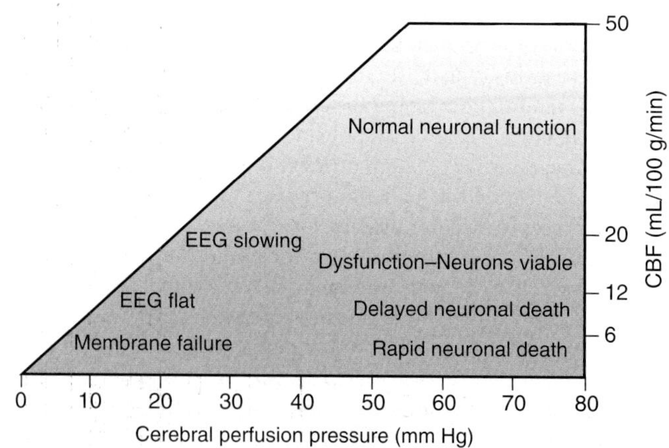

Figure 13-14 Relationships between cerebral perfusion, cerebral blood flow (CBF), the electroencephalogram (EEG), and the functional status/viability of neurons. Note that in the approximate CBF range of 6 to 12 mL/kg/min, the energy supply is insufficient to support electrophysiologic activity (i.e., EEG flat) but can prevent complete membrane failure and neuronal death for extended periods (see Fig. 13-15). These areas are referred to as the ischemic penumbra.[247] The data are derived from studies on the cerebral cortex of barbiturate-anesthetized baboons[247,248] and unanesthetized monkeys.[249] The CBF and mean arterial pressure thresholds may vary with anesthetic and species.[250]

N_2O, the CBF threshold for the initial EEG change[252] is similar to that observed in the animal investigations.

Models of Cerebral Ischemia

Much has been made of the difference between complete cerebral ischemia, as occurs during cardiac arrest, and incomplete cerebral ischemia, as may occur during occlusion of a major cerebral vessel or severe hypotension. However, from the clinician's vantage, the important difference is that the residual blood flow during incomplete ischemia may result in enough delivery of oxygen to allow some generation of ATP and thereby stave off the catastrophic irreversible membrane failure that occurs within minutes during normothermic complete cerebral ischemia. This difference in the rate of failure of the energy supply[253,254] (Fig. 13-15) can result in much greater apparent tolerance for focal or incomplete ischemia than for complete global ischemia (e.g., cardiac arrest).

Energy Failure and Excitotoxicity

Energy failure is the central event that occurs during cerebral ischemia.[255] ATP is required for maintenance of the normal membrane ionic gradient, and energy failure is rapidly attended by membrane depolarization and influx of sodium and calcium into the neuron. Voltage-dependent calcium channels are then activated and calcium gains entry into the cytosol. Depolarization of presynaptic terminals also results in the release of massive quantities of excitatory neurotransmitters, particularly glutamate, into the synaptic cleft. Activation of glutamatergic receptors, the NMDA and α-amino-3-hydroxy-5-methyl-4-isoxazopropionic acid (AMPA) receptors, adds to the influx of Na^+ and Ca^{2+} (Fig. 13-16). Initiation of cellular signaling by activation of metabotropic receptors leads to the release of stored Ca^{2+} from the endoplasmic reticulum via inositol 1,4,5-triphosphate (IP_3) receptors. Ionic influx is accompanied by influx of water, and neuronal swelling occurs rapidly after membrane depolarization. The injury that is initiated by excessive glutamate receptor activity is referred to as excitotoxicity.

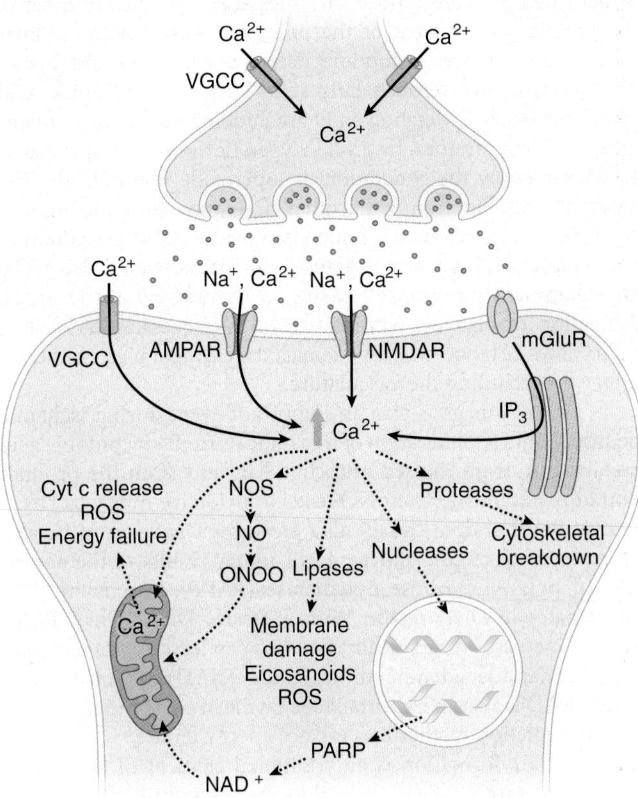

Figure 13-16 During ischemia, depletion of adenosine triphosphate leads to neuronal depolarization and the subsequent release of supranormal quantities of neurotransmitters, especially glutamate. Excessive stimulation of ligand-gated channels and the simultaneous opening of voltage-dependent Ca^{2+} channels permit rapid entry of Ca^{2+} into neurons. Stimulation of metabotropic glutamate receptors generates inositol 1,4,5-triphosphate (IP_3), which causes release of Ca^{2+} from the endoplasmic reticulum (ER)/mitochondria. Activation of the α-amino-3-hydroxy-5-methyl-4-isoxazopropionic acid receptor (AMPAR)-gated subset of glutamate receptors also permits excessive entry of sodium (Na^+). Excessive free Ca^{2+} results in activation of numerous enzymes: protease activation causes breakdown of the cytoskeleton of the neuron; lipases damage plasma membrane lipids and release arachidonic acid, which is metabolized by cyclooxygenases and lipooxygenases to yield free radicals and other mediators of cell injury; activation of nitric oxide synthase (NOS) leads to release of nitric oxide (NO) and, in turn, the generation of peroxynitrite (ONOO), a highly reactive free radical; and activated endonucleases damage DNA, thereby rendering the neuron susceptible to apoptosis. Injury to mitochondria leads to energy failure, generation of free radicals, and release of cytochrome *c* (Cyt c) from the mitochondria; the latter is one of the means by which neuronal apoptosis is initiated. mGluR, metabotropic glutamate receptor; NAD^+, oxidized form of nicotinamide adenine dinucleotide; NMDAR, *N*-methyl-D-aspartate receptor; PARP, poly-ADP-ribose polymerase; ROS, reactive oxygen species; VGCC, voltage-gated calcium channels.

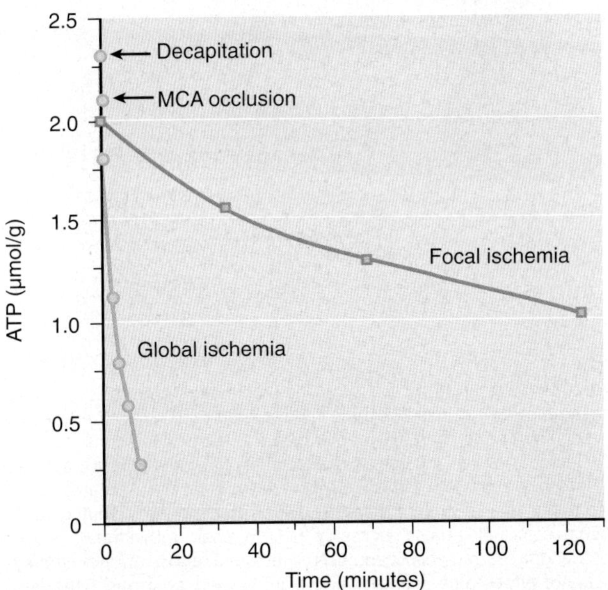

Figure 13-15 Comparison of rates of failure of energy supply (adenosine triphosphate) in complete global ischemia (produced by decapitation in dogs[254]) and in incomplete focal ischemia (middle cerebral artery [MCA] occlusion in monkeys[253]). In the presence of residual CBF, energy supply failure is substantially delayed.

Calcium is a ubiquitous second messenger in cells, and it is a cofactor required for the activation of a number of enzyme systems. The rapid, uncontrolled increase in cytosolic Ca^{2+} levels initiates the activation of a number of cellular processes that contribute to injury. Cytoskeletal proteins such as actin are cleaved by activated proteases. These enzymes also degrade a number of the protein constituents of the neuron. Lipases attack cellular lipids and produce membrane damage. An important lipase, phospholipase A_2, releases fatty acids such as arachidonic acid from membranes. Metabolism of arachidonic acid to prostaglandins and leukotrienes by cyclooxygenase and lipoxygenase is accompanied by the generation of superoxide free radicals. The latter, in combination with other free radicals generated in response to mitochondrial injury, can lead to lipid peroxidation and membrane injury. Prostaglandins and leukotrienes also evoke an inflammatory response and are powerful chemotactic drugs. Activation of platelets within cerebral microvessels, as well as influx of white blood cells into damaged areas, aggravates ischemic injury by occluding the vasculature.

DNA damage is also an important event during ischemic neuronal injury. Generation of free radicals from arachidonic acid metabolism, from injured mitochondria, and from the production of peroxynitrite from NO leads to oxidative injury to DNA. Activation of endonucleases also produces DNA strand breaks. Under normal circumstances, DNA injury results in the activation of poly-ADP-ribose polymerase (PARP), an enzyme that participates in DNA repair. With excessive DNA injury, PARP activity increases dramatically, and this can lead to the depletion of nicotinamide adenine dinucleotide (NAD), a substrate of PARP. NAD is also an important coenzyme in energy metabolism, and its depletion further exacerbates energy failure.

Lactate formation is an additional element of the pathophysiologic process. Lactic acid is formed as a result of the anaerobic glycolysis that takes place after failure of the supply of oxygen. The associated decline in pH contributes to deterioration of the intracellular environment. An increased preischemic serum glucose level may accelerate this process by providing additional substrate for anaerobic glycolysis.

NO, which has emerged as a probable mediator of CBF changes in many normal physiologic states (see the preceding sections), is also of relevance to the pathophysiology of ischemia. NO is, in fact, a weak free radical that in turn leads to the generation of a more reactive species (peroxynitrite), and it is a "killer substance" used by macrophages. In cerebral ischemia, NO is probably both friend and foe. It is likely that during a period of focal ischemia, the vasodilating effect of NO (probably constitutively elaborated NO of endothelial origin) serves to augment collateral CBF. However, in the postischemic phase, NO (probably derived from neurons or macrophages) contributes to neuronal injury.

Collectively, the simultaneous and unregulated activation of a number of cellular pathways overwhelms the reparative and restorative processes within the neuron and ultimately leads to neuronal death.

Nature of Neuronal Death

Neuronal death that occurs in response to these processes has been categorized as necrotic or apoptotic in nature (see Chapter 98). Necrotic death of neurons, mediated by excitotoxic injury, is characterized by rapid cellular swelling, condensation and pyknosis of the nucleus, and swelling of the mitochondria and endoplasmic reticulum. A characteristic of these necrotic neurons is the presence of acidophilic cytoplasm.[256] Necrotic neuronal death results in local infiltration of the brain by inflammatory cells. A consequence of this inflammation is a considerable amount of collateral damage.

Neuronal apoptosis, a form of cellular suicide, has also been demonstrated in a variety of models of cerebral ischemia. Apoptosis is characterized by chromatin condensation, involution of the cell membrane, swelling of mitochondria, and cellular shrinkage. In the later stages of apoptosis, neurons fragment into several apoptotic bodies, which are then cleared from the brain.[256] The lack of a substantial inflammatory response to apoptotic death limits injury to surrounding neurons that have survived the initial ischemic insult.

A number of biochemical pathways that lead to apoptosis have been described. Initiation of apoptosis by the release of cytochrome *c* from injured mitochondria has been studied the most (Fig. 13-17). Cytochrome *c* is restricted from the cytoplasm by the outer mitochondrial membrane.[257] When mitochondria are injured, pores within the outer membrane allow cytochrome *c* to be released into the cytoplasm, where it interacts with procaspase-9 and apoptosis-activating factor (APAF) to produce an apoptosome. Procaspase-9 undergoes activation by proteolytic cleavage. Activated caspase-9 then activates caspase-3. The latter serves as an executor of apoptosis by cleaving a number of protein substrates that are essential in DNA repair (such as PARP). Activation of caspase-3 can also occur by inflammatory signaling via tumor necrosis factor-α (TNF-α) and activation of caspase-8.[258] It should be noted that the neuronal injury that occurs in response to ischemia cannot easily be divided into necrosis or apoptosis. The

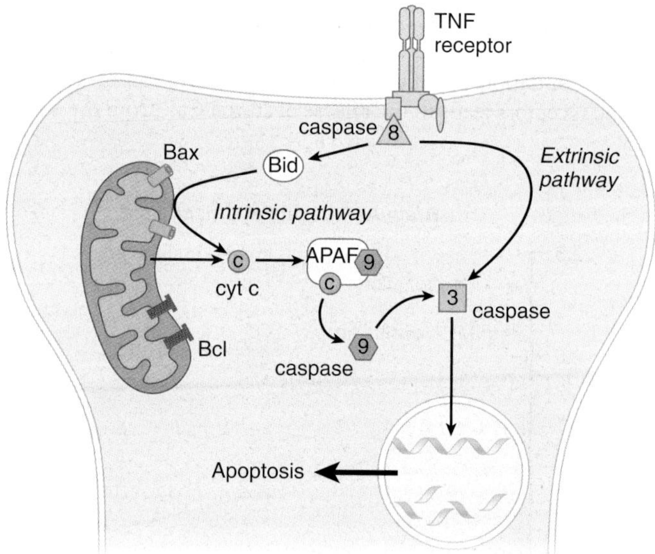

Figure 13-17 Cellular processes that lead to neuronal apoptosis. Cytochrome *c* (cyt c), which is normally restricted to the space between the inner and outer mitochondrial membranes, is released in response to mitochondrial injury. Cytochrome *c*, in combination with apoptosis-activating factor (APAF), activates caspase-9 by proteolytic cleavage. Activated caspase-9 then leads to activation of caspase-3. This enzyme cleaves a number of substrates, including those necessary for DNA repair. Within the mitochondria, Bax augments and Bcl prevents the release of cytochrome *c*. Release of cytochrome *c* can also be initiated by Bid, a substance that is activated by caspase-8 via tumor necrosis factor (TNF) signaling. In addition, caspase-8 can directly activate caspase-3. Excessive activation of poly-ADP-ribose polymerase (PARP), an enzyme integral to DNA repair, depletes cellular stores of oxidized nicotinamide adenine dinucleotide (NAD^+). Depletion of NAD^+ further exacerbates the energy failure because of its critical role in energy metabolism.

nature of neuronal death probably encompasses a spectrum in which some neurons undergo necrosis or apoptosis whereas others undergo cell death that has features of both necrosis and apoptosis.

Timing of Neuronal Death

The traditional concept of ischemic injury was that neuronal death was restricted to the time of ischemia and during the early reperfusion period. However, more recent data indicate that postischemic neuronal injury is a dynamic process in which neurons continue to die for a long period after the initiating ischemic insult (Fig. 13-18).[259] This delayed neuronal death, which was first demonstrated in models of global cerebral ischemia, has been demonstrated during focal ischemia as well. The extent of delayed neuronal death depends on the severity of the ischemic insult. With severe ischemia, most neurons undergo rapid death. With more moderate insults, neurons that survive the initial insult undergo delayed death. This ongoing neuronal loss contributes to the gradual expansion of cerebral infarction after focal ischemia. In experimental studies, evidence of cerebral inflammation, which can theoretically contribute to further injury, has been demonstrated even 6 to 8 months after the primary ischemia.

The occurrence of delayed neuronal death has important implications for the evaluation of studies in which neuroprotective strategies are being investigated. A wide variety of interventions have shown neuroprotective efficacy in studies in which the extent of injury is evaluated within 3 to 4 days after ischemia. However, this neuroprotective efficacy may not be sustained. Recent data indicate that cerebral infarction undergoes gradual expansion and that a reduction in injury attributed to a particular therapeutic intervention is no longer apparent when the injury is evaluated after a long postischemic recovery period.[259] Long-term (>1 month) evaluation of the efficacy of a particular intervention is therefore important.

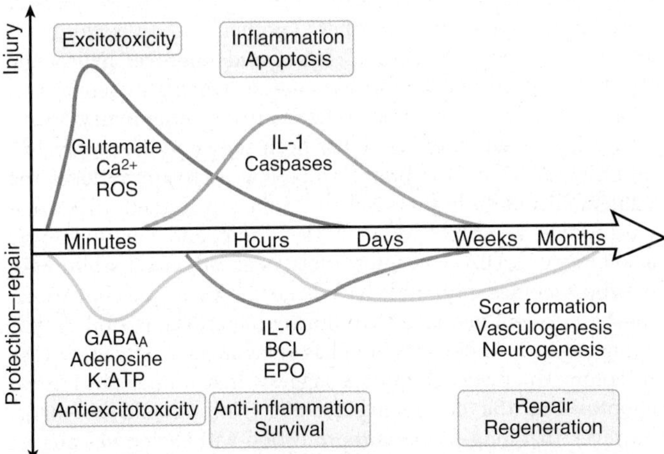

Figure 13-18 Time course of neuronal death. Excitotoxic (glutamate-mediated) injury results in neuronal death within the first few hours after the onset of ischemia. Brain tissue injury elicits an inflammatory response, an important process in removal of injured tissue and in healing, that leads to a substantial amount of collateral damage. Inflammation-mediated neuronal death can continue for several days. Neuronal apoptosis can occur in injured neurons that survived the initial insult. Apoptotic neuronal death has been demonstrated to occur for many days after the initiating ischemic insult. It is now apparent that ischemic neuronal death is a dynamic process in which neurons continue to die for a long period. *(Adapted from Dirnagl U, Iadecola C, Moskowitz M: Pathobiology of ischaemic stroke: An integrated view. Trends Neurosci 22:391-397, 1999.)*

Brain Protection

The literature on cerebral ischemia and brain protection is vast, and a detailed discourse on this topic is beyond the scope of the present discussion. A number of excellent recent reviews on the subject are available.[256,260-262]

Considerations Relevant to Complete Global Ischemia (Cardiac Arrest)

Maintenance of adequate perfusion pressure after cardiac arrest is of considerable importance. Hypotension developing after resuscitation from cardiac arrest may aggravate the microcirculatory and vasospastic processes occurring at this time and increase brain damage. A late phase of intracranial hypertension may occur and is due to the development of extensive cerebral edema, probably both vasogenic and cytotoxic in etiology, associated with brain necrosis. Attempts to control this type of intracranial hypertension with osmotherapy usually fail. ICP monitoring is not generally used because the patients in whom these delayed increases in ICP develop have sustained massive tissue damage.

Both barbiturates and calcium channel blockers have been administered after cardiac arrest. The former are ineffective.[263] In a small cohort (51 patients) of cardiac arrest victims, nimodipine was shown to improve CBF but not neurologic outcome.[264] In a second trial in approximately 150 cardiac arrest victims, no overall benefit in neurologic outcome was observed.[265] However, a subset of patients in whom initiation of advanced life support was delayed for more than 10 minutes demonstrated improved survival. This single study cannot serve as justification for the administration of nimodipine after cardiac arrest, especially in the face of the unequivocally negative results of the multicenter lidoflazine cardiac arrest study.[266] Once again, the important therapeutic objectives are maintenance of normocapnia and normotension, normalization of systemic pH, avoidance of hyperthermia, and prevention and treatment of seizures.

Induced mild hypothermia is effective in reducing mortality and morbidity in patients who sustain a cardiac arrest.[267] Induction of mild hypothermia in the range of 32°C to 34°C for a period of about 24 hours improved neurologic outcome and survival 6 months after cardiac arrest in comparison to a normothermic group. Mild hypothermia was induced without difficulty. Passive rewarming of patients was accomplished slowly over a period of 8 hours. The incidence of complications was similar to that in the control normothermic group. This important study is one of the first to demonstrate the feasibility and efficacy of induced hypothermia as a treatment to prevent injury from global ischemia. Undoubtedly, induced hypothermia will now be added to the armamentarium for the treatment of cerebral complications of cardiac arrest.

Considerations Relevant to Focal (Incomplete) Ischemia

Before discussing individual anesthetics, it should be noted that a general theme that can be extracted from the protection-by-anesthetics literature, in particular for anesthesia with volatile anesthetics, is that anesthesia per se is protective. It appears that for undefined reasons, reducing the level of systemic stress associated with a standardized experimental insult results in an improved outcome.[268,269] In reviewing the protection-by-anesthetics literature, readers should be conscious of the possibility that the protective benefit ascribed to an intervention with an anesthetic drug may in fact be the product of exaggeration of the injury in a high-stress control state, such as N_2O "sedation."

BARBITURATES. There have been numerous demonstrations of the protective efficacy of barbiturates in focal cerebral ischemia in animals[270-272] and a single demonstration of effectiveness in a human.[273] The effect has been attributed principally to suppression of CMR. However, the effects of CBF redistribution and free radical scavenging[274] have been suggested to contribute, and there is evidence that CMR suppression is not the sole mechanism.[275] Suppression of CMR might logically be expected to be of benefit to brain regions in which oxygen delivery is inadequate to meet normal demands but is sufficient to allow energy consumption by some on-going electrophysiologic activity (i.e., in which the EEG was abnormal but not flat). Such regions are likely to be limited in size in the setting of focal ischemia, yet several of the animal investigations suggest a very substantial protective effect.[270,271] Review of these experiments reveals that the methods used to monitor and maintain temperature, though accepted at the time, were below the standards that have evolved from more recent understanding of the effects of both deliberate[276,277] and inadvertent hypothermia. Unrecognized cerebral hypothermia may well have been a factor in some of the cited investigations, and it is therefore possible that the protective efficacy of barbiturates may have been overestimated. Although more recent publications involving suitable temperature control methods do in fact indicate a protective effect by barbiturates,[275,278,279] the magnitude of that effect was modest when compared with the results of earlier studies. Barbiturate-induced EEG suppression in an already anesthetized patient may still be logical therapy when it can be applied before or early in the course of a period of temporary focal ischemia (e.g., temporary occlusion during aneurysm surgery). However, the decision to institute such therapy should be made only after consideration of the risk of the occlusive event, the patient's cardiovascular status, and the physician's willingness to accept the possible prolongation of arousal, together with an objective view of the probable magnitude of the protective effect.

Numerous investigations in animals and humans have failed to demonstrate any protective effect of barbiturates in the setting of global cerebral ischemia (e.g., cardiac arrest).[263]

Because CMR suppression has been the presumed mechanism of effect, barbiturates have traditionally been administered to produce maximal reduction of CMR (which is nearly complete when EEG burst suppression has been achieved). However, data presented by Warner and colleagues[275] demonstrated that the same protective benefit (expressed as reduction of infarct volume) could be achieved with a third of the burst-suppression dose. This raises a clinically important issue. The various barbiturates (thiopental, thiamylal, methohexital, pentobarbital) have similar effects on CMR and have generally been assumed to have equal protective efficacy. However, if the mechanism of protection is a pharmacologic effect other than reduction in CMR, is it reasonable to assume equivalence among the barbiturates? Recent data suggest that the neuroprotective efficacy of barbiturates is not similar. In a direct comparison of three clinically used barbiturates, methohexital and thiopental, but not pentobarbital, reduced injury in an animal model of focal ischemia.[280] These data suggest that mechanisms other than or at least in addition to metabolic suppression may contribute to the protective effect of barbiturates.

VOLATILE ANESTHETICS. Isoflurane is also a potent suppressant of CMR in the cerebral cortex, and EEG evidence suggestive of a protective effect in humans has been reported.[250] In comparison to the awake or N_2O-fentanyl–anesthetized state, isoflurane is neuroprotective in models of hemispheric,[281] focal,[282] and nearly complete ischemia.[283,284] Of interest is the recent observation that isoflurane's neuroprotective efficacy is not sustained.[285] When injury is evaluated 2 days after ischemia, a robust reduction in injury is observed with isoflurane anesthesia. However, by 14 days this reduction in injury was not apparent. These data indicate that neuronal injury continues well into the postischemic recovery period and that the neuroprotection that is evident shortly after ischemia may not persist for the long term. More recent data have shown that long-term neuroprotection with isoflurane is achievable under conditions in which the severity of ischemia is limited and restoration of blood flow after ischemia is complete.[286] The neuroprotective effect of isoflurane is not substantially different from that of other volatile anesthetics. Sevoflurane reduces ischemic injury in animal models of focal[287] and hemispheric ischemia[288]; its efficacy is not different from that of halothane. Desflurane also reduces neuronal injury to the same extent that isoflurane does.[289] The available data therefore suggest that adequate anesthesia per se may have a protective effect[268,269] versus the awake state, but there does not appear to be any difference in neuroprotective efficacy among the volatile anesthetics.

XENON. The inert gas xenon exerts its anesthetic action by noncompetitive blockade of NMDA receptors. As such, it is logical to suspect that it might provide neuroprotection against excitotoxic injury. The neuroprotective efficacy of xenon has been demonstrated against oxygen-glucose deprivation in vitro,[290] focal ischemia in vivo in mice,[291] and cardiopulmonary bypass–induced cognitive dysfunction in rats.[292] Of interest are observations that simultaneous administration of *subanesthetic* doses of xenon in combination with either hypothermia[293] or isoflurane[294] significantly reduces neuronal injury and improves neurologic function in a neonatal rodent model of hypoxia-ischemia; this protective effect was apparent as late as 30 days after injury. Moreover, administration of xenon has been shown to have a preconditioning effect on the brain[295]; previous exposure reduces the vulnerability of the brain to ischemic injury. Anesthetic drugs that have activity at NMDA receptors (ketamine) and γ-aminobutyric acid type A ($GABA_A$) receptors (volatile anesthetics, barbiturates, benzodiazepines, propofol) have been shown to cause neuronal injury in rodent neonatal pups during the critical period of synaptogenesis.[296] Although xenon has antagonist activity at NMDA receptors, the evidence to date suggests that it does not lead to apoptosis in the developing brain.[297] Note should be made, however, that long-term neuroprotection with xenon has not yet been demonstrated in adult experimental subjects. The specific use of xenon for the purpose of neuroprotection awaits results from outcome studies in humans.

PROPOFOL. EEG suppression can also be achieved with clinically feasible doses of propofol. Anecdotal information suggests that it is being used to provide "protection" during both aneurysm surgery[298] and carotid endarterectomy. In experimental models of cerebral ischemia, the extent of neurologic injury in propofol-anesthetized animals was similar to that in halothane-anesthetized animals.[299] Given the previous demonstration that halothane can reduce injury, these data provide indirect evidence of propofol's neuroprotective efficacy. In a more recent investigation, cerebral infarction was significantly reduced in propofol-anesthetized animals in comparison to awake animals.[300] Direct comparison of propofol to pentobarbital has also demonstrated that cerebral injury after focal ischemia is similar in animals anesthetized with the two drugs.[301] Similar to the situation with volatile anesthetics, initial investigations revealed that propofol protection is not sustained.[302] Durable protection with propofol is achievable if the severity of the ischemic insult is mild.[303] Collectively, these data are consistent with the premise that propofol can reduce ischemic cerebral injury.

Etomidate. Etomidate was proposed as a potential protective anesthetic in the setting of aneurysm surgery.[304] It too produces CMR suppression to an extent equivalent to barbiturates, and like the barbiturates, etomidate is an agonist at the (inhibitory) $GABA_A$ receptor. To the contrary, in an experimental model of focal ischemia, the volume of injury was not reduced by etomidate relative to a 1.2 MAC halothane-anesthetized control group. In fact, the volume of injury with etomidate was significantly larger than that in the control group. In patients subjected to temporary intracranial vessel occlusion, administration of etomidate results in greater tissue hypoxia and acidosis than equivalent desflurane anesthesia does. The aggravation of injury produced by etomidate (an imidazole) may be related to direct binding of NO as a consequence of etomidate-induced hemolysis[305] combined with direct inhibition of the NO synthase enzyme by etomidate. Therefore, there is no scientific support for the current use of etomidate for "cerebral protection."

Calcium Channel Blockers. It is now established clinical practice to administer nimodipine orally (the intravenous preparation is not approved for clinical use in North America) for 21 days beginning as soon as possible after subarachnoid hemorrhage.[306] However, it has not yet become standard practice to administer nimodipine or any other calcium channel blocker routinely after neurologic stroke occurring in the operating room or in any other environment. Despite favorable results in small trials, not all investigations in stroke victims have confirmed the benefits of nimodipine.[307]

Other Anesthetics. A remarkable number of anesthetics have shown neuroprotective efficacy in animal studies. However, to date, large-scale randomized trials of a variety of anesthetics in patients with stroke have not demonstrated neuroprotection for any drug. With the exception of tissue plasminogen activator (tPA) for thrombolysis and the calcium channel blockers nimodipine and nicardipine for the management of subarachnoid hemorrhage, pharmacologic neuroprotective anesthetics are not available for the treatment of patients with cerebral ischemia. Details about drugs that have undergone clinical trials and those that are currently being investigated in humans can be found at the Stroke Trials Registry (www.strokecenter.org/trials/TrialDetail.aspx?tid=338) of Washington University, St. Louis, MO.

Cerebral Ischemia: Influence of Physiologic Variables

Cerebral Perfusion Pressure. Measures designed to augment CBF (an important determinant of energy supply) are also important. In the "ischemic penumbra" (described earlier), small improvements in CBF have the potential to prolong neuronal survival substantially. Maintenance of high-normal CPP can augment collateral perfusion pressure and maintain CBF[308] and has been shown to result in improvement in various neurophysiologic parameters, including neurologic function.[309,310] By contrast, hypotension can reduce CBF and exacerbate injury. In trials of nimodipine in patients with acute stroke, a reduction in blood pressure of 10% to 20% increased the probability of an adverse outcome (either death or dependency) fourfold,[311] thus emphasizing the adverse impact of blood pressure reduction on an injured brain. Therefore, in patients with cerebral ischemia, hypotension should be treated promptly and normotension restored. Although it is quite obvious that the target MAP should be based on knowledge of a patient's preexisting blood pressure, there are insufficient data in humans to provide specific guidelines. In the majority of patients, maintenance of MAP in the 70- to 80-mm Hg range should be adequate. The available data provide support for reducing blood pressure to less than 180/105 mm Hg in patients with stroke who have been treated with tPA in the hope of reducing the incidence of hemorrhage into the ischemic brain.[312] In addition, blood pressure augmentation to a systolic pressure of 180 to 220 mm Hg in patients with subarachnoid hemorrhage–induced vasospasm and to a CPP of greater than 60 mm Hg in patients with traumatic brain injury is reasonable.[312] Note, however, that augmentation of CPP in the high-normal range carries the inadequately explored risks of increased edema and hemorrhagic infarction if used as support during more than brief periods of ischemia, particularly when several hours has elapsed since the onset of ischemia.

Carbon Dioxide Tension. Hypercapnia has the potential to cause intracerebral steal and may worsen intracellular pH. Despite some support for the occurrence of a favorable so-called Robin Hood or inverse steal,[313] hypocapnia has not generally proved effective in either laboratory or clinical settings.[314-316] Pending further information and in the absence of a means of verifying the perfusion response to manipulation of $Pa{CO_2}$, normocapnia remains standard practice.

Temperature. Hypothermia is firmly and justifiably established as the principal cerebral protective technique for circulatory arrest procedures (see Chapter 48). It unequivocally enhances cerebral tolerance for episodes of ischemia. For deep hypothermia, this effect has been presumed to be largely a function of the reduction in CMR. Although pharmacologic drugs such as barbiturates reduce only the component of CMR associated with electrophysiologic "work" (about 60% of $CMRO_2$ in the awake state), hypothermia causes a reduction in both electrophysiologic energy consumption and the energy utilization related to maintenance of cellular integrity, and mild hypothermia may preferentially suppress the latter.[317,318] Recently, there has been a surge of interest in *mild* hypothermia as a cerebral protective technique. A substantial number of laboratory studies have demonstrated that mild degrees of hypothermia (2°C to 4°C) during an episode of ischemia can confer substantial protection as measured histologically.[276,277] In addition, there is also evidence from animal studies that hypothermia initiated in the immediate postischemic period confers a protective benefit.[319,320]

In light of this dramatic protective effect of mild hypothermia, its use in the operating room setting has been advocated. Proponents of its use argue that hypothermia is readily achieved and not accompanied by significant myocardial depression or arrhythmias. In addition, the patient can easily be rewarmed in the operating room after the risk of ischemia has subsided. Results of a pilot study clearly demonstrated a trend toward improved neurologic outcome in hypothermic patients undergoing intracranial aneurysm clipping.[321] Unfortunately, the subsequent definitive trial did not demonstrate any improvement in outcome that could be attributable to hypothermia.[322] However, it should be noted that the majority of the patients in that study had subarachnoid hemorrhage of grades I, II, and III. In addition, the number of patients who had temporary clips applied in excess of 20 minutes was quite small (five to six patients). Consequently, an argument has been made that mild hypothermia may well be of benefit in patients with high-grade aneurysms or in those in whom the complexity of the aneurysm clipping is such that prolonged temporary clipping may be required. Given that temperature reduction takes some time, the decision to induce hypothermia must be made in advance. Therefore, the therapeutic use of hypothermia may be considered in such "high-risk" patients.

The application of mild hypothermia after head injury reduced ICP[323] and improved neurologic outcome[324] in pilot trials. Of note is the finding that complications attributable to hypothermia were not observed. A subsequent multicenter trial of hypothermia in head-injured patients, however, failed to confirm the findings of the pilot studies.[325] Induction of mild hypothermia did not improve long-term neurologic outcome. Note should be made, however, of the post hoc finding that outcome in patients younger than 45 years who were initially hypothermic was worse if these patients were rewarmed; these data suggest that such patients should be rewarmed over a prolonged period.

A number of clinical trials of induced hypothermia in a limited number of stroke patients have been conducted. To date, these trials have demonstrated the feasibility of inducing hypothermia in the range of 33°C to 35°C, even in patients who are not subjected to endotracheal intubation and mechanical ventilation.[326] Hypothermia was associated with improved ICP and CPP. However, complications, particularly thrombocytopenia, bradycardia, ventricular ectopy, hypotension, and infection, are frequent. In addition, an intractable increase in ICP can occur during rewarming, even if the elevation in temperature is gradual and accomplished over a period of several hours. These side effects attest to the need to conduct proper randomized trials to properly evaluate the efficacy of mild hypothermia in stroke patients. Such trials are currently under way.

Data regarding the application of mild hypothermia in survivors of cardiac arrest are more positive. Two recent trials have demonstrated that induction of hypothermia (32°C to 34°C) after successful resuscitation from cardiac arrest resulted in a significantly better neurologic outcome 6 months after the arrest.[267,327] These studies demonstrate the clinical efficacy of hypothermia for purposes of reducing ischemic cerebral injury and provide support for the use of intraoperative hypothermia in patients who are considered to be at high risk.

By contrast, increases in brain temperature during and after ischemia aggravate injury.[328] An increase of as little as 1°C can dramatically increase injury. Ischemia that normally results in scattered neuronal necrosis produces cerebral infarction when body temperature is elevated. It therefore seems prudent to avoid hyperthermia in patients who have suffered an ischemic insult or in those who are risk for cerebral ischemia. In the operating room, hyperthermia is seldom a problem (witness our efforts to prevent hypothermia). One situation in which body temperature is often allowed to increase is during rewarming after hypothermic cardiopulmonary bypass. In that situation, hyperthermia (core body temperature in excess of 38°C) is not uncommon. The suggestion that increases in temperature in excess of 37°C to 38°C are detrimental has some merit given the recent information regarding the deleterious effect of hyperthermia.

Glucose. Withholding of glucose-containing solutions in situations in which cerebral ischemia may occur is now an established practice. The practice is based on numerous demonstrations in animal models of brain and spinal cord ischemia that elevation of plasma glucose before episodes of either complete or incomplete ischemia results in aggravation of neurologic injury. However, it should be noted that the majority of investigations have involved adult animals and that there is less certainty about the adverse effects of hyperglycemia in immature subjects, such as neonates.[329] Furthermore, it should be noted that only some[330,331] and not all[332] of the investigations in humans have provided confirmation of an independent effect of serum glucose on neurologic outcome. Nonetheless, in long-term outcome studies, hyperglycemia (diabetic and nondiabetic) has been shown to be an independent predictor of poor outcome.[331] In the National Institutes of Health–sponsored recombinant tPA stroke trial, hyperglycemia was associated with significantly lower odds for desirable clinical outcomes and a higher incidence of intracranial hemorrhage.[333] These data prompted a randomized clinical trial of the efficacy of insulin administration to patients with acute stroke. Although the trial was underpowered, the results showed that administration of insulin to control blood glucose levels in stroke patients did not improve outcome 3 months after stroke.[334] A recurrent theme in the discussion of these studies is that glucose elevation may be the *result* of the stress associated with a severe insult, either ischemic or traumatic, rather than its *cause*. In addition, the inevitable questions of whether and how quickly immediate prerisk treatment of an elevated plasma glucose level with insulin reduces risk to normoglycemic levels have not been examined thoroughly. It is our opinion that at this juncture, acute insulin administration (with its attendant risk of hypoglycemia) in patients with modest glucose elevation (~150 mg/dL) in the operating room setting is not yet justified.

By contrast, hypoglycemia is also associated with cerebral injury. With a gradual reduction in blood glucose values of about 40 mg/dL, a shift in EEG frequencies from α and β toward δ and θ occurs.[335] Below a blood glucose level of 20 mg/dL, suppression of the EEG (flat) is observed. Persistence of this level of hypoglycemia results in seizure activity and neuronal injury, particularly to the hippocampus.

Seizures, pH. Normalization of systemic pH, prevention and treatment of seizures, which dramatically increase CMR, and control of ICP and CPP are all, though mundane and lacking in appeal of the pharmacologic silver bullet, important elements of brain protection and resuscitation.

Volume/Hematocrit Manipulation. Although hemodilution has not proved effective in studies of human stroke, both laboratory and human data support the practice, and it is an established part of management of the ischemia associated with vasospasm. However, the data do not currently justify routine hemodilution (a hematocrit of 30% to 35% is the theoretical optimum) in patients in whom focal ischemia *might* occur in the operating room.[336] On the other hand, the potentially deleterious effects of hemoconcentration should help further suppress the out-of-date notion that neurosurgical patients should be "run dry." An elevated hematocrit, because of viscosity effects, reduces CBF.[7] It is our unsubstantiated opinion that in anticipation of a procedure wherein incomplete ischemia might occur, such as carotid endarterectomy, a hematocrit in excess of 55% should be lowered by preoperative phlebotomy.

Summary of Anesthetics and Neuroprotection

In comparison to the awake or lightly sedated state, the vulnerability of the brain to ischemic injury is reduced under anesthesia. Volatile anesthetics, barbiturates, propofol, xenon, and ketamine have all been shown to reduce injury in experimental models, and there is support for the premise that administration of any of these anesthetics reduces injury in comparison to a pure nitrous oxide–narcotic anesthetic. However, direct comparison has not demonstrated the superiority of any one agent (or combination) over another. Therefore, based on the available data, use of a specific anesthetic or anesthetic regimen for the purpose of brain protection in the clinical setting cannot be advocated. A possible exception is barbiturate administration. In the setting of cardiac surgery under cardiopulmonary bypass, administration of barbiturates has been shown to reduce cerebral injury in humans.[273] The cardiovascular depression and hemodynamic instability attendant on the use of barbiturates have significantly restricted their use clinically. Of considerable importance is the observation that the neuroprotective efficacy of anesthetic drugs is achieved only by strict attention to maintenance of physiologic homeostasis; in fact, the potential for exacerbation of cerebral injury, either traumatic or ischemic, with physiologic mismanagement is significantly greater than the modest protection afforded by pharmacologic drugs. Accordingly, with respect to brain protection, efforts should be focused on maintenance of physiologic parameters (perfusion pressure, oxygenation, normocapnia, temperature management, control of hyperglycemia, and seizure prophylaxis) within the appropriate range and less on pharmacologic or anesthetic drugs to reduce cerebral injury.

Deferring Elective Procedures after Stroke

The risk of extension of cerebral infarction in the event of subsequent anesthesia and surgery has not been studied systematically. In patients who have suffered a stroke, CBF undergoes marked changes. Areas of both high and low CBF occur, and stabilization of regional CBF and CMR is apparent after about 2 weeks.[337] Loss of normal vasomotor responses (CO_2 responsiveness, autoregulation) in the early postinsult period is very common,[338-340] and these changes persist beyond 2 weeks in a small percentage of stroke victims.[339,340] BBB abnormalities, as reflected by accumulation of CT contrast material or brain scan isotopes, are still present 4 weeks after the insult,[341] and the histologic resolution of large infarcts is not complete for several months. The information available does not allow a definite statement regarding how long elective procedures should be deferred. A 6-week delay should give some assurance of the probable recovery of autoregulation, CO_2 responsiveness, and BBB integrity. However, the size and location of the infarction should be weighed. A small infarction in silent cortex may give wider latitudes than a large lesion that has resulted in a paresis that is still resolving. A small prospective study suggested that in patients with nondisabling stroke, early carotid endarterectomy can be safely performed within 2 weeks of the stroke.[342] However, in patients with larger strokes, pending other information, it seems reasonable to defer elective surgery for at least 4 weeks after a cerebral vascular accident and preferably for 6 weeks from the point at which a stable postinsult neurologic state has been achieved.

Chronic Arterial Hypertension

A recurrent concern is that of acceptable levels of blood pressure reduction in chronically hypertensive patients. Firm guidelines have not been established. However, from the vantage of cerebral well-being, limiting elective MAP reduction to 30% to 35% of resting mean levels seems appropriate for both hypertensive and normotensive patients. It is reasonable that the same guidelines might apply in both populations because in chronic hypertension, both the lower and upper limits of autoregulation are shifted to the right with apparently little distortion.[343]

The rationale for a limit of 30% to 35% is as follows. It has been demonstrated that MAP reductions of 50% in nonanesthetized patients, both normotensive and hypertensive, will commonly produce reversible symptoms of cerebral hypoperfusion.[343-345] Although even greater reductions will probably be tolerated provided that exposures are brief, the hematocrit is reasonable, and the cerebral vasculature is patent, we counsel against it. A reduction in MAP of this magnitude will significantly increase the probability of CPP being close to or below the LLA, thereby reducing cerebrovascular reserve. It has been demonstrated that a 25% reduction in MAP will bring both normotensive and hypertensive patients to the LLA.[343] As the reduction in MAP exceeds 25% of baseline, CBF values will be below normal, albeit in subjects free of occlusive vascular disease, but above the threshold for neurophysiologic dysfunction or injury (see Fig. 13-4). However, physiologic reserve is being encroached upon, thereby leaving little margin for error or for other causes of impaired cerebral oxygen delivery (low hematocrit, unrecognized cerebrovascular disease).

It has been demonstrated in animals that treatment of chronic hypertension can restore the LLA to normal.[346,347] A similar phenomenon has been observed in humans by Strandgaard, although restoration was incomplete and had failed to occur after as long as 12 months of treatment in some subjects.[343] It is an unexplored possibility that the extent of restoration of the LLA with antihypertensive therapy is agent dependent. Some may restore the LLA more effectively than others do. In particular, angiotensin-converting enzyme inhibitors have been shown to decrease the LLA acutely in both normotensive and hypertensive subjects.[348,349]

Intracranial Hypertension

Control of intracranial hypertension is discussed in detail in Chapter 63.

Brain Tumors

There are few data regarding the physiology of intracranial tumors. Arbit and colleagues[350] measured CBF in cerebral tumors with laser-Doppler technology. In general, they found that tumors had lower CBF than normal brain did. Autoregulation was occasionally apparent. Vascular responsiveness to changes in $Pa{O_2}$[351] and $Pa{CO_2}$[352] are generally preserved in patients with gliomas. However, in some circumstances, hyperventilation can at times be associated with paradoxical increases in MCA flow velocity ipsilateral to the tumor.[353] Measurement of regional CBF in the area of the tumor might also be a useful predictor of the grade of intracranial gliomas; both regional CBF and regional CBV are greater with higher-grade gliomas.[354] There is often considerable edema in association with intracranial tumors, and the radiologic extent of the edema (which presumably represents the extent of abnormal vessel leakiness) correlates with the severity of the elevation in ICP that occurs in association with intubation-related hypertension.[355] Edema formation in the peritumoral region can be characterized as either vasogenic with leakage of plasma proteins from the vascular space, hydrocephalic secondary to obstruction of CSF flow, or static as a result of venous obstruction by tumor.[356] Although the precise mechanisms by which edema formation occurs are not clear, loss of integrity of the tight junctions of components of the BBB, increased permeability induced by vascular endothelial growth factor expressed by tumors, and increased expression of leukotriene C_4 in peritumoral fluid probably play a role.[357] Osmotherapy with mannitol will effect a reduction in edema; however, with a permeable BBB, mannitol can diffuse into the peritumoral space and lead to rebound edema formation.[356] For acute reduction of ICP in the operating room, this is not a significant concern. Dexamethasone remains the mainstay of treatment of tumor edema; it causes a reduction in edema formation with little effect on edema reabsorption, a reduction in permeability of the BBB that can be seen as rapidly as 1 hour after administration,[358] and a modest reduction in tumor size. See Chapter 63 for a complete discussion.

Coma and Epilepsy

Regardless of its etiology, coma is associated with reductions in brain metabolism. In the case of lesions occurring in the reticular activating system, the reduction in CMR probably represents a normal physiologic adjustment to reduced functional activity. During generalized seizure activity, CMR and CBF may increase dramatically.[200] The intensive motor and brain activity associated with generalized seizures leads to the development of systemic and cerebral acidosis, often accompanied by a reduction in arterial oxygenation, an increase in Pa_{CO_2}, and peripheral lactic acidosis. If generalized seizure activity continues unabated, arterial hypotension ensues. With muscular relaxation and measures ensuring adequate oxygenation and ventilation, the systemic acidosis and hypotension can be avoided and the severity of the cerebral acidosis diminished. During relatively brief episodes of continuous seizures, the brain seems able to meet the high metabolic demands.[214] However, even with effective ventilation and maintenance of perfusion pressure, when seizures continue for a prolonged period, they can lead to the development of irreversible neuronal damage.[359] Therapy aimed at interrupting the seizure and restoring a normal balance between cerebral metabolic demand and blood flow is indicated. Barbiturates, benzodiazepines, or other potent anticonvulsants are appropriate. Adequate ventilation, oxygenation, and maintenance of blood pressure are important adjunctive measures. Muscle relaxants must be viewed as purely symptomatic therapy because they do not alter the abnormal cerebral electrical activity.

The potentially injurious nature of seizures justifies attention to prevention. Practices vary. However, patients who have sustained a severe head injury or subarachnoid hemorrhage and any patient in whom a substantial cortical incision is planned are at risk, and prophylactic anticonvulsants should be considered.

References

1. Drummond JC, Todd MM, U HS: The effect of high dose sodium thiopental on brain stem auditory and median nerve somatosensory evoked responses in humans. Anesthesiology 63:249-254, 1985.
2. Peterson DO, Drummond JC, Todd MM: Effects of halothane, enflurane, isoflurane, and nitrous oxide on somatosensory evoked potentials in humans. Anesthesiology 65:35-40, 1986.
3. Michenfelder JD: Anesthesia and the Brain: Clinical, Functional, Metabolic, and Vascular Correlates. New York, Churchill Livingstone, 1988.
4. Drummond JC: The lower limit of autoregulation: Time to revise our thinking? Anesthesiology 86:1431-1433, 1997.
5. Branston NM: Neurogenic control of the cerebral circulation. Cerebrovasc Brain Metab Rev 7:338-349, 1995.
6. Gupta MM, Bithal PK, Dash HH, et al: Effects of stellate ganglion block on cerebral haemodynamics as assessed by transcranial Doppler ultrasonography. Br J Anaesth 95:669-673, 2005.
7. Harrison MJ: Influence of haematocrit in the cerebral circulation. Cerebrovasc Brain Metab Rev 1:55-67, 1989.
8. Cole DJ, Drummond JC, Patel PM, et al: Effects of viscosity and oxygen content on cerebral blood flow in ischemic and normal rat brain. J Neurol Sci 124:15-20, 1994.
9. Aichner FT, Fazekas F, Brainin M, et al: Hypervolemic hemodilution in acute ischemic stroke: The Multicenter Austrian Hemodilution Stroke Trial (MAHST). Stroke 29:743-749, 1998.
10. Akopov S, Simonian N: Comparison of isradipine and enalapril effects on regional carotid circulation in patients with hypertension with unilateral carotid artery stenosis. J Cardiovasc Pharmacol 30:562-570, 1997.
11. Rogers AT, Stump DA, Gravlee GP, et al: Response of cerebral blood flow to phenylephrine infusion during hypothermic cardiopulmonary bypass: Influence of Pa_{CO_2} management. Anesthesiology 69:547-551, 1988.
12. Nemoto EM, Klementavicius R, Melick JA, et al: Norepinephrine activation of basal cerebral metabolic rate for oxygen ($CMRO_2$) during hypothermia in rats. Anesth Analg 83:1262-1267, 1996.
13. Bryan RM Jr: Cerebral blood flow and energy metabolism during stress. Am J Physiol 259:H269-H280, 1990.
14. Artru AA, Nugent M, Michenfelder JD: Anesthetics affect the cerebral metabolic response to circulatory catecholamines. J Neurochem 36:1941-1946, 1981.
15. King BD, Sokoloff L, Wechsler RL: The effects of L-epinephrine and L-norepinephrine upon cerebral circulation and metabolism in man. J Clin Invest 31:273-279, 1952.
16. Madsen PL, Vorstrup S, Schmidt JF, et al: Effect of acute and prolonged treatment with propranolol on cerebral blood flow and cerebral oxygen metabolism in healthy volunteers. Eur J Clin Pharmacol 39:295-297, 1990.
17. Schroeder T, Schierbeck J, Howardy P, et al: Effect of labetalol on cerebral blood flow and middle cerebral arterial flow velocity in healthy volunteers. Neurol Res 13:10-12, 1991.
18. Bandres J, Yao L, Nemoto EM, et al: Effects of dobutamine and dopamine on whole brain blood flow and metabolism in unanesthetized monkeys. J Neurosurg Anesthesiol 4:250-256, 1992.
19. Townsend JB, Ziedonis DM, Bryan RM, et al: Choroid plexus blood flow: Evidence for dopaminergic influence. Brain Res 290:165-169, 1984.
20. Prielipp RC, Wall MH, Groban L, et al: Reduced regional and global cerebral blood flow during fenoldopam-induced hypotension in volunteers. Anesth Analg 93:45-52, 2001.
21. Zornow MH, Maze M, Dyck JB, et al: Dexmedetomidine decreases cerebral blood flow velocity in humans. J Cereb Blood Flow Metab 13:350-353, 1993.
22. Prielipp RC, Wall MH, Tobin JR, et al: Dexmedetomidine-induced sedation in volunteers decreases regional and global cerebral blood flow. Anesth Analg 95:1052-1059, 2002.
23. Drummond JC, Dao AV, Roth DM, et al: The effect of dexmedetomidine on cerebral blood flow velocity, cerebral metabolic rate and CO_2 response in normal humans. Anesthesiology 108:225-232, 2008.
24. Meyer JS, Terayama Y, Takashima S: Cerebral circulation in the elderly. Cerebrovasc Brain Metab Rev 5:122-146, 1993.
25. Todd MM, Weeks J: Comparative effects of propofol, pentobarbital, and isoflurane on cerebral blood

flow and blood volume. J Neurosurg Anesth 8:296-303, 1996.
26. Powers WJ, Raichle ME: Positron emission tomography and its application to the study of cerebrovascular disease in man. Stroke 16:361-376, 1985.
27. Gibbs JM, Wise RJ, Leenders KL, et al: Evaluation of cerebral perfusion reserve in patients with carotid-artery occlusion. Lancet 1:310-314, 1984.
28. Ferrari M, Wilson DA, Hanley DF, et al: Effects of graded hypotension on cerebral blood flow, blood volume, and mean transit time in dogs. Am J Physiol 262:H1908-H1914, 1992.
29. Lanier WL, Warner DO: Intracranial elastance versus intracranial compliance: Terminology should agree with that of other disciplines. Anesthesiology 77:403-404, 1992.
30. Artru AA: Relationship between cerebral blood volume and CSF pressure during anesthesia with isoflurane or fentanyl in dogs. Anesthesiology 60:575-579, 1984.
31. Archer DP, Labrecque P, Tyler JL, et al: Cerebral blood volume is increased in dogs during administration of nitrous oxide or isoflurane. Anesthesiology 67:642-648, 1987.
32. Weeks JB, Todd MM, Warner DS, et al: The influence of halothane, isoflurane, and pentobarbital on cerebral plasma volume in hypocapnic and normocapnic rats. Anesthesiology 73:461-466, 1990.
33. Renou AM, Vernhiet J, Macrez P, et al: Cerebral blood flow and metabolism during etomidate anaesthesia in man. Br J Anaesth 50:1047-1051, 1978.
34. Jobes DR, Kennell EM, Bush GL, et al: Cerebral blood flow and metabolism during morphine–nitrous oxide anesthesia in man. Anesthesiology 47:16-18, 1977.
35. Vernhiet J, Macrez P, Renou AM, et al: [Effects of high doses of morphinomimetics (fentanyl and fentathienyl) on the cerebral circulation in normal subjects.] Ann Anesthesiol Fr 18:803-810, 1977.
36. Stephan H, Groger P, Weyland A, et al: [The effect of sufentanil on cerebral blood flow, cerebral metabolism and the CO_2 reactivity of the cerebral vessels in man.] Anaesthesist 40:153-160, 1991.
37. Paris A, Scholz J, von Knobelsdorff G, et al: The effect of remifentanil on cerebral blood flow velocity. Anesth Analg 87:569-7563, 1998.
38. Cotev S, Shalit MN: Effects on diazepam on cerebral blood flow and oxygen uptake after head injury. Anesthesiology 43:117-122, 1975.
39. Forster A, Juge O, Morel D: Effects of midazolam on cerebral blood flow in human volunteers. Anesthesiology 56:453-455, 1982.
40. Pierce EC, Lambertsen CJ, Deutsch S, et al: Cerebral circulation and metabolism during thiopental anesthesia and hyperventilation in man. J Clin Invest 41:1664-1671, 1962.
41. Takeshita H, Okuda Y, Sari A: The effects of ketamine on cerebral circulation and metabolism in man. Anesthesiology 36:69-75, 1972.
42. Stephan H, Sonntag H, Schenk HD, et al: [Effect of Disoprivan (propofol) on the circulation and oxygen consumption of the brain and CO_2 reactivity of brain vessels in the human.] Anaesthesist 36:60-65, 1987.
43. Kofke WA, Attaallah AF, Kuwabara H, et al: The neuropathologic effects in rats and neurometabolic effects in humans of large dose remifentanil. Anesth Analg 94:1229-1236, 2002.
44. Zornow MH, Fleischer JE, Scheller MS, et al: Dexmedetomidine, an alpha 2 adrenergic agonist, decreases cerebral blood flow in the isoflurane anesthetized dog. Anesth Analg 70:624-630, 1990.
45. Ogura K, Takayasu M, Dacey RG Jr: Differential effects of pentobarbital on intracerebral arterioles and venules of rats in vitro. Neurosurgery 28:537-541, 1991.
46. Michenfelder JD: The interdependency of cerebral functional and metabolic effects following massive doses of thiopental in the dog. Anesthesiology 41:231-236, 1974.
47. Stullken EH Jr, Milde JH, Michenfelder JD, et al: The nonlinear responses of cerebral metabolism to low concentrations of halothane, enflurane, isoflurane, and thiopental. Anesthesiology 46:28-34, 1977.
48. Astrup J, Rosenorn J, Cold GE, et al: Minimum cerebral blood flow and metabolism during craniotomy. Effect of thiopental loading. Acta Anaesthesiol Scand 28:478-481, 1984.
49. Gronert GA, Michenfelder JD, Sharbrough FW, et al: Canine cerebral metabolic tolerance during 24 hours deep pentobarbital anesthesia. Anesthesiology 55:110-113, 1981.
50. Sawada Y, Sugimoto H, Kobayashi H, et al: Acute tolerance to high-dose barbiturate treatment in patients with severe head injuries. Anesthesiology 56: 53-54, 1982.
51. Vandesteene A, Trempont V, Engelman E, et al: Effect of propofol on cerebral blood flow and metabolism in man. Anaesthesia 43(Suppl):42-43, 1988.
52. Kaisti KK, Metsahonkala L, Teras M, et al: Effects of surgical levels of propofol and sevoflurane anesthesia on cerebral blood flow in healthy subjects studied with positron emission tomography. Anesthesiology 96:1358-1370, 2002.
53. Kaisti KK, Langsjo JW, Aalto S, et al: Effects of sevoflurane, propofol, and adjunct nitrous oxide on regional cerebral blood flow, oxygen consumption, and blood volume in humans. Anesthesiology 99:603-613, 2003.
54. Alkire MT, Haier RJ, Barker SJ, et al: Cerebral metabolism during propofol anesthesia in humans studied with positron emission tomography. Anesthesiology 82:393-403, 1995.
55. Petersen KD, Landsfeldt U, Cold GE, et al: Intracranial pressure and cerebral hemodynamic in patients with cerebral tumors. Anesthesiology 98:329-336, 2003.
56. Fox J, Gelb AW, Enns J, et al: The responsiveness of cerebral blood flow to changes in arterial carbon dioxide is maintained during propofol–nitrous oxide anesthesia in humans. Anesthesiology 77:453-456, 1992.
57. Craen RA, Gelb AW, Murkin JM, et al: Human cerebral autoregulation is maintained during propofol air/O_2 anesthesia [abstract]. J Neurosurg Anesthesiol 4:298, 1992.
58. Matta BF, Mayberg TS, Lam AM: Direct cerebrovasodilatory effects of halothane, isoflurane and desflurane during propofol-induced isoelectric electroencephalogram in humans. Anesthesiology 83:980-985, 1995.
59. Cold GE, Eskesen V, Eriksen H, et al: CBF and $CMRO_2$ during continuous etomidate infusion supplemented with N_2O and fentanyl in patients with supratentorial cerebral tumour. A dose-response study. Acta Anaesthesiol Scand 29:490-494, 1985.
60. Kofke WA, Dong ML, Bloom M, et al: Transcranial Doppler ultrasonography with induction of anesthesia for neurosurgery. J Neurosurg Anesth 6:89-97, 1994.
61. Bingham RM, Procaccio F, Prior PF, et al: Cerebral electrical activity influences the effects of etomidate on cerebral perfusion pressure in traumatic coma. Br J Anaesth 57:843-848, 1985.
62. Modica PA, Tempelhoff R: Intracranial pressure during induction of anaesthesia and tracheal intubation with etomidate-induced EEG burst suppression. Can J Anaesth 39:236-241, 1992.
63. Dearden NM, McDowall DG: Comparison of etomidate and althesin in the reduction of increased intracranial pressure after head injury. Br J Anaesth 57:361-368, 1985.
64. Hoffman WE, Charbel FT, Edelman G, et al: Comparison of the effect of etomidate and desflurane on brain tissue gases and pH during prolonged middle cerebral artery occlusion. Anesthesiology 88:1188-1194, 1998.
65. Levy ML, Aranda M, Zelman V, et al: Propylene glycol toxicity following continuous etomidate infusion for the control of refractory cerebral edema. Neurosurgery 37:363-369; discussion 369-371, 1995.
66. Moyer JH, Pontius R, Morris G, et al: Effect of morphine and *n*-allylnormorphine on cerebral hemodynamics and oxygen metabolism. Circulation 15:379-384, 1957.
67. Jobes DR, Kennell E, Bitner R, et al: Effects of morphine–nitrous oxide anesthesia on cerebral autoregulation. Anesthesiology 42:30-34, 1975.
68. Murkin JM, Farrar JK, Tweed WA, et al: Relationship between cerebral blood flow and O_2 consumption during high-dose narcotic anesthesia for cardiac surgery [abstract]. Anesthesiology 63:A44, 1985.
69. Firestone LL, Gyulai F, Mintun M, et al: Human brain activity response to fentanyl imaged by positron emission tomography. Anesth Analg 82:1247-1251, 1996.
70. McPherson RW, Krempasanka E, Eimerl D, et al: Effects of alfentanil on cerebral vascular reactivity in dogs. Br J Anaesth 57:1232-1238, 1985.
71. Schregel W, Schafermeyer H, Muller C, et al: [The effect of halothane, alfentanil and propofol on blood flow velocity, blood vessel cross section and blood volume flow in the middle cerebral artery.] Anaesthesist 41:21-26, 1992.
72. Mayberg TS, Lam AM, Eng CC, et al: The effect of alfentanil on cerebral blood flow velocity and intracranial pressure during isoflurane–nitrous oxide anesthesia in humans. Anesthesiology 78:288-294, 1993.
73. Marx W, Shah N, Long C, et al: Sufentanil, alfentanil, and fentanyl: Impact on cerebrospinal fluid pressure in patients with brain tumors. J Neurosurg Anesthesiol 1:3-7, 1989.
74. Jung R, Shah N, Reinsel R, et al: Cerebrospinal fluid pressure in patients with brain tumors: Impact of fentanyl versus alfentanil during nitrous oxide–oxygen anesthesia. Anesth Analg 71:419-422, 1990.
75. Moss E: Alfentanil increases intracranial pressure when intracranial compliance is low. Anaesthesia 47:134-136, 1992.
76. Markovitz BP, Duhaime AC, Sutton L, et al: Effects of alfentanil on intracranial pressure in children undergoing ventriculoperitoneal shunt revision. Anesthesiology 76:71-76, 1992.
77. Souter MJ, Andrews PJ, Piper IR, et al: Effects of alfentanil on cerebral haemodynamics in an experimental model of traumatic brain injury. Br J Anaesth 79:97-102, 1997.
78. Herrick IA, Gelb AW, Manninen PH, et al: Effects of fentanyl, sufentanil and alfentanil on brain retractor pressure. Anesth Analg 72:359-363, 1991.
79. From RP, Warner DS, Todd MM, et al: Anesthesia for craniotomy: A double blind comparison of alfentanil, fentanyl and sufentanil. Anesthesiology 73:896-904, 1990.

80. Keykhah MM, Smith DS, Carlsson C, et al: Influence of sufentanil on cerebral metabolism and circulation in the rat. Anesthesiology 63:274-277, 1985.
81. Werner C, Hoffman WE, Baughman VL, et al: Effects of sufentanil on cerebral blood flow, cerebral blood flow velocity and metabolism in dogs. Anesth Analg 72:177-181, 1991.
82. Murkin JM, Farrar JK, Tweed WA: Sufentanil anaesthesia reduces cerebral blood flow and cerebral oxygen consumption [abstract]. Can J Anaesth 35:S131, 1988.
83. Mayer N, Weinstabl C, Podreka I, et al: Sufentanil does not increase cerebral blood flow in healthy human volunteers. Anesthesiology 73:240-243, 1990.
84. Weinstabl C, Mayer N, Spiss CK: Sufentanil decreases cerebral blood flow velocity in patients with elevated intracranial pressure. Eur J Anaesthesiol 9:481-484, 1992.
85. Weinstabl C, Mayer N, Richling B, et al: Effect of sufentanil on intracranial pressure in neurosurgical patients. Anaesthesia 46:837-840, 1991.
86. Werner C, Kochs E, Hoffman WE, et al: Sufentanil does not change cerebral hemodynamics and ICP in head injured patients [abstract]. J Neurosurg Anaesthesiol 4:313, 1992.
87. Jamali S, Ravussin P, Archer D, et al: The effects of bolus administration of opioids on cerebrospinal fluid pressure in patients with supratentorial lesions. Anesth Analg 82:600-606, 1996.
88. Lauer KK, Connolly LA, Schmeling WT: Opioid sedation does not alter intracranial pressure in head injured patients. Can J Anaesth 44:929-933, 1997.
89. Sperry RJ, Bailey PL, Reichman MV, et al: Fentanyl and sufentanil increase intracranial pressure in head trauma patients. Anesthesiology 77:416-420, 1992.
90. Werner C, Kochs E, Bause H, et al: Effects of sufentanil on cerebral hemodynamics and intracranial pressure in patients with brain injury. Anesthesiology 83:721-726, 1995.
91. Bristow A, Shalev D, Rice B, et al: Low-dose synthetic narcotic infusions for cerebral relaxation during craniotomies. Anesth Analg 66:413-416, 1987.
92. Shupak RC, Harp JR: Comparison between high-dose sufentanil-oxygen and high-dose fentanyl-oxygen for neuroanaesthesia. Br J Anaesth 57: 375-381, 1985.
93. Warner DS, Hindman BJ, Todd MM, et al: Intracranial pressure and hemodynamic effects of remifentanil versus alfentanil in patients undergoing supratentorial craniotomy. Anesth Analg 83: 348-353, 1996.
94. Ostapkovich N, Baker KZ, Fogerty-Mack P, et al: Cerebral blood flow and CO_2 reactivity is similar during remifentanil/N_2O and fentanyl/N_2O anesthesia. Anesthesiology 89:358-363, 1998.
95. Wagner K, Wiloch F, Kochs E, et al: Dose-dependent regional cerebral blood flow changes during remifentanil infusion in humans. Anesthesiology 94:732-739, 2001.
96. Lorenz I, Kolbitsch C, Hormann C, et al: The influence of nitrous oxide and remifentanil on cerebral hemodynamics in conscious human volunteers. Neuroimage 17:1056-1064, 2002.
97. Kofke WA, Blissitt PA, Rao H, et al: Remifentanil-induced cerebral blood flow effects in normal humans: Dose and ApoE genotype. Anesth Analg 105:167-175, 2007.
98. Ostapkovich ND, Baker KZ, Fogerty-Mack P, et al: Cerebral blood flow and CO_2 reactivity is similar during remifentanil/N_2O and fentanyl/N_2O anesthesia. Anesthesiology 89:358-363, 1998.
99. Forster A, Juge O, Louis M, et al: Effects of a specific benzodiazepine antagonist (RO 15-1788) on cerebral blood flow. Anesth Analg 66:309-313, 1987.
100. Veselis RA, Reinsel RA, Beattie BJ, et al: Midazolam changes cerebral blood flow in discrete brain regions: an $H_2{}^{15}O$ positron emission tomography study. Anesthesiology 87:1106-1117, 1997.
101. Forster A, Juge O, Morel D: Effects of midazolam on cerebral hemodynamics and cerebral vasomotor responsiveness to carbon dioxide. J Cereb Blood Flow Metab 3:246-249, 1983.
102. Wolf J, Friberg L, Jensen J, et al: The effect of the benzodiazepine antagonist flumazenil on regional cerebral blood flow in human volunteers. Br J Anaesth 34:628-631, 1990.
103. Knudsen L, Cold GE, Holdgard HO, et al: Effects of flumazenil on cerebral blood flow and oxygen consumption after midazolam anaesthesia for craniotomy. Br J Anaesth 67:277-280, 1991.
104. Chiolero RL, Ravussin P, Anderes JP, et al: The effects of midazolam reversal by RO 15-1788 on cerebral perfusion pressure in patients with severe head injury. Intensive Care Med 14:196-200, 1988.
105. Misfeldt BB, Jorgensen PB, Spotoft H, et al: The effects of droperidol and fentanyl on intracranial pressure and cerebral perfusion pressure in neurosurgical patients. Br J Anaesth 48:963-968, 1976.
106. Michenfelder JD, Theye RA: Effects of fentanyl, droperidol, and Innovar on canine cerebral metabolism and blood flow. Br J Anaesth 43:630-636, 1971.
107. Strebel S, Kaufmann M, Maitre L, et al: Effects of ketamine on cerebral blood flow velocity in humans. Influence of pretreatment with midazolam or esmolol. Anaesthesia 50:223-228, 1995.
108. Cavazzuti M, Porro CA, Biral GP, et al: Ketamine effects on local cerebral blood flow and metabolism in the rat. J Cereb Blood Flow Metab 7:806-811, 1987.
109. Vollenweider FX, Leenders KL, Oye I, et al: Differential psychopathology and patterns of cerebral glucose utilisation produced by (*S*)- and (*R*)-ketamine in healthy volunteers using positron emission tomography (PET). Eur Neuropsychopharmacol 7:25-38, 1997.
110. Vollenweider FX, Leenders KL, Scharfetter C, et al: Metabolic hyperfrontality and psychopathology in the ketamine model of psychosis using positron emission tomography (PET) and [^{18}F] fluorodeoxyglucose (FDG). Eur Neuropsychopharmacol 7:9-24, 1997.
111. Holcomb HH, Lahti AC, Medoff DR, et al: Sequential regional cerebral blood flow brain scans using PET with $H_2{}^{15}O$ demonstrate ketamine actions in CNS dynamically. Neuropsychopharmacology 25:165-172, 2001.
112. Schmidt A, Ryding E, Akeson J: Racemic ketamine does not abolish cerebrovascular autoregulation in the pig. Acta Anesthesiol Scand 47:569-575, 2003.
113. Mayberg TS, Lam AM, Matta BF, et al: Ketamine does not increase cerebral blood flow velocity or intracranial pressure during isoflurane/nitrous oxide anesthesia in patients undergoing craniotomy. Anesth Analg 81:84-89, 1995.
114. Strebel S, Kaufmann M, Maître L, et al: Effects of ketamine on cerebral blood flow velocity in humans. Influence of pretreatment with midazolam or esmolol. Anaesthesia 50:223-228, 1995.
115. Sakai K, Cho S, Fukusaki M, et al: The effects of propofol with and without ketamine on human cerebral blood flow velocity and CO_2 response. Anesth Analg 90:377-382, 2000.
116. Albanese J, Arnaud S, Rey M, et al: Ketamine decreases intracranial pressure and electroencephalographic activity in traumatic brain injury patients during propofol sedation. Anesthesiology 87:1328-1334, 1997.
117. Sakabe T, Maekawa T, Ishikawa T, et al: The effects of lidocaine on canine cerebral metabolism and circulation related to the electroencephalogram. Anesthesiology 40:433-441, 1974.
118. Astrup J, Sorensen PM, Sorensen HR: Inhibition of cerebral oxygen and glucose consumption in the dog by hypothermia, pentobarbital, and lidocaine. Anesthesiology 55:263-268, 1981.
119. Lam AM, Donlon E, Eng CC, et al: The effect of lidocaine on cerebral blood flow and metabolism during normocapnia and hypocapnia in humans [abstract]. Anesthesiology 79:A202, 1993.
120. Bedford RF, Persing JA, Pobereskin L, et al: Lidocaine or thiopental for rapid control of intracranial hypertension? Anesth Analg 59:435-437, 1980.
121. Michenfelder JD, Milde JH: Influence of anesthetics on metabolic, functional and pathological responses to regional cerebral ischemia. Stroke 6:405-410, 1975.
122. Michenfelder JD, Sundt TM, Fode N, et al: Isoflurane when compared to enflurane and halothane decreases the frequency of cerebral ischemia during carotid endarterectomy. Anesthesiology 67:336-340, 1987.
123. Todd MM, Drummond JC: A comparison of the cerebrovascular and metabolic effects of halothane and isoflurane in the cat. Anesthesiology 60:276-282, 1984.
124. Lutz LJ, Milde JH, Milde LN: The cerebral functional, metabolic, and hemodynamic effects of desflurane in dogs. Anesthesiology 73:125-131, 1990.
125. Scheller MS, Tateishi A, Drummond JC, et al: The effects of sevoflurane on cerebral blood flow, cerebral metabolic rate for oxygen, intracranial pressure, and the electroencephalogram are similar to those of isoflurane in the rabbit. Anesthesiology 68:548-551, 1988.
126. Michenfelder JD, Cucchiara RF: Canine cerebral oxygen consumption during enflurane anesthesia and its modification during induced seizures. Anesthesiology 40:575-580, 1974.
127. Drummond JC, Todd MM, Scheller MS, et al: A comparison of the direct cerebral vasodilating potencies of halothane and isoflurane in the New Zealand white rabbit. Anesthesiology 65:462-467, 1986.
128. Hansen TD, Warner DS, Todd MM, et al: Distribution of cerebral blood flow during halothane versus isoflurane anesthesia in rats. Anesthesiology 69:332-337, 1988.
129. Lenz C, Rebel A, Klaus V, et al: Local cerebral blood flow, local cerebral glucose utilization, and flow-metabolism coupling during sevoflurane versus isoflurane anesthesia in rats. Anesthesiology 89: 1480-1488, 1998.
130. Heath KJ, Gupta S, Matta BF: The effects of sevoflurane on cerebral hemodynamics during propofol anesthesia. Anesth Analg 85:1284-1287, 1997.
131. Wollman H, Alexander SC, Cohen PJ, et al: Cerebral circulation of man during halothane anesthesia. Anesthesiology 25:180-184, 1964.
132. Murphy FL, Kennell EM, Johnstone RE, et al: The effects of enflurane, isoflurane, and halothane on cerebral blood flow and metabolism in man [abstract]. Paper presented at the Annual Meeting of the American Society of Anesthesiologists, October 1974, pp 62-63.
133. Todd MM, Drummond JC, Shapiro HM: Comparative cerebrovascular and metabolic effects of

halothane, enflurane, and isoflurane [abstract]. Anesthesiology 57:A332, 1982.
134. Mielck F, Stephan H, Weyland A, et al: Effects of one minimum alveolar anesthetic concentration sevoflurane on cerebral metabolism, blood flow, and CO_2 reactivity in cardiac patients. Anesth Analg 89:364-369, 1999.
135. Mielck F, Stephan H, Buhre W, et al: Effects of 1 MAC desflurane on cerebral metabolism, blood flow and carbon dioxide reactivity in humans. Br J Anaesth 81:155-160, 1998.
136. Sakabe T, Maekawa T, Fujii S, et al: Cerebral circulation and metabolism during enflurane anesthesia in humans. Anesthesiology 59:532-536, 1983.
137. Johnson J, Sperry RJ, Lam A, et al: A phase III, randomized, open-label study to compare sevoflurane and isoflurane in neurosurgical patients. Anesth Analg 80(Suppl):S214, 1995.
138. Ornstein E, Young WL, Fleischer LH, et al: Desflurane and isoflurane have similar effects on cerebral blood flow in patients with intracranial mass lesions. Anesthesiology 79:498-502, 1993.
139. Fraga M, Maceiras P, Rodino S, et al: The effects of isoflurane and desflurane on intracranial pressure, cerebral perfusion pressure, and cerebral arteriovenous oxygen content differences in normocapnic patients with supratentorial brain tumors. Anesthesiology 98:1085-1090, 2003.
140. Alkire MT, Haier RJ, Shah NK, et al: Positron emission tomography study of regional cerebral metabolism in humans during isoflurane anesthesia. Anesthesiology 86:549-557, 1997.
141. Kaisti K, Metsahonkala L, Teras M, et al: Effects of surgical levels of propofol and sevoflurane anesthesia on cerebral blood flow in healthy subjects studied with positron emission tomography. Anesthesiology 96:1358-1370, 2002.
142. Ornstein E, Young WL, Ostapkovich N, et al: Comparative effects of desflurane and isoflurane on cerebral blood flow [abstract]. Anesthesiology 75:A209, 1991.
143. Algotsson L, Messeter K, Rosen I, et al: Effects of nitrous oxide on cerebral haemodynamics and metabolism during isoflurane anaesthesia in man. Acta Anaesthesiol Scand 36:46-52, 1992.
144. Reinstrup P, Ryding E, Algotsson L, et al: Regional cerebral blood flow (SPECT) during anaesthesia with isoflurane and nitrous oxide in humans. Br J Anaesth 78:407-411, 1997.
145. Bundgaard H, von Oettingen G, Larsen KM, et al: Effects of sevoflurane on intracranial pressure, cerebral blood flow and cerebral metabolism. A dose-response study in patients subjected to craniotomy for cerebral tumours. Acta Anaesthesiol Scand 42:621-627, 1998.
146. Madsen JB, Cold GE, Hansen ES, et al: The effect of isoflurane on cerebral blood flow and metabolism in humans during craniotomy for small supratentorial cerebral tumors. Anesthesiology 66:332-336, 1987.
147. Kolbitsch C, Lorenz IH, Hormann C, et al: Sevoflurane and nitrous oxide increase regional cerebral blood flow (rCBF) and regional cerebral blood volume (rCBV) in a drug-specific manner in human volunteers. Magn Reson Imaging 19:1253-1260, 2001.
148. Kolbitsch C, Lorenz IH, Hormann C, et al: A subanesthetic concentration of sevoflurane increases regional cerebral blood flow and regional cerebral blood volume and decreases regional mean transit time and regional cerebrovascular resistance in volunteers. Anesth Analg 91:156-162, 2000.
149. Alkire MT, Pomfrett CJ, Haier RJ, et al: Functional brain imaging during anesthesia in humans: Effects of halothane on global and regional cerebral glucose metabolism. Anesthesiology 90:701-709, 1999.
150. Young WL, Prohovnik I, Ornstein E, et al: The effect of arteriovenous malformation resection on cerebrovascular reactivity to carbon dioxide. Neurosurgery 27:257-267, 1990.
151. Kuroda Y, Murakami M, Tsuruta J, et al: Blood flow velocity of middle cerebral artery during prolonged anesthesia with halothane, isoflurane, and sevoflurane in humans. Anesthesiology 87:527-532, 1997.
152. Sanders RD, Maze M: Xenon: From stranger to guardian. Curr Opin Anaesthesiol 18:405-411, 2005.
153. Franks NP, Dickinson R, de Sousa SL, et al: How does xenon produce anaesthesia? Nature 396:324, 1998.
154. Gruss M, Bushell TJ, Bright DP, et al: Two-pore-domain K^+ channels are a novel target for the anesthetic gases xenon, nitrous oxide, and cyclopropane. Mol Pharmacol 65:443-452, 2004.
155. Laitio RM, Kaisti KK, Laangsjo JW, et al: Effects of xenon anesthesia on cerebral blood flow in humans: A positron emission tomography study. Anesthesiology 106:1128-1133, 2007.
156. Rex S, Schaefer W, Meyer PH, et al: Positron emission tomography study of regional cerebral metabolism during general anesthesia with xenon in humans. Anesthesiology 105:936-943, 2006.
157. Schmidt M, Marx T, Papp-Jambor C, et al: Effect of xenon on cerebral autoregulation in pigs. Anaesthesia 57:960-966, 2002.
158. Schmidt M, Marx T, Armbruster S, et al: Effect of xenon on elevated intracranial pressure as compared with nitrous oxide and total intravenous anesthesia in pigs. Acta Anaesthesiol Scand 49:494-501, 2005.
159. Reinelt H, Schirmer U, Marx T, et al: Diffusion of xenon and nitrous oxide into the bowel. Anesthesiology 94:475-477; discussion 6A, 2001.
160. Milde LN, Milde JH: Cerebral effects of sufentanil in dogs with reduced intracranial compliance. Anesth Analg 68(Suppl):S196, 1989.
161. Maksimow A, Kaisti K, Aalto S, et al: Correlation of EEG spectral entropy with regional cerebral blood flow during sevoflurane and propofol anaesthesia. Anaesthesia 60:862-869, 2005.
162. Boarini DJ, Kassell NF, Coester HC, et al: Comparison of systemic and cerebrovascular effects of isoflurane and halothane. Neurosurgery 15:400-409, 1984.
163. Reinstrup P, Ryding E, Algotsson L, et al: Distribution of cerebral blood flow during anesthesia with isoflurane or halothane in humans. Anesthesiology 82:359-366, 1995.
164. Maekawa T, Tommasino C, Shapiro HM, et al: Local cerebral blood flow and glucose utilization during isoflurane anesthesia in the rat. Anesthesiology 65:144-151, 1986.
165. Eintrei C, Leszniewski W, Carlsson C: Local application of ^{133}xenon for measurement of regional cerebral blood flow (rCBF) during halothane, enflurane, and isoflurane anesthesia in humans. Anesthesiology 63:391-394, 1985.
166. Adams RW, Cucchiara RF, Gronert GA: Isoflurane and cerebrospinal fluid pressure in neurosurgical patients. Anesthesiology 54:97, 1981.
167. Grosslight K, Foster R, Colohan AR, et al: Isoflurane for neuroanesthesia: Risk factors for increases in intracranial pressure. Anesthesiology 63:533, 1985.
168. Campkin TV, Flinn RM: Isoflurane and cerebrospinal fluid pressure—a study in neurosurgical patients undergoing intracranial shunt procedures. Anaesthesia 44:50-54, 1989.
169. Scheller MS, Todd MM, Drummond JC: A comparison of the ICP effects of isoflurane and halothane after cryogenic brain injury in rabbits. Anesthesiology 67:507-512, 1987.
170. Warner DS, Boarini DJ, Kassell NF: Cerebrovascular adaptation to prolonged halothane anesthesia is not related to cerebrospinal fluid pH. Anesthesiology 63:243-248, 1985.
171. Albrecht RF, Miletich DJ, Madala LR: Normalization of cerebral blood flow during prolonged halothane anesthesia. Anesthesiology 58:26-31, 1983.
172. Fleischer LH, Young WL, Ornstein E, et al: Cerebral blood flow in humans does not decline over time during isoflurane or desflurane anesthesia [abstract]. Anesthesiology 77:A167, 1992.
173. Madsen JB, Cold GE, Hansen ES, et al: The effect of isoflurane on cerebral blood flow and metabolism in humans during craniotomy for small supratentorial cerebral tumors. Anesthesiology 66:332, 1987.
174. Drummond JC, Todd MM: The response of the feline cerebral circulation to $Paco_2$ during anesthesia with isoflurane and halothane and during sedation with nitrous oxide. Anesthesiology 62:268-273, 1985.
175. Gupta S, Heath K, Matta BF: Effect of incremental doses of sevoflurane on cerebral pressure autoregulation in humans. Br J Anaesth 79:469-472, 1997.
176. Vavilala MS, Lee LA, Lee M, et al: Cerebral autoregulation in children during sevoflurane anaesthesia. Br J Anaesth 90:636-641, 2003.
177. Lu H, Werner C, Englehard K, et al: The effects of sevoflurane on cerebral blood flow autoregulation in rats. Anesth Analg 87:854-858, 1998.
178. Field LM, Dorrance DE, Krzeminska EK, et al: Effect of nitrous oxide on cerebral blood flow in normal humans. Br J Anaesth 70:154-159, 1993.
179. Lam AM, Mayberg TS, Eng CC, et al: Nitrous oxide–isoflurane anesthesia causes more cerebral vasodilation than an equipotent dose of isoflurane in humans. Anesth Analg 78:462-468, 1994.
180. Eng C, Lam AM, Mayberg TS, et al: The influence of propofol with and without nitrous oxide on cerebral blood flow velocity and CO_2 reactivity in humans. Anesthesiology 77:872-879, 1992.
181. Henriksen HT, Jorgensen PB: The effect of nitrous oxide on intracranial pressure in patients with intracranial disorders. Br J Anaesth 45:486-492, 1973.
182. Pelligrino DA, Miletich DJ, Hoffman WE, et al: Nitrous oxide markedly increases cerebral cortical metabolic rate and blood flow in the goat. Anesthesiology 60:405-412, 1984.
183. Phirman JR, Shapiro HM: Modification of nitrous oxide–induced intracranial hypertension by prior induction of anesthesia. Anesthesiology 46:150-151, 1977.
184. Misfeldt BB, Jorgensen PB, Rishoj M: The effect of nitrous oxide and halothane upon the intracranial pressure in hypocapnic patients with intracranial disorders. Br J Anaesth 46:853-858, 1974.
185. Jung R, Reinsel R, Marx W, et al: Isoflurane and nitrous oxide: Comparative impact on cerebrospinal fluid pressure in patients with brain tumors. Anesth Analg 75:724-728, 1992.
186. Wilson-Smith E, Karsli C, Luginbuehl IA, et al: The effect of nitrous oxide on cerebral blood flow velocity in children anesthetized with propofol. Acta Anaesthesiol Scand 47:307-311, 2003.
187. Manohar M, Parks C: Porcine regional brain and myocardial blood flows during halothane-O_2 and halothane–nitrous oxide anesthesia: Comparisons

with equipotent isoflurane anesthesia. Am J Vet Res 45:465-473, 1984.
188. Drummond JC, Todd MM, Schubert A, et al: Effect of the acute administration of high dose pentobarbital on human brain stem auditory and median nerve somatosensory evoked responses. Neurosurgery 20:830-835, 1987.
189. Todd MM: The effects of $Paco_2$ on the cerebrovascular response to nitrous oxide in the halothane-anesthetized rabbit. Anesth Analg 66:1090-1095, 1987.
190. Strebel S, Kaufmann M, Anselmi L, et al: Nitrous oxide is a potent cerebrovasodilator in humans when added to isoflurane. A transcranial Doppler study. Acta Anaesthesiol Scand 39:653-658, 1995.
191. Lam AM, Mayberg TS, Eng CC, et al: Nitrous oxide–isoflurane anesthesia causes more cerebral vasodilation than an equipotent dose of isoflurane in humans. Anesth Analg 78:462-468, 1994
192. Reinstrup P, Ryding E, Ohlsson T, et al: Cerebral blood volume (CBV) in humans during normo- and hypocapnia: Influence of nitrous oxide (N_2O). Anesthesiology 95:1079-1082, 2001.
193. Baughman VL, Hoffman WE, Miletich DJ, et al: Cerebrovascular and cerebral metabolic effects of N_2O in unrestrained rats. Anesthesiology 73:269-272, 1990.
194. Wollman H, Alexander C, Cohen PJ, et al: Cerebral circulation during general anesthesia and hyperventilation in man.: Thiopental induction to nitrous oxide and D-tubocurarine. Anesthesiology 26:329-334, 1965.
195. Drummond JC, Scheller MS, Todd MM: The effect of nitrous oxide on cortical cerebral blood flow during anesthesia with halothane and isoflurane, with and without morphine, in the rabbit. Anesth Analg 66:1083-1089, 1987.
196. Tarkkanen L, Laitinen L, Johansson G: Effects of *d*-tubocurarine on intracranial pressure and thalamic electrical impedance. Anesthesiology 40:247-251, 1974.
197. Schramm WM, Papousek A, Michalek-Sauberer A, et al: The cerebral and cardiovascular effects of cisatracurium and atracurium in neurosurgical patients. Anesth Analg 86:123-127, 1998.
198. Stirt JA, Grosslight KR, Bedford RF, et al: "Defasciculation" with metocurine prevents succinylcholine induced increases in intracranial pressure. Anesthesiology 67:50, 1987.
199. Lanier WL, Milde JH, Michenfelder JD: The cerebral effects of pancuronium and atracurium in halothane-anesthetized dogs. Anesthesiology 63:589-597, 1985.
200. Tateishi A, Fleischer JE, Drummond JC, et al: Nimodipine does not improve neurologic outcome after 14 minutes of cardiac arrest in cats. Stroke 20:1044-1050, 1989.
201. Standaert FG: Magic bullets, science, and medicine. Anesthesiology 63:577-578, 1985.
202. Lanier WL, Iaizzo PA, Milde JH, et al: The cerebral and systemic effects of movement in response to a noxious stimulus in lightly anesthetized dogs. Possible modulation of cerebral function by muscle afferents. Anesthesiology 80:392-401, 1994.
203. Kovarik WD, Mayberg TS, Lam AM, et al: Succinylcholine does not change intracranial pressure, cerebral blood flow velocity, or the electroencephalogram in patients with neurologic injury. Anesth Analg 78:469-473, 1994.
204. Artru AA: Relationship between cerebral blood volume and CSF pressure during anesthesia with halothane or enflurane in dogs. Anesthesiology 58:533-539, 1983.
205. Artru AA: Isoflurane does not increase the rate of CSF production in the dog. Anesthesiology 60:193-197, 1984.
206. Artru AA: Effects of halothane and fentanyl anesthesia on resistance to reabsorption of CSF. J Neurosurg 60:252-256, 1984.
207. Artru AA, Nugent M, Michenfelder JD: Enflurane causes a prolonged and reversible increase in the rate of CSF production in the dog. Anesthesiology 57:255-260, 1982.
208. Maktabi MA, Elbokl FF, Faraci FM, et al: Halothane decreases the rate of production of cerebrospinal fluid. Possible role of vasopressin V_1 receptors. Anesthesiology 78:72-82, 1993.
209. Artru AA: Rate of cerebrospinal fluid formation, resistance to reabsorption of cerebrospinal fluid, brain tissue water content, and electroencephalogram during desflurane anesthesia in dogs. J Neurosurg Anesthesiol 5:178-186, 1993.
210. Johansson BB, Linder LE: Do nitrous oxide and lidocaine modify the blood-brain barrier in acute hypertension in the rat? Acta Anaesthesiol Scand 24:65-68, 1980.
211. Forster A, Van Horn K, Marshall LF, et al: Anesthetic effects on blood-brain barrier function during acute arterial hypertension. Anesthesiology 49:26-30, 1978.
212. Modica PA, Tempelhoff R, White PF: Pro- and anticonvulsant effects of anesthetics (Part I). Anesth Analg 70:303-315, 1990.
213. Modica PA, Tempelhoff R, White PF: Pro- and anticonvulsant effects of anesthetics (Part II). Anesth Analg 70:433-444, 1990.
214. Kreisman NR, Magee JC, Brizzee BL: Relative hypoperfusion in rat cerebral cortex during recurrent seizures. J Cereb Blood Flow Metab 11:77-87, 1991.
215. Neigh JL, Garman JK, Harp JR: The electroencephalographic pattern during anesthesia with Ethrane: Effects of depth of anesthesia, $Paco_2$, and nitrous oxide. Anesthesiology 35:482-487, 1971.
216. Wollman H, Smith AL, Hoffman JC: Cerebral blood flow and oxygen consumption in man during electroencephalographic seizure patterns induced by anesthesia with Ethrane [abstract]. Fed Proc 28:356, 1967.
217. Flemming DC, Fitzpatrick J, Fariello RG, et al: Diagnostic activation of epileptogenic foci by enflurane. Anesthesiology 52:431-433, 1980.
218. Opitz A, Brecht S, Stenzel E: [Enflurane anaesthesia for epileptic patients (author's transl).] Anaesthesist 26:329-332, 1977.
219. Kruczek M, Albin MS, Wolf S, et al: Postoperative seizure activity following enflurane anesthesia. Anesthesiology 53:175-176, 1980.
220. Hymes JA: Seizure activity during isoflurane anesthesia. Anesth Analg 64:367-368, 1985.
221. Harrison JL: Postoperative seizures after isoflurane anesthesia. Anesth Analg 65:1235-1236, 1986.
222. Kofke WA, Young RS, Davis P, et al: Isoflurane for refractory status epilepticus: A clinical series. Anesthesiology 71:653-659, 1989.
223. Komatsu H, Nogaya J, Ogli K: Volatile anaesthetics as central nervous system excitants. Ann Acad Med Singapore 23:130-138, 1994.
224. Kaisti K, Jaaskelainen S, Rinne JO, et al: Epileptiform discharges during 2 MAC sevoflurane anesthesia in two healthy volunteers. Anesthesiology 91:1952-1955, 1999.
225. Hisada K, Morioka T, Fukui K, et al: Electrocorticographic activities in patients with temporal lobe epilepsy. J Neurosurg Anesthesiol 13:333-337, 2001.
226. Hilty CA, Drummond JC: Seizure-like activity on emergence from sevoflurane anesthesia. Anesthesiology 93:1357-1358, 2000.
227. Terasako K, Ishii S: Postoperative seizure-like activity following sevoflurane anesthesia. Anesth Analg 96:1239-1240, 2003.
228. Archer DP, McKenna JM, Morin L, et al: Conscious-sedation analgesia during craniotomy for intractable epilepsy: A review of 354 consecutive cases. Can J Anaesth 35:338-344, 1988.
229. Todd MM, Drummond JC, U HS: The hemodynamic consequences of high-dose methohexital anesthesia in humans. Anesthesiology 61:495-501, 1984.
230. Bennett DR, Madsen JA, Jordan WS, et al: Ketamine anesthesia in brain-damaged epileptics. Electroencephalographic and clinical observations. Neurology 23:449-460, 1973.
231. Ferrer-Allado T, Brechner VL, Dymond A, et al: Ketamine-induced electroconvulsive phenomena in the human limbic and thalamic regions. Anesthesiology 38:333-344, 1973.
232. Steen PA, Michenfelder JD: Neurotoxicity of anesthetics. Anesthesiology 50:437-453, 1979.
233. Hirshman CA, Krieger W, Littlejohn G, et al: Ketamine-aminophylline–induced decrease in seizure threshold. Anesthesiology 56:464-467, 1982.
234. Ghoneim MM, Yamada T: Etomidate: A clinical and electroencephalographic comparison with thiopental. Anesth Analg 56:479-485, 1977.
235. Laughlin TP, Newberg LA: Prolonged myoclonus after etomidate anesthesia. Anesth Analg 64:80-82, 1985.
236. Ebrahim ZY, DeBoer GE, Luders H, et al: Effect of etomidate on the electroencephalogram of patients with epilepsy. Anesth Analg 65:1004-1006, 1986.
237. Gancher S, Laxer KD, Krieger W: Activation of epileptogenic activity by etomidate. Anesthesiology 61:616-618, 1984.
238. Samra SK, Sneyd JR, Ross DA, et al: Effects of propofol sedation on seizures and intracranially recorded epileptiform activity in patients with partial epilepsy. Anesthesiology 82:843-851, 1995.
239. Lowson S, Gent JP, Goodchild CS: Convulsive thresholds in mice during the recovery phase from anaesthesia induced by propofol, thiopentone, methohexitone and etomidate. Br J Pharmacol 102:879-882, 1991.
240. Rampton AJ, Griffin RM, Stuart CS, et al: Comparison of methohexital and propofol for electroconvulsive therapy: Effects on hemodynamic responses and seizure duration. Anesthesiology 70:412-417, 1989.
241. Drummond JC, Iragui-Modoz VJ, Alksne JF, Kalkman CJ: Masking of epileptiform activity by propofol during seizure surgery. Anesthesiology 77:837-838, 1992.
242. Murkin JM, Moldenhauer CC, Hug CC Jr, et al: Absence of seizures during induction of anesthesia with high-dose fentanyl. Anesth Analg 63:489-494, 1984.
243. Smith NT, Westover CJ Jr, Quinn M, et al: An electroencephalographic comparison of alfentanil with other narcotics and with thiopental. J Clin Monit 1:236-244, 1985.
244. Smith NT, Dec-Silver H, Sanford TJ Jr, et al: EEGs during high-dose fentanyl-, sufentanil-, or morphine-oxygen anesthesia. Anesth Analg 63:386-393, 1984.
245. Tempelhoff R, Modica PA, Bernardo KL, et al: Fentanyl-induced electrocorticographic seizures in patients with complex partial epilepsy. J Neurosurg 77:201-208, 1992.

246. Cascino GD, So EL, Sharbrough FW, et al: Alfentanil-induced epileptiform activity in patients with partial epilepsy. J Clin Neurophysiol 10:520-525, 1993.
247. Astrup J, Symon L, Branston NM, et al: Cortical evoked potential and extracellular K^+ and H^+ at critical levels of brain ischemia. Stroke 8:51-57, 1977.
248. Branston NM, Symon L, Crockard HA, et al: Relationship between the cortical evoked potential and local cortical blood flow following acute middle cerebral artery occlusion in the baboon. Exp Neurol 45:195-208, 1974.
249. Jones TH, Morawetz RB, Crowell RM, et al: Thresholds of focal cerebral ischemia in awake monkeys. J Neurosurg 54:773-782, 1981.
250. Michenfelder JD, Sundt TM, Fode N, et al: Isoflurane when compared to enflurane and halothane decreases the frequency of cerebral ischemia during carotid endarterectomy. Anesthesiology 67:336-340, 1987.
251. Hossmann KA: Viability thresholds and the penumbra of focal ischemia. Ann Neurol 36:557-565, 1994.
252. Sundt TM Jr, Sharbrough FW, Piepgras DG, et al: Correlation of cerebral blood flow and electroencephalographic changes during carotid endarterectomy with results of surgery and hemodynamics of cerebral ischemia. Mayo Clin Proc 56:533-543, 1981.
253. Michenfelder JD, Sundt TM Jr: Cerebral ATP and lactate levels in the squirrel monkey following occlusion of the middle cerebral artery. Stroke 2:319-326, 1971.
254. Michenfelder JD, Theye RA: The effects of anesthesia and hypothermia on canine cerebral ATP and lactate during anoxia produced by decapitation. Anesthesiology 33:430-439, 1970.
255. Siesjo BK: Pathophysiology and treatment of focal cerebral ischemia. Part I: Pathophysiology. J Neurosurg 77:169-184, 1992.
256. Lipton P: Ischemic cell death in brain neurons. Phys Rev 79:1431-1568, 1999.
257. Fiskum G, Murphy AN, Beal MF: Mitochondria in neurodegeneration: Acute ischemia and chronic neurodegenerative diseases. J Cereb Blood Flow Metab 19:351-369, 1999.
258. Velier JJ, Ellison JA, Kikly KK, et al: Caspase-8 and caspase-3 are expressed by different populations of cortical neurons undergoing delayed cell death after focal stroke in the rat. J Neurosci 19:5932-5941, 1999.
259. Kawaguchi M, Kimbro JR, Drummond JC, et al: Isoflurane delays but does not prevent cerebral infarction in rats subjected to focal ischemia. Anesthesiology 92:1335-1342, 2000.
260. Zauner A, Daugherty WP, Bullock MR, et al: Brain oxygenation and energy metabolism: Part I—biological function and pathophysiology. Neurosurgery 51:289-301, 2002.
261. Mattson MP, Duan W, Pedersen WA, et al: Neurodegenerative disorders and ischemic brain diseases. Apoptosis 6:69-81, 2001.
262. Dirnagl U, Iadecola C, Moskowitz M: Pathobiology of ischaemic stroke: An integrated view. Trends Neurosci 22:391-397, 1999.
263. Abramson NA: Randomized clinical study of thiopental loading in comatose survivors of cardiac arrest. N Engl J Med 314:397-403, 1986.
264. Forsman M, Aarseth HP, Nordby HK, et al: Effects of nimodipine on cerebral blood flow and cerebrospinal fluid pressure after cardiac arrest: Correlation with neurologic outcome. Anesth Analg 68:436-443, 1989.
265. Roine RO, Kaste M, Kinnunen A, et al: Nimodipine after resuscitation from out-of-hospital ventricular fibrillation. A placebo-controlled, double-blind, randomized trial. JAMA 264:3171-3177, 1990.
266. A randomized clinical study of a calcium-entry blocker (lidoflazine) in the treatment of comatose survivors of cardiac arrest. Brain Resuscitation Clinical Trial II Study Group. N Engl J Med 324:1225-1231, 1991.
267. Hypothermia after Cardiac Arrest Study Group: Mild therapeutic hypothermia to improve the neurologic outcome after cardiac arrest. N Engl J Med 346:549-656, 2002.
268. Hoffman WE, Cheng MA, Thomas C, et al: Clonidine decreases plasma catecholamines and improves outcome from incomplete ischemia in the rat. Anesth Analg 73:460-464, 1991.
269. Hoffman WE, Thomas C, Albrecht RF: The effect of halothane and isoflurane on neurologic outcome following incomplete cerebral ischemia in the rat. Anesth Analg 76:279-283, 1993.
270. Smith AL, Hoff JT, Nielsen SL, et al: Barbiturate protection in acute focal cerebral ischemia. Stroke 5:1-7, 1974.
271. Michenfelder JD, Milde JH, Sundt TM: Cerebral protection by barbiturate anesthesia. Arch Neurol 33:345-350, 1976.
272. Nehls DG, Todd MM, Spetzler RF, et al: A comparison of the cerebral protective effects of isoflurane and barbiturates during temporary focal ischemia in primates. Anesthesiology 66:453-464, 1987.
273. Nussmeier NA, Arlund C, Slogoff S: Neuropsychiatric complications after cardiopulmonary bypass: Cerebral protection by a barbiturate. Anesthesiology 64:165-170, 1986.
274. Shapiro HM: Barbiturates in brain ischaemia. Br J Anaesth 57:82-95, 1985.
275. Warner DS, Takaoka S, Wu B, et al: Electroencephalographic burst suppression is not required to elicit maximal neuroprotection from pentobarbital in a rat model of focal cerebral ischemia. Anesthesiology 84:1475-1484, 1996.
276. Busto R, Dietrich WD, Globus MY, et al: Small differences in intraischemic brain temperature critically determine the extent of ischemic neuronal injury. J Cereb Blood Flow Metab 7:729-738, 1987.
277. Sano T, Drummond JC, Patel PM, et al: A comparison of the cerebral protective effects of isoflurane and mild hypothermia in a rat model of incomplete forebrain ischemia. Anesthesiology 76:221-228, 1992.
278. Warner DS, Zhou J, Ramani R, et al: Reversible focal ischemia in the rat: Effects of halothane, isoflurane, and methohexital anesthesia. J Cereb Blood Flow Metab 11:794-802, 1991.
279. Drummond JC, Cole DJ, Patel PM, et al: Focal cerebral ischemia during anesthesia with etomidate, isoflurane, or thiopental: A comparison of the extent of cerebral injury. Neurosurgery 37:742-748; discussion 748-749, 1995.
280. Cole DJ, Cross LM, Drummond JC, et al: Thiopentone and methohexital, but not pentobarbitone, reduce early focal cerebral ischemic injury in rats. Can J Anaesth 48:807-814, 2001.
281. Baughman VL, Hoffman WE, Miletich DJ, et al: Neurologic outcome in rats following incomplete cerebral ischemia during halothane, isoflurane or N_2O. Anesthesiology 69:192-198, 1988.
282. Soonthan-Brant V, Patel PM, Drummond JC, et al: Fentanyl does not increase brain injury after focal cerebral ischemia in rats. Anesth Analg 88:49-55, 1999.
283. Mackensen GB, Nellgard B, Kudo M, et al: Periischemic cerebral blood flow (CBF) does not explain beneficial effects of isoflurane on outcome from near complete forebrain ischemia in rats. Anesthesiology 93:1102-1106, 2000.
284. Nellgard B, Mackensen GB, Pineda J, et al: Anesthetic effects on cerebral metabolic rate predict histologic outcome from near-complete forebrain ischemia in the rat. Anesthesiology 93:431-436, 2000.
285. Kawaguchi M, Kimbro JR, Drummond JC, et al: Effects of isoflurane on neuronal apoptosis in rats subjected to focal ischemia. J Neurosurg Anesthesiol 12:385, 2000.
286. Sakai H, Sheng H, Yates RB, et al: Isoflurane provides long-term protection against focal cerebral ischemia in the rat. Anesthesiology 106:92-99; discussion 8-10, 2007.
287. Warner DS, McFarlane C, Todd MM, et al: Sevoflurane and halothane reduce focal ischemic brain damage in the rat. Anesthesiology 79:985-992, 1993.
288. Werner C, Mollenberg O, Kochs E, et al: Sevoflurane improves neurological outcome after incomplete cerebral ischaemia in rats. Br J Anaesth 75:756-760, 1995.
289. Engelhard K, Werner C, Reeker W, et al: Desflurane and isoflurane improve neurological outcome after incomplete cerebral ischaemia in rats. Br J Anaesth 83:415-421, 1999.
290. Wilhelm S, Ma D, Maze M, et al: Effects of xenon on in vitro and in vivo models of neuronal injury. Anesthesiology 96:1485-1491, 2002.
291. Homi HM, Yokoo N, Ma D, et al: The neuroprotective effect of xenon administration during transient middle cerebral artery occlusion in mice. Anesthesiology 99:876-881, 2003.
292. Ma D, Yang H, Lynch J, et al: Xenon attenuates cardiopulmonary bypass–induced neurologic and neurocognitive dysfunction in the rat. Anesthesiology 98:690-698, 2003.
293. Ma D, Hossain M, Chow A, et al: Xenon and hypothermia combine to provide neuroprotection from neonatal asphyxia. Ann Neurol 58:182-193, 2005.
294. Ma D, Hossain M, Rajakumaraswamy N, et al: Combination of xenon and isoflurane produces a synergistic protective effect against oxygen-glucose deprivation injury in a neuronal-glial co-culture model. Anesthesiology 99:748-751, 2003.
295. Ma D, Hossain M, Pettet GK, et al: Xenon preconditioning reduces brain damage from neonatal asphyxia in rats. J Cereb Blood Flow Metab 26:199-208, 2006.
296. Jevtovic-Todorovic V, Beals J, Benshoff N, et al: Prolonged exposure to inhalational anesthetic nitrous oxide kills neurons in adult rat brain. Neuroscience 122:609-616, 2003.
297. Williamson PB, Ma D, Hossain M, et al: Xenon does not cause apoptotic neurodegeneration in the neonatal rat and protects against isoflurane-induced apoptosis [abstract]. Anesthesiology 101(Suppl):A864, 2004.
298. Ravussin P, de Tribolet N: Total intravenous anesthesia with propofol for burst suppression in cerebral aneurysm surgery: Preliminary report of 42 patients. Neurosurgery 32:236-240; discussion 240, 1993.
299. Ridenour TR, Warner DS, Todd MM, et al: Comparative effects of propofol and halothane on outcome from temporary middle cerebral artery occlusion in the rat. Anesthesiology 76:807-812, 1992.
300. Gelb AW, Bayona NA, Wilson JX, et al: Propofol anesthesia compared to awake reduces infarct size in rats. Anesthesiology 96:1183-1190, 2002.

301. Pittman JE, Sheng H, Pearlstein RD, et al: Comparison of the effects of propofol and pentobarbital on neurologic outcome and cerebral infarction size after temporary focal ischemia in the rat. Anesthesiology 87:1139-1144, 1997.
302. Bayona NA, Gelb AW, Jiang Z, et al: Propofol neuroprotection in cerebral ischemia and its effects on low-molecular-weight antioxidants and skilled motor tasks. Anesthesiology 100:1151-1159, 2004.
303. Engelhard K, Werner C, Eberspacher E, et al: Influence of propofol on neuronal damage and apoptotic factors after incomplete cerebral ischemia and reperfusion in rats: A long-term observation. Anesthesiology 101:912-917, 2004.
304. Batjer HH, Frankfurt AI, Purdy PD, et al: Use of etomidate, temporary arterial occlusion, and intraoperative angiography in surgical treatment of large and giant cerebral aneurysms. J Neurosurg 68:234-240, 1988.
305. Nebauer AE, Doenicke A, Hoernecke R, et al: Does etomidate cause haemolysis? Br J Anaesth 69:58-60, 1992.
306. Pickard JD, Murray GD, Illingworth R, et al: Effect of oral nimodipine on cerebral infarction and outcome after subarachnoid haemorrhage: British Aneurysm Nimodipine Trial. BMJ 298:636-642, 1989.
307. Randomised, double-blind, placebo-controlled trial of nimodipine in acute stroke. Trust Study Group. Lancet 336:1205-1209, 1990.
308. Drummond J, Oh Y-S, Cole D, et al: Phenylephrine-induced hypertension decreases the area of ischemia following middle cerebral artery occlusion in the rat. Stroke 20:1538-1544, 1989.
309. Wise G, Sutter R, Burkholder J: The treatment of brain ischemia with vasopressor drugs. Stroke 3:135-140, 1972.
310. Young WL, Solomon RA, Pedley TA, et al: Direct cortical EEG monitoring during temporary vascular occlusion for cerebral aneurysm surgery. Anesthesiology 71:794-799, 1989.
311. Ahmed N, Nasman P, Wahlgren NG: Effect of intravenous nimodipine on blood pressure and outcome after acute stroke. Stroke 31:1250-1255, 2000.
312. Rose JC, Mayer SA: Optimizing blood pressure in neurological emergencies. Neurocrit Care 1:287-299, 2004.
313. Artru AA, Merriman HG: Hypocapnia added to hypertension to reverse EEG changes during carotid endarterectomy. Anesthesiology 70:1016-1018, 1989.
314. Waltz AG, Sundt TM Jr, Michenfelder JD: Cerebral blood flow during carotid endarterectomy. Circulation 45:1091-1096, 1972.
315. Christensen MS, Paulson OB, Olesen J, et al: Cerebral apoplexy (stroke) treated with or without prolonged artificial hyperventilation: 1. Cerebral circulation, clinical course and cause of death. Stroke 4:568, 1973.
316. Ruta TS, Drummond JC, Cole DJ: The effect of acute hypocapnia on local cerebral blood flow during middle cerebral artery occlusion in isoflurane anesthetized rats. Anesthesiology 78:134-140, 1993.
317. Nemoto EM, Klementavicius R, Melick JA, et al: Suppression of cerebral metabolic rate for oxygen ($CMRO_2$) by mild hypothermia compared with thiopental. J Neurosurg Anesthesiol 8:52-59, 1996.
318. Klementavicius R, Nemoto EM, Yonas H: The Q_{10} ratio for basal cerebral metabolic rate for oxygen in rats. J Neurosurg 85:482-487, 1996.
319. Boris-Moller F, Smith ML, Siesjo BK: Effects of hypothermia on ischemic brain damage: A comparison between preischemic and postischemia cooling. Neurosci Res Commun 5:87-94, 1989.
320. Buchan A, Pulsinelli WA: Hypothermia but not the *N*-methyl-D-aspartate antagonist, MK-801, attenuates neuronal damage in gerbils subjected to transient global ischemia. J Neurosci 10:311-316, 1990.
321. Hindman BJ, Todd MM, Gelb AW, et al: Mild hypothermia as a protective therapy during intracranial aneurysm surgery: A randomized prospective pilot trial. Neurosurgery 44:23-32; discussion 32-33, 1999.
322. Todd MM, Hindman BJ, Clarke WR, et al: Mild intraoperative hypothermia during surgery for intracranial aneurysm. N Engl J Med 352:135-145, 2005.
323. Shiozaki T, Sugimoto H, Taneda M, et al: Effect of mild hypothermia on uncontrollable intracranial hypertension after severe head injury. J Neurosurg 79:363-368, 1993.
324. Clifton GL, Allen S, Barrodale P, et al: A phase II study of moderate hypothermia in severe brain injury. J Neurotrauma 10:263-271, 1993.
325. Clifton GL, Miller ET, Choi SC, et al: Lack of effect of induction of hypothermia after acute brain injury. N Engl J Med 344:556-563, 2001.
326. Kammersgaard LP, Rasmussen BH, Jorgensen HS, et al: Feasibility and safety of inducing modest hypothermia in awake patients with acute stroke through surface cooling: A case-control study. Stroke 31:2251-2256, 2000.
327. Bernard SA, Gray TW, Buist MD, et al: Treatment of comatose survivors of out-of-hospital cardiac arrest with induced hypothermia. N Engl J Med 346:557-563, 2002.
328. Wass CT, Lanier WL, Hofer RE, et al: Temperature changes of > or = 1 degree C alter functional neurologic outcome and histopathology in a canine model of complete cerebral ischemia. Anesthesiology 83:325-335, 1995.
329. Vannucci RC, Brucklacher RM, Vannucci SJ: The effect of hyperglycemia on cerebral metabolism during hypoxia-ischemia in the immature rat. J Cereb Blood Flow Metab 16:1026-1033, 1996.
330. Mullner M, Sterz F, Binder M, et al: Blood glucose concentration after cardiopulmonary resuscitation influences functional neurological recovery in human cardiac arrest survivors. J Cereb Blood Flow Metab 17:430-436, 1997.
331. Weir CJ, Murray GD, Dyker AG, et al: Is hyperglycaemia an independent predictor of poor outcome after acute stroke? Results of a long-term follow up study. BMJ 314:1303-1306, 1997.
332. Matchar DB, Divine GW, Heyman A, et al: The influence of hyperglycemia on outcome of cerebral infarction. Ann Intern Med 117:449-456, 1992.
333. Bruno A, Levine SR, Frankel MR, et al: Admission glucose level and clinical outcomes in the NINDS rt-PA Stroke Trial. Neurology 59:669-674, 2002.
334. Gray CS, Hildreth AJ, Sandercock PA, et al: Glucose-potassium-insulin infusions in the management of post-stroke hyperglycaemia: the UK Glucose Insulin in Stroke Trial (GIST-UK). Lancet Neurol 6:397-406, 2007.
335. Auer RN: Hypoglycemic brain damage. Metab Brain Dis 19:169-175, 2004.
336. Archer DP: The role of bloodletting in the prevention and treatment of asthenic apoplexy. J Neurosurg Anesthesiol 6:51-53, 1994.
337. Lenzi GL, Frackowiak RS, Jones T: Cerebral oxygen metabolism and blood flow in human cerebral ischemic infarction. J Cereb Blood Flow Metab 2:321-335, 1982.
338. Paulson OB: Regional cerebral blood flow in apoplexy due to occlusion of the middle cerebral artery. Neurology 20:63-77, 1970.
339. Agnoli A, Fieschi C, Bozzao L, et al: Autoregulation of cerebral blood flow. Studies during drug-induced hypertension in normal subjects and in patients with cerebral vascular diseases. Circulation 38:800-812, 1968.
340. Fieschi C, Agnoli A, Prencipe M, et al: Impairment of the regional vasomotor response of cerebral vessels to hypercarbia in vascular diseases. Eur Neurol 2:13-30, 1969.
341. Olsen TS: Regional cerebral blood flow after occlusion of the middle cerebral artery. Acta Neurol Scand 73:321-337, 1986.
342. Ballotta E, Da Giau G, Baracchini C, et al: Early versus delayed carotid endarterectomy after a non-disabling ischemic stroke: A prospective, randomized study. Surgery 131:287-293, 2002.
343. Strandgaard S: Autoregulation of cerebral blood flow in hypertensive patients. The modifying influence of prolonged antihypertensive treatment on the tolerance to acute, drug-induced hypotension. Circulation 53:720-727, 1976.
344. Finnerty FA Jr, Witkin L, Fazekas JF: Cerebral hemodynamics during cerebral ischemia induced by acute hypotension. J Clin Invest 33:1227-1232, 1954.
345. Njemanze PC: Critical limits of pressure-flow relation in the human brain. Stroke 23:1743-1747, 1992.
346. Vorstrup S, Barry DI, Jarden JO, et al: Chronic antihypertensive treatment in the rat reverses hypertension-induced changes in cerebral blood flow autoregulation. Stroke 15:312-318, 1984.
347. Toyoda K, Fujii K, Ibayashi S, et al: Attenuation and recovery of brain stem autoregulation in spontaneously hypertensive rats. J Cereb Blood Flow Metab 18:305-310, 1998.
348. Larsen FS, Olsen KS, Hansen BA, et al: Transcranial Doppler is valid for determination of the lower limit of cerebral blood flow autoregulation. Stroke 25:1985-1988, 1994.
349. Waldemar G, Schmidt JF, Andersen AR, et al: Angiotensin converting enzyme inhibition and cerebral blood flow autoregulation in normotensive and hypertensive man. J Hypertens 7:229-235, 1989.
350. Arbit E, DiResta GR, Bedford RF, et al: Intraoperative measurement of cerebral and tumor blood flow with laser-Doppler flowmetry. Neurosurgery 24:166-170, 1989.
351. Julien C, Payen JF, Tropres I, et al: Assessment of vascular reactivity in rat brain glioma by measuring regional blood volume during graded hypoxic hypoxia. Br J Cancer 91:374-380, 2004.
352. Packard SD, Mandeville JB, Ichikawa T, et al: Functional response of tumor vasculature to $Pa{CO_2}$: Determination of total and microvascular blood volume by MRI. Neoplasia 5:330-338, 2003.
353. Schregel W, Geissler C, Winking M, et al: Transcranial Doppler monitoring during induction of anesthesia: Effects of propofol, thiopental, and hyperventilation in patients with large malignant brain tumors. J Neurosurg Anesthesiol 5:86-93, 1993.
354. Shin JH, Lee HK, Kwun BD, et al: Using relative cerebral blood flow and volume to evaluate the histopathologic grade of cerebral gliomas: preliminary results. AJR Am J Roentgenol 179:783-789, 2002.

355. Bedford RF, Morris L, Jane JA: Intracranial hypertension during surgery for supratentorial tumor: Correlation with preoperative computed tomography scans. Anesth Analg 61:430-433, 1982.
356. Kaal EC, Vecht CJ: The management of brain edema in brain tumors. Curr Opin Oncol 16:593-600, 2004.
357. Stummer W: Mechanisms of tumor-related brain edema. Neurosurg Focus 22:E8, 2007.
358. Shapiro WR, Hiesiger EM, Cooney GA, et al: Temporal effects of dexamethasone on blood-to-brain and blood-to-tumor transport of ^{14}C-alpha-aminoisobutyric acid in rat C6 glioma. J Neurooncol 8:197-204, 1990.
359. Wasterlain CG: Mortality and morbidity from serial seizures. An experimental study. Epilepsia 15:155-176, 1974.

J. A. Jeevendra Martyn

14 Neuromuscular Physiology and Pharmacology

Key Points

1. The neuromuscular junction provides a rich array of receptors and substrates for drug action. Several drugs used clinically have multiple sites of action, and muscle relaxants are not exceptions to the rule that most drugs have more than one site or mechanism of action. The major actions seem to occur by the mechanisms and at the sites described for decades: agonistic and antagonistic actions at postjunctional receptors for depolarizing and nondepolarizing relaxants. This description of neuromuscular drug action is a simplistic one. Neuromuscular transmission is impeded by nondepolarizers because they prevent access of acetylcholine to its recognition site on the postjunctional receptor.
2. If the concentration of nondepolarizer is increased, another, noncompetitive action—block of the ion channel—is superimposed. The paralysis is also potentiated by prejunctional actions of the relaxant, which prevents release of acetylcholine. The latter can be documented as fade that occurs with increased frequency of stimulation. A more accurate description of the effects of relaxants recognizes that the neuromuscular junction is a complex and dynamic system in which the phenomena produced by drugs are composites of actions that vary with drug, dose, activity in the junction and muscle, time after administration, presence of anesthetics or other drugs, and the age and condition of the patient.
3. Inhibition of postjunctional acetylcholinesterase by anticholinesterases increases the concentration of acetylcholine, which can compete with and displace the nondepolarizer and thus reverse the paralysis. These anticholinesterases also have other effects, including those on nerve terminals and on the receptor, by an allosteric mechanism. Cyclodextrins are a new class of compounds that reverse paralysis of only steroidal muscle relaxants by directly binding to them.
4. Depolarizing compounds initially react with the acetylcholine recognition site and, like the transmitter, open ion channels and depolarize the end-plate membrane. Unlike the transmitter, they are not subject to hydrolysis by acetylcholinesterase and therefore remain in the junction. Soon after administration of the drug, some receptors are desensitized and, although occupied by an agonist, they do not open to allow current to flow to depolarize the area.
5. If the depolarizing relaxant is applied in high concentration and allowed to remain at the junction for a long time, other effects occur, including entry of the drug into the channel to obstruct it or to pass through it into the cytoplasm. Depolarizing relaxants also have effects on prejunctional structures, and the combination of prejunctional and postjunctional effects plus secondary ones on muscle and nerve homeostasis results in the complicated phenomenon known as phase II blockade.
6. Intense research in the area of neuromuscular transmission continues at a rapid pace. Newer observations on receptors, ion channels, membranes, and prejunctional function reveal a much broader range of sites and mechanisms of action for agonists and antagonists.
7. Some of the other drugs used clinically (e.g., botulinum toxin) have effects on the nerve and therefore indirectly on muscle. Systemic infection with clostridial toxins (*Clostridium tetanus*, *Clostridium botulinum*) can lead to systemic paralysis as a result of decreased release of acetylcholine from the nerve terminal. Nondepolarizing muscle relaxants administered even for 12 hours or for prolonged periods can have effects on the postsynaptic receptor and simulate denervation (chemical denervation). In recognizing these sites and mechanisms, we begin to bring our theoretical knowledge closer to explaining the phenomena observed when these drugs are administered to living humans.
8. The most recent work seems to be focused on the postjunctional membrane and control of acetylcholine receptor expression in normal and diseased states. The presence or absence of mature and immature isoforms seems to complicate matters further. In certain pathologic states (e.g., stroke, sepsis, burns, immobilization, chronic use of relaxants), acetylcholine

receptors are upregulated, usually with expression of the immature isoform. More recently, another isoform of the acetylcholine receptor, previously described in neuronal tissues only, the α7 neuronal acetylcholine receptor, has been identified in muscle. These receptors have different functional and pharmacologic properties than conventional muscle postsynaptic receptors do. The altered functional and pharmacologic characteristics of the immature (γ-subunit) and neuronal (α7-subunit) receptors result in increased sensitivity to succinylcholine with hyperkalemia and resistance to nondepolarizers.

9. An area of increasing attention is control of the expression of mature versus the other two receptor isoforms. Re-expression of the immature γ and α7 receptors is probably related to aberrant growth factor signaling. Mutations in the acetylcholine receptor that result in prolonged open-channel time, similar to that seen with the immature receptor, can lead to a myasthenia-like state, even in the presence of normal receptor numbers. The weakness is usually related to the prolonged open-channel time. The role of the immature isoform of the receptor in the muscle weakness associated with critical illness such as burns is unknown.

10. Despite the fact that the neuromuscular junction is the most studied receptor, complete knowledge of its workings has not been achieved. This is an area of continuing interest for many researchers worldwide.

The physiology of neuromuscular transmission could be analyzed and understood at the most simple level by using the classic model of nerve signaling to muscle through the acetylcholine receptor (AChR). The mammalian neuromuscular junction is the prototypical and most extensively studied synapse. Research has provided more detailed information on processes that, within the classic scheme, can modify neurotransmission and response to drugs. One example is the role of qualitative or quantitative changes in AChRs that modify neurotransmission and response to drugs.[1-3] In myasthenia gravis, for example, the decrease in AChRs results in decreased efficiency of neurotransmission (and therefore muscle weakness)[4] and altered sensitivity to neuromuscular relaxants.[3] Another example is the importance of nerve-related (prejunctional) changes that alter neurotransmission and response to drugs.[3,5] At still another level is evidence that muscle relaxants act in ways that are not encompassed by the classic scheme of a unitary site of action. The observation that muscle relaxants can have prejunctional effects[6] or that some nondepolarizers can also have agonist-like stimulatory actions on the receptor[7] whereas others have effects not explainable by purely postsynaptic events[8] has provided new insight into some previously unexplained observations. Although muscle relaxants are known to have effects on the presynaptic and postsynaptic receptors of the neuromuscular junction, recent evidence indicates that they can react with nicotinic and muscarinic AChRs other than those in muscle, including receptors on the carotid sinus, on the vagus to the heart, and on bronchial smooth muscle.[9-11] Although this multifaceted action-response scheme makes the physiology and pharmacology of neurotransmission more complex, these added insights also bring experimentally derived knowledge much closer to clinical observations.

Crucial to the seminal concepts that have developed relative to the neurotransmitter acetylcholine and its receptor systems has been the introduction of powerful and contemporary techniques in molecular biology, immunology, and electrophysiology, as well as more elegant techniques for observation of the neuromuscular junction in vivo.[12] These techniques have augmented the more traditional pharmacologic, protein chemical, morphologic, and cytologic approaches.[13,14] Research has elucidated the manner in which the nerve ending regulates the synthesis and release of transmitter and the release of trophic factors, both of which control muscle function, and how these processes are influenced by exogenous and endogenous substances.[14-17] Research continues into how receptors are synthesized and anchored at the end plate, the role of the nerve terminal in the maturation process, and synthesis and control of acetylcholinesterase, the enzyme that breaks down acetylcholine. Several reviews that provide detailed insight into these areas are available.[15-19]

Neuromuscular Transmission

Neuromuscular transmission occurs by a fairly simple and straightforward mechanism. The nerve synthesizes acetylcholine and stores it in small, uniformly sized packages called vesicles. Stimulation of the nerve causes these vesicles to migrate to the surface of the nerve, rupture, and discharge acetylcholine into the cleft separating nerve from muscle. AChRs in the end plate of the muscle respond by opening their channels for influx of sodium ions into the muscle to depolarize the muscle. The end-plate potential created is continued along the muscle membrane by the opening of sodium channels present throughout the muscle membrane to initiate a contraction.[17] The acetylcholine immediately detaches from the receptor and is destroyed by the enzyme acetylcholinesterase, which is also present in the cleft. Drugs, notably depolarizing relaxants or nicotine and carbachol (a synthetic analog of acetylcholine not destroyed by acetylcholinesterase), can also act on these receptors to mimic the effect of acetylcholine and cause depolarization of the end plate. These drugs are therefore called agonists of the receptor because to a greater or lesser extent, they stimulate the receptor, at least initially. Nondepolarizing muscle relaxants (NDMRs) also act on the receptors, but they prevent acetylcholine from binding to the receptor and thus prevent depolarization by agonists. Because these nondepolarizers prevent the action of agonists (e.g., acetylcholine, carbachol, succinylcholine), they are referred to as antagonists of the AChR. Other compounds, frequently called reversal agents or antagonists of neuromuscular paralysis (e.g., neostigmine, prostigmine), inhibit acetylcholinesterase and therefore impair the hydrolysis of acetylcholine. The increased accumulation of undegraded acetylcholine can compete with NDMRs effectively and thereby displace the latter from the receptor (i.e., law of mass action) and antagonize the effects of NDMRs.

Morphology

The neuromuscular junction is specialized on the nerve side and on the muscle side to transmit and receive chemical messages.[12-17] Each motor neuron runs without interruption from the ventral horn of the spinal cord or medulla to the neuromuscular junction as a large, myelinated axon (Fig. 14-1A). As it approaches the muscle, it branches repeatedly to contact many muscle cells and gather them into a functional group known as a motor unit (see Fig. 14-1B). The architecture of the nerve terminal is quite different from that of the rest of the axon. As the terminal reaches the muscle fiber, it loses its myelin, forms a spray of terminal branches against the muscle surface, and is covered by Schwann cells. This arrangement conforms to the architecture on the synaptic area of the muscle membrane (see Fig. 14-1C). The nerve is separated from the surface of the muscle by a gap of approximately 20 nm, called the junctional or synaptic cleft. The nerve and muscle are held in tight alignment by protein filaments called basal lamina that span the cleft between the nerve and end plate. The muscle surface is heavily corrugated, with deep invaginations of the junctional cleft—the primary and secondary clefts—between the folds in the muscle membrane; thus, the end plate's total surface area is very large. The depths of the folds also vary between muscle types and species. Human neuromuscular junctions, relative to muscle size, are smaller than those of the mouse, although the junctions are located on muscle fibers that are much larger. Human junctions have longer junctional foldings and deeper gutters.[12] The functional significance of these folds is unclear. The shoulders of the folds are densely populated with AChRs, about 5 million of them in each junction. AChRs are sparse in the depths between the folds. Instead, these deep areas contain sodium channels (see Fig. 14-1D).

The trophic function of the nerve is vital for the development and maintenance of adequate neuromuscular function. Before birth, each muscle cell commonly has contacts with several nerves and has several neuromuscular junctions.[17,19] At birth, all but one of the nerves retract, and a single end plate remains. Once

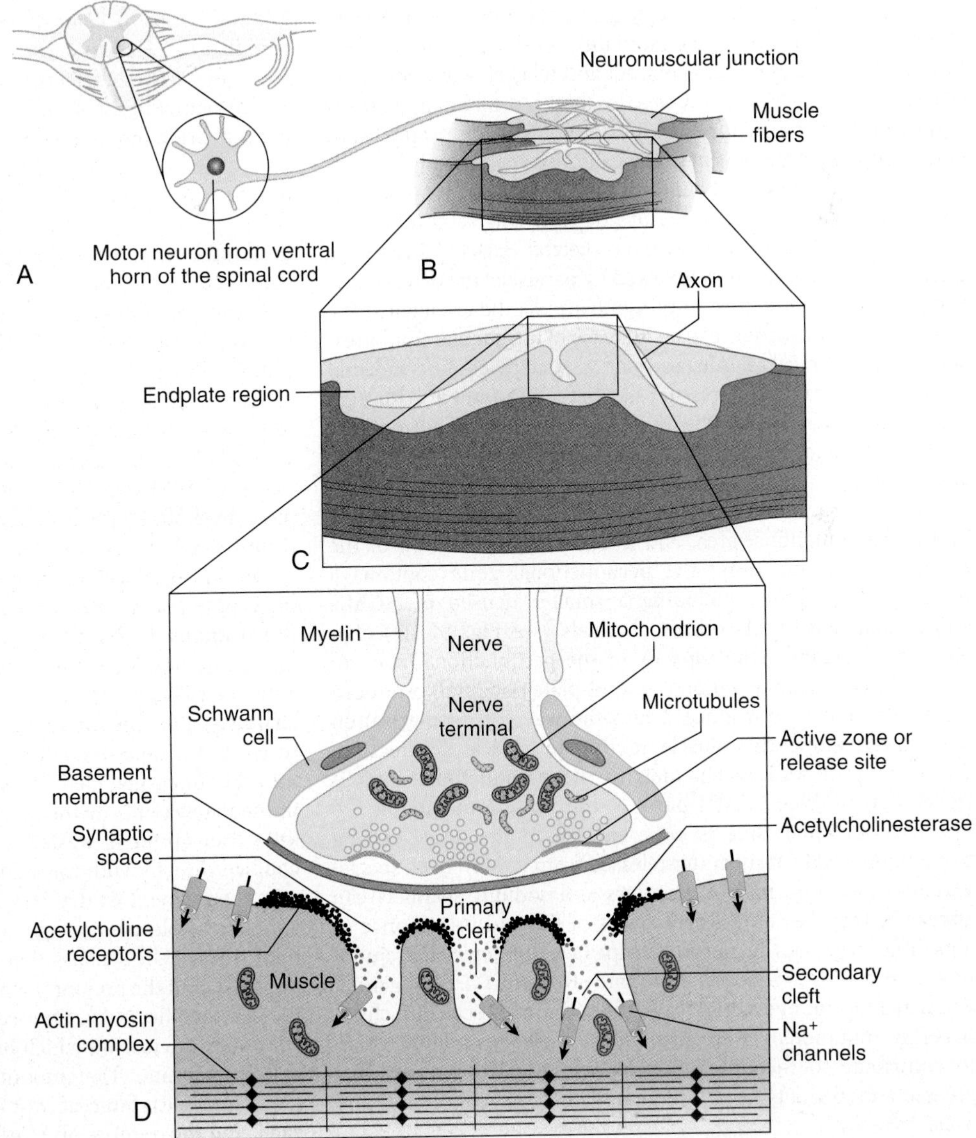

Figure 14-1 Structure of the adult neuromuscular junction showing the three cells that constitute the synapse: the motor neuron (i.e., nerve terminal), muscle fiber, and Schwann cell. **A,** The motor nerve originates in the ventral horn of the spinal cord or brainstem. **B,** As the nerve approaches its muscle fibers and before attaching itself to the surface of the muscle fiber, the nerve divides into branches that innervate many individual muscle fibers. **C,** Each muscle receives only one synapse. The motor nerve loses its myelin and further subdivides into many presynaptic boutons to terminate on the surface of the muscle fiber. **D,** The nerve terminal, covered by a Schwann cell, has vesicles clustered about the membrane thickenings, which are the active zones, toward its synaptic side and mitochondria and microtubules toward its other side. A synaptic gutter or cleft made up of a primary and many secondary clefts separates the nerve from the muscle. The muscle surface is corrugated, and dense areas on the shoulders of each fold contain acetylcholine receptors. Sodium channels are present at the bottom of the clefts and throughout the muscle membrane. The acetylcholinesterase and proteins and proteoglycans that stabilize the neuromuscular junction are present in the synaptic clefts.

formed, the nerve-muscle contact, especially the end plate, is durable. Even if the original nerve dies, the one replacing it innervates exactly the same region of the muscle. The nerve endings on fast muscles are larger and more complicated than those on slow muscles. The reason for this is unclear. These differences in the nerve endings on muscle surfaces may play a role in the difference in response of fast- and slow-twitch muscle fibers to muscle relaxants.

Because all the muscle cells in a unit are excited by a single neuron, stimulation of the nerve electrically or by an action potential originating from the ventral horn or by any agonist, including depolarizing relaxants (e.g., succinylcholine), causes all muscle cells in the motor unit to contract synchronously. Synchronous contraction of the cells in a motor unit is called *fasciculation* and often is vigorous enough to be observed through the skin. Although most adult human muscles have only one neuromuscular junction per cell, an important exception is some of the cells in extraocular muscles. The extraocular muscles are "tonic" muscles, and unlike other mammalian striated muscles, they are multiply innervated, with several neuromuscular junctions strung along the surface of each muscle cell.[20,21] Quite in contrast to other muscles, even the adult ocular muscle contains mature and immature fetal receptors (see "Postjunctional Acetylcholine Receptors") segregated into distinct synapses on different fibers.[20] The ocular muscles contract and relax slowly rather than quickly as other striated muscles do; they can maintain a steady contraction, or contracture, the strength of which is proportional to the stimulus received. Physiologically, this specialization apparently holds the eye steadily in position. These muscles are important to an anesthesiologist because depolarizing relaxants affect them differently than they do most skeletal muscles. Instead of causing a brief contraction followed by paralysis, the drugs cause a long-lasting contracture response that pulls the eye against the orbit and could contribute to an increase in intraocular fluid pressure.[22] The clinical significance of a succinylcholine-induced increase in intraocular pressure has been questioned. Although many textbooks invoke the reported extrusion of intraocular content with succinylcholine, the basis for this effect seems to be anecdotal.[23]

The perijunctional zone is the area of muscle immediately beyond the junctional area, and it is critical to function of the neuromuscular junction. The perijunctional zone contains a mixture of receptors, including a smaller density of AChRs and a high density of sodium channels (see Fig. 14-1D). The admixture enhances the capacity of the perijunctional zone to respond to the depolarization (i.e., end-plate potential) produced by AChRs and to transduce it into the wave of depolarization that travels along the muscle to initiate muscle contraction. The density of sodium channels in the perijunctional area is richer than in more distal parts of the muscle membrane.[17,24] The perijunctional zone is close enough to the nerve ending to be influenced by transmitter released from it. Moreover, special variants (i.e., isoforms) of receptors and sodium channels can appear in this area at different stages of life and in response to abnormal decreases in nerve activity (see "Biology of Prejunctional and Postjunctional Nicotinic Receptors"). Congenital abnormalities in the AChR[4,5] or in the sodium and calcium channels (i.e., mutations)[25,26] are also known. These variabilities seem to contribute to the differences in response to relaxants that are seen in patients with different pathologic conditions and ages.[1-3,27]

Quantal Theory

The contents of nerve ending are not homogeneous. As shown in Figures 14-1 and 14-2, vesicles are congregated in the portion toward the junctional surface, whereas microtubules, mitochondria, and other support structures are located toward the opposite side. The vesicles containing transmitter are ordered in repeating clusters alongside small, thickened, electron-dense patches of membrane referred to as active zones or release sites. This thickened area is a cross section of a band running across the width of the synaptic surface of the nerve ending that is believed to be the structure to which vesicles attach (active zones) before they rupture into the junctional cleft (see "Process of Exocytosis"). High-resolution scanning electron micrographs reveal small protein particles arranged alongside the active zone between vesicles. These particles are believed to be special channels—voltage-gated calcium channels—that allow calcium to enter the nerve and cause the release of vesicles.[28,29] The rapidity with which the neurotransmitter is released (200 μsec) suggests that voltage-gated calcium channels are close to the release sites. Proteomic studies suggest that at least 26 genes encode presynaptic proteins, and mutations in 12 of them cause defects in presynaptic structure that can lead to decreased acetylcholine release and muscle weakness.[30] These defects can be related to exocytosis, endocytosis, formation of active and periactive zones, vesicle transport, and neuropeptide modulation.[30]

When observing the electrophysiologic activity of a skeletal muscle, small, spontaneous depolarizing potentials at neuromuscular junctions can be seen. These potentials have only one hundredth the amplitude of the evoked end-plate potential produced when the motor nerve is stimulated. Except for amplitude, these potentials resemble the end-plate potential in the time course and manner in which they are affected by drugs. These small-amplitude potentials are called miniature end-plate potentials (MEPPs). Statistical analysis led to the conclusion that they are unitary responses; that is, there is a minimum size for the MEPP, and the sizes of all MEPPs are equal to or multiples of this minimum size. Because MEPPs are too big to be produced by a single molecule of acetylcholine, it was deduced that they are produced by uniformly sized packages, or quanta, of transmitter released from the nerve (in the absence of stimulation). The stimulus-evoked end-plate potential is the additive depolarization produced by the synchronous discharge of quanta from several hundred vesicles. The action potential that is propagated to the nerve ending allows entry of calcium into the nerve through voltage-gated calcium channels, and this causes vesicles to migrate to the active zone, fuse with the neural membrane, and discharge their acetylcholine into the junctional cleft.[28,29] Because the release sites are located immediately opposite the receptors on the postjunctional surface, little transmitter is wasted, and the response of the muscle is coupled directly with the signal from the nerve.[17,28]

Alignment of the presynaptic receptor site is achieved by adhesion molecules or specific cell-surface proteins located on both sides of the synapse that grip each other across the synaptic cleft and hold the prejunctional and postjunctional synaptic apparatuses together.[15,31-33] One such protein implicated in synapse adhesion is neurexin, which binds to neuroligins on the postsynaptic membrane. The amount of acetylcholine released by each nerve impulse is large, at least 200 quanta of about 5000 molecules each, and the number of AChRs activated by transmitter released by a nerve impulse is also large, about 500,000 molecules. The ions (mostly Na^+ and some Ca^{2+}) that flow through the channels of activated AChRs cause maximum depolarization of the end plate, which results in an end-plate potential that is greater than the threshold for stimulation of the muscle. This system is very vigorous. The signal is carried by more molecules of transmitter than are needed, and they evoke a response that is greater than needed. At the same time, only a small fraction of the available vesicles and receptors or channels are used to send each signal. Consequently, transmission has a substantial margin of safety, and at the same time the system has substantial capacity in reserve.[34]

The Neuromuscular Junction

Formation of Neurotransmitter at Motor Nerve Endings

The axon of the motor nerve carries electrical signals from the spinal cord to muscles and has all of the biochemical apparatus needed to transform the electrical signal into a chemical one. All the ion channels, enzymes, other proteins, macromolecules, and membrane components needed by the nerve ending to synthesize, store, and release acetylcholine and other trophic factors are made in the cell body and transmitted to the nerve ending by axonal transport (Fig. 14-2).[19,31,33] The simple molecules choline and acetate are obtained from the environment of the nerve ending, the former by a special system that transports it from extracellular fluid to the cytoplasm and the latter in the form of acetyl coenzyme A from mitochondria. The enzyme choline acetyltransferase brings about the reaction of choline and acetate to form acetylcholine; the acetylcholine is stored in cytoplasm until it is transported into vesicles, which are in a better position for release.

Nerve Action Potential

During a nerve action potential, sodium from outside flows across the membrane, and the resulting depolarizing voltage opens calcium channels, which allows entry of calcium ions into the nerve and causes acetylcholine to be released. A nerve action potential is the normal activator that releases the transmitter acetylcholine. The number of quanta released by a stimulated nerve is greatly influenced by the concentration of ionized calcium in extracellular fluid. If calcium is not present, depolarization of the nerve, even by electrical stimulation, will not produce release of transmitter. Doubling the extracellular calcium results in a 16-fold increase in the quantal content of an end-plate potential.[35]

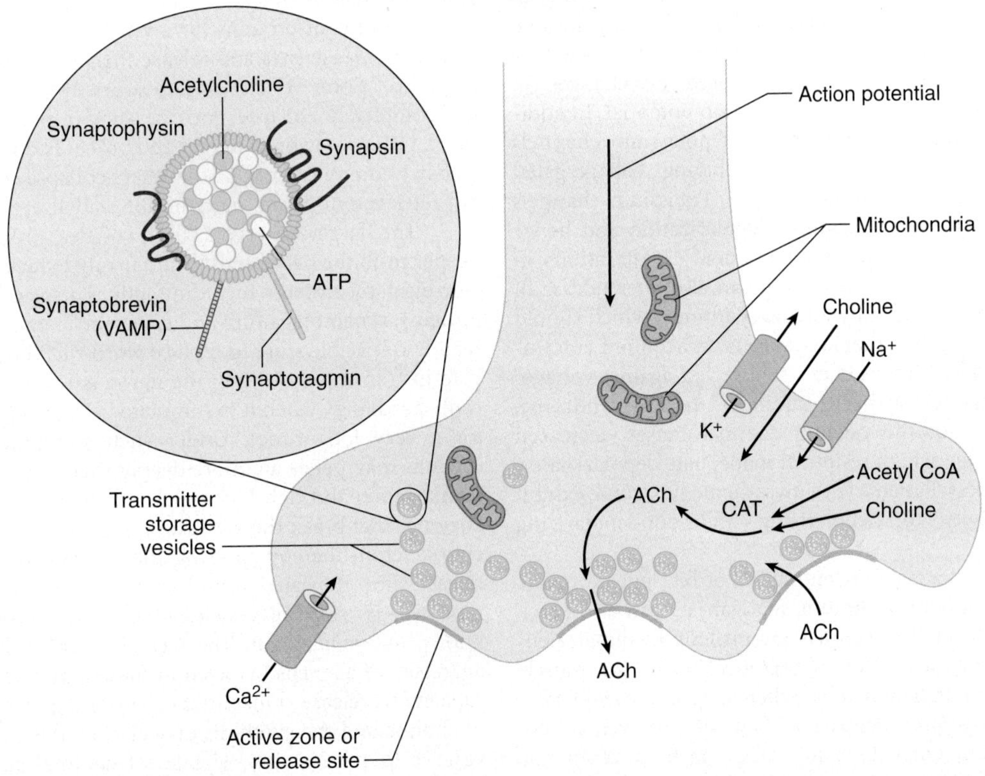

Figure 14-2 The working of a chemical synapse, the motor nerve ending, including some of the apparatus for synthesis of transmitter. The large intracellular structures are mitochondria. Acetylcholine (ACh), synthesized from choline and acetate by acetyl coenzyme A (acetyl CoA), is transported into coated vesicles, which are moved to release sites. A presynaptic action potential that triggers influx of calcium through specialized proteins (Ca^{2+} channels) causes the vesicles to fuse with the membrane and discharge transmitter. Membrane from the vesicle is retracted from the nerve membrane and recycled. Each vesicle can undergo various degrees of release of contents—from incomplete to complete. The transmitter is inactivated by diffusion, catabolism, or reuptake. The *inset* provides a magnified view of a synaptic vesicle. Quanta of ACh together with adenosine triphosphate (ATP) are stored in the vesicle and covered by vesicle membrane proteins. Synaptophysin is a glycoprotein component of the vesicle membrane. Synaptotagmin is the vesicle's calcium sensor. Phosphorylation of another membrane protein, synapsin, facilitates vesicular trafficking to the release site. Synaptobrevin (vesicle-associated membrane protein [VAMP]) is a SNARE protein involved in attaching the vesicle to the release site (see also Fig. 14-3). CAT, choline acetyltransferase.

The calcium current persists until the membrane potential is returned to normal by outward fluxes of potassium from inside the nerve cell. Along with calcium channels on the nerve terminal are potassium channels, including the voltage-gated and calcium-activated potassium channels, whose function is to limit entry of calcium into the nerve and therefore depolarization.[31,36] The calcium current can be prolonged by potassium channel blockers (e.g., 4-aminopyridine, tetraethylammonium), which slow or prevent the efflux of potassium out of the nerve. The increase in quantal content produced in this way can reach astounding proportions.[25,37] An effect of increasing calcium in the nerve ending is also seen clinically as the so-called post-tetanic potentiation, which occurs after a nerve of a patient paralyzed with an NDMR is stimulated at high, tetanic frequencies. Calcium enters the nerve with every stimulus, but because it cannot be excreted as quickly as the nerve is stimulated, it accumulates during the tetanic period. Because the nerve ending contains more than the normal amount of calcium for some time after the tetanus, a stimulus applied to the nerve during this time causes the release of more than the normal amount of acetylcholine. The abnormally large amount of acetylcholine antagonizes the relaxant and causes the characteristic increase in size of the twitch.

Calcium enters the nerve through specialized proteins called calcium channels.[15,25] Of the several types of calcium channels, two seem to be important for release of transmitter: P channels and the slower L channels. P channels, probably the type responsible for normal release of transmitter, are found only in nerve terminals.[13,38] In motor nerve endings, they are located immediately adjacent to the active zones (see Fig. 14-2). They are voltage dependent and opened and closed by changes in membrane voltage caused by the nerve action potential. In addition to calcium channels, several forms of potassium channels are present in the nerve terminal, including voltage-gated and calcium-activated potassium channels. Potassium channels limit the duration of nerve terminal depolarization and hence entry of calcium and release of transmitter.[25,31] Alterations in entry of calcium into the nerve ending can also alter release of transmitter. Eaton-Lambert myasthenic syndrome, which should not be confused with myasthenia gravis, is an acquired autoimmune disease in which antibodies are directed against voltage-gated calcium channels at nerve endings.[39] In this syndrome, decreased function of the calcium channel causes decreased release of transmitter, which results in inadequate depolarization and muscle weakness. Patients with myasthenic syndrome exhibit increased sensitivity to depolarizing and nondepolarizing relaxants.[3,4,31]

Higher than normal concentrations of bivalent inorganic cations (e.g., magnesium, cadmium, manganese) can also block entry of calcium through P channels and profoundly impair neuromuscular transmission. This is the mechanism for muscle weakness in the mother and fetus when magnesium sulfate is administered to treat preeclampsia. P channels, however, are not affected by calcium entry–blocking drugs such as verapamil, diltiazem, and nifedipine. These drugs have profound effects on the slower L channels present in the cardiovascular system. As a result, the L-type calcium channel blockers have no significant effect at therapeutic doses on the normal release of acetylcholine or on the strength of normal neuromuscular transmission. There have been a few reports, however, that calcium entry–blocking drugs may increase the block in neuromuscular transmission induced by NDMRs. The effect is small, and not all investigators have been able to observe it. The explanation may lie in the fact that nerve endings also contain L-type calcium channels.

Synaptic Vesicles and Recycling

There seem to be two pools of vesicles that release acetylcholine, a readily releasable pool and a reserve pool, sometimes called VP2 and VP1, respectively.[40,41] Vesicles in the former are a bit smaller and limited to an area very close to the nerve membrane, where they are bound to the active zones. These vesicles are the ones that ordinarily release transmitter. Electron microscopic studies have demonstrated that the majority of synaptic vesicles (VP1) are sequestered in the reserve pool and tethered to the cytoskeleton in a filamentous network composed mainly of actin, synapsin (an actin-binding protein), synaptotagmin, and spectrin.[40-42]

Release seems to occur when calcium ion enters the nerve through the P channels lined up on the sides of the active zones by SNARE proteins.[40-42] The SNARE (soluble *N*-ethylmaleimide–sensitive attachment protein receptors) proteins are involved in fusion, docking, and release of acetylcholine at the active zone. Calcium needs to move only a very short distance (i.e., a few atomic radii) to encounter a vesicle and activate the proteins in the vesicle wall involved in a process known as docking (see "Process of Exocytosis").[43] The reactivated proteins seem to react with the nerve membrane to form a pore through which the vesicle discharges its acetylcholine into the junctional cleft. Studies using fluorescent proteins have visualized how synaptic vesicles fuse with release sites and release their contents, which are then retrieved.[41] Some vesicles stay open briefly before retrieval and do not completely collapse into the surface membrane ("kiss and run"). Others stay open longer and probably do not collapse completely ("compensatory"). Still others collapse completely and are not retrieved until another stimulus is delivered ("stranded").[41]

The larger reserve (VP1) vesicles, from their position deeper from the nerve ending and firmly tethered to the cytoskeleton by many proteins, including actin, synapsin (an actin-binding protein), synaptotagamin, and spectrin,[40-42] may be moved to the readily releasable store to replace worn-out vesicles or to participate in transmission when the nerve is called on to work especially hard (e.g., when it is stimulated at very high frequencies or for a very long time). Under such strenuous circumstances, calcium may penetrate more deeply than normal into the nerve or may enter through L channels to activate calcium-dependent enzymes that break the synapsin links holding the vesicles to the cytoskeleton, thereby allowing the vesicles to be moved to the release sites. Repeated stimulation requires the nerve ending to replenish its store of vesicles filled with transmitter, a process known as *mobilization*. The term is commonly applied to the aggregate of all steps involved in maintaining the nerve ending's capacity to release transmitter—everything from the acquisition of choline and the synthesis of acetate to the movement of filled vesicles to release sites. Uptake of choline and the activity of choline acetyltransferase, the enzyme that synthesizes acetylcholine, are probably the rate-limiting steps.[13,29,38]

Process of Exocytosis

The readily releasable pool of synaptic vesicles constitutes the vesicles directly available for release. During an action potential

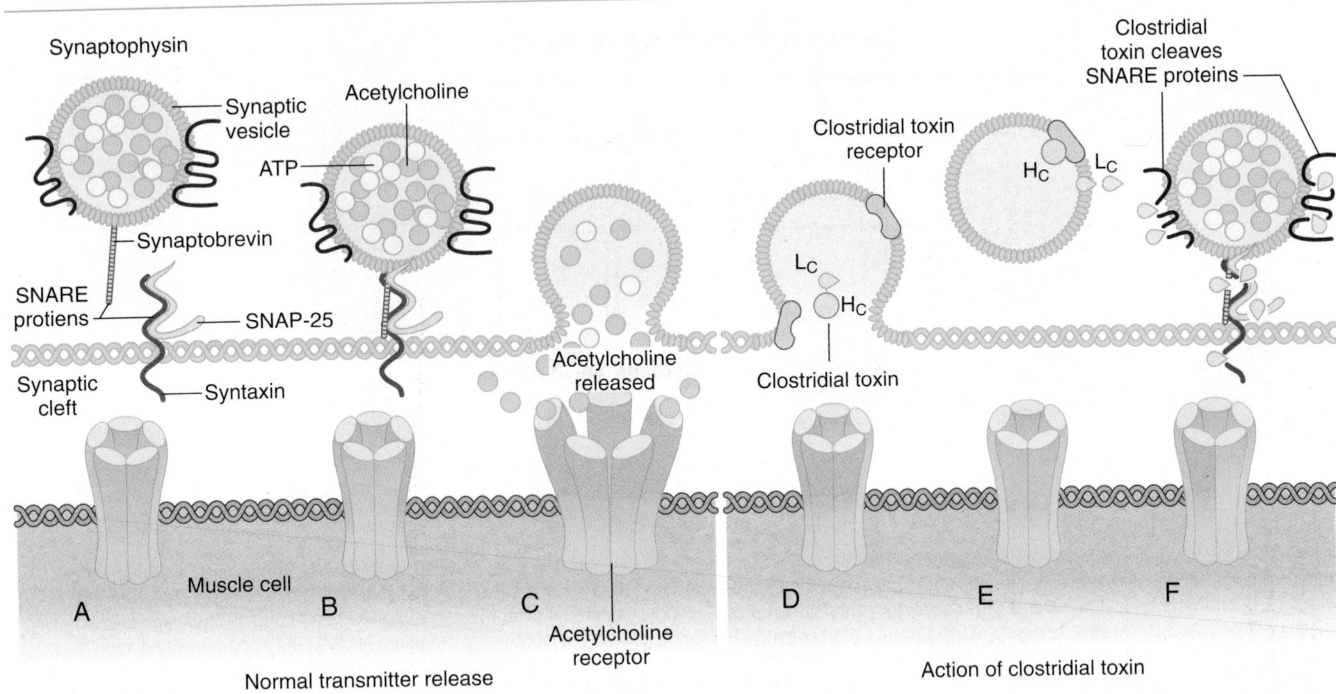

Figure 14-3 Model of protein-mediated membrane fusion and exocytosis. **A,** Release of acetylcholine from vesicles is mediated by a series of proteins collectively called SNARE proteins. Synaptotagmin is the neuronal calcium receptor that detects entry of calcium. Synaptobrevin (i.e., vesicle-associated membrane protein [VAMP]) is a filament-like protein on the vesicle. **B,** During depolarization and entry of calcium, synaptobrevin on the vesicle unfolds and forms a ternary complex with syntaxin/SNAP-25. This process is facilitated by phosphorylation of synapsin, also present on the vesicle membrane. **C,** Assembly of the ternary complex forces the vesicle in close apposition to the nerve membrane at the active zone with release of its contents, acetylcholine. The fusion is disassembled, and the vesicle is recycled. Clostridial toxins, including tetanus and botulinum, inhibit the release of acetylcholine and cause paralysis of muscles. The toxin consists of a light (L_c) and heavy (H_c) chain. **D,** The first stage in intoxication is interaction of the toxin with a thus far unidentified receptor. **E,** This is followed by internalization of the toxin within the vesicle and release of the light chain from the vesicle. The liberated L_c cleaves a variety of SNARE proteins, depending on the type of toxin released, thereby preventing assembly of the fusion complex and thus blocking release of acetylcholine.

and calcium influx, neurotransmitter is released. Studies have shed some light on the inner workings by which the vesicle releases its contents. The whole process is called *exocytosis.* The SNAREs include the synaptic-vesicle protein synaptobrevin and the plasmalemma-associated proteins syntaxin and synaptosome-associated protein of 25 kd (SNAP-25).[42] The current model of protein-mediated membrane fusion in exocytosis is as follows. Syntaxin and SNAP-25 are complexes attached to the plasma membrane. After initial contact, the synaptobrevin on the vesicle forms a ternary complex with syntaxin and SNAP-25. Synaptotagmin is the protein on the vesicular membrane that acts as a calcium sensor, localizes the synaptic vesicles to synaptic zones rich in calcium channels, and stabilizes the vesicles in the docked state.[44] Assembly of the ternary complex forces the vesicle close to the underlying nerve terminal membrane (i.e., the active zone), and the vesicle is then ready for release (Fig. 14-3). An action potential in the nerve terminal allows the entry of calcium. The close proximity of release sites, calcium channels, and synaptic vesicles and use of the calcium sensor lead to a burst of release of new transmitter synchronous with the stimulus.[42,44] The vesicle can release part or all of its contents, some of which can be recycled to form new vesicles as described previously (kiss and run, etc.).[40,41]

Botulinum toxin and tetanus neurotoxins, which selectively digest one or all of these SNARE proteins, block exocytosis of the vesicles.[45,46] The result is muscle weakness or paralysis. These toxins in effect produce a partial or complete chemical denervation. Botulinum toxin is used therapeutically to treat spasticity or spasm in several neurologic and surgical diseases and cosmetically to correct wrinkles.[47,48] Botulinum toxin consists of two protein segments known as heavy and light chains. The heavy chain interacts with lipid molecules called polysialogangliosides in the cell membrane and synaptotagmin on the vesicle to enter the vesicle. Once in the vesicle, the light chain inactivates neuromuscular transmission by breakdown and thereby inhibits the function of SNARE proteins (Fig. 14-4). Recent reports indicate an increased incidence of clostridial infections in both Canada and the United States, with *Clostridium botulinum* infection being particularly common after traumatic injuries, in drug abusers, and after musculoskeletal allografts.[49] Thus, systemic paralysis can occur after clostridial infection. Local injection for therapeutic purposes will usually result in localized paresis, although systemic effects have been reported.[50]

Acetylcholinesterase

The acetylcholine released from the nerve diffuses across the junctional cleft and reacts with specialized receptor proteins in the end plate to initiate muscle contraction. Transmitter molecules that do not react immediately with a receptor or those released after binding to the receptor are destroyed almost instantly by acetylcholinesterase in the junctional cleft. Acetyl-

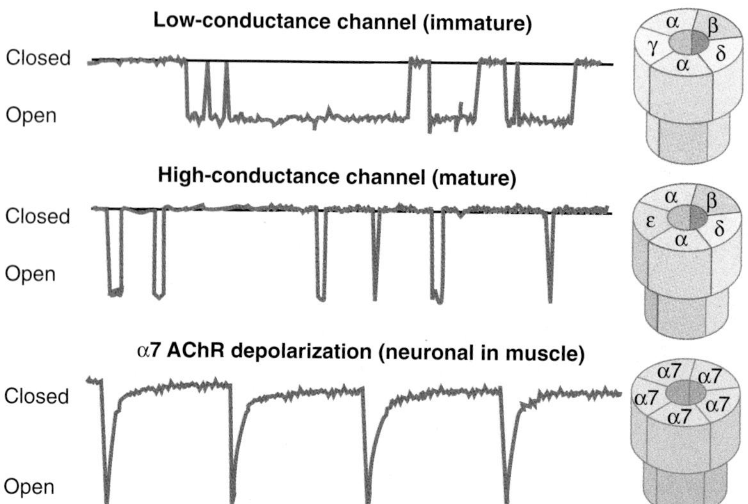

Figure 14-4 Sketch of acetylcholine receptor (AChR) channels (*right*) and tracings of cell-patch records of receptor channel openings (*left*). The mature, or junctional, receptor consists of two α-subunits and one each of β-, δ-, and ε-subunits. The immature, extrajunctional or fetal, form consists of two α- and one each of β, δ, and γ-subunits. The latter is thus called the γ-subunit receptor. Recently, a neuronal receptor consisting of five α7-subunits has been described in muscle. All the subunits are arranged around the central cation channel. The immature isoform containing the γ-subunit has long open times and low-amplitude channel currents. The mature isoform containing the ε-subunit has shorter open times and high-amplitude channel currents during depolarization. Substitution of the ε-subunit for the γ-subunit gives rise to the fast-gated, high-conductance channel type. As expected, application of acetylcholine to the α7 AchR also results in a fast, rapidly decaying inward current. All these depolarizing events are insensitive to treatment with atropine but sensitive to treatment with α-bungarotoxin or muscle relaxants, which block the flow of current.

cholinesterase at the junction is the asymmetric or A12-form protein made in the muscle, under the end plate. Acetylcholinesterase (enzyme classification 3.1.1.7) is a type B carboxylesterase enzyme. There is a smaller concentration of it in the extrajunctional area. The enzyme is secreted from the muscle but remains attached to it by thin stalks of collagen fastened to the basement membrane.[13,17] Most of the molecules of acetylcholine released from the nerve initially pass between the enzymes to reach the postjunctional receptors, but as they are released from the receptors, they invariably encounter acetylcholinesterase and are destroyed. Under normal circumstances, a molecule of acetylcholine reacts with only one receptor before it is hydrolyzed. Acetylcholine is a potent messenger, but its actions are very short lived because it is destroyed in less than 1 millisecond after it is released.

Some congenital and acquired diseases are caused by altered activity of acetylcholinesterase. Congenital absence of the secreted enzyme (in knock-out mice) leads to impaired maintenance of the motor neuronal system and organization of nerve terminal branches.[51] Many syndromes caused by congenital abnormalities in cholinesterase function have been described and result in neuromuscular disorders whose symptoms and signs usually resemble those of myasthenia gravis or myasthenic syndromes.[52,53] Denervation decreases acetylcholinesterase at the junctional and extrajunctional areas.[31] Other acquired diseases involving cholinesterases are related to chronic inhibition of acetylcholinesterase by organophosphate pesticides or nerve gas (e.g., sarin) or to chronic pyridostigmine therapy given as prophylaxis against nerve gas poisoning.[54,55] Symptoms ranging from chronic fatigue to muscle weakness have been attributed to chronic cholinesterase inhibition, thus underscoring the importance of acetylcholinesterase in normal and abnormal neuromuscular function.

Postjunctional Acetylcholine Receptors

The similarity of AChRs among many species and the abundance of AChRs from *Torpedo* electric fish have greatly facilitated research in this area. The availability of messenger RNA from humans and other species and DNA has allowed study of the receptor in artificial systems such as oocytes from frogs and in mammalian cells that do not express the receptor, such as COS or fibroblast cells. It is also possible to mutate receptors by molecular techniques so that they simulate pathologic states and then study receptor function in these artificial systems. By using these and related techniques, much has been learned about the synthesis, composition, and biologic function and the mechanisms that underlie physiologic and pharmacologic responses in AChRs.[56-59] Three isoforms of postjunctional nicotinic AChRs exist, a junctional or mature receptor, an extrajunctional or immature (fetal) receptor, and the most recently described neuronal α7 receptor (see "Biology of Prejunctional and Postjunctional Nicotinic Receptors").[1-3] The differences between receptor subtypes, however, can be neglected in a general discussion of the role of receptors in neuromuscular transmission.

AChRs are synthesized in muscle cells and are anchored to the end-plate membrane by a special 43-kd protein known as rapsyn. This cytoplasmic protein is associated with the AChR in a 1:1 ratio.[31] The receptors, formed of five subunit proteins, are arranged like the staves of a barrel into a cylindrical receptor with a central pore for ion channeling. The key features are sketched in Figure 14-4. The receptor protein has a molecular mass of about 250,000 daltons. Each receptor has five subunits. The mature receptor consists of α, β, δ, and ε and the fetal (immature, extrajunctional) receptor, α, β, δ, and γ; there are two subunits of α and one of each of the others. The neuronal α7 AChR consists of five α7-subunits.[2] Each of all receptor subunits consists of approximately 400 to 500 amino acids. The receptor-protein complex passes entirely through the membrane and protrudes beyond the extracellular surface of the membrane and into the cytoplasm. The binding site for acetylcholine is on each of the α-subunits, and these are the sites of competition between receptor agonists and antagonists. Agonists and antagonists are attracted to the binding site, and either may occupy the site, which is located near cysteine residues (unique to the α-chain) at amino acid positions 192-193 of the α-subunit.[60] Radiolabeled α-bungarotoxin from the cobra, used to quantitate the receptor, binds to heptapeptide region 189-199 of the α-subunit.[61] Motor neuron–derived neuregulin-1β (NRβ-1), originally described as acetylcholine receptor–inducing activity (ARIA), induces AChR gene transcription in subsynaptic myonuclei by activating ErbB receptors.[62]

Synthesis and Stabilization of Postjunctional Receptors

Muscle tissue is formed from the mesoderm and initially appears as myoblasts. Myoblasts fuse to produce myotubes, which therefore have multiple nuclei. As the myotubes mature, the sarcomere, which is the contractile element of the muscle consisting of actin and myosin, develops.[63] The protein β-integrin seems to be essential for myoblast fusion and sarcomere assembly.[63] Shortly afterward, motor nerve axons grow into the developing muscle, and these axons bring in nerve-derived signals (i.e., growth factors), including agrin and neuregulins (NRβ-1 and NRβ-2), which are key to maturation of myotubes to muscle.[62] Agrin is a protein from the nerve that stimulates postsynaptic differentiation by activating muscle-specific kinase (MuSK), a tyrosine kinase expressed selectively in muscle. With signaling from agrin, the AChRs, which have been scattered throughout the muscle membrane, cluster at the area immediately beneath the nerve. Agrin together with other growth factors (neuregulins, etc.) also induce the clustering of other critical muscle-derived proteins, including MuSK, rapsyn, and ErbB proteins, all of which are necessary for maturation and stabilization of AChRs at the junction (Fig. 14-5). In addition to effects on postsynaptic differentiation, agrin and MuSK display effects on presynaptic differentiation as well. Agrin and MuSK induce retrograde signals that instruct axons to undergo neuron outgrowth and terminal differentiation.[19] Current understanding of presynaptic development of the neuromuscular junction, however, is much less advanced than understanding of postsynaptic development. Just before and shortly after birth, the immature, γ-subunit–containing AChRs are converted to the mature, ε-subunit–containing receptors. Although the mechanism of this change is unclear, a neuregulin, NRβ-1, also called ARIA, that binds to one of the ErbB receptors seems to play a role.[44,62-65]

Basic Electrophysiology of Neurotransmission

Progress in electrophysiologic techniques has moved at an equal pace with advances in molecular approaches for studying prejunctional and postjunctional receptors. Patch-clamping is a technique in which a glass micropipette is used to probe the membrane surface until a single functional receptor is encompassed. The tip of the pipette is pressed into the lipid of the membrane, and the electronic apparatus is arranged to keep the membrane potential clamped (i.e., fixed) and measure the current that flows through the channel of the receptor. The solution in the pipette can contain acetylcholine, muscle relaxant, another drug, or a mixture of drugs. By application of these drugs to the receptor through the micropipette, electrical changes can be monitored.

Figure 14-5 illustrates the results of the classic depolarizing action of acetylcholine on end-plate receptors. Normally, the pore of the channel is closed by approximation of the cylinders (i.e., subunits). When an agonist occupies both α-subunit sites, the protein molecule undergoes a conformational change in which a channel is formed in the center through which ions can flow along a concentration gradient. When the channel is open, sodium and calcium flow from the outside of the cell to the inside and

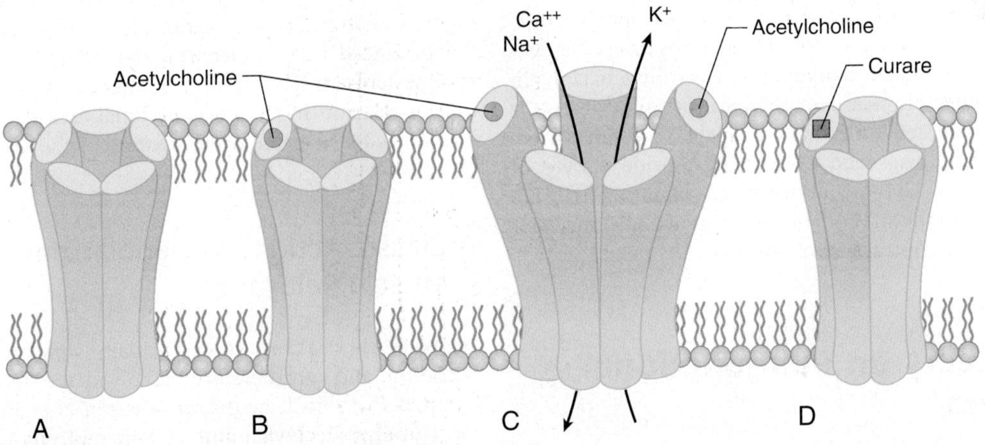

Figure 14-5 Actions of acetylcholine or curare on end-plate receptors. **A,** The ion channel is inactive and does not open in the absence of acetylcholine. **B,** Even binding of one acetylcholine molecule (*filled circle*) to one of two binding sites does not open the channel. **C,** When acetylcholine binds to the recognition sites of both α-subunits simultaneously (*filled circles*), a conformation change is triggered that opens the channel and allows ions to flow across the membrane. **D,** Action of antagonists such as curare (*filled square*). Acetylcholine is in competition with tubocurarine for the receptor's recognition site but may also react with acetylcholinesterase. Tubocurarine is a prototypical nondepolarizing muscle relaxant. Inhibiting the enzyme increases the lifetime of acetylcholine and the probability that it will react with a receptor. When one of the two binding (recognition) sites is occupied by curare, the receptor will not open, even if the other binding site is occupied by acetylcholine.

potassium flows from the inside to the outside. The channel in the tube is large enough to accommodate many cations and electrically neutral molecules, but it excludes anions (e.g., chloride). The current carried by the ions depolarizes the adjacent membrane. The net current is depolarizing and creates the end-plate potential that stimulates the muscle to contract. In this instance, downward-going (i.e., depolarizing) current can be recorded by the electrophysiologic technique described previously (see Fig. 14-4).

The pulse stops when the channel closes and one or both agonist molecules detach from the receptor. The current that passes through each open channel is minuscule, only a few picoamperes (about 10^4 ions/msec). However, each burst of acetylcholine from the nerve normally opens about 500,000 channels simultaneously, and the total current is more than adequate to produce depolarization of the end plate and contraction of muscle. Opening of a channel causes conversion of chemical signals from a nerve to flow of current to end-plate potentials, thereby leading to muscle contraction. We are used to thinking of the end-plate potential as a graded event that may be reduced in magnitude or extended in time by drugs, but in reality, the end-plate potential is the summation of many all-or-nothing events occurring simultaneously at myriad ion channels. It is these tiny events that are affected by drugs.

Receptors that do not have two molecules of agonist bound remain closed. Both α-subunits must be occupied simultaneously by agonist; if only one of them is occupied, the channel remains closed (see Fig. 14-5). This is the basis for prevention of depolarization by antagonists. NDMRs typified by tubocurarine act by binding to either or both α-subunits and thus preventing acetylcholine from binding and opening the channel. This interaction between agonists and antagonists is competitive, and the outcome—transmission or block—depends on the relative concentrations and binding characteristics of the drugs involved (see "Drug Effects on Postjunctional Receptors").

Individual channels are also capable of a wide variety of conformations.[66-68] They may open or stay closed and thereby affect total current flow across the membrane, but they can do more. They may open for a longer or shorter time than normal, open or close more gradually than usual, open briefly and repeatedly (i.e., chatter), or pass fewer or more ions per opening than they usually do. Their function is also influenced by drugs, changes in fluidity of the membrane, temperature, electrolyte balance in the milieu, and other physical and chemical factors.[68] Receptor channels are dynamic structures that are capable of a wide variety of interactions with drugs and of entering a wide variety of current-passing states. All these influences on channel activity are ultimately reflected in the strength or weakness of neuromuscular transmission and the contraction of a muscle.

Drug Effects on Postjunctional Receptors

Classic Actions of Nondepolarizing Muscle Relaxants

Neurotransmission occurs when acetylcholine released by the nerve action potential binds to AChRs. All NDMRs impair or block neurotransmission by competitively preventing the binding of acetylcholine to its receptor. The final outcome (i.e., block or transmission) depends on the relative concentrations of the chemicals and their comparative affinities for the receptor. Figure 14-5 shows a system exposed to acetylcholine and tubocurarine. One receptor has attracted two acetylcholine molecules and opened its channel, where current will flow to depolarize that segment of membrane. Another has attracted one tubocurarine molecule; its channel will not open, and no current will flow, even if one acetylcholine molecule binds to the other site. The third receptor has acetylcholine on one α-subunit and nothing on the other. What will happen depends on which of the molecules binds. If acetylcholine binds, the channel will open and the membrane will be depolarized; if tubocurarine binds, the channel will stay closed and the membrane will not be depolarized. At other times, one or two tubocurarine molecules may attach to the receptor, in which case the receptor is not available to agonists; no current flow is recorded. In the presence of moderate concentrations of tubocurarine, the amount of current flowing through the entire end plate at any instant is reduced from normal, which results in a smaller end-plate potential and, if carried far enough, a block in neurotransmission or production of neuromuscular paralysis.

Normally, acetylcholinesterase destroys acetylcholine and removes it from competition for a receptor, so tubocurarine has a better chance of inhibiting transmission. If, however, an inhibitor of acetylcholinesterase such as neostigmine is added, the cholinesterase cannot destroy acetylcholine. The concentration of agonist in the cleft remains high, and this high concentration shifts the competition between acetylcholine and tubocurarine in favor of the former, thereby improving the chance of two acetylcholine molecules binding to a receptor even though tubocurarine is still in the environment. Cholinesterase inhibitors overcome the neuromuscular paralysis produced by NDMRs by this mechanism. The channel opens only when acetylcholine attaches to both recognition sites. A single molecule of antagonist, however, is adequate to prevent depolarization of that receptor. This modifies the competition by biasing it strongly in favor of the antagonist. Mathematically, if the concentration of tubocurarine is doubled, the concentration of acetylcholine must be increased fourfold if acetylcholine is to remain competitive. Paralysis produced by high concentrations of antagonist is more difficult to reverse than that produced by low concentrations. After large doses of NDMRs, cholinesterase inhibitors may be ineffective until the concentration of relaxant in the perijunctional area decreases to a lower level by redistribution or elimination of the drug.

Classic Actions of Depolarizing Muscle Relaxants

Depolarizing relaxants, at least initially, simulate the effect of acetylcholine and can therefore be considered agonists despite the fact that they block neurotransmission after initial stimulation. Structurally, succinylcholine is two molecules of acetylcholine bound together. It is thus not surprising that it can mimic the effects of acetylcholine. Succinylcholine or decamethonium can bind to the receptor, open the channel, pass current, and depolarize the end plate. These agonists, similar to acetylcholine, attach only briefly; each opening of a channel is of very short duration, 1 millisecond or less. The response to acetylcholine, however, is over in milliseconds because of its rapid degradation by acetylcholinesterase, and the end plate resets to its resting state long before another nerve impulse arrives. In contrast, the depolarizing relaxants characteristically have a biphasic action on muscle—an initial contraction, followed by relaxation lasting minutes to hours. Because they are not susceptible to hydrolysis by acetylcholinesterase, the depolarizing relaxants are not eliminated from the junctional cleft until after they are eliminated from plasma. The time required to clear the drug from the body is the principal determinant of how long the drug effect lasts. Whole-body clearance of the relaxant is very slow in comparison to acetylcholine, even when plasma cholinesterase is normal. Because relaxant molecules are not cleared from the cleft quickly, they react repeatedly with receptors, attaching to one almost immediately after separating from another, thereby repeatedly depolarizing the end plate and opening channels.

The quick shift from excitation of muscle contraction to blockade of transmission by depolarizing relaxants occurs because the end plate is continuously depolarized. This comes about as a result of juxtaposition of the edge of the end plate with the muscle membrane—a different kind of ion channel, the sodium channel, that does not respond to chemicals but opens when exposed to a transmembrane voltage change. The sodium channel is also a cylindrical transmembrane protein through which sodium ions can flow. Two parts of its structure act as gates that allow or stop the flow of sodium ions.[69] Both gates must be open if sodium is to flow through the channel; closing of either cuts off the flow. Because these two gates act sequentially, a sodium channel has three functional conformational states and can move progressively from one state to another (Fig. 14-6).

When the sodium channel is in its resting state, the lower gate (i.e., the time-dependent or inactivation gate) is open, but the upper gate (i.e., the voltage-dependent gate) is closed, and sodium ions cannot pass. When the molecule is subjected to a sudden change in voltage by depolarization of the adjacent membrane, the top gate opens, and because the bottom (time-dependent) gate is still open, sodium flows through the channel. The voltage-dependent gate stays open as long as the molecule is experiencing a depolarizing influence from the membrane around it; it will not close until the depolarization disappears. However, shortly after the voltage-dependent gate opens, the bottom gate closes and again cuts off the flow of ions. It cannot open again until the voltage-dependent gate closes. When depolarization of the end plate stops, the voltage-dependent gate closes, the time-dependent gate opens, and the sodium channel returns to its resting state. This whole process is short lived when depolarization occurs with acetylcholine. The initial response of a depolarizing muscle relaxant resembles that of acetylcholine, but because the relaxant is not hydrolyzed rapidly, depolarization of the end plate is not brief.

Depolarization of the end plate by the depolarizing relaxant initially causes the voltage gate in adjacent sodium channels to open, thereby producing a wave of depolarization that sweeps along the muscle and generates a muscle contraction. Shortly after the voltage-dependent gate opens, the time-dependent inactivation gate closes. Because the relaxant is not removed from the cleft, the end plate continues to be depolarized. Because the sodium channels immediately adjacent to the end plate are influenced by depolarization of the end plate, their voltage-dependent gates stay open and their inactivation gates stay closed. Since sodium cannot flow through a channel that has a closed inactivation gate, the perijunctional muscle membrane does not depolarize. When the flow of ions through sodium channels in the perijunctional zone stops because of closure of the inactivation gates, the channels downstream (beyond the perijunctional zone) are freed of depolarizing influence. In effect, the perijunctional zone becomes a buffer that shields the rest of the muscle from events at the end plate. Consequently, the muscle membrane is separated into three zones: the end plate, which is depolarized by succinylcholine; the perijunctional muscle membrane, in which the sodium channels are frozen in an inactivated state; and the rest of the muscle membrane, in which the sodium channels are in the resting state. Because a burst of acetylcholine from the nerve cannot overcome the inactivated sodium channels in the perijunctional zone, neuromuscular transmission is blocked. This phenomenon is also called *accommodation*. During accommodation, when the synapse is inexcitable through the nerve (transmitter), direct electrical stimulation of muscle causes muscle contraction because the sodium channels beyond the junctional area are in the resting excitable state.

The extraocular muscles contain tonic muscle, which is multiply innervated and chemically excitable along most of its surface.[20,21] Despite its innervation, the ocular muscles express both mature and fetal receptors.[20] Accommodation does not occur, and these muscles can undergo a sustained contracture in the presence of succinylcholine. The tension thus developed forces the eye against the orbit and accounts for part of the increase in intraocular pressure produced by depolarizing relaxants. There is also evidence that the extraocular muscles contain a special type of receptor that does not become desensitized (discussed later) during the continued presence of acetylcholine or other agonists.[21] Whether it is the immature γ-subunit AChR or the α7 AChR that plays a role in this resistance to desensitization in the ocular muscles is unknown.

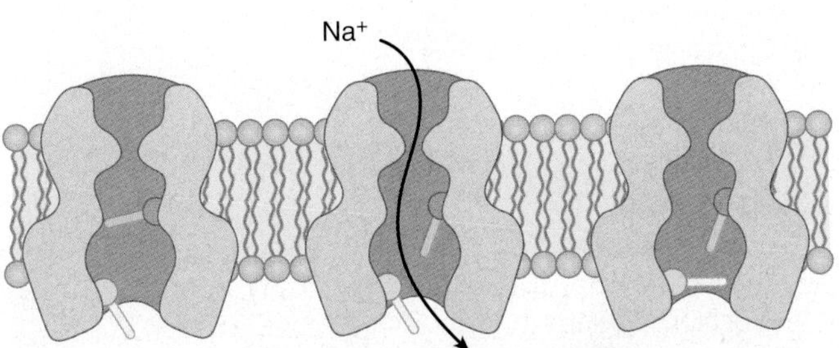

Figure 14-6 Sketch of a sodium channel. The *bars* represent parts of the molecule that act as gates. The *upper bar* is voltage dependent; the *lower bar* is time dependent. The left side of the drawing represents the resting state. Once activated by a change in voltage, the molecule and its gates progress as illustrated (left to right). See text for details.

Nonclassic and Noncompetitive Actions of Neuromuscular Drugs

Several drugs can interfere with the receptor, directly or through its lipid environment, and change transmission. These drugs react with the neuromuscular receptor to change its function and impair transmission but do not act through the acetylcholine binding site. These reactions cause drug-induced changes in the dynamics of the receptor, and instead of opening and closing sharply, the modified channels are sluggish. They open more slowly and stay open longer, or they close slowly and in several steps, or both. These effects on channels cause corresponding changes in the flow of ions and distortions of the end-plate potential. The clinical effect depends on the molecular events. For example, procaine, ketamine, inhaled anesthetics, or other drugs that dissolve in the membrane lipid may change the opening or closing characteristics of the channel.[70,71] If the channel is prevented from opening, transmission is weakened. If, however, the channel is prevented from or slowed in closing, transmission may be enhanced. These drugs do not fit the classic model, and the impaired neuromuscular function is not antagonized by increasing perijunctional acetylcholine concentrations with cholinesterase inhibitors. Such drugs can be involved in two clinically important reactions: receptor desensitization and channel blockade. The former occurs in the receptor molecule, whereas the latter occurs in the ion channel.

Desensitization Block

The AChR, as a result of its flexibility and the fluidity of the lipid around it, is capable of existing in a number of conformational states.[68-73] Because the resting receptor is free of agonist, its channel is closed. The second state exists when two molecules of agonist are bound to the α-subunit of the receptor and the receptor has undergone the conformation change that opens the channel and allows ions to flow. These reactions are the bases of normal neuromuscular transmission. Some receptors that bind to agonists, however, do not undergo the conformational change to open the channel. Receptors in these states are called desensitized (i.e., they are not sensitive to the channel-opening actions of agonists). They bind agonists with exceptional avidity, but the binding does not result in opening of the channel. The mechanisms by which desensitization occurs are not known. The receptor macromolecule, 1000 times larger by weight than most drugs or gases, provides many places at which the smaller molecules may act. The interface between lipid and receptor protein provides additional potential sites of reaction. Several different conformations of the protein are known, and because acetylcholine cannot cause the ion channel to open in any of them, they all are included in the functional term *desensitization*. Some evidence suggests that desensitization is accompanied by phosphorylation of a tyrosine unit in the receptor protein.[74,75]

Although agonists (e.g., succinylcholine) induce desensitization, the receptors are in a constant state of transition between resting and desensitized states, regardless of whether agonists are present. Agonists do promote transition to a desensitized state or, because they bind very tightly to desensitized receptors, trap a receptor in a desensitized state. Antagonists also bind tightly to desensitized receptors and can trap molecules in these states. This action of antagonists is not competitive with that of acetylcholine; it may be augmented by acetylcholine if the latter promotes the change to a desensitized state. Desensitization can lead to significant misinterpretation of data. Superficially, the preparation seems to be normal, but its responsiveness to agonists or antagonists is altered. One variety occurs very rapidly, within a few milliseconds after application of an agonist. This may explain the increased sensitivity to nondepolarizers after prior administration of succinylcholine. There is also a phenomenon caused by prolonged administration of depolarizing relaxants that is known as *phase II block* (see "Phase II Block"). It is frequently referred to as a desensitization block but should not be because desensitization of receptors is only one of many phenomena that contribute to the process.

Many other drugs used by anesthetists also promote the shift of receptors from a normal state to a desensitized state.[70-73] These drugs, some of which are listed in Box 14-1, can weaken neuromuscular transmission by reducing the margin of safety that normally exists at the neuromuscular junction, or they can cause an apparent increase in the capacity of nondepolarizing agents to block transmission. These actions are independent of the classic effects based on competitive inhibition of acetylcholine. The presence of desensitized receptors means that fewer receptor channels than usual are available to carry transmembrane current. The production of desensitized receptors decreases the efficacy of neuromuscular transmission. If many receptors are desensitized, insufficient normal ones are left to depolarize the

Box 14-1 Drugs That Can Cause or Promote Desensitization of Nicotinic Cholinergic Receptors

- Volatile anesthetics
  - Halothane
  - Sevoflurane
  - Isoflurane
- Antibiotics
  - Polymyxin B
- Cocaine
- Alcohols
  - Ethanol
  - Butanol
  - Propanol
  - Octanol
- Barbiturates
  - Thiopental
  - Pentobarbital
- Agonists
  - Acetylcholine
  - Decamethonium
  - Carbachol
  - Succinylcholine
- Acetylcholinesterase inhibitors
  - Neostigmine
  - Pyridostigmine
  - Difluorophosphate
  - Edrophonium
- Local anesthetics
  - Dibucaine
  - Lidocaine
  - Prilocaine
  - Etidocaine
- Phenothiazines
  - Chlorpromazine
  - Trifluoperazine
  - Prochlorperazine
- Phencyclidine
- Calcium channel blockers
  - Verapamil

motor end plate, and neuromuscular transmission will not occur. Even if only some receptors are desensitized, neuromuscular transmission will be impaired, and the system will be more susceptible to block by conventional antagonists such as tubocurarine or pancuronium.

Channel Block

Local anesthetics and calcium entry blockers prevent the flow of sodium or calcium through their respective channels, thus explaining the term *channel-blocking drugs*. Similarly, block of the flow of ions can occur at the AChR with concentrations of drugs used clinically and may contribute to some of the phenomena and drug interactions seen at the receptor. Two major types, closed-channel and open-channel block, can occur.[76,77] In a closed-channel block, certain drugs can occupy the mouth of the channel and prevent ions from passing through the channel to depolarize the end plate. The process can take place even when the channel is not open. In an open-channel block, a drug molecule enters a channel that has been opened by reaction with acetylcholine but does not necessarily penetrate all the way through. Open-channel blockade is a use-dependent block, which means that molecules can enter the channel only when it is open. In open- and closed-channel blocks, the normal flow of ions through the receptor is impaired, thereby resulting in prevention of depolarization of the end plate and a weaker or blocked neuromuscular transmission. However, because the action is not at the acetylcholine recognition site, it is not a competitive antagonism of acetylcholine and is not relieved by anticholinesterases that increase concentrations of acetylcholine. Increasing the concentration of acetylcholine may cause the channels to open more often and consequently become more susceptible to blockade by use-dependent compounds. There is evidence that neostigmine and related cholinesterase inhibitors can act as channel-blocking drugs.[76]

Channel block is believed to play a role in some of the antibiotic, cocaine, quinidine, piperocaine, tricyclic antidepressant, naltrexone, naloxone, and histrionicotoxin-induced alterations in neuromuscular function. Muscle relaxants, in contrast, can bind to the acetylcholine recognition site of the receptor and occupy the channel. Pancuronium preferentially binds to the recognition site. Gallamine seems to act equally at the two sites. Tubocurarine is in between; at low doses, those that produce minimal blockage of transmission clinically, the drug is essentially a pure antagonist at the recognition site; at larger doses, it also enters and blocks channels. Decamethonium and succinylcholine, as agonists, can open channels and, as slender molecules, also enter and block them. Decamethonium and some other long, thin molecules can penetrate all the way through the open channel and enter the cytoplasm of muscle cells. Whether prolonged administration of NDMRs, as in the intensive care situation, can result in entry of the relaxant, occupation of the channel, and entry of drug into the cytosol is unknown. This effect may partially explain the muscle weakness associated with relaxant therapy in the intensive care unit.

Phase II Block

A phase II block is a complex phenomenon that occurs slowly at junctions continuously exposed to depolarizing agents. The junction is depolarized by the initial application of a depolarizing relaxant, but then the membrane potential gradually recovers toward normal, even though the junction is still exposed to drug. Neuromuscular transmission usually remains blocked throughout the exposure. Several factors are involved. The repeated opening of channels allows a continuous efflux of potassium and influx of sodium, and the resulting abnormal electrolyte balance distorts the function of the junctional membrane. Calcium entering the muscle through the opened channels can cause disruption of receptors and the sub–end-plate elements themselves. The activity of the sodium-potassium adenosine triphosphatase pump in the membrane increases with increasing intracellular sodium and, by pumping sodium out of the cell and potassium into it, works to restore the ionic balance and membrane potential toward normal. As long as the depolarizing drug is present, the receptor channels remain open and ion flux through them remains high.[78]

Factors influencing the development of a phase II block include the duration of exposure to the drug, the particular drug used and its concentration, and even the type of muscle (i.e., fast or slow twitch). Interactions with anesthetics and other agents also affect the process. All of these drugs may also have prejunctional effects on the rate and amount of transmitter released and mobilized. With so many variables involved in the interference with neuromuscular transmission, a phase II block is a complex and ever-changing phenomenon. The reversal response of a phase II block produced by a depolarizing muscle relaxant to administration of cholinesterase inhibitors is difficult to predict. It is therefore best that reversal by cholinesterase inhibitors not be attempted, although the response to tetanus or train-of-four stimulation resembles that produced by nondepolarizers.

Biology of Prejunctional and Postjunctional Nicotinic Acetylcholine Receptors

Postjunctional Conventional Acetylcholine Receptors in Muscle versus Neuronal Acetylcholine Receptors in Muscle

Currently, three variants of postjunctional AChRs have been identified. The AChR isoform present in the innervated, adult neuromuscular junction is referred to as the adult, mature, or junctional receptor. Another AChR isoform is expressed when there is decreased activity in muscle, as seen in the fetus before innervation or after chemically or physically induced immobilization; after lower or upper motor neuron injury, burns, or sepsis; or after other events that cause increased muscle protein catabolism, including sepsis or generalized inflammation.[1-3] To contrast with the mature or junctional receptors, the other isoform is referred to as the immature, extrajunctional, or fetal form of AChR. Some evidence suggests that the immature isoform is not seen in the muscle protein catabolism and wasting that occur with malnutrition.[79] Differences in the protein structure of the two isoforms cause significant qualitative variations in the responses of individual patients to relaxants and seem to be responsible for some of the anomalous results observed when administering relaxants to particular individuals. These qualitative differences in isoforms can also cause variations in function of the muscle.[52,53]

In addition to their structural compositions, the two isoforms have other characteristics that are different.[1-3,31] At the molecular level, both types of receptors consists of five subunits (see Fig. 14-4). The mature junctional receptor is a pentamer of two α-subunits and one each of the β-, δ-, and ε-subunits. The immature receptor consists of two α-subunits and one each of the β-, δ-, and γ-subunits; that is, in the immature receptor the γ-subunit is present instead of the ε-subunit. The γ- and ε-subunits differ from each other very little in amino acid homology, but the differences are great enough to affect the physiology and pharmacology of the receptor and its ion channel. Although the names junctional and extrajunctional imply that each is located in the junctional and extrajunctional areas, this is not strictly correct. Junctional receptors are always confined to the end plate (perijunctional) region of the muscle membrane. The immature, or extrajunctional, receptor may be expressed anywhere in the muscle membrane. Despite the name extrajunctional, they are not excluded from the end plate. During development and in certain pathologic states, junctional and extrajunctional receptors can coexist in the perijunctional area of the muscle membrane (Fig. 14-7).

Quite in contrast to the conventional muscle AChRs consisting of α1, β1, δ, and ε/γ subunits described earlier, receptors formed of α7 AChR subunits have recently been found in skeletal muscle during development and denervation.[80,81] Preliminary evidence (Martyn JAJ, abstract ASA 2007) suggests increased protein expression (by Western blotting) of α7 AChRs in muscle after burn injury and immobilization. These α7 AChRs are homomeric (i.e., formed of the same subunits) channels arranged as pentameres (see Fig. 14-4). Ligand (drug) binding pockets are thought to be formed at negative and positive faces of the α7-subunit assembly interphases. As expected, the endogenous agonist acetylcholine binds to α7 AChRs, and each of the five subunits has the potential to bind acetylcholine or succinylcholine molecules.[82,83] Other agonists, including nicotine and choline, and antagonists, including muscle relaxants, pancuronium, cobra toxin, and α-bungarotoxin, also bind to the α7 AChR.[81-83]

The α7 AChRs in muscle display unusual functional and pharmacologic characteristics when compared with conventional muscle (α1, β1, δ, ε/γ) AChRs or neuronal α7 AChRs in the brain. Choline, a precursor and metabolite of acetylcholine (and succinylcholine), is an extremely weak agonist of conventional muscle AChRs but is a full agonist of muscle α7 AChRs; that is, concentrations of choline that do not open conventional AChR channels will open α7 AChR channels.[81] Furthermore, no desensitization of the α7 AChR occurs even during the continued presence of choline,[81] thus allowing a greater chance for potassium to efflux from within the cell (approximately 145 mEq/L in the cell) to the extracellular space, including plasma (approximately 4.5 mEq/L), down its concentration gradient. The chemical α-conotoxin GI specifically inhibits the conventional (mature and immature) AChRs in muscle but does not inhibit α7 AChRs. Muscle α7 AChRs are different from neuronal (autonomic ganglia and brain) α7 AChRs in that the former are not strongly inhibited by methyllycaconitine, a selective antagonist of neuronal α7 AChRs. The α7 AChRs expressed in neuronal tissue are also readily desensitized with choline,[83] a feature that contrasts with muscle α7 AChRs, which do not desensitize with choline.[81] The α7 AChR in muscle also has lower affinity for its antagonists, including pancuronium

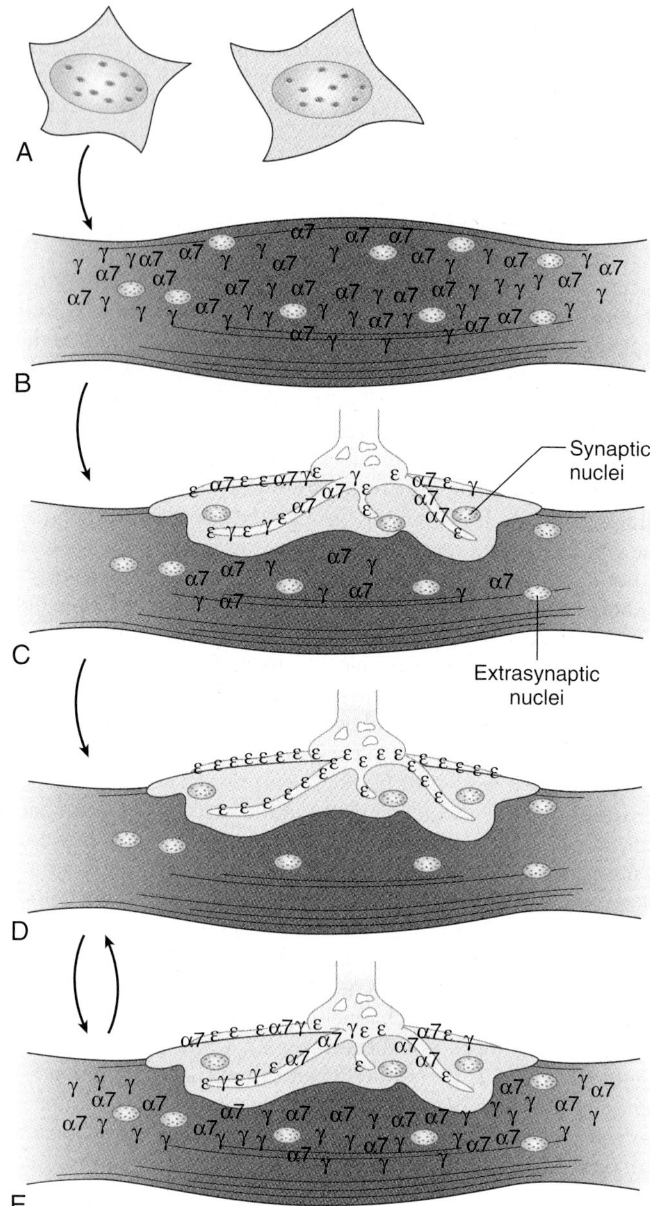

Figure 14-7 Distribution of acetylcholine receptors in developing adult, mature, denervated muscle or in immobilized or inflammation-induced catabolic muscle. **A** and **B,** In the early fetal stage, mononucleated myoblasts, derived from the mesoderm, fuse with each other to form multinucleated myotubes. The γ-subunit–containing immature acetylcholine receptors and the neuronal α7 acetylcholine receptors are scattered throughout the muscle membrane before innervation. **C,** As the nerve makes contact with muscle, clustering of the receptors occurs at the synapse and is associated with some loss of extrasynaptic receptors. **D,** Maturation of the junction is said to occur when ε-subunit–containing receptors replace the γ-subunit– and α7-containing acetylcholine receptors at the neuromuscular junction. Even mature muscle is multinucleated, but it is devoid of extrasynaptic acetylcholine receptors. **E,** Denervation and some other pathologic states, even without anatomic denervation (e.g., burns, immobilization, chronic muscle relaxant therapy, stroke, sepsis), lead to re-expression of the γ-subunit– and α7-containing acetylcholine receptors at the junctional and extrajunctional areas. The latter changes are potentially reversible if muscle immobilization/catabolism/inflammation is restored to normal.

and α-bungarotoxin; higher concentrations of these drugs are therefore required to block agonist-induced depolarization in α7 AChRs than in conventional muscle AChRs (α1, β1, δ, ε/γ).[81] In the conventional AChRs, binding of even one of the α1-subunits by an antagonist results in inactivation of that receptor because acetylcholine needs both α1-subunits of the AChR for its activation. In the α7 AChR, however, even when three subunits are bound by an antagonist (e.g., muscle relaxant), two other subunits are still available for binding to agonist and causing depolarization. This feature may account for the resistance of α7 AChRs, as opposed to conventional AChRs, to the blocking effects of drugs such as pancuronium.[2]

The clinical pharmacology of the muscle α7 AChR has not been studied yet, but its basic pharmacology provides some insight into succinylcholine-related hyperkalemia. Chemical or physical denervation of muscle results in not only upregulation and qualitative (ε-subunit → γ-subunit) changes in AChRs but also upregulation of α7 AChRs in muscle. Succinylcholine, a synthetic analog of acetylcholine that consists of two molecules of acetylcholine joined together, is capable of depolarizing not only conventional AChRs but also α7 AChRs in muscle.[83] In addition, the metabolite of succinylcholine, choline, can depolarize α7 AChRs with little desensitization. The depolarizing effects of succinylcholine and choline on the upregulated α7 AChRs can result in continued leakage of intracellular potassium and flooding of extracellular fluid, including plasma, thereby leading to hyperkalemia.

Maintenance of Mature Neuromuscular Junctions

Quite unlike other cells, muscle cells are unusual in that they have many, usually hundreds, of nuclei per cell. Each of these nuclei has the genes to make both types of receptors. Multiple factors, including electrical activity, growth factor signaling (e.g., insulin, agrin, neuregulins), and the presence or absence of innervation, control expression of the three types of receptor isoforms.[19,31] This is most clearly seen in the developing embryo as the neuromuscular junction is formed. Before they are innervated, the muscle cells of a fetus synthesize only immature and α7 AChRs—hence the term fetal isoform for the former receptor. Synthesis is directed by nearly all the nuclei in the cell, and the receptors are expressed throughout the membrane of the muscle cell (see Fig. 14-7). As the fetus develops and the muscles become innervated, muscle cells begin to synthesize the mature isoform of receptors, which are inserted exclusively into the developing (future) end-plate area. The nerve releases several growth factors that influence the synthetic apparatus of the nearby nuclei. First, nerve-supplied factors induce the subsynaptic nuclei to increase synthesis of AChRs. Next, the nerve-induced electrical activity results in repression of receptors in the extrajunctional area. Nerve-derived growth factors, including agrin and ARIA/neuregulin, cause the receptors to cluster in the subsynaptic area and prompt expression of the mature isoform (Fig. 14-8).[62-65] In conditions associated with insulin resistance, there seems to be a proliferation of AChRs beyond the junctional area. Conditions in which insulin resistance (i.e., decreased growth factor signaling) has been observed include immobilization, burns, and denervation.[84-86] In such conditions, there is associated upregulation of AChRs and expression of the immature and α7 AChR isoforms.[1-3] Therefore, agrin and neuregulin signaling may be important for suppression of α7 AChRs.

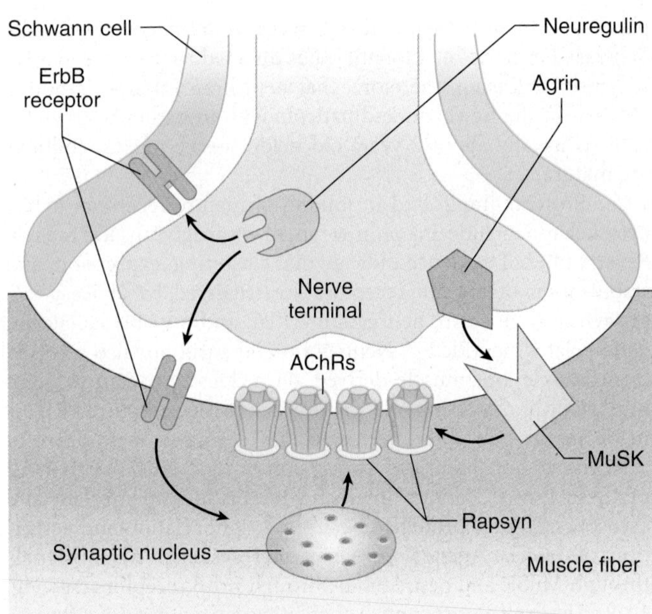

Figure 14-8 Diagram of agrin- and ARIA (acetylcholine receptor–inducing activity)/neuregulin-dependent events during maturation of the neuromuscular junction. After establishment of a nerve on the muscle, growth factors, including agrin and neuregulins, are released. Neuregulin signaling is essential for Schwann cell survival, and Schwann cells are essential for axonal maintenance. Agrin interacting with its receptor MuSK (muscle-specific kinase) enhances the clustering of synaptic proteins, including acetylcholine receptors (AChRs), rapsyn, and ErbB receptors. ARIA/neuregulin is the best candidate for involvement in the conversion of γ-subunit–containing immature receptor to ε-subunit–containing mature (innervated) receptor, which is synapse specific and therefore not inserted in the extrajunctional area.

Before innervation, AChRs are present throughout the muscle membrane. After innervation, AChRs become more and more concentrated at the postsynaptic membrane and are virtually absent in the extrasynaptic area at birth. The innervation process progresses somewhat slowly during fetal life and matures during infancy and early childhood.[15,27,33] With time, the immature receptors diminish in concentration and disappear from the peripheral part of the muscle. In active, adult, normal innervated muscle, just the nuclei under and very near the end plate direct the synthesis of receptor; only the genes for expressing mature receptors are active. Nuclei beyond the junctional area are not active, and therefore no receptors are expressed anywhere in the muscle cells beyond the perijunctional area. Conversion of all of the γ-subunit– to ε-subunit–containing AChRs in the perijunctional area continues to take place after birth. In the rodent, it takes about 2 weeks.[15] In humans, this process takes longer. The timeframe for disappearance of α7 AChRs in the fetus or newborn is also unknown.

At birth, the postsynaptic membrane itself is also not as specialized; the newborn junction has simplified synaptic folds, a widened synaptic space, and reduced numbers of AChRs. Morphologically, the postsynaptic membrane of the newborn and that from a patient with myasthenia gravis are not too different. In patients with myasthenia gravis, receptor numbers are usually decreased because of autoantibodies directed against the AChR.[4] It is not surprising, therefore, that neurotransmission is not as efficient in the newborn and patients with myasthenia gravis. A child is usually about 2 years old before nerve-muscle contacts are mature.[27]

Proteins implicated in linking of mature receptors to the cytoskeleton include utrophin, α- and β-dystroglycan, and rapsyn. Several lines of evidence indicate that clustering, expression, and stabilization of mature receptors are triggered by at least two growth factors: agrin, neuregulin/ARIA, and possibly calcitonin gene–related peptide.[62-65] Neuregulin and agrin are also released from muscle, but muscle-derived agrin does not seem to be as important in clustering and maturation of the receptor. ARIA is made in the nerve and seems to play a role in maturation of vesicular arrangement and conversion of the γ-to-ε switch.[65] All of these growth factors interact with distinct membrane and cytosolic receptor proteins to cause phosphorylation and activation of nuclear (gene) transcriptional systems. Agrin signals through MuSK and neuregulins through ErbB receptors (see Fig. 14-8). These receptors control qualitative and quantitative changes at the junction. Once begun, the process is very stable, and nuclei in the junctional area continue to express mature receptors.

Re-expression of Immature (Fetal) γ-Subunit and α7-Subunit AChRs in Adult Life

The extrajunctional immature receptors can reappear soon after upper and lower motor denervation and in certain pathologic states (e.g., burns, immobilization, chronic muscle relaxant therapy, loss of electrical activity). Stimulation of a denervated muscle with an external electrical stimulus can prevent the appearance of immature receptors. It has been suggested that the calcium that enters the muscle during activity is important in the suppression process.[16,17] In the pathologic states previously enumerated, if the process is severe and prolonged, extrajunctional receptors are inserted all over the surface of the muscle, including the perijunctional area (see Fig. 14-7). The junctional nuclei also continue to make mature receptors. The end plates consist of mature and immature receptors. The synthesis of immature receptors is initiated within hours of inactivity, but it takes several days for the whole muscle membrane to be fully covered with receptors. This upregulation of receptors has implications for the use of depolarizing and nondepolarizing relaxants. The changes in α7 AChRs seem to parallel the expression of immature receptors, although this has not been well studied.

The changes in subunit composition (γ versus ε) in the receptor confer certain changes in electrophysiologic (functional), pharmacologic, and metabolic characteristics.[1,33] Mature receptors are metabolically stable, with a half-life approximating 2 weeks, whereas immature receptors have a metabolic half-life of less than 24 hours. Immature receptors have a smaller single-channel conductance and a 2- to 10-fold longer mean channel open time than mature receptors do (see Fig. 14-4). The changes in subunit composition may also alter the sensitivity or affinity, or both, of the receptor for specific ligands. Depolarizing or agonist drugs such as succinylcholine and acetylcholine depolarize immature receptors more easily, thereby resulting in cation fluxes; doses one tenth to one hundredth of those needed for mature receptors can effect depolarization.[2] The potency of nondepolarizers is also reduced, as demonstrated by the resistance to nondepolarizers documented in patients with burns, denervation, and immobilization.[1,3] This resistance may be related to decreased affinity of the immature and α7 AChRs to NDMRs and to the upregulation of receptors in the perijunctional area. Data suggest that some NDMRs may also cause a partial agonist response in immature receptors, thus explaining the decreased potency.[7] The altered sensitivities for cholinergic ligands may also result from changes in composition of the lipid membrane surrounding the receptor that is known to occur in some pathologic states.[68]

The altered sensitivity to muscle relaxants may occur in just certain parts of the body or certain muscles if only some muscles are affected by the diminution in nerve activity (e.g., after a stroke). Sensitivity to relaxants can begin to change between 24 and 72 hours after an injury or hospitalization. The most serious side effect with the use of succinylcholine in the presence of upregulated AChRs in one or more muscles is hyperkalemia.[1-3] In these subjects, the receptors can be scattered over a large surface of the muscle. The AChR channels opened by the agonist (succinylcholine) allow potassium to escape from the muscle and enter the blood. If a large part of the muscle surface consists of upregulated (immature) receptor channels, each of which stays open for a longer time, the amount of potassium that moves from muscle to blood can be considerable. The resulting hyperkalemia can cause dangerous disturbances in cardiac rhythm, including ventricular fibrillation. Moreover, it is difficult to prevent the hyperkalemia by prior administration of NDMRs because the extrajunctional receptors are not very sensitive to blockade by NDMRs in the usual doses.[1] Larger than normal doses of NDMRs may attenuate the increase in blood potassium but cannot completely prevent it. However, hyperkalemia and cardiac arrest can occur after the administration of succinylcholine, even in the absence of denervation states. This is seen in certain congenital muscle dystrophies in which the muscle membrane is prone to damage by the potassium released into the circulation by succinylcholine.[87]

Prejunctional Acetylcholine Receptors

AChRs exist in a variety of forms apart from that seen in muscle.[6,88] These receptors are expressed in peripheral neurons, autonomic and sensory ganglia, and the central nervous system. There is also direct and indirect evidence of their existence in lymphocytes, fibroblasts, chondrocytes, macrophages, and granulocytes.[14] Diverse genes encode the heterogeneous AChRs, and the ion channel is formed of multiple subunits (multimers). Seventeen AChR genes have been cloned from vertebrates. They include various combinations of α-subunits (α1 through α10) and β-subunits (β1 through β4) and one each of γ-, δ-, and ε-subunits. The γ-, δ-, and ε-subunits are found only in muscle.

Prejunctional or nerve terminal–associated cholinergic receptors have been demonstrated pharmacologically and by molecular biologic techniques, but their form and functions are not as completely understood as those in the postjunctional area. Many drugs with an abundance of potential targets for drug action can affect the capacity of the nerve terminal to carry out its functions. The trophic function to maintain nerve-muscle contact involves release and replenishment of acetylcholine together with trophic factors that require signaling through many receptors, of which the prejunctional nicotinic AChR is just one. Succinylcholine produces fasciculations that can be prevented by NDMRs. Because a fasciculation is, by definition, the simultaneous contraction of the multitude of muscle cells in a single motor unit and because only the nerve can synchronize all the muscles in its motor unit, it became apparent that succinylcholine must also act on nerve endings also. Because NDMRs prevent fasciculation, it was concluded that they acted on the same prejunctional receptor. Since then it has been shown many times that very small doses of cholinergic agonists (e.g., succinylcholine) and antagonists (e.g., NDMRs) affect nicotinic receptors on the nerve ending, the former by depolarizing the ending and sometimes inducing repetitive firing of the nerve and the latter by preventing the action of agonists.[6]

Another clue to differences between prejunctional and postjunctional AChRs was the finding that prejunctional AChRs can bind β-bungarotoxin only, whereas postjunctional receptors can also bind to α-bungarotoxin. Additional clues were found in the many demonstrations of quantitative differences in the reaction of prejunctional and postjunctional nicotinic receptors to cholinergic agonists and antagonists.[82,88] For instance, it was known that tubocurarine binds very poorly to the recognition sites of ganglionic nicotinic cholinoceptors and is not a competitive antagonist of acetylcholine at this site. Decamethonium is a selective inhibitor of the muscle receptor, and hexamethonium is a selective inhibitor of nicotinic receptors in the autonomic ganglia.[89,90] Instead, D-tubocurarine and hexamethonium can block the opened channels of these receptors and owe their ability to block ganglionic transmission to this property. The functional characteristics of prejunctional receptor channels may also be different. For example, the depolarization of motor nerve endings initiated by administration of acetylcholine can be prevented by tetrodotoxin, a specific blocker of sodium flux with no effect on the end plate.

Specific information on the molecular organization of neuronal nicotinic receptors on the motor neuron terminal is still lacking. Some of the subunit composition is similar, but other subunits do not resemble those of the postjunctional receptor. Of the 16 different nicotinic AChR gene products identified, only 12 (α2 to α10 and β2 to β4) are thought to contribute nicotinic receptors expressed on neurons. Most strikingly, nervous tissue does not contain genes for γ-, δ-, or ε-receptor subunits; it contains genes only for the α- and β-subunits. The α- and β-subunit genes in nerve and muscle are not exactly the same; they are variants. Muscle contains the genes for each of the α1 and α7 subunits. In contrast, nervous tissue does not contain α1 subunit gene but instead contains a number of related genes designated α2 through α10. To emphasize the distinction between neural and muscle nicotinic receptors, the former are sometimes designated Nn and the latter Nm. With so many different subunits available, there are many possible combinations, and it is not known which combinations are found in motor nerves. Their physiologic roles have also not been completely characterized. Expression of neuronal nicotinic AChRs in in vitro systems has confirmed that muscle relaxants and their metabolites can bind to some of these neuronal AChRs.[89,90]

The nicotinic receptor on the junctional surface of the nerve senses transmitter in the cleft and, by means of a positive-feedback system, causes the release of more transmitter. In other parts of the nervous system, this positive feedback is complemented by a negative-feedback system that senses when the concentration of transmitter in the synaptic cleft has increased appropriately and shuts down the release system. It is believed that tetanic fade and train-of-four fade during neuromuscular blockade with NDMRs arise from presynaptic cholinergic autoreceptors at the motor nerved ending.[58,59] The neuronal AChR subtype on the nerve terminal that causes fade has been identified as α3β2.[90-93] Quite in contrast, succinylcholine does not inhibit the presynaptic α3β2 autoreceptor at clinically relevant concentrations.[59,93] This may be reason for the typical lack of fade during succinylcholine-induced neuromuscular block. Succinylcholine, however, does not interact with α3β4 AChR found in autonomic ganglia.[59] It has also been shown that NDMRs reduce the hypoxic ventilatory response in partially paralyzed humans,[94] and the mechanism behind the depression might be related to inhibition of nicotine receptors on the carotid body.[9] The motor nerve terminal is also known to bear several other receptors, such as opioid, adrenergic, dopamine, purine, and adenosine receptors, as well as receptors for endogenous hormones, neuropeptides, and a variety of proteins. The physiologic roles of these receptors and the effects of anesthetics on them are unknown.

Antagonism of Neuromuscular Blockade

Mechanism of Antagonism

The NDMRs block neuromuscular transmission predominantly by competitive antagonism of acetylcholine at the postjunctional receptor. The most straightforward way to overcome their effects is to increase the competitive position of acetylcholine. Two factors are important, the first of which is the concentration of acetylcholine. Increasing the number of molecules of acetylcholine in the junctional cleft changes the agonist-to-antagonist ratio and increases the probability that agonist molecules will occupy recognition sites of the receptor. It also increases the probability that an unoccupied receptor will become occupied. Normally, only about 500,000 of the 5 million available receptors are activated by a single nerve impulse, and a large number of receptors are in "reserve" and could be occupied by an agonist. The second factor important to the competitive position of acetylcholine is the length of time that acetylcholine is in the cleft. Acetylcholine must wait for the antagonist to dissociate spontaneously before it can compete for the freed site. NDMRs bind to the receptor for slightly less than 1 millisecond, which is longer than the normal lifetime of acetylcholine. The destruction of acetylcholine normally takes place so quickly that most of it is destroyed before any significant number of antagonist molecules have dissociated from the receptor. Prolonging the time during which acetylcholine is in the junction allows time for the available acetylcholine to bind to receptor when the antagonist dissociates from the receptors.

Classes of Drugs Used

Three classes of drugs, potassium channel–blocking drugs, acetylcholinesterase inhibitors, and γ-cyclodextrin derivatives, can be used clinically to reverse nondepolarizer-induced paralysis.[95,96] The best known of the potassium-blocking drugs is 4-aminopyridine. Its actions are predominantly prejunctional; it impedes efflux of potassium from the nerve ending. Because efflux of potassium is the event that normally ends the action potential of the nerve ending, this action prolongs depolarization of the nerve. Because the flux of calcium into the nerve continues for as long as the depolarization lasts, drugs of this class indirectly increase the flux of calcium into the nerve ending. The nerve releases more acetylcholine and for a longer time than usual, conditions that are effective in antagonizing NDMRs. Because they act prejunctionally, these drugs can antagonize a block produced by certain antibiotics that act on the nerve ending, notably the polymyxins. Although 4-aminopyridine and drugs like it can be used clinically, their use is severely restricted because they are not specific. They affect the release of transmitters by all nerve endings, including motor nerves, autonomic nerves, and central nervous system components. Their use is accompanied by a variety of undesirable effects, and in practice they are used only in special circumstances. A most serious side effect of potassium channel blockers is seizures.

The more commonly used antagonists of neuromuscular block (e.g., neostigmine, pyridostigmine, edrophonium) inhibit acetylcholinesterase by mechanisms that are similar but not identical.[95] Neostigmine and pyridostigmine are attracted by an electrostatic interaction between the positively charged nitrogen in the molecules and the negatively charged catalytic site of the enzyme. This produces a carbamylated enzyme that is not capable of further action (i.e., the catalytic site is blocked and the enzyme is inhibited). Edrophonium has neither an ester nor a carbamate group, but it is attracted and bound to the catalytic site of the enzyme by the electrostatic attraction between the positively charged nitrogen in the drug and the negatively charged acetylcholinesterase site of the enzyme. Edrophonium also seems to have prejunctional effects that enhance release of acetylcholine from the nerve terminal. This effect is therefore useful when deep neuromuscular block needs reversal. Of the three commonly used anticholinesterases, edrophonium shows far greater selectivity than acetylcholinesterase and butyrylcholinesterase, the serum esterase that hydrolyzes succinylcholine and mivacurium. It greatly favors the former enzyme and therefore seems to be the most desirable agent to reverse mivacurium. However, if the patient has normal serum esterase, pharmacokinetic factors are the principal determinants of the duration of block, and the activity of serum esterase or the lack of it plays only a minor role in recovery. There is little reason to prefer one or another reversal drug on these grounds. Anticholinesterases are administered for prolonged periods for the treatment of myasthenia gravis[4] and as prophylaxis in cases of nerve gas poisoning.[54,55] Ironically, prolonged administration of cholinesterase inhibitors can also lead to a myasthenia-like state with muscle weakness.[97]

Cholinesterase inhibitors act preferentially at the neuromuscular junction but also act at other synapses that use the same transmitter, including muscarinic receptors. An atropine-like drug should be administered with the cholinesterase inhibitor to counter the effects of the acetylcholine that accumulates in the muscarinic synapses of the gut, bronchi, and cardiovascular system. The three anticholinesterase inhibitors do not affect synapses in the central nervous system because all are quaternary ammonium ions that do not easily penetrate the blood-brain barrier. A quaternary ammonium derivative of atropine such as glycopyrrolate, which does not diffuse through the blood-brain barrier, is frequently used to limit the anticholinergic effects to the periphery. Other cholinesterase inhibitors, notably physostigmine and tacrine, are not quaternary ammonium compounds and they have profound effects on the central nervous system. They may be antagonized by atropine but not by its quaternary ammonium analog derivatives. Unlike the other cholinesterase inhibitors, physostigmine and tacrine are also potent inhibitors of the enzyme phosphodiesterase, which plays an important role in the regulation of transmitter release at many synapses in the central nervous system. This action may be related to the reported efficacy of these two drugs in the treatment of Alzheimer's dementia.

Cholinesterase inhibitors also have actions at the postjunctional membrane independent of their effects on the enzyme. Several of these compounds contain methyl groups on a positively charged nitrogen, and they can act as agonists on receptor channels by initiating flow of ions and enhancing neuromuscular transmission. Neostigmine, physostigmine, and certain organophosphates can increase the frequency of MEPPs and the quantal content of end-plate potentials, but the importance of the increased release of transmitter to reversal of neuromuscular blockade is not clear. Continuous exposure to carbamate- or organophosphate-containing inhibitors causes degeneration of prejunctional and postjunctional structures, apparently because these structures accumulate toxic amounts of calcium.[54,55] Calcium channel blockers such as verapamil prevent the neural actions of these drugs. All the drugs of this class also act in or on receptors to influence the kinetics of the open-close cycle and block the ion channel.[76,77] The clinical significance of the drugs on reversal of NDMRs is not known.

A new approach to reversing residual neuromuscular blockade is by direct binding of the relaxant by means of chemical interaction. Antidote drugs that work by binding other drugs include protamine, citrate anticoagulation, lead or copper chelators, and RNA molecules recombinantly engineered to bind drugs. Cyclodextrins (i.e., small, cyclic polysaccharides) are one such compound synthesized from starch by bacteria as early as 1891. The γ-cyclodextrin derivative ORG25969 (sugammadex) binds steroidal relaxants with very high affinity, which results in inactive muscle relaxants. The kidney then removes these complexes. Sugammadex has the potential to dramatically change clinical patterns of use of neuromuscular blocking drugs and their antagonists (i.e., neostigmine).[96]

References

1. Martyn JAJ, Fukushima Y, Chon JY, Yang S: Up-and-down regulation of skeletal muscle acetylcholine receptors. Intl Anesthesiol Clin 44:123, 2006.
2. Martyn JAJ, Richtsfeld M: Succinylcholine-induced hyperkalemia in acquired pathologic states: Etiologic factors and molecular mechanisms. Anesthesiology 104:158, 2006.
3. Martyn JAJ, White DA, Gronert GA, et al: Up-and down-regulation of skeletal muscle acetylcholine receptors. Anesthesiology 26:872, 1992.
4. Conti-Fine BM, Milani M, Kaminski HJ: Myasthenia gravis: Past, present, and future. J Clin Invest 116:2843, 2006.
5. Vincent A, Dalton P, Clover L, et al: Antibodies to neuronal targets in neurological and psychiatric diseases. Ann N Y Acad Sci 992:48, 2003.
6. Johnson WC, Prior C, Marshall IG: Presynaptic receptors in the neuromuscular junction. Ann N Y Acad Sci 604:69, 1990.
7. Fletcher GH, Steinbach JH: Ability of depolarizing neuromuscular blocking drugs to act as partial agonists at fetal and adult mouse muscle nicotinic receptors. Mol Pharmacol 49:938, 1996.
8. Paul M, Kindler CH, Fokt RM, et al: Isobolographic analysis of non-depolarising muscle relaxant interactions at their receptor site. Eur J Pharmacol 438:35, 2002.
9. Jonsson M, Wyon N, Lindahl SGE: Neuromuscular blocking agents block carotid body neuronal nicotinic acetylcholine receptors. Eur J Pharmacol 497:173, 2004.
10. Jooste E, Zhang Y, Emala CW: Neuromuscular blocking agents' differential bronchoconstrictive potential in Guinea pig airways. Anesthesiology 106:763, 2007.
11. Fryer AD, Maclagan J: Pancuronium and gallamine are antagonists for pre- and post-junctional muscarinic receptors in the guinea-pig lung. Naunyn Schmiedebergs Arch Pharmacol 335:367, 1987.
12. Lichtman JW, Conchello JA: Fluorescence microscopy. Nat Methods 2:910, 2005.
13. Kelly RB: The cell biology of the nerve terminal. Neuron 1:431, 1988.
14. Kalamida D, Poulas K, Avramopoulou V, et al: Muscle and neuronal nicotinic acetylcholine receptors: Structure, function and pathogenicity. FEBS Lett 274:3799, 2007.
15. Sanes JR, Lichtman JW: Induction, assembly, maturation and maintenance of a postsynaptic apparatus. Nat Rev Neurosci 2:791, 2001.
16. Bruneau EG, Akaaboune M: The dynamics of recycled acetylcholine receptors at the neuromuscular junction in vivo. Development 133:4485, 2006.
17. Cohen-Cory S: The developing synapse: Construction and modulation of synaptic structures and circuits. Science 298:770, 2002.
18. Aldunate R, Casar JC, Brandan E, Inestrosa NC: Structural and functional organization of synaptic acetylcholinesterase. Brain Res Brain Res Rev 47:96, 2004.
19. Song Y, Panzer JA, Wyatt RM, Balice-Gordon RJ: Formation and plasticity of neuromuscular synaptic connections. Int Anesthesiol Clin 44:145, 2006.
20. Fraterman S, Khurana TS, Rubinstein NA: Identification of acetylcholine receptor subunits differentially expressed in singly and multiply innervated fibers of extraocular muscles. Invest Ophthalmol Vis Sci 47:3828, 2006.
21. Buttner-Ennever JA, Horn AK: Oculomotor system: A dual innervation of the eye muscles from the abducens, trochlear, and oculomotor nuclei. Mov Disord 2:S2, 2002.
22. Durant NN, Katz RL: Suxamethonium. Br J Anaesth 54:195, 1982.
23. Vachon CA, Warner DO, Bacon DR: Succinylcholine and the open globe. Tracing the teaching. Anesthesiology 99:220, 2003.
24. Betz WJ, Caldwell JH, Kinnamon SC: Increased sodium conductance in the synaptic region of rat skeletal muscle fibers. J Physiol (Lond) 352:189, 1984.
25. Engel AG: The therapy of congenital myasthenic syndromes. Neurotherapeutics 4:252, 2007.
26. Yu FH, Catterall WA: Overview of the voltage-gated sodium channel family. Genome Biol 4:207, 2003.
27. Goudsouzian NG, Standaert FG: The infant and the myoneural junction. Anesth Analg 65:1208, 1986.
28. Heuser JE, Reese TS: Structural changes after transmitter release at the frog neuromuscular junction. J Cell Biol 88:564, 1981.
29. Rash JE, Walrond JP, Morita M: Structural and functional correlates of synaptic transmission in the vertebrate neuromuscular junction. J Electron Microsc Tech 10:153, 1988.
30. Sieburth D, Ch'ng Q, Dybbs M, et al: Systematic analysis of genes required for synapse structure and function. Nature 436:510, 2005.
31. Naguib M, Flood P, McArdle JJ, Brenner HR: Advances in neurobiology of the neuromuscular junction: Implications for the anesthesiologist. Anesthesiology 96:202, 2002.
32. Littleton JT, Sheng M: Neurobiology: Synapses unplugged. Nature 424:931, 2003.
33. Hall Z, Merlie JR: Synaptic structure and development: The neuromuscular junction. Cell 72:99, 1993.
34. Rich MM: The control of neuromuscular transmission in health and disease. Neuroscientist 12:134, 2006.
35. Wang X, Engisch KL, Li Y, et al: Decreased synaptic activity shifts the calcium dependence of release at the mammalian neuromuscular junction in vivo. J Neurosci 24:10687, 2004.
36. Ryan AM, Matthews E, Hanna MG: Skeletal-muscle channelopathies: Periodic paralysis and nondystrophic myotonias. Curr Opin Neurol 20:558, 2007.
37. Katz B, Miledi R: Estimates of quantal content during "chemical potentiation" of transmitter release. Proc R Soc Lond [Biol] 215:369, 1979.
38. Uchitel OD, Protti DA, Sanchez V, et al: P-type voltage dependent calcium channel mediates presynaptic calcium influx and transmitter release in mammalian synapses. Proc Natl Acad Sci U S A 89:3330, 1992.
39. Vincent A: Immunology of disorders of neuromuscular transmission. Acta Neurol Scand Suppl 183:1, 2006.
40. Sudhof TC: Synaptic vesicles: An organelle comes of age. Cell 127:671, 2006.
41. Rizolli SO, Betz WJ: All change at the synapse. Nature 423:591, 2003.
42. Lang T, Jahn R: Core proteins of the secretory machinery. Handb Exp Pharmacol 184:107, 2008.
43. Valtorta F, Jahn R, Fesce R, et al: Synaptophysin (p38) at the frog neuromuscular junction: Its incorporation into the axolemma and recycling after intense quantal secretion. J Cell Biol 107:2717, 1988.
44. Heidelberger R: Neuroscience: Sensors and synchronicity. Nature 450:623, 2007.
45. Turton K, Chaddock JA, Acharya KR: Botulinum and tetanus neurotoxins: Structure, function and therapeutic utility. Trends Biochem Sci 27:552, 2002.
46. Schiavo G: Structural biology: Dangerous liaisons on neurons. Nature 444:1019, 2006.
47. Schurch B: The role of botulinum toxin in neurourology. Drugs Today (Barc) 40:205, 2004.
48. Lowe NJ: Overview of botulinum neurotoxins. J Cosmet Laser Ther 9(Suppl 1):11, 2007.
49. Frick CG, Richtsfeld M, Martyn JAJ, et al: Long-term effects of botulinum toxin on neuromuscular function. Anesthesiology 106:1139, 2007.
50. Lange DJ, Rubin M, Gelb DJ, et al: Distant effects of locally injected botulinum toxin: A double-blind study of single fiber EMG changes. Muscle Nerve 14:672, 1991.
51. Heeroma JH, Plomp JJ, Roubos EW, Verhage M: Development of the mouse neuromuscular junction in the absence of regulated secretion. Neuroscience 120:733, 2003.
52. Engel AG, Ohno K, Sine SM: Congenital myasthenic syndromes: Progress over the past decade. Muscle Nerve 27:4, 2003.
53. Engel AG, Sine SM: Current understanding of congenital myasthenic syndromes. Curr Opin Pharmacol 5:308, 2005.
54. Abraham RB, Rudick V, Weinbroum AA: Practical guidelines for acute care of victims of bioterrorism: Conventional injuries and concomitant nerve agent intoxication. Anesthesiology 97:989, 2002.
55. Karwa M, Currie B, Kvetan V: Bioterrorism: Preparing for the impossible or the improbable. Crit Care Med 33:S75, 2005.
56. Gu Y, Forsayeth JR, Verall S: Assembly of the mammalian muscle acetylcholine receptor in transfected COS cells. J Cell Biol 114:799, 1991.
57. Kopta C, Steinbach JH: Comparison of mammalian adult and fetal nicotinic acetylcholinic receptors stably expressed in fibroblasts. J Neurosci 14:3922, 1994.
58. Jonsson M, Gulrey D, Dabrowski M, et al: Distinct pharmacologic properties of neuromuscular blocking agents on human neuronal nicotinic acetylcholine receptors: A possible explanation for the train-of-four fade. Anesthesiology 105:521, 2006.
59. Jonsson M, Dabrowski M, Gurley DA, et al: Activation and inhibition of human muscular and neuronal nicotinic acetylcholine receptors by succinylcholine. Anesthesiology 104:724, 2006.
60. Pedersen SE, Cohen JB: D-Tubocurarine binding sites are located at alpha-gamma and alpha-delta subunit interfaces of the nicotinic acetylcholine receptor. Proc Natl Acad Sci U S A 87:2785, 1990.
61. Griesmann GE, McCormick DJ, De Aizpurua HJ, et al: α-Bungarotoxin binds to human acetylcholine receptor α-subunit peptide 185-199. J Neurochem 54:1541, 1990.
62. Escher P, Lacazette E, Courtet M, et al: Synapses form in skeletal muscles lacking neuregulin receptors. Science 308:1920, 2005.
63. Gullberg D: Cell biology: The molecules that make muscle. Nature 424:138, 2003.
64. Missias AC, Chu GC, Klocke BJ, et al: Maturation of the acetylcholine receptor in skeletal muscle: Regulation of the AChR γ-to-ε switch. Dev Biol 179:223, 1996.
65. Tansey MG, Chu GC, Merlie JP: ARIA/HRG regulates AChR epsilon subunit gene expression at the neuromuscular synapse via activation of phosphatidylinositol 3-kinase and Ras/MAPK pathway. J Cell Biol 134:46, 1996.
66. Lukas RJ, Bencherif M: Heterogeneity and regulation of nicotinic acetylcholine receptors. Int Rev Neurobiol 34:25, 1992.

67. McCarthy MP, Stroud RM: Conformational states of the nicotinic acetylcholine receptor from *Torpedo californica* induced by the binding of agonist, antagonists, and local anesthetics. Equilibrium measurements using tritium-hydrogen exchange. Biochemistry 28:40, 1989.
68. Karlin A, DiPaola M, Kao PN, Lobel P: Functional sites and transient states of the nicotinic acetylcholine receptor. *In* Hille B, Fambrough DM (eds): Proteins of Excitable Membranes. Society of General Physiologists. New York, Wiley Interscience, 1987, p 43.
69. Yamaoka K, Vogel SM, Seyama I: Na^+ channel pharmacology and molecular mechanisms of gating. Curr Pharm Des 12:429, 2006.
70. Raines DE: Anesthesia and nonanesthetic volatile compounds have dissimilar activities on nicotinic acetylcholine receptor desensitization kinetics. Anesthesiology 84:663, 1996.
71. Sine SM: The nicotinic receptor ligand binding domain. J Neurobiol 53:431, 2002.
72. Gage PW: Ion channels and postsynaptic potentials. Biophys Chem 29:951, 1988.
73. Gage PW, Hammill OP: Effects of anesthetics on ion channels in synapses. Int Rev Neurophysiol 25:3, 1981.
74. Swope SL, Qu Z, Huganir RL: Phosphorylation of nicotinic acetylcholine receptor by protein tyrosine kinases. Ann N Y Acad Sci 757:197, 1995.
75. Plested CP, Tang T, Spreadbury I, et al: AChR phosphorylation and indirect inhibition of AChR function in seronegative MG. Neurology 59:1682, 2002.
76. Albuquerque EX, Alkondon M, Pereira EF, et al: Properties of neuronal nicotinic acetylcholine receptors: Pharmacologic characterization and modulation of synaptic function. J Pharmacol Exp Ther 280:1117, 1997.
77. Maelicke A, Coban T, Storch A, et al: Allosteric modulation of *Torpedo* nicotinic acetylcholine receptor ion channel activity by noncompetitive agonists. J Receptor Signal Transduc Res 17:11, 1997.
78. Creese R, Head SD, Jenkinson DF: The role of the sodium pump during prolonged end-plate currents in guinea-pig diaphragm. J Physiol 384:377, 1987.
79. Ibebunjo C, Martyn JAJ: Thermal injury induces greater resistance to D-tubocurarine in local than in distant muscles in the rat. Anesth Analg 91:1243, 2000.
80. Fischer U, Reinhardt S, Albuquerque EX, Maelicke A: Expression of functional alpha7 nicotinic acetylcholine receptor during mammalian muscle development and denervation. Eur J Neurosci 11:2856, 1999.
81. Tsuneki H, Salas R, Dani JA: Mouse denervation increases expression of alpha 7 nicotinic receptor with unusual pharmacology. J Physiol 547:169, 2003.
82. Lindstrom JM: Nicotinic acetylcholine receptors of muscles and nerves: Comparison of their structures, functional roles, and vulnerability to pathology. Ann N Y Acad Sci 998:41, 2003.
83. Placzek AN, Grassi F, Papke T, et al: A single point mutation confers properties of the muscle-type nicotinic acetylcholine receptor to homomeric alpha7 receptors. Mol Pharmacol 66:169, 2004.
84. Hirose M, Kaneki M, Martyn JAJ, et al: Immobilization depresses insulin signaling in skeletal muscle. Am J Physiol 279:E1235, 2000.
85. Sugita H, Kaneki M, Martyn JAJ, et al: Burn injury impairs insulin-stimulated Akt/PKB activation in skeletal muscle. Am J Physiol Endocrinol Metab 288:E585, 2005.
86. Hirose M, Kaneki M, Martyn JAJ, et al: Long-term denervation impairs insulin receptor substrate (IRS)-1-mediated insulin signaling in skeletal muscle. Metabolism 50:216, 2001.
87. Gronert GA: Cardiac arrest after succinylcholine: Mortality greater with rhabdomyolysis than receptor upregulation. Anesthesiology 94:523, 2001.
88. Lukas RJ, Changeux J-P, Novère NL, et al: International union of pharmacology. XX. Current status of the nomenclature for nicotinic acetylcholine receptors and their subunits. Pharmacol Rev 51:397, 1999.
89. Chiodini F, Charpantier E, Muller D, et al: Blockade and activation of the human neuronal nicotinic acetylcholine receptors by atracurium and laudanosine. Anesthesiology 94:643, 2001.
90. Vizi ES, Lendvai B: Side effects of nondepolarizing muscle relaxants: Relationship to their antinicotinic and antimuscarinic actions. Pharmacol Ther 73:75, 1997.
91. Tsuneki H, Kimura I, Dezaki K, et al: Immunohistochemical localization of neuronal nicotinic receptor subtypes at the pre- and postjunctional sites in mouse diaphragm muscle. Neurosci Lett 196:13, 1995.
92. Faria M, Oliveira L, Timoteo MA, et al: Blockade of neuronal facilitatory nicotinic receptors containing alpha 3 beta 2 subunits contribute to tetanic fade in the rat isolated diaphragm. Synapse 49:77, 2003.
93. Martyn J, Durieux ME: Succinylcholine: New insights into mechanisms of action of an old drug. Anesthesiology 104:633, 2006.
94. Eriksson LI: Reduced hypoxic chemosensitivity in partially paralysed man. A new property of muscle relaxants? Acta Anaesthesiol Scand 40:520, 1996.
95. Taylor P: Anticholinesterase agents. *In* Bruton LL, Lazo JS, Parker KL (eds): Goodman & Gilman's Pharmacological Basis of Therapeutics, 11th ed. New York, McGraw Hill, 2006, p 201.
96. de Boer HD, Driessen JJ, Marcus MA, et al: Reversal of rocuronium-induced (1.2 mg/kg) profound neuromuscular block by sugammadex: A multicenter, dose-finding and safety study. Anesthesiology 107:239, 2007.
97. Richtsfeld M, Blobner M, Martyn JAJ: Chronic administration of pyridostigmine leads to a myasthenia-like state with down-regulation of acetylcholine receptors. Young Investigator Award for abstract presented at ASCCA at the ASA Annual Meeting of the American Society of Anesthesiologists, October 2003, San Francisco.

Göran Hedenstierna

15 Respiratory Physiology

Key Points

1. Removal of CO_2 is determined by alveolar ventilation, not by total, minute ventilation.
2. Dead space ventilation can be dramatically increased in patients with chronic obstructive pulmonary disease and pulmonary embolism to more than 80% to 90% of minute ventilation in the extreme case.
3. Breathing at low lung volume increases airway resistance and promotes closure of airways.
4. Hypoxemia can be caused by alveolar hypoventilation, diffusion impairment, ventilation-perfusion mismatch, and right-to-left shunt.
5. Almost all anesthetics reduce muscle tone, which in turn lowers functional residual capacity (FRC) to close to awake residual volume.
6. Lowered FRC during anesthesia together with ventilation with a high O_2 concentration causes atelectasis.
7. Preoxygenation before and during induction of anesthesia is a major cause of atelectasis.
8. General anesthesia causes ventilation-perfusion mismatch (airway closure) and shunt (atelectasis).
9. Hypoxic pulmonary vasoconstriction is blunted by most anesthetics, thereby enhancing any ventilation-perfusion mismatch.
10. Respiratory work is increased during anesthesia, a consequence of reduced respiratory compliance (reduced lung volume available for ventilation?) and increased airway resistance (lowered FRC and subsequent decrease in airway dimensions?).

Respiratory Function in Waking Subjects

The major task of the lung is to oxygenate the blood and eliminate carbon dioxide from it. This is accomplished by exchanging gas between alveoli and pulmonary capillary blood. Air is brought down to the alveoli by cyclic breathing, and oxygen in the inspired gas diffuses through the alveolar epithelial wall, the interstitial tissue, and the capillary endothelial wall, as well as through the plasma, and finally reaches the hemoglobin inside red blood cells. Carbon dioxide diffuses in the opposite direction, from the blood cells and plasma to the alveolar gas phase, and is expired. To establish gas exchange in the human lung, there must be ventilation of the alveoli, diffusion through the alveolar-capillary membranes, and circulation or perfusion of the pulmonary capillary bed.

The lung is regularly affected by anesthesia and mechanical ventilation. This occurs even in healthy volunteers or patients with no cardiopulmonary disease, and sometimes the dysfunction can be severe enough to cause life-threatening hypoxemia. In patients with preexisting lung disease, gas exchange will be further compromised in comparison to the awake state. Knowledge of the functional impairment that will ensue during anesthesia and mechanical ventilation will make possible ventilatory support that should, in the large majority of patients, prevent any disastrous impairment in gas exchange.

Ventilation

Dead Space and Alveolar Ventilation

Fresh air is brought into the lungs by cyclic breathing. A normal tidal breath at rest in an adult subject is approximately 0.5 to 0.6 L, and the respiratory frequency is around 16 breaths/min, with a range of 12 to 22 breaths/min. Metabolic demand and pulmonary function will determine the magnitude and rate, provided that the respiratory center in the brainstem is intact and functioning. This results in ventilation of approximately 7 to 8 L/min.[1]

All that is inspired does not reach the alveoli. Approximately 100 to 150 mL will be confined in the airways and does not participate in gas exchange. This "dead space" is approximately

30% of tidal volume; that is, the V_{DS}/V_T ratio is 0.3 (see Fig. 15-1 for different forms of dead space).[2] The remaining part of ventilation reaches the alveoli and respiratory bronchioles (with some alveoli tapered on the airway wall). Thus, "alveolar ventilation" is around 5 L/min, similar to cardiac output, which is also 5 L/min. The overall alveolar ventilation-perfusion ratio accordingly is 1.

There are several causes of increased minute ventilation, such as physical exercise, reduced inspired oxygen concentration (or rather, partial pressure of O_2), increased dead space ventilation, and metabolic acidosis.

Increased Dead Space Ventilation

If dead space is increased, ventilation must be raised to account for the "losses" and to maintain Pa_{CO_2} at a normal level. Dead space is increased when ventilation is performed through a mouthpiece and a valve or through a facemask. This "apparatus dead space" is something between 25 and a few hundred mL, as compared with the 100 to 150 mL that the natural airways make up ("anatomic dead space").[3] Bronchiectasis increases anatomic dead space, but it adds only little to the total figure. A much larger increase can be caused by ventilation of alveoli that are not perfused, such as a pulmonary embolus stopping blood flow in a lung unit ("alveolar dead space") (Fig. 15-1). A worst case is plugging of the right or left main pulmonary artery, thereby leaving one lung essentially unperfused. In this case, the dead space fraction is doubled from the normal 0.3 to 0.6 or so.[4] Patients suffering from recurrent emboli, or pulmonary embolism, often have high V_{DS}/V_T ratios that can exceed 0.7 to 0.8, which means that to maintain an ordinary alveolar ventilation of 5 L/min, minute ventilation must be raised from 7 to 8 to 20 L/min. Patients with recurrent emboli also frequently complain of dyspnea, even in the absence of severe hypoxemia. The increased ventilatory demand may be the reason. Other patients who suffer from increased dead space are those with obstructive lung disease, including asthma, chronic bronchitis, and emphysema. Their major difficulty is that some regions are poorly ventilated because of airway obstruction, so these regions are underventilated in relation to their perfusion, commonly called a ventilation-perfusion mismatch ("$\dot{V}_A/\dot{Q}$" mismatch signified by low $\dot{V}_A/\dot{Q}$ ratios).[5] This forces inspired air to other regions, which may be ventilated in excess of their perfusion. Such opposite $\dot{V}_A/\dot{Q}$ mismatch (signified by high $\dot{V}_A/\dot{Q}$ ratios) has the same effect on gas exchange as an increase in dead space does and is also measured as dead space (see Fig. 15-1). Indeed, patients with advanced chronic bronchitis may have as high a $\dot{V}_A/\dot{Q}$ ratio as 0.8 to 0.9. Such patients would have to ventilate some 30 to 50 L/min to maintain normal Pa_{CO_2}, a difficult task to perform even for a short period with healthy lungs. It should therefore come as no surprise that Pa_{CO_2} is increasing as a result of alveolar "hypoventilation." This has led us to say, erroneously, that bronchitic patients are hypoventilating when in fact they are hyperventilating! Some help to these patients comes from the fact that CO_2 can be excreted by half the "normal" alveolar ventilation if Pa_{CO_2} is doubled, as can be inferred from the alveolar gas equation (Box 15-1).

Because all subjects, even those with healthy lungs, do have some $\dot{V}_A/\dot{Q}$ mismatch, the sum of the anatomic and alveolar dead space, whether attributable to emboli or uneven ventilation and perfusion, is called "physiologic dead space."

Hyperventilation and Exercise

It is possible to voluntarily increase minute ventilation to a maximum that is almost 20-fold higher than resting ventilation, to above 100 L/min in women and above 150 L/min in men, but only for a brief period of half a minute or so.[1] In addition, hyperventilation without a simultaneous increase in metabolic demand

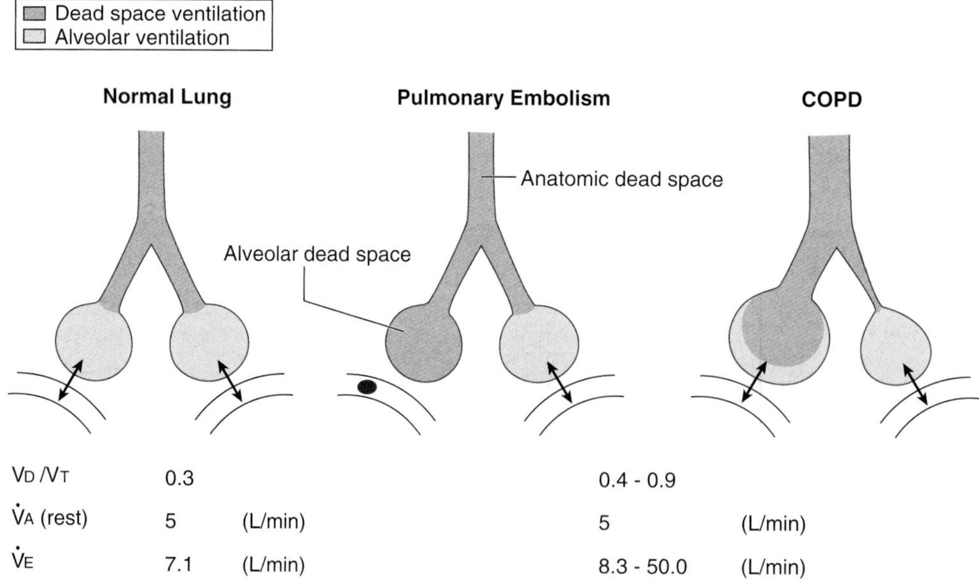

Figure 15-1 Dead space and alveolar ventilation in normal and diseased lungs. Note that both cessation of blood flow and excessive alveolar ventilation relative to perfusion cause an increase in dead space as measured by the conventional CO_2 elimination technique. See also the marked increase in minute ventilation that is required to maintain alveolar ventilation when dead space is increased. COPD, chronic obstructive pulmonary disease; $\dot{V}_A$, alveolar ventilation; V_D/V_T, dead space–to–tidal volume ratio; $\dot{V}_E$, minute ventilation (sum of dead space and alveolar ventilation). *(Courtesy of the editor of the BMJ series Respiratory Measurement.)*

Box 15-1 Alveolar Gas Equations

Alveolar Oxygen Tension (P_{AO_2})

$$P_{AO_2} = P_{IO_2} - \frac{P_{ACO_2}}{R} + \left[P_{ACO_2} \times F_{IO_2} \times \frac{1-R}{R}\right]$$

where P_{IO_2} is inspired oxygen tension, P_{ACO_2} is alveolar CO_2 tension (assumed to equal arterial P_{CO_2}), R is the respiratory exchange ratio (normally in the range of 0.8 to 1.0), and F_{IO_2} is the inspired oxygen fraction.

The term within brackets compensates for the larger O_2 uptake than CO_2 elimination over the alveolar capillary membranes.

A simplified equation can be written without the compensation term:

$$P_{AO_2} = P_{IO_2} - \frac{P_{ACO_2}}{R}.$$

Alveolar Ventilation

Alveolar ventilation ($\dot{V}_A$) can be expressed as

$$\dot{V}_A = f \times (V_T - V_{DS})$$

where f is breaths/min, V_T is tidal volume, and V_{DS} is physiologic dead space.

Alveolar ventilation can also be derived from

$$\dot{V}_{CO_2} = c \times \dot{V}_A \times F_{ACO_2}$$

where $\dot{V}_{CO_2}$ is CO_2 elimination, c is a conversion constant, and F_{ACO_2} is the alveolar CO_2 concentration.

If $\dot{V}_A$ is expressed in L/min, $\dot{V}_{CO_2}$ in mL/min, and F_{ACO_2} is replaced by P_{ACO_2} in mm Hg, $c = 0.863$. By rearranging,

$$\dot{V}_A = \frac{\dot{V}_{CO_2} \times 0.863}{P_{ACO_2}}.$$

will lower Pa_{CO_2} and affect consciousness. In respiratory tests of ventilatory capacity it is therefore necessary to perform the test during rebreathing of expired gas or add CO_2 to the respiratory gas so that Pa_{CO_2} is maintained at a normal or nearly normal level. The increase in ventilation is brought about by an increase in V_T to approximately two thirds of vital capacity (VC) (see later), or 2.5 to 4 L, and an increase in frequency to 40 breaths/min or greater. However, during maximum physical exercise, minute ventilation increases less, to around two thirds of maximum capacity, which means an increase to 65 to 100 L/min in normally fit women and men. In athletes, ventilation may exceed 150 L/min.

Lung Volumes

Functional Residual Capacity

There is a certain amount of air in the lungs after an ordinary expiration. This volume is called functional residual capacity (FRC) (Fig. 15-2). It amounts to approximately 3 to 4 L and is dependent on sex, age, height, and weight. FRC goes up with height and age and down with weight and is smaller in women than in men.[1,6] The balance of the inward force of the lung and the outward force of the chest wall determines the volume. The inward force of the lung, or "elastic recoil," consists of the elastic fibers of the lung tissue, as well as the contractile forces of airway smooth muscles and the surface tension of alveoli. The outward force of the chest wall is exerted by the ribs, joints, and muscles. It can be asked why any gas volume persists in the lung after expiration. There are two good reasons, at the least. One is that if alveoli collapse during expiration, much more effort would have to be spent to reopen them again than during a normal breath with no collapse because less resistance is encountered when expanding an alveolar wall in an open lung with a liquid-gas interphase unit than expanding a collapsed alveolus with a liquid-liquid interphase. The other reason is that the inspired air mixes with the remaining gas in the lung, thereby leveling off the variation in O_2 and CO_2 concentrations that occur during the respiratory cycle. With just little air in the lung, the gas variations in alveoli would be much greater, and they would cause a similarly varying Pa_{O_2} and Pa_{CO_2} in blood. This can indeed be observed in patients with reduced lung volumes (see later).

With increased ventilation, as during exercise, V_T is raised by increasing both inspiration and expiration so that FRC is lowered by approximately 0.5 L. However, in the presence of airway obstruction, as in asthma, for example, expiration is slowed down so that the end-expiratory level is elevated instead of being lowered.[7] This is called air trapping and is a means of reducing the resistance to gas flow in the narrowed airways (Fig. 15-2). However, it has to be paid for because the increased level of breathing increases the elastic work of breathing.

FRC increases with age because of loss of elastic lung tissue, which lessens the contractile force of the lung and moves the balancing point between the outward force of the chest wall and the inward force of the lung to higher lung volume. In patients with chronic obstructive pulmonary disease (COPD), FRC increases faster over the years than in normal subjects because of an effect of chronic air trapping and more severe loss of elastic tissue (in particular in emphysema).[1]

FRC is reduced in lung diseases characterized by fibrosis of the lung, such as idiopathic fibrosis, pneumoconiosis, and different forms of granulomatosis and vasculitis.[7] In extreme cases, the reduction can be down to 1.5 to 2 L (see Fig. 15-2). Obviously, pulmonectomy (e.g., for treatment of lung cancer) will also reduce FRC. However, the remaining lung will expand and fill in some of the space left after resection of lung tissue, sometimes called "compensatory emphysema."

Total Lung Capacity and Subdivisions

The gas volume in the lung after a maximum inspiration is called *total lung capacity* (TLC). It is typically 6 to 8 L.[1] TLC can be increased in patients with COPD either by overexpansion or "hyperinflation" of essentially normal alveoli or by destruction of the alveolar wall with loss of elastic tissue, as in emphysema (see Fig. 15-2).[7] In extreme cases, TLC can be increased by 50%, or up to 11 to 12 L. In restrictive disorders, TLC is reduced in proportion to the severity of the fibrotic process and may be as low as 3 to 4 L (see Fig. 15-2).[7]

Even after a maximum expiratory effort, some air is left in the lung and no region normally collapses. This persisting gas volume is called *residual volume* (RV) and amounts to 2 to 2.5 L.

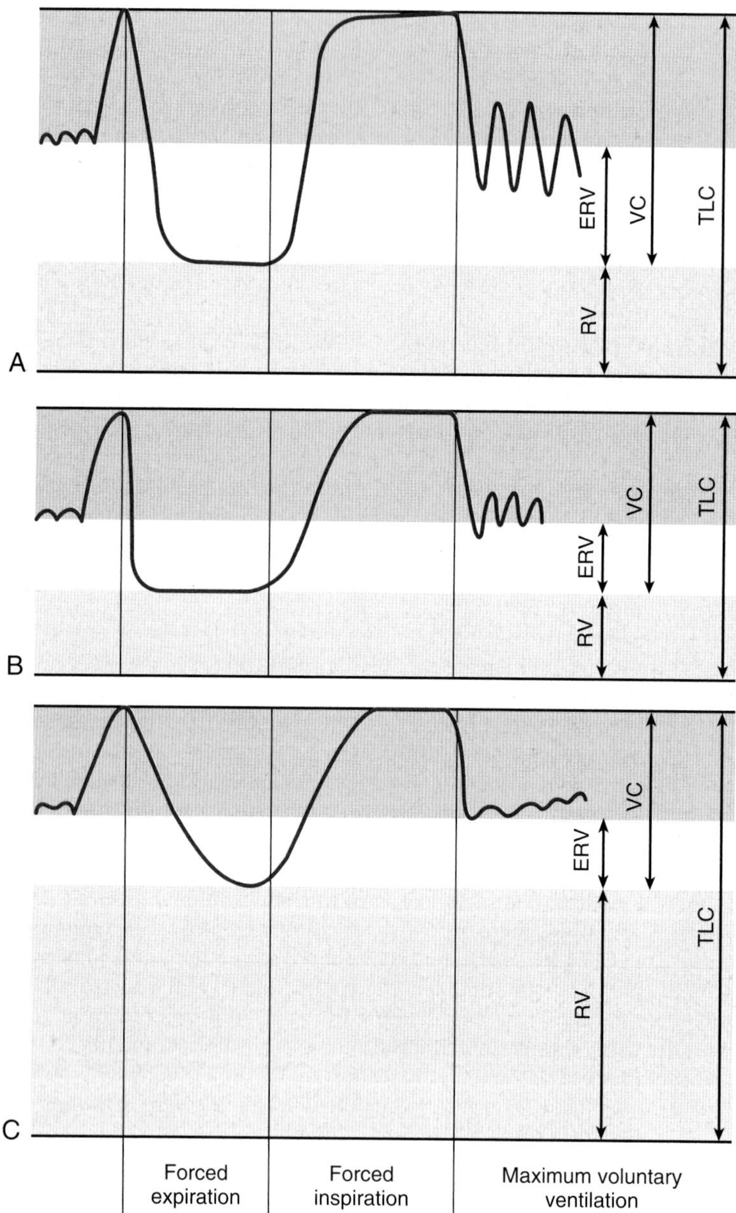

Figure 15-2 Ventilation and lung volumes in a healthy subject with normal lungs (**A**), a patient with restrictive lung disease (**B**), and a patient with chronic obstructive lung disease (**C**). Note the decrease in vital capacity (VC) and the increased expiratory flow (steeper than the normal slope of the forced expiratory curve) in the patient with lung fibrosis. Note also the increased residual volume (RV), reduction in VC, and the slow forced expiration in the obstructive, emphysematous patient. The latter patient demonstrates air trapping during hyperventilation. ERV, expiratory reserve volume; TLC, total lung capacity. *(Courtesy of the editor of the BMJ series: Respiratory Measurement.)*

The reason that expiration stops before all gas has been evacuated seems to be twofold. First, distal airways 2 mm or less in diameter close before alveoli collapse.[8] This trapping of gas will thus prevent the alveoli from being squeezed to emptiness. Second, the chest wall, rib cage, and diaphragm cannot be distorted to the point that all gas in the lung will be expelled. The advantage of not allowing lung tissue to collapse was presented earlier (see Fig. 15-2).

The maximum volume that can be inspired and expired is called *vital capacity*. VC is thus the difference between TLC and RV and is around 4 to 6 L. It is reduced in restrictive lung diseases, frequently before a decrease in RV. What may not be equally clear is that VC is also reduced in obstructive lung disease. This is an effect of the chronic "air trapping" that increases RV, mainly at the expense of VC.[7] However, as said earlier, TLC may also increase, but not in proportion to the rise in RV. The net effect can be a TLC of 12 L made up of an RV of 11 L and a VC as small as 1 L, in an extreme example of emphysema.

Respiratory Mechanics

Understanding the mechanics of the respiratory system serves at least two purposes. One, it gives a clue to what governs the distribution of inspired air, and second, recording of the mechanics can be used as a diagnostic and prognostic tool in lung disease. Here, we will begin with an analysis of the elastic and resistive forces that have to be overcome during breathing and how these forces are affected by pulmonary disorders. We will then continue to analyze the influence of respiratory mechanics on the distribution of inspired air.

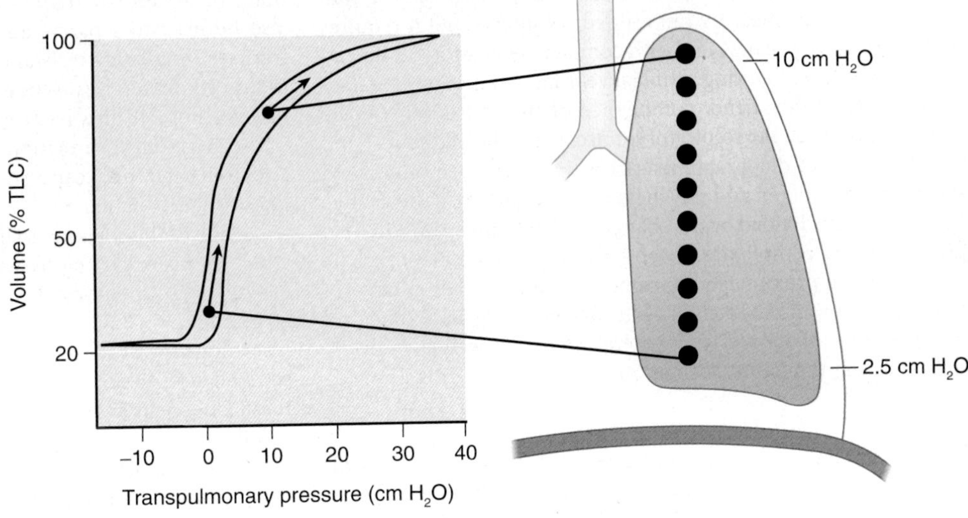

Figure 15-3 Pressure-volume relationships of the lung. Note the curved relationship, which is typical of an elastic structure. Note also the lower (more subatmospheric) pleural pressure in the upper regions. Regional transpulmonary pressure (mouth minus pleural pressure) is thus higher for apical lung units than for basal ones in an upright subject. This results in different positions of the upper and lower lung regions on the pressure-volume curve. The consequence will be that the lower lung regions expand more for a given increase in transpulmonary pressure than the upper units do. Thus, ventilation goes preferably to the lower lung regions.

Compliance of the Respiratory System

The lung recoils like an elastic rubber balloon. Thus, a certain pressure is required to keep it inflated. The pressure needed to keep the lung inflated at a certain volume is pleural minus alveolar pressure, or "transpulmonary pressure" (Ptp). It will be seen that more and more pressure is required for a given increment in volume the more the lung is inflated (Fig. 15-3).[9] Such a curved pressure-volume relationship is typical of elastic structures, and a similar curved force-length relationship will also be seen for a rubber band.

The elastic behavior of the lung is often analyzed in terms of compliance, which is the inverse of elastance. Thus, compliance is expressed as change in lung volume divided by the change in pressure required to cause the increment in volume (or the decrease in pressure that is accompanying a decrement in volume). Normal lung compliance is around 0.2 to 0.3 L/cm H_2O (2 to 3 L/kPa).[9] It varies with lung volume, as can be seen in Figure 15-3, and decreases with an increase in lung volume. Thus, compliance is critically dependent on the lung volume at which it is measured. This should be remembered if one does repeated recordings to monitor the progress of a disease. In addition, if a lung is resected or part of it, the measured compliance is reduced despite the fact that the remaining lung tissue is unaltered.

In fibrotic lung disease, compliance is reduced and the pressure-volume curve is flatter and shifted to the right, as shown in Figure 15-4 (obviously, the direction of a change in the pressure-volume curve depends on which axis is denoted pressure and which is volume; the figure shows the standard drawing).[9] Although the curve is sensitive to changes in the elastic properties of the lung, it is not good at discriminating between different diseases. Thus, idiopathic fibrosis, alveolar proteinosis, a granulomatosis-like sarcoidosis, and interstitial and alveolar edema will all reduce compliance and cause a flattening and right shift of the pressure-volume curve.

Loss of elastic lung tissue, as in emphysema, causes a steeper curve that is shifted to the left (see Fig. 15-4).[9] Similar changes are not seen in chronic bronchitis or asthma. Thus, recording of the pressure-volume curve can help in establishing the diagnosis of emphysema, which cannot easily be done with a conventional chest radiograph. The overaeration that can be seen on conventional chest radiographs does not enable a distinction between obstructive lung disease with and without loss of elastic tissue. High-resolution computed tomography (CT), however, enables visualization of the delicate lung structure and can be used for differential diagnosis.[10]

The chest wall itself also exerts an elastic impedance to breathing that goes undetected during spontaneous breathing

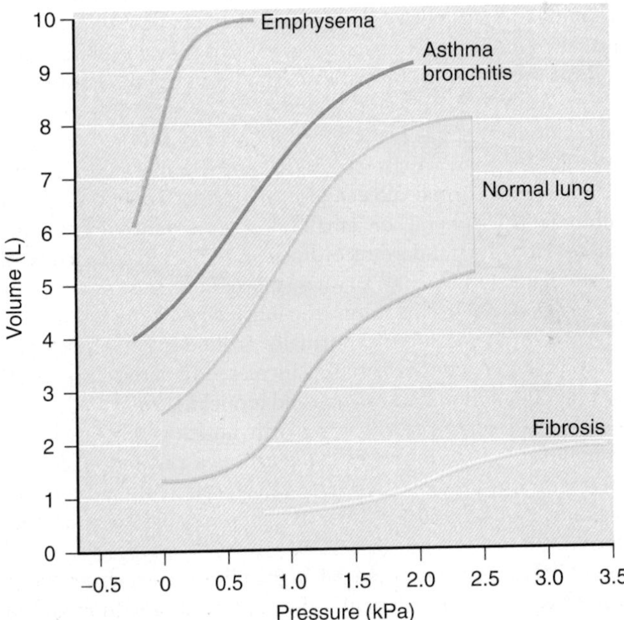

Figure 15-4 Examples of pressure-volume curves of the lung in health and lung disease. Note the much flatter slope of the curve in fibrotic lung disease, which reflects a considerable increase in pressure variation and respiratory work. Also, note the parallel shift in the pressure-volume curve of an asthmatic and bronchitic patient, which shows that compliance need not change in these diseases, although lung volume may have increased. Finally, note the steep slope of the curve of an emphysematous patient. This indicates loss of elastic tissue and might even suggest reduced respiratory work. However, such patients, as well as asthmatic and bronchitic patients, have increased airway resistance, which causes elevated respiratory work. *(Courtesy of the editor of the BMJ series: Respiratory Measurement.)*

because the chest wall is part of the pump itself. Chest wall mechanics can be measured in trained volunteers, but it requires tricky respiratory maneuvers with complete relaxation of the respiratory muscles.[11] During artificial ventilation and muscle relaxation, on the other hand, compliance of the chest wall can be measured because the respiratory muscles are allowed to rest and the rib cage and diaphragm exert elastic impedance only when the lungs are inflated and the chest wall is expanded. The change in lung volume divided by the change in pleural pressure will then give chest wall compliance. It can be seen that compliance of the chest wall is approximately the same magnitude as compliance of the lungs, around 0.2 L/cm H_2O. It may go down in obesity and in conditions associated with general edema, as well as in disorders affecting the joints, such as ankylosing spondylitis.[11]

Resistance of the Respiratory System

Pressure is required to overcome the resistance to gas flow through the airways during respiration. In addition, sliding of different components of lung tissue and the chest wall during inspiration and expiration exerts resistance.[12] This resistance is calculated as forcing pressure divided by gas flow. Flow can be measured at the airway opening, the mouth or nose, and is assumed to apply to the calculation of all three types of resistance (in airways, lung tissue, and the chest wall). The forcing pressure for airway resistance is mouth (or nose) pressure minus alveolar pressure, whereas the other driving pressures will be part of the changes in transpulmonary and pleural pressure.

Gas flow can be turbulent, with a disorderly pattern signified by vortices, or laminar, with a streamlined unidirectional flow pattern. Turbulent flow is proportional to the square of the pressure, and laminar flow, which is less pressure demanding, is linearly related to the pressure. Flow is turbulent in larger airways and at bifurcations and irregularities of the bronchi. It is laminar in the smaller airways. Thus, most of the energy, or pressure, involved in creating flow of gas is expended on overcoming resistance in the larger airways.[12] Only about 20% of the measured airway resistance, in a normal subject, is located in the small bronchi. A doubling of "peripheral" or "small" airway resistance may be difficult to detect by standard recording techniques. The difficulty in detecting changes in small airways, approximately 2 mm wide or less, has coined the expression "the lung's silent zone."

Airflow resistance is normally around 1 cm H_2O/L/sec. With obstructive lung disease it is increased to about 5 cm H_2O/L/sec in mild to moderate asthma and bronchitis and greater than 10 in more severe cases.[13] It is worth noticing that breathing through a size 8 endotracheal tube causes a resistance of 5 cm H_2O/L/sec at a flow of 1 L/sec and that a size 7 tube increases resistance to 8 cm H_2O/L/sec (i.e., comparable to moderate asthma).[14]

Airflow resistance can be higher during expiration than during inspiration, in particular during forced breathing and in patients with obstructive lung disease because the expiratory muscle effort will act not only on alveoli, to empty them, but also on airways, to make them smaller.[12] The inspiratory effort, on the other hand, helps dilate airways within the thorax by lowering pleural pressure, which acts on the outside of the airway wall. Finally, airways that are not in the thoracic cavity, specifically the pharynx, larynx, and trachea, are subject to lower pressure inside than outside their wall during inspiration because they are surrounded by atmospheric pressure, whereas luminal pressure is below atmospheric (otherwise no air would be sucked into that point of the airway tree).[12] These physiologic consequences can also be used to separate an increase in extrathoracic resistance from an increased resistance in other airways. If resistance is increased during inspiration, it is probably caused by narrowing of extrathoracic airways (e.g., sucking of a paralytic vocal chord into the lumen). Retraction of the upper airways and resultant strenuous breathing can also be seen in a neonate with respiratory distress (see Chapter 84).

Resistance of lung tissue and the chest wall has been studied to a lesser extent. Lung tissue resistance amounts to around 1 cm H_2O/L/sec in the normal case and can be increased threefold to fourfold in chronic lung disease.[15] Even less has been studied regarding chest wall resistance. However, it seems as though the sum of lung tissue and chest wall resistance is increased, and markedly so, in acute respiratory failure demanding mechanical ventilation.[16]

Respiratory resistance, in particular airway resistance, is dependent on lung volume. When it comes to airways, it can be understood that during inspiration, airways as well as alveoli are expanded and resistance in the airways will decrease. During expiration, the airways get narrower and resistance will accordingly increase. This is shown in Figure 15-5. Airway resistance may be around 1 cm H_2O/L/sec at the FRC level and is reduced further, although to a small extent, when breathing at higher lung volumes. In contrast, expiration down from FRC rapidly increases resistance, which may be 5 to 8 cm H_2O/L/sec when approaching RV. Indeed, a resistance-versus-lung volume plot as shown in Figure 15-5 approaches infinity at the end of a maximal expiration. This must be realized when taking airway resistance measurements at different lung volumes. One example is when resistance is compared between the waking state and during anesthesia. In the latter situation, FRC is reduced, as will be discussed later.

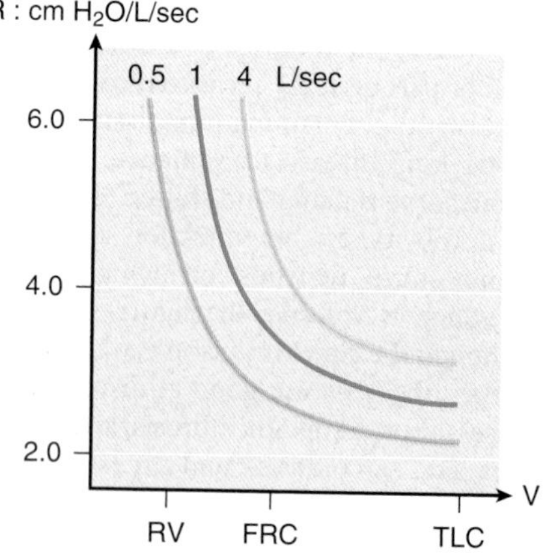

Figure 15-5 Schematic drawing of resistance against lung volume at different flow rates. Note that resistance increases with decreasing lung volume and more so below functional residual capacity (FRC) than at higher lung volume. Note also that resistance increases with an increase in flow rate. Note that at low lung volume, resistance is as high as can be seen in moderate to severe asthma (6 to 8 cm H_2O/L/sec). RV, residual volume; TLC, total lung capacity.

Inertia or Acceleration of Gas and Tissue

There is finally one additional component of the total impedance to breathing, and that is inertance, or the pressure required to accelerate air and tissue during inspiration and expiration. This component, however, is minor and can hardly be measured under normal breathing, regardless of whether the lungs are healthy. During very rapid breathing, such as during high-frequency oscillation in intensive care or the yogi exercise of rapid shallow breathing of around four breaths/sec, acceleration becomes more important and can contribute 5% to 10% of the total impedance to breathing.[17]

Gas Distribution

Distribution of Inspired Gas: Effect of Compliance, Resistance, and Airway Closure

The air that is inspired will not be evenly distributed in the lung. During quiet breathing, most gas goes to the lower, dependent regions—the basal, diaphragmatic areas in the upright or sitting position and the dorsal units in the supine position.[18] This also means that the lower part of the left lung will receive most of the air if the subject is in the left lateral position and that the right lung will be preferentially ventilated in the right position. The reason for this seemingly gravitational orientation of something as light as gas is the combined effect of the curved pressure-volume relationship of the lung tissue and the increasing pleural pressure down the lung. This topic will be discussed at some length in the next paragraph.

First, the curved pressure-volume curve, typical of an elastic tissue as stated earlier, means that with increasing lung volume, more and more pressure is required to inflate the lung with a given increment in volume (there may be a linear pressure-volume relationship for some distance). Second, the increasing pleural pressure, at constant alveolar pressure all over the lung, causes transpulmonary pressure to decrease from the top to the bottom of the lung. In the upright position, the apical lung regions are exposed to higher transpulmonary pressure than the dependent, basal ones are. Thus, the upper and lower lung regions are positioned at different levels of the pressure-volume curve (see Fig. 15-3). During inspiration, pleural pressure is lowered, which causes the lower lung regions to inflate more than the upper ones with a similar change in transpulmonary pressure (it is assumed that pleural pressure changes uniformly in the pleural space).[18] Thus, in a healthy subject, ventilation goes preferentially to the basal regions, as can be inferred from Figure 15-3 (the larger arrow in the lower, basal part of the lung indicates more ventilation than in the upper, apical regions with the subject in the upright position; Fig. 15-6). The pleural pressure gradient is oriented in a vertical, gravitational direction, which is why the distribution of ventilation changes with body position.

What causes the pleural pressure gradient? The major factor is the weight of the lung itself, with less lung tissue exerting pressure at a level higher up in the thoracic cavity than at a lower lung level. This pressure is exerted in all directions, including the pleural space. The specific density of an air-filled and perfused lung is on average approximately 0.3, and this causes the pleural pressure to increase by 0.3 cm H_2O/cm vertical distance. If the lung is heavier, as when it is suffering from edema, the pleural pressure gradient will increase, as does the vertical difference in alveolar size. If weight is reduced or eliminated, as in zero gravity or microgravity, there should be no vertical pleural pressure gradient, and lung expansion as well as gas distribution should be more even. During short parabolic flights causing very low gravity, inspiration and expiration of gases with different characteristics showed reduced inhomogeneity of the distribution of ventilation.[19] However, some inhomogeneity persisted, thus indicating that nongravitational factors also contribute to the distribution of ventilation. Such factors may be uneven convectional and diffusional flow in small lung units and may be related to differences in the anatomic structure of the airways (and parenchyma?).[20]

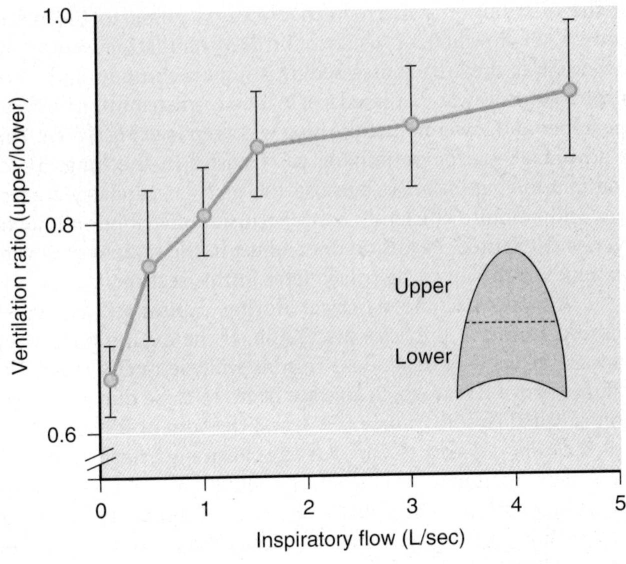

Figure 15-6 Ratio of ventilation to the upper and lower lung regions with a change in inspiratory flow. Note that the distribution of ventilation goes to the lower lung regions at a low flow rate. However, this is replaced by a more even distribution with increasing flow, as, for example, during exercise. This ensures more efficient use of lung tissue and the alveolar-capillary membranes for gas transfer (provided that pulmonary blood flow shows a similar distribution pattern). *(Redrawn from data in Bake B, Wood L, Murphy B, et al: Effect of inspiratory flow-rate on regional distribution of inspired gas. J Appl Physiol 37:8-17, 1974.)*

The vertical pleural pressure gradient may be smaller in the prone position than when supine.[21] This may be due to the weight of the heart, which is compressing the dependent parts of the lung in the supine position and permitting the nondependent regions to expand. In the prone position, the heart is resting on the sternum with less effect on the shape of the lung. The only force that can distort the lung is the weight of the lung itself. Moreover, as discussed earlier, differences in airway anatomy may contribute to differences in the distribution of ventilation when supine and prone. A more even distribution of inspired gas in the prone position has also been demonstrated by isotope technique.[22,23]

Thus far we have dealt with the distribution of inspired gas during, from a technical and purist point of view, static conditions (which, however, would not result in any gas flow). The distribution will be essentially the same during quiet breathing, up to a flow rate of 0.5 L/sec or so. However, with an increasing flow rate, regional differences in airway resistance (and in lung tissue and possibly to some extent chest wall resistance; they will be disregarded here) will play an increasing role in determining gas distribution. Because lung tissue, both alveoli and airways, is more expanded in the upper than in the lower regions, resistance to gas flow is less in the upper part of the lung. This results in a change in the distribution pattern, with more gas going to the upper units.[24] At a flow of 0.3 L/sec, two thirds of ventilation went to the lower half of the lung as assessed by isotope technique, and when inspiratory flow was increased to 4 to 5 L/sec, distribution between the upper and lower half of the lung was even (see Fig. 15-6). This is advantageous for optimizing gas transfer in the lung, as for example during exercise, because the alveolar-capillary surface area will be more efficiently used. Perfusion distribution may be evenly distributed. Perfusion does adjust in the same way as ventilation, which will be discussed later in this section.

Airways become narrower during expiration, as can be inferred from the previous discussion. If the expiration is deep enough, airways in dependent regions will eventually close. The volume above RV at which airways begin to close during expiration is called *closing volume* (CV), and the sum of RV and CV is called *closing capacity* (CC).[25] Airway closure is a normal physiologic phenomenon and is the effect of increasing pleural pressure during expiration. When pleural pressure becomes "positive" (or rather, above atmospheric), it will exceed the pressure inside the airway, which is just or nearly atmospheric at a low flow rate. The higher pressure outside than inside will compress the airway and may close it. Because pleural pressure is higher in dependent regions than higher up, closure of airways begins in the bottom of the lung. The crucial point is thus the creation of "positive" pleural pressure (Fig. 15-7). In young subjects it may not occur until they have expired to RV. However, with increasing age, pleural pressure becomes "positive" at higher and higher lung volume, and at an age of 65 to 70 years, airway closure may occur above FRC.[26] This means that in elderly subjects, dependent lung regions are intermittently closed during the breath. These regions will reopen during inspiration, when lung volume exceeds CC. The impediment to ventilation that closure of airways causes seems to be the major explanation of why arterial oxygenation decreases with age (see Chapter 71).

Airway closure plays an even greater role in the supine position because FRC is reduced whereas CC is not affected by body position. Closure of airways may occur above FRC, even at an age of 45 to 50, and in a 70-year-old subject, the airways may be continuously closed if CC exceeds FRC plus VT. This is illustrated in Figure 15-8.

Airway closure occurs at higher lung volumes in patients with obstructive lung disease. Secretions, edema of the airway wall, and increased bronchial muscle tone all reduce the lumen of the airway and facilitate premature closure.[25] Because these changes are thought to begin in the small airways, recording of CV has been considered an ideal test for early detection of airway disease. However, use of CV is not as popular as it was earlier because its reproducibility is not as good as that of conventional spirometry. However, even if recording of airway closure as a diagnostic and quantitative measure of lung disease may not have been as successful as hoped for, it should not obscure the fact that airway closure is a most important phenomenon. Its detection has taught us a lot of the physiologic principles governing the distribution of ventilation.

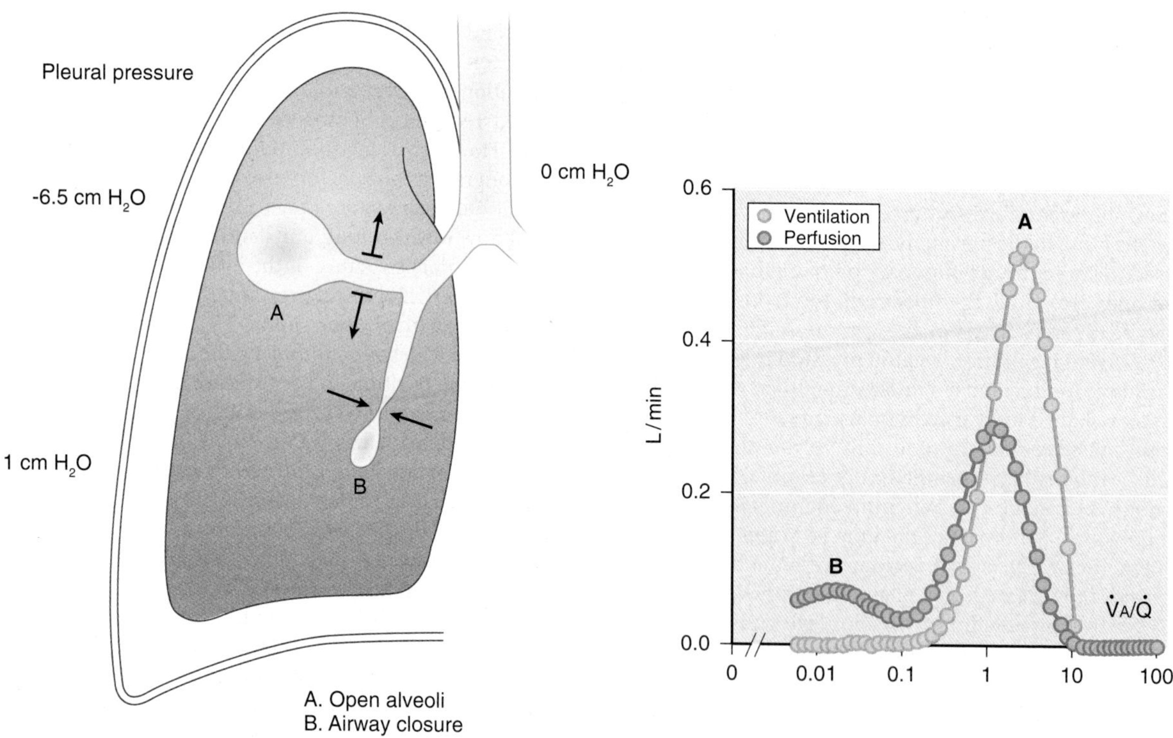

Figure 15-7 Schematic drawing of regional alveolar and airway volume at an upper (A) and a lower (B) lung level, *left panel*. There is a vertical pleural pressure gradient with a difference of approximately 7.5 cm H_2O between the uppermost and lowermost regions. This causes a transpulmonary pressure gradient with higher pressure inside the airway and alveolus in the upper part and higher pressure outside the alveolus and airway in the lower part. This results in closure of the airways with the potential for slow alveolar gas adsorption behind the occluded airway. The *right panel* shows a distribution of ventilation and perfusion ratios as obtained by the multiple inert gas elimination technique. A "normal" mode of ventilation and blood flow (A) can be seen corresponding to the open and ventilated alveoli in the upper parts of the lung. In addition, there is a mode of low $\dot{V}A/\dot{Q}$ ratios with more perfusion than ventilation (B). This could apply to an elderly healthy subject with intermittent airway closure during breathing.

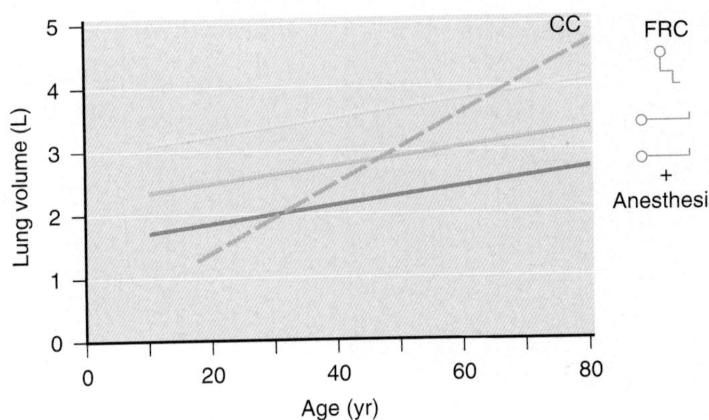

Figure 15-8 Resting lung volume (functional residual capacity [FRC]), upright and supine, and closing capacity (CC, unaffected by body position) at different ages in healthy subjects. Note the lower FRC, by approximately 0.7 to 0.8 L, in the supine position (an effect of cranial displacement of the diaphragm by the abdominal organs). As can be seen, there is also a slight increase in FRC with age at constant height and weight. This is an effect of the loss of elastic tissue with aging. Finally, observe the more rapid increase in CC with age. This results in airway closure above FRC in upright subjects at ages of 65 to 70 years or older. In the supine position, airways may close during breathing even at the age of 45 to 50 years! This relationship between CC and FRC is a likely explanation for the decreasing oxygenation of blood with age. The effect of anesthesia can also be seen with lowering of FRC so that airways may close already at 30-year-old subjects (see section on "Lung Volume and Respiratory Mechanics during Anesthesia"). The curves are based on pooled data from different studies.

As mentioned earlier, secretions, edema, and spasm reduce the airway lumen. This will affect gas distribution as well by decreasing or eliminating ventilation in regions that are affected by airway obstruction and by increasing it in other, less obstructed areas.

Expiring against resistance, such as against half-closed lips ("pursed-lips breathing"), is a technique sometimes taught to a patient with chronic obstructive disease. This may make breathing easier. Devices are also available to breathe out through that act as resistance. These devices build up higher pressure inside the airway, which prevents it from closing during expiration; this is the reason why breathing is more comfortable. Thus, the device "stabilizes" the airway and facilitates expiration.[27] Although the result may be the desired one, the explanation is wrong. The higher airway pressure can be generated only by increasing the expiratory effort, and this increases pleural pressure to the same extent as airway pressure. The decrease in pressure across the airway wall will be the same as without the expiratory resistance, and this will not make the airway more stable. What may explain a beneficial result is that the expiratory resistance increases lung volume and slows down expiration. The former (increase in lung volume) is the only way of increasing transpulmonary and transairway pressure, and this stabilizes the airway. Simultaneously, there is a general increase in airway caliber that further reduces resistance, as discussed earlier. The latter (slowed expiration) reduces the decrease in pressure from the alveoli toward the mouth because lower flow requires less driving pressure. By this means the point along the airway tree where pressure inside the airway has dropped to below that outside the airway (equal to pleural pressure) is moved toward the mouth (Fig. 15-9). Thus, slow expiratory flow may make it possible to move the "equal pressure point," where inside and outside airway pressure is equal, up to the larger airways or the mouth, which will prevent floppy airways from collapsing.[28]

Diffusion of Gas

Diffusion in Airways and Alveoli

Gas flow is convective in the larger and medium-sized airways, down to approximately the 14th generation. Airways at this level begin to be tapered with alveoli and participate in gas exchange with pulmonary blood. In the latter airway generations, from 15 to 23, the total cross-sectional area of the airway tree grows rapidly, from 2.5 cm^2 in the trachea, to 70 cm^2 in the 14th generation entering the acinus, to 0.8 m^2 in the 23rd generation.[29] The total alveolar surface is approximately 140 m^2. Gas flow velocity will decrease as the area increases. For an ordinary breath the average velocity of gas in the trachea will be around 0.7 m/sec, but at the alveolar surface it is no higher than 0.001 mm/sec. This is much slower than the diffusion rate of O_2 and CO_2 in the airway tree and the alveoli. Transport of O_2 and CO_2 is therefore accomplished by diffusion in the peripheral airways and in the alveoli, not by convective flow. CO_2 can be detected in the mouth after a few seconds of breath-holding. However, this is the result not only of diffusion but also of convection brought about by the beating heart, which acts as a mixing pump. Yet even in the absence of heartbeats, CO_2 appears within seconds at the airway opening. This rapid diffusion has an implication when measuring dead space by recording of the expiratory CO_2 curve—an inspiratory breath-hold reducing the measured dead space down to zero, if the breath is held for just a few seconds.

It has often been discussed whether gas mixing is complete in the alveoli of a normal lung during normal breathing or whether there are concentration gradients, often called "stratified inhomogeneity." Many consider alveolar concentrations to be homogeneous. However, if the alveolar dimensions grow, by expansion or confluence of several alveoli as in emphysema, the diffusion distance can be too great to allow complete mixing of inspired and alveolar gas during ordinary breathing. This will cause stratified inhomogeneity of respiratory gas concentrations within the alveolar unit and has an impeding effect on gas exchange, similar to uneven distribution of ventilation by other means.[30]

Diffusion Across Alveolar-Capillary Membranes

Oxygen diffuses passively from the alveolar gas phase into plasma and red cells, where it binds to hemoglobin. Carbon dioxide diffuses in the opposite direction, from plasma to the alveoli. The amount that can diffuse over the membranes for a given period is determined by (1) the surface area available for diffusion, (2) the thickness of the membranes, (3) the pressure difference of the gas across the barrier, (4) the molecular weight of the gas, and (5) the solubility of the gas in the tissues that it has to traverse.[31] These factors are discussed in the following paragraphs.

Surface Area. Lung volume will obviously be of importance. The smaller the lung, the less the overall diffusion. To this should be added that the lung surface can be used for diffusion only if there is circulating blood on the capillary side. Thus, pulmonary capillary blood volume is an important determinant of diffusion. The relative influence of membrane area and characteristics, as well as capillary blood volume, can be analyzed separately by performing a diffusion or transfer test at two different inspired oxygen concentrations. Carbon monoxide (CO) is normally used as the test gas. CO is inspired at a small concentration (0.3%) to TLC after a previous maximum expiration, and the

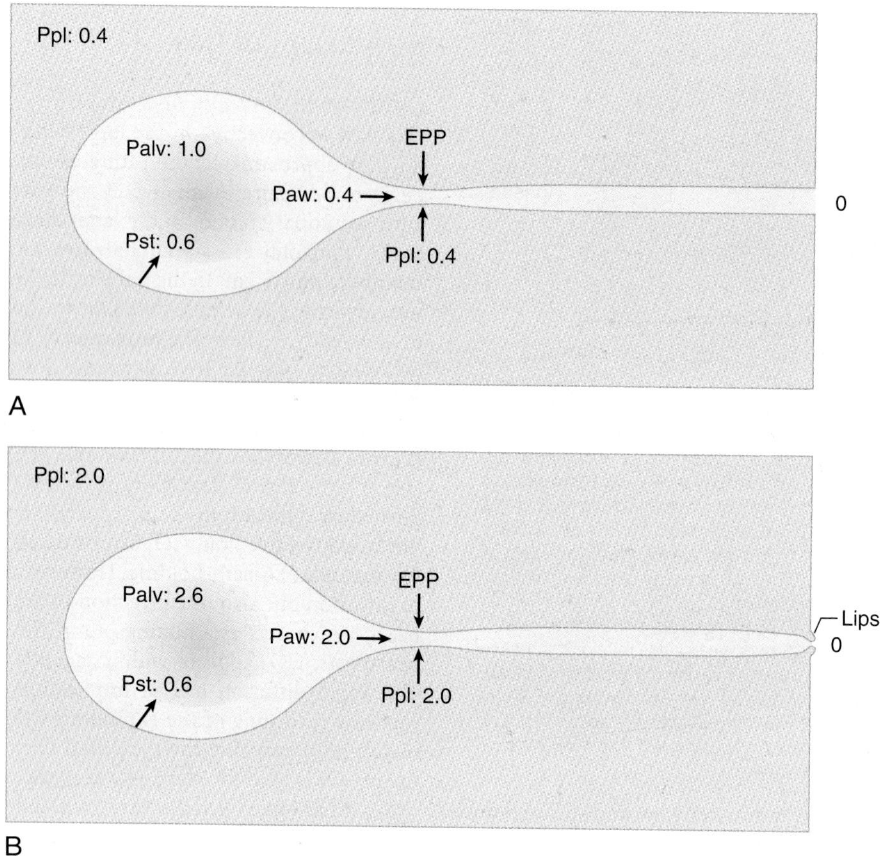

Figure 15-9 Schematic drawings of the "equal pressure point" (EPP) concept and dynamic compression of airways. **A,** Slightly forced expiration during otherwise normal conditions. With the application of some expiratory muscle effort, pleural pressure (Ppl) is positive, 4 cm H_2O (0.4 kPa). The elastic recoil pressure (Pst) of the alveoli (6 cm H_2O) and the pleural pressure add together to yield intra-alveolar pressure (Palv) (10 cm H_2O). This causes expiratory flow. At some point downstream toward the airway opening, airway pressure (Paw) has dropped by 6 cm H_2O, so intraluminal pressure and pleural, extraluminal pressure are the same. This is the EPP. From this point to the mouth, intraluminal airway pressure is lower than the surrounding, extraluminal pressure and the airway may be compressed. **B,** An attempt to stabilize the airway by so-called "pursed-lip" breathing. The increased resistance to expiratory flow requires increased expiratory effort to maintain gas flow. Thus, pleural pressure is increased in comparison to the normal conditions (Ppl = 20 cm H_2O). Alveolar elastic recoil pressure (Pst) is the same as in the earlier condition, provided that lung volume is the same. If expiratory flow is of the same magnitude as during normal breathing, pressure along the airway falls to the same extent as during normal breathing. Thus, the EPP will have the same location as during normal breathing, and no stabilization of the airway has been achieved. The two ways of moving the EPP toward the mouth and to less collapsible airways is by raising alveolar recoil pressure (Pst) by an increase in lung volume or by lowering the expiratory flow rate so that the pressure drop along the airway tree is slowed down.

breath is held for 10 seconds, followed by a deep expiration to RV. The amount of CO that has been taken up can be calculated from the difference between inspired and expired gas. Most of this CO has diffused to blood, where it binds easily to hemoglobin. However, a certain amount of the difference in concentration is due to dilution in the gas volume that was not expired (RV). This can be accounted for by inspiring another tracer gas that is poorly soluble or almost insoluble, such as helium. The dilution of helium (and CO) can be calculated, as can the diffusion or transfer factor of CO. Because oxygen and CO compete for binding to hemoglobin, measurement of diffusion at two different inspired oxygen concentrations as just described may enable distinction between capillary blood volume and the membrane in calculating the diffusion capacity or transfer factor. It is beyond the scope of this chapter to go into further details, but interested readers are referred to an article by Hughes and Bates.[32]

MEMBRANE THICKNESS. The thicker the membrane, the longer the diffusion distance and the lower the diffusion capacity. In addition, solubility for O_2 (and CO_2) is lower in fibrotic tissue than in water. Thickening of the membranes may therefore impede diffusion even more than the increase in diffusion distance does.

PRESSURE GRADIENT. The larger the O_2 or CO_2 tension difference between the gas phase in the alveolus and plasma in the capillary, the greater the diffusion. The mixed venous blood entering the pulmonary capillary has a Po_2 of 40 mm Hg (5.3 kPa), and alveolar Po_2 is approximately 100 mm Hg (13.3 kPa), thus creating a driving pressure of 60 mm Hg (8 kPa). When blood flows through the capillary, it takes up oxygen (and delivers CO_2), but because oxygen pressure builds up in capillary blood, the diffusion rate slows down and becomes zero when pressure is equilibrated over the alveolar-capillary wall (Fig. 15-10). In a normal lung at low cardiac output, equilibrium has been reached within 25% to 30% of the capillary distance, and no or little gas transfer takes place in the remaining capillary. When cardiac output is increased, as during exercise, blood passes through the capillary faster, and a longer distance of the capillary is therefore required before equilibrium is reached, equilibration time being much the

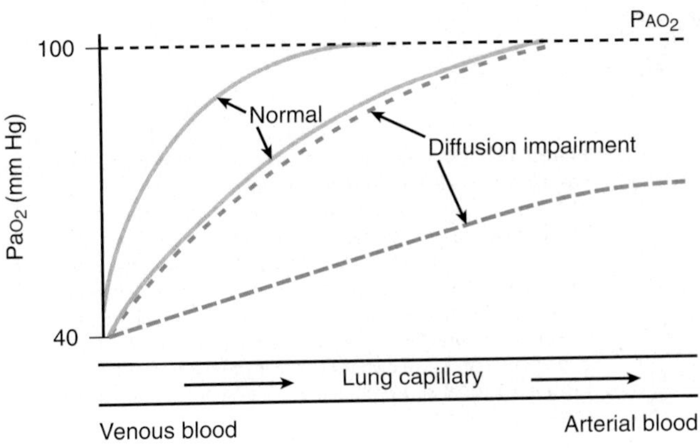

Figure 15-10 Oxygenation of pulmonary capillary blood at rest and during exercise in a normal subject and in a patient with fibrotic lung disease with impaired diffusion. In a normal subject, equilibration of oxygen tension in capillary blood with that in alveolar gas is rapid. This has been achieved within one third of the capillary distance. However, during exercise, most of the capillary distance must be used to reach equilibration between alveolar and pulmonary capillary oxygen tension. This is an effect of the shorter transit time of red blood cells caused by the increased cardiac output. Distention and recruitment of pulmonary capillaries may to some extent offset the effect of raised cardiac output on velocity of blood through the capillaries. With impaired diffusion, equilibration takes a longer time, but full equilibration may still be reached at rest. However, with increased blood velocity during exercise, equilibration of oxygen may be far from complete at the end of the pulmonary capillary, thereby causing desaturation of arterial blood, which may at times be severe.

same as during resting conditions (lower venous Po_2 speeds diffusion up in the beginning). Thickened alveolar-capillary membranes will prolong the equilibration process with the possible effect of causing hypoxemia.

It should also be mentioned that most of the oxygen that dissolves in plasma diffuses into the red cell and binds to hemoglobin. One gram of hemoglobin can bind 1.36 mL O_2 (numbers between 1.34 and 1.39 are used). This means that 1 L of blood with a hemoglobin content of 150 g/L can bind 204 mL of O_2 if fully saturated. With a saturation of 98%, which is normally achieved in arterial blood, the hemoglobin-bound oxygen amounts to 200 mL/L of blood. This should be compared with the mere 3 mL of O_2 that is physically dissolved in 1 L of blood at a Pao_2 of 100 mm Hg (13.3 kPa). The hemoglobin-bound oxygen creates no pressure in plasma, which is important because it allows much more oxygen to diffuse over the membranes before a pressure equilibration is reached. Anemia reduces and polycythemia increases diffusion capacity.

Molecular Weight. Diffusion is inversely related to the square root of the molecular weight of the gas. Thus, the larger the molecule, the more difficult it will be to pass through the membranes. O_2 is a relatively light gas with a molecular weight of 32. CO_2 is heavier with a molecular weight of 44 and should therefore be more limited in diffusion than O_2. However, taking the square root of the weights reduces the difference between the gases, and in practice, CO_2 is much more diffusible than O_2, as explained in the next paragraph.

Solubility. Diffusion is linearly related to solubility in tissue. It is usually set equal to that of water. CO_2 is almost 30 times more soluble in water than O_2 is and diffuses more than 20 times faster (the net effect of all previously mentioned factors).[31] In practice, this means that there is no lung disease compatible with life that causes measurable impairment in CO_2 diffusion.

Pulmonary Perfusion

Pressure-Flow Relationship

In contrast to the systemic circulation, the pulmonary circulation is a low-pressure system. The typical pulmonary artery pressure of 20 mm Hg systolic and 8 mm Hg diastolic is about 6 to 10 times lower than pressure in the systemic arteries. The lower pressure is achieved by the larger vascular diameter and shorter distance of the pulmonary vessels than the systemic ones. In particular, a large vascular lumen decreases the demand on driving pressure. According to Poiseuille's law, an increase in vascular radius reduces the pressure demand by an exponent of 4 to maintain a certain flow, if flow is linear. With turbulent flow, the dependence on vascular dimensions will be even higher. As a consequence of the lower resistance, pulmonary capillary blood flow is pulsatile, contrary to the steady flow in systemic capillaries.[33] Another, presumably more important consequence of the low pressure is that the capillary and alveolar walls can be made very thin without causing any leakage of plasma, and this facilitates diffusion of O_2 and CO_2. A sudden increase in pulmonary artery pressure to above a mean of 30 mm Hg causes effusion of plasma into the interstitial and alveolar spaces, thereby promoting lung edema. A slower increase in pressure, over a period of months or years, stimulates the growth of vascular smooth muscle ("vascular remodeling") with thickening of the vascular wall.[34] Edema is prevented better, despite even severe pulmonary hypertension, but diffusion capacity will be impaired.

Distribution of Lung Blood Flow

Blood flow through the lung is governed by driving pressure and vascular resistance. If these factors are unevenly distributed, perfusion may also be uneven. This seems to be the case. What the perfusion distribution looks like and the mechanisms behind it have become an interesting issue during recent years. Thus, the previously generally accepted explanation of a gravitational orientation of perfusion as demonstrated in the pioneering work by Permutt, West, Hughes and others (for a review, see Reference 35) has been challenged by others who propose a "fractal" distribution with gravity playing only a minor role.[36] Here we will first deal with the "gravitational" concept and then proceed to the "fractal" concept.

Gravitational Distribution of Blood Flow in the Lung

Pulmonary artery pressure increases down the lung, an effect of the hydrostatic pressure that builds up on the way from the top to the bottom of the lung. This pressure increases by 1 cm H_2O/cm distance down the lung (or 0.74 mm Hg/cm vertical distance; blood has a density close to 1, or 1.04). This causes a pressure difference in the pulmonary arterial vessels between the apex and the base of 11 to 15 mm Hg, depending on the height of the lung. There is thus less driving pressure to the top of the lung. Because mean pulmonary artery pressure is approximately 12 mm Hg at the level of the heart, it may approach zero in the apex of the lung in the upright position. Moreover, if alveolar pressure is increased, as during positive-pressure ventilation, it may exceed that in the pulmonary artery and compress the pulmonary capillaries. No blood will then flow through the vessels. That part of the lung is called zone I, according to the nomenclature introduced by West and associates (Fig. 15-11).[35] If arterial pressure and capillary pressure exceed alveolar pressure, as it will farther down the lung

$$\text{Pulmonary vascular resistance (PVR)} = \frac{\bar{P}_{PA} - P_{LA}}{\dot{Q}_T}$$

(true only if lung is in zone III)

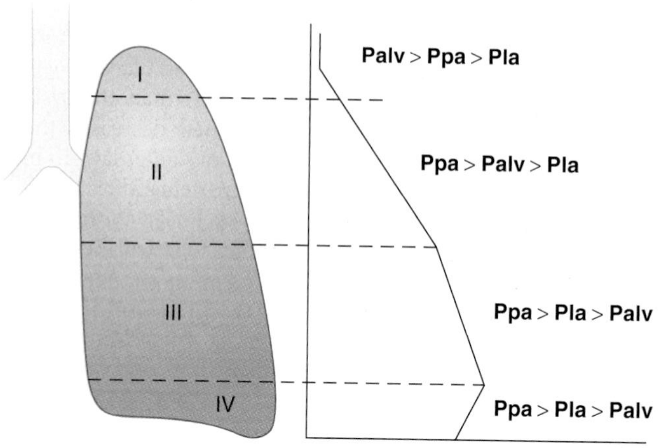

Figure 15-11 Vertical distribution of blood flow in the lung. The so-called zones I, II, III, and IV are indicated. As can be seen, zone I corresponds to a region in which alveolar pressure exceeds vascular pressure, which results in essentially no perfusion. Zone II is characterized by pulmonary artery pressure exceeding alveolar pressure, which in turn exceeds venous pressure. The driving pressure will then be arterial minus alveolar pressure. Farther down in zone III, both arterial pressure and venous pressure exceed alveolar pressure. The difference between arterial and venous pressure creates the driving force through this zone. In the bottom of the lung there is a decrease in blood flow that is explained by increasing interstitial pressure compressing extra-alveolar vessels. For further details see text. $\dot{Q}_T$, cardiac output; Palv, alveolar pressure; Pla, left atrial pressure; Ppa, pulmonary artery pressure.

because of the addition of hydrostatic pressure, blood flow will be established. Perfusion pressure will be arterial minus alveolar pressure, as long as the latter pressure exceeds that of the pulmonary veins. This is different from the systemic circulation, where perfusion pressure is arterial minus venous pressure. Moreover, the increasing pulmonary arterial pressure down the lung and the constant alveolar pressure increase the perfusion pressure down this part of the lung, called zone II. Blood flow therefore increases down this zone. Farther down the lung, both arterial pressure and venous pressure exceed that in the alveoli, so perfusion pressure is arterial minus venous pressure. This part of the lung is called zone III. Because both arterial pressure and venous pressure increase to the same extent down zone III, with hydrostatic pressure adding to both sides, perfusion pressure does not increase down the zone. Nonetheless, perfusion increases downward, albeit possibly less than the increase in zone II. The explanation proposed is that the increasing vascular pressure dilates the vessels down the lung and by this means reduces vascular resistance.[35]

A few years after these initial observations, it was noticed that blood flow decreases in the bottom of the lung, so a zone IV had to be added to the model of lung perfusion.[35] This called for a new explanation in which it was suggested that the increasing interstitial pressure down the lung presses on the extra-alveolar vessels and makes them narrower. The vertical distribution of blood flow could accordingly be explained by the influence of gravitation on vascular, alveolar, and interstitial pressure.

The homogeneity of blood flow distribution has also been tested during shuttle flights at zero gravity or microgravity. By using indirect techniques based on analysis of the variation in expired gas concentrations that are synchronous with heartbeats ("cardiogenic oscillations"), more uniform lung blood flow distribution has been recorded.[37]

Nongravitational Inhomogeneity of Blood Flow Distribution

In dog experiments, groups at the Mayo Clinic and subsequently in Seattle noticed that the vertical lung blood flow distribution was nearly even and did not change when position was altered between supine and prone.[36] This made the Seattle group conclude that gravity was of minor importance in determining the distribution of perfusion. The same group also showed that perfusion at a given vertical level is unevenly distributed on that horizontal plane, with an inhomogeneity far exceeding that in the vertical direction (Fig. 15-12). In carefully repeated experiments they could reproduce the same pattern of inhomogeneity.[38] This suggests that there are morphologic or functional differences (or both) between lung vessels that also—and perhaps more importantly than gravity—determine blood flow distribution. As an example, vascular resistance seems to be lower in the dorsal regions of horse lungs than in the anterior part.[39] Thus, in an animal that is standing or resting on its four legs most of the time, the vascular tree has adjusted to that position and, by increasing resistance in its anterior parts, has made blood flow more evenly distributed.

Other groups have also made observations that suggest an uneven distribution of blood flow that cannot be explained by gravity, with more blood going to the core of the lung and less to the periphery.[40] A longer distance to the peripheral bed was suggested as an explanation for the larger vascular resistance toward the periphery. However, others found less difference between central and peripheral lung regions. The application of positive end-expiratory pressure (PEEP) in anesthetized and mechanically ventilated dogs forced perfusion of the lung toward the periphery.[41] As always, the reliability of the techniques used is critical. It seems that the spatial distribution of blood flow as measured by single photon emission computed tomography (SPECT), a technique that has been used in some studies, suffers from reconstruction artifacts. Still others have used a microspheres technique and measured the distribution in excised lungs. Although it may suffer from other limitations, one may dare to conclude that enough evidence has accumulated to believe in a nongravitational inhomogeneity of lung perfusion.

Hypoxic Pulmonary Vasoconstriction

Hypoxic pulmonary vasoconstriction (HPV) seems to be a compensatory mechanism aimed at reducing blood flow in hypoxic

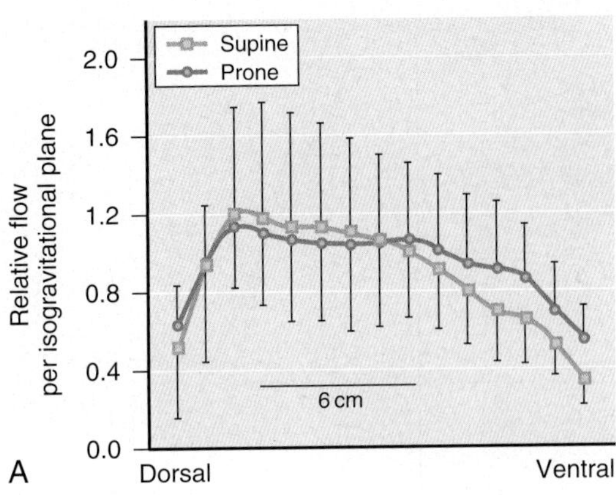

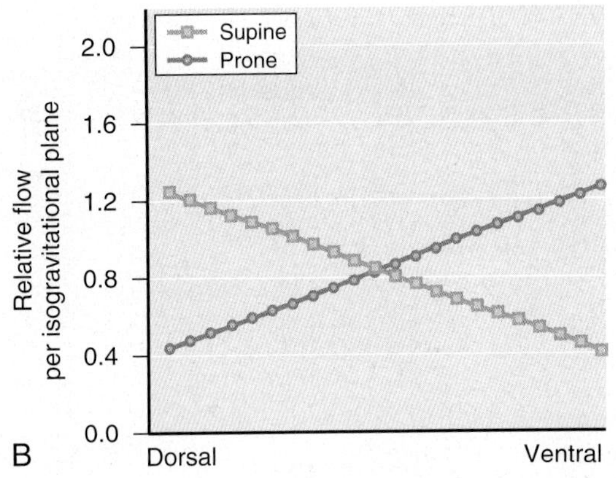

Figure 15-12 Distribution of blood flow from ventral to dorsal lung regions in a canine experiment with the animal supine and prone. Note the similar distributions from ventral to dorsal irrespective of posture. This may suggest that the distribution of perfusion in the vertical direction is determined by anatomic differences in the vasculature rather than by gravity. The *bars* show the spread of perfusion around the mean value. As can be seen, this nongravitational inhomogeneity is larger than that caused in the gravitational orientation. *(From Glenny RW, Lamm WJE, Albert RK, et al: Gravity is a minor determinant of pulmonary blood-flow distribution. J Appl Physiol 71:620-629, 1991.)*

lung regions. The major stimulus for HPV is low alveolar oxygen tension, whether caused by hypoventilation or by breathing gas with a low PO_2. The stimulus of mixed venous PO_2 is much weaker.[42,43] The strength of the constriction is also dependent on the size of the lung segment exposed to the hypoxia, being stronger the smaller the region. Thus, in humans studied during intravenous anesthesia that was assumed to not affect the HPV, one-lung hypoxia with 8% and 4% O_2 during contralateral hyperoxia (FIO_2 of 1.0) caused blood flow to be diverted away from the hypoxic to the other, hyperoxic lung, from 52% to 40% and 30% of cardiac output.[44]

Pulmonary hypertension and pulmonary edema may develop in humans at high altitude because of more general pulmonary vasoconstriction.[45] Chronic lung disease with hypoxemia also causes HPV, but the slow progress of the disease allows time for remodeling of the pulmonary vascular wall, with thickening of the wall preventing edema formation.[32]

Causes of Hypoxemia and Hypercapnia

In the previous sections we discussed ventilation, gas distribution, and the respiratory mechanics that govern distribution, diffusion, and pulmonary perfusion. All these components of lung function can affect the oxygenation of blood, and all except diffusion can also measurably affect CO_2 elimination. The different mechanisms behind hypoxemia and CO_2 retention, or hypercapnia or hypercarbia, have been touched on in previous paragraphs but will be analyzed in more detail here.

Causes of hypoxemia can suitably be classified as hypoventilation, $\dot{V}A/\dot{Q}$ mismatch, impaired diffusion, and right-to-left shunt. Hypercapnia can be caused by hypoventilation, $\dot{V}A/\dot{Q}$ mismatch, and shunt, although in practice hypoventilation is the only cause of real importance (Tables 15-1 and 15-2).

Hypoventilation

If ventilation is low in proportion to metabolic demand, elimination of CO_2 will be inadequate and it will accumulate in the alveoli, blood, and other body tissues. Hypoventilation is often defined as ventilation that results in a $PaCO_2$ above 45 mm Hg (6 kPa). With this definition, hypoventilation can be present even when minute ventilation is high if the metabolic demand or dead space ventilation is increased more than minute ventilation.

The increased alveolar PCO_2 reduces the space available for oxygen in the alveoli. PAO_2 can be estimated by the alveolar gas equation, shown in Box 15-1. A simplified form is derived here. Thus, assuming a normal respiratory exchange ratio, PAO_2 can be calculated as

$$PAO_2 = PIO_2 - (1.25 \times PACO_2)$$

The factor 1.25 is correct if the respiratory exchange ratio is 0.8, and this can reasonably be assumed under resting conditions. $PACO_2$ can be assumed to equal $PaCO_2$. Thus, with a PIO_2 of 149 mm Hg (19.9 kPa) and a $PaCO_2$ of 40 mm Hg (5.3 kPa), PAO_2 is 99 mm Hg (13.2 kPa), and during hypoventilation with a $PaCO_2$ of 60 mm Hg (8 kPa), PAO_2 is 74 mm Hg (9.9 kPa). That gives the highest possible PaO_2 that can exist at that level of alveolar ventilation. Thus, whether a low PaO_2 can be explained by hypoventilation can easily be tested with this simple formula. If there is a gap between the estimated PAO_2 and the measured PaO_2, another or an additional cause of hypoxemia must be sought. It is also

Table 15-1 Causes of Hypoxemia

Disturbance	PaO_2 (breathing air) at Rest	PaO_2 (breathing oxygen) at Rest	PaO_2 (breathing air) with Exercise (Versus Rest)	$PaCO_2$
Hypoventilation	Reduced	Normal	No change or further decrease	Increased
$\dot{V}A/\dot{Q}$ mismatch	Reduced	Normal	No or minor increase or decrease	Normal
Shunt	Reduced	Reduced	No change or further decrease	Normal
Diffusion impairment	Reduced	Normal	Small to large decrease	Normal

Table 15-2 Mechanisms of Hypoxemia in Different Lung Disorders

Disorder	Hypoventilation	Diffusion Impairment	$\dot{V}_A/\dot{Q}$ Mismatch	Shunt
Chronic bronchitis	(+)	–	++	–
Emphysema	+	++	+++	–
Asthma	–	–	++	–
Fibrosis	–	++	+	+
Pneumonia	–	–	+	++
Atelectasis	–	–	–	++
Pulmonary edema	–	+	+	++
Pulmonary emboli	–	–	++	+
Acute respiratory distress syndrome	–	–	+	+++

obvious that the decrease in Pa_{O_2} that is caused by hypoventilation is easily overcome by increasing PI_{O_2} (which on the other hand, may decrease the stimulus to breath and cause further retention of CO_2).

Ventilation-Perfusion Mismatch

For optimum gas exchange, ventilation and perfusion must match each other in all lung regions. At rest, both ventilation and perfusion increase down the lung. Perfusion increases more than ventilation, the difference between the uppermost and lowermost 5-cm segments being 3 times for ventilation and 10 times for perfusion. This results in a mean $\dot{V}_A/\dot{Q}$ ratio of approximately 1 somewhere in the middle of the lung and a range of $\dot{V}_A/\dot{Q}$ ratios from 0.5 in the bottom of the lung to 5.0 in nondependent regions, as illustrated in Figure 15-13, upper panel (the perfusion distribution being a simplified drawing of what is shown in Fig. 15-11). Another way of showing the matching between ventilation and blood flow is by making a multicompartmental analysis of the ventilation distribution of blood flow against $\dot{V}_A/\dot{Q}$ ratios. This can be achieved by a multiple inert gas elimination technique (MIGET).[46] In short, MIGET is based on the constant infusion of a number (usually six) of inert gases with different solubilities in blood. When passing the lung, the different gases will be eliminated via alveoli and expired in proportion to their solubility. A poorly soluble gas will leave the bloodstream and be more or less completely eliminated (e.g., sulfur hexafluoride). A gas of medium solubility will be retained to some extent (e.g., halothane), and a gas with a very high solubility in blood will be retained to an almost full extent (e.g., acetone). This means that the concentration of the different gases in arterial blood will differ, with higher concentrations of gases with high solubility. Retention can be calculated as the ratio between arterial and mixed venous blood concentrations. Similarly, the ratio of expired gas concentration and mixed venous gas concentration can also be calculated and gives the excretion for each gas. With knowledge of the retention, excretion, and solubility of each gas, an essentially continuous distribution of blood flow against $\dot{V}_A/\dot{Q}$ ratios can be constructed. The lower panel in Figure 15-13 shows an example from a healthy subject. Note that ventilation and blood flow are well matched, being distributed to a limited number of compartments

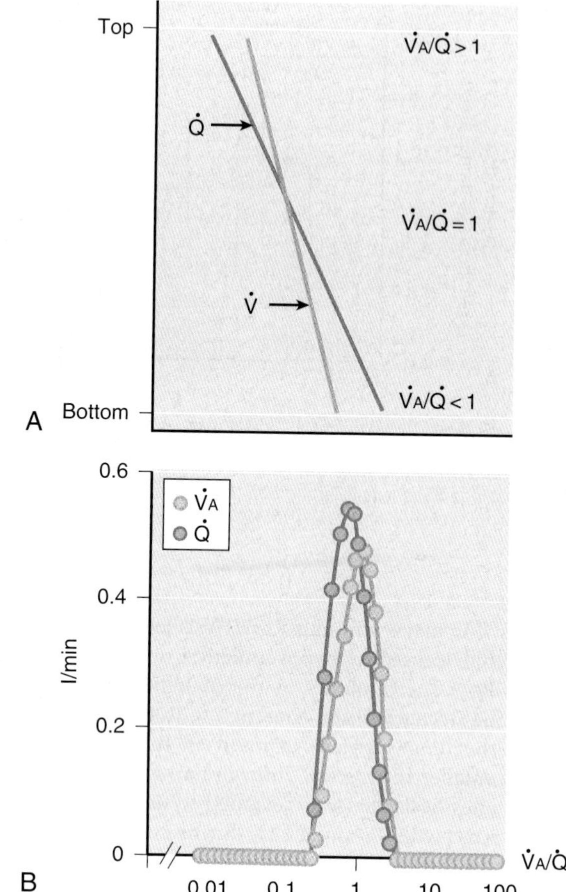

Figure 15-13 Schematic drawing of the vertical distributions of ventilation ($\dot{V}$) and blood flow through the lung ($\dot{Q}$) (**A**) and the resulting ventilation-perfusion distribution ($\dot{V}_A/\dot{Q}$) (**B**). Note the moderate increase in ventilation down the lung and the faster increase in perfusion. The $\dot{V}_A/\dot{Q}$ distribution is centered on a ratio of 1, which corresponds to the intersection of the ventilation and perfusion distribution curves. The slightly larger ventilation than perfusion in the upper lung regions contributes to the high $\dot{V}_A/\dot{Q}$ ratios above 1, whereas the larger perfusion than ventilation in the lower part of the lung is the cause of the lower $\dot{V}_A/\dot{Q}$ ratios, below 1.

centered on a $\dot{V}_A/\dot{Q}$ ratio of 1. MIGET has a high discriminatory capacity of detecting different ventilation/perfusion disturbances but does not have the potential of localizing where in the lung the impairment or variations are located. It is more like looking at a fingerprint of ventilation/perfusion match or mismatch. A number of variables that reflect the degree of mismatch can be calculated and are shown in Table 15-3. In the following paragraphs, examples of $\dot{V}_A/\dot{Q}$ mismatch are discussed.

If ventilation and perfusion are not matched, gas exchange will be affected. The most common cause of impaired oxygenation is indeed $\dot{V}_A/\dot{Q}$ mismatch. Low $\dot{V}_A/\dot{Q}$ will impede oxygenation because ventilation is too small to fully oxygenate the blood. The degree of impairment is dependent on the degree of mismatch, and even normally existing lung regions with a $\dot{V}_A/\dot{Q}$ ratio between 0.5 and 1 are unable to completely saturate the blood. Thus, Pa_{O_2} is seldom equal to alveolar P_{O_2}, but a difference ($PA_{O_2} - Pa_{O_2}$) of about 3 to 5 mm Hg (0.4 to 0.7 kPa) exists in the normal lung. With more $\dot{V}_A/\dot{Q}$ mismatch, the $PA_{O_2} - Pa_{O_2}$ difference is further increased. The $\dot{V}_A/\dot{Q}$ mismatch can account for all the hypoxemia seen in a severely obstructive patient.[47]

Table 15-3 Mean (SD) Ventilation-Perfusion Relationships with No Cardiopulmonary Disease (normal, $n = 45$), Awake and During General Anesthesia and Muscle Paralysis

	$\dot{Q}$mean	log SD$\dot{Q}$	$\dot{V}$mean	log SD$\dot{V}$	Shunt (% $\dot{Q}$T)	Dead Space (% VT)	Pa_{O_2}/FI_{O_2}* (kPa)
Awake	0.76 (0-33)	0.68 (0.28)	1.11 (0.52)	0.52 (0.15)	0.5 (1.0)	34.8 (14.2)	59.5 (8.1)
Anesthetized	0.65 (0.34)	1.04 (0.36)	1.38 (0.76)	0.76 (0.31)	4.8 (4.1)	35.0 (9.9)	50.9 (15.2)

*FI_{O_2} (inspired oxygen fraction): awake, 0.21; anesthetized, 0.42.
log SD$\dot{Q}$, standard deviations of the logarithmic distribution of perfusion; log SD$\dot{V}$, standard deviations of the logarithmic distribution of ventilation; $\dot{Q}$mean, mean $\dot{V}A/\dot{Q}$ of the perfusion distribution; $\dot{V}$mean, mean $\dot{V}A/\dot{Q}$ of ventilation distribution.

Shunt, which is often claimed to exist in patients with COPD, is mostly absent when analyzed with more sophisticated technique such as MIGET. Indeed, shunt in an obstructive patient should be considered indicative of a complicating factor in the disease (Fig. 15-14, lower left panel).

In severe asthma it is common to see a distinct mode of low $\dot{V}A/\dot{Q}$ ratios when using MIGET.[48] Thus, a bimodal distribution of $\dot{V}A/\dot{Q}$ ratios can be seen (Fig. 15-14, upper right panel). The explanation is probably that alveoli behind completely obstructed airways (edema, mucous plug, spasm) can still be ventilated through alveolar pores and interbronchial communications, so-called collateral ventilation. This may also explain why shunting is not normally seen in patients with COPD. However, with standard techniques, such as calculation of shunt by the oxygen equation, low $\dot{V}A/\dot{Q}$ cannot be separated from shunt. One should rather use the expression "venous admixture" in this case.

Airway obstruction is unevenly distributed over the lung, and a large variation in $\dot{V}A/\dot{Q}$ ratios can be seen in a single patient. Indeed, ventilation is redistributed from regions with high airway resistance to other regions that may become overventilated in proportion to their perfusion. This causes high $\dot{V}A/\dot{Q}$ ratios. There are normally regions in the upper part of the lung that have $\dot{V}A/\dot{Q}$ ratios of up to 5, but in obstructive patients ratios of up to 100 or greater can be seen, thus making them practically indistinguishable from true dead space. This is what causes the increase in "physiologic" dead space in obstructive lung disease. The effect of high $\dot{V}A/\dot{Q}$ is also the same as for airway dead space, that is, ventilation that seems to not participate in gas exchange ("wasted ventilation"). Consequently, at the same time an obstructive patient suffers from low $\dot{V}A/\dot{Q}$, which causes hypoxemia, and high $\dot{V}A/\dot{Q}$, which mimics dead space ventilation and impedes CO_2 elimination. However, the complexity of MIGET makes it essentially a research tool, and for clinical purposes and many scientific studies, calculation of dead space must rely on measurement of expired CO_2. Derivation of the CO_2 dead space is shown in Box 15-2.

$\dot{V}A/\dot{Q}$ mismatch exists to varying degree in all patients with COPD and can, as said earlier, explain all hypoxemia in most of these patients. Hypoventilation may be a contributing factor, whereas impaired diffusion (to the extent that it causes hypoxemia) and shunt are less common (see later).

Pulmonary vessels can be affected by lung disease and cause $\dot{V}A/\dot{Q}$ mismatch by impeding regional blood flow. Systemic diseases with vascular involvement such as periarteritis nodosa, disseminated lupus erythematosus, scleroderma, and rheumatoid diseases may cause severe pulmonary dysfunction with $\dot{V}A/\dot{Q}$ mismatch, impaired diffusion, and shunt. $\dot{V}A/\dot{Q}$ mismatch causes most of the hypoxemia that can be seen in pulmonary fibrosis at rest.[49] In addition, hypoxemia can be caused by impaired diffusion (in particular, during exercise, when it may dominate) and a varying degree of shunt (see later). Pulmonary emboli cause $\dot{V}A/\dot{Q}$ mismatch because the occluded vascular bed forces blood flow to other, open regions, thus making these regions overperfused in relation to their ventilation. This, again, causes low $\dot{V}A/\dot{Q}$. Shunt may be small unless pulmonary artery pressure is markedly increased.[50]

Pneumonia and various forms of acute respiratory failure are signified by shunt and to a varying extent by $\dot{V}A/\dot{Q}$ mismatch (Fig. 15-14, lower right panel). This can easily be understood from the presence of atelectasis, fluid filling, and consolidation seen with these diseases.[51]

Is CO_2 removal less affected than oxygenation of blood by $\dot{V}A/\dot{Q}$ mismatch? It is perhaps if the CO_2 content of blood is more linearly related to CO_2 tension than the O_2 content is related to P_{O_2}, according to the oxygen dissociation curve. However, this is not true. Elimination of CO_2 is even more limited by $\dot{V}A/\dot{Q}$ mismatch than O_2 transfer is.[31] Still, it is rare to see hypercapnia caused by mismatch because any increase in CO_2 tension stimulates increased ventilation to bring Pa_{CO_2} back toward normal. If alveolar ventilation is already impaired and cannot be increased, the addition of $\dot{V}A/\dot{Q}$ mismatch may make matters worse.

Impaired Diffusion

Impaired diffusion to the extent that it reduces Pa_{O_2} can occur if the alveolar-capillary membranes are thickened, as in fibrosis and systemic vascular diseases. Diffusion is slowed down and the whole capillary distance may be required before the capillary blood has been fully oxygenated, even in resting conditions. On

Box 15-2 Derivation of the Physiologic Dead Space Equation

$$F\bar{E} \times VT = FA(VT - VDS) + (FI \times VDS)$$

By rearranging,

$$\frac{VDS}{VT} = \frac{FA - F\bar{E}}{FA - FI}$$

If FI = 0, F replaced by P, and PA replaced by Pa, for CO_2,

$$\frac{VDS}{VT} = \frac{Pa_{CO_2} - P\bar{E}_{CO_2}}{Pa_{CO_2}}$$

where F$\bar{E}$, FA, and FI are mixed expired, alveolar, and inspired gas concentration, respectively, and VT, VDS, and VA are tidal volume, dead space, and part of the tidal volume to perfused alveoli, respectively.

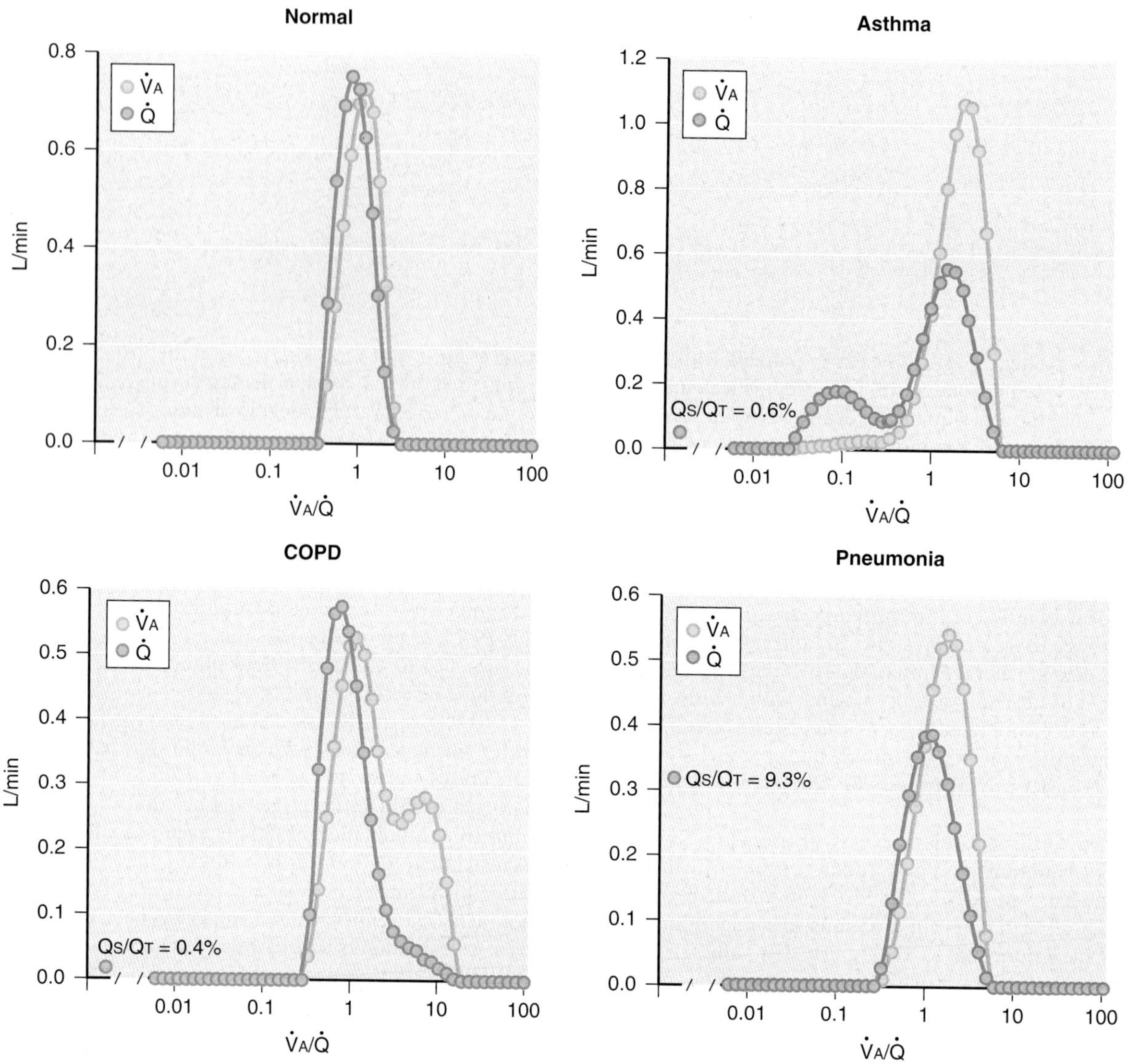

Figure 15-14 Ventilation-perfusion distributions in a normal subject (*upper left panel*), in a patient with asthma (*upper right panel*), in a patient with chronic obstructive pulmonary disease (COPD) (*lower left panel*), and in a patient with pneumonia (*lower right panel*). Note the good matching between ventilation and perfusion with a mode centered around a $\dot{V}_A/\dot{Q}$ ratio of 1 in the normal subject. This results in nearly optimal oxygenation of blood, as well as CO_2 removal. The asthmatic patient has broader distribution of $\dot{V}_A/\dot{Q}$ ratios, with some regions being ventilated well in excess of perfusion ($\dot{V}_A/\dot{Q}$ of 10 and higher), and there is another distinct mode of "low" $\dot{V}_A/\dot{Q}$ ratios centered around a $\dot{V}_A/\dot{Q}$ ratio of 0.1. This mode can reasonably be explained by collateral ventilation that maintains certain gas exchange behind otherwise occluded airways. Finally, no shunt can be seen. The chronic bronchitis patient may have a pattern that is not that different from the asthmatic patient, but there can also be a more clear "high"-$\dot{V}_A/\dot{Q}$ mode that adds to the dead space–like ventilation. A shunt cannot be seen, but if visible in the COPD patient, it indicates a complicating dysfunction (pneumonia, atelectasis, or something else?). The $\dot{V}_A/\dot{Q}$ pattern shown in the figure should not result in any considerable hypoxemia. The patient suffering from pneumonia shows minor widening of the $\dot{V}_A/\dot{Q}$ distribution, and the major finding is a pure shunt that is caused by consolidation of lung tissue that is still perfused but not ventilated. Q_S/Q_T, ratio of shunt blood flow to cardiac output.

the other hand, this means that a diffusion barrier may not cause hypoxemia as long as there is enough time and capillary distance to allow equilibration (see Fig. 15-10). However, when all reserve has been spent, Pa_{O_2} begins to fall. This is particularly noticeable in patients with pulmonary fibrosis, who may have normal Pa_{O_2} at rest but show dramatic decreases during exercise, down to 40 to 45 mm Hg (≈5 to 6 kPa).[31,49] There is almost no other condition that can cause such a decrease and, if found, should bring impaired diffusion into consideration. Obstructive lung disease does not cause such impairment of oxygenation; Pa_{O_2} changes only a little and can even improve! The only condition that can lower Pa_{O_2} to a similar extent is the appearance of or increase in right-to-left shunting in the heart, such as an atrial septal defect with a left-to-right shunt at rest that reverses during exercise because of increasing pulmonary hypertension.

Right-to-Left Shunt

If blood passes through the lung without coming into contact with ventilated alveoli, the blood will not be oxygenated or release CO_2. This is a shunt that lowers Pa_{O_2} and increases, although less easy to observe, Pa_{CO_2}. A small shunt of 2% to 3% of cardiac output can be seen in normal subjects and is caused by the thebesian veins that drain the heart and empty into the left atrium. In pathologic states, shunt may amount to anything between nearly normal to above 50% of cardiac output. Shunt may be considered an extreme of mismatch, with a $\dot{V}_A/\dot{Q}$ of zero. However, there are clear differences between the concepts of mismatch and shunt. First, the anatomic basis differs. Regions with low $\dot{V}A/\dot{Q}$ are caused by airway and vascular narrowing. This reduces ventilation and blood flow in some regions and increases them in others. Examples are obstructive lung disease and vascular disorders. Shunt is caused by the complete cessation of ventilation in a region, usually as a result of collapse (atelectasis) or consolidation (pneumonia, edema, obliterative processes). Contrary to what is normally said, asthma, bronchitis, and emphysema do not cause a shunt.[47] If a shunt is found, it indicates a complication. Second, the effect of "low $\dot{V}A/\dot{Q}$" on oxygenation of blood can essentially be overcome by adding more oxygen to the inspired air. Even in a poorly ventilated lung unit, P_{AO_2} can be increased almost as much as in normal regions, the difference being caused by the higher P_{ACO_2} in the poorly ventilated units. The effect of a moderate shunt can be reduced, but not eliminated, by giving more oxygen because the nonventilated region cannot be reached by the inspired gas. Thus, shunt will always lower Pa_{O_2} at any P_{IO_2}, as compared with what would have been measured without shunt. When the shunt increases to 25%, the rise in Pa_{O_2} will be small, and with a shunt of 30% or greater, almost no effect of added O_2 can be seen.[51] This is the net effect of mixing blood with normal pulmonary end-capillary P_{O_2} and shunt blood with mixed venous P_{O_2}. If the latter is a large enough fraction of total lung blood flow, the additional O_2 that can be physically dissolved by the raised P_{IO_2} is so small that it is almost immeasurable. The shunt is said to be refractory.

Respiratory Function During Anesthesia

Anesthesia causes an impairment in pulmonary function, whether the patient is breathing spontaneously or is ventilated mechanically after muscle paralysis. Impaired oxygenation of blood occurs in most subjects who are anesthetized.[52] It has therefore become routine to add oxygen to the inspired gas so that the inspired oxygen fraction (F_{IO_2}) is maintained at around 0.3 to 0.4. Despite these measures, mild to moderate hypoxemia, defined as an arterial oxygen saturation of between 85% and 90%, may occur in approximately half of all patients undergoing elective surgery, and the hypoxemia can last from a few seconds to up to 30 minutes. About 20% of patients may suffer from severe hypoxemia, or oxygen saturation below 81% for up to 5 minutes.[53] Lung function remains impaired postoperatively, and clinically significant pulmonary complications can be seen in 1% to 2% after minor surgery in up to 20% after upper abdominal and thoracic surgery.[54]

In this section, the effect of anesthesia and mechanical ventilation on lung function will be described. The order of the different paragraphs will follow an order that relates to the sequence of events that affect the lung's ability to oxygenate the blood and to remove carbon dioxide. Thus, the first phenomenon that might be seen with anesthesia is loss of muscle tone with a subsequent change in the balance between outward forces (i.e., respiratory muscles) and inward forces (i.e., elastic tissue in the lung) leading to a fall in FRC. This causes or is paralleled by an increase in the elastic behavior of the lung (reduced compliance) and an increase in respiratory resistance. The decrease in FRC affects the patency of lung tissue with the formation of atelectasis (made worse with the use of high concentrations of inspired oxygen) and airway closure. This alters the distribution of ventilation and matching of ventilation and blood flow and impedes oxygenation of blood and removal of carbon dioxide.

Lung Volume and Respiratory Mechanics During Anesthesia

Lung Volume

Resting lung volume, or FRC, is reduced by 0.8 to 1.0 L by changing body position from upright to supine, and there is another 0.4- to 0.5-L decrease when anesthesia has been induced.[55] End-expiratory lung volume is thus reduced from approximately 3.5 to 2 L, the latter being close or equal to RV. The anesthesia per se causes a fall in FRC despite maintenance of spontaneous breathing,[56,57] and the decrease in FRC occurs regardless of whether the anesthetic is inhaled or given intravenously.[58] Muscle paralysis and mechanical ventilation cause no further decrease in FRC. The average reduction corresponds to around 20% of awake FRC and may contribute to an altered distribution of ventilation and impaired oxygenation of blood, as discussed later.

The decrease seems to be related to loss of respiratory muscle tone, which shifts the balance between the elastic recoil force of the lung and the outward force of the chest wall to a lower chest and lung volume. Maintenance of muscle tone, as during ketamine anesthesia, does not reduce FRC.[58] The influence of body position and anesthesia on FRC is shown in Figure 15-8. As can be seen in the figure, FRC increases with age if weight and height remain unaltered over the years.

The decrease in FRC is caused by a cranial shift of the diaphragm and a small decrease in the transverse thoracic area in a majority of studies as evidenced by repeated CT scanning.[58,59] However, somewhat conflicting results have been reported regarding the diaphragm, with only minor displacement of the diaphragm and the anterior part even being shifted caudally.[60] Such caudal displacement could in theory occur if the ribs are tilted downward during anesthesia.

Compliance and Resistance of the Respiratory System

Static compliance of the total respiratory system (lungs and chest wall) is reduced on average from 95 to 60 mL/cm H_2O during anesthesia.[61] Several studies on lung compliance have been carried out during anesthesia, and the vast majority of studies indicate a decrease in comparison to the awake state (e.g., static lung compliance fell from a mean of 187 mL/cm H_2O awake to 149 mL/cm H_2O during anesthesia when data from several studies were pooled).[61]

There are also studies on resistance of the total respiratory system and the lungs during anesthesia, most of them showing a considerable increase during both spontaneous breathing and mechanical ventilation.[61] However, the studies on resistance during anesthesia have been hampered by different experimental conditions during the awake and anesthetized situations. Thus, a study that enables comparison of resistance under both isovolume and isoflow conditions is still awaited. The possibility remains that the increased lung resistance merely reflects reduced FRC during anesthesia (Fig. 15-15).

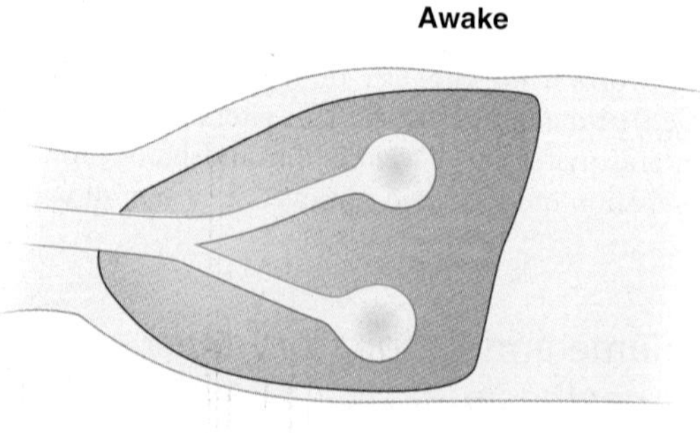

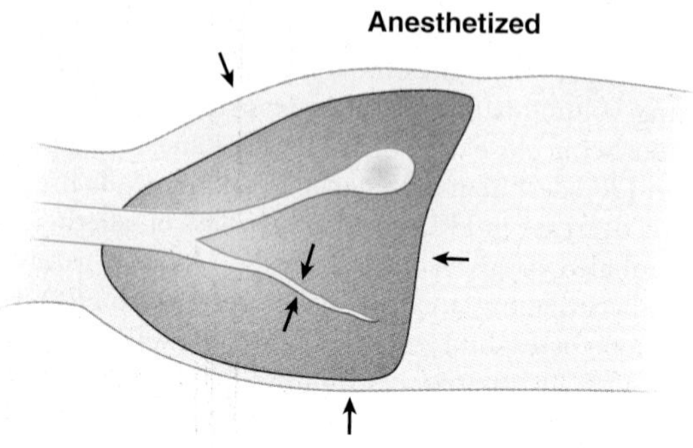

Figure 15-15 Cranial shift of the diaphragm and a decrease in transverse diameter of the thorax contribute to lowered functional residual capacity (FRC) during anesthesia. Decreased ventilated volume (atelectasis and airway closure) is a possible cause of reduced lung compliance (CL). Decreased airway dimensions by the lowered FRC should contribute to increased airway resistance (Raw).

Atelectasis and Airway Closure During Anesthesia

Atelectasis

In their classic paper, Bendixen and coworkers proposed "a concept of atelectasis" as a cause of impaired oxygenation during anesthesia.[62] They had observed a successive decrease in compliance of the respiratory system and a similar successive decrease in arterial oxygenation in both anesthetized humans and experimental animals. This was interpreted as formation of atelectasis. However, other research groups who were unable to reproduce their findings noticed a more prompt fall in compliance and Pa_{O_2} on induction of anesthesia. Moreover, atelectasis could not be shown on conventional chest radiography.

In the mid-eighties, new observations were made that may explain the altered function of the lung during anesthesia. On CT with transverse exposure of the chest, prompt development of densities in the dependent regions of both lungs could be shown during anesthesia. For a review with references from before 1990, see the ISPOCD1 study.[53] Morphologic studies of these densities in various animals supported the diagnosis of atelectasis. An example of atelectasis as seen on a CT scan is shown in Figure 15-16.

Atelectasis appears in approximately 90% of all patients who are anesthetized.[63] It is seen during spontaneous breathing and after muscle paralysis and whether intravenous or inhaled anesthetics are used.[58] The atelectatic area on a CT cut near the diaphragm is around 5% to 6% of the total lung area but can easily exceed 15% to 20%. It should also be remembered that the amount of tissue that is collapsed is even larger, the atelectatic area consisting of mainly lung tissue and the aerated lung consisting of only 20% to 40% tissue, the rest being air. Thus, 15% to 20% of the lung is regularly collapsed at the base of the lung during uneventful anesthesia, before any surgery has even been done! Abdominal surgery does not add much to the atelectasis, but it can remain for several days in the postoperative period.[64] It is likely that it is a focus of infection and can contribute to pulmonary complications.[65] It may also be mentioned that after thoracic surgery and cardiopulmonary bypass, more than 50% of the lung can be collapsed even several hours after surgery.[66] The amount of atelectasis decreases toward the apex, which is mostly spared (fully aerated) (Fig. 15-17).

There is a weak correlation between the size of the atelectasis and body weight or body mass index (BMI),[58,67] with obese patients showing larger atelectatic areas than lean ones do. Although this was expected, it came as a surprise that the atelectasis is independent of age, with children and young people showing as much atelectasis as elderly patients.[63] Another unexpected observation was that patients with COPD showed less or even no atelectasis during the 45 minutes of anesthesia that they were studied.[68] The mechanism that prevents the lung from collapse is not clear but may be airway closure occurring before alveolar collapse takes place, or it may be an altered balance between the chest wall and the lung that counters a decrease in lung dimensions.

There is good correlation between the amount of atelectasis and pulmonary shunt as measured by MIGET. A regression equation based on a total of 45 patients studied during anesthesia with inhaled anesthetics has been calculated as shunt = 0.8 × atelectasis + 1.7 ($r = .81$, $P < .01$), with atelectasis expressed as the percentage of lung area just above the diaphragm on CT scan and shunt expressed as the percentage of cardiac output. Interestingly, shunt did not increase with age.[63] By combining CT scanning and SPECT, the distribution of shunt and its location within the atelectatic area were confirmed (Fig. 15-18).[69]

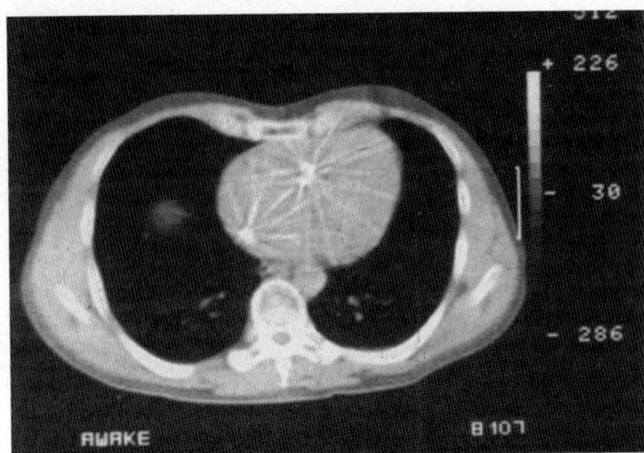

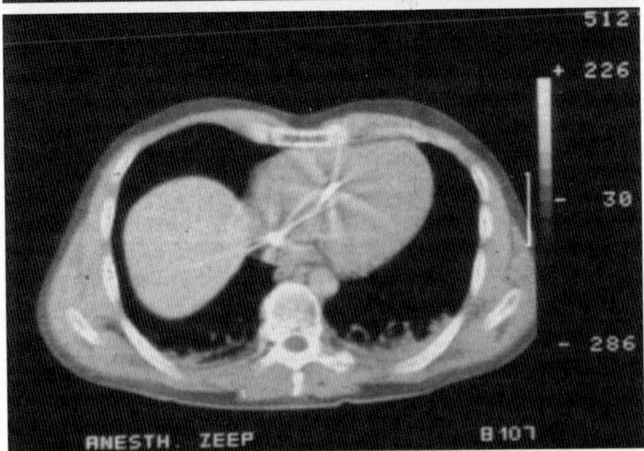

Figure 15-16 Computed tomography with transverse exposure of the chest when the subject is awake (*upper panel*) and then anesthetized (*lower panel*). Note the well-aerated lung in the awake condition. A few pulmonary vessels can be seen in the lower lung regions. The radiating beams in the heart are caused by a catheter that is positioned with its tip in the pulmonary artery. During anesthesia, atelectasis has developed in the most dependent regions of both lungs (seen as gray/white irregular areas). The large gray/white area in the middle of the right lung field is caused by a cranial shift of the diaphragm and the underlying liver. The exposure levels of the two scans are the same relative to the spine.

Prevention of Atelectasis During Anesthesia

Several interventions can help prevent atelectasis or even reopen collapsed tissue, as discussed in the following paragraphs.

Positive End-Expiratory Pressure. The application of 10-cm H_2O PEEP has been tested in several studies and will consistently reopen collapsed lung tissue. This is more likely an effect of increased inspiratory airway pressure than of PEEP per se.[58] However, some atelectasis persists in most patients. Whether a further increase in the PEEP will reopen this tissue was not analyzed in these studies. PEEP, however, does not appear to be the ideal procedure. First, shunt is not reduced proportionately, and arterial oxygenation may not improve significantly. Hewlett and coworkers warned even in 1974 of the "indiscriminate use of PEEP in routine anesthesia."[70] The persistence of shunt may be explained by a redistribution of blood flow toward more dependent parts of the lungs when intrathoracic pressure is increased by PEEP (Fig. 15-19). Under such circumstances, any persisting atelectasis in the bottom of the lung receives a larger share of the pulmonary blood flow than without PEEP.[71] Furthermore, increased intrathoracic pressure will impede venous return and

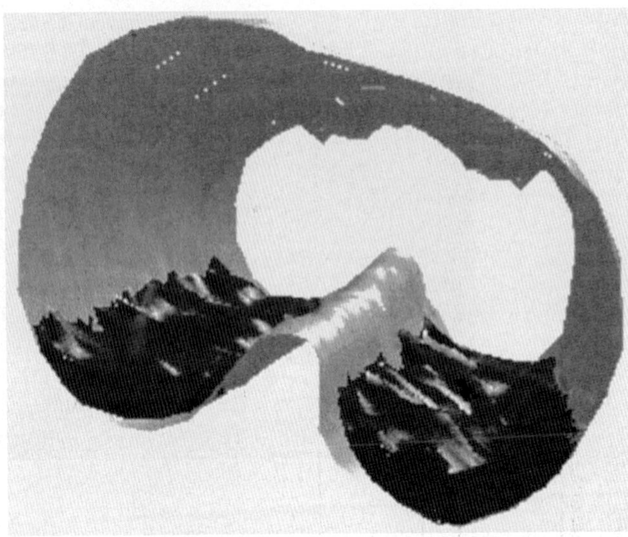

Figure 15-17 Three-dimensional reconstruction of the thorax of an anesthetized patient with atelectasis in the dependent regions of both lungs. Note the irregular shape of the atelectasis. There is a slight decrease in the amount of atelectasis toward the apex, which is at the distal end of the chest wall on the image. *(Redrawn from data in Reber A, Nylund U, Hedenstierna G: Position and shape of the diaphragm: Implications for atelectasis formation. Anaesthesia 53:1054-1061, 1998.)*

decrease cardiac output. This results in a lower venous oxygen tension for a given oxygen uptake and reduces arterial oxygen tension. Second, the lung recollapses rapidly after discontinuation of PEEP. Within 1 minute after cessation of PEEP, the collapse is as large as it was before the application of PEEP.[58]

Maintenance of Muscle Tone. Use of an anesthetic that allows maintenance of respiratory muscle tone will prevent atelectasis from forming. Ketamine does not impair muscle tone and does not cause atelectasis. This is the only anesthetic thus far tested that does not cause collapse. However, if muscle relaxation is required, atelectasis will appear as with other anesthetics.[58]

Another technique used in an attempt to restore respiratory muscle tone is pacing of the diaphragm. This was tested by applying phrenic nerve stimulation, which did reduce the atelectatic area.[72] The effect was small, however, and this technique is certainly too complicated to be used routinely during anesthesia and surgery.

Recruitment Maneuvers. The use of a sigh maneuver, or a double V_T, has been advocated to reopen any collapsed lung tissue.[73] However, the atelectasis is not decreased by a double V_T or by a sigh up to an airway pressure of 20 cm H_2O.[67] Not until an airway pressure of 30 cm H_2O is reached does the atelectasis decrease to approximately half the initial size. For complete reopening of all collapsed lung tissue, an inflation pressure of 40 cm H_2O is required (Fig. 15-20). Such a large inflation corresponds to a maximum spontaneous inspiration, and it can thus be called a VC maneuver.

Because a VC maneuver may result in adverse cardiovascular events, the dynamics in resolving atelectasis during such a procedure was analyzed.[74] It was found that in adults with healthy lungs, inflation of the lungs to +40 cm H_2O maintained for no more than 7 to 8 seconds may re-expand all previously collapsed lung tissue.

Minimizing Gas Resorption. Ventilation of the lungs with pure oxygen after a VC maneuver that had reopened previ-

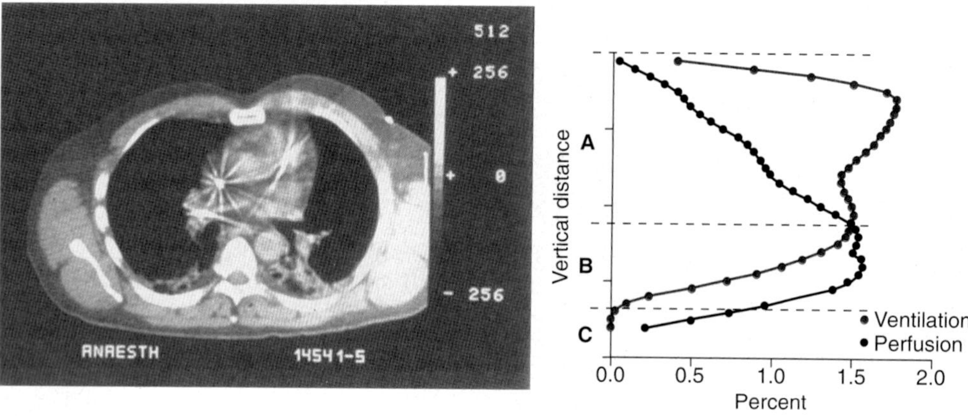

Figure 15-18 Transverse computed tomography (CT) scan with atelectasis visible in the dependent parts of both lungs (*left panel*) and corresponding vertical distributions of ventilation and lung blood flow (*right panel*) in an anesthetized subject. Note that ventilation is distributed preferentially to the upper lung regions, contrary to what is seen in an awake subject. Ventilation exceeds perfusion at that level, and this results in a dead space–like effect, or wasted ventilation (zone A in the *right panel*). Note also the decreasing ventilation in the lower half of the lung such that perfusion is larger at that level. This results in so-called low $\dot{V}_A/\dot{Q}$ and causes impaired oxygenation of blood. Intermittent airway closure is the probable mechanism behind the reduced ventilation (zone B). There is complete cessation of ventilation in the bottom, which corresponds to the atelectatic area. However, there is still perfusion producing a shunt (zone C). It can also be seen that perfusion increases down the lung, except for the bottom-most region, where a decrease can be seen. This so-called zone IV may be caused by increased interstitial lung pressure compressing extra-alveolar vessels and hypoxic pulmonary vasoconstriction. *(Redrawn from data in Tokics L, Hedenstierna G, Svensson L, et al: V/Q distribution and correlation to atelectasis in anesthetized paralyzed humans. J Appl Physiol 81:1822-1833, 1996.)*

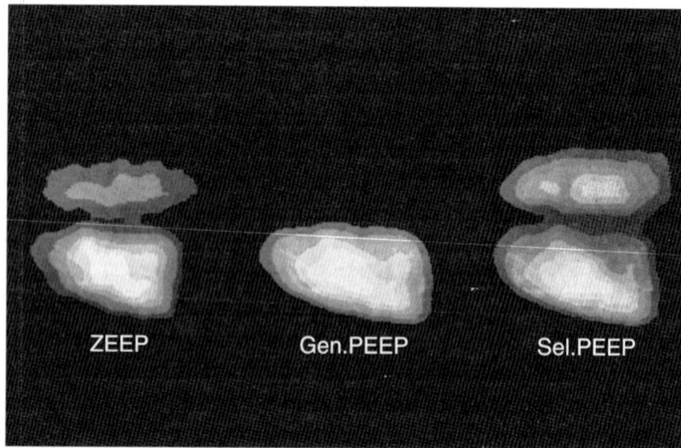

Figure 15-19 Gamma camera images of the distribution of lung blood flow in an anesthetized subject in the lateral position. During mechanical ventilation with zero end-expiratory pressure (ZEEP), perfusion goes mainly to the lower lung, but there is still perfusion of the upper lung, with the average distribution to the upper lung being 33% to 40% of total lung perfusion. With a general PEEP of 10 cm H_2O, perfusion is squeezed down to the lower lung, and in this particular example there is almost no perfusion at all in the upper lung. This causes a dramatic dead space–like effect. If, on the other hand, PEEP is applied selectively to the lower lung, in this example 10 cm H_2O, perfusion might be redistributed to the upper lung so that a more even distribution between the two lungs can be seen. It should be clear that the size of the upper and lower lungs, as shown on the image, does not reflect lung volume but perfused lung tissue. The upper lung should be expected to be larger than the lower lung in the lateral position. *(From Hedenstierna G, Baehrendtz S, Klingstedt C, et al: Ventilation and perfusion of each lung during differential ventilation with selective PEEP. Anesthesiology 61:369-376, 1984.)*

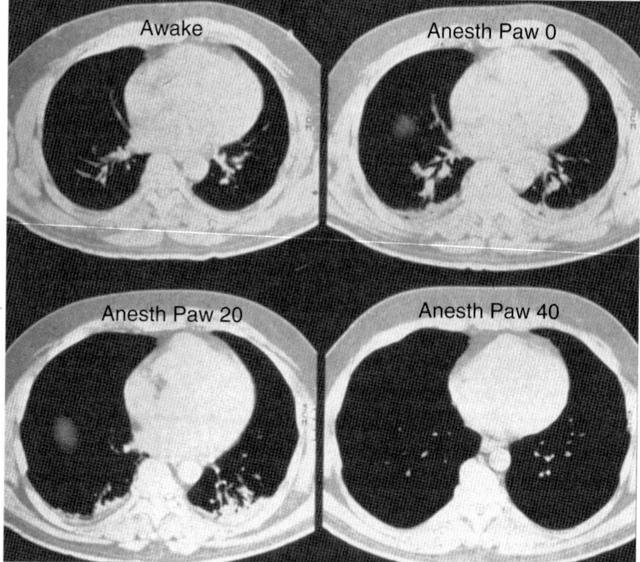

Figure 15-20 Computed tomography scans in a subject when awake (*upper left panel*); during anesthesia at zero end expiratory pressure (*upper right panel*); during anesthesia and an airway pressure of 20 cm H_2O, which corresponds to a double tidal volume (*lower left panel*); and during anesthesia at maximal inflation of the lungs to an airway pressure of 40 cm H_2O (*lower right panel*). Note that there is no atelectasis in the awake subject; only vessels can be seen in the lower part of the lung. During anesthesia with zero airway pressure, atelectasis can be seen in the dependent parts of both lungs. Inflation to 10 cm H_2O, corresponding to a regular tidal volume, does not open any tissue (not shown here). Inflation to 20 cm H_2O still did not open any lung tissue. Not until inflation to 30 cm H_2O (not shown here) did collapsed lung tissue start to open. A maximum inflation of 40 mm Hg airway pressure (Paw) was required to fully open the lung. Thus, a "vital" capacity maneuver was required to open the lung (the volume inflated corresponded to the maximum breath by the awake subject before anesthesia). *(From Rothen HU, Sporre B, Engberg G, et al: Reexpansion of atelectasis during general anaesthesia: A computed tomography study. Br J Anaesth 71:788-795, 1993.)*

ously collapsed lung tissue resulted in rapid reappearance of the atelectasis.[75] If, on the other hand, 40% O_2 in nitrogen is used for ventilation of the lungs, atelectasis reappears slowly, and 40 minutes after the VC maneuver only 20% of the initial atelectasis had reappeared. Thus, ventilation during anesthesia should be done with a moderate fraction of inspired oxygen (e.g., FIO_2 of 0.3 to 0.4) and should be increased only if arterial oxygenation is compromised.

The striking effects of oxygen during anesthesia raised the question of whether "preoxygenation" during induction of anesthesia has an effect on the formation of atelectasis. Breathing of 100% O_2, just for a few minutes before and during commencement of anesthesia, increases the safety margin in the event of difficult intubation of the airway with prolonged apnea. However, there turned out to be a price for it. Avoidance of the preoxygenation procedure (ventilation with 30% O_2) eliminated atelectasis formation during induction and subsequent anesthesia.[76] In a subsequent study, 12 patients were breathing 100% O_2 during induction of anesthesia, another 12 were breathing 80% O_2, and still another 12 breathed 60% O_2.[77] Atelectasis appeared in all patients receiving 100% O_2, was much smaller in the 80% O_2 group, and was almost absent in the 60% O_2 group (Fig. 15-21).

Preoxygenation can also be provided without producing atelectasis if undertaken with continuously increased airway pressure, as with continuous positive airway pressure (CPAP). By applying CPAP of 10 cm H_2O, Rusca and associates could induce anesthesia on 100% O_2 without any substantial atelectasis formation.[78] This technique might provide the greatest safety without atelectasis formation but it requires a tight system and might be complicated in clinical practice.

Postanesthetic Oxygenation. Preoxygenation promotes not only the formation of atelectasis but also the so-called postanesthetic oxygenation at the end of the surgery. This procedure is often combined with suctioning of the airway tree, and it is difficult to see how any other technique can be invented that is so likely to produce atelectasis as suctioning together with postanesthetic oxygenation! This will most likely deliver a patient to the postoperative ward with more atelectasis than at any other moment during anesthesia and surgery. Postanesthetic oxygenation (100% O_2) 10 minutes before termination of anesthesia together with a VC maneuver at the end of anesthesia did not protect against atelectasis at the end of anesthesia.[79] This is most likely the effect of first reopening collapsed tissue and then, under the influence of 100% O_2, derecruiting previously opened lung tissue. A VC maneuver followed by a lower O_2 concentration, 40%, kept the lung open after recruitment until the end of anesthesia. This is not unexpected in view of the findings earlier in the anesthesia procedure.

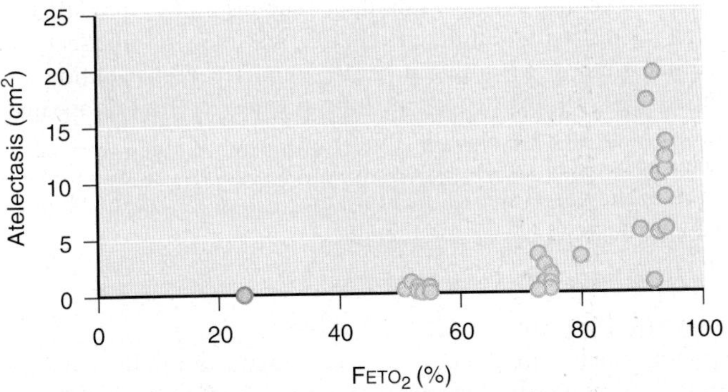

Figure 15-21 Formation of atelectasis in anesthetized subjects whose anesthesia has been induced with different inspired oxygen concentrations during the preoxygenation period. Twelve subjects were given 100% O_2, another 12 subjects 80%, and still another 12 subjects 60% O_2. The graph shows the expired oxygen concentration, which explains why the individual symbols are not at 60%, 80%, and 100%. Note the much larger atelectasis with preoxygenation of 100% (although there is large scatter) than at 80% and 60%, with almost no atelectasis at 60% preoxygenation. The *blue circle* at around an end-tidal oxygen concentration ($FETO_2$) of 25% corresponds to data obtained by Rothen and colleagues, who induced anesthesia in subjects given 30% O_2. *(From Rothen HU, Sporre B, Engberg G, et al: Prevention of atelectasis during general anesthesia. Lancet 345:1387-1391, 1995.)*

Airway Closure

In addition to atelectasis, intermittent closure of airways can be expected to reduce the ventilation of dependent lung regions. Such lung regions may then become "low-$\dot{V}A/\dot{Q}$" units if perfusion is maintained or not reduced to the same extent as ventilation. Airway closure increases with age[25] (see also Fig. 15-7), as does perfusion to "low-$\dot{V}A/\dot{Q}$" regions.[47] Because anesthesia causes a reduction in FRC of 0.4 to 0.5 L,[55] it may be anticipated that airway closure will become even more prominent in an anesthetized subject. There is accumulating evidence that such is the case.[80,81] The reduced ventilation in the lower half of the lung, just above the atelectasis, that can be seen in Figure 15-18 is reasonably explained by airway closure. It can also be seen that ventilation is smaller than perfusion, thereby causing "low-$\dot{V}A/\dot{Q}$" regions. These regions contribute to impaired oxygenation during anesthesia.

As much as 74% of the impaired arterial oxygenation can be explained by atelectasis and airway closure taken together, according to the following equation[57]:

$$PaO_2\,(mm\,Hg) = 218 - 22 \cdot \ln \text{atelectasis}\,(cm^2) - 0.06\,(CV - ERV)(mL)$$

($r = .86$, $P < .001$), where (CV – ERV) indicates the amount of airway closure occurring above FRC and ERV is expiratory reserve volume. A simple three-compartment lung model can be constructed to explain the impaired oxygenation during anesthesia. The model consists of one compartment with "normal" ventilation and perfusion, one compartment with airway closure that impedes ventilation, and a final compartment of collapsed lung with no ventilation at all. This is shown in Figure 15-22, left panel, together with the subsequent impact on $\dot{V}A/\dot{Q}$ distribution.

Distribution of Ventilation and Blood Flow During Anesthesia

Distribution of Ventilation

Redistribution of inspired gas away from dependent to nondependent lung regions has been observed in anesthetized supine humans by isotope techniques. With the use of a radiolabeled aerosol and SPECT, ventilation was shown to be distributed mainly to the upper lung regions, and there was a successive decrease down the lower half of the lung.[69] Moreover, there was no ventilation at all in the bottom of the lung, a finding

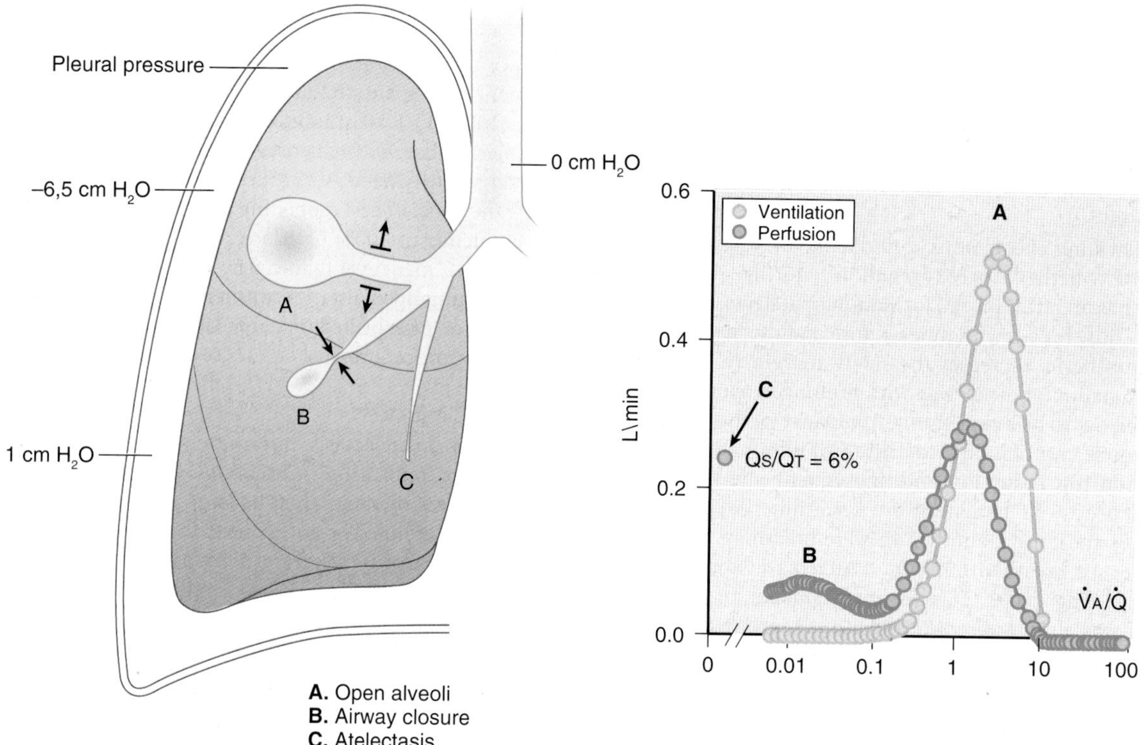

Figure 15-22 Three-compartment model of the lung in an anesthetized subject. In the upper part of the lung, the alveoli and airways are open (zone A). In the middle and lower parts of the lung, the airways are intermittently closed and impede ventilation (zone B), and in the bottom of the lung, the alveoli have collapsed (atelectasis, zone C). Compare with Figure 15-7. The corresponding ventilation-perfusion distribution as assessed by the multiple inert gas elimination technique can be seen in the *right panel*. Modes A and B correspond to a well-ventilated and perfused lung region and a region with intermittent airway closure, respectively, and are similar to what was shown in Figure 15-7. In addition, there is a shunt that is caused by perfusion of the atelectatic zone (C) in the bottom of the lung.

corresponding to the distribution of atelectasis that was simultaneously observed by CT (see Fig. 15-18).

PEEP increases dependent lung ventilation in anesthetized subjects in the lateral position, so the distribution of ventilation is more similar to that in the awake state.[82] Similar findings of more even distribution between the upper and lower lung regions have also been made in supine anesthetized humans after previous inflation of the lungs, similar to PEEP.[83] Thus, restoration of overall FRC toward or beyond the awake level returns gas distribution toward the awake pattern. It is reasonably an effect of the recruitment of collapsed, dependent lung regions (atelectasis), of reopening of closed airways in the lower lung regions, and possibly of increased expansion of the upper lung regions so that they become less compliant (and less ventilated).

Distribution of Lung Blood Flow

As discussed earlier, the distribution of lung blood flow has been studied by injection of radioactively labeled macroaggregated albumin and SPECT in anesthetized, mechanically ventilated patients.[69] A successive increase in perfusion down the lung, from the ventral to the dorsal aspect, was seen, with some reduction in the lowermost region. Thus, the lowermost portion of the lung, which was atelectatic as evidenced by simultaneous CT, was still perfused (see Fig. 15-18).

PEEP will impede venous return to the right heart and therefore reduce cardiac output. It may also affect pulmonary vascular resistance, although this may have less of an effect on cardiac output. In addition, PEEP causes a redistribution of blood flow toward dependent lung regions.[71,83] By this means, upper lung regions may be poorly perfused, thereby causing a dead space–like effect. Moreover, forcing blood volume downward to the dorsal side of the lungs may increase fractional blood flow through an atelectatic region.

Hypoxic Pulmonary Vasoconstriction

Several inhaled anesthetics have been found to inhibit HPV in isolated lung preparations. However, no such effect has been seen with intravenous anesthetics (barbiturates).[84] Results from human studies vary, reasonably explained by the complexity of the experiment, which causes several variables to change at the same time. The HPV response may thus be obscured by simultaneous changes in cardiac output, myocardial contractility, vascular tone, blood volume distribution, blood pH and CO_2 tension, and lung mechanics. In studies with no gross changes in cardiac output, isoflurane and halothane depress the HPV response by 50% at a minimum alveolar concentration (MAC) of 2 (Fig. 15-23).[85]

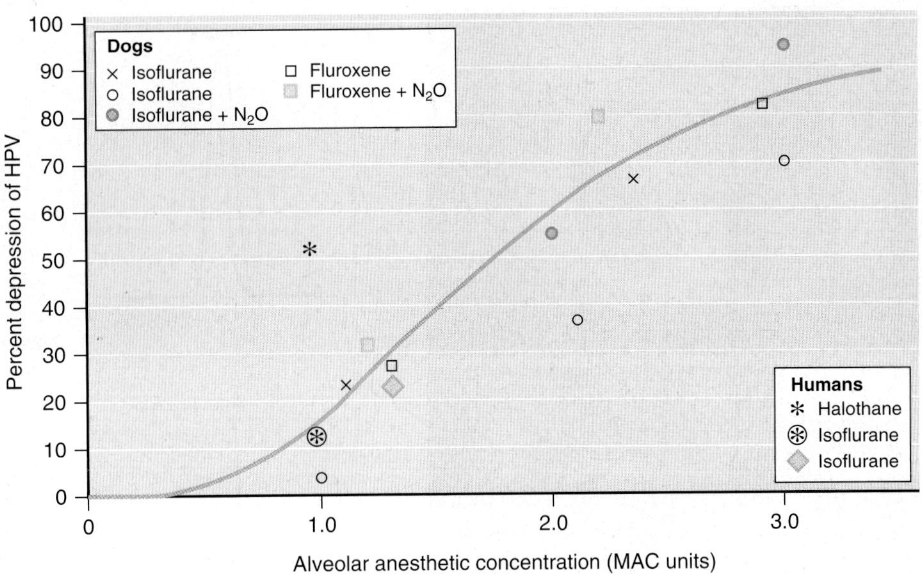

Figure 15-23 Attenuation of hypoxic pulmonary vasoconstriction (HPV) plotted against minimal alveolar anesthetic concentration (MAC units). Note that during anesthesia with different inhaled anesthetics at a MAC of 1, a depression of HPV of about 20% to 30% can be seen, and with higher anesthetic concentrations, HPV can be blunted much more. The consequence is that perfusion through a nonventilated region, as in atelectasis, will not be reduced at higher anesthetic concentrations. *(From Marshall BE. Hypoxic pulmonary Vasoconstriction. Acta Anaesthesiol Scand 94:37-41, 1990.)*

Ventilation-Perfusion Matching During Anesthesia

Dead Space, Shunt, and Ventilation-Perfusion Relationships

Both CO_2 elimination and oxygenation of blood are impaired in most patients during anesthesia. The impeded CO_2 elimination can be attributed to increased dead space ventilation. Single-breath washout recordings have demonstrated that "anatomic" dead space is unchanged, indicating that the "alveolar" or parallel dead space must have increased during anesthesia.[73] By MIGET, the increased CO_2 dead space during anesthesia is not really dead space but poorly perfused lung regions that are signified by so-called high $\dot{V}_A/\dot{Q}$ ratios (Fig. 15-24). Such "high $\dot{V}_A/\dot{Q}$" can be explained by the tiny perfusion of corner vessels in interalveolar septa in the upper lung regions (where alveolar pressure may exceed pulmonary vascular pressure [zone I]).[52] The impaired CO_2 elimination is most easily corrected by increasing the ventilation and is seldom a problem in routine anesthesia with mechanical ventilation.

The impairment in arterial oxygenation during anesthesia is generally considered to be more severe at higher ages, obesity worsens the oxygenation of blood, and smokers show more impairment in gas exchange than nonsmokers do.[86,87] Venous admixture, as calculated according to the standard oxygen "shunt" equation, is also increased during anesthesia to approximately 10% of cardiac output. However, the venous admixture includes not only perfusion of nonventilated lung tissue (true shunt) but also regions that are poorly ventilated or perfused in excess of their ventilation ("low-$\dot{V}_A/\dot{Q}$ regions"). The extent to which the venous admixture includes low-$\dot{V}_A/\dot{Q}$ regions depends on the inspired oxygen fraction (F_{IO_2}). The higher the inspired oxygen fraction, the less there are of the low-$\dot{V}_A/\dot{Q}$ regions. However, with high F_{IO_2}, regions with low $\dot{V}_A/\dot{Q}$ may collapse because of gas adsorption and be transformed to shunt regions.[88] A good correlation between venous admixture and the sum of "true" shunt and perfusion of "low-$\dot{V}_A/\dot{Q}$ regions" was seen in a study involving 45 anesthetized subjects (Fig. 15-25).[63] Derivation of the "oxygen shunt" or venous admixture is shown in Box 15-3.

In young healthy volunteers during anesthesia with thiopental and methoxyflurane, both ventilation and perfusion were distributed to wider ranges of $\dot{V}_A/\dot{Q}$ ratios, which can be expressed as an increase in the logarithmic standard deviation of the perfusion distribution (log SDQ). In a similar group of patients studied during halothane anesthesia and muscle paralysis, log SDQ was almost doubled, from 0.43 when awake to 0.80 during anesthesia. In addition, true shunt was increased to a mean of 8%. A similar increase in shunt from 1% awake to a mean of 9% during anesthesia was recorded in a study on middle-aged (37 to 64 years) surgical patients, and there was a widening of the $\dot{V}_A/\dot{Q}$ distribution (log SDQ of 0.47 when awake and 1.01 during anesthesia). In elderly patients with more severe impairment of lung function, halothane anesthesia with muscle paralysis, with or without nitrous oxide, caused considerable widening of the $\dot{V}_A/\dot{Q}$ distribution, with log SDQ increasing from 0.87 when awake to 1.73 during anesthesia. In addition, shunt increased to a mean of 15%, with large variation between patients (0% to 30%). Thus, the most consistent findings during anesthesia are an increased $\dot{V}_A/\dot{Q}$ mismatch, expressed as an increased log SDQ, and an increase in shunt. For review, see the article by Hedenstierna.[52]

Effects of Anesthetics on Respiratory Drive

Spontaneous ventilation is frequently reduced during anesthesia. Thus, inhaled anesthetics,[89] as well as barbiturates for intravenous use,[90] reduce sensitivity to CO_2. The response is dose dependent and entails decreasing ventilation with deepening anesthesia. Anesthesia also reduces the response to hypoxia. Attenuation of the hypoxic response may be attributed to an effect on the carotid body chemoreceptors.[91]

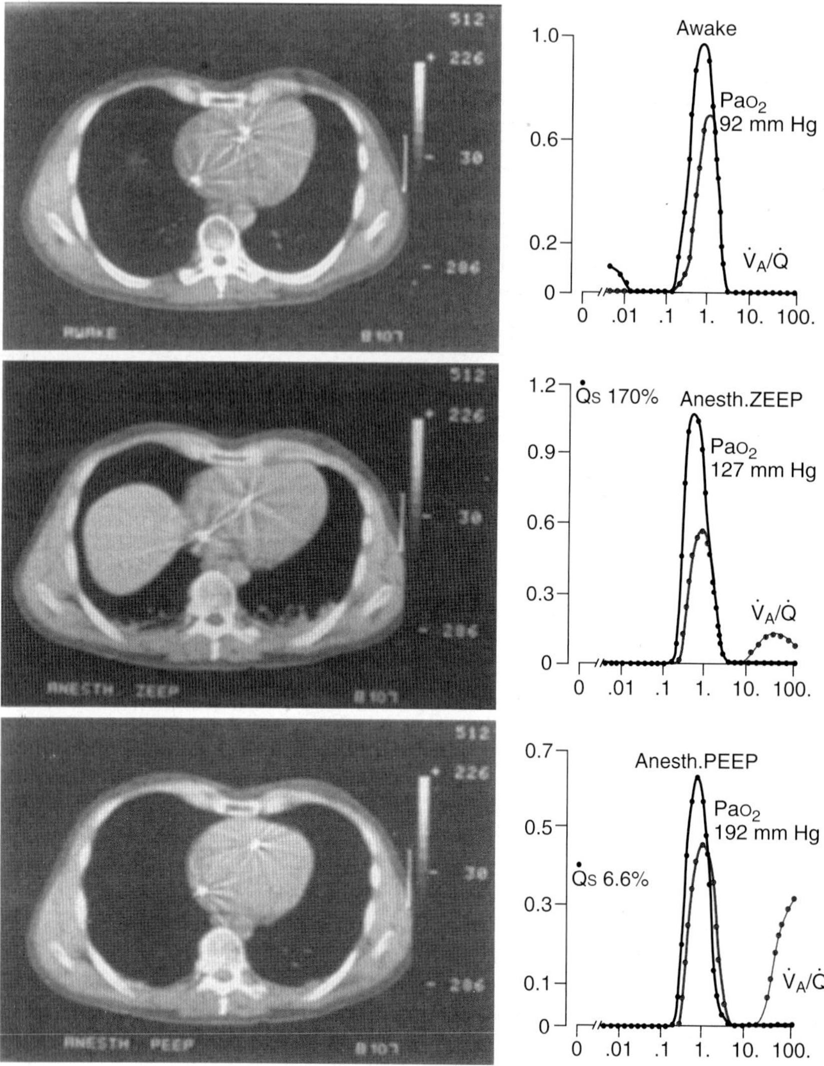

Figure 15-24 Computed tomography scans and $\dot{V}_A/\dot{Q}$ distributions in a lung-healthy subject when awake, during anesthesia with zero end-expiratory pressure (ZEEP), and during anesthesia with 10-cm H_2O positive end-expiratory pressure (PEEP). Note the absence of any atelectasis in the awake condition and the corresponding $\dot{V}_A/\dot{Q}$ distribution with a minor low-$\dot{V}_A/\dot{Q}$ mode that might be explained by intermittent airway closure. During anesthesia with ZEEP, atelectasis can be seen in the bottom of the lung, as well as the diaphragm in the middle of the right lung area (the diaphragm has been pushed cranially during anesthesia). A large shunt can be seen, whereas the "low" $\dot{V}_A/\dot{Q}$ has more or less disappeared, probably by conversion to atelectasis and shunt. Moreover, a small "high"-$\dot{V}_A/\dot{Q}$ mode can be seen that might reflect alveolar dead space in the upper lung regions. With PEEP, the collapsed lung tissue has been recruited and the shunt has been considerably reduced. Moreover, the "high"-$\dot{V}_A/\dot{Q}$ mode has increased in size and may reflect a further increase in nonperfused upper lung regions that has caused a dead space–like effect.

The effect of an anesthetic on respiratory muscles is nonuniform. Rib cage excursions diminish with deepening anesthesia.[92] The normal ventilatory response to CO_2 is produced by the intercostal muscles,[93,94] with no clear increase in rib cage motion with CO_2 rebreathing during halothane anesthesia. Thus, the reduced ventilatory response to CO_2 during anesthesia is due to impeded function of the intercostal muscles.

Factors That Influence Respiratory Function During Anesthesia

Spontaneous Breathing

Most studies on lung function have been performed on anesthetized, mechanically ventilated subjects or animals. Relatively few data have been obtained during spontaneous breathing. FRC is reduced to the same extent during anesthesia, regardless of whether a muscle relaxant is used,[56,58] and atelectasis occurs to almost the same extent in anesthetized spontaneously breathing subjects as during muscle paralysis.[95] Furthermore, the cranial shift of the diaphragm, as reported by Froese and Bryan in their classic paper,[96] was of the same magnitude both during general anesthesia with spontaneous breathing and with muscle paralysis, even though a difference in movement of the diaphragm from the resting position was noted. Thus, during spontaneous breathing, the lower, dependent portion of the diaphragm moved the most, whereas with muscle paralysis, the upper, nondependent part showed the largest displacement.

All these findings have raised the question of whether regional ventilation is different between spontaneous breathing and mechanical ventilation and whether mechanical ventilation worsens $\dot{V}_A/\dot{Q}$ as a consequence of poor ventilation of well-perfused, dependent lung regions. However, there is not much support for worsening of gas exchange by muscle paralysis in the literature, and there is also no support from the few studies on $\dot{V}_A/\dot{Q}$ distribution that have been performed. Dueck and coworkers[97] found the same increase in $\dot{V}_A/\dot{Q}$ mismatch in anesthetized sheep during anesthesia whether they were spontaneously breathing or mechanically ventilated. The log SDQ, indicating the degree of $\dot{V}_A/\dot{Q}$ mismatch, increased from 0.66 to 0.83 and 0.89 from awake to inhaled anesthesia with spontaneous breathing and mechanical ventilation, respectively. Shunt also increased with no significant difference between the two anesthesia conditions (from 1% awake to 11% and 14% during anesthesia with spontaneous breathing and mechanical ventilation). In a

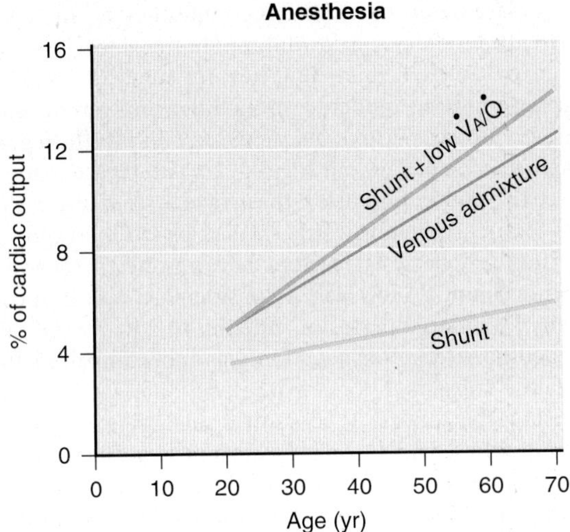

Figure 15-25 Influence of age on shunt, shunt + low $\dot{V}_A/\dot{Q}$, and venous admixture in anesthetized subjects. There is a slight and insignificant increase in shunt with age, whereas shunt + low $\dot{V}_A/\dot{Q}$ increases rapidly. Note also that venous admixture is more similar to shunt + perfusion of low $\dot{V}_A/\dot{Q}$ regions than to shunt alone. *(From Gunnarsson L, Tokics L, Gustavsson H, et al: Influence of age on atelectasis formation and gas-exchange impairment during general-anesthesia. Br J Anaesth 66:423-432, 1991.)*

study of anesthetized human subjects, shunt and log SDQ increased from 1% and 0.47 while awake to 6% and 1.03 during anesthesia with spontaneous breathing and 8% and 1.01 during mechanical ventilation.[52] Thus, most of the gas exchange effects of anesthesia can be seen even during spontaneous breathing, with little or no further derangement added by muscle paralysis and mechanical ventilation.

Increased Oxygen Fraction

In the studies cited thus far, an inspired oxygen fraction (F_{IO_2}) of around 0.4 was used. Anjou-Lindskog and associates[98] induced anesthesia on air (F_{IO_2} of 0.21) in middle-aged to elderly patients during intravenous anesthesia before elective lung surgery and found only small shunts of 1% to 2%, although log SDQ increased from 0.77 to 1.13. When F_{IO_2} was increased to 0.5, an increase in shunt of 3% to 4% was noticed. In another study on elderly patients during halothane anesthesia (see Hedenstierna[52]), an increase in F_{IO_2} from 0.53 to 0.85 caused an increase in shunt from 7% to 10% of cardiac output. Thus, a certain dependence on F_{IO_2} appears to exist, possibly explained by attenuation of the HPV response with increasing F_{IO_2}[85] or further development of atelectasis and shunt in lung units with low $\dot{V}_A/\dot{Q}$ ratios.[88]

Box 15-3 Derivation of the Venous Admixture ("Shunt") Equation

$$Ca \times \dot{Q}_T = (Cc' \times \dot{Q}c) + (C\bar{v} \times \dot{Q}s) \quad (1)$$

$$\dot{Q}c = \dot{Q}_T - \dot{Q}s \quad (2)$$

By inserting Equation 2 into Equation 1,

$$Ca \times \dot{Q}_T = (Cc \times [\dot{Q}_T - \dot{Q}s]) + (C\bar{v} \times \dot{Q}s)$$

Rearranging,

$$\frac{\dot{Q}s}{\dot{Q}_T} = \frac{Cc' - Ca}{Cc' - C\bar{v}}$$

where Cc′, Ca, and $C\bar{v}$ are oxygen content in pulmonary end-capillary, arterial, and mixed venous blood, respectively; $\dot{Q}_T$ is cardiac output; $\dot{Q}c$ is capillary flow; and $\dot{Q}s$ is shunt.

Body Position

Because FRC is dramatically reduced by the combined effect of the supine position and anesthesia (see Chapter 36), it might be advantageous to choose a more upright position in an anesthetized subject to preserve FRC. This was tested by Heneghan and colleagues[99] in lung-healthy patients who underwent general anesthesia. However, no clear improvement in oxygenation was noticed when the patient was semirecumbent as opposed to the supine position. It is likely that pulmonary blood flow is impeded by the semirecumbent position because of a possible decrease in cardiac output and enhanced inhomogeneity of blood flow distribution. Fractional perfusion of the most dependent lung regions, which may still be poorly or not at all ventilated, may have been increased in the semirecumbent position. In the lateral position, differences in lung mechanics, resting lung volumes, and atelectasis formation between the dependent and nondependent portions of the lung have been demonstrated[100] and shown to result in further disturbance of the ventilation-perfusion match, with severe impairment in arterial oxygenation in some patients. However, there are large and unpredictable interindividual variations.[101] With the use of isotope techniques, an increase in $\dot{V}_A/\dot{Q}$ mismatch was also demonstrated in anesthetized, paralyzed patients in the lateral position,[102] and an improvement was noticed in the prone position.[103] There are findings suggesting that the vertical inhomogeneity of the distribution of perfusion is less obvious in the prone position.[104] This may indicate that there are regional differences in vascular configuration that promote perfusion of dorsal lung regions, regardless of whether they are in a dependent or nondependent position. It is also worthy of note that the ventilation distribution was more uniform in anesthetized subjects who were in the prone position.[105]

Age

It is well known that arterial oxygenation is further impeded with increasing age of the patient (see Chapters 71 and 82).[73] As mentioned earlier, formation of atelectasis does not increase with age in adults, and the sparse number of babies who have been studied in the CT scanner during anesthesia appear to have a larger percentage of atelectasis in the transthoracic area than patients of other ages do.[63] Similarly, shunt is independent of age in the tested range of 23 to 69 years. In contrast, there appears to be increasing $\dot{V}_A/\dot{Q}$ mismatch with age, with enhanced perfusion of low-$\dot{V}_A/\dot{Q}$ regions both in awake subjects and when they are subsequently anesthetized. Figure 15-25 shows the relationship between shunt, perfusion of low-$\dot{V}_A/\dot{Q}$ regions, and age of the patient. Thus, the major cause of impaired gas exchange during anesthesia at ages younger than 50 years is shunt, whereas at higher ages mismatch (increased log SDQ) becomes increasingly important. Because the correlation between log SDQ and age during anesthesia is almost parallel with that during the awake state, it can be said that anesthesia worsens the match of ventilation and blood flow by as much as 20 years of aging. Hopefully, log SDQ returns to the preanesthesia level after surgery!

Obesity

Obesity worsens the oxygenation of blood (see Chapter 64).[106,107] A major explanation appears to be a markedly reduced FRC, which promotes airway closure to a greater extent than in a normal subject.[108] The use of high inspired oxygen concentrations will promote rapid atelectasis formation behind closed airways.[57,77] Correlations between BMI and the size of atelectasis during anesthesia and postoperatvely[67,109] and between BMI and pulmonary shunt have been presented (Fig. 15-26).[108] Preventing a fall in FRC by CPAP during induction of anesthesia most likely prevents or reduces atelectasis formation and helps keep arterial oxygenation at a higher level.[87,110,111] The shorter time until desaturation during induction of anesthesia, as observed in morbidly obese patients, may also be prevented by PEEP or CPAP.[112] This can be explained by the increase in lung volume by PEEP or CPAP so that more oxygen is available for diffusion into the capillary blood.

The use of high inspired oxygen concentrations, regularly 100%, to keep an acceptable level of oxygenation during anesthesia and surgery may be the simplest but not necessarily the best method. It will promote further atelectasis formation,[75] and if the shunt is larger than 30%, which may well be the case in these patients, further oxygen will add little to arterial oxygenation.[51] The application of PEEP has been advocated as well. If high enough, PEEP may reduce the atelectasis[86,108,110] but will also have adverse effects such as reduced cardiac output and redistribution of blood flow toward dependent, still collapsed lung regions. Ventilation with near-VC inflations to reopen collapsed tissue, followed by PEEP ventilation, is another option. Body position may have a substantial effect on lung volume and should be considered to the extent that surgery allows.[113]

Preexisting Lung Disease

Smokers and patients with lung disease have more severe impairment of gas exchange in the awake state than healthy subjects do, and this difference also persists during anesthesia.[73] Interestingly, smokers with moderate airflow limitation may have less shunt as measured by MIGET than lung-healthy subjects do. Thus, in patients with mild to moderate bronchitis who were to undergo lung surgery or vascular reconstructive surgery in the leg, only a small shunt was noticed, but log SDQ was increased (for references, see the publication list in the article by Hedenstierna[52]). In patients with chronic bronchitis studied by MIGET and CT, no or very limited atelectasis developed during anesthesia and no or only minor shunt.[68] However, a considerable $\dot{V}_A/\dot{Q}$ mismatch was seen with a large perfusion fraction to low-$\dot{V}_A/\dot{Q}$ regions. Consequently, arterial oxygenation was more impaired than in lung-healthy subjects, but the cause was different from that in normal subjects. A possible reason for the absence of atelectasis and shunt in these patients may be chronic hyperinflation, which changes the mechanical behavior of the lungs and their interaction with the chest wall such that the tendency to collapse is reduced. It should be kept in mind that a patient with obstructive lung disease may have large regions with low $\dot{V}_A/\dot{Q}$ ratios that can be converted over time to resorption atelectasis. Thus, the "protection" against atelectasis formation during anesthesia by the obstructive lung disease need not last long. Regions with low $\dot{V}_A/\dot{Q}$ may be replaced by atelectasis as a result of slow resorption of gas behind occluded airways later during surgery and in the postoperative period.

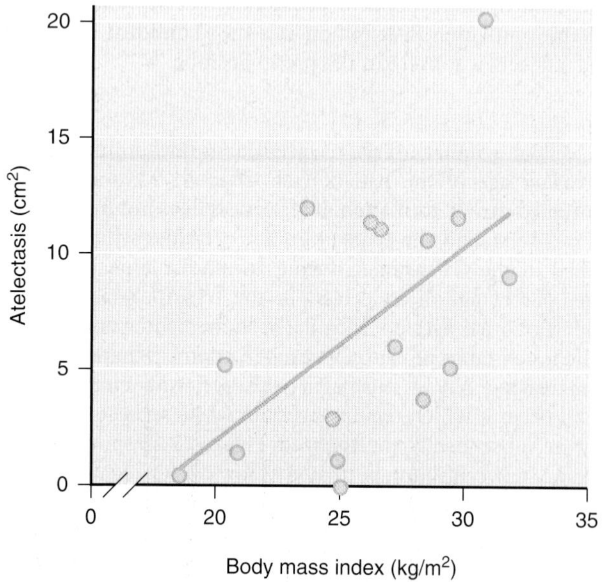

Figure 15-26 Plot of atelectasis during anesthesia versus body dimensions expressed as body mass index (BMI). Note that the larger the body mass index, the larger the atelectasis. *(From Rothen HU, Sporre B, Engberg G, et al: Reexpansion of atelectasis during general anaesthesia: A computed tomography study. Br J Anaesth 71:788-795, 1993.)*

Regional Anesthesia

The ventilatory effects of regional anesthesia depend on the type and extension of motor blockade (see Chapters 51 and 52). With extensive blocks that include all of the thoracic and lumbar segments, inspiratory capacity is reduced by 20% and expiratory reserve volume approaches zero.[114,115] Diaphragmatic function, however, is often spared, even in cases of inadvertent extension of subarachnoid or epidural sensory block up to the cervical segments.[114] Skillfully handled regional anesthesia affects pulmonary gas exchange only minimally. Arterial oxygenation and carbon dioxide elimination are well maintained during spinal and epidural anesthesia. This is in line with the findings of an unchanged relationship of CC and FRC[116] and unaltered distributions of ventilation-perfusion ratios assessed by MIGET during epidural anesthesia.[52]

Lung Function After Cardiac Surgery

Cardiac surgery produces the largest atelectasis in the postoperative period (see Chapter 60).[117] Cardiac surgery is generally undertaken with both lungs collapsed and the patient connected to an extracorporeal pump and oxygenator. If no precautions are taken in the immediate postoperative period, the lung will recruit slowly, and more than half the lung may be collapsed 1 to 2 days later with a shunt that is around 20% to 30% of cardiac output.[118,119] A recruitment maneuver consisting of inflating the lungs to an airway pressure of 30 cm H_2O for a 20-second period is sufficient to reopen the collapsed lung.[118] This lower airway pressure will do the same job as 40 cm H_2O in patients undergoing abdominal surgery because the maneuver is undertaken with an open chest before closure and return to mechanical ventilation. The clinical feasibility and effects on arterial oxygenation of doing such maneuvers were then tested in different clinical trials.[120-122] A few studies will be detailed. Dyhr and coworkers[123] studied 30 patients after cardiac surgery, with (1) one group receiving a lung recruitment maneuver (LRM consisting of four 10-second insufflations to an airway pressure of 45 cm H_2O) and subsequent zero end-expiratory pressure (ZEEP) ventilation, (2) a 12-cm H_2O PEEP group, and (3) an LRM plus PEEP group. The patients were monitored for 75 minutes. Only transient improvement in PaO_2 and end-expiratory lung volume (EELV) was observed in the LRM group. In the PEEP group, no improvement in PaO_2 was seen, although EELV increased by more than 50%. Finally, in the LRM plus PEEP group, PaO_2 more than doubled, EELV increased by 75% to 80%, and both were maintained at these levels throughout the study period. The inspired oxygen fraction was 1.0. Application of 12-cm H_2O PEEP in the study by Dyhr and colleagues resulted in a considerable increase in EELV (+55%), but it was less than when both LRM and PEEP were applied (+80%). Respiratory compliance increased promptly with the recruitment maneuver but increased gradually over a 1-hour period in the PEEP group. These findings may suggest that the recruitment maneuver resulted in true opening of collapsed lung tissue whereas PEEP alone caused hyperinflation of already open alveoli but with slow recruitment over the following hour.

Pasquina and collaborators compared the effect of 30-minute periods four times a day of CPAP ventilation and noninvasive pressure support ventilation (NIPSV) after cardiac surgery.[124] They studied a large group of 150 patients equally distributed between the two treatment protocols. PEEP of 5 cm H_2O was used in both groups, and V_T was 8 to 10 mL/kg in the NIPSV group. Chest radiography showed a decrease in atelectasis in 60% of the patients on NIPSV versus 40% in the CPAP group. However, there was no difference in arterial oxygenation, any pulmonary function test, or length of stay between the groups. The authors concluded that there appears to be no clinical benefit with NIPSV. Nonetheless, it seems that the inspired oxygen fraction was adjusted according to the blood gas data, and with high FIO_2, a PEEP of 5 cm H_2O, as used in the present study, might be inappropriate to gain full effect on atelectasis formation. On the other hand, the patients might not have accepted a higher CPAP.

Miranda and colleagues focused on another potential effect of recruitment maneuvers after cardiac surgery—the possible increase in right ventricular afterload.[125] They used their open-lung concept technique with vigorous recruitment attempts at a peak airway pressure of 46 cm H_2O to achieve a PaO_2/FIO_2 of greater than 50 kPa. Moreover, to keep the lung open (i.e., without deterioration in PaO_2), PEEP of 17 cm H_2O was required. Despite this strong recruitment, neither pulmonary vascular resistance nor right ventricular ejection fraction changed significantly during the succeeding 3-hour observation period.

Another approach to cardiac surgery that is developing is off-pump coronary bypass grafting. Tschernko and coworkers[126] showed that patients who underwent surgery off-pump had a smaller increase in shunt. Moreover, the hospital stay was shorter in the off-pump group (7.5 versus 10.3 days in on-pump patients with a VC recruitment maneuver). Interestingly, a control group that did not receive any VC maneuver had an even longer hospital stay (12.6 days).

Respiratory Function During One-Lung Ventilation

In lung surgery, oxygenation may be a challenge even during anesthesia. One lung is nonventilated but still perfused, and in the postoperative period, restoration of lung integrity and ventilation/perfusion matching may take time (see Chapter 59).[127]

The technique of one-lung anesthesia and ventilation means that only one lung is ventilated and provides oxygenation of blood, as well as elimination of carbon dioxide from the blood. Persisting perfusion through the nonventilated lung causes a shunt and decreased PaO_2 (Fig. 15-27). Measures can be taken to reduce this blood flow by both mechanical and pharmacologic means, as summarized in a short review.[128] However, the dependent, ventilated lung will also contribute to the impeded oxygenation by formation of atelectasis in the dependent regions.[101] There are reasons to also consider a recruitment maneuver in one-lung ventilation (OLV). Tusman and colleagues[129] tested an "alveolar recruitment strategy" (ARS) in 10 patients who were undergoing open lobectomy first during two-lung ventilation and

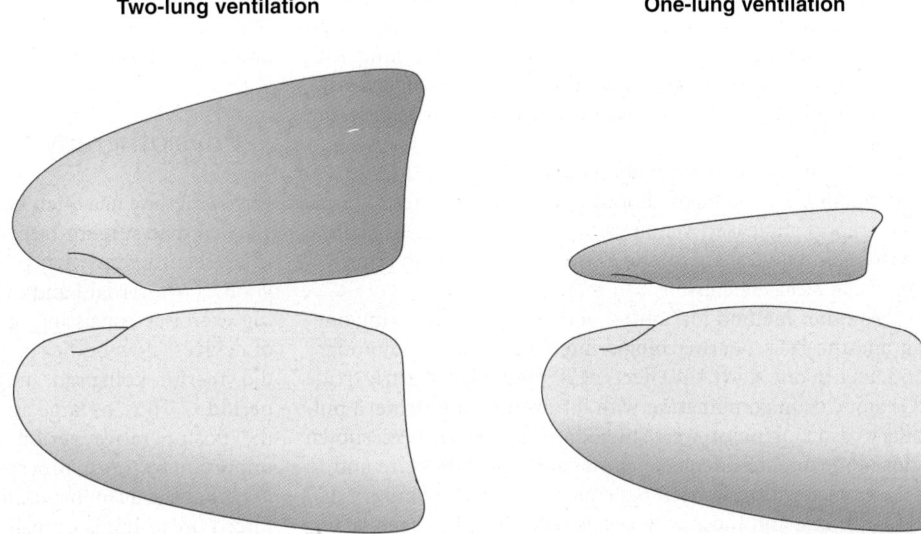

Figure 15-27 Schematic drawing of the distribution of shunt during anesthesia with two-lung ventilation and one-lung ventilation. The shunt region is indicated by the *dark area*, which can be seen in the lower lung during two-lung ventilation but in both the lower lung and in all of upper lung during one-lung ventilation. That the upper, nonventilated lung will act as a shunt region is well known, but one should not forget that the lower part of the dependent lung will also contribute to the shunting.

then during OLV before and then after ARS. The ARS maneuver was executed by increasing peak airway pressure minute by minute from 25 to 30, 35, and finally 40 cm H_2O and simultaneously increasing PEEP from 5 to 10, 15, and finally 20 cm H_2O. Airway pressure was then reduced to a peak of 25 and PEEP to 5 cm H_2O. This resulted in an increase in $Pa{O_2}$ from 217 to 470 mm Hg after ARS. This substantial improvement in oxygenation suggests that more of the shunt is located in the dependent lung than is generally considered.

In another study by Tusman and associates, the effect of ARS on gas exchange and ventilation efficiency was studied, with a particular focus on dead space ventilation.[130] Again, ARS improved oxygenation. Moreover, dead space decreased and the slope of the CO_2 curve during a tidal expiration (phase III) was flatter, indicative of a more even distribution of inspired gas in relation to regional alveolar volume (or more synchronous alveolar emptying). The effect lasted for the total OLV period of 50 to 105 minutes. Thus, a secondary effect of recruiting collapsed lung tissue is more even distribution of ventilation and a decrease in the dead space fraction. If anything, this should facilitate the use of a smaller V_T.

Ishikawa and coworkers studied the effect of compressing the nondependent lung in patients who underwent esophagectomy.[131] By means of an intra-arterial sensor for continuous recording of arterial blood gas values, they noticed that by applying a retractor to expose the nonventilated right lung and subjecting it to compression, $Pa{O_2}$ was increased, more so in some patients than in others. The mechanism has been proposed to be a shift of blood flow from the nondependent, nonventilated lung to the other lung. The clinical importance of the study is that it might indicate the value of deliberate compression of the nondependent lung during surgery to reduce shunting and improve oxygenation. However, whether manual compression of the nonventilated lung has any advantage over complete absorption atelectasis can be discussed.[132]

Patients who underwent OLV for thoracic surgery were receiving either ZEEP to the ventilated lung or PEEP adjusted to achieve the best respiratory compliance.[133] The PEEP that was applied was on average 4.3 cm H_2O during two-lung ventilation, 6.2 cm H_2O during closed-chest OLV, and 6.0 cm H_2O during open-chest OLV. This resulted in an average 10% higher compliance in the PEEP group, but $Pa{O_2}$ was better in the ZEEP group (11.7 versus 10.5 kPa on an $F{IO_2}$ of 0.5). The opposing findings may not appear too surprising; PEEP should redistribute blood flow away from that lung to the other nonventilated lung with certain impairment of oxygenation. The rationale for identifying and using optimum PEEP has also been discussed by Slinger and associates.[134]

Other studies on oxygenation during OLV have focused on the sympatholytic effect of thoracic epidural anesthesia. Some studies report increased venous admixture and decreased $Pa{O_2}$ with thoracic epidural anesthesia,[135] no effect,[136,137] or an improvement.[138] No clear conclusions can therefore be drawn.

Another method for control of deoxygenation during one-lung anesthesia is pharmacologic interference with pulmonary blood flow. In one study, the effects of 20 ppm inhaled nitric oxide (NO) alone or in combination with intravenous almitrine, a pulmonary vasoconstrictor, were studied. Almitrine has been shown to dose-dependently increase pulmonary artery pressure and to increase oxygenation in both patients with acute respiratory distress syndrome and those with sepsis. The effect has been attributed to enhancement of HPV, reduction of blood flow in nonventilated lung regions, and an improved ventilation-perfusion relationship. Little effect of NO alone was seen,[139] but oxygenation was significantly improved when NO was combined with almitrine.[140,141] The effect of almitrine alone during OLV has also been studied.[142] A significant improvement in oxygenation and a reduction in venous admixture in the almitrine group versus placebo were seen. Pulmonary artery pressure or cardiac output did not change at the dose of almitrine given.

Whether intravenous almitrine can be used to treat hypoxia has also been studied, and a moderate positive effect was observed.[143]

Careful analysis of the mechanical obstruction caused by kinking of pulmonary vessels and by HPV has shown that HPV is the important determinant of diversion of blood flow away from nonventilated lung (though not complete).[144] Moreover, positioning of the patient can affect the degree of shunting.[145]

The effects of selective vasodilation of the pulmonary circulation in OLV and in cardiac surgery have been reviewed in more detail in different publications, and two are referred to here.[146,147]

Pneumoperitoneum

Laparoscopic operations are becoming increasingly popular. They are usually performed by insufflation of CO_2 into the abdominal cavity (see Chapter 68). However, insufflation of CO_2 may interfere with cardiac and circulatory function, as well as respiratory function. CO_2 pneumoperitoneum may cause hypercapnia and acidosis.[148,149] The direct effects of carbon dioxide and acidosis lead to decreased cardiac contractility, sensitization of the myocardium to the arrhythmogenic effects of catecholamines, and systemic vasodilation.[150] There may even be long-lasting postoperative effects on breathing control. [151]

Pneumoperitoneum may also cause several respiratory changes, such as decreased FRC and VC,[152] formation of atelectasis,[153] reduced respiratory compliance,[154] and increased peak airway pressure.[155] Nonetheless, shunt is reduced and arterial oxygenation is mostly improved during CO_2 pneumoperitoneum.[156] This seeming paradox, more atelectasis and less shunt, suggests efficient redistribution of blood flow away from collapsed lung regions. CO_2 may enhance HPV, which may be the mechanism and explanation of the paradox.

Physiotherapy

Physiotherapy has often been debated after surgery, not the least after cardiac surgery (see Chapter 93). It has even been claimed in a recent review that physiotherapy may do more harm than good.[157] Westerdahl and colleagues showed with CT that breathing exercises consisting of maximum inspirations with the help of devices (flow bottle) or without (spontaneous VC maneuvers) did recruit collapsed lung tissue promptly after an exercise period.[158] Thus, as large an inspiration as possible and as early in the postoperative period as possible are presumably the two important factors in preventing postoperative lung complications. Whether the deep inspiration is done with or without a device for forced breathing is probably of little importance.

Normal Sleep

Ventilation is affected by sleep.[159] A significant reduction in VT and inspiratory drive has been shown, and minute ventilation falls by approximately 5% to 16%, depending on the sleep stage, with the most marked fall occurring during rapid eye movement (REM) sleep. Lung volume is also reduced during sleep and manifested as a decrease in FRC.[160] The reduction in FRC occurs almost immediately after the onset of sleep, with the most marked fall taking place in REM sleep, during which time it amounts to approximately 0.3 L, or 10% of the awake value.[161]

The fall in FRC during sleep is accompanied by reduced aeration in the dependent lung regions, as shown in a CT study in healthy volunteers.[162] The loss of aeration was as marked as in anesthetized patients who were breathing gas with a moderate concentration of oxygen (FIO_2 of 0.3). When the anesthetized patients were switched to 100% O_2, atelectasis developed rapidly.[75] It is tempting to assume that normal sleep while breathing pure oxygen would also lead to the formation of atelectasis.

References

1. Quanjer PH, Tammeling GJ, Cotes JE, et al: Lung volumes and forced ventilatory flows. Report Working Party "Standardization of Lung Function Tests." European Community for Steel and Coal. Eur Respir J Suppl 16:5-40, 1993.
2. Astrom E, Niklason L, Drefeldt B, et al: Partitioning of dead space—a method and reference values in the awake human. Eur Respir J 16:659-664, 2000.
3. Broughton SJ, Sylvester KP, Page CM, et al: Problems in the measurement of functional residual capacity. Physiol Meas 27:99-107, 2006.
4. Hogg K, Dawson D, Tabor T, et al: Respiratory dead space measurement in the investigation of pulmonary embolism in outpatients with pleuritic chest pain. Chest 128:2195-2202, 2005.
5. Wilschut FA, van der Grinten CPM, Lamers RJS, et al: Intrapulmonary gas mixing and the sloping alveolar plateau in COPD patients with macroscopic emphysema. Eur Respir J 14:166-171, 1999.
6. Roca J, Burgos F, Barbera JA, et al: Prediction equations for plethysmographic lung volumes. Respir Med 92:454-460, 1998.
7. Pellegrino R, Brusasco V: On the causes of lung hyperinflation during bronchoconstriction. Eur Respir J 10:468-475, 1997.
8. Leith D, Mead J: Mechanisms determining residual volume of the lungs in normal subjects. J Appl Physiol 23:221-227, 1967.
9. Grassino AE, Roussos C: Static properties of the lung and chest wall. *In* Crystal RG, West JB, Weibel ER, Barnes PJ (eds): The Lung: Scientific Foundations, 2nd ed. Philadelphia, Lippincott-Raven, 1997, pp 1187-1202.
10. Goldin JG: Quantitative CT of the lung. Radiol Clin North Am 40:145-162, 2002.
11. Van-Lith P, Johnson FN, Sharp JT. Respiratory elastances in relaxed and paralyzed states in normal and abnormal men. J Appl Physiol 23:475-486, 1967.
12. Pedley TJ, Kamm RD: Dynamics of gas flow and pressure-flow relationships. *In* Crystal RG, West JB, Weibel ER, Barnes PJ (eds): The Lung: Scientific Foundations, 2nd ed. Philadelphia, Lippincott-Raven, 1997, pp 1365-1380.
13. Slats AM, Janssen K, van Schadewijk A, et al: Bronchial inflammation and airway responses to deep inspiration in asthma and chronic obstructive pulmonary disease. Am J Respir Crit Care Med 176:121-128, 2007.
14. Holst M, Striem J, Hedenstierna G: Errors in tracheal pressure recording in patients with a tracheostomy tube—a model study. Intensive Care Med 16:384-389, 1990.
15. Verbeken EK, Cauberghs M, Mertens I, et al: Tissue and airway impedance of excised normal, senile, and emphysematous lungs. J Appl Physiol 72:2343-2353, 1992.
16. Tantucci C, Corbeil C, Chasse M, et al: Flow and volume dependence of respiratory system flow resistance in patients with adult respiratory-distress syndrome. Am Rev Respir Dis 145:355-360, 1992.
17. Frostell C, Pande J, Hedenstierna G: Effects of high frequency breathing on pulmonary ventilation and gas exchange. J Appl Physiol 55:1374-1378, 1983.
18. Milic Emili J: Ventilation distribution. *In* Hammid Q, Shannon J, Martin J (eds): Physiologic Bases of Respiratory Disease. Hamilton, Ontario, BC Decker, 2005, pp 133-141.
19. Guy HJB, Prisk GK, Elliott AR, et al: Inhomogeneity of pulmonary ventilation during sustained microgravity as determined by single-breath washouts. J Appl Physiol 76:1719-1729, 1994.
20. Prisk GK: Physiology of a microgravity environment, microgravity and the lung. J Appl Physiol 89:385-396, 2000.
21. Ganesan S, Lai-Fook S: Finite element analysis of regional lung expansion in prone and supine positions: Effect of heart weight and diaphragmatic compliance. Physiologist 32:191, 1989.
22. Mayo JR, MacKay AL, Whittall KP, et al: Measurement of lung water content and pleural pressure gradient with magnetic resonance imaging. J Thorac Imaging 10:73-81, 1995.
23. Petersson J, Sánchez-Crespo A, Rohdin M, et al: Physiological evaluation of a new quantitative SPECT method measuring regional ventilation and perfusion. J Appl Physiol 96:1127-1136, 2004.
24. Bake B, Wood L, Murphy B, et al: Effect of inspiratory flow-rate on regional distribution of inspired gas. J Appl Physiol 37:8-17, 1974.
25. Milic-Emili J, Torchio R, D'Angelo E: Closing volume: A reappraisal (1967-2007). Eur J Appl Physiol 99:567-583, 2007.
26. Teculescu DB, Damel MC, Costantino E, et al: Computerized single-breath nitrogen washout: Predicted values in a rural French community. Lung 174:43-55, 1996.
27. Nield MA, Hoo GWS, Roper JM, et al: Efficacy of pursed-lips breathing—a breathing pattern retraining strategy for dyspnea reduction. J Cardiopulm Rehabil Prev 27:237-244, 2007.
28. Mead J, Turner JM, Macklem PT, Little JB: Significance of relationship between lung recoil and maximum expiratory flow. J Appl Physiol 22:95-108, 1967.
29. Haefeli-Bleuer B, Weibel ER: Morphometry of the human pulmonary acinus. Anat Rec 220:401-414, 1988.
30. Adaro F, Piiper J: Limiting role of stratification in alveolar exchange of oxygen. Respir Physiol 26:195-206, 1976.
31. West JB: Respiratory Physiology—The Essentials, 4th ed. Baltimore, Williams & Wilkins, 1990.
32. Hughes JMB, Bates DV: Historical review: The carbon monoxide diffusing capacity (DLCO) and its membrane (D-M) and red cell (Theta $\dot{V}$) components. Respir Physiol Neurobiol 138:115-142, 2003.
33. Dawson CA, Linehan JH: Dynamics of blood flow and pressure-flow relationships. *In* Crystal RG, West JB, Weibel ER, Barnes PJ (eds): The Lung: Scientific Foundations, 2nd ed. Philadelphia, Lippincott-Raven, 1997, pp 1503-1522.
34. Jeffery PK: Remodeling and inflammation of bronchi in asthma and chronic obstructive pulmonary disease. Proc Am Thorac Soc 1:176-183, 2004.
35. Hughes JMB. Distribution of pulmonary blood flow. *In* Crystal RG, West JB, Weibel ER, Barnes PJ (eds): The Lung: Scientific Foundations, 2nd ed. Philadelphia, Lippincott-Raven, 1997, pp 1523-1536.
36. Glenny RW, Lamm WJE, Albert RK, et al: Gravity is a minor determinant of pulmonary blood-flow distribution. J Appl Physiol 71:620-629, 1991.
37. Dutrieue B, Paiva M, Verbanck S, et al: Tidal volume single-breath wash-in of SF6 and CH4 in transient microgravity. J Appl Physiol 94:75-82, 2003.
38. Glenny RW, Bernard S, Robertson HT, et al: Gravity is an important but secondary determinant of regional pulmonary blood flow in upright primates. J Appl Physiol 86:623-632, 1999
39. Hlastala MP, Bernard SL, Erickson HH, et al: Pulmonary blood flow distribution in standing horses is not dominated by gravity. J Appl Physiol 81:1051-1061, 1996.
40. Hakim TS, Lisbona R, Dean GW: Gravity-independent inequality in pulmonary blood-flow in humans. J Appl Physiol 63:1114-1121, 1987.
41. Hedenstierna G, White FC, Wagner PD: Spatial-distribution of pulmonary blood-flow in the dog with peep ventilation. J Appl Physiol 47:938-946, 1979.
42. Marshall BE, Hanson CW, Frasch F, et al: Role of hypoxic pulmonary vasoconstriction in pulmonary gas-exchange and blood-flow distribution 2. Pathophysiology. Intensive Care Med 20:379-389, 1994.
43. Moudgil R, Michelakis ED, Archer SL: Hypoxic pulmonary vasoconstriction. J Appl Physiol 98:390-403, 2005.
44. Hambraeus-Jonzon K, Bindslev L, Jolin Mellgård Å, et al: Hypoxic pulmonary vasoconstriction in human lungs. Anesthesiology 86: 308-315, 1997.
45. Sartori C, Allemann Y, Scherrer U. Pathogenesis of pulmonary edema: Learning from high-altitude pulmonary edema. Respir Phys Neurobiol 159:338-349, 2007.
46. Roca J, Wagner PD: Contribution of multiple inert gas elimination technique to pulmonary medicine. 1. Principles and information content of the multiple inert gas elimination technique. Thorax 49:815-824, 1994.

47. Agustí AG, Barberà JA: Contribution of multiple inert gas elimination technique to pulmonary medicine. 2. Chronic pulmonary diseases: Chronic obstructive pulmonary disease and idiopathic pulmonary fibrosis. Thorax 49:924-932, 1994.
48. Rodriguez-Roisin R, Roca J: Contributions of multiple inert gas elimination technique to pulmonary medicine. 3. Bronchial asthma. Thorax 49:1027-1033, 1994.
49. Agustí AG, Roca J, Gea J, et al: Mechanisms of gas-exchange impairment in idiopathic pulmonary fibrosis. Am Rev Respir Dis 143:219-225, 1991.
50. Manier G, Castaing Y: Contribution of multiple inert gas elimination technique to pulmonary medicine. 4. Gas exchange abnormalities in pulmonary vascular and cardiac disease. Thorax 49:1169-1174, 1994.
51. Melot C: Contribution of multiple inert gas elimination technique to pulmonary medicine. 5. Ventilation-perfusion relationships in acute respiratory failure. Thorax 49:1251-1258, 1994.
52. Hedenstierna G: Contribution of multiple inert gas elimination technique to pulmonary medicine. 6. Ventilation-perfusion relationships during anesthesia. Thorax 50:85-91, 1995.
53. Moller JT, Cluitmans P, Rasmussen LS, et al: Long-term postoperative cognitive dysfunction in the elderly: ISPOCD1 study. Lancet 351:857-861, 1998.
54. Kroenke K, Lawrence VA, Theroux JF, et al: Postoperative complications after thoracic and major abdominal-surgery in patients with and without obstructive lung-disease. Chest 104:1445-1451, 1993.
55. Wahba RWM: Perioperative functional residual capacity. Can J Anaesth 38:384-400, 1991.
56. Westbrook PR, Stubbs SE, Sessler AD, et al: Effects of anesthesia and muscle paralysis on respiratory mechanics in normal man. J Appl Physiol 34:81-86, 1973.
57. Rothen HU, Sporre B, Engberg G, et al: Airway closure, atelectasis and gas exchange during general anaesthesia. B J Anaesth 81:681-686, 1998.
58. Hedenstierna G, Edmark L: The effects of anesthesia and muscle paralysis on the respiratory system. Intensive Care Med 31:1327-1335, 2005.
59. Reber A, Nylund U, Hedenstierna G: Position and shape of the diaphragm: Implications for atelectasis formation. Anaesthesia 53:1054-1061, 1998.
60. Warner DO, Warner MA, Ritman EL: Atelectasis and chest wall shape during halothane anesthesia. Anesthesiology 85:49-59, 1996.
61. Don H: The mechanical properties of the respiratory system during anesthesia. Int Anesthesiol Clin 15:113-126, 1977.
62. Bendixen HH, Hedleywhyte J, Laver MB: Impaired oxygenation in surgical patients during general anesthesia with controlled ventilation—a concept of atelectasis. N Engl J Med 269:991-996, 1963.
63. Gunnarsson L, Tokics L, Gustavsson H, et al: Influence of age on atelectasis formation and gas-exchange impairment during general-anesthesia. Br J Anaesth 66:423-432, 1991.
64. Lindberg P, Gunnarsson L, Tokics L, et al: Atelectasis and lung-function in the postoperative period. Acta Anaesthesiol Scand 36:546-553, 1992.
65. van Kaam AH, Lachmann RA, Herting E, et al: Reducing atelectasis attenuates bacterial growth and translocation in experimental pneumonia. Am J Respir Crit Care Med 169:1046-1053, 2004.
66. Tenling A, Hachenberg T, Tyden H, et al: Atelectasis and gas exchange after cardiac surgery. Anesthesiology 89:371-378, 1998.
67. Rothen HU, Sporre B, Engberg G, et al: Reexpansion of atelectasis during general anaesthesia: A computed tomography study. Br J Anaesth 71:788-795, 1993.
68. Gunnarsson L, Tokics L, Lundquist H, et al: Chronic obstructive pulmonary-disease and anesthesia-formation of atelectasis and gas-exchange impairment. Eur Respiry J 4:1106-1116, 1991.
69. Tokics L, Hedenstierna G, Svensson L, et al: V/Q distribution and correlation to atelectasis in anesthetized paralyzed humans. J Appl Physiol 81:1822-1833, 1996.
70. Hewlett AM, Hulands GH, Nunn JF, et al: Functional residual capacity during anesthesia III: Artificial ventilation. Br J Anaesth 46:495-503, 1974.
71. West JB, Dollery CT, Naimark A: Distribution of blood flow in isolated lung—relation to vascular + alveolar pressures. J Appl Physiol 19:713-724, 1964.
72. Hedenstierna G, Tokics L, Lundquist H, et al: Phrenic-nerve stimulation during halothane anesthesia. Anesthesiology 80:751-760, 1994.
73. Nunn JF: Nunn's applied respiratory physiology, 4th ed. London, Butterworth Heinemann, 1993.
74. Rothen HU, Neumann P, Berglund JE, et al: Dynamics of re-expansion of atelectasis during general anaesthesia. B J Anaesth 82:551-556, 1999.
75. Rothen HU, Sporre B, Engberg G, et al: Influence of gas-composition on recurrence of atelectasis after a reexpansion maneuver during general-anesthesia. Anesthesiology 82:832-842, 1995.
76. Rothen HU, Sporre B, Engberg G, et al: Prevention of atelectasis during general anesthesia. Lancet 345:1387-1391, 1995.
77. Edmark L, Kostova-Aherdan K, Enlund M, et al: Optimal oxygen concentration during induction of general anesthesia. Anesthesiology 98:28-33, 2003.
78. Rusca M, Proietti S, Schnyder P, et al: Prevention of atelectasis formation during induction of general anesthesia. Anesth Analg 97:1835-1839, 2003.
79. Benoît Z, Wicky S, Fischer JF, et al: The Effect of increased FIO_2 before tracheal extubation on postoperative atelectasis. Anesth Analg 95:1777-1781, 2002.
80. Dueck R, Prutow RJ, Davies NJH, et al: The lung-volume at which shunting occurs with inhalation anesthesia. Anesthesiology 69:854-861, 1988.
81. Hedenstierna G: Alveolar collapse and closure of airways: Regular effects of anaesthesia. Clin Physiol Funct Imaging 23:123-129, 2003.
82. Hedenstierna G, Baehrendtz S, Klingstedt C, et al: Ventilation and perfusion of each lung during differential ventilation with selective PEEP. Anesthesiology 61:369-376, 1984.
83. Hulands GH, Greene R, Iliff LD, et al: Influence of anaesthesia on regional distribution of perfusion and ventilation in lung. Clin Sci 38:451-460, 1970.
84. Marshall BE: Effects of anesthetics on pulmonary gas exchange. *In* Stanley TH, Sperry RJ (eds): Anesthesia and the Lung. London, Kluwer Academic, 1989, pp 117-125.
85. Marshall BE: Hypoxic pulmonary vasoconstriction. Acta Anaesthesiol Scand 94:37-41, 1990.
86. Pelosi P, Ravagnan I, Giurati G, et al: Positive end-expiratory pressure improves respiratory function in obese but not in normal subjects during anesthesia and paralysis. Anesthesiology 91:1221-1231, 1999.
87. Coussa M, Proietti S, Schnyder P, et al: Prevention of atelectasis formation during the induction of general anesthesia in morbidly obese patients. Anesth Analg 98:1491-1495, 2004.
88. Dantzker DR, Wagner PD, West JB: Instability of lung units with low $\dot{V}A/\dot{Q}$ ratios during O_2 breathing. J Appl Physiol 38:886-895, 1975.
89. Sakai EM, Connolly LA, Klauck JA: Inhalation anesthesiology and volatile liquid anesthetics: Focus on isoflurane, desflurane, and sevoflurane. Pharmacotherapy 25:1773-1788, 2005.
90. von Ungern-Sternberg BS, Frei FJ, Hammer J, et al: Impact of depth of propofol anaesthesia on functional residual capacity and ventilation distribution in healthy preschool children. Br J Anaesth 98;503-508, 2007.
91. Ide T, Sakurai Y, Aono M, Nishino T: Contribution of peripheral chemoreception to the depression of the hypoxic ventilatory response during halothane anesthesia in cats. Anesthesiology 90:1084-1091, 1999.
92. Morton CP, Drummond GB: Change in chest wall dimensions on induction of anaesthesia: A reappraisal. Br J Anaesth 73:135-139, 1994.
93. Warner DO, Warner MA: Human chest wall function while awake and during halothane anesthesia. II. Carbon dioxide rebreathing. Anesthesiology 82:20-31, 1995.
94. Warner DO, Joyner MJ, Ritman EL: Anesthesia and chest wall function in dogs. J Appl Physiol 76:2802-2813, 1994.
95. Strandberg A, Tokics L, Brismar B, et al: Atelectasis during anesthesia and in the postoperative period. Acta Anaesthesiol Scand 30:154-158, 1986.
96. Froese AB, Bryan CH: Effects of anesthesia and paralysis on diaphragmatic mechanics in man. Anesthesiology 41:242-255, 1974.
97. Dueck R, Rathbun M, Greenburg AG: Lung-volume and $\dot{V}a/\dot{Q}$ distribution response to intravenous versus inhalation anesthesia in sheep. Anesthesiology 61:55-65, 1984.
98. Anjou-Lindskog E, Broman L, Broman M, et al: Effects of intravenous anesthesia on $\dot{V}a/\dot{Q}$ distribution—a study performed during ventilation with air and with 50-percent oxygen, supine and in the lateral position. Anesthesiology 62:485-492, 1985.
99. Heneghan CPH, Bergman NA, Jones JG: Changes in lung-volume and (PAO_2–PaO_2) during anesthesia. B J Anaesth 56:437-445, 1984.
100. Klingstedt C, Hedenstierna G, Lundquist H, et al: The influence of body position and differential ventilation on lung dimensions and atelectasis formation in anesthetized man. Acta Anaesthesiol Scand 34:315-322, 1990.
101. Klingstedt C, Hedenstierna G, Baehrendtz S, et al: Ventilation-perfusion relationships and atelectasis formation in the supine and lateral positions during conventional mechanical and differential ventilation. Acta Anaesthesiol Scand 34:421-429, 1990.
102. Landmark SJ, Knopp TJ, Rehder K, et al: Regional pulmonary perfusion and V-Q in awake and anesthetized-paralyzed man. J Appl Physiol 43:993-1000, 1977.
103. Mure M, Glenny RW, Domino KB, et al: Pulmonary gas exchange improves in the prone position with abdominal distension. Am J Respir Crit Care Med 157:1785-1790, 1998.
104. Glenny RW, Robertson HT: Fractal modeling of pulmonary blood-flow heterogeneity. J Appl Physiol 70:1024-1030, 1991.
105. Mure M, Nyrén S, Radell P, et al: Regional lung perfusion is more uniform in the prone than in the supine posture in healthy subjects during anesthesia and mechanical ventilation. (Abstract). Paper presented at the 9th Congress of the World Federation of Societies of Intensive and Critical Care Medicine, 2006, Buenos Aires, Argentina.
106. Brooks-Brunn JA: Predictors of postoperative pulmonary complications following abdominal surgery. Chest 111:564-571, 1997.
107. Yoshino J, Akata T, Takahashi S: Intraoperative changes in arterial oxygenation during volume-controlled mechanical ventilation in modestly obese patients undergoing laparotomies with general anesthesia. Acta Anaesthesiol Scand 47:742-750, 2003.

108. Pelosi P, Croci M, Ravagnan I, et al: The effects of body mass on lung volumes, respiratory mechanics, and gas exchange during general anesthesia. Anesth Analg 87:654-660, 1998.
109. Eichenberger A, Proietti S, Wicky S, et al: Morbid obesity and postoperative pulmonary atelectasis: An underestimated problem. Anesth Analg 95: 1788-1792, 2002.
110. Cressey DM, Berthoud MC, Reilly CS: Effectiveness of continuous positive airway pressure to enhance pre-oxygenation in morbidly obese women. Anaesthesia 56:680-684, 2001.
111. Gander S, Frascarolo P, Suter M, et al: Positive end-expiratory pressure during induction of general anesthesia increases duration of nonhypoxic apnea in morbidly obese patients. Anesth Analg 100:580-584, 2005.
112. Berthoud MC, Peacock JE, Reilly CS: Effectiveness of preoxygenation in morbidly obese patients. B J Anaesth 67:464-466, 1991.
113. Mynster T, Jensen LM, Jensen FG, et al: The effect of posture on late postoperative oxygenation. Anaesthesia 51:225-227, 1996.
114. Warner DO, Warner MA, Ritman EL. Human chest wall function during epidural anesthesia. Anesthesiology 85:761-773, 1996.
115. Yamakage M, Namiki A, Tsuchida H, et al: Changes in ventilatory pattern and arterial oxygen-saturation during spinal-anesthesia in man. Acta Anaesthesiol Scand 36:569-571, 1992.
116. McCarthy GS: Effect of thoracic extradural analgesia on pulmonary gas distribution, functional residual capacity and airway-closure. B J Anaesth 48:243-248, 1976.
117. Hachenberg T, Brussel T, Roos N, et al: Gas-exchange impairment and pulmonary densities after cardiac-surgery. Acta Anaesthesiol Scand 36:800-805, 1992.
118. Tenling A, Hachenberg T, Tyden H, et al: Atelectasis and gas exchange after cardiac surgery. Anesthesiology 89:371-378, 1998.
119. Hachenberg T, Tenling A, Hansson HE, et al: The ventilation-perfusion relation and gas exchange in mitral valve disease and coronary artery disease—implications for anesthesia, extracorporeal circulation, and cardiac surgery. Anesthesiology 86:809-817, 1997.
120. Murphy GS, Szokol JW, Curran RD, et al: Influence of a vital capacity maneuver on pulmonary gas exchange after cardiopulmonary bypass. J Cardiothorac Vasc Anesth 15:336-340, 2001.
121. Dyhr T, Laursen N, Larsson A: Effects of lung recruitment maneuver and positive end-expiratory pressure on lung volume, respiratory mechanics and alveolar gas mixing in patients ventilated after cardiac surgery. Acta Anaesthesiol Scand 46:717-725, 2002.
122. Claxton BA, Morgan P, McKeague H, et al: Alveolar recruitment strategy improves arterial oxygenation after cardiopulmonary bypass. Anaesthesia 58:111-116, 2003.
123. Dyhr T, Nygard E, Laursen N, et al: Both lung recruitment maneuver and PEEP are needed to increase oxygenation and lung volume after cardiac surgery. Acta Anaesthesiol Scand 48:187-197, 2004.
124. Pasquina P, Merlani P, Granier JM, et al: Continuous positive airway pressure versus noninvasive pressure support ventilation to treat atelectasis after cardiac surgery. Anesth Analg 99:1001-1008, 2004.
125. Miranda DR, Gommers D, Struijs A, et al: The open lung concept: Effects on right ventricular afterload after cardiac surgery. B J Anaesth 93:327-332, 2004.
126. Tschernko EM, Bambazek A, Wisser W, et al: Intrapulmonary shunt after cardiopulmonary bypass: The use of vital capacity maneuvers versus off-pump coronary artery bypass grafting. J Thorac Cardiovasc Surg 124:732-738, 2002.
127. Benumof JL: One-lung ventilation and hypoxic pulmonary vasoconstriction—implications for anesthetic management. Anesth Analg 64:821-833, 1985.
128. Hedenstierna G, Reber A: Manipulating pulmonary blood flow during one-lung anaesthesia. Acta Anaesthesiol Scand 40:2-4, 1996.
129. Tusman G, Bohm SH, Melkun F, et al: Alveolar recruitment strategy increases arterial oxygenation during one-lung ventilation. Ann Thorac Surg 73:1204-1209, 2002.
130. Tusman G, Bohm SH, Sipmann FS, et al: Lung recruitment improves the efficiency of ventilation and gas exchange during one-lung ventilation anesthesia. Anesth Analg 98:1604-1609, 2004.
131. Ishikawa S, Nakazawa K, Makita K: Progressive changes in arterial oxygenation during one-lung anaesthesia are related to the response to compression of the non-dependent lung. Br J Anaesth 90:21-26, 2003.
132. Ishikawa S, Nakazawa K, Makita K: Acute lung injury following one-lung anaesthesia. Br J Anaesth 91:153-154, 2003.
133. Mascotto G, Bizzarri M, Messina M, et al: Prospective, randomized, controlled evaluation of the preventive effects of positive end-expiratory pressure on patient oxygenation during one-lung ventilation. Eur J Anaesthesiol 20:704-710, 2003.
134. Slinger PD, Kruger M, McRae K, et al: Relation of the static compliance curve and positive end-expiratory pressure to oxygenation during one-lung ventilation. Anesthesiology 95:1096-1102, 2001.
135. Garutti I, Quintana B, Olmedilla L, et al: Arterial oxygenation during one-lung ventilation: Combined versus general anesthesia—in response. Anesth Analg 89:1332, 1999.
136. Garutti I, Cruz P, Olmedilla L, et al: Effects of thoracic epidural meperidine on arterial oxygenation during one-lung ventilation in thoracic surgery. J Cardiothorac Vasc Anesth 17:302-305, 2003.
137. Chow MYH, Goh MH, Boey SK, et al: The effects of remifentanil and thoracic epidural on oxygenation and pulmonary shunt fraction during one-lung ventilation. J Cardiothorac Vasc Anesth 17:69-72, 2003.
138. Von Dossow V, Welte M, Zaune U, et al: Thoracic epidural anesthesia combined with general anesthesia: The preferred anesthetic technique for thoracic surgery. Anesth Analg 92:848-854, 2001.
139. Schwarzkopf K, Klein U, Schreiber T, et al: Oxygenation during one-lung ventilation: The effects of inhaled nitric oxide and increasing levels of inspired fraction of oxygen. Anesth Analg 92:842-847, 2001.
140. Moutafis M, Liu N, Dalibon N, et al: The effects of inhaled nitric oxide and its combination with intravenous almitrine on Pa_{O_2} during one-lung ventilation in patients undergoing thoracoscopic procedures. Anesth Analg 85:1130-1135, 1997.
141. Silva-Costa-Gomes T, Gallart L, Vallès J, et al: Low- vs high-dose almitrine combined with nitric oxide to prevent hypoxia during open-chest one-lung ventilation. B J Anaesth 95:410-416, 2005.
142. Moutafis M, Dalibon N, Liu N, et al: The effects of intravenous almitrine on oxygenation and hemodynamics during one-lung ventilation. Anesth Analg 94:830-834, 2002.
143. Dalibon N, Moutafis M, Liu N, et al: Treatment of hypoxemia during one-lung ventilation using intravenous almitrine. Anesth Analg 98:590-594, 2004.
144. Friedlander M, Sandler A, Kavanagh B, et al: Is hypoxic pulmonary vasoconstriction important during single lung ventilation in the lateral decubitus position? Can J Anesth 41:26-30, 1994.
145. Choi Y, Bang S, Shim J, et al: Effects of head-down tilt on intrapulmonary shunt fraction and oxygenation during one-lung ventilation in the lateral decubitus position. J Thorac Cardiovasc Surg 134:613-618, 2007.
146. Dembinski R, Henzler R, Roissant R: Modulating the pulmonary circulation: An update. Minerva Anesthsiol 70:239-243, 2004.
147. Schilling T, Kozian A, Huth C, et al: The pulmonary immune effects of mechanical ventilation in patients undergoing thoracic surgery. Anesth Analg 101:957-965, 2005.
148. McMahon AJ, Fischbacher CM, Frame SH, et al: Impact of laparoscopic cholecystectomy: A population-based study. Lancet 356:1632-1637, 2000.
149. Neudecker J, Sauerland S, Neugebauer E, et al: The European Association for Endoscopic Surgery clinical practice guideline on the pneumoperitoneum for laparoscopic surgery. Surg Endosc Other Intervent Tech 16:1121-1143, 2002.
150. Gutt CN, Oniu T, Mehrabi A, et al: Circulatory and respiratory complications of carbon dioxide insufflation. Dig Surg 21:95-105, 2004.
151. Bablekos GD, Michaelides SA, Roussou T, et al: Changes in breathing control and mechanics after laparoscopic vs open cholecystectomy. Arch Surg 141:16-22, 2006.
152. Hirvonen EA, Nuutinen LS, Kauko M: Ventilatory effects, blood-gas changes, and oxygen-consumption during laparoscopic hysterectomy. Anesth Analg 80:961-966, 1995.
153. Andersson LE, Baath M, Thorne A, et al: Effect of carbon dioxide pneumoperitoneum on development of atelectasis during anesthesia, examined by spiral computed tomography. Anesthesiology 102:293-299, 2005.
154. Makinen MT, Yli-Hankala A: Respiratory compliance during laparoscopic hiatal and inguinal hernia repair. Can J Anaesth 45:865-870, 1998.
155. Sharma KC, Brandstetter RD, Brensilver JM, et al: Cardiopulmonary physiology and pathophysiology as a consequence of laparoscopic surgery. Chest 110:810-815, 1996.
156. Andersson L, Lagerstrand L, Thorne A, et al: Effect of CO_2 pneumoperitoneum on ventilation-perfusion relationships during laparoscopic cholecystectomy. Acta Anaesthesiol Scand 46:552-560, 2002.
157. Pasquina P, Tramer MR, Walder B: Prophylactic respiratory physiotherapy after cardiac surgery: Systematic review. BMJ 327:1379-1381, 2003.
158. Westerdahl E, Lindmark B, Eriksson T, et al: Deep-breathing exercises reduce atelectasis and improve pulmonary function after coronary artery bypass surgery. Chest 128:3482-3488, 2005.
159. Douglas NJ, White DP, Pickett CK, et al: Respiration during sleep in normal man. Thorax 37:840-844, 1982.
160. Hudgel DW, Devadatta P: Decrease in functional residual capacity during sleep in normal humans. J Appl Physiol 57:1319-1322, 1984.
161. Ballard RD, Irvin CG, Martin RJ, et al: Influence of sleep on lung-volume in asthmatic-patients and normal subjects. J Appl Physiol 68:2034-2041, 1990.
162. Appelberg J, Pavlenko T, Bergman H, et al: Lung aeration during sleep. Chest 131:122-129, 2007.

Lena S. Sun and Johanna C. Schwarzenberger

16 Cardiac Physiology

Key Points

1. The cardiac cycle is the sequence of electrical and mechanical events during the course of a single heartbeat.
2. Cardiac output is determined by the heart rate, myocardial contractility, and preload and afterload.
3. The majority of cardiomyocytes consist of myofibrils, which are rodlike bundles that form the contractile elements within the cardiomyocyte.
4. The basic working unit of contraction is the sarcomere.
5. Gap junctions are responsible for electrical coupling of small molecules between cells.
6. Action potentials have four phases in the heart.
7. The key player in cardiac excitation-contraction coupling is the ubiquitous second messenger calcium.
8. β-Adrenoreceptors stimulate chronotropy, inotropy, lusitropy, and dromotropy.
9. Hormones with cardiac action can be synthesized and secreted by cardiomyocytes or produced by other tissues and delivered to the heart.
10. Cardiac reflexes are fast-acting reflex loops between the heart and central nervous system that contribute to regulation of cardiac function and maintenance of physiologic homeostasis.

The modern concept of circulation and that the heart is the generator for the circulation was initially advanced by Harvey in 1628. Since that time, the field of cardiac physiology has developed to now include the physiology of the heart as a pump, cellular and molecular biology of the cardiomyocyte, and regulation of cardiac function by neural and humoral factors. Moreover, we now appreciate that physiology of the heart is only a component of the interrelated and integrated cardiovascular and circulatory physiology. This chapter discusses only the physiology of the heart. It begins with the physiology of the intact heart. The second part of the chapter focuses on cellular cardiac physiology. Finally, we briefly discuss the various factors that regulate cardiac function.

The basic anatomy of the heart consists of two atria and two ventricles that provide two separate circulations in series. The pulmonary circulation, a low-resistance and high-capacitance vascular bed, receives output from the right side of the heart, and its chief function is bidirectional gas exchange. The left side of the heart provides output for the systemic circulation. It functions to deliver oxygen and nutrients and remove CO_2 and metabolites from various tissue beds.

Physiology of the Intact Heart

To understand the mechanical performance of the intact heart, it is important to have knowledge of the phases of the cardiac cycle and determinants of ventricular function.

Cardiac Cycle

The cardiac cycle is the sequence of electrical and mechanical events during the course of a single heartbeat. Figure 16-1 illustrates (1) the electrical events of a single cardiac cycle represented by the electrocardiogram (ECG) and (2) the mechanical events of a single cardiac cycle represented by left atrial and left ventricular pressure pulses correlated in time with aortic flow and ventricular volume.[1]

The cardiac cycle begins with initiation of the heartbeat. Intrinsic to the specialized cardiac pacemaker tissues is automaticity and rhythmicity. The sinoatrial (SA) node is usually the pacemaker; it can generate impulses at the greatest frequency and is the natural pacemaker.

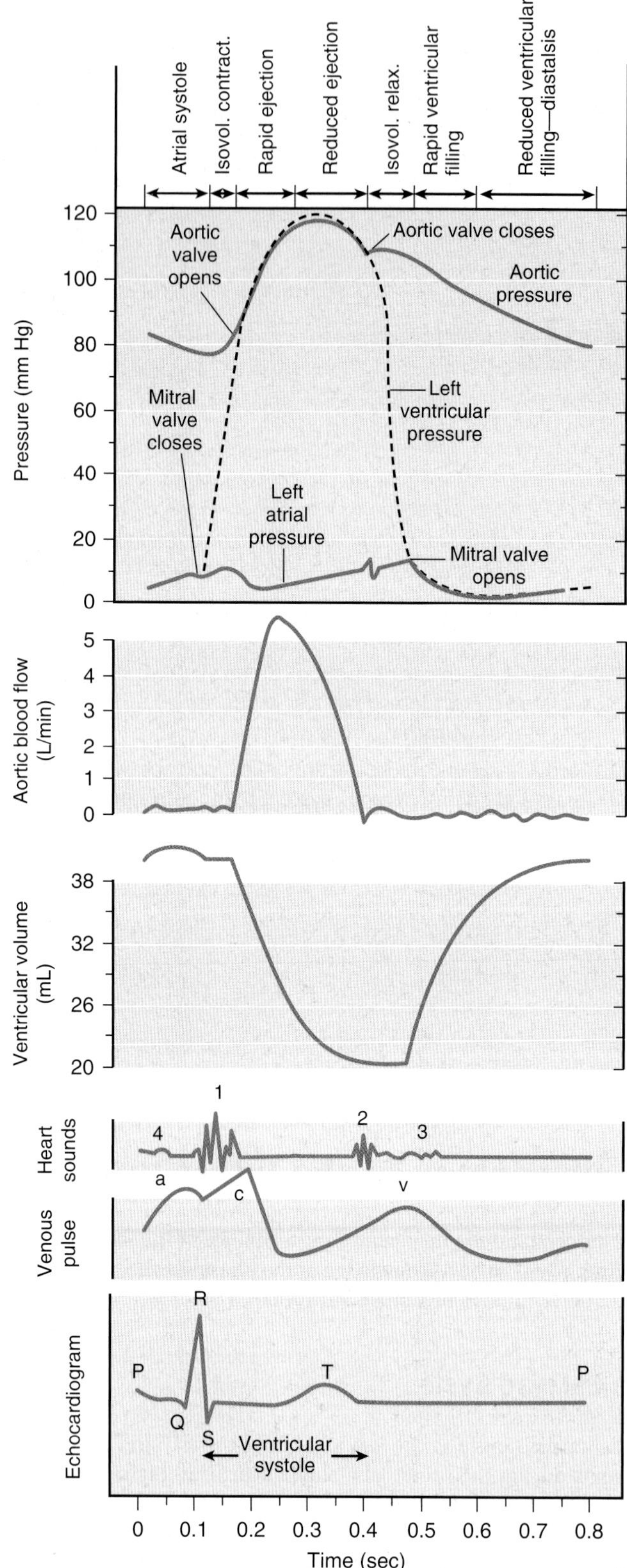

Figure 16-1 Electrical and mechanical events during a single cardiac cycle. Shown are the pressure curves of aortic blood flow, ventricular volume, venous pulse, and the electrocardiogram. *(From Berne RM, Levy MN: The cardiac pump. In Cardiovascular Physiology, 8th ed. St Louis, CV Mosby, 2001, pp 55-82.)*

Electrical Events and the Electrocardiogram

Electrical events of the pacemaker and the specialized conduction system are represented by the ECG at the body surface (also see Chapters 42 and 43). It is the result of differences in electrical potential generated by the heart at sites of the surface recording. The action potential initiated at the SA node is propagated to both atria by specialized conduction tissue, and it leads to atrial systole (contraction) and the P wave of the ECG. At the junction of the interatrial and interventricular septa, specialized atrial conduction tissue converges at the atrioventricular (AV) node, which is connected distally to the His bundle. The AV node is an area of relatively slow conduction, and a delay between atrial and ventricular contraction normally occurs at this locus. The PR interval can be used to measure the delay between atrial and ventricular contraction at the level of the AV node. From the distal His bundle, an electrical impulse is propagated through large left and right bundle branches and finally to the Purkinje system fibers, which are the smallest branches of the specialized conduction system. Finally, electrical signals are transmitted from the Purkinje system to individual ventricular cardiomyocytes. The spread of depolarization to the ventricular myocardium is manifested as the QRS complex on the ECG. Depolarization is followed by ventricular repolarization and appearance of the T wave on the ECG.[2]

Mechanical Events

The mechanical events of a cardiac cycle begin with return of blood to the right and left atria from the systemic and pulmonary circulation, respectively. As blood accumulates in the atria, atrial pressure increases until it exceeds the pressure within the ventricle, and the AV valve opens. Blood first flows passively into the ventricular chambers, and such flow accounts for approximately 75% of total ventricular filling.[3] The remainder of the blood flow is mediated by active atrial contraction or systole, known as the atrial "kick." The onset of atrial systole is coincident with depolarization of the sinus node and the P wave. While the ventricles fill, the AV valves are displaced upward and ventricular contraction (systole) begins with closure of the tricuspid and mitral valves, which corresponds to the end of the R wave on the ECG. The first part of ventricular systole is known as isovolumic or isometric contraction. The electrical impulse traverses the AV region and passes through the right and left bundle branches into the Purkinje fibers. This leads to contraction of ventricular myocardium and a progressive increase in intraventricular pressure. When intraventricular pressure exceeds pulmonary artery and aortic pressure, the pulmonic and aortic valves open and ventricular ejection occurs, which is the second part of ventricular systole.

Ventricular ejection can be further separated into the rapid ejection phase and the reduced ejection phase. During the rapid ejection phase, forward flow is maximal, and pulmonary artery and aortic pressure is maximally developed. In the reduced ejection phase, flow and great artery pressure taper with progression of systole. Pressure in both ventricular chambers falls as blood is ejected from the heart, and ventricular diastole begins with closure of the pulmonic and aortic valves. The initial period of ventricular diastole consists of the isovolumic/isometric relaxation phase. This phase is concomitant with repolarization of the ventricular myocardium and corresponds to the end of the T wave on the ECG. The final portion of ventricular diastole involves a rapid decrease in intraventricular pressure until it falls below that of the right and left atria, at which point the AV valve reopens, ventricular filling occurs, and the cycle repeats itself.

Ventricular Structure and Function

Ventricular Structure

The specific architectural order of the cardiac muscles provides the basis for the heart to function as a pump. The ellipsoid shape of the left ventricle (LV) is a result of the laminar layering of spiraling bundles of cardiac muscles (Fig. 16-2). The orientation of the muscle bundle is longitudinal in the subepicardial myocardium and circumferential in the middle segment and again becomes longitudinal in the subendocardial myocardium. Because of the ellipsoid shape of the LV, there are regional differences in wall thickness that result in corresponding variations in the cross-sectional radius of the LV chamber. These regional differences may serve to accommodate the variable loading conditions of the LV.[4] In addition, such anatomy allows the LV to eject blood in a corkscrew-type motion beginning from the base and ending at the apex. The architecturally complex structure of the LV thus allows maximal shortening of myocytes, which results in increased wall thickness and generation of force during systole. Moreover, release of the twisted LV may provide a suction mechanism for filling of the LV during diastole. The LV free wall and the septum have similar muscle bundle architecture. As a result, the septum moves inward during systole in a normal heart. Regional wall thickness is a commonly used index of myocardial performance that can be assessed clinically, such as by perioperative echocardiography or magnetic resonance imaging.

Unlike the LV, which needs to pump against the higher-pressure systemic circulation, the right ventricle (RV) pumps against a much lower pressure circuit in the pulmonary circulation. Consequently, wall thickness is considerably less in the RV. In contrast to the ellipsoidal form of the LV, the RV is crescent shaped, as a result of which the mechanics of RV contraction are more complex. Inflow and outflow contraction is not simultaneous, and much of the contractile force seems to be recruited from interventricular forces of the LV-based septum.

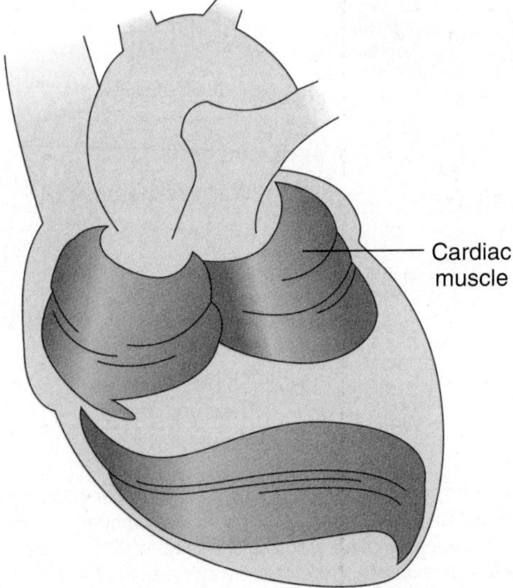

Figure 16-2 Muscle bundles. *(From Marieb EN: Human Anatomy & Physiology, 5th ed. San Francisco, Peason Benjamin Cummings, 2001, p 684.)*

An intricate matrix of collagen fibers form a scaffold of support for the heart and adjacent vessels. This matrix provides enough strength to resist tensile stretch. The collagen fibers are made up of mostly the thick collagen type I fiber, which cross-links with the thin collagen type III fiber, the other major type of collagen.[5] In close proximity to the collagen fibers are elastic fibers that contain elastin. They account for the elasticity of the myocardium.[6]

Systolic Function

The heart provides the driving force for delivering blood throughout the cardiovascular system to supply nutrients and remove metabolic waste. Because of the complexity of RV anatomy, the traditional description of systolic function is usually limited to the LV. Systolic performance of the heart is dependent on loading conditions and contractility. Preload and afterload are two interdependent factors extrinsic to the heart that govern cardiac performance.

Preload and Afterload

Preload is defined as the ventricular load at the end of diastole, before contraction has started. First described by Starling, a linear relationship exists between sarcomere length and myocardial force (Fig. 16-3). In clinical practice, surrogate representatives of LV volume such as pulmonary wedge pressure or central venous pressure are used to estimate preload.[3] With the development of transesophageal echocardiography, a more direct measure of ventricular volume is available.

Afterload is defined as systolic load on the LV after contraction has begun. Aortic compliance is an additional determinant of afterload.[1] Aortic compliance is the ability of the aorta to give way to systolic forces from the ventricle. Changes in the aortic wall (dilation or stiffness) can alter aortic compliance and thus afterload. Examples of pathologic conditions that alter afterload are aortic stenosis and chronic hypertension. Both impede ventricular ejection, thereby increasing afterload. Aortic impedance, or aortic pressure divided by aortic flow at that instant, is an accurate means of gauging afterload. However, clinical measurement of aortic impedance is invasive. Echocardiography can estimate aortic impedance noninvasively by determining aortic blood flow at the time of its maximal increase. In more general clinical practice, measurement of systolic blood pressure is adequate to approximate afterload, provided that aortic stenosis is not present.

Preload and afterload can be thought of as the wall stress that is present at the end of diastole and during LV ejection, respectively. Wall stress is a useful concept because it includes preload, afterload, and the energy required to generate contraction. Wall stress and heart rate are probably the two most relevant indices that account for changes in myocardial oxygen demand. The law of Laplace states that wall stress (σ) is the product of pressure (P) and radius (R) divided by wall thickness (h)[3]:

$$\sigma = P \times R/2h$$

The ellipsoid shape of the LV allows the least amount of wall stress such that as the ventricle changes its shape from ellipsoid to spherical, wall stress is increased. By using the ratio of the long axis to the short axis as a measure of the ellipsoid shape, a decrease in this ratio would signify a transition from ellipsoid to spherical.

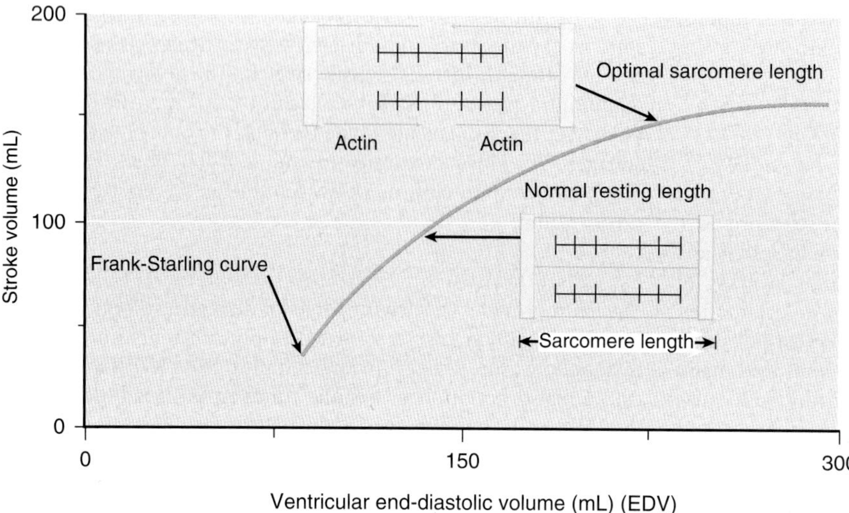

Figure 16-3 Frank-Starling relationship. The relationship between sarcomere length and tension developed in cardiac muscles is shown. In the heart, an increase in end-diastolic volume is the equivalent of an increase in myocardial stretch; therefore, according to Starling's law, increased stroke volume is generated.

Thickness of the LV muscle is an important modifier of wall stress. For example, in aortic stenosis, afterload is increased. The ventricle has to generate far higher pressure to overcome the increased load opposing systolic ejection of blood. To generate such high performance, the ventricle increases its wall thickness (LV hypertrophy). By applying Laplace's law, increased LV wall thickness will decrease wall stress despite the necessary increase in LV pressure to overcome the aortic stenosis (Fig. 16-4).[7] In a failing heart, the radius of the LV increases, thus increasing wall stress.

Frank-Starling Relationship

The Frank-Starling relationship is an intrinsic property of myocardium by which stretching of the myocardial sarcomere results in enhanced myocardial performance for subsequent contractions (see Fig. 16-3). Otto Frank first noted in 1895 that in skeletal muscle, the change in tension was directly related to its length and that in the heart, as pressure changed, a corresponding change in volume occurred.[8] E. H. Starling, using an isolated heart-lung preparation as a model, observed in 1914 that "the mechanical energy set free on passage from the resting to the contracted state is a function of the length of the muscle fiber."[9] If a strip of cardiac muscle is mounted in a muscle chamber under isometric conditions and stimulated at a fixed frequency, an increase in sarcomere length results in an increase in twitch force. Starling concluded that the increased twitch force was the result of a greater interaction of muscle bundles.

Electron microscopy has demonstrated that sarcomere length (2.0 to 2.2 μm) is positively related to the amount of actin and myosin cross-bridging and that there is an optimal sarcomere length at which the interaction is maximal. This concept is based on the assumption that the increase in cross-bridging is equivalent to an increase in muscle performance. Although this theory continues to hold true for skeletal muscle, the force-length relationship in cardiac muscle is more complex. When comparing force-strength relationships between skeletal and cardiac muscle, it is noteworthy that the reduction in force is only 10% even if cardiac muscle is at 80% sarcomere length.[8] The cellular basis of the Frank-Starling mechanism is still being investigated and will be discussed briefly later. A common clinical application of Starling's law is the relationship of left ventricular end-diastolic volume (LVEDV) and stroke volume. The Frank-Starling mechanism may remain intact even in a failing heart.[10] However, ventricular remodeling after injury or in heart failure may modify the Frank-Starling relationship.

Contractility

Each Frank-Starling curve specifies a level of contractility, or the inotropic state of the heart, which is defined as the work performed by cardiac muscle at any given end-diastolic fiber. Factors that modify contractility will create a family of Frank-Starling curves with different contractility (Fig. 16-5).[7] Among factors known to modify contractility are exercise, adrenergic

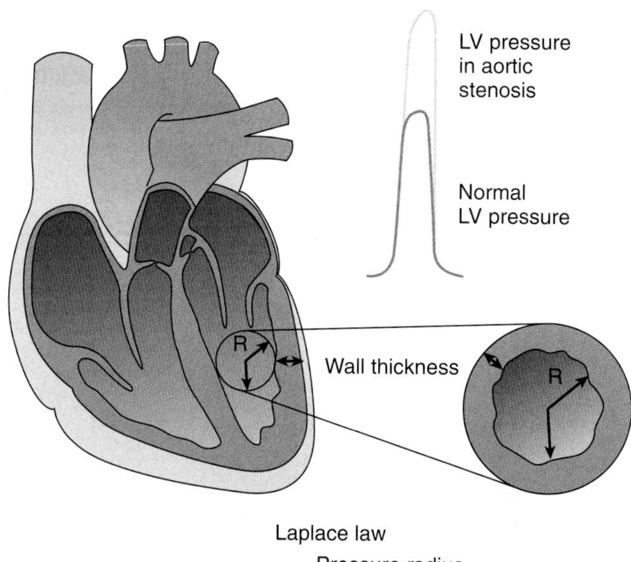

Figure 16-4 In response to aortic stenosis, left ventricular (LV) pressure increases. To maintain wall stress at control levels, compensatory LV hypertrophy develops. According to Laplace's law, wall stress = pressure × radius ÷ (2 × wall thickness). Therefore, the increase in wall thickness offsets the increased pressure, and wall stress is maintained at control levels. *(From Opie LH: Ventricular function. In The Heart. Physiology from Cell to Circulation, 4th ed. Philadelphia, Lippincott-Raven, 2004, pp 355-401.)*

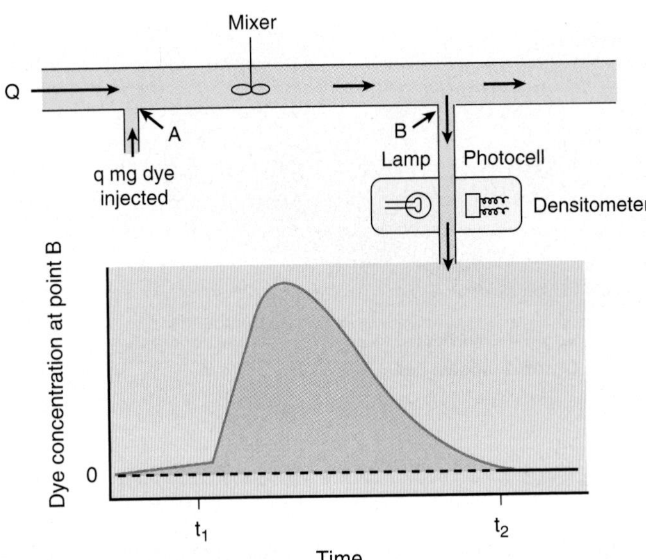

Figure 16-8 Illustration demonstrating the principle of determining cardiac output with the indicator dilution technique. This model assumes that there is no recirculation. A known amount of dye (q) is injected at point A into a stream flowing at $\dot{Q}$ (mL/min). A mixed sample of the fluid flowing past point B is withdrawn at a constant rate through a densitometer. The change in dye concentration over time is depicted in a curve. Flow may be measured by dividing the amount of indicator injected upstream by the area under the downstream concentration curve. *(From Berne RM, Levy MN: The cardiac pump. In Cardiovascular Physiology, 8th ed. St Louis, CV Mosby, 2001, pp 55-82.)*

delivered to the pulmonary capillaries from the alveoli (q_2). Because $q_1 + q_2 = q_3$,

$$\dot{Q}(Cpao_2) + q_2 = \dot{Q}(Cpvo_2)$$

$$q_2 = \dot{Q}(Cpvo_2) - \dot{Q}(Cpao_2)$$

$$q_2 = \dot{Q}(Cpvo_2) - Cpao_2$$

$$\dot{Q} = q_2/(Cpvo_2 - Cpao_2)$$

Thus, if the O_2 concentration in the pulmonary artery ($Cpao_2$), the O_2 concentration in the pulmonary vein ($Cpvo_2$), and O_2 consumption (q_2) are known, cardiac output can be determined.

The indicator dilution technique is another method for determining cardiac output, and it is also based on the law of conservation of mass. The two most commonly used indicator dilution techniques are the dye dilution and the thermodilution methods. Figure 16-8 illustrates the principles of the dye dilution method.[1]

Cellular Cardiac Physiology

Cellular Anatomy

At the cellular level, the heart consists of three major components: cardiac muscle tissue (contracting cardiomyocytes), conduction tissue (conducting cells), and extracellular connective tissue. A group of cardiomyocytes with its connective tissue support network or extracellular matrix make up a myofiber (Fig. 16-9). Adjacent myofibers are connected by strands of collagen. The extracellular matrix is the synthetic product of fibroblasts and is made up of collagen, which is the main determinant of myocardial stiffness, and other major matrix proteins. One of the matrix proteins, elastin, is the chief constituent of elastic fibers. The elastic fibers account for, in part, the elastic properties of the myocardium.[6] Other matrix proteins include the glycoproteins or proteoglycans and matrix metalloproteins. Proteoglycans are proteins with short sugar chains, and they include heparan sulfate, chondroitin, fibronectin, and laminin. Matrix metalloproteins are enzymes that degrade collagen and other extracellular proteins. The balance between accumulation of extracellular matrix proteins by synthesis and their breakdown by matrix metalloproteins contributes to the mechanical properties and function of the heart.[6]

Cardiomyocyte Structure and Function

Individual contracting cardiomyocytes are large cells between 20 μm (atrial cardiomyocytes) and 140 μm (ventricular cardiomyocytes) in length. Approximately 50% of the cell volume in a contracting cardiomyocyte is made up of myofibrils, and the remainder consists of mitochondria, nucleus, sarcoplasmic reticulum (SR), and the cytosol. The myofibril is the rodlike bundle that forms the contractile elements within cardiomyocytes. Within each contractile element are contractile proteins, regulatory proteins, and structural proteins. Contractile proteins make up about 80% of the myofibrillar protein, with the remainder being regulatory and structural proteins.[16,17] The basic unit of contraction is the sarcomere, which will be described later.

The sarcolemma, or the outer plasma membrane, separates the intracellular and extracellular space. It surrounds the cardiomyocyte and invaginates into the myofibrils through an extensive tubular network known as transverse or T tubules, and it also forms specialized intercellular junctions between cells.[18,19]

Transverse or T tubules are in close proximity to an intramembrane system and the SR, which plays an important role in the calcium metabolism that is critical in excitation-contraction coupling (ECC) of the cardiomyocyte. The SR can be further divided into the longitudinal (or network) and the junctional SR. The longitudinal SR is involved in the uptake of calcium for initiation of relaxation. The junctional SR contains large calcium release channels (ryanodine receptors) that release SR calcium stores in

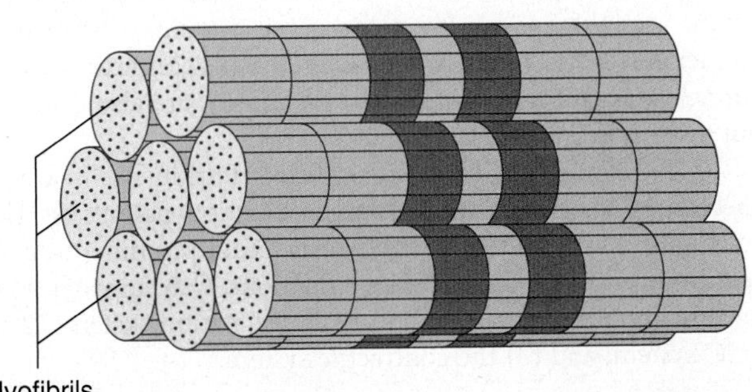

Figure 16-9 Organization of cardiomyocytes. Fifty percent of cardiomyocyte volume is made up of myofibrils; the remainder consists of mitochondria, nucleus, sarcoplasmic reticulum, and cytosol.

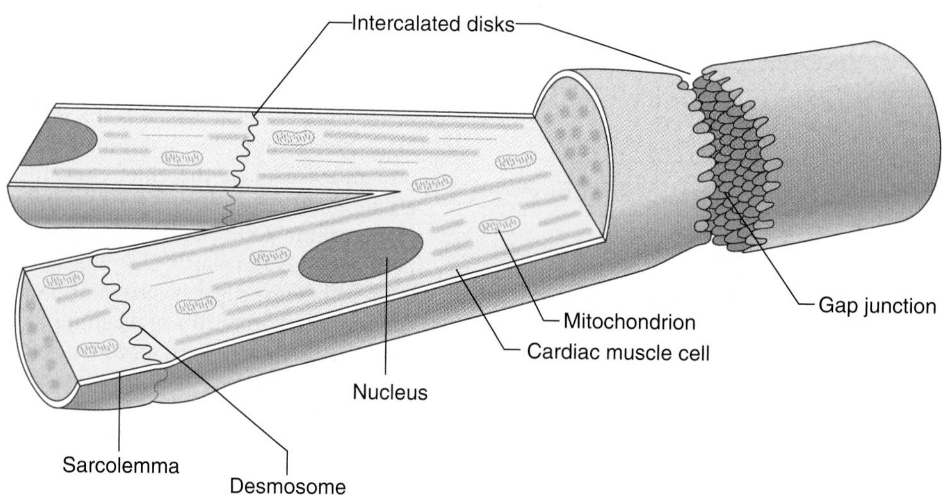

Figure 16-10 The sarcolemma that envelops cardiomyocytes becomes highly specialized to form the intercalated disks where ends of neighboring cells are in contact. The intercalated disks consist of gap junctions and "spot" and "sheet" desmosomes.

response to depolarization-stimulated calcium influx through the sarcolemmal calcium channels. The ryanodine receptors not only are calcium release channels but they also form the scaffolding proteins that anchor many of the key regulatory proteins.[20]

Mitochondria are found immediately beneath the sarcolemma, wedged between myofibrils within the cell. They contain enzymes that promote the generation of adenosine triphosphate (ATP), and they are the energy powerhouse for the cardiomyocyte. In addition, mitochondria can also function to accumulate calcium and thereby contribute to regulation of the cytosolic calcium concentration. Nearly all of the genetic information is found within the centrally located nucleus. The cytosol is the fluid-filled microenvironment within the sarcolemma, exclusive of the organelles and the contractile apparatus and proteins.

Cardiac muscle cells contain three different types of intercellular junctions: gap junctions, "spot" desmosomes, and "sheet" desmosomes (or fasciae adherens) (Fig. 16-10).[19,21] Gap junctions are responsible for electrical coupling and transfer of small molecules between cells, whereas desmosome-like junctions provide mechanical linkage. The adhesion sites formed by "spot" desmosomes anchor the intermediate filament cytoskeleton of the cell; those formed by the fasciae adherens anchor the contractile apparatus. Gap junctions consist of clusters of plasma membrane channels directly linking the cytoplasmic compartments of neighboring cells. Gap junction channels are constructed from connexins, a multigene family of conserved proteins. The principal connexin isoform of the mammalian heart is connexin 43; other connexins, notably connexins 40, 45, and 37, are also expressed, but in smaller quantities.[20,21]

The conducting cardiomyocytes, or Purkinje cells, are cells specialized for conducting propagated action potentials. These cells have a low content of myofibrils and a prominent nucleus and contain an abundance of gap junctions. Cardiomyocytes can be functionally separated into (1) the excitation system, (2) the ECC system, and (3) the contractile system.

Excitation System

The cellular action potential originating in the specialized conduction tissue is propagated to individual cells where it initiates the intracellular event that leads to contraction of the cell through the sarcolemmal excitation system.

Action Potential

Ion fluxes across plasma membranes result in depolarization (attaining a less negative membrane potential) and repolarization (attaining a more negative membrane potential). They are mediated by membrane proteins with ion-selective pores. Because these ion channel proteins open and close the pores in response to changes in membrane potential, the channels are voltage gated. In the heart, sodium, potassium, calcium, and chloride channels have been found to contribute to the action potential.

The types of action potential in the heart can be separated into two categories: fast-response action potentials, which are found in the His-Purkinje system and atrial or ventricular cardiomyocytes, and slow-response action potentials, which are found in the pacemaker cells in the SA and AV nodes. A typical tracing of an action potential in the His-Purkinje system is depicted in Figure 16-11.[12] The electrochemical gradient for potassium across the plasma membrane is the determinant for the resting membrane potential. Mostly as a result of the influx of Na^+, the membrane potential becomes depolarized, which leads to an extremely rapid upstroke (phase 0). As the membrane potential reaches a critical level, or threshold, during depolarization, the action potential is propagated. The rapid upstroke is followed by a transient repolarization (phase 1). Phase 1 is a period of brief and limited repolarization that is largely due to the activation of a transient outward potassium current, i_{to}. The plateau phase (phase 2) occurs with a net influx of Ca^{2+} through L-type calcium channels and efflux of K^+ through several potassium channels: the inwardly rectifying i_k, the delayed rectifier i_{k1}, and i_{to}. Repolarization (phase 3) is brought about when efflux of K^+ from the three outward potassium currents exceeds the influx of Ca^{2+}, thus returning the membrane to the resting potential. Very little ionic flux occurs during diastole (phase 4) in a fast-response action potential.

In contrast, during diastole (phase 4), pacemaker cells that show slow-response action potentials have the capability of spontaneous diastolic depolarization and generate the automatic

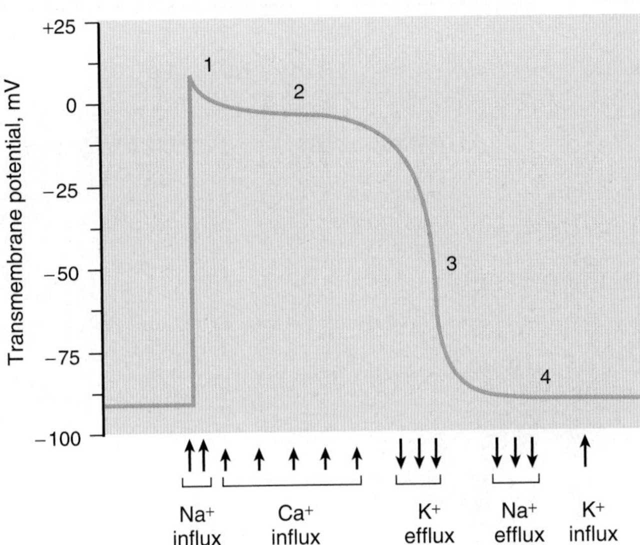

Figure 16-11 Phases of cellular action potentials and major associated currents in ventricular myocytes. The initial phase 0 spike and overshoot (1) are caused by a rapid inward Na^+ current, the plateau phase (2) by a slow Ca^{2+} current through L-type Ca channels, and repolarization (phase 3) by outward K^+ currents. Phase 4, the resting potential (Na^+ efflux, K^+ influx), is maintained by Na^+-K^+-ATPase. The Na^+-Ca^{2+} exchanger is mainly responsible for extrusion of Ca^{2+}. In specialized conduction system tissue, spontaneous depolarization takes place during phase 4 until the voltage resulting in opening of the Na channel is reached. *(From LeWinter MM, Osol G: Normal physiology of the cardiovascular system. In Fuster V [ed]: Hurst's The Heart, 10th ed. New York, McGraw-Hill, 2001, pp 63-94.)*

cardiac rhythm. Pacemaker currents during phase 4 are the result of an increase in the three inward currents and a decrease in the two outward currents. The three inward currents that contribute to spontaneous pacemaker activity include two carried by calcium, i_{CaL} and i_{CaT}, and one that is a mixed cation current, I_f. The two outward currents are the delayed rectifier potassium current i_k and the inward rectifying potassium current i_{k1}. When compared with the fast-response action potential, phase 0 is much less steep, phase 1 is absent, and phase 2 is indistinct from phase 3 in the slow-response action potential.[22]

During the cardiac action potential, movement of Ca^{2+} into the cell and Na^+ out of the cell creates an ionic imbalance. The Na^+-Ca^{2+} exchanger restores cellular ionic balance by actively transporting Ca^{2+} out of the cell against a concentration gradient while moving Na^+ into the cell in an energy-dependent manner.

Excitation-Contraction Coupling

Structures that participate in cardiac ECC include the sarcolemma, transverse tubules, SR, and myofilaments (Fig. 16-12A).[23] The process of ECC begins with depolarization of the plasma membrane and spread of electrical excitation along the sarcolemma of cardiomyocytes. Calcium enters through plasma membrane channels concentrated at the T tubules, and such entry triggers the release of calcium from the SR, which in turn stimulates myofibrillar contraction.[24]

The ubiquitous second messenger calcium is the key player in cardiac ECC (see Fig. 16-12B).[23] Cycling of calcium within the structures that participate in ECC initiates and terminates contraction. Activation of the contractile system depends on an increase in free cytosolic calcium and its subsequent binding to contractile proteins. Influx of calcium through the voltage-gated L-type calcium channels (dihydropyridine receptors) causes an initial small increase in intracellular calcium. The local increase in Ca^{2+} concentration as a result of entry of Ca^{2+} through the voltage-gated L-type calcium channels activates the calcium release channels (ryanodine receptors), induces further release of calcium from subsarcolemmal cisternae in the SR, and thus leads to a large increase in intracellular calcium. The increase in intracellular calcium, however, is transient inasmuch as calcium is removed by (1) active uptake by the SR calcium pump adenosine triphosphatase (ATPase), (2) extrusion of calcium from the cytosol by the Na^+-Ca^{2+} exchanger, and (3) binding of calcium to proteins.[25]

The SR provides the anatomic framework and is the major organelle for the cycling of calcium. It is the depot for intracellular calcium stores. The cyclic release plus reuptake of calcium by the SR regulates the cytosolic calcium concentration and couples excitation to contraction. The physical proximity between L-type calcium channels and ryanodine receptors at the SR membrane makes calcium-induced calcium release occur easily. The "foot" region of the ryanodine receptor is the part that extends from the SR membrane to the T tubules, where the L-type calcium channels are located.[16,25,26]

The SR is also concerned with the reuptake of calcium that initiates relaxation or terminates contraction. Sarcoplasmic/endoplasmic reticulum Ca^{2+}-ATPase (SERCA) is the ATP-dependent pump that actively pumps the majority of the calcium back into the SR after its release. SERCA makes up close to 90% of all of the SR proteins, and it is inhibited by the phosphoprotein phospholamban at rest. Phospholamban is an SR membrane protein that is active in the dephosphorylated form. Phosphorylation by a variety of kinases as a result of β-adrenergic stimulation or other stimuli inactivates phospholamban and releases its inhibitory action on SERCA. Positive feedback ensues and leads to further phospholamban phosphorylation and greater SERCA activity. Active reuptake of calcium by SERCA then promotes relaxation.[16,25,26]

Once taken up into the SR, calcium is stored until it is released during the next cycle. Calsequestrin and calreticulin are two storage proteins in the SR. Calsequestrin is a highly charged protein located in the cisternal component of the SR near the T tubules. Because it lies close to the calcium release channels, the stored calcium can be quickly discharged for release once the calcium release channels are stimulated.

Cytosolic calcium can also be removed by extrusion through the sarcolemmal calcium pump and the activity of the sodium-calcium exchanger. An important "sensor" and regulator of intracellular calcium is the protein calmodulin.[18]

Contractile System

Contractile Elements

The basic working unit of contraction is the sarcomere. A sarcomere is defined as the distance between Z lines (Z is an abbreviation for the German *Zuckung*, or "contraction"), which join the sarcomeres in series. Each sarcomere consists of a central A band that is separated by half of an I band from the Z lines on each side because the Z line bisects the I band. A schematic representation is depicted in Figure 16-13.[12] Within each sarcomere are two principal contractile proteins (see the next section) and one noncontractile protein, titin.[25] The two contractile proteins are actin, the thin filament, and myosin, the thick filament. Actin filaments and titin are both tethered to the Z line, but myosin

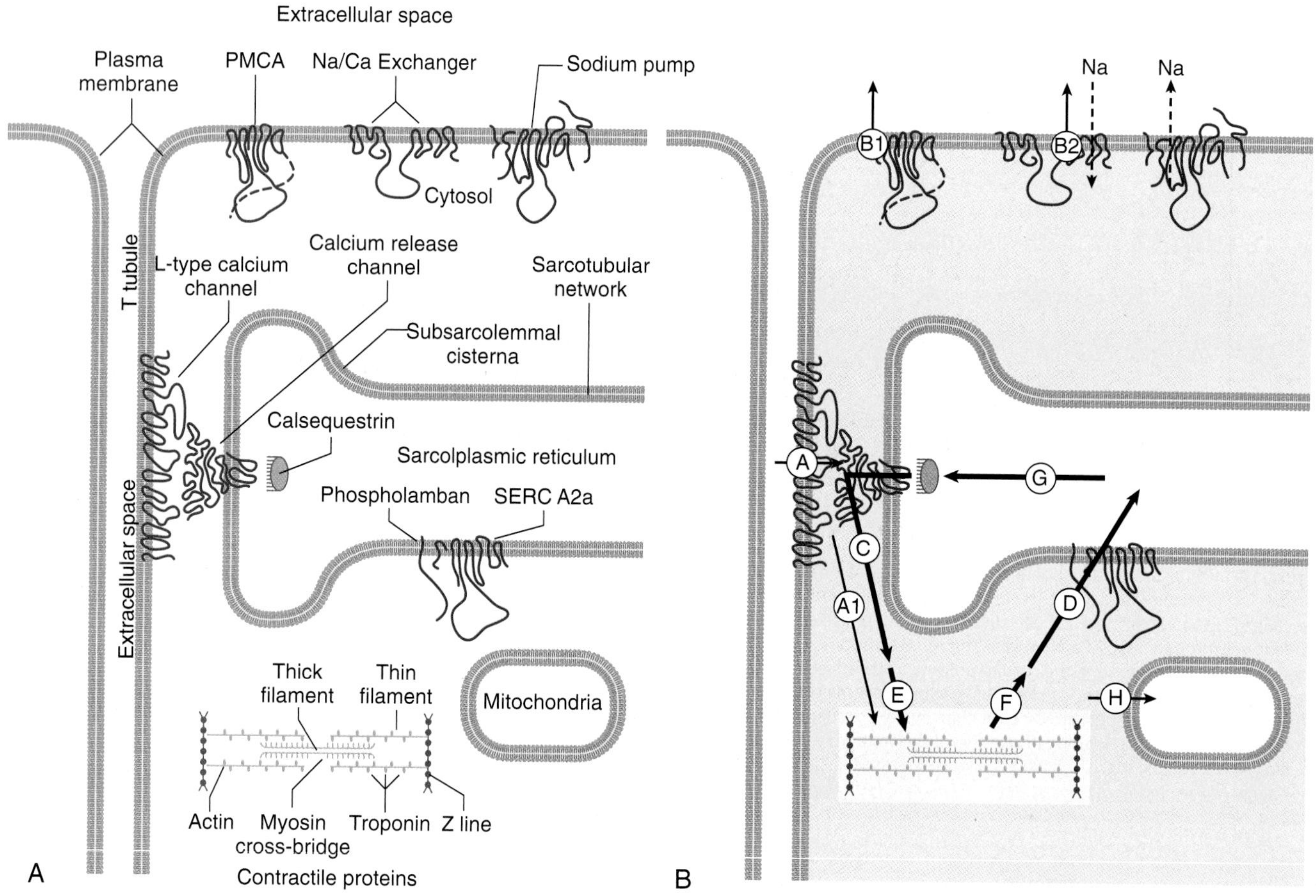

Figure 16-12 A, Diagram depicting the components of cardiac excitation-contraction coupling. Calcium pools are noted in **bold** letters. **B,** Extracellular (*arrows A, B1, B2*) and intracellular calcium flux (*arrows C, D, E, F, G*) is shown. The thickness of the *arrows* indicates the magnitude of the calcium flux, and the vertical orientations describe their energetics: *downward-pointing arrows* represent passive calcium flux, whereas *upward-pointing arrows* represent energy-dependent calcium transport. Calcium entering the cell from extracellular fluid through L-type calcium channels triggers release of calcium from the sarcoplasmic reticulum (SR). Only a small portion directly activates the contractile proteins (A1). *Arrow B1* depicts active transport of calcium into extracellular fluid by means of the plasma membrane pump ATPase and the Na^+-Ca^{2+} exchanger. Sodium that enters the cell in exchange for calcium (*dashed line*) is pumped out of the cytosol by the sodium pump. SR regulates calcium efflux from the subsarcolemmal cisternae (*arrow C*) and calcium uptake into the sarcotubular network (*arrow D*). *Arrow G* represents calcium that diffuses within the SR. Calcium binding to (*arrow E*) and dissociation from (*arrow F*) high-affinity calcium binding sites of troponin C activate and inhibit interactions of the contractile proteins. *Arrow H* depicts movement of calcium into and out of mitochondria to buffer the cytosolic calcium concentration. *(From Katz AM: Calcium fluxes.* In *Physiology of the Heart, 3rd ed. Philadelphia, Lippincott-Raven, 2001, pp 232-233.)*

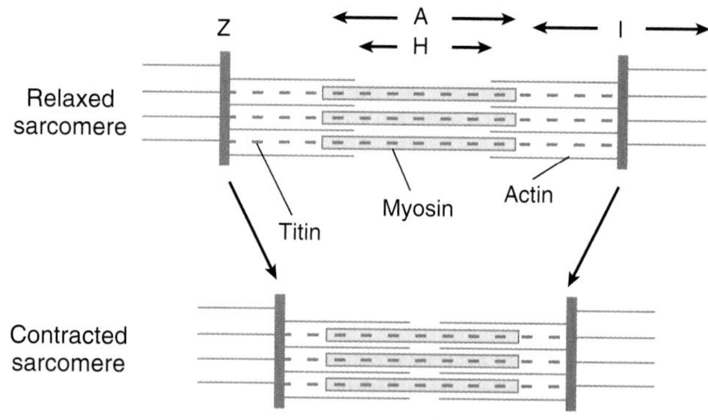

Figure 16-13 The basic unit of contraction is the sarcomere. A contracted and a relaxed sarcomere is depicted. Z lines are located at the ends of the sarcomere. The A band is the site of overlap between myosin and actin filaments. The I band is located on either side of the A band and contains only actin filament. The H zone is located in the center of the A band, and only myosin is present.

filaments do not actually reach the Z lines. Titin, the third filament protein, tethers the myosin thick filament to the Z line. The Z lines at the two ends of the sarcomere are brought closer together during contraction as the thick myosin filament heads interact with the thin actin filaments and slide over each other.[27,28]

Familial hypertrophic cardiomyopathy is an inherited autosomal dominant sarcomeric disease[29] that is the most common cause of sudden death in otherwise healthy individuals. Its clinical features are LV hypertrophy and myocyte/myofibrillar disarray. Mutations in at least eight different genes encoding sarcomere proteins have been identified to be the molecular basis for the disorder. These genes are β-cardiac myosin heavy chain, cardiac troponin T (TnT), α-tropomyosin, cardiac myosin binding protein C, essential or regulatory myosin light chain, cardiac troponin I (TnI), α-cardiac actin, and titin.[29]

Contractile Proteins

The contractile apparatus within the cardiomyocyte consists of contractile and regulatory proteins.[18,30,31] The thin-filament actin and the thick-filament myosin are the two principal contractile proteins. Actin contains two helical chains. Tropomyosin, a double-stranded α-helical regulatory protein, winds around the actin array and forms the backbone for the actin thin filament. The myosin thick filament is made up of 300 myosin molecules. Each myosin molecule has two functional domains: the body or filament and the bilobar myosin head. The myosin head is composed of one heavy chain and two light chains. The heavy head chain has two domains: the larger one interacts with actin at the actin cleft and has an ATP binding pocket where myosin ATPase is located, and the other smaller one is flexible and attached to the two light chains. The regulatory troponin heterotrimer complex is found at regular intervals along tropomyosin. The heterotrimer troponins are made up of troponin C (TnC), the Ca^{2+} receptor; TnI, an inhibitor of actin-myosin interaction; and TnT, which links the troponin complex to tropomyosin. Tropomodulin is another regulatory protein. It is located at the end of the actin thin filament and caps the end to prevent any excessive elongation of the thin filament.[27,28]

Myocyte Contraction and Relaxation

At rest, cross-bridge cycling and generation of force do not occur because either the myosin heads are blocked from physically reacting with the thin filament or they are only weakly bound to actin (Fig. 16-14).[16] Cross-bridge cycling is initiated on binding of calcium to TnC, which increases TnC-TnI interaction and decreases the inhibitory TnI-actin interaction. These events that ensue from binding of Ca^{2+} to TnC lead to conformational changes in tropomyosin and permit attachment of the myosin head to actin. Cross-bridging involves detachment of the myosin head from actin and reattachment of myosin to another actin on hydrolysis of ATP by myosin ATPase. Binding of ATP to the

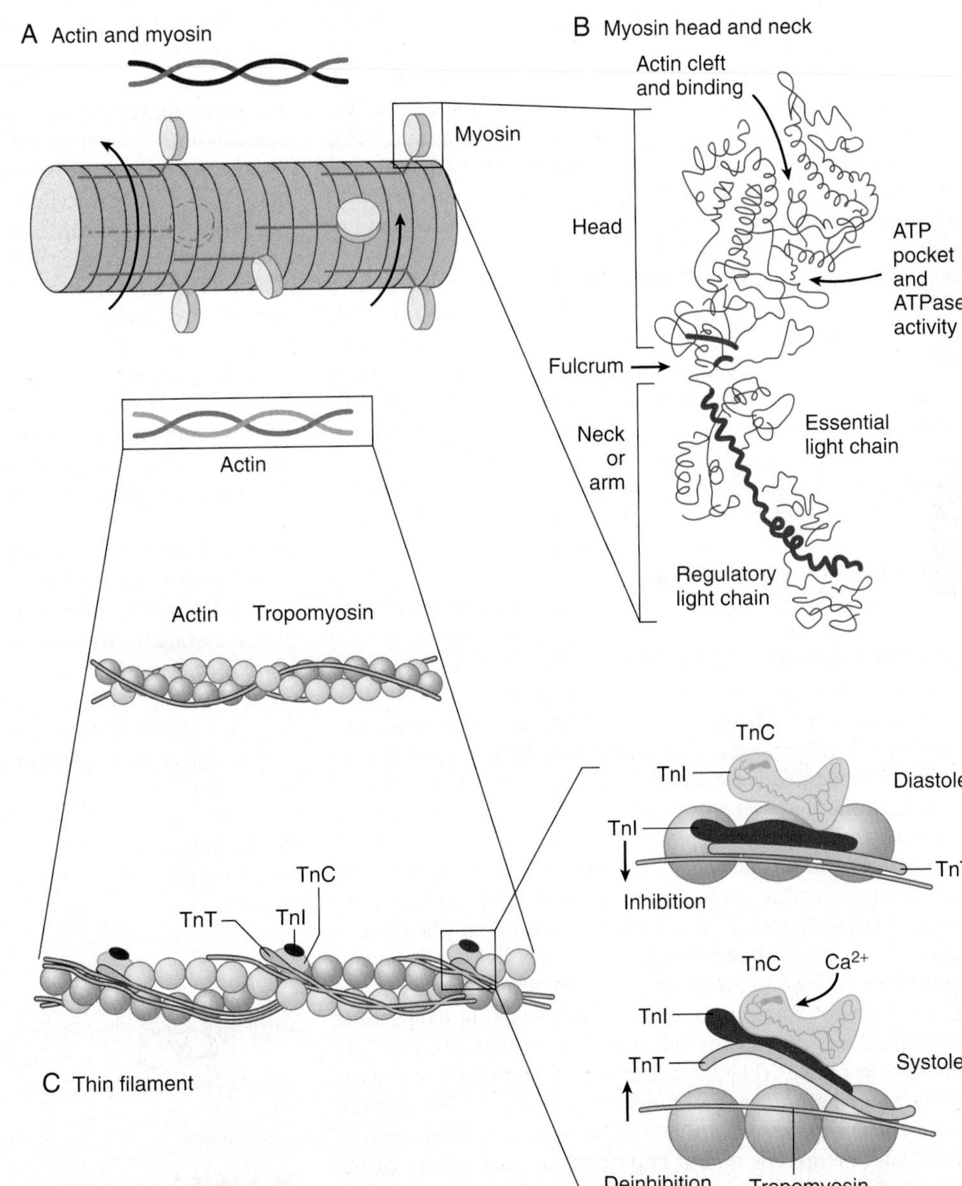

Figure 16-14 Molecules of the contractile system. TnC, TnI, TnT, troponin C, I, T. *(From Opie LH: Myocardial contraction and relaxation. In The Heart. Physiology from Cell to Circulation, 3rd ed. Philadelphia, Lippincott-Raven, 1998, pp 209-231.)*

nucleotide pocket of the myosin head leads to the activation of myosin ATPase,[26-28] ATP hydrolysis, and changes in configuration of the myosin head, all of which facilitate binding of the myosin head to actin and generation of the power stroke of the myosin head. Based on this model, it is apparent that the rate of cross-bridge cycling is dependent on the activity of myosin ATPase.[31] Turnoff of cross-bridge cycling is largely initiated by the fall in cytosolic calcium.

Myocyte relaxation is an energy-dependent process because restoration of cytosolic calcium to resting levels requires the expenditure of ATP. The fall in cytosolic calcium occurs through active reuptake of calcium into the SR by SERCA and extrusion of calcium by the Na^+-Ca^{2+} exchanger. This activity results in release of binding of Ca^{2+} to TnC and separation of the myosin-actin cross-bridge. Myocyte relaxation is dependent on the kinetics of cross-bridge cycling, the affinity of Ca^{2+} for TnC, and the activity of the calcium reuptake mechanisms. Relaxation is enhanced by the increased kinetics of cross-bridge cycling, decreased Ca^{2+} affinity for TnC, and increased activity of calcium reuptake mechanisms.[25]

Titin is a giant stringlike protein that acts as the third filament within the sarcomere. A single titin molecule spans half the sarcomere. Structurally, titin consists of an inextensible anchoring segment and an extensible elastic segment. Its two main functions involve muscle assembly and elasticity. Titin is the principal determinant of the passive properties of the myocardium at low ventricular volume.[32]

The Frank-Starling relationship states that an increase in end-diastolic volume results in enhanced systolic function.[33,34] At the cellular level, the key component for the Frank-Starling relationship is a length-dependent shift in Ca^{2+} sensitivity.[35-37] Several possible mechanisms for this change in Ca^{2+} sensitivity have been implicated, including (1) Ca^{2+} sensitivity as a function of myofilament lattice spacing, (2) Ca^{2+} sensitivity involving positive cooperativity in cross-bridge binding to actin, and (3) dependence of Ca^{2+} sensitivity on strain of the elastic protein titin.[31,36]

Cytoskeleton Proteins

The cytoskeleton is the protein framework within the cytoplasm that links, anchors, or tethers structural components inside the cell.[17,18] Microfilaments (actin filaments), microtubules, and intermediate filaments are three classes of cytoskeleton proteins found in the cytoplasm. Microfilament proteins are actin filaments, either sarcomeric or cortical, depending on their location. Sarcomeric actin filaments are the thin filaments in the contractile machinery that have already been described. Cortical actin filaments are found below the plasma membrane at the cell surface and are linked to several other microfilament proteins, including dystrophin, vinculin, and ankyrin. Microtubules assemble by polymerization of the α- and β-dimers of tubulin. They play a major role in intracellular transport and cell division.[38] Attachment of the ends of microtubules to cellular structures causes the microtubules to expand and contract, thereby pulling and pushing these structures around the cell. The intermediate filaments are relatively insoluble. They have been demonstrated to be important in normal mitochondrial function and behavior. The desmin intermediate filament in cardiomyocytes connects the nucleus to the plasma membrane and is important in transmission of the stress and strain of contractile force between cells.[39] The cytoskeleton provides the organization of microenvironments within the cell for enzyme/protein activity and interaction.

Whereas familial hypertrophic cardiomyopathy is a genetic sarcomeric disease, familial dilated cardiomyopathy (FDCM) is a disease of cytoskeleton proteins. The genetic basis of FDCM includes two genes for X-linked FDCM (dystrophin, G4.5) and four genes for the autosomal dominant form (actin, desmin, lamin A/C, δ-sarcoglycan).[17]

Control of Cardiac Function

Neural Regulation of Cardiac Function

The two limbs of the autonomic nervous system provide opposing input to regulate cardiac function.[40] The neurotransmitter of the sympathetic nervous system is norepinephrine, which provides positive chronotropic (heart rate), inotropic (contractility), and lusitropic (relaxation) effects. The parasympathetic nervous system has a more direct inhibitory effect in the atria and has a negative modulatory effect in the ventricles. The neurotransmitter of the parasympathetic nervous system is acetylcholine. Norepinephrine and acetylcholine both bind to seven-transmembrane–spanning G protein–coupled receptors to transduce their intracellular signals and effect their functional responses (Fig. 16-15).[41] At rest, the heart has a tonic level of parasympathetic cardiac nerve firing and little, if any, sympathetic activity. Therefore, the major influence on the heart at rest is parasympathetic. During exercise or stress, however, the sympathetic neural influence becomes more prominent.

Parasympathetic innervation of the heart is through the vagal nerve. Supraventricular tissue receives much greater vagal innervation than the ventricles do. The principal parasympathetic target neuroeffectors are the muscarinic receptors in the heart.[42,43] Activation of muscarinic receptors reduces pacemaker activity, slows AV conduction, decreases atrial contractile force directly, and exerts inhibitory modulation of ventricular contractile force. A total of five muscarinic receptors have been cloned.[44] M_2 receptors are the predominant subtype found in the mammalian heart. In the coronary circulation, M_3 receptors have been identified. Moreover, non-M_2 receptors have also been reported to exist in the heart. In general, for intracellular signaling, M_1, M_3, and M_5 receptors couple to $G_{q/11}$ protein and activate the phospholipase C–diacylglycerol–inositol phosphate system. On the other hand, the M_2 and M_4 receptors couple to the pertussis toxin–sensitive G protein $G_{i/o}$ to inhibit adenylyl cyclase. M_2 receptors can couple to certain K^+ channels and influence the activity of calcium channels, I_f current, phospholipase A_2, phospholipase D, and tyrosine kinases.

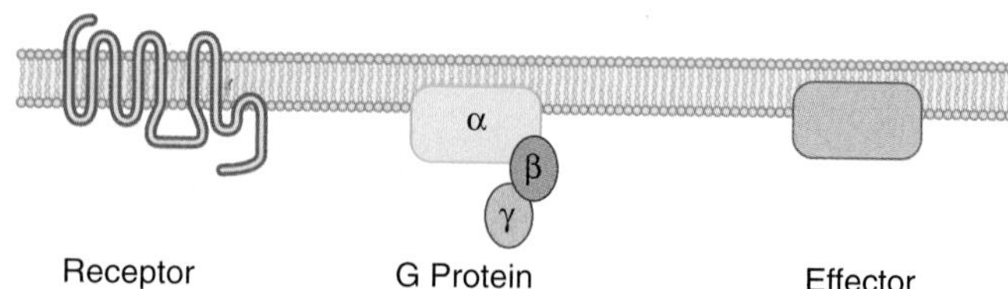

Figure 16-15 General scheme for a G protein–coupled receptor consisting of receptor, the heterotrimeric G protein, and the effector unit. *(Reprinted by permission from Bers DM: Cardiac excitation-contraction coupling. Nature 415:198-205, 2002. Copyright MacMillan Magazines Ltd.)*

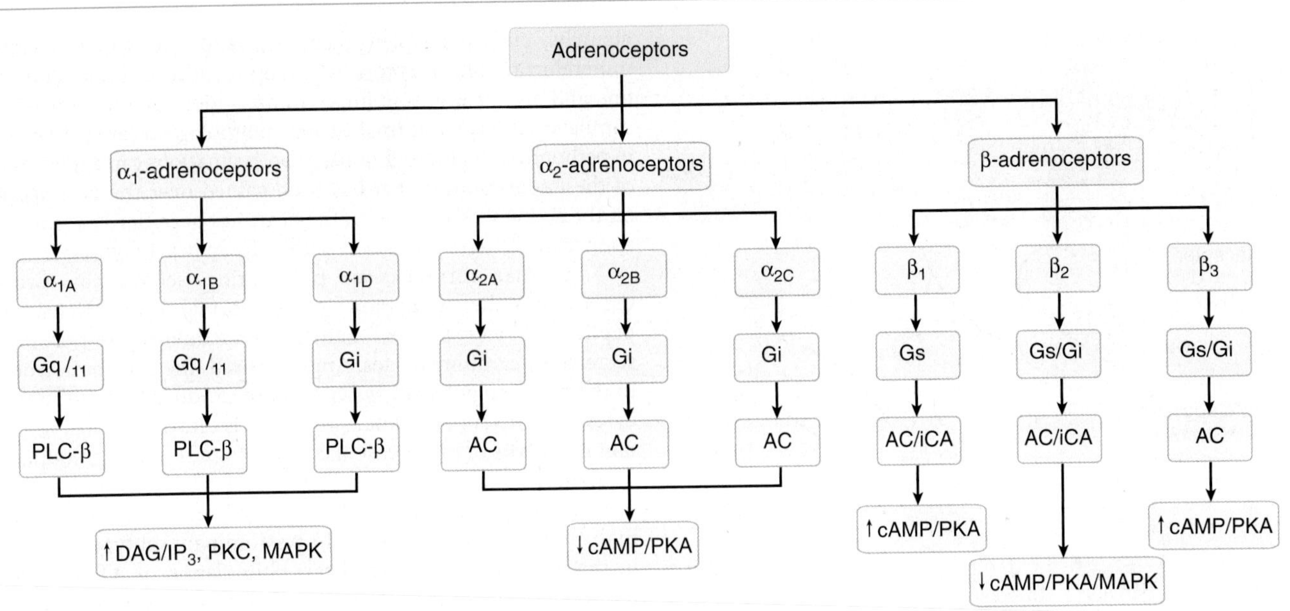

Figure 16-16 Adrenoceptor signaling cascades involving G proteins and effectors (AC, adenylyl cyclase; i_{CaL}, L-type calcium current; PLC-β, phospholipase β) in the heart. The intracellular signals are DAG (diacylglycerol), IP_3 (inositol 1,4,5-triphosphate), PKC (protein kinase C), cAMP (cyclic adenosine monophosphate), PKA (protein kinase A), and MAPK (mitogen-activated protein kinase).

In contrast to vagal innervation, sympathetic innervation of the heart is more predominant in the ventricle than in the atrium. Norepinephrine released from sympathetic nerve terminals stimulates adrenergic receptors (adrenoreceptors [ARs]) located in the heart. The two major classes of ARs are α and β, both of which are G protein–coupled receptors that transduce their intracellular signals by means of specific signaling cascades (Fig. 16-16).

βARs can be further divided into subpopulations of β_1, β_2, and β_3.[43,45] Although most mammalian hearts contain β_1ARs and β_2ARs, β_3ARs have also been demonstrated in many mammalian ventricular tissues. The relative contribution of each βAR subtype to modulation of cardiac function varies among species. In humans, β_1ARs are the predominant subtype in both the atria and ventricle, but a substantial proportion of β_2ARs are located in the atria and approximately 20% of β_2ARs are found in the LV. Much less is known about β_3ARs, but their existence has been documented in the human ventricle. Despite the fact that the β_1AR population is greater than the β_2AR population, the cardiostimulant effect is not proportional to the relative densities of these two subpopulations, which is largely attributable to the tighter coupling of β_2ARs than β_1ARs to the cyclic adenosine monophosphate (cAMP) signaling pathway. Both β_1ARs and β_2ARs activate a pathway that involves the stimulatory G protein (G_s), activation of adenylyl cyclase, accumulation of cAMP, stimulation of cAMP-dependent protein kinase A, and phosphorylation of key target proteins, including L-type calcium channels, phospholamban, and TnI.

Although traditional teaching is that both β_1ARs and β_2ARs are coupled to the G_s-cAMP pathway, more recent experimental evidence has indicated that β_2ARs also couple to the inhibitory G protein G_i to activate non–cAMP-dependent signaling pathways. Additionally, β_2ARs can couple to G protein–independent pathways to modulate cardiac function. βAR stimulation increases both contraction and relaxation, as summarized in Figure 16-17.

The two major subpopulations of αARs are α_1 and α_2. α_1ARs and α_2ARs can be further subdivided into different subtypes. α_1ARs are G protein–coupled receptors and include the α_{1A}, α_{1B}, and α_{1D} subtypes. The α_1AR subtypes are products of separate genes and differ in structure, G protein coupling, tissue distribution, signaling, regulation, and function. Both α_{1A}ARs and α_{1B}ARs mediate positive inotropic responses. However, the positive inotropic effect mediated by α_1ARs is believed to be of minor importance in the heart. α_1ARs are coupled to phospholipase C, phospholipase D, and phospholipase A_2; they increase intracellular Ca^{2+} and myofibrillar sensitivity to Ca^{2+}.

Cardiac hypertrophy is primarily mediated by α_{1A}ARs.[46,47] Cardiac hypertrophic responses to α_1AR agonists involve activation of protein kinase C and mitogen-activated protein kinase through G_q signaling mechanisms. Three subtypes of α_2ARs are recognized: α_{2A}, α_{2B}, and α_{2C}. In the mammalian heart, α_2ARs in the atrium play a role in the presynaptic inhibition of norepinephrine release. These prejunctional α_2ARs are believed to belong to the α_{2C} subtype.

Neural regulation of cardiac function involves a complex interaction between the different classes and subpopulations of adrenoceptors and their signaling pathways. Targeted therapeutics in cardiovascular medicine will involve the clinical application and manipulation of our basic understanding of adrenoceptor pharmacology.

Hormones Affecting Cardiac Function

Many hormones have direct and indirect actions on the heart (Table 16-1). Hormones with cardiac actions can be synthesized and secreted by cardiomyocytes or produced by other tissues and delivered to the heart. They act on specific receptors expressed in cardiomyocytes. The great majority of these hormone receptors are plasma membrane G protein–coupled receptors (GPCRs). Non-GPCRs include the natriuretic peptide receptors, which are

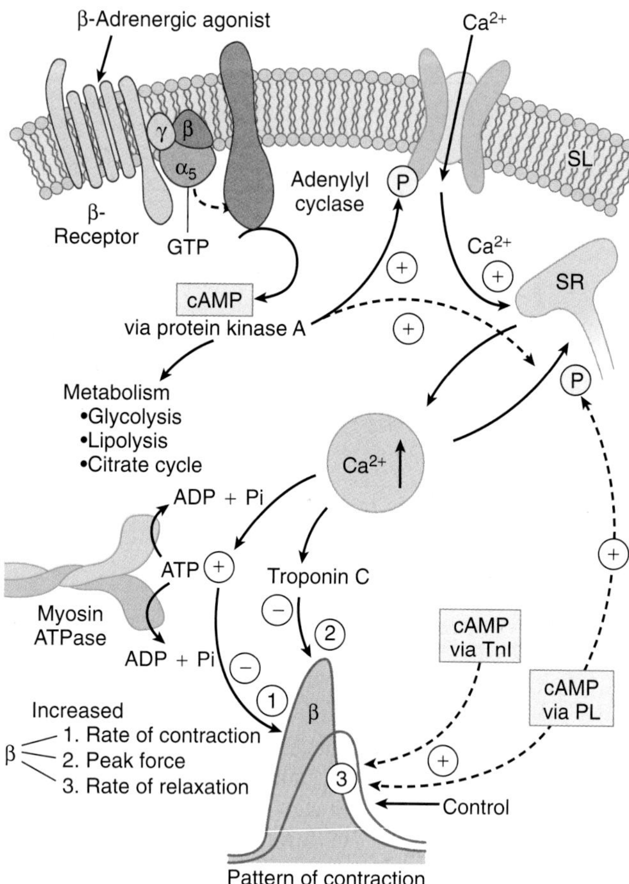

Figure 16-17 The β-adrenoceptor signaling system leads to an increased rate and force of contraction and increased relaxation. ADP, adenosine diphosphate; ATP, adenosine triphosphate; cAMP, cyclic adenosine monophosphate; GTP, guanosine triphosphate; PL, phospholipase; SL, sarcolemma; SR, sarcoplasmic reticulum; TnI, troponin I. *(From Opie LH: Receptors and signal transduction. In The Heart. Physiology from Cell to Circulation, 3rd ed. Philadelphia, Lippincott-Raven, 1998, p 195.)*

guanylyl cyclase–coupled receptors, and the glucocorticoid/mineralocorticoid receptors, which bind androgens and aldosterone and are nuclear zinc finger transcription factors. Hormones can have activity in normal cardiac physiology or are active only in pathophysiologic conditions, or both situations can apply. Much of the understanding that has been gained over the past decade on the action of hormones in the heart has been derived from the endocrine changes associated with chronic heart failure.

Cardiac hormones are polypeptides secreted by cardiac tissues into the circulation in the normal heart. Natriuretic peptides,[51,52] aldosterone,[53] and adrenomedullin[54] are hormones secreted by cardiomyocytes. Angiotensin II, the effector hormone in the renin-angiotensin system, is also produced by cardiomyocytes.[55,56] The renin-angiotensin system is one of the most important regulators of cardiovascular physiology. It is a key modulator of cardiac growth and function. Angiotensin II stimulates two separate receptor subtypes, AT_1 and AT_2, both of which are present in the heart. AT_1 receptors are the predominant subtype expressed in the normal adult human heart. Stimulation of AT_1 receptors induces a positive chronotropic and inotropic effect. Angiotensin II also mediates cell growth and proliferation in cardiomyocytes and fibroblasts and induces release of the growth factors aldosterone and catecholamines through stimulation of AT_1 receptors. Activation of AT_1 receptors is directly involved in the development of cardiac hypertrophy and heart failure, as well as adverse remodeling of the myocardium. In contrast, AT_2 receptor activation is counter-regulatory and is generally antiproliferative. Expression of AT_2 receptors, however, is relatively scant in the adult heart because they are most abundant in the fetal heart and decline with development. In response to injury and ischemia, AT_2 receptors become upregulated. The precise role of AT_2 receptors in the heart remains to be defined.

The beneficial effects of blockade of the renin-angiotensin system with angiotensin-converting enzyme inhibitors in the treatment of heart failure have been attributed to inhibition of AT_1 receptor activity. In addition to the renin-angiotensin system,

Table 16-1 Actions of Hormones on Cardiac Function

Hormone	Receptor	Cardiac Action	Increase with CHF
Adrenomedullin	GPCR	+Inotropy/+chronotropy	+
Aldosterone	MR	?	+
Angiotensin	GPCR	+Inotropy/+chronotropy	+
Endothelin	GPCR	?	+
Natriuretic peptides	GCCR		
ANP (ANF)			+
BNP			+
Neuropeptide Y[48,49]	GPCR	−Inotropy	+
Vasopressin	GPCR	+Inotropy/+chronotropy	+
Vasoactive intestinal peptide[50]	GPCR	+Inotropy	No
Sex steroid hormones			
Estrogen	ERR-α/ERR-β	Indirect	No
Testosterone	AR	Indirect	No
Progesterone	PR	Indirect	No

ANF, atrial natriuretic factor; ANP, atrial natriuretic peptide; AR, androgen receptor; BNP, B-type natriuretic peptide; CHF, congestive heart failure; ERR, estrogen-related receptor; GCCR, guanylyl cyclase–coupled receptor; GPCR, G protein–coupled receptor; MR, cytosolic or nuclear mineralocorticoid receptor; PR, progesterone receptor.

other cardiac hormones that have been shown to play pathogenic roles in the promotion of cardiomyocyte growth and cardiac fibrosis, development of cardiac hypertrophy, and progression of congestive heart failure include aldosterone,[53] adrenomedullin,[57-59] natriuretic peptides,[51,52] angiotensin,[60,61] endothelin,[62] and vasopressin.[63,64]

Increased stretch of the myocardium stimulates the release of atrial natriuretic protein (ANP) and B-type natriuretic protein (BNP) from the atria and ventricles, respectively. Both ANP and BNP bind to natriuretic peptide receptors to generate the second messenger cyclic guanosine monophosphate and represent part of the cardiac endocrine response to hemodynamic changes caused by pressure or volume overload. They also participate in organogenesis of the embryo heart and cardiovascular system.[51,52] In patients with chronic heart failure, elevation of serum ANP and BNP levels has been documented to be a predictor of mortality.

Adrenomedullin is a recently discovered cardiac hormone that was originally isolated from pheochromocytoma tissue. It increases accumulation of cAMP and has direct positive chronotropic and inotropic effects.[54,57,58] Adrenomedullin, with interspecies and regional variations, has also been shown to increase nitric oxide production and it functions as a potent vasodilator.

Aldosterone is one of the cardiac-generated steroids, although its physiologic significance remains to be defined. It binds to mineralocorticoid receptors and can increase the expression or activity (or both) of cardiac proteins involved in ionic homeostasis or regulation of pH, such as cardiac Na^+/K^+-ATPase, the Na^+-K^+ cotransporter, Cl^--HCO_3^{2+}, and the Na^+-H^+ antiporter.[53] Aldosterone modifies cardiac structure by inducing cardiac fibrosis in both ventricular chambers and thereby leads to impairment of cardiac contractile function.

Sex Steroid Hormones and the Heart

Cardiac contractility is greater in premenopausal women than in age-matched men, and withdrawal of hormone replacement therapy in postmenopausal women leads to a reduction in cardiac contractile function. The gender dimorphism in heart function and its adaptive responses to injury and disease states are in part mediated by sex steroid hormones.

The most extensively studied sex steroid hormones are estradiol-17β (E2) and its bioactive metabolites. They bind and act on the two subtypes of estrogen receptors in the heart: ERα and ERβ. Progesterone and testosterone (two other sex steroid hormones) and the enzyme aromatase, which converts testosterone to estrogen, are much less well investigated. Progesterone and testosterone bind and act on their respective progesterone receptors and androgen receptors in the heart. Sex steroid hormones interact with their receptors to effect postsynaptic target cell responses and influence presynaptic sympathoadrenergic function. Cardiomyocytes are not only targets for the action of sex steroid hormones but are also the source of synthesis and site of metabolism of these hormones.[65]

E2 is derived from testosterone and is primarily metabolized in the liver to form hydroxyestradiols, catecholestradiol, and methoxyestradiols. Estradiol metabolism also takes place in vascular smooth muscle cells, cardiac fibroblasts, endothelial cells, and cardiomyocytes. Cardiomyocytes express nuclear steroid hormone receptors that modulate gene expression and non-nuclear receptors for the nongenomic effects of sex steroid hormones. They interact with many different coregulators to confer tissue and temporal specificity in their transcriptional actions. These cell-specific coactivator and corepressor proteins are known as estrogen-related receptors.[66] Sex steroid hormones can activate rapid signaling pathways without changing gene expression (Fig. 16-18). One such example is stimulation of vascular endothelial nitric oxide synthase to mediate vascular dilatation. Estrogen's vasodilatory effect might explain the lower systolic blood pressures of premenopausal women than age-matched men. In men, aromatase-mediated conversion of testosterone to estrogen maintains normal vascular tone. In addition to sex steroid hormone stimulation of nuclear or non-nuclear receptors, sex steroid hormone receptors could also induce rapid signaling of growth factor pathways in the absence of ligands.

There are gender differences in cardiac electrophysiologic function. The modulatory actions of estrogen on calcium channels might be responsible for sex-based differences in repolarization of the heart, such as the faster resting heart rate of women, as well as the higher propensity of women to have prolonged QT syndrome.[67] Estrogen, through the activation of ERβ receptors, confers protection after ischemia and reperfusion in murine models of myocardial infarction. In contrast, testosterone, in the same model, has the opposite effect. Aromatase also has protective effects, probably through its action to increase estrogen and decrease testosterone.

Gender differences in cardiac physiology should include consideration of the cellular physiology of sex steroid hormones in males and females; intrinsic differences in the physiology of cardiomyocytes, vascular smooth muscle cells, and endothelial cells between males and females; and gender-based differences in the autonomic modulation of cardiac physiology.

Cardiac Reflexes

Cardiac reflexes are fast-acting reflex loops between the heart and central nervous system (CNS) that contribute to regulation of cardiac function and maintenance of physiologic homeostasis. Specific cardiac receptors elicit their physiologic responses by various pathways. Cardiac receptors are linked to the CNS by myelinated or unmyelinated afferent fibers that travel along the vagus nerve. Cardiac receptors can be found in the atria, ventricles, pericardium, and coronary arteries. Extracardiac receptors are located in the great vessels and carotid artery. Sympathetic and parasympathetic nerve input is processed in the CNS. After central processing, efferent fibers to the heart or the systemic circulation will provoke a particular reaction. The response of the cardiovascular system to efferent stimulation varies with age and duration of the underlying condition that elicited the reflex in the first instance.

Baroreceptor Reflex (Carotid Sinus Reflex)

The baroreceptor reflex is responsible for maintenance of blood pressure. This reflex is capable of regulating arterial pressure around a preset value through a negative-feedback loop (Fig. 16-19).[68,69] In addition, the baroreceptor reflex is capable of establishing a prevailing set point for blood pressure when the preset value has been reset because of chronic hypertension. Changes in blood pressure are monitored by circumferential and longitudinal stretch receptors located in the carotid sinus and aortic arch. The nucleus solitarius, located in the cardiovascular center of the

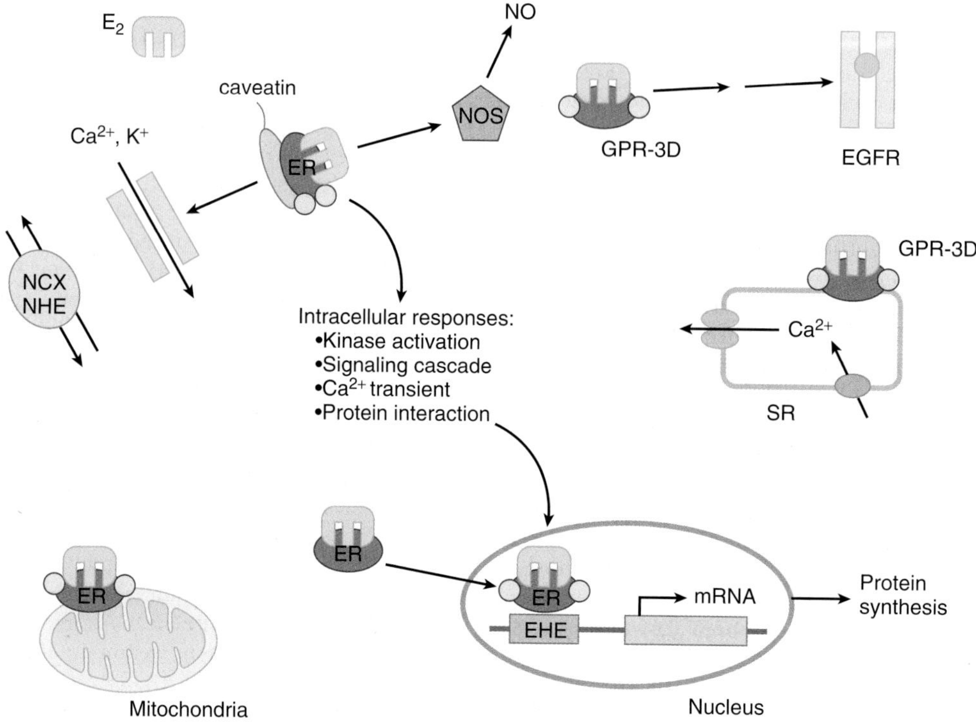

Figure 16-18 Signaling mechanism of nuclear and non-nuclear localized estrogen receptor (ER) and the estrogen binding receptor GPR-30. Nuclear ER influences the transcription of target genes by binding to an ER response element (ERE) within the promotor region of target genes. E2, estrogen; EGFR, epidermal growth factor receptor; NCX, Na^+-Ca^{2+} exchanger; NHE, Na^+-H^+ exchanger; NO, nitric oxide; NOS, nitric oxide synthase. *(From Du XJ, Fang L, Kiriazis H: Sex dimorphism in cardiac pathophysiology: Experimental findings, hormonal mechanisms, and molecular mechanisms. Pharmacol Ther 111:434-475, 2006.)*

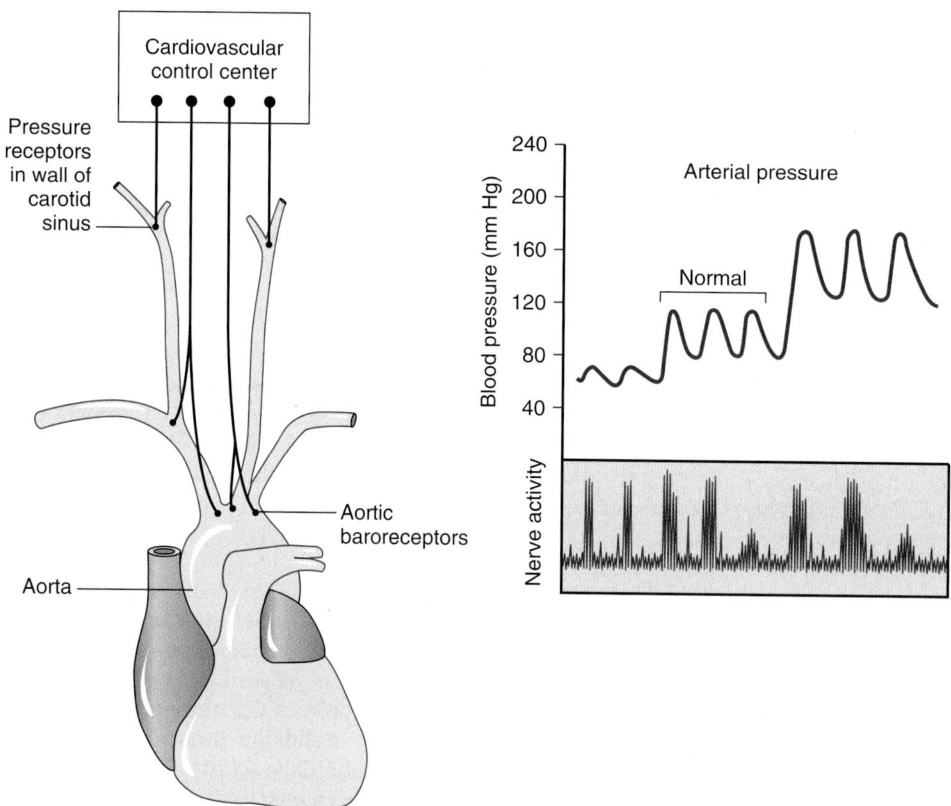

Figure 16-19 Anatomic configuration of the baroreceptor reflex. Pressure receptors in the wall of the carotid sinuses and aorta detect changes in arterial pressure in the circulation. These signals are conveyed to afferent receptive regions of the medulla through the Hering and vagus nerves. Output from effector portions of the medulla modulates peripheral tone and heart rate. The increase in blood pressure results in increased activation of the reflex (*right*), which effects a decrease in blood pressure. *(From Campagna JA, Carter C: Clinical relevance of the Bezold-Jarisch reflex. Anesthesiology 98:1250-1260, 2003.)*

medulla, receives impulses from these stretch receptors through afferents of the glossopharyngeal and vagus nerves. The cardiovascular center in the medulla consist of two functionally different areas: the area responsible for increasing blood pressure is located laterally and rostrally, whereas the area responsible for lowering arterial blood pressure is located centrally and caudally. The latter area also integrates impulses from the hypothalamus and the limbic system. Typically, stretch receptors are activated if systemic blood pressure is greater than 170 mm Hg. The response of the depressor system includes decreased sympathetic activity leading to a decrease in cardiac contractility, heart rate, and vascular tone. In addition, activation of the parasympathetic system further decreases the heart rate and myocardial contractility. Reverse effects are elicited with the onset of hypotension.

The baroreceptor reflex plays an important role during acute blood loss and shock. However, the reflex arch loses its functional capacity at a blood pressure lower than 50 mm Hg. Hormonal status and therefore sex differences have been implicated in altered baroreceptor responses.[70] Furthermore, volatile anesthetics (particularly halothane) inhibit the heart rate component of this reflex.[71] Concomitant use of calcium channel blockers, angiotensin-converting enzyme inhibitors, or phosphodiesterase inhibitors will lessen the cardiovascular response of raising blood pressure through the baroreceptor reflex. This lessened response is achieved by either their direct effects on the peripheral vasculature or, more importantly, their interference with CNS signaling pathways (calcium, angiotensin).[72] Patients with chronic hypertension often exhibit perioperative circulatory instability as a result of a decrease in their baroreceptor reflex response.

Chemoreceptor Reflex

Chemosensitive cells are located in the carotid bodies and the aortic body. These cells respond to changes in pH status and blood oxygen tension. At an arterial partial oxygen pressure (PaO_2) of less than 50 mm Hg or in conditions of acidosis, the chemoreceptors send their impulses along the sinus nerve of Hering (a branch of the glossopharyngeal nerve) and the 10th cranial nerve to the chemosensitive area of the medulla. This area responds by stimulating the respiratory centers and thereby increasing ventilatory drive. In addition, activation of the parasympathetic system ensues and leads to a reduction in heart rate and myocardial contractility. In the case of persistent hypoxia, the CNS will be directly stimulated, with a resultant increase in sympathetic activity.

Bainbridge Reflex

The Bainbridge reflex is elicited by stretch receptors located in the right atrial wall and the cavoatrial junction. An increase in right-sided filling pressure sends vagal afferent signals to the cardiovascular center in the medulla. These afferent signals inhibit parasympathetic activity, thereby increasing the heart rate. Acceleration of the heart rate also results from a direct effect on the SA node by stretching the atrium. The changes in heart rate are dependent on the underlying heart rate before stimulation.

Bezold-Jarisch Reflex

The Bezold-Jarisch reflex responds to noxious ventricular stimuli sensed by chemoreceptors and mechanoreceptors within the LV wall by inducing the triad of hypotension, bradycardia, and coronary artery dilatation.[69] The activated receptors communicate along unmyelinated vagal afferent type C fibers. These fibers reflexively increase parasympathetic tone. Because it invokes bradycardia, the Bezold-Jarisch reflex is thought of as a cardioprotective reflex. This reflex has been implicated in the physiologic response to a range of cardiovascular conditions such as myocardial ischemia or infarction, thrombolysis, or revascularization and syncope. Natriuretic peptide receptors stimulated by endogenous ANP or BNP may modulate the Bezold-Jarisch reflex. Thus, the Bezold-Jarisch reflex may be less pronounced in patients with cardiac hypertrophy or atrial fibrillation.[73]

Valsalva Maneuver

Forced expiration against a closed glottis produces increased intrathoracic pressure, increased central venous pressure, and decreased venous return. Cardiac output and blood pressure will be decreased after this (Valsalva) maneuver. This decrease will be sensed by baroreceptors and reflexively will result in an increase in heart rate and myocardial contractility through sympathetic stimulation. When the glottis opens, venous return increases and causes the heart to respond by vigorous contraction and an increase in blood pressure. This increase in blood pressure will in turn be sensed by baroreceptors, thereby stimulating the parasympathetic efferent pathways to the heart.

Cushing Reflex

The Cushing reflex is a result of cerebral ischemia caused by increased intracranial pressure. Cerebral ischemia at the medullary vasomotor center induces initial activation of the sympathetic nervous system. Such activation will lead to an increase in heart rate, blood pressure, and myocardial contractility in an effort to improve cerebral perfusion. As a result of the high vascular tone, reflex bradycardia mediated by baroreceptors will ensue.

Oculocardiac Reflex

The oculocardiac reflex is provoked by pressure applied to the globe of the eye or traction on the surrounding structures. Stretch receptors are located in the extraocular muscles. Once activated, stretch receptors will send afferent signals through the short and long ciliary nerves. The ciliary nerves will merge with the ophthalmic division of the trigeminal nerve at the ciliary ganglion. The trigeminal nerve will carry these impulses to the gasserian ganglion, thereby resulting in increased parasympathetic tone and subsequent bradycardia. The incidence of this reflex during ophthalmic surgery ranges from 30% to 90%. Administration of an antimuscarinic drug such as glycopyrrolate or atropine reduces the incidence of bradycardia during eye surgery (also see Chapter 75).

References

1. Berne RM, Levy MN: The cardiac pump. *In* Cardiovascular Physiology, 8th ed. St Louis, CV Mosby, 2001, pp 55-82.
2. Berne RM, Levy MN: Electrical activity of the heart. *In* Cardiovascular Physiology, 8th ed. St Louis, CV Mosby, 2001, pp 7-32.
3. Katz AM: The heart as a muscular pump. *In* Physiology of the Heart, 3rd ed. Philadelphia, Lippincott-Raven, 2001, pp 408-417.

4. Takayama Y, Costa KD, Covell JW: Contribution of laminar myofiber architecture to load-dependent changes in mechanics of LV myocardium. Am J Physiol Heart Circ Physiol 282:H1510-H1520, 2002.
5. Katz AM: Structure of the heart. *In* Physiology of the Heart, 3rd ed. Philadelphia, Lippincott-Raven, 2001, pp 1-38.
6. Opie LH: Heart cells and organelles. *In* The Heart. Physiology from Cell to Circulation, 4th ed. Philadelphia, Lippincott-Raven, 2004, pp 42-69.
7. Opie LH: Ventricular function. *In* The Heart. Physiology from Cell to Circulation, 4th ed. Philadelphia, Lippincott-Raven, 2004, pp 355-401.
8. Frank O: Zur Dynamik des Herzmuskels. Z Biol 32:370, 1895.
9. Starling EH: Linacre Lecture on the Law of the Heart. London, Longmans Green, 1918.
10. Holubarsch C, Ruf T, Goldstein D, et al: Existence of the Frank-Starling mechanism in the failing human heart. Circulation 94:683-689, 1996.
11. Katz AM: The working heart. *In* Physiology of the Heart, 3rd ed. Philadelphia, Lippincott-Raven, 2001, pp 418-443.
12. LeWinter MM, Osol G: Normal physiology of the cardiovascular system. *In* Fuster V (ed): Hurst's The Heart, 10th ed. New York, McGraw-Hill, 2001, pp 63-94.
13. Opie LH: Mechanisms of cardiac contraction and relaxation. *In* Braunwald E (ed): Heart Disease, 6th ed. Philadelphia, WB Saunders, 2001, pp 443-478.
14. Little WC: Assessment of normal and abnormal cardiac function. *In* Braunwald E (ed): Heart Disease, 6th ed. Philadelphia, WB Saunders, 2001, pp 479-502.
15. Zile MR, Brutsaert DL: New concepts in diastolic dysfunction and diastolic heart failure. Circulation 105:1387-1393, 2002.
16. Opie LH: Myocardial contraction and relaxation. *In* The Heart. Physiology from Cell to Circulation, 4th ed. Philadelphia, Lippincott-Raven, 2004, pp 221-245.
17. Roberts R: Principles of molecular cardiology. *In* Fuster V (ed): Hurst's The Heart, 10th ed. New York, McGraw-Hill, 2001, pp 95-112.
18. Katz AM: Contractile proteins and cytoskeleton. *In* Physiology of the Heart, 3rd ed. Philadelphia, Lippincott-Raven, 2001, pp 123-150.
19. Severs NJ: The cardiac muscle cell. Bioessays 22:188-199, 2000.
20. Yeager M: Structure of cardiac gap junction intercellular channels. J Struct Biol 121:231-245, 1998.
21. Severs NJ: Intercellular junctions and the cardiac intercalated disk. Adv Myocardiol 5:223-242, 1985.
22. Fill M, Copello JA: Ryanodine receptor calcium release channels. Physiol Rev 82:893-922, 2002.
23. Kumar NM, Gilula NB: The gap junction communication channel. Cell 84:381-388, 1996.
24. Katz AM: The cardiac action potential. *In* Physiology of the Heart, 3rd ed. Philadelphia, Lippincott-Raven, 2001, pp 478-516.
25. Katz AM: Calcium fluxes. *In* Physiology of the Heart, 3rd ed. Philadelphia, Lippincott-Raven, 2001, pp 232-233.
26. Bers DM: Cardiac excitation-contraction coupling. Nature 415:198-205, 2002.
27. de Tombe PP: Cardiac myofilaments: Mechanics and regulation. J Biomech 36:721-730, 2003.
28. Opie LH: Excitation-contraction coupling. *In* The Heart. Physiology from Cell to Circulation, 4th ed. Philadelphia, Lippincott-Raven, 2004, pp 159-185.
29. Bonne G, Carrier L, Richard P, et al: Familial hypertrophic cardiomyopathy, from mutations to functional defect. Circ Res 83:580-593, 1998.
30. Solaro RJ, Rarick HM: Troponin and tropomyosin. Circ Res 83:417-480, 1998.
31. Fuchs F, Smith SH: Calcium, cross-bridges, and the Frank-Starling relationship. News Physiol Sci 16:5-10, 2001.
32. Trinick J, Tskhovrebova L: Titin: A molecular control freak. Trends Cell Biol 9:377-380, 1999.
33. Moss RL, Fitzsimons DP: Frank-Starling relationship. Circ Res 90:11-13, 2002.
34. Alvarez BV, Perez NG, Ennis IL, et al: Mechanisms underlying the increase in force and Ca^{2+} transient that follow stretch of cardiac muscle. Circ Res 85:716-722, 1999.
35. Fukuda N, Sasaki D, Ishiwata S, Kurihara S: Length dependence of tension generation in rat skinned cardiac muscle. Circulation 104:1639-1645, 2001.
36. Konhilas JP, Irving TC, de Tombe PP: Myofilament calcium sensitivity in skinned rat cardiac trabeculae. Circ Res 90:59-65, 2002.
37. Konhilas JP, Irving TC, de Tombe PP: Length-dependent activation in three striated muscle types of the rat. J Physiol 544:225-236, 2002.
38. Capetanaki Y: Desmin cytoskeleton: A potential regulator of muscle mitochondrial behavior and function. Trends Cardiovasc Med 12:339-348, 2002.
39. Howard J, Hyman AA: Dynamics and mechanics of the microtubule plus end. Nature 422:753-758, 2003.
40. Opie LH: Receptors and signal transduction. *In* The Heart. Physiology from Cell to Circulation, 4th ed. Philadelphia, Lippincott-Raven, 2004, p 187.
41. Rockman HA, Koch WJ, Lefkowitz RJ: Seven-transmembrane-spanning receptors and heart function. Nature 415:206-212, 2002.
42. Mendelowitz D: Advances in parasympathetic control of heart rate and cardiac function. News Physiol Sci 14:155-161, 1999.
43. Brodde OE, Michel MC: Adrenergic and muscarinic receptors in the human heart. Pharm Rev 51:651-689, 1999.
44. Dhein S, Van Koppen CJ, Brodde OE: Muscarinic receptors in the mammalian heart. Pharm Res 44:161-182, 2001.
45. Kaumann AJ, Molenaar P: Modulation of human cardiac function through 4 β-adrenoceptor populations. Naunyn Schmiedebergs Arch Pharmacol 355:667-681, 1997.
46. Endoh M: Cardiac α_1-adrenoceptors that regulate contractile function: Subtypes and subcellular signal transduction mechanisms. Neurochem Res 21:217-229, 1996.
47. Artega GM, Kobayashi T, Solaro RJ: Molecular actions of drugs that sensitize cardiac myofilaments to Ca^{2+}. Ann Med 34:248-258, 2002.
48. Maisel AS, Scott NA, Motulsky HJ, et al: Elevation of plasma neuropeptide Y levels in congestive heart failure. Am J Med 86:43-48, 1989.
49. Grundemar L, Hakanson R: Multiple neuropeptide Y receptors are involved in cardiovascular regulation. Peripheral and central mechanisms. Gen Pharmacol 24:785-796, 1993.
50. Henning RJ, Sawmiller DR: Vasoactive intestinal peptide: Cardiovascular effects. Cardiovasc Res 49:27-37, 2001.
51. de Bold AJ, Bruneau BG, Kuroski de Bold M: Mechanical and neuroendocrine regulation of the endocrine heart. Cardiovasc Res 31:7-18, 1996.
52. Cameron VA, Ellmers LJ: Minireview: Natriuretic peptides during development of the fetal heart and circulation. Endocrinology 144:2191-2194, 2003.
53. Delcayre C, Silvestre JS: Aldosterone and the heart: Towards a physiological function? Cardiovasc Res 42:7-12, 1999.
54. Martinez A: Biology of adrenomedullin. Microsc Res Tech 57:1-2, 2002.
55. Schuijt MP, Jan Danser AH: Cardiac angiotensin II: An intracrine hormone? Am J Hypertens 15:1109-1116, 2002.
56. Dinh DT, Frauman AG, Johnston CI, Fabiani ME: Angiotensin receptors: Distribution, signalling and function. Clin Sci 100:481-492, 2001.
57. Kitamura K, Kangawa K, Eto T: Adrenomedullin and PAMP: Discovery, structures, and cardiovascular functions. Microsc Res Tech 57:3-13, 2002.
58. Minamino N, Kikumoto K, Isumi Y: Regulation of adrenomedullin expression and release. Microsc Res Tech 57:28-39, 2002.
59. Smith DM, Coppock HA, Withers DJ, et al: Adrenomedullin: Receptor and signal transduction. Biochem Soc Trans 30:432-437, 2002.
60. Opie LH, Sack MN: Enhanced angiotensin II activity in heart failure. Circ Res 88:654-658, 2001.
61. De Mello WC: Cardiac arrhythmias: The possible role of the renin-angiotensin system. J Mol Med 79:103-108, 2001.
62. Kramer BK, Ittner KP, Beyer ME, et al: Circulatory and myocardial effects of endothelin. J Mol Med 75:886-890, 1997.
63. Walker BR, Childs ME, Adamas EM: Direct cardiac effects of vasopressin: Role of V_1 and V_2 vasopressinergic receptors. Am J Physiol 255:H261-H265, 1988.
64. Chandrashekhar Y, Prahash AJ, Sen A, et al: The role of arginine vasopressin and its receptors in the normal and failing rat heart. J Mol Cell Cardiol 35:495-504, 2003.
65. Mendelsohn ME: Molecular and cellular basis of cardiovascular gender differences. Science 308:1583-1587, 2005.
66. Du XJ, Fang L, Kiriazis H: Sex dimorphism in cardiac pathophysiology: Experimental findings, hormonal mechanisms, and molecular mechanisms. Pharmacol Ther 111:434-475, 2006.
67. Pham TV, Rosen MR: Sex, hormones and repolarization. Cardiovasc Res 53:740-751, 2002.
68. Parlow JL, Bégou G, Sagnard P, et al: Cardiac baroreflex during the postoperative period in patients with hypertension. Anesthesiology 90:681-692, 1999.
69. Campagna JA, Carter C: Clinical relevance of the Bezold-Jarisch reflex. Anesthesiology 98:1250-1260, 2003.
70. Huikuri HV, Pikkujamsa SM, Airaksinen KE, et al: Sex-related differences in autonomic modulation of heart rate in middle-aged subjects. Circulation 94:122-125, 1996.
71. Keyl C, Schneider A, Hobbhahn J, Bernadi L: Sinusoidal neck suction for evaluation of baroreflex sensitivity during desflurane and sevoflurane anesthesia. Anesth Analg 95:1629-1636, 2002.
72. Devlin MG, Angus JA, Wilson KM, et al: Acute effects of L- and T-type calcium channel antagonists on cardiovascular reflexes in conscious rabbits. Clin Exp Pharmacol Physiol 29:372-380, 2002.
73. Thomas CJ, Woods RL: Guanylyl cyclase receptors mediate cardiopulmonary vagal reflex actions of ANP. Hypertension 41:279-285, 2003.

Phillip S. Mushlin and Simon Gelman

17 Hepatic Physiology and Pathophysiology

Key Points

1. Roughly 25% of cardiac output flows through the liver via a dual blood supply. The portal vein conveys 75% of total hepatic blood flow; the hepatic artery provides the rest. Each vessel, however, delivers about 50% of the total hepatic oxygen supply.
2. Hepatic sinusoids are the capillaries of the liver. Blood reaches the sinusoids via terminal branches of the portal vein and hepatic artery; it exits the sinusoids via hepatic venules (i.e., central veins) and travels through a venous network before draining in the inferior vena cava. Postsinusoidal vessels are a major source of total hepatic vascular resistance.
3. The acinus is the functional microvascular unit of the liver. It has three circulatory zones, defined by hepatocellular proximity to the portal axis. Blood perfusing zone 1 hepatocytes (periportal) is rich in oxygen and nutrients. By contrast, zone 3 hepatocytes (centrilobular) are perfused with effluent blood from zones 1 and 2, which is relatively oxygen poor.
4. Hepatocytes of zone 3, which have the highest density of cytochrome P450 proteins, are the most susceptible to injury from drug metabolism, oxidative stress, severe hypotension, or hypoxia.
5. The hepatic arterial buffer response (HABR) is the main intrinsic regulator of liver blood flow. Since the liver lacks pressure-flow autoregulation (in the fasted state), low systemic arterial pressure leads to low portal venous flow. HABR induces a compensatory increase of hepatic arterial flow, thereby preserving hepatic oxygen delivery despite decreases of total hepatic blood flow. Pathologic disruptions of HABR increase the susceptibility of the liver to hypoxic injury.
6. The liver is integral to the splanchnic blood reservoir, which can transfer up to 1 L of whole blood to the systemic circulation within 30 seconds of sympathoadrenal activation in healthy, euvolemic adults. If this reservoir is dysfunctional, abrupt, yet mild losses of intravascular volume (10% to 15%) may cause severe hypotension.
7. The liver regulates the pathways of intermediary metabolism. When hepatic glycogen is depleted (e.g., due to prolonged fasting), the body depends on hepatic gluconeogenesis to supply blood glucose. Stress induces catabolic changes, including increased lipolysis, fatty acid oxidation, and hepatic ketone production. Ketosis develops. But ketosis triggers insulin release, thereby decreasing substrate (fatty acids) availability for ketogenesis. Thus, stress-induced ketosis tends to be self-limited, except in insulin-deficient states, when diabetic ketoacidosis may occur.
8. Hepatocytes play a central role in nitrogen metabolism. They remove nitrogen from various molecules, incorporate it into ammonia, and convert ammonia to urea. If liver failure occurs (without severe renal dysfunction), blood urea nitrogen levels typically remain low, while nitrogenous wastes accumulate in blood and other tissues.
9. Albumin is the most abundant hepatic protein. It is the main determinant of plasma oncotic pressure and an essential plasma transporter of exogenous substances and endogenous compounds, such as unconjugated bilirubin and free fatty acids.
10. Liver produces most of the molecular participants in coagulation pathways (besides factors III, IV, VIII). Hepatic proteins—such as factors II, VII, IX, X, proteins C and protein S—require vitamin K–dependent, posttranslational modifications, which enables their extrahepatic activation and subsequent involvement in the coagulation cascade.
11. Hepatocytes make, and regulate production of, bile salts. These natural ionic detergents have many physiologic roles, including enteric absorption, transport, and secretion of lipids. Disruption of biliary circulation predisposes to vitamin K deficiency; hepatocytes continue to synthesize procoagulants but cannot γ-carboxylate them. Parenteral vitamin K therapy should therefore correct the coagulopathy of cholestasis, unless liver failure has supervened.

12. The liver is the main site of xenobiotic biotransformation. Multifarious, complex chemical reactions of hepatic drug disposition fit in at least one of three broad metabolic categories (or phases): Phase 1 oxidizes drugs via cytochrome P450-mediated redox reactions; phase 2 produces conjugates of endogenous polar molecules and drugs (or their metabolites); phase 3 uses adenosine triphosphate transport proteins to facilitate biliary elimination of endogenous and exogenous substances.
13. The liver is the largest reticuloendothelial organ in the human body. Kupffer cells (macrophages) account for nearly 10% of the liver's mass. These macrophages filter the venous effluent of the gastrointestinal tract and in the process phagocytose microbes, destroy toxins, process antigens, modulate immunity, and regulate inflammatory responses. Kupffer cells, activated by such processes, release nitro-radicals, reactive oxygen species, proteases, chemokines, and cytokines, which recruit neutrophils to the liver and intensify the hepatic inflammation. If uncontrolled, these activated macrophages can damage normal hepatic parenchyma.
14. Portosystemic shunting (as occurs with cirrhosis-induced portal hypertension) circumvents the hepatic filtering mechanism and thereby allows drugs, nitrogenous waste, and toxins to enter the central circulation. Some of these substances are putative mediators of hepatic encephalopathy.
15. Standard liver function tests are used to screen for hepatobiliary diseases and identify categories of pathologic events within the hepatobiliary system, such as hepatocellular injury or biliary dysfunction.
16. The onset of portal hypertension signals depletion of the normal physiologic reserve of the liver. At this stage, severe pathophysiologic derangements develop and can give rise to life-threatening complications such as variceal hemorrhage, hepatic encephalopathy, and renal failure.
17. The cardiovascular hallmark of cirrhosis and portal hypertension is a hyperdynamic circulation in which cardiac output increases, total peripheral resistance decreases, and systemic blood pressure is slightly below normal. The hemodynamic profile is reminiscent of a large arteriovenous fistula because of extensive arteriovenous communications within the splanchnic vasculature and in organs throughout the body. Splanchnic vasculature may be engorged with blood even though effective plasma volume is perilously low. Cardiovascular responses to physiologic and pharmacologic vasoconstrictors are attenuated because of a plethora of endogenous vasodilators, dysfunction of the splanchnic reservoir, and occasionally, cardiac failure (e.g., cirrhotic cardiomyopathy).

Overview

The liver is the largest internal organ and largest gland in the human body. It accounts for about 2% of the total mass of healthy adults and 5% of neonates.[1] Its location within the thoracic portion of the abdominal cavity reflects its physiologic importance as an interface between the gastrointestinal tract and pulmonary/systemic circulation. It filters, excretes, or modifies an enormity of gut-derived substances—it destroys bacteria, inactivates antigens, and detoxifies chemicals that might otherwise injure the heart, lungs, or other vital organs. The liver is at the epicenter of intermediary metabolism, with versatile and massive biochemical pathways for molecular transformations. Such pathways work to maintain homeostatic blood levels of nutrients during feast and famine. As described in this chapter, the multiple and diverse functions of the liver have an impact on every tissue in the body. A fundamental knowledge of hepatic anatomy and physiology is therefore a prerequisite for understanding liver disease, its clinical manifestations, and its therapeutic challenges.

Hepatic Anatomy

Macroscopic Anatomy

The liver is a reddish brown boomerang-shaped gland that occupies the right hypochondrium, most of the epigastrium, and a variable portion of the left hypochondrium (Fig. 17-1). In the right midaxillary line, the liver spans from the 7th to the 11th ribs; the gallbladder lies beneath to the 9th costal cartilage. The liver is highly vascular, friable, and easily lacerated. Because of its sponginess, it conforms to the contours of less malleable, adjacent structures. Based on postmortem studies—using chemicals to harden the liver in situ—the organ is shaped like a right-angled triangular prism (wedge), with a rounded right angle. The three faces of this prism are the superior, inferior, and posterior surfaces of the liver; they provide frames of reference for gross anatomy (Figs. 17-2 and 17-3).

The hepatic ligaments are connective tissue bands that attach the liver to adjacent tissues. Most of these bands are overlapping folds of peritoneal membranes (i.e., membranous ligaments), but two are fibrous cords derived from obliterated fetal vessels, namely, the umbilical vein (ligamentum teres or round ligament) and the ductus venosus (ligamentum venosum). Although a couple of ligaments attach to nearby viscera (e.g., the hepatogastric and hepatoduodenal ligaments, which connect to the lesser curvature of the stomach and duodenum, respectively), most serve to tether the liver to the anterior abdominal wall or the underside of the diaphragm. Among the latter group are the coronary, left lateral, right lateral, falciform, and round ligaments.

Several factors maintain the liver in proper anatomic position. For example, the main posterior supports are (1) the diaphragm, via the coronary and triangular ligaments and the matrix of connective tissue on the bare area, and (2) the inferior vena cava, hepatic veins, and embedded connective tissue. The superior surface of the liver is form-fitted to the underside of the dia-

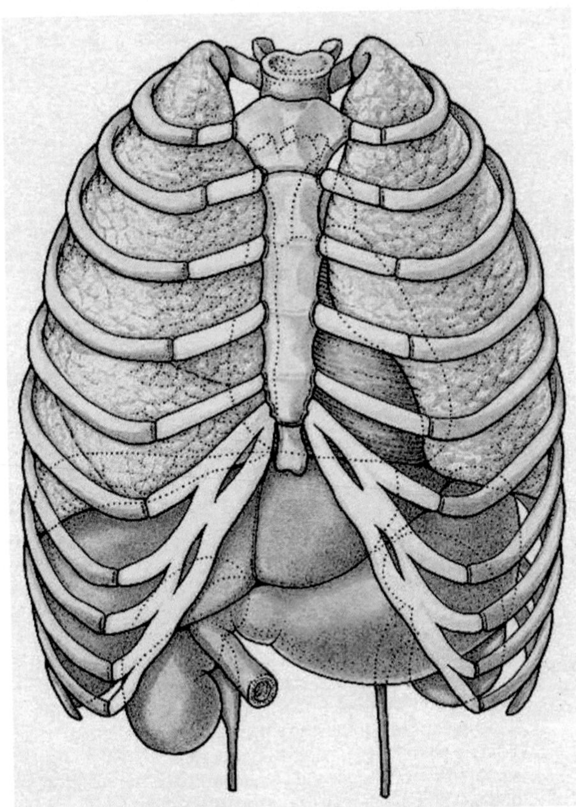

Figure 17-1 Anterior view of the liver and thoracic cage. The liver resides in the thoracic portion of the abdominal cavity; it occupies most of the right hypochondrium, much of the epigastrium, and a variable portion of the left hypochondrium. *(Reproduced © DK Images. Available from http://.dkimages.com/discover/previews/832/20113049.jpg/ Accessed October 23, 2008.)*

phragm, which could keep these structures in apposition at atmospheric pressure. Because abdominal viscera fill the abdominal cavity, the muscular walls of the abdomen remain in a state of tonic contraction. This tonic contraction generates positive intra-abdominal pressure, which pushes the liver against the underside of the diaphragm and keeps their surfaces together, even as the subatmospheric pressure of the thoracic cavity exerts upward pressure on the diaphragm. Because of its laxity, the falciform ligament does little to anchor the liver, although it may limit its lateral displacement.

Traditional Anatomy

Traditional or classic liver anatomy uses topologic landmarks to partition the liver into four lobes: the left, right, caudate, and quadrate.[2] On the superior hepatic surface, the falciform ligament separates the left and right lobes (see Fig. 17-2). Demarcations on posterior-inferior hepatic surfaces (Fig. 17-3) results from (1) the left sagittal fossa (ligamenta venosum and teres hepaticus), which separates left and right lobes; (2) the transverse fissure (porta hepatis), which is a shared border of quadrate and caudate lobes; (3) fossae for the umbilical vein and gallbladder, which border the quadrate lobe; (4) fossae for the ductus venosus (ligamentum venosum) and inferior vena cava fossa, which further delineate the caudate lobe.[3]

Internal Anatomy

After ascending to the porta hepatis (hilum), the portal vein and proper hepatic artery divide into their first-order branches—the left and right portal veins and the left and right hepatic arteries. These vessels enter the liver and travel in parallel as they ramify within the organ (Fig. 17-4). Their terminal branches drain into sinusoids of liver (i.e., the hepatic capillaries). Blood egresses from the sinusoids through intralobular (central) veins; it is conveyed via a series of larger conduits (i.e., the sublobular, interlobular, and lobular veins) to the right, middle, or left hepatic veins. The hepatic veins connect to the inferior vena cava (see Fig. 17-4).

The intrahepatic flow of bile occurs in a direction opposite the flow of afferent blood within the liver. Hepatic parenchymal cells produce bile; they secrete it into canaliculi that connect to bile ductules of the portal areas. Bile egresses from the portal canals and flows via a series of ducts to the left or right hepatic bile duct. These ducts unite to form the common hepatic bile duct, which descends from the porta hepatis and gives rise to the cystic duct and the common bile duct.

Physiologic Anatomy

Physiologic anatomy—also called functional, segmental, modern, or surgical anatomy—focuses on singular, independent segments of the liver (Fig. 17-5). Each independent segment has its own afferent blood supply and routes for venous and biliary drainage,

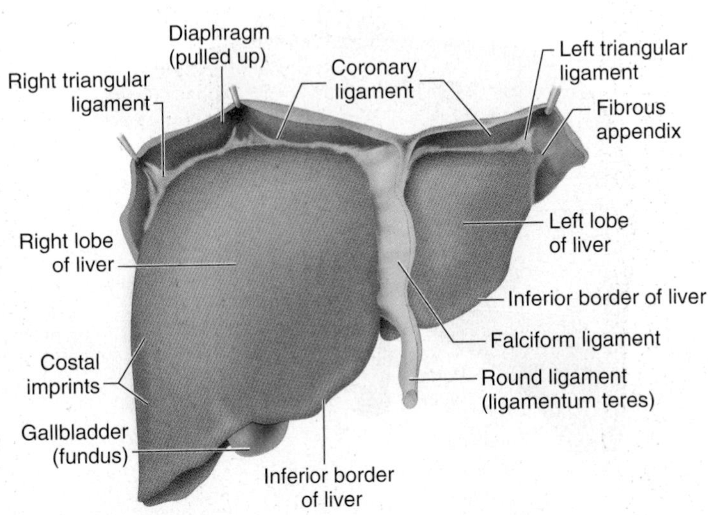

Figure 17-2 Superior hepatic surface: frontal view. The anterior hepatic edge (i.e., the inferior border of the liver) delineates the superior and inferior surfaces of the liver. A sickle-shaped peritoneal fold (falciform ligament) divides the liver into two parts of unequal size, the right lobe and the left lobe. Within the free margin or base of the falciform are paraumbilical veins and the round ligament (ligamentum teres), the latter being the remnant of the obliterated umbilical vein. *(From Strunk H, Stuckmann G, Textor J, et al: Limitations and pitfalls of Couinaud's segmentation of the liver in transaxial imaging. Eur Radiol 13:2472-2482, 2003.)*

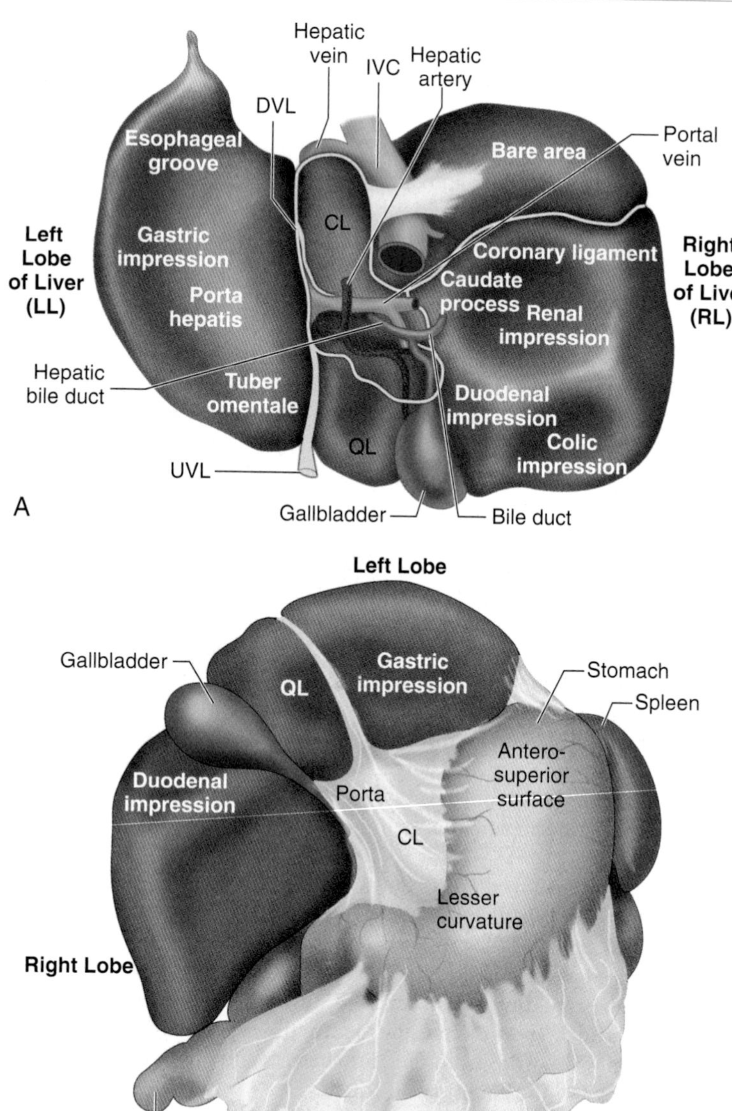

Figure 17-3 **A,** Posterior and inferior hepatic surfaces showing the relationship between four hepatic lobes: left lobe (LL), caudate lobe (CL), quadrate lobe (QL), right lobe (RL). They are delineated by five structures: the ductus venosus ligament (DVL), umbilical vein ligament (UVL), porta hepatis (PH), inferior vena cava (IVC), and gallbladder (GB). These structures can be envisaged as forming the letter H: • The two-part, left vertical bar (DVL in the back, UVL in the front) separates the LL from all the other lobes. • The three-part, right vertical bar (IVC in the back, caudate process in the middle, GB in the front) separates the RL from the others lobes. The caudate process, which connects the RL and CL, forms the upper boundary of the epiploic foramen (of the peritoneum). • The crossbar is the PH (or transverse fissure), which separates the CL in the back from the QL in the front. Notable anatomic features (left to right) are the narrow LL but broad and rounded RL. Protuberances and impressions (imp) on the hepatic surfaces result from contiguous viscera: the LL has an esophageal groove, gastric impression, and tuber omentale; the RL has duodenal, suprarenal, renal, and colic impressions. The vertebral column and crura of the diaphragm produce the deep concavity to the left of IVC. The omental bursa (upper part) lies between the papillary process (an elevation of the CL) and diaphragm. The surfaces of the liver are covered by peritoneum, with a few exceptions. Uncovered areas include (1) the GB attachment site; (2) the porta hepatis, with vessels and ducts splitting the two layers of the lesser omentum; (3) the right suprarenal impression; and (4) nonperitoneal surface (bare area of the liver) bounded by the coronary ligament (upper and lower lines of reflection), which is in direct contact with the diaphragm. **B,** Inferior (visceral) hepatic surface. The gastric impression on the liver molds to the convex, anterosuperior gastric surface. The tuber omentale (hepatic protuberance) fits in the concave, lesser curvature of stomach; it lies superficial to the anterior layer of lesser omentum and connects to the duodenum via the hepatogastric ligament. *(From Human Anatomy. http://theodora.com/anatomy/the_liver.html. Accessed February 11, 2009.)*

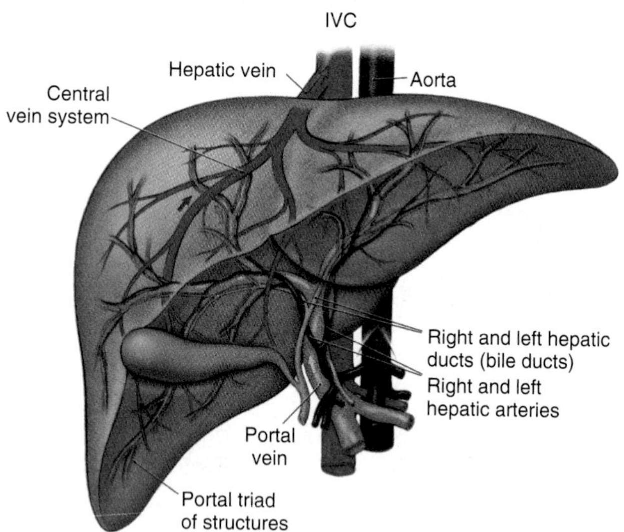

Figure 17-4 Internal anatomy of the liver. The portal vein (*lavender*) and proper hepatic artery (*red*) ascend to the porta hepatics (hilum), where they divide into their left and right main branches. These branches ramify within the liver before emptying into sinusoids. Blood exiting sinusoids is conveyed via central vein system to into hepatic veins (*blue*), which drain directly into the inferior vena cava (IVC; blue). Hepatocytes produce bile and secrete it into canaliculi; bile exits the liver flows though ductules of the portal triads, which drain into a series of intrahepatic ducts, and drains into the common hepatic bile duct (*gray*); the latter exits the liver at the porta hepatis and descends between peritoneal layers of the lesser omentum. *(© MediVisuals, Inc.)*

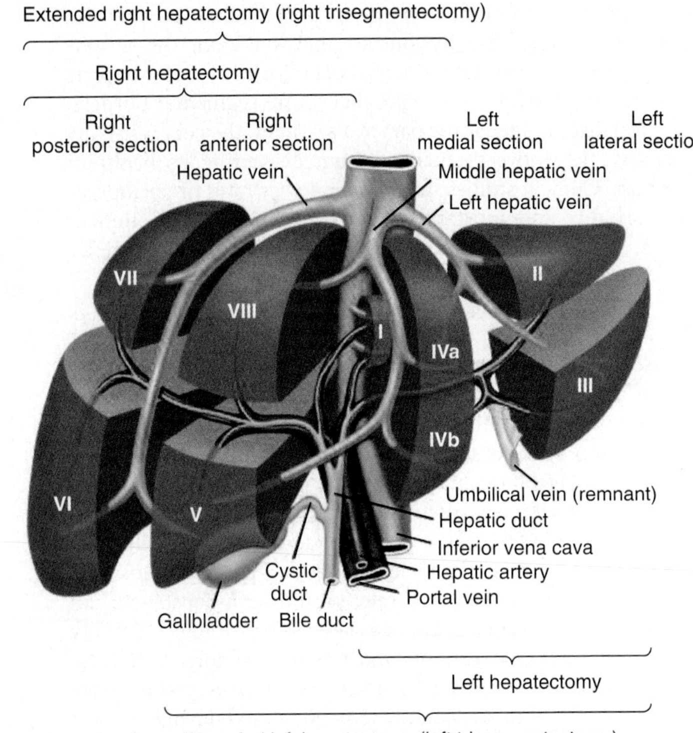

Figure 17-5 Schematic depiction of Couinaud segmental liver anatomy and the normal portal venous structures. Bracketed text shows hepatic segments resected during partial hepatectomies. *(Reproduced from Functional segments of the liver (Segmental_anatomy_of_liver). Management of potentially resectable colorectal cancer liver metastases. Alan P Venook, MD. Steven A Curley, MD, FACS.©2007 UpToDate.)*

allowing it to remain functionally intact after surgical resection of neighboring segments. Owing to the manifold variations in branching patterns of the portal vein, hepatic artery, and hepatic bile duct, there is no universally accepted classification of segmental anatomy.[4] The most widely used classifications—such as those of Couinaud or Bismuth—are based on the anatomy of the portal and hepatic veins. The Couinaud system, for example, uses third-generation branches of the portal vein to partition the liver into eight physiologically independent segments (Fig. 17-5).[4] The geometry of dividing the liver into sectors and segments in accord with Bismuth's method is shown in Figure 17-6.[4]

Physiologic anatomy facilitates both planning and performance of hepatic surgery. For example, surgical incisions through the center of a segment would be likely to devitalize the

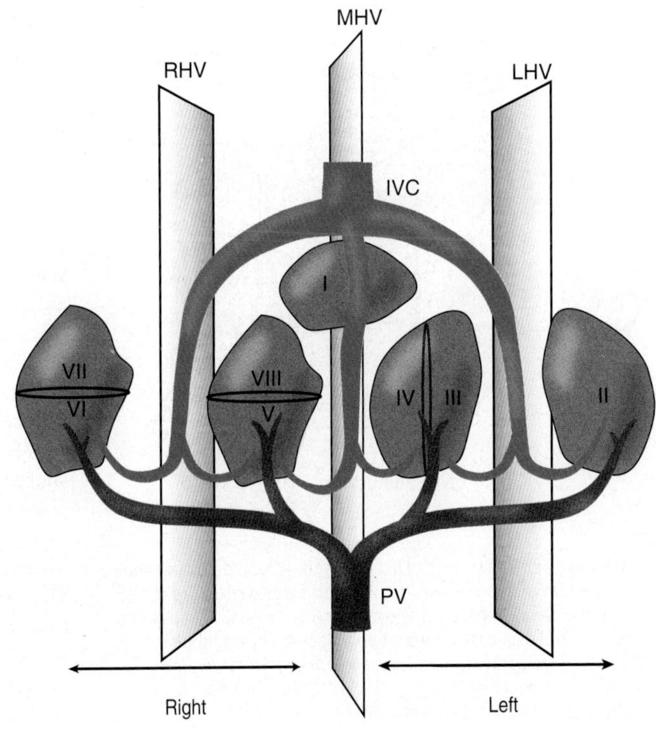

Figure 17-6 Physiologic liver anatomy: Bismuth classification. Three parallel planes host a single hepatic vein (right, RHV; middle, MHV; or left, LHV); each plane is split by a transverse plane (not shown) cutting through the right or left main portal veins (PV); this creates four sectors with portal pedicels (i.e., portal sectors). MHV divides the liver into a left and right hemiliver: LHV splits the former (into one lateral (II) and two medial (III, IV) segments) and RHV splits the latter (into two anterior (VI, VII) and two posterior (V, VIII) segments). In contrast to any other segment, segment I (the caudate lobe) gets its blood supply from both left and right main portal veins; and, its venous outflow—instead of entering a major hepatic vein—drains directly into the inferior vena cava (IVC). *(The authors are grateful to Jennifer Mushlin for designing and crafting this figure.)*

entire segment because therein lies the portal triads (portal vein, hepatic artery, bile duct). By contrast, incisions along the periphery of segments minimize unintentional injuries of major hepatic veins, which generally run in parallel to the segmental borders. If surgical disease affects any part of a segment, the goal is usually to remove the entire segment without disrupting its healthier neighbors. Clinical studies have shown lower rates of perioperative morbidity and mortality when liver surgery (resection of tumors, repair of traumatic injuries) is guided by the principles of physiologic anatomy.[5-7]

Real Anatomy

Because the human liver has so many anatomic variations, knowledge of an individual's real physiologic anatomy derives from advanced imaging techniques, such as contrast-enhanced helical computed tomography scans. These scans provide accurate information on the relationships of surface landmarks and internal hepatic anatomy. In fact, such scan data, when superimposed on normalized computer images of Couinaud segments, yield a data set with enough information to construct a three-dimensional model of a patient's liver. Accurate, see-through constructs can impart an instantaneous grasp of a patient's physiologic anatomy by detailing anatomic variants and precise locations of hepatic lesions. In addition, recent advances in ultrasonography have enabled real physiologic anatomy to be identified during surgical procedures.

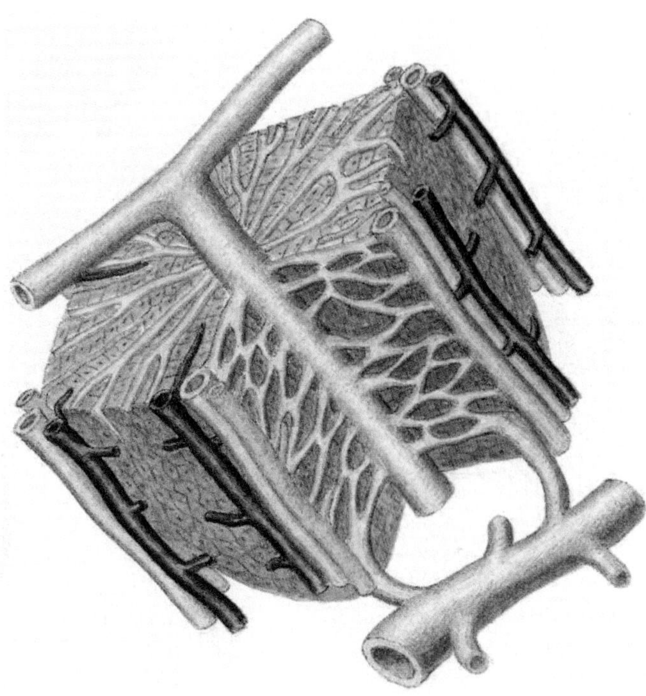

Figure 17-8 Idealized representation of a classic liver lobule. *(© DK Images.)*

Microanatomy

Classic Liver Lobule

The basic unit of the liver can be viewed as a classic lobule, a portal lobule, or a liver acinus; Figure 17-7 shows how these arbitrary units relate to one another. An idealized classic liver lobule is a hexagonal prism with a central vein at its center and six vertically aligned portal canals (Fig. 17-8). Each portal canal includes a connective tissue matrix, surrounding nerve fibers, lymphatic vessels, and a portal triad. The latter contains terminal branches of the portal vein and hepatic artery and a bile ductule.

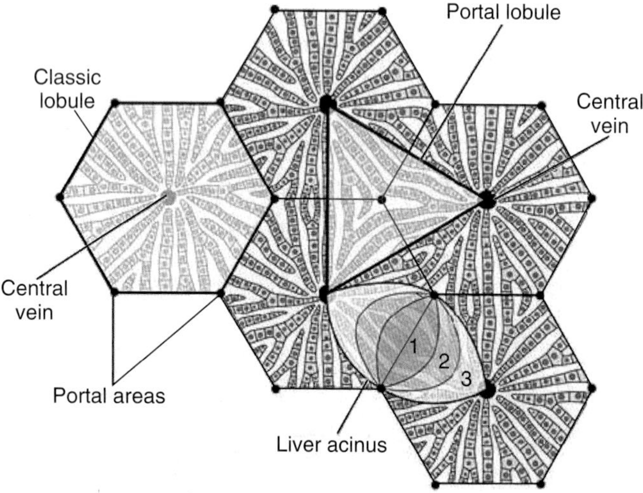

Figure 17-7 Schematic classifications of liver units: liver lobule, portal lobule, and liver acinus. Lobular units have well demarcated central structures (central vein or portal canal), whereas the liver acinus (zones 1, 2, 3; see Fig. 17-10) contains a central axis derived from two adjacent classic lobules. *(From Henrickson R, Kaye GI, Mazurkiewicz J: Liver and gallbladder. In Henrickson R, Kaye GI, Mazurkiewicz [eds]: NMS Histology, 3rd ed. Philadelphia, Lippincott Williams & Wilkins, 1997.)*

A transverse section of a liver lobule shows an array of anastomosing cords of cuboidal hepatocytes separated by vascular channels (lacunae) that radiate from the portal areas and converge on the central vein (see Fig. 17-8). The lacunar labyrinth permeates the entire lobule; it is confined, however, at the periphery of the lobule by a limiting plate of hepatocytes that form a nearly continuous wall. This wall separates the interior of the lobule from the portal canals. Only the tiniest branches of the hepatic artery, portal vein, and bile duct are able to penetrate fenestrae within the limiting plate.

Microscopic examination of the human liver, however, shows a lack of well-defined classic lobules because of a dearth of well-developed connective tissue between lobules. Indeed, the search for lobular boundaries led to the discovery of circumferential terminal hepatic arterioles, portal venules, and bile ductules (Fig. 17-9). This finding is fundamental to the acinar lobe concept, which posits that vessels encircling lobar peripheries, rather than those within portal canals, are the most immediate source of afferent blood to hepatocytes (Fig. 17-10; also see Fig. 17-7). In other words, blood flow to lobules originates along shared borders of classic lobules, which lie between two central veins (see Fig. 17-10).

The Liver Acinus

The acinus is the functional microvascular unit of the liver. It forms around a vertical axis (the portal canal) consisting of a portal venule, hepatic arteriole, bile ductule, lymph vessels, and nerves. Flow of blood within acini is directed radially toward the central veins and vertically to the portal canal.

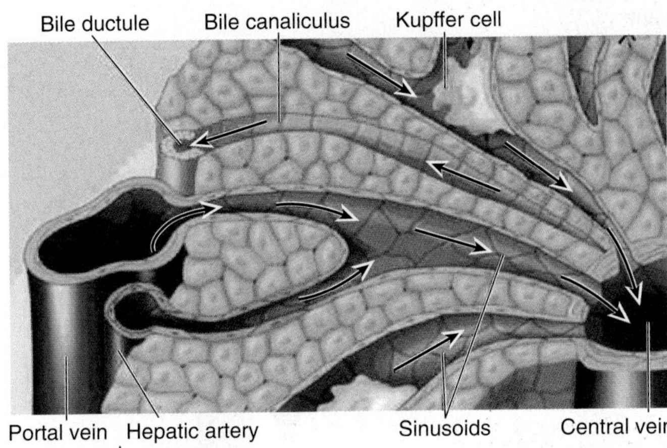

Figure 17-9 Diagram of a portal triad in cross section. Blood enters sinusoids (*blue, black arrows*) and egresses via a central vein (*blue*). Sinusoids contain Kupffer cells (*yellow*). Hepatocytes (*pinkish tan*) produce bile and secrete it into bile canaliculi (*green*, with *black arrows*), which drain into a bile ductule of the portal triad. *(From The Internet Encyclopedia of Science. http://daviddarling.info/encyclopedia/L/liver.html. Accessed February 11, 2009.)*

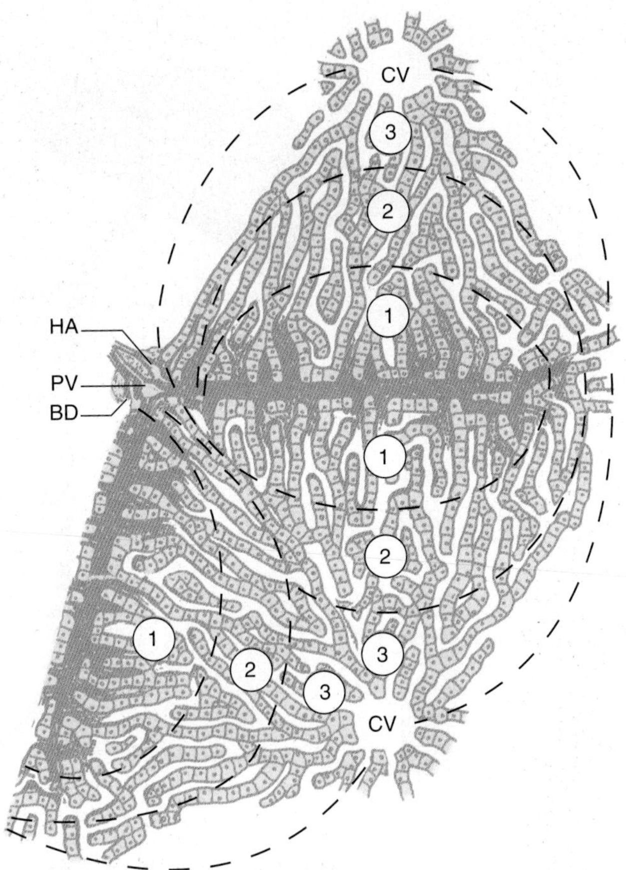

Figure 17-10 Blood supply of a liver acinus. Oxygen tensions and nutrient levels within sinusoids continuously decrease as blood flows from zone 1 through zone 3. The lower part of this figure shows zones 1, 2, and 3 of a neighboring acinus. BD, bile ductule; CV, central vein; HA, hepatic artery; PV, portal vein. *(Reprinted with permission from Jones AL: Anatomy of the normal liver.* In *Zakim D, Boyer T [eds]: Hepatology: A Textbook of Liver Disease, 3rd ed. Philadelphia, WB Saunders, 1996, p 3.)*

Microcirculation

The acinus has three heterogeneous circulatory zones[1] (see Fig. 17-10): zone 1 is periportal, zone 2 is the midzone, and zone 3 is pericentral. Blood supplied to zone 1, which is near the origin of the sinusoid, is rich in oxygen and nutrients. In contrast, zone 3, at the periphery of the acinus, receives blood that is oxygen poor because this blood has already perfused hepatocytes of zones 1 and 2 before it reaches zone 3.

The microvascular architecture of the acinus allows increases in the efficiency of substrate utilization and excretion of waste products.[8,9] Urea cycle enzymes are localized in zones 1 and 2. Hepatocytes within these zones convert amino acids to ketoacids and ammonia; the urea cycle (high capacity, low affinity) captures the ammonia and incorporates it into urea. Any ammonia that eludes the urea cycle is likely to encounter glutamine synthetase, which is expressed only in zone 3. This enzyme facilitates the capture of ammonia within the glutamine substrate. If glutamine substrate were present in zones 1 or 2, it would compete with urea cycle enzymes for ammonia and thereby decrease the liver's capacity to eliminate ammonia. By having glutamine synthetase localized in zone 3, pericentral hepatocytes more efficiently scavenge the ammonia that would otherwise reach the central circulation.[8]

Periportal hepatocytes have the highest density of mitochondria and are the major site of oxidative metabolism and glycogen synthesis. In contrast, pericentral hepatocytes—which have an abundance of smooth endoplasmic reticulum, reduced nicotinamide adenine dinucleotide phosphate (NADPH), and cytochrome P450 (CYP) proteins—are the major site of anaerobic metabolism and xenobiotic biotransformation. Not surprisingly, pericentral hepatocytes bear the brunt of injuries induced by reactive xenobiotic metabolites or hypoxic episodes. The clinical message is that ischemic injury or necrosis of the centrilobular region decreases the liver's capacity to excrete many drugs and other xenobiotics.

Splanchnic Circulation and Hepatic Blood Flow

Hepatic Blood Flow

The liver is at the hub of the splanchnic circulation. Hepatic blood flow is inextricably linked to and hence varies with the effects of intrinsic, extrinsic, and extrahepatic influences on the splanchnic vasculature. The liver receives roughly 25% of the total cardiac output (1 mL of blood per 1 g of liver) via a dual vascular supply. Arterial blood is supplied via the proper hepatic artery—a branch of the common hepatic artery that has its origin at the celiac trunk of the abdominal aorta (Fig. 17-11).[2,3] On the other hand, the portal vein has as its tributaries the superior mesenteric and splenic veins, which carry the entire venous drainage of the preportal splanchnic beds. The portal vein conveys about three fourths and the hepatic artery about one fourth of total hepatic blood flow. Each vessel, however, delivers about half of the total

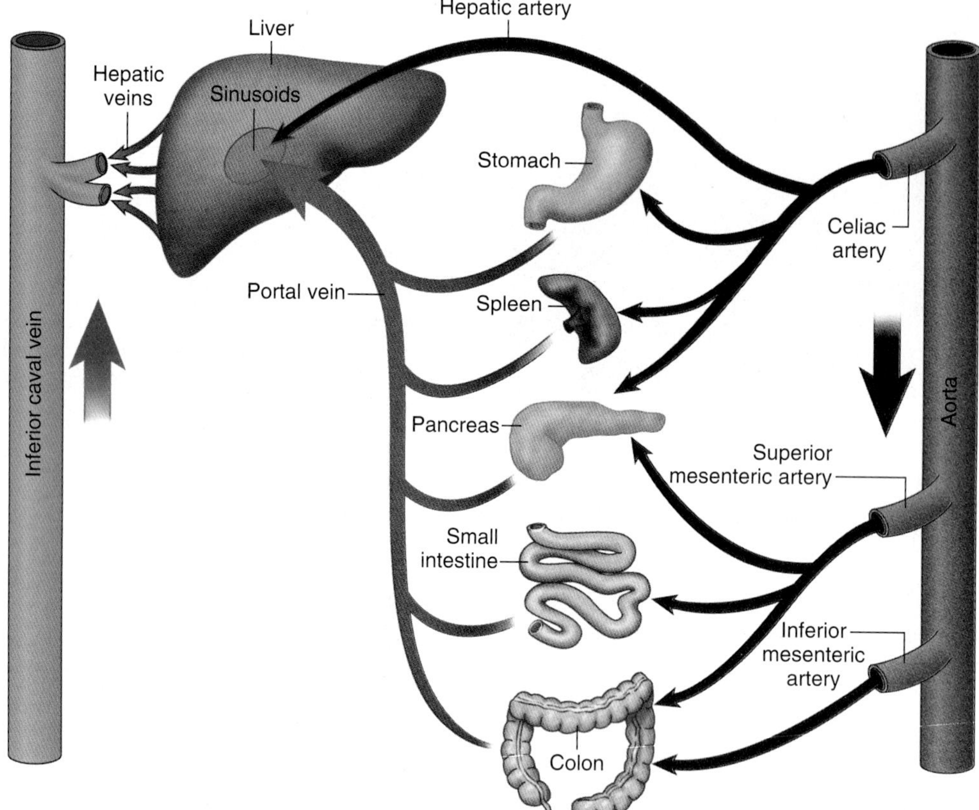

Figure 17-11 The splanchnic circulation. *(Redrawn with permission from Gelman S, Mushlin PS: Catecholamine induced changes in the splanchnic circulation affecting systemic hemodynamics. Anesthesiology 100:434-439, 2004.)*

oxygen supply because arterial blood carries much more oxygen than portal venous blood does.[10]

Splanchnic Reservoir

The vasculature of the splanchnic organs can retain up to 15% of the total blood volume rendering it the largest physiologic reservoir of whole blood in the human body.[11] Generally, 20% of blood volume resides in arterial vessels, 10% in capillaries, and 70% in veins.[10] Therefore, the effects of neuroendocrine, pharmacologic, and pathophysiologic factors on venous capacitance and resistance vessels determine, to a large extent, the instantaneous volume within the splanchnic reservoir. For example, increases in resistance within the postsinusoidal veins of the liver can promote transudation of plasma into lymphatic vessels and the peritoneal cavity (through Glisson's capsule) and thereby result in edema, ascites, and hypovolemia. Indeed, minor changes in hepatic venous pressure can have major consequences on the effective circulatory volume.[3,12]

Regulation of Hepatic Blood Flow

Intrinsic and extrinsic mechanisms play important roles in the regulation of hepatic blood flow. Intrinsic mechanisms—such as the hepatic arterial buffer response (HABR), metabolic control, and pressure-flow autoregulation—work independently of neurohumoral factors.

Intrinsic Regulation

Hepatic Arterial Buffer Response The HABR is the most important intrinsic mechanism. With an intact HABR, changes in portal venous flow cause reciprocal changes in hepatic arterial flow.[13] That is, when portal venous flow decreases, the HABR compensates by increasing hepatic arterial flow, and vice versa. The HABR mechanism involves the synthesis and washout of adenosine (i.e., a vasodilator) from periportal regions.[14] When portal venous flow decreases, adenosine accumulates in the periportal regions, which lowers arteriolar resistance and thereby increases hepatic arterial flow. Conversely, when portal venous flow increases, adenosine is washed out of the periportal regions, which increases arteriolar resistance and decreases hepatic arterial flow. At a maximum, the HABR can double hepatic arterial flow. Therefore, it cannot fully restore hepatic blood flow when portal venous flow falls by more than 50%. Yet because hepatic arterial blood carries more oxygen than portal venous blood does, the HABR more effectively preserves hepatic oxygen supply than hepatic blood flow does. Various disorders (e.g., endotoxemia, splanchnic hypoperfusion) may decrease or even abolish the HABR and render the liver more vulnerable to hypoxic injury.[15,16]

Metabolic Control Many constituents of blood affect hepatic arterial and portal venous blood flow.[17] Decreases in oxygen tension or the pH of portal venous blood typically lead to increases in hepatic arterial flow. Postprandial hyperosmolarity increases hepatic arterial and portal venous flow.[17] The underlying metabolic and respiratory status (e.g., hypercapnia, alkalosis, arterial hypoxemia) also modulates the distribution of blood flow within the liver.

Pressure-Flow Autoregulation Pressure-flow autoregulation enables tissue-specific regulators to govern organ blood flow despite fluctuations in systemic arterial pressure. The mechanism involves myogenic responses of vascular smooth muscle to stretch. For example, a hypertensive episode increases transmural pressure, thereby stretching arterial smooth muscle. The resultant increase in myogenic tone (i.e., vasoconstriction) prevents the increases in organ blood flow that would otherwise occur. Conversely, transient hypotension lowers transmural pressure and myogenic tone (i.e., vasodilation), which helps sustain organ perfusion during systemic hypotension.

The hepatic artery exhibits pressure-flow autoregulation in metabolically active liver (postprandial) but not in the fasting state, which is the most prevalent status of surgical patients.[18] Pressure-flow autoregulation is nonexistent in the portal circulation. Thus, decreases in systemic blood pressure—as often occur during anesthesia—typically lead to proportional decreases in portal venous flow.[19,20] Bottom line, pressure-flow autoregulation has little if any role as an intraoperative regulator of hepatic blood flow, with the possible exception of emergency surgery on patients in the fed state.

Extrinsic Regulation

Neural Control Fibers of the vagus, phrenic, and splanchnic nerves (postganglionic sympathetic fibers from T6 through T11) enter the liver at the hilum; they course through the liver alongside the afferent hepatic blood vessels and bile ducts. The fibers form an intercommunicating plexus that innervates the terminal arterioles and venules. The sympathetic nervous system is an important regulator of the splanchnic vasculature. When sympathetic tone decreases, splanchnic reservoir volume increases. On the other hand, sympathoadrenal stimulation translocates blood volume from the splanchnic reservoir to the central circulation. Within seconds of splanchnic nerve stimulation, up to 80% of the hepatic blood volume (400 to 500 mL) could be transferred to the central circulation in dogs.[10,21] Vagal stimulation alters the tone of the presinusoidal sphincters[22]; the net effect is a redistribution of intrahepatic blood flow without changing total hepatic blood flow.

Humoral Control The hepatic arterial bed has α_1-, α_2-, and β_2-adrenergic receptors, whereas the portal vein has only α-receptors (Fig. 17-12).[3,23] Direct injection of epinephrine into the hepatic artery induces a biphasic response: vasoconstriction (α-receptor stimulation) followed by vasodilation (β-receptor stimulation). However, an injection of epinephrine into the portal vein causes only vasoconstriction (α-receptor response). The dopamine released during sympathoadrenal activation has weak vasoactive effects in the liver that are dwarfed by those of epinephrine and norepinephrine.[17,23]

Glucagon induces dose-dependent relaxation of hepatic arterial smooth muscle and blocks the effects of physiologic vasoconstrictors on the hepatic artery.[24] By contrast, angiotensin II constricts the hepatic arterial and portal venous beds.[25] Pharmacologic doses of angiotensin II can cause hepatic blood flow to plummet because of its ability to markedly decrease both mesenteric arterial and portal venous flow. Vasopressin, on the other hand, elevates splanchnic arterial resistance, but it lowers portal venous resistance. Because of its vascular profile, vasopressin may have efficacy in treating portal hypertension.[26]

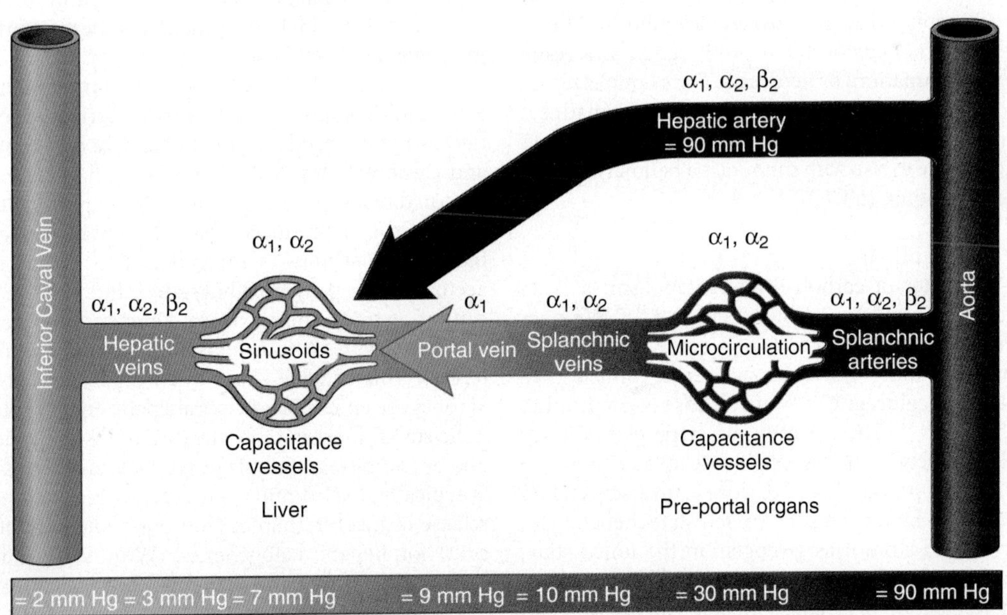

Figure 17-12 Adrenoceptor subtypes (α_1, α_2, β_2) and intravascular pressure within the splanchnic circulation. The splanchnic arteries represent the arterial supply to all preportal organs; the splanchnic veins represent the pooled venous blood from all these organs. *(Redrawn with permission from Gelman S, Mushlin PS: Catecholamine induced changes in the splanchnic circulation affecting systemic hemodynamics. Anesthesiology 100:434-439, 2004.)*

Biochemical and Physiologic Functions of the Liver

Intermediary Metabolism

Protein Metabolism

The liver plays a central role in the production and breakdown of amino acids, peptides, and proteins. Hepatocytes metabolize amino acids to keto acids, glutamine, and ammonia via transamination and oxidative deamination reactions. The Krebs-Henseleit cycle is the major pathway for removing ammonia and other nitrogenous wastes from the body. This pathway captures nitrogen in the form of urea. Thus, with a failing liver (and normal renal function), blood urea nitrogen remains low whereas nitrogenous wastes such as ammonia accumulate in blood and other tissues.

Liver-derived proteins have an impact on every organ in the body. Such proteins include procoagulants, hormones, cytokines, chemokines, acute-phase reactants, and transport proteins. The most abundant of them is albumin, which accounts for roughly 15% of the liver's total protein production. Healthy adults produce 12 to 15 g of albumin every day; the total-body pool of albumin has a mass of about 500 g.[27] Factors that modulate the synthesis of albumin include plasma oncotic pressure,[28] dietary amino acids,[29] and hormones.[30] The main regulator of intravascular albumin is oncotic pressure. Albumin binds to and transports a wide variety of substances—free fatty acids, unconjugated bilirubin, hormones, xenobiotics, and metals. In this way, albumin affects the biologic activity and clearance of a multiplicity of substances.

α-Fetoprotein (AFP) resembles albumin both genetically and functionally. AFP comes mainly from the yolk sac, hepatocytes, and enterocytes.[31] During fetal and neonatal life, AFP has importance as a transport protein and is the major determinant of plasma oncotic pressure. By the postpartum age of 1 year, albumin has largely replaced AFP. Thus, an elevation in AFP in later life typically reflects hepatocellular proliferation as a result of hepatic injury, inflammation, or neoplasia. For example, elevations in AFP occur in nearly all patients with acute hepatitis.[32] However, large, progressive increases in plasma AFP—levels above 400 ng/mL that continue to rise with time—are a hallmark feature of hepatocellular carcinoma (HCC).

Carbohydrate Metabolism

The liver is the epicenter of carbohydrate metabolism. It is an important homeostatic regulator of blood glucose.[33-35] Whether the liver is a net producer or consumer of glucose is dependent on many factors, including the neuroendocrine milieu (i.e., insulin, catecholamines, glucagon)[36-41] and glucose concentration in sinusoidal blood.[9,42-44] The severity of hyperglycemia or hypoglycemia also influences the rate of glucose uptake or release by hepatocytes. Hepatic production of glucose is inversely related to glycogen production by the liver. In the fed state, hepatocytes polymerize glucose and store it as glycogen; in the unfed state, hepatocytes depolymerize glycogen to glucose and release it into the bloodstream. Regulation of glycogen metabolism involves two rate-limiting enzymes: (1) glycogen synthase, which catalyzes the synthesis of glycogen from monomers of uridine diphosphate (UDP) glucose, and (2) glycogen phosphorylase, which catalyzes the sequential cleavage of glycogen to monomers of glucose 1-phosphate.

When liver glycogen stores are depleted—as is likely after prolonged exercise or a 24-hour fast—the body depends on hepatic gluconeogenesis to replenish blood glucose. Substrates for gluconeogenesis include (1) lactate; (2) glycerol from the hydrolysis of triglycerides; and (3) glucogenic amino acids such as alanine and glutamine, which are derived from protein catabolism in skeletal muscle.[9,45] Endocrine modulators of gluconeogenesis include glucagon, catecholamines, and insulin. Both glucagon and catecholamines stimulate gluconeogenesis. Glucagon works via cyclic adenosine monophosphate (cAMP)-dependent protein kinase, and catecholamines use both cAMP-dependent and cAMP-independent mechanisms.[46,47] By contrast, insulin inhibits gluconeogenesis, and it blocks the stimulatory effects of catecholamines and glucagon on this pathway.

Lipid Metabolism

The liver produces, takes up, retains, releases, and oxidizes fatty acids in accord with nutritional and endocrine influences.[48-52] Dietary fatty acids absorbed in the small intestines reach the liver via blood and the lymphatics, mainly in the form of chylomicrons. When replete with glycogen, hepatocytes convert glucose to fatty acids—and may store them as triglycerides (fat). Thus, the major sources of intrahepatic fatty acids include (1) free fatty acids extracted from blood, (2) de novo lipogenesis, (3) hydrolysis of cytoplasmic triglycerides, and (4) hepatocellular uptake and metabolism of blood-borne lipoproteins.[48]

Esterification and β-oxidation pathways have pivotal roles in the hepatic disposition of fatty acids. Esterification of glycerol and fatty acids produces triglycerides—the main storage form of free fatty acids. The liver may either retain triglycerides or package them into lipoproteins, primarily very-low-density lipoproteins (VLDLs), for transport to other tissues. Free fatty acids regulate VLDL production, but endocrine and nutritional factors govern VLDL secretion.[48,53] β-Oxidation is the pathway of fatty acid catabolism. Glucagon activates this pathway, whereas insulin inhibits it. β-Oxidation sequentially cleaves fatty acids to yield monomers of acetyl coenzyme A (acetyl CoA).

Acetyl CoA is at the epicenter of intermediary metabolism. It is a building block for lipids (triglycerides, phospholipids, cholesterol) and a product of the oxidative breakdown of fatty acids and carbohydrates. Mitochondria oxidize acetyl groups to yield carbon dioxide, water, and adenosine triphosphate (ATP). If more acetyl CoA is produced than the tricarboxylic acid cycle can handle, the surplus is metabolized to ketone bodies—namely, acetoacetate, β-hydroxybutyrate, and acetone.[9] Hepatocytes cannot extract energy from ketones, however, because they lack ketoacyl CoA transferase (acetoacetate:succinyl-CoA transferase). This enzyme exists in all organs except the liver.[8] Thus, ketones are an important extrahepatic energy source during catabolic states, most notably starvation. Insulin modulates ketogenesis by inhibiting lipolysis in adipocytes.[54] Stress-induced ketosis is typically a self-limited process because ketones stimulate the release of insulin, thereby limiting availability of substrate (fatty acid) for hepatic ketogenesis.[45] Without insulin, this feedback loop is nonexistent and diabetic ketoacidosis may ensue.[9]

Bile Metabolism and the Enterohepatic Circulation

Daily production of bile ranges from 600 to 800 mL. Although bile contains many different substances (e.g., electrolytes, organic anions, lipids), bile salts (also called bile acids) account for about 85% of biliary solids.[55] Bile salts are natural ionic detergents with important roles in absorption, transport, and secretion of lipids.[56,57] They activate lipases (bile acid dependent), promote micelle formation, and enable the intestinal uptake of fat-soluble vitamins, cholesterol, and other lipids. Bile salts also facilitate the excretion of numerous lipophilic substances, including exogenous compounds such as xenobiotics and endogenous molecules such as bilirubin, cholesterol, and amphipathic steroid hormonal derivatives.

Bile salts are end products of cholesterol synthesis and regulators of lipid metabolism. Bile salts produce their regulatory effects by binding to and activating farnesoid X receptor (FXR). When activated, hormone nuclear receptors (such as FXR) are transferred from cytoplasm to the nucleus; they bind to hormone response elements on DNA to induce either expression or transrepression of specific gene products. An important effect of FXR activation is to decrease the transcription of cholesterol 7α-hydroxylase (CYP7A1), which catalyzes the rate-limiting step in the conversion of cholesterol to bile salts. Bile salts modulate plasma lipid levels by regulating the expression of lipoprotein receptors that enable hepatocytes to remove lipoprotein cholesterol from the bloodstream.[56,58]

The body avidly conserves bile salts by recycling them around 20 to 30 times daily in the enterohepatic circulation. Hepatocellular transport proteins (transporters) regulate both the uptake (from sinusoids) and secretion (into canalicular spaces) of bile salts. Activated transporters on canalicular surfaces overcome large osmotic gradients to pump bile salts into the intrahepatic bile ducts. As bile flows through the ductular collecting system, it is diluted and alkalinized.[55] After reaching the common hepatic bile duct, bile either enters the cystic duct (for storage in the gallbladder) or passes through the common bile duct into the small intestine. The terminal ileum (using sodium-dependent bile salt transporters) reclaims 95% of the bile salts, which it returns to the liver in the portal circulation. These bile salts are taken up by transporters on the sinusoidal surfaces of hepatocellular plasma membranes. Sometime later, the same bile salts are again pumped into the canalicular space, thereby completing one cycle of the enterohepatic circulation. Of note, opioid analgesics (μ-agonists) can disrupt bile flow by inducing intense, painful spasms of the bile ducts and sphincter of Oddi.[59] Fortunately, this opioid effect is usually rapidly reversed by medications, including glucagon, opioid antagonists (naloxone), smooth muscle relaxants (nitroglycerin), antimuscarinic drugs (atropine), and volatile anesthetics.

Coagulation

Coagulants and Procoagulants

Hepatocytes make most of the procoagulants, with notable exceptions such as factors III (tissue thromboplastin), IV (calcium), and VIII (von Willebrand factor). The liver also makes protein regulators of coagulation and the fibrinolytic pathways. Such regulators include protein S, protein C, protein Z, plasminogen activator inhibitor (PAI), and antithrombin III. To further elaborate, protein Z facilitates the degradation of factor Xa, and protein S is a cofactor of activated protein C that inactivates factor VIIIa-Va complexes; a deficiency of protein S increases the risk for venous thrombosis. PAI-1 is an indirect inhibitor of fibrinolysis. This serine protease inhibitor blocks the effects of plasminogen activators, such as urokinase or tissue plasminogen activator, to convert plasminogen to plasmin; a deficiency of PAI increases the risk for uncontrolled fibrinolysis. To summarize, hepatocytes make most of the procoagulants and many proteins that modulate the consumption of clotting factor.[60]

Vitamin K Cofactor and γ-Carboxylation

The vitamin K–dependent proteins include factors II, VII, IX, and X and proteins C and S. These proteins undergo a vitamin K–dependent, post-translational modification; the process involves carboxylation of the γ-position of glutamate residues at the amino terminus and produces the amino acid carboxyglutamate.[45,61] This modification (called γ-carboxylation) enables procoagulants to form complexes with calcium or other divalent cations.[62] Thus, γ-carboxylated procoagulants are primed for activation to serine proteases (e.g., via extrahepatic phospholipids) and for participation in the clotting cascade.[45,63]

The γ-carboxylation pathway holds the key to understanding how warfarin exerts its anticoagulant effect. γ-Carboxylation occurs in two stages.[63] The first involves γ-carboxylation of precursor proteins via vitamin K–dependent γ-carboxylase and the oxidation of vitamin K cofactor (naphthol hydroquinone) to 2,3-epoxide vitamin K. The second stage regenerates the vitamin K cofactor via reactions catalyzed by vitamin K 2,3-epoxide reductase.[64-67] Warfarin targets the second stage. It inhibits vitamin K epoxide reductase and thereby traps vitamin K in the epoxide form. This eventually depletes vitamin K cofactor and shuts down the γ-carboxylation pathway. Warfarin inhibits γ-carboxylation almost immediately after its absorption from the gut, but its anticoagulant effect takes longer than 1 day to develop. This disparity reflects low clearance of the prothrombin complex from the circulation (i.e., half-life of about 14 hours) and the insensitivity of the prothrombin time (PT) to falling blood levels of procoagulants. As a rule, the PT stays in the normal range until the prothrombin complex in blood is at least 70% below the lower limit of normal.

Therapeutic use of vitamin K may help uncover the cause of an unexplained prolongation in PT. For example, PT abnormalities caused by malnutrition or warfarin are correctable with enteral or parenteral vitamin K therapy. When PT abnormalities result from malabsorption syndromes, parenteral vitamin K is superior to oral therapy. However, if PT abnormalities result from liver dysfunction (acute hepatitis, cirrhosis), vitamin K will be ineffective because the problem is not a deficiency of vitamin K but rather a deficiency of hepatic procoagulants.

Erythropoiesis and Erythrocytosis

Heme Metabolism

The liver is the main site of erythrocyte production during fetal life through early infancy. As the bone marrow matures, hematopoietic cells begin to disappear from the liver; occasionally, however, they persist or reappear as a result of disorders such as congenital hemolytic anemias, bone marrow failure, or myeloproliferative diseases. Most of the protein in erythrocytes exists as globulin chains of hemoglobin; the heme portion of hemoglobin contains protoporphyrin IX and ferrous iron. In healthy adults, 20% of the total heme production is from liver; the rest comes from bone marrow. The biochemical pathways that make heme are similar in the two organs.[64,68,69]

Heme synthesis begins with the condensation of glycine and succinyl CoA to produce 5-aminolevulinic acid (ALA). This reaction, catalyzed by ALA synthase, is the rate-limiting step in the heme pathway. Heme inhibits ALA synthase and thereby regulates its own synthesis. ALA is made in mitochondria; it diffuses into the cytoplasm and encounters ALA dehydratase. This enzyme joins two ALA molecules together to form porphobilinogen (PBG). PBG molecules are positioned in a linear arrangement by PBG deaminase to form hydroxymethylbilane (HMB). HMB is transformed to uroporphyrinogen III, which is the precursor of coproporphyrinogen III. The latter is taken up by mitochondria and converted—via coproporphyrinogen oxidase and protoporphyrin oxidase—to protoporphyrin IX. In the final step of the pathway, ferrochelatase catalyzes the formation of a complex of ferrous iron and protoporphyrin IX to produce heme.

Porphyrias Porphyrinogens exposed to O_2 are readily oxidized to the corresponding porphyrins. Accumulation of porphyrins in tissues leads to porphyrias. Porphyrias are rare, genetic diseases characterized by aberrations in heme production. Patients with these disorders are typically asymptomatic until some stressor (exogenous or endogenous) induces a porphyric crisis.[70] The clinical syndrome includes recurrent, dramatic, and occasionally fatal neurologic reactions, accompanied by abdominal pain (90%) and dark urine (80%).

Acute intermittent porphyria (AIP) is the most common porphyria. Its prevalence in the general population is about 1 in 10,000, but it may reach 1 in 500 in psychiatric patients. AIP has a fivefold higher frequency in women than in men.

Substances known to trigger porphyric crises include sex hormones, glucocorticoids, cigarette smoke, and various medications, most notably barbiturates and other CYP inducers.[57,71] Recall that induction of CYP entails the production of CYP hemoproteins. When heme is inserted into these newly minted CYP proteins, intracellular levels of heme decline.[71-74] The result is less feedback inhibition of ALA synthetase and therefore more ALA production.[75] Defects in the heme pathway cause the precursors of heme—made proximal to the site of the block—to accumulate. Consider, for example, patients with a genetic deficiency of PBG deaminase; when ALA synthetase activity increases, so too do tissue levels of ALA and PBG. These heme precursors, which have chemical structures similar to the inhibitory neurotransmitter γ-aminobutyric acid (GABA), are likely contributors to the neurotoxic effects of porphyrias.

Bilirubin Metabolism

The main source of serum bilirubin is heme metabolism. Healthy adults make about 300 mg of bilirubin daily, 80% of which is derived from phagocytosis of senescent erythrocytes by macrophages in the spleen, liver, and bone marrow. These reticuloendothelial cells extract protein from hemoglobin and convert heme to bilirubin.[57] The first step is rate limiting. Heme oxygenase (HO), with O_2 as a substrate, oxidatively cleaves the porphyrin macrocycle of heme to yield biliverdin-IXα, carbon monoxide (CO), and free divalent iron in equimolar amounts.

Most of the endogenous CO production is derived from HO reactions. Thus, the biologic importance of HO may extend beyond the breakdown of heme. To clarify, CO has many physiologic roles, including regulation of vascular tone (vasodilator), platelet aggregation, vascular myocyte proliferation, and neurotransmitter release.[76] Furthermore, CO exerts cytoprotective, antiapoptotic, and antioxidant effects in organs throughout the body.[77,78] Biliverdin also confers protection from oxidative stress[77]; it is rapidly converted to bilirubin by cytoplasmic reductases.[79]

After release from reticuloendothelial cells, bilirubin becomes tightly bound to plasma albumin. Hepatocytes avidly extract this bilirubin from albumin. They produce conjugates of bilirubin (through the action of glucuronic acid and bilirubin UDP-glucuronosyltransferase) and secrete these conjugates into canalicular bile. Although the gut excretes most of this bilirubin, a small amount returns to the liver in the enterohepatic circulation. Thus, the bloodstream normally has a modicum of bilirubin conjugates, which arrive directly via the enterohepatic circulation or indirectly from the bile ducts and lymphatics.

Endocrine Physiology

The liver is the largest gland in human beings and it plays important roles in the metabolism of hormones and hormone-binding proteins.[60] Hepatocytes produce a wide variety of endocrine substances, including angiotensinogen, thrombopoietin, and insulin-like growth factor I (IGF-I).[80] They take up thyroxine (T_4), the major product of the thyroid gland, and may activate it to triiodothyronine (T_3) or inactivate it. The liver inactivates many other hormones, including aldosterone, antidiuretic hormone, estrogens, androgens, and insulin. Nearly half of the insulin released by the pancreas may not reach the systemic circulation because of hepatic degradation.[81]

Immune and Inflammatory Responses

The liver is the largest reticuloendothelial organ in the human body. Hepatic macrophages (Kupffer cells) account for nearly 10% of the total liver mass. Kupffer cells protect and defend the body against foreign intrusions. Before splanchnic venous blood enters the central circulation, it is filtered by Kupffer cells, which degrade toxins, process antigens, and phagocytose bacteria.[82] In addition, Kupffer cells are important modulators of inflammation[83]: they attenuate inflammatory responses by removing inciting substances from the bloodstream; but they can also induce and intensify inflammation by producing and releasing proinflammatory mediators and recruiting neutrophils to the liver.[83] Among these mediators are various cytokines, chemokines, leukotrienes, proteases, nitro-radicals, and reduced oxygen species. If not properly controlled, these same mediators can induce or aggravate injuries to parenchymal and other liver cells.[83-87] For example, endothelial cells of the sinusoids and terminal hepatic veins—because of their low glutathione content—are highly vulnerable to oxidative stress and drug-induced vascular injury.[88] Stellate cells reside mainly in the perisinusoidal spaces and are the liver's major source of matrix deposition. When activated by oxidative stress or toxic chemicals, stellate cells may be transformed to collagen-synthesizing myofibroblasts, which can cause extensive fibrosis of the liver (e.g., methotrexate-induced hepatic fibrosis).

Xenobiotic (Drug) Metabolism and Excretion

Although xenobiotics may be in tissues through the body (lung, liver, kidney, intestines, skin); the liver is the epicenter for biotransformation reactions. Most oral medications contain lipophilic regions that increase their gastrointestinal absorption, membrane penetrability, and biologic activity. Lipid solubility also lowers drug excretion rates and increases drug retention by the body. Whereas the kidney readily excretes most small polar molecules, it cannot efficiently eliminate most lipophilic substances. Lipophilic molecules often bind tightly to plasma proteins, thereby evading glomerular filtration. Even when the glomerulus filters such molecules, the renal tubules usually reabsorb them. The liver, on the other hand, chemically transforms drugs in ways that increase their water solubility. Generally, hepatic biotransformations not only increase drug excretion but also inactivate or attenuate the biologic activity of drugs. However, xenobiotic metabolism produces reactive chemicals that cause severe liver damage (either directly or indirectly by immune sensitization, as is probably involved in the pathogenesis of halothane hepatitis).[89-91]

Pathways of Drug Metabolism

The myriad chemical reactions that hepatocytes use to eliminate drugs fit into three broad categories (or phases). Phase 1 metabolism uses CYP and mixed-function oxidases to increase the polarity of drugs. Phase 2 metabolism increases the polarity of drugs (or their metabolites) by conjugating them with endogenous water-soluble substrates. Phase 3 elimination uses energy-dependent transporters to excrete drugs into canalicular bile. The hepatic clearance of drugs involves at least one of these phases.[90,92,93]

Phase 1 Metabolism Phase 1 reactions (e.g., oxidations, reductions, hydrolysis) convert drugs to more polar compounds by inserting polar groups (e.g., OH, NH_2, SH) or removing nonpolar groups. Generally, the products of phase 1 metabolism are more readily excreted in bile or urine than their precursors are. Such products may also be substrates for phase 2 conjugations.

MICROSOMAL OXIDASES AND CYTOCHROME P450. More than 90% of drug biotransformations involve microsomal oxidases and hemoproteins of the CYP gene superfamily. The human liver has more than 20 different CYP isozymes[90-94] that mediate redox reactions in diverse pathways, including steroid, lipid, and bile salt metabolism. Zone 3 (centrilobular) has the highest total CYP content. In fact, the acinar location of specific isozymes of CYP may clarify relationships between drug metabolism and liver injury.[90] For example, centrilobular necrosis is the classic acetaminophen-induced injury; the probable explanation is that CYP2E—the CYP isoform involved in acetaminophen metabolism—is localized in zone 3.

CYP reactions generate metabolites that are highly reactive and potentially toxic. In brief, the CYP reaction cycle begins with oxygen binding to heme iron; this oxygen becomes activated after receiving an electron from a flavoprotein reductase—NADPH: hemoprotein oxidoreductase (CYP).[91-94] Insertion of activated oxygen into lipophilic molecules (e.g., xenobiotics) produces substrates for mixed-function oxidase reactions. These oxidases transfer a singlet oxygen atom from O_2 to the target molecule; another substrate (e.g., NADPH) simultaneously delivers electrons that reduce the residual oxygen singlet, thereby enabling its incorporation into water. To summarize, oxidases promote the formation of highly active chemicals, including reduced oxygen species and free radical intermediates, which can cause or aggravate liver injury.[95]

A plethora of substances—drugs, nutritional supplements, contaminants, insecticides—alter hepatic microsomal drug metabolism.[91] Some chemicals, such as phenobarbital and phenytoin, induce many different CYP isoforms. Other chemicals are much more selective.[91-94] For example, alcohol selectively induces CYP2E1 and CYP3A4[90,96]; smoke from cigarettes or cannabis increases CYP1A2[97]; isoniazid increases CYP2E1; and rifampicin and hypericum (active ingredient of St. John's wort) selectively induce CYP3A4.[98] With long-term use, CYP inducers often increase their own metabolism while stimulating alkaline phosphatase (AP) and γ-glutamyl transpeptidase (GGTP) production. The latter effect which occurs via activation of transcriptional regulators of nuclear orphan receptors as part of the "hepatic adaptation" to chronic drug administration.[90]

MOLECULAR GENETIC BASIS OF CYP INDUCTION. Studies of CYP3A4—the predominant CYP isoform in human liver—have clarified the molecular genetics of CYP induction.[99] For example, rifampin, a potent inducer of CYP3A4, activates the pregnane X receptor (PXR), which is a transcriptional regulator of the orphan nuclear receptor family. PXR works in concert with another xenobiotic nuclear receptor, constitutive androstane receptor (CAR), to coordinate protective hepatic responses to potentially toxic stimuli.[100] Activated PXR and the analogous CAR bind to cognate nucleotide sequences upstream of the CYP3A4 structural gene within a "xenobiotic responsive enhancer module" (XREM).[99,101] Such binding activates the CYP3A4 promoter (downstream) and thereby induces the synthesis of mRNA for CYP3A4 protein. Similar mechanisms are involved in regulating other CYP pathways.[99,101]

Phase 2 Metabolism Phase 2 reactions conjugate xenobiotics (or their metabolites) with endogenous hydrophilic molecules such as glucuronic acid, acetate, sulfates, amino acids, and glutathione.[90,102] Many conjugations involve glucuronic acid and UDP-glucuronosyltransferase. Other conjugations are catalyzed by sulfatases, glutathione-*S*-transferases, acetyl-*N*-transferases, or amino acid *N*-transferases. When compared with their precursors, conjugated xenobiotics are usually less efficacious, less toxic, more hydrophilic, and more readily excreted in bile or urine.

Phase 3 Elimination Phase 3 reactions involve specific molecular transporters—known as ATP-binding cassette (ABC) transport proteins—that facilitate the excretion of xenobiotics and endogenous compounds. These proteins use ATP hydrolysis to drive molecular transport. Major ABC transport proteins include cystic fibrosis transmembrane conductance regulator (CFTR), canalicular copper transporters, and multidrug resistance protein (MDR). MDR-1 (formerly called P-glycoprotein) resides on the canalicular surfaces of hepatocytes and enables biliary excretion of cationic compounds, including anticancer drugs.[103,104]

Another family of ABC proteins—multidrug resistance-related protein (MRP)—excretes conjugated molecules. MRP-1, located on the lateral surfaces of hepatocytes, can transport drug conjugates into the sinusoids. MRP-2 (formerly, canalicular multispecific organic anion transporter [cMOAT]), on the canalicular surfaces of hepatocytes, secretes conjugates of drugs and endogenous wastes (e.g., bilirubin diglucuronide, glutathionyl-leukotriene conjugates) into canalicular bile. Thus, dysfunction of ABC transport proteins can disrupt the flow of bile, impair excretion of xenobiotics and endogenous compounds, and induce cholestatic liver injury.[105,106]

Determinants of Drug Metabolism

Dose-related responses to drugs often vary considerably within individuals and populations. Much of this variability is due to the heterogeneity of drug disposition and metabolism, which is mainly influenced by genetic and environmental factors. Genetics control the expression of CYP isozymes. Environmental factors (e.g., drugs, other chemicals) modify genetic expression and thereby alter drug biotransformation.[90,92,93] Numerous conditions and disorders are capable of altering the production of CYP proteins.[107] For example, obesity, fasting, and diabetes mellitus may lead to upregulation of CYP2E1.[90,92,93] On the other hand, conditions that may result in downregulation of CYP include systemic inflammatory disorders,[108] fever,[109] nitrogen-free solutions,[110] nitrogen-rich solutions,[111] and hepatic cirrhosis.[92,93] Hypothyroidism and hypopituitarism may selectively downregulate CYP1A and CYP3A4, respectively.[92,93]

Pharmacokinetics

Perfusion models of drug elimination generally focus on three major parameters: intrinsic hepatic clearance, hepatic blood flow, and protein binding. The intrinsic hepatic clearance of a drug divided by hepatic blood flow is the drug's extraction ratio (ER); ER provides a measure of the relative efficiency with which the liver extracts or eliminates a given drug.[112-116] Box 17-1 shows a compilation of drugs with high and low ERs.[116] Such information enables general rules to be made about pharmacologic categories and intrinsic clearances. For example, hepatocytes are efficient extractors of calcium channel blockers, β-adrenoceptor blockers (except atenolol), opioid analgesics, tricyclic antidepressants, and organic nitrates. On the other hand, the liver poorly extracts warfarin, aspirin, alcohol, and many anticonvulsants. For low-ER drugs, hepatic elimination rates are capacity limited. Such rates often change when protein binding or intrinsic hepatic clearance changes, but they are insensitive to fluctuations in hepatic blood flow. For high-ER drugs, hepatic elimination rates are flow dependent. These elimination rates are highly dependent on and directly related to liver blood flow; they are unaffected by changes in either protein binding or the activity of drug-metabolizing enzymes (Table 17-1).

Box 17-1 Drugs that are Efficiently Versus Poorly Extracted from Blood Flowing through the Liver

Efficiently Extracted Drugs	Poorly Extracted Drugs
Amitriptyline	Acetaminophen
Desipramine	Amobarbital
Imipramine	Antipyrine
Labetalol	Aspirin
Lidocaine	Clindamycin
Meperidine	Diazepam
Metoprolol	Digitoxin
Morphine	Ethanol
Nortriptyline	Hexobarbital
Pentazocine	Phenobarbital
Propoxyphene	Phenytoin
Propranolol	Tolbutamide
Ranitidine	Valproic acid
Verapamil	Warfarin
Zidovudine	

Evaluation of the Liver

Clinical Assessment

The only clues to liver disease may be mild, nonspecific symptoms, such as loss of appetite, easy fatigability, malaise, altered sleep patterns, or subtle changes in personality. The history addresses major risk factors for liver disease: (1) alcoholism; (2) illicit drug use; (3) sexual promiscuity; (4) blood transfusions; (5) occupational exposure to hepatotoxins; (6) prior bouts of jaundice, particularly after anesthesia; and (7) genetic diseases such as hemochromatosis, α_1-antitrypsin (α_1-AT) deficiency, and Wilson's disease. Clinical findings consistent with liver disease include nonspecific symptoms (as just mentioned), pruritus, abdominal pain, indigestion, and changes in urine or stool color. The physical examination focuses on stigmata of advanced liver disease, such as icterus, jaundice, ascites, spider angiomas, xanthelasma, encephalopathy, palmar erythema, and fetor hepaticus.

Table 17-1 Flow-Dependent Versus Capacity-Limited Elimination of Drugs by the Liver

Type of Hepatic Elimination	Extraction Ratio (ER)	Rate of Hepatic Drug Metabolism
Flow-dependent elimination	*High ER*: At clinically relevant concentrations, most of the drug in the afferent hepatic blood is eliminated on first pass through the liver	*Rapid*: Because drugs with a high ER are metabolized so rapidly, their hepatic clearances roughly equal their rates of transport to the liver (i.e., hepatic blood flow)
Capacity-limited elimination (also referred to as dose-dependent, nonlinear, saturable, or zero-order elimination)	*Low ER*: Hepatic elimination of these drugs is determined by their plasma concentration	*Slow*: When the capacity of the liver to eliminate a drug is less than the dosing rate, a steady state is unachievable; plasma levels of drug will continue to rise unless the dosing rate is decreased. Drug clearance has no real meaning in such settings

Standard Laboratory Tests

Standard test panels used to evaluate hepatobiliary status are often called "liver function tests" (Table 17-2).[27,117] To be precise, this terminology is a misnomer because none of the tests measure any specific liver function. Instead, they point to broad categories of hepatobiliary pathology: hepatitis, hepatobiliary dysfunction, or insufficient protein synthesis. These categories include large subsets of diseases—for example, all possible causes of hepatitis.

Detection of Hepatocellular Injury

Aminotransferases Hepatocellular injury is the usual cause of elevated serum levels of alanine aminotransferase (ALT) and aspartate aminotransferase (AST), formerly named serum glutamic-pyruvic transaminase (SGPT) and serum glutamic-oxaloacetic transaminase (SGOT), respectively. Both enzymes are involved in gluconeogenesis. They catalyze the transfer of an amine group to α-ketoglutarate to yield glutamate and either pyruvate (via ALT) or oxaloacetate (via AST). ALT is mainly a cytoplasmic liver enzyme. In contrast, cytoplasmic and mitochondrial isozymes of AST are found in most extrahepatic tissues, including the heart, skeletal muscle, brain, kidney, pancreas, adipose tissue, and blood. It is rare to encounter concomitant elevations in AST and ALT when the liver is normal and disease free. In those rare instances, the elevations in AST and ALT levels would most likely result from muscle injury.[117]

Elevated ALT and AST levels are sometimes described in qualitative terms: mild (100 to 249 IU/L), moderate (250 to 999 IU/L), large (1000 to 1999 IU/L), and extreme (>2000 IU/L). Mild elevations in AST and ALT may arise from any disorder that injures hepatocytes. Common causes include steatosis, medications, alcohol consumption, hemochromatosis, cholestasis, chronic viral hepatitis, neoplasms, and cirrhosis. Moderate ALT and AST elevations are characteristic of acute viral hepatitis, drug-induced liver injury, and flare-ups of chronic liver disease (e.g., viral hepatitis, steatohepatitis). Large elevations often reflect acute hepatitis superimposed on chronic active liver disease. Extreme elevations signify massive hepatic necrosis. Typical causes are fulminant viral hepatitis, severe drug-induced liver injury (e.g., from acetaminophen), shock liver or hypoxic hepatitis, and in rare instances, autoimmune hepatitis or acute biliary obstruction.[117]

Ratios of aminotransferases may hold keys to the diagnosis of hepatic disorders. For example, when both AST and ALT are elevated, an AST-to-ALT ratio higher than 4 is characteristic of Wilson's disease, ratios between 2 and 4 are typical of alcoholic liver disease, and a ratio below 1 suggests nonalcoholic steatohepatitis (without cirrhosis). When elevations of AST and ALT are mild, ratios above 2 are consistent with alcoholic liver disease or cirrhosis of any etiology.[117] If the ratio is elevated and ALT is normal, the elevation in AST is most likely from an extrahepatic source of AST.

Although concomitant elevations in AST and ALT are a reliable indicator of hepatocellular injury, aminotransferase levels by themselves seldom reveal the extent of liver damage. For instance, patients with florid liver failure can have normal enzyme levels—when the liver damage is so extensive that too few viable hepatocytes remain to bring about increases in ALT or AST. In addition, chronic, smoldering liver diseases such as hepatitis C can destroy the liver, slowly and silently, without overt increases in ALT or AST.

Lactate Dehydrogenase Elevated serum lactate dehydrogenase (LDH) levels may reflect hepatocellular injury, extrahepatic disorders, or both. Extreme increases signify massive liver damage, which may result from fulminant viral hepatitis, drug-induced liver failure, or hypoxic hepatitis. Prolonged, concurrent elevations in LDH and AP suggest malignant infiltration of the liver. Notable extrahepatic disorders that cause moderate elevations in LDH include hemolysis, rhabdomyolysis, tumor necrosis, renal

Table 17-2 Liver Blood Tests and the Differential Diagnosis of Hepatobiliary Disorders

	Predominant Abnormality		
Blood Test	**Bilirubin Overload (Hemolysis)**	**Hepatocellular Injury**	**Cholestasis**
Aminotransferases	Normal	Increased—may be normal or decreased in advanced stages	Normal—may be increased in advanced stages
Serum albumin	Normal	Decreased—may be normal in acute fulminant hepatic failure	Normal—may be decreased in advanced stages
Prothrombin time*	Normal	Prolonged	Normal—may be prolonged in advanced stages
Bilirubin (main form present)	Unconjugated (also mild increase in conjugates)	Conjugated	Conjugated
Alkaline phosphatase	Normal	Normal—may be increased by hepatic infiltrative disease	Increased
γ-Glutamyl transpeptidase 5′-nucleotidase	Normal	Normal	Increased
Blood urea nitrogen	Normal—may be increased by renal dysfunction	Normal—may be decreased by severe liver disease and normal kidney function	Normal
BSP/ICG (dye)	Normal	Retention of dye	Normal or retention of dye

*Used interchangeably with the international normalized ratio.
BSP/ICG, bromsulphalein/indocyanine green.

infarction, acute cerebrovascular accident, and myocardial infarction. Such disorders cause more pronounced LDH elevations in patients with acute liver injury (e.g., severe preeclampsia). An elevation in LDH that is solely due to hepatocellular injury is typically accompanied by elevations in AST and ALT. Thus, LDH rarely yields information about liver injury beyond that already provided by AST and ALT.[27,117]

Glutathione-S-Transferase Glutathione-*S*-transferase (GST) is a sensitive and specific test for some patterns of drug-induced liver injury.[118] The enzyme has a brief plasma half-life (90 minutes) and is released rapidly into the circulation after hepatocellular injury. Thus, serial GST measurements can reveal the time course of hepatic injury, from its onset to its resolution. In contrast to AST and ALT, which reside in acinar zone 1, GST localizes in acinar zone 3 (centrilobular region).[119] The zone contains the hepatocyte population with the highest susceptibility to injury from hypoxia or reactive drug metabolites. Accordingly, GST would be more sensitive than AST or ALT as a marker of centrilobular necrosis in its incipient stages.

Assessment of Hepatic Protein Synthesis

Serum Albumin Serum albumin yields information about hepatocellular function (i.e., protein synthesis) and is used to evaluate chronic liver disease—with notable caveats. First, hypoalbuminemia has many causes besides low rates of albumin synthesis; examples include renal losses of albumin, increased albumin catabolism, expansion of plasma volume, and maldistribution of total body albumin. In fact, the total body mass of albumin (in the exchangeable pool) is often normal in patients with liver cirrhosis, ascites, and hypoalbuminemia.[120] Second, there is no clear relationship between serum albumin and the instantaneous rate of albumin synthesis because plasma albumin has a half-life of nearly 3 weeks. Thus, if hepatic protein synthesis came to an abrupt and permanent halt, this change would not be reflected as a decrease in the serum albumin level for at least a few days.

Prothrombin Time When compared with albumin, liver-derived procoagulants have short half-lives, which range from 4 hours for factor VII to 4 days for fibrinogen. Plasma levels of such procoagulants start to descend shortly after the liver begins to fail. PT (or the international normalized ratio [INR]) is widely used to evaluate and monitor patients with acute liver dysfunction. A prolonged PT secondary to liver failure generally reflects a low blood level of factor VIIa, which has the shortest plasma half-life of hepatic coagulant factors.[117] Besides diagnostic utility, PT is used as a prognostic indicator. It is a common parameter of models or algorithms designed to facilitate timely, yet correct decisions about the need for liver transplantation. In this regard, PT is of value for patients with drug-induced liver failure[121] or those with active liver disease and a surgical condition that needs immediate attention.[122]

Detection of Cholestatic Disorders

Alkaline Phosphatase Serum AP is used to screen for disorders of the liver or biliary tree, including hepatitis, malignancies, and cholestatic diseases. Because AP isoenzymes exist in plasma membranes throughout the body, AP lacks specificity for hepatobiliary disease.[117] Mild, transient increases in AP may occur in up to a third of those subjected to routine laboratory testing. Major sources of AP include bone, intestine, kidney, leukocytes, placenta (third trimester of gestation), and neoplasms. Increased metabolic activity in one or more of these tissues may lead to elevations in AP. Increased serum AP usually reflects increased production or release of AP rather than decreased clearance of AP. For example, fatty meals increase serum AP by inducing the release of AP isozymes from the plasma membranes of enterocytes in the small bowel.

The AP elevations in cholestatic disorders may reflect the action of bile salt on the plasma membranes of hepatocytes. Serum AP may remain normal for a couple of days after the onset of biliary obstruction—not increasing until hepatocytes produce (and release) more AP. Because it has a half-life of nearly a week, serum AP may remain elevated for days after bile flow is restored.[117] Extreme increases in AP suggest (1) a major block in biliary flow as a result of disorders such as primary biliary cirrhosis and choledocholithiasis or (2) a hepatic malignancy (primary or metastatic) that is compressing small intrahepatic bile ducts. Multifocal blocks of intrahepatic ducts can increase serum AP without increasing serum bilirubin. On the other hand, AP may be normal despite extensive hepatic metastasis or large duct obstruction. The bottom line is that serum AP does not reliably distinguish between bile duct obstruction (intrahepatic or extrahepatic) and malignant infiltration of the liver.[117]

IDENTIFYING THE SOURCE OF INCREASED ALKALINE PHOSPHATASE. Finding the origin of an elevated AP level seldom requires more than a history, physical examination, and imaging studies. The history helps sort through the usual extrahepatic sources of increased AP, including (1) normal bone, especially during puberty and growth spurts; (2) placenta, mainly in the third trimester of pregnancy; (3) bone disorders such as Paget's disease, rickets, and osteomalacia; and (4) intestines (see Table 17-2).

5′-Nucleotidase and γ-Glutamyl Transpeptidase Laboratory tests used to distinguish between hepatic and extrahepatic sources of AP include 5′-nucleotidase (5′-NT) or leucine aminopeptidase (LAP) and GGTP. With regard to 5′-NT, it is as sensitive as AP in detecting hepatobiliary disorders, and it is a much more specific test for such disorders. Although 5′-NT exists in many tissues—placenta, bone, brain, intestine, heart, blood vessels, endocrine pancreas—most of the serum 5′-NT is derived from the hepatobiliary tree. One explanation is that release of 5′-NT from the plasma membranes of hepatocytes requires the detergent action of bile salts. Changes in AP that are secondary to hepatobiliary disease are usually followed by commensurate changes in 5′-NT.[117]

However, increases in AP and 5′-NT have differing time courses—most notably during onset and resolution of biliary disease. For example, shortly after bile flow becomes disrupted, serum AP and GGTP begin to increase in tandem, whereas 5′-NT may not change for days.[117] In this regard, GGTP is preferable to 5′-NT because it more closely tracks AP. However, GGTP also has disadvantages. First, it is an inducible microsomal enzyme (e.g., by alcohol, anticonvulsants, warfarin), which may confound interpretation of elevations in serum GGTP. Second, GGTP is less specific than 5′-NT for hepatobiliary disease. Serum GGTP may come from many extrahepatic sites, including the kidney, spleen, pancreas, heart, lung, and brain. Bone, however, contains very little GGTP. Thus, serum GGTP may be used to distinguish between osseous and hepatobiliary sources of AP.[117]

Serum Bilirubin Serum bilirubin is the most widely used test for hepatic excretory dysfunction. Total bilirubin is normally below 1 mg/dL, but up to 10% of healthy adults have higher levels, mainly in the form of unconjugated bilirubin. This is usually a benign condition (Gilbert's syndrome) that reflects genetically low levels of bilirubin UDP-glucuronosyltransferase. Serum bilirubin levels above 4 mg/dL are discernible on physical examination as jaundice—a yellowish discoloration of body tissues. With natural light, scleral icterus is detectable at bilirubin levels of or below 3 mg/dL.[117,123]

Conjugated hyperbilirubinemia generally results from one or two fundamental problems: (1) flow of bile is blocked within the hepatobiliary tree, or (2) hepatocytes produce more bilirubin conjugates than they can efficiently transport into the canalicular space. Massive hemolysis causes unconjugated and conjugated hyperbilirubinemia. Increases in unconjugated bilirubin occur because hepatocytes are presented with more bilirubin than they can conjugate. Increases in conjugated bilirubin result because hepatocytes conjugate bilirubin faster than hepatocellular transporters can secrete them into canalicular bile. Bilirubinuria usually reflects conjugated hyperbilirubinemia. The kidneys readily excrete bilirubin conjugates, whereas unconjugated bilirubin, which binds tightly to plasma albumin, is neither filtered nor excreted by normal kidneys.[117,123]

Testing for Specific Diseases

Targeted testing is used to identify specific hepatic or biliary diseases. Examples include (1) serologic testing to identify viral, microbial, and autoimmune causes[124,125]; (2) genetic testing to diagnose heritable metabolic disorders; and (3) tumor marker assays to detect hepatic malignancies.

Identifying viral markers—antibodies, antigens, and genetic material—is the key for diagnosis of hepatitis from hepatotropic viruses (A, B, C, E) and herpesviruses such as cytomegalovirus and Epstein-Barr virus.[32] Patients infected with hepatitis B or C virus often have markers of immune pathology, including anti–smooth muscle antibodies, antinuclear antibodies, and mixed cryoglobulins.[32,126] Autoimmune hepatitis and hepatitis A virus infection are commonly associated with anti–asialoglycoprotein receptor antibodies. Autoimmune cholangitides have distinctive serologic profiles.[127] For example, antimitochondrial antibodies usually develop with primary biliary cirrhosis[125,128-130] but are typically absent with primary sclerosing cholangitis. Characteristic findings of primary sclerosing cholangitis include anti–smooth muscle and antinuclear antibodies.[125,131,132]

Special tests are needed to confirm diagnoses of inborn errors of metabolism. Tests for α_1-AT deficiency include serum α_1-AT and phenotype analysis. Hallmarks of Wilson's disease (an autosomal recessive disorder of copper overload) include low serum ceruloplasmin and high urinary copper levels, particularly after the administration of penicillamine.

Markers for hepatic malignancy include AFP and des-γ-carboxylated prothrombin.[60,133-136] As a test for HCC, plasma AFP is 90% specific; its sensitivity ranges from 50% to 90%, depending on population subgroups.[60] Another test for HCC is the plasma γ-carboxylated prothrombin level. HCC cells usually make procoagulants without γ-carboxylating them.[133,136] High levels of des-γ-carboxylated, vitamin K–dependent proteins occur in up to 91% of patients with HCC. In at least two thirds of these patients, levels are above 300 ng/mL, which far exceeds the typical value in patients with liver cirrhosis or acute hepatitis. After surgical removal of HCC, levels of des-γ-carboxylated factors begin to decrease. Subsequent increases suggest tumor recurrence.[137]

Quantitative Liver Tests

Total hepatocellular mass can be estimated by measuring the clearance of a substance that is avidly extracted by the liver, such as bromsulphalein, indocyanine green (ICG), and rose Bengal.[138] However, these are rough estimations because clearance is subject to many influences and unknowns. For example, hepatic clearance of highly extracted substances (1) changes in direct proportion to variations in liver blood flow, (2) is altered by extrahepatic retention or clearance of the substance, and (3) may be affected by anomalous hepatobiliary function.

Drug-metabolizing capacity of the liver can be measured by several methods, such as caffeine clearance, galactose elimination capacity, aminopyrine breath test, antipyrine clearance, and monoethylglycinexylidide (MEGX).[117,139-142] Techniques are available for measuring caffeine clearance noninvasively.[140] For example, subjects take an oral dose of caffeine (150 to 300 mg), and caffeine metabolites in saliva are measured for up to 24 hours. MEGX is an invasive method that has recently gained popularity for measuring liver blood flow in critically ill patients. Fifteen minutes after an intravenous injection of lidocaine (1 mg/kg), a blood sample is obtained and assayed for MEGX, the major metabolite of lidocaine. Currently, quantitative tests are in the domain of research tools; when compared with standard liver chemistry tests, they are expensive and time consuming, with no compelling evidence of being superior, either diagnostically or prognostically.

Measurement of Liver Blood Flow

Methods used to measure hepatic blood flow fall into three broad categories: clearance techniques, indicator dilution techniques, and direct measurements.

Clearance Techniques

Extraction methods using the indirect Fick principle closely approximate hepatic blood flow and are valid for substances with high intrinsic hepatic clearance and total body clearance. Such substances include ICG dye, propranolol, lidocaine, and colloidal particles. Constant infusion of ICG is among the most reliable extraction methods. Hepatocytes take up nearly all of the ICG infused and excrete it unchanged in bile. Clearance methods may also be based on the ability of Kupffer cells to avidly phagocytose radiolabeled colloidal particles such as gold 198. After injecting such particles, one can compute the area under the initial curve (of radioactivity versus time) to obtain a valid measurement of hepatic blood flow—assuming that the reticuloendothelial system is functioning normally.[143] The bottom line is that severe liver disease renders clearance techniques unreliable because of indeterminable disease-related effects on liver blood flow and hepatic capacity to eliminate substances. The latter decreases in direct proportion to the loss of hepatocellular mass.[144]

Indicator Dilution Techniques

Unlike clearance methods, measurements of liver blood flow by indicator dilution techniques are unaffected by liver disease. After a radiolabeled indicator (e.g., iodinated albumin) is injected into the spleen, hepatic flow is computed from indicator dilution curves. These curves are obtained by continuous sampling from one of the hepatic veins or by external γ-scintillation counting. For this technique to be valid, the indicator must be uniformly mixed upon injection and resistant to hepatic clearance.[145]

Direct Measurements

Electromagnetic flow probes provide direct measurements of blood flow through the hepatic artery or portal vein.[146] However, the surgical procedures used to implant the probes can themselves alter hepatic blood flow. Thus, the probes are often left in place after the implantation procedure, and blood flow is subsequently measured via telemetry.

Radiologic and Endoscopic Methods

Radiologic and endoscopic techniques offer therapeutic alternatives to surgery. Endoscopic retrograde cholangiopancreatography (ERCP) and percutaneous transhepatic cholangiography (PTHC) are used to evaluate hepatobiliary disorders. ERCP provides intraductal access to the biliary tree and pancreatic duct. Its main use is to diagnose and treat extrahepatic biliary disorders such as gallstones, tumors, inflammatory strictures, or postsurgical anastomotic leaks. Successful endoscopic papillotomy can obviate surgical removal of stones in the common bile duct.[147] ERCP is less invasive than surgery, but it too can lead to major complications, most notably pancreatitis. Radionuclide and ultrasonic scanning detect space-occupying lesions of the hepatobiliary tree.[147,148] PTHC provides a means of evaluating the intrahepatic bile ducts of patients with unexplained intrahepatic cholestasis or jaundice. Dilated intrahepatic bile ducts on PTHC indicate mechanical blockage of intrahepatic ducts. When no such blockage exists, the most likely cause of intrahepatic cholestasis is hepatic parenchymal disease.

Esophagogastroscopy is an important technique for evaluating and treating submucosal varices in patients with cirrhosis and portal hypertension. Splenoportography provides information about the status of the splenic and portal veins. Portal venography, via three-dimensional computed tomography with a multidetector row technique, can render vascular maps that are superior to those obtained by classic angiography.[149] Such vascular maps show the extent and location of portosystemic collateral communications, which may include abnormalities in gastric, paraumbilical, and abdominal wall veins; esophageal varices; and splenorenal and gastrorenal shunts.

Hepatic Pathophysiology

Mechanisms of Cell Death

Necrosis

Hepatocellular death often results from hypoxia or anoxia. Hypoxia decreases intracellular ATP. This stimulates breakdown of glycogen and anaerobic glycolysis, which raises lactic acid levels and lowers intracellular pH. Sudden, precipitous decreases in ATP initiate a series of events that may culminate in hepatocellular necrosis. Such events include abrupt failure of the energy-dependent ion pumps that regulate intracellular fluid and electrolyte homeostasis. Plasma membranes become dysfunctional, and hepatocytes swell rapidly and then rupture and extrude their contents. This cellular debris, which contains hepatic enzymes and reactive chemicals such as aldehydes, lipid peroxides, and eicosanoids, incites an inflammatory response. The release of cytokines and chemoattractants recruits circulating neutrophils to the liver and augments the hepatic inflammation.

Apoptosis

In contrast to necrosis, apoptosis is an energy-dependent process. Most agents of liver disease (toxins, viruses, oxidants) can activate proapoptotic intracellular signaling pathways or proapoptotic cell-surface receptors such as Fas, tumor necrosis factor receptor (TNFR), and other members of the TNFR superfamily.

Apoptosis has several ultrastructural hallmarks, including (1) a shrunken cell and nucleus; (2) condensed, marginated nuclear chromatin; (3) blebs on the plasma membrane; and (4) apoptotic bodies, which consist of membrane-bound cellular fragments and intact organelles. Epithelial and mesenchymal cells engulf the apoptotic bodies, and their lysosomes digest and recycle the contents of apoptotic bodies, such as intact mitochondria and nucleic acids. Apoptosis and necrosis may be related events at opposite ends of a spectrum of overlapping morphologic and mechanistic cell death processes.[85,150]

Oxidative Stress and the Glutathione System

Hepatocytes continuously produce reactive oxygen species. During aerobic metabolism, mitochondria work nonstop transferring electrons from reduced substrates to molecular oxygen (O_2). This process involves the tetravalent reduction of O_2; the reduced oxygen atoms are incorporated into water. However, small amounts of O_2 undergo univalent or divalent reductions that give rise to superoxide and hydrogen peroxide.[151] Nonparenchymal cells in the liver—Kupffer cells, endothelial cells, polymorphonuclear leukocytes, macrophages—can also generate large amounts of reduced oxygen species and nitro-radicals.[86,152-154]

In health, hepatocytes have many ways to keep oxidant concentrations within a safe range (<1 μM).[90,155] Their defenses against oxidative injury include (1) micronutrients, such as vitamins C and E; (2) metal-sequestering proteins, such as ferritin; (3) enzymes that dispose of reactive oxygen species, such as catalase and superoxide dismutase; (4) enzymes that detoxify lipid peroxides, such as glutathione peroxidase; and (5) thiol-rich peptides, most notably glutathione (γ-glutamyl-cysteine-glycine). Glutathione is the single most important intracellular antioxidant.[150,156-160]

The liver is the main site of glutathione synthesis. Accordingly, hepatocytes have high cytoplasmic concentrations of glutathione, ranging from 5 to 10 mmol/L.[90] Glutathione serves as a cofactor for major enzymes involved in the elimination of oxidants—notably glutathione peroxidase and thiol/disulfide exchangers. Glutathione peroxidase plays a key role as a detoxifier of organic peroxides and free radicals. Another enzyme, GST, helps eliminate toxic electrophiles by attaching them to the free thiol of reduced glutathione (GSH). GSH also participates in nonenzymatic detoxification reactions, which yield oxidized glutathione (GSSG) and mixed disulfides of glutathione and protein.

GSH is the predominant form of glutathione under normal conditions; it is the main determinant of the redox capacity of hepatocytes. Oxidative stress decreases GSH levels by converting GSH to GSSG. The enzyme glutathione reductase helps regenerate GSH and restore the normal redox state. NADPH is the cofactor for glutathione reductase, and its synthesis requires ATP. High-energy phosphates are also needed to actively transport GSH into mitochondria. Disruption of this transport process leads to mitochondrial damage.[150] Thus, conditions that decrease ATP render hepatocytes more susceptible to oxidative injury.[156] Adverse conditions, such as malnutrition, hepatitis, and chemically induced liver injury, can quickly exhaust hepatic GSH. In such instances, therapy with thiol-rich agents such as cysteamine (mercaptoethylamine) or *N*-acetylcysteine may be lifesaving. The beneficial effects of thiol-rich agents relate to their ability to increase glutathione synthesis, replenish the intracellular GSH pool, and restore the capacity of the liver to combat oxidative stress.[156]

Ischemia-Reperfusion Injury

Ischemia-reperfusion (I/R) injury results from both hypoxia during an ischemic episode and cytotoxic events during reperfusion.[153,161-163] Reperfusion induces the production of highly reactive chemicals that can cause necrosis or apoptosis, such as superoxide, hydrogen peroxide, and hydroxyl radicals. After relatively brief ischemic intervals, most of the injury is due to reperfusion. With more prolonged ischemia, hypoxia accounts for a larger fraction of the overall injury from I/R.

Role of Xanthine Dehydrogenase/Xanthine Oxidase

The liver and intestines contain large amounts of xanthine dehydrogenase/xanthine oxidase (XDH/XO).[164] XDH catalyzes the rate-limiting step in nucleic acid degradation by using nicotinamide adenine dinucleotide (NAD) rather than O_2 as the electron acceptor. Thus, no oxygen radicals are produced in healthy tissue. However, ischemic conditions transform XDH to XO. Because XO reactions involve O_2, they produce free radicals. During reperfusion, XO-derived oxidants increase the production and release of leukotriene B_4 and platelet-activating factor, which promote neutrophil adherence and migration. When activated, neutrophils can wreak havoc on the microvascular circulation as they release proteases and physically disrupt the endothelial barrier. Liver injury, independent of the cause, imperils extrahepatic tissue because damaged hepatocytes spew out XO and other inflammatory mediators.[151,155,165-170] XO enters the bloodstream and binds to vascular endothelial cells in many organs.[164,171-173] Endothelial cells produce superoxide, which reacts with nitric oxide (NO·) to form peroxynitrite ($OONO^-$).[152,174] Peroxynitrite is intensely reactive and can increase the severity of injuries to local and remote tissues.

Therapeutic agents that may confer protection from I/R-induced injury include (1) antioxidants, (2) oxygen radical scavengers such as superoxide dismutase and dimethyl sulfoxide, (3) inhibitors of leukocyte adherence and migration,[175-177] and (4) inhibitors of XO. For example, laboratory studies show that allopurinol (inhibits XO) treatment before induction of I/R prevents the usual I/R-related increases in microvascular permeability and epithelial cell necrosis.[175,178]

Hepatic Injury from Liver Transplantation

Preservation Injury. The University of Wisconsin solution protects the donor liver for about 1 day. However, use of this solution for more than 24 hours may lead to microcirculatory disturbances (e.g., leukocyte and platelet adhesion) after liver transplantation. The adverse effects result from (1) depletion of hepatocellular antioxidants over time and (2) biochemical changes that lead to a profusion of reactive oxidants during reperfusion of the transplanted liver.[178] Hypothermic preservation solutions also induce apoptotic changes in endothelial cells, which may engineer their destruction after graft implantation.

The pathogenesis of I/R injury is complex.[179-182] Characteristic events include (1) Kupffer cell activation[183,184]; (2) XO formation[170,185]; (3) profusion of oxidants—superoxide, nitric oxide, peroxynitrite, and hydroxyl radicals; (4) release of proinflammatory cytokines into the bloodstream[186]; and (5) destruction of endothelial cells.[187-190] Flushing grafts (after storage in preservation solution) with various rinse solutions can decrease Kupffer cell activation, reduce endothelial cell damage, and improve graft survival.[191] Contents of the Carolina rinse solution include antioxidants, adenosine, a calcium channel blocker, energy substrates, and glycine, at pH 6.5. Another way to improve graft survival might be through downregulation of Kupffer cells with agents such as pentoxifylline, gadolinium, or calcium channel blockers.

Bacterial, Viral, and Immune Injury

Endotoxins are lipopolysaccharide complexes of the outer membranes of gram-negative bacteria. All endotoxins have a common lipid component (lipid A), a core R antigen, and two variable polysaccharide regions—bacterial strain-specific O-antigen. Lipid A binds to high-density lipoproteins in blood and other tissues, and it mediates the biologic actions common to endotoxins. Endotoxins bind more extensively to Kupffer cells than to hepatic parenchyma. They can induce hepatocellular or cholestatic injury directly or indirectly via activation of Kupffer cells and release of proinflammatory mediators (e.g., cytokines, eicosanoids).[192]

Like endotoxins, viruses may cause direct and indirect hepatocellular injury. Hepatotropic viruses and some herpesviruses can induce cytokine production leading to lymphocyte- or macrophage-dependent cytotoxicity. Antigens on hepatocellular membranes may be primary targets of cell-mediated injury. Antibodies to such antigens are often increased selectively in patients with autoimmune hepatitis and primary biliary cirrhosis. Other potential antigenic focuses for cell-mediated cytotoxicity include liver-specific lipoproteins and hepatic lectins, which may be targets in hepatitis B and other liver diseases.

Drug-Induced Liver Injury

Adverse reactions to drugs fall into two general categories: dose-related toxicity and idiosyncratic drug-induced injury. The former is predictable and develops in all individuals with escalation of the drug dose. The latter is a rare event, inducible with subclinical doses of the drug; it is most likely an immune-mediated injury that occurs in just a tiny fraction of those receiving the drug.

Although obvious differences exist between the two categories of drug reactions, there are also remarkable similarities. For example, both categories involve covalent binding of drugs (or their metabolites) to endogenous macromolecules. Such binding can lead to inactivation of important enzymes, depletion of intracellular antioxidants, and peroxidation of membrane lipids. The body's response to such molecular perturbations determines whether a drug-induced injury is categorized as dose related or idiosyncratic. When drug-induced subcellular damage induces immune sensitization, re-exposure to even a very low dose of the sensitizing drug can cause severe liver injury (e.g., halothane hepatitis).

The hepatotoxic effects of drugs and environmental substances usually involve CYP-mediated production of oxidants such as reduced oxygen species, carbon-based radicals, and nitroradicals. Examples include (1) carbon tetrachloride metabolism via CYP, which yields trichloromethyl radical—a highly toxic intermediate that induces centrilobular necrosis; and (2) metabolism of nitrofurantoin or other aromatic compounds, which generates free radical intermediates that induce hepatic injury. Similar to CYP of the smooth endoplasmic reticulum, mitochondrial electron transporters transform xenobiotics to reactive metabolites. For example, the nitro-radicals that form during cocaine or nitrofurantoin metabolism[90,150] reduce O_2 via flavoprotein reductases to yield superoxide and other oxidizing species. Redox cycling, as occurs with anthracycline chemotherapeutics and imidazole antimicrobials, is yet another source of toxic oxidizing species.

Oxidant formation during drug metabolism contributes to or causes liver injury by weakening the antioxidant defenses of hepatocytes. For example, acetaminophen and bromobenzene cause dose-related decreases in hepatocellular GSH, rendering the liver increasingly susceptible to necrosis.[193,194] This increases the likelihood of oxidants damaging (1) proteins and enzymes, (2) phospholipids in membranes, and (3) nucleotides via activation of proteases, phospholipases, and endonucleases. Oxidative stress can also induce pathologic increases in cytosolic Ca^{2+} by increasing Ca^{2+} uptake by hepatocytes while inducing release of Ca^{2+} from the endoplasmic reticulum or mitochondria. These events can lead to apoptosis, necrosis, or both.

Occasionally, conjugation reactions generate hepatotoxic by-products.[95,195-197] For example, phase 2 metabolism of carboxylate drugs yields acyl glucuronides. These molecules can induce hepatic injury as they covalently bind to and inactivate nucleophiles, thiol-rich proteins, and nucleic acids. Intermediates of phase 2 metabolism can also deplete hepatocellular antioxidants and promote the formation of neoantigens and autoantigens, which trigger immune-mediated liver injury after re-exposure to the inciting agent.

Drug-Induced Apoptosis

Apoptotic pathways can be activated by drug-induced mitochondrial injury.[150,156,198] The sequence of events may be as follows: (1) drug metabolism produces oxidants and depletes GSH; (2) oxidants induce mitochondrial injury, with release of cytochrome *c* and initiation of the mitochondrial membrane permeability transition; and (3) caspase is activated and triggers apoptosis.[198-201] The hepatic pathology of Reye's syndrome may involve mitochondrial injury from drugs such as tetracycline, aspirin, valproic acid, and nucleoside analogs (e.g., zidovudine).[201] Mitochondrial enzymes are likely to be pathogenic targets of *N*-acetyl-*p*-benzoquinone imine (NAPQI), the acetaminophen metabolite associated with hepatocellular necrosis. Whether mitochondrial injury will lead to apoptosis or necrosis depends on the intracellular energy state and the severity of the injury.[150]

Immunopathology

Immunopathology often underlies idiosyncratic adverse drug reactions, such as halothane hepatitis. The clinical syndrome often includes fever, rash, lymphadenopathy, eosinophilia, and inflammatory infiltrates in the liver. Characteristically, the syndrome has a delayed onset after the first-ever dose of the drug, but with subsequent exposures, the onset is more rapid and the syndrome is more severe. Immunopathologic events may include (1) production of antibodies that lyse hepatocytes via molecular mimicry with host enzymes[202]; (2) antibody-dependent cell-mediated immunity, as with diclofenac[203]; (3) dysregulation of the immune system; and (4) drug-induced autoimmunity.[204,205]

According to the altered-antigen concept, drugs (or their metabolites) chemically react with and thereby modify certain intracellular proteins, which gives rise to neoantigens or antigenic drug-protein adducts. The pathogenesis of halothane hepatitis, for example, seems to involve trifluoroacylated (TFA) adducts that form during exposure to halogenated anesthetics.[206] Patients recovering from halothane-induced liver injury typically have circulating antibodies directed against TFA protein adducts. Yet the specificity and pathogenicity of these antibodies remain unclear[206] because such antibodies develop in most individuals after halothane anesthesia without liver injury developing.

Dysregulation of the immune system contributes to the formation of autoantibodies. Some lack tissue specificity (e.g., antinuclear and smooth muscle antibodies). Others are organ specific, such as the liver-kidney microsomal (LKM) antibodies that target microsomal enzymes; halothane hepatitis is associated with LKM antibodies directed against CYP2E1.

Alcohol-Induced Disease

Alcoholism (five or more drinks per day) induces several patterns of liver injury—notably steatosis (fatty liver), alcoholic hepatitis, and cirrhosis. Steatosis develops in nearly everyone who drinks excessively, but cirrhosis develops in only 10% to 20% of these individuals.[207] When compared with the general population, people with alcoholic liver disease have a higher prevalence of health-related disorders—malnutrition, immune incompetence, fluid and electrolyte imbalance. Such individuals are at increased risk for postoperative morbidity secondary to hemorrhage, sepsis, or cardiopulmonary decompensation (from alcoholic or cirrhotic cardiomyopathy).[208]

Characteristic pathologic findings of alcoholic liver disease include (1) acetaldehyde-induced subcellular injury, (2) abnormalities in metabolism, (3) microvascular hypoxia, (4) increased oxygen and nitrogen radical formation, and (5) depletion of antioxidant defenses. Alcohol metabolism is integral to the pathology of alcoholic liver disease.[209-213] The rate-limiting step in ethanol metabolism is catalyzed by alcohol dehydrogenase (ADH). This polymorphic zinc metalloenzyme has more than 20 different isozymes.[207,214] Although it exists in many tissues, hepatocytes metabolize more than 95% of the alcohol consumed. Genetic polymorphisms of ADH explain much of the variability in the relationship between ethanol consumption (dose) and liver disease (response).[214-216] For example, the risk of alcoholic cirrhosis developing relates directly to polymorphisms at the *ADH2* gene locus (i.e., high frequency of the B allele).[217]

Cytoplasmic ADH is the main enzyme involved in oxidizing ethanol to acetaldehyde. Liver disease can decrease ADH activity and cause a higher proportion of ethanol oxidation to occur in peroxisomes via catalase and in endoplasmic reticulum via ethanol-induced CYP2E1.[218] Liver disease can also depress the mitochondrial enzyme aldehyde dehydrogenase (ALDH), which catalyzes the conversion (detoxification) of acetaldehyde to acetate.[215,218,219] Deficiency of ALDH leads to increased acetaldehyde levels in blood and other tissues, which amplifies the intrahepatic and extrahepatic toxicity of alcohol.[220] Acetaldehyde may induce tissue injury by (1) forming adducts with intracellular proteins,[221] (2) binding to GSH, (3) depleting intracellular antioxidant levels,[222] (4) altering plasma membranes to increase superoxide formation,[223] (5) promoting collagen production and fibroplasia,[224] and (6) stimulating the release of chemotactic agents that recruit neutrophils to the liver.[224,225]

Similarities in Hepatic Injuries from Hypoxia and Ethanol

Hepatic injuries from hypoxic episodes and ingestion of ethanol are similar in many respects. Hypoxic injuries promote the release of proinflammatory cytokines, tumor necrosis factor-α, and interleukin-1 and interleukin-6. These signaling molecules lead to increased expression of adhesion molecules, decreased velocity and increased margination of neutrophils, increased platelet adherence, and decreased hepatic blood flow.[226] Hepatoenteric ischemia releases cytokines and XO and leads to activation of complement. This intensifies the local inflammation and can induce systemic inflammatory responses, with subsequent pulmonary and cardiac injury.[151,155,227,228]

Similarly, alcoholic-related liver injury promotes the release of proinflammatory mediators.[229] Alcohol ingestion can markedly increase hepatic oxygen consumption, which would predispose to hypoxic injury.[207,230] The earliest manifestations of ethanol-induced injury occur in acinar zone 3 (the centrilobular region), which has the highest ADH content and the lowest oxygen supply.[90,218,231,232] Prolonged ethanol use leads to increased expression of NO· synthase, increased NO· production, and vasodilation. Such effects of alcohol on the nitric oxide pathway may represent a microcirculatory adaptive response to ethanol-induced vasoconstriction.[233,234]

The notion that ethanol imposes a significant oxidant stress on hepatocytes is strongly supported by indirect (lipid peroxidation)[235] and direct (electron spin resonance data) evidence.[236] Alcohol stimulates the formation of oxidants, and it disrupts antioxidant defenses. It increases consumption of antioxidants while decreasing their production.[213,235] Alcohol use can decrease the genetic expression of antioxidant enzymes because of its intrinsic hepatotoxicity or because of alcohol-related disorders such as malnutrition.[237] The major source of oxidant formation after alcohol intake is alcohol metabolism rather than alcohol itself. Metabolism of alcohol via microsomal and cytosolic oxidases yields superoxide and other reactive compounds. Such chemicals activate inflammatory cells (including Kupffer cells),[238] which stimulates nitric oxide synthetase (iNOS) and peroxynitrite formation[174] in hepatic parenchymal cells, macrophages, endothelial cells, and vascular myocytes.[239] Peroxynitrite—the product of NO· and $O_2 \cdot^-$ reactions—is an unstable anion that oxidizes and nitrosylates lipids and proteins.[240-244] When intracellular antioxidants such as GSH and α-tocopherol are depleted, alcohol metabolism becomes a more potent inducer of liver injury.[235,245]

Cirrhosis and Portal Hypertension

Liver cirrhosis is a chronic disease in which normal hepatic tissue is replaced by fibrotic scar tissue or regenerative nodules. With advancing hepatic fibrosis, there is progressive loss of liver function, and portal hypertension develops. The usual causes of cirrhosis include alcoholism, viral hepatitis, and metabolic disorders, although many other causes exist.[246] Although the etiologic agents of cirrhosis are disparate, the patterns of injury that they produce are remarkably similar and thus suggest similar or overlapping subsets of molecular mechanisms. Alcoholic- and nonalcoholic steatohepatitis–related cirrhosis involves similar patterns of fibrosis despite its overtly disparate etiologic categories.

Characteristic precirrhotic changes include cellular hypertrophy, fatty metamorphosis, mitochondrial and lysosomal dysfunction, disrupted transport and storage processes, and increased fibroplasia. When hepatocytes throughout the liver are encircled by fibrous tissue, cirrhosis exists.[247]

Cirrhosis can develop and progress in an insidious, indolent manner. Indeed, this is prerequisite for cryptogenic cirrhosis and is characteristic of hepatitis C–induced cirrhosis, which often remains clinically silent while destroying up to 70% of the liver. What enables this to happen is the substantial physiologic reserve of the liver, which compensates well for the progressive loss of viable hepatocytes. The development of portal hypertension signals depletion of this reserve. Signs and symptoms include anorexia, nausea, vomiting, abdominal discomfort, weakness, jaundice, spider nevi, ascites, splenomegaly, a firm liver, esophageal varices, and portosystemic encephalopathy. The pathophysiology of this condition can lead to sudden, devastating complications, including massive hemorrhage, sepsis, renal failure, coma, and death.[248]

Pulmonary Dysfunction

Advanced liver disease often leads to pulmonary dysfunction. Hypoxemia may develop for several reasons.[249,250] First, extensive intrapulmonary arteriovenous communications are common. Second, impairment of hypoxic pulmonary vasoconstriction develops secondary to disease-related increases in endogenous vasodilators such as NO·, glucagon, adenosine, and prostacyclin. Third, erythrocyte 2,3-diphosphoglycerate levels often increase and shift the oxyhemoglobin dissociation curve rightward. Fourth, ventilation-perfusion mismatching occurs because of atelectasis or restrictive pulmonary pathophysiology—secondary to ascites or pleural effusions. In fact, hepatic hydrothorax (pleural effusions without coexisting cardiopulmonary disease) develops in up to 10% of patients with cirrhosis.[251]

Renal Dysfunction

Renal dysfunction typically develops in patients with cirrhosis and portal hypertension. The glomerular filtration rate (GFR) steadily decreases, and the renal tubules avidly retain sodium, with no overt glomerular or tubular injury. Urinalysis is unremarkable except for a low urine sodium level.

The main causes of acute renal failure (ARF) in this patient population are prerenal failure and acute tubular necrosis (ATN).

Prerenal failure usually results from hypovolemia, sepsis, or type 1 hepatorenal syndrome (HRS).[252-255] End-stage liver disease puts patients at high risk for systemic hypovolemia as a result of (1) the formation of profuse ascites, (2) aggressive diuretic therapy, (3) gastrointestinal hemorrhage, and (4) sequestration of blood in the splanchnic vasculature. Therapy for prerenal ARF is straightforward; all that is generally required is to restore renal blood flow.

The most common cause of ATN is prerenal ARF—when it is protracted and severe enough to cause ischemic renal tubular injury. Other causes of ATN include nephrotoxic substances such as radiocontrast agents and nonsteroidal anti-inflammatory drugs. Unlike prerenal ARF, there is no specific therapy for ATN; treatment is mainly supportive.[256]

Prerenal failure secondary to type I HRS has a poor prognosis. In many instances, the only effective therapy is liver transplantation. Interventions that may transiently improve renal performance in such patients include (1) intravenous vasoconstrictors, notably terlipressin, norepinephrine, and midodrine, in combination with octreotide, and (2) devices or procedures that support the liver, such as a molecular adsorbent recirculation system (MARS) or transjugular intrahepatic portosystemic shunt (TIPS).[256-258]

Hematologic Dysfunction

Coagulopathies and other hematologic abnormalities are common with end-stage liver disease.[60] Anemia often develops for many reasons, including gastrointestinal bleeding, hemolysis, hypersplenism, malnutrition, vitamin deficiencies, bone marrow depression, and plasma volume expansion. As the liver begins to fail, it cannot make enough vitamin K–dependent procoagulants. When factor VII drops by 70% of the normal level, the PT becomes prolonged. Thrombocytopenia and thrombopathy develop as a result of (1) splenic sequestration syndrome, (2) bone marrow suppression secondary to alcoholism or medications such as interferon, or (3) platelet destruction from immune-mediated, platelet-associated IgG. Dysfibrinogenemia—the activation of fibrinolysis—may develop. Laboratory results typically include increased D-dimer levels, increased fibrin degradation products, and normal or nearly normal fibrinogen levels. However, before attributing any fibrinolytic disorder to liver failure, it is essential to conduct a thorough search for all possible reversible causes of disseminated intravascular coagulation.

Gastrointestinal Complications

Gastrointestinal hemorrhage is always a concern; nearly a third of cirrhosis-related deaths are due to ruptured esophagogastric varices. Portal hypertensive gastropathy, esophageal varices, or gastric varices develop in most patients with cirrhosis and portal hypertension.[259] Hemorrhage from esophageal varices occurs more often than hemorrhage from gastric varices, but the latter is generally more severe than the former. Variceal size is a good predictor of when varices will rupture, and rates of variceal enlargement parallel the severity of liver disease. Less than 2 years after cirrhosis and portal hypertension are diagnosed, 20% to 30% of patients suffer a variceal hemorrhage.[259] The first hemorrhage is acutely lethal in about 7% of cases, with a 6-week mortality rate of around 30%. Untreated survivors of variceal hemorrhage have a 60% chance of rebleeding within 2 years; if this should occur, the death rate would be 40% to 50%.

Endocrinopathies

Because the liver produces, processes, and metabolizes many endocrine substances, advanced liver disease leads to endocrine abnormalities. For example, plasma levels of glucagon and growth hormone increase with liver disease and contribute to insulin resistance. IGF-I decreases in children with liver disease and adversely affects their growth and development.[80] Gonadal dysfunction develops in men and women because of disruptions in the metabolism of sex hormones. Men undergo feminization, with the development of gynecomastia, testicular atrophy, infertility, and impotence. In women, oligomenorrhea, amenorrhea, and infertility are common.

Central Nervous System Dysfunction

Hepatic encephalopathy is a complex neuropsychiatric syndrome that develops in 50% to 70% of patients with cirrhosis.[252] Pathophysiologic phenomena that contribute to the syndrome include (1) hepatobiliary dysfunction, (2) decreased hepatic blood flow, and (3) extrahepatic diversion of portal venous flow through collateral vessels (i.e., portacaval blood flow). Various gut-derived chemicals, including mercaptans, phenols, ammonia, short-chain fatty acids, and manganese, may play a role in the pathogenesis of hepatic encephalopathy. Central nervous system depression may result from false neurotransmitters (e.g., octopamine) or endogenous ligands that increase central inhibitory outflow, such as activators of GABA benzodiazepine receptors. Other possible contributors to encephalopathy are disruptions of the blood-brain barrier and defective cerebral energy metabolism. The pathogenesis and management of hepatic encephalopathy are described in detail elsewhere.[60,252]

Cardiovascular Dysfunction

A hyperdynamic circulation, with high cardiac output and low total peripheral resistance, is a hallmark of cirrhosis and portal hypertension.[260] Generally, systemic arterial pressure is slightly below normal, the heart rate is mildly increased, and central filling pressure is normal. Mixed venous O_2 saturation is elevated, and the arteriovenous O_2 content gap is low. Overall, the hemodynamic profile resembles a peripheral arteriovenous (AV) fistula. Indeed, advanced liver disease causes extensive, widespread AV communications (collateral vessels) within the splanchnic organs, lungs, muscle, and skin. High blood flow through these collateral vessels may result from cirrhosis-induced increases in endogenous vasodilators, such as glucagon, NO·, vasoactive intestinal polypeptide (VIP), and ferritin.[261-265]

Endogenous vasodilators may also explain why severe liver disease diminishes cardiovascular responses to physiologic and pharmacologic vasoconstrictors.[266] Laboratory studies show that NO·, by itself, can induce quintessential cardiovascular and renal hallmarks of cirrhosis and portal hypertension.[267,268] Experimental models of chronic portal hypertension—via partial portal vein ligation or CCl_4-induced cirrhosis—show that NO· induces elevations in cyclic guanosine monophosphate (cGMP), which correlate directly with peripheral arterial dilation.[268,269] Inhibitors of NO· synthase can (1) prevent the characteristic increases in cardiac output and decreases in vascular resistance, (2) restore plasma aldosterone and arginine vasopressin levels, and (3) correct the derangements in sodium and water excretion. In addition, clinical studies comparing healthy subjects and patients with liver cirrhosis show a positive correlation between exhaled NO· and the cardiac index.[270]

Pathogenesis of Portal Hypertension

Characteristic features of cirrhosis-induced portal hypertension include (1) high resistance to intrahepatic blood flow, (2) high preportal blood flow, and (3) high blood flow through portacaval collateral vessels. The pathogenesis of cirrhosis-induced portal hypertension is complex. Putative mechanisms include the "backward" and "forward" concepts, which are not mutually exclusive. According to the backward concept, proliferating intrahepatic fibrosis leads to increased resistance to the flow of blood through the portal vein; this elevates portal venous pressure (i.e., at constant rates of portal venous flow). Experimental narrowing of the portal vein induces portal hypertension characterized by (1) increased mesenteric vascular resistance, (2) decreased mesenteric blood flow, (3) decreased splanchnic venous oxygen saturation, and (4) an increased AV oxygen content gap of mesenteric blood. However, such changes are exactly opposite those that occur when portal hypertension develops in patients with cirrhosis. The forward concept regarding vasodilation may explain this[271]; portal hypertension develops because of cirrhosis-induced changes in the systemic and splanchnic arterial circulations. The hypothesis is supported by observations in cirrhotic patients, including (1) increased blood levels of endogenous vasodilators, (2) widespread AV shunt formation, and (3) high cardiac output with low total peripheral resistance. Putative mediators of the hyperdynamic circulation include NO·, glucagon, prostacyclin, adenosine, CO, and hydrogen sulfide.[272] These substances not only induce direct vasodilation but may also support the formation and patency of extensive AV shunts (AV fistulas) in the intestines, spleen, and other organs. Activation of K_{ATP} channels in arterial smooth muscle cells may mediate increased blood flow in the systemic and splanchnic arterial circulations.[272]

Control of Circulatory Volume

Avid renal retention of sodium is integral to the pathophysiology of cirrhosis and portal hypertension. Volume receptors that detect low effective plasma volume stimulate the sympathetic nervous system and lead to release of renin from the kidney.[273] This increases the production of angiotensin II and aldosterone, which enhances renal tubular uptake of sodium. Norepinephrine levels in blood correlate inversely with renal blood flow. Both norepinephrine and angiotensin II redistribute intrarenal blood flow in a manner that increases retention of sodium by the kidney. Additional factors that may augment sodium retention include the kallikrein-kinin system and some extremely potent renal vasoconstrictors, such as $F_{2\alpha}$-isprostanes[274] and endothelin. Renal vasoconstrictors are likely inducers of the renal dysfunction that accompanies cirrhosis and ascites. In such settings, endogenous vasodilators (e.g., prostaglandins) become increasingly important to counteract the intense vasoconstriction and protect renal blood flow. Accordingly, inhibitors of prostaglandin synthesis can significantly decrease renal plasma flow and GFR and thereby increase the risk for acute renal injury.

Pathogenesis of Ascites

Cirrhosis-induced portal hypertension leads to massive increases in total body water, edema, and ascites formation.[275] The problem can be traced to excessive sodium retention by the kidney (Fig. 17-13).[2,276] However, the principal driver of the sodium retention is unclear. One explanation—the overflow model—is that hepatic cirrhosis gives rise to chemicals that stimulate the kidney to retain sodium. A second explanation—the underfill model—is that renal retention of sodium is a normal physiologic response to a low effective blood volume.[273]

The essence of the overflow model is that excessive renal retention of sodium causes intravascular volume to expand, with two major and direct consequences: (1) plasma oncotic pressure decreases, with the liver unable to produce sufficient albumin to correct the hypoalbuminemia, and (2) portal hydrostatic pressure increases (i.e., portal hypertension). The combination of low oncotic pressure and portal hypertension accelerates the formation of edema and ascites. A pivotal assumption of the overflow model is that a cirrhosis-induced mediator causes normal kidneys to retain sodium and water despite an overfilled intravascular compartment. At present, no such mediator (or process) has been identified.

The underfill model recognizes that homeostatic reflexes work in concert with the kidney to tightly regulate intravascular volume. This model posits that cirrhosis causes the effective plasma volume to decrease, which activates homeostatic mechanisms to retain sodium and water. As Schrier and Abraham point out,[273] "the integrity of the arterial circulation, as determined by cardiac output and peripheral arterial resistance, is the primary determinant of renal sodium and water excretion." That is, with decreases in arterial volume, whether from arterial dilation or low cardiac output, the kidney is instructed to retain sodium and water. Cirrhosis-induced decreases in effective plasma (or arterial) volume can result from arterial dilation or intravascular volume depletion, or both. Although the latter has many possible causes, edema and ascites formation from unbalanced Starling forces are sufficient to significantly decrease intravascular volume. The overflow and underfill models are not mutually exclusive; a primary defect in sodium excretion could be the major factor in earlier stages of cirrhosis, whereas a low effective plasma volume could be the more important factor in progression to end-stage liver disease.[275]

Cholestatic Disease

Cholestasis refers to impaired biliary flow and has a complex pathogenesis[106,277-295] (Box 17-2). The usual cause of intrahepatic cholestasis, whether inherited or acquired, is dysfunction of the bile transporter.[295,296] In contrast, extrahepatic cholestasis most often results from mechanical blockage of the biliary tree. With cholestasis, there are high blood levels of biliary constituents, including hepatocellular enzymes (AP, GGTP, 5′-NT, LAP),

Box 17-2 Etiology of Intrinsic Cholestatic Disorders

- Drugs[106,279,280]
- Alcoholism[281]
- Pregnancy[282,283]
- Inflammation[284]
- Sepsis[285-287]
- Parenteral nutrition[288,289]
- Primary biliary cirrhosis[290]
- Primary sclerosing cholangitis[291]
- Genetic cholestatic liver diseases[292-295]

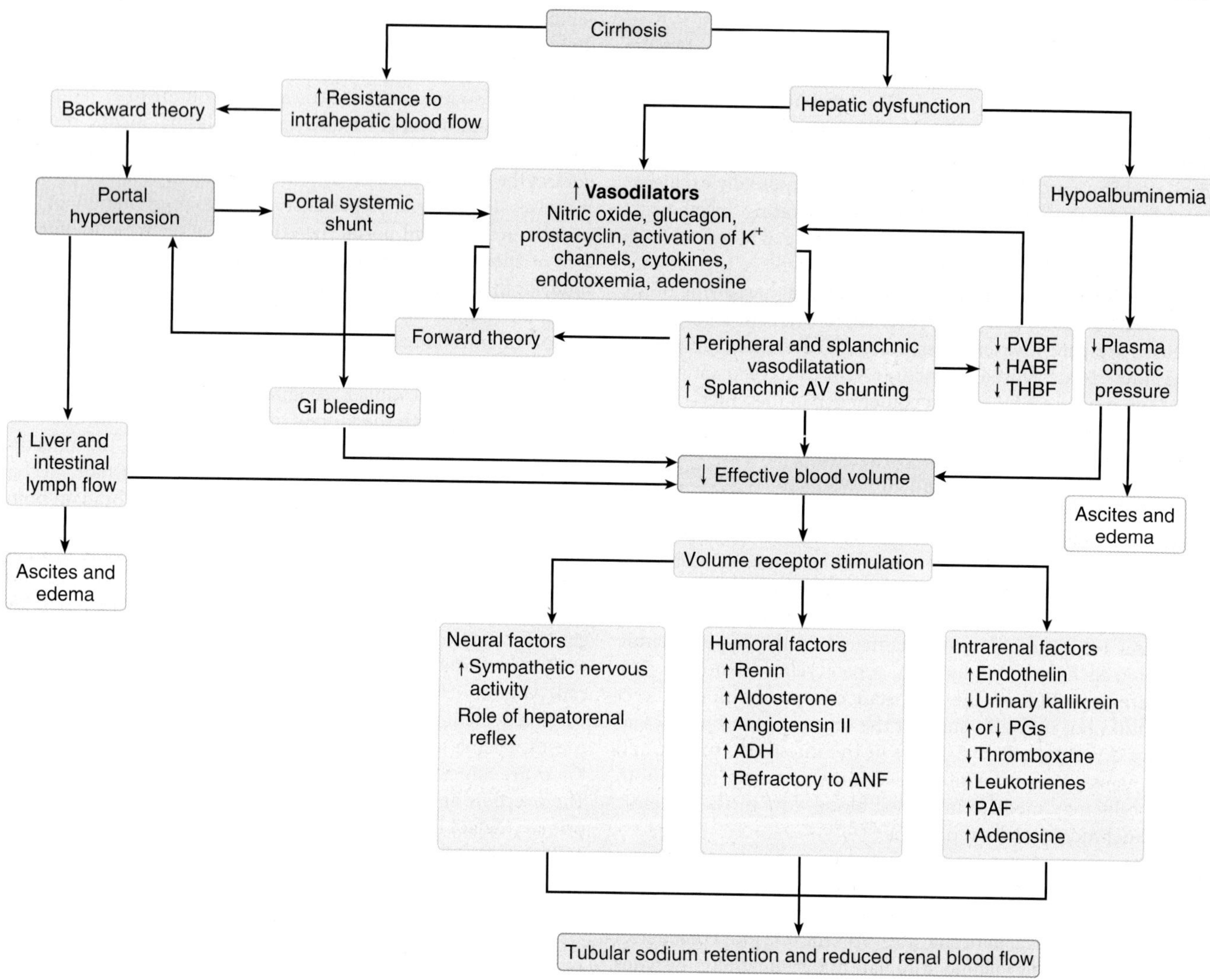

Figure 17-13 Schematic of pathways for cirrhosis-induced portal hypertension: the forward and backward theories. Cirrhosis and portal hypertension induce circulatory changes that decrease effective blood volume. This activates volume receptors and stimulates neurohumoral and intrarenal reflexes, which decreases renal blood flow and increases renal retention of sodium. ADH, antidiuretic hormone; ANF, atrial natriuretic factor; AV, arteriovenous; HABF, hepatic arterial blood flow; PAF, platelet-activating factor; PGs, prostaglandins; PVBF, portal venous blood flow; THBF, total hepatic blood flow. *(Reprinted with permission from Mushlin PS, Gelman S: Anesthesia and the liver.* In *Barash PG, Cullen BF, Stoelting RK [eds]: Clinical Anesthesia, 4th ed. Philadelphia, Lippincott Williams & Wilkins, 2001, p 1088.)*

immunoglobulin A, cholesterol, and various forms of bile salts and bilirubin. The most toxic of these is unconjugated bilirubin; high concentrations of unconjugated bilirubin cause membrane dysfunction and disrupt major metabolic pathways such as the tricarboxylic acid cycle and oxidative phosphorylation. Patients with cholestatic syndromes typically have marked increases in serum bile salts, but normal or slightly elevated serum bilirubin.

The clinical findings in cholestatic syndromes are dependent on the severity of the cholestatic disorder and its pathogenesis.[297-301] Pruritus is a hallmark feature and results mainly from retained bile salts.[277,284,302,303] As cholestatic disorders increase in severity, jaundice develops.[304] The stool becomes lighter in color and the urine darkens as bile pigments are diverted from the gut to the kidney for excretion.

Coagulation Disorders

Enteric absorption of lipids such as vitamin K requires bile salts and an intact enterohepatic circulation. With cholestasis-induced coagulopathies, the liver continues to make procoagulants. However, without vitamin K, hepatocytes cannot add the γ-carboxyl glutamate residues that these procoagulants need for subsequent activation. Parenteral vitamin K should correct this coagulopathy, but if it does not, there must be another cause of the problem. Prolonged cholestasis can induce liver dysfunction and a coagulopathy that would not be cured by vitamin K therapy.

Renal Dysfunction

Cholestatic disorders can cause dysfunction of the splanchnic reservoir. Because the reservoir cannot effectively transfer blood volume to the central circulation, severe hypotension and renal hypoperfusion can result from even mild losses of plasma volume. This predisposes to prerenal ARF and ATN from the prerenal ARF. If liver dysfunction supervenes, ATN may result from unconjugated bilirubin, which can directly cause renal tubular injury.

Cardiovascular Dysfunction

Cholestatic syndromes induce hemodynamic changes that are similar, but less severe than the changes associated with cirrhosis and portal hypertension. Cardiac output increases and peripheral vascular resistance decreases. Portal venous blood flow may decrease as portal venous resistance increases. Yet the mechanisms by which cholestasis alters cardiovascular parameters are incompletely understood and challenging to study for several reasons. First, bile is a heterogeneous fluid with variable compositions and many different forms of bile salts and bilirubin. Second, individual constituents of bile exert dissimilar cardiovascular effects. Third, differing causes of cholestatic syndromes lead to disparate pathophysiologic conditions, which can confound the direct and indirect cardiovascular actions of specific constituents of bile.

The direct cardiac effects of bile salts (primary, conjugated, and secondary) have been studied in isolated heart preparations to obviate concern about the indirect cardiovascular effects of biliary constituents. In isolated ventricular muscle, bile salts, at concentrations similar to those in patients with cholestatic jaundice, exert negative inotropic effects. They decrease (1) peak tension, (2) the maximum rate of tension development, (3) the duration of contraction, and (4) the action potential duration. Electrophysiologic actions of sodium taurocholate, ascertained from voltage clamping of ventricular myocytes, include decreases in the slow inward current and slight increases in the outward potassium current. Taken collectively, these data suggest that bile salts directly induce negative inotropic effects, which could result from altered membrane currents.[305]

Experiments in animals show that high blood levels of bile salts (cholemia) can block the cardiovascular effects of agents such as norepinephrine, angiotensin II, and isoproterenol. It is possible that cholemia exerts such effects by disrupting receptor complexes in plasma membranes.[305-307] On the other hand, acute cholestasis can decrease cardiac contractility without affecting cardiac β-adrenoceptors, as shown in animal studies in which acute cholestasis was induced by bile duct ligation.[306] After experiencing 3 days of extrahepatic cholestasis, myocardial contractility was impaired globally, but β-adrenoceptors were intact.

Studies in animals show that cholestasis can alter homeostatic circulatory reflex responses.[307] For example, removal of 10% of the blood volume of healthy rats had little effect on their arterial blood pressure, whereas removing this same volume of blood from rats with cholestasis caused a 50% decrease in blood pressure. Healthy animals compensated for the blood loss by mobilizing 15% of the blood volume of the pulmonary and splanchnic vasculature; however, animals with cholestasis mobilized only 7% of their pulmonary blood volume, with no contribution from the splanchnic reservoir.[307] These data show that cholestasis induces dysfunction of physiologic blood reservoirs. Whether such laboratory findings are relevant for patients with cholestasis is unclear. A final note of caution about patients with cholestatic disorders is warranted: decompression of the biliary tract, by itself, may lead to significant cardiovascular depression.[308]

References

1. Jones AL: Anatomy of the normal liver. *In* Zakim D, Boyer T (eds): Hepatology: A Textbook of Liver Disease, 3rd ed. Philadelphia, WB Saunders, 1996, p 3.
2. Mushlin PS, Gelman S: Anesthesia and the Liver. *In* Barash PG, Cullen BF, Stoelting RK (eds): Clinical Anesthesia, 4th ed. Philadelphia, Lippincott Williams & Wilkins, 2001, p 1067.
3. Gelman S, Mushlin PS: Catecholamine induced changes in the splanchnic circulation affecting systemic hemodynamics. Anesthesiology 100:434, 2004.
4. Rutkauskas S, Gedrimas V, Pundzius J, et al: Clinical and anatomical basis for the classification of the structural parts of liver. Medicina (Kaunas) 42:98, 2006.
5. Parks RW, Chrysos E, Diamond T: Management of liver trauma. Br J Surg 86:1121, 1999.
6. Gazelle GS, Lee MJ, Mueller PR: Cholangiographic segmental anatomy of the liver. Radiographics 14:1005, 1994.
7. Heriot AG, Karanjia ND: A review of techniques for liver resection. Ann R Coll Surg Engl 84:371, 2002.
8. Cooper AJL: Role of the liver in amino acid metabolism. *In* Zakim D, Boyer T (eds): Hepatology: A Textbook of Liver Disease, 3rd ed. Philadelphia, WB Saunders, 1996, p 563.
9. Zakim D: Metabolism of glucose and fatty acids by the liver. *In* Zakim D, Boyer T (eds): Hepatology: A Textbook of Liver Disease, 3rd ed. Philadelphia, WB Saunders, 1996, p 58.
10. Greenway C, Lautt W: Hepatic Circulation: Handbook of Physiology—The Gastrointestinal System, Motility and Circulation. Bethesda, MD, American Physiology Society, 1989.
11. Campra JL, Reynolds TB: The hepatic circulation. *In* Arias IM, Jakoby WB, Popper H, et al (eds): The Liver: Biology and Pathobiology. New York, Raven Press, 1988, p 911.
12. Greenway CV, Innes IR, Scott GD: Pre- and post-sinusoidal origin of hepatic exudate in anesthetized cats. Can J Physiol Pharmacol 69:1914, 1991.
13. Lautt WW: Mechanism and role of intrinsic regulation of hepatic arterial blood flow: Hepatic arterial buffer response. Am J Physiol 249:G549, 1985.
14. Lautt WW: The 1995 Ciba-Geigy Award Lecture. Intrinsic regulation of hepatic blood flow. Can J Physiol Pharmacol 74:223, 1996.
15. Jakob SM: Splanchnic blood flow in low-flow states. Anesth Analg 96:1129, 2003.
16. Jakob SM: Clinical review: Splanchnic ischaemia. Crit Care (Lond) 6:306, 2002.
17. Richardson PD: Physiological regulation of the hepatic circulation. Fed Proc 41:2111, 1982.
18. Norris CP, Barnes GE, Smith EE, et al: Autoregulation of superior mesenteric flow in fasted and fed dogs. Am J Physiol 237:H174, 1979.
19. Richardson PD, Withrington PG: Liver blood flow. II. Effects of drugs and hormones on liver blood flow. Gastroenterology 81:356, 1981.
20. Richardson PD, Withrington PG: Liver blood flow. I. Intrinsic and nervous control of liver blood flow. Gastroenterology 81:159, 1981.
21. Carneiro JJ, Donald DE: Change in liver blood flow and blood content in dogs during direct and reflex alteration of hepatic sympathetic nerve activity. Circ Res 40:150, 1977.
22. Rappaport AM, Schneiderman JH: The function of the hepatic artery. Rev Physiol Biochem Pharmacol 76:129, 1976.
23. Richardson PD, Withrington PG: The role of beta-adrenoceptors in the responses of the hepatic arterial vascular bed of the dog to phenylephrine, isoprenaline, noradrenaline and adrenaline. Br J Pharmacol 60:239, 1977.
24. Richardson PD, Withrington PG: Glucagon inhibition of hepatic arterial responses to hepatic nerve stimulation. Am J Physiol 233:H647, 1977.
25. Cohen MM, Sitar DS, McNeill JR, et al: Vasopressin and angiotensin on resistance vessels of spleen, intestine, and liver. Am J Physiol 218:1704, 1970.
26. Richardson PD, Withrington PG: The effects of intra-arterial and intraportal injections of vasopressin on the simultaneously perfused hepatic arterial and portal venous vascular beds of the dog. Circ Res 43:496, 1978.
27. Friedman LS, Martin P, Munoz SJ: Liver function tests and the objective evaluation of the patient with liver disease. *In* Zakim D, Boyer T (eds): Hepatology: A Textbook of Liver Disease, 3rd ed. Philadelphia, WB Saunders, 1996, p 791.
28. Schreiber G, Urban J: The synthesis and secretion of albumin. Rev Physiol Biochem Pharmacol 82:27, 1978.
29. Kirsch R, Frith L, Black E, et al: Regulation of albumin synthesis and catabolism by alteration of dietary protein. Nature 217:578, 1968.
30. Kelman L, Saunders SJ, Frith L, et al: Effects of amino acids and hormones on the fractional catabolic rate of albumin by the isolated perfused rat liver. J Nutr 102:1045, 1972.
31. Kew MC: Hepatic tumors and cysts. *In* Feldman M, Friedman LS, Sleisenger MH (eds): Sleisenger & Fordtran's Gastrointestinal and Liver Disease:

Pathophysiology/Diagnosis/Management, 7th ed. St Louis, WB Saunders, 2002, p 1577.
32. Seeff LB: Diagnosis, therapy, and prognosis of viral hepatitis. *In* Zakim D, Boyer T (eds): Hepatology: A Textbook of Liver Disease, 3rd ed. Philadelphia, WB Saunders, 1996, p 1067.
33. Tirone TA, Brunicardi FC: Overview of glucose regulation. World J Surg 25:461, 2001.
34. Galassetti P, Coker RH, Lacy DB, et al: Prior exercise increases net hepatic glucose uptake during a glucose load. Am J Physiol 276:E1022, 1999.
35. Nordlie RC, Foster JD, Lange AJ: Regulation of glucose production by the liver. Annu Rev Nutr 19:379, 1999.
36. Satake S, Moore MC, Igawa K, et al: Direct and indirect effects of insulin on glucose uptake and storage by the liver. Diabetes 51:1663, 2002.
37. Chu CA, Sindelar DK, Igawa K, et al: The direct effects of catecholamines on hepatic glucose production occur via alpha(1)- and beta(2)-receptors in the dog. Am J Physiol 279:E463, 2000.
38. Gustavson SM, Chu CA, Nishizawa M, et al: Interaction of glucagon and epinephrine in the control of hepatic glucose production in the conscious dog. Am J Physiol 284:E695, 2003.
39. Chu CA, Galassetti P, Igawa K, et al: Interaction of free fatty acids and epinephrine in regulating hepatic glucose production in conscious dogs. Am J Physiol 284:E291, 2003.
40. Chu CA, Sherck SM, Igawa K, et al: Effects of free fatty acids on hepatic glycogenolysis and gluconeogenesis in conscious dogs. [erratum appears in Am J Physiol Endocrinol Metab 2002 Oct;283(4):section E following table of contents]. Am J Physiol 282:E402, 2002.
41. Cardin S, Walmsley K, Neal DW, et al: Involvement of the vagus nerves in the regulation of basal hepatic glucose production in conscious dogs. Am J Physiol 283:E958, 2002.
42. Rashid S, Shi ZQ, Niwa M, et al: Beta-blockade, but not normoglycemia or hyperinsulinemia, markedly diminishes stress-induced hyperglycemia in diabetic dogs. Diabetes 49:253, 2000.
43. Cardin S, Emshwiller M, Jackson PA, et al: Portal glucose infusion increases hepatic glycogen deposition in conscious unrestrained rats. J Appl Physiol 87:1470, 1999.
44. Hsieh PS, Moore MC, Neal DW, et al: Importance of the hepatic arterial glucose level in generation of the portal signal in conscious dogs. Am J Physiol 279:E284, 2000.
45. Stolz A: Liver physiology and metabolic function *In* Feldman M, Friedman LS, Sleisenger MH (eds): Sleisenger & Fordtran's Gastrointestinal and Liver Disease: Pathophysiology/Diagnosis/Management, 7th ed. St Louis, WB Saunders, 2002, p 1202.
46. Riou JP, Claus TH, Pilkis SJ: Stimulation of glucagon of in vivo phosphorylation of rat hepatic pyruvate kinase. J Biol Chem 253:656, 1978.
47. Sharma RJ, Rodrigues LM, Whitton PD, et al: Control mechanisms in the acceleration of hepatic glycogen degradation during hypoxia. Biochim Biophys Acta 630:414, 1980.
48. Lewis GF: Fatty acid regulation of very low density lipoprotein production. Curr Opin Lipidol 8:146, 1997.
49. Lewis GF, Vranic M, Harley P, et al: Fatty acids mediate the acute extrahepatic effects of insulin on hepatic glucose production in humans. Diabetes 46:1111, 1997.
50. Lewis GF, Vranic M, Giacca A: Role of free fatty acids and glucagon in the peripheral effect of insulin on glucose production in humans. Am J Physiol 275:E177, 1998.
51. Taghibiglou C, Rashid-Kolvear F, Van Iderstine SC, et al: Hepatic very low density lipoprotein–ApoB overproduction is associated with attenuated hepatic insulin signaling and overexpression of protein-tyrosine phosphatase 1B in a fructose-fed hamster model of insulin resistance. J Biol Chem 277:793, 2002.
52. Lam TK, Carpentier A, Lewis GF, et al: Mechanisms of the free fatty acid–induced increase in hepatic glucose production. Am J Physiol 284:E863, 2003.
53. Chan L, Jackson RL, O'Malley BW, et al: Synthesis of very low density lipoproteins in the cockerel. Effects of estrogen. J Clin Invest 58:368, 1976.
54. Miles JM, Haymond MW, Gerich JE: Suppression of glucose production and stimulation of insulin secretion by physiological concentrations of ketone bodies in man. J Clin Endocrinol Metab 52:34, 1981.
55. Fitz JG: Cellular mechanisms of bile secretion. *In* Zakim D, Boyer T (eds): Hepatology: A Textbook of Liver Disease, 3rd ed. Philadelphia, WB Saunders, 1996, p 362.
56. Dawson PA: Bile secretion and the enterohepatic circulation of bile acids. *In* Feldman M, Friedman LS, Sleisenger MH (eds): Sleisenger & Fordtran's Gastrointestinal and Liver Disease: Pathophysiology/Diagnosis/Management, 7th ed. St Louis, WB Saunders, 2002, p 1051.
57. Leonis MA, Balistreri WF: Inherited metabolic disorders of the liver. *In* Feldman M, Friedman LS, Sleisenger MH (eds): Sleisenger & Fordtran's Gastrointestinal and Liver Disease: Pathophysiology/Diagnosis/Management, 7th ed. St Louis, WB Saunders, 2002, p 1240.
58. Vlahcevic ZR, Heuman DM, Hylemon PB: Physiology and pathophysiology of enterohepatic circulation of bile acids. *In* Zakim D, Boyer T (eds): Hepatology: A Textbook of Liver Disease, 3rd ed. Philadelphia, WB Saunders, 1996, p 376.
59. Radnay PA, Duncalf D, Novakovic M, et al: Common bile duct pressure changes after fentanyl, morphine, meperidine, butorphanol, and naloxone. Anesth Analg 63:441, 1984.
60. Fitz JG: Hepatic encephalopathy, hepatopulmonary syndromes, hepatorenal syndrome, coagulopathy, and endocrine complications of liver disease. *In* Feldman M, Friedman LS, Sleisenger MH (eds): Sleisenger & Fordtran's Gastrointestinal and Liver Disease: Pathophysiology/Diagnosis/Management, 7th ed. St Louis, WB Saunders, 2002, p 1543.
61. Nelsestuen GL, Shah AM, Harvey SB: Vitamin K–dependent proteins. Vitam Horm 58:355, 2000.
62. Sunnerhagen M, Drakenberg T, Forsen S, et al: Effect of Ca^{2+} on the structure of vitamin K–dependent coagulation factors. Haemostasis 26:45, 1996.
63. Berkner KL: The vitamin K–dependent carboxylase. J Nutr 130:1877, 2000.
64. Dowd P, Ham SW, Naganathan S, et al: The mechanism of action of vitamin K. Annu Rev Nutr 15:419, 1995.
65. Furie BC, Furie B: Structure and mechanism of action of the vitamin K–dependent gamma-glutamyl carboxylase: Recent advances from mutagenesis studies. Thromb Haemost 78:595, 1997.
66. Suttie JW: Synthesis of vitamin K–dependent proteins. FASEB J 7:445, 1993.
67. Sugiura I, Furie B, Walsh CT, et al: Propeptide and glutamate-containing substrates bound to the vitamin K–dependent carboxylase convert its vitamin K epoxidase function from an inactive to an active state. Proc Natl Acad Sci U S A 94:9069, 1997.
68. Ponka P: Cell biology of heme. Am J Med Sci 318:241, 1999.
69. Ferreira GC, Gong J: 5-Aminolevulinate synthase and the first step of heme biosynthesis. J Bioenerg Biomembr 27:151, 1995.
70. Daniell WE, Stockbridge HL, Labbe RF, et al: Environmental chemical exposures and disturbances of heme synthesis. Environ Health Perspect 105:37, 1997.
71. Jensen NF, Fiddler DS, Striepe V: Anesthetic considerations in porphyrias. Anesth Analg 80:591, 1995.
72. Ashley EM: Anaesthesia for porphyria. Br J Hosp Med 56:37, 1996.
73. James MF, Hift RJ: Porphyrias. Br J Anaesth 85:143, 2000.
74. Baker SD, Taylor B: Anaesthesia is also risky in patients with porphyria. BMJ 321:1023, 2000.
75. Marks GS, McCluskey SA, Mackie JE, et al: Disruption of hepatic heme biosynthesis after interaction of xenobiotics with cytochrome P-450. FASEB J 2:2774, 1988.
76. Wu L, Wang R: Carbon monoxide: Endogenous production, physiological functions, and pharmacological applications. Pharmacol Rev 57:585, 2005.
77. Bauer M, Bauer I: Heme oxygenase-1: Redox regulation and role in the hepatic response to oxidative stress. Antioxid Redox Signal 4:749, 2002.
78. Morse D, Choi AM: Heme oxygenase-1: The "emerging molecule" has arrived. Am J Respir Cell Mol Biol 27:8, 2002.
79. Shibahara S, Kitamuro T, Takahashi K: Heme degradation and human disease: Diversity is the soul of life. Antioxid Redox Signal 4:593, 2002.
80. Moller S, Becker U: Insulin-like growth factor 1 and growth hormone in chronic liver disease. Dig Dis 10:239, 1992.
81. Rojdmark S, Bloom G, Chou MC, et al: Hepatic insulin and glucagon extraction after their augmented secretion in dogs. Am J Physiol 235:E88, 1978.
82. Laskin DL: Nonparenchymal cells and hepatotoxicity. Semin Liver Dis 10:293, 1990.
83. Dhainaut JF, Marin N, Mignon A, et al: Hepatic response to sepsis: Interaction between coagulation and inflammatory processes. Crit Care Med 29:S42, 2001.
84. Bosch-Morell F, Flohe L, Marin N, et al: 4-Hydroxynonenal inhibits glutathione peroxidase: Protection by glutathione. Free Radic Biol Med 26:1383, 1999.
85. Lemasters JJ: V. Necrapoptosis and the mitochondrial permeability transition: Shared pathways to necrosis and apoptosis. Am J Physiol 276:G1, 1999.
86. Bautista AP, Spitzer JJ: Role of Kupffer cells in the ethanol-induced oxidative stress in the liver. Front Biosci 4:D589, 1999.
87. Bailey SM, Reinke LA: Antioxidants and gadolinium chloride attenuate hepatic parenchymal and endothelial cell injury induced by low flow ischemia and reperfusion in perfused rat livers. Free Radic Res 32:497, 2000.
88. DeLeve LD, McCuskey RS, Wang X, et al: Characterization of a reproducible rat model of hepatic veno-occlusive disease. Hepatology 29:1779, 1999.
89. Mushlin PS, Mushlin SB, Olson RD: Acute liver dysfunction and anesthesia-induced hepatitis. *In* Lobato EB, Gravenstein N, Kirby RR (eds): Complications in Anesthesiology. Philadelphia, Lippincott Wiliams & Wilkens, 2008, p 590.
90. Farrell GC: Liver disease caused by drugs, anesthetics, and toxins. *In* Feldman M, Friedman LS, Sleisenger MH (eds): Sleisenger & Fordtran's Gastrointestinal and Liver Disease: Pathophysiology/Diagnosis/Management, 7th ed. St Louis, WB Saunders, 2002, p 1403.

91. Vessey DA: Metabolism of xenobiotics by the human liver. *In* Zakim D, Boyer T (eds): Hepatology: A Textbook of Liver Disease, 3rd ed. Philadelphia, WB Saunders, 1996, p 257.
92. Estabrook R: An introduction to the cytochrome P450s. Mol Aspects Med 20:5, 1999.
93. Murray M: Induction and inhibition of CYPs and implications for medicine. Mol Aspects Med 20:24, 1999.
94. Hasler JA: Pharmacogenetics of cytochromes P450. Mol Aspects Med 20:12, 1999.
95. Sies H: Oxidative stress: From basic research to clinical application. Am J Med 91:31S, 1991.
96. Sinclair JF, Szakacs JG, Wood SG, et al: Acetaminophen hepatotoxicity precipitated by short-term treatment of rats with ethanol and isopentanol: Protection by triacetyloleandomycin. Biochem Pharmacol 59:445, 2000.
97. Sesardic D, Boobis AR, Edwards RJ, et al: A form of cytochrome P450 in man, orthologous to that formed in the rat, catalyses the *O*-deethylation of phenacetin and is inducible by cigarette smoking. Br J Clin Pharmacol 26:363, 1988.
98. Moore LB, Goodwin B, Jones SA, et al: St. John's wort induces hepatic drug metabolism through activation of the pregnane X receptor. Proc Natl Acad Sci U S A 97:7500, 2000.
99. Goodwin B, Hodgson E, Liddle C: The orphan human pregnane X receptor mediates the transcriptional activation of CYP3A4 by rifampicin through a distal enhancer module. Mol Pharmacol 56:1329, 1999.
100. Moore LB, Parks DJ, Jones SA, et al: Orphan nuclear receptors constitutive androstane receptor and pregnane X receptor share xenobiotic and steroid ligands. J Biol Chem 275:15122, 2000.
101. del Castillo-Olivares A, Gil G: Role of FXR and FTF in bile acid–mediated suppression of cholesterol 7α-hydroxylase transcription. Nucleic Acids Res 28:3587, 2000.
102. Meech R, Mackenzie PI: Structure and function of uridine diphosphate glucuronosyltransferases. Clin Exp Pharmacol Physiol 24:907, 1997.
103. Lee J, Boyer JL: Molecular alterations in hepatocyte transport mechanisms in acquired cholestatic liver disorders. Semin Liver Dis 20:373, 2000.
104. Trauner M, Meier PJ, Boyer JL: Molecular pathogenesis of cholestasis. N Engl J Med 339:1217, 1998.
105. Huang L, Smit JW, Meijer DK, et al: Mrp2 is essential for estradiol-17β(β-D-glucuronide)–induced cholestasis in rats. Hepatology 32:66, 2000.
106. Stieger B, Fattinger K, Madon J, et al: Drug- and estrogen-induced cholestasis through inhibition of the hepatocellular bile salt export pump (Bsep) of rat liver. Gastroenterology 118:422, 2000.
107. George J, Byth K, Farrell GC: Influence of clinicopathological variables on CYP protein expression in human liver. J Gastroenterol Hepatol 11:33, 1996.
108. Whitehouse MW, Beck FJ: Impaired drug metabolism in rats with adjuvant-induced arthritis: A brief review. Drug Metab Dispos 1:251, 1973.
109. Elin RJ, Vesell ES, Wolff SM: Effects of etiocholanolone-induced fever on plasma antipyrine half-lives and metabolic clearance. Clin Pharmacol Ther 17:447, 1975.
110. Alvares AP, Anderson KE, Conney AH, et al: Interactions between nutritional factors and drug biotransformations in man. Proc Natl Acad Sci U S A 73:2501, 1976.
111. Pantuck EJ, Pantuck CB, Weissman C, et al: Effects of parenteral nutritional regimens on oxidative drug metabolism. Anesthesiology 60:534, 1984.
112. Wilkinson GR, Schenker S: Drug disposition and liver disease. Drug Metab Rev 4:139, 1975.
113. Wilkinson GR, Shand DG: Commentary: A physiological approach to hepatic drug clearance. Clin Pharmacol Ther 18:377, 1975.
114. Williams RL, Mamelok RD: Hepatic disease and drug pharmacokinetics. Clin Pharmacokinet 5:528, 1980.
115. Williams RL: Drug administration in hepatic disease. N Engl J Med 309:1616, 1983.
116. Adedoyin A, Branch RA: Pharmacokinetics. *In* Zakim D, Boyer T (eds):Hepatology: A Textbook of Liver Disease, 3rd ed. Philadelphia, WB Saunders, 1996, p 307.
117. Davern TJ, Scharschmidt BF: Biochemical liver tests. *In* Feldman M, Friedman LS, Sleisenger MH (eds): Sleisenger & Fordtran's Gastrointestinal and Liver Disease: Pathophysiology/Diagnosis/Management, 7th ed. St Louis, WB Saunders, 2002, p 1227.
118. Hussey AJ, Aldridge LM, Paul D, et al: Plasma glutathione *S*-transferase concentration as a measure of hepatocellular integrity following a single general anaesthetic with halothane, enflurane or isoflurane. Br J Anaesth 60:130, 1988.
119. Redick JA, Jakoby WB, Baron J: Immunohistochemical localization of glutathione *S*-transferases in livers of untreated rats. J Biol Chem 257:15200, 1982.
120. Rothschild MA, Oratz M, Zimmon D, et al: Albumin synthesis in cirrhotic subjects with ascites studied with carbonate-^{14}C. J Clin Invest 48:344, 1969.
121. Sussman NL: Fulminant hepatic failure. *In* Zakim D, Boyer T (eds): Hepatology: A Textbook of Liver Disease, 3rd ed. Philadelphia, WB Saunders, 1996, p 618.
122. Aranha GV, Greenlee HB: Intra-abdominal surgery in patients with advanced cirrhosis. Arch Surg 121:275, 1986.
123. Roy-Chowdhury J, Jansen PLM: Bilirubin metabolism and its disorders. *In* Zakim D, Boyer T (eds): Hepatology: A Textbook of Liver Disease, 3rd ed. Philadelphia, WB Saunders, 1996, p 323.
124. Zamanou A, Tsirogianni A, Terzoglou C, et al: Anti–smooth muscle antibodies (ASMAs) and anti-cytoskeleton antibodies (ACTAs) in liver diseases: A comparison of classical indirect immunofluorescence with ELISA. J Clin Lab Anal 16:194, 2002.
125. Strassburg CP, Manns MP: Autoimmune tests in primary biliary cirrhosis. Best Pract Res Clin Gastroenterol 14:585, 2000.
126. Nocente R, Ceccanti M, Bertazzoni G, et al: HCV infection and extrahepatic manifestations. Hepatogastroenterology 50:1149, 2003.
127. Invernizzi P, Crosignani A, Battezzati PM, et al: Comparison of the clinical features and clinical course of antimitochondrial antibody–positive and –negative primary biliary cirrhosis. Hepatology 25:1090, 1997.
128. Long SA, Van de Water J, Gershwin ME: Antimitochondrial antibodies in primary biliary cirrhosis: The role of xenobiotics. Autoimmun Rev 1:37, 2002.
129. Jones DE: Autoantigens in primary biliary cirrhosis. J Clin Pathol 53:813, 2000.
130. Nishio A, Bass NM, Luketic VA, et al: Primary biliary cirrhosis: From induction to destruction. Semin Gastrointest Dis 12:89, 2001.
131. Lacerda MA, Ludwig J, Dickson ER, et al: Antimitochondrial antibody–negative primary biliary cirrhosis. Am J Gastroenterol 90:247, 1995.
132. Czaja AJ: Autoimmune hepatitis. *In* Feldman M, Friedman LS, Sleisenger MH (eds): Sleisenger & Fordtran's Gastrointestinal and Liver Disease: Pathophysiology/Diagnosis/Management, 7th ed. St Louis, WB Saunders, 2002, p 1462.
133. Ajisaka H, Shimizu K, Miwa K: Immunohistochemical study of protein induced by vitamin K absence or antagonist II in hepatocellular carcinoma. J Surg Oncol 84:89, 2003.
134. Fujioka M, Nakashima Y, Nakashima O, et al: Immunohistologic study on the expressions of alpha-fetoprotein and protein induced by vitamin K absence or antagonist II in surgically resected small hepatocellular carcinoma. Hepatology 34:1128, 2001.
135. Cui R, He J, Zhang F, et al: Diagnostic value of protein induced by vitamin K absence (PIVKAII) and hepatoma-specific band of serum gamma-glutamyl transferase (GGTII) as hepatocellular carcinoma markers complementary to alpha-fetoprotein. Br J Cancer 88:1878, 2003.
136. Sugimoto H, Takeda S, Inoue S, et al: Des-gamma-carboxy prothrombin (DCP) ratio, a novel parameter measured by monoclonal antibodies MU-3 and 19B7, as a new prognostic indicator for hepatocellular carcinoma. Liver Int 23:38, 2003.
137. Yamanaka J, Yamanaka N, Nakasho K, et al: Clinicopathologic analysis of stage II-III hepatocellular carcinoma showing early massive recurrence after liver resection. J Gastroenterol Hepatol 15:1192, 2000.
138. Barnes P, Lunzer M, O'Halloran M: Comparative sensitivity of serum cholylglycine concentration and bromsulphalein retention in patients with early and late alcoholic liver disease. Aust N Z J Med 16:785, 1986.
139. Denaro CP, Jacob P 3rd, Benowitz NL: Evaluation of pharmacokinetic methods used to estimate caffeine clearance and comparison with a Bayesian forecasting method. Ther Drug Monit 20:78, 1998.
140. Jover R, Carnicer F, Sanchez-Paya J, et al: Salivary caffeine clearance predicts survival in patients with liver cirrhosis. Am J Gastroenterol 92:1905, 1997.
141. Wahllander A, Mohr S, Paumgartner G: Assessment of hepatic function. Comparison of caffeine clearance in serum and saliva during the day and at night. J Hepatol 10:129, 1990.
142. Schnegg M, Lauterburg BH: Quantitative liver function in the elderly assessed by galactose elimination capacity, aminopyrine demethylation and caffeine clearance. J Hepatol 3:164, 1986.
143. Szabo G, Benyo I, Sandor J, et al: Estimation of the hepatic blood flow in the dog with the Xe^{133} and hydrogen wash-out Au^{190}-colloid uptake techniques and with the electromagnetic flowmeter. Res Exp Med 169:69, 1976.
144. Kraul H, Truckenbrodt J, Sigusch H, et al: [Comparison of ICG elimination with biotransformation of model substances and histological features of liver biopsy in liver diseases.] Gastroenterol J 51:123, 1991.
145. Huet PM, Lavoie P, Viallet A: Simultaneous estimation of hepatic and portal blood flows by an indicator dilution technique. J Lab Clin Med 82:836, 1973.
146. Hopkinson BR, Schenk WG Jr: The electromagnetic measurement of liver blood flow and cardiac output in conscious dogs during feeding and exercise. Surgery 63:970, 1968.
147. Whitcomb DC: Hereditary and childhood disorders of the pancreas, including cystic fibrosis. *In* Feldman M, Friedman LS, Sleisenger MH (eds): Sleisenger & Fordtran's Gastrointestinal and Liver Disease: Pathophysiology/Diagnosis/Management, 7th ed. St Louis, WB Saunders, 2002, p 881.
148. Ostroff JW, LaBerge JM: Endoscopic and radiologic treatment of biliary disease. *In* Feldman M, Fried-

man LS, Sleisenger MH (eds): Sleisenger & Fordtran's Gastrointestinal and Liver Disease: Pathophysiology/Diagnosis/Management, 7th ed. St Louis, WB Saunders, 2002, p 1167.
149. Kang HK, Jeong YY, Choi JH, et al: Three-dimensional multi-detector row CT portal venography in the evaluation of portosystemic collateral vessels in liver cirrhosis. Radiographics 22:1053, 2002.
150. Kaplowitz N: Mechanisms of liver cell injury. J Hepatol 32:39, 2000.
151. Nielsen VG, McCammon AT, Tan S, et al: Xanthine oxidase inactivation attenuates postocclusion shock after descending thoracic aorta occlusion and reperfusion in rabbits. J Thorac Cardiovasc Surg 110:715, 1995.
152. Jaeschke H, Gores GJ, Cederbaum AI, et al: Mechanisms of hepatotoxicity. Toxicol Sci 65:166, 2002.
153. Carden DL, Granger DN: Pathophysiology of ischaemia-reperfusion injury. J Pathol 190:255, 2000.
154. Arai M, Thurman RG, Lemasters JJ: Ischemic preconditioning of rat livers against cold storage–reperfusion injury: Role of nonparenchymal cells and the phenomenon of heterologous preconditioning. Liver Transpl 7:292, 2001.
155. Weinbroum A, Nielsen VG, Tan S, et al: Liver ischemia-reperfusion increases pulmonary permeability in rat: Role of circulating xanthine oxidase. Am J Physiol 268:G988, 1995.
156. Kaplowitz N, Tsukamoto H: Oxidative stress and liver disease. Prog Liver Dis 14:131, 1996.
157. Ursini F, Maiorino M, Roveri A: Phospholipid hydroperoxide glutathione peroxidase (PHGPx): More than an antioxidant enzyme? Biomed Environ Sci 10:327, 1997.
158. Doroshow JH, Akman S, Chu FF, et al: Role of the glutathione–glutathione peroxidase cycle in the cytotoxicity of the anticancer quinones. Pharmacol Ther 47:359, 1990.
159. Michiels C, Raes M, Toussaint O, et al: Importance of Se-glutathione peroxidase, catalase, and Cu/Zn-SOD for cell survival against oxidative stress. Free Radic Biol Med 17:235, 1994.
160. Luo GM, Ren XJ, Liu JQ, et al: Towards more efficient glutathione peroxidase mimics: Substrate recognition and catalytic group assembly. Curr Med Chem 10:1151, 2003.
161. Kim JS, Qian T, Lemasters JJ: Mitochondrial permeability transition in the switch from necrotic to apoptotic cell death in ischemic rat hepatocytes. Gastroenterology 124:494, 2003.
162. Sawaya DE Jr, Brown M, Minardi A, et al: The role of ischemic preconditioning in the recruitment of rolling and adherent leukocytes in hepatic venules after ischemia/reperfusion. J Surg Res 85:163, 1999.
163. Kurose I, Argenbright LW, Wolf R, et al: Ischemia/reperfusion-induced microvascular dysfunction: Role of oxidants and lipid mediators. Am J Physiol 272:H2976, 1997.
164. Yokoyama Y, Beckman JS, Beckman TK, et al: Circulating xanthine oxidase: Potential mediator of ischemic injury. Am J Physiol 258:G564, 1990.
165. Nielsen VG, Tan S, Weinbroum A, et al: Lung injury after hepatoenteric ischemia-reperfusion: Role of xanthine oxidase. Am J Respir Crit Care Med 154:1364, 1996.
166. Nielsen VG, Tan S, Baird MS, et al: Gastric intramucosal pH and multiple organ injury: Impact of ischemia-reperfusion and xanthine oxidase. Crit Care Med 24:1339, 1996.
167. Nielsen VG, Tan S, Baird MS, et al: Xanthine oxidase mediates myocardial injury after hepatoenteric ischemia-reperfusion. Crit Care Med 25:1044, 1997.
168. Nielsen VG, Tan S, Kirk KA, et al: Halothane and xanthine oxidase increase hepatocellular enzyme release and circulating lactate after ischemia-reperfusion in rabbits. Anesthesiology 87:908, 1997.
169. Nielsen VG, Tan S, Brix AE, et al: Hextend (hetastarch solution) decreases multiple organ injury and xanthine oxidase release after hepatoenteric ischemia-reperfusion in rabbits. Crit Care Med 25:1565, 1997.
170. Pesonen EJ, Linder N, Raivio KO, et al: Circulating xanthine oxidase and neutrophil activation during human liver transplantation. Gastroenterology 114:1009, 1998.
171. Tan S, Yokoyama Y, Dickens E, et al: Xanthine oxidase activity in the circulation of rats following hemorrhagic shock. Free Radic Biol Med 15:407, 1993.
172. Radi R, Rubbo H, Bush K, et al: Xanthine oxidase binding to glycosaminoglycans: Kinetics and superoxide dismutase interactions of immobilized xanthine oxidase–heparin complexes. Arch Biochem Biophys 339:125, 1997.
173. Adachi T, Fukushima T, Usami Y, et al: Binding of human xanthine oxidase to sulphated glycosaminoglycans on the endothelial-cell surface. Biochem J 289:523, 1993.
174. Beckman JS, Koppenol WH: Nitric oxide, superoxide, and peroxynitrite: The good, the bad, and ugly. Am J Physiol 271:C1424, 1996.
175. Toledo-Pereyra LH: Liver preservation: Experimental and clinical observations. Transplant Proc 20:965, 1988.
176. Jamieson NV, Sundberg R, Lindell S, et al: The 24- to 48-hour preservation of canine liver by simple cold storage using UW lactobionate solution. Transplant Proc 21:1292, 1989.
177. Marsh DC, Vreugdenhil PK, Mack VE, et al: Glycine protects hepatocytes from injury caused by anoxia, cold ischemia and mitochondrial inhibitors, but not injury caused by calcium ionophores or oxidative stress. Hepatology 17:91, 1993.
178. Adkison D, Hollwarth ME, Benoit JN, et al: Role of free radicals in ischemia-reperfusion injury to the liver. Acta Physiol Scand 548:101, 1986.
179. Jaeschke H, Lemasters JJ: Apoptosis versus oncotic necrosis in hepatic ischemia/reperfusion injury. Gastroenterology 125:1246, 2003.
180. Sindram D, Rudiger HA, Upadhya AG, et al: Ischemic preconditioning protects against cold ischemic injury through an oxidative stress dependent mechanism. J Hepatol 36:78, 2002.
181. Lehnert M, Arteel GE, Smutney OM, et al: Dependence of liver injury after hemorrhage/resuscitation in mice on NADPH oxidase–derived superoxide. Shock 19:345, 2003.
182. Schemmer P, Connor HD, Arteel GE, et al: Reperfusion injury in livers due to gentle in situ organ manipulation during harvest involves hypoxia and free radicals. J Pharmacol Exp Ther 290:235, 1999.
183. Lee YG, Lee SH, Lee SM: Role of Kupffer cells in cold/warm ischemia-reperfusion injury of rat liver. Arch Pharmacol Res 23:620, 2000.
184. Schauer RJ, Bilzer M, Kalmuk S, et al: Microcirculatory failure after rat liver transplantation is related to Kupffer cell–derived oxidant stress but not involved in early graft dysfunction. Transplantation 72:1692, 2001.
185. Radi R, Cassina A, Hodara R: Nitric oxide and peroxynitrite interactions with mitochondria. Biol Chem 383:401, 2002.
186. Warle MC, Farhan A, Metselaar HJ, et al: In vitro cytokine production of TNFα and IL-13 correlates with acute liver transplant rejection. Hum Immunol 62:1258, 2001.
187. Imamura H, Sutto F, Brault A, et al: Role of Kupffer cells in cold ischemia/reperfusion injury of rat liver. Gastroenterology 109:189, 1995.
188. Kerkweg U, Jacob M, De Groot H, et al: Cold-induced apoptosis of rat liver endothelial cells: Contribution of mitochondrial alterations. Transplantation 76:501, 2003.
189. Doeppner TR, Grune T, de Groot H, et al: Cold-induced apoptosis of rat liver endothelial cells: Involvement of the proteasome. Transplantation 75:1946, 2003.
190. Sindram D, Porte RJ, Hoffman MR, et al: Platelets induce sinusoidal endothelial cell apoptosis upon reperfusion of the cold ischemic rat liver. Gastroenterology 118:183, 2000.
191. Lemasters JJ, Thurman RG: Reperfusion injury after liver preservation for transplantation. Annu Rev Pharmacol Toxicol 37:327, 1997.
192. Shedlofsky SI, Israel BC, McClain CJ, et al: Endotoxin administration to humans inhibits hepatic cytochrome P450–mediated drug metabolism. J Clin Invest 94:2209, 1994.
193. Gerson RJ, Casini A, Gilfor D, et al: Oxygen-mediated cell injury in the killing of cultured hepatocytes by acetaminophen. Biochem Biophys Res Commun 126:1129, 1985.
194. Casini A, Giorli M, Hyland RJ, et al: Mechanisms of cell injury in the killing of cultured hepatocytes by bromobenzene. J Biol Chem 257:6721, 1982.
195. Tang W, Stearns RA, Bandiera SM, et al: Studies on cytochrome P-450–mediated bioactivation of diclofenac in rats and in human hepatocytes: Identification of glutathione conjugated metabolites. Drug Metab Dispos 27:365, 1999.
196. Wang M, Dickinson RG: Disposition and covalent binding of diflunisal and diflunisal acyl glucuronide in the isolated perfused rat liver. Drug Metab Dispos 26:98, 1998.
197. Tang W, Borel AG, Abbott FS: Conjugation of glutathione with a toxic metabolite of valproic acid, (E)-2-propyl-2,4-pentadienoic acid, catalyzed by rat hepatic glutathione-S-transferases. Drug Metab Dispos 24:436, 1996.
198. Patel T: Apoptosis in hepatic pathophysiology. Clin Liver Dis 4:295, 2000.
199. Fau D, Lekehal M, Farrell G, et al: Diterpenoids from germander, an herbal medicine, induce apoptosis in isolated rat hepatocytes. Gastroenterology 113:1334, 1997.
200. Haouzi D, Lekehal M, Moreau A, et al: Cytochrome P450–generated reactive metabolites cause mitochondrial permeability transition, caspase activation, and apoptosis in rat hepatocytes. Hepatology 32:303, 2000.
201. Lewis W, Dalakas MC: Mitochondrial toxicity of antiviral drugs. Nat Med 1:417, 1995.
202. Gut J, Christen U, Huwyler J, et al: Molecular mimicry of trifluoroacetylated human liver protein adducts by constitutive proteins and immunochemical evidence for its impairment in halothane hepatitis. Eur J Biochem 210:569, 1992.
203. Kretz-Rommel A, Boelsterli UA: Cytotoxic activity of T cells and non-T cells from diclofenac-immunized mice against cultured syngeneic hepatocytes exposed to diclofenac. Hepatology 22:213, 1995.
204. Bourdi M, Larrey D, Nataf J, et al: Anti-liver endoplasmic reticulum autoantibodies are directed against human cytochrome P-450IA2. A specific marker of dihydralazine-induced hepatitis. J Clin Invest 85:1967, 1990.
205. Lecoeur S, Bonierbale E, Challine D, et al: Specificity of in vitro covalent binding of tienilic acid metabo-

lites to human liver microsomes in relationship to the type of hepatotoxicity: Comparison with two directly hepatotoxic drugs. Chem Res Toxicol 7:434, 1994.

206. Mushlin PS, Gelman S: Liver dysfunction after anesthesia. *In* Benumof JL, Saidman LJ (eds): Anesthesia & Perioperative Complications, 2nd ed. St Louis, CV Mosby, 1999, p 441.

207. Bardag-Gorce F, French BA, Li J, et al: The importance of cycling of blood alcohol levels in the pathogenesis of experimental alcoholic liver disease in rats. Gastroenterology 123:325, 2002.

208. Tonnesen H, Kehlet H: Preoperative alcoholism and postoperative morbidity. Br J Surg 86:869, 1999.

209. Nanji AA, Su GL, Laposata M, et al: Pathogenesis of alcoholic liver disease—recent advances. Alcohol Clin Exp Res 26:731, 2002.

210. Lieber CS: Alcoholic liver injury: Pathogenesis and therapy in 2001. Pathol Biol 49:738, 2001.

211. Lieber CS: Microsomal ethanol-oxidizing system (MEOS): The first 30 years (1968-1998)—a review. Alcohol Clin Exp Res 23:991, 1999.

212. Lieber CS: Cytochrome P-4502E1: Its physiological and pathological role. Physiol Rev 77:517, 1997.

213. Zima T, Fialova L, Mestek O, et al: Oxidative stress, metabolism of ethanol and alcohol-related diseases. J Biomed Sci 8:59, 2001.

214. Bosron WF, Li TK: Genetic polymorphism of human liver alcohol and aldehyde dehydrogenases, and their relationship to alcohol metabolism and alcoholism. Hepatology 6:502, 1986.

215. Ehrig T, Bosron WF, Li TK: Alcohol and aldehyde dehydrogenase. Alcohol Alcohol 25:105, 1990.

216. Ramchandani VA, Bosron WF, Li TK: Research advances in ethanol metabolism. Pathol Biol 49:676, 2001.

217. Sherman DI, Ward RJ, Warren-Perry M, et al: Association of restriction fragment length polymorphism in alcohol dehydrogenase 2 gene with alcohol induced liver damage. BMJ 307:1388, 1993.

218. Panes J, Soler X, Pares A, et al: Influence of liver disease on hepatic alcohol and aldehyde dehydrogenases. Gastroenterology 97:708, 1989.

219. Poupon RE, Nalpas B, Coutelle C, et al: Polymorphism of alcohol dehydrogenase, alcohol and aldehyde dehydrogenase activities: Implication in alcoholic cirrhosis in white patients. The French Group for Research on Alcohol and Liver. Hepatology 15:1017, 1992.

220. Crabb DW, Edenberg HJ, Bosron WF, et al: Genotypes for aldehyde dehydrogenase deficiency and alcohol sensitivity. The inactive ALDH2(2) allele is dominant. J Clin Invest 83:314, 1989.

221. Thiele GM, Miller JA, Klassen LW, et al: Long-term ethanol administration alters the degradation of acetaldehyde adducts by liver endothelial cells. Hepatology 24:643, 1996.

222. Shaw S, Rubin KP, Lieber CS: Depressed hepatic glutathione and increased diene conjugates in alcoholic liver disease. Evidence of lipid peroxidation. Dig Dis Sci 28:585, 1983.

223. Williams AJ, Barry RE: Superoxide anion production and degranulation of rat neutrophils in response to acetaldehyde-altered liver cell membranes. Clin Sci 71:313, 1986.

224. Holt K, Bennett M, Chojkier M: Acetaldehyde stimulates collagen and noncollagen protein production by human fibroblasts. Hepatology 4:843, 1984.

225. Roll FJ, Bissell DM, Perez HD: Human hepatocytes metabolizing ethanol generate a non-polar chemotactic factor for human neutrophils. Biochem Biophys Res Commun 137:688, 1986.

226. Granger DN, Korthuis RJ: Physiologic mechanisms of postischemic tissue injury. Annu Rev Physiol 57:311, 1995.

227. Carden DL, Young JA, Granger DN: Pulmonary microvascular injury after intestinal ischemia-reperfusion: Role of P-selectin. J Appl Physiol 75:2529, 1993.

228. Mulligan MS, Smith CW, Anderson DC, et al: Role of leukocyte adhesion molecules in complement-induced lung injury. J Immunol 150:2401, 1993.

229. McClain C, Hill D, Schmidt J, et al: Cytokines and alcoholic liver disease. Semin Liver Dis 13:170, 1993.

230. Mezey E: Commentary on the hypermetabolic state and the role of oxygen in alcohol-induced liver injury. Recent Dev Alcohol 2:135, 1984.

231. Ito D, Ishii H, Kato S, et al: Significance of alcohol dehydrogenase (ADH) as a marker of hepatic centrilobular injury: A biochemical and immunohistochemical study. Alcohol Alcohol Suppl 1:523, 1987.

232. Nanji AA, Zakim D: Alcoholic liver disease. *In* Zakim D, Boyer T (eds): Hepatology: A Textbook of Liver Disease, 3rd ed. Philadelphia, WB Saunders, 1996, p 891.

233. Oshita M, Takei Y, Kawano S, et al: Endogenous nitric oxide attenuates ethanol-induced perturbation of hepatic circulation in the isolated perfused rat liver. Hepatology 20:961, 1994.

234. Nanji AA, Greenberg SS, Tahan SR, et al: Nitric oxide production in experimental alcoholic liver disease in the rat: Role in protection from injury. Gastroenterology 109:899, 1995.

235. Nordmann R: Alcohol and antioxidant systems. Alcohol Alcohol 29:513, 1994.

236. Reinke LA, Kotake Y, McCay PB, et al: Spin-trapping studies of hepatic free radicals formed following the acute administration of ethanol to rats: In vivo detection of 1-hydroxyethyl radicals with PBN. Free Radic Biol Med 11:31, 1991.

237. Nanji AA, Griniuviene B, Sadrzadeh SM, et al: Effect of type of dietary fat and ethanol on antioxidant enzyme mRNA induction in rat liver. J Lipid Res 36:736, 1995.

238. Rosser BG, Gores GJ: Liver cell necrosis: Cellular mechanisms and clinical implications. Gastroenterology 108:252, 1995.

239. Wang JF, Greenberg SS, Spitzer JJ: Chronic alcohol administration stimulates nitric oxide formation in the rat liver with or without pretreatment by lipopolysaccharide. Alcohol Clin Exp Res 19:387, 1995.

240. Skinner KA, White CR, Patel R, et al: Nitrosation of uric acid by peroxynitrite. Formation of a vasoactive nitric oxide donor. J Biol Chem 273:24491, 1998.

241. Beckman JS: Protein tyrosine nitration and peroxynitrite. FASEB J 16:1144, 2002.

242. Beckman JS: -OONO: Rebounding from nitric oxide. Circ Res 89:295, 2001.

243. Reiter CD, Teng RJ, Beckman JS: Superoxide reacts with nitric oxide to nitrate tyrosine at physiological pH via peroxynitrite. J Biol Chem 275:32460, 2000.

244. Beckman JS, Beckman TW, Chen J, et al: Apparent hydroxyl radical production by peroxynitrite: Implications for endothelial injury from nitric oxide and superoxide. Proc Natl Acad Sci U S A 87:1620, 1990.

245. Lauterburg BH, Davies S, Mitchell JR: Ethanol suppresses hepatic glutathione synthesis in rats in vivo. J Pharmacol Exp Ther 230:7, 1984.

246. Quinn PG, Johnston DE: Detection of chronic liver disease: Costs and benefits. Gastroenterologist 5:58, 1997.

247. McCaughan GW, Gorrell MD, Bishop GA, et al: Molecular pathogenesis of liver disease: An approach to hepatic inflammation, cirrhosis and liver transplant tolerance. Immunol Rev 174:172, 2000.

248. Chung RT, Jaffe DL, Friedman LS: Complications of chronic liver disease. Crit Care Clin 11:431, 1995.

249. Rakela J, Krowka MJ: Cardiovascular and pulmonary complications of liver disease. *In* Zakim D, Boyer T (eds): Hepatology: A Textbook of Liver Disease, 3rd ed. Philadelphia, WB Saunders, 1996, p 675.

250. Daoud FS, Reeves JT, Schaefer JW: Failure of hypoxic pulmonary vasoconstriction in patients with liver cirrhosis. J Clin Invest 51:1076, 1972.

251. Lazaridis KN, Frank JW, Krowka MJ, et al: Hepatic hydrothorax: Pathogenesis, diagnosis, and management. Am J Med 107:262, 1999.

252. Jalan R, Hayes PC: Hepatic encephalopathy and ascites. Lancet 350:1309, 1997.

253. Arroyo V, Gines P: Mechanism of sodium retention and ascites formation in cirrhosis. J Hepatol 17:S24, 1993.

254. Moreau R: Hepatorenal syndrome in patients with cirrhosis. J Gastroenterol Hepatol 17:739, 2002.

255. Moore KP, Wong F, Gines P, et al: The management of ascites in cirrhosis: Report on the consensus conference of the International Ascites Club. Hepatology 38:258, 2003.

256. Moreau R, Lebrec D: Acute renal failure in patients with cirrhosis: Perspectives in the age of MELD. Hepatology 37:233, 2003.

257. Lotterer E, Wengert A, Fleig WE: Transjugular intrahepatic portosystemic shunt: Short-term and long-term effects on hepatic and systemic hemodynamics in patients with cirrhosis. Hepatology 29:632, 1999.

258. Wolff B, Machill K, Schumacher D, et al: MARS dialysis in decompensated alcoholic liver disease: A single-center experience. Liver Transpl 13:1189, 2007.

259. de Franchis R, Primignani M: Natural history of portal hypertension in patients with cirrhosis. Clin Liver Dis 5:645, 2001.

260. Vaughan RB, Chin-Dusting JP: Current pharmacotherapy in the management of cirrhosis: Focus on the hyperdynamic circulation. Expert Opin Pharmacother 4:625, 2003.

261. Silva G, Navasa M, Bosch J, et al: Hemodynamic effects of glucagon in portal hypertension. Hepatology 11:668, 1990.

262. Cerini R, Koshy A, Hadengue A, et al: Effects of glucagon on systemic and splanchnic circulation in conscious rats with biliary cirrhosis. J Hepatol 9:69, 1989.

263. Moller S, Bendtsen F, Henriksen JH: Vasoactive substances in the circulatory dysfunction of cirrhosis. Scand J Clin Lab Invest 61:421, 2001.

264. Moller S, Bendtsen F, Henriksen JH: Splanchnic and systemic hemodynamic derangement in decompensated cirrhosis. Can J Gastroenterol 15:94, 2001.

265. Cahill PA, Redmond EM, Sitzmann JV: Endothelial dysfunction in cirrhosis and portal hypertension. Pharmacol Ther 89:273, 2001.

266. Bomzon A, Blendis LM: Vascular reactivity in experimental portal hypertension. Am J Physiol 252:G158, 1987.

267. Martin PY, Gines P, Schrier RW: Nitric oxide as a mediator of hemodynamic abnormalities and sodium and water retention in cirrhosis. N Engl J Med 339:533, 1998.

268. Martin PY, Ohara M, Gines P, et al: Nitric oxide synthase (NOS) inhibition for one week improves

renal sodium and water excretion in cirrhotic rats with ascites [published erratum appears in J Clin Invest 1998 Aug 1;102(3):inside back cover]. J Clin Invest 101:235, 1998.
269. Niederberger M, Martin PY, Gines P, et al: Normalization of nitric oxide production corrects arterial vasodilation and hyperdynamic circulation in cirrhotic rats. Gastroenterology 109:1624, 1995.
270. Matsumoto A, Ogura K, Hirata Y, et al: Increased nitric oxide in the exhaled air of patients with decompensated liver cirrhosis. Ann Intern Med 123:110, 1995.
271. Witte CL, Witte MH: Splanchnic circulatory and tissue fluid dynamics in portal hypertension. Fed Proc 42:1685, 1983.
272. Ebrahimkhani MR, Mani AR, Moore K: Hydrogen sulphide and the hyperdynamic circulation in cirrhosis: A hypothesis. Gut 54:1668, 2005.
273. Schrier RW, Abraham WT: Hormones and hemodynamics in heart failure. N Engl J Med 341:577, 1999.
274. Garcia-Estan J, Ortiz MC, Lee SS: Nitric oxide and renal and cardiac dysfunction in cirrhosis. Clin Sci 102:213, 2002.
275. Heneghan MA, Harrison PM: Pathogenesis of ascites in cirrhosis and portal hypertension. Med Sci Monit 6:807, 2000.
276. Levy M, Wexler MJ: Renal sodium retention and ascites formation in dogs with experimental cirrhosis but without portal hypertension or increased splanchnic vascular capacity. J Lab Clin Med 91:520, 1978.
277. Kullak-Ublick GA, Meier PJ: Mechanisms of cholestasis. Clin Liver Dis 4:357, 2000.
278. Strazzabosco M: Transport systems in cholangiocytes: Their role in bile formation and cholestasis. Yale J Biol Med 70:427, 1997.
279. Velayudham LS, Farrell GC: Drug-induced cholestasis. Expert Opin Drug Saf 2:287, 2003.
280. Levy C, Lindor KD: Drug-induced cholestasis. Clin Liver Dis 7:311, 2003.
281. Tung BY, Carithers RL Jr: Cholestasis and alcoholic liver disease. Clin Liver Dis 3:585, 1999.
282. Mullally BA, Hansen WF: Intrahepatic cholestasis of pregnancy: Review of the literature. Obstet Gynecol Surv 57:47, 2002.
283. Reyes H, Sjovall J: Bile acids and progesterone metabolites in intrahepatic cholestasis of pregnancy. Ann Med 32:94, 2000.
284. Trauner M, Fickert P, Stauber RE: Inflammation-induced cholestasis. J Gastroenterol Hepatol 14:946, 1999.
285. Gilroy RK, Mailliard ME, Gollan JL: Gastrointestinal disorders of the critically ill. Cholestasis of sepsis. Best Pract Res Clin Gastroenterol 17:357, 2003.
286. Hirata K, Ikeda S, Honma T, et al: Sepsis and cholestasis: Basic findings in the sinusoid and bile canaliculus. J Hepatobiliary Pancreat Surg 8:20, 2001.
287. Moseley RH: Sepsis and cholestasis. Clin Liver Dis 3:465, 1999.
288. Sandhu IS, Jarvis C, Everson GT: Total parenteral nutrition and cholestasis. Clin Liver Dis 3:489, 1999.
289. Teitelbaum DH, Tracy T: Parenteral nutrition–associated cholestasis. Semin Pediatr Surg 10:72, 2001.
290. Jansen PL: The pathophysiology of cholestasis with special reference to primary biliary cirrhosis. Best Pract Res Clin Gastroenterol 14:571, 2000.
291. Casali AM, Carbone G, Cavalli G: Intrahepatic bile duct loss in primary sclerosing cholangitis: A quantitative study. Histopathology 32:449, 1998.
292. Luketic VA, Shiffman ML: Benign recurrent intrahepatic cholestasis. Clin Liver Dis 3:509, 1999.
293. Trauner M, Fickert P, Stauber RE: Hepatocellular bile salt transport: Lessons from cholestasis. Can J Gastroenterol 14:99D, 2000.
294. Jansen PL, Muller M: Genetic cholestasis: Lessons from the molecular physiology of bile formation. Can J Gastroenterol 14:233, 2000.
295. Thompson R, Strautnieks S: BSEP: Function and role in progressive familial intrahepatic cholestasis. Semin Liver Dis 21:545, 2001.
296. Shaffer EA: Cholestasis: The ABCs of cellular mechanisms for impaired bile secretion—transporters and genes. Can J Gastroenterol 16:380, 2002.
297. Carulli N, Manenti F, Ponz de Leon M, et al: Alteration of drug metabolism during cholestasis in man. Eur J Clin Invest 5:455, 1975.
298. Richter E, Breimer DD, Zilly W: Disposition of hexobarbital in intra- and extrahepatic cholestasis in man and the influence of drug metabolism–inducing agents. Eur J Clin Pharmacol 17:197, 1980.
299. Miguet JP, Vuitton D, Deschamps JP, et al: Cholestasis and hepatic drug metabolism. Comparison of metabolic clearance rate of antipyrine in patients with intrahepatic or extrahepatic cholestasis. Dig Dis Sci 26:718, 1981.
300. Kawata S, Imai Y, Inada M, et al: Selective reduction of hepatic cytochrome P450 content in patients with intrahepatic cholestasis. A mechanism for impairment of microsomal drug oxidation. Gastroenterology 92:299, 1987.
301. Chen J, Farrell GC: Bile acids produce a generalized reduction of the catalytic activity of cytochromes P450 and other hepatic microsomal enzymes in vitro: Relevance to drug metabolism in experimental cholestasis. J Gastroenterol Hepatol 11:870, 1996.
302. Basso D, Fabris C, Plebani M, et al: Alterations in bilirubin metabolism during extra- and intrahepatic cholestasis. Clin Invest 70:49, 1992.
303. Glasova H, Beuers U: Extrahepatic manifestations of cholestasis. J Gastroenterol Hepatol 17:938, 2002.
304. Berk PD, Javitt NB: Hyperbilirubinemia and cholestasis. Am J Med 64:311, 1978.
305. Binah O, Rubinstein I, Bomzon A, et al: Effects of bile acids on ventricular muscle contraction and electrophysiological properties: Studies in rat papillary muscle and isolated ventricular myocytes. Naunyn Schmiedebergs Arch Pharmacol 335:160, 1987.
306. Jacob G, Nassar N, Hayam G, et al: Cardiac function and responsiveness to beta-adrenoceptor agonists in rats with obstructive jaundice. Am J Physiol 265:G314, 1993.
307. Bomzon A, Monies-Chass I, Kamenetz L, et al: Anesthesia and pressor responsiveness in chronic bile-duct–ligated dogs. Hepatology 11:551, 1990.
308. Tamakuma S, Wada N, Ishiyama M, et al: Relationship between hepatic hemodynamics and biliary pressure in dogs: Its significance in clinical shock following biliary decompression. Jpn J Surg 5:255, 1975.

Robert N. Sladen

18 Renal Physiology

Key Points

1. To cross the filtration barrier between plasma and tubular fluid, a molecule must pass in succession through the endothelial fenestrations, the glomerular basement membrane, and the epithelial slit diaphragm. The capillary endothelium restricts the passage of cells, but the basement membrane filters plasma proteins. All three layers contain negatively charged glycoproteins, which retard the passage of other negatively charged proteins. Thus, the filtration barrier is size selective and charge selective.[1]
2. A primary determinant of glomerular filtration rate (GFR) is the glomerular filtration pressure, which depends not only on the renal artery perfusion pressure but also on the balance between afferent and efferent arteriolar tone. In the presence of decreased afferent arteriolar pressure or blood flow, low levels of catecholamines, angiotensin, and arginine vasopressin (AVP) induce preferential efferent arteriolar constriction, which maintains glomerular filtration pressure. This is reflected by an increase in calculated filtration fraction (FF), which is the GFR expressed as a fraction of the renal plasma flow (RPF), that is, FF = GFR/RPF. High levels of catecholamines and angiotensin (but not AVP) increase afferent arteriolar tone and decrease glomerular filtration pressure (and GFR) out of proportion to RPF, and FF decreases (see Fig. 18-4).
3. Tubuloglomerular feedback may be a primary mechanism in renal autoregulation.[3] When GFR is increased, distal tubular NaCl delivery is enhanced. The increase in chloride is sensed by the macula densa, which triggers the release of renin from the adjacent afferent arteriole. Angiotensin is elaborated and arteriolar constriction ensues, which decreases GFR. When the thick ascending loop becomes ischemic, reabsorption of NaCl ceases, the ability of the tubule to concentrate urine is lost, and, theoretically, intractable polyuria should result. Thurau and Boylan[5] suggested that the increased delivery of NaCl to the macula densa triggers angiotensin-mediated arteriolar constriction, which decreases GFR, induces oliguria, conserves intravascular volume, and protects the organism from dehydration—so-called acute renal success.
4. Autoregulation enables the kidney to maintain solute and water regulation independently of wide fluctuations of arterial blood pressure. It is noteworthy that urinary flow rate is not subject to autoregulation. Tubular water reabsorption determines urinary flow rate and is closely related to the hydrostatic pressure in the peritubular capillaries. Hypotension, whether induced or inadvertent, results in decreased urinary flow rate that may be correctable only when the arterial blood pressure is restored toward normal.
5. The tubule has an enormous capacity for reabsorption of water and NaCl. Each day, 180 L of protein-free glomerular ultrafiltrate is formed, of which almost 99% of the water and 99% of the sodium is reabsorbed. Many other filtered substances are completely reabsorbed, but some, such as glucose, have a maximum rate of tubular reabsorption (tubular maximum). Tubular reabsorption of glucose increases at a rate equal to that of the filtered load.
6. The ability of the kidney to concentrate urine is dependent on the interaction of at least three processes: (1) the generation of a hypertonic medullary interstitium by the countercurrent mechanism and urea recycling, (2) concentration and then dilution of tubular fluid in the loop of Henle, and (3) the action of antidiuretic hormone (now known as arginine vasopressin [AVP]) in increasing water permeability in the last part of the distal tubule and collecting ducts.
7. Serum creatinine reflects the balance between creatinine production by muscle and creatinine excretion by the kidney, which is dependent on the GFR. Creatinine generation rate varies with muscle mass, physical activity, protein intake, and catabolism. However, when these processes are in equilibrium and renal function is stable, serum creatinine is a useful marker of GFR. The relationship between serum creatinine and GFR is inverse and exponential. A doubling of the serum creatinine implies a halving of the GFR. An increase in serum creatinine from 0.8 to 1.6 mg/dL may not generate much attention, but it indicates a 50% decrease in GFR. A much larger increase from 4 to 8 mg/dL also

represents a 50% decrease in GFR, but by this time renal insufficiency is well established (see Fig. 18-11). After a transient renal insult (e.g., suprarenal aortic cross-clamping), serum creatinine may increase for a few days while GFR is actually recovering.

8. The juxtaglomerular apparatus consists of three groups of specialized tissues. In the afferent arteriole, modified fenestrated endothelial cells produce renin; in the juxtaposed distal tubule, cells of the macula densa act as chemoreceptors; and in the glomerulus, mesangial cells have contractile properties (see Fig. 18-3). Together these provide an important regulating system for blood pressure, salt, and water homeostasis.[46]

9. Hypothalamic osmoreceptors are sensitive to increases in serum osmolality of as little as 1% above normal. As illustrated in Figure 18-21A, the threshold for AVP secretion (and the sensation of thirst) is between 280 and 290 mOsm/kg. When this is exceeded, the secretion rate has a very steep gain.[52] Even mild dehydration results in a rapid antidiuresis, and urine osmolality can increase from 300 to 1200 mOs/kg as plasma AVP levels rise from 0 to 5 pg/mL (see Fig. 18-21B). Decreases in intravascular volume also stimulate AVP secretion, mediated by stretch receptors with vagal afferents in the left atrium and pulmonary veins. Hypovolemia-induced secretion of AVP overrides osmolar responses and contributes to the perioperative syndrome of inappropriate antidiuretic hormone secretion (SIADH): fluid retention, hypo-osmolality, and hyponatremia. The situation is exacerbated by administration of large volumes of hypotonic solutions that decrease serum osmolality. Psychic stress, via cortical input, also induces AVP release and can override osmotic and volume sensors.

10. All anesthetic techniques and drugs tend to decrease GFR and intraoperative urine flow. Some drugs also decrease renal blood flow (RBF), but filtration fraction is usually increased, which implies that angiotensin-induced efferent arteriolar constriction limits the decrease in GFR. However, these effects are much less significant than those caused by surgical stress or aortic cross-clamping and after emergence from anesthesia usually resolve promptly. Any anesthetic technique that induces hypotension will result in decreased urine flow because of altered peritubular capillary hydrostatic gradients, even if renal autoregulation is preserved (as it usually is during anesthesia). Permanent injury seldom results, unless the kidneys are abnormal to begin with or the hypovolemic insult is prolonged and exacerbated by nephrotoxic injury.

11. Clinically significant renal injury with the use of low-flow sevoflurane anesthesia has not been reported in patients, even with moderate preexisting renal dysfunction. The relationship between compound A formation, biochemical injury, and clinically relevant renal dysfunction remains unclear and unproven. Nonetheless it appears prudent to follow current FDA guidelines, which recommend a fresh gas flow of at least 2 L/min to inhibit compound A formation and its rebreathing and to enhance its washout.

12. Regardless of the position of the aortic cross-clamp, RBF is decreased to 50% of normal during surgical preparation of the aorta, presumably due to direct compression or reflex spasm of the renal arteries. After release of the suprarenal cross-clamp, RBF increases above normal (reflex hyperemia), but GFR remains depressed to one third of control for up to 2 hours. After 24 hours, GFR is still only two thirds of control. Tubular functions (concentrating ability, sodium, and water conservation) are markedly impaired, but urine flow is maintained. Myers and Moran[106] observed that these changes resemble an attenuated form of acute tubular necrosis. In the above study all patients received mannitol pretreatment, which probably limited the tubular insult because oliguria was uncommon and recovery was relatively rapid. Cross-clamp times longer than 50 minutes are associated with prolonged depression of GFR and transient azotemia.[107]

13. In contrast to dopamine, there does appear to be increasing evidence to support a renoprotective effect for infusion of low-dose fenoldopam infusion (0.1-0.3 μg/kg/min) during cardiac surgery. A meta-analysis of 13 randomized and case-matched studies on 1059 patients found that fenoldopam infusion is associated with a significant decrease in dialysis requirement, intensive care unit length of stay, and in-hospital mortality.[136] Most studies have been relatively small and identified improved serum creatinine and creatinine clearance rather than renal outcome.[137,138] The most convincing evidence thus far comes from a randomized, double-blinded study in 193 high-risk patients by Cogliati and associates.[139] Risk factors included elevated preoperative serum creatinine (>1.5 mg/dL), age older than 70 years, diabetes, and previous cardiac surgery. Patients who received fenoldopam had a decreased incidence of acute kidney injury (12.6 versus 27.6%, $P = .02$) and requirement for dialysis (0 versus 8.2%, $P = .004$).

14. The beneficial effect of AVP on renal function in sepsis may in part be due to its ability to increase low renal perfusion pressure back into the autoregulatory range. Another important factor is that, unlike norepinephrine, even at high local concentrations AVP preferentially constricts the efferent arteriole, thereby improving filtration fraction and GFR.[53] However, in a large, prospective, randomized, blinded trial in 778 patients with severe septic shock, low-dose AVP (0.01-0.03 unit/min) did not provide a mortality benefit or decrease the requirement for dialysis when compared with an infusion of norepinephrine (5-15 μg/min).[194]

The kidneys contain approximately 2 million nephrons, each of which consists of a glomerulus and a tubule, which empties into a collecting duct. Together they regulate intravascular volume, osmolality, and acid-base and electrolyte balance and excrete end products of metabolism and drugs. Urine is formed by the combination of glomerular ultrafiltration and tubular reabsorption and secretion. The nephron also elaborates hormones that contribute to fluid homeostasis (renin, prostaglandins, kinins), bone metabolism (1,25-dihydroxycholecalciferol), and hematopoiesis (erythropoietin). The function of the nephron is closely integrated with the vascular supply of the kidney (Fig. 18-1).

Anatomy and Physiology

The Glomerulus (Renal Corpuscle)

The glomerulus consists of five distinct components: capillary endothelium, glomerular basement membrane, visceral epithelium (which together make up the filtration barrier), parietal epithelium (Bowman's capsule), and mesangium (interstitial cells).[1,2] The glomerular tuft, a highly convoluted series of capillary loops, is fed by the afferent arteriole and drains into the efferent arteriole (Fig. 18-2).

The capillary endothelium synthesizes nitric oxide and endothelin-1, which, by governing vasodilation and vasoconstriction, control renal blood flow. The endothelium has fenestrations about 70 to 100 nm in diameter and lies atop the glomerular basement membrane, which has a total cross section of about 350 nm. The visceral epithelium, which is applied to the underside of the basement membrane, consists of podocytes with filamentous, interdigitating foot processes that contain contractile actin filaments. Filtration slits form 25- to 60-nm gaps between the foot processes and are bridged by a protein membrane slit diaphragm, whose size and permeability are altered by contraction of the foot processes.

The blind parietal epithelial sac of the renal tubule is invaginated around the capillary tuft as Bowman's capsule and meets the visceral epithelium at the vascular pole of the glomerulus. Bowman's space, between the visceral and parietal layers of the capsule, becomes the lumen of the proximal tubule at the urinary pole of the glomerulus, and the parietal endothelium merges with the cuboidal cells of the proximal tubule.

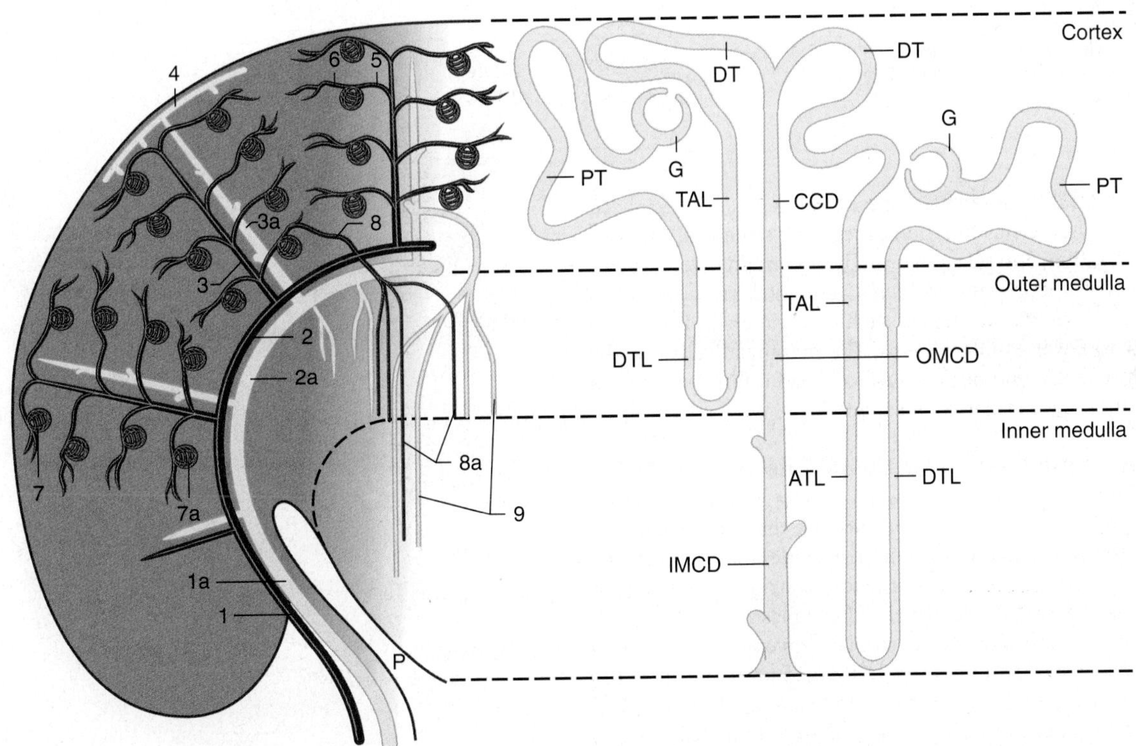

Figure 18-1 Anatomic relationships of the nephron and the renal vasculature. The left side of the diagram represents the renal vasculature as distributed through the inner medulla, outer medulla, and cortex. Arteries are drawn as *solid lines*, veins as *hollow tubes*. The renal artery divides serially into interlobar arteries (1), arcuate arteries (2), and interlobular arteries (3). The afferent arterioles (5) branch off laterally and provide the capillary tufts of the renal glomeruli in the outer cortex (7), whose efferent arterioles (6) supply the cortical capillary network (not shown). In the juxtamedullary zone (7a), the efferent arterioles become the vasa recta, which are closely applied to the long loops of Henle (8, 8a, 9). The venous drainage consists of stellate veins (4), interlobular veins (3a), arcuate veins (2a), and interlobar veins (1a). The right side of the diagram represents two nephrons. On the left is the more numerous superficial cortical nephron with a short loop of Henle. On the right is the juxtamedullary nephron with a long loop of Henle, which dives deep into the inner medulla to generate the hyperosmotic interstitium required for tubular urine concentration. ATL, ascending thin loop of Henle; CCD, cortical collecting duct; DT, distal tubule; DTL, descending thin loop of Henle; G, glomerulus; IMCD, inner medullary collecting duct; OMCD, outer medullary collecting duct; PT, proximal tubule; TAL, thick ascending loop. *(From Kriz W: A standard nomenclature for structures of the kidney. Kidney Int 33:1-7, 1988.)*

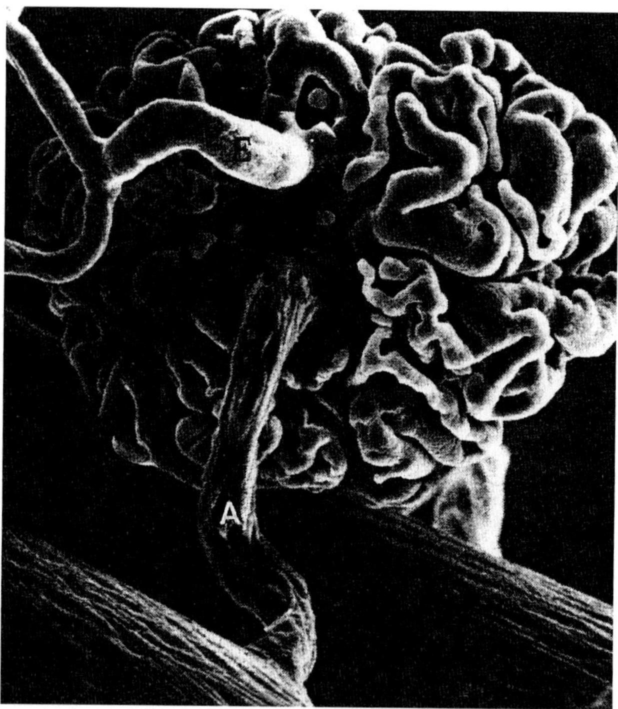

Figure 18-2 Photomicrograph of a cast of a glomerulus without Bowman's capsule. At lower left the afferent arteriole (A) originates from an interlobular artery and enters the glomerulus with its many capillary loops. At upper left the efferent arteriole (E) leaves the glomerulus and branches to form the peritubular capillary plexus (×300). (*From Tisher CC, Madsen KM: Anatomy of the kidney.* In *Brenner BM [ed]: Brenner & Rector's The Kidney, 6th ed. Philadelphia, WB Saunders, 2000, pp 3-67.*)

The central or interstitial mesangial cells are specialized pericytes with numerous functions, including structural support, matrix elaboration, and phagocytosis. They contain myofilament-like threads of actin and myosin. Mesangial contraction in response to vasoactive substances such as angiotensin II restricts blood flow to fewer capillary loops. The mesangial cells thereby regulate the effective glomerular surface area for filtration and, as a consequence, glomerular permeability.[3]

Formation of the Glomerular Ultrafiltrate

To cross the filtration barrier between plasma and tubular fluid, a molecule must pass in succession through the endothelial fenestrations, the glomerular basement membrane, and the epithelial slit diaphragm. The capillary endothelium restricts the passage of cells, but the basement membrane filters plasma proteins. All three layers contain negatively charged glycoproteins, which retard the passage of other negatively charged proteins. Thus, the filtration barrier is both size selective and charge selective.[1] Molecules with an effective radius of less than 1.8 nm (e.g., water, sodium, urea, glucose, inulin) are freely filtered. Molecules larger than 3.6 nm (e.g., hemoglobin, albumin) are not filtered. Filtration of molecules between 1.8 and 3.6 nm depends on their electrical charge. Cations are filtered, whereas anions are not. In glomerulonephritis, the negatively charged glycoproteins are destroyed, polyanionic proteins are filtered, and proteinuria ensues.

Glomerular ultrafiltration is governed by the balance of Starling forces regulating fluid flux across the filtration barrier.[4] Glomerular filtration rate (GFR) depends on the permeability of the filtration barrier and the net difference between the hydrostatic forces pushing fluid into Bowman's space and the osmotic forces keeping fluid in the plasma:

$$GFR = K_{uf}\left[\left(P_{gc} - P_{bs}\right) - \left(\pi_{gc} - \pi_{bs}\right)\right]$$

where uf = ultrafiltration, gc = glomerular capillary, and bs = Bowman's space.

The ultrafiltration coefficient, K_{uf}, reflects capillary permeability and glomerular surface area. Renal arterial pressure determines the hydrostatic pressure in the glomerular capillary, P_{gc}. Afferent arteriolar plasma flow determines the plasma oncotic pressure (π_{gc}): rapid blood flow washes out osmotically effective molecules and lowers π_{gc}, and vice versa.

The Juxtaglomerular Apparatus

The juxtaglomerular apparatus provides a remarkable integration of tubular and glomerular structure and function (Fig. 18-3). A modified portion of the thick ascending limb, the macula densa, is applied to the glomerulus at the vascular pole between the afferent and efferent arterioles.[1] The cells of the macula densa are chemoreceptors and sense the tubular concentration of sodium chloride (NaCl). The juxtaposed segments of the afferent and efferent arterioles contain modified smooth muscle cells (granular cells), which produce renin. The arterioles are innervated by sympathetic nerve fibers and contain baroreceptors that respond

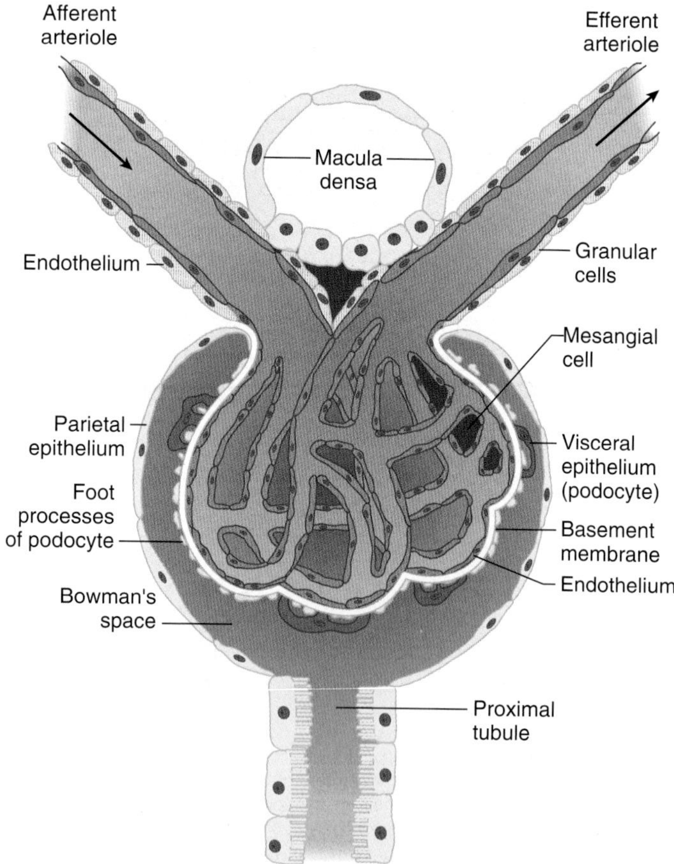

Figure 18-3 The juxtaglomerular apparatus. (*From Stanton BA, Koeppen BM: Elements of renal function.* In *Berne RM, Levy MN [eds]: Physiology, 4th ed. St. Louis, Mosby, 1998, pp 677-698.*)

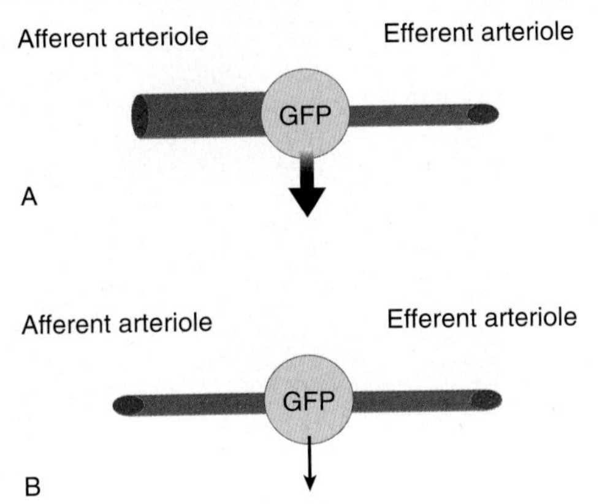

Figure 18-4 Afferent and efferent arteriolar control mechanisms. *(From Sladen RN, Landry D: Renal blood flow regulation, autoregulation, and vasomotor nephropathy. Anesthesiol Clin North Am 18:791-807, ix, 2000.)*

to changes in intraluminal blood pressure. Renin catalyzes the formation of angiotensin, which modulates efferent and afferent arteriolar tone and GFR (see later).

Afferent and Efferent Arteriolar Control Mechanisms

A primary determinant of GFR is the glomerular filtration pressure, which depends not only on the renal artery perfusion pressure but also on the balance between afferent and efferent arteriolar tone. In the presence of decreased afferent arteriolar pressure or blood flow, low levels of catecholamines, angiotensin, and arginine vasopressin (AVP) induce preferential efferent arteriolar constriction, which maintains glomerular filtration pressure (Fig. 18-4A). This is reflected by an increase in calculated filtration fraction (FF), which is the GFR expressed as a fraction of the renal plasma flow (RPF), that is, FF = GFR/RPF. High levels of catecholamines and angiotensin (but not AVP) increase afferent arteriolar tone and decrease glomerular filtration pressure (and GFR) out of proportion to RPF, and FF decreases (Fig. 18-4B).

Tubuloglomerular Feedback

Tubuloglomerular feedback may be a primary mechanism in renal autoregulation.[3] When GFR is increased, distal tubular NaCl delivery is enhanced. The increase in chloride (Cl^-) is sensed by the macula densa, which triggers the release of renin from the adjacent afferent arteriole. Angiotensin is elaborated and arteriolar constriction ensues, which decreases GFR.

When the thick ascending loop becomes ischemic, reabsorption of NaCl ceases, the ability of the tubule to concentrate urine is lost and, theoretically, intractable polyuria should result. Thurau and Boylan[5] suggested that the increased delivery of NaCl to the macula densa triggers angiotensin-mediated arteriolar constriction, which decreases GFR, induces oliguria, conserves intravascular volume, and protects the organism from dehydration—so-called acute renal success.

Renal Autoregulation

Autoregulation enables the kidney to maintain solute and water regulation independently of wide fluctuations of arterial blood pressure. In 1951, the classic dog studies of Shipley and Study[6] demonstrated that the kidney maintains a constant renal blood flow and GFR through an arterial pressure range of 80 to 180 mm Hg (Fig. 18-5). Urinary flow rate is not subject to autoregulation. Tubular water reabsorption determines urinary flow rate and is closely related to the hydrostatic pressure in the peritubular capillaries. Hypotension, whether induced or inadvertent, results in decreased urinary flow rate that may be correctable only when the arterial blood pressure is restored toward normal.

There is considerable evidence to support two major mechanisms for renal autoregulation.[3] As mean arterial pressure decreases, renal vascular resistance decreases and renal blood flow (RBF) is maintained. The most plausible explanation is a myogenic response, that is, the arterioles constrict in response to increased arterial pressure and vice versa. Tubuloglomerular feedback via the juxtaglomerular apparatus also plays a role.[3,4,7] When arterial pressure increases through the autoregulatory range, delivery of sodium chloride is enhanced to the chemosensors of the macula densa, which generate adenosine triphosphate (ATP) and adenosine that stimulate the adenosine A_1 receptor and induce afferent arteriolar constriction (Fig. 18-6). This, in turn, decreases RBF and GFR back to the previous levels. The opposite effect occurs when arterial pressure declines. Local release of nitric oxide attenuates tubuloglomerular feedback, whereas release of angiotensin II enhances it.[4]

Autoregulation is impaired by calcium channel blockade, implying that a calcium-dependent mechanism is involved but not by most anesthetic agents. It is reset in chronic hypertension and may be lost in the diabetic kidney. There is experimental evidence that autoregulation is lost in acute renal failure[8]; in part this may be due to endothelial dysfunction through excessive nitric oxide because inducible nitric oxide synthase is activated by renal ischemia-reperfusion injury.[9] Pressure-dependence of RBF is observed during cardiopulmonary bypass (CPB)[10] and in severe sepsis,[11] but this may simply be due to hypotension below the autoregulatory range, rather than abnormal autoregulation

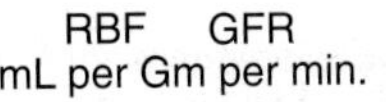

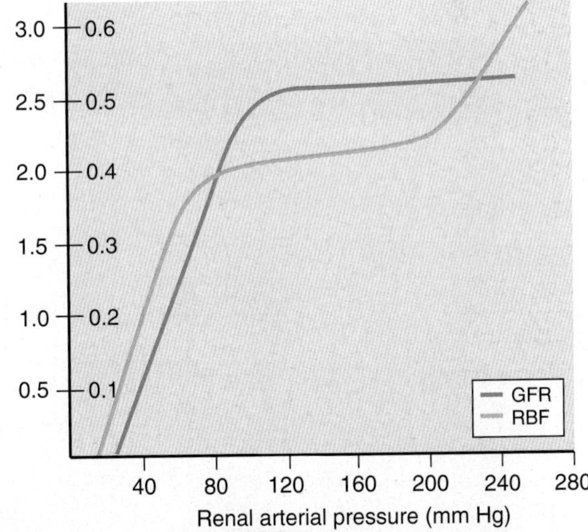

Figure 18-5 Autoregulation of glomerular filtration rate (GFR) and renal blood flow (RBF). GFR and RBF remain constant between renal arterial pressures of 80 and 180 mm Hg. *(Based on the original work of Shipley and Study.[5] From Pitts RF: Physiology of the Kidney and Body Fluids. Chicago, Year Book Medical Publishers, 1974.)*

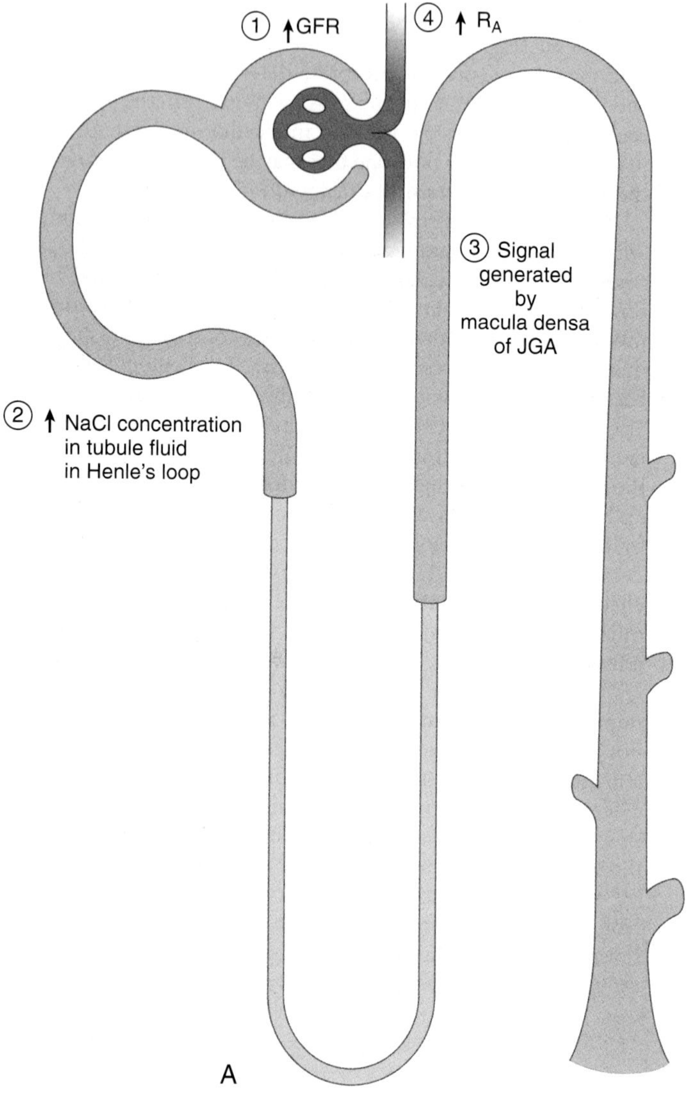

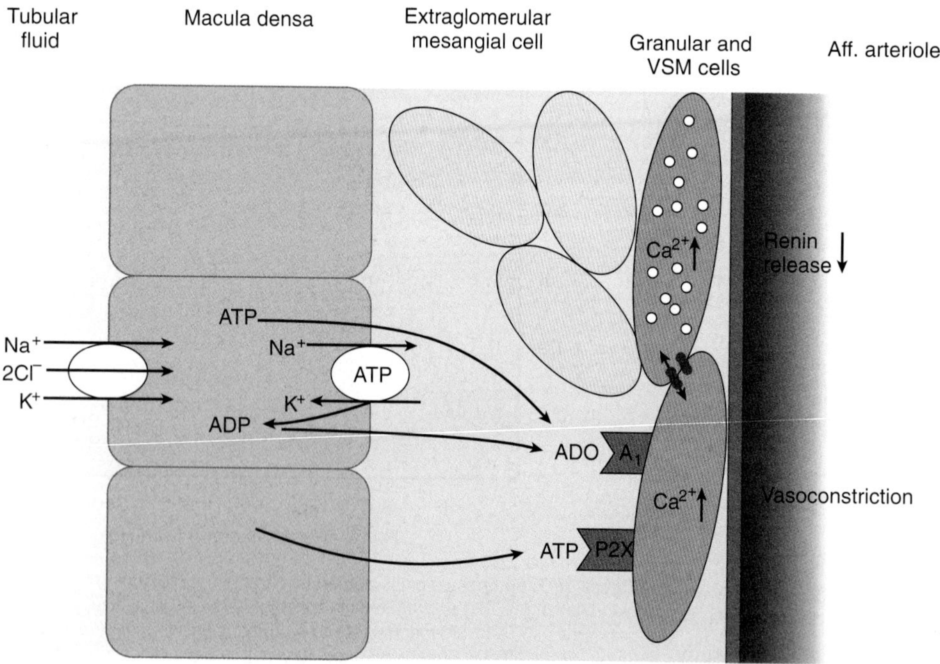

Figure 18-6 A and **B,** Tubuloglomerular feedback. An increase in glomerular filtration rate (GFR) (1) increases sodium chloride (NaCl) concentration in the tubular fluid in the loop of Henle. This is sensed by chemosensors in the modified distal tubular cells of the macula densa in the juxtaglomerular apparatus (JGA) (3). The cells of the macula densa generate adenosine triphosphate (ATP) and adenosine (ADO) that induces afferent arteriolar constriction and increases its resistance (R_A) (4). This returns the GFR to its former level. A decline in the GFR has the opposite effect. (*From Koeppen BM, Stanton BA: Glomerular filtration and renal blood flow.* In *Koeppen BM, Stanton BA [eds]: Renal Physiology, 4th ed. Philadelphia, Mosby Elsevier, 2007, pp 31-46.*)

per se. Normalization of renal perfusion pressure improves RBF, even if this is achieved by vasoconstrictor therapy.

The Tubule

The tubule has four distinct segments: the proximal tubule, the loop of Henle, the distal tubule, and the connecting segment. The loop of Henle itself is divided into the pars recta (the straight portion of the proximal tubule), the descending and ascending thin limb segments, and the thick ascending limb. Each distal tubule drains into a collecting duct, which courses through the cortex, outer medulla, and inner medulla before entering the renal pelvis at the papilla (see Fig. 18-1).

There are two populations of nephrons. The cortical nephrons populate the outer and middle renal cortex, are far more numerous, receive about 85% of the renal blood flow, and have short loops of Henle. The juxtamedullary nephrons populate the inner renal cortex, receive about 10% of the RBF, and have larger glomeruli and long loops of Henle, which dive deeply into the inner medulla.[2] Their efferent arterioles drain into elongated vascular conduits, the vasa recta, which are closely applied to the loops of Henle. Although the vasa recta receive less than 1% of the RBF, they play an important role in generating the countercurrent mechanism for medullary hypertonicity and renal concentrating ability (see later).

Tubular Reabsorption and Secretion

The tubule has an enormous capacity for reabsorption of water and NaCl. Each day, 180 L of protein-free glomerular ultrafiltrate is formed, of which almost 99% of the water and 99% of the sodium is reabsorbed.

Many other filtered substances are completely reabsorbed, but some, such as glucose, have a maximum rate of tubular reabsorption (tubular maximum). Tubular reabsorption of glucose increases at a rate equal to that of the filtered load. If the GFR is constant, the rate is directly proportional to the plasma glucose. Once plasma glucose exceeds the tubular maximum (375 mg/dL), no further glucose is reabsorbed and glycosuria results. Thereafter, the amount of glucose excreted in the urine increases in direct proportion to the filtered load.

Many important endogenous and exogenous solutes are secreted into the tubular lumen from the capillary blood. Some also have a tubular maximum for secretion, such as *p*-aminohippurate (PAH), which is used to calculate RPF. There is a striking relationship between the structure and function of the different segments of the tubule (Fig. 18-7). The most metabolically active components of the tubule are the proximal tubule, the thick ascending loop of Henle, and the first part of the distal tubule.

Figure 18-8 illustrates a tubular cell in the thick ascending loop of Henle, which encompasses all the major mechanisms of reabsorption and secretion. From each apical cell membrane pro-

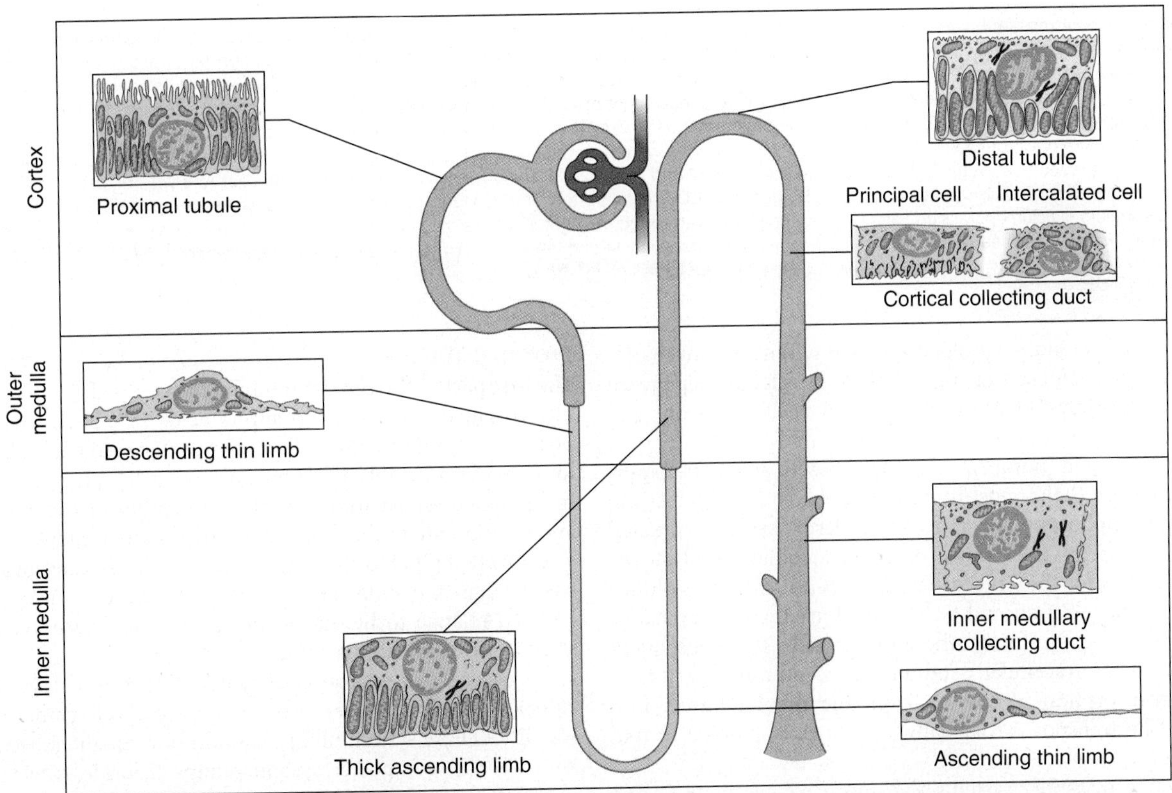

Figure 18-7 Structure-function relationships in the renal tubule. The most metabolically active components of the tubule are the proximal tubule, the thick ascending loop of Henle, and the first part of the distal tubule. Their cells are large, and on the capillary surface (basolateral membrane) there are many invaginations rich in mitochondria. The cells of the proximal tubule have a brush-border on the luminal surface (apical cell membrane), whereas the cells of the descending and thin ascending loops of Henle are flattened with few mitochondria. The second part of the distal tubule and collecting duct are intermediate in nature. The intercalated cells of the distal tubule have many mitochondria; the principal cells are few. *(From Stanton BA, Koeppen BM: Elements of renal function. In Berne RM, Levy MN [eds]: Physiology, 4th ed. St. Louis, Mosby, 1998, pp 677-698.)*

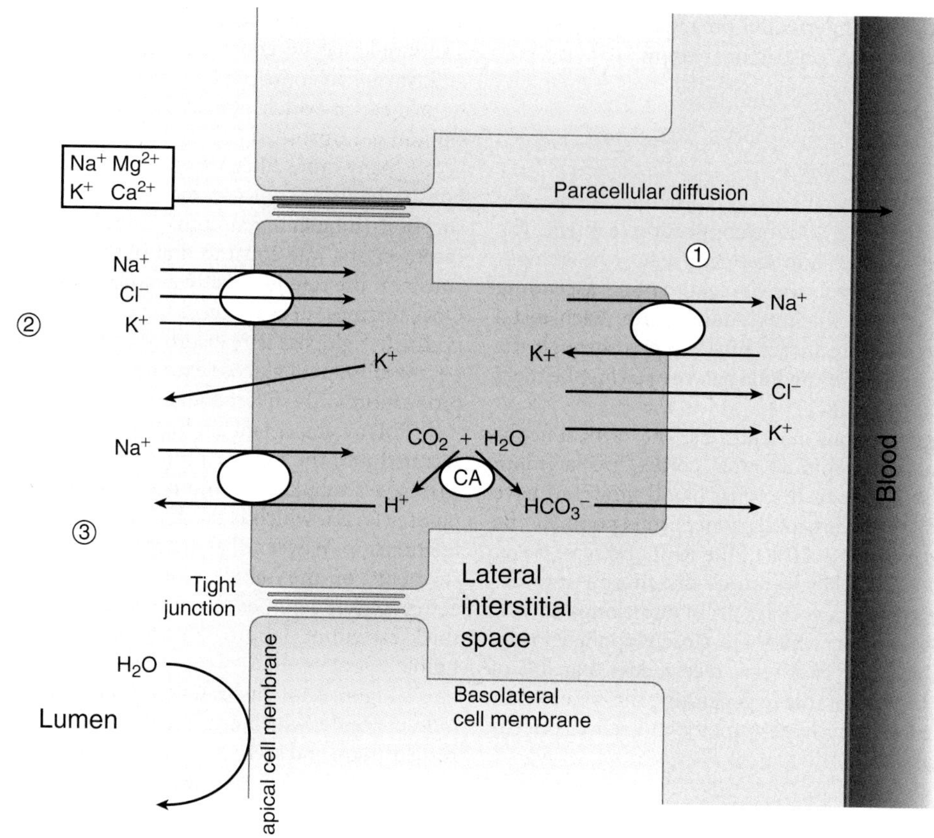

Figure 18-8 Mechanisms of tubular secretion and reabsorption. This tubular cell in the thick ascending loop of Henle encompasses the major mechanisms of secretion and reabsorption, one or more of which is used by various segments of the tubule. The most ubiquitous and important transport mechanism is the energy-requiring Na^+-K^+-ATPase pump in the basolateral cell membrane (1), which pumps sodium out into the interstitium against its concentration gradient and maintains a low intracellular concentration. This favors inward movement of sodium from the tubular lumen, facilitated by a sodium chloride symporter system on the apical cell membrane (2), which creates enough potential energy to draw in potassium against its concentration gradient and which is the primary inhibitory site of action of loop diuretics. An Na^+-H^+ antiporter system on the apical cell membrane (3) aids sodium reabsorption and extrudes H^+, thereby promoting reaction of water with carbon dioxide to form H^+ and HCO_3^- under the influence of carbonic anhydrase (CA). HCO_3^- diffuses out into the capillary. Sodium reabsorption is thereby coupled to H^+ loss and HCO_3^- reabsorption. The transport proteins create a positive charge in the lumen, which drives ions such as sodium, calcium, potassium, and magnesium passively through the tight junctions by paracellular diffusion. The thick ascending loop of Henle is uniquely highly water impermeable so that luminal osmolality progressively falls to less than 150 mOsm/kg (the "diluting segment"). *(Modified from Stanton BA, Koeppen BM: Elements of renal function.* In *Berne RM, Levy MN [eds]: Physiology, 4th ed. St. Louis, Mosby, 1998, pp 677-698.)*

trudes a primary cilium equipped with a flow-sensitive mechanosensor and a chemosensor, both linked to calcium-dependent signaling pathways that control kidney cell function and apoptosis.[1]

There are a number of protein-based active transport systems. Of these, the most important is the sodium-potassium adenosine triphosphatase (Na^+-K^+-ATPase) system, situated in the basolateral membrane. It pumps sodium out of the tubular cell into the interstitial fluid (and capillary blood) against a concentration and an electrical gradient, in exchange for potassium from inside the tubular cell. The consequent decrease in intracellular sodium concentration facilitates passive reabsorption of sodium from the tubular lumen into the cell. The transport of virtually all solutes is coupled to that of sodium.

Active transport systems that move solutes in the same direction into or out of the cell are called symporter systems, whereas those that move solutes in opposite directions are called antiporter systems. Solutes are transported by active and passive mechanisms, but water always diffuses passively along an osmotic gradient.

Proximal Tubule

The first part of the proximal tubule reabsorbs about 100% of the filtered glucose, lactate, and amino acids as well as some phosphate by coupling with sodium-symporter systems.[12] Hydrogen ions are extruded into the tubule by an Na^+/H^+ antiporter system in exchange for bicarbonate. The absorption of organic anions and bicarbonate in the first part of the proximal tubule results in a relatively high chloride concentration downstream, promoting passive ingress of chloride. This leaves the tubular fluid positively charged relative to blood, further promoting the movement of sodium from the tubular fluid into the cell.

Most NaCl is absorbed transcellularly by an Na^+/H^+ and chloride-based antiporter system in the apical cell membrane. The Na^+/K^+-ATPase system pumps sodium into the interstitial space, and a K^+/Cl^- symporter system pumps chloride. The resulting increase in osmolality draws water across as well. In all, about two thirds of the filtered water, chloride, and potassium are reabsorbed by the proximal tubule, coupled with, and strongly influenced by, sodium absorption.[12]

The proximal tubule is also an important site of secretion of many endogenous anions (bile salts, urate), cations (creatinine, dopamine), and drugs (diuretics, penicillin, probenecid, cimetidine). Organic ions compete with each other for protein transport systems. Thus, administration of probenecid impairs tubular secretion of penicillin and prolongs its action. In chronic renal insufficiency there is an accumulation of organic acids that competes with drugs such as furosemide for secretor proteins, thereby conferring an apparent "resistance" to loop diuretics.

Thick Ascending Loop of Henle

The metabolically active component of the loop of Henle is the thick ascending loop, which reabsorbs about 20% of the filtered sodium, chloride, potassium, and bicarbonate. Only the descending loop is permeable to water. In the water-impermeable thick ascending loop, sodium is actively reabsorbed, but water remains. In this so-called diluting segment of the kidney, tubular fluid osmolality decreases to less than 150 mOsm/kg H_2O.

As in the proximal tubule, the Na+/K+-ATPase pump in the basolateral membrane is the engine that drives the resorptive capacity of the thick ascending loop.[12] Sodium moves from the tubular lumen by passive diffusion along its concentration gradient. An Na^+/H^+ antiporter system in the apical cell membrane mediates the net secretion of H^+ and reabsorption of bicarbonate.

An important symporter protein system couples the reabsorption of sodium, chloride, and potassium (the latter against its concentration gradient) across the apical membrane. Blockade of this system is the major site of action of loop diuretics in inhibiting NaCl reabsorption in the thick ascending loop of Henle.

Oxygen Balance in the Medullary Thick Ascending Loop

The kidneys receive 20% of the total cardiac output but extract relatively little oxygen. The renal arteriovenous oxygen difference $[(a\text{-}v)O_2]$ is only 1.5 mL/dL. However, there is a marked discrepancy between the renal cortex and medulla with regard to blood flow, oxygen delivery, and oxygen consumption (Fig. 18-9 and Table 18-1). The medulla receives only 6% of the RBF and has an

Table 18-1 Distribution of Renal Blood Flow Between Cortex and Medulla

	Cortex	Medulla
Percent of renal blood flow	94	6
Blood flow (mL/min/g)	5.0	0.03
Po_2 (mm Hg)	50	8
O_2 extraction ratio (Vo_2/Do_2)	0.18	0.79

The renal medulla receives only a small fraction of the total renal blood flow, and flow rates are extremely slow. As a result, the tissue oxygen tension is extremely low and the medulla extracts almost 80% of the oxygen delivered to it. A very mild reduction in total and cortical renal blood flow may therefore induce ischemia and hypoxia in the renal medulla.

Do_2, oxygen delivery; O_2, oxygen; Vo_2, oxygen consumption; Po_2, oxygen tension.

Data from Brezis M, et al: The pathophysiological implications of medullary hypoxia. Am J Kidney Dis 13:253-258, 1989.

average oxygen tension (Po_2) of 8 mm Hg. Thus, it is possible that severe hypoxia could develop in the medulla despite a relatively adequate total RBF, and the metabolically active medullary thick ascending loop of Henle is particularly vulnerable.[13]

The medullary thick ascending loop is also a potential site for nephrotoxic injury. Intrarenal blood flow is regulated by endogenous vasoactive compounds. In the outer cortex, at variance to its vasodilator actions elsewhere, adenosine induces vasoconstriction by stimulation of the adenosine A_1 receptor. In the deep juxtamedullary zone, endogenous prostaglandins and nitric oxide promote vasodilation. The net effect is to direct as much available blood flow to the medulla as possible. Drugs that inhibit prostaglandin synthesis, such as nonsteroidal anti-inflammatory agents (NSAIDs), can upset this compensatory mechanism and result in medullary ischemia.

Stress (pain, trauma, hemorrhage, hypoperfusion, sepsis, congestive heart failure) activates the sympathoadrenal system and results in renal cortical constriction and potential tubular ischemia. The kidney is relatively devoid of β_2-receptors so epinephrine release induces predominant vasoconstriction through α-receptor or angiotensin activation.

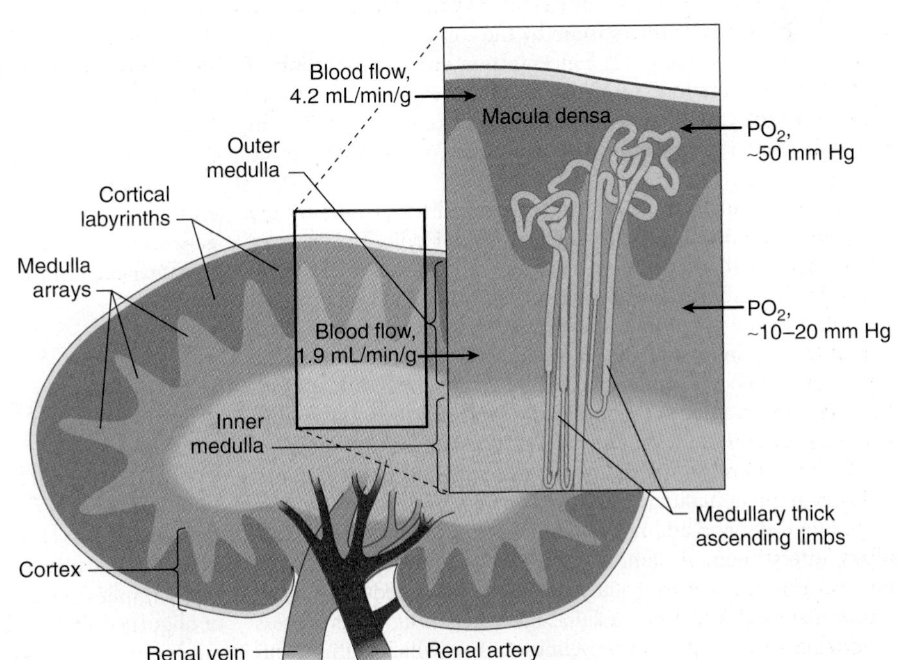

Figure 18-9 Medullary oligemia. To generate and maintain the countercurrent exchange that provides urinary concentrating ability, medullary blood flow must be slow. The juxtamedullary and medullary regions are zones of low blood flow and relative tissue hypoxia. Components of the nephron that have high oxygen consumption such as the medullary thick ascending limb (mTAL) are at high risk of oxygen supply-demand imbalance and ischemic injury. *(From Brezis M, Rosen S: Hypoxia of the renal medulla—its implications for disease. N Engl J Med 332:647-655, 1995.)*

In hemodynamically mediated renal injury, the initial response to renal hypoperfusion is increased active NaCl absorption in the thick ascending limb. This increases oxygen consumption in the presence of decreased oxygen delivery. Subsequent sympathoadrenal responses and renal cortical vasoconstriction may be a compensatory attempt to redistribute blood flow to the medulla. Ultimately, ATP stores become depleted and active NaCl reabsorption winds down. This increases the NaCl concentration in tubular fluid reaching the macula densa in the distal tubule, resulting in angiotensin release and afferent arteriolar constriction (i.e., tubuloglomerular feedback). Teleologically, the resultant decrease in GFR benefits renal oxygen balance by decreasing solute reabsorption and oxygen consumption in the medullary thick ascending loop of Henle.[13]

This hypothesis implies that ischemic or nephrotoxic insults to the renal tubules could be alleviated by the administration of loop diuretics or dopaminergic agents. These drugs inhibit active sodium reabsorption in the thick ascending limb, thereby decreasing oxygen consumption and enhancing tubular oxygen balance.

Distal Tubule and Collecting Duct

Sodium reabsorption is mediated by an apical cell membrane NaCl symporter system, which is the site of action of thiazide diuretics.[12] The last part of the distal tubule is composed of two types of cells. Principal cells reabsorb sodium and water and secrete potassium via the Na^+/K^+-ATPase pump, and intercalated cells secrete H^+ and reabsorb bicarbonate by an H^+-ATPase pump in the apical cell membrane.

Regulatory Mechanisms in Salt and Water Reabsorption

Osmotic Equilibrium

The ability of the kidney to concentrate urine is dependent on the interaction of at least three processes: (1) the generation of a hypertonic medullary interstitium by the countercurrent mechanism and urea recycling, (2) concentration and then dilution of tubular fluid in the loop of Henle, and (3) the action of antidiuretic hormone (now known as arginine vasopressin [AVP]) in increasing water permeability in the last part of the distal tubule and collecting ducts.

The medullary interstitium is rendered hypertonic by the countercurrent multiplier effect of the loop of Henle. The primary mechanism is the separation of solute from water (the single effect) by the combination of NaCl reabsorption and water impermeability in the ascending limb. This results in increased NaCl concentration and osmolality in the medullary interstitium. The descending limb is freely permeable to water, which diffuses into the interstitium along the osmotic gradient; and the tubular fluid becomes progressively hyperosmotic at the bend of the loop.

The vasa recta, which are closely applied to the long loops of Henle of juxtamedullary nephrons, maintain this condition by removing water and adding solute as they pass through the medullary interstitium. A standing osmotic gradient is thereby set up between the cortex (300 mOsm/kg), juxtamedullary zone (600 mOsm/kg), and deep medulla (1200 mOsm/kg). This process is enhanced by the passive recycling of urea, which diffuses out of the inner medullary collecting duct into the interstitium and thence into the distal loop of Henle. These processes are summarized in Figure 18-10.

Tubular Concentration and Dilution

Hypovolemia

Contraction of the extracellular volume (hypovolemia) activates a series of vasoconstrictor, salt-retaining neurohormonal systems: the sympathoadrenal system, the renin-angiotensin-aldosterone axis, and AVP. Initially, the GFR and filtered load of sodium decrease. Sodium reabsorption in the proximal tubule is increased from about 66% to 80% by sympathetic activity and angiotensin II as well as by the decline in peritubular capillary pressure induced by renal vasoconstriction. Sodium delivery to the thick ascending loop of Henle, distal tubule, and collecting duct is decreased, but aldosterone promotes reabsorption of sodium at these sites. Under the influence of AVP, water is also avidly reabsorbed in the collecting duct so that the urine becomes highly concentrated (osmolality, 600 mOsm/kg) but with virtually no sodium (10 mEq/L).

Diuretics abolish the kidney's ability to concentrate urine by washing out the hypertonic medulla. They do this either by an osmotic effect that prevents water reabsorption (e.g., mannitol) or by inhibition of active NaCl transport in the thick ascending loop (e.g., furosemide) or the first part of the distal tubule (e.g., hydrochlorothiazide). An early and important manifestation of acute tubular necrosis is the loss of urinary concentrating ability caused by the breakdown of the energy-requiring Na^+/K^+-ATPase pump in the thick ascending loop of Henle.

Hypervolemia

Expansion of the extracellular volume or hypervolemia is controlled by a series of vasodilator, salt-excreting neuropeptides, of which atrial, or A-type, natriuretic peptide (ANP) is predominant. The GFR and filtered sodium load increase because of a combination of reflex decreases in sympathetic and angiotensin II activity and the release of ANP. Together with the increase in peritubular capillary hydrostatic pressure, these responses cause sodium reabsorption in the proximal tubule to decrease from 67% to 50%. The decline in plasma aldosterone decreases sodium absorption from the thick ascending loop of Henle to the collecting duct. The presence of ANP and absence of AVP impairs water absorption at the collecting duct so that dilute urine (osmolality, 300 mOsm/kg) with abundant sodium (80 mEq/L) is produced.

Loop diuretics, which depress tubular resorptive capacity, and acute tubular necrosis, which abolishes it completely, may generate an identical urinary profile (low osmolality, high urinary sodium) even in the presence of hypovolemia.

Evaluation of Renal Function

Clinical Markers of Renal Function

Urine Output

Perioperative oliguria is common, is almost always prerenal, and rarely implies acute renal failure. On the other hand, the absence of oliguria does not exclude it. Perioperative oliguria is defined as a urine flow rate less than 0.5 mL/kg/hr and is often interpreted as a sign of renal dysfunction. However, in the perioperative

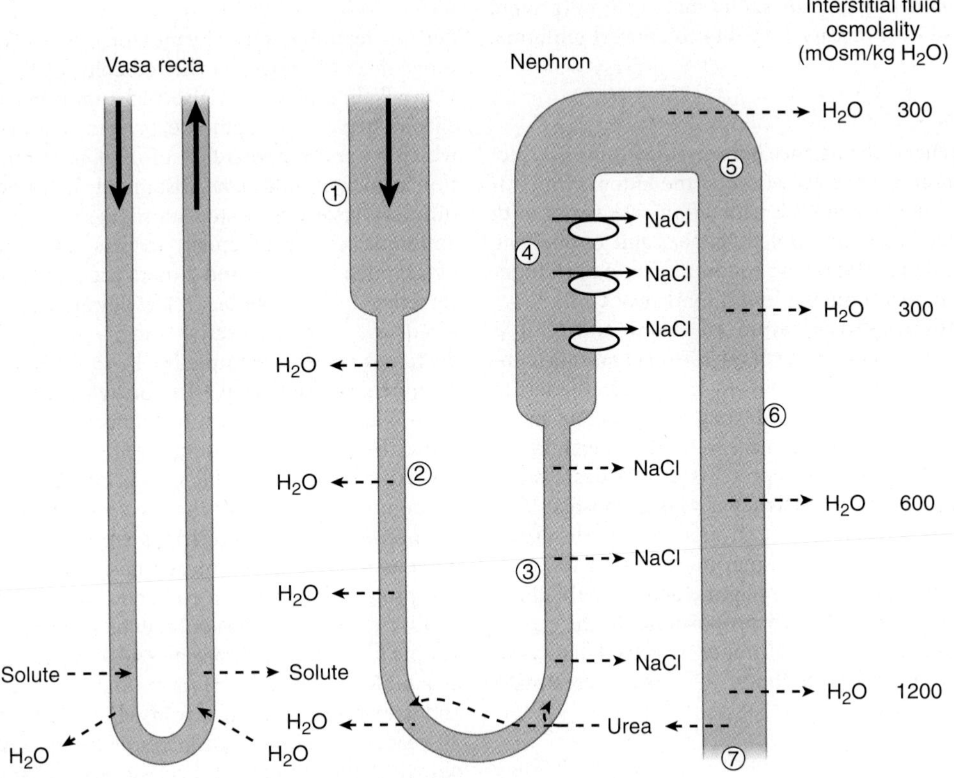

Figure 18-10 Tubular concentration of urine. The juxtamedullary nephrons have long loops of Henle associated with the vasa recta. *Dashed arrows* represent passive movement of fluid or solutes along concentration or osmolar gradients; *solid arrows* represent active transport. (1) Tubular fluid enters the distal proximal tubule iso-osmotic with plasma (300 mOsm/kg). In the descending limb of Henle (2), water rapidly diffuses out into the increasingly hypertonic medulla and is removed by the vasa recta so that the tubular fluid becomes hypertonic, owing largely to concentration of sodium chloride (NaCl). Urea diffuses in from the hypertonic interstitium, further increasing tubular fluid osmolality (1200 mOsm/kg). In the thin ascending loop of Henle (3), NaCl passively diffuses into the interstitium along its concentration gradient but water is trapped in the water-impermeable tubule, which progressively decreases tubular fluid osmolality. Urea passively diffuses into the tubular fluid (urea recycling). Tubular dilution is accelerated by active reabsorption of NaCl in the thick ascending loop (the diluting segment) and proximal distal tubule (4). The fluid entering the distal tubule is quite hypo-osmotic (100 mOsm/kg). In the collecting segment (5), the osmolality of the tubular fluid returns to that of plasma (300 mOsm/kg) but, unlike the contents of the proximal tubule, the solute component consists largely of urea, creatinine, and other excreted compounds. Increased plasma antidiuretic hormone renders the cortical and medullary collecting ducts (6) permeable to water, which passively diffuses into the hypertonic medullary interstitium. Even though some urea diffuses out into the medulla, the maximal osmolality of concentrated urine (7) approaches that of the hypertonic medullary interstitium, about 1200 mOsm/kg. In the absence of antidiuretic hormone, the collecting ducts remain impermeable to water and the urine is diluted. (*From Stanton BA, Koeppen BM: Control of body fluid osmolality and volume. In Berne RM, Levin HR [eds]: Physiology, 4th ed. St. Louis, Mosby, 1998, pp 715-743.*)

period, oliguria is almost inevitable. It is induced by hypotension, occurs as an (appropriate) prerenal response to intravascular hypovolemia, or is a manifestation of the physiologic response to surgical stress[14] (see "Neurohormonal Regulation of Renal Function").

Complete, often abrupt cessation of urine flow suggests a postrenal obstruction, which could occur at the level of the renal pelvis, ureters, bladder, urethra, or urinary catheter. However, subtotal obstruction may also develop into acute renal failure even though urine flow persists, albeit at a decreased rate.

Urine flow rate is an unreliable marker of acute renal failure and may vary from anuric (zero flow), to oliguric (urinary flow rate <15 mL/hr), to nonoliguric (15-80 mL/hr), to polyuric (>80 mL/hr). An attempt has been made to unify the definition of acute kidney injury by the RIFLE criteria, based on changes in serum creatinine and urine flow.[15] The first three categories (Risk, Injury, Failure) are defined in part by oliguria (<0.5 mL/kg/hr) for 6, 12, and 24 hours, respectively. However, this does not take into consideration that nonoliguric renal failure is the most common manifestation of perioperative acute kidney injury.

Blood Urea Nitrogen

Urea is continuously formed by the metabolism of ammonia in the liver. Hepatic deamination implies the splitting off of amide ($-NH_2$) groups from amino acids, and their conversion to ammonia, which enters the arginine cycle and is converted to urea. Urea nitrogen is a small, uncharged molecule, not protein bound, that is rapidly cleared from the blood by glomerular filtration. It subsequently undergoes reabsorption by the tubules so the blood urea nitrogen (BUN) does not correlate directly with GFR.

The normal range of BUN is 5 to 10 mg/dL; given the normal range of serum creatinine (0.5-1.0 mg/dL), the normal ratio of BUN to serum creatinine is about 10 : 1. An increase in BUN to serum creatinine ratio of greater than 20 : 1 implies the existence of a prerenal syndrome (prerenal azotemia). However, elevation of BUN out of proportion to decreases in GFR occurs whenever there is increased protein catabolism and formation of urea nitrogen. This scenario occurs with absorption of blood from the gastrointestinal tract, corticosteroid therapy, major trauma, and sepsis. In contrast, the BUN may be misleadingly low when its production is impaired by severe malnutrition (protein depletion) or severe liver disease (inability to convert ammonia to urea).

Serum Creatinine

Serum creatinine reflects the balance between creatinine production by muscle and creatinine excretion by the kidney, which is dependent on the GFR. Creatinine generation rate varies with muscle mass, physical activity, protein intake, and catabolism. However, when these processes are in equilibrium and renal function is stable, serum creatinine is a useful marker of GFR.

The relationship between serum creatinine and GFR is inverse and exponential. A doubling of the serum creatinine concentration implies a halving of the GFR. An increase in the serum creatinine value from 0.8 to 1.6 mg/dL may not generate much attention, but it indicates a 50% decrease in GFR. A much larger increase from 4 to 8 mg/dL also represents a 50% decrease in GFR, but by this time renal insufficiency is well established (Fig. 18-11). After a transient renal insult (e.g., suprarenal aortic cross-clamping), the serum creatinine level may increase for a few days while GFR is actually recovering. In oliguric acute renal failure, the serum creatinine value is directly proportional to the creatinine generation rate. Creatinine clearance is reliably low but is associated with a wide variability of serum creatinine concentration.

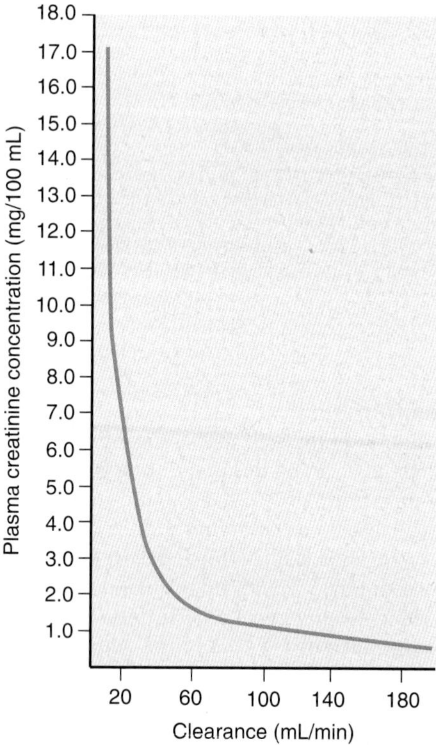

Figure 18-11 Relationship between serum creatinine and GFR. The relationship between serum creatinine and GFR as measured by creatinine clearance is reciprocal and exponential. Doubling of the serum creatinine corresponds to halving of the GFR. Relatively large declines in GFR from normal are associated with small increases in serum creatinine until GFR decreases below 60 mL/min; further decrements are associated with large increases in serum creatinine. *(From Alfrey AC, Chan L: Chronic renal failure: Manifestations and pathogenesis.* In *Schrier RW [ed]: Renal and Electrolyte Disorders, 4th ed. Boston, Little, Brown, 1992, p 541.)*

Limitations to Serum Creatinine as a Reflection of GFR

Serum creatinine is usually measured by the Jaffé reaction, a chromogenic assay based on the red color of the creatinine complex with alkaline picrate. It also picks up other normally occurring chromogens, such as glucose, protein, ketones, and ascorbic acid, which represent about 14% of total creatinine when renal function is normal, although substantially less when the serum creatinine level is elevated. Ketoacidosis, barbiturates, and cephalosporin antibiotics may artifactually increase the serum creatinine level by as much as 100%, and cimetidine and trimethoprim block its secretion by the tubule. *N*-acetylcysteine, an antioxidant advocated as a renoprotective agent in contrast nephropathy,[16] decreases serum creatinine levels, which may in part account for its apparently beneficial effect on renal function.[17]

The serum creatinine concentration does not increase above the normal range until the GFR declines below 50 mL/min, and large declines in GFR may occur above this level without a concomitant increase in the serum creatinine value. The creatinine generation rate is relatively consistent in a given individual, but it varies with muscle mass, rate of catabolism, physical activity, and protein intake.[18] In a cachectic patient with very low muscle mass, creatinine generation may be so feeble that the serum creatinine level remains "normal" (<0.9 mg/dL) even in the presence of a GFR less than 25 mL/min. The GFR declines progressively and predictably with age, from about 125 mL/min in a healthy 20-year old to about 60 mL/min in an 80-year old (or a 60-year old with atherosclerosis). Because these changes occur at a GFR greater than 50 mL/min, the impairment induced by aging is not reflected by the serum creatinine concentration.

Creatinine is soluble, freely distributes through the total body water, and is diluted by the 10% to 15% increases in total body water that occur with fluid administration and retention during major surgery. It is not uncommon for the serum creatinine concentration to be decreased from baseline on the first postoperative day (e.g., 1.5 to 1.2 mg/dL). Subsequently, when total body water is decreased by fluid mobilization and diuresis, the serum creatinine value increases (e.g., from 1.2 to 1.5 mg/dL). This does not necessarily imply acute kidney injury and a decline in GFR but may simply represent hemoconcentration and a re-equilibration to baseline.

Serum creatinine is a useful marker of stable renal function, but it is unreliable when GFR is rapidly changing.[18] If there are no changes in its volume of distribution (see earlier), the serum creatinine concentration represents an equilibrium between the creatinine generation rate, dependent on muscle mass and catabolic activity, and the creatinine excretion rate, dependent on (and reflective of) the GFR. An intervention such as suprarenal aortic cross-clamping causes instantaneous cessation of renal blood flow, GFR, and urinary creatinine excretion. However, measured serum creatinine would still be at baseline and would not detectably increase for several hours. Because it may take up to 48 hours for GFR to return to baseline, in the postoperative period the serum creatinine value may still increase for a few days while GFR is actually recovering.

Cystatin C

There is great interest in defining endogenous plasma markers that provide a more reliable, early indicator of changing GFR, especially in acute kidney injury.[19] One that has received prominence is cystatin C, a cysteine-protease inhibitor that is released into the circulation by all nucleated cells. It is completely filtered by the glomerulus and not secreted by the tubular epithelium so that its serum levels bear a close relationship to serum creatinine, and thereby GFR.[20] Unlike creatinine, however, serum cystatin C is not affected by muscle mass, age, or gender and in certain clinical situations appears to be a more accurate predictor of low GFR than serum creatinine does.[21,22] However, there is also evidence that factors such as cigarette smoking, inflammation (elevated C-reactive protein), and immunosuppressive therapy affect cystatin C levels independently of GFR.[23] At this stage, cystatin C remains an investigational marker and has not supplemented serum creatinine in clinical practice.

Assessment of Glomerular Filtration Rate

Serum Creatinine–Based Nomograms

In clinical investigation, nomograms based on population studies are commonly used to estimate GFR while avoiding the necessity of a timed urine collection. One example is that formulated by Cockroft and Gault utilizing age, weight, serum creatinine concentration, and gender:

$$\text{GFR}\left(\text{in mL/min}\right) = (140 - \text{age}) \times \text{weight in kg/serum creatinine} \times 72$$

For females, the result is multiplied by 0.85 to obtain the derived GFR.

In this formula, the body weight that is used may substantially alter the derived GFR. In obese or edematous patients, the total body weight is much greater than the lean body mass from which creatinine is derived, and GFR is overestimated. In cachectic patients with depleted lean body mass, creatinine production is so low that serum creatinine is frequently less than 1.0 mg/dL and overestimates the true GFR. Robert and associates[24] adjusted the Cockroft-Gault equation to incorporate ideal body weight from a nomogram and serum creatinine concentration corrected to 1.0 mg/dL (if < 1.0 mg/dL). Using this modification they found that single measurements in hemodynamically stable patients correlate more closely with inulin clearance than either a 30-minute or a 24-hour creatinine clearance.

A more complex nomogram, based on a study called Modification of Diet in Renal Disease (MDRD),[25] is independent of body weight:

$$\text{GFR}\left(\text{in mL/min}\right) = 170 \times \text{serum creatinine}^{-0.999} \times \text{age}^{-0.176} \times \text{BUN}^{-0.170}\ \text{albumin}^{0.318}$$

For females, the derived GFR is multiplied by 0.762; and for black patients, by 1.18.

When renal function is rapidly changing, serum creatinine–based nomograms are subject to the same limitations as serum creatinine itself. In fact, serum creatinine levels do not begin to increase above normal until the GFR declines below 50 mL/min/1.73 m^2, and occasionally they will remain normal even when the GFR dips as low as 20 to 40 mL/min/1.73 m^2.

Renal Clearance Techniques

Clearance is the most commonly used technique to estimate GFR, using compounds that are predominantly filtered by the glomerulus and neither secreted nor reabsorbed by the renal tubules.[26] Based on the Fick principle, the amount of substance x excreted by the kidney equals the amount delivered in the arterial supply minus the amount in the venous return:

$$\text{Excretion}_x = \text{delivery}_x - \text{return}_x$$

Therefore,

$$\text{Delivery}_x = \text{return}_x + \text{excretion}_x$$

The amount of substance x delivered to the kidney is the product of the arterial plasma concentration (Pa_x) and RBF. The amount returning from the kidney is the product of the venous plasma concentration (Pv_x) and RBF. The urinary excretion rate of substance x is the product of its urinary concentration (U_x) and the urine flow rate in milliliters per minute (V).

Therefore,

$$\left(Pa_x \times \text{RBF}\right) = \left(Pv_x \times \text{RBF}\right) + \left(U_x \times V\right)$$

However, in practice, RBF and venous return are not measured. Instead, the removal of substance x from the plasma by the kidney is expressed in the concept of clearance. Clearance (C) is defined as the virtual volume of plasma cleared of substance x per unit time, in milliliters per minute. This allows the urinary excretion rate of x to be equated to its renal arterial plasma concentration:

$$Pa_x \times C = U_x \times V$$

If the assumption is made that the concentration of x in renal arterial and venous plasma is identical, the clearance of substance x may be calculated using a urine sample, arm venous sample, and measured urinary flow rate:

$$C_x \times = U_x \times Pa_x / V$$

Inulin Clearance

Inulin is an inert polyfructose sugar that is completely filtered by the glomerulus and is neither secreted nor reabsorbed by the renal tubules. The volume in milliliters of plasma cleared of inulin per minute represents the GFR (in mL/min). After an intravenous loading dose of 30 to 50 mg/kg, a continuous infusion of inulin is given to establish a steady-state plasma concentration of 15 to 20 mg/dL. The bladder is usually flushed with air to eliminate any pooled urine. After a carefully timed urine collection (which can be as short as 30 minutes), urine and plasma inulin concentration (U_{IN}, P_{IN}) are measured and inulin clearance (C_{IN}) is calculated:

$$\text{GFR} = C_{IN} = U_{IN} \times V / P_{IN}$$

Normal values for inulin clearance are 110 to 140 mL/min/1.73 m^2 (males) and 95 to 125 mL/min/1.37 m^2 (females).

Although inulin clearance is the "gold standard" for measurement of GFR, it is seldom used clinically because its accurate measurement is laborious and requires meticulous attention to detail. Large changes in blood glucose during the test may interfere with its measurement. The predicted variability of inulin clearance is 20% when measurements are compared at two different times in the same individual and 40% when measurements are compared between two individuals.[26]

Sodium iothalamate, a radiocontrast dye, has been substituted for inulin and facilitates accurate assessment of rapid changes in GFR in acute kidney injury.[27]

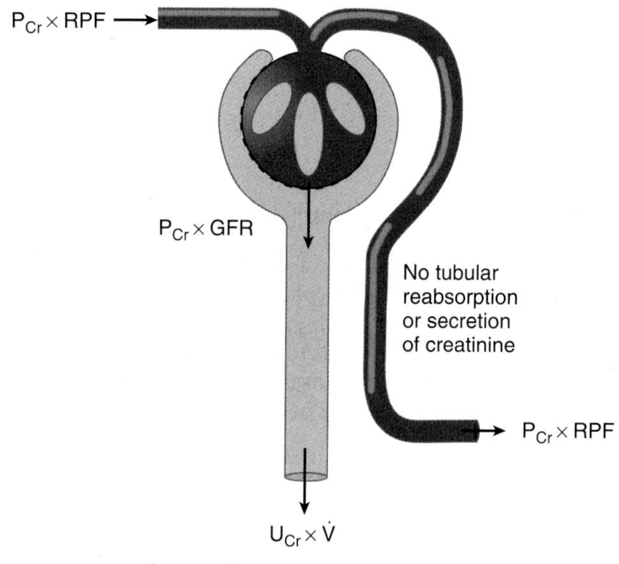

Figure 18-12 Renal handling of creatinine. Creatinine is freely filtered by the glomerulus and there is normally an inconsequential amount secreted or reabsorbed by the tubules. Thus, the amount of creatinine filtered is equivalent to the amount excreted in the urine. For a more detailed explanation, see text. P_{Cr}, plasma creatinine concentration; RPF, renal plasma flow; U_{Cr}, urinary concentration of creatinine; V, urine flow rate. *(From Koeppen BM, Stanton BA: Glomerular filtration and renal blood flow In Koeppen BM, Stanton BA [eds]: Renal Physiology, 4th ed. Philadelphia, Mosby Elsevier, 2007, pp 31-46.)*

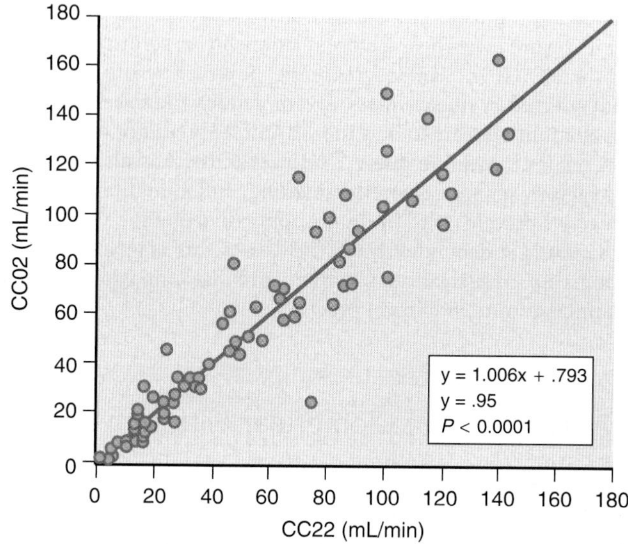

Figure 18-13 Creatinine clearance: 2-hour versus 22-hour values. There is a close and significant correlation in creatinine clearance estimation from a 2-hour and a 22-hour urine collection. CC02, 2-hour urine collection; CC22, 22-hour urine collection. *(From Sladen RN, Endo E, Harrison T: Two-hour versus 22-hour creatinine clearance in critically ill patients. Anesthesiology 67:1013-1016, 1987.)*

Creatinine Clearance

Creatinine, the endogenous end product of creatine phosphate metabolism, is normally generated from muscle at a very uniform rate and is handled by the kidney in a manner similar to that of inulin (Fig. 18-12). Thus, creatinine clearance (C_{CR}) provides a simple, inexpensive bedside estimate of GFR. A single blood sample is drawn at the midpoint of a carefully timed urine collection, and urine and plasma creatinine (U_{CR}, P_{CR}) and urinary flow rate in mL/min (V) are used to calculate GFR:

$$GFR = C_{CR} = U_{CR} \times V / P_{CR}$$

The creatinine clearance is far more accurate in tracking rapid alterations in GFR than the serum creatinine alone, because changes in GFR immediately alter the *creatinine excretion rate,* which is incorporated into the equation above as $U_{CR} \times V$.

The precise timing, not the duration, of the urine collection is the critical issue. If a brisk urine flow is induced by diuresis, and care is taken to empty the bladder, the variability of creatinine clearance is no greater with a 1-hour urine collection than with a 24-hour collection. In catheterized patients with urine flow rates of more than 15 mL/hr, creatinine clearance obtained with a 2-hour urine collection gives values equivalent to those obtained with a 22-hour collection.[28] In the previous example, a 2-hour creatinine clearance obtained at the beginning and end of the 24-hour period would truly reflect the halving of GFR represented by a doubling of the serum creatinine value from 1 to 2 mg/dL. In critically ill patients, a changing GFR can be closely tracked by serial estimations of using a short, carefully timed urine collection (Figs. 18-13 to 18-15). In trauma patients, a 1-hour creatinine clearance of less than 25 mL/min determined within 6 hours of surgery reliably predicted postoperative acute renal failure, despite the absence of oliguria.[29]

There is considerable variation in the normal range of creatinine clearance. Tobias and associates reported a variation in creatinine clearance between 88 and 148 mL/min and in serum creatinine concentration between 0.9 and 1.5 mg/dL in a single healthy individual over 5 years. There is also a diurnal variation, with higher values in the afternoon and a variance of up to 25% around mean values. It is prudent to obtain short-collection creatinine clearance estimations at the same time each day to minimize diurnal variability. "Normal" creatinine clearance is related to body surface area and weight, so values may fluctuate widely in patients with cachexia or edema.

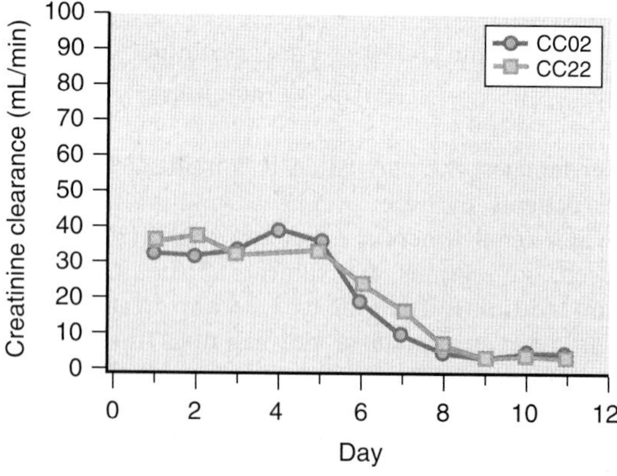

Figure 18-14 New-onset acute renal failure. In a patient developing acute renal failure in the intensive care unit, the exponential decline in creatinine clearance is tracked equally well whether a 2-hour (CC02) or a 22-hour (CC22) urine collection is used. However, data from the 2-hour collection are available well before those from the 22-hour collection.

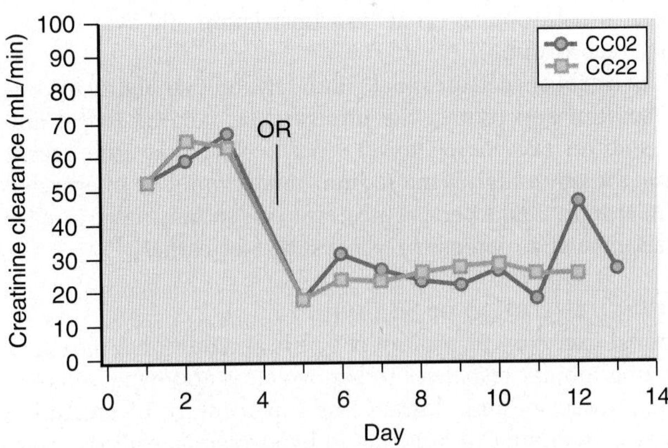

Figure 18-15 Renal revascularization. A patient with renovascular hypertension and renal insufficiency was admitted to the intensive care unit for preoperative monitoring and stabilization. Bilateral renal revascularization was performed, and after return from the operating room there was a substantial decline in renal function. These changes were tracked equally well by creatinine clearance derived from a 2-hour (CC02) and a 22-hour (CC22) collection.

Creatinine clearance has a number of inherent limitations even if collection error is carefully avoided. First, it is subject to many of the limitations imposed by the measurement of creatinine itself (see earlier). Unlike inulin, about 20% of creatinine is secreted by the proximal tubule, so that creatinine clearance overestimates GFR, and the ratio between the clearance of creatinine and inulin is 1.2:1. As the GFR declines, tubular secretion of creatinine increases. When GFR is less than 40 mL/min/1.73 m^2, a creatinine:inulin clearance ratio as high as 1.81 to 2.51 may be achieved. In patients with normal renal function, the underestimate of GFR induced by the Jaffé reaction is balanced by the overestimate of GFR induced by tubular creatinine secretion, and creatinine clearance provides a reasonable representation of GFR. However, widely used drugs such as trimethoprim, H_2-antagonists, and salicylates block tubular secretion of creatinine and may elevate serum creatinine and decrease creatinine clearance. When serum levels of creatinine are very high, it is excreted into the gut and undergoes extrarenal metabolism by intestinal organisms.

Given these constraints, an isolated creatinine clearance estimation may not reveal early renal dysfunction. Nonetheless, serial estimations of creatinine clearance provide a useful clinical guide to alterations in renal function and prognosis. Postoperatively, daily measurement of creatinine clearance is useful in guiding the dosing of renally excreted, potentially nephrotoxic aminoglycoside antibiotics (gentamicin, tobramycin, amikacin) or calcineurin antagonists (cyclosporine, tacrolimus). Because the GFR may decline to less than 50% of normal before serum creatinine increases above the normal range, an observed decrease in creatinine clearance may allow down-adjustment of drug dosing before nephrotoxicity becomes established and the drug accumulates even further.

The variability of creatinine clearance diminishes as GFR declines; in fact, loss of variability is a clue to deteriorating renal function. Directional changes between creatinine clearance and inulin clearance show good agreement. At low levels of GFR, a creatinine:inulin clearance ratio as high as 2:1 (e.g., 12 versus 6 mL/min) would induce little actual difference in clinical management.

Plasma Clearance

Measurement of the rate of disappearance (plasma clearance) of a substance that is completely eliminated by glomerular filtration is an alternate method for measuring GFR without the need for a simultaneous urine collection. It involves an intravenous bolus dose and/or infusion of the marker, followed by measurement of multiple plasma levels to calculate its disappearance rate. The methodology does depend on the achievement of a steady-state plasma concentration of the marker, which is difficult to achieve with rapid changes in GFR.[27]

Numerous markers are used, including nonradioactive inulin and iothalamate, as well as radioisotopes such as ^{51}Cr-ethylenediaminetetraacetic acid (EDTA), ^{99m}Tc-diethylenetriamine pentaacetic acid (DTPA), and ^{125}I-iothalamate. The latter two markers, which utilize measurement of decay in radiation, have shown promise in the rapid assessment of GFR.

Tubular Function Tests

Tests of renal tubular function measure urinary concentrating ability and sodium and urea handling. As such, they can distinguish oliguria due to dehydration (prerenal syndrome) from that due to tubular injury (acute tubular necrosis).

In prerenal oliguria, tubular function is preserved; in fact, it is "switched on" to retain salt and water, resulting in concentrated urine that is low in sodium. With the exception of refractory prerenal states such as severe sepsis and end-stage liver failure (see later), normalization of hemodynamic status reverses oliguria and tubular activation. The administration of potent diuretics may override tubular conservation, resulting in dilute urine that is high in sodium (natriuresis), indistinguishable from acute tubular necrosis (see later). However, if intravascular hypovolemia is severe enough, tubular sodium retention and low urinary sodium may persist despite the administration of diuretics such as low-dose dopamine.[30]

In established acute tubular necrosis, concentrating ability and sodium conservation are lost, resulting in dilute urine with high sodium that is not reversed by restoration of normal RBF. However, in nonoliguric renal failure, which accounts for as much as 75% of cases of acute tubular necrosis encountered clinically,[31] the changes in tubular function are less distinct from those of the prerenal syndrome.

Urinary Concentrating Ability

Concentrating ability is a very sensitive barometer of tubular function. In prerenal states, urinary osmolar concentration is markedly increased. In acute tubular necrosis, the ability to concentrate urine may be lost 24 to 48 hours before serum creatinine or BUN starts to increase.

Urine-to-Plasma Osmolar Ratio

The normal tubular response to dehydration or hypovolemia is to concentrate the urine and increase urine osmolality above 450 mOs/kg, compared with a normal serum or plasma osmolality of 280 to 300 mOs/kg. Thus, a prerenal syndrome is indicated by a urine-to-plasma osmolar ratio ($U:P_{OSM}$) of greater than 1.5. Loss of concentrating ability, or isosthenuria ($U:P_{OSM} = 1.0$), in the presence of oliguria implies tubular damage and established acute renal failure. However, isosthenuria can be induced in a prerenal state when diuretics are administered (see earlier).

Free Water Clearance

Free water clearance (CH_2O) is a measure of renal water regulation by tubular dilution or concentration of urine. In essence, free water is cleared by the tubules in response to hypervolemia ("positive free water clearance") or retained in response to hypovolemia ("negative free water clearance"). The kidney's capacity for water regulation is enormous, and CH_2O can vary from +18 L to −8 L/day.[32] CH_2O is calculated by distinguishing the renal clearance of solute from that of free water.

The solute or osmolar clearance (C_{OSM}) is calculated by standard methods, using urine osmolality in mOs/kg (U_{osm}), plasma osmolality in mOs/kg (P_{OSM}), and urine flow in mL/min (V):

$$C_{OSM} = \left(U_{OSM} \cdot V\right)/P_{OSM} \ (\text{in mL/min})$$

Then, the osmolar clearance is subtracted from the urine flow rate to give free water clearance:

$$C_{H_2O} = V - C_{OSM} \ (\text{in mL/min})$$

This implies that when urine is diluted and flow is greater than osmolar clearance, CH_2O is positive, and when urine is concentrated and flow is less than osmolar clearance, CH_2O is negative. Negative free water clearance (i.e., free water retention) is also known as tubular conservation of water (TCH_2O) and represents the volume of fluid that would have to be added to the urine to make its osmolality equivalent to that of plasma.[32]

With the onset of acute tubular necrosis and loss of concentrating ability, the urine becomes isosmotic, and CH_2O approaches zero (± 0.25 mL/min). However, in distinguishing between prerenal and intrarenal oliguria, CH_2O does not really provide any more information about concentrating ability than $U{:}P_{OSM}$, and, in addition, it requires a timed urine collection.

Water Conservation

Urine-to-Plasma Creatinine Ratio

The urine-to-plasma creatinine ratio ($U{:}P_{CR}$) represents the proportion of water filtered by the glomerulus that is abstracted by the entire tubule. Normally, about 98% of water is abstracted and urine creatinine is much greater than plasma creatinine. The ratio can increase 100-fold in severe prerenal states. When tubular function is lost, the ratio declines to less than 20:1.

For example, two patients have oliguria with a serum creatinine elevated to 2.0 mg/dL. In patient A, the urine creatinine is 100 mg/dL, and in patient B, it is 20 mg/dL. Patient A likely has a prerenal state because tubular water abstraction is high (U:P creatinine = 50:1), whereas patient B likely has acute tubular necrosis because tubular water abstraction is impaired (U:P creatinine = 10:1).

Sodium and Urea Conservation

Urine Sodium

Dehydration or hypovolemia markedly stimulates tubular sodium reabsorption at the medullary thick ascending limb and distal tubule. In the prerenal syndrome, oliguria is characterized by a very low urine sodium (U_{Na}) value, less than 20 mEq/L. Typically, this response is reversed by restoration of intravascular volume. However, in two situations, severe sepsis and the hepatorenal syndrome of liver failure, refractory oliguria with low urine sodium persists despite aggressive fluid resuscitation. The pathogenesis is multifactorial, but common to both syndromes is endotoxemia, which induces renal vasoconstriction and avid tubular sodium reabsorption.

In established acute renal failure, the tubular ability to conserve sodium and protect the intravascular volume is lost and urine sodium exceeds 60 to 80 mEq/L. Note that after recent diuretic therapy a high urine sodium value cannot be interpreted as tubular injury but a persistently low urine sodium value implies the existence of an intense prerenal state (see earlier).[30]

Fractional Excretion of Sodium

Fractional excretion of sodium (FE_{Na}) is an additional means of evaluating tubular responses to hypovolemia and hypervolemia. FE_{Na} expresses sodium clearance as a percentage of creatinine clearance. The implication is that in hypovolemia, sodium clearance (and thus FE_{Na}) declines to reflect tubular sodium conservation; in hypervolemia, the opposite occurs.

FE_{Na} is calculated as follows:

$$FE_{Na} = \left(\text{sodium clearance/creatinine clearance}\right) \times 100\%$$

Based on the relationship expressed earlier:

$$FE_{Na} = \left(U_{Na} \cdot V/P_{Na}\right)/\left(U_{Cr} \cdot V/P_{Cr}\right) \times 100\%$$

Urine flow rate (V) is identical in the numerator and denominator and it cancels out:

$$FE_{Na} = \left(U_{Na}/P_{Na}\right)/\left(U_{Cr}/P_{Cr}\right) \times 100\%$$

Thus, FE_{Na} may be calculated from a spot sample of blood and urine without requiring a timed urine collection.

During dehydration or hypovolemia, sodium clearance and FE_{Na} are decreased to less than 1% of creatinine clearance. When tubular ability to conserve sodium is lost in acute renal failure, FE_{Na} increases to more than 3%. However, FE_{Na} increases with normal tubular function after diuretic therapy and during postoperative sodium mobilization. Sequential increases in FE_{Na} associated with a declining creatinine clearance provide a more reliable indicator of deteriorating renal function than an isolated high FE_{Na}.

Fractional Excretion of Urea Nitrogen

Unlike sodium, handling of urea in the ascending loop of Henle and distal tubule is subject to passive forces and is little influenced by loop diuretic therapy. Fractional excretion of urinary nitrogen (FE_{UN}) is related to water reabsorption in the proximal tubules, which increases to compensate for impaired renal perfusion in a prerenal state. Urea is also reabsorbed, leading to an increased BUN:SCr ratio and decreased FE_{UN}. It has been suggested that the FE_{UN} is more sensitive and specific than the FE_{Na} in differentiating oliguria due to acute tubular necrosis from a prerenal syndrome, especially in the presence of loop diuretic therapy.[33] The FE_{UN} is calculated identically to FE_{Na}:

$$FE_{UN} = \left(U_{UN}/BUN\right)/\left(U_{Cr}/P_{Cr}\right) \times 100\%$$

where U_{UN} is the urinary urea nitrogen, U_{Cr} is urine creatinine, and P_{Cr} is plasma creatinine.

In oliguric patients, an FE_{UN} of less than 35% indicates a prerenal syndrome, whereas an FE_{UN} of 50% to 65% suggests established acute renal failure, even in the presence of loop diuretic therapy.[33]

The major limitation to the FE_{UN} is the concomitant administration of proximal tubule diuretics such as acetazolamide and of osmotic diuretics such as mannitol. These agents impair water reabsorption in the proximal tubule and ameliorate a decrease in FE_{UN} in a prerenal state. Excessive urea production in highly catabolic states may itself induce an osmotic diuresis and render the FE_{UN} inaccurate.

Indices of Tubular Injury

β_2-Microglobulin

β_2-Microglobulin is a small protein component of the major histocompatibility complex that is present on the surface of almost all cells. It is normally filtered by the glomerulus and then undergoes partial tubular reabsorption. The ratio of β_2-microglobulin between serum and urine may help distinguish glomerular from tubular injury, although the relationship between increased urinary β_2-microglobulin and subsequent acute tubular necrosis has not been characterized.

In glomerular injury, serum β_2-microglobulin levels increase and urine levels decrease. This assessment has been utilized as an early sign of rejection in renal transplantation.[34]

In primary tubular injury, reabsorption of β_2-microglobulin is impaired, so urinary levels increase and serum levels decline. In a study in which CPB with pulsatile flow was used, there was a significant decrease in plasma renin activity but urinary β_2-microglobulin increased on CPB with pulsatile or nonpulsatile flow.[35] The implication is that although pulsatile flow maintains better renal perfusion it does not prevent a subclinical renal tubular injury.

Urinary N-Acetyl-β-D-glucosaminidase

The assay of increased urinary concentrations of the tubular enzyme *N*-acetyl-β-D-glucosaminidase (NAG) is a well-established method of identifying subclinical tubular injury. Urinary NAG levels, or the ratio of its isoenzymes, have been used in the early detection of rejection in transplant patients or to follow the course of chronic renal disease (e.g., lupus nephritis).[36] However, there are few data on the relationship between tubular enzymuria and clinical indices of perioperative renal outcome, such as the need for renal replacement therapy.

Neutrophil Gelatinase-Associated Lipocalin

Neutrophil gelatinase-associated lipocalin (NGAL) is a small 25-kDA polypeptide expressed in proximal tubular cells whose mRNA undergoes dramatic upregulation after ischemic tubular injury.[37] Upregulation can be detected within minutes of ischemia-reperfusion injury and increases threefold to fourfold within 2 to 3 hours and up to 10,000-fold by 24 hours. NGAL is protease resistant and is readily detected in tiny (micromilliliter) amounts of urine almost immediately after renal injury, preceding the appearance of NAG and β_2-microglobulin.

Urinary NGAL has been demonstrated to increase significantly within 2 hours of CPB in pediatric or adult patients who subsequently went on to develop a 50% increase in postoperative serum creatinine, whose peak was delayed until 1 to 3 days after surgery.[38,39] Aprotinin is an antifibrinolytic kallikrein inhibitor that is associated with acute kidney injury.[40] In a study on 369 patients undergoing cardiac surgery, urinary NGAL levels were 18 times higher 3 hours after CPB in the 205 patients given aprotinin compared with those who had received ε-aminocaproic acid.[41] These data suggest that urinary NGAL may represent an early, sensitive, noninvasive urinary biomarker for ischemic and nephrotoxic renal injury.

Renal Hemodynamics

Renal Plasma Flow and Renal Blood Flow

p-Aminohippurate Clearance

p-Aminohippurate (PAH) is an organic anion filtered by the glomerulus and secreted by the tubule that is almost completely cleared from the plasma in a single pass through the kidney. Thus, clearance of PAH (C_{PAH}) represents RPF.

Like inulin clearance, the test is laborious and requires intravenous and urinary catheters. A PAH infusion is set up to maintain a steady-state PAH concentration of about 2 mg/dL, together with a carefully timed catheter urine collection.[26] Because 10% of the RPF bypasses the peritubular capillaries, C_{PAH} underestimates the true RPF and is referred to as *effective* RPF.

$$\text{Effective RPF} = C_{PAH} = U_{PAH} \times V / P_{PAH}$$

In young healthy adults, effective RPF is 660 mL/min/1.73 m^2.

Effective renal blood flow (RBF) may be derived if the hematocrit level (Hct) is known and expressed as a decimal (i.e., 35% = 0.35):

$$\text{Effective RBF} = \text{Effective RPF}/1 - \text{Hct}$$

As an example, if effective RPF is 600 mL/min and Hct is 30% (0.3), effective RBF is 600/0.7, i.e., 860 mL/min.

Unfortunately, C_{PAH} is an unreliable indicator of RPF during surgical stress because hypovolemia and oliguria induce sequestration of PAH in the kidney. Ironically, the most important limitation of C_{PAH} is renal injury, because about 80% of PAH is cleared by tubular secretion. In the presence of proximal tubular injury, PAH secretion declines and C_{PAH} underestimates RPF.[42]

These errors can be overcome if renal vein sampling is accessible (e.g., during major abdominal vascular surgery). Measurement of the difference between arterial and renal vein PAH allows calculation of the renal extraction of PAH (E_{PAH}), an index of proximal tubular function:

$$E_{PAH} = \text{arterial PAH} - \text{renal vein PAH}/\text{arterial PAH}$$

When renal function is normal, renal vein PAH is close to zero and E_{PAH} approaches 100% (1.0). With worsening proximal tubular function, renal vein PAH concentration progressively increases and E_{PAH} progressively declines.

True RPF is calculated by dividing PAH clearance by PAH extraction:

$$\text{RPF} = C_{PAH}/E_{PAH}$$

Filtration Fraction

The fraction of the RPF that is filtered by the glomerulus is called the filtration fraction (FF) and can be measured indirectly via the C_{PAH} and C_{IN}:

$$\text{FF} = \text{GFR}/\text{RPF} = C_{IN}/C_{PAH}$$

Normally, GFR is about 125 mL/min and RPF is about 660 mL/min, so that the filtration fraction approximates 125/660, or about 0.2. Changes in filtration fraction are considered to represent changes in periglomerular arteriolar tone (see "'Afferent and Efferent Arteriolar Control Mechanisms," earlier). An increase in filtration fraction indicates that GFR is increased relative to RPF. This could be achieved by efferent arteriolar constriction or afferent arteriolar dilation and maintains glomerular filtration pressure in the presence of decreased RPF. Conversely, a decrease in filtration fraction implies that GFR is decreased relative to RPF by afferent arteriolar constriction or efferent arteriolar dilation.

Total Renal Blood Flow

Flow Probes

Flow measurement by electromagnetic flow probes is based on the creation of a magnetic field around the circumference of the vessel. The field is disrupted by blood flow, and a voltage output proportional to blood velocity is generated. Ultrasonic flow probes use the Doppler technique, in which high-frequency sound is transmitted across the lumen of the vessel. A shift in sound frequency is created by the movement of blood and is proportional to blood velocity.

$$\text{Flow}\left(\text{in mL/min}\right) = \text{blood velocity}\left(\text{in cm/min}\right) \times \text{area of vessel}\left(\text{in cm}^2\right)$$

Flow-probe placement is invasive and requires direct surgical exposure of the renal arteries. Probes must be calibrated in vitro before and after measurements. However, they are generally accurate.

Thermodilution Estimation of Renal Vein Effluent

Schaer and associates[43] used a double-lumen pigtail catheter with a thermistor placed in the renal vein of dogs under direct vision or with fluoroscopy. RBF was calculated by thermodilution with cold saline, which allowed repeated measurements in conscious animals. The effect of the presence of the probe itself on RBF is unknown. A similar technique was used by Haywood and associates[44] to measure RBF for the assessment of renal oxygen delivery and consumption during septic shock in pigs.

Contrast Ultrasonography

Aronson and coworkers[45] attempted to measure RBF in vivo using contrast ultrasonography. They injected sonicated albumin microspheres into the aorta of anesthetized dogs and then recorded simultaneous ultrasonograpic images of the kidney and aorta and calculated RBF using a mathematical model. RBF was altered by means of a renal artery occluder or vasoactive drugs (dopamine or fenoldopam), and the results were compared with direct measurements by electromagnetic flow probe. Although the correlation between ultrasonography and flow probe measurements of RBF was reasonable (0.84), there was a large bias (in many cases greater than 200 mL/min) and variance. Ultrasonography tended to overestimate RBF, especially when cardiac output was changing. The authors concluded that this method allows estimation of trends in RBF and may be helpful in the qualitative assessment of regional distribution of blood flow between the renal cortex and medulla.

Neurohormonal Regulation of Renal Function

Two mutually dependent but opposing neurohormonal systems maintain blood pressure, intravascular volume, and salt and water homeostasis (Fig. 18-16). The sympathoadrenal axis, the renin-angiotensin-aldosterone system, and AVP defend against hypotension and hypovolemia by promoting vasoconstriction and salt and water retention. The prostaglandins and natriuretic peptides defend against hypertension and hypervolemia by promoting vasodilation and salt and water excretion (Fig. 18-17).

Anesthesia does not perturb these systems to any substantial degree. In the intact organism, anesthetics appear to affect renal function through extrarenal circulatory changes rather than by their direct actions on the kidney. Surgical or traumatic injury, on the other hand, induces profound vasoconstriction and salt and water retention, which may persist for several days. The clinical sequel is postoperative oliguria and edema. Renal vasoconstriction also predisposes the kidney to further perioperative ischemic and nephrotoxic insults. Release of endogenous natriuretic peptides by atrial and ventricular stretch reinforces the notion that renal vasoconstriction can be prevented or modified by maintenance of normal or increased intravascular volume.

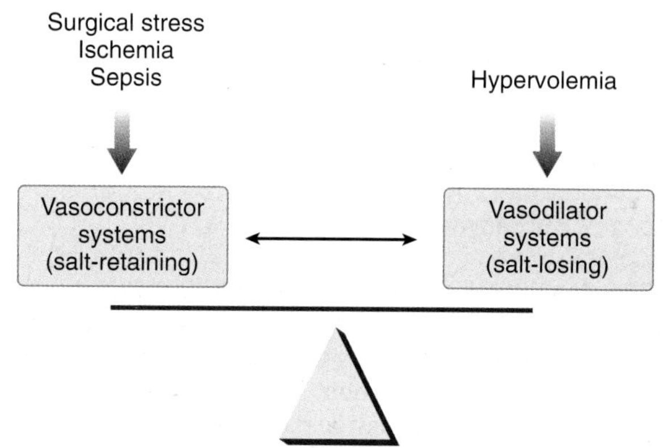

Figure 18-16 Neurohormonal regulation of renal function. Normally, there is a balance between those systems promoting renal vasoconstriction and sodium retention versus those systems promoting renal vasodilation and sodium excretion. Surgical stress, ischemia, and sepsis tip the balance in favor of vasoconstriction and sodium retention. On the other hand, hypervolemia (or the induction of atrial stretch) tips the balance in favor of vasodilation and sodium excretion.

Vasoconstrictor Systems	Vasodilator Systems
Sympathoadrenal system Renin-angiotensin system Aldosterone Antidiuretic hormone (ADH)	Prostaglandins Kinins Atrial natriuretic peptide (ANP)
↓ RBF ↓ GFR ↓ Urine flow ↓ Na excretion	↑ RBF ↑ GFR ↑ Urine flow ↑ Na excretion

Figure 18-17 Neurohormonal renal regulatory systems. GFR, glomerular filtration rate; Na, sodium; RBF, renal blood flow; ↓, decreased; ↑, increased. *(Modified from Sladen RN: Effect of anesthesia and surgery on renal function. Crit Care Clin 3:380, 1987.)*

Systems Promoting Vasoconstriction and Salt Retention

The Sympathoadrenal Axis

Sympathetic effects on the kidney are mediated by circulating epinephrine and neuronal release of norepinephrine. The renal cortex has a dense plexus of autonomic nerve fibers derived from the T12 to L4 spinal segments via the celiac plexus. The primary stimulus to the sympathetic response is a decrease in arterial blood pressure sensed by baroreceptors in the aortic arch, carotid sinus, and afferent arteriole. Afferent fibers travel via the vagus nerve and decrease impulse transmission rate to the mediating centers in the hypothalamus, which results in increased adrenergic nerve activity. The kidney does not have any parasympathetic innervation.

A G protein–coupled phospholipase-C receptor populates vascular smooth muscle and the mesangium and responds to α-adrenergic stimulation by epinephrine and norepinephrine. It also mediates vasoconstriction induced by a variety of other hormones and peptides, including angiotensin II, vasopressin, endothelin, platelet-activating factor, and leukotrienes.[3] The receptor subunit in the cell membrane is coupled through G_q protein to phospholipase C, which hydrolyzes phosphatidylinositol biphosphate (PIP_2) to inositol triphosphate (IP_3) and diacylglycerol (DAG). In turn, DAG activates protein kinase, opening up a calcium channel in the membrane, and IP_3 triggers the release of calcium from the sarcoplasmic or endoplasmic reticulum. Both mechanisms result in a rapid increase in intracellular calcium, which binds with calmodulin and thereby activates myosin light-chain kinase, resulting in smooth muscle contraction. The calcium-calmodulin complex simultaneously activates phospholipase A_2, resulting in the production of vasodilator prostaglandins (see later).

Mild α-adrenergic stimulation appears to cause preferential efferent arteriolar constriction, which preserves the filtration fraction. Severe α-adrenergic stimulation causes predominant afferent arteriolar constriction and decreases filtration fraction. Thus, the adrenergic response to a moderate decrease in renal perfusion (e.g., general anesthesia) favors the preservation of the GFR. In contrast, the adrenergic response to shock exacerbates the decrease in GFR already induced by renal hypoperfusion (see Fig. 18-4).

Adrenergic nerves also supply the proximal tubule, thick ascending limb of the loop of Henle, and collecting duct, and their stimulation enhances NaCl reabsorption at these sites. Gas tracer studies suggested that sympathetic activation caused sodium retention by intrarenal redistribution of RBF from the outer cortex to salt-retaining juxtamedullary nephrons, but this was not confirmed by microsphere studies.

There is a close relationship between sympathetic stimulation and activation of the renin-angiotensin system. Adrenergic stimulation releases renin from the juxtaglomerular apparatus, and adrenergically induced vasoconstriction can be blocked by angiotensin-converting enzyme (ACE) inhibitor drugs such as captopril.

The effects of the administration of exogenous adrenergic drugs depend on their agonist activity. Drugs with predominantly α-adrenergic effects, such as norepinephrine, epinephrine, phenylephrine, and high-dose dopamine (>10 μg/kg/min) exacerbate the endogenous sympathetic responses to hypotension. Drugs with predominantly β_1- and β_2-adrenergic activity, such as dobutamine or isoproterenol, cause marked increases in cardiac output and thus RBF, but it is difficult to ascertain their intrarenal effects. Dopaminergic agonists (Table 18-2) selectively increase RBF and may oppose α-adrenergic renal vasoconstriction.[43]

Table 18-2 Dopamine and its Analogs

Receptor	DA_1	DA_2	β_1	β_2	α_1
Dopamine	+++	++	++	±	+++
Dobutamine	0	0	+++	++	±
Dopexamine	++	+	±	+++	0
Fenoldopam	++++	0	0	0	0

Dobutamine, dopexamine, and fenoldopam are all pharmacologic analogs of dopamine. However, dobutamine is devoid of dopaminergic activity; dopexamine has about one third of the dopaminergic activity of dopamine; and fenoldopam is a pure, selective dopamine$_1$-receptor agonist. α_1, alpha$_1$-receptor; β_1, beta$_1$-receptor; β_2, beta$_2$-receptor; DA_1, dopamine$_1$-receptor; DA_2, dopamine$_2$-receptor.

The Renin-Angiotensin-Aldosterone System

Renin and Angiotensin

The juxtaglomerular apparatus consists of three groups of specialized tissues. In the afferent arteriole, modified fenestrated endothelial cells produce renin; in the juxtaposed distal tubule, cells of the macula densa act as chemoreceptors; and in the glomerulus, mesangial cells have contractile properties (see Fig. 18-3). Together these provide an important regulating system for blood pressure, salt, and water homeostasis.[46]

Renin secretion is stimulated by hypovolemia that may be overt (hemorrhage, diuresis, sodium loss or restriction) or covert (positive-pressure ventilation, congestive heart failure, sepsis, or cirrhosis with ascites). A decrease in renal artery perfusion pressure triggers baroreceptors in the afferent arterioles. Sympathetic nerve stimulation and circulating catecholamines act on β-adrenergic receptors in the afferent arterioles. An increase in chloride concentration in the distal tubular fluid activates the cells of the macula densa, which trigger renin release from the afferent arteriole. This tubuloglomerular feedback appears to play a role in modulating GFR during normal and abnormal renal function through a continuous feedback loop.[4,5]

Renin acts on angiotensinogen, a large circulating glycoprotein released from the liver, and cleaves off a decapeptide, angiotensin I. In the kidney and in the lung angiotensin I is further cleaved by endothelial-based ACE to form an octapeptide, angiotensin II, a potent vasoconstrictor (Fig. 18-18). Renin is the rate-limiting enzyme in the production of angiotensin II.[47]

Activation of modest amounts of angiotensin II causes renal cortical vasoconstriction predominantly at the level of the efferent arterioles (see Fig. 18-4). This acts to maintain glomerular filtration fraction in the presence of mild to moderate decreases in RBF or perfusion pressure. The importance of this protective mechanism is emphasized by the deterioration in GFR that occurs when angiotensin-converting enzyme inhibitors are administered to patients with hypotension, renal insufficiency, or unilateral renal artery stenosis.[48,49] Severe stress induces the release of high levels of angiotensin II, which constricts the glomerular mesangial cells and decreases the glomerular filtration fraction. Angiotensin II promotes systemic vasoconstriction at about one tenth of its renal effect. The effect of angiotensin II in causing salt and

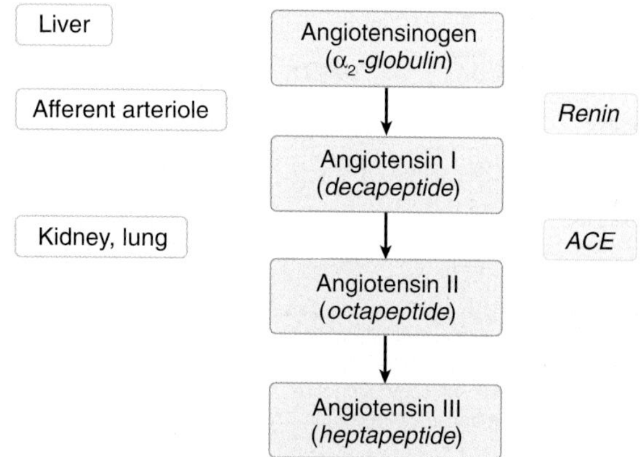

Figure 18-18 Renin-angiotensin system. For explanation, see text. ACE, angiotensin-converting enzyme.

water retention is enhanced by its actions in stimulating aldosterone secretion by the adrenal cortex, AVP secretion by the posterior pituitary, and NaCl reabsorption by the proximal tubule.[46]

Angiotensin II triggers a number of responses that modulate or oppose its own actions. It inhibits renin secretion by a negative feedback mechanism. Blockade of angiotensin formation by ACE inhibitors causes vasodilation but increases plasma renin levels. Angiotensin II activates phospholipase A_2, which triggers the synthesis of intrarenal prostaglandins. Vasodilator prostaglandins modulate the action of angiotensin II and may be responsible for its preferential activity on the efferent arteriole at low plasma levels.[47] Angiotensin-induced vasoconstriction increases atrial pressure and releases ANP, which opposes the renin-angiotensin-aldosterone system.

The consequences of ACE inhibition on renal function depend on the patient's volume status, systemic hemodynamics, and baseline renal perfusion. In the long-term treatment of hypertension and congestive heart failure, especially in diabetics, the administration of ACE inhibitors decreases renal vascular resistance and appears to benefit renal function. Short-term pretreatment with captopril may prevent a decrease in RBF and GFR and preserve sodium excretion during CPB.[50] However, deterioration in renal function and hyperkalemia have been reported with the use of ACE inhibitors in patients with hypotension, renal insufficiency, or unilateral renal artery stenosis, probably related to the blockade of compensatory angiotensin-mediated efferent arteriolar constriction.[49] It may be prudent to avoid their use when hemodynamics are unstable in the immediate perioperative period.

Aldosterone

Aldosterone is a steroid hormone secreted by the zona glomerulosa of the adrenal cortex in response to hyperkalemia or hyponatremia. Angiotensin II and adrenocorticotropic hormone (ACTH) also trigger its release. It acts at the thick ascending limb of the loop of Henle, the principal cells of the distal tubule, and the collecting duct to increase active absorption of sodium and passive absorption of water, culminating in an expanded blood volume. Sodium retention in vessel walls appears to enhance their response to vasoconstrictor agents.

In contrast to the immediate sympathetic angiotensin II response to hypovolemia, there is a delay of 1 to 2 hours from the secretion of aldosterone to its action on sodium reabsorption. As illustrated in Figure 18-19, aldosterone forms a complex with a receptor at the cell membrane in the principal cells of the distal tubule. The aldosterone-receptor complex travels to the cell nucleus, where it induces cytoplasmic transcription of messenger ribonucleic acid (mRNA). This fosters synthesis of proteins that form sodium channels in the apical cell membrane and enhance the Na+/K+-ATPase pump in the basolateral cell membrane.[51] Sodium is transported from the tubular fluid into the peritubular capillary in exchange for potassium. Long-standing stimulation of aldosterone secretion, characteristically induced by the intravascular volume depletion of chronic ascites, culminates in potassium depletion and hypokalemic alkalosis.

Arginine Vasopressin

Arginine vasopressin (AVP), previously known as antidiuretic hormone (ADH), regulates urinary volume and osmolality and controls diuresis and antidiuresis. It is a 9-amino-acid peptide, 8-arginine vasopressin, that is synthesized in the supraoptic and paraventricular nuclei of the anterior hypothalamus.[51] These nuclei are essentially the cell bodies of neurons whose axons extend down into nerve terminals in the posterior pituitary, together comprising the neurohypophysis (Fig. 18-20). When

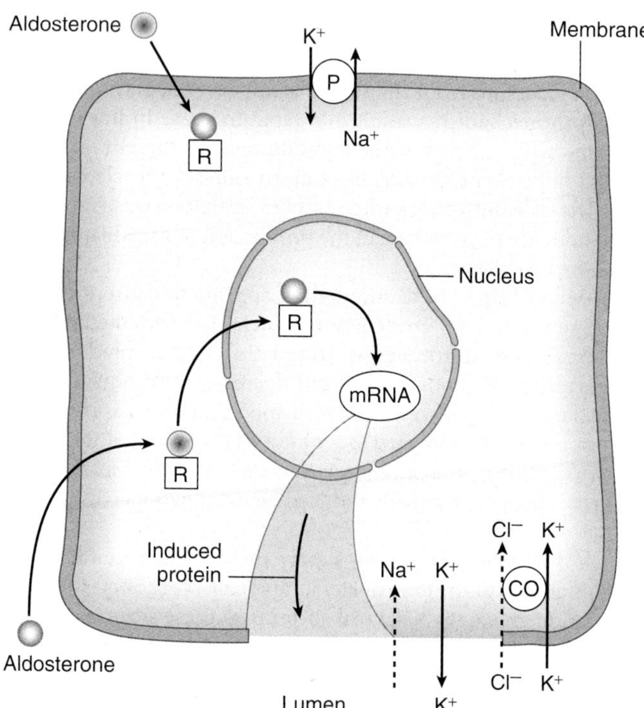

Figure 18-19 Action of aldosterone. Aldosterone enters the distal tubular cytoplasm and attaches to a receptor, then migrates to the nucleus where it induces the formation of a messenger RNA (mRNA). The mRNA in turn induces the synthesis of a protein that enhances the permeability of the apical (luminal) membrane to sodium and potassium. The reabsorption of sodium stimulates the basolateral membrane Na-K-ATPase pump, the intracellular concentration of potassium rises, and it follows its concentration gradient out into the lumen. The net effect of aldosterone's action is sodium reabsorption and potassium loss. Cl^-, chloride; CO, cotransporter (= symporter); K^+, potassium; mRNA, messenger ribonucleic acid; Na^+, sodium; P, sodium-potassium ATPase pump; R, receptor. (*From Wingard LB, Brody TM, Larner J, Schwartz A: Diuretics: Drugs that increase excretion of water and electrolytes.* In *Wingard LB, Brody TM, Larner J, Schwartz A [eds]: Human Pharmacology: Molecular-to-Clinical. London, Wolfe Publishing, 1991, p 249.*)

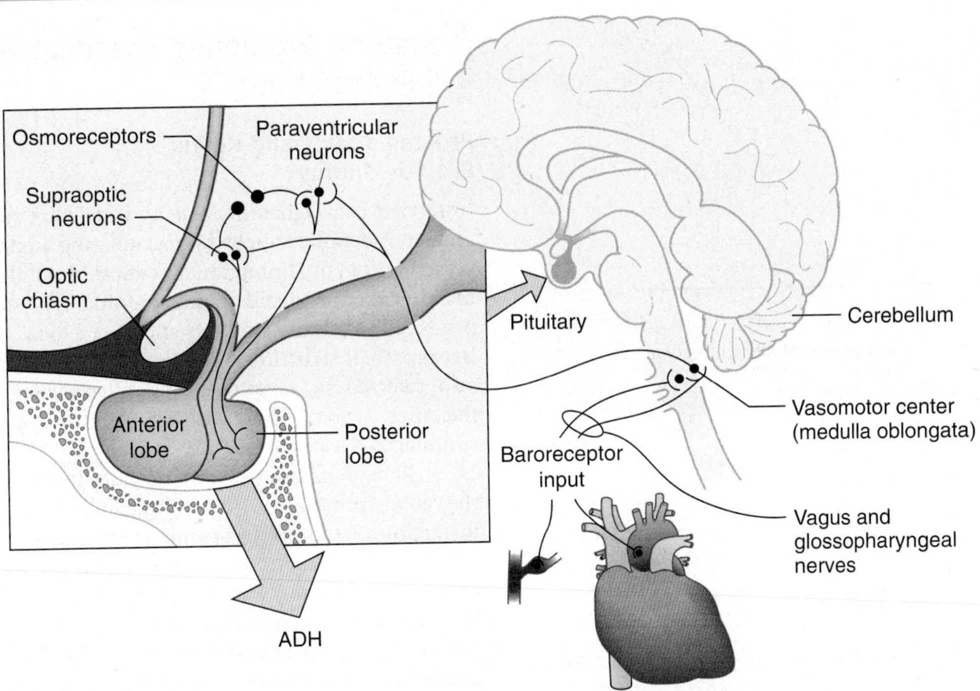

Figure 18-20 Elaboration and control of arginine vasopressin (AVP). *Osmotic control.* An increase in serum osmolality is detected by osmoreceptors in the supraoptic and paraventricular neurons of the hypothalamus. Granules of AVP are elaborated and axonally transported to the posterior lobe of the pituitary gland. From there they are released into the circulation to reach the V_2 receptors in the distal tubule, where they retain water and restore the serum osmolality. *Hemodynamic control.* Decreases in venous volume are sensed by stretch receptors in the atria and great veins, and decreases in arterial pressure are sensed by baroreceptors in the aortic arch and carotid sinus. The afferent arc is via the vagal and glossopharyngeal nerves to the solitary nucleus in the medulla oblongata (vasomotor center). The efferent arc, from the vasomotor center to the hypothalamic nuclei, induces AVP release. At low levels (< 5 pg/mL), AVP stimulation of V_2 receptors may cause inappropriate water retention. At high levels (> 20 pg/mL), AVP stimulation of V_{1a} receptors causes vasoconstriction and participates in the baroreceptor reflex. (*From Koeppen BM, Stanton BA: Regulation of body fluid osmolality: regulation of water balance.* In *Koeppen BM, Stanton BA [eds]: Renal Physiology, 4th ed. Philadelphia, Mosby Elsevier, 2007, pp 71-90.*)

AVP is synthesized it undergoes neuroaxonal transport to the posterior pituitary gland, where it is stored in granules. Neural stimulation of the cell bodies triggers exocytosis of AVP from the terminal vesicles into the circulation.

AVP acts on specific V_2-receptors in the collecting ducts to induce water reabsorption and a decreased flow of concentrated urine. It also increases NaCl reabsorption from the thick ascending loop of Henle into the medullary interstitium, which maintains its hypertonicity and facilitates movement of water out of the collecting duct along the osmotic gradient. This results in tubular conservation of water and free water retention (i.e., negative free water clearance). The net effect is that AVP increases urine osmolality and decreases plasma osmolality, without significant alteration in solute excretion.

The V_2-receptor on the basolateral cell membrane of the collecting duct responds to AVP via a receptor mechanism analogous to the β-adrenergic receptor.[51] Through activation of G protein–coupled adenylyl cyclase, ATP is converted to cyclic adenosine monophosphate (cAMP). This, in turn, activates a protein kinase that causes preformed vesicles containing aquaporin-2 water channels to migrate and fuse with the apical cell membrane. This results in a dramatic increase in membrane permeability to water, which is reabsorbed into the cell and thence into the peritubular capillary. AVP has a short plasma half-life of between 5 and 15 minutes, and this process rapidly reverses as plasma AVP levels decline.

Regulation of AVP Secretion

Hypothalamic osmoreceptors are sensitive to increases in serum osmolality of as little as 1% above normal. As illustrated in Figure 18-21A, the threshold for AVP secretion (and the sensation of thirst) is between 280 and 290 mOsm/kg. Once this is exceeded, the secretion rate has a very steep gain.[52] Even mild dehydration results in a rapid antidiuresis, and urine osmolality can increase from 300 to 1200 mOs/kg as plasma AVP levels rise from 0 to 5 pg/mL (see Fig. 18-21B).

Decreases in intravascular volume also stimulate AVP secretion, mediated by stretch receptors with vagal afferents in the left atrium and pulmonary veins. Hypovolemia-induced secretion of AVP overrides osmolar responses and contributes to the perioperative syndrome of inappropriate antidiuretic hormone secretion (SIADH): fluid retention, hypo-osmolality, and hyponatremia. The situation is exacerbated by administration of large volumes of hypotonic solutions that decrease serum osmolality. Psychic stress, via cortical input, also induces AVP release and can override osmotic and volume sensors.

By far, the most potent trigger for AVP release is systemic arterial hypotension, mediated by aortic and carotid baroreceptors. It overrides all other triggers, and plasma AVP may reach levels 10- to 1000-fold greater than normal (see Fig. 18-21C). At these concentrations AVP acts as a vasoconstrictor, especially in the outer renal cortex. It does so by stimulating the V_{1a} receptor, which exists on vascular smooth muscle, glomerular mesangial

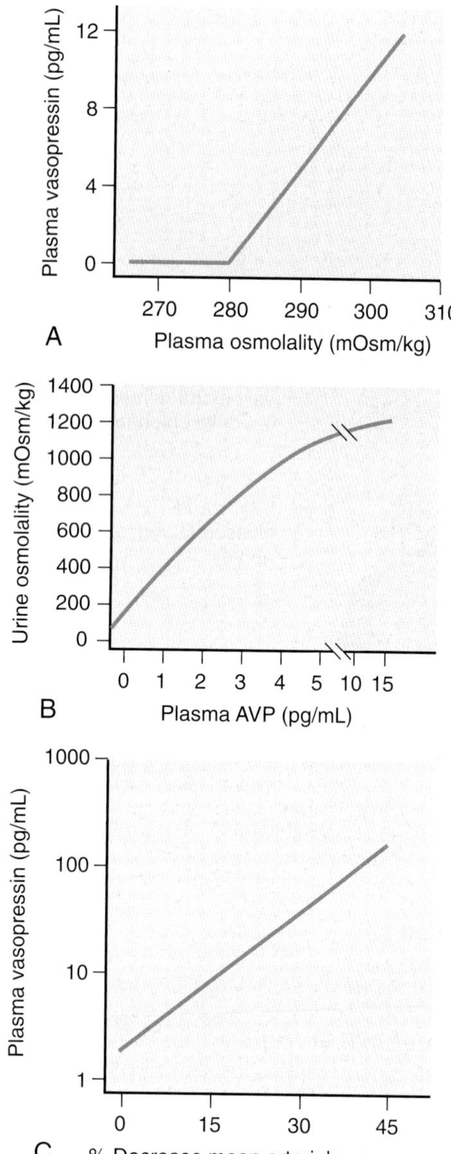

Figure 18-21 **A** to **C**, Physiologic regulation of arginine vasopressin (AVP). For explanation, see text. *(From Landry DW: Vasopressin deficiency and hypersensitivity in vasodilatory shock: Discovery of a new clinical syndrome. P & S Med Rev 3:3-7, 1996.)*

cells, and the vasa recta and promotes vasoconstriction via the phosphatidylinositol pathway.[52] AVP maintains effective glomerular filtration pressure because it is an extremely potent constrictor of the efferent arteriole and, unlike catecholamines and angiotensin, it has little effect on the afferent arteriole even at high plasma levels.[53]

Anesthetic agents have little direct effect on AVP secretion, except via the changes that they induce in arterial blood pressure, venous volume, and serum osmolality. Surgical stimulation is a major stimulus to AVP secretion. This stress response, whether mediated by pain or by volume changes, is profound and lasts at least 2 to 3 days after the surgical procedure.

Systems Promoting Vasodilation and Salt Excretion

Prostaglandins and Kinins

Prostaglandins

Intrarenal prostaglandins play an important role in endogenous renal protection, largely by vasodilating juxtamedullary blood vessels and maintaining inner cortical blood flow.[54] Prostaglandins are called autocoids because unlike true hormones they are produced in minute amounts and have a local, evanescent action. Because their structure is based on a 20-carbon fatty acid they are also referred to as eicosanoids, after *eicosa*, the Greek word meaning "twenty." The synthesis of intrarenal prostaglandins is summarized in Figure 18-22.

Phospholipase A_2, which resides in the inner lipid layer of the cell membrane, controls prostaglandin production through its formation of the prime precursor arachidonic acid. It is stimulated by ischemia and hypotension and also by norepinephrine, angiotensin II, and AVP. Thus, the factors that induce and mediate the stress response simultaneously activate prostaglandins, which defend the kidney against their actions. Cyclooxygenase-1 acts on arachidonic acid to form prostaglandin G_2, the precursor of the family of vasodilator prostaglandins that includes prostaglandins D_2, E_2, and I_2 (prostacyclin). They induce vasodilation through activation of cyclic adenosine monophosphate (AMP), which blocks distal tubule sodium reabsorption, and they oppose the actions of norepinephrine, angiotensin II, and AVP. Prostaglandins may be particularly important in decreasing the vasoconstrictor activity of angiotensin II on the afferent arteriole and glomerular mesangial cells.[47] Production of prostaglandins promotes renal vasodilation, maintains intrarenal hemodynamics, and enhances sodium and water excretion. The renal vasodilator response to mannitol during hypoperfusion appears to be mediated through prostaglandin activation.[55] At the same time, prostaglandins also stimulate renin secretion so that there is a constant "yin and yang" between the two systems.[56]

Cyclooxygenase-2 forms derivatives of arachidonic acid that induce inflammation and renal vasoconstriction and are important in pathologic states. Thromboxane (TXA_2) is derived from cyclic endoperoxides by the action of thromboxane synthetase. It induces vasoconstriction and platelet aggregation, and in the kidney it causes mesangial cell contraction. This decreases GFR by diminishing the effective glomerular surface area and filtration constant (K_f). Renal levels of thromboxane are increased in experimental acute renal failure and sepsis. In animal experiments, the administration of a specific thromboxane synthetase inhibitor prevents the deterioration in renal function induced by the injection of endotoxin.[57] Another vasoconstrictor prostaglandin, PGF_2, which acts on the thromboxane receptor, is formed when arachidonic acid is oxidized by free radicals liberated by leukostasis during acute inflammation. The leukotrienes, which are arachidonic acid derivatives formed by lipooxygenase, are also released from endotoxin-activated leukocytes. Like thromboxane, leukotrienes C_4 and D_4 induce mesangial cell contraction and decrease GFR.

Kinins

Kinins act as vasodilators that interact with and enhance the actions of prostaglandins while modulating the renin-angiotensin system.[58,59] For example, kinins stimulate phospholipase A_2 and

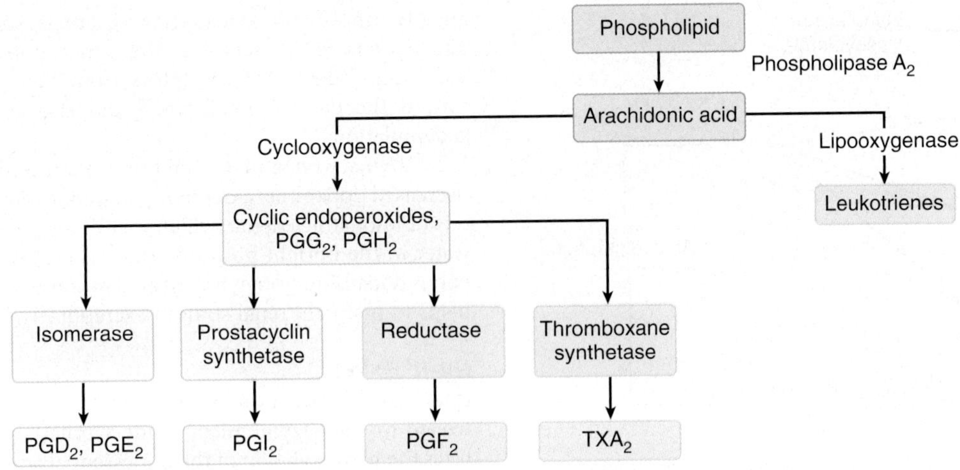

Figure 18-22 Synthesis of renal prostaglandins. Phospholipase A_2 is stimulated by ischemia, norepinephrine, and angiotensin II and cleaves arachidonic acid from its bond with membrane phospholipid. Cyclooxygenase acts on arachidonic acid to form evanescent cyclic endoperoxides (prostaglandins G_2 and H_2). Action of isomerase and prostacyclin synthetase culminates in the formation of vasodilator prostaglandins D_2, E_2, and I_2 (prostacyclin), which oppose the actions of the renin-angiotensin system on the kidney and protect against ischemic stress. Inhibition of cyclooxygenase by nonsteroidal anti-inflammatory drugs predisposes the kidney to damage. Under hypoxic or ischemic conditions, cyclic endoperoxides undergo reduction to the vasoconstrictor PGF_2, which acts on thromboxane receptors. Endotoxin increases the activity of leukocyte lipooxygenase and thromboxane synthetase. Leukotrienes (especially C_4 and D_4) and thromboxane (TXA_2) induce renal vasoconstriction and contribute to the vasomotor nephropathy of sepsis.

prostacyclin formation as well as endothelial nitric oxide formation. Kininase, which controls intrarenal kinin concentration, is blocked by angiotensin-converting enzyme inhibitors, resulting in increased bradykinin levels. This may be beneficial in diseases such as diabetes and hypertension, because two important intrarenal kinins, bradykinin and kallidin, decrease renal vasoconstriction and sodium retention induced by adrenergic hormones and angiotensin II.

Natriuretic Peptides

In 1972, Gorfinkel and colleagues[59a] demonstrated a profound difference in the canine renal response to shock depending on concomitant atrial pressure. Hypovolemic shock resulted in rapid diminution of RBF to 10% of control, whereas in cardiogenic shock RBF was preserved at 75% of control. The primary difference was that in cardiogenic shock atrial pressures were elevated, suggesting that atrial distention caused the release of a renal protective hormone. In 1981, de Bold and associates[60] confirmed the existence of ANP by demonstrating that an extract of atrial tissues caused natriuresis in rats, and the important actions of ANP on renal hemodynamics and sodium excretion were characterized.[61,62]

Subsequently, an entire series of peptides with a similar precursor was identified, with a common 25 to 32 amino acid core. These include ANP (atrial or A-type natriuretic peptide), released from electron-dense granules in atrial myocytes in response to local wall stretch and increased atrial volume, BNP (brain or B-type natriuretic peptide), released from the ventricles when they are distended, CNP (C-type natriuretic peptide) released from the endothelium of major vessels, and urodilatin, a natriuretic peptide produced in the lower urinary tract.[63] Human recombinant analogs have been developed for exogenous administration, including anaritide, derived from ANP, and nesiritide, derived from BNP. All these compounds induce arterial and venous dilation, increase RBF and GFR, and suppress the actions of norepinephrine, angiotensin, and endothelin.[64]

Natriuretic peptides dilate vascular smooth muscle through activation of guanylate cyclase and formation of cyclic guanosine monophosphate (GMP). At the phospholipase C-linked receptor, natriuretic peptides competitively block norepinephrine and noncompetitively block angiotensin II, thus reversing vascular smooth muscle constriction. They cause a prompt, sustained increase in GFR and glomerular filtration fraction, even when RBF is not increased or when arterial pressure is decreased. This suggests that natriuretic peptides promote afferent arteriolar dilation with or without efferent arteriolar constriction. The increased GFR increases the filtered load of sodium, but natriuresis may be due to increased medullary blood flow, which washes out the concentration gradient.

Natriuretic peptides appear to have a mutually antagonistic interaction with endothelin, the endogenous vasoconstrictor peptide produced by vascular endothelium.[47] They oppose the renin-angiotensin-aldosterone system on several fronts (Fig. 18-23). Natriuretic peptides inhibit renin secretion and decrease angiotensin-stimulated aldosterone release. They also inhibit aldosterone release directly at the zona glomerulosa of the adrenal cortex and block the salt-retaining action of aldosterone at the distal tubule and collecting duct. Through cyclic GMP activation, they inhibit NaCl reabsorption at the medullary portion of the collecting duct.[12] Natriuretic peptides also promote diuresis by inhibiting AVP secretion from the posterior pituitary and antagonizing its effect on the antidiuretic V_2-receptor in the collecting duct.

The renal protective role of endogenous ANP was elucidated by Shannon and colleagues,[65] who noticed that patients undergoing mitral valve replacement had lower urine output after cardiac surgery than those undergoing aortic valve replacement or coronary revascularization. They discovered that patients whose postoperative mean left atrial pressure declined by more than 7 mm Hg from preoperative values (which commonly occurs with correction of mitral valve disease) had significantly decreased postoperative urine sodium excretion and flow rate. Furthermore,

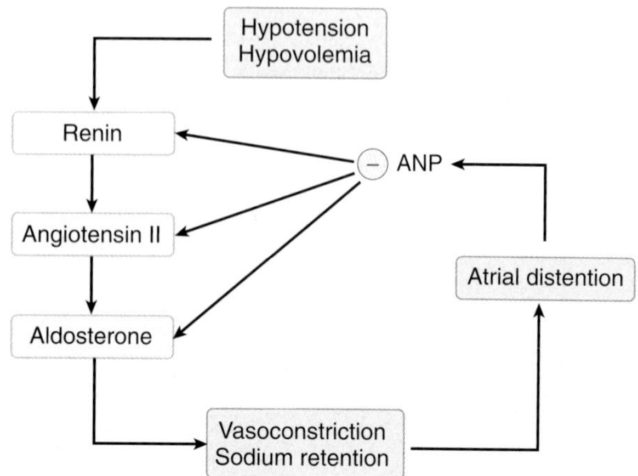

Figure 18-23 Interactions between ANP and the renin-angiotensin-aldosterone system. Hypotension or hypovolemia triggers release of renin from the afferent arteriole, causing the formation of angiotensin II, which stimulates release of aldosterone from the adrenal cortex. Angiotensin II and aldosterone cause vasoconstriction and sodium retention, ultimately resulting in reexpansion of the intravascular volume; this causes atrial distention, which triggers release of ANP. ANP inhibits release of renin, renin's action on angiotensinogen to form angiotensin II, angiotensin- induced vasoconstriction, stimulation of aldosterone secretion by angiotensin II, and the actions of aldosterone on the collecting duct. Thus, the actions of ANP promote vasodilation and sodium excretion. Therapeutic administration of fluids to distend the atrium and release ANP is an important intervention to curtail renal vasoconstriction and sodium retention. ANP, atrial natriuretic pressure.

there was a direct correlation between the quantitative decrease in left atrial pressure and a postoperative decline in circulating ANP levels (Fig. 18-24). In other words, patients with mitral valve disease and high left atrial pressure have a constant stimulus to ANP release. Valve replacement or repair results in decreased left atrial pressure, decreased ANP, and therefore decreased sodium excretion and urinary flow rate.

The Dopaminergic System

There are two subtypes of dopaminergic (DA) receptors (see Chapter 12).[66] At the end organ, DA_1-receptors occur not only on the renal and splanchnic vasculature but also on the proximal tubule itself.[67] Stimulation of the DA_1-receptor activates cyclic AMP and induces renal vasodilation, increased RBF and GFR, natriuresis, and diuresis. However, natriuresis can occur independently of increases in RBF and GFR and is abolished by specific DA_1 receptor antagonists.[68] In the proximal tubule, dopamine inhibits the Na^+/H^+ antiporter system at the brush-border membrane. In the medullary thick ascending limb, it also inhibits the Na^+/K^+-ATPase pump at the basolateral membrane.[68]

Neuronal DA_2-receptors exist on the presynaptic terminal of postganglionic sympathetic nerves. Stimulation inhibits the release of norepinephrine from presynaptic vesicles, a mechanism analogous to stimulation of the presynaptic α_2-receptor. Through inhibition of norepinephrine, DA_2-receptor activation facilitates vasodilation.

The dopaminergic system plays an integral role in the endogenous vasodilator-natriuresis system and the maintenance of normal blood pressure. Endogenous dopamine appears to constitutively activate the DA_2-receptor, which synergistically enhances the activation of the DA_1-receptor.[69] It acts as an autocrine and paracrine natriuretic factor by inhibiting tubular Na^+/K^+-ATPase activity, especially when sodium intake is increased.[70] It also opposes the anti-natriuretic effects of norepinephrine, angiotensin II and aldosterone. There is some evidence that endogenous ANP acts via the renal dopamine system by recruiting "silent" DA_1-receptors from the interior of the cell toward the plasma membrane[70] and also enhances dopamine accumulation.[71]

Urinary dopamine excretion is increased with salt loading; decreased dopaminergic activity may contribute to the pathogenesis of idiopathic edema, which manifests as retention of salt and water in the upright position. There is evidence that the endogenous dopamine system is activated in compensated cirrhosis and helps to maintain renal sodium excretion.[72]

Nitric Oxide

Endogenous formation of nitric oxide (see Chapter 31) is controlled by the enzyme nitric oxide synthase (NOS), which catalyzes the hydroxylation of the nonessential amino acid L-arginine to L-citrulline.[73] Most actions of nitric oxide are mediated through its activation of soluble guanylate cyclase, which catalyzes the

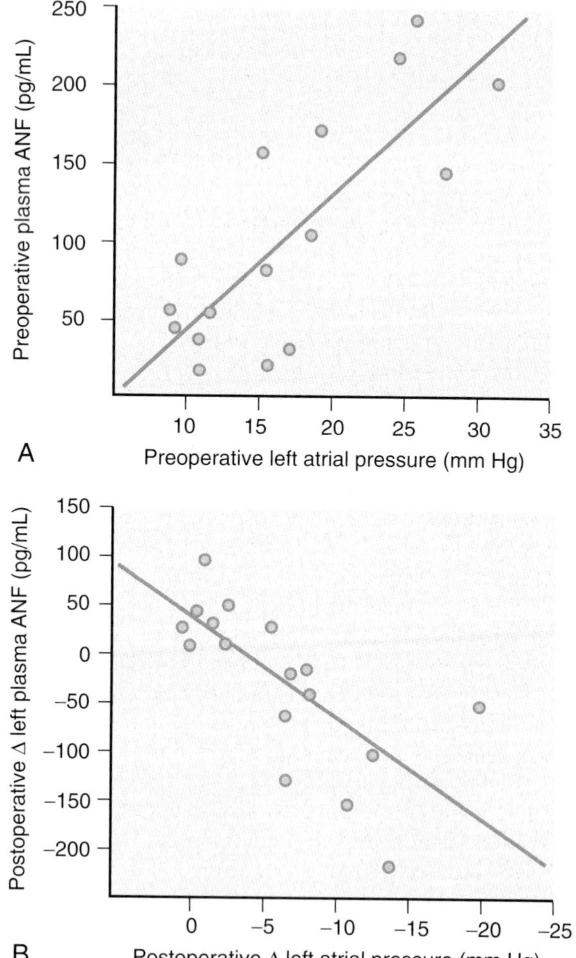

Figure 18-24 Correlation between left atrial pressure and plasma ANP in a group of patients undergoing cardiac surgery. **A,** There is significant correlation ($r = 0.8$, $P < .001$) between absolute preoperative left atrial pressure and plasma ANP. **B,** There is a significant correlation ($r = 0.72$, $P < .002$) between the postoperative decrease in left atrial pressure and postoperative decrease in plasma ANP. ANF, atrial natriuretic factor, synonymous with ANP; ANP, atrial natriuretic pressure; Δ, change. (*From Shannon RP, Libby E, Elahi D, et al: Impact of acute reduction in chronically elevated left atrial pressure on sodium and water excretion. Ann Thorac Surg 46:430-437, 1988.*)

conversion of guanidine triphosphate (GTP) to cyclic GMP. Cyclic GMP has two major actions: relaxation of vascular smooth muscle and suppression of the inflammatory response. It inhibits leukocyte adhesion, platelet activation and aggregation, and cellular proliferation. Cyclic GMP is converted to GMP by phosphodiesterase I and V. Thus, the local action of nitric oxide can be enhanced by the administration of a selective phosphodiesterase V inhibitor, such as sildenafil. Nitric oxide itself is rapidly inactivated by binding to intracellular heme and heme proteins (oxyhemoglobin, oxymyoglobin, guanylate cyclase, cyclooxygenase, cytochrome P_{450}).

Nitric Oxide Synthase (NOS)

There are several distinct subtypes of NOS that determine the site and function of nitric oxide synthesis. Constitutive NOS is calcium and calmodulin dependent and releases small amounts of nitric oxide for short periods of time ("tonic" release). Constitutive NOS has two subtypes: neuronal NOS, which acts as a peripheral neurotransmitter and induces cerebral vasodilation, and endothelial NOS, which exists in the vascular endothelium and mediates the activity previously ascribed to endothelium derived relaxing factor (EDRF). The latter is an important modulator of systemic and pulmonary vascular resistance. In the kidney, endogenous nitric oxide preserves blood flow to the oligemic juxtamedullary cortex and medulla and may also provide endogenous protection against ischemic and nephrotoxic medullary injury.[74-76]

Inducible NOS is calcium and calmodulin independent and is induced by cytokines predominantly in inflammatory cells (macrophages, granulocytes) but also in vascular smooth muscle. At low levels of activation, inducible NOS enhances the response to infection and promotes inflammation and wound healing. In severe sepsis, inducible NOS produces huge amounts of nitric oxide for protracted periods of time ("phasic" release) and is largely responsible for the characteristically profound systemic vasodilation that is refractory to norepinephrine.[77] High levels of nitric oxide, and its reactive products nitrogen dioxide and peroxynitrite, induce lipid peroxidation and denaturation of proteins that drive the systemic inflammatory response syndrome (SIRS) and its attendant acute renal injury.

Duality of Nitric Oxide in Renal Function and Injury

Goligorsky and coworkers[78] have framed the hypothesis that an imbalance between the expression and activity of constitutive and inducible NOS plays an important role in the pathophysiology of acute renal failure. In experimental models of sepsis, nonselective inhibitors of both constitutive and inducible NOS improve blood pressure but worsen overall perfusion, including renal perfusion. Selective inhibitors of inducible NOS show promise in suppressing severe inflammation and vasodilation while maintaining tonic perfusion to vital organs, including the kidneys.[79]

The Renal Adenosine System

Adenosine Receptors

Adenosine, the endogenous degradation product of ATP, is produced by every mammalian cell type and is normally thought of as a potent vasodilator. However, in the kidney, it plays an essential role in regulating intrarenal blood flow by inducing outer cortical vasoconstriction and preserving juxtamedullary perfusion. This variance in function is explained by the identification of at least four subtypes of adenosine receptor: A_1, A_{2a}, A_{2b}, and A_3 (Table 18-3). Activation of the A_1 adenosine receptor induces outer cortical vasoconstriction; it also decreases renin release and inhibits diuresis and natriuresis. In contrast, A_{2a} adenosine receptors increase medullary renal blood flow and enhance renin release, diuresis, and natriuresis.

Table 18-3 Adenosine Receptor Subtypes and Functions

Receptor	Agonist Function	Ischemic Injury
A_1	Outer cortical vasoconstriction	Highly protective
	Decreased renin release	
	Inhibition of diuresis and natriuresis	
A_{2a}	Juxtamedullary vasodilation	Highly protective
	Increased renin release	
	Promotion of diuresis and natriuresis	
A_{2b}	Unknown	
A_3	Unknown	Potentiates injury

From Fozard JR, Hannon JP: Adenosine receptor ligands: potential as therapeutic agents in asthma and COPD. Pulm Pharmacol Ther 12:111-114, 1999.

Perioperative Ischemic and Nephrotoxic Injury

This section will review perioperative agents and events that may disrupt normal renal physiology. If the disruption is severe enough or occurs in susceptible individuals, it may induce ischemic or nephrotoxic acute tubular necrosis, the most common form of perioperative acute kidney injury.

Pathogenesis

Ischemia-Reperfusion Injury

In many clinical situations (e.g., hypovolemic shock, suprarenal aortic-cross clamping) the kidney is subject to a classic ischemia-reperfusion injury that involves several distinct phases.[80] Acute injury to the tubular epithelium and vascular endothelium initiates a rapid decline in GFR. The injury is extended by epithelial and endothelial cell apoptosis and necrosis. The injury becomes stabilized during the maintenance phase, with the beginning of cellular reorganization that culminates in the recovery phase. The initiation phase is often transient, so the extension phase is the most important "window of opportunity" for therapeutic intervention that might reverse acute kidney injury. This emphasizes the importance of early, sensitive detection of rapid declines in GFR.[27]

Nephrotoxic Injury

The putative mechanisms of nephrotoxic tubular injury have been previously discussed (see "Oxygen Balance in the Medullary Thick Ascending Loop"). The risk of nephrotoxic acute kidney injury is exponentially related to the number of nephrotoxic insults.[13] An isolated nephrotoxin (e.g., radiocontrast dye) is unlikely to cause acute kidney injury when the kidney is well perfused. In animal models of nephrotoxic acute tubular necrosis, injection of radiocontrast dye predictably injures more than 50% of the renal medullary thick ascending limb only when the kidney is previously "primed" by a sequence of three other insults: dehydration, LMMA (a nitric oxide synthase inhibitor), and indomethacin (a prostaglandin synthesis inhibitor).[81]

Anesthetic Drugs

The choice of an anesthetic technique to preserve renal function during and after surgery is predicated on the preservation of RBF and perfusion pressure, the suppression of vasoconstrictor, salt-retaining stress responses to surgical stimulation and postoperative pain, and the avoidance or curtailment of nephrotoxic insults. No single anesthetic drug alone meets these criteria.

Regional Anesthesia

Spinal or epidural anesthesia that achieves sympathetic blockade of the fourth through tenth thoracic segments (see Chapters 51 and 52) is extremely effective in suppressing the sympathoadrenal stress response and release of catecholamines, renin, and AVP. During major surgery, RBF and GFR are preserved as long as adequate renal perfusion pressure is maintained.[82] This implies careful titration of the block, especially in elderly patients with cardiovascular disease, and may necessitate a 25% to 50% increase in intraoperative fluid administration. However, Gamulin and coworkers[83] found that renal sympathetic blockade obtained by epidural anesthesia did not block increases in renal vascular resistance induced by infrarenal aortic cross-clamping, nor did it prevent postoperative decreases in creatinine clearance. Combined spinal-epidural anesthesia for nephrectomy in living related donors appeared to promote graft renal blood flow more than general anesthesia, but there was no difference in renal function or outcome in recipients.[84]

General Anesthesia

The overall effect on renal function of anesthetic drugs in common use has been well reported.[85,86] All anesthetic techniques and agents tend to decrease GFR and intraoperative urine flow. Some drugs also decrease RBF, but filtration fraction is usually increased, which implies that angiotensin-induced efferent arteriolar constriction limits the decrease in GFR. However, these effects are much less significant than those caused by surgical stress or aortic cross-clamping and after emergence from anesthesia usually resolve promptly. Any anesthetic technique that induces hypotension will result in decreased urine flow because of altered peritubular capillary hydrostatic gradients, even if renal autoregulation is preserved (as it usually is during anesthesia). Permanent injury seldom results, unless the kidneys are abnormal to begin with or the hypovolemic insult is prolonged and exacerbated by nephrotoxic injury (see Chapter 24).

Halothane, enflurane, or isoflurane with nitrous oxide induce mild to moderate reductions in RBF and GFR, primarily due to their effects on the central circulation (myocardial depression, peripheral pooling).[85] These effects can be attenuated by prior hydration. High-dose opioid techniques using fentanyl or sufentanil do not depress myocardial contractility and have minimal effect on RBF and GFR. They are also considerably more effective in suppressing the release of catecholamines, angiotensin II, aldosterone, and AVP during surgery than are volatile agents. However, during CPB both AVP and catecholamine levels rise markedly despite high-dose opioid anesthesia. Intravenous agents such as thiopental and diazepam cause minor changes in renal function, about 10% to 15% deviation from control. Ketamine increases RBF but decreases urine flow rate, possibly through sympathetic activation; it preserves RBF during hemorrhagic hypovolemia.[86]

Nephrotoxicity of Volatile Anesthetics

The potential nephrotoxicity of volatile anesthetics (see Chapter 24) is due to their metabolic breakdown to free fluoride ions, which cause a tubular lesion that results in loss of concentrating ability and polyuric acute renal failure. Toxicity is exacerbated by aminoglycosides or prior renal dysfunction. Peak fluoride levels less than 50 μm/L seldom induce injury, whereas levels greater than 150 μm/L are associated with a high incidence of polyuric acute renal failure.[87] Administration of methoxyflurane at more than one minimum alveolar concentration (MAC) for more than 2 hours is capable of generating a peak fluoride level greater than 100 μm/L and for this reason this anesthetic is no longer used. Enflurane is metabolized more rapidly, and most studies indicated that peak fluoride levels seldom rose above 25 μm/L. The antituberculotic agent isoniazid enhances fluoride production, but only isolated reports of fluoride-induced nephrotoxicity due to enflurane ever appeared. Isoflurane produces peak fluoride levels less than 4 μm/L, and halothane is not metabolized to fluoride at all.[88]

The potential nephrotoxicity of sevoflurane remains controversial. Although its metabolism generates more fluoride than enflurane does, clinically significant fluoride-induced nephrotoxicity has not been detected. Compound A, a vinyl ether formed by degradation of sevoflurane at low flow through carbon dioxide absorbents, is capable of inducing renal injury in rats. Although acute renal failure has not been reported in humans, Eger and associates reported evidence of transient renal injury (albuminuria, tubular enzymuria) in volunteers subjected to 8 hours of 1.25 MAC sevoflurane at 2 L/min gas flow.[89] There were no changes in urinary concentrating ability, serum creatinine, or BUN. Subsequently, Eger and associates[90] described a dose-response relationship between biochemical markers of glomerular and tubular injury (urinary albumin, α-glutathione-S-transferase) and compound A exposure expressed as parts per million-hours (ppm/h). They suggested that the threshold of renal injury is 80 to 168 ppm/h based on their observation of altered biochemical markers with 1.25 MAC sevoflurane at 2 L/min for 4 hours, which was not seen after 2 hours, and not seen at all with desflurane.

Other laboratories have disputed Eger's findings. Bito and coworkers compared 6-hour patient exposure to low- and high-flow sevoflurane with exposure to low-flow isoflurane and found no differences in BUN, creatinine, or tubular enzymes for 3 days postoperatively.[91] Kharasch and coworkers[92] had similar results with the use of sevoflurane or isoflurane at 1 L/min in 73 patients undergoing procedures lasting longer than 2 hours, and they concluded that moderate duration of low-flow sevoflurane anesthesia, even with the formation of compound A, is as safe as low-flow isoflurane anesthesia. Ebert and associates[93] attempted to duplicate the original 8-hour Eger sevoflurane study in volunteers at two sites with blinded laboratory analyses. Biochemical derangements were minimal and transient, and there were no significant changes in BUN, creatinine, or creatinine clearance. Despite the similarity in experimental design, the mean level of compound A was about 25% lower, and the mean arterial pressure was about

10% higher than the Eger study and may have accounted for the difference in results.

In summary, clinically significant renal injury with the use of low-flow sevoflurane anesthesia has not been reported in patients, even with moderate preexisting renal dysfunction. The relationship between compound A formation, biochemical injury, and clinically relevant renal dysfunction remains unclear and unproven. Nonetheless it appears prudent to follow current U.S. Food and Drug Administration (FDA) guidelines, which recommend a fresh gas flow of at least 2 L/min to inhibit compound A formation and its rebreathing and to enhance its washout.

Volatile Anesthetics and Ischemia-Reperfusion Injury

There is experimental evidence that volatile anesthetics can ameliorate ischemia-reperfusion injury in the kidney. In a murine model, Lee and Emala demonstrated that anesthesia with desflurane, sevoflurane, isoflurane, and halothane significantly attenuated the rise in serum creatinine compared with pentobarbital or ketamine.[94] The mechanism appears to be independent of K^+-ATP channels but related to suppression of the proinflammatory cytokine and chemokine activation in response to ischemia-reperfusion.

Mechanical Ventilation

Mechanical ventilation (see Chapter 93) and positive end-expiratory pressure (PEEP) may cause decreased RBF, GFR, sodium excretion, and urine flow rate or even acute renal injury.[95] Transmission of increased airway and intrapleural pressures to the intravascular space leads to decreases in venous return, transmural (i.e., effective) cardiac filling pressures, and cardiac output. Transmission may actually be attenuated in acute lung injury because of poor lung compliance. High levels of mean airway pressure may compress the pulmonary arterial circulation, increase right ventricular afterload, and induce the intraventricular septum to shift into the left ventricle and decrease its filling and cardiac output.[96] Positive-pressure ventilation increases inferior vena caval pressure and renal venous pressure and may increase tubular sodium reabsorption by increases in peritubular capillary pressure.

The decrease in cardiac output and systemic arterial pressure results in a carotid and aortic baroreceptor-mediated increase in sympathetic nerve tone to the kidney, with renal vasoconstriction, antidiuresis, and anti-natriuresis. Volume receptors in the atria respond to decreased filling by decreased ANP secretion, resulting in increased sympathetic tone, renin activation, and AVP activity.

Salt and water retention during airway pressure therapy was originally thought to be due to an AVP effect,[97] but it is now considered that sympathetic responses are more important and that sodium retention is largely the result of decreased sodium delivery to the tubules. The renin-angiotensin-aldosterone system undoubtedly augments the renal responses to positive-pressure ventilation. Annat and coworkers[98] found that 15 cm H_2O PEEP depressed cardiac output, RBF, GFR, and urine volume by 20% to 30% and was associated with increases in renin and aldosterone but not AVP. The impairment in renal function induced by airway pressure therapy can be prevented or reversed by preserving normal circulatory status, either by hydration[99] or by use of dopamine.[100]

Although theoretically the extent of depression of renal function depends on the mean airway pressure, there appears to be no difference in creatinine clearance and FE_{Na} whether volume-control ventilation or pressure-support ventilation is used.[101] Therapeutic maneuvers used in severe acute lung injury such as permissive hypercapnia or permissive hypoxemia may promote renal vasoconstriction.[95]

Finally, in experimental lung injury there is evidence that an injurious ventilatory mode induces acute inflammation associated with renal epithelial cell apoptosis and dysfunction.[102] These findings appear to be in keeping with the clinical observation of multiorgan dysfunction in patients with acute respiratory distress syndrome and with its amelioration when a lung protective strategy of mechanical ventilation is used.[95]

Induced Hypotension

During anesthesia with induced hypotension, substantial reduction of GFR and urine flow rate is common. However, when the duration of hypotension is less than 2 hours, no permanent impairment of renal function occurs, even in elderly patients.[103] Vasodilator agents used to induce hypotension differ in their effect on RBF. Administration of sodium nitroprusside decreases renal vascular resistance but tends to shunt blood flow away from the kidney. Moreover, its administration is associated with marked renin-angiotensin activation and catecholamine release, which results in rebound hypertension if the infusion is suddenly discontinued. Nitroglycerin decreases RBF less than sodium nitroprusside.[104] The selective DA_1-dopaminergic agonist fenoldopam is capable of providing induced hypotension without any significant decrease in RBF.[105]

Aortic Cross-Clamping

The relative effects of suprarenal and infrarenal aortic cross-clamping (see Chapter 62) on renal function in patients undergoing major vascular surgery have been studied. Regardless of the position of the aortic cross-clamp, RBF is decreased to 50% of normal during surgical preparation of the aorta, presumably owing to direct compression or reflex spasm of the renal arteries. After release of the suprarenal cross-clamp, RBF increases above normal (reflex hyperemia) but GFR remains depressed to one third of control for up to 2 hours. After 24 hours, GFR is still only two thirds of control. Tubular functions (concentrating ability, sodium, and water conservation) are markedly impaired, but urine flow is maintained. Myers and Moran[106] observed that these changes resemble an attenuated form of acute tubular necrosis. In this study all patients received mannitol pretreatment, which probably limited the tubular insult because oliguria was uncommon and recovery was relatively rapid. Cross-clamp times longer than 50 minutes are associated with prolonged depression of GFR and transient azotemia.[107]

In animal models, suprarenal aortic cross-clamping induces a decrease in renal endothelial nitric oxide; nitric oxide synthesis and cortical blood flow are enhanced by the administration of its substrate arginine.[108] Whether this intervention might attenuate the renal consequences of cross-clamping awaits further investigation.

Infrarenal aortic cross-clamping may also impair RBF and GFR by inducing decreases in cardiac output in response to increased systemic vascular resistance.[109] Atheromatous embolism of the renal arteries may be induced by cross-clamping or manipulation in areas of dense aortic plaque. Partial or complete cortical necrosis may occur, which is usually irreversible.

Renal Protection During Aortic Cross-Clamping

Mannitol has been used for more than 40 years to provide renal protection during aortic cross-clamping (see Chapter 62). Its protective effects have been clearly demonstrated in animal models of ischemic acute tubular necrosis,[110] but few prospective controlled human studies exist. Low-dose dopamine has commonly been used during major vascular surgery. In a canine study of thoracic aortic cross-clamping, RBF, GFR, and urine flow remained impaired for a considerable time after cross-clamp release. This delay was not prevented by prophylactic administration of dopamine.[111] In a human study of infrarenal cross-clamping, Paul and colleagues[112] compared diuretic therapy with a combination of mannitol and dopamine versus fluid loading with saline to a pulmonary artery occlusion pressure (PAOP) of 12 to 15 mm Hg. Although mannitol and dopamine substantially increased urine flow and sodium excretion during cross-clamping, they were no better than saline in attenuating residual GFR depression after cross-clamp release.

Fenoldopam, a synthetic phenolated dopamine analog that is a selective agonist of the DA1-receptor, increases renal blood flow in a dose-dependent manner.[113] Infusion of fenoldopam has demonstrated a renoprotective effect in experimental suprarenal aortic cross-clamping.[114] In a controlled, randomized, blinded study in 28 patients undergoing infrarenal aortic cross-clamping, fenoldopam, 0.1 μg/kg/min, or placebo was infused intravenously before surgical skin incision and continued until release of the aortic cross-clamp.[115] Fenoldopam significantly attenuated the decrease in creatinine clearance and increase in serum creatinine observed in patients who received placebo. Larger studies with this agent appear warranted.

Cardiopulmonary Bypass

The incidence of acute renal failure is very low (< 2%) after uncomplicated cardiac surgery in patients with previously normal renal function. It increases with the complexity of surgery (e.g., combined procedures versus simple revascularization). In a prospective review of more than 4000 cases at the Cleveland Clinic, Higgins and associates observed that the risk of renal morbidity and mortality increases exponentially when the preoperative serum creatinine value is greater than 1.9 mg/dL.[116] When it does occur after cardiac surgery, acute renal failure has a devastating effect on mortality, increasing it 15-fold with acute kidney injury (peak postoperative SCr > 1 mg/dL) and 30-fold when renal replacement therapy is required.[117] During CPB (see Chapter 60), hypotension with nonpulsatile flow promotes renal vasoconstriction and decreases RBF. Norepinephrine levels increase progressively during bypass, and the renin-angiotensin system is activated. Acute renal failure has been associated with persistent elevation of plasma renin levels.[106] Thromboxane, released from activated platelets, and vascular elaboration of endothelin could add to renal vasoconstriction during extracorporeal circulation. Tubular enzymuria and microalbuminuria, an index of subclinical injury to the nephron, is consistently observed during CPB.[118]

Renal Protection during Cardiopulmonary Bypass

Pulsatile Perfusion During CPB

In animal and human studies, pulsatile perfusion during CPB enhances renal cortical blood flow and decreases circulating catecholamines, endothelin, and cytokine activation (see Chapter 60).[119,120] However, these physiologic advantages have not translated into clinical benefit. Although plasma renin activity is suppressed by pulsatile perfusion, evidence of glomerular injury (in this case, microalbuminuria) persists.[35] In a randomized prospective study on 215 pediatric patients undergoing repair of congenital heart disease, the use of pulsatile flow during CPB was associated with decreased inotropic requirement, shorter intensive care unit and hospital length of stay, and greater urine output, but there was no difference in serum creatinine value.[121] Intra-aortic balloon counterpulsation was used to provide pulsatile flow during CPB in a randomized, prospective study on 100 adult patients undergoing cardiac surgery.[122] Pulsatile flow attenuated the decline in GFR, but there was no difference in urine flow or renal outcome. In a large nonrandomized observational study, pulsatile flow was provided during CPB in 915 of 1820 patients but did not appear to provide increased protection against perioperative renal injury.[123]

Avoidance of CPB

The benefit to renal function of off-pump coronary artery bypass (OPCAB, also known as beating heart surgery) also remains equivocal. In low-risk patients, there appears to be little difference in the incidence of acute kidney injury whether or not CPB is used.[124] Most published studies to date have been small (<60 patients), and although they demonstrate that OPCAB is associated with less evidence of acute kidney injury, as manifested by lower levels of serum creatinine, cystatin C, microalbuminuria, and NAG, this has not translated into a benefit to renal outcome, morbidity, or mortality.[125,126] In a larger study on 201 patients, the use of CPB resulted in a significant increase in acute kidney injury, defined as a greater than 50% increase in postoperative serum creatinine concentration (27.7 versus 14.0%, $P < .03$).[127] Although the OPCAB technique was identified as the only independent factor associated with a lower incidence of acute kidney injury, the study was not randomized and all procedures were performed by the same experienced surgeon.

Perfusion Pressure During CPB

It has been observed in animal studies of CPB that RBF is dependent on renal perfusion pressure and that infusion of dopamine does not increase RBF during low-pressure states.[10] This suggests that autoregulation may be impaired during CPB. However, Hilberman and colleagues[128] found no relationship between low flow (<50 mL/kg/min) and low mean arterial pressure (<50 mm Hg) and postoperative acute renal failure. Instead, the severity of postoperative renal dysfunction and its outcome correlated with the severity of cardiac dysfunction after CPB.[129]

Dopaminergic and Diuretic Drugs

In a study comparing equi-inotropic doses of dopamine and dobutamine after cardiac surgery, the two agents had similar effects on GFR, RBF, renal vascular resistance, and filtration fraction but dopamine caused greater urine flow rate, natriuresis, FE_{Na}, and potassium excretion, indicating a diuretic effect independent of changes in RBF and GFR.[130] However, there is no evidence that the "prophylactic" administration of low doses of dopamine has a protective role during CPB in patients with previously normal[131,132] or impaired renal function.[124,133]

In part, the lack of benefit may be due to the variable pharmacokinetic effect of dopamine. In a study on normal volunteers, McGregor and coworkers found a 30-fold intersubject variability in plasma dopamine levels.[134] Some subjects given an infusion of "low dose" dopamine had plasma levels consistent with those associated with doses in the high, α-adrenergic range. Even at low doses it can cause unwanted tachycardia, and its postoperative infusion is associated with a higher incidence of supraventricular and ventricular arrhythmias.[135]

In contrast to dopamine, there does appear to be increasing evidence to support a renoprotective effect for infusion of low-dose fenoldopam infusion (0.1-0.3 µg/kg/min) during cardiac surgery. A meta-analysis of 13 randomized and case-matched studies on 1059 patients found that fenoldopam infusion is associated with a significant decrease in dialysis requirement, intensive care unit length of stay, and in-hospital mortality.[136] Most studies have been relatively small and identified improved serum creatinine and creatinine clearance rather than renal outcome.[137,138] The most convincing evidence thus far comes from a randomized, double-blinded study in 193 high-risk patients by Cogliati and colleagues.[139] Risk factors included elevated preoperative serum creatinine (>1.5 mg/dL), age older than 70 years, diabetes, and previous cardiac surgery. Patients who received fenoldopam had a decreased incidence of acute kidney injury (12.6 versus 27.6%, $P = .02$) and requirement for dialysis (0 versus 8.2%, $P = .004$).

Prophylactic administration of diuretics during CPB may actually be harmful: in a study on 126 patients undergoing elective cardiac surgery, perioperative infusion of furosemide (0.5 µg/kg/min) worsened serum creatinine level compared with low-dose dopamine and placebo.[131]

Natriuretic Peptides

Exogenous administration of anaritide (human recombinant ANP) decreases systemic blood pressure through arterial and venous dilation. There has been considerable interest in the ability of infused anaritide to reverse established acute renal failure ("renal rescue"). Animal studies of ischemic and nephrotoxic acute tubular necrosis,[140] as well as preliminary clinical studies,[141] offered promise. A large prospective study demonstrated significantly greater dialysis-free survival with anaritide infusion in oliguric acute renal failure, but in nonoliguric acute renal failure survival actually worsened.[31] Subsequently, a randomized, double-blind, placebo-controlled trial on 222 patients with oliguric acute renal failure found no differences in dialysis requirement, dialysis-free survival, or 60-day mortality between anaritide and placebo.[142] However, patients receiving anaritide had significantly more hypotension during infusion of the study drug.

Infusion of anaritide has been studied during CPB.[143] Compared with controls, patients who received anaritide had significantly lower plasma levels of renin, angiotensin II, and aldosterone and higher GFR and urine output.

Nesiritide (human recombinant BNP) is approved by the FDA for the parenteral treatment of advanced decompensated congestive heart failure. It decreases elevated cardiac preload and afterload, enhances cardiac function, and promotes diuresis and relieves symptoms related to pulmonary congestion and edema.[144] The major adverse effect is dose-related hypotension, which if excessive, can impair renal function.[145] A meta-analysis of studies of nesiritide infusion in patients with advanced decompensated heart failure suggested that its use is associated with worsening serum creatinine.[146] However, there is evidence that perioperative infusion of low doses (0.01 µg/kg/min) of nesiritide in high-risk patients undergoing cardiac surgery may have a renoprotective effect.[147] In a prospective, randomized, blinded study of 279 patients with left ventricular dysfunction (ejection fraction < 40%) undergoing coronary revascularization or mitral valve surgery, patients who received nesiritide had increased urine output, an attenuated postoperative increase in serum creatinine concentration, and improved survival 6 months after surgery. Further studies of nesiritide appear warranted.

N-Acetylcysteine

N-Acetylcysteine is an antioxidant that directly scavenges reactive oxygen species, and there is considerable evidence to support its use to prevent radiocontrast nephropathy (see later). However, a similar benefit has not been demonstrated by its perioperative administration in cardiac surgery. In two prospective, blinded randomized studies, neither intermittent injection[148] nor continuous infusion[149] of *N*-acetylcysteine had any impact on renal function or outcome after cardiac surgery. A large study on 254 patients with chronic renal insufficiency (GFR < 60 mL/min) was similarly unable to demonstrate any significant benefit from intermittent injection of *N*-acetylcysteine.[150]

Nephrotoxic Insults

Drug-Induced Nephrotoxicity

Nephrotoxic injury by drugs or contrast dyes seldom occurs without the presence of coexisting risk factors,[13] including shock, hypovolemia, congestive heart failure or advanced age, diabetes, or chronic renal insufficiency. The risk of nephrotoxicity increases exponentially with the number of risk factors and nephrotoxic combinations.

Nephrotoxic acute renal failure is usually nonoliguric, with loss of concentrating ability and slowly progressive azotemia. As GFR declines, accumulation of renally excreted drugs exacerbates nephrotoxicity, unless drug levels are carefully monitored and dosage is repeatedly adjusted. However, the prognosis for recovery is good if these agents are discontinued in time and when no coexistent organ failure exists.[151]

Aminoglycosides

Aminoglycosides (gentamicin, tobramycin, amikacin) are polycationic compounds that are filtered into the proximal tubule, where they bind to anionic brush-border membrane phospholipids. Their nephrotoxicity is directly related to their polycationic status, so that neomycin (six cationic sites) is more destructive than gentamicin (five sites) or streptomycin (three sites).[152] They are absorbed into intracellular lysosomes by endocytosis and thence released into the cytosol. Within the cell they induce the formation of reactive oxygen metabolites that injure lysosomes, plasma membranes, and mitochondria and, in particular, inhibit oxidative phosphorylation and the synthesis of high-energy phosphate compounds such as ATP. Aminoglycoside-induced nephrotoxicity is directly related to sustained high trough serum levels, especially when associated with advanced age, preexisting renal disease, renal vasoconstrictive states (sepsis, hypovolemia, liver disease, congestive heart failure), adjuvant drug therapy (loop diuretics, vancomycin, cephalosporins, NSAIDs, cyclosporine, amphotericin B), and electrolyte disorders (hypokalemia, hypomagnesemia, hypercalcemia, and metabolic acidosis).[153]

Prevention of aminoglycoside nephrotoxicity depends on maintenance of adequate hydration, avoidance or removal of the risk factors just listed, and careful monitoring of serum aminoglycoside levels. A daily 2-hour creatinine clearance can also be helpful in the early detection of aminoglycoside-induced nephrotoxicity and appropriate dose adjustment for GFR. Once-daily administration of aminoglycosides to achieve a high therapeutic level with an adequate trough period for renal recovery may limit the occurrence of nephrotoxicity.[154]

Nonsteroidal Anti-inflammatory Drugs

Cyclooxygenase-1 is inhibited by NSAIDs (see Chapter 26) such as indomethacin, meclofenamate, and ketorolac for about 8 to 24 hours. A single dose of aspirin causes its irreversible acetylation. In platelets, the impact lasts for the lifetime of these cells (7 to 10 days), but the kidney resynthesizes cyclooxygenase within 24 to 48 hours. The renal protective function of prostaglandins is "switched on" by injury, illustrated by the fact that NSAIDs cause nephrotoxicity in ischemic but not in normal kidneys. During conditions of stress, impaired prostaglandin activity results in decreased RBF and GFR, increased renal vascular resistance, attenuated diuretic responsiveness, and hyperkalemia.

Adverse effects of NSAIDs and aspirin occur in animal models of hemorrhage, endotoxemia, increased venous pressure, and low cardiac output and in humans with mild underlying renal dysfunction who also have congestive heart failure, ascites, or systemic lupus erythematosus.[155] Postoperative analgesia with a single analgesic such as ketorolac is extremely unlikely to cause injury in a relatively young, healthy, well-hydrated patient. The risk of nephrotoxic injury increases exponentially with the addition of concomitant nephrotoxins (e.g., contrast dye, aminoglycosides) in the presence of acute or chronic cardiovascular instability.

NSAIDs selective for cyclooxygenase-2 (celecoxib, rofecoxib, valdecoxib) appear to be less likely to cause gastric irritation and erosion. However, there is no evidence that they decrease the risk of nephrotoxic injury compared with nonselective cyclooxygenase inhibitors.[156] Their use has been severely curtailed after reports of increased adverse cardiovascular events in clinical trials.

Calcineurin Antagonists (Cyclosporine, Tacrolimus)

Cyclosporine is a remarkably potent immunosuppressive agent and, together with corticosteroids and azathioprine, is routinely used to prevent rejection after organ transplantation. Indeed, heart, lung, and liver transplantation increased exponentially after its release in 1981. It causes renal injury, in part because it induces sympathetic hyperreactivity, hypertension, and renal vasoconstriction. Preexisting renal dysfunction, hypovolemia, and other nephrotoxic insults exacerbate its nephrotoxic effects. Many transplant patients must tolerate a moderately elevated serum creatinine (1.5-2 mg/dL) to sustain adequate immunosuppression. A related calcineurin immunosuppressive agent, tacrolimus (FK506), is somewhat less nephrotoxic than cyclosporine and has largely replaced it in liver transplantation.

In patients undergoing cadaveric renal transplantation, the calcium channel blocker diltiazem was added to the graft preservative solution, infused into the donor for 48 hours, and then given orally.[157] The incidence of transplant acute tubular necrosis decreased from 41% to 10%, and when acute renal failure did occur, hemodialysis requirement was significantly less. Diltiazem impairs cyclosporine metabolism so that plasma cyclosporine levels are higher, with fewer episodes of early acute rejection, but it protects against cyclosporine nephrotoxicity.[158] Cyclosporine dosage may be reduced by 30% to achieve the same drug levels, representing a substantial savings to patients.

An alternative approach that is gaining some traction is to replace cyclosporine or tacrolimus with the non-calcineurin agent sirolimus, which appears to have similar immunosuppressive effects with considerably less potential to induce renal injury.[159]

Radiocontrast Nephropathy

The nephrotoxicity of contrast dyes (see Chapter 79) probably involves microvascular obstruction by crenated red cells as well as direct tubular toxicity by release of free oxygen radicals. The risk is markedly increased in diabetic renal insufficiency, hypovolemia, congestive heart failure, and myeloma.[160] Radiocontrast dyes are hypertonic and cause an osmotic diuresis, which induces a false sense of security but exacerbates hypovolemia and renal damage. Azotemia commences 24 to 48 hours after exposure and peaks at 3 to 5 days. Surgery performed during this period greatly increases the risk of perioperative acute renal failure.

Prevention of radiocontrast nephropathy depends on adequate hydration (e.g., 1 mL/kg normal saline initiated at least 4 hours before and continued for 12 hours after radiocontrast administration).[161] Elective surgical procedures should be deferred until the effects of the dye have been evaluated and treated.[162] Nonionic, low-, or iso-osmolar radiocontrast media are less nephrotoxic but are expensive and offer optimal cost-benefit ratio when used in high-risk situations only (e.g., diabetic nephropathy).[154]

A number of pharmacologic agents have possible roles in preventing or attenuating contrast nephropathy but none replaces hydration as first-line protection. Intravenous mannitol has been used for many years but may exacerbate injury if it induces dehydration though excessive osmotic diuresis.

N-Acetylcysteine

Tepel and associates reported that prophylactic administration of the antioxidant *N*-acetylcysteine (600 mg orally twice daily) attenuated renal injury in a study on 83 patients with chronic renal insufficiency (mean serum creatinine, 2.4 mg/dL) undergoing contrast radiography.[163] Only 2% of patients receiving *N*-acetylcysteine had an increase in serum creatinine of more than 0.5 mg/dL, compared with 21% of patients receiving saline placebo, and mean serum creatinine concentrations actually decreased. Subsequent studies either did not confirm these results[164] or found that *N*-acetylcysteine provided better protection than saline alone only when a low dose of contrast dye was used.[165] Moreover, there is evidence that *N*-acetylcysteine itself decreases serum creatinine levels.[17] However, in a study on 354 patients undergoing primary angioplasty, *N*-acetylcysteine significantly decreased the incidence of radiocontrast nephropathy, dialysis requirement, and hospital mortality in a dose-dependent manner.[166]

Fenoldopam

Preliminary evidence demonstrated that fenoldopam infusion prevented the decrease in RPF induced by radiocontrast media.[167] However, a large, multicenter randomized clinical trial on 315 patients with preexisting renal insufficiency (creatinine clearance < 60 mL/min) showed that it had no benefit on renal function compared with placebo.[168]

Pigment Nephropathy

Pigment nephropathy implies acute renal injury due to the nephrotoxic effect of the heme pigments myoglobin, hemoglobin, and bilirubin.

Rhabdomyolysis and Myoglobinemia

Muscle necrosis (rhabdomyolysis) occurs most commonly with direct trauma involving major crush or thermal injury (see Chapter 72). However, it also occurs with acute muscle ischemia induced by vascular disease or injury or by prolonged immobilization. Compartment syndromes exacerbate rhabdomyolysis. They are particularly likely to occur with major hemorrhage in an extremity or when vascular insufficiency coexists with tissue edema (e.g., femoral placement of an intra-aortic balloon after vein harvesting). Dramatic increases in metabolic rate (severe exercise, prolonged fever, status epilepticus, or myoclonus), severe hypophosphatemia, or direct proteolysis (acute pancreatitis) can all precipitate rhabdomyolysis.[169]

Myoglobin, the oxygen-carrying heme pigment of muscle, is released into the bloodstream (myoglobinemia) and rapidly excreted by the glomerulus at a plasma threshold of 0.03 mg/dL. Delivery of myoglobin to the proximal tubule is greater in a well-muscled individual with normal GFR than in a cachectic patient with low GFR. At a urine pH less than 5.6, myoglobin is transformed into ferrihematin, which precipitates in the proximal tubule.[170] Renal damage is facilitated by hypovolemia (i.e., low tubular flow) and acidic urine. Because of the associated hypercatabolic state, oliguria is associated with acute hyperkalemia, hypocalcemia, anion-gap metabolic acidosis, and rapid azotemia. Serum creatinine and BUN increase very rapidly (1.0-1.5 mg/dL/day and 20-30 mg/dL/day, respectively).

The most important aid to the diagnosis of rhabdomyolysis is a high index of suspicion. The affected muscle may be obviously ischemic or swollen, painful, and edematous. Urine myoglobin often tests positive without reddish urine. The serum is clear because of the low renal threshold for myoglobin excretion, whereas hemoglobinemia is associated with pink serum. Serial total creatinine phosphokinase (CPK) is a helpful guide to the severity of rhabdomyolysis (i.e., CPK-MM release).[171] Renal damage is much more likely when total CPK exceeds 10,000 units/L.

Prevention of acute nephrotoxic tubular necrosis is dependent on the maintenance of high RBF and tubular flow. Urine flow should be kept between 100 to 150 mL/hr by osmotic diuresis with intravenous mannitol, 6.25 to 12.5 g every 6 hours, with or without intravenous furosemide, 10 to 20 mg as required.[172] Urine pH should be kept above pH 5.6 with intravenous sodium bicarbonate, 50 mEq intravenously, as required, and/or acetazolamide, 250 mg every 6 hours. However, because there are no prospective data that confirm the beneficial effect of urinary alkalinization, urine pH should not be increased at the expense of causing significant acid-base imbalance. Calcium should be given to treat hyperkalemia only.

Hemolysis and Hemoglobinemia

Acute intravascular hemolysis (see Chapter 52) due to mismatched blood transfusion (ABO incompatibility) represents a direct and devastating renal insult. Renal damage is thought to be predominantly due to red blood cell stroma rather than to free hemoglobin. Management is essentially the same as for rhabdomyolysis.

Jaundice and Bilirubinemia

There is a direct correlation between the degree of preoperative obstructive jaundice and postoperative renal dysfunction.[173] When cholestasis causes the conjugated bilirubin to increase above 8 mg/dL, bile salt excretion effectively ceases, resulting in portal septicemia and renal damage. This situation is analogous to hepatorenal syndrome and sepsis, in which circulating endotoxins induce renal vasoconstriction and damage (vasomotor nephropathy).

Administration of preoperative oral bile salts (e.g., sodium taurocholate) or intravenous mannitol may provide perioperative renal protection in patients with severe obstructive jaundice. In a prospective, randomized study in patients with obstructive jaundice undergoing surgery, Plusa and Clark[174] found no difference in renal outcome between these two regimens. However, mannitol provokes a brisk osmotic diuresis and it is important to replace urinary losses appropriately. Diuresis-induced hypovolemia negates the protective effect of mannitol.[175]

Sepsis

Sepsis is the most common cause of new-onset acute renal failure in the postoperative period (see Chapters 91 and 92). Renal function may deteriorate progressively without defined episodes of hypotension. In addition, sepsis predisposes the kidney to further ischemic and nephrotoxic insults (e.g., from concomitant aminoglycoside usage).[176] Acute renal failure itself and hemodialysis perpetuate sepsis by activating leukocytes. There is a reasonable amount of evidence to suggest that renal autoregulation may be impaired in sepsis and that RBF and GFR decline pari passu with systemic vascular resistance and mean arterial pressure. Hypotension sets off a cascade of neurohormonal responses (sympathoadrenal activity; renin-angiotensin, vasopressin, and thromboxane activation) that result in decreased RBF, GFR, sodium excretion, and urine flow. The severity of renal dysfunction is directly related to the severity of sepsis and the degree of plasma renin activation.[177]

Renal dysfunction in sepsis is characterized as a vasomotor nephropathy, which implies renal vasoconstriction in the presence of increased total cardiac index. Renal vasoconstriction, mesangial cell contraction, decreased ultrafiltration coefficient, and decreased GFR are induced by endotoxin and by compounds activated in sepsis.[178] These include endothelin and eicosanoids, such as thromboxane, prostaglandin F_2, and the leukotrienes C4 and D4. Prostaglandin F_2, which mimics the action of thromboxane, is formed during leukostasis when arachidonic acid is oxidized by free oxygen radicals.

It has been estimated that 10% to 26% of septic patients receiving aminoglycoside antibiotics will develop nephrotoxic renal insufficiency.[153] Aminoglycoside nephrotoxicity is enhanced by the interaction of fever, renal vasoconstriction, hypovolemia, and endotoxin. In the presence of these and other risk factors (see earlier), alternative non-nephrotoxic antibiotics should be considered to treat gram-negative infections, including penicillins (ticarcillin), cephalosporins (ceftazidime), carbapenems (imipenem), or monobactams (aztreonam).

Renal Protection in Septic Shock

Anti-inflammatory Agents

Cumming and coworkers[179] demonstrated a marked renal protective effect of a selective thromboxane synthetase inhibitor (U63557A) in laparotomy on a volume-loaded sheep peritonitis model. Administration of the selective inhibitor either before or 30 minutes after surgery prevented deterioration in creatinine clearance, urinary sodium excretion, and urine flow rate. Beneficial effects have also been observed with aprotinin, perhaps through its anti-inflammatory action.[57] In contrast, nonselective cyclooxygenase inhibition by NSAIDs worsens renal function in sepsis by decreasing the synthesis of the renal vasodilator prostacyclin.[180]

The use of pharmacologic doses of methylprednisolone in septic shock was discredited by two large multicenter studies showing no beneficial effect on outcome.[181,182] Moreover, patients who received corticosteroids had significant increases in BUN but not in serum creatinine concentration, suggesting a prerenal state induced by increased protein catabolism.[183] Other potentially adverse effects of high-dose corticosteroids include impaired mitochondrial function, impaired leukocyte function, and inhibition of phospholipase A_2, resulting in decreased synthesis of intrarenal vasodilator prostaglandins.

Supranormal Oxygen Delivery

Over the past decade there has been considerable controversy in the concept of supranormal oxygen delivery to the tissues to overcome the defect that exists in oxygen utilization by septic tissues.[184] This approach utilizes inotropic support and blood transfusion to drive global oxygen delivery (Do_2) to one of three end points: a Do_2 level consistently found in survivors (600 mL/min/m^2), or when global oxygen consumption (Vo_2) no longer increases with increasing Do_2 (consumption independence), or when blood lactate levels start to decline. The benefits on outcome of supranormal oxygen delivery have been disputed, and high-dose inotropic and vasopressor support may themselves have adverse consequences. Moreover, renal Do_2 and Vo_2 differ markedly from systemic indices. Renal Vo_2 is largely determined by tubular metabolic function, which is regulated by fluid and electrolyte changes. In a volume-loaded septic porcine model, inotropic support with dobutamine increased systemic Do_2 and Vo_2 but did not increase renal indices.[44] Furthermore, decreased global renal Do_2 does not appear to cause tubular damage, possibly because tubular work and Vo_2 are decreased when GFR declines.[185]

Dopaminergic Agents

Low-dose dopamine (1-3 μg/kg/min) is frequently administered to septic patients in the belief that it confers renal protection through renal vasodilation or perhaps by inhibition of the Na^+/K^+-ATPase pump and decreases in renal tubular Vo_2.

In patients with sepsis syndrome (signs of sepsis without hypotension), low-dose dopamine infusion doubled urine flow rate and increased creatinine clearance by 60% without any change in systemic hemodynamics.[186] However, the renal response to dopamine decreased significantly after 48 hours of dopamine infusion, possibly owing to downregulation of the renal dopaminergic receptors or diuresis-induced contraction of the intravascular volume. In patients with established septic shock who required catecholamines for blood pressure support, low-dose dopamine did not alter systemic hemodynamics or renal function.

The prophylactic administration of low-dose dopamine in sepsis appears to have been laid to rest by a large prospective controlled study conducted by the Australian and New Zealand Intensive Care Society (ANZICS). They randomized 328 patients with signs of the systemic inflammatory response syndrome (SIRS) and early renal dysfunction (oliguria or increasing serum creatinine) to dopamine, 2 μg/kg/min, or placebo. They found no differences in serum creatinine, dialysis requirement, intensive care unit or hospital length of stay or overall mortality.[187]

The potential role of dopexamine in septic shock remains speculative. Most studies have examined its role in splanchnic and hepatic perfusion rather than in renal protection. In animal models of sepsis, dopexamine has improved splanchnic and hepatic Do_2, but its β_2-adrenergic activity in causing tachycardia and hypotension may limit its application in clinical sepsis. Smithies and colleagues[188] administered dopexamine to patients with sepsis syndrome, acute respiratory failure, and at least one other organ system failure. Cardiac index increased and gastric intramucosal pH (an index of splanchnic perfusion) improved significantly.

Norepinephrine

In patients with septic shock, profound hypotension, and oliguria, vasopressor therapy with norepinephrine may actually improve renal function by enhancing renal perfusion pressure. Desjars and coworkers[11] evaluated a group of septic patients who remained oliguric despite volume resuscitation and the use of dopamine up to doses of 15 μg/kg/min. The addition of norepinephrine and reduction of dopamine to a low-dose level resulted in an improvement in mean arterial pressure from 50 to 70 mm Hg, a tripling of urine flow, and a doubling of creatinine clearance. Norepinephrine increased the systemic vascular resistance (SVR) with little change in cardiac index or Do_2. Subsequent studies have confirmed that the use of norepinephrine to keep mean arterial pressure greater than 60 mm Hg results in improved cardiac function (increase in stroke volume and decrease in heart rate) and GFR without deleterious effects on cardiac index, Vo_2, or oxygen extraction.[189] Large doses of norepinephrine may be required to achieve these goals, because in septic shock, the peripheral vasculature is notoriously refractory to norepinephrine-induced vasoconstriction. This occurs because of massive inducible nitric oxide release as well as vasopressin deficiency (see later). Nonetheless, these findings strongly support the concept that renal autoregulation is impaired in sepsis and that maintenance of adequate renal perfusion pressure is an important component of renal protection.

Arginine Vasopressin

Patients in vasodilatory shock have inappropriately low plasma levels of AVP and marked vascular sensitivity to its exogenous administration at low doses.[190] Vasodilatory shock is defined as hypotension, increased cardiac index, and low systemic vascular resistance refractory to pressors such as norepinephrine. Septic shock is its most common manifestation, but it is also characteristic of the contact activation syndrome induced by CPB or ventricular assist devices.[191]

Landry and coworkers[192] observed unusual sensitivity to the vasoconstrictor effects of infused AVP in patients with septic shock with profound hypotension despite catecholamine infusion. Infusion of AVP at doses of 2.4 units/hr, less than one tenth of those used in the treatment of bleeding esophageal varices, resulted in a dramatic increase in systolic blood pressure from 92 ± 4 to 146 ± 4 mm Hg (mean ± SEM, $P < .001$), and catecholamine infusions were able to be discontinued. In an associated report,[193] the authors observed that urine flow increased concomitantly in three of five patients, from an average of 30 mL/hr to 110 mL/hr.

Plasma AVP levels were remarkably low (3.1 ± 1.0 pg/mL) and significantly lower than in a cohort of patients in cardiogenic shock also receiving catecholamines (22.7 ± 2.2 pg/mL, $P < .001$).[192] It has been postulated that this "AVP deficiency" may be the result of excessive baroreceptor-mediated AVP release from sustained hypotension. This is strongly supported by a canine study demonstrating almost complete depletion of radiolabeled AVP in the posterior pituitary after 1 hour of hemorrhagic shock.[190]

A second mechanism for sensitivity to AVP in septic patients is explained by its effect on the potassium-ATP (K_{ATP}) channel.[190] Intracellular acidosis, lactic acid accumulation, and ATP depletion close K_{ATP} channels in the sarcolemma of vascular smooth muscle. This traps potassium outside the cell and hyperpolarizes the membrane, which in turn closes calcium channels essential for norepinephrine-induced vasoconstriction. AVP binds at the K_{ATP} channel and opens it, reversing membrane hyperpolarization and restoring sensitivity to norepinephrine.

The beneficial effect of AVP on renal function in sepsis may in part be due to its ability to increase low renal perfusion pressure back into the autoregulatory range. Another important factor is that, unlike norepinephrine, even at high local concentrations, AVP preferentially constricts the efferent arteriole, thereby improving filtration fraction and GFR.[53] However, in a large, prospective, randomized, blinded trial in 778 patients with severe septic shock, low-dose AVP (0.01-0.03 unit/min) did not provide a mortality benefit or decrease the requirement for dialysis when compared with an infusion of norepinephrine (5-15 μg/min).[194]

References

1. Koeppen BM, Stanton BA: Structure and function of the kidneys. *In* Koeppen BM, Stanton BA (eds): Renal Physiology, 4th ed. Philadelphia, Mosby Elsevier, 2007, pp 19-30.
2. Madsen KM, Nielsen S, Tisher CC: Anatomy of the kidney. *In* Brenner BM (ed): Brenner & Rector's The Kidney, 8th ed. Philadelphia, Saunders Elsevier, 2008, pp 25-90.
3. Gong R, Dworkin LD, Brenner BM, et al (eds): The renal circulations and glomerular ultrafiltration. *In* Brenner BM (ed): Brenner & Rector's The Kidney, 8th ed. Philadelphia, Saunders Elsevier, 2008, pp 91-129.
4. Koeppen BM, Stanton BA: Glomerular filtration and renal blood flow. *In* Koeppen BM, Stanton BA (eds): Renal Physiology, 4th ed. Philadelphia, Mosby Elsevier, 2007, pp 31-46.
5. Thurau K, Boylan JW: Acute renal success: The unexpected logic of oliguria in acute renal failure. Am J Med 61:308-315, 1976.
6. Shipley RE, Study RS: Changes in renal blood flow, extraction of inulin, glomerular filtration rate, tissue pressure and urine flow with acute alterations of renal artery pressure. Am J Physiol 167:676-688, 1951.
7. Aukland K, Oien AH: Renal autoregulation: models combining tubuloglomerular feedback and myogenic response. Am J Physiol 252:F768-F783, 1987
8. Kelleher SP, Robinette JB, Miller F, et al: Effect of hemorrhagic reduction in blood pressure on recovery from acute renal failure. Kidney Int 31:725-730, 1987.
9. Guan Z, Gobe G, Willgoss D, et al: Renal endothelial dysfunction and impaired autoregulation after ischemia-reperfusion injury result from excess nitric oxide. Am J Physiol Renal Physiol 291:F619-F628, 2006.
10. Mackay JH, Feerick AE, Woodson LC, et al: Increasing organ blood flow during cardiopulmonary bypass in pigs: comparison of dopamine and perfusion pressure. Crit Care Med 23:1090-1098, 1995.
11. Desjars PH, Pinaud M, Bugnon D, et al: Norepinephrine has no deleterious renal effects in human septic shock. Crit Care Med 17:426-429, 1989.
12. Koeppen BM, Stanton BA: Renal transport mechanisms: NaCl and water reabsorption along the nephron. In Koeppen BM, Stanton BA (eds): Renal Physiology, 4th ed. Philadelphia, Mosby Elsevier, 2007, pp 47-70.
13. Brezis M, Rosen S: Hypoxia of the renal medulla—its implications for disease. N Engl J Med 332:647-655, 1995.
14. Sladen RN: Oliguria in the ICU: systematic approach to diagnosis and treatment. Anesthesiol Clin North Am 18:739-752, viii, 2000.
15. Bellomo R, Ronco C, Kellum JA, et al: Acute renal failure—definition, outcome measures, animal models, fluid therapy and information technology needs: The Second International Consensus Conference of the Acute Dialysis Quality Initiative (ADQI) Group. Crit Care 8:R204-R212, 2004.
16. Tepel M, Zidek W: *N*-Acetylcysteine in nephrology; contrast nephropathy and beyond. Curr Opin Nephrol Hypertens 13:649-654, 2004.
17. Hoffmann U, Fischereder M, Kruger B, et al: The value of *N*-acetylcysteine in the prevention of radiocontrast agent–induced nephropathy seems questionable. J Am Soc Nephrol 15:407-410, 2004.
18. Moran SM, Myers BD: Course of acute renal failure studied by a model of creatinine kinetics. Kidney Int 27:928-937, 1985.
19. Trof RJ, Di Maggio F, Leemreis J, et al: Biomarkers of acute renal injury and renal failure. Shock 26:245-253, 2006.
20. Uchida K, Gotoh A: Measurement of cystatin-C and creatinine in urine. Clin Chim Acta 323:121-128, 2002.
21. Ylinen EA, Ala-Houhala M, Harmoinen AP, et al: Cystatin C as a marker for glomerular filtration rate in pediatric patients. Pediatr Nephrol 13:506-509, 1999.
22. Hojs R, Bevc S, Ekart R, et al: Serum cystatin C as an endogenous marker of renal function in patients with mild to moderate impairment of kidney function. Nephrol Dial Transplant 21:1855-1862, 2006.
23. Rule AD, Bergstralh EJ, Slezak JM, et al: Glomerular filtration rate estimated by cystatin C among different clinical presentations. Kidney Int 69:399-405, 2006.
24. Robert S, Zarowitz BJ, Peterson EL, et al: Predictability of creatinine clearance estimates in the critically ill. Crit Care Med 21:1487-1495, 1993.
25. Levey AS, Bosch JP, Lewis JB, et al: A more accurate method to estimate glomerular filtration rate from serum creatinine: A new prediction equation. Modification of Diet in Renal Disease Study Group. Ann Intern Med 130:461-470, 1999
26. Kasiske BL, Keane WF: Laboratory assessment of renal disease: Clearance, urinalysis and renal biopsy. *In* Brenner BM (ed): Brenner & Rector's The Kidney, 6th ed. Philadelphia, WB Saunders, 2000, pp 1129-1170.
27. Dagher PC, Herget-Rosenthal S, Ruehm SG, et al: Newly developed techniques to study and diagnose acute renal failure. J Am Soc Nephrol 14:2188-2198, 2003.
28. Sladen RN, Endo E, Harrison T: Two-hour versus 22-hour creatinine clearance in critically ill patients. Anesthesiology 67:1013-1016, 1987.
29. Shin B, Mackenzie C, Helrich M: Creatinine clearance for early detection of posttraumatic renal dysfunction. Anesthesiology 64:605-609, 1986.
30. Bryan AG, Bolsin SN, Vianna PTG, et al: Modification of the diuretic and natriuretic effects of a dopamine infusion by fluid loading in preoperative cardiac surgical patients. J Cardiothorac Vasc Anesth 9:158-163, 1995.
31. Allgren RL, Marbury TC, Rahman SN, et al: Anaritide in acute tubular necrosis. Auriculin Anaritide Acute Renal Failure Study Group. N Engl J Med 336:828-834, 1997.
32. Koeppen BM, Stanton BA: Regulation of body fluid osmolality: regulation of water balance. *In* Koeppen BM, Stanton BA (eds): Renal Physiology, 4th ed. Philadelphia, Mosby Elsevier, 2007, pp 71-90.
33. Carvounis CP, Nisar S, Guro-Razuman S: Significance of the fractional excretion of urea in the differential diagnosis of acute renal failure. Kidney Int 62:2223-2229, 2002.
34. Garcia-Garcia M, Garcia-Valero J, Mourad G, et al: Urinary and serum beta 2-microglobulin in living

related kidney donors and in renal failure. Contrib Nephrol 112:77-82, 1995.

35. Canivet JL, Larbuisson R, Damas P, et al: Plasma renin activity and urine beta 2-microglobulin during and after cardiopulmonary bypass: pulsatile vs non-pulsatile perfusion. Eur Heart J 11:1079-1082, 1990.
36. Price RG: Urinary *N*-acetyl-beta-D-glucosaminidase (NAG) as an indicator of renal disease. Curr Probl Clin Biochem (9):150-163, 1979.
37. Mishra J, Ma Q, Prada A, et al: Identification of neutrophil gelatinase-associated lipocalin as a novel early urinary biomarker for ischemic renal injury. J Am Soc Nephrol 14:2534-2543, 2003.
38. Mishra J, Dent C, Tarabishi R, et al: Neutrophil gelatinase-associated lipocalin (NGAL) as a biomarker for acute renal injury after cardiac surgery. Lancet 365:1231-1238, 2005.
39. Wagener G, Jan M, Kim M, et al: Association between increases in urinary neutrophil gelatinase-associated lipocalin and acute renal dysfunction after adult cardiac surgery. Anesthesiology 105:485-491, 2006.
40. Mangano DT, Tudor IC, Dietzel C: The risk associated with aprotinin in cardiac surgery. N Engl J Med 354:353-365, 2006.
41. Wagener G, Gubitosa G, Wang S, et al: Increased incidence of acute kidney injury with aprotinin use during cardiac surgery detected with urinary NGAL. Am J Nephrol 28:576-582, 2008.t
42. Stanton BA, Koeppen BM: Elements of renal function. *In* Berne RM, Levy MN (eds): Physiology, 4th ed. St. Louis, Mosby, 1998, pp 677-698.
43. Schaer GL, Fink MP, Parrillo JE: Norepinephrine alone versus norepinephrine plus low-dose dopamine: Enhanced renal blood flow with combination pressor therapy. Crit Care Med 13:492-496, 1985.
44. Haywood GA, Tighe D, Moss R, et al: Goal directed therapy with dobutamine in a porcine model of septic shock: Effects on systemic and renal oxygen transport. Postgrad Med J 67(S1):S36, 1991.
45. Aronson S, Wiencek JG, Feinstein SB, et al: Assessment of renal blood flow with contrast ultrasonography. Anesth Analg 76:964, 1993.
46. Levens NR, Peach MJ, Carey RM: Role of the intrarenal renin-angiotensin system in the control of renal function. Circ Res 48:157-167, 1981.
47. Ballerman BJ, Zeidel ML, Gunning ME, et al: Vasoactive peptides and the kidney. *In* Brenner BM, Rector FCJ (eds): The Kidney, 4th ed. Philadelphia, WB Saunders, 1991, pp 510-583.
48. Hricik D, Browning P, Kopelman R, et al: Captopril-induced functional renal insufficiency in patients with bilateral renal-artery stenoses or renal-artery stenosis in a solitary kidney. N Engl J Med 308:373-376, 1983.
49. Wynckel A, Ebikili B, Melin JP, et al: Long-term follow-up of acute renal failure caused by angiotensin converting enzyme inhibitors. Am J Hypertens 11:1080-1086, 1998.
50. Colson P, Ribstein J, Mimran A, et al: Effect of angiotensin converting enzyme inhibition on blood pressure and renal function during open heart surgery. Anesthesiology 72:23-27, 1990.
51. Genuth SM: The adrenal glands. *In* Berne RM, Levy EM (eds): Physiology, 4th ed. St. Louis, Mosby, 1998, pp 930-964.
52. Baylis PH: Posterior pituitary function in health and disease. Clin Endocrinol Metab 12:747-770, 1983.
53. Edwards RM, Trizna W, Kinter LB: Renal microvascular effects of vasopressin and vasopressin antagonists. Am J Physiol 256: F274-F278, 1989.
54. Levenson DJ, Simmons CEJ, Brenner BM: Arachidonic acid metabolites, prostaglandins and the kidney. Am J Med 72:354-374, 1982.
55. Johnston PA, Bernard DB, Perrin NS, et al: Prostaglandins mediate the vasodilatory effect of mannitol in the hypoperfused rat kidney. J Clin Invest 68:127-133, 1981.
56. Gerber JG, Olsen RD, Nies AS: Interrelationship between prostaglandins and renin release. Kidney Int 19:816-821, 1981.
57. Cumming AD: Acute renal failure and sepsis: Therapeutic approaches. Nephrol Dialysis Transplant 4:159-163, 1994.
58. Licker M, Morel DR: Inhibitors of the renin angiotensin system: Implications for the anaesthesiologist. Curr Opin Anaesthesiol 11:321-326, 1998.
59. Madeddu P, Emanueli C, El-Dahr S: Mechanisms of disease: The tissue kallikrein-kinin system in hypertension and vascular remodeling. Nat Clin Pract Nephrol 3:208-221, 2007.

59a. Gorfinkel HJ, Szidon JP, Hirsch LJ, et al: Renal performance in experimental cardiogenic shock. Am J Physiol 222:1260-1268, 1972.

60. de Bold AJ, Borenstein HB, Veress AT, et al: A rapid and potent natriuretic response to intravenous injection of atrial myocardial extract in rats. Life Sci 28:89-94, 1981.
61. Laragh J: Atrial natriuretic hormone, the renin-angiotensin axis, and blood-pressure electrolyte homeostasis. N Engl J Med 313:1330-1340, 1985.
62. Maack T, Camargo MJF, Kleinert HD, et al: Atrial natriuretic factor: structure and functional properties. Kidney Int 27:607-615, 1985.
63. Baughman KL: B-type natriuretic peptide—a window to the heart. N Engl J Med 347:158-159, 2002.
64. Baxter GF: The natriuretic peptides. Basic Res Cardiol 99:71-75, 2004.
65. Shannon RP, Libby E, Elahi D, et al: Impact of acute reduction in chronically elevated left atrial pressure on sodium and water excretion. Ann Thorac Surg 46:430-437, 1988.
66. Goldberg L, Rajfer S: Dopamine receptors: Applications in clinical cardiology. Circulation 72:245-248, 1985.
67. Bello-Reuss E, Higashi Y, Kaneda Y: Dopamine decreases fluid reabsorption in the straight portions of the rabbit proximal tubule. Am J Physiol 242:(Renal Fluid Electrolyte Physiol): F634-F640, 1982.
68. Olsen NV: Effects of dopamine on renal haemodynamics tubular function and sodium excretion in normal humans. Dan Med Bull 45:282-297, 1998.
69. Eklof AC: The natriuretic response to a dopamine DA1 agonist requires endogenous activation of dopamine DA2 receptors. Acta Physiol Scand 160:311-314, 1997.
70. Holtbäck U, Kruse MS, Brismar H, et al: Intrarenal dopamine coordinates the effect of antinatriuretic and natriuretic factors. Acta Physiol Scand 168:215-218, 2000.
71. Correa AH, Choi MR, Gironacci M, et al: Atrial natriuretic factor decreases renal dopamine turnover and catabolism without modifying its release. Regul Pept 146:238-242, 2008.
72. Sansoe G, Ferrari A, Baraldi E, et al: Dopaminergic control of renal tubular function in patients with compensated cirrhosis. Dig Dis Sci 47:392-400, 2002.
73. Steudel W, Hurford WE, Zapol WM: Inhaled nitric oxide: Basic biology and clinical applications. Anesthesiology 91:1090-1121, 1999.
74. Brezis M, Heyman SN, Dinour D, et al: Role of nitric oxide in renal medullary oxygenation: studies in isolated and intact rat kidneys. J Clin Invest 88:390-395, 1991.
75. Ito S, Carretero OA, Abe K: Nitric oxide in the regulation of renal blood flow. New Horizons 3:615-623, 1995.
76. Lieberthal W: Biology of ischemic and toxic renal tubular cell injury: Role of nitric oxide and the inflammatory response. Curr Opin Nephrol Hypertens 7:289-295, 1998.
77. Landin L, Lorente JA, Renes E, et al: Inhibition of nitric oxide synthesis improves the vasoconstrictive effect of noradrenaline in sepsis. Chest 106:250-256, 1994.
78. Goligorsky MS, Noiri E: Duality of nitric oxide in acute renal injury. Semin Nephrol 19:263-271, 1999.
79. Noiri E, Peresleni T, Miller F, et al: In vivo targeting of inducible NO synthase with oligodeoxynucleotides protects rat kidney against ischemia. J Clin Invest 97:2377-2383, 1996.
80. Molitoris BA: Transitioning to therapy in ischemic acute renal failure. J Am Soc Nephrol 14:265-267, 2003.
81. Agmon Y, Peleg H, Greenfeld Z, et al: Nitric oxide and prostanoids protect the renal outer medulla from radiocontrast toxicity in the rat. J Clin Invest 94:1069-1075, 1994.
82. Ecoffey C, Edouard A, Pruszczynski W, et al: Effects of epidural anesthesia on catecholamines, renin activity and vasopressin changes induced by tilt in elderly men. Anesthesiology 62:294-297, 1985.
83. Gamulin Z, Forster A, Simonet F, et al: Effects of renal sympathetic blockade on renal hemodynamics in patients undergoing major aortic abdominal surgery. Anesthesiology 65:688-692, 1986.
84. Sener M, Torgay A, Akpek E, et al: Regional versus general anesthesia for donor nephrectomy: Effects on graft function. Transplant Proc 36:2954-2958, 2004.
85. Gelman S, Gowler KC, Smith LR: Regional blood flow during isoflurane and halothane anesthesia. Anesth Analg 63:557-565, 1984.
86. Priano LL: Alteration of renal hemodynamics by thiopental, diazepam and ketamine in conscious dogs. Anesth Analg 61:853-862, 1982.
87. Cousins MJ, Mazze RI: Methoxyflurane nephrotoxicity: A study of dose response in man. JAMA 225:1611-1616, 1973.
88. Mazze RI, Cousins MJ, Barr GA: Renal effects and metabolism of isoflurane in man. Anesthesiology 40:536-542, 1974.
89. Eger EI, Koblin DD, Bowland T, et al: Nephrotoxicity of sevoflurane versus desflurane anesthesia in volunteers. Anesth Analg 84:160-168, 1997.
90. Eger EI, Gong D, Koblin DD, et al: Dose-related biochemical markers of renal injury after sevoflurane versus desflurane anesthesia in volunteers. Anesth Analg 85:1154-1163, 1997.
91. Bito H, Ikeuchi Y, Ikeda K: Effects of low-flow sevoflurane anesthesia on renal function. Anesthesiology 86:1231-1237, 1997.
92. Kharasch ED, Frink EJJ, Zager R, et al: Assessment of low-flow sevoflurane and isoflurane effects on renal function using sensitive markers of tubular toxicity. Anesthesiology 86:1238-1253, 1997.
93. Ebert TJ, Frink EJ, Kharasch ED: Absence of biochemical evidence for renal and hepatic dysfunction after 8 hours of 1.25 minimum alveolar concentration sevoflurane anesthesia in volunteers. Anesthesiology 88:601-610, 1998.
94. Lee HT, Ota-Setlik A, Fu Y, et al: Differential protective effects of volatile anesthetics against renal

ischemia-reperfusion injury in vivo. Anesthesiology 101:1313-1324, 2004.

95. Kuiper JW, Groeneveld AB, Slutsky AS, et al: Mechanical ventilation and acute renal failure. Crit Care Med 33:1408-1415, 2005.
96. Jardin F, Forest JC, Boisante L, et al: Influence of positive end-expiratory pressure on left ventricular performance. N Engl J Med 304:387-392, 1981.
97. Sladen A, Laver MB, Pontoppidan H: Pulmonary complications and water retention in prolonged mechanical ventilation. N Engl J Med 279:448-453, 1968.
98. Annat G, Viale JP, Xuan BB, et al: Effect of PEEP ventilation on renal function, plasma renin, aldosterone, neurophysins and urinary ADH, and prostaglandins. Anesthesiology 58:136-141, 1983.
99. Venus B, Mathru M, Smith RA, et al: Renal function during application of positive end-expiratory pressure in swine: Effects of hydration. Anesthesiology 62:765-769, 1985.
100. Hemmer M, Suter PM: Treatment of cardiac and renal effects of PEEP with dopamine in patients with acute respiratory failure. Anesthesiology 50:399-403, 1979.
101. Botha J, Mudholkar P, Le Blanc V: The effect of changing from pressure support ventilation to volume control ventilation on renal function. Crit Care Resusc 7:303-309, 2005.
102. Imai Y, Parodo J, Kajikawa O, et al: Injurious mechanical ventilation and end-organ epithelial cell apoptosis and organ dysfunction in an experimental model of acute respiratory distress syndrome. JAMA 289:2104-2112, 2003.
103. Thompson GE, Miller RD, Stevens WC, et al: Hypotensive anesthesia for total hip arthroplasty: A study of blood loss and organ function, brain, heart, liver and kidneys. Anesthesiology 48:91-96, 1978.
104. Colley PS, Silvarjan M: Regional blood flow in dogs during halothane anesthesia and controlled hypotension produced by nitroprusside or nitroglycerin. Anesth Analg 63:503-510, 1984.
105. Aronson S, Goldberg LI, Glock D, et al: Effects of fenoldopam on renal blood flow and systemic hemodynamics during isoflurane anesthesia. J Cardiothorac Vasc Anesth 5:29-32, 1991.
106. Myers BD, Moran SM: Hemodynamically mediated acute renal failure. N Engl J Med 314:97-105, 1986.
107. Kudo FA, Nishibe T, Miyazaki K, et al: Postoperative renal function after elective abdominal aortic aneurysm repair requiring suprarenal aortic cross-clamping. Surg Today 34:1010-1013, 2004.
108. Myers SI, Wang L, Liu F, et al: Suprarenal aortic clamping and reperfusion decreases medullary and cortical blood flow by decreased endogenous renal nitric oxide and PGE_2 synthesis. J Vasc Surg 42:524-531, 2005.
109. Gamulin Z, Forster A, Morel D, et al: Effects of infra-renal aortic cross-clamping on renal hemodynamics in humans. Anesthesiology 61:394-399, 1984.
110. Burke TJ, Cronin RE, Duchin KL, et al: Ischemia and tubule obstruction during acute renal failure in dogs: Mannitol in protection. Am J Physiol 238:F305-F314, 1980.
111. Pass LJ, Eberhart RC, Brown JC, et al: The effect of mannitol and dopamine on the renal response to thoracic aortic cross-clamping. J Thorac Cardiovasc Surg 95:608-612, 1988.
112. Paul MD, Mazer CD, Byrick RJ, et al: Influence of mannitol and dopamine on renal function during elective infrarenal aortic clamping in man. Am J Nephrol 6:427-434, 1986.
113. Mathur VS, Swan SK, Lambrecht LJ, et al: The effects of fenoldopam, a selective dopamine receptor agonist, on systemic and renal hemodynamics in normotensive subjects. Crit Care Med 27:1832-1837, 1999.
114. Miller Q, Peyton BD, Cohn EJ, et al: The effects of intraoperative fenoldopam on renal blood flow and tubular function following suprarenal aortic cross-clamping. Ann Vasc Surg 17:656-662, 2003.
115. Halpenny M, Rushe C, Breen P, et al: The effects of fenoldopam on renal function in patients undergoing elective aortic surgery. Eur J Anaesthesiol 19:32-39, 2002.
116. Higgins TL, Estafanous FG, Loop FD, et al: Stratification of morbidity and mortality outcome by preoperative risk factors in coronary artery bypass patients: A clinical severity score. JAMA 267:2344-2348, 1992.
117. Conlon PJ, Stafford-Smith M, White WD, et al: Acute renal failure following cardiac surgery. Nephrol Dialysis Transplant 14:1158-1162, 1999.
118. Ip-Yam PC, Murphy S, Baines M, et al: Renal function and proteinuria after cardiopulmonary bypass: The effects of temperature and mannitol. Anesth Analg 78:842-847, 1994.
119. Nakamura K, Harasaki H, Fukumura F, et al: Comparison of pulsatile and non-pulsatile cardiopulmonary bypass on regional renal blood flow in sheep. Scand Cardiovasc J 38:59-63, 2004.
120. Sezai A, Shiono M, Nakata K, et al: Effects of pulsatile CPB on interleukin-8 and endothelin-1 levels. Artif Organs 29:708-713, 2005.
121. Alkan T, Akcevin A, Undar A, et al: Benefits of pulsatile perfusion on vital organ recovery during and after pediatric open heart surgery. Asaio J 53:651-654, 2007.
122. Onorati F, Presta P, Fuiano G, et al: A randomized trial of pulsatile perfusion using an intra-aortic balloon pump versus nonpulsatile perfusion on short-term changes in kidney function during cardiopulmonary bypass during myocardial reperfusion. Am J Kidney Dis 50:229-238, 2007.
123. Abramov D, Tamariz M, Serrick CI, et al: The influence of cardiopulmonary bypass flow characteristics on the clinical outcome of 1820 coronary bypass patients. Can J Cardiol 19:237-243, 2003.
124. Woo EB, Tang AT, el-Gamel A, et al: Dopamine therapy for patients at risk of renal dysfunction following cardiac surgery: Science or fiction? Eur J Cardiothorac Surg 22:106-111, 2002.
125. Abu-Omar Y, Mussa S, Naik MJ, et al: Evaluation of Cystatin C as a marker of renal injury following on-pump and off-pump coronary surgery. Eur J Cardiothorac Surg 27:893-898, 2005.
126. Loef BG, Epema AH, Navis G, et al: Off-pump coronary revascularization attenuates transient renal damage compared with on-pump coronary revascularization. Chest 121:1190-1194, 2002.
127. Massoudy P, Wagner S, Thielmann M, et al: Coronary artery bypass surgery and acute kidney injury—impact of the off-pump technique. Nephrol Dial Transplant 2008 Apr 3 [Epub ahead of print].
128. Hilberman M, Myers B, Carrie G, et al: Acute renal failure following cardiac surgery. J Thorac Cardiovasc Surg 77:880-888, 1979.
129. Hilberman M, Derby GC, Spencer RJ, et al: Sequential pathophysiological changes characterizing the progression from renal dysfunction to acute renal failure following cardiac operation. J Thorac Cardiovasc Surg 79:838-844, 1980.
130. Hilberman M, Maseda J, Stinson E, et al: The diuretic properties of dopamine in patients after open-heart operation. Anesthesiology 61:489-494, 1984.
131. Lassnigg A, Donner E, Grubhofer G, et al: Lack of renoprotective effects of dopamine and furosemide during cardiac surgery. J Am Soc Nephrol 11:97-104, 2000.
132. Myles PS, Buckland MR, Schenk NJ, et al: Effect of "renal-dose" dopamine on renal function following cardiac surgery. Anaesth Intensive Care 21:56-61, 1993.
133. Costa P, Ottino GM, Matani A, et al: Low-dose dopamine during cardiopulmonary bypass in patients with renal dysfunction. J Cardiothorac Anesth 4:469-473, 1990.
134. MacGregor DA, Smith TE, Prielipp RC, et al: Pharmacokinetics of dopamine in healthy male subjects. Anesthesiology 92:338-346, 2000.
135. Chiolero R, Borgeta A, Fisher A: Postoperative arrhythmias and risk factors after open heart surgery. Thorac Cardiovasc Surg 39:81-84, 1991.
136. Landoni G, Biondi-Zoccai GG, Marino G, et al: Fenoldopam reduces the need for renal replacement therapy and in-hospital death in cardiovascular surgery: A meta-analysis. J Cardiothorac Vasc Anesth 22:27-33, 2008.
137. Caimmi PP, Pagani L, Micalizzi E, et al: Fenoldopam for renal protection in patients undergoing cardiopulmonary bypass. J Cardiothorac Vasc Anesth 17:491-494, 2003.
138. Ranucci M, Soro G, Barzaghi N, et al: Fenoldopam prophylaxis of postoperative acute renal failure in high-risk cardiac surgery patients. Ann Thorac Surg 78:1332-1337; discussion 1337-1338, 2004.
139. Cogliati AA, Vellutini R, Nardini A, et al: Fenoldopam infusion for renal protection in high-risk cardiac surgery patients: A randomized clinical study. J Cardiothorac Vasc Anesth 21:847-850, 2007.
140. Seki G, Suzuki K, Nonaka T, et al: Effects of atrial natriuretic peptide on glycerol induced acute renal failure in the rat. Jpn Heart J 33:383-393, 1992.
141. Rahman SN, Kim GE, Mathew AS, et al: Effects of atrial natriuretic peptide in clinical acute renal failure. Kidney Int 45:1731-1738, 1994.
142. Lewis J, Salem MM, Chertow GM, et al: Atrial natriuretic factor in oliguric acute renal failure. Anaritide Acute Renal Failure Study Group. Am J Kidney Dis 36:767-774, 2000.
143. Sezai A, Shiono M, Orime Y, et al: Low-dose continuous infusion of human atrial natriuretic peptide during and after cardiac surgery. Ann Thorac Surg 69:732-738, 2000.
144. Mills RM, LeJemtel TH, Horton DP, et al: Sustained hemodynamic effects of an infusion of nesiritide (human b-type natriuretic peptide) in heart failure: A randomized, double-blind, placebo-controlled clinical trial. Natrecor Study Group. J Am Coll Cardiol 34:155-162, 1999.
145. Colucci WS: Nesiritide for the treatment of decompensated heart failure. J Card Fail 7:92-100, 2001.
146. Sackner-Bernstein JD, Skopicki HA, Aaronson KD: Risk of worsening renal function with nesiritide in patients with acutely decompensated heart failure. Circulation 111:1487-1491, 2005.
147. Mentzer RM Jr, Oz MC, Sladen RN, et al: Effects of perioperative nesiritide in patients with left ventricular dysfunction undergoing cardiac surgery: The NAPA Trial. J Am Coll Cardiol 49:716-726, 2007.
148. Burns KE, Chu MW, Novick RJ, et al: Perioperative *N*-acetylcysteine to prevent renal dysfunction in high-risk patients undergoing CABG surgery: A randomized controlled trial. JAMA 294:342-350, 2005.
149. Haase M, Haase-Fielitz A, Bagshaw SM, et al: Phase II, randomized, controlled trial of high-dose *N*-acetylcysteine in high-risk cardiac surgery patients. Crit Care Med 35:1324-1331, 2007.

150. Sisillo E, Ceriani R, Bortone F, et al: *N*-acetylcysteine for prevention of acute renal failure in patients with chronic renal insufficiency undergoing cardiac surgery: A prospective, randomized, clinical trial. Crit Care Med 36:81-86, 2008.
151. Pannu N, Nadim MK: An overview of drug-induced acute kidney injury. Crit Care Med 36:S216-S223, 2008.
152. Wardle N: Acute renal failure in the 1980s: The importance of septic shock and of endotoxemia. Nephron 30:193-200, 1982.
153. Zager RA: Endotoxemia, renal hypoperfusion, and fever: Interactive risk factors for aminoglycoside and sepsis-associated acute renal failure. Am J Kidney Dis 20:223-230, 1992.
154. Wetzels JF, Burke TJ, Schrier RW: Prevention and attenuation of acute renal failure. Curr Opin Nephrol Hypertens 1:133-140, 1992.
155. Clive D, Stoff J: Renal syndromes associated with nonsteroidal anti-inflammatory drugs. N Engl J Med 310:563-572, 1984.
156. Ahmad SR, Kortepeter C, Brinker A, et al: Renal failure associated with the use of celecoxib and rofecoxib. Drug Saf 25:537-544, 2002.
157. Kunzendorf U, Walz G, Brockmoeller J, et al: Effects of diltiazem upon metabolism and immunosuppressive action of cyclosporine in kidney graft recipients. Transplantation 52:280-284, 1991.
158. Neumayer HH, Kunzendorf U, Schreiber M: Protective effects of calcium antagonists in human renal transplantation. Kidney Int Suppl 36:87-93, 1992.
159. Raichlin E, Bae JH, Khalpey Z, et al: Conversion to sirolimus as primary immunosuppression attenuates the progression of allograft vasculopathy after cardiac transplantation. Circulation 116:2726-2733, 2007.
160. Parfrey PS, Griffiths SM, Barrett BJ, et al: Contrast material–induced renal failure in patients with diabetes mellitus, renal insufficiency or both: A prospective, controlled study. N Engl J Med 320:143, 1989.
161. Morcos SK: Prevention of contrast media nephrotoxicity—the story so far. Clin Radiol 59:381-389, 2004.
162. Eisenberg RL, Bank WO, Hedgecock MW: Renal failure after major angiography can be avoided with hydration. Am J Radiol 136:859, 1981.
163. Tepel M, van der Giet M, Schwarzfeld C, et al: Prevention of radiographic-contrast-agent–induced reductions in renal function by acetylcysteine. N Engl J Med 343:180-184, 2000.
164. Allaqaband S, Tumuluri R, Malik AM, et al: Prospective randomized study of *N*-acetylcysteine, fenoldopam, and saline for prevention of radiocontrast-induced nephropathy. Cathet Cardiovasc Interv 57:279-283, 2002.
165. Briguori C, Manganelli F, Scarpato P, et al: Acetylcysteine and contrast agent–associated nephrotoxicity. J Am Coll Cardiol 40:298-303, 2002.
166. Marenzi G, Assanelli E, Marana I, et al: *N*-acetylcysteine and contrast-induced nephropathy in primary angioplasty. N Engl J Med 354:2773-2782, 2006.
167. Tumlin JA, Wang A, Murray PT, et al: Fenoldopam mesylate blocks reductions in renal plasma flow after radiocontrast dye infusion: A pilot trial in the prevention of contrast nephropathy. Am Heart J 143:894-903, 2002.
168. Stone GW, McCullough PA, Tumlin JA, et al: Fenoldopam mesylate for the prevention of contrast-induced nephropathy: A randomized controlled trial. JAMA 290:2284-2291, 2003.
169. Gabow PA, Kaehny WD, Kelleher SP: The spectrum of rhabdomyolysis. Medicine (Baltimore) 61:141, 1982.
170. Clyne DH, Kant KS, Pesce AJ, et al: Nephrotoxicity of low molecular weight serum proteins: Physicochemical interactions between myoglobin, hemoglobin, Bence-Jones protein and Tamm-Horsfall mucoprotein. Curr Prob Clin Biochem 9:299, 1979.
171. Ellinas PA, Rosner F: Rhabdomyolysis: Report of eleven cases. J Natl Med Assoc 84:617-624, 1992.
172. Ron D, Taitelman U, Michaelson M, et al: Prevention of acute renal failure in traumatic rhabdomyolysis. Arch Intern Med 144:277, 1984.
173. Wait RB, Kahng KU: Renal failure complicating obstructive jaundice. Am J Surg 157:256-263, 1989.
174. Plusa SM, Clark NW: Prevention of postoperative renal dysfunction in patients with obstructive jaundice: A comparison of mannitol-induced diuresis and oral sodium taurocholate. J R Coll Surg Edinb 36:303-305, 1991.
175. Gubern JM, Martinez-Rodenas F, Sitges-Serra A: Use of mannitol as a measure to prevent postoperative renal failure in patients with obstructive jaundice. Am J Surg 159:444-445, 1990.
176. Zager RA: Sepsis-associated acute renal failure: Some potential pathogenetic and therapeutic insights. Nephrol Dial Transplant 4:164-167, 1994.
177. Cumming AD, Driedger AA, McDonald JW, et al: Vasoactive hormones in the renal response to systemic sepsis. Am J Kidney Dis 11:23-32, 1988.
178. Badr KF: Sepsis-associated renal vasoconstriction: Potential targets for future therapy. Am J Kidney Dis 20:207-213, 1992.
179. Cumming AD, McDonald JW, Lindsay RM, et al: The protective effect of thromboxane synthetase inhibition on renal function in systemic sepsis. Am J Kidney Dis 13:114-119, 1989.
180. Garella S, Matarese RA: Renal effects of prostaglandins and clinical adverse effects of nonsteroidal anti-inflammatory agents. Medicine 63:165-181, 1984.
181. Bone RC, Fisher CJ, Clemmer TP, et al: A controlled clinical trial of high-dose methylprednisolone in the treatment of severe sepsis and septic shock. N Engl J Med 317:653-658, 1987.
182. Veteran's Administration Systemic Sepsis Cooperative Study Group: Effect of high-does glucocorticoid therapy on mortality in patients with clinical signs of systemic sepsis. N Engl J Med 317:659-665, 1987.
183. Slotman GJ, Fisher CJJ, Bone RC, et al: Detrimental effects of high-dose methylprednisolone sodium succinate on serum concentrations of hepatic and renal function indicators in severe sepsis and septic shock. The Methylprednisolone Severe Sepsis Study Group. Crit Care Med 21:191-195, 1993.
184. Rudis MI, Basha MA, Zarowitz BJ: Is it time to reposition vasopressors and inotropes in sepsis? Crit Care Med 24:525-537, 1996.
185. Weber A, Schwieger IM, Poinsot O, et al: Sequential changes in renal oxygen consumption and sodium transport during hyperdynamic sepsis in sheep. Am J Physiol 262 (RFEP 31):F965, 1992.
186. Lherm T, Troche G, Rossignol M, et al: Renal effects of low-dose dopamine in patients with sepsis syndrome or septic shock treated with catecholamines. Intens Care Med 22:213-219, 1996.
187. Bellomo R, Chapman M, Finfer S, et al: Low-dose dopamine in patients with early renal dysfunction: A placebo-controlled randomised trial. Australian and New Zealand Intensive Care Society (ANZICS) Clinical Trials Group. Lancet 356:2139-2143, 2000.
188. Smithies M, Yee TH, Jackson L, et al: Protecting the gut and the liver in the critically ill: Effects of dopexamine. Crit Care Med 22:789-795, 1994.
189. Hesselvik JF, Brodin B: Low-dose norepinephrine in patients with septic shock and oliguria: Effects on afterload, urine flow and oxygen transport. Crit Care Med 17:179-180, 1989.
190. Landry DW, Oliver JA: The pathogenesis of vasodilatory shock. N Engl J Med 345:588-595, 2001.
191. Argenziano M, Choudri AF, Oz MC, et al: A prospective randomized trial of arginine vasopressin in the treatment of vasodilatory shock after left ventricular assist device placement. Circulation 96[Suppl II]:II-286-II-290, 1997.
192. Landry DW, Levin HR, Gallant EM, et al: Vasopressin deficiency contributes to the vasodilation of septic shock. Circulation 95:1122-1125, 1997.
193. Landry DW, Levin HR, Gallant EM, et al: Vasopressin pressor hypersensitivity in vasodilatory septic shock. Crit Care Med 25:1279-1282, 1997.
194. Russell JA, Walley KR, Singer J, et al: Vasopressin versus norepinephrine infusion in patients with septic shock. N Engl J Med 358:877-887, 2008.

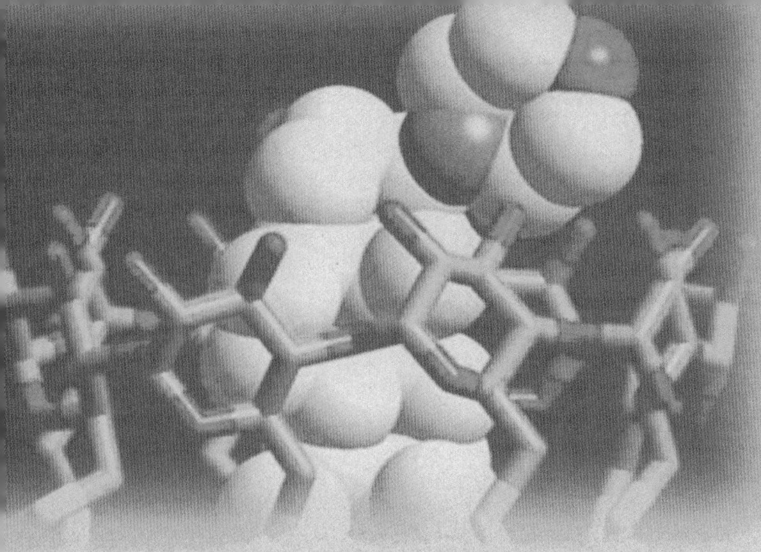

Anesthetic Pharmacology

Section III

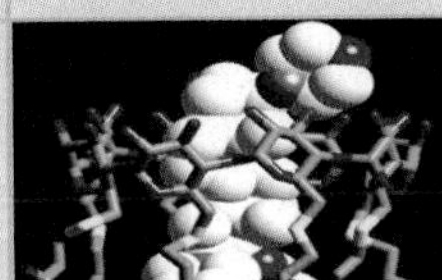

Steven L. Shafer, Pamela Flood, and Debra A. Schwinn

19 Basic Principles of Pharmacology

Key Points

1. The fundamental pharmacokinetic processes are dilution into volumes of distribution and clearance. These processes are governed by the physical properties of the drug and the metabolic capacity of the patient. Anesthetic drugs tend to be highly bound to protein in plasma and highly bound to lipid in peripheral tissues. Most anesthetic drugs are metabolized in the liver.
2. The pharmacokinetics of anesthetic drugs are typically described by mathematical models with a central compartment and one or two peripheral compartments. These compartments do not directly correspond to any anatomic or physiologic structures. Computer simulations can be used to predict the time course of plasma concentration and drug effect after any dose.
3. Drugs exert their effects through binding to receptors. The fraction bound is determined by the law of mass action, which yields a sigmoidal relationship between fractional occupancy and drug concentration.
4. Drugs can be agonists, partial agonists, neutral antagonists, or inverse agonists. Receptors can exist in many states, but for simplicity, one can think of them as having just two states: activated and inactivated. The intrinsic efficacy of a drug is determined by the extent to which it stabilizes the active form of the receptor (agonists) or the inactive form (inverse agonists) or simply displaces agonists from the binding site without favoring either form (neutral antagonists).
5. A fraction of receptors are in the activated state when drug is present. Thus, a "baseline effect" in the absence of drug does not represent the true baseline if all receptors are inactivated. This can be observed only by giving an inverse agonist that forces nearly all receptors into the inactivated state.
6. Four main receptor types of relevance in anesthesia are G protein–coupled receptors (opioids, catecholamines), ligand-gated ion channels (hypnotics, benzodiazepines, muscle relaxants, ketamine), voltage-gated ion channels (local anesthetics), and enzymes (neostigmine, amrinone, caffeine). The first three are located in cell membranes. Enzymes can be located anywhere.
7. Many drugs act through second messengers, which amplify drug action. Common second messengers are G proteins, which can release stimulating or inhibitory subunits in response to drug binding at the receptor; cyclic adenosine monophosphate, which is frequently a target of G protein stimulation or inhibition; inositol 1,4,5-triphosphate and diacylglycerol, also targets of G-protein regulation; and intracellular ions, especially calcium.
8. Advances in molecular pharmacology are helping identify the specific function of individual receptors, the role of individual amino acids in mediating receptor action, and the specific sites of action of many anesthetic drugs. Tools to explore the mechanism of drug action include site-directed mutagenesis to create "designer" receptors and knock-out/knock-down (underexpressed) or transgenic (overexpressed) murine models to understand the physiologic action of individual receptors.
9. The fundamental properties of the concentration-versus-response relationship are potency and efficacy. Potency is the concentration associated with a 50% drug effect. Efficacy is the maximal possible drug effect.
10. Drugs can interact both pharmacokinetically, through enzymatic induction or inhibition, or pharmacodynamically, through synergy or antagonism. Anesthetic techniques typically take advantage of the synergy between hypnotics and opioids to produce the anesthetic state at far lower doses of each drug than would be required if they were used alone.
11. Pharmacogenetics is gradually explaining some of the variability in response to drugs. Genetic variability in pharmacokinetics can be attributed to variability in hepatic cytochromes (e.g., CYP2D6, CYP2C19), circulating enzymes (e.g., pseudocholinesterase), or transporters. Genetic variability in pharmacodynamics can be attributed to alterations in receptors, as has been demonstrated for multiple adrenergic receptor variants. Malignant hyperthermia has been clearly linked to variability in the ryanodine receptor.

12. Variability in response to drugs can also be attributed to nongenetic causes, such as aging, disease, exposure to environmental toxins, and the pharmacokinetic or pharmacodynamic influence of other drugs. Variability is also introduced through continuous exposure to a single drug, which can trigger desensitization (tolerance) or, if the drug is an antagonist, increased receptor sensitivity to the agonist.

Anesthesiologists administer drugs to produce hypnosis, amnesia, analgesia, and muscle relaxation, and to support physiologic homeostasis while minimizing side effects and toxicity. Anesthesiologists select appropriate doses through a combination of scientifically guided administration and empirical titration. Both approaches are enhanced by a thorough understanding of the basic principles of pharmacology.

This chapter is divided into three major sections: pharmacokinetic principles, pharmacodynamic principles, and the principles that underlie variability in drug response. Pharmacokinetics is the relationship between drug administration and drug concentration at the site of action. The fundamental concepts include volumes of distribution, drug clearance, transfer of drugs between plasma and tissues, and binding of drugs to circulating plasma proteins. The section on pharmacokinetics introduces both the physiologic processes that determine pharmacokinetics and the mathematical models used to relate dose to concentration. Pharmacodynamics is the relationship between drug concentration and pharmacologic effect. The broad areas of transduction of biologic signals, fundamental receptor theory and structure, the role of new developments in molecular biology, and clinical evaluation of drug effects are all presented. The last section explores processes that contribute to variability in drug response, including pharmacogenetics, the influence of patient physiology on pharmacokinetics and pharmacodynamics, and drug interactions.

Pharmacokinetics

Pharmacokinetics is the relationship between drug dose and drug concentration in plasma or at the site of drug effect. The processes of absorption, distribution, and clearance govern this relationship. Absorption is not relevant to intravenously administered drugs but is relevant to all other routes of drug delivery. The time course of intravenously administered drugs is a function of volumes of distribution and clearance. We will first discuss the physiologic basis of pharmacokinetics and then review pharmacokinetic models that relate dose to plasma or tissue concentration.

Fundamental Pharmacokinetic Concepts

Volume of Distribution

The distribution of a drug throughout plasma and tissues can be viewed as a process of dilution from the highly concentrated solution in the syringe to the dilute concentration in plasma. This dilution follows the mixing of drug into blood and transfer into tissues. The pharmacokinetic concept of volume is simply the apparent size of the tank required to explain the observed drug concentration. Figure 19-1 shows the dilution of administered drug into a tank of fluid. By definition, the concentration in the tank is the amount of drug administered divided by the volume of the tank. If we do not know the volume beforehand but can measure the concentration, we can rearrange the definition of concentration to calculate the volume of the tank:

$$\text{Volume} = \frac{\text{Amount (or dose)}}{\text{Concentration}} \quad (1)$$

As soon as the volume of the tank is known, the concentration after any bolus of drug can be calculated as the dose per volume. Just as the tank has a volume regardless of whether there is drug in it, the volume of distribution of a drug is an intrinsic property of the drug and individual regardless of whether any drug has been given.

Central Volume of Distribution

If we assume that the drug is injected into an arm vein and that the initial concentration is measured in an artery, the central volume of distribution reflects the volume of the heart, great vessels, and the venous volume of the upper part of the arm. It also reflects drug uptake by the lungs. For example, alfentanil is less lipophilic than fentanyl or sufentanil, which results in less pulmonary uptake and a smaller central volume for alfentanil than fentanyl or sufentanil. The central volume also reflects any metabolism that occurs between the venous injection site and the arterial sample.

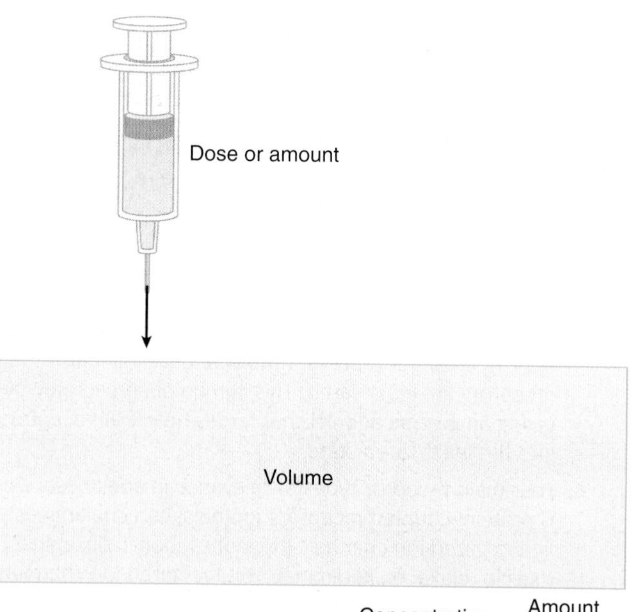

Figure 19-1 Volume represents the dilution of drug from the more concentrated form in the syringe to the dilute form in blood.

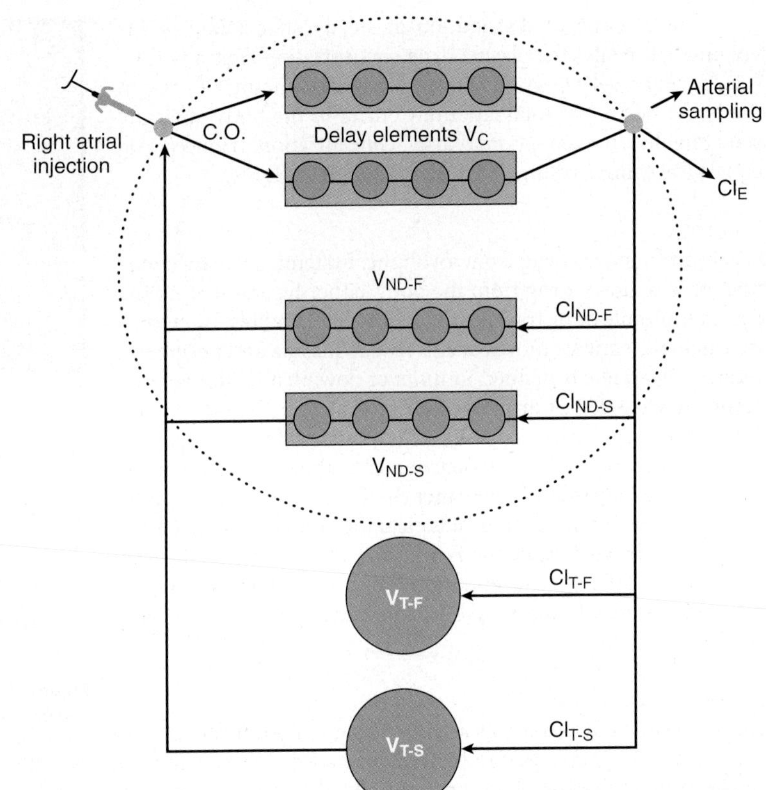

Figure 19-2 A recirculatory model accounting for cardiac output (C.O.), transit delays and pulmonary uptake (Delay Elements V_C), and nondistributive mixing pathways (V_{ND} and Cl_{ND}).[1] All the components within the *dashed circle* are required to accurately model the central volume of distribution. In most situations, this complexity is not required, and the simpler approach of assuming instantaneous mixing within the central volume is an adequate approximation. Cl_{ND-F} and Cl_{ND-S}, fast and slow nondistributive clearance; Cl_{T-F} and Cl_{T-S}, fast and slow tissue clearance; V_{ND-F} and V_{ND-S}, fast and slow nondistributive volume; V_{T-F} and V_{T-S}, fast and slow tissue volume. *(From Krejcie TC, Avram MJ, Gentry WB, et al: A recirculatory model of the pulmonary uptake and pharmacokinetics of lidocaine based on analysis of arterial and mixed venous data from dogs. J Pharmacokinet Biopharm 25:169-190, 1997.)*

The central volume of distribution is the most problematic pharmacokinetic concept. The central volume assumes that an intravenous bolus instantly mixes in this volume, with the peak concentration occurring at the moment of injection. Obviously, mixing is not instantaneous, and drug appears in the arterial circulation 30 to 40 seconds after injection. This 30- to 40-second delay is of no consequence outside anesthesia, but within the field of anesthesia the pharmacokinetic determinants of anesthetic induction are clinically important. The mathematics of the true time course, including the time delay and recirculatory peaks, have been worked out in detail by Henthorn, Avram, and Krejcie, as shown in Figure 19-2.[1]

Despite the assumption of instantaneous mixing, the concept of central volume of distribution is useful. The central volume represents the backward (and upward) extrapolation of the concentration-versus-time curve from its peak at about 30 seconds to the *y* axis. It can be thought of as the initial concentration, had circulation been infinitely fast. Because of this backward extrapolation, estimates of central volume are highly influenced by study design. A study with arterial samples will have higher initial concentrations and thus estimate a smaller central volume than a study with venous samples will. The timing of blood samples also influences estimation of the central volume of distribution. Over the first few minutes after bolus injection, the concentration of anesthetic drugs falls very rapidly, possibly by an order of magnitude. If the first sample is drawn at 30 seconds, backward extrapolation of the concentration-versus-time curve to the *y* axis predicts a high concentration at time 0 and thus a small central volume. If the first sample is drawn at 5 minutes, backward extrapolation of the concentration-versus-curve to the *y* axis predicts a much lower concentration and thus a larger central volume.

Peripheral Volumes of Distribution

Anesthetic drugs distribute extensively into peripheral tissues. This distribution into the periphery is represented pharmacokinetically as additional volumes of distribution that are attached to the central volume. Peripheral volumes are linked to the central compartment (plasma) by blood flow, a process called "intercompartmental clearance." The linkage of peripheral volumes to a central volume is called a "mammillary" model. This name refers to the structure of the plumbing: peripheral piglets suckling off a central (mother) pig. At least that is how the term was explained to us.

The size of the peripheral volumes of distribution reflects the drug's solubility in tissue relative to blood or plasma. The more soluble a drug is in peripheral tissue relative to blood or plasma, the larger the peripheral volumes of distribution. Because tissue solubility depends on simple physiochemical constants, it would seem likely that variability in peripheral volumes of distribution reflects differences in body habitus.

Peripheral volumes of distribution explain the apparent dilution of the drug into all body tissues. However, we usually do not know the actual solubility of drugs in peripheral tissues, nor do we care. The convention in pharmacokinetics is to assume that the solubility of the drug in tissue is the same as the solubility in plasma. This assumption does not compromise the role of peripheral compartments in characterizing the dilution of drugs into tissues, but it does lead to very large volumes of distribution for highly soluble drugs (e.g., 5000 L for propofol).

The volume of distribution at steady state (Vd_{ss}) is the volume that relates the plasma drug concentration at steady state (i.e., during a very long infusion) to the total amount of drug in the body. Vd_{ss} is the total amount of drug in the body at steady state divided by the plasma drug concentration. Hence, Vd_{ss} equals the central volume plus the peripheral volumes.

Clearance

Clearance removes drug from a volume. Systemic clearance permanently removes drug from the body, either by eliminating the parent molecule or by transforming it into metabolites. Intercompartmental clearance moves drug between plasma and peripheral tissues. Clearance is defined in units of flow, that is, the volume completely cleared of drug per unit of time (e.g., liters/minute). Clearance is most easily envisioned as flow to a clearing organ, as shown in Figure 19-3.[2] Clearance describes the body's capacity to remove drug, regardless of whether there is any drug in the body. The actual rate of drug removal is clearance times the concentration of the drug. If clearance is 1 L/min, the actual rate of drug elimination is 0 if the concentration is 0, 1 mg/min if the concentration is 1 mg/L, 10 mg/min if the concentration is 10 mg/L, and so on.

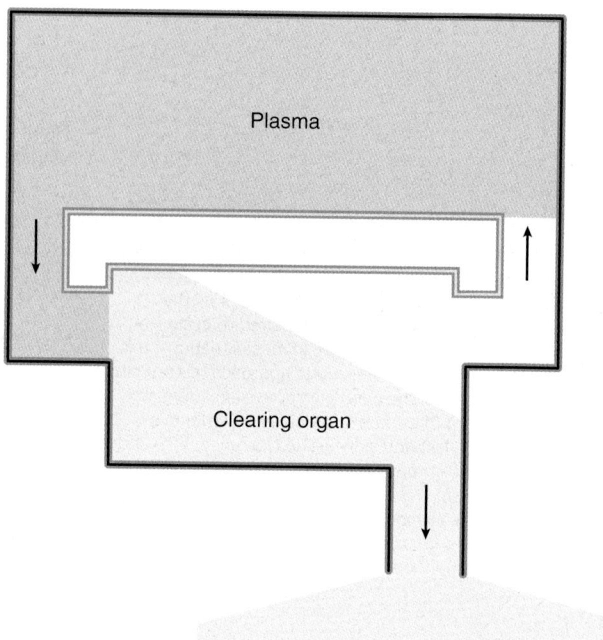

Figure 19-3 Clearance represents the flow of blood or plasma that is completely cleared of drug. If all of the drug is extracted by the clearing organ (i.e., extraction ratio ≈ 1), clearance is simply the flow to the organ, as illustrated here. *(Modified from Shafer S: Principles of pharmacokinetics and pharmacodynamics.* In *Longnecker DE, Tinker JH, Morgan GE [eds]: Principles and Practice of Anesthesiology, 2nd ed. St. Louis, Mosby–Year Book, 1997.)*

Hepatic Clearance

Most anesthetic drugs are cleared by hepatic biotransformation. The synthetic pathways for biotransformation are covered in detail in many biochemistry texts. Briefly, the liver metabolizes drugs through oxidation, reduction, hydrolysis, or conjugation. Oxidation and reduction occur in the cytochrome P450 system. These enzymes can be induced by exposure to certain drugs and increase the liver's intrinsic metabolic capacity. On the other hand, drugs or hepatic disease can inhibit these enzymes. Routes of oxidative metabolism include hydroxylation, dealkylation, deamination, desulfuration, epoxidation, and dehalogenation. Conjugation and hydrolysis often occur outside the P450 system, although glucuronidation involves the P450 system as well. The effect of conjugation is to transform hydrophobic molecules into water-soluble molecules through the addition of polar groups and thus render the metabolites easier to excrete via the kidneys. The metabolites generated by the liver are generally inactive, although some drugs (e.g., morphine, midazolam) have metabolites that are as potent as the parent drug. Genetic polymorphism can occur in all of these pathways, and this accounts for part of the variability in clearance in the population, as discussed in detail in the last section of this chapter.

Although most anesthetic drugs are cleared by hepatic metabolism, remifentanil, succinylcholine, and esmolol are cleared in the plasma and tissues by ester hydrolysis, and pancuronium is cleared via the kidney. The relationship between metabolism and clearance is complex. The following exploration of this relationship will assume hepatic metabolism, although the principles apply to the metabolism of drug in any tissue.

The rate of metabolism for most anesthetic drugs is proportional to the concentration of drug distributed via circulation to the liver. As will be shown later, this means that metabolic clearance is usually constant and independent of dose. This is such a common and fundamental assumption for anesthetic pharmacokinetics that we will explore the conditions that must be satisfied for it to be valid.

It cannot be true that metabolism is always proportional to concentration because the metabolic capacity of the liver is not infinite. At some rate of drug flow into the liver the metabolic capacity becomes saturated, and the rate of metabolism is no longer proportional to concentration. To understand the rate of metabolism quantitatively, we will start with a simple observation of mass balance: the rate at which drug flows *out* of the liver must be the rate at which drug flows *into* the liver minus the rate of metabolism. The rate at which drug flows into the liver is liver blood flow, $\dot{Q}$, times the concentration of drug flowing in, C_{inflow}. The rate at which drug flows out of the liver is liver blood flow, $\dot{Q}$, times the concentration of drug flowing out, $C_{outflow}$. Putting this together, the rate of hepatic metabolism by the liver, R, is the difference between the drug concentration flowing into the liver and the drug concentration flowing out of the liver, times the rate of liver blood flow:

$$\text{Rate of drug metabolism} = R = \dot{Q}\left(C_{inflow} - C_{outflow}\right) \quad (2)$$

This relationship is illustrated in Figure 19-4. Because hepatic metabolism does not have infinite capacity, the relationship between the rate of hepatic metabolism, R, and concentration must be saturable. The saturation equation shows up repeatedly in pharmacokinetics and pharmacodynamics, so we will inspect it carefully:

$$\text{Response} = \frac{C}{C_{50} + C} \quad (3)$$

"Response" in this equation varies from 0 to 1, depending on the value of C. When C is 0, the response is 0. If C is greater than 0 but much less than C_{50}, the response is nearly proportional to C: $\text{Response} \approx \frac{C}{C_{50}}$. If C equals C_{50}, the

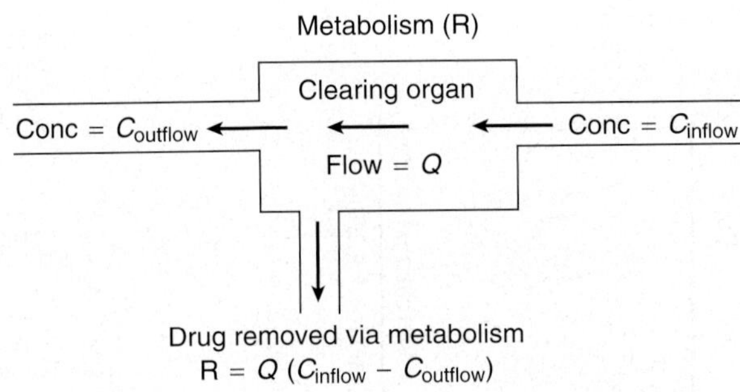

Figure 19-4 The rate of metabolism can be computed as the rate of liver blood flow times the difference between the inflowing and outflowing drug concentrations. This is a common approach to analyzing metabolism or tissue uptake across an organ in mass-balance pharmacokinetic studies.

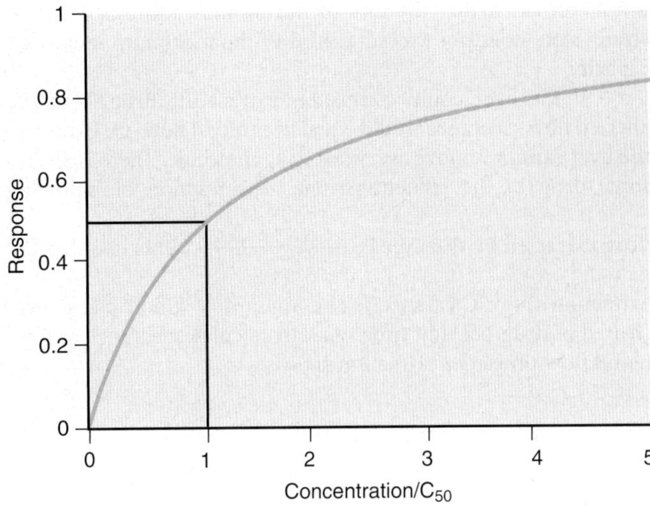

Figure 19-5 The saturation equation, response = $C/(C_{50} + C)$, shows the decreasing incremental response as the system approaches saturation. Variations of this equation show up repeatedly in pharmacokinetics and pharmacodynamics.

response is $\frac{C_{50}}{C_{50}+C_{50}}$, which is simply 0.5. This is where the term "C_{50}" comes from; that is, it is the concentration associated with a 50% response. As C becomes much greater than C_{50}, the equation approaches $\frac{C}{C}$, which is 1.0. The shape of this relationship is shown in Figure 19-5. It is linear at low concentrations, but at high concentrations the response saturates at 1.

We can model the relationship between hepatic metabolism and drug concentration by using the saturation equation, but what concentration determines the rate of metabolism: the concentration flowing into the liver, the average concentration within the liver, or the concentration flowing out of the liver? All three have been used, but the most widely used model of metabolism views the rate of metabolism as a function of the concentration flowing *out* of the liver, $C_{outflow}$. This is discussed extensively by Wagner.[3]

We can expand our equation of metabolism to include the observation that the rate of metabolism, R, approaches saturation at the maximum metabolic rate, V_m, as a function of $C_{outflow}$:

$$\text{Rate of drug metabolism} = R = \dot{Q}\left(C_{inflow} - C_{outflow}\right) = V_m \frac{C_{outflow}}{K_m + C_{outflow}} \quad (4)$$

V_m is the maximum possible metabolic rate. The saturation part of this equation, $\frac{C_{outflow}}{K_m + C_{outflow}}$, determines the fraction of the maximum metabolic rate. K_m, also called the Michaelis constant, is the outflow concentration at which the metabolic rate is 50% of the maximum rate (V_m). This relationship is shown graphically in Figure 19-6. The *x* axis is the outflow concentration, $C_{outflow}$, as a fraction of K_m, the concentration that yields 50% of the maximum metabolic rate. The *y* axis is the rate of drug metabolism as a fraction of V_m, the maximum rate of drug metabolism. By normalizing $C_{outflow}$ to K_m and the metabolic rate to V_m, the relationship in Figure 19-6 is true for all values of V_m and K_m. Figure 19-6 shows that as long as the outflow concentration is less than half of K_m, there is a nearly proportional change in metabolic rate with a proportional change in outflow concentration. For most anesthetic drugs, the clinical concentrations do not exceed half of K_m, and thus metabolism of anesthetic drugs is nearly proportional to concentration. We can also interpret Figure 19-6 in terms of the metabolic rate (*y* axis). As long as the metabolic rate is less than a third of the maximum metabolic capacity, the rate of metabolism increases proportionally with concentration. The clinical message is that metabolism will be proportional to concentration and therefore the pharmacokinetics will remain

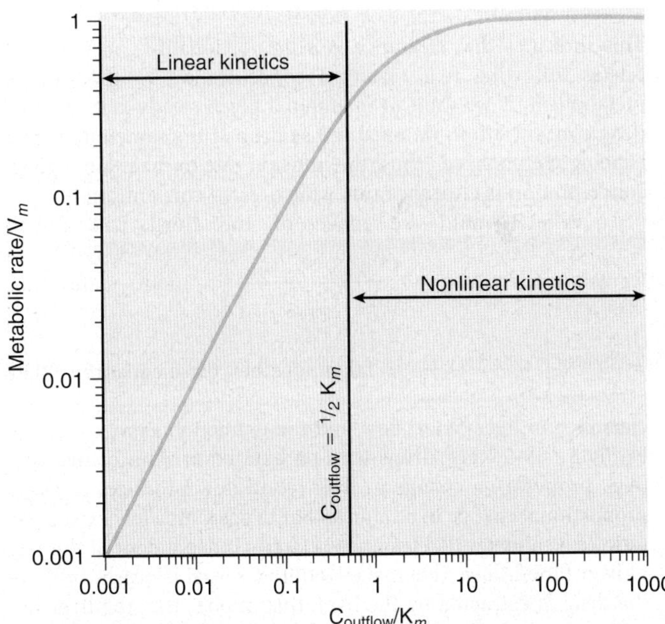

Figure 19-6 Relationship between concentration as a fraction of K_m (Michaelis constant) and drug metabolism as a fraction of V_m (maximum rate). As long as the outflow concentration is less than half K_m, a change in concentration is matched by a proportional change in metabolic rate. This is true of nearly all anesthetic drugs. *(From Shafer S: Principles of pharmacokinetics and pharmacodynamics.* In *Longnecker DE, Tinker JH, Morgan GE [eds]: Principles and Practice of Anesthesiology, 2nd ed. St. Louis, Mosby–Year Book, 1997.)*

linear, provided that the rate of intravenous administration at steady state does not exceed a third of the maximum metabolic capacity.

If the liver could completely extract the drug from the afferent flow, clearance would equal liver blood flow, $\dot{Q}$. However, the liver cannot remove every last drug molecule. There is always some drug in the effluent plasma. The fraction of inflowing drug extracted by the liver is $\frac{C_{inflow} - C_{outflow}}{C_{inflow}}$. This is called the extraction ratio. Clearance is the amount of blood completely cleared of drug per unit time. We can calculate clearance as liver blood flow times the extraction ratio:

$$\text{Clearance} = \dot{Q} \times \text{ER} = \dot{Q}\left(\frac{C_{inflow} - C_{outflow}}{C_{inflow}}\right) \quad (5)$$

With this basic understanding of clearance, let us divide each part of Equation 4 by C_{inflow}:

$$\frac{\text{Rate of drug metabolism}}{C_{inflow}} = \frac{R}{C_{inflow}} = \dot{Q}\left(\frac{C_{inflow} - C_{outflow}}{C_{inflow}}\right) = \frac{C_{outflow}}{C_{inflow}}\left(\frac{V_m}{K_m + C_{outflow}}\right) \quad (6)$$

The third term is clearance as defined in Equation 5: $\dot{Q}$ times the extraction ratio. Thus, each term must be clearance. Consider the first term, $\text{Clearance} = \frac{\text{Rate of drug metabolism}}{C_{inflow}}$. This indicates that clearance is a proportionality constant that relates inflowing (e.g., arterial) concentration to the rate of metabolism. If we want to maintain a given steady-state arterial drug concentration, we must infuse drug at the same rate that it is being metabolized. Thus, the infusion rate to maintain a given concentration is clearance times the desired concentration.

What should we make of the third and fourth terms, $\text{Clearance} = \dot{Q}\left(\frac{C_{inflow} - C_{outflow}}{C_{inflow}}\right)$ and $\text{Clearance} = \frac{C_{outflow}}{C_{inflow}}\left(\frac{V_m}{K_m + C_{outflow}}\right)$? Taken together, these equations relate clearance to liver blood flow and the extraction ratio, as shown in Figure 19-7.[4] For drugs with an extraction ratio of nearly 1 (e.g., propofol), a change in liver blood flow produces a nearly proportional change in clearance. For drugs with a low extraction ratio (e.g., alfentanil), clearance is nearly independent of the rate of liver blood flow. This makes intuitive sense. If nearly 100% of the drug is extracted by the liver, this implies that the liver has tremendous metabolic capacity for the drug. In this case, the rate-limiting step in metabolism is flow of drug to the liver, and such drugs are said to be "flow limited." Any reduction in liver blood flow, such as usually accompanies anesthesia, can be expected to reduce clearance. However, moderate changes in hepatic metabolic function per se will have little impact on clearance because hepatic metabolic capacity is overwhelmingly in excess of demand.

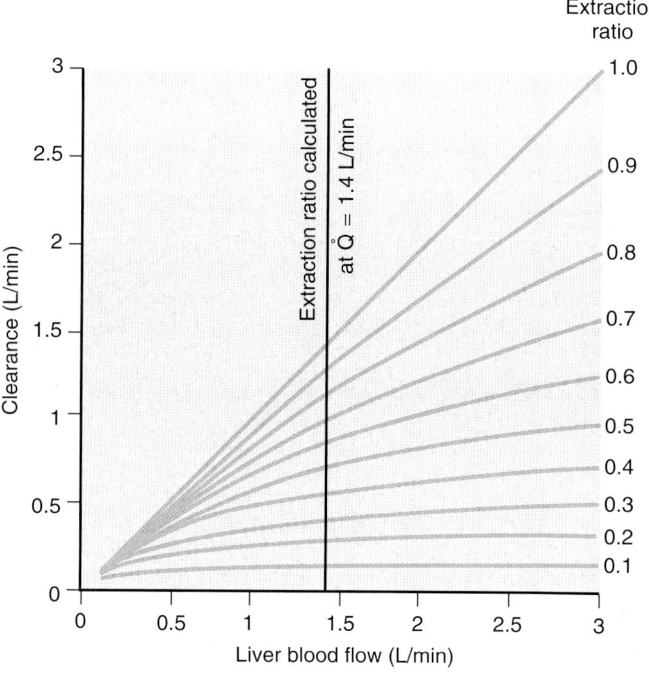

Figure 19-7 Relationship between liver blood flow ($\dot{Q}$), clearance, and extraction ratio. For drugs with a high extraction ratio, clearance is nearly identical to liver blood flow. For drugs with a low extraction ratio, changes in liver blood flow have almost no effect on clearance. *(Adapted from Wilkinson GR, Shand DG: Commentary: A physiological approach to hepatic drug clearance. Clin Pharmacol Ther 18:377-390, 1975.)*

For many drugs (e.g., alfentanil), the extraction ratio is considerably less than 1. For these drugs, clearance is limited by the capacity of the liver to take up and metabolize the drug. These drugs are said to be "capacity limited." Clearance will change in response to any change in the capacity of the liver to metabolize such drugs, as might be caused by liver disease or enzymatic induction. However, changes in liver blood flow, as might be caused by the anesthetic state itself, usually have little influence on clearance because the liver handles only a fraction of the drug that it sees anyway.

The last two components of Equation 6 can also be used to show how the extraction ratio governs the response of clearance to changes in metabolic capacity (V_m). Figure 19-8 shows the clearance of drugs with an extraction ratio ranging from 0.1 to 1, based on a liver blood flow of 1.4 L/min. The extraction ratios were calculated for a V_m of 1. Changes in V_m, as might be caused by liver disease (reduced V_m) or enzymatic induction (increased V_m), have little effect on drugs with a high extraction ratio. However, drugs with a low extraction ratio have a nearly linear change in clearance with a change in intrinsic metabolic capacity (V_m).

Inasmuch as V_m and K_m are often not known, it is occasionally useful to condense them into a single term that summarizes hepatic metabolic capacity: "intrinsic clearance." Because $\text{clearance} = \frac{C_{outflow}}{C_{inflow}}\left(\frac{V_m}{K_m + C_{outflow}}\right)$, consider what happens if hepatic blood flow increases to infinity with no change in hepatic

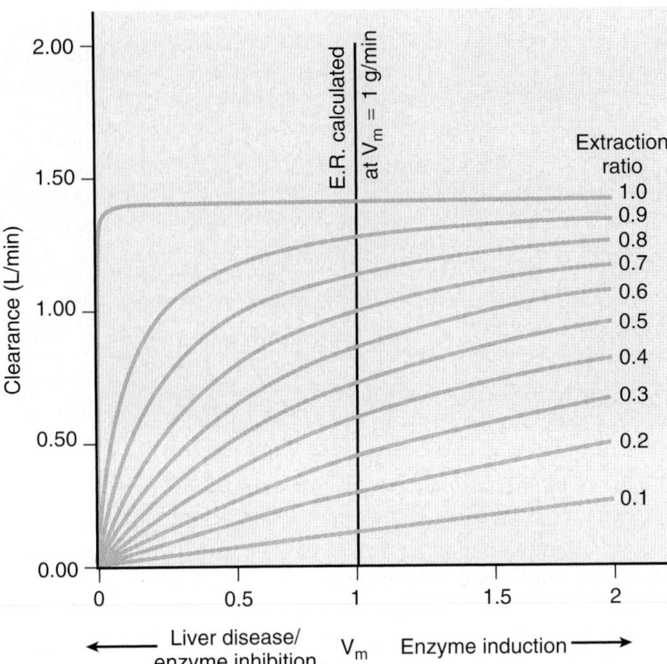

Figure 19-8 Corollary to Figure 19-7 showing the relationship between metabolic capacity, clearance, and extraction ratio (E.R.). Changes in maximum metabolic velocity (V_m) have little effect on drugs with a high extraction ratio, but they cause a nearly proportional decrease in clearance of drugs with a low extraction ratio.

metabolic capacity. $C_{outflow}$ becomes indistinguishable from C_{inflow} because the finite hepatic capacity metabolizes only an infinitesimal fraction of the drug flowing through the liver. As a result, clearance becomes $\frac{V_m}{K_m + C_{inflow}}$. We can solve for this in the "linear range" by finding clearance when $C_{inflow} = 0 : \frac{V_m}{K_m}$. This is the intrinsic clearance, Cl_{int}. In brief, it can be readily demonstrated (although we will spare you the details) from the definition of Cl_{int} that in the linear range, Cl_{int} is directly related to the extraction ratio:

$$\text{Extraction ratio} = \frac{Cl_{int}}{\dot{Q} + Cl_{int}} \tag{7}$$

Combining this with Equation 6 yields the relationship between hepatic clearance and Cl_{int}:

$$\text{Hepatic clearance} = \frac{\dot{Q}\,Cl_{int}}{\dot{Q} + Cl_{int}} \tag{8}$$

The relationship between intrinsic clearance and extraction ratio is shown in Figure 19-9 and was calculated at a hepatic blood flow of 1400 mL/min. In general, true hepatic clearance and extraction ratio are more useful concepts for anesthetic drugs than intrinsic clearance is. However, intrinsic clearance is introduced here because it is occasionally used in pharmacokinetic analysis of anesthetic drugs.

Thus far we have focused on linear pharmacokinetics, that is, the pharmacokinetics of drugs whose metabolic rate at clinical doses is less than $V_m/3$. Clearance of such drugs is generally expressed as a constant (e.g., propofol clearance = 1.6 L/min). Some drugs, such as phenytoin, exhibit saturable pharmacokinetics (i.e., have such low V_m that typical doses exceed the linear portion of Fig. 19-6). Clearance of drugs with saturable metabolism is a function of drug concentration rather than a constant.

Renal Clearance

The kidneys clear drug from plasma by filtration at the glomerulus and direct transport into the tubules. Renal blood flow is inversely correlated with age, as is creatinine clearance, which can be predicted from age and weight according to the equation of Cockroft and Gault[5]:

Men:

$$\text{Creatinine clearance (mL/min)} = \frac{(140 - \text{Age [yr]} \times \text{Weight [kg]})}{72 \times \text{Serum creatinine (mg\%)}} \tag{9}$$

Women:

85% of the above.

Equation 9 shows that age is an independent predictor of creatinine clearance. Thus, elderly patients have decreased creatinine clearance, even in the presence of normal serum creatinine levels. Inhaled anesthetics also decrease renal blood flow. Decreased renal clearance will delay the offset of effect for renally excreted drugs or their metabolites.

Tissue Clearance

Some anesthetic drugs are cleared in other tissues, such as blood, muscle, and the lungs. For example, remifentanil is cleared by nonspecific esterases located primarily in muscle and intestines, with the lungs, liver, kidneys, and blood each contributing minimally to clearance of remifentanil. Succinylcholine, mivacurium, and 2-chloroprocaine are all metabolized by plasma butyrylcho-

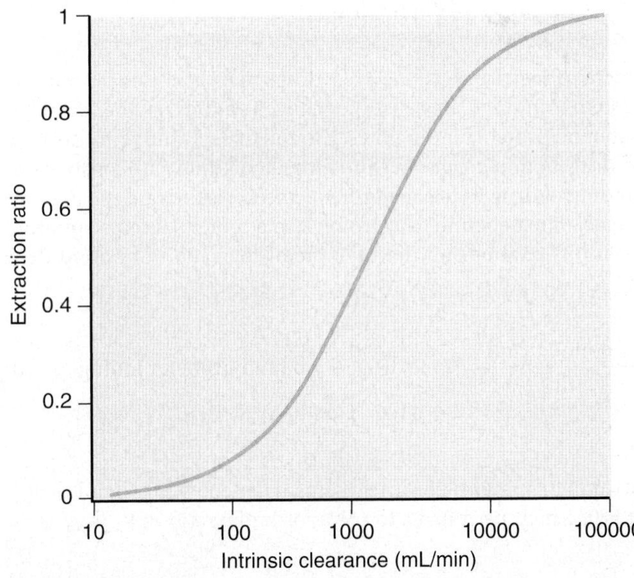

Figure 19-9 Relationship between intrinsic clearance and extraction ratio, calculated for a liver blood flow of 1400 mL/min.

linesterases (formerly called pseudocholinesterase). The half-life of succinylcholine, mivacurium, and 2-chloroprocaine in plasma is about 3 minutes, 5 minutes, and 25 seconds, respectively. About half of atracurium's metabolism is hepatic, and the balance occurs in blood via nonspecific cholinesterases (but not by butyrylcholinesterases). Hofmann degradation is a spontaneous process in plasma at normal pH and temperature and does not depend on any circulating esterases. Hofmann degradation is a minor route of metabolism of atracurium but is the major route of metabolism of cisatracurium, an isomer of atracurium. This is an important distinction: unlike atracurium and mivacurium, metabolism of cisatracurium is unaffected by disease or genetic variants of cholinesterase metabolism.

Clearance by tissues other than blood can be analyzed by using models similar to those for hepatic clearance. Tissue clearance can be flow limited, capacity limited, or both. Clearance within the blood itself cannot be flow limited and thus is entirely dependent on the intrinsic metabolic capacity of the blood.

Distribution Clearance

Distribution clearance is the transfer of drug between blood or plasma and peripheral tissues. Unlike metabolic clearance, distribution clearance does not permanently remove drug from the body. Distribution clearance is a function of cardiac output, tissue blood flow, and permeability of the capillary walls to the drug. For a drug that readily crosses into peripheral tissues, such as propofol, the sum of metabolic clearance and distribution clearance approaches cardiac output. For drugs that are metabolized directly in plasma or in many peripheral tissues, such as succinylcholine and remifentanil, the sum of metabolic clearance and distribution clearance can exceed cardiac output.

Protein Binding

Many drugs are bound to plasma proteins, particularly to albumin and α_1-acid glycoprotein. The relationship between drugs and their binding proteins can be described as

$$[\text{Free drug}] + [\text{Unbound protein binding sites}] \underset{k_{off}}{\overset{k_{on}}{\rightleftharpoons}} [\text{Bound drug}]$$

where [Free drug] is the free drug concentration, [Unbound protein binding sites] is the concentration of the available unbound protein binding sites, [Bound drug] is the concentration of drug bound to plasma proteins, k_{on} is the rate constant for binding of drug to plasma protein, and k_{off} is the rate constant for dissociation of bound drug from plasma protein. It can be inferred from this relationship that the rate of formation of bound drug is

$$\frac{d[\text{Bound drug}]}{dt} = [\text{Free drug}][\text{Unbound protein binding sites}]k_{on} - [\text{Bound drug}]k_{off} \tag{10}$$

At equilibrium (which is nearly instantaneous), d[Bound drug]/dt = 0, which permits us to solve for k, the ratio of k_{on}/k_{off}, as

$$k = \frac{k_{on}}{k_{off}} = \frac{[\text{Bound drug}]}{[\text{Free drug}][\text{Unbound protein binding sites}]} \tag{11}$$

Plasma proteins may have more than one binding site. Therefore, the total number of binding sites is the protein concentration, [Protein], times n, the average number of binding sites per protein molecule. For drugs used in anesthesia, the number of binding sites actually bound is only a trivial fraction of the total available binding sites, and thus we can reasonably approximate [Unbound protein binding sites] by n [Protein]. Because n, the number of binding sites per molecule, is constant, we can fold it into our rate constant k by defining the association constant K_a as

$$K_a = n\frac{k_{on}}{k_{off}} = \frac{[\text{Bound drug}]}{[\text{Free drug}][\text{Protein}]} \tag{12}$$

Let us define f_u as the free fraction of drug:

$$f_u = \frac{[\text{Free drug}]}{[\text{Bound drug}] + [\text{Free drug}]} \tag{13}$$

By combining Equations 12 and 13, we can solve for f_u in terms of the unbound drug concentration:

$$f_u = \frac{1}{1 + K_a[\text{Protein}]} \tag{14}$$

Two observations can be drawn from Equation 14. First, the fraction bound to plasma protein solely depends on the protein concentration, not on the drug concentration, provided that [Bound drug] << n[Protein]. This approximation is always true for anesthetic drugs because of their high potency. Even for thiopental, possibly the least potent drug used in contemporary anesthetic practice, [Bound drug] << n[Protein], and protein binding is independent of the concentration of thiopental. Second, if we solve Equation 14 for $f_u = 0.5$, we find that

$$K_a = \frac{1}{[\text{Protein}]_{50}} \tag{15}$$

where $[\text{Protein}]_{50}$ is the concentration of protein at which 50% of the drug is bound. Thus, another way of thinking about the association constant is that it is the inverse of the protein concentration associated with 50% binding. If we substitute $\frac{1}{[\text{Protein}]_{50}}$ for K_a in Equation 14, we get the relationship

$$f_u = \frac{[\text{Protein}]_{50}}{[\text{Protein}]_{50} + [\text{Protein}]} \tag{16}$$

This relationship is shown graphically in Figure 19-10. On the left side of Figure 19-10, [Protein] is much smaller than $[\text{Protein}]_{50}$. In this situation the drug has little affinity for protein binding, so there is far less protein around than required to bind 50% of the drug. The drug is mostly free, and f_u is nearly 1. On the right side of Figure 19-10, [Protein] is much greater than $[\text{Protein}]_{50}$. This means that there is far more protein present than would be required to bind 50% of the drug. The result is that drug will be mostly bound to plasma proteins, and f_u will be nearly 0.

The association constant K_a and its inverse $[\text{Protein}]_{50}$ reflect the affinity of the drug for plasma protein. They should not change in the presence of disease. However, [Protein] can change with disease, age, or concurrent drugs. Figure 19-11 shows the relationship between changes in protein concentration and

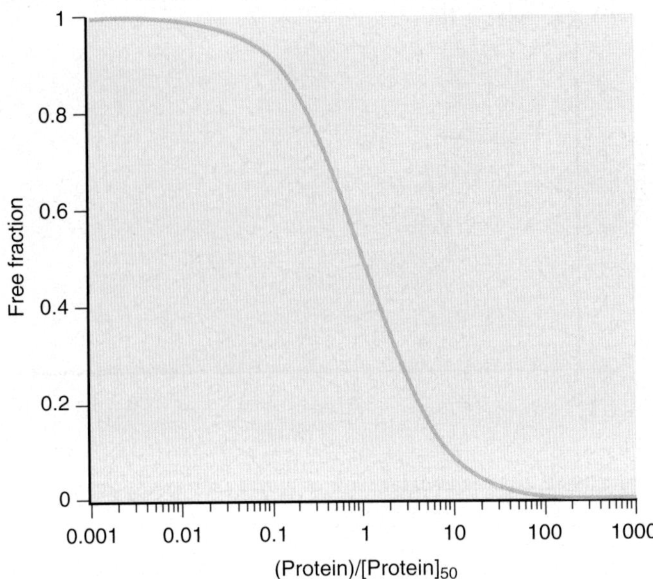

Figure 19-10 Relationship between plasma protein concentration as a fraction of the concentration associated with 50% binding and the fraction of drug that is unbound. This is another example of the saturation equation shown in Figure 19-5.

changes in the free fraction of drug for drugs with different degrees of protein binding in normal clinical use. The lines on the graph correspond to different drugs whose free fraction in normal plasma ranges from 1.0 (horizontal line) to approximately 0.0 (straight diagonal line).

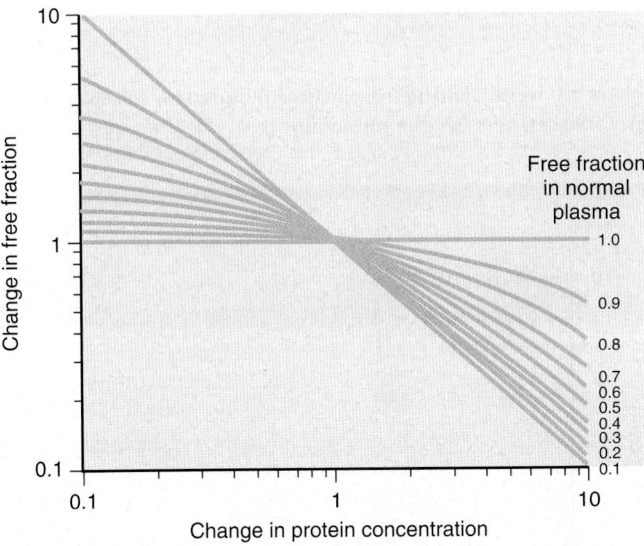

Figure 19-11 Relationship between changes in protein concentration and changes in free fraction. The relationship depends on the free fraction in normal plasma at typical clinical doses. For a drug that is not bound (free fraction ≈ 1), there is no change in free fraction with a change in protein concentration. For a highly bound drug with a free fraction that is nearly 0, any change in protein causes a nearly inversely proportional change in free fraction. *(From Shafer S: Principles of pharmacokinetics and pharmacodynamics.* In *Longnecker DE, Tinker JH, Morgan GE [eds]: Principles and Practice of Anesthesiology, 2nd ed. St. Louis, Mosby–Year Book, 1997.)*

For drugs that are not bound (free fraction = 1.0), there is no relationship between free fraction and protein concentration, as indicated by the flat horizontal line. For drugs whose free fraction is typically 90%, there will be a small change in free drug concentration with changes in protein concentration. For drugs that are highly protein bound, the free drug concentration changes nearly inversely with the change in protein concentration. As the proportion of binding approaches 100% (free drug → 0.0), the relationship between change in protein concentration and change in free fraction becomes inversely proportional. Note that there is never a greater than proportional change in free drug concentration with a change in plasma concentration. For example, the most that a 10% change in protein concentration would produce is a 10% change in free drug concentration, and that would be the case only if the drug were nearly 100% bound to plasma protein.

The in vitro observation that changing protein concentration results in changing free drug concentration, as shown in Figure 19-11, does not necessarily apply to the in vivo situation. It is the free (e.g., unbound) drug that equilibrates between plasma and tissues. If plasma protein binding is decreased, the free drug concentration gradient between plasma and peripheral tissues will increase. As a result, when protein binding decreases, equilibrium is achieved between plasma and the tissue free drug concentration at a lower total plasma drug concentration. This lower concentration gives the appearance that the drug has distributed into a larger total space. Thus, decreased protein binding causes an increase in the apparent volume of distribution when referenced to total, rather than free, drug concentration.

The increased volume of distribution at steady state, Vd_{ss}, seen with decreased plasma protein binding is mostly an illusion. Were only the unbound drug concentration measured, there would be almost no change in the apparent volume of distribution for lipophilic drugs (such as most of those in anesthesia practice) because it is partitioning of drug within peripheral tissues that primarily governs the free concentration of lipophilic drugs.

Changes in protein binding may affect the clearance of drugs. If a drug has a high extraction ratio, the liver is going to remove nearly all the drug flowing to it, regardless of the extent of protein binding. However, if the drug has a low hepatic extraction ratio, an increase in the free fraction of drug will result in an increase in the driving gradient along with an associated increase in clearance. Protein binding also affects the apparent potency of a drug when referenced to the total plasma drug concentration. An increase in free fraction increases the driving pressure to the site of drug effect. Thus, a change in free fraction will increase the concentration at the effect site. Because of this change in apparent potency, decreased protein binding may decrease the dose required to produce a given drug effect, even in the absence of other pharmacokinetic changes.

Stereochemistry

Typical pharmacokinetic analyses describe fictitious drugs. For example, the pharmacokinetics and pharmacodynamics of thiopental, ketamine, and bupivacaine describe drugs that do not exist. The reason is that many anesthetic drugs are chiral and supplied as racemic mixtures. The body is a chiral environment, and drugs interact stereospecifically with enzymes, proteins, and receptors. The pharmacokinetics and pharmacodynamics of the enantiomers may differ. The enantiomers of bupivacaine and ketamine have been particularly well studied, and the levo-isomer of bupivacaine is available commercially as levobupivacaine. Although the importance of studying the pharmacokinetics and pharmacodynamics of individual stereoisomers is widely appreciated, the difficulty of performing such studies has precluded widespread use.

Pharmacokinetic Models

Zero- and First-Order Processes

The body's consumption of oxygen and production of carbon dioxide are processes continuing at a constant rate. These are called zero-order processes. The rate of change (dx/dt) for a zero-order process is

$$\frac{dx}{dt} = k \quad (17)$$

Equation 17 states that the rate of change is constant. If x represents an amount of drug and t represents time, the unit of k is amount/time. If we want to know the value of x at time t, x(t), we can compute it as the integral of Equation 17 from time 0 to time t:

$$x(t) = x_0 + k \times t \quad (18)$$

where x_0 is the value of x at time 0. This is the equation of a straight line with a slope of k and an intercept of x_0.

Many processes occur at a rate proportional to the amount. For example, the interest payment on a loan is proportional to the outstanding balance, and the rate at which water drains from a bathtub is proportional to amount (height) of water in the tub. These are examples of first-order processes. The rate of change in a first-order process is only slightly more complex than that for a zero-order process:

$$\frac{dx}{dt} = k \times x \quad (19)$$

Here, the unit of k is 1/time because the x on the right-hand side already includes the unit for amount. If we want to know the value of x at time t, x(t), it can be computed as the integral from time 0 to time t:

$$x(t) = x_0 \times e^{kt} \quad (20)$$

where x_0 is the value of x at time 0. If k is greater than 0, x(t) increases exponentially. If k is less than 0, x(t) decreases exponentially. In pharmacokinetics, k is negative because concentrations decrease over time. For clarity, the minus sign is usually explicit, so k is expressed as a positive number. Thus, the identical equation for pharmacokinetics, with the minus sign explicitly written, is

$$x(t) = x_0 \times e^{-kt} \quad (21)$$

Figure 19-12 shows the relationship between x and time, as described by Equation 21. In Figure 19-12, x continuously decreases over time. However, the slope of the curve continuously increases (i.e., becomes less negative). Taking the natural logarithm of both sides of Equation 21 gives

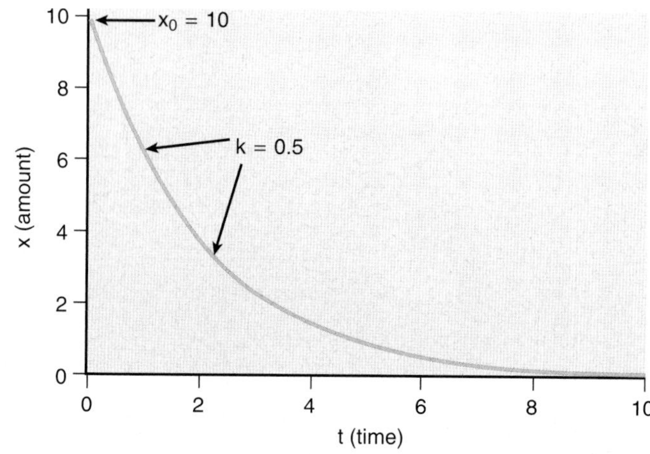

Figure 19-12 Exponential decay curve, as given by $x(t) = x_0e^{-kt}$, plotted on standard axes, with $x_0 = 10$ and $k = 0.5$.

$$\begin{aligned} \ln(x[t]) &= \ln(x_0 \times e^{-kt}) \\ &= \ln(x_0) + \ln(e^{-kt}) \\ &= \ln(x_0) - (k \times t) \end{aligned} \quad (22)$$

This is the equation of a straight line, as shown in Figure 19-13, where the vertical axis is ln(x[t]), the horizontal axis is *t*, the intercept is $\ln(x_0)$, and the slope of the line is $-k$.

How long will it take for x to go from a certain value, x_1 to half that value, $(x_1/2)$? Because k is the slope of a straight line relating ln(x) to time,

$$k = \frac{\Delta \ln(x)}{\Delta t} = \frac{\ln(x_1) - \ln\left(\frac{x_1}{2}\right)}{t_{1/2}} \quad (23)$$

where $t_{1/2}$ is the "half-life", or the time required for a 50% decrease in *x*. We can simplify the numerator to

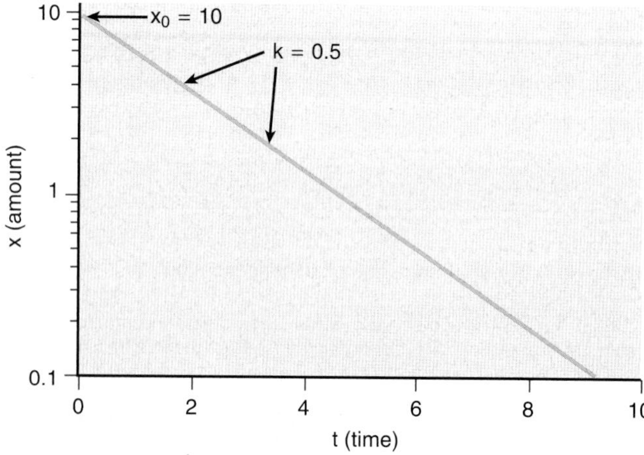

Figure 19-13 The same exponential decay curve, $x(t) = x_0 e^{-kt}$, as in Figure 19-12, but now plotted on a log *y* axis.

$$\ln(x_1) - \ln\left(\frac{x_1}{2}\right) = \ln\left(\frac{x_1}{\frac{x_1}{2}}\right) = \ln(2) \approx 0.693 \tag{24}$$

This succinctly relates slope (or "rate constant"), k, to half-life, $t_{½}$:

$$k = \frac{0.693}{t½} \tag{25}$$

Thus, if we measure the time that it takes for x to fall by 50%, $t_{½}$, we know the rate constant k. If we know k, we can easily calculate from Equation 25 the time that it will take for x to fall by 50%:

$$t½ = \frac{0.693}{k} \tag{26}$$

Physiologic Pharmacokinetic Models

It is possible to analyze volumes and clearances for each organ in the body and construct models of pharmacokinetics by assembling the organ models into physiologically and anatomically accurate models of the entire animal. Figure 19-14 shows such a model for thiopental in rats.[6] Subsequent studies have shown that individual tissue volumes and blood flow can be scaled up from rats to humans to result in accurate models of human pharmacokinetics.[7] This illustrates the potential utility of physiologically based pharmacokinetic models in developing human pharmacokinetic models from animal models.

Models that work with individual tissues are mathematically cumbersome and do not offer a better prediction of plasma drug concentration than models that lump the tissues into a few compartments. If the goal is to determine how to give drugs to obtain therapeutic plasma drug concentrations, all that is needed is to mathematically relate dose to plasma concentration. For this purpose, conventional "compartmental" models are usually adequate.

Compartmental Pharmacokinetic Models

Compartmental models are built on the same basic concepts as physiologic models, but with gross simplifications. The "one-compartment model" seen in Figure 19-15 contains a single volume and a single clearance, as though we were built like buckets. For anesthetic drugs, we resemble several buckets connected by pipes. These are usually modeled by two- or three-compartment models, also shown in Figure 19-15. The volume to the right in the two-compartment model—and in the center of the three-compartment model—is the central volume. The other volumes are peripheral volumes. The sum of the all volumes is the volume of distribution at steady state, Vd_{ss}. Clearance in which the central compartment is left for the outside is the "central" or "metabolic" clearance. Clearances between the central compartment and the peripheral compartments are the "intercompartmental" clearances.

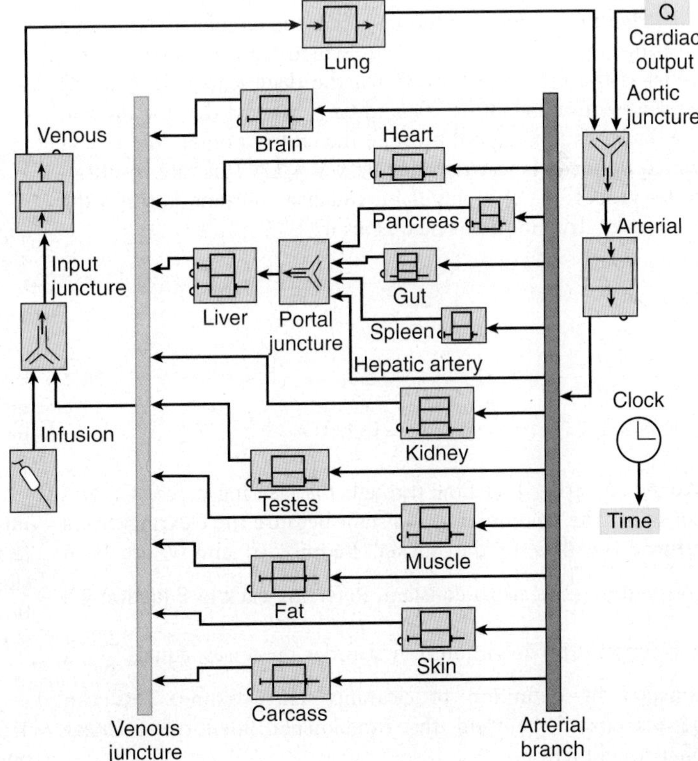

Figure 19-14 Physiologic model for thiopental in rats. The pharmacokinetics of distribution into each organ has been determined individually. The components of the model are linked by zero-order (flow) and first-order (diffusion) processes. *(From Ebling WF, Wada DR, Stanski DR: From piecewise to full physiologic pharmacokinetic modeling: Applied to thiopental disposition in the rat. J Pharmacokinet Biopharm 22:259-292, 1994.)*

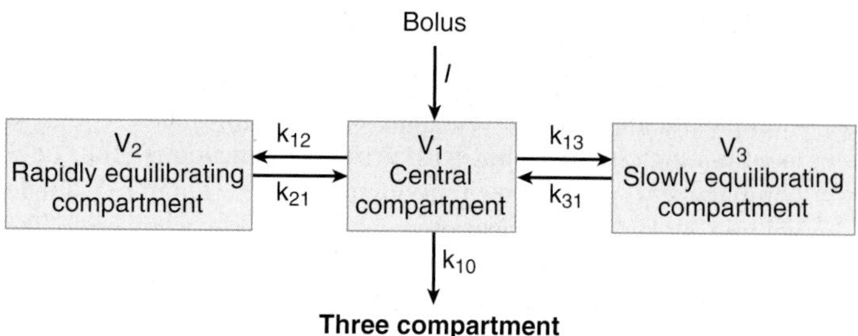

Figure 19-15 One-, two-, and three-compartment mammillary models.

One-Compartment Model

BOLUS PHARMACOKINETICS. Think of the body as a bucket into which we pour drug. Let us call the amount of drug that we pour into the bucket x_0 (x at time 0). The initial concentration is x_0/V, where V is the volume of fluid within the bucket. Returning to Equation 1, if we know the concentration that we want to achieve, C_T (target concentration), and V, the volume in the bucket, we can calculate the dose to achieve C_T by rearranging the definition of concentration: Dose = $C_T \times V$.

Let us assume that the fluid is being circulated through a clearing organ at a constant rate, which we call clearance, Cl. What is the rate, dx/dt, by which the drug leaves the bucket? Because concentration is x/V and Cl is the rate that the fluid in the bucket is flowing out through the clearing organ, the rate at which the drug is leaving must be x/V × Cl. This rate is a first-order process if—and only if—it equals a constant, *k*, times the amount of drug in the bucket. Does it?

$$\begin{aligned}\frac{dx}{dt} &= \frac{x}{V}Cl \\ &= \frac{Cl}{V}x \\ &= kx?\end{aligned} \tag{27}$$

We stated earlier that flow through the clearing organ, Cl, was constant. The volume, V, is constant because the clearing organ returns the flow to the bucket. Because Cl and V are both constants, $\frac{Cl}{V}$ is also a constant. Referring back to Equation 27, k, a constant by definition of first-order processes, equals $\frac{Cl}{V}$, a constant by definition of clearance and volume. This can be rearranged to yield the fundamental identity of linear pharmacokinetics:

$$\begin{aligned}\text{Cl (clearance)} = \text{k (rate constant)} \\ \times \text{V (volume of distribution)}\end{aligned} \tag{28}$$

What does this identity tell us about the relationship between half-life, volume, and clearance? Rearranging the above as $k = \frac{Cl}{V}$ and remembering that $t\frac{1}{2} = \frac{0.693}{k}$, we can conclude that half-life is proportional to volume and inversely proportional to clearance:

$$\begin{aligned}t\tfrac{1}{2} &= 0.693\frac{V}{Cl} \\ t\tfrac{1}{2} &\propto \frac{V}{Cl}\end{aligned} \tag{29}$$

Figure 19-16 shows a one-compartment model with an identical clearance but a bigger volume than is seen in Figure 19-3. It takes longer to clear drug from this bigger volume, so the half-life will increase, as predicted by Equation 29. Figure 19-17 shows a one-compartment model with an identical volume but faster clearance than is seen in Figure 19-3. The concentrations will fall more quickly (shorter half-life) with the larger clearance, as predicted by Equation 29.

Because this is a first-order process, $\frac{dx}{dt} = k\,x$, and the integral of this process gives us the amount of drug at time t in terms of the amount at time 0, $x(t) = x_0\, e^{-kt}$. If we divide both sides by V and remember that x/V is the definition of concentration, we get the equation that relates concentration after an intravenous bolus to time and initial concentration:

$$C(t) = C_0 e^{-kt} \tag{30}$$

This equation defines the "concentration-over-time" curve for a one-compartment model and has the log-linear shape seen in

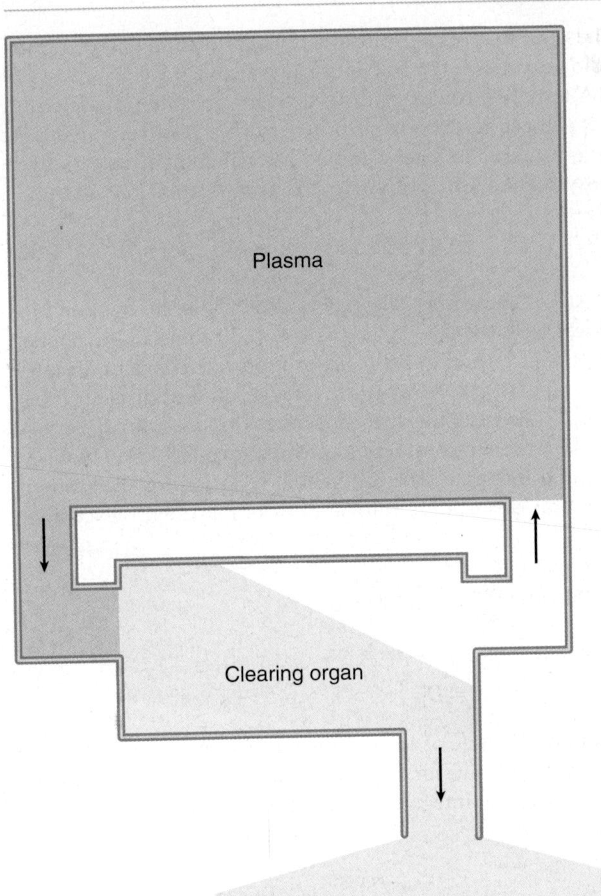

Figure 19-16 A one-compartment model similar to Figure 19-3, but with an increased volume of distribution. After drug administration, concentrations will fall more slowly in this model than in the model shown in Figure 19-3.

Figure 19-13. We can calculate the clearance, Cl, in one of two ways. First, we can calculate V by rearranging the definition of concentration, V = dose/initial concentration = dose/C_0. Referring back to Equation 28, if we measure the slope, –k, we can calculate clearance as k × V. A more general solution is to consider the integral of the concentration-over-time curve, Equation 30, known in pharmacokinetics as the area under the curve (AUC):

$$\begin{aligned} AUC &= \int_0^\infty C_0 e^{-kt} dt \\ &= \int_0^\infty \frac{x_0}{V}\left(e^{-\frac{Cl}{V}t}\right) dt \,(\text{substituting for } C_0 \text{ and } k) \\ &= \frac{x_0}{V} \times \frac{V}{Cl} (\text{evaluating the above integral}) \\ &= \frac{x_0}{Cl} \end{aligned} \tag{31}$$

We can rearrange Equation 31 to solve for clearance, Cl:

$$Cl = \frac{x_0}{AUC} \tag{32}$$

Because x_0 is the dose of drug, clearance equals the dose divided by AUC. This fundamental property of *linear* pharmacokinetic models applies to one-compartment models, multicompartment models, and any type of intravenous drug dosing (provided that the *total* dose administered systemically is used as the numerator). It directly follows that AUC is proportional to dose for linear models (i.e., models in which Cl is constant).

INFUSION PHARMACOKINETICS. If we give an infusion at a rate of I (for input), the plasma concentration will rise as long as the rate of drug going in the body, I, exceeds the rate at which drug leaves the body, C × Cl, where C is the drug concentration. When I = C × Cl, drug is going in and coming out at the same rate, and the body is at steady state. We can calculate the concentration at steady state by observing that the rate of drug going in must equal the rate of drug coming out. From Equation 6 we know that rate of drug metabolism at steady state is

$$\text{Metabolic rate} = C_{ss} \times Cl \tag{33}$$

where C_{ss} is the arterial concentration at steady state. Because by definition at steady state the infusion rate must equal the metabolic rate, the infusion rate, I, at steady state must be I = C_{ss} × Cl. Solving this for the concentration at steady state, C_{ss}, gives $\frac{I}{Cl}$. Thus, the steady state concentration during an infusion is the rate of drug input divided by clearance. It follows that if we want to calculate the infusion rate that will achieve a given target concentration, C_T, at steady state, the infusion rate must be C_T × Cl.

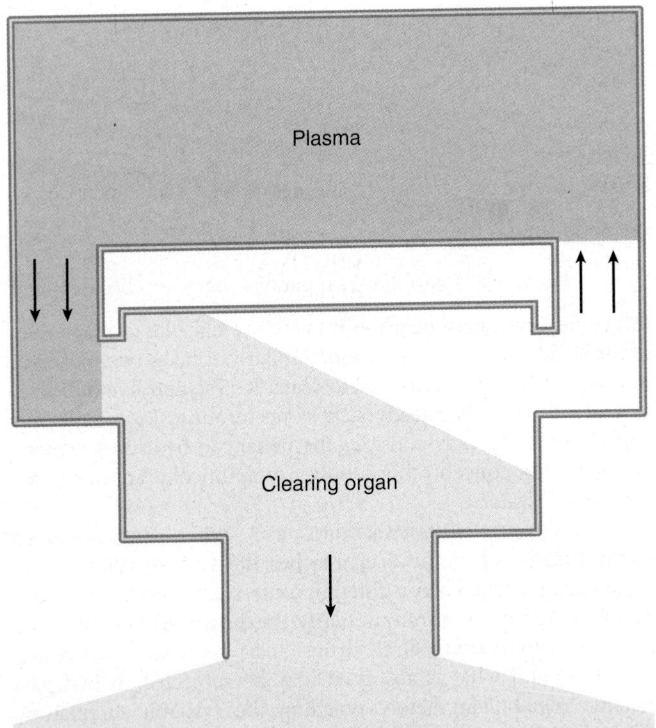

Figure 19-17 A one-compartment model similar to Figure 19-3, but with increased clearance. After drug administration, concentrations will fall faster in this model than in the model shown in Figure 19-3.

$C_\infty = \frac{I}{Cl}$ is similar in form to the equation describing the concentration after a bolus injection: $C_0 = \frac{X_0}{V}$. Thus, volume is a scalar relating bolus to initial concentration, and clearance is a scalar relating infusion rate to steady-state concentration. It follows that the initial concentration after a bolus is independent of clearance and that the steady-state concentration during a continuous infusion is independent of volume.

During an infusion, the rate of change in the amount of drug, x, is rate of inflow, I, minus the rate of outflow, k × x.

$$\frac{dx}{dt} = I - kx \tag{34}$$

We can calculate x at any time t as the integral from time 0 to time *t*. Assuming that $x_0 = 0$ (i.e., we are starting with no drug in the body), the result is

$$x(t) = \frac{I}{k}\left(1 - e^{-kt}\right) \tag{35}$$

As $t \to \infty$, $e^{-kt} \to 0$, and Equation 35 reduces to

$$x_{ss} = \frac{I}{k} \tag{36}$$

How long does it take to reach 50% of the final steady-state concentration (i.e., to reach a concentration of $\frac{x_{ss}}{2}$) during an infusion? From Equation 36 we know that $\frac{x_{ss}}{2} = \frac{I}{2k}$. Substituting $\frac{I}{2k}$ for x(t) in Equation 35, we get

$$\frac{I}{2k} = \frac{I}{k}\left(1 - e^{-kt}\right) \tag{37}$$

Solving Equation 37 for t, we get $\frac{\ln(2)}{k}$. In Equation 26 we found that the half-life, $t_{½}$, after a bolus injection was $\frac{\ln(2)}{k}$. Here, we again have a parallel between boluses and infusions. During an infusion it takes one half-life to reach 50% of the steady-state concentration. Similarly, it takes two half-lives to reach 75%, three half-lives to reach 87.5%, and five half lives to reach 97% of the steady-state concentration. By four to five half-lives we typically consider the patient to be at steady state, although the concentrations only asymptotically approach the steady-state value.

Absorption Pharmacokinetics. When drugs are given intravenously, all of the drug reaches the systemic circulation. When drugs are given by a different route, such as orally, transdermally, epidurally, or intramuscularly, the drug must first reach the systemic circulation. Oral drugs may be only fractionally absorbed, and what is absorbed may be subjected to first-past hepatic metabolism before reaching the systemic circulation. Transdermally applied drugs may be sloughed off with the stratum corneum without being absorbed. We cannot assume that the dose given to the patient is the same as the dose that reaches the systemic circulation when using alternative routes of drug delivery. The dose that reaches the systemic circulation is the administered dose times f, the fraction "bioavailable."

Alternative routes of drug delivery are often modeled by assuming that the drug is absorbed from a reservoir or depot, which is usually modeled as an additional compartment with a monoexponential rate of transfer to the systemic circulation:

$$A(t) = f \times D_{oral} \times k_a \times e^{-k_a t} \tag{38}$$

where A(t) is the absorption rate at time t, f is the fraction bioavailable, D_{oral} is the dose taken orally (or intramuscularly, applied to the skin, etc.), and k_a is the absorption rate constant. Because the integral of $k_a \times e^{-k_a t}$ is 1, the total amount of drug absorbed is f × D_{oral}. To compute the concentrations over time, we first reduce the problem to differential equations, (e.g., Equations 19 and 34) and integrate. The differential equation for the amount, x, with oral absorption into a one-compartment disposition model is

$$\begin{aligned}\frac{dx}{dt} &= \text{inflow} - \text{outflow} \\ &= A(t) - k \times x \\ &= D_{oral} \times f \times k_a \times e^{-k_a t} - k \times x\end{aligned} \tag{39}$$

This is simply the rate of absorption at time t, A(t), minus the rate of exit, k × x. To solve for the amount of drug, x, in the compartment at time t, we integrate this from 0 to time t, knowing that $x(0) = 0$:

$$x(t) = \frac{D_{oral} \times f \times k_a}{k - k_a}\left(e^{-k_a t} - e^{-kt}\right) \tag{40}$$

Equation 40 describes the amount of drug in the systemic circulation after first-order absorption from a depot, such as the stomach, an intramuscular injection, the skin, or even an epidural dose. To describe concentrations rather than amounts of drug, it is necessary to divide both sides of Equation 40 by V, the volume of distribution.

This covers the standard pharmacokinetic equations for one-compartment models. The one-compartment model introduces the concepts of rate constants and half-lives and relates them to the physiologic concepts of volume and clearance. Unfortunately, none of the drugs used in anesthesia can be accurately characterized by one-compartment models. The distribution of anesthetic drugs into and out of peripheral tissues plays a crucial role in the time course of anesthetic drug effect. To describe intravenous anesthetics, we must extend the one-compartment model to account for distribution into tissues.

Multicompartment Models

Plasma concentrations over time after an intravenous bolus resemble the curve in Figure 19-18. In contrast to Figure 19-13, Figure 19-18 is not a straight line, even though it is plotted on a log *y* axis. This curve has the characteristics common to most drugs when given by intravenous bolus. First, the concentrations continuously decrease over time. Second, the rate of decline is initially steep but continuously becomes less steep, until we get to a portion that is "log-linear."

For many drugs, three distinct phases can be distinguished, as suggested by Figure 19-18. There is a "rapid-distribution" phase (solid line in Fig. 19-18) that begins immediately after injection

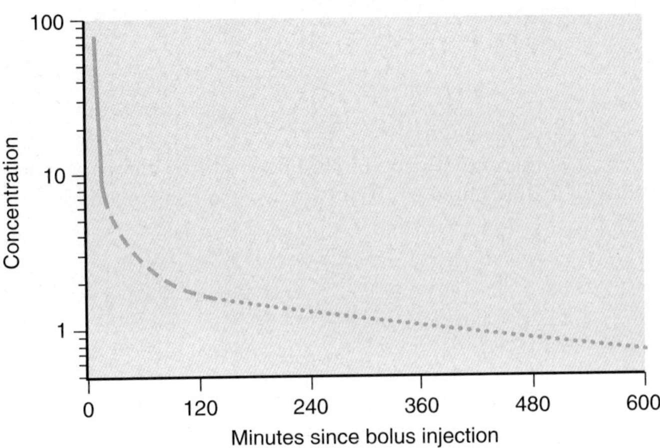

Figure 19-18 Concentration-versus-time relationship showing a very rapid initial decline after injection of a bolus. The terminal log-linear portion is seen only after most of the drug has left the plasma. This is characteristic of most anesthetic drugs. Different line types highlight the rapid, intermediate, and slow (log-linear) portions of the curve.

of the bolus. Very rapid movement of the drug from plasma to the rapidly equilibrating tissues characterizes this phase. Frequently there is a second "slow-distribution" phase (dashed line in Fig. 19-18) that is characterized by movement of drug into more slowly equilibrating tissues and return of drug to plasma from the most rapidly equilibrating tissues. The terminal phase (dotted line in Fig. 19-18) is a straight line when plotted on a semilogarithmic graph. The terminal phase is often called the "elimination phase" because the primary mechanism for decreasing drug concentration during the terminal phase is elimination of drug from the body. The distinguishing characteristic of the terminal elimination phase is that the plasma concentration is lower than tissue concentrations and the relative proportion of drug in plasma and peripheral volumes of distribution remains constant. During this "terminal-phase" drug returns from the rapid- and slow-distribution volumes to plasma and is permanently removed from plasma by metabolism or excretion.

The presence of three distinct phases after bolus injection is a defining characteristic of a mammillary model with three compartments. It is possible to develop hydraulic models, as shown in Figure 19-19, for intravenous drugs.[8] In this model, there are three tanks corresponding (from left to right) to the slowly equilibrating peripheral compartment, the central compartment (the plasma, into which drug is injected), and the rapidly equilibrating peripheral compartment. The horizontal pipes represent intercompartmental clearance or (for the pipe draining onto the page) metabolic clearance. The volumes of each tank correspond to the volumes of the compartments for fentanyl. The cross-sectional areas of the pipes correlate with fentanyl systemic and intercompartmental clearance. The height of water in each tank corresponds to drug concentration.

By using this hydraulic model we can follow the processes that decrease drug concentration over time after bolus injection. Initially, drug flows from the central compartment to both peripheral compartments via intercompartmental clearance and completely out of the model via metabolic clearance. Because there are three places for drug to go, the concentration in the central compartment decreases very rapidly. At the transition between the solid line and the dashed line, there is a change in the role of the most rapidly equilibrating compartment. At this transition, the concentration in the central compartment falls below the concentration in the rapidly equilibrating compartment, and the direction of flow between them is reversed. After this transition (dashed line), drug in plasma has only two places to go: into the slowly equilibrating compartment or out the drain pipe. These processes are partly offset by the return of drug to plasma from the rapidly equilibrating compartment. The net effect is that once the rapidly equilibrating compartment has come to equilibration, the concentration in the central compartment falls far more slowly than before.

Once the concentration in the central compartment falls below both the rapidly and slowly equilibrating compartments (dotted line), the only method of decreasing the plasma concentration is metabolic clearance, the drain pipe. Return of drug from both peripheral compartments to the central compartment greatly slows the rate of decrease in plasma drug concentration.

Curves that continuously decrease over time, with a continuously increasing slope (i.e., curves that look like Figs. 19-18 and 19-19), can be described by a sum of negative exponentials. In pharmacokinetics, one way of denoting this sum of exponentials is to say that the plasma concentration over time is

$$C(t) = Ae^{-\alpha t} + Be^{-\beta t} + Ce^{-\gamma t} \tag{41}$$

where t is the time since the bolus, C(t) is the drug concentration after a bolus dose, and A, α, B, β, C, and γ are parameters of a pharmacokinetic model. A, B, and C are called coefficients, whereas α, β, and γ are called exponents. After a bolus injection, all six of the parameters in Equation 41 will be greater than 0.

The main reason that polyexponential equations are used is that they describe the plasma concentrations observed after

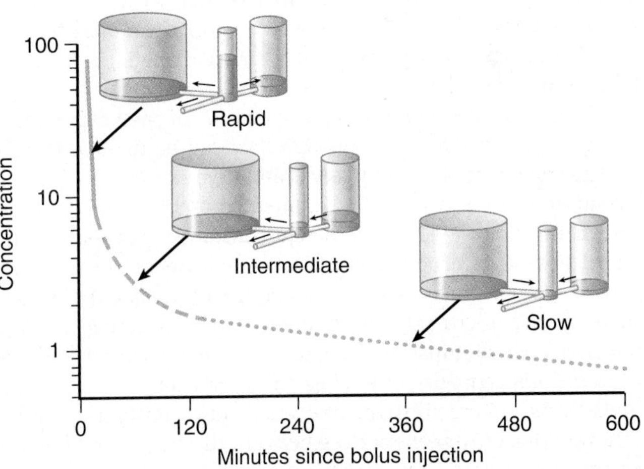

Figure 19-19 Hydraulic model of fentanyl pharmacokinetics. Drug is administered into the central tank, from which it can distribute into two peripheral tanks, or it may be eliminated. The volume of the tanks is proportional to the volumes of distribution. The cross-sectional area of the pipes is proportional to clearance. *(Modified from Youngs EJ, Shafer SL: Basic pharmacokinetic and pharmacodynamic principles.* In White PF [ed]: *Textbook of Intravenous Anesthesia. Baltimore, Williams & Wilkins, 1997, p 10.)*

bolus injection, except for the mis-specification in the first few minutes mentioned previously. Compartmental pharmacokinetics is strictly empirical: the models describe the data, not the processes by which the observations came to be. Fortunately, polyexponential equations permit us to use the one-compartment ideas just developed, with some generalization of the concepts. This involves translating Equation 41 into a model of volumes and clearances that has an appealing, though inaccurate physiologic flavor.

Equation 41 says that concentrations over time are the algebraic sum of three separate functions, $Ae^{-\alpha t}$, $Be^{-\beta t}$, and $Ce^{-\gamma t}$. Typically $\alpha > \beta > \gamma$ by about 1 order of magnitude. We can describe each of these functions separately as graphs, as well as their sum, as shown in Figure 19-19. At time 0 (t = 0), Equation 41 reduces to

$$C_0 = A + B + C \tag{42}$$

The sum of the coefficients A, B, and C, equals the concentration immediately after a bolus. It follows that A + B + C = bolus amount V_1.

Special significance is often ascribed to the smallest exponent. This exponent determines the slope of the final log-linear portion of the curve. When the medical literature refers to the half-life of a drug, unless otherwise stated, the half-life will be the terminal half-life (i.e., 0.693/smallest exponent). However, the terminal half-life for drugs with more than one exponential term is nearly uninterpretable. The terminal half-life sets an upper limit on the time required for the concentrations to decrease by 50% after drug administration. Usually, the time needed for a 50% decrease will be much faster than that upper limit. This is discussed further in Chapter 28.

Constructing pharmacokinetic models represents a trade-off between accurately describing the data, having confidence in the results, and mathematical tractability. Adding exponents to the model generally provides a better description of the observed concentrations. However, adding more exponent terms usually decreases our confidence in how well we know each coefficient and exponential and greatly increases the mathematical burden of the models. This is why most pharmacokinetic models are limited to two or three exponents.

Part of the continuing popularity of polyexponential models of pharmacokinetics is that they can be mathematically transformed from the admittedly unintuitive exponential form in Equation 41 to a more easily intuited compartmental form, as shown in Figure 19-15. Micro rate constants, expressed as k_{ij}, define the rate of drug transfer from compartment i to compartment j. Compartment 0 is the compartment outside the model, so k_{10} is the micro rate constant for processes acting through metabolism or elimination that irreversibly remove drug from the central compartment (analogous to k for a one-compartment model). The intercompartmental micro rate constants (k_{12}, k_{21}, etc.) describe movement of drug between the central and peripheral compartments. Each peripheral compartment has at least two micro rate constants, one for drug entry and one for drug exit. The micro rate constants for the two- and three-compartment models can be seen in Figure 19-15. The differential equations describing the rate of change for the amount of drugs in compartments 1, 2, and 3 follow directly from the micro rate constants. For the two-compartment model, the differential equations for each compartment are

$$\begin{aligned} \frac{dx_1}{dt} &= I + x_2 k_{21} - x_1 k_{10} - x_1 k_{12} \\ \frac{dx_2}{dt} &= x_1 k_{12} - x_2 k_{21} \end{aligned} \tag{43}$$

where I is the rate of drug input. For the three-compartmental model, the differential equations for each compartment are

$$\begin{aligned} \frac{dx_1}{dt} &= I + x_2 k_{21} + x_3 k_{31} - x_1 k_{10} - x_1 k_{12} - x_1 k_{13} \\ \frac{dx_2}{dt} &= x_1 k_{12} - x_2 k_{21} \\ \frac{dx_3}{dt} &= x_1 k_{13} - x_3 k_{31} \end{aligned} \tag{44}$$

An easy way to model pharmacokinetics is to convert these differential equations to difference equations so that dx becomes Δx and dt becomes Δt. With a Δt of 1 second, the error from linearizing the differential equations is less than 1%. In this way, desktop computers can easily simulate pharmacokinetics by using a spreadsheet.

For the one-compartment model, k was both the rate constant and the exponent. For multicompartment models, the relationships are more complex. The interconversion between micro rate constants and exponents becomes exceedingly complex as more exponents are added because every exponent is a function of every micro rate constant and vice versa. Individuals interested in such interconversions can find them in the Excel spreadsheet convert.xls, which can be downloaded from http://www.opentci.org/doku.php?id=code:code.

The Time Course of Drug Effect

The plasma is not the site of drug effect for anesthetic drugs. There is a time lag between plasma drug concentration and effect-site drug concentration. For example, one significant difference between fentanyl and alfentanil is the more rapid onset of alfentanil's drug effect. The orange bar in the top graph of Figure 19-20 shows the duration of a fentanyl infusion.[9] Rapid arterial samples document the rise in fentanyl concentration. The time course of the electroencephalographic effect (spectral edge) lags 2 to 3 minutes behind the rapid rise in arterial concentration. This lag is called hysteresis. The plasma concentration peaks at the moment that the infusion is turned off. After the peak plasma concentration (and the "Mickey Mouse" silhouette that appears at the peak plasma concentration), the fentanyl concentration decreases rapidly. However, the offset of fentanyl drug effect again lags well behind the decrease in concentration. The lower graph in Figure 19-20 shows the same study design in a patient receiving alfentanil. Because of alfentanil's rapid blood-brain equilibration, there is less hysteresis with alfentanil than with fentanyl.

Typically, the relationship between plasma and the site of drug effect is modeled with an "effect-site" model, as shown in Figure 19-21. The site of drug effect is connected to plasma by a first-order process. The equation that relates effect-site concentration to plasma concentration is

$$\frac{dCe}{dt} = k_{e0} \times Cp - k_{e0} \times Ce \tag{45}$$

where Ce is the effect-site concentration, Cp is the plasma drug concentration, and k_{e0} is the rate constant for elimination of drug

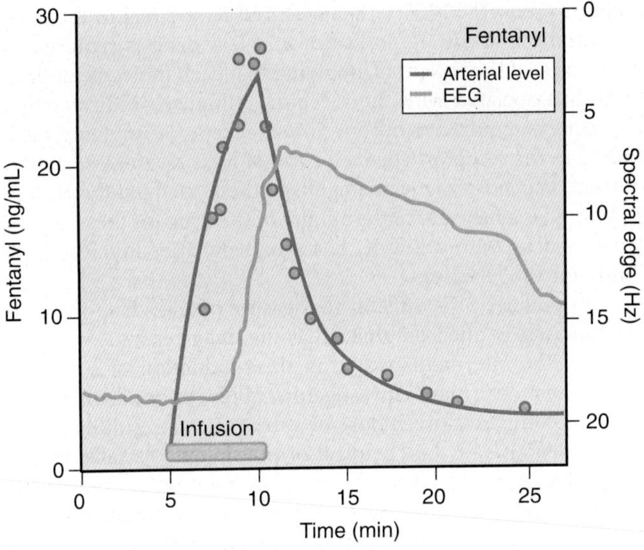

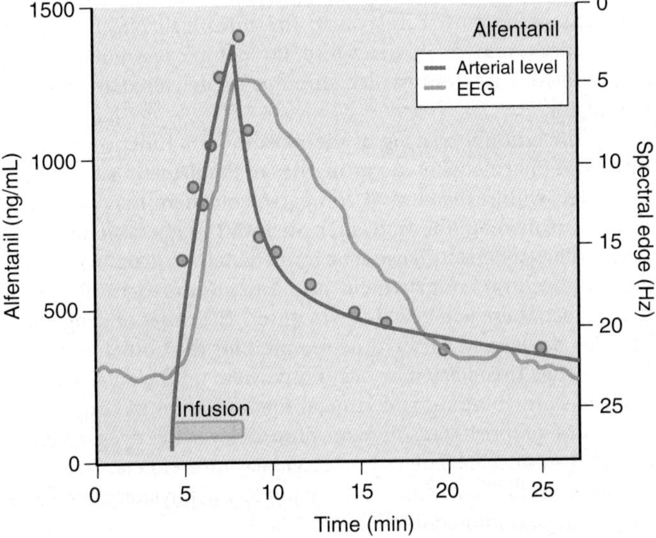

Figure 19-20 Fentanyl and alfentanil arterial concentrations (*circles*) and electroencephalographic (EEG) response (*irregular line*) to an intravenous infusion. With each drug there is a time lag between the rise and fall in arterial concentration and the EEG response, but the time lag is much greater for fentanyl than for alfentanil. *(Modified from Scott JC, Ponganis KV, Stanski DR: EEG quantitation of narcotic effect: The comparative pharmacodynamics of fentanyl and alfentanil. Anesthesiology 62:234-241, 1985.)*

from the effect site. It is most easily understood in terms of its reciprocal, $0.693/k_{e0}$, the half-time for equilibration between plasma and the site of drug effect.

The constant k_{e0} has a large influence on the rate of rise in drug effect, the rate of offset of drug effect, and the dose that is required to produce the desired drug effect. The mathematical basis of these relationships is explored in Chapter 28.

Summary

Pharmacokinetics involves fundamental physiologic processes, including metabolism, protein binding, tissue distribution, and drug transport to the site of drug effect. Pharmacokinetic models are mathematical relationships between dose and concentration, either in plasma or at the site of drug effect. Such models can be used to determine how best to give drugs to achieve a therapeutic objective, but only when the relationship between drug concentration and drug effect is understood. This is the subject of the next section.

Pharmacodynamics

Pharmacodynamics describes the relationship between plasma drug concentration and pharmacologic effect. Simply stated, pharmacokinetics describes what the body does to the drug, whereas pharmacodynamics describes what the drug does to the body. Although the study of clinically important drug effects is multifaceted, we will divide pharmacodynamics into three general areas: transduction of biologic signals (receptor theory and structure), developments in molecular pharmacology, and clinical evaluation of drug effects.

Transduction of Biologic Signals

Receptor Theory

Definition

In the broadest sense, a receptor is a component of a cell that interacts selectively with an extracellular compound to initiate a cascade of biochemical events that culminate in the pharmacologic effects of the compound. Binding of a drug to a receptor

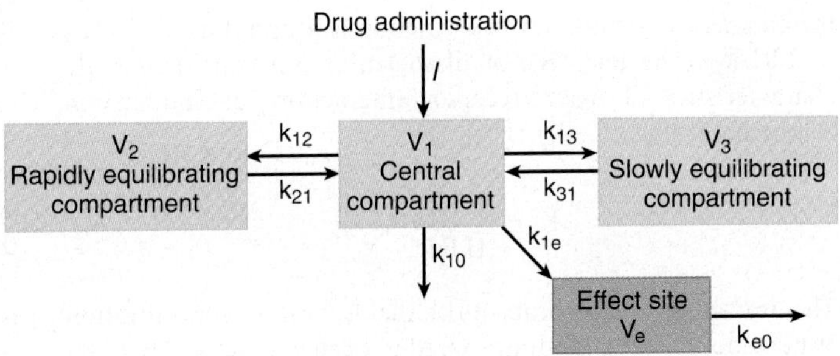

Figure 19-21 A three-compartment model with an added effect site to account for the delay in equilibration between the rise and fall in arterial drug concentrations and the onset and offset of drug effect. The effect site is assumed to have a negligible volume.

determines (1) the quantitative relationship between a given dose of a drug and the resulting effect, (2) the selectivity of a given drug's activity and effect, and (3) the pharmacologic activity of receptor agonists, antagonists, and inverse agonists. Receptors therefore serve to mediate and amplify the effect of a drug on the biologic system.

Historical Perspective

Although the overall concept of receptors is generally attributed to Paul Erhlich (1854-1915), earlier work performed by Claude Bernard (1813-1878) paved the way for receptor theory. This earlier work is of particular interest to anesthesiologists because it centered on elucidation of the mechanism of action of curare in poisoned arrows. In his experiments, Claude Bernard ligated vessels leading to one hind limb of a frog while leaving nerve input intact. He then administered intravenous curare. Pinching the paralyzed hind limb produced reflex movements in the opposite unparalyzed vessel-ligated hind limb. These experiments and others demonstrated for the first time the separation between the sensory and motor nervous systems and also revealed that circulating "substances" produce selective effects on organ systems, a concept important in the development of receptor theory.

The concept of selectivity of effect eventually led Paul Erhlich to his conclusion that "agents cannot act unless they are bound," a cornerstone of receptor theory. Erhlich's contemporary, J. N. Langley (1852-1926), coined the phrase "receptive substance." Langley showed that nicotine and curare have mutually antagonistic effects on the same receptive substance and that the substance was neither nerve nor muscle. Today, we recognize this "receptive substance" as the nicotinic acetylcholine receptor in the neuromuscular junction. Several decades of research has refined receptor theory to the point that receptors are now recognized as discrete excitable proteins.

Classic Receptor Theory

Binding of a ligand, L, to its receptor, R, follows the laws of mass action and can be summarized by the relationship

$$[L]+[R] \underset{k_{off}}{\overset{k_{on}}{\rightleftarrows}} [LR] \tag{46}$$

where k_{on} is the rate constant for binding of the ligand to the receptor, k_{off} is the rate constant for the dissociation of the ligand from the receptor, [L] is the concentration of the ligand, [R] is the concentration of the unbound receptor, and [LR] is the concentration of the bound receptor. Note that the units for k_{on} are $\text{time}^{-1} \cdot$ units of $[L]^{-1}$. The units of L are typically nanomoles per liter. The units for k_{off} are time^{-1}. The rate of formation of [LR] is $\frac{d[LR]}{dt} = [L][R]k_{on} - [LR]k_{off}$. At steady state, which is nearly instantaneous, the net rate of formation is 0, and thus $[L]\ [R]\ k_{on} = [LR]\ k_{off}$. The term K_d, or dissociation constant, defines the characteristics of ligand/receptor interactions at equilibrium. Mathematically,

$$K_d = \frac{[L][R]}{[LR]} = \frac{k_{off}}{k_{on}} \tag{47}$$

The units of K_d are the units of [L], that is, units of concentration. When enough drug is administered to occupy exactly 50% of the receptors (i.e., [R] = [LR]), the measured K_d is equal to the drug concentration. A low K_d indicates that less drug is required to occupy 50% of the receptors, implying that each molecule of drug is tightly associated with the receptor. A high K_d indicates that more drug is required to occupy 50% of receptors, implying weak binding to the receptor. The reciprocal of K_d is K_a, the association constant, which is exactly analogous to the K_a defined for protein binding. K_a is a measure of the affinity of the drug for the receptor. Hence, a drug with a low K_d has a high K_a and therefore high affinity for the receptor.

In practice, it is difficult to measure precise drug-receptor occupancy. It is often assumed that the drug-receptor complex represents an intermediate step in the production of a specific effect. Therefore, many investigators apply pharmacodynamic theory to compare a given dose of a drug with a resulting effect. An effect can be any biochemical or physiologic variable that is measurable. A measured effect can be an alteration in a biochemical compound or an enzyme level, a physiologic variable such as heart rate or blood pressure, or a response to any graded input into the biologic system. For example, in evaluating the pharmacodynamics of muscle relaxants, the measured effect is not a direct measurement of drug-receptor complexes, but rather a response to a neuromuscular stimulus as delivered by a nerve stimulator.

The amount of drug at the receptor is a function of dose, time, and pharmacokinetic properties of the drug. If the receptor is located within the central compartment, there may be nearly instantaneous equilibration after an intravenous injection, and hence the peak effect may occur immediately. If drug must cross from the central compartment into a tissue to reach the site of drug effect, there will be a delay in onset. The onset of drug effect can also be delayed by the time required for the body to respond to the drug. This delay may occur anywhere on the path between drug-receptor binding and clinical manifestation of drug effect. Examples of post-transduction time delays are drug-receptor complex–induced changes in secondary messengers, increased enzyme synthesis, and the time required for physiologic change (e.g., reduced fluid content).

Receptor Agonists and Antagonists. Drugs that are agonists mimic endogenous hormones or neurotransmitters when bound to a receptor. This effect may be excitatory or inhibitory. As described earlier, the term *affinity* as related to a given agonist is a measure of the attraction between the given drug and receptor. A drug with low affinity for a given receptor tends not to bind to the receptor and hence produces little or no effect. An agonist that binds avidly (or with high affinity) to a given receptor produces the receptor-determined effect at a lower given dose.

Full agonists completely activate a receptor, whereas partial agonists only partially activate a receptor, even at very high concentrations (Fig. 19-22). The difference between full and partial agonists results from differing intrinsic efficacy for each drug. Efficacy should not be confused with affinity. Two drugs can have identical affinity for a receptor (and therefore bind to the same extent at a given drug concentration), yet they may produce different levels of activation of the receptor. Both are agonists, but the drug that produces maximal receptor activation is called a full agonist and has high efficacy, whereas the drug that produces less than maximal receptor activation is called a partial agonist with less intrinsic efficacy. The mechanisms underlying whether a drug is a full versus a partial agonist are unclear, but they may be related to the ability of the drug to stabilize the high-activity state

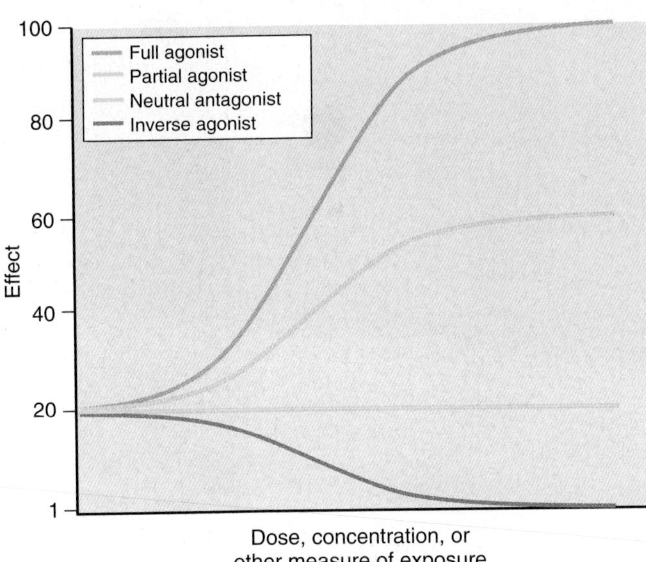

Figure 19-22 Effect of various types of ligands on receptor responses. A full agonist produces complete (100%) activation of a receptor at high concentrations, whereas partial agonist binding results in less than 100% activation, even at very high concentrations. A neutral antagonist has no activity of its own. However, note that in the absence of drug there is still a 20% effect because some receptors are in the activated state in the absence of drug. Inverse agonists can be thought of as "super antagonists" inasmuch as binding of these ligands produces a response below the baseline response measured in the absence of drug because nearly all of the receptors are forced into the unactivated state by the inverse agonist. If the physiologic effect of the baseline levels of activated receptor is small, antagonists and inverse agonists may not be clinically distinguishable.

of the receptor (described under the next heading, "Receptor States").

Drugs that are competitive antagonists inhibit or prevent receptor-mediated agonist effects by competing for the binding site at the receptor. A competitive antagonist can generally be displaced from the receptor complex by the administration of a large enough concentration of receptor agonist, thus permitting the agonist to produce the expected effect despite the presence of antagonist. A noncompetitive antagonist usually binds irreversibly to the receptor complex and produces loss of the expected effect that cannot be compensated by administration of high concentrations of receptor agonist. For example, vecuronium is a competitive antagonist of acetylcholine. Acetylcholine mediates muscle contraction via the postsynaptic nicotinic acetylcholine receptor at the neuromuscular junction. When vecuronium occupies the postsynaptic acetylcholine receptor, acetylcholine agonism is blocked, and neuromuscular transmission is inhibited. The result is flaccid paralysis. Neuromuscular transmission may be reinstated by administering an acetylcholine esterase inhibitor. Acetylcholine esterase inhibitors prevent the breakdown of acetylcholine, thereby effectively raising the concentration of the agonist, acetylcholine, at the receptor, which then displaces vecuronium from the receptor complex. When enough vecuronium is displaced, muscle contraction is reinstated. Most antagonist drugs used in clinical medicine are competitive antagonists.

Inverse agonists can be thought of as "superantagonists" because they decrease receptor responses to less than the "baseline" (see Fig. 19-22) response seen in the absence of drug. Figure 19-23 shows the electroencephalographic response to four different benzodiazepines.[10] Midazolam is a full agonist, whereas RO

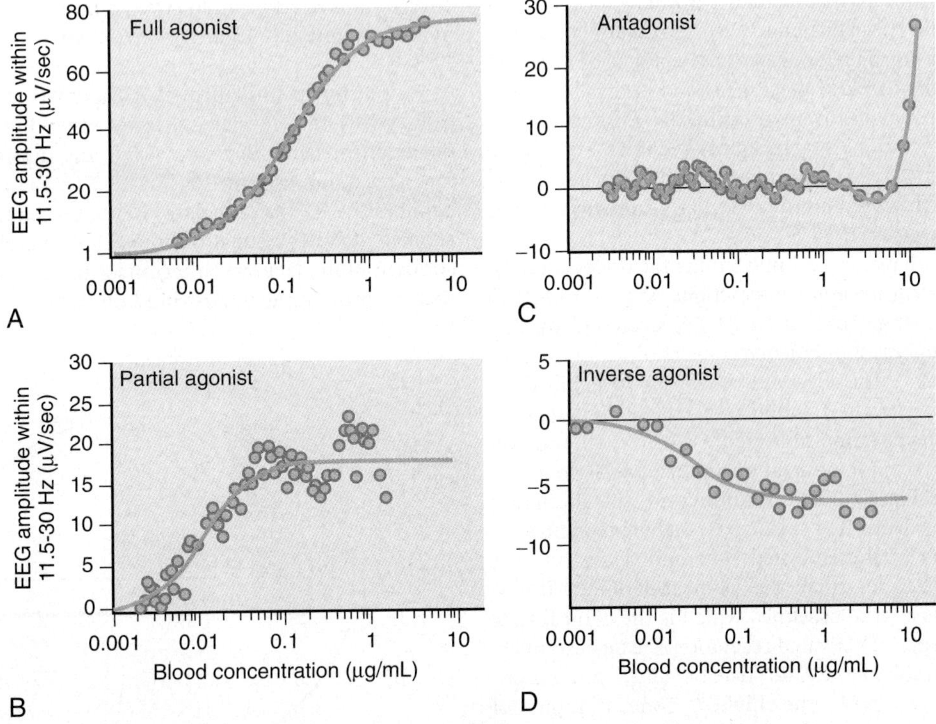

Figure 19-23 The concentration-electroencephalographic (EEG) response relationship for four benzodiazepines: midazolam (full agonist) (**A**), bretazenil (partial agonist) (**B**), flumazenil (antagonist) (**C**), and RO 19-4063 (an inverse agonist) (**D**). The maximum effect seen on the electroencephalogram correlates with clinical action (full agonist > partial agonist > antagonist > inverse agonist). *(From Shafer S: Principles of pharmacokinetics and pharmacodynamics. In Longnecker DE, Tinker JH, Morgan GE [eds]: Principles and Practice of Anesthesiology, 2nd ed. St Louis, Mosby–Year Book, 1997; based on Mandema JW, Kuck MT, Danhof M: Differences in intrinsic efficacy of benzodiazepines are reflected in their concentration-EEG effect relationship. Br J Pharmacol 105:164-170, 1992.)*

19-4063 is an inverse agonist. Note that in Figure 19-22, the "baseline" effect in the absence of drug is 20% effect because some receptors are in the activated state. Only in the presence of the inverse agonist are nearly all of the receptors forced into the unactivated state, thereby revealing the physiologic response in the complete absence of receptor activation.

Receptor States. Classic receptor theory describes the interaction between ligand and receptor according to the laws of mass action. At a molecular level, this interaction has been interpreted over the years to suggest that binding of agonist to receptor initiates a change in receptor conformation that converts the receptor from an inactive (R) to an activated (R*) state (Fig. 19-24). In this model the change in receptor conformation facilitates coupling of activated receptor to intermediary proteins (e.g., guanine nucleotide [G] proteins) or second messengers (effectors, E), which then initiate a rapid cascade of cellular responses.

Transgenic animal experiments have shed light on ligand and receptor interactions. In an elegant set of experiments, β_2-adrenergic receptors (β_2ARs) were massively overexpressed in mouse myocardium.[11] Second messenger responses were increased in the absence of ligand when compared with normal mouse myocardium. In fact, adenylyl cyclase activity (the second messenger most commonly studied for β_2ARs) was the same at baseline in transgenic animals (in the absence of drug) as in normal mice stimulated with isoproterenol (a β_2AR agonist). Furthermore, stimulation of transgenic animals with isoproterenol failed to further increase adenylyl cyclase activity higher than this elevated baseline. This finding suggests that a subpopulation of receptors was already fully activated in the transgenic animals.

These findings imply that a small percentage of receptors spontaneously exist in the activated (R*) state. Because a fraction of the receptors are normally activated, the activity of these R* receptors is part of the baseline effect measured in the absence of drug. However, after massive overexpression of β_2ARs in a transgenic animal, this fraction of total receptors becomes a very large number of activated receptors. This mimics the effect of a maximal dose of agonist, which would produce similar numbers of receptors in the R* state.

These findings have broad implications for understanding receptor states and drug-receptor interactions. Instead of ligand binding causing a change from R to R* (as suggested by Fig. 19-24), these data suggest spontaneous conversion from the R to the R* state (Fig. 19-25). The effect of the ligand is to stabilize the R* state, which increases the fraction of activated receptors. In most tissues, the concentration of R* represents a small fraction of the total overall receptor population (hence the large arrow pointing toward R in Fig. 19-25). This finding explains the action of inverse agonists as drugs that stabilize R, thereby reducing the number of receptors in the activated state and decreasing the physiologic response to less than the "clinical baseline." It also suggests that there is a "true baseline," which is the clinical state in the complete absence of activated receptors. The biggest differences between "clinical baseline" and "true baseline" would probably occur in tissues with the highest concentrations of spontaneous R*. Inverse agonists would therefore be most efficacious in such tissues.

Figure 19-23D illustrates a tissue, the central nervous system (CNS), with enough activated type A γ-aminobutyric acid ($GABA_A$) ligand-gated ion channels (R*) to see electroencephalographic changes with an inverse agonist. Finally, it is important to note that the discussion thus far assumes only two receptor states, R (completely inactive) and R* (fully activated). There may be many transition states between R and R* (hence the use of curved lines in addition to straight lines in Fig. 19-25). However, in the interest of simplicity, this chapter discusses only R and R*.

As shown in Figure 19-26, agonists stabilize (or energetically favor) the R* state, thereby removing the receptor from instantaneous equilibration with R and driving (by mass action) more receptors toward R* (Fig. 19-27). Hence the probability of being in the R* state increases in the presence of agonist. Inverse agonists drive the equation to the left, thereby stabilizing the R configuration. Neutral antagonists bind equally to R and R*, thereby preventing agonist binding without altering the equilib-

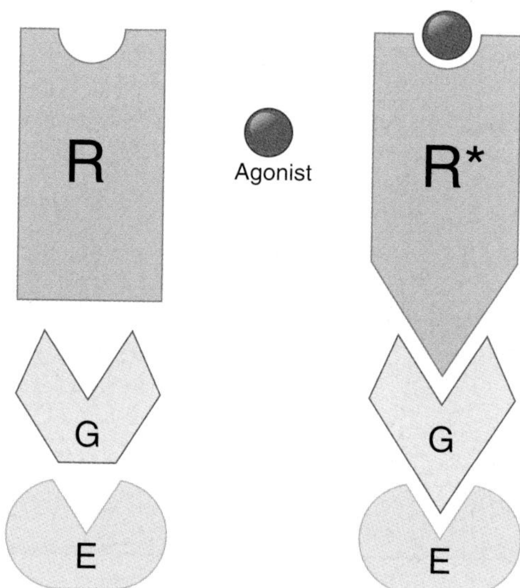

Figure 19-24 Schematic of classic receptor activation. For years, binding of ligand was thought to cause receptors to change from an inactive state (R) to an activated state (R*). The activated receptor then interacts with intermediary guanine nucleotide (G) proteins or directly with second messenger cascades (effectors, E), or with both. More recent information suggests a more complicated equilibrium between R and R*, as shown in Figures 19-25 to 19-27.

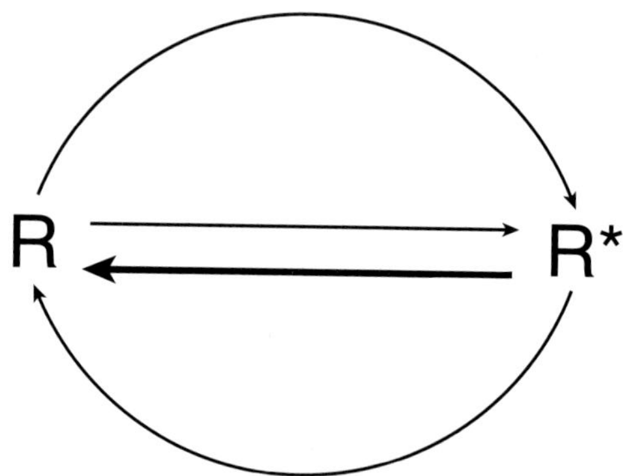

Figure 19-25 Spontaneous conversion of receptors from an inactive (R) to an active (R*) state. In most tissues, R* represents a small fraction of the total receptor population.

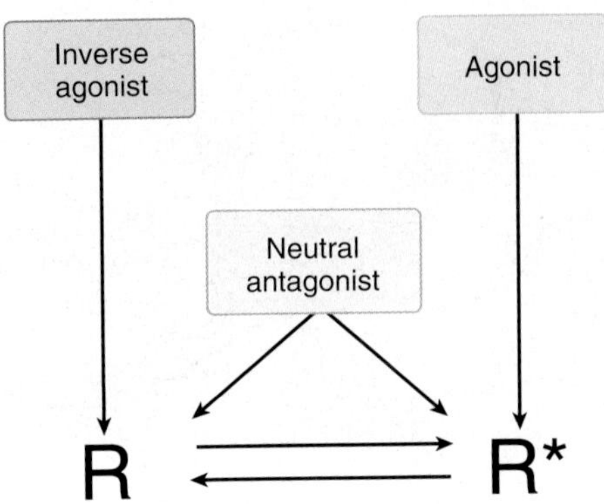

Figure 19-26 Ligand stabilization of receptor states. Agonists stabilize active receptors (R*), inverse agonists stabilize inactive receptors (R), and neutral antagonists bind equally to R and R* without affecting the equilibrium between the two receptor states.

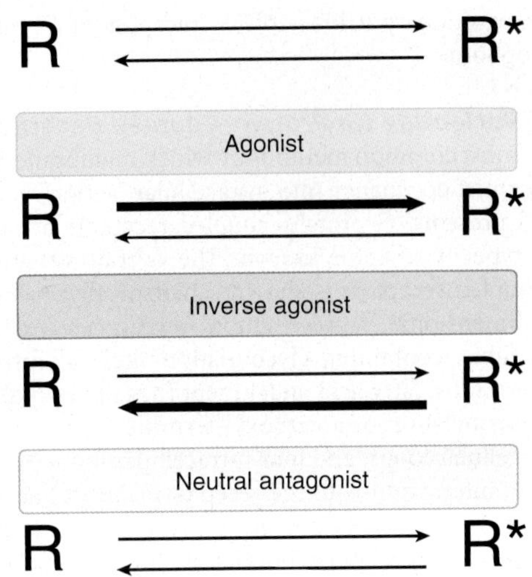

Figure 19-27 Equilibrium between inactive receptors (R) and active receptors (R*) is tissue specific and depends on the type of ligand administered. By stabilizing R*, agonists drive the equilibrium to the right. In contrast, inverse agonists stabilize R, which drives the equilibrium to the left. Because neutral antagonists bind equally to R and R*, they do not affect tissue-specific equilibrium between R and R*.

rium between R and R*. Hence, neutral antagonists do not change the observed baseline response (see Fig. 19-22).

Many classic "antagonists" have been found to be inverse agonists rather than neutral antagonists. For example, the common used β_2AR antagonists, metoprolol and bisoprolol, show significant inverse agonist activity. Carvedilol has weaker inverse agonist properties at β_2ARs and displays neutral antagonist activity at β_1ARs. Alprenolol has even weaker (20%) inverse agonist activity at β_2ARs. Xamoterol displays partial agonist activity at β_1ARs.[12,13] Because inverse agonists may have theoretical advantages in treating certain diseases (e.g., seizures, congestive heart failure), clinicians should critically evaluate recent pharmacologic data before using an antagonist to distinguish whether the drug is a neutral antagonist or an inverse agonist.

Receptor Structure

Receptors are ubiquitous in the cell, being present in cell membranes, cytoplasm, intracellular organelle membranes, and the nucleus. The overall physical structure of a receptor depends on the type of receptor and its location. Cytoplasmic and nuclear receptors bind ligands that readily traverse cell membranes. These ligands must therefore contain significant hydrophobic (lipophilic) components. Examples of cytoplasmic and nuclear receptors include steroid and thyroid hormone receptors. In contrast, the receptors of most interest to anesthesiologists are located on the cell membrane and include membrane receptors, ligand-gated ion channels, and voltage-gated ion channels (Fig. 19-28). Receptors on the cell membrane bind water-soluble ligands that are typically unable to cross lipid bilayers and mediate a cellular response via intermediary proteins (e.g., G protein–coupled receptors) or by causing changes in ion flux (e.g., ligand-gated ion channels). Each of these types of membrane receptor has a role in mediating the action of various drugs important in anesthesiology. It is beyond the scope of this chapter to list all currently identified receptor proteins. However, prototypical examples are used to illustrate important pharmacodynamic principles.

Structure-activity relationships between drug and the three-dimensional configuration of the receptor binding site are critically important in determining binding properties. Though perhaps obvious, the chemical structure of a drug must match the three-dimensional configuration of the binding area of a receptor. Hence, subtle changes in drug structure may dramatically alter the ability of a drug to bind to a specific receptor population. In addition, two drugs with seemingly unrelated two-dimensional chemical structures may bind to the same receptor if their three-dimensional structures and charged areas are similar. The three-dimensional components of a ligand that interact with

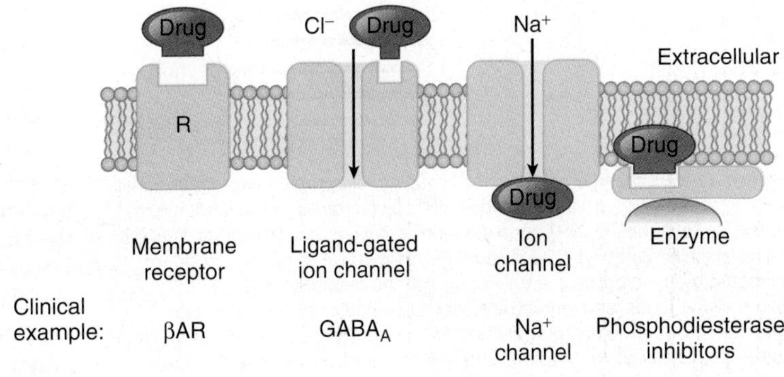

Figure 19-28 Schematic of four types of membrane-associated drug targets in anesthesia: membrane (G protein–coupled) receptor, ligand-gated ion channel, voltage-sensitive ion channel, and an enzyme. Potential sites of drug action are shown. βAR, β-adrenergic receptor; $GABA_A$, γ-aminobutyric acid.

ligand recognition portions of a receptor are called the "pharmacophore."

Guanine Nucleotide (G) Protein–Coupled Receptors

One of the most common methods by which membrane receptors translate agonist occupancy into intracellular "action" is via intermediary G proteins. G protein–coupled receptors are the most abundant type of receptor known. The overall structure of G protein–coupled receptors is shown schematically in Figure 19-29. Two-dimensional representation reveals an extracellular amino terminus containing glycosylation sites, an intracellular carboxyl terminus, fatty acid attachment (usually via palmitoylation or myristoylation of a carboxyl-terminal cysteine residue), three extracellular loops, and four intracellular loops. Major sites of G protein interaction with the receptor occur in the third and fourth (and to a lesser extent the second) intracellular loops, whereas major sites of phosphorylation (often correlated with desensitization [or dampening of receptor responses]) generally occur in the third intracellular loop and carboxyl terminus.

Even though a two-dimensional schematic is shown in Figure 19-29, it is important to remember that G protein–coupled receptors are three-dimensional structures with transmembrane segments coalescing around a central binding pocket (Fig. 19-30).[14] Although transmembrane amino acids must be hydrophobic overall (to be energetically favored in the lipid membrane), side chains on individual amino acids may be charged to act as counter ions for anchoring charged (water-soluble) hormone or drug to the receptor.

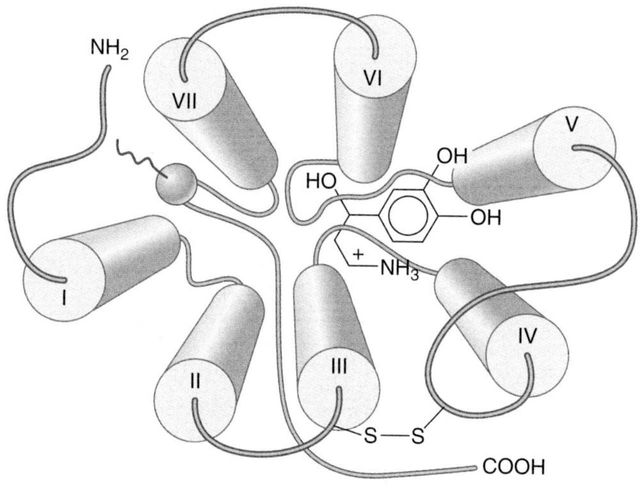

Figure 19-30 Schematic of the three-dimensional structure of the β_2-adrenergic receptor (a prototypical G protein–coupled receptor), looking from the outside of the cell inward. Transmembrane domains (denoted by *cylinders* and numbered with *Roman numerals*) coalesce to form a binding pocket. The correct orientation of the agonist norepinephrine is shown. Note that agonist affinity is determined by specific amino acids located in transmembranes III, IV, and VII. These critical sites in transmembrane domains have been determined experimentally via chimeric receptor and mutagenesis approaches combined with sophisticated computer modeling techniques. Ultimate confirmation of these structures will require crystallographic data. This is currently being attempted by several laboratories. *(From Stapelfeldt WH: The autonomic nervous system. In Schwinn DA [ed]: Scientific Principles of Anesthesia, vol 2. Philadelphia, Current Medicine, 1998.)*

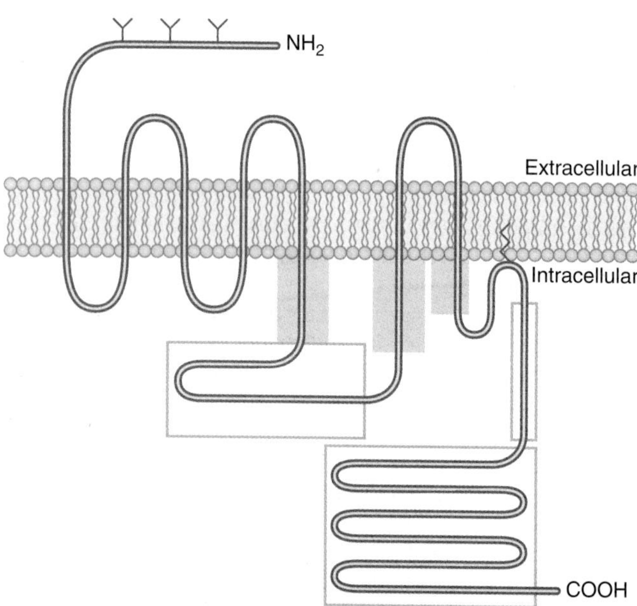

Figure 19-29 Schematic of G protein–coupled receptors. A two-dimensional version of receptor structure is shown with seven transmembrane domains, an extracellular amino (NH_2) terminus (with associated glycosylation sites [Y]), an intracellular carboxyl (COOH) terminus, palmitoylated cysteine residue (denoted by the *crooked line* extending into the membrane), three extracellular loops, and four intracellular loops. Major sites of G protein interactions with the receptor are *speckled*; potential sites of phosphorylation in the third intracellular loop and carboxyl terminus are enclosed in *boxes*.

Ion Channels

Some anesthetic drugs target voltage-gated ion channels. These receptors mediate neural signaling by modulating ion permeability in electrically excitable membranes in response to changes in membrane potential. Voltage-gated ion channels such as the sodium channel have charged regions that span the cell membrane. The formation of ion pairs between many positive and negative charges helps stabilize the ion-conducting pore. Voltage-dependent gating of the sodium channel is made possible by the presence of a voltage sensor, a collection of charges that move under the influence of the cell-membrane electrical field, hence the name voltage-gated ion channel. During depolarization, positively charged sodium ions move intracellularly. The change in membrane potential causes a conformational change in the central pore consisting of rearrangement of ion pairs that favors sodium permeability. Local anesthetics work by blocking voltage-gated sodium channels, as discussed in detail in Chapter 30.

The ligand-gated ion channel is a combination of a classic receptor protein and an ion channel. Ligand-gated ion channels permit certain drugs to directly alter membrane potentials. Many anesthetic drugs act on ligand-gated ion channels, such as the nicotinic acetylcholine receptor and the $GABA_A$ receptor. The structure of the $GABA_A$ receptor is shown in Figure 19-31.[15,16] Ligand-gated ion channels have both hydrophobic and charged transmembrane regions. The hydrophobic regions stabilize the structure in the membrane, whereas the centrally charged region serves as the pore for ion flux. Binding of drugs to ligand-gated ion channels usually enhances or dampens an already existing neurotransmitter-induced ion flux. For example, the neurotransmitter GABA binds to its receptor within the $GABA_A$ ligand-

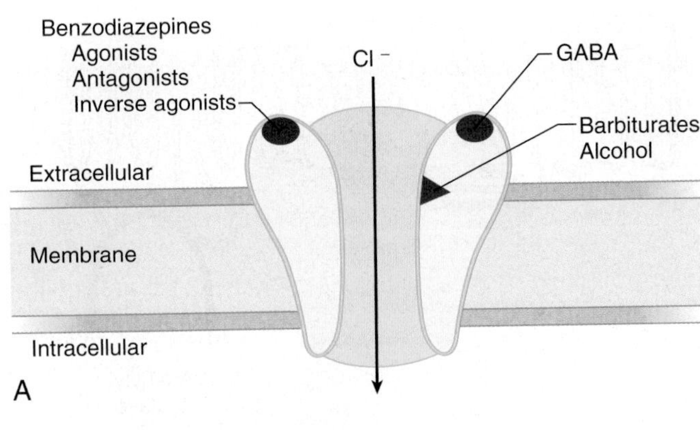

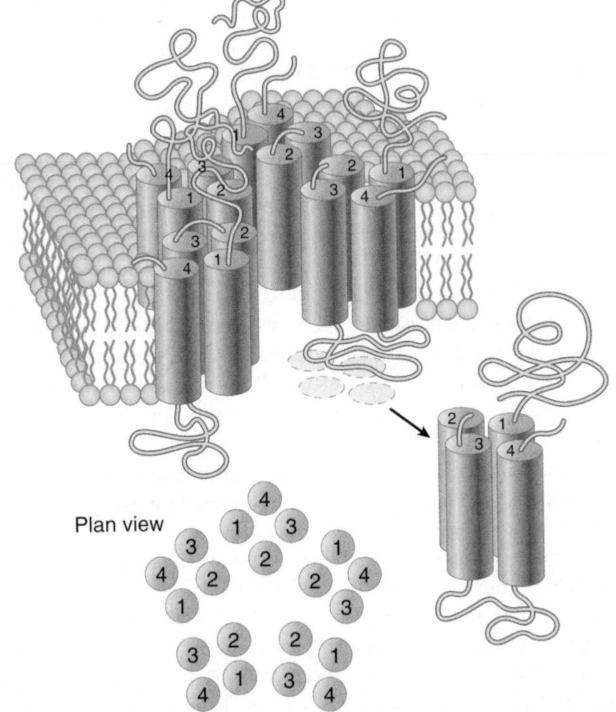

Figure 19-31 Cross section of a schematized γ-aminobutyric acid (GABA)-benzodiazepine receptor complex (a prototypical ligand-gated ion channel complex). Binding of benzodiazepine agonists to the $GABA_A$ ligand-gated ion channel facilitates the action of endogenous GABA. This results in increased inhibitory chloride ion flux in the central nervous system. **A,** Schematic of the $GABA_A$ ligand-gated ion channel complex showing receptor sites for benzodiazepines and GABA, as well as distinct receptor sites for barbiturates and alcohol. **B,** Model of the $GABA_A$ receptor–chloride ion channel protein complex composed of a hetero-oligomer of five subunits, including α, β, and γ, as well as δ or ρ polypeptides. Each subunit has four putative membrane-spanning domains (numbered 1 to 4, represented by *cylinders*). *(**A,** From Berkowitz DE: Cellular signal transduction. In Schwinn DA [ed]: Scientific Principles of Anesthesia, vol 2. Philadelphia, Current Medicine, 1998; **B,** from Firestone L, Quinlan J, Gyulai F: Mechanisms of anesthetic action. In Schwinn DA [ed]: Scientific Principles of Anesthesia, vol 2. Philadelphia, Current Medicine, 1998.)*

gated ion channel complex and causes the intracellular flux of chloride ions. This action results in hyperpolarization of the membrane potential, a hallmark of inhibitory neurotransmission. Drugs binding to other sites on the $GABA_A$ receptor facilitate the action of the endogenous ligand GABA (see Fig. 19-31). Most hypnotics (benzodiazepines, barbiturates, propofol, etomidate, and possibly the hypnotic action of inhaled anesthetics) act through potentiation of endogenous GABA at the $GABA_A$ ligand-gated ion channel.

Ion Pumps

Another type of excitable membrane protein is the ion pump. The sodium-potassium–adenosine triphosphatase (ATPase) pump is perhaps the most familiar ion pump to the anesthesiologist because it is inhibited by digitalis. Extracellular fluid is high in sodium and low in potassium, whereas intracellular fluid is high in potassium and low in sodium. Because the nerve at rest is selectively permeable to potassium but not to sodium, potassium moves extracellularly and creates a net positive extracellular charge and a net negative intracellular charge. Action potentials activate sodium channels, thereby allowing sodium to flux intracellularly along a combined chemical and electrical gradient. The sodium-potassium-ATPase pump then rapidly pumps sodium out of the cell in exchange for potassium, thereby returning the cell to its original cation composition and electrical gradient. Drugs that act on ion pumps alter intracellular/extracellular cation ratios, which results in altered membrane resting potential.

Digitalis acts by inhibiting the sodium-potassium-ATPase pump. This is of special importance in the myocardial cell, where sodium-potassium-ATPase exchange is replaced by slower sodium-calcium exchange, thereby increasing intracellular calcium concentrations. Because calcium increases myocardial contractility, improved myocardial pump function results.

Second Messengers

Binding of a ligand to a receptor does not instantly produce its clinical effects. Instead, a series of rapid biochemical events couples receptor binding to ultimate clinical effects. These biochemical events are called second messengers. Because alterations in second messenger coupling can change the effectiveness of a drug, it is important that the anesthesiologist understand the general principles of second messenger action.

Many membrane receptors couple to their second messenger through G proteins, which are intermediate regulatory molecules. Coupling of G proteins to receptor-hormone complexes requires energy in the form of guanosine triphosphate (GTP). The hydrolysis of G protein–associated GTP to guanosine diphosphate (GDP) is regulated by yet another set of proteins called *RGS proteins.* Once the receptor interacts with the G protein, the biochemical reaction in the effector cascade is triggered. There are stimulating (e.g., G_s, G_q) and inhibitory (e.g., G_i, G_o) G proteins. The physiologic effect is determined by the specific G protein and subsequent cellular response. G proteins are heterotrimeric, composed of three subunits—α, β, and γ. Receptor–G protein interactions result in dissociation of the G protein subunits into α and βγ. The α-subunit of most G proteins confers specificity between receptor and effectors. Although βγ-subunits were originally thought to simply anchor G proteins to the cell membrane, it is now clear that dissociated βγ-subunits are capable of directly stimulating second messengers. In addition, βγ-subunits play a role in anchoring regulatory kinases to the cell membrane, which leads to enhanced phosphorylation of membrane receptors.

One of the best-understood second messenger systems is the adenylyl cyclase system. In this system, stimulatory G protein–

receptor-hormone complexes increase activity of the enzyme adenylyl cyclase, which results in increased levels of cyclic adenosine 3′,5′-monophosphate (cAMP) in the cell (Fig. 19-32). Inhibitory G protein–receptor-hormone complexes decrease the activity of adenylyl cyclase, thereby resulting in decreased levels of cellular cAMP. In general, intracellular cAMP activates protein kinases that phosphorylate various proteins, ion channels, and second messenger enzymes.

Another example of a second messenger system is the phosphatidylinositol system. Here, hydrolysis of phosphatidylinositol 4,5-bisphosphate (PIP_2) in the cell membrane, catalyzed by activation of phospholipase C by G_q, generates two main second messenger molecules, inositol 1,4,5-trisphosphate (IP_3) and 1,2-diacylglycerol (DAG). IP_3 then mobilizes intracellular calcium from nonmitochondrial intracellular stores by interacting with distinct IP_3 receptors on the surface of these organelles. The resulting increase in intracellular calcium levels produces biologic effects such as smooth muscle contraction. α_1-Adrenergic agonists, endothelin, and muscarinic (M_1, M_3, M_5) agonists all mediate hydrolysis of phosphatidylinositol.

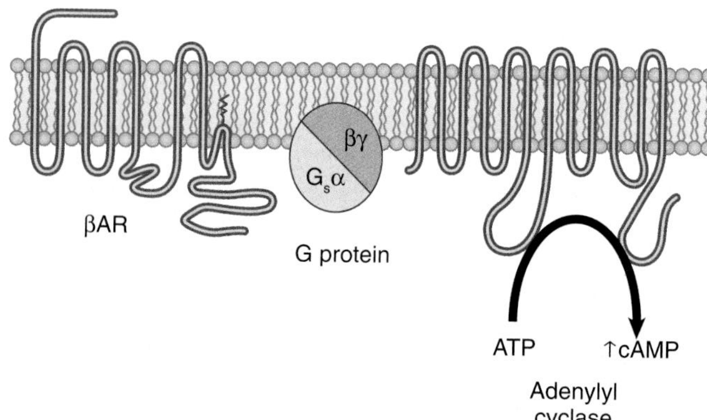

Figure 19-32 Schematic of the β-adrenergic receptor signal transduction cascade. βAR, β-adrenergic receptor; ATP, adenosine triphosphate; cAMP, cyclic adenosine monophosphate; $G_s\alpha$, α subunit of the stimulatory G protein (G_s); βγ, stimulatory G protein, βγ-subunit.

Stimulation of receptors and second messengers ultimately leads to physiologic effects in a given tissue. The physiologic effects produced depend on the presence of specific receptor subtypes, G proteins, and second messengers within that tissue. An example of the wide-ranging cardiovascular effects produced by the predominant sympathetic neurotransmitter norepinephrine can be seen in Figure 19-33.

Developments in Molecular Pharmacology

The field of molecular pharmacology has advanced our understanding of excitable membrane proteins and their mechanisms of action. Novel molecular techniques provide unique opportunities to learn more about receptors, including their structure and function down to the DNA level. Hitherto unknown receptors and receptor subtypes continue to be discovered, paving the way for future development of receptor-specific pharmacologic agents. We will briefly review the general field of molecular pharmacology because future drugs for perioperative use will probably target receptor and receptor subtypes discovered by such molecular approaches.

Molecular pharmacology takes advantage of the finding that all proteins, including excitable membrane proteins, are encoded in the human genome as nucleic acids. Every amino acid present in a protein is encoded by a specific combination of three nucleotides in DNA. Therefore, if the DNA sequence that encodes a receptor protein can be determined, the putative primary structure (amino acid sequence) of the receptor can be deduced. In addition, encoding DNA sequences (i.e., genes) can be inserted into special cells that will express (manufacture, assemble, and deliver to the appropriate location in the cell) the receptor protein in high quantity. This approach has several advantages.

First, studies on the receptor itself can be performed. By changing (mutating) nucleotide sequences, an abnormal (synthetic or "designer") receptor can be created. This abnormal receptor can then be compared with the original receptor to see whether the changes made affect binding of drug to the receptor or coupling of it to second messengers. In this manner, the function of each portion of the receptor can be studied. This type of

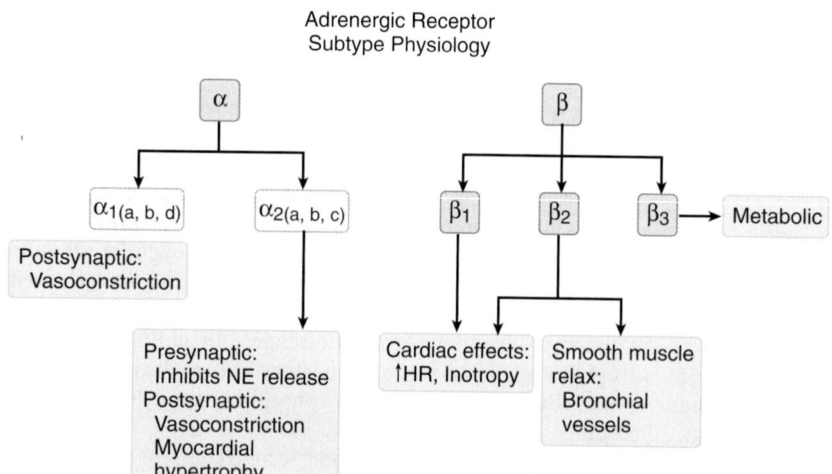

Figure 19-33 Adrenergic receptor subtype physiology. HR, heart rate; NE, norepinephrine.

information is often called structure-activity relationships. G proteins and second messengers can be investigated in a similar manner. More recently, naturally occurring human receptor variants have been investigated and tested for alterations in pharmacologic properties (see the later section "Pharmacogenetics").

The second advantage of using molecular techniques in pharmacology is that new receptors and receptor subtypes can be discovered by searching the genome for DNA sequences similar to those of known receptors. Once these new receptors are discovered, they can easily be characterized because high expression in cells enables them to be screened by various pharmacologic agents. The recent availability of DNA sequences for the full human genome has accelerated the discovery of new receptors through DNA homology searching.

Finally and perhaps the most immediately clinically relevant, new investigational drugs can be rapidly screened for effects on a spectrum of native and variant receptors. In this way, the pharmacologic effects of individual receptors can be studied in a controlled manner, isolated from other receptors and receptor subtypes. Such studies have the potential to lead to the development of new drugs for use in the perioperative period, as well as understanding of the effects of these drugs in patients with receptor variants.

Although there are many advantages to using molecular approaches for understanding the physiologic pathways of individual receptors and for drug discovery, there are also some disadvantages. Cell lines are not integrated organisms, so the function of the receptor protein in a network of physiologic systems cannot be assessed. An approach to understanding the function of previously identified and new gene products that is now classic is to develop mouse (murine) models in which the gene of interest has been eliminated (knock-out mice) or overexpressed (transgenic mice). The physiologic consequence of such altered protein expression is then examined. Although details of these technologies are beyond the scope of this chapter, they have become standardized and are widely available. The transgenic and knock-out mouse models are robust and useful, but they also have important limitations. First, the genetic background of the animals created must be examined carefully. If not carefully controlled, altered phenotypes may result from differences in animal "strain" (or genetic background) rather than from an overexpressed or knocked-out gene product. Second, elimination of specific receptors may be compensated by alterations in other gene products. In this case, the final phenotype represents not only the effect of the absent gene but also the compensatory expression of other genes. Compensation is of particular concern when elimination of a gene is lethal because surviving progeny by definition have compensated in a way that enhances survival and therefore may not be representative of the results of the single gene that was knocked-out. Finally, some receptors and proteins have different tissue localization in humans versus other animal species. Therefore, results from transgenic and knock-out animal studies should be extrapolated cautiously to humans.

Despite these potential limitations, transgenic and knock-out animal models have proved very important in elucidating novel functions of receptors and proteins. Many unexpected physiologic roles for gene products have been discovered, and important physiologic questions have been answered and confirmed with these approaches. Table 19-1 lists conclusions drawn from transgenic and knock-out mice based on alterations in adrenergic receptors and their signal transduction cascade. Novel functions for specific adrenergic receptor subtypes (e.g., the role of α_{2A}ARs in sedation and CNS-mediated hypotension, α_{2B}ARs in mediating vasoconstriction, and α_{2C}ARs in temperature control) have been discovered. Table 19-1 illustrates that alterations in adrenergic receptor signal transduction pathways and modulating kinases have physiologic consequences in the whole animal.

As a result of these advances, we now know the precise location of action of many anesthetic drugs (Table 19-2).[17] This includes identifying the receptor, characterizing the binding site, and studying the downstream consequences of receptor binding responsible for the drug effect. For example, Jurd and colleagues have demonstrated that etomidate and propofol both bind to the same pocket of the β_3-subunit of the $GABA_A$ receptor and have created a genetically altered mouse that is relatively resistant to the hypnotic effects of both drugs.[18] Although most hypnotics and sedatives act by potentiating the action of GABA (the most important inhibitory neurotransmitter in the CNS), the search for the site of action continues for inhaled anesthetics.

Clinical Evaluation of Drug Effects

General Principles

Once pharmacologic agents have exerted their actions on a molecular level, stimulated their targets, and produced a physiologic effect, it is important to evaluate the effect on the whole organism. This section focuses on methods of evaluating clinical drug effects such as dose-response curves, efficacy, potency, the median effective dose (ED_{50}), the median lethal dose (LD_{50}), and the therapeutic index.

Concentration-Versus-Response Relationships

The standard comparison of a drug with its clinical effect is the concentration-versus-response curve, shown in Figure 19-34. The relationship illustrated is the time-independent relationship between dose, concentration, or some other measure of exposure to the drug (*x* axis) and the measured effect (*y* axis). The measured effect can be an absolute response (e.g., twitch height), a normalized response (e.g., percentage of twitch height depression), or a population response (e.g., fraction of subjects moving upon incision). The standard equation for this relationship is the "Hill" equation, sometimes called the "sigmoid-E_{max} relationship":

$$\text{Effect} = E_0 + (E_{max} - E_0)\frac{C^\gamma}{C_{50}{}^\gamma + C^\gamma} \qquad (48)$$

This is another example of the saturation equation shown in Figure 19-5. In this equation, E_0 is the baseline effect in the absence of drug and E_{max} is the maximum possible drug effect. C is typically concentration or dose, although other measures of drug exposure (e.g., peak concentration, area under the concentration-versus-time curve) can be used. C_{50} is the concentration associated with 50% of peak drug effect and is a measure of drug potency. The exponent γ, also called the "Hill coefficient," relates to the sigmoidicity and steepness of the curve. If γ is less than 1 and the curve is plotted on a standard *x* axis, the curve appears hyperbolic (see Figure 19-5). If γ is greater than 1, the curve appears sigmoidal, as in Figure 19-34. If the *x* axis is plotted on

Table 19-1 Summary of Results from Knock-Out and Transgenic Mice in Which Various Portions of Adrenergic Receptor Signaling Pathways were Targeted (Emphasis on Cardiovascular Effects)

Model	Target	Result
Transgenic	↑β_2AR	↑Basal AC, ↑LV fn, ↑atrial contractility, ↑supraventricular premature beats, ↓HR variability
Knock-out	↓β_2AR	No observable effects (except mild exercise effects)
Transgenic	↑β_1AR	Dilated cardiomyopathy and early death, fibrosis
Knock-out	↓β_1AR	70% prenatal death rate, survivors: nl AC, ↓ISO-stim
Transgenic	↑AC-V	↑HR, ↑fractional shortening, no ISO-stim effects
Transgenic	↑GRK2	↓AC activity, ↓fn βARs, ↓ISO-stim (rescued with βARK-ct peptide, which inhibits GRK2)
Transgenic	↑GRK5	Enhanced βAR desensitization, but not angiotensin II desensitization
Transgenic	↑GRK2 inhibitor	Enhanced cardiac contractility with ISO (functional ↓GRK2)
Knock-out	↓GRK2	Lethal phenotype, gestational hyperplasia of LV, LVEF ↓70% in embryos
Transgenic	↑$G_s\alpha$	No Δ baseline EF, ↑ ISO-stim, myocardial fibrosis
Knock-out	↓Phospholamban	↓βAR-mediated contractile responses
Transgenic	↑α_{1A}AR	Hypertension, ↑inotropy
Transgenic	↑α_{1B}AR	Myocardial hypertrophy, hypertension, nociception, memory (constitutively active)
Transgenic	↑α_{1B}AR	No myocardial hypertrophy, hypertension (wild type)
Transgenic	↑α_{1D}AR	Nociception, memory
Transgenic	↑G_q	Myocardial hypertrophy ≈4-fold overexpression, higher expression give heart failure
Transgenic	↑G_q inhibitor	Prevention of myocardial hypertrophy (functional ↓G_q)
Knock-out	↓α_{2A}AR	Presynaptic α_2AR, mediates sedation/hypnosis, ↓BP (central hypotension), analgesia, regulation of DA/5-HT, antiepileptogenic effects of NE
Knock-out	↓α_{2B}AR	Mediates ↑BP (peripheral vasoconstriction)
Knock-out	↓α_{2C}AR	Mediates hypothermia, DA synthesis/metabolism, presynaptic α_2AR also (low-frequency stimulation)

AC, adenylyl cyclase; AR, adrenergic receptor; βARK-ct, c terminal fragment of the, β-adrenergic receptor kinase; BP, blood pressure; DA, dopamine; EF, ejection fraction; fn, function; HR, heart rate; 5-HT, 5-hydroxytryptamine; ISO, isoproterenol; LV, left ventricle; GRK, G protein–coupled receptor kinase; LVEF, left ventricular ejection fraction; NE, norepinephrine.

a log scale, the curve will always appear sigmoidal regardless of the value of γ.

Potency and Efficacy

Considerable confusion exists around the definition of potency because of competing definitions of the term. One use of potency is to describe the effect of a given dose of the drug. Consider two different oral preparations of an identical drug: one that dissolves quickly in the stomach and is rapidly absorbed and one that never completely dissolves and is poorly absorbed. A given dose of the rapidly absorbed formulation would produce a more profound drug effect and thus be considered more potent than an identical dose of the slowly absorbed formulation. Consequently, from a therapeutic perspective, potency is often defined in terms of the dose-versus-response relationship.

However, from a pharmacologic perspective, potency is best described in terms of the concentration-versus-response relationship. As shown in Figure 19-34, a drug with a left-shifted concentration-versus-response curve (i.e., lower C_{50}) is considered more potent, whereas a right-shifted dose-versus-response curve renders it less potent. To be precise, potency should be defined in terms of a specific drug effect (e.g., 50% of maximal effect). This is particularly important if the two drugs have different Hill coefficients or efficacies (E_{max}).

Efficacy is a measure of the intrinsic ability of a drug to produce a given physiologic or clinical effect (Fig. 19-35). For example, in G protein–coupled receptors, efficacy is influenced by coupling of receptor to G proteins, activation of second messengers, and the ability to generate maximal physiologic responses. The scale used to describe intrinsic efficacy at a given receptor ranges from 0 to 1. Efficacy is 1.0 for full agonists, 0 for neutral antagonists, and between 0 and 1.0 for partial agonists. In contrast, the term *potency* refers to the quantity of drug that must be administered to produce a specific effect. Two drugs may have the same efficacy, but if one drug produces the maximum effect at 1 mg whereas the second drug produces the maximum effect only at 100 mg, the second drug is less potent. The difference between a full agonist and a partial agonist (see Figs. 19-22 and 19-23) represents a difference in efficacy.

Effective Dose and Lethal Dose

The ED_{50} is the dose of a drug required to produce a specific effect in 50% of individuals to whom it is administered. The LD_{50} is the dose of a drug required to produce death in 50% of patients (or,

Table 19-2 Site of Action of Sedatives and Hypnotics

Anesthetic	$GABA_A$	Glycine	Neuronal nAChR	$5\text{-}HT_3$	AMPA (GluR1-4)	NMDA
Barbiturates	+++	+/0	–––	–/0	–––	0
Chloroform	+++	+++	–––	Unknown	–––	0
Diethyl ether	+++	+++	–––	+++	–––	–––
Enflurane	+++	+++	–––	+++	–––	–/0
Etomidate	+++	+/0	–/0	0	Unknown	Unknown
Halothane	+++	+++	–––	+++	–––	–/0
Isoflurane	+++	+++	–––	+++	–––	–/0
Ketamine	+/0	0	–––	+/0	0	–––
Methoxyflurane	+++	+++	–––	+++	Unknown	Unknown
Nitrous oxide	+++	+/0	Unknown	Unknown	–/0	–––
Propofol	+++	+++	–/0	0	–/0	–/0
Sevoflurane	+++	+++	–––	Unknown	Unknown	Unknown
Steroidal anesthetics	+++	0	–/0	–/0	0	0
Xenon	0	Unknown	Unknown	Unknown	0	–––

AMPA, α-amino-3-hyudroxy-5-methyl-4-isoxazoleproprionate; GABA, γ-aminobutyric acid; 5-HT, 5-hydroxytryptamine; nAChR, nicotinic acetylcholine receptor; NMDA, *N*-methyl-D-aspartate; +++, potentiation of the agonist; –––, inhibition of the agonist; +/0 and –/0, little potentiation or inhibition, except at concentrations well in excess of the clinical range; 0, no effect at any concentration.
From Krasowski MD, Harrison NL: General anaesthetic actions on ligand-gated ion channels. Cell Mol Life Sci 55:1278-1303, 1999.

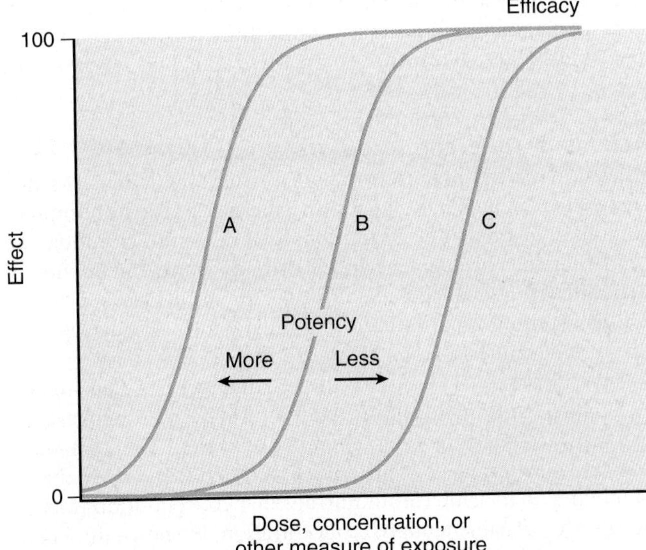

Figure 19-34 Dose- or concentration-versus-response relationships. A sigmoidal concentration-response curve is generated when the log drug concentration is plotted against the clinical response or effect. The concentration-response curve is shifted to the right (B→C) in the presence of a competitive antagonist after desensitization. Curve C might also represent an agonist with lower receptor affinity (K_a) or potency than curve B (or both). Curve A represents an agonist with higher receptor affinity or potency than curve B.

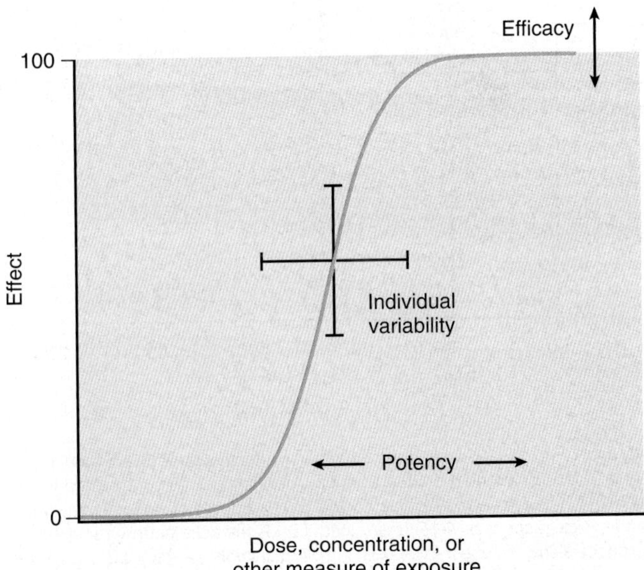

Figure 19-35 Relationship among efficacy, potency, and individual variability as they relate to a typical sigmoidal dose- or concentration-versus-response curve.

more often, animals) to whom it is administered. The therapeutic index of a drug is the ratio between the LD_{50} and the ED_{50} (LD_{50}/ED_{50}). The larger the therapeutic index of a drug, the safer the drug for clinical administration. The relationship among ED_{50}, LD_{50}, and therapeutic index is shown in Figure 19-36.

Drug Interactions

Actions at the Same Receptor

Agonists and antagonists modify dose-response relationships for concurrently administered drugs. If two agonists have identical affinity (K_a) for a given receptor and identical effectiveness in coupling to second messengers, their resultant dose-response curves should be superimposable. However, if two agonists have different receptor affinities despite identical effectiveness in coupling to second messengers, their dose-response curves will be parallel (with the rightward-shifted curve corresponding to the drug with lower receptor affinity; see Fig. 19-34, curves B and C). When two agonists are administered simultaneously, the clinical effect depends on the total amount of drug-receptor complexes generated.

As stated earlier, full agonists produce maximal responses, whereas partial agonists produce less than maximal response at the same receptor occupancy. The precise molecular mechanism that explains this blunting of the maximal response by partial agonists is not known, but it may relate to the ability of full agonists to stabilize the activated state, R*, most effectively. Partial agonists shift the dose-response curve of the agonist to the right (B → C in Fig. 19-34).

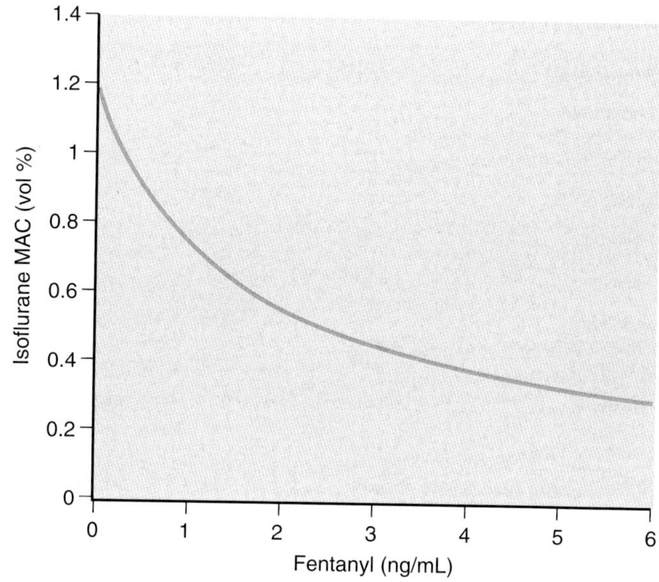

Figure 19-37 Influence of fentanyl on the minimum alveolar concentration (MAC) of isoflurane associated with a 50% probability of movement on incision. Modest amounts of fentanyl greatly reduce the MAC of isoflurane, but a ceiling in MAC reduction is quickly reached. Even with large opioid doses, some isoflurane is required to ablate the movement response. *(Adapted from McEwan AI, Smith C, Dyar O, et al: Isoflurane minimum alveolar concentration reduction by fentanyl. Anesthesiology 78:864-869, 1993.)*

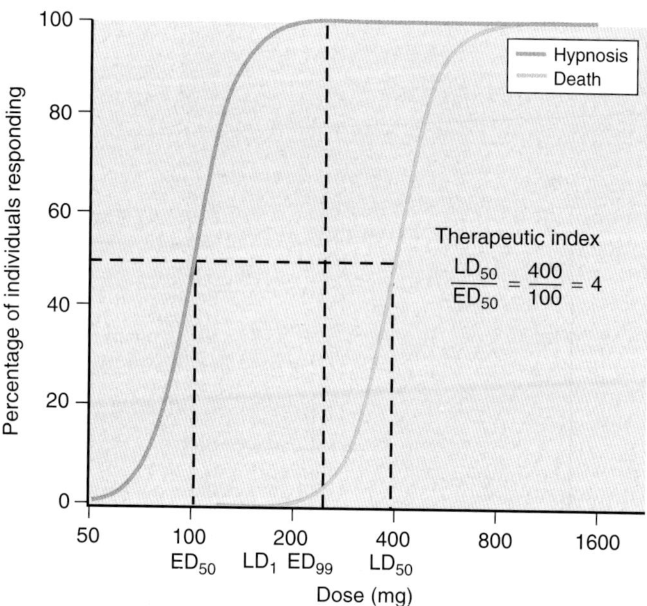

Figure 19-36 Relationship between median effective dose (ED_{50}), median lethal dose (LD_{50}), and therapeutic index. These curves were generated from data in which animals were injected with varying doses of a sedative-hypnotic and clinical responses were determined. ED_{50} is the dose of drug required to produce a specific effect (hypnosis) in 50% of animals to which it is administered (*left curve*). LD_{50} is the dose of drug required to produce death in 50% of animals to which the drug is administered (*right curve*). The therapeutic index of the drug is the ratio between LD_{50} and ED_{50} (LD_{50}/ED_{50}). LD_1 is the lethal dose in 1% of the population. ED_{99} is the effective dose in 99% of the population. As drawn, LD_1 is less than ED_{99}, which would not be clinically acceptable.

The addition of a competitive antagonist also shifts the dose-response curve to the right (B → C in Fig. 19-34). By contrast, the addition of a noncompetitive agonist shifts the dose response curve to the right and reduces the efficacy of the agonist because maximal response cannot be achieved at any agonist dose since blockade of effect (noncompetitive antagonism) cannot be reversed.

Actions at Different Receptors

Anesthesia is the practice of applied drug interactions. As discussed in Chapter 39, general anesthesia is, at a minimum, a combination of hypnosis, immobility, and antinociception. As such, there has been extensive work looking at the interaction of hypnotic drugs, which include inhaled anesthetics and GABA agonists (propofol, barbiturates, etomidate, and benzodiazepines), muscle relaxants, and analgesic drugs.

A prototypical study of the relationship between inhaled anesthetics and opioids is the study of McEwan and colleagues, who characterized the interaction between isoflurane and fentanyl.[19] The isoflurane concentration associated with a 50% chance of moving on incision (minimum alveolar concentration [MAC]) versus the plasma fentanyl concentration is shown in Figure 19-37. Initially, the interaction is profound, with a 50% reduction in isoflurane MAC at a plasma fentanyl concentration of 1.7 ng/mL and a 63% reduction in isoflurane MAC associated with a plasma fentanyl concentration of 3 ng/mL. Beyond 3 ng/mL, there is very little benefit from additional fentanyl. The first clinical implication of this interaction is that a modest amount of opioid dramatically reduces the concentration of inhaled anesthetic required to prevent movement. The second clinical implication is that even with huge doses of opioids, some hypnotic component must be added to the anesthetic to prevent movement.

Similar work has been done for propofol. In a series of elegant studies, Vuyk and colleagues characterized the interaction of propofol with alfentanil.[20] As shown in Figure 19-38, the interaction is markedly synergistic, with modest amounts of alfentanil greatly decreasing the amount of propofol associated with a 50% chance of response to intubation or surgical incision. Vuyk and colleagues also documented the interaction of propofol and alfentanil on return of consciousness, likewise shown in Figure 19-38. As discussed in Chapter 28, studies such as these provide the basis for rational selection of opioids and design of optimal opioid infusion regimens.

Hendrickx and colleagues have recently surveyed the interaction of anesthetic drugs that affect nociception, analgesia, and hypnosis.[21] They examined two end points: "hypnosis," defined as loss of consciousness in humans and loss of the righting reflex in animals, and immobility, defined as loss of the movement response to noxious stimulation in a nonparalyzed subject.[21] As shown in Figure 19-39, the interaction between pairs of intravenous drugs and between intravenous drugs and inhaled anesthetics is typically synergistic. The exception is the *N*-methyl-D-aspartate (NMDA) antagonists, ketamine and nitrous oxide, which demonstrate synergy, additivity, or infra-additivity in different models. By contrast, the inhaled anesthetics are strictly additive in their interactions with other inhaled anesthetics, suggesting a common mechanism of action.

Classic interaction studies such as those just described examine the concentrations associated with a particular response (such as a 50% chance of moving) for two drugs evaluated separately and in combination. However, a more general view is that any combination of two drugs is associated with a response. This is best viewed as a "response surface" in which the *x* and *y* axes of the surface are concentrations (or doses) of drugs A and B and the *z* axis is the response to the particular combination. Minto and colleagues have proposed a mathematical framework for response surfaces for a variety of interaction surfaces of interest to anesthesiologists.[22] Figure 19-40 shows six examples of possible response surfaces, depending on the nature of the interaction.

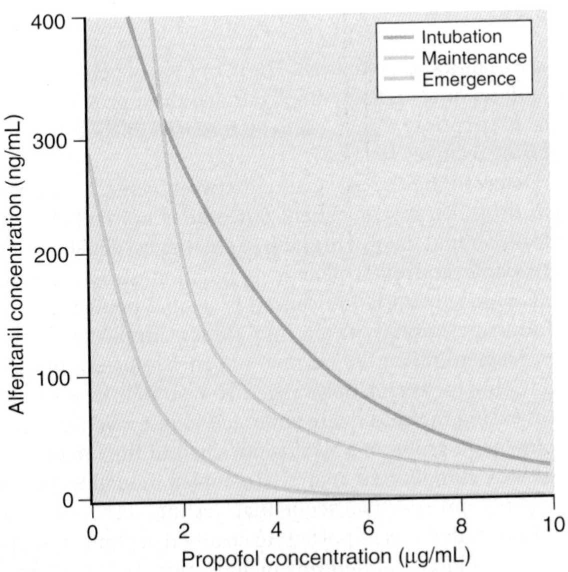

Figure 19-38 Influence of alfentanil on the concentration of propofol associated with a 50% probability of response to intubation and incision, as well as a 50% probability of awakening at the end of surgery. Moderate doses of alfentanil greatly reduce the dose of propofol required to ablate the response to noxious stimulation. However, below propofol concentrations of approximately 2 μg/mL, even large doses of alfentanil cannot reliably ablate the response to noxious stimulation. *(Adapted from Vuyk J, Lim T, Engbers FH, et al: The pharmacodynamic interaction of propofol and alfentanil during lower abdominal surgery in women. Anesthesiology 83:8-22, 1995.)*

Variability in Drug Response

Anesthesiologists observe individual variation in clinical response to administered drugs every day. This variability can occur as a result of differences in pharmacokinetic processes such as absorption, distribution, metabolism, and excretion of a drug. Individual variation can also be due to differences in pharmacodynamics, such as intrinsic differences in receptor sensitivity, upregulation and downregulation, and alterations in other targets that affect drug action. The relationship between patient variability and a typical dose-response curve is shown in Figure 19-35. Sources of pharmacokinetic and pharmacodynamic variability include genetics, patient physiology, and drug interactions.

Pharmacogenetics

The field of pharmacology that describes effects of genetic variation on drug action is called *pharmacogenetics*. Pharmacogenetics refers to genetic diversity in the body's absorption, metabolism, and distribution of drugs (inborn pharmacokinetic variability) or in the body's response to the drug, as might be caused by differences in receptor structure or patient physiology (inborn pharmacodynamic variability). To understand the effect of genetic variation on pharmacokinetics and pharmacodynamics, it is important to first define genetic variants, or polymorphisms.

Genetic polymorphism refers to any type of variation in a gene. More precise language is used to describe each specific type of genetic variant. When one nucleotide is exchanged for another, this variant is called a *single-nucleotide polymorphism* (SNP). The rare substituted nucleotide is defined as the minor allele, whereas the more common "wild-type" nucleotide is defined as the major allele. Most SNPs are biallelic, with only two nucleotides possible, either the minor or the major allele. In rare cases, SNPs can be triallelic, with two possible minor alleles and three total possible nucleotides present. With four total nucleotides available in DNA, it is theoretically possible to have each of the four nucleotides represented, but this almost never happens. We will confine our discussion to biallelic SNPs because they are the most common.

Allele frequency refers to the frequency of the minor allele, notated $f(-)$. The frequency of the major allele is therefore $1-f(-)$. Because this is the minor allele, by definition $f(-)$ is less than 0.5. Individuals have two copies of each allele, so there are three possible combinations of biallelic SNPs: AA, Aa, aa, in which A is a major allele and a is a minor allele. The Hardy-Weinberg equation provides the frequency of each of these combinations based on the generally correct assumption that paring of alleles is random:

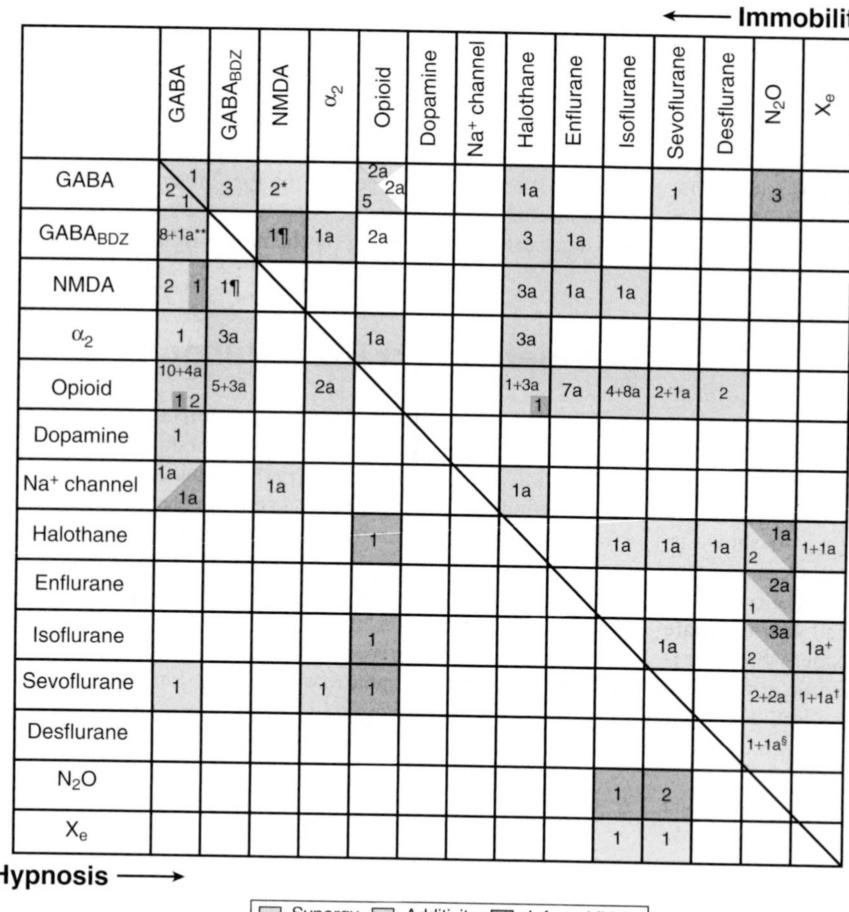

	GABA	$GABA_{BDZ}$	NMDA	α_2	Opioid	Dopamine	Na^+ channel	Halothane	Enflurane	Isoflurane	Sevoflurane	Desflurane	N_2O	X_e
GABA	2 / 1 / 1	3	2*		2a / 2a / 5			1a			1		3	
$GABA_{BDZ}$	8+1a**		1¶	1a	2a			3	1a					
NMDA	2 / 1	1¶						3a	1a	1a				
α_2	1	3a			1a			3a						
Opioid	10+4a / 1 / 2	5+3a		2a				1+3a / 1	7a	4+8a	2+1a	2		
Dopamine	1													
Na^+ channel	1a / 1a		1a					1a						
Halothane					1					1a	1a	1a	1a / 2	1+1a
Enflurane													2a / 1	
Isoflurane					1						1a		3a / 2	1a⁺
Sevoflurane	1			1	1								2+2a	1+1a†
Desflurane													1+1a§	
N_2O										1	2			
X_e										1	1			

Figure 19-39 Summary of drug interactions in humans and animals for hypnosis (loss of consciousness in humans, loss of righting reflex in animals) and immobility (loss of movement response to noxious stimulation). The numbers in each cell refer to the number of papers supporting the finding. γ-Aminobutyric acid (GABA) = propofol, thiopental, methohexital, etomidate; $GABA_{BDZ}$ = midazolam, diazepam; *N*-methyl-D-aspartate (NMDA) = ketamine; α_2 = dexmedetomidine, clonidine; opioid = morphine, alfentanil, fentanyl, sufentanil, remifentanil; dopamine = droperidol, metoclopramide; Na^+ channel = lidocaine, bupivacaine. *(From Hendrickx JFA, Eger EI, Sonner JM, Shafer SL: Is synergy the rule? A review of anesthetic interactions producing hypnosis and immobility. Anesth Analg 107:494-506, 2008.)*

aa (homozygous minor allele): $f(-)^2$
AA (homozygous major allele): $(1-f[-])^2$
Aa (heterozygous): $2\,f(-)\,(1-f[-])$

The sum of these frequencies is 1.

In addition to SNPs, other types of genetic variants include insertions/deletions, in which stretches of genomic DNA are missing or added, and microsatellite repeats, in which several nucleotides repeat (e.g., the dinucleotide repeat GCGCGCGC [n = 4 GC repeats] or the trinucleotide repeat TACTACTACTACTACTAC [n = 6 TAC repeats]). The number of repeats in a microsatellite correlates with some diseases and can be used in genome-wide scans to identify chromosome regions associated with disease.

Catastrophic DNA changes often include DNA deletions or insertions that are not multiples of three in the coding region. Such changes result in a frameshift in the triplet nucleotide sequence used to encode amino acids in proteins, with the probable result being a nonsense protein. SNPs that change an encoded amino acid to a stop codon may also be catastrophic because they could result in a truncated protein.

Not all genetic variants have biologic consequences. Just as differences in eye color or fingerprint pattern do not have medical consequences, many genetic variants provide "background" variation without overt biologic consequences. In fact, genetic variants with biologic/medical effects represent the minority of all genetic variants known to exist. The sum total of genetic variation (with and without biologic implications) does provide a unique genetic fingerprint, a fact used in forensic science to identify suspects or relatives (or both).

Determining the association between genetic variants and disease, drug therapy, or patient outcome is not straightforward and ideally should involve the help of a statistical geneticist. Clinical covariants and even genetic population structure (loosely defined as genetic variation caused by global population movement) must be carefully taken into account in pharmacogenetic studies. Depending on the number of genes to be examined, statistical testing for association ranges from straightforward simple analyses (using the chi-square approach to test whether a variant or haplotype [a group of SNPs] is enriched in the target population) to very complicated analyses (complex modeling, permutation testing, prospective sequential testing, etc.). In clinical association studies it is important to ensure that clinical end point data are reproducible and ideally include intermediate end points such as protein levels or enzyme activity. As more clinically relevant human genetic variants become known, our knowledge of the role of genetics in drug response and patient outcome should be significantly enhanced.

Genetic Variability in Pharmacokinetics

Naturally occurring genetic variants can affect the activity of enzymes responsible for drug metabolism, most often by altering

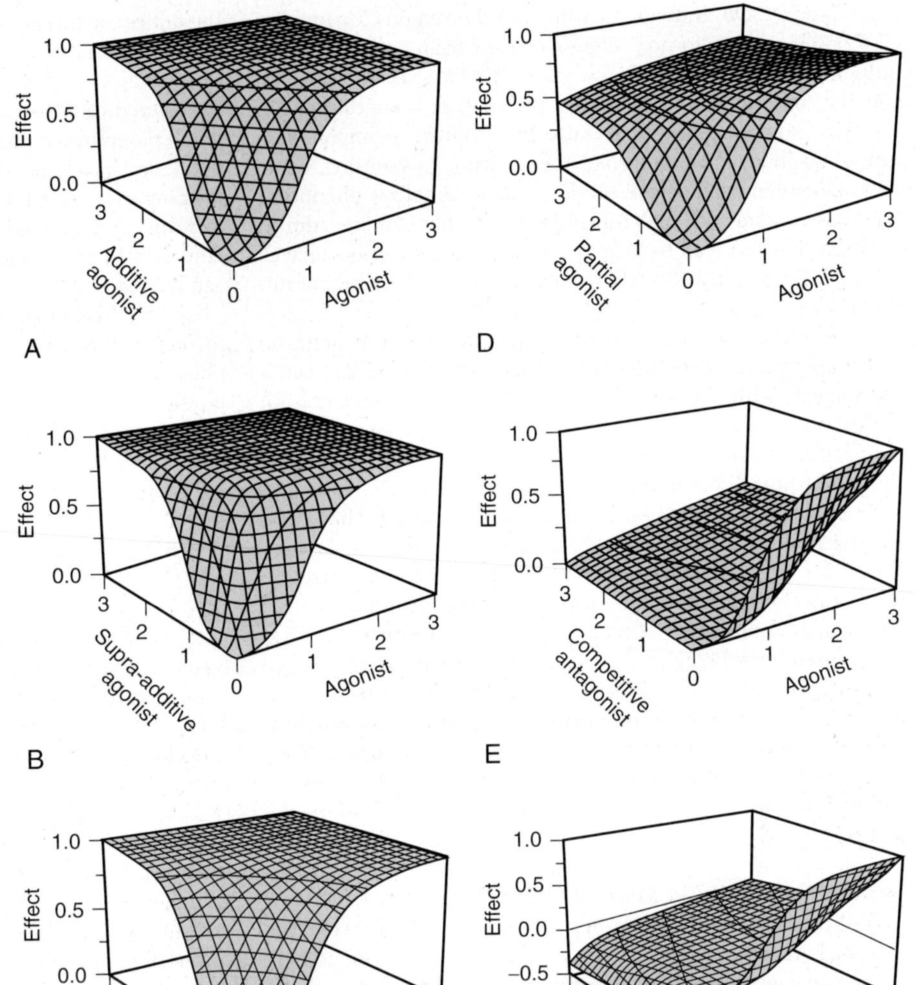

Figure 19-40 Response surfaces for potential pharmacodynamic interactions of anesthetic drugs. **A,** Additive interaction between two agonists that have the same mechanism of action (e.g., interaction of fentanyl and alfentanil). **B,** Supra-additive interaction between two agonists (e.g., isoflurane and fentanyl). **C,** Infra-additive interaction between two agonists (reported for cyclopropane and nitrous oxide). **D,** Partial agonist and full agonist (e.g., hypothetical interaction of nalbuphine and fentanyl). **E,** Competitive antagonist and full agonist (e.g., naloxone and fentanyl). **F,** Inverse agonist and full agonist (e.g., RO 19-4063 and midazolam).

a key amino acid in or near the site of enzymatic action. In practical terms, this enzymatic diversity is rarely evident in the absence of drug therapy. In the presence of drug therapy, pharmacogenetic variation in metabolism is evident as unexpected toxicity, duration of action, or lack of efficacy of administered drugs.

Of particular interest to anesthesiologists is the activity of cytochrome P450 (CYP) 3A4. This is the most abundant cytochrome in the liver and intestines and is responsible for the metabolism of almost half of all drugs, including many important drugs in anesthesia: opioids (fentanyl, alfentanil, sufentanil, methadone), benzodiazepines (diazepam, midazolam, alprazolam, triazolam), local anesthetics (cocaine, lidocaine, ropivacaine), steroids, calcium channel blockers, haloperidol, and halothane. Of the many described genetic mutants of the CYP3A4 enzyme, however, only two alter enzyme activity, with CYP3A4*18 decreasing and CYP3A4*19 increasing drug turnover.[23,24] It is important to note that most of these CYP3A4 studies have examined only heterozygous (Aa genotype) individuals thus far. This enzyme is readily inducible and inhibited by multiple substances. CYP3A4 induction and inhibition significantly overshadow the effects of currently described genetic variants.

In contrast to the lack of genetically important CYP3A4 variants, a different story exists for CYP2C19, the enzyme system responsible for metabolizing mephenytoin, omeprazole, diazepam, proguanil, propranolol, and certain antidepressants. Newly described SNPs in this gene, expressed most commonly in African Americans, appear to decrease the metabolism of these drugs in vitro.[25] Effects on drug plasma concentrations, clinical efficacy, and toxicity need further testing in prospective human clinical trials.

One of the best-studied pharmacogenetic variants is CYP2D6, also called “debrisoquine hydroxylase” or “sparteine oxygenase.” About 7% to 10% of white individuals are homozygous for an inactive variant of CYP2D6. This alters metabolism for at least 40 drugs. For example, codeine is a prodrug with no intrinsic analgesic efficacy. Codeine, oxycodone, and hydrocodone all undergo *O*-demethylation to morphine, oxymorphone, and hydromorphone, their more pharmacologically active metabolites, via CYP2D6. Individuals who are homozygous for inactive CYP2D6 have little to no analgesic efficacy from codeine.[26] Such individuals are likely to receive very little anesthesia from oral codeine and need to be rescued by another analgesic agent. CYP2D6 polymorphisms have also been shown to impair dextromethorphan and metoprolol metabolism. In contrast, other CYP2D6 polymorphisms result in a rapid metabolizer phenotype that is associated with high morphine levels after codeine administration that can lead to toxicity. When patients can be assayed for CYP2D6 activity, this will become a useful screen before initiating pain therapy with opioids.

Anesthesiologists are familiar with the role of genetics in determining butyrylcholinesterase (pseudocholinesterase) activity. Subjects with abnormal butyrylcholinesterase are at risk for prolonged paralysis from succinylcholine and exaggerated systemic effects from ester-based local anesthetics. Not surprisingly, there are ethnic differences in cholinesterase activity. For example, individuals of Middle Eastern descent are likely to have less butyrylcholinesterase activity than those of European descent. Molecular approaches have permitted extensive characterization of plasma cholinesterase variants. Most of these variants are not "all or none" but rather reflect a spectrum of enzymatic activity.

There may be an evolutionary explanation for pharmacogenetic variability in metabolism. It is probable that variability in drug metabolism is a natural adaptive response to an environment that can present a huge variety of toxins. Enzymatic diversity is probably maintained through natural selection to ensure survival when we are confronted with novel environmental toxins.

Genetic Variability in Pharmacodynamics

In addition to variants that affect drug pharmacokinetics, it is now well recognized that genetic variants can alter drug activity by pharmacodynamic mechanisms. Biologically active genetic polymorphisms have been found in numerous receptors, second messenger systems, and ion channels. One of the most intensively studied receptors in this regard is β_2AR. Several β_2AR SNPs have particular relevance to this discussion.[27] One variant, located at −47(T/C) in the 5′-untranslated sequence (referred to as the 5′-leader cistron), increases levels of normal (nonvariant) β_2AR mRNA and protein by 72%. This increase in airway wild-type β_2AR expression is protective against methacholine challenge. Another β_2AR SNP present in the amino terminus is Arg16Gly. Expression of Gly at position 16 increases sensitivity to agonists[28] and enhances agonist-promoted downregulation.[29] Because β_2AR stimulation in vessels is important in mediating vasodilation, an SNP such as Gly16 that enhances desensitization (and therefore dampens receptor responsiveness) is not surprisingly associated with a higher incidence of higher blood pressure, hypertension, and cardiomyopathy. In contrast, patients who are homozygous for Arg at position 16 are poorly responsive to β-agonist therapy for asthma.[30] Interestingly Arg16Gly usually travels together with yet another β_2AR, Gln27Glu, such that Gly16 usually occurs with Glu27. The Glu27 variant is also associated with enhanced responsiveness to β_2AR agonists.[29] This region of the β_2AR is said to be in linkage disequilibrium, with the three SNPs defining a haplotype (regions of DNA that travel together). Gly16, Arg19 (another SNP variant), and Glu27 or Arg16, Cys19, and Gln27 are the two possible haplotypes. This has practical implications because only one of the SNPs in the haplotype needs to be genotyped to infer the entire haplotype. This greatly enhances power and decreases cost in genetic association studies. Finally, another β_2AR SNP (Thr164Ile), located in the fourth membrane-spanning domain, has altered catecholamine binding (lower affinity for isoproterenol, epinephrine, and norepinephrine), along with markedly depressed basal and agonist-stimulated adenylyl cyclase activity in comparison to wild-type Thr164. This poorer coupling appears to result in depressed myocardial function and congestive heart failure, with the variant particularly enriched in heart transplant candidates.

It is likely that many forms of genetically based variability in response to drugs reflect the interaction of many polymorphisms that subtly affect receptor structure, cellular function, and physiologic response. Understanding the interaction of multiple genes on the variability of drug response presents daunting technical challenges in pharmacogenetic research.

Patient Physiology

Age

Total body water is decreased in the elderly. One pharmacokinetic result is a reduced initial mixing volume. This smaller central volume of distribution leads to higher peak concentrations after a bolus or during the early part of an infusion in elderly patients. A decreased central volume of distribution partly accounts for the increased sensitivity of elderly patients to many anesthetic drugs (also see Chapter 71).

Aging is also associated with decreased lean body mass and increased body fat. Because the lipid content of elderly patients is higher than that of young patients, elderly patients have more potential for lipophilic drugs to accumulate in peripheral volumes of distribution, which may be one factor behind the increased duration of effect for many anesthetic drugs seen in the elderly.

Liver volume, liver blood flow, and hepatic metabolic capacity decrease with advanced age. These changes in hepatic physiology account for the decreased clearance of opioids, hypnotics, benzodiazepines, and muscle relaxants and contribute to the increased sensitivity of elderly subjects to anesthetic drugs.

Age per se only modestly reduces cardiac output in the absence of hypertension, coronary artery disease, valvular heart disease, or other cardiovascular pathology. Advancing age can thus be expected to modestly reduce intercompartmental clearance of anesthetic drugs. The effect of decreased intercompartmental clearance is to increase initial plasma concentrations during drug administration. After termination of drug administration, the role of decreased intercompartmental clearance is complex. In general, plasma concentrations will decrease more rapidly after long infusions when intercompartmental clearance is decreased.

Albumin and α_1-acid glycoprotein are the primary sites of protein binding. The albumin concentration decreases with advancing age, hepatic disease, and malnutrition. In contrast, the α_1-acid glycoprotein concentration increases with advancing age and acute disease. Thus, the effects of age and disease on protein binding depend on which protein binds the drug. For example, because diazepam binds primarily to albumin, the free fraction of diazepam increases in elderly patients. This may partly explain the increased sensitivity in elderly subjects. In contrast, lidocaine binds primarily to α_1-acid glycoprotein. In elderly patients, increased α_1-acid glycoprotein reduces the free fraction of lidocaine, which may contribute to reduced lidocaine clearance.

Although important age-related pharmacokinetic differences have been investigated in detail, there is a paucity of data addressing pharmacodynamic differences between age groups. Overall, the presence or absence of age-related pharmacodynamic differences appears to depend on the drug. For example, both antiepileptic agents and digoxin have been examined in adults and children, and the effective plasma concentration is the same. This finding suggests that for these two types of drugs, no age-related differences in pharmacodynamic responses occur. However many drugs with CNS effects (e.g., thiopental,[31] midazolam,[32] opioids,[33,34] propofol[35]) appear to be intrinsically more potent in the elderly, and this change in potency has been quantitated in pharmacodynamic models. Understanding the biologic basis of increased sensitivity in the elderly to anesthetic and perioperative drugs is an area of active investigation by many researchers.

Disease States

Various diseases contribute to variation in drug response. Although diseases frequently result in pharmacokinetic variations (e.g., decreased liver perfusion in heart failure or decreased elimination in renal failure), pharmacodynamic variation is also observed. Conditions such as diabetes, thyroid disease, adrenal disease, myasthenia gravis, and hypertension alter receptor function and therefore represent pharmacodynamic effects. Some diseases directly affect drug receptors. For example, in patients with myasthenia gravis, antibodies to the postsynaptic nicotinic acetylcholine receptor effectively decrease the number of receptors present. Muscle weakness characterizes the disease. As a result, these patients have less reserve at the neuromuscular junction and are exquisitely sensitive to muscle relaxants that act on the nicotinic acetylcholine receptor.

Drug Interactions

Pharmacokinetic Interactions

Historically, certain foods and drugs were known to inhibit drug metabolism. The inhibition of CYP3A4 by grapefruit juice is among the more dramatic of such interactions. As previously mentioned, CYP3A4 is responsible for nearly half of all drug metabolism. Ingestion of grapefruit juice has been shown to increase the plasma concentration of drugs metabolized by CYP3A4.[36] Many drugs also inhibit CYP3A4, including the antifungal drugs ketoconazole and itraconazole; the protease inhibitors ritonavir, indinavir, and saquinavir; the antibiotics troleandomycin, clarithromycin, erythromycin; and the selective serotonin reuptake inhibitors (SSRIs) fluoxetine and sertraline. Propofol also inhibits CYP3A4, although it is unclear whether there is any clinical consequence. Conversely, several drugs induce CYP3A4, thereby increasing the metabolism of 3A4 substrates. Such drugs include rifampin, rifabutin, tamoxifen, glucocorticoids, carbamazepine, and barbiturates and the herb Saint John's wort.

CYP2D6, responsible for the conversion of codeine to morphine, is also subject to inhibition. In particular, quinidine and the SSRIs fluoxetine and paroxetine produce significant inhibition at standard clinical doses. Thus, codeine, oxycodone, or hydrocodone would be relatively poor analgesic choices for patients taking SSRIs.

Anesthetics also interact pharmacokinetically with many drugs by reducing cardiac output and hepatic blood flow. The reduction in cardiac output probably decreases intercompartmental clearance of most drugs, whereas the reduction in hepatic blood flow would be expected to decrease the metabolic clearance of drugs with high hepatic extraction ratios.

Pharmacodynamic Drug Interactions

Drug-Time Interaction: Desensitization

Desensitization is broadly defined as waning of physiologic responsiveness to a drug over time. For example, acute desensitization ("tachyphylaxis") typically occurs to sodium nitroprusside. Therefore, it is often necessary to increase the nitroprusside infusion rate over time to maintain the desired amount of vasodilation.

In general, stimulation of receptor pathways results in the activation of kinases (e.g., protein kinase A, G protein–coupled receptor kinases, protein kinase C) that phosphorylate specific regions of the receptor and thereby prevent further interaction of the receptor with G proteins or second messengers, or with both. Thus, continuous stimulation of a receptor provides a negative-feedback mechanism for receptor stimulation that results in desensitization. Although desensitization was initially thought to occur only at the receptor level, it is now well recognized that alterations in G proteins and second messengers also occur in response to agonist stimulation. Effectively, desensitization shifts the dose-response curve to the right (e.g., Fig. 19-34, curve B → C) or decreases the maximal drug effect (or both). Thus, both efficacy and potency can be diminished by desensitization.

Desensitization of receptor responses is a feature of many diseases present in the aging population and is therefore relevant to consider during the perioperative period. Common diseases in which desensitization is important include congestive heart failure, hypertension, and diabetes. A hallmark of each of these diseases is elevation of hormone (agonist) concentrations. In the case of congestive heart failure, poor cardiac output induces compensatory sympathetic nervous system stimulation, which often results in a doubling of circulating catecholamine concentrations (in particular, the sympathetic neurotransmitter norepinephrine). On a long-term basis, this results in desensitization of the myocardial βAR signal transduction pathway; specifically, β_1AR density and function decrease (75%) with relative sparing of β_2ARs (25%). G_i levels also increase without a change in G_s. Furthermore, G protein–coupled receptor kinase concentrations increase and modulation of adenylyl cyclase isoforms occurs. The physiologic effects of changes important in desensitization of myocardial βARs have been examined with the use of transgenic and knock-out mice (see Table 19-1 and the earlier discussion of molecular pharmacology). To break the cycle of elevated agonist exposure and resultant desensitization, cardiologists now cautiously use long-term, low-dose βAR antagonists (approximately a 10th the usual dose for hypertension or myocardial ischemia) in patients with congestive heart failure. This therapy has been shown to improve functional classification and longevity.

Drug-Time Interaction: Increased Receptor Sensitivity

The opposite of desensitization is increased receptor sensitivity. Long-term exposure to a drug often results in compensatory responses by the receptor system. For example, when a receptor antagonist is administered on a long-term basis, receptor number (density) often increases. If the receptor antagonist is suddenly discontinued, exaggerated responsiveness to agonist may occur. This is the rationale for continuing long-term βAR antagonists during the perioperative period. Abrupt discontinuation of these drugs leaves the myocardium vulnerable to an exaggerated heart rate and inotropic responses to routine procedures such as tracheal intubation, thereby potentially leading to myocardial ischemia and infarction. Finally, a much-feared anesthetic example of increased receptor sensitivity is the upregulation of nicotinic receptors at the neuromuscular junction in patients with spinal cord injuries, burns, or prolonged immobilization. The potential for such patients to have a life-threatening hyperkalemic response to succinylcholine is described in detail in Chapter 29.

Drug-Drug Interactions

There are a huge variety of mechanisms by which drugs can interact pharmacodynamically. The nature of pharmacodynamic drug-drug interactions is so diverse that an anesthesiologist can safely assume that there will be some interaction between anesthetic drugs and virtually all drugs that have action on either the CNS or the cardiovascular system.

Some of these drug interactions, such as those between opioids and hypnotics, are fundamental to the practice of anesthesia and were discussed earlier. An example of interactions between anesthetics and nonanesthetics is the influence of nonanesthetic drugs on the MAC of inhaled anesthetics. Drugs that increase central catecholamines in general increase MAC. This has been clearly demonstrated for amphetamines (acute exposure), ephedrine, and monoamine oxidase inhibitors. Conversely, drugs that decrease central catecholamines decrease MAC. This has been shown for methyldopa, reserpine, and α_2-adrenergic agonists. It has also been demonstrated for chronic amphetamine use.

Summary

This chapter reviews general pharmacology by examining the basic principles of pharmacokinetics, pharmacodynamics, and sources of pharmacologic variability. Careful consideration of these principles should permit the anesthesiologist to understand drug movement from the site of administration through various body compartments to the site of action and the mechanisms by which drugs act on receptors to bring about the desired clinical effect. Many factors may alter the pharmacokinetic and pharmacodynamic processes by which drugs exert their effects, including genetics, age, disease, and concurrent drug therapy. Understanding basic pharmacologic processes and how they may differ between individuals should facilitate drug titration for each patient. There is a biologic basis for finding just the right drug in just the right dose to provide safe and effective care of perioperative patients. Our knowledge of the biologic basis for finding the right dose of the right drug for each individual is currently in its infancy but is rapidly growing with new discoveries.

Suggested Reading

Boroujerdi M: Pharmacokinetics. New York, McGraw-Hill, 2002.

Bowdle TA, Horita A, Kharasch ED: The Pharmacologic Basis of Anesthesiology. New York, Churchill Livingstone, 1994.

Chalmers DT, Behan DP: The use of constitutively active GPCRs in drug discovery and functional genomics. Nat Rev Drug Discov 1:599-608, 2002.

Clarke WP, Bond RA: The elusive nature of intrinsic efficacy. Trends Pharmacol Sci 19:270-276, 1998.

Conti-Tronconi BM, McLane KE, Raftery MA, et al: The nicotinic acetylcholine receptor: Structure and autoimmune pathology. Crit Rev Biochem Mol Biol 29:69-123, 1994.

Eckhart AD, Koch WJ: Transgenic studies of cardiac adrenergic receptor regulation. J Pharmacol Exp Ther 299:1-5, 2001.

Eger EI: Anesthetic Uptake and Action. Baltimore, Williams & Wilkins, 1974.

Freedman NJ, Lefkowitz RJ: Desensitization of G protein–coupled receptors. Recent Prog Horm Res 51:319-351, 1996.

Greco WR, Bravo G, Parsons JC: The search for synergy: A critical review from a response surface perspective. Pharmacol Rev 47:331-385, 1995.

Hamm HE: The many faces of G protein signaling. J Biol Chem 273:669-672, 1998.

Jenkinson DH, Barnard EA, Hoyer D, et al: International Union of Pharmacology Committee on Receptor Nomenclature and Drug Classification. IX. Recommendations on terms and symbols in quantitative pharmacology. Pharmacol Rev 47:255-266, 1995.

Kalow W: Pharmacogenetics in biological perspective. Pharmacol Rev 49:369-379, 1997.

Kenakin T: Inverse, protean, and ligand-selective agonism: Matters of receptor conformation. FASEB J 15:598-611, 2001.

Kenakin T: Efficacy at G-protein–coupled receptors. Nat Rev Drug Discov 1:102-110, 2002.

Kenakin T, Onaran O: The ligand paradox between affinity and efficacy: Can you be there and not make a difference? Trends Pharmacol Sci 23:275-280, 2002.

Krumins AM, Barber R: The stability of the agonist beta$_2$-adrenergic receptor–G$_s$ complex: Evidence for agonist-specific states. Mol Pharmacol 52:144-154, 1997.

Lambert JJ, Belelli D, Hill-Venning C, et al: Neurosteroid modulation of native and recombinant GABA$_A$ receptors. Cell Mol Neurobiol 6:155-174, 1996.

Landry Y, Gies JP: Heterotrimeric G proteins control diverse pathways of transmembrane signaling, a base for drug discovery. Mini Rev Med Chem 2:361-372, 2002.

Liu JG, Anand KJ: Protein kinases modulate the cellular adaptations associated with opioid tolerance and dependence. Brain Res Rev 38:1-19, 2001.

Perry SJ, Lefkowitz RJ: Arresting developments in heptahelical receptor signaling and regulation. Trends Cell Biol 12:130-138, 2002.

Pierce KL, Premont RT, Lefkowitz RJ: Seven-transmembrane receptors. Nat Rev Mol Cell Biol 3:639-650, 2002.

Rathz DA, Gregory KN, Fang Y, et al: Hierarchy of polymorphic variation and desensitization permutations relative to beta-1 and beta-2 adrenergic signaling. J Biol Chem 278:10784-10789, 2003.

Rescigno A: Foundations of Pharmacokinetics. New York, Kluwer Academic/Plenum, 2003.

Rockman HA, Koch WJ, Lefkowitz RJ: Cardiac function in genetically engineered mice with altered adrenergic receptor signaling. Am J Physiol 272:H1553-H1559, 1997.

Rogers JF, Nafziger AN, Bertino JS Jr: Pharmacogenetics affects dosing, efficacy, and toxicity of cytochrome P450–metabolized drugs. Am J Med 113:746-750, 2002.

Ross EM, Kenakin TP: Pharmacodynamics: Mechanisms of drug action and the relationship between drug concentration and effect. *In* Hardman JG, Limbird LE (eds): The Pharmacological Basis of Therapeutics, 10th ed. New York, McGraw-Hill, 2002.

Rowland M, Tozer TN: Clinical Pharmacokinetics: Concepts and Applications, 3rd ed. Baltimore, Williams & Wilkins, 1995.

Schwinn DA (ed): Scientific Principles of Anesthesia, vol 2. Philadelphia, Current Medicine, 1997.

Shuldiner AR: Transgenic animals. N Engl J Med 334:653-655, 1996.

Skiba NP, Hamm HE: How G$_s\alpha$ activates adenylyl cyclase. Nat Struct Biol 5:88-92, 1998.

Svoboda P, Novotny J: Hormone-induced subcellular redistribution of trimeric G proteins. Cell Mol Life Sci 59:501-512, 2002.

Tang WJ, Hurley JH: Catalytic mechanism and regulation of mammalian adenylyl cyclases. Mol Pharmacol 54:231-240, 1998.

Tucek S, Michal P, Vlachova V: Modelling the consequences of receptor–G-protein promiscuity. Trends Pharmacol Sci 23:171-176, 2002.

Vaughan M: Signaling by heterotrimeric G proteins minireview series. J Biol Chem 273:17297, 1998.

Watson J, Gilman M, Witkowski J, et al: Recombinant DNA, 3rd ed. New York, Scientific American, 2007.

Weinshilboum R: Inheritance and drug response. N Engl J Med 348:529-537, 2003.

Wilkinson GR: Pharmacokinetics: The dynamics of drug absorption, distribution, and elimination. *In* Hardman JG, Limbird LE (eds): The Pharmacological Basis of Therapeutics, 10th ed. New York, McGraw-Hill, 2002.

References

1. Krejcie TC, Avram MJ, Gentry WB, et al: A recirculatory model of the pulmonary uptake and pharmacokinetics of lidocaine based on analysis of arterial and mixed venous data from dogs. J Pharmacokinet Biopharm 25:169-190, 1997.
2. Shafer S: Principles of pharmacokinetics and pharmacodynamics. *In* Longnecker DE, Tinker JH, Morgan GE (eds): Principles and Practice of Anesthesiology, 2nd ed. St Louis, Mosby–Year Book, 1997.
3. Wagner JG: Pharmacokinetics for the Pharmaceutical Scientist. Lancaster, PA, Technomic Publishing, 1993.
4. Wilkinson GR, Shand DG: Commentary: A physiological approach to hepatic drug clearance. Clin Pharmacol Ther 18:377-390, 1975.
5. Cockcroft DW, Gault MH: Prediction of creatinine clearance from serum creatinine. Nephron 16:31-41, 1976.
6. Ebling WF, Wada DR, Stanski DR: From piecewise to full physiologic pharmacokinetic modeling: Applied to thiopental disposition in the rat. J Pharmacokinet Biopharm 22:259-292, 1994.
7. Bjorkman S, Wada DR, Stanski DR: Application of physiologic models to predict the influence of changes in body composition and blood flows on the pharmacokinetics of fentanyl and alfentanil in patients. Anesthesiology 88:657-667, 1998.
8. Youngs EJ, Shafer SL: Basic pharmacokinetic and pharmacodynamic principles. *In* White PF (ed): Textbook of Intravenous Anesthesia. Baltimore, Williams & Wilkins, 1997, p 10.
9. Scott JC, Ponganis KV, Stanski DR: EEG quantitation of narcotic effect: The comparative pharmacodynamics of fentanyl and alfentanil. Anesthesiology 62:234-241, 1985.
10. Mandema JW, Kuck MT, Danhof M: Differences in intrinsic efficacy of benzodiazepines are reflected in their concentration-EEG effect relationship. Br J Pharmacol 105:164-170, 1992.
11. Milano CA, Allen LF, Rockman HA, et al: Enhanced myocardial function in transgenic mice overexpressing the beta 2-adrenergic receptor. Science 264:582-586, 1994.
12. Engelhardt S, Grimmer Y, Fan G-H, Lohse MJ: Constitutive activity of the human β_1-adrenergic receptor in β_1-receptor transgenic mice. Mol Pharmacol 60:712-717, 2001.
13. Liu X, Callaerts-Vegh Z, Evans KLJ, Bond RA: Chronic infusion of β-adrenoceptor antagonist and inverse agonists decreases elevated protein kinase A activity in transgenic mice with cardiac-specific overexpression of human β_2ARs. J Cardiovasc Pharmacol 40:448-455, 2002.
14. Stapelfeldt WH: The autonomic nervous system. *In* Schwinn DA (ed): Scientific Principles of Anesthesia, vol 2. Philadelphia, Current Medicine, 1998.
15. Berkowitz DE: Cellular signal transduction. *In* Schwinn DA (ed): Scientific Principles of Anesthesia, vol 2. Philadelphia, Current Medicine, 1998.
16. Firestone L, Quinlan J, Gyulai F: Mechanisms of anesthetic action. *In* Schwinn DA (ed): Scientific Principles of Anesthesia, vol 2. Philadelphia, Current Medicine, 1998.
17. Krasowski MD, Harrison NL: General anaesthetic actions on ligand-gated ion channels. Cell Mol Life Sci 55:1278-1303, 1999.
18. Jurd R, Arras M, Lambert S, et al: General anesthetic actions in vivo strongly attenuated by a point mutation in the GABA(A) receptor beta3 subunit. FASEB J 17:250-252, 2003.
19. McEwan AI, Smith C, Dyar O, et al: Isoflurane minimum alveolar concentration reduction by fentanyl. Anesthesiology 78:864-869, 1993.
20. Vuyk J, Lim T, Engbers FH, et al: The pharmacodynamic interaction of propofol and alfentanil during lower abdominal surgery in women. Anesthesiology 83:8-22, 1995.
21. Hendrickx JFA, Eger EI, Sonner JM, Shafer SL: Is synergy the rule? A review of anesthetic interactions producing hypnosis and immobility. Anesth Analg 107:494-506, 2008.
22. Minto CF, Schnider TW, Short TG, et al: Response surface model for anesthetic drug interactions. Anesthesiology 92:1603-1616, 2000.
23. Lamba JK, Lin YS, Thummel K, et al: Common allelic variants of cytochrome P4503A4 and their prevalence in different populations. Pharmacogenetics 12:121-132, 2002.
24. Dai D, Tang J, Rose R, et al: Identification of variants of CYP3A4 and characterization of their abilities to metabolize testosterone and chlorpyrifos. J Pharmacol Exp Ther 299:825-831, 2001.
25. Blaisdell J, Mohrenweiser H, Jackson J, et al: Identification and functional characterization of new potentially defective alleles of human CYP2C19. Pharmacogenetics 12:703-711, 2002.
26. Poulsen L, Brosen K, Arendt-Nielsen L, et al: Codeine and morphine in extensive and poor metabolizers of sparteine: Pharmacokinetics, analgesic effect and side effects. Eur J Clin Pharmacol 51:289-295, 1996.
27. Johnson JA, Terra SG: β-Adrenergic receptor polymorphisms: Cardiovascular disease associations and pharmacogenetics. Pharm Res 19:1779-1787, 2002.
28. Large V, Hellstrom L, Reynisdottir S, et al: Human beta-2 adrenoceptor gene polymorphisms are highly frequent in obesity and associate with altered adipocyte beta-2 adrenoceptor function. J Clin Invest 100:3005-3013, 1997.
29. Dishy V, Sofowora GG, Xie HG, et al: The effect of common polymorphisms of the beta2-adrenergic receptor on agonist-mediated vascular desensitization. N Engl J Med 345:1020-1035, 2002.
30. Israel E: Genetics and the variability of treatment response in asthma. J Allergy Clin Immunol 115:S532-S538, 2005.
31. Homer TD, Stanski DR: The effect of increasing age on thiopental disposition and anesthetic requirement. Anesthesiology 62:714-724, 1985.
32. Bell GD, Spickett GP, Reeve PA, et al: Intravenous midazolam for upper gastrointestinal endoscopy: A study of 800 consecutive cases relating dose to age and sex of patient. Br J Clin Pharmacol 23:241-243, 1987.
33. Scott JC, Stanski DR: Decreased fentanyl and alfentanil dose requirements with age. A simultaneous pharmacokinetic and pharmacodynamic evaluation. J Pharmacol Exp Ther 240:159-166, 1987.
34. Minto CF, Schnider TW, Egan TD, et al: Influence of age and gender on the pharmacokinetics and pharmacodynamics of remifentanil. I. Model development. Anesthesiology 86:10-23, 1997.
35. Schnider TW, Minto CF, Shafer SL, et al: The influence of age on propofol pharmacodynamics. Anesthesiology 90:1502-1516, 1999.
36. Bailey DG, Malcolm J, Arnold O, Spence JD: Grapefruit juice–drug interactions. Br J Clin Pharmacol 46:101-110, 1998.

Misha Perouansky, Robert A. Pearce, and Hugh C. Hemmings Jr.

20 Inhaled Anesthetics: Mechanisms of Action

Key Points

1. Anesthesia consists of separable and independent components or substates, each of which involves distinct, but possibly overlapping, mechanisms at different sites in the central nervous system.
2. The potency of general anesthetics correlates with their solubility in oil, indicating the importance of their interaction with hydrophobic targets.
3. General anesthetics act by binding directly to amphiphilic cavities in proteins. Binding sites are being identified by a combination of site-directed mutagenesis and high-resolution structural analysis of anesthetic binding.
4. The effects of inhaled anesthetics cannot be explained by a single molecular mechanism. Rather, multiple targets contribute to the effects of each agent.
5. The immobilizing effect of inhaled anesthetics involves a site of action in the spinal cord, whereas sedation/hypnosis and amnesia involve supraspinal mechanisms.
6. Volatile inhaled anesthetics enhance inhibitory synaptic transmission postsynaptically by potentiating ligand-gated ion channels activated by γ-aminobutyric acid (GABA) and glycine, extrasynaptically by enhancing GABA receptors and leak currents, and presynaptically by enhancing basal GABA release.
7. Inhaled anesthetics suppress excitatory synaptic transmission presynaptically by reducing glutamate release (volatile agents) and postsynaptically by inhibiting excitatory ionotropic receptors activated by glutamate (gaseous agents).
8. No comprehensive theory of anesthesia describes the sequence of events leading from the interaction between an anesthetic molecule and its targets to the behavioral effects.

Despite widespread clinical use, current understanding of the molecular and cellular mechanisms of general anesthetic action is incomplete. This critical gap in the pharmacology of one of medicine's most important drug classes not only impedes rational use of available anesthetics but also hinders the development of newer agents to selectively achieve the desirable end points of anesthesia with fewer adverse cardiovascular, respiratory, and neuropsychological side effects. Although major progress has been made in understanding the pharmacology of the intravenous anesthetics by molecular genetic approaches (see Chapter 26), the actions of the inhaled anesthetics at the molecular and cellular levels are more enigmatic. It is still not possible to trace precisely the sequence of events that leads from inhaled anesthetic-target interactions, through ascending levels of biologic complexity, to the various behavioral effects that characterize the composite state of clinical anesthesia in humans. Nevertheless, investigations continue to reveal fundamental principles of action and have led to a framework for understanding anesthetic effects at different organizational levels. The focus of this chapter is on the mechanisms involved in the principal therapeutic effects (anesthesia) and on the side effects of the inhaled anesthetics (Fig. 20-1), a chemically and pharmacologically diverse group that includes the potent halogenated ether (isoflurane, sevoflurane, desflurane, enflurane) and alkane (halothane) volatile anesthetics and the gaseous anesthetics (nitrous oxide and xenon). This critical summary of the current state of knowledge begins with an historical overview and a review of the behavioral end points of anesthesia. We then trace, where possible, inhaled anesthetic effects through ascending levels of organization from molecules, cells, circuits, networks, and organs to mammalian behavior; an overview is provided in Table 20-1. A large body of work on anesthetic effects in model organisms, for which the correct anesthetic end points are unclear, is touched on briefly.[1]

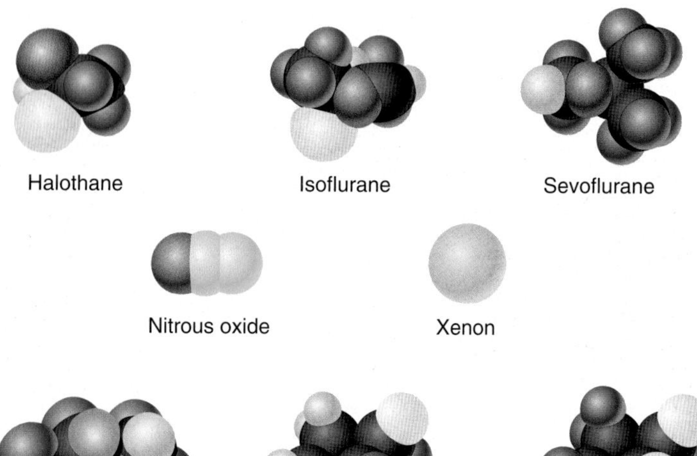

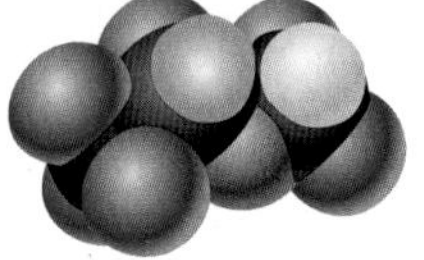

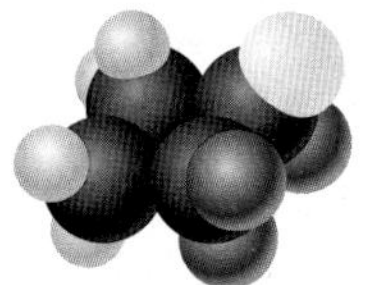

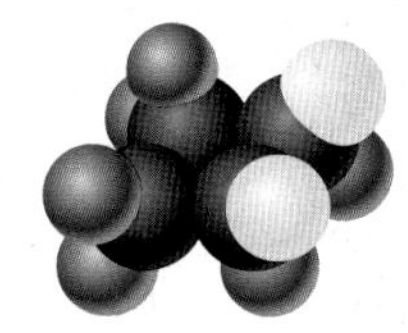

Figure 20-1 Structure of representative general anesthetics and a nonimmobilizer shown as space-filling models.

History

Unitary, Lipid-Based Theories

Inhaled general anesthetics were first used clinically more than 160 years ago, and interest in the mechanisms responsible for their remarkable effects was immediately kindled. The affinity of anesthetic drugs for lipids was soon recognized, which led to early lipid-based hypotheses of anesthetic action. The formulation of the Meyer-Overton correlation at the end of the 19th century was a watershed event, introducing a rigorous scientific approach into anesthesia research. Meyer concluded in 1899 that "All chemically indifferent substances that are soluble in fat are anesthetics … their relative potency as anesthetics will depend on their affinity to fat on the one hand and water on the other hand, that is, on the fat/water partition coefficient,"[2] a conclusion that was reached

Table 20-1 Overview of Proposed Sites of Anesthetic Action

	Site	Effect	Target(s)
Proteins	Amphiphilic binding sites	Conformational flexibility, ligand binding	Ion channels, receptors, signaling proteins
Action Potential	Nervous system Cardiovascular system	Small reduction in amplitude Reduced amplitude, duration	Na^+ channels Ca^{2+} channels, K^+ channels
Synaptic Transmission			
Inhibitory	Presynaptic terminal Postsynaptic receptors	Enhanced transmitter release Enhanced transmitter effects	? Glycine, $GABA_A$ receptors
Excitatory	Presynaptic terminal Postsynaptic receptors	Reduced transmitter release Reduced transmitter effects	Na^+ channels, K_{2P} channels NMDA receptors, nicotinic acetylcholine receptors
Neuronal Networks	Neuronal circuit Neuronal integration	Altered LTP/LTD Altered rhythmicity, coherence	Synaptic plasticity HCN channels, K_{2P} channels, extrasynaptic $GABA_A$ receptors, etc.
Central Nervous System	Neocortex, hippocampus, amygdala	Sedation, amnesia	θ-rhythms, γ-rhythms, synchrony
	Diencephalon (thalamus), brainstem (reticular formation)	Unconsciousness	γ-band transfer entropy?
	Spinal cord	Immobility	Thalamic deafferentation? Nocifensive reflex
Cardiovascular System			
	Myocardium Conduction system Vasculature	Negative inotropy Dysrhythmias Vasodilation	Excitation-contraction coupling Action potential Direct and indirect vasoregulation

independently by Overton.[3] The striking simplicity of the Meyer-Overton correlation (Fig. 20-2A) of anesthetic potency with solubility in olive oil led to the conclusion that lipids must be the anesthetic target. This focused attention on anesthetic effects on the bulk physical properties of cell membranes, which were known at that time to consist primarily of lipid molecules. Such nonspecific or "unitary" anesthetic mechanisms dominated the field for the ensuing decades.

Minimum Alveolar Concentration: A Bridge Between Past and Present

The introduction of the minimum alveolar concentration (MAC) concept as a universal measure for inhaled anesthetic potency in the 1960s had far-reaching implications for both clinical anesthesia and anesthesia research. The potencies of inhaled anesthetics for immobilization were established in the classic studies of Eger and colleagues,[4,5] who defined the "minimum alveolar concentration" of an inhaled anesthetic at atmospheric pressure required to prevent movement in response to a noxious stimulus in 50% of subjects. Because inhaled anesthetic concentrations reflect concentrations in other organs after equilibration, which is most rapidly achieved for well-perfused organs such as the brain and heart, MAC is analogous to the plasma EC_{50} (concentration for 50% effect) for intravenous anesthetics. In clinical applications, MAC is usually expressed as volume percent, which varies considerably with temperature due to changes in aqueous solubility, whereas the equivalent liquid-phase molar concentration is temperature-independent.[6] The MAC concept provided researchers and clinicians with a universal standard to measure a defined anesthetic end point (immobility), making meaningful comparisons of experimental results possible and accelerating laboratory and clinical research into anesthetic mechanisms. Today, a more nuanced understanding of MAC takes into account the structural and functional diversity of the biologic substrates of the different components of the anesthetic state.

Evolution from Lipid- to Protein-Centered Mechanisms

The formulation of the MAC concept was followed by evidence that proteins are plausible alternatives to lipids as anesthetic targets. Noncompetitive inhibition of the soluble firefly enzyme luciferase[7] demonstrated direct interference by anesthetics with the function of a lipid-free protein. Accurate measurements of anesthetic potency also revealed contradictions in lipid-based theories of anesthetic action such as the cutoff in anesthetic potency in homologous series of long-chain anesthetic alcohols and the identification of drugs that do not obey the Meyer-Overton correlation.[8,9] A focus on protein targets gained momentum in the 1980s owing largely to the work of Franks and Lieb,[10] who convincingly demonstrated that protein targets are also compatible with the Meyer-Overton correlation (see Fig. 20-2B) and proposed that anesthetics competitively antagonize protein function.[11] The enantiomeric selectivity of several anesthetics further strengthened the case for specific binding sites on proteins, such as ion channels, as the principal molecular targets of inhaled anesthetics.[12] Today, there is widespread (but not universal) acceptance of the notion that critical signaling proteins (e.g., ion channels and receptors) are the relevant molecular targets of anesthetic action even though the mechanisms of their modulation by anesthetics are debated, and much of the current work in

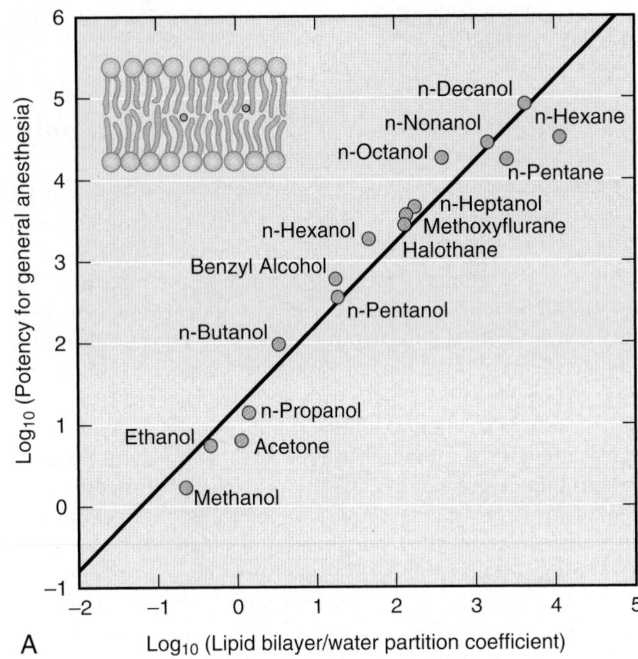

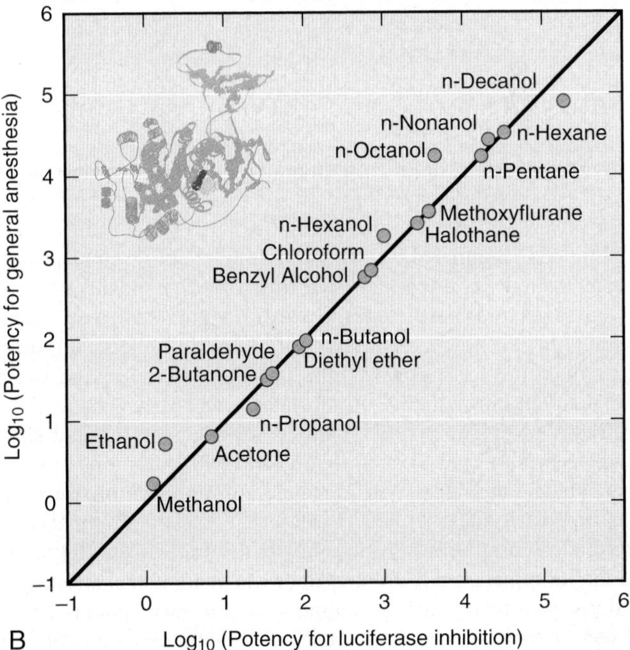

Figure 20-2 General anesthetics act by binding directly to proteins. **A,** The iconic Meyer-Overton correlation (c. 1900) was initially interpreted as evidence that lipids of nerve membranes were the principal anesthetic target sites based on the correlation between anesthetic potency and lipid-water partition coefficient. **B,** Progress in the 20th century showed that general anesthetic potencies correlate equally well with their ability to inhibit activity of the soluble firefly enzyme luciferase. The crystal structure of luciferase is shown in the *inset* with bound anesthetic in *red*. *(Reprinted with permission from Franks NP, Lieb WR: Molecular and cellular mechanisms of general anesthesia. Nature 367:607-614, 1994.)*

the field seeks to determine which proteins contribute to which anesthetic end points.

A Confusing Diversity of Anesthetic Targets

At high concentrations in vitro, most inhaled anesthetics affect multiple proteins, many of which can be plausibly connected to the anesthetic state. However, when considering a specific end point, anesthetics are effective in vivo over a quite narrow concentration range. This makes the concentration at which an effect is observed a critical consideration.[13] The mechanistic relevance of subtle effects observed in vitro at relevant concentrations is less clear, that is, what effect is too small to be considered relevant to anesthesia.[13-15] Whether anesthesia results from the sum of minor perturbations at multiple sites that are amplified in cascades across multiple levels of integration to produce the macroscopic effect or from strong effects on a small number of targets should be resolved as results of reductionist molecular studies are integrated into more complex molecular and cellular networks and as genetic studies are extended to encompass inhaled anesthetics. The emerging realization of the complexity of anesthesia is consistent with the modern concept that multiple cellular and molecular targets in distinct brain regions are involved in their desired and their adverse effects.

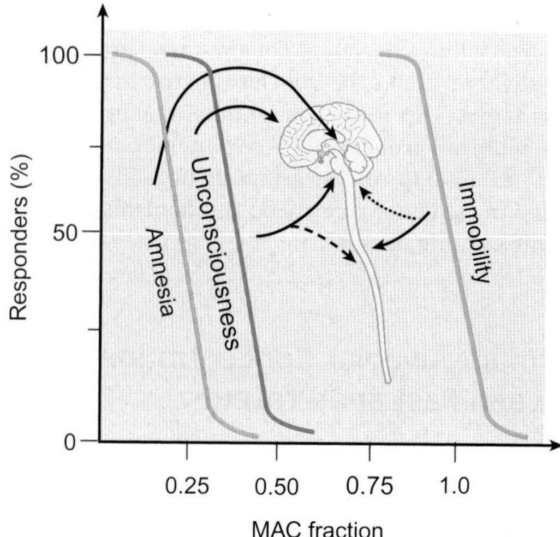

Figure 20-3 Multiple behavioral end points and sites of action underlie inhaled anesthetic action. Amnesia, the most sensitive anesthetic end point, probably involves the hippocampus, amygdala, mediotemporal lobe, and possibly other cortical structures. Unconsciousness likely involves the cerebral cortex, thalamus, and reticular formation. Sedation and hypnosis are part of the consciousness-unconsciousness continuum and are not shown. Immobility occurs by anesthetic action in the spinal cord, although supraspinal effects (*dotted arrow*) are likely important for some anesthetics. Anesthetic action in the spinal cord blunts ascending impulses arising from noxious stimulation and might indirectly contribute to anesthetic-induced unconsciousness and amnesia (*dashed arrow*). Cardiovascular responses occur at even greater MAC fractions (not shown). (*Courtesy of Joseph Antognini, University of California, Davis.*)

Anesthesia: A Complex Composite State

Along with progress in identifying the molecular mechanisms of anesthesia, our understanding of the nature of the anesthetic state has evolved. Whereas a coma-like state of general anesthesia can be induced by inhaled anesthetics administered at appropriate concentrations (approximately 1.3 times MAC, equivalent to the EC_{95} of a volatile anesthetic), the use of such high concentrations is fraught with short- and possibly long-term side effects. It is now clear that anesthesia consists of separable and at least partially independent components or substates, each of which involves distinct, but possibly overlapping, mechanisms at different sites in the central nervous system (CNS) and with variations in relative potencies between specific agents.[16] Immobilization, the core measure of MAC, is mediated largely at the level of the spinal cord by inhaled anesthetics[17,18] but not by barbiturates.[19] On the other hand, the spinal cord is unlikely to be the major site of anesthetic actions, producing such phenomena as amnesia, sedation, and unconsciousness, which are associated with cerebral cortical function (Fig. 20-3). A functional separation between amnesia and sedation has been demonstrated for intravenous anesthetics[20] and is likely for inhaled anesthetics as well. These and similar findings have led to the concept that general anesthesia consists of multiple independent components that are experimentally and clinically identifiable. Theoretically, each component can be preferentially induced in a concentration and agent-specific manner employing individual cellular/molecular pathways in various regions of the CNS. For example, injections of pentobarbital into discrete sites in the mesopontine tegmentum induce an anesthetic state,[21] whereas sedation induced by systemic administration of propofol can be reversed by microinjections of $GABA_A$ receptor antagonists into the tuberomammillary nucleus, a sleep-regulating nucleus in the hypothalamus.[22] Thus, general anesthetics produce separate identifiable anesthetic substates via agent-specific actions at discrete anatomic sites in the CNS by different molecular targets. An important consequence of this complexity is that MAC, which is based exclusively on the motor response, might not proportionately reflect other components of anesthesia. Although this heterogeneity of anesthetic action complicates a mechanistic understanding, it does open the possibility of developing substate-specific drugs.

Integrated Effects on Central Nervous System Function

Immobility

Failure to find a correlation between quantitative measures of electroencephalographic activity and immobility in response to noxious stimulation spawned the somewhat radical (at the time) hypothesis that immobility was not a "cerebral" phenomenon.[23] Experimental demonstration that volatile anesthetics act on the spinal cord to suppress movement[17,18] supported this hypothesis and was a major factor leading to the contemporary separation of anesthetic substates, of which immobility requires the highest anesthetic concentrations (see Fig. 20-3). Taking advantage of the unusual blood supply to the goat CNS that allows separate perfusion of brain and spinal cord, Antognini and coworkers showed that immobility requires anesthetic delivery to the spinal cord because selective delivery of isoflurane or halothane only to the brain required 2.5- to 4-fold higher concentrations.[17,24] Surgical separation of the forebrain from the spinal cord in rats confirmed

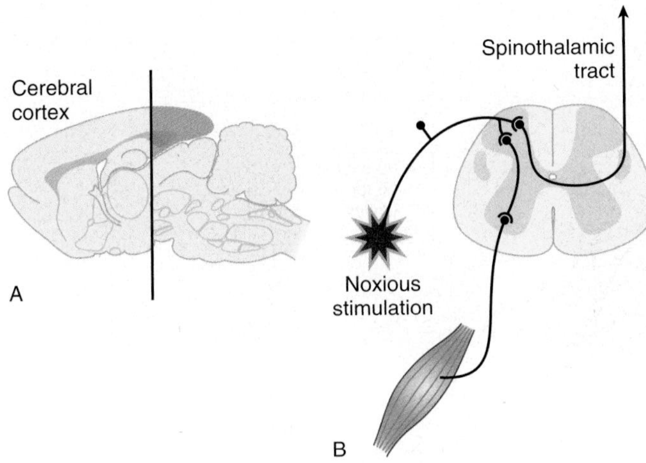

Figure 20-4 Inhaled anesthetics produce immobility at the spinal level. **A,** Decerebration by removal of the forebrain rostral to the *heavy black line* does not alter the MAC of isoflurane in rats, indicating that volatile anesthetic immobilization does not depend on the cerebral cortex. **B,** Anesthetics suppress the nocifensive withdrawal reflex response to noxious stimulation transmitted to the dorsal horn by sensory nerves at the spinal level. Current efforts are focused on identifying the molecular, cellular, and anatomic substrates for this effect. (***A** modified from Rampil IJ, Mason P, Singh H: Anesthetic potency [MAC] is independent of forebrain structures in the rat. Anesthesiology 78:707-712, 1993.*)

that immobilization involves primarily suppression of the nocifensive withdrawal reflex arc at the level of the spinal cord (Fig. 20-4).[18]

Recent studies have focused on the mechanisms by which inhaled anesthetics produce immobility. A pharmacologic approach to identify receptor-level contributions to MAC involves intrathecal administration of selective antagonists of neurotransmitter receptors in vivo. This strategy revealed that actions at spinal *N*-methyl-D-aspartate (NMDA)–type glutamate receptors[25] and glycine receptors[26] contribute to isoflurane-induced immobilization, whereas actions at $GABA_A$ receptors appear to be unimportant.[27] Glycine and $GABA_A$ receptors also appear to play little role in immobilization by cyclopropane,[26] which derives at least in part from antagonism of NMDA receptors.[28] Complementary research strategies have excluded other possible targets. Sensitivity to nonimmobilizer compounds excluded a role for inhibition of nicotinic acetylcholine receptors in immobilization,[29] and anesthetic-resistant transgenic mice confirmed that $GABA_A$ receptors containing α_1- or α_3-subunits do not contribute to the immobilizing action of isoflurane.[30,31] In contrast, mutant mice lacking the TASK-1, TASK-3, and TREK-1 K_{2P} channels have higher MAC values for volatile anesthetics but not intravenous anesthetics,[32-34] indicating a role for these channels, possibly by a presynaptic mechanism.[35] Even though the gross anatomic site for immobility has been identified and specific molecular targets have been implicated, an integrated hypothesis of the mechanism of inhaled anesthetic-induced immobility is still lacking (see reference 36 for review).

Unconsciousness

Consciousness, as a quality of the mind, is easy to recognize but difficult to define (see Chapter 39). As a neurobiologic process realized in the brain, it is within the reach of objective science but is currently poorly understood. Loss of consciousness (or hypnosis) is a hallmark of the onset of anesthesia, which raises the exciting possibility that anesthetic drugs will be useful as tools for understanding consciousness by defining the "neural correlates of consciousness" (NCC).[37] Although there is no universally accepted scientific definition, consciousness consists of inner, qualitative, subjective states of "sentience or awareness"[38] or "explicit awareness."[39]

Understanding how anesthetics ablate consciousness is entwined with theories of how consciousness is generated, many of which lack either experimental support or testable predictions. In contrast, neuroscientific approaches to consciousness are experimentally tractable. The "thalamic theory" of anesthesia proposes a somatosensory deafferentation by anesthetic action in the thalamus as a mechanism of unconsciousness.[40] In support of this hypothesis, isoflurane hyperpolarizes and shunts thalamic neurons,[41] an action consistent with impaired thalamic transfer of information observed in vivo.[42] Functional human brain imaging shows preferential suppression of thalamic activity by some, but not all, anesthetics, and this has led to the "thalamic switch" hypothesis.[43] However, loss of consciousness occurs within a very narrow range of anesthetic concentrations,[44,45] typically at less than 0.5 MAC,[46,47] whereas quantifiable effects in the thalamus occur above this concentration range and are typically incremental (dimmer-like) rather than sudden (switch-like). A comprehensive theory of anesthetic-induced unconsciousness must be more inclusive than a simple block of information transfer through the thalamus to be compatible with existing evidence[48] and must also explain the suppression of endogenous cortical activity that is generated without external stimulation.

Contemporary neuroscience has replaced the cartesian view of an anatomically discrete brain structure as the center of consciousness with the concept that consciousness requires integration of information between multiple brain regions across large-scale cerebral networks.[49,50] Anesthetic interference with the operational synchronicity and coherence of these networks with consequent disruption of cortical functional connectivity, as observed during natural sleep[51] and vegetative states, could result in "cognitive unbinding"[52] with loss of consciousness.[38] Unconsciousness[53] would be characterized not by the absence but by the disintegration of cortical processing.[39] Although the mechanism of "binding" (i.e., creating the unity of perception) is uncertain, synchronicity of neuronal activity in the 40- to 90-Hz range across functionally connected cortical areas (commonly referred to as 40 Hz- or γ-rhythm) is a viable candidate. Animal[54-56] and human[44] data implicate activity in the γ-band throughout the cortex as a network-level target of general anesthetics. Anesthetic actions on cortical information processing probably consist not merely of suppression of responses but of reduced complexity and variability reflected counterintuitively in increased reliability and precision of evoked responses.[57]

Learning and Memory

Anterograde amnesia, one of the core desirable anesthetic effects, is achieved at lower anesthetic concentrations (~0.25 MAC) than those required for unconsciousness (~0.5 MAC). Perhaps the closest analog in rodents to explicit memory in humans is hippocampus-dependent spatial learning. This can be tested by a variety of experimental paradigms, including fear conditioning to

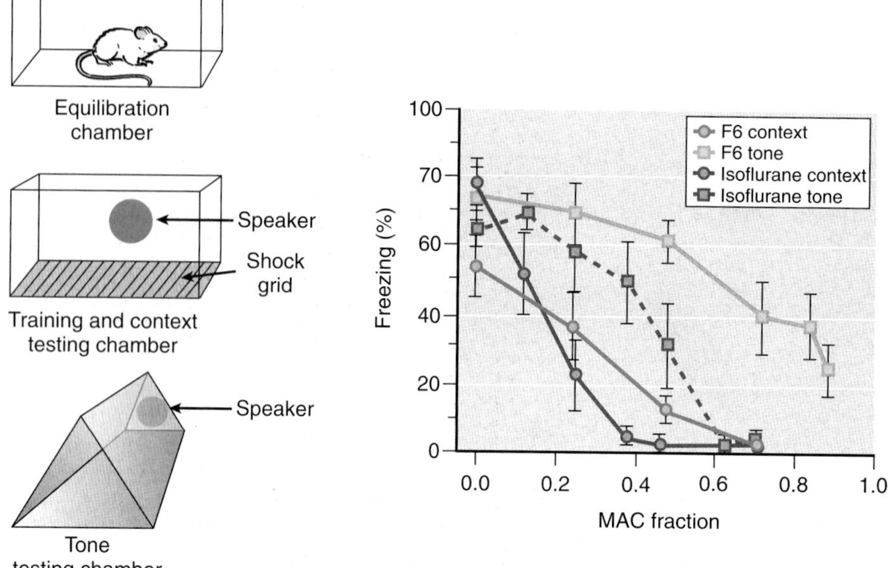

Figure 20-5 Differential sensitivity of different types of learning to anesthetics and nonimmobilizers. Freezing in anticipation of a noxious stimulus is a measure of learning in rats; less freezing indicates less learning. **Left,** The learning protocol involves pre-equilibration of rats in the equilibration chamber to isoflurane or the nonimmobilizer F6 at the desired concentration before placement into the training chamber. For testing of memory to context, training and test chamber are identical. For testing of memory to tone, training and testing take place in different chambers. **Right,** Hippocampus-dependent learning (fear conditioning to context, *closed symbols*) is inhibited by isoflurane (*purple circles*) at lower concentrations than hippocampus-independent learning (fear conditioning to tone, *purple squares*). This differential sensitivity is mirrored by the non-immobilizer F6 (*blue circles* and *yellow squares* for context and tone, respectively). *(**Left panel** adapted with permission from Eger EI 2nd, et al: Isoflurane antagonizes the capacity of flurothyl or 1,2-dichlorohexafluorocyclobutane to impair fear conditioning to context and tone. Anesth Analg 96: 1010-1018, 2003; **Right panel** data points reconstructed from Dutton RC, et al: Short-term memory resists the depressant effect of the nonimmobilizer 1-2-dichlorohexafluorocyclobutane (2N) more than long-term memory. Anesth Analg 94:631-639, 2002, and Dutton RC, et al: The concentration of isoflurane required to suppress learning depends on the type of learning. Anesthesiology 94:514-519, 2001.)*

context (Fig. 20-5). Other learning paradigms, such as fear conditioning to tone, are, by contrast, independent of the hippocampus. Isoflurane and the nonimmobilizer F6 both inhibit hippocampus-dependent learning at about half the concentration necessary for hippocampus-independent learning.[58] Because anesthetic concentrations that inhibit explicit memory in humans are similarly lower than concentrations that impair implicit memory,[47] anesthetic effects on hippocampal function are implicated in explicit memory suppression. Effects on other structures, such as the amygdala, may be crucial to anesthetic impairment of implicit or other types of memory.[59]

Comparison of the amnesic potency of five inhaled anesthetics using the inhibitory avoidance paradigm revealed that nitrous oxide was the most potent and halothane the least potent amnestic (expressed in MAC fractions), with the halogenated ethers of intermediate potency.[60] Because inhaled anesthetics affect multiple cellular targets at amnesic concentrations, it is difficult to attribute amnesia to specific cellular mechanisms. It is also unclear whether inhibition of learning and memory by drugs known to have different receptor affinities shares common mechanisms at some level of integration. Comparison with more selective drugs provides some insight. Abundant evidence indicates that θ-rhythms (4-12 Hz) are important for hippocampus-dependent learning and memory.[61] Benzodiazepines[62] and cannabinoids[63] slow and suppress hippocampal θ-rhythms in proportion to their ability to impair hippocampus-dependent learning. Isoflurane and the nonimmobilizer F6 have comparable effects on θ-rhythms at amnesic concentrations while having different receptor-level profiles and opposite effects on sedation.[56] Thus, alterations in neuronal synchrony provide a common network-level substrate for memory impairment. The synchronization between amygdalar and hippocampal θ-rhythms that occurs during fear memory retrieval indicates that this principle might also apply to other forms of memory and their impairment by anesthetics.[64] As with other components of the anesthetic state, the precise mechanisms of memory impairment by anesthetics, and of memory itself, remain to be fully elucidated.

Sedation

Sedation (defined as a decrease in activity, alertness, arousal, and/or vigilance) and its behavioral continuum hypnosis are achieved at low anesthetic concentrations (<0.5 MAC), near those that produce amnesia. There is no clear mechanistic or clinical separation between sedation and hypnosis. By contrast, even though sedation can be difficult to separate from amnesia, evidence obtained for intravenous anesthetics supports separate but overlapping substrates for these two end points.[20,65] The mechanisms involved in these behavioral effects probably resemble those of less promiscuous drugs, for which genetic approaches have been informative. An amino acid knock-in mutation (H101R) in mice that renders the α_1 $GABA_A$ receptor subunit insensitive to modulation by benzodiazepines produces resistance to the sedative and amnesic effects of benzodiazepines while maintaining other behavioral effects, among them anxiolysis.[66] The α_1 subunit is abundantly expressed in the CNS, mainly in cortical areas and thalamus. Volatile anesthetics have qualitatively similar effects on α_1-containing $GABA_A$ receptors (but also those containing other subunits) at low concentrations. The observation that the nonimmobilizer F6, which is devoid of sedative properties,[56] is amnesic[67] but does not modulate benzodiazepine-sensitive α_1-containing $GABA_A$ receptors[68,69] is compatible with a role for α_1-containing receptors in volatile anesthetic-induced sedation, because few other targets are affected at purely sedative concentrations. Possible targets for the sedative effects of the gaseous anesthetics nitrous oxide and xenon, which do not affect $GABA_A$ receptors, include NMDA receptor antagonism[70,71] and K_{2P} channel activation.[72] Consistent with this distinct pharmacologic profile, nitrous oxide has strikingly different effects from benzodiazepines in behavioral tests aimed at evaluating sedation in mice.[73]

Recognizing that there may be more than a superficial similarity between natural sleep and anesthetic-induced sedation and hypnosis, some anesthetics apparently "hijack" natural sleep mechanisms by directly activating discrete sleep-promoting nuclei in the hypothalamus.[22,74] The observations that electroencephalographic patterns during natural slow-wave sleep and anesthesia show some similarities[75] and that recovery from sleep deprivation can occur during propofol anesthesia[76] support this concept. Anesthetic effects on other cortical[77] and subcortical structures[21] also contribute to anesthetic-induced sedation and hypnosis.

Anesthetic Neurotoxicity and Neuroprotection

Recent animal experiments indicate that general anesthetics can cause persistent neurologic effects beyond their classic reversible production of anesthesia (see Chapter 46). The clinical significance of these changes is largely unknown, but attention has been drawn to the potential for adverse effects.[78] Possible anesthetic damage to the developing rodent CNS has attracted particular scrutiny recently, although clinical evidence in humans is lacking. Postnatal exposure of the developing rodent brain to high doses of commonly used anesthetic drugs, in isolation or in combination, for a period of several hours, can induce apoptotic cell death with potentially long-term functional consequences.[79] However, this appears not to occur with postnatal exposure in precocial species.[80] It is also unclear whether anesthetics contribute to the clinical syndrome of postoperative cognitive dysfunction in the aged brain, primarily owing to difficulty in establishing a robust animal model. More evidence supports a deleterious effect of nitrous oxide than of volatile anesthetics in aged animals.[81] Recent evidence also points to immune-mediated changes triggered by surgical trauma as a potential mechanism of postoperative cognitive dysfunction (see also Chapter 89).[82]

Pharmacologic neuroprotection from cerebral ischemia is a rapidly evolving area of research that is characterized by great potential but comparable disappointments as promising animal studies have failed to translate into clinical benefits. Despite considerable research, clinical evidence for ischemic brain protection by inhaled anesthetics remains controversial.[83] Ischemic neuronal injury results from early excitotoxic cell death mediated by excessive release of excitatory amino acid transmitters such as glutamate together with delayed cell death due to apoptosis.[84,85] Volatile anesthetics (e.g., isoflurane) and xenon exhibit early neuroprotection in animal models that is sustained only for mild insults. This is consistent with a beneficial effect on excitotoxicity but minimal effects on delayed cell death due to apoptosis. A therapeutic strategy to extend this early neuroprotection is suggested by the finding that isoflurane combined with caspase inhibitors to prevent apoptosis results in more sustained neuroprotection.[86] In contrast, xenon appears to have an intrinsic antiapoptotic action that contributes to its neuroprotective properties consistent with its distinct molecular mechanisms.[87] In addition, volatile anesthetics probably protect by suppression of brain energy requirements due to inhibition of excitatory transmission and potentiation of inhibitory receptors and ion channels.[84] The potential for beneficial effects from anesthetic-induced cardiac preconditioning has also received considerable recent attention (see the following section).

Integrated Effects on the Cardiovascular and Respiratory Systems

The cardiovascular effects of the volatile anesthetics are classically recognized as deleterious and undesired side effects that limit their use in the critically ill, but recent studies indicate direct cardioprotective effects of inhaled anesthetics.[88] All volatile anesthetics produce agent- and dose-dependent reductions in myocardial contractility, systemic vascular resistance, and cardiac preload with consequent reduction in mean arterial pressure, but significant differences exist in the relative potencies of these effects among agents (see Chapter 23).[89] Volatile anesthetics depress contractility by reducing Ca^{2+} availability and/or Ca^{2+} sensitivity of the contractile apparatus.[90] The major targets responsible for the negative inotropic effects of volatile anesthetics are cardiac Ca^{2+} channels, sarcoplasmic Ca^{2+} handling, and the contractile apparatus. Inhibition of depolarization-induced increases in myoplasmic Ca^{2+} concentration occur primarily via inhibition of cardiac L-type voltage-gated Ca^{2+} currents and shortening of action potential duration.[91] Volatile anesthetics also inhibit the sarco-endoplasmic Ca^{2+} ATPase (SERCA), while halothane, but not isoflurane or sevoflurane, opens sarcoplasmic reticulum (SR) Ca^{2+} release channels (ryanodine receptors), depleting SR Ca^{2+} content and reducing excitation-evoked SR Ca^{2+} release.[90] The resulting negative inotropic effect of this reduced Ca^{2+} availability is enhanced by reductions in the Ca^{2+} sensitivity of myofibrils. In contrast, xenon has no effects on ventricular contractility, conduction, or major cation currents,[91,92] consistent with its lack of significant cardiovascular effects. Nitrous oxide causes mild reductions in ventricular function[92] by poorly characterized effects on Ca^{2+} availability. This is usually accompanied by sympathetic nervous system stimulation that increases vascular resistance and counteracts the myocardial depression.[93,94]

Volatile anesthetics can produce vasodilation at clinical concentrations.[95] The vascular effects of volatile anesthetics are multifactorial and tissue specific, and the precise cellular mechanisms are poorly understood.[96,97] Peripheral vasodilation is mediated both by direct endothelium-independent vasodilating effects on vascular smooth muscle cells and indirect effects involving the sympathetic nervous system and the vascular endothelium. The mechanisms of these effects involve agent-specific effects on presynaptic norepinephrine release, inhibition of smooth muscle Ca^{2+} influx via L-type Ca^{2+} channels, activation of hyperpolarizing K_{ATP} and K_{Ca} channels, and endothelium-dependent factors, including nitric oxide.[98]

As with the CNS, cardiovascular function depends on the integrated function of multiple ion channels, many of which are expressed in both of these excitable tissues. Volatile anesthetics have agent-specific effects on heart rate and induction of arrhythmias due to actions on cardiac ion channels. Because multiple cardiac ion channels are sensitive to volatile anesthetics at clinical concentrations, and because most manipulations of cardiac ion channel function are potentially proarrhythmic, it is difficult to link anesthetic arrhythmogenicity to actions on specific channels.[99] Electrophysiologic studies indicate that cardiac L-type Ca^{2+} channels, which are critical to the plateau phase of the cardiac action potential and electromechanical coupling, are inhibited by volatile anesthetics, leading to shortening of the refractory period. Multiple voltage-gated K^+ channels are also inhibited and might predispose to arrhythmias by delaying repolarization. On the other hand, inhaled anesthetics can protect the heart against ischemia and reperfusion injury, possibly involving antioxidant, anti-inflammatory, and/or preconditioning mechanisms.[100,101] Volatile anesthetics[102] and xenon[103] can mimic the strong cardioprotective effects produced by ischemic preconditioning (termed *anesthetic preconditioning* by analogy) through activation of various cytoprotective G-protein–coupled receptors and protein kinases, including protein kinase C (PKC), mitogen-activated protein kinases (MAP kinases), extracellular signal-regulated kinases (ERK), Akt (protein kinase B), and tyrosine kinases.[88,104] Although not entirely clarified, sarcolemmal and putative mitochondrial adenosine triphosphate (ATP)-sensitive K^+ (K_{ATP}) channel activation, involving PKC activation and increased formation of free radicals and nitric oxide, are the likely end effectors of anesthetic preconditioning in the heart.

Inhaled anesthetics also have important effects on the respiratory system. All volatile anesthetics cause significant respiratory depression at concentrations necessary for surgical anesthesia. The peripheral chemoreflexes and upper airway patency are particularly sensitive to subanesthetic concentrations of volatile anesthetics.[105] The mechanisms involved in these potentially serious effects involve depression of central respiratory networks mediated by depression of excitatory and facilitation of inhibitory transmission. The precise molecular targets responsible for the exquisite sensitivity of these networks to low concentrations of volatile anesthetics remain to be elucidated (see Chapter 22).

Identification of Molecular Sites of Anesthetic Action

Criteria for Identifying Sites Relevant to Anesthesia

Specific criteria have been proposed to evaluate the relevance of the many potential molecular targets of anesthetics.[106] These criteria include:

1. Reversible alteration of target function at clinically relevant concentrations. This criterion requires comparable in vivo and in vitro sensitivity and depends on the anesthetic end point under consideration. For example, targets involved in immobility must be sensitive to anesthetics near MAC, whereas targets mediating memory impairment must be affected at a fraction of MAC. Recent evidence for persistent effects of inhaled anesthetics demonstrable in the absence of continued anesthetic exposure is challenging the notion of reversibility for certain effects.
2. Expression of the target in appropriate anatomic locations to mediate the specific anesthetic end point. For example, immobilization by inhaled agents appears to involve primarily depression of reflex pathways in the spinal cord independent of drug actions in the brain.
3. Concordant stereoselectivity of anesthetic effects in vivo and on the target in vitro. In the absence of a specific pharmacologic antagonist of anesthesia, correlation between the stereoselective actions of general anesthetics in vivo and in vitro is a useful test of pharmacologic relevance of putative molecular targets. Stereoselectivity data correlating in vivo potency and in vitro receptor actions implicate $GABA_A$ receptors as a target for the anesthetic actions of etomidate, pentobarbital, neurosteroid anesthetics, and possibly isoflurane and the NMDA receptor for the actions of ketamine.
4. Appropriate sensitivity or insensitivity to model anesthetic and nonanesthetic compounds. Anesthetic halogenated cyclobutanes together with structural analogs that do not produce anesthesia at concentrations predicted to be anesthetic by the Meyer-Overton correlation (nonimmobilizers) can be used to discriminate relevant volatile anesthetic targets in vitro. For example, the anesthetic F3 (1-chloro-1,2,2-trifluorocyclobutane), but not the structurally similar nonanesthetic F6 (1,2-dichlorohexafluorocyclobutane), affect $GABA_A$, glycine, AMPA, kainate, and 5-HT_3 receptors, and Na^+ channels, consistent with a role in immobility, whereas both F3 and F6 affect neuronal nicotinic, M1 muscarinic, 5-HT_{2C}, and mGluR5 receptors, indicating that these targets are not involved in immobility. F6 is interesting in that it lacks sedative and immobilizing effects but does possess amnesic effects, hence the more accurate term "nonimmobilizer", thus making it a useful pharmacologic tool for discriminating targets for these actions.

Physicochemical Properties of Anesthetic Binding Sites

A convergence of x-ray crystallography, molecular modeling, and structure-function data indicate that inhaled anesthetics bind in hydrophobic cavities formed within proteins.[107] The lipophilic (or hydrophobic) nature of these binding sites explains their adherence to the Meyer-Overton correlation. An element of amphiphilicity (possessing both polar and nonpolar characteristics) is also required for effective interaction with these cavities, as indicated by improvements in the Meyer-Overton correlation with more polar solvents.

From Model Proteins to Receptors

Identifying inhaled anesthetic binding sites on plausible target proteins is difficult due to their low-affinity interactions and the paucity of atomic resolution structures of pharmacologically rel-

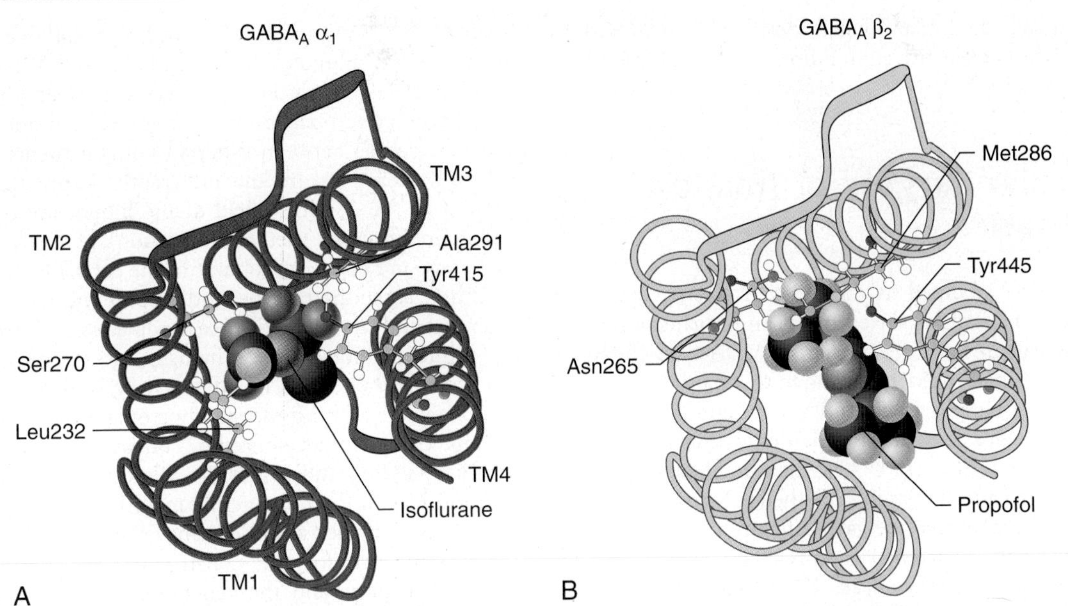

Figure 20-6 Putative anesthetic binding sites on GABA$_A$ receptors. **A,** Model of rat GABA$_A$ α$_1$-subunit with Leu232, Ser270, Ala291, and Tyr415 rendered in ball-and-stick. A molecule of isoflurane built at the same scale is positioned in the putative binding site. The transmembrane (TM) α-helices are numbered 1-4. **B,** Corresponding model of GABA$_A$ β$_2$-subunit with Asn265, Met286, and Tyr445 rendered in ball-and-stick. A model of propofol built at the same scale is positioned in the putative binding site. *(From Hemmings HC Jr, Akabas MH, Goldstein PA, et al: Emerging molecular mechanisms of general anesthetic action. Trends Pharmacol Sci 26:503-510, 2005.)*

evant target proteins. Consequently, most anesthetic binding sites have been identified in well-characterized model proteins for which three-dimensional atomic resolution structures are available, such as luciferase and albumin.[107] These studies indicate that anesthetics bind in pockets with both nonpolar and polar noncovalent chemical interactions. Binding involves weak hydrogen bond interactions with polar amino acid residues and water molecules, nonpolar van der Waals interactions, and a polarizing effect of the amphiphilic binding cavity on the relatively hydrophobic anesthetic molecules. Internal cavities are important for the conformational flexibility involved in ion channel gating and ligand-induced signal transduction of receptor proteins. Occupation of a critical volume within these cavities by anesthetics provides a plausible mechanism for alteration of receptor and ion channel function by selective stabilization of a particular confirmation (e.g., an open or inactivated state of an ion channel). Anesthetics also obtain binding energy from the entropy generated by displacing bound water from these relatively promiscuous binding sites. Studies of glycine, GABA$_A$, and NMDA receptors provide convincing evidence for the existence of anesthetic binding sites in critical neuronal signaling proteins.[108] Amino acid residues critical for volatile anesthetic actions and, by inference, binding have been identified in the α-subunit of the GABA$_A$ receptor.[108-110]

Molecular modeling based on structurally homologous proteins has also been used to identify putative anesthetic binding sites in the transmembrane domains of GABA$_A$ and glycine receptors (Fig. 20-6).[111] This model suggests that different drugs might either bind in different orientations within a single amphiphilic cavity or occupy different cavities within the protein, causing similar functional effects. Refinement of these molecular models will continue to provide new insights in the molecular basis for general anesthetic action that can be experimentally tested. Potential sites of interaction of xenon and isoflurane with the NMDA receptor have also been identified using this approach. One site, which can contain up to three xenon atoms or one molecule of isoflurane, overlaps the known binding site for the co-agonist glycine in the NR1 subunit (Fig. 20-7).[112] This suggests

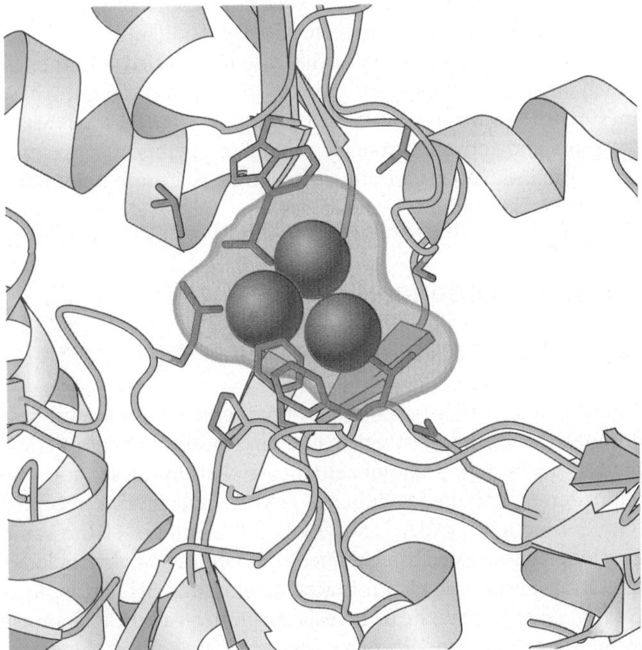

Figure 20-7 Crystal structure of the ligand binding domain of the *NMDA receptor* showing xenon binding sites predicted by molecular modeling. The *red spheres* represent xenon atoms at the center of the density clusters that comprise the binding sites. The predicted xenon binding sites occupy the site normally occupied by glycine. The same site is also large enough to accommodate isoflurane. *(Modified from Dickinson R, Peterson BK, Banks P, et al: Competitive inhibition at the glycine site of the N-methyl-D-aspartate receptor by the anesthetics xenon and isoflurane. Anesthesiology 107:756-767, 2007.)*

that two chemically dissimilar inhaled anesthetics inhibit NMDA receptors by direct competitive inhibition of agonist binding.

Molecular Targets of Inhaled Anesthetics

Ion channels have emerged as the most promising molecular targets for inhaled anesthetics. Neurotransmitter-gated ion channels, in particular $GABA_A$, glycine, and NMDA-type glutamate receptors, are leading candidates owing to their appropriate CNS distributions, essential physiologic roles in inhibitory and excitatory synaptic transmission, and sensitivities to clinically relevant concentrations of anesthetics.[16,113,114] Other ion channels that are sensitive to inhaled anesthetics include the HCN (hyperpolarization-activated cyclic nucleotide-gated) family of channels that give rise to pacemaker currents[115] and regulate dendritic excitability, two-pore domain (K_{2P}) "leak" K^+ channels that maintain resting membrane potential in many cells,[116] and voltage-gated Na^+ and Ca^{2+} channels.[117]

Inhaled anesthetics can be divided into two classes based on their distinct pharmacologic properties. The first class is the potent inhaled (volatile) anesthetics, which exhibit positive modulation of $GABA_A$ receptors, also produce significant, anesthesia-compatible effects on a number of other receptors/channels, including enhancement of inhibitory glycine receptors, inhibition of excitatory NMDA and neuronal nicotinic acetylcholine receptors, activation of K_{2P} channels, and inhibition of presynaptic Na^+ channels. Intravenous anesthetics such as propofol and etomidate represent more potent and specific positive modulators of $GABA_A$ receptors. The second class is the gaseous inhaled anesthetics, which include cyclopropane, nitrous oxide, and xenon. These anesthetics are inactive at $GABA_A$ receptors, but block NMDA receptors and activate certain K_{2P} channels at clinical concentrations. The intravenous anesthetic ketamine is a more potent and specific blocker of NMDA receptors.

Ligand-Gated Ion Channels

Potentiation of Inhibitory $GABA_A$ and Glycine Receptors

The ether anesthetics (including isoflurane, sevoflurane, and desflurane), the alkane anesthetic halothane, most intravenous anesthetics (including propofol, etomidate, barbiturates), and the neurosteroid anesthetics enhance $GABA_A$ and glycine receptor (GlyR) function. $GABA_A$ and GlyRs are members of the same Cys-loop ligand-gated ion channel superfamily that also includes the cation-permeable nicotinic acetylcholine and $5HT_3$ receptors. $GABA_A$ receptors are the principal transmitter-gated Cl^- channels in the neocortex and allocortex, whereas GlyRs fulfill this function in the spinal cord, with some overlap in the diencephalon and brainstem. Activated receptors conduct chloride ions, driving the membrane potential toward the Cl^- equilibrium potential. Both receptors are considered to be inhibitory because the Cl^- equilibrium potential is usually more negative than the normal resting potential. Channel opening also reduces membrane resistance and "shunts" excitatory responses. Most functional $GABA_A$ and GlyRs are heteropentamers, typically consisting of three different $GABA_A$ subunits (e.g., two α, two β, and one γ or δ) or two different GlyR subunits (three α and two β).[118] The subunit composition of $GABA_A$ receptors determines their physiologic and pharmacologic properties and varies between and within brain areas as well as between different compartments of individual neurons. Examples are the preferential expression of the α_5-subunit in the dendritic field of the hippocampal CA1 area (a region important for memory formation), of the α_4-subunit in the thalamus, and of the α_6-subunit in the cerebellum. Presence of a γ-subunit is required for benzodiazepine modulation of $GABA_A$ receptors and can also influence modulation by inhaled anesthetics. While the molecular mechanisms of receptor modulation by inhaled anesthetics are not definitively settled, these receptors have been key to our understanding of anesthetic-receptor interactions. Using chimeric receptor constructs between anesthetic-sensitive $GABA_A$ and insensitive GlyR subunits, specific amino acid residues in the transmembrane domains 2 and 3 critical to the action of inhaled anesthetics have been identified.[119] This laid the groundwork for the construction of anesthetic-resistant $GABA_A$ receptors and the generation of transgenic mice with altered anesthetic sensitivity (see later).

The related cation-permeable 5-hydroxytryptamine (serotonin)-3 ($5HT_3$) receptors are similarly potentiated by volatile anesthetics.[120-122] $5HT_3$ receptors are involved with autonomic reflexes and probably contribute to the emetogenic properties of volatile anesthetics (see Chapter 86).

Inhibition of Excitatory Acetylcholine and Glutamate Receptors

Neuronal nicotinic acetylcholine receptors (nnAChRs), like the other members of the Cys-loop family, are heteropentameric. They are composed of α- and β-subunits, but functional homomeric receptors can be formed by certain α-subunits. In the CNS, nnAChRs are localized primarily presynaptically.[123] Homomeric α_7-receptors have high permeability to Ca^{2+} that can exceed that of NMDA receptors.[123] In contrast to $GABA_A$ and GlyRs, nnAChRs pass cations when activated and therefore depolarize the membrane potential. Receptors containing $\alpha_4\beta_2$ subunits are very sensitive to block by isoflurane and propofol.[124,125] Relevance of nnAChR block to immobilization, sedation, and unconsciousness by inhaled anesthetics is unlikely because nnAChRs are also blocked by nonimmobilizers, although it is possible that they do contribute to amnesia.[9]

NMDA (*N*-methyl-D-aspartate) receptors are a major postsynaptic receptor subtype of ionotropic receptors for glutamate, the principal excitatory neurotransmitter in the mammalian CNS.[126] Typical NMDA receptors, defined pharmacologically by their selective activation by the exogenous agonist NMDA, are heteromers consisting of an obligatory NR1 subunit and modulatory NR2 subunits. Channel opening requires glutamate (or another agonist such as NMDA) binding to the NR2 subunit while the co-agonist glycine binds to the NR1 subunit. NMDA receptors also require membrane depolarization to relieve the voltage-dependent block by Mg^{2+}. The depolarization is typically provided by binding of glutamate to non-NMDA glutamate receptors (see later). Because of this "dual" requirement (transmitter release and postsynaptic depolarization), synaptic NMDA receptors function as coincidence detectors, and this characteristic is thought to be central to their role in learning and memory. NMDA receptors are also involved in the development of chronic pain, perhaps due to similar mechanisms underlying synaptic

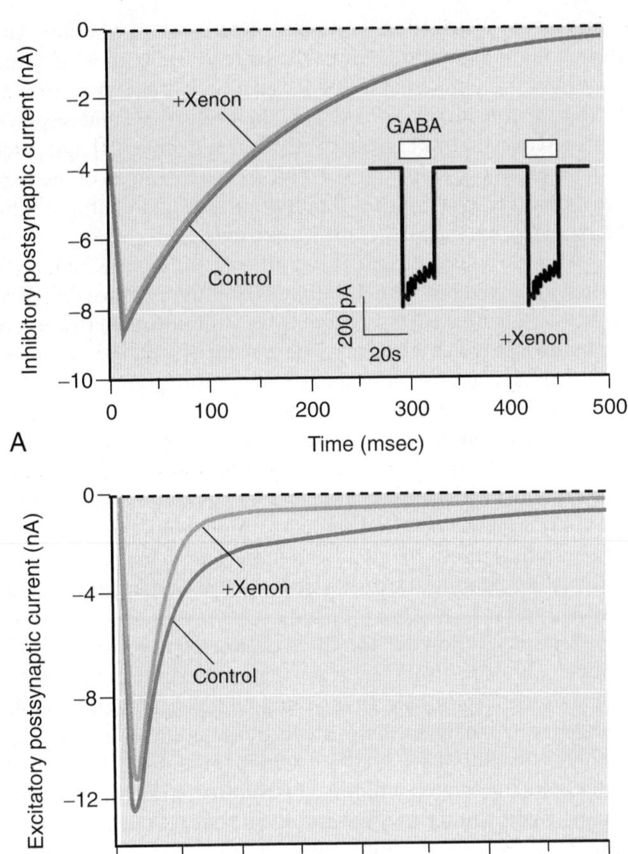

Figure 20-8 The actions of xenon on inhibitory GABAergic and excitatory glutamatergic synapses in cultured rat hippocampal neurons. Xenon (3.4 mM, ~1 MAC) has no significant effect on the inhibitory postsynaptic current (**A**) but greatly depresses the excitatory glutamatergic synaptic current, almost exclusively the slow NMDA receptor-mediated component of the current (**B**). In contrast, the principal effects of ~1 MAC isoflurane are a prolongation in the inhibitory current decay and a reduction in excitatory current peak height with little change in time course (not shown, see Fig. 20-10). *(Reprinted in modified form by permission from de Sousa SLM, et al: Contrasting synaptic activity of the inhalational general anesthetics isoflurane and xenon. Anesthesiology 92:1055-1066, 2000.)*

plasticity, and in ischemia-induced excitotoxicity by virtue of their capacity to allow entry of the ubiquitous intracellular signal Ca^{2+} on activation. The nonhalogenated inhaled anesthetics xenon, nitrous oxide, and cyclopropane, as well as the intravenous anesthetic ketamine, have minimal effects on $GABA_A$ receptors but depress excitatory glutamatergic synaptic transmission postsynaptically via NMDA glutamate receptor blockade (Figs. 20-7 and 20-8).[70,71,127] Volatile anesthetics can also inhibit isolated NMDA receptors at higher concentrations.[128] Along with presynaptic inhibition of glutamate release, this might contribute to their depression of NMDA receptor–mediated excitatory transmission.

A second class of ionotropic glutamate receptors includes the non-NMDA receptors, which are subdivided into AMPA and kainate receptors based again on their sensitivities to selective exogenous agonists.[126] Inhaled anesthetics only weakly inhibit AMPA receptors, so this action is unlikely to be important in their actions.[129] Interestingly, kainate receptors are enhanced by inhaled anesthetics, but this is unlikely to be involved in immobility because MAC is not altered in mice deficient in the GluR6 receptor subunit.[130] Most evidence suggests that the principal mechanism for depression of glutamatergic transmission by volatile anesthetics is presynaptic, with minor contributions from postsynaptic receptor blockade[117,131-133] (see "Cellular Mechanisms").

Voltage-Gated and Other Ion Channels

Na^+ Channels

Voltage-gated Na^+ channels are critical to axonal conduction, synaptic integration, and neuronal excitability. In contrast to findings in invertebrate giant axons,[134] axonal conduction in small (0.1-0.2 μm) unmyelinated hippocampal axons is depressed by volatile anesthetics[135,136] and small reductions in preterminal action potential amplitude significantly depress transmitter release and hence postsynaptic responses at a mammalian synapse.[137]

Heterologously expressed mammalian voltage-gated Na^+ channels are sensitive to clinically relevant concentrations of volatile anesthetics. The Na^+ channel family consists of nine homologous pore-forming α-subunits with distinct cellular and subcellular distributions.[138] Isoflurane and other volatile anesthetics inhibit the major mammalian Na^+ channel isoforms, including neuronal ($Na_v1.2$), skeletal muscle ($Na_v1.4$), and cardiac ($Na_v1.5$) channels, but the peripheral isoform $Na_v1.8$ is apparently resistant.[139] Volatile anesthetics, but not nonimmobilizers, also inhibit native neuronal and nerve terminal Na^+ channels,[140-143] lending support to the notion that Na^+ channel blockade contributes to the depression of synaptic neurotransmitter release.[143] In contrast, xenon has no detectable effect on Na^+, Ca^{2+}, or K^+ channels in isolated cardiomyocytes.[92] The recent demonstration that NaChBac, a prokaryotic homolog of voltage-gated Na^+ channels, is also inhibited by volatile anesthetics opens the way for structure-function studies of these channels.[141]

Ca^{2+} Channels

Multiple cellular functions depend on the tightly controlled concentration of intracellular free Ca^{2+} ($[Ca^{2+}]_i$), which is determined by the integrated activity of voltage-gated Ca^{2+} channels, capacitative Ca^{2+} channels, plasma membrane and sarco/endo-plasmic reticulum Ca^{2+}-ATPases (pumps), Na^+/Ca^{2+} exchangers, and mitochondrial Ca^{2+} sequestration. Alteration of any of these mechanisms by anesthetics could affect the many cellular processes regulated by the second messenger actions of Ca^{2+}, including synaptic transmission, gene expression, cytotoxicity, and muscle excitation-contraction coupling. Excitable cells translate their electrical activity into action by Ca^{2+} fluxes mediated primarily by voltage-gated Ca^{2+} channels in the plasma membrane. Distinct Ca^{2+} subtypes are expressed in various cells and tissues and are classified pharmacologically and functionally by the degree of depolarization required to gate the channel, such as low voltage–activated (LVA; T-type) and high voltage–activated (HVA; L-, N-, R-, and P/Q-type) channels. More recently, the molecular identity of their pore-forming α-subunits has been used for classification.[144] There is convincing evidence that volatile anesthetics inhibit certain Ca^{2+} channel isoforms but not others (for review see reference 145).

Inhibition of the presynaptic voltage-gated Ca^{2+} channels coupled to transmitter release has been proposed as a mechanism by which volatile anesthetics reduce excitatory transmission.[146]

Indeed, N-type ($Ca_v2.2$) and P-type ($Ca_v2.1$) channels, which mediate Ca^{2+} entry coupled to neurotransmitter release, are modestly sensitive to volatile anesthetics[147,148] but not in all neuron types,[149] suggesting the importance of auxiliary subunits, post-translation modification, or other potential modulators of anesthetic sensitivity. A modest contribution of R-type Ca^{2+} channels ($Ca_v2.3$) to anesthesia is suggested by its sensitivity to volatile anesthetics and a small increase in MAC produced by its genetic deletion in mice.[150] T-type Ca^{2+} channels are particularly sensitive to volatile anesthetics[151] and nitrous oxide.[152] However, mutant mice lacking a major neuronal T-type Ca^{2+} channel isoform ($Ca_v3.1$) have normal volatile anesthetic sensitivity, although the onset of anesthesia is delayed.[153] Thus, the role that inhibition of these or other Ca^{2+} channels plays in the CNS effects of inhaled anesthetics is unclear.

By contrast, a role for Ca^{2+} channel inhibition in the negative inotropic effects of volatile anesthetics, prominent at higher doses, is well established. The force of myocardial contraction is determined by the magnitude of cytosolic Ca^{2+} increase after electrical excitation, the responsiveness of the contractile proteins to Ca^{2+}, and sarcomere length. Negative inotropic effects of volatile anesthetics are mediated by reductions in Ca^{2+} availability, Ca^{2+} sensitivity of the contractile proteins, and the rate of cytosolic Ca^{2+} clearance. Volatile anesthetics reduce the Ca^{2+} transient and shorten action potential duration in cardiomyocytes primarily by inhibiting L-type ($Ca_v1.2$) Ca^{2+} currents, resulting in a negative inotropic effect and arrhythmogenicity.[90,99,154] In contrast, xenon does not depress myocardial function or inhibit L-type Ca^{2+}, Na^+, or K^+ currents in isolated cardiomyocytes.[91,92] Inhibition of transsarcolemmal Ca^{2+} influx through cardiac L-type Ca^{2+} channels plays a major role in the negative inotropic effects of volatile anesthetics, greatest for halothane, along with contributions from effects on myofilament Ca^{2+} sensitivity and sarcolemmal Ca^{2+} release.[99,155]

In contrast to voltage-gated Ca^{2+} channels that regulate the influx of extracellular Ca^{2+}, intracellular Ca^{2+} channels regulate Ca^{2+} release from intracellular stores, particularly the endoplasmic reticulum (ER) and sarcoplasmic reticulum (SR). These include 1,4,5-trisphosphate receptors (IP_3Rs), regulated by the second messenger IP_3, and ryanodine receptors (RyRs), which mediate the rapid release of intracellular Ca^{2+} critical to excitation-contraction coupling in muscle. Volatile anesthetic-induced Ca^{2+} leak occurs via both IP_3R and RyR channels, which leads to depletion of intracellular Ca^{2+} stores from the SR and ER. This blunts changes in intracellular Ca^{2+} in response to stimulation and also contributes to the smooth muscle–relaxing properties of volatile anesthetics that underlie bronchodilation and vasodilation.[156] Malignant hyperthermia susceptibility is a pharmacogenetic disorder that manifests as a potentially fatal hypermetabolic crisis triggered by volatile anesthetics, particularly halothane. It is often associated with mutations in RyR1 and the physically associated L-type Ca^{2+} channel ($Ca_v1.1$) that functions as the voltage sensor.[157] Volatile anesthetics activate the abnormal RyRs, resulting in uncontrolled intracellular Ca^{2+} release, muscle contraction, and metabolic activity[158] (see also Chapter 37.)

K^+ Channels and HCN Channels

Potassium (K^+) channels are an extremely diverse ion channel family noted for their varied modes of activation. They regulate electrical excitability, muscle contractility, and neurotransmitter release and are important in determining the input resistance and in driving repolarization and thus determine excitability and action potential duration. Given the large diversity in K^+ channel structure, function, and anesthetic sensitivity, it is not surprising that there is considerable diversity in their sensitivity and response to inhaled anesthetics[159]: from relatively insensitive (voltage-gated K^+ channels $K_v1.1$, K_v3)[160] to sensitive (some members of the two-pore domain K^+ channels [K_{2P}] family), resulting in either inhibition, activation, or no effect on K^+ currents.

Volatile anesthetic activation of certain "leak" K^+ channels was first observed in the snail *Lymnaea*,[161] although the molecular identity of the affected ion channels was unknown. Activation of K_{2P} channels by volatile and gaseous anesthetics, including xenon, nitrous oxide, and cyclopropane, was subsequently observed in mammals.[162] Increased K^+ conductance can hyperpolarize neurons, reducing responsiveness to excitatory synaptic input and altering network synchrony. Targeted deletion of the TASK-1, TASK-3, and TREK-1 K_{2P} channels in mice reduces sensitivity to immobilization by volatile anesthetics, implicating these channels as anesthetic targets in vivo.[32-34] Other members of this large family of K^+ channels are also sensitive to xenon and volatile anesthetics.[163]

The recognition that inherited channelopathies are arrhythmogenic and constitute an important contributor to sudden cardiac death,[164] particularly in young children,[165] highlights the importance of analyzing anesthetic modulation of cardiac ion channels. Recombinant HERG (human ether-a-go-go related) channels are moderately inhibited by halothane, and their depression likely contributes to arrhythmogenic effects of volatile anesthetics.[99,166] HERG channels are also involved in acquired (drug-induced) and inherited long QT syndrome. Cardiac inward-rectifying (K_{IR}), voltage-gated (K_v), and Ca^{2+}-activated K^+ channels are generally relatively insensitive to clinical concentrations of volatile anesthetics and xenon.[91,99,167] In contrast, there is considerable evidence that volatile anesthetics and xenon activate cardiac mitochondrial and sarcolemmal K_{ATP} channels,[100] an effect that plays a critical role in anesthetic preconditioning. Direct electrophysiologic effects of anesthetics with preconditioning properties have been demonstrated on both mitochondrial and sarcolemmal K_{ATP} channels, although the precise mechanisms remain to be clarified.

Volatile anesthetics also inhibit HCN "pacemaker" channels, reducing the rate of rise of pacemaker potentials and the bursting frequency of certain neurons showing autorhythmicity. They decrease I_h conductance in neurons[168] and modulate recombinant HCN1 and HCN2 channel isoforms at clinically relevant concentrations.[169] Because HCN channels contribute to resting membrane potential, control action potential firing, dendritic integration, neuronal automaticity, and temporal summation, and determine periodicity and synchronization of oscillations in many neuronal networks,[170] the anesthetic modulation of these channels could play an important role in anesthetic effects on neuronal integrative functions.

Intracellular Signaling Mechanisms

Cell signaling mechanisms are critical to all phases of organ function and have been attractive targets for the broad effects of general anesthetics. Anesthetics have poorly understood actions on intracellular cell signaling pathways, which include processes downstream from cell surface receptors and ion channels, such as effects of second messengers, protein phosphorylation pathways, and other regulatory mechanisms.[171]

G Protein–Coupled Receptors

A variety of signals, including hormones, neurotransmitters, cytokines, pheromones, odorants, and photons, produce their intracellular actions by interactions with metabotropic receptors that activate heterotrimeric guanine nucleotide (GTP)-binding proteins (G proteins). In contrast to the ionotropic receptors that directly couple to ion-selective channels, G proteins act as indirect molecular switches to relay information from activated plasma membrane receptors to appropriate intracellular targets. Heterotrimeric G proteins consist of a large α-subunit and a smaller β/γ-subunit dimer, each expressed as multiple isoforms with distinct properties and downstream targets. G proteins regulate a plethora of downstream effectors to control the levels of cytosolic second messengers such as Ca^{2+}, cyclic adenosine monophosphate (cAMP), and inositol triphosphate (IP_3). These, in turn, regulate effector proteins such as ion channels and enzymes, either directly or via second messenger–regulated protein phosphorylation pathways. Drugs that act through G protein-coupled receptors (GPCRs), such as agonists for μ opioid and α_2-adrenergic receptors, can affect anesthetic sensitivity (reduce MAC). Inhaled anesthetics can also directly affect signaling via GPCRs.[172] For example, volatile anesthetics activate multiple rat olfactory GPCRs in vivo in a receptor- and agent-selective manner.[173] Analogous effects on related GPCRs more relevant to critical anesthetic end points are possible but remain to be demonstrated. The observation that both volatile anesthetics and nonimmobilizers inhibit mGluR5 glutamate receptors, $5\text{-}HT_{2A}$ serotonin receptors, and muscarinic acetylcholine receptors suggest that these GPCR effects do not contribute to anesthetic immobilization.[174-176]

Protein Phosphorylation

Phosphorylation of proteins on specific serine, threonine, or tyrosine hydroxyl groups, a post-translational modification involved in the regulation of many anesthetic-sensitive receptors and ion channels, is pivotal to synaptic plasticity (e.g., LTP). Phosphorylation is controlled by the balance of activity between protein kinases and phosphatases, several of which are plausible anesthetic targets. The protein kinase C (PKC) family of multifunctional protein kinases is activated by the lipid signaling molecule diacylglycerol and is involved in the regulation of many ion channels and receptors. Halothane[177] and sevoflurane[178] enhance the activity of some PKC isoforms and stimulate phosphorylation of specific PKC substrates. Structural studies have identified a potential binding site in the diacylglycerol binding domain of PKCδ, consistent with the ability of certain anesthetics to mimic this natural regulator by binding to the activating site.[179] A specific role for a direct pharmacologically relevant effect mediated by anesthetic activation of PKC or of any other kinase has yet to be demonstrated. Intrathecal injection of isoform-specific inhibitors of PKC does not affect sensitivity to halothane in vivo.[180] Knockout mice lacking the PKCγ isoform show normal sensitivity to halothane and desflurane while isoflurane MAC was increased,[181] suggesting that PKC is not critical to volatile anesthetic immobilization.

An important role for effects of volatile anesthetics and xenon on cell signaling mechanisms has been discovered for anesthetic-induced preconditioning of heart (see Chapter 23) and brain against ischemic damage.[83,87,102] Anesthetic-induced and ischemic cardiac preconditioning share critical signaling mechanisms, including activation of multiple GPCRs (e.g., adenosine, opioid, adrenergic) and protein kinases (e.g., src kinase, PKCδ, PKCε, Akt, mitogen-activated protein kinases [MAPKs]) and their downstream targets, particularly sarcolemmal and/or mitochondrial K_{ATP} channels, possibly initiated by changes in reactive oxygen species as the critical second messenger.[88] Volatile anesthetics and xenon share cardioprotective and neuroprotective effects involving these signaling pathways.[102]

The effects of anesthetics on the phosphorylation of individual residues in specific substrates can be studied using phosphorylation state-specific antibodies that are able to detect the phosphorylated form of kinase substrates. A comparison of the effects of three mechanistically diverse anesthetics (isoflurane, propofol, and ketamine) on critical intracellular protein phosphorylation signaling pathways that are known to integrate multiple second messenger systems reveals both shared and agent-specific actions in vivo.[182] All three anesthetics reduce phosphorylation of activating sites on NMDA (S897) and AMPA (S831) glutamate receptors and of the downstream extracellular signal-regulated kinase ERK2, which are involved in synaptic plasticity, consistent with depression of normal glutamatergic synaptic transmission in the anesthetized mouse cerebral cortex. This effect is somewhat selective in that several other PKA substrates examined are not affected, indicating a substrate-specific effect rather than a general inhibition of PKA activity.[183] Additional studies will be required to determine which anesthetic effects on kinase pathways represent direct effects, as occurs with PKC, and which are indirect due to anesthetic-induced alterations in signaling molecules known to regulate protein kinase and phosphatase activity such as Ca^{2+} and other second messengers.

Gene Expression

The ability of general anesthetics to alter gene expression in the brain was first observed for the highly reactive acute early genes *c-fos* and *c-jun*.[184] Anesthetic effects on gene expression have since been observed for multiple anesthetics and organs.[185] In the hippocampus of aged rats, changes in gene expression persisted for up to 2 days in rats exposed to isoflurane and nitrous oxide,[186] and changes in protein expression have been observed 3 days after exposure to desflurane.[187] The significance of these changes in gene and protein expression persisting after recovery from the classic signs of anesthesia remains to be established (see reference 78 for review).

Cellular Mechanisms

Neuronal Excitability

Neuronal excitability is determined by resting membrane potential, threshold for action potential initiation, and input resistance (an indication of overall channel activity), which can differ between compartments within an individual neuron owing to subcellular specializations (e.g., soma versus dendrite). High concentrations of volatile anesthetics hyperpolarize hippocampal pyramidal cells in slice preparations by less than 5 mV at more than five times MAC.[188,189] At relevant concentrations, neither resting membrane potential nor input resistance is significantly affected in hippocampal[190] or spinal cord neurons.[191] Anesthetic effects on the firing properties of hippocampal neurons are complex: increased or decreased thresholds (for enflurane) have been reported.[190,192] By contrast, thalamic neurons hyperpolarize in the presence of isoflurane and are less likely to fire action potentials due to a decrease in input resistance (increased shunting), attributed to increased K^+ conductance.[193] Similar effects are observed in hypoglossal motor neurons and neurons from the locus coeruleus, where a TASK-type K_{2P} channel has been causally implicated.[115]

A role for $GABA_A$ receptors located at extrasynaptic sites has been suggested recently for volatile anesthetic effects (Fig. 20-9). Extrasynaptic $GABA_A$ receptors, which differ from synaptic receptors in their subunit composition, mediate tonic inhibition (as opposed to phasic inhibition mediated by synaptic $GABA_A$ receptors) and are remarkably sensitive to many general anesthetics. Extrasynaptic $GABA_A$ receptors have a high affinity for GABA, desensitize slowly, and are tonically exposed to low ambient GABA concentrations,[194] at which the potentiating effect of anesthetics is most significant. The effects of anesthetics on tonic inhibition have been characterized in the hippocampus, which is critically involved in learning and memory. Hippocampal neurons generate a robust tonic current via activation of α_5-subunit–containing $GABA_A$ receptors[195-199] that is highly sensitive to etomidate, propofol, midazolam, and isoflurane. $GABA_A$ receptors containing the α_5-subunit are highly sensitive to low concentrations of propofol and isoflurane that produce amnesia but not unconsciousness. Thus, these receptors provide a potential substrate for the amnesic properties of anesthetics.

Presynaptic versus Postsynaptic Effects on Synaptic Transmission

General anesthetics have potent and specific effects on synaptic transmission, including presynaptic actions (by altering transmitter release) and postsynaptic actions (by altering the responses of neurons to specific transmitters). The relative contributions of presynaptic versus postsynaptic anesthetic effects on synaptic transmission have been difficult to resolve, probably because the effects are transmitter- and synapse-specific.[117] The net effect of anesthetics on synaptic transmission is determined by the relative magnitude and direction of both their presynaptic and postsynaptic effects.

Synaptic excitation is decreased by volatile anesthetics (Fig. 20-10). Experiments in various slice preparations indicate that reduced excitation is primarily due to presynaptic mechanisms (Fig. 20-11).[131,191,200-202] A postsynaptic mechanism is also involved because neuronal excitation to directly applied glutamate is reduced to some degree.[202-204] Volatile anesthetics have inconsistent effects on cloned AMPA or NMDA glutamate receptors but potentiate kainate receptors,[112,205-207] which is consistent with a predominantly presynaptic mechanism for inhibition of glutamatergic synapses, whereas the effects of the nonhalogenated inhaled anesthetics (xenon, nitrous oxide, cyclopropane) are mediated primarily by inhibition of postsynaptic NMDA receptors (see earlier). In contrast, augmentation of GABAergic inhibition by most general anesthetics is mediated both by presynaptic and postsynaptic mechanisms. Enhancement of postsynaptic and extrasynaptic $GABA_A$ receptors is well recognized.[113] Remarkably, however, volatile anesthetics also increase spontaneous GABA release and inhibitory postsynaptic current (IPSC) frequency,[208-212] that is, their presynaptic effects at GABAergic terminals are distinct from those at glutamatergic synapses.

The mechanisms for the presynaptic effects of inhaled anesthetics, like those for their postsynaptic effects, are complex and involve multiple targets. Although a synapse-specific contribution of presynaptic Ca^{2+} channels is likely, presynaptic Na^+ channels are more sensitive than the Ca^{2+} channels coupled to glutamate release. This is consistent with observations that the predominant Ca^{2+} channel coupled to neurotransmitter release at hippocampal glutamatergic synapses (P/Q-type) is insensitive to isoflurane.[149] Other presynaptic mechanisms have been proposed, including actions on the vesicle fusion process as demonstrated in the model organism *Caenorhabditis elegans*.[213,214] However, isoflurane effects on exocytosis in rat hippocampal neurons occur primarily upstream of vesicle fusion[137,245] (see reference 117 for review).

The general effects of inhaled anesthetics are to increase inhibitory synaptic transmission and to inhibit excitatory synaptic transmission (Fig. 20-12). The relative importance of anesthetic effects on excitatory versus inhibitory synaptic transmission, and the mechanisms of these effects, are likely to differ for different anesthetics and for specific synapses and networks.[105,215] This concept extends to other putative targets and mechanisms and is incorporated in "agent-specific multiple-site" hypotheses of anesthesia.[215,216]

Simple Circuits and Complex Networks

Simple Circuit Phenomena

To reach a mechanistic understanding of phenomena involving multiple elements of a complex circuit, anatomically reduced (in vitro) or physiologically simplified (in vivo) preparations have been complemented by models with simulations (in silico). These approaches will be essential for integrating reductionist observations of the multiple molecular effects of anesthetics into functional models relevant to behavioral end points. Anatomically, simplified preparations containing native circuitry typically consist of isolated tissue slices. Anesthetic effects have been studied in acute brain slice preparations from various regions of the CNS (hippocampus, amygdala, cortex, thalamus, brainstem, spinal cord). Acute slices preserve native connections but usually lack natural inputs and outputs. Slices from developing mammalian brain can be cultured in vitro. These "organotypic slice cultures" preserve a high degree of synaptic connectivity and display spontaneous network activity, typically absent from acute slices. Physiologically, simplified preparations involve phenomena (typically evoked responses) with *relatively* well understood circuitry. Examples include paired-pulse depression (PPD), synaptic plasticity (long-term potentiation [LTP] and long-term depression [LTD]), and certain sensory-evoked responses. Computer models and simulations can assist in generating hypotheses for experimental testing and test hypotheses based on experimental data.

Synaptic Plasticity

Paired-pulse depression (PPD) and paired-pulse facilitation (PPF) are examples of short-term plasticity in response to exter-

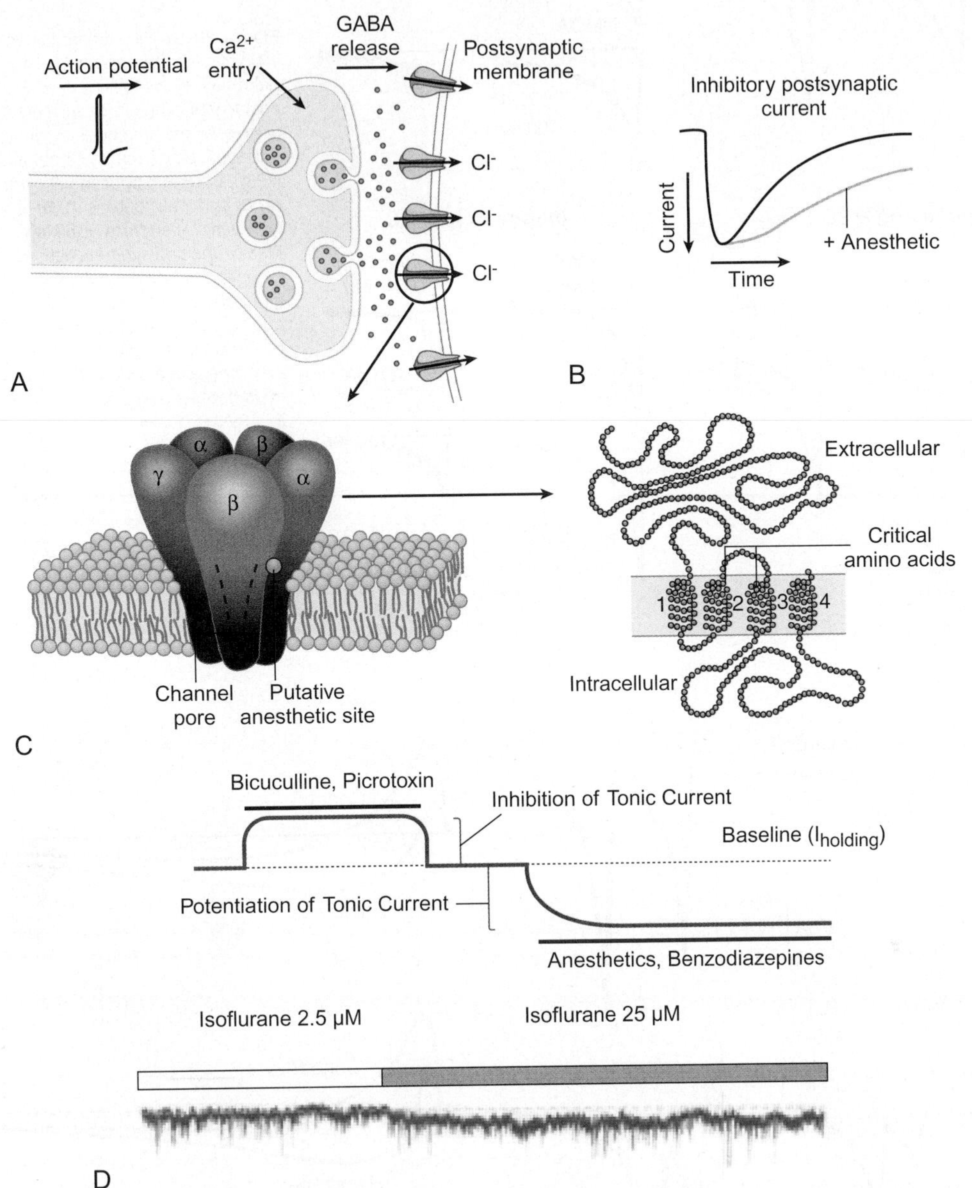

Figure 20-9 Synaptic and extrasynaptic $GABA_A$ receptors are targets for inhaled anesthetics. **A,** On binding of GABA (γ-aminobutyric acid) to the $GABA_A$ receptor, its chloride-permeable channel opens, leading to hyperpolarization. Volatile anesthetics have a relatively low potency but high efficacy at synaptic $GABA_A$ receptors and a high potency and low efficacy at extrasynaptic $GABA_A$ receptors. **B,** General anesthetics prolong channel opening and increase postsynaptic inhibition. The cartoon illustrates the prolongation of miniature inhibitory synaptic currents (mIPSCs) by the slowing of current decay. **C,** A pentameric $GABA_A$ receptor complex in the lipid bilayer membrane (*left*), with a blow-up of a single subunit showing the location of residues critical to anesthetic efficacy in the second and third transmembrane dornains (*right*). **D,** A tonic inhibitory conductance is revealed by the application of a $GABA_A$ receptor antagonist (bicuculline or picrotoxin), as shown by the upward shift in the baseline current. Anesthetics and benzodiazepines increase the tonic conductance as indicated by the inward shift in the current. (*Modified from Hemmings HC Jr, Akabas MH, Goldstein PA, et al: Emerging molecular mechanisms of general anesthetic action. Trends Pharmacol Sci 26:503-510, 2005.*)

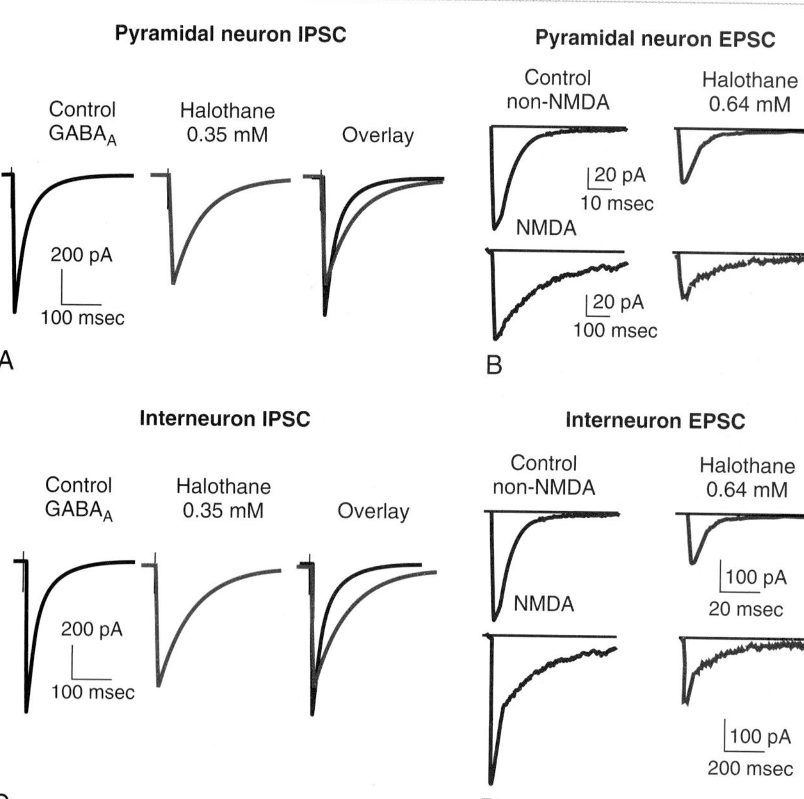

Figure 20-10 Halogenated anesthetics enhance inhibitory and depress excitatory synaptic transmission. Halothane slows the decay of GABA$_A$ receptor–mediated postsynaptic inhibitory currents (IPSCs, **A**) and depresses the amplitude of glutamatergic excitatory postsynaptic currents without affecting the decay (EPSC, **B**, **D**) in hippocampal pyramidal neurons (**A**, **B**) and interneurons (**C**, **D**). *(Panels A and C redrawn with permission from Nishikawa K, MacIver MB: Membrane and synaptic actions of halothane on rat hippocampal pyramidal neurons and inhibitory interneurons. J Neurosci 20:5915-5923, 2000. Panels B and D redrawn with permission from Perouansky M, et al: Effects of halothane on glutamate receptor-mediated excitatory postsynaptic currents: A patch-clamp study in adult mouse hippocampal slices. Anesthesiology 83:109-119, 1995.)*

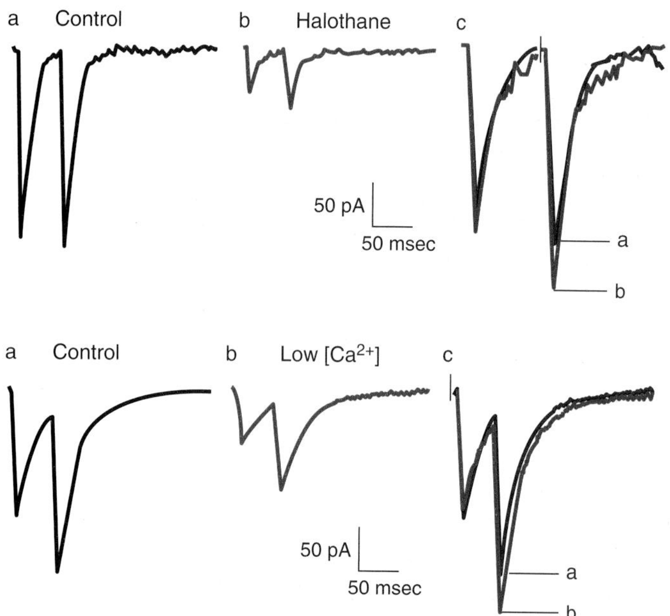

Figure 20-11 Excitatory synaptic transmission is depressed by a presynaptic action. In the paired-pulse facilitation paradigm, halothane (0.64 mM; ~2 MAC) increases the amplitude of the second paired response, an effect similar to that produced by reducing extracellular Ca^{2+} (low Ca^{2+}), indicating a presynaptic site of action. Responses to exogenous, iontophoretically applied AMPA or NMDA are much less sensitive than the presynaptic reduction in transmitter release (not shown). *(Redrawn with permission from Kirson ED, et al: Presynaptic and postsynaptic actions of halothane at glutamatergic synapses in the mouse hippocampus. Br J Pharmacol 124:1607-1614, 1998.)*

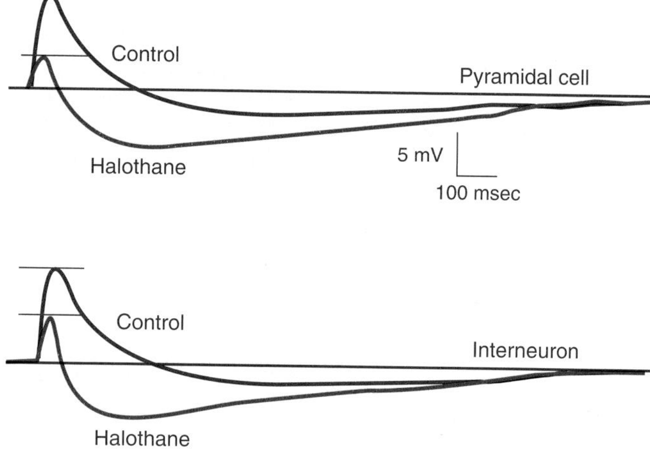

Figure 20-12 Anesthetics affect excitation and inhibition simultaneously. Halothane depresses the excitatory depolarization and augments the inhibitory hyperpolarization in both hippocampal pyramidal cells and interneurons. The net result will depend on the underlying circuitry and its function. *(Redrawn with permission form Nishikawa K, MacIver MB: Membrane and synaptic actions of halothane on rat hippocampal pyramidal neurons and inhibitory interneurons. J Neurosci 20:5915-5923, 2000.)*

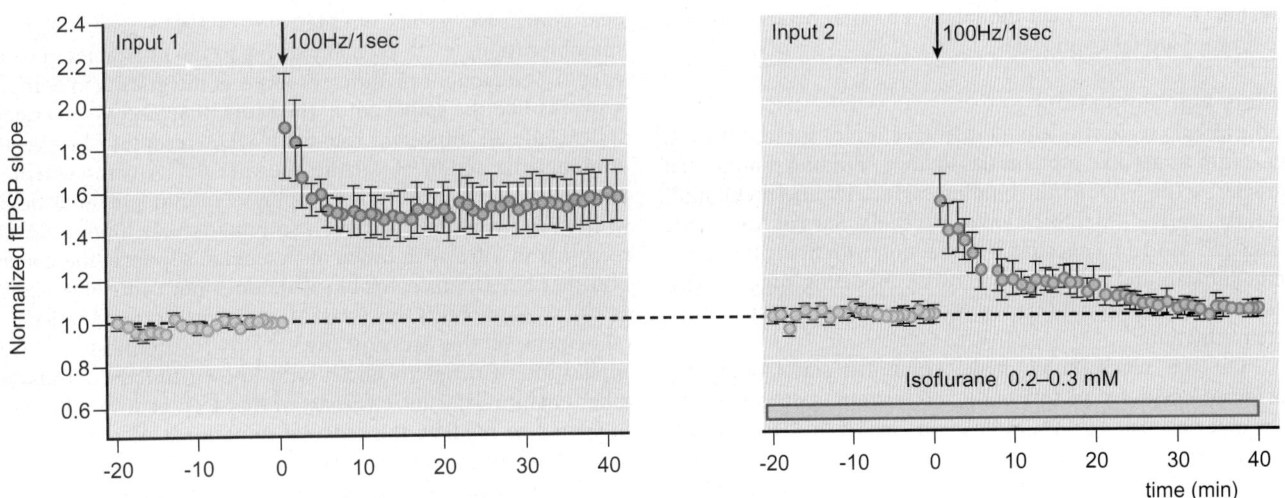

Figure 20-13 Isoflurane blocks the induction of synaptic plasticity (an in-vitro model of learning and memory). Long-term potentiation (an increase in synaptic strength) in hippocampal slices evoked by tetanic stimulation of excitatory synapses is blocked by 200-300 μM of isoflurane. *(Redrawn with permission from Simon W, et al: Isoflurane blocks synaptic plasticity in the mouse hippocampus. Anesthesiology 94:1058-1065, 2001.)*

nal stimulation. Synaptic inhibition is prolonged by volatile anesthetics in vivo[217] and in vitro[218], in general agreement with the notion that anesthetics enhance functional inhibition in the CNS. Enhancement of PPF has been attributed to the presynaptic depressant effect of volatile agents (see Fig. 20-11).[131,201]

LTP (a cellular model of learning and memory) consists of use-dependent strengthening of excitatory synaptic connections mediated by glutamate receptors (see Chapter 11).[219] The few experiments investigating volatile anesthetic effects on LTP have yielded somewhat inconsistent results: halothane, enflurane, and isoflurane do not block LTP induction in vivo, whereas ketamine does.[217] By contrast, isoflurane blocks LTP in the hippocampal slice by enhancing $GABA_A$ receptor–mediated inhibition (Fig. 20-13).[220] LTD, a use-dependent weakening of excitatory connections that is effectively a homeostatic counterpart of LTP, is also blocked by isoflurane.[220] The discrepancy between these findings in vivo and in vitro could reflect differences in the balance between excitatory and inhibitory circuitry activated by the electrical stimuli employed. Etomidate, at amnesic concentrations, blocks LTP by enhancing specific subtypes of $GABA_A$ receptors,[199] whereas ketamine blocks LTP in urethane-anesthetized animals by blocking NMDA receptors.[221,222]

Spontaneously Active Circuits

Spontaneous neuronal activity is decreased by a range of volatile anesthetics both in vivo and in cortical brain slices. This effect is largely $GABA_A$ receptor dependent and marked even at low "sedative" concentrations.[77] Because the cultured slice lacks subcortical input, these results suggest that volatile anesthetics can cause some effects (e.g., sedation) via direct cortical action. However, changes in raw neuronal firing rates might not be a precise quantitative measure of higher cognitive function. Anesthetic effects have also been tested on the circuitry underlying locomotion, a well-studied central pattern generator. Results with isoflurane in the in vitro lamprey spinal cord preparation support the spinal cord as the primary target for volatile anesthetic-induced immobility.[223]

Rhythms and Simulations

Brains perpetually generate complex electrical rhythms that range in frequency from fractions to hundreds of Hertz. Although their physiologic roles are not clear, the prevailing notion is that they reflect, subserve, or constitute fundamental higher-order processing in mammalian brains. Their modulation by anesthetics therefore deserves scrutiny. Two rhythms that have been investigated both in vitro and in vivo in the context of anesthetic mechanisms are γ-rhythms and θ-rhythms.

γ-Rhythms

Isoflurane slows the frequency of evoked γ-oscillations (30-90 Hz, also known as "40 Hz" rhythms) in humans.[224] Studies of γ-oscillations in vitro suggest that their frequency depends on the time constant of decay of $GABA_A$ receptor–mediated synaptic currents in inhibitory networks.[225] Isoflurane slows γ-rhythms in hippocampal[226] and neocortical brain slices[227] to a comparable degree as in humans,[224] providing a tentative link between receptor and circuit-level effects. However, the interaction between anesthetics and behaviorally relevant network effects is unlikely to be unitary, because flash-evoked γ-oscillations in the primary visual cortex are not affected by inhaled agents[54] whereas feedback information transfer at γ frequencies between the visual and frontal cortices is disrupted.[228]

θ-Rhythms

θ-rhythms, present in various cortical structures, are most prominent in the hippocampus where they signal its "online state." They are associated with sensorimotor and mnemonic functions in awake, behaving animals.[229] One component of the θ-rhythm (type I or atropine-resistant) can be affected by amnesic concentrations of isoflurane as well as by the amnestic nonimmobilizer F6,[56] indicating a potential network-level signature effect for anesthetic-induced amnesia. Type II θ-rhythm (atropine-sensitive) can be evoked under anesthesia and is slowed and potentiated by halothane.[230] The γ- and θ-rhythms are interlinked in complex ways, but the nature of their modulation by anesthetics as well as its relevance are far from clear.

Models and Simulations

On the atomic scale, modeling the interaction of anesthetic molecules with target-like proteins has defined "binding motifs" that characterize the amphiphilic binding cavities for anesthetic molecules (see earlier, "Identification of Molecular Sites of Anesthetic Action").[107] Modeling anesthetic interaction with firefly luciferase using gaussian and anisotropic network modeling suggests that anesthetics act by disrupting the modes of motion essential for protein function.[231]

On the macroscopic scale, computer simulations can provide an integrated picture of the modulation of dynamic neuronal and network activity. Simulations based on two different strategies have been published in anesthesia research. A "bottom-up," neuron-by-neuron approach is based on computational models of individual neurons, known anesthetic effects on intrinsic and synaptic membrane conductances, and simple network models. Computer simulations of anesthetic effects on integrated outputs can be generated (e.g., the firing of pacemaker neurons).[232] These models obviously rely on the accuracy of the derived characteristics of real neurons and networks, and the scale of simulations is limited by the complexity of its elements. An alternative is a "top-down" approach such as mean-field modeling in which individual accuracy is sacrificed in favor of global dynamics. Global cortical phenomena, such as anesthetic-induced seizures,[233] are modeled as phase transitions based on mean interactions between populations of averaged neurons (analogous to the EEG signal that also averages the signals of neuronal populations). This approach can be extended to other global cortical phenomena such as consciousness.[234] Neuronal modeling and computer simulations will likely gain importance in the future as bridges between theoretical and experimental studies of anesthesia.

Research Strategies for the Future

The search for anesthetic mechanisms is driven by advances in the basic sciences. Some strategies that should facilitate understanding of anesthetic mechanisms include use of agonists/antagonists in vivo, nonanesthetics/nonimmobilizers, transgenic animals, and high-resolution imaging of the functioning brain.

Pharmacologic

Agonists/Antagonists and Experimental Anesthetics

Use of receptor-specific agonists and antagonists provides a pharmacologic approach to bridging in-vitro with in-vivo studies. A receptor implicated in a specific end point (e.g., immobility) is selected according to the criteria presented earlier, for example the strychnine-sensitive glycine receptor (GlyR). A contribution of spinal GlyRs to isoflurane-induced immobility is indicated if a selective GlyR antagonist applied to the spinal cord in vivo affects immobilization by isoflurane more than immobilization by an anesthetic that is inactive at GlyRs in vitro. This approach did not yield conclusive results for the roles of $GABA_A$ and GlyR for immobilization,[27,235,236] probably owing to the intricacies of drug-receptor interactions on different levels of integration in complex networks like the spinal cord. The same pharmacologic strategy did exclude an important role for NMDA receptor block in the immobilizing action of volatile anesthetics.[28] A complementary pharmacologic approach that employs experimental anesthetics, which are structurally diverse compounds that inhibit NMDA receptors in vitro with different potencies, supports the conclusion that NMDA receptor blockade does not contribute significantly to immobility by conventional volatile anesthetics.[28] A refinement of this strategy involves the anatomically discrete application of drugs to nuclei with known function. Thus, the tuberomammillary nucleus (part of the sleep pathway) has been suggested to mediate the sedative component of anesthesia for some intravenous anesthetics (e.g., propofol).[22] A discrete "general anesthesia site" for GABAergic drugs in the mesopontine tegmentum has also been proposed based on this strategy.[21,234]

Nonimmobilizers

Nonimmobilizers are compounds with physicochemical characteristics similar to those of conventional inhaled anesthetics but predicted anesthetizing concentrations (based on their lipid solubility and the Meyer-Overton correlation: MAC_{pred}) of these drugs do not induce immobility (Fig. 20-14).[8] Initially termed *nonanesthetics,* the terminology was revised when it was discovered that they cause amnesia at similar MAC_{pred} fractions as classic volatile anesthetics.[67] If a molecular or cellular process is affected in

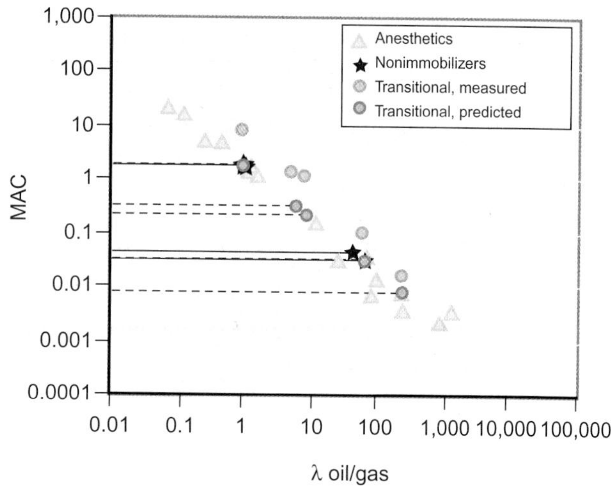

Figure 20-14 Nonimmobilizers disobey the Meyer-Overton correlation. Lipid solubility correlates well with MAC for conventional inhaled anesthetics (*green triangles*), but underestimates experimentally determined MAC for transitional compounds (*orange circles*). *Blue circles* and *dashed drop lines* show MAC values predicted based on lipid solubility for transitional compounds, and *black stars* with *solid drop lines* show predicted MAC values based on lipid solubility for nonimmobilizers. Note that predicted MAC is lower than experimentally determined MAC for transitional compounds, while it can only be calculated for nonimmobilizers, because these drugs do not immobilize at experimentally testable concentrations. MAC values (in volume %) determined in rodents. *(Data for transitional compounds and nonimmobilizers from Koblin DD, et al: Polyhalogenated and perfluorinated compounds that disobey the Meyer-Overton hypothesis. Anesth Analg 79:1043-1048, 1994.)*

similar ways by an anesthetic and a nonimmobilizer, that process is not relevant for the anesthetic state, with the notable exception of amnesia. Despite this elegant rationale, only a limited number of receptors have been excluded because, compared with volatile anesthetics, nonimmobilizers are relatively target-selective. These compounds have the potential to provide insights beyond the initially envisaged receptor-level studies by allowing the separation of sedation from amnesia for the study of underlying network activity in vivo.[56]

Genetic

Genetic strategies take two forms known as "forward" and "reverse" genetics.[238] Reverse genetics approaches focus on a particular gene, chosen because there are reasons to believe that its product might be important to anesthesia. Examples of this strategy are targeted mutations that alter the sensitivity of specific neurotransmitter receptors to anesthetics.[119] Initially, these mutations were used to identify anesthetic binding sites. Subsequently, transgenic animals rendered resistant to anesthetics, either by deletion of a putative target protein from the genome or by expressing a target receptor engineered to be insensitive to an anesthetic, were used to test behavioral relevance of the altered gene product for the anesthetic phenotype. Forward genetics, by contrast, involves the study of randomly generated mutations (either experimentally induced or naturally occurring polymorphisms) in a population that affect the phenotype of interest.

Knock-out and Knock-in Approaches

In the knock-out approach, expression of the gene encoding a protein of interest is disrupted by a specific deletion or insertion. A well-recognized problem with the global knock-out approach is that sometimes extensive compensatory changes can be induced in the proteome of the animal, from anomalies that are lethal in utero to insidious but experimentally confounding differences from wild-type. A complementary strategy is the conditional knock-out, in which the genetic deletion takes place in a restricted fashion—either anatomically (limited to certain brain regions) or temporally (that is, a gene is deleted at a known point in time). These strategies can minimize developmental anomalies and reduce the likelihood of compensatory changes. In the knock-in approach, a mutation, usually of a single amino acid residue, is targeted to produce a protein with altered sensitivity to a drug of interest. Ideally, this mutation remains completely silent in the absence of the drug, that is, it does not perturb the normal expression and function of the protein of interest or alter the expression of other genes.

$GABA_A$ Receptors

Results from transgenic animals illustrate both the utility and the difficulties of the genetic approach with respect to inhaled agents. The conditional forebrain-restricted $GABA_A$ receptor α_1-subunit knock-out mouse is less sensitive to isoflurane-induced amnesia than the wild-type, leading to the conclusion that action at these receptors contributes to its amnesic effects.[239] By contrast, a mouse harboring a mutation of the $GABA_A$ receptor α_1-subunit that renders the receptor insensitive to isoflurane in vitro did not show reduced sensitivity to either the amnesic or the immobilizing effects of isoflurane, leading to the conclusion that this subunit does not mediate the impairment of learning and memory by isoflurane.[31] Similar experiments indicate that action at the $GABA_A$ receptor β_3-subunit does not mediate immobility or amnesia by isoflurane.[30] This "bottom-up" genetic approach is a work-intensive but powerful tool that has yielded clear results with the receptor-specific intravenous anesthetics[16] but has proved more challenging to apply to the more promiscuous inhaled agents.

Two-Pore Domain K^+ Channels

Use of mice harboring knock-out mutations of several two-pore domain K^+ channel (K_{2P}) family members (TASK-1, TASK-3, TREK-1) has demonstrated a role for these channels in volatile anesthesia.[32-34] For example, TREK-1 knock-out mice are partially resistant to all volatile anesthetics tested with respect to both loss of righting reflex (a measure of consciousness) and immobility, but anesthesia can still be induced, albeit at higher anesthetic concentrations. Interestingly, responses to pentobarbital are unaffected, indicating that the mutation does not cause a generalized resistance to anesthesia.

Forward and Population Genetics

The nematode *Caenorhabditis elegans* and the fruit fly *Drosophila melanogaster,* with 300 and 100,000 neurons, respectively, have also been used as model organisms in anesthesia research. The genomes of both organisms have been sequenced and homologous genes in higher organisms can be identified for many genes. Mutations in a number of *C. elegans* genes affect sensitivity to volatile anesthetics, such as *unc64,*[214] *stomatin,*[240] and *gas1*. Mutations in the latter gene confer hypersensitivity to enflurane. Cloning of this gene revealed that it encodes the worm homolog of a subunit of NADH hydrogenase expressed in neurons.[241] Yeasts have also been used as model organisms, with even more obvious limitations with respect to identification of appropriate anesthetic end points.

Sensitivity to anesthetics is a quantitative trait (varying continuously in a population). Quantitative genetics is the study of the heritability of continuous traits. These traits are controlled by genes represented in quantitative trait loci (QTLs). A top-down population-based approach has been used to localize QTLs that govern susceptibility of individuals to anesthetics, in higher as well as lower organisms. Starting from the observation that inbred mouse strains vary in their sensitivity to isoflurane, microsatellite-based linkage analysis on one hand and single nucleotide polymorphism-based analysis of genetic variation on the other hand localized a QTL for isoflurane immobilization to the proximal part of mouse chromosome 7.[242] This type of analysis promises to assist in defining the genetic basis for variability in the susceptibility to both primary anesthetic end points and to side effects.

Imaging

Identification of the anatomic substrates for anesthetic effects on consciousness, memory, and immobility is now approachable with improved functional imaging techniques. Imaging is based on mapping of either hemodynamic or metabolic changes as surrogate measures of neuronal activity, as in positron emission tomography (PET) and functional MRI (fMRI), or on mapping the electrical activity with high-density EEG and low-resolution brain electromagnetic tomography (LORETA). Properties of receptors can also be probed with radioactive ligands (PET). These techniques have the capacity to identify neuroanatomic substrates of drug action, with method-specific limitations. Results from functional PET imaging suggest that propofol suppresses episodic memory by targeting prefrontal and posterior parietal cortex as opposed to the medial temporal lobe[243] and that suppression of consciousness is due to anesthetic action in the thalamus, parts of the medial and posterior parietal cortex, and/or the posterior cingulate and medial parietal cortex (see reference 244 for review). Although observations of regionally specific and global suppressive effects of anesthetics on metabolic activity are unlikely to provide a definitive mechanistic understanding, such information can facilitate hypotheses and experimentally testable predictions.

Summary

The nut of "inhaled anesthetic mechanisms" has proved more difficult to crack than envisaged a generation ago, when the paradigm shifted from lipids to amphiphilic cavities in proteins as anesthetic targets. Despite a remarkable accumulation of factual knowledge, a comprehensive *theory of general anesthetic action* has not yet been formulated. Why has progress toward this goal been so difficult? Important pharmacologic characteristics of inhaled anesthetics that have impeded identification of their relevant molecular targets are their low potency (millimolar), their promiscuous activity at multiple targets, and the lack of specific antagonists. The situation is different for intravenous anesthetics that exhibit more conventional receptor pharmacology. Moreover, accumulating evidence indicates that no universal target exists to explain the actions of every general anesthetic, or even of a single anesthetic agent. It is now clear that the composite state of anesthesia and its core components (i.e., amnesia, sedation/unconsciousness, immobility) are separable behavioral states in vivo that have limited reproducibility in vitro. Resolution of these phenomena at the molecular and cellular levels represents the cutting edge of contemporary neuroscience. Of the multiple molecular and cellular anesthetic effects identified, it is unclear which are critical for the desired behavioral end points, which are harmless or beneficial side effects (e.g., preconditioning), and which, if any, could have long-lasting or delayed undesirable consequences (e.g., cell death, cognitive dysfunction). Progress in identifying the molecular targets of general anesthetics provides a foundation for identification of the network and systems level effects relevant to their behavioral and peripheral end points. As the biologic foundations of behaviors once thought to be exclusively the realm of psychology are unraveled, for which anesthetics provide a valuable investigative tool, a comprehensive theory of anesthesia will also develop.

References

1. Humphrey JA, Sedensky MM, Morgan PG: Understanding anesthesia: Making genetic sense of the absence of senses. Hum Mol Genet 11:1241-1249, 2002.
2. Meyer H: Welche Eigenschaft der Anästhetica bedingt ihre narkotische Wirkung? Arch Exp Pathol Pharmakol 42:109-118, 1899.
3. Overton E: Studien über die Narkose. Jena, Gustav Fischer, 1901.
4. Eger EI: A brief history of the origin of minimum alveolar concentration (MAC). Anesthesiology 96:238-239, 2002.
5. Eger EI, Saidman LJ, Brandstater B: Minimum alveolar anesthetic concentration: A standard of anesthetic potency. Anesthesiology 26:756-763, 1965.
6. Franks NP, Lieb WR: Temperature dependence of the potency of volatile general anesthetics: Implications for in vitro experiments. Anesthesiology 84:716-720, 1996.
7. Ueda I, Kamaya H: Kinetic and thermodynamic aspects of the mechanism of general anesthesia in a model system of firefly luminescence in vitro. Anesthesiology 38:425-436, 1973.
8. Koblin DD, Chortkoff BS, Laster MJ, et al: Polyhalogenated and perfluorinated compounds that disobey the Meyer-Overton hypothesis. Anesth Analg 79:1043-1048, 1994.
9. Raines DE, Miller KW: On the importance of volatile agents devoid of anesthetic action. Anesth Analg 79:1031-1033, 1994.
10. Franks NP, Lieb WR: Seeing the light: Protein theories of general anesthesia: 1984. Anesthesiology 101:235-237, 2004.
11. Franks NP, Lieb WR: Do general anaesthetics act by competitive binding to specific receptors? Nature 310:599-601, 1984.
12. Hall AC, Lieb WR, Franks NP: Stereoselective and non-stereoselective actions of isoflurane on the $GABA_A$ receptor. Br J Pharmacol 112:906-910, 1994.
13. Eger EI 2nd, Fisher DM, Dilger JP, et al: Relevant concentrations of inhaled anesthetics for in vitro studies of anesthetic mechanisms. Anesthesiology 94:915-921, 2001.
14. Eckenhoff RG, Johansson JS: On the relevance of "clinically relevant concentrations" of inhaled anesthetics in in-vitro experiments. Anesthesiology 91:856-860, 1999.
15. Eckenhoff RG, Johansson JS: What are "relevant" concentrations? Anesthesiology 95:1537-1539, 2001.
16. Rudolph U, Antkowiak B: Molecular and neuronal substrates for general anaesthetics. Nat Rev Neurosci 5:709-720, 2004.
17. Antognini JF, Schwartz K: Exaggerated anesthetic requirements in the preferentially anesthetized brain. Anesthesiology 79:1244-1249, 1993.
18. Rampil IJ, Mason P, Singh H: Anesthetic potency (MAC) is independent of forebrain structures in the rat. Anesthesiology 78:707-712, 1993.
19. Stabernack C, Zhang Y, Sonner JM, et al: Thiopental produces immobility primarily by supraspinal actions in rats. Anesth Analg 100:128-136, 2005.
20. Veselis RA, Reinsel RA, Feshchenko VA: Drug-induced amnesia is a separate phenomenon from sedation—electrophysiologic evidence. Anesthesiology 95:896-907, 2001.
21. Devor M, Zalkind V: Reversible analgesia, atonia, and loss of consciousness on bilateral intracerebral microinjection of pentobarbital. Pain 94:101-112, 2001.
22. Nelson LE, Guo TZ, Lu J, et al: The sedative component of anesthesia is mediated by GABA(A) receptors in an endogenous sleep pathway. Nat Neurosci 5:979-984, 2002.
23. Rampil IJ, Laster MJ: No correlation between quantitative electroencephalographic measurements and movement response to noxious stimuli during isoflurane anesthesia in rats. Anesthesiology 77:920-925, 1992.
24. Antognini JF, Carstens E, Atherley R: Does the immobilizing effect of thiopental in brain exceed that of halothane? Anesthesiology 96:980-986, 2002.
25. Stabernack C, Sonner JM, Laster M, et al: Spinal *N*-methyl-D-aspartate receptors may contribute to the immobilizing action of isoflurane. Anesth Analg 96:102-107, 2003.
26. Zhang Y, Laster MJ, Hara K, et al: Glycine receptors mediate part of the immobility produced by inhaled anesthetics. Anesth Analg 96:97-101, 2003.
27. Zhang Y, Sonner JM, Eger EI, et al: Gamma-aminobutyric acidA receptors do not mediate the immobility produced by isoflurane. Anesth Analg 99:85-90, 2004.
28. Eger EI, Liao M, Laster MJ, et al: Contrasting roles of the *N*-methyl-D-aspartate receptor in the production of immobilization by conventional and aromatic anesthetics. Anesth Analg 102:1397-1406, 2006.
29. Raines DE, Claycomb RJ, Forman SA: Nonhalogenated anesthetic alkanes and perhalogenated nonimmobilizing alkanes inhibit alpha(4)beta(2) neuronal nicotinic acetylcholine receptors [comment] [erratum appears in Anesth Analg 2002 95:869]. Anesth Analg 95:573-577, 2002.
30. Liao M, Sonner JM, Jurd R, et al: Beta-3-containing gamma-aminobutyric acid A receptors are not major targets for the amnesic and immobilizing actions of isoflurane. Anesth Analg 101:412-418, 2005.

31. Sonner JM, Werner DF, Elsen FP, et al: Effect of isoflurane and other potent inhaled anesthetics on minimum alveolar concentration, learning, and the righting reflex in mice engineered to express alpha1 gamma-aminobutyric acid type A receptors unresponsive to isoflurane. Anesthesiology 106:107-113, 2007.
32. Heurteaux C, Guy N, Laigle C, et al: TREK-1, a K(+) channel involved in neuroprotection and general anesthesia. EMBO J 23:2684-2695, 2004.
33. Linden AM, Aller MI, Leppa E, et al: The in vivo contributions of TASK-1-containing channels to the actions of inhalation anesthetics, the alpha(2) adrenergic sedative dexmedetomidine, and cannabinoid agonists. J Pharmacol Exp Ther 317:615-626, 2006.
34. Linden AM, Sandu C, Aller MI, et al: TASK-3 knockout mice exhibit exaggerated nocturnal activity, impairments in cognitive functions, and reduced sensitivity to inhalation anesthetics. J Pharmacol Exp Ther 323:924-934, 2007.
35. Westphalen RI, Krivitski M, Amarosa A, et al: Reduced inhibition of cortical glutamate and GABA release by halothane in mice lacking the K(+) channel, TREK-1. Br J Pharmacol 152:939-945, 2007.
36. Sonner JM, Antognini JF, Dutton RC, et al: Inhaled anesthetics and immobility: Mechanisms, mysteries, and minimum alveolar anesthetic concentration. Anesth Analg 97:718-740, 2003.
37. Crick F, Koch C: A framework for consciousness. Nat Neurosci 6:119-126, 2003.
38. Searle JR: Consciousness. Annu Rev Neurosci 23:557-578, 2000.
39. Mashour GA: Integrating the science of consciousness and anesthesia. Anesth Analg 103:975-982, 2006.
40. Angel A: Central neuronal pathways and the process of anesthesia. Br J Anesth 71:148-163, 1993.
41. Ries CR, Puil E: Mechanism of anesthesia revealed by shunting actions of isoflurane on thalamocortical neurons. J Neurophysiol 81:1795-1801, 1999.
42. Detsch O, Vahle-Hinz C, Kochs E, et al: Isoflurane induces dose-dependent changes of thalamic somatosensory information transfer. Brain Res 829:77-89, 1999.
43. Alkire MT, Haier RJ, Fallon JH: Toward a unified theory of narcosis: Brain imaging evidence for a thalamocortical switch as the neurophysiologic basis of anesthetic-induced unconsciousness [see comments]. Conscious Cogn 9:370-386, 2000.
44. John ER, Prichep LS, Kox W, et al: Invariant reversible QEEG effects of anesthetics. Conscious Cogn 10:165-183, 2001.
45. Veselis RA: Anesthesia—a descent or a jump into the depths? Conscious Cogn 10:230-235, 2001.
46. Chortkoff BS, Eger EI 2nd, Crankshaw DP, et al: Concentrations of desflurane and propofol that suppress response to command in humans. Anesth Analg 81:737-743, 1995.
47. Dwyer R, Bennett HL, Eger EI 2nd, et al: Effects of isoflurane and nitrous oxide in subanesthetic concentrations on memory and responsiveness in volunteers. Anesthesiology 77:888-898, 1992.
48. Hudetz AG: Suppressing consciousness: Mechanisms of general anesthesia. Semin Anesth 25:196-204, 2006.
49. Tononi G: An information integration theory of consciousness. BMC Neurosci 5:42, 2004.
50. Varela F, Lachaux JP, Rodriguez E, et al: The brainweb: Phase synchronization and large-scale integration. Nat Rev Neurosci 2:229-239, 2001.
51. Massimini M, Ferraretti F, Huber R, et al: Breakdown of cortical effective connectivity during sleep. Science 309:2228-2232, 2005.
52. Mashour GA: Consciousness unbound—Toward a paradigm of general anesthesia. Anesthesiology 100:428-433, 2004.
53. Lydic R, Biebuyck JF: Sleep neurobiology: Relevance for mechanistic studies of anaesthesia. Br J Anaesth 72:506-508, 1994.
54. Imas OA, Ropella KM, Ward BD, et al: Volatile anesthetics enhance flash-induced gamma oscillations in rat visual cortex. Anesthesiology 102:937-947, 2005.
55. Imas OA, Ropella KM, Wood JD, et al: Isoflurane disrupts anteroposterior phase synchronization of flash-induced field potentials in the rat. Neurosci Lett 402:216-221, 2006.
56. Perouansky M, Hentschke H, Perkins M, et al: Amnesic concentrations of the nonimmobilizer 1,2-dichlorohexafluorocyclobutane (F6, 2N) and isoflurane alter hippocampal theta oscillations in vivo. Anesthesiology 106:1168-1176, 2007.
57. Ter Mikaelian M, Sanes DH, Semple MN: Transformation of temporal properties between auditory midbrain and cortex in the awake Mongolian gerbil. J Neurosci 27:6091-6102, 2007.
58. Dutton RC, Maurer AJ, Sonner JM, et al: The concentration of isoflurane required to suppress learning depends on the type of learning. Anesthesiology 94:514-519, 2001.
59. Alkire MT, Nathan SV: Does the amygdala mediate anesthetic-induced amnesia? Basolateral amygdala lesions block sevoflurane-induced amnesia. Anesthesiology 102:754-760, 2005.
60. Alkire MT, Gorski LA: Relative amnesic potency of five inhalational anesthetics follows the Meyer-Overton rule. Anesthesiology 101:417-429, 2004.
61. Vertes RP: Hippocampal theta rhythm: A tag for short-term memory. Hippocampus 15:923-935, 2005.
62. Pan WX, McNaughton N: The medial supramammillary nucleus, spatial learning and the frequency of hippocampal theta activity. Brain Res 764:101-108, 1997.
63. Robbe D, Montgomery SM, Thome A, et al: Cannabinoids reveal importance of spike timing coordination in hippocampal function. Nat Neurosci 9:1526-1533, 2006.
64. Seidenbecher T, Laxmi TR, Stork O, et al: Amygdalar and hippocampal theta rhythm synchronization during fear memory retrieval. Science 301:846-850, 2003.
65. Pryor KO, Murphy E, Reinsel RA, et al: Heterogeneous effects of intravenous anesthetics on modulatory memory systems in humans. Anesthesiology 107. 2007.
66. Rudolph U, Crestani F, Benke D, et al: Benzodiazepine actions mediated by specific gamma-aminobutyric acid(A) receptor subtypes. Nature 401:796-800, 1999.
67. Kandel L, Chortkoff BS, Sonner J, et al: Nonanesthetics can suppress learning. Anesth Analg 82:321-326, 1996.
68. Mihic SJ, McQuilkin SJ, Eger EI 2nd, et al: Potentiation of gamma-aminobutyric acid type A receptor–mediated chloride currents by novel halogenated compounds correlates with their abilities to induce general anesthesia. Mol Pharmacol 46:851-857, 1994.
69. Zarnowska ED, Pearce RA, Saad AA, et al: The gamma-subunit governs the susceptibility of recombinant gamma-aminobutyric acid type A receptors to block by the nonimmobilizer 1,2-dichlorohexafluorocyclobutane (F6, 2N). Anesth Analg 101:401-406, 2005.
70. Jevtovic-Todorovic V, Todorovic SM, Mennerick S, et al: Nitrous oxide (laughing gas) is an NMDA antagonist, neuroprotectant and neurotoxin. Nat Med 4:460-463, 1998.
71. Mennerick S, Jevtovic-Todorovic V, Todorovic SM, et al: Effect of nitrous oxide on excitatory and inhibitory synaptic transmission in hippocampal cultures. J Neurosci 18:9716-9726, 1998.
72. Gruss M, Bushell TJ, Bright DP, et al: Two-pore-domain K^+ channels are a novel target for the anesthetic gases xenon, nitrous oxide, and cyclopropane. Mol Pharmacol 65:443-452, 2004.
73. Gries DA, Condouris GA, Shey Z, et al: Anxiolytic-like action in mice treated with nitrous oxide and oral triazolam or diazepam. Life Sci 76:1667-1674, 2005.
74. Nelson LE, Lu J, Guo T, et al: The alpha-2-adrenoreceptor agonist dexmedetomidine converges on an endogenous sleep-promoting pathway to exert its sedative effects. Anesthesiology 98:428-436, 2003.
75. Lydic R: Sleep and anesthesia. *In* Hemmings HC Jr, Hopkins PM (eds): Foundations of Anesthesia, 2nd ed. London, Elsevier, 2006, pp 373-383.
76. Tung A, Bergmann BM, Herrera S, et al: Recovery from sleep deprivation occurs during propofol anesthesia. Anesthesiology 100:1419-1426, 2004.
77. Hentschke H, Schwarz C, Antkowiak B: Neocortex is the major target of sedative concentrations of volatile anaesthetics: Strong depression of firing rates and increase of $GABA_A$ receptor-mediated inhibition. Eur J Neurosci 21:93-102, 2005.
78. Perouansky M: Liaisons dangereuses? General anaesthetics and long-term toxicity in the CNS. Eur J Anaesthesiol 24:107-115, 2007.
79. Jevtovic-Todorovic V, Hartman RE, Izumi Y, et al: Early exposure to common anesthetic agents causes widespread neurodegeneration in the developing rat brain and persistent learning deficits. J Neurosci 23:876-882, 2003.
80. Slikker W Jr, Zou X, Hotchkiss CE, et al: Ketamine-induced neuronal cell death in the perinatal rhesus monkey. Toxicol Sci 98:145-158, 2007.
81. Culley DJ, Raghavan SV, Waly M, et al: Nitrous oxide decreases cortical methionine synthase transiently but produces lasting memory impairment in aged rats. Anesth Analg 105:83-88, 2007.
82. Wan Y, Xu J, Ma D, et al: Postoperative impairment of cognitive function in rats: A possible role for cytokine-mediated inflammation in the hippocampus. Anesthesiology 106:436-443, 2007.
83. Kitano H, Kirsch JR, Hurn PD, et al: Inhalational anesthetics as neuroprotectants or chemical preconditioning agents in ischemic brain. J Cereb Blood Flow Metab 27:1108-1128, 2006.
84. Fukuda S, Warner DS: Cerebral protection. Br J Anaesth 99:10-17, 2007.
85. Kawaguchi M, Furuya H, Patel PM: Neuroprotective effects of anesthetic agents. J Anesth 19:150-156, 2005.
86. Inoue S, Drummond JC, Davis DP, et al: Combination of isoflurane and caspase inhibition reduces cerebral injury in rats subjected to focal cerebral ischemia. Anesthesiology 101:75-81, 2004.
87. Preckel B, Weber NC, Sanders RD, et al: Molecular mechanisms transducing the anesthetic, analgesic, and organ-protective actions of xenon. Anesthesiology 105:187-197, 2006.
88. Zaugg M, Lucchinetti E, Uecker M, et al: Anaesthetics and cardiac preconditioning: I. Signalling and cytoprotective mechanisms. Br J Anaesth 91:551-565, 2003.
89. Pagel PS, Warltier DC: Ventricular function. *In* Warltier DC (ed): Anesthetics and Left Ventricular Function. Baltimore, Williams & Wilkins, 1995, pp 213-252.

90. Hanley PJ, ter Keurs HE, Cannell MB: Excitation-contraction coupling in the heart and the negative inotropic action of volatile anesthetics. Anesthesiology 101:999-1014, 2004.
91. Huneke R, Jungling E, Skasa M, et al: Effects of the anesthetic gases xenon, halothane, and isoflurane on calcium and potassium currents in human atrial cardiomyocytes. Anesthesiology 95:999-1006, 2001.
92. Stowe DF, Rehmert GC, Kwok WM, et al: Xenon does not alter cardiac function or major cation currents in isolated guinea pig hearts or myocytes. Anesthesiology 92:516-522, 2000.
93. Ebert TJ, Kampine JP: Nitrous oxide augments sympathetic outflow: Direct evidence from human peroneal nerve recordings. Anesth Analg 69:444-449, 1989.
94. Stowe DF, Monroe SM, Marijic J, et al: Effects of nitrous oxide on contractile function and metabolism of the isolated heart. Anesthesiology 73:1220-1226, 1990.
95. Pagel PS, Kampine JP, Schmeling WT, et al: Alteration of left ventricular diastolic function by desflurane, isoflurane, and halothane in the chronically instrumented dog with autonomic nervous system blockade. Anesthesiology 74:1103-1114, 1991.
96. Tanaka K, Kawano T, Nakamura A, et al: Isoflurane activates sarcolemmal adenosine diphosphate-sensitive potassium channels in vascular smooth muscle cells—A role for protein kinase A. Anesthesiology 106:984-991, 2007.
97. Yoshino J, Akata T, Izumi K, et al: Multiple actions of halothane on contractile response to noradrenaline in isolated mesenteric resistance arteries. Naunyn Schmied Arch Pharmacol 371:500-515, 2005.
98. Vulliemoz Y: The nitric oxide-cyclic 3′,5′-guanosine monophosphate signal transduction pathway in the mechanism of action of general anesthetics. Toxicol Lett 100-101:103-108, 1998.
99. Huneke R, Fassl J, Rossaint R, et al: Effects of volatile anesthetics on cardiac ion channels. Acta Anaesthesiol Scand 48:547-561, 2004.
100. Stadnicka A, Marinovic J, Ljubkovic M, et al: Volatile anesthetic-induced cardiac preconditioning. J Anesth 21:212-219, 2007.
101. Suleiman MS, Zacharowski K, Angelini GD: Inflammatory response and cardioprotection during open-heart surgery: The importance of anaesthetics. Br J Pharmacol 153:21-33, 2008.
102. Pratt PF Jr, Wang C, Weihrauch D, et al: Cardioprotection by volatile anesthetics: new applications for old drugs? Curr Opin Anaesth 19:397-403, 2006.
103. Weber NC, Toma O, Awan S, et al: Effects of nitrous oxide on the rat heart in vivo—Another inhalational anesthetic that preconditions the heart? Anesthesiology 103:1174-1182, 2005.
104. Tanaka K, Ludwig LM, Kersten JR, et al: Mechanisms of cardioprotection by volatile anesthetics. Anesthesiology 100:707-721, 2004.
105. Stuth EAE, Krolo M, Tonkovic-Capin M, et al: Effects of halothane on synaptic neurotransmission to medullary expiratory neurons in the ventral respiratory group of dogs. Anesthesiology 91:804-814, 1999.
106. Franks NP, Lieb WR: Molecular and cellular mechanisms of general anaesthesia. Nature 367:607-614, 1994.
106. Franks NP, Lieb WR: Volatile general anaesthetics activate a novel neuronal K+ current. Nature 333:662-664, 1988.
107. Bertaccini EJ, Trudell JR, Franks NP: The common chemical motifs within anesthetic binding sites. Anesth Analg 104:318-324, 2007.
108. Jenkins A, Greenblatt EP, Faulkner HJ, et al: Evidence for a common binding cavity for three general anesthetics within the GABAA receptor. J Neurosci 21:RC136, 2001.
109. Koltchine VV, Finn SE, Jenkins A, et al: Agonist gating and isoflurane potentiation in the human gamma-aminobutyric acid type A receptor determined by the volume of a second transmembrane domain residue. Mol Pharmacol 56:1087-1093, 1999.
110. Wick MJ, Mihic SJ, Ueno S, et al: Mutations of gamma-aminobutyric acid and glycine receptors change alcohol cutoff: Evidence for an alcohol receptor? Proc Natl Acad Sci U S A 95:6504-6509, 1998.
111. Trudell JR, Bertaccini E: Comparative modeling of a GABAA alpha1 receptor using three crystal structures as templates. J Mol Graph Model 23:39-49, 2004.
112. Dickinson R, Peterson BK, Banks P, et al: Competitive inhibition at the glycine site of the *N*-methyl-D-aspartate receptor by the anesthetics xenon and Isoflurane. Anesthesiology 107:756-767, 2007.
113. Hemmings HC Jr, Akabas MH, Goldstein PA, et al: Emerging molecular mechanisms of general anesthetic action. Trends Pharmacol Sci 26:503-510, 2005.
114. Krasowski MD, Harrison NL: General anaesthetic actions on ligand-gated ion channels. Cell Mol Life Sci 55:1278-1303, 1999.
115. Sirois JE, Lei Q, Talley EM, et al: The TASK-1 two-pore domain K^+ channel is a molecular substrate for neuronal effects of inhalation anesthetics. J Neurosci 20:6347-6354, 2000.
116. Patel AJ, Honore E, Lesage F, et al: Inhalational anesthetics activate two-pore-domain background K^+ channels. Nat Neurosci 2:422-426, 1999.
117. Perouansky M, Hemmings HC: Presynaptic actions of general anesthetics. *In* Antognini JF, Carlens E, Raines D (eds): Neural Mechanisms of Anesthesia. Totowa, NJ, Humana Press, 2003, pp 345-370
118. Lynch JW: Molecular structure and function of the glycine receptor chloride channel. Physiol Rev 84:1051-1095, 2004.
119. Mihic SJ, Ye Q, Wick MJ, et al: Sites of alcohol and volatile anaesthetic action on GABA(A) and glycine receptors. Nature 389:385-389, 1997.
120. Jenkins A, Franks NP, Lieb WR: Actions of general anaesthetics on 5-HT3 receptors in N1E-115 neuroblastoma cells. Br J Pharmacol 117:1507-1515, 1996.
121. Machu TK, Harris RA: Alcohols and anesthetics enhance the function of 5-hydroxytryptamine(3) receptors expressed in *Xenopus laevis it* oocytes. J Pharmacol Exp Ther 271:898-905, 1994.
122. Solt K, Stevens RJ, Davies PA, et al: General anesthetic-induced channel gating enhancement of 5-hydroxytryptamine type 3 receptors depends on receptor subunit composition. J Pharmacol Exp Ther 315:771-776, 2005.
123. Role LW, Berg DK: Nicotinic receptors in the development and modulation of CNS synapses. Neuron 16:1077-1085, 1996.
124. Flood P, Ramirez-Latorre J, Role L: Alpha 4 beta 2 neuronal nicotinic acetylcholine receptors in the central nervous system are inhibited by isoflurane and propofol, but alpha 7-type nicotinic acetylcholine receptors are unaffected. Anesthesiology 86:859-865, 1997.
125. Violet JM, Downie DL, Nakisa RC, et al: Differential sensitivities of mammalian neuronal and muscle nicotinic acetylcholine receptors to general anesthetics. Anesthesiology 86:866-874, 1997.
126. Dingledine R, Borges K, Bowie D, et al: The glutamate receptor ion channels. Pharmacol Rev 51:7-61, 1999.
127. Franks NP, Dickinson R, de Sousa SL, et al: How does xenon produce anaesthesia? Nature 396:324, 1998.
128. Solt K, Eger EI, Raines DE: Differential modulation of human *N*-methyl-D-aspartate receptors by structurally diverse general anesthetics. Anesth Analg 102:1407-1411, 2006.
129. Harris RA, Mihic SJ, Dildy-Mayfield JE, et al: Actions of anesthetics on ligand-gated ion channels: Role of receptor subunit composition. FASEB J 9:1454-1462, 1995.
130. Sonner JM, Vissel B, Royle G, et al: The effect of three inhaled anesthetics in mice harboring mutations in the GluR6 (kainate) receptor gene. Anesth Analg 101:143-148, 2005.
131. MacIver MB, Mikulec AA, Amagasu SM, et al: Volatile anesthetics depress glutamate transmission via presynaptic actions. Anesthesiology 85:823-834, 1996.
132. Perouansky M, Hemmings HC Jr, Pearce RA: Anesthetic effects on glutamatergic neurotransmission: Lessons learned from a large synapse. Anesthesiology 100:470-472, 2004.
133. Winegar BD, MacIver MB: Isoflurane depresses hippocampal CA1 glutamate nerve terminals without inhibiting fiber volleys. BMC Neurosci 7:5, 2006.
134. Haydon DA, Urban BW: The effects of some inhalation anaesthetics on the sodium current of the squid giant axon. J Physiol (Lond) 341:429-439, 1983.
135. Berg-Johnsen J, Langmoen IA: The effect of isoflurane on unmyelinated and myelinated fibres in the rat brain. Acta Physiol Scand 127:87-93, 1986.
136. Mikulec AA, Pittson S, Amagasu SM, et al: Halothane depresses action potential conduction in hippocampal axons. Brain Res 796:231-238, 1998.
137. Wu XS, Sun JY, Evers AS, et al: Isoflurane inhibits transmitter release and the presynaptic action potential. Anesthesiology 100:663-670, 2004.
138. Yu FH, Catterall WA: The VGL-chanome: A protein superfamily specialized for electrical signaling and ionic homeostasis. Sci STKE 2004:re15, 2004.
139. Shiraishi M, Harris RA: Effects of alcohols and anesthetics on recombinant voltage-gated Na^+ channels. J Pharmacol Exp Ther 309:987-994, 2004.
140. OuYang W, Hemmings HC Jr: Depression by isoflurane of the action potential and underlying voltage-gated ion currents in isolated rat neurohypophysial nerve terminals. J Pharmacol Exp Ther 312:801-808, 2005.
141. OuYang W, Jih T-Y, Zhang T-T, et al: Isoflurane inhibits NaChBac, a prokaryotic voltage-gated sodium channel. J Pharmacol Exp Ther 322:1076-1083, 2007.
142. Ouyang W, Hemmings HC Jr: Isoform-selective effects of isoflurane on voltage-gated Na^+ channels. Anesthesiology 107:91-98, 2007.
143. Ratnakumari L, Vysotskaya TN, Duch DS, et al: Differential effects of anesthetic and nonanesthetic cyclobutanes on neuronal voltage-gated sodium channels. Anesthesiology 92:529-541, 2000.
144. Catterall WA: Structure and regulation of voltage-gated Ca^{2+} channels. Annu Rev Cell Dev Biol 16:521-555, 2000.
145. Topf N, Recio-Pinto E, Blanck TJ, et al: Actions of general anesthetics on voltage-gated ion channels. *In* Antognini JF, Carlens E, Raines D (eds): Neural Mechanisms of Anesthesia. Totowa, NJ, Humana Press, 2003, pp 299-318.

146. Miao N, Frazer MJ, Lynch C 3rd: Volatile anesthetics depress Ca^{2+} transients and glutamate release in isolated cerebral synaptosomes. Anesthesiology 83:593-603, 1995.
147. Kameyama K, Aono K, Kitamura K: Isoflurane inhibits neuronal Ca^{2+} channels through enhancement of current inactivation. Br J Anaesth 82:402-411, 1999.
148. Study RE: Isoflurane inhibits multiple voltage-gated calcium currents in hippocampal pyramidal neurons [see comments]. Anesthesiology 81:104-116, 1994.
149. Hall AC, Lieb WR, Franks NP: Insensitivity of P-type calcium channels to inhalational and intravenous general anesthetics. Anesthesiology 81:117-123, 1994.
150. Takei T, Saegusa H, Zong S, et al: Increased sensitivity to halothane but decreased sensitivity to propofol in mice lacking the N-type Ca^{2+} channel. Neurosci Lett 350:41-45, 2003.
151. Joksovic PM, Brimelow BC, Murbartian J, et al: Contrasting anesthetic sensitivities of T-type Ca^{2+} channels of reticular thalamic neurons and recombinant Ca(v)3.3 channels. Br J Pharmacol 144:59-70, 2005.
152. Todorovic SM, Jevtovic-Todorovic V, Mennerick S, et al: Ca(v)3.2 channel is a molecular substrate for inhibition of T-type calcium currents in rat sensory neurons by nitrous oxide. Mol Pharmacol 60:603-610, 2001.
153. Petrenko AB, Tsujita M, Kohno T, et al: Mutation of alpha(1G) T-type calcium channels in mice does not change anesthetic requirements for loss of the righting reflex and minimum alveolar concentration but delays the onset of anesthetic induction. Anesthesiology 106:1177-1185, 2007.
154. Rithalia A, Hopkins PM, Harrison SM: The effects of halothane, isoflurane, and sevoflurane on Ca^{2+} current and transient outward K^+ current in subendocardial and subepicardial myocytes from the rat left ventricle. Anesth Analg 99:1615-1622, 2004.
155. Davies LA, Gibson CN, Boyett MR, et al: Effects of isoflurane, sevoflurane, and halothane on myofilament Ca^{2+} sensitivity and sarcoplasmic reticulum Ca^{2+} release in rat ventricular myocytes. Anesthesiology 93:1034-1044, 2000.
156. Pabelick CM, Prakash YS, Kannan MS, et al: Effects of halothane on sarcoplasmic reticulum calcium release channels in porcine airway smooth muscle cells. Anesthesiology 95:207-215, 2001.
157. Roberts MC, Mickelson JR, Patterson EE, et al: Autosomal dominant canine malignant hyperthermia is caused by a mutation in the gene encoding the skeletal muscle calcium release channel (*RYR1*). Anesthesiology 95:716-725, 2001.
158. Mickelson JR, Louis CF: Malignant hyperthermia: Excitation-contraction coupling, Ca^{2+} release channel, and cell Ca^{2+} regulation defects. Physiol Rev 76:537-592, 1996.
159. Yost CS: Potassium channels: Basic aspects, functional roles, and medical significance. Anesthesiology 90:1186-1203, 1999.
160. Friederich P, Benzenberg D, Trellakis S, et al: Interaction of volatile anesthetics with human Kv channels in relation to clinical concentrations. Anesthesiology 95:954-958, 2001.
161. Franks NP, Lieb WR: Volatile general anesthetics activate a novel neuronal K^+ current. Nature 333:662-664, 1988.
162. Franks NP, Honore E: The TREK K-2P channels and their role in general anaesthesia and neuroprotection. Trends Pharmacol Sci 25:601-608, 2004.
163. Patel AJ, Honore E: Anesthetic-sensitive 2P domain K^+ channels. Anesthesiology 95:1013-1021, 2001.
164. Farwell D, Gollob MH: Electrical heart disease: Genetic and molecular basis of cardiac arrhythmias in normal structural hearts. Can J Cardiol 23(Suppl A):16A-22A, 2007.
165. Antzelevitch C: Molecular biology and cellular mechanisms of Brugada and long QT syndromes in infants and young children. J Electrocardiol 34(Suppl):177-181, 2001.
166. Li J, Correa AM: Kinetic modulation of HERG potassium channels by the volatile anesthetic halothane. Anesthesiology 97:921-930, 2002.
167. Davies LA, Hopkins PM, Boyett MR, et al: Effects of halothane on the transient outward K(+) current in rat ventricular myocytes. Br J Pharmacol 131:223-230, 2000.
168. Sirois JE, Lynch C III, Bayliss DA: Convergent and reciprocal modulation of a leak K^+ current and I(h) by an inhalational anaesthetic and neurotransmitters in rat brainstem motoneurones. J Physiol 541:717-729, 2002.
169. Chen X, Sirois JE, Lei Q, et al: HCN subunit-specific and cAMP-modulated effects of anesthetics on neuronal pacemaker currents. J Neurosci 25:5803-5814, 2005.
170. Robinson RB, Siegelbaum SA: Hyperpolarization-activated cation currents: From molecules to physiological function. Annu Rev Physiol 65:453-480, 2003.
171. Girault JA, Hemmings HC Jr: Cell signaling. *In* Hemmings HC Jr, Hopkins PM (eds): Foundations of Anesthesia, 2nd Edition. London, Mosby, 2005, pp 31-50.
172. Rebecchi MJ, Pentyala SN: Anaesthetic actions on other targets: protein kinase C and guanine nucleotide-binding proteins. Br J Anaesth 89:62-78, 2002.
173. Peterlin Z, Ishizawa Y, Araneda R, et al: Selective activation of G-protein–coupled receptors by volatile anesthetics. Mol Cell Neurosci 30:506-512, 2005.
174. Minami K, Gereau RW, Minami M, et al: Effects of ethanol and anesthetics on type 1 and 5 metabotropic glutamate receptors expressed in *Xenopus laevis* oocytes. Mol Pharmacol 53:148-156, 1998.
175. Minami K, Minami M, Harris RA: Inhibition of 5-hydroxytryptamine type 2A receptor-induced currents by n-alcohols and anesthetics. J Pharmacol Exp Ther 281:1136-1143, 1997.
176. Minami K, Vanderah TW, Minami M, et al: Inhibitory effects of anesthetics and ethanol on muscarinic receptors expressed in *Xenopus* oocytes. Eur J Pharmacol 339:237-244, 1997.
177. Hemmings HC Jr: General anesthetic effects on protein kinase C. Toxicol Lett 100:89-95, 1998.
178. Hasegawa J, Takekoshi S, Nagata H, et al: Sevoflurane stimulates MAP kinase signal transduction through the activation of PKC alpha and betaII in fetal rat cerebral cortex cultured neuron. Acta Histochem Cytochem 39:163-172, 2006.
179. Das J, Addona GH, Sandberg WS, et al: Identification of a general anesthetic binding site in the diacylglycerol-binding domain of protein kinase C-delta. J Biol Chem 279:37964-37972, 2004.
180. Shumilla JA, Sweitzer SM, Eger EI 2nd, et al: Inhibition of spinal protein kinase C-epsilon or -gamma isozymes does not affect halothane minimum alveolar anesthetic concentration in rats. Anesth Analg 99:82-84, 2004.
181. Sonner JM, Gong D, Li J, et al: Mouse strain modestly influences minimum alveolar anesthetic concentration and convulsivity of inhaled compounds. Anesth Analg 89:1030-1034, 1999.
182. Snyder GL, Galdi S, Hendrick JP, et al: General anesthetics selectively modulate glutamatergic and dopaminergic signaling via site-specific phosphorylation in vivo. Neuropharmacology 53:619-630, 2007.
183. Hemmings HC Jr, Adamo AI: Effects of halothane and propofol on purified brain protein kinase C activation. Anesthesiology 81:147-155, 1994.
184. Marota JJ, Crosby G, Uhl GR: Selective effects of pentobarbital and halothane on c-fos and jun-B gene expression in rat brain. Anesthesiology 77:365-371, 1992.
185. Hamaya Y, Takeda T, Dohi S, et al: The effects of pentobarbital, isoflurane, and propofol on immediate-early gene expression in the vital organs of the rat. Anesth Analg 90:1177-1183, 2000.
186. Culley DJ, Yukhananov RY, Xie ZC, et al: Altered hippocampal gene expression 2 days after general anesthesia in rats. Eur J Pharmacol 549:71-78, 2006.
187. Fütterer CD, Maurer MH, Schmitt A, et al: Alterations in rat brain proteins after desflurane anesthesia. Anesthesiology 100:302-308, 2004.
188. Nicoll RA, Madison DV: General anesthetics hyperpolarize neurons in the vertebrate central nervous system. Science 217:1055-1057, 1982.
189. Southan AP, Wann KT: Inhalation anaesthetics block accommodation of pyramidal cell discharge in the rat hippocampus. Br J Anaesth 63:581-586, 1989.
190. Fujiwara N, Higashi H, Nishi S, et al: Changes in spontaneous firing patterns of rat hippocampal neurones induced by volatile anaesthetics. J Physiol (Lond) 402:155-175, 1988.
191. Kullmann DM, Martin RL, Redman SJ: Reduction by general anaesthetics of group Ia excitatory postsynaptic potentials and currents in the cat spinal cord. J Physiol (Lond) 412:277-296, 1989.
192. MacIver MB, Roth SH: Inhalation anaesthetics exhibit pathway-specific and differential actions on hippocampal synaptic responses in vitro. Br J Anaesth 60:680-691, 1988.
193. Ries CR, Puil E: Ionic mechanism of isoflurane's actions on thalamocortical neurons. J Neurophysiol 81:1802-1809, 1999.
194. Semyanov A, Walker MC, Kullmann DM, et al: Tonically active GABA(A) receptors: Modulating gain and maintaining the tone. Trends Neurosci 27:262-269, 2004.
195. Bai D, Zhu G, Pennefather P, et al: Distinct functional and pharmacological properties of tonic and quantal inhibitory postsynaptic currents mediated by γ-aminobutyric $acid_A$ receptors in hippocampal neurons. Mol Pharmacol 59:814-824, 2001.
196. Bieda MC, MacIver MB: Major role for tonic $GABA_A$ conductances in anesthetic suppression of intrinsic neuronal excitability. J Neurophysiol 92:1658-1667, 2004.
197. Caraiscos VB, Elliott EM, You T, et al: Tonic inhibition in mouse hippocampal CA1 pyramidal neurons is mediated by α5 subunit-containing gamma-aminobutyric acid type A receptors. Proc Natl Acad Sci U S A 101:3662-3667, 2004.
198. Caraiscos VB, Newell JG, You T, et al: Selective enhancement of tonic GABAergic inhibition in murine hippocampal neurons by low concentrations of the volatile anesthetic isoflurane. J Neurosci 24:8454-8458, 2004.
199. Cheng VY, Martin LJ, Elliott EM, et al: $Alpha5GABA_A$ receptors mediate the amnestic but not sedative-hypnotic effects of the general anesthetic etomidate. J Neurosci 26:3713-3720, 2006.

200. Berg-Johnsen J, Langmoen IA: The effect of isoflurane on excitatory synaptic transmission in the rat hippocampus. Acta Anaesthesiol Scand 36:350-355, 1992.
201. Kirson ED, Yaari Y, Perouansky M: Presynaptic and postsynaptic actions of halothane at glutamatergic synapses in the mouse hippocampus. Br J Pharmacol 124:1607-1614, 1998.
202. Richards CD, Smaje JC: Anaesthetics depress the sensitivity of cortical neurones to L-glutamate. Br J Pharmacol 58:347-357, 1976.
203. Wakamori M, Ikemoto Y, Akaike N: Effects of two volatile anesthetics and a volatile convulsant on the excitatory and inhibitory amino acid responses in dissociated CNS neurons of the rat. J Neurophysiol 66:2014-2021, 1991.
204. Yang J, Zorumski CF: Effects of isoflurane on *N*-methyl-D-aspartate gated ion channels in cultured rat hippocampal neurons. Ann NY Acad Sci 625:287-289, 1991.
205. de Sousa SLM, Dickinson R, Lieb WR, et al: Contrasting synaptic actions of the inhalational general anesthetics isoflurane and xenon. Anesthesiology 92:1055-1066, 2000.
206. Dildy-Mayfield JE, Eger EI 2nd, Harris RA: Anesthetics produce subunit-selective actions on glutamate receptors. J Pharmacol Exp Ther 276:1058-1065, 1996.
207. Minami K, Wick MJ, Stern-Bach Y, et al: Sites of volatile anesthetic action on kainate (Glutamate receptor 6) receptors. J Biol Chem 273:8248-8255, 1998.
208. Banks MI, Pearce RA: Dual actions of volatile anesthetics on GABA(A) IPSCs: Dissociation of blocking and prolonging effects. Anesthesiology 90:120-134, 1999.
209. Murugaiah KD, Hemmings HC Jr: Effects of intravenous general anesthetics on [^{3}H]GABA release from rat cortical synaptosomes. Anesthesiology 89:919-928, 1998.
210. Nishikawa K, MacIver MB: Agent-selective effects of volatile anesthetics on GABA(A) receptor-mediated synaptic inhibition in hippocampal interneurons. Anesthesiology 94:340-347, 2001.
211. Westphalen RI, Hemmings HC: Selective depression by general anesthetics of glutamate versus GABA release from isolated cortical nerve terminals. J Pharmacol Exp Ther 304:1188-1196, 2003.
212. Westphalen RI, Hemmings HC Jr: Volatile anesthetic effects on glutamate versus GABA release from isolated rat cortical nerve terminals: basal release. J Pharmacol Exp Ther 316:208-215, 2006.
213. Nagele P, Mendel JB, Placzek WJ, et al: Volatile anesthetics bind rat synaptic snare proteins. Anesthesiology 103:768-778, 2005.
214. van Swinderen B, Saifee O, Shebester L, et al: A neomorphic syntaxin mutation blocks volatile-anesthetic action in *Caenorhabditis elegans*. Proc Natl Acad Sci U S A 96:2479-2484, 1999.
215. Pittson S, Himmel AM, MacIver MB: Multiple synaptic and membrane sites of anesthetic action in the CA1 region of rat hippocampal slices. BMC Neurosci 5:52, 2004.
216. Eckenhoff ME, Chan K, Eckenhoff RG: Multiple specific binding targets for inhaled anesthetics in the mammalian brain. J Pharmacol Exp Ther 300:172-179, 2002.
217. Pearce RA, Stringer JL, Lothman EW: Effect of volatile anesthetics on synaptic transmission in the rat hippocampus. Anesthesiology 71:591-598, 1989.
218. Pearce RA: Volatile anaesthetic enhancement of paired-pulse depression investigated in the rat hippocampus in vitro. J Physiol 492:823-840, 1996.
219. Malenka RC, Bear MF: LTP and LTD: An embarrassment of riches. Neuron 44:5-21, 2004.
220. Simon W, Hapfelmeier G, Kochs E, et al: Isoflurane blocks synaptic plasticity in the mouse hippocampus. Anesthesiology 94:1058-1065, 2001.
221. Desmond NL, Colbert CM, Zhang DX, et al: NMDA receptor antagonists block the induction of long-term depression in the hippocampal dentate gyrus of the anesthetized rat. Brain Res 552:93-98, 1991.
222. Maren S, Baudry M, Thompson RF: Differential effects of ketamine and MK-801 on the induction of long-term potentiation. Neuroreport 2:239-242, 1991.
223. Jinks SL, Atherley RJ, Dominguez CL, et al: Isoflurane disrupts central pattern generator activity and coordination in the lamprey isolated spinal cord. Anesthesiology 103:567-575, 2005.
224. Munglani R, Andrade J, Sapsford DJ, et al: A measure of consciousness and memory during isoflurane administration: The coherent frequency. Br J Anaesth 71:633-641, 1993.
225. Traub RD, Spruston N, Soltesz I, et al: Gamma-frequency oscillations: A neuronal population phenomenon, regulated by synaptic and intrinsic cellular processes, and inducing synaptic plasticity. Prog Neurobiol 55:563-575, 1998.
226. Dickinson R, Awaiz S, Whittington MA, et al: The effects of general anaesthetics on carbachol-evoked gamma oscillations in the rat hippocampus in vitro. Neuropharmacology 44:864-872, 2003.
227. Antkowiak B, Hentschke H: Cellular mechanisms of gamma rhythms in rat neocortical brain slices probed by the volatile anaesthetic isoflurane. Neurosci Lett 231:87-90, 1997.
228. Imas OA, Ropella KM, Ward BD, et al: Volatile anesthetics disrupt frontal-posterior recurrent information transfer at gamma frequencies in rat. Neurosci Lett 387:145-150, 2005.
229. Buzsaki G: Theta oscillations in the hippocampus. Neuron 33:325-340, 2002.
230. Bland BH, Bland CE, Colom LV, et al: Effect of halothane on type 2 immobility-related hippocampal theta field activity and theta-on/theta-off cell discharges. Hippocampus 13:38-47, 2003.
231. Szarecka A, Xu Y, Tang P: Dynamics of firefly luciferase inhibition by general anesthetics: gaussian and anisotropic network analyses. Biophys J 93:1895-1905, 2007.
232. Gottschalk A, Haney P: Computational aspects of anesthetic action in simple neural models. Anesthesiology 98:548-564, 2003.
233. Wilson MT, Sleigh JW, Steyn-Ross DA, et al: General anesthetic-induced seizures can be explained by a mean-field model of cortical dynamics. Anesthesiology 104:588-593, 2006.
234. Steyn-Ross ML, Steyn-Ross DA, Sleigh JW: Modelling general anaesthesia as a first-order phase transition in the cortex. Prog Biophys Mol Biol 85:369-385, 2004.
235. Zhang Y, Stabernack C, Sonner J, et al: Both cerebral GABA(A) receptors and spinal GABA(A) receptors modulate the capacity of isoflurane to produce immobility. Anesth Analg 92:1585-1589, 2001.
236. Zhang Y, Wu S, Eger EI 2nd, et al: Neither GABA(A) nor strychnine-sensitive glycine receptors are the sole mediators of MAC for isoflurane. Anesth Analg 92:123-127, 2001.
237. Sukhotinsky I, Zalkind V, Lu J, et al: Neural pathways associated with loss of consciousness caused by intracerebral microinjection of GABA A-active anesthetics. Eur J Neurosci 25:1417-1436, 2007.
238. Nash HA: In vivo genetics of anaesthetic action. Br J Anaesth 89:143-155, 2002.
239. Sonner JM, Cascio M, Xing Y, et al: Alpha 1 subunit–containing GABA type A receptors in forebrain contribute to the effect of inhaled anesthetics on conditioned fear. Mol Pharmacol 68:61-68, 2005.
240. Sedensky MM, Siefker JM, Morgan PG: Model organisms: New insights into ion channel and transporter function: Stomatin homologues interact in *Caenorhabditis elegans*. Am J Physiol Cell Physiol 280:C1340-C1348, 2001.
241. Kayser EB, Morgan PG, Sedensky MM: GAS-1: A mitochondrial protein controls sensitivity to volatile anesthetics in the nematode *Caenorhabditis elegans*. Anesthesiology 90:545-554, 1999.
242. Cascio M, Xing Y, Gong D, et al: Mouse chromosome 7 harbors a quantitative trait locus for isoflurane minimum alveolar concentration. Anesth Analg 105:381-385, 2007.
243. Veselis RA, Reinsel RA, Feshchenko VA, et al: A neuroanatomical construct for the amnesic effects of propofol. Anesthesiology 97:329-337, 2002.
244. Alkire MT, Miller J: General anesthesia and the neural correlates of consciousness. Prog Brain Res 150:229-244, 2005.
245. Hemmings HC Jr, Yan-W, Westphalen RI, Ryan TA: The general anesthetic isoflurane depresses synaptic vesicle exocytosis, Mol Pharmacol 67: 1591-1599, 2005.

Edmond I Eger II

21 Inhaled Anesthetics: Uptake and Distribution

Key Points

1. During induction and maintenance of anesthesia, ventilation, the first of five factors that govern the pulmonary inhaled anesthetic concentration, delivers anesthetic to the lung and thereby increases the alveolar concentration.
2. Uptake of anesthetic by blood passing through the lung opposes the effect of ventilation by drawing anesthetic from the lung.
3. An increased inspired concentration of anesthetic decreases the effect of uptake (the concentration effect), and at 100% inspired concentration, uptake no longer opposes the effect of ventilation.
4. Metabolism of anesthetics can increase uptake.
5. Anesthetic uptake may be enhanced by movement of anesthetic between tissues (intertissue diffusion), especially from highly perfused tissues (e.g., intestine) to poorly perfused tissues with a great capacity for anesthetic (e.g., mesenteric fat).
6. Three factors determine uptake by blood: solubility (the blood-gas partition coefficient), pulmonary blood flow (cardiac output), and the difference in anesthetic partial pressure between the lungs and venous blood returning to the lungs.
7. Solubility differentiates one anesthetic from another in that lower solubility translates to faster recovery from anesthesia.
8. Changes in ventilation and the distribution of ventilation, cardiac output (and its distribution), and inflow rate each influence anesthetic concentration in predictable ways.

The modern anesthetist expeditiously develops and then sustains anesthetic concentrations in the central nervous system that are sufficient for surgery, doing so with agents and techniques that usually permit rapid recovery from anesthesia. Producing a sufficient concentration requires delivery of anesthetic that is adequate but does not impose excessive depression. Knowledge of the factors that govern the relationship between the delivered anesthetic and brain (or heart or muscle) concentrations enhances the optimum conduct of anesthesia.

The Inspired-to-Alveolar Anesthetic Relationship

Of the steps between delivered and brain anesthetic partial pressure, none is more pivotal than that between the inspired and alveolar gases. Alveolar partial pressure governs the partial pressure of anesthetic in all body tissues: all must approach and ultimately equal alveolar partial pressure. With use of high inflow rates (and hence conversion to a non-rebreathing system), the anesthetist can precisely control the partial pressure of anesthetic that is inspired.

The Effect of Ventilation

Two factors determine how quickly the alveolar concentration of an anesthetic (FA) rises toward the concentration being inspired (FI): the inspired concentration itself (see "The Concentration Effect") and alveolar ventilation. Ventilation exerts a powerful effect. On induction, the unopposed effect of ventilation rapidly increases the alveolar concentration (i.e., FA/FI quickly approaches 1). This occurs with oxygen during the course of preoxygenation. Normally, 95% or greater washin of oxygen occurs in 2 minutes or less when a non-rebreathing (or high inflow rate) system is used (Fig. 21-1).

However, the FA/FI ratio for inhaled anesthetics does not mimic the FA/FI ratio for oxygen. In contrast to oxygen, appreci-

Table 21-1 Partition Coefficients at 37°C

Anesthetic	Blood-Gas	Brain-Blood	Liver-Blood	Kidney-Blood	Muscle-Blood	Fat-Blood
Desflurane	0.45	1.3	1.4	1.0	2.0	27
Nitrous oxide	0.47	1.1	0.8	—	1.2	2.3
Sevoflurane	0.65	1.7	1.8	1.2	3.1	48
Isoflurane	1.4	1.6	1.8	1.2	2.9	45
Enflurane	1.8	1.4	2.1	—	1.7	36
Halothane	2.5	1.9	2.1	1.2	3.4	51
Diethyl ether	12	2.0	1.9	0.9	1.3	5
Methoxyflurane	15	1.4	2.0	0.9	1.6	38

Data from references 1 through 8.

able quantities of anesthetics are taken up because the solubilities of anesthetics far exceed the solubility of oxygen (or nitrogen). At low inspired concentrations, the balance between delivery of anesthetic by ventilation and removal of anesthetic by uptake determines the FA/FI ratio. The relationship is a simple one. For example, if uptake removes a third of the inspired anesthetic molecules, FA/FI equals two thirds; if uptake removes two thirds of the inspired molecules, FA/FI equals a third.

Anesthetic Uptake Factors

Three factors determine anesthetic uptake: solubility (λ), cardiac output (Q), and alveolar-to-venous partial pressure difference (PA – Pv).[1] Uptake equals the product of these factors: λ × Q × (PA – Pv) divided by barometric pressure.

Because uptake is the product of these factors rather than a sum, if any factor approaches zero, uptake must approach zero, and ventilation rapidly drives the FA/FI ratio to 1.0. Thus, if solubility is low (as in the case of oxygen), if cardiac output approaches zero (as in profound myocardial depression or death), or if the alveolar-to-venous difference becomes inconsequential (as might occur after an extraordinarily long course of anesthesia), uptake would be minimal, and FA/FI would equal 1.

Solubility

A partition coefficient describes the relative affinity of an anesthetic for two phases and hence how that anesthetic partitions itself between the two phases when equilibrium has been achieved. The blood-gas partition coefficient (λ, or "blood solubility") describes the partitioning of an anesthetic between blood and gas. For example, isoflurane has a blood-gas partition coefficient of 1.4, which means that at equilibrium, the concentration of isoflurane in blood is 1.4 times its concentration in the gas (alveolar) phase. "Equilibrium" means that no difference in partial pressure exists (i.e., a blood-gas partition coefficient of 1.4 does not indicate that the partial pressure in blood is 1.4 times that in the gas phase). The partition coefficient may be thought of in another way—it indicates the relative capacity of the two phases. Thus, a value of 1.4 means that each milliliter of blood holds 1.4 times as much isoflurane as a milliliter of alveolar gas does.

A larger blood-gas partition coefficient produces greater uptake and hence a lower FA/FI ratio. Because the partial pressure of an anesthetic in the alveoli is transmitted to arterial blood and thence to all tissues (especially the central nervous system), development of an adequate central nervous system anesthetic partial pressure may be delayed in the case of highly blood-soluble agents such as ether and methoxyflurane (Table 21-1).[1-8] Indeed, the delay in development of an anesthetizing cerebral partial pressure has contributed to the elimination of such highly blood-soluble agents from anesthetic practice. Even the moderate solubility of isoflurane could slow induction of anesthesia were it not for the use of anesthetic overpressure—that is, we compensate for the uptake of anesthetic by delivering a higher concentration than we hope to achieve in the alveoli, perhaps 2% isoflurane to produce an alveolar concentration of 1%.

Cardiac Output

The effect of altering cardiac output is intuitively obvious. If more blood passes through the lungs, more blood is available to remove anesthetic and thereby lower the FA/FI ratio. To the student of

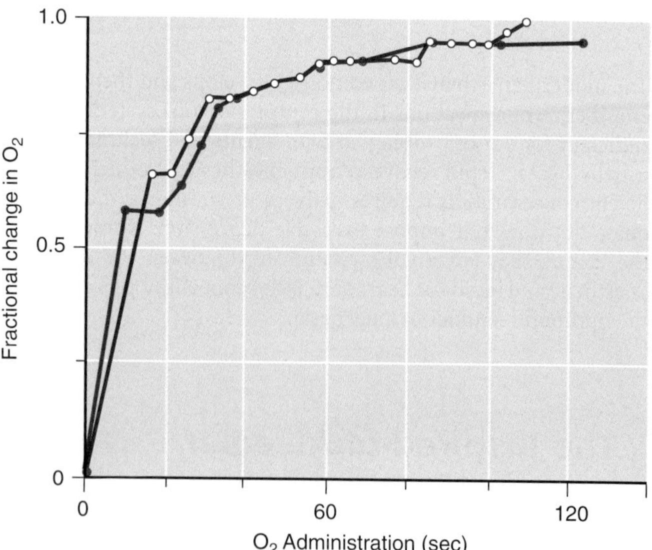

Figure 21-1 Washin of oxygen was determined in two patients breathing from a mask. A 63% change was obtained in about 30 seconds, an 86% change in about 1 minute, and a 95% to 98% change in 2 minutes. *(From Eger EI II [unpublished data].)*

uptake and distribution, this may appear to produce a conflict. It would seem that if more agent were taken up and delivered more rapidly to tissues, the tissue anesthetic partial pressure would rise more rapidly. In one sense this is true: an increase in cardiac output does hasten the equilibration of tissue anesthetic partial pressures with the partial pressure in arterial blood.[9] This reasoning, however, ignores the lower FA/FI ratio found with normal cardiac output. The partial pressure in the central nervous system cannot exceed that in blood, and thus a lower FA/FI ratio produces a lower anesthetic partial pressure in the brain—although that lower partial pressure might be achieved more rapidly.

The effect of a change in cardiac output is analogous to the effect of a change in solubility. As already noted, doubling solubility doubles the capacity of the same volume of blood to hold anesthetic. Doubling cardiac output would also double capacity, but in this case by doubling the volume of blood exposed to anesthetic.

The Alveolar-to-Venous Anesthetic Gradient

The alveolar-to-venous anesthetic partial pressure gradient, or the difference between partial pressure in the alveoli and that in venous blood, results from tissue uptake of anesthetic. Were there no tissue uptake, the venous blood returning to the lungs would contain as much anesthetic as it had when it left the lungs as arterial blood. That is, the alveolar (which equals arterial)-to-venous partial pressure difference would be zero. The presumption that alveolar and arterial anesthetic partial pressures are equal is reasonable in normal patients who have no barrier to diffusion of anesthetic from the alveoli to pulmonary capillary blood and who do not have ventilation-perfusion abnormalities. Later, we shall consider the effect of ventilation-perfusion abnormalities on anesthetic uptake.

Factors that determine the fraction of anesthetic removed from the blood traversing a given tissue parallel the factors that govern uptake at the lungs: tissue solubility, tissue blood flow, and arterial-to-tissue anesthetic partial pressure difference. Again, uptake is the product of these three factors. If any single factor approaches zero, so does uptake. The succeeding paragraphs discuss the characteristics of each of these factors and then how uptake by individual tissues can be summed to give the venous component of the alveolar-to-venous anesthetic partial pressure difference.

Blood-gas partition coefficients span values ranging from 0.45 for desflurane to 15 for methoxyflurane (see Table 21-1), a 33-fold difference. In contrast, tissue-blood partition coefficients (i.e., tissue solubility) lie between 1 and 2 for all lean tissue except muscle, for which the values for potent anesthetics lie between 2 and 3.4 (see Table 21-1)—that is, different lean tissues have similar capacity per milliliter of tissue. Put another way, a given anesthetic has roughly the same affinity for lean tissue and blood. As with blood-gas partition coefficients, tissue-blood partition coefficients define the concentration ratio of anesthetic at equilibrium between the two phases. For example, an isoflurane brain-blood partition coefficient of 1.6 means that 1 cm^3 of brain can hold 1.6 times as much isoflurane as 1 cm^3 of blood can with the same isoflurane partial pressure.

Lean tissues differ in the volume of tissue relative to the volume of blood passing that tissue. A larger volume of tissue relative to flow (as with muscle) has two implications. First, the large tissue capacity increases the transfer of anesthetic (more is lost) from blood to tissue. Second, it takes longer to fill up a tissue with a large capacity (i.e., the tissue takes longer to equilibrate with the anesthetic partial pressure being delivered in arterial blood). Thus, a large tissue volume relative to blood flow sustains the arterial-to-tissue anesthetic partial pressure difference (and hence uptake) for a longer time. In contrast, with its high perfusion per cubic centimeter of tissue, brain equilibrates rapidly with the anesthetic partial pressure. Per cubic centimeter of tissue, muscle has about a 20th the perfusion of brain, and this factor alone means that muscle takes 20 times longer than brain to equilibrate. The muscle-blood partition coefficient relative to the brain-blood partition coefficient causes a further delay. For example, the 3.1 muscle-blood partition coefficient for sevoflurane means that each 100 cm^3 of muscle has the capacity of 310 mL of blood, whereas the brain-blood partition coefficient is 1.7. Thus, equilibration is not simply 20 times longer, it is $20 \times 3.1/1.7$, or 36 times longer than with brain.

The tissue-blood coefficient for fat greatly exceeds 1 for more potent anesthetics (see Table 21-1). Fat-blood coefficients range from 2.3 (nitrous oxide) to 48 (sevoflurane). That is, each cubic centimeter of fat tissue contains 2.3 times more nitrous oxide or 48 times more sevoflurane than does a milliliter of blood with the same nitrous oxide or sevoflurane partial pressure. This enormous capacity of fat for potent inhaled anesthetics means that most of the anesthetic contained in the blood perfusing fat is transferred to the fat. Although most of the anesthetic moves from blood to fat, the anesthetic partial pressure in fat rises slowly because fat has a large capacity and low perfusion per cubic centimeter of fat.

Tissue Groups

The algebraic sum of uptake by individual tissues determines the alveolar-to-venous partial pressure difference and hence uptake at the lungs. However, we do not need to analyze the effect of individual tissues to arrive at the algebraic sum; instead, we can group tissues in terms of their perfusion and solubility characteristics (i.e., in terms of features that define the duration of a substantial arterial-to-tissue anesthetic partial pressure difference). Four tissue groups result from such an analysis (Table 21-2).[1]

The brain, heart, splanchnic bed (including the liver), kidney, and endocrine glands make up the vessel-rich group (VRG). These organs account for less than 10% of body weight but receive 75% of cardiac output. This high perfusion confers several features. The large blood flow permits the VRG to receive and remove a relatively large volume of anesthetic in the earliest moments of induction. However, the small volume of tissue relative to perfusion produces rapid equilibration of this tissue group with the anesthetic delivered in arterial blood. The time to half-equilibration (i.e., the time at which the VRG anesthetic partial pressure equals half that in arterial blood) varies from about 1 minute for nitrous oxide to 2 minutes for sevoflurane. The longer time to equilibration with sevoflurane results from its higher tissue-blood partition coefficients (see Table 21-1). Equilibration of the VRG with the anesthetic partial pressure in arterial blood is more than 90% complete in 4 to 8 minutes. Thus, after 8 minutes, uptake by the VRG is too small (i.e., the arterial-to-VRG anesthetic partial pressure difference is too small) to significantly influence the alveolar concentration. For a substantial period after 8 minutes, the muscle group (MG) determines most of uptake.

Muscle and skin, which make up the MG, have similar blood flow and solubility (lean tissue) characteristics. The lower perfusion (about 3 mL of blood per 100 cm^3 of tissue per minute)

Table 21-2 Tissue Group Characteristics

	Group			
	Vessel Rich	Muscle	Fat	Vessel Poor
Percentage of body mass	10	50	20	20
Perfusion as a percentage of cardiac output	75	19	6	0

Adapted from Eger EI II: Uptake of inhaled anesthetics: The alveolar to inspired anesthetic difference. *In* Eger EI II: Anesthetic Uptake and Action. Baltimore, Williams & Wilkins, 1974, pp 77-96.

distinguishes the MG from the VRG (70 mL per 100 cm^3 per minute). Although the MG represents about half of the body's bulk, it receives only 1 L/min blood flow at rest. That is, the amount of anesthetic delivered to the MG is a quarter of that delivered to the VRG, and initially the MG takes up only a quarter as much anesthetic. The large bulk relative to perfusion means two things: (1) during induction, most of the anesthetic delivered to the MG is removed from the MG blood flow, and (2) the MG continues to remove anesthetic from its blood supply for a long time. The time to half-equilibration ranges from 20 to 25 minutes (nitrous oxide) to 70 to 80 minutes (sevoflurane or isoflurane). Thus, long after equilibration of the VRG has taken place, the MG continues to take up substantial quantities of anesthetic and requires 2 to 4 hours to approach equilibration.

Once MG equilibration is complete, only fat (i.e., the fat group [FG]) serves as an effective depot for uptake. In a normal lean patient, the FG occupies a fifth of the body's bulk and receives a blood flow of about 400 mL/min (i.e., the perfusion per 100 cm^3 of fat nearly equals the perfusion per 100 cm^3 of resting muscle). Thus, during the initial delivery of anesthetic to tissues, the FG receives only 40% as much anesthetic as delivered to the MG (i.e., blood flow to the FG is 40% of that to the MG). The FG has far greater affinity than the MG for anesthetic, a property that greatly lengthens the time over which it absorbs anesthetic. The half-time to equilibration of fat ranges from 70 to 80 minutes for nitrous oxide to 30 hours for sevoflurane and isoflurane. Equilibration with fat does not occur in the course of anesthesia with any potent inhaled anesthetic.

One tissue group, the vessel-poor group (VPG), remains to be defined. The VPG consists of ligaments, tendons, bone, and cartilage (i.e., lean tissues that have little or no perfusion). The absence of significant blood flow means that the VPG does not participate in the uptake process despite the fact that it represents a fifth of the body's mass.

Synthesis of Factors Governing the Rise in FA/FI Ratio

Now consider the combined impact of ventilation, tissue volume, solubility, and blood flow distribution on the rate of rise in FA/FI. The initial rate is rapid for all agents, regardless of their solubility (Fig. 21-2).[10,11] At the start of anesthesia, this rapidity results from the absence of an alveolar-to-venous anesthetic partial pressure difference (there is no anesthetic present in the lung to create a gradient) and hence absence of uptake. Without uptake, the effect of ventilation to generate a sudden rise in FA/FI is unopposed, and the rise initially parallels that noted for oxygen (see Fig 21-1). As ventilation delivers anesthetic to the alveoli, a progressively greater alveolar-to-venous partial pressure difference develops. The resulting rise in uptake increasingly opposes the effect of ventilation to drive the alveolar concentration upward. Ultimately, a rough balance is struck between anesthetic input by ventilation and its removal by uptake. The height of the FA/FI ratio at which the balance is struck depends on the solubility factor in the uptake equation (see the earlier equation for anesthetic uptake). Greater solubility increases uptake for a given alveolar-to-venous partial pressure difference. Hence, the initial rapid rise in FA/FI is halted at a lower level with a more soluble agent. This results in the first "knee" in the curve—higher for desflurane than for sevoflurane, higher for sevoflurane than for isoflurane, and higher for isoflurane than for methoxyflurane. The position of nitrous oxide is discussed later (see "The Concentration Effect"). At 1 minute of anesthetic administration, the FA/FI ratio is approximately 0.6 for desflurane, which indicates that the FA/FI ratio still has 40% to rise (i.e., uptake is removing 40% of the desflurane delivered by ventilation). In contrast, the FA/FI ratio for methoxyflurane has risen only 6.5%, thus indicating that 93.5% of the methoxyflurane delivered by ventilation is taken up.

The balance struck between ventilation and uptake does not remain constant. FA/FI continues to rise, albeit at a slower rate than seen in the first minute. This rise results from the progressive decrease in uptake by the VRG, a decrease to an inconsequential amount after 8 minutes. Thus, by about 8 minutes, three quarters of the cardiac output returning to the lungs (i.e., the blood from the VRG) contains nearly as much anesthetic as it did when it left the lungs. The consequent rise in venous anesthetic partial pressure decreases the alveolar-to-venous partial pressure difference and hence uptake, thereby allowing ventilation to drive the alveolar concentration upward to a second knee at roughly 8 minutes.

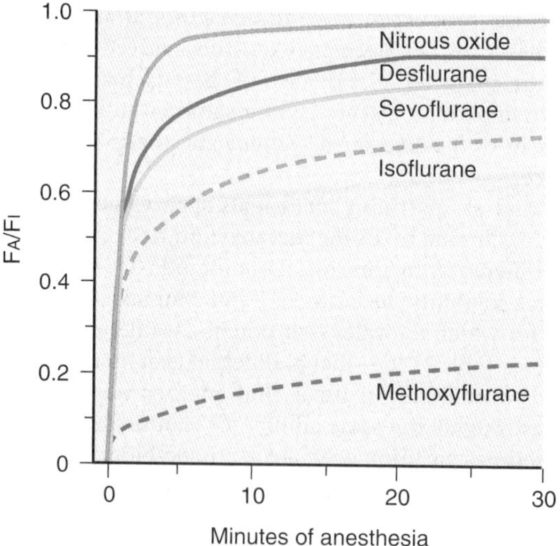

Figure 21-2 The rise in alveolar (FA) anesthetic concentration toward the inspired (FI) concentration is most rapid with the least soluble anesthetic, nitrous oxide, and slowest with the most soluble anesthetic, methoxyflurane. All data are from human studies. *(Data from Yasuda N, Lockhart SH, Eger EI II, et al: Kinetics of desflurane, isoflurane, and halothane in humans. Anesthesiology 74:489-498, 1991; and Yasuda N, Lockhart SH, Eger EI II, et al: Comparison of kinetics of sevoflurane and isoflurane in humans. Anesth Analg 72:316-324, 1991.)*

With the termination of effective uptake by the VRG, the MG and FG become the principal determinants of tissue uptake. The slow rate of change in the anesthetic partial pressure difference between arterial blood and MG or FG produces the gradual ascent of the terminal portion of the FA/FI ratio as the MG and, slower still, the FG progressively equilibrate with the arterial anesthetic partial pressure. If the graphs were extended for several hours, a third knee would be found that indicates equilibration of the MG. After that time, uptake would principally depend on the partial pressure gradient between arterial blood and fat.

The Concentration Effect

The previous analysis ignores the impact of the concentration effect on FA/FI. The inspired anesthetic concentration influences both the rate of rise and the height of the FA/FI ratio.[12] Increasing the inspired concentration accelerates the rate of rise. At an inspired concentration of 100%, the rate of rise is dictated solely by the rate at which ventilation washes gas into the lung; that is, at 100% inspired concentration, uptake no longer opposes the level to which FA/FI may rise. The cause of this extreme effect is readily perceived. At 100% inspired concentration, uptake of anesthetic creates a void that draws sufficient gas down the trachea to replace the gas taken up. Because the replacement gas concentration is 100%, uptake cannot modify the alveolar concentration. This explains why the rise in nitrous oxide shown in Figure 21-2 is more rapid than the rise in desflurane despite their nearly equal blood-gas partition coefficients: the nitrous oxide was given at an inspired concentration of 70%, whereas that of desflurane was 2%.

The concentration effect results from two factors, a concentrating effect and augmentation of inspired ventilation (Fig. 21-3).[13] The first rectangle (see Fig. 21-3A) represents a lung containing 80% (volumes per 100 volumes) nitrous oxide. If half this gas is taken up, the remaining 40 volumes exist in a total of 60 volumes, for a concentration of 67% (see Fig. 21-3B). That is, uptake of half the nitrous oxide does not halve the concentration because the remaining gases are "concentrated" in a smaller volume. If the void created by the uptake of 40 volumes is filled by drawing an equal volume of gas into the lungs (an augmentation of inspired ventilation), the final concentration equals 72% (see Fig. 21-3C).

This explanation has been criticized as being overly simplistic and ignoring the realities of some aspects of ventilation.[14] For example, if ventilation is controlled with a volume-limited respirator, an augmentation in inspired ventilation is limited to the period of the expiratory pause. Spontaneous ventilation minimizes this limitation. In any event, the reader needs to be aware that although Figure 21-3 describes the basic factors governing the concentration (and second gas effects—see the next section), the actual situation is more complex.

The impact of the concentration effect on FA/FI may be thought of as being identical to the impact of a change in solubility[15]: as the inspired concentration increases, the effective solubility decreases. Thus, at 50% inspired nitrous oxide, FA/FI rises as rapidly as the FA/FI of an anesthetic that has half the solubility of nitrous oxide and is given at a 1% inspired concentration, and 75% inspired nitrous oxide acts as an anesthetic given at 1% that has a quarter the solubility of nitrous oxide.

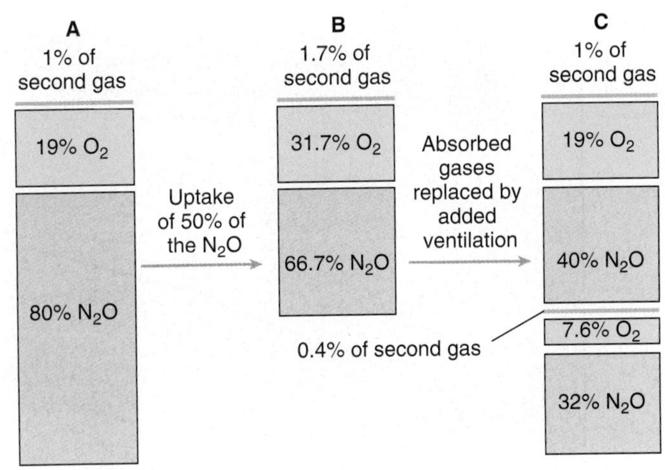

Figure 21-3 The rectangle to the left (**A**) represents a lung filled with 80% nitrous oxide plus 1% of a second gas. Uptake of 50% of the nitrous oxide does not halve the concentration of nitrous oxide (**B**) because the reduction in volume thereby increases its concentration, as well as the concentrations of all "second" gases (the oxygen and the second gas). Restoration of lung volume by the addition of gas with the same concentration as that introduced into the rectangle in **A** will increase the nitrous oxide concentration and add to the amount of second gas present in the lung (**C**). *(Modified from Stoelting RK, Eger EI II: An additional explanation for the second gas effect: A concentrating effect. Anesthesiology 30:273-277, 1969.)*

The Second Gas Effect

The factors that govern the concentration effect also influence the concentration of any potent anesthetic given concurrently.[13] The loss of volume associated with the uptake of nitrous oxide concentrates the potent anesthetic (see Fig. 21-3B). Replacement of the gas taken up by an increase in inspired ventilation augments the amount of potent anesthetic present in the lung (see Fig. 21-3C).

Experiments in dogs[16] and humans[17] demonstrate both the concentration and second gas effects. Humans given 4% desflurane with 5% or 65% nitrous oxide have a more rapid increase in FA/FI for both nitrous oxide and desflurane when 65% nitrous oxide is given (Fig. 21-4).[17]

Hendrickx and colleagues[18] confirmed the presence of the second gas effect but found, further, that the effect persists long after the majority of the uptake of nitrous oxide has ceased. They did not provide an explanation for this finding. An explanation would follow from an assumption of ventilation-perfusion abnormalities. Imagine that half the lung is poorly ventilated and the other half is well ventilated with both sides equally perfused. In the poorly ventilated half, uptake of oxygen will increase the concentration of nitrous oxide, possibly even above the inspired concentration. The increased concentration of nitrous oxide will augment its uptake and thus produce both factors that underlie the concentration and second gas effects (see Fig. 21-3). Furthermore, the half of the lung that is poorly ventilated is usually hypoventilated because of increased airway resistance. The increased airway resistance causes the poorly ventilated lung to empty last, which produces the characteristic upward sloping curve for expired carbon dioxide in patients with chronic obstructive pulmonary disease. Thus, the poorly ventilated lung would provide the increased recorded (literally the end-tidal) values for both nitrous oxide and the second gas.

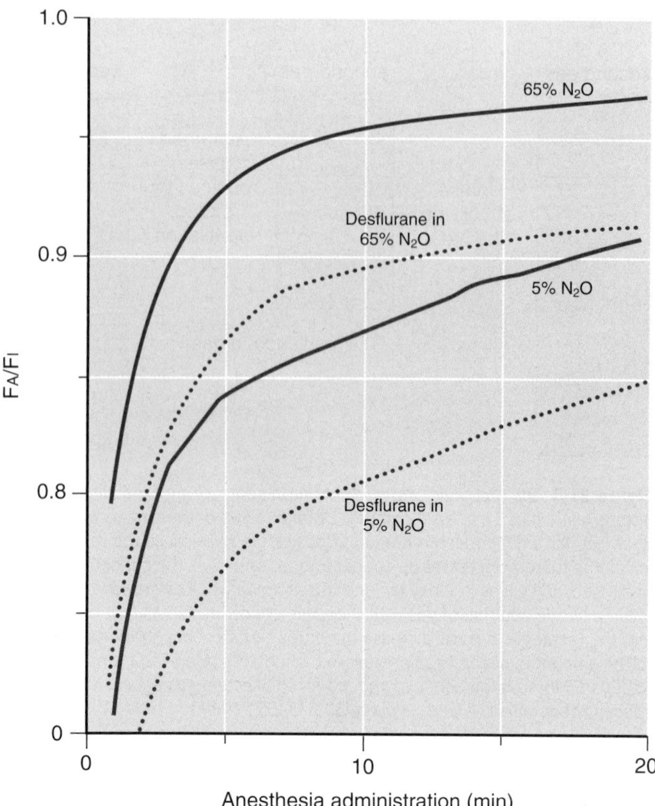

Figure 21-4 In humans, administration of 65% nitrous oxide produces a more rapid rise in the FA/FI ratio of nitrous oxide than does the administration of 5% (concentration effect, *continuous two curves*). The FA/FI ratio for 4% desflurane rises more rapidly when given with 65% nitrous oxide than when given with 5% (second gas effect, *dashed two curves*). *(Modified from Taheri S, Eger EI II: A demonstration of the concentration and second gas effects in humans anesthetized with nitrous oxide and desflurane. Anesth Analg 89:774-780, 1999.)*

Percutaneous and Visceral Anesthetic Loss

Anesthetics may be lost via three routes other than the lungs: (1) transcutaneous movement, (2) transvisceral movement, and (3) metabolism. Although transcutaneous movement does occur, such movement is small.[19-21] The greatest loss per alveolar anesthetic percent occurs with nitrous oxide. Loss of nitrous oxide might equal 5 to 10 mL/min with an alveolar concentration of 70%. Movement of anesthetic across visceral or pleural surfaces during abdominal or pulmonary surgery is greater than movement across skin, but such visceral losses are usually small relative to total uptake.[22]

Metabolism of Anesthetics

Although percutaneous loss of anesthetic may not appreciably affect anesthetic uptake, loss of anesthetic by biodegradation can significantly change uptake, particularly with agents that undergo extensive biodegradation. Carpenter and coworkers[23] found that as much as half of the halothane and three quarters of the methoxyflurane that are taken up undergo biodegradation. They speculated that such biodegradation could explain the finding that the alveolar concentration of halothane decays more rapidly on recovery from anesthesia than does the alveolar concentration of isoflurane, an anesthetic that is significantly less soluble in blood.[24,25] Two reasons suggest that agents such as isoflurane and desflurane are less likely to be affected: first, they are not metabolized as readily as halothane or methoxyflurane,[24,25] and second, anesthetizing concentrations appear to saturate the enzymes responsible for metabolism of the anesthetic.[26] Saturation of enzymes in particular may limit the impact of metabolism during the washin as opposed to the washout of anesthetic. The combined effect of these factors remains to be determined, but it appears that metabolism is not a significant determinant of FA/FI during anesthesia with isoflurane or desflurane.[10,11] A small influence on the kinetics of sevoflurane may exist and thus explain why there is a more substantial difference between the FA/FI for desflurane versus sevoflurane during induction and maintenance of anesthesia than for the parallel washout curves (F_A/F_{A_0}) during recovery.[11]

Intertissue Diffusion

Carpenter and associates[24] examined the washin and washout of isoflurane, enflurane, halothane, and methoxyflurane given simultaneously for fixed times to healthy young patients. Washout was examined for several days after discontinuation of administration of the anesthetics. Analysis suggested that a model with five compartments best explained the resulting data for all the anesthetics (i.e., the model was independent of solubility and metabolism of the anesthetics). Four of these compartments had half-times consistent with the model described earlier in this chapter: compartments related to washin and washout of the lungs, the VRG, the MG, and the FG.

The additional, fifth, compartment was more difficult to explain. This compartment had a half-time of roughly 300 minutes, which is between that for muscle and fat. This additional compartment was important because it accounted for almost a third of the anesthetic taken up. Part of the compartment could be explained by uptake by highly perfused fat, such as that found in bone marrow. However, perfusion of marrow fat alone could not account for the amount of uptake by this compartment. Carpenter and coauthors[24] speculated that this uptake resulted from diffusion of anesthetic from lean tissues to adjacent thin layers of fat tissue. Such diffusion could be from the heart to pericardial fat, from the kidney to perirenal fat, from the intestine to mesenteric and omental fat, and from the dermis to subcutaneous fat. Yasuda and coworkers[10,11] confirmed these findings and extended them to desflurane and sevoflurane.

Factors Modifying the Rate of Rise in FA/FI

Alteration of the factors that govern the rate of delivery of anesthetic to or removal from the lungs changes the alveolar concentration of anesthetic. We have seen the importance of differences in solubility (see Fig. 21-2). The succeeding sections examine the impact of differences in ventilation and circulation and the interaction of these differences with factors such as solubility.

The Effect of Ventilatory Changes

By augmenting delivery of anesthetic to the lungs, increased ventilation accelerates the rate of rise in FA/FI (Fig. 21-5).[1,27] A change in ventilation produces a greater relative change in FA/FI with a more soluble anesthetic. In Figure 21-5, a doubling of ventilation increases the methoxyflurane concentration at 10 minutes of anesthetic administration by 75%, increases the isoflurane concentration by 18%, and increases the desflurane concentration by only 6%.

The impact of solubility may be explained as follows. With a poorly soluble agent such as desflurane, FA/FI increases rapidly, even with hypoventilation. Because FA normally cannot exceed FI, there is little room for augmentation of ventilation to further increase FA/FI. With a highly soluble agent such as methoxyflurane, most of the anesthetic delivered to the lungs is taken up, so if uptake at 4-L/min ventilation equaled x, uptake at 8 L/min would approach 2x. Thus, if cardiac output is held constant, ventilation at 8 L/min produces an arterial methoxyflurane concentration that is nearly twice the concentration produced by ventilation at 4 L/min. Because arterial and alveolar concentrations are in equilibrium, our example suggests that doubling ventilation must nearly double the concentration of a highly soluble anesthetic in the alveoli or blood.

These observations imply that imposed alterations in ventilation (e.g., an increase produced by conversion from spontaneous to controlled ventilation) produce greater changes in anesthetic concentration (and thus effect) with more soluble agents. Because such effects include both anesthetic depth and depression of circulation, greater caution must be exercised when ventilation is augmented during anesthesia produced with a highly soluble agent.

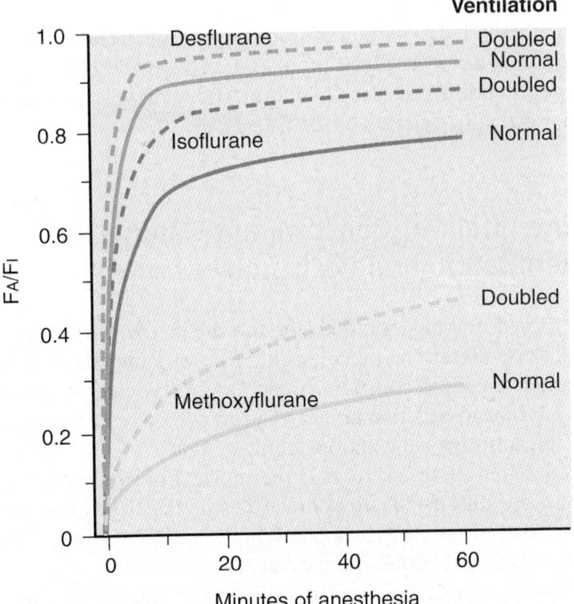

Figure 21-5 The FA/FI ratio rises more rapidly if ventilation is increased, in this case doubled. Solubility modifies this impact of ventilation: the effect on the anesthetizing partial pressure is greatest with the most soluble anesthetic (methoxyflurane) and least with the least soluble anesthetic (desflurane). *(Derived from simulations using GAS MAN from Philip JH: GAS MAN Computer Program. Chestnut Hill, MA, Med Man Simulations, Inc., 2002.)*

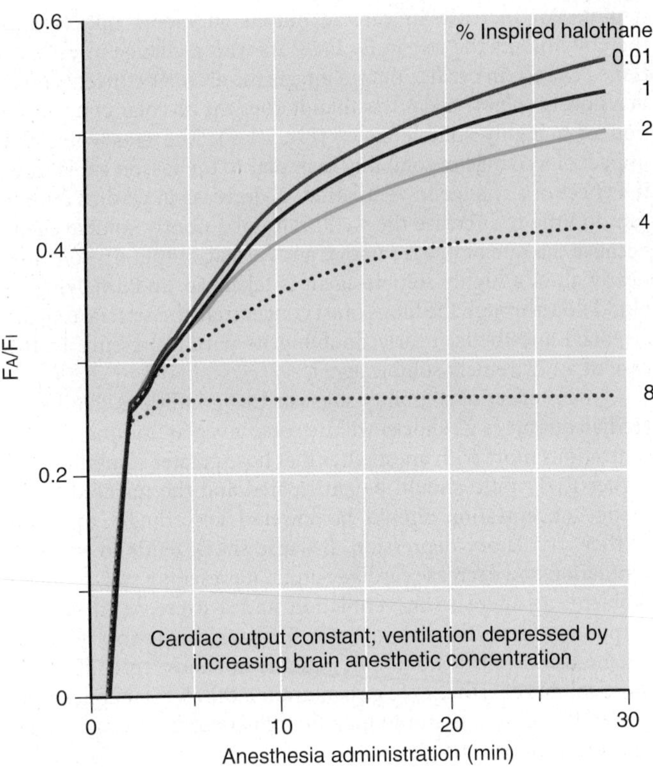

Figure 21-6 An increase in the inspired halothane concentration does not produce a proportional increase in the alveolar concentration because of the progressively greater depression of ventilation that occurs as alveolar halothane is increased. The initial "overshoot" seen with 10% to 20% inspired halothane results from the delay in transfer of alveolar halothane partial pressure to the brain (i.e., time must pass before the brain receives and is depressed by the very great concentrations attained in the lungs). *(From Munson ES, Eger EI II, Bowers DL: Effects of anesthetic-depressed ventilation and cardiac output on anesthetic uptake. Anesthesiology 38:251-259, 1973.)*

Anesthetics themselves may alter ventilation and thereby alter their own uptake.[9,28] Modern potent agents (desflurane, halothane, isoflurane, sevoflurane) are profound respiratory depressants whose capacity to depress ventilation is directly related to anesthetic dose.[29-32] At some concentration, all inhaled anesthetics probably produce apnea, a feature that must limit the maximum alveolar concentration (MAC) that can be obtained with spontaneous ventilation.

Thus, administration of an anesthetic concentration that produces significant respiratory depression decreases delivery of anesthetic to the alveoli.[9,33] As a result, doubling the inspired concentration does not double the alveolar concentration attained at a given point in time. At high inspired concentrations, further increases in inspired concentration produce little absolute change in alveolar concentration (Fig. 21-6). Anesthetics can thereby exert a negative-feedback effect on their own alveolar concentration, an effect that increases the safety of spontaneous ventilation by limiting the maximum concentration that is attained in the alveoli.

The Effect of Changes in Cardiac Output

The previous section assumed constant cardiac output and examined the effect of changes in ventilation; in this section we assume constant ventilation and examine the effect of changes in cardiac output. An increase in cardiac output augments uptake and thereby hinders the rise in FA/FI.[1,33] As with a change in ventilation, a change in cardiac output affects the alveolar concentration of a poorly soluble agent less than it does the alveolar concentration of a highly soluble agent (Fig. 21-7). The reason for the impact of a change in solubility is similar to the reason explaining the effect of a change in ventilation. A decrease in cardiac output can do little to increase the FA/FI ratio of a poorly soluble agent because the rate of rise is rapid at any cardiac output. In contrast, nearly all of a highly soluble agent is taken up, and a halving of blood flow through the lungs must concentrate the arterial (equals alveolar) anesthetic, nearly doubling its partial pressure in the case of an extremely soluble agent.

This effect of solubility suggests that conditions that lower cardiac output (e.g., shock) will increase alveolar anesthetic concentrations more with anesthetics that have greater solubility. The higher FA/FI ratio should be anticipated and the inspired anesthetic concentration should be lowered accordingly to avoid further circulatory depression. Because shock tends to increase ventilation and decrease cardiac output, it presents a two-pronged problem: an increase in ventilation and a decrease in cardiac output accelerate the rise in FA/FI. Perhaps this is an argument for the use of nitrous oxide in patients in shock. In contrast to more soluble anesthetics (e.g., isoflurane), the alveolar concentration of nitrous oxide would be little influenced by the associated cardiorespiratory changes.

Anesthetics also affect the circulation. They can depress cardiac output.[34] In contrast to the negative feedback that results from respiratory depression, circulatory depression produces a positive feedback: depression decreases uptake, and this increases the alveolar concentration, which in turn further decreases uptake.

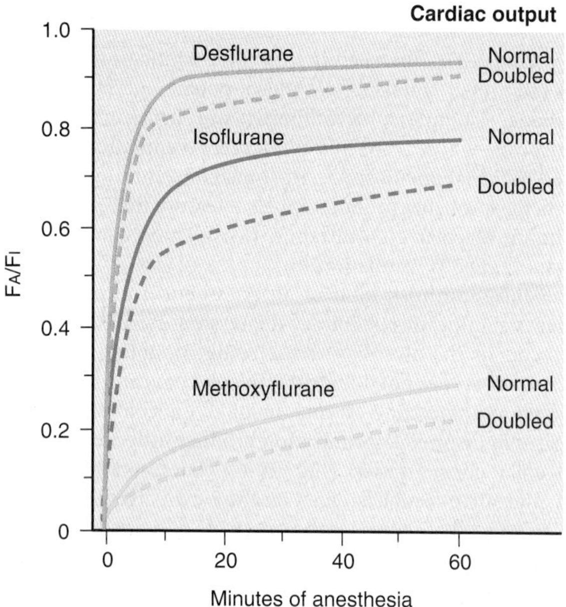

Figure 21-7 If unopposed by a concomitant increase in ventilation, an increase in cardiac output will decrease alveolar anesthetic concentration by augmenting uptake. The resulting alveolar anesthetic change is proportionately greatest (i.e., as a fraction of the "normal" curve; the "doubled" curve is least) with the most soluble anesthetic. *(Derived from simulations using GAS MAN from Philip JH: GAS MAN Computer Program. Chestnut Hill, MA, Med Man Simulations, Inc., 2002.)*

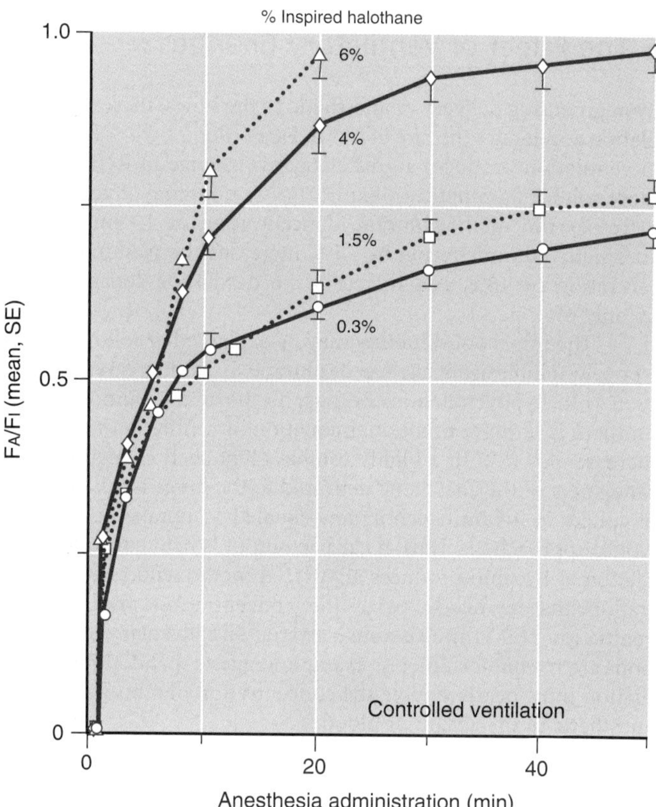

Figure 21-8 Dogs given constant ventilation demonstrate different rates of rise in FA/FI. The rates of rise depend on the inspired halothane concentration. The two greatest concentrations accelerate the rate of rise by depressing cardiac output and thereby decreasing uptake. *(Modified from Gibbons RT, Steffey EP, Eger EI II: The effect of spontaneous versus controlled ventilation on the rate of rise of alveolar halothane concentration in dogs. Anesth Analg 56:32-34, 1977.)*

A potentially lethal acceleration of the rise in FA/FI results from the depression of cardiac output (Fig. 21-8).[9,28,35] The impact of this acceleration increases in importance with increasing anesthetic solubility.

The Effect of Concomitant Changes in Ventilation and Perfusion

The preceding considerations of the effects of ventilatory and circulatory alterations presume that one variable changed while the other remained constant. In fact, both may change concomitantly. If both ventilation and cardiac output increase proportionately, an intuitive expectation might be that FA/FI would not be altered. After all, uptake equals the product of solubility, cardiac output, and the alveolar-to-venous anesthetic partial pressure difference (see the anesthetic uptake equation earlier). In the absence of other changes, doubling cardiac output doubles uptake, and this should exactly balance the influence of doubling of ventilation on FA/FI. That is, a doubling of both delivery of anesthetic to the lungs and removal of anesthetic from the lungs should produce no net change in alveolar concentration.

This reasoning ignores one other factor in the equation that defines uptake. An increase in cardiac output increases tissue blood flow and thereby accelerates the rate at which tissue equilibration occurs. Thus, an increase in cardiac output accelerates the narrowing of the alveolar-to-venous partial pressure difference[36] and consequently reduces the impact of the increase in cardiac output on uptake. The net result is that a proportional increase in ventilation and cardiac output increases the rate of rise in FA/FI.

The magnitude of acceleration of the rise in FA/FI depends in part on the distribution of the increase in cardiac output. If the increase is distributed proportionately to all tissues (e.g., if a doubling of output doubles flow to all tissues), the increase is fairly small (Fig. 21-9).[36,37] Thus, conditions such as hyperthermia and thyrotoxicosis only slightly influence the development of an anesthetizing anesthetic concentration through their influence on FA/FI. However, if the increase in cardiac output is diverted to the VRG, a greater effect is seen. Perfusion of the VRG is normally high and the VRG normally equilibrates rapidly. Further increases in perfusion can hasten the rate of equilibration, but the process is rapid for both normal and accelerated equilibration. Because blood returning from the VRG soon has the same partial pressure that it had leaving the lungs, it cannot remove more anesthetic from the lungs. Thus, after a few minutes, the increase in ventilation is not matched, even in part, by an increase in uptake. The result is a considerable acceleration in the rise in FA/FI. This effect may be seen in a comparison of the FA/FI curves for children and adults (Fig. 21-10). Children (especially infants) have relatively greater perfusion of the VRG and consequently show a significantly faster rise in FA/FI.[6,38,39] A clinical result of this accelerated rise is more rapid development of anesthesia in young patients. The higher perfusion of the brain further accelerates the development of anesthesia.

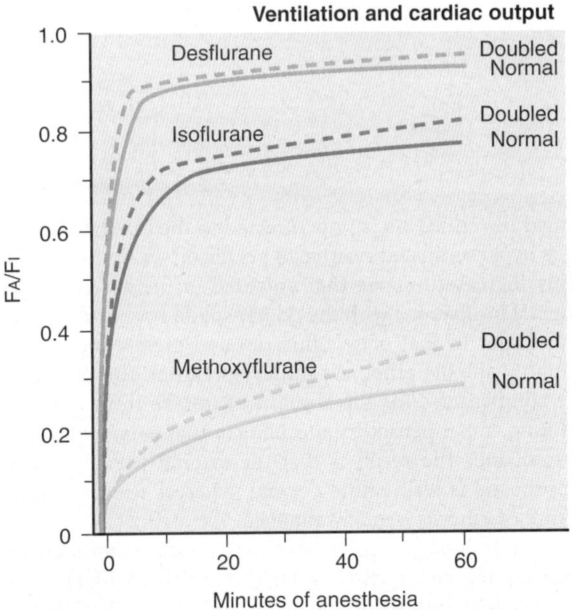

Figure 21-9 Proportional increases in alveolar ventilation (VA) and cardiac output (Q) will increase the rate at which FA/FI rises.[37] As indicated in the illustration, the effect is relatively small if the increase in cardiac output is distributed proportionately to all tissues (i.e., if cardiac output is doubled, all tissue blood flows are doubled). The greatest effect occurs with the most soluble anesthetic. *(Derived from simulations using GAS MAN from Philip JH: GAS MAN Computer Program. Chestnut Hill, MA, Med Man Simulations, Inc., 2002.)*

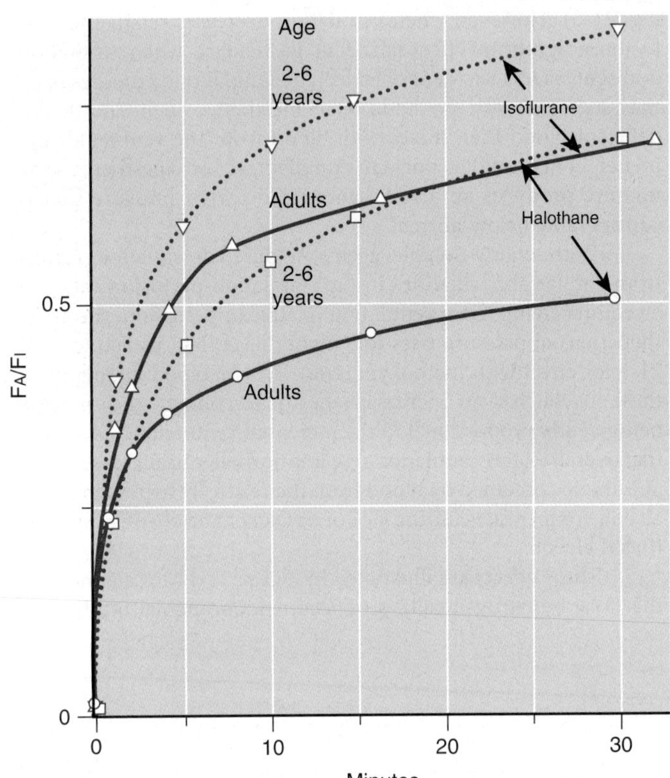

Figure 21-10 The alveolar rate of rise in halothane is more rapid in children (*upper curve*) than in adults (*lower curve*). The difference probably results from the greater ventilation and perfusion per kilogram of tissue in children and the fact that a disproportionate amount of the increased perfusion is devoted to the vessel-rich group. *(Modified from data from several sources.[6,38,39])*

Ventilation-Perfusion Abnormalities

Up to this point I have assumed that alveolar and arterial anesthetic partial pressures are equal (i.e., that the alveolar gases completely equilibrate with the blood passing through the lungs). For normal patients, this assumption is approximately correct, but diseases such as emphysema and atelectasis, as well as congenital cardiac defects, produce substantial deviations in equilibration. The associated abnormality in the ventilation-perfusion ratio does two things: (1) it increases the alveolar (end-tidal) anesthetic partial pressure and (2) it decreases the arterial anesthetic partial pressure (i.e., a partial pressure difference appears between alveolar gas and arterial blood). The relative change depends on the solubility of the anesthetic. With a poorly soluble agent, the end-tidal concentration is slightly increased, but the arterial partial pressure is significantly reduced. The opposite occurs with a highly soluble anesthetic.[40]

The considerable decrease in arterial anesthetic partial pressure that occurs with poorly soluble agents may be explained as follows. Abnormalities in the ventilation-perfusion ratio increase ventilation relative to perfusion of some alveoli, whereas in other alveoli, the reverse occurs. With a poorly soluble anesthetic, an increase in ventilation relative to perfusion does not appreciably increase the alveolar or arterial anesthetic partial pressure issuing from those alveoli (see effect for desflurane in

Fig. 21-5). However, when ventilation decreases relative to perfusion, a significant effect can occur, particularly when ventilation is absent, as in a segment of atelectatic lung. Blood emerges from that segment with no additional anesthetic. Such anesthetic-deficient blood then mixes with blood from the ventilated segments containing a normal complement of anesthetic. The mixture produces an arterial anesthetic partial pressure that is considerably below normal.

With highly soluble agents, a different situation results from similar abnormalities in the ventilation-perfusion ratio. In alveoli receiving more ventilation relative to perfusion, the anesthetic partial pressure rises to a higher level than usual (see Fig. 21-5 for effect with methoxyflurane). That is, blood issuing from these alveoli has an increased anesthetic content, the increase being nearly proportional to the increased ventilation. Assuming that overall (total) ventilation remains normal, this increase in the anesthetic contained by blood from the relatively hyperventilated alveoli compensates for the lack of uptake of anesthetic in unventilated alveoli.

These effects are illustrated in Figure 21-11 for a condition that may be iatrogenically produced, endobronchial intubation.

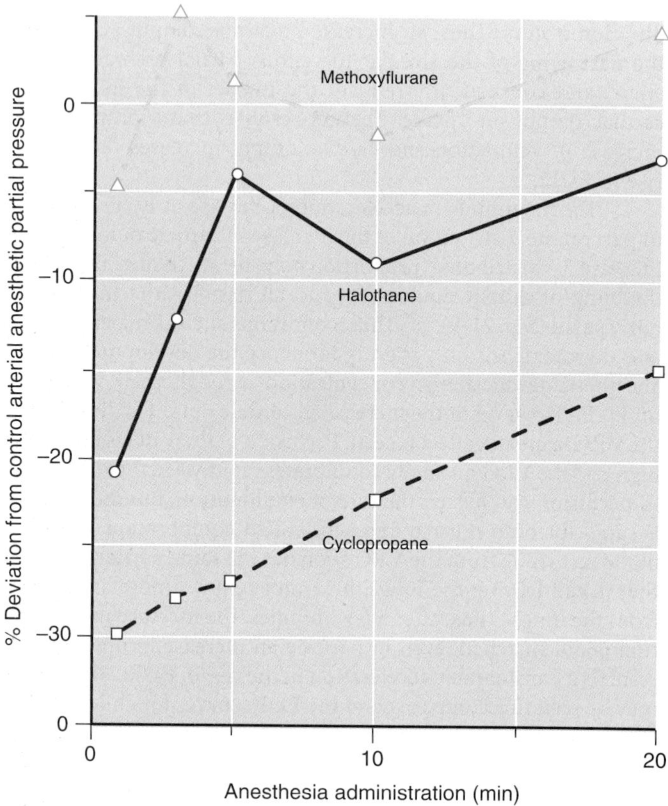

Figure 21-12 In dogs, when only the right lung was ventilated, the increase in the very soluble anesthetic methoxyflurane in arterial blood was normal (i.e., did not deviate from control), whereas the increase in the poorly soluble anesthetic cyclopropane (a blood-gas partition coefficient similar to that of sevoflurane) was significantly slowed. *(From Stoelting RK, Longnecker DE: Effect of right-to-left shunt on rate of increase in arterial anesthetic concentration. Anesthesiology 36:352-356, 1972.)*

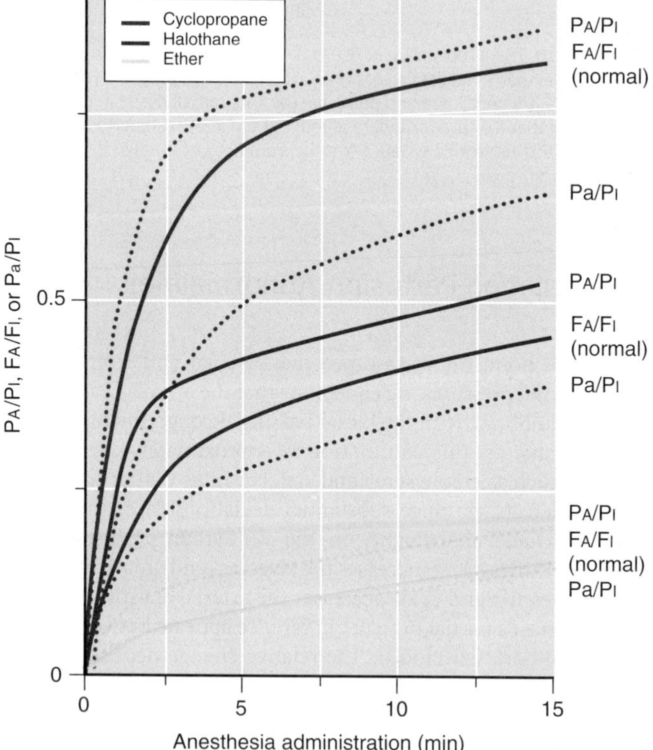

Figure 21-11 When no ventilation-perfusion abnormalities exist, the alveolar (PA or PET) and arterial (Pa) anesthetic partial pressures rise together (*continuous lines*) toward the inspired partial pressure (PI). Shunting of 50% of cardiac output through the lungs accelerates the rate of rise in end-tidal partial pressure (*dashed lines*) and retards the rate of rise in arterial partial pressure (*dot-dashed lines*). The greatest retardation of the rise in Pa/PI is found with the least soluble anesthetic, cyclopropane, and the least with the very soluble anesthetic ether. *(From Eger EI II, Severinghaus JW: Effect of uneven pulmonary distribution of blood and gas on induction with inhalation anesthetics. Anesthesiology 25:620-626, 1964.)*

Because all ventilation is now directed to the intubated lung, this lung is hyperventilated relative to perfusion. FA/FI for this lung is slightly increased (above that obtained in the absence of endobronchial intubation) with the poorly soluble cyclopropane (solubility similar to that of sevoflurane) and greatly increased with the highly soluble ether. As indicated earlier, the increase with ether compensates for the absence of uptake from the unventilated lung, a compensatory mechanism that is not available with cyclopropane. The result is that the arterial partial pressure of cyclopropane is well below normal, whereas the arterial partial pressure of ether is scarcely changed.

These concepts have been confirmed experimentally by comparing the rate of rise in arterial anesthetic with and without endobronchial intubation in dogs.[41] Endobronchial intubation significantly slowed the arterial rate of rise in cyclopropane but did not influence the rise with methoxyflurane. An intermediate result was obtained with halothane (Fig. 21-12). These data suggest that in the presence of ventilation-perfusion ratio abnormalities, the anesthetic effect of agents such as nitrous oxide, desflurane, and sevoflurane may be delayed more than the anesthetic effect of isoflurane.

The Effect of Nitrous Oxide on Closed Gas Spaces

Volume Changes in Highly Compliant Spaces

During the course of anesthetic administration, appreciable volumes of nitrous oxide can move into closed gas spaces. Although such transfer does not influence FA/FI, it may have important functional consequences. There are two types of closed gas spaces in the body, those enclosed by compliant walls and those enclosed by noncompliant walls. The former (bowel gas, pneumothorax, pneumoperitoneum, or air emboli) are subject to changes in volume secondary to transfer of nitrous oxide into these spaces.[42] These spaces normally contain nitrogen (from air), a gas whose low solubility (blood-gas partition coefficient of 0.015) limits its removal by blood. The far greater solubility of nitrous oxide in blood (blood-gas partition coefficient of 0.47) enables blood to carry more nitrous oxide to the enclosed space than it can carry away nitrogen, and the result is an increase in volume. The theoretical limit to the increase in volume is a function of the alveolar nitrous oxide concentration because this is the concentration ultimately achieved in the closed gas space. That is, at equilibrium, the concentration of nitrous oxide in the closed gas space must equal its concentration in the alveoli. An alveolar concentration of 50% might double the gas space volume, and a 75% concentration might produce a fourfold increase.

These theoretical limits may be approached if equilibrium is achieved rapidly, as with pneumothorax or gas emboli. Administration of 75% nitrous oxide in the presence of pneumothorax may double the volume of the pneumothorax by 10 minutes and may triple it by 30 minutes (Fig. 21-13).[42] Because this increase in volume may seriously impair cardiorespiratory function,[43] the use of nitrous oxide is contraindicated in the presence of a significant pneumothorax.

A still more rapid expansion of volume occurs if air inadvertently enters the bloodstream in a patient anesthetized with nitrous oxide. Expansion may be complete in seconds rather than minutes. The volume of an air embolus that is lethal decreases in animals breathing nitrous oxide as opposed to air,[44] doing so by an amount that would be predicted from the maximum theoretical expansion (Fig. 21-14). These results suggest caution in the use of nitrous oxide for procedures in which air embolization is a risk (e.g., posterior fossa craniotomies, laparoscopy). They also suggest that if air embolization is suspected, administration of nitrous oxide should be discontinued immediately. Conversely, a nitrous oxide "challenge" may be used to test whether air embolization has occurred.[45]

An endotracheal tube cuff filled with air is also susceptible to expansion by nitrous oxide[46]; 75% nitrous oxide surrounding such a cuff can double or triple the volume of the cuff. The result may be an unwanted increase in pressure exerted on the tracheal mucosa. Similarly, nitrous oxide may expand the cuffs of balloon-tipped (e.g., Swan-Ganz) catheters[47] when the balloons are inflated with air. The expansion is rapid, and a doubling of volume may occur within 10 minutes, a concern if the cuff lies within the pulmonary artery. Finally, entry of nitrous oxide into the air-filled cuff of a laryngeal mask airway can increase the volume and pressure of gas within the cuff.[48]

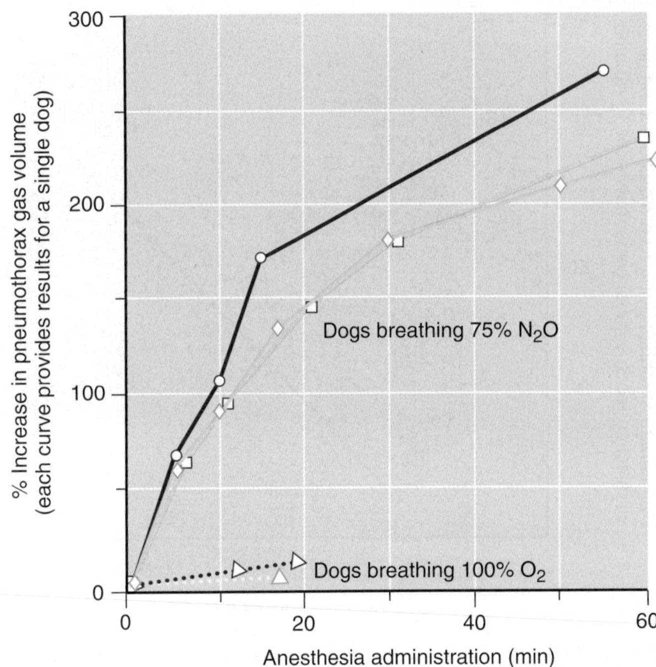

Figure 21-13 The volume of a pneumothorax created by air injection is little affected when oxygen is subsequently breathed (*filled triangle* and *circles*). However, if 75% nitrous oxide is breathed, the volume doubles in 10 minutes and triples in a half-hour (*open circles*, *squares*, and *triangles*). *(From Eger EI II, Saidman LJ: Hazards of nitrous oxide anesthesia in bowel obstruction and pneumothorax. Anesthesiology 26:61-66, 1965.)*

Pressure Changes in Poorly Compliant Spaces

Entrance of nitrous oxide into gas cavities surrounded by poorly compliant walls can increase intracavity pressure. Administration of nitrous oxide may impose untoward increases in intraocular pressure after intravitreal injection of sulfur hexafluoride.[49] Other examples include the gas space created by pneumoencephalography (now rare as a deliberate procedure) and the natural gas space in the middle ear. Pressure in the head or middle ear may rise by 20 to 50 mm Hg because of the ingress of nitrous oxide.[50,51] Recognition of this problem has decreased the use of nitrous oxide for tympanoplasty because the increased pressure may displace the graft. An increase in middle ear pressure may cause adverse postoperative effects on hearing.[52] The capacity of nitrous oxide to expand the gas in the middle ear has also been used to elevate an adherent atelectatic tympanic membrane off the promontory and ossicles.[53]

Anesthetic Circuitry

The previous discussions generally considered that the alveolar anesthetic concentration (FA) was moving toward a constant inspired anesthetic concentration (FI). In practice, the inspired concentration is not usually constant because a non-rebreathing system is not used. The rebreathing that results from the use of an anesthetic circuit causes the inspired concentration to be less than that in the gas delivered from the anesthetic machine. The

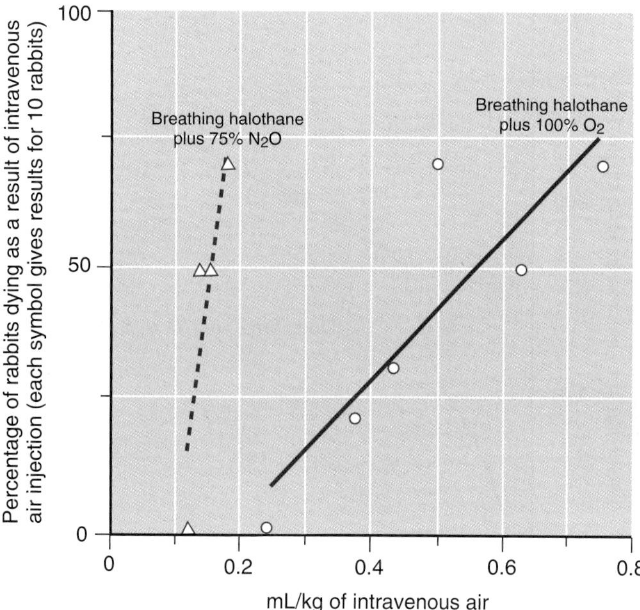

Figure 21-14 An intravenous air embolus equaling 0.55 mL/kg administered to rabbits killed half the rabbits when they breathed oxygen. If they breathed 75% nitrous oxide, only 0.16 mL/kg was required to kill half the animals. *(Modified from Munson ES, Merrick HC: Effect of nitrous oxide on venous air embolism. Anesthesiology 27:783-787, 1966.)*

inspired concentration is thus influenced by the delivered concentration, by the need to "wash in" the circuit, and by the depletion of anesthetic in rebreathed gases produced by uptake of anesthetic.

Washin of the Circuit

To begin anesthesia, anesthetic must be washed into the volume of the circuit. At inflow rates of 1 to 5 L/min and a circuit volume of 7 L (3-L bag, 1-L carbon dioxide absorber, 1 L of various fittings, and 2 L of corrugated hoses), washin of the circuit is 75% to 100% complete in 10 minutes (Fig. 21-15). Higher inflow rates accelerate the rise in inspired concentration, which suggests that induction can be accelerated and made more predictable with the use of high inflow rates.

Loss of Anesthetic to Plastic and Soda Lime

Uptake of anesthetic by several circuit components can also constitute a hindrance to the development of an adequate inspired anesthetic concentration. The rubber or plastic components of the circuit could remove significant amounts of some older anesthetics. However, uptake of nitrous oxide, desflurane, or sevoflurane by circuit components is too insignificant to materially hinder development of the inspired anesthetic concentration.[54,55]

Older normal (moist) carbon dioxide absorbents (e.g., soda lime) containing 13% to 15% water can degrade sevoflurane and thereby slightly increase requirements for sevoflurane.[56] Degradation removes hydrogen fluoride and produces an unsaturated compound (compound A). Nitrous oxide, desflurane, and isoflurane are not materially degraded. Degradation of sevoflurane has been a concern because compound A is nephrotoxic.[57] However, toxicity results only from prolonged sevoflurane administration at high concentrations and appears to require degradation by the obsolete absorbent Baralyme.[58] Some new absorbents, those lacking monovalent bases (e.g., NaOH), do not degrade sevoflurane.[59]

In contrast to normal (moist) carbon dioxide absorbents, older desiccated absorbents materially degrade all potent inhaled anesthetics.[60] Desiccated older absorbents degrade all anesthetics containing the CHF_2-O- moiety (i.e., desflurane and isoflurane) to carbon monoxide.[60] Degradation by soda lime is minimal at hydrations approximately 10% or greater than those found in normal soda lime.[60] Some new absorbents (again, those lacking monovalent bases) do not produce clinically important concentrations of carbon monoxide, even when completely dry.[61]

The Effect of Rebreathing

Inspired gas contains two gases: that delivered from the anesthetic machine and that previously exhaled by the patient and subsequently rebreathed. Because the patient removes (takes up) anesthetic from the rebreathed gas, the amount taken up and the amount rebreathed influence the inspired anesthetic concentration. An increase in uptake or rebreathing lowers the inspired concentration of a highly soluble gas more than the inspired concentration of a poorly soluble gas. This effect of uptake can be diminished by increasing the inflow rate to decrease rebreathing. An inflow rate that equals or exceeds minute ventilation eliminates rebreathing.[62]

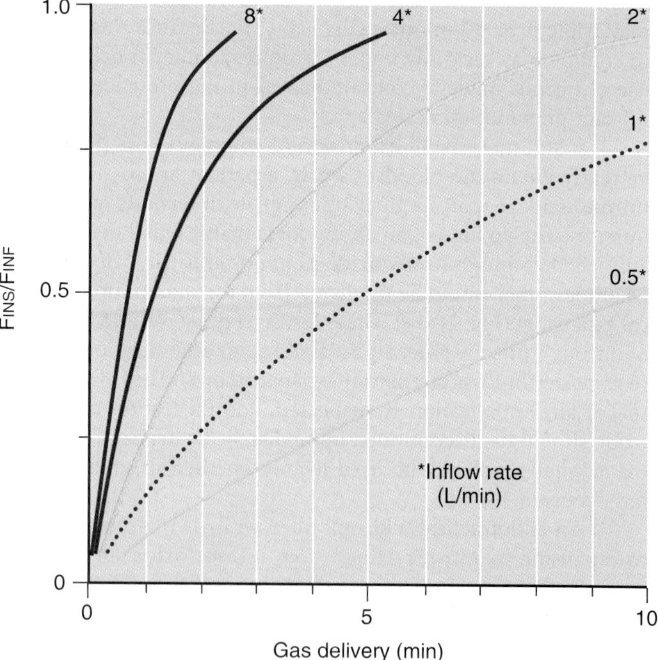

Figure 21-15 The inflow rate and circuit volume determine the rate at which the inspired anesthetic concentration (FINS) rises toward the inflowing concentration (FINF). In the case illustrated here, the circuit volume is 7 L. *(From Eger EI II: Effect of anesthetic circuit on alveolar rate of rise.* In *Eger EI [ed]: Anesthetic Uptake and Action. Baltimore, Williams & Wilkins, 1974, pp 192-205.)*

High inflow rates (i.e., ≥5 L/min) have the advantage of increasing the predictability of the inspired anesthetic concentration but the disadvantages of being wasteful and increasing atmospheric pollution. High inflow rates may be unacceptably costly because they increase consumption of expensive volatile anesthetics. High inflow rates may also dry inspired gas and make it difficult to estimate ventilation from excursions of the rebreathing bag. These several disadvantages prompt the use of low inflow rates.

Low-Flow or Closed-Circuit Delivery of Anesthesia

Much of the previous discussion assumed the use of a nonrebreathing system and a fixed inspired concentration of anesthetic. Although this approach does not invalidate the principles described earlier, it also does not reflect the variety of approaches applied in practice. Practice often deviates in two ways: (1) most anesthetists use lower inflow (fresh gas flow) rates to provide more economical delivery of anesthesia (Fig. 21-16), and (2) most anesthetists apply a constant alveolar rather than a constant inspired concentration because a constant alveolar concentration more closely reflects a constant level of anesthesia.

A low inflow rate provides several advantages and a few disadvantages, the latter particularly applying to kinetics. The advantages of low-inflow administration (defined as fresh gas flow of less than half the minute volume, usually less than 3 L/min) or closed-circuit anesthesia (defined as delivery of gases in amounts sufficient to replace only the gases—oxygen and anesthetic—removed by the patient) include lower cost, increased humidification, reduced heat loss, decreased release of anesthetic to the environment, and better capacity to assess physiologic variables such as ventilation. On the debit side, one must be more concerned about oxygen levels (especially if nitrous oxide is used because the patient also contributes nitrogen from stores in the body, and such nitrogen can slightly decrease the inspired concentration of oxygen). However, the debit of most immediate concern is the lack of control that low flow and especially closed circuits offer.

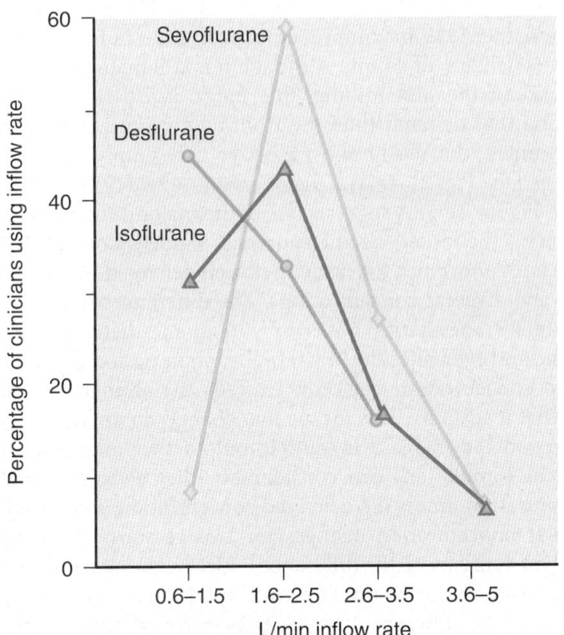

Figure 21-16 In 2005, anesthetists were surveyed regarding the inflow rates that they commonly used for maintenance of anesthesia. The responses varied broadly, but the majority used low-flow systems in which inflow rates of 2 L/min or less were applied. *(Unpublished data from Inform Research Flow Rate Tracking Study, May 2005, supplied as a personal communication by Baxter Healthcare Corp. to E. I. Eger II.)*

Closed-Circuit Anesthesia

Use of a closed circuit represents an extreme of anesthetic administration, one infrequently used because few systems completely eliminate leakage of gas from the circuit. Indeed, anesthetists often draw off approximately 200 mL/min for analysis of oxygen, carbon dioxide, and anesthetic levels.

Usually, closed-circuit anesthesia requires replacement of three gases: (1) oxygen, (2) nitrous oxide, and (3) a potent volatile anesthetic. Each replacement implies somewhat different considerations. Oxygen replacement remains constant unless metabolism changes as a result of a sympathetic response to stimulation, alteration in body temperature, or shivering. Replacement of nitrous oxide follows a fairly predictable course, in part because the concentration applied does not usually vary. Furthermore, nitrous oxide is the least soluble of anesthetics, especially in fat, and is the most prone to percutaneous loss (a constant value). Of most interest and potential variability is uptake of the potent inhaled anesthetics.

Uptake of potent anesthetics may be estimated from the values (constants) obtained by Yasuda and colleagues[10,11] in human volunteers. These values may be applied to achieve uptake at a constant alveolar concentration. To provide an appropriate level for comparison, I have assumed an alveolar concentration equal to MAC. The resulting figure (Fig. 21-17) reveals parallel shapes for each anesthetic, shapes dictated by the perfusion and solvent characteristics of the three major tissue compartments (plus intertissue diffusion). Thus, the large initial uptake rapidly decreases to a much lower level in 5 to 10 minutes as a result of the high initial uptake in the VRG (high because of its large perfusion) and the rapid decrease in uptake imposed by a short time constant (the time constant is obtained by taking the ratio of the capacity of a system to the flow through the system; it is useful in that it indicates the time for a 63% change to take place in the system). The subsequent slower decrease primarily results from the longer time constant of the MG, which dominates this period until its uptake declines below that provided by fourth compartment and the FG.

Although the curves for each anesthetic do not differ in shape, they differ in position. The height of each curve (i.e., uptake) is directly proportional to two factors: solubility and MAC. This relationship tends to minimize differences among anesthetics because solubility and MAC tend to move inversely. For example, although the MAC for desflurane is five times that for isoflurane, its uptake is less than twice that of isoflurane because of its lower solubility in blood and tissues.

Uptake may be estimated from the "square-root-of-time rule," first proposed by Severinghaus[63] and expanded greatly by

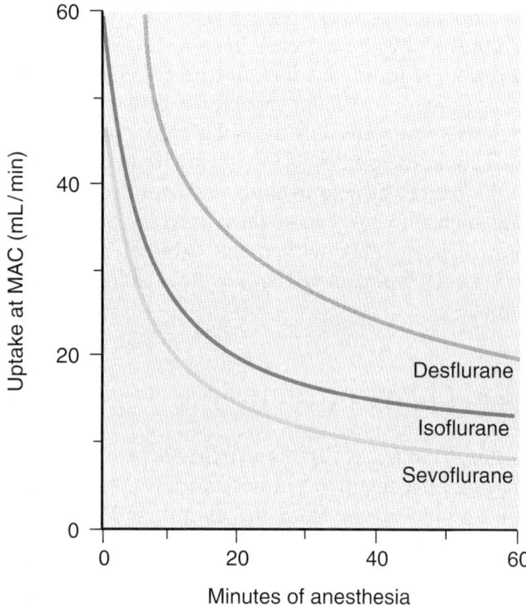

Figure 21-17 The uptake (in milliliters per minute), as illustrated in this graph, resulted from the application of constants calculated by Yasuda and coworkers[10,11] from their measurements in human volunteers. The application also assumed that alveolar concentration equals the minimum alveolar concentration (MAC) required to produce immobility in 50% of patients subjected to a surgical incision. Uptake is a function of both MAC and solubility of the anesthetic in blood and tissues. Thus, the fivefold higher MAC for desflurane than isoflurane is offset by a threefold lower solubility, which produces less than a twofold difference in uptake at any point in time. Uptake for all anesthetics initially declines rapidly as a function of the rate at which the vessel-rich group equilibrates. The further decline after 5 to 10 minutes is a function of the approach to equilibration of the muscle group. *(Data from Yasuda N, Lockhart SH, Eger EI II, et al: Kinetics of desflurane, isoflurane, and halothane in humans. Anesthesiology 74:489-498, 1991; and Yasuda N, Lockhart SH, Eger EI II, et al: Comparison of kinetics of sevoflurane and isoflurane in humans. Anesth Analg 72:316-324, 1991.)*

Lowe and Ernst[64] in their classic description of closed-circuit anesthesia. This rule states that uptake at any point in time may be estimated as uptake during the first minute of anesthesia divided by the square root of time in minutes. Making certain assumptions permits an estimate of uptake during the first minute. In general, uptake equals the product of blood solubility, cardiac output, and alveolar-to-venous anesthetic partial pressure difference. Several sources supply standard values for solubility and cardiac output, and the alveolar-to-venous anesthetic partial pressure difference may be estimated if we determine what alveolar partial pressure we wish and assume that the venous anesthetic partial pressure is inconsequential. At the start of anesthesia, an inconsequential venous partial pressure is reasonable because no anesthetic can appear in venous blood before recirculation (about 30 seconds), and even the anesthetic that appears is small in amount because tissue uptake is maximal during the first minute. Thus, we might estimate isoflurane uptake in a normal adult as $1.4 \times 5400 \times 0.0115$, or 87 mL, where 1.4 is the blood-gas partition coefficient, 5400 is cardiac output, and 0.0115 is MAC as a fraction of 1 atm. By 4 minutes, uptake would equal 87 mL/2; by 9 minutes, 87 mL/3; and by 64 minutes, 87 mL/8.

Hendrickx and associates[65] questioned the accuracy of the square-root-of-time rule and suggested that the rule overestimates the decrease in uptake with the passage of time. This author[66] considered whether the evidence provided by Hendrickx and colleagues overturned the square-root-of-time rule, and the matter continues to be debated.

Replacement of the anesthetic taken up may be accomplished by infusion of liquid anesthetic directly into the anesthetic circuit, either continuously or as boluses. Bolus injection from a syringe has an elegant simplicity but two disadvantages: (1) the circuit concentration modestly oscillates, and (2) the anesthetist is required to remember when and how much to inject. An alternative solution applies a variable bypass (Tec-type) vaporizer, one capable of accurate delivery of a range of concentrations at low inflow rates (e.g., 200 mL/min). This solution may not be applicable in the initial delivery of anesthesia because the demand for vapor may exceed the capability of presently available vaporizers. For example, the maximum output of a conventional isoflurane vaporizer is 5%, and at a 200-mL/min flow of oxygen, only approximately 10 mL of isoflurane vapor can be produced per minute, far less than the 87 mL estimated earlier. Even after 1 hour of anesthesia, an isoflurane vaporizer is barely capable of meeting the demand for anesthetic (Fig. 21-18A). This difficulty may be overcome in several ways. If a concentration less than MAC is acceptable, less delivery of vapor is required. Thus, the concurrent use of nitrous oxide decreases demand on the vaporizer. In addition, the use of nitrous oxide also increases the total fresh gas flow to compensate for the considerable uptake of nitrous oxide. If fresh gas flow increases to 1500 mL/min, 79 mL of isoflurane vapor can be produced. Another solution is to select an anesthetic with a vaporizer capability closer to demand. Such a solution tends to be available for less soluble anesthetics. For example, we calculate the uptake of desflurane in the first minute of anesthesia to be $0.45 \times 5400 \times 0.06$, or 146 mL. At a 200-mL/min flow of oxygen, the 18% maximum output of a desflurane vaporizer permits delivery of 44 mL. Although it is still inadequate to meet demand in the first minute, this figure is 2.6 times closer to meeting that demand than the isoflurane vaporizer, and within 10 minutes, the desflurane vaporizer can supply the required volume (see Fig. 21-18A).

Figure 21-18A suggests one of the major difficulties associated with the closed-circuit approach, namely, control. Clearly, there is an enormous difference between delivered (i.e., vaporizer dial) and alveolar concentrations. The differences decrease with less soluble anesthetics, but even with an anesthetic such as desflurane and even after the initial high-uptake period is passed, the dialed concentration markedly exceeds the alveolar concentration that it sustains. This means that changes in uptake (e.g., secondary to the increase in cardiac output that may result from surgical stimulation) can considerably alter alveolar anesthetic concentration unless the delivered concentration is changed. The alveolar concentration changes for two reasons: (1) assuming constant ventilation, the difference between alveolar and inspired concentrations varies directly with uptake (e.g., greater uptake increases the difference), and (2) because of rebreathing, the inspired concentration varies inversely with uptake (e.g., increased uptake lowers the inspired concentration). Thus, the sum of these effects either decreases or increases the alveolar concentration. A closed circuit has an inherent element of instability not present in an open circuit.

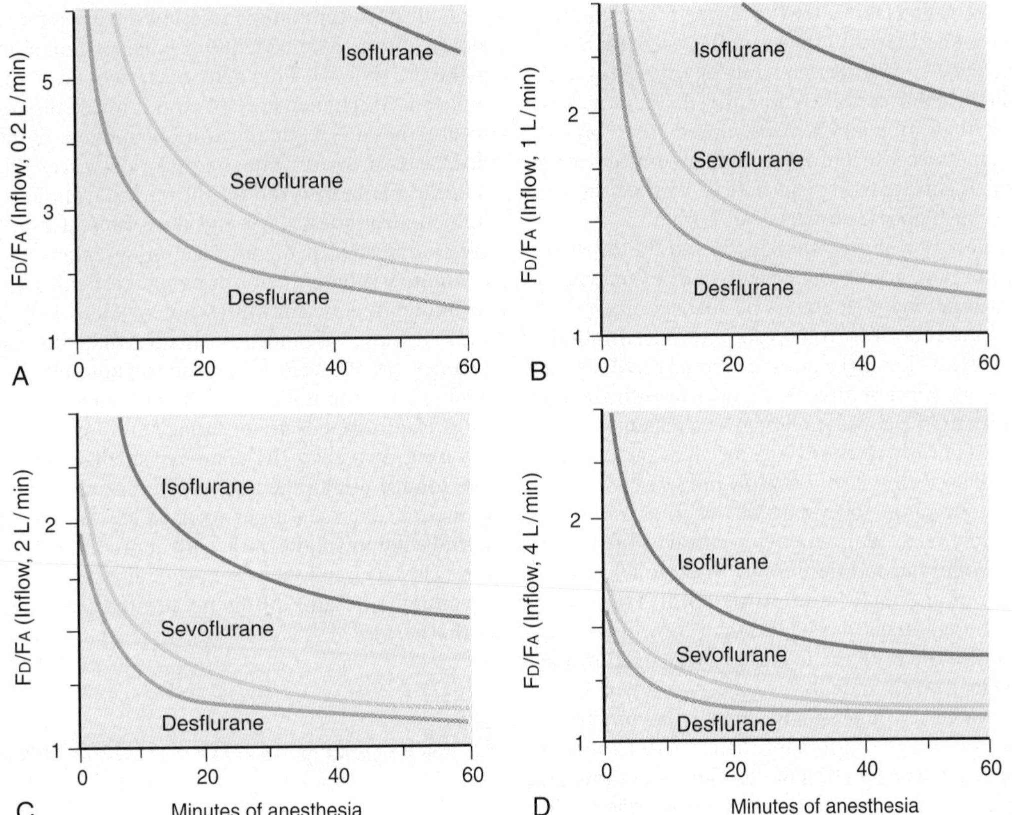

Figure 21-18 A to **D,** The ratio of delivered to alveolar concentrations (FD/FA) required to sustain the alveolar concentration constant at, for example, the minimum alveolar concentration (MAC) is a function of several factors. First, it is determined by uptake (see Fig. 21-17) and thus is greatest with the most soluble anesthetic, isoflurane. Second, it is determined by rebreathing and thus decreases with increasing inflow rates. Although these graphs have the same shape, the concentrations at any point in time progressively decrease as the inflow rate increases. The lowest values for any anesthetic result from a non-rebreathing system (i.e., when the inflow rate equals or exceeds minute ventilation).

Low-Flow Anesthetic Delivery

The instability of the closed circuit may be greatly mitigated by the use of low-flow (less than half minute ventilation) anesthetic delivery. Low-flow delivery may provide most of the advantages of closed systems while retaining considerable advantages over open systems in economy, maintenance of humidification and temperature, and limitation of atmospheric pollution. Low-flow delivery also diminishes the disadvantages of the closed circuit in the areas of constancy of oxygen and anesthetic levels and elimination of carbon monoxide and toxic anesthetic breakdown products.

In a low-flow delivery system, two factors control the relationship between the concentration delivered from a vaporizer (FD) and that in the alveoli (FA), a relationship that may best be described as the ratio of the two variables (FD/FA). First, we have already seen that uptake governs this ratio in a closed system (see Fig. 21-18A). Thus, FD/FA is higher for more soluble anesthetics, and regardless of solubility, the ratio is highest early in anesthetic administration and decreases rapidly in the first 5 to 10 minutes of anesthesia (as uptake by the VRG of tissues decreases to the point of near-equilibration) and more slowly thereafter (as uptake by tissue groups with longer time constants, such as muscle, the fourth compartment, and fat, decreases).

Second, the inflow rate also governs FD/FA. The relationship is inverse: the higher the inflow rate, the lower the ratio (compare Fig. 21-18B to D with Fig. 21-16A). An increase in inflow rate decreases FD/FA by decreasing rebreathing. Rebreathing is important because uptake of anesthetic depletes the concentration of anesthetic in rebreathed gases, and hence the concentration in delivered gases (FD) must be sufficient to compensate for this depletion. The higher the inflow rate, the less the compensation required because rebreathing is less.

However, increases in the inflow rate do not produce proportional decreases in FD/FA. The greatest reduction in FD/FA is achieved with modest increases in the inflow rate. Thus, a large decrease occurs when the inflow rate is changed from that needed for a closed circuit (Fig. 21-18A) to a 1-L/min inflow rate (Fig. 21-18B), whereas only a small decrease occurs when the inflow rate is increased from 2 to 4 L/min (Fig. 21-18C and D). Once the inflow rate exceeds minute ventilation (i.e., a non-rebreathing system exists), further increases in inflow rate have no effect on FD/FA, and FD/FA is the same as the ratio of inspired concentration (FI) to alveolar concentration (i.e., FD/FA = FI/FA).

I have used the term *anesthetic tether* as a metaphor for the FD/FA ratio.[67] A large ratio equates to a long tether, one permitting considerable variability in the alveolar concentration. With a long tether, changes in uptake secondary to changes in physiologic variables (e.g., an increase in cardiac output consequent to surgical stimulation) can appreciably alter the alveolar concentration and thus the level of anesthesia. In the example just cited, there is positive feedback because by increasing uptake, surgical stimulation decreases the alveolar concentration and thereby increases the perception of that stimulation. Most anesthetists prefer a short anesthetic tether because it provides tighter control over the level of anesthesia. A shorter tether is produced by the use of less soluble anesthetics or higher inflow rates, or both.

Another benefit of a short tether accrues to the rare anesthetist who does not have access to an agent-specific analyzer. In the absence of such an analyzer, some anesthetists may rely on the dial setting of the vaporizer to indicate the concentration of anesthetic in the patient's lungs (i.e., would assume that FD equals FA). Although the vaporizer setting may correlate with the concentration in the lungs, the correlation may be a distant one. The correlation is poor (1) early in anesthesia for all agents, (2) later in anesthesia with closed circuits or very low inflow rates, and (3) later in anesthesia for more soluble agents, such as isoflurane, even at higher inflow rates. Note that with poorly soluble anesthetics, such as sevoflurane and desflurane, by 30 to 60 minutes after the inception of anesthetic administration, the concentration delivered by the vaporizer may be less than 20% greater than that in the alveoli (i.e., the FD/FA ratio is 1.2), even at inflow rates of 1 to 2 L/min (Fig. 21-18B and C).

Economic concerns increasingly dictate the practice of anesthesia. The reader may wish to appreciate the differences in anesthetic consumption as a function of the choice of inflow rate, the duration of anesthesia, and the choice of anesthetic. The reports by Yasuda and coauthors[10,11] provide constants that may be used to estimate the uptake of commonly available potent inhaled anesthetics. By using the gas laws and published values for specific gravities, values for uptake of vapor may be converted to milliliters of liquid taken up. Combining this information with knowledge of the function of circuit rebreathing systems[68] allows an estimate of the amount of liquid in milliliters that must be delivered at various inflow rates to provide a constant alveolar concentration equal to MAC (Table 21-3).[68] The relative costs of anesthesia may be estimated by applying the price of the anesthetic of interest to the number of milliliters needed to sustain anesthesia.

Table 21-3 Milliliters of Liquid Anesthetic at Various Inflow Rates Needed to Sustain an Alveolar Concentration Equal to Minimum Alveolar Concentration

Anesthetic	Anesthetic Duration (min)	Inflow Rate (L/min, Not Including Anesthetic)				
		0.2	1.0	2.0	4.0	6.0
Halothane	30	3.0	4.1	5.4	8.0	10.5
	60	4.6	6.5	9.0	13.9	18.8
Isoflurane	30	4.0	5.8	8.0	12.3	16.7
	60	6.3	9.6	13.9	22.3	30.7
Sevoflurane	30	3.3	6.3	10.1	17.6	25.2
	60	4.9	10.9	18.2	33.0	47.8
Desflurane	30	6.7	14.8	25.0	45.2	65.4
	60	10.1	26.1	46.0	85.8	126

Modified from Weiskopf RB, Eger EI II: Comparing the costs of inhaled anesthetics. Anesthesiology 79:1413-1418, 1993.

If both economy and a low FD/FA ratio are desirable, the aforementioned considerations suggest that a good compromise is the use of a low-flow delivery system after an initial period of higher flow. Higher flow (4 to 6 L/min) might be applied early in anesthesia (i.e., at the time of highest uptake) and then be decreased progressively as uptake decreases. Flow rates of 2 to 4 L/min might be given for the period from 5 to 15 minutes after induction of anesthesia, and flow rates of 1 to 2 L/min may be given thereafter. If the average inflow rate were 2 L/min, 1 hour of anesthesia with the four potent anesthetics listed in Table 21-3 would require the administration of 9.0 to 46.0 mL of liquid. This fivefold range of values is smaller than the eightfold range of potency (MAC) values because the amount of anesthetic delivered must account for more than potency. The amount delivered must also compensate for uptake and loss of anesthetic through the overflow valve. The relatively smaller uptake and loss of the less soluble desflurane and sevoflurane are what accounts for the reduction from eightfold to fivefold. An even smaller range is found at lower inflow rates, with approximately twofold decreases for a closed circuit. However, such flows should not be used with sevoflurane because of the greater concentrations of compound A that result.

Recovery from Anesthesia

Nearly all the factors that govern the rate at which the alveolar anesthetic concentration rises on induction apply to recovery. Thus, the immediate decline is extremely rapid because the washout of functional residual capacity by ventilation is as rapid as the washin. Only 2 minutes is required to eliminate 95% to 98% of nitrogen from the lungs when pure oxygen is breathed.

Nitrogen, however, is a poorly soluble gas relative to the inhaled anesthetics. As ventilation sweeps anesthetic from the alveoli, an anesthetic partial pressure gradient develops between the partial pressure in the returning venous blood and the partial pressure in the alveoli. This gradient drives anesthetic into the alveoli, thereby opposing the tendency of ventilation to lower the alveolar concentration. The effectiveness of the venous-to-alveolar gradient in opposing the tendency of ventilation to decrease the alveolar anesthetic partial pressure is in part determined by the solubility of the anesthetic such that an agent with greater solubility, such as isoflurane, opposes the elimination produced by ventilation more than an agent with lesser solubility does, such as desflurane and sevoflurane, because a greater reserve exists in blood for the more soluble anesthetics. Thus, the fall in the alveolar partial pressure of isoflurane is slower than the fall with desflurane and sevoflurane. The rapidity of recovery largely depends on the solubility of the anesthetic.[69]

Differences Between Induction and Recovery

Recovery differs from induction in two crucial ways. First, on induction, the effect of solubility to hinder the rise in alveolar anesthetic concentration could be overcome by increasing the inspired anesthetic concentration (i.e., by applying overpressure). No such luxury is available during recovery; the inspired concen-

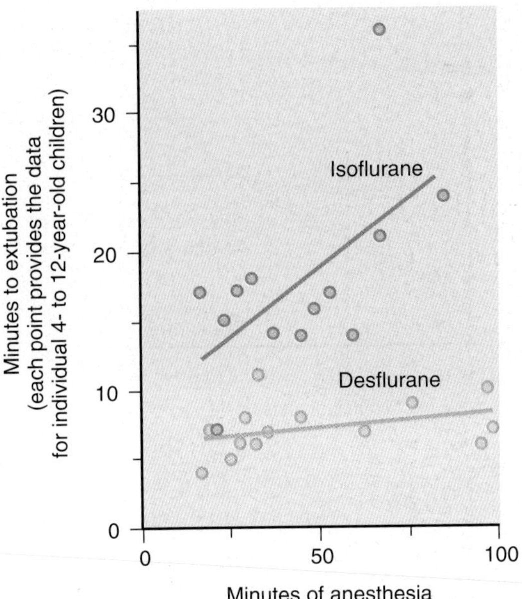

Figure 21-19 Solubility and duration of anesthesia affect the decrease in alveolar concentration on recovery and hence the time needed to recover from anesthesia. The time to tracheal extubation after anesthesia with anesthetics that have different solubilities illustrates these two aspects of recovery.[72] The time to extubation is longer after anesthesia in children anesthetized with isoflurane (the more soluble anesthetic) than in those anesthetized with desflurane. In addition, the duration of anesthesia has less impact on the time to extubation after anesthesia with the less soluble desflurane because most of the desflurane is cleared at the lung (does not recirculate to delay recovery.) *(Data from Nordmann GR, Read JA, Sale SM, et al: Emergence and recovery in children after desflurane and isoflurane anaesthesia: Effect of anaesthetic duration. Br J Anaesth 96:779-785, 2006.)*

tration cannot be reduced below zero. Second, on induction, all the tissues initially have the same anesthetic partial pressure—zero. On recovery, the tissue partial pressures are variable. The VRG has a pressure that usually equals that required for anesthesia; that is, the VRG has come to equilibrium with the alveolar anesthetic partial pressure. The MG may or may not have the same partial pressure as that found in the alveoli. A longer anesthetic course (2 to 4 hours) might permit equilibrium to be approached, but a shorter one would not. The high capacity of fat for all anesthetics except nitrous oxide precludes equilibration of the FG with the alveolar anesthetic partial pressure until hours or even days after anesthesia.

The failure of muscle and fat to equilibrate with the alveolar anesthetic partial pressure means that these tissues cannot initially contribute to the transfer of anesthetic back to the lungs. In fact, as long as an anesthetic partial pressure gradient exists between arterial blood and tissue blood, that tissue will continue to take up anesthetic. Thus, for the first several hours of recovery from anesthesia, fat continues to take up anesthetic and by so doing accelerates the rate of recovery. Only after the alveolar (equals arterial) anesthetic partial pressure falls below that in a tissue can the tissue contribute anesthetic to the alveoli.

The failure of several tissues to reach equilibration with the alveolar anesthetic partial pressure means that the rate of decrease in alveolar anesthetic on recovery is more rapid than its rate of increase on induction and that recovery depends in part on the duration of anesthesia.[70,71] A longer duration of anesthesia puts more anesthetic into the slowly filling muscle and fat depots. Obviously, these reservoirs can supply more anesthetic to the blood returning to the lungs when they are filled than when they are empty and can thereby prolong the time to recovery.[69]

Solubility influences the effect of duration of anesthesia on the rate at which the alveolar anesthetic partial pressure declines.[71] The decline in partial pressure of a poorly soluble agent is rapid in any case, and thus the acceleration imparted by a less than complete tissue equilibration cannot significantly alter the rate of recovery. The approach to equilibration becomes important with increasing solubility. With a more soluble anesthetic, recovery may be rapid after a short duration of anesthesia but may be slow after a prolonged duration. Recovery from anesthesia with desflurane and sevoflurane is more rapid and less influenced by the duration of anesthesia than with isoflurane.[69] For example, in children the time to extubation is longer after anesthesia with isoflurane than after anesthesia with desflurane (Fig. 21-19).[72] In addition, the duration of anesthesia minimally affects the time to extubation after desflurane anesthesia but has a substantial effect after isoflurane anesthesia (see Fig. 21-19).[72] Similarly, in volunteers anesthetized with 1.25 MAC desflurane versus sevoflurane, response to command and orientation occur sooner after desflurane, and duration has less of an impact on the time to respond and be oriented (Fig. 21-20).[73]

The importance of solubility and duration of anesthesia on the rate of recovery may be appreciated with the use of context-dependent times, or times to reach particular levels of washout of the alveoli or the VRG after the administration of anesthetics of specific duration.[74,75] Regardless of the duration of anesthesia, the alveolar concentrations of poorly soluble anesthetics (nitrous oxide, desflurane, sevoflurane) and a moderately soluble anesthetic (isoflurane) decrease by 60% in roughly the same period

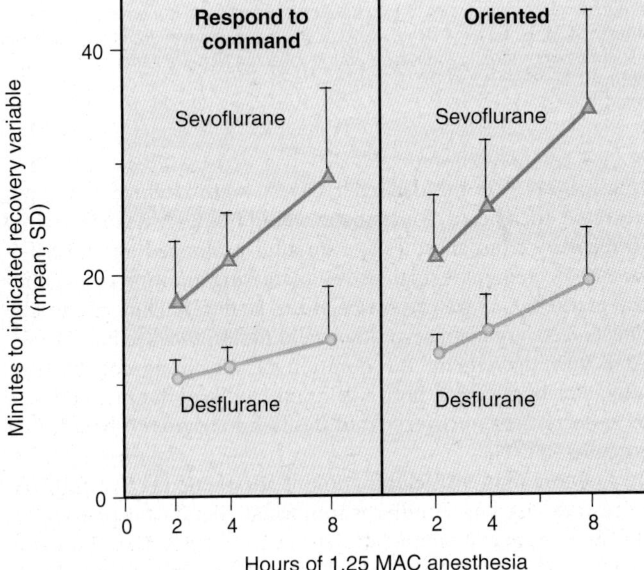

Figure 21-20 A differential time to awakening and a differential effect of anesthetic duration is shown after 2, 4, or 8 hours of anesthesia at 1.25 minimum alveolar concentration (MAC) for desflurane versus sevoflurane. Awakening to respond to a command or to orientation is more rapid after anesthesia with the less soluble desflurane, and the duration of anesthesia has less of an impact. *(From Eger EI II, Gong D, Koblin DD, et al: Effect of anesthetic duration on kinetic and recovery characteristics of desflurane vs. sevoflurane [plus compound A] in volunteers. Anesth Analg 86:414-421, 1998.)*

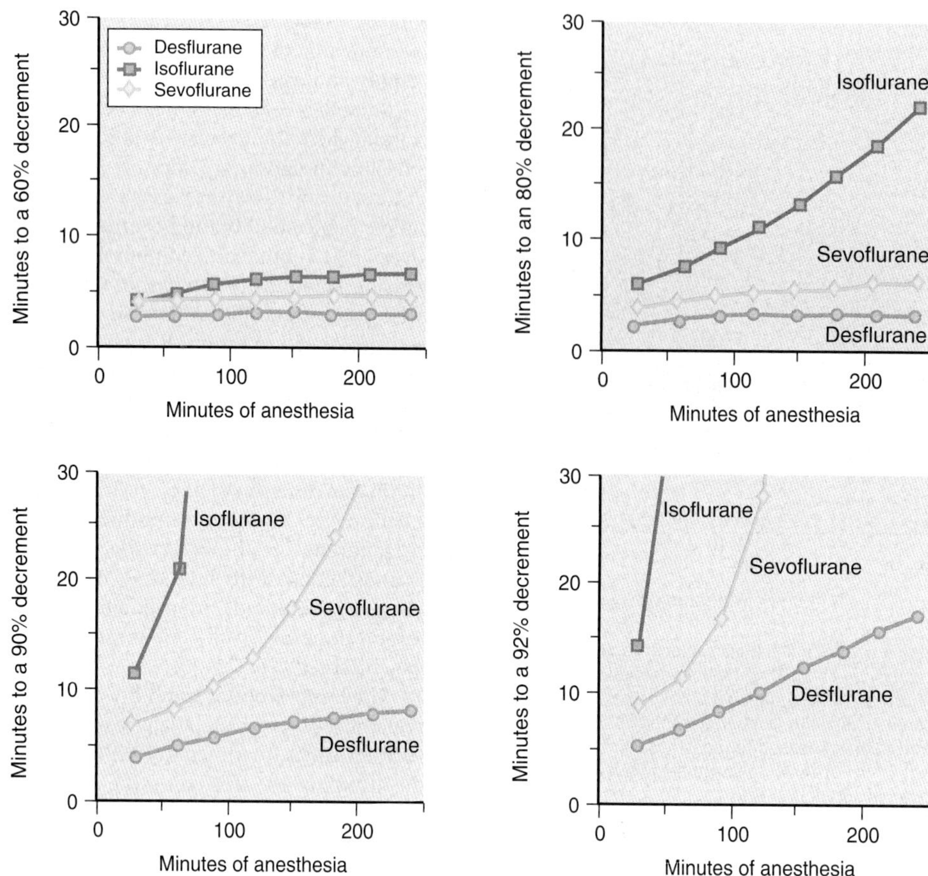

Figure 21-21 The time to decrease partial pressure in the alveoli or vessel-rich group by a certain fraction directly depends on several factors, primary among which are the solubility of the anesthetic and the duration of anesthesia. If a decrement of 60% is needed, little difference in time to recovery will be found for a comparison of isoflurane, sevoflurane, and desflurane. If an 80% decrement is needed to permit awakening, awakening from isoflurane will be delayed for progressively longer times as the duration of anesthesia is increased, but awakening from desflurane or sevoflurane will be minimally affected. If 90% of the anesthetic must be eliminated, awakening from both sevoflurane and isoflurane will be delayed more and more as the duration of anesthesia increases (isoflurane more than sevoflurane), but awakening from desflurane will be minimally affected. At a 92% decrement, the duration of anesthesia will also affect recovery from desflurane. *(Modified from Eger EI II, Shafer SL: Tutorial: Context-sensitive decrement times for inhaled anesthetics. Anesth Analg 101:688-696, 2005.)*

(Fig. 21-21).[75] If the desired recovery were attained at a 60% decrease, the choice of anesthetic would matter little on the time to recovery from anesthesia, even after prolonged anesthesia. If an 80% decrement is required, an increasing duration of anesthesia markedly affects recovery from isoflurane but minimally affects recovery from sevoflurane and desflurane (see Fig. 21-21). At a 90% decrement, the duration of anesthesia considerably affects recovery from both isoflurane and sevoflurane, and at a 92% decrement, recovery from desflurane begins to be affected (see Fig. 21-21).

More than 90% elimination of anesthetic may be required to restore pharyngeal reflexes to normal. Significant pharyngeal dysfunction may be found at 25% of MAC-awake (i.e., 5% to 8% of MAC).[76] At such small MAC values, context-sensitive decrement times become of increasing importance to recovery. McKay and associates[77] found that the capacity to drink 20 mL of water without coughing or drooling occurred sooner after desflurane than after sevoflurane (Fig. 21-22).

Pharmacodynamics adds to the determination of recovery. If immobility is accomplished with an inhaled anesthetic, the concentration exceeds MAC. Recovery sets a different goal, namely, awakening—that is, reaching MAC-awake, the concentration of anesthetic allowing appropriate response to command in 50% of subjects. MAC-awake differs among anesthetics. As a fraction of MAC, the MAC-awake of nitrous oxide (65% of MAC) exceeds that of desflurane isoflurane, and sevoflurane (approximately 33% of MAC).[78-80] The MAC-awake of propofol is still less (20%).[81] A lower MAC-awake value correlates with a greater capacity to provide amnesia: propofol is most potent and nitrous oxide least potent. However, a high MAC-awake means that awakening will occur at a higher anesthetic concentration relative to that required for anesthesia. All other factors being equal, awakening from nitrous oxide anesthesia is more rapid than awakening from anesthesia with desflurane, isoflurane, or sevoflurane.

Can I Have My Cake and Eat It Too?

The less soluble new inhaled anesthetics desflurane and sevoflurane offer more rapid recovery from anesthesia than with more soluble older anesthetics, such as isoflurane. However, this rapid recovery comes at a price: the new anesthetics are more expensive. Might it be possible to have the best of both worlds by using isoflurane for the major portion of anesthesia and reserve desflurane

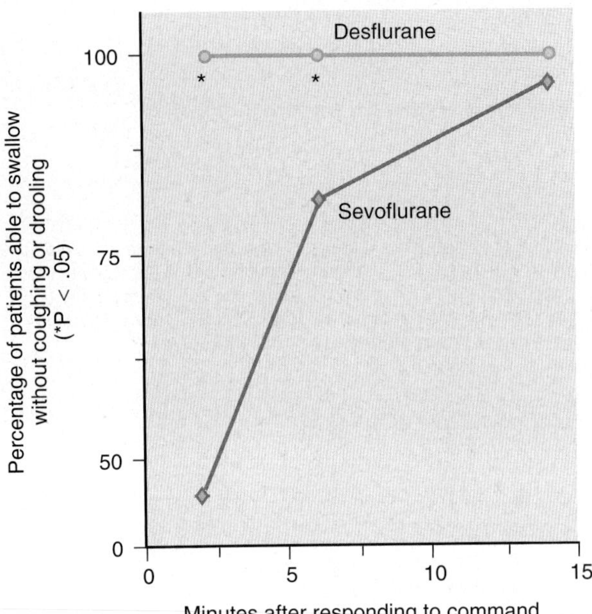

Figure 21-22 Recovery of function of pharyngeal muscles may require a decrement of 92% to 95% in anesthetic concentration.[76] At such substantial amounts of elimination, context-sensitive decrement times would suggest the possibility of more rapid recovery of airway reflexes with the less soluble desflurane, even though both anesthetics are poorly soluble. McKay and colleagues[77] measured the time from responding to command to the time that patients could swallow 20 mL of water without coughing or drooling. All patients anesthetized with desflurane could swallow 20 mL of water without coughing or drooling 2 minutes after responding to command, but fewer than 50% of patients anesthetized with sevoflurane could do so. At 6 minutes after responding to command, a significant percentage of patients given sevoflurane still could not swallow the water without coughing or drooling.

(or sevoflurane) for the final minutes? The premise would be that such an approach would provide the economy of isoflurane and the rapid recovery of desflurane. Neumann and colleagues[82] tested this premise. Volunteers were anesthetized for 2 hours on three occasions: once with 1.25 MAC isoflurane, once with 1.25 MAC desflurane, and once with 1.5 hours of 1.25 MAC isoflurane followed by 0.5 hours of a combination of desflurane and isoflurane ("crossover"). The combination provided a total of 1.25 MAC (i.e., desflurane was added as the isoflurane was eliminated, the addition being sufficient to sustain a total of 1.25 MAC). To ensure economy, all anesthetics were delivered at an inflow rate of 2 L/min. The premise was not realized. Recovery after crossover was no faster than recovery after isoflurane alone (Fig. 21-23). Recovery after desflurane alone was considerably faster than recovery after either isoflurane or the crossover from isoflurane to desflurane.

Impact of Metabolism

Saturation of the enzymes responsible for the metabolism of anesthetics may limit the ability of metabolism to significantly alter the rate at which the alveolar anesthetic partial pressure rises. This limitation does not exist on recovery, and metabolism may be an important determinant of the rate at which the alveolar anesthetic partial pressure declines. However, such metabolism applies significantly only to obsolete anesthetics such as halothane and methoxyflurane.[23] Sevoflurane is only slightly metabolized and desflurane and isoflurane undergo so little metabolism that such degradation cannot affect their kinetics.[10,11]

Diffusion Hypoxia

Uptake of large volumes of nitrous oxide on induction of anesthesia gives rise to the concentration and second gas effects. On recovery from anesthesia, the outpouring of large volumes of nitrous oxide can produce what Fink[83] called diffusion anoxia. These volumes may cause hypoxia (Fig. 21-24) in two ways. First, they may directly affect oxygenation by displacing oxygen.[83] Second, by diluting alveolar carbon dioxide, they may decrease respiratory drive and hence ventilation.[83,84] Both these effects require that large volumes of nitrous oxide be released into the alveoli. Because large volumes of nitrous oxide are released only during the first 5 to 10 minutes of recovery, this is the period of greatest concern. This concern is enhanced by the fact that the first 5 to 10 minutes of recovery may also be the time of greatest respiratory depression. For these reasons, many anesthetists administer 100% oxygen for the first 5 to 10 minutes of recovery. This procedure may be particularly indicated in patients with preexisting lung disease or in those in whom postoperative respiratory depression is anticipated (e.g., after nitrous oxide–narcotic anesthesia).

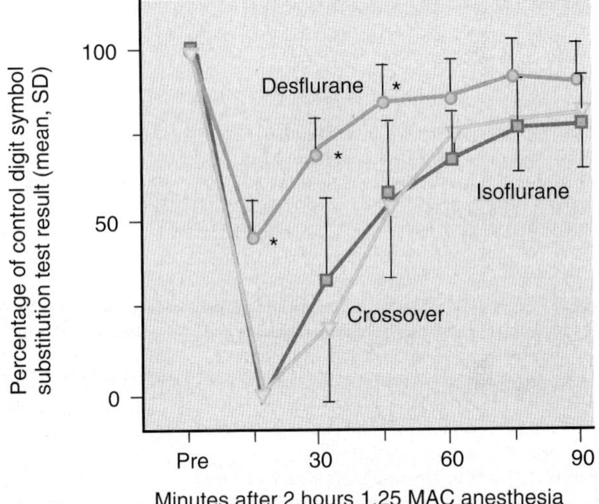

Figure 21-23 Volunteers were anesthetized for 2 hours on three occasions: once with 1.25 minimum alveolar concentration (MAC) isoflurane; once with 1.25 MAC desflurane; and once with 1.5 hours of 1.25 MAC isoflurane, followed by 0.5 hour of a combination of desflurane and isoflurane ("crossover"). The combination provided a total of 1.25 MAC (i.e., desflurane was added as the isoflurane was eliminated, the addition being sufficient to sustain a total of 1.25 MAC). All anesthetics were delivered at a 2-L/min inflow rate. At the end of 2 hours, anesthetic administration was discontinued and a non-rebreathing system was applied. The digit symbol substitution test (DSST) was applied at 15-minute intervals and the results were displayed as a percentage of the control (preanesthesia) results. Recovery of judgment and cognition as defined by the DSST was more rapid at 15, 30, and 45 minutes with desflurane given alone (*asterisks* indicate significant differences from isoflurane or crossover results), and recovery was less affected by the duration of anesthesia with desflurane. *(Data from Neumann MA, Weiskopf RB, Gong DH, et al: Changing from isoflurane to desflurane towards the end of anesthesia does not accelerate recovery in humans. Anesthesiology 88:914-921, 1998.)*

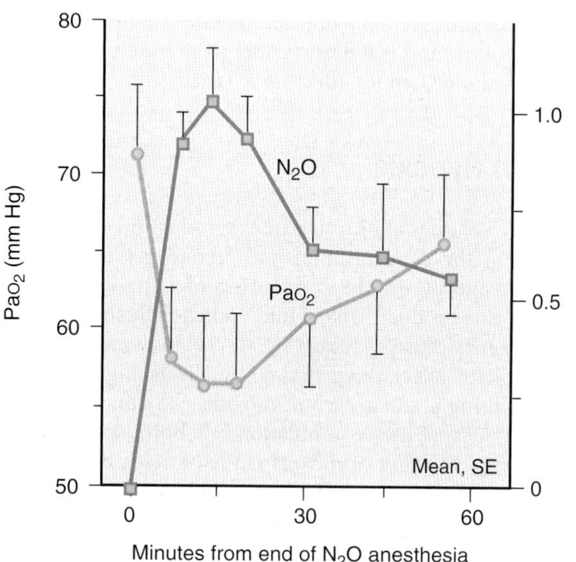

Figure 21-24 At time zero, the inspired gas was changed from 21% oxygen/79% nitrous oxide to 21% oxygen/79% nitrogen. Arterial oxygen subsequently fell in association with the outpouring of nitrous oxide. *(Modified from Sheffer L, Steffenson JL, Birch AA: Nitrous-oxide–induced diffusion hypoxia in patients breathing spontaneously. Anesthesiology 37:436-439, 1972.)*

Impact of the Anesthetic Circuit

The anesthetic circuit may limit the rate of recovery just as it limits induction. If not disconnected from the circuit on cessation of anesthetic delivery, the patient may continue to inspire anesthetic. To reduce the inspired level to zero or nearly zero, two factors must be taken into account: the anesthetic within the circuit must be washed out, and the patient's exhaled air, which contains anesthetic, must not be rebreathed. The effect of each of these factors on raising the inspired anesthetic concentration can be overcome with the use of high inflow rates of oxygen (i.e., 5 L/min or greater).

References

1. Eger EI II: Uptake of inhaled anesthetics: The alveolar to inspired anesthetic difference. *In* Eger EI II (ed): Anesthetic Uptake and Action. Baltimore, Williams & Wilkins, 1974, pp 77-96.
2. Eger EI II: Partition coefficients of I-653 in human blood, saline, and olive oil. Anesth Analg 66:971-973, 1987.
3. Eger RR, Eger EI II: Effect of temperature and age on the solubility of enflurane, halothane, isoflurane and methoxyflurane in human blood. Anesth Analg 64:640-642, 1985.
4. Eger EI II, Shargel RO, Merkel G: Solubility of diethyl ether in water, blood and oil. Anesthesiology 24:676-678, 1963.
5. Eger EI II, Shargel R: The solubility of methoxyflurane in human blood and tissue homogenates. Anesthesiology 24:625-627, 1963.
6. Cromwell TH, Eger EI II, Stevens WC, Dolan WM: Forane uptake, excretion and blood solubility in man. Anesthesiology 35:401-408, 1971.
7. Yasuda N, Targ AG, Eger EI II: Solubility of I-653, sevoflurane, isoflurane, and halothane in human tissues. Anesth Analg 69:370-373, 1989.
8. Lerman J, Schmitt-Bantel BI, Gregory GA, et al: Effect of age on the solubility of volatile anesthetics in human tissues. Anesthesiology 65:307-311, 1986.
9. Munson ES, Eger EI II, Bowers DL: Effects of anesthetic-depressed ventilation and cardiac output on anesthetic uptake. Anesthesiology 38:251-259, 1973.
10. Yasuda N, Lockhart SH, Eger EI II, et al: Kinetics of desflurane, isoflurane, and halothane in humans. Anesthesiology 74:489-498, 1991.
11. Yasuda N, Lockhart SH, Eger EI II, et al: Comparison of kinetics of sevoflurane and isoflurane in humans. Anesth Analg 72:316-324, 1991.
12. Eger EI II: The effect of inspired concentration on the rate of rise of alveolar concentration. Anesthesiology 24:153-157, 1963.
13. Stoelting RK, Eger EI II: An additional explanation for the second gas effect: A concentrating effect. Anesthesiology 30:273-277, 1969.
14. Korman B, Mapleson WW: Concentration and second gas effects: Can the accepted explanation be improved? Br J Anaesth 78:618-625, 1997.
15. Eger EI II, Smith RA, Koblin DD: The concentration effect can be mimicked by a decrease in blood solubility. Anesthesiology 49:282-284, 1978.
16. Epstein RM, Rackow H, Salanitre E, Wolf GL: Influence of the concentration effect on the uptake of anesthetic mixtures: The second gas effect. Anesthesiology 25:364-371, 1964.
17. Taheri S, Eger EI II: A demonstration of the concentration and second gas effects in humans anesthetized with nitrous oxide and desflurane. Anesth Analg 89:774-780, 1999.
18. Hendrickx JF, Carette R, Lemmens HJ, De Wolf AM: Large volume N_2O uptake alone does not explain the second gas effect of N_2O on sevoflurane during constant inspired ventilation. Br J Anaesth 96:391-395, 2006.
19. Cullen BF, Eger EI II: Diffusion of nitrous oxide, cyclopropane, and halothane through human skin and amniotic membrane. Anesthesiology 36:168-173, 1972.
20. Lockhart SH, Yasuda Y, Peterson N, et al: Comparison of percutaneous losses of sevoflurane and isoflurane in humans. Anesth Analg 72:212-215, 1991.
21. Fassoulaki A, Lockhart S, Freire BA, et al: Percutaneous loss of desflurane, isoflurane and halothane in humans. Anesthesiology 74:479-483, 1991.
22. Laster MJ, Tahari S, Eger EI II, et al: Visceral losses of desflurane, isoflurane, and halothane in swine. Anesth Analg 73:209-212, 1991.
23. Carpenter RL, Eger EI II, Johnson BH, et al: The extent of metabolism of inhaled anesthetics in humans. Anesthesiology 65:201-205, 1986.
24. Carpenter RL, Eger EI II, Johnson BH, et al: Pharmacokinetics of inhaled anesthetics in humans: Measurements during and after the simultaneous administration of enflurane, halothane, isoflurane, methoxyflurane, and nitrous oxide. Anesth Analg 65:575-582, 1986.
25. Carpenter RL, Eger EI II, Johnson BH, et al: Does the duration of anesthetic administration affect the pharmacokinetics or metabolism of inhaled anesthetics in humans. Anesth Analg 66:1-8, 1987.
26. Halsey MJ, Sawyer DC, Eger EI II, et al: Hepatic metabolism of halothane, methoxyflurane, cyclopropane, Ethrane and Forane in miniature swine. Anesthesiology 35:43-47, 1971.
27. Yamamura H, Wakasugi B, Okuma Y, Maki K: The effects of ventilation on the absorption and elimination of inhalation anaesthetics. Anaesthesia 18:427-438, 1963.
28. Fukui Y, Smith NT: Interactions among ventilation, the circulation, and the uptake and distribution of halothane—use of a hybrid computer multiple model: I. The basic model. Anesthesiology 54:107-118, 1981.
29. Doi M, Ikeda K: Respiratory effects of sevoflurane. Anesth Analg 66:241-244, 1987.
30. Fourcade HE, Stevens WC, Larson CP Jr, et al: The ventilatory effects of Forane, a new inhaled anesthetic. Anesthesiology 35:26-31, 1971.
31. Munson ES, Larson CP Jr, Babad AA, et al: The effects of halothane, fluroxene and cyclopropane on ventila-

tion: A comparative study in man. Anesthesiology 27:716-728, 1966.

32. Lockhart S, Rampil IJ, Yasuda N, et al: Depression of ventilation by desflurane in humans. Anesthesiology 74:484-488, 1991.
33. Yamamura H: The effect of ventilation and blood volume on the uptake and elimination of inhalation anesthetic agents. *In* Progress in Anaesthesiology. Proceedings of the Fourth World Congress of Anesthesiologists. Amsterdam, Excerpta Medica, International Congress Series 200, 1968, pp 394-399.
34. Eger EI II, Smith NT, Stoelting RK, et al: Cardiovascular effects of halothane in man. Anesthesiology 32:396-409, 1970.
35. Gibbons RT, Steffey EP, Eger EI II: The effect of spontaneous versus controlled ventilation on the rate of rise of alveolar halothane concentration in dogs. Anesth Analg 56:32-34, 1977.
36. Eger EI II, Bahlman SH, Munson ES: Effect of age on the rate of increase of alveolar anesthetic concentration. Anesthesiology 35:365-372, 1971.
37. Wahrenbrock EA, Eger EI II, Laravuso RB, Maruschak G: Anesthetic uptake—of mice and men (and whales). Anesthesiology 40:19-23, 1974.
38. Munson ES, Eger EI II, Tham MK, Embro WJ: Increase in anesthetic uptake, excretion and blood solubility in man after eating. Anesth Analg 57:2221-2231, 1978.
39. Gallagher TM, Black GW: Uptake of volatile anaesthetics in children. Anaesthesia 40:1073-1077, 1985.
40. Eger EI II, Severinghaus JW: Effect of uneven pulmonary distribution of blood and gas on induction with inhalation anesthetics. Anesthesiology 25:620-626, 1964.
41. Stoelting RK, Longnecker DE: Effect of right-to-left shunt on rate of increase in arterial anesthetic concentration. Anesthesiology 36:352-356, 1972.
42. Eger EI II, Saidman LJ: Hazards of nitrous oxide anesthesia in bowel obstruction and pneumothorax. Anesthesiology 26:61-66, 1965.
43. Hunter AR: Problems of anaesthesia in artificial pneumothorax. Proc R Soc Med 48:765, 1955.
44. Munson ES, Merrick HC: Effect of nitrous oxide on venous air embolism. Anesthesiology 27:783-787, 1966.
45. Shapiro HM, Yoachim J, Marshall LF: Nitrous oxide challenge for detection of residual intravascular pulmonary gas following venous air embolism. Anesth Analg 61:3021-3026, 1982.
46. Stanley TH, Kawamura R, Graves C: Effects of nitrous oxide on volume and pressure of endotracheal tube cuffs. Anesthesiology 41:256-262, 1974.
47. Kaplan R, Abramowitz MD, Epstein BS: Nitrous oxide and air-filled balloon-tipped catheters. Anesthesiology 55:71-73, 1981.
48. Algren JT, Gursoy F, Johnson TD, Skjonsby BS: The effect of nitrous oxide diffusion on laryngeal mask airway cuff inflation in children. Paediatr Anaesth 8:31-36, 1998.
49. Wolf GL, Capuano C, Hartung J: Nitrous oxide increases intraocular pressure after intravitreal sulfur hexafluoride injection. Anesthesiology 59:547-548, 1983.
50. Thomsen KA, Terkildsen K, Arnfred J: Middle ear pressure variations during anesthesia. Arch Otolaryngol 82:609-611, 1985.
51. Saidman LJ, Eger EI II: Change in cerebrospinal fluid pressure during pneumoencephalography under nitrous oxide anesthesia. Anesthesiology 26:67-72, 1965.
52. Waun JE, Sweitzer RS, Hamilton WK: Effect of nitrous oxide on middle ear mechanics and hearing acuity. Anesthesiology 28:846-850, 1987.
53. Graham MD, Knight PR: Atelectative tympanic membrane reversal by nitrous oxide supplemented general anesthesia and polyethylene ventilation tube insertion. A preliminary report. Laryngoscope 41:1469, 1981.
54. Eger EI II, Ionescu P, Gong D: Circuit absorption of halothane, isoflurane and sevoflurane. Anesth Analg 86:1070-1074, 1998.
55. Targ AG, Yasuda N, Eger EI II: Solubility of I-653, sevoflurane, isoflurane, and halothane in plastics and rubber composing a conventional anesthetic circuit. Anesth Analg 68:218-225, 1989.
56. Strum DP, Johnson BH, Eger EI II: Stability of sevoflurane in soda lime. Anesthesiology 67:779-781, 1987.
57. Higuchi H, Sumita S, Wada H, et al: Effects of sevoflurane and isoflurane on renal function and on possible markers of nephrotoxicity. Anesthesiology 89:307-322, 1998.
58. Eger EI II, Gong D, Koblin DD, et al: Dose-related biochemical markers of renal injury after sevoflurane vs. desflurane anesthesia in volunteers. Anesth Analg 85:1154-1163, 1997.
59. Kobayashi S, Bito H, Obata Y, et al: Compound A concentration in the circle absorber system during low-flow sevoflurane anesthesia: Comparison of Dragersorb Free, Amsorb, and Sodasorb II. J Clin Anesth 15:33-37, 2003.
60. Fang ZX, Eger EI II, Laster MJ, et al: Carbon monoxide production from degradation of desflurane, enflurane, isoflurane, halothane, and sevoflurane by soda lime and Baralyme. Anesth Analg 80:1187-1193, 1995.
61. Knolle E, Heinze G, Gilly H: Small carbon monoxide formation in absorbents does not correlate with small carbon dioxide absorption. Anesth Analg 95:650-655, 2002.
62. Harper M, Eger EI II: A comparison of the efficiency of three anesthesia circle systems. Anesth Analg 55:7221-7229, 1976.
63. Severinghaus JW: The rate of uptake of nitrous oxide in man. J Clin Invest 33:1183-1189, 1954.
64. Lowe HJ, Ernst EA: The Quantitative Practice of Anesthesia: Use of Closed Circuit. Baltimore, Williams & Wilkins, 1981.
65. Hendrickx JFA, Soetens M, VanderDonck A, et al: Uptake of desflurane and isoflurane during closed-circuit anesthesia with spontaneous and controlled mechanical ventilation. Anesth Analg 84:413-418, 1997.
66. Eger EI II: Complexities overlooked: Things may not be what they seem. Anesth Analg 84:239-240, 1997.
67. Eger EI II: Desflurane (Suprane). A Compendium and Reference. Rutherford, NJ, Healthpress Publishing, 1993, pp 1-119.
68. Weiskopf RB, Eger EI II: Comparing the costs of inhaled anesthetics. Anesthesiology 79:1413-1418, 1993.
69. Eger EI II, Johnson BH: Rates of awakening from anesthesia with I-653, halothane, isoflurane, and sevoflurane: A test of the effect of anesthetic concentration and duration in rats. Anesth Analg 66:977-982, 1987.
70. Mapleson WW: Quantitative prediction of anesthetic concentrations. *In* Papper EM, Kitz RJ (eds): Uptake and Distribution of Anesthetic Agents. New York, McGraw-Hill, 1963, pp 1021-1119.
71. Stoelting RK, Eger EI II: The effects of ventilation and anesthetic solubility on recovery from anesthesia: An in vivo and analog analysis before and after equilibration. Anesthesiology 30:290-296, 1969.
72. Nordmann GR, Read JA, Sale SM, et al: Emergence and recovery in children after desflurane and isoflurane anaesthesia: Effect of anaesthetic duration. Br J Anaesth 96:779-785, 2006.
73. Eger EI II, Gong D, Koblin DD, et al: Effect of anesthetic duration on kinetic and recovery characteristics of desflurane vs. sevoflurane (plus compound A) in volunteers. Anesth Analg 86:414-421, 1998.
74. Bailey JM: Context-sensitive half-times and other decrement times of inhaled anesthetics. Anesth Analg 85:681-686, 1997.
75. Eger EI II, Shafer SL: Tutorial: Context-sensitive decrement times for inhaled anesthetics. Anesth Analg 101:688-696, 2005.
76. Sundman E, Witt H, Sandin R, et al: Pharyngeal function and airway protection during subhypnotic concentrations of propofol, isoflurane, and sevoflurane. Volunteers examined by pharyngeal videoradiography and simultaneous manometry. Anesthesiology 95:1125-1132, 2001.
77. McKay RE, Large MJC, Balea MC, McKay WR: Airway reflexes return more rapidly after desflurane anesthesia than after sevoflurane anesthesia. Anesth Analg 100:697-700, 2005.
78. Katoh T, Suguro Y, Nakajima R, et al: Blood concentration of sevoflurane and isoflurane on recovery from anaesthesia. Br J Anaesth 69:259-262, 1992.
79. Dwyer R, Bennett HL, Eger EI II, Heilbron D: Effects of isoflurane and nitrous oxide in subanesthetic concentrations on memory and responsiveness in volunteers. Anesthesiology 77:888-898, 1992.
80. Katoh T, Suguro Y, Ikeda T, et al: Influence of age on awakening concentrations of sevoflurane and isoflurane. Anesth Analg 76:348-352, 1993.
81. Chortkoff BS, Eger EI II, Crankshaw DP, et al: Concentrations of desflurane and propofol that suppress response to command in humans. Anesth Analg 81:737-743, 1995.
82. Neumann MA, Weiskopf RB, Gong DH, et al: Changing from isoflurane to desflurane towards the end of anesthesia does not accelerate recovery in humans. Anesthesiology 88:914-921, 1998.
83. Fink BR: Diffusion anoxia. Anesthesiology 16:511-519, 1955.
84. Rackow H, Salanitre E, Frumin MJ: Dilution of alveolar gases during nitrous oxide excretion in man. J Appl Physiol 16:723-728, 1961.

Neil E. Farber, Paul S. Pagel, and David C. Warltier

22 Pulmonary Pharmacology

Key Points

1. Inhaled anesthetics affect every facet of pulmonary physiology, from the variety of forces controlling ventilation and pulmonary blood flow to surface tension, secretion of mucus, airway smooth muscle tone, and lung inflammatory responses.
2. The bronchodilatory actions of volatile anesthetics occur through several complex mechanisms that involve both a decrease in intracellular calcium concentration and a reduction in calcium sensitivity. Volatile anesthetics increase baseline pulmonary dynamic compliance, but these agents are more effective at attenuating increases in pulmonary airway resistance caused by chemical or mechanical stimuli. Inhaled anesthetics preferentially dilate the distal airways rather than the proximal airways.
3. Inhaled anesthetics diminish the rate of mucus clearance by decreasing ciliary beat frequency, disrupting metachronism, or altering the characteristics of mucus.
4. Pulmonary surfactant decreases the work of breathing by reducing alveolar surface tension. Volatile anesthetics cause progressive, yet reversible reductions in phosphatidylcholine, the main lipid component of surfactant. The roles of depressed mucociliary function and alterations in type II alveolar cell function in postoperative pulmonary complications after the administration of a volatile agent are unknown.
5. The multiple sites of actions of inhaled anesthetics on the pulmonary parenchyma and vasculature complicate direct assessment of anesthetic-induced alterations in pulmonary vascular resistance. Volatile anesthetics cause a biphasic contraction-relaxation response in pulmonary vascular smooth muscle that is mediated at multiple sites through a Ca^{2+}-mediated signaling pathway. Overall, the net effect of inhaled anesthetic–induced changes in pulmonary vascular resistance is relatively small.
6. Hypoxic pulmonary vasoconstriction (HPV) is an important mechanism by which pulmonary blood is preferentially redistributed away from poorly ventilated lung regions to those with adequate alveolar ventilation. Most inhaled anesthetics attenuate HPV in vitro and exert relatively modest inhibitory effects on HPV, shunting, or oxygenation in vivo.
7. Inhaled anesthetics (with the exception of xenon) reduce tidal volume and minute ventilation and cause tachypnea in a dose-related fashion. The relative effect of inhaled anesthetics in increasing arterial carbon dioxide tension (as an index of respiratory depression) is enflurane > desflurane = isoflurane > sevoflurane = halothane > nitrous oxide.
8. Inhaled anesthetics affect the inspiratory and expiratory respiratory muscles to varying degrees, possibly as a result of the differential sensitivity of bulbospinal inspiratory and expiratory neurons.
9. All inhaled anesthetics depress the ventilatory responses to hypercapnia and hypoxia by altering central and peripheral chemoreceptor function in a dose-dependent fashion. The effects of subanesthetic concentrations of inhaled agents on hypercapnic responses are controversial. Inhibition of hypoxic responses by subanesthetic concentrations of volatile agents depends on the agent used and perhaps the baseline state of central nervous system arousal. These findings may have important clinical implications during the perioperative period.
10. Volatile anesthetics may exhibit proinflammatory actions and worsen acute lung injury. Alternatively, volatile anesthetics have been shown to reduce inflammation and improve both chemical and physiologic pulmonary function in acute lung injury.

This chapter describes the pulmonary pharmacology of inhaled anesthetics. The lungs are unique in their exposure to a wide variety a physical forces, including ventilation, blood flow, and surface tension, and inhaled anesthetics selectively modulate each of these properties. Specific sections of this chapter focus on airway tone, pulmonary vascular resistance (PVR), mucociliary function, surfactant production, ventilatory control, and acute lung injury. The actions of volatile anesthetics on each of these systems are discussed.

Bronchomotor Tone

Transient increases in airway resistance may be caused, at least in part, by an increase in bronchiolar smooth muscle tone. Patients without recent symptoms of asthma have a very low frequency of perioperative respiratory complications, yet perioperative bronchospasm develops in approximately 6% of patients with asthma. Prospective studies have demonstrated that 1.7% of patients with asthma experience a poor respiratory outcome[1] and that 25% wheeze after the induction of anesthesia.[2] Of the 40 cases of bronchospasm resulting in settled malpractice claims reported by the American Society of Anesthesiologists Closed Claims Project,[3] 88% involved brain damage or death, and only half of these patients had a history of asthma or chronic obstructive pulmonary disease (COPD). Because significant bronchospasm may occur in normal subjects without underlying lung disease, understanding of the physiologic effects of inhaled agents on bronchial smooth muscle is very important.

Pharmacology of Bronchial Smooth Muscle

Pinto-Pereira and colleagues[4] summarized the mechanisms by which increases in airway resistance might occur. Airway smooth muscle extends as far distally as the terminal bronchioles and is affected by autonomic nervous system activity and nonadrenergic, noncholinergic mechanisms. Parasympathetic nerves originating in vagal centers within the central nervous system mediate baseline airway tone and reflex bronchoconstriction. Changes in intracellular calcium (ICa^{2+}) levels and Ca^{2+} influx may be caused by alterations in cyclic nucleotides within bronchial smooth muscle. Agonist-induced contraction is mediated by an increase in myosin light chain kinase activity, phosphorylation of the 20-kd regulatory myosin light chain, and an increase in Ca^{2+} sensitivity.[5] Exogenous administration of acetylcholine or stimulation of the vagus nerve increases the level of cyclic guanosine monophosphate (cGMP) relative to cyclic adenosine monophosphate (cAMP) and results in bronchial smooth muscle contraction. Activation of bronchial smooth muscle cells by agonist also involves the second messenger cyclic adenosine diphosphate ribose, which indirectly releases Ca^{2+} from the sarcoplasmic reticulum (SR) by activating ryanodine channels.[6] Agonist-induced stimulation of particulate guanylyl cyclase relaxes bronchial smooth muscle by decreasing Ca^{2+} current. In contrast, stimulation of soluble guanylyl cyclase by substances such as nitric oxide (NO) reduces ICa^{2+} concentration and Ca^{2+} sensitivity.[7]

Release of histamine in the airway or various forms of mechanical or chemical stimulation may increase afferent vagal activity and produce reflex bronchoconstriction. This increase in bronchomotor tone is attenuated by the cholinergic antagonist atropine. M_2 and M_3 muscarinic receptors on airway smooth muscle mediate bronchoconstriction by increasing Ca^{2+} sensitivity.[8] Presynaptic M_2 muscarinic receptors have also been identified that inhibit release of acetylcholine, and thus drugs that preferentially inhibit M_2 receptors (e.g., ipratropium bromide) may paradoxically produce bronchoconstriction,[9] although this effect is not commonly observed in patients.

Adrenergic receptors in bronchial smooth muscle are classified into α and β_2 types. α-Receptors have been characterized in the human bronchial tree, but their activity may be clinically insignificant. In contrast, the β_2-receptor subtypes play an important role in bronchiolar smooth muscle responsiveness. Stimulation of β_2-adrenoreceptors causes cAMP-mediated relaxation via activation of protein kinase A and subsequent efflux of Ca^{2+} out of the cell and into the SR. Notably, asthma, as well as allergy- and methacholine-induced bronchospasm, does not appear to be genetically linked to a dominant β_2-adrenoceptor gene.[10]

Respiratory epithelium releases substances that modulate bronchial smooth muscle tone. Epithelial removal enhances contractile responses to acetylcholine, histamine, and serotonin in large airways and decreases relaxation responses to isoproterenol in small airways. These actions are analogous to the effect of endothelial damage on vascular smooth muscle tone. However, porcine bronchiolar epithelium–mediated bronchomotor activity is not significantly affected by cardiopulmonary bypass, in contrast with the vascular endothelium–mediated smooth muscle dysfunction seen in this situation.[11] Although endogenous epithelial factors have been identified, NO may play an important vasodilatory role in respiratory epithelium, similar to that of vascular endothelium. Endothelin-1 is also a potent endogenous bronchoconstrictor, as well as vasoconstrictor, that functions by activation of the inositol triphosphate (IP_3) pathway.[12]

Volatile Anesthetics

Volatile anesthetics are all bronchodilators, but some controversy remains about which volatile anesthetic exerts the most potent bronchodilation. In many studies using animal models, it appears that halothane has the most pronounced effect of relaxing airway smooth muscle. It is important to eliminate the indirect effects of arterial carbon dioxide tension when examining the actions of volatile agents on bronchial tone, especially during spontaneous ventilation, because hypercapnia-induced bronchodilation and hypocapnia-induced bronchoconstriction are both attenuated by isoflurane.[13] What may be interpreted as a dose-dependent effect of deepening the level of anesthesia with volatile anesthetics may actually be due to an indirect action mediated by a progressive increase in carbon dioxide tension. Isoflurane and halothane (1.5 minimum alveolar concentration [MAC]) produce similar reductions in airway resistance in a canine model of bronchospasm induced by aerosolized *Ascaris* antigen. Similar results were obtained with volatile agents during methacholine-induced airway constriction. Taken together, these data suggest that isoflurane and halothane produce direct bronchodilation and depress airway reflexes. Isoflurane appears to share significant bronchodilating properties with halothane and enflurane, but halothane increases dynamic compliance (a measure of small airway resistance) to a greater extent than isoflurane does. This finding may be particularly important in view of the fact that isoflurane preferentially relaxes bronchioles rather than bronchi in vitro.[14] The structure of the respiratory epithelium changes from pseudostratified columnar cells of the large airways to thinner, cuboidal cells of the bronchioles, and thus a relatively large amount of histologic heterogeneity exists between these regions. Although all volatile anesthetics bronchodilate, their specific effects on bronchioles depend on the location in and structure of the respiratory tree. Park and colleagues[15] demonstrated that isoflurane and halothane dilate fourth-order bronchi at equivalent MAC values. Halothane, isoflurane, sevoflurane, and desflurane, at concentrations of up to 1 MAC, similarly attenuated methacholine-induced bronchoconstriction in open-chest, pentobarbital-anesthetized rats.[16]

Using computed tomography (CT), Brown and coworkers[17,18] showed that halothane causes greater bronchodilation than isoflurane does at low concentrations (Fig. 22-1). Halothane also had a more pronounced relaxing effect than isoflurane did at a similar MAC in intact airway smooth muscle as measured by high-resolution CT.[19] All volatile agents, including sevoflurane[20,21] and desflurane,[22,23] relax airway smooth muscle. Sevoflurane (1 MAC) reduced respiratory system resistance (determined via an isovolume technique) by 15% in patients undergoing elective surgery. In contrast, desflurane did not significantly alter resistance.[24] Halothane, desflurane, and isoflurane appear to relax the distal airways (i.e., bronchioles) to a greater extent than the proximal airways (i.e., bronchi).[22] Similarly, isoflurane and sevoflurane had greater inhibitory effects on bronchial than on tracheal smooth muscle contraction.[25] These differential effects appear to be related to the type of voltage-dependent Ca^{2+} channels (VDCs) present in these regions. Administration of volatile anesthetics to children undergoing elective imaging studies resulted in progressive reductions in the cross-sectional area of the upper airway musculature and subsequent pharyngeal airway collapse.[26] As observed with isoflurane and halothane in animal models, the effects of sevoflurane in children were not uniformly distributed along the upper airway (also see Chapter 82).

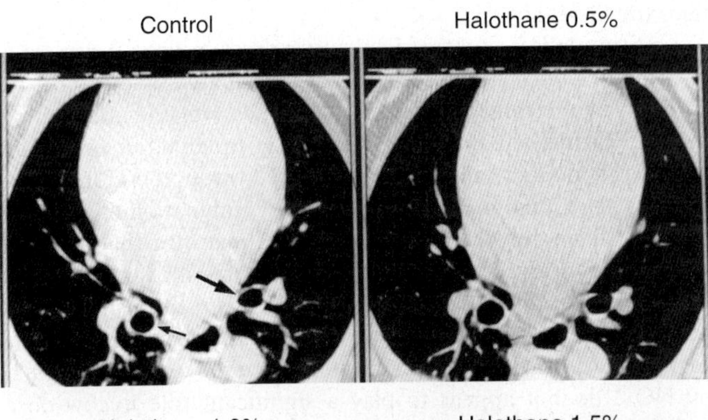

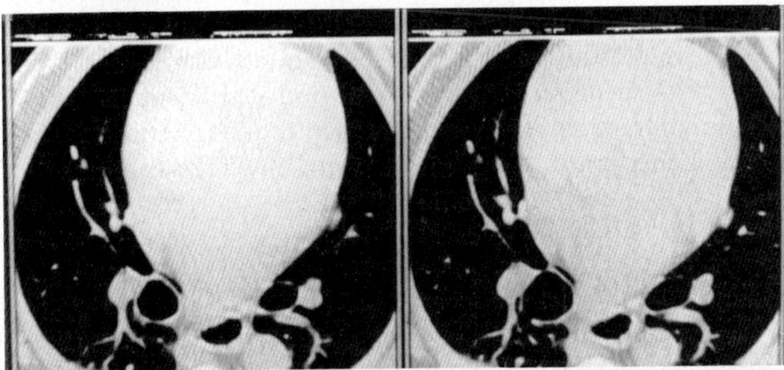

Figure 22-1 High-resolution computed tomography scan from one dog. **Upper left,** control; **upper right,** during 0.5% halothane; **lower left,** during 1.0% halothane; **lower right,** during 1.5% halothane. Note the progressive dilation of the airways as indicated by the *arrows*. *(Reproduced from Brown RH, Mitzner W, Zerhouni E, et al: Direct in vivo visualization of bronchodilation induced by inhalational anesthesia using high-resolution computed tomography. Anesthesiology 78:295, 1993, with permission.)*

Inhalation of 1 or 2 MAC halothane, enflurane, sevoflurane, or isoflurane does not alter baseline pulmonary resistance and dynamic pulmonary compliance. However, these anesthetics significantly attenuated increases in pulmonary resistance and decreases in dynamic pulmonary compliance in response to intravenous histamine. Halothane was most effective in altering indices of bronchodilation, whereas responses to isoflurane, enflurane, and sevoflurane were nearly identical.[21] In contrast, desflurane produced bronchodilation at 1 MAC but increased airway resistance at 2 MAC.[27] Halothane, enflurane, and sevoflurane were found to be equivalent in dilating third- or fourth-generation bronchi as measured directly with a fiberoptic bronchoscope in vivo.[28]

Mechanisms of Action

Volatile anesthetics relax airway smooth muscle by directly depressing smooth muscle contractility. This action appears to result from direct effects on bronchial epithelium and airway smooth muscle cells and indirect inhibition of reflex neural pathways. The mechanisms responsible for the direct relaxation effects involve decreases in ICa^{2+}, an important regulator of smooth muscle reactivity. Several intracellular mediators responsible for mobilization of Ca^{2+} are potential sites for the action of volatile anesthetics, but the predominant mechanism appears to be inhibition of cell-membrane–associated VDCs, an action that reduces entry of Ca^{2+} into the cytosol.[29] Volatile anesthetic–induced increases in cAMP concentration cause decreases in free ICa^{2+} by stimulating efflux of Ca^{2+} and increasing uptake of Ca^{2+} into the SR. This action contributes to airway smooth muscle relaxation.[30] In addition to the decrease in ICa^{2+} levels, volatile anesthetic–induced decrease in calcium sensitivity as a result of inhibition of protein kinase C activity[31] and inhibition of G protein function are also reported mechanisms.[32] It has been suggested that volatile anesthetics differentially modify pulmonary resistance by altering the density of the gas mixture (Fig. 22-2).[31] In a laboratory lung model with fixed resistance, high concentrations of volatile agents increased the density of the gas mixture and the calculated resistance, with desflurane having the greatest increase at all MAC values studied.

The effects of volatile anesthetics on proximal versus distal airways may be related to differential effects on VDCs and the relative distribution of these channels. Long-lasting (L-type) VDCs appear to be the predominant mechanism for entry of Ca^{2+} into tracheal smooth muscle, whereas both transient (T-type) and L-type VDCs are present in bronchial smooth muscle cells.[25,33] Yamakage and associates[25] demonstrated that isoflurane and sevoflurane inhibit both types of VDCs in a dose-dependent fashion but that their effects on T-type VDCs in bronchial smooth muscle were much greater (Fig. 22-3). The differential effects of volatile anesthetics on tracheal as opposed to bronchial smooth muscle may also be related to effects on Ca^{2+}-activated chloride

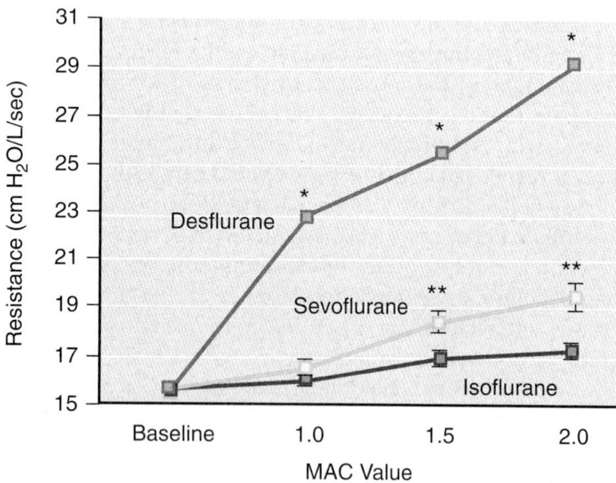

Figure 22-2 Comparison of the effect of different volatile anesthetics at equivalent concentrations on total pulmonary resistance. At 1 minimum alveolar concentration (MAC), only desflurane significantly increased pulmonary resistance when compared with isoflurane and sevoflurane. At 1.5 and 2 MAC, sevoflurane significantly increased total pulmonary resistance when compared with isoflurane, whereas desflurane caused a more pronounced increase than the other two agents did. *Increased pulmonary resistance in comparison to sevoflurane and isoflurane; **increased pulmonary resistance in comparison to isoflurane. *(Reproduced from Nyktari VG, Papaioannou AA, Prinianakis G, et al: Effect of the physical properties of isoflurane, sevoflurane and desflurane on pulmonary resistance in a laboratory lung model. Anesthesiology 104:1202, 2006, with permission.)*

channel activity[34,35] or differential sensitivity of K^+ channel subtypes.[34] Early studies proposed that volatile anesthetics relax airway smooth muscle by opening adenosine triphosphate (ATP)-sensitive potassium channels (K_{ATP}). However, halothane was found to exert minimal effects on tracheal smooth muscle K_{ATP} channels.[36]

The proposed signaling pathways underlying volatile anesthetic-induced bronchodilation are depicted in Figure 22-4. In addition to effects on VDCs, halothane reduces ICa^{2+} by depleting SR Ca^{2+}.[37,38] Halothane-induced reductions in SR Ca^{2+} appear to occur through enhancement of IP_3 and ryanodine receptor channels,[38] but whether halothane exerts direct effects on IP_3 concentrations remains controversial. Warner and coworkers[39] also demonstrated that halothane attenuates acetylcholine-induced Ca^{2+} sensitization in canine tracheal smooth muscle to a greater extent than isoflurane or sevoflurane does. These findings are analogous to the differential effects of volatile anesthetics on relaxing airway smooth muscle. Halothane may reduce free Ca^{2+} in the cytoplasm or limit influx of Ca^{2+} across the cell membrane. Alterations in Ca^{2+} sensitivity are an important mechanism by which volatile anesthetics cause smooth muscle relaxation. This effect appears to be mediated, at least in part, by an increase in smooth muscle protein phosphatase[40] and modulation of G proteins that exert actions on cGMP, specifically G_q and G_i.[32,41] Volatile anesthetics affect the function of G proteins in a variety of tissues, but halothane-induced relaxation of airway smooth muscle occurs independent of pertussis toxin–sensitive inhibitory G proteins, which are sensitive to the relaxation effects of β-adrenoceptor agonists.[42] Volatile anesthetics interact with the muscarinic receptor–heterotrimeric G protein complex to prevent agonist-promoted nucleotide exchange at the Gα subunit of the G protein.[43] It is perhaps through this mechanism that volatile anesthetics inhibit signaling proteins such as phospholipase C, protein kinase C, and ion channels. In addition to the role of volatile anesthetics as inhibitors of muscarinic agonist–induced guanine nucleotide exchange, they also appear to exert direct effects on the G protein–receptor complex.[42] The final pathway in airway smooth muscle contraction is the generation of force and shortening of smooth muscles regulated by myosin cross-bridge number and kinetics. Isoflurane modulated both cross-bridge number and the cycling rates of isolated rat airway smooth muscle.[44]

The bronchoconstricting effects of low inhaled concentrations of carbon dioxide were attenuated by inhaled but not by intravenous halothane, thus suggesting a direct action on airway musculature or local neural reflex arcs rather than centrally controlled reflex pathways. Halothane-, isoflurane-, sevoflurane-, and desflurane-induced dilatation of distal bronchial segments partially depends on the presence of bronchial epithelium.[15,45] A prostanoid (e.g., prostaglandin E_2 or I_2) or NO may mediate the bronchodilatory effects of these volatile anesthetics. For example, isoflurane-mediated bronchodilation appears to more dependent on NO than on prostanoids, but the converse is true for halothane. Focal epithelial damage or inflammation may occur in the small airways of patients with asthma or after exposure to allergen, and as a consequence, the bronchodilatory response to volatile anesthetics may be reduced.[46] The greatest bronchodilatory action of volatile agents in patients with chronic reactive airway disease occurs primarily in the proximal rather than the distal airways.

Stimulation of intrinsic airway nerves in vitro produces a cholinergic contractile response that is inhibited by atropine. In addition to the direct effects just described, volatile anesthetic–induced bronchodilation also occurs via modulation of airway cholinergic neural transmission mediated through prejunctional and postjunctional mechanisms.[47,48] The combination of atropine and halothane did not increase airway caliber over that attained with either drug alone. These findings suggest that halothane dilates airways by blocking vagal tone during unstimulated conditions.[17] Release of histamine and the nonadrenergic, noncholinergic bronchodilatory neural reflex, believed to be mediated by NO,[49] do not appear to play a significant role in low-dose halothane-induced bronchodilation. Potent tracheal constriction occurs in response to the endogenously produced polypeptide endothelin-1. Administration of isoflurane at a clinically relevant dose (2%) depressed endothelin-1–induced airway smooth muscle contraction in rat tracheal rings, thus suggesting another potential mechanism for airway smooth muscle relaxation.[50]

Effects of Inhaled Anesthetics on Bronchomotor Tone in Humans

Volatile anesthetics may be an effective method of treating status asthmaticus when other more conventional treatments have failed.[51] One percent halothane administered to 12 patients in status asthmaticus rapidly improved bronchospasm, reduced the incidence of barotrauma, and enhanced arterial blood gas ten-

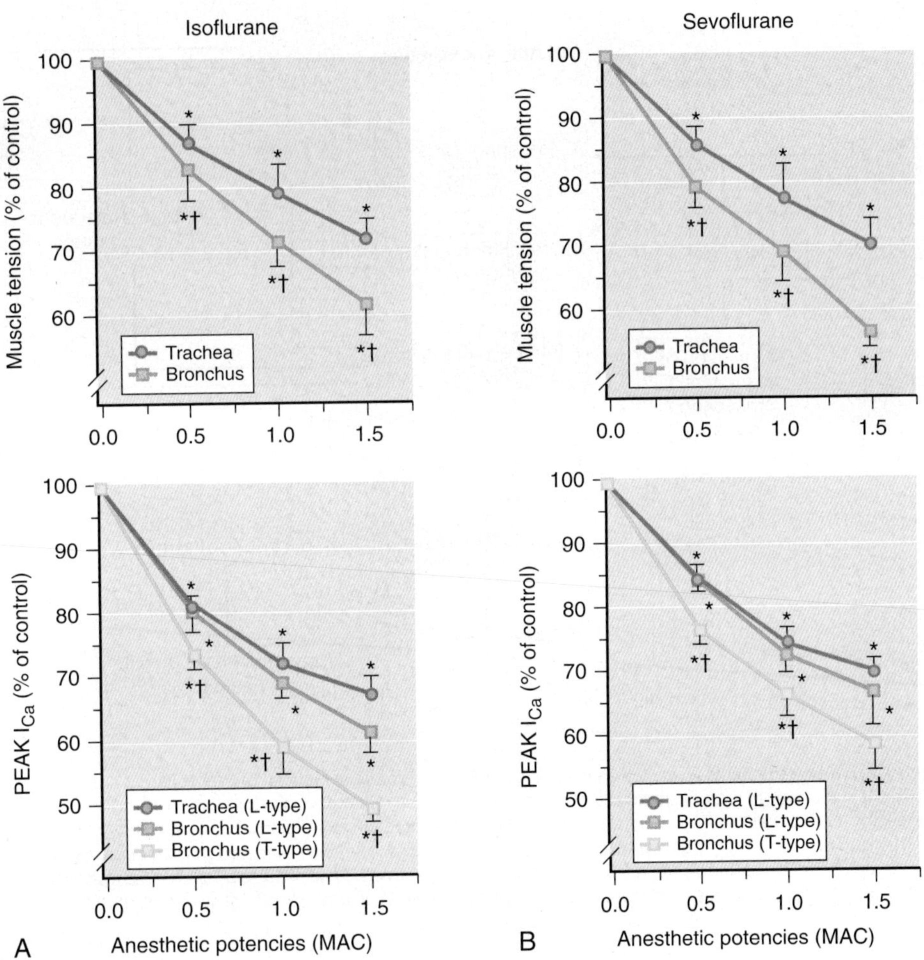

Figure 22-3 Effect of isoflurane and sevoflurane on porcine tracheal versus bronchial smooth muscle tension or inward Ca^{2+} current (I_{Ca}) through T- and L-type voltage-dependent Ca^{2+} channels (VDCs). There were no differences in the inhibition of L-type VDCs. Both anesthetics had greater inhibitory effects on T-type VDCs in bronchial smooth muscle. Symbols represent means ± SD. *$P < .05$ versus 0 MAC. †$P < .05$ versus tracheal smooth muscle in **A** and †$P < .05$ versus L-type VDCs in **B**. *(Reproduced from Yamakage M, Chen X, Tsuijiguchi N, et al: Different inhibitory effects of volatile anesthetics on T- and L-type voltage-dependent Ca^{2+} channels in porcine tracheal and bronchial smooth muscles. Anesthesiology 94:683, 2001, with permission.)*

sions in the absence of adverse hemodynamic effects.[52] However, the possibility of cardiac arrhythmias, depression of myocardial contractility, and lack of availability in the United States suggest that other agents may be preferred in the treatment of status asthmaticus.

Rooke and associates[53] compared the bronchodilating effects of halothane, isoflurane, sevoflurane, and thiopental/nitrous oxide in 66 healthy patients undergoing induction of anesthesia and tracheal intubation (Fig. 22-5). In contrast to thiopental or nitrous oxide, all volatile anesthetics significantly reduced respiratory system resistance. At equivalent MAC, sevoflurane and halothane decreased resistance to a similar degree, whereas isoflurane produced substantially less bronchodilation in vivo. Previously described animal studies demonstrating equal potency of sevoflurane and isoflurane and relatively greater potency of halothane for bronchodilation must be extrapolated with caution because *Ascaris*- or histamine-mediated experimental bronchospasm may not precisely mimic tracheal intubation–induced bronchospasm in humans. In contrast to these findings in experimental animals, Arakawa and colleagues[51] showed that similar inspired concentrations of halothane, isoflurane, and sevoflurane produce nearly identical reductions in airway resistance in patients with status asthmaticus.

Although the use of β-adrenoceptor agonists may be beneficial for the treatment of bronchospasm in patients anesthetized with halothane,[42,54] this may not be the case with other inhaled agents. The β_2-adrenergic agonist fenoterol lowered respiratory system resistance after endotracheal intubation but did not reduce resistance further when administered in the presence of 1.3% isoflurane.[55] These data should be interpreted with caution because the technique used to determine respiratory system resistance may be partially responsible for these results inasmuch as this index incorporates alterations in lung and chest wall resistance, as well as tissue viscosity.

The actions of volatile anesthetics on bronchomotor tone are dependent on the agent eliciting contraction in vitro.[19] Relaxation of tracheal smooth muscle by halothane and isoflurane is greater in the presence of the endogenous mediator serotonin (potentially representing anaphylactoid or immunologic reactions) than in the presence of acetylcholine (representing the

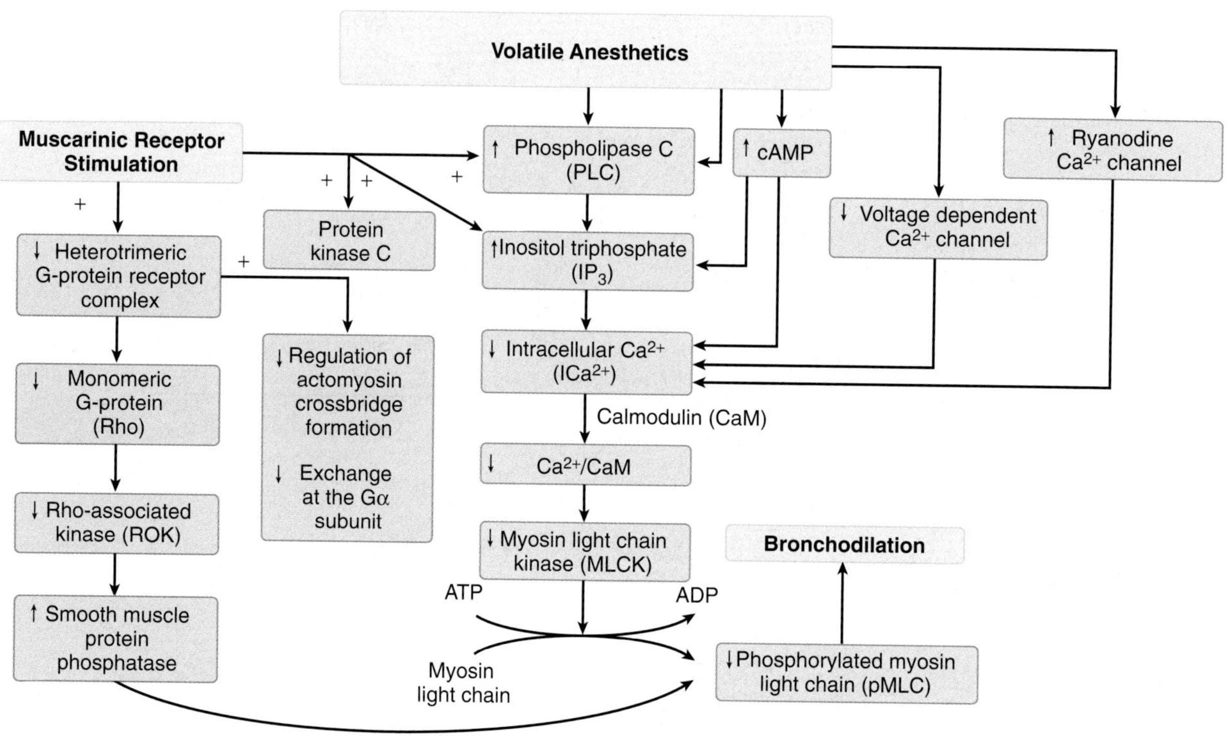

Figure 22-4 Proposed signaling pathways underlying volatile anesthetic (specifically, halothane)-induced bronchodilation or inhibition (or both) of muscarinic agonist–induced contraction of airway smooth muscle. +, excitatory action of muscarinic receptor agonist; ↑, activation or increase attributable to the volatile anesthetic; ↓, inhibition or decrease attributable to the volatile anesthetic. Signal transduction along pathway A is supported by work from Warner and coworkers on a role of halothane in decreasing Ca^{2+} sensitivity rather than a change in ICa^{2+} content. *(Adapted from Pabelick CM, Prakash YS, Kannan MS, et al: Effects of halothane on sarcoplasmic reticulum calcium release channels in porcine airway smooth muscle cells. Anesthesiology 95:207, 2001; and Hanazaki M, Jones KA, Perkins WJ, et al: Halothane increases smooth muscle protein phosphatase in airway smooth muscle. Anesthesiology 94:129, 2001, with permission.)*

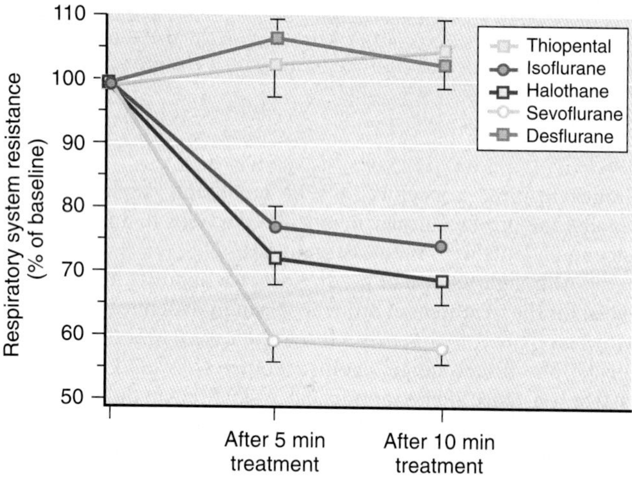

Figure 22-5 Percent change in respiratory system resistance in patients after 5 and 10 minutes of maintenance anesthesia with either 0.25 mg/kg/min thiopental plus 50% nitrous oxide or 1.1 minimum alveolar concentration (MAC) sevoflurane, halothane, or isoflurane or approximately 1 MAC desflurane. All volatile anesthetics except desflurane decreased resistance. Sevoflurane decreased resistance more than isoflurane did. *(Modified from Rooke GA, Choi J-H, Bishop MJ: The effect of isoflurane, halothane, sevoflurane, and thiopental/nitrous oxide on respiratory system resistance after tracheal intubation. Anesthesiology 86:1294, 1997; and Goff MJ, Arain SR, Ficke DJ, et al: Absence of bronchodilation during desflurane anesthesia: A comparison to sevoflurane and thiopental. Anesthesiology 93:404, 2000, with permission.)*

neurally derived mediator of reflex bronchospasm). Inhaled anesthetics may remain effective bronchodilators even with severe serotonin- or histamine-induced bronchospasm that is refractory to β_2-adrenoceptor therapy.

Volatile anesthetic–induced decreases in bronchomotor tone and neurally mediated airway reflexes may be partially opposed by a simultaneous reduction in functional residual capacity (FRC) in anesthetized patients. This decrease in FRC increases airway resistance. An increased risk for morbidity and mortality during the perioperative period has been well established in patients with asthma and may be partially attributed to these FRC-mediated increases in airway resistance. Exposure of airway smooth muscle to low temperatures may abolish the inhibitory effects of volatile anesthetics on carbachol-induced contraction.[56] These findings suggest that intraoperative hypothermia also may attenuate volatile anesthetic–induced bronchodilation.

Bronchospasm may occur with respiratory diseases other than asthma. For example, healthy patients undergoing surgical stimulation of the pulmonary parenchyma or airways (including tracheal stimulation by an endotracheal tube) are at risk for bronchospasm. The choice of preoperative medication, induction agent, muscle relaxant, and type of inhaled agent are important factors in determining the development of bronchospasm in patients with known reactive airway disease. Recently, Iwasaki and coworkers[29] demonstrated that sevoflurane-induced relaxation of airway smooth muscle and VDCs was dependent on the type of hyperreactive airway model. Sevoflurane had smaller effects in a chronic cigarette-smoking model (enlarged alveolar ducts and lesser muscarinic hyperreactivity) than in an acute ovalbumin-sensitized (antigen–acute asthmatic) model. Morphologic changes in the peripheral airways may be responsible to some degree for the decrease in bronchodilator efficacy of volatile anesthetics in cigarette smokers, but sevoflurane and isoflurane decrease respiratory system resistance in patients with COPD.[57] In contrast with an acute asthmatic model characterized by eosinophilic inflammation and airway wall changes, the inflammation in chronic asthma involves many other cell types, including mast cells, macrophages, epithelial cells, and bronchial smooth muscle cells. In addition, chronic inflammation is associated with remodeling of bronchial epithelium to produce smooth muscle hypertrophy, gland hyperplasia, and neovascularization. In a murine model of chronic asthma, administration of sevoflurane acted at the airway level and lung periphery to reduce resistive and viscoelastic pressure, as well as lung static resistance, when compared with animals anesthetized with pentobarbital.[58]

Although halothane may be a more potent bronchodilator than other inhaled anesthetics, the often-profound respiratory irritation produced in the upper airways (even though better tolerated than isoflurane and desflurane) may have outweighed the benefit of a direct bronchodilatory action. Thus, subtle differences in the bronchodilating effects of volatile anesthetics certainly exist, but avoiding or minimizing airway irritation and maintaining adequate depth of anesthesia are probably of greater clinical importance.

Advances in manufacturing technology and scavenging systems have made the use of xenon more economically feasible[59] (also see Chapter 21). Clinical use of xenon remains limited in the United States. Xenon may have important neuroprotective and cardiovascular advantages over volatile anesthetics.[60] The effects of xenon on airway resistance differ markedly from those of volatile agents because this anesthetic gas has higher density and viscosity than air.[61-63] In pentobarbital-anesthetized pigs, baseline airway resistance was significantly greater during 70% xenon-oxygen than during 70% nitrous oxide–oxygen anesthesia, although measured peak and mean airway pressure was unaffected. In contrast, airway pressure and resistance were moderately increased during xenon anesthesia and methacholine-induced bronchoconstriction.[62] In addition, pulmonary resistance during inhalation of 50% xenon was similar to that observed during inhalation of 50% nitrous oxide or 70% nitrogen in methacholine-treated dogs.[64] A randomized, double-blind comparison of xenon and nitrous oxide showed that although both agents similarly increased expiratory lung resistance, fewer patients receiving xenon experienced decreases in oxygen saturation.[65] Administration of 33% xenon to long-term mechanically ventilated patients may transiently, but significantly elevate peak airway pressure.[61] This increase in airway pressure may be attenuated by reducing the inspiratory flow rate. The higher density and viscosity of xenon lead to increases in the Reynolds number and probably cause the zone of transition from turbulent to laminar gas flow to move more distally to smaller airways. Theoretically, this action may result in exacerbation of bronchospasticity in patients with preexisting small airway disease or a decrease in arterial oxygen tension. Other studies have shown that arterial oxygen and carbon dioxide tension is unaffected during administration of xenon and nitrous oxide mixtures,[66] but caution has nevertheless been suggested when using xenon in patients with bronchospastic or obstructive pulmonary disease.

Mucociliary Function and Surfactant

Normal Mucociliary Function

Foreign particulate matter, microorganisms, and dead cells are removed by the upward clearance of mucus from the tracheobronchial tree as a primary pulmonary defense mechanism. Ciliated respiratory epithelium extends throughout the respiratory tract as far as the terminal bronchioles and decreases in density from trachea to alveoli. Ciliary motion consists of a rapid stroke in a cephalad direction, followed by a slower recovery stroke in the opposite direction. Movements of cilia are closely coordinated in a proximal-to-distal direction to move matter toward the trachea efficiently. This resulting wave of motion is known as *metachronism*. The bending of individual cilia results from ATP-dependent sliding of two parallel fibers within the ciliary filament.

Mucus is a mixture of water, electrolytes, and macromolecules (e.g., lipids, mucins, enzymes) secreted by goblet cells and mucosal glands. Thicker layers of mucus slow the removal of surface particles from the airway, whereas low-viscosity mucus promotes more rapid ciliary transport. The amount and physical properties of the mucus layer may also promote the coordination of ciliary beats.[67] Mucociliary function may be assessed by high-speed videomicroscopy to examine the ciliary beat frequency. In vivo techniques in experimental animals have used a tracheal window model. The velocity of mucus movement has been measured with radioactive markers or fiberoptic bronchoscopy in humans.

Impaired mucociliary function in the upper airways correlates with low levels of nasal NO, but the clinical significance of this finding remains to be defined.[68] Maintenance of bronchial perfusion is also critically important to preservation of normal mucociliary function.[69] Although nervous control of ciliary coordination has not been demonstrated in vertebrates, mucociliary clearance is closely related to autonomic nervous system activity, most likely related to changes in the physical characteristics of respiratory secretions.[67]

Postoperative hypoxemia and atelectasis are common causes of perioperative morbidity. Many factors can affect mucociliary function in mechanically ventilated patients and potentially contribute to these complications. Poorly humidified inspired gases are known to reduce ciliary movement and desiccate mucus. The flow rate of mucus was maintained within the normal range during a 40-minute exposure to an inspired air temperature higher than 32°C in dogs. However, 3 hours of inhalation of dry air resulted in complete cessation of the flow of tracheal mucus, which was restored by the subsequent use of inspired gases with 100% relative humidity at 38°C. Several anesthesia-related factors also reduce the rate of mucus movement, including administration of a high inspired oxygen concentration, adjuvant medications (cortisone, atropine, β-receptor blockers), the presence of a cuffed endotracheal tube, and positive-pressure ventilation.[70]

Effects of Inhaled Anesthetics on Mucociliary Function

Volatile anesthetics and nitrous oxide may diminish rates of mucus clearance by decreasing ciliary beat frequency, disrupting metachronism, or altering the physical characteristics or quantity of mucus. Halothane, enflurane, isoflurane, and sevoflurane, in contrast to many intravenous anesthetics,[71,72] reduced ciliary movement and beat frequency in vitro.[73-75] Among the volatile anesthetics, sevoflurane exhibited the weakest cilia-inhibitory effects in rat cultured tracheal epithelial cells in vitro (Fig. 22-6).[75]

Gamsu and colleagues[76] compared the rate of tantalum clearance from the lungs of postoperative patients who had undergone general anesthesia for either intra-abdominal or lower extremity operations. Tantalum is a powder that adheres to airway mucus and can be used to study mucociliary transport. Retention of tantalum was demonstrated for as long as 6 days after intra-abdominal surgery, with an average retention time three times greater than that observed in the control group. Tantalum retention was closely correlated with retention of mucus (Fig. 22-7). Teflon disks placed on the tracheal mucosa and observed with fiberoptic bronchoscopy were used to study tracheal mucus velocity in young women undergoing gynecologic surgery.[77] Administration of halothane (1% to 2%) and nitrous oxide (60%) rapidly decreased the rate of mucus movement. Little or no mucus motion was observed after 90 minutes' exposure to halothane-N_2O. The inspired gases were humidified, but high-inspired concentrations of oxygen, a cuffed endotracheal tube, and positive-pressure ventilation were confounding factors in this study. Bronchial mucosal transport velocity was also determined with the use of radiolabeled albumin microspheres deposited distally in the mainstem bronchi via fiberoptic bronchoscopy in healthy patients.[78] In contrast to the findings of the study with halothane, mucus velocity was unchanged during the administration of isoflurane (1.5 MAC). Whether this relative lack of effect of isoflurane on mucus transport was specifically related to the type of volatile agent was unclear. However, mucus pooling has been observed during and after anesthesia, and impaired bronchial mucus transport velocity is associated with increased pulmonary complications.

Konrad and colleagues[79] have shown that smokers have significantly slower bronchial mucus transport velocity and more frequent pulmonary complications than do nonsmokers undergoing abdominal or thoracic surgery. The specific effects of volatile anesthetics on mucus movement in smokers has not been well studied, but one may presume that there would be a further decrement in mucus transport. Impairment of mucociliary function also occurs after lung transplantation. The mechanism for this dysfunction may be related to alterations in the surface properties of mucus and marked impairment of mucociliary transport distal to the bronchial transection and reanastomosis.[80] The effects of volatile anesthetics on mucus transport in pulmonary transplant patients have not been described; however, the baseline reductions in mucociliary movement would predispose patients to postoperative respiratory complications.

The effects of sevoflurane and remifentanil on bronchial mucus transport were compared with those of total intravenous anesthesia (consisting of propofol and remifentanil) in patients undergoing general surgery.[81] In contrast to the in vitro results,[75] bronchial mucus transport velocity was significantly reduced 30 minutes after endotracheal intubation in patients receiving sevoflurane. The data indicate that pulmonary therapy directed at enhancing clearance of secretions from the airways may be beneficial in the immediate postoperative period regardless of the type of inhaled anesthetic chosen.

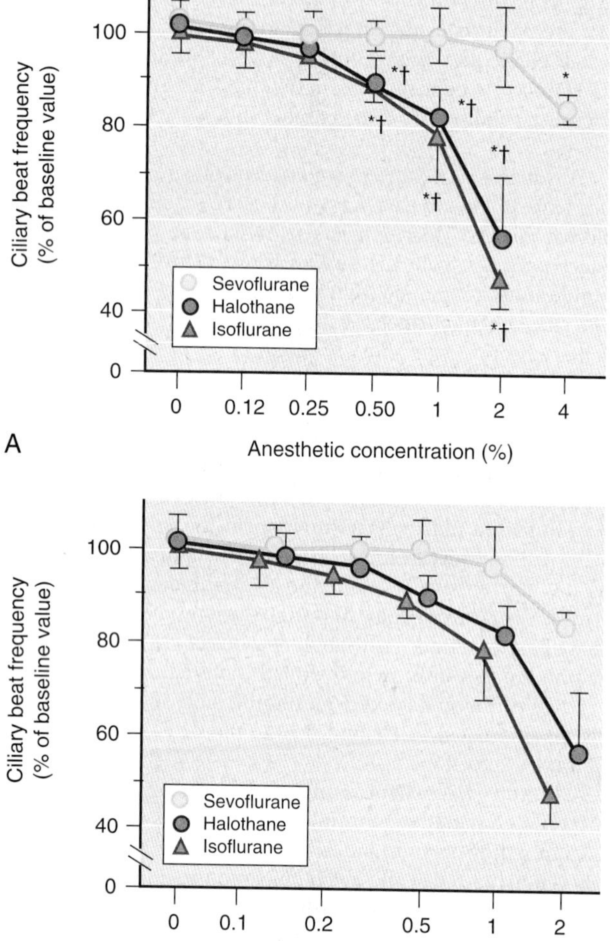

Figure 22-6 Effects of sevoflurane, halothane, and isoflurane on ciliary beat frequency (CBF) in cultured rat tracheal epithelial cells. CBF was measured at baseline and 30 minutes after exposure to various anesthetic concentrations. Values represent means ± SD. **A,** Plot of percent baseline CBF versus anesthetic concentration. *$P < .05$ versus 0% vehicle and †$P < .05$ versus sevoflurane at the same concentration. **B,** Percent baseline CBF versus minimum alveolar concentration (MAC). *(Modified from Matsuura S, Shirakami G, Iada H, et al: The effect of sevoflurane on ciliary motility in rat cultured tracheal epithelial cells: A comparison with isoflurane and halothane. Anesth Analg 102:1703, 2006, with permission.)*

Effects of Inhaled Anesthetics on Surfactant

Pulmonary surfactant decreases the work of breathing by reducing surface tension at the fluid-gas interface. Surfactant is a mixture of proteins and phospholipids synthesized by alveolar type II cells. Similar to mucus, surfactant plays a role in removing foreign particles from airways while also enhancing the bactericidal actions of alveolar macrophages. Both halothane[82] and iso-

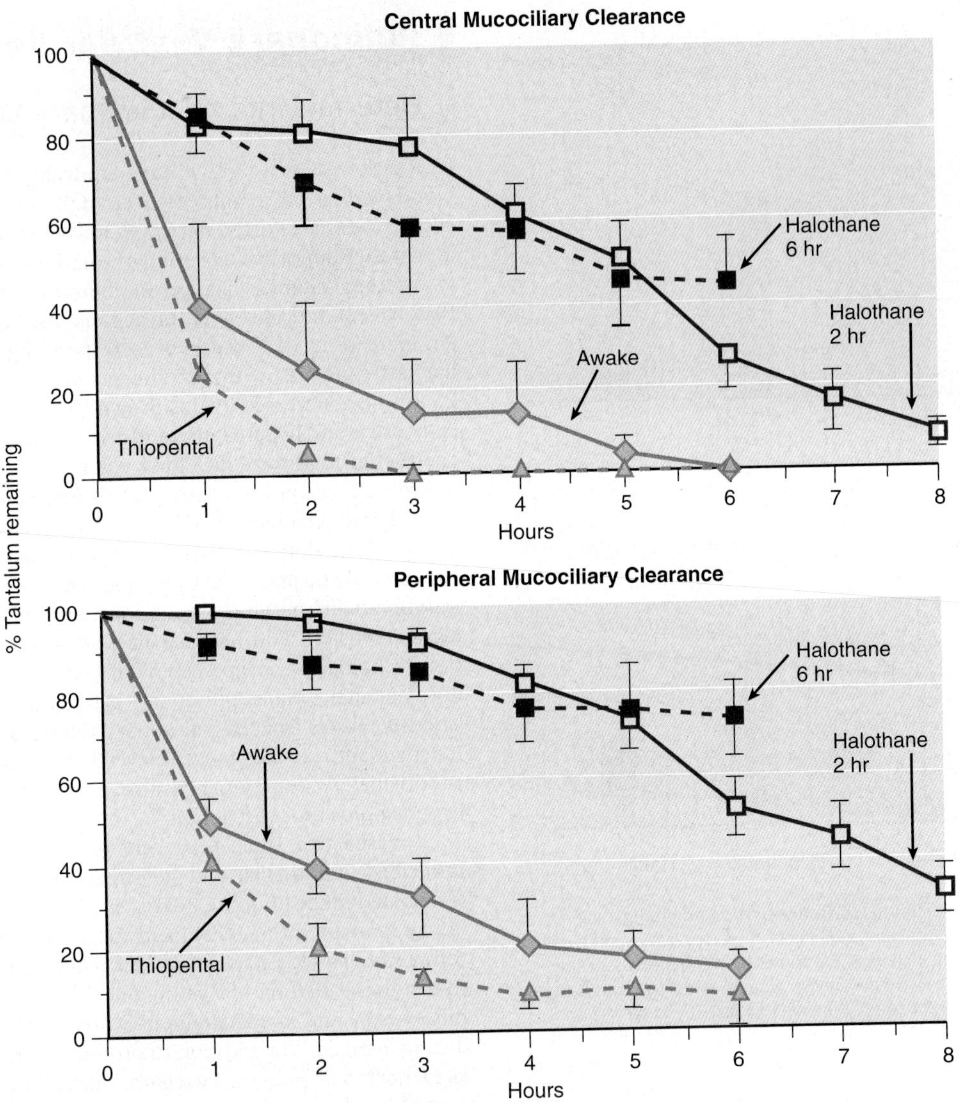

Figure 22-7 Mucociliary clearance measured as tantalum clearance in patients undergoing surgery under either general or local anesthesia (awake). Note the decrease in mucociliary clearance in both the peripheral and central airways during halothane anesthesia. *(Modified from Forbes AR, Gamsu G: Mucociliary clearance in the canine lung during and after general anesthesia. Anesthesiology 50:26, 1979, with permission.)*

flurane[83] transiently reduced phosphatidylcholine synthesis by alveolar cells in a dose-dependent manner during a 4-hour exposure. High concentrations of halothane also disrupted the energy metabolism of cultured alveolar cells as indicated by reduced ATP content and enhanced glycolytic metabolism. Halothane and isoflurane potentiated the hydrogen peroxide–mediated reduction of phosphatidylcholine in alveolar type II cells,[83,84] possibly via halothane-specific effects on cell energetics. Halothane decreased Na^+/K^+-adenosine triphosphatase (ATPase) and Na^+ channel activity in alveolar type II cells, an effect that was probably related to alterations in ICa^{2+} concentrations or ATP depletion.[85] A similar decrease in type II alveolar cell Na^+/K^+-ATPase has been shown after treatment with isoflurane.[86] Transepithelial Na^+ transport helps regulate alveolar fluid balance, and thus significant impairment in such transport may promote alveolar edema. This observation is particularly important because halothane and isoflurane decrease alveolar epithelial fluid clearance.[87] The phospholipid makeup of surfactant is critical to its functional integrity. However, the hydrophobic surfactant-associated protein C, which is synthesized exclusively by alveolar type II cells, confers the properties of rapid surface adsorption and reduction of surface tension to phospholipids, facilitates the adsorption and spreading of phospholipids to form the surfactant monolayer, and enhances lipid uptake in alveolar type II cells. In addition, exogenous surfactant that contains surfactant-associated protein C is effective in decreasing rates of barotrauma and mortality in vivo. Clinically relevant concentrations of halothane increased surfactant-associated protein C mRNA in vitro but exerted the converse effect in mechanically ventilated rats.[88] In contrast, thiopental administration increased the content of surfactant-associated protein C mRNA in both in vitro and in vivo (mechanically ventilated) models (Fig. 22-8).[88] Extrapolation of these findings to patients undergoing anesthesia should be done with caution, but these results suggest a potentially additive and deleterious role of halothane and mechanical ventilation on surfactant production and homeostasis of the alveolar space, particularly in the presence

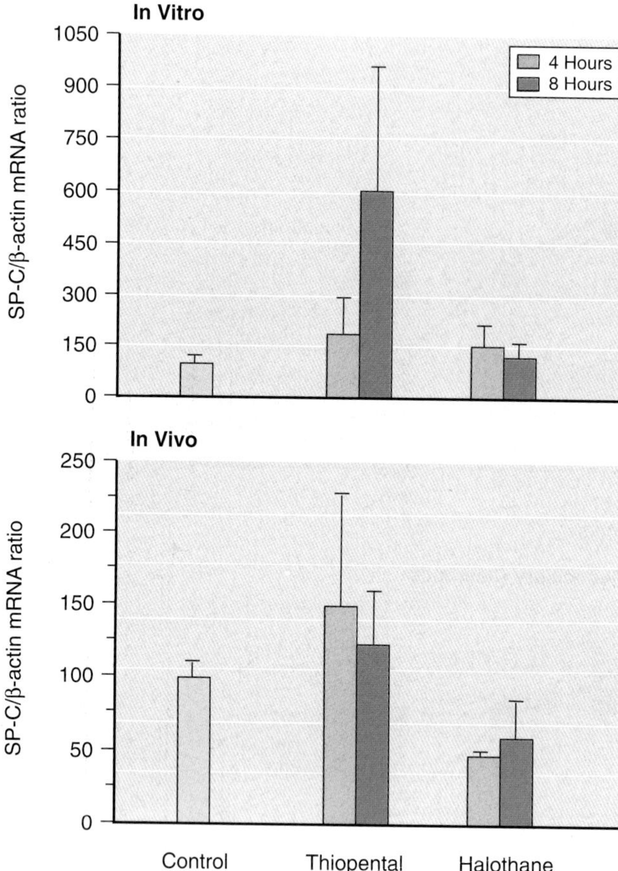

Figure 22-8 Halothane increases surfactant-associated protein C (SP-C) mRNA in vitro but exerts the opposite effects in mechanically ventilated rats. Thiopental administration increased the content of surfactant-associated protein C mRNA in both in vitro and in vivo models. *(Modified from Paugam-Burtz C, Molliex S, Lardeux B, et al: Differential effects of halothane and thiopental on surfactant protein C messenger RNA in vivo and in vitro in rats. Anesthesiology 93:805, 2000, with permission.)*

of acute lung injury. The actions of desflurane and sevoflurane on pulmonary surfactant metabolism have yet to be evaluated.

The specific roles of depressed mucociliary function and alterations in type II alveolar cells on pulmonary complications remain unclear, but impairment of ciliary motility, bronchial mucus transport, and surfactant production may play a significant role in perioperative morbidity. As discussed later, inhaled anesthetics may also play an important immunomodulatory role on type II alveolar cells during lung injury.

Prolonged administration of inhaled anesthetics may lead to mucus pooling and adversely alter alveolar cell surfactant metabolism. These actions may result in deleterious effects on pulmonary function, including atelectasis and infection. Patients at greatest risk appear to include those with excessive or abnormal mucus or surfactant production and those with acute lung injury (e.g., chronic bronchitis, asthma, cystic fibrosis, and chronic mechanical ventilation). Nevertheless, controlled studies of the effects of inhaled anesthetics on mucociliary function, surfactant metabolism, and immunomodulation in patients with or animal models of compromised pulmonary performance have yet to be performed.

Pulmonary Vascular Resistance

Determinants of Pulmonary Vascular Tone

PVR is lowest at a lung volume equivalent to FRC. Pulmonary blood vessels are compressed at high lung volumes, whereas vessels become shorter, narrower, and more tortuous because of loss of the supportive tethering of surrounding lung parenchyma at low lung volumes. Changes in pulmonary arterial pressure and PVR have significant effects on gas and fluid exchange in the lung. An increase in PVR causes a corresponding increase in pulmonary arterial pressure that promotes interstitial fluid transudation. PVR is also increased by positive end-expiratory pressure, alveolar hypoxia and hypercapnia, and critical closing pressure. Inhaled anesthetics tend to reduce lung volume and may therefore have indirect effects on PVR through this mechanism as well.

Direct changes in pulmonary vascular tone alter PVR by changing the slope of the pressure-flow relationship. Such direct changes may be produced by a rapid rise in ICa^{2+} or by alterations in sympathetic nervous system tone, arterial oxygen and carbon dioxide tension, acid-base balance, or circulating concentrations of catecholamines. Hypercapnia at constant pH (i.e., isohydria) does not alter isolated pulmonary arterial tone, but normocapnic acidosis relaxes isolated pulmonary arteries by an endothelium-independent mechanism.[89] Nevertheless, pulmonary arterial endothelial dysfunction has also been reported to potentiate hypercapnic vasoconstriction.[90]

Vasoactive substances can affect vascular tone as well. Inducible, endothelial, and neuronal NO synthases are widely distributed in the lung, are extensively involved in vascular homeostasis, and are intimately linked to the pulmonary oxygen environment (also see Chapter 31). NO synthase appears to play little role in the regulation of PVR in a healthy, normoxic lung,[91,92] but this enzyme and its metabolite NO are critical mediators of PVR during hypoxia.[93] In addition to producing vasodilation in ventilated, normoxic pulmonary regions during one-lung hypoxia, NO may also release an endogenous inhibitor of NO synthase that vasoconstricts nonventilated, hypoxic regions.[94] NO may be beneficial in the treatment of high-altitude pulmonary edema[95] and neonatal pulmonary hypertension resulting from a variety of congenital heart diseases, hypoplastic lung, and meconium aspiration. NO is also beneficial in the treatment of adult pulmonary hypertension as long as the resistance is not "fixed," such as in acute severe mitral regurgitation, congestive heart failure, and heart or lung transplantation. However, inhalation of NO during acute bronchospasm may paradoxically worsen the hypoxemia.[96] Whether this adverse action is mediated by direct bronchodilatory actions on less constricted peripheral airways or by worsening intrapulmonary shunt is unclear. The pulmonary endothelial dysfunction associated with cardiopulmonary bypass impairs endothelium-dependent vasodilation.[97] Nonetheless, use of NO in pediatric and adult cardiac surgical patients has become a common means of reducing PVR in this setting. Similar to NO, carbon monoxide (CO) stimulates guanylyl cyclase and increases cGMP levels in pulmonary arterial vascular smooth muscle cells to regulate vascular tone. Inhaled CO also attenuates the hypoxemia-induced increases in PVR through this mechanism.[98] Prostacyclin is another endogenous vasodilatory substance released from endothelium that elicits smooth muscle relaxation through stimulation of adenylyl cyclase and production of cAMP.

More recently, a role for endothelium-derived hyperpolarizing factor (EDHF) was identified as a third pathway for endothelium-mediated vasorelaxation.[99] EDHF produces relaxation by hyperpolarizing vascular smooth muscle in a process involving activation of potassium channels. Production of EDHF may be elicited by endothelial agonists or alterations in wall shear stress.[99] Although EDHF appears to be an important regulator of pulmonary blood flow, its role in modulating PVR has not been well defined.

Mechanism of Hypoxic Pulmonary Vasoconstriction

Regional alterations in PVR affect the regional distribution of blood flow within the lung, produce changes in ventilation-perfusion matching, and simultaneously affect gas exchange (also see Chapter 15). The distribution of pulmonary blood flow and ventilation in the lung, which was once thought to primarily be a gravity-mediated phenomenon, now appears to also be due to regional heterogeneity caused by asymmetric branching of the airways and blood vessels.[100] An increase in PVR occurring within an area of atelectasis causes localized tissue hypoxia but optimizes overall gas exchange (e.g., decreases the alveolar-arterial oxygen tension gradient [$P_{AO_2} - P_{aO_2}$]) by shifting blood flow away from the atelectatic segment to well-ventilated regions of the lung. This phenomenon, termed hypoxic pulmonary vasoconstriction (HPV), is unique to the pulmonary circulation in that other vascular beds (e.g., coronary, cerebral) dilate in response to hypoxia. Thus, HPV maintains oxygenation, and drugs (including anesthetics) that interfere with HPV may adversely affect gas exchange.

HPV is a locally mediated phenomenon that occurs when alveolar oxygen tension falls below 100 mm Hg and is maximal when oxygen tension is approximately 30 mm Hg. The specific mechanisms underlying HPV and the precise location of oxygen sensors remain unclear.[101,102] Mixed venous oxygen tension may influence HPV in the atelectatic lung because alveolar oxygen tension approaches venous oxygen tension under these conditions. Hypercapnia-induced acidosis increases PVR in intact animals and isolated, perfused lungs. Acidosis-induced increases in PVR are relatively minor at normal alveolar oxygen tensions but are dramatically enhanced during alveolar hypoxia. Local acidosis and increases in alveolar carbon dioxide tension may augment HPV and further improve arterial oxygenation in healthy lungs. High carbon dioxide concentrations reduce NO levels,[103] but whether this action is responsible for hypercapnia-induced improvements in the ratio of ventilation to perfusion is unknown.[104]

Inhaled Anesthetics and Hypoxic Pulmonary Vasoconstriction

All volatile anesthetics vasodilate the pulmonary vascular bed. Akata[105] presented a thorough review of the mechanisms by which inhaled anesthetics produce this vasodilation, including a reduction in free cytosolic calcium and inhibition of myofilament calcium sensitivity. Although nitrous oxide increases PVR, the pulmonary vasodilator effect of volatile agents is relatively small in normal lungs. The limited decreases in PVR produced by volatile anesthetics are frequently offset by a concomitant reduction in cardiac output in vivo. The net effect of these actions results in little if any change in pulmonary artery pressure and a small decrease in total pulmonary blood flow. In contrast with their direct vasodilatory actions, halothane, isoflurane, enflurane, and desflurane attenuate K_{ATP} channel– and endothelin-mediated pulmonary vasodilation in chronically instrumented dogs.[106-108] Inhibition of pulmonary vasodilation is not a uniform observation during administration of volatile anesthetics under all conditions. For example, isoflurane and halothane, but not enflurane, enhance isoproterenol-mediated vasodilation.[109,110] Unlike the findings with other volatile agents, K_{ATP} channel–mediated pulmonary vasodilation in response to lemakalim is preserved during sevoflurane anesthesia.[108] Indeed, there is evidence that halothane, enflurane, and isoflurane but not sevoflurane differentially modulate pulmonary vascular tension through calcium-activated or voltage-sensitive K^+ channels, at least in isolated rabbit lungs.[111] In isolated lungs, halothane- and enflurane-induced constriction of pulmonary vessels was potentiated by Kv channel inhibition. Vasoconstriction during halothane administration was also attenuated by K_{Ca} channel blockade. Isoflurane did not affect pulmonary vessels when Kv channels were inhibited. In contrast to the findings with halothane and enflurane, sevoflurane dilated pulmonary vessels and the dilation was not influenced by K^+ channel subtype inhibitors (Fig. 22-9). Isoflurane also attenuated hypotension-induced pulmonary vasoconstriction.[112]

Rather than causing pure vasodilation, volatile anesthetics produced a paradoxical initial dose-dependent increase in force in isolated pulmonary arterial strips because of release of Ca^{2+} from intracellular stores. Subsequently, a decrease in force (associated with activation of Ca^{2+}-calmodulin–dependent protein kinase II) occurs (Fig. 22-10).[113,114] Extrapolation of these results to humans in vivo must be approached with caution, but these studies suggest that vasodilatory responses may be more profound in patients with reduced SR Ca^{2+} stores (e.g., neonates) or those with depressed protein kinase activity (e.g., primary pulmonary hypertension).

Several mechanisms contribute to the diminished FRC, reduced oxygenation, and increased alveolar-arterial oxygen gradient during anesthesia. Volatile anesthetics contribute to this process by affecting HPV. The effects of volatile agents on HPV are multifactorial and involve direct actions on the pulmonary vasculature combined with indirect effects mediated by systemic hemodynamics, the autonomic nervous system, and humoral actions. In general, in vitro studies have demonstrated that all known inhaled anesthetics attenuate HPV to some degree in isolated perfused lungs or in in situ preparations with constant perfusion (Fig. 22-11), whereas most intravenous anesthetics do not. Addition of the Ca^{2+} channel blocker verapamil to a volatile anesthetic further reduces HPV by an additional 35% to 40%, thus suggesting that volatile anesthetics and Ca^{2+} channel antagonists may inhibit HPV through different sites of action. The mechanism of the direct inhibitory action of volatile anesthetics on HPV is unclear but may be related to enhancement of arachidonic acid metabolism[115] or other endothelial-derived vasodilating factors.[116] Conversely, other evidence suggests that anesthetic-induced inhibition of HPV may occur independent of the presence of pulmonary vascular endothelium, NO, or guanylate cyclase.[117-119]

Volatile anesthetics also disrupt Ca^{2+} homeostasis in vascular smooth muscle and thereby interfere with pulmonary vasoconstriction. Halothane and isoflurane attenuated

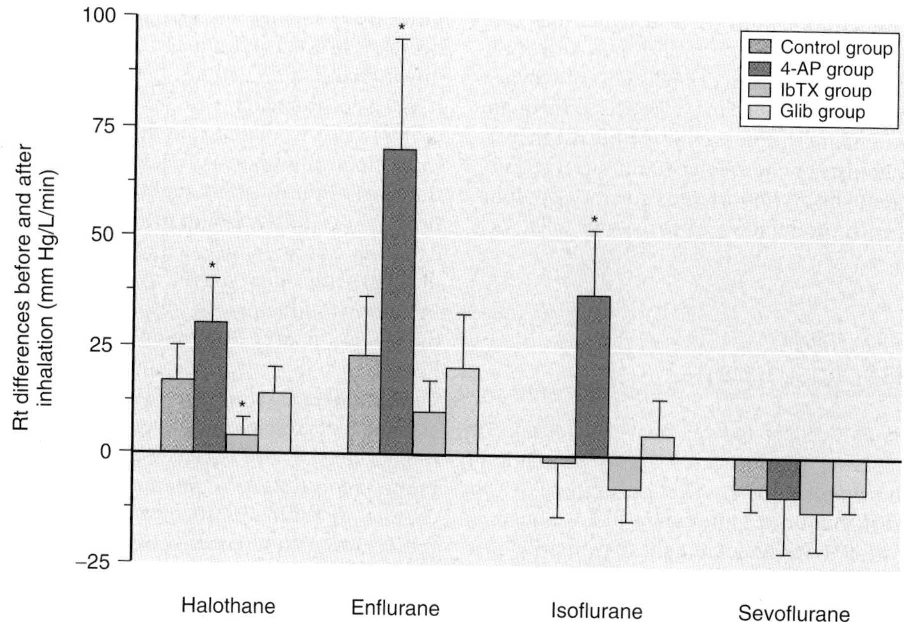

Figure 22-9 Total pulmonary vascular resistance (Rt) before and after anesthetic inhalation. Data are means ± SD. *$P < .01$ versus control group. 4AP, voltage-sensitive K^+ channel inhibitor; Glib, glibenclamide, an adenosine triphosphate–sensitive K^+ channel inhibitor; IbTX, calcium-activated K^+ channel inhibitor; Rt difference, resistance after administration of anesthetic minus resistance before administration of anesthetic. *(Modified from Liu R, Ishibe Y, Okazaki N, et al: Volatile anesthetics regulate pulmonary vascular tension through different potassium channel subtypes in isolated rabbit lungs. Can J Anaesth 50:301, 2003, with permission.)*

endothelium-dependent vasodilation by inhibiting accumulation of cGMP[119] and K_{ATP} channel–mediated interaction between NO and prostacyclin in isolated canine pulmonary artery rings.[120] In contrast, isoflurane modulated the HPV response, at least in part, through Ca^{2+}-activated and voltage-sensitive K^+ but not K_{ATP} channels in isolated rabbit lungs. Attenuation of HPV by sevoflurane occurred independent of K^+ channel function.[121] Rats with liver cirrhosis exhibited a blunted HPV response and arterial hypoxemia. These cirrhotic rats demonstrated increased NO and reduced endothelin concentrations, but the blunted HPV response observed in these animals did not involve these systems and was mediated instead by activation of Ca^{2+}-activated K^+ channels.[122]

The action of volatile anesthetics on HPV in vivo have been poorly delineated, in part because of several factors that are known to impair HPV, including temperature, pH, carbon dioxide tension, relative degree of hypoxia, size of the hypoxic area, surgical trauma, and concomitant medications. During one-lung ventilation, the direct inhibitory effects of volatile anesthetics on HPV may increase perfusion in the nonventilated lung. This enhanced perfusion potentially leads to an increase in shunt fraction and a reduction in arterial oxygenation. However, volatile anesthetics may also affect HPV, lung perfusion, and oxygenation by indirect actions on cardiac output and mixed venous oxygen saturation.[123] The direct effects of anesthetics on HPV, as opposed to indirect actions mediated through alterations in pulmonary perfusion, must be appreciated. The efficacy of HPV varies inversely with pulmonary arterial blood flow, and a direct inhibition of HPV by anesthetics may be opposed by a simultaneous reduction in cardiac output such that HPV may appear to be unaffected. Thus, the net HPV response to volatile anesthetics remains unchanged when cardiac output is reduced, but it may be fully intact or only minimally attenuated when pulmonary blood flow is preserved. A reduction in cardiac output also decreases mixed venous oxygenation, which leads to pulmonary vasoconstriction. These data emphasize the flow dependence of HPV during administration of a volatile anesthetic. Baseline pulmonary blood flow and pressure also modulate the effects of HPV. Elevated pulmonary artery pressure may cause passive distention of constricted vascular beds and thus reverse the HPV. Alternatively, reflex pulmonary and systemic vasoconstriction in response to hypotension may increase PVR in healthy lung segments, thereby leading to a shift of pulmonary blood flow to hypoxic areas of lung.

Early studies suggested that nitrous oxide attenuates HPV in animal models in vivo. In contrast, clinically relevant concentrations of halothane, isoflurane, enflurane, sevoflurane, and desflurane appear to have minimal effects on HPV in vivo (Fig. 22-12).[124,125] As opposed to the findings with isoflurane,[115] inhibition of HPV was not observed during sevoflurane or desflurane anesthesia[124] in chronically instrumented dogs subjected to gradual occlusion of the right main pulmonary artery. Nitrous oxide,[126] desflurane, and isoflurane,[127] but not xenon,[126] reduced mixed venous oxygen saturation, cardiac output, and arterial oxygenation during one-lung ventilation in pigs. However, nitrous oxide,[126] xenon,[126] desflurane,[127,128] and isoflurane[127,129] did not alter perfusion of the nonventilated lung or reduce the shunt fraction during one-lung ventilation. In animals with a preexisting gas exchange defect as a result of pneumoperitoneum, sevoflurane but not isoflurane caused more pronounced abnormalities in gas exchange than did propofol.[130] Thus, although reductions in HPV by inhaled anesthetics, as predicted by in vitro studies, have been relatively small in vivo, coexisting pulmonary disease may worsen anesthetic-induced gas exchange abnormalities.

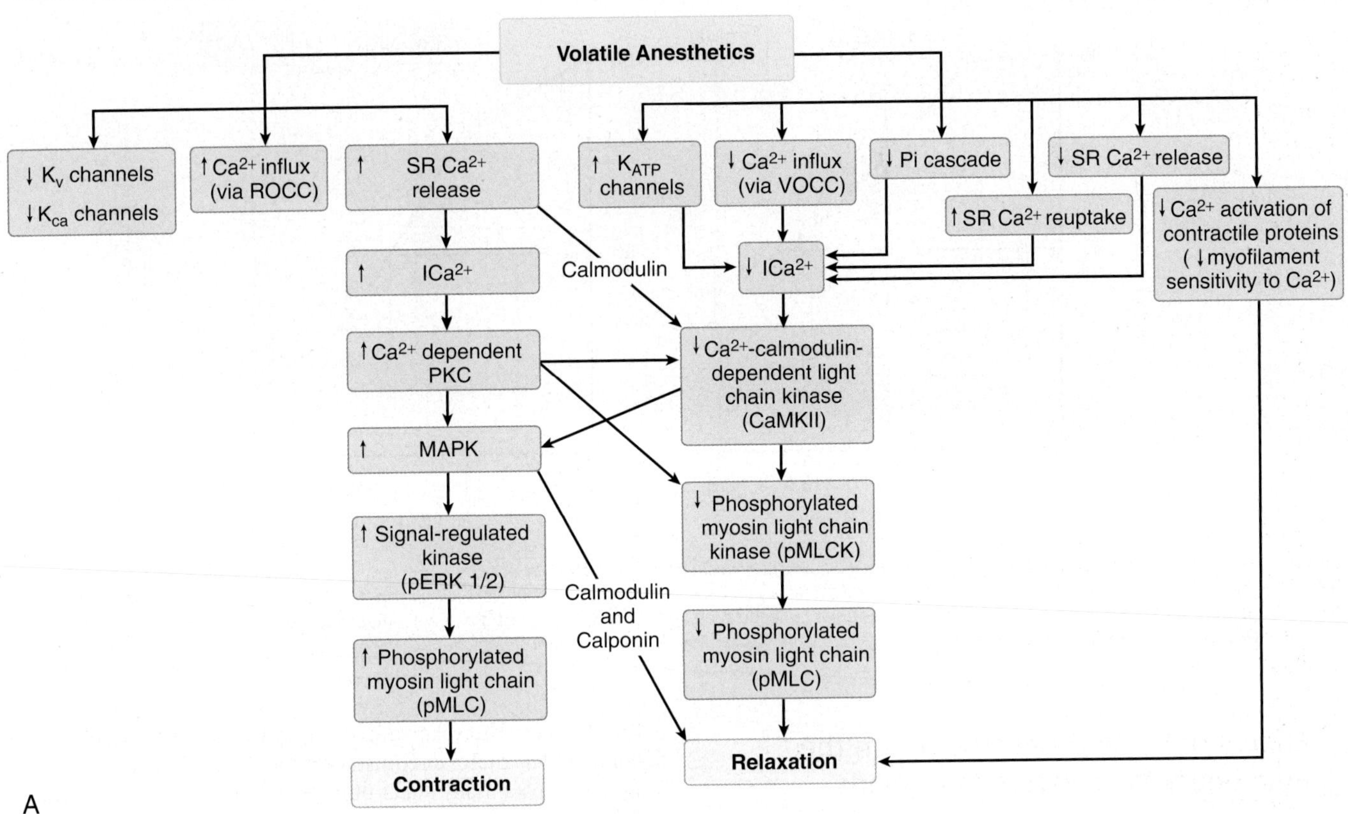

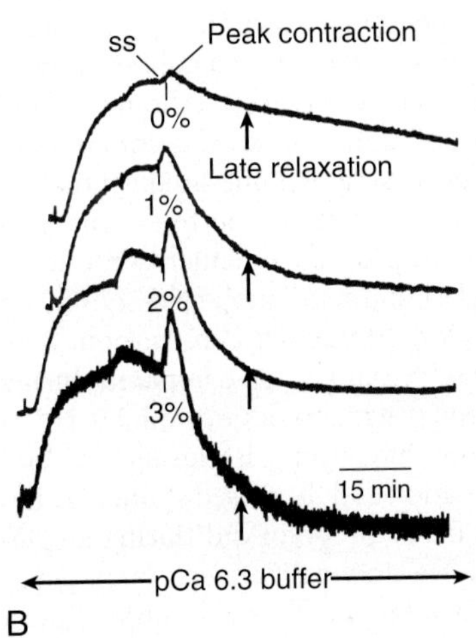

Figure 22-10 A, Proposed signaling pathways underlying volatile anesthetic–induced contraction and relaxation in pulmonary artery smooth muscle. Intracellular calcium (ICa^{2+}) may be increased by release from the sarcoplasmic reticulum (SR), by inhibition of voltage-sensitive (K_v) or calcium-activated (K_{Ca}) potassium channels, or by receptor-operated Ca^{2+} channels. Increased ICa^{2+} results in an initial dose-dependent increase in force (associated with activation of protein kinase C and increased mitogen-activated protein kinase [MAPK]). Volatile anesthetics also decrease ICa^{2+} by activating K_{ATP} channels, thereby inhibiting Ca^{2+} influx via voltage-operated Ca^{2+} channels (VOCC), decreasing SR-induced release of Ca^{2+}, inhibiting the phosphatidylinositol (Pi) cascade, and enhancing SR-mediated reuptake of Ca^{2+}. The resultant decrease in force is associated with activation of Ca^{2+}-calmodulin–dependent protein kinase II. It is important to note that there are many agent-specific effects of volatile anesthetics on each component of these pathways. **B,** Example of a biphasic (contraction/relaxation) effect of halothane on pulmonary arterial smooth muscle. 0%, 1%, 2%, and 3%, halothane concentrations; ss, control force at steady state before halothane. Halothane dose-dependently enhanced Ca^{2+}-activated peak force, as well as late relaxation. *(Modified from Akata[105], Su and Vo[113], and Zhong and Su,[114] with permission.)*

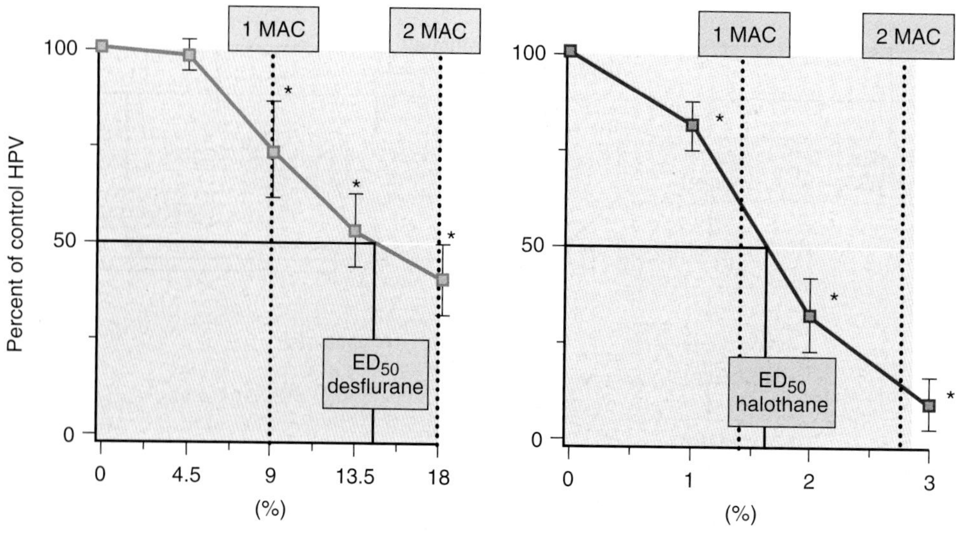

Figure 22-11 Concentration-dependent inhibition of hypoxic pulmonary vasoconstriction (HPV) in isolated rabbit lungs by desflurane (*blue squares*) and halothane (*red squares*), Values are means ± SEM and expressed as a percentage of control. **P* < .05 versus control HPV. The half-maximum inhibiting effect (ED_{50}) values were within the range of 1 and 2 minimum alveolar concentration (MAC) (for rabbits) for both agents. *(Reproduced from Loer SA, Scheeren T, Tarnow J: Desflurane inhibits hypoxic pulmonary vasoconstriction in isolated rabbit lungs. Anesthesiology 83:552, 1995, with permission.)*

Effects of Inhaled Anesthetics on the Pulmonary Vasculature in Humans

Isoflurane does not alter pulmonary shunt function in healthy patients, even at concentrations that produce systemic hypotension.[131] Most clinical thoracic surgery is usually undertaken with the patient in the lateral position with an open chest, which dramatically alters the relative distribution of ventilation and perfusion. Under these circumstances, a diseased nondependent lung may substantially affect pulmonary vascular responsiveness to hypoxia, as may surgical manipulation of the lung itself. Most observations in experimental animals or patients undergoing single-lung ventilation fail to demonstrate clinically significant attenuation of HPV during administration of a volatile anesthetic. There do not appear to be significant differences in shunt fraction, PVR, or oxygenation between isoflurane and sevoflurane anesthesia in patients with lung cancer undergoing one-lung ventilation for lobectomy.[132] Two studies demonstrated that the shunt fraction is similar in patients receiving propofol or either isoflurane[133] or sevoflurane[134] during single-lung ventilation. No significant differences in shunt fraction or arterial oxygen tension were observed when pulmonary gas exchange was compared during intravenous infusion of ketamine (which does not inhibit HPV) and administration of enflurane. In contrast, isoflurane[135,136] and sevoflurane[136] impaired oxygenation and decreased shunt fraction more than intravenous infusion of propofol did during single-lung ventilation in humans. However, the differences in oxygenation observed in these studies were small and of little clinical relevance. Interpretation of the differences in findings between these intravenous and volatile anesthetics observed in studies may be complicated by the depth of anesthesia. In contrast, the doses of propofol and sevoflurane selected were based on similar depth of anesthesia (determined with a bispectral index [BIS] monitor), and comparable reductions in arterial oxygenation were observed in patients undergoing one-lung ventilation.[137] Similar and rather modest changes in shunt fraction and oxygenation were shown to occur with halothane,[138] isoflurane,[132,138,139] desflurane,[139] and sevoflurane[132] in patients undergoing thoracotomy and single-lung ventilation (Fig. 22-13).

There is convincing evidence that all volatile anesthetics may be used safely in patients undergoing thoracotomy and single-lung ventilation (also see Chapter 59). The increase in shunt and decrease in oxygenation caused by halothane or isoflurane[138] was consistent with an approximately 20% inhibition of

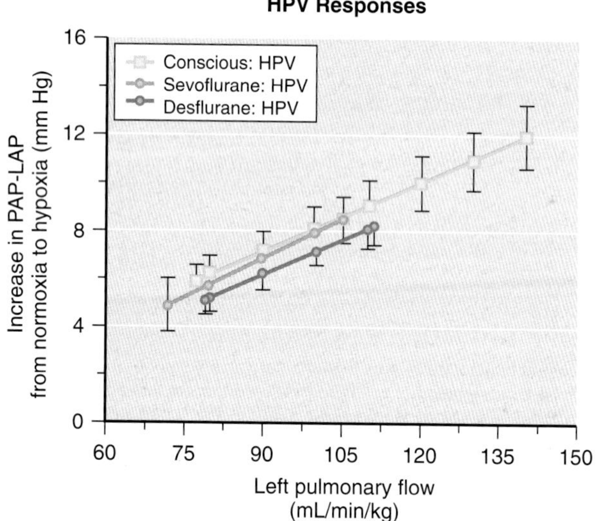

Figure 22-12 Composite hypoxic pulmonary vasoconstriction (HPV) responses (increase in pulmonary artery pressure [PAP] minus left atrial pressure [LAP]) as a function of left pulmonary flow in the same seven chronically instrumented dogs in the conscious state and during sevoflurane and desflurane anesthesia. Neither anesthetic affected the magnitude of HPV when compared with the response in the conscious state. *(From Lesitsky MA, Davis S, Murray PA: Preservation of hypoxic pulmonary vasoconstriction during sevoflurane and desflurane anesthesia compared to the conscious state in chronically instrumented dogs. Anesthesiology 89:1501, 1998, with permission.)*

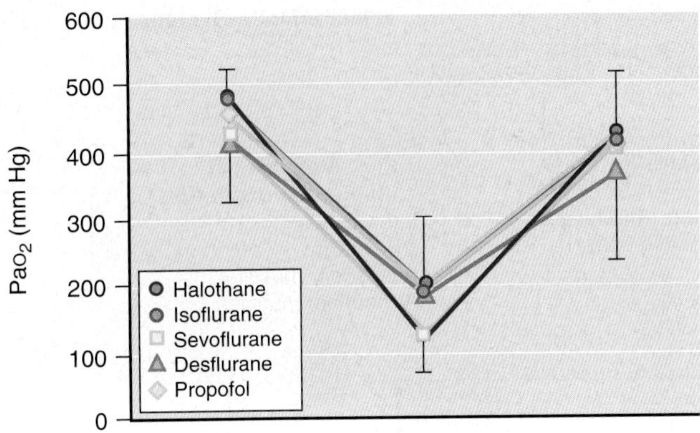

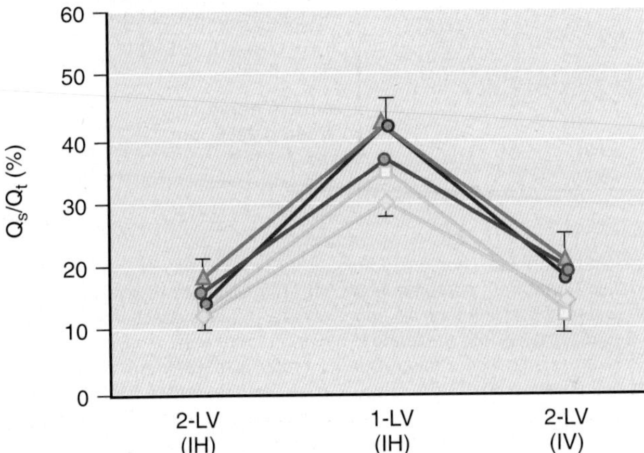

Figure 22-13 Arterial oxygenation (Pa_{O_2}) and intrapulmonary shunt (Q_s/Q_t) in patients with both lungs ventilated (2-LV) or with one lung ventilated (1-LV). Patients received an inhaled agent (IH)—halothane, isoflurane, sevoflurane, or desflurane—or the intravenous anesthetic propofol. Note the minimal effect on Pa_{O_2} and shunt that occurs when changing from a volatile anesthetic to an intravenous agent. *(Adapted from Abe et al.,[132,136] Benumof et al.,[138] and Pagel et al.,[139] with permission.)*

HPV at 1 MAC. Instead of a 50% reduction in pulmonary blood flow in a hypoxic lung in the absence of a volatile agent, blood flow decreases by 40% during hypoxia in the presence of 1 MAC isoflurane. This change in flow corresponds to an increase in pulmonary shunt by about 4% of cardiac output. Carlsson and colleagues[140] applied multiple inert gas elimination techniques to measure the true shunt fraction in humans anesthetized with volatile agents and demonstrated a 2% to 3% increase in shunt fraction corresponding to approximately 20% HPV inhibition with 1.5% isoflurane. There were also no significant effects on arterial oxygenation with clinically relevant concentrations of isoflurane or enflurane. Indeed, the use of total intravenous anesthesia with propofol and alfentanil as opposed to a volatile anesthetic did not decrease the risk for hypoxemia during single-lung ventilation.[133] Not only does isoflurane appear to be safe to use during single-lung ventilation, but administration of isoflurane before pulmonary ischemia also protects against ischemia-reperfusion injury. Isoflurane attenuated increases in PVR and reductions in the coefficient of filtration and the wet-to-dry ratio in isolated rabbit lungs subjected to ischemia and reperfusion.[141]

Marked increases in shunting have been demonstrated by the administration of pulmonary vasodilators (e.g., sodium nitroprusside, nitroglycerin) in dogs with oleic acid–induced pulmonary edema. Theoretically, volatile anesthetics may produce a similar response in patients with adult respiratory distress syndrome or with other types of pulmonary pathology associated with large right-to-left intrapulmonary shunts, but this hypothesis has yet to be comprehensively examined. Isoflurane did not attenuate the enhanced pulmonary vasoconstrictor response to sympathetic α-adrenoreceptor activation or influence pulmonary vascular tone in the presence of increased PVR secondary to endothelin-mediated receptor activation[142] after single-lung transplantation.[143] These findings may have important implications for the intraoperative anesthetic management of patients with similar abnormalities in pulmonary vasoregulation because volatile anesthetics may produce smaller reductions in PVR than might be expected.

The precise effects of inhaled anesthetics on HPV and pulmonary shunt in patients with preexisting pulmonary disease remain to be defined, but the action of these agents on the pulmonary vasculature itself must be considered when evaluating causes of hypoxemia during anesthesia. Clinical observations suggest that volatile anesthetics exert only mild, if any inhibitory effects on HPV and oxygenation. This relatively minor inhibition of HPV by volatile anesthetics should not significantly influence clinical decision-making, especially given the efficacy of continuous positive airway pressure in improving oxygenation of the nondependent lung. Thus, the net effect of volatile anesthetics on HPV is multifactorial and not only depends on the direct effects of these agents on pulmonary vasomotor tone but is also determined by indirect actions that commonly occur during anesthesia and surgery.

Control of Ventilation

Many different stimuli interact in a complex manner to control ventilation in humans. The traditional approach to studying the effects of drugs on ventilation has been to measure ventilatory responsiveness (e.g., expired minute volume, respiratory frequency, arterial carbon dioxide tension) before and after drug administration. A complete description of ventilatory control is beyond the scope of this chapter, and several excellent reviews of this subject already exist.[144-150] However, an understanding of normal ventilatory responses and control mechanisms is necessary to appreciate the actions of anesthetics and the methods by which these effects are measured.

Control of Breathing—Central Controllers, Sensors, Effectors

A control system that modulates ventilation is required to maintain the stability of arterial blood gas tension and acid-base status, as well as to integrate the respiratory rate and tidal volume to minimize the work of breathing in response to variations in total ventilatory requirements (Fig. 22-14). The system responsible for receiving and integrating input signals and ultimately producing movement of air in and out of the lungs is composed of the following:

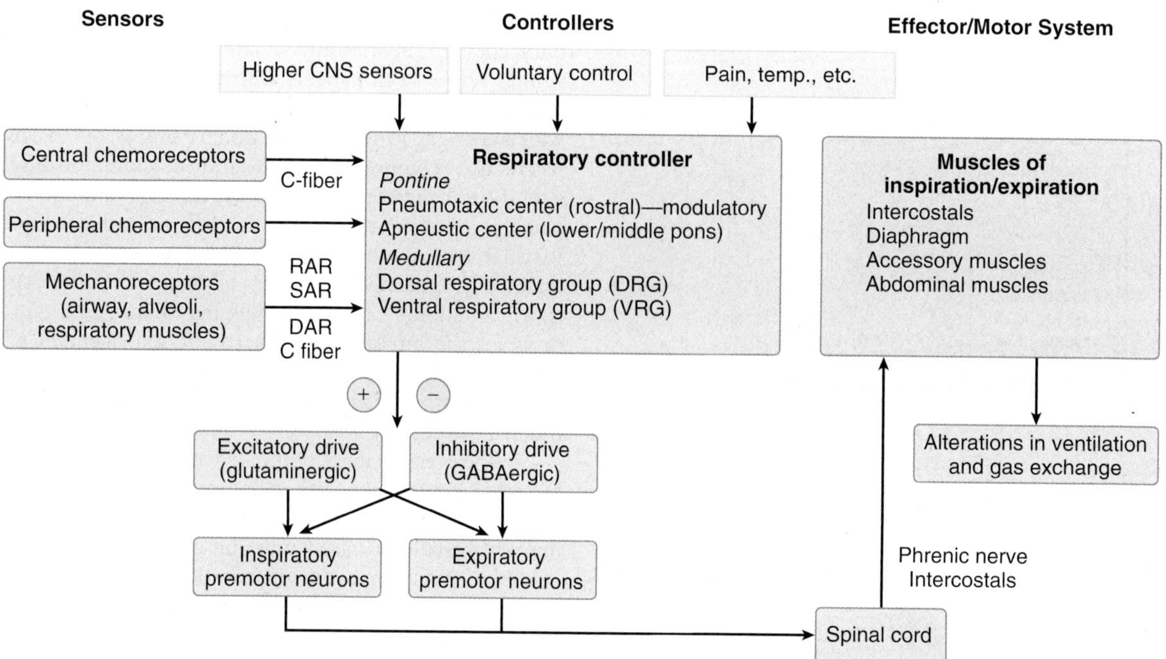

Figure 22-14 Some aspects of the reflex control of ventilation. Sensors include central and peripheral chemoreceptors, as well as a variety of mechanoreceptors. Input from these many sources interacts to alter ventilatory controller output from pontomedullary sites to muscles of respiration, thus altering ventilation and ultimately gas exchange. Central and peripheral chemoreceptors transmit information via nonmyelinated C fibers. Mechanoreceptors, such as rapidly (RAR) and slowly (SAR) adapting stretch receptors and deflation-activated receptors (DAR) are found in airway smooth muscle, alveoli, and respiratory muscle. C fibers may also transmit information from mechanoreceptors. Inspiratory bulbospinal neurons in the medulla are premotor neurons that drive phrenic and intercostal motoneurons and ultimately the diaphragm and muscles of inspiration. Excitatory drive to these motoneurons is mediated by glutaminergic neurotransmission. The neurons of timing and pattern generation, as well as premotor neurons, are also subject to tonic γ-aminobutyric acid (GABA)-mediated inhibition.

The *sensory system* may be chemical (i.e., peripheral and central chemoreceptors) or mechanical (i.e., distortion receptors located in airways, alveoli, and respiratory muscles).

The *respiratory control system* integrates the signal input from receptor sites, centers of consciousness, and other influences (e.g., pain) and subsequently produces nerve traffic to the muscles of respiration.

The *motor system* is composed of the chest wall, intercostal, diaphragmatic, and abdominal muscles, all of which respond to signals from the control center through phrenic and spinal nerves.

The respiratory rhythm generator resides within the brainstem and consists of two primary types of respiratory neurons: the dorsal respiratory group (DRG), chiefly associated with inspiration, and the ventral respiratory group (VRG), which contains inspiratory and expiratory neurons. The cortex is able to override these brainstem centers if voluntary control is desired. Other parts of the brain, such as the hypothalamus and limbic system, may modulate ventilation during certain emotional states. The precise mechanism of rhythm generation remains unknown, but regions in the ventrolateral medulla (including the rostral VRG) contain rhythm-generating, self-oscillating neurons. Central terminations of afferent airway sensory fibers are found in the caudal portion of the nucleus tractus solitarius. Second-order neurons then innervate neurons located in respiratory-related regions of the pons, medulla, and spinal cord. Medullary regions involved in the generation and modulation of respiratory and sympathetic nervous system vasomotor output, such as the retrotrapezoid nucleus, may also contain neurons functioning as central oxygen detectors.[151] The rostral pons contains the pneumotaxic center, which has inspiratory and expiratory neurons and plays a critical modulating role by fine-tuning respiratory rhythm and integrating vagal and chemoreceptive input. The apneustic center, located in the lower portion of the pons, appears to have an excitatory effect on the inspiratory area of the medulla. Whether this center plays an important role in normal respiration is unclear. Central respiratory control mechanisms regulate tidal volume and inspiratory and expiratory times to achieve adequate ventilation and gas exchange. Excitatory drive to bulbospinal inspiratory neurons of the caudal VRG is mediated by tonic input (acting through *N*-methyl-D-aspartate [NMDA] receptors) and phasic input (primarily consisting of non-NMDA glutamate receptors).[152,153] Neurotransmission in bulbospinal expiratory neurons is mediated via NMDA-type glutamate receptor input and modulated by γ-aminobutyric acid type A ($GABA_A$) receptors.[152]

Input signals originate from chemoreceptors and mechanoreceptors in the upper airways, lungs, and chest wall and are transmitted by the vagus and spinal nerves. Extensive discussion of these receptors and their physiologic consequences is beyond the scope of the current chapter. However, because volatile anesthetics may differentially affect pulmonary sensory receptors, a basic understanding of the types, function, and location of these receptors is important. Traditionally, lung sensory receptors were divided into three groups: slowly and rapidly adapting stretch receptors (SARs and RARs, respectively) and bronchopulmonary C fibers. SARs lie within airway smooth muscle, discharge regularly during sustained inflation, and demonstrate little adaptation. Stimulation of these receptors by lung inflation results in slowing of the respiratory rate because of an increase in expiratory time. The opposite effect is observed during lung deflation, which initiates inspiratory activity. This phenomenon, known as the Hering-Breuer reflex, is largely inactive in adult humans but appears to be active and potentially important in neonates. Activation of SARs by persistent elevations in end-expiratory lung volume produced an inhibitory effect on central drive (i.e., an increase in the apneic threshold) and an attenuated ventilatory response to progressive hypercapnia.[154] RARs, also known as irritant receptors, lie between airway epithelial cells and are stimulated by dust, cold air, and other noxious airway irritants. These receptors initially discharge vigorously and cause bronchoconstriction and hyperpnea, but their responses are extinguished rapidly.[147] RARs in the bronchi are more chemosensitive than those located in the more proximal airway but will also cause coughing, mucus secretion, bronchoconstriction, and laryngospasm. In addition, RARs in the bronchi stimulate hyperventilation.[155] C fiber receptors are nonmyelinated chemosensors but may also respond to lung inflation at high thresholds. Activation of these receptors results in tachypnea, bronchoconstriction, and secretion of mucus. Several other receptor types have been described, including Aδ-nociceptors, "cough" receptors, J receptors, deflation-activated receptors (DARs), and a variety of mechanically driven receptors in the upper airways, intercostal muscles, and diaphragm.[146,148]

Changes in chest wall position produce alterations in efferent impulses from stretch receptors in intercostal muscle spindles that act to maintain relatively constant tidal volume during variations in inspiratory resistance. Increases in spindle discharge enhance motor activity to muscle fibers until muscle shortening relieves tension in the spindles. With increased inspiratory resistance, the muscle spindles detect a failure of shortening by the appropriate amount and increase afferent signals to the motor neuron pool. Accessory muscles of inspiration may also be recruited. This reflex increase in inspiratory effort sustains tidal volume and minute ventilation despite a greater inspiratory resistive load. These and other forces maintain normal ventilation with changes in body position, inspiratory resistance, and compliance. Extrapolation of these data obtained from experimental animals to humans should be approached with caution. For example, tension receptors in the diaphragm, not the muscle spindles, induce reflex inhibition of inspiratory intercostal activity associated with a decrease in inspiratory duration in dogs, but not humans. This effect appears to be mediated at the supraspinal level.[156]

Central and peripheral chemoreceptors respond to changes in the chemical composition of blood or the surrounding fluid. A complete discussion of chemical control of ventilation may be found in several excellent reviews.[157-160] Briefly, central and peripheral chemoreceptors are critical to chemical control of respiration. Central chemoreceptors are located near the ventrolateral medulla and other brainstem sites and respond to changes in the hydrogen ion (H^+) concentration in cerebrospinal fluid and not to arterial carbon dioxide tension or pH. Unlike H^+, carbon dioxide diffuses rapidly through the blood-brain barrier. Central chemoreceptors are more profoundly affected by respiratory than by metabolic alterations in arterial carbon dioxide tension. In contrast, peripheral chemoreceptors, located in the carotid bodies, are sensitive to changes in arterial carbon dioxide tension, pH, and most importantly, arterial oxygen tension. The mechanisms by which peripheral chemoreceptive cells respond to hypoxia and hypercapnia appear to be separate and synergistic because hypoxemia potentiates the chemical drive to a carbon dioxide challenge. Peripheral chemoreceptors appear to contribute about a third to total resting minute ventilation at normocapnia and normoxia as determined by respiratory functional testing. This contribution falls to 15% during hyperoxic normocapnia, thus suggesting that central chemoreceptors control 85% of the carbon dioxide drive during hyperoxia. Both stimuli cause membrane depolarization and activation of afferent nerve transmission.

Changes in ventilation secondary to alterations in arterial carbon dioxide tension are mediated principally at the level of the medulla. Patients whose peripheral chemoreceptors have been denervated by bilateral carotid endarterectomy demonstrate a modestly attenuated increase in ventilation in response to inhaled carbon dioxide. Inspiration of carbon dioxide in normal subjects increases minute ventilation by approximately 3 L/min/mm Hg of arterial carbon dioxide tension. This observation demonstrates high gain from central chemoreceptors in response to variations in arterial carbon dioxide tension. The slope of the relationship between minute ventilation and arterial carbon dioxide tension is an index of ventilatory drive, provided that hypoxic conditions are avoided to minimize peripheral chemoreceptor stimulation. NO is increased in the carotid bodies during hypoxia,[161] plays an inhibitory role in both the peripheral and central chemoreflex pathways during hypoxia,[162] and may act as a respiratory stimulant under normoxic conditions.[163] Experiments to determine the relationship between minute ventilation and arterial carbon dioxide tension require interpretation with these potential confounding variables in mind.

A biphasic response to hypoxia exists in humans. Adults and neonates display a similar initial hypoxia-induced increase in ventilation, but neonates exhibit a more pronounced ventilatory decline in response to hypoxic oxygen concentrations than adults do. This reaction may represent a balance between active inhibition of brainstem neuronal activities and augmentation of peripheral chemoreceptor function. Acute hypoxemia stimulates oxygen-sensitive (type I—glomus) cells in the carotid bodies to initiate a cascade of responses, including closure of K^+ channels and resultant membrane depolarization. Reactive oxygen species generated by reduced nicotinamide adenine dinucleotide phosphate (NADPH) oxidase, mitochondria, or heme oxygenase have been proposed as mediators of this response.[158] Release of ATP subsequently activates chemoafferent fibers of the carotid sinus nerve to relay the information to the brainstem respiratory control centers.[160] Similarly, release of ATP by central chemoreceptors on the ventral surface of the medulla after hypercapnic stimulation immediately precedes an increase in respiratory drive.[160]

General Ventilatory Effects of Anesthetics

In general, all volatile anesthetics decrease tidal volume in a dose-dependent manner. A concomitant increase in respiratory rate only partially offsets the depression of minute ventilation. As a result, an increase in resting arterial carbon dioxide tension takes place (Fig. 22-15). Early studies demonstrated that isoflurane produces more profound respiratory depression than halothane does, but in contrast to halothane, isoflurane did not progressively increase the respiratory rate.[164] Like halothane, enflurane reduces tidal volume and minute ventilation concomitant with compensatory tachypnea in a dose-related manner.[165] Prolonged administration (3 to 7 hours) of halothane or enflurane decreases the

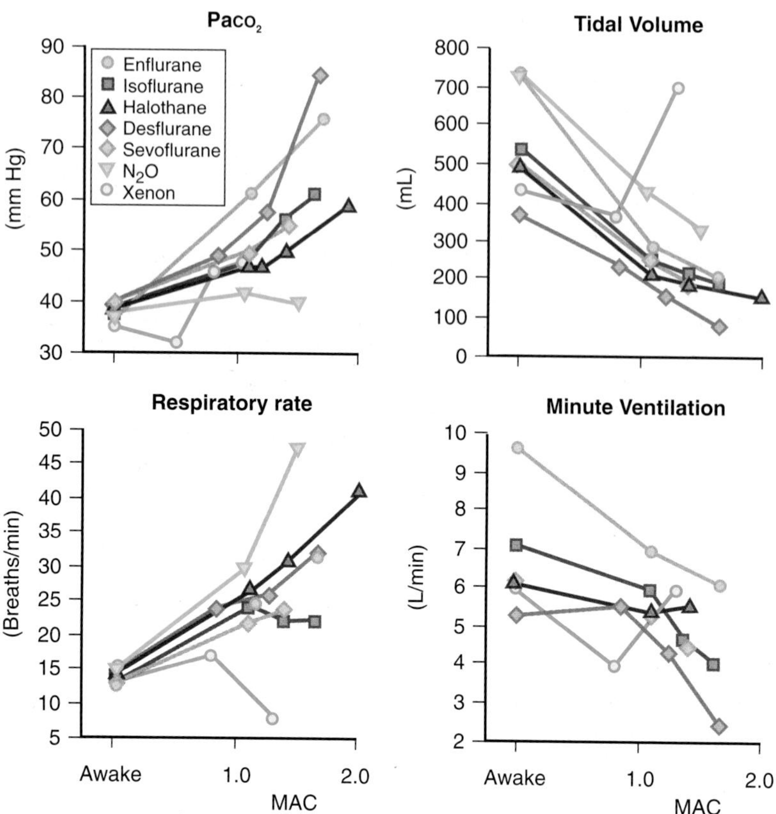

Figure 22-15 Comparison of mean changes in resting Pa_{CO_2}, tidal volume, respiratory rate, and minute ventilation in patients anesthetized with either halothane, isoflurane, enflurane, sevoflurane, desflurane, nitrous oxide, or xenon. Anesthetic-induced tachypnea compensates in part for the ventilatory depression caused by all volatile anesthetics (decrease in minute ventilation and tidal volume and concomitant increase in Pa_{CO_2}). Desflurane results in the greatest increase in Pa_{CO_2} with corresponding reductions in tidal volume and minute ventilation. Isoflurane, like all other inhaled agents, increases the respiratory rate; however, isoflurane does not result in dose-dependent tachypnea. MAC, minimum alveolar concentration. *(Data from references 164-169. Note that the data for xenon have been extrapolated from several sources[63,170,171] because there have been no well-controlled studies measuring all variables.)*

degree of respiratory depression as indicated by resting arterial carbon dioxide tension.[165,172]

Desflurane and sevoflurane also exhibit dose-related ventilatory depression, primarily by reducing tidal volume.[166,167,173] Unlike isoflurane, sevoflurane and desflurane cause dose-related increases in the respiratory rate. Thus, desflurane does not significantly reduce minute ventilation at concentrations less than 1.6 MAC. The reduction in respiratory rate produced by desflurane at higher concentrations was less than that caused by halothane. The relative effect of inhaled anesthetics (<1.24 MAC) in increasing arterial carbon dioxide tension (as an index of respiratory depression) is enflurane > desflurane = isoflurane > sevoflurane = halothane > nitrous oxide. Halothane and sevoflurane also cause similar respiratory changes in spontaneously breathing children. Nevertheless, potentially important differences between these two agents have been identified and include reduced minute ventilation and respiratory rate, a delay in the timing of peak inspiratory flow, and an earlier occurrence of peak expiratory flow during sevoflurane than during halothane anesthesia.[174] The ventilatory depression produced by higher concentrations of desflurane and sevoflurane is similar to that caused by enflurane and isoflurane, respectively. Isoflurane-induced respiratory depression is reduced by surgical stimulation (Fig. 22-16).[175] The respiratory depression observed during desflurane or sevoflurane anesthesia is reduced in the presence of nitrous oxide at equivalent MAC values.[176] This phenomenon is principally related to the reduction in volatile anesthetic required when nitrous oxide is added to the inspired gas mixture. The alteration in ventilatory pattern caused by anesthetics has been attributed to relative sensitization of pulmonary stretch receptors that subsequently produce tachypnea and low tidal volumes. The presence of a volatile anesthetic increased vagal afferent discharge at varying lung volumes in decerebrate cats (i.e., sensitization of pulmonary stretch receptors),[177] but little evidence exists of such a mechanism in humans. Halothane-induced tachypnea is primarily a suprapontine effect that may occur in cats, but the mechanism of

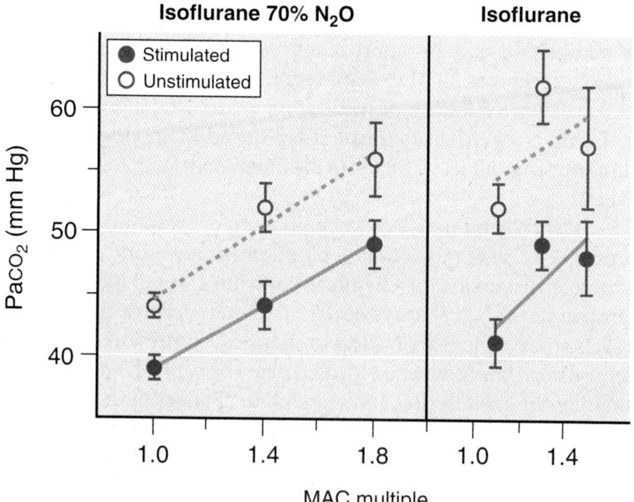

Figure 22-16 Effect of surgical stimulation on the ventilatory depression of inhaled anesthesia with isoflurane in the presence and absence of nitrous oxide. Surgical stimulation increased alveolar ventilation and decreased Pa_{CO_2} at all depths of anesthesia examined. MAC, minimum alveolar concentration. *(Modified from Eger EI, Dolan WM, Stevens WC, et al: Surgical stimulation antagonizes the respiratory depression produced by Forane. Anesthesiology 36:544, 1972, with permission.)*

production of tachypnea with decreased tidal volume in anesthetized humans remains unclear.

The respiratory depressant effects of xenon were first described more than 50 years ago. Xenon (1 MAC) causes a reduction in minute ventilation and a rise in arterial carbon dioxide tension. However, unlike other inhaled anesthetics, the decrease in minute ventilation is due to decreases in the respiratory rate, which are partially compensated by increases in tidal volume.[170] At lower concentrations of xenon (33% or approximately 0.5 MAC), the decrease in respiratory rate may be entirely offset by an increase in tidal volume. Depression of the pontine pneuomotaxic center may be the mechanism for this "xenon effect." Minute ventilation may actually increase and arterial carbon dioxide tension remain the same or decrease in healthy humans.[171]

Lung and Airway Receptors

The receptors responsible for eliciting protective airway reflexes are nonuniformly distributed. Sensitivity to airway irritation appears to be greater at the larynx and trachea than at the more peripheral airways in spontaneously breathing anesthetized patients in the presence of a laryngeal mask airway (LMA). Increasing concentrations of sevoflurane had little effect in altering these responses. The direct effects of halothane, isoflurane, and enflurane on pulmonary and laryngeal irritant receptors and tracheobronchial SARs have been investigated in spontaneously breathing and vagotomized, paralyzed dogs.[178,179] Volatile anesthetics increase the activity of laryngeal irritant receptors[178] and inhibit pulmonary irritant receptors.[179] Volatile anesthetics also elevate the excitation threshold and increase the sensitivity of low-threshold stretch receptors. Halothane and, to a lesser extent, sevoflurane attenuate the end-expiratory discharge frequency of SARs.[179,180] These agents may not affect or may even augment inspiratory activity. The clinical implications of these findings have yet to be precisely determined, but these anesthetic-induced changes in SAR function may play a role in the reduction of bronchomotor tone observed with volatile anesthetics. The severity of airway hyperreactivity was determined in 123 children breathing spontaneously through LMAs and undergoing either isoflurane or sevoflurane anesthesia.[181] Isoflurane was associated with greater airway hyperreactivity and more adverse airway events during LMA removal. An ongoing debate lingers in the anesthesiology literature regarding comparisons of upper airway reactivity between sevoflurane and desflurane. Sevoflurane (1 MAC) may provide greater suppression of responses to tracheal[182] and LMA[183] stimulation than desflurane does in elective surgical patients (Fig. 22-17). Higher concentrations (1.8 MAC) of these agents produce similar attenuation of coughing, tachycardia, and hypertension associated with tracheal stimulation, yet desflurane may irritate the respiratory tract at concentrations exceeding 1 MAC. Nevertheless, there were no differences in airway irritation with the use of an LMA in elective surgical patients receiving low concentrations of either desflurane or sevoflurane.[184] However, a significant increase in airway irritation was observed in smokers independent of the type of volatile agent.[185] The concomitant use of propofol and fentanyl in these patients and the relatively lower concentrations of desflurane than sevoflurane may have limited the ability to detect differences between these two anesthetic

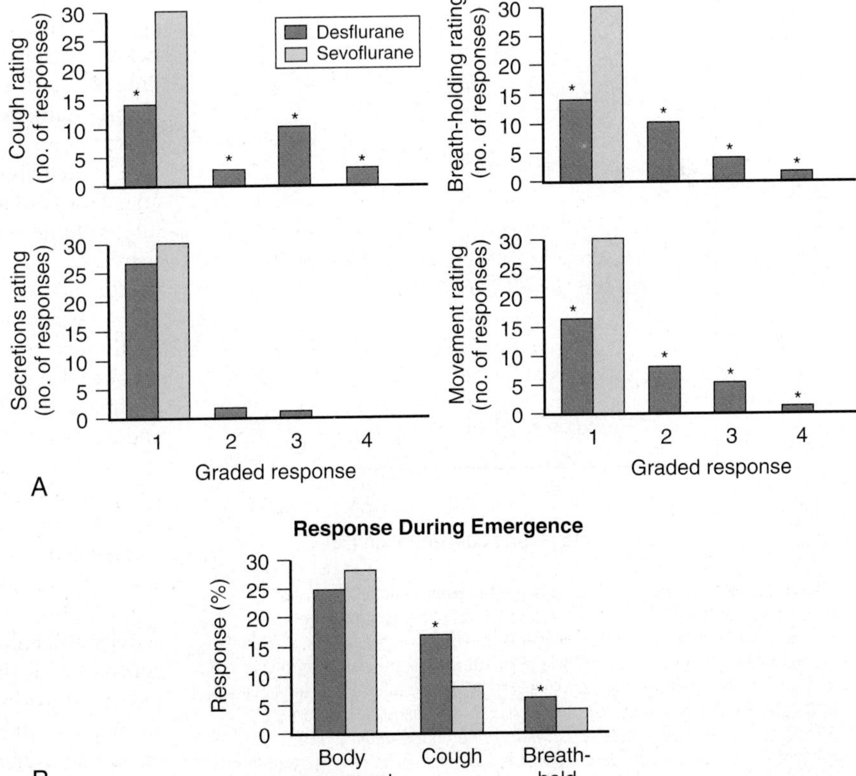

Figure 22-17 A, Graded responses to body movement, coughing, breath-holding, and secretions during transition to 2 minimum alveolar concentration (MAC) desflurane and sevoflurane anesthesia. **B,** Percentage of patients experiencing body movement, coughing, and breath-holding during emergence associated with sevoflurane and desflurane. *Desflurane caused more events than sevoflurane did in elective surgical patients. *(Modified from Arain S, Shankar H, Ebert TJ: Desflurane enhances reactivity during the use of the laryngeal mask airway. Anesthesiology 103:495, 2005, with permission.)*

agents in this study. The profound cardiovascular stimulation induced by rapid increases in the concentration of desflurane is due to activation of tracheopulmonary RARs.[186]

Volatile anesthetics produce a greater magnitude of depression of upper airway electromyographic[187] or nerve activity[188] than diaphragmatic activity in anesthetized, spontaneously breathing (Fig. 22-18) or paralyzed, ventilated, vagotomized cats. The extent to which this depression of upper airway motor neuron activity occurs as a result of anesthetic-induced inhibition of the reticular activating system is unknown. Upper airway caliber represents a balance between dilating and constricting forces. Outward-dilating forces are produced by neurogenic activity in the genioglossus, posterior cricoarytenoid, and hyoid muscles, whereas during inspiration, subatmospheric intraluminal pressure causes an inward collapsing force. It has been suggested that volatile anesthetics may cause relaxation of the genioglossus muscle with resultant posterior tongue displacement, a reduction in airway caliber, and consequent upper airway obstruction. Halothane, isoflurane and sevoflurane have all been shown to relax the upper airway musculature. Inhibition of upper airway muscle activity by isoflurane was independent of dose, and even subanesthetic concentrations totally abolished genioglossus activity.[189] In contrast, sevoflurane-induced changes in upper airway caliber was dose-dependent in children[26] (Fig. 22-19) and primarily occurred in an anterior-posterior dimension. In addition to these direct effects of sevoflurane on airway musculature, sevoflurane may also increase upper airway resistance by reducing lung volumes (which causes rostral tracheal displacement) or by increasing pharyngeal constrictor muscle activity.[26] Interestingly, whereas propofol predominantly caused narrowing in the hypopharynx at the level of the epiglottis,[190] sevoflurane more profoundly reduced airway caliber at the level of the soft palate. Respiratory premotor neurons are inhibited by the effects of volatile anesthetics through enhancement of GABAergic inhibitory activity and simultaneous depression of excitatory glutaminergic mechanisms.[153,191] However, hypoglossal motor neurons (which innervate all tongue muscles and are intimately involved in maintaining airway patency during inspiration) are extremely sensitive to subanesthetic concentrations of volatile anesthetics.[192] This inhibition of inspiratory hypoglossal motor neurons by volatile anesthetics is not related to actions at a K^+ leak channel but may be due to an enhancement of a tonic modulatory inhibition (Fig. 22-20).

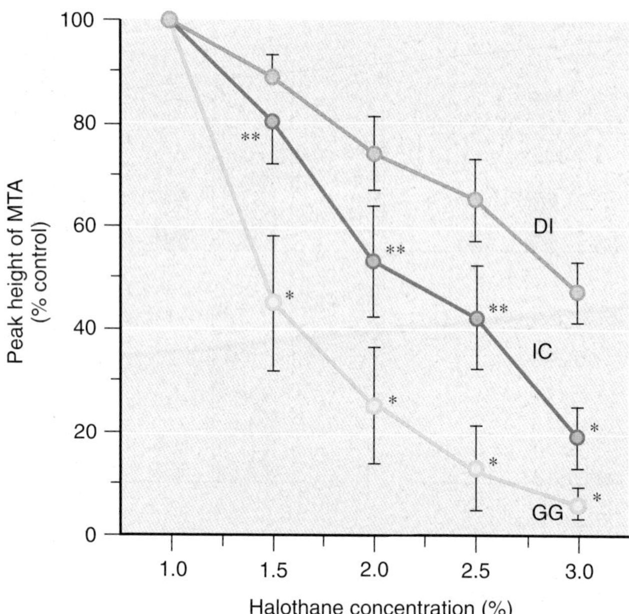

Figure 22-18 Decrease in phasic inspiratory muscle activity expressed as peak height of the moving time average (MTA), in percent change from control (1% halothane), during halothane anesthesia in adult cats. Values are means ± SEM. IC, intercostal muscle. *$P < .05$ versus the diaphragm (DI); **$P < .05$ versus the genioglossus muscle (GG). Note the differential sensitivities of these respiratory muscles. *(From Ochiai R, Guthrie RD, Motoyama EK: Effects of varying concentrations of halothane on the activity of the genioglossus, intercostals, and diaphragm in cats: An electromyographic study. Anesthesiology 70:812, 1989, with permission.)*

Ventilatory Mechanics and Mechanoreceptors in the Chest Wall

Induction of general anesthesia reduces FRC. Loss of tonic parasternal intercostal muscle activity,[193,194] development of phasic expiratory activity of respiratory muscles (Fig. 22-21),[194] alteration in diaphragm position,[193] and changes in thoracic blood volume have been proposed as mechanisms responsible for anesthetic-induced decreases in FRC. In contrast to intercostal muscle function, diaphragmatic activity is relatively spared during halothane anesthesia.[194] A change in diaphragmatic shape occurs during anesthesia, with dependent regions shifting cephalad and nondependent regions shifting caudad (Fig. 22-22).[195] Anesthesia-enhanced expiratory muscle activity results in inward displacement of the rib cage, an action that contributes to the reduction in FRC. In contrast, inspiratory rib cage expansion may remain relatively well preserved because of phasic inspiratory activity of the scalene muscles despite the attenuation of parasternal intercostal muscle activity.[193] Areas of atelectasis in dependent lung regions frequently occur in anesthetized, spontaneously ventilating humans and may be related to alterations in respiratory muscle tone but not specifically to any single chest wall structure.[195] There is no direct correlation between changes in FRC and anesthesia-induced atelectasis.[196] As a result of the reduction in lung volume secondary to decreases in FRC, airway resistance increases. This action may partially counteract the direct bronchodilatory effects of volatile anesthetics.

Reasons for the differential effects of inhaled anesthetics on inspiratory and expiratory respiratory muscles are unknown but may be related to direct actions on brainstem control mechanisms or differential sensitivity of premotor and motor neurons. Stuth and coworkers[197-199] showed that bulbospinal respiratory neurons are more resistant than phrenic nerve activity to the depressant effects of volatile anesthetics in vagotomized, decerebrate dogs. The inhibition of expiratory premotor neurons by volatile agents is mediated by presynaptic reduction of glutaminergic excitation and enhancement of $GABA_A$ergic inhibitory receptor function (Fig. 22-23).[152,153,191] Sevoflurane also depressed phrenic nerve activity and enhanced the overall inhibition of inspiratory motor neurons to a greater extent than halothane did. Increases in carbon dioxide drive only partially compensated for these anesthetic-induced depressant actions. There appears to be less halothane-induced depression of expiratory than inspiratory bulbospinal premotor neurons. These findings suggest that the effects

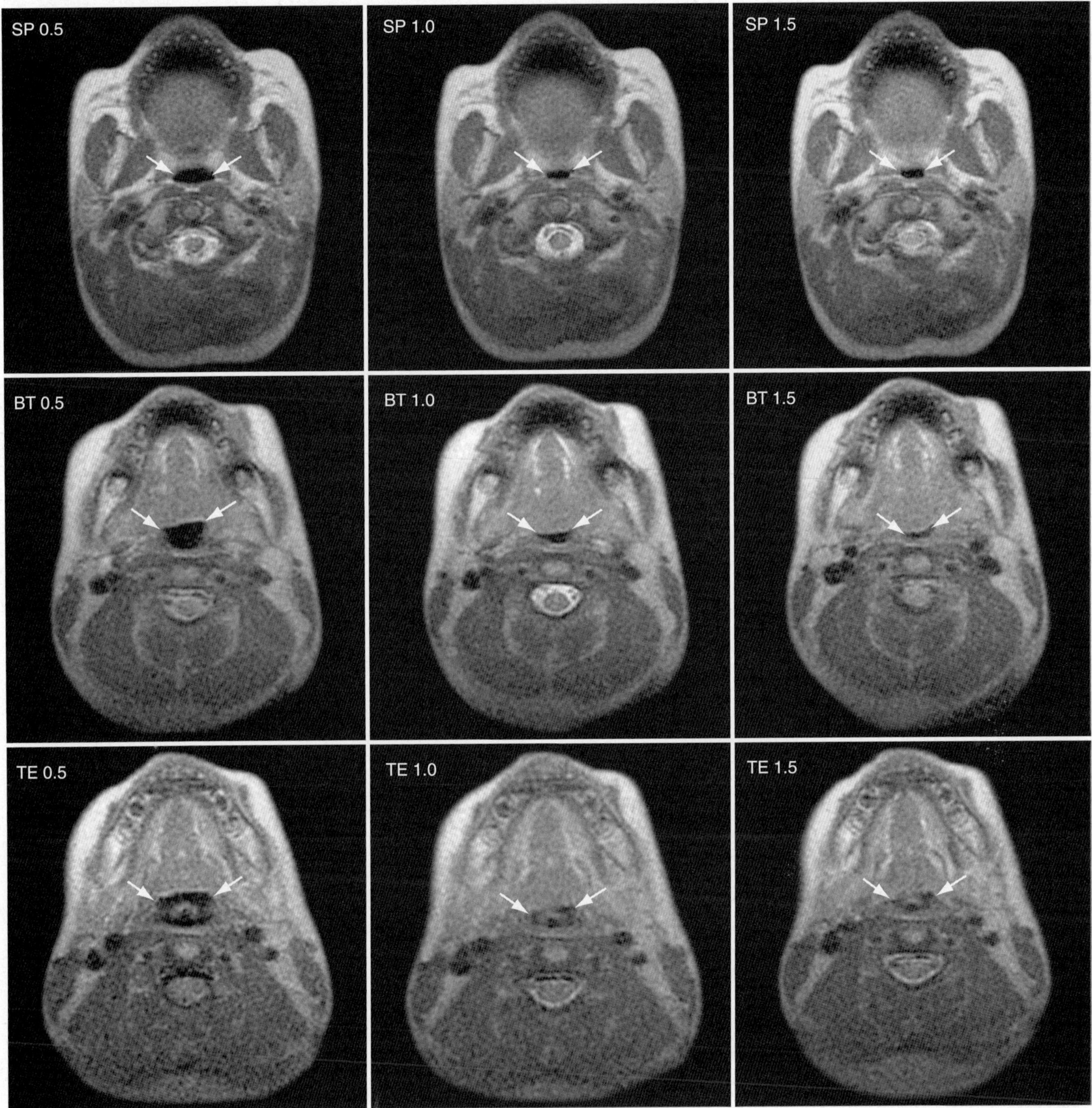

Figure 22-19 Magnetic resonance images at the level of the soft palate (SP), base of the tongue (BT), and tip of the epiglottis (TE) of a child in early expiration demonstrating a progressive reduction in cross-sectional area with increasing concentration of sevoflurane (0.5, 1, 1.5 minimum alveolar concentration). *Arrows* show the site of the collapsible pharyngeal airway. *(From Crawford MW, Arrica M, Macgowan CK, Yoo S-J: Extent and localization of changes in upper airway caliber with varying concentrations of sevoflurane in children. Anesthesiology 105:1147, 2006, with permission.)*

of volatile agents on respiratory muscle function may be due to a relatively greater influence on motor efferent pathways (including spinal respiratory motor neurons) than on brainstem-mediated mechanisms (Fig. 22-24).[198]

Volatile anesthetics differentially depress neuromuscular transmission and skeletal muscle contractility. Halothane impairs excitation-contraction coupling and neuromuscular transmission to equivalent degrees, whereas isoflurane, sevoflurane, and enflurane depress diaphragmatic contraction primarily through alterations in neuromuscular transmission.[200,201] Isoflurane, enflurane, and sevoflurane depress diaphragmatic tension in response to phrenic nerve stimulation. These results may partially explain clinical observations in humans, but a wide range of species variations also exist that make extrapolation of results obtained from experimental animals to humans difficult. Similar to volatile agents, nitrous oxide affects chest wall function and breathing by

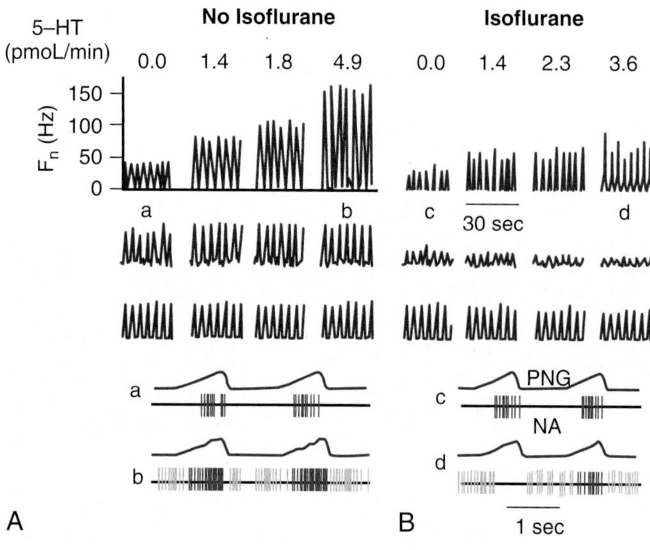

Figure 22-20 Inhibition of inspiratory hypoglossal motoneurons (XII) by a subanesthetic concentration (0.3 minimum alveolar concentration) of isoflurane in the absence and presence of graded doses of serotonin (5-HT). This inhibition in the presence of 5-HT rules out a major contribution of K^+ leak channels. Note the significant decline in hypoglossal nerve activity (≈60%) with isoflurane as opposed to phrenic nerve activity (PNG) (<10%). F_n represents the neurons' spontaneous peak discharge frequency. The letters a to d indicate the records for which time-enlarged views are shown. NA, neuronal activity. *(From Brandes IF, Zuperku EJ, Stucke AG, et al: Isoflurane depresses the response of inspiratory hypoglossal motoneurons to serotonin in vivo. Anesthesiology 106:736, 2007, with permission.)*

changing the distribution and timing of the neural drive to the respiratory muscles.[202] Nitrous oxide decreases tidal volume as a result of a reduction in rib cage motion and increased phasic expiratory activity in humans. In contrast, xenon does not affect transdiaphragmatic pressure or diaphragmatic electromyography

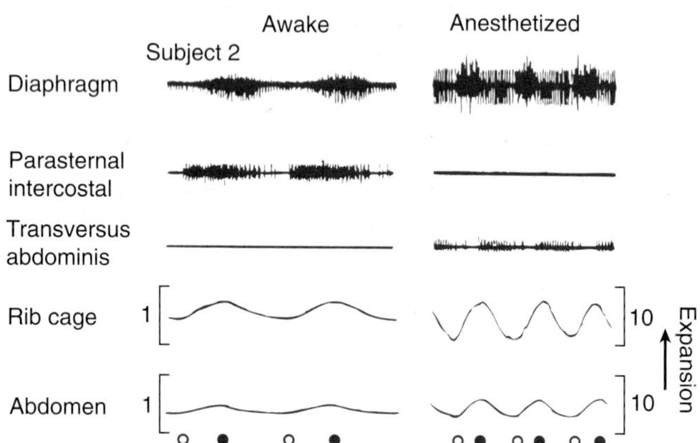

Figure 22-21 Representative record from one subject while awake and during halothane anesthesia. The *upper* three tracings are electromyograms. The *lower* tracings represent rib cage and abdominal dimensions measured by respiratory impedance plethysmography. *Open circles* and *closed circles* denote the beginning and end of inspiration, respectively. Note that the amplitude of rib cage and abdominal excursions diminishes during halothane anesthesia but the relationship between their amplitudes is preserved. *(From Warner DO, Warner MA, Ritman EL: Human chest wall function while awake and during halothane anesthesia. I. Quiet breathing. Anesthesiology 82:6, 1995, with permission.)*

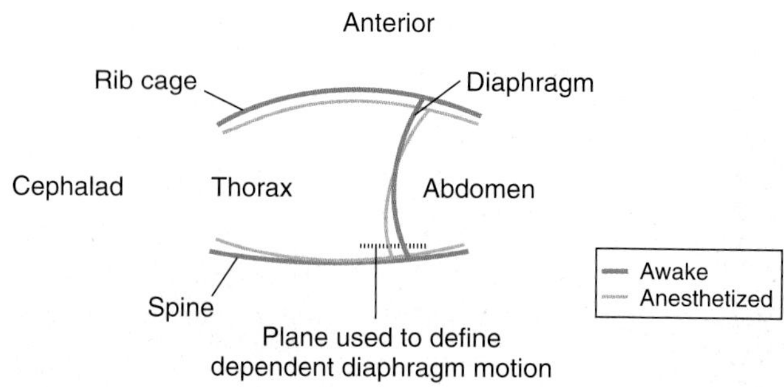

Figure 22-22 Diagram of a midsagittal section of the thorax while awake (*blue lines*) and while anesthetized (*yellow lines*) with a 1.2 minimum alveolar concentration of halothane. The chest wall configuration was determined by using images of the thorax obtained by three-dimensional fast computed tomography. *(Adapted from Warner DO, Warner MA, Ritman EL: Atelectasis and chest wall shape during halothane anesthesia. Anesthesiology 85:49, 1996, with permission.)*

because this anesthetic noble gas preserves neuromuscular transmission.[63]

The work of breathing expressed in joules is defined as pressure or force multiplied by the tidal volume during inspiration. The respiratory work of the lung is further broken down into elastic work (required to overcome recoil of the lung) and resistive work (required to overcome airway flow resistance and the viscoelastic resistance of pulmonary tissue in the absence or presence of an airway apparatus). The work of breathing is usually derived from transpulmonary pressure–tidal volume curves. Volatile anesthetics increase the work of breathing in adults and children. Sevoflurane anesthesia increased viscoelastic and elastic pressure in the lung, findings indicative of a reduction in pulmonary compliance mediated at the lung periphery rather than at the airway level in normal rats.[203] This finding was supported histologically by the observation of increased areas of alveolar collapse alternating with hyperinflation. In contrast, most studies in humans demonstrate that low concentrations of volatile anesthetics significantly reduce upper and lower respiratory system resistance (Fig. 22-25).[204] In a murine model of chronic asthma, sevoflurane anesthesia significantly decreased resistance in the central and distal airways in addition to lowering resistance in the lung periphery.[58] These data suggest that sevoflurane exerts a beneficial action in the presence of chronic airway obstruction and implies that volatile agents reduce the work of breathing (Fig. 22-26).

Expiration is passively affected by the recoil characteristics of the lung during normal breathing. In anesthetized patients, the ventilatory response to expiratory resistance is reduced to a greater extent than the response to inspiratory resistance. Conscious and anesthetized humans exhibit decreases in the respiratory rate during expiratory resistive loads, but the rib cage–abdominal wall motion asynchrony that causes less effective ventilation and increases in carbon dioxide is seen only in anesthetized subjects.[205] This concept may be particularly important in spontaneously breathing, anesthetized patients who demonstrate expiratory obstruction, such as may occur with partial occlusion of a breathing circuit, asthma, emphysema, or airway secretions. Interestingly, the ventilation-perfusion inhomogeneity caused by volatile anesthetics has been proposed as a new mechanism by which nitrous oxide produces a second gas effect in the presence of sevoflurane.[206]

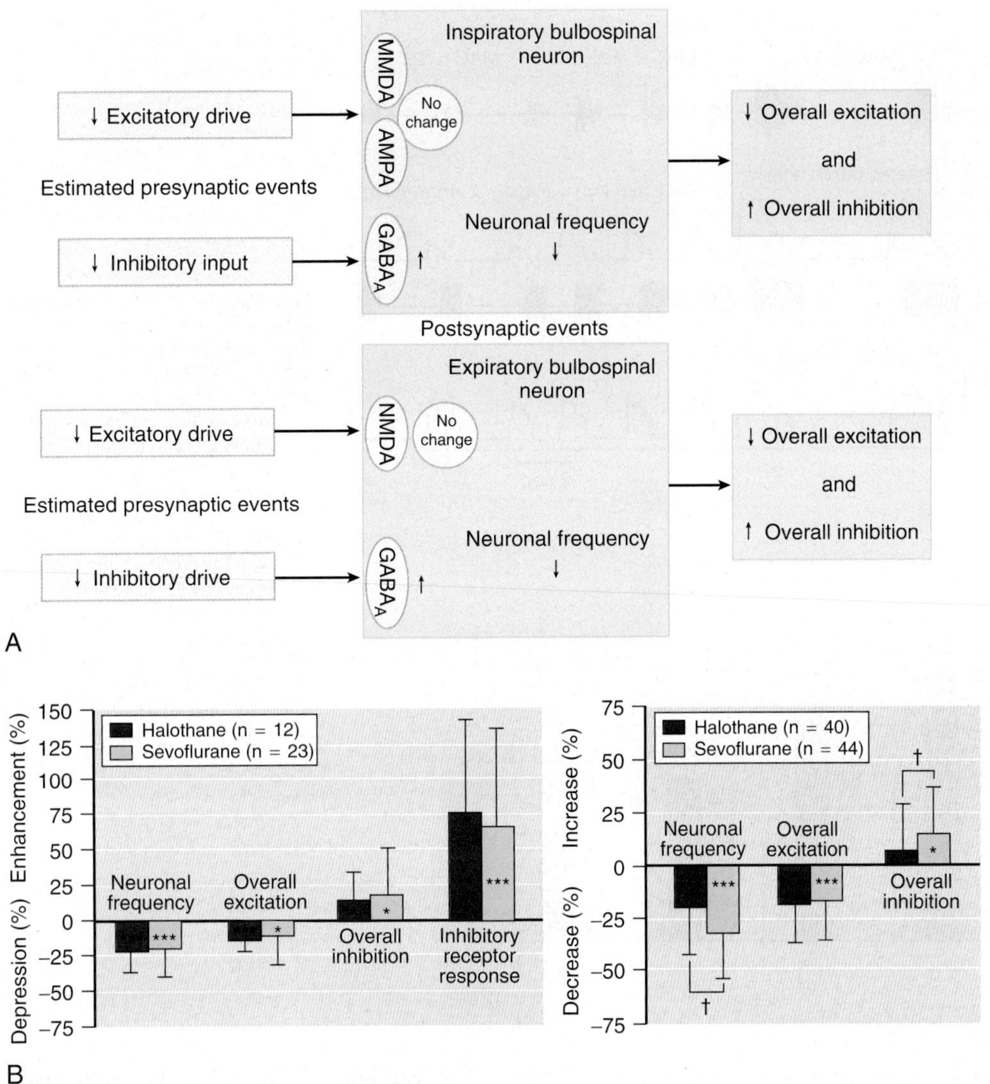

Figure 22-23 **A,** Schematic diagram of the effects of volatile anesthetics on synaptic transmission to expiratory and inspiratory premotor neurons in the caudal ventral respiratory group. In expiratory neurons, the overall glutaminergic excitatory drive is reduced without affecting N-methyl-D-aspartate (NMDA) receptor function, and overall inhibition is increased because of an increase in type A γ-aminobutyric acid ($GABA_A$) receptor function. The presynaptic inhibitory drive is also reduced and leads to a decrease in the control discharge frequency of the premotor neuron. In inspiratory neurons, there is a reduction in overall glutaminergic excitation with an increase in overall inhibitory input. Postsynaptic α-amino-3-hydroxy-5-methylisoxazole-4-propionate (AMPA) and NMDA receptor responses were not changed, thus suggesting that the presynaptic excitatory drive is diminished. **B,** Effects of halothane and sevoflurane on excitatory and inhibitory neurotransmission to canine medullary expiratory (left graph) and inspiratory (right graph) neurons. Values are mean changes ± SD for neuronal control frequency, overall excitation, overall inhibition, and inhibitory receptor response by a 1 minimum alveolar concentration of halothane and sevoflurane. There were no differences in anesthetic-induced changes between halothane and sevoflurane in expiratory neurons. †$P < 0.05$ sevoflurane enhanced overall inhibition and depressed neuronal frequency more than halothane did in inspiratory neurons. *$P < .05$, **$P < .01$, ***$P < .001$ versus no change. *(Adapted from Stucke and colleagues[152,153,189] with permission.)*

Effects of Anesthetics on Ventilatory Response to Chemical Stimuli

The effects of inhaled anesthetics on respiratory drive are typically characterized by the ventilatory response to alterations in arterial carbon dioxide tension or hypoxia. Arterial carbon dioxide tension is the most important stimulus for ventilation. The apneic threshold, defined as the highest arterial carbon dioxide tension at which a subject remains apneic, is approximately 4 or 5 mm Hg below resting arterial carbon dioxide tension. There are no significant agent-specific or depth-related effects of ether, halothane, or isoflurane on the relationship between apneic thresholds and resting arterial carbon dioxide tension in humans. Volatile anesthetic–induced ventilatory depression increases resting carbon dioxide tension and the apneic threshold to similar degrees. Thus, *assisted* ventilation, which lowers arterial carbon dioxide tension below the apneic threshold during anesthesia, ultimately becomes *controlled* ventilation. Return of spontaneous ventilation in a mechanically hyperventilated patient is dependent on return of carbon dioxide tension toward the apneic threshold after cessation of positive-pressure ventilation. The duration of apnea required before a patient will begin to breathe spontaneously is dependent on anesthetic depth. Continuation of positive-pressure ventilation (or intentional hyperventilation) to eliminate volatile agents and maintenance of relative hypercapnia during

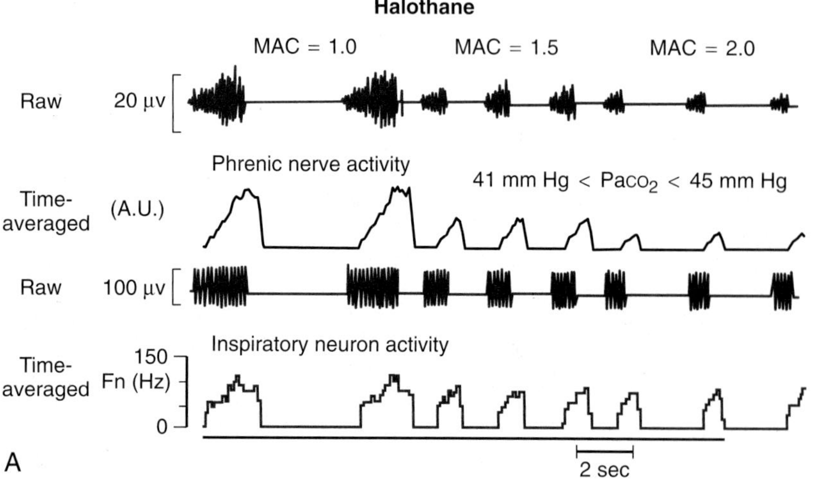

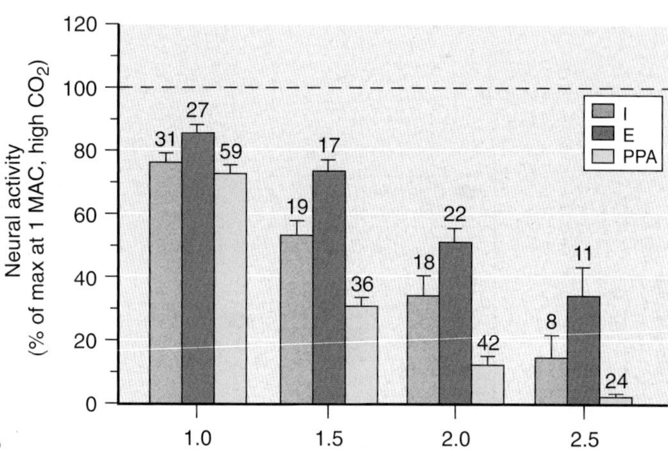

Figure 22-24 Effect of increasing halothane on phrenic nerve and neuron activity. With increasing anesthetic depth, both peak phrenic nerve (PPA) and peak neuron activities are depressed. PPA shows the greatest sensitivity to halothane. **A,** Phrenic nerve activity and the discharge frequency of an inspiratory bulbospinal neuron. Inspiratory (phrenic burst) duration decreases with increasing anesthetic depth. **B,** Peak expiratory neuron (E) activity, peak inspiratory neuron (I) activity, and PPA. Expiratory neuronal activity was most resistant to the effects of halothane. *Bars* show normalized means ± SEM, and the numbers above the *bars* indicate the numbers of neurons studied for each condition. Raw, airway resistance. *(Adapted from Stuth EAE, Tonkovic-Capin M, Kampine JP, et al: Dose-dependent effects of halothane on expiratory and inspiratory bulbospinal neurons and the phrenic nerve activities in dogs. Anesthesiology 81:1470, 1994, with permission.)*

mechanical ventilation are two commonly used clinical strategies to shorten the emergence time. Such maneuvers decrease the apneic threshold or increase resting arterial carbon dioxide tension and reduce emergence time during isoflurane, desflurane, or sevoflurane anesthesia (Fig. 22-27).[207,208] Rebreathing of carbon dioxide[209] or gradual increases in the concentration of sevoflurane[210] may reduce the incidence of apnea during induction with inhaled anesthetics. The activity of expiratory brainstem neurons may be temporarily "switched off" during rapid increases in anesthetic concentration and thereby contribute to apnea under these conditions.[210]

Carbon Dioxide Response Curves

Volatile anesthetics depress the ventilatory response to hypercapnia in a dose-dependent fashion. Moderate concentrations (<1 MAC) of volatile agents markedly attenuate or entirely eliminate hypercapnia-induced increases in ventilatory drive. Even low concentrations of nitrous oxide may substantially affect responses to hypercapnia. The slope of the minute ventilation–arterial carbon dioxide tension relationship returns toward normal after 6 hours of halothane anesthesia, but ventilatory responsiveness to carbon dioxide nevertheless remains profoundly depressed. The addition of nitrous oxide to halothane depresses ventilation less than equivalent-MAC halothane alone does, but the carbon dioxide–ventilatory response slope was unaltered when either a nitrous oxide–desflurane combination or desflurane alone was used.[166] Interestingly, the response to hypercapnia was more profoundly depressed during desflurane than during isoflurane or sevoflurane anesthesia at 0.5 MAC in C3 mice (C3 mice have a blunted response to hypercapnia and hypoxia at baseline).[211]

Subanesthetic concentrations (<0.2 MAC) of volatile anesthetics may depress the peripheral chemoreflex loop and inhibit the ventilatory response to hypercapnia.[212,213] At higher concentrations, central chemoreceptors may also be affected. In contrast, Pandit and colleagues[214] showed that subanesthetic concentrations of sevoflurane did not affect the response to acute or sustained hypercapnia. The apparent discrepancies between these results may be related to the sustained nature of the hypercapnic responses or differences in the state of central nervous system arousal under baseline conditions. A review of all published studies investigating the effect of low concentrations of volatile anesthetics on hypercapnic drive suggests a relative lack of any substantial inhibitory effect.[166]

Depression of ventilatory responsiveness to inhaled carbon dioxide is clinically important. Accumulation of carbon dioxide and concomitant acidemia may cause dysfunction in several organ systems, including the heart (e.g., arrhythmias), lungs (e.g., pulmonary hypertension), and brain (e.g., increased intracranial

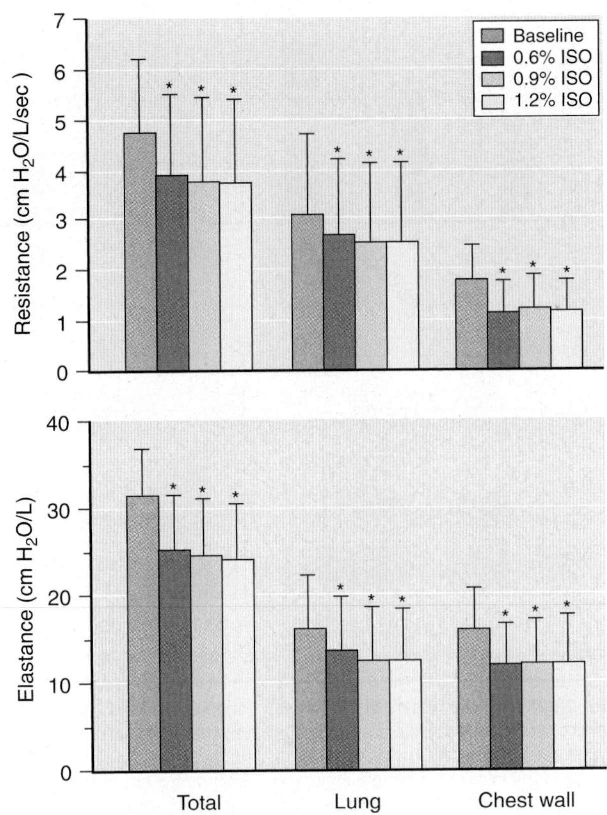

Figure 22-25 Isoflurane at 0.6% reduced respiratory system elastance (E in cm H_2O/L) and resistance (R in cm H_2O/L/sec). "Total" represents the total respiratory system (lung + chest wall). Values are means ± SD. *$P < .05$ versus baseline. There were no further reductions with increasing concentrations of isoflurane. *(Adapted from Ruiz P, Chartrand D: The effect of isoflurane 0.6% on respiratory mechanics in anesthetized-paralyzed humans is not increased at concentrations of 0.9% and 1.2%. Can J Anaesth 50:67, 2003, with permission.)*

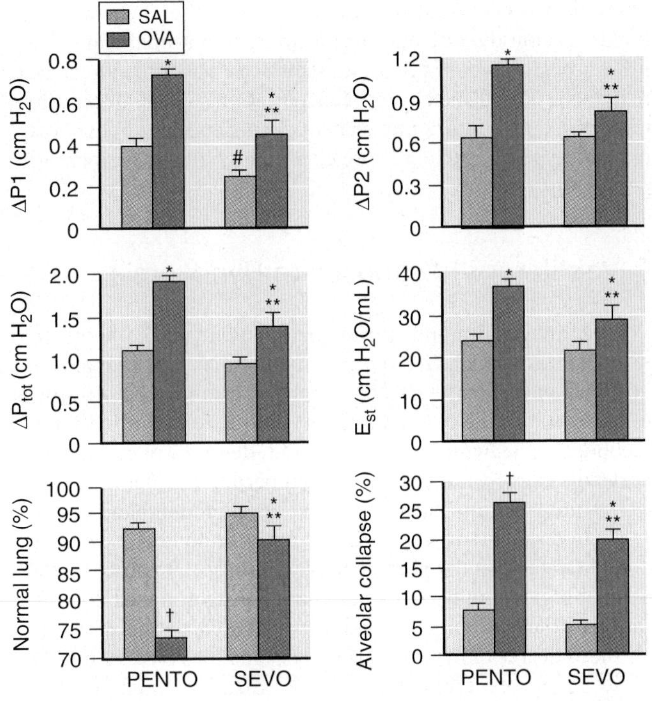

Figure 22-26 Mean ± SEM for ΔP1 (pressure to overcome airway resistance), ΔP2 (viscoelastic lung properties), ΔP_{tot} (total of ΔP1 and ΔP2), and E_{st}, static lung elastance. Also shown are percent normal area and percent alveolar collapse in mice repeatedly challenged with intratracheal instillation of saline (SAL) or ovalbumin (OVA). Animals were anesthetized with pentobarbital sodium (PENTO) or sevoflurane (SEVO), 1 minimum alveolar concentration. *$P < .05$ versus the corresponding SAL group. **$P < .001$ versus the OVA-PENTO group. #$P < .05$ versus the SAL-PENTO group. †$P < .001$ versus the SAL-PENTO group. *(Adapted from Burburan SM, Xisto D, Ferreira HC, et al: Lung mechanics and histology during sevoflurane anesthesia in a model of chronic allergic asthma. Anesth Analg 104:631, 2007, with permission.)*

pressure) in patients with or without coexisting disease. Inadequate respiratory system compensation for elevations in arterial carbon dioxide tension may occur in response to rebreathing of carbon dioxide from malfunctioning anesthetic circuits, from abdominal carbon dioxide insufflation during laparoscopic surgery, or as a result of increased metabolic production of the gas during anesthesia. The reduction in ventilatory drive induced by hypercapnia may also occur in the immediate postoperative period and can contribute to significant morbidity, especially in patients with chronic lung disease.

Experimental studies have shown that rebreathing carbon dioxide recruits expiratory respiratory muscles, including the internal intercostals, but is incapable of reversing the profound depression of parasternal intercostal muscle activity produced by halothane.[215] The peripheral chemoreceptor transduction (i.e., phrenic nerve response) to acute, severe carbon dioxide stimulation was also depressed by halothane in paralyzed, vagotomized dogs in a dose-related manner.[216] Carbon dioxide sensitivity was diminished, but not abolished, by concentrations of halothane usually required for surgical anesthesia. Furthermore, halothane depressed peripheral and central carbon dioxide sensitivity to similar degrees, but the peripheral chemoreceptors contributed only approximately 15% of the total carbon dioxide sensitivity.

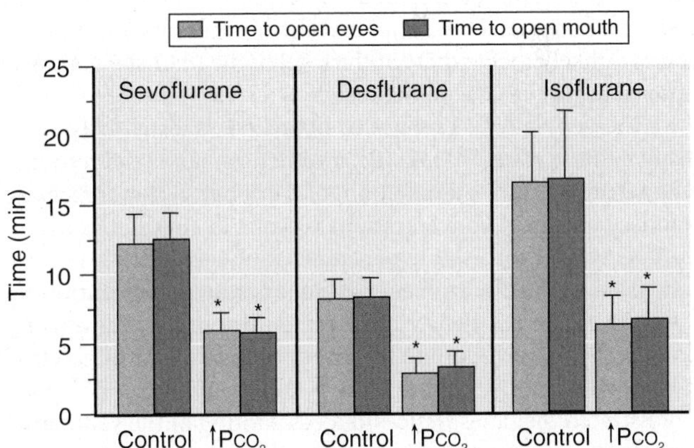

Figure 22-27 Average time between turning off the vaporizer and patients opening their eyes or mouth during the control condition (mild hypocapnia) and during hypercapnia (↑P_{CO_2}). Patients were anesthetized with either isoflurane, sevoflurane, or desflurane. Data are means ± SD. *$P < .05$ versus control—hypocapnia). *(Adapted from Sakata DJ, Golapakrishnan NA, Orr JA, et al: Rapid recovery from sevoflurane and desflurane with hypercapnia and hyperventilation. Anesth Analg 105:79, 2007; and Sakata DJ, Golapakrishnan NA, Orr JA, et al: Hypercapnic hyperventilation shortens emergence time from isoflurane anesthesia. Anesth Analg 104:587, 2007, with permission.)*

These data suggest that the response of peripheral chemoreceptors to carbon dioxide may appear to be of minimal clinical significance. However, if the response of peripheral chemoreceptors to hypoxia is abolished by low concentrations of volatile anesthetics, marked respiratory impairment during episodes of hypercapnia and hypoxia (such as those encountered in the perioperative period) may occur.

Ventilatory Responses to Hypoxemia

Volatile anesthetics and nitrous oxide attenuate the ventilatory response to hypoxia in experimental animals and humans in a dose-dependent manner.[217,218] Peripheral chemoreceptors appear to be the major site of this inhibitory action. Rapid inhibition (30 seconds) of the hypoxic response and reductions in carotid sinus nerve discharge were observed when peripheral chemoreceptors were stimulated during the administration of halothane (0.5% to 1.0%) to decerebrate cats.[219] Alternatively, Stuth and coworkers[220] demonstrated that the phrenic nerve response to hypoxia is attenuated, but not abolished, by halothane in vagotomized dogs. The cause of these differences may be attributed to the more pronounced degree of hypoxia (arterial oxygen tension < 40 mm Hg) achieved in experimental animals than in humans ($Pa{O_2}$ ~50 mm Hg). Volatile anesthetics attenuated the usual synergistic effect of hypoxia and hypercapnia on ventilation, but the ventilatory response to hypoxia depends on the degree to which arterial carbon dioxide tension exceeds the peripheral chemoreflex threshold rather than its elevation above resting partial pressure.[221] The response is also influenced by the presence of NO (and presumably fully functional pulmonary arterial endothelium).[222] This latter role of NO may be more complex because in addition to local release, NO is also released in the ventrolateral medulla after activation of peripheral chemoreceptors during hypoxia in response to sympathoexcitation.[223]

Halothane also produced a biphasic ventilatory response (similar to that observed in newborns) in kittens that have previously attained an adult-like hyperventilatory hypoxic response.[224] Whether the cause of this altered response during halothane anesthesia is mediated by peripheral chemoreceptors is unknown, but it is unlikely that activity at the level of the brainstem is solely responsible for this phenomenon.[225]

The ventilatory response to hypoxia is substantially more sensitive to the effects of volatile anesthetics than is the response to hypercapnia.[217,226] Attenuation of peripheral chemoreceptor responses occurs at concentrations of volatile anesthetics as low as 0.1 MAC. As with the hypercapnic ventilatory drive, controversy exists about the influence of subanesthetic concentrations of volatile agents on the hypoxic ventilatory drive. Administration of 0.1 MAC sevoflurane[227] or isoflurane has little to no effect on the hypoxic drive in humans.[228] Other investigators[229] have demonstrated that anesthetic-induced blunting of the ventilatory response to acute hypoxemia occurs with all volatile anesthetics except desflurane.[230] In analyzing studies on the effect of low concentrations of volatile anesthetics on hypoxic ventilatory responses (including negative studies), Pandit[231] proposed the following order of sensitivity: halothane (most depressant, 42%) > enflurane (52%) > isoflurane (71%) > sevoflurane (72%) > desflurane (96%) (Fig. 22-28). Notably, subanesthetic concentrations of desflurane decrease hypoxic sensitivity during hypercapnia, thus suggesting that this agent exerts an effect at the peripheral chemoreceptors.[230] The reasons for inconsistencies between many of these studies may be related to differences in the state of patient arousal during administration of the subanesthetic concentrations of volatile agent, the specific agent administered, the rate of application of the hypoxic stimulus, and the presence or absence of simultaneous hypercapnia. Attenuation of the acute hypoxic ventilatory response appears to be agent specific inasmuch as the effects of isoflurane, but not halothane or sevoflurane, were blunted in the presence of audiovisual stimulation.[217] The mechanisms by which low concentrations of volatile anesthetics attenuate the hypoxic ventilatory drive is unknown despite extensive study. Interestingly, administration of antioxidants to healthy volunteers reversed the attenuation of the hypoxic ventilatory response to halothane and isoflurane.[218] These results suggest that volatile anesthetics may depress the hypoxic response by influencing the oxidation-reduction state of oxygen-sensing elements in the carotid bodies (Fig. 22-29). How antioxidants mediate this response is unclear but may be related to actions on the mitochondrial electron transport chain, volatile anesthetic binding sites, or potassium channel function.

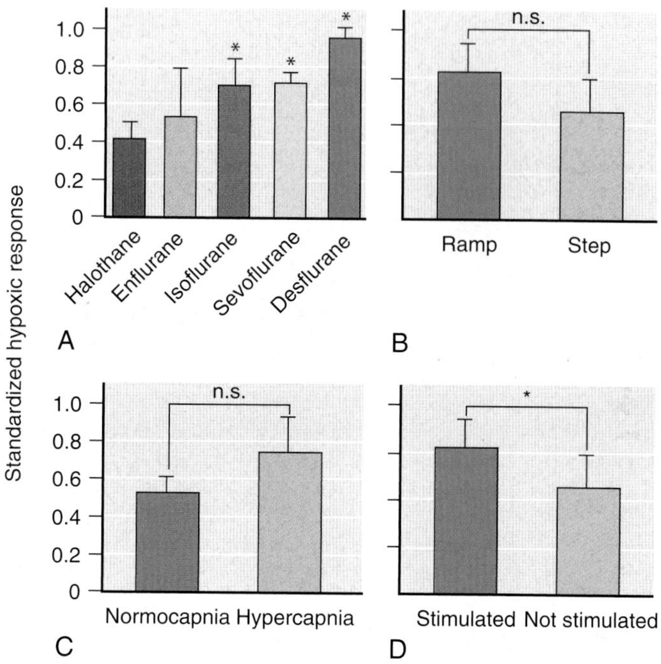

Figure 22-28 Analysis of data groups from 37 separate studies investigating the effect of low-dose volatile anesthetics on the acute ventilatory response to hypoxia in humans. **A,** Anesthetics depress the hypoxic ventilatory response in the order halothane > enflurane > isoflurane > sevoflurane > desflurane. $^*P < 0.05$ versus halothane. **B,** Data grouped according to the speed of the hypoxic stimulus. **C,** Data grouped according to background carbon dioxide. **D,** Data grouped according to whether the hypoxic challenge occurred in the presence or absence of subject stimulation. $^*P < .05$. *Error bars* represent 95% confidence intervals. *(Adapted from Pandit JJ: The variable effect of low-dose volatile anaesthetics on the acute ventilatory response to hypoxia in humans: A quantitative review. Anaesthesia 57:632, 2002, with permission.)*

The profound depression of hypoxic responsiveness produced by volatile anesthetics (with the exception of desflurane as noted earlier) suggests that patients may manifest a diminished ventilatory response to hypoxemia in the recovery room for some time after use of the agent has been discontinued. Audiovisual stimulation may attenuate the effects of low residual concentra-

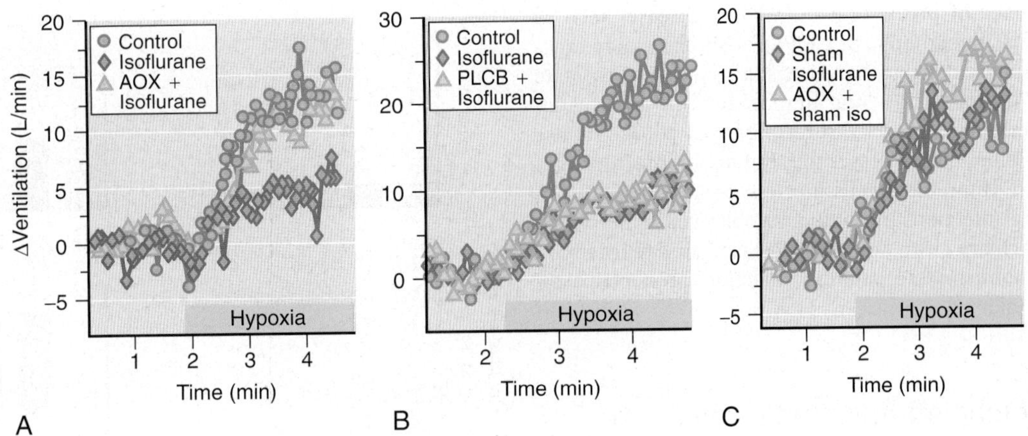

Figure 22-29 Effect of (sham) isoflurane, antioxidants (AOXs), and placebo on the acute hypoxic response in one individual. **A,** Depression of the hypoxic response by isoflurane and its reversal by antioxidants. **B,** Isoflurane reduces the hypoxic response, but placebo (PLCB) does not reverse it. **C,** Sham isoflurane or antioxidants do not significantly alter the hypoxic response. *(From Teppema LJ, Romber RR, Dahan A: Antioxidants reverse reduction of the human hypoxic ventilatory response by subanesthetic isoflurane. Anesthesiology 102:747, 2005, with permission.)*

tions of anesthetics in postoperative patients. In contrast, pain appears to be a poor stimulus to blunt the hypoxic ventilatory response to volatile agents. This phenomenon may be especially important in patients who depend to some degree on a hypoxic drive to establish their level of ventilation (e.g., those with chronic respiratory failure). In these circumstances, the ability of these patients to maintain adequate spontaneous ventilation in the presence of a volatile anesthetic may be severely impaired. Although there appear to be few clinically relevant differences between volatile anesthetics in hypoxia-induced depression of the ventilatory response in normal subjects, the effects in patients with pulmonary disease have not been studied extensively.

Hypoxia may occur postoperatively for several reasons. Diffusion hypoxia is well known and may occur during recovery from nitrous oxide anesthesia. Rapid elimination of nitrous oxide from blood to the alveoli combined with slower nitrogen diffusion reduces the alveolar oxygen concentration. In contrast, diffusion hypoxia may not occur during xenon anesthesia because the blood-gas partition coefficient of the noble gas (0.12) is similar to that of nitrogen and thus diffusion into alveoli may be slower.[66] The specific actions of xenon on the hypoxic ventilatory drive have not been clearly defined.

Acute Lung Injury

Mechanisms of Acute Lung Injury

Acute lung injury and acute respiratory distress syndrome are inflammatory disorders characterized by excessive infiltration of neutrophils, release of inflammatory mediators, and destruction of the alveolar-capillary membrane (also see Chapters 91 and 93). This series of events results in compromised gas exchange and pulmonary edema. There are a variety of causes of acute lung injury, including sepsis and positive-pressure ventilation. Endotoxin-induced lung injury is typified by hypoxemia resulting from a ventilation-perfusion mismatch with shunting through collapsed alveoli. This clinical condition associated with sepsis may be modeled in the laboratory by injection or inhalation of lipopolysaccharide, a component of the outer membrane of gram-negative bacteria. Lipopolysaccharides bind to Toll-like receptor 4 to activate nuclear factor κB, upregulate adhesion molecules, and stimulate cytokine-induced neutrophil migration into the pulmonary parenchyma. The alveolar epithelium, which may be injured by endotoxin, plays a critical role in maintaining alveolar homeostasis by the production of specific proteins, including surfactant and a variety of cytokines, and by clearing excess alveolar liquid. Notably, failure of the alveolar epithelium is even associated with increased mortality.[232]

Acute ventilator-induced lung injury is manifested as severe distention of and damage to bronchoalveolar structures, lung overinflation, and bronchiectasis.[233] Caveolae are flask-shaped invaginations of the plasma membrane that are involved in endocytosis, signal transduction, and transendothelial albumin transport. Caveolin-1, an integral membrane protein and component of endothelial caveolae, regulates the endothelial uptake and transport of albumin.[234] Inflammatory cytokines, including tumor necrosis factor-α, interleukin-1β, and macrophage inflammatory protein 2, may be released from alveolar epithelial cells, neutrophils, and macrophages. Cytokines are important mediators of leukocyte recruitment and activation. In general, attenuation of the cytokine response is considered beneficial in terms of reducing potential lung injury. Alternatively, in certain clinical situations such as immunocompromised patients, blunting of the release of inflammatory mediators and failure of neutrophil migration into the inflamed lung may predispose to a greater risk for pulmonary infections. Unfortunately, release of cytokines is highly variable and depends on experimental conditions. For example, altering the ventilation strategy alone may modify lung cytokine responses to lipopolysaccharide,[231] and positive-pressure ventilation in the absence of anesthesia may exacerbate the inflammatory responses.[235] The molecular mechanisms mediating acute lung injury have not been well defined. Nitric oxide, derived from inducible nitric oxide synthase (iNOS) in response to inflammation and endotoxin, appears to play an important role in acute lung injury inasmuch as inhibition of iNOS substantially reduced pulmonary lymph filtration and improved oxygenation during endotoxemia in conscious sheep.[236]

The presence of preexisting pulmonary disease, such as chronic bronchitis, pneumonia, or COPD, or smoking may exacerbate the pulmonary damage that occurs in response to an acute lung injury.[185] As with acute lung injury, smoking induces an inflammatory state. In contrast to acute lung injury, tobacco abuse increases the number but decreases the response of macrophages and neutrophils. Thus, these cells are less capable of releasing cytokines during infection. In addition, goblet cell hyperplasia, decreased mucociliary clearance, and increased airway reactivity occur and also contribute to potential infection, bronchospasm, and acute lung injury.[237]

Effects of Inhaled Anesthetics on Acute Lung Injury

Previous studies suggested that volatile anesthetics may augment the inflammatory response during mechanical ventilation,[238-240] but results of another investigation indicated that short-term positive-pressure ventilation with high tidal volumes does not affect systemic proinflammatory or anti-inflammatory cytokines in the lungs of healthy, isoflurane-anesthetized patients.[241] Volatile anesthetics have been shown to promote macrophage aggregation, enhance gene expression of proinflammatory cytokines,[238,242] (Fig. 22-30) exacerbate the extent of lung injury, and increase mortality after experimental aspiration.[240] Halothane also caused DNA and cell damage, nuclear fragmentation, and apoptotic-like changes in isolated pulmonary epithelial cells.[243] One mechanism by which volatile anesthetics may worsen acute lung injury is through an increase in alveolar membrane permeability. Halothane and isoflurane were found to transiently increase pulmonary vascular endothelial damage on radionuclide scanning.[244] Isoflurane also enhanced alveolar epithelial permeability in patients undergoing surgery.[245] Desflurane increased lipid peroxidation as measured in bronchoalveolar lavage samples from healthy surgical patients.[246] These data suggest that desflurane may promote pulmonary alveolar membrane injury. In contrast, sevoflurane caused less pronounced effects in this model, thus suggesting that this agent may exert a protective effect. Furthermore, isoflurane but not sevoflurane increased albumin permeability and transport in isolated rat lungs.[234] This deleterious action appeared to be related to enhancement of caveolin-1–mediated albumin uptake. Similarly, pretreatment with isoflurane but not sevoflurane enhanced neurogenic pulmonary edema in rats.[247] The proinflammatory response and enhanced cytokine levels in patients were also more pronounced after desflurane than after sevoflurane anesthesia.[242] In contrast to the transient effects of halothane and isoflurane, there were no significant effects on alveolar integrity or ultrastructure after high concentrations of sevoflurane were administered to pigs.[248] However, administration of sevoflurane to pigs[238] and healthy surgical patients[242] moderately enhanced inflammatory mediators such as leukotriene C_4, nitrate, nitrite, tumor necrosis factor-α, interleukin-1β, and interleukin-6. Inhalation of volatile anesthetics, including sevoflurane, was associated with an increase in proinflammatory cytokine protein from and gene expression in macrophages obtained from mechanically ventilated rats.[239] As with previous studies, sevoflurane appeared to produce relatively less pronounced effects than other volatile agents did. Oleic acid–induced lung injury was associated with impaired pulmonary gas exchange because of a ventilation-perfusion mismatch and shunting in mechanically ventilated dogs. Low concentrations of isoflurane exacerbated this impairment and worsened oxygen delivery.[249]

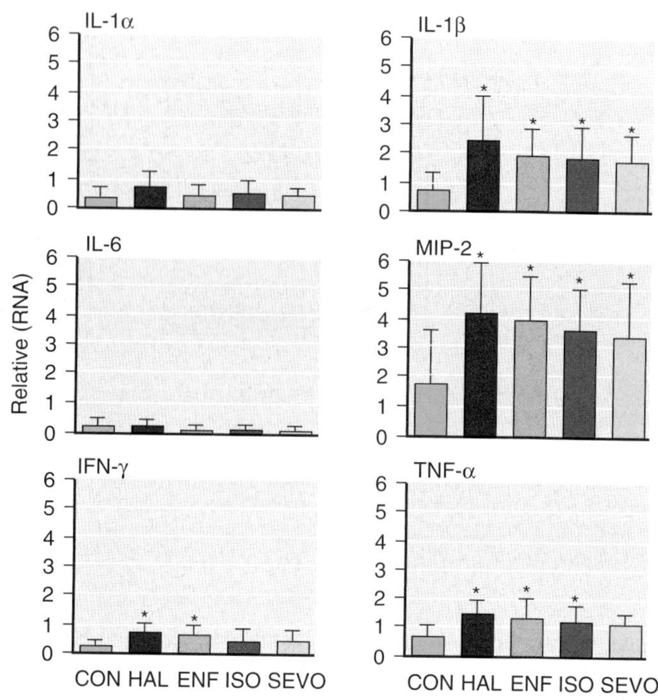

Figure 22-30 Changes in expression of proinflammatory cytokines from macrophages during mechanical ventilation without (CON, control) and with volatile anesthetics (HAL, halothane, ENF, enflurane, ISO, isoflurane, SEVO, sevoflurane). Values are the ratio of cytokine mRNA to β-actin mRNA and are presented as means ± SD. *$P < .05$ versus the control group (mechanical ventilation without volatile anesthetics). Gene expression for interleukin-1β (IL-1β), macrophage inflammatory protein 2 (MIP-2), interferon-γ (IFN-γ), and tumor necrosis factor-α (TNF-α) all increased significantly in comparison to mechanical ventilation alone. *(Adapted from Kotani N, Takahashi S, Sessler DI, et al: Volatile anesthetics augment expression of proinflammatory cytokines in rat alveolar macrophages by mechanical ventilation. Anesthesiology 91:187, 1999, with permission.)*

The actions of volatile anesthetics on lung inflammatory reactions are not clear. Under certain conditions, volatile anesthetics appear to play an anti-inflammatory and protective role in lung injury. One determinant of whether volatile anesthetics reduce or exacerbate pulmonary cytokine formation appears to be the cell types studied and the conditions under which the cytokine expression is measured. Volatile anesthetics increase the secretion and gene expression of some cytokines in alveolar macrophages but decrease the formation of proinflammatory cytokines in alveolar type II cells.[235,250,251] When compared with thiopental anesthesia, pigs anesthetized with sevoflurane exhibited reduced expression of tumor necrosis factor and interleukin-1β in lung tissue.[252] Pretreatment with 1.1% sevoflurane also significantly reduced the inflammatory response by alveolar type II cells exposed to lipopolysaccharide and attenuated the endotoxin-induced chemotaxis of neutrophils.[253] The latter data suggested another potential role of volatile agents in mediating inflammatory responses.

Under controlled conditions, volatile anesthetics tend to increase cytokine formation and appear to enhance inflammatory responses. In contrast, in models of lung acutely injured by stimulation with lipopolysaccharide, *Escherichia coli* endotoxin, or

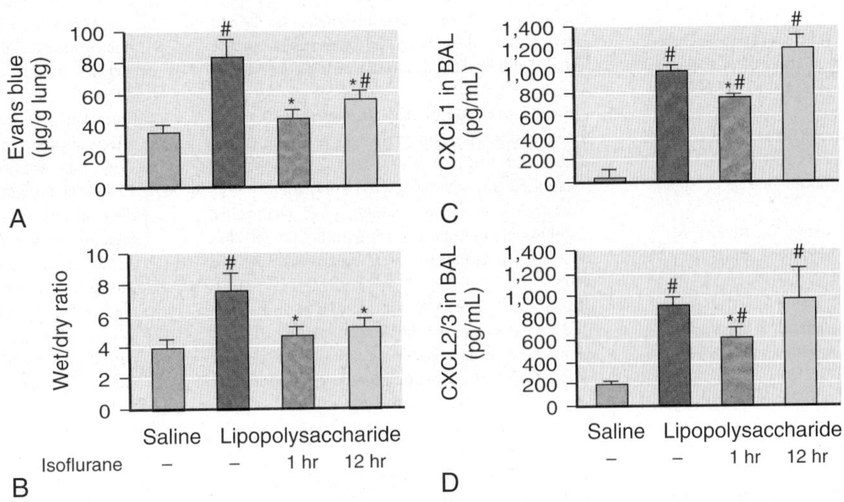

Figure 22-31 Capillary protein leakage measured by extravasation of Evans blue dye (**A**) and formation of lung edema measured by the ratio of wet to dry lung weight (**B**) in mice receiving saline, lipopolysaccharide, or isoflurane 1 or 12 hours before lipopolysaccharide. Endotoxin aerosol induced a significant increase in both capillary protein leakage and edema formation, which was reduced by pretreatment with isoflurane. **C** and **D,** Alveolar release of the two most important neutrophil-attracting chemokines CXCL1 and CXCL2/3 measured with an enzyme-linked immunosorbent assay 2 hours after receipt of lipopolysaccharide. Early, but not late (12 hour) isoflurane pretreatment reduced chemokine secretion significantly. Data are means ± SD. #Significant change between control and endotoxin-treated mice. *Significant difference between animals with and without isoflurane treatment. *(Adapted from Reutershan J, Chang D, Hayes JK, Ley K: Protective effects of isoflurane pretreatment in endotoxin-induced lung injury. Anesthesiology 104:511, 2006, with permission.)*

interleukin-1β, volatile anesthetics appear to exert anti-inflammatory effects, including inhibition of cytokine formation, reduction of neutrophil migration into the lung interstitium and alveolar space, and attenuation of protein leakage and pulmonary edema (Fig. 22-31).[235,250,251] Peri-ischemic inhalation of low concentrations of sevoflurane appears to provide endothelial protection in humans subjected to forearm ischemia-reperfusion injury.[254] Inhibition of leukocyte adhesion has been postulated as a mechanism for this protection. Isoflurane, given after the initiation of ischemia, also protects against warm ischemia-reperfusion injury in an isolated, perfused rat lung model.[255] This protective effect may be related to modulation of potassium channels and prevention of excessive intracellular calcium overload. Hypoxia induces a series of responses, including erythropoiesis, angiogenesis, and glycolysis, to maintain homeostasis. Under hypoxic conditions, hypoxia inducible factor is responsible for the activation of hypoxia-responsive genes, such as iNOS, heme oxygenase, and vascular endothelial growth factor, in the lung. Exposure of isolated cells to isoflurane resulted in significant increases in hypoxia inducible factor 1α, and enhanced gene expression for hypoxia-responsive genes.[256] Whether these actions are involved in the protective effects of volatile anesthetics in acute lung injury remains unknown. The specific effects of nitrous oxide or xenon on pulmonary inflammatory reactions or acute lung injury remain to be examined.

Summary

Inhaled anesthetics have potent and clinically significant effects on respiratory function. Volatile anesthetics reduce bronchial smooth muscle tone, adversely affect mucociliary function, and dilate the pulmonary vasculature. Volatile anesthetics also alter the activity of respiratory sensors, the central nervous system, and muscles of respiration. These actions are mediated by direct effects on pulmonary parenchyma and indirect actions on afferent, central, and efferent neural pathways. The depressant effects of these volatile anesthetics are further enhanced in patients with pulmonary disorders. The inhaled anesthetics nitrous oxide and xenon also affect the respiratory system. Although many actions of xenon have not been as well described, this agent is unusual in that it increases tidal breathing and decreases the respiratory rate, an action opposite that of other anesthetics. The effects of volatile anesthetics on acute lung injury have been described as both proinflammatory and anti-inflammatory. Further investigations are needed to determine the precise role of these agents as friend or foe. An understanding of the multifactorial actions of inhaled anesthetics on the respiratory system is critical to the safe delivery of anesthesia.

References

1. Forrest JB, Rehder K, Cahalan MK, et al: Multicenter study of general anesthesia. III Predictors of severe perioperative adverse outcomes. Anesthesiology 76:3, 1992.
2. Pizov R, Brown RH, Weiss YS, et al: Wheezing during induction of general anesthesia in patients with and without asthma. A randomized, blinded trial. Anesthesiology 82:1111, 1995.
3. Cheney FW, Posner KL, Caplan RA: Adverse respiratory events infrequently leading to malpractice suits. A closed system analysis. Anesthesiology 75:932, 1991.
4. Pinto-Pereira LM, Orrett A, Balbirsingh M: Physiological perspectives of therapy in bronchial hyperreactivity. Can J Anaesth 43:700, 1996.
5. Kai T, Yoshimura H, Jones KA, et al: Relationship between force and regulatory myosin light chain phosphorylation in airway smooth muscle.

Am J Physiol Lung Cell Mol Physiol 279:L52, 2000.

6. Prakash YS, Kannan MS, Walseth TF, et al: Role of cyclic ADP ribose in the regulation of $[Ca^{2+}]i$ in porcine tracheal smooth muscle. Am J Physiol Cell Physiol 274:C1653, 1998.
7. Rho EH, Perkins WJ, Lorenz RR, et al: Differential effects of soluble and particulate guanylyl cyclase on Ca^{2+} sensitivity in airway smooth muscle. J Appl Physiol 92:257, 2002.
8. Hirshman CA, Lande B, Croxton TL: Role of M_2 muscarinic receptors in airway smooth muscle contraction. Life Sci 64:443, 1999.
9. Groeben H, Brown RH: Ipratropium decreases airway size in dogs by preferential M_2 muscarinic receptor blockade in vivo. Anesthesiology 85:867, 1996.
10. Emala CW, McQuitty CK, Eleff SM, et al: Asthma, allergy, and airway hyperresponsiveness are not linked to the beta(2)-adrenoceptor gene. Chest 121:722, 2002.
11. Park KW, Sato K, Dai HB, et al: Epithelium-dependent bronchodilatory activity is preserved in pig bronchioles after normothermic cardiopulmonary bypass. Anesth Analg 90:778, 2000.
12. Fehr JJ, Hirshman CA, Emala CW: Cellular signaling by the potent bronchoconstrictor endothelin-1 in airway smooth muscle. Crit Care Med 28:1884, 2000.
13. D'Angelo E, Calderini IS, Tavola M: The effects of CO_2 on respiratory mechanics in anesthetized paralyzed humans. Anesthesiology 94:604, 2001.
14. Mazzeo AJ, Cheng EY, Stadnicka A, et al: Topographic differences in the direct effects of isoflurane on airway smooth muscle. Anesth Analg 78:948, 1994.
15. Park KW, Dai HB, Lowenstein E, et al: Isoflurane- and halothane-mediated dilation of distal bronchi in the rat depends on the epithelium. Anesthesiology 86:1078, 1997.
16. Habre W, Petak F, Sly PD, et al: Protective effects of volatile agents against methacholine-induced bronchoconstriction in rats. Anesthesiology 94:348, 2001.
17. Brown RH, Mitzner W, Zerhouni E, et al: Direct in vivo visualization of bronchodilation induced by inhalational anesthesia using high-resolution computed tomography. Anesthesiology 78:295, 1993.
18. Brown RH, Zerhouni E, Hirshman CA: Comparison of low concentrations of halothane and isoflurane as bronchodilators. Anesthesiology 78:1097, 1993.
19. Yamamoto K, Morimoto N, Warner DO, et al: Factors influencing the direct actions of volatile anesthetics on airway smooth muscle. Anesthesiology 78:1102, 1993.
20. Mitsuhata H, Saitoh J, Shimizu R, et al: Sevoflurane and isoflurane protect against bronchospasm in dogs. Anesthesiology 81:1230, 2004.
21. Katoh T, Ikeda KCJA: A comparison of sevoflurane with halothane, enflurane, and isoflurane on bronchoconstriction caused by histamine. Can J Anaesth 41:1214, 1994.
22. Cheng EY, Mazzeo AJ, Bosnjak ZJ, et al: Direct relaxant effects of intravenous anesthetics on airway smooth muscle. Anesth Analg 83:162, 1996.
23. Mazzeo AJ, Cheng EY, Bosnjak ZJ, et al: Differential effects of desflurane and halothane on peripheral airway smooth muscle. Br J Anaesth 76:841, 1996.
24. Goff MJ, Arain SR, Ficke DJ, et al: Absence of bronchodilation during desflurane anesthesia: A comparison to sevoflurane and thiopental. Anesthesiology 93:404, 2000.
25. Yamakage M, Chen X, Tsuijiguchi N, et al: Different inhibitory effects of volatile anesthetics on T- and L-type voltage-dependent Ca^{2+} channels in porcine tracheal and bronchial smooth muscles. Anesthesiology 94:683, 2001.
26. Crawford MW, Arrica M, Macgowan CK, Yoo S-J: Extent and localization of changes in upper airway caliber with varying concentrations of sevoflurane in children. Anesthesiology 105:1147, 2006.
27. Dikmen Y, Eminoglou E, Salihoglou Z, Demiroluk S: Pulmonary mechanics during isoflurane, sevoflurane and desflurane anesthesia. Anaesthesia 58:745, 2003.
28. Hashimoto Y, Hirota K, Ohtomo N, et al: In vivo direct measurement of the bronchodilating effect of sevoflurane using a superfine fiberoptic bronchoscope: Comparison with enflurane and halothane. J Cardiothorac Vasc Anesth 10:213, 1996.
29. Iwasaki S, Yamakage M, Satoh J-I, Namiki A: Different inhibitory effects of sevoflurane on hyperreactive airway smooth muscle contractility in ovalbumin-sensitized and chronic cigarette-smoking guinea pig models. Anesthesiology 105:753, 2006.
30. Yamakage M: Direct inhibitory mechanisms of halothane on canine tracheal smooth muscle contraction. Anesthesiology 77:546, 1992.
31. Nyktari VG, Papaioannou AA, Prinianakis G, et al: Effect of the physical properties of isoflurane, sevoflurane and desflurane on pulmonary resistance in a laboratory lung model. Anesthesiology 104:1202, 2006.
32. Kai T, Jones KA, Warner DO: Halothane attenuates calcium sensitization in airway smooth muscle by inhibiting G-proteins. Anesthesiology 89:1543, 1998.
33. Janssen LJ: T-type and L-type Ca^{2+} currents in canine bronchial smooth muscle: Characterization and physiological roles. Am J Physiol Cell Physiol 272:C1757, 1997.
34. Chen X, Yamakage M, Namiki A: Inhibitory effects of volatile anesthetics on K^+ and Cl^- channel currents in porcine tracheal and bronchial smooth muscle. Anesthesiology 96:458, 2002.
35. Yamakage M, Chen X, Kimura A, et al: The repolarizing effects of volatile anesthetics on porcine tracheal and bronchial smooth muscle cells. Anesth Analg 94:84, 2002.
36. Fukushima T, Hirasaki A, Jones KA, et al: Halothane and potassium channels in airway smooth muscle. Br J Anaesth 76:847, 1996.
37. Pabelick CM, Prakash YS, Kannan MS, et al: Effect of halothane on intracellular calcium oscillations in porcine tracheal smooth muscle cells. Am J Physiol Lung Cell Mol Physiol 276:L81, 1999.
38. Pabelick CM, Prakash YS, Kannan MS, et al: Effects of halothane on sarcoplasmic reticulum calcium release channels in porcine airway smooth muscle cells. Anesthesiology 95:207, 2001.
39. Kai T, Bremerich DH, Jones KA, Warner DO: Drug-specific effects of volatile anesthetics on Ca^{2+} sensitization in airway smooth muscle. Anesthesiology 87:425, 1998.
40. Hanazaki M, Jones KA, Perkins WJ, et al: Halothane increases smooth muscle protein phosphatase in airway smooth muscle. Anesthesiology 94:129, 2001.
41. Jones KA, Wong GY, Jankowski CJ, et al: cGMP modulation of Ca^{2+} sensitivity in airway smooth muscle. Am J Physiol Lung Cell Mol Physiol 276:L35, 1999.
42. Morimoto N, Yamamoto K, Jones KA, et al: Halothane and pertussis toxin–sensitive G proteins in airway smooth muscle. Anesth Analg 78:328, 1994.
43. Sakihara C, Perkins WJ, Warner DO, Jones KA: Anesthetics inhibit acetylcholine-promoted guanine nucleotide exchange of heterotrimeric G proteins of airway smooth muscle. Anesthesiology 101:120, 2004.
44. Duracher C, Blanc F-X, Gueugniaud P-Y, et al: The effects of isoflurane on airway kinetics in Fisher and Lewis rats. Anesth Analg 101:136, 2005.
45. Park KW, Dai HB, Lowenstein E, et al: Epithelial dependence of the bronchodilatory effect of sevoflurane and desflurane in rat distal bronchi. Anesth Analg 86:646, 1998.
46. Mougdil GC: The patient with reactive airways disease. Can J Anaesth 44:R77, 1997.
47. Warner DO, Brichant J-F, Rehder K: Direct and neurally mediated effects of halothane on pulmonary resistance in vivo. Anesthesiology 72:1057, 1990.
48. Wiklund CU, Lim S, Lindsten U, et al: Relaxation by sevoflurane, desflurane and halothane in the isolated guinea-pig trachea via inhibition of cholinergic neurotransmission. Br J Anaesth 83:422, 1999.
49. Lindeman KS, Baker SG, Hirshman CA: Interaction between halothane and the nonadrenergic, noncholinergic inhibitory system in porcine trachealis muscle. Anesthesiology 81:641, 1994.
50. Akhtar S, Brull SJ: Effect of isoflurane on endothelin-1 mediated airway smooth muscle contraction. Pulm Pharmacol Ther 11:227, 1998.
51. Arakawa H, Takizawa T, Tokuyama K, et al: Efficacy of inhaled anticholinergics and anesthesia in treatment of a patient in status asthmaticus. J Asthma 39:77, 2002.
52. Saulnier FF, Durocher AV, Deturck RA, et al: Respiratory and hemodynamic effects of halothane in status asthmaticus. Intensive Care Med 16:104, 1990.
53. Rooke GA, Choi J-H, Bishop MJ: The effect of isoflurane, halothane, sevoflurane, and thiopental/nitrous oxide on respiratory system resistance after tracheal intubation. Anesthesiology 86:1294, 1997.
54. Tobias JD, Hirshman CA: Attenuation of histamine-induced airway constriction by albuterol during halothane anesthesia. Anesthesiology 72:105, 1990.
55. Wu RSC, Wu KC, Wong TKM, et al: Isoflurane anesthesia does not add to the bronchodilating effect of a beta 2-adrenergic agonist after tracheal intubation. Anesth Analg 83:238, 1996.
56. Yamakage M, Tsujiguchi N, Hattori J-I, et al: Low-temperature modification of the inhibitory effects of volatile anesthetics on airway smooth muscle contraction in dogs. Anesthesiology 93:179, 2000.
57. Volta CA, Alvisi V, Petrini S, el al: The effect of volatile anesthetics on respiratory system resistance in patients with chronic obstructive pulmonary disease. Anesth Analg 100:348, 2005.
58. Burburan SM, Xisto D, Ferreira HC, et al: Lung mechanics and histology during sevoflurane anesthesia in a model of chronic allergic asthma. Anesth Analg 104:631, 2007.
59. Goto T, Nakata Y, Morita, S: Will xenon be a stranger or a friend? The cost, benefit, and future of xenon anesthesia. Anesthesiology 98:1, 2003.
60. Preckel B, Weber NC, Sanders RD, et al: Molecular mechanisms transducing the anesthetic, analgesic, and organ-protective actions of xenon. Anesthesiology 105:187, 2006.
61. Rueckoldt H, Vangerow B, Marx G, et al: Xenon inhalation increases airway pressure in ventilated patients. Acta Anaesthesiol Scand 43:1060, 1999.
62. Calzia E, Stahl W, Handschuh T, et al: Respiratory mechanics during xenon anesthesia in pigs: Comparison with nitrous oxide. Anesthesiology 91:1378, 1999.

63. Fujii Y: Respiratory effects of xenon. Int Anesthesiol Clin 39:95, 2001.
64. Zhang P, Ohara A, Mashimo T, et al: Pulmonary resistance in dogs: A comparison of xenon with nitrous oxide. Can J Anaesth 42:547, 1995.
65. Lachmann B, Armbruster S, Schairer W, et al: Safety and efficacy of xenon in routine use as an inhalational anaesthetic. Lancet 335:1413, 1995.
66. Calzia E, Stahl W, Handschuh T, et al: Continuous arterial Po_2 and Pco_2 measurements in swine during nitrous oxide and xenon elimination: Prevention of diffusion. Anesthesiology 90:829, 1999.
67. Lund V: Nasal physiology: Neurochemical receptors, nasal cycle, and ciliary action. Allergy Asthma Proc 17:179, 1996.
68. Lindberg S, Cervin A, Runer T: Low levels of nasal nitric oxide (NO) correlate to impaired mucociliary function in the upper airways. Acta Otolaryngol 117:728, 1997.
69. Wagner EM, Foster WM: Importance of airway blood flow on particle clearance from the lung. J Appl Physiol 81:1878, 1996.
70. Keller C, Brimacombe J: Bronchial mucus transport velocity in paralyzed anesthetized patients: A comparison of the laryngeal mask airway and cuffed tracheal tube. Anesth Analg 86:1280, 1998.
71. Raphael JH, Butt MW: Comparison of isoflurane with propofol on respiratory cilia. Br J Anaesth 79:473, 1997.
72. Iida H, Matsuura S, Tanimoto K, Fukuda K: Differential effects of intravenous anesthetics on ciliary motility in cultured rat tracheal epithelial cells. Can J Anaesth 53:242, 2006.
73. Raphael JH, Selwyn DA, Mottram SD, et al: Effects of 3 MAC of halothane, enflurane and isoflurane on cilia beat frequency of human nasal epithelium in vitro. Br J Anaesth 76:116, 1996.
74. Raphael JH, Stupish J, Selwyn DA, et al: Recovery of respiratory depression by inhalation anaesthetic agents: An in vitro study using nasal turbinate explants. Br J Anaesth 76:854, 1996.
75. Matsuura S, Shirakami G, Iada H, et al: The effect of sevoflurane on ciliary motility in rat cultured tracheal epithelial cells: A comparison with isoflurane and halothane. Anesth Analg 102:1703, 2006.
76. Gamsu G, Singer MM, Vincent HH, et al: Postoperative impairment of mucous transport in the lung. Am Rev Respir Dis 114:673, 1976.
77. Lichtiger M, Landa JF, Hirsch JA: Velocity of tracheal mucus in anesthetized women undergoing gynecologic surgery. Anesthesiology 42:753, 1975.
78. Konrad F, Marx T, Schraag M, et al: Combination anesthesia and bronchial transport velocity. Effects of anesthesia with isoflurane, fentanyl, vecuronium and oxygen–nitrous oxide breathing on bronchial mucus transport. Anaesthesist 46:403, 1997.
79. Konrad FX, Shreiber T, Brecht-Kraus D, et al: Bronchial mucus transport in chronic smokers and nonsmokers during general anesthesia. J Clin Anesth 5:375, 1993.
80. Rivero DH, Lorenzi-Filho G, Pazetti R, et al: Effects of bronchial transection and reanastomosis on mucociliary system. Chest 119:1510, 2001.
81. Ledowski T, Paech MJ, Patel B, Schug SA: Bronchial mucus transport velocity in patients receiving propofol and remifentanil versus sevoflurane and remifentanil anesthesia. Anesth Analg 102:1427, 2006.
82. Molliex S, Cresani B, Dureuil B, et al: Effects of halothane on surfactant biosynthesis by rat alveolar type II cells in primary culture. Anesthesiology 81:668, 1994.
83. Yang T, Li Y, Liu Q, et al: Isoflurane aggravates the decrease of phosphatidylcholine synthesis in alveolar type II cells induced by hydrogen peroxide. Drug Metab Drug Interact 18:243, 2001.
84. Patel AB, Sokolowski J, Davidson BA, et al: Halothane potentiation of hydrogen peroxide–induced inhibition of surfactant synthesis: The role of type II cell energy status. Anesth Analg 94:943, 2002.
85. Molliex S, Dureuil B, Aubier M, et al: Halothane decreases Na,K-ATPase, and Na channel activity in alveolar type II cells. Anesthesiology 88:1606, 1998.
86. Li Y, Yang T, Liu Q, et al: Effect of isoflurane on proliferation and Na^+, K^+-ATPase activity of alveolar type II cells injured by hydrogen peroxide. Drug Metabl Drug Interact 20:175, 2004.
87. Rezaiguai-Delclaux S, Jayr C, Feng Luo D, et al: Halothane and isoflurane decrease alveolar epithelial fluid clearance in rats. Anesthesiology 88:751, 1998.
88. Paugam-Burtz C, Molliex S, Lardeux B, et al: Differential effects of halothane and thiopental on surfactant protein C messenger RNA in vivo and in vitro in rats. Anesthesiology 93:805, 2000.
89. Sweeney M, Beddy D, Honner V, et al: Effects of changes in pH and CO_2 on pulmonary arterial wall tension are not endothelium dependent. J Appl Physiol 85:2040, 1998.
90. Myers JL, Wizorek JJ, Myers AK, et al: Pulmonary arterial endothelial dysfunction potentiates hypercapnic vasoconstriction and alters the response to inhaled nitric oxide. Ann Thorac Surg 62:1677, 1996.
91. Hampl V, Herget J: Role of NO in the pathogenesis of chronic pulmonary hypertension. Physiol Rev 80:1337, 2000.
92. Johns RA: New mechanisms for inhaled NO: Release of an endogenous NO inhibitor? Anesthesiology 95:3, 2001.
93. Wang T, El Kabir D, Blaise G: Inhaled nitric oxide in 2003: A review of its mechanisms of action. Can J Anaesth 50:315, 2003.
94. Hambraeus-Jonzon K, Chen L, Freden F, et al: Pulmonary vasoconstriction during regional nitric oxide inhalation. Evidence of a blood-borne regulator of nitric oxide synthase activity. Anesthesiology 95:102, 2001.
95. Scherrer U, Vollenweider L, Delabays A, et al: Inhaled nitric oxide for high-altitude pulmonary edema. N Engl J Med 334:624, 1996.
96. Takahashi Y, Kobatashi H, Tanaka N, et al: Worsening of hypoxemia with nitric oxide inhalation during bronchospasm in humans. Respir Physiol 112:113, 1998.
97. Zanaboni P, Murray PA, Simon BA, et al: Selective endothelial dysfunction in conscious dogs after cardiopulmonary bypass. J Appl Physiol 82:1776, 1997.
98. Nachar RA, Pastene CM, Herrera EA, et al: Low-dose inhaled carbon monoxide reduces pulmonary vascular resistance during acute hypoxemia in adult sheep. High Alt Med Biol 2:377, 2001.
99. Bryan RM Jr, You J, Golding EM, Marrelli SP: Endothelium-derived hyperpolarizing factor. Anesthesiology 102:1261, 2005.
100. Galvin I, Drummond GB, Nirmalan M: Distribution of blood flow and ventilation in the lung: Gravity is not the only factor. Br J Anaesth 98:420, 2007.
101. Preston JR: Clinical perspective of hypoxia-mediated pulmonary hypertension. Antioxid Redox Signal 9:711, 2007.
102. Weissmann N, Sommer N, Schermuly RT, et al: Oxygen sensors in hypoxic pulmonary vasoconstriction. Cardiovasc Res 71:620, 2006.
103. Adding LC, Agvald P, Persson MG, et al: Regulation of pulmonary nitric oxide by carbon dioxide is intrinsic to the lung. Acta Anaesthesiol Scand 167:167, 1999.
104. Yamamoto Y, Nakano H, Ide H, et al: Role of airway nitric oxide on the regulation of pulmonary circulation by carbon dioxide. J Appl Physiol 91:1121, 2001.
105. Akata T: General anesthetics and vascular smooth muscle. Direct actions of general anesthetics on cellular mechanisms regulating vascular tone. Anesthesiology 106:365, 2007.
106. Gambone LM, Fujiwara Y, Murray PA: Endothelium-dependent pulmonary vasodilation is selectively attenuated during isoflurane anesthesia. Am J Physiol Heart Circ Physiol 272:H290, 1997.
107. Seki S, Sato K, Nakayama M, et al: Halothane and enflurane attenuate pulmonary vasodilation mediated by adenosine triphosphate–sensitive potassium channels compared to the conscious state. Anesthesiology 86:923, 1997.
108. Nakayama M, Kondo U, Murray PA: Pulmonary vasodilator response to adenosine triphosphate–sensitive potassium channel activation is attenuated during desflurane but preserved during sevoflurane anesthesia compared with the conscious state. Anesthesiology 88:1023, 1998.
109. Lennon PF, Murray PA: Isoflurane and the pulmonary vascular pressure-flow relation at baseline and during sympathetic α- and β-adrenoceptor activation in chronically instrumented dogs. Anesthesiology 82:723, 1995.
110. Sato K, Seki S, Murray PA: Effects of halothane and enflurane anesthesia on sympathetic β-adrenoreceptor–mediated pulmonary vasodilation in chronically instrumented dogs. Anesthesiology 97:478, 2002.
111. Liu R, Ishibe Y, Okazaki N, et al: Volatile anesthetics regulate pulmonary vascular tension through different potassium channel subtypes in isolated rabbit lungs. Can J Anaesth 50:301, 2003.
112. Fujiwara Y, Murray PA: Effects of isoflurane anesthesia on pulmonary vascular response to K^+ ATP cannel activation and circulatory hypotension in chronically instrumented dogs. Anesthesiology 90:799, 1999.
113. Su JY, Vo AC: Ca^{2+}-calmodulin–dependent protein kinase II plays a major role in halothane-induced dose-dependent relaxation in the skinned pulmonary artery. Anesthesiology 97:207, 2002.
114. Zhong L, Su JY: Isoflurane activates PKC and Ca^{2+}-calmodulin–dependent protein kinase II via MAP kinase signaling in cultured vascular smooth muscle cells. Anesthesiology 96:148, 2002.
115. Lennon PF, Murray PA: Attenuated hypoxic pulmonary vasoconstriction during isoflurane anesthesia is abolished by cyclooxygenase inhibition in chronically instrumented dogs. Anesthesiology 84:404, 1996.
116. Johns RA: Endothelium, anesthetics, and vascular control. Anesthesiology 79:1381, 1993.
117. Marshall C, Marshall BE: Endothelium-derived relaxing factor is not responsible for inhibition of hypoxic pulmonary vasoconstriction by inhalational anesthetics. Anesthesiology 73:441, 1990.
118. Marshall C, Marshall BE: Inhalational anesthetics directly inhibit hypoxic pulmonary vasoconstriction. Anesthesiology 79:A1238, 1993.
119. Yoshida K, Tewari S, Kirby T, et al: Halothane attenuates acetylcholine-induced vasorelaxation and cyclic GMP accumulation in human pulmonary artery. Anesthesiology 87:A1104, 1997.
120. Gambone LM, Murray PA, Flavahan NA: Isoflurane anesthesia attenuates endothelium-dependent

pulmonary vasorelaxation by inhibiting the synergistic interaction between nitric oxide and prostacyclin. Anesthesiology 86:936, 1997.
121. Liu R, Ueda M, Okazaki N, et al: Role of potassium channels in isoflurane- and sevoflurane-induced attenuation of hypoxic pulmonary vasoconstriction in isolated perfused rabbit lungs. Anesthesiology 95:939, 2001.
122. Carter EP, Sato K, Morio Y, et al: Inhibition of K_{Ca} channels restores blunted hypoxic pulmonary vasoconstriction in rats with cirrhosis. Am J Physiol Lung Cell Mol Physiol 279:L903, 2000.
123. Eisenkraft JB: Effects of anaesthetics on pulmonary circulation. Br J Anaesth 65:63, 1990.
124. Lesitsky MA, Davis S, Murray PA: Preservation of hypoxic pulmonary vasoconstriction during sevoflurane and desflurane anesthesia compared to the conscious state in chronically instrumented dogs. Anesthesiology 89:1501, 1998.
125. Kerbaul F, Guidon C, Stephanazzi J, et al: Sub-MAC concentrations of desflurane do not inhibit hypoxic pulmonary vasoconstriction in anesthetized piglets. Can J Anaesth 48:760, 2001.
126. Schwarzkopf K, Shreiber T, Gaser E, et al: The effects of xenon or nitrous oxide supplementation on systemic oxygenation and pulmonary perfusion during one-lung ventilation in pigs. Anesth Analg 100:335, 2005.
127. Schwarzkopf K, Shreiber T, Preussler NP, et al: Lung perfusion, shunt fraction, and oxygenation during one-lung ventilation in pigs: The effects of desflurane, isoflurane, and propofol. J Cardiothorac Vasc Anesth 17:73, 2003.
128. Karzai W, Haberstroh J, Priebe HJ: The effects of increasing concentrations of desflurane on systemic oxygenation during one-lung ventilation in pigs. Anesth Analg 89:215, 1999.
129. Schwarzkopf K, Shreiber T, Bauer R, et al: The effects of increasing concentrations of isoflurane and desflurane on pulmonary perfusion and systemic oxygenation during one-lung ventilation in pigs. Anesth Analg 93:1434, 2001.
130. Kleinsasser A, Lindner KA, Hoermann C, et al: Isoflurane and sevoflurane anesthesia in pigs with a preexistant gas exchange defect. Anesthesiology 95:1422, 2001.
131. Nishiwaki K, Nyhan DP, Rock P, et al: *N*-nitro-L-arginine and pulmonary vascular pressure-flow relationship in conscious dogs. Am J Physiol Heart Circ Physiol 262:H1331, 1992.
132. Abe K, Mashimo T, Yoshiya I: Arterial oxygenation and shunt fraction during one-lung ventilation: A comparison of isoflurane and sevoflurane. Anesth Analg 86:266, 1998.
133. Reid CW, Slinger PD, Lenis S: A comparison of the effects of propofol-alfentanil versus isoflurane anesthesia on arterial oxygenation during one-lung ventilation. J Cardiothorac Vasc Anesth 10:860, 1996.
134. Beck DH, Doepner UR, Sinemus C, et al: Effects of sevoflurane and propofol on pulmonary shunt fraction during one-lung ventilation for thoracic surgery. Br J Anaesth 86:38, 2001.
135. Kellow NH, Scott AD, White SA, Feneck RO: Comparison of the effects of propofol and isoflurane anaesthesia on right ventricular function and shunt fraction during thoracic surgery. Br J Anaesth 75:578, 1995.
136. Abe K, Shimizu T, Takashina M, et al: The effects of propofol, isoflurane and sevoflurane on oxygenation and shunt fraction during one-lung ventilation. Anesth Analg 87:1164, 1998.
137. Pruszkowski O, Dalibon N, Moutafis M, et al: Effects of propofol vs sevoflurane on arterial oxygenation during one-lung ventilation. Br J Anaesth 98:539, 2007.
138. Benumof JL, Augustine SD, Gibbons JA: Halothane and isoflurane only slightly impair arterial oxygenation during one-lung ventilation in patients undergoing thoracotomy. Anesthesiology 67:910, 1987.
139. Pagel P, Fu FL, Damask MC, et al: Desflurane and isoflurane produce similar alterations in systemic and pulmonary hemodynamics and arterial oxygenation in patients undergoing one-lung ventilation during thoracotomy. Anesth Analg 87:800, 1998.
140. Carlsson AJ, Bindslev L, Hedenstierna G: Hypoxia-induced pulmonary vasoconstriction in the human lung: The effect of isoflurane anesthesia. Anesthesiology 66:312, 1987.
141. Liu R, Ishibe Y, Ueda M, et al: Isoflurane administration before ischemia and during reperfusion attenuates ischemia/reperfusion-induced injury of isolated rabbit lungs. Anesth Analg 89:561, 1999.
142. Doi S, Smedira N, Murray PA: Pulmonary vasoregulation by endothelin in conscious dogs after left lung transplantation. J Appl Physiol 88:210, 2000.
143. Lennon PF, Murray PA: Pulmonary vascular effects of isoflurane anesthesia after left lung autotransplantation in chronically instrumented dogs. Anesthesiology 85:592, 1996.
144. Forster HV, Pan L, Lowry TF, et al: Important role of carotid chemoreceptor afferents in control of breathing of adult and neonatal mammals. Respir Physiol 119:199, 2000.
145. Widdicombe J: Reflexes from the lungs and airways: Historical perspective. J Appl Physiol 101:628, 2006.
146. Yu J: Airway mechanosensors. Respir Physiol Neurobiol 148:217, 2005.
147. Kubin L, Alheid G, Zuperku EJ, McCrimmon DR: Central pathways of pulmonary and lower airway vagal afferents. J Appl Physiol 101:618, 2006.
148. Taylor-Clark T, Undem BJ: Transduction mechanisms in airway sensory nerves. J Appl Physiol 101:950, 2006.
149. Horner RL, Bradley TD: Update in sleep and control of ventilation 2006. Am J Respir Crit Care Med 175:426, 2007.
150. Ward DS, Temp JA: Neuropharmacology of the control of ventilation. *In* Yaksh TL, Lynch C III, Zapol WM, et al (eds): Anesthesia: Biologic Foundations. Philadelphia, Lippincott-Raven, 1997.
151. Solomon IC: Excitation of phrenic and sympathetic output during acute hypoxia: Contribution of medullary oxygen detectors. Respir Physiol 121:101, 2000.
152. Stucke AG, Zuperku EJ, Tonkovic-Capin V, et al: Sevoflurane depresses glutaminergic neurotransmission to brainstem inspiratory premotor neurons but not postsynaptic receptor function in a decerebrate dog model. Anesthesiology 103:50, 2005.
153. Stucke AG, Zuperku EJ, Krolo M, et al: Sevoflurane enhances γ-aminobutyric acid type A receptor function and overall inhibition of inspiratory premotor neurons in a decerebrate dog model. Anesthesiology 103:57, 2005.
154. Carl ML, Schelegle ES, Hollstein SB, et al: Control of ventilation during lung volume changes and permissive hypercapnia in dogs. Am J Respir Crit Care Med 158:742, 1998.
155. Sant'Ambrogia G, Widdecombe J: Reflexes from airway rapidly adapting receptors. Respir Physiol 125:33, 2001.
156. De Troyer A, Brunko E, Leduc D, et al: Reflex inhibition of canine inspiratory intercostals by diaphragmatic tension receptors. J Physiol 514:255, 1999.
157. Burton MD, Kazemi H: Neurotransmitters in central respiratory control. Respir Physiol 122:111, 2000.
158. Gonzalez C, Agapitoa M, Rochera A, et al: Chemoreception in the context of the general biology of ROS. Respir Physiol Neurobiol 157:30, 2007.
159. Parkes MJ: Breath-holding and its breakpoint. Exp Physiol 91:1, 2005.
160. Gourine AV: On the peripheral and central chemoreception and control of breathing: An emerging role of ATP. J Physiol 568:715, 2005.
161. Fung ML, Ye JS, Fung PC: Acute hypoxia elevates nitric oxide generation in rat carotid body in vitro. Pflugers Arch 442:903, 2001.
162. Teppema L, Berkenbosch A, Olievier C: Effect of *N* omega-nitro-L-arginine on ventilatory response to hypercapnia in anesthetized cats. J Appl Physiol 82:292, 1997.
163. Iturriaga R: Nitric oxide and carotid body chemoreception. Biol Res 34:135, 2001.
164. Fourcade HE, Stevens WC, Larson CPJ, et al: The ventilatory effects of Forane, a new inhaled anesthetic. Anesthesiology 35:26, 1971.
165. Calverley RK, Smith NT, Jones CW, et al: Ventilatory and cardiovascular effects of enflurane anesthesia during spontaneous ventilation in man. Anesth Analg 57:610, 1978.
166. Lockhart SH, Rampil IJ, Yasuda N, et al: Depression of ventilation by desflurane in humans. Anesthesiology 74:484, 1991.
167. Doi M, Ikeda K: Respiratory effects of sevoflurane. Anesth Analg 66:241, 1987.
168. Hickey RF, Severinghaus JW: Regulation of breathing: Drug effects. *In* Hornbein TF (ed): Regulation of Breathing. Lung Biology in Health and Disease, vol 17. New York, Marcel Dekker, 1981.
169. Eger EII: Isoflurane: A review. Anesthesiology 55:559, 1981.
170. Winkler SS, Nielsen A, Mesina J: Respiratory depression in goats by stable xenon: Implications for CT studies. J Comput Assist Tomogr 11:496, 1987.
171. Holl K, Nemati N, Kohmura E, et al: Stable-xenon-CT: Effects of xenon inhalation on EEG and cardiorespiratory parameters in the human. Acta Neurochir 87:129, 1987.
172. Fourcade HE, Larson C, Hickey RF, et al: Effects of time on ventilation during halothane and cyclopropane anesthesia. Anesthesiology 36:83, 1972.
173. Warltier DC, Pagel PS: Cardiovascular and respiratory actions of desflurane: Is desflurane different from isoflurane? Anesth Analg 75:517, 1992.
174. Brown K, Aun C, Stocks J, et al: A comparison of the respiratory effects of sevoflurane and halothane in infants and young children. Anesthesiology 89:86, 1998.
175. Eger EI, Dolan WM, Stevens WC, et al: Surgical stimulation antagonizes the respiratory depression produced by Forane. Anesthesiology 36:544, 1972.
176. Einarsson S, Bengtsson A, Stenqvst O, et al: Decreased respiratory depression during emergence from anesthesia with sevoflurane/N_2O than with sevoflurane alone. Can J Anaesth 46:335, 1999.
177. Whittenridge D, Bulbring E: Changes in the activity of pulmonary receptors in anesthesia and their influence on respiratory behavior. J Pharmacol Exp Ther 81:340, 1944.
178. Nishino T, Anderson JW, Sant'Ambrogio G: Effects of halothane, enflurane, and isoflurane on laryngeal receptors in dogs. Respir Physiol 91:247, 1993.
179. Nishino T, Anderson JW, Sant'Ambrogio G: Responses of tracheobronchial receptors to halo-

thane, enflurane, and isoflurane in anesthetized dogs. Respir Physiol 95:281, 1994.

180. Moores C, Davies AS, Dallak M: Sevoflurane has less effect than halothane on pulmonary afferent activity in the rabbit. Br J Anaesth 80:257, 1998.
181. Pappas AL, Sukhani R, Lurie J, et al: Severity of airway hyperreactivity associated with laryngeal mask airway removal: Correlation with volatile anesthetic choice and depth of anesthesia. J Clin Anesth 13:498, 2001.
182. Klock PAJ, Czeslick EG, Klafta JM, et al: The effect of sevoflurane and desflurane on upper airway reactivity. Anesthesiology 94:963, 2001.
183. Arain S, Shankar H, Ebert TJ: Desflurane enhances reactivity during the use of the laryngeal mask airway. Anesthesiology 103:495, 2005.
184. Eshima RW, Maurer A, King T, et al: A Comparison of airway responses during desflurane and sevoflurane administration via a laryngeal mask airway for maintenance of anesthesia. Anesth Analg 96:701, 2003.
185. McKay RE, Bostrom A, Balea MC, McKay WR: Airway responses during desflurane versus sevoflurane administration via a laryngeal mask airway in smokers. Anesth Analg 103:1147, 2006.
186. Weiskopf RB, Eger EI III, Daniel M, Noorani M: Cardiovascular stimulation induced by rapid increases in desflurane concentration in humans results from activation of tracheopulmonary and systemic receptors. Anesthesiology 83:1173, 1995.
187. Ochiai R, Guthrie RD, Motoyama EK: Effects of varying concentrations of halothane on the activity of the genioglossus, intercostals, and diaphragm in cats: An electromyographic study. Anesthesiology 70:812, 1989.
188. Nishino T, Kochi T, Yonezawa T, et al: Responses of recurrent laryngeal, hypoglossal, and phrenic nerves to increasing depths of anesthesia with halothane or enflurane in vagotomized cats. Anesthesiology 63:404, 1985.
189. Eastwood PR, Szollosi I, Platt PR, Hillman DR: Collapsibility of the upper airway during anesthesia with isoflurane. Anesthesiology 97:786, 2002.
190. Evans RG, Crawford MW, Noseworthy MD, Yoo S-J: Effect of increasing depth of propofol anesthesia on upper airway configuration in children. Anesthesiology 99:596, 2003.
191. Stucke AG, Stuth EAE, Tonkovic-Capin V, et al: Effects of halothane and sevoflurane on inhibitory neurotransmission to medullary expiratory neurons in a decerebrate dog model. Anesthesiology 96:955, 2002.
192. Brandes IF, Zuperku EJ, Stucke AG, et al: Isoflurane depresses the response of inspiratory hypoglossal motoneurons to serotonin in vivo. Anesthesiology 106:736, 2007.
193. Warner DO, Warner MA, Ritman EL: Mechanical significance of respiratory muscle activity in humans during halothane anesthesia. Anesthesiology 84:309, 1996.
194. Warner DO, Warner MA, Ritman EL: Human chest wall function while awake and during halothane anesthesia. I. Quiet breathing. Anesthesiology 82:6, 1995.
195. Warner DO, Warner MA, Ritman EL: Atelectasis and chest wall shape during halothane anesthesia. Anesthesiology 85:49, 1996.
196. Warner DO: Diaphragm function during anesthesia: Still crazy after all these years. Anesthesiology 97:295, 2002.
197. Stuth EAE, Tonkovic-Capin M, Kampine JP, et al: Dose-dependent effects of isoflurane on the CO_2 responses of expiratory medullary neurons and the phrenic nerve activities in dogs. Anesthesiology 76:763, 1992.
198. Stuth EAE, Tonkovic-Capin M, Kampine JP, et al: Dose-dependent effects of halothane on expiratory and inspiratory bulbospinal neurons and the phrenic nerve activities in dogs. Anesthesiology 81:1470, 1994.
199. Stucke AG, Stuth EAE, Tonkovic-Capin V, et al: Effects of sevoflurane on excitatory neurotransmission to medullary expiratory neurons and on phrenic nerve activity in a decerebrate dog model. Anesthesiology 95:485, 2001.
200. Kochi T, Ide T, Isono S, et al: Different effects of halothane and enflurane on diaphragmatic contractility in vivo. Anesth Analg 70:1990.
201. Ide T, Kochi T, Isono S, et al: Diaphragmatic function during sevoflurane anaesthesia in dogs. Can J Anaesth 38:116, 1991.
202. Warner DO, Warner MA, Joyner MJ, et al: The effect of nitrous oxide on chest wall function in humans and dogs. Anesth Analg 86:1058, 1998.
203. Correa FCF, Ciminelli PB, Falcao H, et al: Respiratory mechanics and lung histology in normal rats anesthetized with sevoflurane. J Appl Physiol 91:803, 2001.
204. Ruiz P, Chartrand D: The effect of isoflurane 0.6% on respiratory mechanics in anesthetized-paralyzed humans is not increased at concentrations of 0.9% and 1.2%. Can J Anaesth 50:67, 2003.
205. Isono S, Nishino T, Sugimori K, et al: Respiratory effects of expiratory flow–resistive loading in conscious and anesthetized humans. Anesth Analg 70:594, 1990.
206. Hendrickx JFA, Carette R, Lemmens HJM, De Wolf AM: Large volume N_2O uptake alone does not explain the second gas effect of N_2O on sevoflurane during constant inspired ventilation. Br J Anaesth 96:391, 2005.
207. Sakata DJ, Golapakrishnan NA, Orr JA, et al: Rapid recovery from sevoflurane and desflurane with hypercapnia and hyperventilation. Anesth Analg 105:79, 2007.
208. Sakata DJ, Golapakrishnan NA, Orr JA, et al: Hypercapnic hyperventilation shortens emergence time from isoflurane anesthesia. Anesth Analg 104:587, 2007.
209. Guracha Boru K, Drummond GB: Comparison of breathing methods for inhalation induction of anaesthesia. Br J Anaesth 83:650, 1999.
210. Pancaro C, Giovannoni S, Toscano A, Peduto VA: Apnea during induction of anesthesia with sevoflurane is related to its mode of administration. Can J Anaesth 52:591, 2005.
211. Groeben H, Meier S, Tankersley CG, et al: Influence of volatile anaesthetics on hypercapnoeic ventilatory responses in mice with blunted respiratory drive. Br J Anaesth 92:697, 2004.
212. Dahan A, van den Elsen MJLJ, Berkenbosch A, et al: Effects of subanesthetic halothane on the ventilatory responses to hypercapnia and acute hypoxia in healthy volunteers. Anesthesiology 80:727, 1994.
213. Dahan A, Teppema L: Influence of low-dose anaesthetic agents on ventilatory control: Where do we stand? Br J Anaesth 83:199, 1999.
214. Pandit JJ, Manning-Fox J, Dorrington KL, et al: Effects of subanaesthetic sevoflurane on ventilation. 1: Response to acute and sustained hypercapnia in humans. Br J Anaesth 83:204, 1999.
215. Warner DO, Warner MA: Human chest wall function while awake and during halothane anesthesia. II. Carbon dioxide rebreathing. Anesthesiology 82:20, 1995.
216. Stuth EAE, Dogas Z, Krolo M, et al: Effects of halothane on the phrenic nerve responses to carbon dioxide mediated by the carotid body chemoreceptors in vagotomized dogs. Anesthesiology 87:1440, 1997.
217. Pandit JJ, Moreau B, Donoghue S, Robbins PA: Effect of pain and audiovisual stimulation on the depression of acute hypoxic ventilatory response by low-dose halothane in humans. Anesthesiology 101:1409, 2004.
218. Teppema LJ, Romber RR, Dahan A: Antioxidants reverse reduction of the human hypoxic ventilatory response by subanesthetic isoflurane. Anesthesiology 102:747, 2005.
219. Davies RO, Edwards MW Jr, Lahiri S: Halothane depresses the response to carotid body chemoreceptors to hypoxia and hypercapnia in the cat. Anesthesiology 57:153, 1982.
220. Stuth EAE, Dogas Z, Krolo M, et al: Dose-dependent effects of halothane on the phrenic nerve responses to acute hypoxia in vagotomized dogs. Anesthesiology 87:1428, 1997.
221. Mohan R, Duffin J: The effect of hypoxia on the ventilatory response to carbon dioxide in man. Respir Physiol 108:101, 1997.
222. Kline DD, Yang T, Huang PL, et al: Altered respiratory responses to hypoxia in mutant mice deficient in neuronal nitric oxide synthase. J Physiol 511:273, 1998.
223. Zanzinger J, Czachurski J, Seller H: Nitric oxide in the ventrolateral medulla regulates sympathetic responses to systemic hypoxia in pigs. Am J Physiol Regul Integr Comp Physiol 275:R33, 1998.
224. Morray JP, Nobel R, Bennet L, et al: The effect of halothane on phrenic and chemoreceptor responses to hypoxia in anesthetized kittens. Anesth Analg 83:329, 1996.
225. Maxova H, Vizek M: Ventilatory response to sustained hypoxia in carotid body denervated rats. Physiol Res 50:327, 2001.
226. Pandit JJ: Effect of low dose inhaled anaesthetic agents on the ventilatory response to carbon dioxide in humans: A quantitative review. Anaesthesia 60:461, 2005.
227. Pandit JJ, Mannington-Fox J, Dorrington KL, et al: Effects of subaenesthetic sevoflurane on ventilation. 2: Response to acute and sustained hypoxia in humans. Br J Anaesth 83:210, 1999.
228. Temp JA, Henson LC, Ward DS: Effect of a subanesthetic minimum alveolar concentration of isoflurane on two tests of the hypoxic ventilatory response. Anesthesiology 80:739, 1994.
229. Nagyova B, Dorrington KL, Poulin MJ, et al: Influence of 0.2 minimum alveolar concentration of enflurane on the ventilatory response to sustained hypoxia in humans. Br J Anaesth 78:707, 1997.
230. Dahan A, Sarton E, van den Elsen M, et al: Ventilatory response to hypoxia in humans. Influences of subanesthetic desflurane. Anesthesiology 85:60, 1996.
231. Pandit JJ: The variable effect of low-dose volatile anaesthetics on the acute ventilatory response to hypoxia in humans: A quantitative review. Anaesthesia 57:632, 2002.
232. Gropper MA, Wiener-Kronsh J: The alveolar epithelium: Suspect or innocent bystander? Anesthesiology 98:3, 2003.
233. Whitehead TC, Zhang H, Mullen B, Slutsky AS: Effect of mechanical ventilation on cytokine response to intratracheal lipopolysaccharide. Anesthesiology 101:52, 2004.
234. Hu G, Schwartz DE, Shajahan AN, et al: Isoflurane, but not sevoflurane, increases transendothelial albumin permeability in the isolated rat lung. Anesthesiology 104:777, 2006.

235. Reutershan J, Chang D, Hayes JK, Ley K: Protective effects of isoflurane pretreatment in endotoxin-induced lung injury. Anesthesiology 104:511, 2006.
236. Koizumi T, Ogasawara H, Yamamoto H, et al: Effect of ONO1714, a specific inducible nitric oxide synthase inhibitor, on lung lymph filtration and gas exchange during endotoxemia in unanesthetized sheep. Anesthesiology 101:59, 2004.
237. Warner DO: Perioperative abstinence from cigarettes: Physiologic and clinical consequences. Anesthesiology 104:356, 2006.
238. Takala RSK, Soukka H, Salo MS, et al: Pulmonary inflammatory mediators after sevoflurane and thiopentone anaesthesia in pigs. Acta Anaesthesiol Scand 48:40, 2004.
239. Kotani N, Takahashi S, Sessler DI, et al: Volatile anesthetics augment expression of proinflammatory cytokines in rat alveolar macrophages by mechanical ventilation. Anesthesiology 91:187, 1999.
240. Nader-Djalal N, Knight P, Bacon MF, et al: Alterations in the course of acid-induced lung injury in rats after general anesthesia: Volatile anesthetics versus ketamine. Anesth Analg 86:141, 1998.
241. Wrigge H, Zinserling J, Stuber F, et al: Effects of mechanical ventilation on release of cytokines into systemic circulation in patients with normal pulmonary function. Anesthesiology 93:1413, 2000.
242. Koksal GM, Sayilgan C, Gungor G, et al: Effects of sevoflurane and desflurane on cytokine response during tympanoplasty surgery. Acta Anaesthesiol Scand 49:835, 2005.
243. Topouzova-Hristova T, Daza P, Garcia-Herdugo G, Stephanova E: Volatile anaesthetic halothane causes DNA damage in A549 lung cells. Toxicology In Vitro 20:585, 2006.
244. Hung CJ, Liu FY, Shaiu YC, et al: Assessing transient pulmonary injury induced by volatile anesthetics by increased lung uptake of technetium-99m hexamethylpropylene amine onime. Lung 181:1, 2003.
245. Hung CJ, Liu FY, Wu RS, et al: The influence of volatile anesthetics on alveolar epithelial permeability measured by noninvasive radionucleotide lung scan. Ann Nucl Med 17:213, 2003.
246. Koksal GM, Sayilgan C, Aydin S, et al: The effects of sevoflurane and desflurane on lipid peroxidation during laparoscopic cholecystectomy. Eur J Anaesthesiol 21:217, 2004.
247. Kandatsu N, Nan Y-S, Feng G-G, et al: Opposing effects of isoflurane and sevoflurane on neurogenic pulmonary edema development in an animal model. Anesthesiology 102:1182, 2005.
248. Takala RSK, Soukka HR, Kirvela OA, et al: Alveolar integrity and ultrastructure in pigs remain undamaged after exposure to sevoflurane. Acta Anaesthesiol Scand 46:1137, 2002.
249. Putensen C, Rasanen J, Putensen-Himmer G, et al: Effect of low isoflurane concentrations on the ventilation-perfusion distribution in injured canine lungs. Anesthesiology 97:652, 2002.
250. Giraud O, Molliex S, Rolland C, et al: Halogenated anesthetics reduce interleukin-1β–induced cytokine secretion by rat alveolar type II cells in primary culture. Anesthesiology 98:74, 2003.
251. Kidani Y, Taniguchi T, Kanakaura H, et al: Sevoflurane pretreatment inhibits endotoxin-induced shock in rats. Anesth Analg 101:1152, 2005.
252. Takala RSK, Soukka HR, Salo MS, et al: Gene expression of pulmonary cytokines after sevoflurane or thiopentone anaesthesia in pigs. Acta Anaesthesiol Scand 50:163, 2006.
253. Suter D, Spahn DR, Blumenthal S, et al: The immunomodulatory effect of sevoflurane in endotoxin-injured alveolar epithelial cells. Anesth Analg 104:638, 2007.
254. Lucchinetti E, Ambrosio S, Aguirre J, et al: Sevoflurane inhalation at sedative concentrations provides endothelial protection against ischemia-reperfusion injury in humans. Anesthesiology 106:262, 2007.
255. Fujinaga T, Nakamura T, Fukuse T, et al: Isoflurane inhalation after circulatory arrest protects against warm ischemia reperfusion injury of the lungs. Transplantation 82:1168, 2006.
256. Fang Q, Wang XR, Yang YW, Su DS: Up-regulation of hypoxia inducible factor 1α by isoflurane in Hep3B cells. Anesthesiology 105:1211, 2006.

Paul S. Pagel, Neil E. Farber, Phillip F. Pratt, Jr., and David C. Warltier

23 Cardiovascular Pharmacology

Key Points

1. In a normal heart, volatile anesthetics produce dose-related depression in left ventricular, right ventricular, and left atrial myocardial contractility; left ventricular diastolic function; and left ventricular–arterial coupling.
2. The negative inotropic effects of volatile anesthetics are related to alterations in intracellular Ca^{2+} homeostasis within the cardiac myocyte.
3. Volatile anesthetics affect the determinants of left ventricular afterload to varying degrees in the presence of normal and dysfunctional myocardium.
4. The systemic hemodynamic effects of volatile anesthetics are complex and determined by the interaction of myocardial effects, direct actions on the arterial and venous vasculature, and alterations in autonomic nervous system activity.
5. Volatile anesthetics sensitize myocardium to the arrhythmogenic effects of epinephrine to varying degrees and may prevent or facilitate the development of atrial or ventricular arrhythmias during myocardial ischemia or infarction, depending on the concentration of the agent, the extent of the injury, and the location affected within the conduction pathway.
6. Volatile anesthetics are relatively weak coronary vasodilators that are not capable of producing coronary steal at typically used clinical concentrations, even in patients with steal-prone coronary artery anatomy.
7. Volatile anesthetics exert important cardioprotective effects against reversible and irreversible myocardial ischemia in experimental animals and humans when administered before, during, or immediately after the onset of coronary artery occlusion and reperfusion.
8. Volatile anesthetics depress baroreceptor reflex control of arterial pressure to varying degrees.
9. Nitrous oxide causes direct negative inotropic effects, does not substantially affect left ventricular diastolic function, and produces modest increases in pulmonary and systemic arterial pressure via a sympathomimetic effect. These actions are dependent to some degree on the baseline anesthetic.
10. Xenon is essentially devoid of cardiovascular effects but has been shown to protect myocardium against infarction in experimental animals.

This chapter comprehensively describes the cardiovascular pharmacology of modern volatile anesthetics (including isoflurane, desflurane, and sevoflurane), nitrous oxide, and xenon. Comparison to older volatile anesthetics (halothane and enflurane) will be made only when necessary because these drugs are no longer clinically available. The actions of inhaled anesthetics on cardiovascular function, cardiac electrophysiology, the coronary circulation, and autonomic nervous system control of the circulation will be examined in detail.

Volatile Anesthetics and Cardiovascular Function

Myocardial Contractility

Isoflurane, desflurane, and sevoflurane depress myocardial contractility in vitro and in vivo. Investigations conducted in the

1960s demonstrated that the older volatile anesthetics halothane and enflurane produce dose-related depression of force-velocity relationships and Frank-Starling curves in isolated cardiac muscle preparations and intact, closed-chest dogs, respectively. These findings supported clinical observations of circulatory depression during halothane and enflurane anesthesia in humans. Isoflurane produces direct negative inotropic effects as indicated by decreases in the maximal velocity of shortening, peak developed force, and maximal rate of force development during isotonic contraction in isolated feline papillary muscles. These reductions in myocardial contractility by isoflurane also contribute to the cardiovascular depression observed with this anesthetic in humans. Similarly, desflurane and sevoflurane depress the intrinsic inotropic state in isolated myocardium, and these actions play an important role in determining the hemodynamic effects of these volatile anesthetics in humans with or without heart disease.

The relative degree of myocardial depression produced by volatile anesthetics in vivo has been more difficult to establish because simultaneous alterations in systemic and pulmonary hemodynamics and autonomic nervous system activity complicate assessment of left ventricular (LV) systolic function. Isovolumic and ejection-phase measures of myocardial contractility demonstrated that halothane and enflurane cause very similar negative inotropic effects in experimental animals and humans. These findings were subsequently confirmed by using the slope (E_{es}) of the LV end-systolic pressure–midaxis diameter relationship as a relatively heart rate– and load-independent index of the inotropic state in chronically instrumented dogs. In contrast, isoflurane produces less myocardial depression in vivo than the older anesthetics do. For example, isoflurane caused smaller reductions in the maximum rate of LV pressure development (dP/dt) than halothane did when identical minimum alveolar concentrations (MACs) were directly compared in the presence and absence of autonomic nervous system function, which suggested that the differences in myocardial depression caused by these anesthetics occur independent of autonomic nervous system activity. Differences in the negative inotropic effects of halothane and isoflurane have been quantified by using the slope (M_w) of the regional preload recruitable stroke work relationship derived from differentially loaded LV pressure–segment length diagrams. In these studies, conducted in chronically instrumented dogs, isoflurane maintained contractility an average of 20% higher than halothane did at identical MAC. Differences in the relative degree of myocardial depression produced by isoflurane and the older volatile anesthetics halothane and enflurane were also inferred in humans by using isovolumic and ejection-phase measures of the contractile state. The negative inotropic actions of all volatile anesthetics are exacerbated by hypocalcemia, calcium (Ca^{2+}) channel blockers, and β_1-adrenoceptor antagonists and may be reversed by the administration of exogenous Ca^{2+}, cardiac phosphodiesterase fraction III inhibitors, β_1-adrenoceptor agonists, Ca^{2+} channel agonists, and myofilament Ca^{2+} sensitizers. The differential effects of isoflurane and the older volatile anesthetics halothane and enflurane on myocardial contractility are maintained during the depression or augmentation of the inotropic state produced by these vasoactive drugs.

Desflurane causes systemic and coronary hemodynamic effects that are remarkably similar to those produced by isoflurane. Desflurane and isoflurane have been shown by isovolumic and ejection-phase measures of contractility to depress myocardial function to equivalent degrees in experimental animals and humans. These observations have been verified by using both end-systolic pressure-volume relationships and preload recruitable stroke work (Fig. 23-1) in the presence and absence of autonomic nervous system activity.[1] However, the unique cardiovascular stimulation associated with rapid increases in inspired desflurane concentration in humans may lead to transient increases in myocardial contractility as a result of augmentation of sympathetic nervous system tone. The effects of sevoflurane on myocardial contractility have also been shown to be virtually indistinguishable from those produced by isoflurane in dogs. Sevoflurane caused less myocardial depression than an equivalent halothane MAC in pigs did and produced less myocardial depression than enflurane did in humans as evaluated by echocardiography. Sevoflurane decreased contractile function to approximately 40% to 45% of control values at 1.75 MAC in the presence and absence of autonomic nervous system tone as determined by regional preload recruitable stroke work in dogs. This magnitude of myocardial depression agreed with previous data for isoflurane and desflurane in an identical experimental model. Thus, the vast

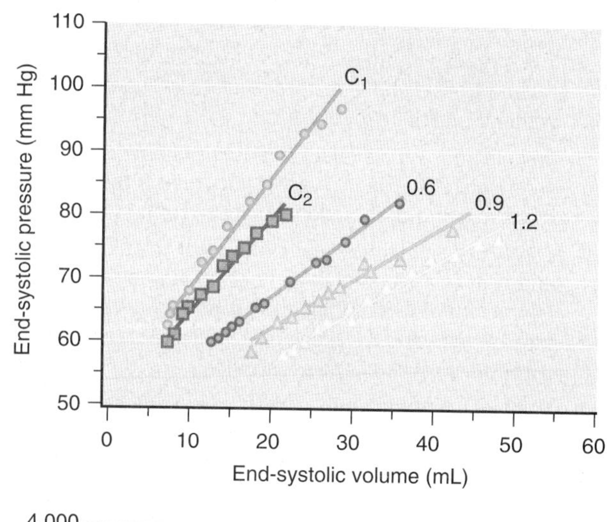

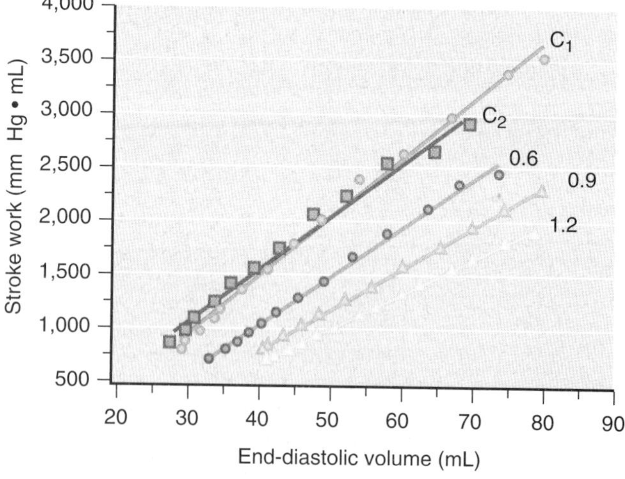

Figure 23-1 End-systolic pressure-volume (*top panel*) and stroke work–end-diastolic volume relationships (*bottom panel*) before (control 1; C_1), during 0.6, 0.9, and 1.2 minimum alveolar concentration, and after isoflurane (control 2; C_2) in an experiment in an open-chest dog. *(Adapted from Hettrick DA, Pagel PS, Warltier DC: Desflurane, sevoflurane, and isoflurane impair canine left ventricular–arterial coupling and mechanical efficiency. Anesthesiology 85:403-413, 1996.)*

majority of evidence collected to date indicates that isoflurane, desflurane, and sevoflurane depress the contractile state to similar degrees in normal ventricular myocardium.

The effects of volatile anesthetics on myocardial contractility in animal models or patients with LV dysfunction have been less extensively studied. An early in vitro study demonstrated that isoflurane causes greater reductions in maximum shortening velocity and the peak rate of force development in feline papillary muscles from failing hearts subjected to chronic pressure overload than in muscles from normal hearts. The older volatile anesthetic halothane also produced more pronounced myocardial depression in ischemic than in normal myocardium. Isoflurane and halothane were shown to cause relatively greater negative inotropic effects in ventricular myocardium obtained from cardiomyopathic hamsters than from normal hamsters (Fig. 23-2).[2] Isoflurane and sevoflurane also produced greater depression of contractility in right ventricular (RV) papillary muscles obtained from ferrets with experimental pressure-overload hypertrophy than from ferrets with normal myocardium.[3] These findings suggested that the myocardial depression caused by volatile anesthetics in failing or hypertrophied myocardium was accentuated and provided indirect evidence that patients with underlying contractile dysfunction may be more sensitive to the negative inotropic effects of volatile anesthetics. This hypothesis has not been comprehensively examined in vivo, however. In contrast, isoflurane, sevoflurane, and desflurane caused similar declines in contractility in ventricular myocytes obtained from rats with and without chemically induced chronic hyperglycemia.[4] These data suggested that volatile anesthetics do not cause a more exaggerated negative inotropic effect in myocardium obtained from this model of diabetes mellitus.

Volatile anesthetic–induced declines in contractile function were well tolerated and did not precipitate frank systolic dysfunction in experimental models of myocardial ischemia or

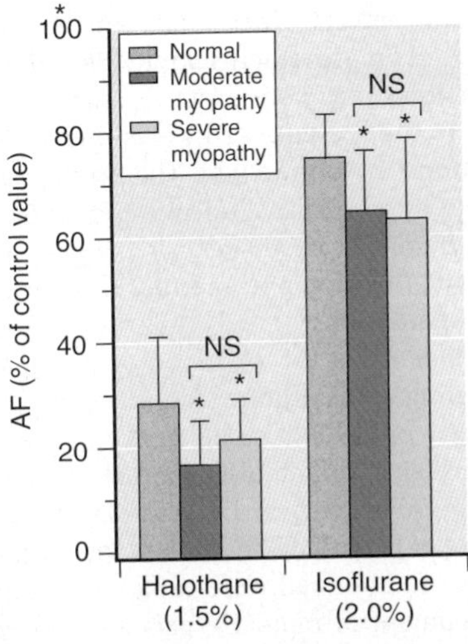

Figure 23-2 Comparison of the effects of halothane (*left*) and isoflurane (right) on isometric active force (AF) of papillary muscles from healthy hamsters (*yellow bars*) and those with cardiomyopathy (*blue and green bars*). Probability values refer to between-group differences. *Significantly ($P < .05$) different from control values. *(Adapted from Vivien B, Hanouz J-L, Gueugniaud P-Y, et al: Myocardial effects of halothane and isoflurane in hamsters with hypertrophic cardiomyopathy. Anesthesiology 87:1406-1416, 1997.)*

infarction. In fact, volatile anesthetics have been shown to exert important beneficial effects on mechanical function during myocardial ischemia and reperfusion injury. Volatile anesthetics reduced experimental myocardial infarct size,[5] preserved metabolic and structural integrity during regional ischemia and reperfusion, enhanced the functional recovery of stunned myocardium, and improved indices of LV diastolic performance during brief coronary artery occlusion. Isoflurane was also shown to produce beneficial decreases in LV preload and afterload in patients with ischemic heart disease. These improvements in loading conditions in patients with compromised LV function may serve to offset the direct negative inotropic effects of anesthetics and contribute to relative maintenance of cardiac performance by optimizing the Starling operating range of the heart or by improving LV diastolic function. Isoflurane produced dose-related depression of myocardial contractility in a canine model of moderate LV dysfunction induced by chronic rapid LV pacing, but isoflurane anesthesia was well tolerated and did not precipitate frank LV failure in this model.[6] These findings with isoflurane were attributed to simultaneous improvements in LV loading conditions and filling dynamics that contributed to relative maintenance of cardiac output in the setting of moderate LV dysfunction despite concomitant reductions in contractility.

Cellular Mechanisms of Myocardial Depression

Volatile anesthetics depress myocardial contractility via alterations in intracellular Ca^{2+} homeostasis at several subcellular targets in the normal cardiac myocyte. Volatile anesthetics caused dose-related inhibition of the transsarcolemmal Ca^{2+} transient by affecting both L- and T-type Ca^{2+} channels. Isoflurane produced less pronounced reductions in the intracellular Ca^{2+} transient than the older volatile anesthetics did. The structural conformation and functional integrity of voltage-dependent Ca^{2+} channels were directly altered by volatile anesthetics as indicated by the attenuated binding of Ca^{2+} channel blockers. The partial inhibition of Ca^{2+} influx via sarcolemmal Ca^{2+} channels has several important consequences, including declines in the availability of Ca^{2+} for contractile activation, depression of Ca^{2+}-dependent release of Ca^{2+} from the sarcoplasmic reticulum (SR), and reduction of the amount of Ca^{2+} that can subsequently be stored in the SR. In contrast to the older volatile anesthetics halothane and enflurane, isoflurane did not stimulate release of Ca^{2+} from the SR nor directly activate ryanodine-sensitive SR Ca^{2+} release channels, thereby reducing SR Ca^{2+} storage. Unlike halothane, isoflurane also did not appear to provoke nonspecific leakage of Ca^{2+} from the SR, an action that contributes to further decreases in accumulation of the Ca^{2+} available for release during contraction in the presence of the older volatile agent. When combined with decreases in transsarcolemmal Ca^{2+} flux, these alterations in SR function represent important mechanisms by which older volatile anesthetics depress the intracellular Ca^{2+} transient and reduce myocardial contractility to a greater extent than with identical MAC concentrations of isoflurane, desflurane, or sevoflurane. In addition, isoflurane and sevoflurane have been shown to inhibit Ca^{2+} transport from the cell through sarcolemmal Ca^{2+}-adenosine triphosphatase (ATPase), an action that partially offsets reductions in SR Ca^{2+} stores. The partial preservation of the myocardial positive frequency staircase effect observed with newer volatile anesthetics at physiologic excitation rates in vitro may also be attributed to this relative maintenance of SR function, in contrast to the findings with halothane or enflurane.

Volatile anesthetics also depress contractile function by inhibiting Na^+-Ca^{2+} exchange and reducing the intracellular Ca^{2+} concentration independent of the voltage-dependent Ca^{2+} channel in vitro. This effect may be particularly important in neonatal myocardium because it is more sensitive to the negative inotropic actions of volatile anesthetics than adult myocardium is. The relative contribution of inhibition of the Na^+-Ca^{2+} exchanger to anesthetic-induced depression of myocardial contractility in the intact heart remains controversial, but a role for inhibition of Na^+-Ca^{2+} exchange in anesthetic preconditioning was demonstrated recently.[7] Volatile anesthetics may also exert direct effects on the contractile apparatus and reduce myofilament Ca^{2+} sensitivity. Volatile anesthetics decreased tension development in skinned cardiac myofibrils and reduced myofibrillar ATPase activity. These actions may contribute to declines in actin-myosin cross-bridge kinetics during contraction, but not through a direct interaction with cardiac cross-bridge mechanics.[8] In addition, volatile anesthetics may modestly reduce myofilament Ca^{2+} sensitivity, but this mechanism probably plays a relatively minor role in the negative inotropic effects of these anesthetics at clinically relevant concentrations in vivo.

The cellular mechanisms responsible for volatile anesthetic–induced depression of myocardial contractility in failing myocardium have not been studied in detail. The most comprehensive investigation published to date examined the effects of isoflurane and sevoflurane on intracellular Ca^{2+} homeostasis in a ferret model of RV pressure-overload hypertrophy.[3] Isoflurane and sevoflurane produced more pronounced reductions in peak intracellular Ca^{2+} concentration and exaggerated decreases in myofilament Ca^{2+} sensitivity in ventricular myocytes obtained from hypertrophied hearts than in normal myocytes.[3] Whether similar alterations in intracellular Ca^{2+} regulation are produced by volatile anesthetics in other forms of heart failure remains to be determined. Profound abnormalities in Ca^{2+} homeostasis are characteristic features of failing myocardium, and it appears highly likely that volatile anesthetics will cause further reductions in contractile function by producing additive or synergistic effects on Ca^{2+} metabolism under these conditions.

Diastolic Function

Definitions of heart failure based solely on contractile dysfunction are inadequate because LV function during diastole significantly influences overall cardiac performance. The heart serves dual roles: it propels blood into the high-pressure arterial vasculature during systole and collects blood from the low-pressure venous circulation during diastole. Thus, heart failure may occur not only as a result of impaired contractility but also as a result of altered LV diastolic function. The timing, rate, and extent of LV filling are determined by several major factors, including the rate and degree of myocardial relaxation, the intrinsic mechanical properties of the left ventricle itself and those imposed by external constraints, and the structure and function of the left atrium, the pulmonary venous circulation, and the mitral valve. Although abnormalities in LV diastolic function may be linked to decreases in myocardial contractility, heart failure may result from primary diastolic dysfunction in the absence of or before the appearance of alterations in LV systolic function in a variety of pathologic conditions, including ischemic heart disease, pressure- or volume-overload hypertrophy, hypertrophic obstructive cardiomyopathy, and restrictive disease processes.

Volatile anesthetics produce dose-related prolongation of LV isovolumic relaxation in vivo. This delay in isovolumic relaxation is associated with declines in early LV filling but is not of sufficient magnitude to affect LV chamber stiffness. Coronary blood flow is highest during isovolumic relaxation, and the delays in relaxation produced by volatile anesthetics contribute to impairment of coronary flow during early diastole. Prolongation of LV relaxation probably occurs as a result of simultaneous depression of myocardial contractility and not because of a direct negative lusitropic effect. In fact, volatile anesthetics modestly enhanced relaxation of isolated ferret myocardium in vitro. Volatile anesthetics cause concentration-related decreases in the rate and extent of early LV filling concomitant with negative inotropic effects. They also reduce LV filling associated with atrial systole.[9] Isoflurane, desflurane, and sevoflurane did not alter invasively derived indices of regional myocardial or chamber stiffness, thus indicating that LV distensibility was unaffected by these volatile anesthetics. The older volatile anesthetic halothane also did not directly alter the intrinsic viscoelastic properties of myocardium despite producing relatively greater negative inotropic effects.

The effects of isoflurane and halothane on LV diastolic function in a canine model of dilated cardiomyopathy were described.[6] In contrast to the findings in dogs with normal LV function, isoflurane improved several indices of LV relaxation and filling in cardiomyopathic dogs despite producing simultaneous negative inotropic effects. In addition, halothane did not exacerbate the preexisting diastolic dysfunction inherent in this experimental model. The findings with isoflurane and halothane were most likely related to favorable reductions in LV preload produced by these volatile anesthetics and were not due to direct positive lusitropic effects. These data further suggested that isoflurane-induced improvements in LV isovolumic relaxation and filling dynamics may contribute to relative maintenance of cardiac output in the presence of LV dysfunction despite simultaneous reductions in contractility. The findings in cardiomyopathic dogs supported earlier clinical observations that patients with severe ischemic heart disease or congestive heart failure tolerate isoflurane or halothane anesthesia without acute hemodynamic decompensation.

The dependence of LV relaxation on afterload is markedly enhanced in failing myocardium. Thus, a reduction in afterload may increase not only LV systolic performance by decreasing impedance to LV ejection but also the rate of LV relaxation and contribute to improvements in LV diastolic filling and compliance. The effects of isoflurane and halothane on the dependence of LV relaxation on afterload were explored in dogs before and after the development of rapid LV pacing–induced cardiomyopathy.[10] The dependence of LV relaxation on afterload was unaffected by isoflurane and halothane anesthesia in dogs with dilated cardiomyopathy (Fig. 23-3), thus further suggesting that these volatile anesthetics do not exert direct actions on LV isovolumic relaxation in failing myocardium independent of negative inotropic effects.

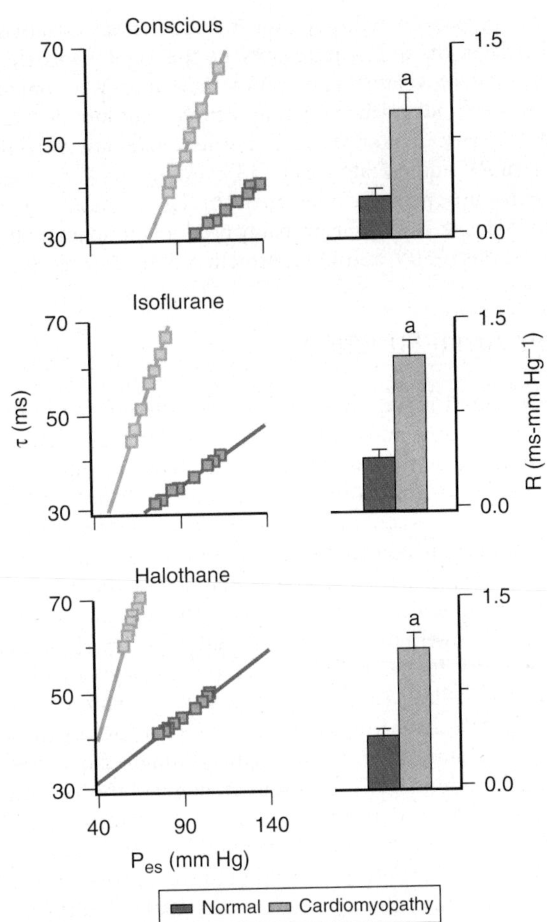

Figure 23-3 Linear relationship between the time constant of isovolumic relaxation (τ) and left ventricular end-systolic pressure (P_{es}) during inferior vena cava occlusion (*left panels*) in a typical dog before (*yellow squares*) and after (*blue squares*) the development of pacing-induced cardiomyopathy in the conscious state and during isoflurane and halothane anesthesia. The histograms on the *right* illustrate the slope (R) of the τ-versus-P_{es} relationship in the conscious state (*top right panel*) and during isoflurane (*middle right panel*) and halothane (*bottom right panel*) anesthesia before (*yellow bars*) and after (*blue bars*) pacing. a, Significantly ($P < .05$) different from normal myocardium. *(Adapted from Pagel PS, Hettrick DA, Kersten JR, et al: Isoflurane and halothane do not alter the enhanced afterload sensitivity of left ventricular relaxation in dogs with pacing-induced cardiomyopathy. Anesthesiology 87:952-962, 1997.)*

Left Ventricular–Arterial Coupling and Mechanical Efficiency

Optimum transfer of stroke volume from the left ventricle to the arterial circulation requires appropriate matching of these mechanical systems. LV-arterial coupling has most often been described by using a series elastic chamber model of the cardiovascular system. The elastances of the contracting left ventricle (E_{es}) and the arterial vasculature (E_a) are determined from LV end-systolic pressure-volume and end-systolic arterial pressure–stroke volume relationships, respectively. The ratio of E_{es} to E_a defines coupling between the left ventricle and the arterial circulation and provides a useful technique for assessment of the actions of drugs, including volatile anesthetics, on LV-arterial matching in vivo. Analysis of the pressure-volume relationship also creates a framework for the study of LV mechanical efficiency as defined by the ratio of stroke work to pressure-volume area. LV-arterial coupling may theoretically be maintained during anesthesia because declines in LV afterload may balance simultaneous reductions in myocardial contractility. Low concentrations of isoflurane (1 MAC), but not halothane, maintained E_{es}/E_a in barbiturate-anesthetized, acutely instrumented dogs, consistent with preservation of mechanical coupling between the left ventricle and the arterial circulation. However, isoflurane decreased E_{es}/E_a at 2 MAC, thus suggesting that the vasodilating effects of this anesthetic were unable to compensate for the relatively greater declines in contractility. Desflurane, sevoflurane, and isoflurane maintained optimum LV-arterial coupling and mechanical efficiency as evaluated by E_{es}/E_a and stroke work–pressure-volume area ratios at low anesthetic concentrations (<0.9 MAC) by producing simultaneous declines in myocardial contractility and LV afterload.[1] However, mechanical matching between the left ventricle and the arterial vasculature and the efficiency of total LV energy transfer to external stroke work degenerate at higher anesthetic concentrations, thus indicating that anesthetic-induced reductions in contractility are not appropriately balanced by declines in afterload. Halothane (<1.0 MAC) but not isoflurane also reduced the ratio of oscillatory to mean hydraulic power in vivo, which indicates that this anesthetic decreases LV mechanical efficiency as well. The detrimental alterations in LV-arterial coupling produced by volatile anesthetics contribute to the reductions in overall cardiac performance observed with higher concentrations of these anesthetics in vivo.

Left Ventricular Afterload

A definition of LV afterload that describes the mechanical properties of the arterial vasculature opposing LV ejection is clear, but quantitative evaluation of afterload in vivo remains a difficult problem whose solution often confuses this clinically intuitive concept. Systemic vascular resistance, calculated as the ratio of mean arterial pressure to cardiac output, is the most commonly used estimate of LV afterload. However, systemic vascular resistance inadequately describes LV afterload because this index ignores the mechanical characteristics of the blood and arterial walls, fails to account for the frequency-dependent, phasic nature of arterial blood pressure and blood flow, and does not consider the potential effects of arterial wave reflection. As a result, systemic vascular resistance cannot be used reliably to quantify changes in LV afterload produced by drugs, including volatile anesthetics, or cardiovascular disease. Aortic input impedance ($Z_{in}[\omega]$) obtained from power spectral or Fourier series analysis of aortic pressure and blood flow waveforms provides a comprehensive description of LV afterload because $Z_{in}(\omega)$ incorporates arterial viscoelasticity, frequency dependence, and wave reflection. However, analysis of $Z_{in}(\omega)$ is conducted in the frequency domain and not as a function of time, and as a result, $Z_{in}(\omega)$ is very difficult to apply in a clinical setting. $Z_{in}(\omega)$ is most often interpreted by using an electrical three-element Windkessel model of the arterial circulation that describes characteristic aortic impedance (Z_c), total arterial compliance (C), and total arterial resistance (R). Z_c represents aortic resistance to LV ejection, C is determined primarily by the compliance of the aorta and represents the energy storage component of the arterial circulation, and R equals the combined resistance of the remaining arterial vasculature. The three-element Windkessel model has been shown to closely approximate $Z_{in}(\omega)$ in a variety of physiologic conditions.

Volatile anesthetics alter $Z_{in}(\omega)$ by affecting the mechanical properties of the arterial vascular tree. In contrast to the results obtained with the older agent halothane, isoflurane produced dose-related decreases in R in a canine model, consistent with the known effects of this drug on systemic vascular resistance. Isoflurane and halothane also caused similar increases in C and Z_c concomitant with reductions in mean arterial pressure. Thus, the major difference between the effects of isoflurane and halothane on LV afterload derived from the Windkessel model of $Z_{in}(\omega)$ was related to R, a property of arteriolar resistance vessels, and not to C or Z_c, the mechanical characteristics of the aorta. In contrast to the findings with sevoflurane, desflurane also reduced R in dogs, thus suggesting that this agent is a more potent peripheral vasodilator. Importantly, the inverse relationship between C and mean arterial pressure remains unchanged by volatile anesthetics, unlike the findings with the arterial vasodilator sodium nitroprusside or the intravenous anesthetic propofol. These data emphasize that volatile anesthetics do not fundamentally affect aortic mechanical characteristics.

Isoflurane and halothane produced alterations in $Z_{in}(\omega)$ in an experimental model of heart failure that are somewhat different from those observed in the normal cardiovascular system. These volatile anesthetics decreased arterial pressure but did not affect C and Z_c in the presence of LV dysfunction. Isoflurane also did not reduce R in the presence of dilated cardiomyopathy, in contrast to the actions of this volatile anesthetic in the presence of normal LV performance. Thus, neither isoflurane nor the older agent halothane reduced arterial hydraulic resistance or favorably improved the rectifying properties of the aorta in the presence of pacing-induced cardiomyopathy. The findings suggest that volatile anesthetics do not exert beneficial actions on LV afterload in the presence of heart failure.

Right Ventricular Function

The crescent-shaped right ventricle is composed of embryologically distinct inflow and outflow tracts that differ in their structure and response to autonomic nervous system activity. Sequential contraction of the RV inflow and outflow tracts establishes regional pressure gradients within the right ventricle during systole and accounts for the peristaltic mechanical action of this pump. True isovolumic relaxation does not occur in the right ventricle. Instead, ejection of blood from the outflow tract into the pulmonary artery continues after the inflow tract has begun to relax. The effects of volatile anesthetics on the function and contraction sequence of the RV inflow and outflow tracts have been incompletely studied. Halothane produced similar depression of contractile function in the RV inflow and outflow tracts when a uniform definition of end-systole and end-diastole was used for both regions of the RV. Halothane also caused dose-related decreases in RV contractility as evaluated by using regional preload recruitable stroke work derived from RV pressure–segment length diagrams in the RV inflow and outflow tracts in the presence and absence of autonomic nervous system reflexes.[11] Importantly, halothane also abolished the normal RV sequential contraction pattern without exerting differential negative inotropic effects on different regions of the right ventricle, thus suggesting that volatile anesthetics may alter RV contraction dynamics by adversely affecting cardiac autonomic nervous system activity. Isoflurane also exerted qualitatively different effects on RV and LV afterload and hydraulic power generation that were also partially mediated by the autonomic nervous system.[12] Hence, isoflurane probably produces fundamentally different actions on RV and LV contraction dynamics in vivo.

Left Atrial Function

The left atrium serves three major roles that exert a profound effect on LV filling and overall cardiovascular performance. The left atrium is a contractile chamber that actively empties immediately before the onset of LV systole and establishes the final LV end-diastolic volume. The left atrium is a reservoir that stores pulmonary venous return during LV contraction and isovolumic relaxation after closure and before opening of the mitral valve. The left atrium is also a conduit that empties its contents into the left ventricle down a pressure gradient after the mitral valve opens and continues to passively transfer pulmonary venous blood flow during LV diastasis. These contraction, reservoir, and conduit functions of the left atrium mechanically facilitate the transition between the almost continuous flow through the pulmonary venous circulation and the intermittent filling of the left ventricle. Advances in the understanding and clinical significance of left atrial (LA) mechanical function were recently reviewed.[9]

The negative inotropic effects of the older volatile anesthetics halothane and methoxyflurane were initially described in rat atrial myocardium in vitro. Volatile anesthetics also depressed the contractile function of atrial human myocardium.[13] These actions have been attributed to reductions in transsarcolemmal Ca^{2+} influx through voltage-dependent Ca^{2+} channels and decreases in Ca^{2+} availability from the SR, mechanisms that are very similar to those responsible for anesthetic-induced depression of LV myocardium. The negative inotropic effects of volatile anesthetics in the intact left atrium were quantified by pressure-volume analysis (Fig. 23-4).[14] Desflurane, sevoflurane, and isoflurane reduced LA contractility (i.e., E_{es}) by approximately 50% at an end-tidal concentration of 1.2 MAC. The magnitude of this effect on LA myocardium was similar to the degree of LV contractile depression produced by these anesthetics as quantified by LV end-systolic pressure-volume relationships.[1] Desflurane, sevoflurane, and isoflurane also impaired LA and LV relaxation to similar degrees. These data indicate that volatile anesthetics produce equivalent alterations in contractility and relaxation in LA and LV myocardium.[14] The magnitude of reductions in the LA inotropic and lusitropic state produced by volatile anesthetics was also similar in the intact left atrium, thus supporting the results obtained in isolated human atrial myocardium.[13]

Desflurane, sevoflurane, and isoflurane altered the passive mechanical behavior of the left atrium.[14] LA reservoir function (V loop area and reservoir volume) was maintained during the administration of anesthetic at concentrations of less than 1.0 MAC. Such preservation of reservoir function contributed to the relative maintenance of LV stroke volume[1] by compensating for decreases in LV filling associated with a reduced contribution of LA contraction. The volatile anesthetics also reduced dynamic LA chamber stiffness, an action that most likely contributed to

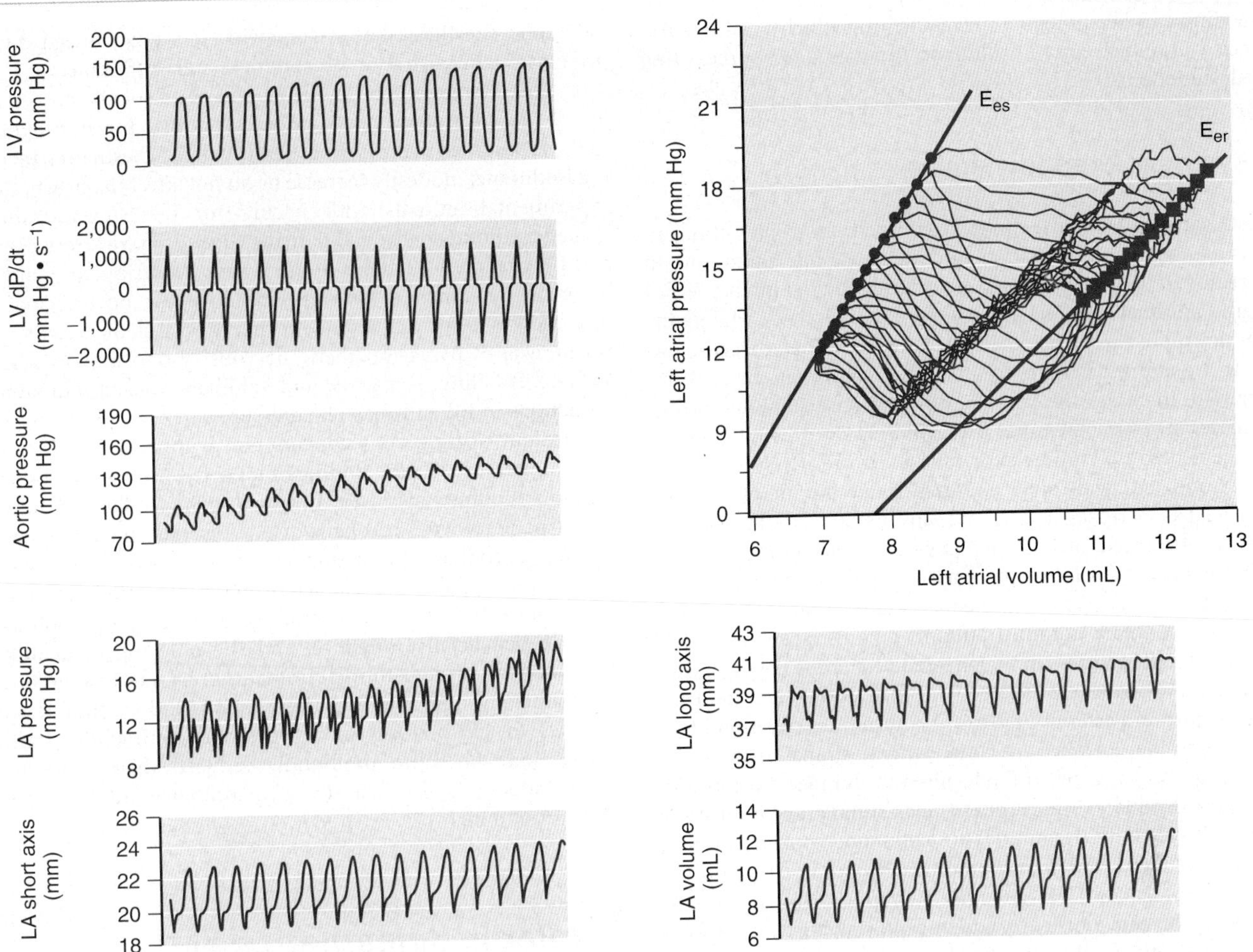

Figure 23-4 Continuous left ventricular (LV) pressure, LV dP/dt, aortic pressure, left atrial (LA) pressure, LA short- and long-axis dimensions, and LA volume waveforms (*left*) and corresponding LA pressure-volume diagrams (*right*) resulting from the intravenous administration of phenylephrine (200 µg) observed in a typical experiment. The maximum LA elastance (*solid dots*) and end-reservoir pressure and volume (*solid squares*) for each pressure-volume diagram were used to obtain the slopes (E_{es} and E_{er}) and extrapolated volume intercepts of the LA end-systolic and end-reservoir pressure-volume relationships to quantify myocardial contractility and dynamic chamber stiffness, respectively. *(Adapted from Gare M, Schwabe DA, Hettrick DA, et al: Desflurane, sevoflurane, and isoflurane affect left atrial active and passive mechanical properties and impair left atrial–left ventricular coupling in vivo. Analysis using pressure-volume relations. Anesthesiology 95:689-698, 2001.)*

the preservation of reservoir function because the delays in LA relaxation and declines in LV systolic function that also occurred would be expected to decrease reservoir function.[15] However, LA reservoir function was reduced during the administration of higher concentrations of volatile anesthetics because further impairment of LA relaxation and LV contractility occurred. Decreases in the ratio of LA stroke work to total pressure-volume diagram area and increases in the ratio of LA conduit to total reservoir volume were also produced by desflurane, sevoflurane, and isoflurane. These data indicate that the LA contribution to LV filling becomes less active and more passive during the administration of volatile anesthetics.

Desflurane, sevoflurane, and isoflurane decreased the ratio of LA to LV elastance (E_{es}/E_{LV}), consistent with impaired mechanical matching between these chambers. As described earlier, volatile anesthetics have been shown to produce LV diastolic dysfunction by delaying LV isovolumic relaxation and impairing early LV filling in association with direct negative inotropic effects. Thus, the attenuation of transfer of kinetic energy from the left atrium to the left ventricle probably resulted from the combination of LA contractile depression and LV systolic and diastolic dysfunction. Volatile anesthetic–induced abnormalities in LA-LV matching were greater than the analogous impairment in LV-arterial coupling evaluated via a similar series elastic chamber model in a previous investigation[1] because these anesthetics produced beneficial alterations in the determinants of LV afterload that partially compensate for simultaneous depression of LV myocardial contractility.

The influence of isoflurane on LA function in the presence of preexisting LV dysfunction has also been examined.[16] Isoflurane depressed LA contractility, impaired LA-LV coupling, and reduced the active LA contribution to LV filling in dogs with pacing-induced cardiomyopathy, findings that were similar in magnitude to those observed in healthy canine hearts.[14] In contrast to the findings in normal dogs,[14] LA reservoir function was reduced in dogs with LV dysfunction at lower isoflurane concentrations (0.6 and 0.9 MAC).[16] These findings indicate that the ability of the left atrium to act as a reservoir for pulmonary venous return is attenuated during isoflurane anesthesia. Such an isoflurane-induced reduction in LA storage ability suggested that the quantity of blood transferred from the left atrium to the left ventricle when the mitral valve opens may be reduced, thereby providing another potential mechanism by which volatile anesthetics can reduce early LV filling in the presence of preexisting LV dysfunction.

Systemic Hemodynamics

Volatile anesthetics cause direct negative chronotropic actions in vitro by depressing sinoatrial node activity, but alterations in heart rate in vivo are primarily determined by the interaction of volatile anesthetics and baroreceptor reflex activity. Halothane does not appreciably change the heart rate in humans because this anesthetic attenuates baroreceptor reflex responses. In contrast, isoflurane increases the heart rate in response to simultaneous decreases in arterial pressure. These findings occur with this volatile agent because baroreceptor reflexes are relatively preserved when compared with older anesthetics. Desflurane also causes dose-related increases in heart rate in humans. Desflurane- and isoflurane-induced tachycardia may be more pronounced in pediatric patients or in the presence of vagolytic drugs and, conversely, may be attenuated in neonates and geriatric patients or by the concomitant administration of opioids (see Chapters 71 and 82). Rapid increases in the inspired desflurane concentration above 1 MAC may be associated with further transient increases in heart rate and arterial pressure as a result of activation of the sympathetic nervous system. Interestingly, similar increases in heart rate also occur when the inspired isoflurane concentration is increased rapidly. The cardiovascular stimulation induced by rapid increases in desflurane or isoflurane concentration in humans resulted from activation of tracheopulmonary and systemic receptors and was attenuated by pretreatment with β_1-adrenoceptor antagonists, α_2-adrenoceptor agonists, or opioids. In contrast to the findings with isoflurane and desflurane, sevoflurane did not alter heart rate or cause cardiovascular stimulation during rapid increases in anesthetic concentration in humans.

All modern volatile anesthetics cause concentration-related decreases in arterial pressure. The mechanism by which these anesthetics reduce arterial pressure differs between anesthetics. The decreases in arterial pressure produced by halothane and enflurane were attributed to reductions in myocardial contractility and cardiac output, whereas isoflurane, desflurane, and sevoflurane decrease arterial blood pressure primarily as a result of reductions in LV afterload. Thus, isoflurane, desflurane, and sevoflurane maintain cardiac output because these anesthetics produce less pronounced reductions in myocardial contractility and greater decreases in systemic vascular resistance in humans than halothane or enflurane does. Isoflurane and desflurane may also preserve autonomic nervous system regulation of the circulation to a greater degree than other volatile anesthetics do. The baroreceptor reflex–mediated tachycardia that occurs during isoflurane and desflurane anesthesia serves to maintain cardiac output despite modest declines in contractility and stroke volume. The declines in arterial pressure produced by volatile anesthetics may be attenuated by surgical stimulation or concomitant administration of nitrous oxide. Volatile anesthetics also cause modest, dose-related increases in right atrial pressure in humans. These effects probably occur as a result of direct negative inotropic actions. The cardiovascular effects of volatile anesthetics are altered by the duration of anesthesia. Increases in myocardial contractility and cardiac output and decreases in LV preload and afterload occur after several hours of constant MAC anesthesia. Recovery from circulatory depression is greatest during halothane anesthesia but is somewhat less pronounced during prolonged administration of isoflurane and desflurane.

The systemic hemodynamic effects of volatile anesthetics in the presence of LV dysfunction are similar but not identical to those observed in the normal heart. Volatile anesthetics, including isoflurane, modestly increase or do not affect the heart rate in experimental animals with pacing- or doxorubicin-induced dilated cardiomyopathy and patients with coronary artery disease and LV dysfunction. These findings may be attributed to altered baroreceptor reflex activity, β_1-adrenoceptor downregulation, increases in central sympathetic nervous system activity, and withdrawal of parasympathetic nervous system tone associated with heart failure. Isoflurane and halothane caused pronounced reductions in LV end-diastolic pressure and chamber dimension in cardiomyopathic dogs concomitant with decreases in mean arterial pressure.[6] These findings supported previously observed declines in pulmonary artery pressure during isoflurane anesthesia in patients with coronary artery disease and heart failure and suggested that venodilation represents a major hemodynamic consequence of this volatile agent in experimental and clinical heart failure. In contrast to the findings in normal dogs, isoflurane did not beneficially influence, and the older agent halothane detrimentally affected, the determinants of LV afterload in cardiomyopathic dogs. As a result of these actions and the simultaneous declines in LV preload and myocardial contractility, cardiac output may be more profoundly reduced during isoflurane or halothane anesthesia in the presence of preexisting LV dysfunction.

Volatile Anesthetics and Cardiac Electrophysiology

Cardiac Conduction

Volatile anesthetics slow the rate of sinoatrial node discharge by direct and indirect effects on sinoatrial node automaticity. These actions may be altered in vivo by vasoactive drugs or autonomic nervous system activity. Older volatile anesthetics and, to a lesser extent, isoflurane shorten the cardiac action potential and the effective duration of the refractory period in normal Purkinje fibers, but volatile anesthetics also prolong His-Purkinje and ventricular conduction times. Halothane, enflurane, and isoflurane also prolong atrioventricular conduction time and refractoriness. When combined with the direct actions of volatile anesthetics on sinoatrial node discharge, these data suggest that volatile anesthetics have the potential to produce bradycardia and atrioventricular conduction abnormalities. However, primary disturbances in atrioventricular conduction leading to second- or third-degree atrioventricular block in humans probably do not occur with volatile anesthetics in the absence of conduction disease or drugs that directly prolong the atrioventricular conduction time.

Volatile anesthetics may have proarrhythmogenic or antiarrhythmogenic actions against the abnormal cardiac electrophysiologic mechanisms produced by myocardial ischemia or infarction. Halothane, enflurane, and isoflurane have been shown to be cardioprotective against ventricular fibrillation produced by coronary artery occlusion and reperfusion. Protective effects against ouabain-induced arrhythmias have also been demonstrated with the older volatile agent halothane. Volatile anesthetics may exert antiarrhythmic effects by opposing subsidiary pacemaker activity in infarcted myocardium. Conversely, halothane and, to a lesser extent, isoflurane may be arrhythmogenic in Purkinje fibers in experimental myocardial infarction by facilitating reentrant activity or increasing temporal dispersion of refractory period recovery. These actions may be related to inhibition of the slow Na^+ current in false tendon fibers and induction of reentry of premature impulses into more refractory Purkinje fibers in the border zone of an ischemic area. Halothane, enflurane, and isoflurane prolong the QT_c interval in humans. These data suggest that patients with idiopathic or acquired long QT syndrome may be at greater risk for the development of torsades de pointes ventricular tachycardia during anesthesia with these agents.

Epinephrine-Induced Arrhythmias

Halothane and, to a lesser extent, other volatile anesthetics sensitize myocardium to the arrhythmogenic effects of epinephrine. Sensitization is the interaction between volatile anesthetics and catecholamines that leads to reductions in the threshold for both atrial and ventricular arrhythmias. Sequentially escalating doses of epinephrine produce premature ventricular contractions and sustained ventricular tachyarrhythmias during halothane anesthesia. Halothane-epinephrine–induced arrhythmias are attenuated by pretreatment with sodium thiopental, presumably via effects on the atrioventricular node or the upper His bundle. A synergistic interaction between α_1- and β-adrenoceptors has been strongly implicated in the pathogenesis of halothane-epinephrine–induced ventricular arrhythmias. Stimulation of the α_{1A}-adrenoceptor in the His-Purkinje system by epinephrine during halothane anesthesia transiently slows Purkinje fiber conduction. This proarrhythmogenic effect is mediated by phospholipase C and the intracellular second messenger inositol triphosphate. Enhanced conduction in the Purkinje–ventricular muscle junction accompanied by simultaneous α_1-adrenoceptor–mediated depression of Purkinje conduction also plays an important role in halothane-epinephrine–induced arrhythmias. The doses of epinephrine required to produce ventricular arrhythmias during desflurane or sevoflurane anesthesia are similar to but significantly less than those observed during administration of isoflurane and halothane. Halothane-catecholamine sensitization also promotes abnormal automaticity of the dominant and latent atrial pacemakers. These effects may produce premature ventricular contractions and arrhythmias originating from the His bundle. Intact sinoatrial node function reduces the incidence of epinephrine-induced ventricular escape during halothane anesthesia and is protective against His bundle arrhythmias.

Volatile Anesthetics and the Coronary Circulation

Coronary Vascular Effects in Vitro

Volatile anesthetics cause direct coronary artery vasodilation in vitro; however, the simultaneous reductions in determinants of myocardial oxygen consumption (MVO_2), including heart rate, preload, afterload, and inotropic state, produced by these anesthetics cause coronary vasoconstriction in vivo via metabolic autoregulation. Volatile anesthetic–induced alterations in coronary blood flow are also affected by the reductions in coronary perfusion pressure produced by these anesthetics. Thus, the combination of direct and indirect actions determines the net effect of volatile anesthetics on coronary vascular tone. Isoflurane and halothane caused vasodilation of isolated coronary arteries. Halothane produced more profound coronary artery dilation than isoflurane did at similar MAC in isolated coronary arteries larger than 2000 μm. In contrast, isoflurane caused vasodilation of predominantly small (<900 μm) canine epicardial coronary arteries. Halothane may produce greater vasodilatory effects in large coronary arteries than isoflurane does because halothane causes more pronounced suppression of the voltage-dependent Ca^{2+} current.

The direct negative inotropic effects of volatile anesthetics caused a reduction in coronary blood flow in isolated, contracting hearts during precise control of ventricular loading conditions via flow-metabolism coupling. Thus, a decrease in myocardial O_2 demand was accompanied by an increase in coronary vascular resistance, findings that may be incorrectly interpreted as suggesting that volatile anesthetics produce coronary vasoconstriction. However, examination of the actions of volatile anesthetics on myocardial O_2 extraction and the ratio of myocardial O_2 delivery to MVO_2 revealed that these drugs are coronary vasodilators. Halothane and isoflurane decreased myocardial O_2 extraction and increased the ratio of O_2 delivery to consumption in isolated, beating hearts.[17] These findings indicate that volatile anesthetics produce direct coronary vasodilation in isolated hearts because myocardial O_2 delivery exceeds MVO_2 and coronary sinus O_2 tension increases. Halothane, isoflurane, and sevoflurane also caused similar reductions in adenosine-induced coronary flow reserve in tetrodotoxin-arrested, isolated hearts. Because mechanical work was not performed in this preparation, these findings supported the hypothesis that volatile anesthetics cause direct coronary vasodilation of similar magnitude.

Coronary Vascular Effects in Vivo

Halothane has variable effects on coronary blood flow and coronary vascular resistance in vivo that occur concomitant with changes in MVO_2. Decreases in MVO_2 caused declines in coronary blood flow with relative maintenance of or modest increases in coronary vascular resistance during halothane anesthesia. Despite the decreases in coronary blood flow, halothane increased coronary sinus O_2 tension and decreased O_2 extraction, thus indicating that halothane is a relatively weak coronary vasodilator. Like halothane, isoflurane variably altered coronary blood flow in vivo.[18,19] Isoflurane reduced MVO_2 and simultaneously decreased O_2 extraction, findings indicative of direct coronary vasodilation.[18] Isoflurane produced mild, transient increases in blood flow independent of changes in MVO_2 and autonomic nervous system activity during induction of anesthesia with inhaled anesthetics. Perfusion of the left anterior descending coronary artery with blood previously equilibrated with isoflurane dramatically increased coronary blood flow,[20] but only mild coronary vasodilation occurred after a period of anesthetic equilibration in a similar experimental model.[19] Isoflurane-induced increases in coronary blood flow were not accompanied by epicardial coronary artery dilation, thus verifying that isoflurane dilates predominantly small coronary arteries. However, adenosine, a potent coronary vasodilator, caused considerably greater vasodilation in coronary microvessels than isoflurane did. The more profound decreases in myocardial O_2 extraction produced by isoflurane than by enflurane indicate that isoflurane is a more potent coronary vasodilator than its structural isomer is.

The influence of desflurane and sevoflurane on coronary blood flow in the intact cardiovascular system has been incompletely examined. Desflurane and isoflurane caused similar increases in the ratio of O_2 delivery to consumption and decreased O_2 extraction, consistent with coronary vasodilation. However, the increases in coronary blood flow produced by desflurane, but not by isoflurane, were attenuated by pharmacologic blockade of the autonomic nervous system, which suggests that isoflurane causes relatively greater direct coronary vasodilation in vivo than desflurane does. Sevoflurane did not produce any significant degree of coronary vasodilation, in contrast to the findings with other volatile anesthetics.

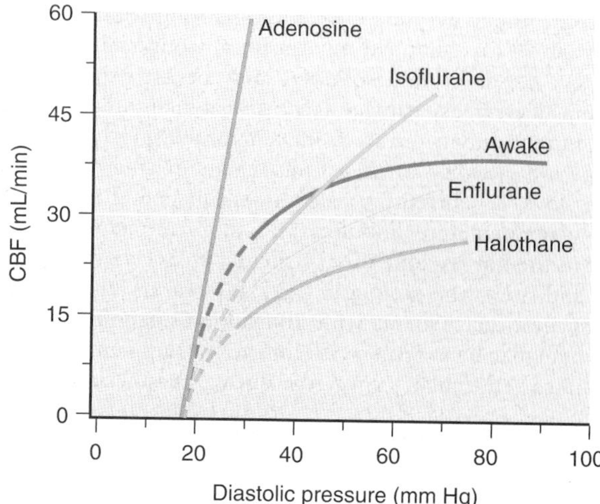

Figure 23-5 Qualitative description of the effects of volatile anesthetics on the coronary blood flow (CBF)–diastolic pressure relationship as compared with the effect of adenosine-induced maximal coronary vasodilation in awake and anesthetized dogs. *Solid lines* are drawn from mean slopes determined by linear regression analysis. *Dashed lines* represent the nonlinear portion of the curve and are estimates. When compared with the findings obtained in awake dogs, the anesthetics affect absolute CBF variably but do not increase the slope of the CBF-pressure plots. *(Adapted from Hickey RF, Sybert PE, Verrier ED, Cason BA: Effects of halothane, enflurane, and isoflurane on coronary blood flow autoregulation and coronary vascular reserve in the canine heart. Anesthesiology 68:21-30, 1988.)*

Coronary Vasodilator Reserve and Autoregulation

Volatile anesthetics alter coronary vasodilator reserve, defined as the ratio of peak coronary blood flow after brief coronary artery occlusion (reactive hyperemia) to baseline flow. Coronary vasodilator reserve was greater during isoflurane than during halothane anesthesia. This observation suggested that the older agent halothane may be a more potent coronary vasodilator than isoflurane because greater baseline coronary vasodilation should be accompanied by a reduced ability to further increase coronary blood flow in response to a brief ischemic episode. However, halothane also reduced the determinants of MVO_2 to a greater degree in vivo than isoflurane did. Peak coronary blood flow during reactive hyperemia and percent flow debt repayment are directly related to the intensity of the ischemic stimulus and the magnitude of the O_2 debt accumulated during coronary artery occlusion. Thus, the differences in coronary vasodilator reserve produced by isoflurane and halothane may reflect differences in the intensity of ischemia during coronary occlusion and not the relative vasodilator efficacy of these volatile anesthetics.

Dilation of coronary arteriolar resistance vessels by volatile anesthetics altered pressure autoregulation in the coronary vasculature.[21] The changes in autoregulation produced by vasoactive drugs, including volatile anesthetics, are typically determined by the slope of the pressure-flow curve generated by progressive constriction of a coronary artery. Changes in these pressure-flow curves demonstrated that autoregulation is disrupted during anesthesia as opposed to the conscious state (Fig. 23-5). Isoflurane produced more profound alterations in autoregulation than the older volatile anesthetics did, as indicated by greater increases in the slope of the pressure-flow relationship. Coronary perfusion pressure also played a more important role in the determination of coronary blood flow during anesthesia. Volatile anesthetics impaired coronary autoregulation to some degree, but these anesthetics did not produce the profound degree of coronary vasodilation and inhibition of autoregulation seen with adenosine or dipyridamole.[21] In contrast to volatile anesthetics, these drugs cause maximal coronary vasodilation and inhibit pressure autoregulation to such a degree that coronary blood flow becomes directly dependent on coronary perfusion pressure. Thus, volatile anesthetics are weak coronary vasodilators.

Mechanisms of Volatile Anesthetic–Induced Coronary Vasodilation

Volatile anesthetics produce direct coronary artery relaxation by affecting intracellular Ca^{2+} regulation at several locations in the vascular smooth muscle cell. Volatile anesthetics inhibited influx of Ca^{2+} through voltage- and receptor-operated Ca^{2+} channels in coronary vascular smooth muscle. Volatile anesthetics also reduced accumulation of Ca^{2+} in and release by the coronary vascular smooth muscle SR, inhibited G proteins linked to phospholipase C, and decreased formation of the second messenger inositol triphosphate. The coronary vasodilating actions of volatile anesthetics are probably not related to the production or release of nitric oxide (NO). Investigations conducted in isolated coronary and aortic vascular preparations and in the intact canine coronary circulation[20] demonstrated that volatile anesthetic–induced coronary vasodilation occurs independent of NO. Some experimental evidence suggested that the direct coronary vasodilator effects of isoflurane may be mediated by the vascular endothelium, but other data indicated that volatile anesthetics, including isoflurane, may adversely affect the release or action of NO.[22] The results of one investigation demonstrated that NO-induced formation of cyclic guanylate monophosphate is partially attenuated by the older agent halothane,[23] whereas other studies have indicated that volatile anesthetics do not affect vasodilation produced by the NO donors sodium nitroprusside or nitroglycerin.[24] Volatile anesthetics may also reduce the stability of NO by generating oxygen-derived free radicals[24] while leaving NO release and its action on vascular smooth muscle unaffected.[22] Whether the results of these later studies conducted in isolated aortic preparations are applicable to the coronary circulation requires further evaluation, but these investigations have provided important information about the potential interactions between NO metabolism and volatile anesthetics in the coronary circulation.

Isoflurane and halothane cause coronary vasodilation by activation of adenosine triphosphate (ATP)-sensitive potassium (K_{ATP}) channels.[25,26] Increases in coronary blood flow in response to halothane and isoflurane were attenuated by the nonselective K_{ATP} channel antagonist glyburide in isolated rat hearts and anesthetized pigs, respectively.[25,26] Glyburide also partially blocked increases in coronary blood flow during intracoronary administration of volatile anesthetic–equilibrated blood in canine hearts in situ.[27] Isoflurane-induced reductions in coronary vascular resistance were attenuated by the selective adenosine$_1$ (A_1) receptor antagonist 8-cyclopentyl-1,3,dipropylxanthine (DPCPX).[28] These data suggest that the coronary vasodilation produced by isoflurane may occur partially as a result of stimulation of A_1 receptors coupled to K_{ATP} channels.[28]

Investigations in dogs with steal-prone anatomy (complete occlusion of a coronary artery with collateral flow from an adjacent vessel with a critical stenosis) have repeatedly demonstrated that isoflurane and halothane do not alter collateral-dependent or ischemic-zone myocardial blood flow, endocardial-to-epicardial coronary blood flow distribution, or electrocardiographic findings when diastolic arterial pressure is held constant. Coronary collateral perfusion was unchanged during isoflurane or halothane anesthesia in dogs at a mean arterial pressure of 50 mm Hg. Coronary steal did not occur in a chronically instrumented canine model of coronary artery disease with the administration of isoflurane,[30] halothane,[31] desflurane,[32] or sevoflurane[33] independent of severe coronary stenosis or the development of coronary collaterals. These findings refuted earlier evidence in dogs with amaroid constrictor–induced augmentation of the coronary collateral circulation in which it was suggested that isoflurane reduces collateral blood flow and causes coronary steal in vivo. These effects of volatile anesthetics were in stark contrast to those obtained with adenosine, a potent coronary vasodilator that produces coronary steal when arterial pressure is maintained at control levels in models of multivessel coronary artery disease (Fig. 23-6).

Volatile Anesthetics and Ischemic Myocardium

Isoflurane and halothane decreased subendocardial blood flow and myocardial lactate extraction, produced contractile dysfunction, and caused electrocardiographic changes in the presence of coronary stenosis concomitant with declines in coronary perfusion pressure. Regional ischemia during isoflurane- or halothane-induced reductions in perfusion pressure was functionally indicated by the appearance of paradoxical systolic lengthening and postsystolic shortening.[29] Contractile dysfunction in the region distal to a critical coronary stenosis was more severe during isoflurane than during halothane anesthesia coincident with higher flow in the normal zone and lower flow in the ischemic zone. These findings suggest that the coronary vasodilation produced by isoflurane may cause a detrimental redistribution of coronary blood flow away from ischemic myocardium if hypotension is allowed to occur ("coronary steal"). However, these potentially adverse effects of volatile anesthetics on ischemic myocardium were avoided if coronary perfusion pressure was restored. Subendocardial blood flow in the perfusion bed distal to a critical coronary stenosis was reduced during isoflurane-induced declines in arterial pressure, but treatment of hypotension with phenylephrine restored subendocardial blood flow to values observed before the administration of isoflurane. The transmural distribution of coronary blood flow between the subendocardium and subepicardium (endo/epi ratio) decreased during isoflurane anesthesia despite control of arterial pressure. Administration of phenylephrine to maintain arterial pressure constant increased subepicardial blood flow more than subendocardial flow. This increase in subepicardial perfusion accounted for the decline in the endo/epi ratio in the absence of an absolute reduction in subendocardial flow. Restoration of coronary perfusion pressure to baseline levels during isoflurane anesthesia also increased coronary collateral blood flow and normalized myocardial oxygen tension in the ischemic zone.[21]

Volatile Anesthetic–Induced Myocardial Protection

Acute Preconditioning by Volatile Anesthetics

The controversy about volatile anesthetic–induced coronary vasodilation and coronary steal has detracted from substantial experimental evidence indicating that volatile anesthetics exert important protective effects during myocardial ischemia and reperfusion injury. The older anesthetic halothane attenuated ST-segment changes caused by brief coronary artery occlusion and decreased ST-segment elevation to a greater extent than propranolol and sodium nitroprusside did despite producing similar hemodynamic effects. Isoflurane and desflurane produced beneficial actions on LV diastolic mechanics during acute regional myocardial ischemia.[29] Isoflurane and sevoflurane decreased myocardial reperfusion injury and improved functional recovery after global ischemia in isolated hearts.[34,35] Volatile anesthetics also enhanced systolic functional recovery of postischemic-reperfused ("stunned") myocardium when these anesthetics were administered before brief periods of myocardial ischemia in vivo. These salutary effects were accompanied by preservation of high-energy phosphate levels.[36] Volatile anesthetics have been shown to attenuate the effect of oxygen-derived free radicals on development of LV pressure in isolated hearts. Halothane also preserved contractile function and ultrastructural integrity during reperfusion after normothermic cardioplegic arrest.[37] In 1997, three research groups independently reported that administration of halothane or isoflurane before prolonged coronary artery occlusion and reperfusion reduces myocardial infarct size in vivo (Fig. 23-7).[5,38,39] Termed "anesthetic preconditioning," this beneficial effect was found to persist despite discontinuation of the volatile anesthetic before coronary artery occlusion.[5] This short-term memory phase was similar to that observed during ischemic preconditioning.

Anesthetic preconditioning has been shown to be dose related in experimental animals[40,41] independent of alterations in

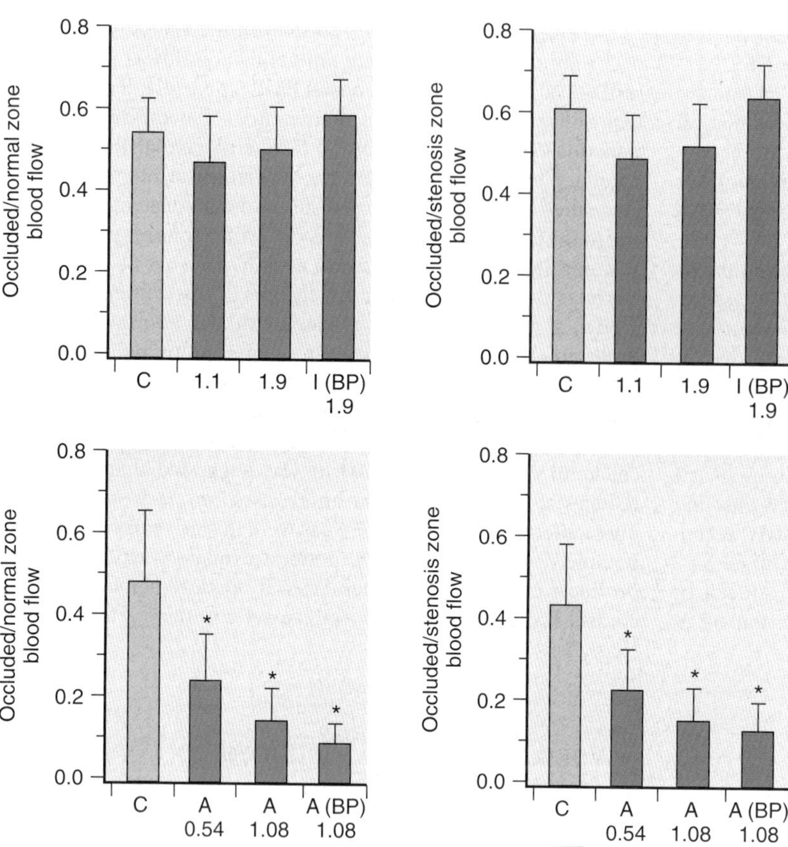

Figure 23-6 Comparison of occluded to normal and occluded to stenotic-zone myocardial blood flow in dogs with steal-prone coronary artery anatomy in the conscious state (C), during administration of isoflurane at 1.1 and 1.9 minimum alveolar concentration (I), during adenosine (A) infusions (0.54 and 1.08 mg/min), and during maintenance of heart rate and arterial pressure at conscious values during the highest doses (BP). Isoflurane does not cause coronary steal, in contrast to the significant (*$P < .05$) reductions in blood flow to collateral-dependent myocardium produced by adenosine. *(Adapted from Hartman JC, Kampine JP, Schmeling WT, Warltier DC: Actions of isoflurane on myocardial perfusion in chronically instrumented dogs with poor, moderate, or well-developed coronary collaterals. J Cardiothorac Anesth 4:715-725, 1990.)*

systemic hemodynamics or coronary collateral blood flow. Isoflurane and sevoflurane also produced dose-dependent preservation of isolated ventricular myocyte viability during ischemia in vitro.[42] Isoflurane elicited cardioprotection when the volatile agent was discontinued 15 or 30 minutes before prolonged coronary artery occlusion and reperfusion in rabbits[43] and dogs,[5] respectively. In contrast, sevoflurane failed to reduce the extent of myocardial infarction if the anesthetic was discontinued 30 minutes before the onset of prolonged ischemia.[44] These data suggest that the memory period of anesthetic preconditioning may differ between volatile anesthetics on the basis of species and pharmacokinetics. Dual as opposed to single exposure to sevoflurane improved anesthetic preconditioning in guinea pig hearts, thus indicating that repetitive administration of a volatile agent appears to confer an additional benefit.[45] The cardioprotection resulting from anesthetic preconditioning was shown to be restricted to a range of ischemia durations between 25 and 40 minutes in Langendorff perfused isolated guinea pig hearts.[46] Accordingly, anesthetic preconditioning may be especially beneficial in patients with ongoing myocardial ischemia of intermediate duration. Interestingly, the mechanism of sevoflurane-induced cardioprotection was independent of the type of ischemic stimulus (hypoxia versus metabolic inhibition) in isolated rat ventricular trabeculae.[47] These results indirectly suggested that anesthetic

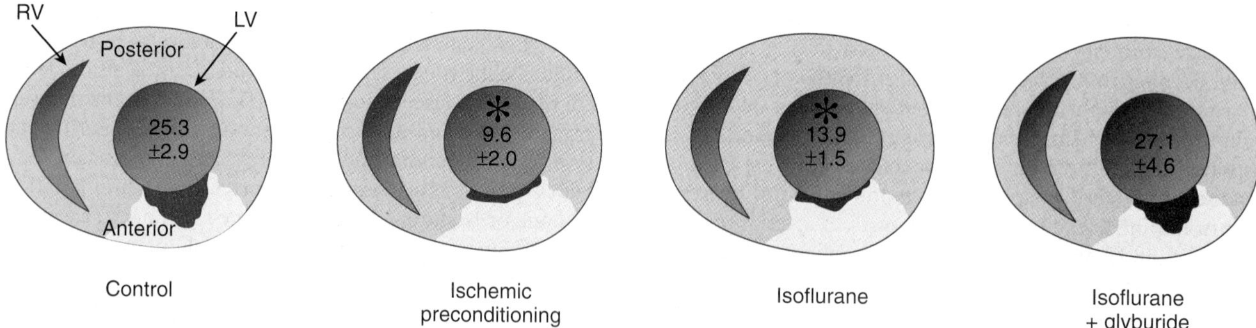

Figure 23-7 Schematic illustration of canine myocardium subjected to 60-minute coronary artery occlusion and reperfusion and then stained to identify the region of myocardial infarction (*dark red area*) within the area of myocardium at risk for infarction (*light yellow area*). Isoflurane decreased the extent of myocardial infarction. The protective effect of isoflurane was equivalent to that produced by ischemic preconditioning and was abolished by pretreatment with glyburide. *Significantly ($P < .05$) different from control. *(Adapted from Kersten JR, Schmeling TJ, Pagel PS, et al: Isoflurane mimics ischemic preconditioning via activation of K_{ATP} channels. Reduction of myocardial infarct size with acute memory phase. Anesthesiology 87:361-370, 1997.)*

preconditioning may be equally effective at preserving myocardial integrity during supply or demand myocardial ischemia in patients with coronary artery disease, but this intriguing hypothesis remains to be formally tested. Advanced age and increased heart size attenuated the efficacy of sevoflurane preconditioning in rats[48] and guinea pigs.[49] These experimental observations may also have important clinical ramifications in elderly patients at risk for the development of myocardial ischemia. In contrast, sevoflurane was capable of exerting cardioprotective effects in ischemic newborn rabbit myocardium.[50]

Volatile anesthetics may also produce beneficial effects on blood flow to and neutrophil interaction with ischemic myocardium. Volatile anesthetics produce coronary vasodilation by activating K_{ATP} channels or by favorably affecting intracellular Ca^{2+} homeostasis in vascular smooth muscle. Decreases in collateral blood flow after coronary artery occlusion have been shown to be less pronounced than declines in flow to normal myocardium in the presence of the older agent halothane. The ratio of myocardial O_2 delivery to MVo_2 was also increased in collateral-dependent myocardium during halothane anesthesia. Halothane inhibited platelet thrombi formation via increases in platelet cyclic adenosine monophosphate concentration and thereby decreased cyclic variations in coronary blood flow associated with a critical coronary artery stenosis. Sevoflurane increased blood flow to collateral-dependent myocardium when arterial pressure was maintained at conscious values mediated by Ca^{2+}-activated potassium (BK_{Ca}) channels.[51] Sevoflurane also improved recovery of coronary vascular reactivity and enhanced endothelial NO release in isolated hearts subjected to global ischemia and reperfusion. Volatile anesthetics attenuated adhesion of neutrophils and platelets in the coronary vasculature after ischemia and reperfusion. Isoflurane pretreatment also inhibited cytokine-induced cell death after ischemia-reperfusion injury in vitro.[52] Furthermore, isoflurane and sevoflurane preconditioned against neutrophil-induced contractile dysfunction in isolated rat hearts through activation of adenosine receptors.[53] Taken together, the results of these investigations suggest that the salutary actions of volatile anesthetics on coronary perfusion and neutrophil function may, to some degree, be responsible for the protection against ischemia-reperfusion injury afforded by these drugs.

The mechanisms responsible for volatile anesthetic–induced protection during myocardial ischemia and reperfusion have been intensively investigated in recent years and are the subject of several major reviews.[54-57] The beneficial effects of volatile anesthetics may be attributed to a favorable reduction in the myocardial oxygen demand required for active contraction along with concomitant preservation of energy-dependent vital cellular processes because these anesthetics cause direct negative inotropic, lusitropic, and chronotropic effects and decrease LV afterload. However, the older agent halothane exerted protective effects during complete functional arrest induced by cardioplegia.[37] Isoflurane, desflurane, and sevoflurane also produced cardioprotection when administered solely during reperfusion.[58] These data indicate that preferential alterations in myocardial oxygen supply-demand relationships are not solely responsible for the anti-ischemic actions of volatile anesthetics. Isoflurane and halothane may significantly lower excessive intracellular Ca^{2+} during reperfusion via a direct decline in the net transsarcolemmal Ca^{2+} transient resulting from partially inhibited Ca^{2+} channel activity or an indirect reduction of oxygen-derived free radical formation. In contrast to this rather nonspecific intracellular Ca^{2+} reduction hypothesis, a large body of very compelling evidence has convincingly demonstrated that cardioprotection by volatile anesthetics occurs as a consequence of the activation of endogenous signal transduction pathways. To date, K_{ATP} channels,[5] G protein–coupled receptor ligands (e.g., adenosine, opioid),[39,59] isoforms of protein kinase C (PKC),[60] protein tyrosine kinase (PTK),[60] reactive oxygen and nitrogen species, nuclear factor κB (NF-κB),[61] and several components of the prosurvival reperfusion injury salvage kinase cascade[62] have all been shown to mediate acute preconditioning by volatile anesthetics. These elements will now be discussed in detail.

Mitochondrial and Sarcolemmal K_{ATP} Channels

The K_{ATP} channel plays a central role in ischemic and anesthetic preconditioning. The K_{ATP} channel is a heteromultimeric complex consisting of an inwardly rectifying K^+ channel (K_{ir}) and a sulfonylurea receptor (SUR).[63] Pharmacologically distinct K_{ATP} channels have been identified in cardiac sarcolemmal and mitochondrial membranes. It was originally proposed that opening of sarcolemmal K_{ATP} channels protects ischemic myocardium by shortening the duration of the action potential and preventing intracellular Ca^{2+} overload. However, subsequent studies performed after discovery of the mitochondrial K_{ATP} channel indicated that the beneficial actions of K_{ATP} channel opening occur independent of the action potential duration. Nevertheless, ischemic preconditioning was not observed in the absence of the sarcolemmal K_{ir} channel in transgenic mice.[64] These data suggest that protection against ischemic injury requires contribution of the sarcolemmal K_{ATP} channel. In contrast, mitochondrial K_{ATP} channels appear to be the primary mediators of ischemic preconditioning.[65] Preservation of mitochondrial bioenergetic function appears to be vital for cellular protection against myocardial ischemia.[66] Mitochondrial K_{ATP} channel openers maintained intracellular Ca^{2+} homeostasis and inhibited mitochondrial Ca^{2+} overload.[67] These actions enhanced myocyte survival by preventing tissue necrosis or apoptosis (programmed cell death).[68] In contrast to the well-known generalized cellular destruction and profound inflammatory response that typify necrosis, the highly regulated, ATP-dependent phenomenon of apoptosis is characterized by selective DNA lysis associated with the formation of apoptotic bodies, appearance of condensed chromatin, absence of inflammation, and preservation of cell membrane structure.[69] Activation of mitochondrial K_{ATP} channels inhibited apoptosis in rat ventricular myocytes by attenuating oxidant stress during reperfusion.[70] Alteration of the mitochondrial oxidation-reduction state by activation of K_{ATP} channels may also promote cellular protection.[71] Experiments conducted in isolated cardiac mitochondria indicated that membrane depolarization, matrix swelling, and uncoupling of ATP synthesis occur as a result of increased oxygen consumption, are associated with opening of mitochondrial K_{ATP} channels, and may mediate cellular viability during ischemic preconditioning.[71] Opening of mitochondrial K_{ATP} channels depolarized the inner mitochondrial membrane and caused transient swelling of the mitochondrial matrix[72] because of a shift in ionic balance.[73] Mitochondrial K_{ATP} channel opening initially reduced ATP production as a result of membrane depolarization[74] but subsequently stimulated a compensatory increase in respiration that optimized the efficiency of oxidative phosphorylation, in part by regulating energy-dependent matrix volume. Influx of potassium into mitochondria occurred as a consequence of the balance between K^+ influx through the mitochondrial K_{ATP}

channel and K^+ efflux produced by the mitochondrial K^+-H^+ antiporter. The mitochondrial K_{ATP} channel agonist diazoxide promoted K^+ influx and caused matrix alkalinization in isolated rat ventricular myocardium.[75] These actions were abolished by 5-hydroxydecanoate (5-HD) and ATP. Thus, a moderate disturbance in mitochondrial homeostasis caused by opening of mitochondrial K_{ATP} channels may promote myocardial tolerance to ischemic stress by altering energetic systems to reduce Ca^{2+} overload, prevent the activation of necrotic or apoptotic pathways, or attenuate oxidant stress.

The endogenous mechanisms involved in anesthetic preconditioning are strikingly similar to those implicated in ischemic preconditioning, although differences between these phenomena have been suggested by microarray gene chip analysis.[76] It is hypothesized that a "trigger" (e.g., a brief ischemic episode, exposure to a volatile anesthetic) initiates a cascade of signaling events leading to activation of an "end-effector" that is responsible for resistance to injury. K_{ATP} channel activation has been implicated as the end-effector in this protective scheme during anesthetic preconditioning. Administration of isoflurane and sevoflurane preserved myocyte viability in a cellular model of ischemia, in contrast to cells that were not exposed to a volatile agent.[42] The selective mitochondrial K_{ATP} channel antagonist 5-HD but not the selective sarcolemmal K_{ATP} channel antagonist HMR-1098 abolished this protective effect.[42] The nonselective K_{ATP} channel blocker glyburide (also known as glibenclamide) attenuated the recovery of contractile function produced by isoflurane in stunned myocardium (Fig. 23-8). Isoflurane-induced reductions in canine myocardial infarct size[5] and the ATP-sparing effects of this agent were also abolished by glyburide. 5-HD inhibited preconditioning by isoflurane in rats,[40] rabbits,[77] and isolated human myocardium.[78] Both HMR-1098 and 5-HD abolished the protective effects of desflurane in dogs,[79] thus supporting a role for both sarcolemmal and mitochondrial K_{ATP} channels in anesthetic acute preconditioning. However, HMR-1098 did not affect desflurane preconditioning of isolated human right atrial myocardium.[80] Thus, controversy continues to exist about the relative importance of sarcolemmal versus mitochondrial K_{ATP} channels in anesthetic preconditioning.

Results from in vitro experiments also strongly suggest that volatile anesthetics produce profound effects on sarcolemmal K_{ATP} channel function. Isoflurane stimulated outward K^+ current through sarcolemmal K_{ATP} channels in isolated ventricular myocytes during patch-clamping.[81] Volatile anesthetics also reduced sarcolemmal K_{ATP} channel sensitivity to inhibition by ATP, thereby increasing the probability of being in the open state.[82] However, other patch-clamp experiments failed to confirm these results and suggested that volatile anesthetics do not open sarcolemmal K_{ATP} channels. For example, isoflurane did not alter sarcolemmal K_{ATP} channel current in human atrial cells[78] and, furthermore, inhibited sarcolemmal K_{ATP} channel activity in rabbit ventricular myocytes.[82] Nevertheless, volatile anesthetics have been shown to enhance sarcolemmal K_{ATP} channel current by facilitating channel opening after initial activation. The ε-isoform of PKC (PKC-ε) was shown to prime the sarcolemmal K_{ATP} channel to open in the presence of isoflurane.[83] Facilitation of sarcolemmal K_{ATP} channel current by isoflurane during reduced intracellular ATP concentrations was also dependent on PKC-dependent signaling.[84] In addition, reactive oxygen species (ROS) contributed to isoflurane-induced sensitization of the sarcolemmal K_{ATP} channel to the opener pinacidil.[85] Isoflurane also directly

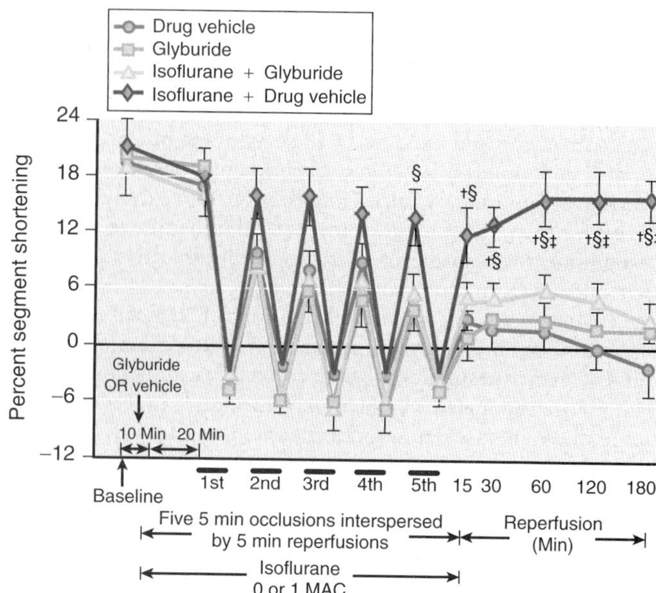

Figure 23-8 Percent segment shortening (%SS) in the intermittently ischemic and reperfused left anterior descending coronary artery (LAD) region. %SS decreases significantly ($P < .05$) from baseline during each 5-minute LAD occlusion and reperfusion in all groups. Significant decreases in %SS during each 5-minute reperfusion and throughout 180 minutes of final reperfusion are observed in dogs pretreated with glyburide, a nonselective K_{ATP} channel antagonist, in the presence or absence of isoflurane. %SS recovers to baseline values after reperfusion in dogs receiving isoflurane alone. †Significantly ($P < .05$) different from dogs pretreated with drug vehicle. ‡Significantly ($P < .05$) different from dogs receiving glyburide and isoflurane. §Significantly ($P < .05$) different from dogs pretreated with glyburide. *(From Kersten JR, Schmeling TJ, Hettrick DA, et al: Mechanism of cardioprotection by isoflurane: Role of adenosine triphosphate–regulated potassium [K_{ATP}] channels. Anesthesiology 85:794-807, 1996.)*

opened sarcolemmal K_{ATP} channels during intracellular acidosis of a magnitude similar to that observed during ischemia.[86] The sarcolemmal K_{ATP} channel acted as an effector during isoflurane preconditioning against oxidative stress in adult ventricular myocytes.[87] The effects of volatile anesthetics on sarcolemmal K_{ATP} channel function may persist beyond the duration of administration,[84] suggesting a cellular basis for the early "memory" phase of anesthetic preconditioning in vivo. Isoflurane preconditioning produced prolonged sensitization of the sarcolemmal K_{ATP} channel to opening by a PKC δ-isoform (PKC-δ)-mediated mechanism[88] or by enhancing induction of sarcolemmal K_{ATP} channel current via a diacylglycerol PKC activator.[84] Isoflurane preconditioning caused persistent reductions in the sensitivity of the sarcolemmal K_{ATP} channel to inhibition by ATP and adenosine 5′-diphosphate.[89] The nucleotide binding domains of the regulatory sulfonylurea receptor SUR2A were shown to play important roles in isoflurane-induced facilitation of sarcolemmal K_{ATP} channel activity during moderate intracellular acidosis, similar to that encountered during early ischemia.[90] These data support the contention that isoflurane directly interacts with subunits of the cardiac sarcolemmal K_{ATP} channel.[90]

It is also clear, based on several experimental studies, that volatile anesthetics directly or indirectly open mitochondrial K_{ATP} channels in vitro. Isoflurane and sevoflurane increased mitochondrial flavoprotein oxidation, an index of mitochondrial K_{ATP} channel activity, in guinea pig cardiac myocytes, and this increase in fluorescence was inhibited by the selective mitochondrial K_{ATP} channel inhibitor 5-HD.[91] Isoflurane also directly activated the mitochondrial K_{ATP} channels reconstituted in lipid bilayers.[92] Isoflurane-induced increases in mitochondrial flavoprotein fluorescence were not inhibited by pretreatment with adenosine, PKC, PTK, or p38 mitogen-activated protein kinase (MAPK) inhibitors, suggesting that isoflurane may directly activate mitochondrial K_{ATP} channels.[93] In contrast, isoflurane and sevoflurane failed to directly enhance flavoprotein fluorescence in rat ventricular myocytes, but these anesthetics did enhance fluorescence induced by the mitochondrial K_{ATP} channel agonist diazoxide.[42] These data suggest that volatile anesthetics may not directly open but, instead, indirectly prime mitochondrial K_{ATP} channels by acting on other intracellular signaling elements that modulate the activity of the channel. Sarcolemmal K_{ATP} channels may also be linked to the function of the inner mitochondrial membrane. The ROS generated by mitochondria may act to open sarcolemmal K_{ATP} channels. An uncoupler of mitochondrial oxidative phosphorylation (2,4-dinitrophenol) reversibly activated sarcolemmal K_{ATP} channel current concomitant with nicotinamide adenine dinucleotide oxidation. These and other data led to the contention that crosstalk may occur between sarcolemmal and mitochondrial K_{ATP} channels during preconditioning phenomena.[94] However, such crosstalk has yet to be specifically demonstrated during anesthetic preconditioning. To summarize, the experimental results collected to date provide somewhat conflicting results about a possible direct action of volatile anesthetics on sarcolemmal and mitochondrial K_{ATP} channel activity. Nevertheless, volatile anesthetics clearly prime the activation of these channels in both sarcolemmal and mitochondrial membranes.

K_{ATP} channels in vascular smooth muscle cells are essential regulators of coronary vascular tone when ATP production is reduced. Volatile anesthetic–induced coronary vasodilation[95] was attenuated by glyburide, thus indicating an important role for K_{ATP} channels in this process. The beneficial actions of anesthetic preconditioning may therefore be partially attributed to increases in myocardial oxygen supply mediated by K_{ATP} channel–dependent coronary vasodilation. However, the fact that sevoflurane caused an increase in coronary collateral blood flow in vivo in the presence of glyburide indicates that this volatile anesthetic may enhance coronary collateral blood flow independent of activation of K_{ATP} channels. Sevoflurane-induced increases in collateral perfusion occur as a result of Ca^{2+}-regulated potassium (BK_{Ca}) and not K_{ATP} channel activation.[51] Thus, the cardioprotection provided by volatile anesthetics is unlikely to be solely related to favorable alterations in coronary vascular tone mediated by K_{ATP} channels.

G Proteins and Their Coupled Receptor Ligands

The sequential activation of several intracellular elements in a transduction pathway may facilitate amplification of the initial signal between other redundant systems. This concept was clearly illustrated by the observation that the direct K_{ATP} channel opener nicorandil enhances the cardioprotective effects of isoflurane.[96] G protein–coupled receptor ligands and their downstream signaling elements have been shown to converge on the K_{ATP} channel during anesthetic preconditioning. Pertussis toxin abolished the reductions in infarct size produced by isoflurane, thus indicating that inhibitory guanine (G_i) nucleotide–binding proteins are linked to the signal transduction pathways that mediate anesthetic preconditioning.[97] In contrast, pertussis toxin did not prevent the beneficial effects of direct K_{ATP} channel opening produced by nicorandil. These data strongly support the contention that volatile anesthetics modulate K_{ATP} channel activity through a second messenger. Halothane-induced protection against infarction was completely abolished by blockade of the adenosine A_1 receptor,[39] and the selective A_1 receptor antagonist DPCPX also partially attenuated the beneficial effects of isoflurane on stunned myocardium.[98] Isoflurane eliminated increases in interstitial adenosine during repetitive periods of coronary artery occlusion and reperfusion as demonstrated via a myocardial microdialysis technique.[98] These findings suggest that ATP preservation and a subsequent reduction in adenosine released into the interstitium occur during isoflurane anesthesia. The results were also very similar to those obtained during ischemic preconditioning and pharmacologic preconditioning with bimakalim. Thus, volatile anesthetics may either directly activate A_1 receptors or indirectly enhance A_1 receptor sensitivity to diminished endogenous adenosine concentrations.[98] The preservation of cardiac myocyte viability during ischemia produced by volatile anesthetics was also sensitive to adenosine receptor– and G_i protein–mediated signaling blockade.[42] Adenosine also enhanced isoflurane preconditioning through both mitochondrial K_{ATP} channel–dependent and channel-independent mechanisms in isolated, buffer-perfused rat hearts.[99]

The nonselective opioid antagonist naloxone also abolished isoflurane-induced preconditioning in the rat.[40] These data indicate an important link between volatile anesthetics and another family of G_i protein–coupled receptors. Volatile anesthetics competitively inhibited the ligand binding site of G_i protein–coupled receptors.[100] Thus, anesthetic preconditioning appears to be associated with the activation of at least two separate receptor-mediated pathways (A_1 and opioid) that are linked to G_i proteins. Interestingly, the combination of isoflurane and a selective δ_1-opioid receptor agonist amplified the preconditioning response in the rat.[59] This effect was synergistic and sensitive to inhibition by glyburide.[59] The combined administration of isoflurane and morphine also markedly reduced infarct size in vivo, and this protective effect was abolished by 5-HD.[40] Hence, combined administration of a volatile anesthetic and an opioid capable of agonist action at the δ_1-opioid receptor may stimulate similar or cooperative signaling cascades that amplify K_{ATP} channel activation to profoundly augment myocardial protection beyond that produced by either drug alone. A G_s protein–coupled receptor ligand system, the β_1-adrenoceptor and its downstream target protein kinase A, was also recently shown to mediate desflurane and sevoflurane but not ischemic preconditioning in rabbits.[101] These data suggest that both G_i and G_s may play important roles in anesthetic preconditioning in vivo.

Protein Kinases

Ischemic preconditioning has been shown to produce translocation and phosphorylation of several protein kinases, most importantly PKC, involved in cardioprotective signal transduction. PKC is an essential component of the signaling pathway involved in protecting myocardium against cell death during ischemia and reperfusion.[102] The diverse PKC isoform family is a large group of serine-threonine protein kinases that are distinguished by variable regulatory domains and cofactors and also display diverse tissue and species distributions. G protein–coupled receptor ligands, including A_1, δ_1-opioid, and bradykinin, have been shown to activate PKC during ischemic preconditioning. Volatile anesthetics stimulated PKC translocation and activity, possibly by interacting with regulatory domain of the enzyme. Inhibition of

PKC partially attenuated isoflurane-induced augmentation of the functional recovery of stunned myocardium in dogs.[103] The beneficial actions of the older agent halothane were entirely blocked by selective inhibition of PKC in rabbits.[39] Colchicine, a drug that depolymerizes microtubule assemblies, prevented isoflurane-induced reductions in myocardial infarct size in rabbits. This interesting result suggests that an intact cytoskeleton is essential for translocation of the PKC to occur. In fact, volatile anesthetic–induced PKC translocation and activation appear to be required to open K_{ATP} channels and produce cardioprotection. For example, the nonselective PKC antagonist chelerythrine abolished sevoflurane-induced increases in mitochondrial K_{ATP} channel activity in rat ventricular myocyte and prevented protection from ischemic damage.[42] Patch-clamp experiments demonstrated that isoflurane does not facilitate K_{ATP} channel opening in excised membranes but enhances K_{ATP} channel current in a whole-cell configuration concomitant with PKC stimulation.[104] These observations were supported by findings that both adenosine and PKC enhance K_{ATP} channel activity during ischemic preconditioning. Specific PKC consensus sites were demonstrated on K_{ATP} channels, thereby suggesting a molecular basis for phosphorylation and activation of the channel by this critical enzyme.[105] Translocation of PKC-δ but not PKC-ε plays an important role in isoflurane preconditioning in isolated perfused rat hearts.[106] Phosphorylation of the serine 643 residue of PKC-δ appeared to mediate transfer of the preconditioning stimulus (exposure to 1.5 MAC isoflurane) to mitochondrial K_{ATP} channels.[106] Both PKC-δ and PKC-ε translocation was implicated in isoflurane (1.0 MAC) preconditioning in rats in vivo, and opening of mitochondrial K_{ATP} channels and generation of ROS were shown to be upstream events that accompanied PKC activation in this model (Fig. 23-9).[60] Another study implicated PKC-ε alone during sevoflurane preconditioning in isolated perfused guinea pig hearts.[107] A role for PKC-ε was also demonstrated in isoflurane preconditioning in rats by another research group,[108] but only at lower concentrations (<0.5 MAC) of the volatile agent. Desflurane preconditioning produced time-dependent translocation of PKC-ε through activation of extracellular signal–regulated kinases 1 and 2 (ERK1/2).[109] In contrast, PKC-δ mediated sevoflurane preconditioning through ROS production independent of mitochondrial K_{ATP} channels in isolated rat trabeculae.[110] Taken as a whole, these experimental data strongly suggest that at least two different isoforms of PKC (ε and δ) appear to be important mediators of anesthetic preconditioning.

PKC has been shown to stimulate PTK[111] and several MAPK moieties[112] during ischemic preconditioning, and some evidence also indicates a role for these proteins in anesthetic-induced cardioprotection independent of receptor activation. The PTK inhibitor lavendustin A and the Src-selective inhibitor PP1 abolished isoflurane preconditioning in rats.[60] In contrast, lavendustin A and another nonselective PTK inhibitor (genistein) did not alter desflurane preconditioning in rabbits.[113] These data suggest that the role of PTK in anesthetic preconditioning may be dependent on the species. The MAPK family of proteins plays important roles in signal transduction from the cell surface to the nucleus and in the initiation and progression of apoptosis. ERK1 and ERK2 are MAPKs that mediate cell division, proliferation, and survival.[62] They were previously implicated in ischemia and opioid-induced preconditioning in rats. The reductions in infarct size and ERK1/2 phosphorylation produced by administration of desflurane before ischemia and reperfusion were abolished by a selective ERK1/2 inhibitor,[109] thereby providing the first evidence suggesting that ERK1/2 mediates anesthetic preconditioning. ERK1/2 was also shown to trigger isoflurane preconditioning in rabbits.[114] In addition, ERK1/2-related signaling proteins control the expression of several genes concerned with cell survival, including hypoxia-inducible factor-1α (HIF-1α), an important DNA-binding complex whose activity is influenced by intracellular oxygen tension. Myocardial hypoxia is a potent inducer of HIF-1α protein expression, and the combination of reduced oxygen tension and activation of ERK1/2 signaling is known to potentiate HIF-1α expression and activity.[115] Furthermore, HIF-1α upregulates transcription of vascular endothelial growth factor (VEGF).[116] This important angiogenic protein plays a central role in coronary collateral development in response to chronic myocardial ischemia,[117] and enhanced expression of both HIF-1α and VEGF occurs during myocardial ischemia in rats.[118] ERK1/2-dependent upregulation of HIF-1α and VEGF has also been shown during ischemic and hypoxic preconditioning.[119] Administration of isoflurane likewise produced temporal upregulation of HIF-1α and VEGF expression by activating ERK1/2 in rabbit myocardium (Figs. 23-10 and 23-11).[114] Another MAPK (p38) strongly implicated in ischemic preconditioning also appeared to mediate anesthetic preconditioning in isolated rat hearts.[120] p38 MAPK has been shown to interact with the actin cytoskeleton through MAPK-activated protein kinase 2 (MAPKAPK-2) and heat shock protein 27 (HSP-27). Isoflurane and xenon preconditioning were recently demonstrated to activate both MAPKAPK-2 and HSP-27 downstream of PKC and p38 MAPK.[121] These exciting data provide another potential link between anesthetic preconditioning and the cytoskeleton, thereby suggesting another mechanism by which signaling elements involved in cardioprotection may be transported to appropriate locations within the cell. Activated protein kinase G (PKG) has been shown to open mitochondrial K_{ATP} channels during ischemic and pharmacologic preconditioning. PKG was recently demonstrated to transmit G_i protein-receptor ligand coupled from the cytosol to the inner mitochondrial membrane by a pathway that includes PKC-ε to produce cardioprotection.[122] Whether PKG also mediates anesthetic preconditioning has yet to be determined.

The prosurvival protein phosphatidylinositol-3′-kinase (PI3K) has been shown to be responsible for the phosphorylation of a variety of subcellular targets implicated in cell survival, protein synthesis, and metabolism. Activation of this kinase pathway not only reduces cell necrosis but also contributes to the preservation of viable myocardium by inhibiting apoptosis and maintaining mitochondrial integrity.[62] PI3K converts phosphatidylinositol 4,5-bisphosphate (PIP_2) to phosphatidylinositol 3,4,5-triphosphate (PIP_3),[123] and PIP_3-stimulated phosphorylation of the serine-threonine kinase Akt by phosphoinositide-dependent kinase 1 (PDK1) subsequently inhibits the formation of several proapoptotic proteins (e.g., Bad, Bax, caspases). PDK1 is a also potent activator of other protein kinases,[123] including PKC and PTK, implicated in anesthetic preconditioning.[56] A role for PI3K signaling in isoflurane preconditioning was recently demonstrated. A selective inhibitor of PI3K (wortmannin) abolished reductions in infarct size and also blocked phosphorylation of the downstream enzyme target Akt that were produced by administration of isoflurane before prolonged coronary artery occlusion in rabbits.[124] Isoflurane preconditioning increased Akt phosphorylation and expression of the antiapoptotic B-cell lymphoma-2 (Bcl-2) protein and reduced expression of the apoptotic protein

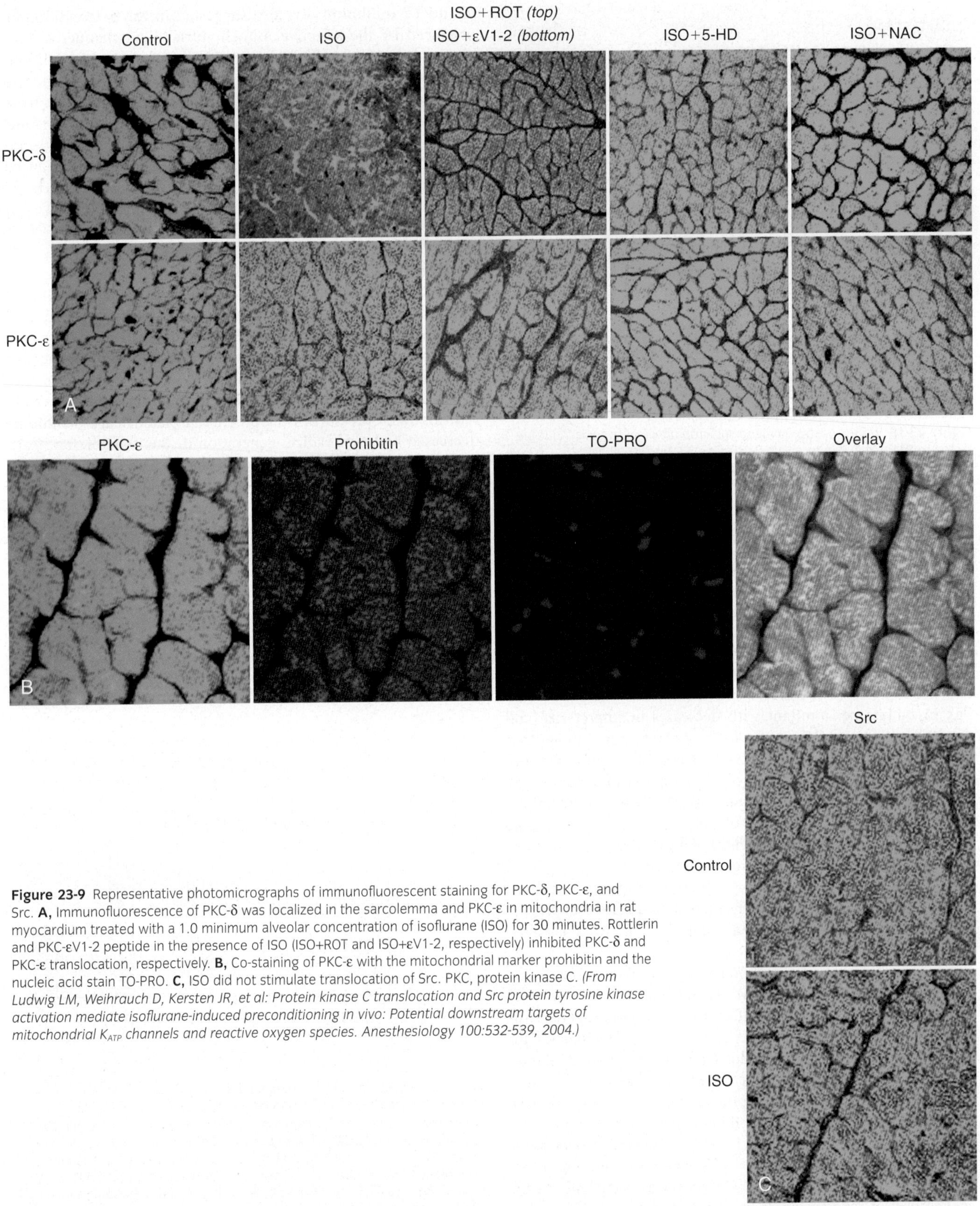

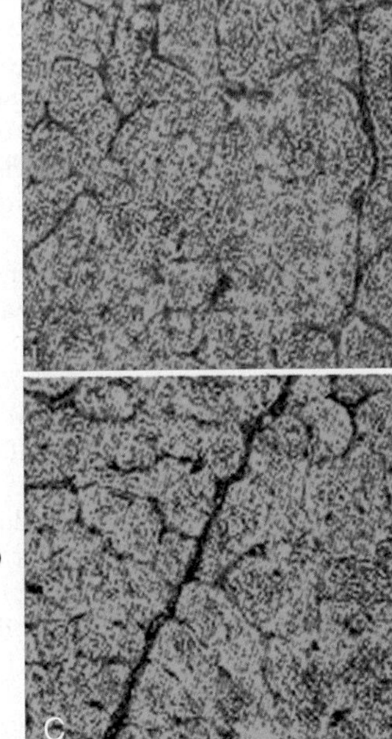

Figure 23-9 Representative photomicrographs of immunofluorescent staining for PKC-δ, PKC-ε, and Src. **A,** Immunofluorescence of PKC-δ was localized in the sarcolemma and PKC-ε in mitochondria in rat myocardium treated with a 1.0 minimum alveolar concentration of isoflurane (ISO) for 30 minutes. Rottlerin and PKC-εV1-2 peptide in the presence of ISO (ISO+ROT and ISO+εV1-2, respectively) inhibited PKC-δ and PKC-ε translocation, respectively. **B,** Co-staining of PKC-ε with the mitochondrial marker prohibitin and the nucleic acid stain TO-PRO. **C,** ISO did not stimulate translocation of Src. PKC, protein kinase C. *(From Ludwig LM, Weihrauch D, Kersten JR, et al: Protein kinase C translocation and Src protein tyrosine kinase activation mediate isoflurane-induced preconditioning in vivo: Potential downstream targets of mitochondrial K_{ATP} channels and reactive oxygen species. Anesthesiology 100:532-539, 2004.)*

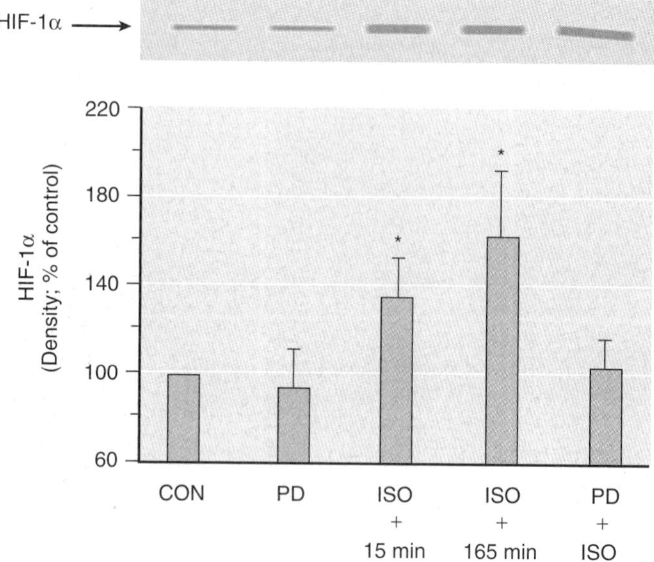

Figure 23-10 Representative immunoblots (*top panel*) of hypoxia-inducible factor-1α (HIF-1α) in rats receiving 0.9% saline (CON), PD 098059 (PD, 1.0 mg/kg), 1.0 minimum alveolar concentration of isoflurane (ISO) administered for 30 minutes, and PD 098059 (1.0 mg/kg) administered before ISO. Left ventricular tissue samples were obtained 15 or 165 minutes after administration of ISO or at a corresponding time point in rats that did not receive the volatile anesthetic. Histograms illustrating HIF-1α expression in each experimental group are depicted in the *lower panel*. All data are means ± SD. *Significantly ($P < .05$) different from CON. *(From Wang C, Weihrauch D, Schwabe DA, et al: Extracellular signal–regulated kinases trigger isoflurane preconditioning concomitant with upregulation of hypoxia-inducible factor-1α and vascular endothelial growth factor in rats. Anesth Analg 103:281-288, 2006.)*

Bax in rabbits concomitant with decreases in infarct size and the number of apoptotic myocytes.[125] Wortmannin and another selective PI3K antagonist (LY294002) abolished these actions, thus indicating that PI3K-induced modulation of proapoptotic and antiapoptotic protein balance plays a role in isoflurane cardioprotection.[125] Activation of Akt by isoflurane was also shown to protect rat atrial and ventricular myocytes against apoptosis in vitro produced by exposure to hypoxia, hydrogen peroxide, or activated neutrophils concomitant with increased expression of Bcl-2.[126] Collectively, these data suggest that prosurvival PI3K signaling plays a central role in anesthetic preconditioning.

A transition in mitochondrial permeability caused by opening of the mitochondrial permeability transition pore (mPTP) may be a critical end-effector in the myocardial necrosis and apoptosis resulting from ischemia-reperfusion injury. This event has been shown to be modulated by PI3K-mediated signaling pathways.[127] The mPTP is located on the inner mitochondrial membrane, and opening of the pore abolishes the mitochondrial membrane potential ($\Delta\Psi_m$), inhibits oxidative phosphorylation, and facilitates the release or activation of several proapoptotic proteins, including cytochrome *c*. These actions rapidly produce cell death. Opening of the mPTP appears to occur specifically at the onset of reperfusion,[128] in part as a consequence of intracellular Ca^{2+} overload and the presence of large quantities of cytotoxic oxygen-derived free radicals. The protective effects of classic[127] and delayed[129] ischemic preconditioning were mediated by inhibition of mitochondrial permeability transition. A role for mPTP inhibition was also suggested in the preconditioning produced by the selective mitochondrial K_{ATP} channel agonist diazoxide.[127] Similar to the findings with ischemic preconditioning, desflurane preconditioning improved mPTP resistance to Ca^{2+}-induced opening in isolated mitochondria obtained from pretreated rabbits.[130] The selective mitochondrial K_{ATP} channel antagonist 5-HD abolished this effect.[130] Isoflurane preconditioning also elicited partial mitochondrial uncoupling and reduced mitochondrial Ca^{2+} uptake in intact ventricular myocytes,[131] presumably mediated through mPTP or mitochondrial K_{ATP} channels.

Reactive Oxygen Species

Reperfusion of ischemic myocardium is associated with the release of large quantities of ROS that disrupt intracellular Ca^{2+} homeostasis, cause lipid peroxidation, damage cell membranes, depress contractility, and produce reversible and irreversible tissue injury.[132] Isoflurane and the older volatile anesthetics have been shown to attenuate the toxic effects of oxygen-derived free radicals on LV pressure development in isolated hearts. Isoflurane decreased hydroxyl radical generation in the ischemic rat heart, and halothane had a similar effect in dogs.[133] The protective effects of sevoflurane were associated with reduced dityrosine formation, an indirect marker of reactive oxygen and nitrogen species.[134] These results supported the contention that volatile anesthetics may reduce the release of deleterious quantities of ROS immediately after coronary artery occlusion and reperfusion.

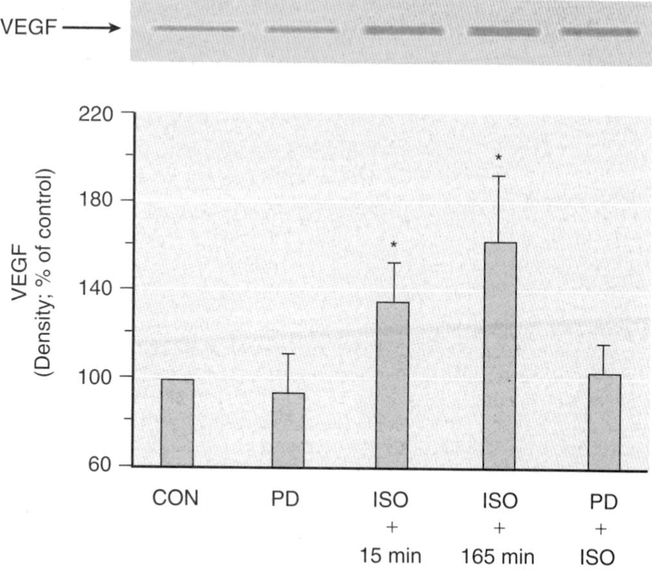

Figure 23-11 Representative immunoblots (*top panel*) of vascular endothelial growth factor (VEGF) in rats receiving 0.9% saline (CON), PD 098059 (PD, 1.0 mg/kg), 1.0 minimum alveolar concentration of isoflurane (ISO) administered for 30 minutes, and PD 098059 (1.0 mg/kg) administered before ISO. Left ventricular tissue samples were obtained 15 or 165 minutes after the administration of ISO or at a corresponding time point in rats that did not receive the volatile anesthetic. Histograms illustrating VEGF expression in each experimental group are depicted in the *lower panel*. All data are means ± SD. *Significantly ($P < .05$) different from CON. *(From Wang C, Weihrauch D, Schwabe DA, et al: Extracellular signal–regulated kinases trigger isoflurane preconditioning concomitant with upregulation of hypoxia-inducible factor-1α and vascular endothelial growth factor in rats. Anesth Analg 103:281-288, 2006.)*

In contrast to these data implicating a pathologic role of large amounts of ROS, a variety of preconditioning stimuli, including brief ischemia, mitochondrial K_{ATP} channel openers, opioids, and volatile anesthetics, stimulate a small burst of ROS that paradoxically appears to initiate downstream signaling events and produce protection from subsequent ischemic injury. Pretreatment with low concentrations of ROS mimicked the beneficial effects of ischemic preconditioning,[135] and free radical scavengers administered before or during ischemia attenuated this cardioprotection.[136] These findings suggest that ischemic preconditioning is mediated by small quantities of ROS released during the preconditioning stimulus. Scavengers of superoxide anion and inhibition of nitric oxide synthase (NOS) abolished the beneficial actions of sevoflurane against ischemic damage.[134] Similarly, desflurane preconditioning was mediated by NO.[137] These results indicate that that superoxide anion may act to trigger anesthetic preconditioning and also suggest that NO may scavenge superoxide anion upon reperfusion to reduce injury. Scavengers of ROS attenuated isoflurane-induced reductions in myocardial infarct size in rabbits[138] (Fig. 23-12) and also inhibited the salutary actions of opening of mitochondrial K_{ATP} channels.[139] Isoflurane was shown with the fluorescent probe dihydroethidium and laser confocal microscopy to directly increase superoxide anion formation in vivo independent of ischemia and reperfusion.[43] Thus, volatile anesthetics may be capable of producing small amounts of superoxide anion that exert protective effects during subsequent ischemia. These data provide compelling evidence that small quantities of ROS play a critical role in anesthetic preconditioning.

ROS act as critical regulatory mediators in many signaling processes that protect the cardiac myocyte from oxidative stress. Activation of PKC[135] and MAPKs[140] by ROS was implicated in ischemic and pharmacologic preconditioning. Hydrogen peroxide activated several MAPK subtypes in neonatal rat ventricular myocytes, but stimulation of p38 MAPK and subsequent phosphorylation of HSP-25/27 appeared to be particularly important in producing cardioprotection. ROS also activated G proteins ($G_i\alpha$ and $G_o\alpha$) that may likewise play a role in preconditioning.[141] Furthermore, there is indirect evidence linking ROS production by volatile anesthetics to activation of protein kinases implicated in the signaling pathways responsible for anesthetic preconditioning. For example, ROS scavengers inhibited isoflurane-induced PKC translocation.[60]

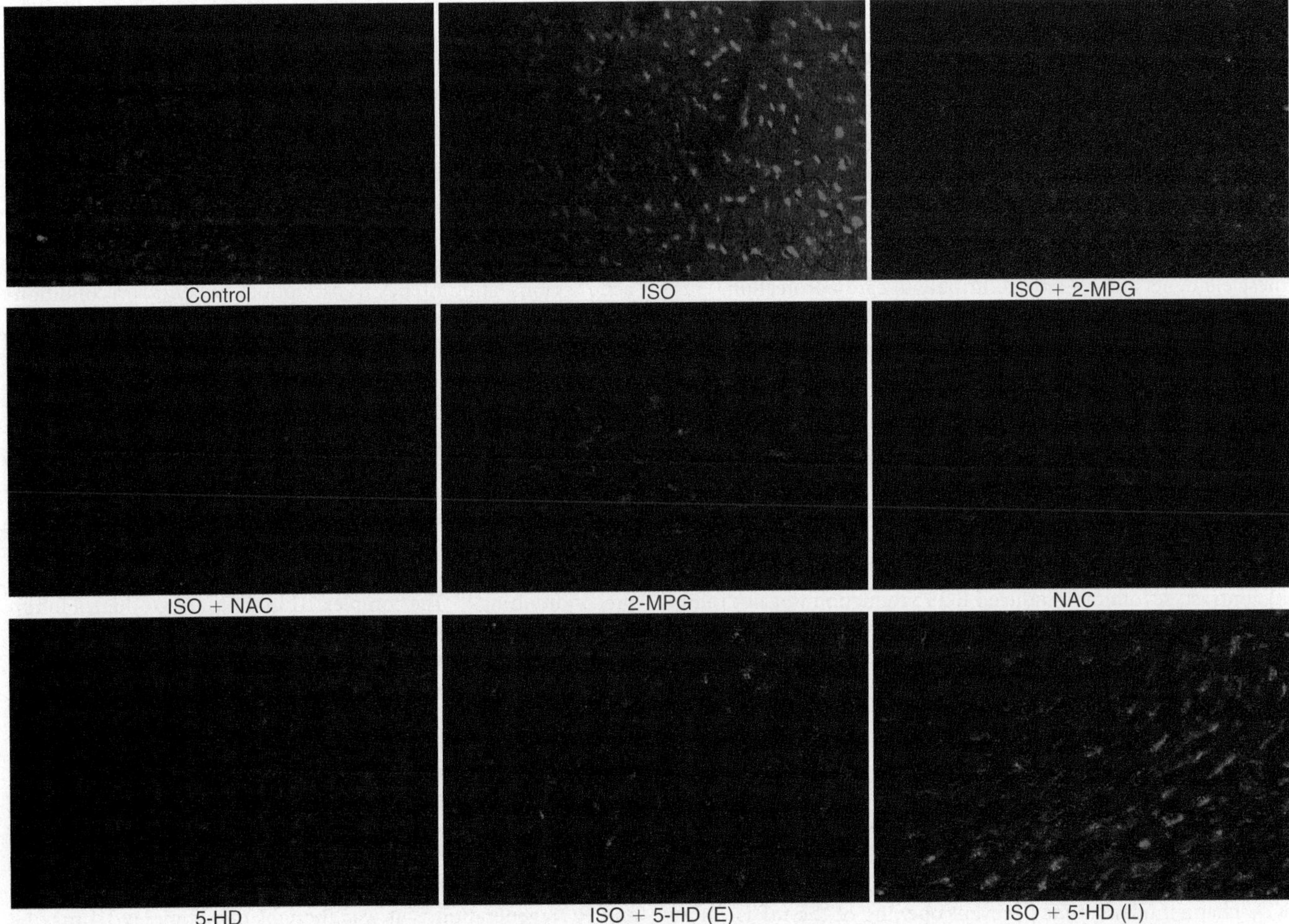

Figure 23-12 Superoxide anion production measured by dihydroethidium fluorescence in control rabbits (CON) and rabbits receiving *N*-acetylcysteine (NAC), *N*-2-mercaptopropionyl glycine (2-MPG), or 5-hydroxydecanoate (5-HD) in the presence and absence of a 1.0 minimum alveolar concentration of isoflurane (ISO). *Significantly ($P < .05$) different from isoflurane. *(From Tanaka K, Weihrauch D, Ludwig LM, et al: Mitochondrial adenosine triphosphate–regulated potassium channel opening acts as a trigger for isoflurane-induced preconditioning by generating reactive oxygen species. Anesthesiology 98:935-943, 2003.)*

The temporal relationship between mitochondrial K_{ATP} channel opening and ROS production during ischemic or pharmacologic preconditioning remains somewhat controversial. Mitochondrial K_{ATP} channels triggered preconditioning by generating ROS.[139] Opening of mitochondrial K_{ATP} channels by selective agonists generated ROS that appeared to be essential for activation of MAPK and the subsequent beneficial effects against ischemic injury. For example, the selective mitochondrial K_{ATP} channel agonist diazoxide enhanced cell viability after hypoxia and reoxygenation in vitro concomitant with the generation of oxygen-derived free radicals.[142] These beneficial actions were attenuated in cells pretreated with 5-HD or ROS scavengers, thus suggesting that the cardioprotection produced by mitochondrial K_{ATP} channel agonists occurs as a result of triggering by ROS. Morphine increased the fluorescence intensity of the hydrogen peroxide–sensitive probe 2′,7′-dichlorofluorescein, an action that was blocked by 5-HD.[143] These data also demonstrated a link between activation of mitochondrial K_{ATP} channels by opioids and ROS production. Diazoxide and another mitochondrial K_{ATP} channel opener (cromakalim) directly caused release of superoxide anion from complex I of the electron transport chain in isolated rat heart mitochondria concomitant with matrix alkalinization.[144] In contrast, other investigations suggested that ROS modulated activity of the mitochondrial K_{ATP} channels. For example, xanthine oxidase–derived superoxide anion–activated mitochondrial K_{ATP} channels from bovine ventricular myocardium reconstituted in lipid bilayers.[145] In addition, ROS triggered opening of mitochondrial K_{ATP} channels, and this event subsequently generated additional quantities of both ROS and NO.[146] Thus, whether mitochondrial K_{ATP} channel opening acts as a trigger or end-effector of ischemic or pharmacologic preconditioning remains unclear.[147] However, a complementary interaction between ROS and mitochondrial K_{ATP} channels appears to exist that may create a positive-feedback interaction between these elements and thereby contribute to cardioprotection.

Whether opening of mitochondrial K_{ATP} channels by volatile anesthetics precedes or follows ROS production during anesthetic preconditioning also remains unclear. Pretreatment with 5-HD or a ROS scavenger (e.g., *N*-acetylcysteine, *N*-2-mercaptoproprionyl glycine) before exposure to isoflurane abolished ROS production in rabbits.[77] However, 5-HD administered after discontinuation of isoflurane but before prolonged coronary artery occlusion only partially attenuated this effect, thus suggesting that mitochondrial K_{ATP} channel opening acted as a trigger for anesthetic preconditioning by producing ROS (Fig. 23-13). In contrast, sevoflurane-induced ROS production was not inhibited by 5-HD pretreatment in isolated guinea pig hearts.[148] Despite the rather equivocal nature of these two studies,[77,148] it is quite evident that ROS play a major role in anesthetic preconditioning in conjunction with mitochondrial K_{ATP} channels. Interestingly, a quantity of ROS that exceeds a critical threshold produced opening of the mPTP and a subsequent burst of ROS[149] that stimulated further release of additional ROS from other mitochondria.[150] This "ROS-induced ROS release" contributed to mPTP-dependent cell death in adult rat myocytes after ischemia-reperfusion.[151] Thus, volatile anesthetics or other mitochondrial K_{ATP} channel openers may prevent opening of the mPTP in an oxidant-sensitive fashion to produce cardioprotection. Desflurane preconditioning increased resistance of Ca^{2+}-induced mPTP opening,[130] but the dependence of this process on ROS has not been examined. Further investigation will be required

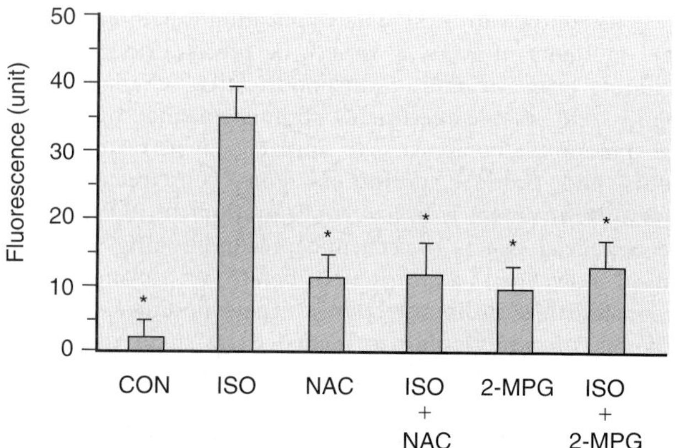

Figure 23-13 Superoxide anion production measured using dihydroethidium fluorescence in rabbits receiving (CON), *N*-acetylcysteine (NAC), or *N*-2-mercaptopropionyl glycine (2-MPG) in the presence and absence of 1.0 minimum alveolar concentration isoflurane (ISO). *Significantly ($P < 0.05$) different from isoflurane. *(From Tanaka K, Weihrauch D, Kehl F, et al: Mechanism of preconditioning by isoflurane in rabbits: a direct role for reactive oxygen species. Anesthesiology 97:1485-1490, 2002.)*

to more clearly define the precise relationship between ROS, mitochondrial K_{ATP} channels, and mPTP during anesthetic preconditioning.

NF-κB is an important transcription factor activated during ischemia-reperfusion injury that is involved in the inflammatory response to oxidative stress. The regulatory protein IκB-α maintains NF-κB in its inactive form under normal conditions, but activation of IκB-α kinase by ROS or inflammatory cytokines during ischemia removes this passive inhibition of NF-κB. Dissociated NF-κB translocates to the nucleus, binds to promoter gene regions, and initiates transcription. Ischemic preconditioning reduces NF-κB activation and blunts the production of inflammatory cytokines, chemokines, and adhesion molecules, thereby contributing to a reduction in myocardial necrosis. Sevoflurane preconditioning also attenuated activation of NF-κB and reduced NF-κB–dependent inflammatory gene expression in isolated rat hearts.[61] These data suggest that inhibition of NF-κB also mediates anesthetic preconditioning. The role of ROS in this process is currently unknown.

ROS derived from mitochondrial oxidative phosphorylation have been shown to mediate ischemic[152] and pharmacologic preconditioning.[143] The complex III inhibitor myxothiazol inhibited hypoxia-[152] and acetylcholine-induced[153] ROS production and abolished preconditioning in vitro. Volatile anesthetics inhibited electron transport chain complexes I and II in isolated cardiac mitochondria.[154,155] Sevoflurane-induced complex I inhibition was attenuated by a superoxide dismutase mimetic[155] and an NOS inhibitor,[156] thus suggesting that ROS, NO, or their reaction products may inhibit mitochondrial respiration through a positive-feedback mechanism to amplify free radical signals for triggering anesthetic preconditioning. Conversely, because myxothiazol, but not a complex I inhibitor, abolished isoflurane cardioprotection and ROS generation,[157] it was thought that complex III may be the source of ROS during anesthetic preconditioning. These data suggested the possibility that volatile anesthetics may modulate multiple sites of the electron transport chain either directly or indirectly through a ROS-mediated feedback mechanism. An inhibitor of cyclooxygenase-2 (COX-2) (celecoxib) but not COX-1 (aspirin) or COX-3 (acetaminophen) blocked isoflurane-induced cardioprotection in rabbits,[158] so selective modulation of arachidonic acid metabolism by volatile anesthetics may represent another potential source of ROS during anesthetic preconditioning. Hence, at least three sources of oxygen- or nitrogen-derived free radicals (mitochondrial electron transport, NOS, and COX-2) have been identified to date, but whether other enzymes (e.g., nicotinamide adenine dinucleotide oxidase, lipoxygenase, xanthine oxidase, cytochrome P450) known to generate such reactive intermediates are involved in anesthetic preconditioning remains unknown.

The precise identity of the ROS involved in anesthetic preconditioning has also not been defined. Superoxide anion directly opened mitochondrial K_{ATP} channels in vitro,[145] thus implicating this reactive intermediate in ischemic preconditioning. Isoflurane directly enhanced ethidium fluorescence in rabbit myocardium independent of subsequent ischemia and reperfusion.[43,77] Dihydroethidium is oxidized by intracellular superoxide anion to produce ethidium, which subsequently binds to DNA, thereby further amplifying its fluorescence. These data strongly suggest that superoxide anion mediates anesthetic preconditioning. Sevoflurane also generated superoxide anion before ischemia and reperfusion in isolated hearts.[148] In contrast to these findings with superoxide anion, another ROS (hydrogen peroxide) stimulated PTK-dependent activation of phospholipase C in mouse embryonic fibroblasts and rendered these cells resistant to stress. Hydrogen peroxide activates G_i and G_o proteins,[141] as well as protein kinases involved in reducing cellular injury.[159] Hydrogen peroxide may also be converted to more reactive species that subsequently modify cysteine residues specific to G proteins and selectively activate these proteins.[160] Thus, hydrogen peroxide or its immediate free radical metabolites represent another group of ROS known to affect many of the signaling molecules implicated in anesthetic preconditioning. Dismutation of superoxide anion leads to the production of hydrogen peroxide, hydroxyl radical, and peroxynitrite, and these radicals may differentially alter channel or protein kinase activity. For example, superoxide anion and hydrogen peroxide enhanced, but peroxynitrite reduced Ca^{2+}-regulated K^+ channel function.[161] Whether anesthetic preconditioning also produces other ROS that activate mitochondrial K_{ATP} channels or inhibit the formation of intermediates that adversely affect these channels, such as peroxynitrite, remains to be elucidated.

Delayed Preconditioning by Volatile Anesthetics

Ischemic preconditioning is characterized by an early phase (limited to 1 to 3 hours after the brief ischemic stimulus) and a late, "delayed," or "second-window" phase of preconditioning that occurs after 24 hours and persists for as long as 72 hours after the ischemic episode.[162] Several protein kinases,[163,164] COX-2,[165] NOS,[166] and NF-κB[167] have been implicated in the signaling responsible for delayed preconditioning. NO donors, G protein–coupled receptor ligands (e.g., δ-opioid, adenosine), and mitochondrial K_{ATP} channel openers mimic the protective effects of delayed preconditioning. Experimental evidence indicates that volatile anesthetics may also be capable of producing late pharmacologic preconditioning. Tonkovic-Capin and colleagues first described delayed preconditioning by isoflurane in isolated perfused neonatal rabbit hearts subjected to a 2-hour exposure to 1% of the volatile agent 24 hours before the onset of ischemia.[168] Remote administration of isoflurane reduced myocardial infarct size and enhanced the recovery of LV pressure development in pretreated rabbit hearts as compared with those that had not previously been exposed to the volatile agent.[168] The magnitude of the delayed cardioprotective effect was similar to that observed during isoflurane preconditioning. The second window of cardioprotection produced by isoflurane was abolished by the mitochondrial K_{ATP} channel antagonist 5-HD and was also partially attenuated by the selective sarcolemmal K_{ATP} channel antagonist HMR-1098.[168] Sevoflurane-delayed preconditioning was also inhibited by pretreatment with 5-HD.[169] These findings established a central role for K_{ATP} channels in anesthetic late preconditioning. Remote exposure to 2.5% sevoflurane for 1 hour decreased infarct size, reduced release of creatine kinase, improved LV function, maintained intracellular ATP concentrations, and preserved intracellular Na^+ and Ca^{2+} homeostasis in isolated rat hearts but not in those not receiving sevoflurane pretreatment.[170] The salutary actions of sevoflurane were more pronounced at 48 than at 24 hours after exposure to the volatile agent.[170] Acute preconditioning with sevoflurane also conferred additional cardioprotection after ischemic late preconditioning in rabbits through activation of mitochondrial K_{ATP} channels.[171]

In contrast to the findings in rabbits and rats, exposure to 1.0 MAC isoflurane for 6 hours did not produce late preconditioning against myocardial infarction in dogs when the volatile agent was administered 24 hours before prolonged coronary artery occlusion and reperfusion in vivo.[172] The results occurred independent of alterations in systemic hemodynamics or coronary collateral perfusion and suggested that delayed cardioprotection by volatile anesthetics may be species specific.[172] Intravenous emulsified sevoflurane produced delayed preconditioning against myocardial infarction in rabbits.[173] The blood concentration of sevoflurane required for this beneficial effect was equivalent to a MAC value of approximately 0.17, suggesting that only a small amount of the volatile agent is required to produce cardioprotection. Similarly, inhalation of subanesthetic (0.5% or 1.0%) concentrations of sevoflurane by healthy volunteers produced time-dependent alterations in gene expression in white blood cells, including several transcripts that have been strongly implicated in late ischemic preconditioning.[174] Sevoflurane also reduced expression of the proinflammatory L-selectin (CD62L) in granulocytes concomitant with increased resistance to inflammatory activation 24 and 48 hours after exposure to the volatile agent.[174] These exciting data provided the first evidence that volatile anesthetics have the potential to produce a second window of cardioprotection in humans.

Several investigations have begun to explore the mechanisms responsible for delayed anesthetic preconditioning in experimental animals. COX-2 mediated late ischemic and δ-opioid–induced pharmacologic preconditioning in rabbits. Delayed ischemic and δ-opioid–induced pharmacologic preconditioning was also shown to increase COX-2 transcription and translation and enhance myocardial concentrations of prostaglandin E_2 (PGE_2) and 6-keto-$PGF_2\alpha$ 24 hours after the initial ischemic stimulus.[165] A role for COX-2 has been demonstrated in the second window of isoflurane preconditioning. Administration of the selective COX-2 antagonist celecoxib after but not before remote isoflurane exposure abolished reductions in myocardial infarct size associated with the volatile agent.[175] These data indicate that COX-2 functions as a mediator but not as a trigger of delayed isoflurane cardioprotection.[175] In contrast to the findings with late ischemic and δ-opioid–induced preconditioning,[165] COX-2 protein expression was unaffected by remote isoflurane administration, suggesting that an increase in COX-2 activity may instead mediate the cardioprotective effect of volatile anesthetics in this setting.[175] Inducible NOS (iNOS) regulates COX-2 activity during the late phase of ischemic preconditioning.[176] NO functions as a trigger and mediator of this second window of ischemic preconditioning.[177] Neuronal NOS (nNOS) may also mediate the late phase of ischemic preconditioning in concert with COX-2.[178] A central role for NO metabolism was described during isoflurane-induced delayed preconditioning in rabbits.[179] Administration of the nonselective NOS antagonist L-arginine methyl ester (L-NAME), but not selective iNOS or nNOS inhibitors, before remote isoflurane exposure or coronary artery occlusion and reperfusion abolished reductions in infarct size produced by the volatile agent.[179] Increases in endothelial NOS (eNOS) but not iNOS transcription and translation were also observed during the second window of isoflurane preconditioning.[179] These data demonstrated that the NO produced by eNOS triggers and mediates late isoflurane preconditioning in rabbits. Administration of isoflurane 24 to 72 hours before global ischemia and reperfusion also reduced infarct size and preserved LV function in isolated rat hearts.[180] In contrast to the findings in rabbits, upregulation and activation of iNOS mediated isoflurane delayed preconditioning in rats.[180] Interestingly, a second window of isoflurane preconditioning did not occur in female rabbits.[181] This gender specificity may be related to an estrogen-related upregulation of eNOS in female rabbits that confers substantial protection against infarction independent of subsequent remote administration of a volatile anesthetic.[181]

A role for reactive oxygen and nitrogen species in isoflurane delayed preconditioning has also been demonstrated in rats.[182] Reductions in infarct size occurred after remote 2-hour inhalation of isoflurane concentrations as low as 0.8%, which confirmed that subanesthetic concentrations of a volatile anesthetic are capable of providing a second window of cardioprotection.[173,174] Pretreatment with a superoxide anion scavenger or a nonselective NOS antagonist abolished the protection produced by remote isoflurane exposure. As observed in isoflurane acute preconditioning,[77] remote administration of the volatile agent increased ethidium fluorescence consistent with the generation of superoxide anion, and pretreatment with an inhibitor of the mitochondrial electron transport chain inhibited this response.[182] Delayed cardioprotection mediated by 12-lipoxygenase expression and activity has been linked to opioid receptor activation.[183] 12-Lipoxygenase was also demonstrated to mediate isoflurane delayed preconditioning in mice.[184] A selective inhibitor of 12-lipoxygenase abolished reductions in infarct size produced by the administration of isoflurane 24 hours before prolonged coronary occlusion and reperfusion. These cardioprotective effects were accompanied by enhanced expression of 12-lipoxygenase localized to the intercalated disk regions adjoining adjacent ventricular myocytes.[184]

Postconditioning by Volatile Anesthetics

The first minutes of reperfusion are critical for salvaging ischemic myocardium, but reperfusion also paradoxically exacerbates the initial damage caused by the ischemic insult.[185] Modulation of conditions during reperfusion favorably affects the extent of ischemic injury. Studies of controlled reperfusion after ischemia have indicated that gradual reperfusion at low intracoronary pressure reduces myocardial damage.[186,187] Such control over coronary hemodynamics during early reperfusion reduced myocardial infarct size, preserved postischemic contractile function, limited endothelial injury, and attenuated myocardial edema. Despite these data, most of the experimental and clinical research examining the adverse consequences of ischemia-reperfusion injury and how they may be minimized has instead focused on interventions performed before the onset of ischemia. Clearly, coronary artery occlusion cannot be temporally predicted in most patients with acute myocardial infarction with any degree of certainty, and as a result, application of preconditioning strategies may be primarily limited to clinical situations in which the precise onset of ischemia is well defined (e.g., inflation of an angioplasty balloon, application of an aortic cross-clamp during cardiopulmonary bypass).

In 2003, Zhao and Vinten-Johansen reported that brief episodes of coronary artery occlusion conducted during early reperfusion after prolonged ischemia reduced myocardial infarct size, attenuated neutrophil accumulation, partially inhibited the generation of cytotoxic reactive oxygen species, decreased endothelial dysfunction, and diminished apoptosis.[187-189] This phenomenon was initially termed “ischemic postconditioning” and later shortened to simply “postconditioning.” The reductions in myocardial infarct size caused by postconditioning were shown to be remarkably similar to those produced by ischemic preconditioning.[189] Activation of ERK1/2 and formation of NO were initially shown to mediate this form of cardioprotection.[189,190] Subsequently, the prosurvival PI3K-Akt signaling cascade, including the downstream enzymes eNOS and target of rapamycin (TOR)/70-kd ribosomal protein s6 kinase (p70s6K), was shown to play a central role in postconditioning.[191] These signaling elements are critical mediators of cellular necrosis and apoptosis via their actions on the balance of proapoptotic and antiapoptotic proteins, the activity of the regulatory enzyme glycogen synthase kinase-3β (GSK-3β), and the transition state of the mPTP (Fig. 23-14).[192,193] Postconditioning has also been shown to occur in the human heart.[194] Administration of a diverse variety of drugs (e.g., G protein–coupled receptor ligands [adenosine, bradykinin, opioids], insulin, statins, urocortin, growth factors [basic fibroblast growth factor, insulin-like growth factor I]) immediately before or during early reperfusion mimics the beneficial actions of postconditioning. Many elements of prosurvival signaling mediate this “pharmacologic postconditioning.”[195]

Although anesthetic preconditioning has been studied extensively and many of the mechanisms responsible for this phenomenon have been characterized in detail, substantially less attention has been directed toward exploration of the possible beneficial effects of volatile anesthetics when administered immediately before or during reperfusion (termed “anesthetic postconditioning”). Nevertheless, some experimental evidence indicates that volatile anesthetics are capable of exerting cardioprotective effects under these conditions. The older volatile agent halothane prevented reoxygenation-induced hypercontracture of cardiac myocytes in vitro, a potential cause of myocyte necrosis during early reperfusion.[196] Halothane also reduced reperfusion injury after regional ischemia in rabbit hearts.[197] Desflurane and sevoflurane reduced infarction size when administered during the first 15 minutes of reperfusion in rabbits.[198] Isoflurane enhanced the functional recovery of isolated rat hearts when administered solely during reperfusion.[58] The salutary actions of sevoflurane during reperfusion were shown to be dose dependent in rats.[199]

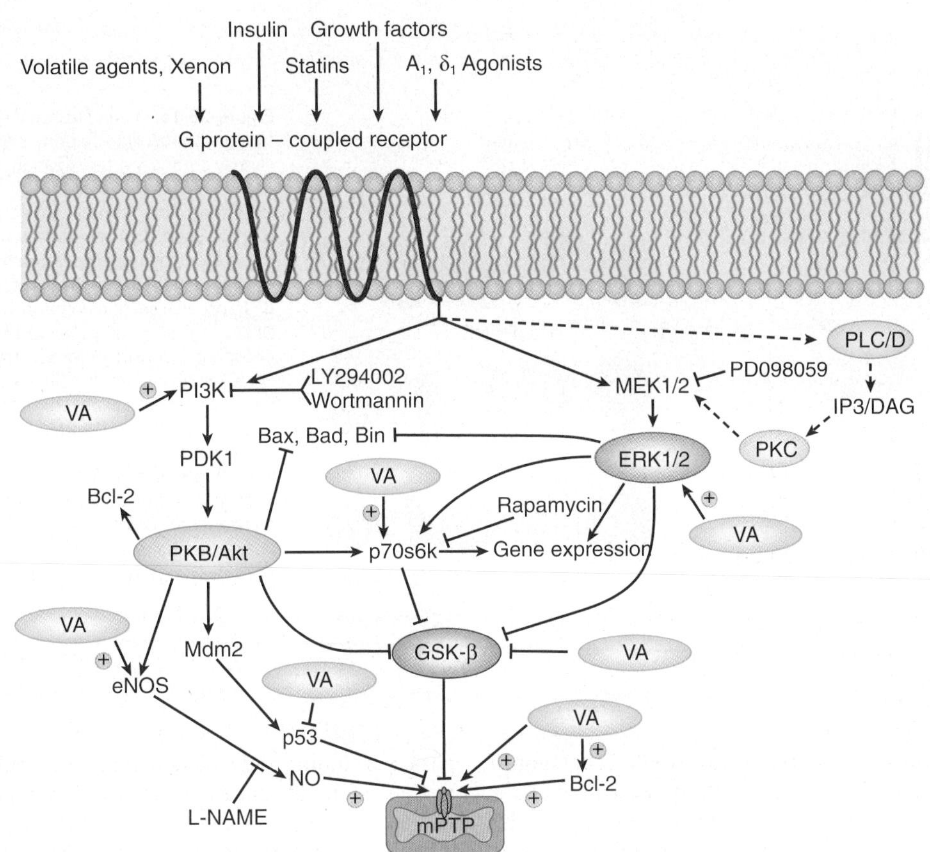

Figure 23-14 Schematic illustration depicting the potential sites of action of volatile anesthetics (VA) on cardioprotective signaling during early reperfusion. G protein–coupled receptor ligands (e.g., adenosine A_1, opioid δ_1), VA, insulin, statins, and growth factors activate parallel phosphoinositol 3-kinase (PI3K) or extracellular signal–regulated kinase (ERK1/2) cascades to produce protection. G protein–coupled activation of protein kinase C (PKC) by phospholipases (PLC/D) through the second messengers diacylglycerol (DAG) and inositol triphosphate (IP3) also contributes to activation of PI3K and ERK1/2. PI3K phosphorylates phosphoinositide-dependent kinase (PDK1), which activates Akt (also known as protein kinase B [PKB]). This moiety stimulates the activity of antiapoptotic proteins (e.g., B-cell lymphoma-2 [Bcl-2]) and simultaneously inhibits the activity of proapoptotic proteins (e.g., Bax, Bad, Bim, caspases). Akt/PKB also inhibits the β-isoform of glycogen synthase kinase (GSK-β) and activates endothelial nitric oxide synthase (eNOS), 70-kd ribosomal protein s6 kinase (p70s6K), and murine double-minute-2 (Mdm2) protein. p70s6K also inhibits GSK-β activity. Nitric oxide (NO) produced by eNOS inhibits whereas Mdm2-induced phosphorylation of the proapoptotic protein p53 opens the mitochondrial permeability transition pore (mPTP). Inhibition of GSK-β and activation of mitochondrial K_{ATP} channels also act to close the mPTP. The transition state of the mitochondrial pore is critical for preservation of mitochondrial integrity and cell viability during ischemia and reperfusion. Activation of ERK1/2 also inhibits GSK-β and blocks the formation of proapoptotic proteins. LY294002 and wortmannin, rapamycin, PD 098059, and L-arginine methyl ester (L-NAME) block the activity of PI3K, p70s6K, ERK1/2, and eNOS, respectively. Volatile anesthetics have been proposed to enhance the activity of PI3K-Akt, p70s6k, ERK1/2, and eNOS. Volatile anesthetics have also been suggested to directly inhibit GSK-β and mPTP concomitant with enhanced expression of Bcl-2 and inhibition of p53. Volatile anesthetic–induced activation of mitochondrial K_{ATP} channels also inhibits mPTP. These actions of volatile anesthetics may contribute to the cardioprotective effects during early reperfusion.

Administration of sevoflurane after ischemia also improved contractile and metabolic function concomitant with reduced myoplasmic Ca^{2+} loading in isolated guinea pig hearts.[200]

The mechanisms by which volatile anesthetics produce cardioprotection during reperfusion have yet to be firmly established. Halothane abolished reoxygenation-induced attenuation of SR-dependent oscillations of intramyoplasmic Ca^{2+} concentration in isolated cardiac myocytes.[196] These[196] and other findings[200] suggested that volatile anesthetics may prevent intracellular Ca^{2+} overload during early reperfusion. Isoflurane and sevoflurane also reduced postischemic adhesion of polymorphonuclear leukocytes.[201] However, the precise mechanisms by which volatile anesthetics act to reduce intracellular Ca^{2+} overload or attenuate the adverse consequences of large quantities of reactive oxygen intermediates during early reperfusion were not elucidated by these previous studies. Although it is certainly tempting to propose that similar signaling pathways mediate anesthetic preconditioning and postconditioning, substantial differences between the genomic responses associated with these phenomena have been demonstrated.[202] These findings suggest that the mechanisms responsible for anesthetic preconditioning and postconditioning may not be identical.

Chiari and coworkers demonstrated that brief exposure to 1.0 MAC isoflurane administered during the final 3 minutes of coronary artery occlusion and the first 2 minutes of reperfusion reduces myocardial infarct size in rabbits.[203] The degree of myocardial preservation observed with isoflurane postconditioning was similar in magnitude to the cardioprotection afforded by isoflurane preconditioning in an identical experimental preparation.[77] Postconditioning with 0.5 MAC isoflurane (a concentration that did not produce cardioprotection alone) also reduced the time threshold required for ischemic postconditioning. The beneficial actions of isoflurane before and during early reperfusion with or without subthreshold ischemic postconditioning

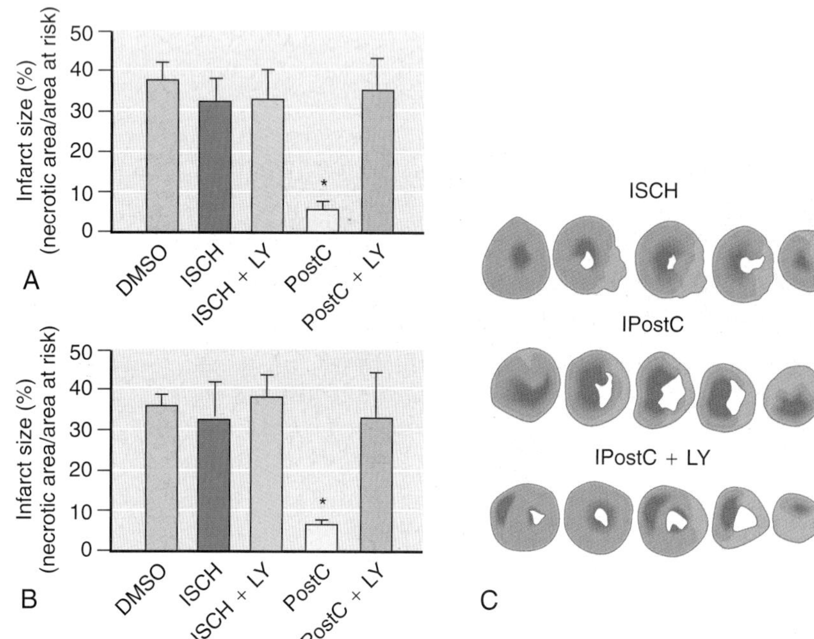

Figure 23-15 Infarct size was determined by 1% triphenyltetrazolium chloride staining. Areas infarcted in vivo by coronary artery ligation were excluded from determination of infarct size (**A**). The scarred chronic infarct resulting from coronary ligation was distinguished from fresh infarcts (*salmon pink*). Release of lactate dehydrogenase during reperfusion (**B**) served as an independent method to estimate infarct size. **C,** Transverse sections of representative experiments. DMSO, dimethyl sulfoxide (<0.1%; used to dissolve the phosphatidylinositol-3′-kinase antagonist LY294002); PostC, ischemic postconditioning; ISCH, unprotected remodeled hearts exposed to ischemia-reperfusion alone; LY, LY294002 (15 μM); PostC, anesthetic postconditioning. Data are given as means ± SD ($n = 5$ in each group). $^*P < 0.05$ versus ISCH. *(From Feng J, Fischer G, Lucchinetti E, et al: Infarct-remodeled myocardium is receptive to protection by isoflurane postconditioning. Role of protein kinase B/Akt signaling. Anesthesiology 104:1004-1014, 2006.)*

were blocked by pretreatment with the selective PI3K antagonist wortmannin. Isoflurane also increased phosphorylation of the PI3K downstream target protein Akt, and this effect was also inhibited by wortmannin pretreatment. These data demonstrated for the first time that activation of the PI3K signaling pathway directly mediates the protective effects of isoflurane postconditioning in vivo.[203] A central role for PI3K-Akt signaling in isoflurane postconditioning was subsequently demonstrated in infarct-remodeled myocardium as well (Fig. 23-15), thus suggesting that postconditioning by volatile anesthetics may also be maintained in diseased myocardium.[204]

Reperfusion after a prolonged ischemic insult initiates or hastens apoptosis.[205] Isoflurane postconditioning reduced cytochrome *c* translocation from mitochondria (an important early marker of apoptosis mediated by PI3K-Akt) and decreased the number of terminal deoxynucleotidyl transferase–mediated dUTP nick end labeling (TUNEL; another indicator of apoptosis)-positive ventricular myocytes in situ.[206] These data provided the first direct evidence indicating that isoflurane postconditioning preserves myocardial integrity, in part by attenuating apoptotic cell death. Volatile anesthetics were previously shown to abolish norepinephrine-induced apoptosis in rat ventricular myocytes as indicated by reductions in TUNEL-positive cell staining, attenuation of increases in annexin V staining (an index of DNA laddering), and inhibition of elevated caspase-9 activity.[207]

When administered in a dose that did not alter infarct size alone, morphine enhanced isoflurane postconditioning against myocardial infarction.[206] The protective effects of the combination of subthreshold doses of morphine and isoflurane during early reperfusion were abolished by pretreatment with wortmannin, thus indicating that the cardioprotection observed was mediated by activation of PI3K. The nonselective opioid antagonist naloxone also inhibited the protective effects of morphine, isoflurane, and their combination during early reperfusion, thus suggesting that opioid receptor activation also mediates isoflurane postconditioning and its augmentation by morphine. Cardioprotection by opioids during reperfusion occurs as a result of activation of δ_1-opioid receptors,[208] and postconditioning against infarction by isoflurane and its potentiation by the clinically relevant opioid morphine may also be mediated by the δ_1-opioid receptor. This hypothesis remains to be tested, but a role for the δ_1-opioid receptor in anesthetic preconditioning was described previously.[59]

Activation of ERK1/2 is a redundant mechanism by which downstream elements of the PI3K cascade may be stimulated to favorably modulate reperfusion injury.[62] ERK1/2 mediates ischemic[209] and pharmacologic[210] postconditioning and also plays an important role in the preconditioning produced by volatile anesthetics.[109,114] Selective inhibition of ERK1/2 abolished the reductions in infarct size produced by isoflurane postconditioning.[211] Both PI3K-Akt and ERK1/2 phosphorylate TOR/p70s6K, an important regulator of protein translation.[62] A selective inhibitor of this enzyme (rapamycin) abolished cardioprotection during ischemic[191] and pharmacologic[208] postconditioning. Isoflurane postconditioning was also inhibited by rapamycin in normal and infarct-remodeled myocardium, thus implicating a role for p70s6K in this phenomenon as well.[211,212]

PI3K-Akt activates eNOS and increases the formation of NO,[191] and a central role for NO has been demonstrated in postconditioning by ischemia[191] or G protein–coupled receptor ligands.[210] A nonselective NOS inhibitor, but not selective iNOS or nNOS inhibitors, abolished reductions in infarct size produced by the administration of isoflurane before and during early reperfusion in rabbits, a finding suggesting that eNOS mediates isoflurane postconditioning.[211] Furthermore, isoflurane inhaled at the onset of reperfusion enhanced the cardioprotective effect of ischemic postconditioning through a NO-dependent mechanism in rabbits.[213] Isoflurane postconditioning also enhanced expression of eNOS in infarct-remodeled rat myocardium, and a selective PI3K antagonist inhibited this isoflurane-induced phosphorylation of eNOS.[204] These data suggest that NO derived from

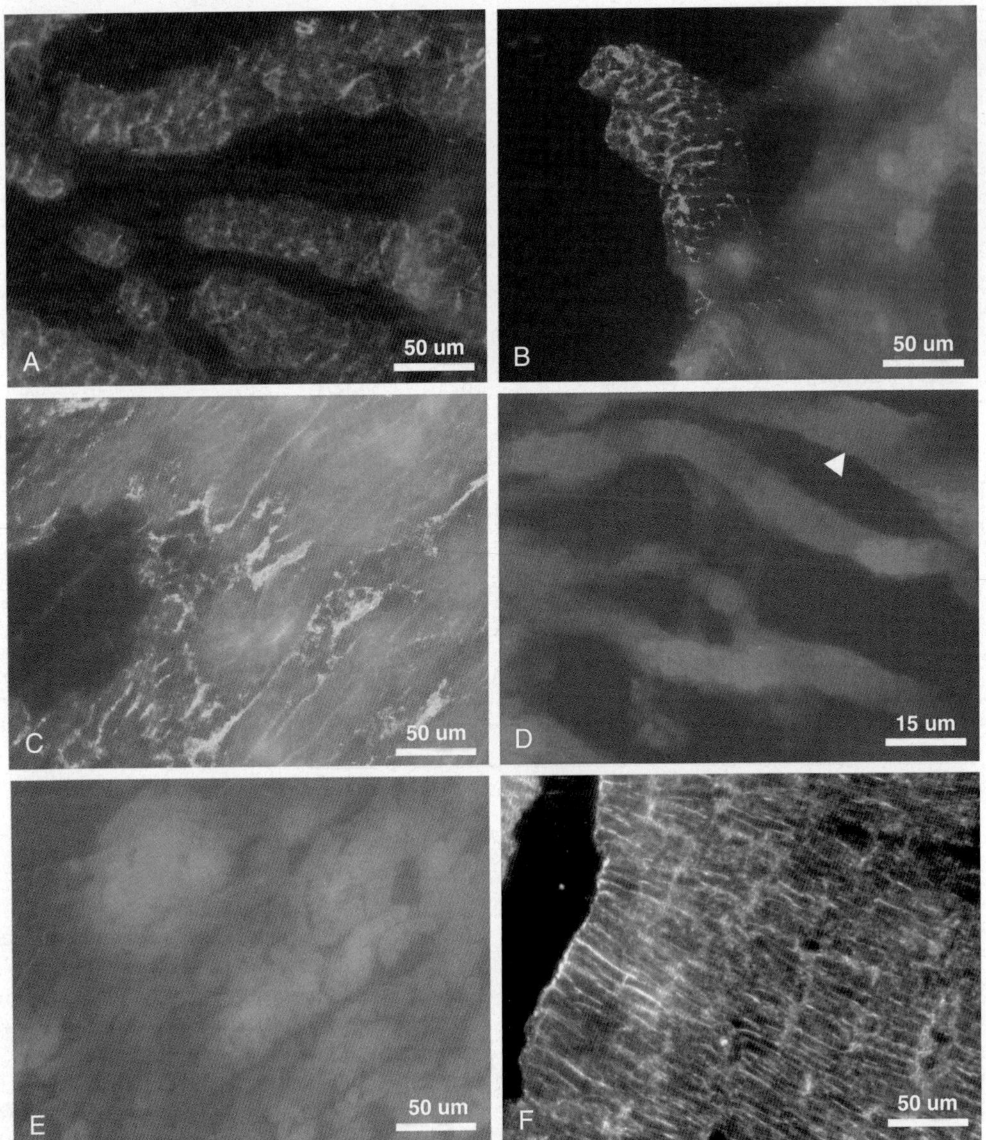

Figure 23-16 Postischemic uptake of MitoTracker Red 580 in the mitochondria of isolated perfused rat hearts. Unprotected hearts show no staining (**A**) except for superficial epicardial layers of the myocardium (**B**). In contrast, postconditioned protected hearts exhibit marked accumulation of MitoTracker Red 580 in tissue (**C** and **D**), similar to control hearts not subjected to ischemia-reperfusion (time-matched perfusion) (**E**). Atractyloside, a direct opener of the mitochondrial permeability transition pore, completely abolished the isoflurane effects (**F**). **A** through **F** are epifluorescence micrographs (*red channel*) merged with phase-contrast images. **D** shows at higher magnification the syncytial net of postconditioned myocytes containing brightly staining mitochondria (*red channel*). The *arrow* indicates intercalated disks. *(From Feng J, Lucchinetti E, Ahuja P, et al: Isoflurane postconditioning prevents opening of the mitochondrial permeability transition pore through inhibition of glycogen synthase kinase 3β. Anesthesiology 103:987-995, 2005.)*

eNOS plays an important role in anesthetic postconditioning in healthy and infarct-remodeled myocardium.

Inhibition of mPTP has been shown to mediate ischemic postconditioning.[214] Isoflurane postconditioning was abolished by the mPTP opener atractyloside and enhanced by the mPTP inhibitor cyclosporine in rabbits.[215] Similarly, atractyloside and a selective PI3K antagonist (LY294002) abolished isoflurane postconditioning in rats.[212] LY294002 also inhibited phosphorylation of the regulatory enzyme GSK-3β and opened the mPTP as determined by nicotinamide adenine dinucleotide measurements (Fig. 23-16).[212] Taken together, these data[212,215] indicate that administration of isoflurane during early reperfusion protects against reperfusion injury by preventing mPTP opening via a PI3K-dependent mechanism through inhibition of GSK-3β.

Experimental evidence has strongly suggested that mitochondrial K_{ATP} channel activation is an end-effector during anesthetic preconditioning.[56] Opening of mitochondrial K_{ATP} channels during ischemic or pharmacologic preconditioning may produce small alterations in intramitochondrial homeostasis that promote protection against subsequent ischemic damage through energy-dependent regulation of mitochondrial matrix volume. Opening of mitochondrial K^+ influx pathways favorably regulated matrix volume and improved function during simulated ischemia and reperfusion.[216] A selective mitochondrial K_{ATP} channel antagonist (5-HD) inhibited isoflurane postconditioning,[215] suggesting that mitochondrial K_{ATP} channel opening by brief administration of isoflurane during early reperfusion may be responsible for cardioprotection in rabbits. Mitochondrial K_{ATP} channels mediate

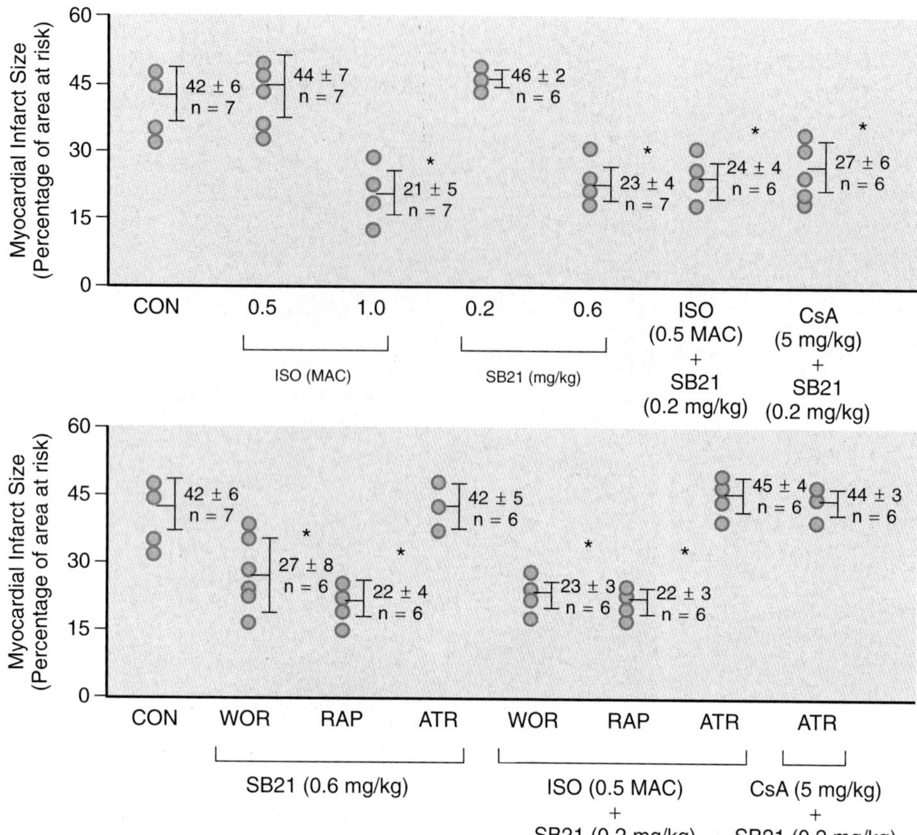

Figure 23-17 Myocardial infarct size depicted as a percentage of the left ventricular area at risk in rabbits receiving 0.9% saline (control, CON), isoflurane (ISO, 0.5 or 1.0 minimum alveolar concentration [MAC]), SB 216763 (SB21, 0.2 or 0.6 mg/kg), 0.5 MAC ISO plus 0.2 mg/kg SB21, or cyclosporine (CsA, 5 mg/kg) plus 0.2 mg/kg SB21 (*top panel*). Infarct sizes in rabbits receiving 0.6 mg/kg SB21 or 0.5 MAC ISO plus 0.2 mg/kg SB21 in the presence of wortmannin (WOR, 0.6 mg/kg), rapamycin (RAP, 0.25 mg/kg), or atractyloside (ATR, 5 mg/kg) are depicted in the *bottom panel*. Infarct sizes in rabbits receiving A (CsA, 5 mg/kg) plus 0.2 mg/kg SB21 in the presence of atractyloside pretreatment are also illustrated in the *bottom panel*. Each point represents a single experiment. All data are means ± SD. *Significantly ($P < .05$) different from CON. *(From Pagel PS, Krolikowski JG, Neff DA, et al: Inhibition of glycogen synthase kinase potentiates isoflurane-induced protection against myocardial infarction during early reperfusion in vivo. Anesth Analg 102:1348-1354, 2006.)*

sevoflurane postconditioning in rats.[217] However, a close interaction between mitochondrial K_{ATP} channels and mPTP was previously identified during diazoxide and desflurane preconditioning.[127,130] Hence, isoflurane postconditioning may not be solely attributable to the actions of the volatile agent on mitochondrial K_{ATP} channels alone but, instead, may be dependent on the interaction between mitochondrial K_{ATP} channel opening and mPTP inhibition.

GSK-3β is an important mediator of cellular function whose activation has been implicated in the pathogenesis of diabetes mellitus and Alzheimer's disease. Inhibition of GSK-3β may play a critical role in protection against myocardial ischemia-reperfusion injury inasmuch as selective blockade of the enzyme mimics the beneficial actions of ischemic preconditioning[218] and opioid postconditioning.[208] GSK-3β was shown to be a central regulator of several prosurvival signaling enzymes (e.g., PI3K, p70s6K, PKC, protein kinase A) during cardioprotection against hypoxia-reoxygenation injury in isolated ventricular myocytes.[192] Selective inhibition of GSK-3β also limited mPTP opening.[192] Thus, many endogenous signaling pathways appear to converge on and regulate the activity of GSK-3β, thereby favorably modulating mitochondrial permeability transition and producing protection against ischemia-reperfusion injury. Administration of isoflurane during early reperfusion phosphorylated and inactivated GSK-3β in a PI3K- and mPTP-dependent fashion concomitant with cardioprotection in isolated perfused rats.[212] A selective inhibitor of GSK-3β (SB 216763) was also shown to lower the threshold of isoflurane postconditioning against infarction in rabbits.[219] The salutary actions of the effects of GSK-3β inhibition were abolished by the mPTP opener atractyloside but not the PI3K or p70s6K antagonists wortmannin or rapamycin.[219] These data suggest that isoflurane postconditioning is mediated by the combined actions of SB 216763 and volatile anesthetic on the mPTP and provide pharmacologic evidence suggesting that isoflurane produces a direct inhibitory effect on GSK-3β independent of its actions on PI3K and p70s6K activity (Fig. 23-17).

Mitochondria are the putative target of several apoptotic proteins that either directly damage mitochondrial membranes or indirectly open the mPTP and lead to release of cytochrome *c*. Phosphorylation of Bad by PI3K results in its sequestration from mitochondria and inhibits apoptosis.[220] Similarly, activation of PI3K prevents Bax-induced apoptosis by inhibiting the critical conformational change required for its translocation to mitochondrial membranes.[221] Activation of PI3K has also been shown to phosphorylate and inactivate procaspase-9 and thereby inhibit this important mediator of apoptotic cell death.[222] The mechanisms by which inhibition of GSK-3β favorably affects the mPTP to cause protection against ischemia-reperfusion injury have not been clearly elucidated. Activated GSK-3β binds to and promotes the actions of p53,[223] a tumor suppressor protein known to interact with and stimulate the disruption of mitochondria during apoptosis.[224] p53 translocates to mitochondria, increases mitochondrial membrane permeability by directly interacting with Bax, abolishes $\Delta\Psi_m$, and causes the release of cytochrome *c*.[225]

A central role for inhibition of p53 in myocardial and neuronal protection against cellular injury has been characterized. Activation of p53 by hypoxia or ROS[226] produces immediate or delayed programmed cell death by stimulating mitochondrial apoptotic pathways and enhancing the transcription of other proapoptotic proteins (e.g., Bax, apoptosis-inducing factor

[AIF]).[227] Enhanced p53 expression was observed after ischemia and reperfusion in isolated rat ventricular myocytes, and ischemic preconditioning substantially reduced this effect.[228] Ischemic preconditioning also attenuated p53 transcription and translation in hippocampal pyramidal neurons in a rat model of global forebrain ischemia and reperfusion.[229] Inhibition of p53 with the selective antagonist pifithrin-α or stimulated degradation of the protein by PI3K-mediated phosphorylation of murine double-minute-2 protein (Mdm2), an oncogenic factor known to facilitate p53 degradation, has previously been shown to protect against ischemic injury in isolated rat hearts.[230] Phosphorylated Mdm2 associates with p53 and inactivates the latter protein by blocking its active site and promoting subsequent degradation of it through ubiquitin complex formation.[231] Thus, ischemic preconditioning may have abrogated the deleterious actions of p53 by PI3K-mediated phosphorylation of the downstream moiety Mdm2.[230] Direct inhibition of p53 with pifithrin-α protected against neuronal cell death produced by ischemia, excitotoxins, or amyloid β-peptide.[232] Targeted deletion of p53 prevented cardiac rupture after infarction in transgenic mice, presumably by simulating the protective actions of ischemic preconditioning via inhibition of apoptotic cell death, thereby preserving myocardial integrity.[233] Inhibition of p53 by pifithrin-α was recently demonstrated to lower the threshold of isoflurane postconditioning in vivo.[234] Blockade of this action by atractyloside indicated that the cardioprotection observed was mediated by actions of the selective p53 inhibitor and the volatile anesthetic on the mPTP. Thus, experimental evidence suggests that administration of isoflurane during early reperfusion may affect the interaction between GSK-3β and p53 to modulate the transition state of the mPTP.

Bcl-2 protein has been identified in the outer mitochondrial membrane, regulates the mPTP, and inhibits apoptosis.[235] Overexpression of Bcl-2 attenuated apoptosis and protected against ischemia-reperfusion injury in transgenic mice.[236] A key interaction between Bcl-2 and mPTP inhibition was previously implicated during delayed ischemic preconditioning.[129] A selective inhibitor (HA14-1) of Bcl-2 abolished isoflurane-induced Bcl-2 expression and attenuated reductions in apoptosis (e.g., cytochrome *c* release, TUNEL staining) in isolated atrial and ventricular myocytes subjected to hypoxia-reoxygenation injury, hydrogen peroxide, or activated neutrophils.[126] HA14-1 also inhibited isoflurane and ischemic postconditioning in vivo but did not affect cardioprotection produced by the direct mPTP inhibitor cyclosporine.[237] Thus, the salutary actions of isoflurane on transient, repetitive ischemia during early reperfusion may also occur as a result of indirect modulation of the mPTP mediated "upstream" by Bcl-2.[237] In fact, PI3K has been shown to phosphorylate and activate Bcl-2 concomitant with inactivation of proapoptotic proteins, including Bad, Bax, and p53.[238] As a result, activation of PI3K signaling by isoflurane postconditioning appears to produce cardioprotection by several redundant mechanisms that affect apoptotic protein homeostasis.

Coronary Vascular Effects of Volatile Anesthetics in Humans

Evaluation of the actions of volatile anesthetics on the human coronary circulation is difficult not only because the methods used to determine coronary blood flow in humans are limited but also because interpretation of clinical findings during anesthesia is complicated by changes in hemodynamics, the impact of surgery, and the use of adjuvant anesthetics or vasoactive drugs. Halothane decreases MV_{O_2} and variably alters coronary blood flow in patients with coronary artery disease, but metabolic or electrocardiographic evidence of ischemia has not been observed during halothane anesthesia. A report published in 1983[239] described the occurrence of myocardial ischemia, as indicated by new electrocardiographic changes and abnormal myocardial lactate extraction, in 10 of 21 patients anesthetized with isoflurane who were undergoing major vascular surgery. Five patients were treated with phenylephrine and pacing to return arterial pressure and heart rate to control values, and after these interventions, the electrocardiographic and metabolic derangements resolved in two of the five patients. Despite the apparent dependence of these new episodes of myocardial ischemia on alterations in systemic hemodynamics, the author[239] proposed that isoflurane had caused coronary steal in these patients, even though no specific evidence of redistribution of blood flow between normal and collateral-dependent zones was presented. The data have not been uniformly supported by subsequent studies. Coronary blood flow remained unchanged during isoflurane anesthesia in patients undergoing coronary artery bypass graft (CABG) surgery, but coronary sinus O_2 content increased consistent with modest coronary vasodilation. Isoflurane alone did not produce electrocardiographic or metabolic evidence of ischemia. Instead, myocardial ischemia occurring during isoflurane anesthesia was most often associated with tachycardia or hypotension. In addition, isoflurane actually increases the tolerance to pacing-induced ischemia in patients with coronary artery disease. Comparison of studies examining the effects of isoflurane on the incidence of intraoperative myocardial ischemia was also complicated by differences in patient age, surgical procedure, operative time, and preoperative LV ejection fraction. Importantly, compelling evidence demonstrating redistribution of coronary blood flow away from ischemic to normal myocardium in humans anesthetized with isoflurane has yet to be reported.

The incidence of intraoperative myocardial ischemia in susceptible patients has been difficult to define. Less than 50% of intraoperative ischemic episodes have been linked to alterations in systemic hemodynamics.[240] The strongest predictor of intraoperative ischemia remains preexisting ischemia on arrival at the operating room and not anesthetic technique.[241] The only hemodynamic event definitively related to intraoperative ischemia in patients undergoing CABG surgery is tachycardia.[241] Perioperative use of β_1-adrenoceptor antagonists to prevent myocardial ischemia strongly supports this contention.[242] Sternotomy caused greater increases in calculated indices of MV_{O_2}, myocardial lactate production, and the incidence of hypertension requiring treatment with vasoactive drugs during morphine than during halothane anesthesia. In contrast, induction of anesthesia with desflurane in patients undergoing CABG surgery may be associated with tachycardia, hypertension, and a greater incidence of ischemia than during induction with sufentanil.[243] Steal-prone anatomy was identified in 23% of patients with coronary artery disease enrolled in the Coronary Artery Surgery Study.[244] However, patients with steal-prone coronary anatomy did not have a greater incidence of ischemia during desflurane anesthesia than did patients with other forms of coronary artery disease.[243] The incidence of myocardial ischemia and adverse cardiac outcomes in cardiac patients undergoing noncardiac surgery has been shown to be similar during sevoflurane and isoflurane anesthesia. New electrocardiographic changes, the incidence of postoperative myocardial infarction, and mortality were similar in patients undergoing CABG surgery independent of anesthetic technique or the presence of steal-prone anatomy.[245] In summary, despite the findings that volatile anesthetics are mild coronary vasodilators, these anesthetics did not cause abnormal redistribution of myocardial perfusion resulting in ischemia when tachycardia and hypotension were avoided in patients with coronary artery disease.

Cardioprotection by Volatile Anesthetics in Humans

Anesthetic preconditioning most likely occurs in human myocardium, but evaluation of this process in patients at risk for myocardial ischemia is complicated by simultaneous alterations in systemic and coronary hemodynamics; the use of other anesthetics, analgesics, or vasoactive drugs; preexisting disease states; and the influence of surgery on cardiovascular homeostasis. Isoflurane[78] and desflurane[80] enhanced the recovery of contractile function in human atrial trabeculae by stimulation of adenosine receptors and activation of K_{ATP} channels. A role for adenosine receptors, MAPKs, and ROS has previously been demonstrated in other forms of preconditioning in human atrial myocytes concomitant with mitochondrial K_{ATP} channel opening. Isoflurane decreased postoperative release of troponin I and the myocardial form of creatine kinase in patients undergoing CABG surgery, thus suggesting a reduction in the severity of myocardial necrosis.[246] Administration of the older agent enflurane before cardioplegic arrest also enhanced postischemic recovery of contractile function in patients undergoing CABG surgery.[247] Sevoflurane, but not the intravenous anesthetic propofol, was shown to preserve myocardial function in patients undergoing CABG surgery or aortic valve replacement concomitant with a reduction in the release of troponin I (Fig. 23-18).[248,249] Desflurane or sevoflurane, but not propofol, maintained contractile function and caused less pronounced release of troponin I after cardiopulmonary bypass in elderly patients with three-vessel coronary artery disease and preexisting LV dysfunction who were undergoing CABG surgery.[250] The beneficial effects of sevoflurane were most apparent when the volatile anesthetic was administered throughout CABG surgery versus before the initiation of cardiopulmonary bypass or after construction of the coronary anastomoses alone.[251] The incidence of atrial fibrillation early after CABG surgery may also be reduced by the intraoperative administration of sevoflurane instead of intravenous anesthetics.[252]

In a double-blind, placebo-controlled study of 72 patients undergoing CABG surgery with cardiopulmonary bypass, sevoflurane preconditioning (inhalation of 4% sevoflurane during the first 10 minutes of cardiopulmonary bypass), but not placebo, reduced postoperative release of brain natriuretic peptide (BNP), a biochemical marker of LV dysfunction, and cystatin C, an indicator of renal dysfunction, concomitant with translocation of PKC-δ and PKC-ε (Fig. 23-19).[253] Postoperative biochemical markers of hepatic injury were also lower with a sevoflurane-based anesthetic technique than with intravenous propofol anesthesia in patients undergoing CABG surgery with cardio-

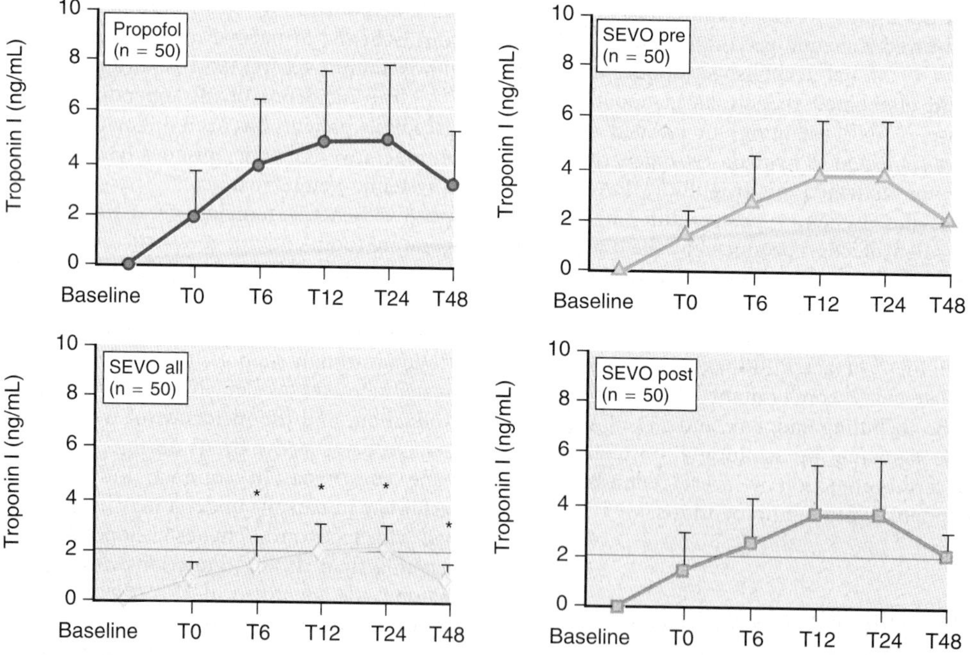

Figure 23-18 Cardiac troponin I concentrations in the four groups before surgery (baseline), at arrival in the intensive care unit (T0), and after 6 (T6), 12 (T12), 24 (T24), and 48 (T48) hours. Data are presented as means ± SD. *Statistically significant difference with the propofol group ($P < .05$). In all groups, a transient increase in troponin I concentrations was observed. Only in the SEVO all group was this increase significantly less than in the propofol group. For the sake of clarity, the SD bars are represented in only one direction. SEVO, sevoflurane. *(From De Hert SG, ten Broecke PW, Mertens E, et al: Sevoflurane but not propofol preserves myocardial function in coronary surgery patients. Anesthesiology 97:42-49, 2002.)*

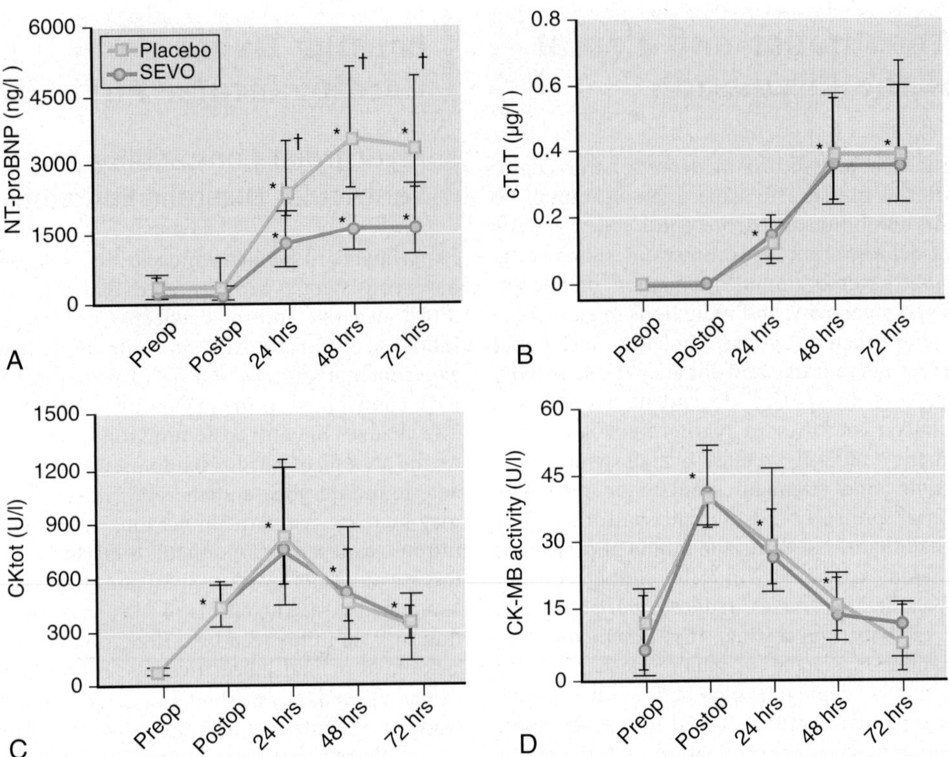

Figure 23-19 Biomarkers of myocardial injury at various time points for the placebo (PLACEBO)- and sevoflurane (SEVO)-treated groups: N-terminal pro–brain natriuretic peptide (NT-proBNP) (**A**), cardiac troponin T (cTnT) (**B**), total creatine kinase (CKtot) (**C**), and creatine kinase-MB (CK-MB) isoenzyme activity (**D**). Two-factor repeated-measures analysis of variance indicated that the groups differed significantly in plasma NT-proBNP concentrations (time effect, $P < .001$; group effect, $P < .001$; group-time interaction, $P = .003$). There was no difference in cTnT, CKtot, and CK-MB concentrations. Multiple *t*-tests with the Bonferroni correction for multiple comparisons were used to compare plasma concentrations of the different biomarkers at each time point with the respective preoperative baseline value within groups and to compare plasma concentrations at each time point between groups. *Significantly increased in comparison to baseline values ($P < 0.05$). †Significant difference between groups ($P < 0.05$). PLACEBO, group with a narrow cap; SEVO, group with a wide cap. The plot shows medians and lower and upper quartiles. *(From Julier K, da Silva R, Garcia C, et al: Preconditioning by sevoflurane decreases biochemical markers for myocardial and renal dysfunction in coronary artery bypass graft surgery: A double-blinded, placebo-controlled multicenter study. Anesthesiology 98:1315-1327, 2003.)*

pulmonary bypass.[254] When compared with placebo, brief (10-minute) administration of 4% sevoflurane reduced platelet–endothelial cell adhesion molecule-1 (PECAM-1/CD31) and increased catalase expression in atrial biopsy specimens concomitant with a reduction in the indices of myocardial injury (e.g., cardiac troponin T, N-terminal pro-BNP) in patients undergoing CABG surgery and cardiopulmonary bypass.[255] The membrane protein PECAM-1 has been shown to play important roles in atherosclerotic plaque instability and migration of leukocytes through the vascular endothelium. Notably, an improvement in 1-year cardiovascular outcome was also observed in sevoflurane-preconditioned patients in this study.[255] These compelling data suggest that volatile anesthetics may exert long-term beneficial effects against ischemic injury in patients with coronary artery disease, in part by favorably modulating transcription of protective and antiprotective proteins.

More recently, low end-tidal concentrations (0.5% to 1.0%) of sevoflurane were shown to protect against endothelial damage in human volunteers undergoing 15-minute forearm ischemia followed by reperfusion.[256] A marked reduction in reactive hyperemic response (an indicator of ischemic injury and endothelial function) and attenuation of leukocyte activation (as measured by CD11a expression) were observed in volunteers pretreated with sevoflurane but not in those who were not.[256] Sevoflurane-induced alterations in genetic regulatory control of myocardial energy metabolism were also recently suggested to predict postoperative cardiac function in patients undergoing off-pump CABG surgery.[257] These data confirmed and extended previous findings indicating that desflurane decreases troponin I release, reduces inotropic drug use, and decreases the number of patients requiring prolonged hospitalization when compared with a propofol-opioid–based intravenous anesthetic technique in patients undergoing off-pump CABG surgery.[258] A meta-analysis of 22 previous studies incorporating more than 2800 patients undergoing CABG surgery suggested that sevoflurane and desflurane anesthesia was associated with reductions in postoperative troponin I release, but whether this decrease in a major index of myocardial necrosis translated into improved long-term outcome was unclear.[259] Thus, clinical investigations conducted to date provide tantalizing evidence suggesting that volatile anesthetics may represent an important therapeutic modality to reduce the risk for perioperative myocardial ischemia and infarction, but this contention will require a large-scale, randomized clinical trial for confirmation.

Volatile Anesthetics and Neural Control of the Circulation

Volatile anesthetics have been shown to depress baroreceptor reflex control of arterial pressure in experimental animals to varying degrees. This inhibition of baroreceptor reflex activity occurs as a result of depression of central nervous system integration of afferent baroreceptor input, attenuation of efferent autonomic nervous system activity, and reductions in ganglionic transmission and end-organ response. Volatile anesthetics increase resting afferent nerve traffic and enhance the sensitivity of arterial baroreceptors by a Ca^{2+}-dependent mechanism. These anesthetic-induced increases in baroreceptor sensitivity and discharge frequency tonically reduce overall sympathetic nervous system activity and attenuate sympathetic responses to declines in arterial pressure.[260] Isoflurane and the older volatile anesthetics halothane and enflurane inhibited preganglionic sympathetic efferent activity at clinically relevant concentrations in vivo. Volatile anesthetics reduced postganglionic sympathetic nerve activity, suggesting that attenuation of ganglionic transmission represents a major mechanism by which volatile anesthetics depress sympathetic nerve traffic. Depression of the sympathetic outflow caused by volatile anesthetics has also been suggested by examination of endogenous plasma norepinephrine kinetics. Isoflurane and halothane decreased plasma concentrations of norepinephrine to varying degrees by causing more pronounced reductions in norepinephrine spillover than clearance. Volatile anesthetics may also attenuate parasympathetic nervous system function. The older agent halothane was shown to depress vagal nerve efferent activity by direct measurement of parasympathetic nerve activity. These findings were supported by the results of several other studies demonstrating that volatile anesthetics inhibit reflex bradycardia in response to increases in arterial pressure. Parasympathetic and sympathetic nervous system outflow appears to be depressed to an equivalent degree during halothane or isoflurane anesthesia.

The effects of volatile anesthetics on neural control of the cardiovascular system have been incompletely examined in healthy humans and have not been described in patients with autonomic nervous system dysfunction. Halothane and enflurane produced greater attenuation of baroreceptor reflex regulation of the heart rate than equivalent MAC concentrations of isoflurane did. Depression of baroreceptor function by these volatile anesthetics may be more profound than with fentanyl, diazepam, and nitrous oxide anesthesia. Baroreceptor-mediated control of peripheral arteriolar tone was also attenuated in young volunteers during halothane anesthesia. Steady-state anesthetic concentrations of sevoflurane were shown to cause greater depression of sympathetic nerve activity measured directly by microneurography than desflurane did at equivalent levels of hypotension.[261] These findings paralleled results demonstrating pronounced sympathetic hyperactivity during rapid increases in inspired desflurane concentration in humans.[262] Importantly, the actions of volatile anesthetics on baroreceptor reflex control of the circulation may be profoundly altered during autonomic dysfunction in elderly patients or in those with essential hypertension, diabetes mellitus, or heart failure.

Nitrous Oxide and Cardiovascular Function

Myocardial Contractility and Left Ventricular Diastolic Function

Experiments in papillary muscle and isolated heart preparations have consistently demonstrated that nitrous oxide produces a direct negative inotropic effect. Conflicting results about the influence of nitrous oxide on contractility have been observed in experimental animals and healthy volunteers. Several problems have contributed to the apparently contradictory results in vivo. The changes in contractile function observed may be influenced by the actions of nitrous oxide on the systemic circulation or by autonomic nervous system reflex effects because nitrous oxide may increase sympathetic nervous system tone.[263] Studies using nitrous oxide alone are difficult to perform and interpret because this gas does not produce total anesthesia at partial pressures of less than 1 atm. The effects of nitrous oxide on contractile function may be influenced by different baseline anesthetics. Finally, lack of use of load-insensitive measures of myocardial contractility has allowed only qualitative assessment of the effects of nitrous oxide on the intrinsic inotropic state in the intact heart.

The regional preload recruitable stroke work relationship demonstrated that nitrous oxide depresses myocardial contractility in dogs anesthetized with isoflurane or sufentanil in the absence of autonomic nervous system activity.[264] Seventy percent nitrous oxide decreased M_w by 28% and 41% during sufentanil and isoflurane anesthesia, respectively. These results indicated that 70% nitrous oxide decreases contractility to approximately the same extent as 1 MAC isoflurane does. Similar findings were reported with the use of LV end-systolic pressure-dimension relationships in acutely instrumented dogs. These nitrous oxide–induced myocardial depressant effects may be offset by concomitant increases in sympathetic nervous system tone. The negative inotropic actions of nitrous oxide may be more pronounced in the presence of preexisting LV dysfunction.[265] In addition, nitrous oxide–induced depression of contractile function appeared to overcome the mild sympathomimetic effect of this anesthetic gas in patients with coronary artery or valvular heart disease and LV dysfunction because increases in baseline sympathetic nervous system activity were not further augmented by nitrous oxide in these clinical conditions.

The actions of nitrous oxide on LV diastolic function have been incompletely studied. Modest increases in maximal lengthening velocity and maximal rate of decline in force were observed in ferret papillary muscle concomitant with decreases in the contractile state.[266] No changes in the rate of isometric or isotonic relaxation were observed, indicating that nitrous oxide does not substantially modify myocardial relaxation. Nitrous oxide modestly increased segmental indices of LV chamber stiffness and reduced early LV filling in acutely instrumented dogs. These findings were supported by evidence indicating that nitrous oxide may produce LV diastolic dysfunction after cardiopulmonary bypass in patients undergoing CABG surgery.[267] Nitrous oxide caused dose-related reductions in the intracellular Ca^{2+} transient in vitro.[268] This finding indicated that nitrous oxide–induced depression of myocardial contractility was related to decreases in the availability of Ca^{2+} for contractile activation. Nitrous oxide did not affect myofibrillar sensitivity to Ca^{2+} or Ca^{2+} uptake and release from the SR. In addition, the diastolic Ca^{2+} transient was unaffected by nitrous oxide, suggesting that this anesthetic gas does not alter myocardial relaxation kinetics.[266,268]

Hemodynamics

Assessment of the hemodynamic effects of nitrous oxide in humans is often complicated by concomitant administration of volatile anesthetics, opioids, or other anesthetic adjuvants in the presence or absence of cardiovascular disease. Typical clinical concentrations of nitrous oxide (e.g., 40% to 70%) caused modest increases in heart rate in healthy volunteers. Small increases in heart rate also occurred when hyperbaric concentrations of nitrous oxide were administered or when this anesthetic gas was added to volatile anesthetics. Declines in heart rate were observed with nitrous oxide in patients with coronary artery disease who were anesthetized with isoflurane. Modest reductions in heart rate have also been reported in patients anesthetized with morphine or fentanyl who were undergoing cardiac surgery. Sixty percent nitrous oxide caused small increases in arterial pressure in humans. Increases in arterial pressure also occurred under hyperbaric conditions or during volatile anesthesia in volunteers, consistent with a mild sympathomimetic effect. Other studies have also indicated that partial substitution of nitrous oxide for a volatile anesthetic either did not affect or modestly increased arterial pressure during isoflurane or desflurane anesthesia in experiments conducted at constant MAC. In contrast, reductions in arterial pressure have been observed in patients with coronary artery disease who received nitrous oxide in the presence and absence of opioids.

Small increases in cardiac output and stroke volume have been observed during the administration of 60% nitrous oxide in oxygen to volunteers, but cardiac output remained unchanged in the presence of hyperbaric nitrous oxide. Cardiac output has been shown to be greater in volunteers anesthetized with nitrous oxide and the older agent halothane than in those receiving halothane alone concomitant with increases in sympathetic nervous system tone. The addition of nitrous oxide to isoflurane or desflurane anesthesia also modestly increased cardiac output. In contrast, nitrous oxide reduced cardiac output and stroke volume in healthy volunteers and patients with cardiac disease receiving opioids. Hyperbaric nitrous oxide (1.5 MAC) caused a modest reduction in systemic vascular resistance. In contrast, systemic vascular resistance was higher during volatile anesthesia in the presence of nitrous oxide than in its absence. Pretreatment with the ganglionic blocker hexamethonium attenuated the relative increase in systemic vascular resistance observed during the administration of halothane and nitrous oxide, findings that may be consistent with a reduction in sympathetic nervous system tone. Nitrous oxide–induced increases in systemic vascular resistance have also been reported in volunteers and patients with cardiac disease who were anesthetized with opioids.

Nitrous oxide increases venous tone and decreases venous capacitance in conscious volunteers. This anesthetic gas has also been shown to modestly increase pulmonary artery pressure and pulmonary vascular resistance in patients with coronary artery disease who are anesthetized with morphine and diazepam or a volatile anesthetic. Thus, the combined effects of enhanced venous return, elevated pulmonary vascular resistance, and depressed contractile function probably contributed to the increases in central venous pressure observed with nitrous oxide in humans. Hyperbaric nitrous oxide also enhanced central venous pressure in association with increases in pulmonary vascular resistance. Nitrous oxide inhibited uptake of norepinephrine by the lung, and subsequent increases in plasma norepinephrine levels detected in the pulmonary vasculature may be partially responsible for the characteristic increases in pulmonary vascular resistance observed during administration of this agent. Nitrous oxide–induced increases in pulmonary vascular resistance may be more pronounced in adults with pulmonary hypertension and children with increased pulmonary blood flow. Increases in pulmonary artery pressure and vascular resistance have also been described during the administration of nitrous oxide to neonatal lambs. Such increases in pulmonary vascular resistance may potentially enhance right-to-left atrial or ventricular shunts and thereby compromise arterial oxygenation in patients with congenital heart disease.

Nitrous Oxide and Cardiac Electrophysiology

Reversible atrioventricular dissociation occurs in humans anesthetized with nitrous oxide and volatile or opioid-based anesthetics. The addition of nitrous oxide to halothane anesthesia lowered the threshold at which arrhythmias occur. This observation may result from a combination of stimulation of the sympathetic nervous system by nitrous oxide and myocardial sensitization by halothane. The incidence of arrhythmias was lower during combined nitrous oxide–opioid anesthesia than during halothane anesthesia alone.

Nitrous Oxide and the Coronary Circulation

Nitrous oxide did not produce direct effects on the coronary vasculature in vitro.[269] This anesthetic gas altered coronary blood flow concomitant with changes in MV_{O_2} in dogs. Nitrous oxide decreased myocardial segment shortening,[270] increased postsystolic shortening, and redistributed transmural coronary blood flow preferentially to the subepicardium (decreased endo/epi ratio) in experimental models of coronary artery disease. Nitrous oxide decreased the recovery of contractile function of canine stunned myocardium[271] and, in contrast to the findings with isoflurane, did not reduce myocardial infarct size in rats.[272] These data suggested that administration of nitrous oxide before or during transient or prolonged coronary artery occlusion and reperfusion is not associated with a cardioprotective effect. Nitrous oxide–induced sympathetic nervous system activation and imbalances in myocardial O_2 supply and MV_{O_2} are potential mechanisms for the absence of any beneficial effect during reversible or irreversible ischemic injury. In the presence of a volatile anesthetic, nitrous oxide decreased MVo_2 and myocardial O_2 extraction and may exacerbate myocardial ischemia during concomitant reductions in arterial pressure in patients with coronary artery disease. However, the addition of nitrous oxide to volatile or opioid anesthetics did not increase the incidence of new regional wall motion abnormalities as assessed by transesophageal echocardiography in this patient population.

Nitrous Oxide and Neural Control of the Circulation

Nitrous oxide caused pupillary dilation, diaphoresis, and increases in systemic vascular resistance, central blood volume, and forearm vascular resistance in volunteers during volatile anesthesia, suggesting that nitrous oxide activates the sympathetic nervous system. A subsequent study demonstrated that nitrous oxide increases sympathetic nerve traffic measured via sympathetic microneurography in human volunteers, especially during the first 15 to 30 minutes of exposure to this anesthetic gas. Baroreceptor reflex–mediated control of heart rate was impaired during the administration of nitrous oxide, but regulation of sympathetic outflow to peripheral blood vessels was preserved.[263] This finding suggested that nitrous oxide does not alter sympathetic vasoconstrictor–induced maintenance of arterial pressure, which may be partially responsible for the relative stability of hemodynamics during nitrous oxide anesthesia.

Xenon

The anesthetic properties of the noble gas xenon were first described more than 50 years ago. Xenon has a blood-gas partition coefficient less than that of nitrous oxide, does not undergo biotransformation, provides rapid induction and emergence from anesthesia,[273] and exerts analgesic effects[274] independent of α_2-adrenergic and opioid receptors.[275] Despite these advantageous properties, xenon has not been routinely used for clinical anesthesia in the United States because it is more expensive than nitrous oxide and volatile anesthetics. In recent years, more efficient manufacturing techniques and the development of low-flow administration and recycling systems have reduced the cost of xenon and rekindled interest in its clinical use. Many of these issues are succinctly summarized in two excellent reviews.[276,277]

Xenon causes minimal systemic and pulmonary hemodynamic effects in vivo,[278] preserves or very modestly reduces myocardial contractility,[279,280] and attenuates alterations in hemodynamics and increases in plasma epinephrine and cortisol concentrations associated with surgical stimulation.[281,282] Xenon did not alter cardiac function or major ion currents in isolated guinea pig hearts and ventricular myocytes.[283] Similar findings were observed in isolated human atrial myocytes.[284] Several studies have recently identified the cardiac and neural protective effects of Xe.[277] The cellular mechanisms responsible for these salutary actions were initially unclear based on data indicating that xenon does not affect the amplitudes of Na^+, L-type Ca^{2+}, and inwardly rectifying K^+ channels in whole-cell patch-clamped myocytes.[283] Xe was initially shown to produce cardioprotection when the anesthetic noble gas was administered early during reperfusion in rabbits.[285] Subsequently, pretreatment with 70% Xe before ischemia was demonstrated to reduce infarct size in rats (from 51% to 28% of the LV area at risk) by activating PKC-ε and its downstream targets p38 MAPK,[286] MAPKAPK-2,[121] and HSP-27.[121] Roles for mitochondrial K_{ATP} channels, PDK1, and ERK1/2 were also implicated in Xe preconditioning,[287,288] suggesting that prosurvival signaling may play an important role in cardioprotection by Xe. Whether Xe preserves myocardial integrity by favorably modulating proteins responsible for the regulation of apoptosis through the mPTP remains unclear. Because Xe and volatile anesthetics exert similar actions on endogenous cardioprotective signal transduction, the reductions in infarct size produced by this noble gas have been assumed to be related to its anesthetic actions.[277] However, other noble gases without anesthetic properties (e.g., helium, neon) also produce cardioprotection by activating prosurvival signaling and inhibiting the mPTP.[289]

The effects of xenon in experimental models of or patients with congestive heart failure have not been studied extensively. Systemic hemodynamics, LV systolic and diastolic function, and the determinants of LV afterload were examined in chronically instrumented dogs before and after the development of rapid LV pacing–induced cardiomyopathy.[279] Xenon was remarkably devoid of hemodynamic effects in normal and cardiomyopathic dogs anesthetized with isoflurane. Xenon did not alter isoflurane-induced reductions in the preload recruitable stroke work slope (M_w) in the presence and absence of pacing-induced LV dysfunction. Xenon caused greater increases in the time constant of isovolumic relaxation in isoflurane-anesthetized, cardiomyopathic dogs than in normal dogs, but indices of early LV filling and chamber compliance remained unchanged, which suggested that xenon does not appreciably influence LV diastolic function during isoflurane anesthesia. Xenon also produced relatively minor alterations in the determinants of LV afterload in dogs before and after pacing. Taken together, these data indicate that xenon produces very subtle cardiovascular effects during isoflurane anesthesia in dogs with and without experimental dilated cardiomyopathy.[1] Finally, 56% xenon (end-tidal concentration) depressed sympathetic and parasympathetic nervous system transmission to a greater extent than did 0.8 MAC isoflurane in healthy patients undergoing elective surgery.

Summary

Volatile anesthetics exert profound effects on the cardiovascular system by altering the inotropic, chronotropic, dromotropic, and lusitropic state of the heart. These anesthetics also have significant actions on both the preload and afterload systems. These pharmacologic effects cause dramatic changes in hemodynamics that may be accentuated in patients with underlying cardiovascular disease. Less profound but equally important effects are observed with nitrous oxide and xenon. Volatile anesthetics and xenon but not nitrous oxide are cardioprotective and directly reduce the sequelae of ischemia and reperfusion injury. The use of inhaled anesthetics requires a clear understanding of their complex cardiovascular pharmacology.

References

1. Hettrick DA, Pagel PS, Warltier DC: Desflurane, sevoflurane, and isoflurane impair canine left ventricular–arterial coupling and mechanical efficiency. Anesthesiology 85:403-413, 1996.
2. Vivien B, Hanouz J-L, Gueugniaud P-Y, et al: Myocardial effects of halothane and isoflurane in hamsters with hypertrophic cardiomyopathy. Anesthesiology 87:1406-1416, 1997.
3. Hannon JD, Cody MJ, Sun DX, et al: Effects of isoflurane and sevoflurane on intracellular calcium and contractility in pressure-overload hypertrophy. Anesthesiology 101:675-686, 2004.
4. Graham M, Qureshi A, Noueihed R, et al: Effects of halothane, isoflurane, sevoflurane and desflurane on contraction of ventricular myocytes from streptozocin-induced diabetic rats. Mol Cell Biochem 261:209-215, 2004.
5. Kersten JR, Schmeling TJ, Pagel PS, et al: Isoflurane mimics ischemic preconditioning via activation of K_{ATP} channels. Reduction of myocardial infarct size with an acute memory phase. Anesthesiology 87:361-370, 1997.
6. Pagel PS, Lowe D, Hettrick DA, et al: Isoflurane, but not halothane, improves indices of diastolic performance in dogs with rapid ventricular, pacing-induced cardiomyopathy. Anesthesiology 85:644-654, 1996.
7. An J, Rhodes SS, Jiang MT, et al: Anesthetic preconditioning enhances Ca^{2+} handling and mechanical and metabolic function elicited by Na^{+}-Ca^{2+} exchange inhibition in isolated hearts. Anesthesiology 105:541-549, 2006.
8. Vivien B, Lecarpentier Y, Riou B, et al: Halothane and isoflurane do not directly interact with cardiac cross-bridge function. Anesthesiology 102:364-370, 2005.
9. Pagel PS, Kehl F, Gare M, et al: Mechanical function of the left atrium: New insights based on analysis of pressure-volume relations and Doppler echocardiography. Anesthesiology 98:975-994, 2003.
10. Pagel PS, Hettrick DA, Kersten JR, et al: Isoflurane and halothane do not alter the enhanced afterload sensitivity of left ventricular relaxation in dogs with pacing-induced cardiomyopathy. Anesthesiology 87:952-962, 1997.
11. Heerdt PM, Pleimann BE: The dose-dependent effects of halothane on right ventricular contraction pattern and regional inotropy in swine. Anesth Analg 82:1152-1158, 1996.
12. Heerdt PM, Gandhi CD, Dickstein ML: Disparity of isoflurane effects on left and right ventricular afterload and hydraulic power generation in swine. Anesth Analg 87:511-521, 1998.
13. Hanouz JL, Massetti M, Guesne G, et al: In vitro effects of desflurane, sevoflurane, isoflurane, and halothane in isolated human right atria. Anesthesiology 92:116-124, 2000.
14. Gare M, Schwabe DA, Hettrick DA, et al: Desflurane, sevoflurane, and isoflurane affect left atrial active and passive mechanical properties and impair left atrial–left ventricular coupling in vivo. Analysis using pressure-volume relations. Anesthesiology 95:689-698, 2001.
15. Barbier P, Solomon SB, Schiller NB, et al: Left atrial relaxation and left ventricular systolic function determine left atrial reservoir function. Circulation 100:427-436, 1999.
16. Kehl F, LaDisa JF Jr, Hettrick DA, et al: Influence of isoflurane on left atrial function in dogs with pacing-induced cardiomyopathy: Evaluation with pressure-volume relations. J Cardiothorac Vasc Anesth 17:709-714, 2003.
17. Stowe DF, Marijic J, Bosnjak ZJ, et al: Direct comparative effects of halothane, enflurane, and isoflurane on oxygen supply and demand in isolated hearts. Anesthesiology 74:1087-1095, 1991.
18. Crystal GJ, Kim S-J, Czinn EA, et al: Intracoronary isoflurane causes marked vasodilation in canine hearts. Anesthesiology 74:757-765, 1991.
19. Hickey RF, Cason BA, Shubayev I: Regional vasodilating properties of isoflurane in normal swine myocardium. Anesthesiology 80:574-581, 1994.
20. Crystal GJ, Kim S-J, Salem MR, et al: Nitric oxide does not mediate coronary vasodilation by isoflurane. Anesthesiology 81:209-220, 1994.
21. Conzen PF, Habazettl H, Vollmar B, et al: Coronary microcirculation during halothane, enflurane, isoflurane, and adenosine in dogs. Anesthesiology 76:261-270, 1992.
22. Blaise G, To Q, Parent M, et al: Does halothane interfere with the release, action, or stability of endothelium-derived relaxing factor/nitric oxide? Anesthesiology 80:417-426, 1994.
23. Hart JL, Jing M, Bina S, et al: Effects of halothane on EDRF/cGMP-mediated vascular smooth muscle relaxations. Anesthesiology 79:323-331, 1993.
24. Yoshida K-I, Okabe E: Selective impairment of endothelium-dependent relaxation by sevoflurane: Oxygen free radicals participation. Anesthesiology 76:440-447, 1992.
25. Larach DR, Schuler HG: Potassium channel blockade and halothane vasodilation in conducting and resistance coronary arteries. J Pharmacol Exp Ther 267:72-81, 1993.
26. Cason BA, Shubayev I, Hickey RF: Blockade of adenosine triphosphate–sensitive potassium channels eliminates isoflurane-induced coronary artery vasodilation. Anesthesiology 81:1245-1255, 1994.
27. Crystal GJ, Gurevicius J, Salem MR, et al: Role of adenosine triphosphate–sensitive potassium channels in coronary vasodilation by halothane, isoflurane, and enflurane. Anesthesiology 86:448-458, 1997.
28. Kersten JR, Schmeling TJ, Hettrick DA, et al: Mechanism of cardioprotection by isoflurane: Role of adenosine triphosphate–regulated potassium (K_{ATP}) channels. Anesthesiology 85:794-807, 1996.
29. Pagel PS, Hettrick DA, Lowe D, et al: Desflurane and isoflurane exert modest beneficial actions on left ventricular diastolic function during myocardial ischemia in dogs. Anesthesiology 83:1021-1035, 1995.
30. Hartman JC, Kampine JP, Schmeling WT, et al: Steal-prone coronary circulation in chronically instrumented dogs: Isoflurane versus adenosine. Anesthesiology 74:744-756, 1991.
31. Hartman JC, Kampine JP, Schmeling WT, et al: Volatile anesthetics and regional myocardial perfusion in chronically instrumented dogs: Halothane versus isoflurane in a single-vessel disease model with enhanced collateral development. J Cardiothorac Anesth 4:588-603, 1990.
32. Hartman JC, Pagel PS, Kampine JP, et al: Influence of desflurane on the regional distribution of coronary blood flow in a chronically instrumented canine model of multivessel coronary artery obstruction. Anesth Analg 72:289-299, 1991.
33. Kersten JR, Brayer AP, Pagel PS, et al: Perfusion of ischemic myocardium during anesthesia with sevoflurane. Anesthesiology 81:995-1004, 1994.
34. Marijic J, Stowe DF, Turner LA, et al: Differential protective effects of halothane and isoflurane against hypoxic and reoxygenation injury in the isolated guinea pig heart. Anesthesiology 73:976-983, 1990.
35. Novalija E, Fujita S, Kampine JP, et al: Sevoflurane mimics ischemic preconditioning effects on coronary flow and nitric oxide release in isolated hearts. Anesthesiology 91:701-712, 1999.
36. Kanaya N, Fujita S: The effects of isoflurane on regional myocardial contractility and metabolism in "stunned" myocardium in acutely instrumented dogs. Anesth Analg 79:447-454, 1994.
37. Lochner A, Harper IS, Salie R, et al: Halothane protects the isolated rat myocardium against excessive total intracellular calcium and structural damage during ischemia and reperfusion. Anesth Analg 79:226-233, 1994.
38. Cason BA, Gamperl AK, Slocum RE, et al: Anesthetic-induced preconditioning. Previous administration of isoflurane decreases myocardial infarct size in rabbits. Anesthesiology 87:1182-1190, 1997.
39. Cope DK, Impastato WK, Cohen MV, et al: Volatile anesthetics protect the ischemic rabbit myocardium from infarction. Anesthesiology 86:699-709, 1997.
40. Ludwig LM, Gross GJ, Kersten JR, et al: Morphine enhances pharmacological preconditioning by isoflurane: Role of mitochondrial K_{ATP} channels and opioid receptors. Anesthesiology 98:705-711, 2003.
41. Kehl F, Krolikowski JG, Mraovic B, et al: Is isoflurane-induced preconditioning dose related? Anesthesiology 96:675-680, 2002.
42. Zaugg M, Lucchinetti E, Spahn DR, et al: Volatile anesthetics mimic cardiac preconditioning by priming the activation of mitochondrial K_{ATP} channels via multiple signaling pathways. Anesthesiology 97:4-14, 2002.
43. Tanaka K, Weihrauch D, Kehl F, et al: Mechanism of preconditioning by isoflurane in rabbits: A direct role for reactive oxygen species. Anesthesiology 97:1485-1490, 2002.
44. Toller WG, Kersten JR, Pagel PS, et al: Sevoflurane reduces myocardial infarct size and decreases the time threshold for ischemic preconditioning in dogs. Anesthesiology 91:1437-1446, 1999.
45. Riess ML, Kevin LG, Camara AK, et al: Dual exposure to sevoflurane improves anesthetic preconditioning in intact hearts. Anesthesiology 100:569-574, 2004.
46. Kevin LG, Katz P, Camara AK, et al: Anesthetic preconditioning: Effects on latency to ischemic injury in isolated hearts. Anesthesiology 99:385-391, 2003.
47. Bouwman RA, van't Hof FN, de Ruijter W, et al: The mechanism of sevoflurane-induced cardioprotection is independent of applied ischaemic stimulus in rat trabeculae. Br J Anaesth 97:307-314, 2006.
48. Sniecinski R, Liu H: Reduced efficacy of volatile anesthetic preconditioning with advanced age in isolated rat myocardium. Anesthesiology 100:589-597, 2004.
49. Riess ML, Camara AK, Rhodes SS, et al: Increasing heart size and age attenuate anesthetic preconditioning in guinea pig isolated hearts. Anesth Analg 101:1572-1576, 2005.
50. Liu H, Wang L, Eaton M, et al: Sevoflurane preconditioning limits intracellular/mitochondrial Ca^{2+} in ischemic newborn myocardium. Anesth Analg 101:349-355, 2005.

51. Kehl F, Krolikowski JG, Tessmer JP, et al: Increases in coronary collateral blood flow produced by sevoflurane are mediated by calcium-activated potassium (BK_{Ca}) channels in vivo. Anesthesiology 97:925-931, 2002.
52. de Klaver MJ, Manning L, Palmer LA, et al: Isoflurane pretreatment inhibits cytokine-induced cell death in cultured rat smooth muscle cells and human endothelial cells. Anesthesiology 97:24-32, 2002.
53. Hu G, Salem MR, Crystal GJ: Role of adenosine receptors in volatile anesthetic preconditioning against neutrophil-induced contractile dysfunction in isolated rat hearts. Anesthesiology 103:287-295, 2005.
54. Zaugg M, Lucchinetti E, Uecker M, et al: Anaesthetics and cardiac preconditioning. Part I. Signaling and cytoprotective mechanisms. Br J Anaesth 91:551-565, 2003.
55. Zaugg M, Lucchinetti E, Garcia C, et al: Anaesthetics and cardiac preconditioning. Part II. Clinical implications. Br J Anaesth 91:566-576, 2003.
56. Tanaka K, Ludwig LM, Kersten JR, et al: Mechanisms of cardioprotection by volatile anesthetics. Anesthesiology 100:707-721, 2004.
57. De Hert SG, Turani F, Mathur S, et al: Cardioprotection with volatile anesthetics: Mechanisms and clinical implications. Anesth Analg 100:1584-1593, 2005.
58. Schlack W, Preckel B, Stunneck D, et al: Effects of halothane, enflurane, isoflurane, sevoflurane and desflurane on myocardial reperfusion injury in the isolated rat heart. Br J Anaesth 81:913-919, 1998.
59. Patel HH, Ludwig LM, Fryer RM, et al: Delta opioid agonists and volatile anesthetics facilitate cardioprotection via potentiation of K_{ATP} channel opening. FASEB J 16:1468-1470, 2002.
60. Ludwig LM, Weihrauch D, Kersten JR, et al: Protein kinase C translocation and Src protein tyrosine kinase activation mediate isoflurane-induced preconditioning in vivo: Potential downstream targets of mitochondrial K_{ATP} channels and reactive oxygen species. Anesthesiology 100:532-539, 2004.
61. Zhong C, Zhou Y, Liu H: Nuclear factor κB and anesthetic preconditioning during myocardial ischemia-reperfusion. Anesthesiology 100:540-546, 2004.
62. Hausenloy DJ, Yellon DM: New directions for protecting the heart against ischaemia-reperfusion injury: Targeting the reperfusion injury salvage kinase (RISK)-pathway. Cardiovasc Res 61:448-460, 2004.
63. Inagaki N, Gonoi T, Clement JP, et al: Reconstitution of IK_{ATP}: An inward rectifier subunit plus the sulfonylurea receptor. Science 270:1166-1170, 1995.
64. Suzuki M, Sasaki N, Miki T, et al: Role of sarcolemmal K_{ATP} channels in cardioprotection against ischemia/reperfusion injury in mice. J Clin Invest 109:509-516, 2002.
65. Sato T, Sasaki N, Seharaseyon J, et al: Selective pharmacological agents implicate mitochondrial but not sarcolemmal K_{ATP} channels in ischemic cardioprotection. Circulation 101:2418-2423, 2000.
66. Dos Santos P, Kowaltowski AJ, Laclau MN, et al: Mechanisms by which opening the mitochondrial ATP-sensitive K^+ channel protects the ischemic heart. Am J Physiol Heart Circ Physiol 283:H284-H295, 2002.
67. Holmuhamedov EL, Wang L, Terzic A: ATP-sensitive K^+ channel openers prevent Ca^{2+} overload in rat cardiac mitochondria. J Physiol 519:347-360, 1999.
68. Green DR, Reed JC: Mitochondria and apoptosis. Science 281:1309-1312, 1998.
69. Gottlieb RA, Engler RL: Apoptosis in myocardial ischemia-reperfusion. Ann N Y Acad Sci 874:412-426, 1999.
70. Ozcan C, Bienengraeber M, Dzeja PP, et al: Potassium channel openers protect cardiac mitochondria by attenuating oxidant stress at reoxygenation. Am J Physiol Heart Circ Physiol 282:H531-H539, 2002.
71. Minners J, Lacerda L, McCarthy J, et al: Ischemic and pharmacological preconditioning in Girardi cells and C2C12 myotubes induce mitochondrial uncoupling. Circ Res 89:787-792, 2001.
72. Halestrap AP: The regulation of the matrix volume of mammalian mitochondria in vivo and in vitro and its role in the control of mitochondrial metabolism. Biochim Biophys Acta 973:355-382, 1989.
73. Garlid KD: Cation transport in mitochondria—the potassium cycle. Biochim Biophys Acta 1275:123-126, 1996.
74. Holmuhamedov EL, Jovanovic S, Dzeja PP, et al: Mitochondrial ATP-sensitive K^+ channels modulate cardiac mitochondrial function. Am J Physiol Heart Circ Physiol 275:H1567-H1576, 1998.
75. Costa AD, Quinlan CL, Andrukhiv A, et al: The direct physiological effects of mitochondrial K_{ATP} opening on heart mitochondria. Am J Physiol Heart Circ Physiol 290:H406-H415, 2006.
76. Sergeev P, da Silva R, Lucchinetti E, et al: Trigger-dependent gene expression profiles in cardiac preconditioning: Evidence for distinct genetic programs in ischemic and anesthetic preconditioning. Anesthesiology 100:474-488, 2004.
77. Tanaka K, Weihrauch D, Ludwig LM, et al: Mitochondrial adenosine triphosphate–regulated potassium channel opening acts as a trigger for isoflurane-induced preconditioning by generating reactive oxygen species. Anesthesiology 98:935-943, 2003.
78. Roscoe AK, Christensen JD, Lynch C 3rd: Isoflurane, but not halothane, induces protection of human myocardium via adenosine A_1 receptors and adenosine triphosphate–sensitive potassium channels. Anesthesiology 92:1692-1701, 2000.
79. Toller WG, Gross ER, Kersten JR, et al: Sarcolemmal and mitochondrial adenosine triphosphate–dependent potassium (K_{ATP}) channels. Mechanism of desflurane-induced cardioprotection. Anesthesiology 92:1731-1739, 2000.
80. Hanouz JL, Yvon A, Massetti M, et al: Mechanisms of desflurane-induced preconditioning in isolated human right atria in vitro. Anesthesiology 97:33-41, 2002.
81. Kwok WM, Martinelli AT, Fujimoto K, et al: Differential modulation of the cardiac adenosine triphosphate–sensitive potassium channel by isoflurane and halothane. Anesthesiology 97:50-56, 2002.
82. Han J, Kim E, Ho WK, et al: Effects of volatile anesthetic isoflurane on ATP-sensitive K^+ channels in rabbit ventricular myocytes. Biochem Biophys Res Commun 229:852-856, 1996.
83. Aizawa K, Turner LA, Weihrauch D, et al: Protein kinase C-ε primes the cardiac sarcolemmal adenosine triphosphate–sensitive potassium channel to modulation by isoflurane. Anesthesiology 101:381-389, 2004.
84. Turner LA, Fujimoto K, Suzuki A, et al: The interaction of isoflurane and protein kinase C–activators on sarcolemmal K_{ATP} channels. Anesth Analg 100:1680-1686, 2005.
85. An J, Stadnicka A, Kwok WM, et al: Contribution of reactive oxygen species to isoflurane-induced sensitization of cardiac sarcolemmal adenosine triphosphate–sensitive potassium channel to pinacidil. Anesthesiology 100:575-580, 2004.
86. Stadnicki A, Bosjnak ZJ: Isoflurane decreases ATP sensitivity of guinea pig cardiac sarcolemmal KATP channel at reduced intracellular pH. Anesthesiology 98:396-403, 2003.
87. Marinovic J, Bosjnak ZJ, Stadnicka A: Distinct roles of sarcolemmal and mitochondial adenosine triphosphate–sensitive potassium channels in isoflurane-induced protection against oxidative stress. Anesthesiology 105:98-104, 2006.
88. Marinovic J, Bosjnak ZJ, Stadnicka A: Preconditioning by isoflurane induces lasting sensitization of the cardiac sarcolemmal adenosine triphosphate–sensitive potassium channel by a protein kinase C-δ–mediated mechanism. Anesthesiology 103:540-547, 2005.
89. Stadnicka A, Marinovic J, Bienengraeber M, et al: Impact of in vivo preconditioning by isoflurane on adenosine triphosphate–sensitive potassium channels in the rat heart: Lasting modulation of nucleotide sensitivity during early memory period. Anesthesiology 104:503-510, 2006.
90. Bienengraeber M, Warltier DC, Bosnjak ZJ, et al: Mechanism of cardiac sarcolemmal adenosine triphosphate–sensitive potassium channel activation by isoflurane in a heterogenous expression system. Anesthesiology 105:534-540, 2006.
91. Kohro S, Hogan QH, Nakae Y, et al: Anesthetic effects on mitochondrial ATP-sensitive K channel. Anesthesiology 95:1435-1440, 2001.
92. Nakae Y, Kwok WM, Bosnjak ZJ, et al: Isoflurane activates rat mitochondrial ATP-sensitive K^+ channels reconstituted in lipid bilayers. Am J Physiol Heart Circ Physiol 284:H1865-H1871, 2003.
93. Nakae Y, Kohro S, Hogan QH, et al: Intracellular mechanism of mitochondrial adenosine triphosphate–sensitive potassium channel activation with isoflurane. Anesth Analg 97:1025-1032, 2003.
94. Gross GJ, Peart JN: K_{ATP} channels and myocardial preconditioning: An update. Am J Physiol Heart Circ Physiol 285:H921-H930, 2003.
95. Crystal GJ, Zhou X, Gurevicius J, et al: Direct coronary vasomotor effects of sevoflurane and desflurane in in situ canine hearts. Anesthesiology 92:1103-1113, 2000.
96. Piriou V, Ross S, Pigott D, et al: Beneficial effect of concomitant administration of isoflurane and nicorandil. Br J Anaesth 79:68-77, 1997.
97. Toller WG, Kersten JR, Gross ER, et al: Isoflurane preconditions myocardium against infarction via activation of inhibitory guanine (G_i) nucleotide binding proteins. Anesthesiology 92:1400-1407, 2000.
98. Kersten JR, Orth KG, Pagel PS, et al: Role of adenosine in isoflurane-induced cardioprotection. Anesthesiology 86:1128-1139, 1997.
99. Wakeno-Takahashi M, Otani H, Nakao S, et al: Adenosine and a nitric oxide donor enhances cardioprotection by preconditioning with isoflurane through mitochondrial adenosine triphosphate–sensitive K^+ channel-dependent and -independent mechanisms. Anesthesiology 100:515-524, 2004.
100. Ishizawa Y, Pidikiti R, Liebman PA, et al: G protein–coupled receptors as direct targets of inhaled anesthetics. Mol Pharmacol 61:945-952, 2002.
101. Lange M, Smul TM, Blomeyer CA, et al: Role of the β_1-adrenergic pathway in anesthetic and ischemic preconditioning against myocardial infarction in the rabbit heart in vivo. Anesthesiology 105:503-510, 2006.
102. Liu H, McPherson BC, Yao Z: Preconditioning attenuates apoptosis and necrosis: Role of protein kinase C-epsilon and -delta isoforms. Am J Physiol Heart Circ Physiol 281:H404-H410, 2001.

103. Toller WG, Montgomery MW, Pagel PS, et al: Isoflurane-enhanced recovery of canine stunned myocardium: Role for protein kinase C? Anesthesiology 91:713-722, 1999.
104. Fujimoto K, Bosnjak ZJ, Kwok WM: Isoflurane-induced facilitation of the cardiac sarcolemmal K_{ATP} channel. Anesthesiology 97:57-65, 2002.
105. Light PE, Bladen C, Winkfein RJ, et al: Molecular basis of protein kinase C–induced activation of ATP-sensitive potassium channels. Proc Natl Acad Sci U S A 97:9058-9063, 2000.
106. Uecker M, Da Silva R, Grampp T, et al: Translocation of protein kinase C isoforms to subcellular targets in ischemic and anesthetic preconditioning. Anesthesiology 99:138-147, 2003.
107. Novalija E, Kevin LG, Camara AK, et al: Reactive oxygen species precede the epsilon isoform of protein kinase C in the anesthetic preconditioning signaling cascade. Anesthesiology 99:421-428, 2003.
108. Obal D, Weber NC, Zacharowski K, et al: Role of protein kinase C-ε in isoflurane-induced cardioprotection. Br J Anaesth 94:166-173, 2005.
109. Toma O, Weber NC, Wolter JI, et al: Desflurane preconditioning induces time-dependent activation of protein kinase C epsilon and extracellular-signal regulated kinase 1 and 2 in the rat heart in vivo. Anesthesiology 101:1372-1380, 2004.
110. Bouwman RA, Musters RJ, van Beek-Harmsen BJ, et al: Reactive oxygen species precede protein kinase C-δ activation independent of adenosine triphosphate–sensitive mitochondrial channel opening in sevoflurane-induced cardioprotection. Anesthesiology 100:506-514, 2004.
111. Baines CP, Wang L, Cohen MV, et al: Protein tyrosine kinase is downstream of protein kinase C for ischemic preconditioning's anti-infarct effect in the rabbit heart. J Mol Cell Cardiol 30:383-392, 1998.
112. Ping P, Zhang J, Cao X, et al: PKC-dependent activation of p44/p42 MAPKs during myocardial ischemia-reperfusion in conscious rabbits. Am J Physiol 276:H1468-H1481, 1999.
113. Ebel D, Mullenheim J, Sudkamp H, et al: Role of tyrosine kinase in desflurane-induced preconditioning. Anesthesiology 100:555-561, 2004.
114. Wang C, Weihrauch D, Schwabe DA, et al: Extracellular signal–regulated kinases trigger isoflurane preconditioning concomitant with upregulation of hypoxia-inducible factor-1α and vascular endothelial growth factor in rats. Anesth Analg 103:281-288, 2006.
115. Bilton RL, Booker GW: The subtle side to hypoxia inducible factor (HIFα) regulation. Eur J Biochem 270:791-798, 2003.
116. Liu Y, Cox SR, Morita T, et al: Hypoxia regulates vascular endothelial growth factor gene expression in endothelial cells. Identification of a 5′ enhancer. Circ Res 77:638-643, 1995.
117. Matsunaga T, Warltier DC, Weihrauch D, et al: Ischemia-induced coronary collateral growth is dependent on vascular endothelial growth factor and nitric oxide. Circulation 102:3098-3103, 2000.
118. Kim CH, Cho YS, Chun YS, et al: Early expression of myocardial HIF-1α in response to mechanical stresses: Regulation by stretch-activated channels and the phosphatidylinositol-3-kinase signaling pathway. Circ Res 90:E25-E33, 2002.
119. Maulik N, Das DK: Potentiation of angiogenic response by ischemia and hypoxic preconditioning of the heart. J Cell Mol Med 6:13-24, 2002.
120. da Silva R, Grampp T, Pasch T, et al: Differential activation of mitogen-activated protein kinases in ischemic and anesthetic preconditioning. Anesthesiology 100:59-69, 2004.
121. Weber NC, Toma O, Wolter JI, et al: Mechanisms of xenon- and isoflurane-induced preconditioning. A potential link to the cytoskeleton via the MAPKAPK-2/HSP27 pathway. Br J Pharmacol 146:445-455, 2005.
122. Costa AD, Garlid KD, West IC, et al: Protein kinase G transmits the cardioprotection signal from cytosol to mitochondria. Circ Res 97:329-336, 2005.
123. Cantley LC: The phosphoinositide 3-kinase pathway. Science 296:1655-1657, 2002.
124. Raphael J, Rivo J, Gozal Y: Isoflurane-induced myocardial preconditioning is dependent on phosphatidylinositol-3-kinase/Akt signaling. Br J Anaesth 95:756-763, 2005.
125. Raphael J, Abedat S, Rivo J, et al: Volatile anesthetic preconditioning attenuates myocardial apoptosis in rabbits after regional ischemia and reperfusion via Akt signaling and modulation of Bcl-2 family proteins. J Pharmacol Exp Ther 318:186-194, 2006.
126. Jamnicki-Abegg M, Weihrauch D, Pagel PS, et al: Isoflurane inhibits cardiac myocyte apoptosis during oxidative and inflammatory stress by activating Akt and enhancing Bcl-2 expression. Anesthesiology 103:1006-1014, 2005.
127. Hausenloy DJ, Maddock HL, Baxter GF, et al: Inhibiting mitochondrial permeability transition pore opening: A new paradigm for myocardial preconditioning? Cardiovasc Res 55:534-543, 2002.
128. Griffiths EJ, Halestrap AP: Mitochondrial non-specific pores remain closed during cardiac ischemia but open upon reperfusion. Biochem J 307:93-98, 1995.
129. Rajesh KG, Sasaguri S, Zhitian Z, et al: Second window of ischemic preconditioning regulates mitochondrial permeability transition pore by enhancing Bcl-2 expression. Cardiovasc Res 59:297-307, 2003.
130. Piriou V, Chiari P, Gateau-Roesch O, et al: Desflurane-induced preconditioning alters calcium-induced mitochondrial permeability transition. Anesthesiology 100:581-588, 2004.
131. Ljubkovic M, Mio Y, Marinovic J, et al: Isoflurane preconditioning uncouples mitochondria and protects against hypoxia-reoxygenation. Am J Physiol Cell Physiol 292:C1583-C1590, 2007.
132. Bolli R, Marban E: Molecular and cellular mechanisms of myocardial stunning. Physiol Rev 79:609-634, 1999.
133. Glantz L, Ginosar Y, Chevion M, et al: Halothane prevents postischemic production of hydroxyl radicals in the canine heart. Anesthesiology 86:440-447, 1997.
134. Novalija E, Varadarajan SG, Camara AK, et al: Anesthetic preconditioning: Triggering role of reactive oxygen and nitrogen species in isolated hearts. Am J Physiol Heart Circ Physiol 283:H44-H52, 2002.
135. Tritto I, D'Andrea D, Eramo N, et al: Oxygen radicals can induce preconditioning in rabbit hearts. Circ Res 80:743-748, 1997.
136. Baines CP, Goto M, Downey JM: Oxygen radicals released during ischemic preconditioning contribute to cardioprotection in the rabbit myocardium. J Mol Cell Cardiol 29:207-216, 1997.
137. Smul TM, Lange M, Redel A, et al: Desflurane-induced preconditioning against myocardial infarction is mediated by nitric oxide. Anesthesiology 105:719-725, 2006.
138. Mullenheim J, Ebel D, Frassdorf J, et al: Isoflurane preconditions myocardium against infarction via release of free radicals. Anesthesiology 96:934-940, 2002.
139. Pain T, Yang XM, Critz SD, et al: Opening of mitochondrial K_{ATP} channels triggers the preconditioned state by generating free radicals. Circ Res 87:460-466, 2000.
140. Kulisz A, Chen N, Chandel NS, et al: Mitochondrial ROS initiate phosphorylation of p38 MAP kinase during hypoxia in cardiomyocytes. Am J Physiol Lung Cell Mol Physiol 282:L1324-L1329, 2002.
141. Nishida M, Maruyama Y, Tanaka R, et al: G alpha(i) and G alpha(o) are target proteins of reactive oxygen species. Nature 408:492-495, 2000.
142. Carroll R, Gant VA, Yellon DM: Mitochondrial K_{ATP} channel opening protects a human atrial-derived cell line by a mechanism involving free radical generation. Cardiovasc Res 51:691-700, 2001.
143. McPherson BC, Yao Z: Morphine mimics preconditioning via free radical signals and mitochondrial K_{ATP} channels in myocytes. Circulation 103:290-295, 2001.
144. Andrukhiv A, Costa AD, West IC, et al: Opening mitoK_{ATP} increases superoxide generation from complex I of the electron transport chain. Am J Physiol Heart Circ Physiol 291:H2067-H2074, 2006.
145. Zhang DX, Chen YF, Campbell WB, et al: Characteristics and superoxide-induced activation of reconstituted myocardial mitochondrial ATP-sensitive potassium channels. Circ Res 89:1177-1183, 2001.
146. Lebuffe G, Schumacker PT, Shao ZH, et al: ROS and NO trigger early preconditioning: Relationship to mitochondrial K_{ATP} channel. Am J Physiol Heart Circ Physiol 284:H299-H308, 2003.
147. Gross GJ, Fryer RM: Mitochondrial K_{ATP} channels: Triggers or distal effectors of ischemic or pharmacological preconditioning? Circ Res 87:431-433, 2000.
148. Kevin LG, Novalija E, Riess M, et al: Sevoflurane exposure generates superoxide but leads to decreased superoxide during ischemia and reperfusion in isolated hearts. Anesth Analg 96:949-955, 2003.
149. Zorov DB, Filburn CR, Klotz LO, et al: Reactive oxygen species (ROS)-induced ROS release: A new phenomenon accompanying induction of the mitochondrial permeability transition in cardiac myocytes. J Exp Med 192:1001-1014, 2000.
150. Zorov DB, Juhaszova M, Sollott SJ: Mitochondrial ROS-induced ROS release: An update and review. Biochim Biophys Acta 1757:509-517, 2006.
151. Kim JS, Jin Y, Lemasters JJ: Reactive oxygen species, but not Ca^{2+} overloading, trigger pH- and mitochondrial permeability transition–dependent death of adult rat myocytes after ischemia-reperfusion. Am J Physiol Heart Circ Physiol 290:H2024-H2034, 2006.
152. Vanden Hoek TL, Becker LB, Shao Z, et al: Reactive oxygen species released from mitochondria during brief hypoxia induce preconditioning in cardiomyocytes. J Biol Chem 273:18092-18098, 1998.
153. Yao Z, Tong J, Tan X, et al: Role of reactive oxygen species in acetylcholine-induced preconditioning in cardiomyocytes. Am J Physiol Heart Circ Physiol 277:H2504-H2509, 1999.
154. Hanley PJ, Ray J, Brandt U, et al: Halothane, isoflurane, and sevoflurane inhibit NADH:ubiquinone oxidoreductase (complex I) of cardiac mitochondria. J Physiol 544:687-693, 2002.
155. Riess ML, Eells JT, Kevin KG, et al: Attenuation of mitochondrial respiration by sevoflurane in isolated cardiac mitochondria is mediated in part by reactive oxygen species. Anesthesiology 100:498-505, 2004.
156. Riess ML, Kevin LG, McCormick J, et al: Anesthetic preconditioning: The role of free radicals in sevoflurane-induced attenuation of mitochondrial electron

transport in Guinea pig isolated hearts. Anesth Analg 100:46-53, 2005.
157. Ludwig LM, Tanaka K, Eells JT, et al: Isoflurane-induced preconditioning is mediated by reactive oxygen species generated from mitochondrial electron transport chain complex III. Anesth Analg 99:1308-1315, 2004.
158. Alcindor D, Krolikowski JG, Pagel PS, et al: Cyclooxygenase-2 mediates ischemic, anesthetic, and pharmacologic preconditioning in vivo. Anesthesiology 100:547-554, 2004.
159. Aikawa R, Komuro I, Yamazaki T, et al: Oxidative stress activates extracellular signal–regulated kinases through Src and Ras in cultured cardiac myocytes of neonatal rats. J Clin Invest 100:1813-1821, 1997.
160. Nishida M, Schey KL, Takagahara S, et al: Activation mechanism of G_i and G_o by reactive oxygen species. J Biol Chem 277:9036-9042, 2002.
161. Liu Y, Gutterman DD: Oxidative stress and potassium channel function. Clin Exp Pharmacol Physiol 29:305-311, 2002.
162. Bolli R: The late phase of preconditioning. Circ Res 87:972-983, 2000.
163. Banerjee S, Tang XL, Qiu Y, et al: Nitroglycerin induced late preconditioning against myocardial stunning via a PKC-dependent pathway. Am J Physiol Heart Circ Physiol 277:H2488-H2494, 1999.
164. Dawn B, Takano H, Tang XL, et al: Role of Src protein tyrosine kinases in late preconditioning against myocardial infarction. Am J Physiol Heart Circ Physiol 283:H549-H556, 2002.
165. Shinmura K, Tang XL, Wang Y, et al: Cyclooxygenase-2 mediates the cardioprotective effects of the late phase of ischemic preconditioning in conscious rabbits. Proc Natl Acad Sci U S A 97:10197-10202, 2000.
166. Takano H, Manchikalapudi S, Tang XL, et al: Nitric oxide synthase is the mediator of late preconditioning against myocardial infarction in conscious rabbits. Circulation 98:441-449, 1998.
167. Xuan YT, Tang XL, Banerjee S, et al: Nuclear factor-κB plays an essential role in the late phase of ischemic preconditioning in conscious rabbits. Circ Res 84:1095-1109, 1999.
168. Tonkovic-Capin M, Gross GJ, Bosnjak ZJ, et al: Delayed cardioprotection by isoflurane: Role of K_{ATP} channels. Am J Physiol Heart Circ Physiol 283:H61-H68, 2002.
169. Masui K, Kashimoto S, Furuya A, et al: Isoflurane and sevoflurane during reperfusion prevent recovery from ischaemia in mitochondrial K_{ATP} channel blocker pretreated hearts. Eur J Anaesthesiol 23:123-129, 2006.
170. Lutz M, Liu H: Inhaled sevoflurane produces better delayed myocardial protection at 48 versus 24 hours after exposure. Anesth Analg 102:984-990, 2006.
171. Mullenheim J, Ebel D, Bauer M, et al: Sevoflurane confers additional cardioprotection after ischemic late preconditioning in rabbits. Anesthesiology 99:624-631, 2003.
172. Kehl F, Pagel PS, Krolikowski JG, et al: Isoflurane does not produce a second window of preconditioning against myocardial infarction in vivo. Anesth Analg 95:1162-1168, 2002.
173. Chiari PC, Pagel PS, Tanaka K, et al: Intravenous emulsified halogenated anesthetics produced acute and delayed preconditioning against myocardial infarction in rabbits. Anesthesiology 101:1160-1166, 2004.
174. Lucchinetti E, Aguirre J, Feng J, et al: Molecular evidence of late preconditioning after sevoflurane inhalation in healthy volunteers. Anesth Analg 105:629-640, 2007.
175. Tanaka K, Ludwig LM, Krolikowski JG, et al: Isoflurane produced delayed preconditioning against myocardial ischemia and reperfusion injury: role of cyclooxygenase-2. Anesthesiology 100:525-531, 2004.
176. Shinmura K, Xuan YT, Tang XL, et al: Inducible nitric oxide synthase modulates cyclooxygenase-2 activity in the heart of conscious rabbits during the late phase of ischemic preconditioning. Circ Res 90:602-608, 2002.
177. Bolli R, Manchikalapudi S, Tang XL, et al: The protective effect of late preconditioning against myocardial stunning in conscious rabbits is mediated by nitric oxide synthase: Evidence that nitric oxide acts both as a trigger and as a mediator of the late phase of ischemic preconditioning. Circ Res 81:1094-1107, 1997.
178. Wang Y, Kodani E, Wang J, et al: Cardioprotection during the final stage of the late phase of ischemic preconditioning is mediated by neuronal NOS in concert with cyclooxygenase-2. Circ Res 95:84-91, 2004.
179. Chiari PC, Bienengraeber MW, Weihrauch D, et al: Role of endothelial nitric oxide synthase as a trigger and mediator of isoflurane-induced delayed preconditioning in rabbit myocardium. Anesthesiology 103:74-83, 2005.
180. Wakeno-Takahashi M, Otani H, Nakao S, et al: Isoflurane induces second window of preconditioning through upregulation of inducible nitric oxide synthase in rat heart. Am J Physiol Heart Circ Physiol 289:H2585-H2591, 2005.
181. Wang C, Chiari PC, Weihrauch D, et al: Gender-specificity of delayed preconditioning by isoflurane in rabbits: potential role of endothelial nitric oxide synthase. Anesth Analg 103:274-280, 2006.
182. Shi Y, Hutchins WC, Su J, et al: Delayed cardioprotection with isoflurane: Role of reactive oxygen and nitrogen. Am J Physiol Heart Circ Physiol 288:H175-H184, 2005.
183. Patel HH, Fryer RM, Gross ER, et al: 12-Lipoxygenase in opioid-induced delayed cardioprotection: Gene array, mass spectrometric, and pharmacological analyses. Circ Res 92:676-682, 2003.
184. Tsutsumi YM, Patel HH, Huang D, et al: Role of 12-lipoxygenase in volatile anesthetic–induced delayed preconditioning in mice. Am J Physiol Heart Circ Physiol 291:H979-H983, 2006.
185. Vinten-Johansen J: Involvement of neutrophils in the pathogenesis of lethal myocardial reperfusion injury. Cardiovasc Res 61:481-497, 2004.
186. Sato H, Jordan JE, Zhao ZQ, et al: Gradual reperfusion reduces infarct size and endothelial injury but augments neutrophil accumulation. Ann Thorac Surg 64:1099-1107, 1997.
187. Vinten-Johansen J, Lefer DJ, Nakanishi K, et al: Controlled coronary hydrodynamics at the time of reperfusion reduces postischemic injury. Coron Artery Dis 3:1081-1093, 1992.
188. Kin H, Zhao ZQ, Sun HY, et al: Postconditioning attenuates myocardial ischemia-reperfusion injury by inhibiting events in the early minutes of reperfusion. Cardiovasc Res 62:74-85, 2004.
189. Zhao ZQ, Corvera JS, Halkos ME, et al: Inhibition of myocardial injury by ischemic postconditioning during reperfusion: Comparison with ischemic preconditioning. Am J Physiol Heart Circ Physiol 285:H579-H588, 2003.
190. Yang XM, Proctor JB, Cui L, et al: Multiple, brief coronary occlusions during early reperfusion protect rabbit hearts by targeting cell signaling pathways. J Am Coll Cardiol 44:1103-1110, 2004.
191. Tsang A, Hausenloy DJ, Mocanu MM, et al: Post-conditioning: A form of "modified reperfusion" protects myocardium by activating the PI3K-Akt pathway. Circ Res 95:230-232, 2004.
192. Juhaszova M, Zorov DB, Kim SH, et al: Glycogen sythase kinase-3b mediates convergence of protection signaling to inhibit the mitochondrial permeability transition pore. J Clin Invest 113:1535-1549, 2004.
193. Gateau-Roesch O, Argaud L, Ovize M: Mitochondrial permeability transition pore and postconditioning. Cardiovasc Res 70:264-273, 2006.
194. Staat P, Rioufol G, Piot C, et al: Postconditioning the human heart. Circulation 112:2143-2148, 2005.
195. Hausenloy D, Yellon D: Survival kinases in ischemic preconditioning and postconditioning. Cardiovasc Res 70:240-253, 2006.
196. Siegmund B, Schlack W, Ladilov YV, et al: Halothane protects cardiomyocytes against reoxygenation-induced hypercontracture. Circulation 96:4372-4379, 1997.
197. Schlack W, Preckel B, Barthel H, et al: Halothane reduces reperfusion injury after regional ischaemia in the rabbit heart in vivo. Br J Anaesth 79:88-96, 1997.
198. Preckel B, Schlack W, Comfere T, et al: Effects of enflurane, isoflurane, sevoflurane and desflurane on reperfusion injury after regional myocardial ischaemia in the rabbit heart in vivo. Br J Anaesth 81:905-912, 1998.
199. Obal D, Preckel B, Scharbatke H, et al: One MAC of sevoflurane provides protection against reperfusion injury in the rat heart in vivo. Br J Anaesth 87:905-911, 2001.
200. Varadarajan SG, An J, Novalija E, et al: Sevoflurane before or after ischemia improves contractile and metabolic function while reducing myoplasmic Ca^{2+} loading in intact hearts. Anesthesiology 96:125-133, 2002.
201. Heindl B, Reichle FM, Zahler S, et al: Sevoflurane and isoflurane protect the reperfused guinea pig heart by reducing postischemic adhesion of polymorphonuclear neutrophils. Anesthesiology 91:521-530, 1999.
202. Lucchinetti E, da Silva R, Pasch T, et al: Anaesthetic preconditioning but not postconditioning prevents early activation of the deleterious cardiac remodelling programme: Evidence of opposing genomic responses in cardioprotection by pre- and postconditioning. Br J Anaesth 95:140-152, 2005.
203. Chiari PC, Bienengraeber MW, Pagel PS, et al: Isoflurane protects against myocardial infarction during early reperfusion by activation of phosphatidylinositol-3-kinase signal transduction: Evidence for anesthetic-induced postconditioning in rabbits. Anesthesiology 102:102-109, 2005.
204. Feng J, Fischer G, Lucchinetti E, et al: Infarct-remodeled myocardium is receptive to protection by isoflurane postconditioning. Role of protein kinase B/Akt signaling. Anesthesiology 104:1004-1014, 2006.
205. Eefting F, Rensing B, Wigman J, et al: Role of apoptosis in reperfusion injury. Cardiovasc Res 61:414-426, 2004.
206. Weihrauch D, Krolikowski JG, Bienengraeber M, et al: Morphine enhances isoflurane-induced postconditioning against myocardial infarction: The role of phosphatidylinositol-3-kinase and opioid receptors in rabbits. Anesth Analg 101:942-949, 2005.
207. Zaugg M, Jamali NZ, Lucchinetti E, et al: Norepinephrine-induced apoptosis is inhibited in adult rat ventricular myocytes exposed to volatile anesthetics. Anesthesiology 93:209-218, 2000.
208. Gross ER, Hsu AK, Gross GJ: Opioid-induced cardioprotection occurs via glycogen synthase kinase β inhibition during reperfusion in intact rat hearts. Circ Res 94:960-966, 2004.

209. Darling CE, Jiang R, Maynard M, et al: Postconditioning via stuttering reperfusion limits myocardial infarct size in rabbit hearts: Role of ERK1/2. Am J Physiol Heart Circ Physiol 289:H1618-H1626, 2005.
210. Yang XM, Krieg T, Cui L, et al: NECA and bradykinin at reperfusion reduce infarction in rabbit hearts by signaling through PI3K, ERK, and NO. J Mol Cell Cardiol 36:411-421, 2004.
211. Krolikowski JG, Weihrauch D, Bienengraeber M, et al: Role of Erk1/2, p70s6K, and eNOS in isoflurane-induced cardioprotection during early reperfusion in vivo. Can J Anesth 53:174-182, 2006.
212. Feng J, Lucchinetti E, Ahuja P, et al: Isoflurane postconditioning prevents opening of the mitochondrial permeability transition pore through inhibition of glycogen synthase kinase 3β. Anesthesiology 103:987-995, 2005.
213. Tessier-Vetzel D, Tissier R, Waintraub X, et al: Isoflurane inhaled at the onset of reperfusion potentiates the cardioprotective effect of ischemic postconditioning through a NO-dependent mechanism. J Cardiovasc Pharmacol 47:487-492, 2006.
214. Argaud L, Gateau-Roesch O, Raisky O, et al: Postconditioning inhibits mitochondrial permeability transition. Circulation 111:194-197, 2005.
215. Krolikowski JG, Bienengraeber M, Weihrauch D, et al: Inhibition of mitochondrial permeability transition enhances isoflurane-induced cardioprotection during early reperfusion: Role of mitochondrial K_{ATP} channels. Anesth Analg 101:1590-1596, 2005.
216. Korge P, Honda HM, Weiss JN: K^+ dependent regulation of matrix volume improves mitochondrial function under conditions mimicking ischemia-reperfusion. Am J Physiol Heart Circ Physiol 289:H66-H77, 2005.
217. Obal D, Dettwiler S, Favoccia C, et al: The influence of mitochondrial K_{ATP}-channels in the cardioprotection of preconditioning and postconditioning by sevoflurane in the rat in vivo. Anesth Analg 101:1252-1260, 2005.
218. Tong H, Imahashi K, Steenbergen C, et al: Phosphorylation of glycogen synthase kinase-3β during preconditioning through phosphatidylinositol-3-kinase–dependent pathway is cardioprotective. Circ Res 90:377-379, 2002.
219. Pagel PS, Krolikowski JG, Neff DA, et al: Inhibition of glycogen synthase kinase potentiates isoflurane-induced protection against myocardial infarction during early reperfusion in vivo. Anesth Analg 102:1348-1354, 2006.
220. Zha J, Harada H, Yang E, et al: Serine phosphorylation of death agonist BAD in response to survival factor results in binding to 14-3-3 not BCL-X(L). Cell 87:619-628, 1996.
221. Tsuruta F, Masuyama N, Gotoh Y: The phosphatidylinositol 3-kinase (PI3K)-Akt pathway suppresses Bax translocation to mitochondria. J Biol Chem 277:14040-14047, 2002.
222. Cardone MH, Roy N, Stennicke HR, et al: Regulation of cell death protease caspase-9 by phosphorylation. Science 282:1318-1321, 1998.
223. Watcharasti P, Bijur GN, Song L, et al: Glycogen synthase kinase-3β (GSK3β) binds to and promotes the actions of p53. J Biol Chem 278:48872-48879, 2003.
224. Hoshi M, Sato M, Kondo S, et al: Different localization of tau protein kinase I/glycogen synthase kinase-3β from glycogen synthase kinase-3α in cerebellum mitochondria. J Biochem (Tokyo) 118:683-685, 1995.
225. Chipuk JE, Kuwana T, Bouchier-Hayes L, et al: Direct activation of Bax by p53 mediates mitochondrial membrane permeabilization and apoptosis. Science 303:1010-1014, 2004.
226. Vousden KH: Activation of the p53 tumor suppressor protein. Biochem Biophys Acta 1602:47-59, 2002.
227. Vousden KH, Lu X: Live or let die: The cell's response to p53. Nat Rev Cancer 2:594-604, 2002.
228. Maulik N, Sasaki N, Addya S, et al: Regulation of cardiomyocyte apoptosis by redox-sensitive transcription factors. FEBS Lett 485:7-12, 2000.
229. Tomasevic G, Shamloo M, Israeli D, et al: Activation of p53 and its target genes p21WAF1/Cip1 and PAG608/Wig-1 in ischemic preconditioning. Brain Res Mol Brain Res 70:304-313, 1999.
230. Mocanu MM, Yellon DM: p53 down-regulation: A new molecular mechanism involved in ischaemic preconditioning. FEBS Lett 555:302-306, 2003.
231. Ogawara Y, Kishishita S, Obata T, et al: Akt enhances Mdm2-mediated ubiquitination and degradation of p53. J Biol Chem 277:21843-21850, 2002.
232. Culmsee C, Zhu X, Yu Q-S, et al: A synthetic inhibitor of p53 protects neurons against death induced by ischemic and excitotoxic insults, and amyloid β-peptide. J Neurochem 77:220-228, 2001.
233. Matsusaka H, Ide T, Matsushima S, et al: Targeted deletion of p53 prevents cardiac rupture after myocardial infarction in mice. Cardiovasc Res 70:457-465, 2006.
234. Venkatapuram S, Wang C, Krolikowski JG, et al: Inhibition of apoptotic protein p53 lowers the threshold of isoflurane-induced cardioprotection during early reperfusion in rabbits. Anesth Analg 103:1400-1405, 2006.
235. Fischer U, Schulze-Osthoff K: New approaches and therapeutics targeting apoptosis in disease. Pharmacol Rev 57:187-215, 2005.
236. Chen Z, Chua CC, Ho YS, et al: Overexpression of Bcl-2 attenuates apoptosis and protects against myocardial I/R injury in transgenic mice. Am J Physiol Heart Circ Physiol 280:H2313-H2320, 2001.
237. Wang C, Neff DA, Krolikowski JG, et al: The influence of B-cell lymphoma 2 protein, an antiapoptotic regulator of mitochondrial permeability transition, on isoflurane-induced and ischemic postconditioning in rabbits. Anesth Analg 102:1355-1360, 2006.
238. Adams JM, Cory S: The Bcl-2 protein family: Arbiters of cell survival. Science 281:1322-1326, 1998.
239. Reiz S: Nitrous oxide augments the systemic and coronary haemodynamic effects of isoflurane in patients with ischaemic heart disease. Acta Anaesthesiol Scand 27:464-469, 1983.
240. Tuman KJ, McCarthy RJ, Spiess BD, et al: Does choice of anesthetic agent significantly affect outcome after coronary artery surgery? Anesthesiology 70:189-198, 1989.
241. Slogoff S, Keats AS: Randomized trial of primary anesthetic agents on outcome of coronary artery bypass operations. Anesthesiology 70:179-188, 1989.
242. Mangano DT, Layug EL, Wallace A, et al: Effect of atenolol on mortality and cardiovascular morbidity after noncardiac surgery. Multicenter Study of Perioperative Ischemia Group. N Engl J Med 335:1713-1720, 1996.
243. Helman JD, Leung JM, Bellows WH, et al: The risk of myocardial ischemia in patients receiving desflurane versus sufentanil anesthesia for coronary artery bypass graft surgery. The S.P.I Research Group. Anesthesiology 77:47-62, 1992.
244. Buffington CW, Davis KB, Gillispie S, et al: The prevalance of steal-prone coronary anatomy in patients with coronary artery disease: An analysis of the Coronary Artery Surgery Study Registry. Anesthesiology 69:721-727, 1988.
245. Slogoff S, Keats AS, Dear WE, et al: Steal-prone coronary anatomy and myocardial ischemia associated with four primary anesthetic agents in humans. Anesth Analg 72:22-27, 1991.
246. Belhomme D, Peynet J, Louzy M, et al: Evidence for preconditioning by isoflurane in coronary artery bypass graft surgery. Circulation 100:II340-II344, 1999.
247. Penta de Peppo A, Polisca P, Tomai F, et al: Recovery of LV contractility in man is enhanced by preischemic administration of enflurane. Ann Thorac Surg 68:112-118, 1999.
248. De Hert SG, ten Broecke PW, Mertens E, et al: Sevoflurane but not propofol preserves myocardial function in coronary surgery patients. Anesthesiology 97:42-49, 2002.
249. Cromheecke S, Pepermans V, Hendrickx E, et al: Cardioprotective properties of sevoflurane in patients undergoing aortic valve replacement with cardiopulmonary bypass. Anesth Analg 103:289-296, 2006.
250. De Hert SG, Cromheecke S, ten Broecke PW, et al: Effects of propofol, desflurane, and sevoflurane on recovery of myocardial function after coronary artery surgery in elderly high-risk patients. Anesthesiology 99:314-323, 2003.
251. De Hert SG, Van der Linden PJ, Cromheecke S, et al: Cardioprotective properties of sevoflurane in patients undergoing coronary surgery with cardiopulmonary bypass are related to the modalities of its administration. Anesthesiology 101:299-310, 2004.
252. Cromheecke S, ten Broecke PW, Hendrickx E, et al: Incidence of atrial fibrillation early after cardiac surgery: Can choice of the anesthetic regimen influence the incidence? Acta Anaesthesiol Belg 56:147-154, 2005.
253. Julier K, da Silva R, Garcia C, et al: Preconditioning by sevoflurane decreases biochemical markers for myocardial and renal dysfunction in coronary artery bypass graft surgery: A double-blinded, placebo-controlled multicenter study. Anesthesiology 98:1315-1327, 2003.
254. Lorsomradee S, Cromheecke S, Lorsomradee S, et al: Effects of sevoflurane on biochemical markers of hepatic and renal dysfunction after coronary artery surgery. J Cardiothorac Vasc Anesth 20:684-690, 2006.
255. Garcia C, Julier K, Bestmann L, et al: Preconditioning with sevoflurane decreases PECAM-1 expression and improves one-year cardiovascular outcome in coronary artery bypass graft surgery. Br J Anaesth 94:159-165, 2005.
256. Lucchinetti E, Ambrosio S, Aguirre J, et al: Sevoflurane inhalation at sedative concentrations provides endothelial protection against ischemia-reperfusion injury in humans. Anesthesiology 106:262-268, 2007.
257. Lucchinetti E, Hofer C, Bestmann L, et al: Gene regulatory control of myocardial energy metabolism predicts postoperative cardiac function in patients undergoing off-pump coronary artery bypass graft surgery: Inhalational versus intravenous anesthetics. Anesthesiology 106:444-457, 2007.
258. Guarracino F, Landoni G, Tritapepe L, et al: Myocardial damage prevented by volatile anesthetics: A multicenter randomized controlled study. J Cardiothorac Vasc Anesth 20:477-483, 2006.
259. Yu CH, Beattie WS: The effects of volatile anesthetics on cardiac ischemic complications and mortality in CABG: A meta-analysis. Can J Anesth 53:906-918, 2006.
260. Ebert TJ, Seagard JL, Hopp FA Jr: Autonomic nervous system: Measurement and response under anesthesia. *In* Yaksh TL, Lynch C III, Zapol WM, et al (eds): Anesthesia: Biologic Foundations. Philadelphia, Lippincott-Raven, 1998, pp 1233-1255.

261. Ebert TJ, Muzi M, Lopatka CW: Neurocirculatory responses to sevoflurane in humans: A comparison to desflurane. Anesthesiology 83:88-95, 1995.
262. Weiskopf RB, Moore MA, Eger II EI, et al: Rapid increase in desflurane concentration is associated with greater transient cardiovascular stimulation than rapid increase in isoflurane concentration in humans. Anesthesiology 80:1035-1045, 1994.
263. Ebert TJ: Differential effects of nitrous oxide on baroreflex control of heart rate and peripheral sympathetic nerve activity in humans. Anesthesiology 72:16-22, 1990.
264. Pagel PS, Kampine JP, Schmeling WT, et al: Effects of nitrous oxide on myocardial contractility as evaluated by the preload recruitable stroke work relationship in chronically instrumented dogs. Anesthesiology 73:1148-1157, 1990.
265. Messina AG, Yao F-S, Canning H, et al: The effect of nitrous oxide on left ventricular pump performance and contractility in patients with coronary artery disease: Effect of preoperative ejection fraction. Anesth Analg 77:954-962, 1993.
266. Carton EG, Wanek LA, Housmans PR: Effects of nitrous oxide on contractility, relaxation and the intracellular calcium transient of isolated mammalian ventricular myocardium. J Pharmacol Exp Ther 257:843-849, 1991.
267. Houltz E, Caidahl K, Hellstrom A, et al: The effects of nitrous oxide on left ventricular systolic and diastolic performance before and after cardiopulmonary bypass: Evaluation by computer-assisted two-dimensional and Doppler echocardiography in patients undergoing coronary artery surgery. Anesth Analg 81:243-248, 1995.
268. Carton EG, Housmans PR: Role of transsarcolemmal Ca^{2+} entry in the negative inotropic effects of nitrous oxide in isolated ferret myocardium. Anesth Analg 74:575-579, 1992.
269. Stowe DF, Monroe SM, Marijic J, et al: Effects of nitrous oxide on contractile function and metabolism of the isolated heart. Anesthesiology 73:1220-1226, 1990.
270. Cason BA, Demas KA, Mazer CD, et al: Effects of nitrous oxide on coronary pressure and regional contractile function in experimental myocardial ischemia. Anesth Analg 72:604-611, 1991.
271. Siker D, Pagel PS, Pelc LR, et al: Nitrous oxide impairs functional recovery of stunned myocardium in barbiturate-anesthetized, acutely instrumented dogs. Anesth Analg 75:539-548, 1992.
272. Weber NC, Toma O, Awan S, et al: Effects of nitrous oxide on the rat heart in vivo. Another inhalational anesthetic that preconditions the heart? Anesthesiology 103:1174-1182, 2005.
273. Goto T, Saito H, Shinkai M, et al: Xenon provides faster emergence from anesthesia than does nitrous oxide–sevoflurane or nitrous oxide–isoflurane. Anesthesiology 86:1273-1278, 1997.
274. Yagi M, Mashimo T, Kawaguchi T, et al: Analgesic and hypnotic effects of subanaesthetic concentrations of xenon in human volunteers: Comparison with nitrous oxide. Br J Anaesth 74:670-673, 1995.
275. Ohara A, Mashimo M, Zhang P, et al: A comparative study of the antinociceptive action of xenon and nitrous oxide. Anesth Analg 85:931-936, 1997.
276. Lynch C III, Baum J, Tenbrinck R: Xenon anesthesia. Anesthesiology 92:865-870, 2000.
277. Preckel B, Weber NC, Sanders RD, et al: Molecular mechanisms transducing the anesthetic, analgesic, and organ-protective actions of xenon. Anesthesiology 105:187-197, 2006.
278. Marx T, Froeba G, Wagner D, et al: Effects on haemodynamics and catecholamine release of xenon anaesthesia compared to total i.v. anaesthesia in the pig. Br J Anaesth 78:326-327, 1997.
279. Hettrick DA, Pagel PS, Kersten JR, et al: Cardiovascular effects of xenon in isoflurane-anesthetized dogs with dilated cardiomyopathy. Anesthesiology 89:1166-1173, 1998.
280. Preckel B, Ebel D, Mullenheim J, et al: The direct myocardial effects of xenon in the dog heart in vivo. Anesth Analg 94:545-551, 2002.
281. Nakata Y, Goto M, Saito H, et al: Plasma concentration of fentanyl with xenon to block somatic and hemodynamic responses to surgical incision. Anesthesiology 92:1043-1048, 2000.
282. Nakata Y, Goto T, Morita S: Effects of xenon on hemodynamic responses to skin incision in humans. Anesthesiology 90:406-410, 1999.
283. Stowe DF, Rehmert GC, Kwok WK, et al: Xenon does not alter cardiac function or major cation currents in isolated guinea pig hearts or myocytes. Anesthesiology 93:1158-1159, 2000.
284. Huneke R, Jugling E, Skasa M, et al: Effects of the anesthetic gases xenon, halothane, and isoflurane on calcium and potassium currents in human atrial cardiomyocytes. Anesthesiology 95:999-1006, 2001.
285. Preckel B, Mullenheim J, Moloschavij A, et al: Xenon administration during early reperfusion reduces infarct size after regional ischemia in the rabbit heart in vivo. Anesth Analg 91:1327-1332, 2000.
286. Weber NC, Toma O, Wolter JI, et al: The noble gas xenon induces pharmacological preconditioning in the rat heart in vivo via induction of PKC-ε and p38 MAPK. Br J Pharmacol 144:123-132, 2005.
287. Weber NC, Stursberg J, Wirthle NM, et al: Xenon preconditioning differently regulates p44/42 MAPK (ERK1/2) and p46/54 MAPK (JNK 1/2 and 3) in vivo. Br J Anaesth 97:298-306, 2006.
288. Weber NC, Toma O, Damla H, et al: Upstream signaling of PKC-ε in xenon-induced pharmacological preconditioning. Implication of mitochondrial K_{ATP} channels and PDK-1. Eur J Pharmacol 539:1-9, 2006.
289. Pagel PS, Krolikowski JG, Venkatapuram S, et al: Noble gases without anesthetic properties protect myocardium against infarction by activating prosurvival signaling kinases and inhibiting mitochondrial permeability transition in vivo. Anesth Analg 105:562-569, 2007.

Jackie L. Martin

24 Inhaled Anesthetics: Metabolism and Toxicity

Key Points

1. The liver is the major site of endogenous and exogenous drug metabolism. The primary result of drug metabolism is the production of more water-soluble and therefore more easily excreted drug metabolites. Drugs are sometimes biotransformed into more reactive metabolites that may lead to toxicity.
2. Most drug metabolism is catalyzed by phase 1 or phase 2 enzymes. The predominant phase 1 enzymes are the cytochrome P450 (CYP) monooxygenases. Approximately 50 of the more than 1000 CYP isoforms are functionally active in humans. The predominant isoform catalyzing the metabolism of inhaled anesthetics is CYP2E1. The major phase 2 enzyme is uridine diphosphate glucuronosyltransferase.
3. Many factors affect drug metabolism. Perhaps the most important are pharmacogenetic factors. Genetics ultimately determines absorption, distribution, metabolism, and excretion. Other important determinants are environmental factors, age, gender, disease states, and other drugs or medications. Induction and inhibition of CYP enzymes because of concurrent medications can have an important impact on therapeutic drug levels and pharmacologic effects.
4. Pharmacogenomics, or the influence of DNA sequence variation on the effect of a drug, provides a basis for understanding the interindividual variation observed in drug responses.
5. Nitrous oxide and xenon are both nonhalogenated anesthetics. Xenon is not currently approved for clinical use; however, aside from the expense associated with its use, it may be the most ideal and environmentally friendly anesthetic agent.
6. The combination of drug-related antibodies, the apparent need for prior sensitization, and the association of fever and eosinophilia all support an immune basis for anesthetic-induced hepatitis.
7. Halothane, enflurane, isoflurane, and desflurane are all metabolized to trifluoroacylated hepatic protein adducts that have been reported to induce liver injury in susceptible patients. The propensity to produce liver injury appears to parallel metabolism of the parent drug; thus, halothane (20%) ⋙ enflurane (2.5%) ≫ isoflurane (0.2%) > desflurane (0.02%). The incidence of halothane hepatitis in the adult population is roughly 1 in 10,000. Sevoflurane does not produce acylated protein adducts.
8. Halothane hepatitis has been reported in the pediatric population. The incidence appears to be approximately 1 in 200,000.
9. Toxicity and liver injury have been reported after repeat exposure on subsequent occasions to different fluorinated anesthetics. This phenomenon of cross-sensitization has also been reported with hydrochlorofluorocarbons, the chlorofluorocarbon replacement agents.
10. Sevoflurane is metabolized to hexafluoroisopropanol, formaldehyde, inorganic fluoride, and carbon dioxide. Although very high fluoride levels have been reported after sevoflurane anesthesia, fluoride-associated renal injury has not been reported.
11. The major base-catalyzed breakdown product of sevoflurane is compound A. Compound A is a nephrotoxic vinyl ether that induces both dose- and time-dependent renal injury. The threshold for renal injury in rats and humans appears to be approximately 150 ppm-hours of exposure to compound A (i.e., 50 ppm for 3 hours). The toxic threshold appears to be reached only under clinical conditions of prolonged sevoflurane anesthesia, and changes in glucosuria and enzymuria are observed. Blood urea nitrogen and creatinine levels remain unchanged. To date, no significant clinical renal toxicity has been associated with the use of sevoflurane.
12. Desiccated carbon dioxide absorbent and inhaled anesthetic interactions can lead to the production of carbon monoxide in the anesthesia circuit (desflurane ⋙ enflurane > isoflurane). Negligible amounts of carbon monoxide are formed from halothane and sevoflurane.
13. New calcium hydroxide–based CO_2 absorbents, such as Amsorb and DragerSorb Free, contain neither NaOH or KOH and thus are chemically inert and do not degrade inhaled anesthetics to carbon monoxide or degrade sevoflurane to compound A.

14. The interaction of inhaled anesthetics with CO_2 absorbents is an exothermic reaction resulting in the production of heat. The temperature of CO_2 canisters during routine clinical use averages 25°C to 45°C but increases inversely with decreased fresh gas flow, and sevoflurane is associated with the greatest production of heat. Hydrogen is an important by-product of this reaction. The high yield of hydrogen, ease of ignition, and low tissue solubility make hydrogen the most likely fuel in anesthesia machine fires because of its reactions with desiccated CO_2 absorbents and sevoflurane. This reaction can be significant and result in fire, toxic gas, and patient injury.
15. There appears to be no risk associated with brief periods of low-level occupational exposure to waste anesthetic gases (operating room, postanesthesia care unit, intensive care unit). Occupational exposure to high concentrations (10^3 ppm) may be correlated with an increased incidence of abortions and decreased fertility. Individuals with vitamin B_{12} deficiency may be at risk for neurologic injury from nitrous oxide.
16. Fluorinated inhaled anesthetics containing bromine and chlorine deplete ozone (halothane ⋙ enflurane > isoflurane) and contribute to the greenhouse gas effect and global warming. N_2O does not deplete ozone, but it does contribute to the greenhouse gas effect and global warming.

Once a drug is administered, it undergoes the processes of absorption, distribution, target interaction, metabolism, and excretion. Unlike most drugs, the inhaled anesthetics are administered in great excess of the amount metabolized, and thus biotransformation has little effect on the pharmacologic activity of anesthetics but may have a significant effect on anesthetic toxicities. It was once thought that the inhaled anesthetics were chemically inert. We now know that many of these anesthetic agents undergo significant metabolism and in many cases biotransform and chemically breakdown to reactive and potentially toxic intermediates. The metabolic processes are affected by many factors, including age, disease, drug-drug interactions, and perhaps most important, genetics. This chapter focuses on the current understanding of mechanisms of anesthetic-associated toxicities, particularly liver injury and the role of drug metabolism in many of these processes. The mechanisms and risks resulting from the interaction of carbon dioxide absorbents with inhaled anesthetics, as well as other side effects of inhaled anesthetics, are also reviewed.

Drug Metabolism and Biotransformation

The Liver and Drug Metabolism

The lipophilic characteristics of drugs that promote their passage through biologic membranes hinder their excretion from the body. Drug metabolism is therefore essential for elimination and termination of the biologic activity of lipophilic drugs because it usually results in the formation of more hydrophilic products that are less pharmacologically active and more readily excreted from the body (Fig. 24-1). Drug metabolism sometimes results in the formation of intermediates whose pharmacologic or toxicologic activity is equal to, greater than, or different from that of the parent drug.[1] Unlike most drugs, the inhaled anesthetics are administered in great excess of the amount metabolized and are excreted mainly by exhalation. Thus, biotransformation has little effect on the pharmacologic activity of anesthetics, but it may have a significant effect on the toxicity of these agents.[2] The inhaled anesthetics are absorbed through the epithelium and mucous membranes of the respiratory tract. Because of the large pulmonary surface area, access to the circulation is rapid, with

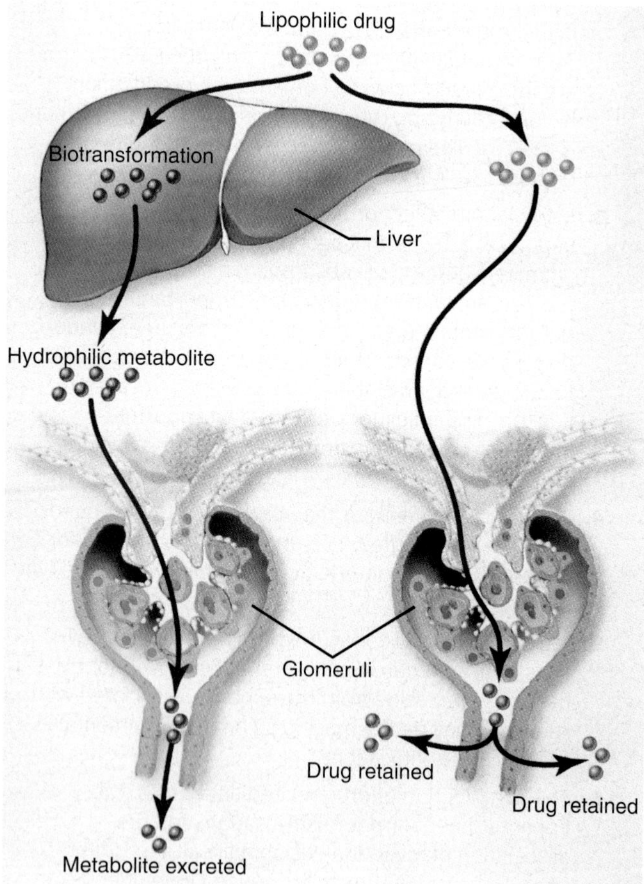

Figure 24-1 Effect of drug metabolism on excretion. Lipophilic (fat-soluble) drugs are metabolized to form relatively more hydrophilic (water-soluble) metabolites than the parent drug, and these metabolites are thus more easily excreted. *(From Weinshilboum R: Inheritance and drug response. N Engl J Med 348:529-557, 2003.)*

almost instantaneous absorption of these agents into blood and avoidance of hepatic first-pass metabolism. Thus, the pharmacologic effects of inhaled anesthetics are quite rapid and less dependent on factors governing the activities of other drugs, such as the amount of drug administered, the extent and rate of absorption, protein binding, excretion, secretion, and metabolism.[3]

The liver is the primary organ of drug metabolism because of its large size, rich concentration of drug-metabolizing enzymes, and unique double blood supply consisting of 70% of flow from the portal vein and 30% from the hepatic artery. Blood in the portal vein comes from the alimentary tract, pancreas, and spleen. Toxic materials absorbed from the alimentary tract are processed by the liver before they enter the systemic circulation. Blood flows through the hepatic sinusoids from the periphery of the hepatic lobule, fed by portal veins and hepatic arteries, to the centrally located hepatic venule or central vein. Hepatocytes, which are bathed by the sinusoidal blood supply, are the major drug-metabolizing cells in the liver and body. Several drug-metabolizing enzyme systems are located within the smooth endoplasmic reticulum of hepatocytes, whereas others are found in the cytosol of these cells. Organs with significant drug-metabolizing activity in addition to the liver are the gastrointestinal tract, kidneys, and lungs.[4,5]

The major enzymatic reactions biotransforming drugs into metabolites are oxidation, hydrolysis, and conjugation. It is very common for a drug to be metabolized into several metabolites. The ratios of various metabolites of a drug depend on enzymatic reaction rates, drug concentration near the enzymes, physicochemical reactions between metabolites and enzymes, competition of multiple drugs or endogenous substrates for the same enzyme, and many other factors.[5] Drug biotransformation reactions are broadly classified into phase 1 functionalization reactions or phase 2 biosynthetic conjugation reactions. Phase 1 reactions are catalyzed by enzymes that introduce or expose a polar functional group such as a hydroxyl or amino moiety in a drug by oxidation and hydrolytic reactions, respectively, whereas phase 2 reactions often lead to enzymatic conjugation of these polar functional groups to very polar molecules. The net effect of these reactions is the formation of molecules that are more easily excreted into urine through the kidneys or into the gastrointestinal tract by biliary excretion. *N*-Acetylation is the exception because it leads to the formation of less water-soluble metabolites.

The phase 1 enzymes most relevant to the metabolism of inhaled anesthetics are the cytochrome P450 (CYP) isoforms. These enzymes are capable of catalyzing several different types of oxidation reactions, including dehalogenation, *N*- and *O*-dealkylation, *N*- and S-oxidation, and deamination reactions. All these reactions require CYP, O_2, and reduced nicotinamide adenine dinucleotide phosphate (NADPH)-dependent cytochrome P450 reductase for activity and occur in the endoplasmic reticulum of cells, particularly hepatocytes. Under conditions of low oxygen tension, these enzymes may catalyze reductive reactions. Approximately 50 of the more than 1000 CYP isoforms are functionally active in humans and are categorized into 17 families and subfamilies. Sequences that are greater than 40% homologous belong to the same family and are identified by an Arabic number. The sequences of subfamily members are at least 55% identical and are distinguished by a capital letter. An Arabic number is used to distinguish individual isoforms within a subfamily. CYP2E1, for example, is a member of the CYP2 family, a large group of isozymes that metabolize many diverse drugs and endogenous compounds.[6] Approximately 10 isoforms in the CYP1, CYP2, and CYP3 families are responsible for the majority of drug metabolism in humans (Fig. 24-2). Most CYP isoforms metabolize multiple drugs, and some overlap in substrate specificity can be seen between the various isoforms. Thus, two or more CYP isoforms may be involved in the overall metabolism of a drug. In human liver, the CYP3A4 and CYP3A5 subfamilies account for as much as 60% of the total CYP present. CYP2E1 is particularly important in the oxidative metabolism of halogenated inhaled anesthetics, and like many CYP isozymes, it is concentrated in perivenular hepatocytes.

In phase 2 reactions, a polar molecule such as glucuronic acid, sulfate, or glycine is conjugated to a drug or its metabolites to produce highly hydrophilic products that are readily excreted into urine or in some cases into bile and the gastrointestinal tract. Glucuronidation is perhaps the most important conjugation reaction, and uridine 5′-diphosphate glucuronosyltransferase (UGT) catalyzes the transfer of glucuronic acid to aromatic and aliphatic alcohols, carboxylic acids, amines, and free sulfhydryl groups to form *O*-, *N*-, and *S*-glucuronides, respectively. UGTs, like CYPs, exist as multiple isoforms with differing substrate specificities and are localized in the endoplasmic reticulum, whereas most other phase 2 enzymes are concentrated in the cytosol. Glucuronidation is also important in the elimination of endogenous steroids, bilirubin, bile acids, and fat-soluble vitamins. Cytosolic sulfation is another important conjugation reaction that involves the catalytic transfer, by various sulfotransferase members, of inorganic sulfate from activated 3′-phosphoadenosine-5′ phosphosulfate to the hydroxyl group of phenols and aliphatic alcohols. Thus, drugs and primary metabolites with a hydroxyl group often form both glucuronide and sulfate conjugates. Two *N*-acetyltransferases, NAT1 and NAT2, are involved in the acylation of amines, hydrazines, and sulfonamides (see Fig. 24-2).

Factors Affecting Drug Metabolism

Various factors may affect drug metabolism, including environmental determinants, disease, age, gender, and genetics. The activity of many drug-metabolizing enzymes may be increased (*induced*) or decreased (*inhibited*) by concomitantly administered substances or drugs. Enzyme induction is due to enhanced gene transcription after prolonged exposure to an induction agent or, in some instances, is due to a decreased rate of enzyme degradation. Induction of CYP isozymes by numerous drugs and environmental agents has been studied extensively.[7] Enzyme inducers are often highly lipophilic drugs and environmental chemicals that are metabolized by the CYP isozymes that they induce. The inducing properties of a drug are unrelated to the nature of its pharmacologic or toxicologic activity and may differ markedly from those of other drugs in the same class. Induction by drugs such as phenobarbital results in proliferation of the smooth endoplasmic reticulum and an increase in liver weight. With this type of inducer, NADPH–cytochrome P450 reductase and specific CYP isozymes are preferentially increased. Although other inducers increase the synthesis of specific CYP isozymes, they do not affect cytochrome P450 reductase or liver weight. The mechanism by which CYP3A4 is induced is shown in Figure 24-3A, and the effect on plasma felodipine concentrations in healthy subjects is shown in Figure 24-3B.[8] Importantly, CYP3A4 induction is the result of de novo protein synthesis, and thus several weeks is needed before steady-state levels are reached. Likewise, once use

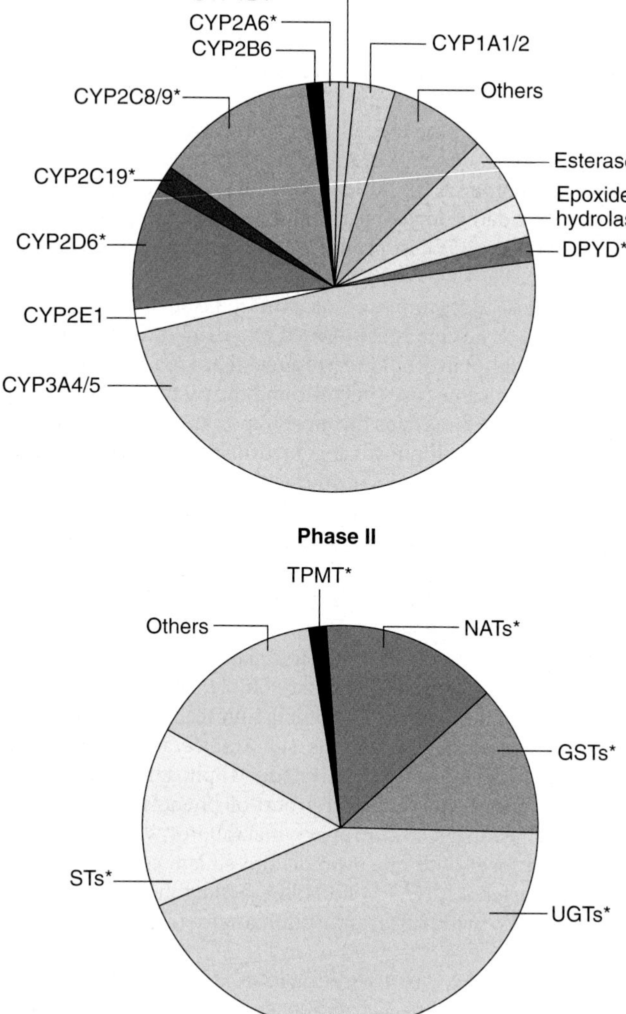

Figure 24-2 Proportion of drugs metabolized by major phase 1 or phase 2 enzymes. The relative size of each pie section indicates the estimated percentage of phase 1 (*top panel*) or phase 2 (*bottom panel*) metabolism that each enzyme contributes to the metabolism of drugs based on literature reports. Enzymes that have functional allelic variants are indicated by an *asterisk*. In many cases, more than one enzyme is involved in a particular drug's metabolism. CYP, cytochrome P450; DPYD, dihydropyridine dehydrogenase; GST, glutathione-S-transferase; NAT, *N*-acetyltransferase; STs, sulfotransferases; TPMT, thiopurine methyltransferase; UGT, uridine diphosphate glucuronosyltransferases. *(Adapted from Wilkinson G: Pharmacokinetics: The dynamics of drug absorption, distribution and elimination.* In *Hardman JG, Limbird LE, Goodman GA [eds]: Goodman and Gilman's The Pharmacological Basis of Therapeutics, 10th ed. New York, McGraw-Hill, 2001.)*

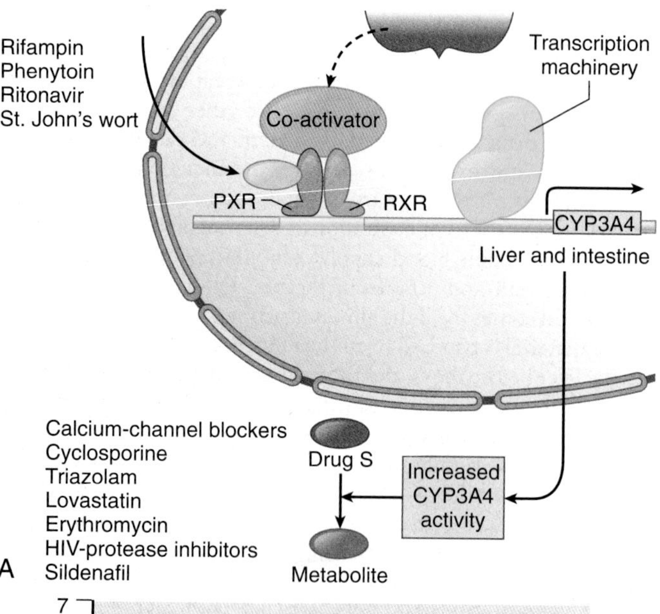

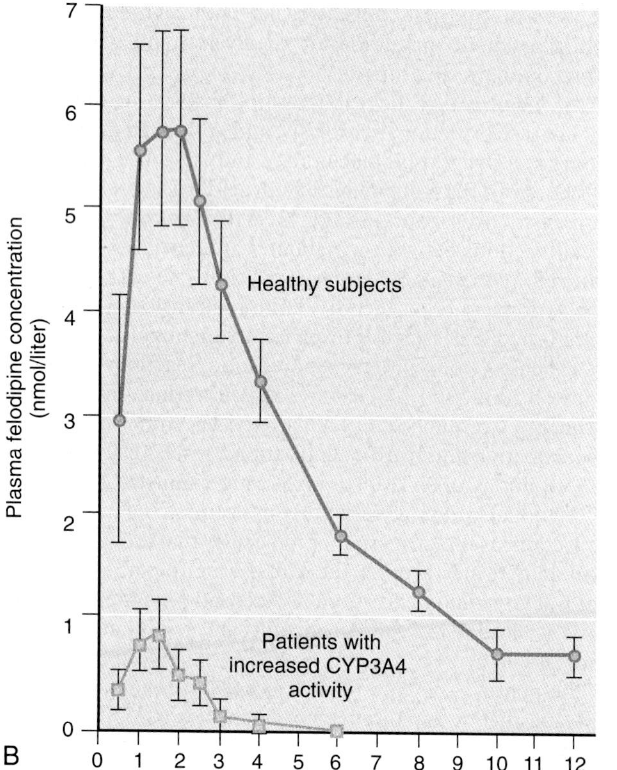

Figure 24-3 Mechanism of induction of CYP3A4-mediated metabolism of drug substrates (**A**) and the resulting reduced plasma drug concentration (**B**). In **A**, an inducing agent (Drug) interacts with the nuclear pregnane X receptor (PXR) to form a heterodimer with the retinoid X receptor (RXR); in turn, the heterodimer binds to cognate recognition sites in the 5′ regulatory region of the CYP3A4 gene. As a result, transcription of DNA is upregulated, which leads to increased synthesis of CYP3A4 enzyme and enhanced oxidative metabolism of its substrates (Drug S). This causes a reduction in the plasma drug concentration as exemplified by felodipine (**B**) and, subsequently, decreased drug effects. The same molecular mechanism is also responsible for the induction of other metabolizing enzymes and membrane transporters important in drug disposition. Comparison of the plasma felodipine concentration-time profiles in **B** with those in **A** indicates the wide range of CYP3A activity that is possible. *I bars* denote standard errors. *(From Wilkinson GR: Drug metabolism and variability among patients in drug response. N Engl J Med 352:2211-2221, 2005.)*

of the inducing drug is discontinued, it may be several weeks before baseline levels of CYP3A4 are established. Many classes of drugs and environmental chemicals, including anesthetics, anticonvulsants, insecticides, sedatives, steroids, tranquilizers, and the anti–human immunodeficiency virus (HIV) agents efavirenz and nevirapine contain one or more compounds thought to be enzyme inducers.[7] St. John's wort is also a known inducer of CYP3A. If the parent compound is toxic, enhanced metabolism may decrease its toxicity. In contrast, when metabolites are more toxic than the parent compound, metabolism increases toxicity. In many cases involving induction, the dosage of an affected drug must be increased to maintain the therapeutic effect. Enzyme-inducing agents have the potential to modify acute and chronic toxicities of anesthetics. In view of the current practice of polypharmacy, enzyme induction may be more common in patients who are undergoing surgery than previously appreciated.

Enzyme inhibition can have as great an effect on therapeutic activity and toxicity as enzyme induction. Enzyme inhibition can lead to an increase in the plasma concentration of the parent drug and a reduction in drug metabolites, as well as exaggerated and prolonged pharmacologic effects and increased potential for toxicity. Many compounds inhibit the activity of drug-metabolizing enzymes and thereby alter the duration and intensity of pharmacologic action and the severity of toxic effects. There are several mechanisms of inhibition. Inhibitors of protein synthesis such as cycloheximide decrease enzyme synthesis and thereby reduce enzyme concentrations. Other agents are reversible inhibitors that compete for the active site of the same enzyme responsible for metabolism of the drug of interest. Still others are irreversible inhibitors that degrade the heme in cytochrome P450. Inhibition of CYP3A is common and important because of the high expression of CYP3A in intestinal epithelium and the fact that oral ingestion is the most common route of entry for drugs. After oral ingestion, bioavailability is potentially increased because of a reduction in first-pass metabolism. Inhibition of CYP3A4, for example, is noted with the ingestion of grapefruit juice. Regular consumption of 250 mL of grapefruit juice will inhibit intestinal CYP3A4 activity. A patient taking oral felodipine with grapefruit juice will experience side effects associated with an overdose of this calcium channel antagonist, such as hypotension and tachycardia, as a result of decreased levels of CYP3A4 (Fig. 24-4).[8] Potent CYP3A inhibitors include ritonavir, diltiazem, nicardipine, verapamil, and several anti-HIV agents (delavirdine, indinavir, ritonavir, and saquinavir). More general CYP inhibitors include amiodarone, cimetidine, and the macrolide antibiotics erythromycin, clarithromycin, and troleandomycin.

Some sex-related differences in drug-metabolizing activity have been observed, particularly for CYP3A, but such differences are minor relative to previously described factors. An exception is the treatment of seizure patients with phenytoin during pregnancy. Because the liver is the major site of drug metabolism, intrinsic liver disease leading to hepatic dysfunction can result in impaired drug metabolism. Diseases such as hepatitis, primary biliary cirrhosis, alcoholic liver disease, cirrhosis, and hepatocarcinoma can lead to a 50% impairment of enzymatic activity. Severe cardiac failure with decreased hepatic perfusion and impaired metabolism can also occur, as evidenced by the twofold difference in loading and maintenance doses of lidocaine for treatment of dysrhythmia in heart failure patients. Moreover, viral infections can lead to the inhibition of CYP-mediated reactions.

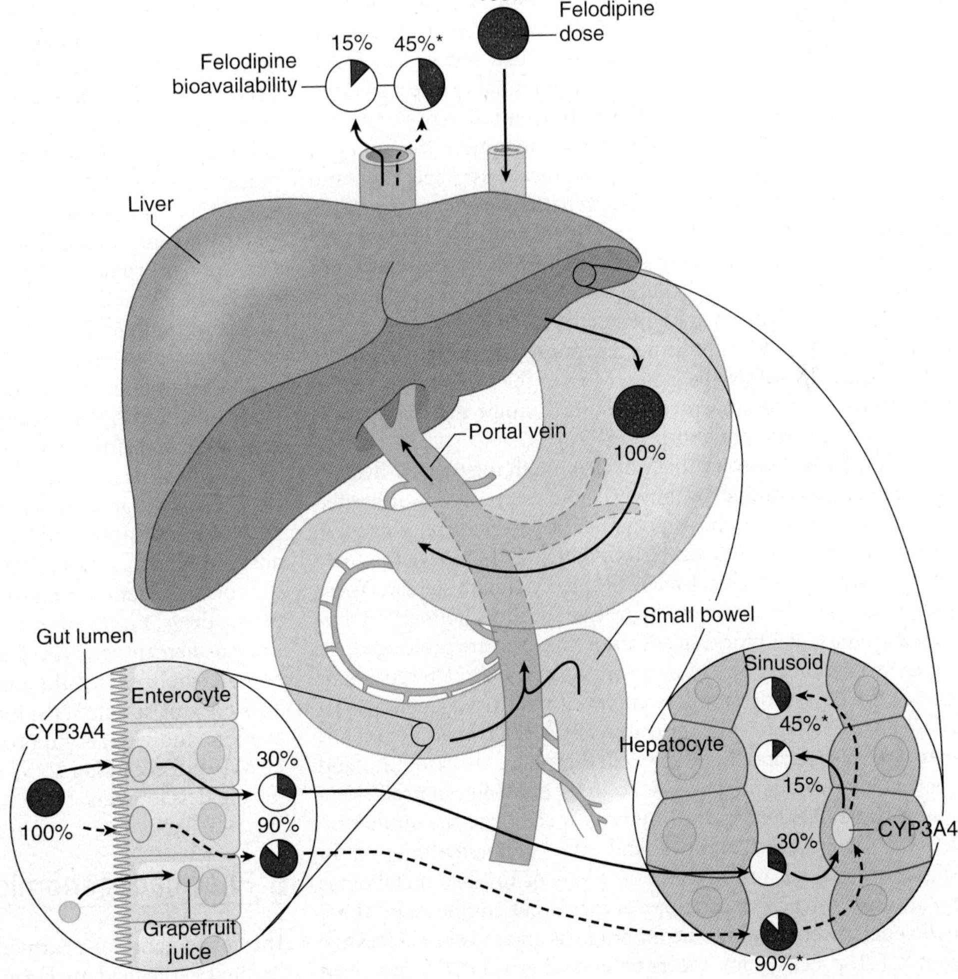

Figure 24-4 First-pass metabolism after the oral administration of a drug, as exemplified by felodipine and its interaction with grapefruit juice. The CYP3A enzymes (e.g., CYP3A4) present in enterocytes of the intestinal epithelium extensively metabolize felodipine during its absorption, and on average only 30% of the dose administered enters the portal vein (*solid line*). Subsequently, CYP3A enzymes in the liver further metabolize the drug so that only 15% of the dose is bioavailable and finally reaches the systemic circulation, where it is able to exert its effects. Grapefruit juice selectively inhibits CYP3A in the enterocyte, with the net result being an increase in the oral bioavailability of felodipine by a factor of 3, denoted by the *asterisks* and the *dashed lines*. *(From Wilkinson GR: Drug metabolism and variability among patients in drug response. N Engl J Med 352:2211-2221, 2005.)*

Developmental Differences in Infants and Children

Both phase 1 and phase 2 enzymes begin to mature during the postnatal period (also see Chapter 82), but the levels may be low enough in some cases to result in toxicity if drug therapy is not carefully monitored. For example, impairment of bilirubin glucuronidation at birth can lead to hyperbilirubinemia of the newborn and the "gray baby" syndrome as a result of high levels of the antibiotic chloramphenicol.[9,10] As children age, phase 1 enzymes appear to be affected to a greater degree than phase 2 enzymes. The predominant isoform expressed in fetal liver is CYP3A7, which peaks shortly after birth and then declines rapidly to levels that are undetectable in most adults.[11] Within hours of birth, CYP2E1 activity increases, followed by CYP2D6, CYP3A4, CYP2C9, and CYP2C19. CYP1A2 is the last isoform to appear at about 2 months of age. CYP2C9 and CYP2C19 are responsible for the biotransformation of phenytoin. The apparent half-life of phenytoin is prolonged to about 75 hours in preterm neonates but decreases to about 20 hours in term neonates during the first week of life and to 8 hours by the second week.[12]

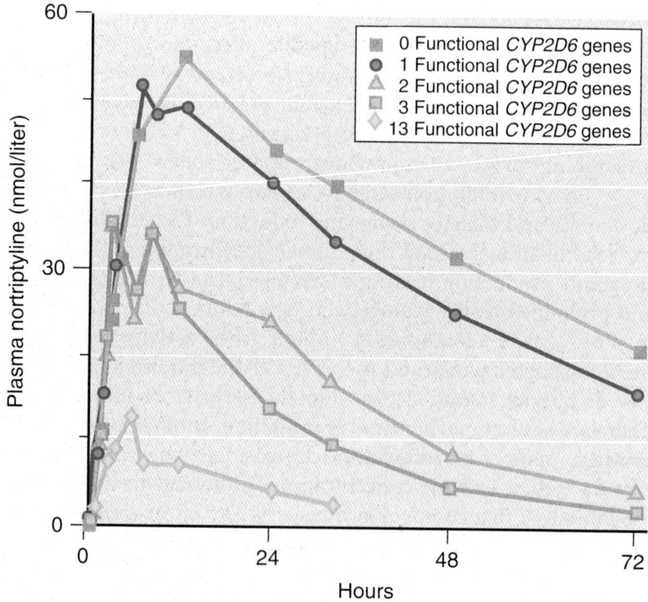

Figure 24-5 Pharmacogenetics of nortriptyline. Mean plasma concentrations of nortriptyline after a single 25-mg oral dose are shown in subjects with 0, 1, 2, 3, or 13 functional CYP2D6 genes. *(Adapted from Weinshilboum R: Inheritance and drug response. N Engl J Med 348:529-537, 2003.)*

Pharmacogenetics of Drug Metabolism

Advances in the field of genetics have had a major impact on drug metabolism and have provided the experimental tools to probe the genetic basis of intersubject variability in human drug pharmacokinetics, metabolism, and toxicity.[13] Although CYPs are most often thought of as being responsible for the deactivation of toxic compounds, they are in fact also responsible for the metabolic activation of drugs and chemicals to toxic forms. Any factor that can influence metabolism has the potential to affect toxicity. As previously discussed, drug biotransformation may be affected by many factors, including route of administration, frequency of administration, exposure to other chemicals, sex, age, diet, and genetics. The concept of pharmacogenetics originated from the clinical observation that there were patients with very low or very high plasma or urinary drug levels, followed by the realization that the biochemical traits leading to this variation were inherited. Soon thereafter, drug-metabolizing enzymes were identified, followed by discovery of the genes encoding the proteins and the DNA sequences within the genes. Most of the early pharmacogenetic traits were monogenic, involving a single gene, and most were due to genetic polymorphism.

The early discovery that impairment in the phase 1 hydrolysis of succinylcholine by butyrylcholinesterase was inherited served as an early stimulus to the development of pharmacogenetics. About 1 in 3500 white individuals is homozygous for a gene encoding an atypical form of butyrylcholinesterase. These individuals have less ability to hydrolyze succinylcholine, and thus the neuromuscular blocking effects of this drug are prolonged.[14,15] More recent studies have demonstrated that CYP2D6 represents one of the best understood examples of pharmacogenetic variation in drug metabolism. Substrates for CYP2D6 include codeine, metoprolol, nortriptyline, dextromethorphan, debrisoquin, and sparteine.[16] Approximately 5% to 10% of white subjects were found to be deficient in the ability to metabolize the antihypertensive drug debrisoquin[16] and the antiarrhythmic drug sparteine,[17] which resulted in low levels of urinary metabolites and high plasma concentrations of the parent compounds. These deficiencies were found to be inherited as an autosomal recessive trait.[17,18] The cDNA for the gene encoding CYP2D6 has been cloned, and a number of genetic variants responsible for the deficient activity of CYP2D6 have been identified. Other subjects have multiple copies of active forms of CYP2D6 that result in rapid elimination of drugs leading to subtherapeutic levels. Such is the case with the antidepressant nortriptyline (Fig. 24-5). Many other examples of poor metabolizers of drugs who have genetic variants of other CYP isoforms have been described. For example, CYP2C9 variants can lead to poor metabolism of warfarin and phenytoin and subsequent toxic levels of these compounds. Similarly, polymorphisms in the phase 2 metabolizing enzyme NAT can lead to bimodal differences in *N*-acetylation and inactivation of the antituberculosis drug isoniazid (Fig. 24-6). More recent molecular cloning studies have shown that there are two NAT genes in humans, *NAT1* and *NAT2*, and that the common genotypic polymorphism responsible for the pharmacogenetic variation in isoniazid metabolism involves the *NAT2* gene.[19] The frequency of each acetylation phenotype is dependent on race but not on sex or age. Fast acetylation is found in the Inuit and Japanese, whereas slow acetylation predominates among Scandinavians and North African white individuals.[20] Another example of the role of genetics in phase 2 metabolism concerns the antineoplastic drug azathioprine, a prodrug that is converted to the active drug 6-mercaptopurine. Thiopurines such as 6-mercaptopurine are metabolized by thiopurine-*S*-methyltransferase (TPMT).[21] This enzymatic activity is inherited in an autosomal codominant fashion. Individuals homozygous for alleles encoding inactive TPMT and receiving standard doses of azathioprine are at risk for the development of severe pancytopenia.

Pharmacogenomics of Drug Metabolism

The convergence of pharmacogenetics and human genomics has resulted in the field of *pharmacogenomics*, a term used to describe

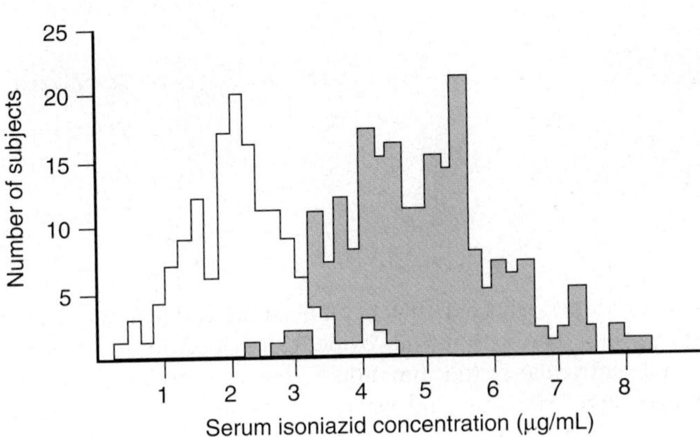

Figure 24-6 Bimodal distribution of serum isoniazid concentrations in a large group of Finnish patients. More than 300 patients were given intravenous injections of 5 mg/kg of isoniazid. Serum drug concentrations were assayed at multiple times after injection. The distribution of serum concentrations of isoniazid is shown 180 minutes after injection. The *blue* histogram represents rapid inactivators and the *black* histogram, slow inactivators. *(From Petri WA Jr: Antimicrobial Mycobacterium complex disease and leprosy. In Hardman JG, Limbird LE, Goodman GA [eds]: Goodman and Gillman's The Pharmacological Basis of Therapeutics, 10th ed. New York, McGraw-Hill, 2001.)*

the influence of variations in DNA sequence on drug responses. Pharmacogenomics holds the promise of personalized medicine: offering patients a precisely targeted drug at a precisely calibrated dose to address a specific condition. The field of pharmacogenomics began with a focus on drug metabolism but has been extended to include the full spectrum of drug disposition, including absorption, transporters, excretion, drug targets, and signal transduction. With completion of the Human Genome Project, the time is rapidly approaching when the sequences of virtually all genes encoding enzymes that catalyze both phase 1 and phase 2 reactions will be known. More than 1.4 million single-nucleotide polymorphisms were identified in the initial screening of the human genome, with over 60,000 in the coding region for genes. Some of these single-nucleotide polymorphisms have already been associated with substantial changes in the metabolism or effects of medications, and some are currently being used to predict clinical response. The potential exists for pharmacogenomics to yield a powerful set of molecular diagnostic tools with which clinicians will select medications and drug doses for individual patients. For example, a growing understanding of pharmacogenomics has led to the implementation of clinical genotyping of certain narrow–therapeutic index drugs such as the thiopurine derivatives azathioprine and 6-mercaptopurine for acute lymphoblastic lymphoma[22] and the colorectal agent irinotecan.[23] The anticoagulant warfarin, which has a narrow therapeutic range and large variations in individual patient dosage requirements, has been studied, and it has been found that mean maintenance doses depend on the CYP2C9 genotype.[24] In reports investigating the genes encoding CYP2C9 and vitamin K epoxide reductase (VKORC1), researchers demonstrated that patients with CYP2C9*2 and CYP2C9*3 allelic variants and the VKORC1 haplotype A/A require lower dosages of warfarin to achieve adequate levels of warfarin with minimal risk of bleeding.[25,26] A more recent report showed that the initial variability in the international normalized ratio (INR) response to warfarin was more strongly associated with genetic variability related to VKORC1 than to CYP2C9.[27] Both the CYP2C9 genotype and the VKORC1 haplotype had a significant influence on the warfarin dose required after the first 2 weeks of therapy. In effect, the maintenance dose of warfarin in persons heterozygous for CYP2C9*2/*3 is lower than the dose in patients who are homozygous for the normal enzyme or in compound heterozygotes. For the homozygous CYP3C9*3 genotype, even smaller doses are required to achieve the desired INR levels for anticoagulation. In the summer of 2007, the Food and Drug Administration found the accumulated evidence related to warfarin dosing compelling enough to warrant a change in the package labeling of warfarin "to highlight the potential relevance of genetic information to prescribing decisions." Predictably, drugs that inhibit CYP2C9, such as amiodarone and fluconazole, when taken with warfarin will result in an enhanced anticoagulant effect and increased risk of bleeding. In contrast, drugs that impair the metabolism of warfarin, such as cimetidine and omeprazole, have only slight potentiating effects on anticoagulation.

Metabolism of Inhaled Anesthetics

Nonhalogenated Inhaled Anesthetics

Nitrous Oxide

Nitrous oxide (N_2O) is the only nonhalogenated anesthetic that currently remains in routine clinical use. This agent is not metabolized in human tissue. However, by means of a physicochemical reaction of N_2O with vitamin B_{12}, N_2O is reductively metabolized by rat and human intestinal bacteria to molecular nitrogen (N_2). Reduction of N_2O in bacteria may occur via a single electron transfer process that results in the formation of nitrogen gas (N_2) and free radicals. N_2O can oxidize vitamin B_{12} and inhibit its coenzyme function. For example, this could affect the activity of methionine synthase, which catalyzes the transmethylation from methyltetrahydrofolate and homocysteine to produce tetrahydrofolate and methionine. Inhibition of methionine synthase has the potential to lead to decreased levels of tetrahydrofolate and methionine and subsequent impairment of DNA synthesis and "carbon 1" metabolic reactions, including methylation. However, such an effect on the activity of vitamin B_{12} would probably be inconsequential with the short courses of exposure to N_2O during anesthesia.

Xenon

The inert noble gases helium, neon, argon, krypton, xenon, and radon have found diverse and expanding applications in clinical medicine.[28] Xenon, krypton, and argon are all chemically inert in most circumstances, and all have anesthetic properties. Xenon is of particular interest because it is the only inert gas that is an anesthetic under normobaric conditions. Xenon was first identified as an anesthetic agent in 1951.[29] Although not approved for clinical use, xenon has been submitted for regulatory medical approval in Europe. Xenon is a normal constituent in atmospheric air at a concentration no greater than 0.086 ppm and thus, unlike all other inhaled anesthetics, it is not an environmental pollutant. The gas cannot be manufactured but is

Table 24-1 Anesthetic Properties of Xenon versus Other Anesthetics

	Xenon	Nitrous Oxide	Isoflurane	Desflurane	Sevoflurane
Oil-gas partition coefficient	1.9	1.4	90	18.7	53.4
Blood-gas partition coefficient	0.14	0.47	1.4	0.42	0.6
Minimum alveolar concentration (%)	71	≈105	1.15	6.0	1.71

recovered in the process of fractional distillation of liquefied air, and after several separation steps, a purity of greater than 99.99% can be obtained. The cost of xenon is presently about $10.00 (U.S.) per liter (100 times more expensive than nitrous oxide), and it may be unlikely to enjoy widespread use because of the expense associated with its extraction from air. If this problem could be overcome, xenon would be the most ideal inhaled anesthetic agent because xenon (minimum alveolar concentration [MAC] of 71%) is more potent than nitrous oxide, can provide surgical anesthesia in 30% oxygen, is very insoluble (blood-gas partition coefficient of 0.14), and has positive medical and environmental effects (Table 24-1). Xenon exhibits minimal cardiovascular and hemodynamic side effects, is not known to be metabolized in the liver or kidney, is not teratogenic, and does not trigger malignant hyperthermia in susceptible swine.[30] Recent evidence suggests both a neuroprotective[31] and a cardioprotective effect after exposure to xenon.[32] Environmental positives are that xenon does not deplete stratospheric ozone or contribute to global warming and the greenhouse effect. The unique combination of analgesia, hypnosis, and lack of cardiovascular depression in this one agent makes xenon a very attractive choice for patients with limited cardiovascular reserve. Xenon has a density of 5.887 g/L, with nitrous oxide and air having densities of 1.53 and 1.00 g/L, respectively. Because of its greater density, xenon does lead to an increase in pulmonary resistance, which results in an increase in the work of breathing.[33] Thus, xenon should be used with caution in patients with moderate to severe chronic obstructive pulmonary disease, the morbidly obese, premature infants, and any other patient in whom an increase in the work of breathing might have adverse effects.

Xenon was first used successfully for general anesthesia in human volunteers and patients in the 1950s,[29,34] was largely forgotten for 40 years, and then was rediscovered in 1990.[35] Over the past 20 years, xenon has been studied intensively in Europe and Japan in a number of clinical trials with very promising results.[36-38] Lachmann and colleagues showed that patients anesthetized with 70% xenon and 30% oxygen required 80% less supplemental fentanyl than did a similar group anesthetized with 70% nitrous oxide and 30% oxygen.[35] In a comparison of 30 American Society of Anesthesiologists (ASA) class I and II patients undergoing total abdominal hysterectomy and receiving either 60% xenon, 60% nitrous oxide with 0.5% isoflurane, or 60% nitrous oxide with 0.7% sevoflurane (all patients had epidurals and received mepivacaine to control the heart rate and blood pressure to within 20% of baseline), Goto and associates found that emergence from xenon anesthesia was two to three times faster than either comparison group.[39] In a randomized controlled multicenter trial, a total of 224 patients from six centers received either 60% xenon in 40% oxygen or 60% nitrous oxide in 0.5% isoflurane, with 1 μg sufentanil administered if indicated by defined criteria.[40] This study demonstrated significantly faster recovery from xenon anesthesia than from isoflurane–nitrous oxide anesthesia. Goto and coworkers showed that hemodynamic stability was better with xenon than with nitrous oxide with respect to maintenance of left ventricular systolic function.[41] More recently, a randomized multicenter trial was undertaken to compare left ventricular function in patients without cardiac disease who were undergoing elective surgery under either xenon or isoflurane anesthesia.[42] Xenon did not reduce contractility, whereas isoflurane decreased the contractile index, suggesting that xenon provides favorable cardiovascular stability in patients without cardiovascular disease. Although it is clear that emergence from xenon anesthesia is more rapid than emergence from desflurane or propofol anesthesia, studies have not found any significant differences in postoperative cognitive measures in patients exposed to these two agents.[43] In a recent study involving ASA III patients undergoing aortic surgery and receiving xenon ($n = 20$) or remifentanil ($n = 19$), no advantage of total intravenous anesthesia over xenon was demonstrated.[44] A recent study that included 40 ASA III and IV patients with known coronary artery disease randomized to either xenon ($n = 20$) or propofol ($n = 20$) anesthesia, both supplemented with remifentanil, showed higher arterial pressure and better left ventricular function, as assessed by echocardiograph indices, with xenon than with propofol.[45] It is certainly too early to know whether xenon anesthesia improves clinical outcomes, particularly in high-risk patients, and thus justifies the additional cost associated with its use in clinical anesthesia.

During xenon anesthesia, nitrogen released from the patient's body accumulates in the anesthesia circuit. Consequently, it is necessary to perform prolonged denitrogenation before starting xenon administration to reduce the risk for hypoxia. Another technical challenge lies in the transition from denitrogenation to closed-circuit xenon anesthesia. One could simply increase fresh gas flow (too expensive) or add xenon to the circuit as oxygen is consumed by the patient. This second method is too slow because patients typically consume only 200 to 250 mL of oxygen per minute. Several investigators use a second anesthesia machine already primed with 4 L of xenon. Thus, xenon must be given with a rebreathing system, low fresh gas flow, or a closed-circuit system. A closed-circuit system is the most economical technique for the clinical use of xenon. In the 2-hour study from Japan by Goto and colleagues, the estimated cost of providing anesthesia per patient was $170.00 for xenon ($17.00/L), $57.00 for isoflurane, and $60.00 for sevoflurane.[39] These differences in cost would be different in the United States, where xenon is $10.00/L, and would become progressively smaller with a longer duration of anesthesia because the rate of xenon consumption declines exponentially as body tissues become saturated in a closed rebreathing system. The total yearly production of xenon is approximately 6 million L, or enough for about 400,000 anesthetic procedures. If delivery systems become available that allow recycling of anesthetic gases, xenon anesthesia may become more economical and accessible to selected patients who might benefit from its lack of adverse systemic effects.

Halogenated Inhaled Anesthetics

Halothane

Approximately 25% of the halothane ($CF_3CHBrCl$) administered is metabolized to trifluoroacetic acid, chloride (Cl^-), and bromide (Br^-) (Fig. 24-7). The major metabolite in humans is trifluoroacetic acid (CF_3COOH), formed from oxidative metabolism primarily by CYP2E1 and to a lesser extent by CYP2A6.[46] The rate-limiting step in oxidative metabolism is breakage of the carbon-hydrogen bond. The first intermediate formed is probably 1,1,1-trifluoro-2-chloro-2-bromoethanol, which would be expected to rapidly decompose and produce hydrogen bromide and the reactive metabolite trifluoroacetyl chloride (TFA-Cl). This latter metabolite reacts with water to produce HCl and trifluoroacetic acid and with phosphatidylethanolamine, a membrane phospholipid, to form *N*-trifluoroacetyl-2-aminoethanol, which has been identified in urine. The TFA-Cl metabolite of halothane also reacts with tissue proteins to form trifluoroacetylated (TFA)-protein adducts, which will be discussed in the section on hepatotoxicity. Although trifluoroethanol has been identified in the urine of experimental animals, this metabolite and its glucuronide conjugate have not been found in human urine. Likewise, trifluoroacetaldehyde, another possible metabolite, has not been isolated from human urine.

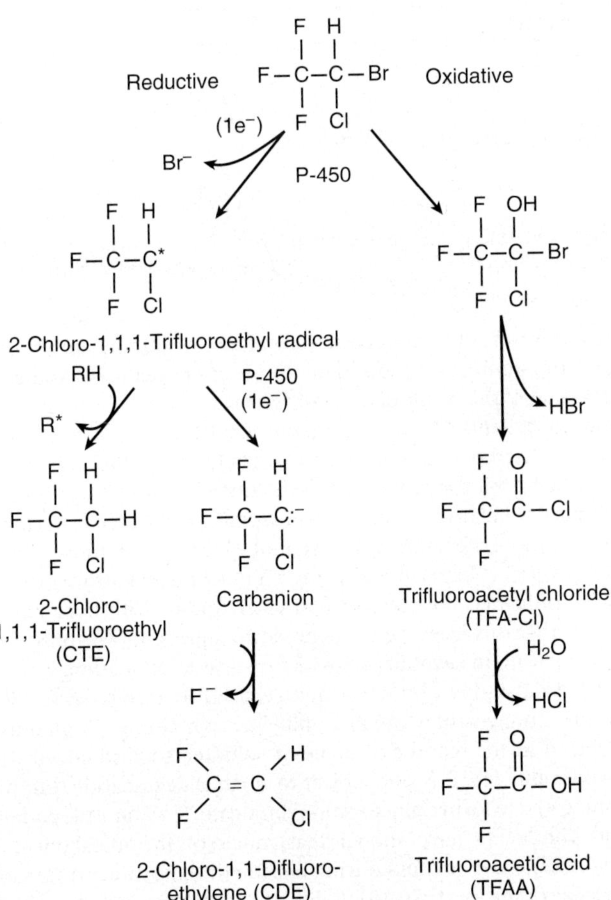

Figure 24-7 Major by-products of oxidative and reductive CYP4502E1-catalyzed halothane metabolism.

An alternative and minor route of halothane metabolism (i.e., <1% of the halothane absorbed) is via a reductive pathway that requires low oxygen tension and can be catalyzed by CYP2A6 and CYP3A4 (see Fig. 24-7).[46] Inorganic Br^- and F^- are end products of this pathway. Two volatile metabolites (2-chloro-1,1-difluoro-ethylene [CDE] and 2-chloro-1,1,1-trifluorethane [CTE]) and a volatile decomposition product of halothane (2-bromo-2-chloro-1,1-difluoroethylene [DBE]) were first identified in the exhaled gases of patients anesthetized with halothane. The formation of CDE and release of F^- probably result from a CYP-mediated two-electron reduction of halothane, whereas the formation of CTE and production of tissue free radicals result from a CYP-mediated one-electron reduction. The suicidal inactivation of CYP observed under hypoxic conditions (<40 torr O_2) is presumably the result of covalent binding of a reactive intermediate of CTE to CYP formed during the metabolism of CTE by CYP. A major pathway of formation of DBE is via the base-catalyzed dehydrofluorination of halothane as a result of its interaction with soda lime. CYP2E1 is inducible by both ethanol and isoniazid and is inhibited by disulfiram.[47] Prolonged exposure to subanesthetic concentrations of halothane results in increased drug metabolism in humans.

Enflurane

Enflurane (CHF_2-O-CF_2-CHClF) is essentially no longer used in the United States, but examination of its metabolism serves to illustrate how relatively minor changes in chemical structure can dramatically affect the extent of metabolism. Approximately 2.5% of the enflurane absorbed is metabolized (Fig. 24-8). Initial oxidation and breaking of the carbon-hydrogen bond may occur at either the chlorofluoromethyl carbon or the difluoromethyl carbon. Studies of the metabolism of enflurane with human hepatic microsomes[48] and isolation of difluoromethoxydifluoroacetic acid from rat liver, human urine, human hepatic microsomes, and cDNA-expressed CYP2E1[48] suggest that primary metabolism occurs at the chlorofluoromethyl carbon. Detection of insignificant amounts of chlorofluoroacetic acid further suggests that there is very little metabolism at the difluorormethyl carbon. The reactive intermediate formed from oxidation at the chlorofluoromethyl carbon can either hydrolyze to produce difluoromethoxydifluoroacetic acid or acetylate tissue protein to produce an adduct with immunogenic potential.[49] In either case, inorganic F^- is a product of these chemical reactions.

Surgical patients treated on a long-term basis with phenobarbital, phenytoin, or diazepam or who consumed ethanol before anesthesia with enflurane did not have elevated serum F^- concentrations when compared with untreated patients. In contrast, about 50% of surgical patients maintained on chronic isoniazid therapy demonstrated significantly elevated serum F^- concentrations.[50] Studies with purified CYP2E1 from humans[51] demonstrate that this CYP isoform is predominantly, if not exclusively, responsible for the defluorination of enflurane in human liver. Isoniazid treatment seems to significantly enhance enflurane metabolism in humans.[51]

Isoflurane

Isoflurane (CHF_2-O-CHCl-CF_3), an isomer of enflurane, is metabolized even more slowly than halothane or enflurane is (≈0.2%) (see Fig. 24-8). The metabolism of isoflurane results from oxidation of the α-carbon by hepatic CYP2E1.[52,53] The initial hydroxylated intermediate can decompose to produce a reactive

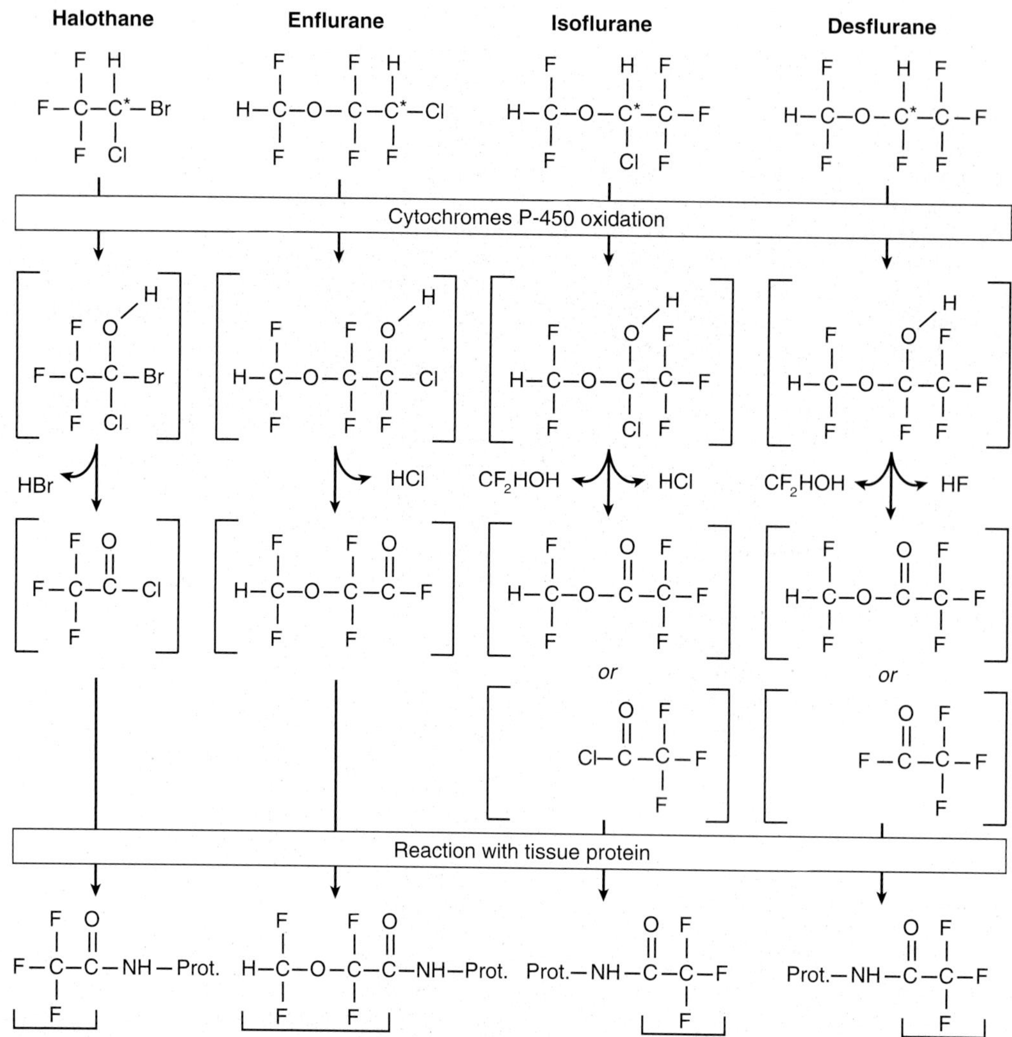

Figure 24-8 Proposed pathways for the CYP4502E1-catalyzed metabolism of halothane, enflurane, isoflurane, and desflurane to acylated hepatic proteins. For halothane, isoflurane, and desflurane, the trifluoroacetylated protein adducts are identical in structure, whereas for enflurane the adduct is immunologically similar.

TFA-Cl metabolite identical to halothane or a reactive trifluoroacetyl ester intermediate. Both these products would be expected to react with water to form trifluoroacetic acid or with protein to produce TFA-protein adducts. Very small amounts of inorganic fluoride would be expected to be formed during this metabolism.

Desflurane

Desflurane (CHF_2-O-CHF-CF_3) is thought to be metabolized in a manner similar to isoflurane because these two molecules differ by only one atom at the α-carbon position, with desflurane having a fluorine atom and isoflurane having a chlorine atom (see Fig. 24-8). However, the fluorine atom substitution decreases metabolism at the α-carbon position significantly so that the F^- and nonvolatile organic fluorine compounds formed from the metabolism of desflurane are considerably less than with isoflurane. Peak serum F^- concentrations are seen immediately after exposure to desflurane.[54]

Sevoflurane

The rate of sevoflurane (CH_2F-O-CH-$[CF_3]_2$) defluorination in vitro is approximately the same as that of methoxyflurane. However, serum F^- concentrations after sevoflurane administration are significantly less than those after methoxyflurane,[55-57] presumably the result of large differences in the blood-gas partition coefficients of the two agents (0.69 for sevoflurane versus 10.2 for methoxyflurane). Approximately 5% of the sevoflurane absorbed is biotransformed.[57,58] The fluoromethoxy C-H bond is the site of oxidative metabolism of sevoflurane, which leads to the formation of hexafluoroisopropanol (HFIP) and inorganic F^- (Fig. 24-9).[59,60] Experiments using CYP2E1 purified from humans have confirmed the results of in vitro studies with liver microsomes that this isozyme is the predominant, if not the only CYP participating in sevoflurane oxidation and F^- formation.

In a study of human volunteers, HFIP accounted for 80% of the nonvolatile organic fluorine-containing compounds detected in the blood and urine of volunteers anesthetized with sevoflurane. HFIP is not subject to further degradation, but it is conjugated to form a glucuronide conjugate.[58,61] Studies in patients and volunteers have shown that much of the metabolism of sevoflurane to F^- occurs during anesthetic exposure, presumably because of the low tissue solubility of sevoflurane and the stability of its metabolites.[62,63] Peak serum F^- concentrations are reached within a few hours of the end of anesthesia.

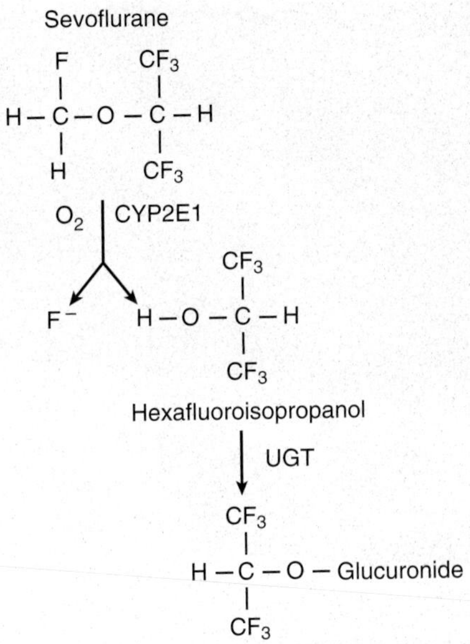

Sevoflurane

O_2 CYP2E1

F^-

Hexafluoroisopropanol

UGT

H–C–O–Glucuronide

Figure 24-9 In vivo metabolism of sevoflurane to inorganic fluoride and hexafluoroisopropanol. UGT, uridine 5′-diphosphate glucuronosyltransferase

Stereoselective Metabolism of Inhaled Anesthetics

Until recently, drug stereochemistry has been an area of relative neglect with regard to the preparation of therapeutic agents. Many drugs, including the fluorinated anesthetics, are commercially prepared and used therapeutically as racemic mixtures. A racemic mixture contains an equal amount of the two enantiomers. Enantiomers are simply nonsuperimposable mirror images, such as your left and right hands. Clinical experience has made it increasingly clear that enantiomeric forms of drugs may differ in their potency, toxicity, and pharmacologic, pharmacokinetic, and pharmacodynamic properties and actions.[64-67] Such nonsuperimposable objects are said to be chiral. The most common chiral origin is the presence of an asymmetric center, a carbon atom attached to four different substitute groups. Enantiomers are optically active; that is, a single enantiomeric form rotates the plane of polarized light passing through an aqueous solution of the enantiomer in a clockwise or counterclockwise direction. The preferred method of the International Union of Pure and Applied Chemistry (IUPAC) for the classification of enantiomers is the Cahn-Perlog-Ingold convention or (*R*/*S*) classification. In this system the four substitutions around the chiral center are assigned priorities that depend on atomic number and atomic mass. When looking down the carbon bond to the substituent with the lowest priority, if the other substituents are ordered from higher to lower in a clockwise direction, the assignment is the (*R*)-configuration; if counterclockwise, the (*S*)-configuration is designated.

The reduced cost of production of purified enantiomeric solutions has made these compounds increasingly available for clinical use. Whether the clinical use of a single stereoisomer provides significant advantages depends on both the pharmacokinetic and the pharmacodynamic properties of the respective enantiomers. For example, (*S*)-penicillamine is used to treat Wilson's disease, cystinuria, and rheumatoid arthritis because of toxicities associated with the racemic drug.[68] The calcium channel blocker (*S*)-verapamil is 10 to 20 times more potent than (*R*)-verapamil and thus appears to be a better antiarrhythmic, antianginal, and antihypertensive agent.[69] The cardiovascular drug (*S*)-propranolol is clinically useful as an antihypertensive and antianginal agent, whereas (*R*)-propranolol, which lacks cardiovascular effects, is useful in the treatment of hypothyroidism.[70,71] Ketamine is provided for clinical use as a racemic mixture, although (*S*)-ketamine has superior efficacy, faster elimination and recovery characteristics, and fewer side effects ranging from restlessness and agitation to emergence reactions than racemic ketamine does.[72] (*S*)-Ketamine is also three times more potent than (*R*)-ketamine as an anesthetic and analgesic agent, and enantiomeric stereoselectivity of the hepatic metabolism of ketamine by microsomal enzymes has been demonstrated.[73] Ropivacaine, the (*S*)-enantiomer of a bupivacaine homolog, and levobupivacaine ([*S*]-bupivacaine) were developed as alternatives to racemic bupivacaine because of its known central nervous system and cardiovascular toxicity. Ropivacaine is less potent than (*S*)-bupivacaine or racemic bupivacaine in blocking sodium channels, although the anesthetic and analgesic effects of the two drugs are similar.[74] Even though both bupivacaine and ropivacaine demonstrate similar plasma protein binding, ropivacaine has lower lipid solubility, higher plasma clearance, and a shorter elimination half-life $(t_{½β})$ than racemic bupivacaine does.[75] Like ropivacaine, levobupivacaine has been shown to have a reduced incidence of toxicity in comparison to its (*R*)-isomer.[76] (*R*)-Cisatracurium offers clinical advantages over racemic atracurium because of its lack of histamine-releasing properties and its higher neuromuscular blocking potency. Ethanol is widely used as a pharmaceutical solvent and has recently been shown to decrease the unbound fraction of (*S*)-warfarin while increasing the unbound portion of (*R*)-warfarin. Perhaps the most infamous example of enantiomeric differences between optical isomers was observed with the drug thalidomide. The (*R*)- and (*S*)-isomers of thalidomide, as well as the racemic mixture, are equally active hypnotics; however, (*S*)-thalidomide is transformed into metabolites that proved to be embryogenic and teratogenic.[77]

Commercial halothane is a racemic mixture of (*R*)- and (*S*)-enantiomers (Fig. 24-10). As discussed previously, metabolic studies have shown that racemic halothane undergoes oxidative metabolism catalyzed by CYP2E1 to TFA-Cl, which covalently binds to several hepatic proteins that are believed to be involved in the immune response leading to halothane hepatotoxicity. To investigate whether CYP2E1 catalyzes the metabolism of halothane in a stereoselective fashion, the enantiomers of halothane were prepared and tested in vivo for their ability to form covalently bound TFA-protein adducts in the liver of mice. It was found that halothane does undergo stereoselective metabolism, with the (*R*)-isomer producing significantly greater amounts of TFA-protein adducts in liver than the (*S*)-isomer does (Fig. 24-11).[78] Because the anesthetic potency of the isomers appears to be equal,[79] these findings suggest that the (*S*)-isomer of halothane might be a safer inhaled anesthetic agent than the (*R*)-isomer or the racemic mixture. This idea is supported by the observation that the hepatotoxicity caused by halothane, enflurane, isoflurane, and desflurane is related to their relative degree

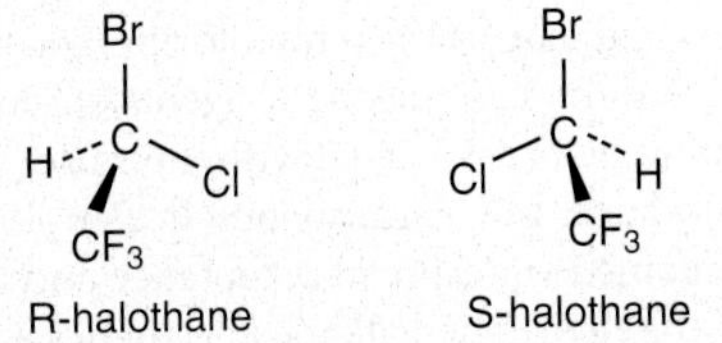

R-halothane S-halothane

Figure 24-10 (*R*)- and (*S*)-enantiomers of halothane

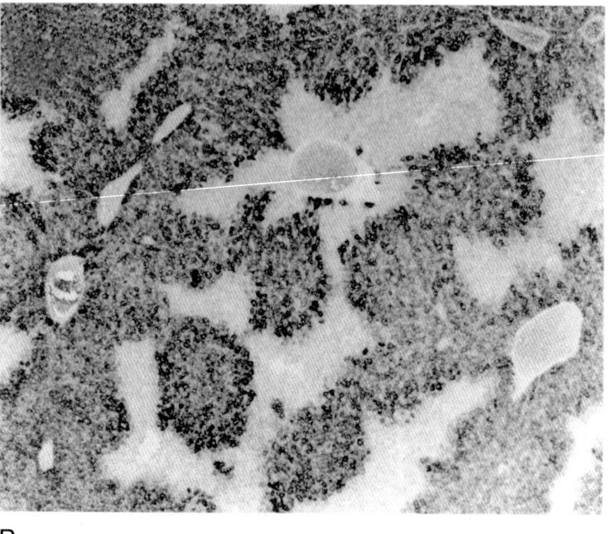

Figure 24-11 Immunochemical detection of trifluoracylated proteins in the livers of mice 24 hours after treatment with (*R*)- or (*S*)-halothane. **A**, From a mouse treated with (*R*)-halothane. **B**, From a mouse treated with (*S*)-halothane (original magnification ×50). *(From Njoku D, Laster MJ, Gong DH, et al: Biotransformation of halothane, enflurane, isoflurane and desflurane to trifluoroacetylated liver proteins: Association between protein acylation and liver injury. Anesth Analg 84:173-178, 1997.)*

of oxidative metabolism in vivo to reactive acyl halide metabolites (see Fig. 24-8). Because enflurane, isoflurane, and desflurane also contain an asymmetric carbon atom, the potential for stereoselective metabolism also exists with these agents. Indeed, other researchers have found that the ratio of (*R*)-enflurane metabolism to (*S*)-enflurane metabolism in human liver microsomes was 1.9:1.[48] It has also been demonstrated that optical isomers of isoflurane exhibit a significant difference in anesthetic potency,[80] differentially increase sleep time in mice,[81] and exhibit modest but significant stereoselectivity at the type A γ-aminobutyric acid ($GABA_A$) receptor.[82-84] Investigations with stereoisomers of anesthetic agents such as etomidate[85] also help provide a better understanding of the mechanisms of action of anesthetic agents. The clinical use of chiral anesthetic drugs as equal mixtures of their enantiomers has been accepted practice in medicine and anesthesia. With increased knowledge and awareness regarding drug toxicities, future anesthetic drugs may be developed and marketed as single, more potent and potentially less toxic optically active isomers.

Toxicity of Inhaled Anesthetics

Hepatitis

Volatile halogenated inhaled anesthetics have been associated with hepatotoxicity since the introduction of chloroform in 1847. Chloroform, as well as carbon tetrachloride and trichloroethylene, were all abandoned as anesthetic agents because of the often observed hepatotoxicity associated with their use. With the introduction of halothane into clinical practice in 1956, this compound quickly gained widespread acceptance and use. Halothane was the first of the fluorinated alkane anesthetics and represented a major advance in general anesthetics because it was safe, nonflammable, nonexplosive, and well tolerated by patients. However within 2 years of its introduction, numerous reports of hepatotoxicity and massive and often fatal hepatic necrosis associated with its use appeared in the medical literature. As a result of continuing reports, a large retrospective analysis was undertaken, "The National Halothane Study," under the auspices of the Committee on Anesthesia of the National Academy of Sciences National Research Council.[86] The purpose of this study was to compare the mortality and incidence of postoperative hepatic necrosis associated with halothane with that of other general anesthetics (ether, cyclopropane, and balanced anesthesia). The study reviewed 865,515 general anesthetics from 1959 to 1962 at 34 medical institutions and identified 82 cases of fatal hepatic necrosis. Drug-induced hepatic injury was suggested in nine of these cases, and seven of the nine patients had received halothane. Furthermore, four of the seven patients had received halothane on more than one occasion during the preceding 6 weeks. The study concluded that the mortality associated with the use of halothane compared favorably with that of other general anesthetics in use at the time and estimated the incidence of fatal hepatic necrosis associated with halothane to be 1 in 10,000 halothane anesthetics. It was further concluded that "unexplained fever and jaundice in a specific patient following the use of halothane should serve as a warning sign to avoid its subsequent use in that patient."[86] These findings provided the impetus for much of the work done over the past 50 years on the etiology of inhaled anesthetic hepatotoxicity, which is now accepted as a distinct clinical entity. Indeed, several hundred cases of hepatotoxicity have been attributed to halothane and approximately 50 cases to enflurane, but the incidence appears to be even lower with isoflurane and desflurane.[87]

Drug-induced liver injury may be caused by intrinsic or idiosyncratic mechanisms. Liver injury that is intrinsic to a particular pharmacologic agent is predictable and largely independent of host influences. Acetaminophen and chloroform are examples of pharmacologic agents that cause an intrinsic form of

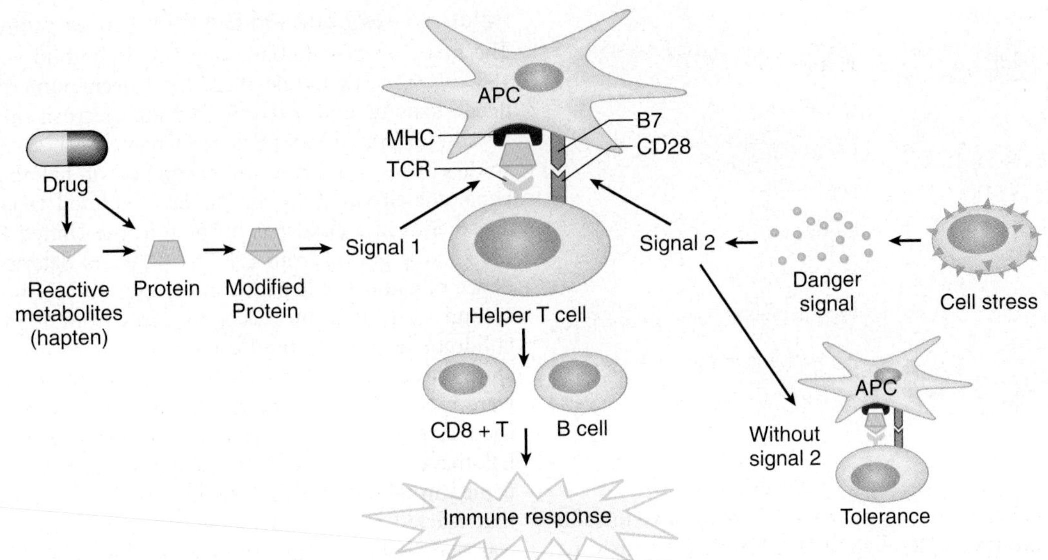

Figure 24-12 Hapten and danger hypotheses. The hapten hypothesis involves a chemically reactive drug or reactive metabolite acting as a hapten by binding to protein, which is then taken up by an antigen-presenting cell (APC) and processed. The processed antigen is presented in the context of the major histocompatibility complex (MHC) to a helper T cell; this represents signal 1. The danger hypothesis involves cell damage or stress (possibly caused by the drug or reactive metabolite) leading to the release of danger signals that result in upregulation of costimulatory factors; this is signal 2. Without signal 2, the result is immune tolerance. *(Redrawn from Uetrecht J: Idiosyncratic drug reactions: Past, present, and future. Chem Res Toxicol 21:84-92, 2008.)*

liver injury. The dose threshold for intrinsic toxicity may be achieved as a result of increased production, altered tissue sequestration, or decreased elimination of toxic metabolites. Moreover, other pharmacologic agents or chemicals, altered physiologic states, or pathologic states may affect the dose threshold for these toxicities. Nonetheless, when the dose threshold is surpassed, tissue injury may be caused by direct actions of the metabolite, which may result in inhibition or modification of the enzymatic and structural systems necessary for maintaining cellular integrity. In contrast to the intrinsic mechanisms of toxicity, many pharmacologic agents produce adverse reactions through an idiosyncratic pathway. These reactions are generally host dependent, relatively rare, and difficult to produce in animals in which the mechanisms can be systematically studied. Many idiosyncratic reactions, including liver injury caused by inhaled anesthetics, may have an immune basis. The injury is not due to the prodrug itself because small molecules are not immunogenic. Instead, reactive metabolites bind irreversibly to tissue proteins and produce a drug-protein adduct (or hapten-carrier conjugate) that can induce an immune response. The hapten hypothesis involves a chemically reactive drug or reactive metabolite acting as a hapten by binding to protein, which is then taken up by an antigen-presenting cell and processed. The processed antigen is presented in the context of the major histocompatibility complex to a helper T cell (signal 1). The danger hypothesis involves cell damage or stress (possibly caused by the drug or reactive metabolite) leading to the release of danger signals that result in the upregulation of costimulatory factors (signal 2). Without signal 2, the result is immune tolerance (Fig. 24-12).[88] In addition to the inhaled anesthetics halothane, enflurane, isoflurane, and desflurane, other examples of well-studied immune-mediated idiosyncratic drug reactions include penicillin and acetaminophen.[89]

Immune-Mediated Halothane Hepatotoxicity

Two distinct types of hepatic injury have been associated with the clinical use of halothane (Table 24-2). Mild injury occurs in 20% of adults who receive halothane, and laboratory tests show mild elevations in alanine aminotransferase (ALT) and aspartate aminotransferase (AST). The second type of injury is the fulminant form, commonly known as halothane hepatitis, which is characterized by elevated ALT, AST, bilirubin, and alkaline phosphatase levels; massive hepatic necrosis; and a fatality rate ranging from 50% to 75%. Because of the potential for halothane-induced hepatitis, halothane is not generally recommended for use in adults. In several medical malpractice cases, injury or death as a result of the use of halothane has been successfully litigated against anesthesia health care providers. Although there are some indications for the use of halothane in adults, they must be clearly evaluated and written in the medical record before each such use.

Table 24-2 Clinical Features of Halothane Hepatitis

Mild Form	Fulminant Form
Incidence, 1 : 5	Incidence, 1 : 10,000
Repeat exposure not necessary	Multiple exposures
Mild elevation of ALT, AST	Marked elevation of ALT, AST, bilirubin, alkaline phosphatase
Focal necrosis	Massive hepatic necrosis
Self-limited	Mortality rate, 50%
	Antibodies to halothane-altered protein antigens

ALT, alanine aminotransferase; AST, aspartate aminotransferase.

Table 24-3 Halothane Antigens

Molecular Mass (kd)	Protein
100	Endoplasmin
82	GRP-78
80	ERP-72
63	Calreticulin
59	Carboxylesterase
58	Protein disulfide isomerase (isoform)
57	Protein disulfide isomerase
54	Cytochrome P450

Halothane hepatotoxicity appears to link reactive metabolite formation and the hapten hypothesis. Halothane is oxidized by CYP2E1 to the reactive TFA-Cl metabolite (see Fig. 24-12). Although the incidence of liver failure is low, most patients in whom halothane hepatitis develops have antibodies against TFA-modified proteins. This implies that modification of protein by the reactive metabolite has led to an immune response. In addition, many patients have antibodies against native proteins. Patients often have a clinical history of multiple anesthetic exposure to halothane and one or more symptoms suggestive of ongoing immune processes, including fever, rash, arthralgia, and eosinophilia.[90-98] There is no evidence that the antibodies observed in halothane hepatitis actually mediate liver damage; it is entirely possible that they are just markers of an immune response. It appears that the TFA-protein adducts (Table 24-3) produced by the oxidative metabolism of halothane induce a cytotoxic T-cell response in sensitized individuals that on subsequent exposure leads to halothane hepatitis (Fig. 24-13).[99,100]

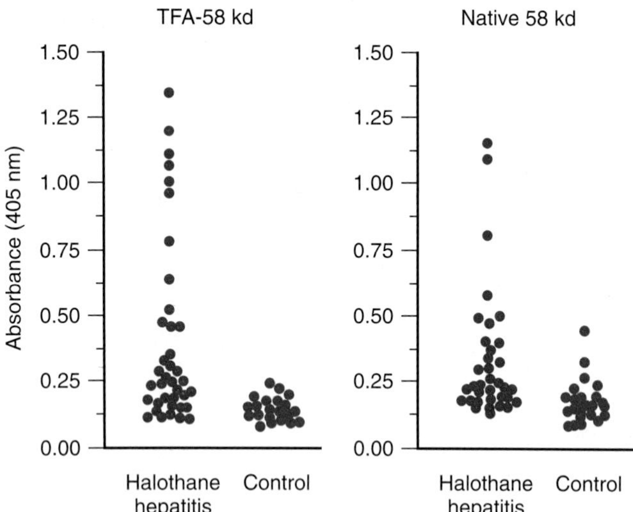

Figure 24-13 Enzyme-linked immunosorbent assay for the sera screening of patients with halothane hepatitis for antibodies that react with trifluoroacetylated 58-kd and native 58-kd proteins. All sera from 40 halothane hepatitis patients and 32 control patients were assayed at a 1 : 100 dilution. *(Adapted from Martin JL, Reed GF, Pohl LR: Association of anti-58 kDa endoplasmic reticulum antibodies with halothane hepatitis. Biochem Pharmacol 46:1247-1250, 1993.)*

Halothane Hepatitis in the Pediatric Population

The first case of halothane hepatitis in a child was reported in 1959.[101] Since that time there have been numerous reports of hepatotoxicity and massive hepatic necrosis after halothane anesthesia in children (also see Chapter 82). Two retrospective studies have examined the incidence of halothane-associated hepatotoxicity in children. The first explored 165,400 halothane anesthetics in a children's hospital in the United Kingdom over the 23-year period from 1957 to 1979 and determined the incidence of halothane hepatitis in children to be 1 in 82,000.[102] The second study examined 200,311 cases from 1958 to 1983 in a children's hospital in the United States. Only one patient in this study was concluded to have halothane hepatitis.[103] In 1987, data were reported describing halothane hepatitis in seven children aged 11 months to 15 years, all of whom had received multiple halothane anesthetics.[104] The diagnosis in this study was confirmed in all but one child by the presence of serum antibodies that reacted with halothane-altered hepatocyte antigens. There was one fatality in this group, and other causes of liver disease were excluded by the investigators. These findings indicate that the clinical syndrome of halothane hepatitis does exist in prepubertal children, although it is much rarer than in adults. The reason for the difference in incidence of halothane hepatitis observed between adults and children is not clear at present because halothane has been found to be metabolized to a similar degree in both adults and children and immune competence is known to exist from birth.

Enflurane, Isoflurane, Desflurane, and Sevoflurane

The incidence of liver injury caused by the fluorinated inhaled anesthetics follows the order of halothane > enflurane > isoflurane > desflurane and correlates with the extent of their oxidative metabolism (see Fig. 24-8), which is halothane (≈20%), enflurane (≈2.5%), isoflurane (≈0.2%), and desflurane (≈0.01%).[105] Because all of these inhaled anesthetics appear to form protein adducts that are identical or related in structure to those of halothane, it seems possible that they may cause liver injury by a mechanism similar to that of halothane, though at an appreciably lower incidence (Fig. 24-14). This lower incidence would be due to the lower levels of potentially immunogenic protein adducts formed from these drugs than from halothane when they are oxidatively metabolized by CYP2E1 (Fig. 24-15).

Enflurane was first used in North America in 1966. Although it is used much less commonly today, during the period of its highest use there were relatively few case reports of liver damage associated with it. In 1986, Eger and coauthors reviewed 10 published reports and several unpublished reports of liver damage after enflurane. Many of the cases were missing critical information on the duration of anesthetic exposure, histologic confirmation of hepatic lesions, and previous exposure to hepatic disease and hepatotoxic agents. In addition, several patients had been hypotensive or severely ill or demonstrated signs of shock and underwent operations with known potential for hepatic dysfunction. Obviously, these investigators had no choice but to conclude that the evidence did not support the existence of enflurane-associated hepatic dysfunction similar to that seen with halothane. Nevertheless, several case reports suggest that enflurane anesthesia given to patients previously anesthetized with or sensitized to halothane can result in hepatotoxicity. For example, it was found that protein adducts of halothane and enflurane, formed in the liver of rats treated separately with these drugs,

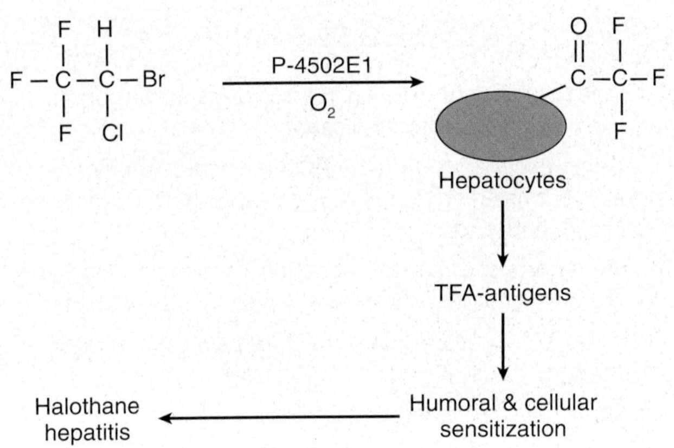

Figure 24-14 Pathway for generation of the immune response after exposure to anesthetic by susceptible patients. Halothane is metabolized to a trifluoroacetylated (TFA) adduct that binds to liver proteins. The altered protein is seen as nonself and generates an immune response, which on subsequent exposure leads to toxicity and cell death. A similar process may occur after exposure to other fluorinated drugs that generate a TFA or similar adduct. *(Adapted from Njoku D, Laster MJ, Gong DH, et al: Biotransformation of halothane, enflurane, isoflurane and desflurane to trifluoroacetylated liver proteins: Association between protein acylation and liver injury. Anesth Analg 84:173-178, 1997.)*

reacted with serum antibodies from patients in whom halothane hepatitis was diagnosed.[106] This apparent cross-reactivity could be explained by the similarity in structure of the protein adducts of halothane and enflurane (see Fig. 24-8).

Isoflurane, the structural isomer of enflurane, became available clinically in 1981. The combination of its minimal oxidative metabolism and low blood-gas solubility contributed to the popularity of this anesthetic agent. Moreover, for several years after its introduction there were no published reports of hepatic injury after the administration of this anesthetic. In 1991, a case report of fulminant hepatic failure after repeated isoflurane exposure was published.[107] In the same patient, the second isoflurane anesthetic for pyloroplasty was administered for a 2-hour period, and the third anesthetic for gastrojejunostomy was isoflurane for 30 minutes, followed by enflurane for 150 minutes. This patient had a far greater serum transaminase and alkaline phosphatase concentration after the second anesthetic than after the third exposure to anesthesia. In 2000, a case of fatal hepatotoxicity after re-exposure to isoflurane was reported in which histologic evidence of centrilobular injury and microvesicular fatty changes were found.[108] Similar histopathologic changes were observed in another case of isoflurane liver injury.[109] In addition, TFA-protein

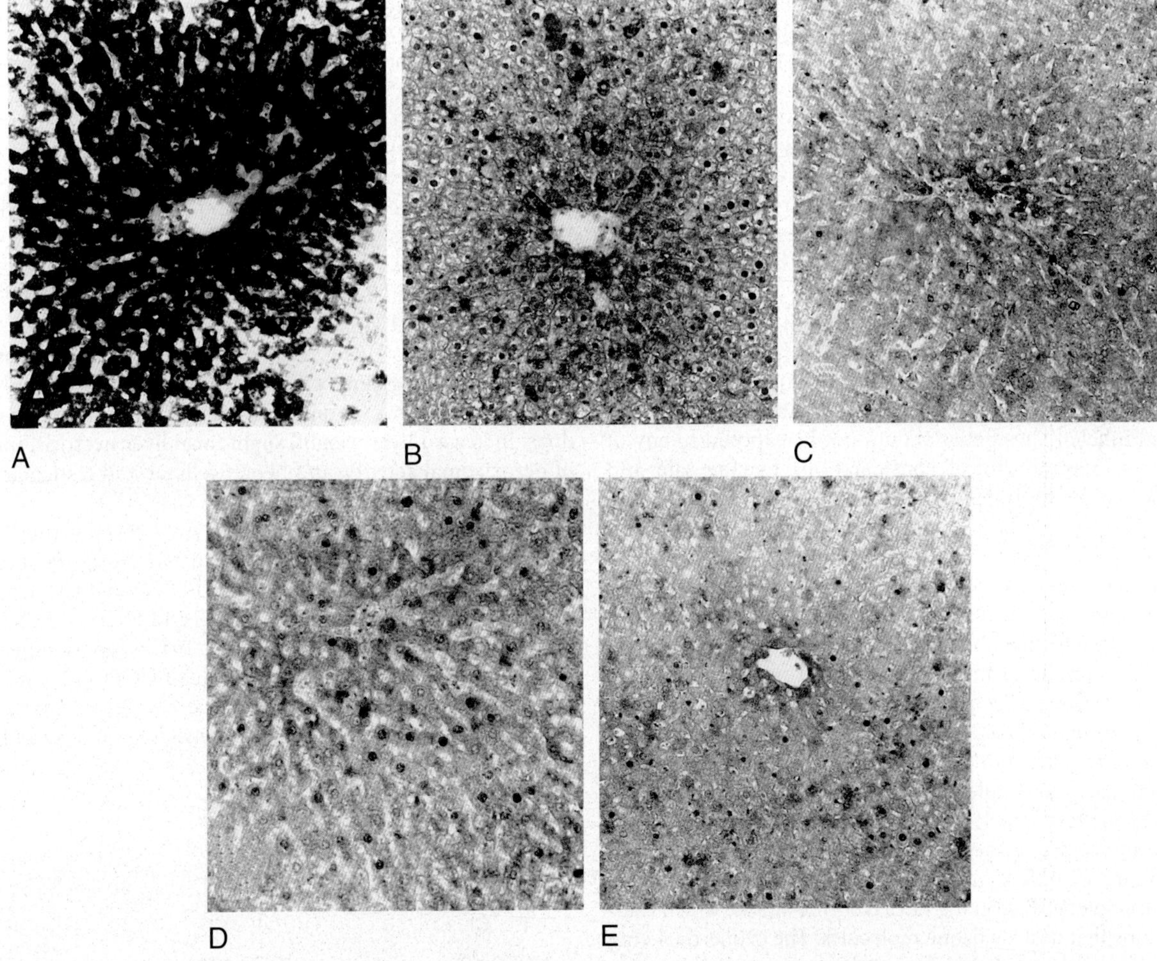

Figure 24-15 Livers from rats exposed to either halothane (**A**), enflurane (**B**), isoflurane (**C**), desflurane (**D**), or oxygen (**E**) were incubated with antitrifluoroacetylated rabbit serum to detect the presence of trifluoroacetylated liver proteins after exposure to anesthetic. Evidence of an immune response to trifluoroacetylated liver proteins can be seen in **A**, **B**, and **C**. No immunoreactivity is evident in **D** or **E**.

adducts were detected in the damaged mitochondria by electron microscopy. This finding suggests that the TFA-protein adducts may have contributed to the mitochondrial injury by a mechanism that was unrelated to an immunopathologic reaction induced by the TFA-protein adducts.

Although earlier studies of patients and volunteers did not suggest that desflurane is associated with hepatotoxicity in humans,[110,111] there are a handful of reports describing postoperative hepatotoxicity after exposure to desflurane. The first was a patient in whom fulminate hepatitis developed 12 days after receiving a desflurane anesthetic.[87] Because this patient had been exposed to halothane 10 and 18 years previously for periods of less than 1 hour, it is possible that the patient may have been sensitized to halothane. After exposure to desflurane, a cross-sensitization reaction may have occurred because both halothane and desflurane can form TFA-protein adducts. A second case has been reported in which a weak association between desflurane exposure and hepatotoxicity was described.[112] More recently, two additional cases were reported; the first was in an adult patient,[113] and the other is the first report of desflurane toxicity in a pediatric patient.[114]

There are several early case reports in the Japanese literature of sevoflurane being associated with postoperative hepatic dysfunction in patients ranging in age from 11 months to 63 years.[115,116] However, in all these reports, the association between sevoflurane exposure and liver injury as manifested by elevations in liver transaminases is extremely weak. In a single recent report from this country, postoperative liver injury was seen after sevoflurane anesthesia for appendectomy. However, this 3-year-old girl was suffering from iatrogenic acetaminophen intoxication, and it may be more likely that her injury was the result of acetaminophen rather than sevoflurane.[117] There has been a single case of fulminant hepatic failure and death attributed to sevoflurane anesthesia.[118] This patient died of multiple organ failure triggered by acute hepatic failure 2 days after open heart surgery with sevoflurane, sufentanil, and propofol anesthesia. Other possible causes of liver failure were excluded. It is worth noting again that sevoflurane is not metabolized to antigenic TFA-adducts, so the mechanism of injury in this case remains unexplained. However, it does reinforce the point that any patient sensitized to any of the fluorinated inhaled anesthetics should not be exposed to any of these agents. Several clinical considerations for the safe and reasonable use of fluorinated anesthetic agents are outlined in Box 24-1.

Hydrochlorofluorocarbons

Until the year 2000, the chlorofluorocarbons (CFCs) were widely used as industrial refrigerants, foam-blowing agents in the manufacture of plastics, aerosol propellants, food preservatives, and cleaning and sterilizing agents. The major source of CFC environmental contamination was the venting of automobile and truck air conditioning units into the atmosphere. CFCs are extremely stable, nontoxic, and nonflammable and were first identified as the compounds responsible for stratospheric ozone depletion in 1985. CFC molecules emitted into the lower atmosphere may take up to 7 years to diffuse upward into the stratosphere, where intense ultraviolet radiation liberates chlorine atoms, which catalyze reactions that destroy ozone molecules. The ozone-depleting potential of all halogenated hydrocarbons is a function of their molecular stability, stratospheric lifetime, and breakdown products (bromide being the most destructive and fluoride the least).

Box 24-1 Clinical Considerations

Halothane should not be used in adult patients without a specific, well-documented indication.

In patients experiencing postoperative hepatotoxicity after fluorinated inhaled anesthetics, these anesthetics should be avoided in the future.

Despite reports of halothane hepatitis in children, halothane remains an acceptable anesthetic choice for use in children.

Enflurane, isoflurane, and desflurane remain safer inhaled anesthetics.

Anesthetic-induced hepatitis remains a diagnosis of exclusion.

Once in place, these compounds may exist for 100 or more years. Depletion of stratospheric ozone may have adverse health effects worldwide, such as increases in the incidence of skin cancer and cataract formation. As a result, recommendations put forth by The Montreal Protocol on Substances That Deplete the Ozone Layer were adopted by the Environmental Protection Agency in the United States and by several other countries. These recommendations called for total elimination of CFCs by the year 2000.

The addition of hydrogen atoms to CFC molecules to form hydrochlorofluorocarbon (HCFC) molecules (Fig. 24-16) allows degradation of these compounds in the lower atmosphere with little effect on stratospheric ozone. HCFC-123 and HCFC-124 are currently used as a CFC replacement. Because of the striking structural similarity between HCFCs and halothane, it seemed possible that the HCFCs would also form TFA-protein adducts similar to halothane (Fig. 25-17) and possibly cause liver injury. In studies in rats, the relative concentrations of TFA-protein adducts formed in the liver after the administration of these compounds were similar between halothane and HCFC-123, much lower for HCFC-124, and nearly undetectable for HCFC-125.[119] Acute exposure to HCFC-123 has been shown to produce severe hepatotoxicity in guinea pigs, which was enhanced by prior glutathione depletion.[120] In subchronic studies performed in rats and dogs, increased liver weight, slight focal liver necrosis, induction of peroxisomal activity, and hepatocellular and testicular adenomas have been found.[121,122]

Human liver microsomes in vitro show a much higher capacity than rat liver microsomes to bioactivate HCFC-123 to reactive metabolites, suggesting that HCFCs might be hepatotoxic to humans. In this regard, HCFC-123 and HCFC-124 have been implicated in liver injury in humans.[123] In this report, nine workers were accidentally exposed to a mixture of HCFC-123 and HCFC-124 repeatedly. All nine exposed workers were affected to varying degrees. For one severely affected worker, liver biopsy and immu-

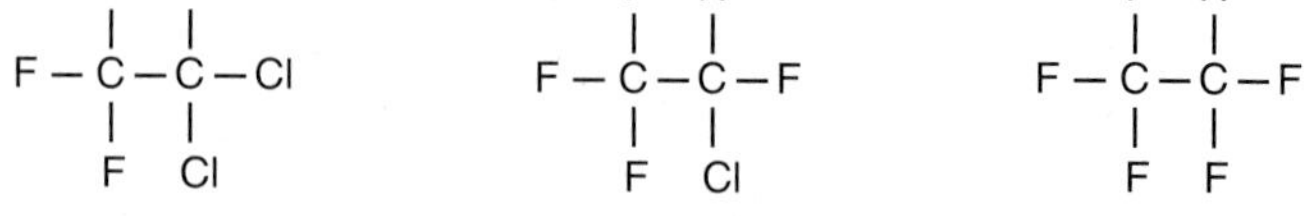

```
   F  H             F  H             F  H
   |  |             |  |             |  |
F—C—C—Cl         F—C—C—F          F—C—C—F
   |  |             |  |             |  |
   F  Cl            F  Cl            F  F

HCFC-123         HCFC-124         HCFC-125
```

Figure 24-16 Chemical structures of the hydrochlorofluorocarbon analogs of halothane, HCFC-123, HCFC-124, and HCFC-125.

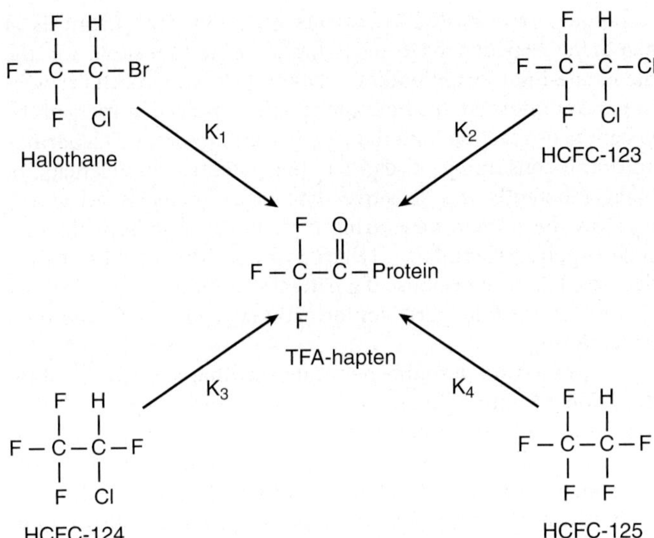

Figure 24-17 Metabolism of halothane and the hydrochlorofluorocarbon replacements HCFC-123, HCFC-124, and HCFC-125 to an identical trifluoroacetyl (TFA) metabolite.

nohistochemical staining for the presence of TFA-protein adducts were performed. The liver biopsy sample showed hepatocellular necrosis that was prominent in perivenular zone 3 and extended focally from portal tracts to portal tracts. TFA-adducted proteins were detected in the surviving hepatocytes. Autoantibodies against CYP2E1 or P58 were found in the sera of five of the nine affected workers. This report demonstrates that repeated exposure of human beings to HCFC-123 and HCFC-124 can result in serious liver injury in a high proportion of the exposed population. By contrast, halothane hepatitis occurs in only a small fraction of individuals repeatedly anesthetized with this compound. A possible explanation for this difference is that halothane is administered acutely to patients, whereas the injured workers were subchronically exposed to the HCFCs. It is possible that protracted formation of TFA-adducted proteins may result in direct toxicity. Alternatively, on the basis of in vitro metabolic studies with human liver CYP2E1, exposure of human beings to HCFC-123 might result in higher concentrations of TFA-adducted liver proteins than produced by halothane.[119] The presence of P58 and CYP2E1 autoantibodies in the serum of the exposed workers indicates that an immune component may have a role in the pathogenesis of HCFC-induced hepatotoxicity.

Presently, HFC-134a is used in virtually all automobile air conditioning units. In 2006, the European Union (EU) agreed to ban any fluorinated gas with global-warming potential (GWP) 150 times greater than an equivalent amount of CO_2 (the GWP of CO_2 is 1). Effectively, HFC-134a will be eliminated in EU countries by 2011. The best replacement candidate to date is a hydrofluoroolefin with a GWP of 4, HFO-1234yf, although unlike HFC-134a, this compound is mildly flammable. Interestingly, beginning in 2011, the German Association for Automotive Industry, which includes Audi, BMW, Daimler, Porsche, and Volkswagen, will begin replacing HFC-134a with CO_2 known in the industry as R-744. The atmospheric burden of CFCs is decreasing as a result of implementation of the Montreal Protocol. The importance of volatile anesthetics on the environment, particularly bromine-containing halothane, continues to be of some concern.

Methoxyflurane

No discussion of immune-mediated hepatotoxicity after inhaled halogenated anesthetics is complete without a brief discussion of methoxyflurane. From a historical perspective, methoxyflurane was introduced into clinical practice in the United States in 1960. There have been a number of reports of hepatic dysfunction and death from hepatic coma after exposure to methoxyflurane. A review of 24 cases of methoxyflurane-associated hepatitis revealed that a syndrome similar to halothane hepatitis may occur.[124] The authors suggested that a rare and indirect immunologic hepatic injury may occur that may have a direct effect on the liver by interfering with the splanchnic circulation. Fortunately, in humans the adverse minor changes in liver function appear to be reversible and may be related to dose, and it is still unclear whether hepatic dysfunction, as measured by bromsulphalein retention and serum hepatic enzyme elevation, was the result of the depth and duration of the anesthetic exposure, the type of operation, the extent of preexisting hepatic disease, or methoxyflurane itself.

Risk Factors for Anesthetic-Induced Hepatitis

The physiologic effects of inhaled halogenated anesthetics on the liver may affect the susceptibility to hepatic dysfunction after their administration. It is well known that inhaled anesthetics can reduce hepatic blood flow to some degree and may in this way contribute to postoperative hepatic dysfunction. However, studies of healthy volunteers found no evidence of hypoxia or anaerobic metabolism in the liver, but hypoxia or abnormalities in hepatic synthetic function may be present in patients with preexisting liver damage or other illnesses. In general, surgical manipulation or disturbance of the surgical site appears to be a more important factor in decreasing hepatic blood flow than the anesthetic agent or technique. In addition, preexisting conditions such as chronic liver disease secondary to alcoholism, viral infection (e.g., viral hepatitis and cytomegalovirus), septicemia, severe burns, nutritional deficiency, and previous or concomitant drug treatment may predispose patients to postoperative hepatic dysfunction. Unfortunately, a patient demonstrating clinical evidence of hepatic dysfunction after exposure to inhaled halogenated anesthetics presents a challenge to the anesthesia care provider because clinical tests to assess hepatic function can be nonspecific and reflect only severe hepatic dysfunction. Even so, traditional measures of hepatic function, such as serum enzymes, aminotransferases, proteins, bilirubin, and alkaline phosphatase, are still used to assess liver damage.

The mortality associated with halothane hepatitis has been reported to range from 40% to 75%. A variety of risk factors have been identified that are commonly associated with this clinical syndrome[125] (Box 24-2). Numerous studies have demonstrated that the risk for halothane hepatitis is greatly increased with use of an increasing number of anesthetics over a short period. Although the basis of this observation is not known, it is possible that increased exposure to TFA-protein adducts as a result of multiple treatments with halothane promotes the chance of a hypersensitivity reaction.

Halothane hepatitis may have a hereditary basis. The low incidence of the disease and the decreasing use of halothane make study of the genetic effects difficult and emphasize the

Box 24-2 Risk Factors for Anesthetic-Induced Hepatitis

Gender
Age
Obesity
Enzyme induction
Prior anesthetic exposure
Genetics

importance of developing an animal model of this disease. Several other associations exist for development of this disease. There is a clear sex difference observed in patients with halothane hepatitis. The disease develops in approximately twice as many females as males, the reason for which is unclear at present. In addition, the vast majority of cases of halothane hepatitis have occurred in middle-aged adults, with relatively few cases reported in prepubertal children,[102,103] and the disease is more common in obese than in nonobese patients. There is currently no evidence to suggest that the incidence of halothane hepatitis is increased in patients with liver disease unrelated to previous halothane exposure. However, because halothane can cause direct hepatotoxicity and other alternatives exist for the provision of general anesthesia, it is prudent to avoid halothane, as well as the other related fluorocarbon inhaled anesthetics, in patients with preexisting hepatic dysfunction.

Assays to Detect Patients Sensitized to Fluorinated Anesthetics

The diagnosis of halothane hepatitis has always been one of exclusion, whereas other potential causes of liver injury, such as hepatitis A, hepatitis B, hepatitis C, cytomegalovirus, Epstein-Barr virus, hepatotoxic drugs, hypotension, and hypoxia, are systematically ruled out as precipitating causes. One of the important goals of halothane hepatitis research is the development of an assay capable of detecting sensitized patients who may be at risk for the development of a hypersensitivity response on re-exposure to halothane or other fluorinated anesthetics, as well as detecting patients with the disease (Box 24-3). The assays that have been developed measure serum antibodies in halothane hepatitis patients. Two general types of immunochemical assays have been reported for detection of these antibodies. The first is immunoblotting. In this procedure, test antigens are microsomal proteins from halothane-treated rats or rabbits that have been separated into constituent polypeptides by sodium dodecyl sulfate–polyacrylamide gel electrophoresis and transferred electrophoretically to the surface of nitrocellulose membranes. With this technique, 42 of 68 (62%) patients with a clinical diagnosis of halothane hepatitis have been found to test positive for the halothane-induced antibodies.[92] Although this approach provides important information about the apparent molecular mass of the neoantigens reacting with the patients' antibodies, it is laborious and time consuming. It also has the potential disadvantage of being inherently less sensitive than other methods because it involves the protein-denaturing conditions of sodium dodecyl sulfate–polyacrylamide gel electrophoresis. This could lead to a decreased level of response if a patient's antibodies were directed against, at least in part, conformational epitopes of the TFA neoantigens.

Box 24-3 Investigation of Postoperative Liver Dysfunction

History and physical examination
Medications
Previous anesthetic exposure
Intraoperative course
Postoperative course
Clinical tests
Antibody screening

The second immunochemical assay that has been used for detection of antibodies in the sera of patients with a clinical diagnosis of halothane hepatitis is based on the more rapid, facile, and potentially more sensitive enzyme-linked immunosorbent assay methodology, in which test antigen is applied directly to the wells of a microtiter plate. One reported enzyme-linked immunosorbent assay procedure uses microsomes from halothane-treated rabbits as test antigen. With this approach, investigators have demonstrated the presence of the antibodies in the sera of 16 of 24 (67%)[126] and 28 of 39 (72%)[126] patients with a clinical diagnosis of halothane hepatitis. In another enzyme-linked immunosorbent assay that uses the TFA hapten as test antigen in the form of TFA–rabbit serum, albumin-positive responses in patients with a clinical diagnosis of halothane hepatitis were found in two of six (33%) patients[127] and five of six patients (83%).[128] More recently, purified proteins from rat liver have been used as test antigens in the enzyme-linked immunosorbent assay. In a study using three of the purified TFA-protein neoantigens (100, 80, and 57 kd), 79% of a group of 24 halothane hepatitis patients tested positive with this assay.[129]

Fluoride-Associated Nephrotoxicity

Evidence suggests that inhaled anesthetics may induce differential effects on renal physiology. For example, halothane and enflurane decrease the glomerular filtration rate and renal blood flow, whereas isoflurane may also decrease the glomerular filtration rate but has minimal effects on renal blood flow. Conversely, the newest inhaled halogenated anesthetics have minimal effects on renal physiology. Nevertheless, despite these physiologic effects, renal autoregulation protects the kidney from decreases in blood flow that may be caused by the inhaled anesthetic. Moreover, it has been suggested that decreases in the glomerular filtration rate caused by decreases in arterial pressure will return to baseline when arterial pressure normalizes. The metabolism of certain inhaled halogenated anesthetics can produce inorganic fluoride, which may be directly nephrotoxic. The potential for fluoride-associated nephrotoxicity after the administration of inhaled halogenated anesthetics is reviewed subsequently.

Methoxyflurane

Methoxyflurane is no longer used in clinical practice; however, nephrotoxicity from inorganic fluoride released after the metabolism of methoxyflurane is discussed as a basis for understanding the nephrotoxic potential of all current and future fluorinated anesthetics. Studies investigating methoxyflurane demonstrated an association with polyuric renal failure as a result of high levels of inorganic fluoride. Patients with inorganic fluoride levels of less than 50 μmol/L had no evidence of renal injury. Levels of 50 to 80 μmol/L were associated with moderate injury and 80 to 120 μmol/L with severe injury. Several patients who had inorganic fluoride levels higher than 120 μmol/L died.

Various mechanisms have been proposed to explain the renal injury from inorganic fluoride after the administration of methoxyflurane. One mechanism involves an inorganic fluoride–induced reduction in adenyl cyclase activity and subsequent effect on antidiuretic hormone.[130] Another mechanism involves effects on the renal countercurrent concentrating system by fluoride-induced increases in renal medullary blood flow. Nonetheless, the mechanism involving intrarenal metabolism of methoxyflurane and subsequent intrarenal production of fluoride ion is believed to be a significant cause of the renal toxicity of methoxyflurane.[131]

Despite the overall correlation between nephrotoxicity and peak serum fluoride concentrations, there is individual variability in the level of nephrotoxicity after methoxyflurane. Genetic heterogeneity, drug interactions, preexisting renal disease, and a host of other factors could account for the differences observed among patients.

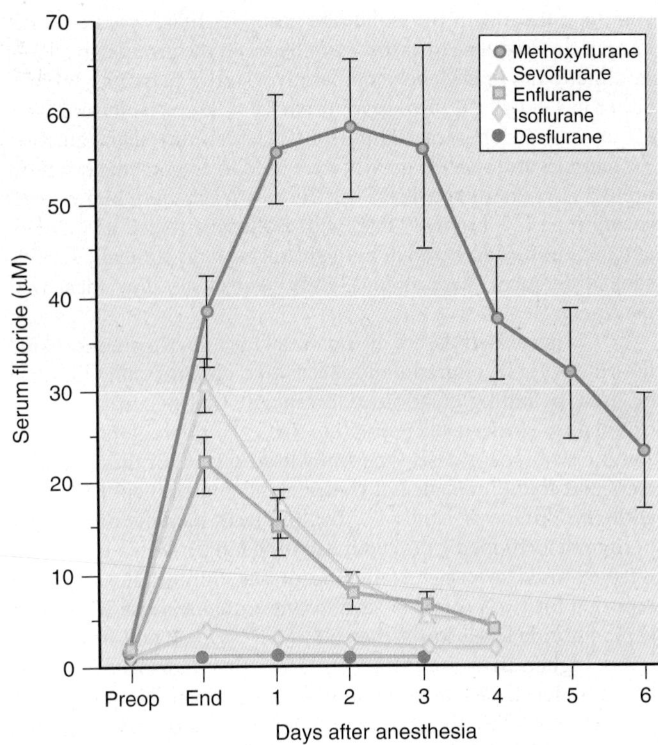

Figure 24-18 Serum inorganic fluoride (F^-) concentration before and after the administration of methoxyflurane, sevoflurane, enflurane, isoflurane, and desflurane anesthesia. After 2 to 3 minimum alveolar concentration (MAC)-hours of methoxyflurane, the mean peak F^- concentration was 61 ± 8 mol/L, which slowly declined. Sevoflurane anesthesia of 3.7 MAC-hours resulted in a mean peak F^- concentration of 30.6 ± 2 mol/L, which declined more rapidly than methoxyflurane but remained elevated for several days. After 2.7 MAC-hours of enflurane, mean peak F^- concentrations were 22.2 ± 2.8 mol/L, which also declined over a period of several days. There was no increase and almost no increase in F^- concentrations after desflurane and isoflurane administration, respectively.

Enflurane

In contrast to the renal effects of methoxyflurane, enflurane has been associated with only transient decreases in renal concentrating ability. When compared with methoxyflurane, serum fluoride concentrations after enflurane anesthesia peak earlier and fall more rapidly, thus emphasizing the important role of lipid solubility in determining total fluoride exposure (Fig. 24-18). Some clinicians have speculated that enflurane administered to patients with significant preexisting renal disease could produce additional renal dysfunction. Such fears have not been borne out, however.

Isoflurane

Isoflurane, an isomer of enflurane, is defluorinated much less than enflurane is. Because of the resistance to defluorination and the decreased likelihood of other toxicities, prolonged isoflurane administration has been investigated for use outside the operating room. Isoflurane was investigated for its effectiveness in long-term sedation of patients maintained on mechanical ventilation.[132,133] In the first study, the highest serum fluoride concentration was measured in a 2-year-old child who received 73 MAC-hours of isoflurane and had a serum fluoride level of 37.4 μmol/L.[134] In the second study, pediatric patients undergoing mechanical ventilation received isoflurane for 13 to 497 MAC-hours. The highest serum F^- concentration was 26.1 μmol/L, with no alterations in serum creatinine or osmolality.[133] From these studies we can safely conclude that isoflurane can be administered for very long periods without producing clinically significant serum fluoride concentrations; however, influences on metabolism and renal and hepatic function should be carefully considered.

Sevoflurane

Sevoflurane is defluorinated through oxidative metabolism (see Fig. 24-9) to approximately the same extent as enflurane.[135] Clinical studies show that serum fluoride concentrations often peak above 50 μmol/L even when sevoflurane is administered during surgery of average duration.[134] Because of sevoflurane's low blood-gas solubility and its rapid elimination, fluoride concentrations fall very quickly after surgery, and renal toxicity is not expected from sevoflurane administration. In vivo studies have shown that although peak fluoride levels are comparable to those with enflurane, sevoflurane has less nephrotoxic potential, as measured by maximum urine-concentrating ability and the production of *N*-acetyl-β-glucosaminidase (NAG), an indicator of renal tubular damage.[136-138]

In a 1994 study, inorganic fluoride levels were also compared after sevoflurane and isoflurane anesthesia.[138] The elimination half-life of fluoride was 8 hours. Mean fluoride levels after sevoflurane were 30 μmol/L, although five of the patients had levels higher than 50 μmol/L. The mean for isoflurane was significantly lower at 3.9 μmol/L. However, despite the high levels in five patients, there was no evidence of renal injury as detected by blood urea nitrogen (BUN) or creatinine in this study. A similar study comparing isoflurane and sevoflurane with longer MAC-hour exposure (13.5 hours) resulted in a longer fluoride elimination half-life of about 58 hours in the sevoflurane patients and dramatically higher mean levels of inorganic fluoride (42.5 μmol/L).[134] Half of all sevoflurane-exposed patients had fluoride levels higher than 50 μmol/L, but again no renal injury was apparent as evidenced by BUN and creatinine measurements. Higuchi and coworkers measured renal concentrating ability after 10.6 MAC-hour sevoflurane or 8.5 MAC-hour isoflurane in surgical patients. Mean peak fluoride levels were 41.9 ± 2.5 μM in the sevoflurane and 5.8 ± 0.4 μM in the isoflurane group.[139] There was no difference in the response to vasopressin between the groups. In a large multinational open-label comparative study, patients received either low-flow (1 L/min) sevoflurane ($n = 98$) or isoflurane ($n = 90$) anesthesia for at least 2 hours. BUN, creatinine, urine glucose, protein pH, and specific gravity were used to assess renal function up to 3 days after exposure. Peak fluoride levels were higher with sevoflurane (40 ±16 μM) than with isoflurane (3 ± 2 μM). BUN and creatinine decreased in both groups, and no clinically significant differences were found with respect to any measured parameter.[140]

To accurately assess the potential for injury from inorganic fluoride with sevoflurane, more sensitive measures may have to be used, including creatinine clearance (CCr), maximal urinary osmolality, urinary excretion of NAG, β_2-microglobulin, and alanine aminopeptidase. One study used several of these parameters and found evidence of transient subclinical nephrotoxicity with sevoflurane anesthesia.[141] In this study, patients underwent peripheral orthopedic procedures lasting longer than 5 hours and were exposed to either isoflurane or sevoflurane. Results were reported for two groups of sevoflurane patients, those with inorganic fluoride levels lower than 50 μM/L ($sevo_{low}$) and those with levels higher than 50 μM/L ($sevo_{high}$). This categorization was based on levels of inorganic fluoride determined 1 hour postoperatively: 4.8 μM/L for isoflurane, 36.8 μM/L for the $sevo_{low}$ group, and 55.8 μM/L for the $sevo_{high}$ group. BUN, creatinine, and CCr were normal in all groups throughout the study. Maximal urine osmolality showed a tendency toward the development of injury in the $sevo_{high}$ group. NAG levels were twice as high as isoflurane levels in the $sevo_{low}$ group and three times higher in the $sevo_{high}$ group, the latter showing evidence of subclinical renal injury. Clinically, transient loss of renal concentrating ability occurred in half the patients in the $sevo_{high}$ group. The dysfunction resolved within 6 days. An accompanying editorial suggested that this study raises the possibility of renal injury with sevoflurane in patients with impaired renal function and cautioned against its use in this patient group.[142] A second report of fluoride-induced renal injury in patients after sevoflurane anesthesia has recently been published.[143] However, a number of clinical reports have demonstrated very high levels of inorganic fluoride in some patients after sevoflurane anesthesia without obvious adverse effects. A report in 1996 described two such patients with refractory status asthmaticus, both treated with prolonged sevoflurane exposure under non-rebreathing conditions.[144] Despite very high inorganic fluoride levels, no obvious injury followed. It appears that the potential for significant renal impairment or injury after sevoflurane anesthesia in healthy patients solely as a result of inorganic fluoride is not an important clinical problem.

However, whether sevoflurane further affects renal tubular function in patients with impaired renal function is a question investigated by several groups. Cozen and associates compared sevoflurane ($n = 21$) with enflurane ($n = 20$) at 4-L/min fresh gas flow rates in patients with chronically impaired renal function (creatinine >1.5 mg/dL). Although peak fluoride levels were significantly higher in the sevoflurane group (25 ± 2.2 μM) than in the enflurane group (13.3 ± 1.1 μM), no difference was found in postoperative renal impairment.[145] Tsukamoto and colleagues compared sevoflurane ($n = 7$) with isoflurane ($n = 7$) in patients with moderately impaired renal function (CCr between 10 and 55 mM/min). Fluoride, urine NAG, γ-glutamyl transpeptidase (γ-GTP), and β_2-microglobulin were measured up to 2 weeks after surgery. With the exception of fluoride levels (sevoflurane group ⋙ isoflurane group), no differences in renal parameters were noted between the groups.[146] In a more recent study, Morita and colleagues[147] evaluated the effect of sevoflurane ($n = 15$) and propofol ($n = 15$) anesthesia on urine concentration and aquaporin-2 (AQP2) levels. AQP2 is an arginine vasopressin (AVP)-regulated water channel protein localized in the apical region of renal collecting duct cells. In both groups, plasma and urinary concentrations of AVP increased, although plasma osmolality remained unchanged. Urinary AQP2 excretion increased in the propofol group along with changes in urinary and plasma AVP. Urinary AQP2 was significantly lower at 90 minutes in the sevoflurane group, and urine osmolality showed a transient but significant decrease in parallel with AQP2 suppression, thus suggesting that sevoflurane may have produced a transient impairment of the APQ2 response to an increase in intrinsic AVP. However, because other inhaled anesthetics were not tested, it is not clear whether this observation applies to sevoflurane alone or is also a characteristic effect of other fluorinated inhaled anesthetic agents.

Desflurane

Clinical studies performed with desflurane thus far show no evidence of nephrotoxicity. Desflurane is extremely resistant to defluorination, and serum fluoride concentrations in surgical patients after exposure to desflurane are not increased above background concentrations.[148] From these findings, desflurane does not appear to be nephrotoxic.

Halothane

Halothane is not significantly defluorinated under normal clinical conditions and is not nephrotoxic. In patients who received about 19 MAC-hours of halothane, peak plasma fluoride levels were much higher in the isoflurane group than in the halothane group.[136]

In summary, fluoride-induced nephrotoxicity is a well-known entity historically associated with methoxyflurane administration and prolonged exposure to enflurane. During the administration of sevoflurane, serum inorganic fluoride levels can exceed 50 μmol/L, the level known to produce nephrotoxicity; however, no correlation with sevoflurane and polyuric renal failure has been documented. Two factors may help explain the differences seen with methoxyflurane and sevoflurane. First, it is not the peak serum fluoride concentration that determines injury but rather the duration of the systemic increase in fluoride (the area under the curve for serum fluoride). In addition, sevoflurane is an order of magnitude less soluble than methoxyflurane and thus is eliminated much more rapidly from the body. Second, the liver is the primary organ of sevoflurane metabolism, whereas both the liver and kidney metabolize methoxyflurane, and it is thought that the high intrarenal fluoride production from methoxyflurane contributes to its nephrotoxicity.

Anesthetic Degradation by Carbon Dioxide Absorbents

Sevoflurane and Compound A

Several decomposition products are formed during the interaction of sevoflurane with carbon dioxide absorbents, and

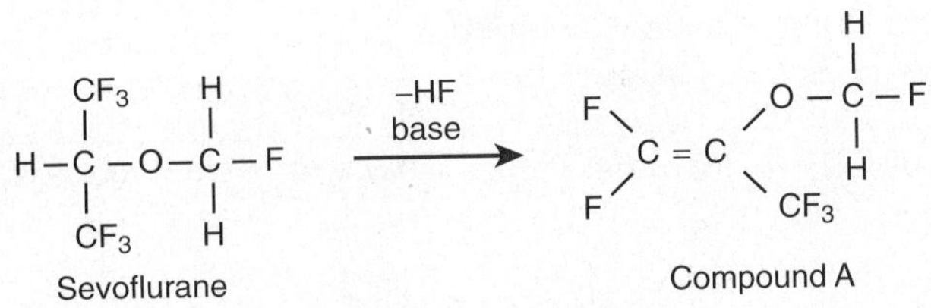

Figure 24-19 Sevoflurane degradation in the presence of base.

fluoromethyl-2-2-difluoro-1-(trifluoromethyl) vinyl ether (compound A) is the major degradation product detected (Fig. 24-19).[149-151] The dehydrofluorination of sevoflurane to form compound A is initiated by soda lime abstraction of a proton from the isopropyl group of sevoflurane in a manner that is similar to the base-catalyzed deprotonation of halothane by soda lime to yield bromochlorodifluoroethane (BCDFE, $F_2C = CBrCl$).

Compound A has been the subject of intense research and debate since the introduction of sevoflurane into clinical practice in the United States in 1995. Morio and coworkers found that high concentrations of compound A could cause renal injury and death in rats.[142] Other investigators have confirmed the findings of Morio and coworkers and have shown further that kidney injury occurs when levels of compound A reach 25 to 50 ppm or greater.[152] Necrosis is found primarily in the proximal tubular cells within the outer strip of the medulla, and the percentage of injured cells was lower 4 days after exposure than 1 day after exposure, consistent with repair after renal injury.[153] These and other studies suggest a threshold for renal injury of 150 to 300 ppm-hours of exposure to compound A, (e.g., 50 ppm of compound A administered for 3 hours).[153,154] Keller and coauthors reported that inspired concentrations of compound A greater than 114 ppm were associated with concentration-dependent increases in BUN, creatinine, and the urinary NAG/creatinine ratio.[153] Moderately severe histopathologic changes were noted at 202 ppm, and all chemical and histopathologic changes reversed within 14 days of exposure. This renal toxicity is both dose and time dependent: the higher the exposures over time, the greater the observed injury. During sevoflurane anesthesia in a closed or semiclosed system at low fresh gas inflow, patients are routinely exposed to compound A.

Several studies in surgical patients and human volunteers have been undertaken to investigate the possible association between sevoflurane anesthesia and renal injury as a result of exposure to compound A during sevoflurane anesthesia. In an early study, Bito and Ikeda exposed 10 patients to sevoflurane for longer than 5 hours under closed-circuit conditions with soda lime used as the absorbent.[149] Peak compound A concentrations were 19.5 ± 5.4 ppm, and serum BUN, creatinine, and electrolytes were essentially unchanged. In a follow-up study by the same investigators, 10 patients were exposed to sevoflurane at 1-L/min fresh gas flow for 10 hours. Mean compound A levels were 24.3 ± 2.4 ppm, and routine tests of renal function showed no change from preoperative values.[155] Frink and associates measured compound A levels in 16 surgical patients during low-flow sevoflurane anesthesia of 3 hours' duration with either soda lime ($n = 8$) or Baralyme ($n = 8$) used as the absorbent.[156] Maximum compound A concentrations averaged 8.16 ± 2.67 ppm with soda lime and 20.28 ± 8.6 ppm with Baralyme. A compound A concentration of 60.8 ppm was found in the breathing circuit of one of eight subjects to whom sevoflurane was administered with Baralyme absorption. In the same study, no compound A level exceeding 50 ppm was found in the eight volunteers in whom soda lime was used to scrub the carbon dioxide.

In a more comprehensive investigation, Bito and Ikeda studied 100 surgical patients undergoing resection of head and neck tumors in which surgery was expected to last longer than 10 hours. Patients received either sevoflurane ($n = 50$) or isoflurane ($n = 50$) anesthesia at low fresh gas inflow (1 L/min).[157] Mean peak compound A concentrations in the sevoflurane group were 24.6 ± 7.2 ppm. Although bilirubin, AST, and ALT levels increased postoperatively in both the sevoflurane and isoflurane groups, there were no significant differences in these parameters between the groups. Preoperative and postoperative BUN and creatinine levels remained unchanged. A number of other reports have used BUN and serum creatinine as markers of renal damage to evaluate renal function after closed-circuit or low-flow sevoflurane anesthesia,[158] and none of these studies demonstrated any change in either of these markers preoperatively and postoperatively.[157-159]

It has been argued that BUN and creatinine are not sensitive enough tests for detecting renal damage after exposure to compound A.[157-160] In an early attempt to address this issue, Kumano and colleagues measured urinary excretion of several renal tubular enzymes as measures of renal injury. Renal excretion of alanine aminopeptidase and NAG (enzymatic markers of renal integrity) increased 7 days after exposure to 7.6 MAC-hours of enflurane, but no increase was observed in patients receiving 9.6 MAC-hours of sevoflurane. Renal excretion of γ-GTP, β_2-microglobulin, BUN, and creatinine was unchanged.[161] Bito and associates studied 48 patients undergoing gastrectomy under both low-flow (1 L/min) ($n = 16$) and high-flow (6 to 10 L/min) ($n = 16$) sevoflurane anesthesia and low-flow isoflurane (1 L/min) ($n = 16$) anesthesia and looked not only at BUN and creatinine but also at CCr, NAG, and alanine aminopeptidase.[162] The average inspired compound A levels were 20 ppm in the $sevo_{low}$ group, and the average duration of exposure to this concentration was 6.11 hours. The only difference noted between the $sevo_{low}$ and the $sevo_{high}$ groups was the degree of compound A formation. Postanesthesia laboratory data showed no significant effects of compound A during sevoflurane anesthesia on any markers of renal function. Postanesthesia BUN and creatinine levels decreased, CCr increased, and urinary excretion of NAG and alanine aminopeptidase increased in all groups in comparison to preanesthesia values, but there was no significant differences observed between any of the groups. Kharasch and colleagues[163] completed a similar study in which 73 surgical patients received either sevoflurane or isoflurane anesthesia at a 1-L/min fresh gas flow. The duration of anesthesia was 3.7 or 3.9 hours, and the maximum inspired concentration of compound A was 27 ppm (range, 10 to 67 ppm). Areas under the inspired and expired compound A concentration-versus-time curves were 79 ppm-hours (range, 10 to 223 ppm-hours) and 53 ppm-hours (range, 6 to 159 ppm-hours), respectively. There were no significant differences between anesthetic groups in postoperative BUN, creatinine or urinary excretion of protein, or glucose (markers of proximal tubular resorptive function) or in NAG, proximal tubular α-glutathione-S-transferase (α-GST), or distal tubular π-GST (markers of tubular cell necrosis). The authors concluded that a moderate duration of low-flow sevoflurane anesthesia during which compound A formation occurs was as safe as low-flow isoflurane

Table 24-4 Percentage of Volunteers with Abnormal Renal Test Results after 8 Hours of 1.25 MAC Sevoflurane Anesthesia

	Eger Study[165]			Ebert Study[166]		
Determination	**Day 1 (%)**	**Day 2 (%)**	**Day 3 (%)**	**Day 1 (%)**	**Day 2 (%)**	**Day 3 (%)**
Glucose	75	50	80	15		
Albumin	88	60	90	31	31	31
α-GST	43	70	70	54	54	
π-GST	25	38	38	*		
MAC-hr exposure	328 ppm/hr			240 ppm/hr		

*The group mean was significantly increased above baseline. No individual data were reported. Blood urea nitrogen and creatinine levels were normal in all patients at all time points.
GST, glutathione-S-transferase; MAC, minimum alveolar concentration.

anesthesia. Nishiyama and associates studied the effect of repeat sevoflurane exposure within 30 to 90 days in neurosurgical patients.[164] Ten patients received sevoflurane at 6-L/min fresh gas flow rates on two occasions. Serum inorganic fluoride was measured 1 day after surgery, and BUN, creatinine, serum and urine β_2-microglobulin, urine NAG, and serum AST, ALT, and total bilirubin were measured 7 days postoperatively. Urine β_2-microglobulin, AST, and ALT all increased to abnormal levels after both anesthetics, with no differences observed between the anesthetics. Thus, the second sevoflurane exposure did not change the hepatic or renal metabolism of sevoflurane. These changes were indicative of mild hepatic and renal injury. The duration of anesthesia for the first and second anesthetics was 4.3 ± 0.6 hours and 4.0 ± 0.6 hours, respectively.

More recent studies in humans that have reported renal changes after the administration of sevoflurane have all occurred under conditions of prolonged sevoflurane exposure. Both Eger and colleagues[165] and Ebert and colleagues[166] exposed human volunteers to 8 hours of 1.25 MAC sevoflurane or desflurane anesthesia at a 2-L/min fresh gas flow rate and investigated pre-exposure and postexposure BUN, creatinine, and enzymatic markers of urinary function for up to 3 days or 5 to 7 days after exposure (Table 24-4). Both investigators found no difference in pre-exposure and postexposure BUN or creatinine levels in either group, but they found significant differences in enzymatic markers of renal integrity (α-GST and π-GST), albuminuria, and glucosuria in the sevoflurane-exposed group. All renal changes were transient, with normal return of renal function by 4 days after exposure in all but one volunteer, whose renal function was normal 2 weeks after exposure. In Eger's volunteers, rebreathing of sevoflurane produced an average inspired compound A concentration of 41 ppm and total exposure to compound A of 328 ppm-hours. In the Ebert study, volunteers were exposed to an average inspired compound A concentration of 27 ppm and a total exposure of 216 ppm-hours. With the exception or BUN and creatinine, both studies showed significant changes in urinary markers, the Ebert volunteers being lower on the compound A toxicity threshold curve and exhibiting less drastic changes in all markers of injury. When Goldberg and coworkers replicated Eger and colleagues' study, they obtained lower average compound A levels (253 ppm-hours) and found similar qualitative renal results.[167] Higuchi and associates[168] found increased excretion of urinary enzymes after average compound A concentrations of 215 ppm-hours. In another study, Higuchi and associates also found proteinuria in patients who were given low-flow (1 L/min) (n = 14) sevoflurane anesthesia and were undergoing orthopedic or dental surgeries, but not in those given high-flow (6 L/min) (n = 14) sevoflurane or low-flow isoflurane (n = 14).[169] Increased urinary NAG excretion was seen in the low-flow and high-flow sevoflurane groups, whereas BUN, creatinine, and CCr were unchanged in all groups. In human volunteers exposed to 1.25 MAC sevoflurane or desflurane for 4 hours (n = 9) or 2 hours (n = 7) at 2-L/min fresh gas flow, Eger and colleagues found average inspired compound A levels of 40 ppm. Relative to desflurane, sevoflurane given for 4 hours resulted in slightly increased urinary albumin and serum creatinine and increased urinary α-GST.[170] In a later study, Ebert and coworkers found that 5 MAC-hours of sevoflurane exposure at 1-L/min fresh gas flow, in which mean peak compound A levels were 39 ppm and total exposure to compound A was 152 ppm-hours, produced no changes in BUN, creatinine, or enzymatic markers of renal or hepatic (AST, ALT, and alkaline phosphatase) injury.[171]

Several studies have examined the use of sevoflurane in the pediatric population (also see Chapter 82). In a recent report, sevoflurane was compared with halothane anesthesia in children with a mean age of 6 years.[172] With comparable exposure, the sevoflurane group had significantly higher inorganic fluoride levels. There were no significant differences in BUN and creatinine levels, and there have been no reports of fluoride-associated renal toxicity in pediatric patients after sevoflurane anesthesia. Other tests of renal integrity were not performed. In another study, ASA class I and II children ranging in age from 3 months to 7 years received 1 MAC sevoflurane exposure at a fresh gas flow rate of 2 L/min.[173] The mean anesthetic exposure was 240 minutes, and fresh carbon dioxide absorbent was used for each patient. The soda lime temperature varied from 23°C to almost 41°C, and the inspired and expired compound A concentrations were 5.4 and 3.7 ppm, respectively. There were no differences in clinical chemical parameters, as reflected by AST, ALT, alkaline phosphatase, bilirubin, BUN, and creatinine. The maximum soda lime temperature correlated with both maximum compound A concentrations and the body surface area of the child. Therefore, to date, there have been no reports of markedly abnormal renal chemical findings in pediatric patients after exposure to sevoflurane.

There is some potential concern in pediatric patients related to HFIP, the major metabolite of sevoflurane, because levels of this metabolite may become relatively high as a result of a deficiency in UGTs that conjugate glucuronic acid to HFIP (see Fig. 24-9). For example, in one study neonatal rats were found to have

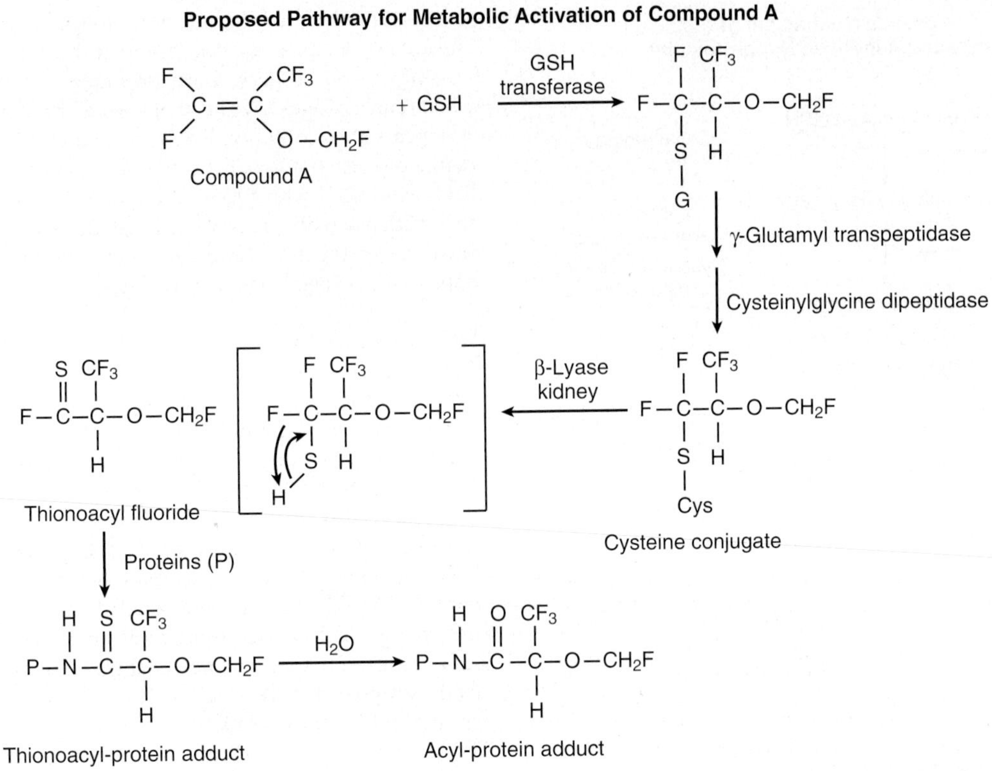

Proposed Pathway for Metabolic Activation of Compound A

Compound A + GSH → (GSH transferase) → glutathione conjugate → (γ-Glutamyl transpeptidase; Cysteinylglycine dipeptidase) → Cysteine conjugate → (β-Lyase kidney) → [intermediate] → Thionoacyl fluoride → (Proteins (P)) → Thionoacyl-protein adduct → (H_2O) → Acyl-protein adduct

Figure 24-20 Proposed pathway for the metabolic activation of compound A showing the formation of an intrahepatic glutathione (GSH) conjugate of compound A that is translocated to the kidney, where γ-glutamyl transpeptidase, cysteinyl glycine dipeptidase, and the renal cysteine conjugate β-lyase catalyze the formation of a nephrotoxic thiol that can acylate kidney proteins. *(Adapted from Martin JL, Kandel L, Laster, MJ, et al: Studies of the mechanism of nephrotoxicity of compound A in rats. J Anesth 11:32-37, 1997.)*

high levels of free HFIP for as long as 21 postnatal days after sevoflurane exposure.[174]

It has been hypothesized that the reason that compound A causes serious injury to kidneys in rats but not humans is because of differences in levels of renal cysteine conjugate β-lyase enzymes,[175] which have been hypothesized to catalyze the conversion of compound A to a reactive thionoacyl fluoride metabolite that can acylate kidney proteins and cause toxicity (Fig. 24-20). Indeed, renal cytosolic and mitochondrial β-lyase enzyme levels in rats are approximately 20 to 30 times higher than those found in humans.[176-178] There is evidence to support the β-lyase theory of compound A–induced nephrotoxicity. Renal β-lyase appears to mediate the renal toxicity produced by several fluorinated alkenes that are structurally similar to compound A,[179-181] and metabolic intermediates of the β-lyase pathway have been identified in the bile and urine of rats and human tissues exposed to compound A.[158,163,177,178,182] Moreover, the glutathione-*S*-conjugate of compound A is nephrotoxic,[183] and the administration of aminooxyacetic acid (AOAA), an inhibitor of β-lyase (Fig. 24-21), protects against the nephrotoxicity of compound A in rats.[184] However, there is some controversy surrounding the relevance of the β-lyase pathway in compound A–induced renal injury.[182,185,186] More recently, Altuntas and coauthors reported an additional pathway of compound A metabolism, sulfoxidation.[187] The investigators showed that compound A cysteine and mercapturic acid conjugates are metabolized both enzymatically and nonenzymatically to sulfoxide metabolites. The enzymatic process was catalyzed by CYP3A1/2 and CYP3A4/5, and there exists a species difference in rat and human liver and kidney microsomes (rat > human and liver > kidney). Sulfoxide conjugates have recently been shown to be more toxic than the corresponding parent cysteine or mercapturic acid compound A conjugate. However, the toxicologic significance of *S*-conjugate sulfoxidation of compound A remains unknown. It represents an alternative route of metabolism to the deacetylation or the β-lyase pathways. Whether sulfoxidation occurs in vivo is uncertain, as is its toxicologic significance.

Investigators have reported that pretreatment of rats with AOAA and acivicin (AT-125), inhibitors of the β-lyase pathway (see Fig. 24-19),[185] did not attenuate the nephrotoxicity produced by compound A but rather was associated with nearly a threefold increase in renal injury, from 19% to 53%. These findings suggest that the β-lyase pathway may actually be a detoxification pathway. In this regard, a report by Kharasch and coworkers[186] showed that pretreatment of rats with AOAA partially protected against compound A–induced diuresis and proteinuria but failed to protect against glucosuria. In another report, AOAA again failed to decrease histologic renal injury, and pretreatment with acivicin significantly increased renal injury.[185] Moreover, using an immunochemical approach, other investigators were unable to detect protein adducts of a thionoacyl fluoride metabolite of compound A in the kidneys of rats after compound A treatment, suggesting that the β-lyase pathway of compound A metabolism in rats either does not occur or is a minor pathway of metabolism. Therefore, these findings suggest that another pathway of metabolism of compound A may be responsible for the nephrotoxicity of compound A.

Higuchi and colleagues studied the effect of low-flow sevoflurane or isoflurane anesthesia (1 L/min) on 17 patients with

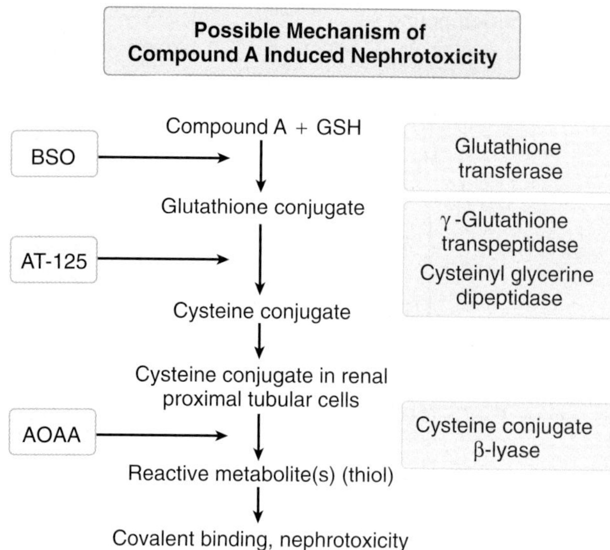

Figure 24-21 Crucial steps in the β-lyase pathway: first, conjugation of compound A with glutathione in the liver mediated by glutathione-S-transferase; this conjugate is then transported to the kidney. Second, the glutathione-S-conjugate is converted to a cysteine-S-conjugate, a process mediated by γ-glutamyl transpeptidase. Finally, the cysteine-S-conjugate of compound A is then converted to a reactive thiol, mediated by the renal cysteine conjugate β-lyase; DL-buthionine-(*S*,*R*)-sulfoximine (BSO) depletes endogenous stores of glutathione in the body, acivicin (AT-125) inhibits the activity of γ-glutamyl transpeptidase, and aminooxyacetic acid (AOAA) inhibits the activity of β-lyase. Compound A, its conjugates, and the reactive thiol have all been postulated to cause the renal necrosis that can occur in rats after the administration of compound A and the glucosuria and enzymuria that can result in rats and humans from the administration of compound A.

stable moderate renal failure (serum creatinine >1.5 mg/dL). They found no difference in BUN or creatinine up to 14 days after exposure or in CCr at 7 days after exposure in either group for patient exposures less than 130 ppm-hours of compound A.[188] In a recent multicenter randomized controlled trial, Conzen and coworkers studied 116 patients with stable renal insufficiency (CCr >1.5 mg/dL) who were administered either low-flow (1 L/min) sevoflurane (n = 59) or isoflurane (n = 57) anesthesia.[189] Total exposure to sevoflurane was 201.3 ± 98 minutes, with an average total compound A exposure of 18.9 ± 7.6 ppm. Isoflurane exposure averaged 213.6 ± 83.4 minutes, and Baralyme was used as the carbon dioxide absorbent. No significant changes above baseline values for serum creatinine, BUN, CCr, urine protein, or glucose were found at 24 or 72 hours after exposure to either anesthetic.

So what does this all mean and how does it translate into clinical care of patients? In a rebreathing system with a carbon dioxide absorber in lime (soda lime or Baralyme), patients exposed to sevoflurane will breathe compound A. The typical levels seen in clinical conditions will vary and are dependent on several factors, the most important being the inspired fresh gas flow rate. The key factor in determining potential toxicity from sevoflurane is total exposure rather than the absolute concentration, with exposure being expressed as the product of concentration and time. It appears from the many studies published to date that the lower threshold for renal changes associated with sevoflurane exposure and compound A is approximately 150 ppm-hours. At a fresh gas inflow of 2 L/min, these levels would be expected to be seen only in conditions of prolonged sevoflurane exposure and are not of concern to the vast majority of patients undergoing anesthesia and surgery. With prolonged sevoflurane exposure, when renal changes have been observed, they have been transient. It appears that compound A is of theoretical concern and academic interest, but to date no significant clinical renal toxicity has been associated with the use of sevoflurane. It is recommended that patients with preexisting renal disease not be exposed to sevoflurane and that sevoflurane be administered according to approved package labeling guidelines.

Halothane and Bromochlorodifluoroethane

Carbon dioxide absorbents also degrade halothane by a dehydrofluorination reaction to form BCDFE (F_2C = CBrCl). The potential nephrotoxicity of BCDFE was compared with that of compound A in a study by Eger and coworkers,[190] who found that (1) BCDFE was 80% less reactive than compound A; (2) halothane degraded to BCDFE 20- to 40-fold less than sevoflurane did to compound A in a standard circle system; (3) BCDFE was 75% less nephrotoxic to rats than compound A was; and (4) compounds that blocked the renal β-lyase pathway either did not change or decreased renal injury from BCDFE, whereas the same blockers either did not change or increased renal injury from compound A (see Fig. 24-21), suggesting that BCDFE and compound A may cause kidney injury by different mechanisms. These studies clearly indicate that the chance of BCDFE causing nephrotoxicity when halothane is being used as an anesthetic is negligible.

Carbon Monoxide and Heat

Carbon monoxide (CO) is an odorless, colorless, gas that is poisonous because it displaces oxygen from hemoglobin in blood and thereby leads to the formation of carboxyhemoglobin. Its affinity for binding hemoglobin is 250 times greater than that of oxygen. All humans have some CO bound to hemoglobin in their blood, on average 1% for nonsmokers and as much as 10% for those who smoke. High levels of CO can produce neuropsychiatric problems in patients, and when levels of carboxyhemoglobin reach 50%, death can occur. The problem of CO poisoning has been reported during clinical anesthesia.[191-196] The difficulty in monitoring CO levels clinically arises from the fact that pulse oximeters have not distinguished between carboxyhemoglobin and oxyhemoglobin. Masimo has just developed such a pulse oximeter that should correct this problem.

All inhaled anesthetics produce some CO as a result of their interaction with the strong bases in relatively dry carbon dioxide (CO_2) absorbents (water content <5%).[197] Several factors influence the level of CO production, including the choice of anesthetic agent, the inspired anesthetic concentration, and the type, temperature, and most important, the degree of dryness of the CO_2 absorbent.[198] Of the inhaled anesthetics, desflurane produces the most CO, followed by enflurane, isoflurane, and negligible amounts from sevoflurane and halothane (Fig. 24-22).[198,199] Intraoperative formation of CO has been reported with desflurane, enflurane, and isoflurane, with CO levels exceeding those established as safe by the U.S. Environmental Protection Agency. Desflurane, enflurane, and isoflurane are all difluoromethyl-ethyl ethers, whereas sevoflurane is a monofluoromethyl ether and halothane is an alkane. The specific mechanism appears to be abstraction of a base-catalyzed difluoromethoxy proton from the anesthetic agent (Fig. 24-23).[199] Furthermore, it has been shown

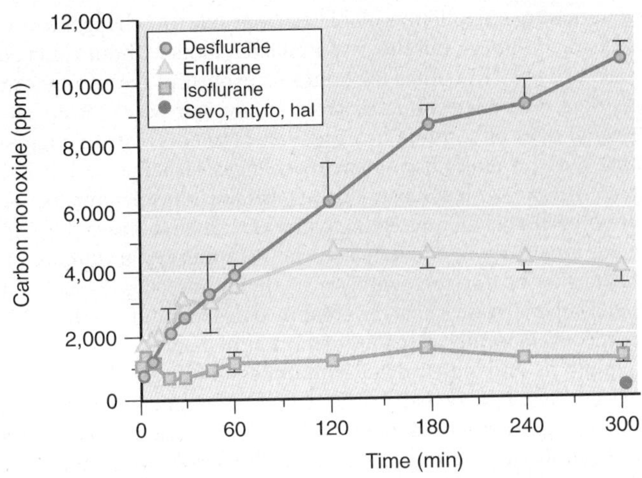

A

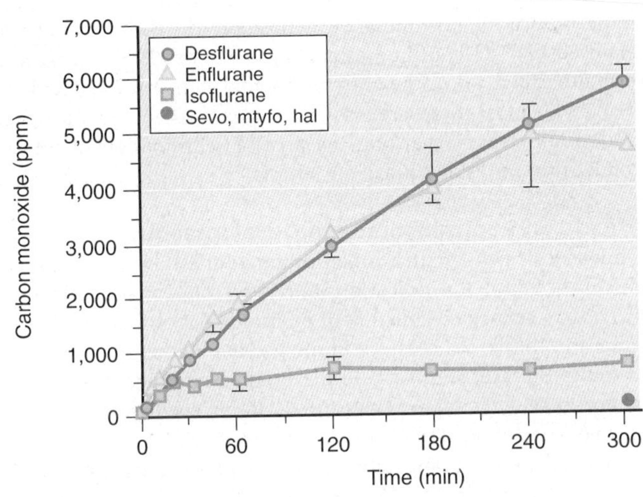

B

Figure 24-22 Anesthetic degradation to carbon monoxide at equivalent minimum alveolar concentrations (1.5 MAC) by barium hydroxide lime (**A**) and soda lime (**B**). Each data point is the mean ± SD ($n = 3$). The single data point at 300 minutes reflects undetectable carbon monoxide from sevoflurane (sevo), methoxyflurane (mtyfo), or halothane (hal). *(Adapted from Baxter PJ, Garton K, Kharasch ED: Mechanistic aspects of carbon monoxide formation from volatile anesthetics. Anesthesiology 89:929-941, 1998.)*

that abstraction of a proton from the difluoromethoxy group is greater with potassium (KOH) than with sodium hydroxide (NaOH).[199,200] Barium hydroxide ($Ba[OH]_2$) contains 4.6% KOH, whereas soda lime contains only 2.5% KOH and 1.5% NaOH. Unlike KOH and NaOH, $Ba(OH)_2$ does not abstract a proton from the difluoromethoxy moiety and catalyze the formation of CO from inhaled anesthetics. Because the divalent $Ca(OH)_2$ and $Ba(OH)_2$ bases are the major active components of the absorbents, the capacity to produce CO is rapidly exhausted, whereas the absorbents retain their capacity to remove CO_2.

New calcium hydroxide–based CO_2 absorbents such as Amsorb and DragerSorb Free contain neither NaOH or KOH and are chemically inert and do not degrade inhaled anesthetics to CO or degrade sevoflurane to compound A.[201] Fully hydrated or rehydrated absorbents do not degrade inhaled anesthetics to CO. Soda lime contains 15% water by weight, and only after this level of hydration has been decreased to about 1.4% will appreciable amounts of CO be formed. In contrast, Baralyme contains 13% water by weight and the threshold of hydration before CO is formed is 4.8%. However, even at these threshold levels, very little CO is actually produced. Production of large amounts of CO requires complete or nearly complete desiccation of the absorbent, a process that requires high flow of dry gas (10 L) for prolonged periods (1 to 2 days). Certain patients had high levels of CO, particularly prevalent in the first case on Mondays.[191] This appeared to be related to the practice of flushing the anesthesia machine with high fresh gas flow over the weekend, which dries out the CO_2 absorbent. Higher temperatures are also associated with increased CO production.

In general, CO toxicity has little clinical significance, regardless of the anesthetic used, as long as simple guidelines to minimize or eliminate CO are observed, including the use of fresh absorbent, the use of soda lime instead of Baralyme, or perhaps better yet, the use of a calcium hydroxide–based CO_2 absorbent. Avoidance of techniques that dehydrate the CO_2 absorbent in the anesthetic circuit is also helpful, such as low fresh gas flow, which is more economical and limits desiccation of the absorbent. Finally, as a last resort the absorbent can be rehydrated simply by adding approximately one cup of water (230 mL) per 1.2 kg of absorbent (standard canister).

The interaction of inhaled anesthetics with CO_2 absorbents is an exothermic reaction that results in the production of heat. The temperature of CO_2 canisters during routine clinical use averages 25°C to 45°C but increases inversely with decreased fresh gas flow; sevoflurane is associated with the greatest production of heat. By-products of this reaction also include HFIP, formaldehyde, methanol, sodium formate, and importantly, hydrogen. The high yield of hydrogen, up to 3 mol of hydrogen per mole of sevoflurane, ease of ignition, and low tissue solubility make it the most likely fuel in anesthesia machine fires because of reactions with desiccated CO_2 absorbents and sevoflurane.[202] These reactions can be significant and result in fires, toxic gases, and patient injury.[203,204] In laboratory settings, prolonged exposure of 1 MAC

$$F_3C{-}CHX{-}O{-}CF_2{-}H + OH^- \rightleftharpoons F_3C{-}CHX{-}O{-}CF_2^- + H_2O$$

$$F_3C{-}CHX{-}O{-}CF_2^- \longrightarrow F_3C{-}C(O){-}H + :CF_2 + X^-$$

$$:CF_2 + H_2O \longrightarrow CO + 2HF$$

$$CF_3CHO + OH^- \longrightarrow CF_3H + HCO_2^-$$

Figure 24-23 Proposed mechanism of carbon monoxide formation from difluoromethyl-ethyl ether anesthetics. Shown is the backbone structure for isoflurane (X = Cl) and desflurane (X = F). Also shown is a putative mechanism for the concomitant formation of trifluoromethane. Water in line 3 may also react as OH^-. *(Adapted from Baxter PJ, Garton K, Kharasch ED: Mechanistic aspects of carbon monoxide formation from volatile anesthetics. Anesthesiology 89:929-941, 1998.)*

sevoflurane to desiccated CO_2 absorbents resulted in canister temperatures in excess of 300°C.[205] At these high temperatures, patient injuries as a result of explosions, fires, and smoldering and melting of the plastic components of anesthesia equipment are all real possibilities. Two recent studies have documented lower concentrations of toxic sevoflurane breakdown products with use of the new-generation CO_2 absorbents.[206,207] Perhaps at some time in the near future the sodium hydroxide– and barium hydroxide–based CO_2 absorbents will be replaced by the nondestructive newer, less reactive calcium hydroxide–based CO_2 absorbents.

Other Toxicities

Nitrous Oxide and Inhaled Anesthetics

Nitrous oxide has been used and abused since its introduction into clinical practice in 1845. It is unique in its ability to oxidize vitamin B_{12} and inactivate methionine synthase and is the only anesthetic known to produce hematologic toxicity and neurotoxicity with long-term administration. Both these toxicities are the result of disruption of several pathways involved in one-carbon chemistry. After several hours of routine anesthesia with N_2O, methionine synthase activity is very low. Methionine synthase catalyzes the conversion of methyltetrahydrofolate and homocysteine to tetrahydrofolate and methionine. Failure to produce these products has a number of biochemical consequences, including reduced synthesis of thymidine, which is an essential DNA base. The reduction in thymidine synthesis takes somewhat longer to develop but lasts several days. The clinical syndrome associated with oxidation of vitamin B_{12} is essentially the same as that seen in pernicious anemia: megaloblastic hematopoiesis and subacute combined degeneration of the spinal cord. The time required to produce megaloblastic hematopoiesis with exposure to N_2O varies among patients. In healthy patients undergoing routine surgery, mild megaloblastic bone marrow changes are not seen after 6 hours, but they are seen after about 12 hours of exposure to 50% N_2O; after 24 hours of exposure, the changes are marked. Complete bone marrow failure can be expected after several days of continuous exposure. Limited evidence suggests that N_2O produces bone marrow changes earlier in seriously ill patients, and evidence also suggests that the bone marrow changes are preventable by pretreating patients with large doses of folinic acid. This drug is converted to the 5,10-methylene tetrahydrofolate needed for the synthesis of thymidine (Fig. 24-24). The neurologic disease, subacute combined degeneration of the spinal cord, develops only after several months of daily exposure to N_2O. Symptoms and signs include numbness and paresthesia in the extremities, loss of balance and unsteady gait, impairment of touch, and muscle weakness. Earlier, the disease was recognized to be similar to vitamin B_{12} deficiency, but treatment with vitamin B_{12} did not alleviate the symptoms or enhance recovery; thus, it occurs in those who abuse N_2O on a long-term basis.[208,209] Sporadic reports of postoperative neurologic disorders in patients exposed to N_2O continue to appear.[210-212] For all of the reasons just described and other environmental concerns that will be discussed later, there are serious discussions in the European Union and Japan regarding the possible elimination of nitrous oxide from modern clinical anesthesia.

Effects on Reproduction and Development

Thousands of pregnant women undergo anesthesia and surgery during gestation for indications unrelated to pregnancy. The incidence of unexpected abortion or premature labor is clearly higher after anesthesia. What is not immediately obvious is whether the patient's disease, surgery, anesthesia, or a combination of these factors is the precipitating cause. Perhaps an even greater concern is that anesthesia during pregnancy may lead to an increased incidence of congenital abnormalities in the offspring of the

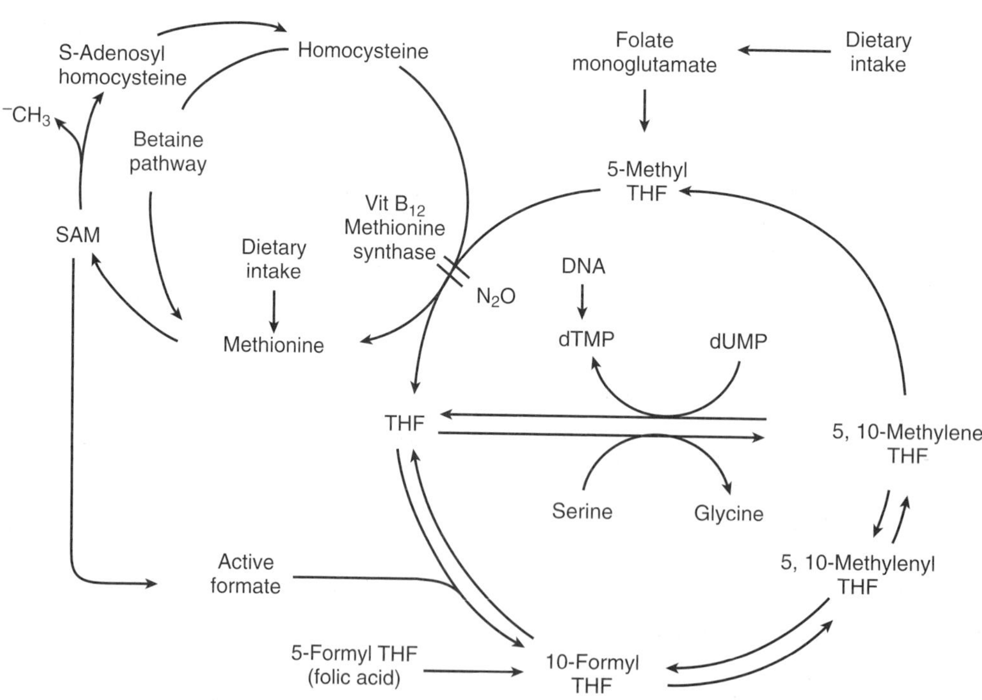

Figure 24-24 Conversion of methyltetrahydrofolate (5-Methyl THF) and homocysteine to tetrahydrofolate and methionine. dTMP, d-thymidine monophosphate; dUMP, d-uridine monophosphate; SAM, s-adenosyl methionine.

patient. A number of studies have been undertaken over the past 40 years to assess the incidence of various anesthesia- and surgery-related hazards occurring during pregnancy. In short, these studies have found that women who underwent surgery did not have an increased incidence of stillbirths or congenital anomalies among offspring. In contrast, the incidence of postnatal death within 7 days of delivery was increased when an operation occurred during the second or third trimester but not during the first trimester. The incidence of low birth weight and premature delivery was increased regardless of the trimester in which an operation occurred. The cause of these hazards was not determined, although the finding that no particular type of operation or anesthesia was associated with a higher incidence of adverse outcomes suggests that the patient's disease played the major role in determining the outcome.

In recent years, the increasing popularity of in vitro fertilization has afforded some opportunity to study the effects of anesthetics on ova. Various anesthetic regimens have been examined for their effects on rates of fertilization and cleavage of oocytes, pregnancy, and carriage to term. The results with general anesthetics have been variable, although there is some consensus that regimens that include inhaled anesthetics produce adverse effects.[213,214] In a well-controlled study of in vitro fertilization, no difference in fertilization or pregnancy rates was found in patients undergoing isoflurane anesthesia with or without N_2O, a finding implying that short exposure to N_2O is not harmful.[215] A publication on transvaginal oocyte retrieval and reproductive outcome[216] reported that general anesthesia with N_2O in combination with opiates, barbiturates, and halothane resulted in significantly lower clinical pregnancy rates (14.5%) than in patients receiving local anesthesia (23.7%) or an epidural block (25.8%). There were no adverse effects reported for oocyte collection, embryo yield, or embryo transfer. Several reports of epidemiologic surveys have been published in which the reproductive performance of operating room and dental personnel exposed to waste gases was examined. Interested readers are referred to a review of these studies.[217] One of the acknowledged shortcomings of many of the earlier published studies was the lack of a quantitative measure of anesthetic exposure, which was addressed in two more recent retrospective analyses[217,218] that attempted to quantitate N_2O exposure in female dental assistants. These investigators reported that in unscavenged dental suites, exposure to more than 5 and 3 hours of N_2O per day, respectively, was associated with reduced fertility and increased spontaneous abortion rates.

In general, N_2O is the only inhaled anesthetic that has been convincingly shown to be directly teratogenic in experimental animals, but only under experimental conditions that are considered extreme. High concentrations (50% to 75%) delivered to rats for 24-hour periods during organogenesis and low concentrations (0.1%) delivered to rats continuously throughout pregnancy result in an increased incidence of fetal resorption and visceral and skeletal abnormalities. A particularly interesting abnormality produced by high N_2O exposure is situs inversus, in which there is a disturbance in the left/right body axis so that organs such as the heart are on the wrong side of the body.[219] Although effects in rodents are seen only after extended periods of continuous exposure, it is not known whether humans are more sensitive than rodents and would show effects after shorter periods of exposure. It appears that lack of methionine rather than lack of thymidine plays the critical role in all the adverse reproductive effects other than situs inversus.[220] With situs inversus, stimulation of α_1-adrenergic receptors by N_2O appears to be the mechanism.[221] The effect is mediated by activation of calmodulin kinase 11.[222] N_2O teratogenesis is actively being investigated, not only because of its relevance to patient and occupational safety but also because N_2O can be used to determine the importance of vitamin B_{12}, folates, one-carbon chemistry, and the adrenergic system in developmental processes. The consensus is that the teratogenic effects observed in animals exposed to inhaled anesthetics are caused by physiologic changes associated with anesthesia rather than by inherent teratologic properties of the anesthetics themselves. Nonetheless, all findings emphasize the potential for anesthetics to interfere with developmental processes regardless of the mechanism.

Human studies have generally focused on the long-term behavioral effects of maternal obstetric medication, including epidural anesthesia. Claims have been made that the medication given at delivery to the mother produces depressed motor skills and impaired language ability in the infant and child for several years. Such claims, however, are controversial. Behavioral abnormalities in offspring whose mothers received inhaled anesthetics at any time during delivery have not been well studied. Furthermore, studies have not been done to assess the neurobehavioral function of children of operating room personnel who have been exposed to waste anesthetic gases. Firm conclusions about the risk for behavioral teratogenesis in the offspring of exposed personnel or in exposed patients therefore await further investigation. Finally, there is no evidence that the modern fluorinated inhaled anesthetics are mutagenic or carcinogenic.

General Anesthetics and Neurotoxicity

The issue of general anesthetics and neurotoxicity is an area of growing concern in the anesthesia community.[223] An increasing body of experimental evidence from animal studies suggests that general anesthetics can be neurotoxic in the developing and senescent brain through a process of accelerated apoptotic neurodegeneration.[224] The present nonclinical data implicate both *N*-methyl-D-aspartate receptor antagonists and drugs that potentiate GABA signal transduction as being potentially damaging to the developing brain.[225] The potential exists for combinations of anesthetic agents that have activity at both receptors to induce greater toxicity. Importantly, recent data suggest that even low nonapoptotic concentrations of anesthetics can perturb neuronal dendritic development and thereby lead to impairment of developing neuronal networks.[226] Moreover, in the rodent, this neurodegeneration is associated with cognitive impairment characterized by learning and memory deficits manifested in adulthood.[227] Several human cohort studies have shown an association between surgery in the neonatal period and poor neurodevelopmental outcomes[228,229] (also see Chapter 82). A large cohort study found a clear association between poor sensineural outcomes and surgery in preterm infants,[230] and more recently, neonates undergoing repair of patent ductus arteriosus were reported to have poorer outcomes.[231] These studies are interesting but are not conclusive evidence of a positive association. Epidemiologic observations suggest that the onset of Alzheimer's disease is related to cumulative anesthetic exposure before the age of 50 years,[232] and both halothane and isoflurane have been shown to increase the generation and toxicity of β-amyloid, a protein strongly implicated in the pathogenesis of Alzheimer's disease. Studies have further confirmed that inhaled anesthetics enhance the production, aggregation, and neurotoxicity of β-amyloid peptides,[233] the appearance of brain plaques, and deficits characteristic of Alzheimer's disease.[234]

The central nervous system seems to be susceptible to anesthetic neurotoxicity at the extremes of ages, and general anesthetics produce neurotoxicity and enduring cognitive impairment in young animals. Extrapolating neurodevelopmental data from animals to humans to examine their clinical applicability is a challenge, and the implications of these findings to clinicians remain unclear. Current evidence is insufficient to recommend substantial changes in current clinical practice. Future animal studies are needed at comparable neurodevelopmental stages and with clinically relevant anesthetic doses and durations in animals exposed to a surgical stimulus and followed with appropriate physiologic monitoring. Further human clinical study is required, and comparison of outcomes in a large cohort study of neonates undergoing surgery under either general or regional anesthesia seems indicated. A study of this type would prove useful in helping to answer this important question, provide data to help guide clinical decisions, and further develop strategies for assessing the safety of anesthetics in neonates and children.

Exposure to Waste Anesthetic Gases

Inhaled anesthetics present a potential for adverse effects in patients administered inhaled anesthetics and in health care personnel exposed to waste anesthetic gases both in and out of the operating room environment. Recognition of postoperative exposure to exhaled waste anesthetic gases in postanesthesia care units (PACUs), intensive care units, and other patient care areas represents a new challenge. The recommended thresholds for trace inhaled anesthetic concentrations are less than 2 ppm for a volatile anesthetic when used alone and less than 0.5 ppm when used with N_2O. The recommended time-weighted average for N_2O is less than 25 ppm, which is much lower than the level of N_2O (1000 ppm) known to produce detectable inactivation of methionine synthase. To control occupational exposure to waste anesthetic gases, it is not sufficient to merely adopt scavenging systems in operating rooms; appropriate work practices, engineering controls, and occupational management protocols are also required throughout the perioperative process in all patient care areas. Many factors affect waste anesthetic gas concentrations, including the efficiency of air handling, room type and size, number of patients in a room or ward, and time spent in a particular patient care area.

Several studies have documented excessive levels of waste anesthetic gases in poorly ventilated PACU areas.[235-239] However, to date, none of these studies have documented any significant long-term adverse health effects.[235,236] An increased incidence of sister chromatid exchange has been found in operating room personnel in three of four recent studies, but the long-term implications of this finding are unknown at present.[240-243] In the only long-term prospective study with or without scavenging of waste anesthetic gases, Spence[244] found no causal relationship between exposure to waste anesthetic gases and adverse health effects.

Environmental Toxicities

The Greenhouse Effect. Solar radiation loads heat energy on the Earth, and to maintain a stable temperature, the Earth returns this load to space via infrared radiation. The primary constituents of the atmosphere, nitrogen and oxygen, are transparent to these rays. In the absence of other gases, the Earth's temperature would be −20°C. Naturally occurring gases such as methane, carbon dioxide, and N_2O absorb the infrared radiation. To overcome this absorption, the Earth has increased its temperature to approximately 15°C—the greenhouse effect. The contribution of major gases to the greenhouse effect is estimated to be 60% for carbon dioxide, 20% for methane, 14% for chlorofluorocarbons, and 6% for N_2O.[245] It is estimated that since the industrial revolution, the number of molecules of CO_2 per million molecules of air has increased from 280 to 385 ppm. *Global warming* is the increase in the average temperature of the Earth's near surface air and oceans since the mid-20th century and its projected continuation. The global air temperature rose 0.74°C during the 100 years ending in 2005. The Intergovernmental Panel on Climate Change (IPCC) concluded that "most of the observed increases in globally averaged temperatures since the mid-twentieth century is very likely due to the observed increase in anthrogenic greenhouse gas concentrations" via the greenhouse effect. The IPCC has predicted an average global rise in temperature of 1.4°C to 5.8°C between 1990 and 2100. Increasing global temperatures will decrease polar ice and thereby cause sea levels to rise and are expected to change precipitation patterns and increase the intensity of severe weather events. As a result, the Kyoto Protocol was negotiated and ratified by 175 countries and came into force on February 16, 2005. The United States is the only major industrialized country that is not a party to this agree-

Table 24-5 Summary of Atmospheric Lifetimes, Relative Input into the Stratosphere, Ozone-Depleting Potential (ODP), and Global-Warming Potential (GWP) Values for CFC-11, CFC-12, and Halogenated Volatile Anesthetics

Compound	M (g/mol)	$T_{1/2}$ (yr)	Input into Stratosphere (%)	ODP	S (cm^2/atm)	GWP
CFC-11	137.5	50	100	1.00	2500	0.033
CFC-12	121.0	102	100	1.55	3300	1.00
Halothane	197.4	6.6	13.2	1.56	1400	0.02
Enflurane	184.5	8.2	16.2	0.04	4800	0.08
Isoflurane	184.5	5.9	14.6	0.03	3900	0.05
Desflurane	168.0	21.4	21.4	0.00	3000	0.14
Sevoflurane	200.0	4.0	12.6	0.00	2550	0.02

CFC, chlorofluorocarbon; S, integrated infrared absorption cross section.

From Langbein T, Sonntag H, Trapp D, et al: Volatile anaesthetics and the atmosphere: Atmospheric lifetimes and atmospheric effects of halothane, enflurane, isoflurane, desflurane and sevoflurane. Br J Anaesth 82:66-73, 1999.

Table 24-6 Global-Warming (GWP) and Ozone-Depleting Potential (PDP) of Anesthetics

Chemical	Formula	Lifetime (yr)	GWP (100-yr integral) in CO_2 Mass Equivalents	ODP (10-yr integral) in CFC-11 Mass Equivalents
Isoflurane	$CHF_2OCHICH$	2.6	350	≈0.02
Sevoflurane	$CH_2FOCH(CF_3)_2$	≈3.7	420	0
Nitrous oxide	N_2O	114	298	<0.01

CFC, chlorofluorocarbon; GWP, global-warming potential; ODP, ozone-depleting potential.
From McGain F: Why anaesthetists should no longer use nitrous oxide. Anaesth Intensive Care 35:808-809, 2007.

ment. The United States is a signatory but has not ratified or withdrawn from the protocol. Essentially, this is an agreement under which industrialized countries will reduce their collective emissions of greenhouse gases by 5.2% relative to the year 1990 via a "cap and trade" system (effectively a 29% decrease over expected emission levels without the cuts). The goal is to lower overall emission of six greenhouse gases: carbon dioxide, methane, nitrous oxide, sulfur hexafluoride, hydrofluorocarbons, and perfluorocarbons, averaged over the period 2008 to 2112. National limitations range from reduction of 8% for the European Union, 7% for the United States, and 6% for Japan. The global-warming and ozone-depleting potential of several halocarbons, including the common fluorinated anesthetics and N_2O, is summarized in Tables 24-5[246] and 24-6.[247] N_2O is extremely stable with an atmospheric lifetime of 100 to 150 years. Its only sink is degradation by ultraviolet radiation outside the ozone layer. N_2O contributes about 5% of the greenhouse gas effect, and medical use of N_2O contributes approximately 0.35% to 2% of this total.[248,249] Like N_2O, in addition to contributing to the greenhouse effect, chlorine-containing compounds such as halothane, enflurane, isoflurane, and desflurane also deplete stratospheric ozone.[246] Present protocols call for elimination of these compounds by 2030. In addition, there is an ongoing movement in Japan[250] and the European Union to reduce and eventually eliminate N_2O from anesthesia. The contribution of anesthetic-released N_2O and chlorinated volatile agents to global warming, the greenhouse effect, and ozone depletion is minor in comparison to that generated by the combustion of fossil fuels and nitrogen-containing fertilizers. N_2O contributes 1% to ozone depletion and 0.05% to the greenhouse effect, whereas the anesthetics contribute 0.01% to ozone depletion and 0.1% to the greenhouse effect. We have reduced the toxicity of anesthetics to patients and health care workers since the inception of modern anesthesia; however, environmental toxicities may prove to be the Achilles heel of these valuable agents. Until such time as these agents are eliminated from practice or better, more stable substitutes become available, we as anesthesia providers can reduce the adverse environmental consequences of these agents by using low-flow anesthesia systems whenever possible and thus can have a small but important positive impact on the environment.

Summary

Volatile anesthetic agents, like most drugs, undergo metabolism in the body and are sometimes associated with toxic reactions. Scientific investigations and industry research have led to the development of more stable anesthetics with more desirable clinical properties. Inhaled agents that are more heavily metabolized are associated with the greatest numbers of reported toxicities. As with most drugs, these toxicities occur when the anesthetics are given as "standard-dose medications"; that is, the appropriate medication and dose are given at the proper time, in the correct manner, to the right patient. Thus, these associated toxicities under most circumstances meet the definition of adverse drug reactions (ADRs). More than 2 million ADRs are reported each year in the United States and result in more than 100,000 deaths. It should be noted that 51% of approved drugs have serious ADRs not detected before approval and that ADRs are responsible for 6% of all hospital admissions, occur in 10% to 20% of hospitalized patients, and are the cause of death in 0.1% of medical and 0.01% of surgical patients. They are the fourth leading cause of death in hospitalized patients (0.32% of hospitalized patients). When compared with most therapeutic agents, the safety of fluorinated inhaled anesthetics is remarkable. Future developments in the field of personalized medicine, in which both the selection of a specific therapeutic agent and its associated dosing are tailored to an individual patient on the basis of individual genetic profiles, will have ramifications for increased efficacy and patient safety. Idiosyncratic toxicities that involve the human immune system continue to present some of the greatest challenges to anesthesia and medicine, but new insight into the structure-toxicity relationships of drugs at the molecular level may provide the necessary tools to solve this puzzle.

The use of any anesthetic agent must be based on specific knowledge of its benefits and risks, how it may produce toxicity, and in which patients it may be most safely administered. Clearly, the perfect anesthetic agent does not exist yet, and individual patient circumstances will continue to dictate the choice and use of inhaled anesthetics in clinical practice. As ongoing research attempts to uncover emerging toxicities, the clinician is challenged to balance new information with current clinical practices and choose the safest, most effective agents for each patient.

Acknowledgment

The author wishes to acknowledge and thank Dolores B. Njoku, M.D., coauthor of this chapter in the sixth edition of *Miller's Anesthesiology*, some of whose text has been retained in this edition.

References

1. Wilkinson G: Pharmacokinetics: The dynamics of drug absorption, distribution and elimination. *In* Hardman J, Limbird LE, Goodman GA (eds): Goodman and Gilman's The Pharmacological Basis of Therapeutics, 10th ed. New York, McGraw-Hill, 2001.
2. Weinshilboum R: Inheritance and drug response. N Engl J Med 348:529-537, 2003.
3. Gibson G, Skett P: Introduction to Drug Metabolism. Cheltenham, UK, Stanley Thornes Publishers, 1999.
4. Krishna DR, Klotz U: Extrahepatic metabolism of drugs in humans. Clin Pharmacokinet 26:144-160, 1994.
5. Lohr JW, Willsky GR, Acara MA: Renal drug metabolism. Pharmacol Rev 50:107-141, 1998.
6. Koop DR: Oxidative and reductive metabolism by cytochrome P450 2E1. FASEB J 6:724-730, 1992.
7. Jana S, Paliwal J: Molecular mechanisms of cytochrome P450 induction: Potential for drug-drug interactions. Curr Protein Pept Sci 8:619-628, 2007.
8. Wilkinson GR: Drug metabolism and variability among patients in drug response. N Engl J Med 352:2211-2221, 2005.
9. Young WS, Lietman PS: Chloramphenicol glucuronyl transferase: Assay, ontogeny and inducibility. J Pharmacol Exp Ther 204:203-211, 1978.
10. Weiss CF, Glazko AJ, Weston JK: Chloramphenicol in the newborn infant. A physiologic explanation of its toxicity when given in excessive doses. N Engl J Med 262:787-794, 1960.
11. Lacroix D, Sonnier M, Moncion A, et al: Expression of CYP3A in the human liver—evidence that the shift between CYP3A7 and CYP3A4 occurs immediately after birth. Eur J Biochem 247:625-634, 1997.
12. Loughnan PM, Greenwald A, Purton WW, et al: Pharmacokinetic observations of phenytoin disposition in the newborn and young infant. Arch Dis Child 52:302-309, 1977.
13. Baillie TA: Metabolism and toxicity of drugs. Two decades of progress in industrial drug metabolism. Chem Res Toxicol 21:129-137, 2008.
14. Kalow W, Gunn DR: The relation between dose of succinylcholine and duration of apnea in man. J Pharmacol Exp Ther 120:203-214, 1957.
15. Kalow W: The Pennsylvania State University College of Medicine 1990 Bernard B. Brodie Lecture. Pharmacogenetics: Past and future. Life Sci 47:1385-1397, 1990.
16. Ingelman-Sundberg M, Oscarson M, McLellan RA: Polymorphic human cytochrome P450 enzymes: An opportunity for individualized drug treatment. Trends Pharmacol Sci 20:342-349, 1999.
17. Sata F, Sapone A, Elizondo G, et al: CYP3A4 allelic variants with amino acid substitutions in exons 7 and 12: Evidence for an allelic variant with altered catalytic activity. Clin Pharmacol Ther 67:48-56, 2000.
18. Kuehl P, Zhang J, Lin Y, et al: Sequence diversity in CYP3A promoters and characterization of the genetic basis of polymorphic CYP3A5 expression. Nat Genet 27:383-391, 2001.
19. Blum M, Grant DM, McBride W, et al: Human arylamine *N*-acetyltransferase genes: Isolation, chromosomal localization, and functional expression. DNA Cell Biol 9:193-203, 1990.
20. Lin HJ, Han Cy, Lin BK, Hardy S: Slow acetylator mutations in the human polymorphic *N*-acetyltransferase gene in 786 Asians, blacks, Hispanics, and whites: Application to metabolic epidemiology. Am J Hum Genet 52:827-834, 1993.
21. Woodson LC, Weinshilboum RM: Human kidney thiopurine methyltransferase. Purification and biochemical properties. Biochem Pharmacol 32:819-826, 1983.
22. Evans WE: Pharmacogenetics of thiopurine *S*-methyltransferase and thiopurine therapy. Ther Drug Monit 26:186-191, 2004.
23. Bosch TM, Meijerman I, Beijnen JH, Schellens JH: Genetic polymorphisms of drug-metabolising enzymes and drug transporters in the chemotherapeutic treatment of cancer. Clin Pharmacokinet 45:253-285, 2006.
24. Daly AK, King BP: Pharmacogenetics of oral anticoagulants. Pharmacogenetics 13:247-252, 2003.
25. Higashi MK, Veenstra DL, Kondo LM, et al: Association between CYP2C9 genetic variants and anticoagulation-related outcomes during warfarin therapy. JAMA 287:1690-1698, 2002.
26. Rieder MJ, Reiner AP, Gage BF, et al: Effect of VKORC1 haplotypes on transcriptional regulation and warfarin dose. N Engl J Med 352:2285-2293, 2005.
27. Schwarz UI, Ritchie MD, Bradford Y, et al: Genetic determinants of response to warfarin during initial anticoagulation. N Engl J Med 358:999-1008, 2008.
28. Harris PD, Barnes R: The uses of helium and xenon in current clinical practice. Anaesthesia 63:284-293, 2008.
29. Cullen SC, Gross EG: The anesthetic properties of xenon in animals and human beings, with additional observations on krypton. Science 113:580-582, 1951.
30. Froeba G, Marx T, Pazhur J, et al: Xenon does not trigger malignant hyperthermia in susceptible swine. Anesthesiology 91:1047-1052, 1999.
31. Laitio RM, Kaisti KK, Låangsjö JW, et al: Effects of xenon anesthesia on cerebral blood flow in humans: A positron emission tomography study. Anesthesiology 106:1128-1133, 2007.
32. Baumert JH, Hein M, Hecker KE, et al: Autonomic cardiac control with xenon anaesthesia in patients at cardiovascular risk. Br J Anaesth 98:722-727, 2007.
33. Zhang P, Ohara A, Mashimo T, et al: Pulmonary resistance in dogs: A comparison of xenon with nitrous oxide. Can J Anaesth 42:547-553, 1995.
34. Morris LE, Knott JR, Pittinger CB: Electro-encephalographic and blood gas observations in human surgical patients during xenon anesthesia. Anesthesiology 16:312-319, 1955.
35. Lachmann B, Armbruster S, Schairer W, et al: Safety and efficacy of xenon in routine use as an inhalational anaesthetic. Lancet 335:1413-1415, 1990.
36. Luttropp HH, Thomasson R, Dahm S, et al: Clinical experience with minimal flow xenon anesthesia. Acta Anaesthesiol Scand 38:121-125, 1994.
37. Hofland J, Gultuna I, Tenbrinck R: Xenon anaesthesia for laparoscopic cholecystectomy in a patient with Eisenmenger's syndrome. Br J Anaesth 86:882-886, 2001.
38. Burov NE, Molchanov IV, Nikolaev LL, Rashchupkin AB: [The method of low-flow xenon anesthesia.] Anesteziol Reanimatol 3:31-34, 2003.
39. Goto T, Saito H, Shinkai M, et al: Xenon provides faster emergence from anesthesia than does nitrous oxide–sevoflurane or nitrous oxide–isoflurane. Anesthesiology 86:1273-1278, 1997.
40. Rossaint R, Reyle-Hahn M, Schulte AM, et al: Multicenter randomized comparison of the efficacy and safety of xenon and isoflurane in patients undergoing elective surgery. Anesthesiology 98:6-13, 2003.
41. Goto T, Hanne P, Ishiguro Y, et al: Cardiovascular effects of xenon and nitrous oxide in patients during fentanyl-midazolam anaesthesia. Anaesthesia 59:1178-1183, 2004.
42. Wappler F, Rossaint R, Baumert J, et al: Multicenter randomized comparison of xenon and isoflurane on left ventricular function in patients undergoing elective surgery. Anesthesiology 106:463-471, 2007.
43. Coburn M, Baumert JH, Roertgen D, et al: Emergence and early cognitive function in the elderly after xenon or desflurane anaesthesia: A double-blinded randomized controlled trial. Br J Anaesth 98:756-762, 2007.
44. Bein B, Turowski P, Renner J, et al: Comparison of xenon-based anaesthesia compared with total intravenous anaesthesia in high risk surgical patients. Anaesthesia 60:960-967, 2005.
45. Baumert JH, Hein M, Hecker KE, et al: Xenon or propofol anaesthesia for patients at cardiovascular risk in non-cardiac surgery. Br J Anaesth 100:605-611, 2008.
46. Kharasch ED, Hankins DC, Fenstamaker K, Cox K: Human halothane metabolism, lipid peroxidation, and cytochromes P(450)2A6 and P(450)3A4. Eur J Clin Pharmacol 55:853-859, 2000.
47. Kharasch ED, Hankins D, Mautz D, Thummel KE: Identification of the enzyme responsible for oxidative halothane metabolism: Implications for prevention of halothane hepatitis. Lancet 347:1367-1371, 1996.
48. Garton KJ, Yuen P, Meinwald J, et al: Stereoselective metabolism of enflurane by human liver cytochrome P450 2E1. Drug Metab Dispos 23:1426-1430, 1995.
49. Christ DD, Satoh H, Kenna JG, Pohl LR: Potential metabolic basis for enflurane hepatitis and the apparent cross-sensitization between enflurane and halothane. Drug Metab Dispos 16:135-140, 1988.
50. Mazze RI, Woodruff RE, Heerdt ME: Isoniazid-induced enflurane defluorination in humans. Anesthesiology 57:5-8, 1982.
51. Thummel KE, Kharasch ED, Podoll T, Kunze K: Human liver microsomal enflurane defluorination catalyzed by cytochrome P-450 2E1. Drug Metab Dispos 21:350-357, 1993.
52. Kharasch ED, Thummel KE: Identification of cytochrome P450 2E1 as the predominant enzyme catalyzing human liver microsomal defluorination of sevoflurane, isoflurane, and methoxyflurane. Anesthesiology 79:795-807, 1993.
53. Kharasch ED, Hankins DC, Cox K: Clinical isoflurane metabolism by cytochrome P450 2E1. Anesthesiology 90:766-771, 1999.
54. Sutton TS, Koblin DD, Gruenke LD, et al: Fluoride metabolites after prolonged exposure of volunteers and patients to desflurane. Anesth Analg 73:180-185, 1991.
55. Cook TL, Beppu WJ, Hitt BA, et al: Renal effects and metabolism of sevoflurane in Fisher 3444 rats: An in-vivo and in-vitro comparison with methoxyflurane. Anesthesiology 43:70-77, 1975.
56. Cook TL, Beppu WJ, Hitt BA, et al: A comparison of renal effects and metabolism of sevoflurane and methoxyflurane in enzyme-induced rats. Anesth Analg 54:829-835, 1975.
57. Holaday DA, Smith FR: Clinical characteristics and biotransformation of sevoflurane in healthy human volunteers. Anesthesiology 54:100-106, 1981.

58. Kharasch ED, Karol MD, Lanni C, Sawchuk R: Clinical sevoflurane metabolism and disposition. I. Sevoflurane and metabolite pharmacokinetics. Anesthesiology 82:1369-1378, 1995.
59. Kharasch ED, Armstrong AS, Gunn K, et al: Clinical sevoflurane metabolism and disposition. II. The role of cytochrome P450 2E1 in fluoride and hexafluoroisopropanol formation. Anesthesiology 82:1379-1388, 1995.
60. Baker MT, Ronnenberg WC Jr, Ruzicka JA, et al: Inhibitory effects of deuterium substitution on the metabolism of sevoflurane by the rat. Drug Metab Dispos 21:1170-1171, 1993.
61. Hoffman J, Konopka K, Buckhorn C, et al: Ethanol-inducible cytochrome P450 in rabbits metabolizes enflurane. Br J Anaesth 63:103-108, 1989.
62. Kikuchi H, Morio M, Fuijii K, et al: Clinical evaluation and metabolism of sevoflurane in patients. Hiroshima J Med Sci 36:93-97, 1987.
63. Frink EJ Jr, Ghantous H, Malan TP, et al: Plasma inorganic fluoride with sevoflurane anesthesia: Correlation with indices of hepatic and renal function. Anesth Analg 74:231-235, 1992.
64. Drayer DE: Pharmacodynamic and pharmacokinetic differences between drug enantiomers in humans: An overview. Clin Pharmacol Ther 40:125-133, 1986.
65. Tucker GT, Lennard MS: Enantiomer specific pharmacokinetics. Pharmacol Ther 45:309-329, 1990.
66. Birkett DJ: Racemates or enantiomers: Regulatory approaches. Clin Exp Pharmacol Physiol 16:479-483, 1989.
67. Ariens EJ, Testa B: Chiral aspects of drug metabolism. Trends Pharmacol Sci 7:60-64, 1986.
68. Howard-Lock HE, Lock CJ, Mewa A, Kean WF: D-Penicillamine: Chemistry and clinical use in rheumatic disease. Semin Arthritis Rheum 15:261-281, 1986.
69. Satoh K, Yanagisawa T, Taira N: Coronary vasodilator and cardiac effects of optical isomers of verapamil in the dog. J Cardiovasc Pharmacol 2:309-318, 1980.
70. Powell JR, Ambre JJ, Rud TI: Drug stereochemistry. *In* Wainer IW, Drayer DE (eds): Analytical Methods and Pharmacology. New York, Dekker, 1988, p 245.
71. Buchinger W, Ober O, Uray G, et al: Synthesis and effects on peripheral thyroid hormone conversion of (*R*)-4-hydroxypropanolol, a main metabolite of (*R*)-propranolol. Chirality 3:145, 1991.
72. Grisslinger G, Hering W, Thomann P, et al: Pharmacokinetics and pharmacodynamics of ketamine enantiomers in surgical patients using a stereoselective analytical method. Br J Anaesth 70:666-671, 1993.
73. Kharasch ED, Labroo R: Metabolism of ketamine stereoisomers by human liver microsomes. Anesthesiology 77:1201-1207, 1992.
74. Brau ME, Branitzki P, Olschewski A, et al: Block of neuronal tetrodotoxin-resistant Na^+ currents by stereoisomers of piperidine local anesthetics. Anesth Analg 91:1499-1505, 2000.
75. Heavner JE: Local anesthetics. Curr Opin Anaesthesiol 20:336-342, 2007.
76. Thomas JM, Schug SA: Recent advances in the pharmacokinetics of local anaesthetics. Long-acting amide enantiomers and continuous infusions. Clin Pharmacokinet 36:67-83, 1999.
77. Blaschke G, Kraft HP, Fickentscher K, Kohler F: Chromatographic separation of racemic thalidomide and teratogenic activity of its enantiomers (author's transl). Arzneimittelforschung 29:1640-1642, 1979.
78. Martin JL, Meinwald J, Radford P, et al: Stereoselective metabolism of halothane enantiomers to trifluoroacetylated liver proteins. Drug Metab Rev 27:179-189, 1995.
79. Kendig JJ, Trudell JR, Cohen EN: Halothane stereoisomers: Lack of stereospecificity in two model systems. Anesthesiology 39:518-524, 1973.
80. Lysko GS, Robinson JL, Castro R, Ferrone RA: The stereospecific effects of isoflurane isomers in vivo. Eur J Pharmacol 263:25-29, 1994.
81. Harris B, Moody E, Skolnick P: Isoflurane anesthesia is stereoselective. Eur J Pharmacol 217:215-216, 1992.
82. Moody EJ, Harris BD, Skolnick P: Stereospecific actions of the inhalation anesthetic isoflurane at the $GABA_A$ receptor complex. Brain Res 615:101-106, 1993.
83. Jones MV, Harrison NL: Effects of volatile anesthetics on the kinetics of inhibitory postsynaptic currents in cultured rat hippocampal neurons. J Neurophysiol 70:1339-1349, 1993.
84. Harris BD, Moody EJ, Basile AS, Skolnick P: Volatile anesthetics bidirectionally and stereospecifically modulate ligand binding to GABA receptors. Eur J Pharmacol 267:269-274, 1994.
85. Tomlin SL, Jenkins A, Lieb WR, Franks NP: Stereoselective effects of etomidate optical isomers on gamma-aminobutyric acid type A receptors and animals. Anesthesiology 88:708-717, 1998.
86. Summary of the national Halothane Study. Possible association between halothane anesthesia and postoperative hepatic necrosis. JAMA 197:775-788, 1966.
87. Martin JL, Plevak DJ, Flannery KD, et al: Hepatotoxicity after desflurane anesthesia. Anesthesiology 83:1125-1129, 1995.
88. Uetrecht J: Idiosyncratic drug reactions: Past, present, and future. Chem Res Toxicol 21:84-92, 2008.
89. Park BK, Kitteringham NR, Maggs JL, et al: The role of metabolic activation in drug-induced hepatotoxicity. Annu Rev Pharmacol Toxicol 45:177-202, 2005.
90. Pohl LR, Pumford NR, Martin JL: Mechanisms, chemical structures and drug metabolism. Eur J Haematol Suppl 60:98-104, 1996.
91. Kenna JG: Immunoallergic drug-induced hepatitis: Lessons from halothane. J Hepatol 26(Suppl 1):5-12, 1997.
92. Kenna JG, Satoh H, Christ DD, Pohl LR: Metabolic basis for a drug hypersensitivity: Antibodies in sera from patients with halothane hepatitis recognize liver neoantigens that contain the trifluoroacetyl group derived from halothane. J Pharmacol Exp Ther 245:1103-1109, 1988.
93. Martin JL, Pumfoprd NR, LaRosa AC, et al: A metabolite of halothane covalently binds to an endoplasmic reticulum protein that is highly homologous to phosphatidylinositol-specific phospholipase C-alpha but has no activity. Biochem Biophys Res Commun 178:679-685, 1991.
94. Butler LE, Thomassen D, Martin JL, et al: The calcium-binding protein calreticulin is covalently modified in rat liver by a reactive metabolite of the inhalation anesthetic halothane. Chem Res Toxicol 5:406-410, 1992.
95. Martin JL, Reed GF, Pohl LR: Association of anti–58 kDa endoplasmic reticulum antibodies with halothane hepatitis. Biochem Pharmacol 46:1247-1250, 1993.
96. Martin JL, Kenna JG, Martin BM, et al: Halothane hepatitis patients have serum antibodies that react with protein disulfide isomerase. Hepatology 18:858-863, 1993.
97. Pumford NR, Martin BM, Thomassen D, et al: Serum antibodies from halothane hepatitis patients react with the rat endoplasmic reticulum protein ERp72. Chem Res Toxicol 6:609-615, 1993.
98. Bourdi M, Demady D, Martin JL, et al: cDNA cloning and baculovirus expression of the human liver endoplasmic reticulum P58: Characterization as a protein disulfide isomerase isoform, but not as a protease or a carnitine acyltransferase. Arch Biochem Biophys 323:397-403, 1995.
99. Pohl LR: An immunochemical approach of identifying and characterizing protein targets of toxic reactive metabolites. Chem Res Toxicol 6:786-793, 1993.
100. Gut J, Christen U, Huwyler J: Mechanisms of halothane toxicity: Novel insights. Pharmacol Ther 58:133-155, 1993.
101. Barton J: Jaundice and halothane. Lancet 1:1097, 1959.
102. Wark HJ: Postoperative jaundice in children. The influence of halothane. Anaesthesia 38:237-242, 1983.
103. Warner LO, Beach TP, Garvin JP, Warner EJ: Halothane and children: The first quarter century. Anesth Analg 63:838-840, 1984.
104. Kenna JG, Neuberger J, Mieli-Vergani G, et al: Halothane hepatitis in children. Br Med J (Clin Res Ed) 294:1209-1211, 1987.
105. Njoku D, Laster MJ, Gong DH, et al: Biotransformation of halothane, enflurane, isoflurane, and desflurane to trifluoroacetylated liver proteins: Association between protein acylation and hepatic injury. Anesth Analg 84:173-178, 1997.
106. Christ DD, Kenna JG, Kammerer W, et al: Enflurane metabolism produces covalently bound liver adducts recognized by antibodies from patients with halothane hepatitis. Anesthesiology 69:833-838, 1988.
107. Brunt EM, White H, Marsh JW, et al: Fulminant hepatic failure after repeated exposure to isoflurane anesthesia: A case report. Hepatology 13:1017-1021, 1991.
108. Turner GB, O'Rourke D, Scott GO, Beringer TR: Fatal hepatotoxicity after re-exposure to isoflurane: A case report and review of the literature. Eur J Gastroenterol Hepatol 12:955-959, 2000.
109. Njoku DB, Shrestha S, Soloway R, et al: Subcellular localization of trifluoroacetylated liver proteins in association with hepatitis following isoflurane. Anesthesiology 96:757-761, 2002.
110. Jones RM, Koblin DD, Cashman JN, et al: Biotransformation and hepato-renal function in volunteers after exposure to desflurane (I-653). Br J Anaesth 64:482-487, 1990.
111. Wrigley SR, Fairfield JE, Jones RM, Black AE: Induction and recovery characteristics of desflurane in day case patients: A comparison with propofol. Anaesthesia 46:615-622, 1991.
112. Berghaus TM, Baron A, Geier A, et al: Hepatotoxicity following desflurane anesthesia. Hepatology 29:613-614, 1999.
113. Anderson JS, Rose NR, Martin JL, et al: Desflurane hepatitis associated with hapten and autoantigen-specific IgG4 antibodies. Anesth Analg 104:1452-1453, 2007.
114. Cote G, Bouchard S: Hepatotoxicity after desflurane anesthesia in a 15-month-old child with Möbius syndrome after previous exposure to isoflurane. Anesthesiology 107:843-845, 2007.
115. Watanabe K, Hatakenaka S, Ikemune K, et al: [A case of suspected liver dysfunction induced by sevoflurane anesthesia.] Masui 42:902-905, 1993.
116. Shichinohe Y, Masuda Y, Takahashi H, et al: [A case of postoperative hepatic injury after sevoflurane anesthesia.] Masui 41:1802-1805, 1992.

117. Bruun LS, ELKjaer S, Bitsch-Larsen D, Anderson O: Hepatic failure in a child after acetaminophen and sevoflurane exposure. Anesth Analg 92(6): 1446-1488, 2001.
118. Lehmann A, Neher M, Kiessling AH: Case report: fatal hepatic failure after aortic valve replacement and sevoflurane exposure. Can J Anaesth 54(11):917-921, 2007.
119. Harris JW, Pohl LR, Martin JL, Anders MW: Tissue acylation by the chlorofluorocarbon substitute 2,2-dichloro-1,1,1-trifluoroethane. Proc Natl Acad Sci U S A 88(4):1407-1410, 1991.
120. Lind RC, Gandolfi AJ, Hall PD: Biotransformation and hepatotoxicity of HCFC-123 in the guinea pig: Potentiation of hepatic injury by prior glutathione depletion. Toxicol Appl Pharmacol 134(1):175-181, 1995.
121. Rusch GM, Trochimonicz HJ, Malley LJ, et al: Subchronic inhalation toxicity studies with hydrochlorofluorocarbon 123 (HCFC 123). Fundam Appl Toxicol 23(2):169-178, 1994.
122. Dekant W: Toxicology of chlorofluorocarbon replacements. Environ Health Perspect 104(Suppl 1):75-83, 1996.
123. Hoet P, Graf ML, Bourdi M, et al: Epidemic of liver disease caused by hydrochlorofluorocarbons used as ozone-sparing substitutes of chlorofluorocarbons. Lancet 350:556-559, 1997.
124. Joshi PH, Conn HO: The syndrome of methoxyflurane-associated hepatitis. Ann Intern Med 80:395-401, 1974.
125. Martin JL: Halothane hepatitis: A possible immune-mediated hepatitis. *In* Newcombe DS, Rose NR, Bloom JC (eds): Clinical Immunotoxicology. New York, Raven Press, 1992, pp 155-175.
126. Kenna JG, Neuberger J, Williams R: Specific antibodies to halothane-induced liver antigens in halothane-associated hepatitis. Br J Anaesth 59: 1286-1290, 1987.
127. Nomura F, Hatano H, Ohnishi K, et al: Effects of anticonvulsant agents on halothane-induced liver injury in human subjects and experimental animals. Hepatology 6:952-956, 1986.
128. Hubbard AK, Roth AK, Gandolfi AJ, et al: Halothane hepatitis patients generate an antibody response toward a covalently bound metabolite of halothane. Anesthesiology 68:791-796, 1988.
129. Martin JL, Kenna JG, Pohl LR: Antibody assays for the detection of patients sensitized to halothane. Anesth Analg 70:154-159, 1990.
130. Njoku D: Effects of halogenated inhalation agents on the liver and kidneys. Probl Anesth Curr Issues Pediatr Anesth 10:478-487, 2000.
131. Kharasch ED, Hankins DC, Thummel KE: Human kidney methoxyflurane and sevoflurane metabolism. Intrarenal fluoride production as a possible mechanism of methoxyflurane nephrotoxicity. Anesthesiology 82:689-699, 1995.
132. Mazze RI, Cousins MJ, Barr GA: Renal effects and metabolism of isoflurane in man. Anesthesiology 40:536-542, 1974.
133. Arnold JH, Truog RD, Rice SA: Prolonged administration of isoflurane to pediatric patients during mechanical ventilation. Anesth Analg 76:520-526, 1993.
134. Kobayashi Y, Ochiai R, Takeda J, et al: Serum and urinary inorganic fluoride concentrations after prolonged inhalation of sevoflurane in humans. Anesth Analg 74:753-757, 1992.
135. Nuscheler M, Conzen P, Peter K: [Sevoflurane: Metabolism and toxicity.] Anaesthesist 47(Suppl 1):S24-S32, 1998.
136. Truog RD, Rice SA: Inorganic fluoride and prolonged isoflurane anesthesia in the intensive care unit. Anesth Analg 69:843-845, 1989.
137. Hara T, Fukusaki M, Nakamura T, Sumikawa K: Renal function in patients during and after hypotensive anesthesia with sevoflurane. J Clin Anesth 10:539-545, 1998.
138. Frink EJ Jr, Malan TP, Isner J, et al: Renal concentrating function with prolonged sevoflurane or enflurane anesthesia in volunteers. Anesthesiology 80:1019-1025, 1994.
139. Higuchi H, Arimura S, Sumikura H, et al: Urine concentrating ability after prolonged sevoflurane anaesthesia. Br J Anaesth 73:239-240, 1994.
140. Groudine SB, Fragen RJ, Kharasch ED, et al: Comparison of renal function following anesthesia with low-flow sevoflurane and isoflurane. J Clin Anesth 11:201-207, 1999.
141. Bito H, Ikeda K: Long-duration, low-flow sevoflurane anesthesia using two carbon dioxide absorbents. Quantification of degradation products in the circuit. Anesthesiology 81:340-345, 1994.
142. Morio M, Fujii K, Satoh N, et al: Reaction of sevoflurane and its degradation products with soda lime. Toxicity of the byproducts. Anesthesiology 77:1155-1164, 1992.
143. Artu A: Renal effects of sevoflurane during conditions of possible increased risk. J Clin Anesth 10:531-538, 1998.
144. Mori N, Nagata H, Ohta S, Suzuki M: Prolonged sevoflurane inhalation was not nephrotoxic in two patients with refractory status asthmaticus. Anesth Analg 83:189-191, 1996.
145. Conzen PF, Nuscheler M, Melotte A, et al: Renal function and serum fluoride concentrations in patients with stable renal insufficiency after anesthesia with sevoflurane or enflurane. Anesth Analg 81:569-575, 1995.
146. Tsukamoto N, Hirabayashi Y, Shimizu R, Mitsuhata H: The effects of sevoflurane and isoflurane anesthesia on renal tubular function in patients with moderately impaired renal function. Anesth Analg 82:909-913, 1996.
147. Morita K, Otsuka F, Ogura T, et al: Sevoflurane anaesthesia causes a transient decrease in aquaporin-2 and impairment of urine concentration. Br J Anaesth 83:734-739, 1999.
148. Smiley RM, Ornstein E, Pantuck EJ, et al: Metabolism of desflurane and isoflurane to fluoride ion in surgical patients. Can J Anaesth 38:965-968, 1991.
149. Bito H, Ikeda K: Closed-circuit anesthesia with sevoflurane in humans. Effects on renal and hepatic function and concentrations of breakdown products with soda lime in the circuit. Anesthesiology 80:71-76, 1994.
150. Cunningham DD, Huang S, Webster J, et al: Sevoflurane degradation to compound A in anaesthesia breathing systems. Br J Anaesth 77:537-543, 1996.
151. Bito H, Ikeda K: Degradation products of sevoflurane during low-flow anaesthesia. Br J Anaesth 74:56-59, 1995.
152. Gonsowski CT, Laster MJ, Eger EI, et al: Toxicity of compound A in rats. Effect of a 3-hour administration. Anesthesiology 80:556-565, 1994.
153. Keller KA, Callan C, Prokocimer P, et al: Inhalation toxicity study of a haloalkene degradant of sevoflurane, compound A (PIFE), in Sprague-Dawley rats. Anesthesiology 83:1220-1232, 1995.
154. Gonsowski CT, Laster MJ, Eger EI, et al: Toxicity of compound A in rats. Effect of increasing duration of administration. Anesthesiology 80:566-573, 1994.
155. Bito H, Ikeda K: Plasma inorganic fluoride and intracircuit degradation product concentrations in long-duration, low-flow sevoflurane anesthesia. Anesth Analg 79:946-951, 1994.
156. Frink EJ Jr, Isner RJ, Malan TP Jr, et al: Sevoflurane degradation product concentrations with soda lime during prolonged anesthesia. J Clin Anesth 6:239-242, 1994.
157. Bito H, Ikeda K: Renal and hepatic function in surgical patients after low-flow sevoflurane or isoflurane anesthesia. Anesth Analg 82:173-176, 1996.
158. Mazze RI, Callan CM, Galvez ST, et al: The effects of sevoflurane on serum creatinine and blood urea nitrogen concentrations: A retrospective, twenty-two–center, comparative evaluation of renal function in adult surgical patients. Anesth Analg 90:683-688, 2000.
159. Kharasch ED, Frink EJ Jr, Artru A, et al: Long-duration low-flow sevoflurane and isoflurane effects on postoperative renal and hepatic function. Anesth Analg 93:1511-1520, 2001.
160. Mazze RI, Jamison RL: Low-flow (1 l/min) sevoflurane: Is it safe? Anesthesiology 86:1225-1227, 1997.
161. Kumano H, Osaka S, Ishimura N, Nishiwada M: [Effects of enflurane, isoflurane, and sevoflurane on renal tubular functions.] Masui 41:1735-1740, 1992.
162. Bito H, Ikeuchi Y, Ikeda K: Effects of low-flow sevoflurane anesthesia on renal function: Comparison with high-flow sevoflurane anesthesia and low-flow isoflurane anesthesia. Anesthesiology 86:1231-1237, 1997.
163. Kharasch ED, Frink EJ Jr, Zager R, et al: Assessment of low-flow sevoflurane and isoflurane effects on renal function using sensitive markers of tubular toxicity. Anesthesiology 86:1238-1253, 1997.
164. Nishiyama T, Hanaoka K: Inorganic fluoride kinetics and renal and hepatic function after repeated sevoflurane anesthesia. Anesth Analg 87:468-473, 1998.
165. Eger EI 2nd, Koblin DD, Rowland T, et al: Nephrotoxicity of sevoflurane versus desflurane anesthesia in volunteers. Anesth Analg 84:160-168, 1997.
166. Ebert TJ, Frink EJ Jr, Kharasch ED: Absence of biochemical evidence for renal and hepatic dysfunction after 8 hours of 1.25 minimum alveolar concentration sevoflurane anesthesia in volunteers. Anesthesiology 88:601-610, 1998.
167. Goldberg ME, Cantillo J, Gratz I, et al: Dose of compound A, not sevoflurane, determines changes in the biochemical markers of renal injury in healthy volunteers. Anesth Analg 88:437-445, 1999.
168. Higuchi H, Wada H, Usui Y, et al: Effects of probenecid on renal function in surgical patients anesthetized with low-flow sevoflurane. Anesthesiology 94:21-31, 2001.
169. Higuchi H, Sumita S, Wada H, et al: Effects of sevoflurane and isoflurane on renal function and on possible markers of nephrotoxicity. Anesthesiology 89:307-322, 1998.
170. Eger EI 2nd, Gong D, Koblin DD, et al: Dose-related biochemical markers of renal injury after sevoflurane versus desflurane anesthesia in volunteers. Anesth Analg 85:1154-1163, 1997.
171. Ebert TJ, Messana LD, Uhrich TD, Staacke TS: Absence of renal and hepatic toxicity after four hours of 1.25 minimum alveolar anesthetic concentration sevoflurane anesthesia in volunteers. Anesth Analg 86:662-667, 1998.
172. Levine MF, Sarner J, Lerman J, et al: Plasma inorganic fluoride concentrations after sevoflurane anesthesia in children. Anesthesiology 84:348-353, 1996.
173. Frink EJ Jr, Green WB Jr, Brown EA, et al: Compound A concentrations during sevoflurane anesthesia in children. Anesthesiology 84:566-571, 1996.
174. Payne AK, Morgan SE, Gandolfi AJ, Brendel K: Biotransformation of sevoflurane by rat neonate liver slices. Drug Metab Dispos 23:497-500, 1995.

175. Iyer RA, Anders MW: Cysteine conjugate beta-lyase–dependent biotransformation of the cysteine *S*-conjugates of the sevoflurane degradation product compound A in human, nonhuman primate, and rat kidney cytosol and mitochondria. Anesthesiology 85:1454-1461, 1996.

176. Spracklin DK, Kharasch ED: Evidence for metabolism of fluoromethyl 2,2-difluoro-1-(trifluoromethyl)vinyl ether (compound A), a sevoflurane degradation product, by cysteine conjugate beta-lyase. Chem Res Toxicol 9:696-702, 1996.

177. Jin L, Baillie TA, Davis MR, Kharasch ED: Nephrotoxicity of sevoflurane compound A (fluoromethyl-2,2-difluoro-1-(trifluoromethyl)vinyl ether) in rats: Evidence for glutathione and cysteine conjugate formation and the role of renal cysteine conjugate beta-lyase. Biochem Biophys Res Commun 210:498-506, 1995.

178. Jin L, Davis MR, Kharasch ED, et al: Identification in rat bile of glutathione conjugates of fluoromethyl 2,2-difluoro-1-(trifluoromethyl)vinyl ether, a nephrotoxic degradate of the anesthetic agent sevoflurane. Chem Res Toxicol 9:555-561, 1996.

179. Commandeur JN, Oostendorp RA, Schoofs PR, et al: Nephrotoxicity and hepatotoxicity of 1,1-dichloro-2,2-difluoroethylene in the rat. Indications for differential mechanisms of bioactivation. Biochem Pharmacol 36:4229-4237, 1987.

180. Vamvakas S, Kremling E, Dekant W: Metabolic activation of the nephrotoxic haloalkene 1,1,2-trichloro-3,3,3-trifluoro-1-propene by glutathione conjugation. Biochem Pharmacol 38:2297-2304, 1989.

181. Green T, Odum J, Nash JA, Foster JR: Perchloroethylene-induced rat kidney tumors: An investigation of the mechanisms involved and their relevance to humans. Toxicol Appl Pharmacol 103:77-89, 1990.

182. Iyer RA, Frink EJ Jr, Ebert TJ, Anders MW: Cysteine conjugate beta-lyase–dependent metabolism of compound A (2-(fluoromethoxy)-1,1,3,3,3-pentafluoro-1-propene) in human subjects anesthetized with sevoflurane and in rats given compound A. Anesthesiology 88:611-618, 1998.

183. Iyer RA, Baggs RB, Anders MW: Nephrotoxicity of the glutathione and cysteine *S*-conjugates of the sevoflurane degradation product 2-(fluoromethoxy)-1,1,3,3,3-pentafluoro-1-propene (compound A) in male Fischer 344 rats. J Pharmacol Exp Ther 283:1544-1551, 1997.

184. Kharasch ED, Thorning D, Garton K, et al: Role of renal cysteine conjugate beta-lyase in the mechanism of compound A nephrotoxicity in rats. Anesthesiology 86:160-171, 1997.

185. Martin JL, Laster MJ, Kandel L, et al: Metabolism of compound A by renal cysteine-*S*-conjugate beta-lyase is not the mechanism of compound A–induced renal injury in the rat. Anesth Analg 82:770-774, 1996.

186. Kharasch ED, Hoffman GM, Thorning D, et al: Role of the renal cysteine conjugate beta-lyase pathway in inhaled compound A nephrotoxicity in rats. Anesthesiology 88:1624-1633, 1998.

187. Altuntas TG, Park SB, Kharasch ED: Sulfoxidation of cysteine and mercapturic acid conjugates of the sevoflurane degradation product fluoromethyl-2,2-difluoro-1-(trifluoromethyl)vinyl ether (compound A). Chem Res Toxicol 17:435-445, 2004.

188. Higuchi H, Adachi Y, Wada H, et al: The effects of low-flow sevoflurane and isoflurane anesthesia on renal function in patients with stable moderate renal insufficiency. Anesth Analg 92:650-655, 2001.

189. Conzen PF, Kharasch ED, Czerner SF, et al: Low-flow sevoflurane compared with low-flow isoflurane anesthesia in patients with stable renal insufficiency. Anesthesiology 97:578-584, 2002.

190. Eger EI 2nd, Ionescu P, Laster MJ, et al: Quantitative differences in the production and toxicity of CF2=BrCl versus CH2F-O-C(=CF2)(CF3) (compound A): The safety of halothane does not indicate the safety of sevoflurane. Anesth Analg 85:1164-1170, 1997.

191. Moon RE: Cause of CO poisoning, relation to halogenated agents still not clear. J Clin Monit 11:67-71, 1995.

192. Woehlck HJ, Dunning M 3rd, Connolly LA: Reduction in the incidence of carbon monoxide exposures in humans undergoing general anesthesia. Anesthesiology 87:228-234, 1997.

193. Berry PD, Sessler DI, Larson MD: Severe carbon monoxide poisoning during desflurane anesthesia. Anesthesiology 90:613-616, 1999.

194. Lentz RE: Carbon monoxide poisoning during anesthesia poses puzzles. J Clin Monit 11:66-67, 1995.

195. Baum J, Sachs G, vd Driesch C, Stanke HG: Carbon monoxide generation in carbon dioxide absorbents. Anesth Analg 81:144-146, 1995.

196. Davies MW, Potter FA: Carbon monoxide, soda lime and volatile agents. Anaesthesia 51:90, 1996.

197. Strum DP, Eger EI 2nd: The degradation, absorption, and solubility of volatile anesthetics in soda lime depend on water content. Anesth Analg 78:340-348, 1994.

198. Wissing H, Kuhn I, Warnken U, Dudziak R: Carbon monoxide production from desflurane, enflurane, halothane, isoflurane, and sevoflurane with dry soda lime. Anesthesiology 95:1205-1212, 2001.

199. Baxter PJ, Garton K, Kharasch ED: Mechanistic aspects of carbon monoxide formation from volatile anesthetics. Anesthesiology 89:929-941, 1998.

200. Stabernack CR, Brown R, Laster MJ, et al: Absorbents differ enormously in their capacity to produce compound A and carbon monoxide. Anesth Analg 90:1428-1435, 2000.

201. Murray JM, Renfrew CW, Bedi A, et al: Amsorb: A new carbon dioxide absorbent for use in anesthetic breathing systems. Anesthesiology 91:1342-1348, 1999.

202. Dunning MB 3rd, Bretscher LE, Arain SR, et al: Sevoflurane breakdown produces flammable concentrations of hydrogen. Anesthesiology 106:144-148, 2007.

203. Fatheree RS, Leighton BL: Acute respiratory distress syndrome after an exothermic Baralyme-sevoflurane reaction. Anesthesiology 101:531-533, 2004.

204. Castro BA, Freedman LA, Craig WL, Lynch C 3rd: Explosion within an anesthesia machine: Baralyme, high fresh gas flows and sevoflurane concentration. Anesthesiology 101:537-539, 2004.

205. Holak EJ, Mei DA, Dunning MB 3rd, et al: Carbon monoxide production from sevoflurane breakdown: Modeling of exposures under clinical conditions. Anesth Analg 96:757-764, 2003.

206. Keijzer C, Perez RS, de Lange JJ: Compound A and carbon monoxide production from sevoflurane and seven different types of carbon dioxide absorbent in a patient model. Acta Anaesthesiol Scand 51:31-37, 2007.

207. Marini F, Bellugi I, Gambi D, et al: Compound A, formaldehyde and methanol concentrations during low-flow sevoflurane anaesthesia: Comparison of three carbon dioxide absorbers. Acta Anaesthesiol Scand 51:625-632, 2007.

208. Shulman RM, Geraghty TJ, Tadros M: A case of unusual substance abuse causing myeloneuropathy. Spinal Cord 45:314-317, 2007.

209. Iwata K, O'Keefe GB, Karanas A: Neurologic problems associated with chronic nitrous oxide abuse in a non-healthcare worker. Am J Med Sci 322:173-174, 2001.

210. El Otmani H, El Moutawakil B, Moutaouakil F, et al: [Postoperative dementia: Toxicity of nitrous oxide.] Encephale 33:95-97, 2007.

211. Cohen Aubart F, Sedel F, Vicart S, et al: [Nitric oxide–triggered neurological disorders in subjects with vitamin B_{12} deficiency.] Rev Neurol (Paris) 163:362-364, 2007.

212. Sethi NK, Mullin P, Torgovnick J, Capasso G: Nitrous oxide "whippit" abuse presenting with cobalamin responsive psychosis. J Med Toxicol 2:71-74, 2006.

213. Hayes MF, Sacco AG, Savoy-Moore RT, et al: Effect of general anesthesia on fertilization and cleavage of human oocytes in vitro. Fertil Steril 48:975-981, 1987.

214. Critchlow BM, Ibrahim Z, Pollard BJ: General anaesthesia for gamete intra-fallopian transfer. Eur J Anaesthesiol 8:381-384, 1991.

215. Rosen MA, Roizen MF, Eger EI, et al: The effect of nitrous oxide on in vitro fertilization success rate. Anesthesiology 67:42-44, 1987.

216. Gonen O, Shulman A, Ghetler Y, et al: The impact of different types of anesthesia on in vitro fertilization–embryo transfer treatment outcome. J Assist Reprod Genet 12:678-682, 1995.

217. Ebi K, Rice S: Reproductive and development toxicity of anesthetics in humans. In Rice S, Fish K (eds): Anesthetic Toxicity. New York, Raven Press, 1994, p 175.

218. Rowland AS, Baird DD, Shore DL, et al: Nitrous oxide and spontaneous abortion in female dental assistants. Am J Epidemiol 141:531-538, 1995.

219. Fujinaga M, Baden JM, Shepard TH, Mazze RI: Nitrous oxide alters body laterality in rats. Teratology 41:131-135, 1990.

220. Baden JM, Fujinaga M: Effects of nitrous oxide on day 9 rat embryos grown in culture. Br J Anaesth 66:500-503, 1991.

221. Fujinaga M, Maze M, Hoffman BB, Baden JM: Activation of alpha-1 adrenergic receptors modulates the control of left/right sidedness in rat embryos. Dev Biol 150:419-421, 1992.

222. Fujinaga M, Hoffman BB, Baden JM: Receptor subtype and intracellular signal transduction pathway associated with situs inversus induced by alpha 1 adrenergic stimulation in rat embryos. Dev Biol 162:558-567, 1994.

223. Soriano SG, Loepke AW: Let's not throw the baby out with the bath water: Potential neurotoxicity of anesthetic drugs in infants and children. J Neurosurg Anesthesiol 17:207-209, 2005.

224. Anand KJ: Anesthetic neurotoxicity in newborns: Should we change clinical practice? Anesthesiology 107:2-4, 2007.

225. Mellon RD, Simone AF, Rappaport BA: Use of anesthetic agents in neonates and young children. Anesth Analg 104:509-520, 2007.

226. Gascon E, Klauser P, Kiss JZ, Vutskits L: Potentially toxic effects of anaesthetics on the developing central nervous system. Eur J Anaesthesiol 24:213-224, 2007.

227. Jevtovic-Todorovic V, Hartman RE, Izumi Y, et al: Early exposure to common anesthetic agents causes widespread neurodegeneration in the developing rat brain and persistent learning deficits. J Neurosci 23:876-882, 2003.

228. Walker K, Holland AJ, Winlaw D, et al: Neurodevelopmental outcomes and surgery in neonates. J Paediatr Child Health 42:749-751, 2006.

229. Chacko J, Ford WD, Haslam R: Growth and neurodevelopmental outcome in extremely-low-birth-

weight infants after laparotomy. Pediatr Surg Int 15:496-499, 1999.

230. Surgery and the tiny baby: Sensorineural outcome at 5 years of age. The Victorian Infant Collaborative Study Group. J Paediatr Child Health 32:167-172, 1996.
231. Kabra NS, Schmidt B, Roberts RS, et al: Neurosensory impairment after surgical closure of patent ductus arteriosus in extremely low birth weight infants: Results from the Trial of Indomethacin Prophylaxis in Preterms. J Pediatr 150:229-234, 234, 2007.
232. Bohnen N, Warner MA, Kokman E, Kurland LT: Early and midlife exposure to anesthesia and age of onset of Alzheimer's disease. Int J Neurosci 77:181-185, 1994.
233. Eckenhoff RG, Johansson JS, Wei H, et al: Inhaled anesthetic enhancement of amyloid-beta oligomerization and cytotoxicity. Anesthesiology 101:703-709, 2004.
234. Xie Z, Dong Y, Maedu U, et al: The inhalation anesthetic isoflurane induces a vicious cycle of apoptosis and amyloid beta-protein accumulation. J Neurosci 27:1247-1254, 2007.
235. Sessler DI, Badgwell JM: Exposure of postoperative nurses to exhaled anesthetic gases. Anesth Analg 87:1083-1088, 1998.
236. McGregor DG, Senjem DH, Mazze RI: Trace nitrous oxide levels in the postanesthesia care unit. Anesth Analg 89:472-475, 1999.
237. Byhahn C, Wilke HJ, Westphal K: Occupational exposure to volatile anaesthetics: Epidemiology and approaches to reducing the problem. CNS Drugs 15:197-215, 2001.
238. Shuhaiber S, Einarson A, Radde IC, et al: A prospective-controlled study of pregnant veterinary staff exposed to inhaled anesthetics and x-rays. Int J Occup Med Environ Health 15:363-373, 2002.
239. Krenzischek DA, Schaefer J, Nolan M, et al: Phase I collaborative pilot study: Waste anesthetic gas levels in the PACU. J Perianesth Nurs 17:227-239, 2002.
240. Sardas S, Cuhruk H, Karakaya AE, Atakurt Y: Sister-chromatid exchanges in operating room personnel. Mutat Res 279:117-120, 1992.
241. Hoerauf K, Lierz M, Wiesner G, et al: Genetic damage in operating room personnel exposed to isoflurane and nitrous oxide. Occup Environ Med 56:433-437, 1999.
242. Hoerauf KH, Wiesner G, Schroegendorfer KF, et al: Waste anaesthetic gases induce sister chromatid exchanges in lymphocytes of operating room personnel. Br J Anaesth 82:764-766, 1999.
243. Bozkurt G, Memis D, Karabogaz G, et al: Genotoxicity of waste anaesthetic gases. Anaesth Intensive Care 30:597-602, 2002.
244. Spence AA: Environmental pollution by inhalation anaesthetics. Br J Anaesth 59:96-103, 1987.
245. Maskell K, Mintzer IM, Callander BA: Basic science of climate change. Lancet 342:1027-1031, 1993.
246. Langbein T, Sonntag H, Trapp D, et al: Volatile anaesthetics and the atmosphere: Atmospheric lifetimes and atmospheric effects of halothane, enflurane, isoflurane, desflurane and sevoflurane. Br J Anaesth 82:66-73, 1999.
247. McGain F: Why anaesthetists should no longer use nitrous oxide. Anaesth Intensive Care 35:808-809, 2007.
248. Sherman SJ, Cullen BF: Nitrous oxide and the greenhouse effect. Anesthesiology 68:816-817, 1988.
249. Ratcliff A, Burns C, Gwinnutt CL: The contribution of medical nitrous oxide to the greenhouse effect. Health Trends 23:119-120, 1991.
250. Yoshimura E, Ushijima K: [The consumption of nitrous oxide used for general anesthesia has been markedly reduced in recent years in our institute.] Masui 54:904-905, 2005.

Russell C. Brockwell and J. Jeff Andrews

25 Inhaled Anesthetic Delivery Systems

Key Points

1. The low-pressure circuit (LPC) is the "vulnerable area" of anesthesia machines because it is most subject to breakage and leaks. The LPC is located downstream from all safety features of anesthesia machines except the oxygen analyzer, and it is the portion of the machine that is missed if an inappropriate LPC leak test is performed.
2. It is mandatory that the LPC be checked for leaks before administering an anesthetic because leaks in the LPC can cause delivery of a hypoxic mixture or patient awareness during anesthesia (or both).
3. Because many GE/Datex-Ohmeda anesthesia machines have a one-way check valve in the LPC, a negative-pressure leak test is required to detect leaks in the LPC. A positive-pressure leak test will not detect leaks in the LPC of most GE/Datex-Ohmeda products.
4. Internal vaporizer leaks can be detected only with the vaporizer turned on.
5. Before administering an anesthetic, the circle system must be checked for leaks and for flow. To test for leaks, the circle system is pressurized to 30 cm H_2O, and the circle system airway pressure gauge is observed (static test). To check for appropriate flow to rule out obstruction and faulty valves, the ventilator and a test lung (breathing bag) are used (dynamic test).
6. Some new anesthesia workstation self-tests do not detect internal vaporizer leaks unless each vaporizer is individually turned on during the self-test.
7. In the event of pipeline crossover, two actions must be taken. The backup oxygen cylinder must be turned "on," and the wall supply sources must be disconnected.
8. Fail-safe valves and proportioning systems help minimize delivery of a hypoxic mixture, but they are not foolproof. Delivery of a hypoxic mixture can result from (1) the wrong supply gas, (2) a defective or broken safety device, (3) leaks downstream from the safety devices, (4) administration of an inert gas, and (5) dilution of the inspired oxygen concentration by high concentrations of inhaled anesthetics.
9. Because of desflurane's low boiling point and high vapor pressure, controlled vaporization of desflurane requires special sophisticated vaporizers such as the Datex-Ohmeda Tec 6 and the Aladin cassette vaporizer.
10. Misfilling a conventional variable-bypass vaporizer with desflurane could theoretically be catastrophic and result in delivery of a hypoxic mixture and a massive overdose of inhaled desflurane anesthetic.
11. Inhaled anesthetics can interact with carbon dioxide absorbents and produce toxic compounds. During sevoflurane anesthesia, compound A can be formed, particularly at low fresh gas flow rates, and during desflurane anesthesia, carbon monoxide can be produced, particularly with desiccated absorbents.
12. Desiccated strong-base absorbents (particularly Baralyme) can react with sevoflurane and produce extremely high absorber temperatures and combustible decomposition products. In combination with the oxygen- or nitrous oxide–enriched environment of the circle system, these effects can produce fires within the breathing system.
13. Anesthesia ventilators with ascending bellows (bellows that ascend during the expiratory phase) are safer than descending bellows because disconnections will be readily manifested by failure ascending bellows to refill.
14. With ascending bellows anesthesia ventilators, fresh gas flow and oxygen flushing during the inspiratory phase contribute to the patient's tidal volume because the ventilator relief valve is closed. Oxygen flushing during the inspiratory phase can cause volutrama and/or barotrauma, (particularly in pediatric patients). Therefore, the oxygen flush should never be activated during the inspiratory phase of mechanical ventilation.

15. New ventilators that use fresh gas decoupling technology virtually eliminate the possibility of barotrauma from oxygen flushing during the inspiratory phase because fresh gas flow and oxygen flush flow are diverted to the reservoir breathing bag. However, if the breathing bag has a leak or is absent, patient awareness under anesthesia and delivery of a lower than expected oxygen concentration could occur because of entrainment of room air.

16. With newer GE/Datex-Ohmeda anesthetic ventilators such as the 7100 and 7900 SmartVent, scavenging of both the patient gas and the drive gas results in substantially increased volumes of scavenged gas. Thus, the scavenging systems must be set appropriately to accommodate the increased volume or pollution of the operating room environment could result.

Over the years, the anesthesia delivery system has evolved from a simple pneumatic device to a complex multisystem workstation, and new technologies continue to advance its development at a rapid pace (Figs. 25-1 and 25-2). These continuing changes to one of the most important pieces of equipment used by anesthesia care providers can make maintaining a current knowledge base (sufficient for their safe use) difficult for many to achieve. To prevent mishaps, providers must be aware of the functional anatomy of the anesthesia workstation. Furthermore, this knowledge base must even include the newer systems as they become available, to the extent that they are represented in an individual's practice. Fortunately, the most basic workstation components are generally fairly consistent from one platform to another. These basic component systems include what was formerly referred to as the anesthesia machine proper (i.e., the pressure-regulating and gas-mixing components), the vaporizers, the anesthesia breathing circuit, the ventilator, the scavenging system, and respiratory and physiologic monitoring systems.

For anesthesia care providers to safely use the many features of today's anesthesia workstation, a thorough understanding of its operation is essential. Because of large-scale education efforts, in addition to improvements in engineering and design of the anesthesia workstation, malpractice claims associated with gas delivery equipment are becoming less frequent. On the other hand, because of the continual development of new volatile anesthetics, aftermarket add-on devices, and even new anesthesia workstation features, equipment-related mishaps are not likely to disappear completely. In fact, in a review of the anesthesia closed-claims literature, Caplan and coworkers found that although claims related to the medical gas delivery system were rare, when they did occur, they were usually severe and death or permanent brain injury frequently resulted.[1]

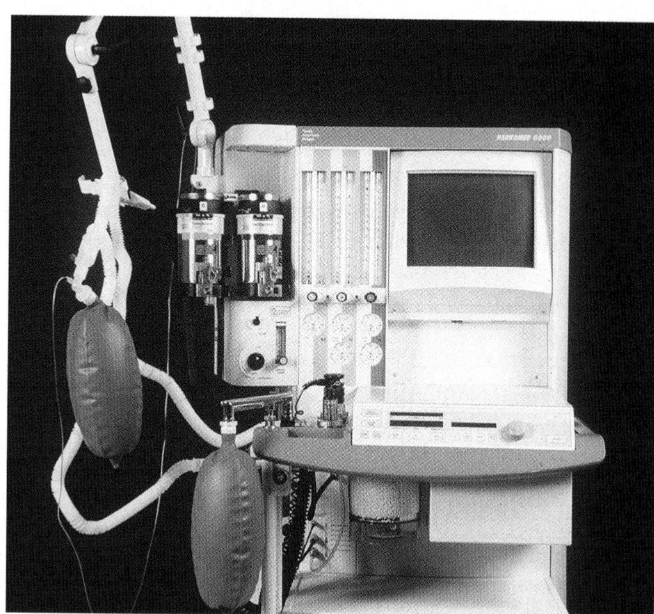

Figure 25-2 Dräger Narkomed 6000 anesthesia workstation.

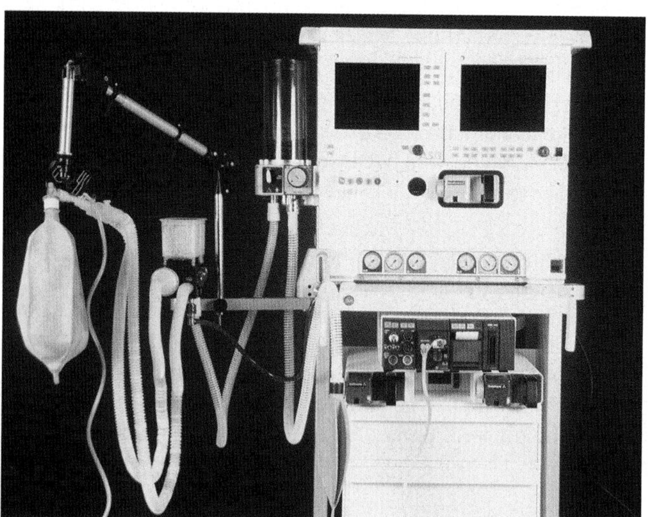

Figure 25-1 GE/Datex-Ohmeda S/5 Anesthesia Delivery Unit (ADU) workstation. *(Courtesy of GE Medical.)*

In this chapter we examine the anesthesia workstation piece by piece. We will describe the normal operation, function, and integration of major anesthesia workstation subsystems. More important, we illustrate potential problems and hazards associated with the various components of the anesthesia delivery system and the appropriate preoperative checks that may help detect and prevent such problems.

Anesthesia Workstation Standards and Pre-use Procedures

A few years ago, fundamental knowledge of basic anesthesia machine pneumatics would suffice for most anesthesia care providers. Today, a detailed understanding of pneumatics, electronics, and even computer science is helpful to fully understand the capabilities and complexities of the anesthesia workstation. Along with changes in the composition of the anesthesia workstation, including more complex ventilation systems and integrated monitoring, recently there has also been increasing divergence between anesthesia workstation designs from different manufacturers. In 1993, a joint effort between the American Society of Anesthesiologists (ASA) and the U.S. Food and Drug Administration (FDA) produced the 1993 FDA Anesthesia Apparatus Checkout Recommendations (Appendix 1). This pre-use checklist was versatile in that it could be applied to most commonly available anesthesia machines equally well, and it did not require users to vary the pre-use procedure significantly from machine to machine.

Today, because of increasing fundamental anesthesia workstation design variations, the 1993 FDA pre-use checklist may no longer be applicable to certain anesthesia workstations. In such cases, anesthesia care providers must be aware of this and follow the original equipment manufacturer's recommended pre-use checklist. Some of the latest workstations even have computer-assisted self-tests that automatically perform all or a part of the pre-use machine checkout procedure. The availability of such automated checkout features further adds to the complexity of constructing a standardized pre-use anesthesia machine checklist such as the one that the anesthesia community has enjoyed in the recent past. Ultimately, the responsibility for performing adequate pre-use testing of the anesthesia workstation falls to the anesthesia care provider. It will be the anesthesia care provider of record who must be aware of which anesthesia workstation components are tested by these automated self-tests and which ones are not. Because of the number of machines available and the variability among their self-testing procedures, we will limit their discussion to general topics related to these systems.

Standards for Anesthesia Machines and Workstations

Standards for anesthesia machines and workstations provide guidelines for manufacturers regarding their minimum performance, design characteristics, and safety requirements. During the past 2 decades, the progression of anesthesia machine standards has been as follows:

- 1979: American National Standards Institute (ANSI) Z79.8-1979[2]
- 1988: American Society for Testing and Materials (ASTM) F1161-88[3]
- 1994: ASTM F1161-94[4] (reapproved in 1994 and discontinued in 2000)
- 2000: ASTM F1850-00[5]

To comply with the 2000 ASTM F1850-00 standard, newly manufactured workstations must have monitors that measure the following parameters: continuous breathing system pressure, exhaled tidal volume, ventilatory carbon dioxide concentration, anesthetic vapor concentration, inspired oxygen concentration, oxygen supply pressure, arterial oxygen saturation of hemoglobin, arterial blood pressure, and continuous electrocardiogram. The anesthesia workstation must have a prioritized alarm system that groups the alarms into three categories: high, medium, and low priority. These monitors and alarms may be automatically enabled and made to function by turning on the anesthesia workstation, or the monitors and alarms can be manually enabled and made functional by following a pre-use checklist.[5]

Checking Your Anesthesia Workstation

A complete anesthesia apparatus checkout procedure must be performed each day before the anesthesia workstation is first used. An abbreviated version should be performed before each subsequent case. Several checkout procedures exist, but the 1993 FDA Anesthesia Apparatus Checkout Recommendations reproduced in Appendix 1 are the most popular and remain applicable to the majority of anesthesia machines in use worldwide.[6-10] Anesthesia care providers should also be aware that many machines have been modified in the field. The addition of aftermarket products may mandate modification of the pre-use checklist. The user must always refer to the original equipment manufacturer's operator's manual for special procedures or precautions related to particular workstations.

Because of the divergent nature of many contemporary anesthesia workstation designs, the philosophy of "one pre-use machine checkout procedure fits all machines" has had to be changed to a philosophy of "not all workstations are created equally." As a result, in 2005 the ASA's Committee on Equipment and Facilities began to develop a revised pre-use checklist that was designed to be more workstation specific and, indeed, was intended to eventually replace the 1993 FDA Anesthesia Apparatus Checkout Recommendations. Instead of the 1993 checklist, which elaborated specific checks and how they should be performed, the new pre-use guideline elaborates only specific systems and subsystems that must be evaluated. It is ultimately up to the user, in conjunction with workstation manufacturers, and local policy to determine the actual mechanisms/specific tests that will be used to accomplish these subsystem evaluations. Appendix 2 contains the most current version of these recommendations. Although the new recommendations also now address who (personnel-wise) may be responsible for performing such machine pre-use evaluations, every anesthesia care provider must be aware that the ultimate responsibility for proper machine pre-use safety checks rests on the provider using the machine to deliver anesthetic care. The current guidelines for developing institution-specific checkout procedures before anesthesia delivery can also be found on the ASA website at www.asahq.org/clinical/fda.htm. Also located at the same website are sample workstation-specific pre-use checklists developed by other institutions that can be adapted/modified for use in other practice settings.

Testing Specific Components of the Anesthesia Delivery System

The three most important preoperative checks are (1) calibration of the oxygen analyzer, (2) the low-pressure circuit leak test, and (3) the circle system tests. Each is discussed in the following paragraphs. Additional details regarding these systems will be presented in subsequent sections describing the anatomy of the anesthesia workstation. For a simplified diagram of a two-gas

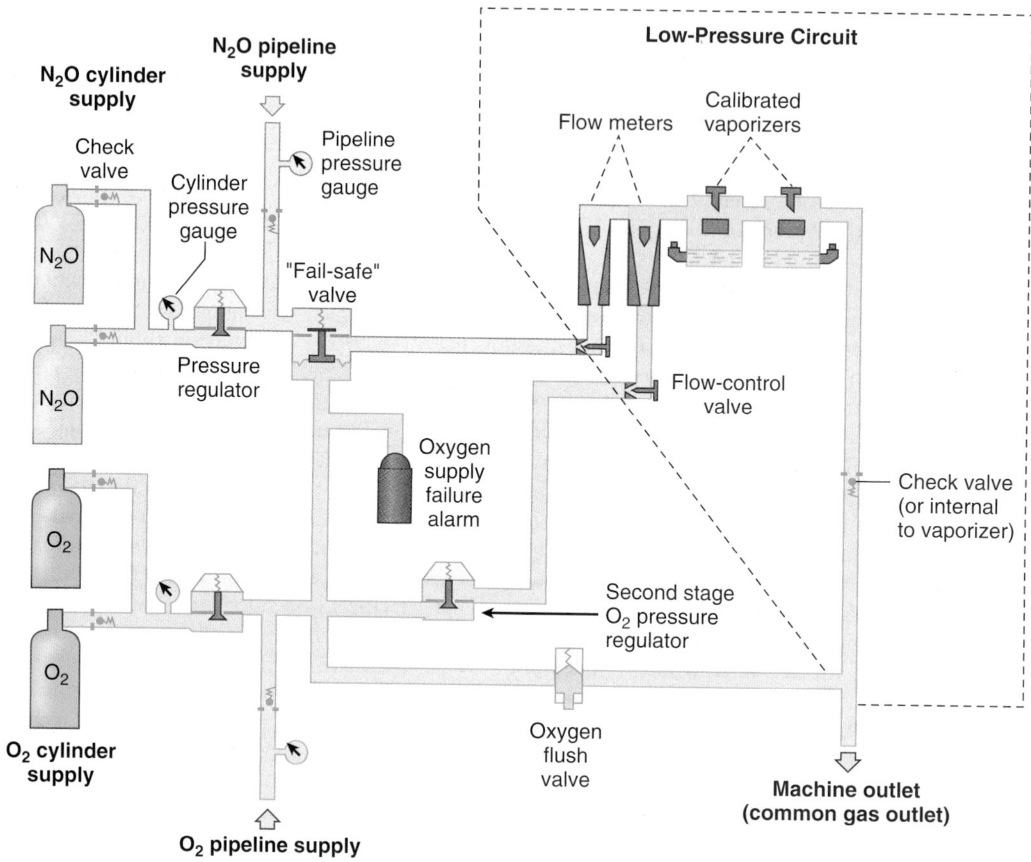

Figure 25-3 Diagram of a generic two-gas anesthesia machine. *(Modified with permission from Check-Out, a Guide for Preoperative Inspection of an Anesthesia Machine. Park Ridge, IL, American Society of Anesthesiologists, 1987.)*

anesthesia machine and the components described in the following discussion, please refer to Figure 25-3. A comprehensive discussion of Figure 25-3 can also be found in the section "Anesthesia Workstation Pneumatics."

Calibration of the Oxygen Analyzer

The oxygen analyzer is one of the most important monitors on the anesthesia workstation. It is the only machine safety device that evaluates the integrity of the low-pressure circuit in an ongoing fashion. Other machine safety devices, such as the fail-safe valve, the oxygen supply failure alarm, and the proportioning system, are all upstream from the flow control valves. The only machine monitor that detects problems downstream from the flow control valves is the oxygen analyzer. Calibration of this monitor is described in Appendix 1 (Anesthesia Apparatus Checkout Recommendations, 1993, No. 9). The actual procedure for calibrating the oxygen analyzer has remained reasonably similar over the recent generations of anesthesia workstations. Generally, the oxygen concentration–sensing element must be exposed to room air for calibration to 21%. This may require manually setting a dial on older machines, but on newer ones, it usually involves only temporary removal of the sensor, selecting and then confirming that the oxygen calibration is to be performed from a set of menus on the workstation's display screen, and finally reinstalling the sensor.

Low-Pressure Circuit Leak Test

The low-pressure leak test checks the integrity of the anesthesia machine from the flow control valves to the common gas outlet. It evaluates the portion of the machine that is downstream from all safety devices except the oxygen analyzer. The components located within this area are *precisely* the ones most subject to breakage and leaks. Leaks in the low-pressure circuit can cause hypoxia and/or patient awareness.[11,12] Flow tubes, the most delicate pneumatic component of the machine, can crack or break. A typical three-gas anesthesia machine has 16 O-rings in the low-pressure circuit. Leaks can occur at the interface between the glass flow tubes and the manifold and at the O-ring junctions between the vaporizer and its manifold. Loose filler caps on vaporizers are a common source of leaks, and these leaks can cause patient awareness under anesthesia.[11,13]

Several different methods have been used to check the low-pressure circuit for leaks, including the oxygen flush test, the common gas outlet occlusion test, the traditional positive-pressure leak test, the North American Dräger positive-pressure leak test, the Ohmeda 8000 internal positive-pressure leak test, the Ohmeda negative-pressure leak test, the 1993 FDA universal negative-pressure leak test, and others. One reason for the large number of methods is that the internal design of various machines differs considerably. The most notable example is that most GE Healthcare/Datex-Ohmeda (hereafter referred to as Datex-

Table 25-1 Check Valves and Manufacturer-Recommended Leak Test

Anesthesia Machine	Machine Outlet Check Valve	Vaporizer Outlet Check Valve	Leak Test Recommended by Manufacturer	
			Positive Pressure	**Negative Pressure (Suction Bulb)**
Dräger Narkomed 2A, 2B, 2C, 3, 4, GS	No	No	X	
Fabius GS	No	No	Self-test	
Narkomed 6000	No	No	Self-test	
Ohmeda Unitrol	Yes	Variable		X
Ohmeda 30/70	Yes	Variable		X
Ohmeda Modulus I	Yes	Variable		X
Ohmeda Modulus II	Yes	No		X
Ohmeda Excel series	Yes	No		X
Ohmeda Modulus II Plus	No	No		X
Ohmeda CD	No	No		X
Datex-Ohmeda Aestiva	Yes	No		X
Datex-Ohmeda S5/ADU	No	No	Self-test	

Data from Ohio Medical Products, Ohmeda, Datex-Ohmeda, North American Dräger, Dräger Medical.

Ohmeda) workstations have a check valve near the common gas outlet whereas Dräger Medical workstations do not. The presence or absence of the check valve profoundly influences which preoperative check is indicated.

Several mishaps have resulted from application of the wrong leak test to the wrong machine.[14-17] It is therefore mandatory that the appropriate low-pressure leak test be performed each day. To do so, it is essential that the exact location and operating principles of the Datex-Ohmeda check valve be understood. Many Datex-Ohmeda anesthesia workstations have a machine outlet check valve located in the low-pressure circuit (see Table 25-1). The check valve is located downstream from the vaporizers and upstream from the oxygen flush valve (Fig. 25-3). It is open (Fig. 25-4, left) in the absence of backpressure. Gas flow from the manifold moves the rubber flapper valve off its seat and allows gas to proceed freely to the common outlet. The valve closes (Fig. 25-4, right) when backpressure is exerted on it.[8] Backpressure sufficient to close the check valve may occur with the following conditions: oxygen flushing, peak breathing circuit pressures generated during positive-pressure ventilation, or use of a positive-pressure leak test.

Generally speaking, the low-pressure circuit of anesthesia workstations without an outlet check valve can be tested with a positive-pressure leak test, and machines with check valves must

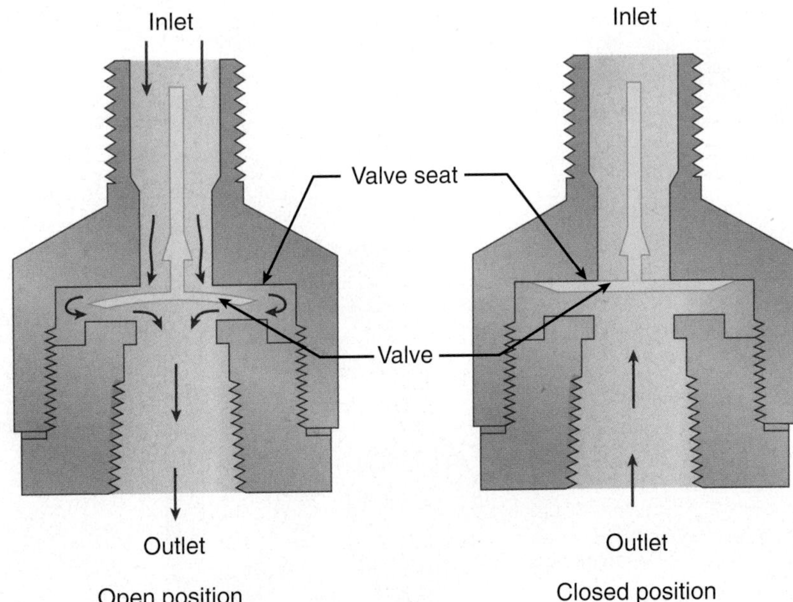

Figure 25-4 Machine outlet check valve. See text for details. *(Reproduced with permission from Bowie E, Huffman LM: The Anesthesia Machine: Essentials for Understanding. Madison, WI, Ohmeda, a Division of BOC Health Care, Inc., 1985.)*

be tested with a negative-pressure leak test. When performing a positive-pressure leak test, the operator generates positive pressure in the low-pressure circuit by using flow from the anesthesia machine or from a positive-pressure bulb to detect a leak. When performing a negative-pressure leak test, the operator creates negative pressure in the low-pressure circuit by using a suction bulb to detect leaks. Two different low-pressure circuit leak tests are described in the following paragraphs.

Oxygen Flush Positive-Pressure Leak Test Historically, older anesthesia machines did not have check valves in the low-pressure circuit. Therefore, it was common practice to pressurize the breathing circuit and the low-pressure circuit with the oxygen flush valve to test for internal anesthesia machine leaks. Because many modern Datex-Ohmeda machines now have check valves in the low-pressure circuit, however, application of a positive-pressure leak test to these machines can be misleading or even dangerous (Fig. 25-5). Inappropriate use of the oxygen flush valve or the presence of a leaking flush valve may lead to inadequate evaluation of the low-pressure circuit for leaks. In turn, this can lull the anesthesia care provider into a false sense of security despite the presence of large leaks.[15-19] Positive pressure from the breathing circuit results in closure of the outlet check valve, and the value on the airway pressure gauge will fail to decline. The system appears to be tight, but in actuality, only the circuitry downstream from the check valve is leak free.[20] Thus, a vulnerable area exists from the check valve back to the flow control valves because this area is not tested by a positive-pressure leak test.

1993 FDA Negative-Pressure Leak Test The 1993 FDA universal negative-pressure leak test[10] (Appendix 1, No. 5) was named "universal" because at that time it could be used to check all contemporary anesthesia machines, regardless of the presence or absence of check valves in the low-pressure circuit. It remains effective for many anesthesia workstations and can be applied to many Datex-Ohmeda machines, Dräger Medical machines, and others. Unfortunately, some newer machines are no longer compatible with this test. The ASA's Committee on Equipment and Facilities in conjunction with the FDA is expected to update the 1993 Anesthesia Apparatus Checkout Recommendations as this chapter comes to press. Until the new recommendations become available, the 1993 guidelines should continue to be followed as closely as possible because they remain applicable to the vast majority of anesthesia workstations in use worldwide.

The 1993 FDA checklist is based upon the Datex-Ohmeda negative-pressure leak test (Fig. 25-6). It is performed with a negative-pressure leak-testing device, which is a simple suction bulb. The machine's master switch, flow control valves, and vaporizers are turned off. The suction bulb is attached to the common fresh gas outlet and squeezed repeatedly until it is fully collapsed. This action creates a vacuum in the low-pressure circuitry. The machine is free of leaks if the hand bulb remains collapsed for at least 10 seconds. A leak is present if the bulb reinflates during this period. The test is repeated with each vaporizer individually turned to the "on" position because internal vaporizer leaks can be detected only with the vaporizer turned on.

The FDA "universal" negative-pressure low-pressure circuit leak test has several advantages.[21] It is quick and simple to perform,

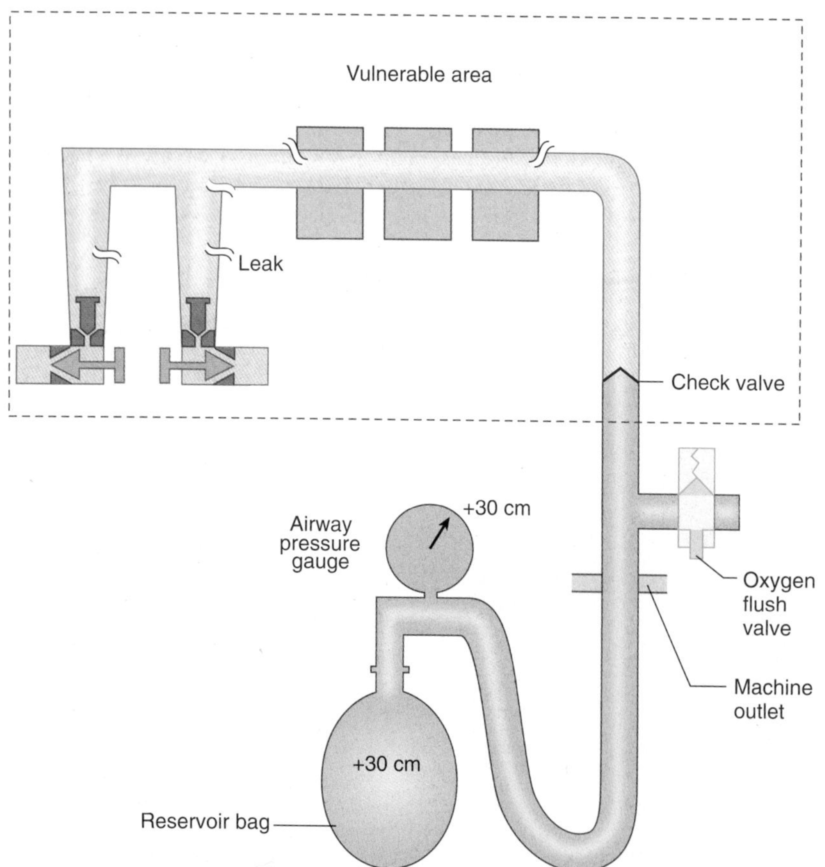

Figure 25-5 Inappropriate use of the oxygen flush valve to check the low-pressure circuit of an Ohmeda machine equipped with a check valve. The area within the *rectangle* is not checked by inappropriate use of the oxygen flush valve. The components located within this area are *precisely* the ones most subject to breakage and leaks. Positive pressure within the patient circuit closes the check valve, and the value on the airway pressure gauge does not decline despite leaks in the low-pressure circuit.

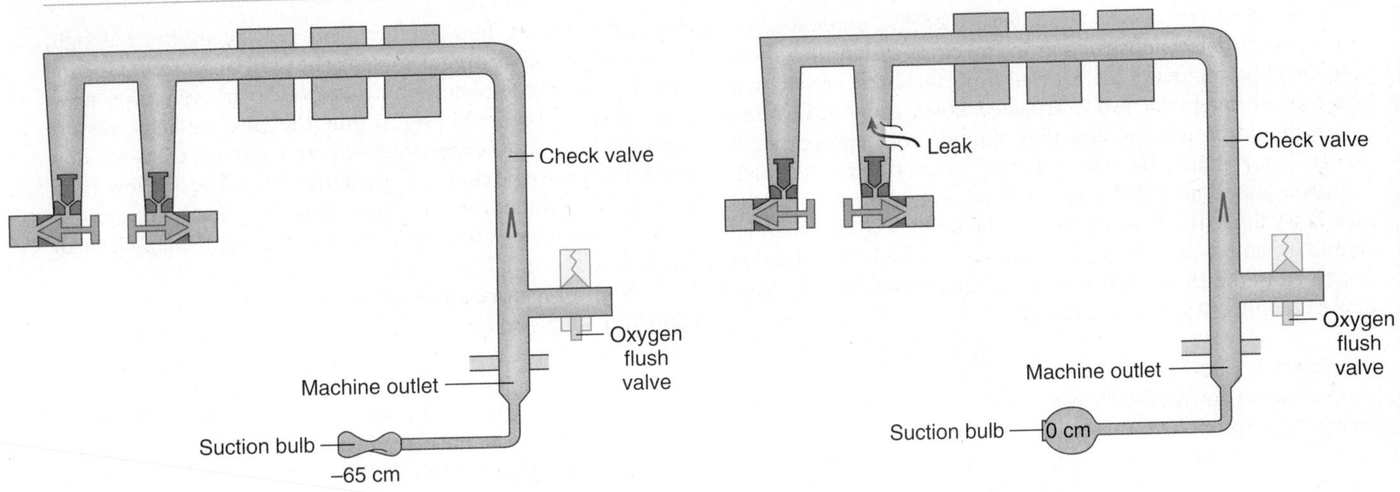

Figure 25-6 Food and Drug Administration negative-pressure leak test. **Left,** A negative-pressure leak-testing device is attached directly to the machine outlet. Squeezing the bulb creates a vacuum in the low-pressure circuit and opens the check valve. **Right,** When a leak is present in the low-pressure circuit, room air is entrained through the leak and the suction bulb inflates. *(Reprinted with permission from Andrews JJ: Understanding anesthesia machines. In 1988 Review Course Lectures. Cleveland, OH, International Anesthesia Research Society, 1988, p 78.)*

has an obvious end point, and may help isolate the problem. For example, if the bulb reinflates in less than 10 seconds, a leak is present somewhere in the low-pressure circuit. Therefore, it differentiates between breathing circuit leaks and leaks in the low-pressure circuit. The "universal" negative-pressure leak test is the most sensitive of all contemporary leak tests because it is not dependent on volume. That is, it does not involve the use of a breathing bag or corrugated hoses whose compliance could mask a significant leak. It can detect leaks as small as 30 mL/min. Finally, the operator does not need detailed or in-depth knowledge of proprietary design differences. If the operator performs the universal test correctly, the leak will be detected.

Circle System Tests

The circle system tests (Appendix 1, Nos. 11 and 12) evaluate the integrity of the circle breathing system, which spans from the common gas outlet to the Y-piece (Fig. 25-7). It has two parts—the *leak test* and the *flow test*. To thoroughly check the circle system for leaks, valve integrity, and obstruction, both tests must be performed preoperatively. The *leak test* is performed by closing the pop-off valve, occluding the Y-piece, and pressurizing the circuit to 30 cm H_2O with the oxygen flush valve. The value on the pressure gauge will not decline if the circle system is leak free, but this does not ensure valve integrity. The value on the gauge will read 30 cm H_2O even if the unidirectional valves are stuck shut or the valves are incompetent.

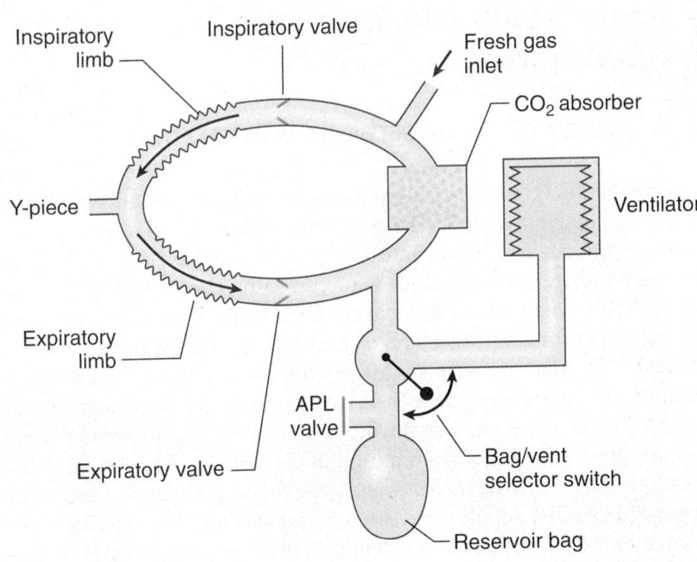

Figure 25-7 Components of the circle system. APL, adjustable pressure-limiting; B, reservoir bag; V, ventilator. *(Reproduced with permission from Brockwell RC: Delivery systems for inhaled anesthesia. In Barash PG [ed]: Clinical Anesthesia, 5th ed. Philadelphia, Lippincott Williams & Wilkins, 2006, p 562.)*

The *flow test* checks the integrity of the unidirectional valves, and it detects obstruction in the circle system. It can be performed by removing the Y-piece from the circle system and breathing through the two corrugated hoses individually. The valves should be present, and they should move appropriately. The operator should be able to inhale but not exhale through the inspiratory limb and able to exhale but not inhale through the expiratory limb. The flow test can also be performed by using the ventilator and a breathing bag attached to the "Y"-piece as described in the 1993 FDA Anesthesia Apparatus Checkout Recommendations (Appendix 1, No. 12).[10]

Workstation Self-Tests

As mentioned previously, many new anesthesia workstations now incorporate technology that allows the machine to either automatically or manually walk the user through a series of self-tests to check for functionality of the electronic, mechanical, and pneumatic components. Tested components commonly include the gas supply system, flow control valves, circle system, ventilator, and, in the case of the Datex-Ohmeda Anesthesia Delivery Unit (ADU), even the Aladin cassette vaporizer. The comprehensiveness of these self-diagnostic tests varies from one model and manufacturer to another. If these tests are to be used, all manufacturer recommendations must be read and strictly followed. Although a thorough understanding of what the particular workstation's self-tests include is very helpful, this information is often difficult to obtain and may vary greatly between devices.

One particularly important point of caution with self-tests should be noted on systems with manifold-mounted vaporizers such as the Dräger Medical Fabius GS and the Narkomed 6000 series. A manifold-mounted vaporizer does not become part of an anesthesia workstation's gas flow stream until its concentration control dial is turned to the "on" position. Therefore, to detect internal vaporizer leaks on this type of system, the "leak test" portion of the self-diagnostic must be repeated separately with each individual vaporizer turned to the "on" position. If this precaution is not taken, large leaks that could potentially result in patient awareness, such as from a loose filler cap or cracked fill indicator, could go undetected.

Anesthesia Workstation Pneumatics

Anatomy of an Anesthesia Workstation

A simplified diagram of a generic two-gas anesthesia machine is presented in Figure 25-3. The pressures within the anesthesia workstation can be divided into three circuits: a high-pressure, an intermediate-pressure, and a low-pressure circuit (see Fig. 25-3). The *high-pressure circuit* is confined to the cylinders and the cylinder primary pressure regulators. For oxygen, the pressure range of the high-pressure circuit extends from a high of 2200 pounds per square inch gauge (psig) to 45 psig, which is the regulated cylinder pressure. For nitrous oxide in the high-pressure circuit, pressures ranges from a high of 750 psig in the cylinder to a low of 45 psig. The *intermediate-pressure circuit* begins at the regulated cylinder supply sources at 45 psig, includes the pipeline sources at 50 to 55 psig, and extends to the flow control valves. Depending on the manufacturer and specific machine design, second-stage pressure regulators may be used to decrease pipeline supply pressure to the flow control valves to an even lower pressure such as 14 or 26 psig within the intermediate-pressure circuit.[22,23] Finally, the *low-pressure circuit* extends from the flow control valves to the common gas outlet. Therefore, the low-pressure circuit includes the flow tubes, vaporizer manifold, vaporizers, and the one-way check valve on most Datex-Ohmeda machines.[22]

Both oxygen and nitrous oxide have two supply sources: a pipeline supply source and a cylinder supply source. The pipeline supply source is the primary gas source for the anesthesia machine. The hospital pipeline supply system provides gas to the machine at approximately 50 psig, which is the normal working pressure of most machines. The cylinder supply source serves as a backup if the pipeline supply fails or as the primary supply if the anesthesia workstation is being used in a location without the availability of pipeline-supplied gases. As previously described, the oxygen cylinder source is regulated from 2200 to approximately 45 psig, and the nitrous oxide cylinder source is regulated from 745 to approximately 45 psig.[22-24]

A safety device traditionally referred to as the *fail-safe* valve is located downstream from the nitrous oxide supply source. It serves as an interface between the oxygen and nitrous oxide supply sources. This valve shuts off or proportionally decreases the supply of nitrous oxide (and other gases) if the oxygen supply pressure declines. To meet ASTM standards, contemporary machines have an alarm device to monitor the oxygen supply pressure. A high-priority alarm is actuated as the declining oxygen supply pressure reaches a predetermined threshold such as 30 psig.[22-24]

Many Datex-Ohmeda machines have a second-stage oxygen regulator located downstream from the oxygen supply source in the intermediate-pressure circuit. It is adjusted to a precise pressure level, such as 14 psig.[23] This regulator supplies a constant pressure to the oxygen flow control valve regardless of fluctuating oxygen pipeline pressures. For example, flow from the oxygen flow control valve will be constant if the oxygen supply pressure is greater than 14 psig.

The flow control valves represent an important anatomic landmark within the anesthesia workstation because they separate the intermediate-pressure circuit from the low-pressure circuit. The low-pressure circuit is the part of the machine that lies downstream from the flow control valves. The operator regulates flow entering the low-pressure circuit by adjusting the flow control valves. The oxygen and nitrous oxide flow control valves are linked mechanically or pneumatically by a proportioning system to help prevent inadvertent delivery of a hypoxic mixture. After leaving the flow tubes, the mixture of gases travels through a common manifold and may be directed to a calibrated vaporizer. Precise amounts of inhaled anesthetic can be added, depending on the vaporizer control dial setting. The total fresh gas flow plus the anesthetic vapor then travel toward the common gas outlet.[22,23]

Many Datex-Ohmeda anesthesia machines have a one-way check valve located between the vaporizer and the common gas outlet in the mixed-gas pipeline. Its purpose is to prevent backflow into the vaporizer during positive-pressure ventilation, thereby minimizing the effects of intermittent fluctuations in downstream pressure on the concentration of inhaled anesthetic (see "Intermittent Backpressure" in the section "Vaporizers"). The presence or absence of this check valve *profoundly* influences which preoperative leak test is indicated (see "Checking Your Anesthesia Workstation"). The oxygen flush connection joins the mixed-gas pipeline between the one-way check valve (when present) and the machine outlet. Thus, when the oxygen flush valve is activated, the pipeline oxygen pressure has a "straight shot" to the common gas outlet.[22,23]

Pipeline Supply Source

Under normal conditions, the pipeline supply serves as the primary gas source for the anesthesia machine. Most hospitals today have a central piping system to deliver medical gases such as oxygen, nitrous oxide, and air to the operating room. The central piping system must supply the correct gases at the appropriate pressure for the anesthesia workstation to function properly. Unfortunately, this does not always occur. Proven as recently as 2002, even large medical centers with huge cryogenic bulk oxygen storage systems are not immune to component failures that may contribute to critical oxygen pipeline supply failures.[25] In this case, rupture of a faulty joint at the bottom of the primary cryogenic oxygen storage tank released 8000 gallons of liquid oxygen to flood the streets in the surrounding area. This mishap suddenly compromised oxygen delivery in a major medical center.

In a survey of approximately 200 hospitals in 1976, 31% reported difficulties with pipeline systems.[26] The most common problem was inadequate oxygen pressure, followed by excessive pipeline pressure. The most devastating reported hazard, however, was accidental crossing of oxygen and nitrous oxide pipelines, which has led to many deaths. This problem caused 23 deaths in a newly constructed wing of a general hospital in Sudbury, Ontario, during a 5-month period.[26,27] More recently, in 2002 two additional hypoxic deaths were reported in New Haven, Connecticut. These deaths resulted from a medical gas system failure in which an altered oxygen flow meter was inadvertently connected to a wall supply source for nitrous oxide.[28]

In the event that a pipeline crossover is ever suspected, the anesthesia care provider must immediately make *two* corrective actions. First, the backup oxygen cylinder should be turned on. Then the pipeline supply must be disconnected. This second step is mandatory because the machine will preferentially use the inappropriate 50-psig pipeline supply source instead of the lower pressure (45 psig) oxygen cylinder source if the wall supply is not disconnected.

Gas enters the anesthesia machine through the pipeline inlet connections (arrows in Fig. 25-3). The pipeline inlet fittings are gas-specific Diameter Index Safety System (DISS) threaded body fittings. The DISS provides threaded noninterchangeable connections for medical gas lines to minimize the risk of misconnection. A check valve located downstream from the inlet prevents reverse flow of gases from the machine to the pipeline or the atmosphere.

Cylinder Supply Source

Anesthesia workstations have E-cylinders for use when a pipeline supply source is not available or the pipeline system fails. As has been shown again in the recent literature, anesthesia care providers can easily become complacent in assuming that backup gas cylinders are in fact present on the back of the anesthesia workstation and, furthermore, if present, that they contain an adequate supply of compressed gas. Any pre-use checklist should contain steps that confirm both.[29]

Medical gases supplied in E-cylinders are attached to the anesthesia machine via the hanger yoke assembly. The hanger yoke assembly orients and supports the cylinder, provides a gas-tight seal, and ensures unidirectional flow of gases into the machine.[22] Each hanger yoke is equipped with the Pin Index Safety System (PISS). The PISS is a safeguard introduced to eliminate cylinder interchanging and the possibility of accidentally placing the incorrect gas on a yoke designed to accommodate another gas. Two metal pins on the yoke assembly are arranged so that that they project into corresponding holes on the cylinder valve. Each gas or combination of gases has a specific pin arrangement.[30]

Once the cylinders are turned on, compressed gases may pass from their respective high-pressure cylinder sources into the anesthesia machine (see Fig. 25-3). A check valve is located downstream from each cylinder if a double-yoke assembly is used. This check valve serves several functions. First, it minimizes transfer of gas from a cylinder at high pressure to one with lower pressure. Second, it allows an empty cylinder to be exchanged for a full one while gas flow continues from the other cylinder into the machine with minimal loss of gas or supply pressure. Third, it minimizes leakage from an open cylinder to the atmosphere if one cylinder is absent.[22,23] A cylinder supply pressure gauge is located downstream from the check valves. The gauge will indicate the pressure in the cylinder with the higher pressure when two reserve cylinders of the same gas are opened at the same time.

Each cylinder supply source has a pressure-reducing valve known as the cylinder pressure regulator. It reduces the high and variable storage pressure present in a cylinder to a lower, more constant pressure suitable for use in the anesthesia machine. The oxygen cylinder pressure regulator reduces the oxygen cylinder pressure from a high of 2200 psig to approximately 45 psig. The nitrous oxide cylinder pressure regulator receives pressure of up to 745 psig and reduces it to approximately 45 psig.[22,23]

The gas supply cylinder valves should be turned off when not in use, except during the preoperative machine checkout period. If the cylinder supply valves are left on, the reserve cylinder supply can be silently depleted whenever the pressure inside the machine decreases to a value lower than the regulated cylinder pressure. For example, oxygen pressure within the machine can decrease below 45 psig with oxygen flushing or possibly even during use of a pneumatically driven ventilator, particularly at high inspiratory flow rates. Additionally, the pipeline supply pressures of all gases can fall to less than 45 psig if problems exist in the central piping system. If the cylinders are left on when this occurs, they will eventually become depleted and no reserve supply may be available if a pipeline failure occurs.[20,23]

The amount of time that an anesthesia machine can operate from E-cylinder supplies is commonly of concern. This is becoming particularly important to anesthesia care providers now that anesthesia machines are being used more frequently in the setting of office-based and remote (outside the operating room) anesthesia care within hospitals. For oxygen, the volume of gas remaining in the cylinder is proportional to cylinder pressure. One author has proposed the following equation to help estimate the time remaining[31]:

$$\text{Approximate remaining time (hr)} \approx \frac{\text{Oxygen cylinder pressure (psig)}}{200 \times \text{Oxygen flow rate (L/min)}}$$

It should be noted that this calculation will provide a gross estimate of the time remaining and may not be exact. Furthermore, users should be cautioned that use of a pneumatically driven mechanical ventilator will dramatically increase oxygen utilization rates, thus decreasing the time remaining until depletion of the cylinder. Hand ventilation at low fresh gas flow rates may consume less than 5% of the amount of oxygen consumed by intermediate flow meter settings coupled with the use of pneumatically powered mechanical ventilation.[25] Because piston-type anesthesia ventilators such as found in the Dräger Medical Fabius GS and Narkomed 6000 series do not affect oxygen consumption rates, they may be preferable to conventional gas-driven ventilators in practice settings that are dependent on the use of compressed gas cylinders as the primary gas source.

Oxygen Supply Pressure Failure Safety Devices

Oxygen and nitrous oxide supply sources existed as independent entities in older models of anesthesia machines, and they were not pneumatically or mechanically interfaced. Therefore, abrupt or insidious oxygen pressure failure had the potential to lead to the delivery of a hypoxic mixture. The 2000 ASTM F1850-00 standard states that "The anesthesia gas supply device shall be designed so that whenever oxygen supply pressure is reduced to below the manufacturer specified minimum, the delivered oxygen concentration shall not decrease below 19% at the common gas outlet."[5] Contemporary anesthesia machines have a number of safety devices that act together in a cascade manner to minimize the risk of delivery of a hypoxic gas mixture as oxygen pressure decreases. Several of these devices are described in the following sections.

Pneumatic and Electronic Alarm Devices

Many older anesthesia machines have a pneumatic alarm device that sounds a warning when the oxygen supply pressure decreases to a predetermined threshold value, such as 30 psig. The 2000 ASTM F1850-00 standard mandates that a medium-priority alarm be activated within 5 seconds when oxygen pressure decreases below a manufacturer-specific pressure threshold.[5] Electronic alarm devices are now used to meet this guideline.

Fail-Safe Valves

A fail-safe valve is present in the gas line supplying each of the flow meters except oxygen. Controlled by oxygen supply pressure, the valve shuts off or proportionally decreases the supply pressure of all other gases (nitrous oxide, air, carbon dioxide, helium, nitrogen) as the oxygen supply pressure decreases. Unfortunately, the misnomer "fail safe" has led to the misconception that the valve prevents administration of a hypoxic mixture. Such is not the case. Machines that either are not equipped with a flow proportioning system (see "Proportioning Systems") or whose system may be disabled by the user can deliver a hypoxic mixture under normal working conditions. On such a system, the oxygen flow control valve can be closed intentionally or accidentally. Normal oxygen pressure will keep the other gas lines open so that a hypoxic mixture can result.[22,23]

Many Datex-Ohmeda machines are equipped with a fail-safe valve known as the pressure sensor shut-off valve (Fig. 25-8). This valve operates in a threshold manner and is either open or closed. Oxygen supply pressure opens the valve, and the valve return spring closes the valve. Figure 25-8 shows a nitrous oxide pressure sensor shut-off valve with a threshold pressure of 20 psig. In Figure 25-8A, an oxygen supply pressure greater than 20 psig is exerted on the mobile diaphragm. This pressure moves the piston and pin upward and the valve opens. Nitrous oxide flows freely to the nitrous oxide flow control valve. In Figure 25-8B, the oxygen supply pressure is less than 20 psig, and the force of the valve return spring completely closes the valve.[23] Nitrous oxide flow stops at the closed fail-safe valve, and it does not advance to the nitrous oxide flow control valve.

North American Dräger uses a different fail-safe valve known as the oxygen failure protection device (OFPD) to interface the oxygen pressure with that of other gases, such as nitrous oxide or other inert gases. In contrast to Datex-Ohmeda's oxygen pressure sensor shut-off valve, the OFPD is based on a proportioning principle rather than a threshold principle. The pressure of all gases controlled by the OFPD will decrease proportionally with the oxygen pressure. The OFPD consists of a seat nozzle

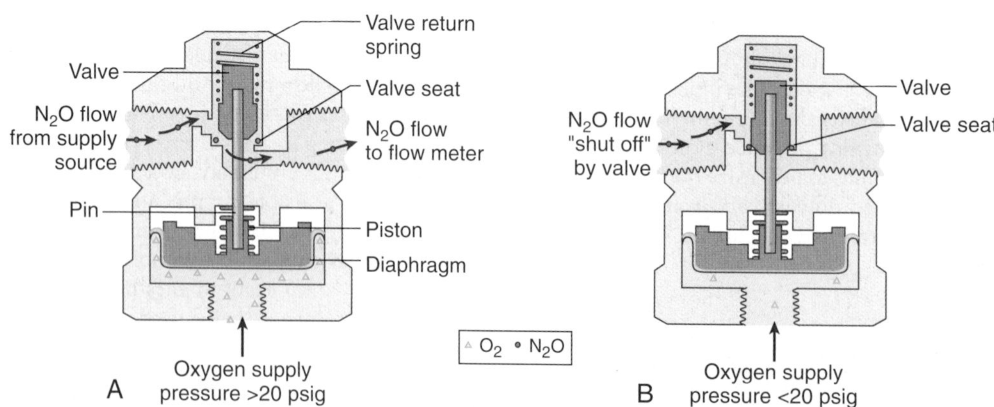

Figure 25-8 Pressure sensor shut-off valve. The valve is open in **A** because the oxygen supply pressure is greater than the threshold value of 20 psig. The valve is closed in **B** because of inadequate oxygen pressure. *(Redrawn with permission from Bowie E, Huffman LM: The Anesthesia Machine: Essentials for Understanding. Madison, WI, Ohmeda, A Division of BOC Health Care, Inc., 1985.)*

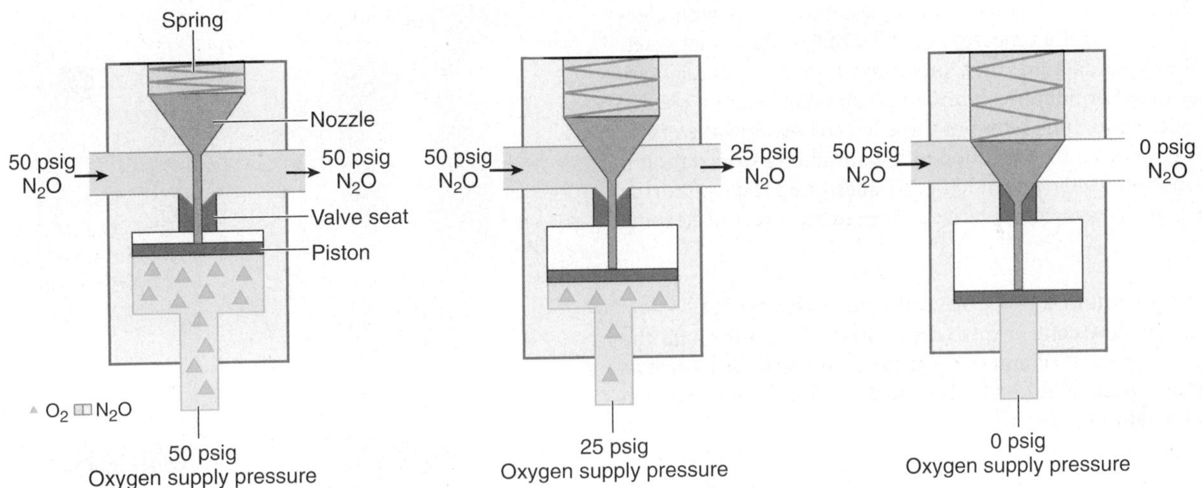

Figure 25-9 An oxygen failure protection device that responds proportionally to changes in oxygen supply pressure. See text for details. *(Redrawn with permission from Narkomed 2A Anesthesia System. Technical Service Manual, 6th ed. Telford, PA, North American Dräger, June 1985.)*

assembly connected to a spring-loaded piston (Fig. 25-9). The oxygen supply pressure in the left panel of Figure 25-9 is 50 psig. This pressure pushes the piston upward, which forces the nozzle away from the valve seat. Nitrous oxide alone or combined with other gases advances toward the flow control valve at 50 psig. The oxygen pressure in the right panel is 0 psig. The spring is expanded and forces the nozzle against the seat, thereby preventing flow through the device. Finally, the center panel shows an intermediate oxygen pressure of 25 psig. The force of the spring partially closes the valve. The nitrous oxide pressure delivered to the flow control valve is 25 psig. There is a continuum of intermediate configurations between the extremes (0 to 50 psig) of oxygen supply pressure. These intermediate valve configurations are responsible for the proportional nature of the OFPD. An important concept to be understood with these particular fail-safe devices is that the Datex-Ohmeda pressure sensor shut-off valve is threshold in nature (all or nothing) whereas the Dräger OFPD is a variable-flow type proportioning system.

Second-Stage Oxygen Pressure Regulator

Most contemporary Datex-Ohmeda workstations have a second-stage oxygen pressure regulator set at a specific value ranging from 12 to 19 psig. Output from the oxygen flow meter is constant when the oxygen supply pressure exceeds the threshold (minimal) value. The pressure sensor shut-off valve of Datex-Ohmeda is set at a higher threshold value (20 to 30 psig) to ensure that oxygen is the last gas flowing if oxygen pressure failure occurs.

Flow Meter Assemblies

The flow meter assembly (Fig. 25-10) precisely controls and measures gas flow to the common gas outlet. With traditional glass flow meter assemblies, the flow control valve regulates the amount of flow that enters a tapered, transparent flow tube known as a Thorpe tube. A mobile indicator float inside the flow tube indicates the amount of flow passing through the associated flow control valve. The quantity of flow is indicated on a scale associated with the flow tube.[22,23] Some newer anesthesia workstations

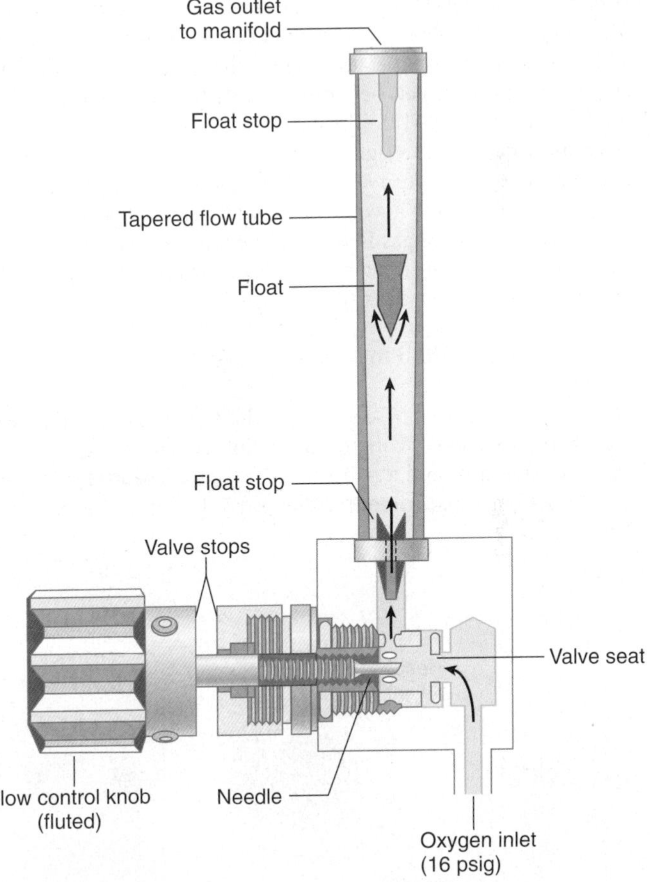

Figure 25-10 Oxygen flow meter assembly. The oxygen flow meter assembly is composed of the flow control valve assembly plus the flow meter subassembly. *(Reproduced with permission from Bowie E, Huffman LM: The Anesthesia Machine: Essentials for Understanding. Madison, WI, Ohmeda, A Division of BOC Health Care, Inc., 1985.)*

have now replaced the conventional glass flow tubes with electronic flow sensors that measure the flow of the individual gases. These flow rate data are then presented to the anesthesia care provider in either numerical format, graphic format, or a combination of the two. Integration of these "electronic flow meters" is an essential step in the evolution of the anesthesia workstation if it is to become fully integrated with anesthesia data-capturing systems such as computerized anesthesia record-keeping systems.

Operating Principles of Conventional Flow Meters

Opening the flow control valve allows gas to travel through the space between the float and the flow tube. This space is known as the annular space (Fig. 25-11). The indicator float hovers freely in an equilibrium position where the upward force resulting from gas flow equals the downward force on the float resulting from gravity at a given flow rate. The float moves to a new equilibrium position in the tube when flow is changed. These flow meters are commonly referred to as *constant-pressure* flow meters because the decrease in pressure across the float remains constant for all positions in the tube.[22,30,32]

Flow tubes are tapered, with the smallest diameter at the bottom of the tube and the largest diameter at the top. The term *variable orifice* designates this type of unit because the annular space between the float and the inner wall of the flow tube varies with the position of the float. Flow through the constriction created by the float can be laminar or turbulent, depending on the flow rate (Fig. 25-12). The characteristics of a gas that influence its flow rate through a given constriction are viscosity (laminar flow) and density (turbulent flow). Because the annular space is tubular at low flow rates, laminar flow is present and *viscosity* determines the gas flow rate. The annular space simulates an orifice at high flow rates, and turbulent gas flow then depends predominantly on the *density* of the gas.[22,32]

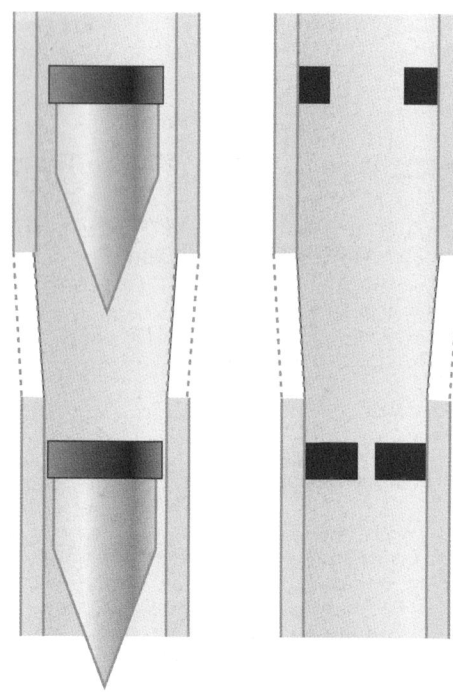

Figure 25-12 Flow tube constriction. The *lower* pair of illustrations represents the lower portion of a flow tube. The clearance between the head of the float and the flow tube is narrow. The equivalent channel is tubular because its diameter is less than its length. Viscosity is dominant in determining the gas flow rate through this tubular constriction. The *upper* pair of illustrations represents the upper portion of a flow tube. The equivalent channel is orificial because its length is less than its width. Density is dominant in determining the gas flow rate through this orificial constriction. *(Redrawn with permission from Macintosh R, Mushin WW, Epstein HG: Physics for the Anaesthetist, 3rd ed. Oxford, Blackwell Scientific, 1963.)*

Components of the Flow Meter Assembly

Flow Control Valve Assembly The flow control valve (see Fig. 25-10) assembly is composed of a flow control knob, a needle valve, a valve seat, and a pair of valve stops.[22] The assembly can receive its pneumatic input either directly from the pipeline source (50 psig) or from a second-stage pressure regulator. The location of the needle valve in the valve seat changes to establish different orifices when the flow control valve is adjusted. Gas flow increases when the flow control valve is turned counterclockwise, and it decreases when the valve is turned clockwise. Extreme clockwise rotation may result in damage to the needle valve and valve seat. Therefore, flow control valves are equipped with valve "stops" to prevent such occurrence.[23]

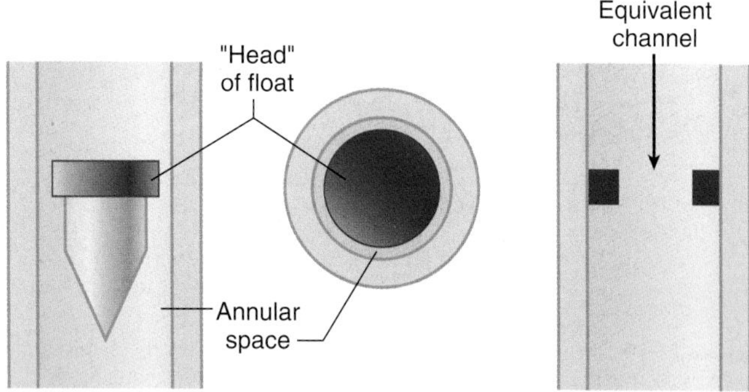

Figure 25-11 The annular space. The clearance between the head of the float and the flow tube is known as the annular space. It can be considered an equivalent to a circular channel of the same cross-sectional area. *(Redrawn with permission from Macintosh R, Mushin WW, Epstein HG: Physics for the Anaesthetist, 3rd ed. Oxford, Blackwell Scientific, 1963.)*

SAFETY FEATURES. Contemporary flow control valve assemblies have numerous safety features. The oxygen flow control knob is physically distinguishable from other gas knobs. It is distinctively fluted, projects beyond the control knobs of the other gases, and is larger in diameter than the flow control knobs of other gases. All knobs are color-coded for the appropriate gas, and the chemical formula or name of the gas is permanently marked on each. Flow control knobs are recessed or protected with a shield or barrier to minimize inadvertent change from a preset position. If a single gas has two flow tubes, the tubes are arranged in series and controlled by a single flow control valve.[5]

Flow Meter Subassembly The flow meter subassembly (see Fig. 25-10) consists of the flow tube, the indicator float with float stops, and the indicator scale.[22]

FLOW TUBES. Contemporary flow tubes are made of glass. Most have a single taper in which the inner diameter of the flow tube increases uniformly from bottom to top. Manufacturers provide double flow tubes for oxygen and nitrous oxide to provide better visual discrimination at low flow rates. A fine flow tube indicates flow from approximately 200 to 1 L/min, and a coarse flow tube indicates flow from approximately 1 to 10 to 12 L/min. The two tubes are connected in series and supplied by a single flow control valve. The total gas flow is that shown on the higher flow meter.

INDICATOR FLOATS AND FLOAT STOPS. Contemporary anesthesia machines use several different types of bobbins or floats, including plumb-bob floats, rotating skirted floats, and ball floats. Flow is read at the top of plumb-bob and skirted floats and at the center of the ball on ball-type floats.[22] Flow tubes are equipped with float stops at the top and bottom of the tube. The upper stop prevents the float from ascending to the top of the tube and plugging the outlet. It also ensures that the float will be visible at maximum flows instead of being hidden in the manifold. The bottom float stop provides a central foundation for the indicator when the flow control valve is turned off.[22,23]

SCALE. The flow meter scale can be marked directly on the flow tube or to the right of the tube.[5] Gradations corresponding to equal increments in flow rate are closer together at the top of the scale because the annular space increases more rapidly than the internal diameter from bottom to top of the tube. Rib guides are used in some flow tubes with ball-type indicators to minimize this compression effect. They are tapered glass ridges that run the length of the tube. There are usually three rib guides spaced equally around the inner circumference of the tube. In the presence of rib guides, the annular space from the bottom to the top of the tube increases almost proportionally with the internal diameter. This results in a nearly linear scale.[22] Rib guides are used on many Dräger Medical flow tubes.

SAFETY FEATURES. The flow meter subassemblies for each gas on the Datex-Ohmeda Modulus I, Modulus II, Modulus II Plus, CD, and Aestiva are housed in independent, color-coded, pin-specific modules. The flow tubes are adjacent to a gas-specific, color-coded backing. The flow scale and the chemical formula (or name of the gas) are permanently etched on the backing to the right of the flow tube. Flow meter scales are individually hand-calibrated to the specific float to provide a high degree of accuracy. The tube, float, and scale make an inseparable unit. The entire set must be replaced if any component is damaged.

Dräger Medical does not use a modular system for its flow meter subassembly. The flow scale, the chemical symbol, and the gas-specific color codes are etched directly onto the flow tube. The scale in use is obvious when two flow tubes for the same gas are used.

Problems with Flow Meters

Leaks Flow meter leaks are a substantial hazard because the flow meters are located downstream from all machine safety devices except the oxygen analyzer.[33] Leaks can occur at the O-ring junctions between the glass flow tubes and the metal manifold or in cracked or broken glass flow tubes, the most fragile pneumatic component of the anesthesia machine. Even though gross damage to conventional glass flow tubes is usually apparent, subtle cracks and chips may be overlooked and result in errors in delivered flow.[34] The use of electronic flow meters and removal of conventional glass flow tubes from some newer anesthesia workstations (Datex-Ohmeda S/5 ADU and the Dräger Fabius) may help eliminate this potential source of leaks (see "Electronic Flow Meters").

Eger and colleagues in 1963[35] demonstrated that in the presence of a flow meter leak, a hypoxic mixture is less likely to occur if the oxygen flow meter is located downstream from all other flow meters.[32] Figure 25-13 is a more contemporary version of the figure in Eger's original publication. The unused airflow tube has a large leak. Nitrous oxide and oxygen flow rates are set at a ratio of 3:1. A potentially dangerous arrangement is shown in Figure 25-13A and B because the nitrous oxide flow meter is located in the downstream position. A hypoxic mixture can result because a substantial portion of the oxygen flow passes through the leak and all nitrous oxide is directed to the common gas outlet. A safer configuration is shown in Figure 25-13C and D. The oxygen flow meter is located in the downstream position. A portion of the nitrous oxide flow escapes through the leak, and the remainder goes toward the common gas outlet. A hypoxic mixture is less likely because all the oxygen flow is advanced by the nitrous oxide.[35] North American Dräger flow meters are arranged as in Figure 25-13C, and Datex-Ohmeda flow meters are arranged as in Figure 25-13D.

A leak in the oxygen flow tube may result in creation of a hypoxic mixture even when oxygen is located in the downstream position (Fig. 25-14).[33,34] Oxygen escapes through the leak and nitrous oxide continues to flow toward the common outlet, particularly at high ratios of nitrous oxide to oxygen flow.

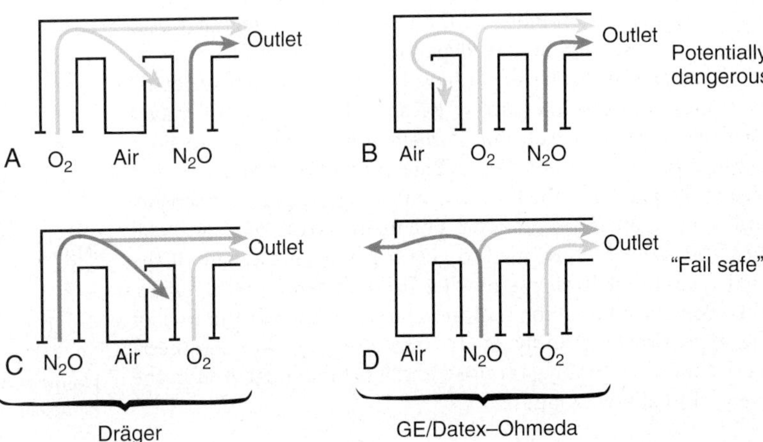

Figure 25-13 The flow meter sequence is a potential cause of hypoxia. In the event of a flow meter leak, a potentially dangerous arrangement exists when nitrous oxide is located in the downstream position (**A** and **B**). The safest configuration exists when oxygen is located in the downstream position (**C** and **D**). See text for details. *(Modified with permission from Eger EI II, Hylton RR, Irwin RH, et al: Anesthetic flow meter sequence—a cause for hypoxia. Anesthesiology 24:396, 1963.)*

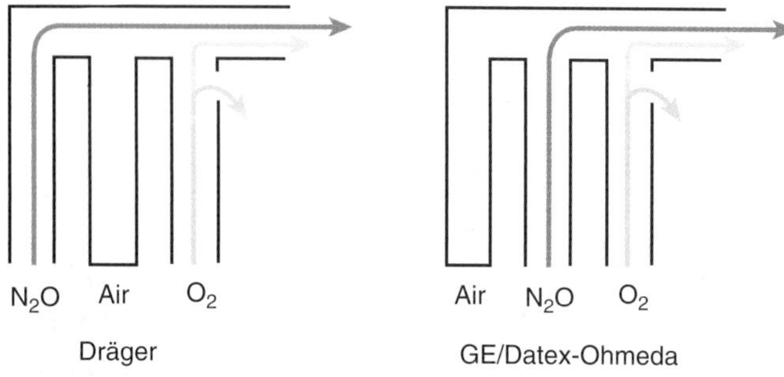

Figure 25-14 An oxygen leak from the flow tube can produce a hypoxic mixture regardless of the arrangement of the flow tubes.

Inaccuracy Flow measurement error can occur even when flow meters are assembled properly with appropriate components. Dirt or static electricity can cause a float to stick, and the actual flow may be higher or lower than that indicated. Sticking of the indicator float is more common in the low flow ranges because the annular space is smaller. A damaged float can cause inaccurate readings because the precise relationship between the float and the flow tube is altered. Backpressure from the breathing circuit can cause a float to drop so that it reads less than the actual flow. Finally, if flow meters are not aligned properly in the vertical position (plumb), readings can be inaccurate because tilting distorts the annular space.[17,22,34]

Ambiguous Scale Before the standardization of flow meter scales and the widespread use of oxygen analyzers, at least two deaths resulted from confusion created by ambiguous scales.[17,34,36] The operator read the float position beside an adjacent, but erroneous scale in both cases. Today, this error is less likely to occur because contemporary flow meter scales are marked either directly on the flow tube or immediately to the right of it.[5] The possibility of confusion is minimized when the scale is etched directly onto the tube.

Electronic Flow Meters

As mentioned earlier, some newer anesthesia workstations such as the Datex-Ohmeda S/5 ADU and the North American Dräger Fabius GS, among others, have conventional control knobs and flow control valves but have electronic flow sensors and digital displays rather than glass flow tubes. The output from the flow control valve is represented graphically, numerically, or by both means in liters per minute on the workstation's integrated user interface. These systems are dependent on electrical power to provide a precise display of gas flow. However, even when electrical power is totally interrupted, because the flow control valves themselves are nonelectronic, oxygen should continue to flow. Because these machines do not have individual flow tubes that physically quantitate the flow of each gas, electronic flow sensors and often a small conventional pneumatic "fresh gas" or "total flow" indicator are provided to give the user an estimate of the total quantity of fresh gas flowing from all flow control valves. This miniature flow tube indicator serves to inform the user of the approximate quantity of gas that is leaving the anesthesia workstation's common gas outlet, and it is functional even in the event of total power failure.

Proportioning Systems

Manufacturers equip anesthesia workstations with proportioning systems in an attempt to prevent the creation and delivery of a hypoxic mixture. Nitrous oxide and oxygen are interfaced mechanically or pneumatically (or both ways) so that the minimum oxygen concentration at the common gas outlet is between 23% and 25%, depending on the manufacturer.

Datex-Ohmeda Link-25 Proportion-Limiting Control System

Conventional Datex-Ohmeda machines use the Link-25 system. The heart of the system is mechanical integration of the nitrous oxide and oxygen flow control valves. It allows independent adjustment of either valve, yet automatically intercedes to maintain a minimum 25% oxygen concentration with a maximum nitrous oxide–oxygen flow ratio of 3:1. The Link-25 automatically increases oxygen flow to prevent delivery of a hypoxic mixture.

Figure 25-15 illustrates the Datex-Ohmeda Link-25 system. The nitrous oxide and oxygen flow control valves are identical. A 14-tooth sprocket is attached to the nitrous oxide flow control valve and a 28-tooth sprocket to the oxygen flow control valve. A chain physically links the sprockets. When the nitrous oxide flow control valve is turned through two revolutions, or 28 teeth, the oxygen flow control valve will revolve once because of the 2:1 gear ratio. The final 3:1 flow ratio results because the nitrous oxide flow control valve is supplied by approximately 26 psig whereas the oxygen flow control valve is supplied by 14 psig. Thus, the combination of the mechanical and pneumatic aspects of the system yields the final oxygen concentration. The Datex-Ohmeda Link-25 proportioning system can be thought of as a system that *increases oxygen flow* when necessary to prevent delivery of a fresh gas mixture with an oxygen concentration of less than 25%.

Recently, a few reports related to failures of the Datex-Ohmeda Link-25 system have been published. The authors of these reports describe failures that either resulted in an inability to administer oxygen without nitrous oxide or allowed creation of a hypoxic mixture. These reported failures of the Link-25 on the Datex-Ohmeda Excel series anesthesia machines should cer-

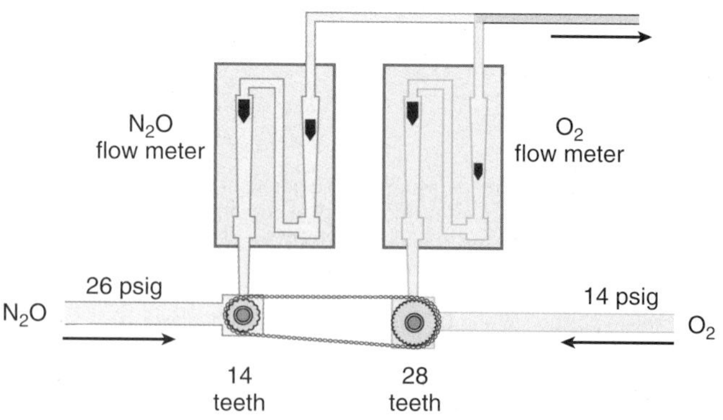

Figure 25-15 Ohmeda Link-25 Proportion-Limiting Control system. See text for details.

tainly raise the awareness of clinicians to the possibility of failure of this type of proportioning system.[36-40]

North American Dräger Oxygen Ratio Monitor Controller/Sensitive Oxygen Ratio Controller System

North American Dräger's proportioning system, the Oxygen Ratio Monitor Controller (ORMC), is used on the North American Dräger Narkomed 2A, 2B, 3, and 4 series. An equivalent system known as the Sensitive Oxygen Ratio Controller (S-ORC) is used on some newer Dräger anesthesia workstations such as the Dräger Fabius GS and Narkomed 6000 series. The ORMC and the S-ORC are pneumatic oxygen–nitrous oxide interlock systems designed to maintain a fresh gas oxygen concentration of at least 25% ± 3%. They maintain the fresh gas oxygen concentration at levels substantially higher than 25% at oxygen flow rates of less than 1 L/min. The ORMC and S-ORC limit nitrous oxide flow to prevent delivery of a hypoxic mixture. This is unlike the Datex-Ohmeda Link-25, which actively increases oxygen flow.

A schematic of the ORMC is shown in Figure 25-16. It is composed of an oxygen chamber, a nitrous oxide chamber, and a nitrous oxide slave control valve. All are interconnected by a mobile horizontal shaft. Pneumatic input into the device is from the oxygen and nitrous oxide flow meters. These flow meters are unique in that they have specific resistors located downstream from the flow control valves. These resistors create backpressure directed to the oxygen and nitrous oxide chambers. The value of the oxygen flow tube resistor is three to four times that of the nitrous oxide flow tube resistor, and the relative value of these resistors determines the value of the controlled fresh gas oxygen concentration. Backpressure in the oxygen and nitrous oxide chambers pushes against rubber diaphragms attached to the mobile horizontal shaft. Movement of the shaft regulates the nitrous oxide slave control valve, which feeds the nitrous oxide flow control valve.

If the oxygen pressure is proportionally higher than the nitrous oxide pressure, the nitrous oxide slave control valve opens wider to allow more nitrous oxide to flow. As the nitrous oxide flow is increased manually, the nitrous oxide pressure forces the shaft toward the oxygen chamber. The valve opening becomes more restrictive and limits flow of nitrous oxide to the flow meter.

Figure 25-16 illustrates the action of a single ORMC/S-ORC under different sets of circumstances. The backpressure exerted on the oxygen diaphragm, in the upper configuration, is greater than that exerted on the nitrous oxide diaphragm. This causes the horizontal shaft to move to the left, thereby opening the nitrous oxide slave control valve. Nitrous oxide is then able to proceed to its flow control valve and out through the flow meter. In the bottom configuration, the nitrous oxide slave control valve is closed because of inadequate oxygen backpressure.[24]

To summarize, in contrast to the Datex-Ohmeda Link-25 system, which actively increases oxygen flow to maintain a fresh gas oxygen concentration greater than 25%, the Dräger ORMC and S-ORC are systems that limit nitrous oxide flow to prevent delivery of a fresh gas mixture with an oxygen concentration of less than 25%.

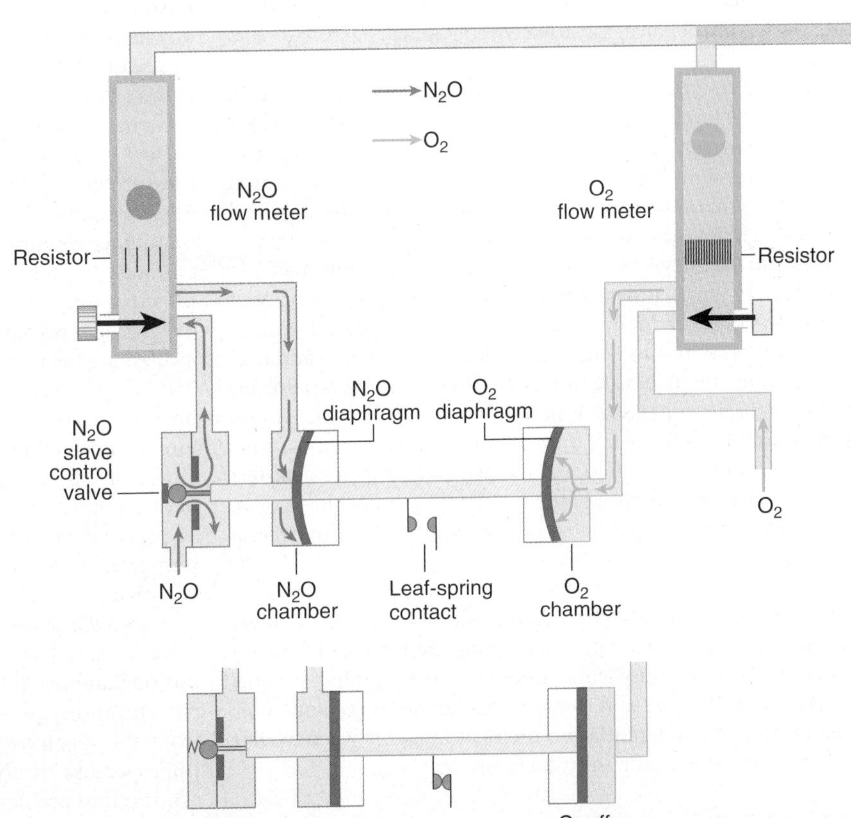

Figure 25-16 North American Dräger Oxygen Ratio Monitor Controller. See text for details. *(Redrawn with permission from Schreiber P: Safety Guidelines for Anesthesia Systems. Telford, PA, North American Dräger, 1984.)*

Limitations

Proportioning systems are not foolproof. Workstations equipped with proportioning systems can still deliver a hypoxic mixture under certain conditions. In the following sections we briefly present some situations in which this can occur.

Wrong Supply Gas Both the Datex-Ohmeda Link-25 and the Dräger ORMC/S-ORC will be fooled if a gas other than oxygen is present in the oxygen pipeline. In the Link-25 system, the nitrous oxide and oxygen flow control valves will continue to be mechanically linked. Nevertheless, a hypoxic mixture can proceed to the common gas outlet. In the case of the Drager ORMC or S-ORC, the rubber diaphragm for oxygen will reflect adequate supply pressure on the oxygen side even though the incorrect gas is present, and flow of both the wrong gas plus nitrous oxide will result. The oxygen analyzer is the only workstation monitor besides an integrated multigas analyzer that would detect this condition in either system.

Defective Pneumatics or Mechanics Normal operation of the Datex-Ohmeda Link-25 and the North American Dräger ORMC/S-ORC is contingent on pneumatic and mechanical integrity.[41] Pneumatic integrity in the Datex-Ohmeda system requires properly functioning second-stage regulators. A nitrous oxide–oxygen ratio other than 3 : 1 will result if the regulators are not precise. The chain connecting the two sprockets must be intact. A 97% nitrous oxide concentration can occur if the chain is cut or broken.[42] In the North American Dräger system, a functional OFPD is necessary to supply appropriate pressure to the ORMC. The mechanical aspects of the ORMC/S-ORC, such as the rubber diaphragms, the flow tube resistors, and the nitrous oxide slave control valve, must likewise be intact.

Leaks Downstream The ORMC/S-ORC and the Link-25 function at the level of the flow control valves. A leak downstream from these devices, such as a broken oxygen flow tube (see Fig. 25-14), can result in delivery of a hypoxic mixture to the common gas outlet. In this situation, oxygen escapes through the leak, and the predominant gas delivered is nitrous oxide. The oxygen monitor and the integrated multigas analyzer are the only machine safety devices that can detect this problem.[33] For the majority of its products, Dräger Medical recommends a preoperative positive-pressure leak test to detect such a leak. However, in addition to this test, for many North American Dräger products, application of the negative-pressure leak test as well may provide a more sensitive way to detect such a leak. Datex-Ohmeda almost universally recommends a preoperative negative-pressure leak test for its workstations because of the frequently present check valve located at the common gas outlet (see "Checking Your Anesthesia Workstation").

Inert Gas Administration Administration of a third inert gas, such as helium, nitrogen, or carbon dioxide, can cause a hypoxic mixture because contemporary proportioning systems link only nitrous oxide and oxygen.[43] Use of an oxygen analyzer is mandatory (or preferentially a multigas analyzer when available) if the operator uses a third inert gas.

Dilution of Inspired Oxygen Concentration by Volatile Inhaled Anesthetics Volatile inhaled anesthetics are added to the mixed gases downstream from both the flow meters and the proportioning system. Concentrations of less potent inhaled anesthetics such as desflurane may account for a larger percentage of the total fresh gas composition than is the case with more potent agents. This can be seen when the maximum vaporizer dial settings of the various volatile agents are examined (e.g., a desflurane maximum dial setting of 18% versus an isoflurane maximum dial setting of 5%). Because significant percentages of these inhaled anesthetics may be added downstream of the proportioning system, the resulting gas-vapor mixture may contain an inspired oxygen concentration less than 21% despite a functional proportioning system. The anesthesia care provider must be aware of this possibility, particularly when high concentrations of less potent volatile inhaled anesthetics are used.

Oxygen Flush Valve

The oxygen flush valve allows direct communication between the oxygen high-pressure circuit and the low-pressure circuit (see Fig. 25-3). Flow from the oxygen flush valve enters the low-pressure circuit downstream from the vaporizers and most importantly downstream from the Datex-Ohmeda machine outlet check valve. The spring-loaded oxygen flush valve stays closed until the operator opens it by depressing the oxygen flush button. Actuation of the valve delivers 100% oxygen at 35 to 75 L/min to the breathing circuit.[23]

The oxygen flush valve can provide a high-pressure oxygen source suitable for jet ventilation under the following circumstances: (1) the anesthesia machine is equipped with a one-way check valve positioned between the vaporizers and the oxygen flush valve, and (2) when a positive-pressure relief valve exists downstream of the vaporizers, this pressure relief valve must be upstream of the outlet check valve. Because the Ohmeda Modulus II has such a one-way check valve and its positive-pressure relief valve is upstream from the check valve, the entire oxygen flow of 35 to 75 L/min is delivered to the common gas outlet at a high pressure of 50 psig. On the other hand, the Ohmeda Modulus II Plus and some Ohmeda Excel machines are not capable of functioning as an appropriate oxygen source for jet ventilation. The Ohmeda Modulus II Plus, which does not have the check valve, provides only 7 psig at the common gas outlet because some oxygen flow travels retrogradely through an internal relief valve located upstream from the oxygen flush valve. The Ohmeda Excel 210, which does have a one-way check valve, also has a positive-pressure relief valve downstream from the check valve and therefore is unsuitable for jet ventilation. Older North American Dräger machines such as the Narkomed 2A (which also does not have an outlet check valve) provide an intermediate pressure of 18 psig to the common gas outlet because some pressure is vented retrogradely through a pressure relief valve located in the vaporizers.[44]

Several hazards have been reported with the oxygen flush valve. A defective or damaged valve can stick in the fully open position and result in barotrauma.[45] A valve sticking in a partially open position can result in patient awareness because oxygen flow from the incompetent valve dilutes the inhaled anesthetic.[19,46] Improper use of normally functioning oxygen flush valves also can result in problems. Overzealous intraoperative oxygen flushing can dilute inhaled anesthetics. Oxygen flushing during the inspiratory phase of positive-pressure ventilation can produce barotrauma if the anesthesia machine does not incorporate fresh

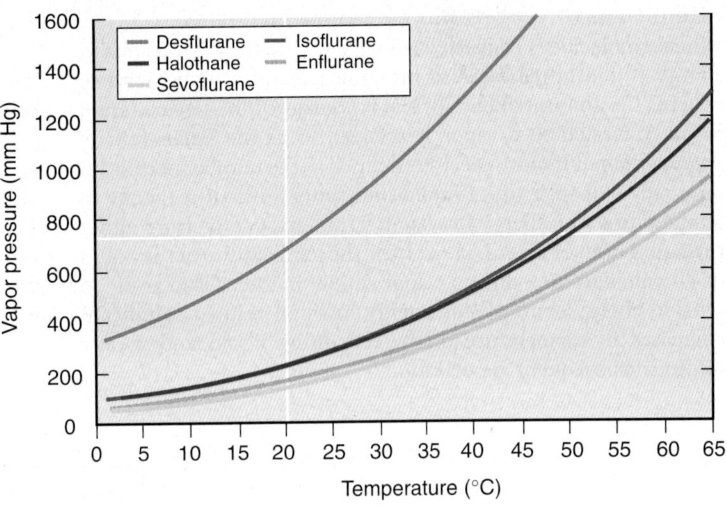

Figure 25-17 Vapor pressure–versus-temperature curves for desflurane, isoflurane, halothane, enflurane, and sevoflurane. The vapor pressure curve for desflurane is both steeper and shifted to higher vapor pressures than the curves for other contemporary inhaled anesthetics are. *(From inhaled anesthetic package insert equations and Susay SR, Smith MA, Lockwood GG: The saturated vapor pressure of desflurane at various temperatures. Anesth Analg 83:864-866, 1996.)*

gas decoupling or an appropriately adjusted inspiratory pressure limiter. Anesthesia systems (Dräger Narkomed 6000 series, Julian, Fabius GS, and Datascope Anestar) with fresh gas decoupling are inherently safer from the standpoint of minimizing the chance of producing barotrauma as a result of inappropriate oxygen flush valve use. These systems physically divorce the fresh gas inflow from either the flow meters or the oxygen flush valve from the delivered tidal volume presented to the patient's lungs (see "Fresh Gas Decoupling"). With traditional anesthesia breathing circuits, excess volume cannot be vented during the inspiratory phase of mechanical ventilation because the ventilator relief valve is closed and the APL valve is either out of circuit or closed.[47] An alternative way to manage this problem can be seen with the Datex-Ohmeda S/5 ADU and Aestiva. These circle systems use an integrated adjustable pressure limiter. If this device is properly adjusted, it functions like the APL valve to limit the maximum airway pressure to a safe level, thereby reducing the possibility of barotrauma.

Some very old anesthesia systems made use of a freestanding vaporizer downstream from the common gas outlet, and with these systems oxygen flushing could rapidly deliver large quantities of inhaled anesthetic to the patient. Finally, inappropriate preoperative use of the oxygen flush to evaluate the low-pressure circuit for leaks can be misleading, particularly on Datex-Ohmeda machines with a one-way check valve at the common outlet.[18] Because backpressure from the breathing circuit closes the one-way check valve air-tight, major low-pressure circuit leaks can go undetected with this leak test (see "Checking Your Anesthesia Workstation").

Vaporizers

As dramatic as the evolution of the anesthesia workstation has been over recent years, vaporizers have also changed from rudimentary ether inhalers and copper kettles to the present temperature-compensated, computer-controlled, and flow-sensing devices that we use today. In 1993, with the introduction of desflurane to the clinical setting, an even more sophisticated vaporizer was introduced to handle the unique physical properties of this agent. Now, a new generation of anesthesia vaporizers blending both "old" copper kettle–like technology and "new" computerized control technology has emerged in the Datex-Ohmeda Aladin cassette vaporizer system. Before discussion of variable-bypass vaporizers, the Datex-Ohmeda Tec 6 desflurane vaporizer and the Datex-Ohmeda Aladin cassette vaporizer, certain physical principles will be reviewed briefly to facilitate understanding of the operating principles, construction, and design of contemporary volatile anesthetic vaporizers.

Physics

Vapor Pressure

Contemporary inhaled volatile anesthetics exist in the liquid state at temperatures below 20°C. When a volatile liquid is in a closed container, molecules escape from the liquid phase to the vapor phase until the number of molecules in the vapor phase is constant. These molecules in the vapor phase bombard the wall of the container and create a pressure known as the *saturated vapor pressure*. As the temperature increases, more molecules enter the vapor phase, and the vapor pressure increases (Fig. 25-17). Vapor pressure is independent of atmospheric pressure and is contingent only on the temperature and physical characteristics of the liquid. The *boiling point* of a liquid is defined as the temperature at which vapor pressure equals atmospheric pressure.[48-50] At 760 mm Hg, the boiling points for desflurane, isoflurane, halothane, enflurane, and sevoflurane are approximately 22.8°C, 48.5°C, 50.2°C, 56.5°C, and 58.5°C, respectively. Unlike other contemporary inhaled anesthetics, desflurane boils at temperatures that may be encountered in clinical settings such as operating rooms for pediatric and burn patients. This unique physical characteristic alone mandates a special vaporizer design to control the delivery of desflurane. If agent-specific vaporizers are inadvertently misfilled with incorrect liquid anesthetic agents, the resulting mixtures of volatile agents may demonstrate properties uniquely different from those of the individual component agents. The altered vapor pressure and other physical properties of the resulting azeotropic mixtures caused by the mixing of various agents may change the output of the anesthetic vaporizer (see "Misfilling" in the section "Variable-Bypass Vaporizers").[51]

Latent Heat of Vaporization

When a molecule is converted from a liquid to the gaseous phase, energy is consumed because the molecules of a liquid tend to cohere. The amount of energy that is consumed for a given liquid to be converted to a vapor is referred to as the *latent heat of vaporization*. It is more precisely defined as the number of calories required to change 1 g of liquid into vapor without a change in temperature. The energy for vaporization must come from either the liquid itself or an outside source. The temperature of the liquid itself will decrease during vaporization in the absence of an outside energy source. This energy loss can lead to significant decreases in temperature of the remaining liquid and greatly diminish subsequent vaporization.[48,50,52]

Specific Heat

The *specific heat* of a substance is the number of calories required to increase the temperature of 1 g of a substance by 1°C.[21,48,50] The substance can be a solid, liquid, or gas. The concept of specific heat is important to the design, operation, and construction of vaporizers because it is applicable in two ways. First, the specific heat for an inhaled anesthetic is important because it indicates how much heat must be supplied to the liquid to maintain a constant temperature when heat is being lost during vaporization. Second, manufacturers select vaporizer component materials that have high specific heat to minimize the temperature changes associated with vaporization.

Thermal Conductivity

Thermal conductivity is a measure of the speed at which heat flows through a substance. The higher the thermal conductivity, the better the substance conducts heat.[48] Vaporizers are constructed of metals that have relatively high thermal conductivity, which helps maintain a uniform internal temperature.

Variable-Bypass Vaporizers

The Datex-Ohmeda Tec 4, Tec 5, and Tec 7, as well as the North American Dräger Vapor 19.n and 20.n vaporizers, are classified as variable-bypass, flow-over, temperature-compensated, agent-specific, out-of-breathing-circuit vaporizers.[48] *Variable bypass* refers to the method of regulating the concentration of anesthetic agent output from the vaporizer. The concentration control dial setting determines the ratio of flow that goes through the bypass chamber and the vaporizing chamber as fresh gas from the flow meters enters the vaporizer inlet. The gas channeled through the vaporizing chamber flows over a wick system saturated with the liquid anesthetic and subsequently also becomes saturated with vapor. Thus, *flow-over* refers to the method of vaporization and is in contrast to the bubble-through system that may be seen in some copper kettle–type vaporizers of old. The Tec 4, Tec 5, Tec 7, and Dräger Vapor 19.n and 20.n are further classified as *temperature compensated*. Each of these vaporizers is equipped with an automatic temperature-compensating device that helps maintain constant vaporizer output over a wide range of operating temperatures. These vaporizers are *agent specific* and *out of circuit* because each is designed to accommodate a single anesthetic agent and to be physically located outside the breathing circuit. Variable-bypass vaporizers are used to deliver halothane, enflurane, isoflurane, and sevoflurane, but not desflurane.

Basic Operating Principles

A diagram of a generic, variable-bypass vaporizer is shown in Figure 25-18. Vaporizer components include the concentration control dial, the bypass chamber, the vaporizing chamber, the filler port, and the filler cap. The operator fills the vaporizing chamber with liquid anesthetic through the filler port. The

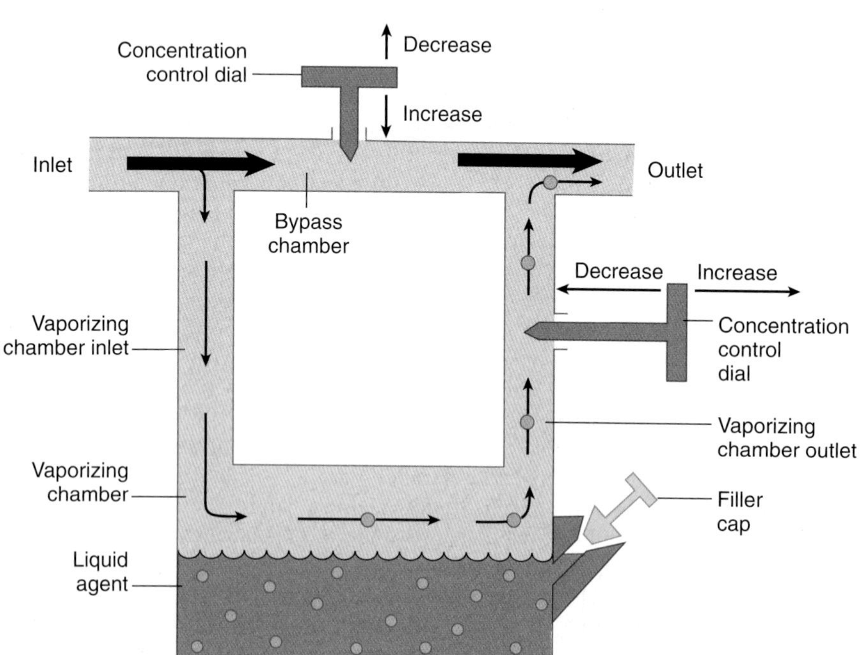

Figure 25-18 Generic variable-bypass vaporizer. See text for details.

maximum safe fill level is predetermined by the position of the filler port, which is situated to minimize the chance of overfilling. If a vaporizer is overfilled or tilted, liquid anesthetic can spill into the bypass chamber. If this were to happen, both the vaporizing chamber flow and the bypass chamber flow could potentially be carrying saturated anesthetic vapor, and an overdose would result. The concentration control dial is a variable restrictor, and it can be located either in the bypass chamber or in the outlet of the vaporizing chamber. The function of the concentration control dial is to regulate the relative flow rates through the bypass and vaporizing chambers.

Flow from the flow meters enters the inlet of the vaporizer. More than 80% of the flow passes straight through the bypass chamber to the vaporizer outlet, and this accounts for the name "bypass chamber." Less than 20% of the flow from the flow meters is diverted through the vaporizing chamber. Depending on the temperature and vapor pressure of the particular inhaled anesthetic, the fresh gases entering the vaporizing chamber entrain a specific flow of the inhaled anesthetic agent. The mixture that exits the vaporizer is the combination of flow through the bypass chamber, flow through the vaporizing chamber, and flow of entrained anesthetic vapor. The final concentration of inhaled anesthetic is the ratio of the flow of the inhaled anesthetic to the total gas flow.[48,53]

The vapor pressure of an inhaled anesthetic depends on the ambient temperature (see Fig. 25-17). For example, at 20°C the vapor pressure of isoflurane is 238 mm Hg, whereas at 35°C the vapor pressure almost doubles (450 mm Hg). Variable-bypass vaporizers have an internal mechanism to compensate for variations in ambient temperature. The temperature-compensating valve of the Datex-Ohmeda Tec 4 is shown in Figure 25-19. At relatively high ambient temperatures, such as those commonly seen in operating rooms designated for the care of pediatric or burn patients, the vapor pressure inside the vaporizing chamber is high. To compensate for this increased vapor pressure, the bimetallic strip of the temperature-compensating valve leans to the right, thereby decreasing resistance to flow through the bypass chamber and allowing more flow to pass through the bypass chamber and less flow to pass through the vaporizing chamber. In contrast, in a cold operating room environment, the vapor pressure inside the vaporizing chamber is reduced. To compensate for this decrease in vapor pressure, the bimetallic strip leans to the left, which increases resistance to flow through the bypass chamber and causes more flow to pass through the vaporizing chamber and less to pass through the bypass chamber. The net effect in both situations is maintenance of relatively constant vaporizer output.

Factors That Influence Vaporizer Output

If an ideal vaporizer existed, with a fixed dial setting its output would be constant regardless of varied flow rates, temperature, backpressure, and carrier gases. Designing such a vaporizer is difficult because as ambient conditions change, the physical properties of gases and vaporizers themselves can change.[53] Contemporary vaporizers approach ideal but still have some limitations. Even though some of the most sophisticated vaporizer systems now available use computer-controlled components and multiple sensors, they have yet to become significantly more accurate than conventional vaporizers. Several factors that affect vaporizer performance in general are described in the following paragraphs.

Flow Rate With a fixed dial setting, vaporizer output can vary with the rate of gas flowing through the vaporizer. This variation is particularly notable at the extremes of flow rates. The output of all variable-bypass vaporizers is less than the dial setting at low flow rates (<250 mL/min) because of the relatively high density of volatile inhaled anesthetics. Insufficient turbulence is generated in the vaporizing chamber at low flow rates to upwardly advance the vapor molecules. At extremely high flow rates, such as 15 L/min, the output of most variable-bypass vaporizers is less than the dial setting. This discrepancy is attributed to incomplete mixing and failure to saturate the carrier gas in the vaporizing chamber.

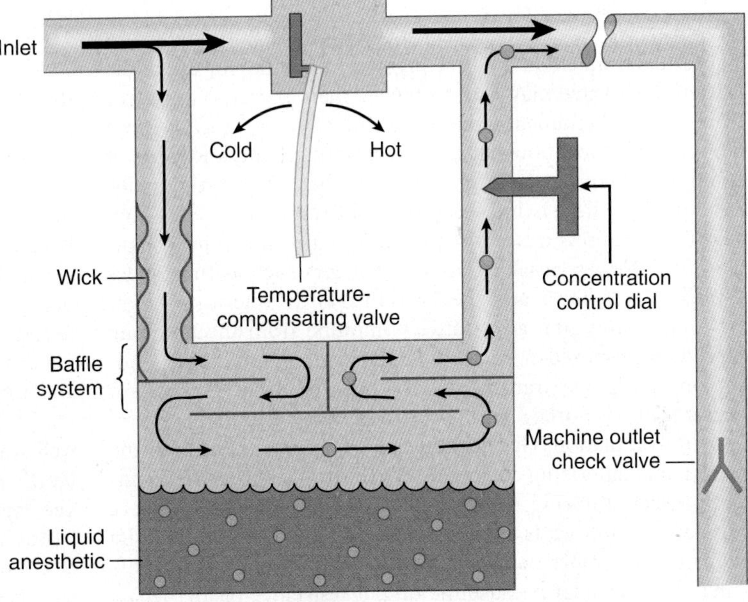

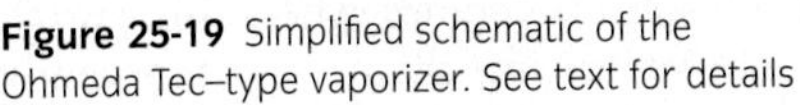

Figure 25-19 Simplified schematic of the Ohmeda Tec–type vaporizer. See text for details

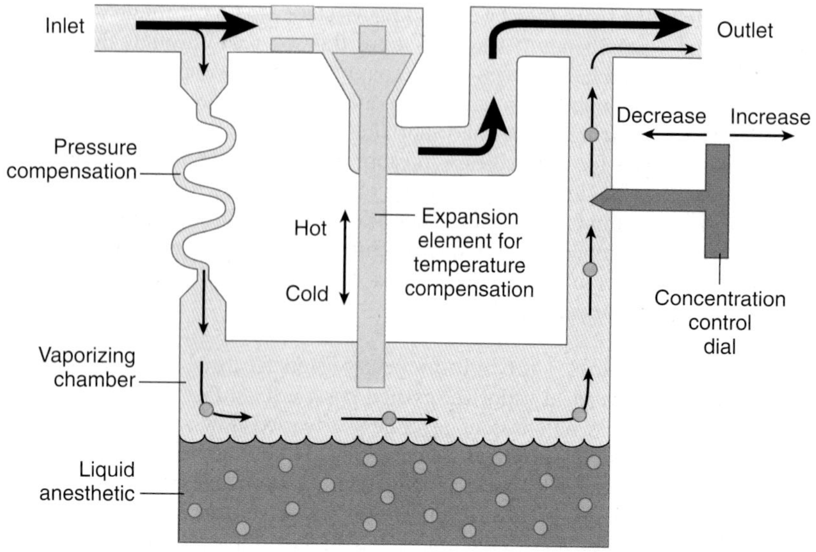

Figure 25-20 Simplified schematic of the North American Dräger Vapor 19.n and 20.n vaporizers. See text for details.

In addition, the resistance characteristics of the bypass chamber and the vaporizing chamber can vary as flow increases. These variations can result in decreased vapor output concentration.[53]

Temperature Because of improvements in design, the output of contemporary temperature-compensated vaporizers is almost linear over a wide range of temperatures. Automatic temperature-compensating mechanisms in the bypass chamber maintain constant vaporizer output with varying temperatures.[23] As previously described, a bimetallic strip (Fig. 25-19) or an expansion element (Fig. 25-20) directs a greater proportion of gas flow through the bypass chamber as temperatures increase.[53] Additionally, the wick systems are placed in direct contact with the metal wall of the vaporizer to help replace energy (heat) consumed during vaporization. The materials that vaporizers are constructed of are chosen because they have a relatively high specific heat and high thermal conductivity. These factors help minimize the effect of cooling during vaporization.

Intermittent Backpressure The intermittent backpressure that results from either positive-pressure ventilation or use of the oxygen flush valve may lead to higher than expected vaporizer output. This phenomenon, known as the *pumping effect*, is more pronounced at low flow rates, low dial settings, and low levels of liquid anesthetic in the vaporizing chamber.[48,53-56] Additionally, the pumping effect is increased by rapid respiratory rates, high peak inspired pressures, and rapid drops in pressure during expiration.[46-50] Newer variable-bypass vaporizers such as the Datex-Ohmeda Tec 4, Tec 5, and Tec 7 and the North American Dräger Vapor 19.n and 20.n are relatively immune from the pumping effect. One proposed mechanism for the pumping effect is dependent on retrograde transmission of pressure from the patient circuit to the vaporizer during the inspiratory phase of positive-pressure ventilation. Gas molecules are compressed in both the bypass and vaporizing chambers. When the backpressure is suddenly released during the expiratory phase of positive-pressure ventilation, vapor exits the vaporizing chamber both through the vaporizing chamber outlet and retrogradely through the vaporizing chamber inlet because the output resistance of the bypass chamber is lower than that of the vaporizing chamber, particularly at low dial settings. The enhanced output concentration results from the increment of vapor that travels in the retrograde direction to the bypass chamber.[53-56]

To decrease the pumping effect, the vaporizing chambers of newer systems are smaller than those of early variable-bypass vaporizers such as the Fluotec Mark II (750 mL).[55] Therefore, no substantial volumes of vapor can be discharged from the vaporizing chamber into the bypass chamber during the expiratory phase. The North American Dräger Vapor 19.n and 20.n vaporizers (see Fig. 25-20) have a long spiral tube that serves as the inlet to the vaporizing chamber.[55] When the pressure in the vaporizing chamber is released, some of the vapor enters this tube but does not enter the bypass chamber because of tube length.[49] The Tec 4 (see Fig. 25-19) has an extensive baffle system in the vaporizing chamber, and a one-way check valve has been inserted at the common gas outlet to minimize the pumping effect. This check valve attenuates but does not eliminate the increase in pressure because gas still flows from the flow meters to the vaporizer during the inspiratory phase of positive-pressure ventilation.[48,57]

Carrier Gas Composition Vaporizer output is influenced by the composition of the carrier gas that flows through the vaporizer.[58-65] During experimental conditions, when the carrier gas is changed rapidly from 100% oxygen to 100% nitrous oxide, a sudden transient decrease in vaporizer output occurs, followed by a slow increase to a new steady-state value (B in Fig. 25-21).[63,64] Because nitrous oxide is more soluble than oxygen in the halogenated liquid within the vaporizer sump, when this switch occurs, the output from the vaporizing chamber is transiently reduced.[63] Once the anesthetic liquid is totally saturated with nitrous oxide, vaporizing chamber output increases somewhat, and a new steady state is established.

The explanation for the new steady-state output value is less well understood.[65] With contemporary vaporizers such as the North American Dräger Vapor 19.n and 20.n and the Ohmeda Tec–type conventional vaporizers, the steady-state output value is less when nitrous oxide is the carrier gas instead of oxygen (see B in Fig. 25-21). Conversely, the output of some older vaporizers is enhanced when nitrous oxide is the carrier gas instead of oxygen.[58,60] The steady-state plateau is achieved more rapidly with

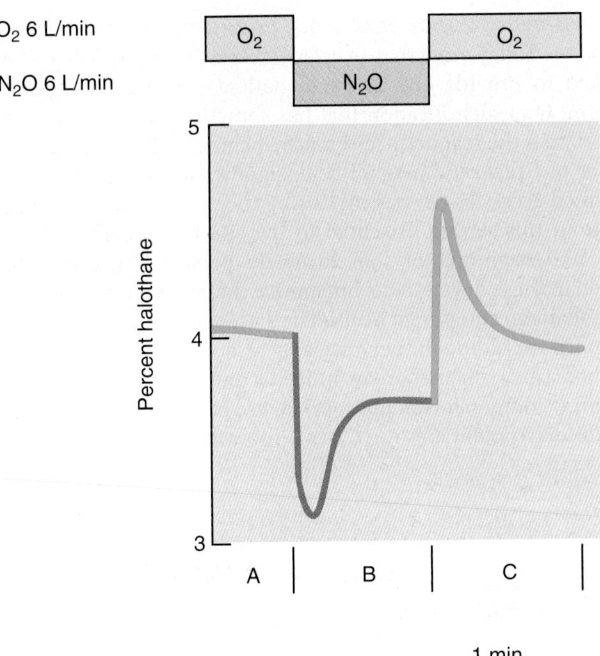

Figure 25-21 Halothane output of a North American Dräger Vapor 19.n vaporizer with different carrier gases. The initial output concentration is approximately 4% halothane when oxygen is the carrier gas at flows of 6 L/min (A). When the carrier gas is quickly switched to 100% nitrous oxide (B), the halothane concentration decreases to 3% within 8 to 10 seconds. A new steady-state concentration of approximately 3.5% is then attained within 1 minute. See text for details. *(Modified with permission from Gould DB, Lampert BA, MacKrell TN: Effect of nitrous oxide solubility on vaporizer aberrance. Anesth Analg 61:939, 1982.)*

increased flow rates, regardless of the ultimate output value.[64] Factors that contribute to the characteristic steady-state response resulting when various carrier gases are used include the viscosity and density of the carrier gas, the relative solubility of the carrier gas in the anesthetic liquid, the flow-splitting characteristics of the specific vaporizer, and the concentration control dial setting.[60,63-65]

Safety Features

Newer generations of anesthesia vaporizers, including the North American Dräger 19.n and 20.n and the Datex-Ohmeda Tec 4, Tec 5, and Tec 7, now have built-in safety features that have minimized or eliminated many hazards once associated with variable-bypass vaporizers. Agent-specific, keyed filling devices help prevent filling a vaporizer with the wrong agent. Overfilling of these vaporizers is minimized because the filler port is located at the maximum safe liquid level. Finally, today's vaporizers are firmly secured to a vaporizer manifold on the anesthesia workstation. Thus, problems associated with vaporizer tipping have become much less frequent. Contemporary interlock systems prevent the administration of more than one inhaled anesthetic.

Hazards

Despite many safety features, some hazards are still associated with contemporary variable-bypass vaporizers.

Misfilling Vaporizers not equipped with keyed fillers have occasionally been misfilled with the wrong anesthetic liquid.[66] A potential for misfilling exists even on contemporary vaporizers equipped with keyed fillers.[67-69] When vaporizer misfilling occurs, either an anesthetic overdose or underdose will result if the anesthesia care provider is depending on the concentration control dial markings to determine the anesthetic dose. The use of supplemental monitoring such as a multigas analyzer may alert the user to such a problem.

Contamination Contamination of anesthetic vaporizer contents has occurred as a result of filling an isoflurane vaporizer with a contaminated bottle of isoflurane. A potentially serious incident was avoided because the operator did not use the contaminated vaporizer after detecting an abnormal acrid odor.[70]

Tipping Tipping of a vaporizer can occur when it is incorrectly "switched out" or moved. However, short of the entire machine being turned over, tipping is unlikely when a vaporizer is attached to the anesthesia workstation manifold. Excessive tipping can allow the liquid agent to enter the bypass chamber and cause an output with an extremely high concentration of agent.[71] The Tec 4 is slightly more immune to tipping than the North American Dräger Vapor 19.n because of its extensive baffle system. However, if either vaporizer is tipped, it should not be used until it has been flushed for 20 to 30 minutes at high fresh gas flow rates. During this procedure, having the vaporizer concentration control dial set at a low concentration maximizes bypass chamber flow and will aid in removal of any residual liquid anesthetic in that area.[48] After this procedure, use of a multigas analyzer is strongly recommended. The Dräger Vapor 20.n series vaporizers now have a transport ("T") dial setting that helps prevent tipping-related problems. When the dial is placed in this position, the vaporizer sump is isolated from the bypass chamber, thereby reducing the likelihood of tipping and resulting in an accidental overdose. Therefore, any time that one of these vaporizers is moved separate from the anesthesia workstation, the control dial should be placed in the "T" position.

The design of the Tec 6 and the Aladin cassette vaporizer systems, both from Datex-Ohmeda, has practically eliminated the possibility of tipping with these products. Because the Aladin cassette vaporizer's bypass chamber is physically separated from the "cassette" and permanently resides in the anesthesia workstation, the possibility of tipping is virtually eliminated, sparing overturning the entire anesthesia workstation. Tipping of the Aladin cassettes themselves when they are not installed in the vaporizer is not problematic.

Overfilling Improper filling procedures combined with failure of the vaporizer sight glass can cause overfilling and patient overdose. Liquid anesthetic enters the bypass chamber, and up to 10 times the intended vapor concentration can be delivered to the common gas outlet.[72] Most modern vaporizers are now relatively immune to overfilling because of side-fill rather than top-fill designs. Side-fill systems largely prevent overfilling.

Underfilling Just as with overfilling, underfilling of anesthetic vaporizers may be problematic. When a Tec 5 sevoflurane vaporizer is in a low fill state and used under conditions of high fresh gas flow rates (>7.5 L/min) and high dial settings (such as seen during inhalational induction), output from the vaporizer may abruptly decrease to less than 2%. The cause of this problem is most likely multifactorial. However, the combination of a low vaporizer fill state (<25% full) and a high vaporizing chamber flow rate can result in a clinically significant and reproducible fall in vaporizer output.[73] Because sevoflurane has become a particularly popular agent for use during inhalational induction, all anesthesia care providers should be aware of this particular hazard.

Simultaneous Administration of Inhaled Anesthetics On some older anesthesia machines from Datex-Ohmeda (equipped with the Select-a-Tec three-vaporizer manifold) that did not use a vapor interlock system, two inhaled anesthetics could be administered simultaneously when the center vaporizer was removed. On such machines, the left or right vaporizer needed to be moved to the central position if the central vaporizer was removed (as indicated by the manifold warning label). Once this was done, the vaporizer's interlock system would operate properly and allow only one agent to be administered at a time. More contemporary Select-a-Tec–type vaporizer manifolds from GE and Dräger Medical have a built-in vapor interlock or vapor exclusion devices that prevent this problem. On these newer two- or three-vaporizer systems, the vaporizers do not necessarily have to be in adjacent positions on the manifold for the vapor exclusion systems to work properly. In one basic type of system used on early GE workstations, a U-shaped plastic device linked the vaporizer extension rods even when the vaporizers were not adjacent to one another on the manifold to prevent simultaneously turning on two vaporizers. On such a system, the manifold and the vaporizers themselves comprise the vapor interlock or vapor exclusion system. This type of system reduced the chance of accidental simultaneous administration of two volatile anesthetic agents.

Leaks Vaporizer leaks occur frequently and can result in patient awareness during anesthesia.[11,15,54,74] A loose filler cap is the most common source of vaporizer leaks. With some key-filled Penlon and Dräger vaporizers, a loose filler screw clamp allows saturated anesthetic vapor to escape.[11] Leaks can occur at the O-ring junctions between the vaporizer and its manifold. To detect a leak within a vaporizer, the concentration control dial must be in the "on" position. Even though vaporizer leaks in Dräger systems can potentially be detected with a conventional positive-pressure leak test (because of the absence of an outlet check valve), a negative-pressure leak test is more sensitive and allows the user to detect even small leaks. Datex-Ohmeda recommends a negative-pressure leak-testing device (suction bulb) to detect vaporizer leaks in the Modulus I, Modulus II, Excel, and Aestiva workstations because of the check valve located just upstream of each machine's fresh gas outlet (see "Checking Your Anesthesia Workstation").

Many newer anesthesia workstations are capable of performing self-testing procedures, which in some cases may eliminate the need for the conventional negative-pressure leak testing. However, it is of vital importance that anesthesia care providers understand that these self-tests may not detect internal vaporizer leaks on systems with add-on vaporizers. For the self-tests to determine whether an internal vaporizer leak is present, the leak test must be repeated with each vaporizer sequentially while its concentration control dial is turned to the "on" position. Recall that when a vaporizer's concentration control dial is set in the "off" position, it may not be possible to detect even major internal leaks such as an absent or loose filler cap.

Anesthesia Vaporizers and Environmental Considerations Today more than ever, anesthesia care providers are being asked to provide anesthesia to patients outside the operating room. One such location that has sometimes proved difficult to work in is the magnetic resonance imaging (MRI) suite. The presence of a powerful magnet field, significant noise pollution, and limited access to the patient during the procedure all complicate care in this setting. Essential to the anesthesia care provider is an understanding of the extremely powerful magnetic fields used in these devices. It is imperative that only nonferrous (MRI-compatible) equipment be used in these settings. Some anesthesia vaporizers, although they may appear nonferrous by testing with a horseshoe magnet, may indeed contain substantial internal ferrous components. Inappropriate use of such devices in an MRI suite may potentially turn them into a dangerous missile if left unsecured.[75]

The Datex-Ohmeda Tec 6 Vaporizer for Desflurane

Because of its unique physical characteristics, controlled vaporization of desflurane required a novel approach to vaporizer design. Datex-Ohmeda developed the Tec 6 vaporizer, the first such system, and released it into clinical use in the early 1990s. The Tec 6 vaporizer is an electrically heated, pressurized device specifically designed to deliver desflurane.[76,77] The vapor pressure of desflurane is three to four times that of other contemporary inhaled anesthetics, and it boils at 22.8°C,[78] which is near room temperature (see Fig. 25-17). Desflurane has minimum alveolar anesthetic concentration (MAC) values of 6% to 7%.[78] Desflurane is valuable because it has a low blood-gas solubility coefficient of 0.45 at 37°C, and recovery from anesthesia is more rapid than with many other potent inhaled anesthetics.[78] In 2004, Dräger Medical received FDA approval for its own version of the Tec 6 desflurane vaporizer. The operating principles described in the following discussion are applicable to either system, even though we refer to the Tec 6 specifically.

Unsuitability of Contemporary Variable-Bypass Vaporizers for Controlled Vaporization of Desflurane

Desflurane's high volatility and moderate potency preclude its use with contemporary variable-bypass vaporizers such as Datex-Ohmeda Tec 4, Tec 5, and Tec 7 or the North American Dräger Vapor 19.n or 20.n for two primary reasons[76]:

1. At 20°C the vapor pressure of desflurane is near 1 atm. The vapor pressures of enflurane, isoflurane, halothane, and desflurane at 20°C are 172, 240, 244, and 669 mm Hg, respectively (see Fig. 25-17).[78] Equal amounts of flow through a traditional vaporizer would vaporize many more volumes of desflurane than any other of these agents. For example, at 1 atm and 20°C, 100 mL/min passing through the vaporizing chamber would entrain 735 mL/min of desflurane versus 29, 46, and 47 mL/min of enflurane, isoflurane, and halothane, respectively.[76] Under these same conditions, to produce a 1% desflurane output, the amount of bypass flow necessary to achieve sufficient dilution of the large volume of desflurane-saturated anesthetic vapor would be approximately 73 L/min versus 5 L/min or less

for the other three anesthetics. Additionally, above 22.8°C at 1 atm, desflurane will boil. The amount of vapor produced would be limited only by the heat energy available from the vaporizer because of its specific heat.[76]

2. Contemporary vaporizers lack an external heat source. The latent heat of vaporization for desflurane is approximately equal to that of enflurane, isoflurane, and halothane; however its MAC is four to nine times higher than those of the other three inhaled anesthetics. Thus, the absolute amount of desflurane vaporized over a given period is considerably greater than that of the other anesthetic drugs. Supplying desflurane via a conventional vaporizer in higher (equivalent MAC) concentrations would lead to excessive cooling of the vaporizer and significantly reduce its output. In the absence of an external heat source, temperature compensation with the traditional mechanical devices would be almost impossible. Because of the broad range of temperatures seen in the clinical setting and because of desflurane's steep vapor pressure–versus-temperature curve (see Fig. 25-17), delivery of desflurane in a conventional anesthetic vaporizer would be at best unpredictable.[767]

Operating Principles of the Tec 6 and Tec 6 Plus

To achieve controlled vaporization of desflurane, Datex-Ohmeda introduced the Tec 6 vaporizer to widespread clinical practice in 1993. This was the first clinically available vaporizer ever to be electrically heated and pressurized. The physical appearance and operation of the Tec 6 and contemporary vaporizers are similar, but some aspects of the internal design and operating principles are radically different. The Tec 6 Plus represents a later version of the original Tec 6. The Tec 6 Plus has the same basic Tec 6 design, but it also incorporates an enhanced audible alarm system not previously available on the Tec 6.

Functionally, operation of the Tec 6 is more accurately described as a dual-gas blender than as a vaporizer. A simplified schematic of the Tec 6 is shown in Figure 25-22. The vaporizer has two independent gas circuits arranged in parallel. The fresh gas circuit is shown in orange, and the vapor circuit is shown in blue. Fresh gas from the flow meters enters at the fresh gas inlet, passes through a fixed restrictor (R1), and exits at the vaporizer gas outlet. The vapor circuit originates at the desflurane sump, which is electrically heated and thermostatically controlled to 39°C, a temperature well above desflurane's boiling point. The heated sump assembly serves as a reservoir of desflurane *vapor*. At 39°C, the vapor pressure in the sump is approximately 1300 mm Hg absolute,[79] or approximately 2 atm absolute (see Fig. 25-17). Just downstream from the sump is the shut-off valve. After the vaporizer warms up, the shut-off valve fully opens when the concentration control valve is turned to the "on" position. A pressure-regulating valve located downstream from the shut-off valve downregulates the pressure to approximately 1.1 atm absolute (74 mm Hg gauge) at a fresh gas flow rate of 10 L/min. The operator controls the output of desflurane by adjusting the concentration control valve (R2), which is a variable restrictor.[76]

The vapor flow through R2 joins the fresh gas flow through R1 at a point downstream from the restrictors. Until this

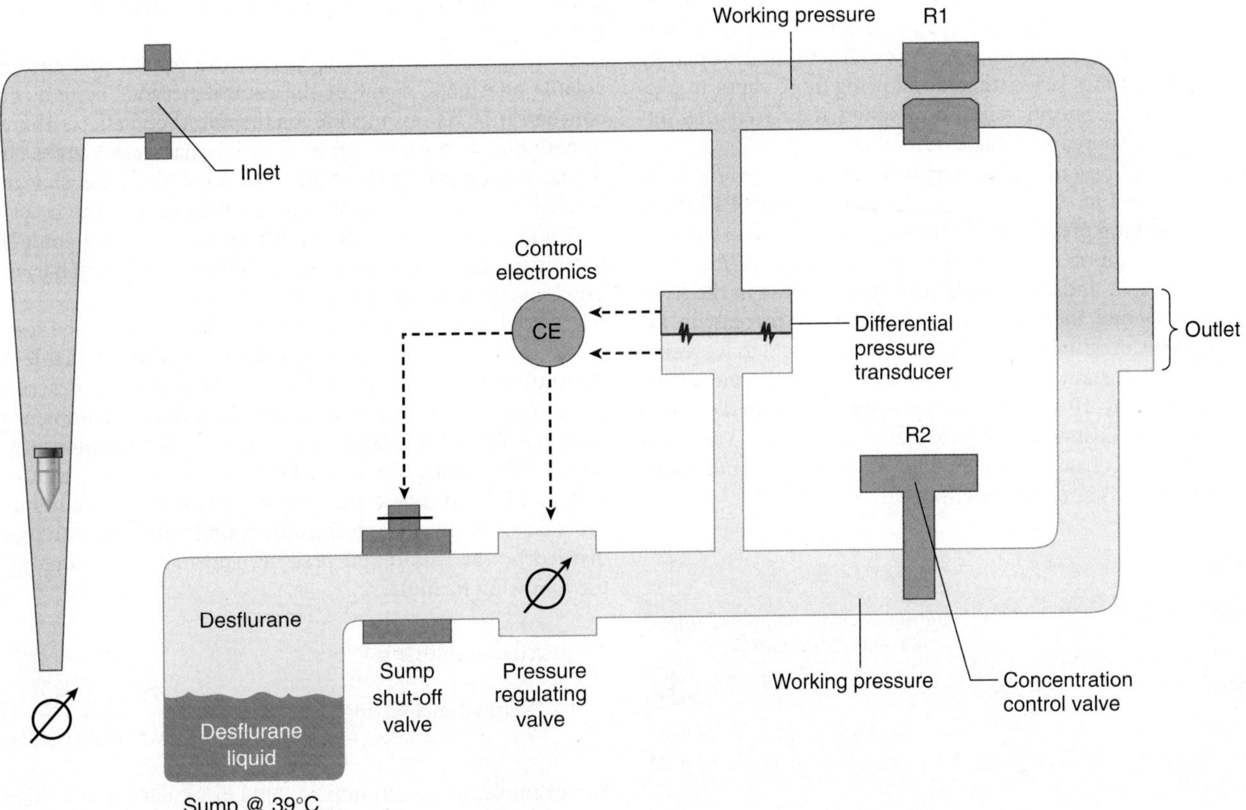

Figure 25-22 Simplified schematic of the Tec 6 desflurane vaporizer. *(From Andrews JJ: Operating Principles of the Ohmeda Tec 6 Desflurane Vaporizer: A Collection of Twelve Color Illustrations. Washington, DC, Library of Congress, 1996, with permission.)*

point, the two circuits are physically divorced. They are interfaced pneumatically and electronically, however, through differential pressure transducers, a control electronics system, and a pressure-regulating valve. When a constant fresh gas flow rate encounters the fixed restrictor R1, a specific backpressure proportional to the fresh gas flow rate pushes against the diaphragm of the control differential pressure transducer. The differential pressure transducer conveys the pressure difference between the fresh gas circuit and the vapor circuit to the control electronics system. The control electronics system regulates the pressure-regulating valve so that the pressure in the vapor circuit equals the pressure in the fresh gas circuit. This equalized pressure supplying R1 and R2 is the working pressure, and the working pressure is constant at a fixed fresh gas flow rate. If the operator increases the fresh gas flow rate, more backpressure is exerted on the diaphragm of the control pressure transducer, and the working pressure of the vaporizer increases.[76]

Table 25-2 shows the approximate correlation between the fresh gas flow rate and working pressure for a typical vaporizer. At a fresh gas flow rate of 1 L/min, the working pressure is 10 millibars, or 7.4 mm Hg gauge. At a fresh gas flow rate of 10 L/min, the working pressure is 100 millibars, or 74 mm Hg gauge. Therefore, there is a linear relationship between the fresh gas flow rate and working pressure. When the fresh gas flow rate is increased 10-fold, the working pressure increases 10-fold.[76]

Listed below are two specific examples to demonstrate the operating principles of the Tec 6.[76]

Example A: *Constant fresh gas flow rate of 1 L/min with an increase in the dial setting.* With a fresh gas flow rate of 1 L/min, the working pressure of the vaporizer is 7.4 mm Hg. That is, the pressure supplying R1 and R2 is 7.4 mm Hg. As the operator increases the dial setting, the opening at R2 becomes larger, thereby allowing more vapor to pass through R2. Specific vapor flow values at different dial settings are shown in Table 25-3.

Example B: *Constant dial setting with an increase in fresh gas flow from 1 to 10 L/min.* At a fresh gas flow rate of 1 L/min, the working pressure is 7.4 mm Hg, and at a dial setting of 6%, the vapor flow rate through R2 is 64 mL/min (see Tables 25-2 and 25-3). With a 10-fold increase in the fresh gas flow rate, there is a concomitant 10-fold increase in the working pressure to 74 mm Hg. The ratio of R2 to R1 resistance is constant at a fixed dial setting of 6%. Because R2 is supplied by 10 times more pressure, the vapor flow rate through R2 increases 10-fold to 640 mL/min. Vaporizer output is constant because both fresh gas flow and vapor flow increase proportionally.

Table 25-2 Fresh Gas Flow Rate Versus Working Pressure

Fresh Gas Flow Rate (L/min)	Working Pressure at R1 and R2 (Gauge) (Gas Inlet Pressure)		
	Millibar	cm H_2O	mm Hg
1	10	10.2	7.4
5	50	51.0	37.0
10	100	102.0	74.0

Reprinted with permission from Andrews JJ, Johnston RV Jr: The new Tec 6 desflurane vaporizer. Anesth Analg 76:1338, 1993.

Table 25-3 Dial Setting Versus Flow through Restrictor R2

Dial Setting (vol%)*	Fresh Gas Flow Rate (L/min)	Approximate Vapor Flow Rate through R2 (mL/min)
1	1	10
6	1	64
12	1	136
18	1	220

$$\text{* Volume percent} = \frac{\text{Vapor flow rate}}{\text{Fresh gas flow rate} + \text{Vapor flow rate}} \times 100\%$$

Reprinted with permission from Andrews JJ, Johnston RV Jr: The new Tec 6 desflurane vaporizer. Anesth Analg 76:1338, 1993.

Factors That Influence Vaporizer Output

Varied altitude and carrier gas composition influence Tec 6 output. Each is discussed in the following paragraphs.

Varied Altitudes Although ambient pressure changes affect conventional vaporizer output significantly in terms of volume percent (%vol/vol; i.e., concentration), their effect on anesthetic potency (partial pressure) is minimal. This effect is illustrated with the example of isoflurane in Table 25-4. With a constant dial setting of 0.89%, at 1 atm, if perfectly calibrated, the %vol/vol delivered would be 0.89%, and the partial pressure of isoflurane would be 6.8 mm Hg. Maintaining the same dial setting and lowering the atmospheric pressure to 0.66 atm or 502 mm Hg (roughly equivalent to an elevation of 10,000 ft) would result in an increase in the concentration output to 1.75% (almost double), but the partial pressure increases to only 8.77 mm Hg (just a 29% increase) because of the proportional decline in ambient pressure.

In general, it is thought that the partial pressure of the volatile anesthetic agent in the central nervous system, not its concentration, is responsible for the anesthetic effect. Therefore, to maintain a constant depth of anesthesia when a gross change in barometric pressure occurs, %vol/vol must be changed in inverse proportion to atmospheric pressure. For the most part, traditional variable-bypass vaporizers automatically compensate for this change, and for practical purposes the effect of barometric pressure can generally be ignored.

This should be considered in stark contrast to the response of the Tec 6 desflurane vaporizer at varied altitudes (Table 25-4). One must remember this device is more accurately described as a dual-gas blender than a vaporizer. Regardless of ambient pressure, the Tec 6 will maintain a constant concentration of vapor output (%vol/vol), not a constant partial pressure. This means that at high altitudes, the partial pressure of desflurane will decrease in proportion to the reduction in atmospheric pressure divided by the calibration pressure (normally 760 mm Hg) per the following formula:

Required dial setting =

$$\text{Normal dial setting (vol\%)} \times \frac{760 \text{ mm Hg}}{\text{Ambient pressure (mm Hg)}}$$

For example, at an altitude of 2000 m or 6564 feet, where the ambient pressure is 608 mm Hg, the operator must advance the concentration control dial from 10% to 12.5% to maintain the required anesthetic partial pressure. In hyperbaric settings, the

Table 25-4 Performance of "Tec"-Type Vaporizers Versus the Tec 6 Desflurane Vaporizer at Varying Ambient Pressure

		Isoflurane Vaporizer with a Dial Setting of 0.89%			Tec 6 Desflurane Vaporizer with a Dial Setting of 6%
Atmospheres	**Ambient Pressure (mm Hg)**	**mL Isoflurane Vapor Entrained by 100 mL O_2**	**Output Concentration (%)**	**Partial Pressure Output (mm Hg)**	**Partial Pressure Output of Desflurane (mm Hg)**
0.66 (2/3)	500 (10,000 ft)	91	1.753	8.77	30
0.74	560	74	1.429	8.0	33.6
0.80	608 (6564 ft)	64.32	1.25	7.6	36.5
1.0	760	46	0.89	6.8	45.6
1.5	1140	26.4	0.515	5.87	68.4
2	1520	19	0.36	5.5	91.2
3	2280	11.65	0.228	5.198	136

Adapted from Ehrenwerth J, Eisenkraft J: Anesthesia vaporizers. *In* Ehrenwerth J, Eisenkraft J (eds): Anesthesia Equipment—Principles and Applications. St Louis, CV Mosby, 1993, pp 69-71.

operator must decrease the dial setting to prevent delivery of an overdose.

Carrier Gas Composition Vaporizer output approximates the dial setting when oxygen is the carrier gas because the Tec 6 vaporizer is calibrated with 100% oxygen. At low flow rates when a carrier gas other than 100% oxygen is used, however, a clear trend toward reduction in vaporizer output emerges. This reduction parallels the proportional decrease in viscosity of the carrier gas. Nitrous oxide has lower viscosity than oxygen does, so the backpressure generated by resistor R1 (see Fig. 25-22) is less when nitrous oxide is the carrier gas, and the working pressure is reduced. At low flow rates and with nitrous oxide used as the carrier gas, vaporizer output is approximately 20% less than the dial setting. This suggests that at clinically useful fresh gas flow rates, gas flow across resistor R1 is laminar, and the working pressure is proportional to both the fresh gas flow rate and the viscosity of the carrier gas.[80]

Safety Features

Because desflurane's vapor pressure is near 1 atm, misfilling contemporary vaporizers with desflurane could theoretically result in both desflurane overdose and creation of a hypoxic gas mixture.[81] Datex-Ohmeda has introduced a unique, anesthetic-specific filling system to minimize occurrence of this potential hazard. The agent-specific filler of the desflurane bottle, known as the "Saf-T-Fill" adapter, is intended to prevent its use with traditional vaporizers. The filling system also minimizes spillage of liquid or vapor anesthetic by maintaining a "closed system" during the filling process. Each desflurane bottle has a spring-loaded filler cap with an O-ring on the tip. The spring seals the bottle until it is engaged in the filler port of the vaporizer. Thus, this anesthetic-specific filling system interlocks the vaporizer and the dispensing bottle and thereby prevents loss of anesthetic to the atmosphere. One recent case report described misfilling of a Tec 6 desflurane vaporizer with sevoflurane. This error was possible because of similarities between a new type of keyed filler for sevoflurane and the desflurane Saf-T-fill adapter. In this case, the desflurane vaporizer detected this error and automatically shut itself off.[69]

Major vaporizer faults cause the shut-off valve located just downstream from the desflurane sump (see Fig. 25-22) to close and produce a no-output situation. The valve is closed and a "no-output" alarm is activated immediately if any of the following conditions occur: (1) the anesthetic level decreases to below 20 mL, (2) the vaporizer is tilted, (3) a power failure occurs, or (4) there is a disparity between the pressure in the vapor circuit and the pressure in the fresh gas circuit that exceeds a specified tolerance.

Summary

The Tec 6 vaporizer is an electrically heated, thermostatically controlled, constant-temperature, pressurized, electromechanically coupled dual-circuit, gas-vapor blender. The pressure in the vapor circuit is electronically regulated to equal the pressure in the fresh gas circuit. At a constant fresh gas flow rate, the operator regulates vapor flow with a conventional concentration control dial. When the fresh gas flow rate increases, the working pressure increases proportionally. For a given concentration setting even when varying the fresh gas flow rate, the vaporizer output is constant because the amount of flow through each circuit remains proportional.[76]

The Datex-Ohmeda Aladin Cassette Vaporizer

The vaporizer system used in the Datex-Ohmeda S/5 ADU is unique in that the single electronically controlled vaporizer is designed to deliver five different inhaled anesthetics, including halothane, isoflurane, enflurane, sevoflurane, and desflurane. The vaporizer consists of a permanent internal control unit housed within the ADU and an interchangeable Aladin agent cassette that contains anesthetic liquid. The Aladin agent cassettes are color-coded for each anesthetic agent, and they are also magnetically coded so that the Datex-Ohmeda ADU can identify which anesthetic cassette has been inserted. The cassettes are filled using agent-specific fillers.[48,82]

Though very different in external appearance, the functional anatomy of the S/5 ADU cassette vaporizer (Fig. 25-23) is very similar to that of the Dräger Vapor 19.n and 20.n and the Datex-Ohmeda Tec 4, Tec 5, and Tec 7 vaporizers. The Aladin

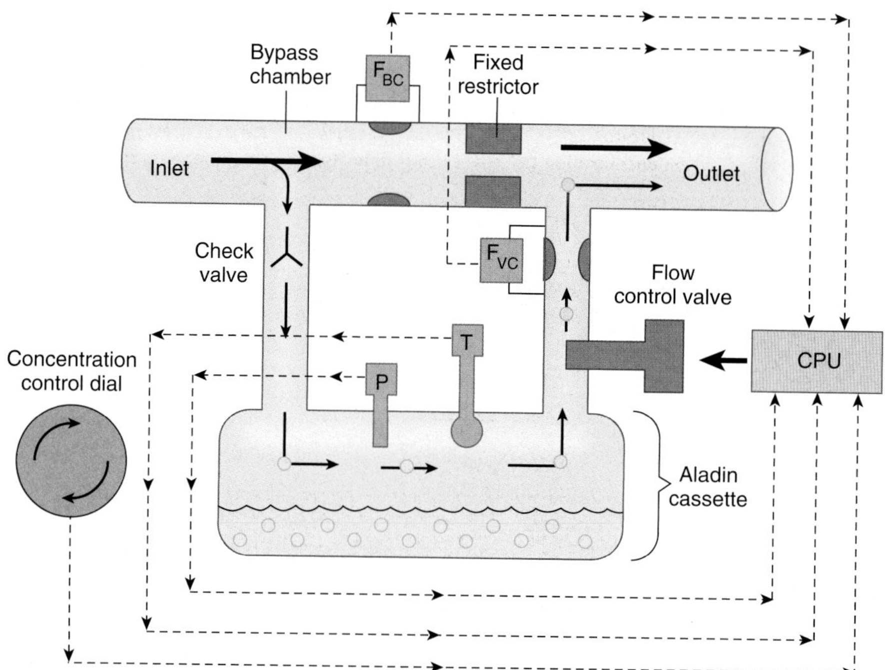

Figure 25-23 Simplified schematic of Datex-Ohmeda Aladin Cassette Vaporizer. The *black arrows* inside the vaporizer represent flow from the flow meters, and the *yellow circles* represent anesthetic vapor. The heart of the vaporizer is the electronically controlled flow control valve located in the outlet of the vaporizing chamber. CPU, central processing unit; F_{BC}, flow measurement unit that measures flow through the bypass chamber; F_{VC}, flow measurement unit that measures flow through the vaporizing chamber; P, pressure sensor; T, temperature sensor. *(Modified from Andrews JJ: Operating Principles of the Datex-Ohmeda Aladin Cassette Vaporizer: A Collection of Color Illustrations. Washington, DC, Library of Congress, 2000.)*

system is functionally similar to these conventional vaporizers because it is also made up of a bypass chamber and vaporizing chamber. A fixed restrictor is located in the bypass chamber, and flow measurement sensors are located both in the bypass chamber and in the outlet of the vaporizing chamber. The heart of the S/5 ADU cassette vaporizer is the electronically regulated flow control valve located in the vaporizing chamber outlet. This valve is controlled by a central processing unit (CPU). The CPU receives input from multiple sources, including the concentration control dial, a pressure sensor located inside the vaporizing chamber, a temperature sensor located inside the vaporizing chamber, a flow measurement unit located in the bypass chamber, and a flow measurement unit located in the outlet of the vaporizing chamber. The CPU also receives input from the flow meters regarding the composition of the carrier gas. By using data from these multiple sources, the CPU is able to precisely regulate the flow control valve to obtain the desired vapor concentration output. Appropriate electronic control of the flow control valve is essential to proper functioning of this vaporizer.[48,83]

A fixed restrictor is located in the bypass chamber, and it causes flow from the vaporizer inlet to split into two flow streams (see Fig. 25-23). One stream passes through the bypass chamber, and the other portion enters the inlet of the vaporizing chamber and passes through a one-way check valve. The presence of this check valve is unique to the Aladin system. This one-way valve prevents retrograde flow of the anesthetic vapor back into the bypass chamber, and its presence is crucial when delivering desflurane if room temperature is higher than the boiling point of desflurane (22.8°C).[48] A precise amount of vapor-saturated carrier gas passes through the flow control valve, which is regulated by the CPU. This flow then joins the bypass flow and is directed to the outlet of the vaporizer.[48]

As mentioned during discussion of the Tec 6, controlled vaporization of desflurane presents a unique challenge, particularly when room temperature is greater than the boiling point of desflurane (22.8°C). At higher temperatures, the pressure inside the vaporizer sump increases, and the sump becomes pressurized. When sump pressure exceeds pressure in the bypass chamber, the one-way check valve located in the vaporizing chamber inlet closes to prevent carrier gas from entering the vaporizing chamber. At this point the carrier gas passes straight through the bypass chamber and its flow sensor. Under these conditions, the electronically regulated flow control valve simply meters in the appropriate flow of pure desflurane vapor needed to achieve the desired final concentration selected by the user. At least one case report has described failure of the vaporizing chamber inlet check valve to function as designed. In this case, an anesthetic overdose occurred as a result of regurgitation of desflurane from the vaporizing chamber in a retrograde fashion back into the bypass chamber. Because of this report, ADU users should be cautious of this potential problem, especially when desflurane is used.[83]

During operating conditions in which high fresh gas flow rates or high dial settings (or both) are used, large quantities of anesthetic liquid are vaporized rapidly. As a result, the temperature of the remaining liquid anesthetic and the vaporizer itself decreases because of energy consumption, or the latent heat of vaporization. To offset this cooling effect, the S/5 ADU is equipped with a fan that forces warmed air from an "agent heating resistor" across the cassette (vaporizer sump) to raise its temperature when necessary. The fan is activated during two common clinical scenarios: (1) desflurane induction and maintenance and (2) sevoflurane induction.

Anesthetic Breathing Circuits

As the prescribed mixture of gases from the flow meters and vaporizer exits the anesthesia workstation at the common gas outlet, it then enters an anesthetic breathing circuit. The function of the anesthesia breathing circuit is not only to deliver oxygen and anesthetic gases to the patient but also to eliminate carbon dioxide. Carbon dioxide can be removed either by washout with adequate fresh gas inflow or by the use of carbon dioxide absorbent media (e.g., soda lime absorption). The following discussion focuses on semiclosed rebreathing circuits and the circle system.

Mapleson Systems

In 1954 Mapleson described and analyzed five different semiclosed anesthetic systems, and they are now classically referred to as the Mapleson systems and are designated with letters A through E (Fig. 25-24).[84] Subsequently, in 1975 Willis and coauthors described the F system that was added to the original five.[85] The Mapleson systems consist of several common components, including a facemask, a spring-loaded pop-off valve, reservoir tubing, fresh gas inflow tubing, and a reservoir bag. Within the Mapleson systems, three distinct functional groups can be seen: A, BC, and DEF groups. The Mapleson A, also known as the Magill circuit, has a spring-loaded pop-off valve located near the facemask, and fresh gas flow enters the opposite end of the circuit near the reservoir bag. In the B and C systems, the spring-loaded pop-off valve is located near the facemask, but the fresh gas inlet tubing is located near the patient. The reservoir tubing and breathing bag serve as a blind limb where fresh gas, dead space gas, and alveolar gas can collect. Finally, in the Mapleson D, E, and F or "T-piece" group, fresh gas enters near the patient, and excess gas is popped off at the opposite end of the circuit.

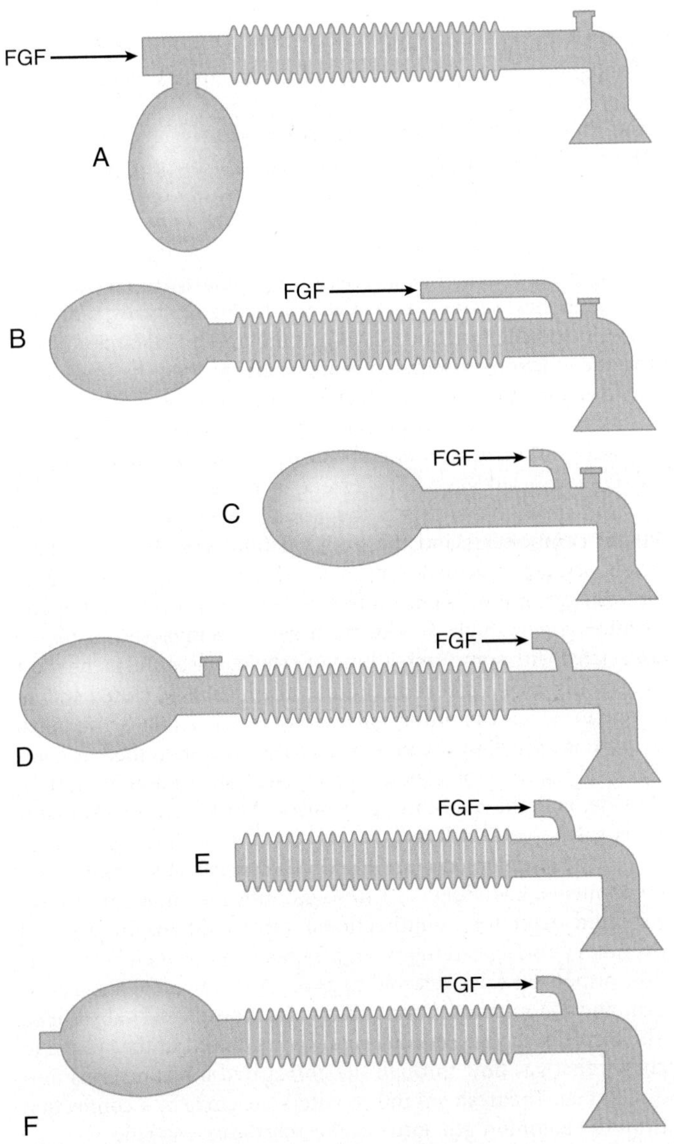

Figure 25-24 Mapleson breathing systems A-F. *(Redrawn with permission from Willis BA, Pender JW, Mapleson WW: Rebreathing in a T-piece: Volunteer and theoretical studies of the Jackson-Rees Modification of Ayer's T-piece during spontaneous respiration. Br J Anesth 47:1239, 1975.)*

Even though the components and their arrangement are simple, functional analysis of the Mapleson systems can be complex.[86,87] The amount of carbon dioxide rebreathing associated with each system is multifactorial, and variables that dictate the ultimate carbon dioxide concentration include the following: (1) the fresh gas inflow rate, (2) minute ventilation, (3) the mode of ventilation (spontaneous or controlled), (4) tidal volume, (5) the respiratory rate, (6) the inspiratory-to-expiratory ratio, (7) the duration of the expiratory pause, (8) the peak inspiratory flow rate, (9) the volume of the reservoir tube, (10) the volume of the breathing bag, (11) ventilation by mask, (12) ventilation through an endotracheal tube, and (13) the CO_2 sampling site.

The performance of the Mapleson systems is best understood by studying the expiratory phase of the respiratory cycle.[88] Illustrations of the various arrangements of Mapleson system component may be found in Figure 25-24. During spontaneous ventilation, the Mapleson A has the best efficiency of the six systems in that it requires a fresh gas inflow rate of only 1 times minute ventilation to prevent rebreathing of carbon dioxide.[89] However, it has the worst efficiency during controlled ventilation because a minute ventilation as high as 20 L/min is needed to prevent rebreathing. Systems DEF are slightly more efficient than systems BC. To prevent rebreathing CO_2, the DEF systems require a fresh gas inflow rate of approximately 2.5 times minute ventilation, whereas the fresh gas inflow rates required for BC systems are somewhat higher.[87]

The following summarizes the relative efficiency of different Mapleson systems with respect to prevention of rebreathing during spontaneous ventilation: A > DFE > CB. During controlled ventilation, DFE > BC > A.[84,87] The Mapleson A, B, and C systems are rarely used today, but the D, E, and F systems are commonly used. In the United States, the most popular representative from the DEF group is the Bain circuit.

Bain Circuit

The Bain circuit is a coaxial circuit and a modification of the Mapleson D system. Fresh gas flows through a narrow inner tube within the outer corrugated tubing.[90] The central fresh gas tubing enters the outer corrugated hose near the reservoir bag, but the fresh gas actually empties into the circuit at the patient end (Fig. 25-25). Exhaled gases enter the corrugated tubing and are vented through the expiratory valve near the reservoir bag. The Bain circuit may be used for both spontaneous and controlled ventilation. The fresh gas inflow rate necessary to prevent rebreathing is 2.5 times minute ventilation.

The Bain circuit has many advantages over other systems. It is lightweight, convenient, easily sterilized, and potentially reusable. Scavenging of gases from the expiratory valve is facilitated because the valve is located away from the patient. Exhaled gases in the outer reservoir tubing add warmth to the inspired fresh

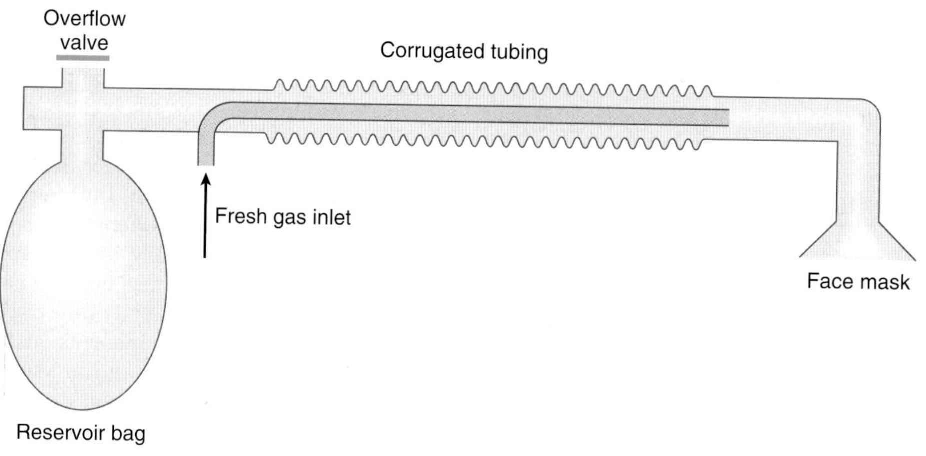

Figure 25-25 The Bain circuit. *(Redrawn with permission from Bain JA, Spoerel WE: A streamlined anaesthetic system. Can Anaesth Soc J 19:426, 1972.)*

gases by countercurrent heat exchange. The main hazards related to use of the Bain circuit are either an unrecognized disconnection or kinking of the inner fresh gas hose. These problems can cause hypercapnia as a result of inadequate gas flow or increased respiratory resistance. As with other circuits, an obstructed antimicrobial filter positioned between the Bain circuit and the endotracheal tube can result in increased resistance in the circuit. This may produce hypoventilation and hypoxemia and may even mimic the signs and symptoms of severe bronchospasm.[91]

The outer corrugated tube should be transparent to allow ongoing inspection of the inner tube. The integrity of the inner tube can be assessed as described by Pethick.[92] With his technique, high-flow oxygen is fed into the circuit while the patient end is occluded until the reservoir bag is filled. The patient end is opened, and oxygen is flushed into the circuit. If the inner tube is intact, the venturi effect occurs at the patient end. This causes a decrease in pressure within the circuit, and as a result, the reservoir bag deflates. Conversely, a leak in the inner tube allows fresh gas to escape into the expiratory limb, and the reservoir bag will remain inflated. This test is recommended as part of the preanesthesia check if a Bain circuit is used.

Circle Breathing Systems

For many years, the overall design of the circle breathing system has changed very little from one anesthesia workstation manufacturer to the next. Both the individual components and the order in which they appeared in the circle system were consistent across major platforms. In recent years, however, with the increasing technologic complexity of the anesthesia workstation, the circle system has undergone some major changes as well. These changes have resulted in part from an effort to improve patient safety (as in the integration of fresh gas decoupling and inspiratory pressure limiters) but have also allowed the deployment of new technologic advances. Two such major new technologies used in some new workstations have been (1) a return to the application of single-circuit piston-type ventilators and (2) the use of new spirometry devices that are located at the Y-connector instead of at the traditional location on the expiratory circuit limb. The following discussion focuses first on the traditional circle breathing system and is then followed by a brief discussion of some variations in the design of newer circle systems.

The Traditional Circle Breathing System

The circle system remains the most popular breathing system in the United States. It is so named because its components are arranged in a circular manner (see Fig. 25-7). One version of the traditional circle system, referred to as either a "universal F" or a "single-limb circuit," has increased in popularity in recent years. Although these systems appear very different externally, they have the same overall functional layout as the traditional circle system, and the following discussion is applicable to both the traditional circle system and the "universal F" system.

The circle system prevents rebreathing of carbon dioxide by use of carbon dioxide absorbents but allows partial rebreathing of other exhaled gases. The extent of rebreathing of the other exhaled gases depends on the arrangement of the breathing circuit components and the fresh gas flow rate. A circle system can be semiopen, semiclosed, or closed, depending on the amount of fresh gas inflow.[93] A semiopen system has no rebreathing and requires a very high flow of fresh gas. A semiclosed system is associated with some rebreathing of exhaled gases and is the most commonly used application in the United States. A closed system is one in which the inflow gas exactly matches that being taken up, or consumed, by the patient. In a closed system there is complete rebreathing of exhaled gases after absorption of carbon dioxide, and the overflow (pop-off or APL) valve or ventilator relief valve remains closed.

The circle system (see Fig. 25-7) consists of seven primary components, including (1) a fresh gas inflow source, (2) inspiratory and expiratory unidirectional valves, (3) inspiratory and expiratory corrugated tubes, (4) a Y-piece connector, (5) an overflow or pop-off valve referred to as the APL valve, (6) a reservoir bag, and (7) a canister containing a carbon dioxide absorbent. The inspiratory and expiratory valves are placed in the system to ensure that gas flow through the corrugated hoses remains unidirectional. The fresh gas inflow enters the circle by a connection from the common gas outlet of the anesthesia machine.

Numerous variations of the circle arrangement are possible, depending on the relative positions of the unidirectional valves, the pop-off valve, the reservoir bag, the carbon dioxide absorber, and the site of fresh gas entry. However, to prevent rebreathing of carbon dioxide *in a traditional circle system*, three rules must be followed: (1) a unidirectional valve must be located between the patient and the reservoir bag on both the inspiratory and expiratory limbs of the circuit, (2) the fresh gas inflow cannot enter the circuit between the expiratory valve and the patient, and (3) the overflow (pop-off) valve cannot be located between the patient and the inspiratory valve. If these rules are followed, any arrangement of the other components will prevent rebreathing of carbon dioxide.[89] Some newer anesthesia workstations now use less traditional circle breathing systems. Two of these systems are discussed in detail later (see "Anesthesia Workstation Variations").

The most efficient circle system arrangement with the highest conservation of fresh gases is one in which the unidirectional valves are near the patient and the pop-off valve is located just downstream from the expiratory valve. This arrangement minimizes dead space gas and preferentially eliminates exhaled alveolar gases. A more practical arrangement, the one used on most conventional anesthesia machines (see Fig. 25-7), is somewhat less efficient because it allows alveolar and dead space gases to mix before they are vented.[94,95]

The main advantages of the circle system over other breathing systems include (1) maintenance of relatively stable inspired gas concentrations, (2) conservation of respiratory moisture and heat, and (3) prevention of operating room pollution. Additionally, the circle system can be used for closed-system anesthesia or semiclosed with very low fresh gas flows. The major disadvantage of the circle system stems from its complex design. Commonly, the circle system may have 10 or more different connections. These multiple connection sites set the stage for misconnections, disconnections, obstructions, and leaks. In a recent closed-claim analysis of adverse anesthetic outcomes arising from gas delivery equipment, more than a third (25/72) of malpractice claims resulted from breathing circuit misconnections or disconnections.[1] Malfunction of the circle system's unidirectional valves can result in life-threatening problems. Rebreathing can occur if the valves stick in the open position, and total occlusion of the circuit can occur if they are stuck shut. If the expiratory valve is stuck in the closed position, breath stacking and barotrauma or volutrauma can result. Obstructed filters located in the expiratory limb of the circle breathing system have caused increased airway pressure, hemodynamic collapse, and bilateral tension pneumothorax. Causes of circle system obstruction and failure include manufacturing defects, debris, patient secretions, and particulate obstruction from other odd sources such as albuterol nebulization.[96-99] Some systems, such as the Datex-Ohmeda 7900 SmartVent, use flow transducers located on both the inspiratory and expiratory limbs of the circle system. In one report, cracks in the flow transducer tubing used by this system produced a leak in the circle system that was difficult to detect.[100]

Carbon Dioxide Absorbents

Much has appeared in the literature lately regarding the issue of adverse chemical reactions between carbon dioxide absorbent materials and anesthetic agents. Some of these undesirable interactions are quite dramatic, such as sevoflurane interacting with desiccated Baralyme and resulting in fires within the breathing system and severe patient injury.[101,102] Although other sources of ignition and fire in the breathing system continue to be described,[103] the Baralyme-sevoflurane problem is somewhat unique in that nothing "unusual" is added to or removed from the breathing system for this to occur. Other reactions such as desflurane or sevoflurane with desiccated strong-base absorbents can produce more insidious patient morbidity and even death from the release of by-products such as carbon monoxide (CO) or compound A.[104] Although absorbent materials may be problematic, they still represent an important component of the circle breathing system. Different anesthesia breathing systems eliminate carbon dioxide with varying degrees of efficiency. The closed and semiclosed circle systems both *require* that carbon dioxide be absorbed from the exhaled gases to avoid hypercapnia. If one could design an ideal carbon dioxide absorbent, its characteristics would include lack of reactivity with common anesthetics, absence of toxicity, low resistance to airflow, low cost, ease of handling, and efficiency in carbon dioxide absorption.

The Absorber Canister

On modern anesthesia machines, the absorber canister (see Fig. 25-7) is composed of one or two clear plastic canisters alone or arranged in series. The canisters can be filled either with loose bulk absorbent or with absorbent supplied by the factory in prefilled plastic disposable cartridges called *prepacks*. Free granules from bulk absorbent can create a clinically significant leak if they lodge between the clear plastic canister and the O-ring gasket of the absorber. Leaks have also been caused by defective prepacks that were larger than factory specifications.[105] Prepacks can also cause total obstruction of the circle system if the clear plastic shipping wrapper is not removed before use.[106]

Chemistry of Absorbents

Two formulations of carbon dioxide absorbents are commonly available today: soda lime and calcium hydroxide lime (Amsorb). Of these agents, the most commonly used is soda lime. All serve to eliminate carbon dioxide from the breathing circuit with varying degrees of efficiency. Formerly, a product known as Baralyme, or barium hydroxide lime, was frequently used. This compound had significant interaction with contemporary volatile anesthetic drugs and was voluntarily removed from the market after several mishaps were reported in the literature (see later).

By weight, the approximate composition of "high-moisture" soda lime is 80% calcium hydroxide, 15% water, 4% sodium hydroxide, and 1% potassium hydroxide (an activator). Small amounts of silica are added to produce calcium and sodium silicate. This addition produces a harder, more stable pellet and thereby reduces dust formation. The efficiency of soda lime absorption varies inversely with its hardness; therefore, little silicate is used in contemporary soda lime. Sodium hydroxide is the catalyst for the carbon dioxide absorptive properties of soda lime.[107,108] Baralyme is a mixture of approximately 20% barium hydroxide and 80% calcium hydroxide. It may also contain some potassium hydroxide. Baralyme is the primary carbon dioxide absorbent implicated as an agent that may produce fires in the breathing system when used with sevoflurane. Calcium hydroxide lime is one of the newest clinically available carbon dioxide absorbents. It consists primarily of calcium hydroxide and calcium chloride and contains two setting agents: calcium sulfate and polyvinylpyrrolidine. The latter two agents serve to enhance the hardness and porosity of the agent.[109] The most significant advantage of calcium hydroxide lime over other agents is its lack of the strong bases sodium and potassium hydroxide. Absence of these chemicals eliminates the undesirable production of CO and the nephrotoxic substance known as compound A, and it may reduce or eliminate the possibility of a fire in the breathing circuit.[110] The most significant disadvantages of calcium hydroxide lime are (1) less absorptive capacity—about 50% less than absorbents containing strong bases—and (2) generally higher cost per unit than other absorbents.[111,112]

The size of the actual absorptive granules has been determined over time by trial and error. The current particle sizes represent a compromise between resistance to airflow and absorptive efficiency.[113] The smaller the granule size, the greater the surface area that is available for absorption. However, as particle size decreases, airflow resistance increases. The granular size of soda lime and Baralyme used in clinical practice is between 4 and 8 mesh, a size at which absorptive surface area and resistance to flow are optimized. Mesh size refers to the number of openings per linear inch in a sieve through which the granular particles can pass. A 4-mesh screen means that there are four quarter-inch openings per linear inch. Likewise, an 8-mesh screen has eight per linear inch.[107]

Absorption of carbon dioxide by absorbents such as soda lime occurs via a series of chemical reactions; it is not a physical process like water soaking into a sponge. Carbon dioxide combines with water to form carbonic acid. Carbonic acid reacts with the hydroxides to form sodium (or potassium) carbonate and water. Calcium hydroxide accepts the carbonate to form calcium carbonate and sodium (or potassium) hydroxide. The equations are as follows:

1. $CO_2 + H_2O \rightleftharpoons H_2CO_3$
2. $H_2CO_3 + 2NaOH\ (KOH) \rightleftharpoons Na_2CO_3\ (K_2CO_3) + 2H_2O +$ Heat
3. $Na_2CO_3\ (K_2CO_3) + Ca(OH)_2 \rightleftharpoons CaCO_3 + 2NaOH\ (KOH)$

Some carbon dioxide may react directly with $Ca(OH)_2$, but this reaction is much slower.

Absorptive Capacity

The maximum amount of carbon dioxide that can be absorbed by soda lime is 26 L of CO_2 per 100 g of absorbent. The absorptive capacity of calcium hydroxide lime is significantly less and has been reported to be 10.2 L per 100 g of absorbent.[109,112] However, as mentioned previously, absorptive capacity is the product of both available chemical reactivity and physical (granule) availability. As the absorbent granules stack up in the absorber canisters, small passageways inevitably form. These small passages channel gases preferentially through low-resistance areas. Because of this phenomenon, the functional absorptive capacity of either soda lime or calcium hydroxide lime may be substantially decreased. In practice, as a result of channeling, the efficiency of soda lime may be reduced such that only 10 to 20 L or less of carbon dioxide can actually be absorbed per 100 g of absorbent.[114]

Indicators

Ethyl violet is the pH indicator added to both soda lime and calcium hydroxide lime to help assess the functional integrity of the absorbent. This compound is a substituted triphenylmethane dye with a critical pH of 10.3.[108] Ethyl violet changes from colorless to violet when the pH of the absorbent decreases as a result of carbon dioxide absorption. When the absorbent is fresh, the pH exceeds the critical pH of the indicator dye, and it exists in its colorless form (Fig. 25-26A). However, as absorbent becomes exhausted, the pH decreases below 10.3, and ethyl violet changes to its violet form (Fig. 25-26B) because of alcohol dehydration. This change in color indicates that the absorptive capacity of the material has been consumed. Unfortunately, in some circumstances ethyl violet may not always be a reliable indicator of the functional status of absorbent. For example, prolonged exposure of ethyl violet to fluorescent light can produce photodeactivation of this dye. When this occurs, the absorbent appears white even though it may have a reduced pH and its absorptive capacity has been exhausted.[115]

Some newer absorbent materials may also include indicators that reveal whether the material has become desiccated. Users should refer to the product manufacturers' literature to determine whether their absorbent material uses this type of indicator.

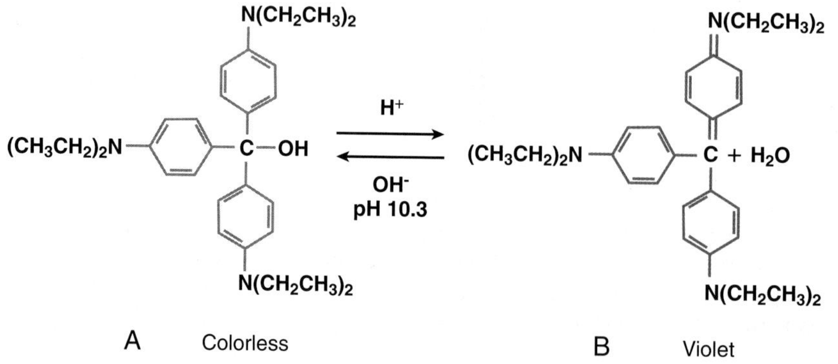

Figure 25-26 **A** and **B**, Ethyl violet. See text for details. *(Reprinted with permission from Andrews JJ, Johnston RV Jr, Bee DE, Arens JF: Photodeactivation of ethyl violet: A potential hazard of Sodasorb. Anesthesiology 72:59, 1990.)*

Interactions of Inhaled Anesthetics with Absorbents

It is important and desirable to have carbon dioxide absorbents that neither release toxic particles or fumes nor produce toxic compounds when exposed to common anesthetics. Soda lime and Baralyme generally fit this description, but inhaled anesthetics do interact with absorbents to some extent. Historically speaking, an uncommon anesthetic, trichloroethylene, reacts with soda lime to produce toxic compounds. In the presence of alkali and heat, trichloroethylene degrades into the cerebral neurotoxin dichloroacetylene, which can cause cranial nerve lesions and encephalitis. Phosgene, a potent pulmonary irritant, is also produced and can cause adult respiratory distress syndrome.[116]

Sevoflurane has been shown to produce degradation products upon interaction with carbon dioxide absorbents.[104,117,118] The major degradation product produced is an olefin compound known as fluoromethyl-2,2-difluoro-1-(trifluoromethyl)vinyl ether, or compound A. During sevoflurane anesthesia, factors apparently leading to an increase in the concentration of compound A include (1) low-flow or closed-circuit anesthetic techniques, (2) use of Baralyme rather than soda lime, (3) higher concentrations of sevoflurane in the anesthetic circuit, (4) higher absorbent temperatures, and (5) fresh absorbent.[117-120] Interestingly, dehydration of Baralyme increases the concentration of compound A, but dehydration of soda lime decreases the concentration of compound A.[121,122] Apparently, the degradation products released during clinical conditions do not commonly result in adverse effects in humans, even during low-flow anesthesia,[119] but further studies are needed to verify this observation.[123-125]

Desiccated strong-base absorbents can also degrade contemporary inhaled anesthetics to clinically significant concentrations of CO, as well as trifluoromethane, which can interfere with monitoring of anesthetic gases.[104] Under certain conditions, this process can produce very high carboxyhemoglobin concentrations that reach 35% or greater.[126] Higher levels of CO are more likely after prolonged contact between absorbent and anesthetics, as well as after disuse of an absorber for at least 2 days, especially over a weekend. Thus, case reports describing CO poisoning have been most common in patients anesthetized on Monday morning, presumably because continuous flow from the anesthesia machine dehydrated the absorbents over the weekend.[127,128] Fresh gas flow rates of 5 L/min or greater through the breathing system and absorbent (without a patient connected) are sufficient to cause critical drying of the absorbent material. The situation is even worse when the breathing bag is left off the breathing circuit. Absence of the reservoir bag facilitates retrograde flow through the circle system (see Fig. 25-7).[126] Because the inspiratory valve leaflet produces some resistance to flow, fresh gas flow takes the retrograde path of least resistance through the absorbent and out the 22-mm breathing bag mount.

Several factors appear to increase the production of CO and resultant elevated carboxyhemoglobin levels, including (1) the inhaled anesthetic used (for a given MAC multiple, the magnitude of CO production from greatest to least is desflurane ≥ enflurane > isoflurane >> halothane = sevoflurane), (2) dryness of the absorbent (completely dry absorbent produces more CO than hydrated absorbent does), (3) the type of absorbent (at a given water content, Baralyme produces more CO than soda lime does), (4) the temperature (increased temperature increases CO production), (5) the anesthetic concentration (more CO is produced with higher anesthetic concentrations),[129] (6) low fresh gas flow rates, and (7) reduced experimental animal (patient) size per 100 g of absorbent.[104,130]

Several interventions have been suggested to reduce the incidence of CO exposure in humans undergoing general anesthesia.[128] Such interventions include (1) educating anesthesia personnel regarding the cause of CO production; (2) turning off the anesthesia machine at the conclusion of the last case of the day to eliminate fresh gas flow, which dries the absorbent; (3) changing the CO absorbent if fresh gas is found to be flowing during the morning machine check; (4) rehydrating desiccated absorbent by adding water to the absorbent[112]; (5) changing the chemical composition of soda lime to reduce or eliminate potassium hydroxide (such products now available include Dragersorb 800 Plus, Sofnolime, and Spherasorb), and (6) using absorbent material that is free of both sodium and potassium hydroxide, such as calcium hydroxide lime. Elimination of sodium and potassium hydroxide from desiccated soda lime diminishes or eliminates degradation of desflurane to CO and sevoflurane to compound A, but it does not compromise carbon dioxide absorption.[110,131]

One extremely rare, but potentially life-threatening complication related to the carbon dioxide absorbent used is the development of fires within the breathing system. Specifically, this can occur as a result of interactions between the strong-base absorbents (particularly Baralyme) and the inhaled anesthetic sevoflurane. In August 2003, Abbott Laboratories changed the package insert for sevoflurane to describe this rare phenomenon and the conditions under which it could occur. Almost 1 year later, in autumn 2004, several case reports describing patient injuries related to this problem were published (all involving Baralyme). It seems that when desiccated strong-base absorbents are exposed to sevoflurane, absorber temperatures of several hundred degrees may result from their interaction.[102] The buildup of very high temperatures, the formation of combustible degradation by-products (formaldehyde, methanol, and formic acid), and the oxygen- or nitrous oxide–enriched environment provide all the substrates necessary for a fire to occur.[104] Avoidance of use of the combination of sevoflurane with strong-base absorbents, particularly Baralyme and especially if it has become desiccated, is the best way to prevent this unusual, potentially life-threatening complication.

Anesthesia Ventilators

The ventilator on the modern anesthesia workstation serves as a mechanized substitute for the hand of the anesthesia care provider in manipulating the reservoir bag of the circle system, the Bain circuit, or another breathing system. As recently as the late 1980s, anesthesia ventilators were mere adjuncts to the anesthesia machine. Today, they have attained a prominent central role in newer anesthesia workstations. In addition to the nearly ubiquitous role of the anesthesia ventilator in today's anesthesia workstation, many advanced intensive care unit (ICU)-style ventilation features have also been integrated into anesthesia ventilators (Fig. 25-27). Anesthesia care providers should be aware that even though more similarities exist between today's anesthesia ventilator and the ICU ventilator than ever before, some fundamental differences in ventilation parameters and control systems still

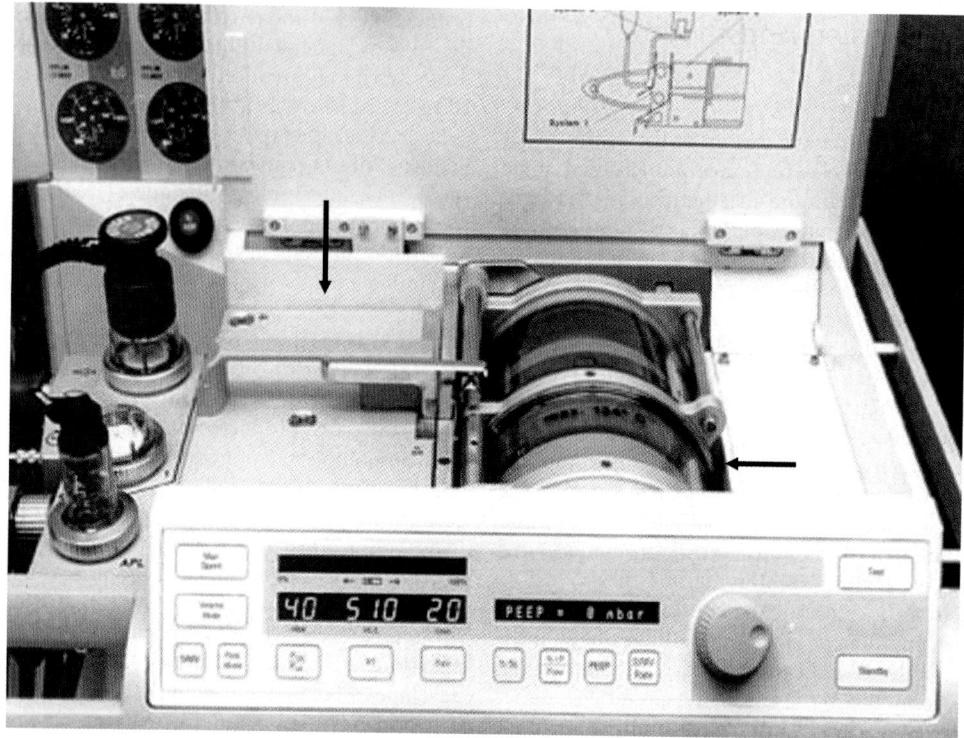

Figure 25-27 The Dräger Medical Narkomed 6000 with its single-circuit ventilator. The *horizontal arrow* indicates the piston cylinder unit of the Divan ventilator. The *vertical arrow* indicates the rectangular valve manifold for fresh gas decoupling.

remain. This discussion focuses on the classification, operating principles, and hazards associated with contemporary anesthesia ventilators.

Classification

Ventilators can be classified according to their power source, drive mechanism, cycling mechanism, and type of bellows.[132,133] The following sections review ventilator classification and terminology before the discussion of specific anesthesia workstation ventilators.

Power Source

The power source required to operate a mechanical ventilator is provided by compressed gas, electricity, or both. Older pneumatic ventilators required only a pneumatic power source to function properly. Contemporary electronic ventilators from Dräger Medical, Datex-Ohmeda, and others require either an electrical-only or both an electrical and a pneumatic power source.

Drive Mechanism and Circuit Designation

Double-circuit ventilators are most commonly used on modern anesthesia workstations. Generally, these conventional ventilators are pneumatically driven. In a double-circuit ventilator, a driving force such as pressurized gas compresses a component analogous to the reservoir bag known as the ventilator bellows. The bellows then in turn delivers ventilation to the patient. The driving gas in the Datex-Ohmeda 7000, 7810, 7100, and 7900 is 100% oxygen. In the North American Dräger AV-E and AV-2+, a venturi device mixes oxygen and air. Some newer pneumatic anesthesia workstations enable the user to select whether compressed air or oxygen is used as the driving gas.

In recent years, with the introduction of circle breathing systems that integrate fresh gas decoupling, a resurgence in the use of mechanically driven anesthesia ventilators has occurred. These "piston"-type ventilators use a computer-controlled stepper motor instead of compressed drive gas to actuate gas movement in the breathing system. In these systems, rather than having dual circuits with patient gas in one and drive gas in another, a single patient gas circuit is present. Thus, they are classified as piston-driven single-circuit ventilators. The piston operates much like the plunger of a syringe to deliver the desired tidal volume or airway pressure to the patient. Sophisticated computerized controls are able to provide advanced types of ventilatory support such as synchronized intermittent mandatory ventilation (SIMV), pressure-controlled ventilation (PCV), and pressure-support assisted ventilation, in addition to the conventional control-mode ventilation. Because the patient's mechanical breath is delivered without the use of compressed gas to actuate a bellows, these systems consume dramatically less compressed gas during ventilator operation than traditional pneumatic ventilators do. This improvement in efficiency may have clinical significance when the anesthesia workstation is used in a setting where no pipeline gas supply is available (e.g., remote locations or office-based anesthesia practices).

Cycling Mechanism

Most anesthesia machine ventilators are time cycled and provide ventilator support in the control mode. The inspiratory phase is initiated by a timing device. Older pneumatic ventilators use a fluidic timing device. Contemporary electronic ventilators use a solid-state electronic timing device and are thus classified as time cycled and electronically controlled. More advanced ventilation modes such as SIMV, PCV, and modes that use a pressure-support option may have an adjustable threshold pressure trigger as well. In these modes, pressure sensors provide feedback to the ventilator control system to allow it to determine when to initiate or terminate the respiratory cycle.

Bellows Classification

The direction of bellows movement during the *expiratory phase* determines the bellows classification. Ascending (standing) bellows ascend during the expiratory phase (Fig. 25-28B), whereas descending (hanging) bellows descend during the expiratory phase. Older pneumatic ventilators and some new anesthesia workstations use weighted descending bellows, but most contemporary electronic ventilators have an ascending bellows design. Of the two configurations, the ascending bellows is generally safer. An ascending bellows will not fill if a total disconnection occurs. However, the bellows of a descending bellows ventilator will continue its upward and downward movement despite patient disconnection. The driving gas pushes the bellows upward during the inspiratory phase. During the expiratory phase, room air is entrained into the breathing system at the site of the disconnection because gravity acts on the weighted bellows. The disconnection pressure monitor and the volume monitor may be fooled even if a disconnection is complete (see "Breathing Circuit Problems").[33] Some contemporary anesthesia workstation designs have returned to the descending bellows to integrate fresh gas decoupling (Dräger Medical Julian and Datascope Anestar). An

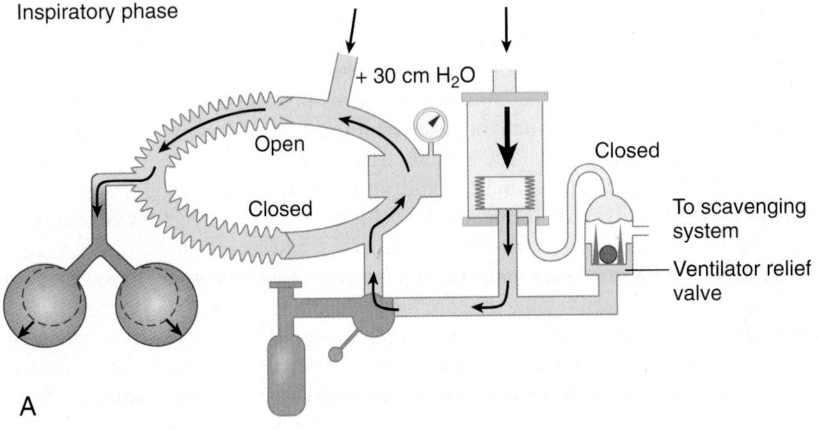

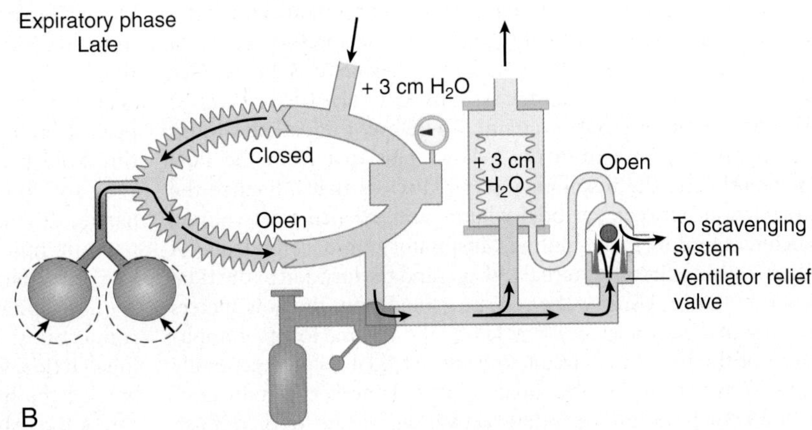

Figures 25-28 Inspiratory (**A**) and expiratory (**B**) phases of gas flow in a traditional circle system with an ascending bellows ventilator. The bellows physically separates the driving gas circuit from the patient gas circuit. The driving gas circuit is located outside the bellows, and the patient gas circuit is inside the bellows. During the inspiratory phase (**A**), the driving gas enters the bellows chamber, which causes the pressure within it to increase. This causes the ventilator relief valve to close, thereby preventing anesthetic gas from escaping into the scavenging system, and the bellows to compress, thereby delivering anesthetic gas within the bellows to the patient's lungs. During the expiratory phase (**B**), pressure within the bellows chamber and the pilot line decreases to zero, which causes the mushroom portion of the ventilator relief valve to open. Gas exhaled by the patient refills the bellows before any scavenging occurs because a weighted ball is incorporated into the base of the ventilator relief valve. Scavenging occurs only during the expiratory phase because the ventilator relief valve is open just during expiration. *(Reprinted with permission from Andrews JJ: The Circle System. A Collection of 30 Color Illustrations. Washington, DC, Library of Congress, 1998.)*

essential safety feature on any anesthesia workstation that uses a descending bellows is an integrated CO_2 apnea alarm that cannot be disabled while the ventilator is in use.

Operating Principles of Ascending Bellows Ventilators

Contemporary examples of ascending bellows, double-circuit, electronic ventilators include the Dräger Medical AV-E and AV-2+ and the Datex-Ohmeda 7000, 7800, and 7900 series. A generic ascending bellows ventilator is illustrated in Figure 25-28. It may be viewed as a breathing bag (bellows) located within a clear plastic box. The bellows physically separates the driving gas circuit from the patient gas circuit. The driving gas circuit is located outside the bellows, and the patient gas circuit is inside the bellows. During the inspiratory phase (see Fig. 25-28A), the driving gas enters the bellows chamber, which causes the pressure within it to increase. This increase in pressure is responsible for two events. First, the ventilator relief valve closes, thereby preventing anesthetic gas from escaping into the scavenging system. Second, the bellows is compressed, and the anesthetic gas within the bellows is delivered to the patient's lungs. This compression action is analogous to the hand of the anesthesiologist squeezing the breathing bag.[48]

During the expiratory phase (see Fig. 25-28B), the driving gas exits the bellows housing. This produces a drop to atmospheric pressure within both the bellows housing and the pilot line to the ventilator relief valve. The decrease in pressure to the ventilator relief valve causes the "mushroom valve" portion of the assembly to open. Exhaled patient gases refill the bellows before any scavenging can begin. The bellows refills first because a weighted ball (like those used in ball-type positive end-expiratory pressure [PEEP] valves) or similar device is incorporated into the base of the ventilator relief valve. Because this ball produces 2 to 3 cm H_2O of backpressure, scavenging occurs only after the bellows fills completely and the pressure inside the bellows exceeds the pressure threshold of the "ball valve." This design causes all ascending bellows ventilators to produce 2 to 3 cm H_2O of PEEP within the breathing circuit when the ventilator is in use. Scavenging occurs just during the expiratory phase because the ventilator relief valve is open only during expiration.[47]

It is important for anesthesia care providers to understand that on most anesthesia workstations, gas flow from the anesthesia machine into the breathing circuit is continuous and independent of ventilator activity. During the inspiratory phase of mechanical ventilation, the ventilator relief valve is closed (see Fig. 25-28A), and the breathing system's APL valve (pop-off valve) is most commonly out of circuit. Therefore, the patient's lungs receive the volume from the bellows plus that from the flow meters during the inspiratory phase. Factors that influence the correlation between set tidal volume and exhaled tidal volume include the flow meter settings, inspiratory time, compliance of the breathing circuit, external leakage, and the location of the tidal volume sensor. Usually, the volume gained from the flow meters during inspiration is counteracted by the volume lost to compliance of the breathing circuit, and the set tidal volume generally approximates the exhaled tidal volume. However, certain conditions such as inappropriate activation of the oxygen flush valve during the inspiratory phase can result in barotrauma or volutrauma (or both) because excess pressure and volume may not be able to be vented from the circle system.[47]

Problems and Hazards

Numerous hazards are associated with anesthesia ventilators, including problems with the breathing circuit, the bellows assembly, and the control assembly.

Traditional Circle System Problems

Breathing circuit misconnections and disconnection are a leading cause of critical incidents in anesthesia.[1,134] The most common disconnection site is at the Y-piece. Disconnections can be complete or partial (leaks). In the past, a common source of leaks with older absorbers was failure to close the APL valve (or pop-off valve) on initiation of mechanical ventilation. On today's anesthesia workstations, the bag/ventilator selector switch has virtually eliminated this problem because the APL valve is usually out of circuit when the ventilator mode is selected. Preexisting undetected leaks can exist in compressed, corrugated, disposable anesthetic circuits. To detect such a leak preoperatively, the circuit must be fully expanded before being checked for leaks.[135] As mentioned previously, disconnections and leaks are manifested more readily with the ascending bellows ventilator systems because they result in a situation in which the bellows will not refill.[33]

Several disconnection monitors exist. The most important monitor is a vigilant anesthesia care provider monitoring breath sounds and chest wall excursion in addition to both the mechanical (spirometers and pressure sensors) and physiologic monitors.

Pneumatic and electronic pressure monitors are helpful in diagnosing disconnections. Factors that influence monitor effectiveness include the disconnection site, the location of the pressure sensor, the threshold pressure alarm limit, the inspiratory flow rate, and the resistance of the disconnected breathing circuit.[136,137] Various anesthesia workstations and ventilators have different locations for the airway pressure sensor and different values for the threshold pressure alarm limit. The threshold pressure alarm limit may be preset at the factory or may be adjustable. An audible or visual alarm is actuated if the peak inspiratory pressure of the breathing circuit does not exceed the threshold pressure alarm limit. When an adjustable threshold pressure alarm limit is available, such as on many workstations from Dräger Medical, the operator should set the pressure alarm limit to within 5 cm H_2O of the peak inspiratory pressure. On systems that have an "autoset" feature, when activated, the threshold limit is automatically set at 3 to 5 cm H_2O pressure below the current peak inspiratory pressure. On such systems, failure to reset the threshold pressure alarm limit may result in either an "apnea pressure" or "threshold low" alert. Figure 25-29 illustrates how a partial disconnection (leak) may be unrecognized by the low-pressure monitor if the threshold pressure alarm limit is set too low or the factory preset value is relatively low.

Respiratory volume monitors are useful in detecting disconnections. Volume monitors may sense exhaled tidal volume, inhaled tidal volume, minute volume, or all three. The user should bracket the high and low threshold volumes slightly above and below the exhaled volumes. For example, if the exhaled minute volume of a patient is 10 L/min, reasonable alarm limits would

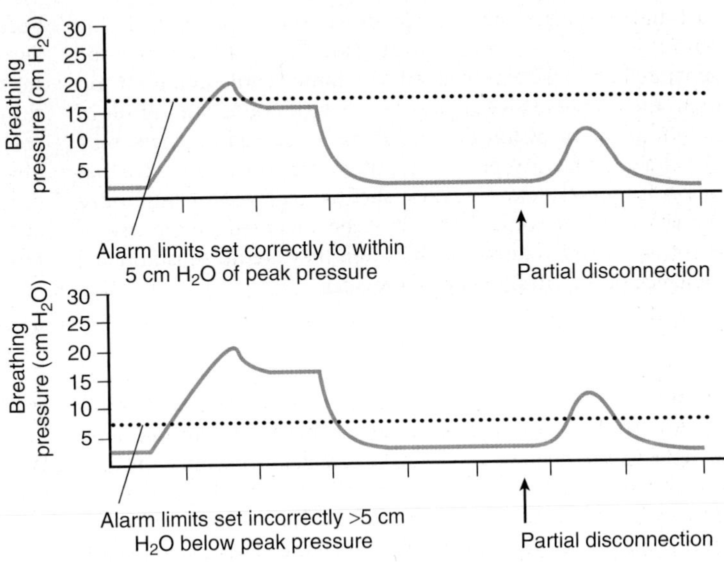

Figure 25-29 Threshold pressure alarm limit. **Top,** The threshold pressure alarm limit (*dotted line*) has been set appropriately. An alarm is actuated when a partial disconnection occurs (*arrow*) because the threshold pressure alarm limit is not exceeded by the breathing circuit pressure. **Bottom,** A partial disconnection is unrecognized by the pressure monitor because the threshold pressure alarm limit has been set too low. *(Redrawn with permission from Baromed Breathing Pressure Monitor. Operator's Instruction Manual. Telford, PA, North American Dräger, August 1986.)*

be 8 to 12 L/min. Many Datex-Ohmeda ventilators are equipped with volume monitor sensors that use infrared light/turbine technology. These volume sensors are usually located in the expiratory limb of the breathing circuit and thus measure exhaled tidal volume. In the case of the Datex-Ohmeda S/5 ADU, a special attachment known as the D-Lite spirometry connector is placed in the breathing circuit. This device is actually placed at or near the level of the patient connection and permits measurement of both inhaled and exhaled volume and pressure (see "Anesthesia Workstation Variations"). With the older infrared-type sensors, exposure to a direct beam of light from the overhead surgical lighting could cause erroneous volume readings if the surgical beam interferes with the infrared sensor.[138] Other types of expiratory volume sensors can be seen in systems such as the Datex-Ohmeda Aestiva, Aespire, and other workstations that incorporate the 7100 ventilator or 7900 SmartVent. These systems generally use differential pressure transduction technology to determine inhaled and exhaled volume, as well as to measure airway pressure. The Dräger Medical Narkomed 6000 series, 2B, and GS workstations commonly use an ultrasonic flow sensor located on the expiratory limb. Still other systems from Dräger measure exhaled volume with "hot-wire" sensor technology. With this type of sensor, a tiny array of two platinum wires is electrically heated to a high temperature. As gas flows past the heated wires, they tend to be cooled. The amount of energy required to maintain the temperature of the wire is proportional to the volume of gas flowing past it. This system has been associated in at least one report with accidental development of a fire in the breathing circuit.[103]

Carbon dioxide monitors are probably the best devices for revealing patient disconnections. The carbon dioxide concentration is measured near the Y-piece either directly (mainstream) or by aspiration of a gas sample to the instrument (sidestream). Either a sudden change in the difference between inspiratory and end-tidal carbon dioxide concentration or the acute absence of measured carbon dioxide indicates a disconnection, a nonventilated patient, or other problems.[33]

Misconnections of the breathing system are unfortunately not uncommon. Despite the efforts of standards committees to eliminate this problem by assigning different diameters to various hoses and hose terminals, they continue to occur. Anesthesia workstations, breathing systems, ventilators, and scavenging systems incorporate many of these diameter-specific connections. The ingenuity of anesthesia care providers in outwitting these "foolproof" systems has led to various hoses being cleverly adapted or forcefully fitted to inappropriate terminals and even to various other solid cylindrically shaped protrusions of the anesthesia machine.[33]

Occlusion (obstruction) of the breathing circuit may occur. Tracheal tubes can become kinked. Hoses throughout the breathing circuit are subject to occlusion by internal obstruction or external mechanical forces that can impinge on flow and have severe consequences. For example, blockage of a bacterial filter in the expiratory limb of the circle system has resulted in bilateral tension pneumothorax.[97] Incorrect insertion of flow direction–sensitive components can result in a no-flow state.[33] Examples of these components include some PEEP valves and cascade humidifiers. Depending on the location of the occlusion relative to the pressure sensor, a high-pressure alarm may alert the anesthesiologist to the problem.

Excess inflow to the breathing circuit from the anesthesia machine during the inspiratory phase can cause barotrauma. The best example of this phenomenon is oxygen flushing. Excess volume cannot be vented from the system during inspiration because the ventilator relief valve is closed and the APL valve is out of circuit.[47] A high-pressure alarm, if present, may be activated when the pressure becomes excessive. With many Dräger Medical systems, both audible and visual alarms are actuated when the high-pressure threshold is exceeded. In the Modulus II Plus System, the Datex-Ohmeda 7810 ventilator automatically switches from the inspiratory to the expiratory phase when the adjustable peak pressure threshold is exceeded.

On workstations equipped with adjustable inspiratory pressure limiters (e.g., the Datex-Ohmeda S/5 ADU and Aestiva and the Dräger Medical Narkomed 6000 series, 2B, 2C, GS, and Fabius GS), maximal inspiratory pressure may be set by the user to a desired peak airway pressure. An adjustable pressure relief valve will open when the predetermined user-selected pressure is reached. This theoretically prevents the generation of excessive airway pressure. Unfortunately, this feature is dependent on the user having preset the appropriate "pop-off" pressure. If the setting is too low, insufficient pressure for ventilation may be generated and result in inadequate minute ventilation; if set too high, the excessive airway pressure may still occur and result in barotrauma. The piston-driven Fabius GS, as well as others, may also include a factory-preset inspiratory pressure safety valve that opens at a preset airway pressure, such as 75 cm H_2O, to minimize the risk of barotrauma. These strategies may reduce the risk of barotrauma and volutrauma; however, they are no substitute for vigilance of the anesthesia care provider.

Bellows Assembly Problems

Leaks can occur in the bellows assembly. Improper seating of the plastic bellows housing can result in inadequate ventilation because a portion of the driving gas is vented to the atmosphere. A hole in the bellows can lead to alveolar hyperinflation and possibly barotrauma in some ventilators because high-pressure driving gas can enter the patient circuit. The oxygen concentration of the patient gas may increase when the driving gas is 100% oxygen, or it may decrease if the driving gas is composed of an air-oxygen mixture.[139]

The ventilator relief valve can cause problems. Hypoventilation occurs if the valve is incompetent because anesthetic gas is delivered to the scavenging system during the inspiratory phase instead of to the patient. Gas molecules preferentially exit into the scavenging system because it represents the path of least resistance, and the pressure within the scavenging system can be subatmospheric. Ventilator relief valve incompetency can result from a disconnected pilot line, a ruptured valve, or a damaged flapper valve.[140,141] A ventilator relief valve stuck in the closed or partially closed position can produce either barotrauma or undesired PEEP.[142] Excessive suction from the scavenging system can draw the ventilator relief valve to its seat and close the valve during both the inspiratory and expiratory phases.[33] In this case, breathing circuit pressure escalates because the excess anesthetic gas cannot be vented. It is worthwhile to note that during the expiratory phase, some newer machines from Datex-Ohmeda (S/5 ADU, 7100 and 7900 SmartVent) scavenge both excess patient gas and the exhausted ventilator drive gas. That is, when the ventilator relief valve opens and waste anesthetic gases are vented from the breathing circuit, the drive gas from the bellows housing joins with it to enter the scavenging system. Under certain conditions, the large volume of exhaust gases could overwhelm the scavenging system and result in pollution of the operating room with waste anesthetic gases (see "Scavenging Systems"). Other mechanical problems that can occur include leaks within the system, faulty pressure regulators, and faulty valves. Unlikely problems such as an occluded muffler on the Dräger AV-E ventilator can result in barotrauma. In this case, obstruction of driving gas outflow closes the ventilator relief valve, and excess patient gas cannot be vented.[143]

Control Assembly and Power Supply Problems

The control assembly can be the source of both electrical and mechanical problems. Electrical failure can be total or partial; the former is the more obvious. As anesthesia workstations are becoming more dependent on integrated computer-controlled systems, power interruptions become more significant. Battery backup systems are designed to continue operation of essential electronics during brief outages (up to several hours). However, even with these systems, in the event of a failure some time may be required for "rebooting" after an electrical outage has occurred. During this time the availability of certain workstation features such as manual or mechanical ventilation can be variable. One cluster of electrical failures that could have potentially resulted in operating room fires was reported early after release of the Dräger Medical Narkomed 6000. Problems with the workstation's power supply printed circuit boards prompted a corrective recall action in November 2002.[144]

Anesthesia Workstation Variations

With the introduction of new technology often comes the need for adaptation of current technology to successfully allow its integration into existing systems. Otherwise, a more comprehensive redesign of an entire anesthesia system from the ground up could be necessary. One such example of adaptation in the anesthesia workstation can be seen with two new design variations of the circle breathing system. The first of these is found on the Datex-Ohmeda S/5 ADU (see Fig. 25-1), and the second is incorporated into the Dräger Narkomed 6000 series (see Fig. 25-2) and Fabius GS workstations. Because use of the circle system is fundamental to day-to-day practice for most anesthesiologists, a comprehensive understanding of these new systems is crucial for their safe use.

The Datex-Ohmeda S/5 ADU

The Datex-Ohmeda S/5 ADU (see Fig. 25-1) debuted as the AS/3 ADU in 1998. Along with its more comprehensive safety features and integrated design that eliminated glass flow tubes and conventional anesthesia vaporizers in exchange for a computer screen with digital fresh gas flow scales and the built-in Aladin Cassette vaporizer system, the machine had a radically different appearance in general. It is not until closer inspection that the other unique properties of the ADU begin to stand out. The principal difference in the ADU's circle system lies in incorporation of the specialized "D-lite" flow and pressure transducer fitting into the circle at the level of the Y-connector. On most traditional circle systems, exhaled tidal volume is measured by a spirometry sensor located in proximity to the expiratory valve. Placement of the D-lite fitting at the Y-connector provides a better location for measuring exhaled volume, allows monitoring of airway gas composition and pressure to be done with a single adapter instead of with multiple fittings added to the breathing circuit, and provides the ability to assess both inspiratory and expiratory gas flow and therefore the generation of complete flow-volume spirometry. Relocation of the spirometer sensor to the Y-connector also makes it possible to move the location of the fresh gas inlet to the "patient" side of the inspiratory valve without adversely affecting the accuracy of exhaled tidal volume measurement.

This atypical circle system arrangement with the fresh gas entering on the patient side of the inspiratory valve is advantageous for several reasons. It is likely to be more efficient in delivering fresh gas to the patient while preferentially eliminating exhaled gases. Importantly, it is also less likely to cause desiccation of the carbon dioxide absorbent (see "Interactions of Inhaled

Anesthetics with Absorbents"). Other notable changes on the S/5 ADU circle system include a compact proprietary carbon dioxide absorbent canister design that can be changed during ventilation without loss of circle system integrity, as well as relocation of the inspiratory and expiratory unidirectional valves from a horizontal position to a vertical position on the "compact block" assembly just below the absorbent canister. Reorientation of the unidirectional valves reduces the breathing circuit resistance encountered by a spontaneously ventilated patient. The vertically oriented unidirectional valves only have to be tipped away from the vertical position to be opened, unlike conventional horizontal valve disks, which have to be physically lifted off the valve seat against gravity to be opened.

The Dräger Medical Narkomed 6000 Series and Fabius GS

Several important differences exist between the traditional circle breathing systems of the newest Dräger products. At first glance, the most notable difference lies in the appearance and design of the ventilators used with these systems. From the inconspicuous horizontally mounted Divan piston ventilator of the Narkomed 6000 series (see Fig. 25-2) to the vertically mounted and visible piston ventilator of the Fabius GS with its absent flow tubes and glowing electronic fresh gas flow indicators, these systems appear drastically different from traditional anesthesia systems. The piston ventilator of the Dräger Narkomed 6000 and Fabius GS anesthesia systems may be classified as electrically powered, piston driven, single circuit, electronically controlled with fresh gas decoupling.

The circle breathing systems used by these Dräger workstations incorporate a feature known as *fresh gas decoupling* (FGD). Incorporation of this patient safety–enhancing technology has required a significant redesign of the traditional circle system. A functional schematic of a circle system similar to the one used by the Dräger Narkomed 6000 series during both the inspiratory and expiratory phases of mechanical ventilation can be seen in Figure 25-30A and B. To understand the operating principles of FGD, it is important to have a good understanding of gas flow in a traditional circle system during both the inspiratory and expiratory phases of mechanical ventilation. A complete discussion of this subject was presented earlier in the section "Operating Principals of Ascending Bellows Ventilators."

The key concept of the FGD breathing system can be illustrated during the inspiratory phase of mechanical ventilation. With the traditional circle system, several events are occurring (see Fig. 25-28A): (1) continuous fresh gas flow from the flow meters or the oxygen flush valve, or from both, is entering the circle system at the fresh gas inlet; (2) the ventilator is delivering the prescribed tidal volume to the patient's lungs; and (3) the ventilator relief valve (ventilator exhaust valve) is closed, so no gas is escaping the circle system except into the patient's lungs.[145] In a traditional circle system, when these events coincide and fresh gas inflow is coupled directly into the circle system, the total volume delivered to the patient's lungs is the sum of the volume from the ventilator plus the volume of gas that enters the circle via the fresh gas inlet. In contrast, when FGD is used, during the inspiratory phase (see Fig. 25-30A) the fresh gas coming from the anesthesia workstation via the fresh gas inlet is diverted into the reservoir bag by a decoupling valve located between the fresh gas source and the ventilator circuit. The reservoir (breathing) bag serves as an accumulator for fresh gas until the expiratory phase begins. During the expiratory phase (see Fig. 25-30B), the decoupling valve opens to allow the accumulated fresh gas in the reservoir bag to be drawn into the circle system to refill the piston ventilator chamber or descending bellows. Because the ventilator exhaust valve also opens during the expiratory phase, excess fresh gas and exhaled patient gas are allowed to escape to the scavenging system.

Current FGD systems are designed with either piston-type or descending bellows–type ventilators. Because the bellows in either of these types of systems refills under slight negative pressure, the accumulated fresh gas from the reservoir bag can be drawn into the ventilator for delivery to the patient during the next ventilator cycle. As a result of this design requirement, it is unlikely that FGD, as described here, can be used with conventional ascending bellows ventilators, which refill under slight positive pressure.

The most significant advantage of circle systems using FGD is a decreased risk for barotrauma and volutrauma. With a traditional circle system, increases in fresh gas flow from the flow meters or from inappropriate use of the oxygen flush valve may contribute directly to tidal volume, which if excessive, may result in pneumothorax or other injury. Because systems with FGD isolate fresh gas coming into the system from the patient while the ventilator exhaust valve is closed, the risk of barotrauma is greatly reduced.

Possibly the greatest disadvantage of the new anesthesia circle systems that use FGD is the possibility of entraining room air into the patient gas circuit. As discussed previously, in an FGD system the bellows or piston refills under slight negative pressure. If the volume of gas contained in the reservoir bag volume plus the returning volume of gas exhaled from the patient's lungs is inadequate to refill the bellows or piston, negative patient airway pressure could develop. To prevent this problem, a negative pressure relief valve is placed in the breathing system (see Fig. 25-30A and B). If breathing system pressure falls below a preset value, such as −2 cm H_2O, the relief valve opens and ambient air is entrained into the patient gas circuit. If this goes undetected, the entrained atmospheric gases could lead to dilution of either or both the inhaled anesthetic agents and the enriched oxygen mixture (lowering the enriched oxygen concentration toward 21%). If unchecked, this could lead to either intraoperative awareness or hypoxia. High-priority alarms with both audible and visual alerts should notify the user that fresh gas flow is inadequate and room air is being entrained.

Another potential problem with an FGD system such as seen on the Narkomed 6000 series lies in its reliance on the reservoir bag to accumulate the incoming fresh gas. If the reservoir bag is removed during mechanical ventilation or if it has a significant leak from poor fit on the bag mount or a perforation, room air may enter the breathing circuit as the ventilator piston unit refills during the expiratory phase. This may also result in dilution of either or both the inhaled anesthetic agents and the enriched oxygen mixture and potentially result in awareness during anesthesia or hypoxia. Furthermore, this type of a disruption could lead to significant pollution of the operating room with anesthetic gases because fresh gases would be allowed to escape into the atmosphere. Other FGD designs, such as those seen in the Dräger Medical Fabius GS and the soon to be released Apollo

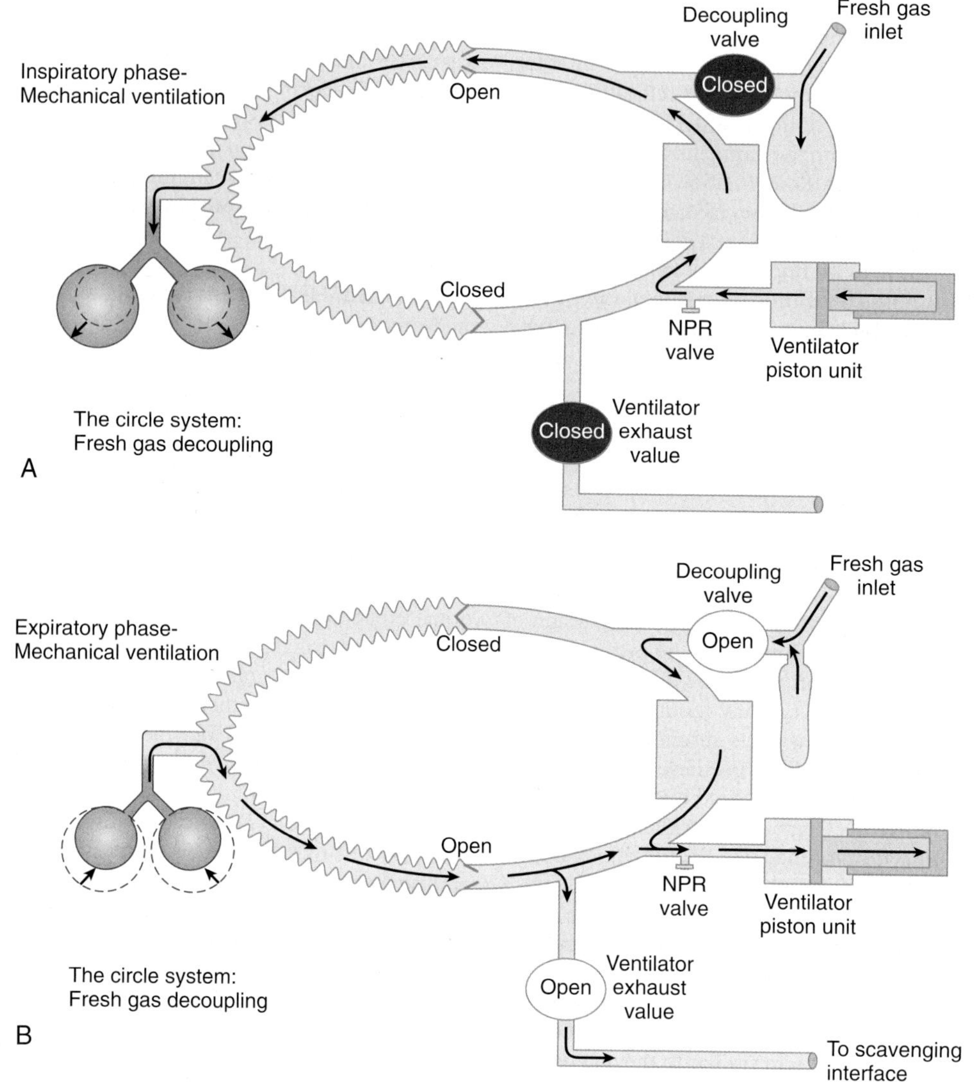

Figures 25-30 A and **B,** Inspiratory- and expiratory-phase gas flows of a Dräger Narkomed 6000 circle system with a piston ventilator and fresh gas decoupling. NPR valve, negative-pressure relief valve. See text for details. *(Reprinted with permission from Andrews JJ: The Circle System. A Collection of 30 Color Illustrations. Washington, DC, Library of Congress, 1998.)*

anesthesia systems, do not use the breathing bag as the fresh gas reservoir but instead have an alternative location for accumulation of fresh gas during the inspiratory phase.

Scavenging Systems

Scavenging is the collection and subsequent removal of waste anesthetic gases from the operating room.[146] In most cases, the amount of gas used to anesthetize a patient for a given anesthetic far exceeds the minimal amount needed. Therefore, scavenging minimizes operating room pollution by removing this excess of gases. In 1977, the National Institute for Occupational Safety and Health (NIOSH) prepared a document titled "Criteria for a Recommended Standard: Occupational Exposure to Waste Anesthetic Gases and Vapors."[147] Although it was maintained that a minimal safe level of exposure could not be defined, the NIOSH proceeded to issue the recommendations shown in Table 25-5.[147] In 1991, ASTM released the ASTM F1343-91 standard titled "Standard Specification for Anesthetic Equipment—Scavenging Systems for Anesthetic Gases."[148] The document provided guidelines for devices that safely and effectively scavenge waste anesthetic gases to reduce contamination in anesthetizing areas.[148] In 1999 the ASA Task Force on Trace Anesthetic Gases developed a booklet titled "Waste Anesthetic Gases: Information for Management in Anesthetizing Areas and the Postanesthesia Care Unit." This publication addresses analysis of the literature, the role of regulatory agencies, scavenging and monitoring equipment, and recommendations.[149]

The two major causes of waste gas contamination in the operating room are the anesthetic technique used and equipment issues.[149,150] Regarding the anesthetic technique, the following factors cause operating room contamination: (1) failure to turn off the gas flow control valves at the end of an anesthetic procedure, (2) poorly fitting masks, (3) flushing the circuit, (4) filling

Table 25-5 NIOSH Recommendations for Trace Gas Levels

Anesthetic Gas	Maximum TWA Concentration (ppm)
Halogenated agent alone	2
Nitrous oxide	25
Combination of halogenated agent plus nitrous oxide	
Halogenated agent	0.5
Nitrous oxide	25
Dental facilities (nitrous oxide alone)	50

Time-weighted average (TWA) sampling, also known as time-integrated sampling, is a sampling method that evaluates the average concentration of anesthetic gas over a prolonged period, such as 1 to 8 hours.
NIOSH, National Institute for Occupational Safety and Health.
Reprinted with permission from US Department of Health, Education, and Welfare: Criteria for a Recommended Standard: Occupational Exposure to Waste Anesthetic Gases and Vapors. Washington DC, US Department of Health, Education, and Welfare, March 1977.

anesthetic vaporizers, (5) use of uncuffed endotracheal tubes, and (6) use of breathing circuits that are difficult to scavenge, such as the Jackson-Rees. Equipment failure or lack of understanding of proper equipment use can also contribute to operating room contamination. Leaks can occur in the high-pressure hoses, the nitrous oxide tank mounting, the high- and low-pressure circuits of the anesthesia machine, or the circle system, particularly at the carbon dioxide absorber assembly. The anesthesia care provider must be certain that the scavenging system is operational and adjusted properly to ensure adequate scavenging. If sidestream carbon dioxide or multigas analyzers are used, the analyzed gas (50 to 250 mL/min) must be directed to the scavenging system or returned to the breathing system to prevent pollution of the operating room.[149,150]

Components

Scavenging systems generally have five components (Fig. 25-31): (1) the gas-collecting assembly, (2) the transfer means, (3) the scavenging interface, (4) the gas disposal assembly tubing, and (5) an active or passive gas disposal assembly.[148] An "active system" uses a central evacuation system to eliminate waste gases. The "weight" or pressure of the waste gas itself produces flow through a "passive system."

Gas-Collecting Assembly

The gas-collecting assembly captures excess anesthetic gas and delivers it to the transfer tubing.[133] Waste anesthetic gases are vented from the anesthesia system either through the adjustable pressure-limiting (APL) valve or through the ventilator relief valve. All excess patient gas is either vented into the room (e.g., from a poor facemask fit or endotracheal tube leak) or exits the breathing system through one of these valves. Gas passing through these valves accumulates in the gas-collecting assembly and is directed to the transfer means. In some newer Datex-Ohmeda systems such as the S/5 ADU and others that incorporate either the 7100 or 7900 ventilators, the ventilator drive gas is also exhausted into the scavenging system. This is significant because under conditions of high fresh gas flow and high minute ventilation, the gases flowing into the scavenging interface may overwhelm the evacuation system. If this occurs, waste anesthetic gases may overflow the system via the positive-pressure relief valve (closed systems) or through the atmospheric vents (open systems) and pollute the operating room. In contrast, most other pneumatic ventilators from both Datex-Ohmeda and Dräger exhaust their drive gas (100% oxygen or oxygen/air mixture) into the operating room through a small vent on the back of the ventilator control housing.

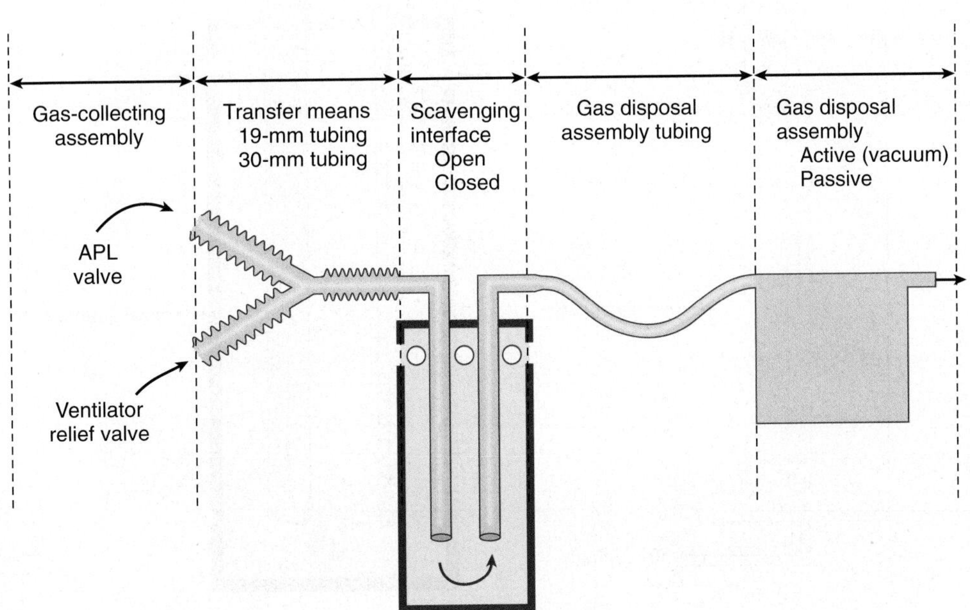

Figure 25-31 Components of a scavenging system. APL valve, adjustable pressure-limiting valve. *(Reproduced with permission from Brockwell RC: Delivery systems for inhaled anesthesia. In Barash PG [ed]: Clinical Anesthesia, 5th ed. Philadelphia, Lippincott Williams & Wilkins, 2006, p 589.)*

Transfer Means

The transfer means carries excess gas from the gas-collecting assembly to the scavenging interface. The tubing must be either 19 or 30 mm, as specified by the ASTM F1343-91 standard.[148] The tubing should be sufficiently rigid to prevent kinking and as short as possible to minimize the chance of occlusion. Some manufacturers color-code the transfer tubing with yellow bands to distinguish it from 22-mm breathing system tubing. Many machines have separate transfer tubes for the APL valve and for the ventilator relief valve. The two tubes frequently merge into a single hose before they enter the scavenging interface. Occlusion of the transfer means can be particularly problematic because it is upstream from the pressure-buffering features of the scavenging interface. If the transfer means is occluded, baseline breathing circuit pressure will increase and barotrauma can occur.

Scavenging Interface

The scavenging interface is the most important component of the system because it protects the breathing circuit or ventilator from excessive positive or negative pressure.[146] The interface should limit the pressure immediately downstream from the gas-collecting assembly to between −0.5 and +10 cm H_2O under normal working conditions.[148] Positive-pressure relief is mandatory, irrespective of the type of disposal system used, to vent excess gas in case of occlusion downstream from the interface. If the disposal system is an "active" system, negative-pressure relief is necessary to protect the breathing circuit or ventilator from excessive subatmospheric pressure. A reservoir is highly desirable with active systems because it stores waste gases until the evacuation system can remove them. Interfaces can be open or closed, depending on the method used to provide positive- and negative-pressure relief.[146]

Open Interfaces An open interface contains no valves and is open to the atmosphere, thereby allowing both positive- and negative-pressure relief. Open interfaces should be used only with active disposal systems that have a central evacuation system. Open interfaces require a reservoir because waste gases are intermittently discharged in surges whereas flow from the evacuation system is continuous.[146]

Many contemporary anesthesia machines are equipped with open interfaces such as those in Figure 25-32A and B.[151] An open canister provides reservoir capacity. The volume of the canister should be large enough to accommodate a variety of waste gas flow rates. Gas enters the system at the top of the canister and travels through a narrow inner tube to the canister base. Gases are stored in the reservoir between breaths. Positive- and negative-pressure relief is provided by holes in the top of the canister. The open interface shown in Figure 25-32A differs somewhat from the one shown in Figure 25-32B. The operator can regulate the vacuum by adjusting the vacuum control valve shown in Figure 25-32B.[151]

The efficiency of an open interface depends on several factors. The vacuum flow rate per minute must equal or exceed the minute volume of excess gases to prevent spillage. The volume of the reservoir and the flow characteristics within the interface are important. Spillage will occur if the volume of a single exhaled breath exceeds the capacity of the reservoir. The flow character-

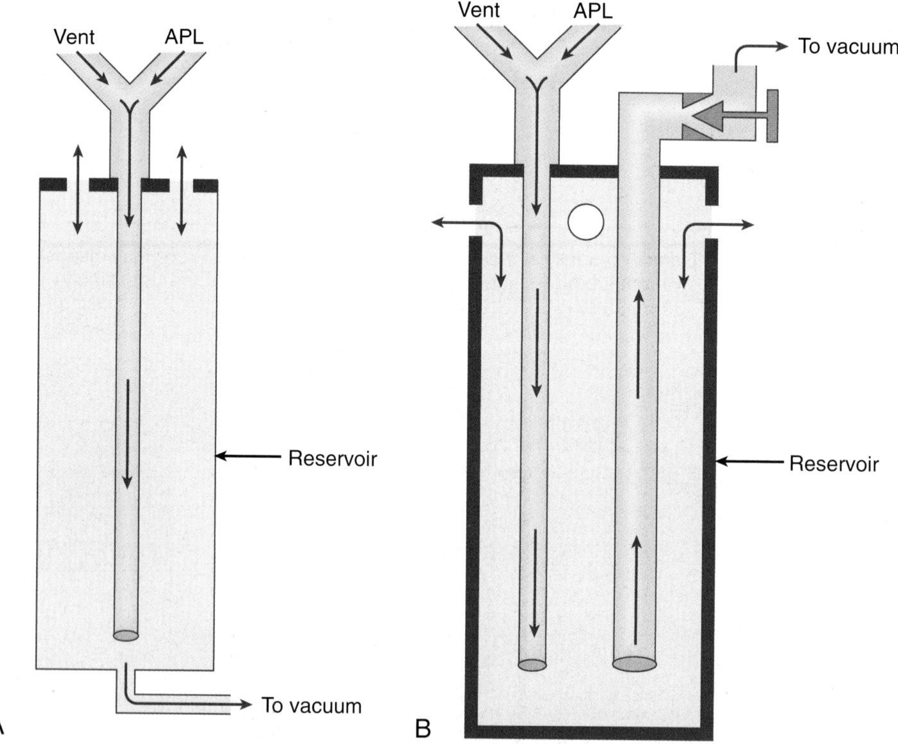

Figure 25-32 **A** and **B,** Two open scavenging interfaces. Each requires an active disposal system. APL, adjustable pressure-limiting valve; Vent, ventilator relief valve. See text for details. *(Modified with permission from Dorsch JA, Dorsch SE: Controlling trace gas levels.* In *Dorsch JA, Dorsch SE* [*eds*]: *Understanding Anesthesia Equipment, 4th ed. Baltimore, Williams & Wilkins, 1999, p 355.)*

istics of the system are important because gas leakage can occur long before the volume of waste gas equals the reservoir volume if significant turbulence occurs within the interface.[152]

Closed Interfaces A closed interface communicates with the atmosphere through valves. All closed interfaces must have a positive-pressure relief valve to vent excess system pressure if obstruction occurs downstream from the interface. A negative-pressure relief valve is mandatory to protect the breathing system from subatmospheric pressure if an active disposal system is used.[146] Two types of closed interfaces are commercially available. One has positive-pressure relief only; the other has both positive- and negative-pressure relief. Each type is discussed in the following paragraphs.

Positive-Pressure Relief Only. This interface (Fig. 25-33, left) has a single positive-pressure relief valve and is designed to be used only with passive disposal systems. Waste gas enters the interface at the waste gas inlets. Transfer of the waste gas from the interface to the disposal system relies on the "weight" or pressure of the waste gas itself because a negative-pressure evacuation system is not used. The positive-pressure relief valve opens at a preset value such as 5 cm H_2O if an obstruction between the interface and the disposal system occurs.[153] On this type of system, a reservoir bag is not required.

Positive- and Negative-Pressure Relief. This interface has a positive-pressure relief valve and at least one negative-pressure relief valve, in addition to a reservoir bag. It is used with active disposal systems. Figure 25-33 (right) is a schematic of Dräger Medical's closed interface for suction systems. A variable volume of waste gas intermittently enters the interface through the waste gas inlets. The reservoir intermittently accumulates excess gas until the evacuation system eliminates it. The operator should adjust the vacuum control valve so that the reservoir bag is properly inflated (A), not overdistended (B) or completely deflated (C). Gas is vented to the atmosphere through the positive-pressure relief valve if the system pressure exceeds +5 cm H_2O. Room air is entrained through the negative-pressure relief valve if the system pressure is more negative than −0.5 cm H_2O. On some systems, a backup negative-pressure relief valve opens at −1.8 cm H_2O if the primary negative-pressure relief valve becomes occluded.

The effectiveness of a closed system in preventing spillage depends on the rate of waste gas inflow, the evacuation flow rate, and the size of the reservoir. Leakage of waste gases into the atmosphere occurs only when the reservoir bag becomes fully inflated and the pressure increases sufficiently to open the positive-pressure relief valve. In contrast, the effectiveness of an open system in preventing spillage depends not only on the volume of the reservoir but also on the flow characteristics within the interface.[152]

Gas Disposal Assembly Conduit The gas disposal assembly conduit (see Fig. 25-31) conducts waste gas from the scavenging interface to the gas disposal assembly. It should be collapse proof and should run overhead, if possible, to minimize the chance of accidental occlusion.[148]

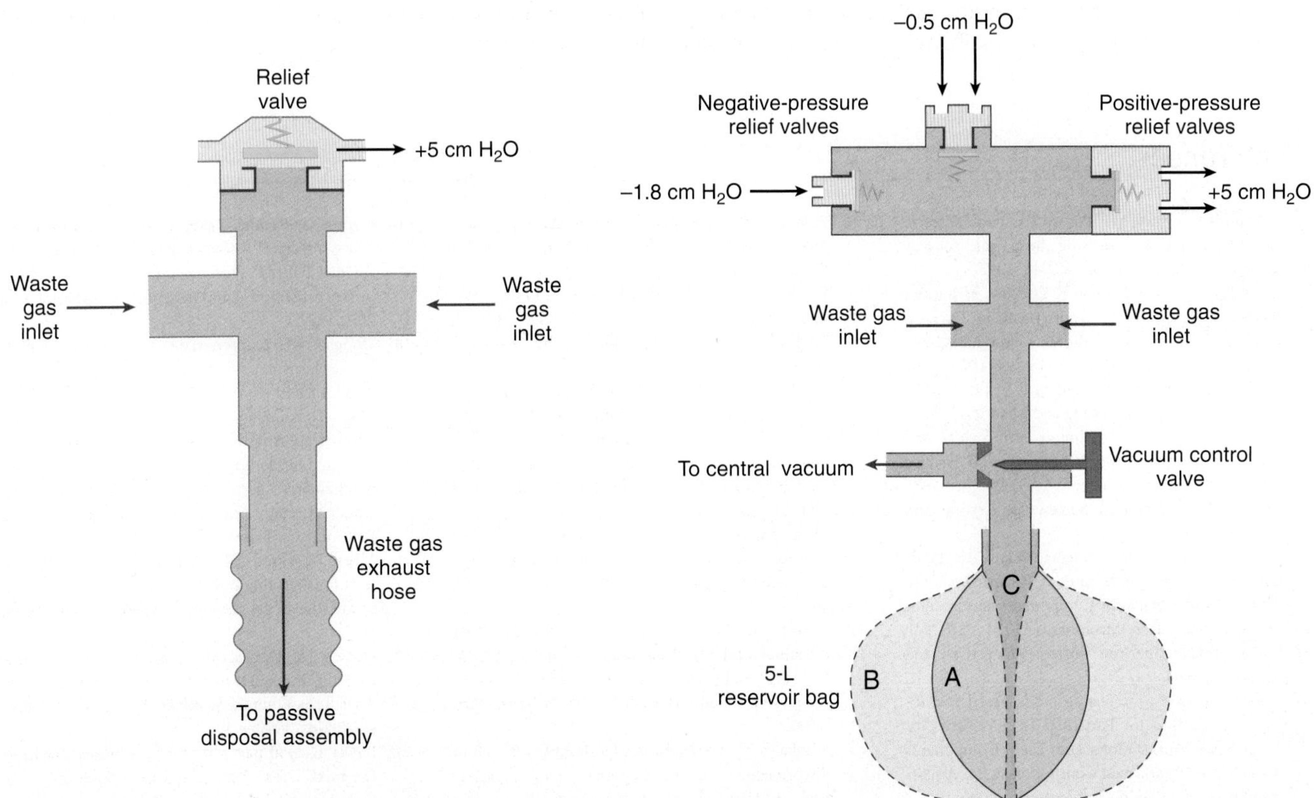

Figure 25-33 Closed scavenging interfaces. **Left,** Interface used with a passive disposal system. **Right,** Interface used with an active system. See text for details. (***Left,*** *Modified with permission from Scavenger Interface for Air Conditioning. Instruction Manual. Telford, PA, North American Dräger, October 1984;* ***right,*** *from Narkomed 2A Anesthesia System. Technical Service Manual. Telford, PA, North American Dräger, 1985.*)

Gas Disposal Assembly The gas disposal assembly ultimately eliminates excess waste gas (see Fig. 25-31). There are two types of disposal systems: active and passive. The most common method of gas disposal is the active assembly, which uses a central evacuation system. A vacuum pump serves as the mechanical flow-inducing device that removes the waste gases, usually to the outside of the building. An interface with a negative-pressure relief valve is mandatory because the pressure within the system is negative. A reservoir is very desirable, and the larger the reservoir, the lower the suction flow rate needed.[146,152]

A passive disposal system does not use a mechanical flow-inducing device. Instead, the "weight" or pressure from the heavier-than-air anesthetic gases produces flow through the system. Positive-pressure relief is mandatory, but negative-pressure relief and a reservoir are unnecessary. Excess waste gases can be eliminated from the operating room suite in a number of ways. Some include venting through the wall, ceiling, or floor or to the room exhaust grill of a non-recirculating air-conditioning system.[146,152]

Hazards

Scavenging systems minimize operating room pollution, yet they add complexity to the anesthesia system. A scavenging system functionally extends the anesthesia circuit all the way from the anesthesia machine to the ultimate disposal site. This extension increases the potential for problems. Obstruction of scavenging pathways can cause excessive positive pressure in the breathing circuit, and barotrauma can occur. Excessive vacuum applied to a scavenging system can result in undesirable negative pressures within the breathing system. Finally, in 2004 another unusual problem that resulted from waste gas scavenging was reported in the *ASA Newsletter* by Lees and coworkers. They reported fires in engineering equipment rooms that house the vacuum pumps used for evacuation of waste anesthetic gases. It seems that in some hospitals, waste gases are not directly vented outside but may be vented into machine rooms that have vents opening to the outside. Because some new anesthesia machines such as the Datex-Ohmeda S/5 ADU and Aestiva, among others, now also scavenge ventilator drive gas (which is 100% oxygen in most cases) in addition to gas from the breathing system, the environments in these machine rooms may become highly enriched with oxygen gas. The result has been the production of fires in these spaces outside the operating room. These sites may contain equipment or materials such as petroleum distillates (pumps/oil/grease) that in the presence of an oxygen-enriched atmosphere could be excessively combustible and a severe fire hazard.[154]

Summary

Rapid advances in technology within the anesthesia workstation industry have made it increasingly difficult for the anesthesia care provider to keep up with latest anesthesia workstation technologies. Nevertheless, a thorough understanding of the anesthesia workstation is mandatory for the safe practice of our specialty. Machines are equipped with dozens of safety features, yet none of them is foolproof. Anesthesia care providers must still check their workstations appropriately before surgery with the correct pre-use checkout procedures to ensure safe delivery of anesthesia for every patient.

References

1. Caplan RA, Vistica MF, Posner KL, et al: Adverse anesthetic outcomes arising from gas delivery equipment. Anesthesiology 87:741, 1997.
2. American National Standards Institute: Minimum Performance and Safety Requirements for Components and Systems of Continuous Flow Anesthesia Machines for Human Use (ANSI Z79.8-1979). New York, American National Standards Institute, 1979.
3. American Society for Testing and Materials: Standard Specification for Minimum Performance and Safety Requirements for Components and Systems of Anesthesia Gas Machines (ASTM F1161-88). Philadelphia, American Society for Testing and Materials, 1988.
4. American Society for Testing and Materials: Standard Specification for Minimum Performance and Safety Requirements for Components and Systems of Anesthetic Gas Machines (ASTM 1161-94). Philadelphia, American Society for Testing and Materials, 1994.
5. American Society for Testing and Materials: Standard Specification for Particular Requirements for Anesthesia Workstations and Their Components (ASTM F1850-00). West Conshohoken, PA, American Society for Testing and Materials, 2000.
6. Cooper JB: Toward prevention of anesthetic mishaps. Int Anesthesiol Clin 22:167, 1984.
7. Spooner RB, Kirby RR: Equipment related anesthetic incidents. Int Anesthesiol Clin 22:133, 1984.
8. Emergency Care Research Institute: Avoiding anesthetic mishaps through pre-use checks. Health Devices 11:201, 1982.
9. Food and Drug Administration: Anesthesia Apparatus Checkout Recommendations, FDA, 8th ed. Rockville, MD, Food and Drug Administration, 1986.
10. Food and Drug Administration: Anesthesia Apparatus Checkout Recommendations. Rockville, MD, Food and Drug Administration, 1993.
11. Lewis SE, Andrews JJ, Long GW: An unexpected Penlon Sigma Elite vaporizer leak. Anesthesiology 90:1221, 1999.
12. Myers JA, Good ML, Andrews JJ: Comparison of tests for detecting leaks in the low-pressure system of anesthesia gas machines. Anesth Analg 84:179, 1997.
13. Dorsch JA, Dorsch SE: Hazards of anesthesia machines and breathing systems. *In* Dorsch JA, Dorsch SE (eds): Understanding Anesthesia Equipment, 4th ed. Baltimore, Williams & Wilkins, 1999, p 399.
14. Yasukawa M, Yasukawa K: Hypoventilation due to disconnection of the vaporizer and negative-pressure leak test to find disconnection. Masui—Jpn J Anesthesiol 41:1345, 1992.
15. Peters KR, Wingard DW: Anesthesia machine leakage due to misaligned vaporizers. Anesth Rev 14:36, 1987.
16. Comm G, Rendell-Baker L: Back pressure check valves a hazard. Anesthesiology 56:227, 1982.
17. Rendell-Baker L: Problems with anesthetic and respiratory therapy equipment. Int Anesthesiol Clin 20:1, 1982.
18. Dodgson BG: Inappropriate use of the oxygen flush to check an anaesthetic machine. Can J Anaesth 35:336, 1988.
19. Mann D, Ananian J, Alston T: Oxygen flush valve booby trap. Anesthesiology 101:558, 2004.
20. Dorsch JA, Dorsch SE: Equipment checking and maintenance. *In* Dorsch JA, Dorsch SE (eds): Understanding Anesthesia Equipment, 4th ed. Baltimore, Williams & Wilkins, 1999, p 937.
21. Myers JA, Good ML, Andrews JJ: Comparison of tests for detecting leaks in the low-pressure system of anesthesia gas machines. Anesth Analg 84:179, 1997.
22. Dorsch JA, Dorsch SE: The anesthesia machine. *In* Dorsch JA, Dorsch SE (eds): Understanding Anesthesia Equipment, 4th ed. Baltimore, Williams & Wilkins, 1999, p 75.
23. Bowie E. Huffman LM: The Anesthesia Machine: Essentials for Understanding. Madison, WI, Ohmeda, BOC Group, Inc, 1985.
24. Cicman JH, Jacoby MI, Skibo VF, et al: Anesthesia systems. Part 1: Operating principles of fundamental components. J Clin Monit 8:295, 1992.

25. Schumacher SD, Brockwell RC, Andrews JJ, et al: Bulk liquid oxygen supply failure. Anesthesiology 100:186, 2004.
26. Feeley TW, Hedley-Whyte J: Bulk oxygen and nitrous oxide delivery systems: Design and dangers. Anesthesiology 44:301, 1976.
27. Pelton DA: Non-flammable medical gas pipeline systems. *In* Wyant GM (ed): Mechanical Misadventures in Anesthesia. Toronto, University of Toronto Press, 1978, p 8.
28. Stassou A: Two Die in Hospital Mix-up. New Haven, CT, WTHN News, 1/16/2002, 11:05 PM. Available at http://www.wtnh.com/Global/story.asp?S=624589. Accessed 11/6/2004.
29. Serlin S: Check your tanks [letter]. Anesth Analg 98:870, 2004.
30. Adriani J: Clinical application of physical principles concerning gases and vapor to anesthesiology. *In* Adriani J (ed): The Chemistry and Physics of Anesthesia, 2nd ed. Springfield, IL, Charles C Thomas, 1962, p 58.
31. Atlas G: A method to quickly estimate remaining time for an oxygen E-cylinder. Anesth Analg 98:1190, 2004.
32. Macintosh R, Mushin WW, Epstein HG: Flowmeters. *In* Macintosh R, Mushin WW, Epstein HG (eds): Physics for the Anaesthetist, 3rd ed. Oxford, Blackwell Scientific, 1963, p 196.
33. Schreiber P: Safety Guidelines for Anesthesia Systems. Telford, PA, North American Dräger, 1984.
34. Eger EI II, Epstein RM: Hazards of anesthetic equipment. Anesthesiology 24:490, 1964.
35. Eger EI II, Hylton RR, Irwin RH, et al: Anesthetic flowmeter sequence—a cause for hypoxia. Anesthesiology 24:396, 1963.
36. Mazze RI: Therapeutic misadventures with oxygen delivery systems. The need for continuous in-line oxygen monitors. Anesth Analg 51:787, 1972.
37. Cheng CJ, Garewal DS: A failure of the chain link mechanism of the Ohmeda Excel 210 anesthetic Machine. Anesth Analg 92:913, 2001.
38. Lohman G: Fault with an Ohmeda Excel 410 machine [letter and response]. Anaesthesia 46:695, 1991.
39. Kidd AG, Hall I: Fault with an Ohmeda Excel 210 anesthetic machine [letter and response]. Anaesthesia 49:83, 1994.
40. Paine GF, Kochan JJ: Failure of the chain link mechanism of the Ohmeda Excel 210 anesthesia machine [letter]. Anesth Analg 94:1374, 2002.
41. Richards C: Failure of a nitrous oxide–oxygen proportioning device. Anesthesiology 71:997, 1989.
42. Abraham ZA, Basagoitia B: A potentially lethal anesthesia machine failure. Anesthesiology 66:589, 1987.
43. Neubarth J: Another hazardous gas supply misconnection [letter]. Anesth Analg 80:206, 1995.
44. Gaughan SD, Benumof JL, Ozaki GT: Can an anesthesia machine flush valve provide for effective jet ventilation? Anesth Analg 76:800, 1993.
45. Anderson CE, Rendell-Baker L: Exposed O_2 flush hazard. Anesthesiology 56:328, 1982.
46. Internal leakage from anesthesia unit flush valves. Health Devices 10:172, 1981.
47. Andrews JJ: Understanding your anesthesia machine and ventilator. *In* 1989 Review Course Lectures. Cleveland, OH, International Anesthesia Research Society, 1989, p 59.
48. Dorsch JA, Dorsch SE; Vaporizers (anesthetic agent delivery devices). *In* Dorsch JA, Dorsch SE (eds): Understanding Anesthesia Machines, 4th ed. Baltimore, Williams & Wilkins, 1999, p 121.
49. Macintosh R, Mushin WW, Epstein HG: Vapor pressure. *In* Macintosh R, Mushin WW, Epstein HG (eds): Physics for the Anaesthetist, 3rd ed. Oxford, Blackwell Scientific, 1963, p 68.
50. Adriani J: Principles of physics and chemistry of solids and fluids applicable to anesthesiology. *In* Adriani J (ed): The Chemistry and Physics of Anesthesia, 2nd ed. Springfield, IL, Charles C Thomas, 1962, p 7.
51. Korman B, Richie IM: Chemistry of halothane-enflurane mixtures applied to anesthesia. Anesthesiology 63:152, 1985.
52. Macintosh R, Mushin WW, Epstein HG: Vaporization. *In* Macintosh R, Mushin WW, Epstein HG (eds): Physics for the Anaesthetist, 3rd ed. Oxford, Blackwell Scientific, 1963, p 26.
53. Schreiber P: Anaesthetic equipment: Performance, Classification, and Safety. New York, Springer-Verlag, 1972.
54. Hill DW, Lowe HJ: Comparison of concentration of halothane in closed and semi-closed circuits during controlled ventilation. Anesthesiology 23:291, 1962.
55. Hill DW: The design and calibration of vaporizers for volatile anaesthesia agents. *In* Scurr C, Feldman S (eds): Scientific Foundations of Anaesthesia, 3rd ed. London, William Heineman, 1982, p 544.
56. Hill DW: The design and calibration of vaporizers for volatile anaesthetic agents. Br J Anaesth 40:648, 1968.
57. Morris LE: Problems in the performance of anesthesia vaporizers. Int Anesthesiol Clin 12:199, 1974.
58. Stoelting RK: The effects of nitrous oxide on halothane output from Fluotec Mark 2 vaporizers. Anesthesiology 35:215, 1971.
59. Diaz PD: The influence of carrier gas on the output of automatic vaporizers. Br J Anaesth 48:387, 1976.
60. Nawaf K, Stoelting RK: Nitrous oxide increases enflurane concentrations delivered by ethrane vaporizers. Anesth Analg 58:30, 1979.
61. Prins L, Strupat J, Clement J: An evaluation of gas density dependence of anaesthetic vaporizers. Can Anaesth Soc J 27:106, 1980.
62. Lin CY: Assessment of vaporizer performance in low-flow and closed-circuit anesthesia. Anesth Analg 59:359, 1980.
63. Gould DB, Lampert BA, MacKrell TN: Effect of nitrous oxide solubility on vaporizer aberrance. Anesth Analg 61:938, 1982.
64. Palayiwa E, Sanderson MH, Hahn CEW: Effects of carrier gas composition on the output of six anaesthetic vaporizers. Br J Anaesth 55:1025, 1983.
65. Scheller MS, Drummond JC: Solubility of N_2O in volatile anesthetics contributes to vaporizer aberrancy when changing carrier gases. Anesth Analg 65:88, 1986.
66. Karis JH, Menzel DB: Inadvertent change of volatile anesthetics in anesthesia machines. Anesth Analg 61:53, 1982.
67. Riegle EV, Desertspring D: Failure of the agent-specific filling device [letter]. Anesthesiology 73:353, 1990.
68. George TM: Failure of keyed agent-specific filling devices. Anesthesiology 61:228, 1984.
69. Broka SM, Gourdange PA, Joucken KL: Sevoflurane and desflurane confusion. Anesth Analg 88:1194, 1999.
70. Lippmann M, Foran W, Ginsburg R, et al: Contamination of anesthetic vaporizer contents. Anesthesiology 78:1175, 1993.
71. Munson WM: Cardiac arrest: A hazard of tipping a vaporizer. Anesthesiology 26:235, 1965.
72. Sinclair A: Vaporizer overfilling. Can J Anaesth 40:77, 1993.
73. Seropian MA, Robins B: Smaller than expected sevoflurane concentrations using the SevoTec 5 vaporizer at low fill states and high fresh gas glows. Anesth Analg 91:834, 2000.
74. Meister GC, Becker KE Jr: Potential fresh gas flow leak through Dräger Vapor 19.1 vaporizer with key-index fill port. Anesthesiology 78:211, 1993.
75. Zimmer C, Janssen M, Treschan T, Peters J: Near-miss accident during magnetic resonance imaging. Anesthesiology 100:1329, 2004.
76. Andrews JJ, Johnston RV Jr: The new Tec 6 desflurane vaporizer. Anesth Analg 76:1338, 1993.
77. Weiskopf RB, Sampson D, Moore MA: The desflurane (Tec 6) vaporizer: Design, design considerations and performance evaluation. Br J Anaesth 72:474, 1994.
78. Eger EI: New inhaled anesthetics. Anesthesiology 80:906, 1994.
79. Susay SR, Smith MA, Lockwood GG: The saturated vapor pressure of desflurane at various temperatures. Anesth Analg 83:864, 1996.
80. Johnston RV Jr, Andrews JJ: The effects of carrier gas composition on the performance of the Tec 6 desflurane vaporizer. Anesth Analg 79:548, 1994.
81. Andrews JJ, Johnston RV Jr, Kramer GC: Consequences of misfilling contemporary vaporizers with desflurane. Can J Anaesth 40:71, 1993.
82. Rupani G: Refilling a Tec 6 desflurane vaporizer [letter]. Anesth Analg 96:1526, 2003.
83. Hendrickx JF, Carette RM, Deloof T, et al: Severe ADU desflurane vaporizing unit malfunction. Anesthesiology 99:1459, 2003.
84. Mapleson WW: The elimination of rebreathing in various semiclosed anaesthetic systems. Br J Anaesth 26:323, 1954.
85. Willis BA, Pender JW, Mapleson WW: Rebreathing in a T-piece: Volunteer and theoretical studies of the Jackson-Rees modification of Ayre's T-piece during spontaneous respiration. Br J Anaesth 47:1239, 1975.
86. Rose DK, Froese AB: The regulation of $Paco_2$ during controlled ventilation of children with a T-piece. Canad Anaesth Soc J 26:104, 1979.
87. Froese AB, Rose DK: A detailed analysis of T-piece systems. *In* Steward DJ (ed): Some Aspects of Paediatric Anaesthesia. Amsterdam, Elsevier North-Holland Biomedical Press, 1982, p 101.
88. Sykes MK: Rebreathing circuits: A review. Br J Anaesth 40:666, 1968.
89. Dorsch JA, Dorsch SE: The breathing system II. The Mapleson systems. *In* Dorsch JA, Dorsch SE (eds): Understanding Anesthesia Equipment, 2nd ed, Baltimore, Williams & Wilkins, 1984, p 182.
90. Bain JA, Spoerel WE: A streamlined anaesthetic system. Can Anaesth Soc J 19:426, 1972.
91. Aarhus D, Holst-Larsen E, Holst-Larsen H: Mechanical obstruction in the anaesthesia delivery-system mimicking severe bronchospasm. Anaesthesia 52:992, 1997.
92. Pethick SL: Letter to the editor. Can Anaesth Soc J 22:115, 1975.
93. Moyers J: A nomenclature for methods of inhalation anesthesia. Anesthesiology 14:609, 1953.
94. Eger EI II: Anesthetic systems: Construction and function. *In* Eger EI II (ed): Anesthetic Uptake and Action. Baltimore, Williams & Wilkins, 1974, p 206.
95. Eger EI II, Ethans CT: The effects of inflow, overflow and valve placement on economy of the circle system. Anesthesiology 29:93, 1968.
96. Smith CR, Otworth JR, Kaluszyk GSW: Bilateral tension pneumothorax due to a defective anesthesia breathing circuit filter. J Clin Anesth 3:229, 1991.

97. McEwan AI, Dowell L, Karis JH: Bilateral tension pneumothorax caused by a blocked bacterial filter in an anesthesia breathing circuit. Anesth Analg 76:440, 1993.
98. Walton JS, Fears R, Burt N, Dorman BH: Intraoperative breathing circuit obstruction caused by albuterol nebulization. Anesth Analg 89:650, 1999.
99. Chacon A, Kuczkowski K, Sanchez R: Unusual case of breathing circuit obstruction: Plastic packaging revisited [letter]. Anesthesiology 100:753, 2004.
100. Dhar P, George I, Sloan P: Flow transducer gas leak detected after induction. Anesth Analg 89:1587, 1999.
101. Kanno T, Aso C, Saito S, et al: A combustive destruction of expiration valve in an anesthetic circuit. Anesthesiology 98:577, 2003.
102. Laster M, Roth P, Eger E II: Fires from the interaction of anesthetics with desiccated absorbent. Anesth Analg 99:769, 2004.
103. Fatheree R, Leighton B: Acute respiratory distress syndrome after an exothermic Baralyme-sevoflurane reaction. Anesthesiology 101:531, 2004.
104. Holak E, Mei D, Dunning M III, et al: Carbon monoxide production from sevoflurane breakdown. Anesth Analg 96:757, 2003.
105. Kshatri AM, Kingsley CP: Defective carbon dioxide absorber as a cause for a leak in a breathing circuit. Anesthesiology 84:475, 1996.
106. Norman PH, Daley MD, Walker JR, et al: Obstruction due to retained carbon dioxide absorber canister wrapping. Anesth Analg 83:425, 1996.
107. Adriani J: Carbon dioxide absorption. *In* Adriani J (ed): The Chemistry and Physics of Anesthesia, 2nd ed. Springfield, IL, Charles C Thomas, 1962, p 151.
108. Dewey & Almy Chemical Division: The Sodasorb Manual of CO_2 Absorption. New York, W. R. Grace and Company, 1962.
109. Murray MM, Renfrew CW, Bedi A, et al: A new carbon dioxide absorbent for use in anesthetic breathing systems. Anesthesiology 91:1342, 1999.
110. Versichelen LF, Bouche MP, Rolly G, et al: Only carbon dioxide absorbents free of both NaOH and KOH do not generate compound-A during in vitro closed system sevoflurane. Anesthesiology 95:750, 2003.
111. Sosis M: Why not use Amsorb alone as the CO_2 absorbent and avoid any risk of CO production [letter]? Anesthesiology 98:1299, 2003.
112. Higuchi H, Adachi Y, Arimura S, et al: The carbon dioxide absorption capacity of Amsorb is half that of soda lime. Anesth Analg 93:221, 2001.
113. Hunt HE: Resistance in respiratory valves and canisters. Anesthesiology 16:190, 1955.
114. Brown ES: Performance of absorbents: Continuous flow. Anesthesiology 20:41, 1959.
115. Andrews JJ, Johnston RV Jr, Bee DE, et al: Photodeactivation of ethyl violet: A potential hazard of Sodasorb. Anesthesiology 72:59, 1990.
116. Case History 39: Accidental use of trichloroethylene (Trilene, Trimar) in a closed system. Anesth Analg 43:740, 1964.
117. Morio M, Fujii K, Satoh N, et al: Reaction of sevoflurane and its degradation products with soda lime. Anesthesiology 77:1155, 1992.
118. Kharasch ED, Powers KM, Artru AA, et al: Comparison of Amsorb, soda lime, Baralyme degradation of volatile anesthetics and formation of carbon monoxide and compound A in swine in vivo. Anesthesiology 96:173, 2002.
119. Frink EJ Jr, Malan TP, Morgan SE, et al: Quantification of the degradation products of sevoflurane in two CO_2 absorbents during low-flow anesthesia in surgical patients. Anesthesiology 77:1064, 1992.
120. Fang ZX, Kandel L, Laster MJ, et al: Factors affecting production of compound-A from the interaction of sevoflurane with Baralyme and soda lime. Anesth Analg 82:775, 1996.
121. Eger EI II, Ion P, Laster MJ et al: Baralyme dehydration increases and soda lime dehydration decreases the concentration of compound A resulting from sevoflurane degradation in a standard anesthetic circuit. Anesth Analg 85:892, 1997.
122. Steffey EP, Laster MJ, Ionescu P, et al: Dehydration of Baralyme increases compound A resulting from sevoflurane degradation in a standard anesthetic circuit used to anesthetize swine. Anesth Analg 85:1382, 1997.
123. Eger EL II, Koblin DD, Bowland T, et al: Nephrotoxicity of sevoflurane versus desflurane anesthesia in volunteers. Anesth Analg 84:160, 1997.
124. Kharasch ED, Frink EJ Jr, Zager R, et al: Assessment of low-flow sevoflurane and isoflurane effects on renal function using sensitive markers of tubular toxicity. Anesthesiology 86:1238, 1997.
125. Bito H, Ikeuchi Y, Ikeda K: Effects of low-flow sevoflurane anesthesia on renal function: Comparison with high-flow sevoflurane anesthesia and low-flow isoflurane anesthesia. Anesthesiology 86:1231, 1997.
126. Berry PD, Sessler DI, Larson MD: Severe carbon monoxide poisoning during desflurane anesthesia. Anesthesiology 90:613, 1999.
127. Baxter PJ, Kharasch ED: Rehydration of desiccated baralyme prevents carbon monoxide formation from desflurane in an anesthesia machine. Anesthesiology 86:1061, 1997.
128. Woehlick HJ, Dunning M, Connolly LA: Reduction in the incidence of carbon monoxide exposures in humans undergoing general anesthesia. Anesthesiology 87:228, 1997.
129. Fang ZX, Eger EI, Laster MJ, et al: Carbon monoxide production from degradation of desflurane, enflurane, isoflurane, halothane, and sevoflurane by soda lime and Baralyme. Anesth Analg 80:1187, 1995.
130. Bonome C, Belda J, Alavarez-Refojo F, et al: Low-flow anesthesia and reduced animal size increase carboxyhemoglobin levels in swine during desflurane and isoflurane breakdown in dried soda lime. Anesth Analg 89:909, 1999.
131. Neumann MA, Laster MJ, Weiskopf RB, et al: The elimination of sodium and potassium hydroxides from desiccated soda lime diminishes degradation of desflurane to carbon monoxide and sevoflurane to compound A but does not compromise carbon dioxide absorption. Anesth Analg 89:768, 1999.
132. Spearman CB, Sanders HG: Physical principles and functional designs of ventilators. *In* Kirby RR, Smith RA, Desautels DA (eds): Mechanical Ventilation. New York, Churchill Livingstone, 1985, p 59.
133. McPherson SP, Spearman CB: Introduction to ventilators. *In* McPherson SP, Spearman CB (eds): Respiratory Therapy Equipment, 3rd ed. St Louis, CV Mosby, 1985, p 230.
134. Cooper JB, Newbower RS, Kitz RJ: An analysis of major errors and equipment failures in anesthesia management. Consideration for prevention and detection. Anesthesiology 60:34, 1984.
135. Reinhart DJ, Friz R: Undetected leak in corrugated circuit tubing in compressed configuration. Anesthesiology 78:218, 1993.
136. Raphael DT, Weller RS, Doran DJ: A response algorithm for the low-pressure alarm condition. Anesth Analg 67:876, 1988.
137. Slee TA, Pavlin EG: Failure of low pressure alarm associated with use of a humidifier. Anesthesiology 69:791, 1988.
138. Sattari R, Reichard PS, Riddle RT: Temporary malfunction of the Ohmeda modulus CD series volume monitor caused by the overhead surgical lighting. Anesthesiology 91:894, 1999.
139. Feeley TW, Bancroft ML: Problems with mechanical ventilators. Int Anesthesiol Clin 20:83, 1982.
140. Khalil SN, Gholston TK, Binderman J: Flapper valve malfunction in an Ohio closed scavenging system. Anaesth Analg 66:1334, 1987.
141. Sommer RM, Bhalla GS, Jackson JM: Hypoventilation caused by ventilator valve rupture. Anesth Analg 67:999, 1988.
142. Bourke D, Tolentino D: Inadvertent positive end-expiratory pressure caused by a malfunctioning ventilator relief valve. Anesth Analg 97:492, 2003.
143. Roth S, Tweedie E, Sommer RM: Excessive airway pressure due to a malfunctioning anesthesia ventilator. Anesthesiology 65:532, 1986.
144. Usher A, Cave D, Finegan B: Critical incident with Narkomed 6000 anesthesia system [letter]. Anesthesiology 99:762, 2003.
145. Dorsch JA, Dorsch SE: Anesthesia ventilators. *In* Dorsch JA, Dorsch SE (eds): Understanding Anesthesia Equipment, 4th ed. Baltimore, Williams & Wilkins, 1999, p 309.
146. Dorsch JA, Dorsch SE: Controlling trace gas levels. *In* Dorsch JA, Dorsch SE (eds): Understanding Anesthesia Equipment, 4th ed. Baltimore, Williams & Wilkins, 1999, p 355.
147. US Department of Health, Education, and Welfare: Criteria for a Recommended Standard: Occupational Exposure to Waste Anesthetic Gases and Vapors. Washington, DC, US Department of Health, Education, and Welfare, March 1977.
148. American Society for Testing and Materials: Standard Specification for Anesthetic Equipment—Scavenging Systems for Anesthetic Gases (ASTM F1343-91). Philadelphia, American Society for Testing and Materials, 1991.
149. McGregor DG (chair): Waste Anesthetic Gases: Information for Management in Anesthetizing Areas and the Postanesthesia Care Unit (PACU). Park Ridge, IL, ASA Task Force on Trace Anesthetic Gases, American Society of Anesthesiologists, 1999, p 3.
150. Kanmura Y, Sakai J, Yoshinaka H, et al: Causes of nitrous oxide contamination in operating rooms. Anesthesiology 90:693, 1999.
151. Open Reservoir Scavenger: Operator's Instruction Manual. Telford, PA, North American Dräger, 1986.
152. Gray WM: Scavenging equipment. Br J Anaesth 57:685, 1985.
153. Scavenger Interface for Air Conditioning: Instruction Manual. Telford, PA, North American Dräger, 1984.
154. Allen M, Lees DE. Fires in medical vacuum pumps: Do you need to be concerned? ASA Newsl 68(10):22, 2004.

Appendix 1

Anesthesia Apparatus Checkout Recommendations, 1993

This checkout, or a reasonable equivalent, should be conducted before administration of anesthesia. These recommendations are valid only for an anesthesia system that conforms to current and relevant standards and includes an ascending bellows ventilator and at least the following monitors: capnograph, pulse oximeter, oxygen analyzer, respiratory volume monitor (spirometer), and breathing system pressure monitor with high- and low-pressure alarms. This is a guideline that users are encouraged to modify to accommodate differences in equipment design and variations in local clinical practice. Such local modifications should undergo appropriate peer review. Users should refer to the operator's manual for the manufacturer's specific procedures and precautions, especially the manufacturer's low-pressure leak test (step 5).

Emergency Ventilation Equipment

*1. **Verify That Backup Ventilation Equipment Is Available and Functioning.**

High-Pressure System

*2. **Check Oxygen Cylinder Supply.**
   a. Open the O_2 cylinder and verify that it is at least half full (≈1000 psi).
   b. Close the cylinder.

*3. **Check Central Pipeline Supplies.**
   a. Check that hoses are connected and pipeline gauges read about 50 psi.

Low-Pressure System

*4. **Check Initial Status of Low-Pressure System.**
   a. Close the flow control valves and turn the vaporizers off.
   b. Check the fill level and tighten the vaporizers' filler caps.

*5. **Perform Leak Check of Machine Low-Pressure System.**
   a. Verify that the machine master switch and flow control valves are OFF.
   b. Attach a "suction bulb" to the common (fresh) gas outlet.
   c. Squeeze the bulb repeatedly until it is fully collapsed.
   d. Verify that the bulb stays *fully* collapsed for at least 10 seconds.
   e. Open one vaporizer at a time and repeat steps c and d as above.
   f. Remove the suction bulb and reconnect the fresh gas hose.

*6. **Turn on Machine Master Switch and All Other Necessary Electrical Equipment.**

*7. **Test Flow Meters.**
   a. Adjust the flow of all gases through their full range while checking for smooth operation of the floats and undamaged flow tubes.
   b. Attempt to create a hypoxic O_2/N_2O mixture and verify correct changes in flow and/or alarm.

Scavenging System

*8. **Adjust and Check Scavenging System.**
   a. Ensure proper connections between the scavenging system and both the APL (pop-off) valve and ventilator relief valve.
   b. Adjust the waste gas vacuum (if possible).
   c. Fully open the APL valve and occlude the Y-piece.
   d. With minimum O_2 flow, allow the scavenger reservoir bag to collapse completely and verify that the absorber pressure gauge reads about zero.
   e. With the O_2 flush activated, allow the scavenger reservoir bag to distend fully and then verify that absorber pressure gauge reads less than 10 cm H_2O.

Breathing System

*9. **Calibrate O_2 Monitor.**
   a. Ensure that the monitor reads 21% in room air.
   b. Verify that the low-O_2 alarm is enabled and functioning.
   c. Reinstall the sensor in the circuit and flush the breathing system with O_2.
   d. Verify that the monitor now reads greater than 90%.

10. **Check Initial Status of Breathing System.**
   a. Set the selector switch to "Bag" mode.
   b. Check that the breathing circuit is complete, undamaged, and unobstructed.
   c. Verify that CO_2 absorbent is adequate.
   d. Install the breathing circuit accessory equipment (e.g., humidifier, positive end-expiratory pressure [PEEP] valve) to be used during the procedure.

11. **Perform Leak Check of Breathing System.**
   a. Set all gas flows to zero (or minimum).
   b. Close the APL (pop-off) valve and occlude the Y-piece.
   c. Pressurize the breathing system to about 30 cm H_2O with an O_2 flush.
   d. Ensure that the pressure remains fixed for at least 10 seconds.
   e. Open the APL (pop-off) valve and ensure that the pressure decreases.

*If an anesthesia provider uses the same machine for successive procedures, these steps need not be repeated or may be abbreviated after the initial checkout.

Manual and Automatic Ventilation Systems

12. Test Ventilation Systems and Unidirectional Valves.
   a. Place a second breathing bag on the Y-piece.
   b. Set the appropriate ventilator parameters for the next patient.
   c. Switch to automatic ventilation (Ventilator) mode.
   d. Turn the ventilator ON and fill the bellows and breathing bag with an O_2 flush.
   e. Set O_2 flow to minimum and other gas flows to zero.
   f. Verify that during inspiration the bellows delivers appropriate tidal volume and that during expiration the bellows fills completely.
   g. Set the fresh gas flow to about 5 L/min.
   h. Verify that the ventilator bellows and simulated lungs fill *and empty* appropriately without sustained pressure at end expiration.
   i. Check for proper action of the unidirectional valves.
   j. Check the breathing circuit accessories to ensure proper function.
   k. Turn the ventilator OFF and switch to manual ventilation (Bag/APL) mode.
   l. Ventilate manually and ensure inflation and deflation of the artificial lungs and appropriate feel of system resistance and compliance.
   m. Remove the second breathing bag from the Y-piece.

Monitors

13. Check, Calibrate, and/or Set Alarm Limits of All Monitors.
   a. Capnometer
   b. Oxygen analyzer
   c. Pressure monitor with high– and low–airway pressure alarms
   d. Pulse oximeter
   e. Respiratory volume monitor (spirometer)

Final Position

14. Check Final Status of Machine.
   a. Vaporizers off
   b. APL valve open
   c. Selector switch to "Bag"
   d. All flowmeters to zero (or minimum)
   e. Patient suction level adequate
   f. Breathing system ready to use

Appendix 2

2007 Guidelines for Preanesthesia Checkout Procedures

Background

Improperly checking anesthesia equipment before use can lead to patient injury and has also been associated with an increased risk for severe postoperative morbidity and mortality.[1,2] In 1993, a preanesthesia checkout (PAC) was developed and widely accepted to be an important step in the process of preparing to deliver anesthesia care.[3] Despite the accepted importance of the PAC, the evidence available suggests that the current version is neither well understood nor reliably used by anesthesia providers.[4-6] Furthermore, anesthesia delivery systems have evolved to the point that one checkout procedure is not applicable to all anesthesia delivery systems currently on the market. For these reasons, a new approach to the PAC has been developed. The goal was to provide guidelines applicable to all anesthesia delivery systems so that individual departments can develop a PAC that can be performed consistently and expeditiously.

General Considerations

The following document is intended to serve not as a PAC itself but rather as a template for developing checkout procedures that are appropriate for each individual anesthesia machine design and practice setting. When using this template to develop a checkout procedure for systems that incorporate automated checkout features, items that are not evaluated by the automated checkout need to be identified and supplemental manual checkout procedures included as needed.

Simply because an automated checkout procedure exists does not mean that it can completely replace a manual checkout procedure or that it can be performed safely without adequate training and thorough understanding of what the automated checkout accomplishes. An automated checkout procedure can be incomplete or misleading, or both. For example, the leak test performed by some current automated checkouts does not test for leaks at the vaporizers. As a result, a loose vaporizer filler cap or a leak at the vaporizer mount could easily be missed.

Ideally, an automated checkout procedure should clearly reveal to the user the functions that are being checked, any deficient function that is found, and recommendations to correct the problem. Documentation of the automated checkout process should preferably be accomplished in a manner that can be recorded on the anesthesia record.

The operator manuals that accompany anesthesia delivery systems include extensive recommendations for checking the equipment out. Although these recommendations are quite extensive and typically not used by anesthesia providers, they are nevertheless important references for developing machine-specific and institution-specific checkout procedures.

Personnel Performing the Preanesthesia Checkout

The previously accepted Anesthesia Apparatus Checkout Recommendation placed all the responsibility for pre-use checkout on the anesthesia provider. This guideline identifies aspects of the PAC that could be completed by a qualified anesthesia or biomedical technician. Using technicians to perform some aspects of the PAC may improve compliance with the PAC. Steps completed by a technician may be part of the morning pre-use check or part of a procedure performed at the end of each day. Critical checkout steps (e.g., availability of backup ventilation equipment) will benefit from intentional redundancy (i.e., having more than one individual responsible for checking the equipment). *Regardless of the level of training and support by technicians, the anesthesia care provider is ultimately responsible for proper function of all equipment used to provide anesthesia care.*

Adaptation of the PAC to local needs, assignment of responsibility for the checkout procedures, and training are the responsibilities of the individual anesthesia department. Training procedures should be documented. Proper documentation should include records of completed coursework (e.g., a manufacturer course) or, for in-house training, a listing of the competency items taught and records of successful completion by trainees.

Objectives for a New Preanesthesia Checkout

- Outline the essential items that need to be available and functioning properly before delivering every anesthetic.
- Identify the frequency with which each of the items needs to be checked.
- Suggest which items may be checked by a qualified anesthesia technician, biomedical technician, or manufacturer-certified service technician.

Basic Principles

- The anesthesia care provider is ultimately responsible for ensuring that the anesthesia equipment is safe and ready for use. This responsibility includes adequate familiarity with the equipment, following relevant local policies for performing and documenting the PAC, and being knowledgeable about these procedures.
- Depending on the staffing resources in a particular institution, anesthesia technicians or biomedical technicians (or both) can participate in the PAC. Biomedical technicians are often trained and certified by manufacturers to perform on-site maintenance of anesthesia delivery systems and can therefore be a useful resource for completing regular checkout procedures. Anesthesia technicians are not commonly trained to perform checkout procedures. Involvement of anesthesia technicians is intended to enhance compliance with the PAC. Each department should decide whether the available technicians can or should be trained to assist with checkout procedures. Formal certification of anesthesia technicians by the American Society of Anesthesia Technicians and Technologists (ASATT) is encouraged but does not necessarily guarantee familiarity with checkout procedures.
- Critical items will benefit from redundant checks to avoid errors and omissions.
- When more than one person is responsible for checking an item, all parties should perform the check if intentional redundancy is deemed important, or either party may be acceptable, depending on the resources available.
- Whoever conducts the PAC should provide documentation of successful performance. The anesthesia provider should include this documentation on the patient chart.
- Whenever an anesthesia machine is moved to a new location, a complete beginning-of-the-day checkout should be performed.
- Automated checks should clearly distinguish the components of the delivery system that are checked automatically from those that require manual checkout.
- Ideally, the date, time, and outcome of the most recent check or checks should be recorded and the information made accessible to the user.
- Specific procedures for pre-use checkout cannot be prescribed in this document because they vary with the delivery systems. Clinicians must learn how to effectively perform the necessary pre-use check for each piece of equipment that they use.
- Each department or health care facility should work with the manufacturer or manufacturers of their equipment to develop pre-use checkout procedures that satisfy both the following guidelines and the needs of the local department.
- Default settings for ventilators, monitors, and alarms should be checked to determine whether they are appropriate.
- These checkout recommendations are intended to replace the preexisting Food and Drug Administration (FDA)-approved Anesthesia Apparatus Checkout Recommendations. They are not intended to be a replacement for required preventive maintenance.
- The PAC is essential for safe care but should not delay initiation of care if patient needs are so urgent that the time taken to complete the PAC could worsen the patient's outcome.

Guidelines for Developing Institution-Specific Checkout Procedures before Anesthesia Delivery

These guidelines describe a basic approach to checkout procedures and rationale to ensure that these priorities are satisfied. They should be used to develop institution-specific checkout procedures designed for the equipment and resources available. (Examples of institution-specific procedures for current anesthesia delivery systems are published at www.ASAHQ.org/clinical/FDA.htm.)

Requirements for Safe Delivery of Anesthesia Care

- Reliable delivery of oxygen at any appropriate concentration up to 100%

- Reliable means of positive-pressure ventilation
- Backup ventilation equipment available and functioning
- Controlled release of positive pressure from the breathing circuit
- Anesthesia vapor delivery (if intended as part of the anesthetic plan)
- Adequate suction
- Means to conform to standards for patient monitoring[7,8]

Specific Items

The following items need to be checked as part of a complete PAC. The intent is to identify what to check, the recommended frequency of checking, and the individual or individuals who could be responsible for the item. For these guidelines, the responsible party would fall into one of four categories: Provider, Technician, Technician or Provider, or Technician and Provider. The designation "Technician and Provider" means that the provider must perform the check regardless of whether it has been completed by a technician. It is not intended to make the use of technician checks mandatory. The intent is not to specify how an item needs to be checked because the specific checkout procedure will depend on the equipment being used.

Item 1: Verify that the auxiliary oxygen cylinder and self-inflating manual ventilation device are available and functioning.

Frequency: Daily.

Responsible Parties: Provider and technician.

Rationale: Failure to be able to ventilate is a major cause of morbidity and mortality related to anesthesia care. Because equipment failure with resulting inability to ventilate the patient can occur at any time, a self-inflating manual ventilation device (e.g., Ambu bag) should be present at every anesthetizing location for every procedure and should be checked for proper function. In addition, a source of oxygen separate from the anesthesia machine and pipeline supply, specifically, an oxygen cylinder with a regulator and a means to open the cylinder valve, should be immediately available and checked. After checking the cylinder pressure, it is recommended that the main cylinder valve be closed to avoid inadvertent emptying of the cylinder through a leaky or open regulator.

Item 2: Verify that patient suction is adequate to clear the airway.

Frequency: Before each use.

Responsible Parties: Provider and technician.

Rationale: Safe anesthetic care requires the immediate availability of suction to clear the airway if needed.

Item 3: Turn on the anesthesia delivery system and confirm that AC power is available.

Frequency: Daily.

Responsible Parties: Provider or technician.

Rationale: Anesthesia delivery systems typically function with backup battery power if AC power fails. Unless the presence of AC power is confirmed, the first obvious sign of power failure can be a complete system shutdown when the batteries can no longer power the system. Many anesthesia delivery systems have visual indicators of the power source showing the presence of both AC and battery power. These indicators should be checked and connection of the power cord to a functional AC power source confirmed.

Desflurane vaporizers require electrical power, and recommendations for checking power to these vaporizers should also be followed.

Item 4: Verify the availability of required monitors and check alarms.

Frequency: Before each use.

Responsible Parties: Provider or technician.

Rationale: Standards for patient monitoring during anesthesia are clearly defined.[7,8] The ability to conform to these standards should be confirmed for every anesthetic. The first step is to visually verify that the appropriate monitoring supplies (blood pressure cuffs, oximetry probes, etc.) are available. All monitors should be turned on and proper completion of power-up self-tests confirmed. Given the importance of pulse oximetry and capnography to patient safety, verifying proper function of these devices before anesthetizing the patient is essential. Capnometer function can be verified by exhaling through the breathing circuit or gas sensor to generate a capnogram or by verifying that the patient's breathing efforts generate a capnogram before the patient is anesthetized. Visual and audible alarm signals should be generated when this is discontinued. Pulse oximeter function, including an audible alarm, can be verified by placing the sensor on a finger and observing for a proper recording. The pulse oximeter alarm can be tested by introducing a motion artifact or removing the sensor.

Audible alarms have also been reconfirmed as essential to patient safety by the American Society of Anesthesiologists (ASA), American Association of Nurse Anesthetists (AANA), Anesthesia Patient Safety Foundation (APSF), and the Joint Commission on Accreditation of Healthcare Organizations (JCAHO). Proper monitor functioning includes visual and audible alarm signals that function as designed.

Item 5: Verify that pressure is adequate in the spare oxygen cylinder mounted on the anesthesia machine.

Frequency: Daily.

Responsible Parties: Provider and technician.

Rationale: Anesthesia delivery systems rely on a supply of oxygen for various machine functions. At a minimum, the oxygen supply is used to provide oxygen to the patient. Pneumatically powered ventilators also rely on a gas supply. The oxygen cylinder or cylinders should be mounted on the anesthesia delivery system and determined to have acceptable minimum pressure. Acceptable pressure depends on the intended use, the design of the anesthesia delivery system, and the availability of piped oxygen.

- Typically, an oxygen cylinder will be used if the central oxygen supply fails.
- If the cylinder is intended to be the primary source of oxygen (e.g., remote-site anesthesia), a cylinder supply sufficient to last for the entire procedure is required. If a pneumatically powered ventilator that uses oxygen as its driving gas will be used, a full "E" oxygen cylinder may provide only 30 minutes of oxygen. In that case, the maximum duration of oxygen supply can be obtained from an oxygen cylinder if it is used to provide only fresh gas to the patient in conjunction with manual or spontaneous ventilation. Mechanical ventilators will consume the oxygen supply if pneumatically powered ventilators

that require oxygen to power the ventilator are used. Electrically powered ventilators do not consume oxygen, so the duration of a cylinder supply will depend only on total fresh gas flow.

- The oxygen cylinder valve should be closed after it has been verified that adequate pressure is present, unless the cylinder is to be the primary source of oxygen (i.e., piped oxygen is not available). If the valve remains open and the pipeline supply should fail, the oxygen cylinder can become depleted while the anesthesia provider is unaware of the oxygen supply problem.
- Other gas supply cylinders (e.g., heliox, CO_2, air, N_2O) need to be checked only if that gas is required to provide anesthetic care.

Item 6: Verify that piped gas pressures are 50 psig or greater.

Frequency: Daily.

Responsible Parties: Provider and technician.

Rationale: A minimum gas supply pressure is required for proper function of the anesthesia delivery system. Gas supplied from a central source can fail for a variety of reasons. Therefore, the pressure in the piped gas supply should be checked at least once daily.

Item 7: Verify that the vaporizers are adequately filled and, if applicable, the filler ports are tightly closed.

Frequency: Before each use.

Responsible Parties: Provider. Technician if redundancy is desired.

Rationale: If delivery of anesthetic vapor is planned, an adequate supply is essential to reduce the risk of light anesthesia or recall, especially if an anesthetic agent monitor with a low-agent alarm is not being used. Partially open filler ports are a common cause of leaks that may not be detected if the vaporizer control dial is not open when a leak test is performed. This source of leakage can be minimized by tightly closing the filler ports. Newer vaporizer designs have filling systems that automatically close the filler port when filling is completed.

High– and low–anesthetic agent alarms are useful to help prevent overdosage or underdosage of anesthetic vapor. Use of these alarms is encouraged, and they should be set to the appropriate limits and enabled.

Item 8: Verify that there are no leaks in the gas supply lines between the flow meters and the common gas outlet.

Frequency: Daily and whenever a vaporizer is changed.

Responsible Parties: Provider or technician.

Rationale: The gas supply in this part of the anesthesia delivery system passes through the anesthetic vaporizer or vaporizers on most anesthesia delivery systems. To perform a thorough leak test, each vaporizer must be turned on individually to check for leaks at the vaporizer mount or inside the vaporizer. Furthermore, some machines have a check valve between the flow meters and the common gas outlet that requires a negative-pressure test to adequately check for leaks. Automated checkout procedures typically include a leak test but may not evaluate leaks at the vaporizer, especially if the vaporizer is not turned on during the leak test. When relying on automated testing to evaluate the system for leaks, the automated leak test would need to be repeated for each vaporizer in place. This test should also be completed whenever a vaporizer is changed. The risk of a leak at the vaporizer depends on the vaporizer design. Vaporizer designs in which the filler port closes automatically after filling can reduce the risk of leaks occurring.

Technicians can provide useful assistance with this aspect of the machine checkout because it can be time consuming.

Item 9: Test for adequate functioning of the scavenging system.

Frequency: Daily.

Responsible Parties: Provider or technician.

Rationale: A properly functioning scavenging system prevents room contamination by anesthetic gases. Proper function depends on correct connections between the scavenging system and the anesthesia delivery system. These connections should be checked daily by a provider or technician. Depending on design of the scavenging system, proper function may also require that the vacuum level be adequate, which should also be confirmed daily. Some scavenging systems have mechanical positive- and negative-pressure relief valves. Positive- and negative-pressure relief is important to protect the patient circuit from pressure fluctuations related to the scavenging system. Proper checkout of the scavenging system should ensure that positive- and negative-pressure relief is functioning properly. Because of the complexity of checking for effective positive- and negative-pressure relief and the variations in scavenging system design, a properly trained technician can facilitate this aspect of the checkout process.

Item 10: Calibrate or verify calibration of the oxygen monitor and check the low-oxygen alarm.

Frequency: Daily.

Responsible Parties: Provider or technician.

Rationale: Continuous monitoring of the inspired oxygen concentration is the last line of defense against delivering hypoxic gas concentrations to the patient. The oxygen monitor is essential for detecting adulteration of the oxygen supply. Most oxygen monitors require calibration once daily, although some are self-calibrating. For self-calibrating oxygen monitors, they should be verified to read 21% when sampling room air. This is a step that is easily completed by a trained technician. When more than one oxygen monitor is present, the primary sensor that will be relied on for oxygen monitoring should be checked.

The low-oxygen concentration alarm should also be checked at this time by setting the alarm above the measured oxygen concentration and confirming that an audible alarm signal is generated.

Item 11: Verify that the carbon dioxide absorbent is not exhausted.

Frequency: Before each use.

Responsible Parties: Provider or technician.

Rationale: Proper function of a circle anesthesia system relies on the absorbent to remove carbon dioxide from rebreathed gas. Exhausted absorbent, as indicated by the characteristic change in color, should be replaced. It is possible for absorbent material to lose the ability to absorb CO_2, yet the characteristic color change may be absent or difficult to see. Some newer absorbents do change color when desiccated. Capnography should be used for every anesthetic, and with use of a circle anesthesia system, rebreathing carbon dioxide as indicated by an inspired CO_2 concentration greater than 0 can also indicate exhausted absorbent (see Note 2).

Item 12: Test for breathing system pressure and leaks.

Frequency: Before each use.

Responsible Parties: Provider and technician.

Rationale: The breathing system pressure and leak test should be performed with the circuit configuration to be used during anesthetic delivery. If any components of the circuit are changed after this test is completed, the test should be performed again. Although the anesthesia provider should perform this test before each use, anesthesia technicians who replace and assemble circuits can also perform this check and add redundancy to this important checkout procedure.

Proper testing will demonstrate that pressure can be developed in the breathing system during both manual and mechanical ventilation and that pressure can be relieved during manual ventilation by opening the adjustable pressure-limiting (APL) valve.

Automated testing is often implemented in the newer anesthesia delivery systems to evaluate the system for leaks and also to determine the compliance of the breathing system. The compliance value determined during this testing will be used to automatically adjust the volume delivered by the ventilator to maintain constant delivery of volume to the patient. It is important that the circuit configuration that is to be used be in place during the test.

Item 13: Verify that gas flows properly through the breathing circuit during both inspiration and exhalation.

Frequency: Before each use.

Responsible Parties: Provider and technician.

Rationale: Pressure and leak testing does not identify all obstructions in the breathing circuit or confirm proper function of the inspiratory and expiratory unidirectional valves. A test lung or second reservoir bag can be used to confirm that flow through the circuit is unimpeded. Complete testing includes both manual and mechanical ventilation. The presence of unidirectional valves can be assessed visually during the PAC; however, proper function of these valves cannot be visually assessed because subtle valve incompetence may not be detected. Checkout procedures to identify valve incompetence that may not be visually obvious can be implemented but are typically too complex for daily testing. A trained technician can perform regular valve competence tests (see Note 4). Capnography should be used during every anesthetic, and the presence of carbon dioxide in the inspired gases can help detect an incompetent valve.

Item 14: Document completion of checkout procedures.

Frequency: Before each use.

Responsible Parties: Provider and technician.

Rationale: Each individual responsible for checkout procedures should document completion of these procedures. Documentation gives credit for completing the job and can be helpful if an adverse event should occur. Some automated checkout systems maintain an audit trail of completed checkout procedures that are dated and timed.

Item 15: Confirm ventilator settings and evaluate readiness to deliver anesthesia care (ANESTHESIA TIME-OUT).

Frequency: Immediately before initiating the anesthetic.

Responsible Parties: Provider.

Rationale: This step is intended to avoid errors resulting from production pressure or other sources of haste. The goal is to confirm that appropriate checks have been completed and that essential equipment is indeed available. The concept is analogous to the "time-out" used to confirm patient identity and the surgical site before incision. Improper ventilator settings can be harmful, especially if a small patient is following a much larger patient or vice versa. Pressure limit settings (when available) should be used to prevent excessive delivery of volume from improper ventilator settings.

Items to check:

- Monitors functional?
- Capnogram present?
- Oxygen saturation by pulse oximetry measured?
- Flow meter and ventilator settings proper?
- Manual/ventilator switch set to manual?
- Vaporizer(s) adequately filled?

Summary of Checkout Recommendations by Frequency and Responsible Party

To Be Completed Daily	**Responsible Party**
Item 1: Verify that the auxiliary oxygen cylinder and self-inflating manual ventilation device are available and functioning	Provider and tech
Item 2: Verify that patient suction is adequate to clear the airway	Provider and tech
Item 3: Turn on the anesthesia delivery system and confirm that AC power is available	Provider or tech
Item 4: Verify the availability of required monitors, including alarms	Provider or tech
Item 5: Verify that pressure is adequate on the spare oxygen cylinder mounted on the anesthesia machine	Provider and tech
Item 6: Verify that piped gas pressures are ≥50 psig	Provider and tech
Item 7: Verify that vaporizers are adequately filled and, if applicable, that filler ports are tightly closed	Provider or tech
Item 8: Verify that there are no leaks in the gas supply lines between the flow meters and the common gas outlet	Provider or tech
Item 9: Test scavenging system function	Provider or tech
Item 10: Calibrate or verify calibration of the oxygen monitor and check the low-oxygen alarm	Provider or tech
Item 11: Verify that the carbon dioxide absorbent is not exhausted	Provider or tech
Item 12: Check for proper breathing system pressure and leaks	Provider and tech
Item 13: Verify that gas flows properly through the breathing circuit during both inspiration and exhalation	Provider and tech

Item 14: Document completion of checkout procedures	Provider and tech
Item 15: Confirm ventilator settings and evaluate readiness to deliver anesthesia care (ANESTHESIA TIME-OUT)	Provider
To Be Completed before Each Procedure	
Item To Be Completed	**Responsible Party**
Item 2: Verify that patient suction is adequate to clear the airway	Provider and tech
Item 4: Verify the availability of required monitors, including alarms	Provider or tech
Item 7: Verify that vaporizers are adequately filled and, if applicable, that filler ports are tightly closed	Provider
Item 11: Verify that the carbon dioxide absorbent is not exhausted	Provider or tech
Item 12: Check for proper breathing system pressure and leaks	Provider and tech
Item 13: Verify that gas flows properly through the breathing circuit during both inspiration and exhalation	Provider and tech
Item 14: Document completion of checkout procedures	Provider and tech
Item 15: Confirm ventilator settings and evaluate readiness to deliver anesthesia care (ANESTHESIA TIME-OUT)	Provider

References

1. Cooper JB, Newbower RS, Kitz RJ: An analysis of major errors and equipment failures in anesthesia management: Considerations for prevention and detection. Anesthesiology 60:34-42, 1984.
2. Arbous MS, Meursing AE, van Kleef JW, de Lange JJ: Impact of anesthesia management characteristics on severe morbidity and mortality. Anesthesiology 102:257-268, 2005.
3. Anesthesia Apparatus Checkout Recommendations, 1993. Available at http://www.fda.gov/cdrh/humfac/anesckot.html.
4. March MG, Crowley JJ: An evaluation of anesthesiologists' present checkout methods and the validity of the FDA checklist. Anesthesiology 75:724-729, 1991.
5. Lampotang S, Moon S, Lizdas DE, et al: Anesthesia machine pre-use check survey—preliminary results [abstract]) Anesthesiology A1195, 2005.
6. Larson ER, Nuttall GA, Ogren BD, et al: A prospective study on anesthesia machine fault identification. Anesth Analg 104:154-156, 2007.
7. American Society of Anesthesiologists: Standards for Basic Anesthetic Monitoring. October 25, 2005. Available at http://www.asahq.org/publicationsAndServices/standards/02.pdf.
8. Scope and standards for nurse anesthesia practice. *In* Professional Practice Manual for the Certified Registered Nurse Anesthetist. Park Ridge, IL, American Association of Nurse Anesthetists, 2006.

Supplement: Additional Notes on Preanesthesia Checkout

Note 1. *Testing the flow meters*: This step is present in the 1993 checkout recommendation and is intended to check the oxygen/nitrous oxide proportioning system. It has been eliminated from the PAC in these guidelines because proper function is verified during preventive maintenance and failures of this system in a properly maintained delivery system are rare.

Note 2. *Desiccated carbon dioxide absorbent*: It has been well established that carbon dioxide absorbents that contain sodium, potassium, or barium hydroxide may become dangerous when desiccated and produce carbon monoxide or excessive heat leading to fires (or both). Unfortunately, it is not possible to reliably identify when the absorbent material has been desiccated. Some departments elect to change all absorbent material on Monday morning to eliminate the possibility of using absorbent exposed to continuous fresh gas flow throughout the weekend. Other departments elect to use absorbent materials that do not pose a risk when desiccated. It is important to have a strategy to prevent hazards related to using absorbents containing the problematic hydroxides that have desiccated. There are no steps that could be included in the checkout recommendation that can reliably identify desiccated absorbent. If a department uses absorbent that may be hazardous when desiccated, it may be prudent to change the absorbent material whenever the duration of exposure to high fresh gas flow cannot be determined and is likely to have been prolonged.

A protocol for preventing absorbent hazards should be part of every department's risk management strategy.

Note 3. *Anesthesia information systems and automated record keepers*: These systems are being adopted by an increasing number of anesthesia departments and are the mainstay of the record-keeping process in these departments. The presence of reliably functioning systems is therefore important to the conduct of anesthesia, though not essential to patient safety in the same fashion as the anesthesia delivery system and patient monitors. For departments that rely on these systems, it would be prudent to have a protocol for checking connections and the proper functioning of associated computers, displays, and network function.

Note 4. *Testing circle system valve competence*: As part of test Item 13 (verify that gas flows properly through the breathing circuit during both inspiration and exhalation), the inspiratory and expiratory valves are visually observed for proper cycling (opening and closing fully). Visual inspection will also detect a missing valve leaflet. Ascertainment of full closure of the valve is subjective. Incompetence of the valve may also be detected during Item 13 by spirometry at the expiratory limb. For malfunction of the expiratory valve, a spirometer with reverse flow detection will signal an alarm when gas flows retrogradely in the expiratory limb. For malfunction of the inspiratory valve, the measured exhaled tidal volume will be less than the expected value. Capnography may also help detect incompetence of the unidirectional valves. Intraoperatively, malfunction of an inspiratory valve may not be indicated by elevation of the inspired CO_2 baseline. If the delivered tidal volume exceeds the volume of gas in the inspiratory limb containing CO_2, rebreathing will appear on the capnogram as a gradual instead of a sharp downstroke. Malfunction of an expiratory valve is indicated by an elevated CO_2 baseline because there is typically a large volume of exhaled gas containing CO_2 that can return to the patient.

J. G. Reves, Peter S. A. Glass, David A. Lubarsky, Matthew D. McEvoy, and Ricardo Martinez-Ruiz

26 Intravenous Anesthetics

Key Points

1. The introduction of thiopental into clinical practice in 1934 marked the advent of modern intravenous (IV) anesthesia. Today, IV anesthetics are used for induction of anesthesia, maintenance of anesthesia, and provision of conscious sedation.
2. The most commonly used IV anesthetic is propofol, an alkylphenol presently formulated in a lipid emulsion. Propofol provides rapid onset and offset with context-sensitive decrement times of approximately 10 minutes when infused for less than 3 hours and less than 40 minutes when infused for up to 8 hours. Its mechanism of action is thought to be potentiation of γ-aminobutyric acid (GABA)–induced chloride currents. At therapeutic doses, propofol produces a moderate depressant effect on ventilation. It causes a dose-dependent decrease in blood pressure primarily through a decrease in cardiac output and systemic vascular resistance. A unique action of propofol is its antiemetic effect, which remains present at concentrations less than those producing sedation. The induction dose is 1 to 2 mg/kg for loss of consciousness with a maintenance infusion of 100 to 200 μg/kg/min. For conscious sedation, rates of 25 to 75 μg/kg/min are usually adequate.
3. Until more recently, the most commonly used IV induction agents were the barbiturates. Thiopental provides rapid onset and offset when used as a single dose, but it accumulates rapidly with prolonged administration and leads to slow recovery. Methohexital has a rapid onset and offset similar to propofol for procedures lasting less than 2 hours. The barbiturates are administered as sodium salts diluted in a water base at an alkaline pH. Similar to propofol, the barbiturates are thought to provide their hypnotic effects largely through action on the $GABA_A$ receptor. Barbiturates provide cerebral protection and are output from induction of anesthesia used primarily for this purpose. They cause a moderate dose-dependent decrease in blood pressure (primarily as a result of peripheral vasodilation) and respiratory drive. The barbiturates are contraindicated in patients with porphyria. The induction dose of thiopental is 4 mg/kg, and the induction dose for methohexital is 2 mg/kg. Methohexital can be used for maintenance of anesthesia at 100 to 200 μg/kg/min or for conscious sedation at 25 to 75 μg/kg/min.
4. The benzodiazepines are used primarily for anxiolysis and amnesia or for conscious sedation. The water-soluble benzodiazepine midazolam is the most frequently used intravenously because of its rapid onset and offset and lack of active metabolites compared with other benzodiazepines (e.g., diazepam). The onset of midazolam is slower than that of propofol and barbiturates, and its offset, especially when used at higher doses or in a prolonged infusion, is considerably longer than that of propofol or methohexital. The benzodiazepines act through the GABA receptor. Flumazenil is a specific benzodiazepine antagonist. It can be used to reverse the effects of benzodiazepines. The benzodiazepines generally produce only a mild decrease in blood pressure and mild-to-moderate respiratory depression. The dose of midazolam for anxiolysis and mild sedation is 0.015 to 0.03 mg/kg intravenously and is generally repeated in 30 to 60 minutes as needed.
5. Ketamine is a phencyclidine derivative that is uniquely different from the above-mentioned hypnotics. It produces a dissociative state of hypnosis and analgesia. It has been used for induction and maintenance of anesthesia. Ketamine acts primarily, but not entirely, through the *N*-methyl-D-aspartate (NMDA) receptor. Ketamine is associated with significant adverse psychological effects at higher doses and several other side effects. It is used now primarily for its analgesic properties. It has rapid onset and relatively rapid offset, even after an infusion of several hours. It has sympathomimetic action that preserves cardiac function. Ketamine has minimal effect on respiration and tends to preserve autonomic reflexes. The induction dose is 2 to 4 mg intravenously. An infusion of ketamine provides analgesia and can be given with propofol in a total IV anesthesia technique. A dose of 10 to 20 mg preoperatively has been shown to provide preemptive analgesia.
6. Etomidate is an imidazole derivative used primarily for induction of anesthesia, especially in elderly patients and

patients who have cardiovascular compromise. It has a rapid onset of effect and a rapid offset even after a continuous infusion. Prolonged infusion results in inhibition of adrenocortical synthesis and potential mortality in intensive care unit (ICU) patients. The major advantage of etomidate is its minimal effect on the cardiovascular and respiratory systems. It is associated with a high incidence of burning on injection, thrombophlebitis, and postoperative nausea and vomiting (PONV), limiting its popularity. The induction dose is 0.2 to 0.3 mg/kg.

7. Dexmedetomidine is the most recently released IV anesthetic. It is a highly selective α_2-adrenergic agonist that produces sedation, hypnosis, and analgesia. Dexmedetomidine is presently approved only for brief (<24 hours) postoperative sedation, although it is finding increasing use in the perioperative period as an adjunct sedative. Its primary action is as an agonist on α_2 receptors in the locus caeruleus. It has minimal effect on respiration. Dexmedetomidine produces a biphasic effect on blood pressure; at low concentrations, mean blood pressure is decreased, and at higher concentrations, blood pressure is increased. Heart rate and cardiac output show a concentration-dependent decrease. Dosing for sedation is a loading dose of 0.25 to 1 mg/kg over a 10-minute period, followed by an infusion of 0.1 to 1 μg/kg/hr.
8. Droperidol, a butyrophenone and major tranquilizer, was initially used to produce a state of neuroleptanesthesia. More recent concern regarding its effect on prolonging the QT interval has resulted in its withdrawal in several countries and its limitation to the treatment of postoperative nausea and vomiting (PONV) with a black box warning in the United States. Because the use of low-dose droperidol (<1.25 mg) for PONV has not been approved by the U.S. Food and Drug Administration (FDA), the black box warning does not relate to this use. Clinically significant prolongation of the QT interval by doses used for PONV (0.625 to 1.25 mg) has been challenged by several editorials, and this effect has not been substantiated by review of the cases reported or any literature. Low-dose droperidol remains an effective antiemetic therapy.

The introduction of thiopental into clinical practice in 1934 marked the advent of modern intravenous (IV) anesthesia. Thiopental and other barbiturates are not ideal IV anesthetics, however, primarily because they provide only hypnosis. The ideal IV anesthetic drug would provide hypnosis, amnesia, analgesia, and muscle relaxation without undesirable cardiac and respiratory depression. Because no single drug is ideal, many newer IV anesthetics, often used together, have been introduced that offer some or all of the desired effects. These drugs were introduced steadily into clinical practice with varying degrees of acceptance. With an increasing number of compounds and superior methods of IV anesthetic drug delivery available (see Chapter 28), the use of IV anesthetics continues to grow.

The future of anesthetic management involves the simultaneous use of several drugs, including inhaled anesthetics. A 1988 survey of mortality in 100,000 cases of anesthesia reveals that the practice of combined anesthetic drug use may be safer than the use of only one or two drugs[1]; the relative odds of dying within 7 days was 2.9 times greater when one or two anesthetic drugs were used than when three or more were used. Although it is exceedingly difficult to interpret these data, the use of several drugs may be beneficial to anesthetic care. The skillful use of multiple IV anesthetics is not only possible, but also preferable. This chapter provides information on the major nonopioid IV anesthetic drugs available for clinical use today.

Propofol

History

Propofol is the most frequently used IV anesthetic today. Work in the early 1970s on substituted derivatives of phenol with hypnotic properties resulted in the development of 2,6-diisopropofol. The first clinical trial, by Kay and Rolly and reported in 1977, confirmed the potential of propofol as an anesthetic to induce anesthesia.[1a] Propofol is insoluble in water and was initially prepared with Cremophor EL (BASF A.G.). Because of anaphylactoid reactions associated with Cremophor EL in this early formulation of propofol, the drug was reformulated in an emulsion. Propofol is used for induction and maintenance of anesthesia and for sedation in and outside the operating room.

Physicochemical Characteristics

Propofol (Fig. 26-1) is one of a group of alkylphenols that have hypnotic properties in animals.[2] The alkylphenols are oils at room temperature and are insoluble in aqueous solution, but they are highly lipid soluble. Numerous formulations are marketed today. The formulation that followed the removal of Cremophor consists of 1% (wt/vol) propofol, 10% soybean oil, 2.25% glycerol, and 1.2% purified egg phosphatide. Following concerns regarding microbial growth in the emulsion, disodium edetate (0.005%) was added as a retardant of bacterial growth. This formulation has a pH of 7 and appears as a slightly viscous, milky white substance. In Europe, a 2% formulation and a formulation in which the emulsion contains a mixture of medium-chain and long-chain triglycerides also are available.

All formulations available commercially are stable at room temperature and are not light sensitive. If a dilute solution of propofol is required, it is compatible with 5% dextrose in water. Changes in the diluent theoretically may result in slight changes in pharmacokinetics, cracking of the emulsion, spontaneous degradation of propofol, and possibly changes in pharmacologic effect. Commercially available formulations of propofol do not have major differences in their clinical utility.

Probably the most interesting formulation likely to be approved soon by the U.S. Food and Drug Administration (FDA) is fospropofol (Aquavan), a phosphorylated prodrug of propofol,

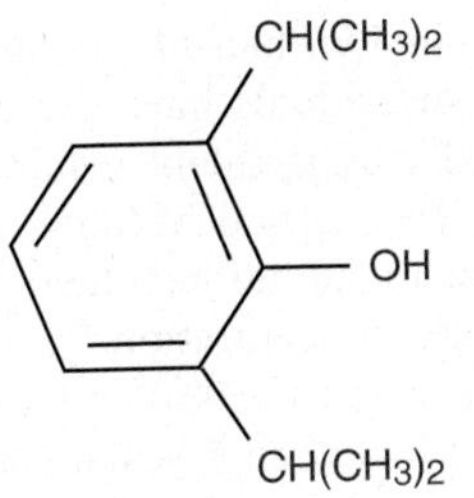

Figure 26-1 Structure of propofol, an alkylphenol derivative.

which produces a unique and distinct pharmacokinetic and pharmacodynamic profile. Compared with propofol emulsion, fospropofol is associated with a slightly longer time to peak effect and a more prolonged pharmacodynamic effect.[3]

Metabolism

Propofol is rapidly metabolized in the liver by conjugation to glucuronide and sulfate[4] to produce water-soluble compounds, which are excreted by the kidneys.[4] Less than 1% propofol is excreted unchanged in urine, and only 2% is excreted in feces.[4] The metabolites of propofol are thought to be inactive. Because clearance of propofol exceeds hepatic blood flow, extrahepatic metabolism or extrarenal elimination has been suggested. Extrahepatic metabolism has been confirmed during the anhepatic phase of patients receiving a transplanted liver.[5] In two more recent studies, the role of the kidneys in propofol metabolism was established, accounting for 30% of total body clearance.[6,7] In in vitro studies with human kidney and small intestine, microsomes in these tissues showed an ability to form propofol glucuronide.[8]

The lungs also may play an important role in this extrahepatic metabolism. The lungs are responsible for approximately 30% of the uptake and first-pass elimination after a bolus dose.[9] During a continuous infusion of propofol, there is a 20% to 30% decrease in propofol concentration measured across the lung in humans and a higher concentration of the metabolite 2,6-diisopropyl 1,4-quinol on the arterial side of the circulation.[10] Other sites of propofol metabolism also are possible. Propofol itself results in a concentration-dependent inhibition of cytochrome P-450 and may alter the metabolism of drugs dependent on this enzyme system (e.g., opiates).[11]

Fospropofol is a prodrug of propofol and is chemically described as phosphono-*O*-methyl-2,6-diisopropylphenol, disodium salt ($C_{13}H_{19}O_5PNa_2$). Phosphono-*O*-methyl prodrugs undergo hydrolysis most notably by endothelial cell surface alkaline phosphatases liberating propofol (the active metabolite), phosphate, and formaldehyde. From the molecular weights of 332.24 D for fospropofol and 178.27 D for propofol, one would expect that 1 mg of fospropofol would liberate 0.54 mg of propofol. When released, propofol undergoes the same metabolic pathway as previously described.[12]

Pharmacokinetics

The pharmacokinetics of propofol has been described by two-compartment and three-compartment models (Table 26-1). After a single bolus injection, whole-blood propofol levels decrease

Table 26-1 Pharmacokinetic Variables for Commonly Used Intravenous Anesthetics

Elimination	Elimination Half-Life (hr)	Clearance (mL/kg/min)	Vd_{ss} (L/kg)
Dexmedetomidine	2-3	10-30	2-3
Diazepam	20-50	0.2-0.5	0.7-1.7
Droperidol	1.7-2.2	14	2
Etomidate	2.9-5.3	18-25	2.5-4.5
Flumazenil	0.7-1.3	5-20	0.6-1.6
Ketamine	2.5-2.8	12-17	3.1
Lorazepam	11-22	0.8-1.8	0.8-1.3
Methohexital	2-6	10-15	1.5-3
Midazolam	1.7-2.6	6.4-11	1.1-1.7
Propofol	4-7	20-30	2-10
Thiopental	7-17	3-4	1.5-3

Vd_{ss}, apparent volume of distribution at steady state.

rapidly as a result of redistribution and elimination (Fig. 26-2). The initial distribution half-life of propofol is 2 to 8 minutes.[4,13] Studies in which the disposition of propofol is described by a three-compartment model give initial and slow distribution half-lives of 1 to 8 minutes and 30 to 70 minutes and an elimination half-life of 4 to 23.5 hours.[14,15] This longer elimination half-life indicates a deep compartment with limited perfusion, which results in a slow return of propofol back to the central compartment. Because of the rapid clearance of propofol from the central compartment, the slow return of propofol from this deep compartment contributes little to the initial rapid decrease in propofol concentrations. The context-sensitive half-time for propofol (Fig. 26-3) for infusions of up to 8 hours is less than 40 minutes.[16]

Because the required decrease in concentration for awakening after anesthesia or sedation with propofol is generally less

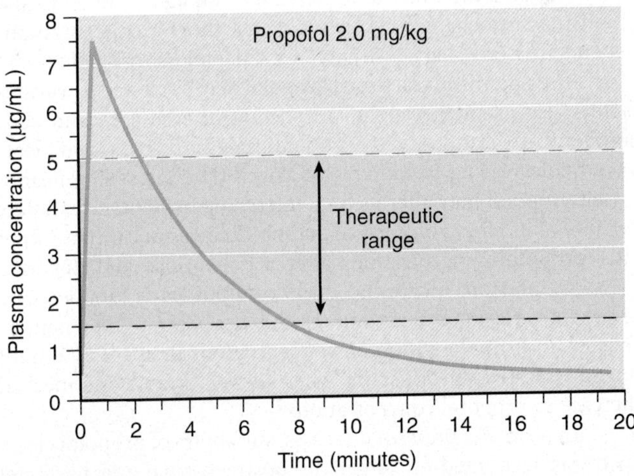

Figure 26-2 Simulated time course of whole blood levels of propofol after an induction dose of 2 mg/kg. Blood levels required for anesthesia during surgery are 2 to 5 µg/mL, with awakening usually occurring at a blood level less than 1.5 µg/mL.

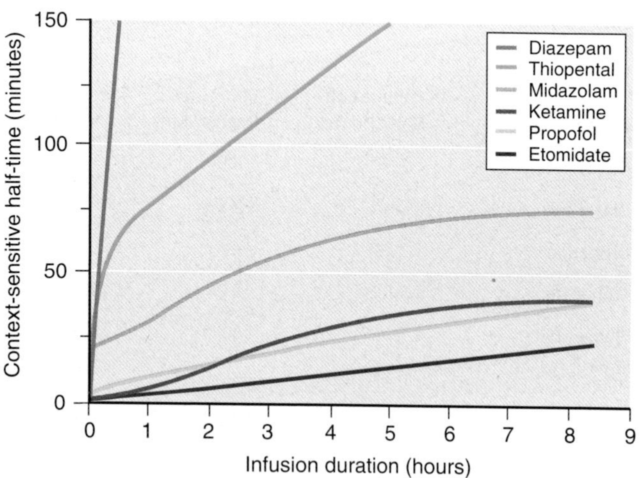

Figure 26-3 The context-sensitive half-times for commonly used IV anesthetic drugs. The context-sensitive half-time is the time for the plasma level of the drug to decrease 50% after cessation of infusion. The duration of infusion is plotted on the horizontal axis. The rapidity with which the drug level decreases is directly related to the time of infusion (i.e., the longer the drug is infused, the longer the half-time). Etomidate, propofol, and ketamine have significantly shorter half-times than thiopental and diazepam, which makes them more suitable for prolonged infusion.

than 50%, recovery from propofol remains rapid even after prolonged infusions. The volume of distribution of the central compartment has been calculated as 20 to 40 L, and the volume of distribution at steady state has been calculated as 150 to 700 L. The clearance of propofol is extremely high—1.5 to 2.2 L/min. As discussed earlier, this exceeds hepatic blood flow, and extrahepatic metabolism has been shown.[5,17]

The equilibrium constant for propofol based on suppression of the electroencephalogram (EEG) (which is strongly correlated with loss of consciousness) is about 0.3 min^{-1}, and the half-life of equilibrium between plasma concentration and EEG effect is 2.5 minutes. The time to peak effect is 90 to 100 seconds.[18] The onset of EEG effect with propofol seems to be independent of age. The onset of decreasing arterial blood pressure is much slower (double the time) and increases with age.[19] For EEG and blood pressure changes, elderly patients show a concentration-dependent increasing sensitivity (see Chapter 71).[19,20]

The pharmacokinetics of propofol may be altered by various factors (e.g., gender, weight, preexisting disease, age, and concomitant medication).[13,21-23] Propofol may impair its own clearance by decreasing hepatic blood flow.[24] Of clinical significance is that propofol may alter its own intercompartmental clearances because of its effects on cardiac output. Changes in cardiac output alter propofol concentrations after a bolus dose and during a constant infusion. Increasing cardiac output leads to a decrease in propofol plasma concentrations and vice versa.[25,26] In a hemorrhagic shock model propofol, concentrations increase 20% until uncompensated shock occurs, when there is a rapid and marked increase in propofol concentrations.[27]

In term and preterm neonates, variability of propofol clearance was accounted for largely by postmenstrual and postnatal age with very fast maturation of clearance in neonatal life. Dosing in these neonates needs to be calculated with extreme care.[28] Women have a larger volume of distribution and higher clearance rates, but the elimination half-life is similar for males and females.[13,22] Elderly individuals have decreased clearance rates, but a smaller central compartment volume.[21,22] During cardiopulmonary bypass, the central volume and initial clearance increase, necessitating higher initial infusion rates to maintain the same propofol plasma concentration.[29] Children have a larger central compartment volume (50%) and a more rapid clearance (25%).[30] In children older than 3 years, volumes and clearances should be weight adjusted.[31] Children younger than 3 years also show weight-proportional pharmacokinetic parameters, but with larger central compartment and systemic clearance values than in adults or older children.[31] This finding explains the larger dosing requirements in this age group (see Chapter 82).[32] Hepatic disease seems to result in a larger steady state and central compartment volumes; clearance is unchanged, but the elimination half-life is slightly prolonged, as is time to recovery.[33]

The effect of fentanyl administration on propofol pharmacokinetic parameters is controversial. Some studies suggest that fentanyl may reduce intercompartmental and total body clearance rates and volumes of distribution.[34] When propofol was administered with alfentanil at similar infusion rates, the measured propofol concentrations were 22% larger than when propofol was administered alone.[35] A separate study found that fentanyl did not alter propofol pharmacokinetics after a single dose of both drugs.[36] Some of these differences in propofol pharmacokinetics when given with an opioid may be explained by studies in cats that showed that pulmonary uptake of propofol is reduced by 30% when propofol is administered immediately after fentanyl, but not if it is administered 3 minutes later.[37] In addition, in vitro studies on human hepatocytes showed that propofol inhibited in a dose-dependent manner the enzymatic degradation of sufentanil and alfentanil.[38] Propofol kinetics is unaltered by renal disease.[23]

The disposition of fospropofol (the parent compound) is best described by a three-compartment model with a relatively small volume of distribution, a fast distribution, and a short terminal half-life of approximately 40 minutes. Fospropofol-delivered propofol has a different pharmacokinetic and pharmacodynamic profile than propofol emulsion, however. Decline of plasma concentrations is slower for fospropofol propofol, and area under the curve values are larger than for a propofol emulsion. Apparent clearance and volume of distribution are much higher in fospropofol propofol than those measured from a propofol emulsion. The peak propofol concentrations from calculated equipotent doses of fospropofol also are higher. Lipid-free formulations of propofol also result in higher peak concentration than equal doses of a lipid emulsion.

Fospropofol also showed a nonlinear relationship between its dose and propofol disposition. Even the propofol maximum concentration was nonlinearly related to dose. Time to maximum concentration of fospropofol was approximately 7 minutes, although at 2 minutes 70% of time to maximum concentration had been reached. Bolus administration of fospropofol achieves loss of response to a verbal command at a similar time and bispectral index (BIS) value as an equipotent amount of propofol emulsion, but shows a longer time to produce a decrease in BIS (almost double) and a more prolonged recovery profile (almost double). Differences in maximum concentration and nonlinearity make simple conversion of dosing from lipid emulsions of propofol to fospropofol difficult.[12,39,40]

Pharmacology

Effects on the Central Nervous System

The hypnotic action of propofol is mostly mediated by enhancing γ-aminobutyric acid (GABA)–induced chloride current through its binding to the β-subunit of $GABA_A$ receptor. Sites on the β_1-subunit (M 286), β_2-subunit (M 286), and β_3-subunit (N265) of the transmembrane domains are crucial for the hypnotic action of propofol.[41,42] The α-subunit and γ_2-subunit subtypes also seem to contribute to modulating the effects of propofol on the GABA receptor.[43] Propofol through its action on $GABA_A$ receptors in the hippocampus inhibits acetylcholine release in the hippocampus and prefrontal cortex.[44] The α_2-adrenoreceptor system also seems to play an indirect role in the sedative effects of propofol.[45] Propofol results in widespread inhibition of the *N*-methyl-D-aspartate (NMDA) subtype of glutamate receptor through modulation of sodium channel gating,[46] an action that also may contribute to the drug's central nervous system (CNS) effects. Studies have shown that propofol has a direct depressant effect on neurons of the spinal cord.[47] In acutely dissociated spinal dorsal horn neurons, propofol acts on $GABA_A$ and glycine receptors.[48] The hypnotic action of propofol is pressure reversible, and it adheres to the correlation exhibited by other general anesthetics between anesthetic potency and octanol/water distribution coefficient.[49] In contrast to barbiturates, propofol is not antianalgesic.

Two notable side effects of propofol are its antiemetic effect and a sense of well-being in patients. Propofol increases dopamine concentrations in the nucleus accumbens (a phenomenon noted with drugs of abuse and pleasure-seeking behavior).[50] Propofol's antiemetic action may be explained by the decrease in serotonin levels it produces in the area postrema, probably through its action on GABA receptors.[51]

The onset of hypnosis after a dose of 2.5 mg/kg is rapid (one arm–brain circulation), with a peak effect seen at 90 to 100 seconds. The median effective dose (ED_{50}) of propofol for loss of consciousness is 1 to 1.5 mg/kg after a bolus. The duration of hypnosis is dose-dependent, being 5 to 10 minutes after 2 to 2.5 mg/kg.[52] Age markedly affects the induction dose, being largest at ages younger than 2 years (ED_{95} 2.88 mg/kg) and decreasing with increasing age.[53] Increasing age decreases the propofol concentration required for loss of consciousness.[54] At subhypnotic doses, propofol provides sedation and amnesia.[55-57] Propofol infusions of at least 2 mg/kg/hr were necessary to provide amnesia in unstimulated volunteers.[58] Awareness during surgery at higher infusion rates has been reported.[59] During surgical procedures, extremely high infusion rates may be necessary to prevent awareness if propofol is used as the sole anesthetic.[54] Propofol also tends to produce a general state of well-being.[60] Hallucinations,[61] sexual fantasies, and opisthotonos[62] have been reported after propofol administration.

The effect of propofol on the EEG as assessed after 2.5 mg/kg followed by an infusion shows an initial increase in alpha rhythm followed by a shift to gamma and theta frequency. High infusion rates produce burst suppression.[63] EEG power analysis indicates that amplitude increases after induction, but is thereafter unaltered at propofol blood concentrations of 3 to 8 μg/mL.[64] At propofol concentrations greater than 8 μg/mL, amplitude markedly decreases, with periods of burst suppression.[64] Propofol causes a concentration-dependent decrease in the BIS, with 50% and 95% of patients unable to respond to a verbal command at a BIS of 63 and 51. The propofol concentration at which 50% of volunteers failed to respond to verbal command was 2.35 μg/mL. Lack of recall was observed in 95% of patients at a BIS value of 77.[65] Propofol produces a decrease in amplitude of the early components of somatosensory evoked potentials,[66] and a small nonsignificant increase in latency of the P_{40} and N_{50} components.[66]

Similar to other IV anesthetics, propofol does not alter brainstem auditory evoked potentials.[67] There are, however, a dose-dependent prolongation of latency and a decrease in amplitude of cortical middle latency auditory potentials, which are concentration-dependent.[67] Propofol effect site concentrations provide similar correlation with decreases in the spectral entropy variable derived from the EEG as it does with BIS, and a similar ability to titrate propofol anesthetic effect.[68] The effect of propofol on epileptogenic EEG activity is controversial. Seizures after propofol administration have been reported, mainly on induction or emergence from anesthesia, rarely during maintenance, and occasionally postoperatively. In various models, a direct anticonvulsant effect of propofol has been shown, which is dose-dependent.[69,70] In a few reports, propofol has been used to treat epileptic seizures.[71] Propofol also results in a shorter duration of motor and EEG seizure activity after electroconvulsive therapy compared with methohexital.[72] Propofol has been associated with grand mal seizures, however, and has been used for cortical mapping of epileptogenic foci.[73,74] There have been a few reports of convulsions after propofol administration that have occurred 6 days after anesthesia. Most of these patients had a history of previous convulsions. The incidence of this adverse effect is rare (1 in 50,000 administrations).

Tolerance to the effects of propofol remains controversial. Repeated dosing to children presenting for radiation therapy showed lack of tolerance for each treatment session,[75] whereas increasingly larger doses were required for repeated electroconvulsive therapy.[76] Of more importance are reports[77] of addiction to propofol. Propofol has been used to treat chronic refractory headache with doses of 20 to 30 mg every 3 to 4 minutes (400 mg maximum).[78]

Propofol decreases intracranial pressure (ICP) in patients with either normal or increased ICP.[79] The decrease in ICP (30% to 50%) is associated with significant decreases in cerebral perfusion pressure (CPP), however. The use of propofol in head-injured patients should be restricted to doses providing mild-to-moderate sedation (i.e., blood concentration of 2 μg/mL, infusion of 25-75 μg/kg/min) (see Chapters 47 and 63).[80] The lesser vasodilatory effects of propofol on the cerebral vasculature compared with volatile anesthetics may provide advantages in certain surgical procedures. Propofol acutely reduces intraocular pressure by 30% to 40%. Compared with thiopental, propofol produces a larger decrease in intraocular pressure and is more effective in preventing an increase in intraocular pressure secondary to succinylcholine and endotracheal intubation (see Chapter 29).[81] Normal cerebral reactivity to carbon dioxide and autoregulation are maintained during a propofol infusion.[82]

The neuroprotective effects of propofol remain controversial. Propofol administered to burst suppression results in significantly better neurologic outcome and less brain tissue injury in an incomplete ischemia model in rats compared with fentanyl.[83] Propofol administered at sedative concentrations started either immediately after or at 1 hour after an ischemic insult significantly reduced infarct size compared with awake controls infused with intralipid.[84] Pretreatment with propofol fails to protect against focal ischemic insult.[85] In a spinal cord injury model, propofol reduced lipid peroxidation without improving ultrastructure at 1 hour after injury compared with thiopental, which reduced both.[86] The neuronal protective effect of propofol may be due to the attenuation of changes in adenosine triphosphate, calcium, sodium, and potassium caused by hypoxic injury[87] and its antioxidant action by inhibiting lipid peroxidation.[88] Current evidence indicates that propofol can protect neurons against ischemic injury caused by excitotoxicity, but neuroprotection may be sustained only if the ischemic insult is relatively mild and is not sustained after a prolonged recovery period.[89] Prolonged propofol sedation in children is associated with adverse neurologic sequelae (see Chapter 82).[90]

Many anesthetic-related drugs decrease the required dose or blood concentrations of propofol's pharmacologic action. The propofol Cp_{50} (blood concentration needed for 50% of subjects to not respond to a defined stimulus) for loss of response to verbal command in the absence of any other drug is 2.3 to 3.5 μg/mL.[54,91,92] The propofol Cp_{50} to prevent movement on skin incision is 16 μg/mL; this is markedly reduced by increasing concentrations of fentanyl or alfentanil.[54,91,92] The propofol Cp_{50} for skin incision when combined with benzodiazepine premedication (lorazepam, 1 to 2 mg) and 66% nitrous oxide is 2.5 μg/mL (venous).[22,92] This concentration is reduced to 1.7 μg/mL when morphine (0.15 mg/kg) rather than lorazepam is used for premedication.[93] The concentration of propofol (when combined with 66% nitrous oxide) required during minor surgery is 1.5 to 4.5 μg/mL,[15,22] and the concentration for major surgery is 2.5 to 6 μg/mL.[54] Awakening usually occurs at concentrations less than 1.6 μg/mL,[15,22,52] and orientation occurs at concentrations less than 1.2 μg/mL[15,22] when the propofol concentration is decreasing. When equilibration between blood and effect site is allowed, however, awakening concentrations (2.2 μg/mL) are much closer to concentrations associated with loss of verbal command.[94]

Effects on the Respiratory System

Apnea occurs after an induction dose of propofol; the incidence and duration of apnea depend on dose, speed of injection, and concomitant premedication. An induction dose of propofol results in a 25% to 30% incidence of apnea.[96] The duration of apnea occurring with propofol may be prolonged to more than 30 seconds, however. The incidence of prolonged apnea (>30 seconds) is increased further by addition of an opiate, either as premedication or just before induction of anesthesia.[96,97] The incidence of apnea with propofol is more frequent than with other commonly used IV induction anesthetics.[96,98] The onset of apnea usually is preceded by marked tidal volume reduction and tachypnea.[97] In volunteers, dose-dependent apnea was more pronounced with propofol emulsion than with fospropofol.[40]

In nearly every clinical setting propofol is used, it is a profound respiratory depressant. A maintenance infusion of propofol (100 μg/kg/min) results in a 40% decrease in tidal volume and a 20% increase in respiratory frequency, with an unpredictable change in minute ventilation.[97] Doubling the infusion rate from 100 to 200 μg/kg/min causes a further moderate decrease in tidal volume (455 to 380 mL), but no change in respiratory frequency.[97] The ventilatory response to carbon dioxide also is decreased during a maintenance infusion of propofol.[97] At 100 μg/kg/min, there is a 58% reduction in the slope of the carbon dioxide-response curve.[97] This is similar to the depression after a brief infusion of 3 mg/kg/min of thiopental. Doubling the infusion rate (and presumably the blood level) of propofol results in only a minimal further decrease in carbon dioxide responsiveness.[97] Propofol, 1.5 to 2.5 mg/kg, results in an acute (13% to 22%) increase in $PaCO_2$ and a decrease in pH. PaO_2 does not change significantly. These changes are similar to the changes seen after an induction dose of thiopental. During a maintenance infusion of propofol (54 μg/kg/min), $PaCO_2$ is moderately increased from 39 to 52 mm Hg. Doubling this infusion rate does not result in a further increase in $PaCO_2$.

Propofol (50 to 120 μg/kg/min) also depresses the ventilatory response to hypoxia, presumably by a direct action on carotid body chemoreceptors.[99] Propofol induces bronchodilation in patients with chronic obstructive pulmonary disease.[100] Propofol attenuates vagal (at low concentrations) and methacholine-induced (at high concentrations) bronchoconstriction,[101] and seems to have a direct action on muscarinic receptors. Propofol inhibits the receptor coupled signal transduction pathway through inositol phosphate generation and inhibition of Ca^{2+} mobilization.[102] The preservative used with propofol seems to be important in its bronchodilator activity. Propofol with metabisulfite (compared with propofol without metabisulfite) does not inhibit vagal or methacholine-induced bronchoconstriction.[103]

Propofol also may have an impact on the pulmonary pathophysiology of adult respiratory distress syndrome. In an animal model of septic endotoxemia, propofol (10 mg/kg/hr) significantly reduced free radical mediated and cyclooxygenase catalyzed lipid peroxidation. In addition, PaO_2 and hemodynamics were maintained closer to baseline.[104] These benefits of propofol have not yet been confirmed in humans. Propofol at therapeutic concentrations also protects mouse macrophages from nitric oxide–induced apoptosis and cell death.[105]

Propofol also attenuates the magnitude of hypoxic pulmonary vasoconstriction.[106] The effect of propofol on pulmonary vasomotor tone inhibits acetylcholine-induced pulmonary vasodilation through nitric oxide and a cytochrome P-450 metabolite (likely endothelium-derived hyperpolarizing factor).[107]

Effects on the Cardiovascular System

The cardiovascular effects of propofol have been evaluated after its use for induction and for maintenance of anesthesia (Table 26-2).[108] The most prominent effect of propofol is a decrease in arterial blood pressure during induction of anesthesia. Independent of the presence of cardiovascular disease, an induction dose of 2 to 2.5 mg/kg produces a 25% to 40% reduction of systolic blood pressure.[108,112,113] Similar changes are seen in mean and diastolic blood pressure. The decrease in arterial pressure is associated with a decrease in cardiac output/cardiac index (±15%),[112,113] stroke volume index (±20%),[113] and systemic vascular resistance (15% to 25%).[112] Left ventricular stroke work index also is decreased (±30%). When looking specifically at right ventricular function, propofol produces a marked reduction in the slope of the right ventricular end-systolic pressure-volume relationship.[114]

In patients with valvular heart disease, pulmonary artery and pulmonary capillary wedge pressure also are reduced, a finding that implies the resultant decrease in pressure is due to a decrease in preload and afterload. Although the decrease in systemic pressure after an induction dose of propofol is due to

Table 26-2 Hemodynamic Changes after Induction of Anesthesia with Nonbarbiturate Hypnotics

	Diazepam	Droperidol	Etomidate*	Ketamine	Lorazepam	Midazolam	Propofol
HR	−9 ± 13%	Unchanged	−5 ± 10%	0-59%	Unchanged	−14 ± 12%	−10 ± 10%
MBP	0-19%	0-10%	0-17%	0 ± 40%	−7-20%	−12-26%	−10-40%
SVR	−22 ± 13%	−5-15%	−10 ± 14%	0 ± 33%	−10-35%	0-20%	−15-25%
PAP	0-10%	Unchanged	−9 ± 8%	+44 ± 47%	—	Unchanged	0-10%
PVR	0-19%	Unchanged	−18 ± 6%	0 ± 33%	Unchanged	Unchanged	0-10%
PAO	Unchanged	+25 ± 50%	Unchanged	Unchanged	—	0-25%	Unchanged
RAP	Unchanged	Unchanged	Unchanged	+15 ± 33%	Unchanged	Unchanged	0-10%
CI	Unchanged	Unchanged	−20 ± 14%	0 ± 42%	0 ± 16%	0-25%	−10-30%
SV	0–8%	0-10%	0-20%	0-21%	Unchanged	0-18%	−10-25%
LVSWI	0-36%	Unchanged	0-33%	0 ± 27%	—	−28-42%	−10-20%
dP/dt	Unchanged	—	0-18%	Unchanged	—	0-12%	Decreased

*The larger deviations are in patients with valvular disease.
CI, cardiac index; dP/dt, first derivative of pressure measured over time; HR, heart rate; LVSWI, left ventricular stroke work index; MBP, mean blood pressure; PAP, pulmonary artery pressure; PVR, pulmonary vascular resistance; PAO, pulmonary artery occluded pressures; RAP, right atrial pressure; SV, stroke volume; SVR, systemic vascular resistance.

vasodilation, the direct myocardial depressant effects of propofol are more controversial. The decrease in cardiac output after propofol administration may be via its action on sympathetic drive to the heart. Propofol at high concentrations (10 μg/mL) abolishes the inotropic effect of α but not β adrenoreceptor stimulation, and enhances the lusitropic (relaxation) effect of β stimulation.[115] Clinically, the myocardial depressant effect and the vasodilation seem to be dose-dependent and plasma concentration–dependent.[116] The vasodilatory effect of propofol seems to be due to a reduction in sympathetic activity,[117] a direct effect on intracellular smooth muscle calcium mobilization,[118] inhibition of prostacyclin synthesis in endothelial cells,[119] reduction in angiotensin II–elicited calcium entry,[120] activation of K^+ adenosine triphosphate channels, and stimulation of nitric oxide. The stimulation of nitric oxide may be modulated by intralipid rather than propofol.[121]

Heart rate does not change significantly after an induction dose of propofol. Propofol either may reset or may inhibit the baroreflex, reducing the tachycardic response to hypotension.[122] Propofol also decreases cardiac parasympathetic tone in a dose-dependent manner.[123] Propofol has a minimal direct effect on sinoatrial node function or on normal atrioventricular and accessory pathway conduction.[124] Propofol attenuates the heart rate response to atropine in a dose-dependent manner. During an infusion of 10 mg/kg/hr of propofol, a cumulative dose of atropine of 30 μg/kg increased heart rate greater than 20 beats/min in only 20% of subjects compared with 100% in the absence of propofol.[125] Propofol suppresses atrial (supraventricular) tachycardias and probably should be avoided during electrophysiologic studies.[126]

In retrospective review of 2406 patients, Reich and colleagues[127] showed that 9% of patients experienced severe hypotension 0 to 10 minutes after induction of general anesthesia. Statistically significant multivariate predictors of hypotension 0 to 10 minutes after anesthetic induction included American Society of Anesthesiologists (ASA) class III through V, baseline mean arterial pressure (MAP) less than 70 mm Hg, age 50 years or older, use of propofol for induction of anesthesia, and increasing induction dosage of fentanyl. The combination of propofol with fentanyl was a particularly potent stimulus for hypotension. A prolonged postoperative stay or death was more common in patients with versus patients without postinduction hypotension; however, the use of propofol per se was not associated with increased morbidity.[127] Limited data indicate that 0.5 mg/kg of ketamine is able to better prevent decreases in hemodynamics after a propofol induction alone or in combination with fentanyl (1 μg/kg).[128]

During maintenance of anesthesia with a propofol infusion, arterial systolic blood pressure also is decreased to 20% to 30% less than preinduction of anesthesia levels. In patients allowed to breathe room air during a maintenance infusion of 100 μg/kg/min of propofol, there is a significant decrease in systemic vascular resistance (30%), but cardiac index and stroke index are unaltered. In contrast, in patients receiving a narcotic premedication and nitrous oxide with an infusion of propofol (54 μg/kg/min and 108 μg/kg/min) for maintenance during surgery, systemic vascular resistance is not significantly decreased from baseline, but cardiac output and stroke volume are decreased. This situation is probably explained by the observation that propofol infusions produce a dose-dependent decrease of sympathetic nerve activity, attenuating the reflex responses to hypotension. In the presence of hypercarbia, the reflex sympathetic responses are better maintained.[129]

Increasing the infusion rate of propofol from 54 to 108 μg/kg/min (blood concentration 2.1 to 4.2 μg/mL) produces only a slightly greater decrease in arterial blood pressure (−10%). The peak plasma concentrations obtained after a bolus dose are substantially higher than the concentrations seen with a continuous infusion. Because the vasodilatory and myocardial depressant effects are concentration-dependent, the decrease in arterial blood pressure from propofol during the infusion phase (maintenance of anesthesia) is much less than that seen after an induction of anesthesia bolus. When propofol was compared with midazolam for sedation after coronary revascularization, propofol resulted in a 17% less frequent incidence of tachycardia, a 28% less frequent incidence of hypertension, and a 17% more frequent incidence in hypotension. These differences in hemodynamic variables resulted in no difference in the number or severity of ischemic events between the two groups. An infusion of propofol results in a significant reduction in myocardial blood flow and myocardial oxygen consumption,[108,111] a finding that suggests that the global myocardial oxygen supply-to-demand ratio is preserved.

The cardioprotective effect of propofol versus volatile anesthetics in patients having cardiac surgery on or off cardiopulmonary bypass is less debatable. In two large studies comparing propofol with sevoflurane in patients undergoing cardiac surgery, postoperative troponin were lower and hemodynamic function better in patients receiving sevoflurane.[130,131] A study comparing desflurane with propofol in patients undergoing off-pump coronary artery bypass showed similar results.[132] In contrast, a small study that administered high-dose propofol (120 µg/kg/min), low-dose propofol (60 µg/kg/min) while on pump, or titrated isoflurane throughout surgery showed improved troponin levels and better hemodynamic function in the large-dose propofol group compared to the isoflurane or low-dose propofol group.[133] This study may indicate that cardioprotection with propofol is dose dependent, but needs confirmation.

Heart rate may increase,[111] decrease,[110] or remain unchanged[109] when anesthesia is maintained with propofol. The extent of hypotension, the ability for the patient to compensate, and the use of any other concomitant drugs are likely the most important factors in determining what happens to the heart rate after propofol administration.

Other Effects

Propofol, similar to thiopental, does not enhance neuromuscular blockade produced by neuromuscular blocking drugs. Propofol produces no effect on the evoked electromyogram or twitch tension; however, good intubating conditions after propofol alone have been reported.[134] Propofol does not trigger malignant hyperthermia and is an appropriate choice in patients with this condition.[135]

Propofol after a single dose or a prolonged infusion does not affect corticosteroid synthesis or alter the normal response to adrenocorticotropic hormone (ACTH) stimulation.[136] Propofol in the emulsion formulation does not alter hepatic, hematologic, or fibrinolytic function. Lipid emulsion per se reduces in vitro platelet aggregation, however.[137] Anaphylactoid reactions to the present formulation of propofol have been reported. In at least some patients, the immune response was entirely due to propofol and not to the lipid emulsion. A high percentage of the patients developing the anaphylactoid response to propofol had a previous history of allergic responses. In patients with multiple drug allergies, propofol should be used with caution.[138] Propofol alone in intralipid does not trigger histamine release.[139] Fospropofol is metabolized to propofol and formate. Formate concentrations do not increase after fospropofol administration.[40]

Propofol also possesses significant antiemetic activity at low (subhypnotic) doses. It has been used successfully to treat postoperative nausea in a bolus dose of 10 mg.[140] The median concentration of propofol that was associated with an antiemetic effect was 343 ng/mL.[141] This concentration can be achieved by a propofol infusion of 10 to 20 mg loading dose followed by 10 µg/kg/min. Propofol used as a maintenance anesthetic during breast surgery was more effective than 4 mg of ondansetron given as prophylaxis in preventing postoperative nausea and vomiting (PONV). In the same study, the maintenance propofol infusion also was superior to adding propofol only at the end of the procedure (sandwich technique).[142] Propofol as an infusion of 1 mg/kg/hr (17 µg/kg/min) also has provided excellent antiemetic action after anticancer chemotherapy. At subhypnotic doses, propofol relieves cholestatic pruritus and is as effective as naloxone in treating pruritus induced by spinal opiates,[143] although not all studies have confirmed this effect of propofol.

Propofol decreases polymorphonuclear leukocyte chemotaxis, but not adherence phagocytosis and killing. This action contrasts with the effect of thiopental, which inhibits all these chemotactic responses.[144] Propofol inhibits phagocytosis and killing of *Staphylococcus aureus* and *Escherichia coli,* however.[145] These findings are particularly pertinent in view of the observation of increased life-threatening systemic infections associated with the use of propofol.[146] In hospitals where these infections occurred, opened vials and syringes of propofol had positive cultures for the offending organisms. The intralipid that acts as the solvent for propofol is an excellent culture medium. Disodium edetate or metabisulfite has been added to the formulation of propofol in an attempt to retard such bacterial growth. Strict aseptic technique still must be observed.

The administration of propofol also has been associated with the development of pancreatitis.[147] The development of pancreatitis seems to be related to hypertriglyceridemia. Patients who developed hypertriglyceridemia tended to be older, had a longer intensive care unit (ICU) stay, and received propofol for a longer duration. It seems prudent, if propofol is being used for prolonged sedation or at higher infusion rates (especially in elderly patients), that serum triglyceride concentrations should be routinely monitored.[148]

Uses

Induction and Maintenance of Anesthesia

Propofol is suitable for the induction and maintenance of anesthesia (Table 26-3). The induction dose is 1 to 2.5 mg/kg. Physiologic characteristics that best determine the induction dose are age, lean body mass, and central blood volume.[149] Premedication with an opiate or a benzodiazepine, or both, markedly reduces the induction dose.[150,151] A dose of 1 mg/kg (with premedication) to 1.75 mg/kg (without premedication) is recommended for inducing anesthesia in patients older than 60 years (see Chapter 71).[152] As noted earlier, older and sicker (ASA class III to IV) patients develop more profound hypotension, especially when propofol is

Table 26-3 Uses and Doses of Intravenous Propofol

Induction of general anesthesia	1-2.5 mg/kg IV dose reduced with increasing age
Maintenance of general anesthesia	50-150 µg/kg/min IV combined with N_2O or an opiate
Sedation	25-75 µg/kg/min IV
Antiemetic	10-20 mg IV, can repeat every 5-10 min or start infusion of 10 µg/kg/min

N_2O, nitrous oxide.

combined with an opiate.[127] To prevent hypotension in sicker patients or in patients presenting for cardiac surgery, a fluid load should be administered as tolerated, and the propofol can be administered in small incremental doses (10 to 30 mg or as an infusion) until the patients lose consciousness. To limit the dose and retain the fastest onset time, an infusion of 80 mg/kg/hr is optimal. Diluting propofol to 0.5 mg/mL further reduces the impact of this induction dose on hemodynamics.[153] For induction in children, the ED_{95} (2 to 3 mg/kg) is increased, primarily because of pharmacokinetic differences (see Chapter 82).[154]

Propofol, when used for induction of anesthesia in briefer procedures, results in a significantly quicker recovery and an earlier return of psychomotor function compared with thiopental or methohexital, regardless of the anesthetic used for maintenance of anesthesia. The incidence of nausea and vomiting when propofol is used for induction also is markedly less than after the use of other IV anesthetics, probably because of the antiemetic properties of propofol.[155]

Because of its pharmacokinetics, propofol provides a rapid recovery and is superior to barbiturates for maintenance of anesthesia, and it seems to be equal to enflurane, isoflurane and sevoflurane.[156] Recovery from desflurane is slightly more rapid than recovery from propofol.[157] Propofol can be given as intermittent boluses or as a continuous infusion for maintenance. After a satisfactory induction dose, a bolus of 10 to 40 mg is needed every few minutes to maintain anesthesia. Because these doses need to be given frequently, it is more suitable to administer propofol as a continuous infusion.

Several infusion schemes have been used to achieve adequate plasma concentrations of propofol.[158] After an induction dose, an infusion of 100 to 200 μg/kg/min is usually needed. The infusion rate is titrated to individual requirements and the surgical stimulus. When combined with propofol, the required infusion rate and concentration of opiates, midazolam, clonidine, or ketamine is reduced. Because opioids alter the concentration of propofol required for adequate anesthesia, the relative dose of either opioid or propofol markedly affects the time from termination of drug to awakening and recovery. The infusion rate required to achieve the combination with the shortest recovery is propofol, 1 to 1.5 mg/kg followed by 140 μg/kg/min for 10 minutes followed by 100 μg/kg/min, and alfentanil, 30 μg/kg followed by an infusion of 0.25 μg/kg/min, or fentanyl, 3 μg/kg followed by 0.02 μg/kg/min. Propofol also has been used as a single mixture with alfentanil, containing 1 mg of alfentanil (2 mL) to 400 mg of propofol (40 mL). When this mixture was administered at infusion rates commonly used for propofol (i.e., 166 μg/kg/min for 10 minutes, 133 μg/kg/min for 10 minutes, and 100 μg/kg/min thereafter), it provided an outcome equal to that obtained by using the two drugs as separate infusions.[159]

Increasing age is associated with a decrease in propofol infusion requirements (see Chapter 71), whereas these requirements are higher in children and infants (see Chapter 82).[30] The blood levels of propofol alone for loss of consciousness are 2.5 to 4.5 μg/mL, and the blood concentrations (when combined with nitrous oxide) required for surgery are 2.5 to 8 μg/mL.[15,22,52,93,160,161] Similar concentrations are necessary when propofol is combined with an opioid for a total IV technique. The knowledge of these levels and of the pharmacokinetics of propofol has enabled the use of pharmacokinetic model–driven infusion systems to deliver propofol as a continuous infusion for the maintenance of anesthesia. A meta-analysis of recovery data after either propofol for maintenance or the newer volatile anesthetics indicated only minor differences in times to reach recovery goals; however, the incidence of nausea and vomiting remained significantly lower in the patients administered propofol for maintenance.[162]

Several studies have investigated the utility of propofol as a maintenance infusion regimen for cardiac surgery. Using reduced and titrated doses of propofol for induction and titrated infusion rates of 50 to 200 μg/kg/min combined with an opioid for maintenance, propofol provided intraoperative hemodynamic control and ischemic episodes similar to those with either enflurane/opioid or a primary opioid technique.[163,164]

Sedation

Propofol has been evaluated for sedation during surgical procedures[55,56,165] and for patients receiving mechanical ventilation in the ICU (see Chapter 92).[166] Propofol by continuous infusion provides the ability to titrate to a desired level of sedation and provide a rapid recovery after infusion is terminated, regardless of the duration of the infusion.[56,168] In a study of patients sedated in the ICU for 4 days with propofol, recovery to consciousness was rapid (±10 minutes). The rate of recovery and the decrease in plasma concentration were similar at 24 hours and at 96 hours, when the infusion was discontinued. In addition, the plasma concentrations required for sedation and for awakening were similar at 24 hours and 96 hours, a finding that implies that tolerance to propofol did not occur.[168] As noted earlier, there have been more recent reports of tolerance with propofol.

Infusion rates required for sedation to supplement regional anesthesia in healthy patients are half or less than the rates required for general anesthesia (i.e., 30 to 60 μg/kg/min).[55] In elderly patients (>65 years old) and in sicker patients, the infusion rates that are necessary are markedly reduced.[55,166,167] It is important to titrate the infusion individually to the desired effect. A 1992 report[169] linked propofol with several deaths in children requiring sedation for mechanical ventilation secondary to upper respiratory tract infections. This rare syndrome (propofol infusion syndrome) also may occur in adults (see later). A potential advantage of propofol for sedation of ICU patients is that it seems to possess antioxidant properties.[170]

Although the pharmacokinetic profile and to a large extent the pharmacology of propofol make it an excellent choice for long-term (days) sedation, this always must be weighed against the hemodynamic effects, the often concomitant need for an analgesic, tolerance, and rare occurrences of hypertriglyceridemia (and potential pancreatitis) or propofol infusion syndrome. Maintaining the lowest possible dose required for the desired level of sedation with potential "sedation holidays" should considered as part of a long-term propofol sedation regimen. In addition, the FDA has specifically recommended against the use of propofol for the prolonged sedation of pediatric patients. The sedation guidelines of the American College of Critical Care Medicine also recommend "that patients receiving propofol for long term sedation should be monitored for unexplained metabolic acidosis or arrhythmias. Alternative sedative agents should be considered for patients with escalating vasopressor or inotrope requirements or cardiac failure during high-dose propofol infusions."[171] The recommended maximal dose of propofol infusion rate is 80 μg/kg/min (<5 mg/kg/hr).[171]

Generally, at propofol infusion rates greater than 30 μg/kg/min, patients are amnesic.[167] Compared with midazolam when used to maintain sedation, propofol provides equal or better control and more rapid recovery.[56,167] In mechanically ventilated patients, more rapid recovery translates to more rapid extubation when sedation is terminated.[167] Propofol also has been used successfully in patient-controlled sedation. Propofol was rated better than midazolam when used by this technique, probably owing to its much more rapid onset and offset.[172] Patient-controlled sedation has been compared with anesthesia provider sedation. Generally, patients use less propofol and recover more quickly, and there are limited differences in patient satisfaction.[173,174]

Side Effects and Contraindications

Induction of anesthesia with propofol is associated with several side effects, including pain on injection, myoclonus, apnea, hypotension, and, rarely, thrombophlebitis of the vein into which propofol is injected. Pain on injection is less than or equal to that with etomidate, equal to that with methohexital, and greater than that after thiopental.[175,154] Pain on injection is reduced by using a large vein, avoiding veins in the dorsum of the hand, and adding lidocaine to the propofol solution or changing the propofol formulation. Multiple other drugs and distraction techniques have been investigated to reduce the pain on injection of propofol. Pretreatment with a small dose of propofol, opiates, nonsteroidal anti-inflammatory drugs, ketamine, esmolol/metoprolol, magnesium, a flash of light, clonidine/ephedrine combination, dexamethasone, and metoclopramide all have been tested with variable efficacy.

Fospropofol causes less pain on injection, but an equal incidence of tingling/discomfort in the genital areas.[40] Myoclonus occurs more frequently after propofol than after thiopental, but less frequently than after etomidate or methohexital.[154] Apnea after induction with propofol is common. The incidence of apnea may be similar to that after thiopental or methohexital; however, propofol produces a greater incidence of apnea lasting longer than 30 seconds.[98,160] The addition of an opiate increases the incidence of apnea, especially prolonged apnea.[95,160]

The most common side effect during induction of anesthesia is hypotension, which is augmented by the concomitant administration of opioids.[113] Conversely, with laryngoscopy and endotracheal intubation, the changes in MAP, heart rate, and systemic vascular resistance are less significant after propofol compared with thiopental.[110,113]

Propofol infusion syndrome is a rare but lethal syndrome associated with infusion of propofol at 4 mg/kg/hr or more for 48 hours or longer. It was first described in children, but subsequently has been observed in critically ill adults. The clinical features of propofol infusion syndrome are acute refractory bradycardia leading to asystole, in the presence of one or more of the following: metabolic acidosis (base deficit >10 mmol/L^{-1}), rhabdomyolysis, hyperlipidemia, and enlarged or fatty liver.[176] Other features include cardiomyopathy with acute cardiac failure, skeletal myopathy, hyperkalemia, hepatomegaly, and lipemia.[151,177] Theories about its causality include mitochondrial toxicity, mitochondrial defects, impaired tissue oxygenation, and carbohydrate deficiency. The major risk factors for its development seem to be poor oxygen delivery, sepsis, serious cerebral injury, and high propofol dosage. In some reports, an increasing lipemia has been noted and was likely to be due to a failure of hepatic lipid regulation, possibly related to poor oxygenation or a lack of glucose or both. In some cases, an increasing lipemia was the first indication of impending propofol infusion syndrome onset, so it should not be viewed as a benign sign.[178]

Barbiturates

History

Thiopental was introduced clinically by Waters and Lundy (Fig. 26-4), and became preferred clinically because of its rapid onset of action and short duration, without the excitatory effects of hexobarbital.[179] Although criticized after many casualties during the attack on Pearl Harbor as "the ideal form of euthanasia in war surgery," the barbiturates continued to be widely used in clinical practice.[180] Although many other barbiturate derivatives have been synthesized throughout the past several decades, none have enjoyed the clinical success and popularity of thiopental.

Physicochemical Characteristics

Chemistry and Formulation

Barbiturates are hypnotically active drugs that are derivatives of barbituric acid (2,4,6-trioxohexahydropyrimidine), a hypnotically inactive pyrimidine nucleus that is formed by the condensation of malonic acid and urea (Fig. 26-5). The two major divisions of barbiturates are those with an oxygen at position 2 and those with a sulfur in position 2—the classes of oxybarbiturates and thiobarbiturates, respectively. Through keto-enol tautomerization, the oxygen or sulfur in position 2 becomes a reactive species in the enol form, allowing for the formation of water-soluble barbiturate salts in alkaline solutions. This solubility permits the IV use of barbiturates. Although tautomerization to the enol form allows for the creation of salts, it is substitution of the hydrogen attached to the carbon atom in position 5 with aryl or alkyl groups that gives the barbiturates their hypnotic activity. Only thiopental and thiamylal, thiobarbiturates, and methohexital, an oxybarbiturate, have been commonly used for induction of anesthesia (Fig. 26-6).

The formulation of barbiturates involves preparing them as sodium salts (mixed with 6% by weight anhydrous sodium carbonate) and then reconstituting with either water or normal saline to produce a 2.5% solution of thiopental, a 2% solution of thiamylal, or a 1% solution of methohexital. The thiobarbiturates are stable for 1 week if refrigerated after reconstitution, and methohexital remains available for use for 6 weeks after reconstitution. A decrease in the alkalinity of the solution can result in precipitation of the barbiturates as free acids, which is why they cannot be reconstituted with lactated Ringer's solution or mixed with other acidic solutions. Examples of drugs that are not to be coadministered or mixed in solution with the barbiturates are pancuronium, vecuronium, atracurium, alfentanil, sufentanil, and midazolam. Studies have shown that in rapid-sequence induction, the mixing of thiopental with vecuronium or pancuronium results in the formation of precipitate that may occlude the IV line.[181]

Structure-Activity Relationships

As noted earlier, substitutions at the 5, 2, and 1 positions confer different pharmacologic activities to the barbiturate nucleus. Sub-

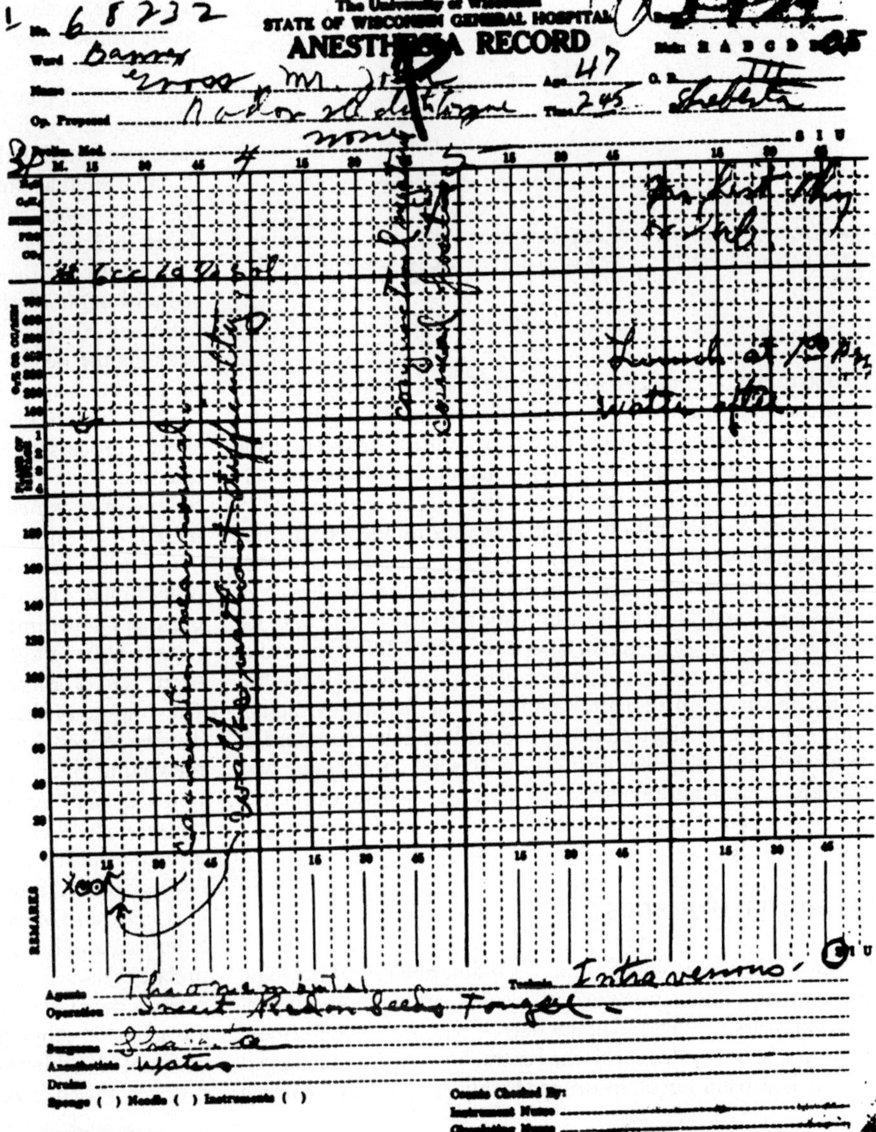

The University of Wisconsin
STATE OF WISCONSIN GENERAL HOSPITAL
ANESTHESIA RECORD

No. 68232
Ward
Name
Op. Proposed
Prelim. Med.
Age 47
Wt. 245
Remarks
Agents
Technic Intravenous
Operation
Surgeons
Anesthetists
Drains
Sponge ( ) Needle ( ) Instruments ( )
Counts Checked By:
Instrument Nurse
Circulating Nurse

Figure 26-4 Reproduction of the first administration of thiopental by Waters on March 8, 1934. *(From Dundee JW, Wyant GM: Intravenous Anaesthesia. Edinburgh, Churchill Livingstone, 1974.)*

stitutions at position 5 with either aryl or alkyl groups produce hypnotic and sedative effects. A phenyl group substitution at C5 produces anticonvulsant activity. An increase in length of one or both side chains of an alkyl group at C5 increases hypnotic potency. Barbiturates used in clinical practice have either an oxygen or sulfur at C2. Substitution of a sulfur at position 2 produces a more rapid onset of action, as with thiopental. The addition of a methyl or ethyl group at position 1 also may produce a more rapid onset of action, but excitatory side effects, including tremor, hypertonus, and involuntary movement, may occur with administration, as with methohexital.

Metabolism

The barbiturates (with the exception of phenobarbital) are hepatically metabolized. The metabolites that are formed are almost all inactive, water-soluble, and excreted in the urine. Barbiturates are biotransformed by four processes: (1) oxidation of the aryl, alkyl, or phenyl moiety at C5; (2) *N*-dealkylation; (3) desulfuration of the thiobarbiturates at C2; and (4) destruction of the barbituric acid ring.[182] Oxidation is the most important pathway, producing polar (charged) alcohols, ketones, phenols, or carboxylic acids. These metabolites are readily excreted in the urine or as glucuronic acid conjugates in the bile. The barbituric acid ring is so stable in vivo that hydrolytic cleavage of the ring is a minimal contribution to the total metabolism of barbiturates. Drugs that induce the oxidative microsomes enhance the metabolism of barbiturates. Long-term administration of barbiturates also induces the enzymes.[182] The hepatic enzyme induction of barbiturates is responsible for the recommendation that they not be administered to patients with acute intermittent porphyria because barbiturates may precipitate an attack by stimulating γ-aminolevulinic acid synthetase, the enzyme responsible for the production of porphyrins.[183]

As mentioned earlier, hepatic metabolism accounts for the elimination of all of the barbiturates with the exception of phenobarbital. Renal excretion is important in the elimination of

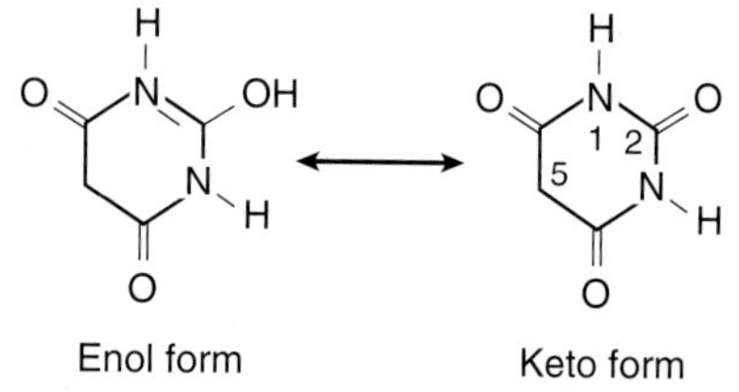

Enol form   Keto form

Figure 26-5 The keto and enol tautomeric forms of barbituric acid with the sites of substitution in the hypnotically active barbiturates identified as 1, 2, and 5.

phenobarbital, accounting for 60% to 90% of drug excretion in an unchanged form. Only trivial amounts of other barbiturates are excreted unchanged by the kidney. The alkalinization of urine with bicarbonate enhances the renal excretion of phenobarbital.

Methohexital is metabolized in the liver by oxidation to an alcohol and *N*-dealkylation. Compared with thiopental, methohexital exhibits similar distribution half-lives, volumes of distribution, and protein bindings. A marked difference exists, however, in plasma disappearance and elimination half-lives (4 hours for methohexital and 12 hours for thiopental). This difference is due to the threefold more rapid rate of hepatic clearance of methohexital (mean 7.8 to 12.5 mL/kg/min).[184] The hepatic extraction ratio of methohexital (clearance to hepatic blood flow) is approximately 0.5, indicating that the liver extracts 50% of the drug presented to it. This ratio contrasts to the lower hepatic extraction ratio of thiopental (0.15).

Pharmacokinetics

Barbiturate pharmacokinetics has been described in physiologic and compartmental models, with the latter gaining more support in recent years.[185] Physiologic models of barbiturates describe a rapid mixing of the drug with the central blood volume followed by a quick distribution of the drug to highly perfused, low-volume tissues (i.e., brain) with a slower redistribution of the drug to lean tissue (muscle), which terminates the effect of the induction dose. In these models, adipose tissue uptake and metabolic clearance (elimination) play only a minor role in the termination of the effects of the induction dose because of the minimal perfusion ratio compared with other tissues and the slow rate of removal. Compartmental model values for thiopental and methohexital, the most commonly used induction barbiturates, are given in Table 26-1.

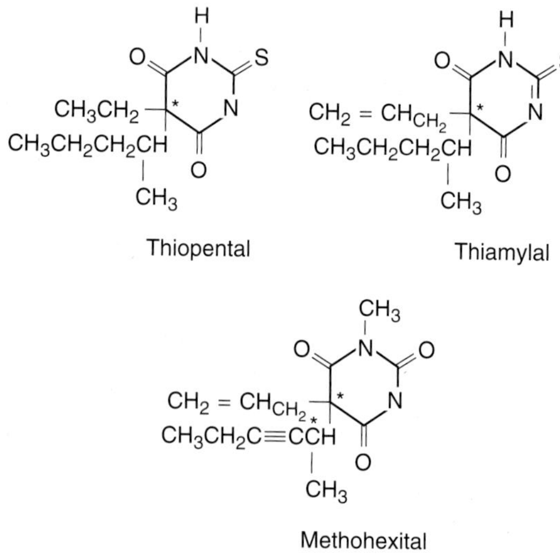

Both of these pharmacokinetic models describe rapid redistribution as the primary mechanism that terminates the action of a single induction dose. The compartmental model explains the delay of recovery when a continuous infusion of a barbiturate is used. This model describes the phenomena whereby the termination of effect becomes increasingly dependent on the slower process of uptake into adipose tissue and elimination clearance through hepatic metabolism. After prolonged infusions, the pharmacokinetics of barbiturate metabolism is best approximated by nonlinear Michaelis-Menten metabolism.

In usual doses (4 to 5 mg/kg), thiopental exhibits first-order kinetics (i.e., a constant *fraction* of drug is cleared from the body per unit time); however, at very high doses of thiopental (300 to 600 mg/kg) with receptor saturation, zero-order kinetics occur (i.e., a constant *amount* of drug is cleared per unit time). The volume of distribution is slightly larger in female patients, causing longer elimination half-lives.[186] Pregnancy also increases the volume of distribution of thiopental, prolonging the elimination half-life.[187] As noted previously, the clearance rate of thiopental is not altered in patients with cirrhosis because the amount of protein available for the drug to bind to is still adequate even at fairly advanced stages of the disease process.[188]

Because of its affinity for fat, relatively large volume of distribution, and low rate of hepatic clearance, thiopental can accumulate in tissues, especially if given in large doses over a prolonged period. The plasma drug level increases when repeat doses of drug are given.[189] Appropriately designed infusion schemes ensure constant blood levels, maintaining the hypnotic effect, although this is not used in routine clinical practice.

Thiopental   Thiamylal

Methohexital

Figure 26-6 Hypnotically active barbiturates commonly used for induction, with their asymmetric centers indicated by an asterisk.

Pharmacology

Mechanism of Action

Much research has been conducted to delineate the mechanisms of action of barbiturates on the CNS, but until more recently, with the exception of their action on $GABA_A$ receptor, these have remained largely unknown.[190,191] Numerous more recent studies have begun to elucidate the role of NMDA receptors in the actions of barbiturates.[192-195] The selectivity of actions of barbiturates on CNS neurophysiologic systems has been grouped into two general categories: (1) enhancement of the synaptic actions of *inhibitory* neurotransmitters, and (2) blockade of the synaptic actions of *excitatory* neurotransmitters.[196]

GABA is the principal inhibitory neurotransmitter in the mammalian CNS, and the $GABA_A$ receptor is the only site that has been proved to be involved in barbiturate-induced anesthesia.[191] The $GABA_A$ receptor is a chloride ion channel that is composed of at least five subunits with specific sites of action for GABA, barbiturates, benzodiazepines, and other molecules.[179] Barbiturate binding to the $GABA_A$ receptor enhances and mimics the action of GABA by increasing chloride conductance through the ion channel, causing hyperpolarization of the cell membrane and increasing the threshold of excitability of the postsynaptic neuron.[197] At low concentrations, barbiturates enhance the effects of GABA, decreasing the rate of dissociation of GABA from its receptor and increasing the duration of GABA-activated chloride ion channel openings. This enhancement of the action of GABA is considered to be responsible for the sedative-hypnotic effects of the barbiturates. At higher concentrations, the barbiturates directly activate the chloride channels without the binding of GABA, acting as the agonist itself. The GABA-mimetic effect at slightly higher concentrations may be responsible for what is termed *barbiturate anesthesia*.[191]

The barbiturates also inhibit synaptic transmission of excitatory neurotransmitters, such as glutamate and acetylcholine.[191] The actions of the barbiturates to block excitatory CNS transmission are specific for synaptic ion channels. Thiopental may exert GABA-independent effects, however, on the glutaminergic-NMDA system.[194] In two studies of rat prefrontal cortex, thiopental was shown to decrease extracellular glutamate levels in the CNS and decrease NMDA-gated currents in a concentration-dependent manner.[192,193] In a similar study in mice, thiopental has GABA-independent actions that inhibit the excitatory activities through inhibition of NMDA receptors.[194]

Effects on Cerebral Metabolism

Barbiturates, similar to other CNS depressants, have potent effects on cerebral metabolism (see Chapters 13 and 63). A dose-related depression of cerebral metabolic oxygen consumption rate ($CMRO_2$), produces a progressive slowing of the EEG, a reduction in the rate of adenosine triphosphate consumption, and protection from incomplete cerebral ischemia.[198] The relationship of depressed metabolism to drug dosage was shown in dogs in which circulation at high thiopental doses was preserved by an extracorporeal circulation pump.[199] When the results of the EEG became isoelectric, a point at which cerebral metabolic activity is roughly 50% of baseline,[200] no further decrements in $CMRO_2$ occurred. These findings support the hypothesis that metabolism and function are coupled. It is the portion of metabolic activity concerned with neuronal signaling and impulse traffic that is reduced by barbiturates, however, not the portion corresponding to basal metabolic function. The only way to suppress baseline metabolic activity concerned with cellular activity is through hypothermia.[200] The effect of barbiturates on cerebral metabolism is maximized at a 50% depression of cerebral function, in which less oxygen is required as $CMRO_2$ is diminished, leaving all metabolic energy to be used for the maintenance of cellular integrity.

With the reduction in $CMRO_2$, there is a parallel reduction in cerebral perfusion, which is seen in decreased cerebral blood flow and ICP. With reduced $CMRO_2$, cerebral vascular resistance increases, and CBF decreases.[201] The ratio of CBF to $CMRO_2$ is unchanged. The reduction in CBF after the administration of barbiturates causes a concurrent decrease in ICP. Even though the MAP decreases, barbiturates do not compromise the overall CPP because the CPP = MAP − ICP. In this relationship, ICP decreases more relative to the decrease in MAP after barbiturate use, preserving CPP.

Pharmacodynamics

Barbiturates produce the clinical effects of sedation and sleep. Sufficient doses produce a CNS depression that is termed *general anesthesia* and is attended by loss of consciousness, amnesia, and respiratory and cardiovascular depression. The response to pain and other noxious stimulation during general anesthesia seems to be obtunded. The results of pain studies reveal that barbiturates may decrease the pain threshold, however.[202] This antanalgesic effect occurs only at low blood levels of barbiturates, such as with small induction doses of thiopental or after emergence from thiopental when the blood levels are low. The amnesic effect of barbiturates has not been well studied, but it is less pronounced than that produced by benzodiazepines.

Onset of Central Nervous System Effects

Drugs with high lipid solubility and low degree of ionization cross the blood-brain barrier rapidly, producing a fast onset of action.[191] Most barbiturates exist in a nonionized form. The degree of lipid solubility of the nonionized form of the drug works in conjunction with the amount of drug that exists in the nonionized form (reflection of pK_a) to determine the rapidity with which a drug crosses the blood-brain barrier. Thiopental and methohexital are more lipid soluble than pentobarbital, which clinically corresponds to the more rapid onset of action of thiopental and methohexital compared with pentobarbital.[203,204]

Only the nonionized form of a drug can directly traverse the cellular membranes. Thiopental has a pK_a of 7.6. Approximately 50% of thiopental is nonionized at physiologic pH, which accounts partly for the rapid accumulation of thiopental in the cerebrospinal fluid (CSF) after IV administration.[205] Methohexital is 75% nonionized at pH 7.4, a fact that may explain the slightly more rapid effect of this drug compared with the effect of thiopental. As pH decreases, with poor perfusion, barbiturates have a larger proportion of nonionized drug available to cross the blood-brain barrier.[204,205]

Protein binding affects the onset of action in the CNS. Barbiturates are highly bound to albumin and other plasma proteins. Because only unbound drug (free drug) can cross the blood-brain barrier, an inverse relationship exists between the degree of plasma protein binding and the rapidity of drug passage across the blood-brain barrier.[206] Drugs have different degrees of protein binding, and generally the thiobarbiturates are more highly bound than are the oxybarbiturates.[207] The degree of protein binding of a drug is influenced by the physiologic pH and disease states, which alter the absolute amount of protein. Most barbiturates tend to experience peak protein binding at or around pH 7.5.

The final factor governing the rapidity of drug penetration of the blood-brain barrier is the plasma drug concentration. Simply as a result of concentration gradient, higher levels of drug concentrations in the plasma produce greater amounts of drug that diffuses into the CSF and brain. The two primary determinants of the plasma concentration are the *dose* administered and the *rate* (speed) of administration. As the dose of thiopental over the same time is increased, an increased percentage of patients are anesthetized.[208] Concerning absolute dose, 2 mg/kg produced anesthesia in 20% of patients, whereas a dose of 2.4 mg/kg produced anesthesia in 80% of patients. Similarly, the speed of injection influences the effect of thiopental.[209] When a fixed initial dose of thiopental of approximately 2.75 mg/kg was used, a significantly ($P < .001$) smaller amount of drug was required to produce anesthesia when the dose rate of the administration was over 5 seconds as opposed to over 15 seconds. The dose *and* rate of IV administration can profoundly affect the onset of barbiturate CNS effect.

Termination of Effect

Because there exists an equilibrium between brain concentration and plasma concentration, factors that determine the rate of onset of barbiturate effects also affect their termination. Lipid solubility, degree of ionization, and CSF drug concentration affect the movement of drugs from the CSF to plasma. As plasma levels decrease, drug levels in the brain and CSF decrease. The most important factors in the termination of drug effect are those that govern plasma disappearance of the drug. These are generally divided into a rapid redistribution phase and a slow metabolic and second redistribution phase.

In a classic pharmacologic study, Brodie and coworkers[210] conclusively showed that awakening from thiopental occurred because the plasma level rapidly declined. They further showed that the cause of the rapid plasma decay of thiopental was *not metabolism* of the drug, but rather was a *redistribution* of the drug to other tissues throughout the body (lean tissue). The role of slow phase distribution to adipose tissue and elimination clearance via metabolism from the plasma was elucidated later.[207] The relationship of the plasma drug level to the onset and termination of effect as it relates to drug redistribution is illustrated in Figure 26-7. Clinically, patients awake from a single dose of thiopental 5 to 10 minutes after administration because the drug level in the brain has decreased (along with the decline in blood level). Drug is redistributed from highly perfused CNS tissues to well-perfused lean tissues. In the case of constant infusion or repeated dosing with saturation of all tissue sites, patients awake at a much delayed rate as first-order hepatic metabolism begins to play a larger role in decreasing plasma levels of the barbiturates. The termination of effect after multiple drug administrations or constant infusion depends on the elimination of the drug from the blood, which becomes more and more dependent on metabolism than redistribution and is a function of its context-sensitive decrement time (see Fig. 26-3).

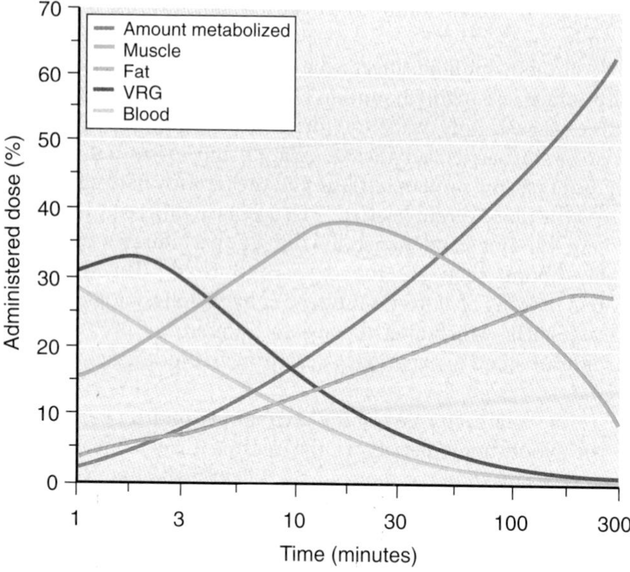

Figure 26-7 After delivery of an IV bolus, the percentage of thiopental remaining in blood rapidly decreases as drug moves from blood to body tissues. The time to attainment of peak tissue levels is a direct function of tissue capacity for barbiturate relative to blood flow. A larger capacity or smaller blood flow is related to a longer time to a peak tissue level. Initially, most thiopental is taken up by the vessel-rich group (VRG) of tissues because of their high blood flow. Subsequently, drug is redistributed to muscle and to a lesser extent to fat. Throughout this period, small but substantial amounts of thiopental are removed and metabolized by the liver. In contrast to removal by tissues, this removal is cumulative. The rate of metabolism equals the early rate of removal by fat. The sum of this early removal by fat and metabolism is the same as the removal by muscle. *(Redrawn from Saidman LJ: Uptake, distribution and elimination of barbiturates.* In *Eger EI [ed]: Anesthetic Uptake and Action. Baltimore, Williams & Wilkins, 1974.)*

Awakening may be delayed in older patients because of increased CNS sensitivity, alterations in metabolism, or decreased central volume of distribution relative to younger adults (see Chapter 71).[211] The initial volume of distribution is less in elderly patients compared with that in young patients, which explains a lower dose requirement for the onset of EEG and hypnotic effects.[211] Pediatric patients (<13 years old) seem to have a more rapid rate of total clearance and a shorter rate of plasma thiopental clearance than do adults, which theoretically might result in earlier awakening, especially after multiple doses of the drug (see Chapter 82).[212]

There is little difference in thiopental and methohexital with regard to distribution, which may explain the similar wake-up time of methohexital and thiopental. There is, however, a difference in the rate of total body clearance, with methohexital being higher. This disparity explains the difference found in the psychomotor skills of patients and the earlier full recovery after methohexital. Sensitive tests of psychomotor skills tend to show better early performance after methohexital than after thiopental use. A driving test reveals, however, abnormal skills for 8 hours after anesthesia, suggesting that despite plasma clearance there is residual CNS impairment for about 1 day.[213] Despite these residual effects, methohexital is cleared more rapidly than thiopental, which explains why methohexital is preferred for use by some clinicians when rapid awakening is desirable, such as in outpatient anesthesia. This prolongation of early and late recovery by the barbiturates is why they have been largely replaced by propofol.

Uses

Barbiturates are used clinically in the practice of anesthesia for induction and maintenance of anesthesia and premedication. Less frequently, barbiturates are used to provide cerebral protection to patients at risk of developing incomplete ischemia. The three barbiturates that are used most commonly in the United States for IV anesthesia and maintenance of anesthesia are thiopental, thiamylal, and methohexital.

Thiopental is an excellent drug to use for induction of anesthesia. The prompt onset (15 to 30 seconds) of action and smooth induction noted with its use make thiopental superior to most other available drugs. The rapid emergence, particularly after single use for induction, also was a reason for the widespread use of thiopental in this setting. Thiopental does not possess analgesic properties, and it must be supplemented with analgesic drugs to obtund reflex responses to noxious stimuli during anesthesia and surgical procedures. Thiopental can be used to maintain general anesthesia because repeated doses reliably sustain unconsciousness and contribute to amnesia. Thiopental is not a perfect choice, however, to use as the hypnotic component of a balanced anesthetic.

Table 26-4 Recommended Doses of Barbiturates for Anesthesia Induction and Maintenance

Drug	Induction Dose (mg/kg)*†	Onset (sec)	Intravenous Maintenance Infusion
Thiopental	3-4	10-30	50-100 mg every 10-12 min
Methohexital	1-1.5	10-30	20-40 mg every 4-7 min

*Adult and pediatric IV doses are roughly the same in milligrams per kilogram.
†Methohexital can be given rectally in pediatric patients as 20-25 mg/kg/dose.

Methohexital is the only IV barbiturate used for induction that offers a serious challenge to thiopental. With a dose of 1 to 2 mg/kg, induction is swift, and so is emergence. Methohexital also may be used as the hypnotic component to maintain anesthesia. Similar to thiopental, it is not an analgesic. Additional opioids or volatile anesthetics are required to provide a balanced technique satisfactory for general anesthesia during surgery. Because methohexital is cleared more rapidly than thiopental, it is superior to thiopental for the maintenance of anesthesia, as accumulation and saturation of peripheral sites takes longer. For brief infusion (<60 minutes), recovery from a methohexital infusion titrated to maintain hypnosis (50 to 150 µg/kg/min) is similar to that provided by propofol. There are probably upper limits of safe infusion doses yet to be defined, but seizures have occurred in neurosurgical patients after large doses of methohexital (24 mg/kg).[214] Finally, some clinicians advocate the use of methohexital in pediatric patients as a rectal premedication drug (see Chapter 82). Methohexital may be given rectally and is absorbed rapidly. Mean peak plasma levels occur within 14 minutes after rectal administration and are associated with a rapid hypnotic effect. The dose recommended for this use is 25 mg/kg rectal instillation (10% solution through a 14F catheter, 7 cm into rectum).[215] With this method of administration, sleep onset is rapid.

Dosing

Dosing for the three most commonly used barbiturates is listed in Table 26-4. The usual doses of thiopental (3 to 4 mg/kg) and thiamylal (3 to 4 mg/kg) are about twice the dose of methohexital (1 to 2 mg/kg). In dose-response studies, the ED_{50} for thiopental ranged from 2.2 to 2.7 mg/kg, and the ED_{50} for methohexital was 1.1 mg/kg.[208] Because the ED_{50} induces anesthesia in only 50% of a given group of patients, higher doses are needed to induce anesthesia reliably in all patients. The usual dose of thiopental is 3 to 4 mg/kg given intravenously over 5 to 15 seconds. There is less interpatient variability in the dose response to barbiturates than to benzodiazepines when used for anesthesia induction, but there still is significant variability in the doses of thiopental required to induce anesthesia.[208]

Interpatient dose variability is related to the presence of hemorrhagic shock, cardiac output, lean body mass, obesity, sex, and age. Hemorrhagic shock, lean body mass, age, and obesity explain variability of patient response owing to a decrease in the central volume of distribution. Less blood volume (patients with shock, patients with dehydration) or less lean body mass (obese patients, elderly patients, female patients) decreases the volume in which the drug is diluted (less blood volume), or decreases the volume into which it is quickly redistributed (less lean body mass). Finally, patients who have severe anemia, burns, malnutrition, widespread malignant disease, uremia, ulcerative colitis, or intestinal obstruction also require lower induction doses of barbiturate.

Side Effects

The effects of barbiturates on various organ systems have been studied extensively. Some side effects occur in unpredictable, varying proportions of patients, whereas cardiovascular and pulmonary side effects are dose related. There are no important differences between the barbiturates with regard to their effects on the various organ systems (respiratory, cardiovascular, gastrointestinal, hepatic, and renal), but there are differences in other complications with these drugs. The complications of injecting barbiturates include a garlic or onion taste (40% of patients), allergic reactions, local tissue irritation, and rarely tissue necrosis. An urticarial rash may develop on the head, neck, and trunk that lasts a few minutes. More severe reactions, such as facial edema, hives, bronchospasm, and anaphylaxis, can occur. Treatment of anaphylaxis is symptomatic.

Thiopental and thiamylal produce fewer excitatory symptoms with induction than methohexital, which produces cough, hiccough, tremors, and twitching approximately five times more often. Tissue irritation and local complications may occur more frequently with the use of thiopental and thiamylal than with methohexital. In comparative studies, pain on injection was shown to be greater with methohexital (12%) than with thiopental (9%). Results also show phlebitis occurs more frequently with methohexital use (8%) than with thiopental use (1%).[216] Tissue and venous irritation are more common if a 5% solution is used, rather than the standard 2% solution.

Rarely, intra-arterial injection can occur. The consequences of accidental arterial injection may be severe. The degree of injury is related to the concentration of the drug. Treatment consists of (1) dilution of the drug by the administration of saline into the artery, (2) heparinization to prevent thrombosis, and (3) brachial plexus block. Overall, the proper administration of thiopental intravenously is remarkably free of local toxicity.

Cardiovascular System

Cardiovascular depression from barbiturates is a result of central and peripheral (direct vascular and cardiac) effects. The hemodynamic changes produced by barbiturates have been studied in healthy subjects and in patients with heart disease.[217,218] The primary cardiovascular effect of barbiturate induction is peripheral vasodilation that results in a pooling of blood in the venous system.[219] A decrease in contractility is another effect, which is related to reduce availability of calcium to the myofibrils. There also is an increase in heart rate.[218] Mechanisms for the decrease in cardiac output include (1) direct negative inotropic action, (2) decreased ventricular filling owing to increased capacitance, and (3) transiently decreased sympathetic outflow from the CNS.[214,220]

The increase in heart rate (10% to 36%) that accompanies thiopental administration probably results from the baroreceptor-mediated sympathetic reflex stimulation of the heart in response to the decrease in output and pressure. Thiopental produces dose-related negative inotropic effects, which seem to result from a decrease in calcium influx into the cells with a resultant diminished amount of calcium at sarcolemma sites. The cardiac index is unchanged or is reduced, and MAP is maintained or is slightly reduced. Thiopental infusions and lower doses tend to be accompanied by smaller hemodynamic changes than the changes noted with rapid bolus injections. In the dose ranges studied, no relationship between plasma thiopental level and hemodynamic effect has been found. A sympathetic discharge in response to intubation increases heart rate and blood pressure and can be attenuated by the administration of fentanyl (1 to 3 μg/kg).

There is little difference in the responses after thiopental and methohexital administration in patients with heart disease. The increase in heart rate (11% to 36%) encountered in patients with coronary artery disease anesthetized with thiopental (1 to 4 mg/kg) is potentially deleterious because of the obligatory increase in myocardial oxygen consumption that accompanies the increased heart rate. In a more recent study in dogs, thiopental prolonged the QT interval, flattened T waves, and increased QT dispersion during and after induction.[221] It is *possible* that thiopental may not be the most appropriate choice for patients with a susceptibility to ventricular dysrhythmias or a prolonged QT interval, such as acidotic patients or patients with conditions that prolong the QT interval, such as long-term dialysis or advanced cirrhosis; however, this remains to be shown in humans. Patients who have normal coronary arteries have no difficulty in maintaining adequate coronary blood flow to meet the increased myocardial oxygen consumption.[222] Thiopental should be avoided in hypovolemic patients because there is a significant reduction in cardiac output (69%) and a significant decrease in blood pressure.[223] Patients without adequate compensatory mechanisms may have serious hemodynamic depression with thiopental induction.

Respiratory System

Barbiturates produce dose-related central respiratory depression. There also is a significant incidence of transient apnea after administration of barbiturates for induction of anesthesia. The evidence for central depression is a correlation between EEG suppression and minute ventilation. With increased anesthetic effect, there is diminished minute ventilation. The time course of respiratory depression has not been fully studied, but it seems that peak respiratory depression (as measured by the slope of carbon dioxide concentration in the blood) and minute ventilation after delivery of thiopental (3.5 mg/kg) occurs 1 to 1.5 minutes after administration. These variables return to predrug levels rapidly, and within 15 minutes the drug effects are barely detectable.[224]

Patients with chronic lung disease are slightly more susceptible to the respiratory depression of thiopental. Apnea occurs during anesthesia induction with thiopental in at least 20% of cases, but the duration of apnea is short, approximately 25 seconds.[225] The usual ventilatory pattern with thiopental induction has been described as "double apnea." The initial apnea that occurs during drug administration lasts a few seconds and is succeeded by a few breaths of reasonably adequate tidal volume, which is followed by a lengthier apneic period. During the induction of anesthesia with thiopental, ventilation must be assisted or controlled to provide adequate respiratory exchange.

Similar to other barbiturates, methohexital is a central respiratory system depressant. Induction doses (1.5 mg/kg) significantly decrease the slope of the ventilatory response to carbon dioxide.[226] Maximal reduction in ventilatory response to carbon dioxide occurred 30 seconds after drug administration and began to approach normal levels within 15 minutes. The peak decrease in tidal volume occurred 60 seconds after methohexital delivery and returned to baseline within 15 minutes. In contrast to the effects on ventilation, patients were awake within about 5 minutes after the administration of methohexital (1.5 mg/kg). There is no difference in the duration of ventilatory depression after methohexital use and after thiopental delivery when the drugs are studied in a similar manner.[224]

Contraindications

Wood has listed the contraindications to IV barbiturate use.[227] (1) When there is respiratory obstruction or an inadequate airway, thiopental may worsen respiratory depression. (2) Severe cardiovascular instability or shock may preclude its use. (3) Status asthmaticus is a condition in which airway control and ventilation may be worsened further by thiopental. (4) Porphyria may be precipitated or acute attacks may be accentuated by the administration of thiopental. (5) Without proper equipment (IV instrumentation) and airway equipment (means of artificial ventilation), thiopental should not be administered.

Benzodiazepines

History

Diazepam (Valium) was synthesized by Sternbach in 1959 in a search for a new and better compound. It was first described for use as an IV anesthetic induction in 1965.[228] Oxazepam (Serax), a metabolite of diazepam, was synthesized in 1961 by Bell. Lorazepam (Ativan), a 2′ chloro-substitution product of oxazepam, was synthesized in 1971 in an attempt to produce a more potent benzodiazepine. The next major achievement was Fryer and Walser's 1976 synthesis of midazolam (Versed), the first clinically used water-soluble benzodiazepine.[229] Midazolam was the first benzodiazepine that was produced primarily for use in anesthesia.[230]

The benzodiazepines have many of the characteristics sought by anesthesiologists. Specific benzodiazepine receptors were described when ligands were found to interact with a central receptor.[231] The discovery and understanding of the mechanism of the benzodiazepine receptor have enabled chemists to develop many agonist compounds and to produce a specific antagonist for clinical use.

Physicochemical Characteristics

Three benzodiazepine receptor agonists are commonly used in anesthesia in the United States: midazolam, diazepam, and lorazepam (Fig. 26-8 and Table 26-5). All these molecules are relatively small and are lipid soluble at physiologic pH. Each milliliter of diazepam solution (5 mg) contains propylene glycol 0.4 mL, alcohol 0.1 mL, benzyl alcohol 0.015 mL, and sodium benzoate/benzoic acid in water for injection (pH 6.2 to 6.9). Lorazepam solution (2 or 4 mg/mL) contains 0.18 mL polyethyl-

Table 26-5 Physicochemical Characterization of Three Benzodiazepines

	Diazepam	Lorazepam	Midazolam
Molecular weight (D)	284.7*	321.2*	362*
pK_a	3.3 (20°)	11.5 (20°)	6.2 (20°)*
Water soluble	No*	Almost insoluble	Yes†
Lipid soluble	Yes*	Yes (less so, however)	Yes†
	Highly lipophilic	Relatively less lipophilic	Highly lipophilic

*Data from Moffet.[581]
†pH dependent: pH >4, lipid soluble; pH <4, water soluble.

ene glycol, with 2% benzyl alcohol as a preservative. Midazolam solution (1 or 5 mg/mL) contains 0.8% sodium chloride and 0.01% disodium edetate, with 1% benzyl alcohol as a preservative. The pH is adjusted to 3 with hydrochloric acid and sodium hydroxide. Midazolam is the most lipid soluble of the three drugs in vivo,[232] but because of its pH-dependent solubility, it is water soluble as formulated in a buffered acidic medium (pH 3.5). The imidazole ring of midazolam accounts for its stability in solution and rapid metabolism. The high lipophilicity of all three accounts for the rapid CNS effect and relatively large volumes of distribution.[233]

Metabolism

Biotransformation of the benzodiazepines occurs in the liver. The two principal pathways involve either hepatic microsomal oxidation (*N*-dealkylation or aliphatic hydroxylation) or glucuronide conjugation. The difference in the two pathways is significant because oxidation is susceptible to outside influences and can be impaired by certain population characteristics (e.g., old age), disease states (e.g., hepatic cirrhosis), or the coadministration of other drugs that can impair oxidizing capacity (e.g., cimetidine). Conjugation is less susceptible to these factors. Midazolam and diazepam undergo oxidation reduction or phase I reactions in the liver. The fused imidazole ring of midazolam is oxidized rapidly by the liver, much more rapidly than the methylene group of the diazepine ring of other benzodiazepines. This fast oxidation accounts for the greater hepatic clearance of midazolam compared with diazepam. Lorazepam is less affected by enzyme induction and some of the other factors known to alter the cytochrome P-450 and other phase I enzymes.

Cimetidine inhibition of oxidative enzyme function impairs the clearance of diazepam,[234] but it has no effect on lorazepam. Age decreases and smoking increases the clearance of diazepam,[235] but neither has a significant effect on midazolam biotransformation. Habitual alcohol consumption increases the clearance of midazolam.[236] Race, because of differences in isoenzymes responsible for hydroxylations, produces genetic differences in drug metabolism.[237] The high frequency of mutated alleles in Asians in the genes coding for CYP2C19 may explain the reduced hepatic biotransformation of diazepam.

The metabolites of the benzodiazepines can be important. Diazepam forms two active metabolites, oxazepam and desmethyldiazepam, which add to and prolong the drug's effects. Midazolam is biotransformed to hydroxymidazolams, which have activity, and when given over a longer time can accumulate.[238] These metabolites are rapidly conjugated and excreted in the urine, however. The α-hydroxymidazolam has an estimated clinical potency 20% to 30% of midazolam.[239] It is excreted largely by the kidneys and can cause profound sedation in patients with renal impairment.[240] The primary hydroxymetabolite is cleared more rapidly[90] than midazolam in healthy patients (Table 26-6). The metabolites are less potent and normally cleared more rapidly than midazolam, making them of little concern in patients with normal hepatic and renal function. Lorazepam has five metabolites, but the principal one is conjugated to glucuronide. This

Table 26-6 Pharmacokinetic and Pharmacodynamic Comparison of Midazolam and Its Active Metabolite*

	EC_{50}^{EEG}	EC_{50}^{SVT}	Clearance	V_{ss}	Clearance Half-Life
Midazolam	1.8 ng/mL	0.9 mg/mL	523 mL/min	60 L	98 min
α-Hydroxymidazolam	10.2 ng/mL	5.3 ng/mL	680 mL/min	69 L	69 min

*All values are significantly ($P < .05$) different between midazolam and α-hydroxymidazolam.
EC_{50}, median effective concentration; EEG, peak electroencephalogram change; SVT, saccadic velocity (eye movement); V_{ss}, volume at steady state.
From Mandema JW, Tuk B, van Steveninck AL, et al: Pharmacokinetic-pharmacodynamic modeling of the central nervous system effects of midazolam and its main metabolite alpha-hydroxymidazolam in healthy volunteers. Clin Pharmacol Ther 51:715-728, 1992.

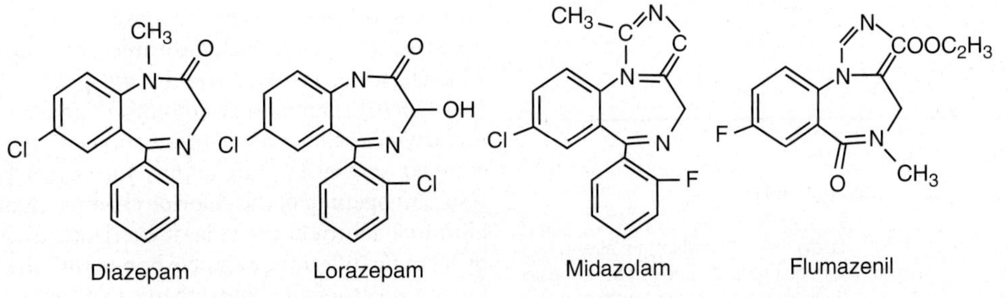

Diazepam Lorazepam Midazolam Flumazenil

Figure 26-8 The structures of four benzodiazepines used in clinical anesthesia practice.

metabolite is inactive, water soluble, and rapidly excreted via the kidney.

Pharmacokinetics

The three benzodiazepines used in anesthesia are classified as short-lasting (midazolam), intermediate-lasting (lorazepam), and long-lasting (diazepam), according to their metabolism and plasma clearance (see Table 26-1). The plasma disappearance curves of all the benzodiazepines can be fitted to a two-compartment or three-compartment model. Protein binding and volumes of distribution are not much different among these three benzodiazepines, but the clearance is significantly different. The clearance rate of midazolam ranges from 6 to 11 mL/kg/min, whereas the clearance of lorazepam is 0.8 to 1.8 mL/kg/min, and the clearance of diazepam is 0.2 to 0.5 mL/kg/min. Because of these differences in clearance, the drugs have predictably different plasma disappearance curves (Fig. 26-9). They also have different context-sensitive half-times (see Fig. 26-3). Although the termination of action of these drugs is primarily a result of redistribution of the drug from the CNS to other tissues after use in anesthesia, after daily (long-term) repeated administration, or after prolonged continuous infusion, midazolam blood levels decrease more rapidly than blood levels of the other drugs because of greater hepatic clearance. Patients given continuous infusions of midazolam or repeated boluses over days should awaken faster than patients given diazepam or lorazepam.

Factors that may influence the pharmacokinetics of benzodiazepines are age, gender, race, enzyme induction, and hepatic and renal disease. Diazepam is sensitive to some of these factors, particularly age. Increasing age tends to reduce the clearance of diazepam[241] significantly and the clearance of midazolam to a lesser degree.[242] Lorazepam is resistant to the effects of age, gender, and renal disease on pharmacokinetics. These drugs all are affected by obesity. The volume of distribution is increased as drug goes from the plasma into the adipose tissue. Although clearance is not altered, elimination half-lives are prolonged, owing to the delayed return of the drug to the plasma in obese patients.[242] Generally, sensitivity to benzodiazepines in some groups, such as elderly patients, is greater despite relatively modest pharmacokinetic effects; factors other than pharmacokinetics must be considered when these drugs are used.

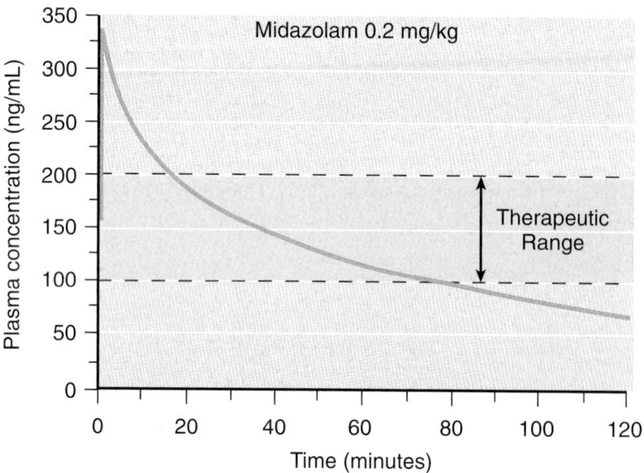

Figure 26-9 Simulated time course of plasma levels of midazolam after an induction dose of 0.2 mg/kg. Plasma levels required for hypnosis and amnesia during surgery are 100 to 200 ng/mL, with awakening usually occurring at levels less than 50 ng/mL.

Pharmacology

All benzodiazepines have hypnotic, sedative, anxiolytic, amnesic, anticonvulsant, and centrally produced muscle-relaxing properties. The drugs differ in their potency and efficacy with regard to each of the pharmacodynamic actions. The chemical structure of each drug dictates its particular physicochemical properties and pharmacokinetics and its receptor binding characteristics. The binding of benzodiazepines to their respective receptors is of high affinity and is stereospecific and saturable; the order of receptor affinity (potency) of the three agonists is lorazepam > midazolam > diazepam. Midazolam is approximately 3 to 6 times,[243] and lorazepam 5 to 10 times, as potent as diazepam.

The mechanism of action of benzodiazepines is reasonably well understood.[244-246] The interaction of ligands with the benzodiazepine receptor is one of the few examples in which the complex systems of biochemistry, molecular pharmacology, genetic mutations, and clinical behavioral patterns can be explained. More is understood about the mechanism of action of benzodiazepines than about the mechanism of action of many other general anesthetics. More recent genetic studies have found the $GABA_A$ subtypes mediate the different effects (amnesic, anticonvulsant, anxiolytic, and sleep).[246] Sedation, anterograde amnesia, and anticonvulsant properties are mediated via $\alpha 1$ receptors,[246] and anxiolysis and muscle relaxation are mediated by the *a2* $GABA_A$ receptor.[246] Drug effect is a function of blood level. By using plasma concentration data and pharmacokinetic simulations, it has been estimated that a benzodiazepine receptor occupancy of less than 20% may be sufficient to produce the anxiolytic effect, sedation is observed with 30% to 50% receptor occupancy, and unconsciousness requires 60% or greater occupation of benzodiazepine agonist receptors.[247]

The benzodiazepine receptors are found in highest densities in the olfactory bulb, cerebral cortex, cerebellum, hippocampus, substantia nigra, and inferior colliculus, but lower densities are found in the striatum, lower brainstem, and spinal cord. Spinal cord benzodiazepine receptors can play an important role in analgesia, however, further elucidating the mechanism of action of this drug class.[248,249] Intrathecal midazolam reduces excitatory GABA-mediated neurotransmission in interneurons, leading to a decrease in the excitability of spinal dorsal horn neurons.[248] Intrathecal midazolam added to a bupivacaine spinal increases analgesia and shortens the time to return of motor function.[249]

A fascinating and therapeutically significant discovery regarding the benzodiazepine receptor is that the pharmacologic spectrum of ligands includes three different types or classes,[244] which have been termed *agonists, antagonists,* and *inverse agonists* (Fig. 26-10), names that connote their actions. Agonists (e.g., midazolam) alter the conformation of the $GABA_A$ receptor complex so that binding affinity for GABA is increased, with a resultant opening of the chloride channel. Agonist and antagonist bind to a common (or at least overlapping) area of the receptor by forming differing reversible bonds with the receptor. The well-known effects of an agonist then occur (anxiolysis, hypnosis, and anticonvulsant action). Antagonists (e.g., flumazenil) occupy the

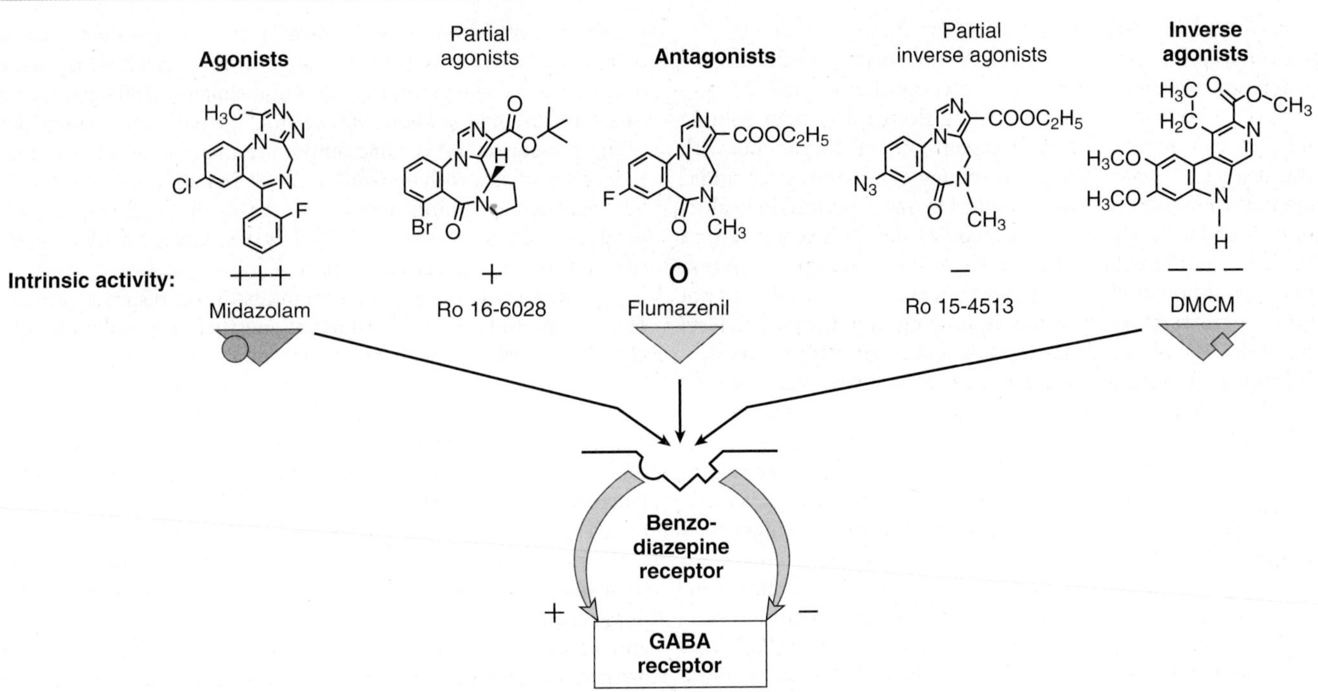

Figure 26-10 Spectrum of the intrinsic activities of benzodiazepine receptor ligands, which range from agonists to inverse agonists. Structures of agonist, partial agonist, antagonist, partial inverse agonist, and inverse agonist compounds are shown. Intrinsic activity is greatest among agonists and is least among inverse agonists. Intrinsic activities are schematically indicated as positive by a plus sign and as negative by a minus sign, with 0 indicating a lack of intrinsic activity. GABA, γ-aminobutyric acid. *(Redrawn with modification from Mohler H, Richards JG: The benzodiazepine receptor: A pharmacological control element of brain function. Eur J Anaesthesiol Suppl 2:15-24, 1988.)*

benzodiazepine receptor, but they produce no activity and block the actions of the agonists and inverse agonists. Inverse agonists reduce the efficiency of GABA-adrenergic synaptic transmission, and because GABA is inhibitory, the result of decreased GABA is CNS stimulation. The potency of the ligand is dictated by its affinity for the benzodiazepine receptor and the duration of effect by the rate of clearance of the drug from the receptor.

Long-term administration of benzodiazepines produces tolerance, which is defined as the decrease of efficacy of the drug over time.[250] Although the mechanism of chronic tolerance is not fully understood, it seems that long-term exposure to benzodiazepines causes decreased receptor binding and function (i.e., downregulation of the benzodiazepine–$GABA_A$ receptor complex). This would explain the increased dose requirements of benzodiazepines for anesthesia in patients who take them on a long-term basis. It seems that after the cessation of long-term use of benzodiazepines, there is upregulation of the receptor complex,[250] which could mean an increased susceptibility to benzodiazepines during a period after recent use.

The onset and duration of action of a bolus IV administration of a benzodiazepine depend on the lipid solubility of the drug, a finding that probably explains the differences in onset and duration of action of midazolam, diazepam, and lorazepam. Midazolam and diazepam have a more rapid onset (usually within 30 to 60 seconds) of action than lorazepam (60 to 120 seconds). The half-life of equilibrium between plasma concentration and EEG effect of midazolam is approximately 2 to 3 minutes and is not affected by age.[251] This is about two times longer[252] than that of diazepam, but compared with diazepam midazolam has a sixfold greater intrinsic potency.[243] Similar data for other benzodiazepines are unavailable. Similar to onset, the duration of effect also is related to lipid solubility and blood level. The more rapid redistribution of midazolam and diazepam compared with lorazepam (presumably because of the lower lipid solubility of lorazepam)[232] accounts for the shorter duration of their actions.

Effects on the Central Nervous System

The benzodiazepines, in a dose-related manner, reduce the $CMRO_2$ and CBF (see Chapters 13, 46, and 63). Midazolam and diazepam maintain a relatively normal ratio of CBF to $CMRO_2$. In healthy human volunteers, midazolam, 0.15 mg/kg, induces sleep and reduces CBF by 34%, despite a slight increase in $Paco_2$ from 34 to 39 mm Hg.[253] Brown and coworkers[254] studied EEG tracings after administration of 10 mg of IV midazolam and showed the appearance of rhythmic beta activity at 22 Hz within 15 to 30 seconds of administration in healthy volunteers. Within 60 seconds, there was a second beta rhythm at 15 Hz. Alpha rhythm started to reappear at 30 minutes; however, after 60 minutes, there was resistant rhythmic beta activity at 15- to 20-μV amplitude. The EEG changes were similar to EEG effects with diazepam and were not typical of light sleep, although the patients were clinically asleep.

Midazolam, diazepam, and lorazepam all increase the seizure initiation threshold to local anesthetics and decrease the mortality rate in mice exposed to lethal doses of local anesthetics.[255] Midazolam and diazepam cause a dose-related protective effect against cerebral hypoxia, shown by extending mouse survival time when mice were placed in 5% oxygen. The protection afforded by midazolam is superior to that of diazepam, but less than that of pentobarbital.[255] Antiemetic effects are not a prominent action of the benzodiazepines.

Effects on the Respiratory System

Benzodiazepines, similar to most IV anesthetics, produce dose-related central respiratory system depression. Lorazepam (2.5 mg) produces a similar but shorter lasting decrease in tidal volume and minute ventilation than diazepam (10 mg) in patients with lung disease.[256] Peak decrease in minute ventilation after midazolam (0.15 mg/kg) is almost identical to that produced in healthy patients given diazepam (0.3 mg/kg), as determined by carbon dioxide response data.[257] The slopes of the ventilatory response curves to carbon dioxide are flatter than normal (control), but not shifted to the right, as with opioids. Judging from the plasma level and steepness of the dose-response effect on $Paco_2$ curves,[258] midazolam is about five to nine times as potent as diazepam.

The peak onset of ventilatory depression with midazolam (0.13 to 0.2 mg/kg) is rapid (about 3 minutes), and significant depression remains for about 60 to 120 minutes.[224] The rate of midazolam administration affects the onset time of peak ventilatory depression; the faster the drug is given, the more quickly this peak depression occurs. The respiratory depression of midazolam is more pronounced and of longer duration in patients with chronic obstructive pulmonary disease, and the duration of ventilatory depression is longer with midazolam (0.19 mg/kg) than with thiopental (3.3 mg/kg).[224,259] Lorazepam (0.05 mg/kg) alone does not depress the carbon dioxide response, but when lorazepam is combined with meperidine, there is predictable respiratory depression.[259] Benzodiazepines and opioids produce additive or supra-additive (synergistic) respiratory depression, even though they act at different receptors.

Apnea occurs with benzodiazepines in a dose-dependent manner. The incidence of apnea after thiopental or midazolam when these drugs are given for induction of anesthesia is similar. Apnea occurred in 20% of 1130 patients given midazolam for induction and 27% of 580 patients given thiopental in clinical trials with midazolam.[230] Apnea is more likely to occur in the presence of opioids. Old age, debilitating disease, and other respiratory depressant drugs probably also increase the incidence and degree of respiratory depression and apnea with benzodiazepines.

Effects on the Cardiovascular System

The benzodiazepines used alone have modest hemodynamic effects. The hemodynamic changes reported with anesthetic induction doses of diazepam, midazolam, and lorazepam are shown in Table 26-2. These values represent the peak hemodynamic effect in the first 10 minutes after administration and are derived from studies of healthy subjects and patients with ischemic and valvular heart diseases.[260-264] The predominant hemodynamic change is a slight reduction in arterial blood pressure, resulting from a decrease in systemic vascular resistance. The mechanism by which benzodiazepines maintain relatively stable hemodynamics involves the preservation of homeostatic reflex mechanisms,[230] but there is evidence that the baroreflex is impaired by midazolam and diazepam.[265] Midazolam causes a slightly larger decrease in arterial blood pressure than the other benzodiazepines, but the hypotensive effect is minimal and about the same as seen with thiopental.[266] Despite the hypotension, midazolam, even in doses of 0.2 mg/kg, is safe and effective for induction of anesthesia even in patients with severe aortic stenosis (see Chapter 60).

The hemodynamic effects of midazolam and diazepam are dose related: the higher the plasma level, the greater the decrease in systemic blood pressure[258]; however, there is a plateau plasma drug effect above which little change in arterial blood pressure occurs. The plateau plasma level for midazolam is 100 ng/mL, and that for diazepam is about 900 ng/mL.[258] Heart rate, ventricular filling pressures, and cardiac output are maintained after induction of anesthesia with benzodiazepines. In patients with elevated left ventricular filling pressures, diazepam and midazolam produce a "nitroglycerin-like" effect by decreasing the filling pressure and increasing cardiac output.

The stresses of endotracheal intubation and surgery are not blocked by midazolam.[260] Adjuvant anesthetics, usually opioids, are often combined with benzodiazepines. The combination of benzodiazepines with opioids and nitrous oxide has been investigated in patients with ischemic and valvular heart diseases.[264,267] The addition of nitrous oxide to midazolam (0.2 mg/kg) and diazepam (0.5 mg/kg) has trivial hemodynamic consequences, whereas the combination of benzodiazepines with opioids does have a supra-additive effect. The combinations of benzodiazepines with opiates produce greater decreases in systemic blood pressure than does each drug alone. The mechanism for this synergistic hemodynamic effect is not completely understood, but it is probably related to a reduction in sympathetic tone when the drugs are given together.[268] There is evidence that diazepam and midazolam decrease catecholamines,[269] a finding consistent with this hypothesis.

Uses

Intravenous Sedation

Benzodiazepines are used for sedation as preoperative premedication, intraoperatively during regional or local anesthesia, and postoperatively. The anxiolysis, amnesia, and elevation of the local anesthetic seizure threshold are desirable benzodiazepine actions. The drugs should be given by titration for this use; end points of titration are adequate sedation or dysarthria (Table 26-7). The onset of action is more rapid with midazolam, usually with peak effect reached within 2 to 3 minutes of administration; time to peak effect is slightly longer with diazepam and is longer still with lorazepam. The duration of action of these drugs depends primarily on the dose used. Although the onset is more rapid with midazolam than with diazepam after bolus administration, the recovery is similar,[270] probably because both drugs have similar early plasma decay (redistribution) patterns (see Fig. 26-9). With lorazepam, sedation and particularly amnesia are slower in onset and are longer lasting than with the other two benzodiazepines.[238,271]

There is often a disparity in the level of sedation compared with the presence of amnesia (patients seem conscious and reasonably coherent, yet they are amnesic for events and instructions) with all three benzodiazepines. Lorazepam is particularly unpredictable with regard to duration of amnesia, and this is undesirable in patients who wish or need to have recall in the immediate postoperative period. The degree of sedation and the reliable amnesia and preservation of respiratory and hemodynamic function are better overall with benzodiazepines than with other sedative-hypnotic drugs used for conscious sedation. When midazolam is compared with propofol for sedation, the two are generally similar except that emergence or wake-up is more rapid with propofol. Propofol requires closer medical supervision because of its respiratory depression,[272] and respiratory function

Table 26-7 Uses and Doses of Intravenous Benzodiazepines

	Midazolam	Diazepam	Lorazepam
Induction	0.05-0.15 mg/kg	0.3-0.5 mg/kg	0.1 mg/kg
Maintenance	0.05 mg/kg prn 1 μg/kg/min	0.1 mg/kg prn	0.02 mg/kg prn
Sedation*	0.5-1 mg repeated 0.07 mg/kg IM	2 mg repeated	0.25 mg repeated

*Incremental doses given until desired degree of sedation is obtained.
prn, as required to keep patient hypnotic and amnestic.

must be monitored when these drugs are used for sedation to prevent undesirable degrees of respiratory depression. There may be a slight synergistic action between midazolam and spinal anesthesia with respect to ventilation.[273] The use of midazolam for sedation during regional and epidural anesthesia requires vigilance with regard to respiratory function, similar to when these drugs are given with opioids.

Sedation for longer periods, such as in the ICU, also is accomplished with benzodiazepines. Prolonged infusion results in accumulation of drug and, in the case of midazolam, significant concentration of the active metabolite. Reviews have pointed out concerns and advantages of benzodiazepine sedation.[238,274,275] The chief advantages are the amnesia and hemodynamic stability, and the disadvantage compared with propofol is the sometimes longer dissipation of effects when infusions are terminated. The superiority of one drug over the other has not been established; both drugs should always be titrated downward to maintain sedation as required. Dosing should not be fixed, but it should be reduced over time to avoid accumulation of parent or metabolites during prolonged infusion.

Finally, two more recent studies have challenged the idea that maternal sedation with midazolam may be unsafe for neonates and infants of breastfeeding mothers (see Chapter 69). Frolich and colleagues[276] showed that a single IV dose of midazolam (0.02 mg/kg) combined with a single IV dose of fentanyl (1 μg/kg) before cesarean section was a safe practice, showing no detriment in Apgar scores, neurobehavioral scores, continuous oxygen saturation, or the ability of the mother to recall the birth events.[276] Nitsun and associates[277] found that 0.005% of the maternal dose of midazolam is transferred into the breast milk during a 24-hour milk collection. Although verification of these findings is needed, they highlight an important clinical use of midazolam that may be safe for mother and infant.

Oral Sedation

For many years, diazepam was given orally for preoperative sedation. It is still used in 5- to 15-mg doses in adults for this purpose. More recently, an oral formulation of midazolam has been used primarily for oral premedication in pediatric patients (see Chapter 82). The dose is 0.5 mg/kg, and one preparation is from the Roche parenteral formulation of 0.5 mg/mL (Roche Laboratories, Inc, Nutley, NJ) mixed in with 10 mg/kg of oral acetaminophen (McNeil-PPC, Inc, Fort Washington, PA).[278] Other preparations have been developed, including strawberry-flavored glucose (pH 4.5) prepared by the pharmacy, which is stable for 8 weeks.[279] The 0.5-mg/kg oral dose is rapid-acting, providing reliable amnesia within 10 minutes and rendering children effectively sedated for anesthesia induction.[278]

Induction and Maintenance of Anesthesia

Midazolam is the benzodiazepine of choice to induce anesthesia. When midazolam is used in appropriate doses (see Table 26-7), induction occurs less rapidly than with thiopental,[230] but the amnesia is more reliable. Numerous factors influence the rapidity of action of midazolam and the other benzodiazepines when used for induction of general anesthesia, including dose, speed of injection, degree of premedication, age, ASA physical status, and concurrent anesthetic drugs.[230,280] In a well-premedicated, healthy patient, midazolam (0.2 mg/kg given in 5 to 15 seconds) induces anesthesia in 28 seconds, whereas induction occurs in 39 seconds with diazepam (0.5 mg/kg given in 5 to 15 seconds).[260] Elderly patients require smaller doses of midazolam than younger patients (Fig. 26-11).[281,282] Patients older than 55 years and patients with ASA physical status greater than III require a 20% or greater reduction in the induction dose of midazolam.[230] The usual induction dose of midazolam in premedicated patients is 0.05 to 0.15 mg/kg. When midazolam is used with other anesthetic drugs (coinduction), there is a synergistic interaction,[254,283] and the induction dose is less than 0.1 mg/kg (Fig. 26-12). The synergy is seen when midazolam is used with opioids or other hypnotics, such as thiopental and propofol.

Awakening after benzodiazepine anesthesia (defined as orientation to time and place) of young, healthy volunteers who received 10 mg of IV midazolam occurred in about 15 minutes,[254] and awakening occurred in about 17 minutes after an induction dose of 0.15 mg/kg.[284] Emergence time is related to the dose of midazolam and to the dose of adjuvant anesthetic drugs.[230] Emergence from midazolam (0.32 mg/kg)/fentanyl anesthesia is about 10 minutes longer than emergence from thiopental (4.75 mg/kg)/fentanyl anesthesia,[262] and is more prolonged than with propofol.[285] This difference accounts for some anesthesiologists' preference for propofol induction for short operations.

Benzodiazepines lack analgesic properties and must be used with other anesthetic drugs to provide sufficient analgesia; however, as maintenance anesthetic drugs during general anesthesia, benzodiazepines provide hypnosis and amnesia. Double-blind studies comparing midazolam and thiopental as the hypnotic component for balanced anesthesia[262,286] have shown that mida-

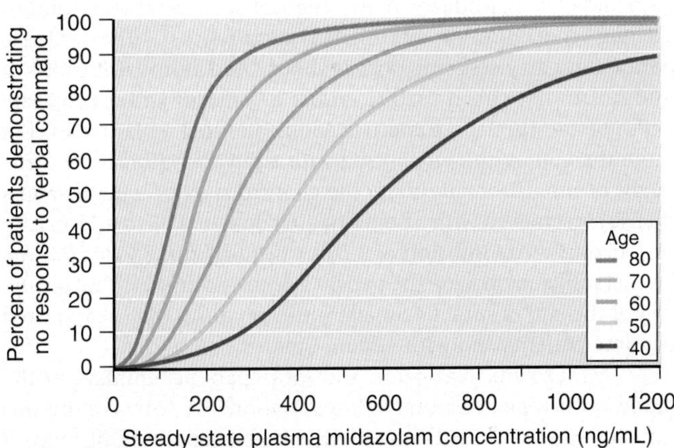

Figure 26-11 Simulated quantal concentration-response curves generated by the parameterized pharmacodynamic model for midazolam. *(Redrawn from Jacobs JR, Reves JG, Marty J, et al: Aging increases pharmacodynamic sensitivity to the hypnotic effects of midazolam. Anesth Analg 80:143-148, 1995.)*

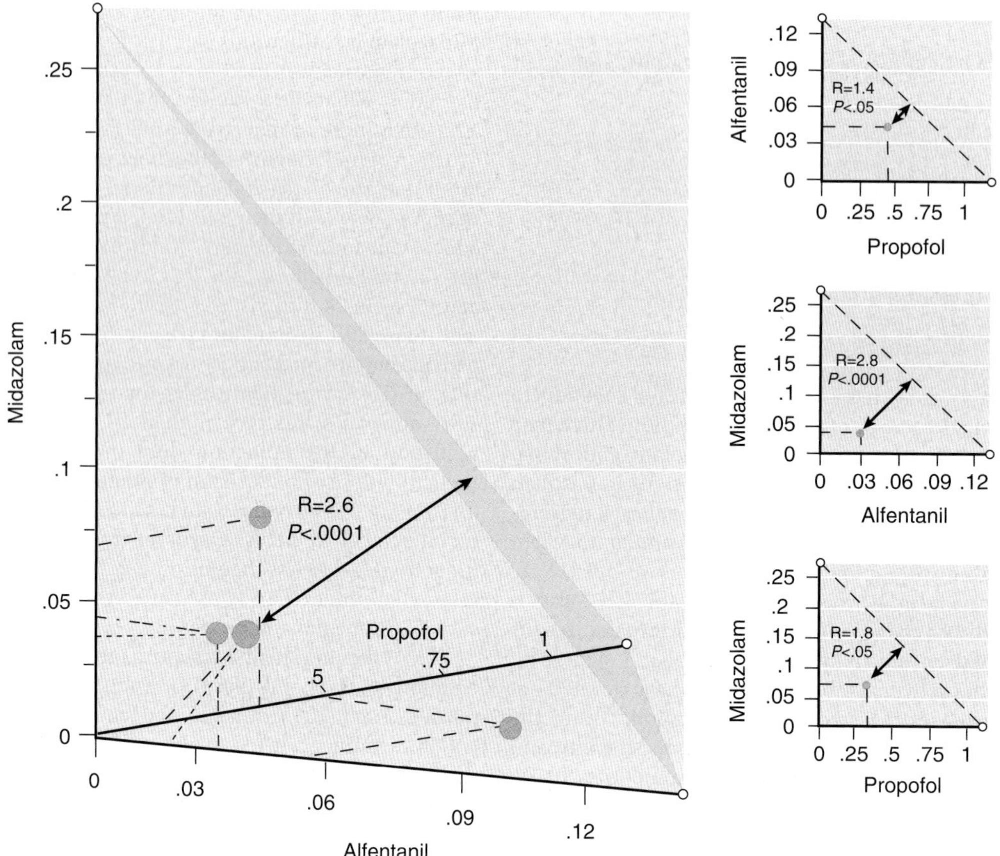

Figure 26-12 Vertical axes all represent drug dose in milligrams per kilogram. On the right, median effective dose (ED_{50}) isobolograms for the hypnotic interactions among midazolam, alfentanil, and propofol are shown. The *dotted lines* are additive effect lines; all combinations fall within the line representing synergism or supra-additive effect. On the left, a triple interaction is depicted. The *shaded area* represents an additive plane passing through three single-drug ED_{50} points (*small open circles*). The largest *closed circle* (with *arrows*) is the ED_{50} point for the triple combination. The smaller *closed circles* are ED_{50} points for the binary combinations. R ratios on all graphs represent the interaction (1.0 indicates an additive effect) of the various drug combinations. The combination of midazolam and alfentanil produces the greatest synergism, but the combination of all three also is synergistic. *P* values denote the significance of the additive effects. *(Redrawn with modification from Vinik HR, Bradley EL Jr, Kissin I: Triple anesthetic combination: Propofol-midazolam-alfentanil. Anesth Analg 76:S450, 1993.)*

zolam is superior for this use because of better amnesia and a smoother hemodynamic course. Opioid requirements are less with midazolam. Midazolam (0.6 mg/kg) decreases the minimum alveolar concentration of inhaled anesthetics.[287] The amnesic period after an anesthetic dose is about 1 to 2 hours. Infusions of midazolam have been used to ensure a constant and appropriate depth of anesthesia.[287] Experience indicates that a plasma level of more than 50 ng/mL when used with adjuvant opioids (e.g., fentanyl) or inhalation anesthetics (e.g., nitrous oxide, volatile anesthetics) is achieved with a bolus loading dose of 0.05 to 0.15 mg/kg and a continuous infusion of 0.25 to 1 µg/kg/min.[283] This plasma level is sufficient to keep the patient asleep and amnesic but arousable at the end of surgery. Smaller infusion doses may be required in some patients and with certain opioids.

Midazolam, diazepam, and lorazepam accumulate in the blood with repeated bolus administrations or with continuous infusion, just as most IV anesthetics do on repeated injection. If the benzodiazepines do accumulate with repeated administrations, prolonged arousal time can be anticipated. This is less of a problem with midazolam than with diazepam and lorazepam because of the shorter context-sensitive half-time and greater clearance of midazolam.

Nausea and Vomiting Prophylaxis

Numerous studies in the past several years have highlighted the role that benzodiazepines, specifically midazolam, may play in the prevention of PONV (see Chapter 86). Jung and colleagues[288] found that in women undergoing middle ear surgery, IV midazolam, 0.075 mg/kg after induction, reduced the incidence of PONV and the need for rescue antiemetics with no difference from placebo in pain intensity or drowsiness. Similarly, Lee and associates[289] found no difference in the incidence of PONV after minor gynecologic or urologic surgery when comparing IV ondansetron, 4 mg, and IV midazolam, 2 mg. Finally, Riad and colleagues[289a] effectively illustrated that IV midazolam, 0.05 mg/kg, reduces PONV after pediatric (4 to 12 years old) strabismus surgery compared with placebo or IV dexamethasone, 0.5 mg/kg. No child vomited with midazolam alone or with the midazolam-dexamethasone combination.

Side Effects and Contraindications

Benzodiazepines have limited allergenic effects and do not suppress the adrenal gland.[290] The most significant problem with midazolam is respiratory depression. The major side effects of lorazepam and diazepam in addition to respiratory depression are venous irritation and thrombophlebitis, problems related to aqueous insolubility and requisite solvents.[230] When used as sedatives or for induction and maintenance of anesthesia, benzodiazepines can produce an undesirable degree or prolonged interval of postoperative amnesia, sedation, and, rarely, respiratory depression. These residual effects can be reversed with flumazenil.

Flumazenil

Flumazenil (Anexate, Romazicon) is the first benzodiazepine antagonist approved for clinical use.[291] Preclinical pharmacologic studies with flumazenil revealed it to be a benzodiazepine receptor ligand with high affinity, great specificity, and by definition minimal intrinsic effect. Flumazenil, similar to the agonists it replaces at the benzodiazepine receptor, interacts with the receptor in a concentration-dependent manner. Because it is a competitive antagonist at the benzodiazepine receptor, its antagonism is reversible and surmountable. Flumazenil has minimal intrinsic activity,[292] which means that its benzodiazepine receptor agonist effects are very weak, significantly less than those of clinical agonists. Flumazenil, similar to all competitive antagonists at receptors, does not displace the agonist, but rather occupies the receptor when an agonist dissociates from the receptor. The half-time (or half-life) of a receptor-ligand bond is a few milliseconds to a few seconds, and new ligand receptor bonds are immediately formed. This dynamic situation accounts for the ability of either an agonist or an antagonist to occupy the receptor readily.

The ratio of agonist to total receptors produces the effects of the agonist drug, but the antagonist can alter this ratio, depending on its concentration and dissociation constant. Flumazenil, which is an avid (high-affinity) ligand, replaces a relatively weak agonist, such as diazepam, as long as it is given in sufficient dose. Flumazenil is cleared rapidly, however, and the proportion of receptors occupied by agonist increases, and the potential for resedation exists (Fig. 26-13). This situation is less likely to occur when flumazenil is used to reverse midazolam, which has a more rapid clearance than other benzodiazepine agonists. Another important finding is that in the presence of extremely high doses of agonist (e.g., when a mistake in dosing has occurred, or suicide is attempted), flumazenil in a low dose attenuates the deep CNS depression (loss of consciousness, respiratory depression) by reducing the fractional receptor occupancy by the agonist without decreasing the agonist effects that occur at low fractional receptor occupancy (drowsiness, amnesia).

Conversely, large doses of flumazenil in the presence of small doses of agonist completely reverse virtually all the agonist effects. Flumazenil can precipitate withdrawal symptoms in animals or in humans physically dependent on a benzodiazepine receptor agonist.[293,294] This is not a problem when flumazenil is used to reverse benzodiazepine receptor agonists in anesthesia.

Physicochemical Characteristics

Flumazenil, synthesized in 1979, is similar to midazolam and other classic benzodiazepines except for the absence of the phenyl group, which is replaced by a carbonyl group (see Fig. 26-8).[295] It

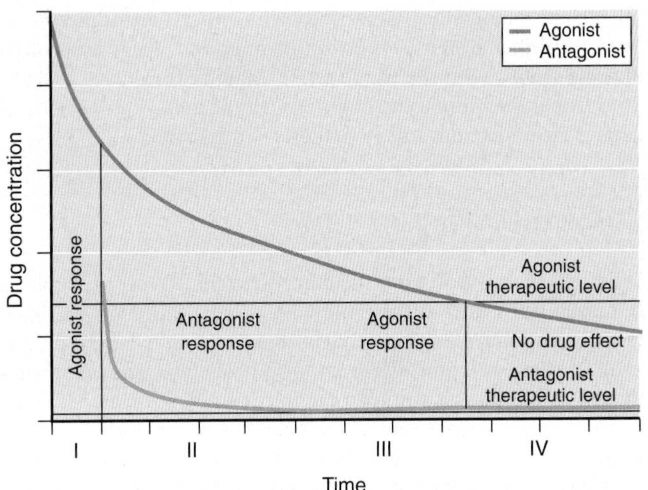

Figure 26-13 Schematic representation of the interaction of a short-acting antagonist with a longer acting agonist resulting in resedation. The *upper curve* shows disappearance of agonist from blood, and the *lower curve* shows disappearance of antagonist from plasma. Four conditions are represented: I, agonist response; II, antagonist response (the antagonist reverses the agonist effect); III, agonist response (resedation or resumption of agonist response with disappearance of short-lasting antagonist); and IV, no drug effect, with disappearance of agonist and antagonist (both drugs are below the therapeutic level).

forms a colorless, crystalline powder; has a dissociation constant of 1.7; and has weak but sufficient water solubility to permit its preparation in aqueous solution. Its octanol/aqueous buffer partition coefficient is 14, showing moderate lipid solubility at pH 7.4.[295]

Metabolism

Flumazenil, similar to the other benzodiazepines, is metabolized in the liver; is rapidly cleared from the plasma; and has three known metabolites, *N*-desmethylflumazenil, *N*-desmethylflumazenil acid, and flumazenil acid.[296] The activities of these metabolites and their corresponding glucuronides are unknown at present. The glucuronides probably are excreted in the urine.

Pharmacokinetics

Flumazenil is a short-lived compound. Table 26-1 includes a summary of its pharmacokinetics, which are described in various clinical settings.[251,296] Compared with benzodiazepine receptor agonists, flumazenil has the most rapid clearance and shortest elimination half-life. The plasma half-life of flumazenil is about 1 hour—it is the shortest lived of all benzodiazepines used in anesthetic practice. The potential exists for the antagonist to be cleared, leaving sufficient concentrations of agonist at the receptor site to cause resedation.[293] To maintain a constant therapeutic blood level over a prolonged time, either repeated administration or a continuous infusion is required. An infusion rate of 30 to 60 μg/min (0.5 to 1 μg/kg/min) has been used for this purpose.[297] The rapid blood clearance of flumazenil approaches hepatic blood flow, a finding that indicates that liver clearance partially depends on hepatic blood flow. Compared with other benzodiazepines, flumazenil has a high proportion of unbound drug; its protein binding is low, with the free fraction ranging from 54% to 64%. This property of flumazenil could contribute to its rapid onset and greater clearance, but this hypothesis is unproved.

Pharmacology

When given in the absence of a benzodiazepine receptor agonist, flumazenil has little discernible CNS effect. Although intrinsic (agonist and inverse agonist) effects have been ascribed to flumazenil,[292] they are clinically unimportant. It has been postulated that in small doses a stimulating effect can be seen, and in high doses a central depressant effect becomes more likely.[298] When given to volunteers and patients in clinically relevant doses, flumazenil has no effect on the EEG or cerebral metabolism.[251,299] In animals, flumazenil has no anticonvulsant properties, and reverses the anticonvulsant properties of benzodiazepines in local anesthetic–induced seizures.[300]

When administered to patients who have benzodiazepine-induced CNS depression, flumazenil produces rapid and dependable reversal of unconsciousness, respiratory depression, sedation, amnesia, and psychomotor dysfunction.[247] Flumazenil can be given before, during, or after the agonist to block or reverse the CNS effects of the agonist. The usual clinical need is to reverse the effects of agonists given before flumazenil. Flumazenil has successfully reversed the effects of midazolam, diazepam, lorazepam, and flunitrazepam. The onset is rapid, with peak effect occurring in 1 to 3 minutes,[247] which coincides with the detection of C-flumazenil in human brain.[301] Flumazenil reverses the agonist by replacing it at the benzodiazepine receptor, and its onset and duration are governed by the law of mass action. A predicted therapeutic plasma level for flumazenil is 20 ng/mL because the relative binding characteristics of agonist and antagonist in part dictate benzodiazepine receptor occupation by the residual agonist, and different doses and plasma levels of flumazenil are required to reverse the effects of particular agonists.

Flumazenil is devoid of the respiratory and cardiovascular depressant effects of benzodiazepine receptor agonists. A large dose of flumazenil (0.1 mg/kg) given to volunteers did not produce significant respiratory depression.[302] When flumazenil is given in the presence of agonists, however, there are significant respiratory effects because it reverses respiratory depression caused by the agonists (e.g., when given to volunteers made apneic with midazolam).[303] The reversal of midazolam-induced (0.13 mg/kg) respiratory depression with flumazenil (1 mg) lasts 3 to 30 minutes. Other agonists and other doses would have different durations of antagonism of respiratory depression. If respiratory depression is related to opioid administration, flumazenil would not reverse it.[304]

Incremental doses, up to 3 mg intravenously, in patients with ischemic heart disease had no significant effect on cardiovascular variables.[303] Administration of flumazenil to patients given agonists is remarkably free of cardiovascular effects,[247,305] in contrast to the experience of opioid reversal with naloxone. Of particular interest is the effect on plasma catecholamines of benzodiazepine receptor agonist reversal with flumazenil because this effect on catecholamines is the suspected mechanism of hyperdynamic response in opioid reversal. Although flumazenil does reverse sedation, it is not associated with significantly higher catecholamines than are found in patients receiving saline,[305] but the increase in catecholamines that accompanies arousal is more rapid after flumazenil.[306]

Table 26-8 Uses and Doses of Flumazenil

Reversal of benzodiazepines*	0.2 mg repeated† up to 3 mg
Diagnosis in coma	0.5 mg repeated up to 1 mg

*The dose required to reverse each benzodiazepine (BZD) depends on residual BZD and the particular BZD (i.e., higher doses are required for more potent BZDs) (see text).

†The degree of reversal should be titrated by repeating 0.2-mg increments every 1-2 min until desired level of reversal is achieved.

Uses and Doses

Uses for a benzodiazepine antagonist (Table 26-8) include the diagnostic and therapeutic reversal of the effects of benzodiazepine receptor agonists. For diagnostic use in suspected benzodiazepine overdose, flumazenil may be given in incremental IV doses of 0.2 to 0.5 mg up to 3 mg. If there is no change in CNS sedation, it is unlikely that CNS depression is based solely on benzodiazepine overdose. More commonly in anesthesia, flumazenil is used to reverse the residual sedation of a patient after administration of a benzodiazepine for conscious sedation or for general anesthesia.

Flumazenil reliably reverses the sedation, respiratory depression, and amnesia of benzodiazepines. There is now evidence, however, of differential reversal effects on the different agonist actions. Flumazenil tends to reverse the hypnotic and respiratory effects more than the amnesic effects of the agonist benzodiazepine.[304,307] Dosage guidelines are given in Table 26-8, but large-scale dosing studies have not been performed yet. The dose varies with the particular benzodiazepine being reversed, and the duration of reversal depends on the kinetics of the agonist and of flumazenil. Surveillance is recommended if a long-lasting benzodiazepine is reversed with a single administration of flumazenil because of the relatively short-lived effect. Flumazenil may be administered by continuous infusion to prevent resedation with longer lasting benzodiazepine receptor agonists.

Side Effects and Contraindications

Flumazenil has been given in large oral and IV doses with remarkably few toxic reactions.[247] It is free of local or tissue irritant properties, and there are no known organotoxicities. Similar to all benzodiazepines, it apparently has a high safety margin, probably higher than the safety margins of agonists, because it does not produce prominent CNS depression. An important caution is that resedation could occur because of the relatively short half-life of the drug.

Phencyclidines (Ketamine)

History

Phencyclidine was the first drug of its class to be used for anesthesia, but had unacceptable side effects. Ketamine (Ketalar) was

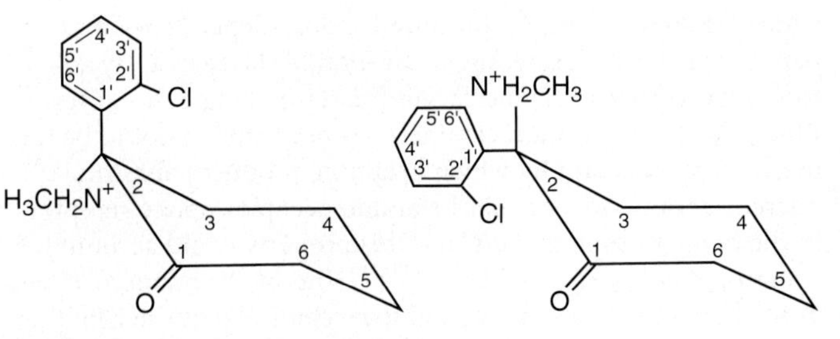

S$_1$(+) Ketamine hydrochloride R$_1$(−) Ketamine hydrochloride

Figure 26-14 Stereoisomers of ketamine as it is formulated.

synthesized in 1962 by Stevens and was first used in humans in 1965 by Corssen and Domino. Ketamine was released for clinical use in 1970 and is still used in various clinical settings. Ketamine differs from most other drugs used to induce anesthesia because it has a significant analgesic effect. It usually does not depress the cardiovascular and respiratory systems,[308] but it does possess some of the adverse psychological effects found with the other phencyclidines. Ketamine consists of two stereoisomers, S(+) and R(−). The S(+) is more potent and is associated with fewer side effects. Interest in ketamine has increased more recently because of its effects on hyperalgesia and opiate tolerance, use in chronic pain states, potential neuroprotective effects, increasing popularity of total IV anesthesia, and the availability (in some countries) of S(+) ketamine.

Physicochemical Characteristics

Ketamine (Fig. 26-14) has a molecular weight of 238 kD, is partially water soluble, and forms a white crystalline salt with a pK_a of 7.5.[308] It has a lipid solubility 5 to 10 times that of thiopental.[309]

Metabolism

Ketamine is metabolized by hepatic microsomal enzymes. The major pathway involves *N*-demethylation to form norketamine (metabolite I), which is then hydroxylated to hydroxynorketamine. These products are conjugated to water-soluble glucuronide derivatives and are excreted in the urine.[308] The activity of the principal metabolites of ketamine has not been well studied, but norketamine (metabolite I) has significantly less (20% to 30%) activity than the parent compound. More recent modeling of norketamine suggests that it does contribute in prolonging the analgesia provided by either a bolus or infusion of ketamine.[310]

Pharmacokinetics

Ketamine pharmacokinetics have been examined after bolus administration of anesthetizing doses (2 to 2.5 mg/kg),[311] after a subanesthetic dose (0.25 mg/kg),[311,312] and after continuous infusion (steady-state plasma level 2000 ng/mL). Regardless of the dose, ketamine plasma disappearance can be described by a two-compartment model.[311] Table 26-1 contains the pharmacokinetic values from bolus administration studies. Of note is the rapid distribution reflected in the relatively brief distribution half-life of 11 to 16 minutes (Fig. 26-15). The high lipid solubility of ketamine is reflected in its large volume of distribution, nearly 3 L/kg. Clearance also is high, 890 to 1227 mL/min, which accounts for the short elimination half-life of 2 to 3 hours. The mean total body clearance (1.4 L/min) is approximately equal to liver blood flow, which means that changes in liver blood flow affect clearance. Low-dose alfentanil increases the volume of distribution and clearance of ketamine. In addition, alfentanil increases the distribution of ketamine into the brain.[313] The pharmacokinetic model of Clements[311] provided the best accuracy when used to administer low-dose ketamine to volunteers using a target-controlled infusion device.[314]

The pharmacokinetics of the two isomers is different. S(+) ketamine has a larger elimination clearance and larger volume of distribution than R(−) ketamine.[315] When the pharmacokinetics of S(+) ketamine was tested in a target-controlled infusion device for procedures of 1 hour and in combination with propofol, the authors found that the accuracy of the pharmacokinetic parameters was improved with a much smaller Vc (167 mL/kg). They also noted that ketamine clearance was not normally distributed, and this was not related to age.[316] The S(+) enantiomer also seems to be more potent in suppressing the EEG than either R(−) or the racemic mixture.[317]

Ketamine is increasingly being given by alternative routes, especially orally and via an intranasal spray. Administration by either of these routes is subject to significant first-pass metabolism. The bioavailability via oral administration is 20% to 30%, and via the intranasal route is approximately 40% to 50%.[318]

Pharmacology

Effects on the Central Nervous System

Ketamine produces dose-related unconsciousness and analgesia. The anesthetized state has been termed *dissociative anesthesia* because patients who receive ketamine alone appear to be in a cataleptic state, in contrast with other states of anesthesia that resemble normal sleep. Patients anesthetized with ketamine have

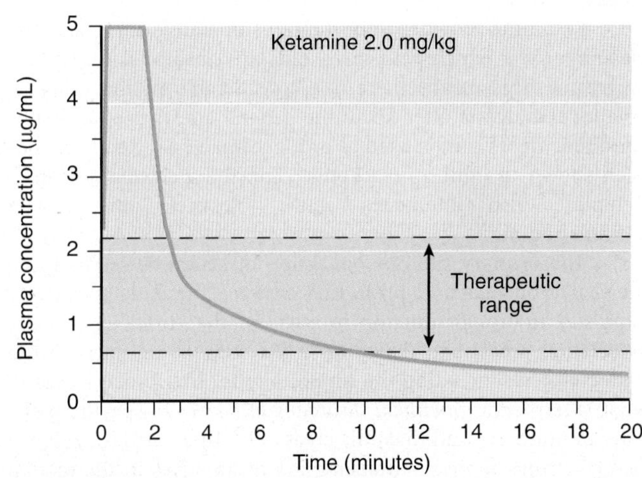

Figure 26-15 Simulated time course of plasma levels of ketamine after an induction dose of 2 mg/kg. Plasma levels required for hypnosis and amnesia during surgery are 0.7 to 2.2 µg/mL, with awakening usually occurring at levels less than 0.5 µg/mL.

profound analgesia, but keep their eyes open and maintain many reflexes. Corneal, cough, and swallow reflexes all may be present, but should not be assumed to be protective. There is no recall of surgery or anesthesia, but amnesia is not as prominent with ketamine as with the benzodiazepines. Because ketamine has a low molecular weight, a pK_a near the physiologic pH, and relatively high lipid solubility, it crosses the blood-brain barrier rapidly and has an onset of action within 30 to 60 seconds of administration. The maximal effect occurs in about 1 minute.

After ketamine administration, pupils dilate moderately, and nystagmus occurs. Lacrimation and salivation are common, as is increased skeletal muscle tone, often with coordinated but seemingly purposeless movements of the arms, legs, trunk, and head. Although there is great interindividual variability, plasma levels of 0.6 to 2 μg/mL are considered the minimum concentrations for general anesthesia; children may require slightly higher plasma levels (0.8 to 4 μg/mL).[319] The duration of ketamine anesthesia after a single IV administration of a general anesthetic dose (2 mg/kg) is 10 to 15 minutes (see Fig. 26-15), and full orientation to person, place, and time occurs within 15 to 30 minutes.

The S(+) enantiomer enables quicker recovery (by a couple of minutes) than the racemic mixture.[320,321] This is thought to be due to the lower dose necessary to produce an equianesthetic effect and to the 10% faster hepatic biotransformation.[321]

The duration of ketamine anesthesia is determined by the dose; larger doses produce more prolonged anesthesia, and the concurrent use of other anesthetics prolongs the time of emergence. Because there is a good correlation between blood level of ketamine and CNS effect, it seems that the relatively short duration of action of ketamine is due to its redistribution from the brain and blood to the other tissues in the body. The termination of effect after a single bolus administration of ketamine is caused by drug redistribution from the well-perfused to the less well-perfused tissues. Concomitant administration of benzodiazepines, a common practice, may prolong the effect of ketamine.[322] When used in combination with a benzodiazepine, the S(+) enantiomer was no different in terms of awareness at 30 minutes, but it was significantly better at 120 minutes than the racemic mixture.[323] Analgesia occurs at considerably lower blood levels than loss of consciousness.

Ketamine provides important postoperative analgesia. The plasma level at which pain thresholds are elevated is 0.1 μg/mL or greater. This means there is a considerable period of postoperative analgesia after ketamine general anesthesia, and subanesthetic doses can be used to produce analgesia. Ketamine has been shown to inhibit nociceptive central hypersensitization.[324] Ketamine also attenuates acute tolerance after opiate administration.[325]

The primary site of CNS action of ketamine seems to be the thalamoneocortical projection system. The drug selectively depresses neuronal function in parts of the cortex (especially association areas) and thalamus, while stimulating parts of the limbic system, including the hippocampus. This process creates what is termed a *functional disorganization* of nonspecific pathways in midbrain and thalamic areas.[326,327] There also is evidence that ketamine depresses transmission of impulses in the medial medullary reticular formation, which is important for transmission of the affective-emotional components of nociception from the spinal cord to higher brain centers.[328] In volunteers experiencing heat pain, functional magnetic resonance imaging (MRI) studies showed ketamine produced a dose-dependent effect on pain processing by decreasing activation of the secondary somatosensory cortex (S2), insula, and anterior cingulate cortex.[329] Blockade of CNS sodium channels has been shown not to be the mechanism of action by which ketamine produces anesthesia.[330] There is some evidence that ketamine occupies opiate receptors in the brain and spinal cord, and this property could account for some of the analgesic effects.[179,308,331] The S(+) enantiomer has been shown to have some opioid μ-receptor activity, accounting for part of its analgesic effect.[332] NMDA receptor interaction may mediate the general anesthetic effects and some analgesic actions of ketamine.[333,334] The spinal cord analgesic effect of ketamine is postulated to be due to inhibition of dorsal horn wide dynamic range neuronal activity.[335] Although some drugs have been used to antagonize ketamine, no specific receptor antagonist is yet known that reverses all the CNS effects of ketamine.

Ketamine increases cerebral metabolism, CBF, and ICP (see Chapter 63). Because of its excitatory CNS effects, which can be detected by generalized EEG development of theta wave activity and by petit mal seizure–like activity in the hippocampus,[336] ketamine increases $CMRO_2$. Although theta wave activity signals the analgesic activity of ketamine, alpha waves indicate its absence. There is an increase in CBF, which appears higher than the increase in $CMRO_2$ would mandate. With the increase in CBF and the generalized increase in sympathetic nervous system response, there is an increase in ICP after ketamine.[337,338] The increase in $CMRO_2$ and CBF can be blocked by the use of thiopental[339] or diazepam.[337,338] Cerebrovascular responsiveness to carbon dioxide seems to be preserved with ketamine; reducing $Paco_2$ attenuates the increase in ICP after ketamine.[337]

In animal models of incomplete cerebral ischemia and reperfusion, ketamine reduces necrosis and improves neurologic outcome.[340] Decreased sympathetic tone and inhibition of NMDA receptor–mediated ion currents were believed to mediate the reduction of necrotic cell death. More recently, S (+) ketamine was found to influence the expression of apoptosis-regulating proteins in rat brains 4 hours after cerebral ischemia/reperfusion.[341] The neuroprotection observed with ketamine may involve anti-apoptotic mechanisms in addition to reducing necrotic cell death.

In contrast, ketamine or other NMDA receptor antagonists accentuate apoptosis in the newborn brain of animals.[342] This has been shown with other anesthetics either at high relative doses or with prolonged exposure. This finding has sparked controversy over the use of ketamine in neonates. An editorial in the journal *Anesthesiology* and the Anesthetic and Life Support Drugs Advisory Committee of the U.S. FDA cautioned changing clinical practice based on present available data.[343]

Ketamine, similar to other phencyclidines, produces undesirable psychological reactions, which occur during awakening from ketamine anesthesia and are termed *emergence reactions*. The common manifestations of these reactions, which vary in severity and classification, are vivid dreaming, extracorporeal experiences (sense of floating out of body), and illusions (misinterpretation of a real, external sensory experience).[344] These incidents of dreaming and illusion are often associated with excitement, confusion, euphoria, and fear.[345] They occur in the first hour of emergence and usually abate within 1 to several hours. It has been postulated that the psychic emergence reactions occur secondary to ketamine-induced depression of auditory and visual relay nuclei, leading to misperception or misinterpretation of auditory and visual stimuli.[308] The incidence ranges from 3%[179,308] to 100%.[344] A clinically relevant range is probably 10% to 30% of adult patients who receive ketamine as a sole or major part of the anesthetic technique.

Factors that affect the incidence of emergence reactions are age,[346] dose,[179] gender, psychological susceptibility,[347] and concurrent drugs. Pediatric patients do not report as high an incidence of unpleasant emergence reactions as do adult patients; men also report a lower incidence compared with women. Larger doses and rapid administration of large doses seem to predispose patients to a higher incidence of adverse effects.[348,349] Finally, certain personality types seem prone to the development of emergence reactions. Patients who score high in psychotism on the Eysenck Personality Inventory are prone to develop emergence reactions,[347] and individuals who commonly dream at home are more likely to have postoperative dreams in the hospital after ketamine.[348] Numerous drugs have been used to reduce the incidence and severity of postoperative reactions to ketamine[179,308]; the benzodiazepines seem to be the most effective group of drugs to attenuate or to treat ketamine emergence reactions. Midazolam,[308] lorazepam,[350] and diazepam[351] are useful in reducing reactions to ketamine. Midazolam reduces the psychotomimetic effect of the S (+) enantiomer.[352]

Effects on the Respiratory System

Ketamine has minimal effects on the central respiratory drive as reflected by an unaltered response to carbon dioxide.[353] There can be a transient (1 to 3 minutes) decrease in minute ventilation after the bolus administration of an induction dose of ketamine (2 mg/kg intravenously). Unusually large doses can produce apnea,[354] but this is seldom seen. Arterial blood gases generally are preserved when ketamine is used alone for anesthesia or analgesia. With the use of adjuvant sedatives or anesthetic drugs, however, respiratory depression can occur. Ketamine has been shown to affect ventilatory control in children and should be considered a possible respiratory depressant when the drug is given to them in bolus doses.[355]

Ketamine is a bronchial smooth muscle relaxant. When it is given to patients with reactive airway disease and bronchospasm, pulmonary compliance is improved.[356] Ketamine is as effective as halothane or enflurane in preventing experimentally induced bronchospasm.[357] The mechanism for this effect is probably a result of the sympathomimetic response to ketamine, but there are isolated bronchial smooth muscle studies showing that ketamine can directly antagonize the spasmogenic effects of carbachol and histamine.[358] Owing to its bronchodilating effect, ketamine has been used to treat status asthmaticus unresponsive to conventional therapy.[359]

A potential respiratory problem, especially in children (see Chapter 82), is the increased salivation that follows ketamine administration. This increased salivation can produce upper airway obstruction, which can be complicated further by laryngospasm. The increased secretions also may contribute to or may complicate further laryngospasm. In addition, although swallow, cough, sneeze, and gag reflexes are relatively intact after ketamine administration, there is evidence that silent aspiration can occur during ketamine anesthesia.

Effects on the Cardiovascular System

Ketamine also has unique cardiovascular effects; it stimulates the cardiovascular system and is usually associated with increases in blood pressure, heart rate, and cardiac output (see Table 26-2). Other anesthetic induction drugs either cause no change in hemodynamic variables or produce vasodilation with cardiac depression. The S(+) enantiomer, despite hope that reducing the dose by half (equianesthetic potency) would attenuate side effects, is equivalent to the racemic mixture regarding hemodynamic response.[352] The increase in hemodynamic variables is associated with increased work and myocardial oxygen consumption. The healthy heart is able to increase oxygen supply by increased cardiac output and decreased coronary vascular resistance, so that coronary blood flow is appropriate for the increased oxygen consumption.[360] The hemodynamic changes are not related to the dose of ketamine (e.g., there is no hemodynamic difference between IV administration of 0.5 mg/kg and 1.5 mg/kg).[361] A second dose of ketamine produces hemodynamic effects less than or even opposite to the effects of the first dose.[362]

The hemodynamic changes after anesthesia induction with ketamine tend to be the same in healthy patients and in patients with various acquired or congenital heart diseases.[361] In patients with congenital heart disease, there are no significant changes in shunt directions or fraction[363] or systemic oxygenation after ketamine induction of anesthesia.[364] In patients who have elevated pulmonary artery pressure (as with mitral valvular and some congenital lesions), ketamine seems to cause a more pronounced increase in pulmonary than systemic vascular resistance.[363]

The mechanism by which ketamine stimulates the circulatory system remains enigmatic. It seems not to be a peripheral mechanism such as baroreflex inhibition, but rather to be central. There is some evidence that ketamine attenuates baroreceptor function via an effect on NMDA receptors in the nucleus tractus solitarius.[365] Ketamine injected directly into the CNS produces an immediate sympathetic nervous system hemodynamic response.[366] Ketamine also causes the sympathoneuronal release of norepinephrine, which can be detected in venous blood. Blockade of this effect is possible with barbiturates, benzodiazepines, and droperidol.[367] Ketamine in vitro probably has negative inotropic effects. Myocardial depression has been shown in chronically instrumented dogs,[368] and isolated canine heart preparations.[369] In isolated guinea pig hearts, ketamine was the least depressant of all the major induction drugs, however.[370] The finding that ketamine may exert its myocardial effects by acting on myocardial ionic currents (which may exert different effects from species to species or among tissue types) may explain the tissue and animal model variances in direct myocardial action.[371]

The centrally mediated sympathetic responses to ketamine usually override the direct depressant effects of ketamine. Some peripheral nervous system actions of ketamine play an undetermined role in the hemodynamic effects of the drug. Ketamine inhibits intraneuronal uptake of catecholamines in a cocaine-like effect,[160,161] and inhibits extraneuronal norepinephrine uptake.[372]

Stimulation of the cardiovascular system is not always desirable, and certain pharmacologic methods have been used to block the ketamine-induced tachycardia and systemic hypertension. Successful methods include use of adrenergic antagonists (α and β), various vasodilators,[373] and clonidine.[374] Probably the most fruitful approach has been prior administration of benzodiazepines. Modest doses of diazepam, flunitrazepam, and midazolam all attenuate the hemodynamic effects of ketamine. It also is possible to decrease the tachycardia and hypertension caused by ketamine by using a continuous infusion technique with or without a benzodiazepine.[375] Inhalation anesthetics[376] and propofol blunt the hemodynamic effect of ketamine. Ketamine can produce hemodynamic depression in the setting of deep anesthesia, when sympathetic responses do not accompany its administration.

Uses

The many unique features of ketamine pharmacology, especially its propensity to produce unwanted emergence reactions, have limited its use for routine anesthesia. Nevertheless, ketamine has an important niche in the practice of anesthesiology when its unique sympathomimetic activity and bronchodilating capabilities are indicated during induction of anesthesia. It is used for premedication, sedation, induction, and maintenance of general anesthesia (Table 26-9). There has been increased interest in the routine use of ketamine in small doses (20 to 60 mg) for preventive analgesia and for the treatment or prevention of opiate tolerance and hyperalgesia.

Induction and Maintenance of Anesthesia

Most candidates for ketamine induction are poor-risk patients (ASA class IV) with respiratory and cardiovascular system disorders (excluding ischemic heart disease), in particular, patients with reactive airway disease or patients with hemodynamic compromise based on either hypovolemia or cardiomyopathy (not coronary artery disease). Ketamine bronchodilation and profound analgesia allowing the use of high oxygen concentrations make ketamine an excellent choice for induction in patients with reactive airway disease. Otherwise healthy trauma victims whose blood loss is extensive also are candidates for rapid-sequence anesthesia induction with ketamine.[377] Patients with septic shock also may benefit from ketamine.[378] The intrinsic myocardial depressant effect of ketamine may manifest in this situation, however, if trauma or sepsis has caused depletion of catecholamine stores before the patient's arrival in the operating room. Use of ketamine in these patients does not obviate the need for appropriate preoperative preparation, including restoration of blood volume.

Other cardiac diseases that can be well managed with ketamine anesthesia are cardiac tamponade and restrictive pericarditis.[379] The finding that ketamine preserves heart rate and right atrial pressure through its sympathetic stimulating effects makes ketamine an excellent anesthetic induction and maintenance drug in this setting. Ketamine also is often used in patients with congenital heart disease, especially patients in whom the propensity for right-to-left shunting exists. Use of ketamine has been reported in a patient susceptible to malignant hyperthermia.[380]

Ketamine combined with propofol or midazolam can be given by continuous infusion to produce satisfactory cardiac anesthesia for patients with valvular and ischemic heart disease. The combination of a benzodiazepine[375] or of a benzodiazepine plus sufentanil[381] with ketamine attenuates or eliminates the unwanted tachycardia and hypertension and postoperative psychological derangements. With this technique, there are minimal hemodynamic perturbations, profound analgesia, dependable amnesia, and an uneventful convalescence. The use of propofol plus low-dose ketamine also has gained increasing popularity as a total IV anesthesia technique for patients undergoing noncardiac surgery. The advantages of this combination are maintenance of stable hemodynamics and minimal ventilatory depression when allowing spontaneous ventilation.

Table 26-9 Uses and Doses of Ketamine

Induction of general anesthesia*	0.5-2 mg/kg IV 4-6 mg/kg IM
Maintenance of general anesthesia	0.5-1 mg/kg IV with N_2O 50% in O_2 15-45 μg/kg/min IV with N_2O 50-70% in O_2 30-90 μg/kg/min IV without N_2O
Sedation and analgesia	0.2-0.8 mg/kg IV over 2-3 min 2-4 mg/kg IM
Preemptive/preventive analgesia	0.15-0.25 mg/kg IV

*Lower doses are used if adjuvant drugs such as midazolam or thiopental also are given.
N_2O, nitrous oxide.

Pain Management

Ketamine administered in small doses decreases postoperative analgesic consumption (see Chapter 87). Several meta-analyses of the use of low-dose ketamine (20 to 60 mg) perioperatively have been done. These meta-analyses showed an overall decrease in opiate use or improved analgesia and a decrease in opiate-induced side effects, especially PONV. Side effects, especially psychotomimetic effects, were minimal, especially if a benzodiazepine also was administered.[382] Ketamine in a 1:1 combination with morphine using an 8-minute lockout interval provided optimal postoperative analgesia for this combination.[383] Alternatively, an initial bolus of 0.5 mg/kg of ketamine followed by a continuous infusion of 3 μg/kg/min during surgery and 1.5 μg/kg/min for 48 hours after surgery has been used successfully in total knee arthroplasty.[384]

The action of ketamine on opiate tolerance and hyperalgesia combined with its direct analgesic activity has prompted increasing use of ketamine in chronic pain states. Ketamine may be effective in the treatment of cancer pain, chronic peripheral and central neuropathic pain, phantom and ischemic limb pain, fibromyalgia, complex regional pain syndrome, visceral pain, and migraine. These indications are based largely on a few short-term trials with limited clinical application or limited nonrandomized trials and case studies.[385] There also have been a limited number of reports that indicate the value of multimodal pain therapy including ketamine in preventing postoperative chronic pain.[386,387]

The epidural/caudal administration of ketamine (0.5 to 1 mg/kg) has been increasingly reported. Although the efficacy of these doses of ketamine seems to be established, the safety of this technique has not yet received regulatory approval. The preservative of racemic mixture is potentially neurotoxic, whereas studies to date indicate preservative-free S(+) ketamine may be safe.[388]

Sedation

Ketamine is particularly suitable for sedation of pediatric patients undergoing procedures outside of the operating room (see Chapter 82). Pediatric patients have fewer adverse emergence reactions[346] than adults, and this feature makes the use of ketamine in pediatric patients more versatile. Ketamine is used for sedation or general anesthesia for the following pediatric procedures: cardiac catheterization, radiation therapy, radiologic studies, dressing changes,[389] and dental work.[322]

Usually, a subanesthetic dose (≤1.0 mg/kg intravenously) is used for dressing changes; this dose provides adequate operating conditions, but a rapid return to normal function, including the resumption of eating, which is important in maintaining proper nutrition in burn patients.[308,179] Often, ketamine is combined with premedication of a barbiturate or benzodiazepine and an antisialagogue (e.g., glycopyrrolate) to facilitate management. The premedications reduce the dose requirement for ketamine, and the antisialagogue reduces the sometimes troublesome salivation.

In adults and children, ketamine can be used as a supplement or an adjunct to regional anesthesia, extending the usefulness of the primary (local anesthetic) form of anesthesia (see Chapter 52). In this setting, ketamine can be used before the application of painful blocks,[390] but more commonly it is used for sedation or supplemental anesthesia during long or uncomfortable procedures. When used for supplementation of regional anesthesia, IV ketamine (0.5 mg/kg) can be combined with IV diazepam (0.15 mg/kg).[391] In outpatients, premedication with midazolam (1 to 2 mg), concurrent low-dose propofol infusion, and intermittent ketamine (for analgesia) in doses less than 3 mg/kg[392] or as an infusion of 0.15 to 0.3 µg/kg/min provides excellent sedation, analgesia, and recovery (see Chapter 78). Ketamine also may be considered for sedation of patients in a critical care unit because of its combined sedative and analgesic properties and favorable effects on hemodynamics. Although controversial, a more recent review on the use of ketamine for patients with brain injury concluded, "Ketamine can be used safely in neurologically impaired patients under conditions of controlled ventilation, coadministration of a GABA receptor agonist, and avoidance of nitrous oxide."[393]

Doses and Routes of Administration

Ketamine has been administered intravenously, intramuscularly, transcutaneously, orally, nasally, and rectally, and as a preservative-free solution epidurally or intrathecally.[394] Most clinical use involves the IV and intramuscular (IM) routes, by which the drug rapidly achieves therapeutic levels. The dose depends on the desired therapeutic effect and on the route of administration. Table 26-9 contains general recommended doses for the IV and IM administration of ketamine for various therapeutic goals.[308] Intranasal administration has an onset closer to IV administration; an oral dose of 3 to 10 mg/kg generates a sedative effect in 20 to 45 minutes.

For sedation, ketamine may be given in an IM dose of 2 to 4 mg/kg. It also has been administered orally in doses of 3 to 10 mg/kg, with 6 mg/kg providing optimal conditions in 20 to 25 minutes in one study and 10 mg/kg providing sedation in 87% of children within 45 minutes in another study.[395,396]

Side Effects and Contraindications

The common psychological emergence reactions were discussed earlier. Contraindications to ketamine relate to specific pharmacologic actions and patient diseases. Patients with increased ICP and with intracranial mass lesions breathing spontaneously should not receive ketamine because it can increase ICP and has been reported to cause apnea.[397] The S (+) enantiomer also increases CBF and is probably similarly contraindicated.[283] In ventilated patients, because ketamine retains the response of CBF to carbon dioxide, its use for sedation in head-injured patients may be valuable owing to its potential neuroprotective effect.[393]

Ketamine may be contraindicated in patients with an open eye injury or other ophthalmologic disorder, in which a ketamine-induced increase in intraocular pressure would be detrimental (see Chapter 75). Because ketamine has a propensity to cause hypertension and tachycardia, with a commensurate increase in myocardial oxygen consumption, it is contraindicated as the sole anesthetic in patients with ischemic heart disease.[398] Likewise, it is unwise to give ketamine to patients with vascular aneurysms because of the possible sudden change in arterial pressure. Psychiatric disease, such as schizophrenia, and a history of adverse reaction to ketamine or one of its congeners also are contraindications.[179] One also should consider carefully using ketamine when there is a possibility of postoperative delirium from other causes (e.g., delirium tremens, possibility of head trauma), and a ketamine-induced psychomimetic effect would confuse the differential diagnosis.

As mentioned earlier, ketamine or other NMDA receptor antagonists accentuate apoptosis in the newborn brain of animals, and the clinical implications of this are unknown. Finally, because ketamine's preservative, chlorobutanol, has been shown to be neurotoxic, this formulation of ketamine for subarachnoid or epidural administration is contraindicated.[399] S(+) ketamine is available in a preservative-free solution. The FDA has not approved the use of intrathecal or epidural ketamine.

Etomidate

History

The properties of etomidate (Amidate, Hypnomidate) include hemodynamic stability, minimal respiratory depression, cerebral protection, and pharmacokinetics enabling rapid recovery after either a single dose or a continuous infusion. In animals, etomidate also provides a wider margin of safety (ED_{50}/LD_{50}) than thiopental (26.4 versus 4.6).[400] These beneficial properties led to widespread use of etomidate for induction, for maintenance of anesthesia, and for prolonged sedation in critically ill patients. Anesthesiologists' enthusiasm for etomidate was tempered, however, by reports that the drug can cause temporary inhibition of steroid synthesis after single doses and infusions.[401,402] This effect, combined with other minor disadvantages (e.g., pain on injection, superficial thrombophlebitis, myoclonus, and a high incidence of nausea and vomiting), led to several editorials[403,404] questioning the role of etomidate in modern anesthetic practice. Use of the drug waned significantly after those editorials, but it has expanded as a result of a rediscovery of etomidate's beneficial physiologic profile combined with a lack of any new reports describing clinically significant adrenocortical suppression after an induction dose or brief infusions.

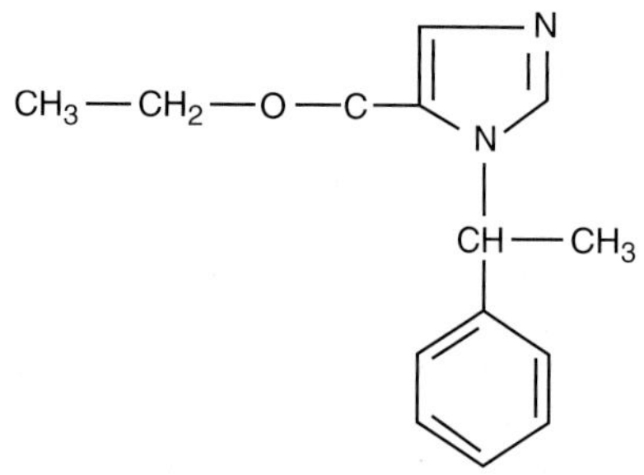

Figure 26-16 Structure of etomidate, an imidazole derivative.

Physicochemical Characteristics

Etomidate is an imidazole derivative (R-(+)-pentylethyl-1H-imidazole-5 carboxylate sulfate). Its chemical structure is illustrated in Figure 26-16. With a molecular weight of 342.36 kD,[179] etomidate exists as two isomers, the (+) isomer being the one active as a hypnotic.[179] Etomidate is water insoluble and is unstable in a neutral solution. It has been formulated with several solvents. In the United States, it is supplied as a 2-mg/mL propylene glycol (35% by volume) solution with a pH of 6.9 and an osmolality of 4640 mOsm/L. In Europe, lipid emulsion has been introduced in an attempt to reduce some of the side effects of etomidate.[405] In contrast to sodium thiopental, when etomidate is mixed with other commonly used anesthetics, such as neuromuscular blockers, vasoactive drugs, or lidocaine, it does not cause precipitation.[406]

Metabolism, Induction, and Maintenance of Anesthesia

Etomidate is metabolized in the liver primarily by ester hydrolysis to the corresponding carboxylic acid of etomidate (major metabolite) or by *N*-dealkylation.[179] The main metabolite is inactive.[406] Only 2% of the drug is excreted unchanged, the rest being excreted as metabolites by the kidney (85%) and bile (13%).[406]

Etomidate has been used for induction and maintenance of anesthesia (Table 26-10). The induction dose of etomidate is 0.2 to 0.6 mg/kg,[407] and it is reduced by premedication with an opiate, a benzodiazepine, or a barbiturate. Onset of anesthesia after a routine induction dose of 0.3 mg/kg of etomidate is rapid (one arm–brain circulation) and is equivalent to anesthesia obtained with an induction dose of thiopental or methohexital.[407] The duration of anesthesia after a single induction dose is linearly related to the dose—each 0.1 mg/kg administered provides about 100 seconds of loss of consciousness.[408] Repeat doses of etomidate by bolus or infusion prolong the duration of hypnosis. Recovery after multiple doses or an infusion of etomidate is still usually rapid.[409-411] The addition of small doses of fentanyl with etomidate for short surgical procedures reduces the required dose of etomidate and allows earlier awakening. In children, induction by rectal administration of etomidate has been obtained with 6.5 mg/kg. Hypnosis occurs in 4 minutes. At this dose, hemodynamics are unaltered, and recovery is still rapid.[412]

Table 26-10 Uses and Doses of Etomidate

Use	Dose
Induction of general anesthesia	0.2-0.6 mg/kg IV
Maintenance of general anesthesia	10 μg/kg/min IV with N_2O and an opiate
Sedation and analgesia	Limited to periods of brief sedation because of inhibition of corticosteroid synthesis

N_2O, nitrous oxide.

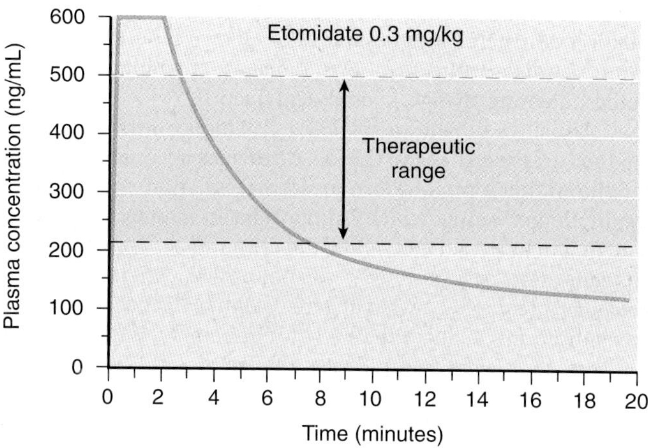

Figure 26-17 Simulated time course of plasma levels of etomidate after an induction dose of 0.3 mg/kg. Plasma levels required for hypnosis during surgery are 300 to 500 ng/mL, with awakening usually occurring at levels less than 225 ng/mL.

Various infusion schemes have been devised to use etomidate as a maintenance anesthetic for the hypnotic component of anesthesia. Most regimens aim to achieve a plasma level of 300 to 500 ng/mL, which is the concentration necessary for hypnosis.[413] Two-stage and three-stage infusions have been used successfully. These consist of an initial rapid infusion of 100 μg/kg/min for 10 minutes followed by 10 μg/kg/min thereafter,[414] or of 100 μg/kg/min for 3 minutes, 20 μg/kg/min for 27 minutes, and 10 μg/kg/min thereafter.[415] Loss of consciousness with these techniques occurs after 100 to 120 seconds.[415] The infusion is usually terminated 10 minutes before desired awakening.[415]

Pharmacokinetics

The pharmacokinetics of etomidate has been calculated after single bolus doses and after continuous infusion (see Table 26-1).[416] The time course of plasma disappearance after a 0.3-mg/kg bolus is shown in Figure 26-17. The kinetics of etomidate is best described by an open three-compartment model. The drug has an initial distribution half-life of 2.7 minutes, a redistribution half-life of 29 minutes, and an elimination half-life of 2.9 to 5.3 hours.[416] Clearance of etomidate by the liver is high (18 to 25 mL/kg/min), with a hepatic extraction ratio of 0.5 ± 0.9 [407,413] Drugs affecting hepatic blood flow alter the elimination half-life. Because redistribution is the mechanism whereby the effect of a bolus of etomidate is dissipated, hepatic dysfunction should not appreciably alter recovery from an induction dose. Etomidate is 75% protein bound.[417] Pathologic conditions altering serum proteins (e.g., hepatic or renal disease) vary the amount of the free (unbound) fraction and may cause a given dose to have an exaggerated pharmacodynamic effect.[417] A hemorrhagic shock model in pigs bled to a mean pressure of 50 mm Hg did not alter etomidate pharmacokinetics or pharmacodynamics.[418] This finding contrasts with the marked changes seen in this same model with other IV anesthetics.

In patients with cirrhosis, the volume of distribution is doubled, whereas clearance is normal; the result is an elimination half-life that is twice normal.[419] The initial distribution half-life and clinical effect are likely unchanged. Increasing age is associated with a smaller initial volume of distribution and a decreased clearance of etomidate.[420] The short elimination half-life and the rapid clearance of etomidate make it suitable for administration in a single dose, in multiple doses, or in a continuous infusion.

Pharmacology

Effects on the Central Nervous System

The primary action of etomidate on the CNS is hypnosis, which is achieved in one arm–brain circulation after a normal induction dose (0.3 mg/kg).[407] Etomidate has no analgesic activity. Plasma levels required for the maintenance of anesthesia are approximately 300 to 500 ng/mL, for sedation are 150 to 300 ng/mL, and for awakening are 150 to 250 ng/mL (see Fig. 26-17).[413,414,416] The mechanism by which etomidate produces hypnosis is not fully elucidated; however, it seems largely (but not solely) related to GABA. Its action may be antagonized by GABA antagonists.[421] Generally, the mechanism of action of etomidate seems to be similar to that established so far for propofol (see earlier).[422] For etomidate, it seems that the β2 and β3 subunits are more important for its hypnotic action than the α1 $GABA_A$ subunit.[42,423]

At a dose of 0.2 to 0.3 mg/kg, etomidate reduces CBF (by 34%) and $CMRO_2$ (by 45%) without altering MAP.[424] CPP is maintained or increased, and there is a beneficial net increase in the cerebral oxygen supply-to-demand ratio.[424] Etomidate given in doses sufficient to produce EEG burst suppression acutely decreases ICP by 50% in patients with already increased ICP, returning increased ICP to almost normal values.[425,426] The decrease in ICP is maintained in the period immediately after intubation.[426] To maintain the effects of etomidate on ICP, high infusion rates (60 µg/kg/min) are necessary.[427] In contrast to the situation with other neuroprotective drugs such as thiopental, reduction of ICP and maintenance of burst suppression are not associated with a decrease in MAP.[426] Because cerebrovascular reactivity is still maintained after etomidate administration,[427] hyperventilation theoretically may reduce ICP further when used in conjunction with etomidate. In animals, etomidate reduced neuronal death after acute cortical ischemic insult.[428,429] Other investigators disagree on the neuroprotective qualities of etomidate.[430] Deeper structures, such as the brainstem, may not be afforded ischemic protection by etomidate.[431]

Etomidate produces changes in the EEG similar to those produced by the barbiturates.[432] There is an initial increase in alpha amplitude with sharp beta bursts followed by mixed delta-theta waves, with delta wave activity predominating before the onset of periodic burst suppression.[432] The absence of beta waves in the initial phase of induction with etomidate is the major difference in EEG changes compared with thiopental.[432] Etomidate has been associated with grand mal seizures[433,434] and produces increased EEG activity in epileptogenic foci. This feature has proved useful for intraoperative mapping of seizure foci before surgical ablation.[434] Etomidate also is associated with a frequent incidence of myoclonic movement.[409,410] Myoclonus is not thought to be associated with seizure-like EEG activity.[432] The myoclonic movement is believed to result from activity either in the brainstem or in deep cerebral structures.

The effect of etomidate on auditory evoked potentials is similar to that produced by the inhaled anesthetics. There is a dose-dependent increase in latency and a decreasing amplitude of the early cortical components (Pa and Nb).[435]

Effects on the Respiratory System

Etomidate has less effect on ventilation than other anesthetics used to induce anesthesia. It does not induce histamine release either in healthy patients or in patients with reactive airway disease.[436] Ventilatory response to carbon dioxide is depressed by etomidate, but the ventilatory drive at any given carbon dioxide tension is greater than that following an equipotent dose of methohexital.[226] Induction with etomidate produces a brief period of hyperventilation, sometimes followed by a similarly brief period of apnea,[437] which results in a slight (±15%) increase in $Paco_2$, but no change in the partial pressure of arterial oxygen (Pao_2).[438] The incidence of apnea is altered by premedication.[439] Hiccups or coughing may accompany etomidate induction, with an incidence similar to that after methohexital induction.[407]

In laboratory models, etomidate seems to be as effective as propofol in relaxing precontracted tracheal rings, but less effective than propofol in preventing tracheal ring contraction by muscarinic agonists.[440] Etomidate's action on pulmonary vascular tone are similar to the actions observed with ketamine and propofol.[441]

Effects on the Cardiovascular System

The minimal effect of etomidate on cardiovascular function sets it apart from other rapid-onset anesthetics (see Table 26-2).[442,443] An induction dose of 0.3 mg/kg of etomidate given to cardiac patients for noncardiac surgery results in almost no change in heart rate, MAP, mean pulmonary artery pressure, pulmonary capillary wedge pressure, central venous pressure, stroke volume, cardiac index, and pulmonary and systemic vascular resistance.[442] A large dose of etomidate, 0.45 mg/kg (which is 50% larger than a normal induction dose),[444] also produces minimal changes in cardiovascular variables. In patients with ischemic heart disease or valvular disease, etomidate (0.3 mg/kg) produces similar minimal alterations in cardiovascular variables.[442] In patients with mitral or aortic valve disease, etomidate may produce greater changes in MAP (an approximate 20% decrease)[438] than in patients without cardiac valvular disease. After induction (18 mg) and infusion (2.4 mg/min), etomidate produces a 50% decrease in myocardial blood flow and oxygen consumption, and a 20% to 30% increase in coronary sinus blood oxygen saturation.[108] The myocardial oxygen supply-to-demand ratio is well maintained. There is minimal effect on the QT interval.[445]

The hemodynamic stability seen with etomidate may be due partly to its unique lack of effect on the sympathetic nervous system and on baroreceptor function.[122] Etomidate lacks analgesic efficacy, however, and needs to be combined with an opiate to prevent hemodynamic perturbations during laryngoscopy and intubation.

Endocrine Effects

Ledingham and Watt[401] in 1983 first raised concerns regarding long-term etomidate infusion in critically ill patients. They pos-

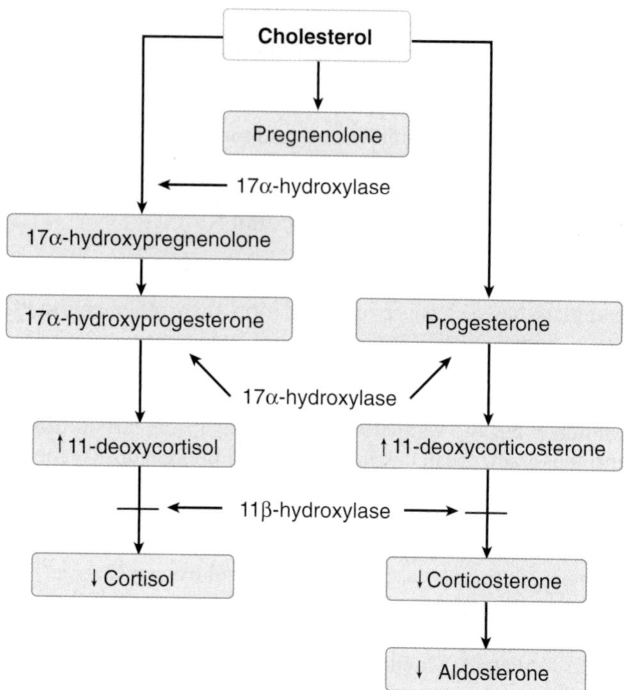

Figure 26-18 Pathway for the biosynthesis of cortisol and aldosterone. The sites at which etomidate affects cortisol-aldosterone synthesis by its action on 11β-hydroxylase (major site) and 17α-hydroxylase (minor site) are illustrated.

tulated that adrenocortical suppression secondary to long-term etomidate infusion was the cause of the increased mortality.[401]

The specific endocrine effects manifested by etomidate are a dose-dependent reversible inhibition of the enzyme 11β-hydroxylase, which converts 11-deoxycortisol to cortisol, and a relatively minor effect on 17α-hydroxylase (Fig. 26-18).[446,447] This activity results in an increase in the cortisol precursors 11-deoxycortisol and 17-hydroxyprogesterone and an increase in ACTH. The blockade of 11β-hydroxylase and, to a lesser extent, 17α-hydroxylase[446] seems to be related to the free imidazole radical of etomidate-binding cytochrome P-450.[447,448] This results in inhibition of ascorbic acid resynthesis, which is required for steroid production in humans.[448] The blockade of the cytochrome P-450–dependent enzyme 11β-hydroxylase also results in decreased mineralocorticoid production and an increase in intermediaries (11-deoxycorticosterone).[402,404] Vitamin C supplementation restores cortisol levels to normal after the use of etomidate.[448] Because minor adrenocortical suppressive effects were shown to follow even single bolus doses,[446] concerns about the use of etomidate for anesthetic induction arose.[403] No large prospective studies have been done, but several smaller studies have provided some insight into the exact nature of adrenocortical suppression after an induction dose.

Duthie and colleagues[449] showed that in otherwise healthy patients undergoing minor peripheral surgery, plasma cortisol levels were slightly depressed from the preinduction levels for 1 hour postoperatively. The nadir of mean cortisol levels did not fall out of the normal range. 11-Deoxycorticosterone, substrate for the etomidate-inhibited 11β-hydroxylase, peaked at very high levels compared with the thiopental control group.[449] In another study, patients undergoing orthopedic surgery were given an etomidate induction followed by an infusion of etomidate (average total dose 68 mg). Temporary adrenocortical suppression, as measured by a reduced response to ACTH stimulation, was documented for 6 hours postoperatively and returned to normal by 20 hours postoperatively. Postoperative cortisol levels in the etomidate study patients were not significantly different from the levels in patients who received a midazolam induction. As in the study by Duthie and colleagues,[449] mean cortisol levels in the etomidate group remained in the normal range at all times postoperatively.[450] Other studies have shown similar results when evaluating etomidate induction doses; none reported adverse outcomes secondary to short-term adrenocortical suppression.[402,446]

In each of the prospective etomidate studies documenting adrenocortical suppression without associated clinical sequelae, a conclusion of safety was not forthcoming. The reason was that these studies did not address high-stress procedures, in which the benefit of a high cortisol level in response to a major stress could be desirable, and etomidate's blockade of the response to ACTH could be detrimental. In 1994, the cortisol levels during and after coronary artery bypass surgery were compared in patients receiving total IV anesthesia with etomidate/fentanyl (mean etomidate dose of 87 ± 3 mg) versus midazolam/fentanyl. Except for the first hour after induction, cortisol levels were the same or higher in the etomidate group compared with the midazolam group, a finding implying that the body's ability to respond to a high surgical stress was still intact despite high doses of etomidate. This finding suggests that etomidate is probably safe for use in major surgery.[451]

Three facts suggest that the issue of temporary adrenocortical suppression after perioperative induction doses of etomidate is not clinically significant: (1) Although there is one questionable case report suggesting acute symptomatic postoperative adrenocortical suppression in a 74-year-old ICU patient,[452] there are no other known reports of any negative clinical outcome associated with an etomidate induction despite millions of uses. (2) After etomidate induction, the nadir of cortisol levels usually remains in the low-normal range, and the adrenocortical suppression is a short-lived phenomenon. (3) High-stress surgery can overcome the temporary adrenocortical suppression caused by etomidate.

Other Effects

Although etomidate provides stable hemodynamics and minimal respiratory depression, it is associated with several adverse effects when used for induction, including nausea and vomiting, pain on injection, myoclonic movement, and hiccups. Etomidate has been associated with a frequent (30% to 40%) incidence of nausea and vomiting.[409-411,439] More recently, etomidate in a lipid emulsion was associated with an equal incidence of postoperative nausea compared with propofol.[453]

Superficial thrombophlebitis of the vein used may occur 48 to 72 hours after etomidate injection.[454] The incidence may be 20% when etomidate is given alone through a small (21-gauge) IV needle. Intra-arterial injection of etomidate is not associated with local or vascular disease. Pain on injection, similar in incidence to pain with propofol,[175] can be essentially eliminated by injecting lidocaine immediately before injection of etomidate; 20 to 40 mg may be enough.[455] Pain on injection is reduced further by using a large vein. The incidence of pain on injection is 0 to 50%. The lipid formulation of etomidate also is associated with a much lower incidence of pain on injection, thrombophlebitis, and histamine release on injection.[456]

The incidence of muscle movement (myoclonus) and of hiccups also is highly variable (0 to 70%), but myoclonus is reduced by premedication with either a narcotic or 0.015 mg/kg of midazolam 90 seconds before induction.[457] Etomidate enhances the neuromuscular blockade of nondepolarizing neuromuscular blockers.[458] In vitro, etomidate inhibits aminolevulinic acid synthetase, but it has been administered to patients with porphyria without inducing an acute attack of porphyria.[459]

The carrier for etomidate, propylene glycol, also has been reported to have some negative effects. Some reports suggest that propylene glycol can be associated with a small degree of hemolysis.[405] Additionally, high-dose prolonged infusion has been reported to result in propylene glycol toxicity (a hyperosmolar state).[460]

Uses

Etomidate is most appropriate in patients with cardiovascular disease, reactive airway disease, intracranial hypertension, or any combination of disorders indicating the need for an induction agent with limited or beneficial physiologic side effects. The hemodynamic stability of etomidate is unique among the rapid-onset anesthetics used to induce anesthesia.

Etomidate has been used primarily in sick patients. In multiple studies, etomidate has been used for induction in patients with a compromised cardiovascular system who are undergoing coronary artery bypass surgery or valve surgery, and in patients requiring induction of general anesthesia for percutaneous transluminal coronary angioplasty, aortic aneurysm repair, and thoracic surgery. When etomidate is used in combination with fentanyl, titrating etomidate up to 0.6 mg/kg maintains blood pressure and heart rate in a narrow range, preserving coronary perfusion pressure in these patients with probable coronary artery disease, while blunting the response to intubation and avoiding unnecessary stress. For cardioversion, the rapid onset, quick recovery, and maintenance of blood pressure in these sometimes hemodynamically tenuous patients, combined with continued spontaneous respiration, make etomidate an acceptable choice,[175] although there is one report of myoclonus interfering with electrocardiographic evaluation.[461]

Although definitive proof of the neuroprotective effect of etomidate in humans is lacking, the combination of animal data and anecdotal reports of successful use of etomidate in neurosurgical procedures such as giant aneurysm clippings makes etomidate a reasonable choice during neurosurgical induction.[414,426,428] In addition, etomidate should be considered as an anesthetic to reduce increased ICP when maintenance of cerebral or coronary perfusion pressure also is important. Trauma patients with questionable volume status may be well served by an etomidate induction. Although the indirect sympathomimetic effect seen with ketamine induction is absent, there is no direct myocardial depression and no confusion in the differential diagnosis of postoperative delirium. This is especially important in patients whose trauma may be related to drug or alcohol use. When using the drug in trauma patients, loss of consciousness by itself can be associated with decreased adrenergic output, and postinduction controlled ventilation by itself can exacerbate a decreased preload (see Chapter 72). Both of these factors may cause a significant decrease in blood pressure at induction despite etomidate having no direct cardiovascular drug effect.

During an infusion, hemodynamic status is well maintained, and adequate spontaneous ventilation is present.[294] The incidence of pain on injection and of myoclonus and thrombophlebitis tends to be less with an infusion technique.[413,462]

Short-term sedation with etomidate is useful in hemodynamically unstable patients, such as patients requiring cardioversion[175] or patients requiring sedation after an acute myocardial infarction or with unstable angina for a minor operative procedure.[463] Etomidate also is useful for intubation in the emergency department and in the ICU. When used during electroconvulsive therapy, etomidate can produce longer seizures compared with other hypnotics.[464] Prolonged sedation for patients in the ICU, although initially popular after the release of etomidate, is now contraindicated owing to inhibition of corticosteroid and mineralocorticoid production, with subsequent increase in morbidity.[401,403,465]

α-Adrenergic Agonists: Dexmedetomidine

History

The α_2-adrenergic agonists provide sedation, anxiolysis, hypnosis, analgesia, and sympatholysis. The initial impetus for the use of α_2 agonists in anesthesia resulted from observations made in patients during anesthesia who were receiving clonidine therapy.[466,467] This was soon followed by a description of the minimum alveolar concentration (MAC) reduction of halothane by clonidine.[468] Dexmedetomidine is a more selective α_2 agonist with a 1600 greater selectivity for the α_2 receptor compared with the α_1 receptor. It was introduced in clinical practice in the United States in 1999 and approved by the FDA only as a short-term (<24 hours) sedative for mechanically ventilated adult ICU patients. Dexmedetomidine is now being used off-label outside of the ICU in various settings, including sedation and adjunct analgesia in the operating room, sedation in diagnostic and procedure units, and for other applications such as withdrawal/detoxification amelioration in adult and pediatric patients.[469,470]

Physicochemical Characteristics

Dexmedetomidine is the d-enantiomer of medetomidine, a substance that has been used for sedation and analgesia in veterinary medicine for many years.[471] It shows a high ratio of specificity for the α_2 receptor (α_2/α_1 1600:1) compared with clonidine (α_2/α_1 200:1), making it a complete α_2 agonist.[472] Dexmedetomidine belongs to the imidazole subclass of α_2 receptor agonists, similar to clonidine, and its structure is illustrated in Figure 26-19. It is freely soluble in water.

Metabolism and Pharmacokinetics

Dexmedetomidine is rapidly distributed and extensively metabolized in the liver and excreted in urine and feces. It undergoes conjugation (41%), n-methylation (21%), or hydroxylation fol-

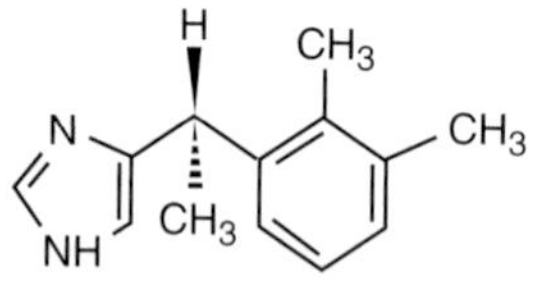

Figure 26-19 Chemical structure of dexmedetomidine.

lowed by conjugation. Dexmedetomidine is 94% protein bound, and its concentration ratio between whole blood and plasma is 0.66. Dexmedetomidine has profound effects on cardiovascular variables and may alter its own pharmacokinetics. With large doses, there is marked vasoconstriction, which probably reduces the drug's volumes of distribution. In essence, dexmedetomidine displays nonlinear pharmacokinetics.[473] Dyck and coworkers[474] found that its pharmacokinetics in volunteers is best described by a three-compartment model (see Table 26-1). These pharmacokinetic parameters apparently are unaltered by age or weight or renal failure, but clearance is a function of height.[473,475] The elimination half-life of dexmedetomidine is 2 to 3 hours, with a context-sensitive half-time ranging from 4 minutes after a 10-minute infusion to 250 minutes after an 8-hour infusion. Postoperative patients sedated with dexmedetomidine display similar pharmacokinetics to the pharmacokinetics seen in volunteers.[476]

Pharmacology

Dexmedetomidine is a nonselective α_2 agonist. Alpha$_2$ adrenoreceptors are membrane-spanning G proteins. Intracellular pathways include inhibition of adenylate cyclase and modulation of ion channels Three subtypes of α_2 adrenoreceptors have been described in humans: α_{2A}, α_{2B}, and α_{2C} (Fig. 26-20).[477] The α_{2A} adrenoreceptors are primarily distributed in the periphery, whereas α_{2B} and α_{2C} are in the brain and spinal cord. Postsynaptic located α_2 adrenoreceptors in peripheral blood vessels produce vasoconstriction, whereas presynaptic α_2 adrenoreceptors inhibit the release of norepinephrine, potentially attenuating the vasoconstriction. The overall response to α_2 adrenoreceptors agonists is related to the stimulation of α_2 adrenoreceptors located in the CNS and spinal cord. These receptors are involved in the sympatholysis, sedation, and antinociception effects of α_2 adrenoreceptors.[478]

Effects on the Central Nervous System

Sedation

The α_2 agonists produce their sedative-hypnotic effect by an action on α_2 receptors in the locus caeruleus and an analgesic action at α_2 receptors within the locus caeruleus and within the spinal cord.[479] The quality of sedation produced by dexmedetomidine seems different compared with that produced by other sedatives acting through the GABA systems. Patients receiving dexmedetomidine infusions as part of their sedation regimen in the postoperative ICU setting have been described as being very easy to wake up and having the ability to follow commands and cooperate while being tracheally intubated. Undisturbed, patients were noted to fall asleep right away.[480] Despite sound levels of sedation with dexmedetomidine, there is limited respiratory depression, providing wide safety margins.[481] This characteristic allows for "daily wake up" tests to be done in a safe fashion. This

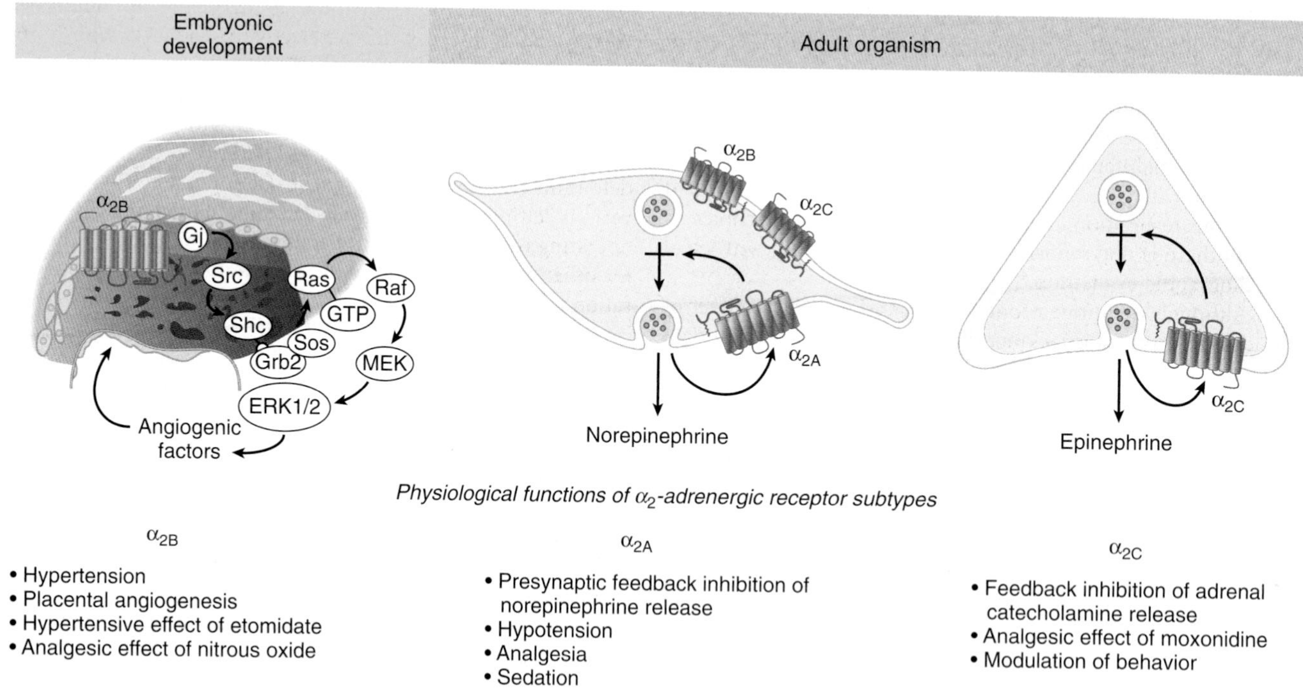

Figure 26-20 The different physiologic functions of α_2 adrenoreceptors. The *top panel* depicts the three α_2 receptor subtypes acting as presynaptic inhibitory feedback receptors to control the release of norepinephrine and epinephrine from peripheral or central adult neurons. Also, a negative feedback loop has been seen in the adrenal gland. Alpha$_{2B}$ receptors have been involved in the development of the placental vascular system during prenatal development. The *lower panel* lists a series of physiologic effects with its associated α_2 adrenoreceptors. *(From Paris A, Tonner PH: Dexmedetomidine in anaesthesia. Curr Opin Anaesthesiol 18:412-418, 2005.)*

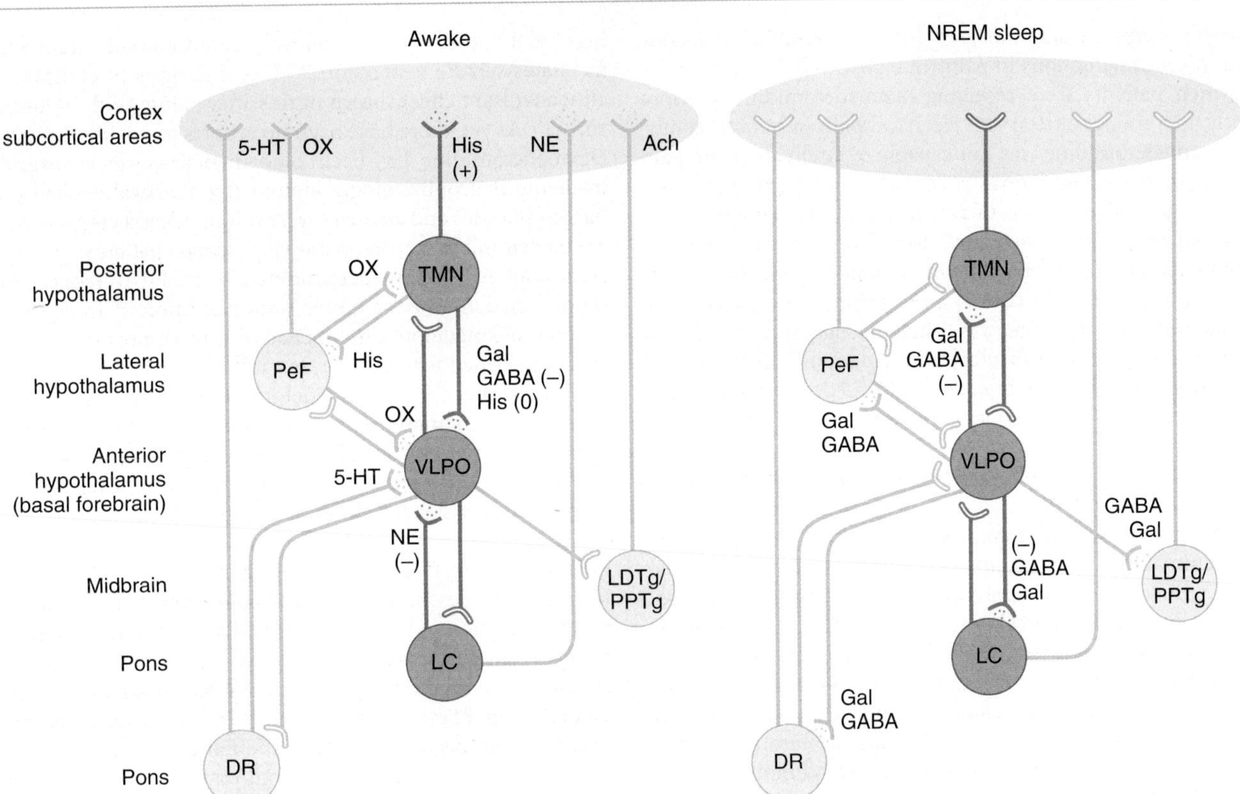

Figure 26-21 Dexmedetomidine has been shown to induce a non–rapid eye movement sleeping pattern (NREM). The stimulation of the locus caeruleus (LC) by dexmedetomidine (*right diagram*) releases the inhibition the LC has over the ventrolateral preoptic nucleus (VLPO). The VLPO subsequently releases γ-aminobutyric acid (GABA) onto the tuberomammillary nucleus (TMN). This inhibits the release of the arousal-promoting histamine on the cortex and forebrain, inducing the loss of consciousness. *(From Ebert T, Maze M: Dexmedetomidine: Another arrow for the clinician's quiver. Anesthesiology 101:569-570, 2004.)*

critical test—when ventilated ICU patients are taken off all sedatives to assess their mental status and titrate sedation—shortens their ventilated and ICU length of stay.[482]

The α_2 agonists act through the endogenous sleep-promoting pathways to exert their sedative effect (Fig. 26-21). Dexmedetomidine produces a decrease in activity of the projections of the locus caeruleus to the ventrolateral preoptic nucleus. This increases GABAergic and galanin release in the tuberomammillary nucleus, producing a decrease in histamine release in cortical and subcortical projections.[483] The α_2 agonists seem to inhibit ion conductance through L-type or P-type calcium channels and facilitate conductance through voltage-gated calcium-activated potassium channels.[484] The similarity between natural sleep (non–rapid eye movement) and dexmedetomidine-induced hypnosis has been speculated to maintain cognitive and immunologic function in the sleep-deprived states (as in the ICU).[485] Dexmedetomidine can produce profound sedation, and it has been used as a total IV anesthetic when given at 10 times the normal sedation concentration range.[486]

The α_2 agonists have the advantage that their effects are readily reversible by α_2-adrenergic antagonists (e.g., atipamezole).[487] Atipamezole is not currently approved for human use. Similar to other adrenergic receptors, the α_2 agonists also show tolerance after prolonged administration.[488] Because dexmedetomidine is approved by the FDA only for short-term sedation (24 hours), tolerance, dependence, or addiction does not seem to be a problem. Dexmedetomidine can be employed for addiction treatment; dexmedetomidine has been described for use in rapid opioid detoxification, cocaine withdrawal, and iatrogenic induced benzodiazepine and opioid tolerance after prolonged sedation.[489] In animals, dexmedetomidine, in contrast to opioids, does not result in hyperalgesia or allodynia after its withdrawal.[490] Rats rendered tolerant to morphine also show a decrease in efficacy of hypnotic and analgesic effects of dexmedetomidine. As tolerance to opioids recovers, there is a more rapid recovery of the hypnotic effect of dexmedetomidine than its analgesic efficacy.[491] These data would tend to indicate a possible cross-tolerance between receptors.

Analgesia

The analgesic effects of dexmedetomidine are complex. Alpha$_2$ agonists do have an analgesic effect when injected via the intrathecal or epidural route.[492] Clonidine injected in the neural axis helps with short-term pain, cancer pain, and neuropathic pain.[493,494] Intrathecally injected dexmedetomidine in sheep reduces blood pressure in 1 minute. When dexmedetomidine is injected into the epidural space, it rapidly diffuses into the CSF (in one study,[495] 22% of the injected dose was identified in the CSF). The effects on blood pressure are slower in onset with an epidural injection than with an intrathecal administration. Epidural effects are seen in 5 to 20 minutes. The primary site of analgesic action is thought to be the spinal cord.[495] Systemic use of dexmedetomidine shows narcotic sparing. In the postoperative ICU setting, narcotic requirements were reduced by 50% when patients were receiving a dexmedetomidine drip compared with placebo.[480]

Some of the systemic analgesic effects have been attributed to the confounding sedative effects.[496] In human pain studies, the results of systemically administered dexmedetomidine are inconsistent. Modest reductions in pain were observed in cold pressor tests when patients were receiving dexmedetomidine.[497] More recently, in a model of heat and electrical pain in human volunteers, dexmedetomidine was not capable of attenuating the pain response in the clinical dose range when subjects were conscious.[485] The analgesic effect of dexmedetomidine has been compared with remifentanil. In a noxious heat versus pain intensity plot obtained in a group of volunteers, dexmedetomidine was less effective in reducing pain (less of a right shift of the curve) than remifentanil. Also, the slope was different, suggesting a different mechanism of action and an effect from sedation.[498] In the clinical setting, when pain is likely to occur, if dexmedetomidine is to be used, the addition of a narcotic seems warranted.

Central Nervous System Protection and Other Central Nervous System Effects

The CNS protective effects are not well defined. Dexmedetomidine in animal models of incomplete cerebral ischemia and reperfusion reduces cerebral necrosis and improves neurologic outcome. In a model of focal ischemia in rabbits, dexmedetomidine, administered at doses that reduced the MAC of halothane by 50%, resulted in less cortical neuronal damage than when halothane was administered alone at equieffective MAC concentrations.[499] In a rat model of unilateral carotid ligation accompanied by systemic hypotension, the administration of dexmedetomidine provided for lower plasma catecholamines with less neurologic and histopathologic damage.[500] The prevalent idea was that dexmedetomidine reduced the intracerebral catecholamine outflow during injury and resulted in less neural tissue damage with better neurologic outcome.[501] Others have found no reduction in cerebral catecholamines after receiving dexmedetomidine during injury.[502] The neuroprotection may be attributed to modulation of proapoptotic and antiapoptotic proteins.[341] Also, the reduction of the excitatory neurotransmitter glutamate during injury may explain some of the protective effects.[503]

The neuroprotective properties of dexmedetomidine in humans have not been investigated. Little is known of the effects of dexmedetomidine alone on ICP and CBF. In patients after pituitary surgery, a target concentration of 600 ng/mL of dexmedetomidine resulted in no increase in lumbar CSF pressure.[504] In dogs, in the presence of volatile anesthetics and dexmedetomidine, CBF was decreased, and oxygen consumption was maintained.[505,506] CBF velocity, as measured by transcranial Doppler, decreased with increasing concentrations of dexmedetomidine in parallel with decreasing MAP and increasing $Pa{CO_2}$.[507] These decreases in CBF are not accompanied by a reduction in $CRMO_2$. Despite the significant reduction in CBF with dexmedetomidine, there was no evidence of cerebral ischemia in a dog model.[551] In a preliminary study in patients undergoing cerebrovascular surgery using dexmedetomidine, there was no evidence of a detrimental effect on local brain tissue oxygenation.[508] More recently, in a study in six normal volunteers, the administration of dexmedetomidine to achieve serum levels of 0.6 ng/mL and 1.2 ng/mL (with and without hyperventilation) produced the predicted reduction of CBF with a concomitant reduction in $CRMO_2$.[509] This finding suggests the maintenance of the cerebral oxygen supply-to-demand relationship; however, further work in injured brains needs to be done.

In a rat seizure model, dexmedetomidine showed significant proconvulsant action, which is consistent with previous findings that inhibition of central noradrenergic transmission facilitates seizure expression.[510] This finding is in contrast to an anticonvulsant effect shown in rats after kainic acid–induced seizures.[511] As yet, there have been no reports of seizures in humans. Dexmedetomidine has been used in neurosurgical procedures involving neurophysiologic monitoring. Cortical evoked potentials amplitudes and latencies were minimally affected when using dexmedetomidine intraoperatively when patients underwent craniotomies.[508] Dexmedetomidine also is able to reduce muscle rigidity after high-dose opioid administration.[512] In resting volunteers, dexmedetomidine increased growth hormone secretion in a dose-dependent manner, but it had no effect on other pituitary hormones.[513,514] Dexmedetomidine ablates memory in a dose-dependent manner. In concentrations used for clinical sedation (i.e., 0.7 ng/mL), recall of picture cards is preserved. Increasing the concentration of dexmedetomidine to 2 ng/mL largely ablates recall and recognition of a picture card.[515]

Effects on the Respiratory System

In volunteers, dexmedetomidine at concentrations producing significant sedation reduces minute ventilation, but retains the slope of the ventilatory response to increasing carbon dioxide.[516] The changes in ventilation appeared similar to those observed during natural sleep. Ebert and colleagues,[515] infusing dexmedetomidine to concentrations of 15 ng/mL in spontaneously breathing volunteers, showed no change in arterial oxygenation or pH. At the highest concentrations, $Pa{CO_2}$ increased by 20%. Respiratory rate increased with increasing concentration from 14 breaths/min to 25 breaths/min.[515] When dexmedetomidine and propofol were titrated to equal sedative end points (BIS of 85), both resulted in no change in respiratory rate.[517] In a study comparing the effects of remifentanil and dexmedetomidine on respiratory parameters in normal volunteers,[518] the hypercapnic ventilatory response was unaffected even at doses that produced unresponsiveness to vigorous stimulation. $Pa{CO_2}$ increased mildly with dexmedetomidine, but it reached a plateau after the first increment. Dexmedetomidine also exhibited a hypercarbic arousal phenomenon, which has been described during normal sleep and is a safety feature. IV or inhaled dexmedetomidine has been implicated in blocking histamine-induced bronchoconstriction in dogs.[519]

Effects on the Cardiovascular System

The basic effects of α_2 agonists on the cardiovascular system are decreased heart rate; decreased systemic vascular resistance; and indirectly decreased myocardial contractility, cardiac output, and systemic blood pressure. By developing highly selective α agonists, it has been hoped to decrease some of these adverse cardiovascular effects and to maximize the desirable hypnotic-analgesic properties. The hemodynamic effects of a bolus of dexmedetomidine in humans have shown a biphasic response. An acute IV injection of 2 μg/kg resulted in an initial increase in blood pressure (22%) and decrease in heart rate (27%) from baseline that occurred at 5 minutes after injection. This initial increase in blood pressure is probably due to the vasoconstrictive effects of dexmedetomidine when stimulating peripheral α_2 receptors. Heart rate returned to baseline by 15 minutes, and blood pressure gradually declined to approximately 15% below baseline by 1 hour. After an IM injection of the same dose, the initial increase in blood pressure was not seen, and heart rate and blood pressure remained within 10% of baseline.[473]

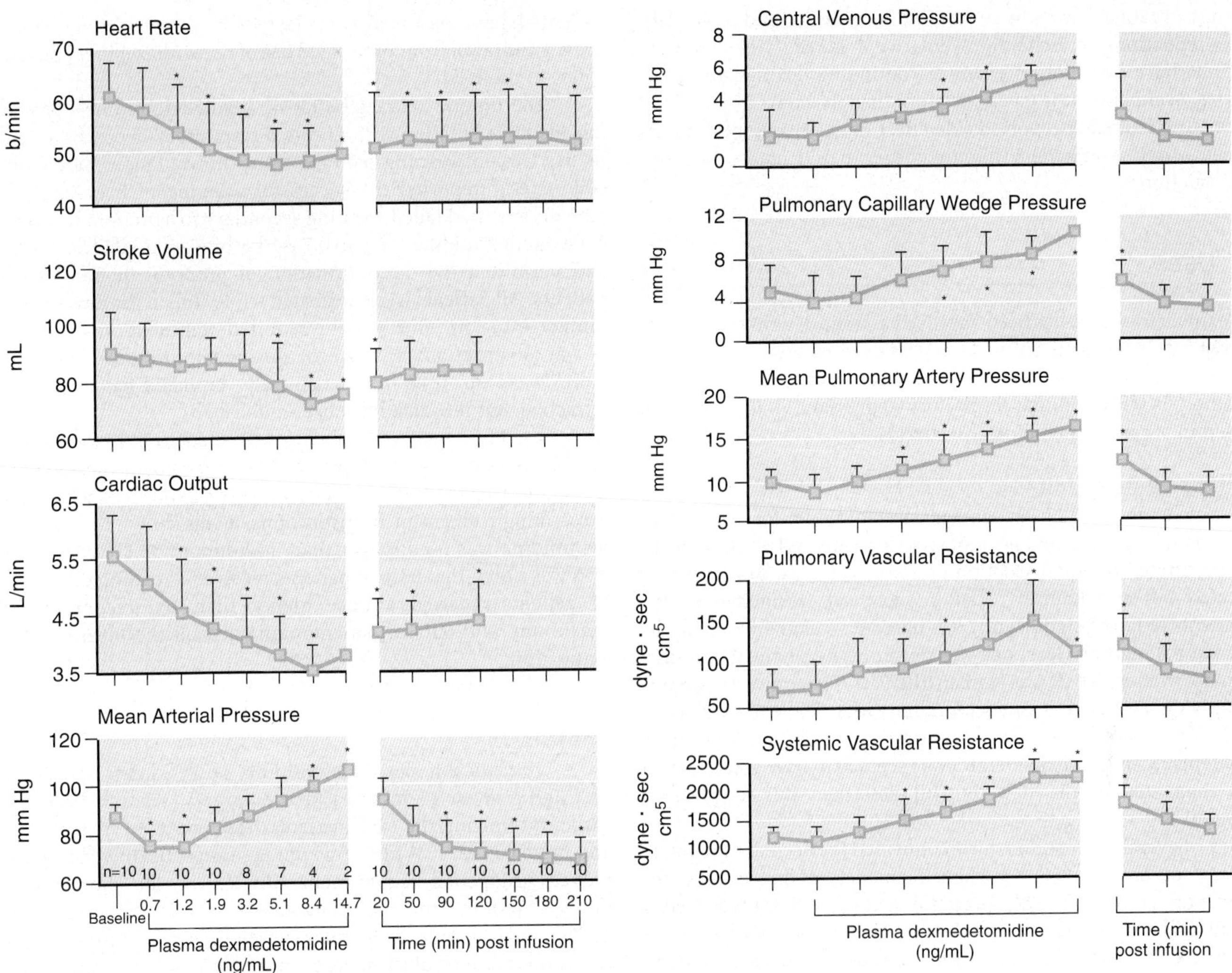

Figure 26-22 Effects of increasing plasma concentrations of dexmedetomidine.

Ebert and colleagues[515] performed an elegant study in volunteers using a target-controlled infusion system to provide increasing concentrations (0.7 to 15 ng/mL) of dexmedetomidine (Fig. 26-22). The lowest two concentrations produced a decrease in MAP (13%) followed by progressive increase (12%). Increasing concentrations of dexmedetomidine also produce progressive decreases in heart rate (maximum 29%) and cardiac output (35%).[515] Infusion of dexmedetomidine in volunteers also has been shown to result in a compensated reduction in systemic sympathetic tone without changes in baroreflex sensitivity. It also blunts the heart rate and systemic sympathetic activation owing to sweating, but is less effective in blunting cardiac sympathetic response to shivering.[520]

The incidence of hypotension and bradycardia may be related to the administration of a loading dose. Omitting the loading dose or not giving more than 0.4 μg/kg reduces the incidence of hypotension, or makes it less pronounced. Giving the loading dose over 20 minutes also minimizes the transient hypertension.[521] In several studies after IM and IV administration, dexmedetomidine caused, in a small percentage of patients, profound bradycardia (<40 beats/min) and occasionally sinus arrest/pause. Generally, these episodes resolved spontaneously or were readily treated without adverse outcome by anticholinergics. It would be expected from its profile that dexmedetomidine would be beneficial to the ischemic myocardium. In animal models, dexmedetomidine showed some beneficial effects on the ischemic heart through decreased oxygen consumption and redistribution of coronary flow from nonischemic zones to ischemic zones after acute brief occlusion.[522] Dexmedetomidine also decreases serum lactate in a dog model of coronary ischemia with an associated decrease in heart rate and measured catecholamines. It also produced an increase in the endocardial/epicardial blood flow ratio by 35%.[523]

The perioperative use of α_2 agonists reduces the incidence of perioperative myocardial ischemia.[524] More recently, Wallace and associates[525] showed that the administration of clonidine in the preoperative period reduces the incidence of perioperative cardiac ischemia from 31% to 14%, and reduces the mortality for 2 years from 29% to 15% compared with placebo. The only data on potential benefits in perioperative ischemia prevention with dexmedetomidine are provided in an underpowered study in vascular surgery patients who received the drug in the perioperative period. Blood pressure and heart rate were lower in the dexmedetomidine group, but these patients also needed the use of more drugs intraoperatively to sustain blood pressure and heart rate. No reductions of ischemic events were noted.[189] No rebound effects have been found when discontinuing dexmedetomidine drips, even when it is given for more than 24 hours.[526]

A frequently reported side effect of dexmedetomidine has been a dry mouth. Dry mouth is due to a decrease in saliva production.[527]

Uses

Dexmedetomidine has been approved as a short-term sedative for adult intubated patients in the ICU. Given its well-documented beneficial effects of anxiolysis, sedation, analgesia, and sympatholysis with minimal respiratory depression, it also has been used in various other clinical scenarios.

Intensive Care Unit

Dexmedetomidine has advantages over propofol for sedation in mechanically ventilated postoperative patients. When both drugs were titrated to equal sedation as assessed by the BIS (approximately 50) and Ramsay sedation score (5), dexmedetomidine patients required significantly less narcotics (alfentanil 2.5 mg/hr versus 0.8 mg/hr). Heart rate was slower in the dexmedetomidine group, whereas MAP was similar. The PaO_2/FIO_2 ratio was significantly higher in the dexmedetomidine group. Time to extubation after discontinuation of the infusion was similar at 28 minutes. Patients receiving dexmedetomidine seemed to have greater recall of their stay in the ICU, but all described this as pleasant overall.[528]

Several other studies have confirmed the decreased requirement for opioids (>50%) when dexmedetomidine is used for sedation compared with propofol or benzodiazepines. Most studies also describe more stable hemodynamics during weaning when dexmedetomidine is used for sedation.[529] This is of obvious benefit in patients with high risk for myocardial ischemia. For sedation in the ICU, loading doses of 0.5 to 1 μg/kg have been used. Omitting the bolus or giving the lower dose has been associated with fewer episodes of severe bradycardia and other hemodynamic perturbations. Infusion rates of 0.1 to 1 μg/kg/hr are generally needed to maintain adequate sedation. Delirium in the ICU is a risk factor for increased length of stay and increased mortality.[530] In a double-blind, randomized controlled trial of sedation in ventilated patients with dexmedetomidine versus lorazepam, it was found that using dexmedetomidine infusions provided more days alive without delirium or coma and a greater amount of time spent at the appropriate sedation level compared with lorazepam.[531]

α_2-adrenoreceptor agonists have been used in the treatment of alcohol and drug withdrawal. In a comparison between clonidine and chlordiazepoxide in the treatment of patients with alcohol withdrawal, clonidine proved to give better anxiolysis with better hemodynamics.[532] Dexmedetomidine has been successfully used in the treatment of withdrawal of narcotics, benzodiazepines, alcohol, and recreational drugs. Maccioli[489] reported the successful use of dexmedetomidine in two adult patients, one with cocaine and alcohol withdrawal symptoms, and another with withdrawal from prolonged use of benzodiazepines and narcotics in the ICU. Dexmedetomidine controlled withdrawal behavior and allowed for successful detoxification of young cardiothoracic patients (spanning the ages of days to 17 years) who developed drug withdrawal from prolonged use of benzodiazepines and narcotics in the ICU.[533]

The unique characteristics of dexmedetomidine—providing adequate sedation with minimal respiratory depression—can be used when weaning patients from the ventilator. Siobal and colleagues[534] reported the successful weaning of five ventilated patients who had failed weaning secondary to agitation. Infusions of dexmedetomidine of 0.5 to 0.7 μg/kg/hr were used (no loading) and permitted the discontinuation of propofol in four of five patients. All patients were extubated while still on the dexmedetomidine infusion. One patient required reintubation for upper airway obstruction. The use of dexmedetomidine to facilitate daily "wake up" tests in mechanically ventilated patients seems attractive, but few data have been published.[535]

The FDA approved the use of dexmedetomidine infusions for 24 hours or less. Multiple studies have shown the safety of using this drug for longer periods, however. In data collected from prescribing patterns in 10 institutions, it was shown that dexmedetomidine was used longer than 24 hours in 33.8% of cases. It also was noted that 33% of patients received a loading dose, 27% of patients received a dose higher than the recommended maximum, and 60% of patients remained on the infusion after extubation.[536]

Anesthesia

As a premedicant, dexmedetomidine, at IV doses of 0.33 to 0.67 μg/kg given 15 minutes before surgery, seems efficacious, while minimizing the cardiovascular side effects of hypotension and bradycardia.[537] Within this dosage range, dexmedetomidine reduces thiopental requirements (by ±30%) for short procedures,[537] reduces the requirements of volatile anesthetics (by ±25%), and more effectively attenuates the hemodynamic response to endotracheal intubation compared with 2 μg/kg of fentanyl.[538] Dexmedetomidine also has been evaluated as an IM injection (2.5 μg/kg) with or without fentanyl administered 45 to 90 minutes before surgery. This regimen was compared with IM midazolam plus fentanyl and was found to provide equal anxiolysis, reduced response to intubation, smaller volatile anesthetic requirements, and a decreased incidence of postoperative shivering but a higher incidence of bradycardia. Atipamezole, a selective α_2 antagonist, at 50 μg/kg was effective in reversing the sedation of dexmedetomidine (2 μg/kg intramuscularly), when used to provide sedation for brief operative procedures.[487] This reversal of effects resulted in a more rapid recovery than occurred after equisedative doses of midazolam.

Dexmedetomidine has been used for sedation for monitored anesthesia care. In a study comparing the efficacy of dexmedetomidine or propofol as a sedative agent in a group of 40 patients receiving local anesthesia or regional blocks, dexmedetomidine (1 μg/kg given over 10 minutes) when used for intraoperative sedation resulted in a slower onset than propofol (75 μg/kg/min for 10 minutes), but similar cardiorespiratory effects when titrated to equal sedation. The average infusion rate of dexmedetomidine intraoperatively to maintain a BIS value of 70 to 80 was 0.7 μg/kg/min. Sedation was more prolonged after termination of the infusion, as was recovery of blood pressure. Smaller doses of opioid were needed in the first hour, however.[517]

Dexmedetomidine sedation has been done successfully in pediatric patients. Two studies, comprising 140 children 1 to 7 years old, reported successful sedation for MRI scans compared with midazolam or propofol.[539,540]

When dexmedetomidine is used as a premedication 10 minutes before general surgery for cataract removal, intraocular pressure is decreased (33%), catecholamine secretion is reduced, perioperative analgesic requirements are less, and recovery is more rapid.[541,542]

For maintenance of anesthesia, dexmedetomidine has been used in patients undergoing multiple types of surgery. In patients given an infusion regimen to achieve a plasma concentration of slightly less than 1 ng/mL, combined with 70% nitrous oxide, dexmedetomidine reduced isoflurane requirements by 90% compared with a control group.[543] One retrospective study and two prospective, randomized controlled trials in bariatric surgical patients have found that a balanced anesthetic with desflurane or propofol plus dexmedetomidine (0.5 to 0.8 µg/kg bolus plus 0.4 µg/kg/hr infusion) reduces postoperative pain scores and morphine consumption, and improves hemodynamics compared with desflurane-fentanyl or propofol-fentanyl anesthetics.[544-546]

In patients presenting for vascular surgery, three infusion rates of dexmedetomidine were compared with a placebo infusion starting 1 hour before surgery and administered until 48 hours after surgery. In the groups receiving dexmedetomidine, more vasoactive agents were required to maintain hemodynamics intraoperatively, but less tachycardia was noted postoperatively. No other significant differences were noted between the groups.[547]

Grant and colleagues[548] described the use of dexmedetomidine when securing the airway with a fiberoptic intubation in three patients undergoing cervical spine surgery. The procedure was well tolerated with no hemodynamic compromise or respiratory depression. Because this drug provides good sedation with minimal respiratory depression, it has been used in patients undergoing awake craniotomies with functional testing and electrocorticography[549] or awake carotid endarterectomies with fewer fluctuations from the desired sedation level and more stable hemodynamics.[550]

Another use of dexmedetomidine has been as an anesthetic adjunct or sedative agent for patients who are susceptible to narcotic-induced respiratory depression or sleep apnea. In a morbidly obese patient, the narcotic-sparing effects of dexmedetomidine were evident intraoperatively and postoperatively after bariatric surgery.[551] The addition of dexmedetomidine infusions to assist on transesophageal echocardiography examination has been described, with better hemodynamic profile and improved patient satisfaction than with benzodiazepine and narcotics alone, with no added respiratory depression.

The use of dexmedetomidine has dramatically increased. This highly selective α_2 agonist has a set of unique effects that include titratable sedation, sympatholysis, and analgesia without significant respiratory depression. Originally approved as a sedative in the ICU, it has found many off-label applications in the ICU, the operating room, and perioperative environment. The off-label use of dexmedetomidine in infants and children is rapidly increasing. More than 800 reports have been published regarding its use in this population.[470]

Droperidol

History

Janssen[552] synthesized haloperidol, the first member of the butyrophenones, which became the primary neuroleptic component in neuroleptanesthesia. In 1959, DeCastro and Mundeleer[553] combined haloperidol with phenoperidine (a meperidine derivative also synthesized by Janssen) in the forerunner to the practice of neuroleptanesthesia. Droperidol, a derivative of haloperidol, and fentanyl (a phenoperidine congener), both synthesized by Janssen, were used by DeCastro and Mundeleer[553] in a combination they reported to be superior to haloperidol and phenoperidine. This neuroleptanesthesia combination produced more rapid onset of analgesia, less respiratory depression, and fewer extrapyramidal side effects. The fixed combination of droperidol and fentanyl, marketed as Innovar in the United States, was the drug primarily used for neuroleptanesthesia.

The use of neuroleptanesthesia has largely disappeared in modern anesthetic practice. The primary use of droperidol in anesthesia has been as an antiemetic and to a lesser extent as a sedative and antipruritic. The present package insert for droperidol in the United States carries a black box warning regarding the potential for fatal arrhythmias and recommendations that it be administered only during continuous electrocardiogram monitoring. With the withdrawal of droperidol in certain countries and more stringent labeling regarding potentially lethal dysrhythmias in others, the use of droperidol has decreased tremendously. The validity of the risk of low-dose droperidol in causing QT prolongation, dysrhythmias, and death has been challenged by numerous editorials, articles, and letters reviewing the cases that prompted this action.[554-559]

Droperidol is a butyrophenone, a fluorinated derivative of phenothiazines (Fig. 26-23).[345] Butyrophenones produce CNS depression, characterized by marked apparent tranquility and cataleptic immobility. They are potent antiemetics. Droperidol is a potent butyrophenone, and, similar to the others, it produces its action centrally at sites where dopamine, norepinephrine, and serotonin act. It has been postulated that butyrophenones may occupy GABA receptors on the postsynaptic membrane, reducing synaptic transmission and resulting in a buildup of dopamine in the intersynaptic cleft.[345,552] In particular, droperidol results in a submaximal inhibition of the $GABA_A$ α_1, β_1, and γ_2 acetylcholine receptors and full inhibition of α_2 acetylcholine receptors. This submaximal inhibition of GABA receptors by droperidol may explain the anxiety, dysphoria, and restlessness that may occur with its administration.[560] An imbalance in dopamine and acetylcholine is thought to occur, which results in alteration in normal transmission of signals in the CNS. The chemoreceptor trigger

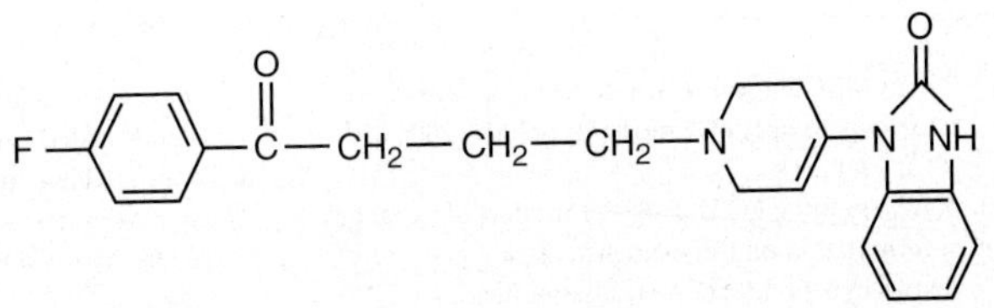

Figure 26-23 Structure of droperidol, a butyrophenone derivative.

zone is the emetic center, and "red" astrocytes transport neurolept molecules from the capillary to dopaminergic synapses in the chemoreceptor trigger zone, where they occupy GABA receptors. This is thought to be the mechanism by which droperidol exerts its antiemetic effect.[561]

Metabolism and Pharmacokinetics

Droperidol is biotransformed in the liver into two primary metabolites.[562] Its plasma decay can be described by a two-compartment model. The pharmacokinetics is shown in Table 26-1.[563]

Pharmacology

Effects on the Central Nervous System

The effects of neuroleptanesthetics on human CBF and $CMRO_2$ have not been studied. In dogs, droperidol causes potent cerebral vasoconstriction, producing a 40% reduction in CBF (see Chapter 13). No significant change in $CMRO_2$ occurs during droperidol administration.[564] The EEG in conscious patients shows some reduction in frequency, with occasional slowing.[565] Low-dose droperidol also has been shown to cause balance disturbances at the time of discharge after doses used for antiemetic prophylaxis.[566] Droperidol may produce extrapyramidal signs and worsens symptoms of Parkinson's disease. It also rarely may precipitate malignant neuroleptic syndrome.

Effects on the Respiratory System

When used alone, droperidol has little effect on the respiratory system.[567] Droperidol (0.044 mg/kg) given to surgical patients produced a slight reduction in respiratory rate,[568] and IV droperidol (3 mg) had no significant effect on tidal volume in volunteers.[569] More detailed respiratory studies are unavailable.

Effects on the Cardiovascular System

Similar to most antipsychotics, droperidol may prolong the QT interval by delaying myocardial repolarization and precipitating torsades de pointes. This seems to be dose dependent and may be of clinical significance when other causes of QT prolongation also are present.[570] Droperidol also may possess some antiarrhythmic effects that are similar to those of quinidine.[571] Droperidol produces vasodilation with a decrease in blood pressure (see Table 26-2). This effect is considered to be a result of moderate α-adrenergic blockade.[562] The dopamine-induced increase in renal blood flow (renal artery flowmeter methodology) is not significantly impaired by administration of droperidol.[572] Droperidol has little effect on myocardial contractility.[571]

Uses

Use of droperidol today in the perioperative period is largely restricted to its antiemetic and sedative effects. It is an effective antiemetic[573]; the dose for this use ranges from 10 to 20 μg/kg (0.6 to 1.25 mg for a 70-kg individual).[574] These doses of droperidol, given at the start of anesthesia for operations lasting 1 hour, reduce the incidence of nausea and vomiting by about 30%. These doses given at induction have little effect on wake-up time, but should they be given at the end of surgery, there could be some residual hypnotic effect. Overall, antiemetic efficacy of droperidol alone is equal to that of ondansetron and results in an equal number of side effects, but droperidol is more cost-effective.[575] The efficacy of droperidol as an antiemetic is enhanced when used in combination with serotonin antagonists or dexamethasone or both.

Droperidol also has been shown to be effective in the treatment and prevention of pruritus secondary to opioid administration. It has been given intravenously and into the epidural space for this purpose.[576,577] When used in this fashion, droperidol also effectively reduces nausea, but it increases sedation. The safety of droperidol administration into the epidural space has not been fully evaluated, however, and it is not approved for administration via this route.

Summary

Many different IV drugs are available for use in the care of patients requiring general anesthesia. The selection of a particular drug must be based on the individual patient's need for hypnosis, amnesia, and analgesia. Drug selection must match the physiology or the pathophysiology or both of the individual patient with the pharmacology of the particular drug. A patient in shock who requires anesthesia induction should receive the drug that would produce rapid onset of effect without causing further hemodynamic compromise. The knowledge of the clinical pharmacology of each of the IV anesthetic drugs enables the clinician to induce and maintain sedation or general anesthesia safely and effectively. There is no single perfect drug for any particular patient, but rather the informed practitioner wisely employs the appropriate drug or drugs in the practice of good anesthesia care.

References

1. Cohen MM, Duncan PG, Tate RB: Does anesthesia contribute to operative mortality? JAMA 260:2859-2863, 1988.

1a. Kay B, Rolly G: I.C.I. 35868—The effect of a change of formulation on the incidence of pain after intravenous injection. Acta Anaesthesiol Belg 28(4:)317-322, 1977.

2. James R, Glen JB: Synthesis, biological evaluation, and preliminary structure-activity considerations of a series of alkylphenols as intravenous anesthetic agents. J Med Chem 23:1350-1357, 1980.

3. Gan TJ: Pharmacokinetic and pharmacodynamic characteristics of medications used for moderate sedation. Clin Pharmacokinet 45:855-869, 2006.

4. Simons P, Cockshott I, Douglas E: Blood concentrations, metabolism and elimination after a subanesthetic intravenous dose of (14)C-propofol (Diprivan) to male volunteers. Postgrad Med J 61:64, 1985.

5. Veroli P, O'Kelly B, Bertrand F, et al: Extrahepatic metabolism of propofol in man during the anhepatic phase of orthotopic liver transplantation. Br J Anaesth 68:183-186, 1992.

6. Takizawa D, Hiraoka H, Goto F, et al: Human kidneys play an important role in the elimination of propofol. Anesthesiology 102:327-330, 2005.

7. Hiraoka H, Yamamoto K, Miyoshi S, et al: Kidneys contribute to the extrahepatic clearance of propofol in humans, but not lungs and brain. Br J Clin Pharmacol 60:176-182, 2005.
8. Raoof AA, van Obbergh LJ, de Ville de Goyet J, Verbeeck RK: Extrahepatic glucuronidation of propofol in man: Possible contribution of gut wall and kidney. Eur J Clin Pharmacol 50:91-96, 1996.
9. Kuipers JA, Boer F, Olieman W, et al: First-pass lung uptake and pulmonary clearance of propofol: Assessment with a recirculatory indocyanine green pharmacokinetic model. Anesthesiology 91:1780-1787, 1999.
10. Dawidowicz AL, Fornal E, Mardarowicz M, Fijalkowska A: The role of human lungs in the biotransformation of propofol. Anesthesiology 93:992-997, 2000.
11. Chen TL, Ueng TH, Chen SH, et al: Human cytochrome P450 mono-oxygenase system is suppressed by propofol. Br J Anaesth 74:558-562, 1995.
12. Fechner J, Ihmsen H, Hatterscheid D, et al: Pharmacokinetics and clinical pharmacodynamics of the new propofol prodrug GPI 15715 in volunteers. Anesthesiology 99:303-313, 2003.
13. Kay NH, Sear JW, Uppington J, et al: Disposition of propofol in patients undergoing surgery: A comparison in men and women. Br J Anaesth 58:1075-1079, 1986.
14. Gepts E, Camu F, Cockshott ID, Douglas EJ: Disposition of propofol administered as constant rate intravenous infusions in humans. Anesth Analg 66:1256-1263, 1987.
15. Schuttler J, Stoeckel H, Schwilden H: Pharmacokinetic and pharmacodynamic modeling of propofol (Diprivan) in volunteers and surgical patients. Postgrad Med J 61:53, 1985.
16. Hughes MA, Glass PS, Jacobs JR: Context-sensitive half-time in multicompartment pharmacokinetic models for intravenous anesthetic drugs. Anesthesiology 76:334-341, 1992.
17. Gray PA, Park GR, Cockshott ID, et al: Propofol metabolism in man during the anhepatic and reperfusion phases of liver transplantation. Xenobiotica 22:105-114, 1992.
18. Dyck J, Varvel J, Hung O: The pharmacokinetics of propofol vs. age. Anesthesiology 75:A315, 1991.
19. Kazama T, Ikeda K, Morita K, et al: Comparison of the effect-site k(eO)s of propofol for blood pressure and EEG bispectral index in elderly and younger patients. Anesthesiology 90:1517-1527, 1999.
20. Schnider TW, Minto CF, Shafer SL, et al: The influence of age on propofol pharmacodynamics. Anesthesiology 90:1502-1516, 1999.
21. Kirkpatrick T, Cockshott ID, Douglas EJ, Nimmo WS: Pharmacokinetics of propofol (diprivan) in elderly patients. Br J Anaesth 60:146-150, 1988.
22. Shafer A, Doze VA, Shafer SL, White PF: Pharmacokinetics and pharmacodynamics of propofol infusions during general anesthesia. Anesthesiology 69:348-356, 1988.
23. Morcos W, Payne J: The induction of anaesthesia with propofol (Diprivan) compared in normal and renal failure patients. Postgrad Med J 61:62-63, 1985.
24. Leslie K, Sessler DI, Bjorksten AR, Moayeri A: Mild hypothermia alters propofol pharmacokinetics and increases the duration of action of atracurium. Anesth Analg 80:1007-1014, 1995.
25. Upton RN, Ludbrook GL, Grant C, Martinez AM: Cardiac output is a determinant of the initial concentrations of propofol after short-infusion administration. Anesth Analg 89:545-552, 1999.
26. Kurita T, Morita K, Kazama T, Sato S: Influence of cardiac output on plasma propofol concentrations during constant infusion in swine. Anesthesiology 96:1498-1503, 2002.
27. Kazama T, Kurita T, Morita K, et al: Influence of hemorrhage on propofol pseudo-steady state concentration. Anesthesiology 97:1156-1161, 2002.
28. Allegaert K, Peeters MY, Verbesselt R, et al: Inter-individual variability in propofol pharmacokinetics in preterm and term neonates. Br J Anaesth 99:864-870, 2007.
29. Bailey JM, Mora CT, Shafer SL: Pharmacokinetics of propofol in adult patients undergoing coronary revascularization. The Multicenter Study of Perioperative Ischemia Research Group. Anesthesiology 84:1288-1297, 1996.
30. Marsh B, White M, Morton N, Kenny GN: Pharmacokinetic model driven infusion of propofol in children. Br J Anaesth 67:41-48, 1991.
31. Kataria BK, Ved SA, Nicodemus HF, et al: The pharmacokinetics of propofol in children using three different data analysis approaches. Anesthesiology 80:104-122, 1994.
32. Murat I, Billard V, Vernois J, et al: Pharmacokinetics of propofol after a single dose in children aged 1-3 years with minor burns: Comparison of three data analysis approaches. Anesthesiology 84:526-532, 1996.
33. Servin F, Desmonts JM, Farinotti R, et al: [Pharmacokinetics of the continuous infusion of propofol in the cirrhotic patient: Preliminary results]. Ann Fr Anesth Reanim 6:228-229, 1987.
34. Benoni G, Cuzzolin L, Gilli E: Pharmacokinetics of propofol: Influence of fentanyl administration. Eur J Anaesthesiol 183:1457, 1990.
35. Pavlin DJ, Coda B, Shen DD, et al: Effects of combining propofol and alfentanil on ventilation, analgesia, sedation, and emesis in human volunteers. Anesthesiology 84:23-37, 1996.
36. Gill SS, Wright EM, Reilly CS: Pharmacokinetic interaction of propofol and fentanyl: Single bolus injection study. Br J Anaesth 65:760-765, 1990.
37. Matot I, Neely CF, Katz RY, Marshall BE: Fentanyl and propofol uptake by the lung: Effect of time between injections. Acta Anaesthesiol Scand 38:711-715, 1994.
38. Janicki PK, James MF, Erskine WA: Propofol inhibits enzymatic degradation of alfentanil and sufentanil by isolated liver microsomes in vitro. Br J Anaesth 68:311-312, 1992.
39. Gibiansky E, Struys MM, Gibiansky L, et al: AQUAVAN injection, a water-soluble prodrug of propofol, as a bolus injection: A phase I dose-escalation comparison with DIPRIVAN (part 1): Pharmacokinetics. Anesthesiology 103:718-729, 2005.
40. Struys MM, Vanluchene AL, Gibiansky E, et al: AQUAVAN injection, a water-soluble prodrug of propofol, as a bolus injection: A phase I dose-escalation comparison with DIPRIVAN (part 2): Pharmacodynamics and safety. Anesthesiology 103:730-743, 2005.
41. Krasowski MD, Nishikawa K, Nikolaeva N, et al: Methionine 286 in transmembrane domain 3 of the GABAA receptor beta subunit controls a binding cavity for propofol and other alkylphenol general anesthetics. Neuropharmacology 41:952-964, 2001.
42. Jurd R, Arras M, Lambert S, Drexler B: General anesthetic actions in vivo strongly attenuated by a point mutation in the $GABA_A$ receptor beta-3 subunit. FASEB J 2002.
43. Lam DW, Reynolds JN: Modulatory and direct effects of propofol on recombinant $GABA_A$ receptors expressed in xenopus oocytes: Influence of alpha- and gamma2-subunits. Brain Res 784:179-187, 1998.
44. Kikuchi T, Wang Y, Sato K, Okumura F: In vivo effects of propofol on acetylcholine release from the frontal cortex, hippocampus and striatum studied by intracerebral microdialysis in freely moving rats. Br J Anaesth 80:644-648, 1998.
45. Kushikata T, Hirota K, Yoshida H, et al: Alpha-2 adrenoceptor activity affects propofol-induced sleep time. Anesth Analg 94:1201-1206, 2002.
46. Lingamaneni R, Birch ML, Hemmings HC Jr: Widespread inhibition of sodium channel-dependent glutamate release from isolated nerve terminals by isoflurane and propofol. Anesthesiology 95:1460-1466, 2001.
47. Antognini J, Wang X, Piercy M, Carstens E: Propofol directly depresses lumbar dorsal horn neuronal responses to noxious stimulation in goats. Can J Anaesth 47:273-279, 2000.
48. Dong XP, Xu TL: The actions of propofol on gamma-aminobutyric acid-A and glycine receptors in acutely dissociated spinal dorsal horn neurons of the rat. Anesth Analg 95:907-914, 2002.
49. Tonner PH, Poppers DM, Miller KW: The general anesthetic potency of propofol and its dependence on hydrostatic pressure. Anesthesiology 77:926-931, 1992.
50. Pain L, Gobaille S, Schleef C, et al: In vivo dopamine measurements in the nucleus accumbens after non-anesthetic and anesthetic doses of propofol in rats. Anesth Analg 95:915-919, 2002.
51. Cechetto DF, Diab T, Gibson CJ, Gelb AW: The effects of propofol in the area postrema of rats. Anesth Analg 92:934-942, 2001.
52. Adam HK, Kay B, Douglas EJ: Blood disoprofol levels in anesthetised patients: Correlation of concentrations after single or repeated doses with hypnotic activity. Anaesthesia 37:536-540, 1982.
53. Aun CS, Short SM, Leung DH, Oh TE: Induction dose-response of propofol in unpremedicated children. Br J Anaesth 68:64-67, 1992.
54. Smith C, McEwan A, Jhaveri R: Reduction of propofol Cp50 by fentanyl. Anesthesiology 77:A340, 1992.
55. Mackenzie N, Grant IS: Propofol for intravenous sedation. Anaesthesia 42:3-6, 1987.
56. Wilson E, Mackenzie N, Grant IS: A comparison of propofol and midazolam by infusion to provide sedation in patients who receive spinal anaesthesia. Anaesthesia 43(Suppl):91-94, 1988.
57. Veselis RA, Reinsel RA, Wronski M, et al: EEG and memory effects of low-dose infusions of propofol. Br J Anaesth 69:246-254, 1992.
58. Zacny JP, Lichtor JL, Coalson DW, et al: Subjective and psychomotor effects of subanesthetic doses of propofol in healthy volunteers. Anesthesiology 76:696-702, 1992.
59. Kelly JS, Roy RC: Intraoperative awareness with propofol-oxygen total intravenous anesthesia for microlaryngeal surgery. Anesthesiology 77:207-209, 1992.
60. McDonald NJ, Mannion D, Lee P, et al: Mood evaluation and outpatient anaesthesia: A comparison between propofol and thiopentone. Anaesthesia 43(Suppl):68-69, 1988.
61. Nelson V: Hallucinations after propofol. Anaesthesia 43:170, 1988.
62. Cameron A: Opisthotonos again. Anaesthesia 42:1124, 1987.
63. Hazeau C, Tisserant D, Vespignani H: Electroencephalographic changes produced by propofol. Ann Fr Anesth Reanim 6:261, 1987.
64. Yate PM, Maynard DE, Major E, et al: Anaesthesia with ICI 35,868 monitored by the cerebral function analysing monitor (CFAM). Eur J Anaesthesiol 3:159-166, 1986.

65. Glass PS, Bloom M, Kearse L, et al: Bispectral analysis measures sedation and memory effects of propofol, midazolam, isoflurane, and alfentanil in healthy volunteers. Anesthesiology 86:836-847, 1997.
66. Maurette P, Simeon F, Castagnera L, et al: Propofol anaesthesia alters somatosensory evoked cortical potentials. Anaesthesia 43(Suppl):44-45, 1988.
67. Savoia G, Esposito C, Belfiore F, et al: Propofol infusion and auditory evoked potentials. Anaesthesia 43(Suppl):46-49, 1988.
68. Vanluchene AL, Vereecke H, Thas O, et al: Spectral entropy as an electroencephalographic measure of anesthetic drug effect: A comparison with bispectral index and processed midlatency auditory evoked response. Anesthesiology 101:34-42, 2004.
69. al-Hader A, Hasan M, Hasan Z: The comparative effects of propofol, thiopental, and diazepam, administered intravenously, on pentylenetetrazol seizure threshold in the rabbit. Life Sci 51:779-786, 1992.
70. Heavner J, Arthur J, Zou J: Propofol vs. thiopental for treating bupivacaine induced seizures in rats. Anesthesiology 77:A802, 1992.
71. Chilvers CR, Laurie PS: Successful use of propofol in status epilepticus. Anaesthesia 45:995-996, 1990.
72. Dwyer R, McCaughey W, Lavery J, et al: Comparison of propofol and methohexitone as anaesthetic agents for electroconvulsive therapy. Anaesthesia 43:459-462, 1988.
73. Hodkinson BP, Frith RW, Mee EW: Propofol and the electroencephalogram. Lancet 2:1518, 1987.
74. Committee on Safety of Medicines: Propofol. Curr Probl 20, 1987.
75. Keidan I, Perel A, Shabtai EL, Pfeffer RM: Children undergoing repeated exposures for radiation therapy do not develop tolerance to propofol: Clinical and bispectral index data. Anesthesiology 100:251-254, 2004.
76. Cohen Y, Feldinger E, Ogorek D, Weinbroum AA: Increased propofol requirement during succeeding administrations for electroconvulsive therapy. J Clin Anesth 16:282-285, 2004.
77. Follette JW, Farley WJ: Anesthesiologist addicted to propofol. Anesthesiology 77:817-818, 1992.
78. Mendes PM, Silberstein SD, Young WB, et al: Intravenous propofol in the treatment of refractory headache. Headache 42:638-641, 2002.
79. Vandesteene A, Trempont V, Engelman E, et al: Effect of propofol on cerebral blood flow and metabolism in man. Anaesthesia 43(Suppl):42-43, 1988.
80. Steiner LA, Johnston AJ, Chatfield DA, et al: The effects of large-dose propofol on cerebrovascular pressure autoregulation in head-injured patients. Anesth Analg 97:572-576, 2003.
81. Mirakhur RK, Shepherd WF, Darrah WC: Propofol or thiopentone: Effects on intraocular pressure associated with induction of anaesthesia and tracheal intubation (facilitated with suxamethonium). Br J Anaesth 59:431-436, 1987.
82. Enns J, Gelb A, Manninen P: Cerebral autoregulation is maintained during propofol-nitrous oxide anaesthesia in humans. Can J Anaesth 39:A43, 1992.
83. Kochs E, Hoffman WE, Werner C, et al: The effects of propofol on brain electrical activity, neurologic outcome, and neuronal damage following incomplete ischemia in rats. Anesthesiology 76:245-252, 1992.
84. Gelb AW, Bayona NA, Wilson JX, Cechetto DF: Propofol anesthesia compared to awake reduces infarct size in rats. Anesthesiology 96:1183-1190, 2002.
85. Bhardwaj A, Castro IA, Alkayed NJ, et al: Anesthetic choice of halothane versus propofol: Impact on experimental perioperative stroke. Stroke 32:1920-1925, 2001.
86. Kaptanoglu E, Sen S, Beskonakli E, et al: Antioxidant actions and early ultrastructural findings of thiopental and propofol in experimental spinal cord injury. J Neurosurg Anesthesiol 14:114-122, 2002.
87. Amorim P, Chambers G, Cottrell J, Kass IS: Propofol reduces neuronal transmission damage and attenuates the changes in calcium, potassium, and sodium during hyperthermic anoxia in the rat hippocampal slice. Anesthesiology 83:1254-1265, 1995.
88. Ergun R, Adkemir G, Sen S, et al: Neuroprotective effects of propofol following global cerebral ischemia in rats. Neurosurg Rev 2001.
89. Kawaguchi M, Furuya H, Patel PM: Neuroprotective effects of anesthetic agents. J Anesth 19:150-156, 2005.
90. Lanigan C, Sury M, Bingham R, et al: Neurological sequelae in children after prolonged propofol infusion. Anaesthesia 47:810-811, 1992.
91. Vuyk J, Engbers FH, Lemmens HJ, et al: Pharmacodynamics of propofol in female patients. Anesthesiology 77:3-9, 1992.
92. Forrest FC, Tooley MA, Saunders PR, Prys-Roberts C: Propofol infusion and the suppression of consciousness: The EEG and dose requirements. Br J Anaesth 72:35-41, 1994.
93. Spelina KR, Coates DP, Monk CR, et al: Dose requirements of propofol by infusion during nitrous oxide anaesthesia in man, I: Patients premedicated with morphine sulphate. Br J Anaesth 58:1080-1084, 1986.
94. Kazama T, Ikeda K, Morita K, Sanjo Y: Awakening propofol concentration with and without blood-effect site equilibration after short-term and long-term administration of propofol and fentanyl anesthesia. Anesthesiology 88:928-934, 1998.
95. Sanderson JH, Blades JF: Multicentre study of propofol in day case surgery. Anaesthesia 43(Suppl):70-73, 1988.
96. Taylor MB, Grounds RM, Mulrooney PD, Morgan M: Ventilatory effects of propofol during induction of anaesthesia: Comparison with thiopentone. Anaesthesia 41:816-820, 1986.
97. Goodman NW, Black AM, Carter JA: Some ventilatory effects of propofol as sole anaesthetic agent. Br J Anaesth 59:1497-1503, 1987.
98. Gold MI, Abraham EC, Herrington C: A controlled investigation of propofol, thiopentone and methohexitone. Can J Anaesth 34:478-483, 1987.
99. Jonsson MM, Lindahl SG, Eriksson LI: Effect of propofol on carotid body chemosensitivity and cholinergic chemotransduction. Anesthesiology 102:110-116, 2005.
100. Conti G, Dell'Utri D, Vilardi V, et al: Propofol induces bronchodilation in mechanically ventilated chronic obstructive pulmonary disease (COPD) patients. Acta Anaesthesiol Scand 37:105-109, 1993.
101. Brown RH, Wagner EM: Mechanisms of bronchoprotection by anesthetic induction agents: Propofol versus ketamine. Anesthesiology 90:822-828, 1999.
102. Lin CC, Shyr MH, Tan PP, et al: Mechanisms underlying the inhibitory effect of propofol on the contraction of canine airway smooth muscle. Anesthesiology 91:750-759, 1999.
103. Brown RH, Greenberg RS, Wagner EM: Efficacy of propofol to prevent bronchoconstriction: Effects of preservative. Anesthesiology 94:851-855, 2001.
104. Basu S, Mutschler DK, Larsson AO, et al: Propofol (Diprivan-EDTA) counteracts oxidative injury and deterioration of the arterial oxygen tension during experimental septic shock. Resuscitation 50:341-348, 2001.
105. Chang H, Tsai S, Chang Y, et al: Therapeutic concentrations of propofol protects mouse macrophages from nitric oxide-induced cell death and apoptosis. Can J Anaesth 49:477, 2002.
106. Kondo U, Kim SO, Murray PA: Propofol selectively attenuates endothelium-dependent pulmonary vasodilation in chronically instrumented dogs. Anesthesiology 93:437-446, 2000.
107. Horibe M, Ogawa K, Sohn JT, Murray PA: Propofol attenuates acetylcholine-induced pulmonary vasorelaxation: Role of nitric oxide and endothelium-derived hyperpolarizing factors. Anesthesiology 93:447-455, 2000.
108. Larsen R, Rathgeber J, Bagdahn A, et al: Effects of propofol on cardiovascular dynamics and coronary blood flow in geriatric patients: A comparison with etomidate. Anaesthesia 43(Suppl):25-31, 1988.
109. Vermeyen KM, Erpels FA, Janssen LA, et al: Propofol-fentanyl anaesthesia for coronary bypass surgery in patients with good left ventricular function. Br J Anaesth 59:1115-1120, 1987.
110. Patrick M, Blair I, Feneck R: A comparison of the haemodynamic effects of propofol (Diprivan) and thiopentone in patients with coronary artery disease. Postgrad Med J 61:23, 1985.
111. Stephan H, Sonntag H, Schenk HD, et al: Effects of propofol on cardiovascular dynamics, myocardial blood flow and myocardial metabolism in patients with coronary artery disease. Br J Anaesth 58:969-975, 1986.
112. Coates D, Prys-Roberts C, Spelina K: Propofol (Diprivan) by intravenous infusion with nitrous oxide: Dose requirements and hemodynamic effects. Postgrad Med J 61:76, 1985.
113. Van Aken H, Meinshausen E, Prien T, et al: The influence of fentanyl and tracheal intubation on the hemodynamic effects of anesthesia induction with propofol/N_2O in humans. Anesthesiology 68:157-163, 1988.
114. Wahr JA, Plunkett JJ, Ramsay JG, et al: Cardiovascular responses during sedation after coronary revascularization: Incidence of myocardial ischemia and hemodynamic episodes with propofol versus midazolam. Institutions of the McSPI Research Group. Anesthesiology 84:1350-1360, 1996.
115. Lejay M, Hanouz JL, Lecarpentier Y, et al: Modifications of the inotropic responses to alpha- and beta-adrenoceptor stimulation by propofol in rat myocardium. Anesth Analg 87:277-283, 1998.
116. Pagel PS, Warltier DC: Negative inotropic effects of propofol as evaluated by the regional preload recruitable stroke work relationship in chronically instrumented dogs. Anesthesiology 78:100-108, 1993.
117. Ebert T, Muzi M, Goff D: Does propofol really preserve baroreflex function in humans? Anesthesiology 77:A337, 1992.
118. Chang KS, Davis RF: Propofol produces endothelium-independent vasodilation and may act as a Ca2+ channel blocker. Anesth Analg 76:24-32, 1993.
119. Yamashita A, Kajikuri J, Ohashi M, et al: Inhibitory effects of propofol on acetylcholine-induced, endothelium-dependent relaxation and prostacyclin synthesis in rabbit mesenteric resistance arteries. Anesthesiology 91:1080-1089, 1999.
120. Samain E, Bouillier H, Marty J, et al: The effect of propofol on angiotensin II-induced Ca(2+) mobilization in aortic smooth muscle cells from normotensive and hypertensive rats. Anesth Analg 90:546-552, 2000.

121. Doursout MF, Joseph PM, Liang YY, et al: Role of propofol and its solvent, intralipid, in nitric oxide-induced peripheral vasodilatation in dogs. Br J Anaesth 89:492-498, 2002.
122. Ebert TJ, Muzi M, Berens R, et al: Sympathetic responses to induction of anesthesia in humans with propofol or etomidate. Anesthesiology 76:725-733, 1992.
123. Kanaya N, Hirata N, Kurosawa S, et al: Differential effects of propofol and sevoflurane on heart rate variability. Anesthesiology 98:34-40, 2003.
124. Sharpe MD, Dobkowski WB, Murkin JM, et al: Propofol has no direct effect on sinoatrial node function or on normal atrioventricular and accessory pathway conduction in Wolff-Parkinson-White syndrome during alfentanil/midazolam anesthesia. Anesthesiology 82:888-895, 1995.
125. Horiguchi T, Nishikawa T: Heart rate response to intravenous atropine during propofol anesthesia. Anesth Analg 95:389-392, 2002.
126. Wu M: Propofol and the supraventricular tachydysrhythmias in children. Anesth Analg 86:914, 1998.
127. Reich DL, Hossain S, Krol M, et al: Predictors of hypotension after induction of general anesthesia. Anesth Analg 101:622-628, 2005.
128. Goh PK, Chiu CL, Wang CY, et al: Randomized double-blind comparison of ketamine-propofol, fentanyl-propofol and propofol-saline on haemodynamics and laryngeal mask airway insertion conditions. Anaesth Intensive Care 33:223-228, 2005.
129. Ebert TJ, Muzi M: Propofol and autonomic reflex function in humans. Anesth Analg 78:369-375, 1994.
130. Conzen PF, Fischer S, Detter C, Peter K: Sevoflurane provides greater protection of the myocardium than propofol in patients undergoing off-pump coronary artery bypass surgery. Anesthesiology 99:826-833, 2003.
131. Tritapepe L, Landoni G, Guarracino F, et al: Cardiac protection by volatile anaesthetics: A multicentre randomized controlled study in patients undergoing coronary artery bypass grafting with cardiopulmonary bypass. Eur J Anaesthesiol 24:323-331, 2007.
132. Guarracino F, Landoni G, Tritapepe L, et al: Myocardial damage prevented by volatile anesthetics: A multicenter randomized controlled study. J Cardiothorac Vasc Anesth 20:477-483, 2006.
133. Xia Z, Huang Z, Ansley DM: Large-dose propofol during cardiopulmonary bypass decreases biochemical markers of myocardial injury in coronary surgery patients: A comparison with isoflurane. Anesth Analg 103:527-532, 2006.
134. McKeating K, Bali IM, Dundee JW: The effects of thiopentone and propofol on upper airway integrity. Anaesthesia 43:638-640, 1988.
135. Denborough M, Hopkinson KC: Propofol and malignant hyperpyrexia. Lancet 1:191, 1988.
136. Van Hemelrijck J, Weekers F, Van Aken H, et al: Propofol anesthesia does not inhibit stimulation of cortisol synthesis. Anesth Analg 80:573-576, 1995.
137. Aviram M, Deckelbaum RJ: Intralipid infusion into humans reduces in vitro platelet aggregation and alters platelet lipid composition. Metabolism 38:343-347, 1989.
138. Laxenaire MC, Mata-Bermejo E, Moneret-Vautrin DA, Gueant JL: Life-threatening anaphylactoid reactions to propofol (Diprivan). Anesthesiology 77:275-280, 1992.
139. Doenicke A, Lorenz W, Stanworth D, et al: Effects of propofol ("Diprivan") on histamine release, immunoglobulin levels and activation of complement in healthy volunteers. Postgrad Med J 61(Suppl 3):15-20, 1985.
140. Borgeat A, Wilder-Smith OH, Saiah M, Rifat K: Subhypnotic doses of propofol relieve pruritus induced by epidural and intrathecal morphine. Anesthesiology 76:510-512, 1992.
141. Gan TJ, Glass PS, Howell ST, et al: Determination of plasma concentrations of propofol associated with 50% reduction in postoperative nausea. Anesthesiology 87:779-784, 1997.
142. Gan TJ, Ginsberg B, Grant AP, Glass PS: Double-blind, randomized comparison of ondansetron and intraoperative propofol to prevent postoperative nausea and vomiting. Anesthesiology 85:1036-1042, 1996.
143. Saiah M, Borgeat A, Wilder-Smith OH, et al: Epidural-morphine-induced pruritus: Propofol versus naloxone. Anesth Analg 78:1110-1113, 1994.
144. Skoutelis A, Lianou P, Papageorgiou E, et al: Effects of propofol and thiopentone on polymorphonuclear leukocyte functions in vitro. Acta Anaesthesiol Scand 38:858-862, 1994.
145. Krumholz W, Endrass J, Hempelmann G: Propofol inhibits phagocytosis and killing of *Staphylococcus aureus* and *Escherichia coli* by polymorphonuclear leukocytes in vitro. Can J Anaesth 41:446-449, 1994.
146. Bennett SN, McNeil MM, Bland LA, et al: Postoperative infections traced to contamination of an intravenous anesthetic, propofol. N Engl J Med 333:147-154, 1995.
147. Donmez A, Arslan G, Pirat A, Demirhan B: Is pancreatitis a complication of propofol infusion? Eur J Anaesthesiol 16:367-370, 1999.
148. Devlin JW, Lau AK, Tanios MA: Propofol-associated hypertriglyceridemia and pancreatitis in the intensive care unit: An analysis of frequency and risk factors. Pharmacotherapy 25:1348-1352, 2005.
149. Kazama T, Morita K, Ikeda T, et al: Comparison of predicted induction dose with predetermined physiologic characteristics of patients and with pharmacokinetic models incorporating those characteristics as covariates. Anesthesiology 98:299-305, 2003.
150. Mclune S, McKay A, Wright P: Synergistic interaction between midazolam and propofol. Br J Anaesth 68:240, 1992.
151. Short TG, Plummer JL, Chui PT: Hypnotic and anaesthetic interactions between midazolam, propofol and alfentanil. Br J Anaesth 69:162-167, 1992.
152. Steib A, Freys G, Beller JP, et al: Propofol in elderly high risk patients: A comparison of haemodynamic effects with thiopentone during induction of anaesthesia. Anaesthesia 43(Suppl):111-114, 1988.
153. Kazama T, Ikeda K, Morita K, et al: Investigation of effective anesthesia induction doses using a wide range of infusion rates with undiluted and diluted propofol. Anesthesiology 92:1017-1028, 2000.
154. Mirakhur RK: Induction characteristics of propofol in children: Comparison with thiopentone. Anaesthesia 43:593-598, 1988.
155. Heath PJ, Kennedy DJ, Ogg TW, et al: Which intravenous induction agent for day surgery? A comparison of propofol, thiopentone, methohexitone and etomidate. Anaesthesia 43:365-368, 1988.
156. Hocker J, Tonner PH, Bollert P, et al: Propofol/remifentanil vs sevoflurane/remifentanil for long lasting surgical procedures: A randomised controlled trial. Anaesthesia 61:752-757, 2006.
157. Van Hemelrijck J, Smith I, White PF: Use of desflurane for outpatient anesthesia: A comparison with propofol and nitrous oxide. Anesthesiology 75:197-203, 1991.
158. Roberts FL, Dixon J, Lewis GT, et al: Induction and maintenance of propofol anaesthesia: A manual infusion scheme. Anaesthesia 43(Suppl):14-17, 1988.
159. Taylor IN, Kenny GN, Glen JB: Pharmacodynamic stability of a mixture of propofol and alfentanil. Br J Anaesth 69:168-171, 1992.
160. Turtle MJ, Cullen P, Prys-Roberts C, et al: Dose requirements of propofol by infusion during nitrous oxide anaesthesia in man, II: Patients premedicated with lorazepam. Br J Anaesth 59:283-287, 1987.
161. Sear JW, Shaw I, Wolf A, Kay NH: Infusions of propofol to supplement nitrous oxide-oxygen for the maintenance of anaesthesia: A comparison with halothane. Anaesthesia 43(Suppl):18-22, 1988.
162. Dexter F, Tinker JH: Comparisons between desflurane and isoflurane or propofol on time to following commands and time to discharge: A metaanalysis. Anesthesiology 83:77-82, 1995.
163. Underwood SM, Davies SW, Feneck RO, Walesby RK: Anaesthesia for myocardial revascularisation: A comparison of fentanyl/propofol with fentanyl/enflurane. Anaesthesia 47:939-945, 1992.
164. Hall RI, Murphy JT, Moffitt EA, et al: A comparison of the myocardial metabolic and haemodynamic changes produced by propofol-sufentanil and enflurane-sufentanil anaesthesia for patients having coronary artery bypass graft surgery. Can J Anaesth 38:996-1004, 1991.
165. Fanard L, Van Steenberge A, Demeire X, van der Puyl F: Comparison between propofol and midazolam as sedative agents for surgery under regional anaesthesia. Anaesthesia 43(Suppl):87-89, 1988.
166. Newman LH, McDonald JC, Wallace PG, Ledingham IM: Propofol infusion for sedation in intensive care. Anaesthesia 42:929-937, 1987.
167. Grounds R, Lalor J, Lumley J: Propofol infusion for sedation in the intensive care unit: Preliminary report. BMJ 294:397, 1987.
168. Beller JP, Pottecher T, Lugnier A, et al: Prolonged sedation with propofol in ICU patients: Recovery and blood concentration changes during periodic interruptions in infusion. Br J Anaesth 61:583-588, 1988.
169. Parke TJ, Stevens JE, Rice AS, et al: Metabolic acidosis and fatal myocardial failure after propofol infusion in children: Five case reports. BMJ 305:613-616, 1992.
170. Murphy PG, Myers DS, Davies MJ, et al: The antioxidant potential of propofol (2,6-diisopropylphenol). Br J Anaesth 68:613-618, 1992.
171. Jacobi J, Fraser GL, Coursin DB, et al: Clinical practice guidelines for the sustained use of sedatives and analgesics in the critically ill adult. Crit Care Med 30:119-141, 2002.
172. Rudkin GE, Osborne GA, Finn BP, et al: Intra-operative patient-controlled sedation: Comparison of patient-controlled propofol with patient-controlled midazolam. Anaesthesia 47:376-381, 1992.
173. Crepeau T, Poincloux L, Bonny C, et al: Significance of patient-controlled sedation during colonoscopy: Results from a prospective randomized controlled study. Gastroenterol Clin Biol 29:1090-1096, 2005.
174. Alhashemi JA, Kaki AM: Anesthesiologist-controlled versus patient-controlled propofol sedation for shockwave lithotripsy. Can J Anaesth 53:449-455, 2006.
175. Canessa R, Lema G, Urzua J, et al: Anesthesia for elective cardioversion: A comparison of four anesthetic agents. J Cardiothorac Vasc Anesth 5:566-568, 1991.
176. Kam PC, Cardone D: Propofol infusion syndrome. Anaesthesia 62:690-701, 2007.
177. Kang TM: Propofol infusion syndrome in critically ill patients. Ann Pharmacother 36:1453-1456, 2002.

178. Ahlen K, Buckley CJ, Goodale DB, Pulsford AH: The "propofol infusion syndrome": The facts, their interpretation and implications for patient care. Eur J Anaesthesiol 23:990-998, 2006.
179. Corssen G, Reves J, Stanley T: Dissociative anesthesia. *In*: Intravenous Anesthesia and Analgesia. Philadelphia, Lea & Febiger, 1988, p 99.
180. Halford F: A critique of intravenous anaesthesia in war surgery. Anaesthesiology 4:67-69, 1943.
181. Mahisekar UL, Callan CM, Derasari M, Kirkpatrick AF: Infusion of large particles of thiopental sodium during anesthesia induction. J Clin Anesth 6:55-58, 1994.
182. Mark L: Metabolism of barbiturates in man. Clin Pharmacol Ther 4:504, 1963.
183. Granik S: Induction of the synthesis of d-aminolevulinic acid synthetase in liver parenchyma cells in culture by chemicals that induce acute porphyria. J Biol Chem 238:PC2247, 1963.
184. Bremier D: Pharmacokinetics of methohexitone following intravenous infusions in humans. Br J Anaesth 48:643, 1976.
185. Henthorn T, Avram M, Krejcie T: Intravascular mixing and drug distribution: The concurrent disposition of thiopental and indocyanine green. Clin Pharmacol Ther 45:46, 1989.
186. Christensen J, Andreasen F, Jansen J: Pharmacokinetics of thiopentone in a group of young women and a group of young men. Br J Anaesth 52:913, 1980.
187. Morgan D, Blackman G, Paull J, Wolf L: Pharmacokinetics and plasma binding of thiopental, II: Studies at cesarean section. Anesthesiology 54:474, 1981.
188. Pandele G, Chaux F, Salvadori C, et al: Thiopental pharmacokinetics in patients with cirrhosis. Anesthesiology 59:123-126, 1983.
189. Toner W, Howard P, McGowan W, Dundee J: Another look at acute tolerance of thiopentone. Br J Anaesth 52:1005, 1980.
190. Downie DL, Franks NP, Lieb WR: Effects of thiopental and its optical isomers on nicotinic acetylcholine receptors. Anesthesiology 93:774-783, 2000.
191. Tomlin SL, Jenkins A, Lieb WR, Franks NP: Preparation of barbiturate optical isomers and their effects on GABA(A) receptors. Anesthesiology 90:1714-1722, 1999.
192. Liu H, Yao S: Thiopental sodium reduces glutamate extracellular levels in rat intact prefrontal cortex. Exp Brain Res 167:666-669, 2005.
193. Liu H, Dai T, Yao S: Effect of thiopental sodium on *N*-methyl-D-aspartate-gated currents. Can J Anaesth 53:442-448, 2006.
194. Ge ZJ, Zhang LC, Zeng YM, et al: Involvement of NMDA receptors in thiopental-induced loss of righting reflex, antinociception and anticonvulsion effects in mice. Pharmacology 80:127-133, 2007.
195. Fredriksson A, Ponten E, Gordh T, Eriksson P: Neonatal exposure to a combination of *N*-methyl-D-aspartate and gamma-aminobutyric acid type A receptor anesthetic agents potentiates apoptotic neurodegeneration and persistent behavioral deficits. Anesthesiology 107:427-436, 2007.
196. Judge S: Effect of general anaesthetics on synaptic ion channels. Br J Anaesth 55:191-200, 1983.
197. Tanelian DL, Kosek P, Mody I, MacIver MB: The role of the $GABA_A$ receptor/chloride channel complex in anesthesia. Anesthesiology 78:757-776, 1993.
198. Michenfelder JD, Milde JH, Sundt TM Jr: Cerebral protection by barbiturate anesthesia: Use after middle cerebral artery occlusion in Java monkeys. Arch Neurol 33:345-350, 1976.
199. Stullken EH Jr, Milde JH, Michenfelder JD, Tinker JH: The nonlinear responses of cerebral metabolism to low concentrations of halothane, enflurane, isoflurane, and thiopental. Anesthesiology 46:28-34, 1977.
200. Baughman VL: Brain protection during neurosurgery. Anesthesiol Clin North Am 20:315-327, 2002.
201. Albrecht RF, Miletich DJ, Rosenberg R, Zahed B: Cerebral blood flow and metabolic changes from induction to onset of anesthesia with halothane or pentobarbital. Anesthesiology 47:252-256, 1977.
202. Dundee J: Alterations in response to somatic pain associated with anaesthesia, II: The effect of thiopentone and pentobarbitone. Br J Anaesth 32:407, 1960.
203. Pancrazio JJ, Frazer MJ, Lynch C 3rd: Barbiturate anesthetics depress the resting K+ conductance of myocardium. J Pharmacol Exp Ther 265:358-365, 1993.
204. Brodie B, Kurz H, Schanker L: The importance of dissociation constant and lipid-solubility in influencing the passage of drugs into the cerebrospinal fluid. J Pharmacol Exp Ther 130:22, 1960.
205. Mark L, Bruns J, Camponmanes C: The passage of thiopental into brain. J Pharmacol Exp Ther 119:35, 1957.
206. Burch P, Stanski D: The role of metabolism and protein binding in thiopental anesthesia. Anesthesiology 58:146, 1983.
207. Saidman L: Uptake, distribution and elimination of barbiturates. *In* Eger E (ed): Anesthetic Uptake and Action. Baltimore, Williams & Wilkins, 1974.
208. Stella L, Torri G, Castiglioni CL: The relative potencies of thiopentone, ketamine, propanidid, alphaxalone and diazepam: A statistical study in man. Br J Anaesth 51:119-122, 1979.
209. Way W, Trevor A: Pharmacology of intravenous nonnarcotic anesthetics. *In* Miller RD (ed): Anesthesia, vol II, 2nd ed. New York, Churchill Livingstone, 1986.
210. Brodie B, Mark L, Papper E: The fate of thiopental in man and method for its estimation in biological material. J Pharmacol Exp Ther 98:85, 1950.
211. Homer TD, Stanski DR: The effect of increasing age on thiopental disposition and anesthetic requirement. Anesthesiology 62:714-724, 1985.
212. Sorbo S, Hudson RJ, Loomis JC: The pharmacokinetics of thiopental in pediatric surgical patients. Anesthesiology 61:666-670, 1984.
213. Korttila K, Ghoneim MM, Jacobs L, Lakes RS: Evaluation of instrumented force platform as a test to measure residual effects of anesthetics. Anesthesiology 55:625-630, 1981.
214. Todd MM, Drummond JC, U HS: The hemodynamic consequences of high-dose thiopental anesthesia. Anesth Analg 64:681-687, 1985.
215. Rodriguez E, Jordan R: Contemporary trends in pediatric sedation and analgesia. Emerg Med Clin North Am 20:199-222, 2002.
216. Kawar P, Dundee JW: Frequency of pain on injection and venous sequelae following the I.V. administration of certain anaesthetics and sedatives. Br J Anaesth 54:935-939, 1982.
217. Tarabadkar S, Kopriva D, Sreenivasan N, et al: Hemodynamic impact of induction in patients with decreased cardiac reserve. Anesthesiology 53:S43, 1980.
218. Seltzer J, Gerson J, Allen F: Comparison of the cardiovascular effects of bolus IV: Incremental administration of thiopentone. Br J Anaesth 52:527, 1980.
219. Eckstein J, Hamilton W, McCammond J: The effect of thiopental on peripheral venous tone. Anesthesiology 22:525, 1961.
220. Kissin I, Motomura S, Aultman DF, Reves JG: Inotropic and anesthetic potencies of etomidate and thiopental in dogs. Anesth Analg 62:961-965, 1983.
221. Dennis SG, Wotton PR, Boswood A, Flaherty D: Comparison of the effects of thiopentone and propofol on the electrocardiogram of dogs. Vet Rec 160:681-686, 2007.
222. Sonntag H, Hellberg K, Schenk HD, et al: Effects of thiopental (Trapanal) on coronary blood flow and myocardial metabolism in man. Acta Anaesthesiol Scand 19:69-78, 1975.
223. Dundee J, Moore J: Thiopentone and methohexital: A comparison as main anesthetic agents for a standard operation. Anaesthesia 16:50, 1961.
224. Gross JB, Zebrowski ME, Carel WD, et al: Time course of ventilatory depression after thiopental and midazolam in normal subjects and in patients with chronic obstructive pulmonary disease. Anesthesiology 58:540-544, 1983.
225. Wyant G, Dobkin A, Aasheim G: Comparison of seven intravenous anaesthetic agents in man. Br J Anaesth 29:194, 1957.
226. Choi SD, Spaulding BC, Gross JB, Apfelbaum JL: Comparison of the ventilatory effects of etomidate and methohexital. Anesthesiology 62:442-447, 1985.
227. Wood M: Intravenous anesthetic agents. *In*: Drugs and Anesthesia: Pharmacology for Anesthesiologists. Baltimore, Williams & Wilkins, 1982.
228. Stovner J, Endresen R: Diazepam in intravenous anesthesia. Lancet 2:1298-1299, 1965.
229. Walser A, Benjamin L, Flynn T: Quinazolines and 1, 4-benzodiazepines. 84: Synthesis and reactions of imidazo (1,5)(1.4)-benzodiazepines. J Org Chem 43:936, 1978.
230. Reves JG, Fragen RJ, Vinik HR, Greenblatt DJ: Midazolam: Pharmacology and uses. Anesthesiology 62:310-324, 1985.
231. Squires R, Braestrup C: Benzodiazepine receptors in rat brain. Nature 266:732, 1977.
232. Greenblatt DJ, Shader RI, Abernethy DR: Drug therapy: Current status of benzodiazepines. N Engl J Med 309:354-358, 1983.
233. Arendt RM, Greenblatt DJ, deJong RH, et al: In vitro correlates of benzodiazepine cerebrospinal fluid uptake, pharmacodynamic action and peripheral distribution. J Pharmacol Exp Ther 227:98-106, 1983.
234. Klotz U, Reimann I: Elevation of steady-state diazepam levels by cimetidine. Clin Pharmacol Ther 30:513-517, 1981.
235. Philip BK, Simpson TH, Hauch MA, Mallampati SR: Flumazenil reverses sedation after midazolam-induced general anesthesia in ambulatory surgery patients. Anesth Analg 71:371-376, 1990.
236. Kassai A, Toth G, Eichelbaum M, Klotz U: No evidence of a genetic polymorphism in the oxidative metabolism of midazolam. Clin Pharmacokinet 15:319-325, 1988.
237. Bertilsson L: Geographical/interracial differences in polymorphic drug oxidation: Current state of knowledge of cytochromes P450 (CYP) 2D6 and 2C19. Clin Pharmacokinet 29:192-209, 1995.
238. Barr J, Donner A: Optimal intravenous dosing strategies for sedatives and analgesics in the intensive care unit. Crit Care Clin 11:827-847, 1995.
239. Mandema JW, Tuk B, van Steveninck AL, et al: Pharmacokinetic-pharmacodynamic modeling of the central nervous system effects of midazolam and its main metabolite alpha-hydroxymidazolam in healthy volunteers. Clin Pharmacol Ther 51:715-728, 1992.
240. Bauer TM, Ritz R, Haberthur C, et al: Prolonged sedation due to accumulation of conjugated metabolites of midazolam. Lancet 346:145-147, 1995.

241. MacLeod SM, Giles HG, Bengert B, et al: Age- and gender-related differences in diazepam pharmacokinetics. J Clin Pharmacol 19:15-19, 1979.
242. Greenblatt DJ, Abernethy DR, Locniskar A, et al: Effect of age, gender, and obesity on midazolam kinetics. Anesthesiology 61:27-35, 1984.
243. Mould DR, DeFeo TM, Reele S, et al: Simultaneous modeling of the pharmacokinetics and pharmacodynamics of midazolam and diazepam. Clin Pharmacol Ther 58:35-43, 1995.
244. Mohler H, Richards JG: The benzodiazepine receptor: A pharmacological control element of brain function. Eur J Anaesthesiol Suppl 2:15-24, 1988.
245. Amrein R, Hetzel W: Pharmacology of Dormicum (midazolam) and Anexate (flumazenil). Acta Anaesthesiol Scand Suppl 92:6-15, 1990.
246. Mohler H, Fritschy JM, Rudolph U: A new benzodiazepine pharmacology. J Pharmacol Exp Ther 300:2-8, 2002.
247. Amrein R, Hetzel W, Hartmann D, Lorscheid T: Clinical pharmacology of flumazenil. Eur J Anaesthesiol Suppl 2:65-80, 1988.
248. Kohno T, Wakai A, Ataka T, et al: Actions of midazolam on excitatory transmission in dorsal horn neurons of adult rat spinal cord. Anesthesiology 104:338-343, 2006.
249. Wu YW, Shiau JM, Hong CC, et al: Intrathecal midazolam combined with low-dose bupivacaine improves postoperative recovery in diabetic mellitus patients undergoing foot debridement. Acta Anaesthesiol Taiwan 43:129-134, 2005.
250. Miller LG: Chronic benzodiazepine administration: From the patient to the gene. J Clin Pharmacol 31:492-495, 1991.
251. Breimer LT, Burm AG, Danhof M, et al: Pharmacokinetic-pharmacodynamic modelling of the interaction between flumazenil and midazolam in volunteers by aperiodic EEG analysis. Clin Pharmacokinet 20:497-508, 1991.
252. Persson MP, Nilsson A, Hartvig P: Relation of sedation and amnesia to plasma concentrations of midazolam in surgical patients. Clin Pharmacol Ther 43:324-331, 1988.
253. Forster A, Juge O, Morel D: Effects of midazolam on cerebral blood flow in human volunteers. Anesthesiology 56:453-455, 1982.
254. Brown CR, Sarnquist FH, Canup CA, Pedley TA: Clinical, electroencephalographic, and pharmacokinetic studies of a water-soluble benzodiazepine, midazolam maleate. Anesthesiology 50:467-470, 1979.
255. de Jong RH, Bonin JD: Benzodiazepines protect mice from local anesthetic convulsions and deaths. Anesth Analg 60:385-389, 1981.
256. Denaut M, Yernault JC, De Coster A: Double-blind comparison of the respiratory effects of parenteral lorazepam and diazepam in patients with chronic obstructive lung disease. Curr Med Res Opin 2:611-615, 1974.
257. Forster A, Gardaz JP, Suter PM, Gemperle M: I.V. midazolam as an induction agent for anaesthesia: A study in volunteers. Br J Anaesth 52:907-911, 1980.
258. Sunzel M, Paalzow L, Berggren L, Eriksson I: Respiratory and cardiovascular effects in relation to plasma levels of midazolam and diazepam. Br J Clin Pharmacol 25:561-569, 1988.
259. Alexander CM, Teller LE, Gross JB: Slow injection does not prevent midazolam-induced ventilatory depression. Anesth Analg 74:260-264, 1992.
260. Samuelson PN, Reves JG, Kouchoukos NT, et al: Hemodynamic responses to anesthetic induction with midazolam or diazepam in patients with ischemic heart disease. Anesth Analg 60:802-809, 1981.
261. Rao S, Sherbaniuk RW, Prasad K, et al: Cardiopulmonary effects of diazepam. Clin Pharmacol Ther 14:182-189, 1973.
262. Reves JG, Samuelson PN, Lewis S: Midazolam maleate induction in patients with ischaemic heart disease: Haemodynamic observations. Can Anaesth Soc J 26:402-409, 1979.
263. Elliott HW, Nomof N, Navarro G, et al: Central nervous system and cardiovascular effects of lorazepam in man. Clin Pharmacol Ther 12:468-481, 1971.
264. Ruff R, Reves JG: Hemodynamic effects of a lorazepam-fentanyl anesthetic induction for coronary artery bypass surgery. J Cardiothorac Anesth 4:314-317, 1990.
265. Marty J, Nitenberg A, Blanchet F, et al: Effects of midazolam on the coronary circulation in patients with coronary artery disease. Anesthesiology 64:206-210, 1986.
266. Lebowitz PW, Cote ME, Daniels AL, et al: Comparative cardiovascular effects of midazolam and thiopental in healthy patients. Anesth Analg 61:771-775, 1982.
267. Heikkila H, Jalonen J, Arola M, et al: Midazolam as adjunct to high-dose fentanyl anaesthesia for coronary artery bypass grafting operation. Acta Anaesthesiol Scand 28:683-689, 1984.
268. Tomichek R, Rosow C, Schneider R: Cardiovascular effects of diazepam-fentanyl anesthesia in patients with coronary artery disease. Anesth Analg 61:217, 1982.
269. Marty J, Gauzit R, Lefevre P, et al: Effects of diazepam and midazolam on baroreflex control of heart rate and on sympathetic activity in humans. Anesth Analg 65:113-119, 1986.
270. Cole SG, Brozinsky S, Isenberg JI: Midazolam, a new more potent benzodiazepine, compared with diazepam: A randomized, double-blind study of preendoscopic sedatives. Gastrointest Endosc 29:219-222, 1983.
271. McNulty SE, Gratch D, Costello D, et al: The effect of midazolam and lorazepam on postoperative recovery after cardiac surgery. Anesth Analg 81:404-407, 1995.
272. Vargo JJ, Zuccaro G Jr, Dumot JA, et al: Gastroenterologist-administered propofol versus meperidine and midazolam for advanced upper endoscopy: A prospective, randomized trial. Gastroenterology 123:8-16, 2002.
273. Gauthier RA, Dyck B, Chung F, et al: Respiratory interaction after spinal anesthesia and sedation with midazolam. Anesthesiology 77:909-914, 1992.
274. Shapiro BA, Warren J, Egol AB, et al: Practice parameters for intravenous analgesia and sedation for adult patients in the intensive care unit: An executive summary. Society of Critical Care Medicine. Crit Care Med 23:1596-1600, 1995.
275. Walder B, Elia N, Henzi I, et al: A lack of evidence of superiority of propofol versus midazolam for sedation in mechanically ventilated critically ill patients: A qualitative and quantitative systematic review. Anesth Analg 92:975-983, 2001.
276. Frolich MA, Burchfield DJ, Euliano TY, Caton D: A single dose of fentanyl and midazolam prior to Cesarean section have no adverse neonatal effects. Can J Anaesth 53:79-85, 2006.
277. Nitsun M, Szokol JW, Saleh HJ, et al: Pharmacokinetics of midazolam, propofol, and fentanyl transfer to human breast milk. Clin Pharmacol Ther 79:549-557, 2006.
278. Kain ZN, Hofstadter MB, Mayes LC, et al: Midazolam: Effects on amnesia and anxiety in children. Anesthesiology 93:676-684, 2000.
279. Funk W, Jakob W, Riedl T, Taeger K: Oral preanaesthetic medication for children: Double-blind randomized study of a combination of midazolam and ketamine vs midazolam or ketamine alone. Br J Anaesth 84:335-340, 2000.
280. Kanto J, Sjovall S, Vuori A: Effect of different kinds of premedication on the induction properties of midazolam. Br J Anaesth 54:507-511, 1982.
281. Gamble JA, Kawar P, Dundee JW, et al: Evaluation of midazolam as an intravenous induction agent. Anaesthesia 36:868-873, 1981.
282. Jacobs JR, Reves JG, Marty J, et al: Aging increases pharmacodynamic sensitivity to the hypnotic effects of midazolam. Anesth Analg 80:143-148, 1995.
283. Theil DR, Stanley TE 3rd, White WD, et al: Midazolam and fentanyl continuous infusion anesthesia for cardiac surgery: A comparison of computer-assisted versus manual infusion systems. J Cardiothorac Vasc Anesth 7:300-306, 1993.
284. Forster A, Gardaz JP, Suter PM, Gemperle M: Respiratory depression by midazolam and diazepam. Anesthesiology 53:494-497, 1980.
285. Norton AC, Dundas CR: Induction agents for day-case anaesthesia: A double-blind comparison of propofol and midazolam antagonised by flumazenil. Anaesthesia 45:198-203, 1990.
286. Crawford ME, Carl P, Andersen RS, Mikkelsen BO: Comparison between midazolam and thiopentone-based balanced anaesthesia for day-case surgery. Br J Anaesth 56:165-169, 1984.
287. Melvin MA, Johnson BH, Quasha AL, Eger EI 3rd: Induction of anesthesia with midazolam decreases halothane MAC in humans. Anesthesiology 57:238-241, 1982.
288. Jung JS, Park JS, Kim SO, et al: Prophylactic antiemetic effect of midazolam after middle ear surgery. Otolaryngol Head Neck Surg 137:753-756, 2007.
289. Lee Y, Wang JJ, Yang YL, et al: Midazolam vs ondansetron for preventing postoperative nausea and vomiting: A randomised controlled trial. Anaesthesia 62:18-22, 2007.
289a. Riad W, Altaf R, Abdulla A, Oudan H: Effect of midazolam, dexamethasone and their combination on the prevention of nausea and vomiting following strabismus repair in children. Eur J Anaesthesiol 24:697-701, 2007.
290. Nilsson A, Persson MP, Hartvig P, Wide L: Effect of total intravenous anaesthesia with midazolam/alfentanil on the adrenocortical and hyperglycaemic response to abdominal surgery. Acta Anaesthesiol Scand 32:379-382, 1988.
291. Brogden RN, Goa KL: Flumazenil: A reappraisal of its pharmacological properties and therapeutic efficacy as a benzodiazepine antagonist. Drugs 42:1061-1089, 1991.
292. File SE, Pellow S: Intrinsic actions of the benzodiazepine receptor antagonist Ro 15-1788. Psychopharmacology (Berl) 88:1-11, 1986.
293. Lauven PM, Schwilden H, Stoeckel H, Greenblatt DJ: The effects of a benzodiazepine antagonist Ro 15-1788 in the presence of stable concentrations of midazolam. Anesthesiology 63:61-64, 1985.
294. Cumin R, Bonetti EP, Scherschlicht R, Haefely WE: Use of the specific benzodiazepine antagonist, Ro 15-1788, in studies of physiological dependence on benzodiazepines. Experientia 38:833-834, 1982.
295. Hunkeler W: Preclinical research findings with flumazenil (Ro15-1788, Anexate): Chemistry. Eur J Anaesthesiol Suppl 2:37, 1988.
296. Klotz U, Kanto J: Pharmacokinetics and clinical use of flumazenil (Ro 15-1788). Clin Pharmacokinet 14:1-12, 1988.
297. Kleinberger G, Grimm G, Laggner A, et al: Weaning patients from mechanical ventilation by benzodi-

azepine antagonist Ro15-1788. Lancet 2:268-269, 1985.

298. Mendelson WB: Neuropharmacology of sleep induction by benzodiazepines. Crit Rev Neurobiol 6:221-232, 1992.
299. Wolf J, Friberg L, Jensen J, et al: The effect of the benzodiazepine antagonist flumazenil on regional cerebral blood flow in human volunteers. Acta Anaesthesiol Scand 34:628-631, 1990.
300. Yokoyama M, Benson KT, Arakawa K, Goto H: Effects of flumazenil on intravenous lidocaine-induced convulsions and anticonvulsant property of diazepam in rats. Anesth Analg 75:87-90, 1992.
301. Samson Y, Hantraye P, Baron JC, et al: Kinetics and displacement of [11C]RO 15-1788, a benzodiazepine antagonist, studied in human brain in vivo by positron tomography. Eur J Pharmacol 110:247-251, 1985.
302. Forster A, Juge O, Louis M, Nahory A: Effects of a specific benzodiazepine antagonist (RO 15-1788) on cerebral blood flow. Anesth Analg 66:309-313, 1987.
303. Rouiller M, Forster A, Gemperle M: [Assessment of the efficacy and tolerance of a benzodiazepine antagonist (Ro 15-1788)]. Ann Fr Anesth Reanim 6:1-6, 1987.
304. Weinbrum A, Geller E: The respiratory effects of reversing midazolam sedation with flumazenil in the presence or absence of narcotics. Acta Anaesthesiol Scand Suppl 92:65-69, 1990.
305. Duka T, Ackenheil M, Noderer J, et al: Changes in noradrenaline plasma levels and behavioural responses induced by benzodiazepine agonists with the benzodiazepine antagonist Ro 15-1788. Psychopharmacology (Berl) 90:351-357, 1986.
306. Nilsson A: Autonomic and hormonal responses after the use of midazolam and flumazenil. Acta Anaesthesiol Scand Suppl 92:51-54, 1990.
307. Ghoneim MM, Dembo JB, Block RI: Time course of antagonism of sedative and amnesic effects of diazepam by flumazenil. Anesthesiology 70:899-904, 1989.
308. White PF, Way WL, Trevor AJ: Ketamine—its pharmacology and therapeutic uses. Anesthesiology 56:119-136, 1982.
309. Cohen MG, Chan SL, Bhargava HN, Trevor AJ: Inhibition of mammalian brain acetylcholinesterase by ketamine. Biochem Pharmacol 23:1647-1652, 1974.
310. Herd DW, Anderson BJ, Holford NH: Modeling the norketamine metabolite in children and the implications for analgesia. Paediatr Anaesth 17:831-840, 2007.
311. Clements JA, Nimmo WS: Pharmacokinetics and analgesic effect of ketamine in man. Br J Anaesth 53:27-30, 1981.
312. Grant IS, Nimmo WS, Clements JA: Pharmacokinetics and analgesic effects of i.m. and oral ketamine. Br J Anaesth 53:805-810, 1981.
313. Edwards SR, Minto CF, Mather LE: Concurrent ketamine and alfentanil administration: pharmacokinetic considerations. Br J Anaesth 88:94-100, 2002.
314. Absalom AR, Lee M, Menon DK, et al: Predictive performance of the Domino, Hijazi, and Clements models during low-dose target-controlled ketamine infusions in healthy volunteers. Br J Anaesth 98:615-623, 2007.
315. Geisslinger G, Hering W, Thomann P, et al: Pharmacokinetics and pharmacodynamics of ketamine enantiomers in surgical patients using a stereoselective analytical method. Br J Anaesth 70:666-671, 1993.
316. White M, de Graaff P, Renshof B, et al: Pharmacokinetics of S(+) ketamine derived from target controlled infusion. Br J Anaesth 96:330-334, 2006.
317. Schuttler J, Stanski DR, White PF, et al: Pharmacodynamic modeling of the EEG effects of ketamine and its enantiomers in man. J Pharmacokinet Biopharm 15:241-253, 1987.
318. Yanagihara Y, Ohtani M, Kariya S, et al: Plasma concentration profiles of ketamine and norketamine after administration of various ketamine preparations to healthy Japanese volunteers. Biopharm Drug Dispos 24:37-43, 2003.
319. Grant IS, Nimmo WS, McNicol LR, Clements JA: Ketamine disposition in children and adults. Br J Anaesth 55:1107-1111, 1983.
320. Adams HA, Thiel A, Jung A, et al: [Studies using S-(+)-ketamine on probands: Endocrine and circulatory reactions, recovery and dream experiences]. Anaesthesist 41:588-596, 1992.
321. Kharasch ED, Labroo R: Metabolism of ketamine stereoisomers by human liver microsomes. Anesthesiology 77:1201-1207, 1992.
322. Okamoto GU, Duperon DF, Jedrychowski JR: Clinical evaluation of the effects of ketamine sedation on pediatric dental patients. J Clin Pediatr Dent 16:253-257, 1992.
323. Doenicke A, Kugler J, Mayer M, et al: [Ketamine racemate or S-(+)-ketamine and midazolam: The effect on vigilance, efficacy and subjective findings]. Anaesthetist 41:610-618, 1992.
324. Chapman V, Dickenson AH: The combination of NMDA antagonism and morphine produces profound antinociception in the rat dorsal horn. Brain Res 573:321-323, 1992.
325. Kissin I, Bright CA, Bradley EL Jr: The effect of ketamine on opioid-induced acute tolerance: Can it explain reduction of opioid consumption with ketamine-opioid analgesic combinations? Anesth Analg 91:1483-1488, 2000.
326. Sparks DL, Corssen G, Aizenman B, Black J: Further studies of the neural mechanisms of ketamine-induced anesthesia in the rhesus monkey. Anesth Analg 54:189-195, 1975.
327. Massopust LC Jr, Wolin LR, Albin MS: Electrophysiologic and behavioral responses to ketamine hydrochloride in the Rhesus monkey. Anesth Analg 51:329-341, 1972.
328. Ohtani M, Kikuchi H, Kitahata LM, et al: Effects of ketamine on nociceptive cells in the medial medullary reticular formation of the cat. Anesthesiology 51:414-417, 1979.
329. Sprenger T, Valet M, Woltmann R, et al: Imaging pain modulation by subanesthetic S-(+)-ketamine. Anesth Analg 103:729-737, 2006.
330. Frenkel C, Urban BW: Molecular actions of racemic ketamine on human CNS sodium channels. Br J Anaesth 69:292-297, 1992.
331. Finck A, Ngai S: A possible mechanism of ketamine-induced analgesia. Anesthesiology 51:S34, 1979.
332. Freye E, Latasch L, Schmidhammer H: [Pharmacodynamic effects of S-(+)-ketamine on EEG, evoked potentials and respiration: A study in the awake dog]. Anaesthetist 41:527-533, 1992.
333. Irifune M, Shimizu T, Nomoto M, Fukuda T: Ketamine-induced anesthesia involves the *N*-methyl-D-aspartate receptor-channel complex in mice. Brain Res 596:1-9, 1992.
334. Oye I, Paulsen O, Maurset A: Effects of ketamine on sensory perception: Evidence for a role of *N*-methyl-D-aspartate receptors. J Pharmacol Exp Ther 260:1209-1213, 1992.
335. Nagasaka H, Nagasaka I, Sato I, et al: The effects of ketamine on the excitation and inhibition of dorsal horn WDR neuronal activity induced by bradykinin injection into the femoral artery in cats after spinal cord transection. Anesthesiology 78:722-732, 1993.
336. Kayama Y, Iwama K: The EEG, evoked potentials, and single-unit activity during ketamine anesthesia in cats. Anesthesiology 36:316-328, 1972.
337. Shapiro H, Wyte S, Harria A: Ketamine anaesthesia in patients with intracranial pathology. Br J Anaesth 44:1200, 1972.
338. Thorsen T, Gran L: Ketamine/diazepam infusion anaesthesia with special attention to the effect on cerebrospinal fluid pressure and arterial blood pressure. Acta Anaesthesiol Scand 24:1-4, 1980.
339. Dawson B, Michenfelder JD, Theye RA: Effects of ketamine on canine cerebral blood flow and metabolism: Modification by prior administration of thiopental. Anesth Analg 50:443-447, 1971.
340. Reeker W, Werner C, Mollenberg O, et al: High-dose S(+)-ketamine improves neurological outcome following incomplete cerebral ischemia in rats. Can J Anaesth 47:572-578, 2000.
341. Engelhard K, Werner C, Eberspacher E, et al: The effect of the alpha 2-agonist dexmedetomidine and the *N*-methyl-D-aspartate antagonist S(+)-ketamine on the expression of apoptosis-regulating proteins after incomplete cerebral ischemia and reperfusion in rats. Anesth Analg 96:524-531, 2003.
342. Mellon RD, Simone AF, Rappaport BA: Use of anesthetic agents in neonates and young children. Anesth Analg 104:509-520, 2007.
343. Anand KJ: Anesthetic neurotoxicity in newborns: Should we change clinical practice? Anesthesiology 107:2-4, 2007.
344. Garfield JM, Garfield FB, Stone JG, et al: A comparison of psychologic responses to ketamine and thiopental–nitrous oxide–halothane anesthesia. Anesthesiology 36:329-338, 1972.
345. Corssen G, Reves J, Stanley T: Neuroleptanalgesia and neuroleptanesthesia. *In*: Intravenous Anesthesia and Analgesia. Philadelphia, Lea & Febiger, 1988, p 175.
346. Sussman DR: A comparative evaluation of ketamine anesthesia in children and adults. Anesthesiology 40:459-464, 1974.
347. Khorramzadeh E, Lotfy AO: Personality predisposition and emergence phenomena with ketamine. Psychosomatics 17:94-95, 1976.
348. Hejja P, Galloon S: A consideration of ketamine dreams. Can Anaesth Soc J 22:100-105, 1975.
349. Wulfsohn NL: Ketamine dosage for induction based on lean body mass. Anesth Analg 51:299-305, 1972.
350. Dundee J, Lilburn J: Ketamine-lorazepam: Attenuation of the psychic sequelae of ketamine by lorazepam. Anaesthesia 37:312, 1977.
351. Kothary S, Zsigmond E: A double-blind study of the effective anti-hallucinatory doses of diazepam prior to ketamine anesthesia. Clin Pharmacol Ther 21:108, 1977.
352. Doenicke A, Angster R, Mayer M, et al: [The action of S-(+)-ketamine on serum catecholamine and cortisol: A comparison with ketamine racemate]. Anaesthetist 41:597-603, 1992.
353. Soliman M, Brinale G, Kuster G: Response to hypercapnia under ketamine anaesthesia. Can Anaesth Soc J 22:486, 1975.
354. Dillon J: Clinical experience with repeated ketamine administration for procedures requiring anesthesia. *In* Kreuscher H (ed): Ketamine. Berlin, Springer-Verlag, 1969.
355. Hamza J, Ecoffey C, Gross JB: Ventilatory response to CO_2 following intravenous ketamine in children. Anesthesiology 70:422-425, 1989.

356. Corssen G, Gutierrez J, Reves JG, Huber FC Jr: Ketamine in the anesthetic management of asthmatic patients. Anesth Analg 51:588-596, 1972.
357. Hirshman CA, Downes H, Farbood A, Bergman NA: Ketamine block of bronchospasm in experimental canine asthma. Br J Anaesth 51:713-718, 1979.
358. Wanna HT, Gergis SD: Procaine, lidocaine, and ketamine inhibit histamine-induced contracture of guinea pig tracheal muscle in vitro. Anesth Analg 57:25-27, 1978.
359. Sarma VJ: Use of ketamine in acute severe asthma. Acta Anaesthesiol Scand 36:106-107, 1992.
360. Sonntag H, Heiss HW, Knoll D, et al: [Myocardial perfusion and myocardial oxygen consumption in patients during the induction of anesthesia using dehydrobenzperidol-fentanyl or ketamine]. Z Kreislaufforsch 61:1092-1105, 1972.
361. Zsigmond E, Domino E: Clinical pharmacology and current uses of ketamine. *In* Aldrete J, Stanley T (eds): Trends in Intravenous Anesthesia. Chicago, Year Book, 1980, p 283.
362. Savege TM, Colvin MP, Weaver EJ, et al: A comparison of some cardiorespiratory effects of althesin and ketamine when used for induction of anaesthesia in patients with cardiac disease. Br J Anaesth 48:1071-1081, 1976.
363. Morray JP, Lynn AM, Stamm SJ, et al: Hemodynamic effects of ketamine in children with congenital heart disease. Anesth Analg 63:895-899, 1984.
364. Greeley WJ, Bushman GA, Davis DP, Reves JG: Comparative effects of halothane and ketamine on systemic arterial oxygen saturation in children with cyanotic heart disease. Anesthesiology 65:666-668, 1986.
365. Ogawa A, Uemura M, Kataoka Y, et al: Effects of ketamine on cardiovascular responses mediated by *N*-methyl-D-aspartate receptor in the rat nucleus tractus solitarius. Anesthesiology 78:163-167, 1993.
366. Ivankovich AD, Miletich DJ, Reimann C, et al: Cardiovascular effects of centrally administered ketamine in goats. Anesth Analg 53:924-933, 1974.
367. Balfors E, Haggmark S, Nyhman H, et al: Droperidol inhibits the effects of intravenous ketamine on central hemodynamics and myocardial oxygen consumption in patients with generalized atherosclerotic disease. Anesth Analg 62:193-197, 1983.
368. Pagel PS, Kampine JP, Schmeling WT, Warltier DC: Ketamine depresses myocardial contractility as evaluated by the preload recruitable stroke work relationship in chronically instrumented dogs with autonomic nervous system blockade. Anesthesiology 76:564-572, 1992.
369. Urthaler F, Walker A, James T: Comparison of the inotropic action of morphine and ketamine studied in canine cardiac muscle. J Thorac Cardiovasc Surg 72:142, 1976.
370. Stowe DF, Bosnjak ZJ, Kampine JP: Comparison of etomidate, ketamine, midazolam, propofol, and thiopental on function and metabolism of isolated hearts. Anesth Analg 74:547-558, 1992.
371. Endou M, Hattori Y, Nakaya H, et al: Electrophysiologic mechanisms responsible for inotropic responses to ketamine in guinea pig and rat myocardium. Anesthesiology 76:409-418, 1992.
372. Salt PJ, Barnes PK, Beswick FJ: Inhibition of neuronal and extraneuronal uptake of noradrenaline by ketamine in the isolated perfused rat heart. Br J Anaesth 51:835-838, 1979.
373. Reves J, Flezzani P, Kissin I: Pharmacology of intravenous anesthetic induction drugs. *In* Kaplan J (ed): Cardiac Anesthesia. Orlando, FL, Grune & Stratton, 1987, p 125.
374. Munro HM, Sleigh JW, Paxton LD: The cardiovascular response to ketamine: The effects of clonidine and lignocaine. Acta Anaesthesiol Scand 37:75-78, 1993.
375. Hatano S, Keane D, Boggs R: Diazepam-ketamine anaesthesia for open heart surgery: A "micro-mini" drip administration technique. Can J Anaesth 23:648, 1976.
376. Bidwal A, Stanley T, Graves C: The effects of ketamine on cardiovascular dynamics during halothane and enflurane anesthesia. Anesth Analg 54:588, 1975.
377. Corssen G, Reves J, Carter J: Neuroleptanesthesia, dissociative anesthesia, and hemorrhage. Int Anesthesiol Clin 12:145, 1974.
378. Van der Linden P, Gilbart E, Engelman E, et al: Comparison of halothane, isoflurane, alfentanil, and ketamine in experimental septic shock. Anesth Analg 70:608-617, 1990.
379. Kingston H, Bretherton K, Holloway A: A comparison between ketamine and diazepam as induction agents for pericardectomy. Anaesth Intensive Care 6:66, 1978.
380. Fletcher JE, Rosenberg H, Lizzo FH: Effects of droperidol, haloperidol and ketamine on halothane, succinylcholine and caffeine contractures: Implications for malignant hyperthermia. Acta Anaesthesiol Scand 33:187-192, 1989.
381. Raza SM, Masters RW, Zsigmond EK: Haemodynamic stability with midazolam-ketamine-sufentanil analgesia in cardiac surgical patients. Can J Anaesth 36:617-623, 1989.
382. Elia N, Tramer MR: Ketamine and postoperative pain—a quantitative systematic review of randomised trials. Pain 113:61-70, 2005.
383. Sveticic G, Gentilini A, Eichenberger U, et al: Combinations of morphine with ketamine for patient-controlled analgesia: A new optimization method. Anesthesiology 98:1195-1205, 2003.
384. Adam F, Chauvin M, Du Manoir B, et al: Small-dose ketamine infusion improves postoperative analgesia and rehabilitation after total knee arthroplasty. Anesth Analg 100:475-480, 2005.
385. Visser E, Schug SA: The role of ketamine in pain management. Biomed Pharmacother 60:341-348, 2006.
386. Lavand'homme P, De Kock M, Waterloos H: Intraoperative epidural analgesia combined with ketamine provides effective preventive analgesia in patients undergoing major digestive surgery. Anesthesiology 103:813-820, 2005.
387. Suzuki M, Haraguti S, Sugimoto K, et al: Low-dose intravenous ketamine potentiates epidural analgesia after thoracotomy. Anesthesiology 105:111-119, 2006.
388. Eisenach JC, Yaksh TL: Epidural ketamine in healthy children—what's the point? Anesth Analg 96:626; author reply 627, 2003.
389. Groeneveld A, Inkson T: Ketamine: A solution to procedural pain in burned children. Can Nurse 88:28-31, 1992.
390. Thompson G, Moore D: Ketamine, diazepam, and Innovar: A computerized comparative study. Anesth Analg 50:458, 1971.
391. Korttila K, Levanen J: Untoward effects of ketamine combined with diazepam for supplementing conduction anaesthesia in young and middle-aged adults. Acta Anaesthesiol Scand 22:640-648, 1978.
392. Friedberg BL: Propofol-ketamine technique. Aesthetic Plast Surg 17:297-300, 1993.
393. Himmelseher S, Durieux ME: Revising a dogma: Ketamine for patients with neurological injury? Anesth Analg 101:524-534, 2005.
394. Fuchs C, Schwabe M: [Rectal premedication using ketamine-dehydrobenzperidol-atropine in childhood]. Anaesthesiol Reanim 15:322-326, 1990.
395. Gutstein HB, Johnson KL, Heard MB, Gregory GA: Oral ketamine preanesthetic medication in children. Anesthesiology 76:28-33, 1992.
396. Tobias JD, Phipps S, Smith B, Mulhern RK: Oral ketamine premedication to alleviate the distress of invasive procedures in pediatric oncology patients. Pediatrics 90:537-541, 1992.
397. Shapiro H: Intracranial hypertension: Therapeutic and anesthetic considerations. Anesthesiology 43:445, 1971.
398. Reves JG, Lell WA, McCracken LE Jr, et al: Comparison of morphine and ketamine anesthetic techniques for coronary surgery: A randomized study. South Med J 71:33-36, 1978.
399. Malinovsky JM, Lepage JY, Cozian A, et al: Is ketamine or its preservative responsible for neurotoxicity in the rabbit? Anesthesiology 78:109-115, 1993.
400. Janssen P, Niemegeers J, Schellekens K: Etomidate, R-(+)-Ethyl-1-(alpha-methyl-benzyl)imidazole-5-carboxylate (R 16659): A potent, short-acting and relatively atoxic intravenous hypnotic agent in rats. Arzneimittelforschung 21:1234, 1971.
401. Ledingham IM, Watt I: Influence of sedation on mortality in critically ill multiple trauma patients. Lancet 1:1270, 1983.
402. Wagner RL, White PF: Etomidate inhibits adrenocortical function in surgical patients. Anesthesiology 61:647-651, 1984.
403. Longnecker DE: Stress free: To be or not to be? Anesthesiology 61:643-644, 1984.
404. Owen H, Spence AA: Etomidate. Br J Anaesth 56:555-557, 1984.
405. Doenicke A, Roizen MF, Nebauer AE, et al: A comparison of two formulations for etomidate, 2-hydroxypropyl-beta-cyclodextrin (HPCD) and propylene glycol. Anesth Analg 79:933-939, 1994.
406. Hadzija BW, Lubarsky DA: Compatibility of etomidate, thiopental sodium, and propofol injections with drugs commonly administered during induction of anesthesia. Am J Health Syst Pharm 52:997-999, 1995.
407. Nimmo W, Miller M: Pharmacology of etomidate. *In* Brown B (ed): New Pharmacologic Vistas in Anesthesia. Philadelphia, FA Davis, 1983, p 83.
408. Dundee J, Zacharias M: Etomidate. *In* Dundee J (ed): Current Topics in Anaesthesia Series 1. London, Arnold, 1979, p 46.
409. Fragen RJ, Caldwell N: Comparison of a new formulation of etomidate with thiopental—side effects and awakening times. Anesthesiology 50:242-244, 1979.
410. Giese JL, Stockham RJ, Stanley TH, et al: Etomidate versus thiopental for induction of anesthesia. Anesth Analg 64:871-876, 1985.
411. Wells JK: Comparison of ICI 35868, etomidate and methohexitone for day-case anaesthesia. Br J Anaesth 57:732-735, 1985.
412. Linton DM, Thornington RE: Etomidate as a rectal induction agent, part II: A clinical study in children. S Afr Med J 64:309-310, 1983.
413. Fragen RJ, Avram MJ, Henthorn TK, Caldwell NJ: A pharmacokinetically designed etomidate infusion regimen for hypnosis. Anesth Analg 62:654-660, 1983.
414. Sear JW, Walters FJ, Wilkins DG, Willatts SM: Etomidate by infusion for neuroanaesthesia: Kinetic and dynamic interactions with nitrous oxide. Anaesthesia 39:12-18, 1984.
415. Fragen R, Shanks C, Molteni A: Effect on plasma cortisol concentration of a single induction dose of etomidate or thiopentone. Lancet 2:625, 1983.

416. Schuttler J, Schwilden H, Stoeckel H: Infusion strategies to investigate the pharmacokinetics and pharmacodynamics of hypnotic drugs: Etomidate as an example. Eur J Anaesthesiol 2:133-142, 1985.
417. Meuldermans W, Heykants J: The plasma protein binding and distribution of etomidate in dog, rat and human blood. Arch Int Pharmacodyn Ther 221:150, 1976.
418. Johnson KB, Egan TD, Layman J, et al: The influence of hemorrhagic shock on etomidate: A pharmacokinetic and pharmacodynamic analysis. Anesth Analg 96:1360-1368, 2003.
419. van Beem H, Manger FW, van Boxtel C, van Bentem N: Etomidate anaesthesia in patients with cirrhosis of the liver: Pharmacokinetic data. Anaesthesia 38(Suppl):61-62, 1983.
420. Arden JR, Holley FO, Stanski DR: Increased sensitivity to etomidate in the elderly: Initial distribution versus altered brain response. Anesthesiology 65:19-27, 1986.
421. Evans RH, Hill RG: The GABA-mimetic action of etomidate [proceedings]. Br J Pharmacol 61:484P, 1977.
422. Lingamaneni R, Hemmings HC Jr: Differential interaction of anaesthetics and antiepileptic drugs with neuronal Na+ channels, Ca2+ channels, and GABA(A) receptors. Br J Anaesth 90:199-211, 2003.
423. Blednov YA, Jung S, Alva H, et al: Deletion of the $alpha_1$ or $beta_2$ subunit of $GABA_A$ receptors reduces actions of alcohol and other drugs. J Pharmacol Exp Ther 304:30-36, 2003.
424. Cold GE, Eskesen V, Eriksen H, et al: CBF and $CMRO_2$ during continuous etomidate infusion supplemented with N_2O and fentanyl in patients with supratentorial cerebral tumour: A dose-response study. Acta Anaesthesiol Scand 29:490-494, 1985.
425. Dearden NM, McDowall DG: Comparison of etomidate and althesin in the reduction of increased intracranial pressure after head injury. Br J Anaesth 57:361-368, 1985.
426. Modica PA, Tempelhoff R: Intracranial pressure during induction of anaesthesia and tracheal intubation with etomidate-induced EEG burst suppression. Can J Anaesth 39:236-241, 1992.
427. Renou A, Vernhiet J, Macrez P: Cerebral blood flow and metabolism during etomidate anaesthesia in man. Br J Anaesth 50:1047, 1978.
428. Tulleken CA, van Dieren A, Jonkman J, Kalenda Z: Clinical and experimental experience with etomidate as a brain protective agent. J Cereb Blood Flow Metab 2(Suppl 1):S92-S97, 1982.
429. Takanobu S, Piyush M, Drummond J: A comparison of the cerebral protective effects of etomidate, thiopental, and isoflurane in a model of forebrain ischemia in the rat. Anesth Analg 76:990, 1993.
430. Drummond JC, Cole DJ, Patel PM, Reynolds LW: Focal cerebral ischemia during anesthesia with etomidate, isoflurane, or thiopental: A comparison of the extent of cerebral injury. Neurosurgery 37:742-748, 1995.
431. Guo J, White J, Batjer H: Limited protective effects of etomidate during brainstem ischemia in dogs. J Neurosurg 82:278, 1995.
432. Ghoneim MM, Yamada T: Etomidate: A clinical and electroencephalographic comparison with thiopental. Anesth Analg 56:479-485, 1977.
433. Lees NW, Hendry JG: Etomidate in urological outpatient anaesthesia: A clinical evaluation. Anaesthesia 32:592-597, 1977.
434. Ebrahim E, DeBoer G, Luders H: Effect of etomidate on the electroencephalogram of patients with epilepsy. Anesth Analg 65:1004, 1986.
435. Thornton C, Heneghan CP, Navaratnarajah M, et al: Effect of etomidate on the auditory evoked response in man. Br J Anaesth 57:554-561, 1985.
436. Guldager H, Sondergaard I, Jensen FM, Cold G: Basophil histamine release in asthma patients after in vitro provocation with Althesin and etomidate. Acta Anaesthesiol Scand 29:352-353, 1985.
437. Morgan M, Lumley J, Whitwam JG: Respiratory effects of etomidate. Br J Anaesth 49:233-236, 1977.
438. Colvin MP, Savege TM, Newland PE, et al: Cardiorespiratory changes following induction of anaesthesia with etomidate in patients with cardiac disease. Br J Anaesth 51:551-556, 1979.
439. Craig J, Cooper GM, Sear JW: Recovery from day-case anaesthesia: Comparison between methohexitone, Althesin and etomidate. Br J Anaesth 54:447-451, 1982.
440. Ouedraogo N, Marthan R, Roux E: The effects of propofol and etomidate on airway contractility in chronically hypoxic rats. Anesth Analg 96:1035-1041, 2003.
441. Ogawa K, Tanaka S, Murray PA: Inhibitory effects of etomidate and ketamine on endothelium-dependent relaxation in canine pulmonary artery. Anesthesiology 94:668-677, 2001.
442. Gooding JM, Weng JT, Smith RA, et al: Cardiovascular and pulmonary responses following etomidate induction of anesthesia in patients with demonstrated cardiac disease. Anesth Analg 58:40-41, 1979.
443. Gooding JM, Corssen G: Effect of etomidate on the cardiovascular system. Anesth Analg 56:717-719, 1977.
444. Criado A, Maseda J, Navarro E, et al: Induction of anaesthesia with etomidate: Haemodynamic study of 36 patients. Br J Anaesth 52:803-806, 1980.
445. Lischke V, Wilke HJ, Probst S, et al: Prolongation of the QT-interval during induction of anesthesia in patients with coronary artery disease. Acta Anaesthesiol Scand 38:144-148, 1994.
446. Allolio B, Dorr H, Stuttmann R: Effect of a single bolus dose of etomidate upon eight major corticosteroid hormones and plasma ACTH. Clin Endocrinol (Oxf) 22:281, 1985.
447. Lamberts SW, Bons EG, Bruining HA, de Jong FH: Differential effects of the imidazole derivatives etomidate, ketoconazole and miconazole and of metyrapone on the secretion of cortisol and its precursors by human adrenocortical cells. J Pharmacol Exp Ther 240:259-264, 1987.
448. Boidin MP: Steroid response to ACTH and to ascorbinic acid during infusion of etomidate for general surgery. Acta Anaesthesiol Belg 36:15-22, 1985.
449. Duthie DJ, Fraser R, Nimmo WS: Effect of induction of anaesthesia with etomidate on corticosteroid synthesis in man. Br J Anaesth 57:156-159, 1985.
450. Crozier TA, Beck D, Schlaeger M, et al: Endocrinological changes following etomidate, midazolam, or methohexital for minor surgery. Anesthesiology 66:628-635, 1987.
451. Crozier TA, Schlaeger M, Wuttke W, Kettler D: [TIVA with etomidate-fentanyl versus midazolam-fentanyl: The perioperative stress of coronary surgery overcomes the inhibition of cortisol synthesis caused by etomidate-fentanyl anesthesia]. Anaesthetist 43:605-613, 1994.
452. Lundy JB, Slane ML, Frizzi JD: Acute adrenal insufficiency after a single dose of etomidate. J Intensive Care Med 22:111-117, 2007.
453. St Pierre M, Dunkel M, Rutherford A, Hering W: Does etomidate increase postoperative nausea? A double-blind controlled comparison of etomidate in lipid emulsion with propofol for balanced anaesthesia. Eur J Anaesthesiol 17:634-641, 2000.
454. Korttila K, Aromaa U: Venous complications after intravenous injection of diazepam, flunitrazepam, thiopentone and etomidate. Acta Anaesthesiol Scand 24:227, 1980.
455. Galloway PA, Nicoll JM, Leiman BC: Pain reduction with etomidate injection. Anaesthesia 37:352-353, 1982.
456. Doenicke AW, Roizen MF, Hoernecke R, et al: Solvent for etomidate may cause pain and adverse effects. Br J Anaesth 83:464-466, 1999.
457. Huter L, Schreiber T, Gugel M, Schwarzkopf K: Low-dose intravenous midazolam reduces etomidate-induced myoclonus: A prospective, randomized study in patients undergoing elective cardioversion. Anesth Analg 105:1298-1302, 2007.
458. Olkkola KT, Tammisto T: Quantitation of the interaction of rocuronium bromide with etomidate, fentanyl, midazolam, propofol, thiopentone, and isoflurane using closed-loop feedback control of infusion of rocuronium. Eur J Anaesthesiol Suppl 9:99-100, 1994.
459. Famewo C, Odugbesan C: Further experience with etomidate. Can Anaesth Soc J 25:130, 1978.
460. Van de Wiele B, Rubinstein E, Peacock W, Martin N: Propylene glycol toxicity caused by prolonged infusion of etomidate. J Neurosurg Anesthesiol 7:259-262, 1995.
461. Shulman MS, Edelmann R: Use of etomidate for elective cardioversion. Anesthesiology 68:656, 1988.
462. Schuttler J, Schwilden H, Stoekel H: Pharmacokinetics as applied to total intravenous anaesthesia: Practical implications. Anaesthesia 38(Suppl):53-56, 1983.
463. de Bruijn NP, Hlatky MA, Jacobs JR, et al: General anesthesia during percutaneous transluminary coronary angioplasty for acute myocardial infarction: Results of a randomized controlled clinical trial. Anesth Analg 68:201-207, 1989.
464. Avramov MN, Husain MM, White PF: The comparative effects of methohexital, propofol, and etomidate for electroconvulsive therapy. Anesth Analg 81:596-602, 1995.
465. Ledingham I, Finlay W, Watt I: Etomidate and adrenocortical function [letter]. Lancet 1434, 1983.
466. Maze M, Tranquilli W: Alpha-2 adrenoceptor agonists: Defining the role in clinical anesthesia. Anesthesiology 74:581-605, 1991.
467. Kaukinen S, Kaukinen L, Eerola R: Preoperative and postoperative use of clonidine with neurolept anaesthesia. Acta Anaesthesiol Scand 23:113-120, 1979.
468. Bloor BC, Flacke WE: Reduction in halothane anesthetic requirement by clonidine, an alpha-adrenergic agonist. Anesth Analg 61:741-745, 1982.
469. Gerlach AT, Dasta JF: Dexmedetomidine: An updated review. Ann Pharmacother 41:245-252, 2007.
470. Tobias JD: Dexmedetomidine: applications in pediatric critical care and pediatric anesthesiology. Pediatr Crit Care Med 8:115-131, 2007.
471. Bhana N, Goa KL, McClellan KJ: Dexmedetomidine. Drugs 59:263-268, 2000.
472. Virtanen R, Savola JM, Saano V, Nyman L: Characterization of the selectivity, specificity and potency of medetomidine as an alpha 2-adrenoceptor agonist. Eur J Pharmacol 150:9-14, 1988.
473. Dyck JB, Maze M, Haack C, et al: Computer-controlled infusion of intravenous dexmedetomidine hydrochloride in adult human volunteers. Anesthesiology 78:821-828, 1993.
474. Dyck JB, Maze M, Haack C, et al: The pharmacokinetics and hemodynamic effects of intravenous and

intramuscular dexmedetomidine hydrochloride in adult human volunteers. Anesthesiology 78:813-820, 1993.
475. De Wolf AM, Fragen RJ, Avram MJ, et al: The pharmacokinetics of dexmedetomidine in volunteers with severe renal impairment. Anesth Analg 93:1205-1209, 2001.
476. Venn RM, Karol MD, Grounds RM: Pharmacokinetics of dexmedetomidine infusions for sedation of postoperative patients requiring intensive caret. Br J Anaesth 88:669-675, 2002.
477. Aantaa R, Jalonen J: Perioperative use of alpha$_2$-adrenoceptor agonists and the cardiac patient. Eur J Anaesthesiol 23:361-372, 2006.
478. Paris A, Tonner PH: Dexmedetomidine in anaesthesia. Curr Opin Anaesthesiol 18:412-418, 2005.
479. Guo TZ, Jiang JY, Buttermann AE, Maze M: Dexmedetomidine injection into the locus ceruleus produces antinociception. Anesthesiology 84:873-881, 1996.
480. Venn RM, Bradshaw CJ, Spencer R, et al: Preliminary UK experience of dexmedetomidine, a novel agent for postoperative sedation in the intensive care unit. Anaesthesia 54:1136-1142, 1999.
481. Venn RM, Hell J, Grounds RM: Respiratory effects of dexmedetomidine in the surgical patient requiring intensive care. Crit Care 4:302-308, 2000.
482. Kress JP, Pohlman AS, O'Connor MF, Hall JB: Daily interruption of sedative infusions in critically ill patients undergoing mechanical ventilation. N Engl J Med 342:1471-1477, 2000.
483. Nelson LE, Lu J, Guo T, et al: The alpha$_2$-adrenoceptor agonist dexmedetomidine converges on an endogenous sleep-promoting pathway to exert its sedative effects. Anesthesiology 98:428-436, 2003.
484. Nacif-Coelho C, Correa-Sales C, Chang LL, Maze M: Perturbation of ion channel conductance alters the hypnotic response to the alpha 2-adrenergic agonist dexmedetomidine in the locus coeruleus of the rat. Anesthesiology 81:1527-1534, 1994.
485. Angst MS, Ramaswamy B, Davies MF, Maze M: Comparative analgesic and mental effects of increasing plasma concentrations of dexmedetomidine and alfentanil in humans. Anesthesiology 101:744-752, 2004.
486. Ramsay MA, Luterman DL: Dexmedetomidine as a total intravenous anesthetic agent. Anesthesiology 101:787-790, 2004.
487. Aho M, Erkola O, Kallio A, et al: Comparison of dexmedetomidine and midazolam sedation and antagonism of dexmedetomidine with atipamezole. J Clin Anesth 5:194-203, 1993.
488. Reid K, Hayashi Y, Guo TZ, et al: Chronic administration of an alpha 2 adrenergic agonist desensitizes rats to the anesthetic effects of dexmedetomidine. Pharmacol Biochem Behav 47:171-175, 1994.
489. Maccioli GA: Dexmedetomidine to facilitate drug withdrawal. Anesthesiology 98:575-577, 2003.
490. Davies MF, Haimor F, Lighthall G, Clark JD: Dexmedetomidine fails to cause hyperalgesia after cessation of chronic administration. Anesth Analg 96:195-200, 2003.
491. Hayashi Y, Guo TZ, Maze M: Hypnotic and analgesic effects of the alpha 2-adrenergic agonist dexmedetomidine in morphine-tolerant rats. Anesth Analg 83:606-610, 1996.
492. Asano T, Dohi S, Ohta S, et al: Antinociception by epidural and systemic alpha(2)-adrenoceptor agonists and their binding affinity in rat spinal cord and brain. Anesth Analg 90:400-407, 2000.
493. Tryba M, Gehling M: Clonidine—a potent analgesic adjuvant. Curr Opin Anaesthesiol 15:511-517, 2002.
494. Eisenach JC, De Kock M, Klimscha W: Alpha(2)-adrenergic agonists for regional anesthesia: A clinical review of clonidine (1984-1995). Anesthesiology 85:655-674, 1996.
495. Eisenach JC, Shafer SL, Bucklin BA, et al: Pharmacokinetics and pharmacodynamics of intraspinal dexmedetomidine in sheep. Anesthesiology 80:1349-1359, 1994.
496. Aho MS, Erkola OA, Scheinin H, et al: Effect of intravenously administered dexmedetomidine on pain after laparoscopic tubal ligation. Anesth Analg 73:112-118, 1991.
497. Hall JE, Uhrich TD, Barney JA, et al: Sedative, amnestic, and analgesic properties of small-dose dexmedetomidine infusions. Anesth Analg 90:699-705, 2000.
498. Cortinez LI, Hsu YW, Sum-Ping ST, et al: Dexmedetomidine pharmacodynamics, part II: Crossover comparison of the analgesic effect of dexmedetomidine and remifentanil in healthy volunteers. Anesthesiology 101:1077-1083, 2004.
499. Maier C, Steinberg GK, Sun GH, et al: Neuroprotection by the alpha 2-adrenoreceptor agonist dexmedetomidine in a focal model of cerebral ischemia. Anesthesiology 79:306-312, 1993.
500. Hoffman WE, Kochs E, Werner C, et al: Dexmedetomidine improves neurologic outcome from incomplete ischemia in the rat: Reversal by the alpha 2-adrenergic antagonist atipamezole. Anesthesiology 75:328-332, 1991.
501. Kuhmonen J, Pokorny J, Miettinen R, et al: Neuroprotective effects of dexmedetomidine in the gerbil hippocampus after transient global ischemia. Anesthesiology 87:371-377, 1997.
502. Engelhard K, Werner C, Kaspar S, et al: Effect of the alpha2-agonist dexmedetomidine on cerebral neurotransmitter concentrations during cerebral ischemia in rats. Anesthesiology 96:450-457, 2002.
503. Talke P, Bickler PE: Effects of dexmedetomidine on hypoxia-evoked glutamate release and glutamate receptor activity in hippocampal slices. Anesthesiology 85:551-557, 1996.
504. Talke P, Tong C, Lee HW, et al: Effect of dexmedetomidine on lumbar cerebrospinal fluid pressure in humans. Anesth Analg 85:358-364, 1997.
505. Karlsson BR, Forsman M, Roald OK, et al: Effect of dexmedetomidine, a selective and potent alpha 2-agonist, on cerebral blood flow and oxygen consumption during halothane anesthesia in dogs. Anesth Analg 71:125-129, 1990.
506. Zornow MH, Fleischer JE, Scheller MS, et al: Dexmedetomidine, an alpha 2-adrenergic agonist, decreases cerebral blood flow in the isoflurane-anesthetized dog. Anesth Analg 70:624-630, 1990.
507. Zornow MH, Maze M, Dyck JB, Shafer SL: Dexmedetomidine decreases cerebral blood flow velocity in humans. J Cereb Blood Flow Metab 13:350-353, 1993.
508. Bekker A, Sturaitis MK: Dexmedetomidine for neurological surgery. Neurosurgery 57:1-10, 2005.
509. Drummond JC, Dao AV, Roth DM, et al: Effect of dexmedetomidine on cerebral blood flow velocity, cerebral metabolic rate, and carbon dioxide response in normal humans. Anesthesiology 108:225-232, 2008.
510. Mirski MA, Rossell LA, McPherson RW, Traystman RJ: Dexmedetomidine decreases seizure threshold in a rat model of experimental generalized epilepsy. Anesthesiology 81:1422-1428, 1994.
511. Halonen T, Kotti T, Tuunanen J, et al: Alpha 2-adrenoceptor agonist, dexmedetomidine, protects against kainic acid-induced convulsions and neuronal damage. Brain Res 693:217-224, 1995.
512. Weinger MB, Segal IS, Maze M: Dexmedetomidine, acting through central alpha-2 adrenoceptors, prevents opiate-induced muscle rigidity in the rat. Anesthesiology 71:242-249, 1989.
513. Schmucker P, van Ackern K, Franke N, et al: [Effect of the intravenous administration of lormetazepam on hemodynamics and arterial blood gases in patients with coronary heart disease]. Anaesthetist 31:557-563, 1982.
514. Karhuvaara S, Kallio A, Koulu M, et al: No involvement of alpha 2-adrenoceptors in the regulation of basal prolactin secretion in healthy men. Psychoneuroendocrinology 15:125-129, 1990.
515. Ebert TJ, Hall JE, Barney JA, et al: The effects of increasing plasma concentrations of dexmedetomidine in humans. Anesthesiology 93:382-394, 2000.
516. Yung-Wei H, Robertson K, Young C, et al: Compare the respiratory effects of remifentanil and dexmedetomidine. Anesthesiology 95:A1357, 2001.
517. Arain SR, Ebert TJ: The efficacy, side effects, and recovery characteristics of dexmedetomidine versus propofol when used for intraoperative sedation. Anesth Analg 95:461-466, 2002.
518. Hsu YW, Cortinez LI, Robertson KM, et al: Dexmedetomidine pharmacodynamics, part I: Crossover comparison of the respiratory effects of dexmedetomidine and remifentanil in healthy volunteers. Anesthesiology 101:1066-1076, 2004.
519. Lou YP, Franco-Cereceda A, Lundberg JM: Variable alpha 2-adrenoceptor-mediated inhibition of bronchoconstriction and peptide release upon activation of pulmonary afferents. Eur J Pharmacol 210:173-181, 1992.
520. Hogue CW Jr, Talke P, Stein PK, et al: Autonomic nervous system responses during sedative infusions of dexmedetomidine. Anesthesiology 97:592-598, 2002.
521. Riker RR, Fraser GL: Adverse events associated with sedatives, analgesics, and other drugs that provide patient comfort in the intensive care unit. Pharmacotherapy 25:8S-18S, 2005.
522. Roekaerts P, Prinzen F, Willingers H: The effect of dexmedetomidine on systemic haemodynamics, regional myocardial function and blood flow during coronary artery stenosis in acute anaesthetized dogs. J Cardiothorac Anesth 8:58, 1994.
523. Willigers HM, Prinzen FW, Roekaerts PM, et al: Dexmedetomidine decreases perioperative myocardial lactate release in dogs. Anesth Analg 96:657-664, 2003.
524. Nishina K, Mikawa K, Uesugi T, et al: Efficacy of clonidine for prevention of perioperative myocardial ischemia: A critical appraisal and meta-analysis of the literature. Anesthesiology 96:323-329, 2002.
525. Wallace AW, Galindez D, Salahieh A, et al: Effect of clonidine on cardiovascular morbidity and mortality after noncardiac surgery. Anesthesiology 101:284-293, 2004.
526. Venn M, Newman J, Grounds M: A phase II study to evaluate the efficacy of dexmedetomidine for sedation in the medical intensive care unit. Intensive Care Med 29:201-207, 2003.
527. Karhuvaara S, Kallio A, Salonen M, et al: Rapid reversal of alpha 2-adrenoceptor agonist effects by atipamezole in human volunteers. Br J Clin Pharmacol 31:160-165, 1991.
528. Venn RM, Grounds RM: Comparison between dexmedetomidine and propofol for sedation in the intensive care unit: Patient and clinician perceptions. Br J Anaesth 87:684-690, 2001.
529. Triltsch AE, Welte M, von Homeyer P, et al: Bispectral index-guided sedation with dexmedetomidine in intensive care: a prospective, randomized, double blind, placebo-controlled phase II study. Crit Care Med 30:1007-1014, 2002.
530. Ely EW, Shintani A, Truman B, et al: Delirium as a predictor of mortality in mechanically ventilated

patients in the intensive care unit. JAMA 291:1753-1762, 2004.
531. Pandharipande PP, Pun BT, Herr DL, et al: Effect of sedation with dexmedetomidine vs lorazepam on acute brain dysfunction in mechanically ventilated patients: The MENDS randomized controlled trial. JAMA 298:2644-2653, 2007.
532. Baumgartner GR, Rowen RC: Transdermal clonidine versus chlordiazepoxide in alcohol withdrawal: A randomized, controlled clinical trial. South Med J 84:312-321, 1991.
533. Baddigam K, Russo P, Russo J, Tobias JD: Dexmedetomidine in the treatment of withdrawal syndromes in cardiothoracic surgery patients. J Intensive Care Med 20:118-123, 2005.
534. Siobal MS, Kallet RH, Kivett VA, Tang JF: Use of dexmedetomidine to facilitate extubation in surgical intensive-care-unit patients who failed previous weaning attempts following prolonged mechanical ventilation: A pilot study. Respir Care 51:492-496, 2006.
535. Maze M, Angst MS: Dexmedetomidine and opioid interactions: Defining the role of dexmedetomidine for intensive care unit sedation. Anesthesiology 101:1059-1061, 2004.
536. Dasta JF, Kane-Gill SL, Durtschi AJ: Comparing dexmedetomidine prescribing patterns and safety in the naturalistic setting versus published data. Ann Pharmacother 38:1130-1135, 2004.
537. Aantaa R, Kanto J, Scheinin M, et al: Dexmedetomidine, an alpha 2-adrenoceptor agonist, reduces anesthetic requirements for patients undergoing minor gynecologic surgery. Anesthesiology 73:230-235, 1990.
538. Aho M, Lehtinen AM, Erkola O, et al: The effect of intravenously administered dexmedetomidine on perioperative hemodynamics and isoflurane requirements in patients undergoing abdominal hysterectomy. Anesthesiology 74:997-1002, 1991.
539. Koroglu A, Demirbilek S, Teksan H, et al: Sedative, haemodynamic and respiratory effects of dexmedetomidine in children undergoing magnetic resonance imaging examination: Preliminary results. Br J Anaesth 94:821-824, 2005.
540. Koroglu A, Teksan H, Sagir O, et al: A comparison of the sedative, hemodynamic, and respiratory effects of dexmedetomidine and propofol in children undergoing magnetic resonance imaging. Anesth Analg 103:63-67, 2006.
541. Jaakola ML, Ali-Melkkila T, Kanto J, et al: Dexmedetomidine reduces intraocular pressure, intubation responses and anaesthetic requirements in patients undergoing ophthalmic surgery. Br J Anaesth 68:570-575, 1992.
542. Scheinin B, Lindgren L, Randell T, et al: Dexmedetomidine attenuates sympathoadrenal responses to tracheal intubation and reduces the need for thiopentone and peroperative fentanyl. Br J Anaesth 68:126-131, 1992.
543. Aho M, Erkola O, Kallio A, et al: Dexmedetomidine infusion for maintenance of anesthesia in patients undergoing abdominal hysterectomy. Anesth Analg 75:940-946, 1992.
544. Feld JM, Hoffman WE, Stechert MM, et al: Fentanyl or dexmedetomidine combined with desflurane for bariatric surgery. J Clin Anesth 18:24-28, 2006.
545. Bakhamees HS, El-Halafawy YM, El-Kerdawy HM, et al: Effects of dexmedetomidine in morbidly obese patients undergoing laparoscopic gastric bypass. Middle East J Anesthesiol 19:537-551, 2007.
546. Dholakia C, Beverstein G, Garren M, et al: The impact of perioperative dexmedetomidine infusion on postoperative narcotic use and duration of stay after laparoscopic bariatric surgery. J Gastrointest Surg 11:1556-1559, 2007.
547. Talke P, Li J, Jain U, et al: Effects of perioperative dexmedetomidine infusion in patients undergoing vascular surgery. The Study of Perioperative Ischemia Research Group. Anesthesiology 82:620-633, 1995.
548. Grant SA, Breslin DS, MacLeod DB, et al: Dexmedetomidine infusion for sedation during fiberoptic intubation: A report of three cases. J Clin Anesth 16:124-126, 2004.
549. Bekker AY, Kaufman B, Samir H, Doyle W: The use of dexmedetomidine infusion for awake craniotomy. Anesth Analg 92:1251-1253, 2001.
550. Bekker AY, Basile J, Gold M, et al: Dexmedetomidine for awake carotid endarterectomy: efficacy, hemodynamic profile, and side effects. J Neurosurg Anesthesiol 16:126-135, 2004.
551. Hofer RE, Sprung J, Sarr MG, Wedel DJ: Anesthesia for a patient with morbid obesity using dexmedetomidine without narcotics. Can J Anaesth 52:176-180, 2005.
552. Janssen P: The pharmacology of haloperidol. Int J Neuropsychiatry 3(Suppl 1):10, 1967.
553. DeCastro J, Mundeleer P: Anesthesie sans barbituriques: la neuroleptanalgesie (R1407, R1625, hydergine, procain). Anesth Analg 42:1022, 1959.
554. Scuderi PE: Droperidol: Many questions, few answers. Anesthesiology 98:289-290, 2003.
555. Dershwitz M: Droperidol: Should the black box be light gray? J Clin Anesth 14:598-603, 2002.
556. White PF: Droperidol: A cost-effective antiemetic for over thirty years. Anesth Analg 95:789-790, 2002.
557. Gan TJ, Alexander R, Fennelly M, Rubin AP: Comparison of different methods of administering droperidol in patient-controlled analgesia in the prevention of postoperative nausea and vomiting. Anesth Analg 80:81-85, 1995.
558. Gan TJ, White PF, Scuderi PE, et al: FDA "black box" warning regarding use of droperidol for postoperative nausea and vomiting: Is it justified? Anesthesiology 97:287, 2002.
559. Bailey P, Norton R, Karan S: The FDA droperidol warning: Is it justified? Anesthesiology 97:288-289, 2002.
560. Flood P, Coates KM: Droperidol inhibits $GABA_A$ and neuronal nicotinic receptor activation. Anesthesiology 96:987-993, 2002.
561. Borison H, Wang S: Physiology and pharmacology of vomiting. Pharmacol Rev 5:193, 1953.
562. Janssen P: Zur Frage des Abbaus und der Ausscheidung der bei Neuroleptanalgesie zur Anwendung kommenden Pharmaka. *In* Henschel W (ed): Die Neuroleptanalgesie. Berlin, Springer-Verlag, 1966.
563. Fischler M, Bonnet F, Trang H, et al: The pharmacokinetics of droperidol in anesthetized patients. Anesthesiology 64:486-489, 1986.
564. Michenfelder JD, Theye RA: Effects of fentanyl, droperidol, and innovar on canine cerebral metabolism and blood flow. Br J Anaesth 43:630-636, 1971.
565. Barker J, Harper A, McDowall D: Cerebral blood flow, cerebrospinal fluid pressure and EEG activity during neuroleptanalgesia induced with dehydrobenzperidol and phenoperidine. Br J Anaesth 40:143, 1968.
566. Song D, Chung F, Yogendran S, Wong J: Evaluation of postural stability after low-dose droperidol in outpatients undergoing gynaecological dilatation and curettage procedure. Br J Anaesth 88:819-823, 2002.
567. Prys-Roberts C, Kelman G: The influence of drugs used in neuroleptanalgesia on cardiovascular and ventilatory function. Br J Anaesth 39:134, 1967.
568. Corssen G, Domino E, Sweet R: Neuroleptanalgesia and anesthesia. Anesth Analg 43:748, 1964.
569. Israel J, Jansen G, Dobkin A: Circulatory and respiratory response to tilt with pentazocine (Win 20, 228), droperidol (R4749), droperidol-fentanyl (Innovar), and methotrimeprazine in normal healthy male subjects. Anesthesiology 26:253, 1965.
570. Wooltorton E: Droperidol: Cardiovascular toxicity and deaths. Can Med Assoc J 166:932, 2002.
571. Yelonsky J, Katz R, Dietrich E: A study of some of the pharmacologic actions of droperidol. Toxicol Appl Pharmacol 6:37, 1964.
572. Birch AA, Boyce WH: Effects of droperidol-dopamine interaction on renal blood flow in man. Anesthesiology 47:70-71, 1977.
573. Wetchler B, Collins I, Jacob L: Antiemetic effects of droperidol on the ambulatory surgery patient. Anesthesiol Rev 9:23, 1982.
574. Pandit SK, Kothary SP, Pandit UA, et al: Dose-response study of droperidol and metoclopramide as antiemetics for outpatient anesthesia. Anesth Analg 68:798-802, 1989.
575. Hill RP, Lubarsky DA, Phillips-Bute B, et al: Cost-effectiveness of prophylactic antiemetic therapy with ondansetron, droperidol, or placebo. Anesthesiology 92:958-967, 2000.
576. Aldrete JA: Reduction of nausea and vomiting from epidural opioids by adding droperidol to the infusate in home-bound patients. J Pain Sympt Manage 10:544-547, 1995.
577. Kjellberg F, Tramer MR: Pharmacological control of opioid-induced pruritus: A quantitative systematic review of randomized trials. Eur J Anaesthesiol 18:346-357, 2001.
578. Cressman WA, Plostnieks J, Johnson PC: Absorption, metabolism and excretion of droperidol by human subjects following intramuscular and intravenous administration. Anesthesiology 38:363-369, 1973.
579. DeRuiter G, Popescu D, DeBoer A: Pharmacokinetics of etomidate in surgical patients. Arch Int Pharmacodyn Ther 249:180, 1981.
580. Breimer LT, Hennis PJ, Burm AG, et al: Pharmacokinetics and EEG effects of flumazenil in volunteers. Clin Pharmacokinet 20:491-496, 1991.
581. Moffet A: Clarke's Isolation and Identification of Drugs, 2nd ed. London, Pharmaceutical Press, 1986.

Kazuhiko Fukuda

27 Opioids

Key Points

1. An increased understanding of the molecular pharmacology of opioid receptors and opioid-induced cellular responses allows the use of innovative techniques for analgesia.
2. Opioids suppress pain by their action in the brain, spinal cord, and peripheral nervous system.
3. Opioids affect many organ systems, including the respiratory and cardiovascular systems, and can cause a variety of adverse effects. Proper dosing and monitoring allow the adverse effects to be minimized.
4. New pharmacokinetic principles have allowed more intelligent use of opioids along with more predictable durations of action.
5. The pharmacokinetic and pharmacodynamic properties of opioids are affected by a variety of factors, such as age, body weight, organ failure, and shock. To appropriately use opioids, these factors should be taken into consideration.
6. During total intravenous anesthesia, the use of opioids is a vital part of providing the analgesic component of anesthesia. Short-acting drugs, such as remifentanil, allow dissipation of total intravenous anesthesia even more rapidly than with inhaled anesthetics.
7. New opioid delivery systems, such as transdermal fentanyl patches, are continually being developed. Such systems allow more flexibility in providing analgesia, both inside and outside the operating room.
8. Opioids can pharmacokinetically or pharmacodynamically interact with drugs used perioperatively. Drug interaction should be understood for proper patient management.

The term *opioid* refers broadly to all compounds related to opium. The word "opium" is derived from *opos*, the Greek word for juice, inasmuch as the drug is derived from the juice of the opium poppy *Papaver somniferum*. Opiates are drugs derived from opium and include the natural products morphine, codeine, and thebaine, as well as many semisynthetic congeners derived from them.

The first undisputed reference to opium is found in the writings of Theophrastus in the third century BC. During the Middle Ages, many of the uses of opium were appreciated. Opium contains more than 20 distinct alkaloids. In 1806, Sertürner reported the isolation of a pure substance in opium that he named morphine after Morpheus, the Greek god of dreams. By the middle of the 19th century, the use of pure alkaloids rather than crude opium preparations began to spread throughout the medical world.

In addition to the remarkable beneficial effects of opioids, the toxic side effects and addictive potential of these drugs have also been known for centuries. Synthetic opioid analgesics without side effects were explored, but many of the synthetic opioids share the side effects of natural opioids. The search for new opioid agonists led to the synthesis of opioid antagonists and compounds with mixed agonist/antagonist properties, which expanded therapeutic options and provided important tools for exploring the mechanisms of opioid actions. Furthermore, new methods of opioid administration, including patient-controlled analgesia (PCA) and computer-based infusion techniques, have been developed.

Pharmacology of Opioids

Classification of Opioid Compounds

Opioids can be classified as naturally occurring, semisynthetic, and synthetic (Box 27-1). The naturally occurring opioids can be divided into two chemical classes, phenanthrenes (morphine and codeine) and benzylisoquinolines (papaverine). The semisynthetic opioids are morphine derivatives in which one of several changes have been made. Synthetic opioids are classified into four groups, the morphinan derivatives (levorphanol), the diphenyl or methadone derivatives (methadone, *d*-propoxyphene), the benzomorphans (phenazocine, pentazocine), and the phenylpiperidine derivatives (meperidine, fentanyl, alfentanil, sufentanil, and remifentanil). Structures of opioid compounds are shown in Figure 27-1[1] and Table 27-1.[1]

Box 27-1 Classification of Opioid Compounds

Naturally Occurring

Morphine

Codeine

Papaverine

Thebaine

Semisynthetic

Heroin

Dihydromorphone/morphinone

Thebaine derivatives (e.g., etorphine, buprenorphine)

Synthetic

Morphinan series (e.g., levorphanol, butorphanol)

Diphenylpropylamine series (e.g., methadone)

Benzomorphan series (e.g., pentazocine)

Phenylpiperidine series (e.g., meperidine, fentanyl, sufentanil, alfentanil, remifentanil)

From Bailey PL, Egan TD, Stanley TH: Intravenous opioid anesthetics. *In* Miller RD (ed): Anesthesia, 5th ed. New York, Churchill Livingstone, 2000, p 276.

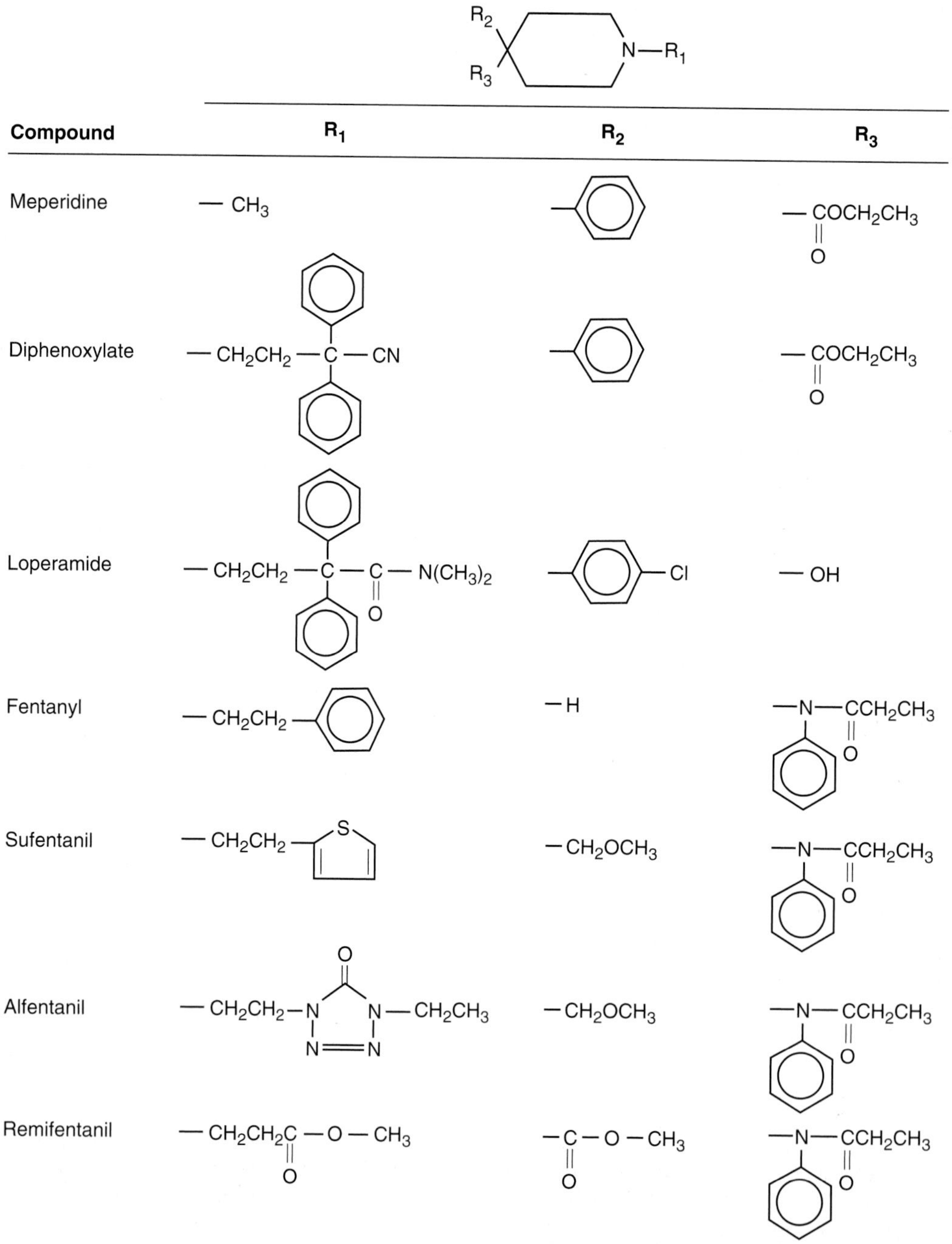

R_2, R_3 — N — R_1

Compound	R_1	R_2	R_3
Meperidine	$—CH_3$		$—COCH_2CH_3$ (=O)
Diphenoxylate	$—CH_2CH_2—C—CN$		$—COCH_2CH_3$ (=O)
Loperamide	$—CH_2CH_2—C—C—N(CH_3)_2$ (=O)	—Cl	—OH
Fentanyl	$—CH_2CH_2—$	—H	$—N—CCH_2CH_3$ (=O)
Sufentanil	$—CH_2CH_2—$ (S)	$—CH_2OCH_3$	$—N—CCH_2CH_3$ (=O)
Alfentanil	$—CH_2CH_2—N$ (O) $N—CH_2CH_3$, N═N	$—CH_2OCH_3$	$—N—CCH_2CH_3$ (=O)
Remifentanil	$—CH_2CH_2C—O—CH_3$ (=O)	$—C—O—CH_3$ (=O)	$—N—CCH_2CH_3$ (=O)

Figure 27-1 Chemical structures of piperidine and phenylpiperidine analgesics. *(From Gutstein HB, Akil H: Opioid analgesics.* In *Hardman JG, Limbird LE [eds]: Goodman and Gilman's The Pharmacological Basis of Therapeutics, 10th ed. New York, McGraw-Hill, 2001, pp 569-619.)*

Table 27-1 Structures of Opioids and Opioid Antagonists Chemically Related to Morphine

MORPHINE

	Chemical Radicals and Position*			
Nonproprietary Name	**3**	**6**	**17**	**Other Changes†**
Morphine	$-OH$	$-OH$	$-CH_3$	—
Heroin	$-OCOCH_3$	$-OCOCH_3$	$-CH_3$	—
Hydromorphone	$-OH$	$=O$	$-CH_3$	(1)
Oxymorphone	$-OH$	$=O$	$-CH_3$	(1), (2)
Levorphanol	$-OH$	$-H$	$-CH_3$	(1), (3)
Levallorphan	$-OH$	$-H$	$-CH_2CH=CH_2$	(1), (3)
Codeine	$-OCH_3$	$-OH$	$-CH_3$	—
Hydrocodone	$-OCH_3$	$=O$	$-CH_3$	(1)
Oxycodone	$-OCH_3$	$=O$	$-CH_3$	(1), (2)
Nalmefene	$-OH$	$=CH_2$	$-CH_2-$◁	(1), (2)
Nalorphine	$-OH$	$-OH$	$-CH_2CH=CH_2$	—
Naloxone	$-OH$	$=O$	$-CH_2CH=CH_2$	(1), (2)
Naltrexone	$-OH$	$=O$	$-CH_2-$◁	(1), (2)
Buprenorphine	$-OH$	$-OCH_3$	$-CH_2-$◁	(1), (4)
Butorphanol	$-OH$	$-H$	$-CH_2-$◇	(1), (2), (3)
Nalbuphine	$-OH$	$-OH$	$-CH_2-$◇	(1), (2)

*The numbers 3, 6, and 17 refer to positions in the morphine molecule, as shown in the line drawing.
†Other changes in the morphine molecule are as follows:
(1) Single instead of double bond between C7 and C8
(2) OH added to C14
(3) No oxygen between C4 and C5
(4) Endoetheno bridge between C6 and C14; 1-hydroxy-1,2,2-trimethylpropyl substitution on C7
From Gutstein HB, Akil H: Opioid analgesics. *In* Hardman JG, Limbird LE (eds): Goodman and Gilman's The Pharmacological Basis of Therapeutics, 10th ed. New York, McGraw-Hill, 2001, pp 569-619.

Opioids can be classified as agonists, partial agonists, mixed agonist-antagonists, and antagonists on the basis of their interaction with opioid receptors.

Opioid Receptors

In 1973, based on radioligand binding assays, three types of opioid receptors were postulated. They were named μ for the morphine type, κ for the ketocyclazocine type, and σ for the SKF10047 (*N*-allylnormetazocine) type. In addition, a high-affinity receptor for enkephalins was found in the mouse vas deferens and designated the δ-receptor. Furthermore, an ε-receptor was proposed as the binding site for β-endorphin in the rat vas deferens. The pharmacologic actions of opioids and the involved receptors have been analyzed (Table 27-2).

Biochemical studies were performed to purify the opioid receptor protein but have not been successful. Since the early 1990s, molecular biologic studies have elucidated the molecular structures and signal transduction mechanisms of the opioid

Table 27-2 Pharmacologic Actions of Opioids and Opioid Receptors in Animal Models

		Actions of	
	Receptor	**Agonists**	**Antagonists**
Analgesia			
Supraspinal	μ, δ, κ	Analgesic	No effect
Spinal	μ, δ, κ	Analgesic	No effect
Respiratory function	μ	Decrease	No effect
Gastrointestinal tract	μ, κ	Decrease transit	No effect
Psychotomimesis	κ	Increase	No effect
Feeding	μ, δ, κ	Increase feeding	Decrease feeding
Sedation	μ, κ	Increase	No effect
Diuresis	κ	Increase	
Hormone secretion			
Prolactin	μ	Increase release	Decrease release
Growth hormone	μ and/or δ	Increase release	Decrease release
Neurotransmitter release			
Acetylcholine	μ	Inhibit	
Dopamine	δ	Inhibit	

receptors. Four different cDNAs have been isolated as members of the opioid receptor family.[2] Three of them correspond to the pharmcacologically defined μ-, δ-, and κ-opioid receptors. The fourth receptor did not bind with opioid ligands with high affinity. Later, a novel peptide named nociceptin/orphanin FQ was identified as an endogenous agonist of the fourth member of the opioid receptor family.[3,4] The characteristics of three opioid receptors and the nociceptin/orphanin FQ receptor are listed in Table 27-3.

The μ-receptors are located in both the brain and spinal cord[5] and mediate a variety of pharmacologic effects of opioids. Further pharmacologic classification of the μ-receptor as μ_1, μ_2, and μ_3 has been proposed. Perhaps post-translational modification of the μ-receptor is the molecular basis of the μ-receptor subtypes. However, the molecular identity of these receptors still remains to be clarified.

Hydropathy analysis of the primary structures of the opioid receptors indicates that the opioid receptors possess seven transmembrane domains (Fig. 27-2), a characteristic structural feature of the G protein–coupled receptor. The μ-, δ-, and κ-opioid receptors and the nociceptin receptor share approximately 50% amino acid sequence homology with each other.

Several single-nucleotide polymorphisms have been identified in the human μ-opioid receptor gene.[6] The A118G mutation, an A-to-G substitution in exon 1 that results in exchange of asparagine at position 40 for aspartate (N40D), is the most common mutation leading to a change in the gene product in the human μ-opioid receptors. It was suggested that cancer patients who were homozygous for the A118G variant required higher doses of oral morphine for long-term treatment of their pain.[7] A118G mutation of the human μ-opioid receptor gene reduces analgesic responses to morphine-6-glucuronide (M6G) but does not significantly affect the respiratory depression induced by M6G.[8] Furthermore, morphine consumption via intravenous PCA after total abdominal hysterectomy was significantly greater in women homozygous for the A118G variant than in other patients.[9]

Endogenous Opioid Peptides

Enkephalin, β-endorphin, and dynorphin were identified as endogenous agonists for the δ-, μ-, and κ-opioid receptors, respectively. After purification of these peptides from mammalian tissues, cDNAs for the precursors of these peptides were cloned. cDNA cloning and amino acid determination of proopiomelanocortin demonstrated that cleavage of this precursor protein produces not only β-endorphin but also several other neuro-

Table 27-3 Characteristics of Opioid Receptors

	μ	δ	κ	**Nociceptin**
Tissue bioassay	Guinea pig ileum	Mouse vas deferens	Rabbit vas deferens	
Endogenous ligand	β-Endorphin	Leu-enkephalin	Dynorphin	Nociceptin
	Endomorphin	Met-enkephalin		
Agonist	Morphine	DPDPE	Buprenorphin	
	Fentanyl	Deltorphin	Pentazocine	
	DAMGO		U50,488	
Antagonist	Naloxone	Naloxone	Naloxone	
	Naltrexone	Naltrindole	NorBNI	
Coupled G-protein	$G_{i/o}$	$G_{i/o}$	$G_{i/o}$	$G_{i/o}$
Adenylate cyclase	Inhibition	Inhibition	Inhibition	Inhibition
Voltage-gated Ca^{2+} channels	Inhibition	Inhibition	Inhibition	Inhibition
Inwardly rectifying K^+ channels	Activation	Activation	Activation	Activation

DPDPE, [D-penicillamine[2], D-penicillamine[5]]enkephalin; DAMGO, [D-Ala[2], MePhe[4], Gly-ol[8]]enkephaline; NorBNI, norbinaltorphimine.

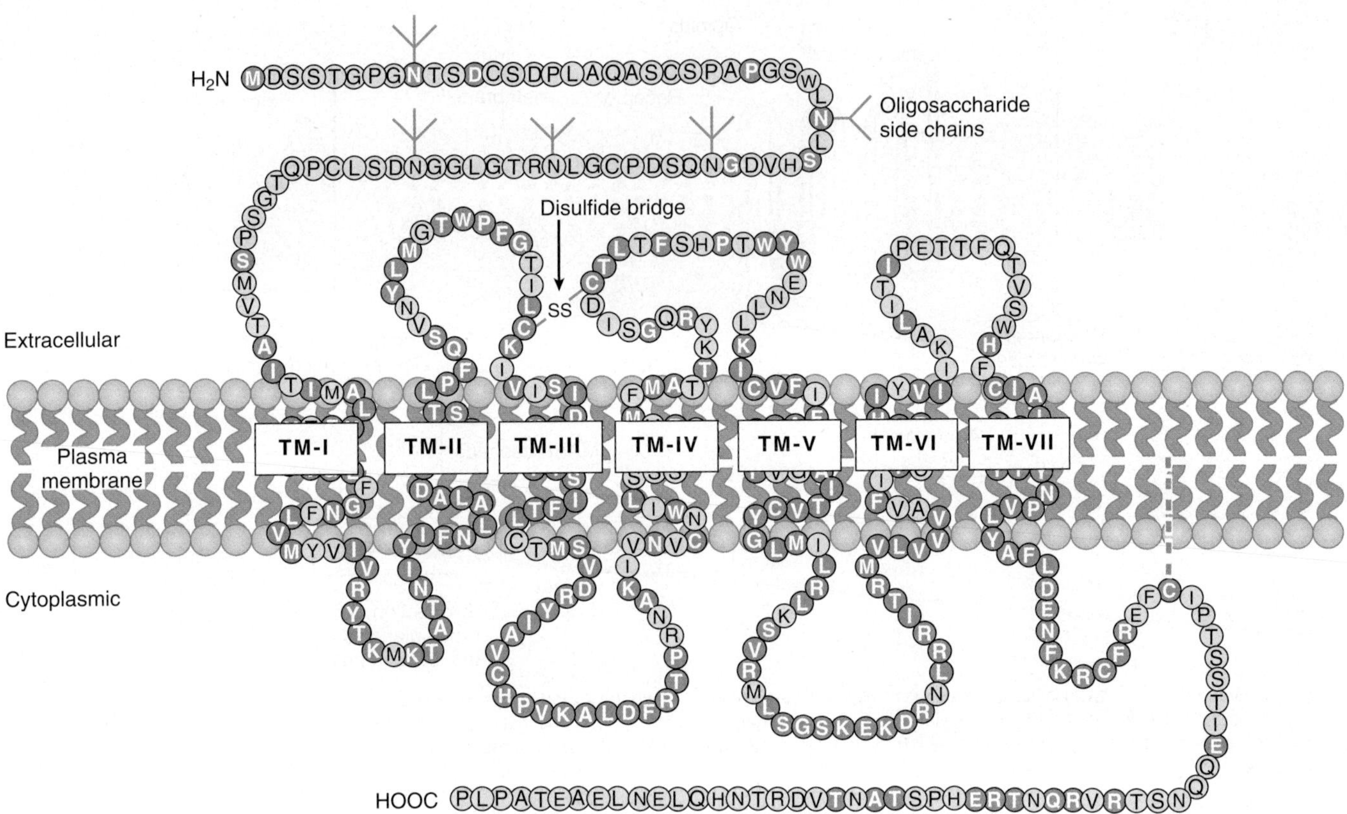

Figure 27-2 Proposed structure of the μ-opioid receptor. *Filled circles* indicate amino acid residues identical in the μ- and δ-opioid receptors. TM-I to TM-VII show putative transmembrane segments composed of hydrophobic amino acid residues.

peptides, including methionine enkephalin, adrenocorticotropic hormone, and α-melanocyte–stimulating hormone. Amino acid sequencing of preproenkephalin indicates that four methionine enkephalins and one leucine enkephalin are cleaved from this precursor. Furthermore, the primary structure of preprodynorphin, the precursor of dynorphin, was determined by cDNA cloning.

A novel endogenous opioid peptide with significant sequence homology to dynorphin was isolated in 1995.[3,4] This peptide was called orphanin FQ or nociceptin because it lowered the pain threshold under certain conditions, in contrast to the other endogenous opioid peptides. Pharmacologic and physiologic studies have demonstrated that orphanin FQ/nociceptin has behavioral and pain modulatory properties distinct from those of the three classic opioid peptides.[10] Studies of the effect of orphanin FQ/nociceptin on pain sensitivity have produced conflicting results, which may suggest that the effects of orphanin FQ/nociceptin on pain sensitivity depend on the underlying behavioral state of the subject. Prepronociceptin, the precursor of orphanin FQ/nociceptin, was cloned, and its amino acid sequence suggested the existence of prepronociceptin-derived neuropeptides other than orphanin FQ/nociceptin.[11]

The search for an endogenous ligand that binds to the μ-receptor with high affinity and high selectivity led to the discovery of a class of novel endogenous opioids termed endomorphin-1 and endomorphin-2.[12] These peptides are tetrapeptides with the sequence Tyr-Pro-Trp-Phe and Tyr-Pro-Phe-Phe, respectively. An endomorphin gene has yet to be cloned, and much remains to be learned about the anatomic distribution, mode of interaction with opioid receptors, function in vivo, and potential existence of other related peptides that are highly selective for each of the opioid receptors.

Intracellular Signal Transduction Mechanism

The opioid receptors belong to the G protein–coupled receptor family. Activation of the opioid receptors leads to activation of the pertussis toxin–sensitive G proteins (G_i and/or G_o). Expression of the cloned opioid receptors in cultured cells by transfection of the cloned cDNA has facilitated analysis of the intracellular signal transduction mechanisms activated by the opioid receptors (Fig. 27-3).[2] Adenylate cyclase is inhibited by activation of the opioid receptor, thereby resulting in a reduction in cellular cyclic adenosine monophosphate (AMP) content. Electrophysiologically, the voltage-gated Ca^{2+} channel is inhibited and the inwardly rectifying K^+ channels are activated by the opioid receptors. As a result, neuronal excitability is reduced by activation of the opioid receptors. In contrast, it was reported that opioids also stimulate the influx of Ca^{2+} into neuronal cultured cells.[13] Recently, it was shown that extracellular signal–related kinase, a class of mitogen-activated protein kinases, is activated by the opioid receptors.[14]

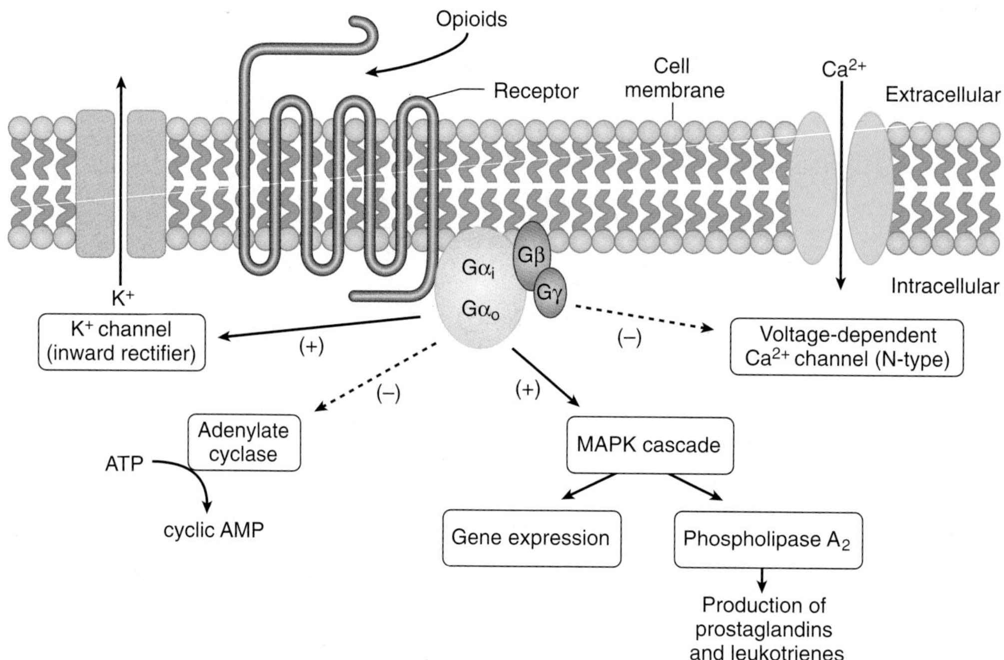

Figure 27-3 Intracellular signal transduction mechanisms linked with the opioid receptors. Binding of opioid agonists with the opioid receptors leads to activation of the G protein. The activity of adenylate cyclase and the voltage-dependent Ca^{2+} channels is suppressed. On the other hand, the inwardly rectifying K^+ channels and mitogen-activated protein kinase (MAPK) cascade are activated. AMP, adenosine monophosphate; ATP, adenosine triphosphate.

Opioid-induced activation of extracellular signal–related kinase can lead to an increase in release of arachidonate[14] and expression of the immediate early genes c-fos and junB.[15]

Chronic exposure of the opioid receptors to agonists induces cellular adaptation mechanisms that may be involved in opioid tolerance, dependence, and withdrawal symptoms. Short-term desensitization probably involves phosphorylation of the opioid receptors via protein kinase C.[16] A number of other kinases have also been implicated, including protein kinase A and β-adrenergic receptor kinase (βARK).[17] BARKs selectively phosphorylate agonist-bound receptors, thereby promoting interactions with β-arrestins, which interfere with G protein coupling and promote receptor internalization. Acute morphine-induced analgesia was enhanced in mice lacking β-arrestin 2, suggesting that this protein contributes to regulation of responsivity to opioids in vivo.[18]

Like other G protein–coupled receptors, the opioid receptors can undergo rapid agonist-mediated internalization via a classic endocytic pathway.[19,20] These processes may be induced differentially as a function of the class of the ligand. For example, certain agonists, such as etorphine and enkephalins, cause rapid internalization of the μ-receptor, whereas morphine, although it decreases adenylyl cyclase activity equally well, does not cause internalization of the μ-receptor.[21] These findings may suggest that different ligands induce different conformational changes in the receptor that lead to divergent intracellular events. Furthermore, they may provide an explanation for differences in the efficacy and abuse potential of various opioids.[22]

Long-term tolerance to opioids has been thought to be associated with superactivation of adenylyl cyclase activity—a counter-regulatory response to the decrease in cyclic AMP levels seen after acute opioid administration.[23] This effect is prevented by pretreatment of cells with pertussis toxin, thus demonstrating the involvement of G proteins (G_i and/or G_o).

Mechanism of Analgesia

Pain control by opioids needs to be considered in the context of brain circuits modulating analgesia and the functions of the various types of receptors in these circuits.[24] The analgesic effects of opioids arise from their ability to directly inhibit ascending transmission of nociceptive information from the spinal cord dorsal horn and to activate pain control circuits that descend from the midbrain, via the rostral ventromedial medulla (RVM), to the spinal cord dorsal horn. Petrovic and colleagues used an experimental pain model and positron emission tomography (PET) to study the mechanisms of action of the short-acting μ-opioid agonist remifentanil and found drug-induced activation of the rostral anterior cingulate cortex, insula, orbitofrontal cortex, and brainstem areas.[25] The latter overlapped with brain areas that have been implicated in pain modulation, such as the periaqueductal gray matter (PAG). Interestingly, placebo analgesia acts similarly on the activity of these brain areas, presumably via endogenous opioid release.[26]

Immunohistochemical studies and in situ hybridization analysis have demonstrated that opioid receptors are expressed in various areas in the central nervous system (CNS),[5] including the amygdala, mesencephalic reticular formation, PAG, and RVM. However, the role of opioid receptors in all these areas has not been completely clarified.

Microinjection of morphine into the PAG or direct electrical stimulation of this area produces analgesia that can be blocked by naloxone. Opioid actions at the PAG influence the RVM, which in turn modulates nociceptive transmission in the dorsal horn of the spinal cord through the action of the descending inhibition pathway. Thus, opioids produce analgesia not only by direct actions on the spinal cord but also by neurally mediated action in regions separate from the site of opioid administration.

The distribution of opioid receptors in descending pain control circuits indicates substantial overlap between μ- and κ-receptors. Interactions between the κ-receptor and the μ-receptor may be important for modulating nociceptive transmission from higher nociceptive centers, as well as in the spinal cord dorsal horn. The μ-receptor produces analgesia within descending pain control circuits, at least in part by the removal of GABAergic (transmitting or secreting γ-aminobutyric acid) inhibition of RVM-projecting neurons in the PAG and spinally projecting neurons in the RVM.[24] The actions of μ-receptor agonists are invariably analgesic, whereas those of κ-receptor agonists can be either analgesic or antianalgesic. The pain-modulating effects of κ-receptor agonists in the brainstem appear to oppose those of μ-receptor agonists.[27]

Local spinal mechanisms, in addition to descending inhibition, underlie the analgesic action of opioids. In the spinal cord, opioids act at synapses either presynaptically or postsynaptically. Opioid receptors are abundantly expressed in the substantia gelatinosa, where release of substance P from the primary sensory neuron is inhibited by opioids.

There is significant opioid receptor-ligand binding and little detectable receptor mRNA expression in the spinal cord dorsal horn but high levels of opioid receptor mRNA in the dorsal root ganglia. This distribution might suggest that the actions of opioid receptor agonists relevant to analgesia at the spinal level are predominantly presynaptic. It is well known that opioids decrease the pain-evoked release of tachykinins from primary afferent nociceptors. However, at least 80% of tachykinin signaling in response to noxious stimulation remains intact after the intrathecal administration of large doses of opioids.[28] These results suggest that although opioid administration may reduce release of tachykinin from primary afferent nociceptors, this reduction has little functional impact on the actions of tachykinin on postsynaptic pain-transmitting neurons.

The actions of opioids in the bulbospinal pathways are critical to their analgesic efficacy. Opioid actions in the forebrain clearly contribute to analgesia because decerebration prevents analgesia when rats are tested for pain sensitivity with the formalin test[29] and microinjection of opioids into several forebrain regions is analgesic in this test.[30] The analgesia induced by systemic administration of morphine in both the tail flick and formalin tests was disrupted either by lesioning or by reversibly inactivating the central nucleus of the amygdala, thus demonstrating that opioid actions in the forebrain contribute to analgesia after tissue damage, as well as after acute phasic nociception.[31,32]

Opioids may also produce analgesia through a peripheral mechanism.[33] Immune cells infiltrating an inflammatory site may release endogenous opioid-like substances that act on opioid receptors located on the primary sensory neuron.[33] However, others do not support this conclusion.[34,35]

Mood Alterations and Rewarding Properties

The mechanisms by which opioids produce euphoria, tranquility, and other alterations in mood (including rewarding properties) are not entirely clear. Behavioral and pharmacologic evidence points to the role of dopaminergic pathways, particularly those involving the nucleus accumbens, in drug-induced reward. Functional magnetic resonance imaging studies have demonstrated that a small intravenous dose (4 mg) of morphine induces positive signal changes in reward structures, including the nucleus accumbens, sublenticular extended amygdala, orbitofrontal cortex, and hippocampus, and decreases signal in cortical areas similar to the action of sedative-hypnotics such as propofol and midazolam.[36] These observations are consistent with results from pharmacologic studies.

The shell of the nucleus accumbens is the site that may be involved directly in the emotional and motivational aspects of drug-induced reward. All three opioid receptor types are present on the nucleus accumbens and are thought to mediate, at least in part, the motivational effects of opiate drugs.[5] Selective μ- and δ-receptor agonists are rewarding when defined by place preference and intracranial self-administration paradigms. Conversely, selective κ-receptor agonists produce aversive effects. The positive motivational effects of opioids are partially mediated by release of dopamine at the level of the nucleus accumbens.

The locus ceruleus contains both noradrenergic neurons and high concentrations of opioid receptors and is postulated to play a critical role in feelings of alarm, panic, fear, and anxiety. Neural activity in the locus ceruleus is inhibited by both exogenous opioids and endogenous opioid peptides.

Analysis of Knock-out Mice

The physiologic roles of the opioid receptors and endogenous opioid peptides have been investigated mainly by pharmacologic and physiologic methods. However, it has been difficult to analyze the functional roles of these proteins. Recently, knock-out mice, in which a specific gene is inactivated by molecular biologic methods, have been produced. By analysis of knock-out mice the physiologic significance of the respective opioid receptors and endogenous opioid peptide precursors can be deteremined.[37]

In μ-receptor knock-out mice, analgesia, the reward effect, and the withdrawal effect of morphine are lost.[38,39] Morphine-induced respiratory depression was not observed in the μ-receptor knock-out mice.[40] Therefore, the μ-receptor is a mandatory component of the opioid system for morphine action. In μ-receptor knock-out mice, ketamine-induced respiratory depression and antinociception are diminished,[41] suggesting that ketamine interacts with the μ-receptor to lead to these phenomena. Furthermore, the significantly higher minimum alveolar concentration (MAC) of sevoflurane in the μ-receptor knock-out mice than in wild-type mice suggest that the μ-receptor is involved in the anesthetic potency of sevoflurane.[40] δ-Receptor knock-out mice display a markedly reduced analgesic effect of opioids selective for δ-receptors at the spinal cord level.[42] However, at the supraspinal level, analgesia can be induced by δ-receptor agonists in δ-receptor knock-out mice, suggesting the existence of a second δ-like analgesic system. Because disruption of the κ-receptor abolishes the analgesic, hypolocomotive, and aversive actions of the κ-receptor agonists and induces hyperreactivity in the abdominal constriction test, the κ-receptor is thought to be involved in the perception of visceral chemical pain.[43]

In mice lacking β-endorphin, morphine induces normal analgesia, but naloxone-reversible stress-induced analgesia cannot be observed.[44] Preproenkephalin knock-out mice are more anxious than wild-type mice, and males display increased offensive aggressiveness.[45] The mutant mice show a marked difference from controls in supraspinal but not in spinal responses to painful stimuli.

Thus, the functional roles of individual components of the opioid system have been elucidated by analysis of knock-out mice. However, many points remain to be clarified.

Actions of Opioids on Targets Other Than Opioid Receptors

Recent progress in molecular pharmacologic analysis has shown that opioids can interact with molecules other than the opioid receptors. In cardiac myocytes, it was shown that morphine can inhibit voltage-dependent Na^+ current in a naloxone-insensitive manner, thus suggesting the existence of a signal transduction mechanism that is not dependent on the opioid receptors.[46] Meperidine is an agonist of both μ- and κ-receptors. In addition, it was demonstrated that meperidine can block voltage-dependent Na^+ channels in amphibian peripheral nerves,[47] as well as in a *Xenopus* oocyte expression system (Fig. 27-4).[48] Furthermore, meperidine exerts agonist activity at the α_{2B}-adrenoreceptor.[49] Yamakura and coworkers have shown that high concentrations of opioids, including meperidine, morphine, fentanyl, codeine, and naloxone, directly inhibit the *N*-methyl-D-aspartate (NMDA) receptor expressed in *Xenopus* oocytes.[50] Methadone is used clinically as a racemic mixture of the *l* and *d* isomers. The opioid-like activity of the racemate seems to be almost entirely due to *l*-methadone, whereas *d*-methadone acts as an NMDA antagonist.[51] The commercially available remifentanil solution Ultiva, which contains glycine, directly activates the NMDA receptor expressed in *Xenopus* oocytes.[52] Furthermore, an electrophysiologic study involving the rat spinal cord showed that remifentanil hydrochloride does not directly activate NMDA receptors, the NMDA current recorded after the application of Ultiva is related to the

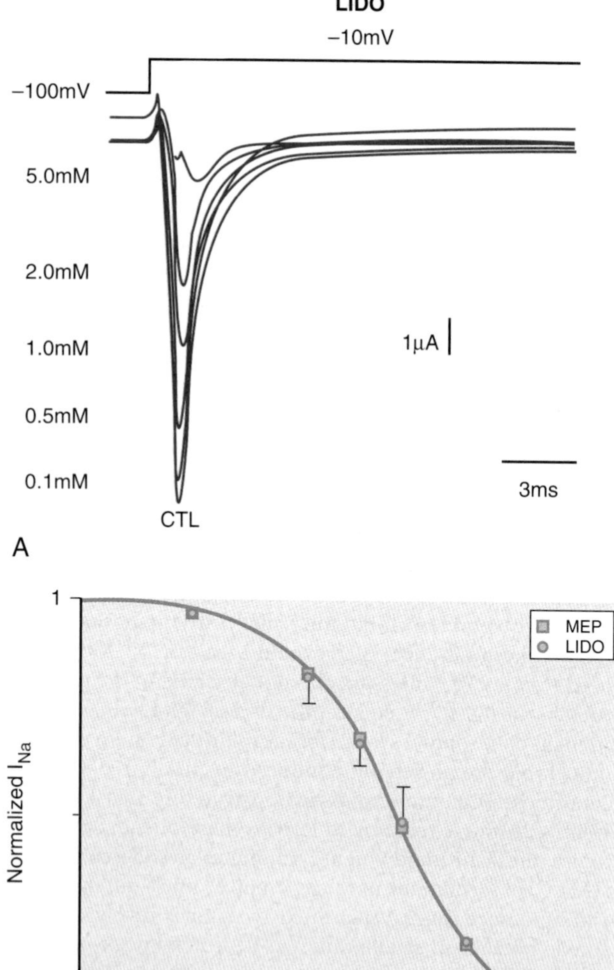

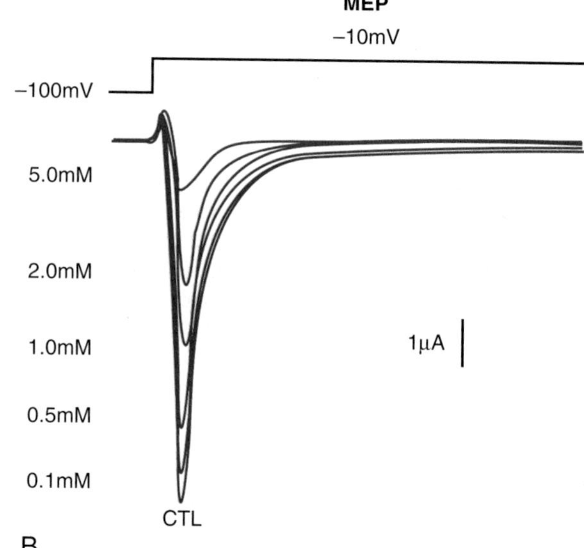

Figure 27-4 Meperidine blocks the Na^+ channels in a similar fashion as lidocaine. Na^+ currents induced by a jump in voltage were recorded from *Xenopus* oocytes expressing Na^+ channels. Lidocaine (LIDO; **A**) and meperidine (MEP; **B**) dose-dependently inhibited the current. *(From Wagner LE 2nd, Eaton M, Sabnis SS, Gingrich KJ: Meperidine and lidocaine block of recombinant voltage-dependent Na^+ channels: Evidence that meperidine is a local anesthetic. Anesthesiology 91:1481-1490, 1999.)*

presence of glycine, and the glycine-induced NMDA current is potentiated by the application of remifentanil hydrochloride through a pathway involving the μ-opioid receptor.[53] The serotonin 5-HT_{3A} receptor, which is directly and indirectly linked to gastrointestinal motility, visceral pain, nausea, and vomiting, was shown to be competitively inhibited by morphine, as well as by naloxone.[54]

Whether these actions of opioids on targets other than the opioid receptor have physiologic or clinical implications is not known.

The Role of Nociceptin/Orphanin FQ in Pain Modulation

Nociceptin/orphanin FQ is a 17–amino acid peptide, the sequence of which resembles that of opioid peptides. Nociceptin/orphanin FQ precursor mRNA and peptide are present throughout the descending pain control circuits. In the spinal cord, there is stronger nociceptin/orphanin FQ receptor mRNA expression in the ventral horn than in the dorsal horn, but higher levels of ligand binding in the dorsal horn. Targeted disruption of the nociceptin/orphanin FQ receptor in mice had little effect on basal pain sensitivity in several measures, whereas targeted disruption of the nociceptin/orphanin FQ precursor consistently elevated basal responses in the tail flick test, suggesting an important role for nociceptin/orphanin FQ in regulating basal pain sensitivity.[55,56] Intrathecal injections of nociceptin/orphanin FQ have been shown to be analgesic[57]; however, supraspinal administration has produced either hyperalgesia, antiopioid effects, or a biphasic hyperalgesic/analgesic response.[58] Nociceptin/orphanin FQ inhibits both pain-facilitating and analgesia-facilitating neurons in the RVM.[59] The effects of nociceptin/orphanin FQ on pain responses appear to depend on the preexisting state of pain in the animal. Yamamoto and Sakashita reported that intrathecal injection of nociceptin/orphanin FQ significantly attenuated the level of mechanical hyperalgesia induced by skin incision, which suggests involvement of the nociceptin/orphanin FQ receptor in maintaining postoperative pain.[57] The physiologic implications of nociceptin/orphanin FQ remain to be elucidated.

Neurophysiologic Effects of Opioids

Analgesic Action of Opioids

In human beings, morphine-like drugs produce analgesia, drowsiness, changes in mood, and mental clouding. A significant feature of opioid analgesia is that it is not associated with loss of consciousness. When morphine in the same dose is given to a normal, pain-free individual, the experience may be unpleasant. Relief of pain by morphine-like opioids is relatively selective in that other sensory modalities are not affected. Patients frequently report that the pain is still present but that they feel more comfortable. It is also important to distinguish between pain caused by stimulation of nociceptive receptors and transmitted over intact neural pathways (nociceptive pain) and pain caused by damage to neural structures, often involving neural supersensitivity (neuropathic pain). Although nociceptive pain is usually responsive to opioid analgesics, neuropathic pain typically responds poorly to opioid analgesics and may require higher doses of drug.[60] Not only is the sensation of pain altered by opioid analgesics, but the affective response is changed as well. However, alteration of the emotional reaction to painful stimuli is not the sole mechanism of analgesia.

The level of antinociception produced by an opioid is determined by the intensity of the nociceptive stimulus and the intrinsic efficacy of the opioid. When opioids are given in combination, the effects can be predicted only on the basis of the nociception experienced when the drugs are administered alone.[61] The antinociceptive effects of opioids are enhanced in animal models of inflammation. The sensitization to opioids is related to a central rather than a peripheral site of action.[62]

Animal and human studies indicate the existence of sex-related differences in opioid-mediated behavior.[63] Sarton and associates examined the influence of morphine on experimentally induced pain in healthy volunteers and demonstrated sex differences in morphine analgesia, with greater morphine potency but slower speed of onset and offset in women.[64] The mechanism of the sex difference remains to be clarified.

The analgesia produced by the peripheral actions of opioids is still a source of controversy. Recent reviews have concluded from meta-analysis that intra-articularly administered morphine has a definite, but mild analgesic effect.[65] It may be dose dependent, and a systemic effect cannot be completely excluded. The addition of opioids to brachial plexus blocks has been reported to improve the success rate and postoperative analgesia.[66,67] In contrast, the addition of sufentanil did not prolong the duration of brachial plexus blockade.[68] Because of its local anesthetic effect on peripheral nerves, meperidine was tested for intravenous regional anesthesia. However, doses of meperidine large enough to produce effective postoperative analgesia cause a significant incidence of side effects.[69]

Opiods As Anesthetics

Cortical acetylcholine originates in the basal forebrain and is essential for maintaining normal cognition and arousal. Injection of morphine into the substantia innominata or intravenous administration of morphine significantly decreased release of acetylcholine within the prefrontal cortex in the rat, which might be the neurochemical basis of opioid-induced change in consciousness.[70] Whether opioids alone are capable of producing anesthesia was a subject of debate in the past.[71] Reports of patient awareness during high-dose fentanyl anesthesia highlighted the potential for this problem (see Chapter 39). The anesthetic potential of opioids was tested by measurement of MAC.[72] Studies in rats demonstrated that opioids reduce the MAC of volatile anesthetics to a greater degree than in other animals. Interspecies differences in opioid actions are significant.[73] Fentanyl can reduce the MAC of isoflurane at skin incision in patients by at least 80%.[74] The relationship between the plasma fentanyl concentration and reduction in MAC is not linear, and there is a sub-MAC ceiling effect of fentanyl on reduction of the MAC of isoflurane. The MAC of sevoflurane was also dose-dependently reduced by fentanyl, with 3 ng/mL resulting in a 61% reduction in MAC (Fig. 27-5).[75] A ceiling effect was observed for MAC, with 6 ng/

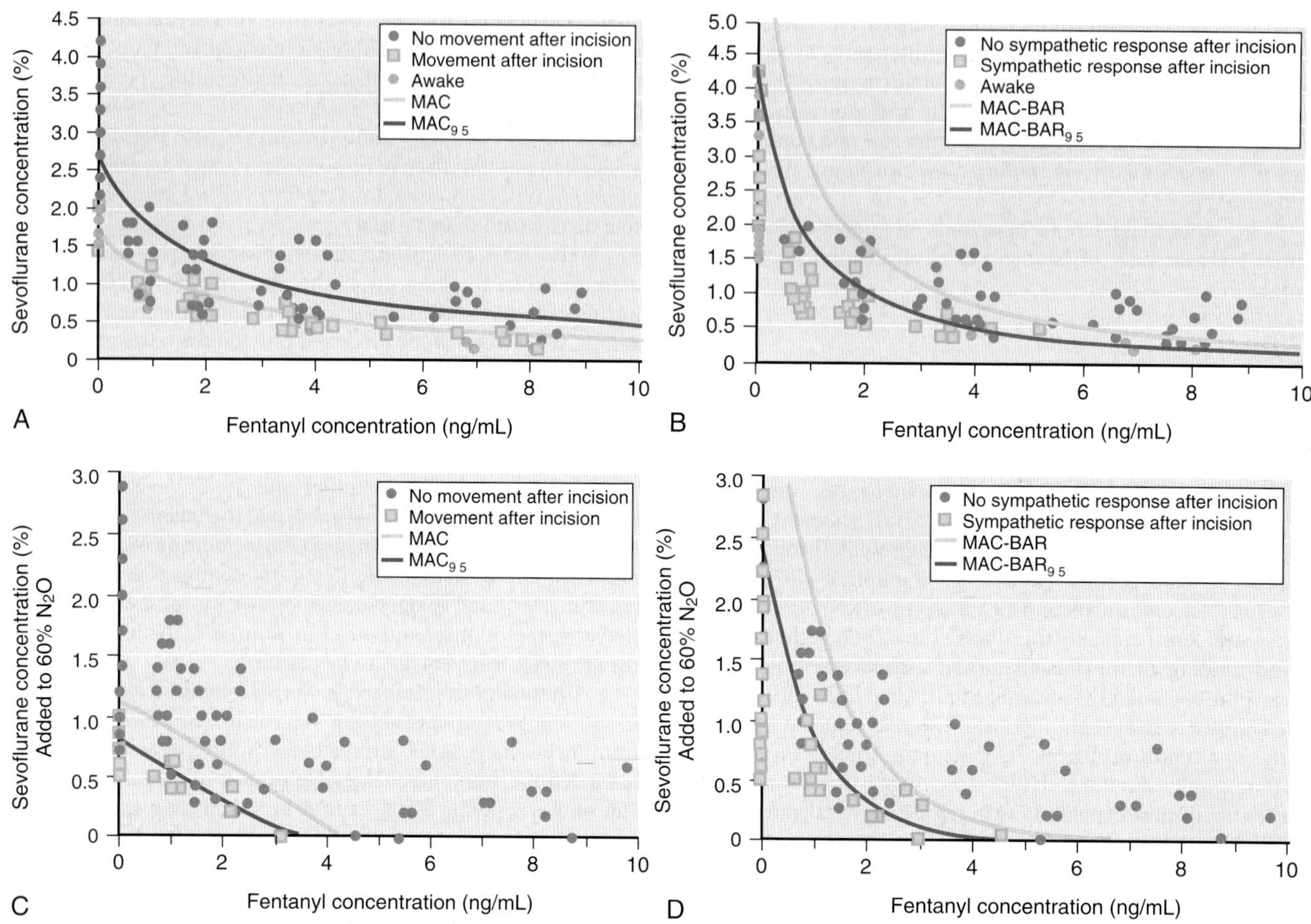

Figure 27-5 Effects of increasing concentration of fentanyl on the minimum alveolar concentration (MAC) and MAC-BAR (MAC that prevents sympathetic responses to surgical incision in 50% of patients) of sevoflurane. **A** and **C,** Reduction of the concentration of sevoflurane by increasing concentrations of fentanyl at which 50% or 95% of patients did not move at skin incision (MAC or MAC_{95}, respectively). **B** and **D,** Reduction of the concentration of sevoflurane by increasing concentrations of fentanyl at which 50% or 95% of patients did not show sympathetic responses (an increase in heart rate or mean arterial pressure >15%) at skin incision (MAC-BAR or $MAC\text{-}BAR_{95}$, respectively). Analysis was performed in the absence or presence of 60% nitrous oxide in **A** and **B** and in **C** and **D,** respectively. *(From Katoh T, Kobayashi S, Suzuki A, et al: The effect of fentanyl on sevoflurane requirements for somatic and sympathetic responses to surgical incision. Anesthesiology 90:398-405, 1999.)*

mL fentanyl providing only an additional 13% reduction in the MAC of sevoflurane. The potency ratios for fentanyl, sufentanil, alfentanil, and remifentanil, based on MAC reduction studies in humans, are approximately 1:12:0.0625:1.2.[76] Esmolol, a short-acting β_1-receptor antagonist, significantly decreased the MAC of isoflurane in the presence of alfentanil, although it did not significantly affect it in the absence of alfentanil.[77] The mechanism of the interaction is unknown. It was demonstrated that epidural fentanyl infusion reduces the awakening concentration of isoflurane more than intravenous fentanyl infusion does despite the lower plasma concentration, possibly by modulating afferent nociceptive input in the spinal cord.[78] The hypnotic effect of midazolam is also significantly enhanced by alfentanil.[79]

The MAC that prevents movement in response to laryngoscopy and tracheal intubation in 50% of patients (MAC-TI) is higher than the MAC that prevents movement in response to surgical incision (MAC). The MAC-TI of sevoflurane was 3.55% and was markedly reduced to 2.07%, 1.45%, and 1.37% by the addition of fentanyl, 1, 2, and 4 μg/kg, with no significant difference in the reduction between 2 and 4 μg/kg, thus showing a ceiling effect.[80] The MAC that prevents sympathetic responses to surgical incision in 50% of patients (MAC-BAR) decreased with increasing concentrations of fentanyl in plasma, and the initial steep reduction was followed by a ceiling effect (see Fig. 27-5).[75] In the presence of nitrous oxide, MAC and MAC-BAR decreased similarly but did not exhibit a ceiling effect.

The bispectral index (BIS) has been proposed as a measure of the effects of anesthetics on the brain (see Chapter 39). In the presence of fentanyl, alfentanil, remifentanil, or sufentanil, loss of consciousness occurred at a lower effect-site concentration of propofol and at a higher BIS value than with propofol alone.[81] This finding suggests that the hypnotic effect of propofol is enhanced by analgesic concentrations of opioids without changes in the BIS value. On the other hand, infusion of remifentanil (effect-site target concentrations of 0.25, 2.5, and 10 ng/mL), combined with propofol infusion adjusted to a BIS of approximately 60, dose-dependently decreased the BIS, thus suggesting a sedative or hypnotic effect of remifentanil.[82] Response surface analysis showed considerable synergy between opioids and hypnotics for sedation and suppression of responses to various noxious stimuli (Fig. 27-6).[83]

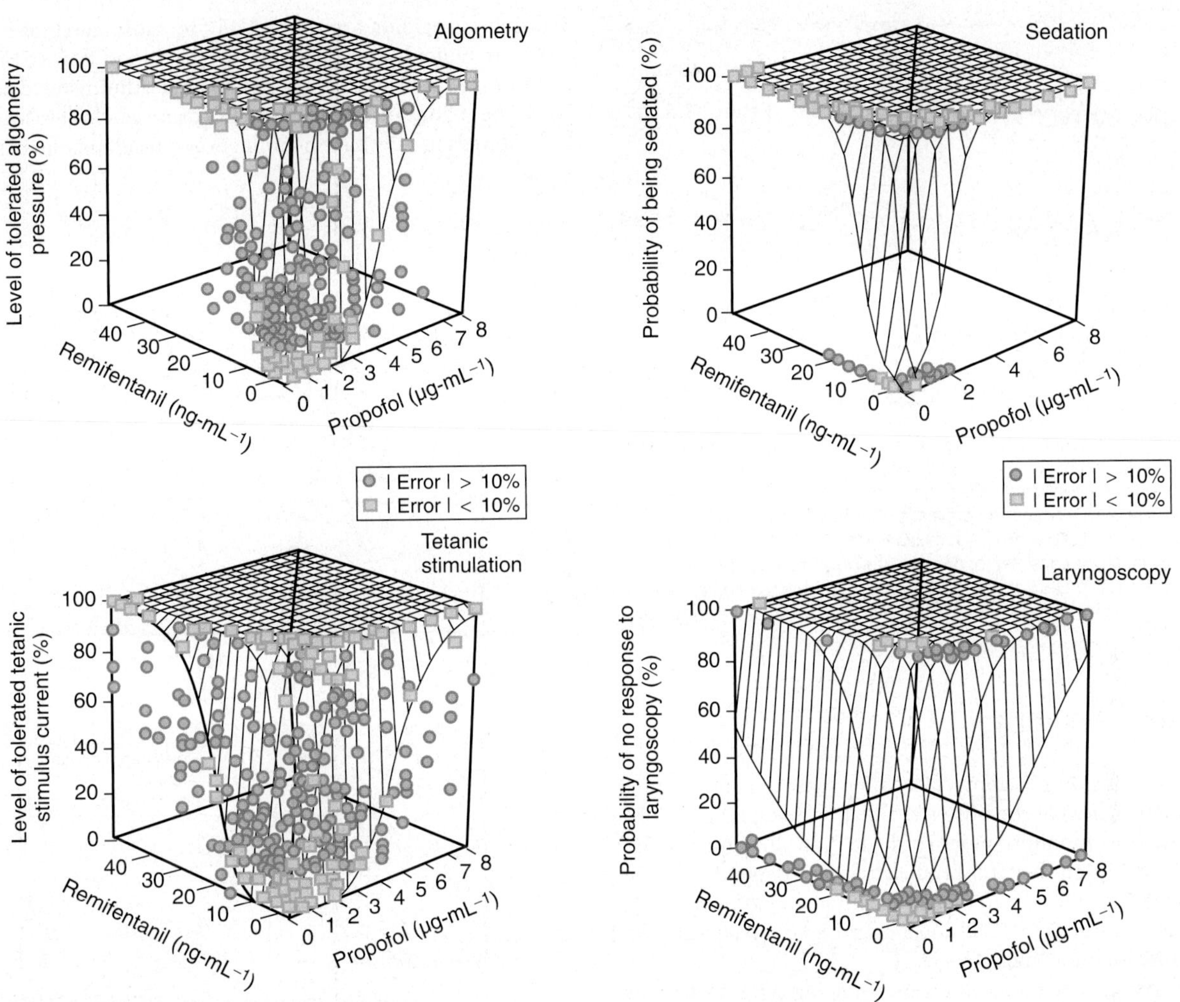

Figure 27-6 Prediction of sedation and blunting of the response to noxious stimuli, including tibial pressure algometry, electrical tetany, and laryngoscopy, by a response surface model. Sedation is indicated by an alertness/sedation score of 0 to 3 as assessed by an observer. Response to the noxious stimuli was based on whether the subjects exhibited withdrawal movement, painful verbalization, or a 20% increase in heart rate over the prestimulus level. The symbols show actual measured responses from the study subjects. *(From Kern SE, Xie G, White JL, Egan TD: A response surface analysis of propofol-remifentanil pharmacodynamic interaction in volunteers. Anesthesiology 100:1373-1381, 2004.)*

Although unconsciousness in humans can be produced with large doses of opioids alone, opioid anesthesia can be unpredictable and inconsistent.[84] Therefore, opioids are not suitable as the sole drug for intravenous induction of anesthesia.[85]

Electroencephalography

Increasing concentrations of inhaled anesthetics produce a continuum of changes on the electroencephalogram (EEG) and eventually result in burst suppression and a flat EEG. In contrast, a ceiling effect is reached with opioids. Increasing opioid dosage, when this ceiling has been attained does not further affect the EEG.[86] Problems with lead placement and signal processing need to be resolved before analysis of the EEG can be used as a routine monitor of the depth of opioid anesthesia.

Although the potency and rate of equilibrium between plasma and brain are different among opioids, the effects of fentanyl, alfentanil, sufentanil, and remifentanil are consistent (Fig. 27-7).[87] Small doses of fentanyl (200 µg) produce minimal changes on the EEG, whereas higher doses (30 to 70 µg/kg) result in high-voltage slow (δ) waves that are suggestive of a state consistent with anesthesia. Although transient isolated (usually frontotemporal) sharp wave activity can be observed after large doses of fentanyl and other opioids, it is not generalized.

As an effect-site measure, the EEG can be used to assess the onset of drug action and drug potency ratios. The spectral edge and serum concentration are closely parallel for remifentanil,[88] whereas significant time lag is found for recovery of the spectral edge for fentanyl and sufentanil (Fig. 27-8).[89] The serum concentration ratio of fentanyl and sufentanil was 12 : 1 at half-maximal slowing of the EEG.[89] Similar studies suggest that fentanyl and remifentanil are 75 and 16 times as potent as alfentanil, respectively.[88] Potency ratios based on the EEG are similar to those obtained from studies determining the plasma drug levels of each opioid necessary to reduce the MAC of isoflurane by 50%. Potency ratios of sufentanil:fentanyl:remifentanil: alfentanil for reducing the MAC of isoflurane are nearly 1 : 1/10 : 1/10 : 1/100.[74,90-92]

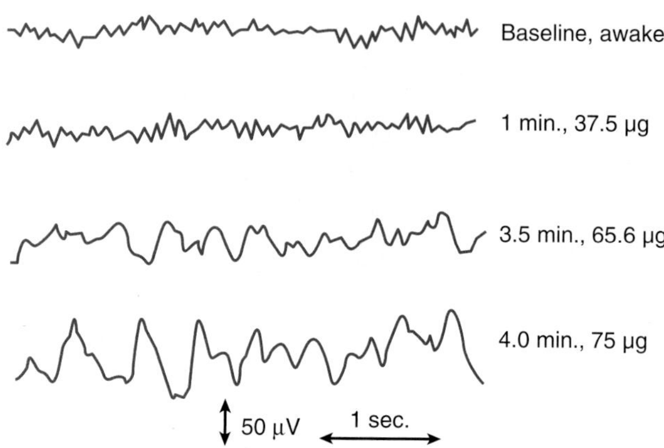

Figure 27-7 Representative 4-second tracings on the electroencephalogram (EEG) during infusion of sufentanil (total dose shown in the *right column*). The awake baseline EEG consists of mixed β and α activity. At 1 minute, the EEG showed loss of β activity and the presence of primarily α waves (8 to 13 Hz). At 3.5 minutes, the EEG consisted of mixed θ (4 to 7 Hz) and δ (<4 Hz) waves, and at 4.0 minutes, it consisted of δ waves of high amplitude. *(From Scott JC, Cooke JE, Stanski DR: Electroencephalographic quantitation of opioid effect: Comparative pharmacodynamics of fentanyl and sufentanil. Anesthesiology 74:34-42, 1991.)*

Evoked Responses

Because opioids do not appreciably alter sensory evoked potentials (SEPs) elicited at the posterior tibial or median nerve, SEPs can be used to monitor spinal cord function during anesthesia with opioids.[93] Remifentanil produced a dose-dependent reduction in auditory evoked potentials.[94] Remifentanil infusion (target plasma concentrations of 1, 2, and 3 ng/mL) did not affect evoked potential amplitudes and latencies.[95]

In healthy human volunteers receiving 3 µg/kg fentanyl, the amplitude and latency of motor evoked responses to transcranial stimulation were not significantly affected.[96] Kawaguchi and coauthors reported that intraoperative monitoring of myogenic motor evoked potentials is feasible during isoflurane or sevoflurane anesthesia with fentanyl.[97]

The middle latency auditory evoked response has been shown to change after the administration of opioids. However, it remains unclear whether these changes are due to a direct depressant effect of opioids on the middle latency auditory evoked response itself or an indirect effect because of their action in attenuating CNS arousal associated with noxious stimuli. Wright and colleagues examined the effect of remifentanil (1 or 3 µg/kg/min) on the middle latency auditory evoked response in intubated and nonintubated patients and showed that remifentanil has an effect on the middle latency auditory evoked response in attenuating the arousal associated with intubation of the trachea but has no effect in the absence of a stimulus.[98]

Cerebral Blood Flow and Cerebral Metabolic Rate

Opioids generally produce modest decreases in the cerebral metabolic rate (CMR) and intracranial pressure, although such changes are influenced by the concomitant administration of other agents and anesthetics, as well as by patient conditions (see Chapter 63). When vasodilation is produced by coadministered anesthetics, opioids are more likely to cause cerebral vasoconstriction. Opioids also decrease cerebral blood flow (CBF) when combined with N_2O. When opioids are administered alone or when the coadministered anesthetics cause cerebral vasoconstriction, opioids usually have no influence or result in a small increase in CBF.

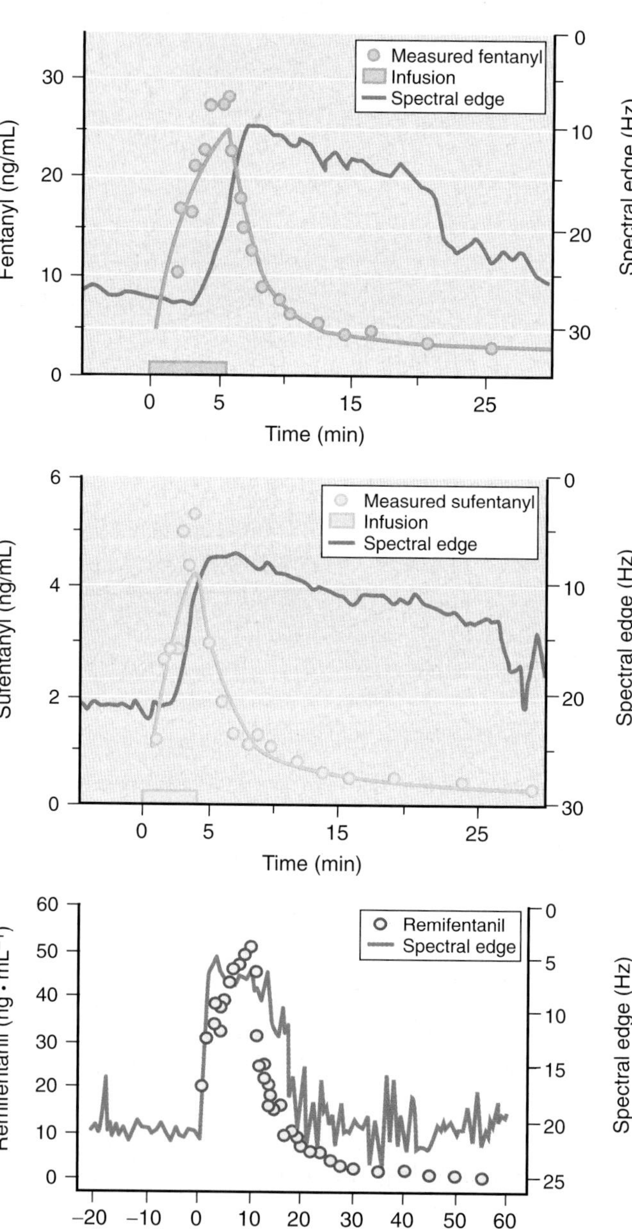

Figure 27-8 Time course of the spectral edge and serum opioid concentration. Fentanyl (*upper panel*) and sufentanil (*middle panel*) were infused at 150 and 18.75 µg/min, respectively. Remifentanil (*lower panel*) was administered at 3 µg/kg/min for 10 minutes. The spectral edge changes lag behind the changes in serum concentration in the case of fentanyl and sufentanil, whereas the spectral edge and serum concentration are closely parallel in the case of remifentanil. *(From Scott JC, Ponganis KV, Stanski DR: EEG quantitation of narcotic effect: The comparative pharmacodynamics of fentanyl and alfentanil. Anesthesiology 62:234-241, 1985; and Egan TD, Minto CF, Hermann DJ, et al: Remifentanil versus alfentanil: Comparative pharmacokinetics and pharmacodynamics in healthy adult male volunteers. Anesthesiology 84:821-833, 1996.)*

Endogenous opioid activity is present in the cerebral arteries, although exogenously administered opioids were found to exert little effect on pial artery diameter in several animal models.[99] Fentanyl (100 μg/kg) causes dose-related reductions in CBF and $CMRO_2$ in rats receiving N_2O. In the piglet, fentanyl, alfentanil, and sufentanil decrease arteriolar diameter in a dose-dependent, naloxone-reversible manner.[100] In human volunteers, PET demonstrated that the CBF changes induced by fentanyl are regionally heterogeneous.[101]

The effect of sufentanil on CBF in the dog may be dose and time dependent. It was reported that sufentanil (20 μg/kg intravenously [IV]) produces 30% to 40% decreases in CBF 5 to 10 minutes after opioid administration.[102] Another report showed that sufentanil (10 to 200 μg/kg) produces transient increases in CBF that peak 2 minutes after drug administration in the dog.[103] In humans, both fentanyl and sufentanil can increase middle cerebral artery blood flow velocity by about 25%.[104] In healthy volunteers, sufentanil (0.5 μg/kg IV) produces no significant effect on CBF.[104] Alfentanil (25 to 50 μg/kg IV), when administered to patients receiving isoflurane (0.4% to 0.6%)-N_2O anesthesia, produces minimal reductions in middle cerebral artery flow velocity.[105]

In the dog, alfentanil and remifentanil decrease regional blood flow by 40% to 50% in the cortex, hippocampus, and caudate.[106] A PET study in human volunteers showed that remifentanil induces dose-dependent changes in relative regional CBF in areas involved in pain processing, such as the lateral prefrontal cortex, inferior parietal cortex, and supplementary motor area.[107] In patients scheduled to undergo supratentorial tumor surgery and receiving N_2O, remifentanil (1 μg/kg/min), similar to fentanyl (2 μg/kg/min), reduced CBF and did not significantly affect cerebrovascular carbon dioxide reactivity.[108]

Opioids usually produce mild to moderate decreases in CMR that remain coupled to CBF. However, opioid-induced neuroexcitation and focal seizure activity can cause regional increases in brain metabolism. Regional increases in glucose utilization induced by high doses of alfentanil in the rat are associated not only with epileptiform activity but also with neuropathic lesions.[109] In humans, PET evaluation demonstrated that a 1- to 3-μg/kg/min infusion of remifentanil induces a significant increase in the CMR of glucose.[110]

Neuroprotection

Although certain early studies suggested potentially adverse effects of μ-opioid agonists on ischemic brain, other studies have documented that at least certain opioid agents, such as the κ-agonists, can be neuroprotective, at least in animal models of focal ischemia.[111,112] It was also shown that activation of δ-opioid receptors increases the survival time of mice during lethal hypoxia.[113,114] An in vitro study involving rat cerebellar brain slices demonstrated that pretreatment with morphine at clinically relevant concentrations induces acute neuroprotection mediated by activation of δ_1-opioid receptors, activation of adenosine triphosphate (ATP)-sensitive K^+ channels, and production of free radicals in mitochondria.[115] In contrast, Charchaflieh and coworkers demonstrated in the rat hippocampal slice model that fentanyl is neither neurotoxic nor protective against anoxic injury to neurons when used in concentrations comparable to those applied in clinical practice.[116] In the rat focal ischemia model, in contrast to isoflurane, fentanyl neither increased nor decreased brain injury when compared with awake unanesthetized rats.[117]

Table 27-4 Potential Problems Associated with Opioid-Induced Rigidity

System	Problem
Hemodynamic	↑CVP, ↑ PAP, ↑ PVR
Respiratory	↓ Compliance, ↓ FRC, ↓ ventilation
	Hypercapnia
	Hypoxemia
Miscellaneous	↑ Oxygen consumption
	↑ Intracranial pressure
	↑ Fentanyl plasma levels

CVP, central venous pressure; FRC, functional residual capacity; PAP, pulmonary artery pressure; PVR, pulmonary vascular resistance.
Modified from Bailey PL, Egan TD, Stanley TH: Intravenous opioid anesthetics. *In* Miller RD (ed): Anesthesia, 5th ed. New York, Churchill Livingstone, 2000, p 291.

Muscle Rigidity

Opioids can increase muscle tone and may cause muscle rigidity. The incidence of rigidity noted with opioid anesthetic techniques varies greatly because of differences in the dose and speed of opioid administration, concomitant use of N_2O, presence or absence of muscle relaxants, and patient age. Opioid-induced rigidity is characterized by increased muscle tone that sometimes progresses to severe stiffness with the potential for serious problems (Table 27-4). Clinically significant opioid-induced rigidity usually begins just as or after a patient loses consciousness. Mild manifestations of rigidity, such as hoarseness, can occur in conscious patients. It has been demonstrated that vocal cord closure is primarily responsible for the difficult ventilation with bag and mask that follows the administration of opioids. Delayed or postoperative rigidity is probably related to the second peaks that can occur in plasma opioid concentrations, similar to the recurrence of respiratory depression.

The precise mechanism by which opioids cause muscle rigidity is not clearly understood. Muscle rigidity is not due to direct action on muscle fibers because it can be decreased or prevented by pretreatment with muscle relaxants. Mechanisms of opioid-induced muscle rigidity involving the CNS have been postulated. Pharmacologic studies using selective agonists and antagonists have suggested that systemic opioid-induced muscle rigidity is primarily due to the activation of central μ-receptors, whereas supraspinal δ_1- and κ_1-receptors may attenuate this effect.[118] Some aspects of opioid-induced catatonia and rigidity (increased incidence with age, muscle movements resembling extrapyramidal side effects) are similar to Parkinson's disease and suggest similarities in neurochemical mechanisms. Parkinsonian patients, particularly if inadequately treated, may experience reactions such as dystonia after opioid administration.[119]

Pretreatment with or concomitant use of nondepolarizing muscle relaxants can decrease the incidence and severity of rigidity. Induction doses of thiopental and subanesthetic doses of diazepam and midazolam prevent, attenuate, or successfully treat rigidity. Persisting in an attempt to mask-ventilate a patient with opioid-induced rigidity will probably result in gastric insufflation and inadequate ventilation or oxygenation until a muscle relaxant is administered. To minimize the occurrence of muscle rigidity and facilitate ventilation and airway management, anesthesiologists should anticipate the need for rapid neuromuscular blockade when doses of opioids are administered that produce rigidity.

Neuroexcitatory Phenomena

Fentanyl causes seizure activity on the EEG in animals, but evidence of seizure activity after fentanyl, alfentanil, and sufentanil is generally lacking in humans. Remifentanil induces generalized tonic-clonic seizure–like activity in otherwise healthy adults.[120] Morphine produces tonic-clonic activity after epidural and intrathecal administration.[121] Focal neuroexcitation on the EEG (e.g., sharp and spike wave activity) occasionally occurs in humans after large doses of fentanyl, sufentanil, or alfentanil.

The mechanisms underlying opioid-induced neuroexcitatory phenomena are not completely clear. Excitatory opioid actions may be related to their coupling to mitogen-activated protein kinase cascades.[122] Local increases in CBF and metabolism are also of theoretical concern because prolonged seizure activity, even if focal, could lead to neuronal injury or cellular death. In large doses in rats, fentanyl, alfentanil, and sufentanil also induce hypermetabolism and histopathologic alterations in the limbic system.[123] Midazolam, naloxone, and phenytoin prevent seizure activity on the EEG and histologically evident brain damage induced by high-dose fentanyl in rats.[124]

Measurement of CBF via magnetic resonance imaging in human volunteers has indicated that the cingulate cortex is the most susceptible to activation by remifentanil (0.05 to 0.2 μg/kg/min) and that susceptibility is affected by the apolipoprotein E genotype.[125] These findings support the notion that neuroactivation of limbic areas via the perioperative use of opioids might have a role in the genesis of postoperative cognitive dysfunction.

Pupil Size

Morphine and most μ- and κ-agonists cause constriction of the pupil by an excitatory action on the parasympathetic nerve innervating the pupil. Opioids abolish cortical inhibition of the Edinger-Westphal nucleus, thereby resulting in papillary constriction. After the intravenous administration of morphine (0.125 mg/kg), there was a 26% decrease in pupil diameter at 1 hour, and longer than 6 hours was necessary for complete recovery of pupil diameter.[126] Alfentanil in a dose-dependent manner attenuates the reflex papillary dilatation that normally follows noxious stimulation in anesthetized individuals.[127] The changes in pupil size associated with opioid action may be too slight to be of clinical utility in assessing the degree of opioid effect.

Thermoregulation and Shivering

Opioid-based anesthesia probably reduces thermoregulatory thresholds to an extent similar to that of the potent inhaled agents (see Chapter 48).[128] However, meperidine is unique among opioids in its ability to effectively terminate or attenuate shivering. The antishivering effect of meperidine is primarily related to a reduction in the shivering threshold[129] and seems to be mediated by meperidine's activity on the κ-receptor.[130] However, the relatively specific κ-receptor agonist nalbuphine did not show significant antishivering activity.[131] Meperidine exerts agonist activity at the α_{2B}-adrenoreceptor subtype, suggesting possible involvement of this novel action in the antishivering action of meperidine.[49] Alfetanil, morphine, and fentanyl are not as effective as meperidine in the treatment of postoperative shivering. Tramadol (0.5 mg/kg) suppressed post–epidural anesthetic shivering in parturients as effectively as meperidine did (0.5 mg/kg),[132] but the incidence of somnolence was lower with tramadol than with meperidine.

Pruritus

Intrathecal morphine–induced itching in monkeys was suggested to be mediated by the μ-receptor.[133] Naloxone reverses opioid-induced itching, and this finding supports a receptor-mediated central mechanism for pruritus. However, opioid antagonists are not ideal therapeutic agents against pruritus because opioid analgesia is also reversed by these agents. Perhaps some mixed opioids with low to medium efficacy at both the μ- and κ-receptors, such as nalbuphine and butorphanol, are useful antipruritics because they may partially antagonize μ actions with intact κ actions to maintain analgesic function.[134,135] Recently, ondansetron has been proposed for the treatment of spinal or epidural morphine–induced pruritus.[136] Tenoxicam, a nonsteroidal anti-inflammatory drug, was reported to be effective for pruritus induced by epidural fentanyl.[137] Intravenous administration of droperidol (1.25 mg), propofol (20 mg), or alizapride (100 mg) reduced the incidence of pruritus induced by the use of morphine, 0.2 mg intrathecally, in patients undergoing cesarean section under spinal anesthesia.[138] Histamine release, once thought to underlie this phenomenon, is not causative because non–histamine-releasing opioids also produce pruritus.

Facial itching may not necessarily be a manifestation of direct opioid action at the level of the trigeminal nucleus; instead, it may be a reflection of opioid-triggered neural transmission at a distant site. It is not known why the face is prone to pruritus even after spinal opioids. Interestingly, pruritus secondary to cholestasis is ameliorated by opioid antagonists.[139]

Respiratory Effects of Opioids

The respiratory depressant actions of opioids are their most serious adverse effect. Although significant adverse events related to opioid-induced respiratory depression are presumably preventable, they persist with a perioperative incidence of approximately 0.1% to 1%, no matter what the route of administration.[140] Even though some early studies indicated both μ- and δ-opioid receptor involvement, a recent report demonstrated that activation of the μ-opioid receptor in the caudal medullary raphe region, which is important for pain regulation and respiratory modulation, inhibits the ventilatory response to hypercapnia in anesthetized rats.[141] Furthermore, administration of morphine or M6G did not produce significant respiratory depression in μ-opioid receptor knock-out mice.[142] Polymorphism of the μ-opioid receptor at nucleotide position 118, which is known to affect M6G-induced analgesia, does not significantly change susceptibility to the respiratory depressive effect of M6G.[8] This result may suggest that analgesia and respiratory depression are mediated by different signal transduction mechanisms activated by the μ-opioid receptor. In dogs, naltrindole, a highly selective antagonist of the δ-opioid receptor, can reverse the sufentanil-induced respiratory depression without significant effect on the analgesic action of sufentanil.[143]

Several studies have reported a depressant effect of morphine on respiratory mucus transport, which is one of the most important defenses against respiratory tract infections. However, morphine had no effect on the beating frequency of nasal cilia in vitro.[144]

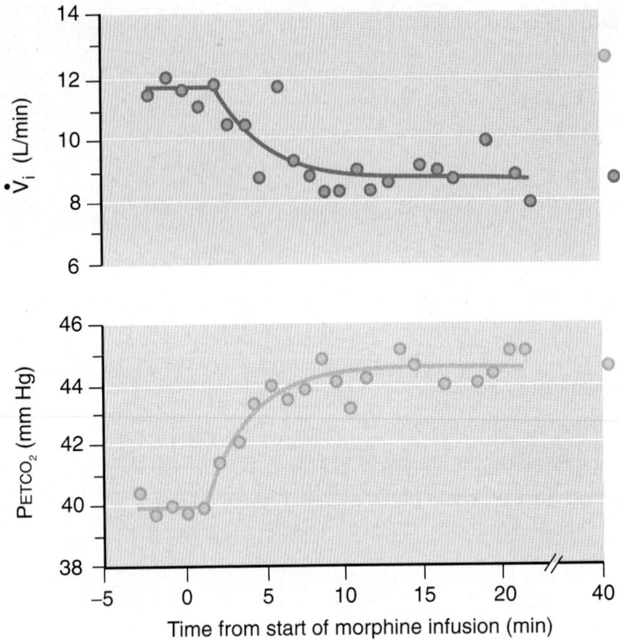

Figure 27-9 Influence of morphine administration (bolus dose of 100 μg/kg given at time t = 0 minutes, followed by a continuous infusion of 30 μg/kg/hr) on resting inspired minute ventilation and resting pressure of end-tidal CO_2 in a single subject. A one-component exponential was fitted to the data. The estimated time constant is 3.0 minutes for the V_I data and 2.6 minutes for the P_{ETCO_2} data. The time delays are between 1 and 2 minutes. *(From Sarton E, Teppema L, Dahan A: Sex differences in morphine-induced ventilatory depression reside within the peripheral chemoreflex loop. Anesthesiology 90:1329-1338, 1999.)*

Therapeutic Effects

Opioids, by decreasing pain and central ventilatory drive, are effective agents in preventing hyperventilation induced by pain or anxiety.[145,146] The lack of adequate pain relief can also cause postoperative respiratory dysfunction. Opioids can be used as postoperative analgesics to prevent respiratory dysfunction. The antitussive actions of opioids are well known and central in origin. However, fentanyl, sufentanil, and alfentanil curiously elicit a brief cough in up to 50% of patients when injected by intravenous bolus.[147] Fentanyl, administered via a peripheral intravenous cannula, provoked cough when injected rapidly, but the incidence was decreased significantly as the injection time was increased[148] or by the administration of 1.5 mg/kg lidocaine 1 minute before fentanyl administration.[149] In addition, current smokers had a lower incidence of cough than nonsmokers did, whereas heavy smokers did not.

Opioids are also excellent agents for depressing upper airway, tracheal, and lower respiratory tract reflexes, but the mechanism is not clear. Although opioids can affect the contractile responses of airway smooth muscles, the clinical significance and relevance of opioid-induced effects on airway resistance remain controversial.[150] Opioids blunt or eliminate somatic and autonomic responses to tracheal intubation. They allow patients to tolerate endotracheal tubes without coughing or "bucking." Opioids can also help avoid increases in bronchomotor tone in asthma. In addition, fentanyl has antimuscarinic, antihistaminergic, and antiserotoninergic actions and may be more effective than morphine in patients with asthma or other bronchospastic diseases.

Nontherapeutic Effects

Opioids activating the μ-receptor cause dose-dependent depression of respiration, primarily through a direct action on brainstem respiratory centers. How the various respiratory centers involved in the ventilatory drive, respiratory rhythm generation, chemoreception, and neural integration are affected by opioids is unclear.

The stimulatory effect of CO_2 on ventilation is significantly reduced by opioids. The hypercapneic response can be separated into central and peripheral components. Morphine-induced changes in the central component were equal in men and women, whereas changes in the peripheral component were larger in women.[151] In addition, the apneic threshold and resting end-tidal P_{CO_2} are increased by opioids (Fig. 27-9). Opioids also decrease the hypoxic ventilatory drive.

The respiratory rate is usually drastically slowed in opioid overdose, although a hypoxic CNS insult can counter this effect. The prolonged expiratory time in the respiratory cycle induced by opioids frequently results in greater reductions in respiratory rate than in tidal volume. Monitoring of breath intervals can sensitively detect fentanyl-induced respiratory depression and can be used as a measure of dynamic opioid effect.[152] High doses of opioids usually eliminate spontaneous respirations without necessarily producing unconsciousness. Patients receiving high doses of opioids may still be responsive to verbal command and often breathe when directed to do so.

The peak onset of respiratory depression after an analgesic dose of morphine is slower than after comparable doses of fentanyl: 30 ± 15 minutes versus 5 to 10 minutes. The respiratory depression induced by small doses of morphine usually lasts longer than after equipotent doses of fentanyl. Sufentanil (0.1 to 0.4 μg/kg) produces shorter-lasting respiratory depression and longer-lasting analgesia than fentanyl does (1.0 to 4.0 μg/kg).[153] Plasma fentanyl concentrations of 1.5 to 3.0 ng/mL are generally associated with significant decreases in CO_2 responsiveness. With higher doses of fentanyl (50 to 100 μg/kg), respiratory depression can persist for many hours. When moderately large (20 to 50 μg/kg or greater) doses of fentanyl are used, the potential need for

Box 27-2 Factors Increasing the Magnitude or Duration of Opioid-Induced Respiratory Depression

- High dose
- Sleep
- Old age
- Central nervous system depressant
  - Inhaled anesthetics, alcohol, barbiturates, benzodiazepines
- Renal insufficiency
- Hyperventilation, hypocapnia
- Respiratory acidosis
- Decreased clearance
  - Reduction of hepatic blood flow
- Secondary peaks in plasma opioid levels
  - Reuptake of opioids from muscle, lung, fat, and intestine
- Pain

postoperative mechanical ventilation should be anticipated. The effects of remifentanil, no matter what the dose, are attenuated rapidly and completely within 5 to 15 minutes after termination of its administration. In healthy humans, the median effective concentration (EC_{50}) causing depression of minute ventilation with remifentanil and alfentanil was 1.17 and 49.4 ng/mL, respectively.[154]

Although the mechanism by which pain modulates ventilatory control is unknown, daily clinical practice provides indirect evidence that pain stimulates ventilation, especially during emergence from anesthesia. Combes and colleagues demonstrated that pain relief via a nerve block in knee surgery patients who had previously been treated with morphine PCA increases the incidence of abnormal respiratory events associated with oxygen desaturation.[155]

Naloxone is standard therapy for opioid-induced respiratory depression. However, there have been reports of naloxone-resistant respiratory depression after intrathecal morphine.[156]

Factors Affecting Opioid-Induced Respiratory Depression

Many factors affect the magnitude and duration of opioid-induced respiratory depression (Box 27-2).

Older patients are more sensitive to the anesthetic and respiratory depressant effects of opioids. They experience higher plasma concentrations of opioids when administered on a weight basis. Morphine can produce greater respiratory depression on a weight basis in neonates than in adults because it easily penetrates the brain in neonates and infants with incomplete blood-brain barriers.

The respiratory depressant effects of opioids are increased or prolonged (or both) when administered with other CNS depressants, including the potent inhaled anesthetics, alcohol, barbiturates, benzodiazepines, and most of the intravenous sedatives and hypnotics.[153] Exceptions are droperidol, scopolamine, and clonidine, which do not enhance the respiratory depressant effects of fentanyl or other opioids.[157]

Although opioid action is usually dissipated by redistribution and hepatic metabolism rather than by urinary excretion, the adequacy of renal function may influence the duration of opioid activity. In renal insufficiency, the respiratory depressant properties of the morphine metabolite M6G would become evident as it accumulated. One study indicated that M6G is a somewhat weaker respiratory depressant than morphine is.[158]

Hypocapnic hyperventilation enhances and prolongs postoperative respiratory depression after fentanyl (10 and 25 μg/kg). Intraoperative hypercapnia produces the opposite effects. Possible explanations for these findings include increased brain opioid penetration (increased un-ionized fentanyl with hypocapnia) and removal (decreased CBF with hypocapnia). In patients who hyperventilate because of anxiety or pain, even small intravenous doses of opioids can result in transient apnea because of acute shifts in apneic thresholds.

Delayed or recurring respiratory depression has been reported with most opioids. Mechanisms for this phenomenon may include augmented release of fentanyl or other opioids from skeletal muscle into the systemic circulation on rewarming, shivering, motion, or any other condition that enhances muscle perfusion.

Cardiovascular Effects of Opioids

Large doses of opioids, administered as the sole or primary anesthetic, result in hemodynamic stability throughout the operative period. The choice of opioid can affect the perioperative hemodynamic profile. For example, alfentanil is less reliable than fentanyl and sufentanil in blocking increases in heart rate and blood pressure during induction of anesthesia, sternotomy, sternal spread, and aortotomy in patients with ischemic heart disease who undergo coronary artery surgery.[159]

Neurologic Mechanisms

Key areas of the brainstem that integrate cardiovascular responses and maintain cardiovascular homeostasis are the nucleus solitarius, the dorsal vagal nucleus, the nucleus ambiguus, and the parabrachial nucleus. The nucleus solitarius and parabrachial nucleus play an important role in the hemodynamic control of vasopressin secretion. Enkephalin-containing neurons and opioid receptors are distributed in these regions. Direct administration of μ-agonists into the CNS of animals most commonly, but not always, produces hypotension and bradycardia.[160] In addition, the ventrolateral PAG region, a key central site mediating opioid analgesia, affects hemodynamic control.[161] Opioids can also modulate the stress response through receptor-mediated actions on the hypothalamic-pituitary-adrenal axis. Most opioids reduce sympathetic and enhance vagal and parasympathetic tone. Patients who are intravascularly volume depleted or individuals depending on high sympathetic tone or exogenous catecholamines to maintain cardiovascular function are predisposed to hypotension after the administration of opioids.

The predominant and usual effect of opioids on the heart rate is to produce bradycardia from stimulation of the central vagal nucleus. Blockade of sympathetic actions may also play a role in opioid-induced bradycardia. Meperidine, in contrast to other opioids, rarely results in bradycardia but can cause tachycardia. Tachycardia after meperidine may be related to its structural similarity to atropine, to normeperidine, its principal metabolite, or to early manifestations of its toxic CNS effects.

Cardiac Mechanisms

The direct cardiac actions of opioids, in particular, the effects on myocardial contractile mechanisms, are significantly less than those of many other intravenous and inhaled anesthetics. However, opioid receptors have been demonstrated in the cardiac myocytes of several species.

Contractility

Some investigators suggest that opioids produce direct positive inotropic effects on the heart.[162] However, others report negative inotropic actions with some agents (meperidine) and no direct effects with others (morphine).[163] Some investigators suggest that local anesthetic–like effects and not receptor-related opioid actions mediate some of the negative inotropic effects of opioids, especially with high drug concentrations.

Morphine decreases Ca^{2+} transients but not cardiac contraction and enhances myofilament Ca^{2+} sensitivity through action on the δ_1-opioid receptor expressed in the heart.[164] In rabbit ventricular myocytes, morphine prolongs the action potential duration by increasing the L-type Ca^{2+} current, an effect mediated by δ- and κ-opioid receptors, and hyperpolarizes cardiac resting membrane potential by increasing the inwardly rectifying K^+ current, which is not mediated by opioid receptors.[165] On the other hand, it was demonstrated that morphine decreases the isometric force of contraction in atrial muscles from nonfailing and failing human hearts through a naloxone-insensitive mechanism.[166] Fentanyl produces little or no change in myocardial contractility.[167] Usually, most hemodynamic variables remain unchanged after large doses of fentanyl. However, fentanyl has positive inotropic effects. Possible mechanisms of the dose-dependent positive inotropic effects of fentanyl, as well as sufentanil, include release of catecholamines or direct myocardial adrenergic activation. Alfentanil, at concentrations achieved in clinical practice, increases contraction in ventricular cells by a mechanism involving an increase in the sensitivity of the contractile apparatus to Ca^{2+}.[168] The negative inotropic effect of tumor necrosis factor-α (TNF-α) and interleukin-1β (IL-1β) on ventricular myocytes caused by disruption of sarcoplasmic reticulum Ca^{2+} handling and the Ca^{2+} transient was ameliorated by alfentanil, but this response may not be mediated by opioid receptors.[169] Studies in dogs have demonstrated little change in hemodynamics with moderate doses (160 μg/kg) of alfentanil and transient cardiac stimulation (increases in left ventricular contractility, aortic blood flow velocity, and acceleration) with very large doses (5 mg/kg). In dogs, remifentanil produces hemodynamic effects that include decreases in contractility and cardiac output, as well as reductions in heart rate and blood pressure.[170]

Heart Rate and Rhythm

Opioid-induced bradycardia is primarily mediated by the CNS. Opioids have direct effects on cardiac pacemaker cells. Alfentanil significantly decreased the frequency of contractions of the right atrial–sinoatrial node in a dose-related manner in isolated cardiac tissue from young adult rabbits.[162] Premedication with or concomitant administration of β-adrenergic or Ca^{2+} channel entry blockers can exacerbate the bradycardia and may result in asystole after the administration of opioids. Periods of asystole, 10 to 12 seconds in duration, may resolve on their own, but they usually respond to atropine (0.4 to 0.8 mg IV).

Cardiac Conduction

Fentanyl may depress cardiac conduction by a mechanism mediated by direct membrane actions as opposed to opioid receptor interactions.[171] During induction of anesthesia in patients undergoing coronary artery bypass graft surgery, the QT interval increased significantly after the injection of fentanyl.[172] In contrast, both sufentanil and alfentanil have been demonstrated to be devoid of electrophysiologic effects on the normal or accessory pathways in patients with Wolff-Parkinson-White syndrome.[173,174] Clinically, cardiac conduction disturbances attributable to opioids are rare, but they may be more likely to occur in the presence of Ca^{2+} channel entry or β-adrenergic blockers.

The overall effect of opioid anesthesia is antiarrhythmogenic.[175] It was reported that naloxone, morphine, and levorphanol protected against arrhythmia induced by coronary artery occlusion in rats.[176] A direct effect on ionic currents in cardiac muscle was suggested as the mechanism of the antiarrhythmogenic activity of opioids. It was also reported that opioid antagonists are more antiarrhythmogenic than agonists in rats.[177] Some of the electrophysiologic actions of opioids resemble those of class III antiarrhythmogenic drugs.

Ischemia

Determining the effects and consequences of opioid action on myocardial ischemia is complex because the results can depend on such factors as the species studied and experimental design. Opioids can mimic ischemic preconditioning. Stimulation of the opioid receptor results in a reduction in infarct size similar to that produced by ischemic preconditioning (Fig. 27-10).[178] Although the preconditioning effect of opioids is mediated mainly by cardiac κ- and δ-opioid receptors,[179] part of the protective effect of remifentanil may be produced by μ-agonist activity outside the heart.[180] Late preconditioning, in which cardioprotective effects can be observed 24 hours after drug administration, can also be produced by morphine-induced activation of the opioid receptor in rat hearts.[181] Remote preconditioning by brief ischemia in other distant organs, such as the intestine, kidney and limb, likewise provides cardioprotection that is as effective as classic ischemic preconditioning. The myocardial κ-opioid receptors were demonstrated to mediate cardioprotection by remote preconditioning.[182] Volatile anesthetics may also be capable of protecting against ischemic injury when administered solely on reperfusion. This anesthetic-induced postconditioning can be enhanced by morphine through the activation of phosphatidyl-3-kinase and opioid receptors.[183]

Stimulation of the δ_1-opioid receptor generates oxygen radicals via mitochondrial ATP-sensitive K^+ channels and thereby results in attenuation of oxidant stress and cell death in cardiomyocytes.[184] Involvement of the adenosine A_1 receptor and protein kinase C in the cardioprotective effect of opioids was also suggested.[185,186] Whether the experimental results showing protective effects of opioid against myocardial ischemia will translate into reductions in morbidity and mortality in patients with coronary

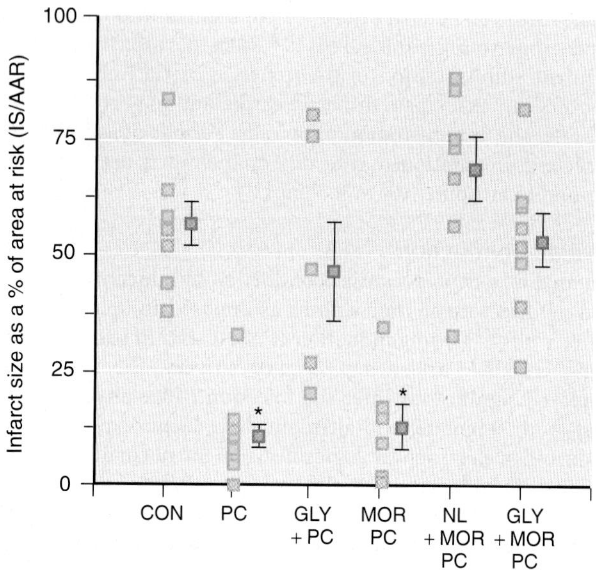

Figure 27-10 Infarct sizes in rat hearts subjected to control conditions (CON), ischemic preconditioning (PC), glibenclamide (0.3 mg/kg intravenously) given 30 minutes before ischemic PC (GLY + PC), morphine-induced PC (3 × 100 μg/kg, 5-minute intravenous infusion) (MOR PC), naloxone (3 mg/kg intravenously) given 10 minutes before morphine-induced PC (NL + MOR PC), and glibenclamide (0.3 mg/kg intravenously) given 30 minutes before morphine-induced PC (GLY + MOR PC). *(From Schultz JE, Hsu AK, Gross GJ: Morphine mimics the cardioprotective effect of ischemic preconditioning via a glibenclamide-sensitive mechanism in the rat heart. Circ Res 78:1100-1104, 1996.)*

artery disease has yet to be established in clinical trials.[187] Clinically, high doses of opioids can maintain myocardial perfusion and the O_2 supply-demand ratio as well as or better than inhalation-based techniques can.[188,189]

Coronary Circulation

Opioids appear to have no significant effect on coronary vasomotion or myocardial metabolism, do not produce steal phenomena, and do not diminish the ability of large coronary arterioles to respond to vasoactive agents.[190] Coronary conductance is regulated by arterial baroreflex control, and a vasodilator response is induced by a rise in aortic pressure. This baroreflex control is enhanced by low plasma concentrations of fentanyl (1 to 2 ng/mL) but appears to be depressed with increasing plasma concentrations of fentanyl.[191] In a study of the effects of opioids and neuroendocrine modulators on porcine coronary arteries, fentanyl, but not sufentanil or morphine, antagonized acetylcholine-induced contractions.[192] The effect of fentanyl was not reversible by naloxone and thus was thought to represent a direct smooth muscle effect.

Circulatory Reflexes

In an experiment examining baroreceptor reflex responses induced by perfusion of the carotid sinus at predetermined levels, baroreceptor reflexes were well preserved with moderate doses of fentanyl, whereas high doses of fentanyl depressed the baroreceptor reflexes.[193] The oculocardiac reflex, which is caused by traction on the extraocular muscles during strabismus surgery, was significantly augmented by fentanyl, sufentanil, and remifentanil.[194] In pediatric patients undergoing strabismus surgery and anesthetized with propofol (12 mg/kg/hr) and alfentanil (0.04 mg/kg/hr), an oculocardiac reflex developed in virtually all patients, and atrioventricular rhythm disorders were frequent.[195]

Histamine Release

Morphine causes release of histamine and sympathoadrenal activation. Codeine and meperidine induce mast cell activation with the release of histamine, probably by a mechanism other than the μ-opioid receptors.[196]

Increases in plasma histamine after morphine cause dilatation of terminal arterioles and direct positive cardiac chronotropic and inotropic actions. The cardiovascular changes after morphine are similar when patients are pretreated with diphenhydramine (histamine H_1-antagonist) or cimetidine (histamine H_2-antagonist). However, in patients pretreated with both H_1- and H_2-antagonists, cardiovascular responses were significantly attenuated despite comparable increases in plasma histamine concentration. Meperidine also causes histamine release more frequently than most other opioids do. Unlike morphine or meperidine, fentanyl, alfentanil, and remifentanil do not produce increases in plasma histamine, and hypotension is less frequent with these opioids.

Vascular Mechanisms

A new pharmacologically defined opioid receptor subtype, designated μ_3, is opiate alkaloid sensitive and opioid peptide insensitive, including peptides previously shown to have affinity for μ-opioid receptors. This receptor is expressed in human endothelial cells and is coupled to vasodilation via production of nitric oxide. Morphine-induced vasodilation may be caused in part by activation of the μ_3-receptor.[197] Pharmacologic studies evaluating alfentanil, fentanyl, and sufentanil in the dog have demonstrated direct peripheral vessel smooth muscle relaxation.[198] Measurement of forearm blood flow after infusion of sufentanil into the brachial artery indicated that sufentanil has a direct vasodilatory effect on human vascular tissue that is probably independent of a neurogenic or systemic mechanism.[199] A supraclinical dose of alfentanil attenuates the phenylephrine-induced contraction via an inhibitory effect on calcium influx by blocking the L-type calcium channels in the rat aortic vascular smooth muscle.[200] Remifentanil can cause transient instability in hemodynamic variables. However, this change may not solely be the result of autonomic or CNS inhibition or centrally mediated vagal stimulation. A pharmacologic study using rat thoracic aortic rings indicated that remifentanil vasodilates by an endothelium-dependent mechanism involving release of prostacyclin and nitric oxide from the endothelium, as well as by an endothelium-independent mechanism probably mediated by suppression of voltage-sensitive Ca^{2+} channels.[201]

Opioids may affect the pulmonary vasculature, as well as the systemic circulation. It was recently shown that phenylephrine-induced contraction of the canine pulmonary artery is mediated primarily by activation of the α_{1B}-adrenergic receptor and is attenuated by fentanyl binding to and directly inhibiting the α_{1B}-adrenergic receptor.[202] Pharmacologic studies in cats have demonstrated that sufentanil and remifentanil have potent vasodepressor activity in the pulmonary vascular bed and that these responses may be mediated by the histamine and opioid receptor–sensitive pathway.[203,204]

Activation of the muscarinic acetylcholine receptors expressed on endothelial cells results in the activation of nitric oxide synthase and release of nitric oxide, which relaxes vascular smooth muscle by activation of 3,5-cyclic guanosine monophosphate. It was shown that fentanyl attenuates acetylcholine-induced relaxation of rat aorta precontracted with phenylephrine via an inhibitory effect at a level proximal to activation of nitric oxide synthase on the pathway involving endothelial M_3 muscarinic receptor activation.[205]

Endocrinologic Effects of Opioids

The main components of the neuroendocrine stress response are the corticotropin-releasing hormone brain centers (e.g., the paraventricular hypothalamic nucleus) and the locus ceruleus–norepinephrine/autonomic nervous system.[206] Increased levels of stress hormones are considered undesirable because they promote hemodynamic instability and intraoperative and postoperative metabolic catabolism. In some circumstances, the hormonal and metabolic responses to surgery are extreme and thought to contribute to operative mortality.[207]

Opioids are capable of reducing the stress response by modulating nociception at several different levels of the neuraxis, as well as by influencing centrally mediated neuroendocrine responses. Opioids are potent inhibitors of the pituitary-adrenal axis.[208] Endogenous opioid peptides may serve as stress hormones themselves and not just as modulators of the secretion of other hormones. This activity is suggested by the finding that β-endorphin and adrenocorticotropic hormone (ACTH) are derived from the same precursor proopiomelanocortin and cosecreted during stress.

Morphine modifies hormonal responses to surgical trauma in a dose-related fashion. Morphine can prevent the release of ACTH, suppress surgically induced increases in plasma cortisol, and attenuate the pituitary-adrenal response to surgical stress. Morphine can increase some stress-responding hormones by increasing plasma histamine release, adrenal medullary release mechanisms, and release of catecholamine from sympathetic nerve endings.

Fentanyl and its congeners are more effective than morphine in modifying hormonal responses to surgery. The efficacy of fentanyl in controlling the hormonal manifestations of the stress response can be dose dependent. Fentanyl doses of 50 μg/kg or greater can help reduce the hyperglycemic response to cardiac surgery in pediatric patients to less than 200 mg/dL throughout surgery.[209] In contrast, neither fentanyl nor sufentanil alone can completely block the sympathetic and hormonal stress responses, and perhaps no dose-response relationship exists for opioid-associated control of the stress response.[71] The stress response to cardiopulmonary bypass (CPB) is difficult to suppress with sufentanil or fentanyl. Alfentanil can suppress increases in plasma cortisol and catecholamines before but not during CPB and may prevent increases in antidiuretic hormone (ADH) and growth hormone throughout coronary artery bypass surgery. A randomized controlled trial showed that remifentanil (0.85 μg/kg/min), when compared with fentanyl (total doses of 15 and 28 μg/kg), blunts the hypertensive responses and cortisol excretion associated with cardiac surgery but is associated with more hypotension.[210]

Stress Reduction and Outcome

Anesthetic techniques or drugs that minimize the stress response may reduce morbidity and mortality in a variety of circumstances. Sufentanil appears to be the most likely opioid to modify stress responses and outcome successfully.[211,212] Anand and Hickey[211] evaluated the impact of sufentanil versus morphine-halothane anesthesia on hormonal and metabolic responses and morbidity and mortality in neonates undergoing cardiac surgery. Most strikingly, a statistically significant difference in postoperative mortality was observed (0 of 30 given sufentanil versus 4 of 15 given halothane plus morphine). Mangano and coauthors[212] also reported that after myocardial revascularization, patients receiving intense postoperative analgesia with sufentanil (1 μg/kg/hr) experience a lower incidence and severity of electrocardiographically documented ischemia than do patients receiving intermittent intravenous morphine (2.2 ± 2.1 mg/hr) for postoperative analgesia. It was also shown that high-dose opioids (remifentanil, 0.85 μg/kg/min, or fentanyl, 28 μg/kg) are associated with a decreased rate of myocardial infarction after cardiac surgery.[210]

Many different hormonal changes induced by surgery have been described. However, the concomitant neural, cellular, immune, and biochemical changes have been less well defined, and little is understood or proven with regard to how modifying hormonal responses alters outcome.[213] Additional studies are necessary for complete elucidation of the relationship between control of surgically induced hormonal responses and outcome.

Opiate Tolerance and Addiction

The mechanisms of dependence and tolerance involve genetic, molecular, cellular, physiologic, and functional factors. In the locus ceruleus, the major noradrenergic nucleus in the brain, long-term opioid exposure results in inhibition of adenylyl cyclase, reduced activity of protein kinase A, and upregulation of the cyclic AMP pathway.[214] The changes in μ-receptor density that occur before or during the development of tolerance do not appear to be essential for the development of opioid tolerance.[215] Possible mechanisms involve protein kinase signal transduction cascades that link extracellular signals to cellular changes by regulating target gene expression. Central glucocorticoid receptors (GRs) have been implicated in the cellular mechanism of neuronal plasticity, which has many cellular steps in common with the mechanism of opioid tolerance. It was shown that the development of tolerance to the antinociceptive effect of morphine was substantially attenuated when a GR antagonist was coadministered with morphine but that the GR agonist dexamethasone facilitated the development of morphine tolerance, suggesting an important role of spinal GRs in the cellular mechanisms of morphine tolerance in rats.[216] Morphine tolerance occurs more rapidly in younger rats than in older rats and is unlikely to be the result of differences in drug metabolism or clearance, an observation suggesting that aging may have an impact on the molecular processes involved in the development of tolerance.[217]

Acute administration of opioids results in analgesia and side effects, whereas tolerance and dependence were thought to occur only after chronic administration. However, tolerance can also develop rapidly after acute opioid exposure in animals and humans.[218-220] Intraoperative remifentanil infusion (0.3 μg/kg/

min) in patients undergoing major abdominal surgery under desflurane anesthesia increased postoperative pain and morphine requirements when compared with low-dose remifentanil (0.1 μg/kg/min), suggesting the development of acute remifentanil tolerance.[221] In contrast, there is a report that target-controlled infusion of alfentanil and remifentanil for postoperative analgesia does not lead to opioid tolerance.[222] In human volunteers, continuous infusion of remifentanil (0.08 μg/kg/min) for 3 hours did not decrease the pain threshold.[223] Thus, the development of acute opioid tolerance in humans remains controversial. Opioids can elicit hyperalgesia in experimental models after repeated opioid administration or continuous delivery.[224] This phenomenon seems to be related to opioid tolerance.[225] In rats, thermal hyperalgesia and mechanical allodynia were observed for several days after cessation of morphine administration (40 mg/kg/day for 6 days).[226] The opioid-induced hyperalgesia is due to spinal sensitization to glutamate and substance P.[227] Furthermore, cholecystokinin and the NMDA–nitric oxide system are responsible for the development of acute tolerance to opioids,[228] which is also affected by spinal serotonin activity.[229] Opioid-induced hyperalgesia and subsequent acute opioid tolerance can be prevented by ketamine, suggesting involvement of the NMDA receptor.[230,231] Methadone is unique in possessing both μ-opioid and NMDA antagonist properties. Opioid-induced hyperalgesia resulted from the presence of *l*-methadone (μ-opioid agonist) in the racemate and was antagonized by the presence of *d*-methadone (NMDA antagonist).[232] Spinal cyclooxygenase-2 (COX-2) is upregulated and release of prostaglandin E_2 in the spinal cord is increased after morphine withdrawal in rats.[233] In humans, hyperalgesia after a 30-minute intravenous infusion of remifentanil (0.1 μg/kg/min) could be prevented by the administration of parecoxib, a COX-2 inhibitor, before the infusion of remifentanil,[234] findings suggesting involvement of COX-2 in opioid-induced hyperalgesia. Genetic analysis in mice suggested that genetic variants of the β_2-adrenergic receptor gene seem to explain some of the differences between various strains of mice in the development of opioid-induced hyperalgesia, and the selective β_2-adrenergic receptor antagonist butoxamine was shown to dose-dependently reverse opioid-induced hyperalgesia.[235] Human data generally support the existence of opioid-induced hyperalgesia in a few specific settings. The conditions under which opioid-induced hyperalgesia is expressed should be clarified and its clinical significance elucidated.[236]

The peripheral effects of morphine have been suggested to be less prone to tolerance.[237] Thus, the method and schedule of drug administration may also affect the development of tolerance.[238] However, modifying an opioid administration schedule to modulate the development of tolerance may not always be useful or effective.[239] Certain patients may appear to be tolerant to opioids but instead suffer from pathophysiologic conditions that are poorly responsive to opioids, such as neuropathies.[240]

Management of Opioid-Dependent Patients

A variety of problems should be taken into consideration in the anesthetic management of opioid-dependent patients.[241] Complications in opioid-addicted patients include cardiopulmonary problems, renal problems, and anemia. Long-term morphine administration causes adrenal hypertrophy and impairs corticosteroid secretion. Viral and nonviral hepatitis, acquired immunodeficiency syndrome, osteomyelitis, muscle weakness, and neurologic complications may be found in addicted patients. Anesthetic management of an opiate-dependent or opiate-addicted patient should include adequate premedication with opioids, administration of supplemental intraoperative and postoperative opioids, and provision of nonopioid analgesics and neural blockade. There is no ideal anesthetic approach for a chronic addict or a patient with an acute opiate overdose. Support of the circulatory system with fluids and monitoring of arterial blood gases and pulmonary function are also important.

Recently, rapid detoxification with a high dose of naloxone or naltrexone has been reported for the treatment of opioid addiction. For such treatment, general anesthesia is induced before the start of opioid antagonism and maintained for several hours to prevent the perception of withdrawal symptoms by the patient.[242,243] Blockade of μ-opioid receptors by naloxone (total dose of 12.4 mg) in opioid-addicted patients induces sympathetic neural activation, including an increase in plasma catecholamine concentration and cardiovascular stimulation, which is abolished by α_2-agonists.[244]

Renal and Urodynamic Effects of Opioids

μ-Receptor activation causes antidiuresis and decreases electrolyte excretion. κ-Receptor stimulation predominantly produces diuresis with little change in electrolyte excretion. The stable dynorphin analog E-2078 causes κ-mediated diuretic effects in the isolated perfused rat kidney.[245] Indirect actions may involve inhibiting or altering the secretion of ADH and atrial natriuretic peptide.[246] The absence of increases in plasma ADH, renin, and aldosterone indicates that fentanyl, sufentanil, alfentanil, and probably remifentanil most likely preserve or minimally alter renal function in humans. If renal function does change during opioid anesthesia and surgery, it is probably due to secondary changes in systemic and renal hemodynamics.

The mechanism by which opioids cause urinary retention is incompletely understood. Effects of opioids on the lower urinary tract include disturbances in micturition characterized by urinary retention, especially after intrathecal opioid administration. Intrathecal administration of morphine and sufentanil caused dose-dependent suppression of detrusor contractility and decreased sensation of urge.[247] Mean times to recovery of normal lower urinary tract function were 5 and 8 hours after 10 and 30 μg sufentanil and 14 and 20 hours after 0.1 and 0.3 mg morphine, respectively. Not all opioid agonists behave similarly, and morphine appears to be particularly potent with regard to producing urodynamic problems. Malinovsky and associates compared the urodynamic effects of intravenously administered morphine (10 mg), buprenorphine (0.3 mg), fentanyl (0.35 mg), and nalbuphine (20 mg).[248] All of the opioids altered bladder sensation, but detrusor contraction decreased only after the administration of fentanyl and buprenorphine. Urinary retention induced by intravenous infusion of remifentanil, 0.15 μg/kg/min, could be reversed by a single intravenous dose of methylnaltrexone, 0.3 mg/kg, or naloxone, 0.01 mg/kg.[249] Reversal of urinary retention by methylnaltrexone indicates that peripheral mechanisms may play a role in opioid-induced bladder dysfunction.

Gastrointestinal Effects of Opioids

Opioids decrease gastrointestinal motility,[250] and this action underlies their use as antidiarrheal agents. Patients receiving parenteral opioid therapy preoperatively are more likely to have "full stomachs" regardless of their "NPO" status.

Several opioid receptor types can be demonstrated on myenteric neurons, and both κ- and μ-receptor agonists regulate cholinergic transmission in the myenteric plexus. κ-Agonists appear to modulate release of acetylcholine more potently than μ-agonists do by inhibition of N-type voltage-sensitive Ca^{2+} channels via a pertussis toxin–sensitive G protein in guinea pig ileum.[251]

The effect of morphine on esophageal motility has not been explored very extensively. Morphine (80 μg/kg) increased the velocity but did not alter the amplitude or duration of primary peristalsis of the esophagus, and it decreased the duration and magnitude of swallow-induced relaxation of the lower esophageal sphincter.[252] Gastric emptying is delayed by opioids via supraspinal (vagus nerve–mediated) and spinal as well as peripheral mechanisms. Intrathecal morphine (0.4 mg) significantly decreased gastroduodenal propagation velocity and acetaminophen absorption, and intramuscular morphine (4 mg) resulted in additional effects.[253] Tramadol (1.25 mg/kg IV) has a measurable but smaller inhibitory effect on gastric emptying than codeine (1 mg/kg IV) and morphine (0.125 mg/kg IV) do.[254] Opioids administered epidurally as well as intrathecally reduce gastrointestinal motility.[255,256] It was reported that translocation of enteric microorganisms from the intestinal tract to extraintestinal sites is promoted by reduction of gut propulsion after morphine treatment in rats.[257] Propofol (0.3- mg/kg bolus and 1.0 mg/kg/hr) abolished the decrease in gastric tone induced by morphine (0.1 mg/kg IV) but did not abolish morphine-induced delay of gastric emptying.[258]

Naloxone reverses opioid-induced delays in gastric emptying. Methylnaltrexone, a quaternary naloxone derivative that does not cross the blood-brain barrier, can attenuate morphine-induced delays in gastric emptying, thus suggesting that a peripheral mechanism is involved in the opioid effect on the gastrointestinal tract.[250] Naloxone (0.7 mg/kg) significantly inhibited gastric emptying of saline and milk in rats.[259] This observation might suggest that opioids can affect the gastrointestinal tract by a mechanism independent of the opioid receptors. Intravenous, but not intramuscular metoclopramide (10 mg) can also reverse morphine-induced delays in gastric emptying.[260]

Opioid effects on the intestine are complex. Transit time from the mouth to the ileum may not be significantly altered by morphine because morphine enhances ileal propulsion before decreasing motility. Opioids increase tone and decrease propulsive activity in most of the intestine. In rats, pretreatment with epidural or intraperitoneal morphine can attenuate ischemia-induced inhibition of bowel motility.[261]

Biliary and Hepatic Effects

Opioid agonists increase biliary duct pressure and sphincter of Oddi (choledochoduodenal sphincter) tone in a dose- and drug-dependent manner through opioid receptor–mediated mechanisms. However, the clinical consequences of opioid-induced biliary tract actions are usually minimal. Although traditional teaching dictates that morphine induces "spasm" in the sphincter of Oddi and should not be used in patients with acute pancreatitis, no studies or evidence exists to indicate that morphine is contraindicated for use in acute pancreatitis.[262] Increases in biliary pressure caused by opioids are, with the exception of meperidine, reversible with naloxone. Oddi sphincter manometry via choledochoscopy demonstrated that the regular dose of morphine could increase common bile duct pressure, whereas pethidine had no effect and tramadol inhibited motility of the sphincter of Oddi.[263] Fragen and colleagues studied the effect of remifentanil (0.1 μg/kg/min) on the flow of dye from the gallbladder into the duodenum and showed that remifentanil delays the drainage of dye from the gallbladder into the duodenum but the delay is shorter than that reported after morphine or meperidine.[264] Opioids produce minimal effects on liver function during anesthesia and surgery.

Nausea and Vomiting

Postoperative nausea/vomiting is a serious problem that often embarrasses patients and anesthesiologists (also see Chapter 86).[265,266] The cause, treatment, and prevention of postoperative nausea and vomiting have been investigated extensively (Fig. 27-11).[267] Intraoperative use of opioids is a well-known risk factor for postoperative nausea and vomiting. Opioids stimulate the chemoreceptor trigger zone in the area postrema of the medulla, possibly through δ-receptors, and thereby lead to nausea and vomiting. When compared with approximately equipotent doses of fentanyl and sufentanil, alfentanil is associated with a lower incidence of postoperative nausea and vomiting.[268]

The use of propofol in balanced or total intravenous anesthesia (TIVA) significantly reduces the incidence of opioid-induced nausea and vomiting.[269] The incidence of postoperative nausea and vomiting can be as low as 5% to 20% after propofol-alfentanil anesthesia.

When opioids are administered, antiemetic prophylaxis should be considered, including drugs with anticholinergic activity, butyrophenones, dopamine antagonists, serotonin antagonists, and acupressure. Ondansetron, a serotonin type 3 receptor antagonist, was found to be effective for postoperative opioid-induced nausea and vomiting.[270] Nausea and vomiting after epidural morphine (3 mg) for post–cesarean section analgesia could be prevented by dexamethasone (8 mg IV) as efficiently as droperidol (1.25 mg IV).[271] Cannabinoid receptor agonists have been demonstrated to be effective antiemetics in some clinical settings. Animal experiments have shown that the cannabinoid agonist suppresses opioid-induced retching and vomiting by activation of the cannabinoid CB1 receptor.[272]

Other Opioid Effects

Obstetrics

Alfentanil and pethidine have been used safely as analgesics during the harvesting of human oocytes for subsequent in vitro

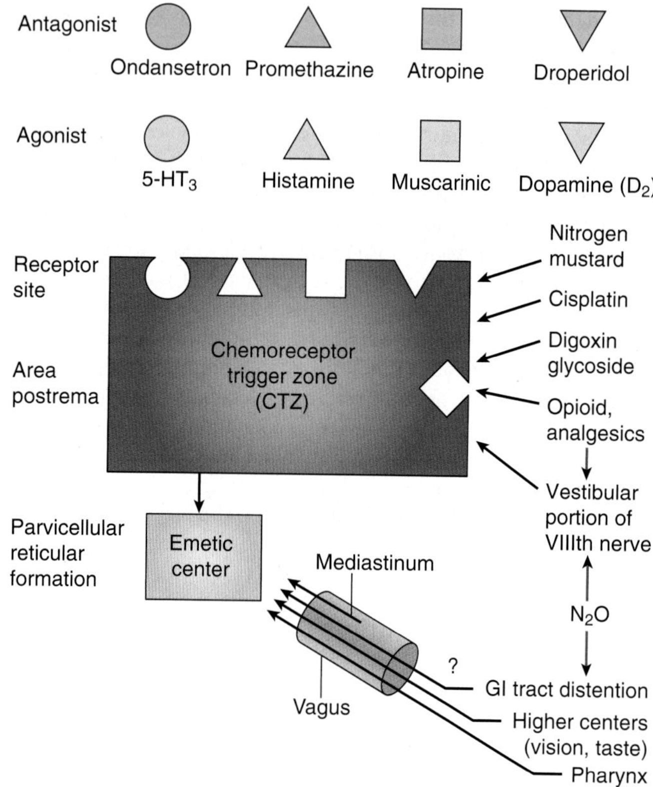

Figure 27-11 The chemoreceptor trigger zone and the emetic center with the agonist and antagonist sites of action of various anesthetic-related agents and stimuli. GI, gastrointestinal. *(From Watcha MF, White PF: Postoperative nausea and vomiting. Its etiology, treatment, and prevention. Anesthesiology 77:162-184, 1992.)*

fertilization.[273,274] The teratogenic actions of opioids, including fentanyl, sufentanil, and alfentanil, appear to be minimal, at least in animal models.

Parenteral administration of opioids before delivery remains a commonly used method of analgesia (also see Chapter 69). Nociception as a result of uterine cervical distention could be suppressed by μ- and κ-agonists in rats,[275] but the analgesic effect of μ-agonist but not κ-agonist was reduced by estrogen.[276] Aortocaval compression and associated hypotension may be exacerbated by parenteral opioids, especially after the use of morphine or meperidine. Fatal manifestations of maternal opioid administration include decreases in heart rate variability. Adverse neonatal effects can occur after the administration of either morphine or meperidine to mothers. Fetal acidosis increases transfer of opioid from the mother. Attempts to minimize the neonatal effects of opioids include restricting opioid administration to the first stage of labor. The short-acting opioid alfentanil administered before cesarean delivery attenuated the maternal stress response but led to a slightly reduced Apgar score.[277]

In sheep, neither intravenous nor epidural injection of sufentanil (50 μg) affected maternal mean arterial pressure, uterine blood flow, maternal heart rate, fetal mean arterial pressure, fetal heart rate, or blood gases and acid-base status in the mother and fetus.[278] Because the fetus is capable of pain perception after the 26th week of gestation, adequate postoperative fetal pain management is essential after fetal surgery. It was shown that the sheep fetus absorbs sufentanil after intra-amniotic instillation and that significantly greater plasma concentrations were achieved in the fetal lamb than in the ewe.[279]

Morphine and meperidine have been found in the breast milk of mothers receiving intravenous opioid analgesia.[280,281] Although both fentanyl and morphine are concentrated in breast milk in milk-to-plasma ratios of 2 : 1 to 3 : 1, newborn exposure is reported to be insignificant. Newborns of addicted mothers can exhibit opioid withdrawal and require observation and appropriate treatment.[282]

Anaphylactoid Reactions

True allergic reactions and systemic anaphylactoid reactions to opioids are rare. More commonly, local reactions caused by preservatives or histamine may occur. In 32% of heroin addicts dying suddenly after injection, the concentration of tryptase was elevated (>10 μg/L), but no correlation was found between IgE levels and tryptase, thus supporting the hypothesis that mast cell degranulation was not mediated by allergic reaction.[283] This report suggests that many heroin fatalities are caused by an anaphylactoid reaction.

Ocular Effects

The use of fentanyl, sufentanil, and alfentanil during induction of anesthesia can help prevent increases in intraocular pressure (see Chapter 75). Fentanyl, alfentanil, and sufentanil doses as low as 2.5, 10, and 0.1 μg/kg, respectively, may be sufficient as long as appropriate anesthetic depth is achieved before tracheal intubation. Remifentanil (1 μg/kg) combined with propofol (2 mg/kg) or thiopental (5 mg/kg) is effective for prevention of changes in intraocular pressure after succinylcholine and tracheal intubation.[284,285]

Immune Effects

It is now firmly established that opioids influence immune regulation. Direct effects of opioid agonists include modulation of immune cellular activity, as well as modulation of specific enzymatic degradation and regulation processes.[286] Several immune cell populations, including T cells, macrophages, and natural killer (NK) cells, serve as targets for the effects of opioids. It was shown that maximal suppression of NK cell activity, proliferation of splenic T and B cells, and interferon-γ production are observed 0.5 to 1 hour after the injection of 15 mg/kg morphine into rats.[287] The time course was nearly concordant with the antinociceptive effect of morphine. Postoperative administration of morphine (10 mg intramuscularly [IM]) did not significantly affect NK cell activity, whereas tramadol (100 mg IM) did enhance NK cell activity.[288] It was reported that intravenously administered fentanyl causes a rapid increase in NK cell cytotoxicity, which was coincident with an increase in the percentage of $CD16^+$ and $CD8^+$ cells in peripheral blood.[289] When compared with fentanyl (1000 μg), administration of morphine (40 mg) as part of a balanced anesthetic technique suppressed several components of the inflammatory response (IL-6, CD11b, CD18, postoperative hyperthermia) to cardiac surgery and CPB.[290]

Table 27-5 Physicochemical and Pharmacokinetic Data for Commonly Used Opioid Agonists

	Morphine	Meperidine	Fentanyl	Sufentanil	Alfentanil	Remifentanil
pK_a	8.0	8.5	8.4	8.0	6.5	7.1
% Un-ionized at pH 7.4	23	<10	<10	20	90	67?
Octanol-H_2O partition coefficient	1.4	39	813	1778	145	17.9
% Bound to plasma protein	20-40	39	84	93	92	80?
Diffusible fraction (%)	16.8	2.2	1.5	1.6	8.0	13.3?
$t_{½\alpha}$ (min)	1-2.5	—	1-2	1-2	1-3	0.5-1.5
$t_{½\beta}$ (min)	10-20	5-15	10-30	15-20	4-17	5-8
$t_{½\gamma}$ (hr)	2-4	3-5	2-4	2-3	1-2	0.7-1.2
Vd_c (L/kg)	0.1-0.4	1-2	0.4-1.0	0.2	0.1-0.3	0.06-0.08
Vd_{ss} (L/kg)	3-5	3-5	3-5	2.5-3.0	0.4-1.0	0.2-0.3
Clearance (mL/min/kg)	15-30	8.18	10-20	10-15	4-9	30-40
Hepatic extraction ratio	0.6-0.8	0.5-0.7	0.8-1.0	0.7-0.9	0.3-0.5	NA

$t_{½}$ α, β, γ are the half-lives of a three-compartment model; Vd_c, volume of distribution of the central compartment; Vd_{ss}, volume of distribution at steady state.
From Bailey PL, Egan TD, Stanley TH: Intravenous opioid anesthetics. *In* Miller RD (ed): Anesthesia, 5th ed. New York, Churchill Livingstone, 2000, p 312.

As a potential mechanism of the immunosuppressive effects of morphine, it was demonstrated that activation of the nuclear factor NF-κB by an inflammatory stimulus was inhibited by morphine-induced activation of μ_3-opioid receptors in a nitric oxide–dependent manner.[291] Several investigators have independently reported direct effects of morphine on apoptosis in cultured human peripheral blood lymphocytes, which may result in compromised immune function.[292,293] However, there is also a report that morphine has no effect on apoptosis-related molecules and does not promote apoptosis of human peripheral blood lymphocytes.[294]

Pharmacokinetics and Pharmacodynamics of Opioids

With the advent of modern drug assay technology and the widespread availability of computers, it is now possible to analyze pharmacologic data with combined pharmacokinetic-pharmacodynamic models to separate drug response into its pharmacokinetic and pharmacodynamic components. Pharmacokinetic parameters govern the relationship between opioid dose and opioid concentrations in blood (or other body fluid). Pharmacodynamic parameters describe the relationship between the opioid concentration in blood (or other fluid) and opioid effect.

Physicochemical Properties

Opioids are weak bases. When dissolved in solution, they are dissociated into protonated and free-base fractions, with the relative proportions depending on the pH and pK_a. The free-base fraction is more lipid soluble than the protonated fraction. High lipid solubility facilitates transport of opioid into the biophase or site of action. Therefore, highly lipid-soluble opioids have a more rapid onset of action. However, because the opioid receptor "recognizes" an opioid molecule in the protonated form, the intensity of opioid effects is closely related to the ionized concentration of drug in the biophase.

All opioids are to some extent bound to plasma proteins, including albumin and α_1-acid glycoprotein. It is only the unionized, unbound fraction that constitutes the diffusible fraction and provides the concentration gradient that promotes diffusion of opioid from blood to the tissue of interest. Thus, the speed of onset of opioid effect is affected by both lipid solubility and protein binding.

Common Pharmacokinetic Features of Opioids

Representative pharmacokinetic parameters for the opioids commonly used in anesthesia are displayed in Table 27-5.

After intravenous injection, arterial plasma concentrations of opioids rise to a peak within one circulation time. Thereafter, they exhibit a rapid redistribution phase and a slower elimination phase typical of drugs whose pharmacokinetics is described by compartmental models. After administration into a central compartment, opioids are either eliminated from the central compartment (by excretion or biotransformation) or distributed to peripheral compartments. In general, opioids are cleared from plasma by biotransformation in the liver. However, extrahepatic metabolism is important for some opioids.

As a rule, because of their high lipid solubility, opioids are widely distributed in body tissues. In pharmacokinetic terms, this means that opioids typically have a high apparent volume of distribution at steady state. Because opioids are distributed so widely and so rapidly to various body tissues, redistribution has a prominent impact on the decline in opioid concentration, particularly

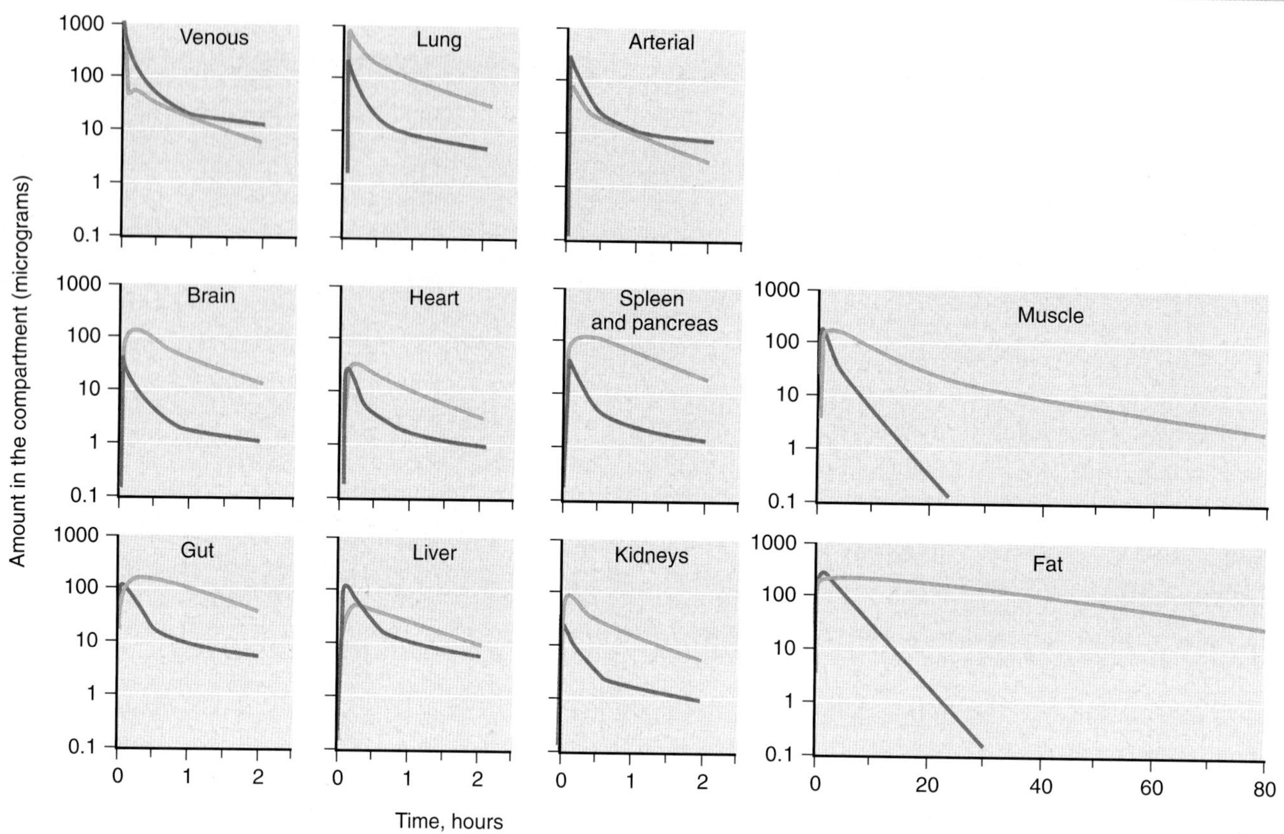

Figure 27-12 Computer simulations of the amounts of fentanyl (*yellow lines*) or alfentanil (*blue lines*) in various organs and tissues in a 70-kg human after a bolus intravenous injection of 1 mg of each drug. *(From Bjorkman S, Stanski DR, Verotta D, Harashima H: Comparative tissue concentration profiles of fentanyl and alfentanil in humans predicted from tissue/blood partition data obtained in rats. Anesthesiology 72:865-873, 1990.)*

in the early period after injection. Figure 27-12 shows a computer simulation of opioids in various organs. The difference in physicochemical properties between fentanyl and alfentanil causes the marked overall difference in disposition. Distribution to muscle and fat is extensive and declines slowly because of limited blood flow.

Opioid uptake by the lung has a significant implication in opioid pharmacokinetics. The time necessary to reach the peak concentration of an opioid is influenced by the degree of pulmonary uptake. Pulmonary uptake of fentanyl is more extensive than the pulmonary uptake of alfentanil, which may be explained by the difference in sequestration into pulmonary endothelial cells. Pulmonary uptake of opioids can affect the pharmacokinetics of other drugs. It was shown that pulmonary uptake of propofol is significantly reduced by the administration of fentanyl 30 seconds before the injection of propofol in cats.

Pharmacokinetic Features of Individual Drugs

Morphine

Morphine pharmacokinetics is notably different from that of the fentanyl congeners. This difference is due in large part to morphine's comparatively low lipid solubility. There is relatively little transient first-pass uptake of morphine by the lung.

The pK_a of morphine (8.0) is greater than physiologic pH, and thus after intravenous injection only a small fraction (10% to 20%) of morphine is un-ionized. Penetration of morphine into and out of the brain is presumably slower than that of other opioids. Approximately 20% to 40% of morphine is bound to plasma proteins, mostly albumin.

Morphine is principally metabolized by conjugation in the liver, but the kidney plays a key role in the extrahepatic metabolism of morphine. Morphine-3-glucuronide (M3G) is the major matabolite of morphine, but it does not bind to opioid receptors and possesses little or no analgesic activity. M3G may actually antagonize morphine, and this effect may contribute to both variability in response and resistance to morphine analgesic therapy. M6G accounts for nearly 10% of the morphine metabolite; it is a more potent μ-receptor agonist than morphine is and has a similar duration of action. It was reported that M6G contributes substantially to morphine's analgesic effects, even in patients with normal renal function. Especially in patients with renal dysfunction, accumulation of M6G can lead to an increased incidence of adverse effects, including respiratory depression. A recent report suggested that a single-nucleotide polymorphism at the μ-opioid receptor affects the susceptibility to M6G-related opioid toxicity. Because the hepatic extraction ratio of morphine is high, the bioavailability of orally administered morphine is significantly lower (20% to 30%) than after intramuscular or subcutaneous injection. It appears that M6G is in fact the primary active compound when morphine is administered orally (Fig. 27-13). In contrast to

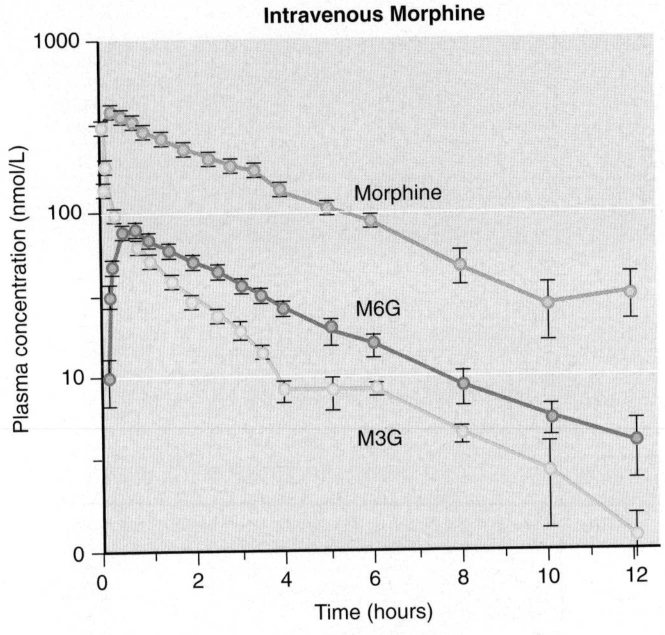

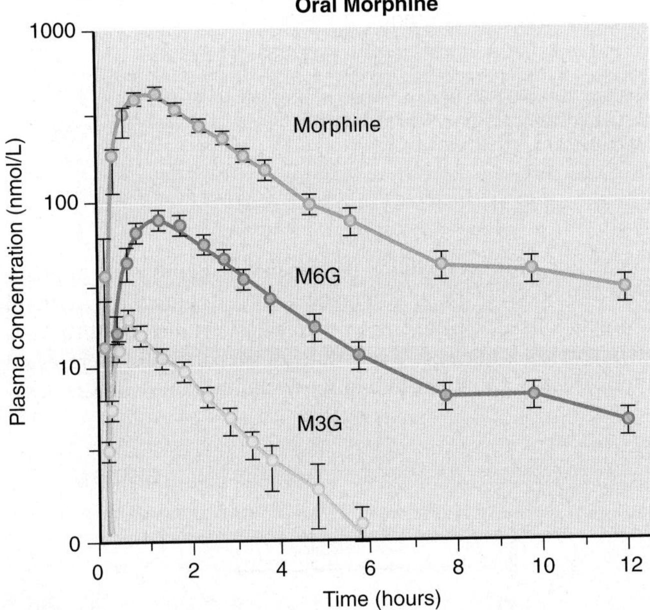

Figure 27-13 Mean plasma concentrations (± SEM) of morphine, morphine-6-glucuronide (M6G), and morphine-3-glucuronide (M3G) after intravenous and oral administration of morphine. *(From Osborne R, Joel S, Trew D, Slevin M: Morphine and metabolite behavior after different routes of morphine administration: Demonstration of the importance of the active metabolite morphine-6-glucuronide. Clin Pharmacol Ther 47:12-19, 1990.)*

reports suggesting a high potency of M6G, others have shown that short-term intravenous administration of M6G does not provide effective analgesia.

Meperidine

Unlike morphine, after intravenous injection, first-pass uptake of meperidine by the lungs is approximately 65%. Meperidine is more highly bound to plasma proteins than morphine is, principally (70%) to α_1-acid glycoprotein. As with morphine, a relatively high hepatic extraction ratio results in biotransformation that is dependent on hepatic blood flow. Normeperidine, the major metabolite, has analgesic activity and is roughly twice as potent as meperidine in producing seizures in animals. The elimination half-life of normeperidine is considerably greater than that of meperidine, and thus repeated doses can easily cause this toxic metabolite to accumulate in patients with renal disease and potentially produce seizures.

Fentanyl

A three-compartment model is typically used to describe decay of plasma fentanyl concentrations. The lungs exert a significant first-pass effect and transiently take up approximately 75% of an injected dose of fentanyl. Approximately 80% of fentanyl is bound to plasma proteins, and significant amounts (40%) are taken up by red blood cells. Fentanyl is relatively long acting, in large part because of this widespread distribution in body tissues.

Fentanyl is primarily metabolized in the liver by *N*-dealkylation and hydroxylation. Metabolites begin to appear in plasma as early as 1.5 minutes after injection. Norfentanyl, the primary metabolite, is detectable in urine for up to 48 hours after intravenous fentanyl in humans.

Alfentanil

After intravenous injection, plasma concentrations of alfentanil are described by either a two-compartment or a three-compartment model. Alfentanil is bound to plasma proteins (mostly glycoproteins) in higher proportions (90%) than fentanyl is. At physiologic pH, it is mostly (90%) un-ionized because of its relatively low pK_a (6.5). Thus, despite more intense protein binding, alfentanil's diffusible fraction is higher than that of fentanyl. This explains, in part, its short latency to peak effect after intravenous injection.

The main metabolic pathways of alfentanil are similar to those of sufentanil and include oxidative *N*-dealkylation and *O*-demethylation, aromatic hydroxylation, and ether glucuronide formation. The degradation products of alfentanil have little, if any, opioid activity. Human alfentanil metabolism may be accomplished predominantly, if not exclusively, by cytochrome P450 3A3/4 (CYP3A3/4). This enzyme is known to display at least an eightfold difference in activity in humans. Alfentanil is also metabolized by human liver microsomal CYP3A5, which shows more than 20-fold pharmacogenetic variability in expression and thus results in significant differences in human liver alfentanil metabolism. An in vitro study demonstrated that propofol in clinically relevant concentrations interferes with oxidative metabolic degradation of alfentanil and sufentanil in the microsomal fraction of pig and human liver.

Sufentanil

The pharmacokinetic property of sufentanil is adequately described by a three-compartment model. After intravenous injection, first-pass pulmonary extraction, retention, and release are similar to those of fentanyl. The pK_a of sufentanil at physiologic pH is the same as that of morphine (8.0), and therefore only a small amount (20%) exists in the un-ionized form. Sufentanil is twice as lipid soluble as fentanyl and is highly bound (93%) to plasma proteins, including α_1-acid glycoprotein.

The major metabolic pathways of sufentanil include *N*-dealkylation, oxidative *O*-demethylation, and aromatic hydroxylation. Major metabolites include *N*-phenylpropanamide.

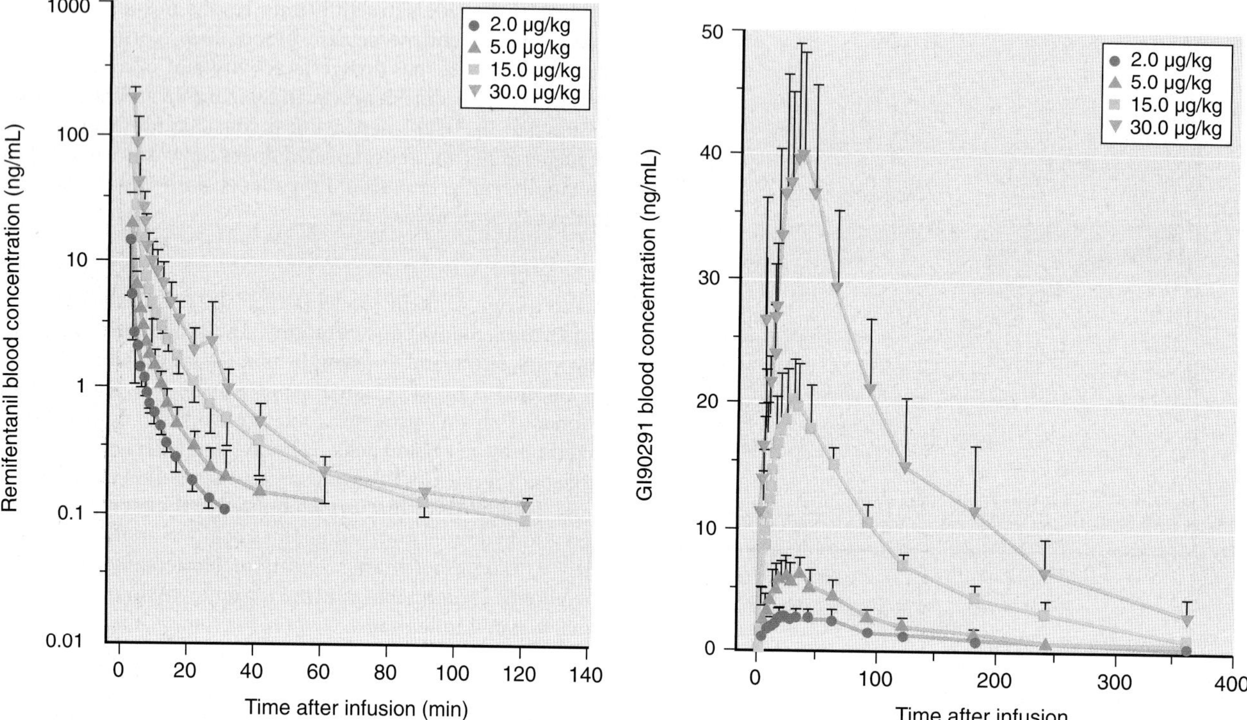

Figure 27-14 Mean (± SD) blood concentration-time curves of remifentanil and its metabolite GI90291 after a 1-minute transfusion of remifentanil of 2, 5, 15, and 30 μg/kg; *n* = 6 for each dose. *(From Westmoreland CL, Hoke JF, Sebel PS, et al: Pharmacokinetics of remifentanil (GI87084B) and its major metabolite (GI90291) in patients undergoing elective inpatient surgery. Anesthesiology 79:893-903, 1993.)*

Remifentanil

Although chemically related to the fentanyl congeners, remifentanil is structurally unique because of its ester linkages. Remifentanil's ester structure renders it susceptible to hydrolysis by blood- and tissue-nonspecific esterases, which results in rapid metabolism and rapid reduction of blood concentrations after cessation of infusion (Fig. 27-14). Remifentanil thus constitutes the first "ultrashort"-acting opioid for use as a supplement to general anesthesia.

The pharmacokinetic properties of remifentanil are best described by a three-compartment model.[88] Its clearance is several times more rapid than normal hepatic blood flow, consistent with widespread extrahepatic metabolism. However, remifentanil is not significantly metabolized or sequestered in the lungs. It is a weak base with a pK_a of 7.07. It is highly lipid soluble with an octanol-water partition coefficient of 19.9 at pH 7.4. Remifentanil is highly bound (70%) to plasma proteins (mostly α_1-acid glycoprotein). The remifentanil free base is formulated with glycine. Because glycine has been shown to act as an inhibitory neurotransmitter that causes a reversible motor weakness when injected intrathecally into rodents, remifentanil is not approved for spinal or epidural use.

The primary metabolic pathway of remifentanil is de-esterification to form a carboxylic acid metabolite, GI90291 (Fig. 27-15), which is 0.003 to 0.001 times as potent as remifentanil. The low in vivo potency of GI90291 can be explained by low affinity to the μ-receptor in combination with poor brain penetration. Excretion of GI90291 is dependent on renal clearance mechanisms. Evidence from dogs suggests that the remifentanil metabolites are, for practical purposes, completely inactive, even in patients with renal failure. Its pharmacokinetics is not appreciably influenced by renal or hepatic failure. In blood, remifentanil is metabolized primarily by enzymes within erythrocytes. Remifentanil is not a good substrate for pseudocholinesterase and therefore is not influenced by pseudocholinesterase deficiency.

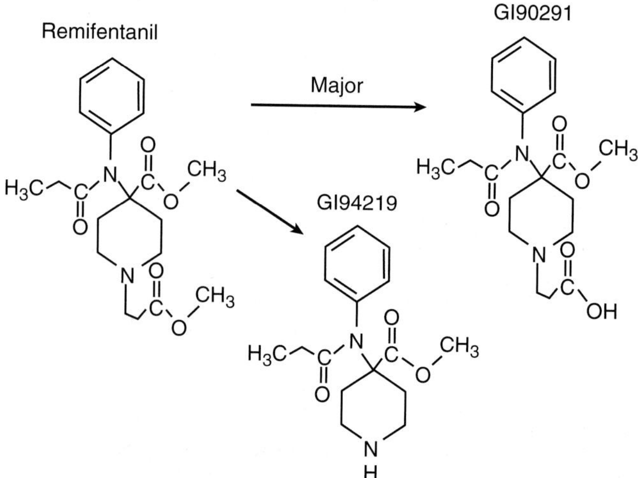

Figure 27-15 Metabolic pathway of remifentanil. De-esterification by nonspecific plasma and tissue esterases to form a carboxylic acid metabolite (GI90291) that has only 1/300 to 1/1000 the potency of the parent compound is the primary metabolic pathway. *N*-Dealkylation of remifentanil to GI94219 is a minor metabolic pathway. *(From Egan TD, Lemmens HJ, Fiset P, et al: The pharmacokinetics of the new short-acting opioid remifentanil [GI87084B] in healthy adult male volunteers. Anesthesiology 79:881-892, 1993.)*

Computerized Delivery Methods in Clinical Practice

Advances in pharmacokinetic modeling and infusion pump technology have made it possible to administer opioids (and other drugs) via a computer-controlled infusion pump (CCIP).[295] The physician operating a CCIP designates a target concentration to achieve rather than specifying an infusion rate. The CCIP then calculates the necessary infusion rates to achieve the targeted concentration.

Delivery of an opioid via a CCIP requires a different approach by clinicians. Rather than setting an infusion rate based on clinical experience and literature recommendations, the anesthesiologist using a CCIP designates a target concentration, and the CCIP calculates the infusion rates necessary to achieve the concentration over time. It has been reported that target-controlled infusion of alfentanil and remifentanil was useful for intraoperative and postoperative analgesia.[296,297] Successful use of a CCIP thus requires knowledge of the therapeutic concentrations appropriate for the clinical setting.

Surrogate Measures of Opioid Potency

Because a high-resolution measure of analgesia is not available, opioid potencies are usually estimated by some surrogate measures. Reduction of the MAC required to produce lack of movement to skin incision has been a frequently used surrogate measure for estimation of opioid potency (Fig. 27-16).[90,92] However, the MAC is not useful as a surrogate measure of opioid potency outside the operating room.

The EEG has been another widely used surrogate measure in estimating opioid potency.[89] The EEG is advantageous because it is noninvasive and can be used as an effect measure when an experimental subject is unconscious or apneic. When processed by Fourier spectral analysis, the raw changes on the EEG translate into a significant decrease in the value of the spectral edge, a parameter that quantitates the frequency below which a given percentage (usually 95%) of the power in the signal of the EEG is found. Although the clinical meaning of the changes on the EEG produced by opioids is unclear, the opioid potencies estimated by using the EEG as a surrogate measure appear to be clinically reliable because they relate to clinically determined potencies in a proportional, reproducible fashion.

For opioids, because the surrogate measures do not always assess the drug effect of clinical interest (analgesia), estimations of potency based on surrogate measures must be interpreted with some caution.

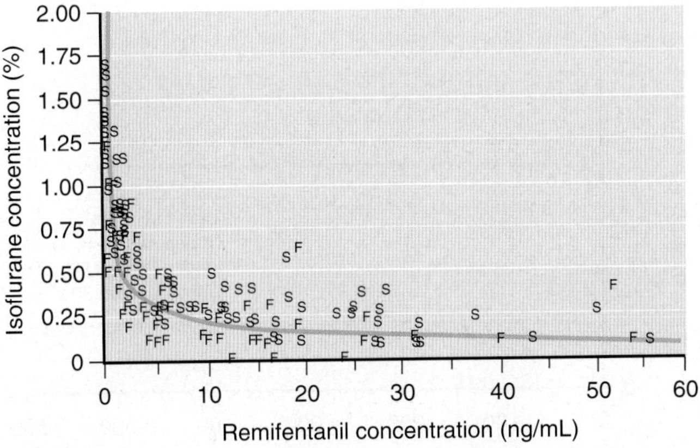

Figure 27-16 The reduction in isoflurane concentration to prevent movement at skin incision in 50% of patients by increasing measured remifentanil whole-blood concentrations. F represents a patient who moved and S a patient who did not move. The *solid line* is the logistic regression solution for a patient 40 years of age. *(From Lang E, Kapila A, Shlugman D, et al: Reduction of isoflurane minimal alveolar concentration by remifentanil. Anesthesiology 85:721-728, 1996.)*

Factors Affecting the Pharmacokinetics and Pharmacodynamics of Opioids

Age

The pharmacokinetics and pharmacodynamics of opioids can be influenced by age (see Chapter 71). It is clear that neonates exhibit a reduced rate of elimination of essentially all opioids,[298] presumably because of immature metabolic mechanisms, including the cytochrome P450 system. The prolonged elimination of opioids observed in the neonatal period quickly normalizes toward adult values within the first year of life.[298]

With advanced age, although pharmacokinetic changes may play a minor role, pharmacodynamic differences are primarily responsible for the decreased dose requirement in the elderly. Age was inversely correlated with the central volume of distribution, clearance, and potency of remifentanil (Fig. 27-17).[299] These combined pharmacokinetic and pharmacodynamic changes mandate a reduction in remifentanil dosage by at least 50% or more in the elderly.

Body Weight

Many opioid pharmacokinetic parameters, especially clearance, appear to be more closely related to lean body mass, which means that opioid dosage regimens may best be based on lean body mass and not total body weight. Total body weight–based dosing in an obese patient results in much higher remifentanil effect-site concentrations than lean body mass–based dosing does.[300] In contrast, for lean patients, the concentrations that result from total body weight–based dosing are not much greater than those based on body mass (Fig. 27-18). Clinically, context-sensitive half-times are not significantly different between obese and lean subjects (Fig. 27-19). Mounting evidence suggests that lean body mass is a better predictor of metabolic capacity than total body weight is. Ideal body weight, a parameter closely related to lean body mass and one that is perhaps more easily estimated by the clinician, is probably an acceptable alternative.

Renal Failure

Renal failure has implications of major clinical importance with respect to morphine and meperidine.[301] For the fentanyl congeners, the clinical importance of renal failure is less marked.

Morphine is an opioid with active metabolites that are dependent on renal clearance mechanisms for elimination. Morphine is principally metabolized by conjugation in the liver, and the water-soluble glucuronides (M3G and M6G) are excreted via the kidney. The kidney also plays a role in the conjugation of morphine and accounts for nearly 40% of its metabolism. Very

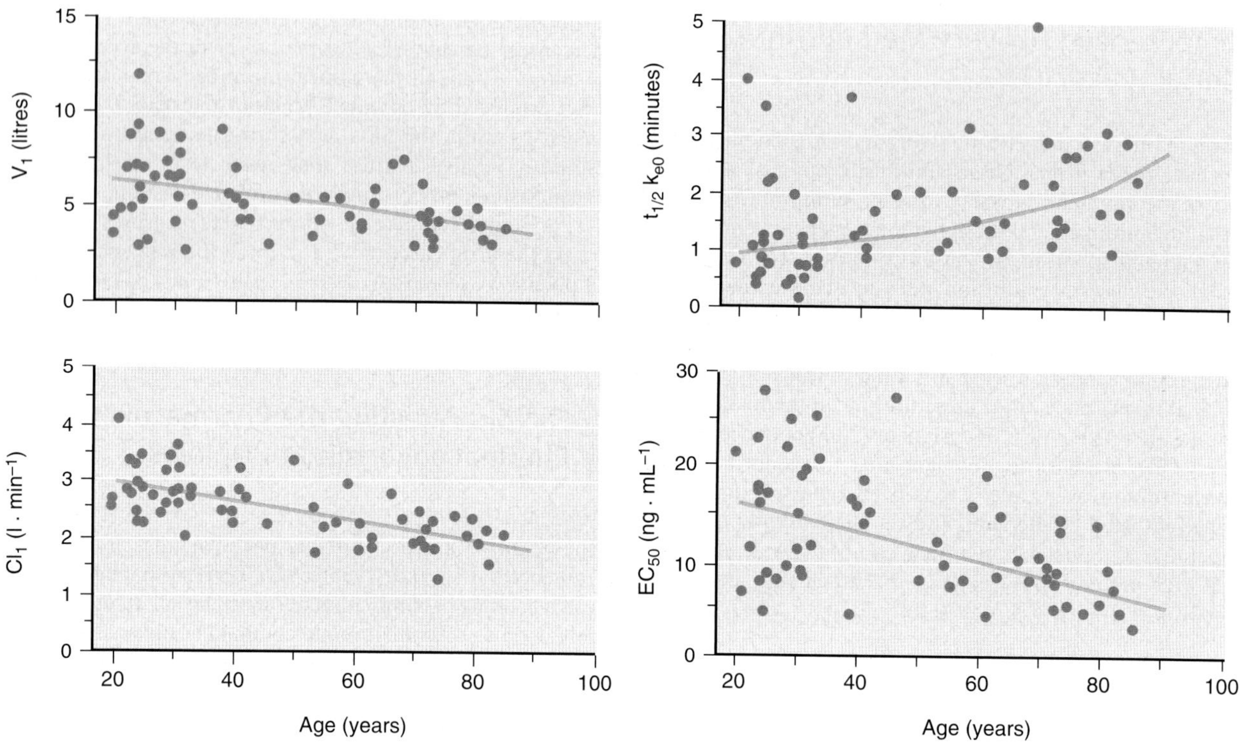

Figure 27-17 Relationship between pharmacokinetic and pharmacodynamic parameters and age for remifentanil. V_1 and Cl_1 are estimated from a three-compartment model. $t_{1/2}k_{e0}$ is a half-life corresponding to k_{e0}, a first-order rate constant for elimination of drug from the effect compartment. *(From Minto CF, Schnider TW, Shafer SL: Pharmacokinetics and pharmacodynamics of remifentanil. II. Model application. Anesthesiology 86:24-33, 1997.)*

high levels of M6G and life-threatening respiratory depression can develop in patients with renal failure (Fig. 27-20).[302] In view of these changes induced by renal failure, morphine may not be a good choice in patients with severely altered renal clearance mechanisms.

The clinical pharmacology of meperidine is also significantly altered by renal failure. Normeperidine, the main metabolite, has analgesic and excitatory CNS effects. Because the active metabolites are subject to renal excretion, this potential CNS toxicity secondary to accumulation of normeperidine is especially a concern in patients with renal failure.

The clinical pharmacology of the fentanyl congeners is not grossly altered by renal failure, although a decrease in plasma protein binding may potentially alter the free fraction of the fentanyl class of opioids.[301] In the presence of renal impairment, fentanyl, alfentanil, sufentanil, and remifentanil do not deliver a

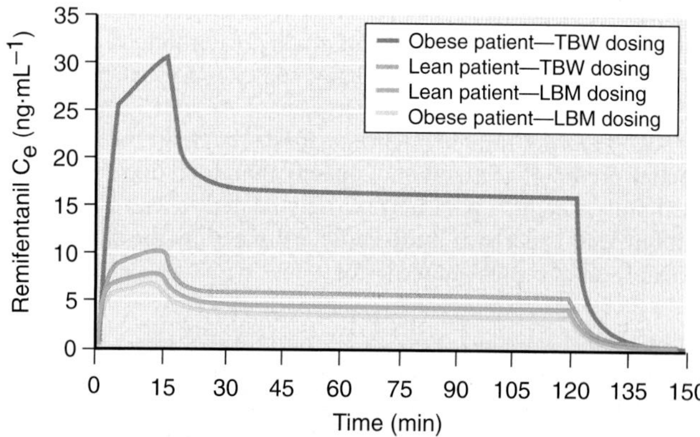

Figure 27-18 Computer simulation of the time course of change in remifentanil concentration when the dosage regimen is calculated according to lean body mass (LBM) or total body weight (TBW) for both obese and lean patients. Note that TBW-based dosing in an obese patient results in dramatically higher concentrations. *(From Egan TD, Huizinga B, Gupta SK, et al: Remifentanil pharmacokinetics in obese versus lean patients. Anesthesiology 89:562-573, 1998.)*

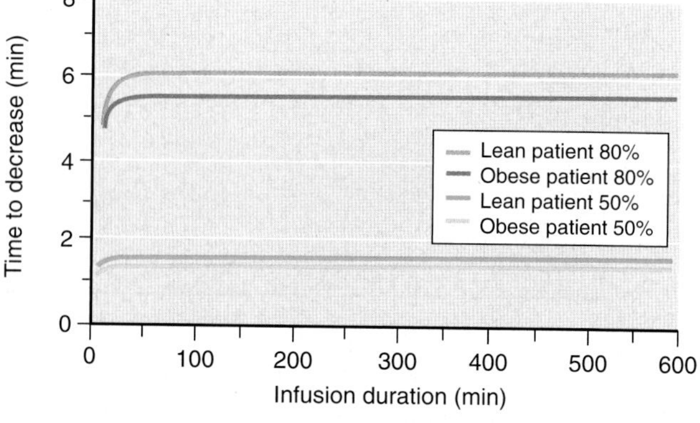

Figure 27-19 Computer simulation of the context-sensitive half-times (50% decrement times) and 80% decrement times of remifentanil in obese versus lean subjects. Note that in clinical terms the curves are not grossly different in obese versus lean subjects. *(From Egan TD, Huizinga B, Gupta SK, et al: Remifentanil pharmacokinetics in obese versus lean patients. Anesthesiology 89:562-573, 1998.)*

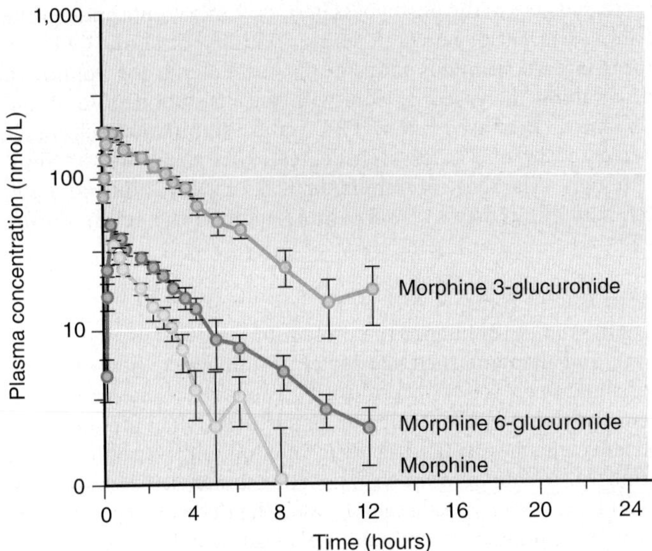

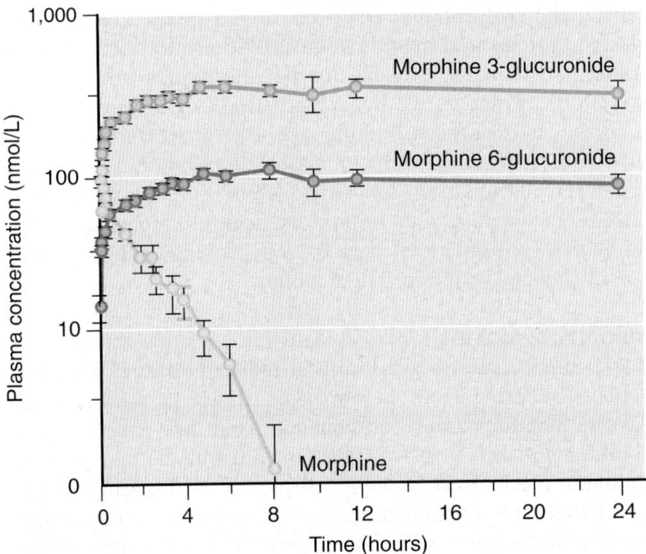

Figure 27-20 Effect of renal failure on the pharmacokinetics of morphine. The graphs show the time-dependent change in serum concentration of morphine and its metabolite in patients with normal renal function (*top*) and those with renal failure (*bottom*) who received 0.1 mg/kg of morphine intravenously. *(From Osborne R, Joel S, Grebenik K, et al: The pharmacokinetics of morphine and morphine glucuronides in kidney failure. Clin Pharmacol Ther 54:158-167, 1993.)*

high active metabolite load or suffer from significantly prolonged clearance.[303] Neither the pharmacokinetics nor the pharmacodynamics of remifentanil is altered by impaired renal function. The levels of GI90291 that develop during remifentanil infusion in patients with renal failure are not likely to produce any clinically significant effects.

Hepatic Failure

Even though the liver is the metabolic organ primarily responsible for opioid biotransformation, the degree of liver failure typically observed in perioperative patients, with the exception of patients undergoing liver transplantation, does not have a major impact on the pharmacokinetics of most opioids. In addition to reduced metabolic capacity (i.e., cytochrome P450 system and conjugation), liver disease may also lead to reductions in hepatic blood flow, hepatocellular mass, and plasma protein binding. The increase in total body water and the edema of advanced liver disease may alter the distribution characteristics of a drug. Enzyme induction, such as that observed in early alcoholism, can actually increase the metabolic capacity of the liver.

The pharmacokinetics of morphine is relatively unchanged by developing liver disease, such as liver cirrhosis and hepatic carcinoma, because of the substantial compensatory extrahepatic metabolism of morphine. A reduction in hepatic blood flow would be expected to slow the decline in morphine plasma concentrations. After liver resection, M6G/morphine and M3G/morphine ratios were significantly reduced and the circulating morphine concentration was increased, mainly as a result of lower morphine clearance.[304] In patients with cirrhosis the metabolism of meperidine is decreased, which leads to accumulation of the parent drug and possible CNS depressive effects similar to hepatic encephalopathy. Although elimination of normeperidine is decreased as well in these patients, the ratio of normeperidine to meperidine is generally low, and the narcotic effects of meperidine usually predominate.[305] The disposition of fentanyl and sufentanil appears to be unaffected by liver disease.[306] The reductions in liver blood flow that result from either liver disease or some other disorder (e.g., shock) can affect the pharmacokinetic parameters of alfentanil, fentanyl, and sufentanil.[307] A significant decrease in clearance of alfentanil was demonstrated in patients with mild to moderate cirrhosis when compared with volunteers from the historical control group.[308] Greater elimination half-lives (3.7 ± 2.6 hours) have also been observed for alfentanil in patients undergoing abdominal aortic surgery.[309] Remifentanil is an opioid whose phamacokinetics is completely unchanged by liver disease (Fig. 27-21). Its kinetics does not change during the anhepatic phase of orthotopic liver transplantation.[310]

Cardiopulmonary Bypass

CPB produces significant alterations in the pharmacokinetics of most opioids (see Chapter 60).[311] These alterations are a result of CPB-induced modifications in distribution volumes (secondary to priming) and changes in acid-base balance, organ blood flow, plasma protein concentrations, and body temperature. Binding of drugs to components of the bypass circuit can also alter opioid pharmacokinetics.

When morphine is given as a premedicant before cardiac anesthesia, its concentrations decline significantly on initiation of CPB.[312] Miller and colleagues examined the effect of CPB on plasma fentanyl concentrations and showed that the total concentration of fentanyl in plasma was significantly decreased and the unbound fraction of fentanyl rose on initiation of CPB.[313] The total fentanyl concentration remained relatively stable during bypass until near the end of CPB, at which time the mean total concentration increased, coincident with rewarming. Population pharmacokinetic modeling applied to concentration-versus-time data from patients undergoing coronary artery bypass grafting with CPB demonstrated that the effect of CPB on fentanyl pharmacokinetics is clinically insignificant and that a simple three-compartment model accurately predicts fentanyl concentrations throughout surgery involving the use of CPB.[314] Elimination of alfentanil is prolonged by CPB primarily because of increased distribution.[315] The volume of distribution in steady state (Vd_{ss}) and the volume of the central compartment for alfentanil were

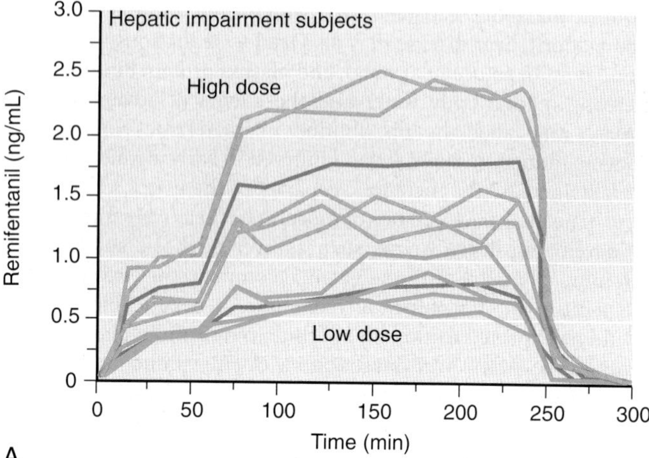

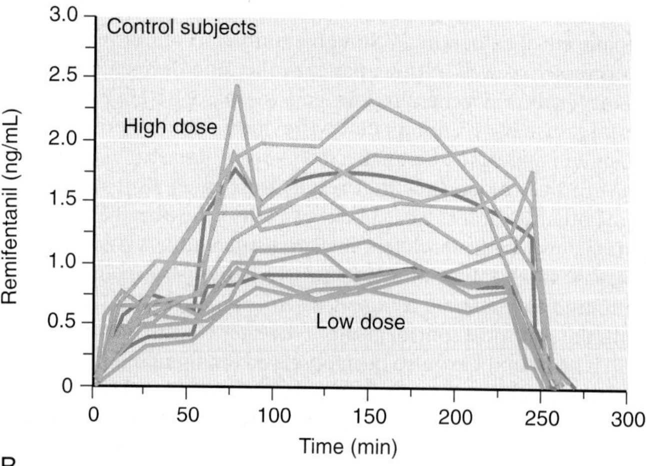

Figure 27-21 Time-dependent changes in the blood concentration of remifentanil in patients with liver disease (*top*) and control subjects (*bottom*). In the low-dose group, remifentanil was infused at 0.0125 μg/kg/min for 1 hour and then at 0.025 μg/kg/min for 3 hours. In high-dose group, the infusion rate of remifentanil was 0.025 μg/kg/min for 1 hour and then 0.05 μg/kg/min for 3 hours. *(From Dershwitz M, Hoke JF, Rosow CE, et al: Pharmacokinetics and pharmacodynamics of remifentanil in volunteer subjects with severe liver disease. Anesthesiology 84:812-820, 1996.)*

significantly greater in the CPB groups than in the nonbypass group.[316] However, the elimination half-life $(T_{1/2\beta})$ of alfentanil did not differ significantly between the normothermic CPB, hypothermic CPB, and nonbypass groups. No significant differences in Vd_{ss}, clearance, or $T_{1/2\beta}$ were found between the normothermic and hypothermic CPB groups. The free fraction of alfentanil during CPB remains constant despite complex changes in binding protein concentrations.[317] In adult patients undergoing elective myocardial revascularization with hypothermic CPB who received continuous infusions of remifentanil, 1.0 to 2.0 μg/kg/min, no evidence of accumulation or sequestration was found. Russell and coauthors reported that normothermic CPB did not significantly affect the clearance of remifentanil but that hypothermic CPB reduced it by an average of 20%, which was attributed to the effect of temperature on blood and tissue esterase activity (Fig. 27-22).[318] In pediatric patients undergoing CPB for repair of atrial septal defects, there was no change in Vd_{ss}, volume of the central compartment, $T_{1/2\alpha}$ and $T_{1/2\beta}$, but clearance values increased 20% in the postbypass period.[319] In patients undergoing coronary artery bypass graft surgery with hypothermic CPB and receiving a continuous infusion of remifentanil, the volume of distribution increased by 86% with the institution of CPB and remained increased after CPB, and elimination clearance decreased by 6.37% for each degree lower than 37°C.[320] Thus, although clearance of remifentanil is reduced during CPB, remifentanil remains a very short-acting drug, even during CPB.

Acid-Base Changes

Changes in pH influence the protein binding of fentanyl, sufentanil, and alfentanil such that protein binding increases with alkalosis and decreases with acidosis.[307] These effects are greater for fentanyl than for sufentanil and for sufentanil than for alfentanil. Relative changes in the free drug fraction with variation in pH from 7.4 to 7.0 were much higher for fentanyl (52%) than for sufentanil (29%) and alfentanil (6%). The dependence of plasma protein binding of the opioids on pH significantly correlates with their partition between an organic and aqueous phase, thus suggesting the hydrophobic character of the interaction between plasma proteins and opioids. Increased ionization decreases the amount of fentanyl available for hepatic metabolism or renal excretion. Intraoperative hyperventilation during surgical procedures can significantly influence the pharmacokinetics of sufentanil and result in an increased distribution volume and prolonged elimination half-time. Thus, both intraoperative respiratory alkalosis and respiratory acidosis, especially in the immediate postoperative period, can prolong and exacerbate opioid-induced respiratory depression.

Hemorrhagic Shock

It is common practice to administer reduced doses of opioids to patients suffering from hemorrhagic shock to minimize any adverse hemodynamic consequences and prevent prolonged opioid effect. This is at least partially attributable to a pharmacokinetic mechanism. Analysis of pigs receiving fentanyl suggested that central clearance and central and second compartment distribution volumes were significantly reduced in hemorrhagic shock, with higher fentanyl concentrations for any given dosage and a prolonged context-sensitive half-time (Fig. 27-23).[321] Hemorrhagic shock also altered the pharmacokinetics of remifentanil, suggesting that less remifentanil would be required to maintain a target plasma concentration (Fig. 27-24).[322] However, because of its rapid metabolism, changes in context-sensitive half-time are small.

Anesthetic Techniques Using Opioids

Analgesia

Opioids are frequently used to relieve pain during monitored anesthesia care and regional anesthesia.

A single bolus of opioids can provide significant pain relief. Morphine is slow in onset and does not allow rapid titration to effect. Meperidine (50 to 100 mg IV) produces variable degrees of pain relief and is not always effective in patients with severe

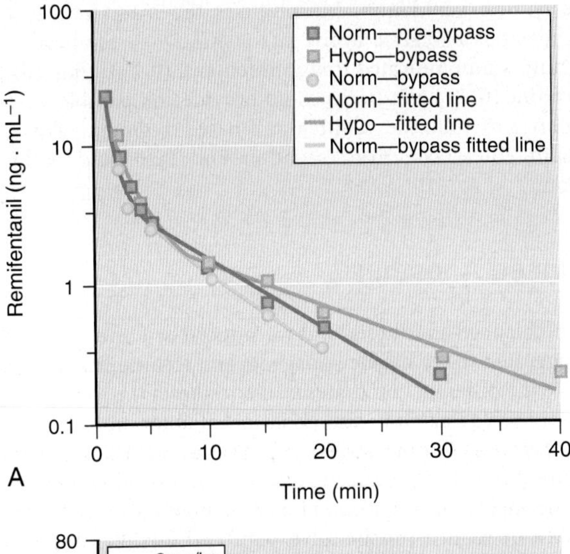

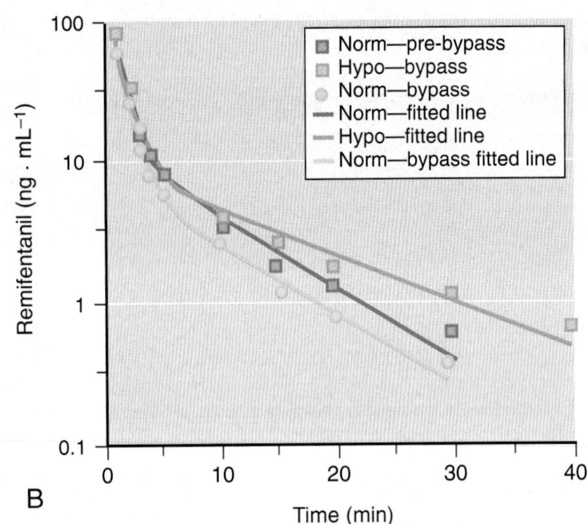

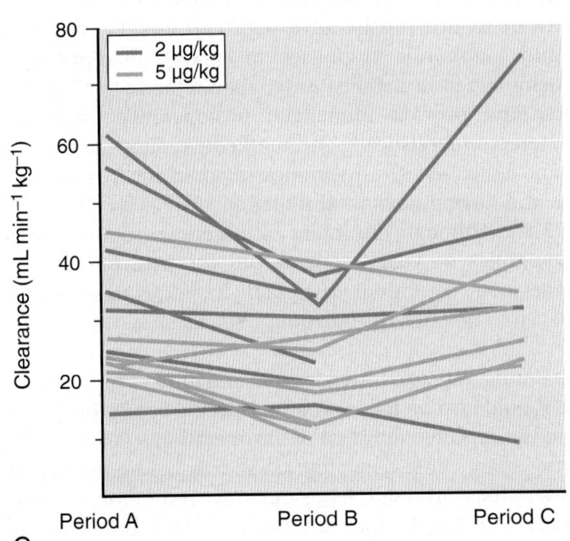

Figure 27-22 Effect of cardiopulmonary bypass (CPB) on the pharmacokinetics of remifentanil. Remifentanil was administered as a bolus of 2 μg/kg (**A**) or 5 μg/kg (**B**), and time-dependent changes in mean blood concentration were assessed. Clearance of remifentanil (**C**) after the administration of 2 or 5 μg/kg was measured during period A (pre-bypass, normothermia), period B (CPB, hypothermia), and period C (CPB, normothermia). Clearance during period B was significantly lower than during period A or C. *(From Russell D, Royston D, Rees PH, et al: Effect of temperature and cardiopulmonary bypass on the pharmacokinetics of remifentanil. Br J Anaesth 79:456-459, 1997.)*

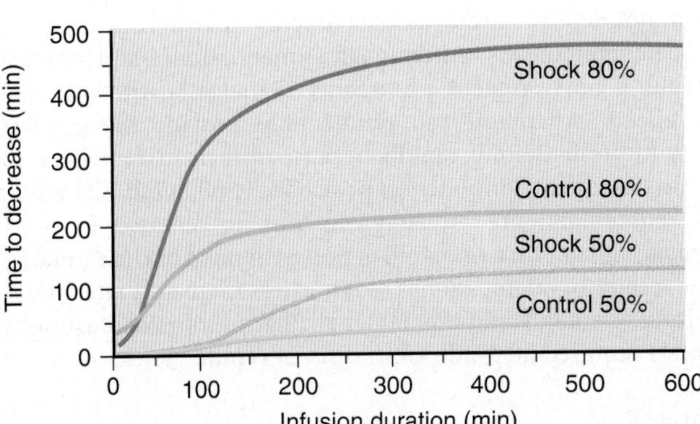

Figure 27-23 Computer simulation of the context-sensitive half-times (50% decrement times) and 80% decrement times of fentanyl in shock versus control animals. *(From Egan TD, Kuramkote S, Gong G, et al: Fentanyl pharmacokinetics in hemorrhagic shock: A porcine model. Anesthesiology 91:156-166, 1999.)*

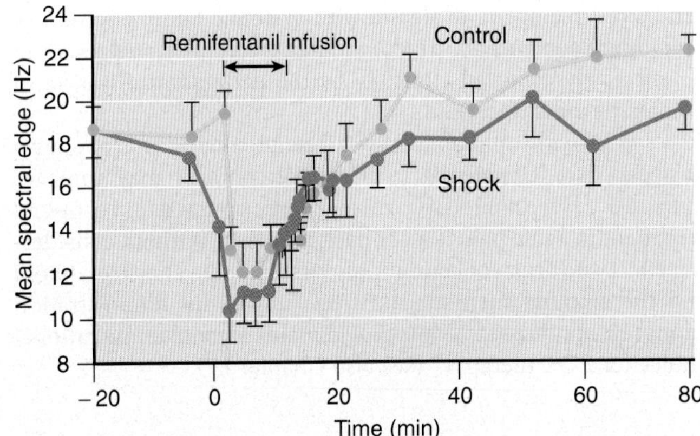

Figure 27-24 Mean spectral edge changes versus time during remifentanil infusion. The *green* and *blue* indicate spectral edge measurements for the control animals and animals with hemorrhagic shock, respectively. *(From Johnson KB, Kern SE, Hamber EA, et al: Influence of hemorrhagic shock on remifentanil: A pharmacokinetic and pharmacodynamic analysis. Anesthesiology 94:322-332, 2001.)*

Table 27-6 Range of Approximate Plasma (or Whole Blood for Remifentanil) Opioid Concentrations (ng/mL)

	Fentanyl	Sufentanil	Alfentanil	Remifentanil
Predominant agent	15-30	5-10	400-800	—
Major surgery	4-10	1-3	200-400	2-4
Minor surgery	3-6	0.25-1	50-200	1-3
Spontaneous ventilation	1-3	<0.4	<200	0.3-0.6
Analgesia	1-2	0.2-0.4	50-150	0.2-0.4

From Bailey PL, Egan TD, Stanley TH: Intravenous opioid anesthetics. *In* Miller RD (ed): Anesthesia, 5th ed. New York, Churchill Livingstone, 2000, p 330.

pain. Intravenous boluses of fentanyl (1 to 3 μg/kg), alfentanil (10 to 20 μg/kg), or sufentanil (0.1 to 0.3 μg/kg) can produce potent and short-lasting analgesia. Infusion rates range from 0.01 to 0.05 μg/kg/min for fentanyl, 0.0015 to 0.01 μg/kg/min for sufentanil, 0.25 to 0.75 μg/kg/min for alfentanil, and 0.05 to 0.25 μg/kg/min for remifentanil. The plasma concentrations of opioids needed for various purposes are listed in Table 27-6.

Changes in the excitability of central neurons play an important role in the establishment of pain. Low doses of fentanyl block the synaptic form of central sensitization in the rat spinal cord in vivo, suggesting the possibility of preemptive analgesia by fentanyl, but larger doses do not have this effect.[323] Reductions in postoperative pain and improved recovery have been attributed to preemptive analgesia with either epidural fentanyl or bupivacaine after radical prostatectomy.[324] In contrast, in patients undergoing transperitoneal tumor nephrectomy, preoperative intravenous administration of a combination of morphine, ketamine, and clonidine failed to exert a clinically relevant effect on postoperative pain.[325] Aida and coauthors reported that the effectiveness of preemptive analgesia varies according to the type of surgery and that preemptive analgesia with epidural morphine was reliably effective in limb and breast surgery but ineffective in abdominal surgery.[326] A meta-analysis demonstrated that the results of preemptive analgesia with systemic administration of opioids are equivocal.[327] Thus, whether preemptive analgesia can be effectively achieved clinically by the early administration of opioids remains uncertain.

PCA with opioids is now a cornerstone of postoperative analgesia (see Chapter 87). PCA with opioids may improve outcome.[328] Nevertheless, pharmacokinetic optimization of opioid treatment in acute pain is a complex matter.[329] Without considering effect-site drug concentrations over time, the choice of opioid and the amount, method, and frequency of its administration cannot be optimized.[329] Morphine remains a popular and rational choice for PCA therapy[330] (see also Chapter 87).

Sedation

Critically ill subjects in the intensive care unit (ICU) often experience anxiety and agitation while being exposed to numerous stressful or noxious stimuli. ICU patients generally require a combination of analgesia and sedation to relieve their state of anxiety, improve adaptation to the endotracheal tube, and aid compliance with mechanical ventilation. Morphine is the most frequently used intravenous analgesic agent in the ICU.[331] A randomized double-blind study indicated that remifentanil (0.15 μg/kg/min) and morphine (0.75 μg/kg/min) could provide comparable levels of sedation and that the remifentanil-based regimen allowed more rapid emergence from sedation and facilitated earlier extubation.[332]

Balanced Anesthesia

The term "balanced anesthesia" was introduced by Lundy in 1926. Lundy suggested that a balance of agents and techniques be used to produce the different components of anesthesia (i.e., analgesia, amnesia, muscle relaxation, and abolition of autonomic reflexes with maintenance of homeostasis). Anesthesia with a single agent can require doses that produce excessive hemodynamic depression.[333] The inclusion of an opioid as a component of balanced anesthesia can reduce preoperative pain and anxiety, decrease somatic and autonomic responses to airway manipulation, improve hemodynamic stability, lower requirements for inhaled anesthetics, and provide immediate postoperative analgesia. Opioids interact synergistically and markedly reduce the dose of propofol and other sedative-hypnotics required for loss of consciousness and during noxious stimulation such as skin incision (Fig. 27-25).[334] Although the intent of combining opioids with sedative-hypnotics or volatile anesthetics (or with both) is to produce anesthetic conditions with stable hemodynamics before as well as after noxious stimulation, this ideal is not always achieved.[335,336]

The timing, rate of administration, and dose of supplemental opioid should also be tailored to the specific condition of the patient and the expected duration of the operation to avoid problems. Giving a large dose of any opioid shortly before the end of surgery is very likely to result in postoperative respiratory depression. However, analgesic concentrations of opioids have little effect on the MAC-awake of inhaled anesthetics.[337]

Choice of Opioid

The ideal opioid would permit rapid titration, successfully prevent unwanted responses to noxious stimuli, require little supplementation, not depress cardiovascular function, permit the return of adequate spontaneous ventilation in a timely manner, and produce residual, if not complete, postoperative analgesia with minimal side effects. Alfentanil and remifentanil provide the greatest ability to titrate opioids rapidly because of their extremely rapid time to onset (1 to 2 minutes) of peak effect. Sufentanil, alfentanil, and remifentanil are arguably superior to fentanyl in most respects. Antagonism of opioid action with naloxone for troublesome respiratory depression is required less frequently after alfentanil and sufentanil than after fentanyl. Pharmacologic antagonism is rarely required after administration of remifentanil.

Fentanyl

Anesthetic induction is usually achieved by combining a loading dose of fentanyl (2 to 6 μg/kg) with a sedative-hypnotic, most commonly thiopental or propofol, and a muscle relaxant. Maintenance of anesthesia can be achieved with N_2O (60% to 70%) in O_2, low concentrations of potent inhaled anesthetics, and additional fentanyl (intermittent boluses of 25 to 50 μg every 15 to 30 minutes or a constant infusion of 0.5 to 5.0 μg/kg/hr).

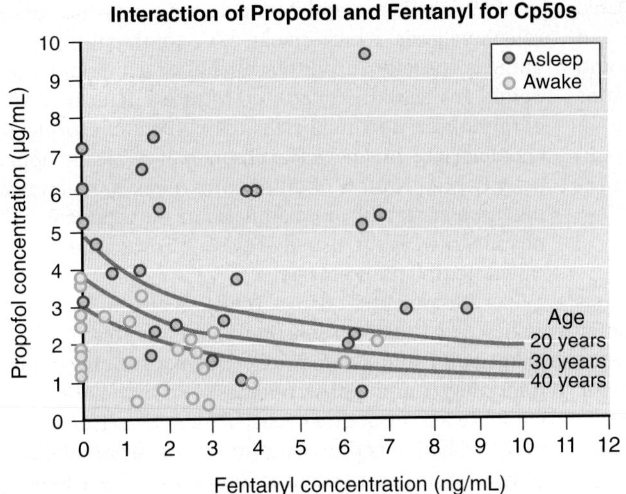

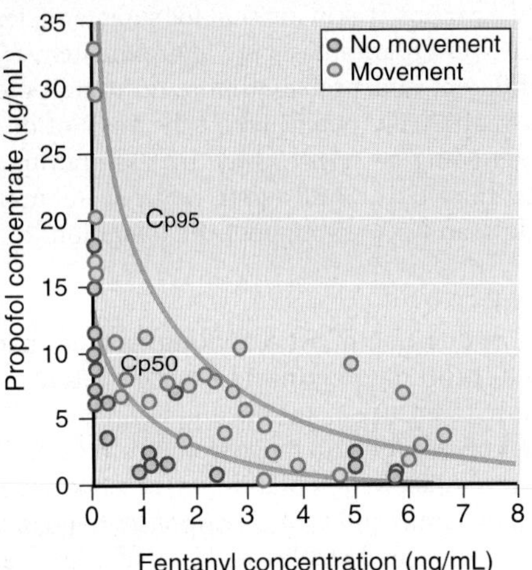

Figure 27-25 **Left,** Measured arterial propofol and fentanyl concentrations at which patients did and did not respond to a verbal command at 10 minutes after initiation of infusion of these drugs. *Solid lines* represent the modeled concentration of propofol according to decade of age when combined with measured fentanyl concentrations at which 50% of patients did not respond to verbal command (Cp_{50}). **Right,** Reduction of the propofol concentration at which 50% or 95% of patients did not move at skin incision by increasing the concentration of fentanyl (Cp_{50} and Cp_{95}, respectively). *Sold lines* represent logistic regression solutions. *(From Smith C, McEwan AI, Jhaveri R, et al: The interaction of fentanyl on the Cp_{50} of propofol for loss of consciousness and skin incision. Anesthesiology 81:820-828, 1994.)*

The plasma concentration of fentanyl required for postoperative analgesia was approximately 1.5 ng/mL,[338] but levels of at least 2 to 3 ng/mL are usually required during surgery if the only inhaled agent is N_2O. In unpremedicated patients anesthetized with a fentanyl infusion and N_2O in O_2, the Cp_{50} (minimal steady-state plasma concentration of an intravenous analgesic/anesthetic required to prevent a somatic response in 50% of patients after skin incision) and Cp_{50}-BAR (minimal plasma concentration of an intravenous analgesic/anesthetic required to prevent either a somatic, hemodynamic, or autonomic response in 50% of patients after skin incision) for fentanyl at skin incision are 3.26 and 4.17 ng/mL, respectively.[339] The MAC of isoflurane at skin incision can be reduced by 50% and 63% with plasma fentanyl concentrations of 1.67 and 3.0 ng/mL, respectively.[74] Increasing plasma fentanyl concentrations from 3.0 to 10 ng/mL only further reduced the MAC of isoflurane from 63% to 82%. The intraoperative requirement for propofol is also reduced by fentanyl. In patients undergoing spine fusion, to keep mean arterial pressure within 15% of the control value when fentanyl was infused to keep the plasma concentration at 0, 1.5, 3.0, and 4.5 ng/mL, average propofol infusion rates were 10.1 ± 2.5 (mean ± SD), 7.5 ± 1.2, 5.7 ± 1.1, and 4.9 ± 1.2 mg/kg/hr, respectively.[340]

Opioid pharmacokinetics and pharmacodynamics vary considerably among patients. It was reported that basing the fentanyl dose on total body weight may cause overdosing in obese patients.[338] Nevertheless, a balanced technique with fentanyl, titrated in anticipation of various stimuli and patient responses with pharmacokinetic guidelines in mind, will often result in a stable hemodynamic course and rapid awakening in a pain-free patient. Repeated doses or continuous infusions of fentanyl are most likely to result in significant depression of spontaneous ventilation.

Alfentanil

Because alfentanil penetrates the brain so rapidly, equilibration of alfentanil between plasma and the CNS can be achieved while plasma alfentanil levels are quite high relative to those of sufentanil and fentanyl. This property explains how low doses (10 to 30 µg/kg) of alfentanil, administered just before or simultaneously with a sedative-hypnotic, are effective.

Alfentanil (25 to 50 µg/kg IV), followed by small titrated sleep doses of any sedative-hypnotic (e.g., 50 to 100 mg sodium thiopental), is usually successful in preventing significant hemodynamic stimulation from laryngoscopy and intubation. Further opioid supplementation can be achieved with an alfentanil infusion (0.5 to 2.0 µg/kg/min) or intermittent boluses of alfentanil (5 to 10 µg/kg) for shorter procedures. In balanced anesthetic techniques in which potent inhaled anesthetics are also administered, relatively low plasma alfentanil concentrations (e.g., 29 ng/mL) can reduce the MAC of isoflurane by approximately 50%.[90] The EC_{50} of alfentanil during propofol anesthesia, in which the plasma concentration of propofol was kept at target concentrations of 3 µg/mL, was 92 ng/mL for intubation, 55 ng/mL for skin incision, 84 ng/mL for opening of the peritoneum, and 66 ± 38 ng/mL for the intra-abdominal portion of the surgery.[341] It was reported that the hemodynamic changes induced by propofol might have an important influence on the pharmacokinetics of alfentanil. Propofol (target concentration, 1.5 µg/mL) decreased the elimination clearance of alfentanil by 15%, rapid distribution clearance by 68%, slow distribution clearance by 51%, and lag time by 62%.[342] Alfentanil infusions or repeated doses should be minimized 15 to 30 minutes before the end of surgery to avoid problematic residual respiratory depression.

Sufentanil

The mean plasma sufentanil concentration reported to be the Cp_{50} for prevention of hemodynamic responses to laryngoscopy and tracheal intubation was 1.08 ng/mL with a range of 0.73 to 2.55. Maintenance of anesthesia can be achieved with N_2O (60% to 70%) in O_2 and additional sufentanil (intermittent boluses of 0.1 to 0.25 µg/kg or a constant infusion of 0.5 to 1.5 µg/kg/hr). The Cp_{50} for sufentanil during skin incision (2.08 ± 0.62 ng/mL) is twice as great as that for intubation in unpremedicated patients.[343] Cp_{50} ratios at skin incision for sufentanil, fentanyl, and alfentanil in N_2O-O_2 anesthesia are approximately 1:2:150 and represent different and probably more accurate potency ratios than those traditionally published on the basis of drug dose. In patients undergoing coronary artery bypass grafting, sufentanil doses greater than 1.25 ± 0.21 ng/mL reduced isoflurane requirements to less than 0.5% throughout the operation.[344]

Remifentanil

The very short duration of action of remifentanil mandates that an infusion (0.1 to 1.0 μg/kg/min) be started before or soon after the bolus dose to ensure a sustained opioid effect. Maintenance infusion rates of remifentanil range from 0.1 to 1.0 μg/kg/min for balanced anesthesia. Remifentanil can reliably suppress autonomic, hemodynamic, and somatic responses to noxious stimulation and allows predictable and rapid emergence from anesthesia.[345]

The use of remifentanil permits rapid (5 to 15 minutes) emergence without postoperative respiratory depression.[346] Infusion rates of 0.1 ± 0.05 μg/kg/min should allow the return of spontaneous ventilation and responsiveness with maintenance of analgesia. A randomized, double-blind, placebo-controlled study demonstrated that the combination of 0.05 to 0.1 μg/kg/min remifentanil and 2 mg midazolam provided effective sedation and analgesia during outpatient surgical procedures performed under local anesthesia.[347] Administration of remifentanil, 1 μg/kg followed by 0.5 μg/kg/min, with propofol and 66% N_2O provided sufficient anesthesia for craniotomy with stable hemodynamics and rapid tracheal extubation.[348]

During emergence from remifentanil anesthesia, the need for alternative analgesic therapies should be anticipated and administered in timely fashion. It was reported that perioperative administration of morphine (0.15 or 0.25 mg/kg IV) or fentanyl (0.15 mg) did not provide entirely adequate immediate postoperative pain control after remifentanil-based anesthesia for major abdominal surgery.[349,350] Administration of ketamine (0.15 mg/kg followed by 2 μg/kg/min) decreased intraoperative remifentanil use during abdominal surgery and postoperative morphine consumption without increasing the incidence of side effects.[351] In children undergoing strabismus surgery, the combination of sevoflurane (2.5%) and remifentanil (1 μg/kg followed by 0.1 to 0.2 μg/kg/min) produced less frequent postoperative vomiting but higher postoperative pain scores than fentanyl did (2 μg/kg followed by 1 μg/kg every 45 minutes).[352]

Postoperative pain relief with low-dose remifentanil infusion was also reported. After general anesthesia with propofol (75 μg/kg/min) and remifentanil (0.5 to 1.0 μg/kg/min) for abdominal or thoracic surgery, continuous infusion of remifentanil (0.05 or 0.1 μg/kg/min) provided adequate analgesia.[353]

Neuroleptanalgesia-Neuroleptanesthesia

In 1949, Laborit and Huygenard introduced the concept of an anesthetic technique that blocked not only cerebrocortical responses but also some cellular, endocrine, and autonomic mechanisms usually activated by surgical stimulation. This state was called "ganglioplegia" or "neuroplegia" (artificial hibernation) and was achieved with the use of a lytic cocktail consisting of chlorpromazine, promethazine, and meperidine. From this idea, in 1959 De Castro and Mundeleer derived the concept of neuroleptanalgesia, which involved the combination of a major tranquilizer (usually the butyrophenone droperidol) and a potent opioid analgesic (fentanyl) to produce a detached, pain-free state of immobilization and insensitivity to pain. Neuroleptanalgesia is characterized by analgesia, absence of clinically apparent motor activity, suppression of autonomic reflexes, maintenance of cardiovascular stability, and amnesia in most patients. The addition of an inhaled agent, usually N_2O, improves amnesia and has been called neuroleptanesthesia.

"Neuroleptic" drugs traditionally include the phenothiazines (e.g., chlorpromazine) and the butyrophenones (e.g., haloperidol and droperidol). Butyrophenones cause sedation, tranquility, immobility, antiemesis, an extrapyramidal syndrome with face and neck dyskinesia, oculogyric crises, torticollis, agitation, and hallucinations. Administering droperidol alone, without analgesics or other sedatives, often produces feelings of discomfort or dysphoria in patients. The cardiovascular effects of droperidol are most often limited to mild hypotension, which is thought to be mediated through α-adrenergic blockade. There is little respiratory depression induced by droperidol, although significant variability exists and respiratory depression may be noted occasionally. Droperidol and other butyrophenones may enhance hypoxic-induced increases in ventilation in humans because of their antidopaminergic effects at the carotid body. Droperidol can be used as a premedicant (0.025 to 0.075 mg/kg IM), an antiemetic (0.01 to 0.02 mg/kg IV), an adjunct for awake intubation (0.025 to 0.1 mg/kg IV), and therapy for agitated, belligerent, or psychotic patients (0.05 to 0.2 mg/kg IV or IM).

Neuroleptanalgesia or neuroleptanesthesia is contraindicated in patients receiving monoamine oxidase inhibitors (MAOIs), in those who abuse drugs or alchohol, or in patients with Parkinson's disease.

Total Intravenous Anesthesia

Many different intravenous compounds can be used in a number of combinations to provide TIVA. Most commonly, an opioid is combined with another drug more likely to provide hypnosis and amnesia. For example, the combination of alfentanil and propofol produces excellent TIVA. Alfentanil provides analgesia and hemodynamic stability while blunting responses to noxious stimuli. On the other hand, propofol provides hypnosis and amnesia and is antiemetic. Profound synergism also exists when more than two agents, such as propofol-alfentanil-midazolam, are combined.[354,355] Induction of anesthesia with alfentanil (25 to 50 μg/kg) and propofol (0.5 to 1.5 mg/kg), followed by infusions of alfentanil at 0.5 to 1.5 μg/kg/min and propofol at 80 to 120 μg/kg/min, will produce anesthesia in patients ventilated with air and O_2 with or without N_2O for a variety of procedures. It is proposed that alfentanil concentrations as low as 85 ng/mL, when combined with a blood propofol concentration of 3.5 μg/mL, can produce both optimal anesthetic conditions and speed of recovery.[355] Stanski and Shafer suggested that bolus doses and initial infusion rates would be 30 μg/kg and 0.35 μg/kg/min for alfentanil and 0.7 mg/kg and 180 μg/kg/min for propofol.[356] Recognizing that these calculations were based on EC_{50} data in patients undergoing only moderately painful procedures, anesthesiologists should adjust these doses accordingly. Premedication before alfentanil-propofol anesthesia can prolong postoperative recovery and should be avoided if appropriate.[357] In patients undergoing ear-nose-throat surgery, TIVA with remifentanil and propofol provided more rapid respiratory recovery after brief surgical procedures than TIVA with alfentanil and propofol did.[358]

The optimal propofol-opioid concentrations that ensure adequate anesthesia and rapid emergence were determined by computer modeling. The optimal propofol concentration decreases in the order of fentanyl > alfentanil > sufentanil ≫ remifentanil. A shorter context-sensitive half-time allows the administration of greater amounts of opioid (and less propofol) during anesthesia without creating prolonged opioid effects.

Maintenance infusions vary according to patient condition and surgical stimuli. Propofol (75 to 125 μg/kg/min) and alfentanil (1.0 to 2.0 μg/kg/min) are initially recommended. Drug infusions should be terminated 10 to 20 minutes before the end of anesthesia if N_2O is used. Otherwise, propofol infusions should be terminated 5 to 10 minutes before anticipated patient awakening. Alfentanil infusion rates do not need to be less than 0.25 to 0.5 μg/kg/min until surgery is terminated. A multicenter evaluation demonstrated that in patients undergoing elective inpatient surgery, remifentanil, 1 μg/kg intravenously, followed by 1.0 μg/kg/min, when combined with propofol, 75 μg/kg/min, effectively controlled responses to tracheal intubation.[346] Reduction of the remifentanil infusion rate to 0.25 to 0.40 μg/kg/min after tracheal intubation was also recommended.

Midazolam-opioid combinations can also provide complete anesthesia. However, midazolam-alfentanil TIVA has not been found to compare favorably with propofol-alfentanil TIVA, even with flumazenil reversal of benzodiazepine action.[359]

TIVA techniques are especially useful when delivery of inhaled agents is compromised. By keeping the goals of balanced anesthesia in mind, combining modern opioids and other drugs, using infusion pumps, and having an increased understanding of pharmacokinetics, clinicians can successfully perform a variety of TIVA techniques. Approximate opioid doses and infusion rates for TIVA are listed in Table 27-7.

Opioid-Based (High-Dose Opioid) Anesthesia for Cardiac Surgery

Opioids can be administered as the primary or sole anesthetic in opioid-based anesthetic techniques. High-dose opioid anesthesia was introduced as a stress-free anesthetic method for cardiac surgery (also see Chapter 60). However, several factors have diminished the popularity of high-dose opioid anesthesia, even in cardiac anesthesia, including the lack of evidence substantiating any significant outcome benefit associated with the use of large doses of opioids, the added drug costs, and the trend toward "fast-track" approaches to cardiac patients that can be impeded by large doses of opioids, especially fentanyl.[212,360] Nonetheless, opioids, particularly when administered by continuous infusion, are still among the most effective anesthetics for patients undergoing cardiac or other extensive operations. High-dose opioid anesthesia was first performed with morphine. However, fentanyl and sufentanil were recommended later.

In an attempt to decrease the cost of cardiac surgery, fast-track programs have become popular. Engoren and associates reported that the more expensive but shorter-acting opioids sufentanil and remifentanil produce equally rapid extubation, similar stays, and similar costs to fentanyl, indicating that any of these opioids can be recommended for fast-track cardiac surgery.[361]

Table 27-7 Approximate Opioid Loading (Bolus) Doses, Maintenance Infusion Rates, and Additional Maintenance Doses for Total Intravenous Anesthesia

	Loading Dose (μg/kg)	Maintenance Infusion Rate	Additional Boluses
Alfentanil	25-100	0.5-2 μg/kg/min	5-10 μg/kg
Sufentanil	0.25-2	0.5-1.5 μg/kg/hr	2.5-10 μg
Fentanyl	4-20	2-10 μg/kg/hr	25-100 μg
Remifentanil	1-2	0.1-1.0 μg/kg/min	0.1-1.0 μg/kg

From Bailey PL, Egan TD, Stanley TH: Intravenous opioid anesthetics. *In* Miller RD (ed): Anesthesia, 5th ed. New York, Churchill Livingstone, 2000, p 335.

Fentanyl

Many different techniques have been used to achieve anesthesia with fentanyl.[360,362] Rapid or slow bolus injections of fentanyl range from 5 to 75 μg/kg. These doses will establish plasma fentanyl concentrations (10 to 30 ng/mL) that are often sufficient to provide stable hemodynamics throughout the induction/intubation sequence. Continuous infusions of fentanyl for cardiac surgery range from 0.1 to 1.0 μg/kg/min up to or continuing through CPB. High-dose fentanyl anesthesia has also proved effective and safe for pediatric heart surgery. It was indicated that fentanyl, 25 to 50 μg/kg, combined with isoflurane, 0.2% to 0.4%, was sufficient to obtund hemodynamic and stress responses in the pre-CPB phase of open heart surgery in infants and young children (Fig. 27-26).[363] On the other hand, high-dose fentanyl, 75 to 100 μg/kg, was shown to cause prolonged suppression of NK cell function.[364] It was reported that 57 of 59 eligible patients were successfully extubated at 34 ± 14 minutes after termination of fentanyl (total dose, 127 ± 64 μg/kg) with naloxone (total bolus, 3.4 ± 2.6 μg/kg) and recovered fully without ventilatory support under the naloxone infusion, which was terminated at 11 ± 7 hours.[365] These results suggest that naloxone infusion with individual dose titration facilitates the use of high-dose opioid anesthesia while maintaining the advantage of this anesthesia. It was recently shown that high-dose fentanyl (50 μg/kg) is not associated with a difference in the incidence of postoperative cognitive dysfunction at 3 or 12 months after coronary artery bypass surgery in the elderly, whereas low-dose fentanyl (10 μg/kg) leads to shorter postoperative ventilation times and may be associated with a greater incidence of postoperative cognitive dysfunction 1 week after surgery.[366]

Alfentanil

Induction of anesthesia with large doses of alfentanil has been applied to cardiac surgery.[367] Large doses of alfentanil (150 μg/kg) may be used with or without thiopental to induce anesthesia. Other investigators claim that anesthesia cannot be reliably induced with alfentanil alone, at least in young and healthy adults.[85] Continuous infusions of alfentanil (2 to 12 μg/kg/min) have been used to maintain moderate to very high plasma alfentanil concentrations (<3000 ng/mL) during cardiac surgery. Enthusiasm for high-dose alfentanil anesthesia techniques is limited by the amount (and cost) of drug required and sugges-

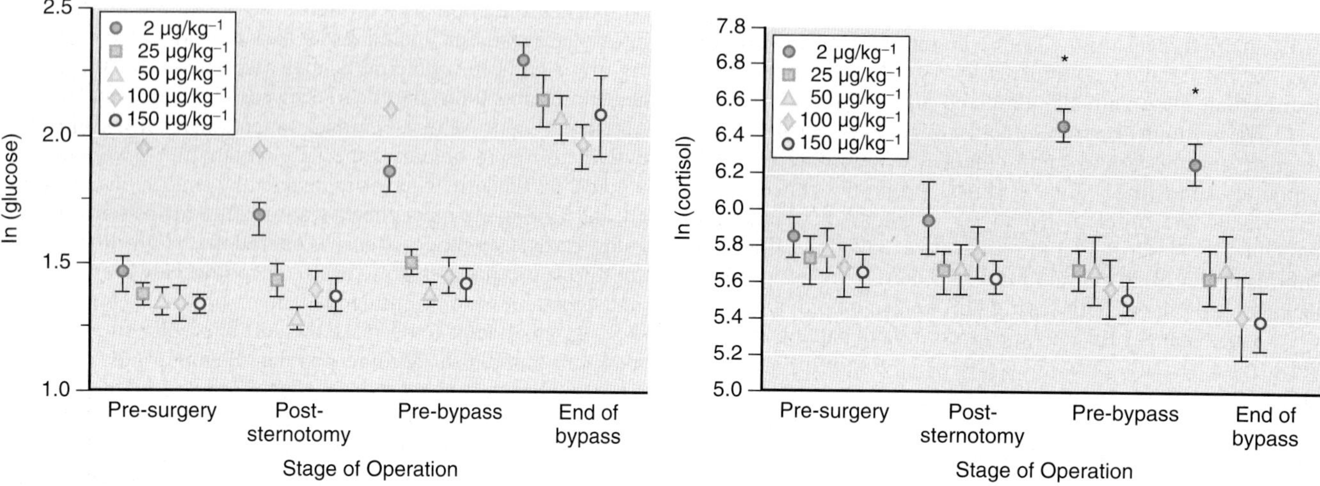

Figure 27-26 Suppression of stress responses in the pre-bypass phase of open heart surgery in infants and young children by fentanyl combined with a low concentration (0.2% to 0.4%) of isoflurane: mean (± SE) ln (glucose) (*left*) or ln (cortisol) (*right*) versus stage of surgery for each dose of fentanyl. The values for the 2-μg/kg group indicated by *asterisks* were significantly higher ($P < .01$) than in the other groups. ln, natural logarithm. *(From Benthuysen JL, Foltz BD, Smith NT, et al: Prebypass hemodynamic stability of sufentanil-O_2, fentanyl-O_2, and morphine-O_2 anesthesia during cardiac surgery: A comparison of cardiovascular profiles. J Cardiothorac Anesth 12:749-757, 1988.)*

tions that alfentanil anesthesia for cardiac surgery is inadequate and associated with more cardiovascular adverse effects than is the case with fentanyl and sufentanil. More modest doses of alfentanil have been successfully administered in combination with sedative-hypnotics such as propofol for cardiac anesthesia.[368]

Sufentanil

Advantages of high-dose sufentanil include more rapid induction, better blunting or elimination of hypertensive episodes, greater reduction in left ventricular stroke work, and higher cardiac output and more stable hemodynamics intraoperatively and postoperatively.[369] Induction doses of sufentanil range from 2 to 20 μg/kg administered as a bolus or infused over a period of 2 to 10 minutes. Total doses of sufentanil used in high-dose techniques usually range from 15 to 30 μg/kg, but no additional benefit could be demonstrated in terms of hemodynamic control or EEG signs by increasing the dose of sufentanil from 3 to 15 μg/kg for induction of anesthesia in patients premedicated with lorazepam.[370] It has been thought that muscle rigidity during induction of anesthesia with high-dose opioid causes difficult ventilation with a mask. However, it was shown that the difficult ventilation during induction of anesthesia with sufentanil, 3 μg/kg, is due to upper airway closure at the level of the glottis or above.[371]

The amount of sufentanil required can be markedly influenced by the supplements administered concomitantly. For patients undergoing coronary artery surgery, induction (0.4 ± 0.2 μg/kg) and total maintenance (2.4 ± 0.8 μg/kg) doses of sufentanil were used in combination with propofol (1.5 ± 1 mg/kg for induction and 32 ± 12 mg/kg total). Interestingly, sufentanil requirements tripled when midazolam was used instead of propofol.[372] Etomidate, combined with an opioid, can provide excellent anesthetic conditions with minimal hemodynamic perturbations. Inducing anesthesia with sufentanil (0.5 to 1.0 μg/kg) and etomidate (0.1 to 0.2 mg/kg) frequently confers hemodynamic stability. Maintenance of anesthesia with an infusion of sufentanil (1.0 to 2.0 μg/kg/hr) in a balanced anesthetic technique achieves the advantages of opioid-based anesthesia and avoids prolonged opioid action into the postoperative period.

Remifentanil

Remifentanil has been used in cardiac anesthesia.[318] It was shown that induction with remifentanil, 2 μg/kg, and propofol and maintenance with remifentanil at 0.25 or 0.5 μg/kg/min provided appropriate anesthesia for minimally invasive coronary artery bypass surgery with rapid awakening and tracheal extubation (Fig. 27-27).[373] Kazmaier and coworkers compared high-dose remifentanil (2.0 μg/kg/min) and remifentanil (0.5 μg/kg/min) combined with propofol (target-controlled infusion aiming at a plasma concentration of 2.0 μg/mL) in patients undergoing elective coronary artery bypass grafting.[374] It was demonstrated that high-dose remifentanil reduces the stroke volume index, heart rate, mean arterial pressure, myocardial blood flow, and myocardial oxygen uptake and that its effects do not differ from those of remifentanil/propofol anesthesia. Geisler and colleagues examined the efficacy and safety of high-dose remifentanil anesthesia in patients undergoing coronary artery bypass graft surgery.[375] It was demonstrated that continuous infusions of remifentanil at 1.0 to 2.0 μg/kg/min in combination with propofol, 3 mg/kg/hr, provided profound suppression of responses to surgical stimuli in the majority of patients, but there was a high incidence of muscle rigidity when remifentanil was used to induce anesthesia. They concluded that there was no apparent advantage in starting the remifentanil infusion rate above 1.0 μg/kg/min and that remifentanil is not suitable for use as a sole induction agent.

Other Applications of Opioids

Transdermal Therapeutic System

Transdermal drug delivery generally requires high solubility in both water and oil, low molecular weight, high potency, and little or no skin irritation. Fentanyl is available in a transdermal therapeutic system (TTS). Potential advantages of delivering fentanyl

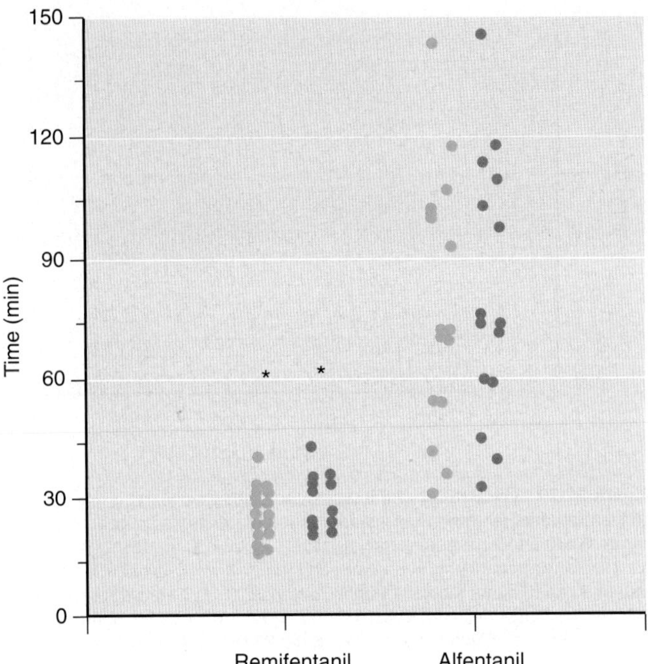

Figure 27-27 Times to awakening (*green circles*) and tracheal extubation (*blue circles*) in patients who underwent minimally invasive direct coronary artery bypass surgery after intravenous anesthesia with remifentanil-propofol or alfentanil-propofol. *(From Ahonen J, Olkkola KT, Verkkala K, et al: A comparison of remifentanil and alfentanil for use with propofol in patients undergoing minimally invasive coronary artery bypass surgery. Anesth Analg 90:1269-1274, 2000.)*

transdermally include no first-pass drug metabolism by the liver; improved patient compliance, convenience, and comfort; and consistent analgesia. Doses of TTS fentanyl include 20, 50, 75, and 100 μg/hr, and blood levels ranging from less than 1.0 to 2.0 ng/mL are achieved, although significant variability exists.[376] The pharmacokinetics of transdermally delivered fentanyl (50 μg/hr) was compared in 10 young adult (25- to 38-year-old) and 8 elderly (64- to 82-year-old) patients.[377] It was shown that the mean half-time (time for plasma concentrations to double after patch application) was 4.2 and 11.1 hours and the mean maximum plasma concentration was 1.9 and 1.5 ng/mL in the younger and elderly groups, respectively. There were no differences in the time at which maximum plasma concentrations occurred or the elimination half-life after patch removal. Elevated body temperature accelerates either release of fentanyl from the patch or distribution from the subcutaneous fat depot. Portenoy and coworkers demonstrated that a steady-state serum concentration was achieved by repeated application of TTS fentanyl and that the apparent half-life following system removal after repeated application was relatively long, presumably because of ongoing absorption from a subcutaneous depot (Fig. 27-28).[378]

The results of clinical trials using the transdermal fentanyl system for postoperative analgesia have demonstrated a high incidence of significant respiratory depression, and this application is not recommended.[376] In cancer pain, TTS fentanyl offers an alternative to oral morphine, and its effectiveness and tolerability for this indication have been demonstrated in a number of trials.[379] Its usefulness in chronic pain of nonmalignant origin remains to be confirmed in controlled trials. In general, TTS fentanyl produces the same adverse effects as other opioids, mainly sedation, nausea, vomiting, and constipation. In comparison to oral morphine, TTS fentanyl causes fewer gastrointestinal adverse events. The risk of hypoventilation is comparatively low in cancer patients. Sufentanil and buprenorphine may also be suitable for transdermal delivery, but clinical results are not yet available. Transdermal morphine is useful only if applied to de-epithelialized skin.

Iontophoresis

Iontophoresis is a technique by which drug passage through the skin is augumented with an external electric current. Clinically significant doses of morphine and fentanyl can be delivered iontophoretically.[380] The fentanyl HCl iontophoretic transdermal system (fentanyl ITS) is a novel PCA system that has been approved in the United States and Europe for the management of acute, moderate to severe postoperative pain.[381] This system allows patients to self-administer preprogrammed doses of fentanyl noninvasively through the use of iontophoretic technology. To assess the efficacy and safety of patient-controlled fentanyl ITS (40-μg infusion over a 10-minute period) versus standard intravenous morphine PCA (1-mg bolus every 5 minutes; maximum of 10 mg/hr), a prospective, randomized, controlled, parallel-group trial was performed.[382] The results indicated that the fentanyl ITS can provide pain control equivalent to that of standard morphine PCA, with a similar incidence of opioid-related adverse events. Fentanyl ITS may offer a number of clinical advantages over existing PCA modalities.[381] Its method of drug delivery avoids the risk of complications from needle-related injuries and infection, and its preprogrammed electronics eliminate the potential for manual programming errors and excessive dosing. In addition, the compact size of the system could enable greater patient mobility after surgery. Patient-controlled fentanyl ITS has the potential to become a valuable option in the management of acute postoperative pain.

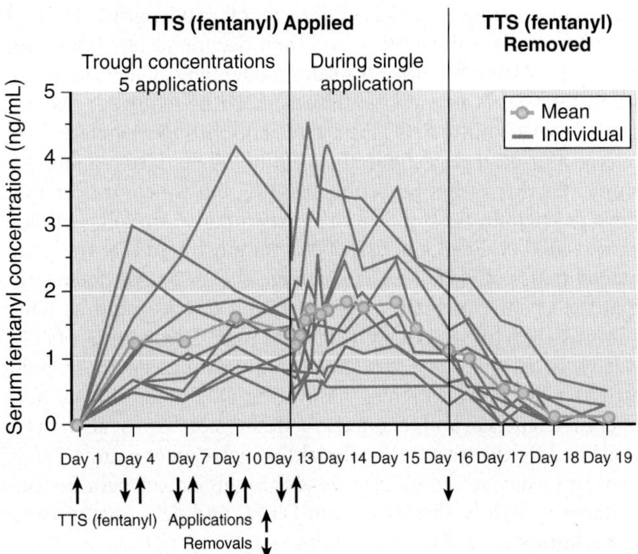

Figure 27-28 Individual and mean (SE) serum fentanyl concentration-time profiles measured in 10 patients during five consecutive applications of the transdermal fentanyl system. *(From Portenoy RK, Southam MA, Gupta SK, et al: Transdermal fentanyl for cancer pain. Repeated dose pharmacokinetics. Anesthesiology 78:36-43, 1993.)*

Transmucosal Drug Delivery

Similar to transdermal drug delivery, transmucosal delivery through the oropharynx and nasopharynx eliminates hepatic first-pass metabolism (drugs are absorbed directly into the systemic circulation) and improves patient comfort, convenience, and compliance.

Buprenorphine, a potent synthetic morphine analog with mixed opioid agonist-antagonist properties and a long half-time, is readily absorbed from sublingual mucosal tissues. The portion of the drug that is swallowed is almost completely metabolized by the liver, and only a small fraction can reach the systemic circulation when swallowed. Systemic bioavailability after sublingual buprenorphine is approximately 50% of that after intravenous administration. In several studies, sublingual buprenorphine (0.4 mg) was compared with conventional intramuscular morphine or meperidine and found to provide comparable and satisfactory analgesia.[383]

The initial experience with buccal morphine for postoperative analgesia had been promising. However, in female patients undergoing lower abdominal surgical procedures, buccal morphine did not significantly reduce postoperative pethidine consumption when compared with placebo, and all patients receiving buccal morphine reported a taste that reduced its acceptability.[384] The low lipid solubility of morphine makes it an unlikely candidate for effective transmucosal absorption. Opioids with high lipid solubility, such as buprenorphine, fentanyl, and methadone, are more effectively absorbed sublingually than those with low lipid solubility, such as morphine.

Oral transmucosal fentanyl citrate (OTFC) is a solid dosage form of fentanyl that consists of fentanyl incorporated into a sweetened lozenge on a stick. A portion of the fentanyl is absorbed through the oral mucosa, and the rest is swallowed and absorbed through the gastrointestinal tract. The swallowed fentanyl has low bioavailability because of hepatic first-pass metabolism. Recommended doses range from 5 to 20 μg/kg.[385,386] OTFC should be administered approximately 30 minutes before surgery (or a painful procedure) to obtain peak effect. Plasma concentrations after administration of OTFC peak at 2.0 ± 0.5 ng/mL 15 to 30 minutes after administration and then decline to less than 1 ng/mL an hour later.[387] Unlike transdermal fentanyl, OTFC leaves no significant depot in mucosal tissues after it is removed. The systemic bioavailability of OTFC is 50%, and this figure reflects both buccal and gastrointestinal absorption. OTFC bioavailability is similar to that of buprenorphine (55%), but much greater than the bioavailability of buccal morphine and other opioids with low lipid solubility. Egan and associates demonstrated that the pharmacokinetics of OTFC did not change with repeated dosing and that the decline in plasma concentration was as rapid as when administered intravenously (Fig. 27-29).[388] Preoperative OTFC was reported to be effective for postoperative analgesia in pediatric tonsillectomy patients.[389] However, OTFC can induce perioperative emesis and respiratory depression. It is also being evaluated for the treatment of breakthrough cancer pain.[390] OTFC may be ideally suited to treat breakthrough cancer pain because fentanyl is rapidly absorbed from OTFC and patients can easily self-administer OTFC.

Delivery of opioids through the nasal mucosa has also been investigated. Pharmacokinetic studies in volunteers have been reported for fentanyl, alfentanil, sufentanil, butorphanol, oxycodone, and buprenorphine.[391] Mean times to achieve maximum serum concentrations vary from 5 to 50 minutes, whereas bioavailability varies from 46% to 71%. Fentanyl, pethidine, and butorphanol have been studied for postoperative pain. Mean onset times vary from 12 to 22 minutes and times to peak effect from 24 to 60 minutes. Transnasal butorphanol provides superior and more prolonged analgesia than do similar doses given intravenously for postoperative pain after cesarean section.[392] PCA with intranasal fentanyl was demonstrated to be effective for postoperative pain management.[393] Side effects of intranasal sufentanil in children include reduced ventilatory compliance (chest wall rigidity), hypoxemia, impaired manual ventilation, and nausea and vomiting.[394,395] It appears that further exploration of the transnasal approach to drug delivery for pain management is merited. Improvements in nasal sprayer devices and opioid formulations may improve the clinical outcome.

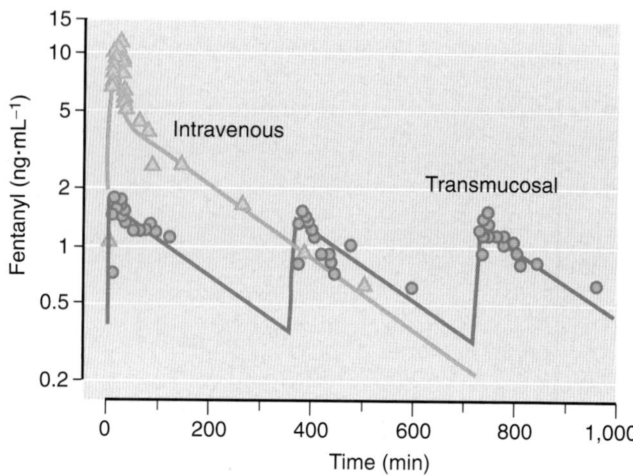

Figure 27-29 Typical result of the time-dependent change in plasma concentration of fentanyl after the application of oral transmucosal fentanyl citrate OTFC) and intravenous administration. Three 800-μg doses of OTFC were administered at 6-hour intervals, and fentanyl was infused at a constant rate of 50 μg/min to a total of 15 μg/kg. *(From Egan TD, Sharma A, Ashburn MA, et al: Multiple dose pharmacokinetics of oral transmucosal fentanyl citrate in healthy volunteers. Anesthesiology 92:665-673, 2000.)*

Inhalation of fentanyl (300 μg) produces a low plasma drug level (0.1 ng/mL) after 15 minutes and analgesia that may be disproportionately greater than expected.[396] Inhaled liposome-encapsulated fentanyl was also demonstrated to be a noninvasive route of administration that provides a rapid increase in and prolonged maintenance of the plasma fentanyl concentration.[397] Inhaled nebulized fentanyl citrate significantly improved patient perception of breathing, the respiratory rate, and oxygen saturation in terminally ill cancer patients.[398] This inexpensive and readily available treatment may offer substantial relief of end-of-life dyspnea. The advent of specialized and efficient pulmonary drug delivery systems has facilitated the evaluation of inhaled opioids, such as morphine and fentanyl, for the management of severe pain associated with surgery or malignant disease.[399]

The rectal mucosa is another site for transmucosal drug delivery. The bioavailability of a 30-mg morphine sulfate controlled-release suppository formulation was significantly greater than that of 30-mg oral controlled-release morphine sulfate tablets, which may be the result of partial avoidance of hepatic biotransformation with rectal administration.[400] The hydrogel formulation of rectal morphine may also be useful for premedication and analgesia in pediatric patients.[401]

Oral Controlled-Release Medications

Despite the high first-pass metabolism of opioid analgesics, morphine has been formulated into an oral, sustained-release tablet (MST) and evaluated for premedication, for postoperative analgesia, and as an analgesic for chronic cancer pain. MST provides unreliable preoperative anxiolysis and postoperative pain relief, possibly because of delayed time to the onset of peak effects (3 to 5 hours), which can be increased by impaired gastric emptying and absorption from the small intestine. As an analgesic for chronic cancer pain, MST was shown to be an excellent choice.[402]

A controlled-release formulation of oxycodone administered every 12 hours for a maximum of 7 days was shown to provide adequate pain control in patients undergoing abdominal, orthopedic, or gynecologic surgery.[403] The relative analgesic potency of single doses of oral controlled-release oxycodone (20 or 40 mg) and oral controlled-release morphine (45 or 90 mg) was compared in a randomized, double-blind trial in women with moderate to severe pain after abdominal hysterectomy.[404] Controlled-release oxycodone at doses of 20 or 40 mg was comparable to controlled-release morphine at doses of 45 or 90 mg, respectively, in total and peak analgesic effects, thus indicating that oral controlled-release oxycodone was twice as potent as oral controlled-release morphine. A randomized, double-blind, crossover trial indicated that controlled-release oxycodone is as safe and effective as controlled-release morphine in the treatment of cancer pain.[405]

Other Opioid Agonists

Codeine (methylmorphine) is half as potent as morphine and has a high oral-parenteral potency ratio (2:3) and a plasma half-life of 2 to 3 hours. Codeine has mild to moderate analgesic but strong cough-suppressant properties after oral administration. CYP2D6 is the enzyme responsible for *O*-demethylation of codeine to morphine.[406] Intravenous codeine produces profound hypotension and is neither approved nor recommended.[407]

Hydromorphone is structurally related to morphine but is approximately 5 to 10 times as potent. Analgesia after hydromorphone lasts 4 to 5 hours.[408] The effects of hydromorphone are essentially indistinguishable from those of heroin.[409] Hydromorphone has been used for both acute and chronic pain conditions in adults and children.[410] It was reported that hydromorphone PCA provided adequate postoperative analgesia with improved mood and that it can be an alternative to morphine PCA.[411]

Levorphanol is an opioid agonist of the morphinan series with a long (12- to 19-hour) half-life. It is five times as potent as morphine with an intramuscular-oral potency ratio of 1:2. Levorphanol may have particular utility in patients who have chronic pain and demonstrate morphine tolerance, perhaps because of differences in opioid receptor activity. The analgesia produced by levorphanol is mediated via its interactions with μ-, δ-, and κ-opioid receptors. Levorphanol is also an NMDA receptor antagonist. The long half-life of the drug increases the potential for drug accumulation.[412]

Methadone has equivalent potency but a longer duration of action than morphine does. The plasma half-life of methadone is very long and variable (13 to 100 hours). Despite this property, many patients require dosing every 4 to 8 hours to maintain analgesic effects. Its major clinical applications are for the prevention of opioid withdrawal symptoms and the treatment of chronic pain. It was shown that the same intravenous dose of methadone (20 mg) that is effective for postoperative pain is also suitable for induction of anesthesia in combination with etomidate and that methadone may have the potential to produce histamine release.[413]

Oxymorphone is a semisynthetic opioid agonist that is specific for the μ-opioid receptor and approved to treat both acute and chronic pain. Because of extensive liver metabolism, oral oxymorphone is contraindicated in patients with moderate to severe hepatic impairment.[414] Oxymorphone, structurally related to morphine, is almost 10 times as potent as morphine but has a similar duration of action. It was shown that in patients with acute moderate to severe postsurgical pain, oral immediate-release oxymorphone, 10, 20, or 30 mg, provided significant dose-related pain relief in comparison to placebo and that this relief was maintained for a period of several days with a safety profile comparable to that of immediate-release oxycodone.[415]

Piritramide, a synthetic opioid structurally related to meperidine, is devoid of emetic activity and is used for postoperative analgesia in several European countries.[416] Pharmacokinetic analysis has shown that piritramide is distributed extensively and eliminated slowly, and intermittent bolus administration is recommended.[417]

Tramadol is a synthetic 4-phenyl-piperidine analog of codeine with a dual mechanism of action. Tramadol stimulates the μ-receptor and, to a lesser extent, the δ- and κ-opioid receptors, and like tricyclic antidepressants, it also activates spinal inhibition of pain by decreasing the reuptake of norepinephrine and serotonin.[418] It is suggested that tramadol may have a direct serotonin-releasing action.[419] Tramadol is one fifth to one tenth as potent as morphine. In rats, tramadol could reduce the MAC of isoflurane in a naloxone-sensitive manner.[420] It was shown that intravenously administered tramadol was effective for post-thoracotomy pain relief.[421] Analgesic doses of tramadol may produce less respiratory depression, in part because of its non–opioid receptor–mediated actions,[422] and have minimal effects on gastrointestinal motor function.[423] Seizures have been reported in patients taking the drug. Caution should be exercised when combining tramadol with MAOIs, neuroleptic agents, and other drugs that lower the seizure threshold. It was suggested that tramadol has local anesthetic properties on peripheral nerves when used alone.[424] Tramadol added to lidocaine for intravenous regional anesthesia provided a shorter time to onset of sensory blockade.[425]

Sameridine possesses both local anesthetic and opioid properties. In patients undergoing arthroscopic knee joint surgery, sameridine was administered intrathecally and provided clinically adequate anesthesia.[426] A large intravenous dose of sameridine depressed resting ventilation and the hypercapnic ventilatory response, whereas a smaller clinical dose did not.[427,428]

M6G is a potent metabolite of morphine. In contrast to morphine, M6G is not metabolized but excreted via the kidneys and exhibits enterohepatic cycling inasmuch as it is a substrate for multidrug resistance transporter proteins in the liver and intestines.[429] M6G exhibits a delay in its analgesic effect (blood effect-site equilibration half-life of 4 to 8 hours), which is partly related to slow passage through the blood-brain barrier and distribution within the brain compartment. In humans, the potency of M6G is just half of that of morphine. Trials to use M6G as an analgesic have been reported. Osborne and colleagues reported that 0.5 to 4 mg of M6G intravenously was effective for cancer pain for 2 to 24 hours without nausea and vomiting.[430] M6G, 100 μg and 125 μg given intrathecally, provided excellent analgesia after total hip replacement, as did intrathecal morphine sulfate, 500 μg.[431]

Agonist-Antagonist Opioid Compounds

Nalorphine, the first agonist-antagonist opioid, was successfully synthesized by Weijland and Erickson in 1942 and found to be strongly antagonistic to almost all the properties of morphine. Although nalorphine was found to possess strong analgesic actions, it was unsuitable for clinical use because of its psychotomimetic effects. Nalorphine was used in lower doses as an opioid antagonist.

Agonist-antagonist opioids are usually produced by alkylation of the piperidine nitrogen and addition of a three-carbon side chain such as a propyl, allyl, or methyl allyl to morphine. Buprenorphine is a partial agonist at the μ-receptor. The other compounds are μ-antagonists and full or partial agonists at the κ-receptor. Agonist-antagonist opioids are less prone (but not immune) to abuse because they cause less euphoria and are associated with less drug-seeking behavior and physical dependence.

Dosing data of these compounds are shown in Table 27-8. Agonist-antagonist compounds depress respiration in a similar manner as morphine, but ceiling effects exist (Table 27-9). Effects on the cardiovascular system differ among these compounds (Table 27-10).

Pentazocine

The analgesia produced by pentazocine is primarily related to stimulation of the κ-receptor. Pentazocine is one half to one fourth as potent as morphine. Ceilings in both analgesia and respiratory depression occur after 30 to 70 mg of pentazocine. Although the potential for abuse is less than with morphine, prolonged use of pentazocine can lead to physical dependence.

Table 27-8 Dosing Data for Agonist-Antagonist Opioids and Morphine

	Equianalgesic Intramuscular Dose (mg)	Duration of Analgesia (hr)	Oral-Intramuscular Efficacy Ratio
Morphine	10	4-5	1:6
Buprenorphine	0.3-0.4	>6	1:2*
Butorphanol	2	3-4	—
Nalbuphine	10	3-6	1:4-5
Pentazocine	40	3	1:3

*Sublingual-intramuscular ratio.

Table 27-9 Respiratory Depressant Effects of Agonist-Antagonists Compared with Morphine*

Drug	Correlation of Respiratory Depression with Dose
Morphine	Increases proportionally with dose
Buprenorphine	Ceiling effect at 0.15-1.2 mg in adults
Butorphanol	Ceiling effect at 30-60 μg/kg
Nalbuphine	Ceiling effect at 30 mg in adults
Pentazocine	Ceiling effect suggested, but difficult to study because of psychotomimetic effects

*Low or moderate naloxone doses readily reverse the respiratory effects produced by therapeutic doses of all the drugs listed except buprenorphine.
From Zola EM, McLeod DC: Comparative effects of analgesic efficacy of the agonist-antagonist opioids. Drug Intell Clin Pharm 17:411, 1983.

Nalorphine-like dysphoric side effects are common, especially after high doses (>60 mg) of pentazocine in the elderly. The dysphoric effects of pentazocine can be reversed with naloxone. Pentazocine depresses myocardial contractility and increases arterial blood pressure, heart rate, systemic vascular resistance, pulmonary artery pressure, and left ventricular work index. Pentazocine also increases blood catecholamine levels.

Pentazocine inhibited gastric emptying and gastrointestinal transit in rats, whereas U50488H, a pure κ-agonist, did not significantly inhibit either.[432] Therefore, it might be speculated that pentazocine affects gastrointestinal function through a mechanism other than the opioid receptors.

Pentazocine has limited application because it is associated with a high incidence of postoperative nausea and vomiting, provides limited analgesia, partially antagonizes other opioids, and can produce undesirable cardiovascular and psychotomimetic effects.

Butorphanol

Butorphanol is an agonist at κ-receptors. Its activity at μ-receptors is either antagonistic or partially agonistic. It is five to eight times as potent as morphine and is available only in parenteral form. After intramuscular injection, the onset of effect is rapid,

Table 27-10 Hemodynamic Effects of Agonist-Antagonist Compounds Compared with Morphine

Drug	Cardiac Workload	Blood Pressure	Heart Rate	Pulmonary Artery Pressure
Morphine	↓	↓	=↓	=↓
Buprenorphine	↓	↓	↓	?
Butorphanol	↑	=↑	=	↑
Nalbuphine	↓	=	=↓	=
Pentazocine	↑	↑	↑	↑

From Zola EM, McLeod DC: Comparative effects of analgesic efficacy of the agonist-antagonist opioids. Drug Intell Clin Pharm 17:411, 1983.

and peak analgesia occurs within 1 hour. Whereas the duration of action of butorphanol is similar to that of morphine, its plasma half-life is only 2 to 3 hours. Although butorphanol (10 mg IM) causes as much respiratory depression as the same dose of morphine, higher doses reach a ceiling. Side effects after butorphanol include drowsiness, sweating, nausea, and CNS stimulation. In healthy volunteers, butorphanol (0.03 or 0.06 mg/kg IV) produces no or minimal cardiovascular changes. However, in patients with cardiac disease, butorphanol causes significant increases in cardiac index, left ventricular end-diastolic pressure, and pulmonary artery pressure.

Because butorphanol decreases the MAC for enflurane by only a small fraction, it cannot serve as an anesthetic agent like the fentanyl congeners. Butorphanol is subject to less abuse and has less addictive potential than morphine or fentanyl does. Acute biliary spasm can occur after butorphanol, but increases in biliary pressure are less than after equipotent doses of fentanyl or morphine. Transnasal butorphanol is effective in relieving migraine and postoperative pain.[433]

Buprenorphine

Buprenorphine is a thebaine derivative, μ-receptor partial agonist and similar in structure to morphine but approximately 33 times more potent. Whereas fentanyl dissociates rapidly from μ-receptors (half-life of 6.8 minutes), buprenorphine has higher affinity and takes much longer (half-life of 166 minutes). The onset of action of buprenorphine is slow, its peak effect may not occur until 3 hours, and its duration of effect is prolonged (<10 hours). The volume of distribution of buprenophine is 2.8 L/kg and its clearance is 20 mL/kg/min. The metabolites of buprenorphine, buprenorphine-3-glucuronide and norbuprenorphine, are significantly less potent and have lower affinity for the μ-receptor.

The subjective effects (e.g., euphoria) of buprenorphine are similar to those of morphine. Buprenorphine produces depression of minute ventilation, which leveled off at doses higher than 3.0 μg/kg to about 50% of baseline, in contrast to fentanyl, in which dose-dependent respiratory depression results in apnea at doses higher than 2.9 μg/kg (Fig. 27-30).[434] Buprenorphine has been used successfully for premedication (0.3 mg IM), as the analgesic component in balanced anesthesia (4.5 to 12 μg/kg), and for postoperative pain control (0.3 mg IM). Buprenorphine, like the other agonist-antagonist compounds, is not acceptable as a sole anesthetic, and its receptor kinetic profile restricts its usefulness if other μ-agonists are used. Opioid withdrawal symptoms develop slowly (5 to 10 days) when buprenorphine is discontinued after long-term use.

Nalbuphine

Nalbuphine is an agonist-antagonist opioid that is structurally related to oxymorphone and naloxone and binds to μ-receptors, as well as to κ- and δ-receptors. Nalbuphine acts as an antagonist at the μ-receptor and as an agonist at the κ-receptor. Activation of supraspinal and spinal κ-receptors results in limited analgesia, respiratory depression, and sedation. Nalbuphine, like other agonist-antagonist compounds, interferes with the analgesia produced by pure μ-agonists. In rats, coadministration of nalbuphine with morphine dose-dependently blocked the development of morphine tolerance and dependence, without attenuation of the antinociceptive effect of morphine.[435] Nalbuphine is available only for parenteral use. The onset of effect is rapid (5 to 10 minutes), and its duration is long (3 to 6 hours) because of an extended plasma elimination half-life (5 hours).

Premedication with nalbuphine (0.1 mg/kg) in patients scheduled for cardiac surgery results in sedation, relief of anxiety, and respiratory depression similar to morphine (0.1 mg/kg), but

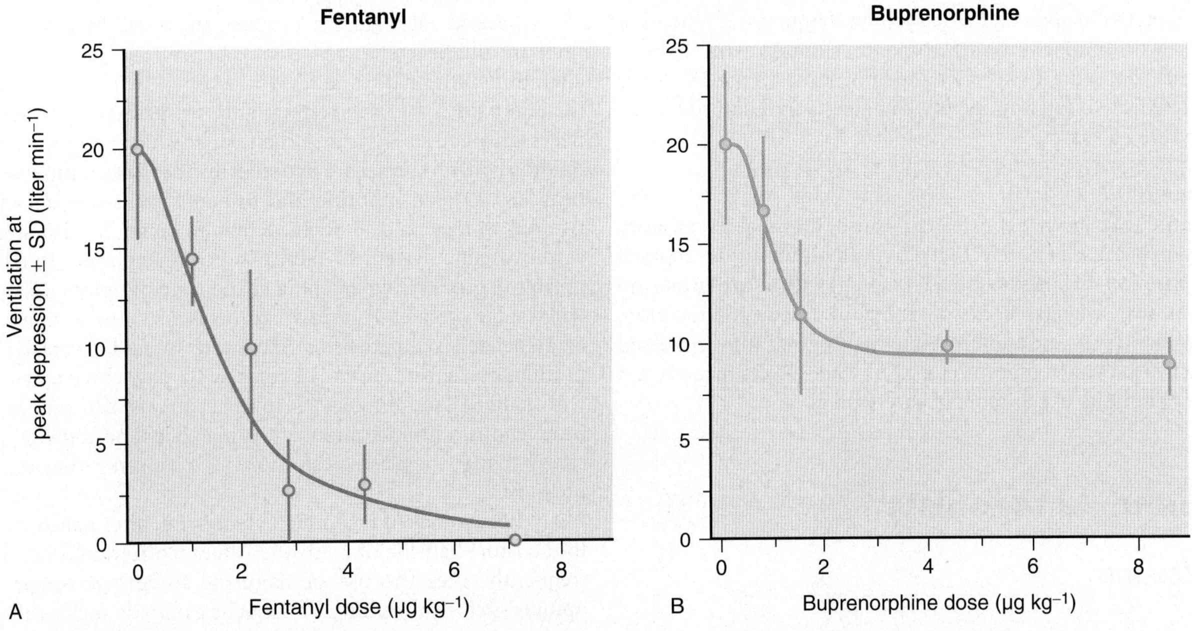

Figure 27-30 Dose-response relationships for reduction of minute ventilation induced by fentanyl (**A**) and buprenorphine (**B**). The response is the peak ventilatory depression at each dose. The line through the data is the fit to the Hill equation; 0 μg/kg is placebo. Data are means ± SD. *(From Dahan A, Yassen A, Bijl H, et al: Comparison of the respiratory effects of intravenous buprenorphine and fentanyl in humans and rats. Br J Anaesth 94:825-834, 2005.)*

it causes no significant hemodynamic changes. Nalbuphine (10 mg) caused no significant changes in systemic, pulmonary arterial, and pulmonary capillary wedge pressure in patients experiencing myocardial infarction.

Nalbuphine has been administered as an analgesic supplement for conscious sedation or balanced anesthesia and as an analgesic for postoperative and chronic pain problems. For postoperative patient-controlled epidural analgesia, the combination of hydromorphone, 0.075 mg/mL, and nalbuphine, 0.04 mg/mL, resulted in a lower incidence of nausea and decreased need for bladder catheterization when compared with hydromorphone alone.[436] In patients undergoing myocardial revascularization, continuous infusion of nalbuphine (0.05 to 0.1 mg/kg/min) and fentanyl (0.15 to 0.3 μg/kg/min) was compared.[437] It was shown that nalbuphine lacks the ability to attenuate cardiovascular and hormonal responses to tracheal intubation and surgical procedures, and it was concluded that continuous infusion of nalbuphine cannot be recommended for anesthesia in patients undergoing myocardial revascularization.

A prospective randomized double-blind study demonstrated that nalbuphine (4 mg IV) was as effective as ondansetron (4 to 8 mg IV) for the prevention of intrathecal morphine–induced pruritus after cesarean delivery.[438] Some reports showed that nalbuphine provides a rapid and potent antishivering effect, similar to meperidine.[439] However, a quantitative systematic review of randomized controlled trials did not support this conclusion.[440]

Other Compounds

Dezocine

Dezocine is slightly more potent and acts faster than morphine; it has a similar duration of action and is a partial agonist at μ- and probably δ-receptors. Its side effects are similar to those of morphine. Although shown to be an effective alternative to fentanyl when administered during outpatient laparoscopy with propofol and nitrous oxide, dezocine was associated with a high incidence of postoperative nausea and a delayed discharge time.[441] In adult patients who underwent arthroscopic surgery with general anesthesia, dezocine (5 mg IV) and morphine (5 mg IV) were similarly effective for postoperative analgesia and showed comparable side effects.[442]

Meptazinol

Meptazinol has been reported to cause minimal respiratory depression because of its selectivity for μ_1 (high-affinity) receptors. In patients receiving meptazinol (2.5 mg/kg) with a barbiturate, no cardiovascular changes were observed at tracheal intubation, whereas blood pressure and heart rate were significantly increased in patients receiving fentanyl (5 μg/kg).[443] Side effects (nausea and vomiting) limit its use to relief of severe pain.

Opioid Antagonists

Naloxone

Clinically, opioid antagonists are used to restore spontaneous ventilation in patients who breathe inadequately after opioid overdose or opioid anesthesia. In addition, opioid antagonists can reduce or reverse opioid-induced nausea and vomiting, pruritus, urinary retention, rigidity, and biliary spasm associated with numerous therapies using opioids, such as neuraxial analgesic techniques. It was reported that the naloxone-nalbuphine potency ratio for antagonism of the pruritic effects of epidural morphine was approximately 40 : 1.[444]

Morphine requirements were significantly less in patients receiving naloxone, thus suggesting that naloxone enhances analgesia.[445] Possible mechanisms proposed for this apparent paradoxical effect of naloxone include enhanced release of endogenous opioids and opioid receptor upregulation.

Although naloxone is generally considered to be a pure opioid receptor antagonist, it delays gastric emptying of saline or milk, as does morphine in the rat.[259] Furthermore, high-dose naloxone possesses partial agonistic activity on μ- and κ-opioid receptors in cultured cells.[446]

Reversal of Respiratory Depression by Naloxone

In the early 1950s, nalorphine and levallorphan were evaluated as opioid antagonists. They were often found unacceptable because of a high incidence of side effects, as well as incomplete reversal. Naloxone was introduced into clinical practice in the late 1960s. There have been reports of side effects (increases in heart rate and blood pressure) and more serious complications (e.g., pulmonary edema). Initial naloxone dose recommendations ranged from 0.4 to 0.8 mg. The onset of action of intravenous naloxone is rapid (1 to 2 minutes), and its half-life and duration of effect are short, approximately 30 to 60 minutes. If intravenous access is not available, naloxone, in doses similar to those given intravenously, is effectively absorbed after intratracheal administration.[447] Reversal with naloxone is limited by high affinity for and slow dissociation from the μ-opioid receptor of buprenorphine and depends on the buprenorphine dose and the correct naloxone dose window (Fig. 27-31).[448] Because respiratory depression from buprenorphine may outlast the effects of naloxone boluses or short infusions, continuous infusion of naloxone may be required to maintain reversal of respiratory depression.[448]

Several mechanisms produce increases in arterial blood pressure and heart rate, as well as other significant hemodynamic alterations, after naloxone reversal of opioids. These mechanisms include pain, rapid awakening, and sympathetic activation not necessarily caused by pain. When patients receiving naloxone for opioid agonist reversal are hypothermic because of intraoperative heat loss, O_2 consumption and minute ventilation can increase twofold to threefold.[449] Such metabolic demands also stress the cardiovascular system by increasing cardiac output. In addition, greater degrees of hypercapnia at the time of opioid antagonism will result in greater degrees of cardiovascular stimulation because of associated sympathetic stimulation. Opioid reversal may be particularly hazardous in patients with pheochromocytoma or chromaffin tissue tumors.[450] However, it was also reported that intravenous administration of 10-mg naloxone did not significantly change the plasma catecholamine concentration and blood pressure.[451]

Recurrence of respiratory depression after naloxone is due to the short half-life of naloxone. "Renarcotization" occurs more frequently after the use of naloxone to reverse longer-acting opioids such as morphine. Short-acting opioids such as alfentanil rarely pose a danger of renarcotization because of a rapid plasma decay curve and weaker opioid receptor binding than with fentanyl and sufentanil.

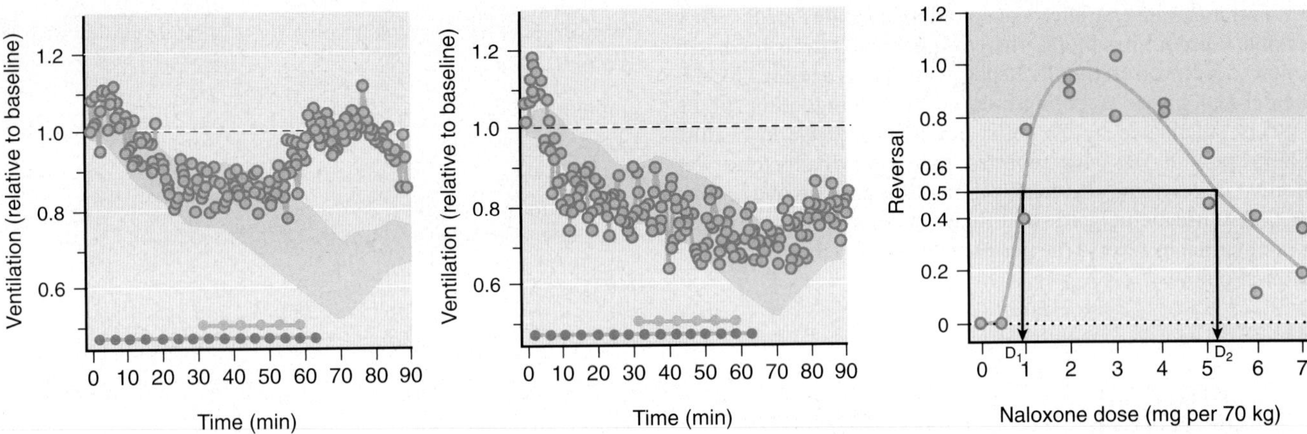

Figure 27-31 Reversal of buprenorphine-induced respiratory depression with naloxone depends on the correct naloxone dose window. Respiratory depression induced by 0.2 mg buprenorphine was reversed by naloxone, 2 mg (**left**) and 6 mg (**middle**), given over a 30-minute period in one subject. The *light blue field* in the background is the result of the placebo group, in which saline was infused instead of naloxone. *Dark blue dots* and *light blue dots* represent buprenorphine and naloxone infusion, respectively. **Right,** Influence of 0 (placebo) and 0.5 to 7 mg naloxone on respiratory depression induced by 0.2 mg intravenous buprenorphine. Reversal was calculated from the naloxone-induced change in ventilation and ranged from 0 (effect not different from placebo) to 1 (reversal to predrug baseline level). *(From van Dorp E, Yassen A, Sarton E, et al: Naloxone reversal of buprenorphine-induced respiratory depression. Anesthesiology 105:51-57, 2006.)*

Naloxone, though active at μ-, δ-, and κ-receptors, has greatest affinity for μ-receptors, which mediate most potent opioid effects, including respiratory depression and analgesia. Careful titration of naloxone can often restore adequate spontaneous ventilation without reversal of adequate analgesia.

Other Applications of Naloxone

Reversal of the effects of alcohol, barbiturates, and benzodiazepines by naloxone has been reported. However, it was also reported that naloxone potentiates the anxiolytic-like action of benzodiazepines and barbiturates in the rat.[452] It is not advisable to try to reverse the effects of overdose of benzodiazepines and barbiturates with naloxone. Although it was suggested that the μ-opioid receptor is involved in the antinociceptive action of ketamine in mice,[41] naloxone did not affect the action of ketamine on secondarty hyperalgesia induced by burn injury in humans.[453]

Evidence indicates that endogenous opioid peptides participate in the control of cardiovascular regulation during hemorrhagic shock. Intracerebroventricular administration of 10 mg of naloxone resulted in a significant increase in the bleeding volume required to lower arterial pressure from 60 to 40 mm Hg in rats.[454] In patients with documented septic shock and resistance to a 1-L fluid challenge, administration of naloxone by an initial bolus of 0.03 mg/kg followed by infusion at a rate of 0.2 mg/kg/hr significantly increased mean arterial pressure but did not affect survival.[455] This effect may be due to centrally mediated increases in sympathetic tone and decreases in parasympathetic output or antagonism of endogenous opioids. However, the clinical usefulness of naloxone in treating shock remains to be determined, and additional randomized clinical trials are needed to assess its usefulness.[456]

It has been reported that naloxone may ameliorate the neurologic deficit after an ischemic or traumatic neurologic insult in animals.[457] In humans, a randomized controlled trial demonstrated that naloxone (a bolus of 5.4 mg/kg, followed by infusion at 4.0 mg/kg/hr for 23 hours) does not improve neurologic recovery after acute spinal cord injury.[458] However, it was reported that combined use of cerebrospinal fluid drainage and naloxone reduces the risk of paraplegia in patients undergoing thoracoabdominal aneurysm repair.[459] Naloxone may also have a therapeutic role in heat stroke disorders[460] and cholestasis-induced pruritus.[461] Although intravenous naloxone has been claimed to produce pain relief in opioid-resistant central poststroke pain, a double-blind trial concluded that intravenous naloxone was of no value in alleviating central poststroke pain.[462]

Other Opioid Antagonists

Naltrexone

Naltrexone is a μ-, δ-, and κ-opioid receptor antagonist. It is longer acting than naloxone (plasma half-life of 8 to 12 versus 0.5 to 1.5 hours), and it is active when taken orally. A double-blind, placebo-controlled study of patients undergoing cesarean section indicated that naltrexone (6 mg) was an effective oral prophylactic against the pruritus and vomiting associated with intrathecal morphine but was associated with a shorter duration of analgesia.[463]

Nalmefene

Nalmefene has a greater preference for μ-receptors than for δ- or κ-receptors. It is equipotent to naloxone.[464] Nalmefene is long acting after oral (0.5 to 3.0 mg/kg) and parenteral (0.2 to 2.0 mg/kg) administration. Bioavailability after oral administration is 40% to 50%, and peak plasma concentrations are reached in 1 to 2 hours. The mean terminal elimination half-life of nalmefene is 8.5 hours as compared with 1 hour for naloxone. Prophylactic administration of nalmefene significantly decreased the need for antiemetics and antipruritic medications in patients receiving intravenous PCA with morphine.[465]

Methylnaltrexone

Methylnaltrexone is the first quarternary ammonium opioid receptor antagonist that does not cross the blood-brain barrier. It can reverse the adverse effects of opioid medications mediated by peripheral opioid receptors, whereas the opioid effects mediated by opioid receptors in the CNS, such as analgesia, are not affected. The delayed gastric emptying induced by 0.09 mg/kg morphine could be attenuated by 0.3 mg/kg methylnaltrexone in healthy volunteers.[250] It was also reported that methylnaltrexone was effective in reversing the constipation from chronic methadone use.[466] Because methylnaltrexone does not cross the dura, it might have potential to reverse the peripherally mediated side effects of epidural opioids.[467]

Drug Interactions with Opioids

Opioids are frequently combined with other anesthetic agents to produce optimal anesthetic conditions. In anesthesia, most concomitantly administered drugs interact. Although some of these interactions are intentionally sought, others are unwanted and adverse. There are three general types of mechanisms of drug interactions: pharmaceutical, pharmacokinetic, and pharmacodynamic.[468]

Pharmaceutical interactions are chemical in nature, as illustrated when an alkaline solution of thiopental and an acidic solution of succinylcholine precipitate when simultaneously administered intravenously.

Pharmacokinetic interactions occur when the administration of one agent alters the pharmacokinetics or disposition of another. The hemodynamic changes induced by one agent can affect the pharmacokinetic behavior of the other agent. Sufentanil, which has a greater hepatic extraction ratio than alfentanil does, is more likely to be affected by decreases in hepatic blood flow. Opioid plasma levels also increase in the presence of propofol.[469] Decreased opioid metabolism by the CYP3A4 isoform of the cytochrome P450 enzyme responsible for the oxidative metabolism of more than 50 drugs may also underlie the pharmacokinetic interactions. A wide range of chemical compounds, including many drugs, can interact with the cytochrome P450 system and cause either increased activity (enzyme induction) or enzyme inhibition (Box 27-3).[468]

Pharmacodynamic interactions between opioids and inhaled anesthetics were assessed by evaluating classic MAC reduction in animals and humans. Although marked synergism between opioids and inhaled anesthetics occurs with analgesic doses of opioids, there is a ceiling effect to MAC reduction by opioids. The pharmacodynamic synergism between opioids and sedative-hypnotics such as propofol is profound. Choosing an opioid with a short context-sensitive half-life allows greater doses of that opioid to be administered, along with reduced doses of propofol, without compromising the time needed for recovery from anesthesia. Thus, the optimal plasma level of propofol is estimated to be approximately 30% less when it is combined with remifentanil instead of alfentanil.[469]

Drug dosing regimens and a plasma concentration of opioid and sedative-hypnotics that provide optimal hemodynamic control during a range of noxious stimuli are necessary. However, complicating our understanding of drug interactions is the observation that the same degree of interaction does not apply across different types of stimuli.

Box 27-3 Drugs That Inhibit or Induce Cytochrome P450 Enzymes

Inhibitors

- Antibiotics
  - Maclorides
    - Troleandromycin
    - Erythromycin
  - Fluoroquinolones
  - Isoniazid
- Azole antifungal drugs
  - Ketoconazole
  - Itraconazole
- Calcium entry blockers
  - Diltiazem
  - Verapamil
- Omeprazole
- Cimetidine
- Propofol
- Grapefruit juice

Inducers

- Barbiturates
- Antiepileptics
  - Carbamazepine
  - Phenytoin
  - Primidone
- Rifampicin
- Dichloralphenazone
- Ethanol
- Tobacco smoke

From Bovill JG: Adverse drug interactions in anesthesia. J Clin Anesth 9:3S, 1997.

Sedative-Hypnotics

Alfentanil was found to reduce the median effective dose (ED_{50}) of midazolam for induction of anesthesia in a dose-dependent fashion. The smallest dose of alfentanil (3 μg/kg) that causes a marked shift in the midazolam dose-response curve to the left along the dose axis (from an ED_{50} of 270 μg/kg to an ED_{50} of 142 μg/kg) represents approximately 2% of the alfentanil ED_{50} for induction of unconsciousness (130 μg/kg).[463] On the contrary, with regard to the antinociceptive effect, interaction between these two types of drugs may be less than additive.[470,471] Midazolam enhances opioid-induced antinociception at the spinal level but inhibits it at the supraspinal level.[472] Many studies reveal that benzodiazepine-opioid interactions for many properties other than analgesia are synergistic (supra-additive). Both the cardiovascular and respiratory actions of opioids can be significantly altered by the concomitant administration of benzodiazepines.[473] In anesthetized rabbits, fentanyl and midazolam synergistically caused depression of phrenic nerve activity.[474] Combinations of benzodiazepines and opioids, though occasionally preserving ventricular function, can result in significant and occasionally profound decreases in blood pressure, cardiac index, heart rate, and systemic vascular resistance. Fluid loading may attenuate the circulatory depression that occurs when benzodiazepines and opioids are combined.

Barbituraes can potentiate or produce hypotension if a large dose is administered with opioids. Hypotension after a barbiturate-opioid combination is due to venodilatation, decreased cardiac filling, myocardial depression, and decreased sympathetic nervous system activity. Reducing induction doses of barbiturates administered concomitantly with opioids is recommended.

The administration of propofol-opioid combinations provides unconsciousness and blocks responses to noxious stimuli. However, when given as an intravenous bolus for induction of anesthesia, propofol can create moderate to severe preintubation hypotension. The addition of 2 to 4 μg/kg fentanyl significantly potentiated the decrease in mean blood pressure induced by 2.0 to 3.5 mg/kg propofol.[475] Propofol-fentanyl and propofol-sufentanil anesthesia for coronary artery bypass surgery may provide acceptable conditions, but mean arterial pressure can decrease to levels that may jeopardize coronary perfusion, especially during induction of anesthesia.[476] In healthy volunteers, the addition of alfentanil (effect-site concentration of 50 or 100 ng/mL) did not affect the changes in BIS induced by propofol but blocked the increase in BIS induced by painful stimuli.[477] In patients undergoing spine fusion, infusion of fentanyl (blood levels of 1.5 to 4.5 ng/mL) reduced the infusion rate of propofol necessary to maintain mean arterial pressure but delayed spontaneous eye opening and recovery of orientation.[340] In patients undergoing ambulatory gynecologic laparoscopy, administration of fentanyl (25 to 50 μg IV) at the time of induction of anesthesia reduced the maintenance propofol requirement but failed to provide effective postoperative analgesia and increased the need for postoperative use of antiemetics.[478] Pharmacokinetic interaction, as well as pharmacodynamic interaction, between propofol and opioids has been reported. Target-controlled infusion of alfentanil (target concentration, 80 ng/mL) was shown to increase the blood propofol concentration by 17% and decrease the elimination clearance, distribution clearance, and peripheral volume of distribution of propofol.[479]

Other anesthetic induction agents such as etomidate and ketamine can be combined in low doses with opioids with little loss of cardiovascular stability. In patients scheduled for coronary artery bypass grafting, etomidate (0.25 mg/kg) plus fentanyl (6 μg/kg) resulted in less hypotension after induction and intubation than propofol (1 mg/kg) plus fentanyl (6 μg/kg) did.[480] As described in the previous section, opioid-induced hyperalgesia and subsequent acute opioid tolerance can be prevented by ketamine in rats, suggesting the usefulness of the combination of ketamine and opioids for postoperative analgesia. However, it was reported that the combination of ketamine (2.5 or 10 mg IV) and alfentanil (0.25 or 1 mg IV) provides no advantage over a larger dose of either drug alone in relieving pain caused by intradermal capsaicin injection in healthy volunteers.[481] Furthermore, the combination of ketamine, 1 mg/mL, and morphine, 1 mg/mL, for PCA did not provide benefit to patients undergoing major abdominal surgery.[482] In contrast, Lauretti and coauthors reported that oral ketamine and transdermal nitroglycerin effectively reduced the daily consumption of oral morphine in patients with cancer pain.[483]

Gabapentin, a structural analog of GABA, is a novel anticonvulsant drug that has analgesic effects in patients with neuropathic pain. It was suggested that pharmacodynamic and pharmacokinetic interaction between morphine and gabapentin leads to increased analgesic effects.[484] Furthermore, intrathecal administration of gabapentin was shown to prevent the development of opioid tolerance induced by repeated intrathecal injection of morphine.[485] $GABA_A$ receptors contribute to inhibitory control at the spinal cord level. Intrathecal administration of muscimol or baclofen, $GABA_A$ and $GABA_B$ receptor agonists, respectively, increased the analgesic action of morphine in intensity and duration.[486]

Inhaled Anesthetics

N_2O produces analgesia that is in part mediated by release of the proenkephalin-derived family of endogenous opioid peptides.[487] This may imply that interaction between opioids and N_2O is neither synergistic nor additive. Combining N_2O with an opioid in a balanced technique may not best take advantage of drug interaction synergism. Although amnesia and intraoperative conditions may be improved somewhat, N_2O does not produce any effects that are not already produced by either an opioid or a sedative-hypnotic. The advent of short-acting intravenous anesthetics and volatile anesthetics with a blood-gas partition coefficient comparable to that of N_2O has decreased the popularity of N_2O in balanced anesthesia.

Volatile anesthetics are frequently combined with opioids to ensure amnesia and promote immobility and hemodynamic stability. Clinical trials of opioids supplemented with newer volatile anesthetics for cardiac surgery demonstrate well-preserved cardiac output and minimal decreases in mean arterial blood pressure.[488,489] Myocardial ischemia may not, however, always be ameliorated by approaches that combine opioids with potent inhaled agents despite apparent "good" hemodynamic control. Some of the potent inhaled anesthetics can increase sympathetic nervous system activity and may increase the risk for myocardial ischemia in cardiac patients.[490,491] Prior administration of fentanyl, in doses as low as 1.5 μg/kg, can markedly attenuate such responses.[490] Alfentanil (10 μg/kg) is also effective in attenuating these effects.

Muscle Relaxants

Pancuronium bromide has been used frequently for muscle relaxation during high-dose opioid anesthesia. It was reported that the vagolytic action of pancuronium can attenuate opioid-induced bradycardia and support blood pressure,[492] but other reports have cautioned against the use of pancuronium with high-dose opioids.[493] In patients undergoing coronary artery bypass grafting and administered sufentanil (3 to 8 μg/kg), pancuronium (120 μg/kg) caused a significant increase in mean arterial pressure, heart rate, and cardiac output but did not induce myocardial ischemia.[494] Pancuronium-induced tachycardia was easily and rapidly treated and caused no differences in ischemia or perioperative myocardial infarction. Many factors alter the impact of pancuronium and other muscle relaxants on hemodynamics when combined with opioids, including the dose, timing, and rate of administration of each relaxant, as well as the premedication, intravascular volume, left ventricular function, and presence of other drugs with autonomic nervous system actions.[492]

Combinations of vecuronium and high doses of opioids produce negative chronotropic and inotropic effects that result in decreases in heart rate, cardiac output, and blood pressure and increases in the need for vasopressor support.[495] In patients scheduled for coronary artery surgery and administered 40 μg/kg sufentanil in combination with vecuronium (0.1 mg/kg), heart rate, mean arterial pressure, and systemic vascular resistance decreased from baseline values after tracheal intubation with neither a significant change in cardiac output nor evidence of new myocardial ischemia.[492]

In patients anesthetized with fentanyl, 50 μg/kg, and scheduled to undergo elective coronary artery bypass grafting, rocuronium, 0.6 mg/kg (approximately equivalent to 2 × ED_{95} doses), was associated with changes of only small magnitude in hemodynamic variables, including increases in stroke volume index (+15%) and cardiac index (+11%) and a decrease in pulmonary capillary wedge pressure (−25%).[496] In patients undergoing coronary artery bypass surgery under fentanyl anesthesia, mivacurium, 0.15 or 0.2 mg/kg, produced decreases in mean arterial pressure and systemic vascular resistance, possibly mediated by histamine release, whereas atracurium (0.5 mg/kg) produced no significant hemodynamic changes.[497] Pipecuronium (150 μg/kg) has been found to be devoid of circulatory actions in patients undergoing coronary artery bypass grafting surgery with midazolam-sufentanil (3 to 8 μg/kg) anesthesia.[494] In patients administered 50 μg/kg fentanyl, doxacurium caused a small decrease in mean arterial pressure.[498]

Miscellaneous

MAOIs can underlie the most serious and potentially fatal interactions of opioid and other drugs. It was reported that the combination of meperidine and an MAOI can induce the serotonin syndrome, which is caused by excess availability of serotonin in the CNS at the 5-HT_{1A} receptor and characterized by confusion, fever, shivering, diaphoresis, ataxia, hyperreflexia, myoclonus, and diarrhea.[499] The phenylpiperidine series opioids, including meperidine, tramadol, and methadone, appear to be weak serotonin reuptake inhibitors and have all been involved in serotonin toxicity reactions with MAOIs, whereas morphine, codeine, oxycodone, and buprenorphine are known to not be serotonin reuptake inhibitors and do not precipitate serotonin toxicity with MAOIs.[500] Alfentanil and remifentanil could be used with MAOIs without complications.[501,502]

Because opioids can inhibit voltage-dependent Ca^{2+} channel activity through the activation of G proteins, it may be possible that opioid action is potentiated by Ca^{2+} channel blockers. Numerous animal studies and few clinical studies have documented that opioid-induced analgesia is potentiated by L-type Ca^{2+} channel blockers. Systemically administered nifedipine was shown to potentiate morphine analgesia in both rats and humans.[503] Furthermore, intrathecal administration of verapamil, diltiazem, and nicardipine enhanced the antinociceptive effect of low-dose morphine in rats.[504] However, there is also a report that L-type Ca^{2+} channel blockers do not potentiate morphine analgesia at clinically relevant doses.[505] N-type Ca^{2+} channels are involved in the release of neurotransmitters from sensory neurons in the spinal cord. It was reported that intrathecal administration of a blocker of this channel, ω-conotoxin GVIA, produces antinociception and interacts synergistically with opioids at the spinal cord level.[506]

Erythromycin can inhibit the metabolism of several compounds. It supposedly reduces the oxidizing activity of cytochrome P450. Alfentanil, but not sufentanil, may have its action prolonged as a result of impaired metabolism in patients receiving erythromycin.[507,508] Cimetidine can prolong opioid effects by decreasing hepatic blood flow or diminishing hepatic metabolism (or by both means). Other drugs that inhibit certain cytochrome systems can increase endogenous morphine production from codeine.[406]

Magnesium has been shown to have antinociceptive effects, probably because of its antagonistic action on the NMDA receptor. Intravenous administration of magnesium sulfate, 50 mg/kg preoperatively and 8 mg/kg/hr intraoperatively, significantly reduced the intraoperative and postoperative fentanyl requirement.[509] However, passage of magnesium across the blood-brain barrier is limited. Intrathecal administration of fentanyl, 25 μg, plus magnesium sulfate, 50 mg, provided significantly prolonged analgesia when compared with fentanyl alone in patients requesting analgesia for labor.[510] It is likely that magnesium can potentiate opioid analgesia by both central and peripheral mechanisms.[511]

Nonsteroidal anti-inflammatory drugs such as ibuprofen, diclofenac, and ketorolac have been administered perioperatively to reduce the opioid requirement. Preoperative administration of ibuprofen (2 × 800 mg) to patients scheduled for lower abdominal gynecologic surgery was shown to reduce postoperative morphine consumption without an increase in side effects.[512] It was also reported that perioperative administration of diclofenac (75 mg twice daily) reduces morphine consumption and the incidence of adverse effects such as sedation and nausea after total abdominal hysterectomy.[513] In healthy volunteers, ketoprofen (1.5 mg/kg IV) reduced the respiratory depression induced by morphine (0.1 mg/kg).[514]

The tricyclic antidepressants are widely used to treat various chronic inflammatory and neuropathic pain conditions. Results in clinical studies were not consistent with respect to interactions between opioids and tricyclic antidepressants. An isobolographic analysis demonstrated that systemic administration of amitriptyline and morphine synergistically inhibits cutaneous orofacial inflammatory pain in rats.[515]

Diphenhydramine, a histamine H_1-receptor antagonist, is used as a sedative, an antipruritic, and an antiemetic drug. When administered alone, it modestly stimulates ventilation by augmenting the interaction of hypoxic and hypercapnic ventilatory drives. Diphenhydramine counteracts the alfentanil-induced decrease in the slope of the ventilatory response to carbon dioxide.[516]

References

1. Gutstein HB, Akil H: Opioid analgesics. *In* Hardman JG, Limbird LE (ed): Goodman and Gilman's The pharmacological basis of therapeutics. New York, McGraw-Hill, 2001, pp 569-619.
2. Minami M, Satoh M: Molecular biology of the opioid receptors: Structures, functions and distributions. Neurosci Res 23:121-145, 1995.
3. Reinscheid RK, Nothacker HP, Bourson A, et al: Orphanin FQ: A neuropeptide that activates an opioidlike G protein–coupled receptor. Science 270:792-794, 1995.
4. Meunier JC, Mollereau C, Toll L, et al: Isolation and structure of the endogenous agonist of opioid receptor–like ORL1 receptor. Nature 377:532-535, 1995.
5. Mansour A, Fox CA, Akil H, Watson SJ: Opioid-receptor mRNA expression in the rat CNS: Anatomical and functional implications. Trends Neurosci 18:22-29, 1995.
6. Lotsch J, Geisslinger G: Are μ-opioid receptor polymorphisms important for clinical opioid therapy? Trends Mol Med 11:82-89, 2005.
7. Klepstad P, Rakvag TT, Kaasa S, et al: The 118 A → G polymorphism in the human μ-opioid receptor gene may increase morphine requirements in patients with pain caused by malignant disease. Acta Anaesthesiol Scand 48:1232-1239, 2004.
8. Romberg RR, Olofsen E, Bijl H, et al: Polymorphism of μ-opioid receptor gene (OPRM1:c.118A → G) does not protect against opioid-induced respiratory depression despite reduced analgesic response. Anesthesiology 102:522-530, 2005.
9. Chou WY, Wang CH, Liu PH, et al: Human opioid receptor A118G polymorphism affects intravenous patient-controlled analgesia morphine consumption after total abdominal hysterectomy. Anesthesiology 105:334-337, 2006.
10. Mogil JS, Pasternak GW: The molecular and behavioral pharmacology of the orphanin FQ/nociceptin peptide and receptor family. Pharmacol Rev 53:381-415, 2001.
11. Nothacker HP, Reinscheid RK, Mansour A, et al: Primary structure and tissue distribution of the orphanin FQ precursor. Proc Natl Acad Sci U S A 93:8677-8682, 1996.
12. Adina JE, Hackler L, Ge LJ, Kastin AJ: A potent and selective endogenous agonist for the μ-opiate receptor. Nature 386:499-502, 1997.
13. Wandless AL, Smart D, Lambert DG: Fentanyl increases intracellular Ca^{2+} concentrations in SH-SY5Y cells. Br J Anaesth 76:461-463, 1996.
14. Fukuda K, Kato S, Morikawa H, et al: Functional coupling of the δ-, μ-, and κ-opioid receptors to mitogen-activated protein kinase and arachidonate release in Chinese hamster ovary cells. J Neurochem 67:1309-1316, 1996.
15. Shoda T, Fukuda K, Uga H, et al: Activation of μ-opioid receptor induces expression of c-fos and junB via mitogen-activated protein kinase cascade. Anesthesiology 95:983-989, 2001.
16. Mestek A, Hurley JH, Bye LS, et al: The human μ opioid receptor: Modulation of functional desensitization by calcium/calmodulin-dependent protein kinase and protein kinase C. J Neurosci 15:2396-2406, 1995.
17. Pei G, Kieffer BL, Lefkowitz RJ, Freedman NJ: Agonist-dependent phosphorylation of the mouse δ-opioid receptor: Involvement of G protein–coupled receptor kinases but not protein kinase C. Mol Pharmacol 48:173-177, 1995.
18. Bohn LM, Lefkowitz RJ, Gainetdinov RR, et al: Enhanced morphine analgesia in mice lacking beta-arrestin 2. Science 286:2495-2498, 1999.
19. Trapaidze N, Keith DE, Cvejic S, et al: Sequestration of the δ opioid receptor. Role of the C terminus in agonist-mediated internalization. J Biol Chem 271:29279-29285, 1996.
20. Gaudriault G, Nouel D, Dal Farra C, et al: Receptor-induced internalization of selective peptidic μ and δ opioid ligands. J Biol Chem 272:2880-2888, 1997.
21. Keith DE, Murray SR, Zaki PA, et al: Morphine activates opioid receptors without causing their rapid internalization. J Biol Chem 271:19021-19024, 1996.
22. Hashimoto T, Saito Y, Yamada K, et al: Enhancement of morphine analgesic effect with induction of μ-opioid receptor endocytosis in rats. Anesthesiology 105:574-580, 2006.
23. Avidor Reiss T, Nevo I, Levy R, et al: Chronic opioid treatment induces adenylyl cyclase V superactivation. Involvement of Gbg. J Biol Chem 271:21309-21315, 1996.
24. Fields HL, Heinricher MM, Mason P: Neurotransmitters in nociceptive modulatory circuits. Annu Rev Neurosci 14:219-245, 1991.
25. Petrovic P, Kalso E, Petersson KM, Ingvar M: Placebo and opioid analgesia—imaging a shared neuronal network. Science 295:1737-1740, 2002.
26. Wager TD, Rilling JK, Smith EE, et al: Placebo-induced changes in FMRI in the anticipation and experience of pain. Science 303:1162-1167, 2004.
27. Pan ZZ, Tershner SA, Fields HL: Cellular mechanism for anti-analgesic action of agonists of the κ-opioid receptor. Nature 389:382-385, 1997.
28. Trafton JA, Abbadie C, Marchand S, et al: Spinal opioid analgesia: How critical is the regulation of substance P signaling? J Neurosci 19:9642-9653, 1999.
29. Matthies BK, Franklin KB: Formalin pain is expressed in decerebrate rats but not attenuated by morphine. Pain 51:199-206, 1992.
30. Manning BH, Morgan MJ, Franklin KB: Morphine analgesia in the formalin test: Evidence for forebrain and midbrain sites of action. Neuroscience 63:289-294, 1994.
31. Manning BH, Mayer DJ: The central nucleus of the amygdala contributes to the production of morphine antinociception in the rat tail-flick test. J Neurosci 15:8199-8213, 1995.
32. Manning BH, Mayer DJ: The central nucleus of the amygdala contributes to the production of morphine antinociception in the formalin test. Pain 63:141-152, 1995.
33. Stein C: The control of pain in peripheral tissue by opioids. N Engl J Med 332:1685-1690, 1995.
34. Heard SO, Edwards WT, Ferrari D, et al: Analgesic effect of intraarticular bupivacaine or morphine after arthroscopic knee surgery: A randomized, prospective, double-blind study. Anesth Analg 74:822-826, 1992.
35. Picard PR, Tramer MR, McQuay HJ, Moore RA: Analgesic efficacy of peripheral opioids (all except intra-articular): A qualitative systematic review of randomised controlled trials. Pain 72:309-318, 1997.
36. Becerra L, Harter K, Gonzalez RG, Borsook D: Functional magnetic resonance imaging measures of the effects of morphine on central nervous system circuitry in opioid-naive healthy volunteers. Anesth Analg 103:208-216, 2006.
37. Kieffer BL: Opioids: First lessons from knockout mice. Trends Pharmacol Sci 20:19-26, 1999.
38. Matthes HW, Maldonado R, Simonin F, et al: Loss of morphine-induced analgesia, reward effect and withdrawal symptoms in mice lacking the μ-opioid-receptor gene. Nature 383:819-823, 1996.
39. Sora I, Takahashi N, Funada M, et al: Opiate receptor knockout mice define μ receptor roles in endogenous nociceptive responses and morphine-induced analgesia. Proc Natl Acad Sci U S A 94:1544-1549, 1997.
40. Dahan A, Sarton E, Teppema L, et al: Anesthetic potency and influence of morphine and sevoflurane on respiration in μ-opioid receptor knockout mice. Anesthesiology 94:824-832, 2001.
41. Sarton E, Teppema LJ, Olievier C, et al: The involvement of the μ-opioid receptor in ketamine-induced respiratory depression and antinociception. Anesth Analg 93:1495-1500, 2001.
42. Zhu Y, King MA, Schuller AG, et al: Retention of supraspinal δ-like analgesia and loss of morphine tolerance in δ opioid receptor knockout mice. Neuron 24:243-252, 1999.
43. Simonin F, Valverde O, Smadja C, et al: Disruption of the κ-opioid receptor gene in mice enhances sensitivity to chemical visceral pain, impairs pharmacological actions of the selective κ-agonist U-50,488H and attenuates morphine withdrawal. EMBO J 17:886-897, 1998.
44. Rubinstein M, Mogil JS, Japon M, et al: Absence of opioid stress-induced analgesia in mice lacking β-endorphin by site-directed mutagenesis. Proc Natl Acad Sci U S A 93:3995-4000, 1996.
45. Konig M, Zimmer AM, Steiner H, et al: Pain responses, anxiety and aggression in mice deficient in pre-proenkephalin. Nature 383:535-538, 1996.
46. Hung CF, Tsai CH, Su MJ: Opioid receptor independent effects of morphine on membrane currents in single cardiac myocytes. Br J Anaesth 81:925-931, 1998.
47. Brau ME, Koch ED, Vogel W, Hempelmann G: Tonic blocking action of meperidine on Na^+ and K^+ channels in amphibian peripheral nerves. Anesthesiology 92:147-155, 2000.
48. Wagner LE 2nd, Eaton M, Sabnis SS, Gingrich KJ: Meperidine and lidocaine block of recombinant voltage-dependent Na^+ channels: Evidence that meperidine is a local anesthetic. Anesthesiology 91:1481-1490, 1999.
49. Takada K, Clark DJ, Davies MF, et al: Meperidine exerts agonist activity at the α_{2B}-adrenoceptor subtype. Anesthesiology 96:1420-1426, 2002.
50. Yamakura T, Sakimura K, Shimoji K: Direct inhibition of the *N*-methyl-D-aspartate receptor channel by high concentrations of opioids. Anesthesiology 91:1053-1063, 1999.
51. Davis AM, Inturrisi CE: *d*-Methadone blocks morphine tolerance and *N*-methyl-D-aspartate–induced hyperalgesia. J Pharmacol Exp Ther 289:1048-1053, 1999.
52. Hahnenkamp K, Nollet J, Van Aken HK, et al: Remifentanil directly activates human *N*-methyl-D-aspartate receptors expressed in *Xenopus laevis* oocytes. Anesthesiology 100:1531-1537, 2004.
53. Guntz E, Dumont H, Roussel C, et al: Effects of remifentanil on *N*-methyl-D-aspartate receptor: An electrophysiologic study in rat spinal cord. Anesthesiology 102:1235-1241, 2005.
54. Wittmann M, Peters I, Schaaf T, et al: The effects of morphine on human $5\text{-}HT_{3A}$ receptors. Anesth Analg 103:747-752, 2006.

55. Nishi M, Houtani T, Noda Y, et al: Unrestrained nociceptive response and disregulation of hearing ability in mice lacking the nociceptin/orphanin FQ receptor. EMBO J 16:1858-1864, 1997.
56. Koster A, Montkowski A, Schulz S, et al: Targeted disruption of the orphanin FQ/nociceptin gene increases stress susceptibility and impairs stress adaptation in mice. Proc Natl Acad Sci U S A 96:10444-10449, 1999.
57. Yamamoto T, Sakashita Y: The role of the spinal opioid receptor like1 receptor, the NK-1 receptor, and cyclooxygenase-2 in maintaining postoperative pain in the rat. Anesth Analg 89:1203-1208, 1999.
58. Grisel JE, Mogil JS, Belknap JK, Grandy DK: Orphanin FQ acts as a supraspinal, but not a spinal, anti-opioid peptide. Neuroreport 7:2125-2129, 1996.
59. Pan Z, Hirakawa N, Fields HL: A cellular mechanism for the bidirectional pain-modulating actions of orphanin FQ/nociceptin. Neuron 26:515-522, 2000.
60. Portenoy RK, Foley KM, Inturrisi CE: The nature of opioid responsiveness and its implications for neuropathic pain: New hypotheses derived from studies of opioid infusions. Pain 43:273-286, 1990.
61. Morgan D, Cook CD, Smith MA, Picker MJ: An examination of the interactions between the antinociceptive effects of morphine and various μ-opioids: The role of intrinsic efficacy and stimulus intensity. Anesth Analg 88:407-413, 1999.
62. Perrot S, Guilbaud G, Kayser V: Differential behavioral effects of peripheral and systemic morphine and naloxone in a rat model of repeated acute inflammation. Anesthesiology 94:870-875, 2001.
63. Kest B, Sarton E, Dahan A: Gender differences in opioid-mediated analgesia: Animal and human studies. Anesthesiology 93:539-547, 2000.
64. Sarton E, Olofsen E, Romberg R, et al: Sex differences in morphine analgesia: An experimental study in healthy volunteers. Anesthesiology 93: 1245-1254, discussion 1246A, 2000.
65. Gupta A, Bodin L, Holmstrom B, Berggren L: A systematic review of the peripheral analgesic effects of intraarticular morphine. Anesth Analg 93:761-770, 2001.
66. Kapral S, Gollmann G, Waltl B, et al: Tramadol added to mepivacaine prolongs the duration of an axillary brachial plexus blockade. Anesth Analg 88:853-856, 1999.
67. Nishikawa K, Kanaya N, Nakayama M, et al: Fentanyl improves analgesia but prolongs the onset of axillary brachial plexus block by peripheral mechanism. Anesth Analg 91:384-387, 2000.
68. Bouaziz H, Kinirons BP, Macalou D, et al: Sufentanil does not prolong the duration of analgesia in a mepivacaine brachial plexus block: A dose response study. Anesth Analg 90:383-387, 2000.
69. Latta KS, Ginsberg B, Barkin RL: Meperidine: A critical review. Am J Ther 9:53-68, 2002.
70. Osman NI, Baghdoyan HA, Lydic R: Morphine inhibits acetylcholine release in rat prefrontal cortex when delivered systemically or by microdialysis to basal forebrain. Anesthesiology 103:779-787, 2005.
71. Philbin DM, Rosow CE, Schneider RC, et al: Fentanyl and sufentanil anesthesia revisited: How much is enough? Anesthesiology 73:5-11, 1990.
72. Michelsen LG, Salmenpera M, Hug CC Jr, et al: Anesthetic potency of remifentanil in dogs. Anesthesiology 84:865-872, 1996.
73. Steffey EP: Isoflurane-sparing effect of fentanyl in swine. Relevance and importance. Anesthesiology 83:446-448, 1995.
74. McEwan AI, Smith C, Dyar O, et al: Isoflurane minimum alveolar concentration reduction by fentanyl. Anesthesiology 78:864-869, 1993.
75. Katoh T, Kobayashi S, Suzuki A, et al: The effect of fentanyl on sevoflurane requirements for somatic and sympathetic responses to surgical incision. Anesthesiology 90:398-405, 1999.
76. Glass PS, Gan TJ, Howell S, Ginsberg B: Drug interactions: Volatile anesthetics and opioids. J Clin Anesth 9:18s-22s, 1997.
77. Johansen JW, Schneider G, Windsor AM, Sebel PS: Esmolol potentiates reduction of minimum alveolar isoflurane concentration by alfentanil. Anesth Analg 87:671-676, 1998.
78. Inagaki Y, Tsuda Y: Contribution of the spinal cord to arousal from inhaled anesthesia: Comparison of epidural and intravenous fentanyl on awakening concentration of isoflurane. Anesth Analg 85:1387-1393, 1997.
79. Kissin I, Vinik HR, Castillo R, Bradley EL Jr: Alfentanil potentiates midazolam-induced unconsciousness in subanalgesic doses. Anesth Analg 71:65-69, 1990.
80. Katoh T, Nakajima Y, Moriwaki G, et al: Sevoflurane requirements for tracheal intubation with and without fentanyl. Br J Anaesth 82:561-565, 1999.
81. Lysakowski C, Dumont L, Pellegrini M, et al: Effects of fentanyl, alfentanil, remifentanil and sufentanil on loss of consciousness and bispectral index during propofol induction of anaesthesia. Br J Anaesth 86:523-527, 2001.
82. Koitabashi T, Johansen JW, Sebel PS: Remifentanil dose/electroencephalogram bispectral response during combined propofol/regional anesthesia. Anesth Analg 94:1530-1533, 2002.
83. Kern SE, Xie G, White JL, Egan TD: A response surface analysis of propofol-remifentanil pharmacodynamic interaction in volunteers. Anesthesiology 100:1373-1381, 2004.
84. Streisand JB, Bailey PL, LeMaire L, et al: Fentanyl-induced rigidity and unconsciousness in human volunteers. Incidence, duration, and plasma concentrations. Anesthesiology 78:629-634, 1993.
85. Jhaveri R, Joshi P, Batenhorst R, et al: Dose comparison of remifentanil and alfentanil for loss of consciousness. Anesthesiology 87:253-259, 1997.
86. Chi OZ, Sommer W, Jasaitis D: Power spectral analysis of EEG during sufentanil infusion in humans. Can J Anaesth 38:275-280, 1991.
87. Gambus PL, Gregg KM, Shafer SL: Validation of the alfentanil canonical univariate parameter as a measure of opioid effect on the electroencephalogram. Anesthesiology 83:747-756, 1995.
88. Egan TD, Minto CF, Hermann DJ, et al: Remifentanil versus alfentanil: Comparative pharmacokinetics and pharmacodynamics in healthy adult male volunteers. Anesthesiology 84:821-833, 1996.
89. Scott JC, Cooke JE, Stanski DR: Electroencephalographic quantitation of opioid effect: Comparative pharmacodynamics of fentanyl and sufentanil. Anesthesiology 74:34-42, 1991.
90. Westmoreland CL, Sebel PS, Gropper A: Fentanyl or alfentanil decreases the minimum alveolar anesthetic concentration of isoflurane in surgical patients. Anesth Analg 78:23-28, 1994.
91. Brunner MD, Braithwaite P, Jhaveri R, et al: MAC reduction of isoflurane by sufentanil. Br J Anaesth 72:42-46, 1994.
92. Lang E, Kapila A, Shlugman D, et al: Reduction of isoflurane minimal alveolar concentration by remifentanil. Anesthesiology 85:721-728, 1996.
93. Langeron O, Lille F, Zerhouni O, et al: Comparison of the effects of ketamine-midazolam with those of fentanyl-midazolam on cortical somatosensory evoked potentials during major spine surgery. Br J Anaesth 78:701-706, 1997.
94. Crabb I, Thornton C, Konieczko KM, et al: Remifentanil reduces auditory and somatosensory evoked responses during isoflurane anaesthesia in a dose-dependent manner. Br J Anaesth 76:795-801, 1996.
95. Haenggi M, Ypparila H, Takala J, et al: Measuring depth of sedation with auditory evoked potentials during controlled infusion of propofol and remifentanil in healthy volunteers. Anesth Analg 99:1728-1736, 2004.
96. Kalkman CJ, Drummond JC, Ribberink AA, et al: Effects of propofol, etomidate, midazolam, and fentanyl on motor evoked responses to transcranial electrical or magnetic stimulation in humans. Anesthesiology 76:502-509, 1992.
97. Kawaguchi M, Sakamoto T, Ohnishi H, et al: Intraoperative myogenic motor evoked potentials induced by direct electrical stimulation of the exposed motor cortex under isoflurane and sevoflurane. Anesth Analg 82:593-599, 1996.
98. Wright DR, Thornton C, Hasan K, et al: The effect of remifentanil on the middle latency auditory evoked response and haemodynamic measurements with and without the stimulus of orotracheal intubation. Eur J Anaesthesiol 21:509-516, 2004.
99. Thorogood MC, Armstead WM: Influence of polyethylene glycol superoxide dismutase/catalase on altered opioid-induced pial artery dilation after brain injury. Anesthesiology 84:614-625, 1996.
100. Monitto CL, Kurth CD: The effect of fentanyl, sufentanil, and alfentanil on cerebral arterioles in piglets. Anesth Analg 76:985-989, 1993.
101. Adler LJ, Gyulai FE, Diehl DJ, et al: Regional brain activity changes associated with fentanyl analgesia elucidated by positron emission tomography. Anesth Analg 84:120-126, 1997.
102. Werner C, Hoffman WE, Baughman VL, et al: Effects of sufentanil on cerebral blood flow, cerebral blood flow velocity, and metabolism in dogs. Anesth Analg 72:177-181, 1991.
103. Milde LN, Milde JH, Gallagher WJ: Effects of sufentanil on cerebral circulation and metabolism in dogs. Anesth Analg 70:138-146, 1990.
104. Mayer N, Weinstabl C, Podreka I, Spiss CK: Sufentanil does not increase cerebral blood flow in healthy human volunteers. Anesthesiology 73:240-243, 1990.
105. Mayberg TS, Lam AM, Eng CC, et al: The effect of alfentanil on cerebral blood flow velocity and intracranial pressure during isoflurane–nitrous oxide anesthesia in humans. Anesthesiology 78:288-294, 1993.
106. Hoffman WE, Cunningham F, James MK, et al: Effects of remifentanil, a new short-acting opioid, on cerebral blood flow, brain electrical activity, and intracranial pressure in dogs anesthetized with isoflurane and nitrous oxide. Anesthesiology 79:107-113, 1993.
107. Wagner KJ, Willoch F, Kochs EF, et al: Dose-dependent regional cerebral blood flow changes during remifentanil infusion in humans: A positron emission tomography study. Anesthesiology 94:732-739, 2001.
108. Ostapkovich ND, Baker KZ, Fogarty-Mack P, et al: Cerebral blood flow and CO_2 reactivity is similar during remifentanil/N_2O and fentanyl/N_2O anesthesia. Anesthesiology 89:358-363, 1998.
109. Kofke WA, Garman RH, Tom WC, et al: Alfentanil-induced hypermetabolism, seizure, and histopathology in rat brain. Anesth Analg 75:953-964, 1992.
110. Kofke WA, Attaallah AF, Kuwabara H, et al: The neuropathologic effects in rats and neurometabolic

effects in humans of large-dose remifentanil. Anesth Analg 94:1229-1236, 2002.
111. Baskin DS, Widmayer MA, Browning JL, et al: Evaluation of delayed treatment of focal cerebral ischemia with three selective κ-opioid agonists in cats. Stroke 25:2047-2053, 1994.
112. Takahashi H, Traystman RJ, Hashimoto K, et al: Postischemic brain injury is affected stereospecifically by pentazocine in rats. Anesth Analg 85:353-357, 1997.
113. Mayfield KP, D'Alecy LG: Delta-1 opioid agonist acutely increases hypoxic tolerance. J Pharmacol Exp Ther 268:683-688, 1994.
114. Bofetiado DM, Mayfield KP, D'Alecy LG: Alkaloid δ agonist BW373U86 increases hypoxic tolerance. Anesth Analg 82:1237-1241, 1996.
115. Lim YJ, Zheng S, Zuo Z: Morphine preconditions Purkinje cells against cell death under in vitro simulated ischemia-reperfusion conditions. Anesthesiology 100:562-568, 2004.
116. Charchaflieh J, Cottrell JE, Kass IS: The effect of fentanyl on electrophysiologic recovery of CA 1 pyramidal cells from anoxia in the rat hippocampal slice. Anesth Analg 87:68-71, 1998.
117. Soonthon Brant V, Patel PM, Drummond JC, et al: Fentanyl does not increase brain injury after focal cerebral ischemia in rats. Anesth Analg 88:49-55, 1999.
118. Vankova ME, Weinger MB, Chen DY, et al: Role of central m, *d-1*, and κ-1 opioid receptors in opioid-induced muscle rigidity in the rat. Anesthesiology 85:574-583, 1996.
119. Mets B: Acute dystonia after alfentanil in untreated Parkinson's disease. Anesth Analg 72:557-558, 1991.
120. Haber GW, Litman RS: Generalized tonic-clonic activity after remifentanil administration. Anesth Analg 93:1532-1533, 2001.
121. Parkinson SK, Bailey SL, Little WL, Mueller JB: Myoclonic seizure activity with chronic high-dose spinal opioid administration. Anesthesiology 72:743-745, 1990.
122. Gutstein HB, Rubie EA, Mansour A, et al: Opioid effects on mitogen-activated protein kinase signaling cascades. Anesthesiology 87:1118-1126, 1997.
123. Kofke WA, Garman RH, Janosky J, Rose ME: Opioid neurotoxicity: Neuropathologic effects in rats of different fentanyl congeners and the effects of hexamethonium-induced normotension. Anesth Analg 83:141-146, 1996.
124. Sinz EH, Kofke WA, Garman RH: Phenytoin, midazolam, and naloxone protect against fentanyl-induced brain damage in rats. Anesth Analg 91:1443-1449, 2000.
125. Kofke WA, Blissitt PA, Rao H, et al: Remifentanil-induced cerebral blood flow effects in normal humans: Dose and ApoE genotype. Anesth Analg 105:167-175, 2007.
126. Knaggs RD, Crighton IM, Cobby TF, et al: The pupillary effects of intravenous morphine, codeine, and tramadol in volunteers. Anesth Analg 99:108-112, 2004.
127. Larson MD, Kurz A, Sessler DI, et al: Alfentanil blocks reflex pupillary dilation in response to noxious stimulation but does not diminish the light reflex. Anesthesiology 87:849-855, 1997.
128. Kurz A, Go JC, Sessler DI, et al: Alfentanil slightly increases the sweating threshold and markedly reduces the vasoconstriction and shivering thresholds. Anesthesiology 83:293-299, 1995.
129. Ikeda T, Sessler DI, Tayefeh F, et al: Meperidine and alfentanil do not reduce the gain or maximum intensity of shivering. Anesthesiology 88:858-865, 1998.
130. Kurz M, Belani KG, Sessler DI, et al: Naloxone, meperidine, and shivering. Anesthesiology 79:1193-1201, 1993.
131. Greif R, Laciny S, Rajek AM, et al: Neither nalbuphine nor atropine possess special antishivering activity. Anesth Analg 93:620-627, 2001.
132. Tsai YC, Chu KS: A comparison of tramadol, amitriptyline, and meperidine for postepidural anesthetic shivering in parturients. Anesth Analg 93:1288-1292, 2001.
133. Ko MC, Naughton NN: An experimental itch model in monkeys: Characterization of intrathecal morphine–induced scratching and antinociception. Anesthesiology 92:795-805, 2000.
134. Cohen SE, Ratner EF, Kreitzman TR, et al: Nalbuphine is better than naloxone for treatment of side effects after epidural morphine. Anesth Analg 75:747-752, 1992.
135. Dunteman E, Karanikolas M, Filos KS: Transnasal butorphanol for the treatment of opioid-induced pruritus unresponsive to antihistamines. J Pain Symptom Manage 12:255-260, 1996.
136. Borgeat A, Stirnemann HR: Ondansetron is effective to treat spinal or epidural morphine–induced pruritus. Anesthesiology 90:432-436, 1999.
137. Colbert S, O'Hanlon DM, Chambers F, Moriarty DC: The effect of intravenous tenoxicam on pruritus in patients receiving epidural fentanyl. Anaesthesia 54:76-80, 1999.
138. Horta ML, Morejon LC, da Cruz AW, et al: Study of the prophylactic effect of droperidol, alizapride, propofol and promethazine on spinal morphine-induced pruritus. Br J Anaesth 96:796-800, 2006.
139. Jones EA, Bergasa NV: The pruritus of cholestasis and the opioid system. JAMA 268:3359-3362, 1992.
140. Etches RC: Respiratory depression associated with patient-controlled analgesia: A review of eight cases. Can J Anaesth 41:125-132, 1994.
141. Zhang Z, Xu F, Zhang C, Liang X: Activation of opioid μ receptors in caudal medullary raphe region inhibits the ventilatory response to hypercapnia in anesthetized rats. Anesthesiology 107:288-297, 2007.
142. Romberg R, Sarton E, Teppema L, et al: Comparison of morphine-6-glucuronide and morphine on respiratory depressant and antinociceptive responses in wild type and μ-opioid receptor deficient mice. Br J Anaesth 91:862-870, 2003.
143. Freye E, Latasch L, Portoghese PS: The δ receptor is involved in sufentanil-induced respiratory depression—opioid subreceptors mediate different effects. Eur J Anaesthesiol 9:457-462, 1992.
144. Selwyn DA, Raphael JH, Lambert DG, Langton JA: Effects of morphine on human nasal cilia beat frequency in vitro. Br J Anaesth 76:274-277, 1996.
145. Jaeckle KA, Digre KB, Jones CR, et al: Central neurogenic hyperventilation: Pharmacologic intervention with morphine sulfate and correlative analysis of respiratory, sleep, and ocular motor dysfunction. Neurology 40:1715-1720, 1990.
146. Tobias JD, Heideman RL: Primary central hyperventilation in a child with a brainstem glioma: Management with continuous intravenous fentanyl. Pediatrics 88:818-820, 1991.
147. Bohrer H, Fleischer F, Werning P: Tussive effect of a fentanyl bolus administered through a central venous catheter. Anaesthesia 45:18-21, 1990.
148. Lin JA, Yeh CC, Lee MS, et al: Prolonged injection time and light smoking decrease the incidence of fentanyl-induced cough. Anesth Analg 101:670-674, 2005.
149. Pandey CK, Raza M, Ranjan R, et al: Intravenous lidocaine suppresses fentanyl-induced coughing: A double-blind, prospective, randomized placebo-controlled study. Anesth Analg 99:1696-1698, 2004.
150. Ruiz Neto PP, Auler Junior JO: Respiratory mechanical properties during fentanyl and alfentanil anaesthesia. Can J Anaesth 39:458-465, 1992.
151. Sarton E, Teppema L, Dahan A: Sex differences in morphine-induced ventilatory depression reside within the peripheral chemoreflex loop. Anesthesiology 90:1329-1338, 1999.
152. Smart JA, Pallett EJ, Duthie DJ: Breath interval as a measure of dynamic opioid effect. Br J Anaesth 84:735-738, 2000.
153. Bailey PL, Streisand JB, East KA, et al: Differences in magnitude and duration of opioid-induced respiratory depression and analgesia with fentanyl and sufentanil. Anesth Analg 70:8-15, 1990.
154. Glass PS, Iselin-Chaves IA, Goodman D, et al: Determination of the potency of remifentanil compared with alfentanil using ventilatory depression as the measure of opioid effect. Anesthesiology 90:1556-1563, 1999.
155. Combes X, Cerf C, Bouleau D, et al: The effects of residual pain on oxygenation and breathing pattern during morphine analgesia. Anesth Analg 90:156-160, 2000.
156. Krenn H, Jellinek H, Haumer H, et al: Naloxone-resistant respiratory depression and neurological eye symptoms after intrathecal morphine. Anesth Analg 91:432-433, 2000.
157. Furst SR, Weinger MB: Dexmedetomidine, a selective α_2-agonist, does not potentiate the cardiorespiratory depression of alfentanil in the rat. Anesthesiology 72:882-888, 1990.
158. Peat SJ, Hanna MH, Woodham M, et al: Morphine-6-glucuronide: Effects on ventilation in normal volunteers. Pain 45:101-104, 1991.
159. Robbins GR, Wynands JE, Whalley DG, et al: Pharmacokinetics of alfentanil and clinical responses during cardiac surgery. Can J Anaesth 37:52-57, 1990.
160. Feldman PD, Parveen N, Sezen S: Cardiovascular effects of Leu-enkephalin in the nucleus tractus solitarius of the rat. Brain Res 709:331-336, 1996.
161. Keay KA, Crowfoot LJ, Floyd NS, et al: Cardiovascular effects of microinjections of opioid agonists into the 'Depressor Region' of the ventrolateral periaqueductal gray region. Brain Res 762:61-71, 1997.
162. Zhang CC, Su JY, Calkins D: Effects of alfentanil on isolated cardiac tissues of the rabbit. Anesth Analg 71:268-274, 1990.
163. Helgesen KG, Ellingsen O, Ilebekk A: Inotropic effect of meperidine: Influence of receptor and ion channel blockers in the rat atrium. Anesth Analg 70:499-506, 1990.
164. Nakae Y, Fujita S, Namiki A: Morphine enhances myofilament Ca^{2+} sensitivity in intact guinea pig beating hearts. Anesth Analg 92:602-608, 2001.
165. Xiao GS, Zhou JJ, Wang GY, et al: In vitro electrophysiologic effects of morphine in rabbit ventricular myocytes. Anesthesiology 103:280-286, 2005.
166. Llobel F, Laorden ML: Effects of morphine on atrial preparations obtained from nonfailing and failing human hearts. Br J Anaesth 76:106-110, 1996.
167. Kawakubo A, Fujigaki T, Uresino H, et al: Comparative effects of etomidate, ketamine, propofol, and fentanyl on myocardial contractility in dogs. J Anesth 13:77-82, 1999.
168. Graham MD, Hopkins PM, Harrison SM: The effects of alfentanil on cytosolic Ca(2+) and contraction in rat ventricular myocytes. Anesth Analg 98:1013-1016, 2004.
169. Duncan DJ, Hopkins PM, Harrison SM: Negative inotropic effects of tumour necrosis factor-alpha

and interleukin-1beta are ameliorated by alfentanil in rat ventricular myocytes. Br J Pharmacol 150:720-726, 2007.
170. James MK, Vuong A, Grizzle MK, et al: Hemodynamic effects of GI 87084B, an ultra-short acting μ-opioid analgesic, in anesthetized dogs. J Pharmacol Exp Ther 263:84-91, 1992.
171. Weber G, Stark G, Stark U: Direct cardiac electrophysiologic effects of sufentanil and vecuronium in isolated guinea-pig hearts. Acta Anaesthesiol Scand 39:1071-1074, 1995.
172. Lischke V, Wilke HJ, Probst S, et al: Prolongation of the QT-interval during induction of anesthesia in patients with coronary artery disease. Acta Anaesthesiol Scand 38:144-148, 1994.
173. Sharpe MD, Dobkowski WB, Murkin JM, et al: Alfentanil-midazolam anaesthesia has no electrophysiological effects upon the normal conduction system or accessory pathways in patients with Wolff-Parkinson-White syndrome. Can J Anaesth 39:816-821, 1992.
174. Sharpe MD, Dobkowski WB, Murkin JM, et al: The electrophysiologic effects of volatile anesthetics and sufentanil on the normal atrioventricular conduction system and accessory pathways in Wolff-Parkinson-White syndrome. Anesthesiology 80:63-70, 1994.
175. Atlee JL 3rd, Bosnjak ZJ: Mechanisms for cardiac dysrhythmias during anesthesia. Anesthesiology 72:347-374, 1990.
176. Sarne Y, Flitstein A, Oppenheimer E: Anti-arrhythmic activities of opioid agonists and antagonists and their stereoisomers. Br J Pharmacol 102:696-698, 1991.
177. McIntosh M, Kane K, Parratt J: Effects of selective opioid receptor agonists and antagonists during myocardial ischaemia. Eur J Pharmacol 210:37-44, 1992.
178. Schultz JE, Hsu AK, Gross GJ: Morphine mimics the cardioprotective effect of ischemic preconditioning via a glibenclamide-sensitive mechanism in the rat heart. Circ Res 78:1100-1104, 1996.
179. Zhang Y, Irwin MG, Wong TM, et al: Remifentanil preconditioning confers cardioprotection via cardiac κ- and δ-opioid receptors. Anesthesiology 102:371-378, 2005.
180. Zhang Y, Irwin MG, Wong TM: Remifentanil preconditioning protects against ischemic injury in the intact rat heart. Anesthesiology 101:918-923, 2004.
181. Frassdorf J, Weber NC, Obal D, et al: Morphine induces late cardioprotection in rat hearts in vivo: The involvement of opioid receptors and nuclear transcription factor κB. Anesth Analg 101:934-941, 2005.
182. Zhang SZ, Wang NF, Xu J, et al: κ-Opioid receptors mediate cardioprotection by remote preconditioning. Anesthesiology 105:550-556, 2006.
183. Weihrauch D, Krolikowski JG, Bienengraeber M, et al: Morphine enhances isoflurane-induced postconditioning against myocardial infarction: The role of phosphatidylinositol-3-kinase and opioid receptors in rabbits. Anesth Analg 101:942-949, 2005.
184. McPherson BC, Yao Z: Signal transduction of opioid-induced cardioprotection in ischemia-reperfusion. Anesthesiology 94:1082-1088, 2001.
185. Kato R, Foex P: Fentanyl reduces infarction but not stunning via δ-opioid receptors and protein kinase C in rats. Br J Anaesth 84:608-614, 2000.
186. Kato R, Ross S, Foex P: Fentanyl protects the heart against ischaemic injury via opioid receptors, adenosine A_1 receptors and K_{ATP} channel linked mechanisms in rats. Br J Anaesth 84:204-214, 2000.
187. Warltier DC, Pagel PS, Kersten JR: Approaches to the prevention of perioperative myocardial ischemia. Anesthesiology 92:253-259, 2000.
188. Helman JD, Leung JM, Bellows WH, et al: The risk of myocardial ischemia in patients receiving desflurane versus sufentanil anesthesia for coronary artery bypass graft surgery. The S.P.I. Research Group. Anesthesiology 77:47-62, 1992.
189. Leung JM, Goehner P, O'Kelly BF, et al: Isoflurane anesthesia and myocardial ischemia: Comparative risk versus sufentanil anesthesia in patients undergoing coronary artery bypass graft surgery. The SPI (Study of Perioperative Ischemia) Research Group. Anesthesiology 74:838-847, 1991.
190. Blaise GA, Witzeling TM, Sill JC, et al: Fentanyl is devoid of major effects on coronary vasoreactivity and myocardial metabolism in experimental animals. Anesthesiology 72:535-541, 1990.
191. Moore PG, Quail AW, Cottee DB, et al: Effect of fentanyl on baroreflex control of circumflex coronary conductance. Clin Exp Pharmacol Physiol 27:1028-1033, 2000.
192. Yamanoue T, Brum JM, Estafanous FG, et al: Effects of opioids on vasoresponsiveness of porcine coronary artery. Anesth Analg 74:889-896, 1992.
193. Lennander O, Henriksson BA, Martner J, Biber B: Effects of fentanyl, nitrous oxide, or both, on baroreceptor reflex regulation in the cat. Br J Anaesth 77:399-403, 1996.
194. Arnold RW, Jensen PA, Kovtoun TA, et al: The profound augmentation of the oculocardiac reflex by fast acting opioids. Binocul Vis Strabismus Q 19:215-222, 2004.
195. Hahnenkamp K, Honemann CW, Fischer LG, et al: Effect of different anaesthetic regimes on the oculocardiac reflex during paediatric strabismus surgery. Paediatr Anaesth 10:601-608, 2000.
196. Blunk JA, Schmelz M, Zeck S, et al: Opioid-induced mast cell activation and vascular responses is not mediated by μ-opioid receptors: An in vivo microdialysis study in human skin. Anesth Analg 98:364-370, 2004.
197. Stefano GB: Autoimmunovascular regulation: Morphine and anandamide and ancondamide stimulated nitric oxide release. J Neuroimmunol 83:70-76, 1998.
198. White DA, Reitan JA, Kien ND, Thorup SJ: Decrease in vascular resistance in the isolated canine hindlimb after graded doses of alfentanil, fentanyl, and sufentanil. Anesth Analg 71:29-34, 1990.
199. Ebert TJ, Ficke DJ, Arain SR, et al: Vasodilation from sufentanil in humans. Anesth Analg 101:1677-1680, 2005.
200. Sohn JT, Park KE, Kim C, et al: Alfentanil attenuates phenylephrine-induced contraction in rat aorta. Eur J Anaesthesiol 24:276-282, 2007.
201. Unlugenc H, Itegin M, Ocal I, et al: Remifentanil produces vasorelaxation in isolated rat thoracic aorta strips. Acta Anaesthesiol Scand 47:65-69, 2003.
202. Sohn JT, Ding X, McCune DF, et al: Fentanyl attenuates α_{1B}-adrenoceptor–mediated pulmonary artery contraction. Anesthesiology 103:327-334, 2005.
203. Kaye AD, Baluch A, Phelps J, et al: An analysis of remifentanil in the pulmonary vascular bed of the cat. Anesth Analg 102:118-123, 2006.
204. Kaye AD, Phelps J, Baluch A, et al: The effects of sufentanil in the feline pulmonary vascular bed. Eur J Pharmacol 534:159-164, 2006.
205. Sohn JT, Ok SH, Kim HJ, et al: Inhibitory effect of fentanyl on acetylcholine-induced relaxation in rat aorta. Anesthesiology 101:89-96, 2004.
206. Chrousos GP, Gold PW: The concepts of stress and stress system disorders. Overview of physical and behavioral homeostasis. JAMA 267:1244-1252, 1992.
207. Anand KJ, Hansen DD, Hickey PR: Hormonal-metabolic stress responses in neonates undergoing cardiac surgery. Anesthesiology 73:661-670, 1990.
208. Delitala G, Trainer PJ, Oliva O, et al: Opioid peptide and α-adrenoceptor pathways in the regulation of the pituitary-adrenal axis in man. J Endocrinol 141:163-168, 1994.
209. Ellis DJ, Steward DJ: Fentanyl dosage is associated with reduced blood glucose in pediatric patients after hypothermic cardiopulmonary bypass. Anesthesiology 72:812-815, 1990.
210. Myles PS, Hunt JO, Fletcher H, et al: Remifentanil, fentanyl, and cardiac surgery: A double-blinded, randomized, controlled trial of costs and outcomes. Anesth Analg 95:805-812, 2002.
211. Anand KJ, Hickey PR: Halothane-morphine compared with high-dose sufentanil for anesthesia and postoperative analgesia in neonatal cardiac surgery. N Engl J Med 326:1-9, 1992.
212. Mangano DT, Siliciano D, Hollenberg M, et al: Postoperative myocardial ischemia. Therapeutic trials using intensive analgesia following surgery. The Study of Perioperative Ischemia (SPI) Research Group. Anesthesiology 76:342-353, 1992.
213. Plunkett JJ, Reeves JD, Ngo L, et al: Urine and plasma catecholamine and cortisol concentrations after myocardial revascularization. Modulation by continuous sedation. Multicenter Study of Perioperative Ischemia (McSPI) Research Group, and the Ischemia Research and Education Foundation (IREF). Anesthesiology 86:785-796, 1997.
214. Nestler EJ, Aghajanian GK: Molecular and cellular basis of addiction. Science 278:58-63, 1997.
215. Chan KW, Duttory A, Yoburn BC: Magnitude of tolerance to fentanyl is independent of μ-opioid receptor density. Eur J Pharmacol 319:225-228, 1997.
216. Lim G, Wang S, Zeng Q, et al: Spinal glucocorticoid receptors contribute to the development of morphine tolerance in rats. Anesthesiology 102:832-837, 2005.
217. Wang Y, Mitchell J, Moriyama K, et al: Age-dependent morphine tolerance development in the rat. Anesth Analg 100:1733-1739, 2005.
218. Kissin I, Brown PT, Robinson CA, Bradley EL Jr: Acute tolerance in morphine analgesia: Continuous infusion and single injection in rats. Anesthesiology 74:166-171, 1991.
219. Chia YY, Liu K, Wang JJ, et al: Intraoperative high dose fentanyl induces postoperative fentanyl tolerance. Can J Anaesth 46:872-877, 1999.
220. Vinik HR, Kissin I: Rapid development of tolerance to analgesia during remifentanil infusion in humans. Anesth Analg 86:1307-1311, 1998.
221. Guignard B, Bossard AE, Coste C, et al: Acute opioid tolerance: Intraoperative remifentanil increases postoperative pain and morphine requirement. Anesthesiology 93:409-417, 2000.
222. Schraag S, Checketts MR, Kenny GN: Lack of rapid development of opioid tolerance during alfentanil and remifentanil infusions for postoperative pain. Anesth Analg 89:753-757, 1999.
223. Gustorff B, Nahlik G, Hoerauf KH, Kress HG: The absence of acute tolerance during remifentanil infusion in volunteers. Anesth Analg 94:1223-1228, 2002.
224. Celerier E, Rivat C, Jun Y, et al: Long-lasting hyperalgesia induced by fentanyl in rats: Preventive effect of ketamine. Anesthesiology 92:465-472, 2000.
225. Mao J, Price DD, Mayer DJ: Mechanisms of hyperalgesia and morphine tolerance: A current view of their possible interactions. Pain 62:259-274, 1995.

226. Li X, Angst MS, Clark JD: Opioid-induced hyperalgesia and incisional pain. Anesth Analg 93:204-209, 2001.
227. Li X, Clark JD: Hyperalgesia during opioid abstinence: Mediation by glutamate and substance p. Anesth Analg 95:979-984, 2002.
228. Kissin I, Bright CA, Bradley EL Jr: Acute tolerance to continuously infused alfentanil: The role of cholecystokinin and *N*-methyl-D-aspartate–nitric oxide systems. Anesth Analg 91:110-116, 2000.
229. Li JY, Wong CH, Huang EY, et al: Modulations of spinal serotonin activity affect the development of morphine tolerance. Anesth Analg 92:1563-1568, 2001.
230. Laulin JP, Maurette P, Corcuff JB, et al: The role of ketamine in preventing fentanyl-induced hyperalgesia and subsequent acute morphine tolerance. Anesth Analg 94:1263-1269, 2002.
231. Kissin I, Bright CA, Bradley EL Jr: The effect of ketamine on opioid-induced acute tolerance: Can it explain reduction of opioid consumption with ketamine-opioid analgesic combinations? Anesth Analg 91:1483-1488, 2000.
232. Holtman JR Jr, Wala EP: Characterization of the antinociceptive and pronociceptive effects of methadone in rats. Anesthesiology 106:563-571, 2007.
233. Dunbar SA, Karamian I, Roberts L, Zhang J: Increased prostaglandin E_2 release and activated Akt/beta-catenin signaling pathway occur after opioid withdrawal in rat spinal cord. Anesthesiology 105:154-159, 2006.
234. Troster A, Sittl R, Singler B, et al: Modulation of remifentanil-induced analgesia and postinfusion hyperalgesia by parecoxib in humans. Anesthesiology 105:1016-1023, 2006.
235. Liang DY, Liao G, Wang J, et al: A genetic analysis of opioid-induced hyperalgesia in mice. Anesthesiology 104:1054-1062, 2006.
236. Angst MS, Clark JD: Opioid-induced hyperalgesia: A qualitative systematic review. Anesthesiology 104:570-587, 2006.
237. Stein C, Pfluger M, Yassouridis A, et al: No tolerance to peripheral morphine analgesia in presence of opioid expression in inflamed synovia. J Clin Invest 98:793-799, 1996.
238. Duttaroy A, Yoburn BC: The effect of intrinsic efficacy on opioid tolerance. Anesthesiology 82:1226-1236, 1995.
239. Ouellet DM, Pollack GM: Pharmacodynamics and tolerance development during multiple intravenous bolus morphine administration in rats. J Pharmacol Exp Ther 281:713-720, 1997.
240. Hanks GW, Forbes K: Opioid responsiveness. Acta Anaesthesiol Scand 41:154-158, 1997.
241. Mitra S, Sinatra RS: Perioperative management of acute pain in the opioid-dependent patient. Anesthesiology 101:212-227, 2004.
242. Kienbaum P, Thurauf N, Michel MC, et al: Profound increase in epinephrine concentration in plasma and cardiovascular stimulation after μ-opioid receptor blockade in opioid-addicted patients during barbiturate-induced anesthesia for acute detoxification. Anesthesiology 88:1154-1161, 1998.
243. Hensel M, Wolter S, Kox WJ: EEG controlled rapid opioid withdrawal under general anaesthesia. Br J Anaesth 84:236-238, 2000.
244. Kienbaum P, Heuter T, Michel MC, et al: Sympathetic neural activation evoked by μ-receptor blockade in patients addicted to opioids is abolished by intravenous clonidine. Anesthesiology 96:346-351, 2002.
245. Salas SP, Roblero JS, Lopez LF, et al: [*N*-methyl-Tyr1,*N*-methyl-Arg7-D-Leu8]-dynorphin-A-(1-8)ethylamide, a stable dynorphin analog, produces diuresis by kappa-opiate receptor activation in the rat. J Pharmacol Exp Ther 262:979-986, 1992.
246. Pesonen A, Leppaluoto J, Ruskoaho H: Mechanism of opioid-induced atrial natriuretic peptide release in conscious rats. J Pharmacol Exp Ther 254:690-695, 1990.
247. Kuipers PW, Kamphuis ET, van Venrooij GE, et al: Intrathecal opioids and lower urinary tract function: A urodynamic evaluation. Anesthesiology 100:1497-1503, 2004.
248. Malinovsky JM, Le Normand L, Lepage JY, et al: The urodynamic effects of intravenous opioids and ketoprofen in humans. Anesth Analg 87:456-461, 1998.
249. Rosow CE, Gomery P, Chen TY, et al: Reversal of opioid-induced bladder dysfunction by intravenous naloxone and methylnaltrexone. Clin Pharmacol Ther 82:48-53, 2007.
250. Murphy DB, Sutton JA, Prescott LF, Murphy MB: Opioid-induced delay in gastric emptying: A peripheral mechanism in humans. Anesthesiology 87:765-770, 1997.
251. Kojima Y, Takahashi T, Fujina M, Owyang C: Inhibition of cholinergic transmission by opiates in ileal myenteric plexus is mediated by kappa receptor. Involvement of regulatory inhibitory G protein and calcium N-channels. J Pharmacol Exp Ther 268:965-970, 1994.
252. Penagini R, Picone A, Bianchi PA: Effect of morphine and naloxone on motor response of the human esophagus to swallowing and distension. Am J Physiol 271:G675-680, 1996.
253. Thorn SE, Wattwil M, Lindberg G, Sawe J: Systemic and central effects of morphine on gastroduodenal motility. Acta Anaesthesiol Scand 40:177-186, 1996.
254. Crighton IM, Martin PH, Hobbs GJ, et al: A comparison of the effects of intravenous tramadol, codeine, and morphine on gastric emptying in human volunteers. Anesth Analg 87:445-449, 1998.
255. Yukioka H, Tanaka M, Fujimori M: Recovery of bowel motility after high dose fentanyl or morphine anaesthesia for cardiac surgery. Anaesthesia 45:353-356, 1990.
256. Thorn SE, Wickbom G, Philipson L, et al: Myoelectric activity in the stomach and duodenum after epidural administration of morphine or bupivacaine. Acta Anaesthesiol Scand 40:773-778, 1996.
257. Runkel NS, Moody FG, Smith GS, et al: Alterations in rat intestinal transit by morphine promote bacterial translocation. Dig Dis Sci 38:1530-1536, 1993.
258. Hammas B, Thorn SE, Wattwil M: Propofol and gastric effects of morphine. Acta Anaesthesiol Scand 45:1023-1027, 2001.
259. Asai T, Power I: Naloxone inhibits gastric emptying in the rat. Anesth Analg 88:204-208, 1999.
260. McNeill MJ, Ho ET, Kenny GN: Effect of i.v. metoclopramide on gastric emptying after opioid premedication. Br J Anaesth 64:450-452, 1990.
261. Matot I, Eimerl D, Rabinovich Y, Udassin R: Effect of morphine on small bowel propulsion after intestinal ischemia. Anesthesiology 100:450-452, 2004.
262. Thompson DR: Narcotic analgesic effects on the sphincter of Oddi: A review of the data and therapeutic implications in treating pancreatitis. Am J Gastroenterol 96:1266-1272, 2001.
263. Wu SD, Zhang ZH, Jin JZ, et al: Effects of narcotic analgesic drugs on human Oddi's sphincter motility. World J Gastroenterol 10:2901-2904, 2004.
264. Fragen RJ, Vilich F, Spies SM, Erwin WD: The effect of remifentanil on biliary tract drainage into the duodenum. Anesth Analg 89:1561-1564, 1999.
265. Fisher DM: The "big little problem" of postoperative nausea and vomiting: Do we know the answer yet? Anesthesiology 87:1271-1273, 1997.
266. Tramer MR, Reynolds DJ, Moore RA, McQuay HJ: Efficacy, dose-response, and safety of ondansetron in prevention of postoperative nausea and vomiting: A quantitative systematic review of randomized placebo-controlled trials. Anesthesiology 87:1277-1289, 1997.
267. Watcha MF, White PF: Postoperative nausea and vomiting. Its etiology, treatment, and prevention. Anesthesiology 77:162-184, 1992.
268. Langevin S, Lessard MR, Trepanier CA, Baribault JP: Alfentanil causes less postoperative nausea and vomiting than equipotent doses of fentanyl or sufentanil in outpatients. Anesthesiology 91:1666-1673, 1999.
269. Raftery S, Sherry E: Total intravenous anaesthesia with propofol and alfentanil protects against postoperative nausea and vomiting. Can J Anaesth 39:37-40, 1992.
270. Rung GW, Claybon L, Hord A, et al: Intravenous ondansetron for postsurgical opioid-induced nausea and vomiting. S3A-255 Study Group. Anesth Analg 84:832-838, 1997.
271. Tzeng JI, Wang JJ, Ho ST, et al: Dexamethasone for prophylaxis of nausea and vomiting after epidural morphine for post-caesarean section analgesia: Comparison of droperidol and saline. Br J Anaesth 85:865-868, 2000.
272. Simoneau II, Hamza MS, Mata HP, et al: The cannabinoid agonist WIN55,212-2 suppresses opioid-induced emesis in ferrets. Anesthesiology 94:882-887, 2001.
273. Stener-Victorin E, Waldenstrom U, Nilsson L, et al: A prospective randomized study of electro-acupuncture versus alfentanil as anaesthesia during oocyte aspiration in in-vitro fertilization. Hum Reprod 14:2480-2484, 1999.
274. Lok IH, Chan MT, Chan DL, et al: A prospective randomized trial comparing patient-controlled sedation using propofol and alfentanil and physician-administered sedation using diazepam and pethidine during transvaginal ultrasound–guided oocyte retrieval. Hum Reprod 17:2101-2106, 2002.
275. Sandner-Kiesling A, Eisenach JC: Pharmacology of opioid inhibition to noxious uterine cervical distension. Anesthesiology 97:966-971, 2002.
276. Sandner-Kiesling A, Eisenach JC: Estrogen reduces efficacy of μ- but not κ-opioid agonist inhibition in response to uterine cervical distension. Anesthesiology 96:375-379, 2002.
277. Gin T, Ngan Kee WD, Siu YK, et al: Alfentanil given immediately before the induction of anesthesia for elective cesarean delivery. Anesth Analg 90:1167-1172, 2000.
278. Vertommen JD, Marcus MA, Van Aken H: The effects of intravenous and epidural sufentanil in the chronic maternal-fetal sheep preparation. Anesth Analg 80:71-75, 1995.
279. Strumper D, Durieux ME, Gogarten W, et al: Fetal plasma concentrations after intraamniotic sufentanil in chronically instrumented pregnant sheep. Anesthesiology 98:1400-1406, discussion 1405A-1406A, 2003.
280. Wittels B, Scott DT, Sinatra RS: Exogenous opioids in human breast milk and acute neonatal neurobehavior: A preliminary study. Anesthesiology 73:864-869, 1990.
281. Spigset O: Anaesthetic agents and excretion in breast milk. Acta Anaesthesiol Scand 38:94-103, 1994.
282. Doberczak TM, Kandall SR, Wilets I: Neonatal opiate abstinence syndrome in term and preterm infants. J Pediatr 118:933-937, 1991.

283. Edston E, van Hage-Hamsten M: Anaphylactoid shock—a common cause of death in heroin addicts? Allergy 52:950-954, 1997.
284. Alexander R, Hill R, Lipham WJ, et al: Remifentanil prevents an increase in intraocular pressure after succinylcholine and tracheal intubation. Br J Anaesth 81:606-607, 1998.
285. Ng HP, Chen FG, Yeong SM, et al: Effect of remifentanil compared with fentanyl on intraocular pressure after succinylcholine and tracheal intubation. Br J Anaesth 85:785-787, 2000.
286. Stefano GB, Scharrer B, Smith EM, et al: Opioid and opiate immunoregulatory processes. Crit Rev Immunol 16:109-144, 1996.
287. Nelson CJ, Dykstra LA, Lysle DT: Comparison of the time course of morphine's analgesic and immunologic effects. Anesth Analg 85:620-626, 1997.
288. Sacerdote P, Bianchi M, Gaspani L, et al: The effects of tramadol and morphine on immune responses and pain after surgery in cancer patients. Anesth Analg 90:1411-1414, 2000.
289. Yeager MP, Procopio MA, DeLeo JA, et al: Intravenous fentanyl increases natural killer cell cytotoxicity and circulating CD16(+) lymphocytes in humans. Anesth Analg 94:94-99, 2002.
290. Murphy GS, Szokol JW, Marymont JH, et al: The effects of morphine and fentanyl on the inflammatory response to cardiopulmonary bypass in patients undergoing elective coronary artery bypass graft surgery. Anesth Analg 104:1334-1342, 2007.
291. Welters ID, Menzebach A, Goumon Y, et al: Morphine inhibits NF-κB nuclear binding in human neutrophils and monocytes by a nitric oxide-dependent mechanism. Anesthesiology 92:1677-1684, 2000.
292. Singhal PC, Kapasi AA, Reddy K, et al: Morphine promotes apoptosis in Jurkat cells. J Leukoc Biol 66:650-658, 1999.
293. Yin D, Mufson RA, Wang R, Shi Y: Fas-mediated cell death promoted by opioids. Nature 397:218, 1999.
294. Ohara T, Itoh T, Takahashi M: Immunosuppression by morphine-induced lymphocyte apoptosis: Is it a real issue? Anesth Analg 101:1117-1122, 2005.
295. Egan TD: Intravenous drug delivery systems: Toward an intravenous "vaporizer." J Clin Anesth 8:8s-14s, 1996.
296. van den Nieuwenhuyzen MC, Engbers FH, Burm AG, et al: Target-controlled infusion of alfentanil for postoperative analgesia: Contribution of plasma protein binding to intra-patient and inter-patient variability. Br J Anaesth 82:580-585, 1999.
297. Murdoch JA, Hyde RA, Kenny GN: Target-controlled remifentanil in combination with propofol for spontaneously breathing day-case patients. Anaesthesia 54:1028-1031, 1999.
298. Olkkola KT, Hamunen K, Maunuksela EL: Clinical pharmacokinetics and pharmacodynamics of opioid analgesics in infants and children. Clin Pharmacokinet 28:385-404, 1995.
299. Minto CF, Schnider TW, Egan TD, et al: Influence of age and gender on the pharmacokinetics and pharmacodynamics of remifentanil. I. Model development. Anesthesiology 86:10-23, 1997.
300. Egan TD, Huizinga B, Gupta SK, et al: Remifentanil pharmacokinetics in obese versus lean patients. Anesthesiology 89:562-573, 1998.
301. Davies G, Kingswood C, Street M: Pharmacokinetics of opioids in renal dysfunction. Clin Pharmacokinet 31:410-422, 1996.
302. Osborne R, Joel S, Grebenik K, et al: The pharmacokinetics of morphine and morphine glucuronides in kidney failure. Clin Pharmacol Ther 54:158-167, 1993.
303. Murphy EJ: Acute pain management pharmacology for the patient with concurrent renal or hepatic disease. Anaesth Intensive Care 33:311-322, 2005.
304. Rudin A, Lundberg JF, Hammarlund-Udenaes M, et al: Morphine metabolism after major liver surgery. Anesth Analg 104:1409-1414, 2007.
305. Danziger LH, Martin SJ, Blum RA: Central nervous system toxicity associated with meperidine use in hepatic disease. Pharmacotherapy 14:235-238, 1994.
306. Tegeder I, Lotsch J, Geisslinger G: Pharmacokinetics of opioids in liver disease. Clin Pharmacokinet 37:17-40, 1999.
307. Scholz J, Steinfath M, Schulz M: Clinical pharmacokinetics of alfentanil, fentanyl and sufentanil. An update. Clin Pharmacokinet 31:275-292, 1996.
308. Baririan N, Van Obbergh L, Desager JP, et al: Alfentanil-induced miosis as a surrogate measure of alfentanil pharmacokinetics in patients with mild and moderate liver cirrhosis. Clin Pharmacokinet 46:261-270, 2007.
309. Hudson RJ, Thomson IR, Burgess PM, Rosenbloom M: Alfentanil pharmacokinetics in patients undergoing abdominal aortic surgery. Can J Anaesth 38:61-67, 1991.
310. Navapurkar VU, Archer S, Frazer NM, et al: Pharmacokinetics of remifentanil during hepatic transplantation. Anesthesiology 83:A382, 1995.
311. Gedney JA, Ghosh S: Pharmacokinetics of analgesics, sedatives and anaesthetic agents during cardiopulmonary bypass. Br J Anaesth 75:344-351, 1995.
312. Kentala E, Kaila T, Arola M, et al: Pharmacokinetics and clinical response of hyoscine plus morphine premedication in connection with cardiopulmonary bypass surgery. Eur J Anaesthesiol 8:135-140, 1991.
313. Miller RS, Peterson GM, McLean S, Moller C: Effect of cardiopulmonary bypass on the plasma concentrations of fentanyl and alcuronium. J Clin Pharm Ther 22:197-205, 1997.
314. Hudson RJ, Thomson IR, Jassal R, et al: Cardiopulmonary bypass has minimal effects on the pharmacokinetics of fentanyl in adults. Anesthesiology 99:847-854, 2003.
315. Hug CC Jr, Burm AG, de Lange S: Alfentanil pharmacokinetics in cardiac surgical patients. Anesth Analg 78:231-239, 1994.
316. Petros A, Dunne N, Mehta R, et al: The pharmacokinetics of alfentanil after normothermic and hypothermic cardiopulmonary bypass. Anesth Analg 81:458-464, 1995.
317. Hynynen M, Hynninen M, Soini H, et al: Plasma concentration and protein binding of alfentanil during high-dose infusion for cardiac surgery. Br J Anaesth 72:571-576, 1994.
318. Russell D, Royston D, Rees PH, et al: Effect of temperature and cardiopulmonary bypass on the pharmacokinetics of remifentanil. Br J Anaesth 79:456-459, 1997.
319. Davis PJ, Wilson AS, Siewers RD, et al: The effects of cardiopulmonary bypass on remifentanil kinetics in children undergoing atrial septal defect repair. Anesth Analg 89:904-908, 1999.
320. Michelsen LG, Holford NH, Lu W, et al: The pharmacokinetics of remifentanil in patients undergoing coronary artery bypass grafting with cardiopulmonary bypass. Anesth Analg 93:1100-1105, 2001.
321. Egan TD, Kuramkote S, Gong G, et al: Fentanyl pharmacokinetics in hemorrhagic shock: A porcine model. Anesthesiology 91:156-166, 1999.
322. Johnson KB, Kern SE, Hamber EA, et al: Influence of hemorrhagic shock on remifentanil: A pharmacokinetic and pharmacodynamic analysis. Anesthesiology 94:322-332, 2001.
323. Benrath J, Brechtel C, Martin E, Sandkuhler J: Low doses of fentanyl block central sensitization in the rat spinal cord in vivo. Anesthesiology 100:1545-1551, 2004.
324. Gottschalk A, Smith DS, Jobes DR, et al: Preemptive epidural analgesia and recovery from radical prostatectomy: A randomized controlled trial. JAMA 279:1076-1082, 1998.
325. Holthusen H, Backhaus P, Boeminghaus F, et al: Preemptive analgesia: No relevant advantage of preoperative compared with postoperative intravenous administration of morphine, ketamine, and clonidine in patients undergoing transperitoneal tumor nephrectomy. Reg Anesth Pain Med 27:249-253, 2002.
326. Aida S, Baba H, Yamakura T, et al: The effectiveness of preemptive analgesia varies according to the type of surgery: A randomized, double-blind study. Anesth Analg 89:711-716, 1999.
327. Ong CK, Lirk P, Seymour RA, Jenkins BJ: The efficacy of preemptive analgesia for acute postoperative pain management: A meta-analysis. Anesth Analg 100:757-773, 2005.
328. Wasylak TJ, Abbott FV, English MJ, Jeans ME: Reduction of postoperative morbidity following patient-controlled morphine. Can J Anaesth 37:726-731, 1990.
329. Upton RN, Semple TJ, Macintyre PE: Pharmacokinetic optimisation of opioid treatment in acute pain therapy. Clin Pharmacokinet 33:225-244, 1997.
330. Plummer JL, Owen H, Ilsley AH, Inglis S: Morphine patient-controlled analgesia is superior to meperidine patient-controlled analgesia for postoperative pain. Anesth Analg 84:794-799, 1997.
331. Shapiro BA, Warren J, Egol AB, et al: Practice parameters for intravenous analgesia and sedation for adult patients in the intensive care unit: An executive summary. Society of Critical Care Medicine. Crit Care Med 23:1596-1600, 1995.
332. Dahaba AA, Grabner T, Rehak PH, et al: Remifentanil versus morphine analgesia and sedation for mechanically ventilated critically ill patients: A randomized double blind study. Anesthesiology 101:640-646, 2004.
333. Andrews DT, Leslie K, Sessler DI, Bjorksten AR: The arterial blood propofol concentration preventing movement in 50% of healthy women after skin incision. Anesth Analg 85:414-419, 1997.
334. Smith C, McEwan AI, Jhaveri R, et al: The interaction of fentanyl on the Cp_{50} of propofol for loss of consciousness and skin incision. Anesthesiology 81:820-828, 1994.
335. Vuyk J, Engbers FH, Burm AG, et al: Pharmacodynamic interaction between propofol and alfentanil when given for induction of anesthesia. Anesthesiology 84:288-299, 1996.
336. Kazama T, Ikeda K, Morita K: Reduction by fentanyl of the Cp_{50} values of propofol and hemodynamic responses to various noxious stimuli. Anesthesiology 87:213-227, 1997.
337. Katoh T, Uchiyama T, Ikeda K: Effect of fentanyl on awakening concentration of sevoflurane. Br J Anaesth 73:322-325, 1994.
338. Shibutani K, Inchiosa MA Jr, Sawada K, Bairamian M: Pharmacokinetic mass of fentanyl for postoperative analgesia in lean and obese patients. Br J Anaesth 95:377-383, 2005.
339. Glass PS, Doherty M, Jacobs JR, et al: Plasma concentration of fentanyl, with 70% nitrous oxide, to prevent movement at skin incision. Anesthesiology 78:842-847, 1993.

340. Han T, Kim D, Kil H, Inagaki Y: The effects of plasma fentanyl concentrations on propofol requirement, emergence from anesthesia, and postoperative analgesia in propofol–nitrous oxide anesthesia. Anesth Analg 90:1365-1371, 2000.
341. Vuyk J, Lim T, Engbers FH, et al: Pharmacodynamics of alfentanil as a supplement to propofol or nitrous oxide for lower abdominal surgery in female patients. Anesthesiology 78:1036-1045, discussion 1023A, 1993.
342. Mertens MJ, Vuyk J, Olofsen E, et al: Propofol alters the pharmacokinetics of alfentanil in healthy male volunteers. Anesthesiology 94:949-957, 2001.
343. Glass PS, Doherty M, Jacobs JR, et al: CP_{50} for sufentanil. Anesthesiology 73:A378, 1990.
344. Thomson IR, Henderson BT, Singh K, Hudson RJ: Concentration-response relationships for fentanyl and sufentanil in patients undergoing coronary artery bypass grafting. Anesthesiology 89:852-861, 1998.
345. Patel SS, Spencer CM: Remifentanil. Drugs 52:417-427, 1996.
346. Hogue CW Jr, Bowdle TA, O'Leary C, et al: A multicenter evaluation of total intravenous anesthesia with remifentanil and propofol for elective inpatient surgery. Anesth Analg 83:279-285, 1996.
347. Avramov MN, Smith I, White PF: Interactions between midazolam and remifentanil during monitored anesthesia care. Anesthesiology 85:1283-1289, 1996.
348. Sneyd JR, Whaley A, Dimpel HL, Andrews CJ: An open, randomized comparison of alfentanil, remifentanil and alfentanil followed by remifentanil in anaesthesia for craniotomy. Br J Anaesth 81:361-364, 1998.
349. Fletcher D, Pinaud M, Scherpereel P, et al: The efficacy of intravenous 0.15 versus 0.25 mg/kg intraoperative morphine for immediate postoperative analgesia after remifentanil-based anesthesia for major surgery. Anesth Analg 90:666-671, 2000.
350. Kochs E, Cote D, Deruyck L, et al: Postoperative pain management and recovery after remifentanil-based anaesthesia with isoflurane or propofol for major abdominal surgery. Remifentanil Study Group. Br J Anaesth 84:169-173, 2000.
351. Guignard B, Coste C, Costes H, et al: Supplementing desflurane-remifentanil anesthesia with small-dose ketamine reduces perioperative opioid analgesic requirements. Anesth Analg 95:103-108, 2002.
352. Eltzschig HK, Schroeder TH, Eissler BJ, et al: The effect of remifentanil or fentanyl on postoperative vomiting and pain in children undergoing strabismus surgery. Anesth Analg 94:1173-1177, 2002.
353. Calderon E, Pernia A, De Antonio P, et al: A comparison of two constant-dose continuous infusions of remifentanil for severe postoperative pain. Anesth Analg 92:715-719, 2001.
354. Vinik HR, Bradley EL Jr, Kissin I: Triple anesthetic combination: Propofol-midazolam-alfentanil. Anesth Analg 78:354-358, 1994.
355. Vuyk J, Lim T, Engbers FH, et al: The pharmacodynamic interaction of propofol and alfentanil during lower abdominal surgery in women. Anesthesiology 83:8-22, 1995.
356. Stanski DR, Shafer SL: Quantifying anesthetic drug interaction. Implications for drug dosing. Anesthesiology 83:1-5, 1995.
357. Richards MJ, Skues MA, Jarvis AP, Prys Roberts C: Total i.v. anaesthesia with propofol and alfentanil: Dose requirements for propofol and the effect of premedication with clonidine. Br J Anaesth 65:157-163, 1990.
358. Wuesten R, Van Aken H, Glass PS, Buerkle H: Assessment of depth of anesthesia and postoperative respiratory recovery after remifentanil- versus alfentanil-based total intravenous anesthesia in patients undergoing ear-nose-throat surgery. Anesthesiology 94:211-217, 2001.
359. Vuyk J, Hennis PJ, Burm AG, et al: Comparison of midazolam and propofol in combination with alfentanil for total intravenous anesthesia. Anesth Analg 71:645-650, 1990.
360. Bell J, Sartain J, Wilkinson GA, Sherry KM: Propofol and fentanyl anaesthesia for patients with low cardiac output state undergoing cardiac surgery: Comparison with high-dose fentanyl anaesthesia. Br J Anaesth 73:162-166, 1994.
361. Engoren M, Luther G, Fenn Buderer N: A comparison of fentanyl, sufentanil, and remifentanil for fast-track cardiac anesthesia. Anesth Analg 93:859-864, 2001.
362. Howie MB, Black HA, Romanelli VA, et al: A comparison of isoflurane versus fentanyl as primary anesthetics for mitral valve surgery. Anesth Analg 83:941-948, 1996.
363. Duncan HP, Cloote A, Weir PM, et al: Reducing stress responses in the pre-bypass phase of open heart surgery in infants and young children: A comparison of different fentanyl doses. Br J Anaesth 84:556-564, 2000.
364. Beilin B, Shavit Y, Hart J, et al: Effects of anesthesia based on large versus small doses of fentanyl on natural killer cell cytotoxicity in the perioperative period. Anesth Analg 82:492-497, 1996.
365. Takahashi M, Sugiyama K, Hori M, et al: Naloxone reversal of opioid anesthesia revisited: Clinical evaluation and plasma concentration analysis of continuous naloxone infusion after anesthesia with high-dose fentanyl. J Anesth 18:1-8, 2004.
366. Silbert BS, Scott DA, Evered LA, et al: A comparison of the effect of high- and low-dose fentanyl on the incidence of postoperative cognitive dysfunction after coronary artery bypass surgery in the elderly. Anesthesiology 104:1137-1145, 2006.
367. Mantz J, Abi Jaoude F, Ceddaha A, et al: High-dose alfentanil for myocardial revascularization: A hemodynamic and pharmacokinetic study. J Cardiothorac Vasc Anesth 5:107-110, 1991.
368. Roekaerts PM, Gerrits HJ, Timmerman BE, de Lange S: Continuous infusions of alfentanil and propofol for coronary artery surgery. J Cardiothorac Vasc Anesth 9:362-367, 1995.
369. Howie MB, Smith DF, Reilley TE, et al: Postoperative course after sufentanil or fentanyl anesthesia for coronary artery surgery. J Cardiothorac Vasc Anesth 5:485-489, 1991.
370. Sareen J, Hudson RJ, Rosenbloom M, Thomson IR: Dose-response to anaesthetic induction with sufentanil: Haemodynamic and electroencephalographic effects. Can J Anaesth 44:19-25, 1997.
371. Abrams JT, Horrow JC, Bennett JA, et al: Upper airway closure: A primary source of difficult ventilation with sufentanil induction of anesthesia. Anesth Analg 83:629-632, 1996.
372. Jain U, Body SC, Bellows W, et al: Multicenter study of target-controlled infusion of propofol-sufentanil or sufentanil-midazolam for coronary artery bypass graft surgery. Multicenter Study of Perioperative Ischemia (McSPI) Research Group. Anesthesiology 85:522-535, 1996.
373. Ahonen J, Olkkola KT, Verkkala K, et al: A comparison of remifentanil and alfentanil for use with propofol in patients undergoing minimally invasive coronary artery bypass surgery. Anesth Analg 90:1269-1274, 2000.
374. Kazmaier S, Hanekop GG, Buhre W, et al: Myocardial consequences of remifentanil in patients with coronary artery disease. Br J Anaesth 84:578-583, 2000.
375. Geisler FE, de Lange S, Royston D, et al: Efficacy and safety of remifentanil in coronary artery bypass graft surgery: A randomized, double-blind dose comparison study. J Cardiothorac Vasc Anesth 17:60-68, 2003.
376. Sandler AN, Baxter AD, Katz J, et al: A double-blind, placebo-controlled trial of transdermal fentanyl after abdominal hysterectomy. Analgesic, respiratory, and pharmacokinetic effects. Anesthesiology 81:1169-1180, 1994.
377. Thompson JP, Bower S, Liddle AM, Rowbotham DJ: Perioperative pharmacokinetics of transdermal fentanyl in elderly and young adult patients. Br J Anaesth 81:152-154, 1998.
378. Portenoy RK, Southam MA, Gupta SK, et al: Transdermal fentanyl for cancer pain. Repeated dose pharmacokinetics. Anesthesiology 78:36-43, 1993.
379. Grond S, Radbruch L, Lehmann KA: Clinical pharmacokinetics of transdermal opioids: Focus on transdermal fentanyl. Clin Pharmacokinet 38:59-89, 2000.
380. Ashburn MA, Streisand J, Zhang J, et al: The iontophoresis of fentanyl citrate in humans. Anesthesiology 82:1146-1153, 1995.
381. Power I: Fentanyl HCl iontophoretic transdermal system (ITS): Clinical application of iontophoretic technology in the management of acute postoperative pain. Br J Anaesth 98:4-11, 2007.
382. Viscusi ER, Reynolds L, Chung F, et al: Patient-controlled transdermal fentanyl hydrochloride vs intravenous morphine pump for postoperative pain: A randomized controlled trial. JAMA 291:1333-1341, 2004.
383. Moa G, Zetterstrom H: Sublingual buprenorphine as postoperative analgesic: A double-blind comparison with pethidine. Acta Anaesthesiol Scand 34:68-71, 1990.
384. Manara AR, Bodenham AR, Park GR: Analgesic efficacy of perioperative buccal morphine. Br J Anaesth 64:551-555, 1990.
385. Friesen RH, Lockhart CH: Oral transmucosal fentanyl citrate for preanesthetic medication of pediatric day surgery patients with and without droperidol as a prophylactic anti-emetic. Anesthesiology 76:46-51, 1992.
386. Goldstein Dresner MC, Davis PJ, Kretchman E, et al: Double-blind comparison of oral transmucosal fentanyl citrate with oral meperidine, diazepam, and atropine as preanesthetic medication in children with congenital heart disease. Anesthesiology 74:28-33, 1991.
387. Streisand JB, Varvel JR, Stanski DR, et al: Absorption and bioavailability of oral transmucosal fentanyl citrate. Anesthesiology 75:223-229, 1991.
388. Egan TD, Sharma A, Ashburn MA, et al: Multiple dose pharmacokinetics of oral transmucosal fentanyl citrate in healthy volunteers. Anesthesiology 92:665-673, 2000.
389. Dsida RM, Wheeler M, Birmingham PK, et al: Premedication of pediatric tonsillectomy patients with oral transmucosal fentanyl citrate. Anesth Analg 86:66-70, 1998.
390. Mystakidou K, Katsouda E, Parpa E, et al: Oral transmucosal fentanyl citrate: Overview of pharmacological and clinical characteristics. Drug Deliv 13:269-276, 2006.
391. Dale O, Hjortkjaer R, Kharasch ED: Nasal administration of opioids for pain management in adults. Acta Anaesthesiol Scand 46:759-770, 2002.
392. Abboud TK, Zhu J, Gangolly J, et al: Transnasal butorphanol: A new method for pain relief in post-

cesarean section pain. Acta Anaesthesiol Scand 35:14-18, 1991.
393. Striebel HW, Oelmann T, Spies C, et al: Patient-controlled intranasal analgesia: A method for noninvasive postoperative pain management. Anesth Analg 83:548-551, 1996.
394. Karl HW, Keifer AT, Rosenberger JL, et al: Comparison of the safety and efficacy of intranasal midazolam or sufentanil for preinduction of anesthesia in pediatric patients. Anesthesiology 76:209-215, 1992.
395. Zedie N, Amory DW, Wagner BK, O'Hara DA: Comparison of intranasal midazolam and sufentanil premedication in pediatric outpatients. Clin Pharmacol Ther 59:341-348, 1996.
396. Worsley MH, MacLeod AD, Brodie MJ, et al: Inhaled fentanyl as a method of analgesia. Anaesthesia 45:449-451, 1990.
397. Hung OR, Whynot SC, Varvel JR, et al: Pharmacokinetics of inhaled liposome-encapsulated fentanyl. Anesthesiology 83:277-284, 1995.
398. Coyne PJ, Viswanathan R, Smith TJ: Nebulized fentanyl citrate improves patients' perception of breathing, respiratory rate, and oxygen saturation in dyspnea. J Pain Symptom Manage 23:157-160, 2002.
399. Farr SJ, Otulana BA: Pulmonary delivery of opioids as pain therapeutics. Adv Drug Deliv Rev 58:1076-1088, 2006.
400. Babul N, Darke AC, Anslow JA, Krishnamurthy TN: Pharmacokinetics of two novel rectal controlled-release morphine formulations. J Pain Symptom Manage 7:400-405, 1992.
401. Lundeberg S, Beck O, Olsson GL, Boreus LO: Rectal administration of morphine in children. Pharmacokinetic evaluation after a single-dose. Acta Anaesthesiol Scand 40:445-451, 1996.
402. Klepstad P, Kaasa S, Jystad A, et al: Immediate- or sustained-release morphine for dose finding during start of morphine to cancer patients: A randomized, double-blind trial. Pain 101:193-198, 2003.
403. Ginsberg B, Sinatra RS, Adler LJ, et al: Conversion to oral controlled-release oxycodone from intravenous opioid analgesic in the postoperative setting. Pain Med 4:31-38, 2003.
404. Curtis GB, Johnson GH, Clark P, et al: Relative potency of controlled-release oxycodone and controlled-release morphine in a postoperative pain model. Eur J Clin Pharmacol 55:425-429, 1999.
405. Bruera E, Belzile M, Pituskin E, et al: Randomized, double-blind, cross-over trial comparing safety and efficacy of oral controlled-release oxycodone with controlled-release morphine in patients with cancer pain. J Clin Oncol 16:3222-3229, 1998.
406. Caraco Y, Tateishi T, Guengerich FP, Wood AJ: Microsomal codeine *N*-demethylation: Cosegregation with cytochrome P4503A4 activity. Drug Metab Dispos 24:761-764, 1996.
407. Parke TJ, Nandi PR, Bird KJ, Jewkes DA: Profound hypotension following intravenous codeine phosphate. Three case reports and some recommendations. Anaesthesia 47:852-854, 1992.
408. Hill HF, Coda BA, Tanaka A, Schaffer R: Multiple-dose evaluation of intravenous hydromorphone pharmacokinetics in normal human subjects. Anesth Analg 72:330-336, 1991.
409. Wallenstein SL, Houde RW, Portenoy R, et al: Clinical analgesic assay of repeated and single doses of heroin and hydromorphone. Pain 41:5-13, 1990.
410. Quigley C, Wiffen P: A systematic review of hydromorphone in acute and chronic pain. J Pain Symptom Manage 25:169-178, 2003.
411. Rapp SE, Egan KJ, Ross BK, et al: A multidimensional comparison of morphine and hydromorphone patient-controlled analgesia. Anesth Analg 82:1043-1048, 1996.
412. Prommer E: Levorphanol: The forgotten opioid. Support Care Cancer 15:259-264, 2007.
413. Bowdle TA, Even A, Shen DD, Swardstrom M: Methadone for the induction of anesthesia: Plasma histamine concentration, arterial blood pressure, and heart rate. Anesth Analg 98:1692-1697, 2004.
414. Chamberlin KW, Cottle M, Neville R, Tan J: Oral oxymorphone for pain management. Ann Pharmacother 41:1144-1152, 2007.
415. Gimbel J, Ahdieh H: The efficacy and safety of oral immediate-release oxymorphone for postsurgical pain. Anesth Analg 99:1472-1477, 2004.
416. Morlion B, Ebner E, Weber A, et al: Influence of bolus size on efficacy of postoperative patient-controlled analgesia with piritramide. Br J Anaesth 82:52-55, 1999.
417. Bouillon T, Kietzmann D, Port R, et al: Population pharmacokinetics of piritramide in surgical patients. Anesthesiology 90:7-15, 1999.
418. Halfpenny DM, Callado LF, Hopwood SE, et al: Effects of tramadol stereoisomers on norepinephrine efflux and uptake in the rat locus coeruleus measured by real time voltammetry. Br J Anaesth 83:909-915, 1999.
419. Bamigbade TA, Davidson C, Langford RM, Stamford JA: Actions of tramadol, its enantiomers and principal metabolite, *O*-desmethyltramadol, on serotonin (5-HT) efflux and uptake in the rat dorsal raphe nucleus. Br J Anaesth 79:352-356, 1997.
420. de Wolff MH, Leather HA, Wouters PF: Effects of tramadol on minimum alveolar concentration (MAC) of isoflurane in rats. Br J Anaesth 83:780-783, 1999.
421. James MF, Heijke SA, Gordon PC: Intravenous tramadol versus epidural morphine for postthoracotomy pain relief: A placebo-controlled double-blind trial. Anesth Analg 83:87-91, 1996.
422. Vickers MD, O'Flaherty D, Szekely SM, et al: Tramadol: Pain relief by an opioid without depression of respiration. Anaesthesia 47:291-296, 1992.
423. Wilder Smith CH, Bettiga A: The analgesic tramadol has minimal effect on gastrointestinal motor function. Br J Clin Pharmacol 43:71-75, 1997.
424. Pang WW, Huang PY, Chang DP, Huang MH: The peripheral analgesic effect of tramadol in reducing propofol injection pain: A comparison with lidocaine. Reg Anesth Pain Med 24:246-249, 1999.
425. Acalovschi I, Cristea T, Margarit S, Gavrus R: Tramadol added to lidocaine for intravenous regional anesthesia. Anesth Analg 92:209-214, 2001.
426. Westman L, Valentin A, Eriksson E, Ekblom A: Intrathecal administration of sameridine to patients subjected to arthroscopic knee joint surgery. Acta Anaesthesiol Scand 42:691-697, 1998.
427. Osterlund Modalen A, Arlander E, Eriksson LI, Lindahl SG: The effects on hypercarbic ventilatory response of sameridine compared to morphine and placebo. Anesth Analg 92:529-534, 2001.
428. Osterlund A, Arlander E, Eriksson LI, Lindahl SG: The effects on resting ventilation of intravenous infusions of morphine or sameridine, a novel molecule with both local anesthetic and opioid properties. Anesth Analg 88:160-165, 1999.
429. van Dorp EL, Romberg R, Sarton E, et al: Morphine-6-glucuronide: Morphine's successor for postoperative pain relief? Anesth Analg 102:1789-1797, 2006.
430. Osborne R, Thompson P, Joel S, et al: The analgesic activity of morphine-6-glucuronide. Br J Clin Pharmacol 34:130-138, 1992.
431. Grace D, Fee JP: A comparison of intrathecal morphine-6-glucuronide and intrathecal morphine sulfate as analgesics for total hip replacement. Anesth Analg 83:1055-1059, 1996.
432. Asai T, Mapleson WW, Power I: Effects of nalbuphine, pentazocine and U50488H on gastric emptying and gastrointestinal transit in the rat. Br J Anaesth 80:814-819, 1998.
433. Zacny JP, Lichtor JL, Klafta JM, et al: The effects of transnasal butorphanol on mood and psychomotor functioning in healthy volunteers. Anesth Analg 82:931-935, 1996.
434. Dahan A, Yassen A, Bijl H, et al: Comparison of the respiratory effects of intravenous buprenorphine and fentanyl in humans and rats. Br J Anaesth 94:825-834, 2005.
435. Lee SC, Wang JJ, Ho ST, Tao PL: Nalbuphine coadministered with morphine prevents tolerance and dependence. Anesth Analg 84:810-815, 1997.
436. Parker RK, Holtmann B, White PF: Patient-controlled epidural analgesia: Interactions between nalbuphine and hydromorphone. Anesth Analg 84:757-763, 1997.
437. Weiss BM, Schmid ER, Gattiker RI: Comparison of nalbuphine and fentanyl anesthesia for coronary artery bypass surgery. Hemodynamics, hormonal response, and postoperative respiratory depression. Anesth Analg 73:521-529, 1991.
438. Charuluxananan S, Kyokong O, Somboonviboon W, et al: Nalbuphine versus ondansetron for prevention of intrathecal morphine-induced pruritus after cesarean delivery. Anesth Analg 96:1789-1793, 2003.
439. Wang JJ, Ho ST, Lee SC, Liu YC: A comparison among nalbuphine, meperidine, and placebo for treating postanesthetic shivering. Anesth Analg 88:686-689, 1999.
440. Kranke P, Eberhart LH, Roewer N, Tramer MR: Pharmacological treatment of postoperative shivering: A quantitative systematic review of randomized controlled trials. Anesth Analg 94:453-460, 2002.
441. Ding Y, White PF: Comparative effects of ketorolac, dezocine, and fentanyl as adjuvants during outpatient anesthesia. Anesth Analg 75:566-571, 1992.
442. Cohen RI, Edwards WT, Kezer EA, et al: Serial intravenous doses of dezocine, morphine, and nalbuphine in the management of postoperative pain for outpatients. Anesth Analg 77:533-539, 1993.
443. Freye E, Levy JV: Reflex activity caused by laryngoscopy and intubation is obtunded differently by meptazinol, nalbuphine and fentanyl. Eur J Anaesthesiol 24:53-58, 2007.
444. Kendrick WD, Woods AM, Daly MY, et al: Naloxone versus nalbuphine infusion for prophylaxis of epidural morphine-induced pruritus. Anesth Analg 82:641-647, 1996.
445. Gan TJ, Ginsberg B, Glass PS, et al: Opioid-sparing effects of a low-dose infusion of naloxone in patient-administered morphine sulfate. Anesthesiology 87:1075-1081, 1997.
446. Fukuda K, Kato S, Shoda T, et al: Partial agonistic activity of naloxone on the opioid receptors expressed from complementary deoxyribonucleic acids in Chinese hamster ovary cells. Anesth Analg 87:450-455, 1998.
447. Kulig K: Initial management of ingestions of toxic substances. N Engl J Med 326:1677-1681, 1992.
448. van Dorp E, Yassen A, Sarton E, et al: Naloxone reversal of buprenorphine-induced respiratory depression. Anesthesiology 105:51-57, 2006.
449. Just B, Delva E, Camus Y, Lienhart A: Oxygen uptake during recovery following naloxone. Relationship with intraoperative heat loss. Anesthesiology 76:60-64, 1992.

450. Mannelli M, Maggi M, De Feo ML, et al: Naloxone administration releases catecholamines. N Engl J Med 308:654-655, 1983.
451. Staessen J, Fagard R, Lijnen P, et al: Influence of opioid antagonism on plasma catecholamines in pheochromocytoma patients. J Cardiovasc Pharmacol 15:386-391, 1990.
452. Belzung C, Barreau S, Agmo A: Naloxone potentiates anxiolytic-like actions of diazepam, pentobarbital and meprobamate but not those of Ro19-8022 in the rat. Eur J Pharmacol 394:289-294, 2000.
453. Mikkelsen S, Ilkjaer S, Brennum J, et al: The effect of naloxone on ketamine-induced effects on hyperalgesia and ketamine-induced side effects in humans. Anesthesiology 90:1539-1545, 1999.
454. Eijgelshoven MH, De Kloet ER, Van den Berg DT, Van Giersbergen PL: Activation of glucocorticoid receptors and the effect of naloxone during hemorrhagic hypotension. Eur J Pharmacol 205:183-189, 1991.
455. Hackshaw KV, Parker GA, Roberts JW: Naloxone in septic shock. Crit Care Med 18:47-51, 1990.
456. Boeuf B, Gauvin F, Guerguerian AM, et al: Therapy of shock with naloxone: A meta-analysis. Crit Care Med 26:1910-1916, 1998.
457. Benzel EC, Khare V, Fowler MR: Effects of naloxone and nalmefene in rat spinal cord injury induced by the ventral compression technique. J Spinal Disord 5:75-77, 1992.
458. Bracken MB, Shepard MJ, Collins WF, et al: A randomized, controlled trial of methylprednisolone or naloxone in the treatment of acute spinal-cord injury. Results of the Second National Acute Spinal Cord Injury Study. N Engl J Med 322:1405-1411, 1990.
459. Acher CW, Wynn MM, Hoch JR, et al: Combined use of cerebral spinal fluid drainage and naloxone reduces the risk of paraplegia in thoracoabdominal aneurysm repair. J Vasc Surg 19:236-246, discussion 247-238, 1994.
460. Romanovsky AA, Blatteis CM: Heat stroke: Opioid-mediated mechanisms. J Appl Physiol 81:2565-2570, 1996.
461. Bergasa NV: Treatment of the pruritus of cholestasis. Curr Treat Options Gastroenterol 7:501-508, 2004.
462. Bainton T, Fox M, Bowsher D, Wells C: A double-blind trial of naloxone in central post-stroke pain. Pain 48:159-162, 1992.
463. Abboud TK, Lee K, Zhu J, et al: Prophylactic oral naltrexone with intrathecal morphine for cesarean section: Effects on adverse reactions and analgesia. Anesth Analg 71:367-370, 1990.
464. Glass PS, Jhaveri RM, Smith LR: Comparison of potency and duration of action of nalmefene and naloxone. Anesth Analg 78:536-541, 1994.
465. Joshi GP, Duffy L, Chehade J, et al: Effects of prophylactic nalmefene on the incidence of morphine-related side effects in patients receiving intravenous patient-controlled analgesia. Anesthesiology 90:1007-1011, 1999.
466. Yuan CS, Foss JF, O'Connor M, et al: Methylnaltrexone for reversal of constipation due to chronic methadone use: A randomized controlled trial. JAMA 283:367-372, 2000.
467. Murphy DB, El Behiery H, Chan VW, Foss JF: Pharmacokinetic profile of epidurally administered methylnaltrexone, a novel peripheral opioid antagonist in a rabbit model. Br J Anaesth 86:120-122, 2001.
468. Bovill JG: Adverse drug interactions in anesthesia. J Clin Anesth 9:3S-13S, 1997.
469. Vuyk J: Pharmacokinetic and pharmacodynamic interations between opioids and propofol. J Clin Anesth 9:23S-26S, 1997.
470. Schwieger IM, Hall RI, Hug CC Jr: Less than additive antinociceptive interaction between midazolam and fentanyl in enflurane-anesthetized dogs. Anesthesiology 74:1060-1066, 1991.
471. Kissin I, Brown PT, Bradley EL Jr: Morphine and fentanyl anesthetic interactions with diazepam: Relative antagonism in rats. Anesth Analg 71:236-241, 1990.
472. Luger TJ, Hayashi T, Weiss CG, Hill HF: The spinal potentiating effect and the supraspinal inhibitory effect of midazolam on opioid-induced analgesia in rats. Eur J Pharmacol 275:153-162, 1995.
473. Bailey PL, Pace NL, Ashburn MA, et al: Frequent hypoxemia and apnea after sedation with midazolam and fentanyl. Anesthesiology 73:826-830, 1990.
474. Ma D, Sapsed-Byrne SM, Chakrabarti MK, Whitwam JG: Synergistic interaction between the effects of propofol and midazolam with fentanyl on phrenic nerve activity in rabbits. Acta Anaesthesiol Scand 42:670-677, 1998.
475. Billard V, Moulla F, Bourgain JL, et al: Hemodynamic response to induction and intubation. Propofol/fentanyl interaction. Anesthesiology 81:1384-1393, 1994.
476. Hall RI, Murphy JT, Moffitt EA, et al: A comparison of the myocardial metabolic and haemodynamic changes produced by propofol-sufentanil and enflurane-sufentanil anaesthesia for patients having coronary artery bypass graft surgery. Can J Anaesth 38:996-1004, 1991.
477. Iselin Chaves IA, Flaishon R, Sebel PS, et al: The effect of the interaction of propofol and alfentanil on recall, loss of consciousness, and the bispectral index. Anesth Analg 87:949-955, 1998.
478. Sukhani R, Vazquez J, Pappas AL, et al: Recovery after propofol with and without intraoperative fentanyl in patients undergoing ambulatory gynecologic laparoscopy. Anesth Analg 83:975-981, 1996.
479. Mertens MJ, Olofsen E, Burm AG, et al: Mixed-effects modeling of the influence of alfentanil on propofol pharmacokinetics. Anesthesiology 100:795-805, 2004.
480. Haessler R, Madler C, Klasing S, et al: Propofol/fentanyl versus etomidate/fentanyl for the induction of anesthesia in patients with aortic insufficiency and coronary artery disease. J Cardiothorac Vasc Anesth 6:173-180, 1992.
481. Sethna NF, Liu M, Gracely R, et al: Analgesic and cognitive effects of intravenous ketamine-alfentanil combinations versus either drug alone after intradermal capsaicin in normal subjects. Anesth Analg 86:1250-1256, 1998.
482. Reeves M, Lindholm DE, Myles PS, et al: Adding ketamine to morphine for patient-controlled analgesia after major abdominal surgery: A double-blinded, randomized controlled trial. Anesth Analg 93:116-120, 2001.
483. Lauretti GR, Lima IC, Reis MP, et al: Oral ketamine and transdermal nitroglycerin as analgesic adjuvants to oral morphine therapy for cancer pain management. Anesthesiology 90:1528-1533, 1999.
484. Eckhardt K, Ammon S, Hofmann U, et al: Gabapentin enhances the analgesic effect of morphine in healthy volunteers. Anesth Analg 91:185-191, 2000.
485. Hansen C, Gilron I, Hong M: The effects of intrathecal gabapentin on spinal morphine tolerance in the rat tail-flick and paw pressure tests. Anesth Analg 99:1180-1184, 2004.
486. Hara K, Saito Y, Kirihara Y, et al: The interaction of antinociceptive effects of morphine and GABA receptor agonists within the rat spinal cord. Anesth Analg 89:422-427, 1999.
487. Finck AD, Samaniego E, Ngai SH: Nitrous oxide selectively releases Met5-enkephalin and Met5-enkephalin-Arg6-Phe7 into canine third ventricular cerebrospinal fluid. Anesth Analg 80:664-670, 1995.
488. Phillips AS, McMurray TJ, Mirakhur RK, et al: Propofol-fentanyl anesthesia: A comparison with isoflurane-fentanyl anesthesia in coronary artery bypass grafting and valve replacement surgery. J Cardiothorac Vasc Anesth 8:289-296, 1994.
489. Searle NR, Martineau RJ, Conzen P, et al: Comparison of sevoflurane/fentanyl and isoflurane/fentanyl during elective coronary artery bypass surgery. Sevoflurane Venture Group. Can J Anaesth 43:890-899, 1996.
490. Weiskopf RB, Eger EI 2nd, Noorani M, Daniel M: Fentanyl, esmolol, and clonidine blunt the transient cardiovascular stimulation induced by desflurane in humans. Anesthesiology 81:1350-1355, 1994.
491. Ebert TJ, Muzi M: Sympathetic hyperactivity during desflurane anesthesia in healthy volunteers. A comparison with isoflurane. Anesthesiology 79:444-453, 1993.
492. Cote D, Martin R, Tetrault JP: Haemodynamic interactions of muscle relaxants and sufentanil in coronary artery surgery. Can J Anaesth 38:324-329, 1991.
493. Thomson IR, MacAdams CL, Hudson RJ, Rosenbloom M: Drug interactions with sufentanil. Hemodynamic effects of premedication and muscle relaxants. Anesthesiology 76:922-929, 1992.
494. Shorten GD, Sieber T, Maslow AD, et al: Left ventricular regional wall motion and haemodynamic changes following bolus administration of pipecuronium or pancuronium to adult patients undergoing coronary artery bypass grafting. Can J Anaesth 42:695-700, 1995.
495. Paulissian R, Mahdi M, Joseph NJ, et al: Hemodynamic responses to pancuronium and vecuronium during high-dose fentanyl anesthesia for coronary artery bypass grafting. J Cardiothorac Vasc Anesth 5:120-125, 1991.
496. McCoy EP, Maddineni VR, Elliott P, et al: Haemodynamic effects of rocuronium during fentanyl anaesthesia: Comparison with vecuronium. Can J Anaesth 40:703-708, 1993.
497. Loan PB, Elliott P, Mirakhur RK, et al: Comparison of the haemodynamic effects of mivacurium and atracurium during fentanyl anaesthesia. Br J Anaesth 74:330-332, 1995.
498. Rathmell JP, Brooker RF, Prielipp RC, et al: Hemodynamic and pharmacodynamic comparison of doxacurium and pipecuronium with pancuronium during induction of cardiac anesthesia: Does the benefit justify the cost? Anesth Analg 76:513-519, 1993.
499. Sporer KA: The serotonin syndrome. Implicated drugs, pathophysiology and management. Drug Saf 13:94-104, 1995.
500. Gillman PK: Monoamine oxidase inhibitors, opioid analgesics and serotonin toxicity. Br J Anaesth 95:434-441, 2005.
501. Ure DS, Gillies MA, James KS: Safe use of remifentanil in a patient treated with the monoamine oxidase inhibitor phenelzine. Br J Anaesth 84:414-416, 2000.
502. Beresford BJ, Glick D, Dinwiddie SH: Combination propofol-alfentanil anesthesia for electroconvulsive therapy in patients receiving monoamine oxidase inhibitors. J ECT 20:120-122, 2004.

503. Carta F, Bianchi M, Argenton S, et al: Effect of nifedipine on morphine-induced analgesia. Anesth Analg 70:493-498, 1990.
504. Omote K, Sonoda H, Kawamata M, et al: Potentiation of antinociceptive effects of morphine by calcium-channel blockers at the level of the spinal cord. Anesthesiology 79:746-752, 1993.
505. Hasegawa AE, Zacny JP: The influence of three L-type calcium channel blockers on morphine effects in healthy volunteers. Anesth Analg 85:633-638, 1997.
506. Omote K, Kawamata M, Satoh O, et al: Spinal antinociceptive action of an N-type voltage-dependent calcium channel blocker and the synergistic interaction with morphine. Anesthesiology 84:636-643, 1996.
507. Bartkowski RR, Goldberg ME, Huffnagle S, Epstein RH: Sufentanil disposition. Is it affected by erythromycin administration? Anesthesiology 78:260-265, 1993.
508. Bartkowski RR, McDonnell TE: Prolonged alfentanil effect following erythromycin administration. Anesthesiology 73:566-568, 1990.
509. Koinig H, Wallner T, Marhofer P, et al: Magnesium sulfate reduces intra- and postoperative analgesic requirements. Anesth Analg 87:206-210, 1998.
510. Buvanendran A, McCarthy RJ, Kroin JS, et al: Intrathecal magnesium prolongs fentanyl analgesia: A prospective, randomized, controlled trial. Anesth Analg 95:661-666, 2002.
511. Kroin JS, McCarthy RJ, Von Roenn N, et al: Magnesium sulfate potentiates morphine antinociception at the spinal level. Anesth Analg 90:913-917, 2000.
512. Plummer JL, Owen H, Ilsley AH, Tordoff K: Sustained-release ibuprofen as an adjunct to morphine patient-controlled analgesia. Anesth Analg 83:92-96, 1996.
513. Ng A, Parker J, Toogood L, et al: Does the opioid-sparing effect of rectal diclofenac following total abdominal hysterectomy benefit the patient? Br J Anaesth 88:714-716, 2002.
514. Moren J, Francois T, Blanloeil Y, Pinaud M: The effects of a nonsteroidal antiinflammatory drug (ketoprofen) on morphine respiratory depression: A double-blind, randomized study in volunteers. Anesth Analg 85:400-405, 1997.
515. Luccarini P, Perrier L, Degoulange C, et al: Synergistic antinociceptive effect of amitriptyline and morphine in the rat orofacial formalin test. Anesthesiology 100:690-696, 2004.
516. Babenco HD, Blouin RT, Conard PF, Gross JB: Diphenylhydramine increases ventilatory drive during alfentanil infusion. Anesthesiology 89:642-647, 1998.

Peter S. A. Glass, Steven L. Shafer, and J. G. Reves

28 Intravenous Drug Delivery Systems

Key Points

1. Anesthetic drugs are described by multicompartmental models. Accurate intravenous drug delivery requires adjusting the dose for accumulation of drug in peripheral tissues.
2. The biophase is the site of action of anesthetic drugs. Initiation, maintenance, and titration of intravenous anesthetics must account for the delay in equilibration between plasma and the site of drug effect.
3. Some drug effects directly reflect the concentration of drug in the biophase (direct-effect models). Other drug effects reflect the alteration of feedback systems by anesthetics (indirect-effect models). The influence of opioids on ventilation reflects the dynamic influence of opioids on the feedback between ventilation and carbon dioxide and is thus an example of an indirect drug effect.
4. The target concentration in the effect site is the same as the target concentration in plasma at steady state. The target concentration is influenced by patient physiology, surgical stimulation, and concurrent drug administration. Typically, one must set a target concentration for the hypnotic (volatile anesthetic or propofol) and the analgesic (opioid) that properly accounts for the synergy between them.
5. To achieve an effective target concentration, the conventional teaching of administering a loading dose calculated as target concentration times volume of distribution, followed by a maintenance rate calculated as target concentration times clearance, is inaccurate. The initial loading dose may be calculated as the target concentration times the volume of distribution at peak effect. Maintenance rates must initially account for distribution of drug in peripheral tissues and are turned down to the target concentration times clearance only after equilibration with peripheral tissues.
6. The terminal half-life does not reflect the clinical time course of drug concentration. The context-sensitive decrement time is the time for a given decrement in drug concentration as a function of the duration of infusion for an infusion that maintains a steady plasma concentration. Context-sensitive decrement times properly incorporate the multicompartmental behavior of intravenous anesthetics. The context-sensitive half-time is the time for a 50% decrement in concentration.
7. Alfentanil, fentanyl, sufentanil, remifentanil, propofol, thiopental, methohexital, etomidate, ketamine, and midazolam can all be given by intravenous infusion. Specific caveats, infusion rates, and titration guidelines are presented in the text.
8. Target-controlled infusions use pharmacokinetic models to titrate intravenous anesthetics to specified plasma or effect-site drug concentrations. The Diprifusor is a propofol target-controlled infusion system that is available worldwide except in North America.
9. Closed-loop drug delivery systems have used the median electroencephalographic frequency, bispectral index, and auditory evoked potentials to control intravenous anesthetic delivery. These systems have generally performed well clinically but remain investigational.

Anesthetic drugs must reach their site of action to be effective. In 1628, William Harvey proved in *Exercitatio Anatomica de Motu Cordis et Sanguinis in Animalibus* that venous blood was transported to the arterial circulation and thus to the organs of the body by the heart. It was recognized almost immediately that drugs injected into veins could be rapidly carried to the entire body. In 1657 Christopher Wren injected opium intravenously by means of a quill and bladder (Fig. 28-1A) into dogs and humans and rendered them unconscious. Eight years later, Sigismund Elsholtz gave an opioid solution for the purpose of rendering subjects insensitive, but it was not until 1874 that Pierre-Cyprien Ore administered chloral hydrate intravenously for a surgical procedure. This landmark event followed unsuccessful attempts by the Russian surgeon Pirogoff to administer ether intravenously in

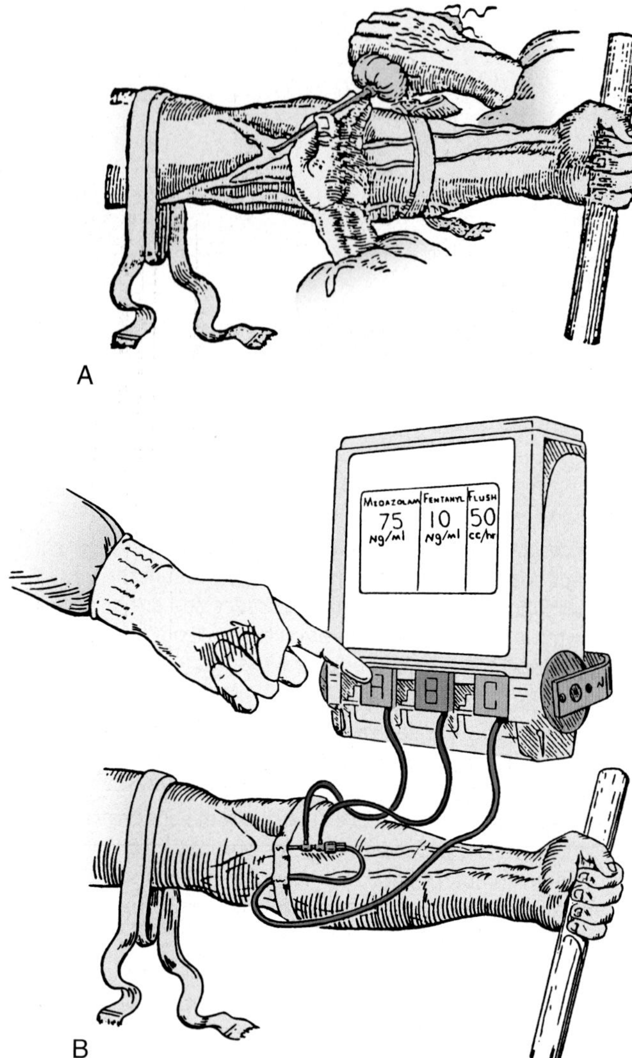

Figure 28-1 Intravenous drug delivery, past and future. **A,** A depiction of the first intravenous injection of opium with a quill and bladder. **B,** The future of intravenous drug delivery. Drugs are delivered with the aid of a small, sophisticated infusion pump, which permits dosing in terms of plasma drug concentration rather than amount.

1846, shortly after Crawford Long and William Morton had independently demonstrated the efficacy of ether inhalation for surgery.[1]

Intravenous methods of anesthetic drug delivery have depended on steady improvement in technology. The quill and bladder used by Wren were not significantly improved until Alexander Wood used a needle and syringe to administer intravenous medications in 1853. The hollow hypodermic needle and a functional syringe were developed by Frances Rynd and Charles Pravaz, respectively.[1] Contemporary needles, catheters, and syringes are descendants of these early devices. A more recent technologic development in intravenous anesthesia was the introduction of computerized pharmacokinetic model–driven continuous-infusion devices (see Fig. 28-1B), first reported by Helmut Schwilden[2] in 1981. Schwilden demonstrated the ability to attain desired plasma levels of an intravenous anesthetic drug by using a computer-controlled infusion pump operated in accordance with the published pharmacokinetics of the drug. These efforts resulted in release of the first commercial target-controlled infusion (TCI) device in Europe, developed by Zeneca specifically for the administration of propofol. The March 1998 issue of the journal *Anaesthesia* was devoted entirely to a review of TCI and the role of TCI devices in clinical practice. Since that time, nearly the rest of the world, with the notable exception of the United States, has approved TCI devices for the delivery of anesthetic drugs.

The ultimate development in anesthetic delivery systems will be devices for closed-loop administration of intravenous drugs during anesthesia. Systems have been developed for closed-loop administration of sodium nitroprusside and muscle relaxants based on defined and measurable end points. The lack of an unequivocal measure of "anesthetic depth" has hindered the development of closed-loop anesthetic delivery systems. Most such systems have been developed with the electroencephalogram (EEG) used as the measure of anesthetic drug effect. Schwilden developed closed-loop systems for infusion of methohexital[3,4] and propofol[5] on the basis of the median EEG frequency. Other investigators have developed closed-loop systems based on other derivatives of the EEG (e.g., auditory evoked potentials[6] or the bispectral index [BIS][7]).

The development of new techniques has coincided with the development of new drugs. Rapid intravenous induction became popular with the introduction of sodium thiopental in 1934. The pharmacokinetics of thiopental, however, prevented its becoming popular for maintenance of anesthesia. During the past 50 years, numerous intravenous hypnotics (methohexital, 1957; propanidid, 1957; althesin, 1971; etomidate, 1973; propofol, 1977), anxiolytics (diazepam, 1966; midazolam, 1978), and analgesics (fentanyl, 1959; ketamine, 1966; sufentanil, 1979; alfentanil, 1980; remifentanil, 1996; dexmedetomidine, 1999) have been introduced. The general trend in the introduction of these newer agents has been to provide drugs with further shortening of the time needed for recovery from drug effect. In this context, the newer intravenous drugs propofol and remifentanil provide a rapid onset of anesthesia, a stable maintenance phase, and rapid recovery.

Before reviewing delivery techniques and devices for intravenous anesthesia, this chapter presents pharmacokinetic and pharmacodynamic principles as background for understanding how to administer intravenous drugs to their best advantage. Specifically, intravenous anesthesia delivery systems can be used to rationally determine the dose of intravenous drugs used in clinical practice. Further discussion of the principles of pharmacokinetics and pharmacodynamics can be found in Chapter 19.

Pharmacokinetic Considerations

The goal of administering anesthetics is to produce the clinically desired time course of anesthetic effect. Usually, such a course includes a rapid onset, smooth maintenance, and rapid recovery after termination of the anesthetic. Conventional pharmacokinetic models assume that a bolus of drug is instantaneously mixed into plasma and produces an immediate peak in its plasma concentration. The concentration then declines continuously until the next bolus. Except for a transient perioperative stimulus (endotracheal intubation, surgical incision, bowel traction), the

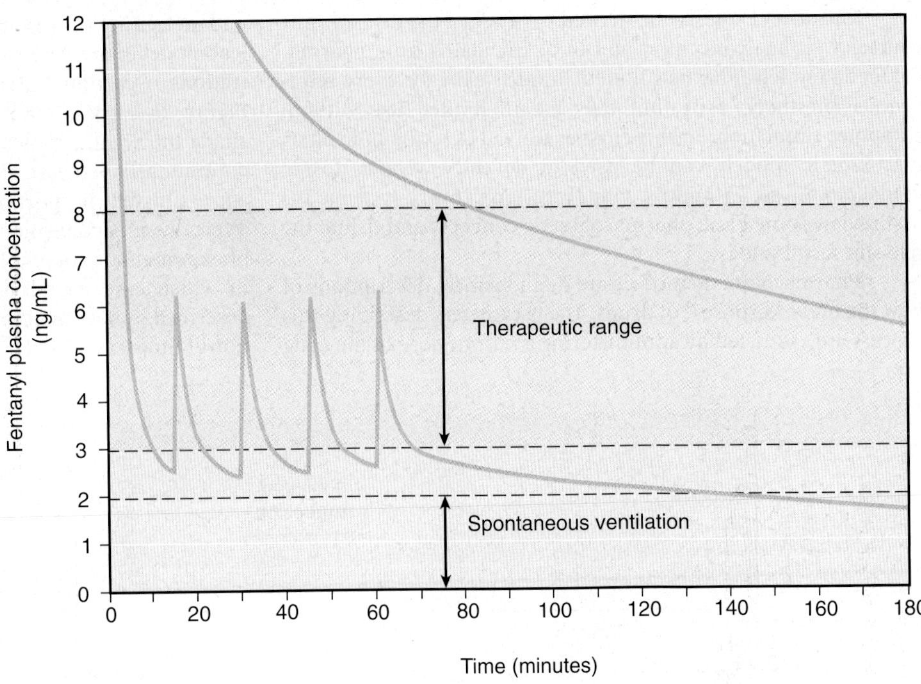

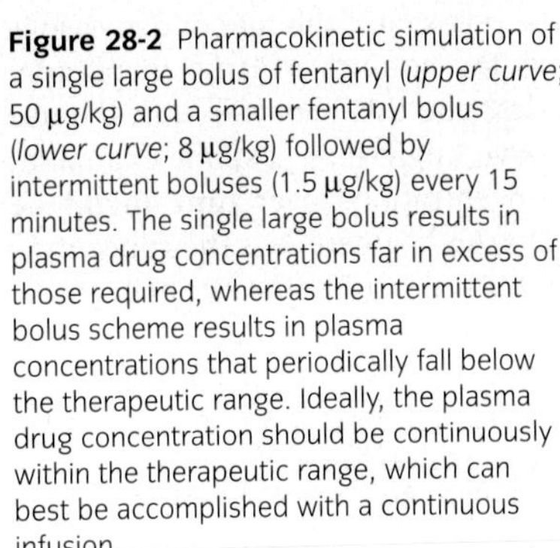

Figure 28-2 Pharmacokinetic simulation of a single large bolus of fentanyl (*upper curve*; 50 µg/kg) and a smaller fentanyl bolus (*lower curve*; 8 µg/kg) followed by intermittent boluses (1.5 µg/kg) every 15 minutes. The single large bolus results in plasma drug concentrations far in excess of those required, whereas the intermittent bolus scheme results in plasma concentrations that periodically fall below the therapeutic range. Ideally, the plasma drug concentration should be continuously within the therapeutic range, which can best be accomplished with a continuous infusion.

patient's anesthetic requirements will probably not follow the saltatory time course of anesthetic effect seen with repeated bolus injections. Thus, the technique of intermittent boluses results in excessive drug effect at the time of the bolus, inadequate drug effect before the next bolus, or both (Fig. 28-2). The technique of giving the entire anesthetic as an initial bolus produces a needlessly huge initial peak and, depending on the dose, grossly excessive or possibly subtherapeutic levels later in the procedure. This technique is well tolerated for opioids in paralyzed patients whose lungs are mechanically ventilated. However, this approach would produce considerable hypotension if attempted with propofol.

To produce a time course of drug effect that follows the time course of anesthetic requirement, a continuous infusion titrated to the perceived anesthetic requirement should be used. Ideally, just enough drug is given to achieve the therapeutic blood or plasma drug concentration, and it is then continuously titrated throughout surgery (Fig. 28-3). This method of drug delivery avoids the peaks and valleys in drug concentration seen with intermittent drug boluses. Theoretical advantages of continuous infusions over intermittent bolus injections include fewer periods of poor anesthetic control, a reduction in the total amount of drug used, and more rapid recovery from anesthesia.[8,9]

Surgical stress map

Stress response or plasma concentration
Intubation
Incision
Theoretical plasma drug concentration for adequate anesthesia
Mount surgery
Lake prep
Anxiety mound
Sleep river
Peritoneal traction
Bowel vascular clamping
Recovery plains
ICU highlands
Duration of surgery

Figure 28-3 Landscape of surgical anesthesia. The stimuli of surgery are not constant; therefore, the plasma concentration of the anesthetic drug should be titrated to match the needs of the patient.

The dose of anesthetic needed to produce the desired time course of plasma concentration can be calculated from pharmacokinetic models. Pharmacokinetic models exist for every intravenous anesthetic drug, but they are of limited use without computer simulation. In this chapter we will describe how pharmacokinetic models can be used to develop rational dosing guidelines for use with intravenous infusion delivery systems. We first review some basic pharmacokinetic concepts and define the relevant terminology.

Pharmacokinetic models are mathematical descriptions of how the body "disposes" of drugs. The parameters describing this process are estimated by administering a known dose of the drug and measuring the resulting plasma concentrations. A mathematical model then relates the input over time, I(t), with the concentrations over time, C(t). These models can take many forms. Figure 28-4 shows concentrations in plasma over time after a single intravenous bolus of drug at time 0. Drug concentrations continuously decrease after the bolus, and the rate of decrease is approximately proportional to the amount of drug in plasma. Typically, it is convenient to describe this behavior with the use of exponential models. The curve might have a single exponent, in which case the plasma concentrations over time might be described by the function $C(t) = Ae^{-kt}$, where A is the concentration at time 0 and k is a constant that describes the rate of decrease

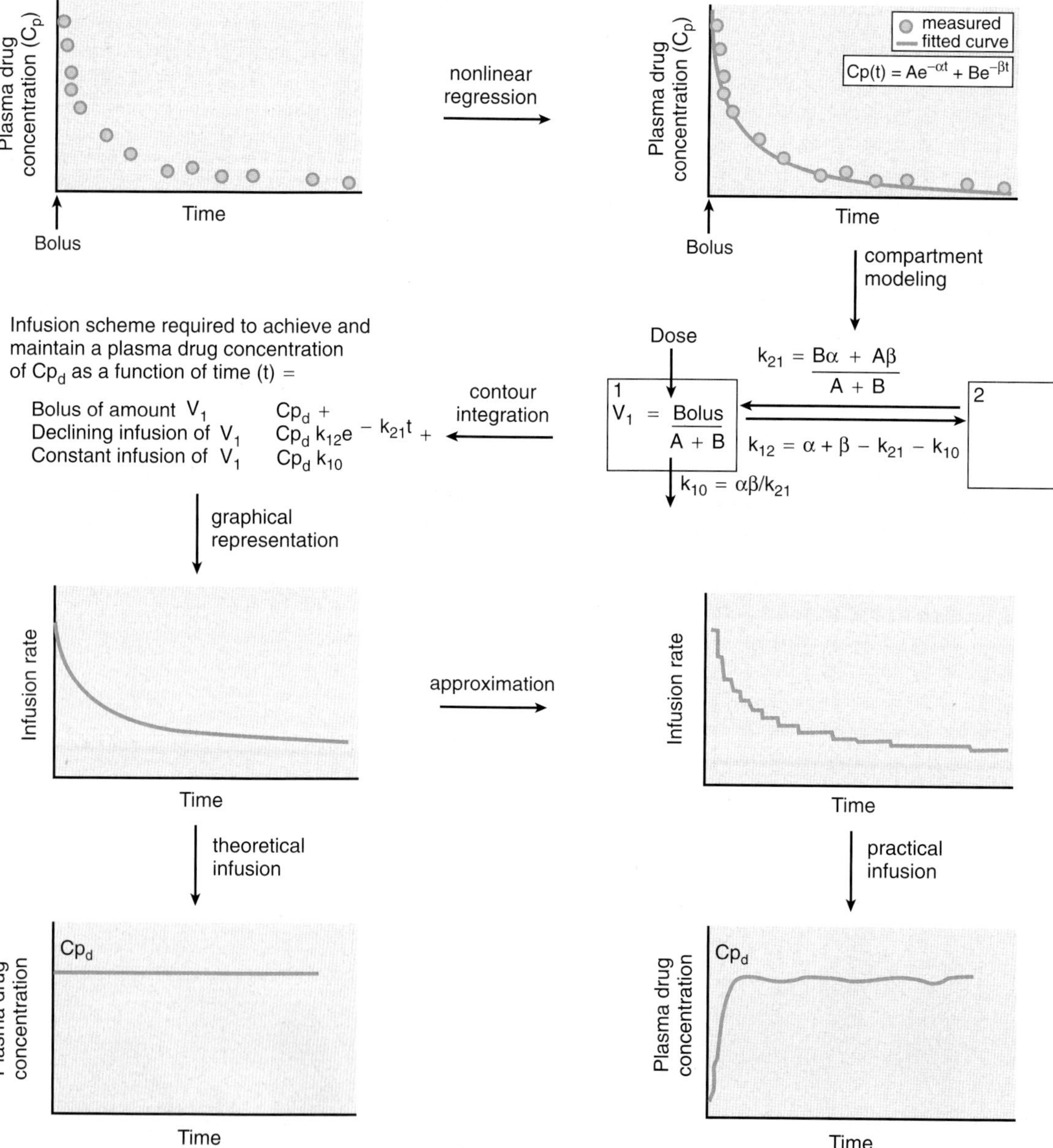

Figure 28-4 Steps involved in pharmacokinetic model–driven infusion. Typically, pharmacokinetic models are derived from experiments in which plasma drug concentrations are measured at intervals after bolus administration of the drug. Nonlinear regression is used to fit a monoexponential, biexponential, or triexponential curve to the resulting concentration-versus-time data. There is an algebraic relationship between the exponential decay curves and a one-, two-, or three-compartment pharmacokinetic model. The "BET" infusion scheme is developed and consists of a bolus, a continuous infusion to replace drug eliminated from the body, and an exponentially declining infusion to replace drug transferred out of plasma to other body compartments. BET infusion results in maintenance of a constant specified plasma drug concentration. Practical implementation of the BET scheme with real infusion pumps and infusion rates that change only at discrete intervals of time results in a plasma drug concentration profile that approximates that resulting from a BET infusion.

in concentration. The relationship appears to be a straight line when graphed as the log of concentration versus time. The pharmacokinetics of intravenous anesthetic drugs is more complex because after the bolus, a period of rapid decline is observed before the terminal "log-linear" portion (e.g., the part that is a straight line when described as log concentration versus time). It is possible to model this process by taking several monoexponential (i.e., one exponent) curves and adding them together. The result is a polyexponential curve. For example, the concentrations after an intravenous bolus might be described by an equation with two exponents, $C(t) = Ae^{-\alpha t} + Be^{-\beta t}$, or an equation with three exponents, $C(t) = Ae^{-\alpha t} + Be^{-\beta t} + Ce^{-\gamma t}$.

There are ways of administering intravenous anesthetic drugs besides single boluses. A more general way to think of pharmacokinetics is to decompose the input into a series of small bits (boluses) and consider each bit of drug separately. The general pharmacokinetic model of drug disposition commonly used in anesthesia considers each bit of drug independently and analyzes its contribution by means of polyexponential decay over time. The formal mathematical description of each bit of drug in terms of polyexponential decay over time is the relationship

$$C(t) = I(t) * \sum_{i=1}^{n} A_i e^{-\lambda_i t} \quad (1)$$

where C(t) is the plasma concentration at time t and I(t) is drug input (i.e., a bolus or infusion). The summation after the asterisk (described later) is the function describing how each bit of drug is disposed of (hence its name the "disposition" function). Note that this is again a sum of *n* exponentials, as described in the previous paragraph.

Pharmacokinetic modeling is the process of estimating the parameters within this function. The integer *n* is the number of exponentials (i.e., compartments) and is usually two or three. Each exponential term is associated with a coefficient A_i and an exponent λ_i. The λ values are inversely proportional to the half-lives (half-life = $0.693/\lambda$), with the smallest λ representing the longest (terminal) half-life. The A values are the relative contribution of each half-life to overall drug disposition. If a drug has a very long terminal half-life but a coefficient that is much smaller than the other coefficients, the long half-life is likely to be clinically meaningless. Conversely, if a drug has a very long half-life with a relatively large coefficient, the drug will be long lasting even after brief administration. The * operator is the mathematical process called "convolution," which is simply the process of breaking the infusion into "bits" of drug and then adding up the results to see the overall concentrations.

The pharmacokinetic model shown has some useful characteristics that account for its enduring popularity in pharmacokinetic analysis. Most important, the model describes observations from studies reasonably well, the sine qua non for models. Second, these models have the useful characteristic of "linearity." Simply stated, if you double the dose, I, (e.g., give a bolus twice as large or an infusion twice as fast), you double the concentrations.

More generally, linearity implies that the system (i.e., the body acting to produce a plasma drug concentration output from a drug dosage input) behaves in accordance with the principle of superposition. The superposition principle states that the response of a linear system with multiple inputs can be computed by determining the response to each individual input and then summing the individual responses. In other words, when the body treats each bit of drug by polyexponential decay over time, the "disposing" of each bit of drug does not influence the disposing of other bits of drug.

The third reason for the continuing popularity of these models is that they can be mathematically transformed from the admittedly unintuitive exponential form shown earlier to a more easily intuitive compartmental form, as shown in Figure 28-5. The fundamental parameters of the compartment model are the volumes of distribution (central, rapidly equilibrating, and slowly equilibrating peripheral volumes) and clearances (systemic, rapid, and slow intercompartmental). The central compartment (V_1) represents a distribution volume and includes the rapidly mixing portion of the blood and first-pass pulmonary uptake. The peripheral compartments are composed of tissues and organs that show a time course and extent of drug accumulation (or dissipation) different from that of the central compartment. In the three-compartment model, the two peripheral compartments may correspond roughly to splanchnic and muscle tissues (rapidly equilibrating) and fat stores (slowly equilibrating). The sum of the compartment volumes is the apparent volume of distribution at steady state (Vd_{ss}) and is the proportionality constant relating the plasma drug concentration at steady state to the total amount of drug in the body. The intercompartmental rate constants (k_{12}, k_{21}, and so on) describe the movement of drug between the central and peripheral compartments. The elimination rate constant (k_{10}) encompasses processes acting through biotransformation or elimination that irreversibly remove drug from the central compartment.

Despite their physiologic flavor, compartmental models are simply mathematical transformations of the polyexponential disposition functions computed from observed plasma concentrations. Thus, physiologic interpretation of volumes and clearances (with the possible exception of systemic clearance and Vd_{ss} [the algebraic sum of the volumes]) is entirely speculative.

The last reason that these models have been popular is that they can be used to design infusion regimens, the point of introducing them in this chapter. If we abbreviate the disposition function

$$\sum_{i=1}^{n} A_i e^{-\lambda_i t} \quad (2)$$

as simply D(t), we can rewrite the relationship among concentration, dose, and the pharmacokinetic model D(t) as

$$C(t) = I(t) * D(t) \quad (3)$$

where * is the convolution operator, as noted earlier. In the usual pharmacokinetic study we know I(t), the dose that we gave the patient, and we measure C(t), the concentrations over time. Our goal is to find D(t), the pharmacokinetic disposition function. Pharmacokinetic analysis can be thought of as a simple rearrangement of Equation 3 to solve for D(t):

$$D(t) = \frac{C(t)}{\underset{\times}{} I(t)} \quad (4)$$

where the symbol $\frac{\ }{\times}$ means deconvolution, the inverse operation of convolution. Deconvolution is like division, but of functions rather than simple numbers. When we design dosing regimens from known pharmacokinetic models and a desired course for the plasma concentration over time, the known values

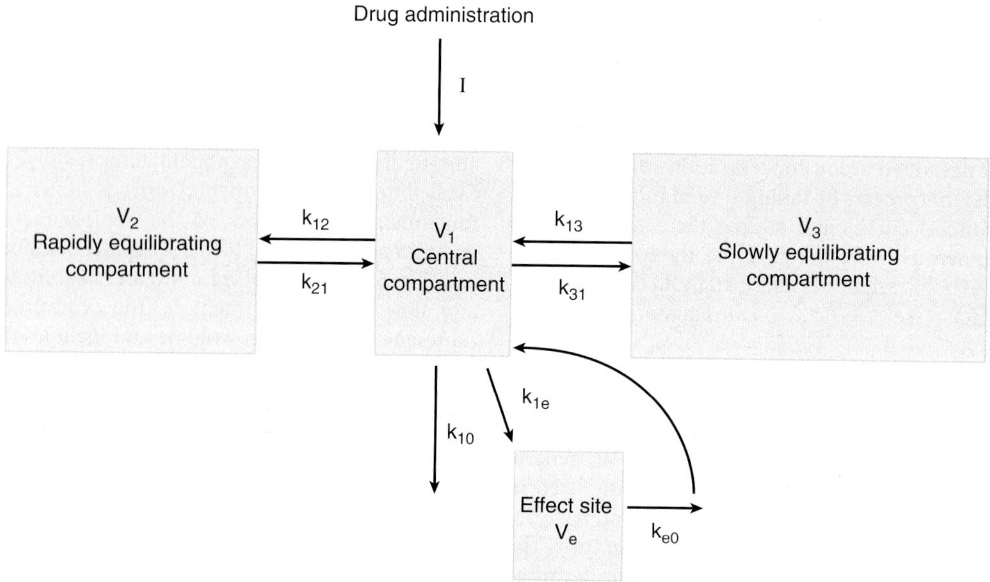

Figure 28-5 Three-compartment model (including the biophase) schematizing the basic pharmacokinetic processes that occur after intravenous drug administration. I, dosing scheme as a function of time; k_{10}, rate constant reflecting all processes acting to irreversibly remove drug from the central compartment; k_{ij}, intercompartmental rate constants; V_1, central compartment volume, usually expressed in liters or liters per kilogram.

are D(t) (the pharmacokinetics) and $C_T(t)$ (the desired target concentrations), and the drug dosing scheme is:

$$I(t) = \frac{C_T(t)}{D(t)} \qquad (5)$$

Thus, one can calculate the necessary infusion rates, I(t), given desired target concentrations, $C_T(t)$, and the pharmacokinetics, D(t), by applying the same tools used to calculate the original pharmacokinetics. Unfortunately, such a solution might require some negative infusion rates, which are obviously impossible. Because we cannot suck drug out of the body (i.e., give negative infusions), we must restrict ourselves to plasma concentrations over time that can be achieved with non-negative infusion rates.

The standard pharmacokinetic model has one glaring shortcoming. It assumes that after a bolus injection there is complete mixing within the central compartment such that the peak concentration occurs precisely at time 0. It actually takes about 30 to 45 seconds for the drug to make its transit from the venous injection site to the arterial circulation. This model misspecification over the first minute or so may not seem significant, but it can cause problems in attempts to relate the drug effect after a bolus to drug concentrations in the body.[10] Researchers are modifying the standard polyexponential pharmacokinetic models to provide more accurate models of plasma drug concentration in the first minute after bolus injection.[11]

Pharmacodynamic Considerations

The Biophase

Although the plasma concentration after an intravenous bolus peaks nearly instantaneously, no anesthesiologist would push an intravenous bolus of hypnotic and immediately intubate the patient's trachea. The reason, of course, is that although the plasma concentration peaks almost instantly, additional time is required for the drug concentration in the brain to rise sufficiently to induce unconsciousness. This delay between peak plasma concentration and peak concentration at the effect site is called *hysteresis.* Hysteresis is the clinical manifestation of the fact that plasma is not the site of anesthetic action, only the mechanism of transport. Drugs exert their pharmacologic effect in the *biophase,* which is also called the "effect site." Physically, the biophase is the immediate milieu in which the drug acts on the body, including membranes, receptors, and enzymes.

The concentration of drug in the biophase cannot be measured for two reasons. First, it is usually inaccessible, at least in human subjects. Second, even if we could take tissue samples, the drug concentration in the microscopic environment of the receptive molecules would not be the same as the concentration measured in, for example, homogenated brain. Although it is not possible to actually measure drug concentration in the biophase, we can characterize the time course of drug effect by using rapid measures of drug effect. Knowing the time course of drug effect, we can characterize the rate of drug flow in and out of the biophase (or "effect site") with the use of mathematical models,[12,13] as well as the apparent drug concentration in the biophase in terms of the steady-state plasma concentration that would produce the same effect.

Measures of effect used to characterize the time course of drug between plasma and the biophase will vary with the drug being evaluated. For neuromuscular blockers, the twitch response is an ideal measure of effect. For opioids and hypnotics, the measure of effect is more challenging. The desired effect for opioids is analgesia, which is a subjective measure that is difficult to monitor and quantify moment by moment. Similarly for hypnotics, until recently there has been no validated monitor of drug effect. For these reasons investigators have turned to the EEG as an objective measure of opioid and hypnotic drug effect. Even if the EEG did not measure the clinically desired effect of opioids and hypnotics, it was assumed that changes in the EEG would at least reflect the time course of clinical effects. Thus, the time course for opioids and hypnotics to equilibrate between plasma and the biophase has largely been defined from the EEG. The validity of this approach has been confirmed by several studies. Glass and colleagues measured the blood concentration of remifentanil and its analgesic response in volunteers.[14] The time course for equilibration between plasma and the biophase calculated in this study was essentially identical to the time course determined by using the spectral edge of the EEG as the measure of effect.[15] Ludbrook and associates measured propofol concentrations in the carotid artery and jugular bulb to establish movement of propofol into and equilibration with the brain.[16] They measured the BIS simultaneously and found close correlation between brain concentration (calculated by mass balance) and changes in the BIS.

Direct-Effect Models

Just as shown for plasma pharmacokinetics earlier, the biophase concentration is the convolution of an input function (in this case, the plasma drug concentration over time) and the disposition function of the biophase. This relationship can be expressed as

$$C_{biophase}(t) = C_{plasma}(t) * D_{biophase}(t) \tag{6}$$

The disposition function of the biophase is typically modeled as a single exponential decay:

$$D_{biophase}(t) = k_{e0}e^{-k_{e0}t} \tag{7}$$

The monoexponential disposition function implies that the effect site is simply an additional compartment in the standard compartmental model that is connected to the plasma compartment (see Fig. 28-5). The effect site is the hypothetical compartment that relates the time course of plasma drug concentration to the time course of drug effect, and k_{e0} is the rate constant of elimination of drug from the effect site. By definition, the effect compartment receives such small amounts of drug from the central compartment that it has no influence on plasma pharmacokinetics.

We cannot directly measure either $C_{biophase}(t)$ or $D_{biophase}(t)$, but we can measure drug effect. Knowing that the observed drug effect is a function of the drug concentration in the biophase, we can predict the drug effect as

$$\text{Effect} = f_{PD}\left[C_{plasma}(t) * D_{biophase}(t), P_{PD}, k_{e0}\right] \tag{8}$$

where f_{PD} is a pharmacodynamic model (typically sigmoidal in shape), P_{PD} represents the parameters of the pharmacodynamic model, and k_{e0} is the rate constant for equilibration between plasma and the biophase. Nonlinear regression programs are used to find values of P_{PD} and k_{e0} that best predict the time course of drug effect. Knowledge of these parameters can then be incorporated into dosing regimens that produce the desired time course of drug effect.[17,18]

If a constant plasma concentration is maintained, the time required for the biophase concentration to reach 50% of the plasma concentration ($t_{1/2}\ k_{e0}$) can be calculated as $0.693/k_{e0}$. After a bolus dose, the time to peak biophase concentration is a function of both plasma pharmacokinetics and k_{e0}. For drugs with a very rapid decline in plasma concentration after a bolus (e.g., adenosine, which has a half-life of several seconds), the effect-site concentration peaks within several seconds of the bolus, regardless of k_{e0}. For drugs with a rapid k_{e0} and a slow decrease in concentration after a bolus injection (e.g., pancuronium), the peak effect-site concentration is determined more by k_{e0} than by plasma pharmacokinetics. The time to peak effect and the $t_{1/2}\ k_{e0}$ for several intravenous anesthetics are listed in Table 28-1.

Table 28-1 Time to Peak Effect and $t_{1/2}\ k_{e0}$ after a Bolus Dose

Drug	Time to Peak Drug Effect (min)	$t_{1/2}\ k_{e0}$ (min)
Fentanyl	3.6	4.7
Alfentanil	1.4	0.9
Sufentanil	5.6	3.0
Remifentanil	1.6	1.3
Propofol	2.2	2.4
Thiopental	1.6	1.5
Midazolam	2.8	4.0
Etomidate	2.0	1.5

$t_{1/2}\ k_{e0} = 0.693/k_{e0}$, the rate constant for transfer of drug from the site of drug effect to the environment.

Indirect-Effect Models

Thus far, effects that are an instantaneous function of drug concentration at the site of drug effect have been discussed, as implied by Equation 8. For example, once hypnotics reach the brain or muscle relaxants reach the muscles, drug action is seen almost instantaneously. On the other hand, some effects are much more complex. For example, consider the effect of opioids on ventilation. Initially, opioids depress ventilation, and as a result of this ventilatory depression, CO_2 starts to accumulate. Accumulation of CO_2 acts to stimulate ventilation, thereby partly counteracting the ventilatory depressant effects of opioids. Ventilatory depression is an example in which there is a direct and indirect drug effect. The direct effect of the opioid is to depress ventilation, and the indirect effect is to increase CO_2. Modeling the time course of opioid-induced ventilatory depression requires consideration of both components. Bouillon and colleagues have developed a model of ventilatory depression that incorporates both direct and indirect effects.[19,20] As is generally the case with indirect-effect models, characterizing drug-induced ventilatory depression requires considering the entire time course of drug therapy, which is embodied by the following differential equation:

$$\frac{d}{dt}Pa_{CO_2} = k_{el} \cdot Pa_{CO_2}(0) - k_{el} \cdot \left[1 - \frac{Cp(t)^{\gamma}}{C_{50}{}^{\gamma} + Cp(t)^{\gamma}}\right] \cdot \left[\frac{P_{biophase}CO_2(t)}{P_{biophase}CO_2(0)}\right]^F \cdot Pa_{CO_2}(t) \tag{9}$$

where Pa_{CO_2} is arterial CO_2, $P_{biophase}CO_2$ is CO_2 in the biophase (i.e., ventilation control centers), k_{el} is the rate constant for elimination of CO_2, C_{50} is the effect-site opioid concentration associated with a 50% reduction in ventilatory drive, and F is the steepness or "gain" of the effect of CO_2 on ventilatory drive.

Dose Implications of the Biophase

The delay in onset has important clinical implications. After a bolus, the plasma concentration peaks nearly instantly and then declines steadily. The effect-site concentration starts at zero and increases over time until it equals the descending plasma concentration. The plasma concentration continues to decline, and after the moment of identical concentrations, the gradient between plasma and the effect site favors removal of drug from the effect site, and the effect-site concentration decreases. The rate at which the effect site rises toward the peak after a bolus dictates how much drug must be injected into plasma to produce a given effect. For alfentanil, its rapid plasma effect-site equilibration (large k_{e0}) causes the effect-site concentration to rise rapidly, with a peak produced in about 90 seconds. At the time of the peak, about 60% of the alfentanil bolus has been distributed into peripheral tissues or eliminated from the body. For fentanyl, the effect site concentration rises much more slowly and peaks 3 to 4 minutes after the bolus.[21] At the time of the peak, more than 80% of the initial bolus of fentanyl has been distributed into tissues or eliminated. As a result of slower equilibration with the effect site, relatively more fentanyl than alfentanil must be injected into plasma, which makes the rate of offset of drug effect after a fentanyl bolus slower than after an alfentanil bolus.

This difference in pharmacokinetics suggests that k_{e0} must be incorporated into dosing strategies. For rapid onset of effect, a drug with a large k_{e0} (short $t_{1/2}$ k_{e0}) should be chosen. For example, for rapid-sequence induction, alfentanil or remifentanil may be the opioid of choice because the peak opioid effect-site concentration coincides with endotracheal intubation. However, for a slower induction in which a nondepolarizing neuromuscular blocking drug is used, it may be appropriate to choose an opioid with a slower onset of drug effect to coincide with the peak effect of the muscle relaxant. In this case, a bolus of fentanyl or sufentanil at the time of induction may be more appropriate. The time to peak effect for the commonly used opioids is shown in Figure 28-6. Knowing k_{e0} (or time to peak effect) also improves titration of the drug by identifying the time at which the clinician should make an assessment of drug effect. For example, midazolam has a slow time to peak effect, and repeat bolus doses should be spaced at least 3 to 5 minutes apart to avoid inadvertent overdosing.

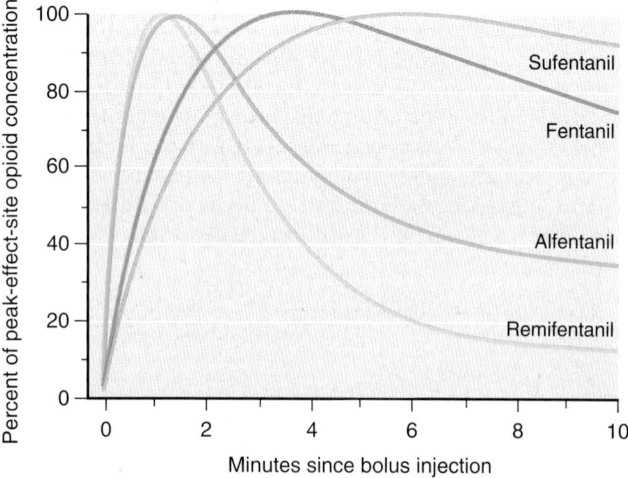

Figure 28-6 Simulated onset and time to peak effect of commonly used opioids based on their k_{e0} and pharmacokinetic parameters. k_{e0}, rate constant for transfer of drug from the site of drug effect to the environment.

Drug Potency

Having established that we can produce almost any desired concentration time course at the effect site, what concentration should we choose? The pharmacokinetics and pharmacodynamics of inhaled anesthetics are greatly simplified by the equilibrium established at the alveolar gas-blood interface, which permits measurement of the minimum alveolar concentration (MAC) associated with a 50% likelihood of movement in response to noxious stimulation.[22] Considerable effort has gone into developing a concept equivalent to MAC for intravenous anesthetic drugs.

The pharmacodynamics of intravenous anesthetics is reported in terms of C_{50}, the concentration that produces 50% of the maximum possible drug effect. There are many ways of thinking about C_{50}. It might be the drug concentration that prevents response (e.g., movement, hypertension, release of catecholamines) to a particular stimulus (e.g., incision, intubation, sternal spreading) in 50% of patients. In this case, each combination of stimulus and response may have a unique C_{50}. For example, Ausems and colleagues defined the C_{50} for alfentanil in the presence of 66% nitrous oxide for several noxious stimuli.[23] When C_{50} is defined as the drug concentration that produces a given response in 50% of patients, it is also the concentration associated with a 50% probability of response in a given patient. Note that defining C_{50} as the concentration that produces a given effect in 50% of individuals implicitly assumes that the effect can be achieved in all individuals. Some drugs exhibit a ceiling effect. For example, there appears to be a ceiling on the ability of opioids to suppress response to noxious stimulation. When a ceiling in drug effect exists, some patients may not exhibit the drug effect even at infinitely high doses. In this case, C_{50} is not the concentration that causes the drug effect in 50% of patients but is the concentration associated with the drug effect in half of whatever fraction of patients are able to respond.

Several studies have been performed to establish appropriate concentrations of intravenous anesthetics. C_{50} values for alfentanil, fentanyl, and remifentanil in the presence of 70% nitrous oxide have been defined for skin incision (Table 28-2). C_{50} values for loss of consciousness and skin incision have also been defined for the hypnotics thiopental,[24,25] propofol,[26-28] and midazolam (see Table 28-2).[29] Defining the C_{50}, like MAC, provides a measure of relative potency between intravenous anesthetics.

Another interpretation of C_{50} is the concentration that produces 50% of the maximum possible physiologic response. For example, the C_{50} for an EEG response is the drug concentration that provides 50% of the maximal EEG effect. The C_{50} for EEG response has been measured for the opioids alfentanil,[30] fentanyl,[30] sufentanil,[31] and remifentanil.[32-34] It has also been determined for thiopental,[24,35,36] etomidate,[37] propofol,[38] and benzodiazepines (see Table 28-2).[39]

Although C_{50} values for all combinations of stimuli and measures have not been determined experimentally for each opioid, they can be estimated accurately by scaling the values of C_{50} determined experimentally for other opioids according to their relative potency.[40] For example, the C_{50} of alfentanil for

Table 28-2 Steady-State Concentrations for Predefined Effects*

Drug	C_{50} for EEG Depression†	C_{50} for Incision or Painful Stimulus‡	C_{50} for Loss of Consciousness§	C_{50} for Spontaneous Ventilation¶	C_{50} for Isoflurane MAC Reduction	MEAC
Propofol (µg/mL)	3-4	4-8	2-3	1.33	Not studied	—
Thiopental (µg/mL)	15-20	35-40	8-16	—	—	—
Midazolam (ng/mL)	250-350	—	125-250	—	—	—
Alfentanil (ng/mL)	500-600	200-300	—	170-230	50	10-30
Fentanyl (ng/mL)	6-10	4-6	—	2-3	1.7	0.5-1
Sufentanil (ng/mL)	0.5-0.75	(0.3-0.4)	—	(0.15-0.2)	0.15	0.025-0.05
Remifentanil (ng/mL)	10-15	4-6	—	2-3	1.2	0.5-1

*Values in parentheses are estimated by scaling to the alfentanil C_{50} (see text for details).
†The C_{50} for depression of the electroencephalogram (EEG) is the steady-state serum concentration that causes a 50% slowing of the maximal EEG, except for midazolam, where the C_{50} is associated with 50% activation of the EEG.
‡The C_{50} for skin incision is the steady-state plasma concentration that prevents a somatic or autonomic response in 50% of patients.
§The C_{50} for loss of consciousness is the steady-state plasma concentration for absence of a response to a verbal command in 50% of patients.
¶The C_{50} for spontaneous ventilation is the steady-state plasma concentration associated with adequate spontaneous ventilation in 50% of patients.
MEAC, minimum effective plasma concentration providing postoperative analgesia.

spontaneous ventilation is about 40% of the C_{50} for EEG response (see Table 28-2). Knowing this, we can estimate the C_{50} of sufentanil for spontaneous ventilation (which has not yet been determined experimentally) as 0.2 to 0.3 ng/mL, that is, 40% of the C_{50} for EEG response (0.7 ng/mL).

To be entirely independent of dosing history, C_{50} must be determined at steady state, which is rarely possible because most anesthetic drugs do not reach steady state during a continuous infusion until many hours have passed. However, if the drug exhibits rapid equilibration between plasma and the effect site and the investigator waits long enough after starting the infusion, this choice can be reasonably satisfactory. For example, in their experiments Ausems and colleagues[23,41] used a continuous infusion of alfentanil, which equilibrated quickly. They also took their measurements after the effect-site concentration had equilibrated with plasma.

A second alternative to performing a true steady-state experiment is to use mathematical modeling to calculate the effect-site concentrations of drug at the time of measurement, as proposed by Hull and colleagues[12] and Sheiner and colleagues.[13] The relationship between effect-site and plasma concentrations is represented graphically in Figure 28-5 and mathematically in Equation 6. Calculating effect-site concentrations is the same as attempting to determine the steady-state plasma concentrations that would produce the observed drug effect. When the C_{50} reflects effect-site concentrations, it is represented as Ce_{50} to distinguish it from values of C_{50} that are based on plasma concentrations, which are then termed Cp_{50}. However, the distinction is artificial. In both cases, C_{50} is intended to represent the steady-state plasma drug concentration associated with a given drug effect.

A third alternative to performing a steady-state experiment is to establish a pseudo–steady state with the use of computer-controlled drug delivery. This has become the state-of-the-art method for determining the C_{50} for anesthetic drugs, and many of the C_{50} values referenced earlier were determined at pseudo–steady state with the use of computer-controlled drug delivery. Typically, maintaining a constant plasma steady-state concentration for four to five plasma effect-site equilibration half-lives (e.g., 10 to 15 minutes for fentanyl) is required. Such a long delay is not necessarily needed when computer-controlled drug delivery is used. For example, computer-controlled infusions can be used to target initially higher plasma target concentrations to provide more rapid achievement of the desired effect-site concentration.[42] This can be automated by having the computer actually target the concentration at the effect-site rather than plasma and thereby rapidly establish plasma–effect site equilibration.[17,18]

Thus, there are several ways to establish C_{50} in terms of steady-state concentrations. C_{50} can be estimated through mathematical effect-site modeling or can be measured experimentally with the use of computer-controlled drug delivery to quickly establish a pseudo–steady state. Either way, when performing studies to define the concentration-effect relationship, equilibrium must exist or be modeled for between the biophase (the site of effect) and plasma or blood (where the concentration is actually measured).

When C_{50} is defined in terms of the concentration associated with a response in half of a population, that same C_{50} is the concentration associated with a 50% probability of response in a typical individual. However, individual patients are not typical individuals but instead will have their own value for C_{50}. Expressed in clinical terms, different patients have different anesthetic requirements for the same stimulus. For example, the minimal effective analgesic concentration of fentanyl is 0.6 ng/mL, but it varies among patients from 0.2 to 2.0 ng/mL.[43] The minimal effective analgesic concentrations of alfentanil[44,45] and sufentanil[46] similarly vary among patients by a factor of 5 to 10. This range encompasses both variability in the intensity of the stimulus and variability of the individual patient. However, this wide range reflects the clinical reality that must be accounted for when dosing regimens are designed. Because of this variability, intravenous anesthetics should be titrated to each patient's unique anesthetic requirement for the given stimulus.

Pharmacodynamic Drug Interactions

Drug interactions cause the C_{50} of one drug to shift in response to administration of a second drug. We have already referred to the ability of opioids to reduce MAC, a clinically useful drug interaction with a long history. In 1901, George Crile suggested that opioids be administered with supplemental drugs for intravenous anesthesia. In 1959, DeCastro and Mundeleer introduced the term "neurolept anesthesia," which consists of a tranquilizer, opioid, and nitrous oxide. Today, the term coined by John Lundy, "balanced anesthesia," is used to describe the concurrent administration of several anesthetic drugs so that no single drug is given in a dosage sufficient to produce toxicity during or after surgery. The interaction of hypnotics and opioids in producing the anesthetic state is complex but predictable.

The MAC of volatile anesthetics appears to be additive when several inhaled anesthetics are administered concurrently.[47,48] The additivity of MAC suggests a uniform mechanism of action for the inhaled anesthetics, although the "unitary theory" of inhalational anesthesia has fallen into disfavor.[49,50] The intravenous anesthetics encompass categories of drugs (hypnotics, opioids, psychotomimetics, anxiolytics, neuroleptics, local anesthetics, and so on) with different receptors and mechanisms of action. In the absence of a uniform mechanism of action, there is no reason to anticipate simple additivity, for example, that maintaining 30% C_{50} of drug A plus 40% C_{50} of drug B will produce the same effect as 70% C_{50} of either drug A or drug B.

The assumption of balanced anesthesia is that drug combinations will be synergistic in anesthetic effect (however defined) but not in toxicity. Such synergism has been demonstrated for a variety of drug combinations but not for others.[51,52] For example, Smith and coworkers[28] found minimal synergy between propofol and fentanyl for the end point loss of consciousness, but profound synergy between propofol and fentanyl for the end point loss of response to skin incision (Fig. 28-7). More profound synergy for such end points related to analgesia and hypnosis has also been demonstrated for the interaction between propofol and alfentanil[27] and for that between sevoflurane and fentanyl.[53] Thus, when anesthetic regimens are designed that rely on synergy to produce the anesthetic state, it is important to distinguish the desired end point—loss of consciousness or ablation of response to noxious stimulation. Different combinations of drugs may be required to achieve each end point.

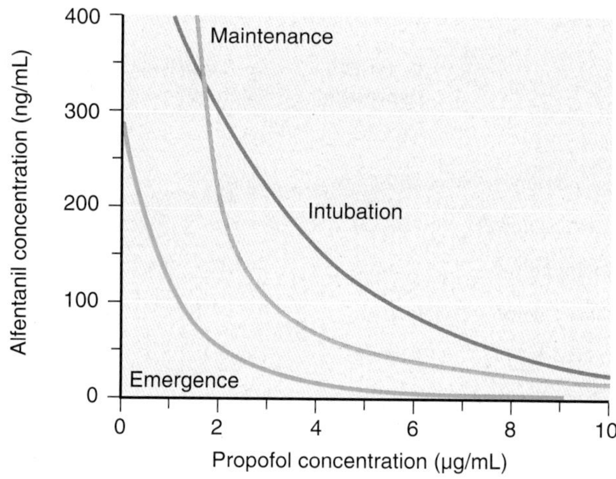

Figure 28-8 Interaction between alfentanil and propofol on three different end points: response to intubation (*blue line*), maintenance of anesthesia (*orange line*), and concentrations associated with emergence from anesthesia (*green line*). The curve shows the concentrations associated with a 50% probability of the respective end point. *(Adapted from Vuyk J, Lim T, Engbers FH, et al: The pharmacodynamic interaction of propofol and alfentanil during lower abdominal surgery in women. Anesthesiology 83:8-22, 1995.)*

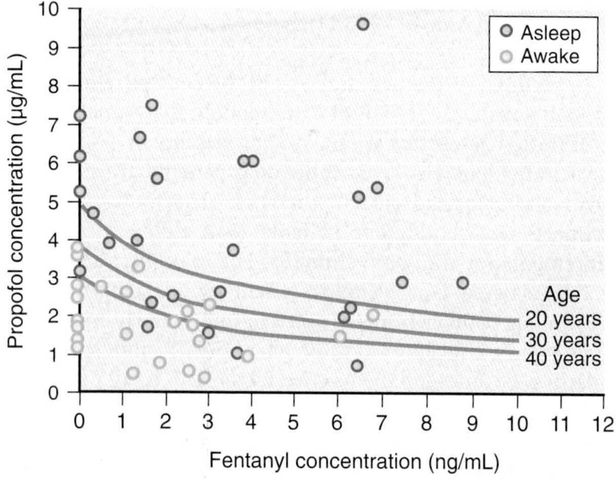

Figure 28-7 Interaction of propofol and fentanyl in preventing a somatic response at skin incision. The *solid line* represents the concentrations of propofol and fentanyl when administered together that are required to prevent purposeful movement in 50% of patients at skin incision. The *dashed line* represents the concentration of propofol and fentanyl when administered together that is required to prevent purposeful movement in 95% of patients at skin incision. *(From Smith C, McEwan AI, Jhaveri R, et al: Reduction of propofol Cp_{50} by fentanyl. Anesthesiology 77:A340, 1992.)*

Vuyk and colleagues characterized the interaction between propofol and alfentanil for several end points: loss of response to intubation, loss of response to intraoperative stimulation, and emergence from anesthesia (Fig. 28-8).[27] The most profound stimulation was tracheal intubation, and abolition of that stimulus required a propofol concentration of at least 2 µg/mL.

MAC is defined as the steady-state alveolar concentration of anesthetic gas that inhibits movement upon incision in 50% of patients. It is a well-established measure of potency. MAC is also a useful guideline for clinical dosage, provided that the clinician remembers that it is the concentration in 50% of patients that inhibits a movement response and that it is defined in terms of an analgesic end point—loss of movement in response to noxious stimulation. To establish the interaction between volatile anesthetics and opioids, the reduction in MAC can be used. When such studies are performed, it is important that both the volatile anesthetic and the opioid be maintained at stable concentrations and have equilibrated with their effect site. For the volatile anesthetic, this is readily achieved with use of a calibrated vaporizer. For the opioid, target-controlled delivery devices described in this chapter are used to maintain constant opioid concentrations within the effect compartment.

Reduction of the MAC of isoflurane by fentanyl,[54] sufentanil,[55] alfentanil,[56] and remifentanil[57] (see also Chapter 27) has been defined for all. The concentrations of these opioids that provide a 50% reduction in MAC are listed in Table 28-2. McEwan and associates[54] demonstrated that the MAC of isoflurane is reduced by 50% at a fentanyl concentration of 1.7 ng/mL (Fig. 28-9). This corresponds with a fentanyl loading dose of 4 µg/kg followed by a 1.75-µg/kg/hr infusion. The minimum effective analgesic concentration of fentanyl is 0.6 ng/mL,[43] and clinically significant respiratory depression may occur with plasma fentanyl concentrations above 2 ng/mL.[58] The steepest reduction in MAC

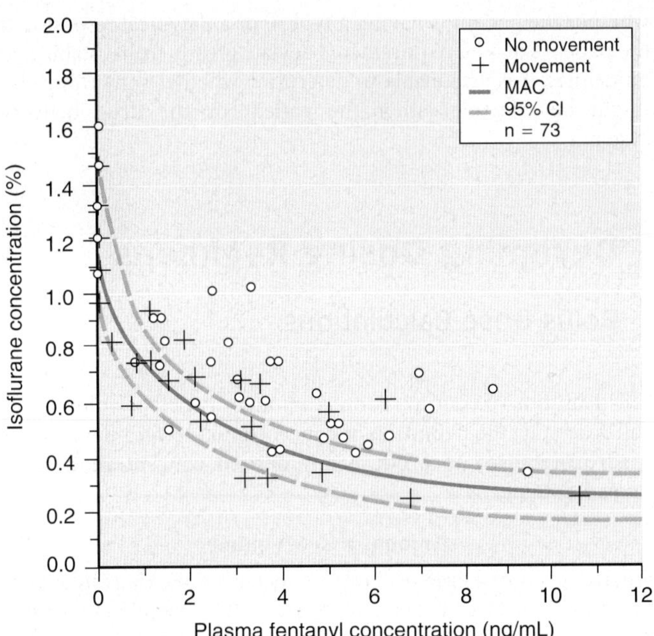

Figure 28-9 Interaction of isoflurane and fentanyl in preventing a somatic response at skin incision (i.e., minimum alveolar concentration [MAC] reduction of isoflurane). The *blue line* represents the concentrations of isoflurane and fentanyl when administered together that are required to prevent purposeful movement in 50% of patients at skin incision. The *yellow lines* represent the 95% confidence interval of the MAC at each combination of fentanyl and isoflurane. *(From McEwan AI, Smith C, Dyar O, et al: Isoflurane MAC reduction by fentanyl. Anesthesiology 78:864-869, 1993.)*

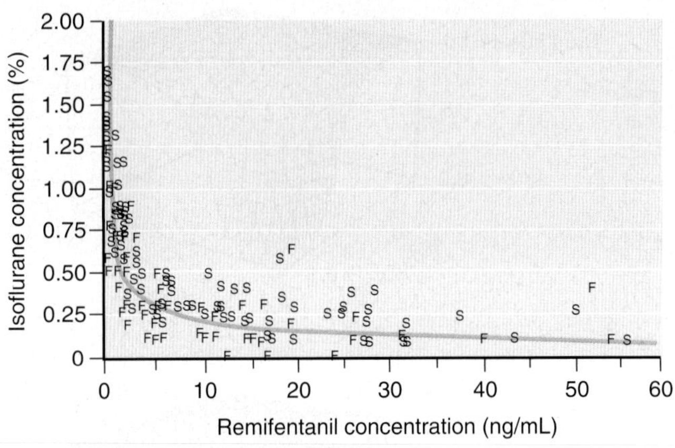

Figure 28-10 Interaction of isoflurane and remifentanil in preventing a somatic response at skin incision (i.e., minimum alveolar concentration [MAC] reduction of isoflurane). The *solid line* represents the concentrations of isoflurane and remifentanil when administered together that are required to prevent purposeful movement in 50% of patients at skin incision. *(From Lang E, Kapila A, Shlugman D, et al: Reduction of isoflurane minimal alveolar concentration by remifentanil. Anesthesiology 85:721-728, 1996.)*

thus occurs within the useful analgesic range for fentanyl (i.e., 0.6 to 2 ng/mL). In other words, by maintaining fentanyl within an analgesic range, the MAC of isoflurane can be reduced by 50%. The study by McEwan and colleagues also demonstrated that beyond a fentanyl plasma concentration of 5 ng/mL, a plateau is seen with a maximum MAC reduction of approximately 80%. The maximum reduction in isoflurane was to a concentration of ±0.3%, that is, a value close to the MAC-awake value for isoflurane.[59]

Alfentanil,[56] sufentanil,[55] and remifentanil[57] produce similar reductions in isoflurane MAC, with an initial steep reduction at lower concentrations and a ceiling effect at higher concentrations. Because remifentanil is metabolized rapidly,[15] it is possible to give huge doses during MAC studies and still awaken patients after surgery. The reduction in isoflurane MAC by remifentanil is shown in Figure 28-10.[57] Even with very high plasma concentrations (>30 ng/mL), a ceiling of opioid effect is observed, and the MAC of isoflurane is not reduced below 0.2% to 0.3%. Similar results have been demonstrated with the other volatile anesthetics and opioids. Thus, there is little clinical benefit in administering opioid at concentrations exceeding those that produce a ceiling in MAC reduction. This occurs at a concentration of 3 to 5 ng/mL for fentanyl and remifentanil, 200 to 400 ng/mL for alfentanil, and 0.25 to 0.5 ng/mL for sufentanil. Keeping the opioid dose within an analgesic range prevents the very slow recovery that is associated with high opioid concentrations.

The relationship between opioids and hypnotics on the C_{50}, the concentration of drug associated with 50% of maximum effect, has been examined. The interaction between two drugs describes a surface in which each drug has its own axis and the third axis is the effect from any combination of the two drugs. Figure 28-11 shows the relationship between the three-dimensional response surfaces and the more commonly shown relationship in two dimensions between the C_{50} of two drugs. Minto and colleagues published "response surfaces" for combinations of midazolam-alfentanil, propofol-alfentanil, and midazolam-propofol associ-

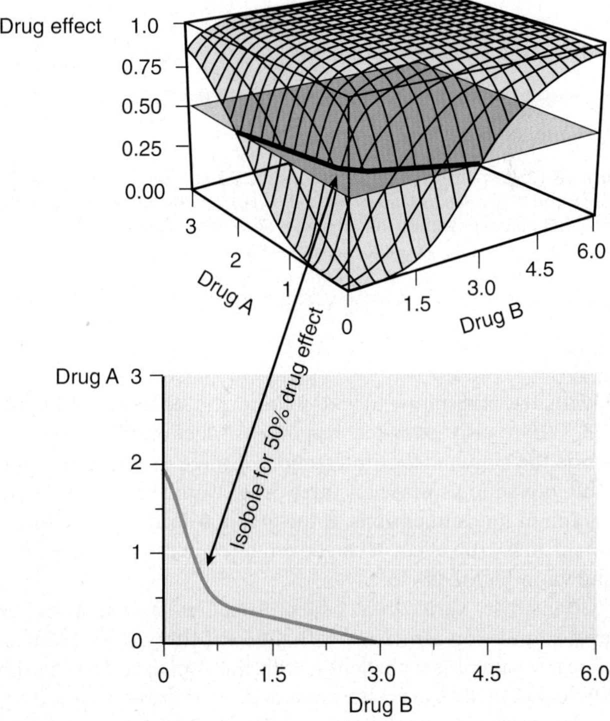

Figure 28-11 Relationship between a response surface and a standard isobologram. Conventional "isobolographic" analysis, whether for doses or concentrations, describes only the concentration of both drugs that yields a 50% drug effect and thus fails to capture the entire response surface. *(From Minto CF, Schnider TW, Short TG, et al: Response surface model for anesthetic drug interactions. Anesthesiology 92:1603-1616, 2000.)*

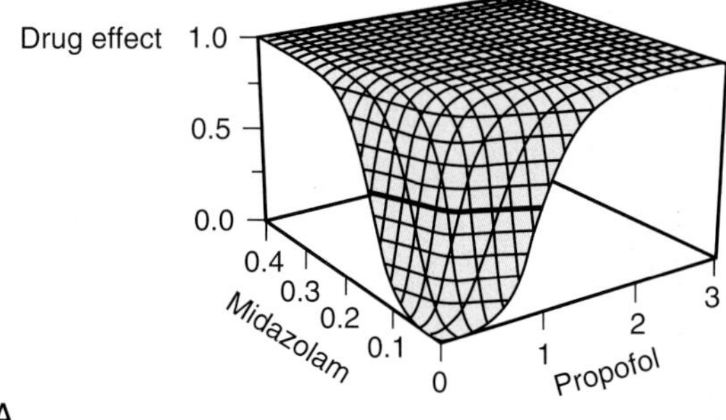

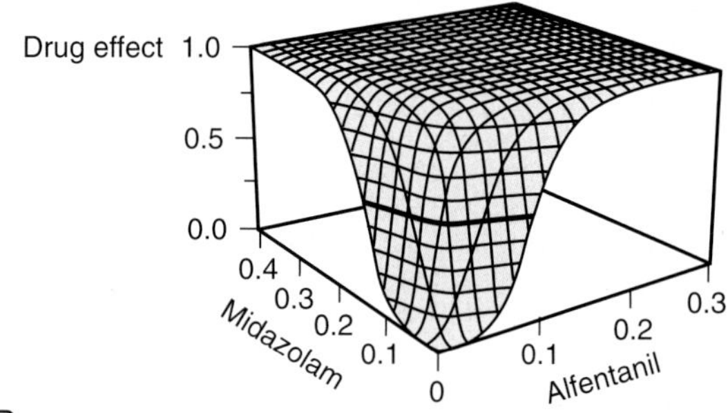

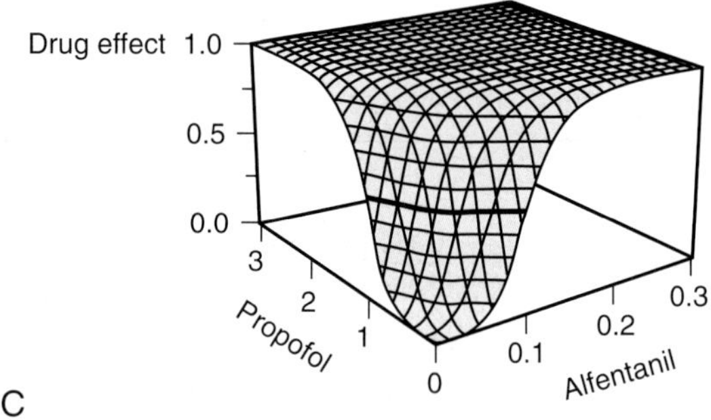

Figure 28-12 Response surface for each of the paired interactions between propofol and midazolam (**A**), alfentanil and midazolam (**B**), and alfentanil and propofol (**C**) on the probability of opening eyes to verbal command. The isoboles for a 10%, 20%, 30%, 40%, 50%, 60%, 70%, 80%, and 90% response are shown. *(From Minto CF, Schnider TW, Short TG, et al: Response surface model for anesthetic drug interactions. Anesthesiology 92:1603-1616, 2000.)*

ated with loss of response to verbal command, as shown in Figure 28-12.[60] They also extended response surface methodology to describe the simultaneous interaction of three drugs. Rendering the full interaction surface for three drugs would require drawing the graph in four dimensions. If the graph is limited to the interaction at 50% drug effect, it can be rendered in three dimensions, as shown in Figure 28-13.

Sensitivity varies from patient to patient, as well as in the level of stimulation associated with different surgical procedures. Thus, each patient is a challenge, with the clinician learning the individual patient's C_{50} for the combination of drugs used during the administration of each anesthetic. Despite this variability, dosing guidelines play an important role in the practice of anesthesia. The concentration ranges of intravenous anesthetics for anesthesia, sedation, and analgesia are given in Table 28-3. These ranges provide starting estimates on which subsequent titration can be based. They also provide a means of estimating whether the patient is having a typical or an atypical response. If the patient's dosing requirements deviate greatly from established guidelines, it is reasonable to determine whether something else might be affecting either the patient or the drug delivery system.

Designing Dosing Regimens

Bolus Dose Calculations

The definition of concentration is amount divided by volume. We can rearrange the definition of concentration to find the amount of drug required to produce any desired concentration for a known volume:

$$\text{Amount} = C_T \times \text{Volume} \tag{10}$$

where C_T is the desired or "target" concentration. Many introductory pharmacokinetic texts suggest using this formula to calculate the loading bolus required to achieve a given concentration. The problem with applying this concept to anesthetic drugs is that there are several volumes: V_1 (central compartment), V_2 and V_3 (the peripheral compartments), and Vd_{ss}, the sum of the individual volumes. V_1 is usually much smaller than Vd_{ss}, and thus it is tempting to say that the loading dose should be something between $C_T \times V_1$ and $C_T \times Vd_{ss}$.

Consider the dose of fentanyl required to attenuate the hemodynamic response to intubation when combined with thiopental. The C_{50} for fentanyl, combined with thiopental for intubation, is approximately 3 ng/mL. The V_1 and Vd_{ss} for fentanyl are 13 and 360 L, respectively. The aforementioned equations can thus be interpreted as suggesting that an appropriate dose of fentanyl to attenuate the hemodynamic response is between 39 μg (3 ng/mL × 13 L) and 1080 μg (3 ng/mL × 360 L). A fentanyl bolus of 39 μg achieves the desired concentration in plasma for an initial instant, but plasma levels almost instantly decrease

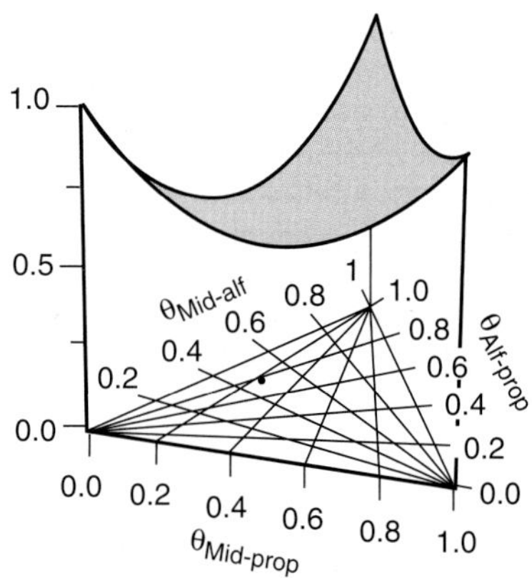

Figure 28-13 Interaction at 50% drug effect between propofol, midazolam, and alfentanil. Downward deflection of the surface represents synergy, in units of fractional reduction in C_{50}. The three edges represent relative amounts of propofol to midazolam ($\theta_{Mid\text{-}prop}$), alfentanil to midazolam ($\theta_{Mid\text{-}alf}$), and alfentanil to propofol ($\theta_{Alf\text{-}prop}$). The surface between the edges represents the relative synergy of all three drugs taken together. *(From Minto CF, Schnider TW, Short TG, et al: Response surface model for anesthetic drug interactions. Anesthesiology 92:1603-1616, 2000.)*

Table 28-3 Plasma Drug Concentration Ranges

Drug*	Skin Incision	Stimulus: Major Surgery	Stimulus: Minor Surgery	Spontaneous Ventilation	Awakening	Analgesia or Sedation
Alfentanil (ng/mL)	200-300	250-450	100-300	<200-250	—	50-100
Fentanyl (ng/mL)	3-6	4-8	2-5	<1-2	—	1-2
Sufentanil (ng/mL)	1-3	2-5	1-3	<0.2	—	0.02-0.2
Remifentanil (ng/mL)	4-8	4-8	2-4	<1-3	—	1-2
Propofol (μg/mL)	2-6	2.5-7.5	2-6	—	0.8-1.8	1.0-3.0
Methohexital (μg/mL)	5-10	5-15	5-10	—	1-3	2-5
Thiopental (μg/mL)	7.5-12.5 (with N_2O) 35-45 (without N_2O)	10-20	10-20	—	4-8	7.5-15.0
Etomidate (ng/mL)	400-600	500-1000	300-600	—	200-350	100-300
Midazolam (ng/mL)	—	50-250 (combined with an opioid)	50-250 (combined with an opioid)	—	15-200 (reduced to 20-70 in the presence of an opioid)	40-100
Ketamine (μg/mL)	—	—	1-2	—	—	0.1-1
Dexmedetomidine† (ng/mL)						0.1-0.6

*Drug levels when combined with 65% to 70% nitrous oxide (N_2O) unless otherwise stated. Effective plasma concentrations may differ markedly, depending on premedication and intraoperative drug combinations.
†Dexmedetomidine provides sedation and mild analgesia at the concentrations listed. It may be combined with other sedatives or analgesics to reduce their C_{50} for the end points listed.

below the desired target. Levels at the effect site will never be close to the desired target concentration of 3 ng/mL. A fentanyl bolus of 1080 μg, not surprisingly, produces a marked overshoot in plasma levels that persists for hours (Fig. 28-14). Additionally, it is absurd to use equations to calculate the fentanyl dose if the resulting recommendation is "pick a dose between 39 and 1080 μg."

The usual dosing guidelines for a bolus dose, presented earlier, are designed to produce a specific plasma concentration. Because plasma is not the site of drug effect, it is illogical to base calculation of the initial bolus on a desired plasma concentration. As pointed out previously, by knowing the k_{e0} of an intravenous anesthetic, we can design a dosing regimen that yields the desired concentration at the site of drug effect. If we do not want to overdose the patient, we should select a bolus that produces the desired peak concentration at the effect site.

The decline in plasma concentration between the initial concentration after the bolus (amount/V_1) and the concentration at the time of peak effect can be thought of as dilution of the bolus into a larger volume than the volume of the central compartment. This introduces the concept of Vd_{pe}, the apparent volume of distribution at the time of peak effect,[17,61] or pseudo-equilibration between plasma and the site of drug effect.[62] The size of this volume can readily be calculated from the observation that the plasma and effect-site concentrations are the same at the time of peak effect:

$$Vd_{pe} = \frac{\text{Bolus amount}}{C_{pe}} \quad (11)$$

where C_{pe} is the plasma concentration at the time of peak effect.

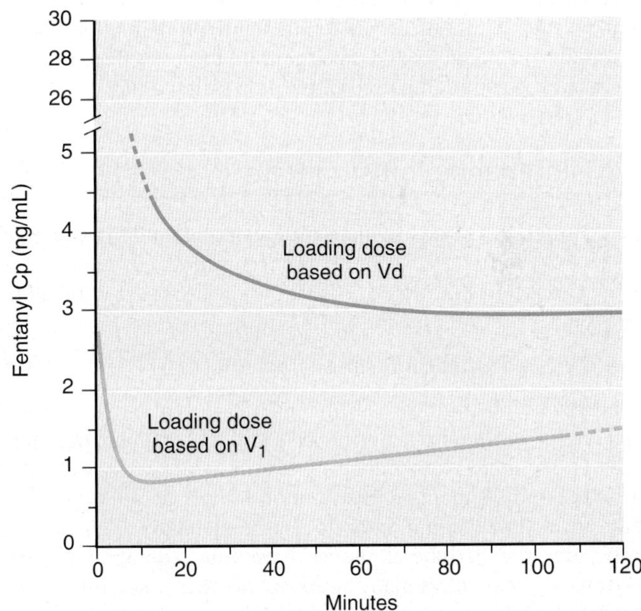

Figure 28-14 Pharmacokinetic simulation demonstrating the limitations of infusion regimens based on simple pharmacokinetic parameters, with fentanyl used as an example. These infusion schemes were designed to achieve a plasma fentanyl concentration of 3 ng/mL. The *upper blue curve* shows that a regimen using a loading dose based on the volume of distribution followed by a constant infusion based on clearance results in a transient period of very high plasma concentrations. If the same maintenance infusion is given but the loading dose is based on the volume of the central compartment, distribution of drug to the peripheral compartments causes the plasma concentration to fall below the desired level until the compartments reach steady-state concentrations, as shown in the *lower yellow curve*. Cp, plasma drug concentration.

Table 28-4 Volume of Distribution at the Time of Peak Effect

Drug	V_1 (L)	Vd_{pe} (L)
Fentanyl	12.7	75
Alfentanil	2.19	5.9
Sufentanil	17.8	89
Remifentanil	5.0	17
Propofol	6.7	37
Thiopental	5.6	14.6
Midazolam	3.4	31

V_1, volume of the central compartment; Vd_{pe}, apparent volume of distribution at the time of peak effect.

Let us assume that our clinical goal is to select the dose required to achieve a certain drug effect without producing an overdose. We can rearrange Equation 11 by substituting C_T, the target concentration (which is the same in plasma and the effect site at the moment of peak effect), for C_{pe} to calculate the size of the initial bolus:

$$\text{Loading dose} = C_T \times Vd_{pe} \tag{12}$$

The Vd_{pe} for fentanyl is 75 L. To achieve a peak fentanyl effect-site concentration of 3.0 ng/mL requires 225 μg, which produces a peak effect in 3.6 minutes. This is a much more reasonable dosing guideline than the previous recommendation of a dose between 39 and 1080 μg. Table 28-4 lists V_1 and Vd_{pe} for fentanyl, alfentanil, sufentanil, remifentanil, propofol, thiopental, and midazolam. Table 28-1 lists the time to peak effect and the $t_{½}\ k_{e0}$ of the commonly used intravenous anesthetics.

Maintenance Infusion Rate

By definition, the rate at which drug exits the body is systemic clearance, Cl_S, times the plasma concentration. To maintain a given target concentration, C_T, drug must be delivered at the same rate that it is exiting the body. Thus,

$$\text{Maintenance infusion rate} = C_T \times Cl_S \tag{13}$$

For drugs with multicompartmental pharmacokinetics, which includes all of the intravenous drugs used in anesthetic practice, drug is distributed into the peripheral tissues as well as cleared from the body. The rate of distribution into tissues changes over time as the tissues equilibrate with plasma. Equation 13 is correct only after the peripheral tissues have fully equilibrated with plasma, which requires many hours. At all other times, this maintenance infusion rate underestimates the infusion rate to maintain a target concentration.

In some situations this simple maintenance rate calculation may be acceptable. For example, if an infusion at this rate is used along with a bolus dose based on Vd_{pe} and the drug has a long delay between the bolus and peak effect, much of the distribution of drug into tissues may have occurred by the time that the effect-site concentration reaches the target concentration. In this case, the maintenance infusion rate calculated as clearance times target concentration may be accurate because Vd_{pe} is sufficiently higher than V_1 to account for the distribution of drug into peripheral tissues. Unfortunately, most drugs used in anesthesia achieve sufficiently rapid equilibration between plasma and the effect site that Vd_{pe} does not adequately encompass the distribution process, thus making this approach unsuitable.

Another example of calculating infusion rates for drugs with multicompartmental pharmacokinetics is the two-step approach proposed by Wagner.[63] In this method, two infusions, Q_1 and Q_2, are administered in sequence. The loading infusion, Q_1, is selected on the basis of convenience and the degree of overshoot in plasma concentration that will be clinically acceptable. The second infusion, Q_2, is calculated as $C_T \times Cl_S$, exactly as noted earlier. The Wagner two-step approach does not consider the time course of drug effect and thus is probably not appropriate for most anesthetic drugs.

Having considered two approaches that do not work very well, we now turn to approaches that are mathematically and clinically sound. Because the net flow of drug into peripheral tissues decreases over time, the infusion rate required to maintain any desired concentration must also decrease over time. If the initial bolus has been based on Vd_{pe}, no infusion need be administered until the effect-site concentrations peak. After the peak in effect-site concentration, the (nearly) correct equation to maintain the desired concentration is

$$\text{Maintenance infusion rate} = C_T \times V_1 \times \left(k_{10} + k_{12}e^{-k_{21}t} + k_{13}e^{-k_{31}t}\right) \tag{14}$$

This equation indicates that a high infusion rate is initially required to maintain C_T. Over time, the infusion rate gradually decreases (see Fig. 28-4). At equilibrium ($t = \infty$), the infusion rate decreases to $C_T \times V_1 \times k_{10}$, which is the same as $C_T \times Cl_S$. Few anesthesiologists would choose to mentally solve such an equation during administration of an anesthetic. Fortunately, there are simple techniques that can be used in place of solving such a complex expression.

Figure 28-15 is a nomogram in which Equation 14 has been solved; the infusion rates at different times necessary to maintain any desired concentration of fentanyl, alfentanil, sufentanil, and propofol are shown. This nomogram is complex, so we will review it in detail. The *y* axis represents the target concentration C_T. The *x* axis is the time since the beginning of the anesthetic (i.e., since the initial bolus). The suggested initial target concentrations (shown in red) are based on the work of Vuyk and colleagues[27] with propofol and alfentanil (see Fig. 28-8) and are scaled to fentanyl and sufentanil according to their relative potencies.[61] The intersections of the target concentration line and the diagonal lines indicate the infusion rate appropriate at each point in time. For example, to maintain a fentanyl concentration of 1.5 ng/mL, the appropriate rates are 4.5 μg/kg/hr at 15 minutes, 3.6 μg/kg/hr at 30 minutes, 2.7 μg/kg/hr at 60 minutes, 2.1 μg/kg/hr at 120 minutes, and 1.5 μg/kg/hr at 180 minutes. Of course, it is possible to select target concentrations and different times of rate adjustment, depending on clinical circumstances and your assessment of how accurately the intravenous drug needs to be titrated.

Another recent approach to manually determine infusion rates for maintenance of anesthesia to a desired target concentration is through the application of concepts involving the use of a slide rule.[64] Figure 28-16 illustrates such a slide rule for propofol. As described by Bruhn and colleagues, "The bolus dose required to reach a given target plasma concentration is the product of the (weight-related) distribution volume and required concentration.

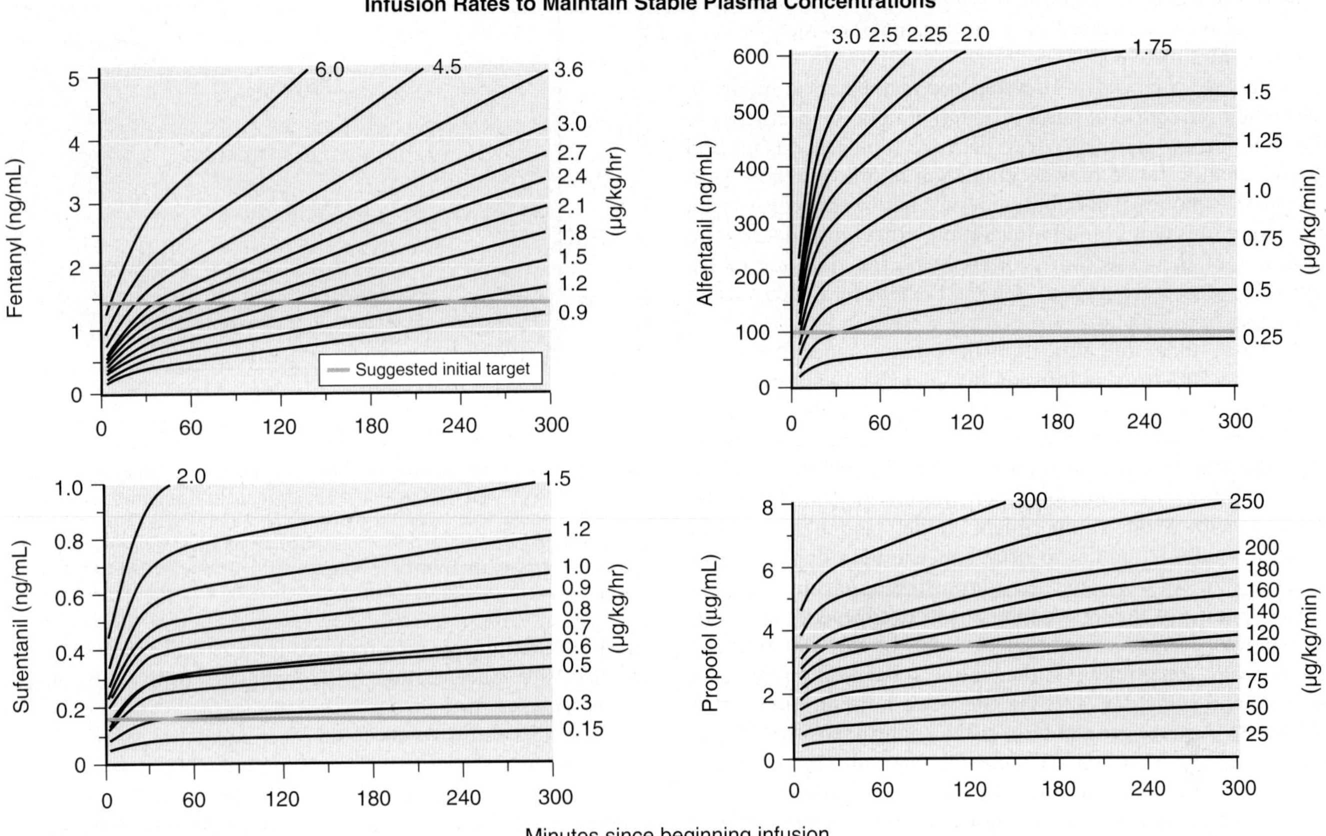

Figure 28-15 Nomogram for calculating maintenance infusion rates to maintain a stable concentration of fentanyl, alfentanil, sufentanil, or propofol. The *y* axis is the desired concentration. The *x* axis is the time relative to the initial bolus. The *diagonal lines* show the infusion rates at different times required to maintain the desired concentration selected on the *y* axis.

Similarly, the infusion rate at a particular time point is the product of target concentration, body weight, and a correction factor that depends on the time elapsed from the start of the initial infusion. This factor can be determined for each time point using a PK simulation program."[64] When compared with computer simulation programs, this manual device performed within an acceptable degree of accuracy (within 7% of the simulated target concentration) for a single target concentration and decreased in accuracy (within 20%) when applied to changing target concentrations.

Recovery from Anesthesia

Recovery from anesthesia is determined by the pharmacokinetic principles that govern the rate of decrease in drug from the effect compartment once drug administration is terminated, as well as by the pharmacodynamics of the drug. Although the terminal elimination half-life is often interpreted as a measure of how short or long lasting a drug is, the rate at which drug decreases is dependent on both elimination and redistribution of the drug from the central compartment. The contribution of both

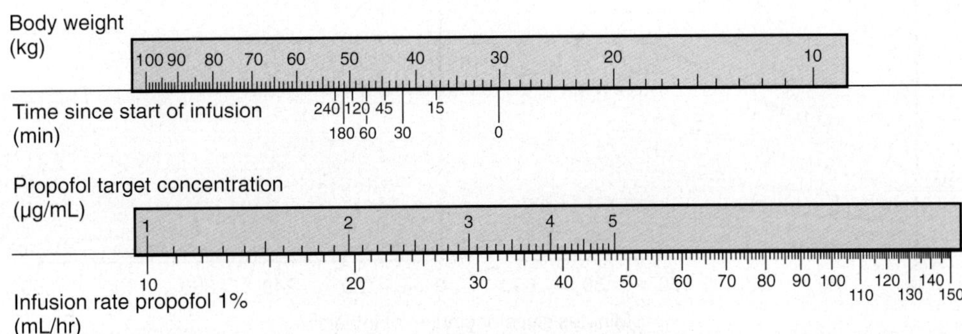

Figure 28-16 Slide rule for calculating the maintenance propofol infusion rate from the patient's weight, the desired target concentration, and the elapsed time. *(Adapted from Bruhn J, Bouillon TW, Ropcke H, Hoeft A: A manual slide rule for target-controlled infusion of propofol: Development and evaluation. Anesth Analg 96:142-147, 2003.)*

redistribution and elimination toward the rate of decrease in drug concentration varies according to the duration for which the drug has been administered.[61,65]

In 1985, Schwilden[66] developed a mathematical model to relate the time course of offset of action of inhaled anesthetics to the duration of anesthetic drug delivery. Similarly, Fisher and Rosen[67] demonstrated how accumulation of muscle relaxants in peripheral volumes of distribution results in slowed recovery with increasing duration of administration. They introduced two measures of the time course of recovery, the time for twitch tension to recover from 5% to 25% and the time for twitch tension to recover from 25% to 75%.

Since then, the time for the plasma concentration to decrease by 50% from an infusion that maintains a constant concentration (e.g., the infusion given by Equation 14) has been termed the "context-sensitive half-time" (Fig. 28-17),[65] with the context being the duration of the infusion. The 50% decrease was chosen both for tradition (e.g., half-lives are the time for a 50% decrease with a one-compartment model) and because, very roughly, a 50% reduction in drug concentration appears to be necessary for recovery after the administration of most intravenous hypnotics at the termination of surgery. Depending on circumstances, decreases other than 50% may be clinically relevant. Additionally, sometimes it is the plasma concentration that is of interest, and sometimes it is the effect-site concentration that is of interest. A more general term is the context-sensitive "decrement time,"[68] in which the decrement in concentration is specifically noted, as is the compartment where the decrease is modeled (plasma or effect site). For example, the relationship between infusion duration and time required for a 70% decrease in fentanyl effect-site concentration is the "context-sensitive 70% effect-site decrement time."

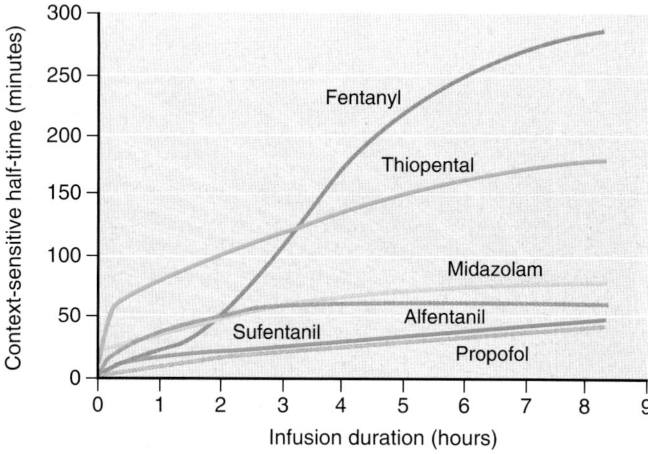

Figure 28-17 Context-sensitive half-times as a function of infusion duration (the "context") derived from pharmacokinetic models of fentanyl, sufentanil, alfentanil, propofol, midazolam, and thiopental. *(From Hughes MA, Glass PSA, Jacobs JR: Context-sensitive half-time in multicompartment pharmacokinetic models for intravenous anesthetic drugs. Anesthesiology 76:334-341, 1992.)*

Context-sensitive effect-site decrement times for varying percent decreases in alfentanil, fentanyl, and remifentanil concentration are illustrated in Figure 28-18. To determine when an infusion should be terminated (to enable awakening of the patient

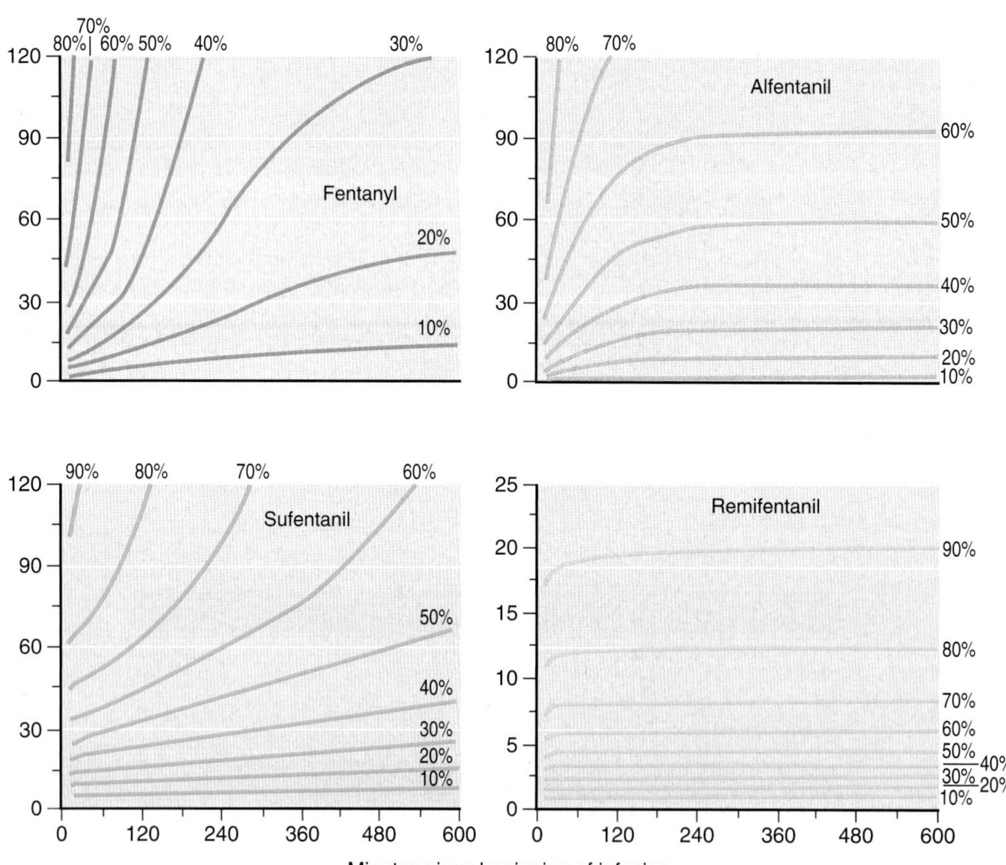

Figure 28-18 Context-sensitive effect-site decrement times for alfentanil, fentanyl, sufentanil, and remifentanil showing the time required for decreases of a given percentage (labeled for each curve) from the maintained effect-site concentration after termination of the infusion.

at the end of surgery), the clinician needs to bear in mind the decrease in concentration necessary for recovery, the duration of the infusion (the context), and the context-sensitive effect-site decrement time required for the necessary decrease.

Context-sensitive decrement times are fundamentally different from the elimination half-life. With monoexponential decay, each 50% decrease in concentration requires the same amount of time, and this time is independent of how the drug is given. This is not true for the context-sensitive half-time. First, as the name is intended to imply, the time needed for a 50% decrease is absolutely dependent on how the drug was given, with infusion duration being the context to which the name refers. In addition, small changes in percent decrement can result in surprisingly large increases in the time required. As can be seen from Figure 28-18, in some situations the time required for a 60% decrease in drug concentration can be more than twice the time required for a 50% decrease.

Context-sensitive decrement times are based on the assumption that plasma or the effect site is maintained at a constant concentration. Such is rarely the case clinically, but maintenance of constant concentrations is a necessary assumption to provide a unique mathematical solution to the time required for a given percent decrement in plasma or effect-site concentration. Because plasma and effect-site concentrations are rarely kept constant, it is important that context-sensitive decrement times be used as general guidelines for interpreting the pharmacokinetics of intravenous drugs and not as absolute predictions for any given case or infusion regimen. Automated drug delivery systems can provide more precise predictions of the time required for the plasma or effect-site concentration to decrease to any desired concentration based on the actual drug dosing in the individual patient. This provides the clinician with guidance for the most appropriate time to terminate the infusion.

Context-sensitive decrement times focus on the role of pharmacokinetics in recovery from anesthesia. Pharmacodynamics plays an important role in recovery as well. Bailey[69] used integrated pharmacokinetic/pharmacodynamic models to define the "mean effect time" as the average time to responsiveness after maintenance of anesthesia at the 90% probability of unresponsiveness. The mean effect time demonstrates that when drugs have a very shallow concentration-versus-response relationship, concentrations must decrease by a significant fraction to provide adequate emergence. This delays recovery from anesthesia. In contrast, recovery is hastened by a steep concentration-versus-response relationship, in which emergence from anesthesia occurs after a relatively small fractional decrease in concentration. Most intravenous hypnotics have a fairly steep concentration-versus-response relationship.

Pharmacodynamic drug interactions also play a role in recovery from anesthesia. Interaction relationships predict that the same anesthetic state can be achieved by different ratios of two drugs. One way of selecting the best ratio might be the combination that offers the most rapid recovery. For example, when an opioid is combined with a hypnotic, recovery from anesthesia depends on the opioid and hypnotic concentrations, the rate of decrease in both drugs, and the relative synergy between them for loss of response to noxious stimulation (i.e., the state maintained during anesthesia) versus the relative synergy for loss of consciousness. Although the time course of decreases in opioid and hypnotic concentrations can be approximately described by their respective context-sensitive decrement times for both drugs

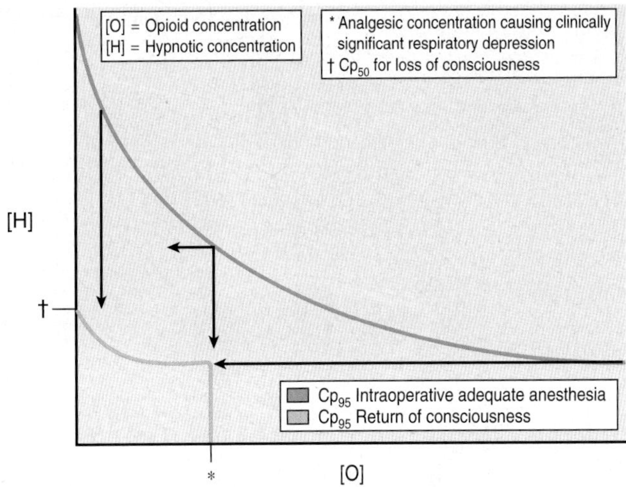

Figure 28-19 Interaction between hypnotics and opioids for prevention of movement after a noxious stimulus and for awakening and adequate spontaneous ventilation at the end of a surgical procedure. From this it can be seen that the time to recover at the end of a procedure is dependent on the concentration of both drugs used during surgery and the time for both to decrease below that required for consciousness and adequate spontaneous ventilation (i.e., their context-sensitive decrement times).

(Fig. 28-19; for propofol/alfentanil, see Fig. 28-8), the influence of relative synergy for different end points must be captured by separate models of the interaction of the drugs for adequate anesthesia and emergence from anesthesia.

Vuyk and coworkers[70] modeled the predicted time to awakening when propofol is combined with fentanyl, sufentanil, alfentanil, or remifentanil on the basis of the interaction between propofol and these opioids to provide adequate anesthesia and the interaction between propofol and opioids on emergence from anesthesia, as seen in Figures 28-20 and 28-21. Recovery times vary with the choice of opioid and the relative balance of opioid and propofol during maintenance of anesthesia. For example, in the upper left of Figure 28-20 is a simulation of emergence from a propofol/fentanyl anesthetic of 10 minutes' duration. The simulations assume a steady concentration of fentanyl and propofol throughout the anesthesia, similar to the underlying assumption of context-sensitive decrement times. The red curve in the lower plane is the interaction curve between fentanyl and propofol; it ranges from no fentanyl and 12 μg/mL of propofol on the left to 6 ng/mL of fentanyl and 1.8 μg/mL of propofol on the right. In theory, any point along this curve would provide equivalent maintenance of anesthesia. When the infusion is turned off after 10 minutes of anesthesia, the concentrations of both drugs decrease. The decreasing concentrations of propofol and fentanyl when the infusion is turned off can be found by the upward lines drawn from different points on the interaction curve, with the distance away from the lower plane representing time. Taken together, these upward lines represent a "recovery surface." The red line drawn on the recovery surface shows the points at which the fentanyl-propofol interaction model predicts emergence.

Figure 28-20 shows that after 10 minutes of maintaining 1.8 μg/mL of propofol and 6 ng/mL of fentanyl (right edge of the interaction curve), approximately 12 minutes is needed for the concentrations of both drugs to decrease enough to permit emergence. However, if one maintains concentrations of 3.5 μg/mL of propofol and 1.5 ng/mL of fentanyl (toward the middle of the

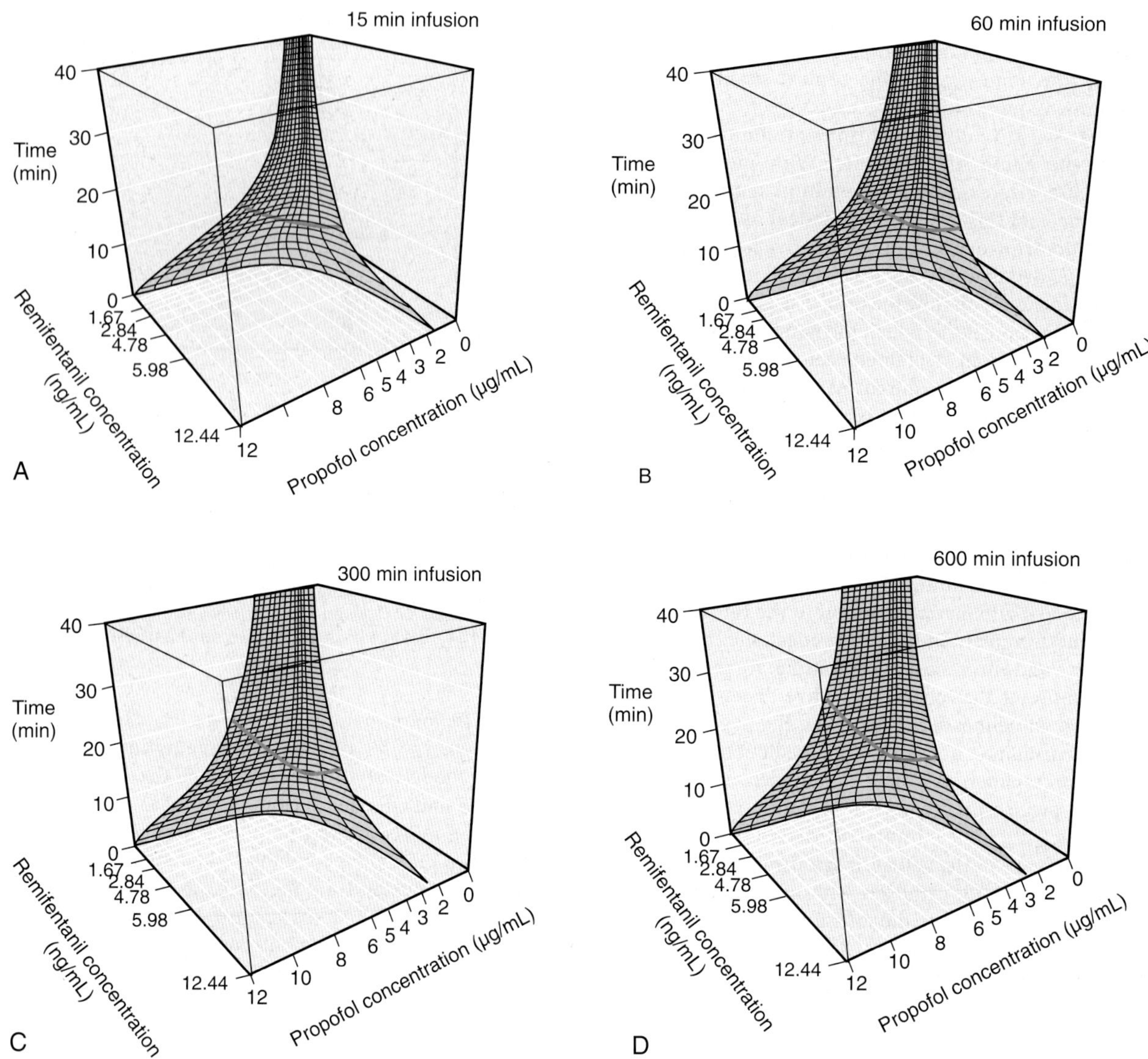

Figure 28-20 Simulation of the interaction of propofol and fentanyl in preventing a somatic response at skin incision and time to recovery. On the *x* axis is the fentanyl concentration, and on the *y* axis, the propofol concentration. The *blue curve* in the lower plane shows the propofol-fentanyl interaction required to provide adequate anesthesia. When the infusion is turned off, the concentrations of each drug decrease, as shown on the *z* axis. The *blue curve* drawn on the recovery surface shows the time to emergence from anesthesia for combinations of fentanyl and propofol after an anesthetic of 15 minutes' (**A**), 60 minutes' (**B**), 180 minutes' (**C**), or 600 minutes' (**D**) duration. Note that the optimal combination for the most rapid recovery is a propofol concentration of 3.0 to 3.5 µg/mL combined with 1.5 ng/mL fentanyl. As the concentration of propofol or fentanyl increases, the time for recovery increases. In addition, the longer the duration of drug infusion, the longer recovery takes, especially if the optimal combination is not used. *(Adapted from Vuyk J, Mertens MJ, Olofsen E, et al: Propofol anesthesia and rational opioid selection: Determination of optimal EC_{50}-EC_{95} propofol-opioid concentrations that assure adequate anesthesia and a rapid return of consciousness. Anesthesiology 87:1549-1562, 1997.)*

interaction curve), emergence can be expected just 8 minutes after the infusions are turned off. Examination of the curves for 60, 300, and 600 minutes of propofol/fentanyl anesthesia suggests that the fentanyl target concentration that provides the most rapid emergence is approximately 1.0 to 1.5 ng/mL, which requires a propofol concentration of approximately 3.0 to 3.5 µg/mL to maintain adequate anesthesia. This is consistent with the earlier observation that most of the MAC reduction benefit of fentanyl occurs within the analgesic range and that exceeding this range is of little benefit during anesthesia. In similar simulations, Vuyk and colleagues demonstrated that maintaining alfentanil and sufentanil concentrations in excess of the analgesic range (i.e., approximately 80 ng/mL for alfentanil and 0.15 ng/mL for sufentanil) is of little clinical benefit but can be expected to delay recovery from anesthesia. A second conclusion from these simulations is that if the patient demonstrates inadequate anesthesia, to prevent prolongation of recovery, it is preferable to increase the hypnotic concentration than to increase the opioid concentration beyond the analgesic range.

The situation is different for remifentanil because of its unusual pharmacokinetic properties (Fig. 28-21). When a remifentanil infusion is terminated, the extraordinary clearance of remifentanil results in very rapid offset of opioid drug effect. In Figure 28-21, the lower plane again shows equivalent anes-

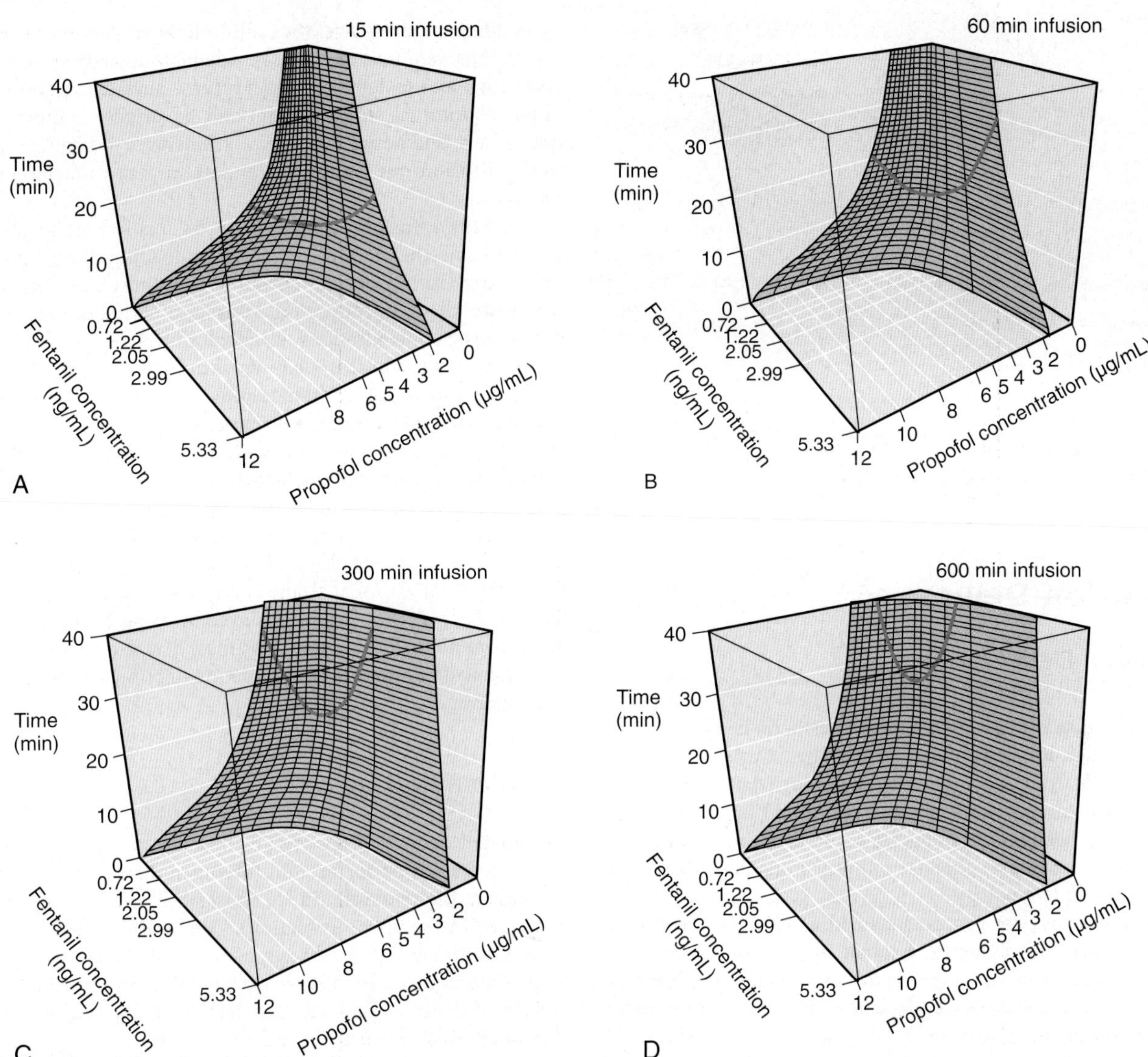

Figure 28-21 Simulation of the interaction of propofol and remifentanil in preventing a somatic response at skin incision and time to recovery. Note that with remifentanil, the optimal combination is a propofol concentration of 2.5 μg/mL and, with remifentanil, 5 to 7 ng/mL; also note that increasing the duration of the infusion has minimal impact on recovery time if the optimal dose of remifentanil is not used. However, if the propofol dose is increased, recovery is prolonged. *(Adapted from Vuyk J, Mertens MJ, Olofsen E, et al: Propofol anesthesia and rational opioid selection: Determination of optimal EC_{50}-EC_{95} propofol-opioid concentrations that assure adequate anesthesia and a rapid return of consciousness. Anesthesiology 87:1549-1562, 1997.)*

thetic states during maintenance with an opioid, remifentanil, and propofol. High doses of remifentanil permit a modest reduction in the dose of propofol needed for adequate anesthesia. However, the recovery surfaces show that high doses of remifentanil, with a modest reduction in the propofol dose, permit considerably faster emergence from anesthesia. For example, it takes approximately 12 minutes to awaken from 600 minutes of anesthesia maintained with 3 μg/mL of propofol and 2.5 ng/mL of remifentanil (Fig. 28-20, lower left graph). If the remifentanil concentration is increased to 5 ng/mL, the propofol concentration can be reduced to 2 to 2.5 μg/mL, and emergence can be anticipated within 6 minutes of discontinuation of the infusions. One might be concerned that such a technique places patients at increased risk for awareness because a propofol concentration of 2 μg/mL is below the C_{50} value for wakefulness.[26,28] Therefore, it is probably reasonable to combine such a technique with intraoperative EEG monitoring to assess anesthetic adequacy.

The offset of isoflurane and sevoflurane is similar to that of propofol. The offset of desflurane is slightly quicker than that of propofol. We can draw some logical extrapolations from these propofol/opioid simulations to anesthesia consisting of volatile anesthetics combined with opioids. When fentanyl, alfentanil, or sufentanil is combined with a volatile anesthetic, the most rapid recovery occurs when the opioid concentration is maintained at an analgesic concentration equivalent to 1 to 1.5 ng/mL of fentanyl (Table 28-5). Concurrently, the volatile anesthetic should be administered at the lowest concentration required to provide adequate anesthesia but no less than an end-tidal concentration of 0.3 MAC, the MAC value for return of consciousness. If the patient demonstrates signs of inadequate anesthesia, it is preferable to increase the volatile anesthetic because this has less of an effect on prolonging the wake-up time than increasing the opioid does (with the exception of remifentanil) and is more likely to ensure that awareness does not occur.

Table 28-5 Infusion Rates for Opioids to Achieve Preset Concentrations

Drug	Target Plasma Concentration (ng/mL)	Bolus (μg/kg)	Infusion Rate (μg/kg/min)
Fentanyl (low)	1	3	0.02
Fentanyl (high)	4	10	0.07
Alfentanil (low)	40	20	0.25
Alfentanil (high)	160	80*	1
Sufentanil (low)	0.15	0.15	0.003
Sufentanil (high)	0.5	0.5	0.01
Remifentanil (low)	2	0.5-1*	0.06-0.1
Remifentanil (high)	10	1-2*	0.3-0.5

*Give as a rapid infusion over a 1- to 2-minute period.

Infusion Devices

Manual Delivery

When an infusion of an intravenous anesthetic is administered, the infusion regimen can be controlled by a variety of mechanisms varying from the simple Cair clamp or Dial-a-Flo (Abbott Laboratories) to complex computer-controlled infusion pumps. Simplicity of mechanical design, however, is not necessarily correlated with ease of use. This has prompted ongoing advances in infusion device technology.

Infusion devices can be classified as either controllers or positive displacement pumps. Explicit in their title, controllers contain mechanisms that control the rate of flow produced by gravity, whereas positive displacement pumps contain active pumping mechanisms.

The most commonly used pumps for administration of intravenous anesthetics are positive displacement syringe pumps that use a variety of mechanisms. These pumps are highly accurate and have several features that make them particularly suitable for anesthetic delivery. An important advance has been the introduction of a calculator feature within the pump so that the clinician can set the weight of the patient, the drug concentration, and the infusion rate in dose/unit weight/unit time and the pump will then calculate the infusion in volume/unit time. These pumps also permit simple application of a staged infusion scheme (e.g., the two-stage approach of Wagner[63]) by allowing a loading dose and a maintenance infusion rate to be programmed into the pump. Numerous syringe pumps also now include automated recognition of syringe size. Further enhancements are drug libraries by class of drug, suggested dosing schemes, and maximal dosing alerts. These modest advances in pump technology and design enable intravenous anesthetics to be delivered conveniently.

Table 28-6 offers recommendations for delivering intravenous anesthetics via conventional infusion pumps based on integrated pharmacokinetic-pharmacodynamic models. However, it is the patient's response, demonstrating adequate or inadequate anesthesia, that ultimately determines the rate of drug administration. Individuals vary markedly in their response to a given drug dose or concentration, and it is therefore essential to titrate to an adequate drug level for each individual patient. Drug concentrations required to provide adequate anesthesia also vary according to the type of surgery (e.g., surface surgery versus upper abdominal surgery). The end of surgery requires lower drug levels, and hence titration often involves judicious lowering of the infusion rate toward the end of surgery to facilitate rapid recovery.

If the infusion rate proves to be insufficient to maintain adequate anesthesia, both an additional loading (bolus) dose and an increase in infusion are required to rapidly raise the plasma (biophase) drug concentration. Various interventions also require greater drug concentrations, usually for brief periods (e.g., laryngoscopy, endotracheal intubation, skin incision) (see Fig. 28-3). Therefore, the infusion scheme should be tailored to provide peak concentrations during these brief periods of intense stimulation. An adequate drug level for endotracheal intubation is often achieved with the initial loading dose, but for procedures such as skin incision, a further bolus dose may be necessary.

Infusion schemes such as those shown in Table 28-6 do not approach the convenience and precision of use associated with the delivery of an inhaled anesthetic via a calibrated vaporizer. This level of precision can be achieved by using TCI devices (such as the commercially available Diprifusor). Such devices go beyond simple calculator pumps to the creation of pumps with automated drug delivery.

Automated Delivery

Automated drug delivery implies that electronic or mechanical instrumentation performs adjustments in dose rate independent of human intervention (in contrast with the manual devices described in the previous section). The desired target (e.g., drug concentration and clinical response) is still chosen by the clinician. Preprogrammed dosing (either bolus or infusion) is the simplest form of automated drug delivery. It consists of a preprogrammed infusion (usually calculated to provide a single target blood or effect concentration) that is automatically implemented by the microprocessor in the pump.[71] Preprogrammed devices are limited in their application for intravenous anesthetic drugs because of their inability to allow the user to vary the target concentration.[72] There are two different methods of automated target-based anesthetic drug delivery: model-based (a form of open-loop control) and closed-loop systems.

Terms and Definitions

Open- and closed-loop systems require a set point (Fig. 28-22).[73] The set point is a quantifiable entity (e.g., plasma concentration, percent T1 of the electromyogram, or BIS value) related to the clinical objective (e.g., level of anesthesia, neuromuscular blockade). Accordingly, the set point is the value (i.e., target) that the automated system is attempting to maintain. The feedback signal is the measured (e.g., percent T1 of the electromyogram) or predicted (e.g., predicted effect-site concentration from pharmacokinetic simulation) value that has resulted from the automated delivery process.

Open-loop model-based drug delivery is most useful when the feedback signal cannot be readily measured and clinical judgment is required to assess drug effect. The model is the mathematical (e.g., pharmacokinetic) relationship between dose and predicted concentration in plasma and at the site of drug effect.

Table 28-6 Manual Infusion Schemes*

	Anesthesia		Sedation or Analgesia	
Drug	**Loading Dose (μg/kg)**	**Maintenance Infusion (μg/kg/min)**	**Loading Dose (μg/kg)**	**Maintenance Infusion (μg/kg/min)**
Alfentanil	50-150	0.5-3	10-25	0.25-1
Fentanyl	5-15	0.03-0.1	1-3	0.01-0.03
Sufentanil	0.5-5	0.01-0.05	0.1-0.5	0.005-0.01
Remifentanil	0.5-1.0	0.1-0.4	†	0.025-0.1
Ketamine	1500-2500	25-75	500-1000	10-20
Propofol	1000-2000	50-150	250-1000	10-50
Midazolam	50-150	0.25-1.5	25-100	0.25-1
Methohexital	1500-2500	50-150	250-1000	10-50
Dexmedetomidine‡			0.5-1 over 10 min	0.2-0.7

*After the loading dose, an initially high infusion rate to account for redistribution should be used and then titrated to the lowest infusion rate that will maintain adequate anesthesia or sedation. When using opiates as part of a nitrous-narcotic technique or for cardiac anesthesia, the dosing scheme listed under anesthesia is used. When the opiate is combined as part of balanced anesthesia, dosing listed for analgesia is needed.

†For analgesia or during sedation, an initial loading dose of remifentanil should not be given because its very rapid onset may result in apnea or muscle rigidity.

Consequently, the accuracy of any model-based control system depends on how well the model represents the process under control. In an open-loop system, it is the clinician who learns about the patient and adapts drug administration to the needs of the individual patient.

In a closed-loop "adaptive" controller, the device itself makes a measurement of drug effect and adjusts the internal model to better represent the individual patient. Closed-loop signals require precisely measured end points. For example, a closed-loop system to control blood pressure with sodium nitroprusside will have an expected dosing regimen that is likely to be quite conservative to avoid profound hypotension. As the system learns about individual patient sensitivity, it will adjust the dosing of sodium nitroprusside to the sensitivity of the individual patient by adapting the internal pharmacokinetic/pharmacodynamic model to better reach the clinical target. In anesthesia, closed-loop systems have typically used some signal derived from the EEG as the basis of adaptive closed-loop control.

Target Control Infusion Systems

Devices

In 1968, Kruger-Thiemer[74] described the infusion regimen theoretically required to quickly achieve and maintain a constant plasma concentration of an intravenously administered drug whose kinetics is described by a two-compartment model. This regimen has become known as the "BET scheme" (see Fig. 28-4) and consists of an initial bolus of $C_T V_1$, infusion at a rate of $C_T Cl_S$ to replace drug eliminated from the body, and an exponentially decreasing infusion at a rate given by Equation 14 to replace drug transferred to the peripheral tissues. The earlier section on designing dosage regimens demonstrates that the bolus portion, calculated as $C_T V_1$, will probably be inadequate for reaching the desired effect-site concentration. Mathematically, the "ET" portion of the BET scheme is identical to the exponentially declining maintenance infusion rate shown in the section "Designing Dosing Regimens." Precise implementation of this complex dosage regimen requires infusion rates that change continuously as a function of time until steady state is achieved.

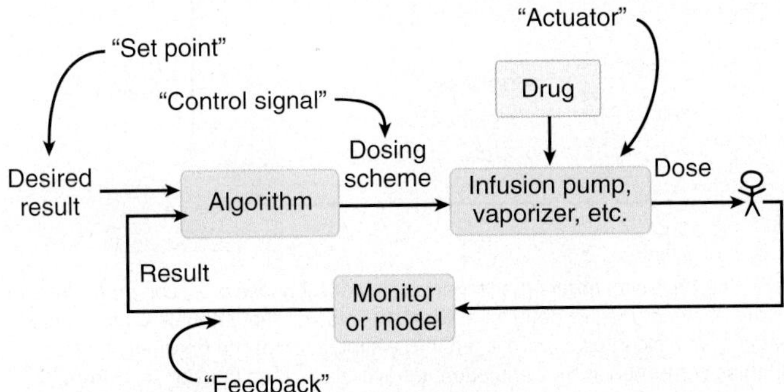

Figure 28-22 Components of a typical automated drug delivery system.

More than a decade after publication of Kruger-Thiemer's classic paper, Schwilden and colleagues[2,75,76] interfaced a microcomputer to an infusion pump and demonstrated clinical application of the BET infusion scheme. Many other groups have since implemented either the BET algorithm or modifications of this algorithm on microcomputers connected to infusion pumps. These algorithms are based on the same polyexponential equations or compartment models described previously and calculate the infusion rates theoretically required to obtain the desired plasma or effect-site drug concentration. In implementing these algorithms it is necessary to consider the physical limitations of the system. For example, infusion rates must be positive or zero. Additionally, some pumps have limitations on precision and accuracy that can reduce the accuracy of the infusion.

Although there are minor differences in the approaches taken by different investigators using pharmacokinetic model–driven infusion systems, all are conceptually similar. Each consists of a microcomputer interfaced to an infusion pump, as seen in Figure 28-23. The microcomputer executes a program that incorporates the pharmacokinetic model. In using the device, the anesthesiologist enters a target plasma or effect-site drug concentration (Fig. 28-24). This target concentration is based on knowledge of the pharmacokinetic-pharmacodynamic relationship of

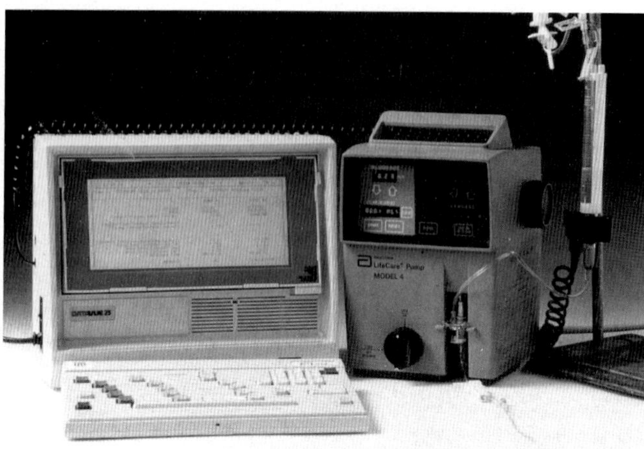

Figure 28-23 The CACI system used at Duke University Medical Center. The CACI consists of a laptop computer electronically linked to an infusion pump. The desired drug plasma or effect-site concentration is entered via the keyboard.

the drug and the desired effect, as well as on the individual responses of the patient. At frequent intervals (e.g., every 9 to 15 seconds), the program compares the target concentration with the current prediction of the plasma or effect-site drug concentration, which is computed by real-time simulation of a pharmacokinetic model of the drug being infused. The computer calculates the infusion rate required to achieve the desired target concentration and transmits this rate to the pump after adjusting the rate to reflect the physical capabilities of the pump. The pump then delivers drug to the patient at the desired rate.

At each step the computer makes sure that the pump has delivered the drug that it was instructed to give and checks for errors reported by the infusion pump (e.g., air in the line, out of drug). The computer then calculates what the pump delivered during the previous interval and updates the internal pharmacokinetic model on the basis of the reported drug delivered. The cycle is completed when the computer calculates the infusion rate required over the next interval to reach the desired target concentration and transmits this rate to the infusion pump. Concurrently, the computer supplies the anesthesiologist with information about the state of the model, the state of the pump, any problems reported by the pump, the anticipated time course for elimination of drug from the patient, the total amount of drug delivered, the current infusion rate, and other information that may be of assistance in providing clinical care.

As a result of the increasing popularity of intravenous anesthesia and continuous-infusion techniques, the inherent reasonableness of pharmacokinetically based drug delivery, and the promising results achieved with automated administration of a variety of drugs by research groups around the world, pharmacokinetic model–driven infusion of propofol has become widely available worldwide except in the United States.[77] This system consists of a commercial pump and software that provides the control algorithm.

Several device companies are now providing TCI pumps that permit users to select from a variety of drugs and patient groups. Pharmacokinetic parameters for various drugs are already programmed into the device, and the devices have the ability to target the plasma concentration or the concentration at the site of drug effect. Such devices are well adapted to the need for rapid titration in anesthesia. The user selects the drug to be infused, enters information about the patient (e.g., weight, age, and gender), and ensures that the infusion setup is primed with drug at a specified concentration. The user titrates the target concentration during anesthesia in the same manner as for adjustment of the inspired concentration of an inhaled anesthetic.

Pharmacokinetic models are being incorporated into the next generation of anesthesia workstations. These workstations could then control many different brands of infusion pumps and provide a common platform for implementing precise titration of intravenous anesthetics in the concentration domain.

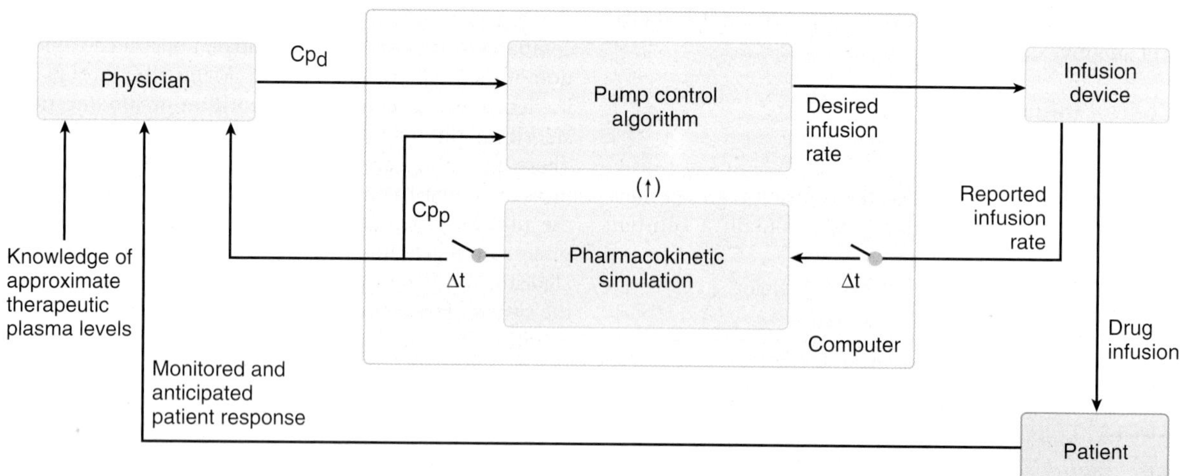

Figure 28-24 Schematic illustration of pharmacokinetic model–driven drug delivery. The physician enters the target plasma or biophase drug concentration (Cp_d). An infusion device control algorithm uses a pharmacokinetic model for the drug being infused to determine what the infusion rate should be for the next infusion interval (e.g., 9 to 15 seconds). The infusion device delivers drug to the patient, and the infusion rate is fed into a simulation of the pharmacokinetic model to compute the current predicted plasma drug concentration (Cp_p). The variables computed in the simulation are available to the infusion algorithm, which then calculates the infusion rate necessary for the next 9 to 15 seconds to achieve the target concentration. On the basis of monitored and anticipated patient responses, knowledge of approximate therapeutic plasma drug concentrations (e.g., Cp_{50}), and Cp_p, the physician can titrate Cp_d as necessary.

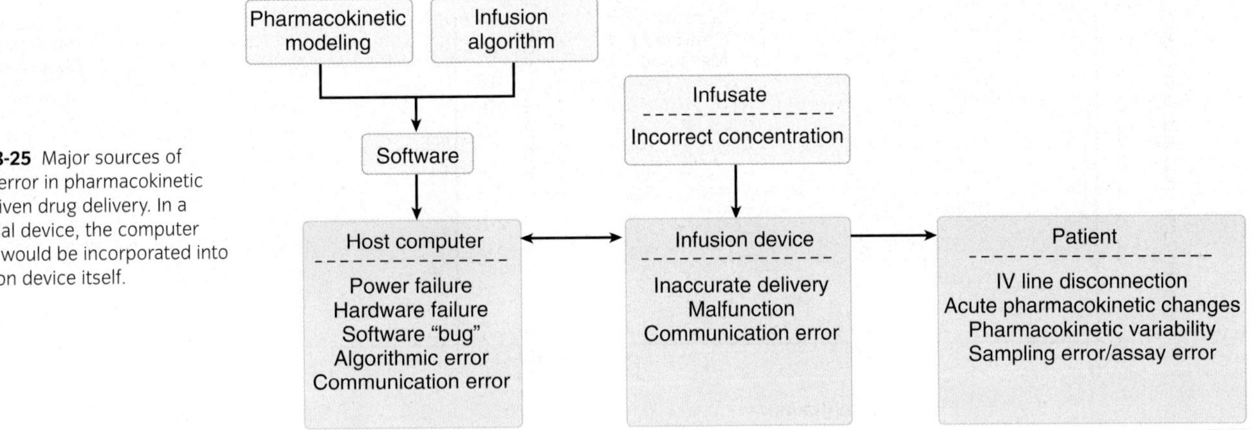

Figure 28-25 Major sources of potential error in pharmacokinetic model–driven drug delivery. In a commercial device, the computer functions would be incorporated into the infusion device itself.

Evaluation of Target-Controlled Drug Delivery

Acceptance of target-controlled drug delivery of intravenous anesthetics requires evaluation of both accuracy, defined as the difference between predicted and measured concentrations, and outcome of patients in whom automated drug delivery has been used. Sources of inaccuracy with pharmacokinetic model–driven devices include the software, the hardware, and pharmacokinetic variability (Fig. 28-25).

Inaccuracy in the software results from incorrect mathematical implementation of the pharmacokinetic model. Computer simulations can be used to test the infusion rates calculated by a software program, and thus software errors are fairly simple to identify and correct.[78] Inaccurate drug delivery from the infusion pump occurs infrequently with present syringe-pump technology and thus contributes little to the overall inaccuracy of these devices. The major cause of inaccuracy is biologic variability, of which there are two sources: (1) the pharmacokinetic model is always wrong, and (2) the pharmacokinetics of the patient is never that programmed into the model. The pharmacokinetic model is always wrong because individuals are far more complex than implied by simple compartmental models, and thus no such model can precisely predict the concentrations, even if the pharmacokinetic parameters in the individual were known with absolute precision. However, even if the pharmacokinetic model truly reflected the underlying biology, the parameters of the model would be average parameters for the population and not the parameters in the individual patient. Even if the parameters are modified to reflect the influence of demographic factors such as age, gender, hypovolemia, and coadministration of other drugs, they will still deviate from the true pharmacokinetic parameters in the individual. Thus, biologic variability fundamentally precludes the possibility of precisely achieving the desired target concentration when automated drug delivery devices are used. It is important to realize that biologic variability always exists, no matter how drugs are given, and that this same biologic variability affects all methods of drug delivery. Indeed, the variability with TCI devices will always be less than the variability observed after a single bolus injection.[79]

Optimization of Target-Controlled Drug Delivery

The performance of computer-controlled drug administration must be interpreted in terms of the therapeutic expectations of the clinician. Possible goals include accurately producing a desired concentration in plasma, precisely titrating the plasma drug concentration, achieving the desired drug effect, and producing the desired time course of drug effect. Over the past decade, investigators have addressed each of these goals and have refined the performance of automated drug delivery devices accordingly.

The ability of an automated drug delivery system to rapidly achieve and then maintain a selected target concentration is a logical measure of the performance of such a device. There are several ways of expressing the difference between the measured and target concentrations. The most simple means is either to diagram a plot of the target and measured concentration of each sample in each individual patient (Fig. 28-26) or to diagram an *xy* plot of the measured to target concentration and observe how much the plots vary from the line of identity (Fig. 28-27).[58] The primary concern is how far the measured concentration is from the predicted one, and this is now most frequently described in terms of performance error, which is the difference between the measured and target concentrations as a percentage of the desired target (i.e., [measured − target]/target × 100%).[80] The median value of the performance error for a patient or a population is referred to as the median performance error (MDPE) and represents the average overshoot or undershoot of the system. The median absolute performance error (MDAPE) is the median of the absolute values of all performance errors. The MDAPE is commonly used as a measure of the inaccuracy of an automated drug delivery device. An MDAPE of zero is perfect performance, and an MDAPE of 20% means that half the plasma concentrations will be within 20% of the target and half will be outside that range. A further assessment of accuracy is whether the system maintains a stable target concentration. This is best measured by the wobble of the system. Varvel and colleagues[80] asked a group of clinicians to evaluate the performance of automated drug delivery devices and demonstrated that the MDAPE best predicted the adequacy of performance of the automated delivery device, as judged by experienced clinicians.

As observed earlier, it is not reasonable to expect all performance errors to be zero. However, it would be desirable if positive and negative errors offset each other so that the MDPE of an automated drug delivery device were 0%. The MDPE does not indicate the range of performance errors (because positive and negative performance errors offset each other), but it does indicate whether the plasma concentrations achieved with the

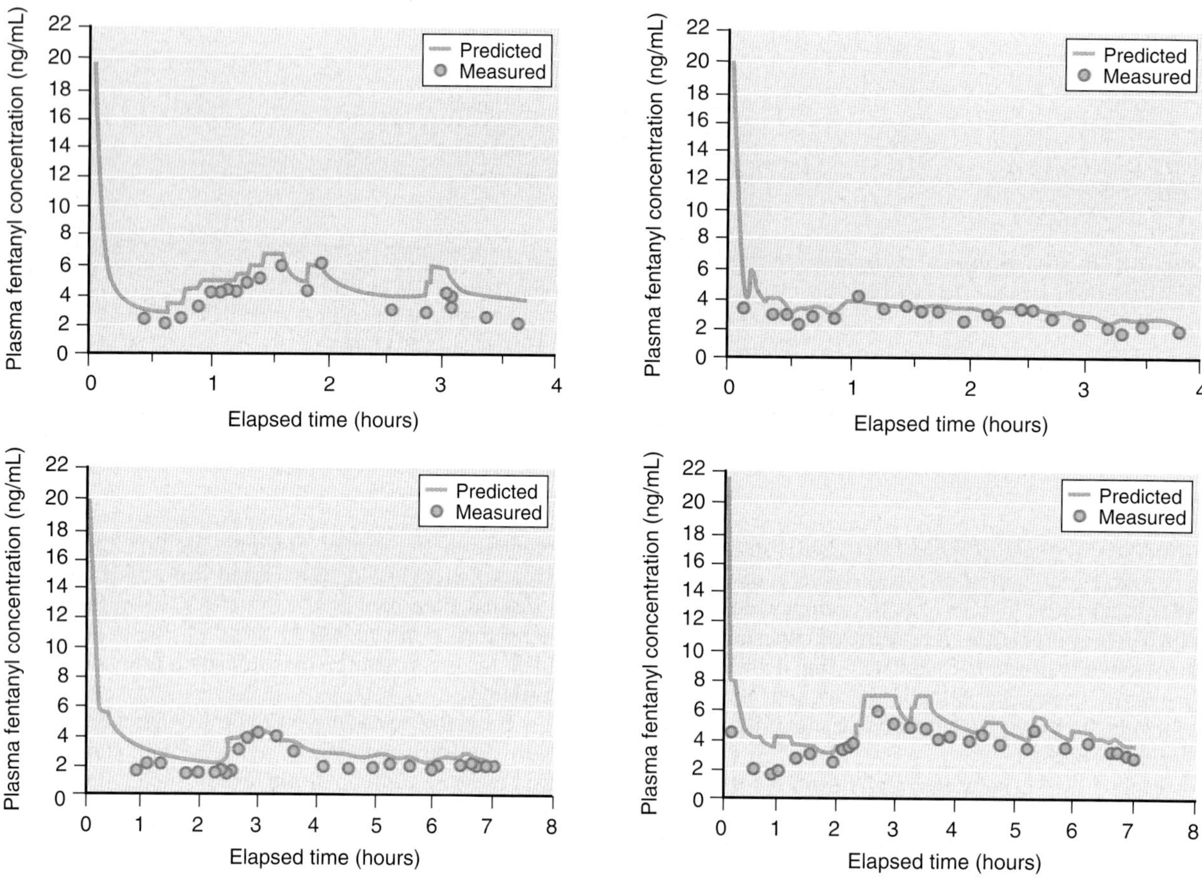

Figure 28-26 Individual plots of the target plasma fentanyl concentration (*solid line*) and measured concentration (*dots*) in four separate patients.

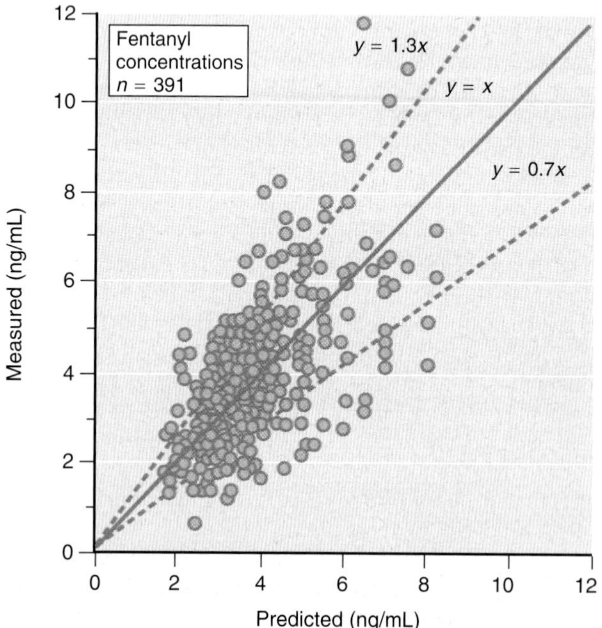

Figure 28-27 Plot of the measured to predicted concentration of fentanyl administered via CACI in 24 patients. The *solid line* represents the line of identity; that is, the target concentration is equal to the measured concentration. The *dashed lines* represent a bias of ±30%.

device tend to overshoot (+MDPE) or undershoot (−MDPE) the desired target.

Many groups have evaluated the accuracy of many different pharmacokinetic sets for virtually all the intravenous analgesics and hypnotics.[23,58,71,81-88] Based on many of these studies the expected performance of such devices, at best, tends to be around 20% to 30% MDAPE. The pharmacokinetics of propofol has been the most frequently tested. Coetzee and coworkers[87] tested the accuracy of three parameter sets and found those of Marsh[88] Tackley[89] and their colleagues to provide the best accuracy in adult patients (Fig. 28-28). To demonstrate the effect of the three different pharmacokinetic parameters on propofol dosing, the infusion rates required to produce a set of target concentrations are plotted in Figure 28-29. The pharmacokinetic parameter set of Marsh and colleagues is the one included in the Diprifusor software. Better accuracy has been obtained in children[81] because they may have less pharmacokinetic variability as a result of their general lack of chronic disease and more narrow distribution of weight at any given age than found in adults.

There are numerous published pharmacokinetic parameter sets for each of the drugs used in anesthesia. The pharmacokinetic parameters within each set may vary considerably depending on a variety of factors, such as the mode of drug administration (e.g., bolus versus infusion), duration of sampling, site of drug sampling (arterial versus venous), sensitivity of the assay, and evalu-

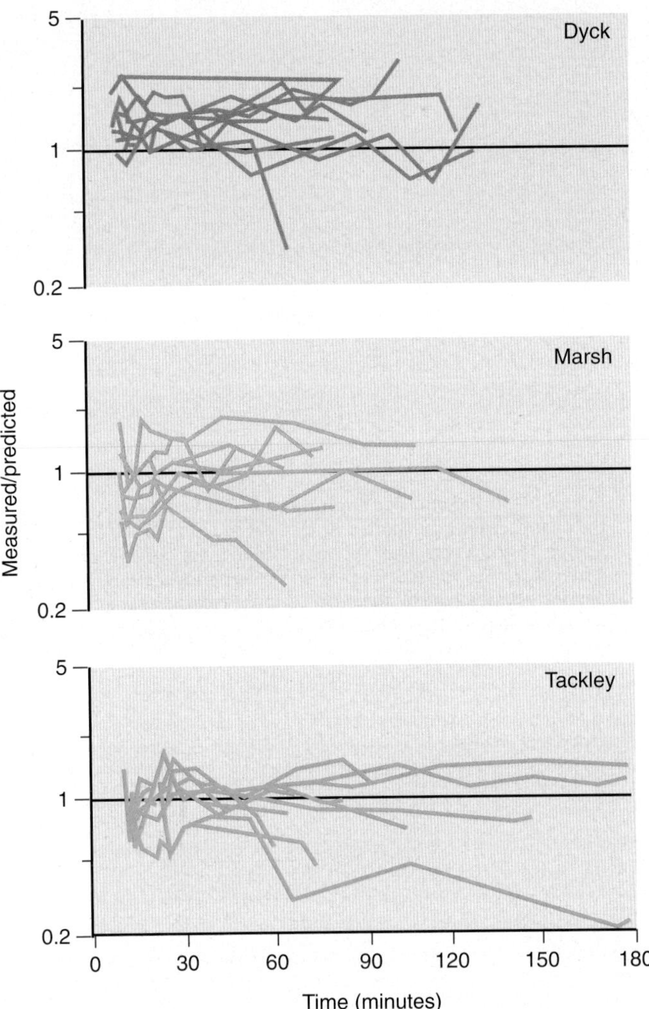

Figure 28-28 Evaluation of three pharmacokinetic parameter sets for propofol. Plotted is the measured-to-predicted ratio for samples obtained during administration of propofol via a target-controlled infusion device programmed with pharmacokinetics derived by Dyck, Marsh, or Tackley (*n* = 10 per group). A ratio of 1 means that measured equals predicted. Note that the pharmacokinetic parameters of Dyck provide a consistently positive bias.

ation of population covariates in determining the model parameters. The implications of such differences are not always obvious and it is therefore important to test the parameter set to determine whether the parameters provide adequate accuracy for clinical use. For example, as shown in Figure 28-30A-C,[85] the accuracy of fentanyl delivered according to the pharmacokinetics reported by Scott and Stanski[30] is much better than the accuracy of fentanyl delivered on the basis of the pharmacokinetics reported by McClain and Hug.[90] Glass and coworkers[58] examined the performance of a pharmacokinetic model–driven infusion device by using the same fentanyl pharmacokinetics described by McClain and Hug.[90] They demonstrated an MDAPE of 21% and an MDPE of +4% (i.e., an almost completely unbiased performance), much better performance than demonstrated by Shafer and associates[85] for the same pharmacokinetic set. This is explained by differences in study methodology, such as arterial versus venous samples, rapid sampling after changes in target concentration versus sampling only when a pseudo–steady state was achieved, and a different set of patients—cardiac versus noncardiac.

With the goal of improving pharmacokinetic model–driven infusion device performance, Shafer and coworkers[85] recalculated the optimal pharmacokinetic parameters of fentanyl directly from the observed concentrations that were obtained when fentanyl was administered via a pharmacokinetic model–driven infusion device by use of the initial pharmacokinetics of McLean and Hug.[90] Figure 28-30C shows the performance errors over time for the optimal fentanyl pharmacokinetics estimated for that population of patients (versus those of McLean and Hug[90] and Scott and associates[30] in the same group of patients). The optimal pharmacokinetic parameter set still had a median residual error of 21% when retrospectively tested against the same group of patients. This represents the limit imposed by pharmacokinetic variability on the possible performance of any fentanyl parameter set for dosing to a similar adult population. In other words, it is unlikely that any fentanyl pharmacokinetic parameter set would produce less than a 21% MDAPE.

Marsh and colleagues[88] took the same approach to optimizing the performance of a pharmacokinetic model–driven infusion device for administration of propofol to children. They initially used a pharmacokinetic parameter set derived from adult subjects in their device and obtained an MDAPE of 25% and an MDPE of −18.5%. They subsequently derived new propofol pharmacokinetics for children and prospectively demonstrated that they had decreased the MDAPE to 16%, with a bias of less than 3%. This is highly accurate performance for a model-based device. Ginsberg and coworkers[91] similarly derived a pharmacokinetic set for fentanyl in children, as did Fiset and associates[92] for alfentanil. Several other studies have also demonstrated that pharmacokinetic parameters vary with certain subsets of patients. For example, the pharmacokinetic parameters of propofol for patients about to undergo open heart surgery are different from the previously verified pharmacokinetic parameters for the general population. These new pharmacokinetic parameters for propofol also vary both during bypass and after bypass.[93] Similarly for patients undergoing liver transplantation, the Marsh pharmacokinetics performs poorly.[94]

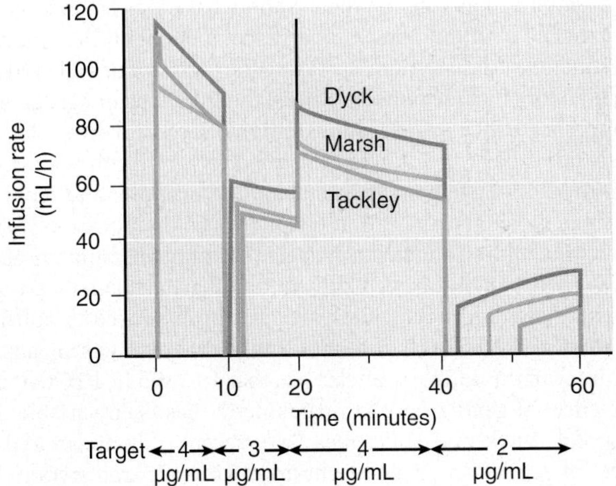

Figure 28-29 Infusion rates (mL/hr) calculated to achieve propofol target concentrations of 4 (10 minutes), 3 (10 minutes), 4 (20 minutes), and 2 μg/mL (20 minutes) based on the three pharmacokinetic parameter sets of Dyck, Marsh, and Tackley.

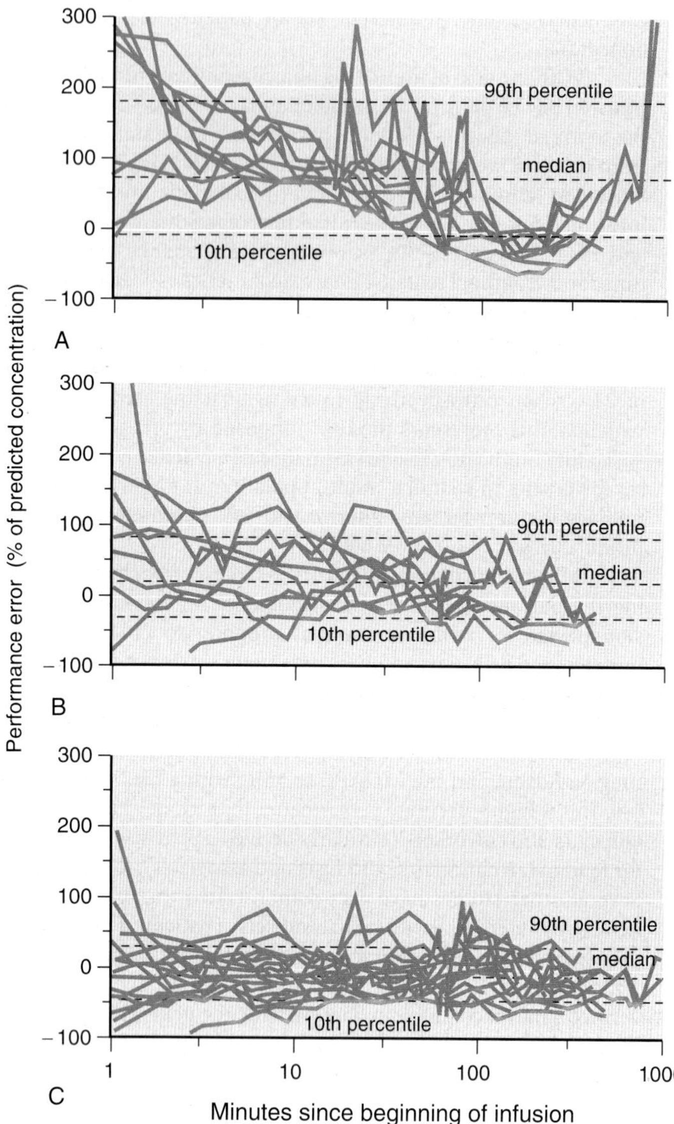

Figure 28-30 Performance errors over time for fentanyl derived from the pharmacokinetics reported by McClain and Hug (**A**) and Scott and Stanski (**B**) and a parameter set derived from these observations (**C**). *(From Shafer SL, Varvel SL, Aziz N, et al: The pharmacokinetics of fentanyl administered by computer controlled infusion pump. Anesthesiology 73:1091-1102, 1990.)*

Interest has recently focused on what other factors may be responsible for alterations in pharmacokinetic with the objective of reducing variability and increasing the accuracy of TCI systems. Such factors include, among others, the influence of age, gender, hemorrhagic shock, and administration of a second drug. Numerous studies have investigated the effect of age (both young and old) on pharmacokinetic parameters. For propofol and fentanyl, it has been shown that an adult pharmacokinetic set performs poorly in children and that age-specific parameters improve accuracy.[88,91] Although it is well known that pharmacokinetic parameters are altered in the elderly, it has not been well established whether these changes are sufficiently different to impact the accuracy of the adult parameter sets that are used in a TCI device. The effect of gender on pharmacokinetics has been variable. For propofol, Vuyk and colleagues have recently demonstrated an effect of gender on propofol pharmacokinetic parameters in the elderly.[95] In a pharmacokinetic analysis of several pooled databases of propofol, Schuttler and Ihmsen found that gender was not a significant covariate.[96] Similarly, there is no clear indication that gender has a significant effect on opioids pharmacokinetic parameters. Several authors have looked at the effect of hemorrhagic shock on pharmacokinetic parameters. In a pseudo–steady-state model of propofol, compensated hemorrhage increased propofol concentrations by only 20%; however, when uncompensated shock was induced, propofol concentrations increased by 375%.[97] Using a non–steady-state model, Egan and associates found that hemorrhagic shock reduced central clearance and central volumes of fentanyl[98] and remifentanil,[99] thereby resulting in higher fentanyl concentrations in animals in shock. Investigators have also focused on the impact of simultaneous administration of a second drug, especially another anesthetic. Propofol, midazolam, and etomidate have been shown in in vitro studies to reduce the clearance of opioids because of an interaction on the cytochrome P450 system. In turn, several studies have shown that alfentanil may alter the pharmacokinetic parameters of propofol.[100-102] The exact mechanism of this interaction is unclear. It is unlikely to be related to any interaction with cytochrome P450 systems because the pharmacokinetics of propofol are limited by liver blood flow and thus are not likely to be affected by modest alterations in hepatic metabolic capacity. The differences may result from alterations in cardiac output or reductions in hepatic blood flow. In contrast with alfentanil, remifentanil at concentrations of 0 to 4 ng/mL did not alter the pharmacokinetics of propofol.[103] However, propofol decreased the central volume of distribution and distributional clearance of remifentanil by 41% and elimination clearance by 15%. Of interest in a study of propofol administered to critically ill patients, two covariates established in the model that best described the pharmacokinetics of these patients were temperature and serum triglyceride concentration for terminal clearance.[104] Not all of the factors that have been shown to alter pharmacokinetic parameters have been associated with a change in outcomes or in the utility of TCI devices. However, some have, and thus in principle, pharmacokinetic sets adapted to the appropriate clinical milieu should be determined for each of the commonly used drugs to enhance the accuracy of TCI drug administration. It is incumbent on users to be aware of which pharmacokinetic set is being used in their TCI system and the reasonableness of this set in providing sufficient accuracy for clinical application in the particular patient in which it is being used.

Not only is there interindividual variability, but there may also be significant intraindividual variability. Hill and colleagues[105] studied volunteers to learn the individual's own pharmacokinetics for morphine and alfentanil. These investigators then used that volunteer's unique pharmacokinetic values to subsequently control a pharmacokinetic model–driven infusion device. With this technique of personalized pharmacokinetics, they reduced the average error to just less than 20%. It appears that studies in which the pharmacokinetics of an individual is used to infuse the same drug to the same individual later result in bias and an MDAPE similar to those seen when an optimal pharmacokinetic set derived from the general population is used. The implication of these data is that although highly specific pharmacokinetic sets are desirable, they may not necessarily improve overall accuracy. They also demonstrate that biologic variability precludes obtaining better than approximately 20% accuracy with TCI devices.

It is unlikely that we will have the opportunity to conduct a full pharmacokinetic study on patients *during a single anesthetic*. However, bayesian forecasting is a statistical technique by which a few measured plasma concentrations from an individual can be incorporated into pharmacokinetic parameters to improve the performance of a pharmacokinetic model–driven infusion device. Maitre and Stanski[106] demonstrated the theoretical improvement in such devices when using bayesian forecasting for alfentanil. In this study, Maitre and Stanski demonstrated that measurement of a single plasma alfentanil concentration could potentially reduce the inaccuracy by half, to a 14% average performance error. Unfortunately, a rapid assay does not exist for any of the intravenous drugs used in anesthetic practice. However, there are rapid assays for lidocaine, and at least one pharmacokinetic model–driven infusion device (STANPUMP, developed by Shafer and Maitre at Stanford and available at http://anesthesia.stanford.edu/pkpd) performs real-time bayesian forecasting from measured lidocaine levels for use in coronary care units.

In the absence of rapid assays for anesthetic drugs, the obvious method to decrease variability is to observe the drug effect and adjust the target to the concentration that produces the desired level of drug effect.[17,18] As discussed earlier under "Pharmacodynamic Considerations," by knowing the rate constant k_{e0}, it is possible to model the concentration at the site of drug effect. Figure 28-31 shows the plasma fentanyl concentrations that could theoretically be obtained over the course of a brief operation. Figure 28-31B shows the fentanyl concentrations at the effect site for the same anesthetic shown in Figure 28-31A. Even if the pump produced precisely the concentrations shown in Figure 28-31A (i.e., had perfect performance), the lag between concentrations in plasma and the site of drug effect would, at best, produce a very slurred response because of the delay in equilibration between plasma and the effect site. Several pharmacokinetic model–driven infusion devices now simultaneously display both plasma and effect-site concentrations. Such devices permit the clinician to target the concentration in the effect site rather than plasma to provide more precise control of drug effect.

By targeting the effect site there is an overshoot in the plasma concentration of the drug. The k_{e0} used to model the effect site for intravenous anesthetics has been derived from surrogate measures of effect (i.e., derivatives of the EEG). Thus, for TCI devices that target the effect site, it is important to establish that the k_{e0} value used actually results in the desired effect. Glass[107] and Struys[108] and their colleagues conducted similar studies in which they targeted either plasma or an effect-site concentration of propofol and then observed the time and plasma versus effect-site concentration at loss of consciousness. In both studies, regardless of whether the effect-site or plasma concentration was targeted,

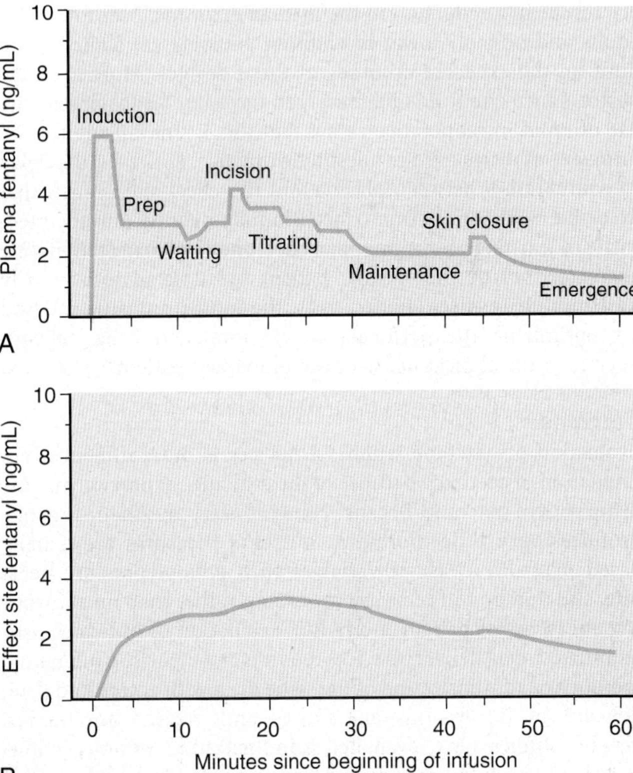

Figure 28-31 A, Simulated plasma fentanyl concentrations over time for a brief anesthetic showing the rapid rise and fall and impression of precise titration that can be created by a target-controlled drug delivery device. **B,** Effect-site concentrations for the same anesthetic course demonstrating that precise control of the plasma concentration does not necessarily translate into precise control at the site of drug effect. *(Adapted from Shafer SL, Gregg K: Algorithms to rapidly achieve and maintain stable drug concentrations at the site of drug effect with a computer controlled infusion pump. J Pharmacokinet Biopharm 20:147-169, 1992.)*

loss of consciousness occurred when the appropriate *effect-site* concentration for loss of consciousness was achieved, thus validating the concept. Two other important observations were made during these studies. First, hemodynamics was not different whether plasma or the effect site was targeted, even though higher plasma concentrations were achieved in the effect-site group. This implies, at least for propofol, that the time course for its hemodynamic effects is similar (or longer)[109] to that for its anesthetic effects. Second, k_{e0} is dependent on the pharmacokinetic set from which it is derived.[110] One cannot take a k_{e0} value from one pharmacokinetic set and use it with another pharmacokinetic set. Just as various demographics may alter the pharmacokinetics, they may also alter k_{e0}. Hence, it is desirable to use the k_{e0} best adapted for the clinical milieu. An ideal test of whether targeting plasma or the effect site is better is to compare their use in a closed-loop system where a measure of effect (e.g., the BIS) is used as the target of control. In a small study of 10 patients per group, Absalom and Kenny showed that maintenance of the targeted BIS (as measured by MDPE, MDAPE, and wobble) was somewhat improved and induction times were significantly shorter when the pharmacokinetic model was for the effect site rather than plasma.[111]

In summary, automated drug delivery devices appear to be able to achieve and maintain desired plasma concentrations with a median expected error of about 20% to 30% of the target. Although pharmacokinetic analysis after automated drug delivery results in a reduction in the median error to closer to 20% in adults and possibly lower in children, biologic variability sets a limit on the expected accuracy of these devices. More accurate performance could be obtained with bayesian feedback and the use of rapid intraoperative assays, but this is unavailable for the intravenous drugs used in anesthetic practice. However, the delay in equilibration between plasma and the effect site is such that excessive focus on plasma concentrations may be unwarranted. Instead, learning about the pharmacokinetic/pharmacodynamic characteristics of the specific patient by titrating to a readily measured drug effect appears to be the most promising method for optimizing the performance of automated drug delivery devices to the clinical needs of the individual patient.

Outcome

Evaluation of outcome with TCI devices is more difficult than evaluation of accuracy because of the difficulty of precisely measuring patient outcome. Because contemporary anesthetic practice produces very little morbidity, outcome measures are usually based on readily measured variables, such as blood pressure, heart rate, and duration of recovery room stay, rather than on substantive measures of patient morbidity. Evaluation of outcome with automated drug delivery devices requires a comparison of manual methods of administration of the same drug with automated drug delivery of intravenous anesthetics and volatile anesthetics. Several studies have evaluated administration of intravenous anesthetics by automated drug delivery devices for both brief and complex surgery, in children and in adults, in short-term sedation, in prolonged sedation (days), and in chronic pain management.

Two decades ago, Ausems and coworkers[9] compared pharmacokinetic model–driven administration with intermittent bolus administration of alfentanil. Automated drug delivery produced fewer episodes of muscular rigidity, hypotension, and bradycardia on induction. Automated drug delivery during maintenance resulted in a significantly lower incidence of hemodynamic response, which resulted in a greater percentage of anesthesia time within 15% of the desired blood pressure and heart rate. Recovery after TCI was associated with significantly less use of naloxone for adequate ventilation.

Pharmacokinetic model–driven infusion of fentanyl during cardiac surgery resulted in better hemodynamic control with fewer additional drug interventions and significantly fewer episodes of either hypotension or hypertension than occurred with bolus dose administration.[86] A small study comparing manual alfentanil administration with pharmacokinetic model–driven infusion of alfentanil showed no statistical differences during maintenance or recovery.[112] Theil and colleagues[113] compared double-blind manual administration of fentanyl/midazolam with pharmacokinetic model–driven infusion of these two anesthetics in a small group of patients undergoing cardiac surgery. Both systems were titrated simultaneously (one containing placebo), with the aim of maintaining hemodynamics within 20% of baseline values. Both systems were equally effective in providing hemodynamic control as dictated by the protocol. The most significant difference between the two modes of delivery was the greater variability in drug plasma concentrations in the manual group. This suggested that pharmacokinetic model–driven infusion maintained patients within a narrower therapeutic range.

Several comparative studies have been performed with the commercial TCI device for propofol. Struys and colleagues[114] ($N = 90$), Russel and colleagues[115] ($N = 160$), and Servin,[116] in a large multicenter study ($N = 562$), found when they compared manual infusion of propofol with TCI administration that there were small differences between the two means of propofol administration. Of interest in the TCI groups, the maintenance infusion rate tended to be higher, which was associated with a lower incidence of patient movement. Both Servin and Russel and their coworkers noted that there was a marked preference of clinicians for the TCI system, even though this was their first use of the device. In contrast, when TCI propofol or manual propofol was titrated to a target BIS, no differences were observed between the two groups.[117] Remifentanil delivered manually and by TCI has also been evaluated in patients undergoing carotid surgery.[118] TCI remifentanil provided improved hemodynamic control both intraoperatively and postoperatively with less remifentanil and similar propofol infusion rates. As discussed, targeting the plasma concentration does not provide optimal control of effect. When manual propofol administration has been compared with target effect-site administration, there was a lower incidence of movement, improved hemodynamic stability, and more rapid recovery with the latter.[119]

Pharmacokinetic model–driven infusion of propofol compares favorably with thiopental/isoflurane anesthesia for general surgery lasting several hours.[120] Induction, maintenance, and recovery were similar between the two groups. Godet and colleagues compared sevoflurane, propofol followed by isoflurane, and TCI propofol in patients undergoing carotid surgery. They found minor differences in hemodynamics that tended to favor TCI propofol and no differences in recovery parameters.[121] Sneyd and coworkers compared TCI propofol with sevoflurane in patients undergoing neurosurgical procedures and similarly found little difference between the two techniques.[122] This implies that given the appropriate means for administration, intravenous anesthetics can be equal to inhaled anesthetics in providing the objectives of anesthesia, that is, rapid induction and recovery with stable maintenance. Suttner and associates examined the cost and recovery characteristics of target-controlled propofol infusion regimens and standard methodologies.[123] They found that "target-controlled infusion/total IV anesthesia was associated with the largest intraoperative costs but allowed the most rapid recovery from anesthesia, was associated with fewest postoperative side effects, and permitted earlier discharge from the postanesthesia care unit."

In noncomparative studies, pharmacokinetic model–driven infusion has been used to administer most of the potent opioids, as well as the hypnotics. Different anesthetic techniques have also been tested with pharmacokinetic model–driven infusion devices, including nitrous-opioid anesthesia, supplementation of volatile anesthetics, total intravenous anesthesia, sedation for monitored anesthesia care, and intensive care unit sedation. In all these studies, outcome, as measured by hemodynamics and recovery, has been within the expectations of normal clinical care. Etomidate, methohexital, midazolam, propofol, thiopental, dexmedetomidine, alfentanil, fentanyl, remifentanil, and sufentanil have all been used with TCI. When these drugs were used with target-controlled drug delivery systems for total intravenous anesthesia or to supplement nitrous oxide or volatile anesthetics, hemodynamics was well maintained during induction and intubation, as well as during maintenance. Recovery milestones were reached at times comparable to those achieved with similar drug combinations used in manual infusion schemes. In none of these studies have authors commented on adverse outcomes resulting from target-controlled drug delivery.

TCI devices have also been used to provide patient-controlled analgesia. Hill and colleagues studied patient-controlled analgesia devices using morphine, fentanyl, or alfentanil[105,124] and demonstrated the clinical utility of such devices.[125-128] Van den Nieuwenhuyzen and colleagues[44] demonstrated advantages of such a system with alfentanil over routine morphine patient-controlled anesthesia.

From the body of literature presently available, it appears that automated drug delivery of intravenous anesthetics is at least equal to manual delivery of these drugs. Intravenous drug administration via target-controlled drug delivery is analogous to inhaled vapor delivery via a calibrated vaporizer. Like the vaporizer, pharmacokinetic model–driven infusion facilitates drug delivery based on plasma or biophase concentration rather than on drug dosage. There is variability with the use of a calibrated vaporizer, including variability in the accuracy of drug delivery with vaporizers, slow equilibration between the fresh gas flow and the circuit at low flow rates, and variable uptake by the patient. This variability does not particularly complicate the titration of inhaled anesthetics. The variability with target-controlled drug delivery is of a similar magnitude and can be demonstrated to be less than the variability associated with vaporizers, and likewise, it does not particularly complicate titration of intravenous anesthetics. Indeed, the time-varying stresses of surgery and the variability in patient response require that the anesthesiologist titrate the administration of potent inhaled anesthetics by using the calibrated vaporizer as a tool. These same factors require that the anesthesiologist vigilantly titrate the infusion of intravenous anesthetic drugs when using automated drug delivery as a tool.

Target-controlled drug delivery has advantages beyond a delivery system to simplify the clinical administration of intravenous anesthetics. Another significant contribution of these delivery devices is their use in research. The pseudo–steady state that can be almost instantly achieved with these devices permits the plasma and effect site to rapidly come into equilibrium. This is critically important in studies examining concentration-response relationships (i.e., C_{50} values) for anesthetic drugs.[9,24,42] In addition, these systems enable interactions involving intravenous drugs to be clearly defined.[54-56] Closed-loop target delivery will eventually enable unbiased and more precise comparisons between drugs. Finally, as noted earlier, target-controlled delivery has provided us with the ability to prospectively test pharmacokinetic parameter sets and modeling approaches and may ultimately provide the most suitable pharmacokinetic parameters for any intravenous drug delivery.[85,88,92,129]

Closed-Loop Drug Delivery Systems

The next step in automated drug delivery is to feed the measured drug effect directly back into the automated drug delivery device so that the model can be updated from observed measures of drug effect, thus providing a closed-loop system.[3-7,130-137] In this instance the set point is the measured effect rather than a particular drug concentration. It has been proposed that closed-loop control of anesthesia may provide several advantages: increased stability of the control variable because of more frequent sampling of the effect with more frequent adjustment of drug delivery; more customized dose delivery to account for interindividual pharmacokinetic and pharmacodynamic differences; and as a result of the first two advantages, improvement in hemodynamic stability, inadvertent awareness, and recovery.[137]

Closed-loop systems fall into two general categories. All controllers are based on measuring the error between the target effect and the observed effect. Conventional "proportional/integral/derivative" (PID) controllers adjust the infusion rates in a manner that is proportional to the magnitude of the error, the integral of the error over time, and the derivative of the error over time. A "model-based" controller has an internal model of the system, typically set up as an integrated pharmacokinetic/pharmacodynamic model relating dose to concentration (pharmacokinetics) and concentration to drug effect (pharmacodynamics). The model is updated to explain the difference between the measured and predicted drug effect.

An example of the model-based approach is the system described by Struys and colleagues in which the response to a loading propofol bolus was used to estimate the sigmoidal concentration-versus-effect relationship for the individual patient.[134] As shown in Figure 28-32, the device starts with a population estimate that a particular concentration, C_1, will produce the desired effect. It then monitors the drug effect in response to the initial bolus of propofol. As shown by point X, the patient did not reach the desired effect at an effect-site concentration of C_1. The device recalculates the shape of the concentration-versus-response relationship and determines that C_2 is the proper target effect-site concentration. The device then raises the target concentration to C_2 to produce the desired effect.

Bayesian optimization is used in pharmacokinetic-dynamic modeling to individualize a drug dosing regimen by combining individual information with the knowledge of an a priori probability density function containing the statistical properties of the parameter to be estimated. These values are adjusted to reflect the patient's own parameters over time based on the observed response of the individual patient under varying circumstances. In a simulation study, De Smet and colleagues compared a PID

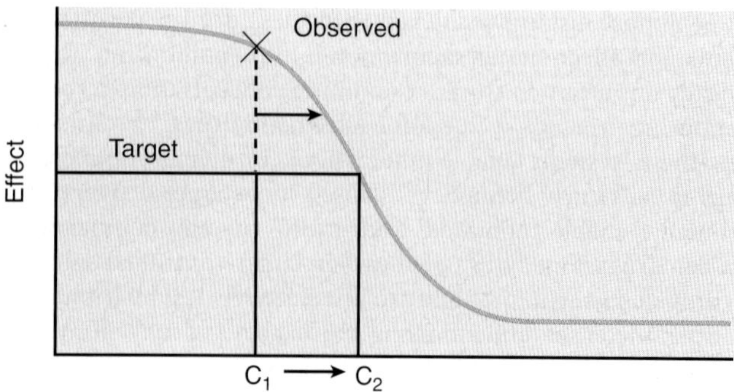

Figure 28-32 Real-time model–based adjustment of the "Hill equation" describing the relationship between propofol concentration and hypnotic effect. The system sets a target concentration and starts out with an assumed value of the effect-site concentration, C_1, needed to reach the effect. After administering an adequate dose, the system discovers that the desired effect has not been reached. It then re-estimates the concentration-versus-effect relationship based on the observed data point (X) and now has a more precise estimation of the concentration, C_2, required to reach the desired effect. *(Adapted from Struys MM, De Smet T, Versichelen LF, et al: Comparison of closed-loop controlled administration of propofol using bispectral index as the controlled variable versus "standard practice" controlled administration. Anesthesiology 95:6-17, 2001.)*

controller with a bayesian model–based controller, both targeting a BIS of 30, 50, and 70.[138] They demonstrated robust performance under a variety of challenging scenarios.

As mentioned earlier, the ability to measure adequacy of anesthesia is limited. Anesthesia is a composite of several effects: hypnosis or loss of consciousness, amnesia, analgesia, lack of movement, and hemodynamic stability. There are now several derivatives of the EEG that show a strong correlation with hypnosis/loss of consciousness. Fortunately, amnesia is also reflected by the EEG signal and appears to precede the derived EEG values associated with drug-induced loss of consciousness. The major component of anesthesia for which we do not have a monitor of effect is analgesia. This continues to constitute an impediment to the general application of closed-loop anesthesia. Noxious stimuli during surgery are extremely variable. Intravenous hypnotics (with the exception of ketamine and dexmedetomidine) have limited or no analgesic activity. Thus, a closed-loop system based solely on a derivative of the EEG may provide perfect hypnosis in the absence of a stimulus, but awakening and movement are likely to occur as soon as a noxious stimulus is administered. To overcome this hurdle, investigators have taken several approaches to test closed-loop systems for anesthesia in patients. They have been used in combination with a regional anesthetic, thereby preventing any painful stimulus from reaching the brain. Most have used a low-dose constant opioid concentration for superficial surgery or a high-dose opioid concentration for more extensive surgery. Another interesting approach is a combination of an analgesic concentration of opioid and application of a noxious stimulus (e.g., tetany) at regular short intervals to minimize oscillations as a result of surgical stimuli.

It is unclear whether closed-loop systems offer any benefits over open-loop TCI systems. Morley and coworkers compared closed-loop administration of isoflurane or a propofol/alfentanil mixture and manual control of these agents to provide a BIS of 50.[139] The closed-loop system used a PID control algorithm. The authors were unable to demonstrate any advantage of their closed-loop system over manual control when intraoperative control of the BIS, hemodynamic stability, intraoperative drug use, or recovery parameters were used as measures of outcome. More recently, Locher and coworkers demonstrated that their closed-loop system for controlling the BIS with isoflurane provided significantly better performance than manual isoflurane administration did in terms of periods of inadequate control (BIS >65 for longer than 3 minutes) or time beyond a BIS of less than 40 or a BIS greater than 60.[140]

Struys and associates also performed a study to determine whether there are any advantages of a closed-loop system over manual administration of propofol for lower abdominal surgery.[134] The closed-loop control group achieved statistically significant better control of both its control variable (BIS, 89% ± 10%) and systolic pressure (51% ± 27%) than the manual group did (systolic pressure, 34% ± 31%; BIS, 49% ± 29%). In addition, recovery was also improved in the closed-loop group (Fig. 28-33). This study does not definitively answer whether closed-loop delivery of anesthesia is better than any manual system, nor does it define what an optimal closed-loop control system is; however, its results are encouraging and should further stimulate work on developing closed-loop anesthetic drug delivery for day-to-day anesthesia.[141]

In a multicenter study of 164 patients randomized to either closed-loop control of propofol or manual TCI propofol with a target BIS of 40 to 60, Lin and colleagues found that the closed-loop system performed significantly better in nearly all performance metrics: lower overall drug dose, BIS closer to the target level throughout anesthesia, and faster recovery.[142] During maintenance the control system made more frequent and smaller adjustments in the propofol dose and enabled more rapid recovery to endotracheal extubation. The performance parameters MDPE, MDAPE, and wobble, as well as the percentage of time that the BIS was maintained between 40 and 60, was significantly better in the closed-loop group. This study demonstrated the feasibility of using a closed-loop system in daily anesthesia practice with a large variation in age and patient comorbid conditions.

Closed-loop control is also a valuable investigative tool. It can be used to determine the unbiased interaction between two drugs. It has been used with neuromuscular blockers to determine their interaction with various anesthetics.[143,144] Similarly, closed-loop control can be used to determine the interaction between opioids and intravenous anesthetics.[145,146] Closed-loop systems may also have the potential to diagnose different pathologic states based on drug dosing. Albrecht and coworkers observed that when using closed-loop sedation with propofol, trauma patients required lower EEG set points and needed more propofol to achieve the same level of sedation.[147] As the number of investigators who have access to closed-loop systems for anesthesia increases, the utility of such devices for research is likely to increase substantially.

Summary

When compared with intermittent bolus administration, continuous infusion of intravenous anesthetic drugs provides greater control of anesthetic depth, thus ensuring (1) better hemodynamic control with fewer episodes of hemodynamic instability, (2) smaller total drug doses, and (3) more rapid return to the awake state. Improved drug administration techniques combined with several new intravenous anesthetic agents have provided greater impetus for the use of intravenous anesthesia in clinical practice. Devices for the administration of intravenous

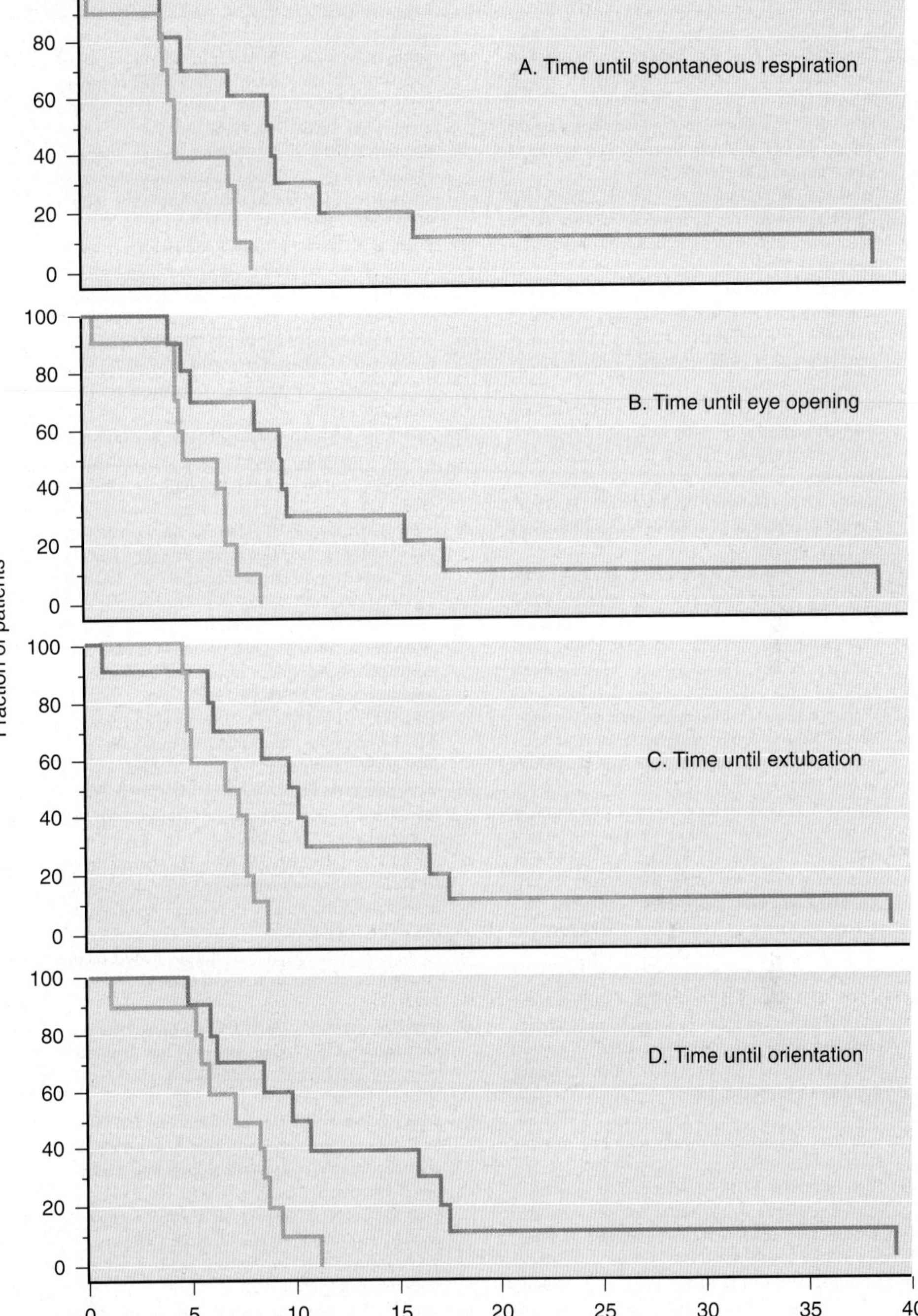

Figure 28-33 Comparison of manual and closed-loop anesthetic control on the time course of return of spontaneous ventilation (**A**), eye opening (**B**), extubation (**C**), and orientation (**D**). In each case, the more rapid curve is the closed-loop control, and the slower curve is the manual control. *(Adapted from Struys MM, De Smet T, Versichelen LF, et al: Comparison of closed-loop controlled administration of propofol using bispectral index as the controlled variable versus "standard practice" controlled administration. Anesthesiology 95:6-17, 2001.)*

anesthetics are continuing to evolve. The introduction of pumps designed specifically for continuous intravenous delivery of anesthetic drugs has enhanced intravenous anesthesia. Automated drug delivery is becoming routine in many countries. There are several theoretical advantages of pharmacokinetic model–driven infusion over manual infusion systems, such as further improvements in hemodynamic control and more predictable rapid awakening. Studies comparing outcomes with automated drug delivery of intravenous anesthetics versus manual methods or inhaled anesthetics have either demonstrated improved outcome or been equivocal. No studies have identified clinical or safety problems with automated anesthetic drug delivery. It thus appears that pharmacokinetic model–driven infusion systems, though limited by the same biologic variability that affects manual drug delivery, are safe and effective in clinical use.

With the advent of monitors of hypnosis and increased understanding of the components of anesthesia, closed-loop drug delivery for anesthesia is showing promise to provide further advantages. Many hurdles still need to be overcome before such devices will come into routine use. However, present knowledge and the results of recent studies are sufficiently encouraging to pursue this goal.

References

1. Corssen G, Reves JG, Stanley T: Intravenous Anesthesia and Analgesia. Philadelphia, Lea & Febiger, 1988.
2. Schwilden H: A general method for calculating the dosage scheme in linear pharmacokinetics. Eur J Clin Pharmacol 20:379-386, 1981.
3. Schwilden H, Schüttler J, Stockel H: Closed-loop feedback control of methohexital anesthesia by quantitative EEG analysis in humans. Anesthesiology 67:341, 1987.
4. Schwilden H, Stoeckel H: Effective therapeutic infusions produced by closed-loop feedback control of methohexital administration during total intravenous anesthesia with fentanyl. Anesthesiology 73:225-229, 1990.
5. Schwilden H, Stoeckel H, Schuttler J: Closed-loop feedback control of propofol anaesthesia by quantitative EEG analysis in humans. Br J Anaesth 62:290-296, 1989.
6. Kenny GNC, Davies FW, Mantzardis H, et al: Closed-loop control of anesthesia. Anesthesiology 77:A328, 1992.
7. Struys M, Desmet T, Audenaert S, et al: Development of a closed loop system for propofol using bispectral analysis and a patient-individual pharmacokinetic-dynamic (PK-PD) model: Preliminary results [abstract]. Br J Anaesthesia 78(Suppl 1):23, 1997.
8. White PF: Use of continuous infusion versus intermittent bolus administration of fentanyl or ketamine during outpatient anesthesia. Anesthesiology 59:294, 1983.
9. Ausems ME, Vuyk J, Hug CC, et al: Comparison of a computer-assisted infusion versus intermittent bolus administration of alfentanil as a supplement to nitrous oxide for lower abdominal surgery. Anesthesiology 68:851-861, 1988.
10. Avram MJ, Krejcie TC: Using front-end kinetics to optimize target-controlled drug infusions. Anesthesiology 99:1078-1086, 2003.
11. Krejcie TC, Avram MJ, Gentry WB, et al: A recirculatory model of the pulmonary uptake and pharmacokinetics of lidocaine based on analysis of arterial and mixed venous data from dogs. J Pharmacokinet Biopharm 25:169-190, 1997.
12. Hull CJ, Van Beem HB, McLeod K, et al: A pharmacodynamic model for pancuronium. Br J Anaesth 50:1113-1123, 1978.
13. Sheiner LB, Stanski DR, Vozeh S, et al: Simultaneous modeling of pharmacokinetics and pharmacodynamics: Application to *d*-tubocurarine. Clin Pharmacol Ther 25:358-371, 1979.
14. Glass PS, Hardman D, Kamiyama Y, et al: Preliminary pharmacokinetics and pharmacodynamics of an ultra-short–acting opioid: Remifentanil (GI87084B). Anesth Analg 77:1031-1040, 1993.
15. Egan TD, Lemmens HJM, Fiset P, et al: The pharmacokinetics of the new short-acting opioid remifentanil (GI87084B) in healthy adult male volunteers. Anesthesiology 79:881-892, 1993.
16. Ludbrook GL, Visco E, Lam AM: Propofol: Relation between brain concentrations, electroencephalogram, middle cerebral artery blood flow velocity, and cerebral oxygen extraction during induction of anesthesia. Anesthesiology 97:1363-1370, 2002.
17. Shafer SL, Gregg K: Algorithms to rapidly achieve and maintain stable drug concentrations at the site of drug effect with a computer controlled infusion pump. J Pharmacokinet Biopharm 20:147-169, 1992.
18. Jacobs JR, Williams EA: Algorithm to control "effect compartment" drug concentrations in pharmacokinetic model–driven drug delivery. IEEE Trans Biomed Eng 40:993-999, 1993.
19. Bouillon T, Schmidt C, Garstka G, et al: Pharmacokinetic-pharmacodynamic modeling of the respiratory depressant effect of alfentanil. Anesthesiology 91:144-155, 1999.
20. Bouillon T, Bruhn J, Radu-Radulescu L, et al: A model of the ventilatory depressant potency of remifentanil in the non steady state. Anesthesiology 99:779-787, 2003.
21. Scott JC, Ponganis KV, Stanski DR: EEG quantitation of narcotic effect: The comparative pharmacodynamics of fentanyl and alfentanil. Anesthesiology 62:234-241, 1985.
22. Eger EID, Saidman LJ, Brandstater B: Minimum alveolar anesthetic concentration: A standard of anesthetic potency. Anesthesiology 26:756-763, 1965.
23. Ausems ME, Stanski DR, Hug CC: An evaluation of the accuracy of pharmacokinetic data for the computer assisted infusion of alfentanil. Br J Anaesth 57:1217-1225, 1985.
24. Hung OR, Varvel JR, Shafer SL, et al: Thiopental pharmacodynamics II. Quantitation of clinical and electroencephalographic depth of anesthesia. Anesthesiology 77:237-244, 1992.
25. Telford RJ, Glass PSA, Goodman D, et al: Fentanyl does not alter the "sleep" plasma concentration of thiopental. Anesth Analg 75:523-529, 1992.
26. Vuyk J, Engbers FHM, Lemmens HJM, et al: Pharmacodynamics of propofol in female patients. Anesthesiology 77:3-9, 1992.
27. Vuyk J, Lim T, Engbers FH, et al: The pharmacodynamic interaction of propofol and alfentanil during lower abdominal surgery in women. Anesthesiology 83:8-22, 1995.
28. Smith C, McEwan AI, Jhaveri R, et al: Reduction of propofol Cp_{50} by fentanyl. Anesthesiology 77:A340, 1992.
29. Jacobs JR, Reves JG, Marty J, et al: Aging increases pharmacodynamic sensitivity to the hypnotic effects of midazolam. Anesth Analg 80:143-148, 1995.
30. Scott JC, Stanski DR: Decreased fentanyl and alfentanil dose requirements with age: A simultaneous pharmacokinetic and pharmacodynamic evaluation. J Pharmacol Exp Ther 240:159-166, 1987.
31. Scott JC, Cooke JE, Stanski DR: Electroencephalographic quantitation of opioid effect: Comparative pharmacodynamics of fentanyl and sufentanil. Anesthesiology 74:34, 1991.
32. Egan TD, Lemmens HJ, Fiset P, et al: The pharmacokinetics of the new short-acting opioid remifentanil (GI87084B) in healthy adult male volunteers. Anesthesiology. 79:881-892, 1993.
33. Egan TD, Minto CF, Hermann DJ, et al: Remifentanil versus alfentanil: Comparative pharmacokinetics and pharmacodynamics in healthy adult male volunteers. Anesthesiology 84:821-833, 1996.
34. Minto CF, Schnider TW, Egan TD, et al: The influence of age and gender on the pharmacokinetics and pharmacodynamics of remifentanil. I. Model development. Anesthesiology 86:10-23, 1997.
35. Homer TD, Stanski DR: The effect of increasing age on thiopental disposition and anesthetic requirement. Anesthesiology 62:714-724, 1985.
36. Stanski DR, Maitre PO: Population pharmacokinetics and pharmacodynamics of thiopental: The effect of age revisited. Anesthesiology 72:412-422, 1990.
37. Arden JR, Holley FO, Stanski DR: Increased sensitivity to etomidate in the elderly: Initial distribution versus altered brain response. Anesthesiology 65:19, 1986.
38. Billard V, Gambus PL, Chamoun N, et al: A comparison of spectral edge, delta power, and bispectral index as EEG measures of alfentanil, propofol, and midazolam drug effect. Clin Pharmacol Ther 61:45-58, 1997.
39. Schnider TW, Minto CF, Fiset P, et al: Semilinear canonical correlation applied to the measurement of the electroencephalographic effects of midazolam and flumazenil reversal. Anesthesiology 84:510-519, 1996.
40. Egan TD, Muir KT, Hermann DJ, et al: The electroencephalogram (EEG) and clinical measure of opioid potency: Defining the EEG–clinical potency relationship ("fingerprint") with application to remifentanil. Int J Pharm Med 15:1-9, 2001.
41. Ausems ME, Hug CC Jr, Stanski DR, et al: Plasma concentrations of alfentanil required to supplement nitrous oxide anesthesia for general surgery. Anesthesiology 65:362-373, 1986.
42. Glass PSA, Doherty M, Jacobs JR, et al: Plasma concentration of fentanyl, with 70% nitrous oxide, to prevent movement at skin incision. Anesthesiology 78:842-847, 1993.
43. Gourlay GK, Kowalski SR, Plummer JL, et al: Fentanyl blood concentration analgesic response relationship in the treatment of postoperative pain. Anesth Analg 67:329-337, 1988.
44. Van den Nieuwenhuyzen MCO, Engbers FHM, Burm AGL, et al: Computer-controlled infusion of alfentanil versus PCA-morphine for postoperative analgesia: A double-blind study. Anesth Analg 40:1112-1118, 1995.
45. Lehmann KA: Patient-controlled analgesia for postoperative pain. Adv Pain Res Ther 14:297, 1990.
46. Lehmann KA, Gerhard A, Horrichs-Haermeyer G, et al: Postoperative patient-controlled analgesia with sufentanil: Analgesic efficacy and minimum effective concentrations. Acta Anaesthesiol Scand 35:221, 1991.
47. Ropcke H, Schwilden H: The interaction of nitrous oxide and enflurane on the EEG median of 2-3 Hz is additive, but weaker than at 1.0 MAC. Anaesthesist 45:819-825, 1996.
48. Gonsowski CT, Eger EI 2nd: Nitrous oxide minimum alveolar anesthetic concentration in rats is greater than previously reported. Anesth Analg 79:710-712, 1994.
49. Deady JE, Koblin DD, Eger EI 2nd, et al: Anesthetic potencies and the unitary theory of narcosis. Anesth Analg 60:380-384, 1981.
50. Targ AG, Yasuda N, Eger EI 2nd, et al: Halogenation and anesthetic potency. Anesth Analg 68:599-602, 1989.
51. Kissin I: General anesthetic action: An obsolete notion? Anesth Analg 76:215-218, 1993.
52. Hendrickx JFA, Eger EI 2nd, Sonner JM, Shafer SL: Is synergy the rule? A review of anesthetic interactions producing hypnosis and immobility. Anesth Analg 107:494-506, 2008.
53. Katoh T, Ikeda I: The effects of fentanyl on sevoflurane requirements for loss of consciousness and skin incision. Anesthesiology 88:18-24, 1998.
54. McEwan AI, Smith C, Dyar O, et al: Isoflurane MAC reduction by fentanyl. Anesthesiology 78:864-869, 1993.

55. Brunner MD, Braithwaite P, Jhaveri R, et al: The MAC reduction of isoflurane by sufentanil. Br J Anaesth 72:42-46, 1994.
56. Westmoreland C, Sebel PS, Groper A, et al: Reduction of isoflurane MAC by fentanyl or alfentanil. Anesthesiology 77:A394, 1992.
57. Lang E, Kapila A, Shlugman D, et al: Reduction of isoflurane minimal alveolar concentration by remifentanil. Anesthesiology 85:721-728, 1996.
58. Glass PSA, Jacobs JR, Smith RL, et al: Pharmacokinetic model–driven infusion of fentanyl: Assessment of accuracy. Anesthesiology 73:1082-1090, 1990.
59. Dwyer R, Bennett HL, Eger EI 2nd, et al: Isoflurane anesthesia prevents unconscious learning. Anesth Analg 75:107-112, 1992.
60. Minto CF, Schnider TW, Short TG, et al: Response surface model for anesthetic drug interactions. Anesthesiology 92:1603-1616, 2000.
61. Shafer SL, Varvel JR: Pharmacokinetics, pharmacodynamics, and rational opioid selection. Anesthesiology 74:53-63, 1991.
62. Henthorn TK, Krejcie TC, Shanks CA, et al: Time-dependent distribution volume and kinetics of the pharmacodynamic effector site. J Pharm Sci 81: 1136, 1992.
63. Wagner JG: A safe method for rapidly achieving plasma concentration plateaus. Clin Pharmacol Ther 16:691-700, 1974.
64. Bruhn J, Bouillon TW, Ropcke H, Hoeft A: A manual slide rule for target-controlled infusion of propofol: Development and evaluation. Anesth Analg 96:142-147, 2003.
65. Hughes MA, Glass PSA, Jacobs JR: Context-sensitive half-time in multicompartment pharmacokinetic models for intravenous anesthetic drugs. Anesthesiology 76:334-341, 1992.
66. Schwilden H: Optimization of the dosage of volatile anesthetics based on pharmacokinetic and dynamic models. Anasth Intensivther Notfallmed 20:307-315, 1985.
67. Fisher DM, Rosen JI: A pharmacokinetic explanation for increasing recovery time following larger or repeated doses of nondepolarizing muscle relaxants. Anesthesiology 65:286-291, 1986.
68. Youngs EJ, Shafer SL: Pharmacokinetic parameters relevant to recovery from opioids. Anesthesiology 81:833-842, 1994.
69. Bailey JM: Technique for quantifying the duration of intravenous anesthetic effect. Anesthesiology 83:1095-1103, 1995.
70. Vuyk J, Mertens MJ, Olofsen E, et al: Propofol anesthesia and rational opioid selection: Determination of optimal EC_{50}-EC_{95} propofol-opioid concentrations that assure adequate anesthesia and a rapid return of consciousness. Anesthesiology 87:1549-1562, 1997.
71. Crankshaw DP, Morgan DJ, Beemer GH, et al: Preprogrammed infusion of alfentanil to constant arterial plasma concentration. Anesth Analg 76:556, 1993.
72. Shafer SL: Constant versus optimal plasma concentrations. Anesth Analg 76:467-469, 1993.
73. Reves JG, Jacobs JR, Glass PSA: Automated drug delivery in anesthesia. In ASA Refresher Course in Anesthesiology. American Society of Anesthesiologists, San Francisco, 1991, p 19.
74. Kruger-Thiemer E: Continuous intravenous infusion and multicompartment accumulation. Eur J Pharmacol 4:317-324, 1968.
75. Schwilden H, Schuttler J, Stoekel H: Pharmacokinetics as applied to total intravenous anaesthesia: Theoretical considerations. Anaesthesia 38(Suppl):51-52, 1983.
76. Schüttler J, Schwilden H, Stoekel H: Pharmacokinetics as applied to total intravenous anaesthesia: Practical implications. Anaesthesia 38(Suppl):53-56, 1983.
77. Bazaral MG, Ciarkowski A: Food and drug administration regulations and computer-controlled infusion pumps. Int Anesthesiol Clin 33:45-63, 1995.
78. Shafer SL, Siegel LC, Cooke JE, et al: Testing computer-controlled infusion pumps by simulation. Anesthesiology 68:261-266, 1988.
79. Hu C, Horstman DJ, Shafer SL: Variability of target-controlled infusion is less than the variability after bolus injection. Anesthesiology 102:639-645, 2005.
80. Varvel JR, Donoho DL, Shafer SL: Measuring the predictive performance of computer-controlled infusion pumps. J Pharmacokinet Biopharm 20:63, 1992.
81. Raemer DB, Buschman A, Varvel JR, et al: The prospective use of population pharmacokinetics in a computer-driven infusion system for alfentanil. Anesthesiology 73:66-72, 1990.
82. Schüttler J, Kloos S, Schwilden H, et al: Total intravenous anaesthesia with propofol and alfentanil by computer-assisted infusion. Anaesthesia 43(Suppl):2-7, 1988.
83. Lemmens HJM, Bovill JG, Burm AGL, et al: Alfentanil infusion in the elderly. Anaesthesia 43:850-856, 1988.
84. Veselis RA, Glass P, Dnistrian A, et al: Performance of computer-assisted continuous infusion at low concentrations of intravenous sedatives. Anesth Analg 84:1049-1057, 1997.
85. Shafer SL, Varvel SL, Aziz N, et al: The pharmacokinetics of fentanyl administered by computer controlled infusion pump. Anesthesiology 73: 1091-1102, 1990.
86. Alvis JM, Reves JG, Govier AV, et al: Computer assisted continuous infusions of fentanyl during cardiac anesthesia: Comparison with a manual method. Anesthesiology 63:41-49, 1985.
87. Coetzee JF, Glen JB, Wium CA, et al: Pharmacokinetic model selection for target controlled infusions of propofol: Assessment of three parameter sets. Anesthesiology 82:1328-1345, 1995.
88. Marsh B, White M, Morton N, et al: Pharmacokinetic model driven infusion of propofol in children. Br J Anaesth 67:41, 1991.
89. Tackley RM, Lewis GTR, Prys-Roberts C, et al: Computer controlled infusion of propofol. Br J Anaesth 62:46, 1989.
90. McClain DA, Hug CC Jr: Intravenous fentanyl kinetics. Clin Pharmacol Ther 28:106-114, 1980.
91. Ginsberg B, Howell S, Glass PSA, et al: Pharmacokinetic model–driven infusion of fentanyl in children. Anesthesiology 85:1268-1275, 1996.
92. Fiset P, Mathers L, Engstrom R, et al: Pharmacokinetics of computer controlled alfentanil administration in children undergoing cardiac surgery. Anesthesiology 83:944-955, 1995.
93. Bailey JM, Mora CT, Shafer SL, et al: Pharmacokinetics of propofol in adult patients undergoing coronary revascularization. Anesthesiology 81: 1288-1297, 1996.
94. Wu J, Zhu SM, He HL, et al: Plasma propofol concentrations during orthotopic liver transplantation. Acta Anaesthesiol Scand 49:804-819, 2005.
95. Vuyk J, Oostwouder CJ, Vletter AA, et al: Gender differences in the pharmacokinetics of propofol in elderly patients during and after continuous infusion. Br J Anaesth 86:183-188, 2001.
96. Schuttler J, Ihmsen H: Population pharmacokinetics of propofol: A multicenter study. Anesthesiology 92:727-738, 2000.
97. Kazama T, Kurita T, Morita K, et al: Influence of hemorrhage on propofol pseudo–steady state concentration. Anesthesiology 97:1156-1161, 2002.
98. Egan TD, Kuramkote S, Gong G, et al: Fentanyl pharmacokinetics in hemorrhagic shock: A porcine model. Anesthesiology 91:156-166, 1999.
99. Johnson KB, Kern SE, Hamber EA, et al: Influence of hemorrhagic shock on remifentanil: A pharmacokinetic and pharmacodynamic analysis. Anesthesiology 94:322-332, 2001.
100. Pavlin DJ, Coda B, Shen DD, et al: Effects of combining propofol and alfentanil on ventilation, analgesia, sedation, and emesis in human volunteers. Anesthesiology 84:23-37, 1996.
101. Kharasch ED, Russell M, Mautz D, et al: The role of cytochrome P450 3A4 in alfentanil clearance. Anesthesiology 87:36-50, 1997.
102. Vuyk J, Mertens MJ, Vletter AA, et al: Alfentanil modifies the pharmacokinetics of propofol in volunteers. Anesthesiology 87:A300, 1997.
103. Bouillon T, Bruhn J, Radu-Radulescu L, et al: Non–steady state analysis of the pharmacokinetic interaction between propofol and remifentanil. Anesthesiology. 97:1350-1362, 2002.
104. Knibbe CA, Zuideveld KP, DeJongh J, et al: Population pharmacokinetic and pharmacodynamic modeling of propofol for long-term sedation in critically ill patients: A comparison between propofol 6% and propofol 1%. Clin Pharmacol Ther 72:670-684, 2002.
105. Hill HF, Saeger L, Bjurstrom R, et al: Steady-state infusions of opioids in human volunteers. I. Pharmacokinetic tailoring. Pain 43:57, 1990.
106. Maitre PE, Stanski DR: Bayesian forecasting improves the prediction of intraoperative plasma concentrations of alfentanil. Anesthesiology 69:652-659, 1988.
107. Wakeling HG, Zimmerman JB, Howell S, Glass PS: Targeting effect compartment or central compartment concentration of propofol: What predicts loss of consciousness? Anesthesiology 90:92-97, 1999.
108. Struys MM, De Smet T, Depoorter B, et al: Comparison of plasma compartment versus two methods for effect compartment–controlled target-controlled infusion for propofol. Anesthesiology 92:399-406, 2000.
109. Kazama T, Ikeda K, Morita K, et al: Comparison of the effect-site k_{e0}s of propofol for blood pressure and EEG bispectral index in elderly and younger patients. Anesthesiology 90:1517-1527, 1999.
110. Minto CF, Schnider TW, Gregg KM, et al: Using the time of maximum effect site concentration to combine pharmacokinetics and pharmacodynamics. Anesthesiology 99:324-333, 2003.
111. Absalom AR, Kenny GNC: Closed-loop control of propofol anaesthesia using bispectral index: Performance assessment in patients receiving computer-controlled propofol and manually controlled remifentanil infusions for minor surgery. B J Anaesth 90:737-741, 2003.
112. Glass PSA, Jacobs J, Alvis M, et al: Computer assisted continuous infusion of alfentanil during noncardiac anesthesia: A comparison with a manual method. Anesthesiology 65:A546, 1986.
113. Theil DR, Stanley TE 3rd, White WD, et al: Midazolam and fentanyl continuous infusion anesthesia for cardiac surgery: A comparison of computer-assisted versus manual infusion systems. J Cardiothorac Vasc Anesth 7:300-306, 1993.
114. Struys M, Versichelen L, Thas O, et al: Comparison of computer-controlled propofol administration with two manual infusion methods [abstract]. Br J Anaesth 76(Suppl 2):87, 1996.

115. Russel D, Wilkes MP, Hunter SC, et al: Manual compared with target-controlled infusion of propofol. Br J Anaesth 75:562-566, 1995.
116. Servin FS: TCI compared with manually controlled infusion of propofol: A multicentre study. Anaesthesia 53(Suppl 1):82-86, 1998.
117. Gale T, Leslie K, Kluger M: Propofol anaesthesia via target controlled infusion or manually controlled infusion: Effects on the bispectral index as a measure of anaesthetic depth. Anaesth Intensive Care 29:579-584, 2001.
118. De Castro V, Godet G, Mencia G, et al: Target-controlled infusion for remifentanil in vascular patients improves hemodynamics and decreases remifentanil requirement. Anesth Analg 96:33-38, 2003.
119. Passot S, Servin F, Allary R, et al: Target-controlled versus manually-controlled infusion of propofol for direct laryngoscopy and bronchoscopy. Anesth Analg 94:1212-1216, 2002.
120. Glass PSA, Ginsberg B, Hawkins ED, et al: Comparison of sodium thiopental/isoflurane to propofol (delivered by means of a pharmacokinetic model–driven device) for the induction, maintenance, and recovery from anesthesia. Anesthesiology 69:A575, 1988.
121. Godet G, Watremez C, El Kettani C, et al: A comparison of sevoflurane, target-controlled infusion propofol, and propofol/isoflurane anesthesia in patients undergoing carotid surgery: A quality of anesthesia and recovery profile. Anesth Analg 93:560-565, 2001.
122. Sneyd JR, Andrews CJ, Tsobokwa T: Comparison of propofol/remifentanil and sevoflurane/remifentanil for maintenance of anaesthesia for elective intracranial surgery. Br J Anaesth 94:778-783, 2005.
123. Suttner S, Boldt J, Schmidt C, et al: Cost analysis of target-controlled infusion-based anesthesia compared with standard anesthesia regimens. Anesth Analg 88:77-82, 1999.
124. Hill HF, Chapman CR, Saeger LS, et al: Steady-state infusions of opioids in human. II. Concentration-effect relationships and therapeutic margins. Pain 43:69-79, 1990.
125. Hill HF, Mather LE: Patient-controlled analgesia: Pharmacokinetic and therapeutic considerations. Clin Pharmacokinet 24:124-140, 1993.
126. Hill H, Mackie A, Coda B, et al: Evaluation of the accuracy of a pharmacokinetically-based patient-controlled analgesia system. Eur J Clin Pharmacol 43:67-75, 1992.
127. Hill HF, Jacobson RC, Coda BA, et al: A computer-based system for controlling plasma opioid concentration according to patient need for analgesia. Clin Pharmacokinet 20:319-330, 1991.
128. Hill HF, Mackie AM, Coda BA, et al: Patient-controlled analgesic administration: A comparison of steady-state morphine infusions with bolus doses. Cancer 67:873-882, 1991.
129. Schnider TW, Gaeta R, Brose W, et al: Derivation and cross-validation of pharmacokinetic parameters for computer-controlled infusion of lidocaine in pain therapy. Anesthesiology 84:1043-1050, 1996.
130. Struys M, Versichelen L, Byttebier G, et al: Clinical usefulness of the bispectral index for titrating propofol target effect-site concentration. Anaesthesia 53:4-12, 1998.
131. Morley AP, Derrick J, Seed PT, et al: Isoflurane dosage for equivalent intraoperative electroencephalographic suppression in patients with and without epidural blockade. Anesth Analg 95:1412-1418, 2002.
132. Gentilini A, Rossoni-Gerosa M, Frei CW, et al: Modeling and closed-loop control of hypnosis by means of bispectral index (BIS) with isoflurane. IEEE Trans Biomed Eng 48:874-889, 2001.
133. Kansanaho M, Olkkola KT: The effect of halothane on mivacurium infusion requirements in adult surgical patients. Acta Anaesthesiol Scand 41:754-759, 1997.
134. Struys MM, De Smet T, Versichelen LF, et al: Comparison of closed-loop controlled administration of propofol using Bispectral Index as the controlled variable versus "standard practice" controlled administration. Anesthesiology 95:6-17, 2001.
135. Kenny GN, Mantzaridis H: Closed-loop control of propofol anaesthesia. Br J Anaesth 83:223-228, 1999.
136. Sakai T, Matsuki A, White PF, Giesecke AH: Use of an EEG-bispectral closed-loop delivery system for administering propofol. Acta Anaesthesiol Scand 44:1007-1010, 2000.
137. Absalom AR, Sutcliffe N, Kenny GN: Closed-loop control of anesthesia using Bispectral index: Performance assessment in patients undergoing major orthopedic surgery under combined general and regional anesthesia. Anesthesiology 96:67-73, 2002.
138. De Smet T, Struys MM, Greenwald S, et al: Estimation of optimal modeling weights for a Bayesian-based closed-loop system for propofol administration using the bispectral index as a controlled variable: A simulation study. Anesth Analg 105:1629-1638, 2007.
139. Morley A, Derrick J, Mainland P, et al: Closed loop control of anaesthesia: An assessment of the bispectral index as the target of control. Anaesthesia 55:953-959, 2000.
140. Locher S, Stadler KS, Boehlen T, et al: A new closed-loop control system for isoflurane using bispectral index outperforms manual control. Anesthesiology 101:591-602, 2004.
141. Glass PS, Rampil IJ: Automated anesthesia: Fact or fantasy? Anesthesiology 95:1-2, 2001.
142. Liu N, Chazot T Genty A, et al: Titration of propofol for anesthetic induction and maintenance guided by the bispectral index: Closed-loop versus manual control: A Prospective, randomized, multicenter study. Anesthesiology 104:686-695, 2006.
143. Kansanaho M, Olkkola KT, Wierda JM: Dose-response and concentration-response relation of rocuronium infusion during propofol–nitrous oxide and isoflurane–nitrous oxide anaesthesia. Eur J Anaesthesiol 14:488-494, 1997.
144. Meretoja OA, Wirtavuori K, Taivainen T, Olkkola KT: Time course of potentiation of mivacurium by halothane and isoflurane in children. Br J Anaesth 76:235-238, 1996.
145. Milne SE, Kenny GN, Schraag S: Propofol sparing effect of remifentanil using closed-loop anaesthesia. Br J Anaesth 90:623-629, 2003.
146. Schwilden H, Schuttler J: [The determination of an effective therapeutic infusion rate for intravenous anesthetics using feedback-controlled dosages.] Anaesthesist 39:603-606, 1990.
147. Albrecht S, Frenkel C, Ihmsen H, Schuttler J: A rational approach to the control of sedation in intensive care unit patients based on closed-loop control. Eur J Anaesthesiol 16:678-687, 1999.

Mohamed Naguib and Cynthia A. Lien

29 Pharmacology of Muscle Relaxants and Their Antagonists

Key Points

1. Two different populations of nicotinic acetylcholine receptors exist at the mammalian neuromuscular junction. In adults, the nicotinic acetylcholine receptor at the postsynaptic (muscular) membrane is composed of $\alpha_2\beta\delta\varepsilon$-subunits. Each of the two α-subunits has an acetylcholine binding site. The presynaptic (neuronal) nicotinic receptor is also a pentameric complex composed of $\alpha_3\beta_2$-subunits.
2. Nondepolarizing muscle relaxants produce neuromuscular blockade by competing with acetylcholine for postsynaptic α-subunits. In contrast, succinylcholine produces prolonged depolarization that results in decreased sensitivity of the postsynaptic nicotinic acetylcholine receptor and inactivation of sodium channels so that propagation of the action potential across the muscle membrane is inhibited.
3. Different forms of neuromuscular stimulation test for neuromuscular blockade at different areas of the motor end plate. Depression of the response to single-twitch stimulation is probably due to blockade of postsynaptic nicotinic acetylcholine receptors, whereas fade in the response to tetanic and train-of-four stimuli results from blockade of presynaptic nicotinic receptors.
4. Succinylcholine is the only available depolarizing neuromuscular blocker. It is characterized by rapid onset of effect and ultrashort duration of action because of its rapid hydrolysis by butyrylcholinesterase.
5. The nondepolarizing neuromuscular blockers available can be classified according to chemical class (steroidal, benzylisoquinolinium, or other compounds) or, alternatively, according to onset or duration of action (long-, intermediate-, and short-acting drugs) of equipotent doses.
6. The speed of onset is inversely proportional to the potency of nondepolarizing neuromuscular blocking agents. With the exception of atracurium, molar potency is highly predictive of a drug's rate of onset of effect. Rocuronium has a molar potency ($ED_{95} \approx 0.54$ μM/kg) that is about 13% that of vecuronium and 9% that of cisatracurium. Its onset of effect is more rapid than that of either of these agents.
7. Neuromuscular blockade develops faster, lasts a shorter time, and is recovered from more quickly in the more centrally located neuromuscular units (e.g., laryngeal adductors, diaphragm, and masseter muscle) than in the more peripherally located adductor pollicis.
8. The long-acting neuromuscular blockers undergo minimal or no metabolism, and they are eliminated, largely unchanged, primarily by renal excretion. Neuromuscular blockers with an intermediate duration of action have more rapid clearance than the long-acting agents do because of multiple pathways of degradation, metabolism, and elimination. Mivacurium, a short-acting neuromuscular blocker, is cleared rapidly and almost exclusively via metabolism by butyrylcholinesterase.
9. After the administration of nondepolarizing neuromuscular blocking agents, it is essential to ensure adequate return of normal neuromuscular function. Residual paralysis decreases upper esophageal tone, coordination of the esophageal musculature during swallowing, and the hypoxic ventilatory drive.

History and Clinical Use

In 1942, Griffith and Johnson[1] suggested that *d*-tubocurarine (dTc) is a safe drug to use during surgery to provide skeletal muscle relaxation. One year later, Cullen[2] described its use in 131 patients who had received general anesthesia for their surgery. In 1954, Beecher and Todd[3] reported a sixfold increase in mortality in patients receiving dTc in comparison with those who had not received a relaxant. The increased mortality was due to a general lack of understanding of the pharmacology of neuromuscular blockers and their antagonism. The effect of residual neuromuscular blockade postoperatively was not appreciated, guidelines for monitoring muscle strength had not been established, and the importance of pharmacologically antagonizing any residual blockade was not understood.

Succinylcholine, introduced by Thesleff[4] and Foldes and colleagues[5] in 1952, changed anesthetic practice drastically. Its rapid onset of effect and ultrashort duration of action permitted rapid endotracheal intubation.

In 1967, Baird and Reid[6] first reported on clinical administration of the synthetic aminosteroid pancuronium.

Development of the intermediate-acting neuromuscular blockers built on the compounds' metabolism and resulted in the introduction of vecuronium,[7] an aminosteroid, and atracurium,[8] a benzylisoquinolinium, into clinical practice in the 1980s.

Mivacurium, the first short-acting nondepolarizing neuromuscular blocker, was introduced into clinical practice in the 1990s,[9] as was rocuronium,[10] an intermediate-acting nondepolarizing blocker with rapid onset of effect.

Other neuromuscular blockers have been introduced into clinical practice since the use of dTc was first advocated. Such blockers include pipecuronium, doxacurium, cisatracurium, and rapacuronium. Although all do not remain in use, each represented an advance or improvement in at least one aspect over its predecessors. Still other neuromuscular blockers, such as gantacurium,[11] are undergoing investigation.

Neuromuscular blockers should be administered only to anesthetized individuals to provide relaxation of skeletal muscles. They should not be administered to stop patient movement because they have no analgesic or amnestic properties. Awareness during surgery[12] and in the intensive care unit (ICU)[13] has been described in multiple publications. Neuromuscular blockers are valuable adjuncts to general anesthetics and should be used as such. As stated by Cullen and Larson, "muscle relaxants given inappropriately may provide the surgeon with optimal [operating] conditions in ... a patient [who] is paralyzed but not anesthetized—a state that [is] wholly unacceptable for the patient." Additionally, "muscle relaxants used to cover up deficiencies in total anesthetic management ... represent an ... inappropriate use of the valuable adjuncts to anesthesia." To administer relaxants for maintenance of neuromuscular blockade intraoperatively, the patient's depth of neuromuscular blockade must be monitored and the depth of anesthesia continuously assessed.

That said, the use of neuromuscular blockers in the operating room is quite common and has been important in the growth and development of anesthesia and surgery. As stated by Foldes and colleagues,[5] "... [the] first use of ... muscle relaxants ... not only revolutionized the practice of anesthesia but also started the modern era of surgery and made possible the explosive development of cardiothoracic, neurologic, and organ transplant surgery." Certainly, neuromuscular blockers are now used routinely to facilitate endotracheal intubation and mechanical ventilation and are commonly used to maintain neuromuscular blockade through any number of different surgical procedures. This chapter reviews the pharmacology and clinical use of neuromuscular blocking agents and anticholinesterases in the anesthesia and intensive care settings. Finally, the economics of providing neuromuscular blockade is considered.

Principles of Action of Neuromuscular Blockers at the Neuromuscular Junction

For a comprehensive overview of neuromuscular blocker effects, see Chapter 14. This section provides a brief introduction to the principles of action of these agents. In the following, a brief introduction is made for the purpose of this chapter.

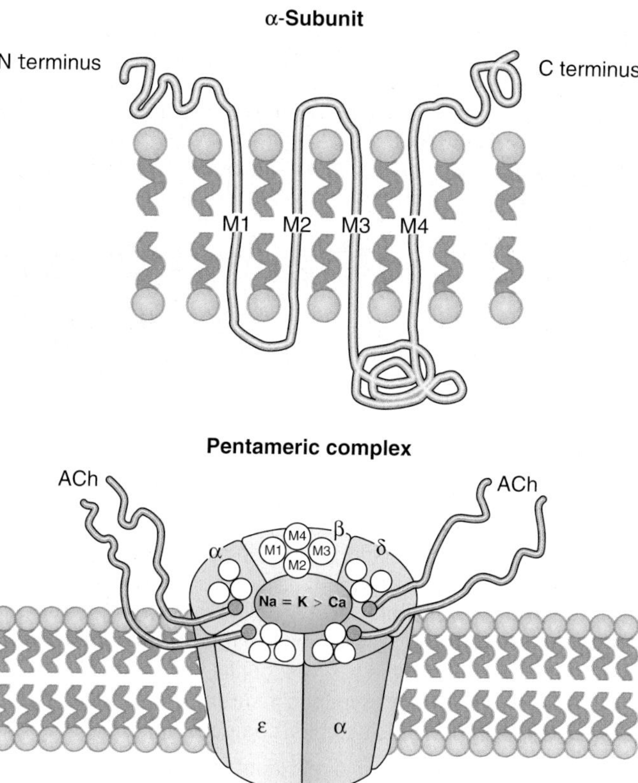

Figure 29-1 Subunit composition of the nicotinic acetylcholine (ACh) receptor (nAChR) in the end-plate surface of adult mammalian muscle. The adult AChR is an intrinsic membrane protein with five distinct subunits ($\alpha_2\beta\delta\varepsilon$). Each subunit contains four helical domains, labeled M1 to M4. The M2 domain forms the channel pore. The *upper panel* shows a single α-subunit with its N and C termini on the extracellular surface of the membrane lipid bilayer. Between the N and C termini, the α-subunit forms four helices (M1, M2, M3, and M4) that span the membrane bilayer. The *lower panel* shows the pentameric structure of the nAChR of adult mammalian muscle. The N termini of two subunits cooperate to form two distinct binding pockets for ACh. These pockets occur at the ε-α– and the δ-α–subunit interface. The M2 membrane-spanning domain of each subunit lines the ion channel. The doubly liganded ion channel has equal permeability to Na^+ and to K^+; Ca^{2+} contributes approximately 2.5% to the total permeability. *(From Naguib M, Flood P, McArdle JJ, Brenner HR: Advances in neurobiology of the neuromuscular junction: Implications for the anesthesiologist. Anesthesiology 96:202-231, 2002, with permission from Anesthesiology.)*

Postjunctional Effects

In adult mammalian skeletal muscle, the nicotinic acetylcholine receptor (nAChR) is a pentameric complex of two α-subunits in association with single β-, δ-, and ε-subunits (Fig. 29-1). These subunits are organized to form a transmembrane pore (i.e., a channel), as well as extracellular binding pockets, for acetylcholine and other agonists or antagonists.[14] Each of the two α-subunits has an acetylcholine binding site. These sites are proteins located in pockets approximately 3.0 nm above the surface membrane at the interfaces of the α_H-ε- and α_L-δ-subunits.[15] α_H and α_L indicate the high- and low-affinity binding sites, respectively, for dTc and probably result from the contribution of the different neighboring subunits.[16] For instance, the binding affinity of dTc for the α_H-ε site is approximately 100 to 500 times higher than that for the α_L-δ site.[16] The fetal nAChR contains a γ-subunit instead of an adult ε-subunit. The mature nAChR has a shorter burst duration and higher conductance for Na^+, K^+, and Ca^{2+} than the fetal nAChR does.[14]

Functionally, the ion channel of the acetylcholine receptor is closed in the resting state. Simultaneous binding of two acetylcholine molecules to the α-subunits initiates conformational changes that open the channel. On the other hand, it is enough for one molecule of a nondepolarizing neuromuscular blocker (i.e., a competitive antagonist) to bind to one subunit to produce blockade. Paul and coworkers[17] found a correlation between the ED_{50} (the dose that produces a 50% depression in twitch tension) and the potency of nondepolarizing blockers at the adult nAChR.

Depolarizing neuromuscular blockers such as succinylcholine produce prolonged depolarization of the end-plate region, which results in (1) desensitization of the nAChR, (2) inactivation of voltage-gated sodium channels at the neuromuscular junction, and (3) increases in potassium permeability in the surrounding membrane. The end result is failure of action potential generation, and blockade ensues. It should be noted that although acetylcholine produces depolarization, it results in muscle contraction under physiologic conditions because it has a very short duration of action (a few milliseconds). Acetylcholine is rapidly hydrolyzed by acetylcholinesterase to acetic acid and choline. Administration of large doses of acetylcholine to experimental animals, however, produces neuromuscular blockade.

The fetal nAChR is a low-conductance channel, in contrast to the high-conductance channel of the adult nAChR. Thus, release of acetylcholine causes brief activation and a reduced probability of opening of the channel.[14] The upregulation of nAChRs found in states of functional or surgical denervation is characterized by the spreading of predominantly fetal-type nAChRs. These receptors are resistant to nondepolarizing neuromuscular blockers and more sensitive to succinylcholine.[18] When depolarized, the immature isoform has a prolonged open channel time that exaggerates the efflux of K^+.[19]

Prejunctional Effects

Prejunctional receptors are involved in modulating the release of acetylcholine in the neuromuscular junction. The existence of both nicotinic and muscarinic receptors on motor nerve endings has been described. Bowman[20] suggested that the prejunctional nicotinic receptors are activated by acetylcholine and function in a positive-feedback control system that serves to maintain the availability of acetylcholine when demand for it is high (e.g., during tetany).[20] Blockade of these receptors by nondepolarizing neuromuscular blockers would explain the "fade" phenomenon seen with tetanic and train-of-four (TOF) stimulation (four stimuli delivered over a period of 2 seconds).[20,21] The G protein–coupled muscarinic receptors are also involved in feedback modulation of acetylcholine release.[22] The prejunctional muscarinic M_1 and M_2 receptors are involved in facilitation and inhibition of acetylcholine release, respectively, via modulation of Ca^{2+} influx.[22] The prejunctional nicotinic receptors are involved in mobilization of acetylcholine but not directly in the release process.[23] Hence, blockade of the prejunctional nicotinic receptors by nondepolarizing neuromuscular blockers prevents acetylcholine from being made available fast enough to support tetanic or TOF stimulation. In contrast, the prejunctional muscarinic receptors are involved in upregulation or downmodulation of the release mechanism.

Monitoring Neuromuscular Function

Details of monitoring neuromuscular function are discussed in Chapter 47. In this chapter, only the general concepts of monitoring as they relate to the clinical use of neuromuscular blockers are presented.

Monitoring of neuromuscular function after the administration of neuromuscular blocking agents is extremely important for appropriate dosing of these agents and for better guaranteeing patient safety. In the operating room or ICU, the depth of neuromuscular blockade is typically monitored by observing the response to stimulation of any superficially located neuromuscular unit. Most commonly, contraction of the adductor pollicis muscle associated with stimulation of the ulnar nerve, either at the wrist or at the elbow, is monitored. In certain circumstances, depending on patient positioning, when access to the patients' arms may be limited or because of the nature of the patient's injury, the peroneal nerve or the facial nerve may be monitored.

The pattern of response to TOF stimulation or a tetanic stimulus varies with the type of neuromuscular blocker administered because of the different mechanisms of action of the two relaxant types, depolarizing and nondepolarizing. With complete blockade, no response to either mode of stimulation should occur. However, during partial neuromuscular blockade, different responses to these modes of stimulation are seen, depending on the agent administered. Nondepolarizing neuromuscular blocking agents are competitive inhibitors of the acetylcholine receptor and compete with acetylcholine for the active, or binding, sites on the α-subunits of the receptor. Because of a decrease in the amount of acetylcholine released from the prejunctional nerve terminal with repetitive or intense stimulation, the response to stimulation fades over time. The fourth response to a TOF stimulus is decreased relative to the first response (Fig. 29-2) because the lesser amount of acetylcholine released into the synaptic cleft with the fourth stimulus cannot overcome the competitive blockade as readily. Similarly, fading is seen in response to tetanic

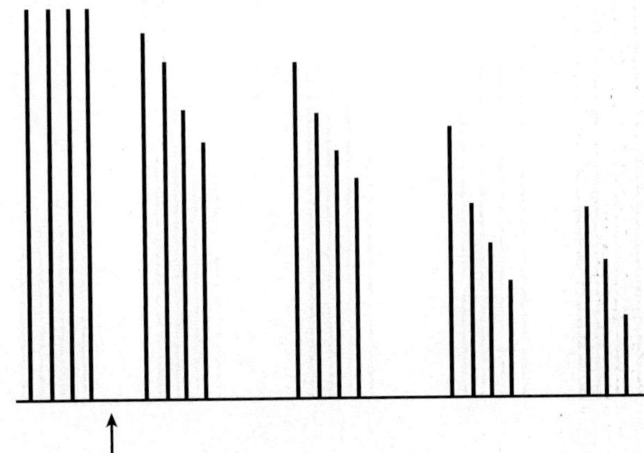

Figure 29-2 Schematic representation of the onset of neuromuscular blockade after the administration of a nondepolarizing neuromuscular blocking agent at the *arrow*. Neuromuscular function is monitored with repetitive train-of-four stimuli (four stimuli 0.5 msec in duration administered over a 2-second period).

stimuli when partial nondepolarizing neuromuscular blockade is present. During neuromuscular blockade with nondepolarizing agents, if one administers a TOF stimulus shortly after a tetanic stimulus, the response to stimulation is augmented and neuromuscular function appears stronger than it did just a couple of minutes earlier. This presumably occurs because with the tetanic stimuli, acetylcholine is mobilized toward the presynaptic portion of the nerve terminal and then, with subsequent stimulation (TOF), an increased amount of acetylcholine is released into the synaptic cleft and the blockade imposed by the nondepolarizing agent is more readily overcome. It may take 1 to 10 minutes for recovery to return to pretetanic or baseline values.[24] In the case of administration of a depolarizing neuromuscular blocking agent such as succinylcholine, the response that has classically been described is quite different. With repetitive TOF stimuli after the administration of doses of succinylcholine that cause 100% paralysis, four equal responses are seen with each stimulus, but there is a weakening of response with each successive TOF stimulus (Fig. 29-3). Similarly, there is no fading or weakening of the response to a tetanic stimulus; however, the entire response will be weaker than it was at baseline. The onset of blockade after the administration of small doses of succinylcholine, 0.05 to 0.3 mg/kg, is accompanied by fading of the TOF response, as has been described for nondepolarizing agents. Interestingly, although one would not necessarily anticipate that there would be posttetanic potentiation after the administration of succinylcholine, it has been described.[25] The reason for this observation has yet to be elucidated.

The neuromuscular blockade develops faster in centrally located muscles, such as the larynx, jaw, and diaphragm, than in more peripherally located muscles, such as the adductor pollicis.[26] In addition to developing more quickly, neuromuscular blockade in these regions, at a given dose, is less profound and recovers more quickly (Fig. 29-4) (for details, see the later section "Neuromuscular Blockers and Tracheal Intubation").[26] Consequently, the choice of monitoring site is important.

To determine the depth of blockade during maintenance and recovery of neuromuscular function, the response of the adductor pollicis to stimulation of the ulnar nerve should be monitored. If recovery in this neuromuscular unit is complete, recovery in the musculature of the airway should also be complete.[26] It is recommended that objective monitoring (e.g., the TOF ratio displayed digitally in real time) be used clinically. Subjective (visual or tactile) evaluation of the evoked muscular response to TOF stimulation is extremely inaccurate.

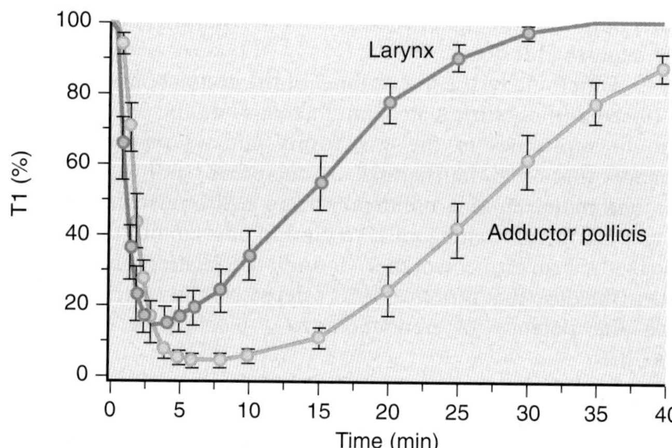

Figure 29-4 Evolution of neuromuscular blockade in the larynx and thumb (adductor pollicis) after a 0.07-mg/kg dose of vecuronium. Onset and recovery from blockade occur more rapidly in the larynx. *(From Donati F, Meistelman C, Plaud B: Vecuronium neuromuscular blockade at the adductor muscles of the larynx and adductor pollicis. Anesthesiology 74:833-837, 1991.)*

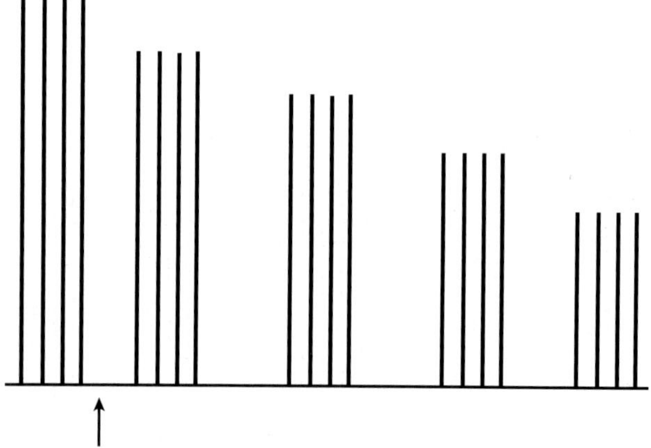

Figure 29-3 Schematic representation of the onset of neuromuscular blockade after the administration of a depolarizing neuromuscular blocking agent at the *arrow*. Neuromuscular function is monitored by repetitive train-of-four stimuli (four stimuli 0.5 msec in duration administered over a 2-second period).

Pharmacology of Succinylcholine

Structure-Activity Relationships

All neuromuscular blockers, being quaternary ammonium compounds, are structurally related to acetylcholine. Positive charges at these sites in the molecules mimic the quaternary nitrogen atom of the transmitter acetylcholine and are the principal reason for the attraction of these drugs to muscle- and neuronal-type nAChRs at the neuromuscular junction. These receptors are also located at other physiologic sites of acetylcholine in the body, such as the neuronal-type nicotinic receptors in autonomic ganglia and as many as five different muscarinic receptors on both the parasympathetic and sympathetic sides of the autonomic nervous system. In addition, populations of neuronal nicotinic and muscarinic receptors are located prejunctionally at the neuromuscular junction.

The depolarizing neuromuscular blocker succinylcholine is composed of two molecules of acetylcholine linked back to back through the acetate methyl groups (Fig. 29-5). As described by Bovet,[27] succinylcholine is a long, thin, flexible molecule. Like acetylcholine, succinylcholine stimulates cholinergic receptors at the neuromuscular junction and at nicotinic (ganglionic) and muscarinic autonomic sites, thereby opening the ionic channel in the acetylcholine receptor.

Pharmacokinetics and Pharmacodynamics

Succinylcholine is the only available neuromuscular blocker with a rapid onset of effect and an ultrashort duration of action. The

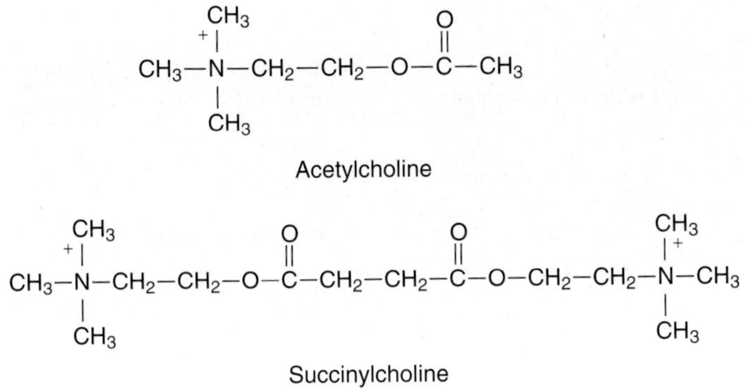

$$CH_3-\overset{+}{N}(CH_3)_2-CH_2-CH_2-O-\overset{O}{\overset{\|}{C}}-CH_3$$

Acetylcholine

$$CH_3-\overset{+}{N}(CH_3)_2-CH_2-CH_2-O-\overset{O}{\overset{\|}{C}}-CH_2-CH_2-\overset{O}{\overset{\|}{C}}-O-CH_2-CH_2-\overset{+}{N}(CH_3)_2-CH_3$$

Succinylcholine

Figure 29-5 Structural relationship of succinylcholine, a depolarizing neuromuscular blocking agent, and acetylcholine. Succinylcholine consists of two acetylcholine molecules linked through the acetate methyl groups. Like acetylcholine, succinylcholine stimulates nicotinic receptors at the neuromuscular junction.

ED_{95} of succinylcholine (the dose causing on average 95% suppression of neuromuscular response) is 0.51 to 0.63 mg/kg.[28] Using cumulative dose-response techniques, Kopman and coworkers[29] estimated that its potency is far greater, with an ED_{95} of less than 0.3 mg/kg.

Administration of 1 mg/kg of succinylcholine results in complete suppression of response to neuromuscular stimulation in approximately 60 seconds.[30] In patients with genotypically normal butyrylcholinesterase (also known as plasma cholinesterase or pseudocholinesterase) activity, recovery to 90% muscle strength after the administration of 1 mg/kg succinylcholine requires 9 to 13 minutes.[31]

The short duration of action of succinylcholine is due to its rapid hydrolysis by butyrylcholinesterase to succinylmonocholine and choline. Butyrylcholinesterase has an enormous capacity to hydrolyze succinylcholine, and only 10% of the administered drug reaches the neuromuscular junction.[32] The initial metabolite, succinylmonocholine, is a much weaker neuromuscular blocking agent than succinylcholine and is metabolized much more slowly to succinic acid and choline. The elimination half-life of succinylcholine is estimated to be 47 seconds.[33]

Because there is little or no butyrylcholinesterase at the neuromuscular junction, the neuromuscular blockade of succinylcholine is terminated by its diffusion away from the neuromuscular junction back into the circulation. Butyrylcholinesterase, therefore, influences the onset and duration of action of succinylcholine by controlling the rate at which the drug is hydrolyzed before it reaches and after it leaves the neuromuscular junction.

Dibucaine Number and Butyrylcholinesterase Activity

Butyrylcholinesterase is synthesized by the liver and found in plasma. The neuromuscular blockade induced by succinylcholine is prolonged by a decreased concentration or activity of the enzyme. The activity of the enzyme refers to the number of substrate molecules (μmol) hydrolyzed per unit of time, often expressed in international units (IU). The normal range of butyrylcholinesterase activity is quite large[31]; significant decreases in butyrylcholinesterase activity result in modest increases in the time required to return to 100% twitch recovery (Fig. 29-6).

Factors that have been described as lowering butyrylcholinesterase activity are liver disease,[34] advanced age,[35] malnutrition, pregnancy, burns, oral contraceptives, monoamine oxidase inhibitors, echothiophate, cytotoxic drugs, neoplastic disease, anticholinesterase drugs,[36] tetrahydroaminacrine,[37] hexafluorenium, and metoclopramide.[38] The histamine type 2 receptor antagonists have no effect on butyrylcholinesterase activity or the duration of succinylcholine's effect.[39] Bambuterol, a prodrug of terbutaline, produces marked inhibition of butyrylcholinesterase activity and causes prolongation of succinylcholine-induced blockade.[40] The β-blocker esmolol inhibits butyrylcholinesterase but causes only minor prolongation of succinylcholine blockade.[41]

Despite all the publications and efforts to identify situations in which normal butyrylcholinesterase enzyme activity may be low, this has not been a major concern in clinical practice because even large decreases in butyrylcholinesterase activity result in only moderate increases in the duration of action of succinylcholine. When butyrylcholinesterase activity is reduced to 20% of normal by severe liver disease, the duration of apnea after the administration of succinylcholine increases from a normal duration of 3 minutes to just 9 minutes. Even when treatment of glaucoma with echothiophate decreased butyrylcholinesterase activity from 49% of control to no activity, the increase in duration of neuromuscular blockade varied from 2 to 14 minutes. In no patient did the total duration of neuromuscular blockade exceed 23 minutes.[42]

Dibucaine Number and Atypical Butyrylcholinesterase Activity

Succinylcholine-induced neuromuscular blockade can be significantly prolonged if the patient has an abnormal genetic variant

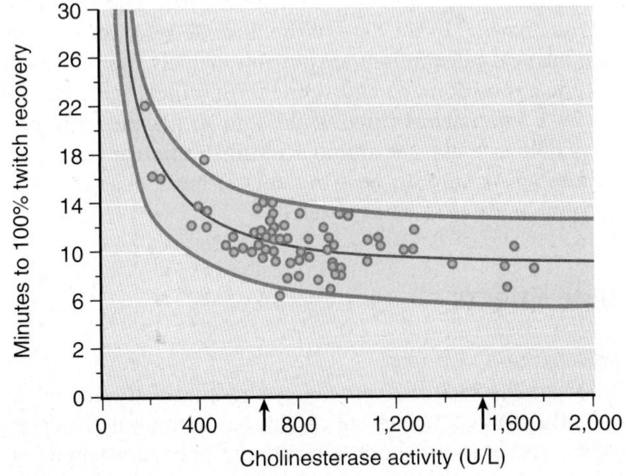

Figure 29-6 Correlation between the duration of succinylcholine neuromuscular blockade and butyrylcholinesterase activity. The normal range of activity lies between the *arrows*. *(From Viby-Mogensen J: Correlation of succinylcholine duration of action with plasma cholinesterase activity in subjects with the genotypically normal enzyme. Anesthesiology 53:517-520, 1980.)*

Table 29-1 Relationship between Dibucaine Number and Duration of Succinylcholine or Mivacurium Neuromuscular Blockade

Type of Butyrylcholinesterase	Genotype	Incidence	Dibucaine Number*	Response to Succinylcholine or Mivacurium
Homozygous typical	$E_1^uE_1^u$	Normal	70-80	Normal
Heterozygous atypical	$E_1^uE_1^a$	1/480	50-60	Lengthened by 50%-100%
Homozygous atypical	$E_1^aE_1^a$	1/3200	20-30	Prolonged to 4-8 hr

*The dibucaine number indicates the percentage of enzyme inhibited.

of butyrylcholinesterase. The variant was found by Kalow and Genest[43] to respond to dibucaine differently than normal butyrylcholinesterase does. Dibucaine inhibits normal butyrylcholinesterase to a far greater extent than it inhibits the abnormal enzyme. This observation led to development of the test for dibucaine number. Under standardized test conditions, dibucaine inhibits expression of the normal enzyme by about 80% and the abnormal enzyme by about 20% (Table 29-1). Subsequently, many other genetic variants of butyrylcholinesterase have been identified, although the dibucaine-resistant variants are the most important. The review by Jensen and Viby-Mogensen[44] can be consulted for more detailed information on this topic.

Although the dibucaine number indicates the genetic makeup of an individual with respect to butyrylcholinesterase, it does not measure the concentration of the enzyme in plasma, nor does it indicate the efficiency of the enzyme in hydrolyzing a substrate such as succinylcholine or mivacurium. Both of the latter factors are determined by measuring butyrylcholinesterase activity, which may be influenced by genotype.

The molecular biology of butyrylcholinesterase is well understood. The amino acid sequence of the enzyme is known, and the coding errors responsible for most genetic variations have been identified.[44] Most variants are due to a single amino acid substitution error or sequencing error at or near the active site of the enzyme. For example, in the case of the "atypical" dibucaine-resistant (A) gene, a mutation occurs at nucleotide 209, where guanine is substituted for adenine. The resultant change in this codon causes substitution of glycine for aspartic acid at position 70 in the enzyme. In the case of the fluoride-resistant (F) gene, two amino acid substitutions are possible, namely, methionine for threonine at position 243 and valine for glycine at position 390. Table 29-1 summarizes three of the known genetic variants of butyrylcholinesterase: the amino acid substitution at position 70 is written as Asp Ø Gly. New variants of butyrylcholinesterase genotypes continue to be discovered.[45]

Side Effects

Cardiovascular Effects

Succinylcholine-induced cardiac dysrhythmias are many and varied. The drug stimulates all cholinergic autonomic receptors: nicotinic receptors on both sympathetic and parasympathetic ganglia[46] and muscarinic receptors in the sinus node of the heart. At low doses, both negative inotropic and chronotropic responses may occur. These responses can be attenuated by prior administration of atropine. With large doses of succinylcholine, these effects may become positive[47] and result in tachycardia. A prominent clinical manifestation of generalized autonomic stimulation is the development of cardiac dysrhythmias, principally manifested as sinus bradycardia, junctional rhythms, and ventricular dysrhythmias. Clinical studies have described these dysrhythmias under various conditions in the presence of the intense autonomic stimulus of tracheal intubation. It is not entirely clear whether the cardiac irregularities are due to the action of succinylcholine alone or to the added presence of extraneous autonomic stimulation. An in vitro study using the ganglionic acetylcholine receptor subtype $\alpha_3\beta_4$ expressed in *Xenopus laevis* oocytes suggested that at clinically relevant concentrations, succinylcholine had no effect on the expressed receptors.[48] Only at high doses of succinylcholine was inhibition of ganglionic acetylcholine receptors noted.[48] The significance of these findings is difficult to extrapolate into clinical practice because the method used (*Xenopus laevis* oocyte expression model) does not match clinical reality.

Sinus Bradycardia. The autonomic mechanism involved in sinus bradycardia is stimulation of cardiac muscarinic receptors in the sinus node. This is particularly problematic in individuals with predominantly vagal tone, such as children who have not received atropine. Sinus bradycardia has also been noted in adults and appears more commonly after a second dose of the drug is given approximately 5 minutes after the first.[49] The bradycardia may be prevented by the administration of thiopental, atropine, ganglion-blocking drugs, and nondepolarizing neuromuscular blockers.[50] The implication of this information is that direct myocardial effects, increased muscarinic stimulation, and ganglionic stimulation may all be involved in the bradycardia response. The higher incidence of bradycardia after a second dose of succinylcholine suggests that the hydrolysis products of succinylcholine (succinylmonocholine and choline) may sensitize the heart to a subsequent dose.

Nodal (Junctional) Rhythms. Nodal rhythms commonly occur after the administration of succinylcholine. The mechanism probably involves relatively greater stimulation of muscarinic receptors in the sinus node, which suppresses the sinus mechanism and allows emergence of the atrioventricular node as the pacemaker. The incidence of junctional rhythm is greater after a second dose of succinylcholine but is prevented by prior administration of dTc.[50]

Ventricular Dysrhythmias. Under stable anesthetic conditions, succinylcholine lowers the threshold of the ventricle to catecholamine-induced dysrhythmias in the monkey and dog. Circulating catecholamine concentrations increase fourfold and potassium concentrations increase by a third after administration of succinylcholine to dogs.[51] Similar increases in catecholamine levels after administration of succinylcholine to humans are also observed.[52] Other autonomic stimuli, such as endotracheal intubation, hypoxia, hypercapnia, and surgery, may be additive to the effect of succinylcholine. The possible influence of drugs such as digitalis, tricyclic antidepressants, monoamine oxidase inhibitors, exogenous catecholamines, and anesthetic drugs such as halothane and cyclopropane, all of which may lower the ventricular threshold for ectopic activity or increase the arrhythmogenic effect of catecholamines, must also be considered. Ventricular escape beats may also occur as a result of severe sinus and atrioventricular nodal slowing secondary to succinylcholine administration. The development of ventricular dysrhythmias is further encouraged by the release of potassium from skeletal muscle as a consequence of the depolarizing action of the drug.

Hyperkalemia

Administration of succinylcholine to an otherwise well individual for an elective surgical procedure increases plasma potassium levels by approximately 0.5 mEq/dL. This increase in potassium is due to the depolarizing action of the relaxant. With activation of the acetylcholine channels, movement of sodium into the cells is accompanied by movement of potassium out of the cells. This slight increase in potassium is well tolerated by most individuals and generally does not cause dysrhythmias.

Several early reports suggested that patients in renal failure may be susceptible to a hyperkalemic response to succinylcholine.[53] Nevertheless, more controlled studies have shown that such patients are no more susceptible to an exaggerated response to succinylcholine than those with normal renal function are.[54] One might postulate that patients who have uremic neuropathy may be susceptible to succinylcholine-induced hyperkalemia, although the evidence supporting this view is scarce.[53,54]

However, severe hyperkalemia may follow the administration of succinylcholine to patients with severe metabolic acidosis and hypovolemia.[55] In rabbits, the combination of metabolic acidosis and hypovolemia results in a high resting potassium level and an exaggerated hyperkalemic response to succinylcholine.[56] In this situation, the potassium originates from the gastrointestinal tract, not from muscle as in the classic hyperkalemic response.[57] In patients with metabolic acidosis and hypovolemia, correction of the acidosis by hyperventilation and administration of sodium bicarbonate should be attempted before administration of succinylcholine. Should severe hyperkalemia occur, it can be treated with immediate hyperventilation, 1.0 to 2.0 mg of calcium chloride intravenously, 1 mEq/kg of sodium bicarbonate, and 10 units of regular insulin in 50 mL of 50% glucose for adults or, for children, 0.15 units of regular insulin per kilogram in 1.0 mL/kg of 50% glucose.

Kohlschütter and associates[58] found that four of nine patients with severe abdominal infections had an increase in serum potassium levels of as much as 3.1 mEq/L after the administration of succinylcholine. These investigators found that in patients with intra-abdominal infections persisting for longer than 1 week, the possibility of a hyperkalemic response to succinylcholine should be considered.

Stevenson and Birch[59] described a single, well-documented case of a marked hyperkalemic response to succinylcholine in a patient with a closed head injury but no peripheral paralysis.

In studying soldiers who had undergone trauma during the Vietnam War, Birch and colleagues[60] found that a significant increase in serum potassium did not occur in 59 patients until about 1 week after the injury, at which time a progressive increase in the serum potassium level was noted after the infusion of succinylcholine. Three weeks after injury, three of these patients with especially severe trauma showed marked hyperkalemia with an increase in serum potassium of greater than 3.6 mEq/L, sufficient to cause cardiac arrest. Birch and coworkers[60] found that prior administration of 6 mg of dTc prevented the hyperkalemic response to succinylcholine. In the absence of infection or persistent degeneration of tissue, a patient is susceptible to the hyperkalemic response for probably at least 60 days after massive trauma or until adequate healing of damaged muscle has occurred.

In addition, patients with any number of conditions that result in the proliferation of extrajunctional acetylcholine receptors, such as neuromuscular disease, are likely to have an exaggerated hyperkalemic response after the administration of succinylcholine. The response of these patients to neuromuscular blocking agents is reviewed in detail later in this chapter. These disease states include cerebrovascular accident with resultant hemiplegia or paraplegia, muscular dystrophies, and Guillain-Barré syndrome (see also Chapter 37). The hyperkalemia occurring after the administration of succinylcholine may be of such an extent that cardiac arrest ensues. For a recent review on succinylcholine-induced hyperkalemia in patients with acquired pathologic states, see Martyn and Richtsfeld.[61]

Increased Intraocular Pressure

Succinylcholine usually causes an increase in intraocular pressure (IOP). The increased IOP is manifested within 1 minute after injection, peaks at 2 to 4 minutes, and subsides by 6 minutes.[62] The mechanism by which succinylcholine increases IOP has not been clearly defined, but it is known to involve contraction of tonic myofibrils or transient dilatation of choroidal blood vessels (or both). Sublingual administration of nifedipine has been reported to attenuate the increase in IOP from succinylcholine, thus suggesting a circulatory mechanism.[63] Despite this increase in IOP, the use of succinylcholine for eye operations is not contraindicated unless the anterior chamber is open. Although Meyers and associates[64] were unable to confirm the efficacy of precurarization in attenuating increases in IOP after the administration of succinylcholine, numerous other investigators have found that prior administration of a small dose of nondepolarizing neuromuscular blocker (such as 3 mg of dTc or 1 mg of pancuronium) will prevent a succinylcholine-induced increase in IOP.[65] Furthermore, Libonati and coauthors[66] described the anesthetic management of 73 patients with penetrating eye injuries who received succinylcholine; no loss of global contents resulted. Thus, despite the potential concerns of Meyers and coworkers,[64] Libonati and colleagues[66] found that the use of succinylcholine in patients with penetrating eye injuries, after pretreatment with a nondepolarizing neuromuscular blocker and with carefully controlled, rapid-sequence induction of anesthesia, is an acceptable technique. Succinylcholine is only one of many factors, such as endotracheal intubation and "bucking" on the tube, that may elevate IOP.[64] Of prime importance is ensuring that the patient is well anesthetized and not straining or coughing. Because nondepolarizing neuromuscular blockers with shorter times to onset of effect are now available, providing an anesthetic that allows the trachea to be intubated rapidly without administering succinylcholine is now an option. Finally, should a patient's anesthesia become too light over the course of intraocular surgery, succinylcholine should not be given to immobilize the patient. Rather, the surgeon should be asked to pause while the anesthesia is deepened. If necessary, the depth of neuromuscular blockade can also be increased with nondepolarizing relaxants.

Increased Intragastric Pressure

Unlike the rather consistent increase in IOP, the increase in intragastric pressure (IGP) caused by succinylcholine is quite variable. The increase in IGP from succinylcholine is presumed to be due to fasciculations of abdominal skeletal muscle. This is not surprising because more coordinated abdominal skeletal muscle activity (e.g., straight-leg raising) may increase IGP to values as high as 120 cm H_2O. In addition to skeletal muscle fasciculations, the acetylcholine-like effect of succinylcholine may be partly responsible for the observed increases in IGP. Greenan[67] noted consistent increases in IGP of 4 to 7 cm H_2O with direct vagal stimulation.

Miller and Way[68] found that 11 of 30 patients had essentially no increase in IGP after the administration of succinylcholine, yet 5 of the 30 had an increase in IGP of greater than 30 cm H_2O. The increase in IGP from succinylcholine appeared to be related to the intensity of the abdominal skeletal muscle fasciculations. Accordingly, when fasciculations were prevented by prior administration of a nondepolarizing neuromuscular blocker, no increase in IGP was observed.

Are the increases in IGP after succinylcholine administration enough to cause incompetence of the gastroesophageal junction? Generally, an IGP of greater than 28 cm H_2O is required to overcome the competence of the gastroesophageal junction. However, when the normal oblique angle of entry of the esophagus into the stomach is altered, as may occur with pregnancy, an abdomen distended by ascites, bowel obstruction, or a hiatal hernia, the IGP required to cause incompetence of the gastroesophageal junction is frequently less than 15 cm H_2O.[68] In these circumstances, regurgitation of stomach contents after the administration of succinylcholine is a distinct possibility, and precautionary measures should be taken to prevent fasciculation. Endotracheal intubation may be facilitated by administration of either a nondepolarizing neuromuscular blocker or a defasciculating dose of a nondepolarizing relaxant before the succinylcholine.

Apparently, succinylcholine does not increase IGP appreciably in infants and children, which may be related to the minimal or absent fasciculations from succinylcholine in these age groups.[69]

Increased Intracranial Pressure

Succinylcholine has the potential to increase intracranial pressure.[70] The mechanisms and clinical significance of this transient increase are unknown, but the rise in intracranial pressure does not occur after pretreatment with nondepolarizing neuromuscular blockers.[70]

Myalgias

The incidence of muscle pain after the administration of succinylcholine varies from 0.2% to 89%.[71] It occurs more frequently after minor surgery, especially in women and in ambulatory rather than bedridden patients.[72] Waters and Mapleson[72] postulated that the pain is secondary to damage produced in muscle by the unsynchronized contractions of adjacent muscle fibers just before the onset of paralysis. That damage to muscle may occur has been substantiated by finding myoglobinemia and increases in serum creatine kinase after succinylcholine administration.[73] Prior administration of a small dose of a nondepolarizing neuromuscular blocker clearly prevents succinylcholine-related fasciculations.[73] However, the efficacy of this approach in preventing muscle pain is questionable. Although some investigators claim that pretreatment with a defasciculating dose of a nondepolarizing neuromuscular blocker has no effect,[71] many believe that the pain from succinylcholine is at least attenuated.[73] Pretreatment with a prostaglandin inhibitor (e.g., lysine acetyl salicylate) has been shown to be effective in decreasing the incidence of muscle pain after succinylcholine.[74] This suggests a possible role for prostaglandins and cyclooxygenases in succinylcholine-induced myalgias. Other investigators have found that myalgias after outpatient surgery occur even in the absence of succinylcholine.[75]

Masseter Spasm

An increase in tone of the masseter muscle is a frequent response to succinylcholine in adults[76] and children.[77] Meakin and coworkers[77] suggested that the high incidence of spasm in children may be due to an inadequate dosage of succinylcholine. In all likelihood, this increase in tone is an exaggerated contractile response at the neuromuscular junction and cannot be used to establish a diagnosis of malignant hyperthermia. Although an increase in tone of the masseter muscle may be an early indicator of malignant hyperthermia, it is not consistently associated with that syndrome.[78] There is currently no indication to change to a "nontriggering" anesthetic in instances of isolated masseter spasm.[79]

Clinical Uses

Despite its many adverse effects, succinylcholine remains in common use. Its popularity is probably due to its rapid onset of effect, the profound depth of neuromuscular blockade that it produces, and its short duration of action. Although it may be less commonly used than in the past for routine endotracheal intubation, it is the neuromuscular blocker of choice for rapid-sequence induction of anesthesia. In a study comparing intubating conditions after the administration of 1 mg/kg of succinylcholine with those after the administration of 0.1 mg/kg of vecuronium or 0.1 mg/kg of pancuronium 30 seconds after administration of the relaxant and at 30-second intervals after that up for 120 seconds, intubation could be accomplished in all patients receiving succinylcholine at 30 seconds, in contrast with the other neuromuscular blockers studied.[80] Furthermore, at all time points studied up to 90 seconds, intubating conditions were better after the administration of succinylcholine than after either of the other neuromuscular blockers. Although 1.0 mg/kg of succinylcholine has long been recommended to facilitate endotracheal intubation at 60 seconds, a recent study indicated that 0.5 to 0.6 mg/kg of succinylcholine should allow adequate intubating conditions 60 seconds after administration.[81] Reduction of the succinylcholine dose from 1.0 mg/kg to 0.6 mg/kg decreased the incidence of hemoglobin saturation from 85% to 65% but did not shorten the time to spontaneous diaphragmatic movement.[82] However, a significant fraction of patients would be at risk if there were failure to intubate and ventilate regardless of whether succinylcholine is administered or the dose of succinylcholine administered.[82]

A small dose of nondepolarizing neuromuscular blocker is commonly given 2 minutes before the intubating dose of succinylcholine. This defasciculating dose of nondepolarizing neuromuscular blocker will attenuate any increases in IGP and intracranial pressure and minimize the incidence of fasciculations in response to succinylcholine. Prior administration of a

Table 29-2 Clinical Characteristics of Phase 1 and Phase 2 Neuromuscular Blockade during Succinylcholine Infusion

Characteristic	Phase 1	Transition	Phase 2
Tetanic stimulation	No fade	Slight fade	Fade
Post-tetanic facilitation	None	Slight	Yes
Train-of-four fade	No	Moderate fade	Marked fade
Train-of-four ratio	>0.7	0.4-0.7	<0.4
Edrophonium	Augments	Little effect	Antagonizes
Recovery	Rapid	Rapid to slow	Increasingly prolonged
Dose requirements (mg/kg)*	2-3	4-5	>6
Tachyphylaxis	No	Yes	Yes

*Cumulative dosage of succinylcholine by infusion under nitrous oxide anesthesia supplemented with intravenous agents. The dosage required to cause a phase 2 block is less in the presence of potent anesthetic vapors, such as isoflurane.
Adapted from Lee C, Katz RL: Neuromuscular pharmacology. A clinical update and commentary. Br J Anaesth 52:173-188, 1980.

nondepolarizing agent will render the muscle relatively resistant to succinylcholine, however, so the succinylcholine dose should be increased by 50%.[83] The use of a defasciculating dose of a nondepolarizing neuromuscular blocker may also slow the onset of succinylcholine and produce less favorable conditions for tracheal intubation.[73]

Typically after administration of succinylcholine for intubation, a nondepolarizing neuromuscular blocker is given to maintain neuromuscular blockade. Succinylcholine given first may enhance the depth of blockade induced by a subsequent dose of nondepolarizing neuromuscular blocker.[84-86] However, the effect on duration of action is variable. Succinylcholine has no effect on the duration of action of pancuronium, pipecuronium, or mivacurium[86,87] but increases that of atracurium and rocuronium.[84,85] The reasons for these differences are not clear.

The changing characteristics of succinylcholine neuromuscular blockade over the course of prolonged administration have been reviewed by Lee and Katz[88] and are summarized in Table 29-2. TOF stimulation is a very safe and useful guide for detecting the transition from a phase 1 to a phase 2 block. A phase 1 block has all the characteristics of a depolarizing block as described previously in the monitoring section. A phase 2 block has the characteristics of a nondepolarizing block. With the administration of large doses of succinylcholine, the nature of the block, as determined by a neuromuscular blockade monitor, changes from that of a depolarizing agent to that of a nondepolarizing agent. Clearly, both the dose and the duration of administration of succinylcholine are important variables, although the relative contribution of each has not been established. In practical terms, if administration of the drug is terminated shortly after TOF fading is clearly evident, rapid return of normal neuromuscular function should ensue. In addition, the decision whether to attempt antagonism of a phase 2 block has always been controversial. However, if the TOF ratio is less than 0.4, administration of edrophonium or neostigmine should result in prompt antagonism. Ramsey and associates[89] recommended that antagonism of a succinylcholine-induced phase 2 block with edrophonium or neostigmine be attempted after spontaneous recovery of the twitch has been observed for 20 to 30 minutes and has reached a plateau phase with further recovery proceeding slowly. These researchers stated that in this situation, edrophonium and neostigmine invariably produce "dramatic" acceleration of the return of the TOF ratio toward normal.[89] In any event, monitoring neuromuscular function via TOF stimuli will help avoid succinylcholine overdose, detect the development of phase 2 blockade, observe its rate of recovery, and assess the effect of edrophonium or neostigmine on recovery.

A recent study showed that post-tetanic potentiation and fade in response to TOF and tetanic stimuli are characteristics of neuromuscular blockade after bolus administration of different doses of succinylcholine.[25] It seems that some characteristics of phase 2 blockade are evident after an initial dose of succinylcholine (i.e., as small as 0.3 mg/kg).[25]

Interactions with Anticholinesterases

Another interaction with succinylcholine involves neostigmine or pyridostigmine. For example, after dTc has been used for intra-abdominal surgery of long duration and the neuromuscular blockade has been reversed by neostigmine, the surgeon announces that another 15 minutes is needed to retrieve a missing sponge. Succinylcholine should not be administered to reestablish neuromuscular blockade because it produces relaxation that will last up to 60 minutes when given soon after the administration of neostigmine. Sunew and Hicks[36] found that the effect of succinylcholine (1 mg/kg) was prolonged from 11 to 35 minutes when given 5 minutes after the administration of neostigmine (5 mg). This can be partly explained by the inhibition of butyrylcholinesterase by neostigmine and, to a lesser extent, by pyridostigmine. Ninety minutes after the administration of neostigmine, butyrylcholinesterase activity will have returned to less than 50% of its baseline value.

Nondepolarizing Neuromuscular Blockers

The use of neuromuscular blocking drugs in anesthesia has its origin in the South American Indians' arrow poisons or curare. Several nondepolarizing neuromuscular blockers are still purified from naturally occurring sources. For example, although dTc can be synthesized, it is still less expensive to isolate from the Amazonian vine *Chondodendron tomentosum*. Similarly, intermediates for the production of metocurine and alcuronium, which are semisynthetic, are obtained from *Chondodendron* and *Strychnos toxifera*. Malouetine, the first steroidal neuromuscular blocking drug, was originally isolated from *Malouetia bequaertiana*, which grows in the jungles of the Democratic Republic of Congo in central Africa. The agents pancuronium, vecuronium, pipecuronium, rocuronium, rapacuronium, atracurium, doxacurium, mivacurium, cisatracurium, gantacurium, and gallamine are entirely synthetic.

The available nondepolarizing neuromuscular blockers can be classified according to chemical class (steroidal, benzylisoquinolinium, or other compounds) or, alternatively, according to

Table 29-3 Classification of Nondepolarizing Neuromuscular Blockers According to Duration of Action (Time to T1 = 25% of Control) after Twice the ED_{95}

	Clinical Duration			
Class of Blocker	**Long-Acting (>50 min)**	**Intermediate-Acting (20-50 min)**	**Short-Acting (15-20 min)**	**Ultrashort-acting (<10-12 min)**
Steroidal compounds	Pancuronium Pipecuronium	Vecuronium Rocuronium		
Benzylisoquinolinium compounds	*d*-Tubocurarine Metocurine Doxacurium	Atracurium Cisatracurium	Mivacurium	
Others				
Asymmetrical mixed-onium chlorofumarates				Gantacurium
Phenolic ether	Gallamine			
Diallyl derivative of toxiferine	Alcuronium			

A majority of nondepolarizing neuromuscular blockers are bisquaternary ammonium compounds. *d*-Tubocurarine, vecuronium, rocuronium, and rapacuronium are monoquaternary compounds, and gallamine is a trisquaternary ammonium compound.

onset or duration of action (long-, intermediate-, and short-acting drugs) of equipotent doses (Table 29-3).

Structure-Activity Relationships

Nondepolarizing neuromuscular blocking drugs were originally classified by Bovet[27] as pachycurares, or bulky molecules having the amine functions incorporated into rigid ring structures. Two extensively studied chemical series of synthetic nondepolarizing neuromuscular blockers are the aminosteroids (steroidal), in which the interonium distance is maintained by an androstane skeleton, and the benzylisoquinolinium series, in which the distance is maintained by linear diester-containing chains or, in the case of curare, by benzyl ethers. For a detailed account of structure-activity relationships, see Lee.[90]

Benzylisoquinolinium Compounds

dTc is a neuromuscular blocker in which the amines are present in the form of two benzyl-substituted tetrahydroisoquinoline structures (Fig. 29-7). The quaternary or tertiary nature of the two amines was initially questioned; however, with the use of nuclear magnetic resonance spectroscopy and methylation-demethylation studies, Everett and coworkers[91] demonstrated that dTc contains only three *N*-methyl groups. One amine is quaternary (i.e., permanently charged with four nitrogen substituents) and the other is tertiary (i.e., pH-dependent charge with three nitrogen substituents). At physiologic pH, the tertiary nitrogen is protonated to render it positively charged. The structure-activity relationships of the bis-benzylisoquinolines (see Fig. 29-7) have been described by Waser[92] and by Hill and associates[93] as follows:

1. The nitrogen atoms are incorporated into isoquinoline ring systems. This bulky molecule favors nondepolarizing rather than depolarizing activity.
2. The interonium distance (distance between charged amines) is approximately 1.4 nm.
3. Both the ganglion-blocking and the histamine-releasing properties of dTc are probably due to the presence of the tertiary amine function.
4. When dTc is methylated at the tertiary amine and at the hydroxyl groups, the result is metocurine, a compound with greater potency (by a factor of 2 in humans) but much weaker ganglion-blocking and histamine-releasing properties than dTc has (see Fig. 29-7). Metocurine contains three additional methyl groups, one of which quaternizes the tertiary nitrogen of dTc; the other two form methyl ethers at the phenolic hydroxyl groups.
5. Bisquaternary compounds are more potent than their monoquaternary analogs. The bisquaternary derivative of dTc, chondocurine, has more than double the potency of dTc (Fig. 29-7).
6. Substitution of the methyl groups on the quaternary nitrogen with bulkier groups causes a reduction in both potency and duration of action.

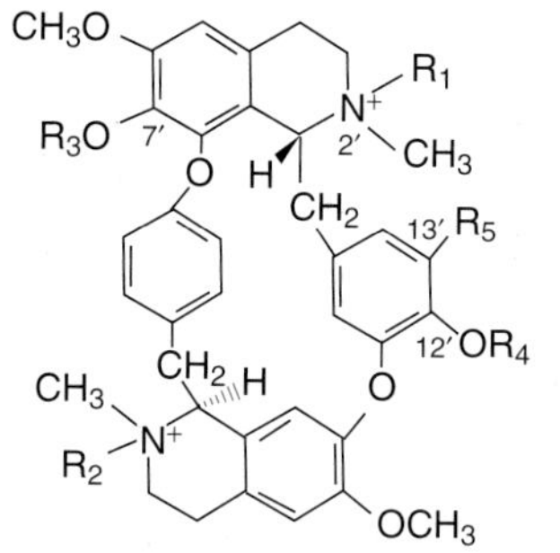

Cyclic benzylisoquinoline

Cyclic benzylisoquinoline derivatives

Name	R_1	R_2	R_3	R_4	R_5	1	1'
d-Tubocurarine	CH_3	H	H	H	H	*S*	*R*
Metocurine	CH_3	CH_3	CH_3	CH_3	H	*S*	*R*
Chondocurine	CH_3	CH_3	H	H	H	*S*	*R*

R and S represent the stereochemical configuration about the designated carbon

Figure 29-7 Chemical structures of *d*-tubocurarine, metocurine, and chondocurine.

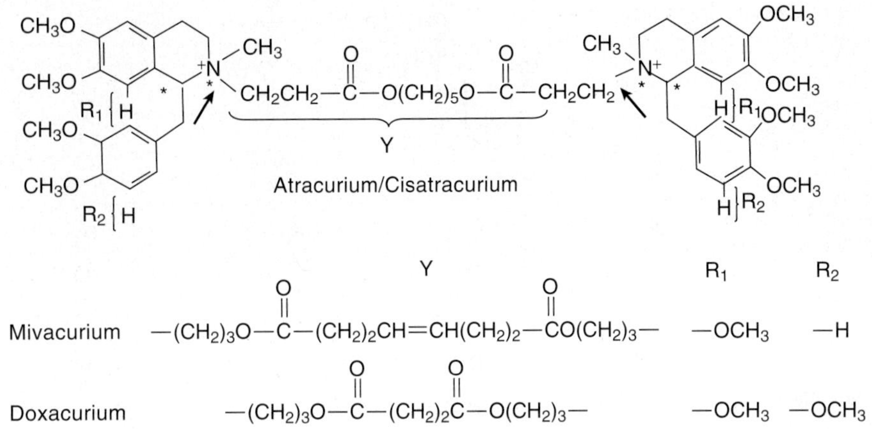

Figure 29-8 Chemical structures of atracurium, cisatracurium, mivacurium, and doxacurium. The *asterisks* indicate chiral centers; *arrows* show cleavage sites for Hofmann elimination.

Atracurium is a bis-benzyltetrahydroisoquinolinium with isoquinolinium nitrogens connected by a diester-containing hydrocarbon chain (Fig. 29-8). The presence (in duplicate) of two-carbon separations between quaternary nitrogen and ester carbonyl provides the basis for a Hofmann elimination reaction.[94] Furthermore, it can undergo ester hydrolysis. In a Hofmann elimination reaction, a quaternary ammonium group is converted to a tertiary amine by cleavage of a carbon-nitrogen bond. This is a pH- and temperature-dependent reaction in which higher pH and temperature favor elimination. The actual structure of the quaternary centers is the laudanosinium moiety, as in metocurine. Atracurium has four chiral centers at each of the adjacent chiral carbons of the two amines. The marketed product has 10 isomers.[94] These isomers have been separated into three geometric isomer groups that are designated *cis-cis*, *cis-trans*, and *trans-trans* according to their configuration about the tetrahydroisoquinoline ring system.[94] The ratio of the *cis-cis*, *cis-trans*, and *trans-trans* isomers is approximately 10:6:1, which corresponds to 50% to 55% *cis-cis*, 35% to 38% *cis-trans*, and 6% to 7% *trans-trans* isomers.

Cisatracurium is the 1R *cis*–1′R *cis* isomer of atracurium and represents about 15% of the marketed atracurium mixture by weight but more than 50% in terms of potency or neuromuscular blocking activity (see Fig. 29-8). R designates the absolute stereochemistry of the benzyl tetrahydroisoquinoline rings and *cis* represents the relative geometry of the bulky dimethoxy and 2-alkyester groups at C(1) and N(1), respectively.[95,96] Cisatracurium is metabolized by Hofmann elimination. It is approximately four times as potent as atracurium, but unlike atracurium, it does not cause release of histamine in the clinical dose range.[95,97] This indicates that the phenomenon of histamine release may be stereospecific.[95,98] Cisatracurium is the second benzylisoquinolinium (after doxacurium) to be largely free of this side effect.

Mivacurium differs from atracurium by the presence of an additional methylated phenolic group (see Fig. 29-8). When compared with other isoquinolinium neuromuscular blockers, the interonium chain of mivacurium is longer (16 atoms).[93] Mivacurium consists of a mixture of three stereoisomers.[99] The two most active are the *trans-trans* and *cis-trans* isomers (57% and 37% wt/wt, respectively), which are equipotent; the *cis-cis* isomer (6% wt/wt) has only a 10th the activity of the others in cats and monkeys.[99] Mivacurium is metabolized by butyrylcholinesterase at 70% to 88% the rate of succinylcholine to a monoester, a dicarboxylic acid.[9]

Doxacurium is a bisquaternary benzylisoquinolinium diester of succinic acid (see Fig. 29-8). The interonium chain is shorter than that of either atracurium or mivacurium. Lee[90] pointed out that the number of methoxy groups on benzylisoquinolinium heads is increased from four (atracurium) and five (mivacurium) to six (doxacurium).[93] This increase was associated with both an increase in potency and a reduction in the propensity to release histamine.[90,93]

Steroidal Neuromuscular Blockers

In the steroidal compounds, it is probably essential that one of two nitrogen atoms in the molecule be quaternized. The presence of acetyl ester (acetylcholine-like moiety) is thought to facilitate its interaction with nAChRs at the postsynaptic muscle membrane.

Pancuronium is characterized by the presence of two acetyl ester groups on the A and D rings of the steroidal molecule. Pancuronium is a potent neuromuscular blocking drug with both vagolytic and butyrylcholinesterase-inhibiting properties (Fig. 29-9).[100] Deacetylation of the 3-OH or 17-OH groups decreases its potency.[101]

Vecuronium is the *N*-demethylated derivative of pancuronium in which the 2-piperidine substituent is not methylated (i.e., vecuronium lacks the *N*-methyl group at position 2) (see Fig. 29-9).[7] At physiologic pH, the tertiary amine is largely protonated, as it is in dTc. The minor molecular modification relative to pancuronium results in (1) a slight change in potency; (2) a marked reduction in vagolytic properties; (3) molecular instability in solution, which explains in part the shorter duration of action of vecuronium than pancuronium; and (4) increased lipid solubility, which results in greater biliary elimination of vecuronium than pancuronium.[93]

Pancuronium and vecuronium are very similar in structure, yet vecuronium is prepared as a lyophilized powder. Vecuronium is degraded by the hydrolysis of acetyl esters at either or both the C3 and C17 positions. Hydrolysis at the C3 position is the primary degradation product. The acetate at position 3 is more susceptible to hydrolysis in aqueous solutions. Vecuronium is less stable in solution because of the group effect of the adjacent basic piperidine at position 2, which facilitates hydrolysis of the 3-acetate. Therefore, vecuronium cannot be prepared as a ready-to-use solution with a sufficient shelf life, even as a buffered solution. In pancuronium, the 2-piperidine is quaternized and no

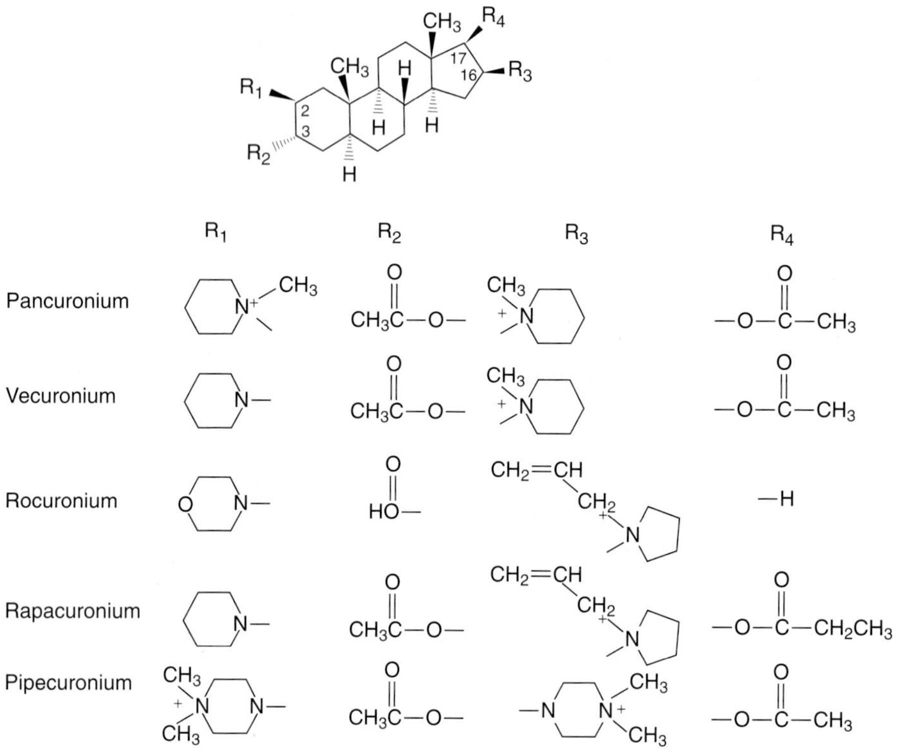

Figure 29-9 Chemical structures of different steroidal neuromuscular blockers.

longer alkaline. Thus, it does not participate in catalysis of the 3-acetate hydrolysis.

Pipecuronium, like pancuronium, is a bisquaternary compound. Pipecuronium has piperazine rings attached to the A and D rings of the steroid nucleus, whereas pancuronium has piperidine rings (see Fig. 29-9).[93] Pipecuronium is a nonvagolytic substitute for pancuronium. Changes in the quaternary groups in which the quaternary nitrogen atoms are placed at the distal (4-position) aspect of the 2,16-β-substitutions lessen the vagolytic effects.[93] As a result, pipecuronium is about 10 times less vagolytic than pancuronium.

Rocuronium lacks the acetyl ester that is found in the steroid nucleus of pancuronium and vecuronium in the A ring (see Fig. 29-9). The introduction of cyclic substituents other than piperidine at the 2- and 16-positions results in a fast-onset compound.[102] The methyl group attached to the quaternary nitrogen of vecuronium and pancuronium is replaced by an allyl group in rocuronium. As a result, rocuronium is about 6 and 10 times less potent than vecuronium and pancuronium, respectively.[102-104] Replacement of the acetyl ester attached to the A ring by a hydroxy group has made it possible to present rocuronium as a stable solution. At room temperature, rocuronium is stable for only 60 days, whereas pancuronium is stable for 6 months. The reason for this difference in shelf life is related to the fact that rocuronium is terminally sterilized in manufacturing and pancuronium is not. Terminal sterilization causes some degree of degradation.

Asymmetric Mixed-Onium Chlorofumarates

Gantacurium (Fig. 29-10) represents a new class of nondepolarizing neuromuscular blockers called asymmetric mixed-onium chlorofumarates. The presence of three methyl groups between the quaternary nitrogen and oxygen atom at each end of the carbon chain suggests that similar to mivacurium, this compound will not undergo Hofmann elimination.[105] Gantacurium has an ultrashort duration of action in human volunteers and in different animal species. A study in anesthetized human volunteers using an earlier formulation of gantacurium estimated the ED_{95} to be 0.19 mg/kg.[106] The pattern of blockade resembled that of succinylcholine. The time to onset of 90% blockade ranged from 1.3 to 2.1 minutes, depending on the dose. Clinical durations ranged from 4.7 to 10.1 minutes and increased with increasing dose. Spontaneous recovery to a TOF of 0.9 develops in the thumb within about 12 to 15 minutes after the administration of doses as large as 0.54 mg/kg (or three times the ED_{95}). Recovery is accelerated by edrophonium. Transient cardiovascular side effects were observed at doses beginning at three times the ED_{95} and were suggestive of histamine release.[106]

Phenolic Ether Derivative

Gallamine is a trisquaternary compound (Fig. 29-11). Its potent vagolytic activity is due to the presence of three positively charged nitrogen atoms. Gallamine was originally synthesized by Bovet[27] as part of an extensive structure-activity study that helped evolve the concepts of "pachycurares" and "leptocurares." Succinylcholine also evolved from this work, for which Bovet received the Nobel Prize.

Diallyl Derivative of Toxiferine

Introduced in 1964, alcuronium is a long-acting agent that is the semisynthetic diallyl derivative of toxiferine (Fig. 29-12). The latter is purified from *Strychnos toxifera*. The advantage of alcuronium at the time of its introduction was a relative lack of side effects. It is mildly vagolytic and is excreted unchanged by the kidney with a minor secondary biliary pathway.

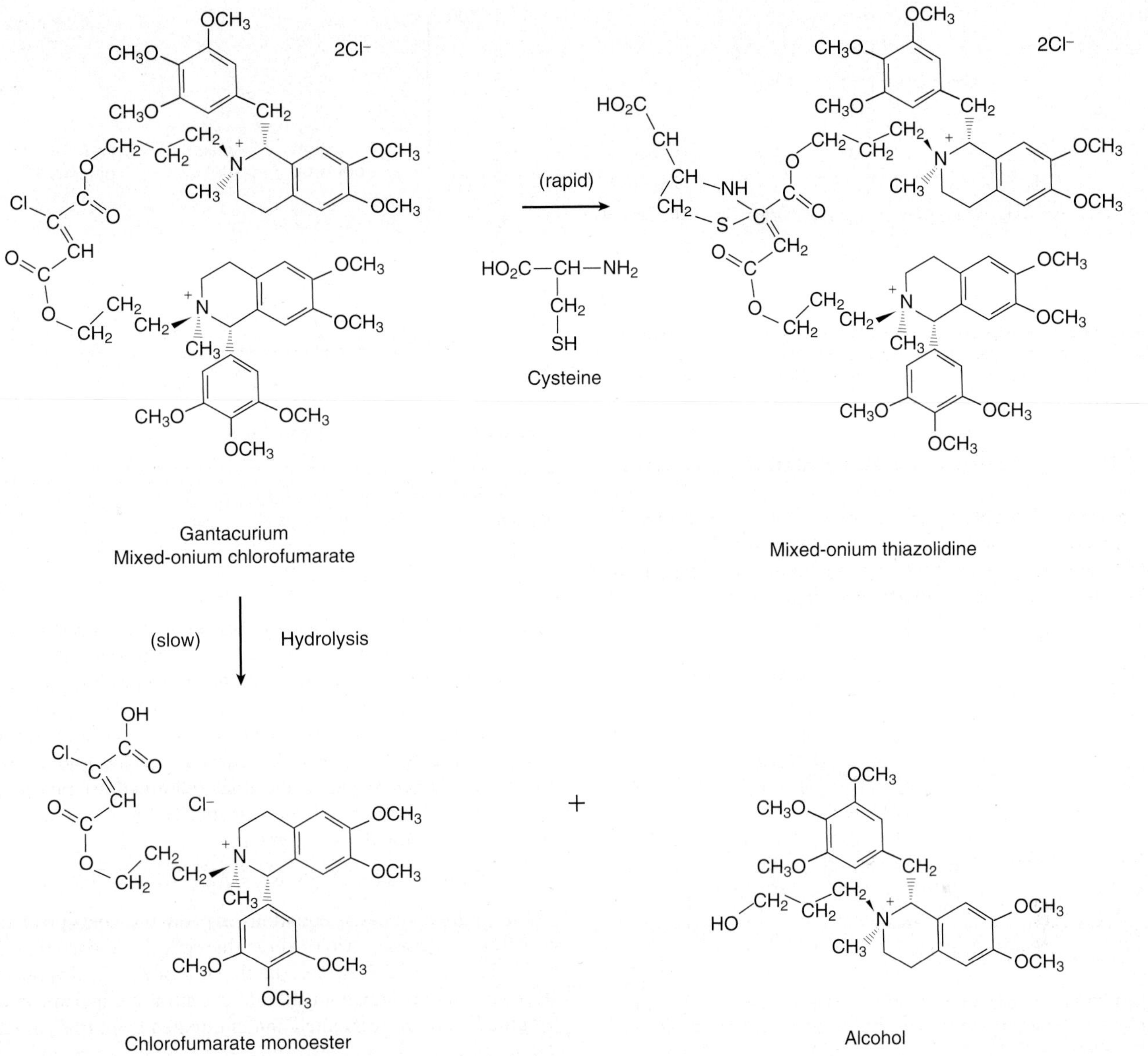

Figure 29-10 Chemical structure of gantacurium (a mixed-onium chlorofumarate). In whole human blood, two pathways of deactivation occur, neither of which is enzymatic: (1) rapid formation of an apparently inactive cysteine adduction product, with cysteine replacing chlorine, and (2) slower hydrolysis of the ester bond adjacent to the chlorine substitution to chlorofumarate monoester and alcohol. *(From Boros EE, Samano V, Ray JA, et al: Neuromuscular blocking activity and therapeutic potential of mixed-tetrahydroisoquinolinium halofumarates and halosuccinates in rhesus monkeys. J Med Chem 46:2502-2515, 2003.)*

Potency of Nondepolarizing Neuromuscular Blockers

Drug potency is commonly expressed by the dose-response relationship. The dose of a neuromuscular blocking drug required to produce an effect (e.g., 50%, 90%, or 95% depression of twitch height, commonly expressed as ED_{50}, ED_{90}, and ED_{95}, respectively) is taken as a measure of its potency.[9,11,103,107-117] The neuromuscular blocking drugs have different potencies, as illustrated in Table 29-4 and Figure 29-13. For factors affecting the potency of neuromuscular blockers, see the section on drug interactions later in this chapter. The dose-response relationship for nondepolarizing neuromuscular blockers is sigmoidal in shape (see Fig. 29-13) and has been derived in various ways. The simplest method is to perform linear regression over the approximately linear portion of a semilogarithmic plot between 25% and 75% neuromuscular blockade. Alternatively, the curve can be subjected to probit or logit transformation to linearize it over its whole length or can be subjected to nonlinear regression using the sigmoid E_{max} model of the form

$$\text{Effect}(e) = .\backslash F\left(\text{dose}_e^{\gamma}, \text{dose}_e^{\gamma} + \text{dose}_{e50}^{\gamma}\right)$$

This can be applied to the raw data.[119] More complex models relating the concentration of neuromuscular blockers at the neuromuscular junction to their pharmacologic effect have been developed, as discussed later.[120,121]

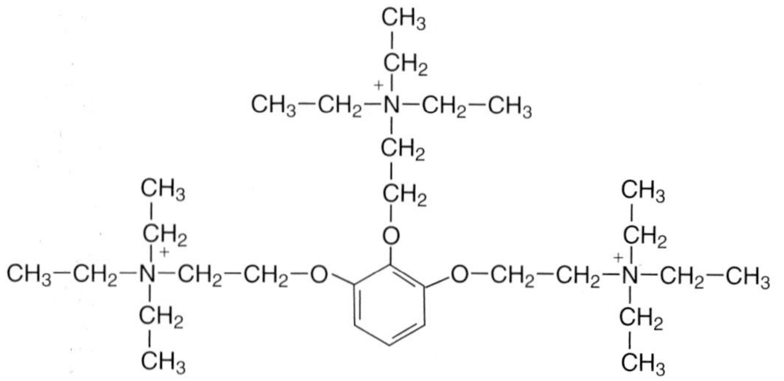

Figure 29-11 Chemical structure of gallamine, a trisquaternary ether of gallic acid. Gallamine is the only trisquaternary compound available. Its strong vagolytic property is probably due to its trisquaternary structure.

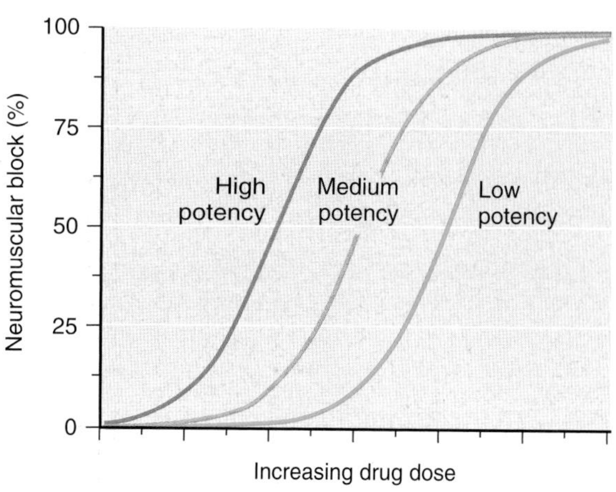

Figure 29-13 Schematic representation of a semilogarithmic plot of a muscle relaxant dose versus neuromuscular blockade. A drug of high potency is doxacurium; one of medium potency, atracurium; and one of low potency, gallamine. The graph illustrates that the relative potencies of muscle relaxants span a range of approximately 2 orders of magnitude.

Pharmacokinetics and Pharmacodynamics

As defined by Wright,[122] pharmacokinetics and pharmacodynamics are "empirical mathematical model[s] ... that [describe] drug effect time course after administration." In pharmacokinetic modeling, the concept of "compartments" represents different organs or tissues (or both) grouped together on the basis of their degree of blood perfusion (high or low). After a neuromuscular blocker is injected into the circulation, its concentration in plasma decreases rapidly at first and then more slowly (Fig. 29-14). The shape of this curve is determined by the processes of distribution and elimination. Classically, this curve is divided into an initial (distribution) phase and a terminal (elimination) phase. This curve can be represented mathematically by biexponential or triexponential equations in the form

$$\text{Concentration (at time t)} = Ae^{-\alpha t} + Be^{-\beta t}(+Pe^{-\pi t})$$

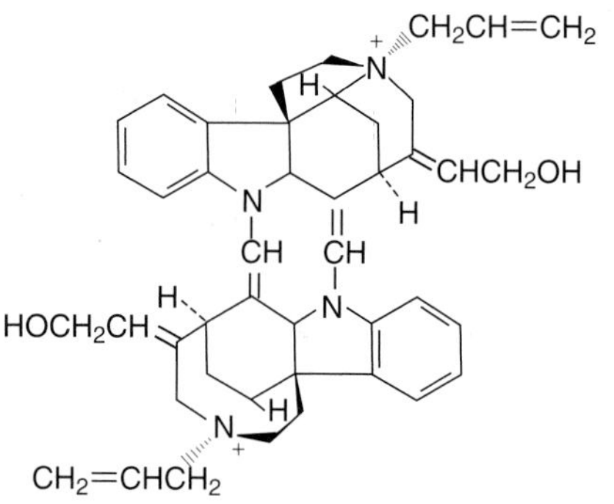

These multiexponential equations express the concept of drug distribution between two or three theoretical compartments.

Figure 29-15 illustrates the classic model, in which the drug is administered intravenously into a central compartment with volume V_1 and is distributed and eliminated from this compartment only. The drug is distributed very rapidly throughout this

Figure 29-12 Chemical structure of alcuronium, the semisynthetic diallyl derivative of toxiferine. The quaternizing allyl groups actually reduce its potency by a factor of 3 to 5.

Table 29-4 Dose-Response Relationships of Nondepolarizing Neuromuscular Blocking Drugs in Human Subjects

	ED_{50} (mg/kg)	ED_{90} (mg/kg)	ED_{95} (mg/kg)	Reference(s)
Long-Acting				
Pancuronium	0.036 (0.022-0.042)	0.056 (0.044-0.070)	0.067 (0.059-0.080)	103, 107
d-Tubocurarine	0.23 (0.16-0.26)	0.41 (0.27-0.45)	0.48 (0.34-0.56)	107
Intermediate-Acting				
Rocuronium	0.147 (0.069-0.220)	0.268 (0.200-0.419)	0.305 (0.257-0.521)	103, 108-110
Vecuronium	0.027 (0.015-0.031)	0.042 (0.023-0.055)	0.043 (0.037-0.059)	107
Atracurium	0.12 (0.08-0.15)	0.18 (0.19-0.24)	0.21 (0.13-0.28)	107
Cisatracurium	0.026 (0.015-0.031)	—	0.04 (0.032-0.05)	11, 111, 112, 118
Short-Acting				
Mivacurium	0.039 (0.027-0.052)	—	0.067 (0.045-0.081)	9, 113-115
Ultrashort-Acting				
Gantacurium	0.09	—	0.19	106

Data are medians and ranges of reported values. ED_{50}, ED_{90}, and ED_{95} are the doses of each drug that produce, respectively, a 50%, 90%, and 95% decrease in the force of contraction or amplitude of the electromyogram of the adductor pollicis muscle after ulnar nerve stimulation.

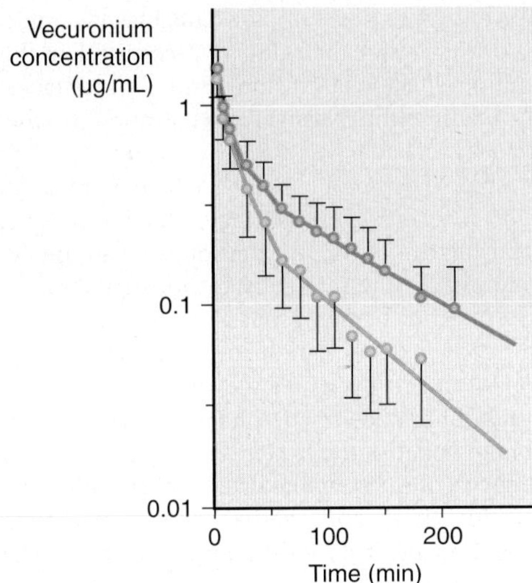

Figure 29-14 Disappearance of vecuronium from plasma after a single bolus dose of 0.2 mg/kg as shown in a semilogarithmic plot of mean concentration versus time for patients with normal hepatic function (*yellow circles*) and cirrhotic patients (*blue circles*). *Error bars* are the standard deviation for that value. *(From Lebrault C, Berger JL, D'Hollander AA, et al: Pharmacokinetics and pharmacodynamics of vecuronium (ORG NC 45) in patients with cirrhosis. Anesthesiology 62:601-605, 1985.)*

central compartment, which includes the plasma volume and the organs of elimination; in the case of neuromuscular blockers, the organs of elimination are the kidneys and liver. The "k" terms are the rate constants for movement of drug between compartments in the direction of the arrows. The peripheral compartments (usually one or two, here represented by V_2 and V_3) can be thought of as the "tissues." The "effect" compartment, which will be discussed later, is the neuromuscular junction. For computational purposes, it has infinitesimal volume and therefore does not influence overall drug distribution. Drug administration and elimination are unidirectional; distribution is bidirectional.

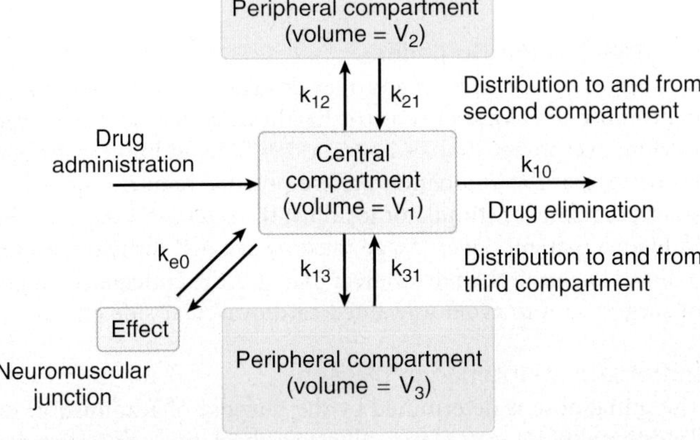

Figure 29-15 Schematic representation of drug disposition into different compartments. These compartments are mathematical concepts only and do not represent real physiologic spaces. The effect compartment in this case would be the neuromuscular junction; for computational purposes, it has infinitesimal volume. The terms k_{nm} are the rate constants for drug movement, in the direction of the *arrow*, between these theoretical compartments. See text for further discussion.

Initially, the drug concentration in the central compartment (i.e., the plasma concentration) will exceed that in the peripheral compartment (i.e., the tissue concentration), and the drug will move from plasma to tissues. Later, as the plasma concentration decreases, it becomes less than the tissue concentration, and the net direction of drug movement is now from tissues to plasma. In general, this conceptual model is appropriate for all the neuromuscular blockers, with the exception of atracurium and cisatracurium, which also undergo elimination (by degradation) from tissues.[123] For simplicity, the following discussion assumes the presence of only one peripheral compartment.

The volume of distribution is the volume to which the drug has distributed when the processes of distribution and elimination are in equilibrium. Elimination is represented by the variable plasma clearance, that is, the volume of plasma from which the drug is irreversibly and completely eliminated per unit time. For most nondepolarizing neuromuscular blockers, the process of distribution is more rapid than the process of elimination, and the initial rapid decline in plasma concentration is due primarily to distribution of the drug to tissues. An exception to this rule is mivacurium, which has such rapid clearance, because of metabolism by butyrylcholinesterase, that elimination is the principal determinant of the initial decline in plasma concentration.

After the initial process of drug distribution to tissues, the plasma concentration falls more slowly (the terminal phase). The rate of decrease in plasma concentration during this terminal phase is often expressed in terms of elimination half-life, which equals the natural logarithm of 2 divided by the rate constant of decline (i.e., the slope of the terminal phase). During this terminal phase, the concentration of drug in the tissue exceeds that in plasma, and the rate of decrease in plasma concentration is determined by two factors: the rate at which drug can move from tissues back into plasma and clearance of drug from plasma. In classic theory for neuromuscular blockers, the drug can move rapidly from tissues into plasma, and its elimination from plasma (i.e., clearance) is the rate-limiting step. For this reason, the terminal portion of the curve is often termed the elimination phase, even though the distribution of drug from tissues into plasma occurs continually throughout. The volume of distribution can also influence the terminal portion of the curve: the greater the volume of distribution, the slower the decline in plasma concentration.

The neuromuscular blockers are polar drugs, and their volume of distribution is classically thought to be limited to a volume roughly equivalent to a portion of the extracellular fluid space, namely, 150 to 450 mL/kg (see Tables 29-13 and 29-14).[124] With this model of drug distribution, the potential rate of drug movement from tissues to plasma exceeds the rate of elimination, and plasma clearance is the process that limits the rate of decline in plasma drug concentration. However, there is evidence that neuromuscular blockers are distributed more widely into tissues with low blood flow (e.g., connective tissue),[125] and the true volume of distribution of dTc has been estimated to be as high as 3.4 L/kg and its elimination half-life as long as 40 hours (compare with values in Tables 29-13 and 29-14).[126] Because the rate of drug movement from such tissues is less than that of plasma clearance, this becomes the limiting step in the rate of decline in plasma drug concentration. This phase becomes obvious only when drug is administered for many days or when sampling is continued for 24 to 96 hours after drug administration. In normal operating room use of neuromuscular blockers, the amount of drug that is

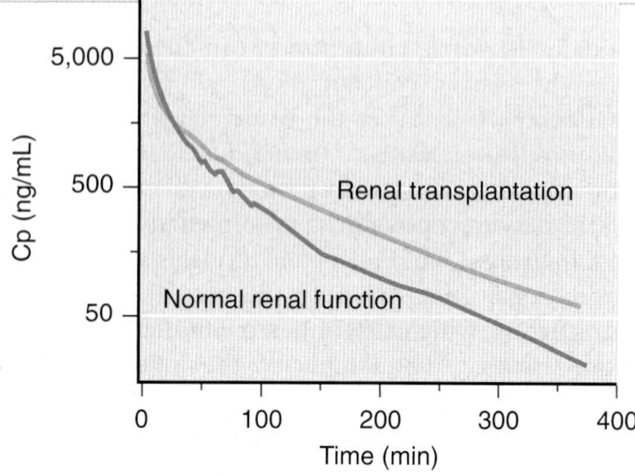

Figure 29-16 "Average" plasma concentration (Cp) versus time after a dose of 0.6 mg/kg rocuronium in patients with normal renal function (*blue line*) or patients undergoing renal transplantation (*yellow line*). *(From Szenohradszky J, Fisher DM, Segredo V, et al: Pharmacokinetics of rocuronium bromide (ORG 9426) in patients with normal renal function or patients undergoing cadaver renal transplantation. Anesthesiology 77:899-904, 1992.)*

distributed to this compartment does not affect clinical response to the drug. In conditions in which clearance of the neuromuscular blocker is reduced, such as renal or hepatic disease, the terminal portion of the plasma concentration-versus-time curve is most affected (see Fig. 29-14).[127] The rate of decline in plasma concentration is slowed, and recovery from paralysis is potentially delayed.[127] In conditions associated with an increased volume of distribution, such as renal or hepatic disease, early plasma concentrations of drug may be less than those observed when organ function is normal: with a greater volume of distribution, the plasma concentration should be less, whereas the total amount of a drug would be greater (Fig. 29-16). Decreased protein binding of a drug results in a larger distribution volume, but because the degree of protein binding of neuromuscular blockers is small, changes in protein binding will have minimal effect on their distribution.[128]

Recovery of neuromuscular function takes place as plasma concentrations decline, and the greater part of this decrease occurs primarily because of distribution. Thus, processes that primarily affect elimination of the drug, such as renal failure, may not be associated with prolonged duration of blockade.[129,130] However, as recovery comes to rely more on drug elimination than on distribution (i.e., from 25% to 75% or greater) or after the administration of larger or repeated doses, the duration of action may be prolonged.[123,131]

After the injection of a neuromuscular blocker, the plasma drug concentration immediately starts to decrease. The effect (neuromuscular blockade) takes approximately 1 minute to begin, increases initially, and does not start to recover for many more minutes despite the continually decreasing plasma concentration of drug. This discrepancy between plasma concentration and drug effect occurs because the action of neuromuscular blockers is not in plasma but at the neuromuscular junction. To produce paralysis, the drug must diffuse from plasma into the neuromuscular junction, and the effect is terminated later by diffusion of drug back into plasma (see Fig. 29-15). Thus, concentrations at the neuromuscular junction lag behind those in plasma, and they are lower during the onset of blockade and greater during recovery. The plasma concentration-effect relationship exhibits hysteresis; that is, for a given level of blockade, plasma concentrations are greater during onset than during recovery. For this reason, a concentration-effect relationship cannot be obtained simply by directly relating the plasma concentration to the level of neuromuscular blockade.

To overcome this problem, pharmacodynamic models have been developed to incorporate a factor for the delay caused by diffusion of drug to and from the neuromuscular junction.[84,120,132-143] This factor, k_{e0}, is the rate constant for equilibration of drug between plasma and the neuromuscular junction. By measuring plasma drug concentrations and neuromuscular blockade during both the onset and recovery phases and using the technique of simultaneous pharmacokinetic/pharmacodynamic modeling, it is possible to collapse the hysteresis in the plasma concentration-effect curve, estimate actual drug concentrations at the neuromuscular junction, and derive true concentration-effect relationships (Ce_{50} and k_{e0}) for the neuromuscular blockers (Table 29-5).[120]

Clinical Management

Neuromuscular blockers are used mainly to facilitate tracheal intubation and provide surgical relaxation. The intensity of neuromuscular blockade required varies with the surgical procedure. Important safety issues arise with the use of neuromuscular blockers: cardiovascular and respiratory side effects and the adequacy of recovery to normal neuromuscular function.

Several clinical alternatives to neuromuscular blockers are available that provide adequate surgical relaxation. It is important to keep them all in mind to avoid relying only on neuromuscular blockade to achieve a desired degree of relaxation. Such options include adjustment of the depth of general anesthesia, the use of regional anesthesia, proper positioning of the patient on the operating table, and proper adjustment of the depth of neuromuscular blockade. The choice of one or several of these options is determined by the estimated remaining duration of surgery, the anesthetic technique, and the surgical maneuver required.

Dosage

General Dosage Guidelines

It is important to select the proper dosage of a nondepolarizing neuromuscular blocker to ensure that the desired effect is achieved without overdosage (Tables 29-6 and 29-7). In addition to general knowledge of the guidelines, precise practice requires the use of a peripheral nerve stimulator to adjust the relaxant dosage for the individual patient. Overdosage must be avoided for two reasons: to limit the duration of drug effect to match the anticipated length of surgery and to avoid unwanted cardiovascular side effects.

Initial and Maintenance Dosage

The initial dose is determined by the purpose of administration. Traditionally, doses used to facilitate tracheal intubation are twice the ED_{95} (this also approximates four times the ED_{50}) (see Table 29-6). If the trachea has already been intubated without the use of a nondepolarizing blocker or with succinylcholine and the purpose is simply to produce surgical relaxation, a dose slightly less than the ED_{95} (see Table 29-7) should be given, with adjustment upward as indicated by responses evoked by peripheral

Table 29-5 Pharmacodynamic Parameters Derived by Simultaneous Pharmacokinetic/Pharmacodynamic Modeling

	Study Group	Adductor Pollicis		Reference
		Ce_{50}* (ng/mL)	k_{eo}† (min^{-1})	
Mivacurium				
Central link		57	0.169	132
Peripheral link		130	0.101	132
Rocuronium	Adult female: Propofol-remifentanil anesthesia, standard model	684	0.329	133
	Recirculatory model	876	0.129	133
	Volunteers: Propofol-fentanyl anesthesia	3510	0.405	134
	Infants	1190	0.25	135
	Children	1650	0.32	135
Cisatracurium, 0.075-3.0 mg/kg	Adults: Propofol-fentanyl anesthesia	126-158	0.07-0.09	135
Atracurium	Infants	363	0.19	137
	Children	444	0.16	137
	Young adults	449	0.13	138
	Elderly adults	436	0.12	138
	Standard model	359	0.12	139
	Threshold model	357	0.12	139
	Young adults	669‡	0.07	140
	Burn patients	2270‡	0.10	140
	No succinylcholine	454‡	0.07	84
	After succinylcholine	305‡	0.09	84
Vecuronium	Young adults	94	—	141
	Young adults	92	0.17	142
	Elderly adults	106	0.17	143
d-Tubocurarine	Normal renal function	370	0.13	120
	Renal failure	380	0.16	120
	Halothane, 0.5%-0.7%	360‡	0.09‡	143§
	Halothane, 1.0%-1.2%	220‡	0.12	143§
	Narcotic anesthesia	600‡	0.15‡	143§
Pancuronium	Young adults	88	—	141

*Ce_{50} is the concentration of each drug at the neuromuscular junction that produces a 50% decrease in the force of contraction or amplitude of the electromyogram of the adductor pollicis muscle after ulnar nerve stimulation.

†k_{eo} is the rate constant for equilibration of drug between plasma and the neuromuscular junction.

‡All groups different from each other.

§k_{eo} values calculated as 0.693/ $t_{½}k_{eo}$.

nerve stimulation. Downward adjustment of the initial dose is necessary in the presence of any of the potent inhaled anesthetics (see the subsection later on drug interactions).

To avoid prolonged residual paralysis, inadequate antagonism of residual blockade, or both, the main goal should be to use the lowest possible dose that will provide adequate relaxation for surgery. Management of individual patients should always be guided by monitoring with a peripheral nerve stimulator. In an adequately anesthetized and monitored patient, there is little reason to completely abolish twitch or TOF responses to peripheral nerve stimulation during maintenance of relaxation. Supplemental (maintenance) doses of neuromuscular blockers should be about one-fourth (in the case of intermediate- and short-acting neuromuscular blockers) to one-tenth (in the case of long-acting neuromuscular blockers) the initial dose and should not be given until there is clear evidence of beginning of recovery from the previous dose.

Maintenance of relaxation by continuous infusion of intermediate- and short-acting drugs can be performed and is useful to keep the relaxation smooth and to rapidly adjust the depth of relaxation according to surgical needs. The depth of blockade in each patient is kept moderate, if possible, to ensure prompt spontaneous recovery or easy reversal at the end of the procedure. Table 29-6 lists the approximate dose ranges that are usually required during infusion to maintain 90% to 95% blockade of the twitch (one twitch visible on TOF stimulation) under nitrous oxide–oxygen anesthesia supplemented with intravenous anesthetics. The infusion dosage is usually decreased by 30% to 50% in the presence of potent inhaled anesthetics.

Neuromuscular Blockers and Tracheal Intubation

The speed of onset of neuromuscular blockade is one of the requirements for rapidly securing the airway, and it is affected by several factors, including the rate of delivery of drug to the

Table 29-6 Guide to Nondepolarizing Relaxant Dosage (mg/kg) with Different Anesthetic Techniques*

	ED_{95} under N_2O/O_2	Dose for Intubation	Supplemental Dose after Intubation	Dosage for Relaxation	
				N_2O	Anesthetic Vapors†
Long-Acting					
Pancuronium	0.07	0.08-0.12	0.02	0.05	0.03
d-Tubocurarine	0.5	0.5-0.6	0.1	0.3	0.15
Intermediate-Acting					
Vecuronium	0.05	0.1-0.2	0.02	0.05	0.03
Atracurium	0.23	0.5-0.6	0.1	0.3	0.15
Cisatracurium	0.05	0.15-0.2	0.02	0.05	0.04
Rocuronium	0.3	0.6-1.0	0.1	0.3	0.15
Short-Acting					
Mivacurium	0.08	0.2-0.25	0.05	0.1	0.08
Continuous Infusion Dosage (μg/kg/min) Required to Maintain 90%-95% Twitch Inhibition under N_2O/O_2 with Intravenous Agents					
Mivacurium	3-15				
Atracurium	4-12				
Cisatracurium	1-2				
Vecuronium	0.8-1.0				
Rocuronium	9-12				

*The suggested dosages provide good intubating conditions under light anesthesia. Satisfactory abdominal relaxation may be achieved at the dosages listed after intubation without a relaxant or with succinylcholine. This table is intended as a general guide to dosage. Individual relaxant requirements should be confirmed with a peripheral nerve stimulator.

†The potentiation of nondepolarizing relaxants by different anesthetic vapors has been reported to vary 20% to 50%. Recent data suggest, however, that this variation may be much less, particularly in the case of intermediate- and short-acting relaxants. Therefore, for the sake of simplicity, this table assumes a potentiation of 40% in the case of all volatile anesthetics.

neuromuscular junction, receptor affinity, plasma clearance, and the mechanism of neuromuscular blockade (depolarizing versus nondepolarizing).[101,155,156] The speed of onset is inversely proportional to the potency of nondepolarizing neuromuscular blockers.[101,155] A high ED_{95} (i.e., low potency) is predictive of rapid onset of effect and vice versa (Fig. 29-17; Table 29-7). Except for atracurium,[157] the molar potency (the ED_{50} or ED_{95} expressed as μM/kg) is highly predictive of a drug's initial rate of onset of effect (at the adductor pollicis).[155] A drug's measured molar potency is the end result of many contributing factors: the drug's intrinsic potency (Ce_{50}—the biophase concentration resulting in 50% twitch depression), the rate of equilibration between plasma and the biophase (k_{e0}), the initial rate of plasma clearance, and probably other factors as well.[158] Rocuronium has a molar potency (ED_{95}) of 0.54 μM/kg, which is about 13% that of vecuronium and only 9% that of cisatracurium. Thus, rapid onset of rocuronium's effect (at the adductor pollicis) is not unexpected.

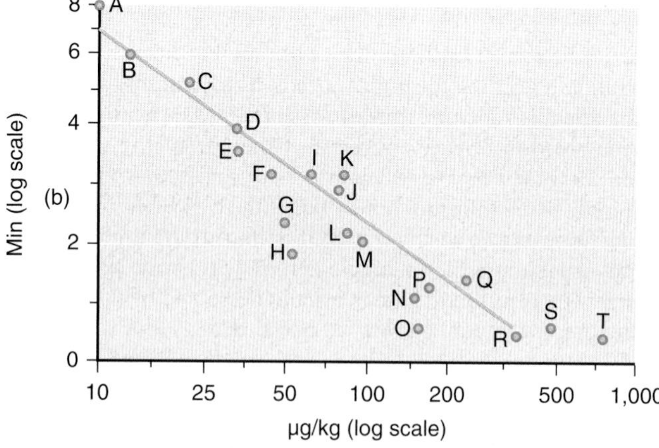

Figure 29-17 Linear regression of the onset of neuromuscular blockade (ordinate) versus potency of a series of steroidal relaxants studied in the cat model by Bowman and colleagues.[101] The data show that onset may be increased in compounds of low potency and encouraged the eventual development of rocuronium and rapacuronium (ORG 9487). A, pipecuronium; C, pancuronium; D, vecuronium.

Donati and Meistelman[156] proposed a model to explain this inverse potency-onset relationship. Nondepolarizing neuromuscular blockers of low potency (e.g., rocuronium) have more molecules to diffuse from the central compartment into the effect compartment. Once in the effect compartment, all molecules act promptly. Weaker binding of the low-potency drugs to receptors prevents buffered diffusion,[156] a process that occurs with more potent drugs. Buffered diffusion causes repetitive binding and unbinding to receptors, which keeps potent drugs in the neighborhood of the effector sites and potentially lengthens the duration of effect.

The times to 95% blockade at the adductor pollicis after administration of the ED_{95} dose of succinylcholine, rocuronium, vecuronium, atracurium, mivacurium, and cisatracurium are shown in Figure 29-18.[117,155,157] This illustration shows that the most potent compound, cisatracurium, has the slowest onset and that the least potent compound, rocuronium, has the most rapid onset.[117,155,157] Bevan[159] also proposed that rapid plasma clearance is associated with a rapid onset of action. The fast onset of succinylcholine's action is related to its rapid metabolism and plasma clearance.

Table 29-7 Pharmacodynamic Effects of Succinylcholine and Nondepolarizing Neuromuscular Blockers

	Anesthesia	Intubating Dose (mg/kg)	Approximate ED_{95} Multiples	Maximum Block (%)	Time to Maximum Block (min)	Clinical Duration* (min)	Reference
Succinylcholine	Narcotic or halothane	0.5	1.7	100	—	6.7	144
Succinylcholine	Desflurane	0.6	2	100	1.4	7.6	145
Succinylcholine	Narcotic or halothane	1.0	2	100	—	11.3	144
Succinylcholine	Desflurane	1.0	3	100	1.2	9.3	145
Succinylcholine	Narcotic	1.0	3	—	1.1	8	146
Succinylcholine	Narcotic	1.0	3	—	1.1	9	147
Succinylcholine	Isoflurane	1.0	3	100	0.8	9	148
Steroidal Compounds							
Rocuronium	Narcotic	0.6	2	100	1.7	36	149
Rocuronium	Isoflurane	0.6	2	100	1.5	37	148
Rocuronium	Isoflurane	0.9	3	100	1.3	53	148
Rocuronium	Isoflurane	1.2	4	100	0.9	73	148
Vecuronium	Isoflurane	0.1	2	100	2.4	41	148
Vecuronium	Narcotic	0.1	2	100	2.4	44	150
Pancuronium	Narcotic	0.08	1.3	100	2.9	86	151
Pancuronium	Narcotic	0.1	1.7	99	4	100	152
Benzylisoquinolinium Compounds							
Mivacurium	Narcotic	0.15	2	100	3.3	16.8	9
Mivacurium	Narcotic	0.15	2	100	3	14.5	149
Mivacurium	Halothane	0.15	2	100	2.8	18.6	153
Mivacurium	Narcotic	0.2	2.6	100	2.5	19.7	9
Mivacurium	Narcotic	0.25	3.3	100	2.3	20.3	9
Mivacurium	Narcotic	0.25	3.3	—	2.1	21	147
Atracurium	Narcotic	0.5	2	100	3.2	46	11
Cisatracurium	Narcotic	0.1	2	99	7.7	46	154
Cisatracurium	Narcotic	0.1	2	100	5.2	45	11
Cisatracurium	Narcotic	0.2	4	100	2.7	68	11
Cisatracurium	Narcotic	0.4	8	100	1.9	91	11
d-Tubocurarine	Narcotic	0.6	1.2	97	5.7	81	152

For atracurium and mivacurium, slower injection (30 seconds) is recommended to minimize circulatory effects.
*Time from injection of the intubating dose to recovery of twitch to 25% of control.

The onset of neuromuscular blockade is much more rapid in the muscles that are relevant to obtaining optimal intubating conditions (laryngeal adductors, diaphragm, and masseter) than in the muscle that is typically monitored (adductor pollicis) (see Fig. 29-4).[160] Thus, neuromuscular blockade develops faster, lasts a shorter time, and recovers more quickly in these muscles (Table 29-8).[26,160-163] These observations may seem contradictory because there is also convincing evidence that the median effective concentration (EC_{50}) for almost all drugs studied is between 50% and 100% higher at the diaphragm or larynx than it is at the adductor pollicis. Fisher and coworkers[164] explain this apparent contradiction by postulating more rapid equilibration (shorter $t_{1/2}k_{e0}$) between plasma and the effect compartment at these central muscles. This accelerated rate of equilibrium probably represents little more than differences in regional blood flow. Therefore, muscle blood flow rather than the drug's intrinsic potency may be more important in determining the onset and offset time of nondepolarizing neuromuscular blockers. More luxuriant blood flow (greater blood flow per gram of muscle) at the diaphragm or larynx would result in delivery of a higher peak plasma concentration of drug to the central muscle in the brief period before rapid redistribution is well under way.

Onset of blockade occurs 1 to 2 minutes earlier in the larynx than at the adductor pollicis after the administration of nondepolarizing neuromuscular blocking agents. The pattern of blockade (onset, depth, and speed of recovery) in the orbicularis oculi is similar to that in the larynx.[165] By monitoring the onset of neuromuscular blockade at the orbicularis oculi, one can predict the quality of intubating conditions. The onset of maximal blockade in the larynx also corresponds to the point at which the adductor pollicis begins to show palpable evidence of weakening. Furthermore, the return of thumb responses to normal suggests that the efferent muscular arc of the protective airway reflexes is intact.

Rapid Tracheal Intubation

Succinylcholine remains the drug of choice when rapid tracheal intubation is needed because it consistently provides muscle relaxation within 60 to 90 seconds. When succinylcholine is considered undesirable or contraindicated, the onset of action of

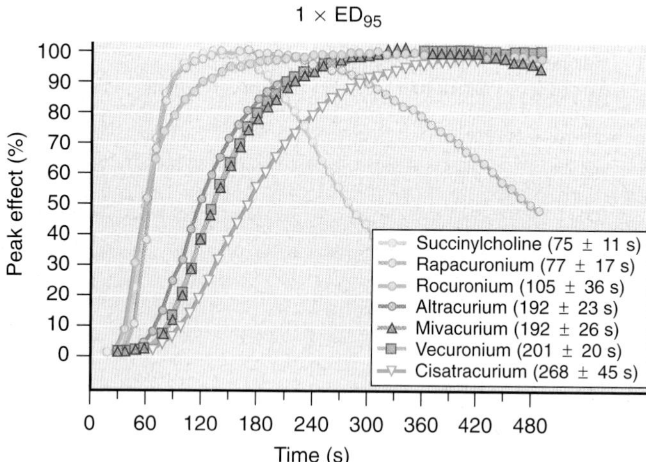

Figure 29-18 Percentages of peak effect after an ED_{95} of succinylcholine, rocuronium, rapacuronium, vecuronium, atracurium, mivacurium, and cisatracurium at the adductor pollicis muscle. Times (mean ± SD) in seconds to 95% of peak effect are shown in parentheses. *(Data from Kopman AF, Klewicka MM, Ghori K, et al: Dose-response and onset/offset characteristics of rapacuronium. Anesthesiology 93:1017-1021, 2000; Kopman AF, Klewicka MM, Kopman DJ, Neuman GG: Molar potency is predictive of the speed of onset of neuromuscular block for agents of intermediate, short, and ultrashort duration. Anesthesiology 90:425-431, 1999; and Kopman AF, Klewicka MM, Neuman GG: Molar potency is not predictive of the speed of onset of atracurium. Anesth Analg 89:1046-1049, 1999.)*

nondepolarizing neuromuscular blocking drugs can be accelerated by preceding the intubating dose with a priming dose of neuromuscular blocker,[166] by using high doses of an individual agent,[148] or by using combinations of neuromuscular blockers.[149] Although some combinations of mivacurium and rocuronium can achieve rapid onset without undue prolongation of action and without undesirable side effects,[149] combination therapy may not consistently result in rapid onset of effect.

THE PRIMING TECHNIQUE. Since the introduction of rocuronium, the use of priming has decreased considerably. Several groups of investigators have recommended that a small subparalyzing dose of the nondepolarizer (about 20% of the ED_{95} or about 10% of the intubating dose) be given 2 to 4 minutes before a large second dose for tracheal intubation.[166] This procedure, termed priming, has been shown to accelerate the onset of blockade for most nondepolarizing neuromuscular blockers by 30 to 60 seconds, which means that intubation can be performed within approximately 90 seconds of the second dose. However, the intubating conditions that occur after priming do not match those that occur after succinylcholine. Moreover, priming carries the risks of aspiration and difficulty swallowing, and the visual disturbances associated with subtle degrees of blockade are uncomfortable for the patient.[167]

THE HIGH-DOSE REGIMEN FOR RAPID TRACHEAL INTUBATION. Larger doses of neuromuscular blockers are usually recommended when intubation must be accomplished in less than 90 seconds. High-dose regimens, however, are associated with a considerably prolonged duration of action and potentially increased cardiovascular side effects (see Table 29-7).[148,168] Increasing the dosage of rocuronium from 0.6 mg/kg (twice the ED_{95}) to 1.2 mg/kg (four times the ED_{95}) shortened the onset time of complete neuromuscular blockade from 89 ± 33 seconds (mean ± SD) to 55 ± 14 seconds but significantly prolonged the clinical duration (i.e., recovery of the first twitch of TOF [T1] to 25% of baseline) from 37 ± 15 minutes to 73 ± 32 minutes.[148]

Whatever technique of rapid-sequence induction of anesthesia and intubation is elected, the following four principles are important: (1) preoxygenation must be performed, (2) sufficient doses of intravenous drugs must be administered to ensure that the patient is adequately anesthetized, (3) intubation within 60 to 90 seconds must be considered acceptable, and (4) cricoid pressure should be applied subsequent to injection of the induction agent.

Low-Dose Relaxants for Tracheal Intubation

The low-dose technique is not suitable for rapid-sequence induction, but several studies have demonstrated that low doses of neuromuscular blocking drugs can be used for routine tracheal intubation. The use of low doses of neuromuscular blockers has advantages: (1) it shortens the time to recovery from

Table 29-8 Time Course of Action and Peak Effect at the Laryngeal Adductors and Adductor Pollicis

		Laryngeal Adductors			Adductor Pollicis			
Dose (mg/kg)	Anesthesia	Onset Time (sec)	Maximum Block (% Depression)	Clinical Duration (min)	Onset Time (sec)	Maximum Block (% Depression)	Clinical Duration (min)	Reference
Succinylcholine, 1.0	Propofol-fentanyl	34 ± 12	100 ± 0	4.3 ± 1.6	56 ± 15	100 ± 0	8 ± 2	161
Rocuronium, 0.25	Propofol-fentanyl	96 ± 6	37 ± 8	—	180 ± 18	69 ± 8	—	160
Rocuronium, 0.4	Propofol-fentanyl	92 ± 29	70 ± 15	—	155 ± 40	99 ± 3	24 ± 7	161
Rocuronium, 0.5	Propofol-fentanyl	84 ± 6	77 ± 5	8 ± 3	144 ± 12	98 ± 1	22 ± 3	160
Vecuronium, 0.04	Propofol-fentanyl	198 ± 6	55 ± 8	—	342 ± 12	89 ± 3	11 ± 2	26
Vecuronium, 0.07	Propofol-fentanyl	198 ± 12	88 ± 4	9 ± 2	342 ± 18	98 ± 1	22 ± 2	26
Mivacurium, 0.14	Propofol- alfentanil	137 ± 20	90 ± 7	5.7 ± 2.1	201 ± 59	99 ± 1	16.2 ± 4.6	162
Mivacurium, 0.2 mg	Propofol- alfentanil	89 ± 26	99 ± 4	10.4 ± 1.5	202 ± 45	99 ± 2	20.5 ± 3.9	163

Clinical duration is the time until T1 recovers to 25% of its control value. Values are means ± SD[161-163] or SEM.[26,160]

neuromuscular blockade and (2) it reduces the requirement for anticholinesterase drugs. Rocuronium has the shortest onset time of all the nondepolarizing neuromuscular blocking agents currently available.[160,161] The maximal effect of either 0.25 or 0.5 mg/kg of rocuronium at the laryngeal muscles occurs after 1.5 minutes.[160] This interval is shorter than the 3.3 minutes reported after the administration of equipotent doses of vecuronium (0.04 or 0.07 mg/kg)[26] and only slightly more than the 0.9 minute reported after 0.25 or 0.5 mg/kg of succinylcholine (see Table 29-8).[169]

With a better understanding of the multiple factors that contribute to satisfactory conditions for intubation, it is now possible to take full advantage of the onset profile for rocuronium. Intubating conditions are related more closely to the degree of neuromuscular blockade of the laryngeal adductor muscles than to the degree of blockade typically monitored at the adductor pollicis. Figure 29-19 demonstrates this principle.[158] Complete blockade at the larynx, diaphragm, or both may not be a prerequisite for satisfactory tracheal intubating conditions.

Kopman and associates[171] noted that 0.5 mg/kg of rocuronium (1.5 times the ED_{95}) provided very satisfactory conditions for intubation (25 intubations were rated excellent and 5 were rated good) in patients anesthetized with 12.5 µg/kg of alfentanil and 2.0 mg/kg of propofol if laryngoscopy were delayed for 75 seconds after drug administration. They estimated that 1.5 times the ED_{95} of rocuronium will produce at least 95% blockade in 98% of the population.[171] A similar or lower multiple of rocuronium's ED_{95} was shown to have a more rapid onset and shorter duration of action than atracurium[172] or cisatracurium.[112] The onset of cisatracurium's effect is too slow to provide good conditions for intubation in less than 2 minutes, even after a dose twice the ED_{95}.

In the vast majority of patients receiving 15 µg/kg of alfentanil followed by 2.0 mg/kg of propofol and 0.45 mg/kg of rocuronium, good to excellent conditions for intubation will be present 75 to 90 seconds after the completion of drug administration.

	Muscle X	Adductor pollicis
EC_{50} (µg/mL)	3.00	1.18
$t_{1/2}k_{e0}$ (min)	1.93	3.85
Hill coefficient	4.00	4.50

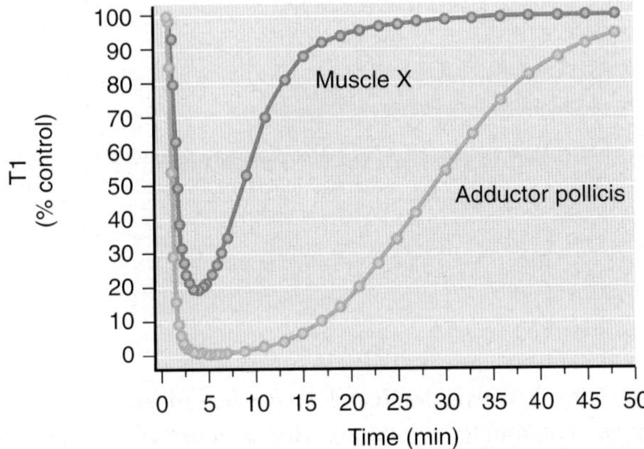

Figure 29-19 Computer simulation based on Sheiner's model[120] and data reported by Wierda and colleagues.[170] The ED_{95} of rocuronium at the adductor pollicis from this model is 0.33 mg/kg. Rocuronium, 0.45 mg/kg, is given as a bolus at time zero. Muscle X represents a muscle (such as the diaphragm or the laryngeal adductors) that is less sensitive to the effects of nondepolarizing relaxants than the adductor pollicis but has greater blood flow. In this example, the concentration of rocuronium producing a 50% block (EC_{50}) of muscle X is 2.5 times that of the adductor pollicis, but the half-life of transport between plasma and the effect compartment ($t_{1/2}k_{e0}$) of muscle X is only half as long. The rapid equilibration between plasma concentrations of rocuronium and muscle X results in more rapid onset of blockade of muscle X than the adductor pollicis. The greater EC_{50} at muscle X explains the faster recovery of this muscle than of the adductor pollicis from neuromuscular blockade. Lower blood concentrations of rocuronium must be achieved at the adductor pollicis than at muscle X before recovery begins. *(From Naguib M, Kopman AF: Low dose rocuronium for tracheal intubation. Middle East J Anesthesiol 17:193-204, 2003.)*

Metabolism and Elimination

The specific pathways of the metabolism (biotransformation) and elimination of neuromuscular blocking drugs are summarized in Table 29-9. Of the nondepolarizing neuromuscular blockers listed, pancuronium, pipecuronium, vecuronium, atracurium, cisatracurium, and mivacurium are the only ones that are metabolized or degraded. Nearly all nondepolarizing neuromuscular blocker molecules contain ester linkages, acetyl ester groups, and hydroxy or methoxy groups. These substitutions, especially the quaternary nitrogen groups, confer a high degree of water solubility with only slight lipid solubility. The hydrophilic nature of relaxant molecules enables easy elimination in urine by glomerular filtration, with no tubular resorption or secretion. Therefore, all nondepolarizing neuromuscular blockers show elimination of the parent molecule in urine as the basic route of elimination; those with a long duration of action thus have a clearance rate that is limited by the glomerular filtration rate (1 to 2 mL/kg/min).

Steroidal Compounds

LONG-ACTING NEUROMUSCULAR BLOCKERS. Pancuronium is cleared largely by the kidney.[173] Its hepatic uptake is limited. A small amount (15% to 20%) is deacetylated at the 3-position in the liver, but this makes a minimal contribution to the total clearance. Deacetylation also occurs at the 17-position, but to such a small extent that it is clinically irrelevant. The three known metabolites have been studied individually in anesthetized humans.[151] The 3-OH metabolite is the most potent of the three, being approximately half as potent as pancuronium, and is the only one present in detectable concentrations in plasma. This metabolite has pharmacokinetics and a duration of action similar to those of pancuronium.[151] In addition, the 3-OH metabolite is most likely excreted largely by the kidney.[151] The parent compound and the 3-OH metabolite are also cleared in small amounts via a minor liver pathway. Total clearance is delayed, and the duration of action is significantly lengthened by severe disorders of renal or hepatic function.[129,174,175]

INTERMEDIATE-ACTING NEUROMUSCULAR BLOCKERS. - Vecuronium, the 2-desmethyl derivative of pancuronium, is more lipid soluble than pancuronium because of absence of the quaternizing methyl group at the 2-position. It undergoes two to three times more metabolism than pancuronium does. Vecuronium is taken up into the liver by a carrier-mediated transport system[176] and then deacetylated at the 3-position by liver microsomes. About 12% of clearance of vecuronium occurs by conversion to 3-desacetylvecuronium,[177] and 30% to 40% is cleared in bile as

Table 29-9 Metabolism and Elimination of Neuromuscular Blocking Drugs

Drug	Duration	Metabolism (%)	Elimination: Kidney (%)	Elimination: Liver (%)	Metabolites
Succinylcholine	Ultrashort	Butyrylcholinesterase (98%-99%)	<2%	None	Monoester (succinyl monocholine) and choline; monoester metabolized much more slowly than succinylcholine
Gantacurium	Ultrashort	Cysteine (fast) and ester hydrolysis (slow)	?	?	Inactive cysteine adduction product, chloroformate monoester, and alcohol
Mivacurium	Short	Butyrylcholinesterase (95%-99%)	<5% (Metabolites eliminated in urine and bile)	None	Monoester and quaternary alcohol. The metabolites are inactive. They are most likely not themselves metabolized any further.
Atracurium	Intermediate	Hofmann elimination and nonspecific ester hydrolysis (60%-90%)	10%-40% (Metabolites eliminated in urine and bile)	None	Laudanosine, acrylates, alcohols, and acids. Although laudanosine has CNS-stimulating properties, the clinical relevance of this effect is negligible.
Cisatracurium	Intermediate	Hofmann elimination (77%?)	Renal clearance is 16% of total		Laudanosine and acrylates. Ester hydrolysis of the quaternary monoacrylate occurs secondarily. Because of the greater potency of cisatracurium, laudanosine quantities produced by Hofmann elimination are 5 to 10 times lower than in the case of atracurium, thus making this not an issue in practice.
Vecuronium	Intermediate	Liver (30%-40%)	40%-50% (Metabolites excreted in urine and bile, ≈40%)	50%-60%	The 3-OH metabolite accumulates, particularly in renal failure. It has about 80% the potency of vecuronium and may be responsible for delayed recovery in ICU patients.
Rocuronium	Intermediate	None	10%-25%	>70%	None
Pancuronium	Long	Liver (10%-20%)	85%	15%	The 3-OH metabolite may accumulate, particularly in renal failure. It is about two thirds as potent as the parent compound.
d-Tubocurarine	Long	None	80% (?)	20%	None

CNS, central nervous system; ICU, intensive care unit.

parent compound.[127] Although the liver is the principal organ of elimination for vecuronium, the drug also undergoes significant (up to 25%) renal excretion, and this combined organ elimination gives it a clearance rate of 3 to 6 mL/kg/min.[177,178]

The principal metabolite of vecuronium, 3-desacetylvecuronium, is a potent (~80% of vecuronium) neuromuscular blocking drug in its own right. The metabolite, though, has slower plasma clearance and a longer duration of action than vecuronium does.[177] 3-Desacetylvecuronium has a clearance rate of 3.5 mL/kg/min, and renal clearance accounts for approximately a sixth of its elimination.[177] In patients in the ICU with renal failure, 3-desacetylvecuronium can accumulate and produce prolonged neuromuscular blockade.[179] Other putative metabolites are 17-desacetylvecuronium and 3,17-bisdesacetylvecuronium, neither of which occurs in clinically significant amounts.

Rocuronium is eliminated primarily by the liver, with a small fraction (~10%) eliminated in urine.[180] It is taken up into the liver by a carrier-mediated active transport system.[181] The putative metabolite, 17-desacetylrocuronium, has not been detected in significant quantities.

Benzylisoquinolinium Compounds

SHORT-ACTING NEUROMUSCULAR BLOCKERS. Mivacurium is hydrolyzed in plasma by butyrylcholinesterase to a monoester and an amino alcohol,[9] which are excreted in urine and bile. The metabolites are positively charged, thus making their entry into the central nervous system (CNS) unlikely. They show less than 1% of the neuromuscular blocking activity of the parent compound and do not affect the autonomic nervous system. Less than 5% is excreted in urine as the parent compound.

Mivacurium consists of three stereoisomers, and clearance rates for the two most pharmacologically active isomers, *cis-trans* and *trans-trans*, are approximately 100 and 50 to 70 mL/kg/min, respectively.[99,182,183] These two isomers show elimination half-lives of 2 to 3 minutes.[99] The third stereoisomer, *cis-cis*, is present as only 4% to 8% of the mivacurium mixture and has less than 10% of the neuromuscular blocking potency of the other two isomers.[99] Consequently, even though it has a much longer elimination half-life (55 minutes) and lower clearance (~4 mL/kg/min) than the two other isomers, it does not contribute significantly to the duration of action of mivacurium.[99] This rapid enzymatic clearance of mivacurium accounts for its short duration of action,[9,99] which is much shorter than that of vecuronium and atracurium but about twice that of succinylcholine.[184] When butyrylcholinesterase activity is severely deficient, however, such as in the rare patients (1/3000) who are homozygous for genetically atypical enzymes, the duration of action of mivacurium is prolonged for up to several hours.[185-188]

Intermediate-Acting Neuromuscular Blockers. Theoretically, atracurium is metabolized by two pathways: Hofmann elimination and ester hydrolysis by nonspecific esterases. Hofmann elimination is a purely chemical process that results in loss of the positive charges by molecular fragmentation to laudanosine (a tertiary amine) and a monoquaternary acrylate, compounds that were thought to have no neuromuscular and little or no cardiovascular activity of clinical relevance.[189] Under the proper chemical conditions, however, these breakdown products may actually be used to synthesize the parent compound.

Because it undergoes Hofmann elimination, atracurium is relatively stable at pH 3.0 and 4°C and becomes unstable when injected into the bloodstream. Early observations of breakdown of the drug in buffer and plasma showed faster degradation in plasma, thus suggesting possible enzymatic hydrolysis of the ester groups. Further evidence suggested that this second pathway, ester hydrolysis, may be more important than originally realized in the breakdown of atracurium.[190] By pharmacokinetic analysis, Fisher and colleagues[191] concluded that a significant amount of clearance of atracurium may be accomplished by routes other than ester hydrolysis and Hofmann elimination. Hence, it appears that atracurium's metabolism is complicated and may not be completely understood.[191]

Laudanosine, a metabolite of atracurium, has CNS-stimulating properties. Unlike atracurium, laudanosine is dependent on the liver and kidney for its elimination and has a long elimination half-life.[192] Laudanosine concentrations are elevated in patients with liver disease[193] and those who have received atracurium for many hours in an ICU.[194] Laudanosine freely crosses the blood-brain barrier.[192] Beemer and coworkers[195] found that patients awakened at a 20% higher arterial concentration of thiopental when atracurium had been given; this was attributed to the CNS-stimulatory effect of laudanosine. These relatively low concentrations of laudanosine, however, did not influence an animal model of epilepsy[196] or lidocaine-induced seizures.[197] In the ICU, blood levels of laudanosine can be as high as 5.0 to 6.0 μg/mL.[186] Though not known in humans, the seizure threshold in animals ranges from 5.0 μg/mL in rabbits[198] to 17 μg/mL in dogs.[199] Thus, adverse effects are unlikely to occur with the use of atracurium in the operating room or ICU.

Laudanosine also has cardiovascular effects. In dogs, hypotension occurs at a blood concentration of about 6 μg/mL,[199] a level higher than that usually found in patients in the ICU. However, there is one case report of a patient who experienced severe hypotension and bradycardia while receiving atracurium, which resolved only when vecuronium was substituted.[200] Laudanosine enhances the stimulation-evoked release of norepinephrine,[201] a finding that may also partly account for its CNS-stimulating effect.

Atracurium is a mixture of 10 optical isomers. Cisatracurium is the 1R *cis*–1′R *cis* isomer of atracurium.[95] Like atracurium, cisatracurium is metabolized by Hofmann elimination to laudanosine and a monoquaternary acrylate.[202,203] In contrast, however, there is no ester hydrolysis of the parent molecule. Hofmann elimination accounts for 77% of the total clearance of 5 to 6 mL/kg/min. Twenty-three percent of the drug is cleared through organ-dependent means, with renal elimination accounting for 16% of this figure.[203] Because cisatracurium is about four or five times as potent as atracurium, about five times less laudanosine is produced, and accumulation of this metabolite is not thought to be of any consequence in clinical practice.

Long-Acting Neuromuscular Blockers. With these agents, there is no active metabolism of dTc. The kidney is the major pathway of elimination, with approximately 50% of a dose being eliminated through renal pathways. The liver is probably a secondary route of elimination. Therefore and because more suitable agents are available, these drugs are not indicated for use in patients with either renal[130] or hepatic failure.

Asymmetric Mixed-Onium Chlorofumarates (Gantacurium)

Gantacurium appears to be degraded by two chemical mechanisms, neither of which is enzymatic: (1) rapid formation of an apparently inactive cysteine adduction product, with cysteine replacing chlorine, and (2) slower hydrolysis of the ester bond adjacent to the chlorine substitution, presumably to inactive hydrolysis products (see Fig. 29-10).[105]

In summary, the only short-acting neuromuscular blocker currently available for clinical use, mivacurium, is cleared rapidly and almost exclusively via metabolism by butyrylcholinesterase, which results in much greater plasma clearance than with any other nondepolarizing neuromuscular blocker.[9] Neuromuscular blockers of intermediate duration, such as vecuronium, rocuronium, atracurium, and cisatracurium, have clearance rates in the range of 3 to 6 mL/kg/min because of multiple pathways of degradation, metabolism, and elimination. Atracurium is cleared two to three times more rapidly than the long-acting drugs.[123,193,204,205] Similar clearance values have been obtained for rocuronium[206-210] and cisatracurium.[202,203,211] Finally, the long-acting neuromuscular blockers undergo minimal or no metabolism, and they are eliminated largely unchanged, mostly by renal excretion. Hepatic pathways are less important in their metabolism.

Adverse Effects of Neuromuscular Blockers

Neuromuscular blocking agents seem to play a prominent role in the incidence of adverse reactions that occur during anesthesia. The Committee on Safety of Medicines in the United Kingdom reported that 10.8% (218 of 2014) of adverse drug reactions and 7.3% of deaths (21 of 286) were attributable to neuromuscular blocking drugs.[212]

Autonomic Effects

Neuromuscular blocking agents may interact with nicotinic and muscarinic cholinergic receptors within the sympathetic and

Table 29-10 Approximate Autonomic Margins of Safety of Nondepolarizing Neuromuscular Blockers*

Drug	Vagus†	Sympathetic Ganglia†	Histamine Release‡
Benzylisoquinolinium Compounds			
Mivacurium	>50	>100	3.0
Atracurium	16	40	2.5
Cisatracurium	>50	>50	None
d-Tubocurarine	0.6	2.0	0.6
Steroidal Compounds			
Vecuronium	20	>250	None
Rocuronium	3.0-5.0	>10	None
Pancuronium	3.0	>250	None

*Number of multiples of the ED_{95} for neuromuscular blockade required to produce the autonomic side effect (ED_{50}).
†In the cat.
‡In human subjects.

parasympathetic nervous systems and with nicotinic receptors at the neuromuscular junction.

Dose-response ratios to compare the neuromuscular blocking potencies of these agents (the ED_{95}) with their potencies in blocking vagal (parasympathetic) or sympathetic ganglionic transmission (the ED_{50}) can be constructed (Table 29-10). These ratios are termed the autonomic margin of safety of the relaxant in question. The higher the dose ratio, the lower the likelihood of or the greater the safety ratio for the occurrence of the particular autonomic effect. The side effect is considered absent (none) in clinical practice if the safety ratio is greater than 5; it is weak or slight if the safety ratio is 3 or 4, moderate if 2 or 3, and strong or prominent if the ratio is 1 or less.

These autonomic responses are not reduced by slower injection of the relaxant. They are dose related and additive over time if divided doses are given. If identical to the original dose, subsequent doses will produce a similar response; that is, no tachyphylaxis will occur. This is not the case, however, when the side effect of histamine release is in question. Cardiovascular responses secondary to histamine release are decreased by slowing the injection rate, and the response undergoes rapid tachyphylaxis. The autonomic effects of neuromuscular blocking drugs are summarized in Table 29-11.

Table 29-11 Clinical Autonomic Effects of Neuromuscular Blocking Drugs

Drug	Autonomic Ganglia	Cardiac Muscarinic Receptors	Histamine Release
Depolarizing Substance			
Succinylcholine	Stimulates	Stimulates	Slight
Benzylisoquinolinium Compounds			
Mivacurium	None	None	Slight
Atracurium	None	None	Slight
Cisatracurium	None	None	None
d-Tubocurarine	Blocks	None	Moderate
Steroidal Compounds			
Vecuronium	None	None	None
Rocuronium	None	Blocks weakly	None
Pancuronium	None	Blocks moderately	None

HISTAMINE RELEASE. Quaternary ammonium compounds such as neuromuscular blockers are generally weaker histamine-releasing substances than tertiary amines such as morphine are. Nevertheless, when large doses of certain neuromuscular blockers are administered rapidly, erythema of the face, neck, and upper part of the torso may develop, as well as a brief decrease in arterial pressure and a slight to moderate increase in heart rate. Bronchospasm in this setting is very rare. The clinical effects of histamine are seen when plasma concentrations increase to 200% to 300% of baseline values, and these effects involve chemical displacement of the contents of mast cell granules containing histamine, prostaglandin, and possibly other vasoactive substances.[213] The serosal mast cell, located in the skin and connective tissue and near blood vessels and nerves, is principally involved in the degranulation process.[213]

The side effect of histamine release is most often noted after administration of the benzylisoquinolinium class of muscle relaxants, although it has also been noted with steroidal relaxants of low potency. The effect is usually of short duration (1 to 5 minutes), is dose related, and is clinically insignificant in healthy patients. Hatano and associates[214] showed that the hypotensive cardiovascular response to 0.6 mg/kg of dTc in humans is prevented not only by antihistamines but also by nonsteroidal anti-inflammatory drugs (e.g., aspirin). These investigators concluded that the final step in dTc-induced hypotension is modulated by prostaglandins that are vasodilators.[214] This side effect can be reduced considerably by using a slower injection rate. It is also prevented by prophylaxis with combinations of $histamine_1$ and $histamine_2$ blockers.[215] If a minor degree of histamine release such as just described occurs after an initial dose of a neuromuscular blocker, subsequent doses will generally cause no response at all, as long as they are no larger than the original dose. This is clinical evidence of tachyphylaxis, an important characteristic of histamine release. A much more significant degree of histamine release occurs during anaphylactic or anaphylactoid reactions; these reactions are very rare.

Clinical Cardiovascular Manifestations of Autonomic Mechanisms

HYPOTENSION. The hypotension seen with the use of atracurium and mivacurium is due to release of histamine, whereas dTc causes hypotension via histamine release and ganglion blockade.[216,217] The effects of dTc occur closer to the dose required to achieve neuromuscular blockade.[116] The safety margin for histamine release is about three times greater for atracurium and mivacurium than it is for dTc.[213,214,217] Rapid administration of atracurium in doses greater than 0.4 mg/kg and mivacurium in doses greater than 0.15 mg/kg has been associated with transient hypotension as a result of release of histamine (Fig. 29-20).

TACHYCARDIA. Pancuronium causes a moderate increase in heart rate and, to a lesser extent, in cardiac output, with little or no change in systemic vascular resistance.[218] Pancuronium-induced tachycardia has been attributed to (1) vagolytic action,[218] probably secondary to inhibition of M_2 receptors, and (2) sympathetic stimulation that involves both direct (blockade of neuronal uptake of norepinephrine) and indirect (release of norepinephrine from adrenergic nerve endings) mechanisms.[219] In studies in humans, Roizen and colleagues[220] surprisingly found decreases in plasma norepinephrine levels after the administration of either pancuronium or atropine. They postulated that the increase in

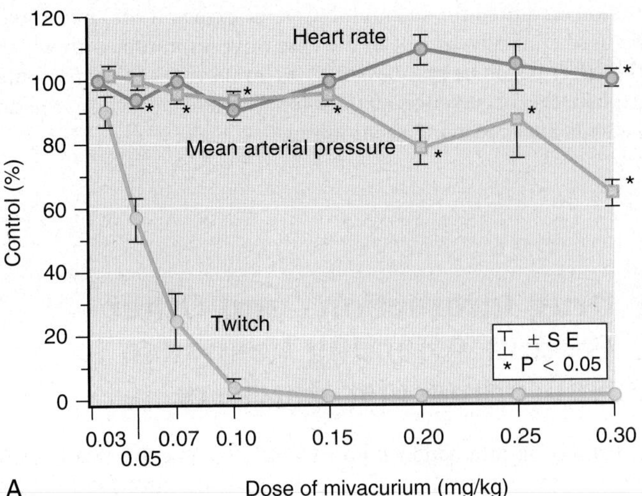

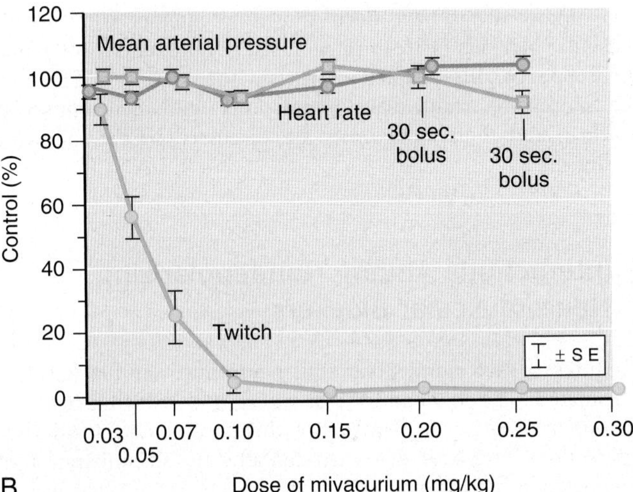

Figure 29-20 Dose response to mivacurium in patients under nitrous oxide–oxygen–opioid anesthesia. Maximum changes at each dose are shown; $n = 9$ subjects per group. **A,** With fast injection, a 15% to 20% decrease in arterial pressure occurred at 2.5 to 3 times the ED_{95} (0.20 to 0.25 mg/kg). **B,** The changes were less than 10% with a slower injection (30 seconds). *(From Savarese JJ, Ali HH, Basta SJ, et al: The cardiovascular effects of mivacurium chloride [BW B1090U] in patients receiving nitrous oxide–opiate–barbiturate anesthesia. Anesthesiology 70:386-394, 1989.)*

heart rate or rate-pressure product occurs because pancuronium (or atropine) acts through baroreceptors to reduce sympathetic outflow.[220] More specifically, the vagolytic effect of pancuronium increases the heart rate and, hence, blood pressure and cardiac output, which in turn influences the baroreceptors to decrease sympathetic tone. Support for this concept is provided by the fact that prior administration of atropine will attenuate or eliminate the cardiovascular effects of pancuronium.[218] However, a positive chronotropic effect that places emphasis on the vagolytic mechanism has not been found in humans.[221] The tachycardia seen with benzylisoquinolinium compounds is due to release of histamine.

DYSRHYTHMIAS. Succinylcholine and dTc actually reduce the incidence of epinephrine-induced dysrhythmias.[222] Possibly because of enhanced atrioventricular conduction,[223] the incidence of dysrhythmias caused by pancuronium appears to increase during halothane anesthesia.[218] Edwards and associates[224] observed a rapid tachycardia (more than 150 beats/min) that progressed to atrioventricular dissociation in two patients anesthetized with halothane who also received pancuronium. The only other factor common to these two patients was that both were taking tricyclic antidepressant agents.

BRADYCARDIA. Several case reports[225,226] have described the occurrence of severe bradycardia and even asystole after the administration of vecuronium or atracurium. All of these cases were also associated with opioid administration. Subsequent studies indicated that administration of vecuronium or atracurium alone does not cause bradycardia.[227] When combined with other drugs that do cause bradycardia (e.g., fentanyl), however, the nonvagolytic relaxants such as vecuronium, cisatracurium, and atracurium allow this mechanism to occur unopposed. Thus, the moderate vagolytic effect of pancuronium is often used to counteract opioid-induced bradycardia.

Respiratory Effects

The muscarinic cholinergic system plays an important role in regulating airway function. Five muscarinic receptors have been cloned,[228] three of which—M_1 to M_3—exist in the airways.[229] M_1 receptors are under sympathetic control, and they mediate bronchodilation.[230] M_2 receptors are located presynaptically (Fig. 29-21) at the postganglionic parasympathetic nerve endings, and they function in a negative-feedback mechanism to limit the release of acetylcholine. M_3 receptors, which are located postsynaptically (Fig. 29-21), mediate contraction of the airway smooth muscles (i.e., bronchoconstriction).[230] Nondepolarizing neuromuscular blockers have different antagonistic activities at both the M_2 and M_3 receptors.[231] For example, blockage of M_3 muscarinic receptors on airway smooth muscle inhibits vagally induced bronchoconstriction (i.e., causes bronchodilation), whereas blockage of M_2 receptors results in increased release of acetylcholine, which will act on M_3 receptors and cause bronchoconstriction.

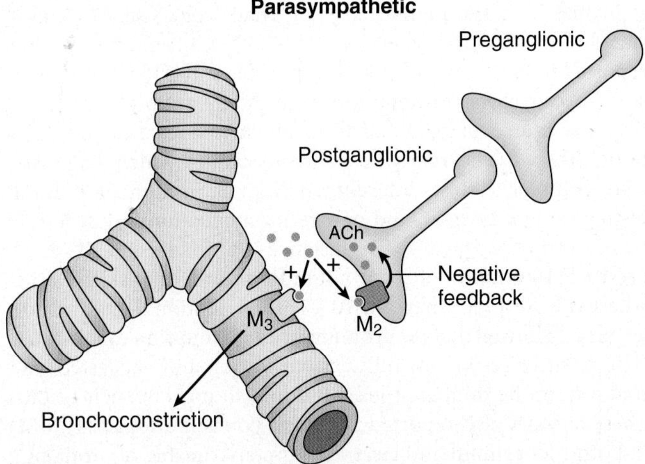

Figure 29-21 The muscarinic M_3 receptors are located postsynaptically on airway smooth muscle. Acetylcholine (ACh) stimulates M_3 receptors to cause contraction. M_2 muscarinic receptors are located presynaptically at the postganglionic parasympathetic nerve endings, and they function in a negative-feedback mechanism to limit the release of ACh.

The affinity of the compound rapacuronium to block M_2 receptors is 15 times higher than its affinity to block M_3 receptors.[231] This explains the high incidence (>9%) of severe bronchospasm[232-234] that was seen with this drug and resulted in its withdrawal from the market.

The administration of benzylisoquinolinium neuromuscular blocking drugs (with the exception of cisatracurium) is associated with histamine release, which may result in increased airway resistance and bronchospasm in patients with hyperactive airway disease.

Allergic Reactions

The frequency of life-threatening anaphylactic (immune-mediated) or anaphylactoid reactions occurring during anesthesia has been estimated to be between 1 in 1000 and 1 in 25,000 anesthetizations, with about a 5% mortality rate.[235,236] In France, the most common causes of anaphylaxis in patients who experienced allergic reactions were reported to be neuromuscular blocking drugs (58.2%), latex (16.7%), and antibiotics (15.1%).[237] Anaphylactic reactions are mediated through immune responses involving immunoglobulin E antibodies fixed to mast cells. Anaphylactoid reactions are not immune mediated and represent exaggerated pharmacologic responses in very rare and very sensitive individuals.

Neuromuscular blocking drugs contain two quaternary ammonium ions, which are the epitopes commonly recognized by specific immunoglobulin E.[238] Cross-reactivity has been reported between neuromuscular blocking drugs and food, cosmetics, disinfectants, and industrial materials.[238] Cross-reactivity is seen in 70% of patients with a history of anaphylaxis to a neuromuscular blocking drug.[237]

Steroidal compounds (e.g., rocuronium, vecuronium, pancuronium) result in no significant histamine release.[217] For example, four times the ED_{95} of rocuronium (1.2 mg/kg) causes no significant release of histamine.[239] Nevertheless, rocuronium and succinylcholine are reportedly associated with a 43.1% and 22.6% incidence of anaphylaxis in France.[237] Rose and Fisher[240] classified rocuronium and atracurium as having intermediate levels of risk for causing allergic reactions. They also noted that the increased number of reports of anaphylaxis with rocuronium is in line with the market share of that drug's use. Watkins[241] stated, "The much higher incidence of rocuronium reactions reported in France is currently inexplicable and is likely to remain so if investigators continue to seek a purely antibody-mediated response as an explanation of all anaphylactoid reaction presentations." There are currently no standards against which diagnostic tests (skin prick test, interdermal test, or immunoglobulin E testing) are performed, and new recommendations are still only in the proposal stage.[242] For instance, Laxenaire and Mertes[243] used a 1 : 10 dilution of rocuronium for interdermal skin testing, whereas Rose and Fisher[240] used a 1 : 1000 dilution. Levy and colleagues[244] showed that rocuronium in a 1 : 10 dilution can produce false-positive results on intradermal testing and suggested that rocuronium be diluted at least 100-fold to prevent such results. These authors also reported that high concentrations ($\geq 10^{-4}$ M) of both rocuronium and cisatracurium are capable of producing a wheal-and-flare response to intradermal testing, which was associated with mild to moderate mast cell degranulation in the cisatracurium group only.[244]

All neuromuscular blocking drugs can cause noncompetitive inhibition of histamine-*N*-methyltransferase, but the concentrations required for such inhibition far exceed those that would be used clinically, except in the case of vecuronium, with which the effect becomes manifested at 0.1 to 0.2 mg/kg.[245] This could explain the occurrence of occasional severe bronchospasm in patients after receiving vecuronium.[246]

Drug Interactions and Other Factors Affecting Response to Neuromuscular Blockers

A drug-drug interaction is an in vivo phenomenon that occurs when the administration of one drug alters the effects or kinetics of another drug. In vitro physical or chemical incompatibilities are *not* considered drug interactions.[247]

Many drugs have been shown to interact with neuromuscular blockers or their antagonists, or both, and it is beyond the scope of this chapter to review them all.[247,248] Some of the more important drug interactions with neuromuscular blockers and their antagonists are discussed in the following sections.

Interactions Among Nondepolarizing Neuromuscular Blockers

Mixtures of two nondepolarizing neuromuscular blockers are considered to be either additive or synergistic. Antagonistic interactions have not been reported in this class of drugs. Additive interactions have been demonstrated after the administration of chemically related agents, such as atracurium and mivacurium,[249] or after the coadministration of various pairs of steroidal neuromuscular blockers.[103] On the other hand, combinations of structurally dissimilar (e.g., a steroidal with a benzylisoquinolinium) neuromuscular blockers, such as pancuronium and dTc,[250] pancuronium and metocurine,[250] rocuronium and mivacurium,[149] or rocuronium and cisatracurium,[112] produce a synergistic response.

The administration of two neuromuscular blockers in combination was first introduced by Lebowitz and coworkers[250] in an attempt to reduce the cardiovascular side effects of neuromuscular blockers by giving smaller doses of each drug as a combination. An additional advantage (rapid onset and short duration) is noted for mivacurium-rocuronium combinations.[149] Although the precise mechanisms underlying a synergistic interaction are not known, hypotheses that have been put forward include the existence of multiple binding sites at the neuromuscular junction (presynaptic and postsynaptic receptors)[251] and the nonequivalence of binding affinities of the two α-subunits (α_H and α_L). Furthermore, inhibition of butyrylcholinesterase by pancuronium results in decreased plasma clearance of mivacurium and marked potentiation of the neuromuscular blockade.[252]

It should be noted that the pharmacodynamic response to the use of two different nondepolarizing blockers during the course of anesthesia depends not only on the specific drugs used but also on the sequence of their administration.[253,254] Approximately three half-lives will be required for a clinical changeover (so that 95% of the first drug has been cleared) and for the duration of the blockade to begin to take on the characteristics of the second drug. After the administration of pancuronium, recovery from the first two maintenance doses of vecuronium is reportedly prolonged, although this effect becomes negligible by the third dose.[253] Similarly, Naguib and coauthors[249] noted that the mean duration of the first maintenance dose of mivacurium to 10% recovery of the first twitch was significantly longer after atracurium (25 minutes) than after mivacurium (14.2 minutes). However, the duration of the second maintenance dose of mivacurium after atracurium (18.3 minutes) was similar to that of mivacurium after mivacurium (14.6 minutes).

The apparent prolongation of action of the first maintenance dose of mivacurium administered after atracurium[249] and the prolongation reported with vecuronium after pancuronium[253,254] are not related to synergism. Combinations of atracurium and mivacurium[249] and vecuronium and pancuronium[103] are simply additive. However, this prolongation of the duration of action could be attributed to the relative concentrations of these drugs at the receptor site. Because most receptors remain occupied by the drug administered initially, the clinical profile depends on the kinetics or dynamics (or both) of the drug administered first rather than on those of the second (maintenance) drug. However, with further incremental doses of the second drug, a progressively larger proportion of the receptors are occupied by that drug, and its clinical profile becomes evident.

Interactions Between Succinylcholine and Nondepolarizing Neuromuscular Blockers

The interaction between succinylcholine and nondepolarizing neuromuscular blockers depends on the order of administration and the doses used.[86,255,256] Small doses of different nondepolarizing neuromuscular blockers administered before succinylcholine to prevent fasciculations have an antagonistic effect on the development of a subsequent depolarizing block produced by succinylcholine.[28,86] Therefore, it is recommended that the dose of succinylcholine be increased after the administration of a defasciculating dose of a nondepolarizing neuromuscular blocker.[28]

Studies on the effects of administration of succinylcholine before nondepolarizing neuromuscular blockers have produced conflicting results. Several investigators reported potentiation of the effects of pancuronium,[255] vecuronium, and atracurium[256] by prior administration of succinylcholine. In contrast, others found no significant influence of succinylcholine on the subsequent administration of pancuronium, rocuronium, or mivacurium.[86,257,258]

Interactions with Inhaled Anesthetics

Deep anesthesia induced with potent volatile anesthetics (in the absence of neuromuscular blockade) may cause a slight reduction in neuromuscular transmission, as measured by depression of sensitive indicators of clinical neuromuscular function, such as tetanus and TOF.[259] Inhaled anesthetics also enhance the neuromuscular blocking effects of nondepolarizing neuromuscular

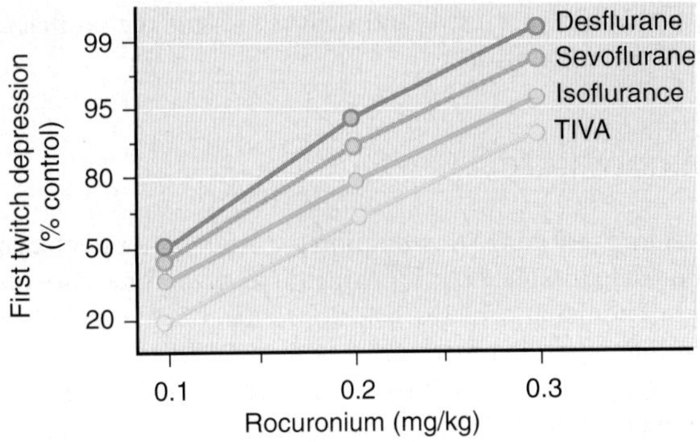

Figure 29-22 Cumulative dose-response curves for rocuronium-induced neuromuscular blockade during 1.5 minimum alveolar concentration (MAC) anesthesia with desflurane, sevoflurane, isoflurane, and total intravenous anesthesia (TIVA). *(From Wulf H, Ledowski T, Linstedt U, et al: Neuromuscular blocking effects of rocuronium during desflurane, isoflurane, and sevoflurane anaesthesia. Can J Anaesth 45:526-532, 1998, with permission from the Canadian Journal of Anaesthesia.)*

blockers. Inhaled anesthetics will decrease the dose of neuromuscular blockers needed, as well as prolong both the duration of action of the blocker and recovery from neuromuscular blockade,[260] depending on the duration of anesthesia,[259,261,262] the specific inhaled anesthetic,[263] and the concentration (dose) given.[264] The rank order of potentiation is desflurane > sevoflurane > isoflurane > halothane > nitrous oxide–barbiturate–opioid or propofol anesthesia (Fig. 29-22).[265-267]

The greater clinical muscle-relaxing effect produced by less potent anesthetics is mainly due to their larger aqueous concentrations.[268] Desflurane and sevoflurane have low blood-gas and tissue-gas solubility, so equilibrium between the end-tidal concentration and the neuromuscular junction is reached more rapidly with these anesthetics than with older inhaled anesthetics.

The interaction between volatile anesthetics and neuromuscular blockers is one of pharmacodynamics, not pharmacokinetics.[143] The proposed mechanisms behind this interaction include (1) a central effect on α motoneurons and interneuronal synapses,[269] (2) inhibition of postsynaptic nAChRs,[270] and (3) augmentation of the antagonist's affinity at the receptor site.[268]

Interactions with Antibiotics

Most antibiotics can cause neuromuscular blockade in the absence of neuromuscular blocking agents. The aminoglycoside antibiotics, the polymyxins, and lincomycin and clindamycin primarily inhibit the prejunctional release of acetylcholine and also depress postjunctional nAChR sensitivity to acetylcholine. The tetracyclines, on the other hand, exhibit postjunctional activity only. When combined with neuromuscular blockers, the aforementioned antibiotics can potentiate neuromuscular blockade.[271] The cephalosporins and penicillins have not been reported to potentiate neuromuscular blockade. Because antagonism of neuromuscular blockade has been reported to be more difficult after the administration of aminoglycosides,[272] ventilation should be controlled until the neuromuscular blockade terminates spontaneously. Calcium should not be used to hasten the recovery of neuromuscular function for two reasons: the antagonism that it produces is not sustained, and it may prevent the antibacterial effect of the antibiotics.

Temperature

Hypothermia prolongs the duration of action of nondepolarizing neuromuscular blockers.[273-275] The force of contraction of the adductor pollicis decreases by 10% to 16% per degree Celsius decline in muscle temperature below 35.2°C.[276,277] To maintain muscle temperature at or above 35.2°C, central temperature must be maintained at 36.0°C.[273] Recovery to 10% twitch height with 0.1 mg/kg of vecuronium increases from 28 minutes at a mean central temperature of 36.4°C to 64 minutes at 34.4°C.[273] The mechanism or mechanisms underlying this prolongation may be pharmacodynamic, pharmacokinetic, or both.[275] They include diminished renal and hepatic excretion, changing volumes of distribution, altered local diffusion receptor affinity, changes in pH at the neuromuscular junction, and the net effect of cooling on the various components of neuromuscular transmission.[273,278] Hypothermia decreases the plasma clearance and prolongs the duration of action of rocuronium and vecuronium.[275] Temperature-related differences in the pharmacodynamics of vecuronium have also been reported: k_{e0} decreases (0.023/min/°C) with lower temperature, suggesting slightly delayed equilibration of drug between the circulation and the neuromuscular junction during hypothermia.[275] The Hofmann elimination process of atracurium is slowed by a decrease in pH and especially by a decrease in temperature.[279] In fact, atracurium's duration of action is markedly prolonged by hypothermia.[274] For instance, the duration of action of a 0.5-mg/kg dose of atracurium is 44 minutes at 37°C but 68 minutes at 34.0°C.

Changes in temperature will also affect interpretation of the results of monitoring neuromuscular blockade. For example, the duration of action of vecuronium measured in an arm cooled to a skin temperature of 27°C is prolonged, and monitoring by post-tetanic count in that arm is unreliable.[280] In the same patient, TOF responses are different if the arms are at different temperatures, and correlation of responses in the two arms becomes progressively poorer as the temperature difference between the arms increases.[281]

The efficacy of neostigmine is not altered by mild hypothermia.[282-284] Hypothermia does not change the clearance, maximum effect, or duration of action of neostigmine in volunteers.[284]

Interactions with Magnesium and Calcium

Magnesium sulfate, given for the treatment of preeclampsia and eclamptic toxemia, potentiates the neuromuscular blockade induced by nondepolarizing neuromuscular blockers (see Chapter 69).[285,286] After a dose of 40 mg/kg of magnesium sulfate, the ED_{50} of vecuronium was reduced by 25%, the onset time was nearly halved, and the recovery time nearly doubled.[286] Neostigmine-induced recovery is also attenuated in patients treated with magnesium.[285] The mechanisms underlying the enhancement of nondepolarizing blockade by magnesium probably involve both prejunctional and postjunctional effects. High magnesium concentrations inhibit calcium channels at the presynaptic nerve terminals that trigger the release of acetylcholine.[14] Furthermore, magnesium ions have an inhibitory effect on postjunctional potentials and cause decreased excitability of muscle fiber membranes. In patients receiving magnesium, the dose of nondepolarizing neuromuscular blocker must be reduced and carefully titrated with a nerve stimulator to ensure adequate recovery of neuromuscular function at the end of surgery.

The interaction between magnesium and succinylcholine is controversial. However, more recent results suggest that magnesium antagonizes the block produced by succinylcholine.[287]

Calcium triggers the release of acetylcholine from the motor nerve terminal and enhances excitation-contraction coupling in muscle.[14] Increasing calcium concentrations decreased the sensitivity to dTc and pancuronium in a muscle-nerve model.[288] In hyperparathyroidism, hypercalcemia is associated with decreased sensitivity to atracurium and thus a shortened time course of neuromuscular blockade.[289]

Interactions with Lithium

Lithium remains the drug of choice for the treatment of bipolar affective disorder (manic-depressive illness). The lithium ion resembles sodium, potassium, magnesium, and calcium ions and may therefore affect the distribution and kinetics of all of these electrolytes.[290] Lithium enters cells via sodium channels and tends to accumulate within the cells.

By its activation of potassium channels, lithium inhibits neuromuscular transmission presynaptically and muscular contraction postsynaptically.[291] The combination of lithium and pipecuronium results in a synergistic inhibition of neuromuscular transmission, whereas the combination of lithium and succinylcholine results in additive inhibition.[291] Prolongation of neuromuscular blockade was reported in patients taking lithium carbonate and both depolarizing[282] and nondepolarizing neuromuscular blockers.[292] Only one report did not demonstrate prolongation of recovery from succinylcholine in patients receiving lithium.[293] In patients who are stabilized on lithium therapy and undergoing surgery, neuromuscular blockers should be administered in incremental and reduced doses and titrated to the degree of blockade required.

Interactions with Local Anesthetic and Antidysrhythmic Drugs

Local anesthetics act on the presynaptic, postsynaptic, and muscle membranes. In large intravenous doses, most local anesthetics block neuromuscular transmission; in smaller doses, they enhance the neuromuscular blockade produced by both nondepolarizing and depolarizing neuromuscular blockers.[294] The ability of neostigmine to antagonize a combined local anesthetic–neuromuscular blockade has not been studied. Procaine also inhibits butyrylcholinesterase and may augment the effects of succinylcholine and mivacurium by decreasing their hydrolysis by the enzyme.

In small intravenous doses, local anesthetics depress post-tetanic potentiation, and this is thought to be a neural prejunctional effect.[295] In larger doses, local anesthetics block acetylcholine-induced muscular contractions, which suggests that local anesthetics have a stabilizing effect on the postjunctional membrane.[296] Procaine displaces calcium from the sarcolemma and thus inhibits caffeine-induced contracture of skeletal muscle.[297] Most of these mechanisms of action probably apply to all of the local anesthetics.

Several drugs used for the treatment of dysrhythmias augment the blockade induced by neuromuscular blockers. Single-fiber electromyography has disclosed that verapamil and amlodipine impair neuromuscular transmission in subjects without neuromuscular disease.[298] Clinical reports have suggested potentiation of neuromuscular block with verapamil[299] and impaired reversal of vecuronium in a patient receiving disopyramide.[300] However, the clinical significance of these interactions is probably minor.

Interactions with Antiepileptic Drugs

Anticonvulsants have a depressant action on release of acetylcholine at the neuromuscular junction.[301] Patients receiving chronic anticonvulsant therapy demonstrated resistance to nondepolarizing muscle blockers (except mivacurium[302] and probably atracurium as well),[301] as evidenced by accelerated recovery from neuromuscular blockade and the need for increased doses to achieve complete neuromuscular blockade. Clearance of vecuronium is increased twofold in patients receiving chronic carbamazepine therapy.[303] Some investigators, however, attribute this resistance to increased binding (i.e., decreased free fraction) of the neuromuscular blockers to α_1-acid glycoproteins or to upregulation of neuromuscular acetylcholine receptors (or to both mechanisms).[204] The latter could also explain the hypersensitivity seen with succinylcholine.[205] The slight prolongation of succinylcholine's action in patients taking anticonvulsants has few clinical implications. On the other hand, the potential hyperkalemic response to succinylcholine in the presence of receptor upregulation is of concern.

Interactions with Diuretics

In patients undergoing renal transplantation, the intensity and duration of dTc neuromuscular blockade is increased after a dose of furosemide (1 mg/kg intravenously).[306] Furosemide reduced the concentration of dTc required to achieve 50% twitch tension depression in the indirectly stimulated rat diaphragm and intensified the neuromuscular blockade produced by dTc and succinylcholine.[307] Furosemide appears to inhibit the production of cyclic adenosine monophosphate. In addition, the breakdown of adenosine triphosphate is inhibited, which results in reduced output of acetylcholine. Acetazolamide antagonizes the effects of anticholinesterases in the rat phrenic-diaphragm preparation.[308] However, in one report, 1 mg/kg of furosemide facilitated recovery of the evoked twitch response after pancuronium.[309] Chronic furosemide treatment had no effect on either dTc- or pancuronium-induced neuromuscular blockade.[310]

In contrast, mannitol appears to have no effect on nondepolarizing neuromuscular blockade. Moreover, increasing urine output by the administration of mannitol or other osmotic or tubular diuretics has no effect on the rate at which dTc and presumably other neuromuscular blockers are eliminated in urine.[126] However, this lack of effect on the excretion of dTc should not be surprising. Urinary excretion of all neuromuscular blockers that are long acting depends primarily on glomerular filtration. Mannitol is an osmotic diuretic that exerts its effects by altering the osmotic gradient within the proximal tubules so that water is retained within them. An increase in urine volume in patients with adequate glomerular filtration, therefore, would not be expected to increase the excretion of neuromuscular blockers.

Interactions with Other Drugs

Dantrolene (see Chapter 37), a drug used for the treatment of malignant hyperthermia, prevents release of calcium from the sarcoplasmic reticulum and blocks excitation-contraction coupling. Although it does not block neuromuscular transmission, the mechanical response to stimulation will be depressed, with subsequent potentiation of the nondepolarizing neuromuscular blockade.[88]

Azathioprine, an immunodepressant drug used in patients undergoing renal transplantation, has a minor antagonistic action on muscle relaxant–induced neuromuscular blockade.[311]

Steroids antagonize the effects of nondepolarizing neuromuscular blockers in both humans[312] and animals.[313] Possible mechanisms for this interaction include facilitation of acetylcholine release because of the effect of steroids on the presynaptic motor nerve terminal[314] and channel blockade of the nAChR.[315] Endogenous steroids act noncompetitively on nAChRs.[316] Prolonged treatment with a combination of corticosteroids and neuromuscular blocking drugs can result in prolonged weakness in critical care patients (see the later section "Neuromuscular Blockers and Weakness Syndromes in the Critically Ill").

Antiestrogenic drugs such as tamoxifen appear to potentiate the effects of nondepolarizing neuromuscular blockers.[317]

Recovery From Neuromuscular Blockade

In the 1970s, Ali and colleagues[318] described a TOF ratio of 0.60 as indicating adequate recovery of neuromuscular strength. Nonetheless, in 1997 a TOF ratio of 0.70 in unanesthetized volunteers was associated with difficulty speaking and swallowing, weakness of the facial musculature, visual disturbances, and inability to sit up without assistance.[319] Also in human volunteers, TOF ratios of 0.6 to 0.7 were associated with decreased upper esophageal tone and decreased coordination of the esophageal musculature during swallowing.[320,321] Fluoroscopic examination of these individuals demonstrated significant pharyngeal dysfunction resulting in a fourfold to fivefold increase in the risk for aspiration. With recovery of the TOF ratio to 0.9, esophageal tone and pharyngeal coordination returned toward baseline.[320,321]

Residual paralysis also decreases the hypoxic ventilatory drive (Fig. 29-23),[322,323] which is due to inhibition of the carotid body's neural response to hypoxia.[324] Vecuronium decreases carotid sinus nerve activity in response to hypoxia in a dose-related fashion, presumably through its interaction with nicotinic chemotransduction of the carotid body.

After the administration of nondepolarizing neuromuscular blocking drugs, adequate return of normal neuromuscular function must be present. Whether that degree of recovery is a

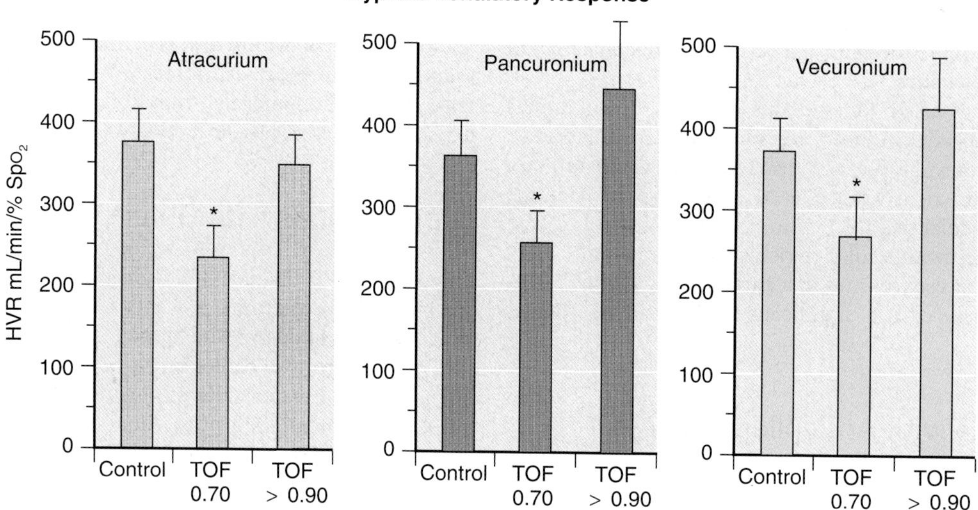

Figure 29-23 Hypoxic ventilatory response (HVR) before (control); during steady-state infusion (train-of-four [TOF] = 0.07) of atracurium, pancuronium, and vecuronium; and after recovery (TOF > 0.90). Data are presented as means ± SD. *P < .01. *(From Eriksson LI: Reduced hypoxic chemosensitivity in partially paralysed man. A new property of muscle relaxants? Acta Anaesthesiol Scand 40:520-523, 1996.)*

TOF ratio of 0.7, 0.8, or 0.9 has been an area of debate, and in a recent international guideline a TOF ratio of 0.9 was recommended as an end point for recovery from a nondepolarizing neuromuscular block. Certainly, the clinician's ability to quantify the degree of residual neuromuscular block is limited. Kopman and colleagues'[319] work in volunteers demonstrated that when they could oppose their incisors to retain a tongue depressor, their TOF ratio was, on average, 0.8 and at least 0.68. This test of muscle strength, though, would have limited usefulness in tracheally intubated patients.

Recommendations for detection and prevention of residual neuromuscular blockade are summarized in Chapter 47.

Recovery from muscle relaxation caused by nondepolarizing neuromuscular blockers depends on several factors. Primarily, it depends on an increase in the acetylcholine concentration relative to that of the relaxant to overcome the competitive neuromuscular blockade. Although neostigmine will increase the acetylcholine concentration, ultimately, the muscle relaxant needs to be eliminated. The relative increase in acetylcholine concentration depends first on the ongoing movement of relaxant from the motor end plate into the central circulation and then on its elimination from the circulating blood volume so that it is not free to move into the synaptic cleft. Ultimately, recovery depends on elimination of the neuromuscular blocker from the body. Neuromuscular blockers may be eliminated through a host of mechanisms, including excretion as unchanged drug in urine, metabolism in the liver, enzymatic hydrolysis, and chemical breakdown. Although it has never been specifically examined, several groups of investigators have, through their ranges of recovery parameters, described wide interpatient variation in the spontaneous recovery of neuromuscular function.[325-327]

Several factors in addition to coexisting disease will affect the speed of spontaneous recovery of neuromuscular function. The presence of volatile anesthetics will potentiate any existing neuromuscular block and, presumably, cause recovery to be more prolonged.[328] If the anesthesiologist observes no or only minimal recovery of neuromuscular function in the presence of a volatile anesthetic, discontinuing or decreasing the concentration of that anesthetic should augment the recovery of neuromuscular function.

As will be discussed later in this section, acidosis, hypokalemia, hypothermia, and concomitant medications all potentiate residual neuromuscular blockade and render pharmacologic antagonism more difficult.

Antagonism of Residual Neuromuscular Blockade

Anticholinesterases act by inhibiting acetylcholinesterase (enzyme classification 3.1.1.7), which is a type B carboxylesterase. At the neuromuscular junction, acetylcholinesterase occurs in the asymmetric or A12 form and consists of three tetramers of catalytic subunits covalently linked to a collagen-like tail. Acetylcholinesterase has a powerful catalytic capacity: it can catalyze 4000 molecules of acetylcholine per active site per second. The active site lies deep inside the enzyme protein. Nearly half of the acetylcholine released is hydrolyzed across the synaptic cleft before reaching the nAChRs. For a detailed account of this enzyme, see the article by Soreq and Seidman.[329]

The active surface of acetylcholinesterase is best viewed as having two sites: the anionic site, which is concerned with binding and orienting the substrate molecule, and the esteratic site, which is responsible for the hydrolytic process. The existence of a second "anionic" site, known as the "peripheral" anionic site, has also been proposed. This topic has been reviewed by Silman and Sussman.[330]

Three anticholinesterases—neostigmine, pyridostigmine, and edrophonium—are used to antagonize residual neuromuscular blockade. They exert their effect primarily by inhibiting acetylcholinesterase and thus increasing the concentration of acetylcholine at the motor end plate. Neostigmine and pyridostigmine are oxydiaphoretic (acid-transferring) inhibitors of acetylcholinesterase. They transfer a carbamate group to acetylcholinesterase and form a covalent bond at the esteratic site. Edrophonium is a prosthetic inhibitor that binds to the anionic site on the acetylcholinesterase by electrostatic attraction and to the esteratic site by hydrogen bonding. In addition, anticholinesterases may increase the release of acetylcholine from presynaptic nerve terminals, block neural potassium channels, and have a direct agonistic effect. For more details, see Bevan and colleagues.[331]

Major Determinants of the Speed and Adequacy of Recovery

Antagonism of nondepolarizing neuromuscular blockade is time dependent. Recovery occurs at a rate that depends primarily on five factors: (1) depth of the blockade when the antagonist is administered, (2) which anticholinesterase is administered, (3) dose of the anticholinesterase, (4) rate of spontaneous recovery from the neuromuscular blocker, and (5) concentration of inhaled anesthetic agent present during reversal.

Depth of the Blockade

Generally, more time is required to antagonize profound levels than lesser levels of blockade.[332] It is interesting that in a study by Bevan and coworkers,[333] antagonism of the blockade induced by doses of vecuronium or rocuronium that were 1.5 times the ED_{95} occurred at the same rate regardless of the timing of administration of 70 µg/kg of neostigmine. Neostigmine shortened the recovery time by approximately 40%, whether it was administered at the time of 1%, 10%, or 25% of spontaneous recovery. However, as shown in Figure 29-24, the time from administration of the neuromuscular blocker to TOF ratios of 0.7 and 0.9 did not decrease as the extent of spontaneous recovery at the time of neostigmine administration increased. Recovery to TOF ratios of 0.7 and 0.9 required, on average, 25 and 30 minutes, respectively. More specifically, should neostigmine be given during a profound (i.e., little or no response to peripheral nerve stimulation) neuromuscular block? Unfortunately, the answer is not clear. Thus, recommendations about the timing of administration of anticholinesterase are equivocal. Instinctively, many experts recommend not administering the anticholinesterase at the earliest degrees of recovery. Kirkegaard and associates[334] recently demonstrated that to recover to a TOF ratio of 0.7 within 10 minutes of administering neostigmine, three or four responses to TOF stimulation had to be present at the time of neostigmine administration. If only one response to TOF stimulation was present, recovery to a TOF ratio of 0.7 required up to 23 minutes.

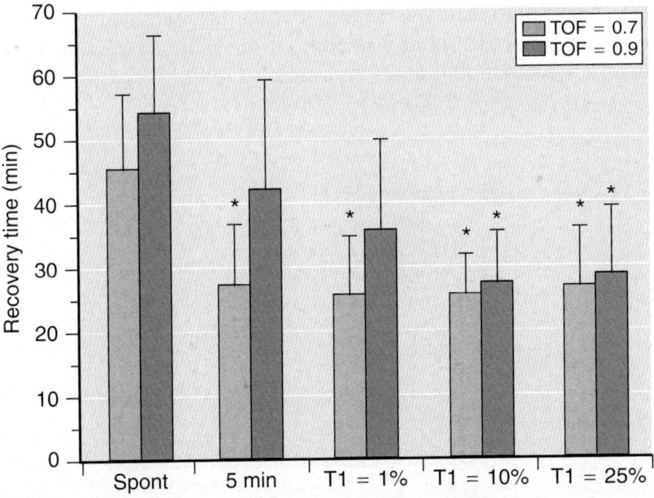

Figure 29-24 Recovery times (mean ± SD) after the administration of a single dose of 0.45 mg/kg (1.5 times the ED_{95}) rocuronium. In one group (Spont), spontaneous recovery was allowed. In the remaining groups, 70 µg/kg of neostigmine was administered 5 minutes after rocuronium or at 1%, 10%, and 25% recovery of the first twitch (T1) from its control value. *$P < .01$ versus spontaneous recovery. Note that the times to attain a train-of-four (TOF) ratio of 0.9 are significantly shorter when neostigmine was administered at T1 = 10% or 25% of control tension. *(From Bevan JC, Collins L, Fowler C, et al: Early and late reversal of rocuronium and vecuronium with neostigmine in adults and children. Anesth Analg 89:333-339, 1999.)*

The maximum antagonistic effect of neostigmine occurs in 10 minutes or less. If adequate recovery does not occur within this time, subsequent recovery is slow and requires ongoing elimination of the neuromuscular blocker from plasma. For profound vecuronium-induced blockade in which no twitch recovery has occurred, administration of 70 µg/kg of neostigmine produces an initial reversal that falls far short of adequate recovery.[327] Subsequent recovery occurs at the same rate as spontaneous recovery and is caused by the decrease in plasma concentration of vecuronium as the drug is eliminated.[327,335] Administration of a second dose of neostigmine has no further effect on recovery[327] because acetylcholinesterase is already maximally inhibited.

If the blockade at the time of neostigmine administration is sufficiently deep that adequate recovery does not occur within 10 minutes, the time at which full recovery of neuromuscular function will occur depends on the inherent duration of action of the neuromuscular blocker.[332] With drugs that have a long duration of action, this period of inadequate neuromuscular function can be 30 to 60 minutes or even longer, whereas with drugs that have an intermediate duration of action, it will be much shorter (e.g., 15 to 30 minutes).[336]

The Anticholinesterase Administered

Under the conditions of a moderate depth of blockade (such as two to three twitches palpable by TOF monitoring), the order of rapidity of antagonism of residual blockade by anticholinesterases is edrophonium > neostigmine > pyridostigmine.[337,338] For this reason and because of its lesser atropine requirement, edrophonium regained popularity as an antagonist during the 1980s.[327] However, Rupp and coworkers[339] found that edrophonium is not as effective as neostigmine in antagonizing profound blockade of more than 90% twitch depression (only one twitch palpable by TOF) whereas increasing the edrophonium dose from 0.5 to 1.0 mg/kg increased its efficacy. Neostigmine remains capable of more complete antagonism.[340] To be equivalent to 40 µg/kg of neostigmine as an antagonist of profound vecuronium blockade, 1.5 mg/kg of edrophonium must be administered.[330]

The relative potencies of edrophonium and neostigmine differ at various intensities of blockade (Fig. 29-25.).[341] Edrophonium becomes less potent relative to neostigmine as the depth of blockade becomes more intense. In other words, the dose-response curves are not parallel and become increasingly divergent as the depth of blockade intensifies. This difference indicates that edrophonium may be less effective than neostigmine when antagonizing very deep levels of blockade.

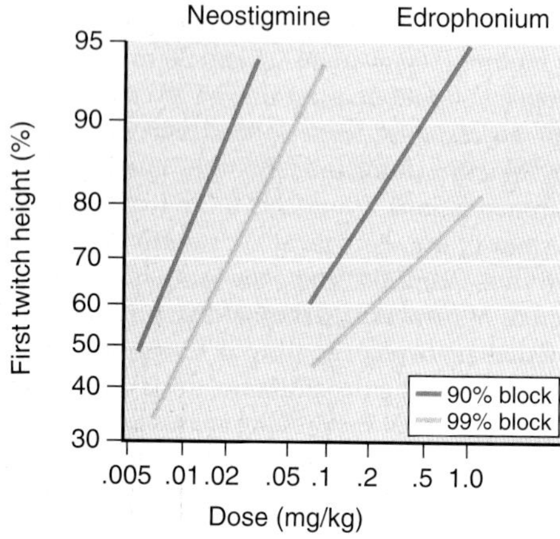

Figure 29-25 First twitch height (logit scale) versus dose (log scale) 10 minutes after the administration of neostigmine and edrophonium given at either 1% (99% block) or 10% (90% block) first twitch recovery. *(From Donati F, Smith CE, Bevan DR: Dose-response relationships for edrophonium and neostigmine as antagonists of moderate and profound atracurium blockade. Anesth Analg 68:13-19, 1989.)*

The Dose of Anticholinesterase

Larger doses of anticholinesterases should antagonize neuromuscular blockade more rapidly and more completely than smaller doses do. This relationship is true up to the point of the maximum effective dose, beyond which additional amounts of anticholinesterase will not produce any further antagonism. For neostigmine, this maximum effective dose is in the 60- to 80-µg/kg range,[327] and for edrophonium, it is in the 1.0- to 1.5-mg/kg range.[339,340]

Mixing or combining antagonists is not advisable. Neostigmine and edrophonium do not potentiate each other; in fact, their effects in combination may not even be additive.[342] Therefore, when inadequate reversal occurs, one should not be tempted to add a different anticholinesterase but should ensure only that the maximum dose of the original drug has been administered. Ventilation should then be supported until adequate neuromuscular function is achieved.

Rate of Spontaneous Recovery from the Neuromuscular Blocker

After administration of an anticholinesterase, two processes contribute to recovery of neuromuscular function. The first is the antagonism induced by the effect of the anticholinesterase at the neuromuscular junction; the second is the natural process of decrease in plasma concentration of the neuromuscular blocker (and hence its effect at the neuromuscular junction).[332,335] Therefore, the more rapid the elimination of the neuromuscular blocker, the faster the recovery of adequate neuromuscular function after the administration of an antagonist (Fig. 29-26).[343] A clear illustration of this principle is the difference in antagonism of the blockade induced by neuromuscular blockers with an intermediate duration of action versus those with a long duration. Plasma concentrations of drugs with an intermediate duration of action decrease more rapidly than those with a long duration of action,[141] and consequently, recovery of neuromuscular function is more rapid. Thus, the incidence of inadequate neuromuscular function in the postoperative period is less with intermediate-acting than with long-acting neuromuscular blockers.[336,344] This difference in speed of reversal between intermediate- and long-acting drugs is due to the effect of different rates of spontaneous recovery and not to a difference in response to neostigmine.[345] When neostigmine is administered to antagonize a stable level of blockade maintained by continuous infusion of either vecuronium or pancuronium, the rate and degree of recovery are similar to those achieved in the case of administration of each neuromuscular blocker alone.[345]

Even though mivacurium is no longer available in the United States, its pharmacology allows better understanding of basic pharmacology. The interaction between spontaneous recovery from and anticholinesterase-induced reversal of mivacurium's effect is more complex. The rate of spontaneous recovery from mivacurium-induced bockade is more rapid than that from any other nondepolarizing neuromuscular blocker. This is a result of its rapid hydrolysis by butyrylcholinesterase. Neostigmine-induced reversal of mivacurium is similar to or faster than that of atracurium.[184,346] During profound (<3% twitch recovery) mivacurium-induced blockade, the administration of neostigmine may prolong recovery.[347] Neostigmine has two major effects relevant to mivacurium. First, it inhibits acetylcholinesterase at the neuromuscular junction, thereby effectively increasing the acetylcholine concentration and facilitating recovery. Second, it inhibits butyrylcholinesterase, the enzyme responsible for metabolism of mivacurium, and slows the normally rapid decrease in the plasma concentration of mivacurium.[348] In contrast, edrophonium is a less potent inhibitor of butyrylcholinesterase[348] and should have little effect on the metabolism of mivacurium. Provided that there is 10% recovery of twitch response (one twitch in the TOF), either 20 to 40 µg/kg of neostigmine or 0.3 to 0.5 mg/kg of edrophonium will accelerate recovery from mivacurium.[346]

It has been suggested that routine administration of an anticholinesterase may often be omitted because spontaneous recovery from mivacurium's effect is so rapid. However, this strategy may lead to inadequate recovery and postoperative weakness unless at least 20 minutes is allowed for spontaneous recovery before the anticholinesterase is administered.[346]

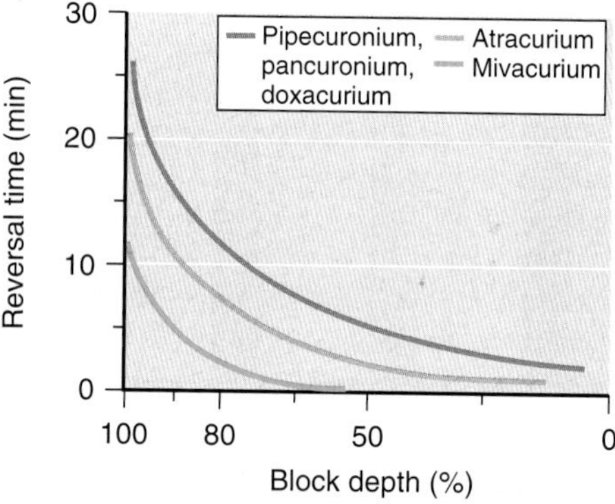

Figure 29-26 Comparative mean speed of antagonism by neostigmine of neuromuscular blockade induced by long-acting agents (doxacurium, pancuronium, pipecuronium), intermediate-acting drugs (atracurium and others), and the short-acting agent mivacurium. Antagonism is more rapid as processes of clearance increase (see text). *(From Savarese JJ: Reversal of nondepolarizing blocks: More controversial than ever?* In *Review Course Lectures, 67th Congress. Cleveland, OH, International Anesthesia Research Society, 1993.)*

Because mivacurium is metabolized by butyrylcholinesterase, administration of exogenous human butyrylcholinesterase can theoretically hasten recovery from mivacurium's effects. Administration of purified human cholinesterase does produce some antagonism of mivacurium-induced blockade,[349] but it is ineffective in profound blockade[348] and no better than edrophonium alone.[350] Administration of purified butyrylcholinesterase to patients who are genetically homozygous for atypical butyrylcholinesterase and have a prolonged blockade may be justified,[188] but this therapy is expensive and has not yet been tested adequately.

Concentration of Inhaled Anesthetic

Several studies have documented that antagonism of residual blockade is actually retarded by anesthetizing concentrations of anesthetic vapors.[351,352] For example, reversal of rocuronium by neostigmine under sevoflurane (and to a lesser extent, isoflurane) anesthesia occurred more slowly than under propofol anesthesia.[352] Sevoflurane may impede neostigmine-induced antagonism more than isoflurane does.[351] When compared with recovery from isoflurane anesthesia, recovery from that produced by desflurane or sevoflurane is prolonged.[343] Withdrawal of the anesthetic vapor at the end of surgery, with subsequent reduction of its enhancement of neuromuscular blockade, will speed pharmacologic reversal.[328]

Clinical Recommendations

When antagonizing deep levels of neuromuscular blockade (about 10% recovery or one twitch in response to TOF stimulation), larger doses of anticholinesterases (e.g., neostigmine, 35 μg/kg) should be administered and adequate time allowed for recovery of neuromuscular function. The time required for recovery to a TOF ratio of 0.7 will be approximately 60 minutes for the long-acting neuromuscular blocking drugs (pancuronium) and 30 minutes for the intermediate-acting ones (rocuronium). To antagonize lesser degrees of blockade, smaller doses of anticholinesterases may be administered, with additional anticholinesterase given if adequate recovery has not occurred in 10 minutes.

It is not advisable to administer additional anticholinesterase if maximal doses of edrophonium (1.5 mg/kg), neostigmine (70 μg/kg), or pyridostigmine (350 μg/kg) fail to antagonize the residual blockade.[340] Giving too much anticholinesterase to antagonize residual neuromuscular blockade may actually render patients weaker.[326,354,355] These doses inhibit acetylcholinesterase completely, and if they fail to fully antagonize the residual blockade, another likely cause of the inadequate antagonism should be sought. Some of these additional potential causes of inadequate antagonism of neuromuscular blockade are described in the following sections.

Acid-Base State

Both metabolic and respiratory acidosis may augment the blockade induced by a nondepolarizing neuromuscular blocker, but only respiratory acidosis prevents adequate antagonism.[338,356] The probability of achieving adequate antagonism of nondepolarizing neuromuscular blockade in the presence of significant respiratory acidosis (partial pressure of carbon dioxide in arterial gas >50 mm Hg) is low. Therefore, attempts to antagonize residual blockade may fail if a patient hypoventilates. Administration of narcotics to relieve pain may, by producing hypoventilation, increase the likelihood of this adverse event. Although metabolic acidosis might also be predicted to prevent antagonism by neostigmine, this hypothesis has not been substantiated.[338,356] Metabolic alkalosis, but not metabolic acidosis, prevents neostigmine's antagonism of dTc and pancuronium.[338,356,357] These results suggest that extracellular pH is not as important as changes in electrolyte concentrations and intracellular pH.

Electrolyte Imbalance

Few data are available on the effect of electrolyte imbalance on antagonism of a nondepolarizing neuromuscular blockade induced by neostigmine. Low extracellular concentrations of potassium enhance the blockade from nondepolarizing neuromuscular blockers and diminish the ability of neostigmine to antagonize the blockade. This effect is caused by the increase in end-plate transmembrane potential that results from a higher ratio of intracellular to extracellular potassium. Thus, a decrease in extracellular potassium causes hyperpolarization and produces resistance to depolarization. Patients with an imbalance in potassium may have other diseases or injuries that alter their response to neuromuscular blockers (e.g., patients with burns). In addition, severe dehydration will concentrate the neuromuscular blocker present in plasma, in effect decreasing the volume of distribution and increasing muscle relaxant activity. In an animal model of chronic hypokalemia, cats were given a diuretic without potassium supplementation for 15 days. Less pancuronium was required for neuromuscular blockade and more neostigmine was required for antagonism.[358] Even though the differences were small, the blockade was always antagonized completely. If we assume that this animal model approximates the clinical situation, changes in potassium appear to be of relatively minor consequence with respect to the clinical question of adequacy of reversal.

Other Factors

The calcium channel blocker verapamil will potentiate nondepolarizing neuromuscular blocking drugs and may render achieving adequate reversal difficult.[359,360] When attempting reversal of neuromuscular blockade in patients receiving verapamil, edrophonium may be more effective than neostigmine.[359,360] Other factors that may interfere with antagonism are hypothermia and the administration of antibiotics, particularly those of the aminoglycoside or polypeptide classes (see the section on drug interactions).[271] In the case of antibiotics, administration of an anticholinesterase may in fact deepen the blockade.

Side Effects of Anticholinesterases

Cardiovascular Effects

Because only the nicotinic effects of edrophonium, neostigmine, and pyridostigmine are desired, the muscarinic effects must be blocked by atropine or glycopyrrolate. Atropine induces its vagolytic effect much more rapidly than glycopyrrolate does. To minimize cardiovascular changes, atropine is better suited for administration with the rapid-acting edrophonium, and glycopyrrolate is better suited for administration with the slower-acting neostigmine and pyridostigmine.[361] In general, 7 to 10 μg/kg of atropine should be given with 0.5 to 1.0 mg/kg of edrophonium.[337] When cardiac dysrhythmias are a concern, glycopyrrolate may be preferable to atropine,[362] and the anticholinesterases and anticholinergics should be administered more slowly (e.g., 2 to 5 minutes) to reduce the incidence and severity of disordered rhythm.

Nausea and Vomiting

Reports on the effect of anticholinesterase administration on postoperative nausea and vomiting are conflicting. Neostigmine has been implicated as a cause of postoperative nausea and vomiting,[363] but it has also been described as having antiemetic properties[364] and as having no effect on the incidence of postoperative nausea and vomiting.[365] A meta-analysis by Tramer and Fuchs-Bader[366] looked at the results of anticholinesterase administration in more than 1100 patients. They found a dose-response relationship for the incidence of nausea and vomiting after the administration of neostigmine: the highest incidence of vomiting after the administration of 1.5 mg of neostigmine was lower than the lowest incidence of vomiting after the administration of 2.5 mg of neostigmine. Discrepancies between the results of other studies may have been at least partly attributable to the use of different dosing regimens. Although vomiting occurs in 17% to 33% of patients after the administration of neostigmine, the authors did not recommend that all patients be allowed to recover spontaneously because of the risk for postoperative residual paralysis.[366] A more recent study demonstrated the hazards of not antagonizing residual neuromuscular blockade at least 2 hours after the administration of a dose twice the ED_{95} of vecuronium, rocuronium, or atracurium.[367]

Pharmacokinetics of Neostigmine, Pyridostigmine, and Edrophonium

The pharmacokinetics of edrophonium, neostigmine, and pyridostigmine is summarized in Table 29-12.[368-371] The data indicate several relevant clinical conclusions:

1. Pyridostigmine has a longer elimination half-life than that of the other anticholinesterases, which probably accounts for its longer duration of action.[368,369]
2. Comparison data on the elimination half-lives in patients with and without renal failure showed that renal excretion accounts for about 50% of the excretion of neostigmine and about 75% of the excretion of pyridostigmine and edrophonium. Renal failure decreases the plasma clearance of neostigmine, pyridostigmine, and edrophonium as much as, if not more than that of the long-acting neuromuscular blockers. Therefore, if proper doses of anticholinesterase drugs are given and overdoses of neuromuscular blockers are avoided, renal failure should not be associated with "recurarization."[368,369] This remote possibility is further diminished if the clinician restricts the relaxants used to the intermediate- or short-acting drugs in patients with renal failure.
3. Edrophonium was once thought to be an unsuitable antagonist in clinical practice because its duration of action was believed to be too short. However, when larger doses (e.g., 0.5 to 1.0 mg/kg) are given, sustained antagonism of nondepolarizing neuromuscular–induced blockade results.[372] In fact, the elimination half-life of edrophonium is similar to that of neostigmine and pyridostigmine (see Table 29-12).[370]

Mild hypothermia (i.e., 34°C to 35°C), which commonly occurs intraoperatively, affects the pharmacokinetics of neostigmine. Its clearance is decreased from 16.2 mL/kg/min at 36.5°C to 13.5 mL/kg/min at 34.5°C.[284] In addition, onset of the peak effect of neostigmine is delayed by mild hypothermia from 4.2 to 5.5 minutes.[284] If hypothermia has any influence on the efficacy of neostigmine-induced reversal, it is more likely to be due to the effect of temperature on the neuromuscular blocker (e.g., prolonged duration of action[273]) than to the pharmacology of neostigmine.

The pharmacokinetics of the anticholinesterases depends on several factors, including distribution, metabolism, and elimination. In the case of neostigmine, a carbamylated complex with acetylcholinesterase is formed, and it is the rate of dissociation of neostigmine from this complex (i.e., its metabolism) that is probably the major determinant of its duration of action. The decrease in the plasma concentration of neostigmine (i.e., its distribution and elimination) may not be as pertinent a determinant of its duration of action.

Table 29-12 Pharmacokinetics of Neostigmine (N), Pyridostigmine (P), and Edrophonium (E) in Patients without and with Renal Failure

	Without Renal Failure			With Renal Failure		
	N	P	E	N	P	E
Distribution half-life ($t_{1/2\alpha}$, min)	3.4	6.7	7.2	2.5	3.9	7.0
Elimination half-life ($t_{1/2\beta}$, min)	77	113	110	181	379	304
Volume of central compartment (L/kg)	0.2	0.3	0.3	0.3	0.4	0.3
Total plasma clearance (mL/kg/min)	9.1	8.6	9.5	4.8	3.1	3.9

Data from Cronnelly et al.[368,369] and Morris et al.[370,371]

Other Antagonists of Nondepolarizing Neuromuscular Blockade

Sugammadex

Sugammadex may be the most exciting drug in clinical neuromuscular pharmacology in the last 50 years. The combination of rocuronium and sugammadex could replace succinylcholine for rapid-sequence induction of anesthesia and completely eliminate residual paralysis in the postanesthetic recovery room.[373]

Sugammadex (ORG 25969) is the first selective relaxant binding agent (*su* refers to *sugar*, and *gammadex* refers to the structural molecule *gamma*-cyclo*dex*trin). A modified γ-cyclodextrin, sugammadex (Fig. 29-27) is a new type of reversal agent.[374] The three natural unmodified cyclodextrins consist of six, seven, and eight cyclic oligosaccharides (i.e., dextrose units joined through one to four glycosyl bonds) and are called α-, β-,

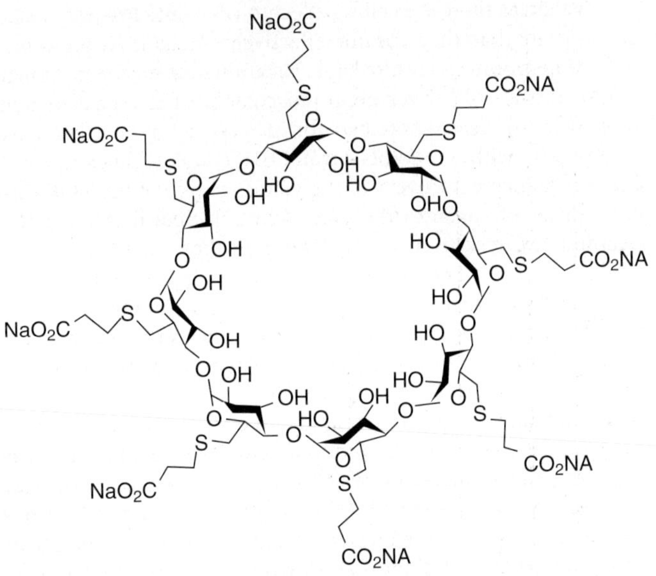

Figure 29-27 Structure of the synthetic γ-cyclodextrin sugammadex (ORG 25969).

and γ-cyclodextrin, respectively. Their three-dimensional structure resembles a hollow truncated cone or a doughnut. The structure has a hydrophobic cavity and a hydrophilic exterior because of the presence of polar hydroxyl groups. Hydrophobic interactions trap the drug in the cyclodextrin cavity (the "doughnut hole"), thereby resulting in the formation of a water-soluble guest-host complex. Although unmodified γ-cyclodextrin possesses a larger lipophilic cavity (7.5 to 8.3 Å) than any other cyclodextrin does, it is still not deep enough to accommodate the larger rigid structure of the rocuronium molecule. Therefore, the cavity was modified by adding eight side chains to extend it to 11 Å for better accommodation of the four hydrophobic steroidal rings of rocuronium and by adding negatively charged carboxyl groups at the end of the side chains to enhance electrostatic binding to the positively charged quaternary nitrogen of rocuronium (Fig. 29-28).[374,375] The stability of the rocuronium-sugammadex complex is the end result of an interplay of intermolecular forces (van der Waals forces), including thermodynamic (hydrogen bonds) and hydrophobic interactions.[376]

Sugammadex exerts its effect by forming very tight complexes in a 1 : 1 ratio with steroidal neuromuscular blocking agents (rocuronium > vecuronium ≫ pancuronium).[374] The guest-host complex exists in an equilibrium with a very high association rate and very low dissociation rate, so the complex is tight.[374] During rocuronium-induced neuromuscular blockade, intravenous administration of sugammadex results in rapid removal of free rocuronium molecules from plasma. This creates a concentration gradient favoring movement of the remaining rocuronium molecules from the neuromuscular junction back into plasma, where they are encapsulated by free sugammadex molecules. These molecules also enter tissues and form a complex with rocuronium. Therefore, the neuromuscular blockade of rocuronium is terminated rapidly by the diffusion of rocuronium away from the neuromuscular junction back into plasma. This results in an increase in the total plasma concentration of rocuronium (free and that bound to sugammadex).[377] Sugammadex therefore acts as a binding agent and has no effect on acetylcholinesterase or any receptor system in the body, thus eliminating the need for anticholinergic drugs and their undesirable side effects.

Pharmacokinetics. During an infusion of rocuronium to maintain a stable depth of neuromuscular blockade, administration of sugammadex increases the measured plasma concentration of rocuronium; the relaxant is redistributed from the effect compartment to the central compartment as it is encapsulated by sugammadex.[377] Recovery of muscle strength can occur despite increasing plasma concentrations of relaxant because the efficacy of sugammadex does not rely on renal excretion of the cyclodextrin-relaxant complex.[378]

When administered by itself to volunteers who had not received a neuromuscular blocking agent, 0.1 to 8.0 mg/kg of sugammadex had a clearance rate of 120 mL/min, an elimination half-life of 100 minutes, and a volume of distribution of 18 L.[379] Approximately 75% of a dose was eliminated in urine. The kinetics of sugammadex appears to be dose dependent in that clearance increases and the elimination half-life decreases as the dose of sugammadex increases from 0.15 to 1.0 mg/kg.[379]

In the absence of sugammadex, rocuronium is eliminated mainly by biliary excretion (>75%) and to a lesser degree by renal excretion (10% to 25%). Plasma clearance of sugammadex alone is approximately three times lower than that of rocuronium alone.[380] In volunteers, plasma clearance of rocuronium was decreased by a factor of greater than 2 after the administration of a 2.0-mg/kg or greater dose of sugammadex.[379] This decreased clearance occurs because the biliary route of excretion becomes unavailable for the rocuronium-sugammadex complex, and rocuronium clearance decreases to a value approaching the glomerular filtration rate (120 mL/min). Because of the soluble

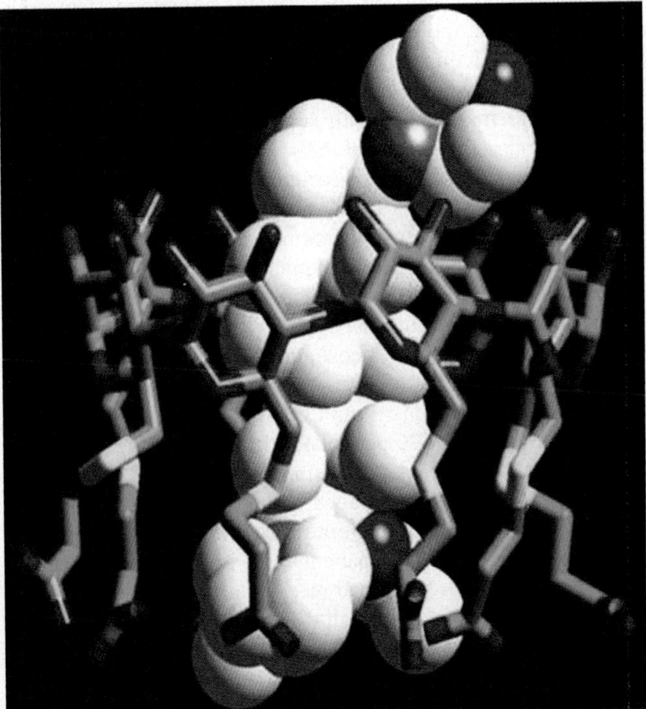

Figure 29-28 The sugammadex-rocuronium complex. *(From Bom A, Bradley M, Cameron K, et al: A novel concept of reversing neuromuscular block: Chemical encapsulation of rocuronium bromide by a cyclodextrin-based synthetic host. Angew Chem 41:266-270, 2002.)*

nature of the rocuronium-cyclodextrin complex, urinary excretion of the complex is the major route of elimination of rocuronium. Renal excretion of rocuronium is increased by more than 100% after the administration of 4 to 8 mg/kg of sugammadex.[380]

As noted earlier, after the administration of sugammadex, the plasma concentration of free rocuronium decreases rapidly, but the total plasma concentration of rocuronium (both free and that bound to sugammadex) increases.[377]

PHARMACODYNAMICS. In male volunteers, administration of 8 mg/kg of sugammadex 3 minutes after the administration of 0.6 mg/kg of rocuronium resulted in recovery of the TOF ratio to 0.9 within 2 minutes.[379] Decreasing the dose of sugammadex to 4 mg/kg resulted in recovery of the TOF ratio to 0.9 in less than 4 minutes.[379] Additionally, in surgical patients who were anesthetized with total intravenous anesthetic agents and had received 0.6 mg/kg of rocuronium, different doses of sugammadex or placebo were administered at reappearance of the second twitch of the TOF response.[381] Sugammadex decreased the median recovery time in a dose-dependent manner from 21.0 minutes in the placebo group to 1.1 minutes in the group given 4.0 mg/kg of sugammadex.[381]

Administration of sugammadex when the TOF count had returned to two detectable responses resulted in a dose-dependent recovery from the neuromuscular blockade induced by either rocuronium (0.60 mg/kg) or vecuronium (0.10 mg/kg).[382] After a dose of 4.0 mg/kg of sugammadex, the mean time to recovery of the TOF ratio to 0.9 was 1.1 minutes and 1.5 minutes after rocuronium and vecuronium, respectively. A sugammadex dose of 0.5 mg/kg is considered to be grossly inadequate for antagonism.[382-384]

One of the features that make sugammadex so different pharmacodynamically from the available anticholinesterases is that it takes effect more quickly and reliably than either neostigmine or edrophonium.[385] In a trial by Sacan and colleagues,[385] patients received 0.6 mg/kg of rocuronium, and neuromuscular blockade was maintained with supplemental doses of rocuronium given at reappearance of the second twitch in the TOF. The reversal agent—70 µg/kg of neostigmine, 1 mg/kg of edrophonium, or 4 mg/kg of sugammadex—was administered at least 15 minutes after the last dose of rocuronium. A 4-mg/kg dose of sugammadex reversed the rocuronium-induced neuromuscular blockade more rapidly than neostigmine or edrophonium did. The average time to achieve a TOF ratio of 0.9 was 10 times longer after the administration of neostigmine than it was after sugammadex (1044 versus 107 seconds) and three times longer after the administration of edrophonium (331 seconds) than after sugammadex. Although 5 of 20 patients in the neostigmine group and 2 of 20 patients in the edrophonium group achieved a TOF ratio of 0.9, all 20 in the sugammadex group achieved this degree of recovery. Furthermore, 5 minutes after the administration of edrophonium, none of the patients who had received edrophonium and 5% of those who had received neostigmine had recovered to a TOF ratio of 0.9, but all the patients in the sugammadex group had.[385] Hence, sugammadex appears to allow more complete recovery of neuromuscular function than the anticholinesterases do, and it does so more quickly than the more conventional agents. Unlike the case with neostigmine or edrophonium,[328,351,353] the choice of anesthetic agent (e.g., propofol versus sevoflurane) does not appear to influence the ability of sugammadex to antagonize rocuronium-induced neuromuscular blockade.[386]

Whereas there is a ceiling effect to what anticholinesterases can do[332] in that they cannot effectively antagonize profound levels of neuromuscular blockade, sugammadex has been shown to do so in trials.[384,387] Deep neuromuscular blockade (post-tetanic count of <10) was maintained for at least 2 hours in patients anesthetized with propofol–nitrous oxide–opioid anesthesia.[387] After spontaneous recovery of the second twitch of the TOF, different doses of sugammadex were administered; increasing the sugammadex dose from 0.5 to 4.0 mg/kg shortened the average recovery time to a TOF of 0.9 from 6.8 minutes (range, 4.8 to 11.4 minutes) to 1.4 minutes (range, 0.95 to 2.3 minutes), respectively.[387] Unexpectedly, the recovery time was longer (2.6 minutes[388]) with a 6.0-mg/kg dose.[387] The reason for this deviation is unclear.

Sugammadex produces rapid and effective reversal of even more profound rocuronium-induced neuromuscular blockade. In one study, sugammadex or placebo was administered 5 minutes after the administration of 1.2 mg/kg of rocuronium.[389] Increasing the dose of sugammadex to 16 mg/kg decreased the mean recovery time to a TOF ratio of 0.9 from 122.1 minutes (spontaneous recovery) to less than 2 minutes.[389]

In another study, patients were randomized to receive an intubating dose of 1.2 mg/kg of rocuronium followed 3 minutes later by 16 mg/kg of sugammadex or an intubating dose of 1.0 mg/kg of succinylcholine.[390] The mean time to 90% recovery of first twitch was significantly faster in the rocuronium-sugammadex group than it was in the succinylcholine group. The mean (± SD) time to 90% recovery of first twitch from the start of sugammadex administration was 2.9 minutes (1.7 minutes).[390] Therefore, the use of rapid-sequence induction with rocuronium can be facilitated by the presence of sugammadex. Administration of 1.2 mg/kg of rocuronium followed 3 minutes later by 16 mg/kg of sugammadex seems to provide a faster onset-offset profile than that seen with 1.0 mg/kg of succinylcholine (Fig. 29-29).[391]

Sugammadex is ineffective against succinylcholine and benzylisoquinolinium neuromuscular blockers such as mivacurium, atracurium, and cisatracurium[392] because it cannot form inclusion complexes with these drugs. Therefore, if neuromuscular blockade must be reestablished after using sugammadex, one of the benzylisoquinolinium neuromuscular blockers should be considered.

SIDE EFFECTS. The ability of sugammadex to form complexes with steroidal and nonsteroidal compounds such as cortisone, atropine, and verapamil is probably clinically insignificant and is 120 to 700 times less than that of rocuronium.[393] In phase I and II studies, the most frequently reported side effects have been hypotension, coughing, movement, nausea, vomiting, dry mouth, parosmia (an abnormal sense of smell), a sensation of a changed temperature, and abnormal levels of *N*-acetyl-glucosaminidase in urine.[379,381,387] Patient movement with the administration of sugammadex may have been due to the unmasking of inadequate anesthesia rather than an adverse response to the reversal agent. In one study, prolongation of the corrected QT interval was noted in five subjects who received placebo and in three who received sugammadex.[379]

Cysteine

Gantacurium undergoes rapid degradation in plasma by chemical hydrolysis and inactivation by cysteine adduction (see Fig. 29-10),[105] which is a novel chemical mechanism of inactivation. Exogenous administration of cysteine can accelerate the

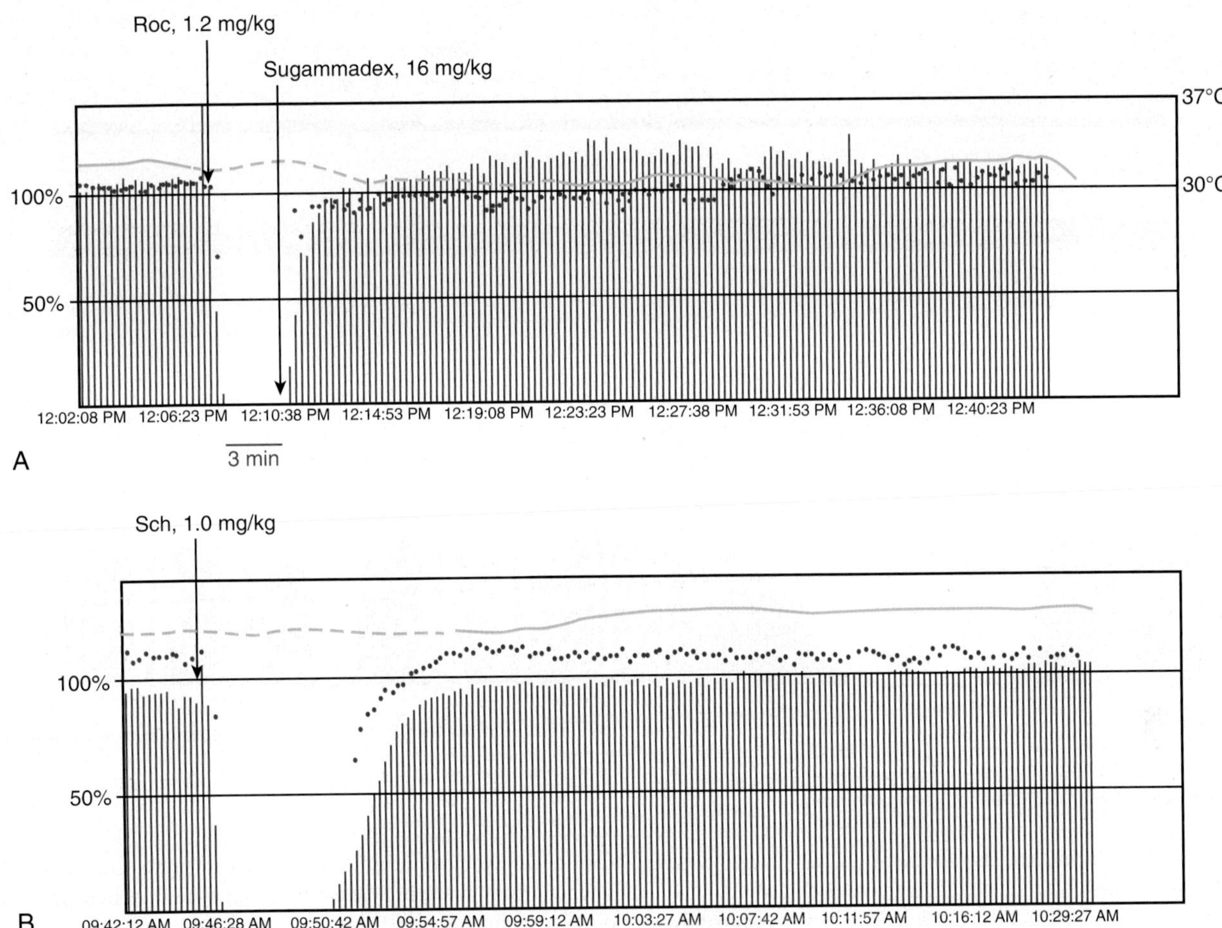

Figure 29-29 **A,** Recovery of twitch height and the train-of-four (TOF) ratio after the administration of 1.2 mg/kg of rocuronium, followed 3 minutes later by 16 mg/kg of sugammadex, both given intravenously. Recovery to a first twitch height (T1) of 90% and a TOF ratio of 0.94 occurred 110 seconds later. The onset-offset time with this sequence (i.e., time from the end of the injection of rocuronium until T1 recovery to 90%) was 4 minutes, 47 seconds. **B,** Effects of administering 1.0 mg/kg of succinylcholine (Sch) with spontaneous recovery to a T1 of 90% occurring after 9 minutes, 23 seconds. *(From Naguib M: Sugammadex: Another milestone in clinical neuromuscular pharmacology. Anesth Analg 104:575-581, 2007.)*

antagonism of gantacurium-induced neuromuscular blockade. As shown in Figure 29-30, after administration of a second 0.2-mg/kg dose of gantacurium, followed less than 1 minute later by 10 mg/kg of cysteine, complete recovery from neuromuscular blockade occurred within 4 minutes.

Special Populations

Pediatric Patients

Development of the neuromuscular junction is not complete at birth.[14] In humans, maturation of neuromuscular transmission probably occurs after the first 2 months of age. Nonetheless, neuromuscular blockers can be used safely in term and preterm infants.

Routine administration of succinylcholine to healthy children should be discontinued. In apparently healthy children, intractable cardiac arrest with hyperkalemia, rhabdomyolysis, and acidosis may occur after succinylcholine administration, particularly in patients with unsuspected muscular dystrophy of the Duchenne type.[394] In response to this report, the U.S. Food and Drug Administration and Glaxo-Wellcome have modified the package insert for succinylcholine to warn against the use of succinylcholine in children except for emergency control of the airway (see the section on complications of succinylcholine).

It is not apparent from older studies whether neonates are more sensitive than adults to nondepolarizing neuromuscular blockers.[395] More recent studies by Fisher and coworkers[137,396,397] on the pharmacokinetics and pharmacodynamics of neuromuscular blockers in infants, children, and adults, however, have made it possible to better understand the clinical pharmacology of these drugs in pediatric patients (see Chapter 82). Neonates and infants are more sensitive than adults to the neuromuscular blocking effects of dTc.[396] A lower plasma concentration of this neuromuscular blocker is required to achieve a desired level of neuromuscular blockade in these young patients. However, the dosage should not be decreased because infants have a larger volume of distribution. The increased volume of distribution and slower clearance (Fig. 29-31) contribute to a longer elimination half-life,[396,398]

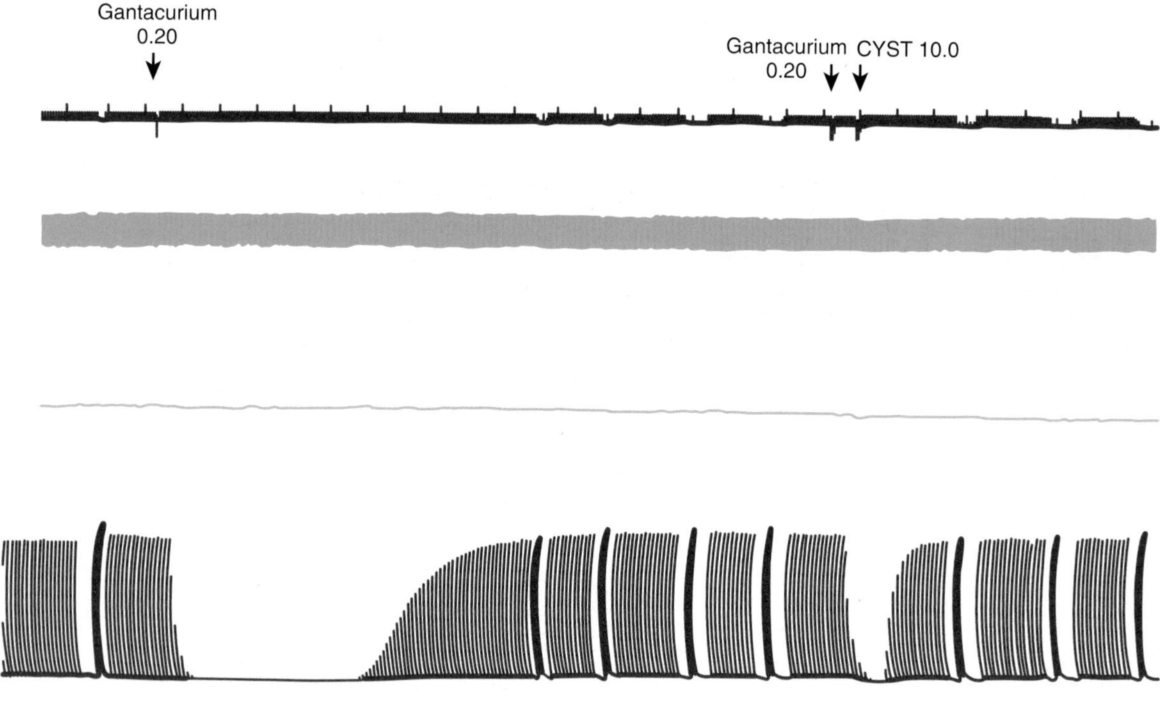

Figure 29-30 Twitch recording from a single monkey demonstrating complete spontaneous recovery from 3.2 times the ED_{95} of gantacurium, 0.2 mg/kg. Complete spontaneous recovery occurred within 10 minutes. Six minutes after complete recovery, a second dose of gantacurium, 0.2 mg/kg, was administered to this animal. Less than 1 minute later, 10 mg/kg of cysteine was administered. With cysteine administration, complete recovery occurred within 4 minutes of administering gantacurium. *(Courtresy of John J. Savarese.)*

which means that in infants, less frequent dosing (longer dosing intervals) of dTc may be required than in older children.

Atracurium, vecuronium, cisatracurium, rocuronium, and mivacurium are commonly administered to children. The popularity of these drugs in children most likely stems from the following points: minimal residual paralysis is seen in the postoperative period, and onset of action is faster in children than in adults.

Atracurium and vecuronium, in comparison, show very different kinetic and dynamic patterns in infants. As with the long-acting neuromuscular blockers, the sensitivity of infants to vecuronium is greater than it is in children (ED_{95} of 0.047 versus 0.081 mg/kg, respectively).[399] The increased duration of action in infants is most likely secondary to the increased volume of distribution of vecuronium because its clearance is unchanged.[397,398] Vecuronium therefore acts as a long-acting neuromuscular blocker in neonates.[397,398]

In contrast, the duration of action of atracurium is not significantly different in pediatric patients and adults.[400] As with vecuronium and dTc, the volume of distribution is increased in infants.[137] However, clearance of atracurium is also more rapid.[137] Therefore, the same dose (0.5 to 0.6 mg/kg) can be used in infants, children, and adults for tracheal intubation without any major difference between the three groups in its duration of action. In children, a dose of 0.1 mg/kg of cisatracurium has an onset of just over 2 minutes and a clinical duration of approximately 30 minutes during balanced or halothane anesthesia.[401] The calculated ED_{95} doses of cisatracurium in infants and children are 43

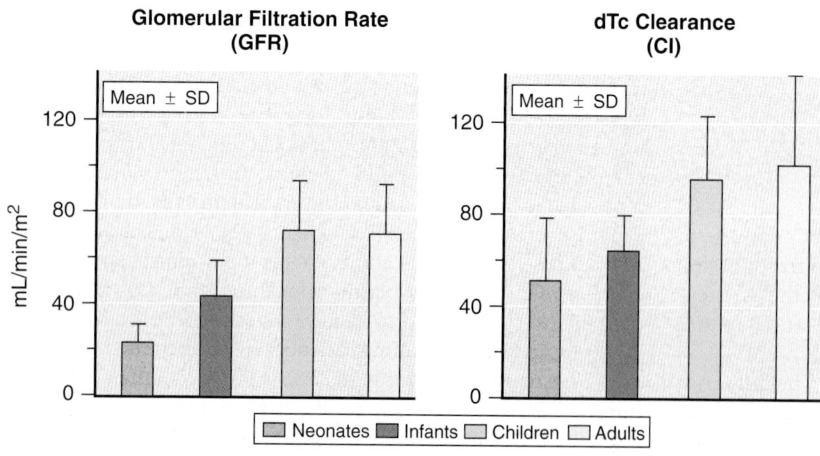

Figure 29-31 Correlation between age, glomerular filtration, and clearance of curare. *(From Fisher DM, O'Keeffe C, Stanski DR, et al: Pharmacokinetics and pharmacodynamics of d-tubocurarine in infants, children, and adults. Anesthesiology 57:203-208, 1982.)*

and 47 mg/kg, respectively.[402] The mean infusion rate necessary to maintain 90% to 99% neuromuscular blockade is also similar in infants and children.[402]

Rocuronium in adults is an intermediate-acting neuromuscular blocker with a fast onset of action, and this is also true in infants and children.[403,404] Its potency is greater in infants than in children, but its onset is faster in the latter age group.[404] In children, 0.6 mg/kg of rocuronium produces better conditions for rapid tracheal intubation than 0.1 mg/kg of vecuronium or 0.5 mg/kg of atracurium does.[403] As with adults, for rapid-sequence intubation (60 seconds) in the presence of a full stomach, a 1.2-mg/kg dose of rocuronium is suggested.

Antagonism of residual neuromuscular blockade in the case of the various nondepolarizers is similar in children and adults. Fisher and coauthors described some minor variations in the neostigmine and edrophonium dosage for pediatric patients. For example, the ED_{50} of neostigmine for antagonism of a dTc-induced 90% blockade of the adductor pollicis twitch was 22.9 µg/kg in adults versus 15.5 µg/kg in infants. In the case of edrophonium, the ED_{50} for antagonism of dTc-induced 90% blockade was 128 µg/kg in adults. In children, the ED_{50} was 233 µg/kg, and in infants it was 145 µg/kg.[405] The rate of recovery from intermediate- or short-acting neuromuscular blockers is faster than that from long-acting drugs in children.[333]

Neostigmine doses of 50 to 60 µg/kg or edrophonium doses of 500 to 1000 µg/kg should be used for antagonism of residual neuromuscular blockade in children. In all cases, tests of clinical recovery, such as head lift, leg lift, and cry, should be performed and documented for pediatric patients and adults.

Elderly Patients

The pharmacodynamics of neuromuscular blockers is altered in elderly patients (see Chapter 71). A number of physiologic changes that accompany the aging process, including decreases in total body water, increases in total body fat, decreases in hepatic and renal blood flow, and decreases in cardiac reserve, account for the altered responses of the elderly to neuromuscular blockers. A number of physiologic and anatomic changes at the neuromuscular junction also occur with aging. Such changes include an increase in the distance between the junctional axon and the motor end plate, flattening of the folds of the motor end plate, decreased concentration of acetylcholine receptors at the motor end plate, a reduction in the amount of acetylcholine in each vesicle in the prejunctional axon, and decreased release of acetylcholine from the preterminal axon in response to a neural impulse.[14] That is, the elderly and young adults have similar degrees of neuromuscular blockade at the same plasma concentration of a neuromuscular blocker. Rather, it appears that in the elderly, decreased splanchnic and renal blood flow, decreased glomerular filtration rate, and decreased hepatic function are responsible for the prolonged durations of action of most neuromuscular blockers. The greater depth of blockade with a given dose of relaxant in elderly patients than in young patients may also be due, in part, to altered volumes of distribution. The effect of aging alone, versus disease states often associated with the aging process, may be difficult to distinguish in identifying mechanisms of altered neuromuscular blocker action in the elderly.

Pancuronium,[406] vecuronium,[325,397] and rocuronium[208] all show altered pharmacodynamics and pharmacokinetics in elderly patients. Decreased clearance of each of these drugs from plasma explains their prolonged duration of action in these patients. These neuromuscular blockers depend on the kidney or the liver (or on both) for their metabolism and elimination.

In the case of drugs whose elimination is independent of hepatic or renal blood flow, pharmacokinetics and pharmacodynamics should be unaffected by age. This is true of atracurium, which depends on Hofmann elimination for its clearance.[138] Cisatracurium, which also undergoes Hofmann elimination, has a delayed onset of effect in elderly patients. The duration of action of the relaxant, however, appears to not be influenced by advanced age. The prolonged elimination half-life of the drug in the elderly is due to an increased volume of distribution. Clearance is not decreased with advanced age.

Butyrylcholinesterase activity in the elderly, though still in the normal range, is approximately 26% lower than it is in young adults.[407] Because mivacurium is metabolized by butyrylcholinesterase, its clearance is likely to be slightly reduced in the elderly; as a result, the duration of action of mivacurium is 20% to 25% longer in elderly patients,[408] and the infusion rate needed to maintain a stable depth of blockade is decreased.

In general, when maintaining neuromuscular blockade with nondepolarizing neuromuscular blockers in elderly patients, one can expect that with the exception of atracurium and cisatracurium, the dosing interval will be increased and fewer doses of neuromuscular blocker will be required to maintain the desired depth of neuromuscular blockade. The choice of drug and monitoring the depth of blockade are exceptionally important in this population because recovery of neuromuscular function is generally delayed in the elderly. Inadequate or incomplete recovery of muscle strength after the use of pancuronium is associated with an increased incidence of perioperative pulmonary complications in this patient population.[336]

Obese Patients

Reports on the effect of obesity on the pharmacodynamics of nondepolarizing neuromuscular blockade are conflicting. Although the duration of action of pancuronium is unaffected by a patient's weight,[409] obese patients recover more slowly from vecuronium-[410] or rocuronium-induced[411] neuromuscular blockade. These findings imply that elimination of these drugs is decreased. Recovery from atracurium-induced neuromuscular blockade, however, is not affected by obesity,[410] most likely because of lack of dependence on end-organ function for elimination.

Neuromuscular blockers should be administered to obese patients on the basis of about 20% more than lean body mass rather than on their actual body weight[412] to ensure that these patients are not receiving relative overdoses.

Severe Renal Disease

Renal failure influences the pharmacologic characteristics of nondepolarizing neuromuscular blockers either by decreased elimination of the drug or its metabolites via the kidney or by decreased activity of butyrylcholinesterase (Table 29-13). Consequently, the duration of action of neuromuscular blockers may be prolonged in patients with renal failure (see Chapters 65 and 67).

Table 29-13 Pharmacokinetics of Neuromuscular Blocking Drugs in Patients with Normal Renal Function or Renal Failure

	Plasma Clearance (mL/kg/min)		Volume of Distribution (mL/kg)		Elimination Half-life (min)		
	Normal Function	**Renal Failure**	**Normal Function**	**Renal Failure**	**Normal Function**	**Renal Failure**	**Reference**
Short-Acting Drugs							
Mivacurium isomers							183
Cis-trans	106	80	278	475	2.0	4.3	
Trans-trans	57	48	211	270	2.3	4.3	
Cis-cis	3.8	2.4a	227	244	68	80	
Intermediate-Acting Drugs							
Atracurium	6.1	6.7	182	224	21	24	204
	5.5	5.8	153	141	19	20	205*†
	10.9	7.8	280	265	17.3	19.7	413
Cisatracurium	5.2	—	31	—	—	—	203
Vecuronium	3.0	2.5	194	239	78	97	414
	5.3	3.1[a]	199	241	53	83[a]	415
Rocuronium	2.9	2.9	207	264[a]	71	97[a]	206
Long-Acting Drugs							
d-Tubocurarine	2.4	1.5	250	250	84	132	120
Pancuronium	74	20*	148	236*	97	475*	129†
	1.7	0.9	261	296*	132	257*	416

*Significant difference between normal renal function and renal failure.
†Values expressed as milliliters per minute, not weight adjusted.

Renal failure does not alter the sensitivity (dose-response relationship) of patients to the neuromuscular blocking action of pancuronium,[130] atracurium,[417] vecuronium,[418] or rocuronium.[419]

All long-lasting muscle relaxants are eliminated predominantly via the kidney, and renal failure is associated with reduced plasma clearance and an increased elimination half-life of these drugs as well.[107] As a consequence of these pharmacokinetic changes, the duration of neuromuscular blockade produced by these drugs is longer and more variable than in patients with normal renal function. Because of the potential for prolonged blockade and the availability of intermediate- and short-acting neuromuscular blockers, there is no longer any reason to recommend the use of the long-acting neuromuscular blockers in patients with renal failure.

The pharmacokinetics and duration of action of atracurium are unaffected by renal failure.[413,420] This lack of effect occurs in part because Hofmann elimination and ester hydrolysis[205] account for 50% of its total clearance.[191] The elimination half-life of laudanosine, the principal metabolite of atracurium, increases in renal failure.[413] Recent evidence suggests, however, that significant concentrations of laudanosine are not achieved during the administration of atracurium in the operating room setting.[413]

In patients with chronic renal failure, the duration of action of cisatracurium is not prolonged.[154] Hofmann elimination accounts for 77% of the total clearance of cisatracurium,[203] and renal excretion accounts for 16% of its elimination.[203] Clearance of the drug is slightly decreased (by 13%) in this patient population.

Vecuronium relies principally on hepatic, not renal, mechanisms for its elimination. However, its clearance is reduced and its elimination half-life is increased in patients with renal failure.[414,415] In one study, the duration of action of 0.1 mg/kg of vecuronium was both longer and more variable in patients with renal failure than in those with normal renal function.[415] In three other studies, the duration of action of 0.05 to 0.14 mg/kg of vecuronium was not prolonged by renal failure, but this result was probably due to the use of relatively small doses or inadequate sample sizes.[414] The principal metabolite of vecuronium, 3-desacetylvecuronium, has 80% of the neuromuscular blocking activity of vecuronium[177]; it may cause prolonged paralysis in patients with renal failure in the ICU.[179] In patients with renal failure, the duration of action and rate of recovery from vecuronium- or atracurium-induced neuromuscular blockade during surgery are similar.[421]

Plasma clearance of rocuronium may be decreased in patients with renal failure and its volume of distribution increased.[206] The duration of action of single and repeated doses, though, is not significantly affected.[419] When rocuronium is administered to patients with renal failure undergoing renal transplantation as opposed to patients with normal renal function, plasma clearance is unchanged (2.89 mL/kg/min), the volume of distribution is increased by 28%, and its elimination half-life is lengthened by 37% (see Fig. 29-16).[206]

Hepatobiliary Disease

Patients with hepatobiliary disease may exhibit prolonged blockade with pancuronium,[175] vecuronium,[127] rocuronium,[207,210] and mivacurium (see Chapters 66 and 67).[182] In the case of pancuronium,[175] vecuronium,[127] and mivacurium,[182] this prolonged action is associated with decreased plasma clearance of the drug. However, this relationship is not consistent, and many studies have described a reduction in clearance without a prolonged duration of action. In the case of atracurium, one study even demonstrated increased clearance in patients with cirrhosis, but the duration of action was normal.[193]

The influence of hepatobiliary disease on the pharmacokinetics of neuromuscular blockers is complex (Table 29-14). In

Table 29-14 Pharmacokinetics of Neuromuscular Blocking Drugs in Patients with Normal Liver Function or Hepatobiliary Disease

	Plasma Clearance (mL/kg/min)		Volume of Distribution (mL/kg)		Elimination Half-life (min)			
	Normal	Disease	Normal	Disease	Normal	Disease	Hepatic Pathology	Reference
Short-Acting Drugs								
Mivacurium isomers							Cirrhosis	182
Cis-trans	95	44*	210	188	1.53	2.48*		
Trans-trans	70	32*	200	199	2.32	11.1*		
Cis-cis	5.2	4.2	266	237	50.3	60.8		
Intermediate-Acting Drugs								
Atracurium	5.3	6.5	159	207*	21	22	Hepatorenal	417
	6.6	8.0*	202	282*	21	25	Cirrhosis	193
Cisatracurium	5.7	6.6*	161	195*	23.5	24.4	Transplantation-related	
Vecuronium	4.26	2.73*	246	253	58	848	Cirrhosis	127
	4.30	2.36*	247	206	58	98*	Cholestasis	422
	4.5	4.4	180	220	58	51	Cirrhosis	178
Rocuronium	2.79	2.41	184	234	87.5	96.0	Cirrhosis	207
	217	217	16.4	23.4*	76.4	111.5*	Mixed	209†
	296	189	151	264*	56	98*	Cirrhosis	423†
	3.70	2.66*	211	248	92	143*	Cirrhosis	210
Long-Acting Drugs								
Pancuronium	123	59*	261	307*	133	267*	Cholestasis	175†
	1.86	1.45*	279	416*	114	2088	Cirrhosis	174
	1.76	1.47	284	425*	141	224*	Cholestasis	424

*Significant difference between normal hepatic function and hepatobiliary disease.
†Values expressed as milliliters per minute or liters, not weight adjusted.

most studies, hepatic disease has been associated with an increased volume of distribution and, as a result, apparent resistance to the effect of dTc,[193] atracurium,[425] pancuronium,[423] and rocuronium.[426] The effect of hepatic disease on the pharmacokinetics of neuromuscular blockers (see Table 29-14) suggests that initial doses may need to be greater than those in patients with normal hepatic function but that once the desired level of blockade has been achieved, subsequent recovery may be slower. This is illustrated in the case of vecuronium, in which doses of up to 0.15 mg/kg have a normal duration of action[178,427] but a dose of 0.2 mg/kg results in prolonged action (see Fig. 29-14).[422]

Hepatic disease can alter the elimination of neuromuscular blockers by several mechanisms. The principal route of metabolism of pancuronium and vecuronium is deacetylation at the 3-position.[173] This metabolic process is presumed to occur in the liver because 10% to 20% of the total dose of pancuronium and 40% of that of vecuronium is found in the liver and bile as both parent drug and metabolite.[173] In hepatic disease, an increased plasma concentration of bile salts can reduce the hepatic uptake of pancuronium and vecuronium,[173] which may be an explanation for the decreased clearance of these drugs observed by some investigators.[174,175] Excretion of vecuronium is diminished in the presence of decreased hepatic function.[397] The duration of action of vecuronium is longer in these patients, and recovery is slower than in young healthy individuals.

Atracurium and cisatracurium share organ-independent modes of elimination.[189,202,203] As a consequence, their clearance should be little affected by hepatic disease. In fact and in contrast with that of all other neuromuscular blockers, plasma clearance of atracurium and cisatracurium is slightly increased in patients with liver disease (see Table 29-14).[193,211] Because elimination of atracurium and cisatracurium occurs outside of as well as from within the central compartment, it has been suggested that a larger volume of distribution should be associated with greater clearance.[203] In two studies,[193,211] the volume of distribution and clearance of the drugs increased with liver disease, thus lending support to this hypothesis.[203] The increased clearance of the relaxant in patients with liver disease is not reflected in a decrease in the drug's duration of action.[193,211]

One concern raised about administering atracurium to patients with hepatic disease was the possible accumulation of laudanosine. Although laudanosine relies principally on hepatic mechanisms for elimination, the concentrations encountered during liver transplantation are unlikely to be associated with clinical sequelae.[428]

In patients with hepatic disease (most commonly cirrhosis), the volume of distribution of rocuronium is increased,[207,209,210,426] and its clearance may be decreased.[210] The duration of action of rocuronium is prolonged in patients with hepatic disease,[207,210,426] and its onset may be prolonged.[207]

In patients with severe liver disease, butyrylcholinesterase activity is decreased because of decreased synthesis of the hepatic enzymes. Consequently, plasma clearance of the isomers of mivacurium is decreased by approximately 50% (see Table 29-14),[182] and its duration of action is prolonged and may be almost tripled.[182]

Burns

After a period of immobilization, burn injury causes upregulation of both fetal ($\alpha_2\beta\gamma\delta$) and mature ($\alpha_2\beta\varepsilon\delta$) nAChRs.[429] This upregulation of nAChRs is usually associated with resistance to nondepolarizing neuromuscular blockers and increased sensitivity to succinylcholine.[430] Causes of upregulation of nAChRs are listed in Box 29-1. A significant increase in the quantal content of evoked acetylcholine release is noted by 72 hours after scald injury in rats.[431] This also contributes to the resistance to nondepolarizing blockers in burn patients. In mice, thermal injury induces changes in diaphragm acetylcholinesterase with respect to total content and specific molecular forms.[432]

Resistance to the effects of nondepolarizing neuromuscular blocking drugs is usually seen in patients with burns over at least 25% of their total body surface area.[140,430] Recovery of neuromuscular function to preburn levels may take several months or even years after the burn injury.[433] The increase in serum potassium concentration that normally follows the administration of succinylcholine is markedly exaggerated in burned victims.[434] Potassium concentrations as high as 13 mEq/L have been reported to result in ventricular tachycardia, fibrillation, and cardiac arrest.[434] The magnitude of the hyperkalemic response does not appear to closely correlate with the magnitude of the burn injury. Potentially lethal hyperkalemia was seen in a patient with only an 8% total body surface area burn.[435] Succinylcholine has been safely administered within 24 hours of a burn injury. After this initial 24 hours, however, sufficient alteration in muscle response may have occurred, and the use of succinylcholine is best avoided.

The time course of abnormal muscle membrane function corresponds with that of the healing process. Once normal skin has regrown and any infection subsides, the normal acetylcholine receptor populations appear to return.[433] Normal responses to succinylcholine have been demonstrated in burn patients studied 3 years after injury.[433] The length of time during which a burn patient may be at risk for a hyperkalemic response is not well defined. A conservative guideline therefore would be to avoid the use of succinylcholine in patients 24 to 48 hours after a thermal injury and for at least 1 or 2 years after the burned skin has healed.

Box 29-1 Conditions Associated with Upregulation and Downregulation of Acetylcholine Receptors

- nAChR upregulation
  - Spinal cord injury
  - Stroke
  - Burns
  - Prolonged immobility
  - Prolonged exposure to neuromuscular blockers
  - Multiple sclerosis
  - Guillain-Barré syndrome
- nAChR downregulation
  - Myasthenia gravis
  - Anticholinesterase poisoning
  - Organophosphate poisoning

nAChR, nicotinic acetylcholine receptor.

From Naguib M, Flood P, McArdle JJ, Brenner HR: Advances in neurobiology of the neuromuscular junction: Implicatifons for the anesthesiologist. Anesthesiology 96:202-231, 2002, with permission from Anesthesiology.

Box 29-2 Reported Indications for the Use of Muscle Relaxants in the Intensive Care Unit

- Facilitate mechanical ventilation
  - Facilitation of endotracheal intubation
  - Enable patients to tolerate mechanical ventilation
  - High pulmonary inflation pressures, e.g., acute respiratory distress syndrome
- Hyperventilation for increased intracranial pressure
- Facilitate therapeutic or diagnostic procedures
- Tetanus
- Status epilepticus
- Reduce oxygen consumption
  - Abolish shivering
  - Reduce work of breathing

Neuromuscular Blockers and Weakness Syndromes in the Critically Ill

Neuromuscular blocking drugs are frequently used in conjunction with sedatives and analgesics in ICUs. Indications for the use of neuromuscular blockers in the ICU are outlined in Box 29-2. Few available data support their use, and evidence for a beneficial effect on pulmonary function or patient oxygenation is inconclusive.[436] Yet nondepolarizing neuromuscular blockers are commonly used for weeks in ICU patients, most of the time without monitoring and frequently at doses exceeding those used in the operating room.[437] The results of two surveys in the United States, including anesthesiologists and nurses with special certificates of competence in critical care, indicated that 98% of those surveyed use neuromuscular blocking drugs at least occasionally.[437]

Of particular concern in intensive care settings is the risk that paralyzed patients will receive inadequate analgesia and sedation.[438] This may be due to the fact that ICU nurses and physicians are unfamiliar with the pharmacology of neuromuscular blocking drugs.[437,438] For instance, pancuronium was thought to be an anxiolytic by 50% to 70% of ICU nurses and house staff, and 5% to 10% thought that it was an analgesic.[438] In the United Kingdom, the erroneous use of neuromuscular blockers as sedatives in intensive care was not uncommon in the 1980s.[439] Approximately 96% of ICU patients received neuromuscular blockers to aid mechanical ventilation in 1980. By 1986, their use had fallen to 16% of ventilated patients.[439] In the United States, neuromuscular blockers are used in less than 20% of all patients requiring mechanical ventilation.[437]

A prolonged ICU stay during critical illness is associated with disorders of neuromuscular function that contribute to morbidity, length of hospital stay, weaning difficulty, and prolonged rehabilitation.[440] Complications of long-term administration of

Box 29-3 Complications of Muscle Paralysis in the Intensive Care Unit

- Short-term use
  - Specific, known drug side effects
  - Inadequate ventilation in the event of ventilator failure or circuit disconnection
  - Inadequate analgesia and/or sedation
- Long-term use
  - Complications of immobility
    - Deep venous thrombosis and pulmonary embolism
    - Peripheral nerve injuries
    - Decubitus ulcers
  - Inability to cough
    - Retention of secretions and atelectasis
    - Pulmonary infection
- Dysregulation of nicotinic acetylcholine receptors
- Prolonged paralysis after stopping relaxants
  - Persistent neuromuscular blockade
  - Critical illness myopathy
  - Critical illness polyneuropathy
  - Combination of the above
- Unrecognized effects of drug or metabolites
  - Succinylcholine and metabolic acidosis/hypovolemia
  - 3-Desacetylvecuronium and neuromuscular blockade
  - Laudanosine and cerebral excitation

neuromuscular blockers in the ICU are outlined in Box 29-3. In the ICU, the duration of mechanical ventilation, sepsis, dysfunction of two or more organs, female sex, administration of steroids, and hypercapnia are known risk factors for the development of neuromuscular dysfunction. Syndromes of weakness in critically ill patients are relatively common and probably polymorphic in origin. In a retrospective study of 92 critically ill patients with clinically diagnosed weakness, electromyographic studies indicated that acute myopathy (critical illness myopathy) is three times as common as acute axonal neuropathy (critical illness neuropathy): 43% versus 13%, respectively.[440] The additional health care cost of one case of persistent weakness was estimated to be approximately $67,000.[441] Conditions to consider in the differential diagnosis of neuromuscular weakness in the ICU are listed in Box 29-4.

Critical Illness Myopathy

Lacomis and colleagues[442] suggested using the term "critical illness myopathy" (CIM) instead of the current terms used in the literature, such as acute quadriplegic myopathy,[443] acute (necrotizing) myopathy of intensive care, thick filament myopathy, acute corticosteroid myopathy, and critical care myopathy.

Most published reports of CIM in the ICU have focused on patients with status asthmaticus.[444] Affected individuals typically have been treated with corticosteroids and nondepolarizing neuromuscular blockers. Nevertheless, myopathy has also been documented in asthmatic patients and those with chronic lung disease without paralysis who received corticosteroids[445] and in critically ill patients with sepsis who received neither corticosteroids nor nondepolarizing neuromuscular blockers.[446] Animal studies have revealed that the number of cytosolic corticosteroid receptors is increased in immobilized muscles relative to contralateral controls.[447] It seems—at least in some patients—that prolonged immobility may be the key risk factor for myopathy in corticosteroid-treated patients[448] and that selective muscle atrophy is a result of changes in glucocorticoid sensitivity.[447]

Sepsis, immobility, and the catabolism associated with negative nitrogen balance may also result in myopathy.[14] Skeletal muscle hypoperfusion is noted in patients with severe sepsis despite normal or elevated whole blood oxygen delivery.[449] Antibodies to nAChRs have been demonstrated in a rodent model of sepsis.[450] Thus, myasthenia-like syndrome is also seen in critically

Box 29-4 Causes of Generalized Neuromuscular Weakness in the Intensive Care Unit

- Central nervous system
  - Septic or toxic-metabolic encephalopathy
  - Brainstem stroke
  - Central pontine myelinolysis
  - Anterior horn cell disorders (e.g., amyotrophic lateral sclerosis)
- Peripheral neuropathies
  - Critical illness polyneuropathy
  - Guillain-Barré syndrome
  - Porphyria
  - Paraneoplasia
  - Vasculitis
  - Nutritional and toxic
- Neuromuscular junction disorders
  - Myasthenia gravis
  - Lambert-Eaton myasthenic syndrome
  - Botulism
  - Prolonged neuromuscular junction blockade
- Myopathies
  - Critical illness myopathy
  - Cachectic myopathy
  - Rhabdomyolysis
  - Inflammatory and infectious myopathies
  - Muscular dystrophies
  - Toxic
  - Acid maltase deficiency
  - Mitochondrial
  - Hypokalemia
  - Hypermetabolic syndromes with rhabdomyolysis (e.g., neuroleptic malignant syndrome)

From Lacomis D: Critical illness myopathy. Curr Rheumatol Rep 4:403-408, 2002.

ill patients. Evidence of local immune activation by cytokine expression in skeletal muscle was reported in patients with CIM.[451]

The major feature of CIM is flaccid weakness that tends to be diffuse and sometimes also includes the facial muscles and diaphragm.[442] The clinical features of CIM overlap with those of critical illness polyneuropathy (CIP) and prolonged neuromuscular blockade.[442] Electrophysiologic studies and increases in serum creatine kinase concentration may differentiate neuropathy from myopathy.[442] Lacomis and coworkers[442] stated that "muscle biopsy should be considered if another myopathic process such as an inflammatory myopathy is suspected or if the histologic findings would affect management."

Critical Illness Polyneuropathy

The polyneuropathy seen in the critically ill has been termed "critical illness polyneuropathy (CIP)." It affects both sensory and motor nerves and occurs in 50% to 70% of patients with multisystem organ failure and systemic inflammatory response syndrome.[452] It has been postulated that systemic inflammatory response syndrome contributes to CIP by releasing cytokines and free radicals that damage the microcirculation of the central and peripheral nervous systems.[451] Dysregulation of the microcirculation may render the peripheral nervous system susceptible to injury.

No specific treatment of weakness syndromes in critically ill patients is available other than physical rehabilitation. Intravenous immunoglobulin and nerve growth factors appear to be promising in CIP syndrome. Recently, intensive insulin therapy during critical illness has been found to decrease the risk for CIP, and maintenance of blood glucose at or below 110 mg/mL in critically ill patients may reduce the risk for CIP.[453]

Outcomes after CIM and CIP appear to be similar.[440] The reported mortality rate of patients with CIP syndrome is about 35%. In one study, 100% (13 of 13) of the patients who survived had abnormal clinical or neurophysiologic findings 1 to 2 years after the onset of CIP syndrome, and quality of life was markedly impaired in all patients.[454]

Clinical Implications

Should Succinylcholine Be Used in ICU Patients?

It is likely that the upregulation of nAChRs induced by immobilization and by prolonged administration of nondepolarizing neuromuscular blockers contributes to (1) the higher incidence of cardiac arrest associated with the use of succinylcholine in ICU patients[455] and (2) increased requirements for nondepolarizing neuromuscular blockers in ICU patients.[456] Upregulation of nAChRs was noted in the muscles of deceased critically ill adults who had received long-term infusions of vecuronium.[455] Therefore, succinylcholine is best avoided in ICU patients in whom total body immobilization exceeds 24 hours.[14] In a survey in U.K. ICUs, 68.7% of respondents indicated that they would use succinylcholine in a clinical scenario suggestive of CIP.[457] This highlights the lack of awareness of the dangers associated with the use of succinylcholine in these patients.[457]

Should Nondepolarizing Neuromuscular Blockers Be Used in ICU Patients? Nondepolarizing neuromuscular blocker–associated persistent weakness appears to be a distinct pathologic entity and is not simply a manifestation of weakness syndromes in the critically ill. In a prospective study, Kupfer and associates[458] showed a 70% incidence of persistent weakness in ICU patients who received neuromuscular blockers for more than 2 days versus a 0% incidence in similar ICU patients who did not receive a neuromuscular blocker. This is compelling evidence for the effects of nondepolarizing neuromuscular blockers in this complication.

Long-term weakness has been described after all commonly used nondepolarizing neuromuscular blockers.[179,459,460] The overall incidence of prolonged paralysis after long-term use of neuromuscular blockers is about 5%. Prolonged weakness developed in approximately 20% of patients who received neuromuscular blockers for more than 6 days,[459] in 15% to 40% of asthmatic patients who also received high-dose steroids,[444] and in 50% of patients with renal failure who received vecuronium.[179] Clinically, it appears that prolonged recovery from neuromuscular blockade occurs more frequently when steroidal neuromuscular blockers are used.[179,459]

However, prolonged weakness was also noted after the use of atracurium in ICU patients.[460] Furthermore, the use of atracurium has raised concern about its metabolite laudanosine. Laudanosine, also detected in the cerebrospinal fluid (CSF) of ICU patients given atracurium,[461] is an analeptic and can trigger seizures in animals.[462] The toxic dose in humans is not known, but there are case reports of patients having seizures while receiving atracurium, and laudanosine has not been ruled out as a cause of these seizures.[463-465] There is also evidence that laudanosine can activate neuronal nicotinic receptors.[466] Cisatracurium is a single isomer of atracurium, and because it is four to five times more potent than atracurium, it is given in smaller doses. Therefore, the risk of laudanosine-related adverse effects should be minimal.[199]

Nondepolarizing neuromuscular blockers are polar molecules and do not cross the blood-brain barrier readily, but vecuronium and its long-acting active metabolite 3-desacetylvecuronium have been detected in the CSF of patients in the ICU. The CNS effects of neuromuscular blockers and their metabolites in humans have not been well studied, but in rats, atracurium, pancuronium, and vecuronium injected into CSF will cause dose-related cerebral excitation culminating in seizures.[462] Cerebral excitation with consequent increased cerebral oxygen demand is undesirable in ICU patients at risk for cerebral ischemia. It has also been suggested that nondepolarizing neuromuscular blockers can gain access to nerves during systemic inflammatory response syndrome and thereby result in direct neurotoxicity.[462]

Combining corticosteroids and nondepolarizing neuromuscular blockers should be avoided. When nondepolarizing neuromuscular blockers are necessary, the use of a peripheral nerve stimulator is recommended, and periodic return of muscle function should be allowed. However, routine monitoring of neuromuscular function alone is insufficient in eliminating prolonged recovery and weakness syndromes in ICU patients.[467] Adjusting the dosage of neuromuscular blockers by peripheral nerve stimulation versus standard clinical dosing in critically ill patients reduces drug requirements, produces faster recovery of neuromuscular function, and results in a total cost savings of $738 per patient.[468] A recent study found that daily interruption of sedative-drug infusions decreases the duration of mechanical ventilation and length of stay in the ICU.[469] The effect of such an approach on weakness syndromes in ICU patients is unknown. When nondepolarizing neuromuscular blockers are used, the guidelines in Box 29-5 may help minimize the incidence of

Box 29-5 Recommendations for the Use of Neuromuscular Blockers in the Intensive Care Unit

Avoid the use of neuromuscular blockers by:
- Maximal use of analgesics and sedatives
- Manipulation of ventilatory parameters and modes

Minimize the dose of neuromuscular blocker:
- Use a peripheral nerve stimulator with train-of-four monitoring.
- Do not administer for more than 2 days continuously.
- Administer by bolus rather than infusion.
- Administer only when required and to achieve a well-defined goal.
- Continually allow recovery from paralysis.

Consider alternative therapies:
- Avoid vecuronium in female patients with renal failure.
- Use isoflurane in place of muscle relaxants in patients with severe asthma.
- Minimize the dose of steroid in patients with asthma.

complications. As stated in the clinical practice guidelines for sustained neuromuscular blockade in adult critically ill patients,[436] "*Independent of the reasons for using neuromuscular blockers, we emphasize that all other modalities to improve the clinical situation must be tried, using neuromuscular blockers only as a last resort.*"

References

1. Griffith HR, Johnson GE: The use of curare in general anesthesia. Anesthesiology 3:418-420, 1942.
2. Cullen SC: The use of curare for improvement of abdominal relaxation during inhalation anesthesia: Report on 131 cases. Surgery 14:261-266, 1943.
3. Beecher HK, Todd DP: A study of deaths with anesthesia and surgery. Ann Surg 140:2-34, 1954.
4. Thesleff S: Farmakologiska och kliniska forsok med L.T. I. (O,O-succinylcholine jodid). Nord Med 46:1045-1051, 1951.
5. Foldes FF, McNall PG, Borrego-Hinojosa JM: Succinylcholine, a new approach to muscular relaxation in anaesthesiology. N Engl J Med 247:596-600, 1952.
6. Baird WL, Reid AM: The neuromuscular blocking properties of a new steroid compound, pancuronium bromide. A pilot study in man. Br J Anaesth 39:775-780, 1967.
7. Savage DS, Sleigh T, Carlyle I: The emergence of ORG NC 45, 1-[2 beta,3 alpha,5 alpha,16 beta,17beta)-3,17-bis(acetyloxy)-2-(1-piperidinyl)-androstan-16-yl]-1-methylpiperidinium bromide, from the pancuronium series. Br J Anaesth 52(Suppl 1):3S-9S, 1980.
8. Stenlake JB, Waigh RD, Dewar GH, et al: Biodegradable neuromuscular blocking agents. Part 4: Atracurium besylate and related polyalkylylene di-esters. Eur J Med Chem 16:515-524, 1981.
9. Savarese JJ, Ali HH, Basta SJ, et al: The clinical neuromuscular pharmacology of mivacurium chloride (BW B1090U). A short-acting nondepolarizing ester neuromuscular blocking drug. Anesthesiology 68:723-732, 1988.
10. Wierda JM, de Wit AP, Kuizenga K, Agoston S: Clinical observations on the neuromuscular blocking action of Org 9426, a new steroidal non-depolarizing agent. Br J Anaesth 64:521-523, 1990.
11. Belmont MR, Lien CA, Quessy S, et al: The clinical neuromuscular pharmacology of 51W89 in patients receiving nitrous oxide/opioid/barbiturate anesthesia. Anesthesiology 82:1139-1145, 1995.
12. On being aware. Br J Anaesth 51:711-712, 1979.
13. Shovelton DS: Reflections on an intensive therapy unit. BMJ 1:737-738, 1979.
14. Naguib M, Flood P, McArdle JJ, Brenner HR: Advances in neurobiology of the neuromuscular junction: Implications for the anesthesiologist. Anesthesiology 96:202-231, 2002.
15. Machold J, Weise C, Utkin Y, et al: The handedness of the subunit arrangement of the nicotinic acetylcholine receptor from *Torpedo californica*. Eur J Biochem 234:427-430, 1995.
16. Willcockson IU, Hong A, Whisenant RP, et al: Orientation of *d*-tubocurarine in the muscle nicotinic acetylcholine receptor–binding site. J Biol Chem 277:42249-42258, 2002.
17. Paul M, Kindler CH, Fokt RM, et al: The potency of new muscle relaxants on recombinant muscle-type acetylcholine receptors. Anesth Analg 94:597-603, 2002.
18. Martyn JA: Basic and clinical pharmacology of the acetylcholine receptor: Implications for the use of neuromuscular relaxants. Keio J Med 44:1-8, 1995.
19. Kallen RG, Sheng ZH, Yang J, et al: Primary structure and expression of a sodium channel characteristic of denervated and immature rat skeletal muscle. Neuron 4:233-242, 1990.
20. Bowman WC: Prejunctional and postjunctional cholinoceptors at the neuromuscular junction. Anesth Analg 59:935-943, 1980.
21. Prior C, Tian L, Dempster J, Marshall IG: Prejunctional actions of muscle relaxants: Synaptic vesicles and transmitter mobilization as sites of action. Gen Pharmacol 26:659-666, 1995.
22. Slutsky I, Wess J, Gomeza J, et al: Use of knockout mice reveals involvement of M_2-muscarinic receptors in control of the kinetics of acetylcholine release. J Neurophysiol 89:1954-1967, 2003.
23. Bowman WC, Prior C, Marshall IG: Presynaptic receptors in the neuromuscular junction. Ann N Y Acad Sci 604:69-81, 1990.
24. Brull SJ, Connelly NR, O'Connor TZ, Silverman DG: Effect of tetanus on subsequent neuromuscular monitoring in patients receiving vecuronium. Anesthesiology 74:64-70, 1991.
25. Naguib M, Lien CA, Aker J, Eliazo R: Posttetanic potentiation and fade in the response to tetanic and train-of-four stimulation during succinylcholine-induced block. Anesth Analg 98:1686-1691, 2004.
26. Donati F, Meistelman C, Plaud B: Vecuronium neuromuscular blockade at the adductor muscles of the larynx and adductor pollicis. Anesthesiology 74:833-837, 1991.
27. Bovet D: Some aspects of the relationship between chemical constitution and curare-like activity. Ann N Y Acad Sci 54:407-437, 1951.
28. Szalados JE, Donati F, Bevan DR: Effect of *d*-tubocurarine pretreatment on succinylcholine twitch augmentation and neuromuscular blockade. Anesth Analg 71:55-59, 1990.
29. Kopman AF, Klewicka MM, Neuman GG: An alternate method for estimating the dose-response relationships of neuromuscular blocking drugs. Anesth Analg 90:1191-1197, 2000.
30. Curran MJ, Donati F, Bevan DR: Onset and recovery of atracurium and suxamethonium-induced neuromuscular blockade with simultaneous train-of-four and single twitch stimulation. Br J Anaesth 59:989-994, 1987.
31. Viby-Mogensen J: Correlation of succinylcholine duration of action with plasma cholinesterase activity in subjects with the genotypically normal enzyme. Anesthesiology 53:517-520, 1980.
32. Gissen AJ, Katz RL, Karis JH, Papper EM: Neuromuscular block in man during prolonged arterial infusion with succinylcholine. Anesthesiology 27:242-249, 1966.
33. Torda TA, Graham GG, Warwick NR, Donohue P: Pharmacokinetics and pharmacodynamics of suxamethonium. Anaesth Intensive Care 25:272-278, 1997.
34. Birch JH, Foldes FF, Rendell-Baker L: Causes and prevention of prolonged apnea with succinylcholine. Anesth Analg 35:609-633, 1956.
35. Lepage L, Schiele F, Gueguen R, Siest G: Total cholinesterase in plasma: Biological variations and reference limits. Clin Chem 31:546-550, 1985.
36. Sunew KY, Hicks RG: Effects of neostigmine and pyridostigmine on duration of succinylcholine action and pseudocholinesterase activity. Anesthesiology 49:188-191, 1978.
37. Lindsay PA, Lumley J: Suxamethonium apnoea masked by tetrahydroaminacrine. Anaesthesia 33:620-622, 1978.
38. Kao YJ, Tellez J, Turner DR: Dose-dependent effect of metoclopramide on cholinesterases and suxamethonium metabolism. Br J Anaesth 65:220-224, 1990.
39. Woodworth GE, Sears DH, Grove TM, et al: The effect of cimetidine and ranitidine on the duration

of action of succinylcholine. Anesth Analg 68:295-297, 1989.

40. Fisher DM, Caldwell JE, Sharma M, Wiren JE: The influence of bambuterol (carbamylated terbutaline) on the duration of action of succinylcholine-induced paralysis in humans. Anesthesiology 69:757-759, 1988.
41. Barabas E, Zsigmond EK, Kirkpatrick AF: The inhibitory effect of esmolol on human plasmacholinesterase. Can Anaesth Soc J 33:332-335, 1986.
42. Pantuck EJ: Ecothiopate iodide eye drops and prolonged response to suxamethonium. Br J Anaesth 38:406-407, 1966.
43. Kalow W, Genest K: A method for the detection of atypical forms of human serum cholinesterase; determination of dibucaine numbers. Can J Biochem 35:339-346, 1957.
44. Jensen FS, Viby-Mogensen J: Plasma cholinesterase and abnormal reaction to succinylcholine: Twenty years' experience with the Danish Cholinesterase Research Unit. Acta Anaesthesiol Scand 39:150-156, 1995.
45. Primo-Parmo SL, Lightstone H, La Du BN: Characterization of an unstable variant (BChE115D) of human butyrylcholinesterase. Pharmacogenetics 7:27-34, 1997.
46. Galindo AHF, Davis TB: Succinylcholine and cardiac excitability. Anesthesiology 23:32-40, 1962.
47. Goat VA, Feldman SA: The dual action of suxamethonium on the isolated rabbit heart. Anaesthesia 27:149-153, 1972.
48. Jonsson M, Dabrowski M, Gurley DA, et al: Activation and inhibition of human muscular and neuronal nicotinic acetylcholine receptors by succinylcholine. Anesthesiology 104:724-733, 2006.
49. Stoelting RK, Peterson C: Heart-rate slowing and junctional rhythm following intravenous succinylcholine with and without intramuscular atropine preanesthetic medication. Anesth Analg 54:705-709, 1975.
50. Schoenstadt DA, Whitcher CE: Observations on the mechanism of succinylcholine-induced cardiac arrhythmias. Anesthesiology 24:358-363, 1963.
51. Leiman BC, Katz J, Butler BD: Mechanisms of succinylcholine-induced arrhythmias in hypoxic or hypoxic:hypercarbic dogs. Anesth Analg 66:1292-1297, 1987.
52. Derbyshire DR: Succinylcholine-induced increases in plasma catecholamine levels in humans. Anesth Analg 63:465-467, 1984.
53. Powell JN, Golby M: The pattern of potassium liberation following a single dose of suxamethonium in normal and uraemic rats. Br J Anaesth 43:662-668, 1971.
54. Walton JD, Farman JV: Suxamethonium hyperkalaemia in uraemic neuropathy. Anaesthesia 28:666-668, 1973.
55. Schwartz DE, Kelly B, Caldwell JE, et al: Succinylcholine-induced hyperkalemic arrest in a patient with severe metabolic acidosis and exsanguinating hemorrhage. Anesth Analg 75:291-293, 1992.
56. Antognini JF, Gronert GA: Succinylcholine causes profound hyperkalemia in hemorrhagic, acidotic rabbits. Anesth Analg 77:585-588, 1993.
57. Antognini JF: Splanchnic release of potassium after hemorrhage and succinylcholine in rabbits. Anesth Analg 78:687-690, 1994.
58. Kohlschütter B, Baur H, Roth F: Suxamethonium-induced hyperkalaemia in patients with severe intra-abdominal infections. Br J Anaesth 48: 557-562, 1976.
59. Stevenson PH, Birch AA: Succinylcholine-induced hyperkalemia in a patient with a closed head injury. Anesthesiology 51:89-90, 1979.
60. Birch AA Jr, Mitchell GD, Playford GA, Lang CA: Changes in serum potassium response to succinylcholine following trauma. JAMA 210:490-493, 1969.
61. Martyn JA, Richtsfeld M: Succinylcholine-induced hyperkalemia in acquired pathologic states: Etiologic factors and molecular mechanisms. Anesthesiology 104:158-169, 2006.
62. Pandey K, Badola RP, Kumar S: Time course of intraocular hypertension produced by suxamethonium. Br J Anaesth 44:191-196, 1972.
63. Indu B, Batra YK, Puri GD, Singh H: Nifedipine attenuates the intraocular pressure response to intubation following succinylcholine. Can J Anaesth 36:269-272, 1989.
64. Meyers EF, Krupin T, Johnson M, Zink H: Failure of nondepolarizing neuromuscular blockers to inhibit succinylcholine-induced increased intraocular pressure, a controlled study. Anesthesiology 48:149-151, 1978.
65. Miller RD, Way WL, Hickey RF: Inhibition of succinylcholine-induced increased intraocular pressure by non-depolarizing muscle relaxants. Anesthesiology 29:123-126, 1968.
66. Libonati MM, Leahy JJ, Ellison N: The use of succinylcholine in open eye surgery. Anesthesiology 62:637-640, 1985.
67. Grennan J: The cardio-oesophageal junction. Br J Anaesth 33:432, 1961.
68. Miller RD, Way WL: Inhibition of succinylcholine-induced increased intragastric pressure by non-depolarizing muscle relaxants and lidocaine. Anesthesiology 34:185-188, 1971.
69. Salem MR, Wong AY, Lin YH: The effect of suxamethonium on the intragastric pressure in infants and children. Br J Anaesth 44:166-170, 1972.
70. Minton MD, Grosslight K, Stirt JA, Bedford RF: Increases in intracranial pressure from succinylcholine: Prevention by prior nondepolarizing blockade. Anesthesiology 65:165-169, 1986.
71. Brodsky JB, Brock-Utne JG, Samuels SI: Pancuronium pretreatment and post-succinylcholine myalgias. Anesthesiology 51:259-261, 1979.
72. Waters DJ, Mapleson WW: Suxamethonium pains: Hypothesis and observation. Anaesthesia 26:127-141, 1971.
73. McLoughlin C, Elliott P, McCarthy G, Mirakhur RK: Muscle pains and biochemical changes following suxamethonium administration after six pretreatment regimens. Anaesthesia 47:202-206, 1992.
74. Naguib M, Farag H, Magbagbeola JA: Effect of pretreatment with lysine acetyl salicylate on suxamethonium-induced myalgia. Br J Anaesth 59:606-610, 1987.
75. Smith I, Ding Y, White PF: Muscle pain after outpatient laparoscopy—influence of propofol versus thiopental and enflurane. Anesth Analg 76:1181-1184, 1993.
76. Leary NP, Ellis FR: Masseteric muscle spasm as a normal response to suxamethonium. Br J Anaesth 64:488-492, 1990.
77. Meakin G, Walker RW, Dearlove OR: Myotonic and neuromuscular blocking effects of increased doses of suxamethonium in infants and children. Br J Anaesth 65:816-818, 1990.
78. Van der Spek AF, Fang WB, Ashton-Miller JA, et al: The effects of succinylcholine on mouth opening. Anesthesiology 67:459-465, 1987.
79. Littleford JA, Patel LR, Bose D, et al: Masseter muscle spasm in children: Implications of continuing the triggering anesthetic. Anesth Analg 72: 151-160, 1991.
80. Clarke RSJ: Intubating conditions and neuromuscular effects following vecuronium bromide. Comparison with suxamethonium chloride and pancuronium bromide. *In* Clinical Experiences with Norcuron. Amsterdam, Excerpta Medica, 1983.
81. Naguib M, Samarkandi A, Riad W, Alharby SW: Optimal dose of succinylcholine revisited. Anesthesiology 99:1045-1049, 2003.
82. Naguib M, Samarkandi AH, Abdullah K, et al: Succinylcholine dosage and apnea-induced hemoglobin desaturation in patients. Anesthesiology 102:35-40, 2005.
83. Miller RD: The advantages of giving *d*-tubocurarine before succinylcholine. Anesthesiology 37:568-569, 1972.
84. Donati F, Gill SS, Bevan DR, et al: Pharmacokinetics and pharmacodynamics of atracurium with and without previous suxamethonium administration. Br J Anaesth 66:557-561, 1991.
85. Dubois MY, Lea DE, Kataria B, et al: Pharmacodynamics of rocuronium with and without prior administration of succinylcholine. J Clin Anesth 7:44-48, 1995.
86. Naguib M, Abdulatif M, Selim M, al-Ghamdi A: Dose-response studies of the interaction between mivacurium and suxamethonium. Br J Anaesth 74:26-30, 1995.
87. Erkola O, Rautoma P, Meretoja OA: Interaction between mivacurium and succinylcholine. Anesth Analg 80:534-537, 1995.
88. Lee C, Katz RL: Neuromuscular pharmacology. A clinical update and commentary. Br J Anaesth 52:173-188, 1980.
89. Ramsey FM, Lebowitz PW, Savarese JJ, Ali HH: Clinical characteristics of long-term succinylcholine neuromuscular blockade during balanced anesthesia. Anesth Analg 59:110-116, 1980.
90. Lee C: Structure, conformation, and action of neuromuscular blocking drugs. Br J Anaesth 87:755-769, 2001.
91. Everett AJ, Lowe LA, Wilkinson S: Revision of the structures of (+)-tubocurarine chloride and (+)-chondocurine. J Chem Soc D 13:1020-1021, 1970.
92. Waser PG: Chemistry and pharmacology of natural curare compounds, Neuromuscular blocking and stimulating agents. *In* Cheymol J (ed): International Encyclopedia of Pharmacology and Therapeutics. Oxford, Pergamon Press, 1972, pp 205-239.
93. Hill SA, Scott RPF, Savarese JJ: Structure-activity relationships: From tubocurarine to the present day. Baillieres Clin Anesthesiol 8:317-348, 1994.
94. Stenlake JB, Waigh RD, Dewar GH, et al: Biodegradable neuromuscular blocking agents. 6. Stereochemical studies on atracurium and related polyalkylene di-esters. Eur J Med Chem 19:441-450, 1984.
95. Wastila WB, Maehr RB, Turner GL, et al: Comparative pharmacology of cisatracurium (51W89), atracurium, and five isomers in cats. Anesthesiology 85:169-177, 1996.
96. Lien CA: The role of stereoisomerism in neuromuscular blocking drugs. Curr Opin Anesthesiol 9: 348-353, 1996.
97. Lien CA, Belmont MR, Abalos A, et al: The cardiovascular effects and histamine-releasing properties of 51W89 in patients receiving nitrous oxide/opioid/barbiturate anesthesia. Anesthesiology 82:1131-1138, 1995.
98. Savarese JJ, Wastila WB: The future of the benzylisoquinolinium relaxants. Acta Anaesthesiol Scand Suppl 106:91-93, 1995.
99. Lien CA, Schmith VD, Embree PB, et al: The pharmacokinetics and pharmacodynamics of the stereoisomers of mivacurium in patients receiving nitrous oxide/opioid/barbiturate anesthesia. Anesthesiology 80:1296-1302, 1994.

100. Stovner J, Oftedal N, Holmboe J: The inhibition of cholinesterases by pancuronium. Br J Anaesth 47:949-954, 1975.
101. Bowman WC, Rodger IW, Houston J, et al: Structure:action relationships among some desacetoxy analogues of pancuronium and vecuronium in the anesthetized cat. Anesthesiology 69:57-62, 1988.
102. Wierda JM, Proost JH: Structure-pharmacodynamic-pharmacokinetic relationships of steroidal neuromuscular blocking agents. Eur J Anaesthesiol Suppl 11:45-54, 1995.
103. Naguib M, Samarkandi AH, Bakhamees HS, et al: Comparative potency of steroidal neuromuscular blocking drugs and isobolographic analysis of the interaction between rocuronium and other aminosteroids. Br J Anaesth 75:37-42, 1995.
104. Goulden MR, Hunter JM: Rapacuronium (Org 9487): Do we have a replacement for succinylcholine? Br J Anaesth 82:489-492, 1999.
105. Boros EE, Samano V, Ray JA, et al: Neuromuscular blocking activity and therapeutic potential of mixed-tetrahydroisoquinolinium halofumarates and halosuccinates in rhesus monkeys. J Med Chem 46:2502-2515, 2003.
106. Belmont MR, Lien CA, Tjan J, et al: Clinical pharmacology of GW280430A in humans. Anesthesiology 100:768-773, 2004.
107. Shanks CA: Pharmacokinetics of the nondepolarizing neuromuscular relaxants applied to calculation of bolus and infusion dosage regimens. Anesthesiology 64:72-86, 1986.
108. Booij LH, Knape HT: The neuromuscular blocking effect of Org 9426. A new intermediately-acting steroidal non-depolarising muscle relaxant in man. Anaesthesia 46:341-343, 1991.
109. Bartkowski RR, Witkowski TA, Azad S, et al: Rocuronium onset of action: A comparison with atracurium and vecuronium. Anesth Analg 77: 574-578, 1993.
110. Bevan DR, Fiset P, Balendran P, et al: Pharmacodynamic behaviour of rocuronium in the elderly. Can J Anaesth 40:127-132, 1993.
111. Savarese JJ, Lien CA, Belmont MR, Wastila WB: [The clinical pharmacology of new benzylisoquinoline-diester compounds, with special consideration of cisatracurium and mivacurium.] Anaesthesist 46:840-849, 1997.
112. Naguib M, Samarkandi AH, Ammar A, et al: Comparative clinical pharmacology of rocuronium, cisatracurium, and their combination. Anesthesiology 89:1116-1124, 1998.
113. Weber S, Brandom BW, Powers DM, et al: Mivacurium chloride (BW B1090U)-induced neuromuscular blockade during nitrous oxide–isoflurane and nitrous oxide–narcotic anesthesia in adult surgical patients. Anesth Analg 67:495-499, 1988.
114. Caldwell JE, Kitts JB, Heier T, et al: The dose-response relationship of mivacurium chloride in humans during nitrous oxide–fentanyl or nitrous oxide–enflurane anesthesia. Anesthesiology 70: 31-35, 1989.
115. Diefenbach C, Mellinghoff H, Lynch J, Buzello W: Mivacurium: Dose-response relationship and administration by repeated injection or infusion. Anesth Analg 74:420-423, 1992.
116. Wierda JM, Beaufort AM, Kleef UW, et al: Preliminary investigations of the clinical pharmacology of three short-acting non-depolarizing neuromuscular blocking agents, Org 9453, Org 9489 and Org 9487. Can J Anaesth 41:213-220, 1994.
117. Kopman AF, Klewicka MM, Ghori K, et al: Dose-response and onset/offset characteristics of rapacuronium. Anesthesiology 93:1017-1021, 2000.
118. Kim KS, Chung CW, Shin WJ: Cisatracurium neuromuscular block at the adductor pollicis and the laryngeal adductor muscles in humans. Br J Anaesth 83:483-484, 1999.
119. Holford NH, Sheiner LB: Understanding the dose-effect relationship: Clinical application of pharmacokinetic-pharmacodynamic models. Clin Pharmacokinet 6:429-453, 1981.
120. Sheiner LB, Stanski DR, Vozeh S, et al: Simultaneous modeling of pharmacokinetics and pharmacodynamics: Application to *d*-tubocurarine. Clin Pharmacol Ther 25:358-371, 1979.
121. Holford NH, Sheiner LB: Kinetics of pharmacologic response. Pharmacol Ther 16:143-166, 1982.
122. Wright PM: Population based pharmacokinetic analysis: Why do we need it; what is it; and what has it told us about anaesthetics? Br J Anaesth 80: 488-501, 1998.
123. Fisher DM, Rosen JI: A pharmacokinetic explanation for increasing recovery time following larger or repeated doses of nondepolarizing muscle relaxants. Anesthesiology 65:286-291, 1986.
124. Bevan DR, Bevan JC, Donati F: Pharmacokinetic principles. In Muscle Relaxants in Clinical Anesthesia. Chicago, Year Book, 1988.
125. Waser PG, Wiederkehr H, Sin-Ren AC, Kaiser-Schonenberger E: Distribution and kinetics of ^{14}C-vecuronium in rats and mice. Br J Anaesth 59:1044-1051, 1987.
126. Matteo RS, Nishitateno K, Pua EK, Spector S: Pharmacokinetics of *d*-tubocurarine in man: Effect of an osmotic diuretic on urinary excretion. Anesthesiology 52:335-338, 1980.
127. Lebrault C, Berger JL, D'Hollander AA, et al: Pharmacokinetics and pharmacodynamics of vecuronium (ORG NC 45) in patients with cirrhosis. Anesthesiology 62:601-605, 1985.
128. Wood M: Plasma drug binding: Implications for anesthesiologists. Anesth Analg 65:786-804, 1986.
129. McLeod K, Watson MJ, Rawlins MD: Pharmacokinetics of pancuronium in patients with normal and impaired renal function. Br J Anaesth 48:341-345, 1976.
130. Miller RD, Matteo RS, Benet LZ, Sohn YJ: The pharmacokinetics of *d*-tubocurarine in man with and without renal failure. J Pharmacol Exp Ther 202:1-7, 1977.
131. Wright PM, Hart P, Lau M, et al: Cumulative characteristics of atracurium and vecuronium. A simultaneous clinical and pharmacokinetic study. Anesthesiology 81:59-68, 1994.
132. Laurin J, Donati F, Nekka F, Varin F: Peripheral link model as an alternative for pharmacokinetic-pharmacodynamic modeling of drugs having a very short elimination half-life. J Pharmacokinet Biopharm 28:7-25, 2001.
133. Kuipers JA, Boer F, Olofsen E, et al: Recirculatory pharmacokinetics and pharmacodynamics of rocuronium in patients: The influence of cardiac output. Anesthesiology 94:47-55, 2001.
134. Wright PM, Brown R, Lau M, Fisher DM: A pharmacodynamic explanation for the rapid onset/offset of rapacuronium bromide. Anesthesiology 90:16-23, 1999.
135. Wierda JM, Meretoja OA, Taivainen T, Proost JH: Pharmacokinetics and pharmacokinetic-dynamic modelling of rocuronium in infants and children. Br J Anaesth 78:690-695, 1997.
136. Bergeron L, Bevan DR, Berrill A, et al: Concentration-effect relationship of cisatracurium at three different dose levels in the anesthetized patient. Anesthesiology 95:314-323, 2001.
137. Fisher DM, Canfell PC, Spellman MJ, Miller RD: Pharmacokinetics and pharmacodynamics of atracurium in infants and children. Anesthesiology 73:33-37, 1990.
138. Kitts JB, Fisher DM, Canfell PC, Sp et al: Pharmacokinetics and pharmacodynamics of atracurium in the elderly. Anesthesiology 72:272-275, 1990.
139. Parker CJ, Hunter JM: Dependence of the neuromuscular blocking effect of atracurium upon its disposition. Br J Anaesth 68:555-561, 1992.
140. Marathe PH, Dwersteg JF, Pavlin EG, et al: Effect of thermal injury on the pharmacokinetics and pharmacodynamics of atracurium in humans. Anesthesiology 70:752-755, 1989.
141. Cronnelly R, Fisher DM, Miller RD, et al: Pharmacokinetics and pharmacodynamics of vecuronium (ORG NC45) and pancuronium in anesthetized humans. Anesthesiology 58:405-408, 1983.
142. Rupp SM, Castagnoli KP, Fisher DM, Miller RD: Pancuronium and vecuronium pharmacokinetics and pharmacodynamics in younger and elderly adults. Anesthesiology 67:45-49, 1987.
143. Stanski DR, Ham J, Miller RD, Sheiner LB: Pharmacokinetics and pharmacodynamics of *d*-tubocurarine during nitrous oxide–narcotic and halothane anesthesia in man. Anesthesiology 51:235-241, 1979.
144. Katz RL, Ryan JF: The neuromuscular effects of suxamethonium in man. Br J Anaesth 41:381-390, 1969.
145. Kopman AF, Zhaku B, Lai KS: The "intubating dose" of succinylcholine: The effect of decreasing doses on recovery time. Anesthesiology 99:1050-1054, 2003.
146. Wierda JM, van den Broek L, Proost JH, et al: Time course of action and endotracheal intubating conditions of Org 9487, a new short-acting steroidal muscle relaxant; a comparison with succinylcholine. Anesth Analg 77:579-584, 1993.
147. Miguel R, Witkowski T, Nagashima H, et al: Evaluation of neuromuscular and cardiovascular effects of two doses of rapacuronium (ORG 9487) versus mivacurium and succinylcholine. Anesthesiology 91:1648-1654, 1999.
148. Magorian T, Flannery KB, Miller RD: Comparison of rocuronium, succinylcholine, and vecuronium for rapid-sequence induction of anesthesia in adult patients. Anesthesiology 79:913-918, 1993.
149. Naguib M: Neuromuscular effects of rocuronium bromide and mivacurium chloride administered alone and in combination. Anesthesiology 81:388-395, 1994.
150. Agoston S, Salt P, Newton D, et al: The neuromuscular blocking action of ORG NC 45, a new pancuronium derivative, in anaesthetized patients. A pilot study. Br J Anaesth 52(Suppl 1):53S-59S, 1980.
151. Miller RD, Agoston S, Booij LH, et al: The comparative potency and pharmacokinetics of pancuronium and its metabolites in anesthetized man. J Pharmacol Exp Ther 207:539-543, 1978.
152. Savarese JJ, Ali HH, Antonio RP: The clinical pharmacology of metocurine: Dimethyltubocurarine revisited. Anesthesiology 47:277-284, 1977.
153. From RP, Pearson KS, Choi WW, et al: Neuromuscular and cardiovascular effects of mivacurium chloride (BW B1090U) during nitrous oxide–fentanyl–thiopentone and nitrous oxide–halothane anaesthesia. Br J Anaesth 64:193-198, 1990.
154. Boyd AH, Eastwood NB, Parker CJ, Hunter JM: Pharmacodynamics of the 1R cis-1'R cis isomer of atracurium (51W89) in health and chronic renal failure. Br J Anaesth 74:400-404, 1995.
155. Kopman AF, Klewicka MM, Kopman DJ, Neuman GG: Molar potency is predictive of the speed of onset of neuromuscular block for agents of intermediate, short, and ultrashort duration. Anesthesiology 90:425-431, 1999.

156. Donati F, Meistelman C: A kinetic-dynamic model to explain the relationship between high potency and slow onset time for neuromuscular blocking drugs. J Pharmacokinet Biopharm 19:537-552, 1991.
157. Kopman AF, Klewicka MM, Neuman GG: Molar potency is not predictive of the speed of onset of atracurium. Anesth Analg 89:1046-1049, 1999.
158. Naguib M, Kopman AF: Low dose rocuronium for tracheal intubation. Middle East J Anesthesiol 17:193-204, 2003.
159. Bevan DR: The new relaxants: Are they worth it? Can J Anaesth 46:R88-R100, 1999.
160. Meistelman C, Plaud B, Donati F: Rocuronium (ORG 9426) neuromuscular blockade at the adductor muscles of the larynx and adductor pollicis in humans. Can J Anaesth 39:665-669, 1992.
161. Wright PM, Caldwell JE, Miller RD: Onset and duration of rocuronium and succinylcholine at the adductor pollicis and laryngeal adductor muscles in anesthetized humans. Anesthesiology 81: 1110-1105, 1994.
162. Plaud B, Debaene B, Lequeau F, et al: Mivacurium neuromuscular block at the adductor muscles of the larynx and adductor pollicis in humans. Anesthesiology 85:77-81, 1996.
163. Hemmerling TM, Schmidt J, Hanusa C, et al: Simultaneous determination of neuromuscular block at the larynx, diaphragm, adductor pollicis, orbicularis oculi and corrugator supercilii muscles. Br J Anaesth 85:856-860, 2000.
164. Fisher DM, Szenohradszky J, Wright PM, et al: Pharmacodynamic modeling of vecuronium-induced twitch depression. Rapid plasma-effect site equilibration explains faster onset at resistant laryngeal muscles than at the adductor pollicis. Anesthesiology 86:558-566, 1997.
165. Donati F, Meistelman C, Plaud B: Vecuronium neuromuscular blockade at the diaphragm, the orbicularis oculi, and adductor pollicis muscles. Anesthesiology 73:870-875, 1990.
166. Mehta MP, Choi WW, Gergis SD, et al: Facilitation of rapid endotracheal intubations with divided doses of nondepolarizing neuromuscular blocking drugs. Anesthesiology 62:392-395, 1985.
167. Engbaek J, Howardy-Hansen P, Ording H, Viby-Mogensen J: Precurarization with vecuronium and pancuronium in awake, healthy volunteers: The influence on neuromuscular transmission and pulmonary function. Acta Anaesthesiol Scand 29:117-120, 1985.
168. Savarese JJ, Ali HH, Basta SJ, et al: The cardiovascular effects of mivacurium chloride (BW B1090U) in patients receiving nitrous oxide-opiate-barbiturate anesthesia. Anesthesiology 70:386-394, 1989.
169. Meistelman C, Plaud B, Donati F: Neuromuscular effects of succinylcholine on the vocal cords and adductor pollicis muscles. Anesth Analg 73:278-282, 1991.
170. Wierda JM, Kleef UW, Lambalk LM, et al: The pharmacodynamics and pharmacokinetics of Org 9426, a new non-depolarizing neuromuscular blocking agent, in patients anaesthetized with nitrous oxide, halothane and fentanyl. Can J Anaesth 38:430-435, 1991.
171. Kopman AF, Klewicka MM, Neuman GG: Reexamined: The recommended endotracheal intubating dose for nondepolarizing neuromuscular blockers of rapid onset. Anesth Analg 93:954-959, 2001.
172. Miguel RV, Soto R, Dyches P: A double-blind, randomized comparison of low-dose rocuronium and atracurium in a desflurane anesthetic. J Clin Anesth 13:325-329, 2001.
173. Agoston S, Vermeer GA, Kertsten UW, Meijer DK: The fate of pancuronium bromide in man. Acta Anaesthesiol Scand 17:267-275, 1973.
174. Duvaldestin P, Agoston S, Henzel D, et al: Pancuronium pharmacokinetics in patients with liver cirrhosis. Br J Anaesth 50:1131-1136, 1978.
175. Somogyi AA, Shanks CA, Triggs EJ: Disposition kinetics of pancuronium bromide in patients with total biliary obstruction. Br J Anaesth 49:1103-1108, 1977.
176. Mol WE, Fokkema GN, Weert B, Meijer DK: Mechanisms for the hepatic uptake of organic cations. Studies with the muscle relaxant vecuronium in isolated rat hepatocytes. J Pharmacol Exp Ther 244:268-275, 1988.
177. Caldwell JE, Szenohradszky J, Segredo V, et al: The pharmacodynamics and pharmacokinetics of the metabolite 3-desacetylvecuronium (ORG 7268) and its parent compound, vecuronium, in human volunteers. J Pharmacol Exp Ther 270:1216-1222, 1994.
178. Arden JR, Lynam DP, Castagnoli KP, et al: Vecuronium in alcoholic liver disease: A pharmacokinetic and pharmacodynamic analysis. Anesthesiology 68:771-776, 1988.
179. Segredo V, Caldwell JE, Matthay MA, et al: Persistent paralysis in critically ill patients after long-term administration of vecuronium. N Engl J Med 327:524-528, 1992.
180. Khuenl-Brady K, Castagnoli KP, Canfell PC, et al: The neuromuscular blocking effects and pharmacokinetics of ORG 9426 and ORG 9616 in the cat. Anesthesiology 72:669-674, 1990.
181. Smit JW, Duin E, Steen H, et al: Interactions between P-glycoprotein substrates and other cationic drugs at the hepatic excretory level. Br J Pharmacol 123:361-370, 1998.
182. Head-Rapson AG, Devlin JC, Parker CJ, Hunter JM: Pharmacokinetics of the three isomers of mivacurium and pharmacodynamics of the chiral mixture in hepatic cirrhosis. Br J Anaesth 73:613-618, 1994.
183. Head-Rapson AG, Devlin JC, Parker CJ, Hunter JM: Pharmacokinetics and pharmacodynamics of the three isomers of mivacurium in health, in end-stage renal failure and in patients with impaired renal function. Br J Anaesth 75:31-36, 1995.
184. Caldwell JE, Heier T, Kitts JB, et al: Comparison of the neuromuscular block induced by mivacurium, suxamethonium or atracurium during nitrous oxide–fentanyl anaesthesia. Br J Anaesth 63:393-399, 1989.
185. Goudsouzian NG, d'Hollander AA, Viby-Mogensen J: Prolonged neuromuscular block from mivacurium in two patients with cholinesterase deficiency. Anesth Analg 77:183-185, 1993.
186. Maddineni VR, Mirakhur RK: Prolonged neuromuscular block following mivacurium. Anesthesiology 78:1181-1184, 1993.
187. Ostergaard D, Jensen FS, Jensen E, et al: Mivacurium-induced neuromuscular blockade in patients with atypical plasma cholinesterase. Acta Anaesthesiol Scand 37:314-318, 1993.
188. Naguib M, el-Gammal M, Daoud W, et al: Human plasma cholinesterase for antagonism of prolonged mivacurium-induced neuromuscular blockade. Anesthesiology 82:1288-1292, 1995.
189. Neill EA, Chapple DJ, Thompson CW: Metabolism and kinetics of atracurium: An overview. Br J Anaesth 55(Suppl 1):23S-25S, 1983.
190. Stiller RL, Cook DR, Chakravorti S: In vitro degradation of atracurium in human plasma. Br J Anaesth 57:1085-1088, 1985.
191. Fisher DM, Canfell PC, Fahey MR, et al: Elimination of atracurium in humans: Contribution of Hofmann elimination and ester hydrolysis versus organ-based elimination. Anesthesiology 65:6-12, 1986.
192. Canfell PC, Castagnoli N Jr, Fahey MR, et al: The metabolic disposition of laudanosine in dog, rabbit, and man. Drug Metab Dispos 14:703-708, 1986.
193. Parker CJ, Hunter JM: Pharmacokinetics of atracurium and laudanosine in patients with hepatic cirrhosis. Br J Anaesth 62:177-183, 1989.
194. Yate PM, Flynn PJ, Arnold RW, et al: Clinical experience and plasma laudanosine concentrations during the infusion of atracurium in the intensive therapy unit. Br J Anaesth 59:211-217, 1987.
195. Beemer GH, Bjorksten AR, Dawson PJ, Crankshaw DP: Production of laudanosine following infusion of atracurium in man and its effects on awakening. Br J Anaesth 63:76-80, 1989.
196. Tateishi A, Zornow MH, Scheller MS, Canfell PC: Electroencephalographic effects of laudanosine in an animal model of epilepsy. Br J Anaesth 62: 548-552, 1989.
197. Lanier WL, Sharbrough FW, Michenfelder JD: Effects of atracurium, vecuronium or pancuronium pretreatment on lignocaine seizure thresholds in cats. Br J Anaesth 60:74-80, 1988.
198. Shi WZ, Fahey MR, Fisher DM, Miller RD: Modification of central nervous system effects of laudanosine by inhalation anaesthetics. Br J Anaesth 63:598-600, 1989.
199. Chapple DJ, Miller AA, Ward JB, Wheatley PL: Cardiovascular and neurological effects of laudanosine. Studies in mice and rats, and in conscious and anaesthetized dogs. Br J Anaesth 59:218-225, 1987.
200. Powles AB, Ganta R: Use of vecuronium in the management of tetanus. Anaesthesia 40:879-881, 1985.
201. Kinjo M, Nagashima H, Vizi ES: Effect of atracurium and laudanosine on the release of ^{3}H-noradrenaline. Br J Anaesth 62:683-690, 1989.
202. Lien CA, Schmith VD, Belmont MR, et al: Pharmacokinetics of cisatracurium in patients receiving nitrous oxide/opioid/barbiturate anesthesia. Anesthesiology 84:300-308, 1996.
203. Kisor DF, Schmith VD, Wargin WA, et al: Importance of the organ-independent elimination of cisatracurium. Anesth Analg 83:1065-1071, 1996.
204. Fahey MR, Rupp SM, Fisher DM, et al: The pharmacokinetics and pharmacodynamics of atracurium in patients with and without renal failure. Anesthesiology 61:699-702, 1984.
205. Ward S, Boheimer N, Weatherley BC, et al: Pharmacokinetics of atracurium and its metabolites in patients with normal renal function, and in patients in renal failure. Br J Anaesth 59:697-706, 1987.
206. Szenohradszky J, Fisher DM, Segredo V, et al: Pharmacokinetics of rocuronium bromide (ORG 9426) in patients with normal renal function or patients undergoing cadaver renal transplantation. Anesthesiology 77:899-904, 1992.
207. Khalil M, D'Honneur G, Duvaldestin P, et al: Pharmacokinetics and pharmacodynamics of rocuronium in patients with cirrhosis. Anesthesiology 80:1241-1247, 1994.
208. Matteo RS, Ornstein E, Schwartz AE, et al: Pharmacokinetics and pharmacodynamics of rocuronium (Org 9426) in elderly surgical patients. Anesth Analg 77:1193-1197, 1993.
209. Magorian T, Wood P, Caldwell J, et al: The pharmacokinetics and neuromuscular effects of rocuronium bromide in patients with liver disease. Anesth Analg 80:754-759, 1995.
210. van Miert MM, Eastwood NB, Boyd AH, et al: The pharmacokinetics and pharmacodynamics of rocuronium in patients with hepatic cirrhosis. Br J Clin Pharmacol 44:139-144, 1997.

211. De Wolf AM, Freeman JA, Scott VL, et al: Pharmacokinetics and pharmacodynamics of cisatracurium in patients with end-stage liver disease undergoing liver transplantation. Br J Anaesth 76:624-628, 1996.
212. Anaesthetists and the reporting of adverse drug reactions. Br Med J (Clin Res Ed) 292:949, 1986.
213. Basta SJ: Modulation of histamine release by neuromuscular blocking drugs. Curr Opin Anaesth 5:572-576, 1992.
214. Hatano Y, Arai T, Noda J, et al: Contribution of prostacyclin to *d*-tubocurarine–induced hypotension in humans. Anesthesiology 72:28-32, 1990.
215. Scott RP, Savarese JJ, Basta SJ, et al: Atracurium: Clinical strategies for preventing histamine release and attenuating the haemodynamic response. Br J Anaesth 57:550-553, 1985.
216. Savarese JJ: The autonomic margins of safety of metocurine and *d*-tubocurarine in the cat. Anesthesiology 50:40-46, 1979.
217. Naguib M, Samarkandi AH, Bakhamees HS, et al: Histamine-release haemodynamic changes produced by rocuronium, vecuronium, mivacurium, atracurium and tubocurarine. Br J Anaesth 75: 588-592, 1995.
218. Miller RD, Eger EI 2nd, Stevens WC, Gibbons R: Pancuronium-induced tachycardia in relation to alveolar halothane, dose of pancuronium, and prior atropine. Anesthesiology 42:352-355, 1975.
219. Docherty JR, McGrath JC: Sympathomimetic effects of pancuronium bromide on the cardiovascular system of the pithed rat: A comparison with the effects of drugs blocking the neuronal uptake of noradrenaline. Br J Pharmacol 64:589-599, 1978.
220. Roizen MF, Forbes AR, Miller RD, et al: Similarity between effects of pancuronium and atropine on plasma norepinephrine levels in man. J Pharmacol Exp Ther 211:419-422, 1979.
221. Reitan JA, Fraser AI, Eisele JH: Lack of cardiac inotropic effects of gallamine in anesthetized man. Anesth Analg 52:974-979, 1973.
222. Wong KC, Wyte SR, Martin WE, Crawford EW: Antiarrhythmic effects of skeletal muscle relaxants. Anesthesiology 34:458-462, 1971.
223. Geha DG, Rozelle BC, Raessler KL, et al: Pancuronium bromide enhances atrioventricular conduction in halothane-anesthetized dogs. Anesthesiology 46:342-345, 1977.
224. Edwards RP, Miller RD, Roizen MF, et al: Cardiac responses to imipramine and pancuronium during anesthesia with halothane or enflurane. Anesthesiology 50:421-425, 1979.
225. Clayton D: Asystole associated with vecuronium. Br J Anaesth 58:937-938, 1986.
226. Starr NJ, Sethna DH, Estafanous FG: Bradycardia and asystole following the rapid administration of sufentanil with vecuronium. Anesthesiology 64: 521-523, 1986.
227. Cozanitis DA, Erkola O: A clinical study into the possible intrinsic bradycardic activity of vecuronium. Anaesthesia 44:648-650, 1989.
228. Bonner TI, Young AC, Brann MR, Buckley NJ: Cloning and expression of the human and rat m_5 muscarinic acetylcholine receptor genes. Neuron 1:403-410, 1988.
229. Mak JC, Barnes PJ: Autoradiographic visualization of muscarinic receptor subtypes in human and guinea pig lung. Am Rev Respir Dis 141:1559-1568, 1990.
230. Coulson FR, Fryer AD: Muscarinic acetylcholine receptors and airway diseases. Pharmacol Ther 98:59-69, 2003.
231. Jooste E, Klafter F, Hirshman CA, Emala CW: A mechanism for rapacuronium-induced bronchospasm: M_2 muscarinic receptor antagonism. Anesthesiology 98:906-911, 2003.
232. Naguib M: How serious is the bronchospasm induced by rapacuronium? Anesthesiology 94: 924-925, 2001.
233. Meakin GH, Pronske EH, Lerman J, et al: Bronchospasm after rapacuronium in infants and children. Anesthesiology 94:926-927, 2001.
234. Kron SS: Severe bronchospasm and desaturation in a child associated with rapacuronium. Anesthesiology 94:923-924, 2001.
235. Laxenaire MC, Moneret-Vautrin DA, Widmer S, et al: [Anesthetics responsible for anaphylactic shock. A French multicenter study.] Ann Fr Anesth Reanim 9:501-506, 1990.
236. Fisher MM, More DG: The epidemiology and clinical features of anaphylactic reactions in anaesthesia. Anaesth Intensive Care 9:226-234, 1981.
237. Mertes PM, Laxenaire MC, Alla F: Anaphylactic and anaphylactoid reactions occurring during anesthesia in France in 1999-2000. Anesthesiology 99: 536-545, 2003.
238. Baldo BA, Fisher MM: Substituted ammonium ions as allergenic determinants in drug allergy. Nature 306:262-264, 1983.
239. Levy JH, Davis GK, Duggan J, Szlam F: Determination of the hemodynamics and histamine release of rocuronium (Org 9426) when administered in increased doses under N_2O/O_2-sufentanil anesthesia. Anesth Analg 78:318-321, 1994.
240. Rose M, Fisher M: Rocuronium: High risk for anaphylaxis? Br J Anaesth 86:678-682, 2001.
241. Watkins J: Incidence of UK reactions involving rocuronium may simply reflect market use. Br J Anaesth 87:522, 2001.
242. Mertes PM, Moneret-Vautrin DA, Leynadier F, Laxenaire MC: Skin reactions to intradermal neuromuscular blocking agent injections: A randomized multicenter trial in healthy volunteers. Anesthesiology 107:245-252, 2007.
243. Laxenaire MC, Mertes PM: Anaphylaxis during anaesthesia. Results of a two-year survey in France. Br J Anaesth 87:549-558, 2001.
244. Levy JH, Gottge M, Szlam F, et al: Wheal and flare responses to intradermal rocuronium and cisatracurium in humans. Br J Anaesth 85:844-849, 2000.
245. Futo J, Kupferberg JP, Moss J, et al: Vecuronium inhibits histamine *N*-methyltransferase. Anesthesiology 69:92-96, 1988.
246. O'Callaghan AC, Scadding G, Watkins J: Bronchospasm following the use of vecuronium. Anaesthesia 41:940-942, 1986.
247. Naguib M, Magboul MM, Jaroudi R: Clinically significant drug interactions with general anesthetics—incidence, mechanims and management. CNS Drugs 8:51-78, 1997.
248. Miller RD: Factors affecting the action of muscle relaxants. *In* Katz RL (ed): Muscle Relaxants. Amsterdam, Excerpta Medica, 1975.
249. Naguib M, Abdulatif M, al-Ghamdi A, et al: Interactions between mivacurium and atracurium. Br J Anaesth 73:484-489, 1994.
250. Lebowitz PW, Ramsey FM, Savarese JJ, et al: Combination of pancuronium and metocurine: Neuromuscular and hemodynamic advantages over pancuronium alone. Anesth Analg 60:12-17, 1981.
251. Paul M, Kindler CH, Fokt RM, et al: Isobolographic analysis of non-depolarising muscle relaxant interactions at their receptor site. Eur J Pharmacol 438:35-43, 2002.
252. Motamed C, Menad R, Farinotti R, et al: Potentiation of mivacurium blockade by low dose of pancuronium: A pharmacokinetic study. Anesthesiology 98:1057-1062, 2003.
253. Kay B, Chestnut RJ, Sum Ping JS, Healy TE: Economy in the use of muscle relaxants. Vecuronium after pancuronium. Anaesthesia 42:277-280, 1987.
254. Rashkovsky OM, Agoston S, Ket JM: Interaction between pancuronium bromide and vecuronium bromide. Br J Anaesth 57:1063-1066, 1985.
255. Katz RL: Modification of the action of pancuronium by succinylcholine and halothane. Anesthesiology 35:602-606, 1971.
256. Ono K, Manabe N, Ohta Y, et al: Influence of suxamethonium on the action of subsequently administered vecuronium or pancuronium. Br J Anaesth 62:324-326, 1989.
257. Katz JA, Fragen RJ, Shanks CA, et al: The effects of succinylcholine on doxacurium-induced neuromuscular blockade. Anesthesiology 69:604-607, 1988.
258. Cooper R, Mirakhur RK, Clarke RS, Boules Z: Comparison of intubating conditions after administration of Org 9246 (rocuronium) and suxamethonium. Br J Anaesth 69:269-273, 1992.
259. Kelly RE, Lien CA, Savarese JJ, et al: Depression of neuromuscular function in a patient during desflurane anesthesia. Anesth Analg 76:868-871, 1993.
260. Saitoh Y, Toyooka H, Amaha K: Recoveries of post-tetanic twitch and train-of-four responses after administration of vecuronium with different inhalation anaesthetics and neuroleptanaesthesia. Br J Anaesth 70:402-404, 1993.
261. Miller RD, Way WL, Dolan WM, et al: The dependence of pancuronium- and *d*-tubocurarine–induced neuromuscular blockades on alveolar concentrations of halothane and forane. Anesthesiology 37:573-581, 1972.
262. Miller RD, Crique M, Eger EI 2nd: Duration of halothane anesthesia and neuromuscular blockade with *d*-tubocurarine. Anesthesiology 44:206-210, 1976.
263. Rupp SM, Miller RD, Gencarelli PJ: Vecuronium-induced neuromuscular blockade during enflurane, isoflurane, and halothane anesthesia in humans. Anesthesiology 60:102-105, 1984.
264. Gencarelli PJ, Miller RD, Eger EI 2nd, Newfield P: Decreasing enflurane concentrations and *d*-tubocurarine neuromuscular blockade. Anesthesiology 56:192-194, 1982.
265. Miller RD, Way WL, Dolan WM, et al: Comparative neuromuscular effects of pancuronium, gallamine, and succinylcholine during forane and halothane anesthesia in man. Anesthesiology 35:509-514, 1971.
266. Wulf H, Ledowski T, Linstedt U, et al: Neuromuscular blocking effects of rocuronium during desflurane, isoflurane, and sevoflurane anaesthesia. Can J Anaesth 45:526-532, 1998.
267. Bock M, Klippel K, Nitsche B, et al: Rocuronium potency and recovery characteristics during steady-state desflurane, sevoflurane, isoflurane or propofol anaesthesia. Br J Anaesth 84:43-47, 2000.
268. Paul M, Fokt RM, Kindler CH, et al: Characterization of the interactions between volatile anesthetics and neuromuscular blockers at the muscle nicotinic acetylcholine receptor. Anesth Analg 95:362-367, 2002.
269. Pereon Y, Bernard JM, Nguyen The Tich, et al: The effects of desflurane on the nervous system: From spinal cord to muscles. Anesth Analg 89:490-495, 1999.
270. Franks NP, Lieb WR: Molecular and cellular mechanisms of general anaesthesia. Nature 367:607-614, 1994.
271. Burkett L, Bikhazi GB, Thomas KC Jr, et al: Mutual potentiation of the neuromuscular effects of antibi-

otics and relaxants. Anesth Analg 58:107-115, 1979.

272. Hasfurther DL, Bailey PL: Failure of neuromuscular blockade reversal after rocuronium in a patient who received oral neomycin. Can J Anaesth 43:617-620, 1996.
273. Heier T, Caldwell JE, Sessler DI, Miller RD: Mild intraoperative hypothermia increases duration of action and spontaneous recovery of vecuronium blockade during nitrous oxide–isoflurane anesthesia in humans. Anesthesiology 74:815-819, 1991.
274. Leslie K, Sessler DI, Bjorksten AR, Moayeri A: Mild hypothermia alters propofol pharmacokinetics and increases the duration of action of atracurium. Anesth Analg 80:1007-1014, 1995.
275. Caldwell JE, Heier T, Wright PM, et al: Temperature-dependent pharmacokinetics and pharmacodynamics of vecuronium. Anesthesiology 92:84-93, 2000.
276. Heier T, Caldwell JE, Sessler DI, et al: The relationship between adductor pollicis twitch tension and core, skin, and muscle temperature during nitrous oxide–isoflurane anesthesia in humans. Anesthesiology 71:381-384, 1989.
277. Heier T, Caldwell JE, Sessler DI, Miller RD: The effect of local surface and central cooling on adductor pollicis twitch tension during nitrous oxide/isoflurane and nitrous oxide/fentanyl anesthesia in humans. Anesthesiology 72:807-811, 1990.
278. Miller RD, Agoston S, van der Pol F, et al: Hypothermia and the pharmacokinetics and pharmacodynamics of pancuronium in the cat. J Pharmacol Exp Ther 207:532-538, 1978.
279. Stenlake JB, Hughes R: In vitro degradation of atracurium in human plasma. Br J Anaesth 59:806-807, 1987.
280. Eriksson LI, Viby-Mogensen J, Lennmarken C: The effect of peripheral hypothermia on a vecuronium-induced neuromuscular block. Acta Anaesthesiol Scand 35:387-392, 1991.
281. Thornberry EA, Mazumdar B: The effect of changes in arm temperature on neuromuscular monitoring in the presence of atracurium blockade. Anaesthesia 43:447-449, 1988.
282. Miller RD, Van Nyhis LS, Eger EI: The effect of temperature on a *d*-tubocurarine neuromuscular blockade and its antagonism by neostigmine. J Pharmacol Exp Ther 195:237-241, 1975.
283. Miller RD, Roderick LL: Pancuronium-induced neuromuscular blockade, and its antagonism by neostigmine, at 29, 37, and 41°C. Anesthesiology 46:333-335, 1977.
284. Heier T, Clough D, Wright PM, et al: The influence of mild hypothermia on the pharmacokinetics and time course of action of neostigmine in anesthetized volunteers. Anesthesiology 97:90-95, 2002.
285. Sinatra RS, Philip BK, Naulty JS, Ostheimer GW: Prolonged neuromuscular blockade with vecuronium in a patient treated with magnesium sulfate. Anesth Analg 64:1220-1222, 1985.
286. Fuchs-Buder T, Wilder-Smith OH, Borgeat A, Tassonyi E: Interaction of magnesium sulphate with vecuronium-induced neuromuscular block. Br J Anaesth 74:405-409, 1995.
287. Tsai SK, Huang SW, Lee TY: Neuromuscular interactions between suxamethonium and magnesium sulphate in the cat. Br J Anaesth 72:674-678, 1994.
288. Waud BE, Waud DR: Interaction of calcium and potassium with neuromuscular blocking agents. Br J Anaesth 52:863-866, 1980.
289. Al-Mohaya S, Naguib M, Abdelatif M, Farag H: Abnormal responses to muscle relaxants in a patient with primary hyperparathyroidism. Anesthesiology 65:554-556, 1986.
290. Price LH, Heninger GR: Lithium in the treatment of mood disorders. N Engl J Med 331:591-598, 1994.
291. Abdel-Zaher AO: The myoneural effects of lithium chloride on the nerve-muscle preparations of rats. Role of adenosine triphosphate–sensitive potassium channels. Pharmacol Res 41:163-178, 2000.
292. Hill GE, Wong KC, Hodges MR: Lithium carbonate and neuromuscular blocking agents. Anesthesiology 46:122-126, 1977.
293. Martin BA, Kramer PM: Clinical significance of the interaction between lithium and a neuromuscular blocker. Am J Psychiatry 139:1326-1328, 1982.
294. Usubiaga JE, Wikinski JA, Morales RL, Usubiaga LE: Interaction of intravenously administered procaine, lidocaine and succinylcholine in anesthetized subjects. Anesth Analg 46:39-45, 1967.
295. Usubiaga JE, Standaert F: The effects of local anesthetics on motor nerve terminals. J Pharmacol Exp Ther 159:353-361, 1968.
296. Kordas M: The effect of procaine on neuromuscular transmission. J Physiol 209:689-699, 1970.
297. Thorpe WR, Seeman P: The site of action of caffeine and procaine in skeletal muscle. J Pharmacol Exp Ther 179:324-330, 1971.
298. Ozkul Y: Influence of calcium channel blocker drugs in neuromuscular transmission. Clin Neurophysiol 118:2005-2008, 2007.
299. van Poorten JF, Dhasmana KM, Kuypers RS, Erdmann W: Verapamil and reversal of vecuronium neuromuscular blockade. Anesth Analg 63:155-157, 1984.
300. Baurain M, Barvais L, d'Hollander A, Hennart D: Impairment of the antagonism of vecuronium-induced paralysis and intra-operative disopyramide administration. Anaesthesia 44:34-36, 1989.
301. Ornstein E, Matteo RS, Schwartz AE, et al: The effect of phenytoin on the magnitude and duration of neuromuscular block following atracurium or vecuronium. Anesthesiology 67:191-196, 1987.
302. Spacek A, Neiger FX, Spiss CK, Kress HG: Chronic carbamazepine therapy does not influence mivacurium-induced neuromuscular block. Br J Anaesth 77:500-502, 1996.
303. Alloul K, Whalley DG, Shutway F, et al: Pharmacokinetic origin of carbamazepine-induced resistance to vecuronium neuromuscular blockade in anesthetized patients. Anesthesiology 84:330-339, 1996.
304. Kim CS, Arnold FJ, Itani MS, Martyn JA: Decreased sensitivity to metocurine during long-term phenytoin therapy may be attributable to protein binding and acetylcholine receptor changes. Anesthesiology 77:500-506, 1992.
305. Melton AT, Antognini JF, Gronert GA: Prolonged duration of succinylcholine in patients receiving anticonvulsants: Evidence for mild up-regulation of acetylcholine receptors? Can J Anaesth 40:939-942, 1993.
306. Miller RD, Sohn YJ, Matteo RS: Enhancement of *d*-tuborcurarine neuromuscular blockade by diuretics in man. Anesthesiology 45:442-445, 1976.
307. Scappaticci KA, Ham JA, Sohn YJ, et al: Effects of furosemide on the neuromuscular junction. Anesthesiology 57:381-388, 1982.
308. Carmignani M, Scoppetta C, Ranelletti FO, Tonali P: Adverse interaction between acetazolamide and anticholinesterase drugs at the normal and myasthenic neuromuscular junction level. Int J Clin Pharmacol Ther Toxicol 22:140-144, 1984.
309. Azar I, Cottrell J, Gupta B, Turndorf H: Furosemide facilitates recovery of evoked twitch response after pancuronium. Anesth Analg 59:55-57, 1980.
310. Hill GE, Wong KC, Shaw CL, Blatnick RA: Acute and chronic changes in intra- and extracellular potassium and responses to neuromuscular blocking agents. Anesth Analg 57:417-421, 1978.
311. Glidden RS, Martyn JA, Tomera JF: Azathioprine fails to alter the dose-response curve of *d*-tubocurarine in rats. Anesthesiology 68:595-598, 1988.
312. Meyers EF: Partial recovery from pancuronium neuromuscular blockade following hydrocortisone administration. Anesthesiology 46:148-150, 1977.
313. Leeuwin RS, Veldsema-Currie RD, van Wilgenburg H, Ottenhof M: Effects of corticosteroids on neuromuscular blocking actions of *d*-tubocurarine. Eur J Pharmacol 69:165-173, 1981.
314. Parr SM, Robinson BJ, Rees D, Galletly DC: Interaction between betamethasone and vecuronium. Br J Anaesth 67:447-451, 1991.
315. Bouzat C, Barrantes FJ: Modulation of muscle nicotinic acetylcholine receptors by the glucocorticoid hydrocortisone. Possible allosteric mechanism of channel blockade. J Biol Chem 271:25835-25841, 1996.
316. Valera S, Ballivet M, Bertrand D: Progesterone modulates a neuronal nicotinic acetylcholine receptor. Proc Natl Acad Sci U S A 89:9949-9953, 1992.
317. Naguib M, Gyasi HK: Antiestrogenic drugs and atracurium—a possible interaction? Can Anaesth Soc J 33:682-683, 1986.
318. Ali HH, Wilson RS, Savarese JJ, Kitz RJ: The effect of tubocurarine on indirectly elicited train-of-four muscle response and respiratory measurements in humans. Br J Anaesth 47:570-574, 1975.
319. Kopman AF, Yee PS, Neuman GG: Relationship of the train-of-four fade ratio to clinical signs and symptoms of residual paralysis in awake volunteers. Anesthesiology 86:765-771, 1997.
320. Eriksson LI, Sundman E, Olsson R, et al: Functional assessment of the pharynx at rest and during swallowing in partially paralyzed humans: Simultaneous videomanometry and mechanomyography of awake human volunteers. Anesthesiology 87:1035-1043, 1997.
321. Sundman E, Witt H, Olsson R, et al: The incidence and mechanisms of pharyngeal and upper esophageal dysfunction in partially paralyzed humans: Pharyngeal videoradiography and simultaneous manometry after atracurium. Anesthesiology 92:977-984, 2000.
322. Eriksson LI: Reduced hypoxic chemosensitivity in partially paralysed man. A new property of muscle relaxants? Acta Anaesthesiol Scand 40:520-523, 1996.
323. Eriksson LI: The effects of residual neuromuscular blockade and volatile anesthetics on the control of ventilation. Anesth Analg 89:243-251, 1999.
324. Igarashi A, Amagasa S, Horikawa H, Shirahata M: Vecuronium directly inhibits hypoxic neurotransmission of the rat carotid body. Anesth Analg 94:117-122, 2002.
325. Lien CA, Matteo RS, Ornstein E, et al: Distribution, elimination, and action of vecuronium in the elderly. Anesth Analg 73:39-42, 1991.
326. Caldwell JE: Reversal of residual neuromuscular block with neostigmine at one to four hours after a single intubating dose of vecuronium. Anesth Analg 80:1168-1174, 1995.
327. Magorian TT, Lynam DP, Caldwell JE, Miller RD: Can early administration of neostigmine, in single or repeated doses, alter the course of neuromuscular recovery from a vecuronium-induced neuromuscular blockade? Anesthesiology 73:410-414, 1990.
328. Baurain MJ, d'Hollander AA, Melot C, et al: Effects of residual concentrations of isoflurane on the

reversal of vecuronium-induced neuromuscular blockade. Anesthesiology 74:474-478, 1991.

329. Soreq H, Seidman S: Acetylcholinesterase—new roles for an old actor. Nat Rev Neurosci 2:294-302, 2001.

330. Silman I, Sussman JL: Acetylcholinesterase: 'classical' and 'non-classical' functions and pharmacology. Curr Opin Pharmacol 5:293-302, 2005.

331. Bevan DR, Donati F, Kopman AF: Reversal of neuromuscular blockade. Anesthesiology 77:785-805, 1992.

332. Beemer GH, Goonetilleke PH, Bjorksten AR: The maximum depth of an atracurium neuromuscular block antagonized by edrophonium to effect adequate recovery. Anesthesiology 82:852-858, 1995.

333. Bevan JC, Collins L, Fowler C, et al: Early and late reversal of rocuronium and vecuronium with neostigmine in adults and children. Anesth Analg 89:333-339, 1999.

334. Kirkegaard H, Heier T, Caldwell JE: Efficacy of tactile-guided reversal from cisatracurium-induced neuromuscular block. Anesthesiology 96:45-50, 2002.

335. Caldwell JE, Robertson EN, Baird WL: Antagonism of vecuronium and atracurium: Comparison of neostigmine and edrophonium administered at 5% twitch height recovery. Br J Anaesth 59:478-481, 1987.

336. Berg H, Roed J, Viby-Mogensen J, et al: Residual neuromuscular block is a risk factor for postoperative pulmonary complications. A prospective, randomised, and blinded study of postoperative pulmonary complications after atracurium, vecuronium and pancuronium. Acta Anaesthesiol Scand 41:1095-1103, 1997.

337. Cronnelly R, Morris RB, Miller RD: Edrophonium: Duration of action and atropine requirement in humans during halothane anesthesia. Anesthesiology 57:261-266, 1982.

338. Miller RD, Van Nyhuis LS, Eger EI 2nd, et al: Comparative times to peak effect and durations of action of neostigmine and pyridostigmine. Anesthesiology 41:27-33, 1974.

339. Rupp SM, McChristian JW, Miller RD, et al: Neostigmine and edrophonium antagonism of varying intensity neuromuscular blockade induced by atracurium, pancuronium, or vecuronium. Anesthesiology 64:711-717, 1986.

340. Engbaek J, Ording H, Ostergaard D, Viby-Mogensen J: Edrophonium and neostigmine for reversal of the neuromuscular blocking effect of vecuronium. Acta Anaesthesiol Scand 29:544-546, 1985.

341. Donati F, Smith CE, Bevan DR: Dose-response relationships for edrophonium and neostigmine as antagonists of moderate and profound atracurium blockade. Anesth Analg 68:13-19, 1989.

342. Naguib M, Abdulatif M: Priming with anti-cholinesterases—the effect of different combinations of anti-cholinesterases and different priming intervals. Can J Anaesth 35:47-52, 1988.

343. Savarese JJ: Reversal of nondepolarizing blocks: More controversial than ever? *In* Review Course Lectures, 67th Congress. Cleveland, OH, International Anesthesia Research Society, 1993.

344. Bevan DR, Smith CE, Donati F: Postoperative neuromuscular blockade: A comparison between atracurium, vecuronium, and pancuronium. Anesthesiology 69:272-276, 1988.

345. Gencarelli PJ, Miller RD: Antagonism of org NC 45 (vecuronium) and pancuronium neuromuscular blockade by neostigmine. Br J Anaesth 54:53-56, 1982.

346. Naguib M, Abdulatif M, al-Ghamdi A, et al: Dose-response relationships for edrophonium and neostigmine antagonism of mivacurium-induced neuromuscular block. Br J Anaesth 71:709-714, 1993.

347. Kao YJ, Le ND: The reversal of profound mivacurium-induced neuromuscular blockade. Can J Anaesth 43:1128-1133, 1996.

348. Naguib M, Selim M, Bakhamees HS, et al: Enzymatic versus pharmacologic antagonism of profound mivacurium-induced neuromuscular blockade. Anesthesiology 84:1051-1059, 1996.

349. Naguib M, Daoud W, el-Gammal M, et al: Enzymatic antagonism of mivacurium-induced neuromuscular blockade by human plasma cholinesterase. Anesthesiology 83:694-701, 1995.

350. Naguib M, Samarkandi AH, Bakhamees HS, et al: Edrophonium and human plasma cholinesterase combination for antagonism of mivacurium-induced neuromuscular block. Br J Anaesth 77: 424-426, 1996.

351. Morita T, Tsukagoshi H, Sugaya T, et al: Inadequate antagonism of vecuronium-induced neuromuscular block by neostigmine during sevoflurane or isoflurane anesthesia. Anesth Analg 80:1175-1180, 1995.

352. Reid JE, Breslin DS, Mirakhur RK, Hayes AH: Neostigmine antagonism of rocuronium block during anesthesia with sevoflurane, isoflurane or propofol. Can J Anaesth 48:351-355, 2001.

353. Lowry DW, Mirakhur RK, McCarthy GJ, et al: Neuromuscular effects of rocuronium during sevoflurane, isoflurane, and intravenous anesthesia. Anesth Analg 87:936-940, 1998.

354. Astley BA, Katz RL, Payne JP: Electrical and mechanical responses after neuromuscular blockade with vecuronium, and subsequent antagonism with neostigmine or edrophonium. Br J Anaesth 59:983-988, 1987.

355. Goldhill DR, Wainwright AP, Stuart CS, Flynn PJ: Neostigmine after spontaneous recovery from neuromuscular blockade. Effect on depth of blockade monitored with train-of-four and tetanic stimuli. Anaesthesia 44:293-299, 1989.

356. Miller RD, Roderick LL: Acid-base balance and neostigmine antagonism of pancuronium neuromuscular blockade. Br J Anaesth 50:317-324, 1978.

357. Miller RD, Van Nyhuis LS, Eger EI 2nd, Way WL: The effect of acid-base balance on neostigmine antagonism of *d*-tubocurarine–induced neuromuscular blockade. Anesthesiology 42:377-383, 1975.

358. Miller RD, Roderick LL: Diuretic-induced hypokalaemia, pancuronium neuromuscular blockade and its antagonism by neostigmine. Br J Anaesth 50:541-544, 1978.

359. Jones RM, Cashman JN, Casson WR, Broadbent MP: Verapamil potentiation of neuromuscular blockade: Failure of reversal with neostigmine but prompt reversal with edrophonium. Anesth Analg 64:1021-1025, 1985.

360. Wali FA: Interaction of verapamil with gallamine and pancuronium and reversal of combined neuromuscular blockade with neostigmine and edrophonium. Eur J Anaesthesiol 3:385-393, 1986.

361. Salem MG, Richardson JC, Meadows GA, et al: Comparison between glycopyrrolate and atropine in a mixture with neostigmine for reversal of neuromuscular blockade. Studies in patients following open heart surgery. Br J Anaesth 57:184-187, 1985.

362. van Vlymen JM, Parlow JL: The effects of reversal of neuromuscular blockade on autonomic control in the perioperative period. Anesth Analg 84:148-154, 1997.

363. Ding Y, Fredman B, White PF: Use of mivacurium during laparoscopic surgery: Effect of reversal drugs on postoperative recovery. Anesth Analg 78:450-454, 1994.

364. Boeke AJ, de Lange JJ, van Druenen B, Langemeijer JJ: Effect of antagonizing residual neuromuscular block by neostigmine and atropine on postoperative vomiting. Br J Anaesth 72:654-656, 1994.

365. Hovorka J, Korttila K, Nelskyla K, et al: Reversal of neuromuscular blockade with neostigmine has no effect on the incidence or severity of postoperative nausea and vomiting. Anesth Analg 85:1359-1361, 1997.

366. Tramer MR, Fuchs-Buder T: Omitting antagonism of neuromuscular block: Effect on postoperative nausea and vomiting and risk of residual paralysis. A systematic review. Br J Anaesth 82:379-386, 1999.

367. Debaene B, Plaud B, Dilly MP, Donati F: Residual paralysis in the PACU after a single intubating dose of nondepolarizing muscle relaxant with an intermediate duration of action. Anesthesiology 98: 1042-1048, 2003.

368. Cronnelly R, Stanski DR, Miller RD, et al: Renal function and the pharmacokinetics of neostigmine in anesthetized man. Anesthesiology 51:222-226, 1979.

369. Cronnelly R, Stanski DR, Miller RD, Sheiner LB: Pyridostigmine kinetics with and without renal function. Clin Pharmacol Ther 28:78-81, 1980.

370. Morris RB, Cronnelly R, Miller RD, et al: Pharmacokinetics of edrophonium in anephric and renal transplant patients. Br J Anaesth 53:1311-1314, 1981.

371. Morris RB, Cronnelly R, Miller RD, et al: Pharmacokinetics of edrophonium and neostigmine when antagonizing *d*-tubocurarine neuromuscular blockade in man. Anesthesiology 54:399-401, 1981.

372. Kopman AF: Edrophonium antagonism of pancuronium-induced neuromuscular blockade in man: A reappraisal. Anesthesiology 51:139-142, 1979.

373. Miller RD: Sugammadex: An opportunity to change the practice of anesthesiology? Anesth Analg 104:477-478, 2007.

375. Bom A, Bradley M, Cameron K, et al: A novel concept of reversing neuromuscular block: Chemical encapsulation of rocuronium bromide by a cyclodextrin-based synthetic host. Angew Chem 41:266-270, 2002.

375. Adam JM, Bennett DJ, Bom A, et al: Cyclodextrin-derived host molecules as reversal agents for the neuromuscular blocker rocuronium bromide: Synthesis and structure-activity relationships. J Med Chem 45:1806-1816, 2002.

376. Baker MT, Naguib M: Propofol: The challenges of formulation. Anesthesiology 103:860-876, 2005.

377. Epemolu O, Bom A, Hope F, Mason R: Reversal of neuromuscular blockade and simultaneous increase in plasma rocuronium concentration after the intravenous infusion of the novel reversal agent Org 25969. Anesthesiology 99:632-637, 2003.

378. de Boer HD, van Egmond J, van de Pol F, et al: Reversal of profound rocuronium neuromuscular blockade by sugammadex in anesthetized rhesus monkeys. Anesthesiology 104:718-723, 2006.

379. Gijsenbergh F, Ramael S, Houwing N, van Iersel T: First human exposure of Org 25969, a novel agent to reverse the action of rocuronium bromide. Anesthesiology 103:695-703, 2005.

380. Sparr HJ, Vermeyen KM, Beaufort AM, et al: Early reversal of profound rocuronium-induced neuromuscular blockade by sugammadex in a randomized multicenter study: Efficacy, safety, and pharmacokinetics. Anesthesiology 106:935-943, 2007.

381. Sorgenfrei IF, Norrild K, Larsen PB, et al: Reversal of rocuronium-induced neuromuscular block by the selective relaxant binding agent sugammadex: A dose-finding and safety study. Anesthesiology 104:667-674, 2006.
382. Suy K, Morias K, Cammu G, et al: Effective reversal of moderate rocuronium- or vecuronium-induced neuromuscular block with sugammadex, a selective relaxant binding agent. Anesthesiology 106:283-288, 2007.
383. Eleveld DJ, Kuizenga K, Proost JH, Wierda JM: A temporary decrease in twitch response during reversal of rocuronium-induced muscle relaxation with a small dose of sugammadex. Anesth Analg 104:582-584, 2007.
384. Groudine SB, Soto R, Lien C, et al: A randomized, dose-finding, phase II study of the selective relaxant binding drug, sugammadex, capable of safely reversing profound rocuronium-induced neuromuscular block. Anesth Analg 104:555-562, 2007.
385. Sacan O, White PF, Tufanogullari B, Klein K: Sugammadex reversal of rocuronium-induced neuromuscular blockade: A comparison with neostigmine-glycopyrrolate and edrophonium-atropine. Anesth Analg 104:569-574, 2007.
386. Vanacker BF, Vermeyen KM, Struys MM, et al: Reversal of rocuronium-induced neuromuscular block with the novel drug sugammadex is equally effective under maintenance anesthesia with propofol or sevoflurane. Anesth Analg 104:563-568, 2007.
387. Shields M, Giovannelli M, Mirakhur RK, et al: Org 25969 (sugammadex), a selective relaxant binding agent for antagonism of prolonged rocuronium-induced neuromuscular block. Br J Anaesth 96:36-43, 2006.
388. Baraka A: Onset of neuromuscular block in myasthenic patients. Br J Anaesth 69:227-228, 1992.
389. de Boer HD, Driessen JJ, Marcus MA, et al: Reversal of rocuronium-induced (1.2 mg/kg) profound neuromuscular block by sugammadex: A multicenter, dose-finding and safety study. Anesthesiology 107:239-244, 2007.
390. Lee C, Jahr JS, Candiotti K, et al: Reversal of profound rocuronium NMB with sugammadex is faster than recovery from succinylcholine [abstract A988]. Presented at the annual meeting of the American Association of Anesthesiologists, San Francisco, 2007.
391. Naguib M: Sugammadex: Another milestone in clinical neuromuscular pharmacology. Anesth Analg 104:575-581, 2007.
392. de Boer HD, van Egmond J, van de Pol F, et al: Sugammadex, a new reversal agent for neuromuscular block induced by rocuronium in the anaesthetized Rhesus monkey. Br J Anaesth 96:473-479, 2006.
393. Zhang MQ: Drug-specific cyclodextrins: The future of rapid neuromuscular block reversal? Drugs Future 28:347-354, 2003.
394. Henderson WA: Succinylcholine-induced cardiac arrest in unsuspected Duchenne muscular dystrophy. Can Anaesth Soc J 31:444-446, 1984.
395. Goudsouzian NG, Ryan JF, Savarese JJ: The neuromuscular effects of pancuronium in infants and children. Anesthesiology 41:95-98, 1974.
396. Fisher DM, O'Keeffe C, Stanski DR, et al: Pharmacokinetics and pharmacodynamics of *d*-tubocurarine in infants, children, and adults. Anesthesiology 57:203-208, 1982.
397. Fisher DM, Castagnoli K, Miller RD: Vecuronium kinetics and dynamics in anesthetized infants and children. Clin Pharmacol Ther 37:402-406, 1985.
398. Fisher DM, Miller RD: Neuromuscular effects of vecuronium (ORG NC45) in infants and children during N_2O, halothane anesthesia. Anesthesiology 58:519-523, 1983.
399. Meretoja OA, Wirtavuori K, Neuvonen PJ: Age-dependence of the dose-response curve of vecuronium in pediatric patients during balanced anesthesia. Anesth Analg 67:21-26, 1988.
400. Goudsouzian NG, Liu LM, Cote CJ, et al: Safety and efficacy of atracurium in adolescents and children anesthetized with halothane. Anesthesiology 59: 459-462, 1983.
401. Meretoja OA, Taivainen T, Wirtavuori K: Cisatracurium during halothane and balanced anaesthesia in children. Paediatr Anaesth 6:373-378, 1996.
402. de Ruiter J, Crawford MW: Dose-response relationship and infusion requirement of cisatracurium besylate in infants and children during nitrous oxide–narcotic anesthesia. Anesthesiology 94:790-792, 2001.
403. Scheiber G, Ribeiro FC, Marichal A, et al: Intubating conditions and onset of action after rocuronium, vecuronium, and atracurium in young children. Anesth Analg 83:320-324, 1996.
404. Taivainen T, Meretoja OA, Erkola O, et al: Rocuronium in infants, children and adults during balanced anaesthesia. Paediatr Anaesth 6:271-275, 1996.
405. Fisher DM, Cronnelly R, Miller RD, Sharma M: The neuromuscular pharmacology of neostigmine in infants and children. Anesthesiology 59:220-225, 1983.
406. Duvaldestin P, Saada J, Berger JL, et al: Pharmacokinetics, pharmacodynamics, and dose-response relationships of pancuronium in control and elderly subjects. Anesthesiology 56:36-40, 1982.
407. Maddineni VR, Mirakhur RK, McCoy EP: Plasma cholinesterase activity in elderly and young adults. Br J Anaesth 72:497, 1994.
408. Maddineni VR, Mirakhur RK, McCoy EP, Sharpe TD: Neuromuscular and haemodynamic effects of mivacurium in elderly and young adult patients. Br J Anaesth 73:608-612, 1994.
409. Soderberg M, Thomson D, White T: Respiration, circulation and anaesthetic management in obesity. Investigation before and after jejunoileal bypass. Acta Anaesthesiol Scand 21:55-61, 1977.
410. Weinstein JA, Matteo RS, Ornstein E, et al: Pharmacodynamics of vecuronium and atracurium in the obese surgical patient. Anesth Analg 67:1149-1153, 1988.
411. Puhringer FK, Khuenl-Brady KS, Mitterschiffthaler G: Rocuronium bromide: Time-course of action in underweight, normal weight, overweight and obese patients. Eur J Anaesthesiol Suppl 11:107-110, 1995.
412. Beemer GH, Bjorksten AR, Crankshaw DP: Effect of body build on the clearance of atracurium: Implication for drug dosing. Anesth Analg 76:1296-1303, 1993.
413. Vandenbrom RH, Wierda JM, Agoston S: Pharmacokinetics and neuromuscular blocking effects of atracurium besylate and two of its metabolites in patients with normal and impaired renal function. Clin Pharmacokinet 19:230-240, 1990.
414. Fahey MR, Morris RB, Miller RD, et al: Pharmacokinetics of Org NC45 (norcuron) in patients with and without renal failure. Br J Anaesth 53:1049-1053, 1981.
415. Lynam DP, Cronnelly R, Castagnoli KP, et al: The pharmacodynamics and pharmacokinetics of vecuronium in patients anesthetized with isoflurane with normal renal function or with renal failure. Anesthesiology 69:227-231, 1988.
416. Somogyi AA, Shanks CA, Triggs EJ: The effect of renal failure on the disposition and neuromuscular blocking action of pancuronium bromide. Eur J Clin Pharmacol 12:23-29, 1977.
417. Ward S, Neill EA: Pharmacokinetics of atracurium in acute hepatic failure (with acute renal failure). Br J Anaesth 55:1169-1172, 1983.
418. Bevan DR, Donati F, Gyasi H, Williams A: Vecuronium in renal failure. Can Anaesth Soc J 31:491-496, 1984.
419. Khuenl-Brady KS, Pomaroli A, Puhringer F, et al: The use of rocuronium (ORG 9426) in patients with chronic renal failure. Anaesthesia 48:873-875, 1993.
420. Hunter JM, Jones RS, Utting JE: Use of atracurium in patients with no renal function. Br J Anaesth 54:1251-1258, 1982.
421. Hunter JM, Jones RS, Utting JE: Comparison of vecuronium, atracurium and tubocurarine in normal patients and in patients with no renal function. Br J Anaesth 56:941-951, 1984.
422. Lebrault C, Duvaldestin P, Henzel D, et al: Pharmacokinetics and pharmacodynamics of vecuronium in patients with cholestasis. Br J Anaesth 58:983-987, 1986.
423. Nana A, Cardan E, Leitersdorfer T: Pancuronium bromide. Its use in asthmatics and patients with liver disease. Anaesthesia 27:154-158, 1972.
424. Westra P, Vermeer GA, de Lange AR, et al: Hepatic and renal disposition of pancuronium and gallamine in patients with extrahepatic cholestasis. Br J Anaesth 53:331-338, 1981.
425. Gyasi HK, Naguib M: Atracurium and severe hepatic disease: A case report. Can Anaesth Soc J 32:161-164, 1985.
426. Servin FS, Lavaut E, Kleef U, Desmonts JM: Repeated doses of rocuronium bromide administered to cirrhotic and control patients receiving isoflurane. A clinical and pharmacokinetic study. Anesthesiology 84:1092-1100, 1996.
427. Bell CF, Hunter JM, Jones RS, Utting JE: Use of atracurium and vecuronium in patients with oesophageal varices. Br J Anaesth 57:160-168, 1985.
428. Lawhead RG, Matsumi M, Peters KR, et al: Plasma laudanosine levels in patients given atracurium during liver transplantation. Anesth Analg 76:569-573, 1993.
429. Ward JM, Rosen KM, Martyn JA: Acetylcholine receptor subunit mRNA changes in burns are different from those seen after denervation: The 1993 Lindberg Award. J Burn Care Rehabil 14:595-601, 1993.
430. Martyn JA, Szyfelbein SK, Ali HH, et al: Increased *d*-tubocurarine requirement following major thermal injury. Anesthesiology 52:352-355, 1980.
431. Edwards JP, Hatton PA, Little RA, et al: Increased quantal release of acetylcholine at the neuromuscular junction following scald injury in the rat. Muscle Nerve 22:1660-1666, 1999.
432. Tomera JF, Lilford K, Martyn JA: Diaphragm acetylcholinesterase multimeric forms in mice in response to burn trauma. J Burn Care Rehabil 14:406-419, 1993.
433. Martyn JA, White DA, Gronert GA, et al: Up-and-down regulation of skeletal muscle acetylcholine receptors. Effects on neuromuscular blockers. Anesthesiology 76:822-843, 1992.
434. Schaner PJ, Brown RL, Kirksey TD, et al: Succinylcholine-induced hyperkalemia in burned patients. 1. Anesth Analg 48:764-770, 1969.
435. Viby-Mogensen J, Hanel HK, Hansen E, Graae J: Serum cholinesterase activity in burned patients. II:

Anaesthesia, suxamethonium and hyperkalaemia. Acta Anaesthesiol Scand 19:169-179, 1975.

436. Murray MJ, Cowen J, DeBlock H, et al: Clinical practice guidelines for sustained neuromuscular blockade in the adult critically ill patient. Crit Care Med 30:142-156, 2002.
437. Hansen-Flaschen JH, Brazinsky S, et al: Use of sedating drugs and neuromuscular blocking agents in patients requiring mechanical ventilation for respiratory failure. A national survey. JAMA 266:2870-2875, 1991.
438. Loper KA, Butler S, Nessly M, Wild L: Paralyzed with pain: The need for education. Pain 37:315-316, 1989.
439. Pollard BJ: Muscle relaxants in critical care. Br J Intensive Care 4:347-353, 1994.
440. Lacomis D, Petrella JT, Giuliani MJ: Causes of neuromuscular weakness in the intensive care unit: A study of ninety-two patients. Muscle Nerve 21:610-617, 1998.
441. Rudis MI, Guslits BJ, Peterson EL, et al: Economic impact of prolonged motor weakness complicating neuromuscular blockade in the intensive care unit. Crit Care Med 24:1749-1756, 1996.
442. Lacomis D, Zochodne DW, Bird SJ: Critical illness myopathy. Muscle Nerve 23:1785-1788, 2000.
443. Showalter CJ, Engel AG: Acute quadriplegic myopathy: Analysis of myosin isoforms and evidence for calpain-mediated proteolysis. Muscle Nerve 20:316-322, 1997.
444. Shee CD: Risk factors for hydrocortisone myopathy in acute severe asthma. Respir Med 84:229-233, 1990.
445. Hanson P, Dive A, Brucher JM, et al: Acute corticosteroid myopathy in intensive care patients. Muscle Nerve 20:1371-1380, 1997.
446. Deconinck N, Van Parijs V, Beckers-Bleukx G, Van den Bergh P: Critical illness myopathy unrelated to corticosteroids or neuromuscular blocking agents. Neuromuscul Disord 8:186-192, 1998.
447. DuBois DC, Almon RR: Disuse atrophy of skeletal muscle is associated with an increase in number of glucocorticoid receptors. Endocrinology 107:1649-1651, 1980.
448. Hund E: Myopathy in critically ill patients. Crit Care Med 27:2544-2547, 1999.
449. Neviere R, Mathieu D, Chagnon JL, et al: Skeletal muscle microvascular blood flow and oxygen transport in patients with severe sepsis. Am J Respir Crit Care Med 153:191-195, 1996.
450. Tsukagoshi H, Morita T, Takahashi K, et al: Cecal ligation and puncture peritonitis model shows decreased nicotinic acetylcholine receptor numbers in rat muscle: Immunopathologic mechanisms? Anesthesiology 91:448-460, 1999.
451. De Letter MA, van Doorn PA, Savelkoul HF, et al: Critical illness polyneuropathy and myopathy (CIPNM): Evidence for local immune activation by cytokine-expression in the muscle tissue. J Neuroimmunol 106:206-213, 2000.
452. Tepper M, Rakic S, Haas JA, Woittiez AJ: Incidence and onset of critical illness polyneuropathy in patients with septic shock. Neth J Med 56:211-214, 2000.
453. van den Berghe G, Wouters P, Weekers F, et al: Intensive insulin therapy in the critically ill patients. N Engl J Med 345:1359-1367, 2001.
454. Zifko UA: Long-term outcome of critical illness polyneuropathy. Muscle Nerve Suppl 9:S49-S52, 2000.
455. Dodson BA, Kelly BJ, Braswell LM, Cohen NH: Changes in acetylcholine receptor number in muscle from critically ill patients receiving muscle relaxants: An investigation of the molecular mechanism of prolonged paralysis. Crit Care Med 23:815-821, 1995.
456. Coursin DB, Klasek G, Goelzer SL: Increased requirements for continuously infused vecuronium in critically ill patients. Anesth Analg 69:518-521, 1989.
457. Hughes M, Grant IS, Biccard B, Nimmo G: Suxamethonium and critical illness polyneuropathy. Anaesth Intensive Care 27:636-638, 1999.
458. Kupfer Y, Namba T, Kaldawi E, Tessler S: Prolonged weakness after long-term infusion of vecuronium bromide. Ann Intern Med 117:484-486, 1992.
459. Op de Coul AA, Lambregts PC, Koeman J, et al: Neuromuscular complications in patients given Pavulon (pancuronium bromide) during artificial ventilation. Clin Neurol Neurosurg 87:17-22, 1985.
460. Tousignant CP, Bevan DR, Eisen AA, et al: Acute quadriparesis in an asthmatic treated with atracurium. Can J Anaesth 42:224-227, 1995.
461. Gwinnutt CL, Eddleston JM, Edwards D, Pollard BJ: Concentrations of atracurium and laudanosine in cerebrospinal fluid and plasma in three intensive care patients. Br J Anaesth 65:829-832, 1990.
462. Szenohradszky J, Trevor AJ, Bickler P, et al: Central nervous system effects of intrathecal muscle relaxants in rats. Anesth Analg 76:1304-1309, 1993.
463. Griffiths RB, Hunter JM, Jones RS: Atracurium infusions in patients with renal failure on an ITU. Anaesthesia 41:375-381, 1986.
464. Beemer GH, Dawson PJ, Bjorksten AR, Edwards NE: Early postoperative seizures in neurosurgical patients administered atracurium and isoflurane. Anaesth Intensive Care 17:504-509, 1989.
465. Eddleston JM, Harper NJ, Pollard BJ, et al: Concentrations of atracurium and laudanosine in cerebrospinal fluid and plasma during intracranial surgery. Br J Anaesth 63:525-530, 1989.
466. Chiodini F, Charpantier E, Muller D, et al: Blockade and activation of the human neuronal nicotinic acetylcholine receptors by atracurium and laudanosine. Anesthesiology 94:643-651, 2001.
467. Prielipp RC, Coursin DB, Scuderi PE, et al: Comparison of the infusion requirements and recovery profiles of vecuronium and cisatracurium 51W89 in intensive care unit patients. Anesth Analg 81:3-12, 1995.
468. Zarowitz BJ, Rudis MI, Lai K, et al: Retrospective pharmacoeconomic evaluation of dosing vecuronium by peripheral nerve stimulation versus standard clinical assessment in critically ill patients. Pharmacotherapy 17:327-332, 1997.
469. Kress JP, Pohlman AS, O'Connor MF, Hall JB: Daily interruption of sedative infusions in critically ill patients undergoing mechanical ventilation. N Engl J Med 342:1471-1477, 2000.

Charles B. Berde and Gary R. Strichartz

30 Local Anesthetics

Key Points

1. Local anesthetics block voltage-gated sodium channels and thereby interrupt initiation and propagation of impulses in axons, but they have a wide variety of other biologic actions, desirable and undesirable.
2. Currently available local anesthetics are of two chemical classes: aminoesters and aminoamides.
3. The low potency and lack of specificity of available local anesthetics are due in part to the very weak structural constraints at their binding site on the sodium channel. Most of their features derive from the requirement for high solubility and rapid diffusion in both aqueous environments and the lipid phases of biologic membranes.
4. Reversible protonation of the tertiary amine group tends to make local anesthetics less charged at more basic pH and more charged at neutral or acidic pH; the neutral base forms are more soluble in lipid environments, whereas the charged acid forms are more soluble in aqueous environments.
5. Aminoesters are metabolized primarily by plasma esterases, and aminoamides are metabolized primarily by hepatic cytochrome P450–linked enzymes.
6. The principal systemic toxicities of local anesthetics involve the heart (including atrioventricular conduction block, arrhythmias, myocardial depression, and cardiac arrest) and the brain (including agitation, lethargy, seizures, and generalized central nervous system depression). Hypoxemia and acidosis exacerbate these toxicities. Resuscitation after bupivacaine overdose is particularly difficult. Therefore, prevention of intravascular injection or overdose is crucial, and major nerve blockade should involve incremental, fractionated dosing.
7. Local anesthetics are directly toxic to nerve at the concentrations supplied in commercial solutions. Intraneural concentrations during regional anesthesia are generally (but not always) below a threshold for toxicity because of spread of solutions through tissues and diffusion gradients from injection sites into nerve. Injection into a constrained tissue space increases the risk for local toxicity.
8. Optimal use of local anesthetics in regional anesthesia requires an understanding of (1) the individual patient's clinical situation; (2) the location, intensity, and duration of regional anesthesia and analgesia required; (3) anatomic factors affecting deposition of drug near nerves; (4) proper drug selection and dosing; and (5) ongoing assessment of clinical effects after administration of a local anesthetic.
9. Recent efforts have led to the development of several new formulations for topical anesthesia. Single-stereoisomer (as opposed to a racemic mixture) formulations have been developed in an effort to reduce systemic toxicity and improve sensory selectivity.
10. Local anesthetics are increasingly being used for postoperative infusions and via both local and systemic administration for the management of chronic pain. Further research and development may lead to safe, more selective agents that will facilitate more prolonged administration in the setting of acute or chronic pain.

Local anesthesia results from the blockade of nerve impulses to abolish sensation. All currently available, clinically useful agents are either aminoesters or aminoamides. These drugs, when applied in sufficient concentration at the site of action, prevent conduction of electrical impulses by the membranes of nerve and muscle. In addition to blockade of impulses, local anesthetics can inhibit various receptors, enhance release of glutamate, and depress the activity of certain intracellular signaling pathways. When local anesthetic agents are given systemically, the functions of cardiac, skeletal, and smooth muscle, as well as transmission of impulses in the central and peripheral nervous systems and within the specialized conducting system of the heart, may all be altered. Local anesthetics may abolish sensation in various parts of the body by topical application, injection in the vicinity of peripheral nerve endings and major nerve trunks, or instillation within the epidural or subarachnoid spaces. Toxicity may be local or systemic. The central nervous and cardiovascular systems are most commonly involved in acute clinical toxicity.

Basic Pharmacology

Chemistry

The Local Anesthetic Molecule

The typical local anesthetic molecule, exemplified by lidocaine and procaine (Fig. 30-1), contains a tertiary amine attached to a substituted aromatic ring by an intermediate chain that almost always contains either an ester ($-\overset{O}{\overset{\|}{C}}-O$) or an amide ($-NH\overset{O}{\overset{\|}{C}}-$) linkage; local anesthetics may therefore be classified as aminoester or aminoamide compounds. The aromatic ring system gives a lipophilic (membrane-liking) character to its portion of the molecule, whereas the tertiary amine end is relatively hydrophilic, particularly since it is partially protonated and thus bears some positive charge in the physiologic pH range (Fig. 30-2). The structures of commonly administered local anesthetics are given in Table 30-1 and their physicochemical properties in Table 30-2.

Structure-Activity Relationships and Physicochemical Properties

The intrinsic potency and duration of action of local anesthetics are clearly dependent on certain features of the molecule.

Lipophilic-Hydrophilic Balance

The lipophilic versus hydrophilic character of a local anesthetic depends on the size of alkyl substituents on or near the tertiary amine and on the aromatic ring. "Lipophilicity" expresses the tendency of a compound to associate with membrane lipids, a property usually approximated by equilibrium partitioning into a hydrophobic solvent such as octanol.[1] Although octanol-buffer partition coefficients are comparable to membrane-buffer partition coefficients for the uncharged species of local anesthetics, they severely underestimate membrane partitioning for the charged, protonated species, octanol being a poor model for the polar regions near the membrane surface where local anesthetics are concentrated.[2] Here we use the term "hydrophobicity," expressed as octanol-buffer partitioning, to describe a physicochemical property of local anesthetics.

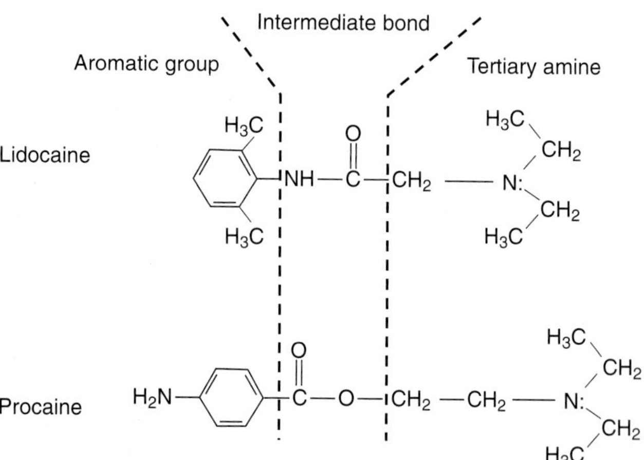

Figure 30-1 Structures of two local anesthetics, the aminoamide lidocaine and the aminoester procaine. In both drugs a hydrophobic aromatic group is joined to a more hydrophilic base, the tertiary amine, by an intermediate amide or ester bond.

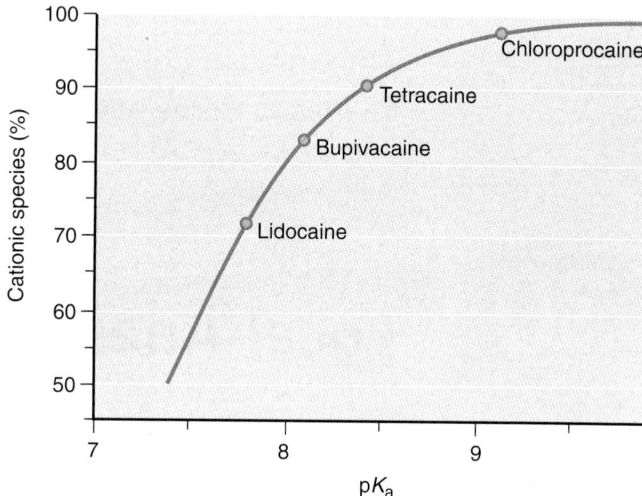

Figure 30-2 Fraction of local anesthetic in the protonated, cationic form of an aqueous solution at physiologic pH (7.4) as a function of the pK_a of the drug. Lidocaine, the drug with the lowest pK_a, has the smallest fraction of its molecules protonated, the largest in the neutral form, and vice versa for chloroprocaine, the local anesthetic with the highest pK_a. Individual drug molecules become protonated and deprotonated in thousandths of a second in solution.

Compounds with a more hydrophobic nature are obtained by increasing the size of the alkyl substituents. These agents are more potent and produce longer-lasting blocks than their less hydrophobic congeners do.[3-5] For example, etidocaine, which has three more carbon atoms than lidocaine does in the amine end of the molecule, is four times as potent and five times as long lasting when compared by impulse blockade in the isolated sciatic nerve.

Hydrogen Ion Concentration

Local anesthetics in solution exist in a very rapid chemical equilibrium between the basic uncharged form (B) and the charged cationic form (BH^+). At a certain hydrogen ion concentration ($\log_{10}^{-1}$ [−pH]) specific for each drug, the concentration of local anesthetic base in solution is equal to the concentration of charged cation. The logarithm of this hydrogen ion concentration is called pK_a. The relationship is defined by

$$\frac{[BH^+]}{[B]} = 10^{pK_a - pH} \tag{1}$$

pK_a values of local anesthetic agents in aqueous solution are listed in Table 30-2. The tendency to be protonated also

Table 30-1 Representative Local Anesthetics in Common Clinical Use

Generic* and Common Proprietary Name	Chemical Structure	Approximate Year of Initial Clinical Use	Main Anesthetic Use	Representative Commercial Preparation
Cocaine	$CH_2-CH-CHCOOCH_3$; $NCH_3-CHOOC_6H_5$; $CH_2-CH-CH_2$ (bridged ring)	1884	Topical	40 mg/mL solution
Benzocaine (Americaine)	$H_2N-C_6H_4-C(=O)-OC_2H_5$	1900	Topical Topical	200 mg/mL 200 mg/mL
Procaine (Novocain)	$H_2N-C_6H_4-COOCH_2CH_2N(C_2H_5)_2$	1905	Infiltration Spinal	10- and 20-mg/mL solutions 100-mg/mL solution
Dibucaine (Nupercaine)	Quinoline ring with OC_4H_9 and $CONHCH_2CH_2N(C_2H_5)_2$	1929	Spinal	0.667-, 2.5-, and 5-mg/mL solutions
Tetracaine (Pontocaine)	$H_9C_4(H)N-C_6H_4-COOCH_2CH_2N(CH_3)_2$	1930	Spinal	Niphanoid crystals—20- and 10-mg/mL solutions
Lidocaine (Xylocaine)	$(CH_3)_2C_6H_3-NHCOCH_2N(C_2H_5)_2$	1948	Infiltration Peripheral nerve blockade Epidural Spinal Topical Topical	5- and 10-mg/mL solutions 10-, 15-, and 20-mg/mL solutions 10-, 15-, and 20-mg/mL solutions 50-mg/mL solution 20 mg/mL jelly, viscous 25, 50 mg/mL ointment
Chloroprocaine (Nesacaine)	$H_2N-C_6H_3(Cl)-COOCH_2CH_2N(C_2H_5)_2$	1955	Infiltration Peripheral nerve blockade Epidural	10-mg/mL solution 10- and 20-mg/mL solutions 20- and 30-mg/mL solutions
Mepivacaine (Carbocaine)	$(CH_3)_2C_6H_3-NHCO-$ (N-CH_3 piperidine ring)	1957	Infiltration Peripheral nerve blockade Epidural	10-mg/mL solution 10- and 20-mg/mL solutions 10-, 15-, and 20-mg/mL solutions

Table 30-1 Representative Local Anesthetics in Common Clinical Use—cont'd

Generic* and Common Proprietary Name	Chemical Structure	Approximate Year of Initial Clinical Use	Main Anesthetic Use	Representative Commercial Preparation
Prilocaine (Citanest)	CH_3; NHCOCH—NH—C_3H_7; CH_3	1960	Infiltration	10- and 20-mg/mL solutions
			Peripheral nerve blockade	10-, 20-, and 30-mg/mL solutions
			Epidural	10-, 20-, and 30-mg/mL solutions
Bupivacaine (Marcaine)	CH_3; NHCO; N; C_4H_9; CH_3	1963	Infiltration	2.5-mg/mL solution
			Peripheral nerve blockade	2.5- and 5-mg/mL solutions
			Epidural	2.5-, 5-, and 7.5-mg/mL solutions
			Spinal	5- and 7.5-mg/mL solutions
Ropivacaine (Naropin)	CH_3; NHCO; N; C_3H_7; CH_3	1992	Infiltration	2.5- and 5-mg/mL solutions
			Peripheral nerve blockade	5- and 10-mg/mL solutions
			Epidural	5- and 7.5-mg/mL solutions

*USP nomenclature.
Modified from Covino B, Vassallo H: Local Anesthetics: Mechanisms of Action and Clinical Use. Orlando, FL, Grune & Stratton, 1976.

depends on environmental factors, such as temperature and ionic strength, and on the medium surrounding the drug. In the relatively apolar milieu of a membrane, the average pK_a of local anesthetics is lower than in solution.[6] This is chemically equivalent to saying that the membrane concentrates the base form of the local anesthetic more than it concentrates the protonated cation form.

The pH of the medium containing the local anesthetic influences drug activity by altering the relative percentage of the base and protonated forms. For example, in inflamed tissues the pH is lower than normal, and local anesthetics are more protonated than in normal tissue and thus penetrate the tissue relatively poorly (see later).

The relationship between pK_a and the percentage of local anesthetic present in the cationic form is shown in Figure 30-2. As described later, there are dual effects of pH on clinical effectiveness, depending on where the local anesthetic is injected and the importance of the base form for tissue penetration.

Anatomy of the Peripheral Nerve

Each peripheral nerve axon possesses its own cell membrane, the axolemma. Nonmyelinated nerves, such as autonomic postganglionic efferent and nociceptive afferent C fibers, contain many axons encased in a single Schwann cell sheath. In contrast, all large motor and sensory fibers are enclosed in many layers of myelin, which consists of the plasma membranes of specialized Schwann cells that wrap themselves around the axon during axonal outgrowth. Myelin greatly increases the speed of nerve conduction by insulating the axolemma from the surrounding conducting salt medium and forcing the "action current" generated by an impulse to flow through the axoplasm to the nodes of Ranvier, which are periodic interruptions in the myelin sheath where the active impulse is regenerated (Fig. 30-3). The Na^+ channels that serve generation and propagation of impulses are highly concentrated at the nodes of Ranvier of myelinated fibers[7] but are

Table 30-2 Relative in vitro Conduction-Blocking Potency and Physiochemical Properties of Local Anesthetic Drugs

Drug	Relative Conduction-Blocking Potency*	Physiochemical Properties	
		pK_a†	Hydrophobicity†
Low Potency			
Procaine	1	8.9	100
Intermediate Potency			
Mepivacaine	1.5	7.7	130
Prilocaine	1.8	8.0‡	129
Chloroprocaine	3	9.1	810
Lidocaine	2	7.8	366
High Potency			
Tetracaine	8	8.4	5822
Bupivacaine	8	8.1	3420
Etidocaine	8	7.9	7320

*Data derived from C fibers of isolated rabbit vagus and sciatic nerve.
†pK_a and hydrophobicity at 36°C; hydrophobicity equals the octanol-buffer partition coefficient of the base. Values are ratios of concentrations.
‡Values at 25°C.
From Strichartz GR, Sanchez V, Arthur GR, et al: Fundamental properties of local anesthetics. II. Measured octanol: buffer partition coefficients and pK_a values of clinically used drugs. Anesth Analg 71:158-170, 1990.

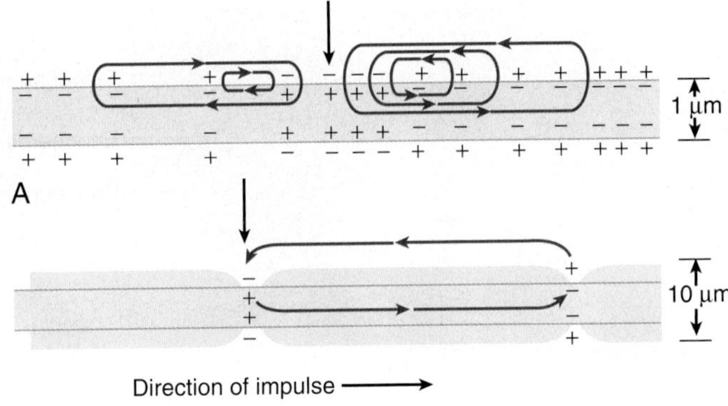

Figure 30-3 Pattern of "local circuit currents" flowing during propagation of an impulse in a nonmyelinated C fiber's axon (**A**) and a myelinated axon (**B**). During propagation of impulses, from left to right, current entering the axon at the initial rising phase of the impulse (*large vertical arrows*) passes through the axoplasm (local circuit current) and depolarizes the adjacent membrane. "Plus" and "minus" signs adjacent to the axon membrane indicate the polarization state of the axon membrane: negative inside at rest, positive inside during active depolarization under the action potential, and less negative in regions where local circuit currents flow. This ionic current passes relatively uniformly across the nonmyelinated axon, but in the myelinated axon it is restricted to entry at the nodes of Ranvier, several of which are simultaneously depolarized during a single action potential.

distributed all along the axon of nonmyelinated fibers (Fig. 30-3). A classification of peripheral nerves according to fiber size and physiologic properties is presented in Table 30-3.

A typical peripheral nerve consists of several axon bundles, or fascicles. Each axon has its own connective tissue covering, the *endoneurium*. Each fascicle of many axons is encased by a second connective tissue layer, the epithelial-like *perineurium*, and the entire nerve is wrapped in a loose outer sheath called the *epineurium* (Fig. 30-4). To reach the nerve axon, a local anesthetic molecule must traverse four or five layers of connective tissue or lipid membranous barriers, or both.

Structure of the Axonal Membrane

Biologic membranes consist of a molecular lipid bilayer containing proteins adsorbed on the surfaces, as well as embedded in or spanning the hydrocarbon core (Fig. 30-5). The character of the bilayer is determined by the phospholipids, which have long hydrophobic fatty acyl tails that lie in the center of the membrane, as well as by the polar hydrophilic head groups, which are usually composed of zwitterionic portions (containing positive and negative charges) that project into the cytoplasm or the extracellular

Table 30-3 Classification of Peripheral Nerves According to Anatomy, Physiology, and Function

Fiber Class	Subclass	Myelin	Diameter (µm)	Conduction Velocity (msec)	Location	Function	Susceptibility to Local Anesthetic Block
A	α	+	6-22	30-120	Efferent to muscles	Motor	++
	β	+	6-22	30-120	Afferent from skin and joints	Tactile, proprioception	++
	γ	+	3-6	15-35	Efferent to muscle spindles	Muscle tone	++++
	δ	+	1-4	5-25	Afferent sensory nerves	Pain, cold temperature, touch	+++
B		+	<3	3-15	Preganglionic sympathetic	Various autonomic functions	++
C	sC	–	0.3-1.3	0.7-1.3	Postganglionic sympathetic	Various autonomic functions	++
	dC	–	0.4-1.2	0.1-2.0	Afferent sensory nerves	Various autonomic functions Pain, warm temperature, touch	+

Modified From Bonica JJ: Principles and Practice of Obstetric Anesthesia and Analgesia. Philadelphia, FA Davis, 1967.

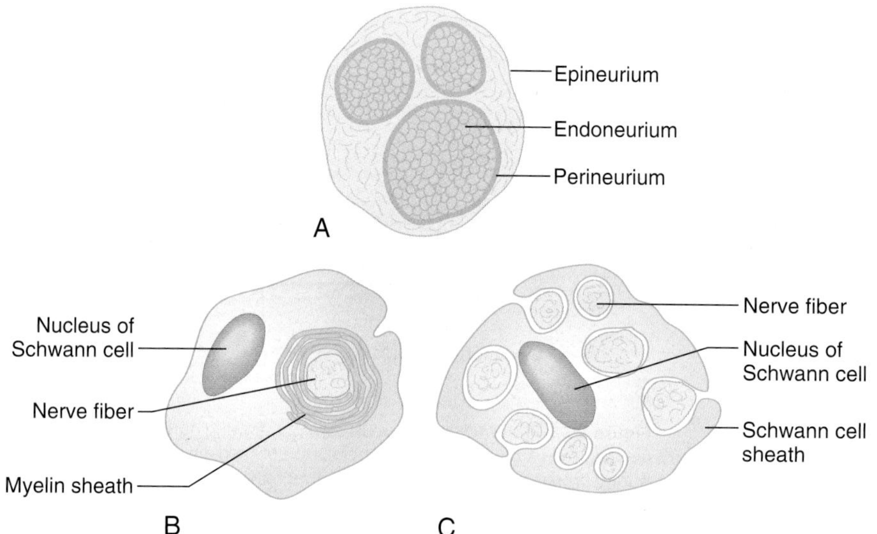

Figure 30-4 Transverse sections of a peripheral nerve (**A**) showing the outermost epineurium; the inner perineurium, which collects nerve axons in fascicles; and the endoneurium, which surrounds each myelinated fiber. Each myelinated axon (**B**) is encased in the multiple membranous wrappings of myelin formed by one Schwann cell, each of which stretches longitudinally more than approximately 100 times the diameter of the axon. The narrow span of axon between these myelinated segments, the node of Ranvier, contains the ion channels that support action potentials. Nonmyelinated fibers (**C**) are enclosed in bundles of 5 to 10 axons by a chain of Schwann cells that tightly embrace each axon with but one layer of membrane.

fluid. Within the membrane there is both lateral and rotational diffusion, which allows lipids and certain proteins to migrate in a fluid mosaic, but most membrane proteins are fixed within specific regions of a membrane, anchored by connections to specific proteins of the cell's cytoskeleton.[7]

A dynamic interaction exists between the cell's membrane and cytoplasm. Although we focus here on the channel-blocking actions of local anesthetics, it is noteworthy that many other cellular activities, including both metabolic and signal transduction pathways, are inhibited by these drugs.

Physiology of Nerve Conduction

The neural membrane is able to maintain a voltage difference of −60 to −90 mV between the intracellular medium and the cell's outside because at rest it is relatively impermeable to sodium ions but selectively permeable to potassium ions. The Na^+/K^+ pump, an active, energy-dependent mechanism, sustains the ion gradients that drive this potential difference by constant extrusion of sodium from within the cell in exchange for a net uptake of potassium, with adenosine triphosphate used as an energy source. Although the membrane is relatively permeable to potassium ions, an intracellular-to-extracellular potassium ratio of 150 to 5 mM, or 30 : 1, is maintained by active removal of potassium as it leaks passively across the plasma membrane.

The nerve at rest behaves largely as a "potassium electrode," according to the Nernst equation:

$$E_m \approx E_K = \left(\frac{-RT}{F}\right)\ln\left(\frac{[K^+]_i}{[K^+]_o}\right) \quad (2)$$

where E_m is the membrane potential, E_K is the potassium equilibrium potential, R is the gas constant, T is temperature (Kelvin), F

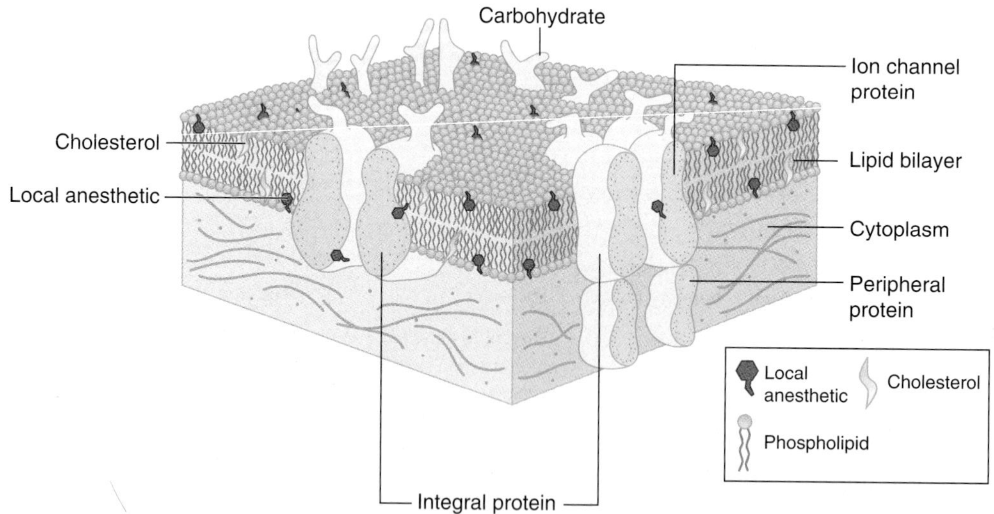

Figure 30-5 A typical plasma membrane has at its core the lipid bilayer, composed of phospholipids and cholesterol molecules (in about a 5 : 1 ratio) embedding the membrane integral proteins, which are most often glycosylated by extracellular carbohydrates and include receptors and ion channels essential for intercellular communication. "Peripheral proteins" regulate the functions of membrane proteins, chaperone them to the plasma membrane, and stabilize them in the cell through interactions with both the cytoskeleton and the extracellular matrix. Probable membrane locations and protein sites for local anesthetics are also shown.

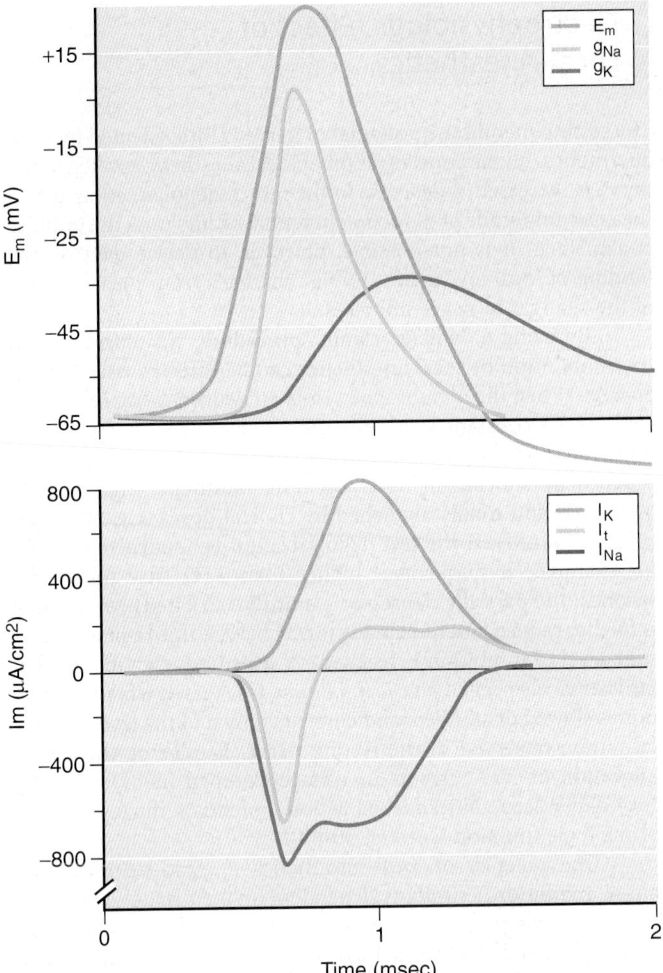

Figure 30-6 Membrane potential (E_m) and the voltage-gated ionic conductance of sodium (g_{Na}) and potassium (g_K), which determine the corresponding membrane currents Im (I_{Na} and I_K) during a propagated action potential. Modeled from the original studies of Hodgkin and Huxley on the squid giant axon (see Hodgkin[8]), these relationships hold for almost all invertebrate and vertebrate nerve fibers. The direction of the total ionic current (i_t), which is the sum of I_{Na} and I_K, is inward (negative values) for the depolarizing phase of the action potential and outward (positive values) for the repolarizing phase.

is Faraday's constant, and [K^+] is the potassium ion concentration inside (i) and outside (o) the cell. For potassium, therefore,

$$E_K = -58 \log 30, \text{ or } -85.7 \text{ mV}$$

An opposite situation exists for Na^+, which is at higher concentration outside the cell and has a Nernst potential, E_{Na}, of about +60 mV. During an action potential, the nerve membrane transiently switches its higher permeability from K^+ to Na^+, thereby changing the membrane potential from negative to positive, and back again.[8] The progress of this potential change and the underlying events are graphed in Figure 30-6. They provide a basis for understanding local anesthetic conduction block.

Permeation of ions through membranes occurs via specialized proteins called ion channels.[9] The conformation of these channels is often sensitive to the membrane potential; both Na^+ and K^+ channels in nerve membranes are activated to an "open" conformation by membrane depolarization. Sodium channels, in addition, close to an "inactivated" conformation after their initial activation. A small membrane depolarization extending along an axon from a region of excited membrane, for example, will begin to open both Na^+ and K^+ channels. The Na^+ channels open faster, however, and the inwardly directed Na^+ current (see Fig. 30-6) depolarizes the membrane further, thereby leading to opening of more Na^+ channels and increasing the inward Na^+ current even further (Fig. 30-7). This sequence of events continues during the *depolarizing phase* until some of the Na^+ channels have become inactivated and enough of the K^+ channels have opened to change the balance of current and result in a net outward current that produces membrane *repolarization* (see Fig. 30-7). After one action potential, the concentrations of Na^+ and K^+ have changed little for the large myelinated fibers but by as much as 10% for the small, nonmyelinated axons. The Na^+ ions entering and K^+ ions leaving the cell as a result of this process are restored by the Na^+/K^+ pump.

Depolarizations too weak to activate enough Na^+ channels to produce a net inward current are below the membrane's excitability *threshold*. The precise value of the threshold varies in different regions of the cell and also changes with time. For example, directly after an impulse, when some Na^+ channels are still inactivated and some K^+ channels are still activated, the threshold is above its "resting" value and the membrane is "refractory" to stimulation. Over time, however, as Na^+ inactivation decays and K^+ channels return to their closed conformation, the original resting threshold value is restored.

The action potential is a wave of depolarization that is propagated along the axon by continuous coupling between excited and nonexcited regions of membrane. Ionic current (the action current) enters the axon in the excited, depolarized region and then flows down the axoplasm and exits through the surrounding membrane, thereby passively depolarizing this adjacent region (see Fig. 30-3). Although this *local circuit current* spreads away from the excited zone in both directions, the region behind the impulse, having just been depolarized, is absolutely refractory and propagation of impulses is thus unidirectional.

The local circuit current spreads rapidly along a length of insulated internode in a myelinated axon (see Fig. 30-3), and

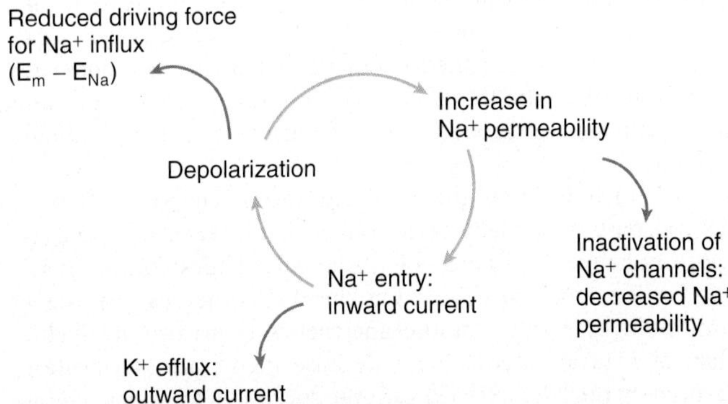

Figure 30-7 The action potential can be understood in terms of the cyclic relationships between factors contributing to the regenerative, depolarizing phase and the passive, repolarizing phase. *Positive* factors (*yellow arrows*) increase the rate of depolarization in a "positive-feedback loop," each element in the cycle favoring the subsequent one. *Negative* factors (*gray arrows*) decrease the depolarization rate by reducing or opposing the related positive factor, with efflux of K^+ eventually dominating the ionic flow and repolarizing the membrane.

many nodes of Ranvier in sequence are depolarized to threshold with little intervening delay. Single impulses do not jump from node to node as separate, discrete events; instead, active depolarization occurs simultaneously along several centimeters of the largest axons (see Fig. 30-3). Indeed, the local circuit current is so robust that it can skip past two completely nonexcitable nodes (e.g., blocked by local anesthetic) and successfully stimulate a third node. If excitability is partially reduced, such as by inhibition of some of the Na^+ channels, the amplitude of impulses in successive nodes falls decrementally, a process that can continue for many centimeters.[10,11] This situation probably occurs during certain phases of local anesthesia, as discussed later. However, when enough of the Na^+ channels are blocked, local circuit current fails to bring the adjacent resting region to threshold, and the impulse is fully extinguished.

Mechanism of Action of Local Anesthetics (Pharmacodynamics)

Active Form

Local anesthetic bases are poorly to sparingly soluble in water but are quite soluble in relatively hydrophobic organic solvents. Therefore, as a matter of chemistry (and to optimize shelf life), most of these drugs are formulated as hydrochloride salts. The pK_a of the drug and tissue pH determine the amount of drug that exists in solution as free base or as positively charged cation when injected into living tissue (see earlier). Furthermore, uptake of the drug by tissue, largely via lipophilic adsorption, will also alter its activity, both by shifting the effective pK_a downward, thereby favoring the neutral base form, and by limiting diffusion of the anesthetic away from the site of injection. Moderately hydrophobic local anesthetics block faster than either hydrophilic or highly hydrophobic ones, delivered at the same concentration, for the following reasons. Moderately hydrophilic molecules, such as lidocaine, are less bound to tissues than very hydrophobic drugs are (e.g., tetracaine) but are still more membrane permeant than very hydrophilic ones (e.g., 2-chloroprocaine). The highly hydrophobic local anesthetics, having higher intrinsic potencies (see Table 30-2), are therefore used in lower concentrations and their diffusion-controlled rate of onset is correspondingly reduced.

Which form of the local anesthetic, charged cation or neutral base, is actually responsible for blockade of impulses? More alkaline solutions of local anesthetics block nerve conduction more effectively. On sheath-free nerves, the rate of inhibition by tertiary amine anesthetics is greater at alkaline than at neutral external pH[12] because membrane permeation, favored by the base over the cationic species, determines the rate of access to the binding site. Direct control of axoplasmic pH (or internal perfusion with permanently charged quaternary amine homologs) shows that the dominant potency derives from the cationic species acting from the cytoplasmic surface.[13,14] The uncharged base also has intrinsic pharmacologic activity, however, which explains the effectiveness of benzocaine as a topical local anesthetic.

Electrophysiologic Effect of Local Anesthetics

The resting membrane potential of nerve is little affected by local anesthetics. As the concentration of local anesthetic applied to the nerve is increased, a decrease in the rate of depolarization and in the peak amplitude of the action potential occurs until the impulse is abolished. It is not possible, however, to derive data on the binding of local anesthetics to Na^+ channels from measurement of the changes in nerve impulses.

By using a "voltage-clamp" procedure, Na^+ currents and their inhibition by local anesthetics can be directly assayed (Fig. 30-8A). When the membrane of isolated neurons is rapidly depolarized to a constant value, the time course of ionic currents is observed. Sodium currents during one initial depolarization are reduced by subclinical doses of local anesthetic (e.g., 0.2 mM lidocaine) and totally abolished by clinical doses (e.g., 1% lidocaine, ≈40 mM). If the test depolarization is applied repeatedly, for example, at frequencies higher than 5 Hz (five pulses per second), the partially depressed (*tonically* inhibited) Na^+ current is further reduced incrementally for each pulse until a new steady-state level of inhibition is reached.[15,16] This frequency-dependent inhibition, also called *phasic inhibition*, is reversed when stimulation is slowed or stopped, and currents return to the level of tonic inhibition observed in the resting nerve. Paralleling the phasic inhibition of Na^+ currents in voltage-clamped membranes is a "use-dependent" blockade of action potentials during normal physiologic function (see Fig. 30-8B).

The potency of local anesthetics to produce tonic and phasic inhibition is similarly dependent on their structure, hydrophobicity, and pK_a. At its simplest, there appears to be a single binding site for local anesthetics on the Na^+ channel, with a "tonic" affinity at rest and increased "phasic" affinity occurring as a result of depolarization. The phasic blocking phenomenon can thus be used to reveal the true kinetics of binding of local anesthetic to the functional receptor, the Na^+ channel itself.

Phasic actions are a manifestation of the selective affinity of local anesthetics for conformations of the Na^+ channel that result from depolarization. Both "open" and "inactivated" states of the channel bind local anesthetics more avidly than the resting state does. Repeated depolarization thus increases the fraction of drug-bound channels; dissociation of these bound drug molecules is usually a slower process than the normal recovery from inactivation (see earlier) and results in the use-dependent accumulation of channels in the blocked condition and the phenomenon of phasic block.

By its selective binding to a channel state, the local anesthetic stabilizes that state. During phasic block, therefore, more inactivated channels become drug bound, and reciprocally, less activation can occur. This relationship between state-dependent affinities and modification of transitions among states through drug binding is known as the "modulated receptor" model.[17] Overall binding of anesthetic is increased by membrane depolarization for two reasons: *more binding sites become accessible* during activation (the "guarded receptor" model) and drug *dissociation* from inactivated channels *is slower* than from resting channels (the modulated receptor model).

The specific binding rates and affinities for the different conformations of the sodium channel depend on the particular local anesthetic drug. When the details of this dependence are

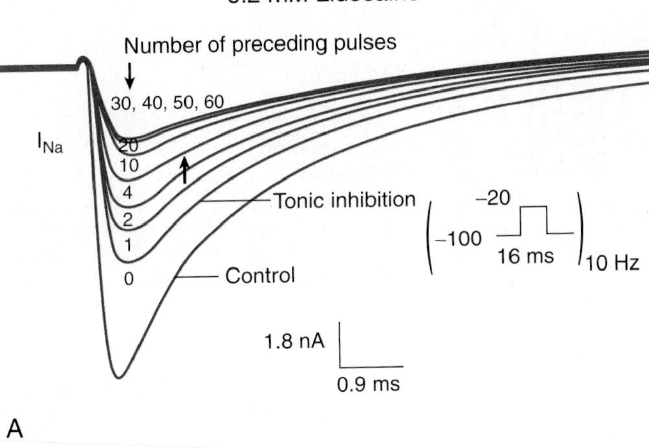

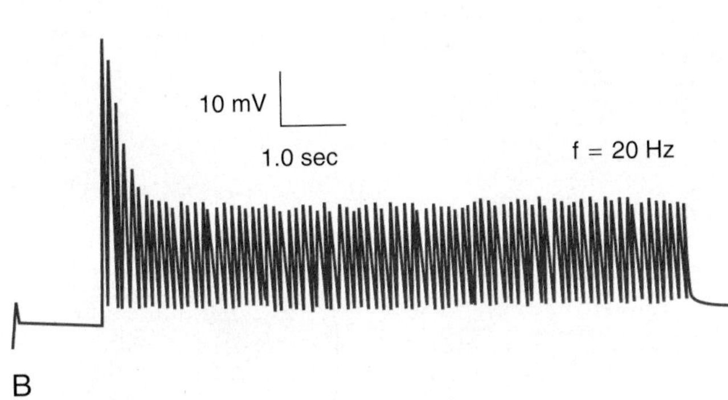

Figure 30-8 "Use-dependent" actions of local anesthetics on excitable membrane properties. **A,** Ionic Na^+ currents measured by a voltage-clamping technique are transiently activated by brief steps of depolarization applied infrequently ("tonic" test) or in a train at 10 times per second ("phasic" test, see E_m pattern in parentheses). After equilibration with 0.2 mM (0.005%) lidocaine, the currents measured tonically are reduced by about 30% from the control currents. Application of the "phasic" train of depolarizations results in a dynamic reduction of currents after each depolarization, with a steady-state value of phasic inhibition reached during the train of 75% of control currents. Recovery of currents to the tonic value occurs within a few seconds when phasic testing stops (not shown). **B,** Action potentials are also inhibited in a phasic manner by local anesthetics. After equilibration with 0.8 mM lidocaine (0.02%), the action potential is tonically reduced by about 20% from its amplitude in drug-free solution (not shown). Stimulation by a train at 20 stimuli per second induces a phasic inhibition that further reduces the amplitude by about 70% from the control value. As with the ionic currents (**A**), phasic inhibition of the action potential recovers rapidly when high-frequency stimulation stops.

correlated with the physicochemical properties of the drug and with the experimental conditions, they provide insight into the molecular features of the local anesthetic binding site.

The Nature of the Local Anesthetic Binding Site

Intentional mutation of specific amino acids of the Na^+ channel has allowed definition of regions that interact directly with local anesthetics. The major functional protein of the Na^+ channel (the α-subunit) is composed of four homologous "domains" (DI to DIV), each of which contains six helical regions (S1 to S6) that span the core of the membrane (Fig. 30-9A). Each domain also has a loop, termed the "P region," that links the extracellular ends of its S5 and S6 transmembrane segments; the P regions extend inward between the transmembrane regions such that when the α-subunit folds together, each P loop contributes a quarter of the cylindrical ion "selectivity pore," the narrowest passage of an open channel (see Fig. 30-9B). Voltage sensitivity derives from the positive charges located on S4 segments, which slide or swing "outward" in response to membrane depolarization. By linkages still unknown, this movement of S4 results in a conformational rearrangement of the S6 segments, which form the inner, cytoplasmic entry to the channel. Closed-to-open channel gating results from movement of the S6 segments, whereas inactivation gating results from binding of the cytoplasmic loop located between D-3 and D-4 to the cytoplasmic opening of the channel.

Local anesthetics bind in the "inner vestibule" of the closed Na^+ channel (see Fig. 30-9C). Amino acid mutations in the S6 segments of D-1, D-3, and D-4 all modify local anesthetic action, thus suggesting either that these regions form a "pharmocophore" small enough to simultaneously contact the drug at three surfaces or that the local anesthetic molecule moves rapidly among these three segments.

The rate constant for binding of local anesthetic to the closed Na^+ channel is larger for the more hydrophobic molecules, which suggest that drug molecules can reach the binding site (and depart from it) through a "hydrophobic" pathway. This path could be movement from the membrane phase laterally, into the channel, or through hydrophobic amino acid residues that limit access through a pathway in the closed pore. The slow block of closed and inactivated channels appears to use such a hydrophobic access and thus accounts for tonic inhibition.

The charged species of local anesthetics dissociates much more slowly from closed and inactivated Na^+ channels than the neutral form does, which suggests that an ionic bond may be involved in drug binding or that the charged molecule moves only slowly along the hydrophobic pathway.

In brief, hydrophobicity delivers the drug to the receptor and charge keeps it there.

Neurophysiologic Aspects of Phasic Inhibition

Different fiber types in the nerve are affected differently during local anesthesia. At least part of this difference arises from pharmacokinetic factors. At the onset of and during recovery from clinical block, in particular, longitudinal and radial diffusion of drug will produce concentration variations within and along the nerve. This variation is superimposed on the dynamic use-dependent inhibition to provide variable propagation, which depends on a fiber's geometry, position within the nerve, and functional as well as electrophysiologic properties.

Different fiber types are also differentially sensitive to local anesthetic blockade. In vivo experiments in which continuous superperfusion of peripheral nerve allows equilibration with drug and experiments in which a drug bolus is delivered by percutaneous injection,[18] analogous to clinical peripheral nerve block, show unequivocally that small myelinated axons (Aγ motor and Aδ sensory fibers) are the most susceptible to impulse annihilation. Next in order of block are the large myelinated (Aα and Aβ) fibers, and the least susceptible are the small, nonmyelinated C

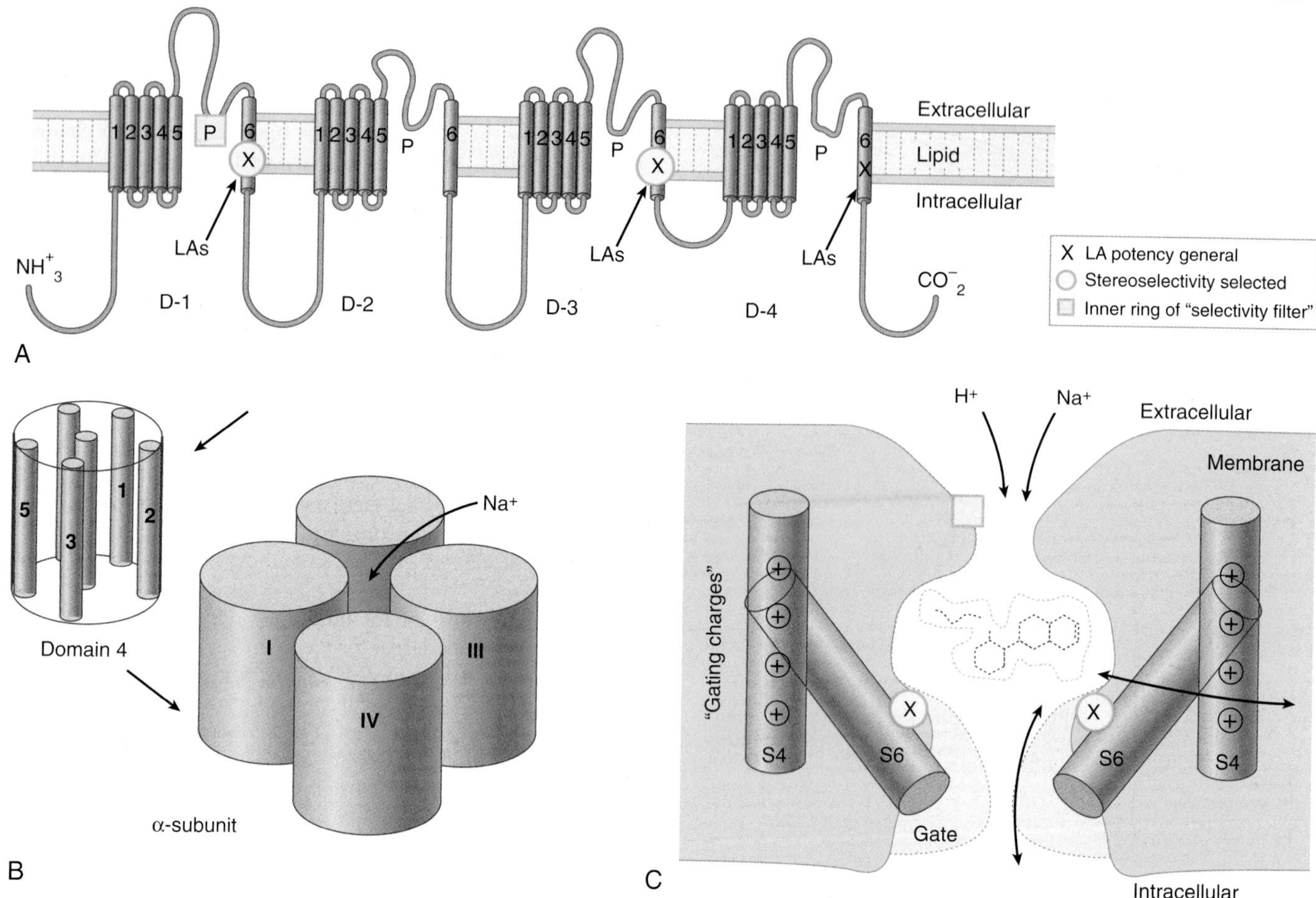

Figure 30-9 Structural features of the Na+ channel that determine local anesthetic (LA) interactions. **A,** Consensus arrangement of the single peptide of the Na+ channel α-subunit in a plasma membrane. Four domains with homologous sequences (D-1 through D-4) each contain six α-helical segments that span the membrane (S1 to S6). Each domain folds within itself to form one cylindrical bundle of segments, and these bundles converge to form the functional channel's quaternary structure (**B**). Activation gating leading to channel opening results from primary movement of the positively charged S4 segments in response to membrane depolarization (see panel **C**). Fast inactivation of the channel follows binding to the cytoplasmic end of the channel of part of the small loop that connects D-3 to D-4. Ions travel through an open channel along a pore defined at its narrowest dimension by the P region formed by partial membrane penetration of the four extracellular loops of protein connecting S5 and S6 in each domain. Intentional, directed mutations of different amino acids on the channel indicate residues that are involved in LA binding in the inner vestibule of the channel (X on S6 segments), at the interior regions of the ion-discriminating "selectivity filter (*square* on the P region), and also are known to influence stereoselectivity for phasic inhibition (*circle*, also on S6 segments). **C,** Schematic cross section of the channel speculating on the manner in which S6 segments, forming a "gate," may realign during activation to open the channel and allow entry and departure of a bupivacaine molecule by the "hydrophilic" pathway. The closed (inactivated) channel has a more intimate association with the LA molecule, whose favored pathway for dissociation is no longer between S6 segments (the former pore) but now, much more slowly, laterally between segments and then through the membrane, the "hydrophobic" pathway. Na+ ions entering the pore will compete with the LA for a site in the channel, and H+ ions, which pass very slowly through the pore, can enter and leave from the extracellular opening, thereby protonating and deprotonating a bound LA molecule and thus regulating its rate of dissociation from the channel.

fibers. In fact, in this last group, impulses in the slowest conducting population (conduction velocity of 0.5 to 0.8 msec) are the most resistant to local anesthetic.[18] The generalized notion that local anesthetics block the smallest fibers first or most is clearly wrong.

Selective Susceptibility of Na+ Channel Isoforms

Ten different Na+ channels have been physiologically identified and biochemically sequenced. At least four of them are found in peripheral neurons, some exclusively associated with nociceptive afferents. Obviously, it would be clinically advantageous to selectively inhibit these channels and thus prevent or reduce pain while sparing other functions. Although selective channel blockade has been attained with naturally occurring small peptide toxins,[19] relatively little selective blockade by local anesthetics has been reported,[20] probably because the local anesthetic pharmacophore is too similar among the different channel isoforms and the local anesthetic molecules themselves have several rotational axes, which makes them poor structural templates for selecting among static binding pockets.

Sodium Channel Isoforms in Human Diseases Characterized by Pain or Pain Insensitivity. Mutations in sodium channel isoform $Na_V1.7$ can produce disease states with either spontaneous pain[21,22] or profound and selective impairment of pain sensitivity.[23] Erythromelalgia is characterized by episodes of severe burning pain, predominantly in the feet and hands. In these subjects, pain is exacerbated by heat and relieved by cold. This disorder may occur as an isolated problem or can coexist with certain rheumatologic disorders. In a small subgroup of these patients the disorder has a clear familial pattern with an autosomal dominant pattern of inheritance. A second autosomal dominant disorder characterized by spontaneous pain is known initially as "familial rectal pain disorder" or "paroxysmal extreme pain disorder." Recent molecular studies have shown that these disorders involve several distinct types of mutations in $Na_V1.7$ sodium channels.[21,22] When these channels are inserted into cells that lack sodium channels, they generate spontaneous, temperature-sensitive inward currents.

Perhaps even more remarkable is the recent report of several consanguineous families in Pakistan in which certain members exhibit profound insensitivity to pain while being neurologically normal in almost all other respects.[23] Genetic, biochemical, and electrophysiologic studies have demonstrated an autosomal recessive pattern of inheritance. Molecular studies have shown that these mutations are of the nonsense type and generate functionally impaired $Na_V1.7$ sodium channels; when placed into cell membranes in vitro, they fail to generate inward currents in response to depolarizing stimuli.

On the other hand, aberrant impulses, which are often considered the hallmarks of various diseases of excitable membranes such as abnormal repetitive firing in neuropathic pain or in certain types of inherited skeletal myotonia, are abolished by systemic lidocaine in doses that do not block normal propagating impulses. Conditions for the sensitivity of such impulses to local anesthetics, such as lidocaine, appear to result from the patterns of impulse spikes superimposed on slow membrane depolarizations caused by abnormal expression of Na^+ channels rather than from selective sensitivity of certain subtypes of channels to these drugs.[24]

Summary of Local Anesthetic Mechanisms

Impulse blockade by local anesthetics may be summarized by the following chronology[4]:

1. Solutions of local anesthetic are deposited near the nerve. Removal of free drug molecules away from this locus is a function of tissue binding, removal by the circulation, and local hydrolysis of aminoester anesthetics. The net result is penetration of the nerve sheath by the remaining free drug molecules.
2. Local anesthetic molecules then permeate the nerve's axon membranes and reside there and in the axoplasm. The speed and extent of these processes depend on a particular drug's pK_a and on the lipophilicity of its base and cation species.
3. Binding of local anesthetic to sites on voltage-gated Na^+ channels prevents opening of the channels by inhibiting the conformational changes that underlie channel activation. Local anesthetics bind in the channel's pore and also occlude the path of Na^+ ions.
4. During onset of and recovery from local anesthesia, impulse blockade is incomplete and partially blocked fibers are further inhibited by repetitive stimulation, which produces an additional, use-dependent binding to Na^+ channels.
5. One local anesthetic binding site on the Na^+ channel may be sufficient to account for the drug's resting (tonic) and use-dependent (phasic) actions. Access to this site may potentially involve multiple pathways, but for clinical local anesthetics, the primary route is the hydrophobic approach from within the axon membrane.
6. The clinically observed rates of onset and recovery from blockade are governed by the relatively slow diffusion of local anesthetic molecules into and out of the whole nerve, not by their much faster binding and dissociation from ion channels. A clinically effective block that may last for hours can be accomplished with local anesthetic drugs that dissociate from Na^+ channels in a few seconds.

Clinical Pharmacology

Successful use of regional anesthesia requires knowledge of the pharmacologic properties of the various local anesthetic drugs, as well as technical skill in performance of the nerve block. Local anesthetic requirements vary considerably, depending on factors such as the type of block, surgical procedure, and physiologic status of the patient.

Commonly used aminoester local anesthetics include procaine, chloroprocaine, tetracaine, and cocaine. Commonly used aminoamides include lidocaine, mepivacaine, prilocaine, bupivacaine (racemic and its levo-enantiomer), ropivacaine, and etidocaine. The ester and amide local anesthetics differ in their chemical stability, locus of biotransformation, and allergic potential. Amides are extremely stable, whereas esters are relatively unstable in solution. Aminoesters are hydrolyzed in plasma by cholinesterase enzymes, but the amides undergo enzymatic degradation in the liver. Two exceptions to this trend include cocaine, an ester that is metabolized predominantly by hepatic carboxylesterase,[25] and articaine, an amide local anesthetic widely used in dentistry that is inactivated by plasma carboxylesterase-induced cleavage of a methyl ester on the aromatic ring.

p-Aminobenzoic acid is one of the metabolites of ester-type compounds that can induce allergic-type reactions in a small percentage of patients. The aminoamides are not metabolized to *p*-aminobenzoic acid, and reports of allergic reactions to these agents are extremely rare.

General Considerations

Clinically important properties of the various local anesthetics include potency, speed of onset, duration of anesthetic action, and differential sensory/motor blockade. As previously indicated, the profile of individual drugs is determined by their physicochemical characteristics (see Table 30-2).

Anesthetic Potency

Hydrophobicity appears to be a primary determinant of intrinsic anesthetic potency[5] because the anesthetic molecule must penetrate into the nerve membrane and bind at a partially hydrophobic site on the Na^+ channel. Clinically, however, the correlation between hydrophobicity and anesthetic potency is not as precise as in an isolated nerve. For example, etidocaine is more potent than bupivacaine in an isolated nerve, whereas etidocaine is actually less potent than bupivacaine in vivo. Differences between in vitro and in vivo potency may be related to a number of factors, including local anesthetic charge and hydrophobicity (which influence partitioning into and transverse diffusion across biologic membranes) and vasodilator or vasoconstrictor properties (which influence the initial rate of vascular uptake from injection sites into the central circulation).

Onset of Action

The onset of conduction block in isolated nerves is related to the physicochemical properties of the individual agents. In vivo latency is also dependent on the dose or concentration of local anesthetic used. For example, 0.25% bupivacaine possesses a rather slow onset of action, but increasing the concentration to 0.75% results in a significant acceleration of its anesthetic effect.[26] Chloroprocaine demonstrates a rapid onset of action in humans despite the fact that its pK_a is approximately 9, its proportion of charged molecules is high (97%), and thus its onset of action in isolated nerves is relatively slow. However, the low systemic toxicity of this agent allows its use in high concentrations (e.g., 3%). Therefore, the rapid onset of chloroprocaine in vivo may be related simply to mass diffusion because of the large number of molecules placed in the vicinity of peripheral nerves. In humans, 1.5% lidocaine produces a more rapid onset of epidural anesthesia than 1.5% chloroprocaine does[27]; however, 3% chloroprocaine results in more rapid onset than 2% lidocaine does.

Duration of Action

The duration of action of the various local anesthetics differs markedly. Procaine and chloroprocaine have a short duration of action. Lidocaine, mepivacaine, and prilocaine produce a moderate duration of anesthesia, whereas tetracaine, bupivacaine, ropivacaine, and etidocaine have the longest durations. For example, with procaine, the duration of brachial plexus blockade is 30 to 60 minutes, but up to approximately 10 hours of anesthesia (or at least analgesia) is common for brachial plexus blockade with bupivacaine or ropivacaine.[28]

In humans, the duration of anesthesia is markedly influenced by the peripheral vascular effects of the local anesthetic drugs. Many local anesthetics have a biphasic effect on vascular smooth muscle; at low concentrations these agents tend to cause vasoconstriction, whereas at higher, clinically administered concentrations, they cause vasodilation.[29] However, differences exist in the degree of vasodilator activity of the various drugs. For example, lidocaine is a more potent vasodilator than mepivacaine or prilocaine is. The effects of local anesthetics on vascular tone and regional blood flow are complex and vary according to concentration, time, and the particular vascular bed near the site of application, among other factors. As a practical example, the topical local anesthetic formulation EMLA (eutectic mixture of the local anesthetics lidocaine and prilocaine) vasoconstricts cutaneous vessels initially and through most of the first hour of application, but vasodilation is observed after 2 or more hours of application.

Differential Sensory/Motor Blockade

Another important clinical consideration is the ability of local anesthetic agents to cause differential inhibition of sensory and motor activity. Bupivacaine became popular in the 1980s for epidural blocks because it was better than the previously available long-acting agents (e.g., etidocaine) in producing adequate antinociception without profound inhibition of motor activity, particularly when dilute solutions are used. Bupivacaine is widely used epidurally for obstetric analgesia and postoperative pain management because it can provide acceptable analgesia with only mild muscle weakness, particularly when used for infusions in concentrations of 0.125% or less (also see Chapters 51, 69 and 87). When given by epidural bolus dosing, bupivacaine produces more effective sensory than motor blockade over a concentration range from 0.25% to 0.75%, whereas etidocaine produces almost equally effective sensory and motor blockade over this concentration range. Additional observations on the sensory selectivity of newer local anesthetics are detailed later in the section on chiral local anesthetics.

Traditional texts often state that small-diameter axons, such as C fibers, are more susceptible to local anesthetic block than larger-diameter fibers are. However, when careful measurements are made of single-impulse annihilation in individual nerve fibers, exactly the opposite differential susceptibility is noted (see earlier).[30,31] Repetitive stimulation, such as occurs during propagation of trains of impulses, produces a further, phasic inhibition of excitability, but it is unclear how this will affect a functionally selective failure of impulses. The length of drug-exposed nerve in the intrathecal space, imposed by anatomic restrictions, can perhaps explain clinically documented differential spinal or epidural blockade,[32] with longer drug-exposed regions yielding block by lower concentrations of local anesthetic.[33] However, this reasoning does not explain the functionally differential loss from peripheral nerve block. Other factors may include actual spread of the drug along the nerve or its selective ability to inhibit Na^+ channels over K^+ channels,[34] which in itself can produce a differential block because these channels are present in very different proportions in different types of nerves. As a result of these confounding factors, clinicians should be discouraged from making conclusions about fiber-type involvement in chronic pain syndromes based on the dose or concentration requirement for pain relief in diagnostic nerve blockade.[35]

Factors Influencing Anesthetic Activity in Humans

Dosage of Local Anesthetic

As the dosage of local anesthetic is increased, the probability and duration of satisfactory anesthesia increase and the time to onset of block is shortened. The dosage of local anesthetic can be increased by administering either a larger volume or a more concentrated solution. For example, increasing the concentration of epidurally administered bupivacaine from 0.125% to 0.5% while maintaining the same volume of injectate (10 mL) resulted in shorter latency, an improved incidence of satisfactory analgesia, and a longer duration of sensory analgesia.[36] The volume per se of anesthetic solution probably influences the spread of anesthesia. For example, 30 mL of 1% lidocaine administered into the epidural space produced a level of anesthesia that was 4.3 dermatomes higher than that achieved when 10 mL of 3% lidocaine was given.[37]

In selecting the volume and concentration for a specific block in a particular patient, clinicians must balance the risk of adverse effects from excessive dosing (systemic toxicity, excessive motor or autonomic blockade, etc.) against the increased risk of block failure if an inadequate volume or concentration is chosen. The degree to which additional volume can compensate for imprecise needle placement varies among different blocks.

With the advent of very precise needle placement using ultrasound-guided blockade, it has become clear that the median effective volume for obtaining successful blockade can be achieved with smaller volumes than have been recommended from some previous clinical series based on traditional methods of needle localization. For example, in a recent dose-finding randomized trial for femoral nerve blockade, the median volumes for 50% or 95% success in obtaining dense sensory and motor block at 30 minutes under ultrasound guidance were 57% and 54% of the corresponding volumes with the use of nerve stimulation.[38] Interested readers will note the very wide confidence intervals found in this study and are encouraged to read recent work on some statistical design issues for dose-response studies involving all types of anesthetics.[39] As limited by toxicity considerations, the aim in most clinical situations should be to choose doses that provide high success rates; that is, a dose effective in 95% of patients (ED_{95}) is generally a more relevant guide to dose selection than an ED_{50} dose. We should not aim for failure 50% of the time.[40]

Addition of Vasoconstrictors

Vasoconstrictors, usually epinephrine (5 μg/mL or 1:200,000), are frequently included in local anesthetic solutions to decrease the rate of vascular absorption, thereby allowing more anesthetic molecules to reach the nerve membrane and thus improve the depth and duration of anesthesia, as well as to provide a marker for inadvertent intravascular injection.[41] Test dosing with epinephrine can generate false negatives and false positives. Some of these sources of error have been described for specific patient groups, such as adults and children under general anesthesia, parturients in labor, and patients receiving β-blockers. Despite these limitations, test dosing has utility in a wide range of clinical situations.[42]

Epinephrine in a concentration of 1:200,000 has been reported to provide the optimal degree of vasoconstriction when used with lidocaine for epidural or intercostal blockade.[43] Other vasoconstrictor agents, such as norepinephrine and phenylephrine, have been used but do not appear to be superior to epinephrine.

The extent to which epinephrine prolongs the duration of anesthesia depends on the specific local anesthetic used and the site of injection. Epinephrine will significantly extend the duration of both infiltration anesthesia and peripheral nerve blockade with shorter-duration agents (e.g., lidocaine); epinephrine produces mild intensification of blockade but only most modest prolongation of epidural or peripheral blocks with bupivacaine.[44] α_2-Adrenergic receptors in the spinal cord are known to activate endogenous analgesic mechanisms, and the increased depth of analgesic action produced by epinephrine and the α_2-agonist clonidine[45] with both epidural and intrathecal local anesthetics may arise from this pharmacodynamic mechanism and from the pharmacokinetic (vasoconstrictive) action.

Site of Injection

The most rapid onset but the shortest duration of action occurs after intrathecal or subcutaneous administration of local anesthetics. The longest latencies and durations are observed after brachial plexus blocks. For example, intrathecal bupivacaine will usually produce anesthesia within 5 minutes that will persist for 3 to 4 hours. However, when bupivacaine is administered for brachial plexus blockade, the onset time is approximately 20 to 30 minutes, and the duration of anesthesia (or at least analgesia) averages 10 hours.[28] These differences in the onset and duration of anesthesia and analgesia are due in part to the particular anatomy of the area of injection, which will influence the rate of diffusion and vascular absorption and, in turn, affect the amount of drug used for various types of regional anesthesia. In the subarachnoid space, for example, the lack of a nerve sheath around the spinal cord and deposition of the local anesthetic solution in the immediate vicinity of the spinal cord are responsible for the rapid onset of action, whereas the relatively small amount of drug used for spinal anesthesia probably accounts for the short duration of conduction block.

In contrast, the onset of brachial plexus blockade is slow because the anesthetic agent is usually deposited at some distance from the nerve and must diffuse through various tissue barriers before reaching the nerve membrane. The prolonged block with brachial plexus blockade may be related to several factors, including comparatively slow rates of vascular absorption from the brachial plexus sheath, larger doses of drug required for this regional anesthetic technique, and comparatively long segments of nerves exposed to local anesthetic.

Carbonation and pH Adjustment of Local Anesthetics

The addition of sodium bicarbonate to a solution of local anesthetic applied to an isolated nerve accelerates the onset and decreases the minimum concentration (C_m) required for conduction blockade.[46] Although the effect of carbon dioxide on local anesthetic activity is easily demonstrable in isolated nerve, controversy exists concerning the clinical utility of carbonated local anesthetic solutions.[47]

The addition of sodium bicarbonate to local anesthetic solutions has also been reported to decrease the onset time of conduction blockade.[47] An increase in the pH of the local anesthetic solution increases the amount of drug in the uncharged base form, which should enhance the rate of diffusion across the nerve sheath and nerve membrane and result in a more rapid onset of anesthesia. Alkalinization of solutions of bupivacaine or lidocaine accelerated the onset of brachial plexus and epidural blockade in some studies[47] but not others.[48]

Mixtures of Local Anesthetics

Mixtures of local anesthetics for regional anesthesia are sometimes used in an effort to compensate for the short duration of action of certain rapidly acting agents such as chloroprocaine and lidocaine and the long latency of longer-acting agents such as tetracaine and bupivacaine. Mixtures of chloroprocaine and bupivacaine theoretically offer significant clinical advantages because of the rapid onset and low systemic toxicity of chloroprocaine and the long duration of action of bupivacaine; however, clinical results in studies of combinations have been mixed.[49] In addition, the use of catheter techniques for many forms of regional anesthesia makes it possible to begin with a rapid-onset local anesthetic such as lidocaine, mepivacaine, or chloroprocaine and then follow with an infusion of either a shorter-acting or longer-acting local anesthetic thereafter. Conversely, clinicians should be cautioned to not use maximum doses of two local anesthetics in combination in the mistaken belief that their toxicities are independent.[50]

In the absence of additional data, the toxicities should be presumed to be additive.

Pregnancy

The spread and depth of epidural and spinal anesthesia are greater in pregnant than in nonpregnant women (also see Chapter 69). The effects of pregnancy on local anesthetic potency may reflect a combined effect of mechanical factors associated with pregnancy (i.e., dilated epidural veins decrease the volume of the epidural and subarachnoid spaces) and direct effects of hormones, especially progesterone, on the susceptibility of nerves to conduction blockade by local anesthetics per se.[51] Hormonal alterations are probably the more important of these two factors because greater spread of epidural anesthesia occurs during the first trimester of pregnancy,[52] before any gross change in vascular dimensions within the epidural or subarachnoid spaces. The dosage of local anesthetics should probably should be reduced in patients in all stages of pregnancy.

Choice of Local Anesthetic for Various Regional Anesthetic Procedures

On the basis of anatomic considerations, regional anesthesia may be divided into infiltration anesthesia, intravenous regional anesthesia, peripheral nerve blockade (including plexus blockade), central neural blockade, and topical anesthesia (also see Chapters 51, 52 , 53, 69, 70, 81, and 87). An additional method of local anesthetic injection, tumescent anesthesia, is included because it is widely used in office plastic surgery practice.

Infiltration Anesthesia

Any local anesthetic may be used for infiltration anesthesia. Onset of action is almost immediate for all agents after intradermal or subcutaneous administration; however, the duration of anesthesia varies (Table 30-4). Epinephrine will prolong the duration of infiltration anesthesia by all local anesthetic drugs, although this effect is most pronounced when epinephrine is added to lidocaine. The choice of a specific drug for infiltration anesthesia largely depends on the desired duration of action.

The dosage of local anesthetic required for adequate infiltration anesthesia depends on the extent of the area to be anesthetized and the expected duration of the surgical procedure. When large surface areas have to be anesthetized, large volumes of dilute anesthetic solutions should be used. These considerations are particularly important when performing infiltration anesthesia in infants and smaller children. As an example, consider a 4-kg infant receiving infiltration anesthesia with the maximum safe dose of lidocaine, 5 mg/kg. Dosing to 5 mg/kg $\times$ 4 kg permits 20 mg, which is 1 mL of a 2% solution or 4 mL of a 0.5% solution. Lidocaine is effective for infiltration in concentrations as dilute as 0.3% to 0.5%, so the more dilute solution can be used more safely to anesthetize a larger area.

Patients frequently experience pain immediately after subcutaneous injection of local anesthetic solutions, in part because of the acidic nature of these solutions. For example, neutralization of lidocaine solutions by the addition of sodium bicarbonate immediately before injection reduces pain on skin infiltration[53] and may improve onset (see earlier).

Intravenous Regional Anesthesia

Intravenous regional anesthesia involves the intravenous administration of a local anesthetic into a tourniquet-occluded limb (i.e., Bier block) (see Chapter 70).[54] The local anesthetic diffuses from the peripheral vascular bed to nonvascular tissue such as axons and nerve endings. Both the safety and the efficacy of this regional anesthetic procedure depend on interruption of blood flow to the involved limb and gradual release of the occluding tourniquet. Intravenous regional anesthesia has been used primarily for surgical procedures on the upper limbs. Shorter procedures on the foot can also be successfully performed under intravenous regional anesthesia. If a lower leg tourniquet is used, it should be applied well below the fibular neck to avoid pressure

Table 30-4 Infiltration Anesthesia

	Plain Solution			Epinephrine-Containing Solution	
Drug	**Concentration (%)**	**Max Dose (mg)**	**Duration (min)**	**Max Dose (mg)**	**Duration (min)**
Short Duration					
Procaine	1-2	500	20-30	600	30-45
Chloroprocaine	1-2	800	15-30	1000	30
Moderate Duration					
Lidocaine	0.5-1	300	30-60	500	120
Mepivacaine	0.5-1	300	45-90	500	120
Prilocaine	0.5-1	350	30-90	550	120
Long Duration					
Bupivacaine	0.25-0.5	175	120-240	200	180-240
Ropivacaine	0.2-0.5	200	120-240	250	180-240

over the superficial peroneal nerve; in general, use of an upper leg tourniquet is preferred over lower leg tourniquets.[55]

Lidocaine has been the drug used most frequently for intravenous regional anesthesia. Prilocaine, mepivacaine, chloroprocaine, procaine, bupivacaine, and etidocaine have also been used successfully. One might suppose a safety advantage with the aminoester-linked compounds because of their hydrolysis in blood; however, thrombophlebitis has been reported in several patients with chloroprocaine. Cardiovascular collapse has occurred after the use of bupivacaine for intravenous regional anesthesia, and this use of bupivacaine is discouraged.[56]

In general, approximately 3 mg/kg (40 mL of a 0.5% solution) of preservative-free lidocaine without epinephrine is used for upper extremity procedures. For surgical procedures on the lower limbs, 50 to 100 mL of a 0.25% lidocaine solution has been used.

Peripheral Nerve Blockade

Regional anesthetic procedures that inhibit conduction in fibers of the peripheral nervous system can be classified together under the general category of peripheral nerve blockade (also see Chapters 52 and 53). This form of regional anesthesia has been arbitrarily subdivided into minor and major nerve blocks. Minor nerve blocks are defined as procedures involving single nerve entities such as the ulnar or radial nerve, whereas major nerve blocks involve the blockade of two or more distinct nerves or a nerve plexus or the blockade of very large nerves at more proximal sites (i.e., the femoral and sciatic nerves).

Most local anesthetic drugs can be used for minor nerve blocks. The onset of blockade is rapid with most drugs, and the choice of drug is determined primarily by the required duration of anesthesia. A classification of the various drugs according to their duration of action is shown in Table 30-5. The duration of both sensory analgesia and motor blockade is prolonged significantly when epinephrine is added to the various local anesthetic solutions in some, but not all applications.[57]

In 1986, a technique of interpleural regional analgesia was described as an alternative to multiple intercostal nerve blocks.[58] This procedure involves the administration of local anesthetic solution into the pleural space, either by percutaneous placement or by placement through the open chest by the surgeon during thoracotomy. The risk of pneumothorax has varied in published case series. Although interpleural analgesia appears to be useful for unilateral postoperative analgesia after cholecystectomy, mastectomy, and nephrectomy, its efficacy for post-thoracotomy pain is doubtful.[59] This technique has been associated with extremely high plasma concentrations of anesthetic, with an associated risk of convulsions. Interpleural analgesia has also been used to provide analgesia for chronic pain conditions as diverse as upper extremity complex regional pain syndromes, pancreatitis, and cancer of the thorax and abdomen. In many centers, interpleural analgesia has largely been supplanted by thoracic epidural analgesia for the majority of thoracic and abdominal procedures.

Two related approaches for unilateral somatic blockade in the thorax are continuous extrapleural catheters[60] (placed by the surgeon through the chest dorsal to the parietal pleura) and continuous thoracic paravertebral somatic blockade.[61] One advantage of these two approaches over interpleural analgesia is that very little of the administered solution leaks out of the chest into chest tubes.

Brachial plexus blockade for upper limb surgery is the most common major peripheral nerve block technique. A significant difference exists between the onset times of various agents when these blocks are used (Table 30-6). In general, agents of intermediate potency exhibit a more rapid onset than the more potent compounds do. Onset times of approximately 14 minutes for lidocaine and mepivacaine have been reported versus approximately 23 minutes for bupivacaine. A variety of approaches to the brachial plexus are available; the choice among these approaches is dictated by several factors, including the site of surgery and the ability of the patient to tolerate spillover to other nerves, including the phrenic nerve; these considerations are detailed in Chapters 52, 53, and 70. Similarly, the lumbar plexus can be approached via several routes, including a posterior approach, an anterior perivascular "3 in 1" approach, and an anterior fascia iliaca compartment approach.[62]

The variation in duration of anesthesia after brachial plexus blockade is also considerably greater than that observed with other types of conduction block. For example, durations of anesthesia varying from 4 to 30 hours have been reported for bupivacaine. It is prudent to warn patients before a major nerve block about the possibility of prolonged sensory and motor block in the involved region, particularly when agents such as bupivacaine, levobupivacaine, and ropivacaine are used.

Table 30-5 Minor Nerve Blocks

		Plain Solutions			Epinephrine-Containing Solutions
Drug	**Usual Concentration (%)**	**Usual Volume (mL)**	**Dosage (mg)**	**Average Duration (min)**	**Average Duration (min)**
Procaine	2	5-20	100-400	15-30	30-60
Chloroprocaine	2	5-20	100-400	15-30	30-60
Lidocaine	1	5-20	50-200	60-120	120-180
Mepivacaine	1	5-20	50-200	60-120	120-180
Prilocaine	1	5-20	50-200	60-120	120-180
Bupivacaine	0.25-0.5	5-20	12.5-100	180-360	240- 420
Ropivacaine	0.2-0.5	5-20	10-100	180-360	240-420

Also see Chapter 52.
Doses refer to 70-kg adults. For pediatric doses, see Chapter 81.

Table 30-6 Major Nerve Blocks

Drug with Epinephrine 1:200,000	Usual Concentration (%)	Usual Volume (mL)	Maximal Dose (mg)	Usual Onset (min)	Usual Duration (min)
Lidocaine	1-2	30-50	500	10-20	120-240
Mepivacaine	1-1.5	30-50	500	10-20	180-300
Prilocaine	1-2	30-50	600	10-20	180-300
Bupivacaine	0.25-0.5	30-50	225	20-30	360-720
Levobupivacaine	0.25-0.5	30-50	225	20-30	360-720
Ropivacaine	0.2-0.5	30-50	250	20-30	360-720

Also see Chapter 52. Doses listed refer to 70-kg adults receiving epinephrine-containing solutions. Doses should be reduced, as detailed in Chapter 81, for children, for patients with specific risk factors, and when non–epinephrine-containing solutions are used.

Central Neural Blockade

Any of the local anesthetic drugs may be used for epidural anesthesia (Table 30-7), although procaine and tetracaine are rarely used because of their long onset times (also see Chapter 51). Drugs of intermediate potency produce surgical anesthesia of 1 to 2 hours' duration, whereas long-acting drugs usually produce 3 to 4 hours of anesthesia. The duration of short- and intermediate-acting drugs is significantly prolonged by the addition of epinephrine (1:200,000), but the duration of long-acting drugs is only minimally affected by epinephrine. The onset of lumbar epidural anesthesia occurs within 5 to 15 minutes after the administration of chloroprocaine, lidocaine, mepivacaine, and prilocaine. Bupivacaine has a slower onset of action.

Bupivacaine bolus doses at a concentration of 0.125% produce adequate analgesia in many clinical settings with only mild motor deficits.[63] Continuous epidural infusions of bupivacaine as dilute as 0.0625% to 0.1% are useful for labor epidural analgesia, especially when administered in combination with opioids and other additives. Bupivacaine 0.25% may be used for more intense analgesia (particularly during combined epidural–light general anesthesia cases) with moderate degrees of motor block. Bupivacaine at concentrations of 0.5% to 0.75% is associated with a more profound degree of motor block, which makes these solutions most suitable for major surgical procedures, particularly when epidural anesthesia is not combined with general anesthesia. It should be emphasized that although high concentrations of local anesthetics may be appropriate for episodic bolus dosing for surgery, these concentrations (i.e., >0.2% for bupivacaine) should generally be avoided for continuous epidural infusions. Bolus injections produce much more cephalocaudad spread than infusions do. When concentrated bupivacaine solutions are used for infusions, they have the potential for excessive local effect with an associated risk for unwanted and very prolonged motor blockade. Etidocaine produces adequate sensory analgesia and profound, long-lasting motor block. Use of etidocaine has decreased in recent years, and at present it is primarily restricted to surgical procedures for which profound muscle relaxation is required.

Drugs available for subarachnoid administration are shown in Table 30-8.

Although lidocaine has long been used for spinal anesthesia as a 5% solution, recent studies of local anesthetic neurotoxicity have led some to question this practice; this issue is discussed later in the chapter in the section on the neurotoxicity of local anesthetics.

Tetracaine is available both as crystals and as a 1% solution, which may be diluted with 10% glucose to obtain a 0.5% hyperbaric solution. Hypobaric solutions of tetracaine (tetracaine in sterile water) may be used for specific operative situations, such as anorectal or hip surgery. Isobaric tetracaine obtained by mixing 1% tetracaine with cerebrospinal fluid or normal saline is useful for lower limb surgical procedures.

Bupivacaine is widely used as a spinal anesthetic, either as a hyperbaric solution at a concentration of 0.75% with 8.25% dextrose or by using the nearly isobaric 0.5% solution. Intrathecal

Table 30-7 Epidural Anesthesia

Drug with Epinephrine 1:200,000	Usual Concentration (%)	Usual Volume (mL)	Total Dose (mg)	Usual Onset (min)	Usual Duration (min)
Chloroprocaine	2-3	15-30	300-900	5-15	30-90
Lidocaine	1-2	15-30	150-500	5-15	
Mepivacaine	1-2	15-30	150-500	5-15	60-180
Prilocaine	1-3	15-30	150-600	5-15	
Bupivacaine	0.25-0.5	15-30	40-225	15-20	180-350
Levobupivacaine	0.25-0.75	15-30	40-250	15-20	180-350
Ropivacaine	0.2-0.75	15-30	40-250	15-20	180-350

Also see Chapter 51. Doses listed refer to 70-kg adults receiving epinephrine-containing solutions. Doses should be reduced, as detailed in Chapter 81, for children, for patients with specific risk factors, and when non–epinephrine-containing solutions are used.

Table 30-8 Spinal Anesthesia*

Drug	Usual Concentration (%)	Usual Volume (mL)	Total Dose (mg)	Baricity	Glucose Concentration (%)	Usual Duration (min)
Procaine	10.0	1-2	100-200	Hyperbaric	5.0	30-60
Lidocaine	1.5, 5.0	1-2	30-100	Hyperbaric	7.5	30-90
Mepivacaine	4	1-2	40-80	Hyperbaric	9.0	30-90
Tetracaine	0.25-1.0	1-4	5-20	Hyperbaric	5.0	90-200
	0.25	2-6	5-20	Hypobaric		90-200
	1.0	1-2	5-20	Isobaric		90-200
Dibucaine	0.25	1-2	2.5-5.0	Hyperbaric	5.0	90-200
	0.5	1-2	5-10	Isobaric		90-200
	0.06	5-20	3-12	Hypobaric		90-200
Bupivacaine	0.5	3-4	15-20	Isobaric		90-200
	0.75	2-3	15-20	Hyperbaric	8.25	90-200
Levobupivacaine	0.5	3-4	15-20	Isobaric		90-200
	0.75	2-3	15-20	Hyperbaric		90-200
Ropivacaine	0.5	3-4	15-20	Isobaric		90-200
	0.75	2-3	15-20	Hyperbaric		90-200

*Dosing refers to a 70-Kg adult. Dosing may be reduced in pregnancy (see Chapter 69) and with advancing age (see Chapter 71). Pediatric dosing is detailed in Chapter 81.

bupivacaine possesses an anesthetic profile similar to that of tetracaine.[64]

The addition of vasoconstrictors may prolong the duration of spinal anesthesia; for example, the addition of 0.2 to 0.3 mg of epinephrine to lidocaine, tetracaine, or bupivacaine solutions will produce a 50% or greater increase in duration.[65,66] The duration of spinal anesthesia produced by tetracaine can also be increased to a similar extent by adding 1 to 5 mg of phenylephrine. The addition of epinephrine to bupivacaine or lidocaine may be more effective in prolonging the duration of spinal anesthesia in lumbosacral segments than in thoracic segments.

Topical Anesthesia

A number of local anesthetic formulations are available for topical anesthesia (Table 30-9), lidocaine, dibucaine, tetracaine, and benzocaine being the drugs used most commonly. In general, these preparations provide effective but relatively short durations of analgesia when applied to mucous membranes or abraded skin. Lidocaine and tetracaine sprays are commonly used for endotracheal anesthesia before intubation or for mucosal analgesia for bronchoscopy or esophagoscopy.

A variety of topical local anesthetic formulations have been developed to penetrate intact skin. EMLA, which is a eutectic mixture of 2.5% lidocaine base and 2.5% prilocaine base, is widely used for venipuncture, intravenous cannulation, skin grafting, and a range of other uses, including circumcision.[67-69] This preparation must be applied under an occlusive bandage for 45 to 60 minutes to obtain effective cutaneous anesthesia; longer application times increase the depth and reliability of skin analgesia. EMLA appears to be quite safe in neonates, and methemoglobinemia with the use of prilocaine is exceedingly uncommon. EMLA is more effective for newborn circumcision than placebo is but less effective than dorsal penile nerve block.[69,89] Several alternative topical local anesthetic formulations also are in use, including tetracaine gel[70] and liposomal lidocaine.[71] Physical methods to accelerate local anesthetic transit across skin, including iontophoresis, local heating, electroporation, and a variety of forms of needle-less pressure injection, may lead to more rapid onset of cutaneous analgesia.[72] Synera (originally studied as S-Caine) is a formulation of lidocaine and tetracaine that was developed with a heating element (activated by opening the package to initiate an oxygen-dependent exothermic reaction). This formulation has a rapid onset and evokes vasodilatation.[73]

Topical anesthesia through cut skin is commonly used in pediatric emergency departments for liquid application into lacerations that require suturing. Historically, this had been provided by a mixture of tetracaine, epinephrine (adrenaline), and cocaine, known as TAC.[74] TAC is usually supplied as tetracaine 0.5%, epinephrine 1:2000, and cocaine 10% to 11.8%, although studies suggest that more dilute concentrations may be almost equally effective and less likely to cause toxicity. The generally recommended safe maximum dose is 3 to 4 mL for adults or 0.05 mL/kg for children. TAC is ineffective through intact skin; in contrast, its rapid absorption from mucosal surfaces can lead to toxic, even fatal reactions.

Because of concerns regarding cocaine toxicity and the potential for diversion and abuse, several groups have investigated alternative cocaine-free topical preparations. Non–cocaine-containing formulations, especially lidocaine-epinephrine-tetracaine (LET) and tetracaine-phenylephrine, have largely supplanted TAC.[75] Similarly, otolaryngologists previously administered cocaine routinely as a solution or aerosol into the nasal passages to provide mucosal analgesia and vasoconstriction. In recent years, cocaine has increasingly been replaced for nasal application by the combined use of an α_1-adrenergic agonist (oxymetazoline or phenylephrine) and a local anesthetic such as 2% to 4% lidocaine, with more dilute solutions being recommended for infants and children (see Chapter 81). Systemic absorption of phenylephrine can cause severe hypertension and reflex bradycardia; oxymetazoline is associated with much less

Table 30-9 Various Preparations Intended for Topical Anesthesia

Anesthetic Ingredient	Concentration (%)	Pharmaceutical Application Form	Intended Area of Use
Benzocaine	1-5	Cream	Skin and mucous membrane
	20	Ointment	Skin and mucous membrane
	20	Aerosol	Skin and mucous membrane
Cocaine	4	Solution	Ear, nose, throat
Dibucaine	0.25-1	Cream	Skin
	0.25-1	Ointment	Skin
	0.25-1	Aerosol	Skin
	0.25	Solution	Ear
	2.5	Suppositories	Rectum
Cyclonine	0.5-1	Solution	Skin, oropharynx, tracheobronchial tree, urethra, rectum
Lidocaine	2-4	Solution	Oropharynx, tracheobronchial tree, nose
	2	Jelly	Urethra
	2.5-5	Ointment	Skin, mucous membrane, rectum
	2	Viscous	Oropharynx
	10	Suppositories	Rectum
	10	Aerosol	Gingival mucosa
Tetracaine	0.5-1	Ointment	Skin, rectum, mucous membrane
	0.5-1	Cream	Skin, rectum, mucous membrane
	0.25-1	Solution	Nose, tracheobronchial tree
EMLA	Lidocaine, 2.5 Prilocaine, 2.5	Cream	Intact skin
TAC	Tetracaine, 0.5 Epinephrine, 1:200,000 Cocaine, 11.8	Solution	Cut skin
LET	Lidocaine, 4% Epinephrine, 1:20,000 Tetracaine, 0.5%	Solution	Cut skin

EMLA, eutectic mixture of lidocaine and prilocaine; LET, lidocaine-epinephrine-tetracaine; TAC, tetracaine-epinephrine-cocaine.
Modified from Covino B, Vassallo H: Local Anesthetics: Mechanisms of Action and Clinical Use. Orlando, FL, Grune & Stratton, 1976, with permission.

systemic effect and has a considerably wider margin of safety. In our view, there is no clinical setting for which the benefits of cocaine clearly outweigh the potential risks when compared with alternative approaches involving combined administration of a local anesthetic and a topical vasoconstrictor such as oxymetazoline.

Tumescent Anesthesia

A technique of local anesthesia most commonly used by plastic surgeons during liposuction procedures involves the subcutaneous injection of large volumes of dilute local anesthetic in combination with epinephrine and other agents. Total doses of lidocaine ranging from 35 to 55 mg/kg have been reported to produce safe plasma concentrations, which may peak more than 8 to 12 hours after infusion.[76] Despite these seemingly huge doses, very good outcomes have been reported in several case series.[77] Conversely, there have been several case series of cardiac arrest and death during plastic surgical procedures in which multiple risk factors, including high local anesthetic concentrations and concomitant use of sedatives, may have contributed to the patients' instability and deterioration.[78] Factors governing uptake and clearance from this method of local anesthetic delivery deserve further study. Clinicians should exercise great caution when administering additional local anesthetics by infiltration or other routes for at least 12 to 18 hours after the use of this technique.

Systemic Local Anesthetics for Neuropathic Pain

A broad variety of local anesthetics, antiarrhythmics, anticonvulsants, and other Na^+ channel blockers are administered intravenously, orally, or both to relieve a number of forms of neuropathic pain (see Chapter 58).[79] Clinical results are unpredictable. Although successful responses from intravenous lidocaine are often taken as a positive indication for oral mexiletine, many patients find mexiletine difficult to tolerate. When the signs of neuropathic pain are reversed by lidocaine infusion, normal nociception and other sensory modalities are unaffected, suggesting that the neurophysiologic correlate of the disease has an unusually high susceptibility to these drugs, present in plasma at concentrations 50 to 100 times lower than that required to block normal impulses in peripheral fibers. Laboratory studies suggest that ectopic impulse activity arising at a site of injury or elsewhere, such as the dorsal root ganglion, contributes to the neuropathic pain and that such impulses are particularly sensitive to use-dependent Na^+ channel blockers. It is noteworthy that relief of preexisting neuropathic pain, both clinically and in animal models,[80] can in some cases persist for days, weeks, or months after a single intravenous infusion of drug (e.g., lidocaine), far beyond the lifetime of the drug in vivo or any nerve block that it might affect. The mechanism of this remarkable action remains a mystery.

Pharmacokinetics

The concentration of local anesthetics in blood is determined by the amount injected, the rate of absorption from the site of injection, the rate of tissue distribution, and the rate of biotransformation and excretion of the specific drug.[81-83] Patient-related factors such as age, cardiovascular status, and hepatic function influence the physiologic disposition and resultant blood concentration of local anesthetics.

Absorption

The systemic absorption of local anesthetics is determined by the site of injection, dosage and volume, addition of a vasoconstrictor agent, and the pharmacologic profile of the agent itself.[81-83] Comparison of the blood concentration of local anesthetics after various routes of administration reveals that the anesthetic drug level is highest after intercostal nerve blockade, followed in order of decreasing concentration by injection into the caudal epidural space, lumbar epidural space, brachial plexus, and subcutaneous tissue.[83] When a local anesthetic solution is exposed to an area of greater vascularity, a greater rate and degree of absorption occur. This relationship is of clinical significance because use of a fixed dose of a local anesthetic agent may be potentially toxic in one area of administration but not in others. For example, the use of 400 mg of lidocaine without epinephrine for an intercostal nerve block results in an average peak venous plasma level of approximately 7 µg/mL, which is sufficiently high to cause symptoms of central nervous system (CNS) toxicity in some patients. By comparison, this same dose of lidocaine used for a brachial plexus block yields a mean maximum blood level of approximately 3 µg/mL, which is rarely associated with signs of toxicity.[83]

The maximum blood concentration of local anesthetic drugs is related to the total dose of drug administered for any particular site of administration. For most drugs there is a proportionality between the amount of drug administered and the resultant peak anesthetic blood concentration.

Local anesthetic solutions frequently contain a vasoconstrictor agent, usually epinephrine, in concentrations varying from 5 to 20 µg/mL. Epinephrine decreases the rate of vascular absorption of certain agents from various sites of administration and thus lowers their potential systemic toxicity. A 5-µg/mL concentration of epinephrine (1:200,000) significantly reduces the peak blood levels of lidocaine and mepivacaine irrespective of the site of administration. Peak blood levels of bupivacaine and etidocaine are minimally influenced by the addition of a vasoconstrictor after injection into the lumbar epidural space. However, epinephrine will significantly reduce the rate of vascular absorption of these drugs when they are used for peripheral nerve blocks such as brachial plexus blockade.

Differences also exist in the rate of absorption of various local anesthetics. In some studies, absorption of local anesthetics from the epidural space has appeared to involve both rapid and slow processes, as described by two-compartment models.[84]

Distribution

The systemic distribution of local anesthetics can be described sufficiently by a two-compartment model.[85] The rapid disappearance phase is believed to be related to uptake by rapidly equilibrating tissues (i.e., tissues that have high vascular perfusion). The slower phase of disappearance from blood is mainly a function of the particular compound.[85]

Local anesthetic drugs are distributed throughout all body tissues, but the relative concentration in different tissues varies. In general, more highly perfused organs show higher concentrations of local anesthetic drug than less well perfused organs do. Because local anesthetics are rapidly extracted by lung tissue, the whole blood concentration of local anesthetics decreases markedly as they pass through the pulmonary vasculature.[86]

Biotransformation and Excretion

The pattern of metabolism of local anesthetic agents varies according to their chemical classification. The ester, or procaine-like, drugs undergo hydrolysis in plasma by the pseudocholinesterase enzymes; clearance of chloroprocaine is especially rapid.[87,88]

The aminoamide drugs undergo enzymatic degradation primarily in the liver. Lidocaine is metabolized somewhat more rapidly than mepivacaine, which in turn is more rapidly metabolized than bupivacaine.[89-91]

Excretion of the metabolites of amide-type local anesthetics occurs via the kidney. Less than 5% of the unchanged drug is excreted via the kidney into urine.

Pharmacokinetic Alterations by Patient Status

Patient age may influence the physiologic disposition of local anesthetics (see Chapters 71 and 81). The half-life of lidocaine after intravenous administration averaged 80 minutes in human volunteers varying in age from 22 to 26 years, whereas volunteers 61 to 71 years of age demonstrated a significantly prolonged lidocaine half-life that averaged 138 minutes.[92]

Newborn infants have immature hepatic enzyme systems and hence prolonged elimination of lidocaine, bupivacaine, and ropivacaine.[93-95] Bupivacaine, for example, has a terminal elimination half-life in adults that averages around 3.5 hours. In neonates and some younger infants, terminal elimination half-lives may be as long as 8 to 12 hours. Prolonged elimination is particularly an issue for continuous infusions of local anesthetics in infants, and seizures have been associated with high bupivacaine infusion rates.[96] Based on analysis of these cases, a maximum infusion rate of 0.4 mg/kg/hr for prolonged bupivacaine infusions has been proposed for children and adults, whereas prolonged infusion rates for neonates and young infants should not exceed 0.2 mg/kg/hr.[97] Even at 0.2 mg/kg/hr, plasma bupivacaine concentrations were found to be rising toward a toxic range in some younger infants after 48 hours.[98] Similarly, prolonged lidocaine infusions in neonates should not exceed 0.8 mg/kg/hr. The potential for toxicity with lidocaine infusions in neonates is also increased by the accumulation of its principal metabolite, monoethylglycinexylidide (MEGX), which can cause seizures. Chloroprocaine may offer unique advantages for epidural infusion in neonates in that it is rapidly cleared from plasma, even in preterm neonates.[99]

Decreased hepatic blood flow or impaired hepatic enzyme function can produce a substantial elevation of blood levels of the aminoamide local anesthetics. An average lidocaine half-life of 1.5 hours was reported in volunteers with normal hepatic function, whereas patients with liver disease demonstrated an average half-life of 5.0 hours.[100] The rate of disappearance of lidocaine from blood has also been shown to be markedly prolonged in patients with congestive heart failure.[101]

Toxicity

Local anesthetic drugs are relatively safe if administered in an appropriate dosage and in the correct anatomic location. However, systemic and localized toxic reactions can occur, usually as a result of accidental intravascular or intrathecal injection or administration of an excessive dose. In addition, specific adverse effects are associated with the use of certain drugs, such as allergic reactions to the aminoester drugs and methemoglobinemia after the use of prilocaine.

Systemic Toxicity

Systemic reactions to local anesthetics primarily involve the CNS and the cardiovascular system (also see Chapters 51 to 53 and 81). In general, the CNS is more susceptible to the actions of systemic local anesthetics than the cardiovascular system is, and thus the dose or blood level of local anesthetic required to produce CNS toxicity is usually lower than that resulting in circulatory collapse.

Central Nervous System Toxicity

The initial symptoms of local anesthetic–induced CNS toxicity are feelings of lightheadedness and dizziness followed frequently by visual and auditory disturbances such as difficulty focusing and tinnitus. Other subjective CNS symptoms include disorientation and occasional feelings of drowsiness. Objective signs of CNS toxicity are usually excitatory in nature and include shivering, muscular twitching, and tremors initially involving muscles of the face and distal parts of the extremities. Ultimately, generalized convulsions of a tonic-clonic nature occur. If a sufficiently large dose or rapid intravenous injection of a local anesthetic is administered, the initial signs of CNS excitation are rapidly followed by a state of generalized CNS depression. Seizure activity ceases, and respiratory depression and ultimately respiratory arrest may occur. In some patients CNS depression is seen without a preceding excitatory phase, particularly if other CNS depressant drugs have been administered.

CNS excitation may be the result of an initial blockade of inhibitory pathways in the cerebral cortex by local anesthetic drugs[102] but can also result from the net stimulation of release of glutamate, an excitatory amino acid neurotransmitter. Blockade of inhibitory pathways allows facilitatory neurons to function in an unopposed fashion, which results in an increase in excitatory activity leading to convulsions. A further increase in the dose of local anesthetic leads to inhibition of activity of both the inhibitory and facilitatory circuits, which results in a generalized state of CNS depression.

In general, a correlation exists between potency of the local anesthetic and intravenous CNS toxicity.[103] Convulsions caused by an inadvertent intravenous bolus of local anesthetic can generally be terminated by small intravenous doses of a benzodiazepine, such as midazolam, or by small intravenous doses of thiopental.

Respiratory or metabolic acidosis increases the risks for CNS toxicity from local anesthetics.[104]

Elevated $Paco_2$ enhances cerebral blood flow and thus the anesthetic is delivered more rapidly to the brain. In addition, diffusion of carbon dioxide into neuronal cells decreases intracellular pH, which facilitates conversion of the base form of the drugs to the cationic form. The cationic form does not diffuse well across the nerve membrane, so ion trapping will occur, which will increase the apparent CNS toxicity of local anesthetics.

Hypercapnia and acidosis also decrease the plasma protein binding of local anesthetic agents.[105] Accordingly, an elevation in $Paco_2$ or a decrease in pH will increase the proportion of free drug available for diffusion into the brain. On the other hand, acidosis increases the cationic form of the local anesthetic, which should decrease the rate of diffusion through lipoid barriers.

The clinical implication of this effect of hypercapnia and acidosis on toxicity deserves emphasis. Seizures produce hypoventilation and a combined respiratory and metabolic acidosis, which further exacerbates the CNS toxicity. In the setting of local anesthetic toxic reactions, it is essential to provide prompt assisted ventilation and circulatory support as needed to prevent or correct hypercapnia and acidosis and to prevent or correct hypoxemia, which also exacerbates CNS toxicity. Based on the preceding discussion, it should be apparent that clinicians performing major conduction blockade should make a routine practice of having the following ready at hand: monitoring equipment; an oxygen tank or wall oxygen outlet; airway equipment, including at minimum, a bag-mask circuit for delivery of positive-pressure ventilation; and drugs to terminate convulsions, such as midazolam, lorazepam, diazepam, or thiopental.

Cardiovascular System Toxicity

Local anesthetics can exert direct actions on both the heart and peripheral blood vessels, as well as indirect actions on the circulation by blockade of sympathetic or parasympathetic efferent activity.

Direct Cardiac Effects

The primary cardiac electrophysiologic effect of local anesthetics is a decrease in the rate of depolarization in the fast conducting tissues of Purkinje fibers and ventricular muscle.[106] This reduction in rate is believed to be due to a decrease in the availability of fast sodium channels in cardiac membranes. Action potential duration and the effective refractory period are also decreased by local anesthetics.

The electrophysiologic effects of various agents differ qualitatively. Bupivacaine depresses the rapid phase of depolarization (Vmax) in Purkinje fibers and ventricular muscle to a greater extent than lidocaine does. In addition, the rate of recovery from a use-dependent block is slower in bupivacaine-treated papillary muscles than in lidocaine-treated muscles. This slow rate of recovery results in incomplete restoration of Na^+ channel availability between action potentials, particularly at high heart rates. These differential effects of lidocaine and bupivacaine have been advanced as explanations of the antiarrhythmic properties of lidocaine and the arrhythmogenic potential of bupivacaine.

Electrophysiologic studies have shown that high blood levels of local anesthetics will prolong conduction time through various parts of the heart, as indicated on the electrocardiogram (ECG) by an increase in the PR interval and duration of the QRS complex. Extremely high concentrations of local anesthetics depress spontaneous pacemaker activity in the sinus node, thereby resulting in sinus bradycardia and sinus arrest.

All local anesthetics exert dose-dependent negative inotropic action on cardiac muscle[107]; the depression of cardiac contractility is roughly proportional to conduction blocking potency. Thus, bupivacaine and tetracaine are more potent cardiodepressants than lidocaine is.

Local anesthetics may depress myocardial contractility by affecting calcium influx and triggered release from the sarcoplasmic reticulum,[108] as well as by inhibiting cardiac sarcolemmal Ca^{2+} currents and Na^+ currents.

Direct Peripheral Vascular Effects

Local anesthetics exert biphasic effects on peripheral vascular smooth muscle.[109] Low concentrations of lidocaine and bupivacaine produced vasoconstriction in the cremaster muscle of rats, whereas high concentrations produced vasodilation in both isolated tissue models and in vivo.

Cocaine is the only local anesthetic that consistently causes vasoconstriction at all concentrations because of its ability to inhibit the uptake of norepinephrine by premotor neurons and thus to potentiate neurogenic vasoconstriction.

Comparative Cardiovascular Toxicity

All local anesthetics, but especially bupivacaine, can cause rapid and profound cardiovascular depression (also see Chapters 51 to 53 and 81). The cardiotoxicity of bupivacaine appears to differ from that of lidocaine in the following manner:

1. The ratio of the dosage required for irreversible cardiovascular collapse (CC) and the dosage that will produce CNS toxicity (convulsions) (i.e., the CC/CNS ratio) is lower for bupivacaine and etidocaine than for lidocaine.[110]
2. Ventricular arrhythmias and fatal ventricular fibrillation may occur more often after the rapid intravenous administration of a large dose of bupivacaine but far less frequently with lidocaine.[111,112] The CNS effects of local anesthetics may contribute to the generation of arrhythmias (see Chapter 61).[113]
3. A pregnant animal or patient may be more sensitive to the cardiotoxic effects of bupivacaine than a nonpregnant animal or patient[114] (see also Chapter 69). The 0.75% solution of bupivacaine is no longer recommended for use in obstetric anesthesia in the United States.
4. Cardiac resuscitation is more difficult after bupivacaine-induced cardiovascular collapse, and acidosis and hypoxia markedly potentiate the cardiotoxicity of bupivacaine.[115]

Many resuscitation drugs, including atropine, epinephrine, bretylium, lidocaine, amrinone, and phenytoin, have been used in animal studies and occasionally in humans for the treatment of bupivacaine overdose and cardiovascular collapse. In our view, beyond the established uses of epinephrine, vasopressin, and atropine in their designated steps in the advanced cardiac life support (ACLS) protocol[116] and beyond the use of Intralipid as detailed later, there is no established role for antiarrhythmic drugs or other traditional resuscitation drugs in the setting of bupivacaine-induced cardiac arrest. It is *not* recommended that bupivacaine-induced ventricular arrhythmias be treated with lidocaine or amiodarone.

The clinical implications for cardiac resuscitation after intravascular injection or overdose of local anesthetic are the following:

1. No medications are uniformly effective in facilitating resuscitation from bupivacaine-induced cardiac arrest or severe ventricular tachycardia (despite our recommendations regarding Intralipid later). Basic principles of cardiopulmonary resuscitation should be emphasized first, including attention to securing the airway, providing oxygenation and ventilation, and performing chest compressions if needed.
2. Because resuscitation after local anesthetic–induced circulatory collapse is so difficult, prevention of massive intravascular injection or excessive dosing is crucial.
3. Negative aspiration of the syringe does not always exclude intravascular placement. Incremental, fractionated dosing should be the rule for all patients undergoing major conduction blockade. Although changes on the ECG are not always present before circulatory collapse, they often are, and continuous attention to the ECG (including changes in QRS morphology, rate, rhythm, or ectopy) may be lifesaving by terminating injection before a lethal dose is administered.
4. Based on animal studies[117] and a growing number of human case reports,[118-120] we recommend that hospitals and clinics that perform major conduction blockade keep available for emergency use a supply of Intralipid 20%. If a patient experiences profound cardiovascular depression or circulatory arrest after the administration of bupivacaine, ropivacaine, or by extrapolation, other local anesthetics, then along with initiation of basic life support and the ACLS protocol we support the recommendation of Weinberg and colleagues[120] that a rapid bolus of Intralipid 20%, 1.5 mL/kg (or roughly 100 mL in adults), be administered without delay, followed if necessary by an infusion of 0.25 mL/kg/min for the next 10 minutes.

Chiral Local Anesthetics: Ropivacaine and Levobupivacaine

Commercial bupivacaine is a racemic mixture of (*R*)- and (*S*)-stereoisomers. In response to the problem of cardiovascular toxicity as a result of accidental intravenous injection of bupivacaine, single enantiomers were developed in the hope that they would be potentially safer local anesthetics. Ropivacaine (Naropin)[121] and levo-(*S*)-bupivacaine (Chirocaine)[122] were formulated to exploit this stereoselectivity. Ropivacaine is a single (*S*)-stereoisomer that differs from levobupivacaine in the substitution of a propyl for the butyl group on the piperidine ring (see Fig. 30-2). With these designed changes in molecular structure, it was hoped that ropivacaine and levobupivacaine would be less intrinsically cardiotoxic. Conversely, it appears that the (*S*)-enantiomers of mepivacaine and bupivacaine are metabolized by the liver more slowly than the corresponding (*R*)-enantiomers, which would lead to somewhat greater systemic accumulation with prolonged infusions.[123]

The cardiovascular toxicity of local anesthetics is complex and involves direct effects on the myocardium, on vascular tissue (both smooth muscle and its neuronal supply), and on the central innervation of the heart. The very slow reversal of Na^+ channel blockade after a cardiac action potential, which is a hallmark of bupivacaine, is considerably faster with ropivacaine. In addition to these electrical differences, the negative inotropic potency of ropivacaine on isolated cardiac tissue appears to be considerably less than that of bupivacaine.[124,125] Both electrical and mechanical differences in the toxic profiles may arise from the selective inhibition of Ca^{2+} currents by bupivacaine.

Do the data support the claim of a greater therapeutic index for ropivacaine than bupivacaine, particularly with regard to cardiotoxicity? In clinical studies comparing potencies of ropivacaine and bupivacaine administered for brachial plexus[126] or lumbar epidural block,[127] the anesthetic profiles of the drugs were almost identical. A third study comparing lumbar epidural 0.5% bupivacaine with 0.75% ropivacaine also found no significant differences in motor or sensory effects between the drugs at these different concentrations.[128] Overall, it appears that ropivacaine is slightly less potent than (1:1.3 to 1:1.5) or equally potent as bupivacaine for regional anesthesia. In some laboratory animal studies and in some human studies, ropivacaine also produced blocks of shorter duration than those induced by bupivacaine. Other studies in animals and humans have found equal durations of sensory and motor block for the two drugs.

At the projected equipotent doses for nerve block, are the drugs equally toxic? The overall impression is that ropivacaine is less cardiotoxic than bupivacaine. Studies in animals have generally found that bupivacaine more readily produces conduction disturbances, cardiac collapse, or ventricular fibrillation than ropivacaine does and that aggressive cardiac resuscitation after an intentional intravenous bolus in dogs leads to effective reversal of the toxic effects far more frequently with ropivacaine than with bupivacaine.[129]

The greater safety of ropivacaine than bupivacaine may be related both to the reduced toxicity of the single (*S*)-isomer and to the difference between the propyl- and butyl-*N*-piperidine substituent. In contrast to bupivacaine, the cardiotoxic profile of ropivacaine in pregnant ewes is the same as the corresponding profile in nonpregnant ewes.[130]

Levobupivacaine has been studied in a range of clinical settings and sites of administration.[131-133] Although a number of publications have compared levobupivacaine with racemic bupivacaine and ropivacaine,[132,133] conclusions differ among studies regarding the relative potency and duration of block of these three drugs at different sites of administration with respect to sensory and motor end points. Clinicians should note that levobupivacaine is formulated as a weight percentage with regard to its free base content, whereas the weight percentage of most other local anesthetics is calculated on the basis of the hydrochloride salt.[134]

Acidosis and Hypoxia

As with CNS toxicity, hypercapnia, acidosis, and hypoxia potentiate the negative chronotropic and inotropic actions of lidocaine and bupivacaine in isolated cardiac tissue, and the combination of hypoxia and acidosis markedly potentiates the cardiodepressant effects of bupivacaine.[135] Hypoxia and acidosis also increased the frequency of cardiac arrhythmias and the mortality rate in sheep after the intravenous administration of bupivacaine. Hypercapnia, acidosis, and hypoxia occur very rapidly in some patients after seizure activity caused by the rapid accidental intravascular injection of local anesthetic agents.[136] Thus, the cardiovascular depression observed in some patients after the accidental intravenous injection of bupivacaine may be related in part to the effect of seizures producing acidosis and hypoxia and thereby leading to an exacerbation of bupivacaine's intrinsic cardiotoxicity.

Indirect Cardiovascular Effects

High levels of spinal or epidural blockade can produce severe hypotension. A follow-up study of closed claims of patients who suffered perioperative cardiac arrest confirmed previous reports of a series of cardiac arrests involving generally healthy patients undergoing spinal or epidural anesthesia.[137] These events frequently occurred in conjunction with high dermatomal levels of blockade, liberal use of sedatives, and progression to cardiac arrest after a period of hypotension accompanied by bradycardia, often involving delays in recognition of the problem, delays in instituting airway support (particularly in sedated patients), and delays in administration of direct-acting combined α- and β-adrenergic agonists, such as epinephrine. Whereas mild to moderate degrees of hypotension generally respond well to indirect-acting sympathomimetics such as ephedrine or incremental dosing of phenylephrine, the combination of severe hypotension and severe bradycardia under spinal anesthesia should in most clinical settings be treated promptly with incremental dosing of epinephrine, initially at doses of 0.1 to 1 μg/kg, or roughly 20- to 200-fold below those used in the ACLS cardiac arrest algorithm.

Methemoglobinemia

A unique systemic side effect associated with a specific local anesthetic is the development of methemoglobinemia after the administration of large doses of prilocaine.[138] In general, 600-mg doses are required for the development of clinically significant levels of methemoglobinemia in adults. Hepatic metabolism of prilocaine generates *O*-toluidine, which oxidizes hemoglobin to methemoglobin. Methemoglobinemia, if severe, may be treated by the intravenous administration of methylene blue. Standard dosing of the topical local anesthetic EMLA (a mixture of lidocaine and prilocaine) in term newborns produced minimal amounts of methemoglobin, and EMLA should be regarded as very safe in the great majority of newborns. Risk may be increased in newborns with rare metabolic disorders or after the concomitant administration of other drugs that impair reduction of methemoglobin.

Allergies

Even though patients receiving local anesthetics may experience a range of local and systemic symptoms, prospective studies indicate that very few of these reactions are confirmed as allergic reactions.[139] Aminoester drugs such as procaine may produce allergic-type reactions more commonly than the aminoamides do, although even with aminoesters, the vast majority of reactions are not allergic. Aminoesters, unlike aminoamides, are derivatives of *p*-aminobenzoic acid, which is known to be allergenic. Some aminoamide solutions may contain a preservative, methylparaben, whose chemical structure is similar to that of *p*-aminobenzoic acid, but for most aminoamides, preservative-free solutions are available. Contamination of vials with latex antigen has been suspected in some allergic reactions, although it has been difficult to confirm. In the very rare patient for whom confirmed allergy to both aminoamides and aminoesters precludes their use for spinal anesthesia, meperidine can be considered as an alternative.[140]

Local Tissue Toxicity

All the clinically used aminoamide and aminoester local anesthetics can produce direct toxicity to nerves if they achieve sufficiently high intraneural concentrations. Conversely, in the great majority of clinical applications, no damage to nerves occurs. Although local anesthetics are usually packaged and injected at concentrations well above their physiologically effective range, in the process of delivery they are generally diluted sufficiently that no harm is done. If such dilution does not occur, however, long-term or permanent neural deficits do result. Thus, the application of 5% (200 mM) lidocaine in viscous, dense solutions through narrow intrathecal catheters has been associated with a high frequency of transient or longer-term radicular symptoms or even cauda equina syndrome.[141] Laboratory investigations have shown that such high concentrations of local anesthetics alone applied directly to bare nerve fibers produce an irreversible conduction block in less than 5 minutes.[142] Indeed, previous studies on ensheathed peripheral nerves in vivo had shown neurologic and histologic changes after infiltration of the space surrounding the nerve with local anesthetics at concentrations as low as 1% to 2%. Clinicians should be aware that the concentrations of formulated local anesthetic solutions are neurotoxic per se and that their dilution, in situ or in tissue, is essential for safe use. A recently published randomized trial has renewed interest in continuous spinal anesthesia,[143] and it may have a favorable risk-benefit ratio for selected high-risk patients.

In the late 1970s and early 1980s, prolonged sensory and motor deficits were reported in some patients after the epidural or subarachnoid injection of large doses of chloroprocaine.[144] Studies in animals have proved somewhat contradictory regarding the potential neurotoxicity of chloroprocaine.[145,146] Some studies suggest that the combination of low pH, sodium bisulfite, and inadvertent intrathecal dosing is responsible in part for the neurotoxic reactions observed after the use of large amounts of chloroprocaine solution; other studies have disputed this claim and note that chloroprocaine itself at high concentrations can also be neurotoxic,[145,146] but these concentrations are probably rarely achieved during properly positioned epidural anesthesia, as opposed to inadvertent spinal anesthesia. The currently available commercial solutions of chloroprocaine do not contain sodium bisulfite. This was initially replaced by ethylene glycol-bis-(β-aminoethyl ether)-*N*,*N*-tetraacetic acid (EGTA), a preservative and high-affinity calcium chelator that was occasionally reported to cause local muscle spasms after epidural administration. More recently, chloroprocaine has become available in an entirely preservative-free preparation. Chloroprocaine has unique utility in situations in which rapid plasma clearance is required to prevent excessive systemic accumulation of local anesthetic. Chloroprocaine has been given by epidural infusion to neonates and young infants in settings in which lidocaine and bupivacaine may not provide an effective therapeutic index,[99] and it has also recently become popular as a short-duration spinal anesthetic.

Single-shot spinal anesthesia with commonly recommended doses and concentrations of many different local anesthetics can produce more limited and transient neurologic symptoms (back pain, paresthesias, radicular pain, or hypoesthesia).[147] Some studies and systematic reviews have found that mepivacaine and lidocaine at a range of dilutions cause more frequent symptoms than bupivacaine and prilocaine do.[148] The risk of transient neurologic symptoms after spinal anesthesia was not diminished by dilution of lidocaine from 5% to 1%-2%. Differences in study design, method of questioning, and criteria for inclusion may be partially responsible for differences in the prevalence of radicular sequelae in various studies. Despite these differences in study design, a meta-analysis concluded that the pooled relative risk for transient neurologic symptoms after spinal anesthesia with lidocaine was 6.7-fold higher than with bupivacaine and 5.5-fold higher than with prilocaine.[148] The addition of vasoconstrictors to local anesthetic solutions may also increase risk.[149] Neurotoxicity appears to be unrelated to conduction block because tetrodotoxin, a highly potent blocker of sodium channels, can produce intense conduction blockade without histologic or behavioral signs of nerve injury.[150]

Intraoperative positioning also appears to be a risk factor. Patients undergoing surgery in the lithotomy position appear to be at increased risk for neurologic symptoms after either spinal or epidural anesthesia. It is unknown at present why this association produces increased risk; nerve compression or stretch or reduced perfusion pressure in the vasa nervorum may possibly exacerbate the toxicity from local anesthetics. The lithotomy position can produce neurologic sequelae and lower extremity compartment syndrome, particularly with prolonged surgery and use of the Trendelenburg position.[151]

Skeletal muscle changes have been observed after the intramuscular injection of local anesthetic agents such as lidocaine, mepivacaine, prilocaine, bupivacaine, and etidocaine. In general, the more potent, longer-acting agents bupivacaine and etidocaine appear to cause more localized skeletal muscle damage than the less potent, shorter-acting agents lidocaine and prilocaine do. This effect on skeletal muscle is reversible, and muscle regeneration occurs rapidly and is complete within 2 weeks after the injection of local anesthetic agents. Local anesthetic–induced myotoxicity may involve actions on mitochondria.[152]

Prolonged Infusions of Local Anesthetics and the Development of Long-Duration Local Anesthetics

Local anesthetics are increasingly being administered by continuous infusion for several days after surgery or for periods of weeks to months for the treatment of chronic malignant and nonmalignant pain (see also Chapters 58 and 87). With prolonged infusions there is the potential for delayed systemic accumulation and toxicity. Continuous bupivacaine infusions of up to 30 mg/hr in adults for as long as 2 weeks produced no overt CNS or cardiac toxicity despite total plasma bupivacaine concentrations in the range of 2 to 5 μg/mL in several patients.[153]

Several methods for producing long-duration nerve blockade are under investigation. Liposomal encapsulation can prolong nerve blockade, depending on the dose and the physical properties of the liposome (surface charge, size, lamellar structure).[154-156] Local anesthetics can be incorporated into biodegradable polymer microspheres for sustained release.[157] These preparations produce peripheral nerve blockade in animal models and human volunteers[158] ranging from 2 to 8 days, depending on the dose, site, and species. Because of the intrinsic neurotoxicity of all aminoamide and aminoester local anesthetics, there is likely to be some irreducible potential for neurotoxicity with most of these approaches to controlled release of aminoamide and aminoester local anesthetics in proximity to major nerve trunks. Thus, these formulations will have the most favorable risk-benefit ratio when used in nonprotective locations, such as intercostal nerve blockade, where prolonged numbness may be a benefit rather than a complication of the intervention. This risk is also likely to be less clinically important for infiltration analgesia.

Prolonged-duration local anesthesia also appears to be feasible with the use of site 1 sodium channel toxins in combination with either local anesthetics or adrenergics.[159] Other site 1 toxins have been used in humans in preliminary case series.[160] A combination of site 1 toxins with either local anesthetics or adrenergics results in prolongation of blockade and improvement in the therapeutic index.[159] Theoretically attractive features of site 1 toxins include their apparent lack of local tissue toxicity on nerves[150] or muscles[161] and their minimal effects on cardiac sodium channels.

Other drugs have been examined for use as local anesthetics, including tricyclic antidepressants,[162] although neurotoxicity may limit the clinical utility of this group of drugs.

It remains to be determined whether prolonged-duration local anesthetics will gain widespread use in clinical practice. If they prove to be safe and effective, they may have potential utility in intercostal blockade and wound infiltration, particularly for surgery on the thorax and abdomen, where protective sensation is comparatively less important than for limb surgery. If agents can be developed that last for weeks or longer, they may have additional applications in the management of chronic pain and cancer pain.

Biologic Mechanisms of Local Anesthetic Failure: Inflammation, Hyperalgesia, Tachyphylaxis, and Genetic Variants

Failure of local anesthesia is commonly ascribed to technical failure of delivery, insufficient volume or concentration of drug, or erroneous clinical decisions in selection of techniques. However, there are a number of clinical situations in which biologic processes contribute to failed local anesthesia, even with proper technique and drug selection. For example, in patients going to the dentist with infections such as a tooth abscess or severe pulpitis, failure rates of standard doses of local anesthetic have been reported to be as high as 70%. Local anesthetic failure at a site of inflammation appears to reflect a combination of pharmacokinetic factors and pharmacodynamic factors. Pharmacokinetic factors include (1) increased local blood flow leading to accelerated removal of drug from perineural injection compartments; (2) local tissue acidosis leading to a greater proportion of the drug in the hydrochloride form, which diffuses more poorly across biologic membranes; and (3) local tissue edema, which increases diffusion distances for drug into nerves. Pharmacodynamic factors include the effects of inflammation on both peripheral sensitization of nerves and central sensitization.[163,164] It is noteworthy that in the setting of an infected mandibular tooth, inferior alveolar nerve block (performed proximally at a site presumably remote from the infected area) also has an unexpectedly high failure rate.

Local anesthetics and regional anesthesia, in turn, can suppress components of inflammatory responses by a complex interplay of local, spinal, and systemic mechanisms.[165,166]

Apparent reductions in the effectiveness of local anesthetic infusions over time may be due to a number of causes unrelated to tolerance per se, including dislodgement of catheters and changes in the dermatomal origin or intensity of nociceptive input. In obstetric patients receiving epidural bolus injections, recurrence of pain before the next injection resulted in a reduction in the intensity and duration of blockade, whereas repeat injection before the return of pain prevented this rapidly occurring form of tolerance, or tachyphylaxis.[167] In postoperative patients, coadministration of systemic opioids prevented regression of segmental block in patients receiving thoracic epidural bupivacaine infusions.[168] Studies in rats suggest that both pharmacokinetic and pharmacodynamic mechanisms are involved. In a rat model, tachyphylaxis was linked to the development of hyperalgesia,[169] and drugs that inhibit hyperalgesia, including *N*-methyl-D-aspartate receptor antagonists and nitric oxide synthase inhibitors,[170] also prevented tachyphylaxis. Conversely, repeated sciatic injections of lidocaine resulted in reduced intraneural lidocaine content along with reduced duration of block.[171]

Occasional patients report that "local anesthetics don't work for me." Although this claim may reflect previous technical failures or a variety of other processes and patient- or procedure-specific factors, it is possible that in some cases these failures may involve genetic variation in local anesthetic responsiveness. For example, a subgroup of patients with the connective tissue disorder Ehlers-Danlos syndrome appears to have diminished responses to topical local anesthesia.[172]

References

1. Sanchez V, Arthur GR, Strichartz GR: Fundamental properties of local anesthetics. I. The dependence of lidocaine's ionization and octanol:buffer partitioning on solvent and temperature. Anesth Analg 66:159-165, 1987.
2. Zhang J, Hadlock T, Gent A, Strichartz GR: Tetracaine-membrane interactions: Effects of lipid composition and phase on drug partitioning, location, and ionization. Biophys J 92:3988-4001, 2007.
3. Gissen AJ, Covino BG, Gregus J: Differential sensitivities of mammalian nerve fibers to local anesthetic agents. Anesthesiology 53:467-474, 1980.
4. Courtney KR: Structure-activity relations for frequency-dependent sodium channel block in nerve by local anesthetics. J Pharmacol Exp Ther 213:114-119, 1980.
5. Courtney K, Strichartz G: Structural elements which determine local anesthetic activity. *In* Schwartz GR (ed): Handbook of Experimental Pharmacology: Local Anesthetics, vol 81. Berlin, Springer-Verlag, 1987, pp 53-89.
6. Schreier S, Frezzatti WA Jr, Araujo PS, et al: Effect of lipid membranes on the apparent pK of the local anesthetic tetracaine. Spin label and titration studies. Biochim Biophys Acta 769:231-237, 1984.
7. Ritchie JM, Rogart RB: Density of sodium channels in mammalian myelinated nerve fibers and nature of the axonal membrane under the myelin sheath. Proc Natl Acad Sci U S A 74:211-215, 1977.
8. Hodgkin A: The Conduction of the Nervous Impulse. Springfield, IL, Charles C Thomas, 1964.
9. Catterall W: From ionic currents to molecular mechanisms. The structure and function of voltage-gated sodium channels. Neuron 26:13-25, 2000.
10. Condouris GA, Goebel RH, Brady T: Computer simulation of local anesthetic effects using a mathematical model of myelinated nerve. J Pharmacol Exp Ther 196:737-745, 1976.
11. Ritchie JM, Ritchie B, Greengard P: The effect of the nerve sheath on the action of local anesthetics. J Pharmacol Exp Ther 150:160, 1965.
12. Hille B: The pH-dependent rate of action of local anesthetics on the node of Ranvier. J Gen Physiol 69:475-496, 1977.
13. Narahashi T, Frazier T, Yamada M: The site of action and active form of local anesthetics. I. Theory and pH experiments with tertiary compounds. J Pharmacol Exp Ther 171:32-44, 1970.
14. Strichartz GR: The inhibition of sodium currents in myelinated nerve by quaternary derivatives of lidocaine. J Gen Physiol 62:37-57, 1973.
15. Courtney KR, Kendig JJ, Cohen EN: Frequency-dependent conduction block: The role of nerve impulse pattern in local anesthetic potency. Anesthesiology 48:111-117, 1978.
16. Chernoff D: Kinetics of Anesthetic Binding to Sodium Channels: Role of p*K*a. Boston, Massachusetts Institute of Technology, 1988.
17. Hille B: Local anesthetics: Hydrophilic and hydrophobic pathways for the drug-receptor reaction. J Gen Physiol 69:497-515, 1977.
18. Gokin AP, Philip B, Strichartz GR: Preferential block of small myelinated sensory and motor fibers by lidocaine: In vivo electrophysiology in the rat sciatic nerve. Anesthesiology 95:1441-1454, 2001.
19. Ekberg J, Jayamanne A, Vaughan CW, et al: μO-conotoxin MrVIB selectively blocks Nav1.8 sensory neuron specific sodium channels and chronic pain behavior without motor deficits. Proc Natl Acad Sci U S A 103:17030-17035, 2006.
20. Chevrier P, Vijajaragavan K, Chahine M: Differential modulation of Nav 1.7 and Nav 1.8 peripheral nerve sodium channels by the local anesthetic lidocaine. Br J Pharmacol 142:576-584, 2004.
21. Fertleman C, Maker M, Parker K, et al: SCN9A mutation in paroxysmal extreme pain disorder: Allelic variants underlie distinct channel defects and phenotypes. Neuron 52:767-774, 2006.
22. Sheets PL, Jackson JO, Waxman SG, et al: A Na 1.7 channel mutation associated with hereditary erythromelalgia contributes to neuronal hyperexcitability and displays reduced lidocaine sensitivity. J Physiol 581:1019-1031, 2007.
23. Cox JJ, Reimann F, Nicholas AK, et al: An SCN9A channelopathy causes congenital inability to experience pain. Nature 444:894-898, 2006.
24. Persaud N, Strichartz G: Micromolar lidocaine selectively blocks propagating ectopic impulses at a distance from their site of origin. Pain 99:333-340, 2002.
25. Pindel EV, Kedishvili NY, Abraham TL, et al: Purification and cloning of a broad substrate specificity human liver carboxylesterase that catalyzes the hydrolysis of cocaine and heroin. J Biol Chem 272:14769-14775, 1997.
26. Scott DB, McClure JH, Giasi RM, et al: Effects of concentration of local anaesthetic drugs in extradural block. Br J Anaesth 52:1033-1037, 1980.
27. Galindo A, Benavides O, De Munos SO, et al: Comparison of anesthetic solutions used in lumbar and caudal peridural anesthesia. Anesth Analg 57:175-179, 1978.
28. Klein SM, Greengrass RA, Steele SM, et al: A comparison of 0.5% bupivacaine, 0.5% ropivacaine, and 0.75% ropivacaine for interscalene brachial plexus block. Anesth Analg 87:1316-1319, 1998.
29. Johns RA, DiFazio CA, Longnecker DE: Lidocaine constricts or dilates rat arterioles in a dose-dependent manner. Anesthesiology 62:141-144, 1985.
30. Fink BR, Cairns AM: Differential slowing and block of conduction by lidocaine in individual afferent myelinated and unmyelinated axons. Anesthesiology 60:111-120, 1984.
31. Fink BR, Cairns AM: Lack of size-related differential sensitivity to equilibrium conduction block among mammalian myelinated axons exposed to lidocaine. Anesth Analg 66:948-953, 1987.
32. Fink BR: 1992 Labat Lecture. Toward the mathematization of spinal anesthesia. Reg Anesth 17:263-273, 1992.
33. Raymond SA, Steffensen SC, Gugino LD, Strichartz GR: The role of length of nerve exposed to local anesthetics in impulse blocking action. Anesth Analg 68:563-570, 1989.
34. Drachman D, Strichartz G: Potassium channel blockers potentiate impulse inhibition by local anesthetics. Anesthesiology 75:1051-1061, 1991.
35. Hogan QH, Abram SE: Neural blockade for diagnosis and prognosis. A review. Anesthesiology 86:216-241, 1997.
36. Littlewood DG, Scott DB, Wilson J, Covino B: Comparative anaesthetic properties of various local anaesthetic agents in extradural block for labour. Br J Anaesth 49:75-79 , 1979.
37. Erdemir HA, Soper LE, Sweet RB: Studies of factors affecting peridural anesthesia. Anesth Analg 44:400-404, 1965.
38. Casati A, Baciarello M, Di Cianni S, et al: Effects of ultrasound guidance on the minimum effective anaesthetic volume required to block the femoral nerve. Br J Anaesth 98:823-827, 2007.
39. Pace NL, Stylianou MP: Advances in and limitations of up-and-down methodology: A précis of clinical use, study design, and dose estimation in anesthesia research. Anesthesiology 107:144-152, 2007.
40. Fisher DM: What if half of your patients moved (or remembered or did something else bad) at incision? Anesthesiology 107:1-2, 2007.
41. Moore DC, Batra MS: The components of an effective test dose prior to epidural block. Anesthesiology 55:693-696, 1981.
42. Tobias J: Caudal epidural block: A review of test dosing and recognition of systemic injection in children. Anesth Analg 93:1156-1161, 2001.
43. Braid D, Scott D: The systemic absorption of local analgesic drugs. Br J Exp Anaesth 37:396, 1965.
44. Eisenach JC, Grice SC, Dewan DM: Epinephrine enhances analgesia produced by epidural bupivacaine during labor. Anesth Analg 66:447-451, 1987.
45. Eisenach JC, Lysak SZ, Viscomi CM: Epidural clonidine analgesia following surgery: Phase I. Anesthesiology 71:640-646, 1989.
46. Wong K, Strichartz GR, Raymond SA: On the mechanisms of potentiation of local anesthetics by bicarbonate buffer: Drug structure-activity studies on isolated peripheral nerve. Anesth Analg 76:131-143, 1993.
47. DiFazio CA, Carron H, Grosslight KR, et al: Comparison of pH-adjusted lidocaine solutions for epidural anesthesia. Anesth Analg 65:760-764, 1986.
48. Bedder MD, Kozody R, Craig DB: Comparison of bupivacaine and alkalinized bupivacaine in brachial plexus anesthesia. Anesth Analg 67:48-52, 1988.
49. Cohen SE, Thurlow A: Comparison of a chloroprocaine-bupivacaine mixture with chloroprocaine and bupivacaine used individually for obstetric epidural analgesia. Anesthesiology 51:288-292, 1979.
50. Badgwell JM, Heavner JE, Kyttä J, Rosenberg PH: Cardiovascular and central nervous system effects of co-administered lidocaine and bupivacaine in piglets. Reg Anesth 16:89-94, 1991.
51. Popitz-Bergez FA, Leeson S, Thalhammer JG, Strichartz GR: Intraneural lidocaine uptake compared with analgesic differences between pregnant and nonpregnant rats. Reg Anesth 22:363-371, 1997.
52. Fagraeus L, Urban BJ, Bromage PR: Spread of epidural analgesia in early pregnancy. Anesthesiology 58:184-187, 1983.
53. McKay W, Morris R, Mushlin P: Sodium bicarbonate attenuates pain on skin infiltration with lidocaine, with or without epinephrine. Anesth Analg 66:572-574, 1987.
54. Harris WH, Slater EM, Bell HM: Regional anesthesia by the intravenous route. JAMA 194:1273-1276, 1965.
55. Hoffmann AC, van Gessel E, Gamulin Z, et al: Quantitative evaluation of tourniquet leak during i.v. regional anaesthesia of the upper and lower limbs in human volunteers. Br J Anaesth 75:269-273, 1995.
56. Albright GA: Cardiac arrest following regional anesthesia with etidocaine or bupivacaine. Anesthesiology 51:285-287, 1979.
57. Liu S, Carpenter RL, Chiu AA, et al: Epinephrine prolongs duration of subcutaneous infiltration of local anesthesia in a dose-related manner. Correlation with magnitude of vasoconstriction. Reg Anesth 20:378-384, 1995.
58. Reiestad F, Strömskag KE: Interpleural catheter in management of post-operative pain: A preliminary report. Reg Anesth 11:88-91, 1986.

59. Rosenberg PH, Scheinin BM, Lepantalo MJ, Lindfors O: Continuous intrapleural infusion of bupivacaine for analgesia after thoracotomy. Anesthesiology 67:811-813, 1987.
60. Liu S, Richman J, Thirlby R, Wu C: Efficacy of continuous wound catheters delivering local anesthetic for postoperative analgesia: A quantitative and qualitative systematic review of randomized controlled trials. J Am Coll Surg 203:914-932, 2006.
61. Marret E, Bazelly B, Taylor G, et al: Paravertebral block with ropivacaine 0.5% versus systemic analgesia for pain relief after thoracotomy. Ann Thorac Surg 79:2109-2113, 2005.
62. Dalens B, Vanneuville G, Tanguy A: Comparison of the fascia iliaca compartment block with the 3-in-1 block in children [erratum appears in Anesth Analg 1990 Apr;70(4):474]. Anesth Analg 69:705-713, 1989.
63. Cohen SE, Yeh JY, Riley RT, et al: Walking with labor epidural analgesia: The impact of bupivacaine concentration and a lidocaine-epinephrine test dose. Anesthesiology 92:387, 2000.
64. Brull SJ, Greene NM: Time-courses of zones of differential sensory blockade during spinal anesthesia with hyperbaric tetracaine or bupivacaine. Anesth Analg 69:342-347, 1989.
65. Chambers WA, Littlewood DG, Logan MR, Scott DB: Effect of added epinephrine on spinal anesthesia with lidocaine. Anesth Analg 60:417-420, 1981.
66. Chambers WA, Littlewood DG, Scott DB: Spinal anesthesia with hyperbaric bupivacaine: Effect of added vasoconstrictors. Anesth Analg 61:49-52, 1982.
67. Hallen B, Uppfeldt A: Does lidocaine-prilocaine cream permit pain free insertion of catheters in children? Anesthesiology 57:340-342, 1982.
68. Ohlsen L, Englesson S, Evers H: An anaesthetic lidocaine/prilocaine cream (EMLA) for epicutaneous application tested for cutting split skin grafts. Scand J Plast Reconstr Surg 19:201-209, 1985.
69. Butler-O'Hara M, LeMoine C, Guillet R: Analgesia for neonatal circumcision: A randomized controlled trial of EMLA cream versus dorsal penile nerve block. Pediatrics 101:E5, 1998.
70. Browne J, Awad I, Plant R, et al: Topical amethocaine (Ametop) is superior to EMLA for intravenous cannulation. Eutectic mixture of local anesthetics. Can J Anaesth 46:1014-1048, 1999.
71. Eichenfield LF, Funk A, Fallon-Friedlander S, Cunningham BB: A clinical study to evaluate the efficacy of ELA-Max (4% liposomal lidocaine) as compared with eutectic mixture of local anesthetics cream for pain reduction of venipuncture in children. Pediatrics 109:1093-1099, 2002.
72. Galinkin JL, Rose JB, Harris, K, Watcha MF: Lidocaine iontophoresis versus eutectic mixture of local anesthetics (EMLA) for IV placement in children. Anesth Analg 94:1484-1488, 2002.
73. Sethna NF, Verghese ST, Hannallah RS, et al: A randomized controlled trial to evaluate S-Caine Patch for reducing pain associated with vascular access in children. Anesthesiology 102:403-408, 2005.
74. Bonadio WA, Wagner V: TAC (tetracaine, adrenaline, cocaine) for the repair of minor dermal lacerations. Pediatr Emerg Care 4:82, 1988.
75. Smith GA, Strausbaugh SD, Harbeck-Weber C, et al: New non–cocaine-containing topical anesthetics compared with tetracaine-adrenaline-cocaine during repair of lacerations. Pediatrics 100:825-830, 1997.
76. Nordström H, Stånge K: Plasma lidocaine levels and risks after liposuction with tumescent anaesthesia. Acta Anaesthesiol Scand 49:1487-1490, 2005.
77. Houseman TS, Lawrence N, Mellen BG, et al: The safety of liposuction: Results of a national survey. Dermatol Surg 28:971-978, 2002.
78. Grazer FM, de Jong RH: Fatal outcomes from liposuction: Census survey of cosmetic surgeons. Plast Reconstr Surg 105:436-466, 2000.
79. Tremont-Lukats IW, Challapalli V, McNicol ED, et al: Systemic administration of local anesthetics to relieve neuropathic pain: A systematic review and meta-analysis. Anesth Analg 101:1738-1749, 2005.
80. Araujo MC, Sinnott CJ, Strichartz GR: Multiple phases of relief from experimental mechanical allodynia by systemic lidocaine: Responses to early and late infusions. Pain 103:21-29, 2003.
81. Tucker GT: Pharmacokinetics of local anesthetics. Br J Anaesth 58:717-731, 2007.
82. Rosenberg PH, Veering BT, Urmey WF: Maximum recommended doses of local anesthetics: A multifactorial concept. Reg Anesth Pain Med 29:564-575, 2004.
83. Wildsmith JA, Tucker GT, Cooper S, et al: Plasma concentrations of local anaesthetics after interscalene brachial plexus block. Br J Anaesth 49:461-466, 1977.
84. McCann ME, Sethna NF, Mazoit J-X, et al: The pharmacokinetics of epidural ropivacaine in infants and young children. Anesth Analg 93:893-897, 2001.
85. Tucker GT, Mather LE: Pharmacology of local anaesthetic agents. Pharmacokinetics of local anaesthetic agents. Br J Anaesth 47:213-224, 1975.
86. Lofstrom JB: Tissue distribution of local anesthetics with special reference to the lung. Int Anesthesiol Clin 16:53-71, 1978.
87. Kuhnert BR, Kuhnert RM, Philipson EH, et al: The half-life of 2-chloroprocaine. Anesth Analg 65:273-278, 1986.
88. Kuhnert BR, Kuhnert PM, Prochaska AL, Gross TL: Plasma levels of 2-chloroprocaine in obstetric patients and their neonates after epidural anesthesia. Anesthesiology 53:21-25, 1980.
89. Arthur GR, Scott DHT, Boyes RN, Scott DB: Pharmacokinetic and clinical pharmacological studies with mepivacaine and prilocaine. Br J Anaesth 51:481-485, 1979.
90. Scott DB, Jebson PJR, Boyes RN: Pharmacokinetic study of the local anaesthetics bupivacaine (Marcaine) and etidocaine (Duranest) in man. Br J Anaesth 45:1010-1012, 1973.
91. Katz JA, Bridenbaugh PO, Knarr DC: Pharmacodynamics and pharmacokinetics of epidural ropivacaine in humans. Anesth Analg 70:16-21, 1990.
92. Nation RL, Triggs EJ, Selig M: Lignocaine kinetics in cardiac patients and aged subjects. Br J Clinl Pharmacol 4:439-448, 1977.
93. Mazoit J, Denson D, Samii K: Pharmacokinetics of bupivacaine following caudal anesthesia in infants. Anesthesiology 68:387-391, 1988.
94. Yaster M, Aronoff D, Kornhauser DM, et al: The pharmacokinetics of lidocaine during caudal anesthesia in children. Anesthesiology 63:A465, 1985.
95. Bösenberg AT, Thomas J, Cronje L, et al: Pharmacokinetics and efficacy of ropivacaine for continuous epidural infusion in neonates and infants. Pediatr Anesth 15:739-749, 2005.
96. Agarwal R, Gutlove DP, Lockhart CH: Seizures occurring in pediatric patients receiving continuous infusion of bupivacaine. Anesth Analg 75:284-286, 1992.
97. Berde CB: Convulsions associated with pediatric regional anesthesia. Anesth Analg 75:164-166, 1992.
98. Larsson BA, Lonnqvist PA, Olsson GL: Plasma concentrations of bupivacaine in neonates after continuous epidural infusion. Anesth Analg 84:501-505, 1997.
99. Henderson K, Sethna NF, Berde CB: Continuous caudal anesthesia for inguinal hernia repair in former preterm infants. J Clin Anesth 5:129-133, 1993.
100. Stenson RE, Constantino RT, Harrison DC: Interrelationships of hepatic blood flow, cardiac output, and blood levels of lidocaine in man. Circulation 43:205-211, 1971.
101. Thomson PD, Melmon KL, Richardson JA, et al: Lidocaine pharmacokinetics in advanced heart failure, liver disease, and renal failure in humans. Ann Intern Med 78:499-508, 1973.
102. Wagman IH, De Jong RH, Prince DA: Effects of lidocaine on the central nervous system. Anesthesiology 28:155-172, 1967.
103. Scott DB: Evaluation of clinical tolerance of local anaesthetic agents. Br J Anaesth 47:328-331, 1975.
104. Englesson S: The influence of acid-base changes on central nervous system toxicity of local anaesthetic agents. I. An experimental study in cats. Acta Anaesthesiol Scand 18:79-87, 1974.
105. Burney RG, DiFazio CA, Foster JA: Effects of pH on protein binding of lidocaine. Anesth Analg 57:478-480, 1978.
106. Clarkson CW, Hondeghem LM: Mechanism for bupivacaine depression of cardiac conduction: Fast block of sodium channels during the action potential with slow recovery from block during diastole. Anesthesiology 62:396-405, 1985.
107. Block A, Covino B: Effect of local anesthetic agents on cardiac conduction and contractility. Reg Anesth 6:55, 1982.
108. Chamberlain BK, Volpe P, Fleischer S: Inhibition of calcium-induced calcium release from purified cardiac sarcoplasmic reticulum vesicles. J Biol Chem 259:7547-5753, 1984.
109. Johns RA, Difazio CA, Longnecker DE: Lidocaine constricts or dilates rat arterioles in a dose dependent manner. Anesthesiology 62:141-144, 1985.
110. de Jong RH, Ronfeld RA, DeRosa RA: Cardiovascular effects of convulsant and supraconvulsant doses of amide local anesthetics. Anesth Analg 61:3-9, 1982.
111. Kotelko DM, Shnider SM, Dailey PA, et al: Bupivacaine-induced cardiac arrhythmias in sheep. Anesthesiology 60:10-18, 1984.
112. Kasten G: High serum bupivacaine concentrations produce rhythm disturbances similar to torsades de pointes in anesthetized dogs. Reg Anesth 11:20, 1986.
113. Heavner JE: Cardiac dysrhythmias induced by infusion of local anesthetics into the lateral cerebral ventricle of cats. Anesth Analg 65:133-138, 1986.
114. Morishima HO, Pedersen H, Finster M, et al: Bupivacaine toxicity in pregnant and nonpregnant ewes. Anesthesiology 63:134-139, 1985.
115. Rosen MA, Thigpen JW, Shnider SM, et al: Bupivacaine-induced cardiotoxicity in hypoxic and acidotic sheep. Anesth Analg 64:1089-1096, 1985.
116. American Heart Association Consensus Group: Part 6: Advanced Cardiovascular Life Support. Circulation 102:I-86, 2000.
117. Weinberg GL, VadeBoncouer T, Ramaraju GA, et al: Pretreatment or resuscitation with a lipid infusion shifts the dose-response to bupivacaine-induced asystole in rats. Anesthesiology 88:1071-1075, 1998.
118. Litz RJ, Popp M, Stehr SN, Koch T: Successful resuscitation of a patient with ropivacaine-induced asys-

tole after axillary plexus block using lipid infusion. Anaesthesia 61:800-801, 2006.

119. Rosenblatt MA, Abel M, Fischer G, et al: Successful use of a 20% lipid emulsion to resuscitate a patient after a presumed bupivacaine-related cardiac arrest. Anesthesiology 105:217-218, 2006.

120. Weinberg G: Lipid rescue resuscitation from local anaesthetic cardiotoxicity. Toxicological Reviews 25:139-145, 2006.

121. Moller R, Covino BG: Cardiac electrophysiologic properties of bupivacaine and lidocaine compared with those of ropivacaine, a new amide local anesthetic. Anesthesiology 72:322-329, 1990.

122. Rutten AJ, Mather LE, McLean CF: Cardiovascular effects and regional clearances of i.v. bupivacaine in sheep: Enantiomeric analysis. Br J Anaesth 67:247-256, 1991.

123. Mather LE: Disposition of mepivacaine and bupivacaine enantiomers in sheep. Br J Anaesth 67:239-246, 1991.

124. Pitkanen M, Feldman HS, Arthur GR, Covino BG: Chronotropic and inotropic effects of ropivacaine, bupivacaine, and lidocaine in the spontaneously beating and electrically paced isolated, perfused rabbit heart. Reg Anesth 17:183-192, 1992.

125. Moller R, Covino BG: Cardiac electrophysiologic properties of bupivacaine and lidocaine compared with those of ropivacaine, a new amide local anesthetic. Anesthesiology 72:322-329, 1990.

126. Hickey R, Hoffman J, Ramamurthy S: A comparison of ropivacaine 0.5% and bupivacaine 0.5% for brachial plexus block. Anesthesiology 74:639-642, 1991.

127. Brown DL, Carpenter RL, Thompson GE: Comparison of 0.5% ropivacaine and 0.5% bupivacaine for epidural anesthesia in patients undergoing lower-extremity surgery. Anesthesiology 72:633-636, 1990.

128. Katz JA, Knarr D, Bridenbaugh PO: A double-blind comparison of 0.5% bupivacaine and 0.75% ropivacaine administered epidurally in humans. Reg Anesth 15:250-252, 1990.

129. Feldman HS, Arthur GR, Pitkanen M, et al: Treatment of acute systemic toxicity after the rapid intravenous injection of ropivacaine and bupivacaine in the conscious dog. Anesth Analg 73:373-384, 1991.

130. Santos AC, Pedersen H, Harmon TW, et al: Does pregnancy alter the systemic toxicity of local anesthetics? Anesthesiology 70:991-995, 1989.

131. Lerman J, Nolan J, Eyres R, et al: Efficacy, safety, and pharmacokinetics of levobupivacaine with and without fentanyl after continuous epidural infusion in children: A multicenter trial. Anesthesiology 99:1166-1174, 2003.

132. Camorcia M, Capogna G, Columb MO: Minimum local analgesic doses of ropivacaine, levobupivacaine, and bupivacaine for intrathecal labor analgesia. Anesthesiology 102:646-650, 2005.

133. Benhamou D, Ghosh C, Mercier FJ: A randomized sequential allocation study to determine the minimum effective analgesic concentration of levobupivacaine and ropivacaine in patients receiving epidural analgesia for labor. Anesthesiology 99:1383-1386, 2003.

134. Rosenberg PH, Schug SA: Levobupivacaine base and levobupivacaine hydrochloride. Br J Anaesth 94:544, 2005.

135. Sage DJ, Feldman HS, Arthur GR, et al: Influence of lidocaine and bupivacaine on isolated guinea pig atria in the presence of acidosis and hypoxia. Anesth Analg 63:1-7, 1984.

136. Moore DC, Crawford RD, Scurlock JE: Severe hypoxia and acidosis following local anesthetic–induced convulsions. Anesthesiology 53:259-260, 1980.

137. Lee LA, Posner KL, Domino KB, et al: Injuries associated with regional anesthesia in the 1980s and 1990s: A closed claims analysis. Anesthesiology 101:143-152, 2004.

138. Lund P, Cwik J: Propitocaine (Citanest) and methemoglobinemia. Anesthesiology 53:259, 1980.

139. Sidhu SK, Shaw S, Wilkinson JD: A 10-year retrospective study on benzocaine allergy in the United Kingdom. Am J Contact Dermatitis 10:57-61, 1999.

140. Norris MC, Honet JE, Leighton BL, Arkoosh VA: A comparison of meperidine and lidocaine for spinal anesthesia for postpartum tubal ligation. Reg Anesth 21:84-88, 1996.

141. Rigler ML, Drasner K, Krejcie TC, et al: Cauda equina syndrome after continuous spinal anesthesia. Anesth Analg 72:275-281, 1991.

142. Lambert LA, Lambert DH, Strichartz GR: Irreversible conduction block in isolated nerve by high concentrations of local anesthetics. Anesthesiology 80:1082-1093, 1994.

143. Arkoosh VA, Palmer CM, Yun EM, et al: A randomized, double-masked, multicenter comparison of the safety of continuous intrathecal labor analgesia using a 28-gauge catheter versus continuous epidural labor analgesia. Anesthesiology 108:286-298, 2008.

144. Reisner LS, Hochman BN, Plumer MH: Persistent neurologic deficit and adhesive arachnoiditis following intrathecal 2-chloroprocaine injection. Anesth Analg 59:452-454, 1980.

145. Wang BC, Hillman DE, Spielholz NI, Turndorf H: Chronic neurological deficits and Nesacaine-CE—an effect of the anesthetic, 2-chloroprocaine, or the antioxidant, sodium bisulfite? Anesth Analg 63:445-447, 1984.

146. Taniguchi M, Bollen AW, Drasner K: Sodium bisulfite: Scapegoat for chloroprocaine neurotoxicity? Anesthesiology 100:85-91, 2004.

147. Freedman JM, Li DK, Drasner K, et al: Transient neurologic symptoms after spinal anesthesia: An epidemiologic study of 1,863 patients [erratum appears in Anesthesiology 1998 Dec;89(6):1614]. Anesthesiology 89:633-641, 1998.

148. Eberhart LH, Morin AM, Kranke P, et al: Transient neurologic symptoms after spinal anesthesia. A quantitative systematic overview (meta-analysis) of randomized controlled studies. Anaesthesist 51:539-546, 2002.

149. Sakura S, Sumi M, Sakaguchi Y, et al: The addition of phenylephrine contributes to the development of transient neurologic symptoms after spinal anesthesia with 0.5% tetracaine. Anesthesiology 87:771-778, 1997.

150. Sakura S, Bollen AW, Ciriales R, Drasner K: Local anesthetic neurotoxicity does not result from blockade of voltage-gated sodium channels. Anesth Analg 81:338-346, 1995.

151. Warner MA, Warner DO, Harper CM, et al: Lower extremity neuropathies associated with lithotomy positions. Anesthesiology 93:938-942, 2000.

152. Irwin W, Fontaine E, Agnolucci A, et al: Bupivacaine myotoxicity is mediated by mitochondria. J Biol Chem 277:12221-12227, 2002.

153. Denson DD, Raj PP, Saldahna F, et al: Continuous perineural infusion of bupivacaine for prolonged analgesia: Pharmacokinetic considerations. Int J Clin Pharmacol Ther Toxicol 21:591-597, 1983.

154. Boogaerts JG, Lafont ND, Carlino S, et al: Biodistribution of liposome-associated bupivacaine after extradural administration to rabbits. Br J Anaesth 75:319-325, 1995.

155. Mowat JJ, Mok MJ, MacLeod BA, Madden TD: Liposomal bupivacaine. Extended duration nerve blockade using large unilamellar vesicles that exhibit a proton gradient. Anesthesiology 85:635-643, 1996.

156. Soderberg L, Dyhre H, Roth B, Bjorkman S: Ultralong peripheral nerve block by lidocaine: prilocaine 1:1 mixture in a lipid depot formulation: Comparison of in vitro, in vivo, and effect kinetics. Anesthesiology 104:110-121, 2006.

157. Curley J, Castillo J, Hotz J, et al: Prolonged regional nerve blockade. Injectable biodegradable bupivacaine/polyester microspheres. Anesthesiology 84:1401-1410, 1996.

158. Kopacz DJ, Lacouture PG, Wu D, et al: The dose response and effects of dexamethasone on bupivacaine microcapsules for intercostal blockade (T9 to T11) in healthy volunteers. Anesth Analg 96:576-582, 2003.

159. Kohane DS, Yieh J, Lu NT, et al: A re-examination of tetrodotoxin for prolonged duration local anesthesia. Anesthesiology 89:119-131, 1998.

160. Rodriguez-Navarro AJ, Lagos N, Lagos M, et al: Neosaxitoxin as a local anesthetic: Preliminary observations from a first human trial. Anesthesiology 106:339-345, 2007.

161. Padera RF, Tse JY, Bellas E, Kohane DS: Tetrodotoxin for prolonged local anesthesia with minimal myotoxicity. Muscle Nerve 34:747-753, 2006.

162. Sudoh Y, Cahoon EE, Gerner P, Wang GK: Tricyclic antidepressants as long-acting local anesthetics. Pain 103:49-55, 2003.

163. Cairns BE, Gambarota G, Dunning PS, et al: Activation of peripheral excitatory amino acid receptors decreases the duration of local anesthesia. Anesthesiology 98:521-529, 2003.

164. Cairns BE, Svensson P, Wang K, et al: Activation of peripheral NMDA receptors contributes to human pain and rat afferent discharges evoked by injection of glutamate into the masseter muscle. J Neurophysiol 90:2098-2105, 2003.

165. Beloeil H, Ababneh Z, Chung R, et al: Effects of bupivacaine and tetrodotoxin on carrageenan-induced hind paw inflammation in rats (Part 1): Hyperalgesia, edema, and systemic cytokines. Anesthesiology 105:128-138, 2006.

166. Beloeil H, Ji RR, Berde CB: Effects of bupivacaine and tetrodotoxin on carrageenan-induced hind paw inflammation in rats (Part 2): Cytokines and p38 mitogen–activated protein kinases in dorsal root ganglia and spinal cord. Anesthesiology 105:139-145, 2006.

167. Bromage PR, Pettigrew RT, Crowell DE: Tachyphylaxis in epidural analgesia: I. Augmentation and decay of local anesthesia. J Clin Pharmacol 9:30-38, 1969.

168. Lund C, Mogensen T, Hjortso NC, Kehlet H: Systemic morphine enhances spread of sensory analgesia during postoperative epidural bupivacaine infusion. Lancet 2:1156-1157, 1985.

169. Lee KC, Wilder RT, Smith RL, Berde CB: Thermal hyperalgesia accelerates and MK-801 prevents the development of tachyphylaxis to rat sciatic nerve blockade. Anesthesiology 81:1284-1293, 1994.

170. Wilder RT, Sholas MG, Berde CB: NG-nitro-L-arginine methyl ester (L-NAME) prevents tachyphylaxis to local anesthetics in a dose-dependent manner. Anesth Analg 83:1251-1255, 1996.

171. Choi RH, Birknes JK, Popitz-Bergez FA, et al: Pharmacokinetic nature of tachyphylaxis to lidocaine: Peripheral nerve blocks and infiltration anesthesia in rats. Life Sci 61:PL177-PL184, 1997.

172. Arendt-Nielsen L, Kaalund S, Bjerring P, Hogsaa B: Insufficient effect of local analgesics in Ehlers Danlos type III patients (connective tissue disorder). Acta Anaesthesiol Scand 34:358-361, 1990.

Fumito Ichinose and Warren M. Zapol

31 Nitric Oxide and Inhaled Pulmonary Vasodilators

Key Points

1. Endogenous nitric oxide (NO) is produced from oxygen and L-arginine by a group of enzymes called nitric oxide synthases with L-citrulline as a by-product.
2. Most of the effects of NO on the cardiovascular system are mediated by activation of the enzyme soluble guanylate cyclase, which catalyzes formation of the second messenger cyclic guanosine monophosphate (cGMP) from guanosine 5′-triphosphate. NO stimulates soluble guanylate cyclase to synthesize cGMP, which in turn activates cGMP-dependent protein kinase and thereby leads to vascular relaxation.
3. Because NO binds rapidly to hemoglobin with high affinity, the vasodilatory effect of inhaled NO is limited to the lung.
4. NO can be safely inhaled when delivered by facemask, nasal cannula, or an endotracheal tube.
5. According to a survey in 2000, 94% of pediatric cardiologists consider inhaled NO to be a clinically proven agent to test pulmonary vasoreactivity in the cardiac catheterization laboratory.[66]
6. Several clinical trials of inhaled NO in patients with acute lung injury demonstrated no effect on mortality or the duration of mechanical ventilation; however, the frequency of progression to severe respiratory failure from milder respiratory failure was decreased by inhaled NO in one study.[78]
7. Inhaled NO has been reported to ameliorate the postoperative pulmonary hypertension of congenital heart disease[91,92] and decrease the need for postoperative extracorporeal membrane oxygenation.[93]
8. The vasodilatory response to inhaled NO is variable in patients with valvular heart disease.[86,95] The variability in dilator response is likely to be related to the balance between pulmonary vascular remodeling and active vasoconstriction.
9. In contrast to therapy with intravenous vasodilators, which often cause systemic hypotension, inhaled NO has been shown in a small group of patients to selectively reduce peripheral vascular resistance and enhance right ventricular stroke work after cardiac transplantation.[98]
10. A trial of inhaled NO is recommended before consideration of implantation of a right ventricular assist device because this invasive procedure may be avoided if there is a salutary response to inhaled NO.[102]
11. Inhaled NO can combine with hemoglobin to form nitrosylhemoglobin, which is rapidly oxidized to methemoglobin. The enzyme methemoglobin reductase rapidly converts methemoglobin to hemoglobin in the red blood cell. Because neonates have reduced activity of this enzyme, they are at greater risk than adults for the development of significant methemoglobinemia after the inhalation of high levels of NO for a prolonged period.[142]

Pulmonary hypertension often complicates patient care intraoperatively, as well as in intensive care units (ICUs). Severe acute pulmonary hypertension may produce right ventricular (RV) failure. Pulmonary hypertension and RV failure may reduce left ventricular (LV) filling, decrease cardiac output, and lead to systemic hypotension. Decreased arterial blood pressure may compromise RV coronary perfusion at a time when RV end-diastolic pressure and RV myocardial oxygen consumption are increased because of increased RV wall tension, thereby leading to RV ischemia.[1] RV ischemia will exacerbate RV failure and cause a further reduction in cardiac output and blood pressure (Fig. 31-1). This vicious cycle may continue unless pulmonary artery pressure is reduced to permit increased RV ejection. Unfortunately, treatment of pulmonary hypertension with intravenous vasodilators may worsen the systemic hypotension. Inhalation of nitric oxide (NO) produces selective pulmonary vasodilation without reducing systemic arterial pressure in patients with acute or chronic pulmonary hypertension. Addi-

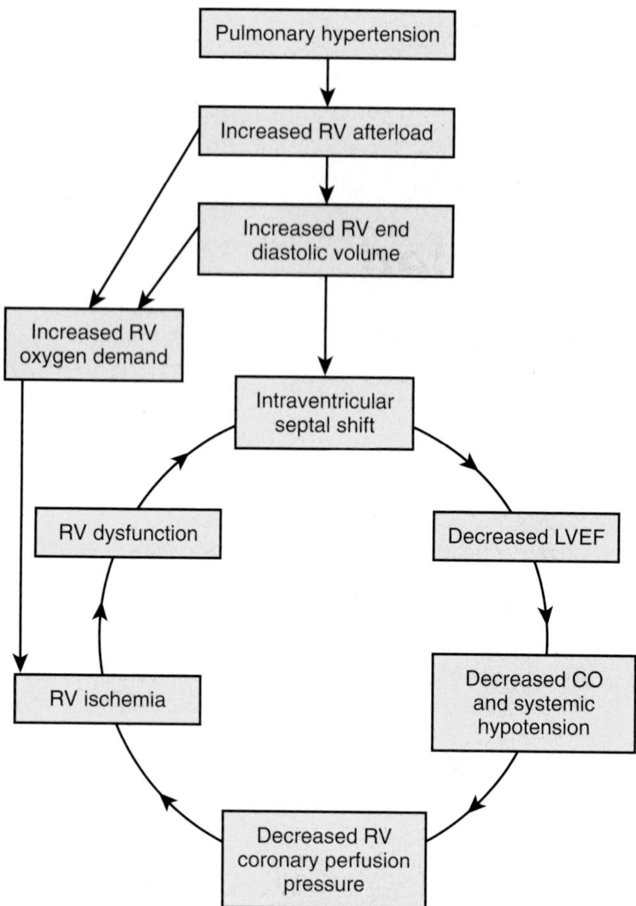

Figure 31-1 Vicious cycle of right ventricular (RV) failure triggered by pulmonary hypertension. CO, cardiac output; LVEF, left ventricular ejection fraction.

tionally, there are now a number of other experimental inhaled pulmonary vasodilators described in the literature that may provide potential alternatives to inhaled NO. In this chapter the theoretical background, current uses, and future therapeutic potential of inhaled NO and other inhaled pulmonary vasodilators are discussed.

Inhaled Nitric Oxide

Since recognition of NO as a key endothelial-derived vasodilator molecule in 1987, the field of NO research has expanded to encompass many areas of biomedical research. It is now well established that NO is an important signaling molecule throughout our body. Endogenous NO is produced from oxygen and L-arginine by a group of enzymes called nitric oxide synthases (NOSs) with L-citrulline as a by-product. Most of the effects of NO on the cardiovascular system are mediated by activation of the enzyme-soluble guanylate cyclase (sGC), which catalyzes formation of the second messenger cyclic guanosine monophosphate (cGMP) from guanosine 5′-triphosphate. Studies also indicate that NO may directly modulate other signaling systems. For example, recent evidence suggests that NO is directly involved in post-translational protein modification, including nitrosylation of proteins (Fig. 31-2).

A therapeutic potential for inhaled NO to act as a selective pulmonary vasodilator was demonstrated by Frostell and colleagues in 1991, who showed that breathing NO gas resulted in rapid and profound pulmonary vasodilation in an awake lamb model of pulmonary hypertension produced by infusion of a stable thromboxane analog (Fig. 31-3).[2] Because NO binds rapidly to hemoglobin (Hb) with high affinity, the vasodilatory effect of inhaled NO is limited to the lung. This is in sharp contrast to intravenously infused vasodilators, which often cause systemic vasodilation and lead to systemic arterial hypotension. This unique ability of inhaled NO to cause highly selective pulmonary vasodilation has prompted a large number of preclinical and clinical studies. The early pilot studies also demonstrated that inhaled NO therapy rapidly improves oxygenation without causing systemic hypotension in critically ill newborns with acute pulmonary hypertension (see Chapter 84).[3,4] Subsequently, the efforts of many research groups studying animals and patients led to approval of inhaled NO by the U.S. Food and Drug Administration in 1999 and by the European Medicine Evaluation Agency and European Commission in 2001.[5-8]

A number of studies now indicate that inhaled NO may play an important role in treating pulmonary hypertension in pediatric and adult patients with respiratory and cardiac failure, in determining the vasodilatory capacity of the pulmonary vas-

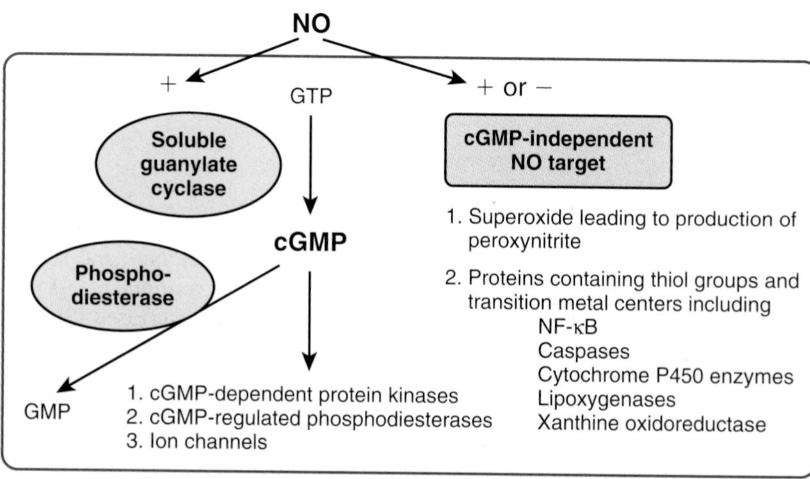

Figure 31-2 Nitric oxide (NO) signaling pathway. cGMP, cyclic guanosine monophosphate; GTP, guanosine triphosphate.

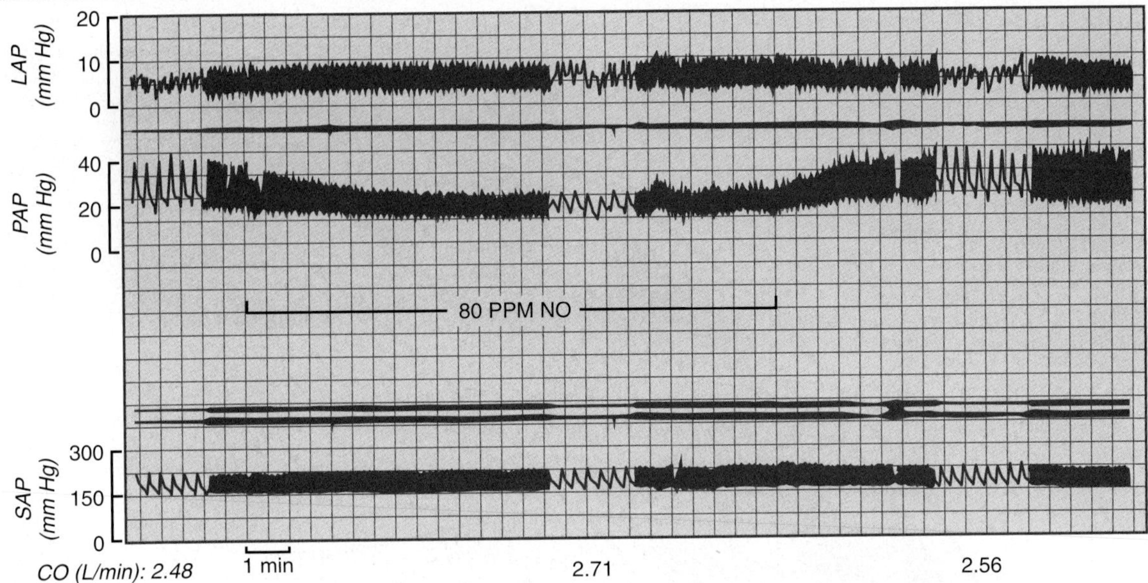

Figure 31-3 Effects of breathing nitric oxide (NO) at 80 ppm in a lamb with pulmonary hypertension induced by an infusion of U46619, a stable thromboxane analog. CO, cardiac output; LAP, left atrial pressure; PAP, pulmonary artery pressure; SAP, systemic artery pressure. Note that breathing NO decreased PAP without affecting LAP and SAP. *(From Frostell C, Fratacci MD, Wain JC, et al: Inhaled nitric oxide. A selective pulmonary vasodilator reversing hypoxic pulmonary vasoconstriction. Circulation 83:2038-2047, 1991, with permission.)*

cular bed, and perhaps in preventing the development of chronic lung disease in infants with lung injury.

Inhaled Nitric Oxide: Physical Properties, Methods of Administration, and Mechanism of Action

Chemistry of Nitric Oxide Gas

NO is a colorless and odorless gas that is only slightly soluble in water.[9] Atmospheric concentrations of NO usually range between 10 and 500 parts per billion by volume (ppb) but can exceed 1.5 parts per million (ppm) in areas of heavy traffic or lightning.[10] In the inhaled smoke of a burning cigarette, NO is produced by oxidation of nitrogen from the atmosphere and nitrogen-containing compounds in tobacco and can reach levels of 1000 ppm.[11] NO is unstable in air and undergoes spontaneous oxidation to form the more toxic nitrogen oxides (NO_2, N_2O_4, etc.). NO is therefore stored in cylinders diluted in an inert gas, usually nitrogen.

Delivery and Monitoring of Inhaled Nitric Oxide

NO can be safely inhaled when delivered by facemask, nasal cannula, or an endotracheal tube. It is important to carefully regulate the concentration of NO and its length of exposure to oxygen, which can be achieved with several commercially available systems. Although NO and NO_2 are more accurately measured by chemiluminescence devices, electrochemical detectors have proved adequate for the measurement of inhaled NO and are integrated components of several clinical delivery systems. Despite concern that ICU workers would passively inhale NO, this has not become a problem because levels of NO in ICU air remain quite low.[12]

Nitric Oxide/Cyclic Guanosine Monophosphate Signal Transduction System

After inhalation, NO diffuses rapidly across the alveolar-capillary membrane into the subjacent smooth muscle of pulmonary vessels (Fig. 31-4). NO stimulates sGC to synthesize cGMP, which in turn activates cGMP-dependent protein kinase and thereby leads to vascular relaxation. The physiologic actions of cGMP are limited by its hydrolysis to GMP and by export from the cell. A family of cyclic nucleotide phosphodiesterases (PDEs) is known to hydrolyze cyclic nucleotides. Of the 11 reported PDE isozymes, PDE5 is considered to be the most active cGMP-hydrolyzing PDE in smooth muscle (for review, see Rybalkin and associates[13]). PDE5 has high affinity for cGMP and is selectively inhibited by PDE inhibitors such as zaprinast, sildenafil, and verdenafil. In addition to its pulmonary vasodilating effects, inhaled NO has several other effects in the lung. For instance, inhaled NO has been shown to cause bronchodilation[14,15] and to possess anti-inflammatory[16] and antiproliferative[17] effects. NO can also elicit effects via cGMP-independent mechanisms, including interactions with heme-containing molecules (in addition to sGC) and with proteins containing reactive thiol groups.[18] NO interacts with the superoxide radical (O_2^-), which limits the bioavailability of NO and results in formation of the potent oxidant peroxynitrite ($ONOO^-$). In the presence of oxygenated Hb, NO is rapidly metabolized to nitrate with the formation of methemoglobin (MetHb). Within red blood cells, electron donors rapidly convert MetHb back to ferrous Hb.

Enhancement of Ventilation-Perfusion Matching by Inhalation of Nitric Oxide

The intrapulmonary distribution of blood flow and ventilation (ventilation-perfusion [$\dot{V}/\dot{Q}$] distribution) is a major determinant of the efficiency of transpulmonary oxygenation and determines the partial pressure of oxygen in arterial blood (Pa_{O_2}). In a normal, healthy lung, the majority of ventilated areas are well perfused (see also Chapter 15). The shunt from the right to the

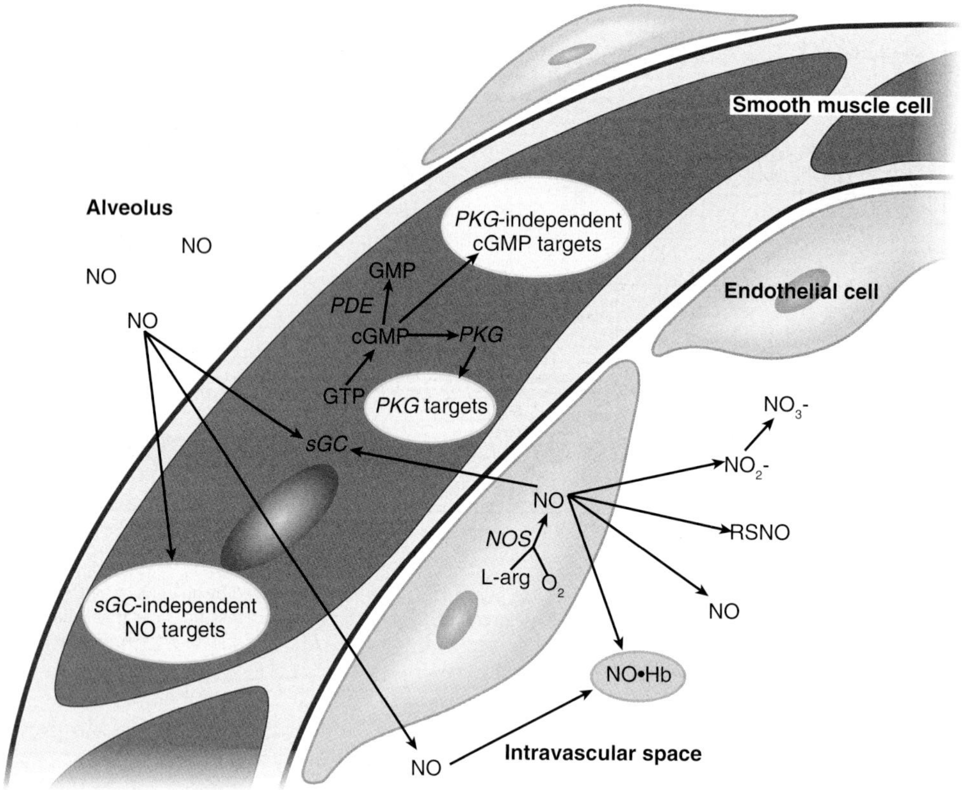

Figure 31-4 Schematic of the nitric oxide (NO) signaling pathway in the lung. NO, formed by endothelial cells or administered by inhalation, diffuses to vascular smooth muscle cells. Numerous targets of NO contribute to the wide variety of effects of this molecule on the cardiovascular system. One of the primary targets for NO is soluble guanylate cyclase (sGC). NO binds to the heme moiety of sGC and stimulates synthesis of the intracellular second messenger cyclic guanosine monophosphate (cGMP). cGMP interacts with a variety of targets, including ion channels, cGMP-regulated phosphodiesterases (PDEs), and cGMP-dependent protein kinases (PKGs). PKGs have been shown to phosphorylate various proteins in vascular smooth muscle cells. cGMP is metabolized to GMP by PDEs. On arrival in the bloodstream, the majority of NO rapidly binds to hemoglobin with high affinity, but small amounts of NO may remain to react with other molecules, including proteins. GTP, guanosine triphosphate; NOS, nitric oxide synthase; RSNO, S-nitrosothiol. *(From Ichinose F, Roberts JD, Zapol WM: Inhaled nitric oxide, a selective pulmonary vasodilator, current uses and therapeutic potential. Circulation 109:3106-3111, 2004, with permission.)*

left side of the circulation is mainly extrapulmonary (e.g., bronchial veins) and is less than 5% to 8% of cardiac output.[19] In a normal lung, local alveolar hypoxia constricts the vascular bed adjacent to hypoxic regions and redistributes blood flow toward lung regions with better ventilation and higher intra-alveolar PO_2. It has been proposed that inhaled NO amplifies this mechanism by increasing blood flow to well-ventilated lung areas, which may, in some diseases, cause increased vasomotor tone. This inhaled vasodilatory effect is in marked contrast to the effect of intravenously administered vasodilators, which produce diffuse dilation of the pulmonary vasculature, increase blood flow to areas of nonventilated lung, and thereby increase intrapulmonary shunting and reduce PaO_2. In contrast, inhaled NO should selectively improve the perfusion of ventilated regions and hence reduce intrapulmonary shunting and improve arterial oxygenation (Fig. 31-5). These beneficial effects of inhaled NO on intrapulmonary shunting and oxygenation have been demonstrated in some adult and pediatric patients with acute respiratory distress syndrome (ARDS).[20,21] Unfortunately, this effect can at times be transient.[22]

Clinical Use of Inhaled Nitric Oxide

Perinatal and Pediatric Uses of Inhaled Nitric Oxide

Nitric Oxide Is an Important Regulatory Molecule in the Perinatal Lung. Several studies indicate that NO has an important role in modulating pulmonary vascular resistance (PVR) at birth. For example, in the developing lungs of several animals, NOS and sGC expression and signaling increase late in gestation, are maximal in the postnatal period, and decrease in adults.[23-25] Moreover, because NOS inhibitors attenuate the reduction in PVR at birth,[26,27] it is likely that NO signaling plays a critical role in transition from the fetal to the newborn pulmonary circulatory system.

Many forms of newborn and infant lung disease are associated with endothelial cell injury and decreased NO/cGMP signaling. Studies in newborns suggest that premature constriction of the ductus arteriosus, septic mediators, and meconium aspiration all cause pulmonary endothelial cell injury. For example, in utero ligation of the ductus arteriosus in the fetal lamb causes flow-

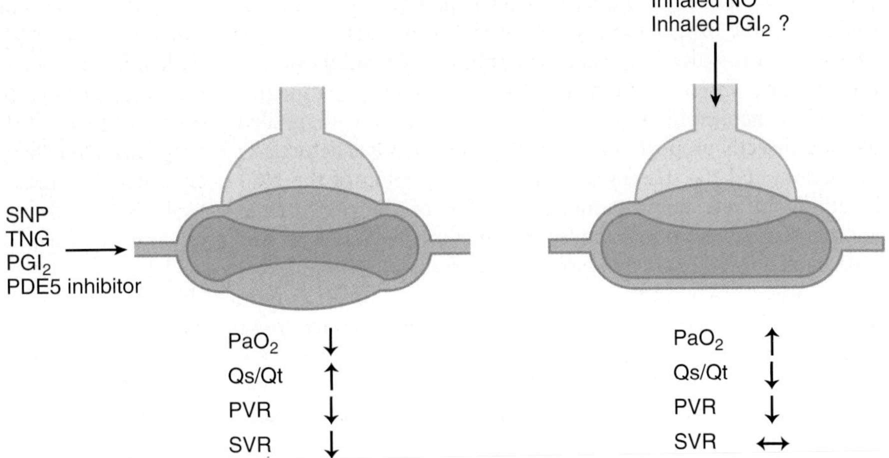

Figure 31-5 Diagram illustrating the differing pathophysiologic effects of inhaled pulmonary vasodilators and intravenous vasodilators. SNP, sodium nitroprusside; TNG, nitroglycerine; PGI_2, prostaglandin I_2; PDE5 inhibitor, phosphodiesterase 5 inhibitor; PaO_2, partial pressure of oxygen in arterial blood; Qs/Qt, right-to-left shunt fraction; PVR, pulmonary vascular resistance; SVR, systemic vascular resistance.

induced endothelial cell dysfunction and decreases the expression of endothelial NOS (NOS3)[28] and vasorelaxation caused by NO.[29] Moreover, cardiac lesions, such as atrial and ventricular septal defects, atrioventricular canals, persistent ductus arteriosus, and transposition of the great vessels without a ventricular septal defect, cause endothelial cell injury, decrease NO-mediated pulmonary vasorelaxant activity, and lead to pulmonary hypertension.[30]

Accumulating evidence suggests that NO/cGMP signaling has an important role in regulating lung development. For example, in mildly hypoxemic newborn NOS3-deficient mice, alveolar development is severely inhibited in a manner that can be improved by inhalation of NO.[31,32] Furthermore, in perinatal models of pulmonary vascular disease, in which NO activity has been observed to be decreased, inhaled NO improves the development of peripheral pulmonary arteries.[33]

Experimental Studies of the Selective Pulmonary Vasodilator Effects of Inhaled Nitric Oxide in the Newborn. Several investigations in newborn animals have demonstrated that inhaled NO decreases pulmonary hypertension. For example, in fetal lambs with an intact placental circulation, inhaled NO decreased PVR.[34] Similarly, in newborn lambs with pulmonary vasoconstriction associated with hypoxemia, inhaled NO was observed to decrease PVR and increase lung cGMP levels in a manner that was not modified by acidosis.[35] Importantly, in the latter study inhaled NO did not cause systemic vasodilation, and breathing up to 80 ppm NO did not decrease either systemic vascular resistance or blood pressure.

Inhaled NO also reversed vasoconstriction in newborn animals with pulmonary vascular remodeling. In newborn lambs with pulmonary vascular disease induced by premature ligation of the ductus arteriosus and associated with muscularization of peripheral arteries in the lung periphery, inhaled NO caused dose-dependent vasodilatation and improved systemic oxygenation and survival rates.[36] Moreover, in lambs with lung hypoplasia caused by congenital diaphragmatic hernia, NO improved systemic oxygenation when inhaled after exogenous surfactant treatment or during partial liquid ventilation.[37] These latter findings suggest that lung volume recruitment is required for inspired NO to effectively reduce pulmonary vasoconstriction in models associated with lung hypoplasia.

Inhaled Nitric Oxide Can Attenuate Pulmonary Disease in Newborn Animals. In newborn rats, lung injury caused, for example, by sustained hypoxia or exposure to endothelial toxins results in pulmonary artery muscularization and hypertension similar to that observed in patients with pulmonary artery hypertension (PAH) and many forms of congenital heart disease. In these models, prolonged inhalation of NO has been reported to attenuate pulmonary vascular remodeling and RV hypertrophy in chronically hypoxic newborns.[33] Importantly, it appears that breathing NO can inhibit pulmonary vascular remodeling even in the absence of pulmonary hypertension. Roberts and colleagues reported that in newborn rats with monocrotaline-induced endothelial injury, inhaled NO decreased the abnormal proliferation of cells in the walls of pulmonary arteries and prevented abnormal pulmonary vascular remodeling even before the development of pulmonary hypertension.[17] These findings suggest that inhaled NO may play an important role in modifying the abnormal vascular development and secondary pulmonary hypertension of the injured newborn lung.

Lung injury decreases alveolar and pulmonary microvascular development in premature lambs and baboons and in newborn mice and rats.[38] Accumulating experimental evidence suggests that inhaled NO promotes the development of the injured maturing lung. For example, prolonged NO inhalation has been observed to increase alveologenesis in chronically ventilated premature baboons[39] and lambs.[40] Moreover, inhaled NO improves alveolar development in mice after hyperoxic lung injury.[41] The mechanisms responsible for the protective effects of inhaled NO in alveologenesis are unknown. Because studies suggest that the pulmonary vasculature importantly regulates alveolar development[42] and inhaled NO protects newborn lung vessels from injury,[33] it is possible that inhaled NO protects the lung via its effects on the microvasculature. This concept is supported by the observation that inhaled NO improves alveolarization in rat pups that have decreased microvascular development.[43] However, it is also possible that NO regulates the homeostasis of other cells or might modulate other signaling systems regulating or contributing to lung development.

Inhaled Nitric Oxide Increases Systemic Oxygenation in Hypoxemic Newborns with Pulmonary Hypertension. Pilot studies revealed that inhalation of NO increases systemic oxygenation in severely hypoxemic newborns with pulmonary hypertension (see Chapter 84).[3,4] The ability of inhaled NO to increase systemic oxygen levels was confirmed in several multicenter randomized controlled studies of term and near-term babies with hypoxemia and pulmonary hypertension.[6,8,44] In one study, systemic oxygenation was observed to increase in nearly half of patients with severe persistent pulmonary hypertension of the newborn who received inhaled NO.[6] Importantly, the magnitude of the increase in oxygen levels in babies treated with inhaled NO was directly proportional to the degree of hypoxia before NO inhalation, and the increased systemic oxygenation of the NO-breathing infants was maintained in 75% of the patients. In another study, the optimal concentration of inhaled NO level was investigated[45]; although the maximum increase in systemic oxygenation was observed in babies breathing 80 ppm NO, as little as 5 to 20 ppm NO increased arterial oxygen levels above those measured in babies not breathing NO. Several studies have reported that inhaled NO decreases the need for extracorporeal membrane oxygenation (ECMO), an invasive procedure requiring systemic heparinization.[6,8,44]

Inhaled Nitric Oxide in Bronchopulmonary Dysplasia. Bronchopulmonary dysplasia (BPD) is an important chronic lung disease of prematurely born infants that results, in part, from the inhibition or disruption of normal pulmonary alveolar and microvascular development as a result of oxygen- and ventilator-induced lung injury.[46] Although an early study suggested that inhaled NO does not decrease the incidence of BPD,[47] a subsequent single-center trial involving 207 premature infants conducted by Schreiber and colleagues suggested that inhaled NO decreases the incidence of BPD and death in prematurely born infants.[48] These observations were supported by results from a later multicenter trial in which inhaled NO was noted to decrease the rate of BPD and death in premature infants with a birth weight of less than 1000 g.[49] In a more recent study of 793 newborns 34 weeks of gestational age or less, Kinsella and coauthors reported that inhaled NO decreased the incidence of BPD in the subset of 129 infants with a birth weight of at least 1000 g.[50] Furthermore, in another multicenter study of 582 premature infants with a birth weight of 1250 g or less in whom inhaled NO was commenced 7 to 21 days after birth, Ballard and coworkers reported that inhalation of NO improved survival and reduced the incidence of BPD.[51] Although these results are encouraging when considered together, additional studies need to be performed before the role of inhaled NO in preventing BPD can be defined.

Safety of Inhaled Nitric Oxide in the Newborn. Even though studies in newborns and infants suggest that prolonged inhalation of NO is safe,[52] the long-term pulmonary and extrapulmonary effects of inhaled NO are unknown. In particular, the effects of chronic NO inhalation on normal pulmonary cell proliferation and differentiation, as well as on alveolar and microvascular development, are unknown.

NO can increase cGMP levels in platelets and inhibit their function (reviewed by Schwarz and colleagues[53]). The potential of inhaled NO to alter platelet function[54] is of particular concern for immature infants because abnormal hemostatic activity might increase the incidence or evolution of intraventricular hemorrhage (IVH) and associated neurologic injury. In one study, breathing NO was associated with increased mortality and rates of IVH in infants weighing 1000 g or less.[49] Nevertheless, data from several other studies suggest that inhaled NO does not increase the incidence or severity of IVH in premature babies.[47,48,51] In fact, in one very large study of premature infants, inhaled NO was reported to decrease the frequency of IVH and its sequelae.[50]

It is uncertain whether the improvement in pulmonary disease in some premature babies who breathed NO is associated with improved neurologic development. In a European multicenter trial of nearly 100 premature babies, inhaled NO was not observed to affect the incidence of death or severe disability at 1 year corrected for postnatal age.[55] On the other hand, a more rigorous evaluation of older premature babies treated in another trial suggested that inhaled NO can improve neurologic outcomes.[56]

Uses of Inhaled Nitric Oxide in Adult Patients with Cardiopulmonary Diseases

Pulmonary Vasoreactivity Testing in the Cardiac Catheterization Laboratory. Demonstration of a positive response to vasodilating agents in patients with pulmonary hypertension correlates with an improved long-term clinical outcome and has been used to guide medical therapy (see Chapter 60).[57] Although a number of vasodilators, including intravenous prostacyclin and calcium channel blockers, have been used for diagnostic testing during cardiac catheterization, such circulating agents produce systemic vasodilation and increase intrapulmonary right-to-left shunting.[58] In contrast, recent studies indicate that inhaled NO is a safe and effective agent to determine the pulmonary circulation's capacity for vasodilation in pediatric[59] and adult patients[60,61] with pulmonary hypertension. In these patients, selective pulmonary vasodilation during NO breathing correlates with a subsequent response to oral and systemically active vasodilators.[62,63] Preoperative hemodynamic evaluation with oxygen and inhaled NO as opposed to a test with oxygen alone is suggested to more accurately identify patients with pulmonary hypertension who will be the most appropriate candidates for corrective cardiac surgery or transplantation.[64] In 1998, inhaled NO was the primary vasodilator used to test pulmonary vascular responsiveness in 32% of U.S. tertiary hospitals.[65] According to a survey in 2000, 94% of pediatric cardiologists consider inhaled NO to be a clinically proven agent to test pulmonary vasoreactivity in the cardiac catheterization laboratory.[66]

Treatment of Chronic Pulmonary Hypertension with Inhaled Nitric Oxide. Even though continuous administration of intravenous prostacyclin (epoprostenol) is associated with improved survival and exercise tolerance,[67] indwelling central venous catheters carry the risk of bacteremia. The feasibility of an ambulatory NO delivery system has been reported in a small number of patients with primary pulmonary hypertension.[68,69] The safety and efficacy of long-term domiciliary NO inhalation require investigation in larger patient populations. On the other hand, clinical trials with newer orally active vasodilators (bosentan,[70] beraprost,[71] and sildenafil[72]) in patients with primary pulmonary hypertension have reported promising results. Although these orally active medications are more convenient for ambulatory patients than intravenous or inhalation therapies are, inhaled NO may prove more effective than these agents. In addition, because these agents may cause systemic hypotension, inhaled NO may prove safer.

Treatment of Cardiogenic Shock Caused by Right Ventricular Myocardial Infarction. RV injury and dysfunction may complicate inferior myocardial infarction (MI) caused by right coronary artery occlusion. If coronary revascularization is delayed, cardiogenic shock may develop despite preserved LV function and is associated with a high frequency of mortality. In a small series of patients with cardiogenic shock caused by right ventricular myocardial infarction (RVMI), Inglessis and colleagues reported that unloading the right ventricle by breathing 80 ppm NO acutely improved the cardiac index by approximately 25%.[73] In RVMI patients with a patent foramen ovale, treatment with inhaled NO markedly reduced right-to-left shunting and improved systemic oxygenation. Further studies are required to determine whether NO inhalation will decrease the morbidity and mortality associated with RVMI.

Acute Respiratory Distress Syndrome in Adults. In clinical studies of patients with severe ARDS, inhaled NO has been shown to produce selective pulmonary vasodilation,[20] decrease pulmonary capillary pressure[74] and pulmonary transvascular albumin flux,[75] and improve oxygenation (see Chapters 92 and 93).[20] Although these clinical studies, as well as a number of studies in animal models of acute lung injury, have demonstrated a physiologic benefit of inhaled NO therapy, subsequent clinical trials reported disappointing results. Two pilot trials were conducted in the United States. Both were randomized, unblinded, controlled, single-center studies with small sample sizes ($n = 40$ and $n = 30$) and demonstrated only transient improvements in oxygenation during the first 24 hours of treatment but no effect of inhaled NO on the mortality rate.[22,76] Subsequently, a randomized, double-blind, placebo-controlled trial of 177 patients (average entry $PaO_2/FIO_2 \approx 129$ mm Hg) treated with various concentrations of inhaled NO (1.25 to 80 ppm) versus placebo failed to find a difference in either the mortality rate or the number of days alive and off mechanical ventilation.[77] A prospective, randomized, unblinded European multicenter trial of inhaled NO in patients with acute lung injury ($n = 286$, average entry $PaO_2/FIO_2 \approx 105$ mm Hg) also demonstrated no effect on mortality or the duration of mechanical ventilation; however, the frequency of progression to severe respiratory failure from milder respiratory failure was decreased by inhaled NO.[78] Although renal failure was identified as a possible adverse effect of NO inhalation in the European trial, this finding remains unexplained and has not been confirmed in other clinical trials.

Several possible explanations why the physiologically beneficial effects of inhaled NO in ARDS were not translated into clinical outcome benefits have been offered: (1) because the majority of patients dying of ARDS suffer from multiple organ failure, the beneficial effects of a lung-selective therapy such as inhaled NO (e.g., improvement in gas exchange and reduced pulmonary artery pressure) may not alter the overall survival rate; (2) the beneficial effects of NO inhalation may be offset by toxic effects such as the formation of peroxynitrite in the presence of inflammation-produced superoxide; and (3) inhalation of NO has a narrow therapeutic range, and the effective dose may have changed over time as patients and their disease states vary.[79] Whether the subgroup of severely hypoxemic ARDS patients will respond more favorably to inhaled NO and have an improved clinical outcome has not yet been conclusively resolved.[80]

Chronic Obstructive Pulmonary Disease. Severe chronic obstructive pulmonary disease (COPD) is frequently complicated by pulmonary hypertension and hypoxemia. Systemic hypoxemia in COPD is primarily caused by ventilation-perfusion mismatching and not by intrapulmonary right-to-left shunting (as in ARDS). Hypoxic pulmonary vasoconstriction diverts venous blood flow to better ventilated lung regions, thereby improving arterial oxygenation. Although inhaled NO is a more potent pulmonary vasodilator than oxygen in patients with COPD, breathing inhaled NO admixed with air may produce vasodilation of poorly ventilated regions of the obstructed lung without receiving sufficient oxygen replenishment. Increasing blood flow with inhaled NO to these hypoventilated lung areas can reduce the transcutaneous arterial oxygen tension[81] and PaO_2.[82] However, when NO gas is breathed in combination with modest oxygen enrichment (1 L/min via facemask),[83] PaO_2 is increased to a greater extent than with oxygen therapy alone. Along these lines, a recent controlled, prospective randomized trial demonstrated that the combined use of supplemental oxygen and inhaled NO for a period of 3 months via a portable inspiratory pulsing device caused greater improvement in pulmonary hemodynamics than supplemental oxygen alone did without worsening the oxygenation of COPD patients.[84] Further studies are needed to determine the effect of long-term ambulatory breathing of pulsed NO and oxygen on the quality of life and mortality rate of patients with severe COPD.

Treatment of Perioperative Pulmonary Hypertension with Inhaled Nitric Oxide

Coronary Artery Bypass Grafting. Pulmonary hypertension often complicates the management of patients during and after cardiac surgery involving cardiopulmonary bypass (CPB) (see Chapter 60). A number of uncontrolled studies have demonstrated that 20 to 40 ppm inhaled NO effectively decreases pulmonary artery pressure after coronary artery bypass grafting (CABG), even in patients without significant preoperative pulmonary hypertension.[85-87] Although these results suggest a role for inhaled NO in treating transient pulmonary hypertension after CPB, whether inhaled NO can improve the clinically important outcomes of patients undergoing CABG is unknown. A large prospective randomized trial would be needed to define a role for inhaled NO in this patient population.

Congenital Heart Disease. Postoperative pulmonary hypertensive crises are an important cause of morbidity and mortality after congenital heart surgery[88,89] and may be precipitated by diminished NO bioavailability because of endothelial dysfunction.[30,90] PAH and subsequent heart failure are associated with certain types of congenital heart defects, particularly those characterized by increased pulmonary blood flow (e.g., ventricular septal defect and atrioventricular canal). Inhaled NO has been reported to ameliorate the postoperative pulmonary hypertension of congenital heart disease[91,92] and decrease the need for postoperative ECMO.[93] In a randomized double-blind study, Miller and colleagues examined the effects of the prophylactic use of inhaled NO in high-risk infants undergoing congenital heart surgery.[94] One hundred twenty-four patients were randomized before surgery, and inclusion in the study did not depend on the presence of pulmonary hypertension. They reported that when compared with placebo, infants who inhaled 10 ppm NO continuously after surgery until just before extubation had fewer pulmonary hypertensive crises and a shorter time to eligibility for extubation. These studies indicate that inhaled NO safely decreases postoperative pulmonary hypertension in patients after surgery for congenital heart disease. Further studies are needed to test if inhaled NO should be used in all patients after CPB for congenital heart disease surgery to decrease their perioperative morbidity and mortality.

Valvular Heart Disease. Patients with chronic mitral valve disease may have preoperative pulmonary hypertension caused by retrograde transmission of elevated left atrial pressure (see Chapter 60). After mitral valve repair or replacement, pulmonary vascular remodeling and vasoconstriction may persist or slowly decrease. It has been reported that the vasodilatory response to inhaled NO is variable in patients with valvular heart disease.[86,95] The variability in dilator response is likely to be related to the balance between pulmonary vascular remodeling and active vasoconstriction. Treatment with inhaled NO after repair of valvular heart disease can relieve the vasoconstrictor component of pulmonary hypertension in these patients.[96] Whether inhaled NO can alter the clinical outcome of patients after valvular heart surgery is unknown.

Cardiac Transplantation. Pulmonary hypertension in cardiac transplant recipients is a major cause of right heart failure and early death. Goals in the management of acute RV failure include preservation of coronary perfusion through maintenance of systemic blood pressure and reduction of RV afterload by decreasing PVR.[97] In contrast to therapy with intravenous vasodilators, which often cause systemic hypotension, inhaled NO has been shown in a small group of patients to selectively reduce PVR and enhance RV stroke work after cardiac transplantation.[98] A positive pulmonary vasodilator response to inhalation of NO has been used as a criterion to select patients for cardiac transplantation.[99]

Insertion of Left Ventricular Assist Devices. RV dysfunction occurs in 20% to 50% of patients after insertion of a left ventricular assist device (LVAD).[100] The ability of the right ventricle to pump sufficient quantities of blood to the LVAD is critically related to the intrinsic contractility of the right ventricle and RV afterload, which is influenced by PVR. PVR is usually elevated in long-standing congestive heart failure and can be further increased in the early postoperative period by the effects of CPB. Inhaled NO has been shown to effectively decrease PVR in the setting of RV dysfunction after LVAD insertion.[101] A trial of inhaled NO is recommended before consideration of implantation of an RV assist device because this invasive procedure may be avoided if there is a salutary response to inhaled NO.[102] In a randomized, double-blind trial, Argenziano and coworkers demonstrated the hemodynamic benefits of inhaled NO (decreased pulmonary artery pressure and increased LVAD flow) in LVAD recipients with pulmonary hypertension.[103]

Treatment of Pulmonary Ischemia-Reperfusion Injury. Ischemia-reperfusion (I-R) injury is one of the major causes of early graft failure after lung transplantation. Adhesion and sequestration of activated leukocytes by activated pulmonary endothelium is believed to be an important mechanism of I-R injury. NO possesses anti-inflammatory properties, and inhaled NO has been shown to attenuate pulmonary I-R injury in preclinical studies.[104] Although two uncontrolled clinical studies suggested that inhaled NO may prevent lung I/R injury,[105,106] a small randomized, placebo-controlled study demonstrated that inhaling 20 ppm NO commencing 10 minutes after reperfusion did not affect the physiologic or clinical outcome of patients after lung transplantation.[107] Additional studies are required to define the therapeutic role of inhaled NO in patients in whom I-R injury develops after lung transplantation.

Experimental Methods to Improve the Efficacy of Inhaled Nitric Oxide

In an important fraction of patients, inhalation of NO fails to reduce PVR, improve oxygenation, or both. Moreover, because the pulmonary vasodilator effects of inhaled NO disappear after NO is discontinued, continuous therapy is required. Use of the lowest effective concentration of NO may decrease the risk for methemoglobinemia, augment matching of ventilation and perfusion, and theoretically, minimize lung toxicity. Based on an understanding of the NO/cGMP signal transduction system, several research groups have developed strategies to augment or prolong the efficacy of inhaled NO (or both). For example, inhibition of PDE5, the cGMP-specific PDE, by intravenous administration of zaprinast prolonged the pulmonary vasodilator effects of NO inhalation in awake adult lambs with U46619-induced pulmonary hypertension[108] and augmented the effects of inhaled NO in perinatal lambs with pulmonary hypertension induced by prenatal ligation of the ductus arteriosus.[109] Delivery of PDE5 inhibitors by inhalation also augmented and prolonged the efficacy of inhaled NO in adult lambs.[110,111] Steinhorn and colleagues have reported that reduction of NO scavenging by superoxide via superoxide dismutase can augment the efficacy of inhaled NO in neonatal pulmonary hypertension.[112] In studies of awake adult lambs with U46619-induced pulmonary hypertension, Evgenov and coauthors reported that agents that sensitize sGC to NO can augment and prolong the pulmonary vasodilator effects of inhaled NO.[113,114]

These observations in animal models have been extended to patients with pulmonary diseases. For example, sildenafil augmented and prolonged the pulmonary vasodilator effects of inhaled NO in patients with PAH secondary to pulmonary vascular disease[115] or congestive heart failure.[116] Importantly, sildenafil was also found to attenuate the pulmonary vascular rebound associated with discontinuing NO inhalation[117] and may facilitate weaning from NO gas in patients with cardiovascular instability.

Extrapulmonary Effects of Breathing Nitric Oxide

Because breathing NO decreased PVR without altering systemic blood pressure, it was initially proposed that the action of inhaled NO was limited to the lungs. It was hypothesized that any NO reaching the bloodstream would be rapidly scavenged by oxygenated Hb and lead to the production of nitrate and MetHb.[2] However, as early as 1993, evidence began to accumulate that inhalation of NO could inhibit platelet function.[54] Subsequently, studies describing a wide range of systemic effects of breathing NO were published, as summarized recently by McMahon and Doctor[118] and highlighted in Table 31-1. In this section, the ability of NO inhalation to decrease I-R injury is reviewed, and circumstances in which breathing NO can modulate systemic vascular tone are discussed. In addition, potential mechanisms by which inhaled NO may exert its systemic effects are outlined.

Inhaled Nitric Oxide and Platelet Function

The ability of NO-donor compounds to inhibit platelet function is well known, but the therapeutic application of their antithrombotic effects is limited by systemic hypotension. In 1993, Hogman and colleagues first reported that breathing NO (30 ppm) could prolong the bleeding time in rabbits and healthy human subjects.[54] Subsequent reports from multiple research groups presented conflicting data, with some investigators reporting that breathing NO increases the bleeding time in neonates and adults

Table 31-1 Biological Effects of Breathing Nitric Oxide with Selected Physiologic Impacts and Potential Therapeutic Applications

Biologic Effect	Impact	Therapeutic Application	References*
Pulmonary vasodilation	Reduction in pulmonary artery pressure	Pulmonary arterial hypertension	2
	Decrease in extrapulmonary right-to-left shunting and improved systemic oxygenation	Pulmonary hypertension of the newborn and congenital heart disease	3, 4, 91
	Decrease in RV afterload	RV failure after LVAD placement	103
		RVMI complicated by cardiogenic shock	73
		RV failure after cardiac surgery	85
Improved matching of lung ventilation and perfusion	Increased systemic oxygenation	Acute lung injury/pneumonia	20, 77, 78
		Chronic pulmonary disease	84
Pulmonary vascular and alveolar development	Decreased vascular SMC hyperplasia and increased alveolarization in the injured developing lung	Prevent or ameliorate pulmonary hypertension in infants with congenital heart disease and chronic lung disease in premature infants	32, 33, 39, 40
Systemic effects of breathing NO	Platelet inhibition	Decrease thrombosis after coronary thrombolysis (dogs)	54, 119
	Leukocyte inhibition	Improve mesenteric blood flow after ischemia and reperfusion (cats)	120
		Decrease infarct size in cardiac ischemia-reperfusion injury	121, 122
	Oxidization of extraerythrocytic hemoglobin	Decrease hemolysis-induced vasoconstriction and renal dysfunction (dogs)	123

*Representative references are included.
LVAD, left ventricular assist device; NO, nitric oxide; RV, right ventricular; RVMI, RV myocardial infarction; SMC, smooth muscle cell.
From Bloch KD, Ichinose F, Robert JD, Zapol WM: Inhaled NO as a therapeutic agent. Cardiovasc Res 75:339-348, 2007, with permission.

and others reporting that NO inhalation does not alter either the bleeding time or platelet function. Prolongation of the bleeding time raised the possibility of increased hemorrhagic complications in patients treated with inhaled NO, particularly neonates at increased risk for intracranial hemorrhage. On the other hand, the observation that breathing NO could decrease platelet function led other investigators to examine in animal models whether NO inhalation could be used to treat vascular diseases associated with platelet activation. For example, Semigran's group reported that in a canine model of coronary thrombosis after thrombolysis, breathing 20 and 80 ppm NO decreased platelet-mediated thrombosis,[119] an effect that was augmented by coadministration of inhibitors of type 5 PDE.[124] In addition, Lee and coworkers observed that breathing 80 ppm NO for 1 or 2 weeks decreased neointimal formation in rat carotid arteries subjected to balloon injury.[125] In both models, breathing NO did not prolong the bleeding time or cause systemic hypotension.

Inhaled Nitric Oxide and Ischemia-Reperfusion Injury of Extrapulmonary Organs

Observations that NO can form stable, biologically active adducts with protein thiol constituents led Kubes' group to examine whether inhaled NO could be used to deliver NO to peripheral tissues.[120] Studying postcapillary venules from cats subjected to intestinal I-R, these investigators observed that breathing 80 ppm NO, but not 20 ppm, prevented the reduction in blood flow, the increase in leukocyte activation (rolling, adherence, and migration), and vascular leakage. The investigators also observed that breathing NO prevented the arteriolar constriction and neutrophil activation induced by the administration of N^G-nitro-L-arginine methyl ester (L-NAME), a NOS inhibitor. Interestingly, because inhaled NO did not alter neutrophil activation or vascular leakage in endotoxin-challenged cats, the investigators proposed that inhaled NO does not affect peripheral tissues with abundant NO (produced by inducible NOS). In contrast, Neviere and coauthors reported that breathing NO (10 ppm) decreased adhesion of leukocytes to the mesenteric venular endothelium of endotoxin-challenged rats.[126] Furthermore, breathing NO prevented endotoxin-induced cardiac dysfunction and leukocyte accumulation. In a subsequent report, Kubes and associates reported that in contrast to NO-donor compounds, inhaled NO did not prevent the increase in mucosal permeability induced by intestinal I-R and suggested that the effects of breathing NO were limited to the vascular compartment.[127]

Based on these observations, Guery and colleagues evaluated the ability of breathing NO to preserve cardiac function after myocardial I-R injury.[128] Hearts from rats that had breathed air with or without 10 ppm NO for 4 hours were isolated and perfused. Coronary perfusion was stopped for 30 minutes, followed by reperfusion for 40 minutes. The investigators observed that pretreatment with inhaled NO led to improved systolic and diastolic function after ischemia and reperfusion. These findings were extended by Hataishi and colleagues, who examined the ability of breathing NO to decrease cardiac I-R injury in intact mice.[121] They observed that breathing NO for the final 20 minutes of ischemia and for 24 hours after reperfusion decreased MI size and improved systolic and diastolic function. Breathing 80 ppm NO decreased MI size similarly after 30, 60, or 120 minutes of ischemia. Breathing 40 and 80 ppm NO decreased myocardial I-R injury equally, but 20 ppm was not effective. Breathing NO decreased cardiac neutrophil accumulation, and leukocyte depletion prevented the beneficial effects of NO on MI size. Observations in rodents have recently been extended to a clinically relevant porcine model of cardiac I-R injury; Liu and colleagues reported that in pigs subjected to 50 minutes of cardiac ischemia and 4 hours of reperfusion, breathing 80 ppm NO decreased MI size and improved myocardial perfusion.[122] The ability of inhaled NO to decrease cardiac I-R injury is further suggested by the observation that breathing NO decreased the release of cardiac enzymes in a small series of patients undergoing CPB.[129] Taken together with the observations of Fox-Robichaud and coworkers,[120] these results suggest that when inhaled, the concentrations of NO required to elicit systemic effects (in vivo) are greater than those required to directly elicit pulmonary vascular effects. Based on these considerations, a randomized clinical trial has been initiated to test whether breathing 80 ppm can decrease MI size in patients with ST-segment elevation MI.

Inhaled Nitric Oxide and Systemic Vascular Tone

Whether breathing NO can modulate systemic vascular tone remains controversial. Clinically significant systemic hypotension has not been observed in adults and babies with a wide variety of disorders treated with NO concentrations of up to 80 ppm. However, breathing 80 ppm NO has been reported to attenuate the ability of L-NAME to increase blood pressure in cats.[127] Cannon and colleagues reported that breathing 80 ppm NO increased forearm blood flow in healthy subjects treated by intrabrachial artery infusion of the NOS inhibitor L-NMMA.[130] In contrast, Hataishi and colleagues observed that breathing NO did not decrease SVR in L-NAME–treated mice or in mice congenitally deficient in NOS3.[131]

The ability of inhaled NO to decrease SVR is perhaps clearest in the case of the endothelial dysfunction associated with hemolysis. Studying dogs with free water–induced hemolysis, Minneci and associates observed that the presence of Hb in plasma induced hypertension and decreased creatinine clearance, probably via scavenging of endothelium-derived NO.[123] Breathing 80 ppm NO attenuated the hemolysis-induced hypertension and renal dysfunction by oxidizing free Hb to MetHb and preventing the scavenging of endogenous NO. The authors proposed that inhalation of NO may attenuate the hypertension, vascular disease, and prothrombotic state characteristic of diseases associated with hemolysis, such as sickle cell anemia.

How Does Inhaled Nitric Oxide Exert Its Systemic Effects?

With the exception of the case of hemolysis, the mechanisms by which NO, once inhaled, is able to induce responses in the periphery remain incompletely understood. One hypothesis is that during NO inhalation, blood cells, including white blood cells and platelets, are exposed to NO before scavenging of the gas by red blood cells and that NO-exposed blood cells are responsible for the systemic effects of inhaled NO. For example, exposure of platelets to NO in the pulmonary circulation may inhibit their activation at the site of vascular injury. However, this hypothesis does not fully account for the dilator effects of breathing NO seen in some vascular beds or the observations of Fox-Robichaud and coworkers,[120] who reported that inhaled NO did not alter the ability of feline blood leukocytes to bind to immobilized platelet monomers ex vivo.

An alternative hypothesis is that some of the inhaled NO escapes scavenging by Hb and is carried in a stable, bioavailable form to the periphery. Loscalzo's group proposed that endogenously synthesized NO reacts with low- and high-molecular-weight thiols in blood, including serum albumin.[132,133] These *S*-nitrosothiols can deliver NO to tissues distant from the site of its synthesis. Stamler and colleagues[132] observed that NO reacts with the thiol group on Cys93 of the Hb β-chain and that *S*-nitrosylation of Hb (SNO-Hb) is dependent on the oxygen tension enabling erythrocytes to load Hb in the rich oxygen environment of the lungs and release low-molecular-weight *S*-nitrosothiols in the relatively hypoxic periphery (reviewed by McMahan and Doctor[118]). NO can be oxidized in blood to nitrite, which regenerates NO in the presence of nitrite reductases, including deoxyhemoglobin (reviewed by Gladwin and colleagues[134]). Erythrocyte SNO-Hb and nitrite have both been implicated as potential mediators of the systemic vasodilation induced by tissue hypoxia. NO may also react with other plasma species that are subsequently capable of regenerating NO, including *N*-nitrosamines, iron-nitrosyls, and nitrated lipids.

Even before it was appreciated that breathing NO could selectively dilate the pulmonary vasculature, several research groups examined the metabolic fate of inhaled NO. In 1975, Oda and colleagues reported that inhalation of NO led to the formation of nitrosyl-Hb in the blood of mice, rats, and rabbits.[135] In 1987, Yoshida and Kasama reported that breathing ^{15}NO (145 ppm for 123 minutes) led to the formation of nitrosyl-Hb, nitrite, and nitrate.[136] More recently, Cannon and coworkers found that in healthy adults breathing 80 ppm NO, nitrosyl-Hb concentrations increased markedly, whereas nitrite increased modestly.[130] Arterial concentrations of both products were greater than venous levels, thus suggesting consumption in peripheral tissues. Cannon and colleagues did not detect an increase in plasma *S*-nitrosothiols or SNO-Hb. In contrast, Ng and coauthors reported that in cats, breathing 80 ppm NO increased plasma levels of *S*-nitrosoalbumin and nitrite, both of which were further increased in the setting of intestinal I-R.[137] Arterial levels of *S*-nitrosoalbumin were higher than venous levels, whereas the converse was true for nitrite levels, which suggested that *S*-nitrosoalbumin was consumed in the periphery and nitrite was generated.

The potential importance of nitrite as a mediator of inhaled NO's impact on I-R injury was highlighted in recent studies of Duranski and colleagues.[138] They observed that small increases in blood nitrite levels were sufficient to decrease I-R injury in the liver and heart. Moreover, in studies of murine I-R injury, Hataishi and coauthors[121] reported that breathing NO increased nitrite concentrations in plasma and blood to levels similar to those demonstrated to be effective by Duranski and associates.

Controversy regarding the identity of the circulating NO-derived products whose levels increase during inhalation of NO may be attributable to differences in the methods used to detect these products. Nonetheless, there appears to be a consensus that bioavailable NO derivatives contribute to the effects of breathing NO on the periphery. However, many questions remain, including the following: Do NO-derived products accumulate in tissues during the inhalation of NO? Are cGMP-dependent or cGMP-independent mechanisms responsible for the systemic effects of inhaled NO?

Safety Issues and Method of Administration

Prolonged inhalation of low levels of NO appears to be safe. The major clinical toxicity is due to the formation of NO_2 and methemoglobinemia. Nitrogen dioxide is rapidly converted to nitric acid in aqueous solution (acid rain) and is highly toxic to the respiratory tract. Increased airway reactivity has been reported

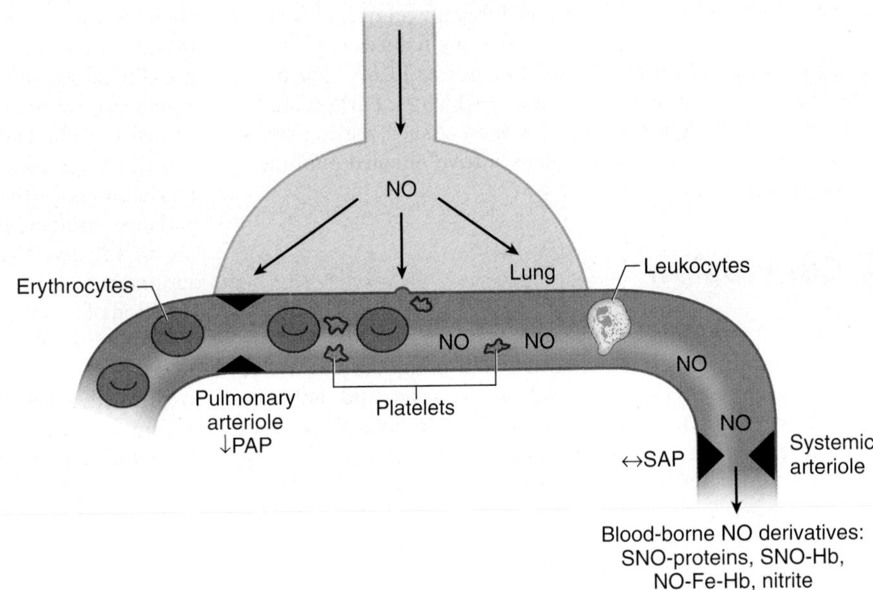

Figure 31-6 Inhaled nitric oxide (NO) is a selective pulmonary vasodilator with actions on the systemic vasculature. A schematic of an alveolar-capillary unit is presented in which the ability of inhaled NO to dilate pulmonary arterioles and reduce pulmonary artery pressure (PAP) is highlighted. Although inhaled NO does not dilate systemic arterioles or alter systemic arterial pressure (SAP) under normal conditions, inhaled NO does have systemic effects (described in text) that may be mediated by circulating cells exposed to NO in the lungs and blood-borne NO derivatives: SNO-proteins or S-nitroso proteins including SNO-albumin; SNO-Hb or S-nitroso-Hb (nitrosylated on Cys93 of the β-chain); NO-Fe-Hb or nitrosyl-Hb; and nitrite. *(From Bloch KD, Ichinose F, Robert JD, Zapol WM: Inhaled NO as a therapeutic agent. Cardiovasc Res 75:339-348, 2007, with permission.)*

in humans after exposure to as low as 1.5 ppm NO_2.[139] At higher inhaled NO_2 concentrations, pulmonary edema is the major toxicologic effect[140] and can result in rapid death after inhalation.[141]

Inhaled NO can combine with Hb to form nitrosyl-Hb, which is rapidly oxidized to MetHb. Rates of uptake and release of NO from ferrous (Fe^{2+}) Hb are 10^5- to 10^6-fold greater than those of oxygen. Tissue hypoxia can be produced at excessive circulating MetHb concentrations. In general, cyanosis does not appear until MetHb levels approach 15% to 20%, and clinical symptoms of hypoxia (such as fatigue and dyspnea) become significant at MetHb levels above 30% of the Hb concentration.[142] The enzyme MetHb reductase rapidly converts MetHb to Hb in red blood cells. Because neonates have reduced activity of this enzyme, they are at greater risk than adults for the development of significant methemoglobinemia after the inhalation of high levels of NO for prolonged periods.[142] Blood MetHb concentrations and inspired NO_2 concentrations were frequently monitored in clinical trials of inhaled NO in adults and neonates.[6,77,143,144] In a large number of adult (n = 120) and newborn patients (n = 351) pooled from several clinical trials, significant methemoglobinemia or NO_2 formation was uncommon in patients breathing NO at doses ranging from 1.25 to 80 ppm (see the summary table in the article by Steudel and coworkers).[19] If MetHb or NO_2 levels increased above predetermined limits, the concentration of inhaled NO was decreased. Discontinuation of NO administration because of excessive NO_2 or MetHb formation was necessary in only 3 of 471 patients (0.6%).

Inhaled NO has been demonstrated to be a selective pulmonary vasodilator in heart failure patients, although breathing NO can be accompanied by an elevation in LV filling pressure in patients with severe LV dysfunction.[58,145] Taken together with the in vitro experimental evidence of a direct negative inotropic action of NO,[146,147] these clinical observations led to concern that inhaled NO may exert clinically important negative inotropic effects in patients with impaired LV function. However, investigators learned that the elevation in LV filling pressure that occurs with breathing NO is due to the augmentation of filling into a relatively noncompliant left ventricle and is not caused by a negative inotropic effect.[148] This concept is supported by an observation in heart failure patients with mechanical LV assistance that inhaled NO increases LV filling pressure only when cardiac output is not assisted.[149] Nonetheless, it is important to be aware of the possibility that inhaled NO can produce pulmonary vasodilation and may overwhelm a failing left ventricle, thereby producing pulmonary edema.

Other Inhaled Pulmonary Vasodilators

Successful clinical use of inhaled NO as a selective pulmonary vasodilator prompted the search for other alternatives, at least in part because of the significant cost of inhaled NO therapy (e.g., $3000/day with a $12,000 monthly cap) in the United States.[150] A wide variety of intravenous vasodilators were clinically tested via the inhaled route, including prostacyclin (prostaglandin I_2 [PGI_2]),[151] milrinone,[152] nitroglycerin,[153] sodium nitroprusside,[154] PGE_1,[155] and iloprost, a stable analog of PGI_2.[156] It was expected that inhalation of intravenous vasodilators would maximize drug levels in the lung while minimizing their systemic effects (Fig. 31-6). Although encouraging results have been reported by some studies, especially with inhaled PGI_2 and iloprost, at the time of this writing, the efficacy and safety profile of these inhaled vasodilators have not been established. For instance, even though very brief exposure to inhaled PGI_2 has been reported to decrease PVR similar to inhaled NO,[157,158] PGI_2 is known to cause hypotension when large doses are inhaled.[158] The plasma half-life of PGI_2 is sufficiently long (5 minutes) to allow systemic effects, and systemic arterial levels of an active metabolite have been measured during the inhalation of even small doses of PGI_2. Furthermore, PGI_2 must be dissolved in a highly viscous and basic glycine diluent (pH = 10.5) that is associated with tracheitis,[159] interstitial pneumonia,[160] and ventilator valve malfunction.[161] Finally, although the drug cost associated with inhaled PGI_2 is claimed to be lower than that of inhaled NO, a robust cost comparison taking into account the impact of prolonged therapy on overall cost has not been done. For example, if one therapy reduces ICU stay by 1 day or the need for an RV assist device or ECMO perfusion, the difference in drug cost would be incidental. Further studies appropriately designed to address these issues are needed to better define the role of other "less selective" inhaled pulmonary vasodilators.

Conclusion

Inhaled NO is the first vasodilator to produce truly selective pulmonary vasodilation. It is characterized by pulmonary vasoselectivity and it also raises arterial oxygenation and enhances pulmonary ventilation-perfusion matching by increasing blood flow to ventilated regions of the lung. A large number of laboratory and clinical research studies have been performed to delineate its biochemistry, physiology, side effects, and clinical efficacy in various diseases of children and adults. Nearly simultaneously, the clinical use of inhaled NO has become widespread. It is estimated that twenty thousand patients are treated with inhaled NO annually in the United States. During the past 16 years, inhaled NO has been used to treat pulmonary hypertension and hypoxemia in more than a hundred thousand pediatric and adult patients worldwide. For many it is lifesaving. The experimental use of inhaled NO continues to be a unique and fascinating approach to studying and treating diseases as diverse as acute rejection of a transplanted lung and sickle cell crisis. In evaluating this complex field, it is critical that our view not become colored by a single study of a particular disease state. As with most medical advances, it is the accumulation of a wide-ranging body of clinical research that will eventually determine the place of NO inhalation therapy in our therapeutic armamentarium for many diseases.

References

1. Vlahakes GJ, Turley K, Hoffman JI: The pathophysiology of failure in acute right ventricular hypertension: Hemodynamic and biochemical correlations. Circulation 63:87-95, 1981.
2. Frostell C, Fratacci MD, Wain JC, et al: Inhaled nitric oxide. A selective pulmonary vasodilator reversing hypoxic pulmonary vasoconstriction. Circulation 83:2038-2047, 1991.
3. Roberts JD Jr, Polaner DM, Lang P, Zapol WM: Inhaled nitric oxide in persistent pulmonary hypertension of the newborn. Lancet 340:818-819, 1992.
4. Kinsella JP, Neish SR, Shaffer E, Abman SH: Low-dose inhalation nitric oxide in persistent pulmonary hypertension of the newborn. Lancet 340:819-820, 1992.
5. Kinsella JP, Truog WE, Walsh WF, et al: Randomized, multicenter trial of inhaled nitric oxide and high-frequency oscillatory ventilation in severe, persistent pulmonary hypertension of the newborn. J Pediatr 131:55-62, 1997.
6. Roberts JD Jr, Fineman JR, Morin FC III, et al: Inhaled nitric oxide and persistent pulmonary hypertension of the newborn. The Inhaled Nitric Oxide Study Group. N Engl J Med 336:605-610, 1997.
7. The Neonatal Inhaled Nitric Oxide Study Group: Inhaled nitric oxide in full-term and nearly full-term infants with hypoxic respiratory failure. N Engl J Med 336:597-604, 1997.
8. Clark RH, Kueser TJ, Walker MW, et al: Low-dose nitric oxide therapy for persistent pulmonary hypertension of the newborn. Clinical Inhaled Nitric Oxide Research Group. N Engl J Med 342:469-474, 2000.
9. Fukuto JM: Chemistry of nitric oxide: Biologically relevant aspects. Adv Pharmacol 34:1-15, 1995.
10. Mourgeon E, Levesque E, Duveau C, et al: Factors influencing indoor concentrations of nitric oxide in a Parisian intensive care unit. Am J Respir Crit Care Med 156:1692-1695, 1997.
11. Norman V, Keith CH: Nitrogen oxides in tobacco smoke. Nature 205:915-917, 1965.
12. Phillips ML, Hall TA, Sekar K, Tomey JL: Assessment of medical personnel exposure to nitrogen oxides during inhaled nitric oxide treatment of neonatal and pediatric patients. Pediatrics 104: 1095-1100, 1999.
13. Rybalkin SD, Yan C, Bornfeldt KE, Beavo JA: Cyclic GMP phosphodiesterases and regulation of smooth muscle function. Circ Res 93:280-291, 2003.
14. Dupuy PM, Shore SA, Drazen JM, et al: Bronchodilator action of inhaled nitric oxide in guinea pigs. J Clin Invest 90:421-428, 1992.
15. Kacmarek RM, Ripple R, Cockrill BA, et al: Inhaled nitric oxide. A bronchodilator in mild asthmatics with methacholine-induced bronchospasm. Am J Respir Crit Care Med 153:128-135, 1996.
16. Kinsella JP, Parker TA, Galan H, et al: Effects of inhaled nitric oxide on pulmonary edema and lung neutrophil accumulation in severe experimental hyaline membrane disease. Pediatr Res 41:457-463, 1997.
17. Roberts JD Jr, Chiche JD, Weimann J, et al: Nitric oxide inhalation decreases pulmonary artery remodeling in the injured lungs of rat pups. Circ Res 87:140-145, 2000.
18. Hare JM, Stamler JS: NO/redox disequilibrium in the failing heart and cardiovascular system. J Clin Invest 115:509-517, 2005.
19. Steudel W, Hurford WE, Zapol WM: Inhaled nitric oxide: Basic biology and clinical applications. Anesthesiology 91:1090-1121, 1999.
20. Rossaint R, Falke KJ, Lopez F, et al: Inhaled nitric oxide for the adult respiratory distress syndrome. N Engl J Med 328:399-405, 1993.
21. Sheridan RL, Zapol WM, Ritz RH, Tompkins RG: Low-dose inhaled nitric oxide in acutely burned children with profound respiratory failure. Surgery 126:856-862, 1999.
22. Michael JR, Barton RG, Saffle JR, et al: Inhaled nitric oxide versus conventional therapy: Effect on oxygenation in ARDS. Am J Respir Crit Care Med 157:1372-1380, 1998.
23. Abman SH, Chatfield BA, Rodman DM, et al: Maturational changes in endothelium-derived relaxing factor activity of ovine pulmonary arteries in vitro. Am J Physiol 260:L280-L285, 1991.
24. Bloch KD, Filippov G, Sanchez LS, et al: Pulmonary soluble guanylate cyclase, a nitric oxide receptor, is increased during the perinatal period. Am J Physiol 272:L400-L406, 1997.
25. Kawai N, Bloch DB, Filippov G, et al: Constitutive endothelial nitric oxide synthase gene expression is regulated during lung development. Am J Physiol 268:L589-L595, 1995.
26. Abman SH, Chatfield BA, Hall SL, McMurtry IF: Role of endothelium-derived relaxing factor during transition of pulmonary circulation at birth. Am J Physiol 259:H1921-H1927, 1990.
27. Moore P, Velvis H, Fineman JR, et al: EDRF inhibition attenuates the increase in pulmonary blood flow due to oxygen ventilation in fetal lambs. J Appl Physiol 73:2151-2157, 1992.
28. Shaul PW, Yuhanna IS, German Z, et al: Pulmonary endothelial NO synthase gene expression is decreased in fetal lambs with pulmonary hypertension. Am J Physiol 272:L1005-L1012, 1997.
29. Steinhorn RH, Russell JA, Morin FC III: Disruption of cGMP production in pulmonary arteries isolated from fetal lambs with pulmonary hypertension. Am J Physiol 268:H1483-H1489, 1995.
30. Celermajer DS, Cullen S, Deanfield JE: Impairment of endothelium-dependent pulmonary artery relaxation in children with congenital heart disease and abnormal pulmonary hemodynamics. Circulation 87:440-446, 1993.
31. Balasubramaniam V, Tang JR, Maxey A, et al: Mild hypoxia impairs alveolarization in the endothelial nitric oxide synthase–deficient mouse. Am J Physiol Lung Cell Mol Physiol 284:L964-L971, 2003.
32. Balasubramaniam V, Maxey AM, Morgan DB, et al: Inhaled NO restores lung structure in eNOS-deficient mice recovering from neonatal hypoxia. Am J Physiol Lung Cell Mol Physiol 291:L119-L127, 2006.
33. Roberts JD Jr, Roberts CT, Jones RC, et al: Continuous nitric oxide inhalation reduces pulmonary arterial structural changes, right ventricular hypertrophy, and growth retardation in the hypoxic newborn rat. Circ Res 76:215-222, 1995.
34. Kinsella JP, McQueston JA, Rosenberg AA, Abman SH: Hemodynamic effects of exogenous nitric oxide in ovine transitional pulmonary circulation. Am J Physiol 263:H875-H880, 1992.
35. Roberts JD Jr, Chen TY, Kawai N, et al: Inhaled nitric oxide reverses pulmonary vasoconstriction in the hypoxic and acidotic newborn lamb. Circ Res 72:246-254, 1993.
36. Zayek M, Wild L, Roberts JD, Morin FC III: Effect of nitric oxide on the survival rate and incidence of

lung injury in newborn lambs with persistent pulmonary hypertension. J Pediatr 123:947-952, 1993.

37. Wilcox DT, Glick PL, Karamanoukian HL, et al: Partial liquid ventilation and nitric oxide in congenital diaphragmatic hernia. J Pediatr Surg 32:1211-1215, 1997.
38. Bourbon J, Boucherat O, Chailley-Heu B, Delacourt C: Control mechanisms of lung alveolar development and their disorders in bronchopulmonary dysplasia. Pediatr Res 57:38R-46R, 2005.
39. McCurnin DC, Pierce RA, Chang LY, et al: Inhaled NO improves early pulmonary function and modifies lung growth and elastin deposition in a baboon model of neonatal chronic lung disease. Am J Physiol Lung Cell Mol Physiol 288:L450-L459, 2005.
40. Bland RD, Albertine KH, Carlton DP, MacRitchie AJ: Inhaled nitric oxide effects on lung structure and function in chronically ventilated preterm lambs. Am J Respir Crit Care Med 172:899-906, 2005.
41. Lin YJ, Markham NE, Balasubramaniam V, et al: Inhaled nitric oxide enhances distal lung growth after exposure to hyperoxia in neonatal rats. Pediatr Res 58:22-29, 2005.
42. Galambos C, Ng YS, Ali A, et al: Defective pulmonary development in the absence of heparin-binding vascular endothelial growth factor isoforms. Am J Respir Cell Mol Biol 27:194-203, 2002.
43. Tang JR, Markham NE, Lin YJ, et al: Inhaled nitric oxide attenuates pulmonary hypertension and improves lung growth in infant rats after neonatal treatment with a VEGF receptor inhibitor. Am J Physiol Lung Cell Mol Physiol 287:L344-L351, 2004.
44. Inhaled nitric oxide and hypoxic respiratory failure in infants with congenital diaphragmatic hernia. The Neonatal Inhaled Nitric Oxide Study Group (NINOS). Pediatrics 99:838-845, 1997.
45. Davidson D, Barefield ES, Kattwinkel J, et al: Inhaled nitric oxide for the early treatment of persistent pulmonary hypertension of the term newborn: A randomized, double-masked, placebo-controlled, dose-response, multicenter study. The I-NO/PPHN Study Group. Pediatrics 101:325-334, 1998.
46. Kinsella JP, Greenough A, Abman SH: Bronchopulmonary dysplasia. Lancet 367:1421-1431, 2006.
47. Kinsella JP, Walsh WF, Bose CL, et al: Inhaled nitric oxide in premature neonates with severe hypoxaemic respiratory failure: A randomised controlled trial. Lancet 354:1061-1065, 1999.
48. Schreiber MD, Gin-Mestan K, Marks JD, et al: Inhaled nitric oxide in premature infants with the respiratory distress syndrome. N Engl J Med 349:2099-2107, 2003.
49. Van Meurs KP, Wright LL, Ehrenkranz RA, et al: Inhaled nitric oxide for premature infants with severe respiratory failure. N Engl J Med 353:13-22, 2005.
50. Kinsella JP, Cutter GR, Walsh WF, et al: Early inhaled nitric oxide therapy in premature newborns with respiratory failure. N Engl J Med 355:354-364, 2006.
51. Ballard RA, Truog WE, Cnaan A, et al: Inhaled nitric oxide in preterm infants undergoing mechanical ventilation. N Engl J Med 355:343-353, 2006.
52. Kinsella JP: Inhaled nitric oxide therapy in premature newborns. Curr Opin Pediatr 18:107-111, 2006.
53. Schwarz UR, Walter U, Eigenthaler M: Taming platelets with cyclic nucleotides. Biochem Pharmacol 62:1153-1161, 2001.
54. Hogman M, Frostell C, Arnberg H, Hedenstierna G: Bleeding time prolongation and NO inhalation. Lancet 341:1664-1665, 1993.
55. Field D, Elbourne D, Truesdale A, et al: Neonatal ventilation with inhaled nitric oxide versus ventilatory support without inhaled nitric oxide for preterm infants with severe respiratory failure: The INNOVO Multicentre Randomised Controlled Trial (ISRCTN 17821339). Pediatrics 115:926-936, 2005.
56. Mestan KKL, Marks JD, Hecox K, et al: Neurodevelopmental outcomes of premature infants treated with inhaled nitric oxide. N Engl J Med 353:23-32, 2005.
57. Rich S, Kaufmann E, Levy PS: The effect of high doses of calcium-channel blockers on survival in primary pulmonary hypertension. N Engl J Med 327:76-81, 1992.
58. Semigran MJ, Cockrill BA, Kacmarek R, et al: Hemodynamic effects of inhaled nitric oxide in heart failure. J Am Coll Cardiol 24:982-988, 1994.
59. Atz AM, Adatia I, Lock JE, Wessel DL: Combined effects of nitric oxide and oxygen during acute pulmonary vasodilator testing. J Am Coll Cardiol 33:813-819, 1999.
60. Krasuski RA, Warner JJ, Wang A, et al: Inhaled nitric oxide selectively dilates pulmonary vasculature in adult patients with pulmonary hypertension, irrespective of etiology. J Am Coll Cardiol 36:2204-2211, 2000.
61. Cockrill BA, Kacmarek RM, Fifer MA, et al: Comparison of the effects of nitric oxide, nitroprusside, and nifedipine on hemodynamics and right ventricular contractility in patients with chronic pulmonary hypertension. Chest 119:128-136, 2001.
62. Sitbon O, Humbert M, Jagot JL, et al: Inhaled nitric oxide as a screening agent for safely identifying responders to oral calcium-channel blockers in primary pulmonary hypertension. Eur Respir J 12:265-270, 1998.
63. Ricciardi MJ, Knight BP, Martinez FJ, Rubenfire M: Inhaled nitric oxide in primary pulmonary hypertension: A safe and effective agent for predicting response to nifedipine. J Am Coll Cardiol 32:1068-1073, 1998.
64. Balzer DT, Kort HW, Day RW, et al: Inhaled nitric oxide as a preoperative test (INOP test I): the INOP Test Study Group. Circulation 106:I76-I81, 2002.
65. Robbins IM, Christman BW, Newman JH, et al: A survey of diagnostic practices and the use of epoprostenol in patients with primary pulmonary hypertension. Chest 114:1269-1275, 1998.
66. Waldman JD: From PediHeart: Inhaled nitric oxide—in clinical trial or in clinical practice? Pediatr Cardiol 21:274, 2000.
67. Barst RJ, Rubin LJ, McGoon MD, et al: Survival in primary pulmonary hypertension with long-term continuous intravenous prostacyclin. Ann Intern Med 121:409-415, 1994.
68. Channick RN, Newhart JW, Johnson FW, et al: Pulsed delivery of inhaled nitric oxide to patients with primary pulmonary hypertension: An ambulatory delivery system and initial clinical tests. Chest 109:1545-1549, 1996.
69. Perez-Penate G, Julia-Serda G, Pulido-Duque JM, et al: One-year continuous inhaled nitric oxide for primary pulmonary hypertension. Chest 119:970-973, 2001.
70. Rubin LJ, Badesch DB, Barst RJ, et al: Bosentan therapy for pulmonary arterial hypertension. N Engl J Med 346:896-903, 2002.
71. Barst RJ, McGoon M, McLaughlin V, et al: Beraprost therapy for pulmonary arterial hypertension. J Am Coll Cardiol 41:2119-2125, 2003.
72. Ghofrani HA, Wiedemann R, Rose F, et al: Sildenafil for treatment of lung fibrosis and pulmonary hypertension: A randomised controlled trial. Lancet 360:895-900, 2002.
73. Inglessis I, Shin JT, Lepore JJ, et al: Hemodynamic effects of inhaled nitric oxide in right ventricular myocardial infarction and cardiogenic shock. J Am Coll Cardiol 44:793-798, 2004.
74. Benzing A, Geiger K: Inhaled nitric oxide lowers pulmonary capillary pressure and changes longitudinal distribution of pulmonary vascular resistance in patients with acute lung injury. Acta Anaesthesiol Scand 38:640-645, 1994.
75. Benzing A, Brautigam P, Geiger K, et al: Inhaled nitric oxide reduces pulmonary transvascular albumin flux in patients with acute lung injury. Anesthesiology 83:1153-1161, 1995.
76. Troncy E, Collet JP, Shapiro S, et al: Inhaled nitric oxide in acute respiratory distress syndrome: A pilot randomized controlled study. Am J Respir Crit Care Med 157:1483-1488, 1998.
77. Dellinger RP, Zimmerman JL, Taylor RW, et al: Effects of inhaled nitric oxide in patients with acute respiratory distress syndrome: Results of a randomized phase II trial. Inhaled Nitric Oxide in ARDS Study Group. Crit Care Med 26:15-23, 1998.
78. Lundin S, Mang H, Smithies M, et al: Inhalation of nitric oxide in acute lung injury: Results of a European multicentre study. The European Study Group of Inhaled Nitric Oxide. Intensive Care Med 25:911-919, 1999.
79. Gerlach H, Keh D, Semmerow A, et al: Dose-response characteristics during long-term inhalation of nitric oxide in patients with severe acute respiratory distress syndrome: A prospective, randomized, controlled study. Am J Respir Crit Care Med 167:1008-1015, 2003.
80. Kaisers U, Busch T, Deja M, et al: Selective pulmonary vasodilation in acute respiratory distress syndrome. Crit Care Med 31:S337-S342, 2003.
81. Katayama Y, Higenbottam TW, Diaz de Atauri MJ, et al: Inhaled nitric oxide and arterial oxygen tension in patients with chronic obstructive pulmonary disease and severe pulmonary hypertension. Thorax 52:120-124, 1997.
82. Barbera JA, Roger N, Roca J, et al: Worsening of pulmonary gas exchange with nitric oxide inhalation in chronic obstructive pulmonary disease. Lancet 347:436-440, 1996.
83. Yoshida M, Taguchi O, Gabazza EC, et al: Combined inhalation of nitric oxide and oxygen in chronic obstructive pulmonary disease. Am J Respir Crit Care Med 155:526-529, 1997.
84. Vonbank K, Ziesche R, Higenbottam TW, et al: Controlled prospective randomised trial on the effects on pulmonary haemodynamics of the ambulatory long term use of nitric oxide and oxygen in patients with severe COPD. Thorax 58:289-293, 2003.
85. Fullerton DA, Jones SD, Jaggers J, et al: Effective control of pulmonary vascular resistance with inhaled nitric oxide after cardiac operation. J Thorac Cardiovasc Surg 111:753-762, 1996.
86. Fullerton DA, Jaggers J, Wollmering MM, et al: Variable response to inhaled nitric oxide after cardiac surgery. Ann Thorac Surg 63:1251-1256, 1997.
87. Lindberg L, Larsson A, Steen S, et al: Nitric oxide gives maximal response after coronary artery bypass surgery. J Cardiothorac Vasc Anesth 8:182-187, 1994.
88. Wheller J, George BL, Mulder DG, Jarmakani JM: Diagnosis and management of postoperative pulmonary hypertensive crisis. Circulation 60:1640-1644, 1979.
89. Hopkins RA, Bull C, Haworth SG, et al: Pulmonary hypertensive crises following surgery for congenital heart defects in young children. Eur J Cardiothorac Surg 5:628-634, 1991.

90. Wessel DL, Adatia I, Giglia TM, et al: Use of inhaled nitric oxide and acetylcholine in the evaluation of pulmonary hypertension and endothelial function after cardiopulmonary bypass. Circulation 88:2128-2138, 1993.
91. Roberts JD Jr, Lang P, Bigatello LM, et al: Inhaled nitric oxide in congenital heart disease. Circulation 87:447-453, 1993.
92. Russell IA, Zwass MS, Fineman JR, et al: The effects of inhaled nitric oxide on postoperative pulmonary hypertension in infants and children undergoing surgical repair of congenital heart disease. Anesth Analg 87:46-51, 1998.
93. Goldman AP, Delius RE, Deanfield JE, et al: Pharmacological control of pulmonary blood flow with inhaled nitric oxide after the fenestrated Fontan operation. Circulation 94:II44-II48, 1996.
94. Miller OI, Tang SF, Keech A, et al: Inhaled nitric oxide and prevention of pulmonary hypertension after congenital heart surgery: A randomised double-blind study. Lancet 356:1464-1469, 2000.
95. Rich GF, Murphy GD Jr, Roos CM, Johns RA: Inhaled nitric oxide. Selective pulmonary vasodilation in cardiac surgical patients. Anesthesiology 78:1028-1035, 1993.
96. Mahoney PD, Loh E, Blitz LR, Herrmann HC: Hemodynamic effects of inhaled nitric oxide in women with mitral stenosis and pulmonary hypertension. Am J Cardiol 87:188-192, 2001.
97. Stobierska-Dzierzek B, Awad H, Michler RE: The evolving management of acute right-sided heart failure in cardiac transplant recipients. J Am Coll Cardiol 38:923-931, 2001.
98. Ardehali A, Hughes K, Sadeghi A, et al: Inhaled nitric oxide for pulmonary hypertension after heart transplantation. Transplantation 72:638-641, 2001.
99. Fojon S, Fernandez-Gonzalez C, Sanchez-Andrade J, et al: Inhaled nitric oxide through a noninvasive ventilation device to assess reversibility of pulmonary hypertension in selecting recipients for heart transplant. Transplant Proc 37:4028-4030, 2005.
100. Frazier OH, Rose EA, Macmanus Q, et al: Multicenter clinical evaluation of the HeartMate 1000 IP left ventricular assist device. Ann Thorac Surg 53:1080-1090, 1992.
101. Macdonald PS, Keogh A, Mundy J, et al: Adjunctive use of inhaled nitric oxide during implantation of a left ventricular assist device. J Heart Lung Transplant 17:312-316, 1998.
102. Yahagi N, Kumon K, Nakatani T, et al: Inhaled nitric oxide for the management of acute right ventricular failure in patients with a left ventricular assist system. Artif Organs 19:557-558, 1995.
103. Argenziano M, Choudhri AF, Moazami N, et al: Randomized, double-blind trial of inhaled nitric oxide in LVAD recipients with pulmonary hypertension. Ann Thorac Surg 65:340-345, 1998.
104. Struber M, Harringer W, Ernst M, et al: Inhaled nitric oxide as a prophylactic treatment against reperfusion injury of the lung. Thorac Cardiovasc Surg 47:179-182, 1999.
105. Date H, Triantafillou AN, Trulock EP, et al: Inhaled nitric oxide reduces human lung allograft dysfunction. J Thorac Cardiovasc Surg 111:913-919, 1996.
106. Ardehali A, Laks H, Levine M, et al: A prospective trial of inhaled nitric oxide in clinical lung transplantation. Transplantation 72:112-115, 2001.
107. Meade MO, Granton JT, Matte-Martyn A, et al: A randomized trial of inhaled nitric oxide to prevent ischemia-reperfusion injury after lung transplantation. Am J Respir Crit Care Med 167:1483-1489, 2003.
108. Ichinose F, Adrie C, Hurford WE, Zapol WM: Prolonged pulmonary vasodilator action of inhaled nitric oxide by zaprinast in awake lambs. J Appl Physiol 78:1288-1295, 1995.
109. Thusu KG, Morin FC III, Russell JA, Steinhorn RH: The cGMP phosphodiesterase inhibitor zaprinast enhances the effect of nitric oxide. Am J Respir Crit Care Med 152:1605-1610, 1995.
110. Ichinose F, Adrie C, Hurford WE, et al: Selective pulmonary vasodilation induced by aerosolized zaprinast. Anesthesiology 88:410-416, 1998.
111. Ichinose F, Erana-Garcia J, Hromi J, et al: Nebulized sildenafil is a selective pulmonary vasodilator in lambs with acute pulmonary hypertension. Crit Care Med 29:1000-1005, 2001.
112. Steinhorn RH, Albert G, Swartz DD, et al: Recombinant human superoxide dismutase enhances the effect of inhaled nitric oxide in persistent pulmonary hypertension. Am J Respir Crit Care Med 164:834-839, 2001.
113. Evgenov OV, Ichinose F, Evgenov NV, et al: Soluble guanylate cyclase activator reverses acute pulmonary hypertension and augments the pulmonary vasodilator response to inhaled nitric oxide in awake lambs. Circulation 110:2253-2259, 2004.
114. Evgenov OV, Kohane DS, Bloch KD, et al: Inhaled agonists of soluble guanylate cyclase induce selective pulmonary vasodilation. Am J Respir Crit Care Med 176:1138-1145, 2007.
115. Lepore JJ, Maroo A, Pereira NL, et al: Effect of sildenafil on the acute pulmonary vasodilator response to inhaled nitric oxide in adults with primary pulmonary hypertension. Am J Cardiol 90:677-680, 2002.
116. Lepore JJ, Maroo A, Bigatello LM, et al: Hemodynamic effects of sildenafil in patients with congestive heart failure and pulmonary hypertension: Combined administration with inhaled nitric oxide. Chest 127:1647-1653, 2005.
117. Namachivayam P, Theilen U, Butt WW, et al: Sildenafil prevents rebound pulmonary hypertension after withdrawal of nitric oxide in children. Am J Respir Crit Care Med 174:1042-1047, 2006.
118. McMahon TJ, Doctor A: Extrapulmonary effects of inhaled nitric oxide: Role of reversible *S*-nitrosylation of erythrocytic hemoglobin. Proc Am Thorac Soc 3:153-160, 2006.
119. Adrie C, Bloch KD, Moreno PR, et al: Inhaled nitric oxide increases coronary artery patency after thrombolysis. Circulation 94:1919-1926, 1996.
120. Fox-Robichaud A, Payne D, Hasan SU, et al: Inhaled NO as a viable antiadhesive therapy for ischemia/reperfusion injury of distal microvascular beds. J Clin Invest 101:2497-2505, 1998.
121. Hataishi R, Rodrigues AC, Neilan TG, et al: Inhaled nitric oxide decreases infarction size and improves left ventricular function in a murine model of myocardial ischemia-reperfusion injury. Am J Physiol Heart Circ Physiol 291:H379-H384, 2006.
122. Liu X, Huang Y, Pokreisz P, et al: Nitric oxide inhalation improves microvascular flow and decreases infarction size after myocardial ischemia and reperfusion. J Am Coll Cardiol 50:808-817, 2007.
123. Minneci PC, Deans KJ, Zhi H, et al: Hemolysis-associated endothelial dysfunction mediated by accelerated NO inactivation by decompartmentalized oxyhemoglobin. J Clin Invest 115:3409-3417, 2005.
124. Schmidt U, Han RO, DiSalvo TG, et al: Cessation of platelet-mediated cyclic canine coronary occlusion after thrombolysis by combining nitric oxide inhalation with phosphodiesterase-5 inhibition. J Am Coll Cardiol 37:1981-1988, 2001.
125. Lee JS, Adrie C, Jacob HJ, et al: Chronic inhalation of nitric oxide inhibits neointimal formation after balloon-induced arterial injury. Circ Res 78:337-342, 1996.
126. Neviere R, Guery B, Mordon S, et al: Inhaled NO reduces leukocyte–endothelial cell interactions and myocardial dysfunction in endotoxemic rats. Am J Physiol Heart Circ Physiol 278:H1783-H1790, 2000.
127. Kubes P, Payne D, Grisham MB, et al: Inhaled NO impacts vascular but not extravascular compartments in postischemic peripheral organs. Am J Physiol 277:H676-H682, 1999.
128. Guery B, Neviere R, Viget N, et al: Inhaled NO preadministration modulates local and remote ischemia-reperfusion organ injury in a rat model. J Appl Physiol 87:47-53, 1999.
129. Gianetti J, Del Sarto P, Bevilacqua S, et al: Supplemental nitric oxide and its effect on myocardial injury and function in patients undergoing cardiac surgery with extracorporeal circulation. J Thorac Cardiovasc Surg 127:44-50, 2004.
130. Cannon RO III, Schechter AN, Panza JA, et al: Effects of inhaled nitric oxide on regional blood flow are consistent with intravascular nitric oxide delivery. J Clin Invest 108:279-287, 2001.
131. Hataishi R, Zapol WM, Bloch KD, Ichinose F: Inhaled nitric oxide does not reduce systemic vascular resistance in mice. Am J Physiol Heart Circ Physiol 290:H1826-H1829, 2006.
132. Stamler JS, Jaraki O, Osborne J, et al: Nitric oxide circulates in mammalian plasma primarily as an *S*-nitroso adduct of serum albumin. Proc Natl Acad Sci U S A 89:7674-7677, 1992.
133. Scharfstein JS, Keaney JF Jr, Slivka A, et al: In vivo transfer of nitric oxide between a plasma protein-bound reservoir and low molecular weight thiols. J Clin Invest 94:1432-1439, 1994.
134. Gladwin MT, Raat NJ, Shiva S, et al: Nitrite as a vascular endocrine nitric oxide reservoir that contributes to hypoxic signaling, cytoprotection, and vasodilation. Am J Physiol Heart Circ Physiol 291:H2026-H2035, 2006.
135. Oda H, Kusumoto S, Nakajima T: Nitrosylhemoglobin formation in the blood of animals exposed to nitric oxide. Arch Environ Health 30:453-456, 1975.
136. Yoshida K, Kasama K: Biotransformation of nitric oxide. Environ Health Perspect 73:201-205, 1987.
137. Ng ES, Jourd'heuil D, McCord JM, et al: Enhanced *S*-nitroso-albumin formation from inhaled NO during ischemia/reperfusion. Circ Res 94:559-565, 2004.
138. Duranski MR, Greer JJ, Dejam A, et al: Cytoprotective effects of nitrite during in vivo ischemia-reperfusion of the heart and liver. J Clin Invest 115:1232-1240, 2005.
139. Frampton MW, Morrow PE, Cox C, et al: Effects of nitrogen dioxide exposure on pulmonary function and airway reactivity in normal humans. Am Rev Respir Dis 143:522-527, 1991.
140. Centers for Disease Control and Prevention (CDC): 1988 NIOSH recommendations for occupational safety and health standards. MMWR Morb Mortal Wkly Rep 37(Suppl 7):1-29, 1988.
141. Clutton-Brock J: Two cases of poisoning by contamination of nitrous oxide with higher oxides of nitrogen during anaesthesia. Br J Anaesth 39:388-392, 1967.
142. Weinberger B, Laskin DL, Heck DE, Laskin JD: The toxicology of inhaled nitric oxide. Toxicol Sci 59:5-16, 2001.
143. Kinsella JP, Truog WE, Walsh WF, et al: Randomized, multicenter trial of inhaled nitric oxide

and high-frequency oscillatory ventilation in severe, persistent pulmonary hypertension of the newborn. J Pediatr 131:55-62, 1997.

144. The Neonatal Inhaled Nitric Oxide Study Group: Inhaled nitric oxide and hypoxic respiratory failure in infants with congenital diaphragmatic hernia. Pediatrics 99:838-845, 1997.

145. Loh E, Stamler JS, Hare JM, et al: Cardiovascular effects of inhaled nitric oxide in patients with left ventricular dysfunction. Circulation 90:2780-2785, 1994.

146. Brady AJ, Warren JB, Poole-Wilson PA, et al: Nitric oxide attenuates cardiac myocyte contraction. Am J Physiol 265:H176-H182, 1993.

147. Finkel MS, Oddis CV, Jacob TD, et al: Negative inotropic effects of cytokines on the heart mediated by nitric oxide. Science 257:387-389, 1992.

148. Dickstein ML, Burkhoff D: A theoretic analysis of the effect of pulmonary vasodilation on pulmonary venous pressure: Implications for inhaled nitric oxide therapy. J Heart Lung Transplant 15:715-721, 1996.

149. Hare JM, Shernan SK, Body SC, et al: Influence of inhaled nitric oxide on systemic flow and ventricular filling pressure in patients receiving mechanical circulatory assistance. Circulation 95:2250-2253, 1997.

150. Lowson SM: Alternatives to nitric oxide. Br Med Bull 70:119-131, 2004.

151. Walmrath D, Schneider T, Pilch J, et al: Aerosolised prostacyclin in adult respiratory distress syndrome. Lancet 342:961-962, 1993.

152. Haraldsson A, Kieler-Jensen N, Ricksten SE: The additive pulmonary vasodilatory effects of inhaled prostacyclin and inhaled milrinone in postcardiac surgical patients with pulmonary hypertension. Anesth Analg 93:1439-1445, 2001.

153. Yurtseven N, Karaca P, Kaplan M, et al: Effect of nitroglycerin inhalation on patients with pulmonary hypertension undergoing mitral valve replacement surgery. Anesthesiology 99:855-858, 2003.

154. Mestan KKL, Carlson AD, White M, et al: Cardiopulmonary effects of nebulized sodium nitroprusside in term infants with hypoxic respiratory failure. J Pediatr 143:640-643, 2003.

155. Sood BG, Delaney-Black V, Aranda JV, Shankaran S: Aerosolized PGE_1: A selective pulmonary vasodilator in neonatal hypoxemic respiratory failure: Results of a phase I/II open label clinical trial. Pediatr Res 56:579-585, 2004.

156. Olschewski H, Walmrath D, Schermuly R, et al: Aerosolized prostacyclin and iloprost in severe pulmonary hypertension. Ann Intern Med 124:820-824, 1996.

157. Walmrath D, Schneider T, Schermuly R, et al: Direct comparison of inhaled nitric oxide and aerosolized prostacyclin in acute respiratory distress syndrome. Am J Respir Crit Care Med 153:991-996, 1996.

158. Haraldsson A, Kieler-Jensen N, Nathorst-Westfelt U, et al: Comparison of inhaled nitric oxide and inhaled aerosolized prostacyclin in the evaluation of heart transplant candidates with elevated pulmonary vascular resistance. Chest 114:780-786, 1998.

159. van Heerden PV, Caterina P, Filion P, et al: Pulmonary toxicity of inhaled aerosolized prostacyclin therapy—an observational study. Anaesth Intensive Care 28:161-166, 2000.

160. Morimatsu H, Goto K, Matsusaki T, et al: Rapid development of severe interstitial pneumonia caused by epoprostenol in a patient with primary pulmonary hypertension. Anesth Analg 99:1205-1207, 2004.

161. Dickstein ML: Con: Inhaled prostaglandin as a pulmonary vasodilator instead of nitric oxide. J Cardiothorac Vasc Anesth 19:403-405, 2005.

Michael Ang-Lee, Chun-Su Yuan, and Jonathan Moss

32 Complementary and Alternative Therapies

Key Points

1. Despite lack of federal oversight, herbal medication use has increased dramatically in the overall population and particularly in preoperative patients.
2. Patients may not volunteer information unless they are specifically queried about herbal medication use.
3. Many commonly used herbs have side effects that affect drug metabolism, bleeding, and neuronal function.
4. Although stopping the use of herbal medication up to 2 weeks preoperatively can eliminate many of these problems, patients often arrive for surgery without a preoperative visit 2 weeks before surgery. Knowledge of specific interactions and metabolism of these herbs can provide practical guidelines to facilitate care.
5. Other complementary therapies, including acupuncture and music therapy, have become increasingly popular, although less is known about their effectiveness.

Complementary and alternative medicine (CAM) has implications for physicians in general but has particular importance for perioperative physicians because of complications associated with the use of certain therapies and their roles as anesthesia adjuvants. In 2002, 35% of Americans used CAM therapies.[1] Visits to CAM practitioners exceed those to American primary care physicians,[2] and CAM is even more widely used in Europe, where herbal medicines are more frequently prescribed than conventional drugs in many situations. Of particular relevance for anesthesiologists is that patients undergoing surgery appear to use CAM more than the general population does.[3,4]

Despite the public enthusiasm for CAM, scientific knowledge in this area is still incomplete and often confusing for practitioners and patients. One recent study confirmed poor knowledge of this subject among physicians.[5] Recommendations for clinicians are often based on small clinical trials, case reports, animal studies, predictions derived from known pharmacology, and expert opinion. Research is essential because CAM therapies are often widely adopted by the public before adequate data are available to support their safety and efficacy. In 1991, Congress established the Office of Alternative Medicine, which became the National Center for Complementary and Alternative Medicine within the National Institutes of Health in 1998. In 2006, more than twice as many CAM-related English-language research articles were published as in 1996.

Practices encompassed by CAM are heterogeneous and evolving as CAM therapies are integrated into conventional medicine (e.g., diet, exercise, behavioral medicine). CAM practices can be classified into five general categories (Box 32-1).[6] This chapter is not intended as a comprehensive review of CAM. Specific therapies relevant to anesthesia are discussed, and we focus primarily on herbal medicines. Nonherbal dietary supplements, acupuncture, and music are also examined.

Herbal Medicines

Preoperative use of herbal medicines has been associated with adverse perioperative events.[3] Surveys estimate that 22% to 32% of patients undergoing surgery use herbal medications.[7-9] As pharmacologically active agents, herbal medicines may affect the perioperative period through several mechanisms: direct effects (i.e., intrinsic pharmacologic effects), pharmacodynamic interactions (i.e., alteration of the action of conventional drugs at effector sites), and pharmacokinetic interactions (i.e., alteration of the absorption, distribution, metabolism, and elimination of conventional drugs). Because approximately 50% of herbal medicine users take multiple herbs concomitantly[8] and 25% of herbal medicine users take prescription drugs,[10] adverse effects are difficult to predict and attribute. For example, PC-SPES, a commercially available combination of eight herbs used by patients with prostate cancer, has been associated with thrombotic (i.e., deep venous thrombosis and pulmonary embolism) and hemorrhagic (i.e., anticoagulation from phytocoumarins) complications.[11]

Herbal medicines are associated with problems not usually found with conventional drugs.[12] Because herbal medicines are classified as dietary supplements, they are not subject to

Box 32-1 Five Major Categories of Complementary and Alternative Medicine

1. Alternative medical systems (e.g., homeopathic medicine, naturopathic medicine, traditional Chinese medicine, ayurveda)
2. Mind-body interventions (e.g., meditation; prayer; art, music, or dance therapy)
3. Biologically based treatments (e.g., herbal medicines, dietary supplements)
4. Manipulative and body-based methods (e.g., chiropractic manipulation, osteopathic manipulation, massage)
5. Energy therapies (e.g., acupuncture, electromagnetic fields, reiki, qi gong)

Adapted from the National Center for Complementary and Alternative Medicine. Available at http://nccam.nih.gov/health/whatiscam/ Accessed August 15, 2003.

preclinical animal studies, premarketing controlled clinical trials, or postmarketing surveillance. Under current law, the burden is shifted to the U.S. Food and Drug Administration (FDA) to prove products unsafe before they can be withdrawn from the market. Commercial herbal medicine preparations may have unpredictable pharmacologic effects resulting from inaccurate labeling, misidentified plants, adulterants, variations in natural potency, and unstandardized processing methods.

In this chapter we discuss the preoperative assessment and management of patients who use herbal medicines and examine nine herbal medicines that have the greatest impact on perioperative patient care: echinacea, ephedra, garlic, *Ginkgo biloba*, ginseng, kava, saw palmetto, St. John's wort, and valerian (Table 32-1). These nine account for 50% of the herbal medicines sold in the United States (Box 32-2).[13] Print and Internet resources for additional information on herbal medicines are provided in Table 32-2.

Preoperative Assessment and Management

Preoperative assessment should address the use of herbal medicines (see Chapter 34). However, 90% of anesthesiologists do not routinely ask about herbal medicine use.[14] Moreover, more than 70% of patients are not forthcoming about their herbal medicine use during routine preoperative assessment.[8] When a positive history of herbal medicine use is elicited, one in five patients is unable to properly identify the preparation being taken.[15] Patients should be asked to bring their herbal medicines and other dietary supplements with them at the time of the preoperative evaluation. A positive history of herbal medicine use should also prompt anesthesiologists to suspect the presence of undiagnosed disorders causing symptoms leading to self-medication. Patients who use herbal medicines may be more likely than those who do not to avoid conventional diagnosis and therapy.[16]

In general, herbal medicines should be discontinued preoperatively. When pharmacokinetic data for the active constituents in an herbal medication are available, the timeframe for preoperative discontinuation can be tailored. For other herbal medicines, 2 weeks is recommended.[17] However, in clinical practice because many patients require nonelective surgery, are not evaluated until the day of surgery, or are noncompliant with instructions to discontinue herbal medications preoperatively, they may take herbal medicines until the day of surgery. In this situation, anesthesia can usually proceed safely at the discretion of the anesthesiologist, who should be familiar with commonly used herbal medicines to avoid or recognize and treat complications that may arise. For instance, recent use of herbal medicines that inhibit platelet function (e.g., garlic, ginseng, *Ginkgo biloba*) may warrant specific strategies for procedures with substantial intraoperative blood loss (e.g., platelet transfusion) and those that alter the risk-benefit ratio of using certain anesthetic techniques (e.g., neuraxial blockade).

Preoperative discontinuation of all herbal medicines may not eliminate complications related to their use. Withdrawal of regular medications is associated with increased morbidity and mortality after surgery.[18] Alcoholics who abstain from drinking alcohol preoperatively may have poorer postoperative outcomes than those who continue drinking preoperatively.[19] The danger of abstinence after long-term use may be similar with herbal medicines such as valerian, which has the potential to produce acute withdrawal after long-term use.

Echinacea

Three species of echinacea, a member of the daisy family, are used for the prophylaxis and treatment of viral, bacterial, and fungal infections, particularly those of upper respiratory origin, although its efficacy in the latter is doubtful.[20] A recent meta-analysis

Box 32-2 Most Commonly Used Herbal Medicines in 2001

1. Echinacea*
2. *Ginkgo biloba**
3. Garlic*
4. Ginseng*
5. Saw palmetto*
6. Noni (*Morinda*)
7. St. John's wort*
8. Soy
9. Ephedra (ma huang)*
10. Milk thistle
11. Valerian*
12. Kava*
13. Grape seed extract
14. Green tea
15. Goldenseal
16. Primrose
17. Black cohosh root
18. Aloe
19. Bilberry
20. Cranberry

*Reviewed in this chapter.
Adapted from the Nutritional Business Journal's herbal and botanical U.S. consumer sales.[13]

Table 32-1 Clinically Important Effects, Perioperative Concerns, and Recommendations for Perioperative Discontinuation of Nine Commonly Used Herbal Medicines

Herbs (Common Names)	Pharmacologic Effects	Perioperative Concerns	Discontinue before Surgery
Echinacea (purple coneflower root)	Activation of cell-mediated immunity	Allergic reactions Decreases effectiveness of immunosuppressants Potential for immunosuppression with long-term use	No data
Ephedra (ma huang)	Increases heart rate and blood pressure through direct and indirect sympathomimetic effects	Risk of myocardial ischemia and stroke from tachycardia and hypertension Ventricular arrhythmias with halothane Long-term use depletes endogenous catecholamines and may cause intraoperative hemodynamic instability Life-threatening interaction with MAO inhibitors	24 hours
Garlic (ajo)	Inhibits platelet aggregation (may be irreversible) Increases fibrinolysis Equivocal antihypertensive activity	May increase risk of bleeding, especially when combined with other medications that inhibit platelet aggregation	7 days
Ginkgo (duck-foot tree, maidenhair tree, silver apricot)	Inhibits platelet-activating factor	May increase risk of bleeding, especially when combined with other medications that inhibit platelet aggregation	36 hours
Ginseng (American ginseng, Asian ginseng, Chinese ginseng, Korean ginseng)	Lowers blood glucose Inhibits platelet aggregation (may be irreversible) Increased PT/PTT in animals	Hypoglycemia May increase risk of bleeding May decrease anticoagulant effect of warfarin	7 days
Kava (awa, intoxicating pepper, kawa)	Sedation Anxiolysis	May increase sedative effect of anesthetics Increase in anesthetic requirements with long-term use unstudied	24 hours
Saw palmetto (dwarf palm, sabal)	Inhibits 5α-reductase Inhibits cyclooxygenase	May increase risk of bleeding	No data
St. John's wort (amber, goat weed, hardhay, hypericum, Klamath weed)	Inhibits neurotransmitter reuptake MAO inhibition unlikely	Induction of cytochrome P450 enzymes; affects cyclosporine, warfarin, steroids, and protease inhibitors; may affect benzodiazepines, calcium channel blockers, and many other drugs Decreased serum digoxin levels Delayed emergence	5 days
Valerian (all heal, garden heliotrope, vandal root)	Sedation	May increase sedative effect of anesthetics Benzodiazepine-like acute withdrawal May increase anesthetic requirements with long-term use	No data

MAO, monoamine oxidase; PT, prothrombin time; PTT, partial thromboplastin time.

showed echinacea's benefit in decreasing the incidence and duration of the common cold.[21] Its pharmacologic activity cannot be attributed to a single compound, although the lipophilic fraction, which contains alkylamides, polyacetylenes, and essential oils, appears to be more active than the hydrophilic fraction.

Echinacea had a number of immunostimulatory effects in preclinical studies.[22] Although no studies have specifically addressed interactions between echinacea and immunosuppressive drugs, expert opinion generally warns against the concomitant use of echinacea and these drugs because of the probability of diminished effectiveness.[22,23] Therefore, patients who may require perioperative immunosuppression, such as those awaiting organ transplantation, should be counseled to avoid echinacea. In contrast to its immunostimulatory effects with short-term use, long-term use of more than 8 weeks is accompanied by the potential for immunosuppression[23] and a theoretically increased risk for certain postsurgical complications such as poor wound healing and opportunistic infections.

Echinacea has also been associated with allergic reactions, including one reported case of anaphylaxis.[24] Therefore, echinacea should be used with caution in patients with asthma, atopy, or allergic rhinitis. Concern for potential hepatotoxicity has also been raised, although documented cases are lacking.[25] In the absence of definitive information, patients with preexisting liver

Table 32-2 Printed and World Wide Web Sources of Herbal Medicine Information

Source	Comments
Physicians' Desk Reference for Herbal Medicines	
Commission E Monographs	
Textbook of Complementary and Alternative Medicine	
Center for Food Safety and Applied Nutrition, Food and Drug Administration: http://vm.cfsan.fda.gov/~dms/supplmnt.html	Clinicians should use this site to report adverse events associated with herbal medicines and other dietary supplements. Sections also contain safety, industry, and regulatory information
National Center for Complementary and Alternative Medicine, National Institutes of Health: http://nccam.nih.gov/	This site contains fact sheets about alternative therapies, consensus reports, and data bases
Agricultural Research Service, U.S. Department of Agriculture: www.ars-grin.gov/duke	The site contains an extensive phytochemical database with search capabilities
Quackwatch: www.quackwatch.com	Although this site addresses all aspects of health care, there is a considerable amount of information covering complementary and herbal therapies
National Council Against Health Fraud: www.ncahf.org	This site focuses on health fraud with a position paper on over-the-counter herbal remedies
HerbMed: www.herbmed.org	This site contains information on numerous herbal medications, with evidence for activity, warnings, preparations, mixtures, and mechanisms of action. There are short summaries of important research publications with Medline links
ConsumerLab: www.consumerlab.com	This site is maintained by a corporation that conducts independent laboratory investigations of dietary supplements and other health products

dysfunction should be cautious in using echinacea. Furthermore, because the pharmacokinetics of echinacea have not been studied, it may be prudent to discontinue this herb as far in advance of surgery as possible when compromise in hepatic function or blood flow is anticipated.

Ephedra

Ephedra, known as ma huang in Chinese medicine, is a shrub native to central Asia. It is used to promote weight loss, increase energy, and treat respiratory conditions such as asthma and bronchitis. Ephedra contains alkaloids, including ephedrine, pseudoephedrine, norephedrine, methylephedrine, and norpseudoephedrine.[26] Commercial preparations may be standardized to a fixed ephedrine content. Publicity about adverse reactions to this herb prompted the FDA to bar its sale in 2004, but ephedra is still widely available via the Internet.

Ephedra causes dose-dependent increases in blood pressure and heart rate. Ephedrine, the predominant active compound, is a noncatecholamine sympathomimetic that exhibits α_1, β_1, and β_2 activity directly at adrenergic receptors and indirectly by releasing endogenous norepinephrine (noradrenaline). These sympathomimetic effects have been associated with more than 1070 reported adverse events, including fatal cardiac and central nervous system complications.[27]

Although ephedrine is widely used as first-line therapy for intraoperative hypotension and bradycardia, the unsupervised preoperative use of ephedra raises certain concerns. Vasoconstriction and, in some cases, vasospasm of coronary and cerebral arteries may cause myocardial infarction and thrombotic stroke.[28] Ephedra may also affect cardiovascular function by causing hypersensitivity myocarditis characterized by cardiomyopathy with myocardial lymphocyte and eosinophil infiltration.[29] Long-term use results in tachyphylaxis from depletion of endogenous catecholamine stores and may contribute to perioperative hemodynamic instability. In these situations, direct-acting sympathomimetics may be preferred as first-line therapy for intraoperative hypotension and bradycardia. Concomitant use of ephedra and monoamine oxidase inhibitors can result in life-threatening hyperpyrexia, hypertension, and coma. Finally, continuous ephedra use has been documented as a very rare cause of radiolucent kidney stones.[30]

The pharmacokinetics of ephedrine has been studied in humans.[31,32] Ephedrine has an elimination half-life of 5.2 hours, with 70% to 80% of the compound excreted unchanged in urine. Based on the pharmacokinetic data and the known cardiovascular risks associated with ephedra, including myocardial infarction, stroke, and cardiovascular collapse from catecholamine depletion, this herb should be discontinued at least 24 hours before surgery.

Garlic

Garlic is one of the most extensively researched medicinal plants. It has the potential to modify the risk for atherosclerosis by reducing blood pressure, thrombus formation, and serum lipid and cholesterol levels.[33] These effects are primarily attributed to its sulfur-containing compounds, particularly allicin and its transformation products. Commercial garlic preparations may be standardized to a fixed alliin and allicin content.

Garlic inhibits platelet aggregation in vivo in a dose-dependent fashion. The effect of one of its constituents, ajoene, appears to be irreversible and may potentiate the effect of other platelet inhibitors such as prostacyclin, forskolin, indomethacin, and dipyridamole.[34] Although these effects have not been consistently demonstrated in volunteers, there is one case in the literature of an octogenarian in whom a spontaneous epidural hematoma developed that was attributed to continuous garlic use.[35] In addition to bleeding concerns, garlic has the potential to decrease systemic and pulmonary vascular resistance in laboratory animals, but this effect is marginal in humans.[36]

Although there are insufficient pharmacokinetic data on garlic's constituents, the potential for irreversible inhibition of platelet function may warrant discontinuation of garlic at least 7 days before surgery, especially if postoperative bleeding is a particular concern or other anticoagulants are given.

Ginkgo

Ginkgo is derived from the leaf of *Ginkgo biloba* and has been used for cognitive disorders, peripheral vascular disease, age-related macular degeneration, vertigo, tinnitus, erectile dysfunction, and altitude sickness. Studies have suggested that ginkgo may stabilize or improve cognitive performance in patients with Alzheimer's disease and multi-infarct dementia[37] but not in healthy geriatric patients.[38] The compounds believed to be responsible for its pharmacologic effects are the terpenoids and flavonoids. The two ginkgo extracts used in clinical trials are standardized to ginkgo-flavone glycosides and terpenoids.

Ginkgo appears to alter vasoregulation, act as an antioxidant, modulate neurotransmitter and receptor activity, and inhibit platelet-activating factor (PAF). Of these effects, inhibition of PAF raises the greatest concern for the perioperative period. Clinical trials in a small number of patients have not demonstrated bleeding complications, but four reported cases of spontaneous intracranial bleeding,[39-42] one case of spontaneous hyphema,[43] and one case of postoperative bleeding after laparoscopic cholecystectomy[44] have been associated with ginkgo use.

Terpenoids are highly bioavailable when administered orally. Glucuronidation appears to be part of the metabolism of flavonoids.[45] The elimination half-lives of the terpenoids after oral administration are between 3 and 10 hours.[46] Based on the pharmacokinetic data and the risk of bleeding in the surgical population, ginkgo should be discontinued at least 36 hours before surgery.

Ginseng

Among the several species used for their pharmacologic effects, Asian ginseng and American ginseng are the most commonly described. Ginseng has been labeled an "adaptogen" because it reputedly protects the body against stress and restores homeostasis.[47,48] Most pharmacologic actions are attributed to the ginsenosides, a group of compounds known as steroidal saponins. Commercially available ginseng preparations may be standardized to ginsenoside content.

Ginseng has a broad but incompletely understood pharmacologic profile because of the many heterogeneous and sometimes opposing effects of different ginsenosides.[49] The underlying mechanism appears to be similar to that classically described for steroid hormones. A potential therapeutic use for this herb lies in its ability to lower postprandial blood glucose in both type 2 diabetics and nondiabetics,[50] an effect that may create unintended hypoglycemia in patients who have fasted before surgery. There is concern about ginseng's effect on coagulation pathways. Ginsenosides inhibited platelet aggregation in vitro[51,52] and prolonged both the thrombin time and the activated partial thromboplastin time in rats.[53] One early study suggested that the antiplatelet activity of panaxynol, a constituent of ginseng, may be irreversible in humans.[54] Although ginseng may inhibit the coagulation cascade, in one case its use was associated with a significant decrease in warfarin anticoagulation.[55] A recent study in volunteers confirmed its ability to interfere with warfarin-induced anticoagulation.[56] Because warfarin is often used after orthopedic or vascular procedures, this drug interaction is more than theoretical in nature.

Studies of the pharmacokinetics of the ginsenosides Rg1, Re, and Rb2 in rabbits found elimination half-lives between 0.8 and 7.4 hours.[57] These data suggest that ginseng should be discontinued at least 24 hours before surgery. Because platelet inhibition by ginseng may be irreversible, it is probably prudent to discontinue ginseng use at least 7 days before surgery.

Kava

Kava is derived from the dried root of the pepper plant *Piper methysticum*. Kava has gained widespread popularity as an anxiolytic and sedative. The kavalactones appear to be the source of kava's pharmacologic activity.[58]

Because of its psychomotor effects, kava was one of the first herbal medications expected to interact with anesthetics. The kavalactones have dose-dependent effects on the central nervous system, including antiepileptic, neuroprotective, and local anesthetic properties. Kava may act as a sedative-hypnotic by potentiating inhibitory neurotransmission of γ-aminobutyric acid (GABA). The kavalactones increased barbiturate sleep time in laboratory animals.[59] This effect may explain the mechanism underlying the report of a coma attributed to an alprazolam-kava interaction.[60] Although kava has abuse potential, whether long-term use can result in addiction, tolerance, and acute withdrawal after abstinence has not been satisfactorily investigated. Continuous kava use may elevate γ-glutamyl transpeptidase levels, thus raising concern about hepatotoxicity.[61] With continuous use, kava produces "kava dermopathy," characterized by reversible scaly cutaneous eruptions.[62]

Peak plasma levels occur 1.8 hours after an oral dose, and the elimination half-life of kavalactones is 9 hours.[58] Unchanged kavalactones and their metabolites undergo renal and fecal elimination.[63] Pharmacokinetic data and the possibility for potentiation of the sedative effects of anesthetics suggest that kava should be discontinued at least 24 hours before surgery. Earlier discontinuation should be considered when surgical procedures are expected to compromise hepatic function or blood flow.

Saw Palmetto

Saw palmetto, which is used by more than 2 million men in the United States to treat symptoms associated with benign prostatic hypertrophy, is ineffective for this purpose.[64] The major constituents of saw palmetto are fatty acids and their glycerides (i.e., triacylglycerides and monoacylglycerides), carbohydrates, steroids, flavonoids, resin, pigment, tannin, and volatile oil. The pharmacologic activity of saw palmetto has not been attributed to a single compound.

The mechanism of action of saw palmetto is not known, but multiple mechanisms have been proposed.[65] In vitro data suggest that saw palmetto extract, like finasteride, inhibits 5α-reductase. However, results of in vivo studies have been inconsistent.[65] Other proposed mechanisms are inhibition of estrogen and androgen receptors, binding of autonomic receptors, blocking of prolactin receptor signal transduction, interference with fibroblast proliferation, induction of apoptosis, inhibition of α_1-adrenergic receptors, and anti-inflammatory effects.

In a patient undergoing craniotomy, saw palmetto was associated with excessive intraoperative bleeding that required termination of the procedure.[66] This complication was attributed to saw palmetto's anti-inflammatory effects, specifically the inhibition of cyclooxygenase and subsequent platelet dysfunction. Because there are no pharmacokinetic data for saw palmetto, specific recommendations for preoperative discontinuation cannot be made.

St John's Wort

St John's wort is the common name for *Hypericum perforatum*. A multicenter clinical trial concluded that St John's wort is not effective in the treatment of major depression.[67] The compounds believed to be responsible for its pharmacologic activity are hypericin and hyperforin.[68] Commercial preparations are often standardized to a fixed hypericin content of 0.3%.

St John's wort exerts its effects by inhibiting reuptake of serotonin, norepinephrine, and dopamine.[69] Concomitant use of this herb with or without serotonin reuptake inhibitors may create a syndrome of central serotonin excess.[70] Although early in vitro data implicated monoamine oxidase inhibition as a possible mechanism of action, a number of later investigations have demonstrated that monoamine oxidase inhibition is insignificant in vivo.[71]

Use of St John's wort can significantly increase the metabolism of many concomitantly administered drugs, some of which are vital to the perioperative care of certain patients. There is induction of the cytochrome P450 3A4 isoform, with approximate doubling of its metabolic activity.[72] Interactions with substrates of the 3A4 isoform, including indinavir sulfate,[73] ethinylestradiol[74] and cyclosporine, have been documented. In one series of 45 organ transplant patients, St John's wort was associated with an average 49% decrease in blood cyclosporine levels.[75] Another group reported two cases of acute heart transplant rejection associated with this particular pharmacokinetic interaction.[76] Other P450 3A4 substrates commonly used in the perioperative period include alfentanil, midazolam, lidocaine, calcium channel blockers, and 5-hydroxytryptamine receptor antagonists. In addition to the 3A4 isoform, the cytochrome P450 2C9 isoform may also be induced. The anticoagulant effect of warfarin, a substrate of the 2C9 isoform, was reduced in seven reported cases.[74] Other 2C9 substrates include the nonsteroidal anti-inflammatory drugs. Furthermore, the enzyme induction caused by St John's wort may be more pronounced when other enzyme inducers, which could include other herbal medications, are taken concomitantly. St John's wort also affects digoxin pharmacokinetics.[77] A recent study in the rat showed that St John's wort could markedly alter intracellular accumulation of irinotecan and its major metabolite (SN-38) in hepatocytes and glucuronidation of SN-38.[78]

The single-dose and steady-state pharmacokinetics of hypericin, pseudohypericin, and hyperforin has been determined in humans.[79,80] After oral administration, peak plasma levels of hypericin and hyperforin are achieved in 6.0 and 3.5 hours, respectively, and their median elimination half-lives are 43.1 and 9.0 hours, respectively. Long half-life and altered metabolism of many drugs make concomitant use of St John's wort a particular risk in the perioperative setting. Pharmacokinetic data suggest that this herbal medication should be discontinued at least 5 days before surgery. Discontinuation is especially important in patients awaiting organ transplantation or in those who may require oral anticoagulation postoperatively. Moreover, these patients should be advised to avoid taking St John's wort postoperatively.

Valerian

Valerian (*Valeian officinalis*) is an herb native to temperate regions of the Americas, Europe, and Asia. It is used as a sedative, particularly in the treatment of insomnia, and virtually all herbal sleep aids contain valerian.[81] Valerian contains many compounds acting synergistically, but the sesquiterpenes are the primary source of valerian's pharmacologic effects. Commercially available preparations may be standardized to valerenic acid.

Valerian produces dose-dependent sedation and hypnosis.[82] These effects appear to be mediated through modulation of GABA neurotransmission and receptor function.[83] Valerian increased barbiturate sleep time in experimental animals.[84] In one patient, valerian withdrawal appeared to mimic an acute benzodiazepine withdrawal syndrome characterized by delirium, cardiac complications after surgery, and attenuation of the symptoms by administration of a benzodiazepine.[85] Based on these findings, valerian should be expected to potentiate the sedative effects of anesthetics and adjuvants that act at the GABA receptor, such as midazolam.

The pharmacokinetics of valerian's constituents has not been studied, although their effects are thought to be short lived. Abrupt discontinuation in patients who may be physically dependent on valerian risks benzodiazepine-like withdrawal. In these individuals, it may be prudent to taper this herbal medication with close medical supervision over the course of several weeks before surgery. If tapering is not feasible, physicians can advise patients to continue taking valerian up until the day of surgery. Based on the mechanism of action and a reported case of efficacy,[85] benzodiazepines can be used to treat withdrawal symptoms should they develop in the postoperative period.

Summary

Although the American Society of Anesthesiologists has no official standards or guidelines on the preoperative use of herbal medications, public and professional educational information released by this organization suggests that herbals be discontinued at least 2 to 3 weeks before surgery.[17,86] Our review of the literature favors a more targeted approach because in practice, evaluating patients 2 to 3 weeks before elective surgery may be impossible. Moreover, some patients require nonelective surgery or are noncompliant with instructions to discontinue herbal medications preoperatively. These factors and the extensive use of herbal medicines may mean that herbal medications are taken until the time of surgery. Pharmacokinetic data on selected active constituents indicate that some herbal medications are eliminated quickly and may be discontinued closer to the time of surgery.

Evidence-based estimates of herbal safety in the perioperative period are limited. One recent study of 601 patients who used traditional Chinese herbal medications suggested a low rate of potential serious complications.[87] Clinicians should be familiar with commonly used herbal medications to recognize and treat any complications that may arise. Table 32-1 summarizes the clinically important effects, perioperative concerns, and recommendations for preoperative discontinuation of the nine herbal medications discussed in this chapter.

Nonherbal Dietary Supplements

Herbal medicines fall into the broader category of dietary supplements that also includes vitamins, minerals, amino acids, enzymes, and animal extracts. Data on the safety of these agents in the perioperative period are scant. High-dose vitamin use, particularly of the fat-soluble vitamins (i.e., A, D, E, and K), can be associated with acute and chronic toxicity. Glucosamine and chondroitin sulfate, which are used for joint disorders by many patients undergoing orthopedic procedures, have not been associated with perioperative complications, although chondroitin sulfate, which belongs to the same group of glycosaminoglycan molecules as heparin, may have minor anticoagulant effects.[88] Whether long-term chondroitin sulfate use can cause thrombocytopenia is unknown. Creatine, a dietary supplement used by athletes to enhance performance, has been associated with renal dysfunction in at least one case.[89] There are preliminary data that exogenous melatonin, a hormone produced by the pineal gland, may be useful in preventing and treating postoperative delirium.[90]

Acupuncture

Mechanism and General Practice

There has been interest in using acupuncture as an aid in diminishing preoperative anxiolysis to reduce intraoperative anesthetic requirements, in supporting cardiovascular function, in controlling postoperative pain, and in reducing postoperative ileus, nausea, and vomiting.[91]

Acupuncture is the stimulation of anatomic locations on the skin by a variety of techniques that can be classified as invasive (e.g., needles, injections) or noninvasive (e.g., transcutaneous electrical stimulation, pressure, laser). Needles inserted into the skin can be stimulated by manual manipulation, moxibustion (i.e., burning a substance to produce heat), pressure, laser, and electricity. There are Chinese, Japanese, Korean, French, and other acupuncture systems for identifying acupuncture points, but little research has compared these different systems. As a result, there are no standard or optimal acupuncture points. Practitioners consider acupuncture an art as much as a science.

The traditional theory of acupuncture is that it corrects disruptions in the flow of energy (i.e., qi) and restores the balance of dual forces (i.e., ying-yang) in the body. Data suggest that there is a scientific basis for acupuncture. Acupuncture stimulates high-threshold, small-diameter nerves leading to the activation of spinal cord, brainstem (i.e., periaqueductal gray area), and hypothalamic (i.e., arcuate) neurons, which trigger endogenous opioid mechanisms.[92] The effect of acupuncture analgesia can be reversed by naloxone.[93] Other mechanisms such as modulation of immune function,[94] inhibition of the inflammatory response,[95] regulation of neuropeptide gene expression,[96] and alterations in hormonal levels[97] have been proposed. The development of neuroimaging tools, such as positron emission tomography (PET)[98] and functional magnetic resonance imaging (fMRI),[99,100] make noninvasive studies of acupuncture's effects on human brain activity possible. Studies using PET have demonstrated that the thalamic asymmetry present in patients suffering from chronic pain was reduced after the patients underwent acupuncture treatment. Other studies, using fMRI, have pointed to relationships between particular acupoints and activation of the visual cortex.[101]

Many of the clinical acupuncture studies that have been published are of poor quality and suffer from insufficient sample size, high dropout rates, inadequate follow-up, and poorly defined illnesses, enrollment criteria, and outcome measures.[92] Acupuncture studies suffer from inherent methodologic problems, including difficulties in blinding patients and acupuncturists, using placebo or sham acupuncture, and choosing between different acupuncture techniques. One of the most promising indications for acupuncture is to prevent postoperative nausea and vomiting (PONV).

Acupuncture for Postoperative Nausea and Vomiting

PONV remains a significant problem that results in patient dissatisfaction, delayed discharge, unanticipated hospital admission, and the use of resources (see Chapter 86). Pharmacologic agents, the mainstay of management, have limited effectiveness, are associated with adverse effects, and can be costly. There is considerable interest in acupuncture for its potential to prevent PONV with minimal adverse effects and expense.

The evidence available suggests that when compared with placebo (e.g., sham acupuncture, no treatment), acupuncture prevents PONV.[91] Acupuncture appears to prevent PONV to approximately the same extent as pharmacologic agents do, including metoclopramide, droperidol, prochlorperazine, and ondansetron. A meta-analysis of studies published before 1998 showed that acupuncture and related techniques prevented PONV in adults, not children, with a calculated absolute reduction in risk of 20% to 25% (i.e., for every four or five patients treated, one case of PONV is avoided).[102] Several subsequent randomized, controlled trials suggested that acupuncture may also prevent PONV in the pediatric population[103-106]; another meta-analysis found that acupuncture was not useful for PONV prophylaxis in children after tonsillectomy.[107] P6 acupressure did not reduce PONV in women who underwent cesarean delivery with spinal anesthesia.[108]

Most PONV acupuncture studies use the P6 (i.e., Nei-Nuan or pericardium) acupuncture point, which is located between the palmaris longus and flexor carpi radialis muscle tendons, 4 cm proximal to the distal wrist crease and 1 cm below the skin (Fig. 32-1). Korean hand acupuncture may be equally effective.[109] Studies often differ on the acupuncture method: duration and timing of stimulation, unilateral versus bilateral stimulation, and type of stimulation (i.e., needles with or without additional stimulation, acupressure, transcutaneous electrical stimulation, cutaneous laser stimulation, injection of a 50% dextrose solution, or capsicum plaster). Data to compare the effectiveness, safety, and costs of different methods of stimulation are inadequate. It is

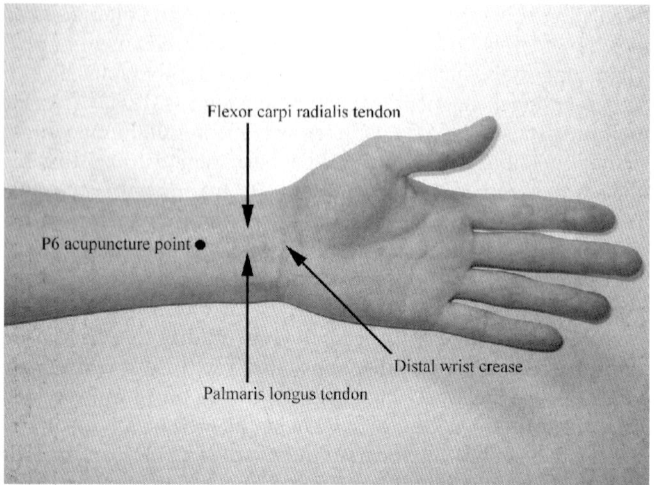

Figure 32-1 The P6 acupuncture point is located between the palmaris longus and flexor carpi radialis muscle tendons, 4 cm proximal to the distal wrist crease and 1 cm below the skin.

typically recommended that stimulation of the acupuncture point be initiated before induction of anesthesia.[110] However, some evidence suggests that postoperative stimulation may be just as or more effective.[111] In children, stimulation immediately before emergence and in the recovery room has been effective. Some anesthesiologists anecdotally report tapping a small needle cap or other piece of smooth plastic over the P6 point as an effective means of acupressure stimulation.

Music Therapy

Music may decrease preoperative anxiety, reduce intraoperative sedative and analgesic requirements, and increase patient satisfaction. Patient-selected music reduced patient-controlled sedative requirements during spinal anesthesia and analgesic requirements during lithotripsy.[112] Music in the preoperative area reduced anxiety without affecting physiologic measures of stress.[113] Music may be part of a low–sensory stimulation strategy to reduce anxiety and increase cooperation in children undergoing induction of anesthesia.[114] Music increased patient satisfaction and reduced systolic blood pressure during cataract surgery performed under a retrobulbar block.[115]

Conclusion

One of the fastest changing aspects of health care is the growing public and scientific interest in CAM. When taken preoperatively, some herbal medicines may adversely affect patient care. Surgery and anesthesia can usually proceed safely if potential complications are predicted and can be avoided. Preliminary data suggest that acupuncture and music may be useful adjuncts in the perioperative period. Although medical schools are beginning to incorporate CAM into their curricula, it is important for anesthesiologists already in practice to stay informed about these alternative therapies.

References

1. Tindle HA, Davis RB, Phillips RS, Eisenberg DM: Trends in use of complementary and alternative medicine by US adults: 1997-2002. Altern Ther Health Med 11:42, 2005.
2. Eisenberg DM, Davis RB, Ettner SL, et al: Trends in alternative medicine use in the United States, 1990-1997. JAMA 280:1569, 1998.
3. Ang-Lee MK, Moss J, Yuan CS: Herbal medicines and perioperative care. JAMA 286:208, 2001.
4. Wang SM, Caldwell-Andrews AA, Kain ZN: The use of complementary and alternative medicines by surgical patients: A follow-up survey study. Anesth Analg 97:1010, 2003.
5. Ashar BH, Rice TN, Sisson SD: Physicians' understanding of the regulation of dietary supplements. Arch Intern Med 167:966, 2007.
6. National Center for Complementary and Alternative Medicine. Available at http://nccam.nih.gov/health/whatiscam/ Accessed August 15, 2003.
7. Tsen LC, Segal S, Pothier M, et al: Alternative medicine use in presurgical patients. Anesthesiology 93:148, 2000.
8. Kaye AD, Clarke RC, Sabar R, et al: Herbal medications: Current trends in anesthesiology practice—a hospital survey. J Clin Anesth 12:468, 2000.
9. Leung JM, Dzankic S, Manku K, et al: The prevalence and predictors of the use of alternative medicine in presurgical patients in five California hospitals. Anesth Analg 93:1062, 2001.
10. Gardiner P, Graham RE, Legedza AT, et al: Factors associated with dietary supplement use among prescription medication users. Arch Intern Med 166:1968, 2006.
11. Weinrobe MC, Montgomery B: Acquired bleeding diathesis in a patient taking PC-SPES. N Engl J Med 347:1213, 2001.
12. De Smet P: Herbal remedies. N Engl J Med 347:2046, 2002.
13. NBJ's herbal and botanical U.S. consumer sales. Available at http://store.yahoo.com/nbj/new2019top75.html/ Accessed November 24, 2003.
14. McKenzie AG, Simpson KR: Current management of patients taking herbal medicines: A survey of anaesthetic practice in the UK. Eur J Anaesthesiol 22:597, 2005.
15. Kassler WJ, Blanc P, Greenblatt R: The use of medicinal herbs by human immunodeficiency virus–infected patients. Arch Intern Med 151:2281, 1991.
16. Cirigliano M, Sun A: Advising patients about herbal therapies. JAMA 280:1565, 1998.
17. Leak JA: Herbal medicines: What do we need to know? ASA Newsl 64:6, 2000.
18. Kennedy JM, van Rij AM, Spears GF, et al: Polypharmacy in a general surgical unit and consequences of drug withdrawal. Br J Clin Pharmacol 49:353, 2000.
19. Tonnesen H, Rosenberg J, Nielsen HJ, et al: Effect of preoperative abstinence on poor postoperative outcome in alcohol misusers: Randomized controlled trial. BMJ 318:1311, 1999.
20. Barrett BP, Brown RL, Locken K, et al: Treatment of the common cold with unrefined echinacea. A randomized, double-blind, placebo-controlled trial. Ann Intern Med 137:939, 2002.
21. Shah SA, Sander S, White CM, et al: Evaluation of echinacea for the prevention and treatment of the common cold: A meta-analysis. Lancet Infect Dis 7:473, 2007.
22. Pepping J: Echinacea. Am J Health Syst Pharm 56:121, 1999.
23. Boullata JI, Nace AM: Safety issues with herbal medicine. Pharmacotherapy 20:257, 2000.
24. Mullins RJ: Echinacea-associated anaphylaxis. Med J Aust 168:170, 1998.
25. Miller LG: Herbal medicinals: Selected clinical considerations focusing on known or potential drug-herb interactions. Arch Intern Med 158:2200, 1998.
26. Gurley BJ, Gardner SF, Hubbard MA: Content versus label claims in ephedra-containing dietary supplements. Am J Health Syst Pharm 57:963, 2000.
27. Nightingale SL: From the Food and Drug Administration. JAMA 278:15, 1997.
28. Haller CA, Benowitz NL: Adverse cardiovascular and central nervous system events associated with dietary supplements containing ephedra alkaloids. N Engl J Med 343:1833, 2000.

29. Zaacks SM, Klein L, Tan CD, et al: Hypersensitivity myocarditis associated with ephedra use. J Toxicol Clin Toxicol 37:485, 1999.
30. Powell T, Hsu FF, Turk J, Hruska K: Ma-huang strikes again: Ephedrine nephrolithiasis. Am J Kidney Dis 32:153, 1998.
31. White LM, Gardner SF, Gurley BJ, et al: Pharmacokinetics and cardiovascular effects of ma-huang (*Ephedra sinica*) in normotensive adults. J Clin Pharmacol 37:116, 1997.
32. Gurley BJ, Gardner SF, White LM, Wang PL: Ephedrine pharmacokinetics after the ingestion of nutritional supplements containing *Ephedra sinica* (ma huang). Ther Drug Monit 20:439, 1998.
33. Stevinson C, Pittler MH, Ernst E: Garlic for treating hypercholesterolemia: A meta-analysis of randomized clinical trials. Ann Intern Med 133:420, 2000.
34. Srivastava KC: Evidence for the mechanism by which garlic inhibits platelet aggregation. Prostaglandins Leukoc Med 22:313, 1986.
35. Rose KD, Croissant PD, Parliament CF, Levin MB: Spontaneous spinal epidural hematoma with associated platelet dysfunction from excessive garlic ingestion: A case report. Neurosurgery 26:880, 1990.
36. Silagy CA, Neil HA: A meta-analysis of the effect of garlic on blood pressure. J Hypertens 12:463, 1994.
37. Le Bars PL, Katz MM, Berman N, et al: A placebo-controlled, double-blind, randomized trial of an extract of *Ginkgo biloba* for dementia. North American Egb Study Group. JAMA 278:1327, 1997.
38. Solomon PR, Adams F, Silver A, et al: Ginko for memory enhancement: A randomized controlled trial. JAMA 288:835, 2000.
39. Rowin J, Lewis SL: Spontaneous bilateral subdural hematomas associated with chronic *Ginkgo biloba* ingestion. Neurology 46:1775, 1996.
40. Vale S: Subarachnoid haemorrhage associated with *Ginkgo biloba*. Lancet 352:36, 1998.
41. Gilbert GJ: Ginkgo biloba. Neurology 48:1137, 1997.
42. Matthews MK Jr: Association of *Ginkgo biloba* with intracerebral hemorrhage. Neurology 50:1933, 1998.
43. Rosenblatt M, Mindel J: Spontaneous hyphema associated with ingestion of *Ginkgo biloba* extract. N Engl J Med 336:1108, 1997.
44. Fessenden JM, Wittenborn W, Clarke L: *Gingko biloba*: A case report of herbal medicine and bleeding postoperatively from a laparoscopic cholecystectomy. Am Surg 67:33, 2001.
45. Watson DG, Oliveira EJ: Solid-phase extraction and gas chromatography–mass spectrometry determination of kaempferol and quercetin in human urine after consumption of *Ginkgo biloba* tablets. J Chromatogr B Biomed Sci Appl 723:203, 1999.
46. Mills S, Bone K (eds): Ginkgo. *In* Mills S, Bone K (eds): Principles and Practice of Phytotherapy. New York, Churchill Livingstone, 2000, pp 404-417.
47. Brekham II, Dardymov IV: New substances of plant origin which increase nonspecific resistance. Annu Rev Pharmacol 9:419, 1969.
48. Soori GS, Bauer B, Sloan J, et al: A pilot, multi-dose, placebo-controlled evaluation of American ginseng (*Panax quinquefolius*) to improve cancer-related fatigue: NCCTG trial N03CA. J Clin Oncol 25:493S, 2007.
49. Attele AS, Wu JA, Yuan CS: Ginseng pharmacology: Multiple constituents and multiple actions. Biochem Pharmacol 58:1685, 1999.
50. Vuksan V, Sievenpiper JL, Koo VY, et al: American ginseng (*Panax quinquefolius* L) reduces postprandial glycemia in nondiabetic subjects and subjects with type 2 diabetes mellitus. Arch Intern Med 160:1009, 2000.
51. Kimura Y, Okuda H, Arichi S: Effects of various ginseng saponins on 5-hydroxytryptamine release and aggregation in human platelets. J Pharm Pharmacol 40:838, 1988.
52. Kuo SC, Teng CM, Lee JC, et al: Antiplatelet components in *Panax ginseng*. Planta Med 56:164, 1990.
53. Park HJ, Lee JH, Song YB, Park KH: Effects of dietary supplementation of lipophilic fraction from *Panax ginseng* on cGMP and cAMP in rat platelets and on blood coagulation. Biol Pharm Bull 19:1434, 1996.
54. Teng CM, Kuo SC, Ko FN, et al: Antiplatelet actions of panaxynol and ginsenosides isolated from ginseng. Biochim Biophys Acta 990:315, 1989.
55. Janetzky K, Morreale AP: Probable interaction between warfarin and ginseng. Am J Health Syst Pharm 54:692, 1997.
56. Yuan CS, Wei G, Dey L: American ginseng reduces warfarin's effect in healthy patients: A randomized, controlled trial. Ann Intern Med 141:23, 2004.
57. Chen SE, Sawchuk RJ, Staba EJ: American ginseng. III. Pharmacokinetics of ginsenosides in the rabbit. Eur J Drug Metab Pharmacokinet 5:161, 1980.
58. Pepping J: Kava: *Piper methysticum*. Am J Health Syst Pharm 56:957, 1999.
59. Jamieson DD, Duffield PH, Cheng D, Duffield AM: Comparison of the central nervous system activity of the aqueous and lipid extract of kava (*Piper methysticum*). Arch Int Pharmacodyn Ther 301:66, 1989.
60. Almeida JC, Grimsley EW: Coma from the health food store: Interaction between kava and alprazolam. Ann Intern Med 125:940, 1996.
61. Brown AC, Onopa J, Holck P, et al: Traditional kava beverage consumption and liver function tests in a predominantly Tongan population in Hawaii. Clin Toxicol (Phila) 45:549, 2007.
62. Norton SA, Ruze P: Kava dermopathy. J Am Acad Dermatol 31:89, 1994.
63. Rasmussen AK, Scheline RR, Solheim E, Hansel R: Metabolism of some kava pyrones in the rat. Xenobiotica 9:1, 1979.
64. Bent S, Kane C, Shinohara K, et al: Saw palmetto for benign prostatic hyperplasia. N Engl J Med 354:557, 2006.
65. Gerber GS: Saw palmetto for the treatment of men with lower urinary tract symptoms. J Urol 163:1408, 2000.
66. Cheema P, El-Mefty O, Jazieh AR: Intraoperative haemorrhage associated with the use of extract of saw palmetto herb: A case report and review of literature. J Intern Med 250:167, 2001.
67. Shelton RC, Keller MB, Gelenberg A, et al: Effectiveness of St. John's wort in major depression. JAMA 285:1978, 2001.
68. Muller WE, Singer A, Wonnemann M, et al: Hyperforin represents the neurotransmitter reuptake inhibiting constituent of *Hypericum* extract. Pharmacopsychiatry 31:16, 1998.
69. Neary JT, Bu Y: *Hypericum* LI 160 inhibits uptake of serotonin and norepinephrine in astrocytes. Brain Res 816:358, 1999.
70. Brown TM: Acute St. John's wort toxicity. Am J Emerg Med 18:231, 2000.
71. Muller WE, Rolli M, Schafer C, Hafner U: Effects of *Hypericum* extract (LI 160) in biochemical models of antidepressant activity. Pharmacopsychiatry 30:102, 1997.
72. Ernst E: Second thoughts about safety of St. John's wort. Lancet 354:2014, 1999.
73. Piscitelli SC, Burstein AH, Chaitt D, et al: Indinavir concentrations and St. John's wort. Lancet 355:547, 2000.
74. Yue QY, Bergquist C, Gerden B: Safety of St. John's wort. Lancet 355:576, 2000.
75. Breidenbach T, Hoffmann MW, Becker T, et al: Drug interaction of St. John's wort with cyclosporin. Lancet 355:1912, 2000.
76. Ruschitzka F, Meier PJ, Turina M, et al: Acute heart transplant rejection due to Saint John's wort. Lancet 355:548, 2000.
77. Johne A, Brockmoller J, Bauer S, et al: Pharmacokinetic interaction of digoxin with an herbal extract from St. John's wort (*Hypericum perforatum*). Clin Pharmacol Ther 66:338, 1999.
78. Hu ZP, Yang XX, Chen X, et al: A mechanistic study on altered pharmacokinetics of irinotecan by St. John's wort. Curr Drug Metab 8:157, 2007.
79. Kerb R, Brockmoller J, Staffeldt B, et al: Single-dose and steady-state pharmacokinetics of hypericin and pseudohypericin. Antimicrob Agents Chemother 40:2087, 1996.
80. Biber A, Fischer H, Romer A, Chatterjee SS: Oral bioavailability of hyperforin from *Hypericum* extracts in rats and human volunteers. Pharmacopsychiatry 31:36, 1998.
81. Houghton PJ: The scientific basis for the reputed activity of valerian. J Pharm Pharmacol 51:505, 1999.
82. Hendriks H, Bos R, Allersma DP, et al: Pharmacological screening of valerenal and some other components of essential oil of *Valeriana officinalis*. Planta Med 42:62, 1981.
83. Ortiz JG, Nieves-Natal J, Chavez P: Effects of *Valeriana officinalis* extracts on [^{3}H]flunitrazepam binding, synaptosomal [^{3}H]GABA uptake and hippocampal [^{3}H]GABA release. Neurochem Res 24:1373, 1999.
84. Leuschner J, Muller J, Rudmann M: Characterization of the central nervous depressant activity of a commercially available valerian root extract. Arzneimittelforschung 43:638, 1993.
85. Garges HP, Varia I, Doraiswamy PM: Cardiac complications and delirium associated with valerian root withdrawal. JAMA 280:1566, 1998.
86. Anesthesiologists warn: If you're taking herbal products, tell your doctor before surgery. Available at: http://www.asahq.org/PublicEduction/herbal.html/ Accessed 10 May 2001.
87. Lee A, Chui PT, Aun CST, et al: Incidence and risk of adverse perioperative events among surgical patients taking traditional Chinese herbal medicines. Anesthesiology 105:454, 2006.
88. Bjornsson TD, Nash PV, Schaten R: The anticoagulant effect of chondroitin-4-sulfate. Thromb Res 27:15, 1982.
89. Pritchard NR, Kalra PA: Renal dysfunction accompanying oral creatine supplements. Lancet 351:1252, 1998.
90. Hanania M, Kitain E: Melatonin for treatment and prevention of postoperative delirium. Anesth Analg 94:338, 2002.
91. Chernyak GV, Sessler DI: Perioperative acupuncture and related techniques. Anesthesiology 102:1031, 2005.
92. Kaptchuk TJ: Acupuncture: Theory, efficacy, and practice. Ann Intern Med 136:374, 2002.
93. Tsunoda Y, Sakahira K, Nakano S, et al: Antagonism of acupuncture analgesia by naloxone in unconscious man. Bull Tokyo Med Dent Univ 27:89, 1980.
94. Mori H, Nishijo K, Kawamura H, et al: Unique immunomodulation by electro-acupuncture in humans possibly via stimulation of the autonomic nervous system. Neurosci Lett 320:21, 2002.

95. Son YS, Park HJ, Kwon OB, et al: Antipyretic effects of acupuncture on the lipopolysaccharide-induced fever and expression of interleukin-6 and interleukin-1 beta mRNAs in the hypothalamus of rats. Neurosci Lett 319:45, 2002.
96. Guo HF, Tian J, Wang X, et al: Brain substrates activated by electroacupuncture (EA) of different frequencies (II): Role of Fos/Jun proteins in EA-induced transcription of preproenkephalin and preprodynorphin genes. Brain Res Mol Brain Res 43:167, 1996.
97. Gerhard I, Postneek F: Auricular acupuncture in the treatment of female infertility. Gynecol Endocrinol 6:171, 1992.
98. Hsieh JC, Tu CH, Chen FP, et al: Activation of the hypothalamus characterizes the acupuncture stimulation at the analgesic point in human: A positron emission tomography study. Neurosci Lett 307:105, 2001.
99. Wu MT, Hsieh JC, Xiong J, et al: Central nervous pathway for acupuncture stimulation: Localization of processing with functional MR imaging of the brain—preliminary experience. Radiology 212:133, 1999.
100. Hui KK, Liu J, Makris N, et al: Acupuncture modulates the limbic system and subcortical gray structures of the human brain: Evidence from fMRI studies in normal subjects. Hum Brain Mapp 9:13, 2000.
101. Shen J: Research on the neurophysiological mechanisms of acupuncture: Review of selected studies and methodological issues. J Altern Complement Med 7:S121, 2001.
102. Lee A, Done ML: The use of nonpharmacologic techniques to prevent postoperative nausea and vomiting: A meta-analysis. Anesth Analg 88:1362, 1999.
103. Rusy LM, Hoffman GM, Weisman SJ: Electroacupuncture prophylaxis of postoperative nausea and vomiting following pediatric tonsillectomy with or without adenoidectomy. Anesthesiology 96:300, 2002.
104. Schlager A, Boehler M, Puhringer F: Korean hand acupressure reduces postoperative nausea and vomiting in children after strabismus surgery. Br J Anaesth 85:267, 2000.
105. Schlager A, Offer T, Baldissera I: Laser stimulation of acupuncture point P6 reduces postoperative vomiting in children undergoing strabismus surgery. Br J Anaesth 81:529, 1998.
106. Wang SM, Kain ZN: P6 acupoint injections are as effective as droperidol in controlling early postoperative nausea and vomiting in children. Anesthesiology 97:359, 2002.
107. Bolton CM, Myles PS, Nolan T, Sterne JA: Prophylaxis of postoperative vomiting in children undergoing tonsillectomy: A systematic review and meta-analysis. Br J Anaesth 97:593, 2006.
108. Habib AS, Itchon-Ramos N, Phillips-Bute BG, Gan TJ, for the Duke Women's Anesthesia (DWA) Research Group: Transcutaneous acupoint electrical stimulation with the ReliefBand for the prevention of nausea and vomiting during and after cesarean delivery under spinal anesthesia. Anesth Analg 102:581, 2006.
109. Boehler M, Mitterschiffthaler G, Schlager A: Korean hand acupressure reduces postoperative nausea and vomiting after gynecological laparoscopic surgery. Anesth Analg 94:872, 2002.
110. Dundee JW, Ghaly RG: Does the timing of P6 acupuncture influence its efficacy as a postoperative antiemetic? Br J Anaesth 63:630, 1989.
111. White PF, Hamza MA, Recart A, et al: Optimal timing of acustimulation for antiemetic prophylaxis as an adjunct to ondansetron in patients undergoing plastic surgery. Anesth Analg 100:367, 2005.
112. Koch ME, Kain ZN, Ayoub C, et al: The sedative and analgesic sparing effect of music. Anesthesiology 89:300, 1998.
113. Wang SM, Kulkarni L, Dolev J, et al: Music and preoperative anxiety: A randomized, controlled study. Anesth Analg 94:1489, 2002.
114. Kain ZN, Wang SM, Mayes LC, et al: Sensory stimuli and anxiety in children undergoing surgery: A randomized, controlled trial. Anesth Analg 92:897, 2001.
115. Cruise CJ, Chung F, Yogendran S, et al: Music increases satisfaction in elderly outpatients undergoing cataract surgery. Can J Anaesth 44:43, 1997.

Anesthesia Management

Section IV

Lee A. Fleisher

33 Risk of Anesthesia

Key Points

1. Perioperative risk is multifactorial and depends on the interaction of anesthesia-, surgery-, and patient-specific factors.
2. Anesthesia-related (and surgery-related) risk includes morbidity and mortality within 30 days, although shorter periods may be relevant, depending on the extent of surgery.
3. Anesthesia and the actions of anesthesiologists may completely or partially cause perioperative morbidity and mortality, but the actions of the anesthesiologist may also decrease or modify risk related to patient disease.
4. In the literature on anesthesia-related risk, rates of morbidity and mortality depend on the wide variety of definitions found.
5. Studies of anesthesia-related risk have found that postanesthesia respiratory depression is the major cause of death and coma totally attributable to anesthesia; this finding prompted the development of postanesthesia care units.
6. Research into anesthesia-related cardiac arrest has found it to be attributable to medication administration, airway management, and technical problems of central venous access.
7. Multivariate modeling using logistic regression equations can be used to determine factors associated with increased risk in the cohort and in individuals and has been used to develop risk indices such as the Cardiac Risk Index.
8. Surveys of maternal mortality suggest that the absolute rate of complications by anesthesia type has not decreased but that the increased use of regional anesthesia has led to improvements in outcome.
9. Medication-related and cardiovascular causes of cardiac arrest were the most common causes in the Pediatric Perioperative Cardiac Arrest Registry.
10. With increases in outpatient surgery, increased surveillance is required to ensure that appropriate procedures are performed in appropriate locations.

Much attention has been focused on the risks associated with anesthesia—surgery-related risks to the patient and occupational risks to the anesthesiologist. From the patient's perspective, it is important to provide an accurate assessment of the probability of complications and to study perioperative morbidity and mortality as a means of quality assurance to improve outcome. Numerous studies have attempted to define the probability of morbidity and mortality, with widely variable results. Risk indices have been developed to identify patients who have a higher probability of complications developing, and it has become evident that individual genetic makeup can affect outcome. In all these areas, as well as in clinical discussions with patients, the key issue is what risk are we attempting to define.

To determine the risk associated with anesthesia, multiple factors have to be entered into the equation. A myopic perspective could include only the morbidity and mortality that occur intraoperatively. From a quality assurance perspective, any death within 48 hours after the use of an anesthetic is evaluated for potential relevancy. Other investigators have evaluated 30-day morbidity and mortality as part of their estimation of anesthesia- and surgery-related risks. However, an important question is the period after anesthesia and surgery at which baseline risk returns to normal, although it is increasingly being recognized that events that take place during the perioperative period may have implications for quite a long time. From the perspective of a shorter timeframe, patients undergoing ambulatory surgery have been shown to have the lowest risk of death the day of surgery as opposed to 1 month later.[1] At the opposite end of the spectrum, asymptomatic release of cardiac enzyme in the perioperative period can have implications for months to years.[2,3] It is therefore important to define the time perspective when evaluating such studies (Table 33-1).

It is also important to differentiate the potential risk that is solely attributable to the administration of anesthesia from the risks that anesthesia may modify. Anesthesia has been touted as the one area of medicine that has achieved very low rates of

Table 33-1 Time Perspective of Anesthetic Morbidity and Mortality Studies

Study	Study Year	Time Perspective
Beecher and Todd	1954	All deaths on the surgical services
Dornette and Orth	1956	Deaths in the operating room or after failure to regain consciousness
Clifton and Hotten	1963	Any death under, attributable to, or without return of consciousness after anesthesia
Harrison	1978	Death within 24 hours
Marx, et al.	1973	Death within 5 days
Hovi-Viander	1980	Death within 3 days
Lunn and Mushin	1982	Death within 6 days
Tiret and Hatton	1986	Complications within 24 hours
Mangano, et al.	1996	Death within 2 years
Monk, et al.	2005	Death within 1 year

Adapted from Derrington MC, Smith G: A review of studies of anaesthetic risk, morbidity and mortality. Br J Anaesth 59:827, 1987.

medical error and complications when the rate of death directly attributable to anesthesia is considered. However, from a quality assurance perspective, a patient with coronary artery disease who experiences a perioperative myocardial infarction would have the primary cause of morbidity assigned to the disease, but tight heart rate control might have prevented the adverse outcome. In this situation, the perioperative infarction might be considered attributable to patient disease rather than the anesthesia, alternatively, it can be considered an event that is partially preventable by anesthesia care. Anesthesiologists must view perioperative organ protection as part of their goals to provide the highest quality of care and reduce perioperative risk. Another example is the use of regional anesthesia to reduce graft thrombosis in patients undergoing infrainguinal arterial reconstruction.[4,5] The importance of anesthesia care on perioperative risk may also be a reflection of the local risk associated with the surgery. For example, benefit from regional anesthesia was found in only two studies; the third study had a much lower rate of graft thrombosis that was not influenced by the type of anesthesia, suggesting that the benefit may be manifested only if the rate of complications is sufficiently large. Assessment of risk therefore depends on the rate of complications.

Traditionally, anesthesiologists and investigators have focused on issues of death and major morbidity such as myocardial infarction, pneumonia, and renal failure. It is becoming increasingly important to include outcomes that affect economic issues, quality of life, and satisfaction for the patient (Table 33-2). For example, a delay in or prevention of discharge home by nausea and vomiting is important from the perspective of economics and quality of life. Readmission to the hospital after outpatient surgery is an important component of outcome studies. Overall satisfaction with care is increasingly being included as an outcome. Further research is required to assess the influence of anesthesia care for nonmorbid outcomes and the importance of these outcomes from a patient-oriented perspective.

Many studies have also looked at what some investigators describe as surrogate end points. For example, nausea and vomiting that do not require treatment or do not delay discharge do not have the same impact as episodes that do affect these outcomes. Myocardial ischemia on the electrocardiogram is another example of a surrogate outcome that may not lead directly to overt morbidity. In determining the risk attributable to anesthesia, it is important to define the outcome of greatest significance.

Finally, many investigators as well as insurers, such as the Centers for Medicare and Medicaid Services, are now evaluating process measures. Examples of process measures include antibiotic timing (did the patient receive antibiotic within 1 hour before surgical incision). These measures are not the outcomes of interest, but there is sufficient evidence that improvement in compliance with these measures should decrease morbidity (e.g., surgical site infections) to warrant measurement and potentially payment for the action. Importantly, compliance with these measures are now publicly reported on websites such as www.hospitalcompare.hhs.gov.

Framework of Perioperative Risk

Perioperative risk is multifactorial and depends on the interaction of anesthesia-, patient-, and surgery-specific factors (Fig. 33-1). With respect to anesthesia, the effects of the agents and the skills of the practitioner are important. Similarly, the surgeon's skills and the surgical procedure itself affect perioperative risk. From the patient's perspective, the question remains whether coexisting disease raises the probability of complications to a level such that the benefit of the surgery is outweighed by the risk. Anesthesiologists frequently have focused on perioperative risk, but the patient is most concerned with management of the disease process. As the specialty focuses on its role in the 21st century, it is important to acknowledge the patient's perspective and desire to undergo procedures that prolong life or improve quality of life. Increasing the ability of the anesthesiologist to affect the decision-making process and overall risk is the future challenge.

Given these various goals, perspectives, and influences, this chapter attempts to define the current state of knowledge in this area. With the increasing interest in evidence-based medicine, it

Table 33-2 Examples of Common Outcome Measures

Outcome	Example
Mortality	
Morbidity	
Major	Myocardial infarction
	Pneumonia
	Pulmonary embolism
	Renal failure/insufficiency
	Postoperative cognitive dysfunction
Minor	Nausea
	Vomiting
	Readmission
Patient satisfaction	
Quality of life	

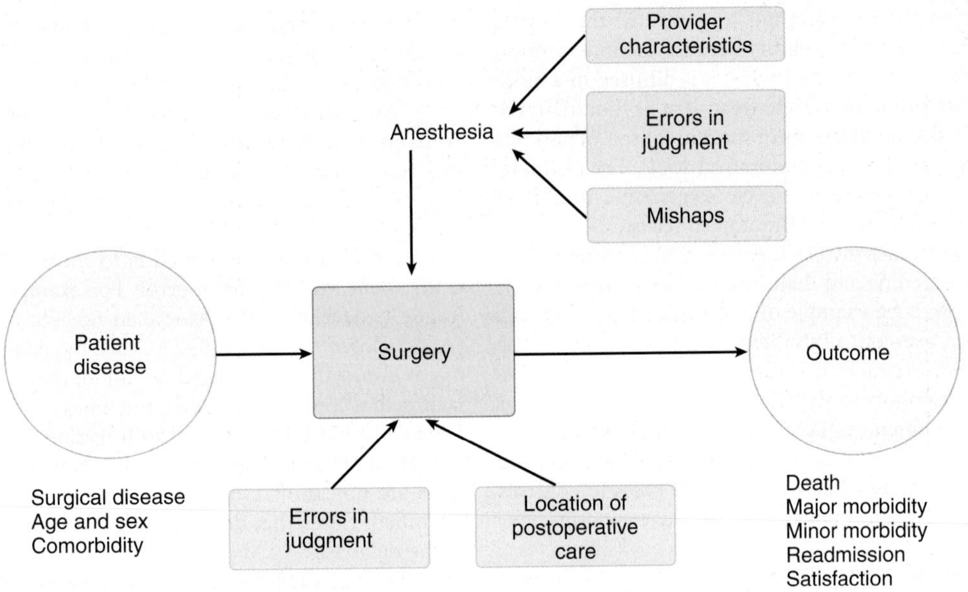

Figure 33-1 Representation of the influences of various components on poor perioperative outcomes. Surgical, anesthetic, and patient characteristics all contribute to outcome. Anesthesia-related contributions can include issues of judgment and mishaps, as well as characteristics of the provider. The surgical procedure itself affects outcome, as does the location of intraoperative and postoperative care.

is important to define what is known and not known. Because it would be unethical to compare operations performed with the use of an "ideal anesthetic" with those using a less ideal or no anesthetic, virtually all studies looking at the factors that contribute to perioperative mortality involve evaluations of large cohorts of patients. However, since the 1990s there have been several well-designed, randomized clinical trials to evaluate different anesthesia regimens, which has advanced the field. This chapter also reviews the literature, with an emphasis on the strength of the evidence for the conclusions.

Issues Related to Study Design

Types of Studies

To interpret the literature, it is important to understand the strengths and limitations of the various study designs. Prospective cohort studies involve the identification of a group of subjects who are monitored over time for the occurrence of an outcome of interest. The goal is to identify patients in whom the outcome develops. For studies of perioperative mortality, individual cases can be reviewed to determine the cause of mortality. Alternatively, data on all patients in the cohort can be obtained, and factors associated with the development of morbidity or mortality can be discerned. An example of a prospective cohort study to identify factors associated with perioperative cardiac morbidity and mortality is that of Goldman and colleagues,[6] which led to development of the Cardiac Risk Index.

Another example of a prospective cohort study is one in which patients with a known disease are studied for the development of predefined outcomes. Such studies provide the natural history of the disease. For example, studies of patients who have sustained a myocardial infarction could be important in determining optimal timing between occurrence of the infarct and surgery.

Although prospective cohort studies have important value in identifying risk factors for the outcome of interest, there are significant limitations. Selection of the cohort of interest can significantly affect the results obtained. The larger the cohort, the more the results can be generalized. A second bias is that many patients may be lost to follow-up. In perioperative studies, this may not be an important issue for short-term outcomes. The importance of a risk factor depends on the completeness of the data. For example, if the presence of severe angina were not included in the database, it could not be considered a risk factor, and other factors may appear to be more important.[6]

A specific example of a prospective cohort study is the randomized clinical trial. Randomized clinical trials represent the standard for evidence of causation. They have defined inclusion and exclusion criteria, treatment protocols, and outcomes of interest. They are usually single- or double-blinded (to patient and physician) studies and are designed to test the effect of a new drug or intervention. They are rarely used as a means of identifying risk, but they may be used to determine whether a risk factor is truly linked by a causal relationship or is simply an association. For example, hypothermia in the perioperative period has been associated with an increased incidence of perioperative ischemia, a surrogate marker for morbidity.[7] In a randomized clinical trial, the use of forced-air warming to maintain normothermia was associated with a significantly lower incidence of perioperative morbid cardiac events.[8] Randomized clinical trials directed at interventions that reduce the frequency of a given risk factor in the population are frequently performed after the results of a prospective cohort study to confirm the findings of an association between poor outcome and that factor.

Randomized clinical trials derive their strength from an evidence-based perspective because of their high degree of internal validity; the randomization scheme and the use of placebo (or accepted alternative treatments) provide strong evidence that the results are related to the intervention. Importantly, these trials have a lower degree of external validity because the intervention may not behave in the same manner when it is diffused in a more heterogeneous population in which treatment is not defined. Additionally, low-risk complications in specific subsets of patients may not be detected in smaller randomized trials. For example, the cardiovascular complications of cyclooxygenase-2 inhibitors were not initially detected in the randomized trials.

Retrospective studies involve identification of patients who have sustained an outcome and definition of risk factors associated with the outcome. An example of a retrospective design is a case-control study. Case-control studies identify patients with the outcome of interest. Frequently, these patients are included as part of a prospective cohort study. The prevalence of a risk factor in patients with the outcome (i.e., cases) is compared with the prevalence of the risk factor in matched controls to maximize the efficiency and power of the results. The ratio of cases to controls can be varied to yield greater power with an increasing number of controls.

Case-control studies are subject to several biases. The exact definitions of cases and controls can influence the analysis. Frequently, patients are matched for age and gender, but other factors may play an important role. It is critical that the exposure precede the outcome, and a dose-response gradient further confirms the relationship.

Problems Inherent in Studying Anesthesia-Related Risk

Several issues related to studying anesthesia-related risk can affect the findings. For example, multiple definitions of perioperative mortality exist. In particular, the timeframe in which a death can be attributed to the surgery and delivery of anesthesia varies. Because in-hospital stays have shortened, many events related to surgery may occur after discharge. For this reason, the National Surgical Quality Improvement Project (NSQIP) requires 30-day follow-up on all patients to develop robust risk-adjusted models of morbidity and mortality. The issue of the time horizon is particularly important with ambulatory or short-stay surgery, for which recovery from anesthesia occurs at home. As we continue to monitor our patients for safety, it will be important to extend follow-up care beyond the traditional hospital setting, and many recent studies have included such an approach.

A major problem in any study of risk is the actual rate of complications in the population of interest. There are multiple sources of data for studying perioperative risk. Although some of the original studies used data from only one or a small group of institutions, such approaches may not be practical in the current era. As demonstrated throughout this chapter, most individuals believe that risk related to anesthesia has decreased over time, although this premise has been questioned.[9] For example, the rate of anesthesia-related mortality described in the Confidential Enquiry into Perioperative Deaths (CEPOD) of 1987 was 1 in 185,000 patients as opposed to the 1 in 2680 cases reported by Beecher and Todd about 30 years earlier.[10,11] In view of the current rate, any study would have to be enormous to detect anesthesia-related mortality. Such a study would require information from a large number of sites or data covering multiple years from a single institution. Because of concern in the United States regarding confidentiality and legal liability, a multicenter study of risk in unselected patients would be difficult to undertake. Such problems may not be inherent in other countries.

Another issue is the effect of the act of studying outcome. As in any study of risk, the actual rate of complications decreases as a result of increased observation. This is frequently observed as a lower than expected rate of complications in the placebo arm of a randomized, controlled trial.

An alternative approach is to identify bad outcomes and study them for patterns of error. For example, Cheney and colleagues[12] developed the American Society of Anesthesiologists (ASA) Closed Claims Study (ACCS). By obtaining the records of major events that led to legal litigation, they were able to identify factors that contributed to bad outcomes. With this methodology, selected morbidities that lead to litigation can be identified. The limitation of this methodology is that the actual rates of complications are not known; only the number of closed legal claims is identified. Cases that do not result in litigation are not included in the database.

Several attempts have been made to establish large epidemiologic databases. One example of such an approach has been the work of Mangano and the Multicenter Study of Perioperative Ischemia group with regard to cardiac surgery. This group used their database to evaluate issues such as the rate and importance of atrial fibrillation after cardiac surgery and the use of aspirin.[13,14] Other approaches include the development of cardiac surgery databases by the Society of Thoracic Surgeons, the U.S. Veterans Administration NSQIP, and the New England Collaborative Project.[15-18] These databases are used to define risk factors for poor outcome, to compare local with national complication rates, and as educational tools. Such databases currently include little or no information regarding anesthesia practice, although many anesthesia specialty societies are in discussion to develop independent databases or join with surgical groups to develop more robust databases. Even though these databases may provide extremely important information to improve care, the ability to generalize results to centers that do not have sufficient infrastructure to participate in such projects (e.g., smaller hospitals) is unknown.

This final issue—the institutional site of the surgery—may have other implications related to the pattern of care at a particular hospital. Although studies frequently categorize risk as related to anesthesia, surgery, or patient disease, postoperative care may have a profound impact on risk. For example, risk for pulmonary embolism may be related to nursing care and the frequency of patient ambulation after surgery.[19] The presence of an intensivist who makes daily rounds and higher nurse staffing ratios may also affect outcome.[20] Variations in the total care provided by a hospital, including anesthesiologists and surgeons, may significantly affect outcomes.

One advance in determining local complication rates is the development of hospital information systems. The use of computer databases in the assessment of risk began with Marx and colleagues[21] in the 1970s. These information systems are now nearly a requirement for survival of the hospital. The ability to query these systems will make large-scale studies of institutional risk much less burdensome in the future. Anesthesia information systems are increasingly becoming common. Reich and coworkers[22] used one such system to identify intraoperative hemodynamic abnormalities, including pulmonary hypertension, hypotension during cardiopulmonary bypass, and pulmonary diastolic hypertension after cardiopulmonary bypass, as independent predictors of mortality, stroke, and perioperative myocardial infarction beyond the effects of other preoperative risk factors.

When extremely large sample sizes are needed, administrative databases may be among the most cost-effective approaches to this issue. Examples of administrative databases include Medicare claims files, private insurance company claims, and hospital electronic records. These databases include a small number of data points for an extremely large number of subjects. For example, the Medicare database includes financial data, disease codes (International Classification of Diseases, 9th revision [ICD-9]), and procedure codes (Current Procedural Terminology [CPT]) for each patient. It also includes information regarding the location of care and provider type. The Medicare claims file is being extensively used to provide benchmarks for rates of mortality and major complications after coronary bypass surgery.[23] Hospitals can compare their rates with those of neighboring and competing hospitals and may use these data as markers for quality of hospital care.[24,25] Silber and associates[26] took an alternative approach to the use of Medicare databases and evaluated perioperative factors that influence failure to rescue. Failure to rescue is the concept whereby the actual rate of complications associated with death is studied rather than the overall death and complication rate.[26] The underlying assumption is that higher quality of care results in a lower rate of fatal outcomes, even among patients who sustain complications. Importantly, the use of administrative databases to study outcomes should be considered as hypothesis generating rather than simply answering specific questions in the same manner as randomized controlled trials.

Mortality Related to Anesthesia

The first report of the delivery of anesthesia (ether) for an operative procedure took place in 1846. Only 2 years later, a death attributable to anesthesia was reported.[27] In that report, Hannah Greener died on induction with chloroform. Since that time there have been numerous investigations into the cause of anesthesia-related deaths. The first formal investigation of anesthesia-related deaths was published by John Snow in 1858.[28] Snow analyzed 50 deaths that occurred during chloroform anesthesia. At that time, mortality occurred principally in healthy patients undergoing minor procedures, suggesting that anesthesia was the principal cause of the mortality. Subsequent studies reported deaths of patients with significant comorbid conditions who were undergoing major surgical procedures; in these cases the cause of mortality was frequently multifactorial.

Surgery Without Anesthesia

Surgical procedures were carried out before the introduction of anesthetics. The key to success was the speed of the procedure, with successful amputations lasting only 30 seconds. Strong assistants and restraints were frequently required. Alternatively, decreased cerebral perfusion by means of bilateral carotid compression was used to decrease sensation during the procedure. Surgical procedures were associated with a significant risk of death and, at a minimum, were associated with severe pain. The development of anesthesia has been heralded as one of the great advances of modern medicine because it allowed surgery to advance.

Early Studies of Anesthesia-Related Mortality

One of the earliest systematic approaches to anesthesia-related risk occurred in 1935, when Ruth[29] helped establish the first anesthesia study commission to analyze perioperative deaths (Table 33-3). The commissioners relied on voluntary submission of cases and determined the cause of death by majority vote. Both

Table 33-3 Estimates of the Incidence of Mortality Related to Anesthesia before 1980

Study	Year	Number of Anesthetics	Primary Cause	Primary and Associated Cause
Beecher and Todd	1954	599,548	1:2680	1:1560
Dornette and Orth	1956	63,105	1:2427	1:1343
Schapira, et al.	1960	22,177	1:1232	1:821
Phillips, et al.	1960	—	1:7692	1:2500
Dripps, et al.	1961	33,224	1:852	1:415
Clifton and Hotton	1963	205,640	1:6048	1:3955
Memery	1965	114,866	1:3145	1:1082
Gebbie	1966	129,336	—	1:6158
Minuck	1967	121,786	1:6766	1:3291
Marx, et al.	1973	34,145	—	1:1265
Bodlander	1975	211,130	1:14,075	1:1703
Harrison	1978	240,483	—	1:4537
Hovi-Viander	1980	338,934	1:5059	1:1412

From Ross AF, Tinker JH: Anesthesia risk. *In* Miller RD (ed): Anesthesia, 3rd ed. New York, Churchill Livingstone, 1990.

these methodologies were deemed inadequate in subsequent years.

From a pragmatic standpoint, determining the cause of anesthesia-related mortality is important if information from the analysis can be used to improve subsequent care. This concept was best voiced by Sir Robert MacIntosh in 1948.[30] He stated that many anesthesia-related deaths were preventable and that improved education was the best means to avoid unnecessary mortality. He went so far as to suggest that all development of new drugs be halted for 5 years to direct more attention to training young anesthetists. He attempted to focus attention on postoperative care by suggesting that more deaths occurred after patients were returned to the ward than intraoperatively. His final comments were related to the need to establish a formal inquiry mechanism for determining the cause of any death because such an analysis could lead to improved practice. In many ways, the CEPOD was the culmination of such a philosophy.

A major advance in the analysis of anesthesia-related risk was the 1954 report by Beecher and Todd[10] of anesthesia-related deaths at 10 institutions. Their study included 599,548 anesthesia procedures. The overall chance of mortality from any cause was 1 per 75 cases. Anesthesia was the primary cause of mortality in 1 in 2680 procedures, and it was a primary or contributory cause of mortality in 1 in 1560 procedures. Surgical error in diagnosis, judgment, or technique was the primary cause of death in 1 in 420 cases, and patient disease was the primary cause in 1 in 95 cases.

Dornette and Orth[31] reported on deaths occurring in the operating room at their institution during a 12-year period from 1943 through 1954. The rate of mortality totally attributable to anesthesia was 1 in 2427 cases, and the rate of mortality totally or partially attributable to anesthesia was 1 in 1343 cases.

Dripps and colleagues[32] at the University of Pennsylvania surveyed their experience during the 10-year period from 1947 through 1957. They identified 1285 operative deaths (i.e., death within 30 days) in approximately 120,000 anesthesia procedures, for a gross mortality rate of 1.1%. This definition includes late deaths, in contrast to many studies that focused on the intraoperative period or the first 48 postoperative hours. After review of hospital records, the investigators determined whether anesthesia was definitely or possibly contributory to each death. Among patients who underwent spinal anesthesia, mortality definitely related to anesthesia occurred in 1 in 1560 procedures, and mortality definitely or possibly related to anesthesia occurred in 1 in 780 procedures. Among those who underwent general anesthesia, mortality was definitely related to anesthesia in 1 in 536 cases and definitely or possibly related in 1 in 259 cases. Mortality was correlated with physical status with use of the ASA physical status classification scoring system. The higher mortality figures than in other reports may be related to the higher physical acuity at this hospital. Importantly, deaths attributable to anesthesia did not occur in any of the 16,000 patients with ASA class 1 physical status.

Dripps and colleagues compared their data with those of Beecher and Todd. The principal intraoperative complications were hypotension and hypoxia. Virtually all patients who underwent spinal anesthesia had intraoperative complications, but postoperative complications were rare in this group. The investigators believed that anesthesia-related mortality had improved since the start of the study, mainly because of improvements in cardiac resuscitation, more rational transfusion therapy, standard use of recovery rooms, and efficient use of mechanical ventilators.

There were a number of reports from individual hospitals or a small group of hospitals during the subsequent 2 decades.[33] The Baltimore Anesthesia Study Committee[34] reviewed 1024 deaths occurring on the day of or the day after a surgical procedure to determine the potential contribution of anesthesia. This short period of observation (48 hours) contrasts with the 30-day period used by Dripps and coworkers. For each case reviewed, the committee determined whether anesthesia was the principal cause or one of several contributing factors. In 196 cases (19.2%), the committee voted that anesthesia management contributed to the death of the patient. Anesthesia was the principal cause of death in approximately one third of the cases (64 of 196), with one half of them being related to improper management of the anesthetic. The researchers estimated that operative mortality occurred in 4 per 10,000 operations by using these data and applying rates of surgery from the National Health Survey. In more than 50% of all cases studied, death occurred in the patient's room, which led the investigators to emphasize the need for routine use of postanesthesia care areas. In an attempt to educate practitioners and prevent duplication of preventable causes of death, each of the perioperative deaths was discussed.

Schapira and coauthors[35] reported on mortality occurring within 24 hours after surgery between the years 1952 and 1956 at Montefiore Hospital in New York. They ascribed 27 deaths to anesthesia, including 18 in which anesthesia was a primary cause and 9 in which it was contributory. The overall prevalence of death partially or totally attributable to anesthesia was 1 in 1232 procedures.

Clifton and Hotton[36] reported 162 deaths associated with anesthesia in 205,640 operations performed at the Royal Prince Alfred Hospital in Sydney, Australia, between 1952 and 1962. They calculated that the incidence of mortality totally attributable to anesthesia was 1 in 3955, that attributable to surgery was 1 in 2311, and that attributable to patient disease was 1 in 1996 procedures. One cause of postoperative mortality was respiratory insufficiency. The researchers argued that many of these complications would have been prevented by the use of a recovery unit. The potential safety advantages of a postanesthesia care unit (PACU) constituted a general theme in reports from the 1960s.

Dinnick[37] reported 600 deaths associated with anesthesia as part of a series of investigations sponsored by the Association of Anaesthetists in London. This represents the second report from this group since a committee was established to collect clinical data in 1949. The first report included a review of 1000 fatalities and concluded that "in the majority of the reports there were departures from accepted practice." The initial report, published in 1956, found that regurgitation or vomiting was the main factor leading to death, whereas the second report, published in 1964, found that low blood volume was more important. Underventilation was the second most common finding and it accounted for 25% of deaths.

Bodlander[38] provided a follow-up report of anesthesia-related mortality at the Royal Prince Alfred Hospital for the years 1963 to 1972. The incidence of mortality totally attributed to anesthesia decreased to 1 in 1702 cases, whereas anesthesia contributed to mortality in 1 in 502 cases as compared with 1 in 1208 for the years 1952 to 1962. The reduction in anesthesia-related deaths was attributed to an increase in the number of qualified staff and the degree of supervision.

Marx and colleagues[21] evaluated the incidence of death within 7 days after surgery in 34,145 consecutive patients at the Bronx Municipal Hospital Center between 1965 and 1969. A total of 645 patients died, and a death report form based on that developed by a committee of the New York Academy of Medicine was constructed. The deaths were then analyzed in relation to perioperative data available from a computer system. The patient's preexisting disease was considered to be the primary cause of death in 83% of cases, surgery in 10%, and anesthesia in only 4% (1 of 1265 cases). Although mortality rose progressively with age, physical status correlated best with the incidence of mortality.

Marx and colleagues also determined the relationship between type of anesthesia and mortality. Regional anesthesia was associated with the lowest incidence of death, local anesthesia with the highest; the incidence for general anesthesia was intermediate. Although this relationship was significantly different between groups, the difference appeared to be related to patient risk factors, a finding supported by a study by Cohen and coworkers.[39]

Farrow and associates[40,41] studied hospital mortality after 108,878 anesthesia procedures in Cardiff, Wales, between 1972 and 1977. The crude mortality rate was 2.2 per 100 patients. Mortality was greatest in patients older than 65 years. The mortality rate also increased with the severity of disease and the need for emergency operations.

Harrison[42] evaluated mortality associated with 240,483 anesthesia procedures performed between 1967 and 1976 at Groote Schuur Hospital in Cape Town, South Africa. Data were collected prospectively, beginning in 1956. Anesthesia was the cause of death or a major contributory factor in 0.22 cases per 1000 procedures, as opposed to 0.33 per 1000 operations in the previous 10 years. Anesthesia contributed to 2.2% of all the deaths associated with surgery. The most common causes of anesthesia-related mortality, in order of frequency, were hypovolemia, respiratory inadequacy after neuromuscular blockade, complications of tracheal intubation, and inadequate postoperative care. Although the improvement in anesthesia-related mortality could not be directly attributed to specific improvements in care, four specific changes did occur: continuing improvement in routine monitoring, an increase in the ratio of consultants to registrars (British system residents), a decrease in the case load per anesthesiologist, and the introduction of recovery rooms and intensive care units (ICUs).

Studies before 1980 demonstrated steady improvements in anesthesia-related mortality. Studies performed throughout the world focused on identifying causative factors for perioperative mortality. Several general themes emerged. Anesthesia represents a small but significant cause of perioperative mortality, perioperative respiratory complications represent a major complication, and elucidation of the causes of perioperative mortality and education about these causes should lead to improved outcomes.

Anesthesia-Related Mortality Studies after 1980

Whereas studies conducted before 1980 typically focused on one institution or a small group of institutions, studies since then have frequently been performed on a national basis. Improvements in anesthesia-related and overall mortality have made analysis of a single institution inadequate because of the small sample size. For example, Holland[43] reported deaths occurring within 24 hours after an anesthesia procedure in New South Wales, Australia. A committee of six anesthesiologists, three surgeons, an obstetrician, a general practitioner, and a medical administrator was established in 1960 and reviewed all such cases except those that occurred during a 3-year period between mid-1980 and mid-1983. Four categories were established to define the relationship of anesthesia to operative morbidity and mortality (Table 33-4). Between 1960 and 1985, information was available on 92% to 96% of all cases. The incidence of anesthesia-attributable deaths decreased from 1 in 5500 procedures performed in 1960 to 1 in 10,250 in 1970 and then to 1 in 26,000 in 1984. Based on these estimates, the investigators asserted that it was at least five times safer to undergo anesthesia in 1984 than in 1960, particularly for healthy individuals. A subsequent follow-up report stated that factors under the control of the anesthesiologist caused or contributed to perioperative mortality at a rate of 1 in 20,000 operations.[44] The latter study demonstrated a preponderance of male over female patients (1.7 : 1). The reason for this finding is unclear, although it confirms other reports. Importantly, 64% of the deaths were deemed inevitable, suggesting that only one third were preventable.

Table 33-4 Edwards Classification of the Relationship of Anesthesia to Operative Morbidity and Mortality

Category	Definition
I	When it is reasonably certain that the event or death was caused by the anesthetic agent or technique of administration or in other ways coming directly within the anesthetist's province
II	Similar to type I cases, but ones in which there is some element of doubt about whether the agent or technique was entirely responsible for the result
III	Cases in which the patient's adverse event or death was caused by the anesthetic and the surgical technique
IV	Events entirely referable to surgical technique

From Holland R: Anaesthetic mortality in New South Wales. Br J Anaesth 59:834, 1987.

The New South Wales study of anesthesia-related mortality evaluated the contribution of the anesthetist to perioperative mortality. Four groups of providers were identified: specialists, nonspecialists, certified registered nurse anesthetists (CRNAs), and residents. The absolute number of anesthesia-related deaths decreased in all groups but was most pronounced for nonspecialists. During the period 1960 through 1969, the resident medical officer frequently provided anesthesia. During this same period it was found that residents contributed significantly to the mortality observed in "good-risk" patients, which led to phasing out of the resident medical officer as a member of the anesthesia workforce.

Under the direction of the French Ministry of Health, Tiret and colleagues[45] carried out a prospective survey of complications associated with anesthesia in France between 1978 and 1982 from a representative sample of 198,103 anesthesia procedures chosen at random from hospitals throughout the country. The sample included a survey of 460 public and private hospitals. The investigators evaluated the occurrence of death or coma within 24

Table 33-5 Incidence of Complications Partially or Totally Related to Anesthesia

Complications	Partially Related	Totally Related	Total*
All complications	1:1887	1:1215	1:739
Death	1:3810	1:13,207	1:1957
Death and coma	1:3415	1:7924	1:2387

*Total number of anesthetics: 198,103.

From Tiret L, Desmonts JM, Hatton F, Vourc'h G: Complications associated with anaesthesia—A prospective survey in France. Can Anaesth Soc J 33:336-344, 1986.

hours after surgery. The opinion of the participating anesthesiologists and the National Committee of Assessors was determined, and the latter was accepted if there was disagreement. In the group studied, 268 patients had major complications, 67 patients died, and 16 patients suffered persistent coma. Death was totally related to anesthesia in 1 in 13,207 procedures and partially related in 1 in 3810 (Table 33-5). Sixty-two percent of the coma cases were deemed totally attributable to anesthesia, with the remainder being partially attributable to anesthesia. The French survey confirmed previous findings that major complications occur more frequently in older patients, those undergoing emergency operations, and those with more extensive comorbid conditions as measured by the ASA physical status classification.

One of the most important findings of the survey was that postanesthesia respiratory depression was the leading cause of death and coma that were totally attributable to anesthesia. Almost all the patients who had respiratory depression leading to a major complication had received narcotics and muscle relaxants that had not been reversed. They also reported a high incidence of anaphylactoid shock, which the investigators contended was caused primarily by the use of Althesin and succinylcholine. There was no category of drug overdose, which might have been a more appropriate label for some of these cases.

The study by Tiret and colleagues had the advantage of collecting data prospectively, thereby allowing more accurate estimation of overall mortality than many of the other studies completed. A major limitation of the study was that only deaths occurring within 24 hours after surgery were included, thus ignoring late deaths that were the direct result of intraoperative complications.

Tikkanen and Hovi-Viander[46] studied deaths associated with anesthesia and surgery in Finland and compared the results in 1986 with those collected in 1975. Mortality related to anesthesia decreased during the 9-year period; the incidence of anesthesia-related mortality was 0.15 per 10,000 procedures in 1986.

Lunn and coworkers[47-50] published two reports on anesthesia-related surgical mortality in the United Kingdom. When a death occurred in a hospital within 6 days after surgery, a questionnaire was sent to the patient's anesthetist and surgeon. For 59.3% of the 4034 reported deaths, both the surgeon and the anesthetist returned the forms. The replies were reviewed anonymously by two assessors, and differences of opinion were determined by arbitration. After review, further details were obtained if the reply indicated that anesthesia was at least partly responsible for the death. The second report was based on an analysis of 197 reports of death within 6 days after anesthesia during 1981. In this report, 43% of the deaths were found by the assessors to have nothing to do with anesthesia, 41% were partly attributable to anesthesia, and 16% were totally attributable to anesthesia. Of the 32 cases for which death was totally attributable to anesthesia, most were caused by faulty anesthesia technique or postoperative respiratory failure.

The pioneering work of Lunn and others led to the development of CEPOD, which assessed almost 1 million cases of anesthesia during a 1-year period in 1987 in three large regions of the United Kingdom. Unique to this study was the establishment of "crown privilege" by the government to allow total confidentiality:

> *The Secretary of State is satisfied that the disclosure of documents about individual cases prepared for the Enquiry into Perioperative Deaths would be against the public interest and would undermine the whole basis of a confidential study. The data or information sent to the Confidential Enquiry into Perioperative Deaths is therefore protected from subpoena ...*

Deaths occurring within 30 days after surgery were included in the study. There were 4034 deaths in an estimated 485,850 operations, for a crude mortality rate of 0.7% to 0.8%. Surgery contributed totally or partially in 30% of all cases. Progression of the present disease contributed to death in 67.5% of the cases, and progression of an intercurrent disease was relevant in 44.3%. Anesthesia was considered the sole cause of death in only three individuals, for a rate of 1 in 185,000 cases, and anesthesia was contributory in 410 deaths, for a rate of 7 in 10,000 cases (Table 33-6).

There are several potential causes for the improvement in mortality between the CEPOD study and previous studies, including cases from the same group. One explanation is that improvement in care led to improvement in outcome. Many of the deaths that would previously have been classified as "anesthesia totally contributory" were later classified as "anesthesia partially contributory."

An important aspect of the CEPOD study was that it established anesthesia- and surgery-related factors that contributed to mortality. The five most common causes of death are shown in Table 33-7. Of the 410 perioperative deaths, there were 9 cases of aspiration or vomiting and 18 cases of cardiac arrest. A large proportion of elderly women had fractures of the femoral neck. The death rate was inversely related to the seniority of the operating surgeon and to preoperative preparation. The operating surgeon was a consultant in only 19% of the orthopedic cases as compared with 47% overall.

The CEPOD study also provided important information regarding anesthesia practice. Patients were seen preoperatively

Table 33-6 Death Totally Attributable to Each Component of Risk in the Confidential Enquiry into Perioperative Deaths

Component	Mortality Rate Contribution
Patient	1:870
Operation	1:2860
Anesthetic	1:185,056

Adapted from Buck N, Devlin HB, Lunn JL: Report of a Confidential Enquiry into Perioperative Deaths, Nuffield Provincial Hospitals Trust. London, The King's Fund Publishing House, 1987.

Table 33-7 Most Common Clinical Causes of Death in the Confidential Enquiry into Perioperative Deaths

Cause of Death	Percentage of Total
Bronchopneumonia	13.5
Congestive heart failure	10.8
Myocardial infarction	8.4
Pulmonary embolism	7.8
Respiratory failure	6.5

Adapted from Buck N, Devlin HB, Lunn JL: Report of a Confidential Enquiry into Perioperative Deaths, Nuffield Provincial Hospitals Trust. London, The King's Fund Publishing House, 1987.

in more than 80% of the cases but postoperatively in less than 50%. Although the electrocardiogram was monitored in 97% of cases, core temperature was assessed in only 7%. Muscle relaxants were used in more than 50% of the cases, but a nerve stimulator was used in only 14%.

The assessors concluded that avoidable factors were present in about 20% of the perioperative deaths. Contributing factors for anesthesiologists and surgeons tended to be failure to act appropriately with existing knowledge (rather than lack of knowledge), equipment malfunction, and fatigue. However, the researchers suggested that inadequate supervision was a problem and that no operation on a patient with an ASA physical status of class 4 or 5 should be performed without direct consultation with the appropriate anesthesia or surgical authority (Table 33-8).

Several large national studies have been published since the CEPOD. Pedersen and colleagues[51] performed a series of studies in the late 1980s in Denmark to look at factors attributable to anesthesia that led to serious morbidity or mortality. They performed a prospective study of 7306 anesthesia procedures. In a method similar to that used in earlier studies, three anesthetists reviewed the records of complications and determined whether the cause was attributable to anesthesia (no distinction was made between totally and partially contributing factors). Complications attributable to anesthesia occurred in 43 patients (1 in 170), and 3 patients (1 in 2500) died. Complications in the 43 patients, in order of incidence, included cardiovascular collapse in 16 (37%), severe postoperative headache after regional anesthesia in 9 (21%), and awareness under anesthesia in 8 (19%). The researchers determined that 37% of the anesthesia-related morbidity was preventable. The three deaths occurred in severely ill patients (ASA class 3 or greater physical status), and two of these deaths were judged to be preventable.

Table 33-8 Grade of Physician According to Time of Surgery in the Confidential Enquiry into Perioperative Deaths

	Anesthetist		Surgeon	
Grade	Day*	Night†	Day*	Night†
Consultant	50	25	45	34
Others	50	75	55	66

*Day represents Monday through Friday, 9 AM to 7 PM.
†Night represents Monday through Friday, 7 PM to 9 AM, and Saturday and Sunday.
Adapted from Buck N, Devlin HB, Lunn JL: Report of a Confidential Enquiry into Perioperative Deaths, Nuffield Provincial Hospitals Trust. London, The King's Fund Publishing House, 1987.

Cohen and coworkers[39] developed a methodology for studying the outcome of anesthesia in four teaching hospitals in Canada. They developed a new anesthesia record to serve as a data collection instrument. Research nurses reviewed all inpatient records within 72 hours after surgery, conducted interviews of the patients with a standardized instrument, and conducted a telephone survey of most of the outpatients. Assessment of the contribution of anesthesia to each complication was determined by using the classification of the New South Wales Committee on Anaesthesia Mortality (see Table 33-4). In a total of 6914 anesthesia procedures in adults, no deaths were directly attributable to anesthesia.

Lagasse[9] reviewed perioperative deaths (i.e., deaths occurring within 2 days after surgery) at a suburban university hospital network between 1992 and 1994 and an urban university hospital network between 1995 and 1999. There were a total of 347 deaths in 184,472 cases. Anesthesia-related mortality (i.e., death to which error by an anesthesia practitioner contributed) occurred in 1 in every 12,641 procedures in the suburban setting and in 1 in 13,322 procedures in the urban setting. Mortality increased with increasing ASA physical status (Fig. 33-2). In reviewing data over the previous decade, the investigators estimated that anesthesia-related mortality had remained stable at approximately 1 death per 13,000 procedures, with wide variation making it impossible to detect trends in anesthesia safety.

The Thai Anesthesia Incidents Study (THAI Study) consists of a prospectively defined cohort of patients who underwent anesthesia from February 1, 2003, to January 31, 2004 (N = 163,403).[52] The incidence of 24-hour perioperative death, death directly related to anesthesia, and death partially related to anesthesia per 10,000 anesthetics was 28.2 (95% confidence interval [CI], 25.7 to 30.8), 1.7 (95% CI, 1.1 to 2.3), and 4.0 (95% CI, 3.1 to 5.0), respectively. Of 462 deaths, 28 cases (6.1%) were directly related to anesthesia, 66 (14.3%) were partially related to anesthesia, 61 (3.3%) were related to surgery, 399 (86.4%) were

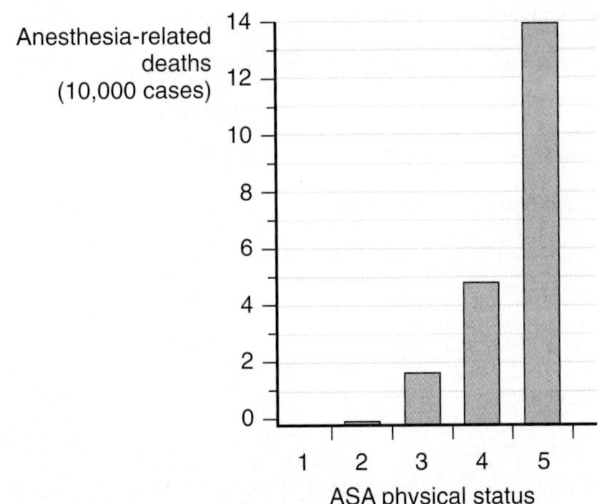

Figure 33-2 Relationship between the American Society of Anesthesiologists (ASA) physical status classification and perioperative mortality (within 2 days of surgery) related to anesthesia provided in urban and suburban institutions. *(Adapted from Lagasse RS: Anesthesia safety: Model or myth? A review of the published literature and analysis of current original data. Anesthesiology 97:1609, 2002.)*

related to patient disease, and 104 (22.5%) were related to the system or management.

Analysis of Intraoperative Cardiac Arrest

Rather than studying perioperative mortality associated with anesthesia, several studies have evaluated intraoperative fatal and nonfatal cardiac arrest (Table 33-9). In this situation there are sufficient numbers of complications to perform an analysis at a single institution. Keenan and Boyan[53] studied the incidence and causes of cardiac arrest related to anesthesia at the Medical College of Virginia during a 15-year period. A total of 27 cardiac arrests occurred during 163,240 procedures, for an incidence of 1.7 per 10,000 cases. Fourteen patients died, for an incidence of 0.9 per 10,000 cases. Pediatric patients had a threefold higher risk of arrest than adults did; emergency cases had a sixfold greater risk. Specific errors in anesthesia management could be identified in 75% of the cases, most commonly inadequate ventilation and absolute overdose of an inhaled anesthetic. The time of day did not appear to influence the rate of anesthesia-related cardiac arrest. From an educational perspective, the investigators identified progressive bradycardia preceding all but one arrest, suggesting that early identification and treatment may prevent complications.

Table 33-9 Cardiac Arrest Series When the Denominator is Greater Than 40,000 Anesthetics

Study	Years	Total No. of Anesthetics	Rate of Arrest
Hanks and Papper	1947-1950	49,728	1:2162
Ehrenhaft, et al.	1942-1951	71,000	1:2840
Bonica	1945-1952	90,000	1:6000
Blades	1948-1952	42,636	1:21,318
Hewlett, et al.	1950-1954	56,033	1:2061
Briggs, et al.	1945-1954	103,777	1:1038
Keenan and Boyan	1969-1978	107,257	1:6704 (P)
Cohen, et al.	1975-1983	112,721	1:1427 (C)
Tiret, et al.	1978-1982	198,103	1:3358 (C)
Tiret, et al.	1978-1982	198,103	1:11,653 (P)
Keenan and Boyan	1979-1988*	134,677	1:9620 (P)
Newland, et al.	1989-1999	72,959	1:14,493 (P)
Newland, et al.	1989-1999	72,959	1:7299 (C)
Olsson, et al.	1967-1984	250,543	1:33,000
Biboulet, et al.	1989-1995	101,769	1:7828
Kawashima, et al.	1994-1998	2,363,038	1:10,000 (P)
Sprung, et al.	1990-2000	518,294	1:20,000 (P)
Braz, et al.	1996-2005	53,718	1.9:10,000 (P)

C, contributory cause; P, primary cause.
*Because pulse oximetry was introduced in 1984, no "preventable respiratory" cardiac arrests have occurred.
Adapted from Brown DL: Anesthesia risk: A historical perspective. *In* Brown DL (ed): Risk and Outcome in Anesthesia, 2nd ed. Philadelphia, JB Lippincott, 1992.

Olsson and Hallen[54] studied the incidence of intraoperative cardiac arrest at the Karolinska Hospital in Stockholm, Sweden, from 1967 to 1984. A total of 170 arrests occurred in 250,543 anesthesia procedures performed. Sixty patients died, for a mortality rate of 2.4 per 10,000 procedures. After elimination of cases of inevitable death (e.g., rupture of a cerebral aneurysm, trauma), the rate of mortality caused by anesthesia was 0.3 per 10,000 procedures. The most common causes of anesthesia-related cardiac arrest were inadequate ventilation (27 patients), asystole after succinylcholine (23 patients), and postinduction hypotension (14 patients). The incidence of cardiac arrest increased with increasing severity of comorbid disease, as assessed by the ASA physical status classification. In evaluating the incidence of intraoperative cardiac arrest over time, there was a considerable decline between 1967 and 1984, coincident with the increased number of anesthesia specialists employed at the clinic.

Biboulet and colleagues[55] studied fatal and nonfatal cardiac arrests encountered during anesthesia and during the first 12 postoperative hours in the PACU or ICU in a single hospital in France. Eleven cardiac arrests related to anesthesia were identified in 101,769 anesthesia procedures (1.1 per 10,000). The mortality rate related to anesthesia was 0.6 per 10,000 cases. The major causes of death were anesthetic overdose, hypovolemia, and hypoxemia; 10 of the 11 cases had at least one human error, and all were classified as avoidable.

Newland and associates[56] reported anesthesia-related cardiac arrests during 72,959 procedures over a 10-year period in a teaching hospital in the United States. They judged that 15 of the 144 cardiac arrests were related to anesthesia (0.69 per 10,000 procedures), and in an additional 10 cases, anesthesia was considered contributory, for a total rate of 1.37 per 10,000 procedures (95% CI, 0.52 to 2.22). The risk of death from perioperative cardiac arrest that was attributable to anesthesia was 0.55 per 10,000 procedures. Most of the arrests were related to medication administration, airway management, or technical problems of central venous access.

Kawashima and colleagues sent confidential questionnaires to all Japan Society of Anesthesiologists Certified Training Hospitals every year from 1994 through 1998.[57] A total of 2,363,038 cases were documented over a 5-year period. The average yearly incidence of cardiac arrest during surgery that was totally attributable to anesthesia was 1.00 (95% CI, 0.88 to 1.12) per 10,000 cases. The average mortality per year in the operating room or within 7 postoperative days that was totally attributable to anesthesia was 0.21 (0.15 to 0.27) per 10,000 cases. The two principal causes of cardiac arrest totally attributable to anesthesia were drug overdose or selection error (15.3%) and serious arrhythmia (13.9%). Preventable human errors caused 53.2% of cardiac arrests and 22.2% of deaths in the operating room that were totally attributable to anesthesia. The outcomes of cardiac arrests totally attributable to anesthesia are shown in Table 33-10.

Sprung and colleagues studied patients who experienced cardiac arrest in the operating room, during transport to the PACU or ICU, or in the PACU after noncardiac surgery between 1990 and 2000.[58] Cardiac arrest occurred in 223 of 518,294 anesthesia procedures (4.3 per 10,000) during the study period. The frequency of arrest in patients receiving general anesthesia

Table 33-10 Cardiac Arrest Totally Attributable to Anesthesia During Anesthesia and Surgery and Its Outcomes, 1994-1998

		Outcomes				
	Number of Arrests	**Uneventful Recovery**	**Death in OR**	**Death within 7 Days**	**Vegetative State**	**Others**
5-year total	237	185	13	15	9	15
Incidence/10,000	1.00	0.78	0.05	0.08	0.04	0.06
95% CI	0.88- ≈1.12	0.66- ≈0.89	0.2- ≈0.08	0.02- ≈0.13	0.03- ≈0.05	0.02- ≈0.10
Ratio	100%	78.1%	5.5%	6.3%	3.8%	6.3%
95% CI		55.3- ≈100	1.7- ≈9.3	3.0- ≈9.7	2.5- ≈5.3	1.7- ≈11.0

N = 2,363,038.
CI, confidence interval; OR, operating room.
Reproduced with permission from Kawashima Y, Takahashi S, Suzuki M, et al: Anesthesia-related mortality and morbidity over a 5-year period in 2,363,038 patients in Japan. Acta Anaesthesiol Scand 47:809-817, 2003.

decreased over time (7.8 per 10,000 during 1990 to 1992; 3.2 per 10,000 during 1998 to 2000). The frequency of arrest during regional anesthesia (1.5 per 10,000) and monitored anesthesia care (0.7 per 10,000) remained consistent (Fig. 33-3). The hospital survival rate was 34.5%. Twenty-four patients (0.5 per 10,000) had cardiac arrest related primarily to anesthesia, 19 of whom (79.2%) survived to hospital discharge. The in-hospital mortality attributable to anesthetic-related cardiac arrest was 0.1 per 10,000 anesthetics. Given the small number of events, no relationship between the type of anesthesia and anesthetic-related cardiac arrest could be determined.

Braz and coworkers studied perioperative cardiac arrest that occurred during 53,718 anesthetics performed between 1996 and 2005 in a Brazilian teaching hospital.[59] One hundred eighty-six cardiac arrests (34.6 per 10,000) and 118 deaths (21.97 per 10,000) were reported. Major risk factors for cardiac arrest were neonates, children younger than 1 year and the elderly, male patients with ASA 3 or poorer physical status, emergency surgery, and general anesthesia. There were 18 anesthesia-related cardiac arrests (3.35 per 10,000), 10 totally attributed (1.86 per 10,000) and 8 partially related to anesthesia (1.49 per 10,000). There were six anesthesia-related deaths (1.12 per 10,000), three totally attributable and three partially related to anesthesia (0.56 per 10,000 in both cases). The main causes of anesthesia-related cardiac arrest were respiratory events (55.5%) and medication-related events (44.5%).

Perioperative Mortality and Morbidity in Outpatient Surgery

It is estimated that 60% of all surgical procedures are performed on an outpatient basis, and this percentage is increasing annually. The type and extent of surgical procedures performed in an outpatient setting are constantly changing, and procedures associated with greater perioperative risk are increasingly being performed on an outpatient basis (see Chapter 78). The value of overnight observation in a hospital setting as opposed to immediate discharge home has been studied for a number of surgical procedures. One of the first procedures advocated to be performed on an ambulatory basis was tonsillectomy. In 1968, a case series of 40,000 outpatient tonsillectomies with no deaths was reported.[60] Details on patient selection and length of postoperative monitoring were vague. Based on insurance company and state mandates, performance of tonsillectomy on an outpatient

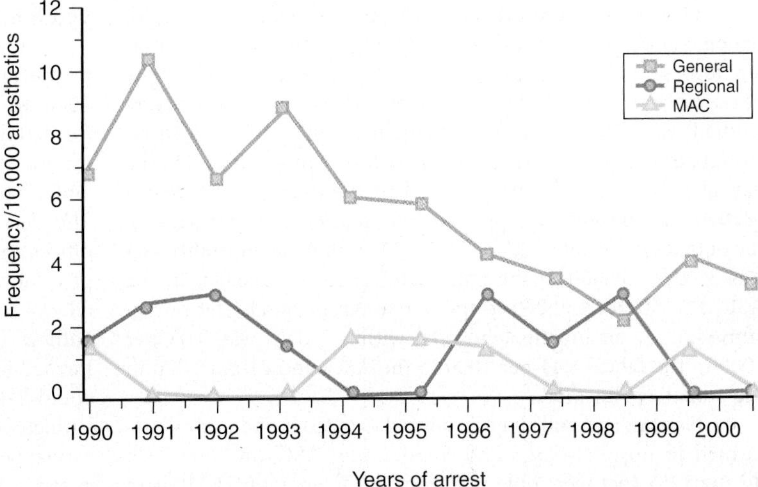

Figure 33-3 Frequency of cardiac arrest by calendar year and type of anesthesia. MAC, monitored anesthesia care. *(From Sprung J, Warner ME, Contreras MG, et al: Predictors of survival following cardiac arrest in patients undergoing noncardiac surgery: A study of 518,294 patients at a tertiary referral center. Anesthesiology 99:259-269, 2003.)*

basis became routine.[61] Beginning in the mid-1980s and continuing in the 1990s, a number of articles evaluated the risk associated with early discharge. For example, Carithers and colleagues[62] at Ohio State University analyzed 3000 tonsillectomies and argued that early discharge might be hazardous and economically unwarranted. The rate of readmission for active bleeding between 5 and 24 hours after surgery was reported to be between 0.2% and 0.5%.[63-66] Although the absolute rate of readmission is low, it represents a substantial risk for children. Whether the benefits of early discharge outweigh the risks is a decision society will have to make.

Another procedure being performed on an outpatient basis is mastectomy. An analysis of Medicare claims demonstrated that the rate of outpatient mastectomy increased from only two procedures reported to Medicare in 1986 to 10.8% of the mastectomies performed in this population in 1995.[67] The investigators compared the rate of readmission within 7 days after surgery for those who had the procedure performed on an inpatient basis versus those treated on an outpatient basis, with adjustment for the severity of disease. Simple mastectomies performed on an outpatient basis had a significantly higher rate of readmission than 1-day stays did, with an adjusted odds ratio (OR) of 1.84. There were 33.8 readmissions per 1000 cases for the outpatient surgeries as compared with 24.2 readmissions for surgeries with 1-day length of hospital stay. When compared with the group treated on an outpatient basis, there were significantly lower rates of readmission after 1-day stays for infection (4.1 versus 1.8 per 1000 cases), nausea and vomiting (1.1 versus 0 per 1000 cases), and pulmonary embolism or deep venous thrombosis (1.1 versus 0 per 1000 cases). Similarly, modified radical mastectomies performed on an outpatient basis had a significantly higher rate of readmission than 1-day stays did, with an adjusted OR of 1.72. The researchers suggested that patients who undergo the procedure on an outpatient basis may wait longer at home until seeking medical care and therefore may have more advanced symptoms initially.

Warner and colleagues[68] at the Mayo Clinic studied major morbidity and mortality occurring within 1 month after ambulatory surgery in 38,598 patients (see Chapter 78). Four patients died, two of myocardial infarction and two in an automobile accident (Fig. 33-4). The two deaths from myocardial infarction occurred at least 1 week after surgery and were not directly attributable to anesthesia. In view of the rate of mortality directly related to anesthesia described in the CEPOD study, no deaths would be expected in a study of this size.

Fleisher and coworkers[1] performed a claims analysis of patients undergoing 16 different surgical procedures in a nationally representative (5%) sample of Medicare beneficiaries for the years 1994 through 1999. A total of 564,267 procedures were studied, with 360,780 in an outpatient hospital, 175,288 in an ambulatory surgery center (ASC), and 28,199 in an office. On the day of surgery, no deaths occurred in the office, but 4 deaths occurred in the ASC (2.3 per 100,000) and 9 deaths occurred in the outpatient hospital (2.5 per 100,000). The 7-day mortality rate was 35 per 100,000 in the office setting, 25 per 100,000 in the ASC, and 50 per 100,000 in the outpatient hospital. The rate of admission to an inpatient hospital within 7 days was 9.08 per 1000 in the office, 8.41 per 1000 in the ASC, and 21 per 1000 in the outpatient hospital.

Fleisher and colleagues analyzed data from operations performed in hospital-based and freestanding ASCs in New York during 1997 that were obtained from the Agency for Healthcare Research and Quality's Healthcare Cost & Utilization Project.[69] Of the 783,558 patients eligible for inclusion in this study, 4351 were discharged directly for short-term hospitalization (1 in 180), and 19 died (1 in 41,240).

Chukmaitov and colleagues compared quality outcomes between ASCs and hospital-based outpatient departments in the state of Florida between the years 1997 and 2004.[70] They used 7- and 30-day mortality and unexpected hospitalization as the outcomes of interest in 12 surgical procedures. The importance of location of care varied by surgical procedure and the number of comorbid conditions included in the analysis. They postulated that the difference in outcomes between the two locations may be related to variations in organizational structure, processes, and strategies. The study, however, is flawed because of extreme selection bias and huge differences in available data between the ASC and hospital-based outpatient department setting. The differences in data sets were evaluated with a limited set and a set using all available data (which differed between settings). Not surprisingly, the results between settings changed with the two types of data.

Interest in performing surgery and providing anesthesia in office-based settings is increasing. There are no good data to determine the safety of such practice, although a number of high-profile cases have occurred in which patients have died during plastic surgery and during dental office procedures. Anesthesia and sedation are frequently provided by individuals other than anesthesiologists or nurse anesthetists in these settings, with reports of office nurses or even clerical help administering anesthetic agents.

There has been an attempt to quantify the incidence of complications in an office-based setting. The American Association for Ambulatory Plastic Surgery Facilities mailed a survey to their members to determine the incidence of complications occurring in office facilities.[71] The overall response rate was 57%. The findings showed that 0.47% of patients had at least one complication, including bleeding, hypertension, infection, and hypotension, and 1 in 57,000 patients died. Assuming that these are very minor procedures performed only on healthy individuals, a rate of mortality that is three times the current estimate for anesthesia-related complications is a concern. Further research and quality assurance mechanisms need to be in place before this practice is generalized. One of the problems inherent in an office-based setting is the inability to perform quality assurance reviews. For example, few surgeons or anesthesiologists would be willing to allow their "competitors" to review their complication rate unless mandated to perform such a review.

Vila and colleagues reviewed all adverse incident reports to the Florida Board of Medicine for procedure dates April 1, 2000, to April 1, 2002.[72] The numbers of office procedures performed during a 4-month period were used to estimate the total number of procedures. Adverse incidents occurred at a rate of 66 and 5.3 per 100,000 procedures in offices and ASCs, respectively. The death rate per 100,000 procedures performed was 9.2 in offices and 0.78 in ASCs. The relative risk for injury and death for procedures performed in the office versus ASCs was 12.4 (95% CI, 9.5 to 16.2) and 11.8 (95% CI, 5.8 to 24.1), respectively. The authors concluded that if all office procedures had been performed in ASCs, approximately 43 injuries and 6 deaths per year could have been prevented. In contrast, Coldiron and colleagues studied office-based surgery in Florida and showed that the greatest danger to patients lies not with surgical procedures in office-based settings per se but with cosmetic procedures that are

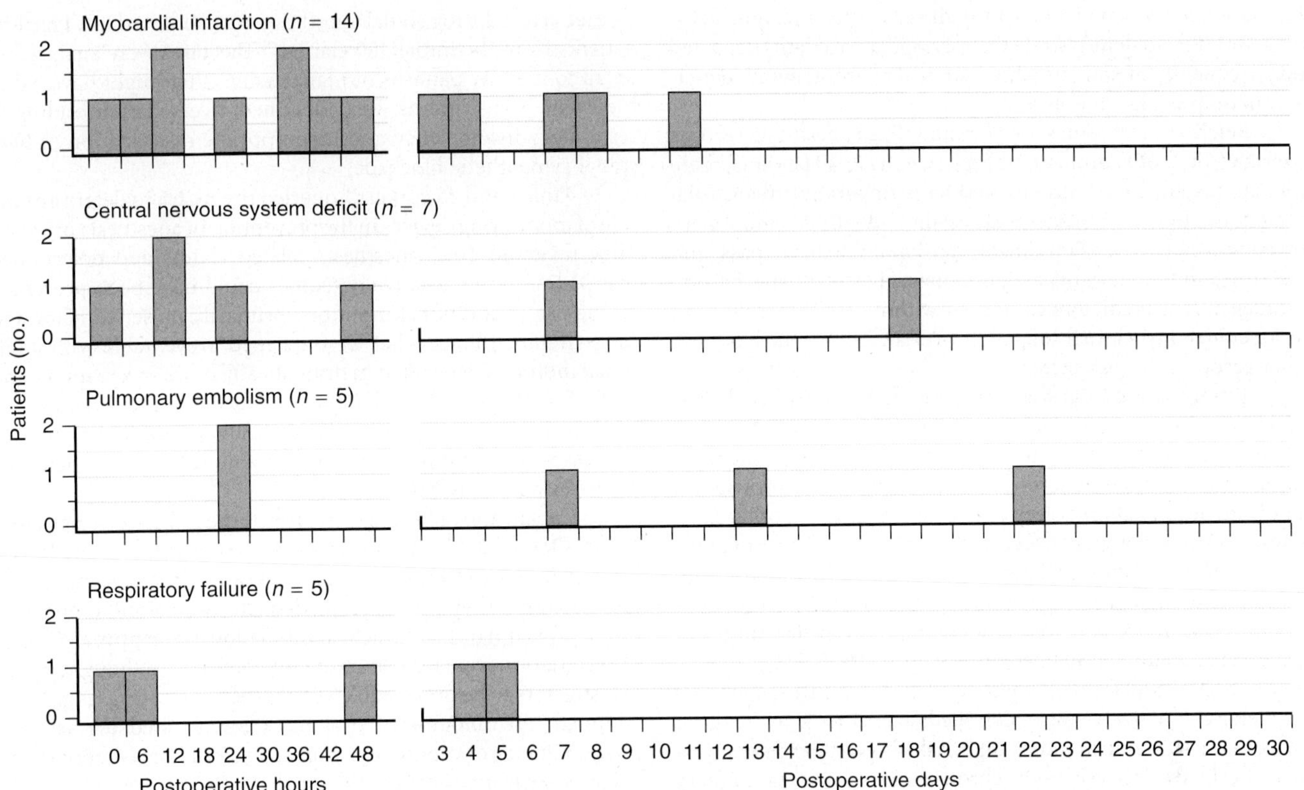

Figure 33-4 Timing of perioperative events in patients undergoing ambulatory surgery. Many of the events occurring within the first 48 hours are probably related to the stress of surgery. A subset of events occurring after this period may be related to background event rates. The overall rate of morbidity was lower than expected for a similar cohort of age-matched nonsurgical patients. *(From Warner MA, Shields SE, Chute CG: Major morbidity and mortality within 1 month of ambulatory surgery and anesthesia. JAMA 270:1437, 1993.)*

performed in office-based settings, particularly when under general anesthesia.[73] Several other groups have analyzed the Florida data and have been unable to document the increased risk in the office setting.[74,75]

Problems in evaluating the risk associated with outpatient surgery include the lack of any large database compiled from a diverse group of settings and the lack of uniform standards for quality assurance. Even though the Joint Commission accredits ASCs, as do two other organizations, accreditation is still not widespread and remains optional. Although ASCs have led the way in performing appropriate follow-up of their patients at home, such follow-up is not uniformly complete. As of 1998, only three states had established regulations for office-based settings, and these regulations vary greatly. The implications of the lack of regulation are unclear, but issues related to emergency plans and resuscitation equipment may be left to the discretion of the local personnel, potentially placing patients at risk.

The decision to perform a procedure in an ambulatory setting is based on the surgeon's preference and the insurance company's mandates. Frequently, a case series by a surgeon or review by an insurance company demonstrates that otherwise healthy individuals can undergo a given procedure safely in an outpatient setting. The need for subsequent medical attention or use of resources at home is not necessarily taken into account. This may lead to insurance company mandates that the procedure be performed in all patients in an ambulatory setting. The generalization from healthy individuals to patients with comorbid disease may not be justified in the absence of data to demonstrate its safety. As an advocate for the patient, the anesthesiologist should continue to evaluate the safety of such practices and determine when the risks of ambulatory surgery outweigh any potential benefits. It is also important to determine whether the insurance companies are in essence transferring the risk of undergoing surgery from the medical system to the patient.

Use of Anesthesia Information Management Systems

Use of computer databases has enhanced the ability of investigators to identify perioperative complications (see Chapter 4). In one of the earliest computer analyses of postanesthesia deaths, Marx and associates[21] identified 645 individuals who died within 7 days after surgery out of a total cohort of 34,145 consecutive surgical patients. More recently, anesthesia information systems have been installed in many operating rooms. The advantage of these systems is the ability to query very large sets of data; however, the limitation is that many of these systems do not link with data from outside the operating room or the PACU. Therefore, the risk related to anesthesia for most of these studies is restricted to intraoperative events. Currently, there are several initiatives to try to link these data, including linking multiple institutions, with validated postoperative data from the NSQIP or Society of Thoracic Surgeons database.

One of the first such analyses was performed by Sanborn and colleagues,[76] who used a computer anesthesia record to identify intraoperative incidents with high sensitivity and specificity. They were able to demonstrate that perioperative deaths occurred more frequently in patients who sustained an intraoperative incident than in those who did not.

Reich and colleagues used computerized anesthesia records to evaluate hemodynamic variables.[22] Among 2149 patients, there were 50 mortalities, 51 strokes, and 85 perioperative myocardial infarctions. By multivariate analysis they identified pulmonary hypertension, hypotension during cardiopulmonary bypass, and post–cardiopulmonary bypass pulmonary diastolic hypertension as independent predictors associated with mortality, stroke, and perioperative myocardial infarction over and above the effects of other preoperative risk factors.

Tremper's group at the University of Michigan used their home-grown information system to identify predictors of perioperative risk. For example, they queried 22,660 attempts at mask ventilation.[77] Limited or severely limited mandibular protrusion, abnormal neck anatomy, sleep apnea, snoring, and a body mass index of 30 kg/m^2 or greater were independent predictors of grade 3 or 4 mask ventilation and difficult intubation. In another publication, a total of 15,102 patients had a normal preoperative creatinine clearance and were undergoing noncardiac surgery.[78] Acute renal failure developed in 121 patients (0.8%), and 14 required renal replacement therapy (0.1%). Seven independent preoperative predictors were identified: age, emergency surgery, liver disease, body mass index, high-risk surgery, peripheral vascular occlusive disease, and chronic obstructive pulmonary disease necessitating chronic bronchodilator therapy. They found that acute renal failure was associated with increased 30-day, 60-day, and 1-year all-cause mortality.

Given the growth in the use of anesthesia information management systems and the ease of collecting large quantities of data and linking them to outcome, it is likely that many more studies documenting associations with outcome will be published.

Other Approaches to Discern the Root Cause of Morbidity and Mortality

The accumulating data clearly demonstrate that risk directly attributable to anesthesia has declined over time (see Chapter 5). The cause of this reduction in mortality is unclear. Numerous factors have been implicated in the improved outcome, including new monitoring modalities, new anesthetic drugs, and changes in the anesthesia workforce. However, it is difficult to document reduced risk related to any one factor (issues related to manpower are addressed later). Although the use of newer monitoring modalities, particularly pulse oximetry, would be expected to improve outcomes, no randomized trial has been able to document such a conclusion. This limitation supports the need for continued monitoring of complications and their root cause with studies such as the ACCS.

Studies similar to the CEPOD have not been performed in the United States, most likely because of the legal system, and information related to perioperative mortality must be obtained from other sources. The Professional Liability Committee of the ASA conducted a nationwide survey of closed insurance claims for major anesthesia mishaps. In the ACCS, fatal and nonfatal outcomes were reviewed. Among the fatal events, unexpected cardiac arrest during spinal anesthesia was observed in 14 healthy patients from the initial 900 claims.[79] The cases were analyzed in detail to identify patterns of management that might have led to the event. Two patterns were identified: oversedation leading to respiratory insufficiency and inappropriate resuscitation of high spinal sympathetic blockade.

Tinker and coworkers[80] queried the ACCS to determine the role of monitoring devices in the prevention of anesthesia mishaps. They reviewed 1097 anesthesia-related claims and determined that 31.5% of the negative outcomes could have been prevented by the use of additional monitors, primarily pulse oximetry and capnography. Injuries that were deemed preventable with additional monitoring resulted in dramatically more severe injury and cost of settlement than did those judged nonpreventable with additional monitoring. In nearly 90% (305 of 346) of the preventable cases, at least one clinical sign of abnormality was identified by the existing monitors.

Caplan and colleagues[81] reviewed the ACCS for respiratory events (Table 33-11). These claims represented the single largest class of injury (34%), with death or brain damage occurring in 85% of cases. They identified inadequate ventilation, esophageal intubation, and difficult tracheal intubation as the primary causes of respiratory events. Most of the outcomes were thought by the investigators to be preventable with better monitoring (Fig. 33-5). Although no randomized trial has demonstrated the value of pulse oximetry or capnography, an analysis of claims supports the value of such monitoring. This analysis also formed part of the basis for the guidelines and algorithm endorsed by the ASA Task Force on Management of the Difficult Airway.

The closed claims analysis has recently focused on such topics as monitored anesthesia care.[82] More than 40% of 121 claims associated with monitored anesthesia care involved death or permanent brain damage. Respiratory depression, after an absolute or relative overdose of sedative or opioid drugs, was the most common (21%, $n = 25$) of the complications.

A similar registry was developed by the Danish Patient Insurance Association.[83] For the period 1996 to 2004, 1256 files were related to anesthesia and 24 deaths were considered to be a result of the anesthetic procedure: 4 deaths were related to airway management, 2 to ventilation management, 4 to central venous catheter placement, 4 as a result of medication errors, 4 from infusion pump problems, and 4 after complications from regional blockade. Severe hemorrhage caused one death, and in one case the cause was uncertain.

Table 33-11 Distribution of Adverse Respiratory Events in the American Society of Anesthesiologists Closed Claims Study

Event	No. of Cases	Percentage of 522 Respiratory Claims
Inadequate ventilation	196	38
Esophageal intubation	94	18
Difficult tracheal intubation	87	17
Inadequate inspired oxygen concentration	11	2

From Caplan RA, Ward RJ, Posner K, Cheney FW: Unexpected cardiac arrest during spinal anesthesia: A closed claims analysis of predisposing factors. Anesthesiology 68:5, 1988.

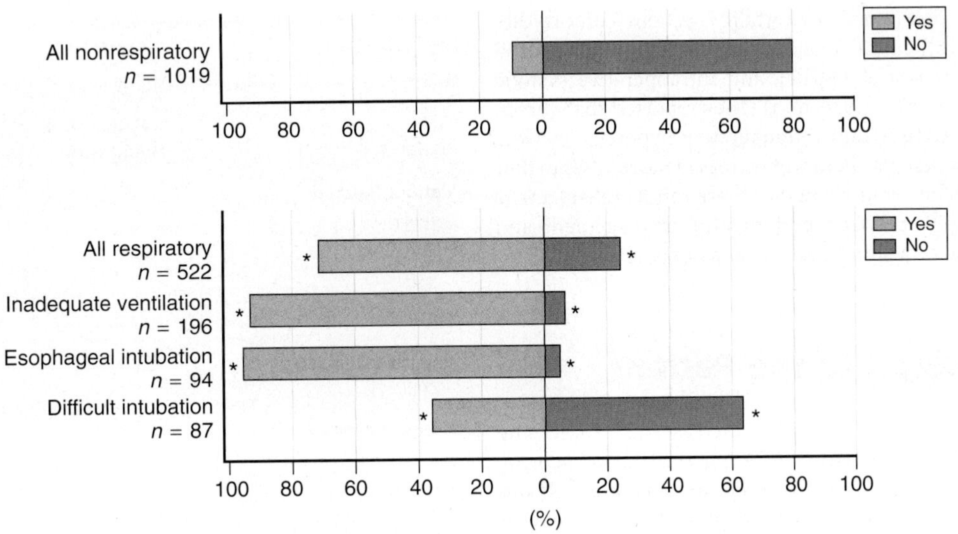

Figure 33-5 Relationship between adverse events in the American Society of Anesthesiologists Closed Claims Study and preventable complications. Preventable events related to respiratory complications were significantly more common than those related to all nonrespiratory complications. Of the respiratory complications, difficult intubation had the least number of preventable complications (*$P < .05$ versus nonrespiratory claims). *(From Caplan RA, Posner KL, Ward RJ, Cheney FW: Adverse respiratory events in anesthesia: A closed claims analysis. Anesthesiology 72:828, 1990.)*

Cooper and colleagues[84-86] approached the problem of sample size for determining perioperative morbidity by identifying critical incidents, which were defined as those that were preventable but could lead to undesirable outcomes. This definition included events that led to no or only transient effects in the patient. The investigation involved collecting data on anesthesia-related human errors and equipment failures from anesthesiologists, residents, and nurse anesthetists. In a series of reports, the authors identified frequent incidents, such as disconnections in breathing circuits, and causes of discovery of errors, such as intraoperative relief. They confirmed that equipment failure was a small cause of anesthesia mishaps (4%), whereas human error was dominant. They suggested that future studies of anesthesia-related mortality and morbidity should classify events according to a strategy for prevention rather than outcome alone.

The Australian Incident Monitoring Study was developed by the Australian Patient Safety Foundation and has been in existence since the early 1990s. It is a method of reporting and analyzing critical incidents so that corrective strategies can be implemented. Similar to the ACCS, there is no rate of occurrence, only an analysis of reported cases. Numerous reports have looked at the cause of critical incidents, including problems with ventilation, with vascular access, and in the PACU.[87-89]

Buffington and coworkers[90] studied the ability of attendees of an anesthesia meeting to identify five faults intentionally created in a standard anesthesia machine. A survey was distributed, and the answer sheets were scored with respect to the number of correct answers. Only 3.4% of the respondents found all five faults. The average number of faults detected was 2.2. The professional background of the participants did not influence the ability to find the faults; distributions were similar between physicians and CRNAs. There was a small improvement in fault-finding ability in those with more than 10 years of experience. Studies such as these highlight the problem of the practitioner's ability to identify conditions that may lead to anesthesia mishaps. Whether improved technology or education can reduce some basal level of mishaps is unknown.

Issues Associated with Anesthesia-Related Mortality

Most of the studies have focused on in-hospital and short-term mortality, but perioperative complications may be the events that directly lead to death. For example, a perioperative stroke or myocardial infarction may lead to death after the period of analysis. Even small myocardial infarctions or unstable angina during the perioperative period has been associated with worse long-term survival in several studies.[91,92] Should these "late" deaths be attributed to anesthesia complications for the purpose of such analyses? Results from several studies add to the dilemma. For example, Mangano and colleagues[93] performed a randomized clinical trial in which 7 days of perioperative β-blockade was compared with placebo in high-risk patients undergoing noncardiac surgery. They reported significantly improved survival at 6 months, which remained significant during the 2 years of follow-up. In a subsequent report regarding this trial, Wallace and coworkers[94] demonstrated that the improved survival in the group receiving β-blockade was associated with a significantly lower incidence of perioperative myocardial ischemia but no difference in perioperative cardiac events. The authors of the original study suggested that atenolol administration led to better plaque stabilization during the perioperative period, which resulted in improved long-term survival. If the hyperdynamic perioperative state is not well controlled, this theory suggests that more plaque becomes destabilized and progresses to acute occlusion and sudden death. If atenolol is not used and patients die within 6 months of surgery, should this be attributed to an error in anesthesia and perioperative management? Part of the answer relies on the strength of this study to support the conclusion that routine use of atenolol does result in improved long-term survival.

The potential effects of anesthesia on long-term survival were suggested by Monk and colleagues.[95] Multivariate Cox proportional hazards modeling identified three variables as significant independent predictors of mortality: patient comorbidity (relative risk, 16.116), cumulative deep hypnotic time (bispectral index <45) (relative risk, 1.244/hr), and intraoperative systolic hypotension (relative risk, 1.036/min). They reported that cumulative deep hypnotic time and intraoperative hypotension were significant, independent predictors of increased mortality. Further work is required to determine whether these results reflect a true pathophysiologic link between perioperative management and long-term outcome or a simple statistical association.

Risks Related to the Patient

Perioperative morbidity and mortality increase with increasing patient comorbidity. The original ASA physical status scoring system was proposed in 1941 and included six categories.[96] It was intended to standardize terminology and allow statistical analysis of outcomes between sites.[97] The original classification avoided the inclusion of surgical variables and was restricted to preoperative patient characteristics. It was revised in 1961 by Dripps and colleagues[32] to five categories, which were then adopted by the ASA.

The simplest example of such a relationship is the incidence of mortality correlated with ASA physical status. In their original study of perioperative mortality, Dripps and coworkers demonstrated that mortality increased as the severity of comorbid disease increased, as assessed by the ASA physical status classification. Several investigators have re-evaluated the relationship between operative mortality and ASA physical status. Studies by Pedersen and Tiret and their colleagues demonstrated such relationships. Vacanti and coworkers[98] also demonstrated the relationship between increasing mortality and decreasing physical status in 68,388 cases.

In Canada, Cohen and colleagues[99] analyzed 100,000 anesthesia procedures and determined mortality within 7 days of surgery by using governmental vital statistics mortality data between the years 1975 and 1984. They established a computer database for each procedure that included age, preoperative conditions, ASA physical status, anesthesia technique, monitors, and other factors. The overall 7-day mortality rate was 71.04 deaths per 10,000 procedures. The mortality rate increased with advanced age, and it showed a marked increase in those older than 80 years. Rates were low for normal, healthy individuals and for those undergoing minor procedures. The investigators developed a multiple logistic regression model to determine the independent predictors of mortality. Significant risk markers for increasing mortality were advanced age, male gender, increasing physical status score, major or intermediate surgery, emergency procedure, having a complication in the operating room, narcotic anesthesia techniques, and having received only one or two anesthetic drugs (Table 33-12).

Table 33-12 Risk Factors Associated with Increased Odds of Dying within 7 Days for All Cases

Variable	All Procedures: Relative Odds of Dying within 7 Days	95% Confidence Limits
Patient Related		
Age (yr)		
60-79/<60	2.32	1.70-3.17
80+/<60	3.29	2.18-4.96
Sex (F/M)	0.77	0.59-1.00
Physical status score (3-5/1-2)	10.65	7.59-14.85
Surgery Related		
Major/minor	3.82	2.50-5.93
Intermediate/minor	1.76	1.24-2.5
Length of anesthesia (≤2 hr/<2 hr)	1.08	0.77-1.50
Emergency/elective	4.44	3.38-5.83
Other Factors		
Year of surgery (1975-1979/1980-1984)	1.75	1.32-2.31
Had a complication in the operating or recovery room (yes/no)	1.42	1.06-1.89
Anesthesia Related*		
Experience of the anesthetist (>600 procedures for ≥8 yr/<600 procedures for <8 yr)	1.06	0.82-1.37
Inhalation with narcotic/ inhalation alone	0.76	0.51-1.15
Narcotic alone/inhalation alone	1.41	1.01-2.00
Narcotic with inhalation/ inhalation alone	0.79	0.47-1.32
Spinal/inhalation alone	0.53	0.29-0.98
No. of anesthetic drugs (1-2/3+)	2.94	2.20-3.84

*All cases performed with the five most frequently used anesthetic techniques.
Adapted from Cohen MM, Duncan PG, Tate RB: Does anesthesia contribute to operative mortality? JAMA 260:2861, 1988.

In an attempt to look at each of the categories of contributing factors independently, Cohen's group constructed receiver-operator characteristic curves. There was no increment in prediction of mortality beyond that based on characteristics of the patient plus surgery. Plots including "other" or anesthesia-related factors showed almost complete overlap with curves including only patient- and surgery-specific factors.

One of the limitations of the ASA physical status classification is that ranking is a subjective measure conferred by the practitioner rather than an objective measure determined by the presence of specific disease states. Owens and coworkers[100] evaluated this hypothesis by asking 255 anesthesiologists to classify 10 hypothetical patients. In six of the cases there was general agreement among the practitioners about classification of the patient; in the other four cases, opinion diverged. The key finding of this study was that the ASA physical status classification is "useful but suffers from a lack of scientific precision."

Rather than evaluating the risk of overall mortality, many studies have attempted to define the patient characteristics associated with morbidity and mortality related to a particular organ system. In evaluating the risk directly related to the patient's condition, it is important to understand the limitations of the methodology. All such studies evaluate the predictive value of a clinical or laboratory risk factor for a defined perioperative complication. In this approach, a cohort of individuals of interest is defined. In the optimal state the study is performed prospectively, and the outcome of interest is assessed in a rigorous, blinded fashion. Unfortunately, many of the studies focus on selected patients and include a retrospective design, methods that greatly limit their generalizability and validity. For example, many studies evaluating risk factors in vascular surgery patients include only patients who are referred for diagnostic testing rather than a consecutive series of patients.

Many studies have adopted the approach of defining a cohort of individuals, determining their clinical and laboratory risk factors, and using multivariate modeling to determine the factors associated with increased risk. Frequently, perioperative risk is used to define intraoperative and postoperative complications. A major limitation in the use of multivariate modeling for this purpose is the assumption that the intraoperative period is a "black box" and that care is not modified by knowledge of the risk factor (Fig. 33-6). However, anesthesiologists do modify their intraoperative care of high-risk patients in an attempt to reduce the risk. Changes in medical care over time and better knowledge about high-risk patients should result in a reduction of the risk related to specified clinical factors. For this reason, many of the indices developed previously may no longer have clinical validity.

In designing a multivariate risk index for perioperative morbidity and mortality, only factors that are included in the analysis and in the patient population of interest can be included in the final model. For example, if the population studied represents a unique referral bias, some risk factors may be overrepresented, and others may not be present in sufficient quantity to study. An example is unstable angina in the original Cardiac Risk Index developed by Goldman and colleagues.[6] Because patients with unstable angina are typically seen only for emergency surgery, that risk factor is rarely represented in many indices.

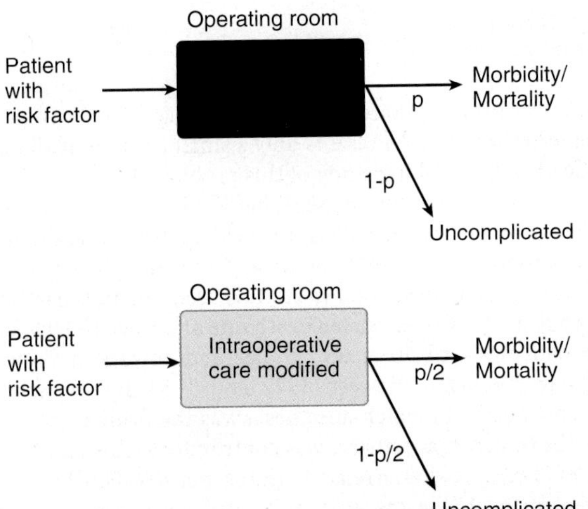

Figure 33-6 The concept of the black box for risk indices. In developing a risk index, patients with a specific risk factor enter the operating room and have a complication at a rate (p). If the anesthesiologist is aware of the importance of the risk factor and can modify care to reduce such risk (p/2), the risk factor may no longer be significant. If the risk factor is ignored, complications may again occur in such patients.

There are numerous specific disease states that increase perioperative risk. Cardiovascular disease has been the most extensively studied, with the goal of identifying patients at greatest risk for fatal and nonfatal myocardial infarction. One of the earliest attempts to define cardiac risk was performed by Goldman and colleagues at the Massachusetts General Hospital. They studied 1001 patients older than 45 years who were undergoing noncardiac surgery, excluding those who underwent transurethral resection of the prostate under spinal anesthesia. Using multivariate logistic regression, they demonstrated nine clinical factors associated with increased morbidity and mortality. Each of these risk factors was associated with a given weight in the logistic regression equation, which was converted into points in the index. An increasing number of points was associated with increasing perioperative cardiac morbidity or mortality.

There have been several attempts to validate the Goldman Cardiac Risk Index. Zeldin[101] prospectively determined the Cardiac Risk Index for 1140 surgical patients and reported that the overall accuracy of the index was as high as in the original study, although the rate of complications in the highest-risk group was less than originally reported. Larsen and coworkers[102] also found that the Cardiac Risk Index demonstrated good accuracy in 2609 consecutive unselected patients older than 40 years. Domaingue and colleagues[103] studied patients undergoing various vascular surgery procedures and reported a higher probability of major cardiac complications than that reported by Goldman and associates; however, they also demonstrated a higher rate of complications with increasing cardiac risk class. The validity of the Cardiac Risk Index is more controversial for vascular surgery patients. Jeffrey and colleagues[104] evaluated the rate of cardiac complications in 99 patients undergoing elective abdominal aortic surgery and demonstrated a similar pattern of increased overall complication rates with increasing cardiac risk. A higher percentage (7%) of patients in the lowest category in their study sustained a cardiac complication. White and associates[105] demonstrated the value of the Goldman Cardiac Risk Index for long-term survival after vascular surgery. Several other studies, however, were unable to demonstrate any relationship between the Cardiac Risk Index and perioperative cardiac complications, with a high incidence of complications found in patients with a Cardiac Risk Index of I or II.[106,107] When the ASA physical status classification was compared with the Goldman Cardiac Risk Index in a cohort of 16,277 patients undergoing noncardiac surgery,[108] both indices demonstrated predictive value, although the objective Goldman Cardiac Risk Index had little increased value over the more subjective ASA physical status classification.

Other investigators have attempted to develop risk indices. Detsky and coworkers[109] studied a cohort of individuals who were referred to an internal medicine service for preoperative evaluation. Many of the factors identified by Goldman were confirmed or slightly modified in the Detsky index, and angina was added to the risk factors. The researchers advocated the calculation of a pretest probability of complications based on the type of surgery, after which the Detsky Modified Risk Index is applied with the use of a nomogram. In this manner, the overall probability of complications can be determined as a function of the surgical procedure and patient disease. The Detsky index was advocated as the starting point for risk stratification in the American College of Physicians guidelines on preoperative evaluation.[110] In an attempt to update the original index, Lee and colleagues[111] at the Brigham and Women's Hospital studied 4315 patients 50 years or older who were undergoing elective major noncardiac procedures in a tertiary care teaching hospital. Six independent predictors of complications were identified and included in a Revised Cardiac Risk Index: high-risk type of surgery, history of ischemic heart disease, history of congestive heart failure, history of cerebrovascular disease, preoperative treatment with insulin, and preoperative serum creatinine level higher than 2.0 mg/dL. The rate of major cardiac complications increased with the number of risk factors.

Numerous risk indices for cardiac surgery have been developed. The goal has been to identify patients who are at greatest risk for adverse perioperative outcomes, not specifically anesthesia-related risk. Many of these indices focus on anatomic considerations for perioperative risk. They are extremely useful in risk adjustment to assess rates of mortality. For example, the state of New York annually publishes data on mortality rates associated with coronary bypass grafting by surgeon and by hospital.[112-114] For comparison of rates across institutions, risk figures must be adjusted so that institutions that perform predominantly high-risk surgery are not penalized.

Vanzetto and coworkers[115] performed a prospective evaluation in which an expanded number of clinical variables were identified in a cohort of patients undergoing major vascular surgery. Cardiovascular morbidity and mortality were determined prospectively in this population. An increasing number of clinical variables was associated with increasing perioperative risk. Most importantly, dipyridamole-thallium imaging was performed only in the subset of patients with two or more clinical variables, and the results of the test were not made available to the clinicians caring for the patients. In this well-performed study, the presence of thallium redistribution identified a cohort who had an incrementally greater perioperative risk than did those with negative scan results and a similar number of clinical variables.

As part of their study of anesthesia-related mortality, Pedersen and colleagues[51] evaluated the occurrence of cardiovascular and pulmonary complications. For a total of 7306 anesthesia procedures, they reported a 6.3% incidence of intraoperative or postoperative cardiovascular complications and a 4.8% incidence of intraoperative or postoperative pulmonary complications. Acute myocardial infarction occurred in 0.16% of the patients. The investigators evaluated a number of characteristics, including gender, age, presence of ischemic heart disease, duration of anesthesia, and type of surgery, and assessed their relationship to cardiovascular and pulmonary complications and overall mortality in the hospital (Table 33-13). Cardiopulmonary complications were associated with advanced age (>70 years), preoperative signs of ischemic heart disease with recent myocardial infarction, chronic heart failure, chronic lung disease, and abdominal surgery, particularly of an emergent nature. They observed that the use of pancuronium was associated with worse perioperative outcome, a finding reminiscent of the curare-related deaths of the 1940s and 1950s.

Numerous studies have evaluated the importance of single variables such as hypertension on perioperative risk. Goldman and Caldera[116] evaluated a cohort of patients undergoing noncardiac surgery under general anesthesia. Hypertension did not denote a group with increased perioperative risk, although the number of patients with diastolic blood pressure greater than 110 mm Hg was insufficient to draw any conclusions. This study highlighted the problems related to generalization of results in that many subsequent researchers have suggested that surgery be delayed in patients with a diastolic blood pressure greater than 110 mm Hg. In one of the few studies to demonstrate a relationship, Hollenberg and coworkers[117] identified hypertension and the presence of left ventricular hypertrophy as predictors of perioperative ischemia, but they did not consider their independent relationship to perioperative major morbidity.

Examples of prospective cohort studies to identify the risk associated with a particular clinical factor include studies of the rate of perioperative reinfarction in patients who had previously sustained a myocardial infarction. Traditionally, risk assessment for noncardiac surgery was based on the time interval between the myocardial infarction and surgery. Multiple studies have demonstrated an increased incidence of reinfarction if the myocardial infarction occurred within 6 months of surgery. With improvements in perioperative care, this difference has decreased.

The previous example of assessing risk illustrates the issue of changes in management over time. The importance of the intervening time interval may no longer be valid in the current era of thrombolytics, angioplasty, and risk stratification after acute myocardial infarction. Although many patients with myocardial infarction continue to have myocardium at risk for subsequent ischemia and infarction, in others, the critical area of coronary stenosis is totally occluded or widely patent. Patients should be evaluated from the perspective of their risk for ongoing ischemia. In their Guidelines for Perioperative Evaluation of Noncardiac Surgery, the American Heart Association/American College of Cardiology Task Force on Assessment of Diagnostic and Therapeutic Cardiovascular Procedures[118] proposed that patients who have experienced a myocardial infarction within less than 30 days be considered the group at highest risk; after that period, risk stratification is based on disease severity and exercise tolerance.

Special Patient Groups

Obstetrics

Maternal mortality is rare, and the anesthesia-related component of maternal delivery represents only a small fraction of all maternal deaths, thus making study of this problem difficult or impossible in any one institution (see Chapter 69). A series of studies were performed between 1974 and 1985 to determine the rate of complications in the United States and England. One of the first reports included the period 1974 to 1978. Kaunitz and coauthors[119] reported an anesthesia-related death rate of 0.6 per 100,000 births with data from all 50 states. Endler and coworkers[120] studied births in Michigan between 1972 and 1984 and reported 15 maternal deaths in which anesthesia was the primary cause and 4 deaths in which anesthesia was contributory. This resulted in a rate of 0.82 anesthesia-related deaths per 100,000 live births. Eleven of the 15 deaths were associated with cesarean section. Obesity and emergency surgery were risk factors in many patients. Complications related to regional anesthesia were problems during the early part of the study, whereas failure to secure a patent airway was the primary cause of mortality in later years. There were no anesthesia-related maternal deaths in the final 2 years of the study. The incidence of anesthesia-related death was

Table 33-13 Factors Associated with Increased Perioperative Complications

Risk Factors	No. of Anesthetics (*N* = 7306)*	Cardiovascular Complications		Pulmonary Complications		Mortality in Hospital	
		%	Odds Ratio	%	Odds Ratio	%	Odds Ratio
Sex							
Female	4587	4.9		3.7		0.7	
Male	2634	8.8†	1.8	6.6†	1.8	2.2†	3.2
Age (yr)							
<50	3965	2.6		2.3		0.3	
50-90	2043	8.2		6.7		1.8	
70-79	886	14.3†		8.9		2.9†	
≥80	293	16.7†		10.2†		5.8†	
Ischemic heart disease	103	29.1†	6.5	8.7	1.9	2.9	2.5
Myocardial infarction							
>1 yr	125	20.8†		7.7		4.0†	
≤1 yr	26	38.5†		10.4†		7.7†	
Chronic heart failure	199	35.2†		15.1†	3.8	9.0†	9.9
Hypertension	380	11.8†	2.1	7.1†	1.6	1.3	1.1
Hypertension (SBP ≤90 mm Hg)	127	16.5†	2.5	17.3†	4.0	9.4†	9.8
Chronic obstructive lung disease	201	12.4†	2.1	12.4	3.0	5.0†	4.7
Renal failure	153	14.4†	2.2	11.8†	2.4	5.9†	5.2
Diabetes mellitus	141	9.2	1.5	7.1	1.5	2.1†	1.8
Neurologic disease	34	5.9	1.0	8.8†	1.9	2.9	2.4
Cancer	1257	7.0	1.1	5.5	1.2	1.1	1.0
Cancer (abdominal)	242	19.8†	3.2	19.4†	4.3	5.0†	5.4
Emergency surgery	2454	7.4†	1.3	6.3†	3.0	2.8†	3.2
Duration of anesthesia (min)							
<30	1774	1.2		0.6		0.1	
30-179	4621	6.8		4.5		1.3	
180-299	470	17.9†		13.4†		3.2†	
≥300	162	20.4†		30.2†		4.9†	
Minor surgery	4916	3.2		1.8		0.3	
Major surgery	2113	13.0†	4.1	10.6	5.8	3.1†	4.9
Total		6.3		4.8		1.2	

SBP, systolic blood pressure.
*The analysis shows the maximum number of patients in the various groups.
†$P < .05$ indicates a statistically significant higher rate of complications and mortality when compared with the rest of the total incidence.
From Pedersen T: Complications and death following anaesthesia: A prospective study with special reference to the influence of patient-, anaesthesia-, and surgery-related risk factors. Dan Med Bull 41:319, 1994.

markedly higher in black women, which the investigators suggested might have been related to an inability to detect cyanosis. Rochat and colleagues[121] studied 19 areas of the United States between 1980 and 1985 and reported 0.98 anesthesia-related deaths per 100,000 live births. They observed that maternal mortality did not decrease over the time of the study.

The Confidential Enquiry into Maternal Deaths in England and Wales has been assessing maternal deaths since 1952.[122] Records of all maternal deaths are sent to a district medical officer, who sends an inquiry form to all health practitioners involved in the care of these patients. These forms are evaluated by a senior obstetrician and an anesthesia assessor. Morgan[122] reported the maternal deaths from anesthesia between 1952 and 1981 (Table 33-14). The total maternal mortality rate decreased over time, but the percentage of deaths related to anesthesia increased, although the absolute number of deaths associated with anesthesia decreased. During the early years of the study, endotracheal intubation was rarely performed during obstetric anesthesia. Later reports advocated the use of endotracheal intubation after thiopental-suxamethonium, and technical difficulties with intubation were identified. The other major finding of this study was that the experience of the anesthetist in obstetric anesthesia was the most important factor in anesthesia-related maternal mortality.

Table 33-14 Maternal Mortality Figures Obtained from the Confidential Enquiry into Maternal Deaths in England and Wales

Years	Maternal Mortality per 1000 Total Births	Number of Deaths from Anesthesia	Percentage of True Maternal Deaths from Anesthesia	Percentage with Avoidable Factors
1952-1954	0.53	49	4.5	—
1955-1957	0.43	31	3.6	77
1958-1960	0.33	30	4.0	80
1961-1963	0.26	28	4.0	50
1964-1966	0.20	50	8.7	48
1967-1969	0.16	50	10.9	68
1970-1972	0.13	37	10.4	76
1973-1975	0.11	31	13.2	90
1976-1978	0.11	30	13.2	93
1979-1981	0.11	22	12.2	100

From Morgan M: Anaesthetic contribution to maternal mortality. Br J Anaesth 59:842, 1987.

Several studies have attempted to define the cause of anesthesia-related maternal deaths. Insight into the cause of maternal mortality can also be elicited from the ACCS. In 1991, Chadwick and coauthors[123] published a report of closed malpractice claims related to 190 obstetric cases—127 cesarean sections and 63 vaginal deliveries. The most frequent complications were maternal death and brain damage in the newborn. There were 15 maternal deaths in patients who underwent regional anesthesia and 26 in patients who had general anesthesia. Because the absolute number of patients who underwent each type of anesthesia was unknown, the risk attributable to anesthesia could not be determined, unlike the subsequent report from Hawkins and coworkers.[124]

Hawkins and associates[124] obtained data from the ongoing National Pregnancy Mortality Surveillance System of the Centers for Disease Control and Prevention. Using state data on births and fetal deaths from 1979 through 1990, three obstetric anesthesiologists reviewed the records to determine the possible risk related to anesthesia. A total of 129 women died of anesthesia-related causes during the study period, most (82%) during cesarean section, and the incidence decreased over time (Table 33-15). The decreased mortality rate appeared to be related to increased use of regional anesthesia. The primary cause of mortality was related to the type of anesthesia. For general anesthesia, 73% of the deaths were related to airway problems. Unlike the Confidential Enquiry into Maternal Deaths in England, the U.S. study lacked the extensive detail for each event, and the absolute cause of mortality therefore remained somewhat in doubt. In particular, the researchers acknowledge that general anesthesia may be used more often in patients with a higher acuity of disease, which may account for the higher mortality rate associated with its use. The availability of national databases should allow accurate tracking of mortality to ensure that appropriate quality assurance and quality improvement systems are in place.

Panchal and colleagues[125] conducted a retrospective case-control study using patients' records from a state-maintained anonymous database of all nonfederal Maryland hospitals that performed deliveries between 1984 and 1997 (Fig. 33-7). Variables studied included patient demographics and ICD-9 (Clinical Modification) diagnosis and procedure codes. Of the 822,591 hospital admissions for delivery during the 14-year study period, there were 135 maternal deaths. The most common diagnoses associated with mortality during hospital admission for delivery were preeclampsia or eclampsia (22.2%); postpartum hemorrhage or obstetric shock (22.2%); pulmonary complications (14%); blood clot or amniotic embolism, or both (8.1%); and anesthesia-related complications (5.2%).

Gibbs and coworkers[126] surveyed 1200 hospitals in 1981 and sent questionnaires to the chiefs of anesthesia and obstetrics. Anesthesiologists were available for obstetric anesthesia in only 21% of all hospitals and at night and on the weekends in just 15%. Hospitals with fewer than 500 deliveries per year had the most

Table 33-15 Numbers, Case Fatality Rates, and Risk Ratios of Anesthesia-related Deaths during Cesarean Section Delivery by Type of Anesthesia in the United States, 1979-1984 and 1985-1990

	Number of Deaths		Case-Fatality Rate		Risk Ratio	
Population	1979-1984	1985-1990	1979-1984	1985-1990	1979-1984	1985-1990
General	33	32	20.0* (95% CI, 17.7-22.7)	32.3* (95% CI, 25.9-49.3)	2.3 (95% CI, 1.9-2.9)	16.7 (95% CI, 12.9-21.8)
Regional	19	9	8.6† (95% CI, 1.8-9.4)	1.9† (95% CI, 1.8-2.0)	Referent	Referent

CI, confidence interval.
*Per million general anesthetics for cesarean section.
†Per million regional anesthetics for cesarean section.
Adapted from Hawkins JL, Gibbs CP, Orleans M, et al: Obstetric anesthesia work force survey, 1981 versus 1992. Anesthesiology 87:135, 1997.

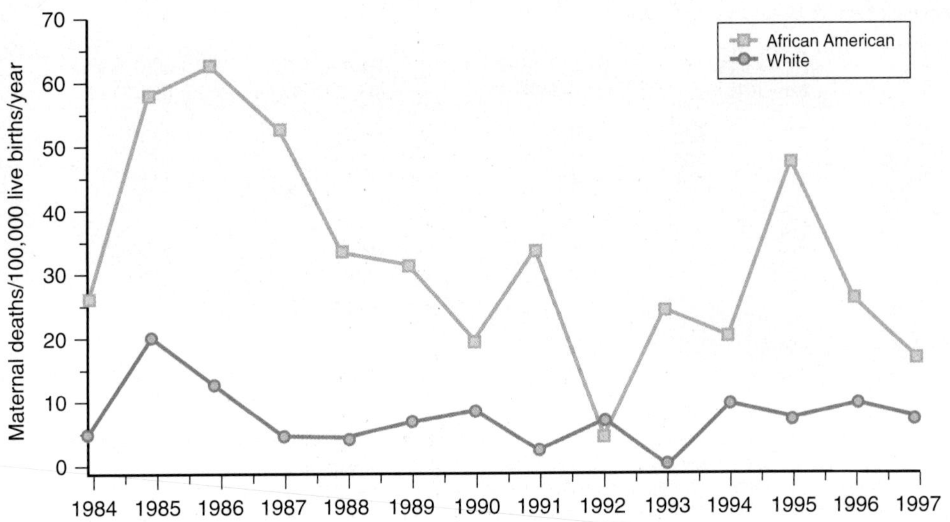

Figure 33-7 Delivery mortality ratios by race in Maryland, from 1984 to 1997, according to discharge summaries. *(From Panchal S, Arria AM, Labhsetwar SA: Maternal mortality during hospital admission for delivery: A retrospective analysis using a state-maintained database. Anesth Analg 93:134, 2001.)*

striking deficiencies in anesthesia personnel. Even for cases in which general anesthesia was provided for cesarean section, an anesthesiologist was involved in care only 44% of the time, whereas hospitals with greater than 1500 deliveries per year had an anesthesiologist present 85% of the time. The researchers did not evaluate the relationship between outcome and staffing models. The survey was performed again in 1992.[127] When compared with 1981, the researchers found a marked increase in the availability of labor analgesia and a decrease in the use of general anesthesia. In more than half of the anesthesia procedures for cesarean section, care was provided by nurse anesthetists without medical direction by an anesthesiologist. How these trends in staffing have affected maternal mortality requires further evaluation.

Mhyre and colleagues reviewed maternal mortality in Michigan between 1985 and 2003.[128] Of 855 pregnancy-associated deaths, 8 were related to anesthesia, and anesthesia was considered to be contributory in 7. All anesthesia-related deaths from airway obstruction or hypoventilation took place during emergence and recovery, not during induction of general anesthesia. Lapses in postoperative monitoring and inadequate supervision by an anesthesiologist seemed to contribute to more than half of the deaths.

Bloom and associates studied anesthesia-related morbidity and mortality as part of a prospective observational study conducted in women ($N = 37{,}142$) with singleton gestations undergoing cesarean delivery in the centers forming the National Institute of Child Health and Human Development Maternal-Fetal Medicine Units Network.[129] There was one maternal death, caused by failed intubation, in which the anesthetic procedure was directly implicated. Importantly, 93% received regional anesthesia.

Pediatrics

There are few studies of anesthesia-related risk in the pediatric population (see Chapters 81 to 84). Two themes emerge from these studies: very young infants are at increased risk, and anesthesia-related risk is reduced in centers with specialized pediatric anesthesia facilities. In the report by Beecher and Todd,[10] there was a "disproportionate number" of anesthesia-related deaths in children younger than 10 years.

Graff and colleagues[130] from the Baltimore Anesthesia Study Committee reported 335 operative deaths in the pediatric age group. Of these, 58 were thought to be primarily or partially attributable to anesthesia. The percentage of operative deaths attributable to anesthesia was relatively constant among age groups at 16.6% to 21.7%. The estimated anesthesia-associated mortality rate was 3.3 deaths per 10,000 operations for those younger than 15 years versus 0.6 for those between 15 and 24 years of age and 11.7 for those older than 64 years. More than half of the patients were categorized as ASA physical status class 1 or 2, suggesting that the majority of deaths occurred in children with good anesthesia risk. Most deaths occurred during tonsillectomy, which probably reflects the fact that tonsillectomy is the most common operation in this age group. The investigators attempted to determine the phase of the operation that was associated with highest risk. Improper management of the anesthetic accounted for approximately half of the cases. Respiratory complications (e.g., underventilation, aspiration of vomitus or blood) were apparent in 82% of the anesthesia-related deaths. The investigators suggested that female patients have a lower operative risk than male patients in all age groups.

Tiret and coauthors[131] published a study of pediatric anesthesia risk in 1988. They prospectively studied major anesthesia-related complications in pediatric patients in 440 hospitals in France between 1978 and 1982. There were 27 major complications in 40,240 cases, which included 12 cardiac arrests and 1 death. The incidence of major complications and cardiac arrest was significantly higher in infants than in older children. The rate of cardiac arrest related to anesthesia was highest in infants (19 per 10,000) and lowest in children (2.1 per 10,000). Most complications in infants involved the respiratory system and consisted predominantly of airway problems and aspiration. Older children experienced respiratory and cardiac complications, which occurred most frequently during induction and recovery.

Cohen and colleagues[132] studied 29,220 anesthesia procedures at the Winnipeg Children's Hospital. Data were collected

Table 33-16 Summary of Perioperative Events by Age Group*

	<1 Month (*n* = 361)	1-12 Months (*n* = 2544)	1-5 Years (*n* = 13,484)	6-10 Years (*n* = 7184)	11+ Years Event (*n* = 5647)
Any intraoperative event	14.96	7.31	7.10	12.22	9.69
Any recovery room event	16.61	7.23	12.20	14.88	15.23
Any postoperative event					
Minor event†	13.57	10.30	20.32	31.49	32.44
Major event‡	23.82	7.51	3.26	3.37	3.33
Any event§					
Among patients seen	48.89	25.92	37.50	50.52	51.33
Among all patients	41.55	23.47	33.16	45.04	45.78

*All figures are given as the percentage of events per total anesthetics.

†Includes nausea and vomiting, sore throat, muscle pain, headache, dental conditions, positional conditions, conditions involving extremities, eye conditions, croup, temperature, behavioral problems, thrombophlebitis, arterial line problem, awareness, and "other" problems.

‡Includes "other respiratory" conditions, cardiovascular disorders, nerve palsy, hepatic disorders, renal disorders, seizures, surgical complications, and death.

§Percentage of total anesthetics in which there was at least one event in the intraoperative, recovery room, or later postoperative period.

Adapted from Cohen MM, Cameron CB, Duncan PG: Pediatric anesthesia morbidity and mortality in the perioperative period. Anesth Analg 70:160, 1990.

from mid-1982 to 1987 and stored in a databank. Data on patients' coexisting medical conditions and postoperative follow-up were obtained within 72 hours. Complications included death, cardiac arrest, drug reactions, airway obstruction, and minor complications such as nausea and vomiting, arrhythmias, and sore throat. Neonates underwent a higher percentage of major vascular or cardiac and intra-abdominal procedures, and older children had a higher incidence of extremity procedures. Intraoperative cardiac arrest occurred most frequently in patients younger than 1 year (4 in 2901 procedures). Postoperatively, minor events such as nausea and vomiting were more common in older children, whereas respiratory events were more common in infants and younger children (Table 33-16). When compared with adult patients, children experienced different complications, which frequently extended well into the postoperative period. In a comparison of 2-year periods between 1982 and 1987, rates of intraoperative events were found to be stable, and the rate of postoperative complications decreased. The researchers suggested that identification of these problems could lead to changes in management that result in improved outcomes.

Flick and associates[132a] studied patients younger than 18 years who underwent surgery at the Mayo Clinic and experienced perioperative cardiac arrest between November 1, 1988, and June 30, 2005, A total of 92,881 anesthetics were administered during the study period, 4242 of which (5%) were for repair of congenital heart malformations. The incidence of perioperative cardiac arrest during noncardiac procedures was 2.9 per 10,000, and the incidence during cardiac procedures was 127 per 10,000. The incidence of perioperative cardiac arrest attributable to anesthesia was 0.65 per 10,000 anesthetics. The incidence of cardiac arrest and mortality was highest in neonates (0 to 30 days of life) undergoing cardiac procedures (incidence, 435 per 10,000; mortality, 389 per 10,000).

Investigators at the Children's Hospital of Boston used an established data registry that included all cardiac arrests from January 2000 through December 2005 related to surgery for congenital heart disease.[133] There were 41 cardiac arrests in 40 patients during 5213 anesthetics over the time period, for an overall frequency of 0.79%. Eleven cardiac arrests (26.8%) were classified as either likely (*n* = 6) or possibly related (*n* = 5) to anesthesia (21.1 per 10,000 anesthetics), but with no mortality; 30 were categorized as being related to the procedure.

In 1994, the Pediatric Perioperative Cardiac Arrest (POCA) Registry[134] was formed to determine the clinical factors and outcomes associated with cardiac arrest in anesthetized children. Institutions included in the registry submitted standardized data from each cardiac arrest occurring in an anesthetized child 18 years or younger. A total of 289 cardiac arrests occurred in the 63 institutions in the database during the first 4 years of the registry, 150 of which were judged to be related to anesthesia (1.4 per 10,000 anesthesia procedures), with a 26% mortality rate. Medication-related causes and cardiovascular causes of cardiac arrest were most common. Anesthesia-related cardiac arrest occurred most often in patients younger than 1 year and in patients with severe underlying disease. The goal of the registry is similar to that of the closed claims studies—to identify the causes in this unique population and thereby formulate preventive strategies.

An update from the POCA Registry was published in 2007.[135] From 1998 to 2004, 193 arrests (49%) were related to anesthesia. Medication-related arrests accounted for 18% of all arrests. Cardiovascular causes of cardiac arrest were the most common (41% of all arrests), with hypovolemia from blood loss and hyperkalemia from transfusion of stored blood being the most common identifiable cardiovascular causes (Fig. 33-8). Among respiratory causes of arrest (27%), airway obstruction from laryngospasm was the most common. Vascular injury incurred during placement of central venous catheters was the most frequent equipment-related cause of arrest. Cardiovascular and respiratory causes occurred most commonly in the surgical and postsurgical phases, respectively.

Geriatrics

Numerous studies have documented the importance of advanced age to perioperative risk (see Chapter 71). In many of the original studies on factors associated with perioperative mortality, the highest rates of death after surgery occurred in the youngest and the oldest patients. Age was implicated as one of the factors in the

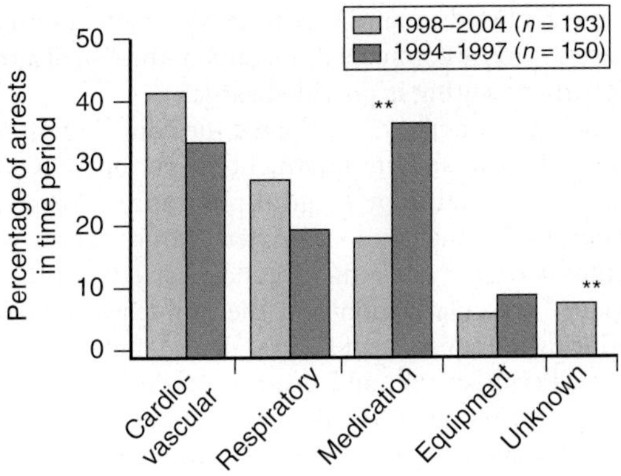

Figure 33-8 Causes of anesthesia-related cardiac arrest in in the Pediatric Perioperative Cardiac Arrest Registry from 1998 to 2004 versus 1994 to 1997. (**$P < .01$ 1998-2004 vs. 1994-1997 by Z test). *(From Bhananker SM, Ramamoorthy C, Geiduschek JM, et al: Anesthesia-related cardiac arrest in children: Update from the Pediatric Perioperative Cardiac Arrest Registry. Anesth Analg 105:344-350, 2007.)*

risk indices developed by Goldman, Detsky, and Pedersen. Age is predominantly analyzed as a dichotomous variable, with many studies focusing on age older than 70 years.

One of the issues regarding mortality rates in the geriatric population is the definition of this group. Multiple definitions have been used for advanced age, including patients older than 65, 70, 80, or 90 years. Denney and Denson[136] evaluated risk associated with surgery in patients older than 90 years. They suggested that the prevailing philosophy in 1972—that surgery might not be appropriate in this cohort in view of their high perioperative risk—was without objective supporting data. They reported 272 patients undergoing 301 operations at the University of Southern California Medical Center and found, contrary to their expectation, that the risk was more than justified in at least 70% of the nonagenarians. They reported that serious bowel obstruction was the only underlying comorbid condition associated with a prohibitive perioperative mortality rate (63%).

Djokovic and Hedley-Whyte[137] studied outcome after surgery in 500 patients older than 80 years at the Harvard University medical system. They found that mortality was predicted by ASA physical status classification, with greater comorbid conditions associated with increasing risk. Myocardial infarction was the leading cause of postoperative death. Patients without significant comorbid diseases (ASA class 1) had a mortality rate of less than 1%. The data suggest that surgery is safe in this cohort and that risk is not a function of age but of coexisting disease.

Del Guercio and Cohn[138] investigated the value of preoperative invasive monitoring in obtaining hemodynamic and cardiopulmonary variables for predicting operative risk in the elderly. A total of 148 consecutive patients older than 65 years were studied preoperatively in an ICU. Only 13.5% had normal physiologic measurements. Advanced and uncorrectable functional deficits were found in 63% of patients, and all in this group who underwent the planned operation died. This further supports the contention that coexisting disease, not age, is the risk.

An elderly patient presents a difficult issue for the anesthesiologist. Atherosclerosis increases with advancing age, and the heart muscle itself ages. Further preoperative evaluation in the elderly usually focuses on the identification of comorbid disease. Based on the accumulating evidence, these factors influence perioperative risk.

Risks Directly Related to the Anesthetic Drug

Numerous studies have evaluated the influence of the choice of anesthetic on outcome, a question that is discussed throughout this book. From a global perspective, there does not appear to be one best anesthesia technique. In a multivariate analysis by Cohen and coworkers[99] of 100,000 anesthesia procedures performed in Canada, the choice of drug did not provide any additional prognostic information for predicting mortality beyond that of patient disease and the surgical procedure. In univariate analysis, monitored anesthesia care did appear to be associated with worse outcomes, but this was attributable to its use in sicker patients (see Table 33-12).

One question that has plagued the anesthesia literature is the issue of inherent toxicity of anesthetics (see Chapter 24). There are important distinctions between undesirable side effects of anesthesia and true toxicity. In the initial reports of the mid-20th century, there was much concern about curare toxicity. Recent discussions of anesthetic toxicity have focused on halothane and sevoflurane. The issues for halothane were fulminant hepatic necrosis and death. The issue for sevoflurane was whether its metabolite compound A was nephrotoxic. After several case reports of hepatic necrosis after halothane anesthesia, a retrospective study of 856,500 anesthesia procedures at 34 institutions was undertaken.[139-141] In all but nine cases, hepatic necrosis could be explained by other causes. Of the remaining nine cases, only seven received halothane. Halothane could be associated with hepatitis and hepatic failure, but the incidence was very low.

Despite concern about the renal toxicity of sevoflurane (see Chapter 24), the overall safety of this drug has been sufficiently established for the U.S. Food and Drug Administration to allow its continued sale in the United States. Some laboratory studies have supported the contention that sevoflurane reacts with soda lime to form compound A and that this metabolite can lead to renal toxicity.[142,143] However, clinical studies have been unable to confirm this potentially detrimental effect.[144,145]

Numerous studies have attempted to define the "safest" anesthetic for high-risk patients. In the late 1980s, there was particular concern that isoflurane caused coronary steal in patients with coronary stenosis and collaterals and that this could result in myocardial ischemia.[146,147] A series of studies were conducted to evaluate the rate of perioperative cardiac morbidity and mortality in patients undergoing coronary artery bypass grafting to determine the importance of the agent used for general anesthesia.[148-151] All these studies demonstrated no difference in outcome, thus supporting the contention that there is no one safest anesthesia technique.

A series of randomized trials demonstrated improved outcome with regional rather than general anesthesia.[152] For lower extremity and pelvic surgery, regional anesthesia was associated with a lower incidence of graft thrombosis and deep venous thrombosis, as well as decreased bleeding. For vascular surgery patients, the primary finding was a lower incidence of graft thrombosis and need for reoperation in patients undergoing infrainguinal bypass surgery; however, the largest of these studies was unable to demonstrate any difference in outcome based on anesthesia technique.[4,153,154] The rate of this complication was low in the total cohort in the largest trial, which made it impossible to detect any difference based on technique.

Rodgers and coworkers[152] published a large meta-analysis of regional versus general anesthesia. Neuraxial blockade was found to reduce postoperative mortality and other serious complications. The magnitude of some of these benefits remained uncertain. Discussion of regional versus general anesthesia is presented in Chapters 51 and 52.

Risks Related to Surgery

The surgical procedure itself significantly influences perioperative risk. In virtually every study performed, emergency surgery is associated with additional risk. For example, in the study of Goldman and colleagues,[6] emergency surgery was associated with the second highest weight (i.e., number of points) after active signs of congestive heart failure. In the same study, intrathoracic and abdominal procedures were determined to have higher risk.

In some cases, the risk related to surgery is a function of the underlying disease processes and the stress related to the surgical procedure. Cardiovascular surgery is associated with the highest risk of any procedure. The risks related to cardiac surgery are reviewed in Chapter 60. Vascular surgery is among the highest-risk group of noncardiac procedures. Although aortic reconstructive surgery has traditionally been considered the procedure with highest risk, infrainguinal procedures have shown a similar rate of cardiac morbidity in several studies.[155,156] In an attempt to analyze the cause of the high complication rate with a relatively peripheral procedure, L'Italien and associates[156] demonstrated that the extent of coronary artery disease is higher in patients undergoing infrainguinal procedures and most likely accounts for the excess morbidity and mortality.

Ashton and colleagues[157] evaluated perioperative morbidity and mortality in a cohort of patients at a Veterans hospital. Although vascular surgery was among the highest-risk procedures, amputation was associated with the highest in-hospital cardiac complication rate within this subgroup. This finding most likely represents the more severe nature of the cardiovascular disease in these patients and the prolonged hospitalization needed to facilitate recuperation. As in the study by Goldman and coworkers,[6] intra-abdominal, thoracic, and orthopedic procedures were associated with increased risk. In another report, Ashton and colleagues[158] evaluated the rate of perioperative myocardial infarction in patients undergoing transurethral resection of the prostate. Despite the high frequency of coronary artery disease in this population, the incidence of perioperative myocardial infarction was only 1%.

Numerous studies have evaluated the perioperative complication rate related to superficial procedures. Backer and associates[159] evaluated the rate of perioperative myocardial reinfarction in patients undergoing ophthalmologic surgery. They demonstrated that the rate of perioperative cardiac morbidity after ophthalmologic surgery was extremely low, even in patients with recent myocardial infarction. Virtually all studies have confirmed that ophthalmologic surgery is very safe under anesthesia.[160] Warner and colleagues[161] studied patients undergoing ambulatory surgery and reported no anesthesia-related deaths in more than 45,000 cases. A more complete discussion of the risk of anesthesia in the outpatient setting is provided earlier.

Eagle and associates[162] evaluated the contribution of coronary artery disease and its treatment to perioperative cardiac morbidity and mortality by surgical procedure. They evaluated patients enrolled in the Coronary Artery Surgery Study who had documented coronary artery disease and received medical therapy or coronary revascularization and then underwent noncardiac surgery during the subsequent 10-year period. Rates of perioperative myocardial infarction and death were determined, and the surgical procedures were divided into three broad categories. Major vascular surgery was associated with the highest risk, with a combined incidence of morbidity and mortality of greater than 5%. Procedures associated with a combined complication rate of 1% to 5% included intra-abdominal, thoracic, and head and neck operations. In all these cases, patients who had previously undergone coronary artery bypass grafting had a significantly lower combined morbidity and mortality rate than did those in the medically treated group. Low-risk procedures included breast, skin, urologic, and orthopedic surgery. These broad groups of surgical procedures were the basis for the definitions of surgical risk published in the guidelines on perioperative cardiovascular evaluation for noncardiac surgery by the American Heart Association/American College of Cardiology Task Force on Assessment of Diagnostic and Therapeutic Cardiovascular Procedures.[163]

Risks Related to the Location of Surgery and Postoperative Monitoring

Perioperative risk varies among hospitals for major procedures such as coronary artery bypass grafting and abdominal aortic aneurysm repair (see Chapters 60 and 62).[164,165] Multiple studies have documented a relationship between surgical volume and mortality. Although surgical skill most certainly plays a role in the rate of complications and mortality, local factors may also play an important role. For example, low surgical volume may lead to less skilled anesthesia and postoperative care. The influence of each of these factors on overall morbidity and mortality is unknown.

Although the value of postoperative monitoring and care in an ICU has never been documented in a randomized clinical trial, many investigators have suggested that such care is one of the primary reasons for the improved morbidity and mortality in recent years. For patients undergoing major vascular surgery, several investigators have suggested that more intense postoperative monitoring could obviate the need for preoperative cardiac testing and revascularization.[163] One potential value of risk assessment is identification of patients who could benefit from referral to centers with more extensive perioperative resources. Patients with a low probability of perioperative morbidity and mortality could have surgery performed locally, and individuals at higher risk could receive benefit from transfer to a larger center.

Risks Related to the Anesthesia Provider

The added risk associated with the provider of anesthesia is an emotionally charged issue, particularly in the United States. Over the history of the specialty, various individuals have provided anesthesia, including anesthesiologists, general medical officers, residents, and CRNAs.

The importance of the anesthesiologist to outcome is best illustrated by the work of Slogoff and Keats.[166] They studied the association of perioperative myocardial ischemia and cardiac morbidity in patients undergoing coronary artery bypass grafting and found that perioperative myocardial infarction occurred significantly more frequently in patients with ischemia before the bypass operation. They then reported the rate of ischemia and infarction by anesthesiologist (identified by number). Anesthesiologist no. 7 had a significantly higher rate of complications than the average for the rest of the group. Operator technique or experience may affect risk. This observation parallels similar findings that surgical volume (and presumably experience) is associated with outcome.[167]

Arbous and coauthors reported a case-control study of major morbidity (coma) and mortality affecting a total of 869,463 procedures over a 1-year period in the Netherlands.[168] Eight hundred seven cases of coma or death within 24 hours of anesthesia were identified and matched by age and sex to randomly selected controls who underwent anesthesia temporally in close proximity to the matched case. The Hospital Characteristics Questionnaire, Procedure Questionnaire, and anesthesia and recovery records were used to examine the intraoperative and postoperative characteristics of cases and controls. Anesthesia practice in the Netherlands is described as a "flexible" system with one-on-one anesthesiologist coverage of induction and emergence, assisted by a nurse anesthetist or resident, and a two-on-one system during maintenance anesthesia, with a nurse or resident present in the room and an anesthesiologist in the vicinity. The authors elected to use multivariate analysis on data sets rather than match cases and controls for anesthesia/physical risk categories or the type of surgical procedure (or both).

Included in analysis were 807 cases and 883 controls. Cases and controls, however, were not comparable for ASA classification, and controls were more likely than cases to have undergone minor elective procedures during regular working hours. Cases more frequently underwent cardiac and major vascular procedures, and controls more often underwent orthopedic, urologic, and ophthalmologic procedures. Of 807 cases, 95% died within 24 hours, and 5% remained comatose, all of whom eventually died in the hospital. Postoperative mortality was 8.8% per 10,000 anesthetics, and postoperative coma occurred in 0.5% of 10,000 anesthetics. Confounding factors were, expectedly, ASA status, type of procedure, anesthetic technique, and hospital. Independent variables that were associated with decreased risk for coma and death in 24 hours were (1) anesthesia equipment check performed with a checklist (OR, 0.61); (2) direct availability of an anesthesiologist during maintenance anesthesia by phone, beeper, or walkie-talkie (OR, 0.46); (3) no change of anesthesiologist during the case (OR, 0.46); (4) presence of a full-time nurse anesthetist versus part-time anesthetist during maintenance anesthesia (OR, 0.41); (5) presence of two persons (anesthesiologist plus resident or nurse anesthetist) versus one person during emergence (OR, 0.69); (6) reversal of muscle relaxant (OR, 0.1); and (7) reversal of muscle relaxant and opioids (OR, 0.29).

This study is one of very few to attempt to identify practice characteristics rather than specific drugs or techniques that have an impact on anesthesia outcomes. The size of this study and the nonambiguity of outcomes followed are important characteristics. The study suffers from several significant problems, however. Study groups were not comparable in very important ways. The estimated incidence of underreporting of coma and death was 13% to 47%, and selective underreporting could have occurred. The finding that a change of anesthesiologist during maintenance anesthesia adversely affected patient outcomes contradicts findings in previous studies and requires further explanation. Confounding variables associated with a change of anesthesiologist during maintenance anesthesia could include case length and the time of day in which cases are performed. An intriguing finding is that practitioner characteristics affect outcomes (better outcomes with more availability of an anesthesiologist and better outcomes when nurse anesthetists practice full-time rather than part-time), and this finding warrants further follow-up.

Several studies have attempted to evaluate the complication rates and risks associated with various care provider models. Bechtoldt,[169] as a member of the North Carolina Anesthesia Study Committee, evaluated 900 perioperative deaths that occurred in an estimated 2 million anesthesia procedures performed in North Carolina between 1969 and 1976. Data were obtained from the medical examiner's report, routine death certificates, and a questionnaire completed by the person who administered the anesthetic. The committee concluded that 90 of these deaths were related to anesthesia. About half of the anesthesia-related deaths took place in the operating room, including 19 that occurred on induction. With information attained from a survey of hospitals, they then determined the relationship between mortality and anesthesia provider based on the total number of procedures administered by each group. The lowest rate of anesthesia-related deaths (1 per 28,166 procedures) occurred in patients who received anesthesia from an anesthesia care team (physician anesthesiologist and CRNA), and the highest rate (1 per 11,432 procedures) was associated with anesthesia administered by a dentist (1 per 11,432); the rate for the nurse anesthetist–only cohort was intermediate (1 per 20,723). The large number of cases in which the care provider was unknown and reliance on hospital estimates of the number of cases performed by each group made interpretation of this study difficult.

The Stanford Center for Health Care Research[170] also evaluated the impact of provider on outcome of care. They prospectively collected data from 8593 patients undergoing 15 surgical procedures over a 10-month period (May 1973 through February 1974). Using a risk adjustment methodology, the actual patient outcome was compared with that predicted by the patient's health status and operative procedure. The investigators reported that death plus severe morbidity was 11% higher than predicted in patients who received their care in a nurse anesthetist–only setting, 3% lower than predicted for physician-only care, and 20% lower than predicted for an anesthesia care team environment. Because of the small sample size, these findings did not reach statistical significance between groups.

The differences in outcome among anesthesia providers are extremely difficult to study from a methodologic standpoint. The impact of specific provider types may be greatest in specific situations. For example, there may be no difference in outcome for healthy individuals, particularly if no complications occur. In contrast, patients with significant comorbid diseases and those who sustain perioperative complications may benefit from having providers with specific skill sets. One way to study such issues is to evaluate the rate of survival after complications. Silber and colleagues[26] at the University of Pennsylvania studied the medical records of 5972 surgical patients randomly selected from 531 hospitals. They evaluated patient and hospital characteristics, including the number and type of physicians, board certification status, and ratio of care providers. The 30-day mortality rate correlated with patient characteristics. Failure to rescue (i.e., prevent death) after an adverse event was inversely associated with the proportion of board-certified anesthesiologists on staff in each facility. Improved perioperative survival was significantly associated with the presence of an increased number of board-certified anesthesiologists.

As a follow-up to this study, Silber and colleagues[171] used an administrative data set to compare the outcomes of surgical patients for whom anesthesia care was or was not personally performed or medically directed by an anesthesiologist. They analyzed all elderly patients in Pennsylvania who underwent general surgical or orthopedic procedures between 1991 and 1994. The 30-day mortality rate and the mortality rate after complications (i.e., failure to rescue) were lower when anesthesiologists directed anesthesia care, even after adjustment for patient and hospital characteristics. Interpretation of the study was limited because the undirected group was small and included a large percentage of procedures in which there was no bill submitted for anesthesia services, thus questioning the validity of the classification. Administrative data sets, such as Medicare claims, allow the investigator to study a large number of patients, but there are significant limitations related to the robustness of the data and potential uncontrolled confounding factors. Therefore, most investigators suggest that such studies are best at generating hypotheses rather than defining best practices.[172]

Silber and colleagues[173] used similar methodology to determine the importance of board certification on perioperative risk. Adjusted ORs for death (1.13; 95% CI, 1.00 to 1.26; $P < .04$) and for failure to rescue (1.13; 95% CI, 1.01 to 1.27; $P < .04$) were greater when care was delivered by noncertified, midcareer anesthesiologists.

Pine and coworkers evaluated mortality after eight specific surgical procedures.[174] Procedure-specific risk adjustment models (including institutional and geographic factors) were derived by stepwise logistic regression. Observed and predicted values by type of provider were not statistically significantly different. Hospitals without anesthesiologists had results similar to those where anesthesiologists provided or directed anesthesia care. The authors did not evaluate failure to rescue or cause of mortality.

Smith and associates[175] performed a systematic review of the available published studies through 2004 on the influence of anesthesia providers. They identified four studies, two smaller observational studies and the two previously described studies using administrative data sets. They concluded that all of the studies had potential confounding factors that limited the validity of the results and that the paucity of high-level primary evidence made it impossible to draw a conclusion regarding differences in patient safety as a function of provider type. Therefore, the relationship of patient outcomes to the type of anesthesia provider has not been conclusively demonstrated. Nurse anesthetists and other nonphysician providers are vital to the delivery of anesthesia care in the United States and elsewhere, and differences, if present, are small or restricted to specific situations.

Risks to the Anesthesiologist

Several potential risks to the anesthesiologist are related to the provision of care (see Chapter 101), including medicolegal risk, the risk of an allergic reaction, and the risk of a needlestick injury and transmission of disease from the patient to the practitioner. Medicolegal risks are described in Chapter 10.

It is increasingly becoming apparent that anesthesiologists are at risk for latex allergy, which can lead to a life-threatening reaction. Many anesthesiologists realize that they are sensitized to latex and apply appropriate precautions. The problem is that many sensitized individuals are asymptomatic. Brown and coworkers[176] studied 168 eligible anesthesiologists and nurse anesthetists working in the anesthesia department of The Johns Hopkins Hospital. The prevalence of latex allergy with clinical symptoms was 2.4% and that of latex sensitization without clinical symptoms was 10.1%. The prevalence of irritant or contact dermatitis was 24%. These data suggest that latex is an important problem to the anesthesiologist and that there is a need to transform the hospital to a latex-free environment.

There has always been concern that anesthesiologists are at risk for contracting a disease from a patient. In the past the risk was primarily hepatitis, but human immunodeficiency virus (HIV) is a greater concern today. In a review of the literature, Berry and Greene[177] reported that at least 20 different pathogens have been transmitted through accidental needlestick injuries.

Among anesthesia personnel in several studies conducted in the United States, hepatitis B seropositivity ranged from 12.7% to 48.6%, a rate at least four times greater than that in the general population.[178-180] The risk of hepatitis B infection after percutaneous exposure to antigen-positive blood is estimated to be 27% to 43%.[181] Development of the hepatitis B vaccine has substantially reduced this risk. Hepatitis C virus has been identified as a major cause of post-transfusion hepatitis. There have been several reports of occupationally acquired hepatitis in health care workers.[182] Because signs of chronic liver infection develop in up to 50% of infected individuals, this represents a potentially serious problem.

Among the greatest fears of health care workers is HIV infection. The risk of acquiring HIV is approximately 0.4% from a single percutaneous exposure to blood or bloody fluid from an HIV-infected patient.[183] There has been at least one case report of an anesthesiologist who was infected with HIV from a needlestick injury during insertion of a central venous catheter into an HIV-positive patient.[184]

Several strategies have been developed to reduce the transmission of communicable diseases (see Chapter 101). Although anesthesiologists traditionally think of the risk to the patient, they must now include the risk to themselves. Widespread adoption of universal precautions should reduce the rate of infection; however, anesthesiologists have not accepted these recommendations widely. In a study of nine hospitals, 59% of the contaminated percutaneous injuries were preventable.[185] In a theoretical model of the risk for HIV infection, it was estimated that the 30-year occupational risk was 0.10% to 0.22% in low-prevalence areas and

8.26% to 13% in high-prevalence areas.[186] The researchers suggested that double-gloving practices may lead to reduced risk.

Improving Anesthesia Safety

Over the past several decades there have been major initiatives to improve the safety of anesthesia. In 1984, Cooper, Kitz, and Ellison hosted the first International Symposium on Preventable Anesthesia Mortality and Morbidity in Boston. Approximately 50 anesthesiologists from around the world attended the meeting and, after much debate, established a series of definitions of outcome, morbidity, and mortality (Box 33-1). These meetings have been held every 2 years since the first symposium. The Anesthesia Patient Safety Foundation was established as a result of the Boston meeting. The society has been active in publishing widely circulated newsletters and awarding annual grants. Similar societies have been established in countries outside the United States, and a National Patient Safety Foundation has been created on the same model.

Starting with the ACCS, there has been much interest in establishing guidelines for the best and safest practice. Practice policies or guidelines are summations by clinicians of the available evidence about the benefits and risks of particular treatment plans. Guidelines are a method of codifying recommendations regarding the use of a given technology. Several types of recommendations fall into the general category of a practice parameter. A standard implies that a therapy or practice should be performed for patients with a particular condition. Standards are approved only if an assessment of the probabilities and utilities of the group indicate that the decision to choose the treatment or a strategy would be virtually unanimous. If a particular therapy or strategy is considered a standard, it is a cost-effective measure for those for whom it is being recommended. Standards are intended to be applied rigidly. The ASA has established standards for intraoperative monitoring, which were developed from safety guidelines adopted by the Harvard University hospital system. Guidelines are intended to be more flexible than standards, but they should be followed in most cases. Depending on the patient, the setting, and other factors, guidelines can and should be tailored to fit individual needs. Like standards, guidelines should be cost-effective methods. A number of specific guidelines have been adopted by the ASA for diverse issues such as a difficult airway,[187] use of the pulmonary artery catheter,[188] and use of blood components.[189] The goal is to define the evidence on which optimal practice can be based.

There is much interest in the use of anesthesia simulators to train and test individuals and their ability to react to simulated crises.[190-194] Standardized scenarios have been developed for making comparisons among individuals. Further research is required to determine how best to use this technology in anesthesia training and recertification. Further discussion of this topic can be found in Chapters 5, 6, and 7.

Box 33-1 Proposed Definitions from the 1994 International Symposium on Preventable Anesthesia Morbidity and Mortality

- Outcome
  - Normal
  - Abandoned procedure
  - Morbidity
  - Death
- Morbidity
  - An unplanned, unwanted, undesirable consequence of anesthesia
- Mortality
  - Death that occurs before recovery from the effects of a drug or drugs given to facilitate a procedure
  - Death that occurs during an attempt to relieve the pain of a condition
  - Death that results from an incident that occurs while the drugs are effective

Adapted from Pierce EC Jr: The 34th Rovenstine Lecture: 40 years behind the mask: Safety revisited. Anesthesiology 84:965, 1996.

Future Directions in Perioperative Risk

The impact of genetics on perioperative risk has been well known since elucidation of the inheritance pattern of malignant hyperthermia. With malignant hyperthermia, there is a clear link between the autosomal dominant disease and an adverse outcome after administration of an anesthetic.[195] Interest in evaluating the impact of genetic polymorphism on overall perioperative outcome is increasing, even if the link to anesthesia is less well defined. For example, apolipoprotein E_4 has been shown to modulate neurologic injury and recovery after a variety of acute ischemic insults, including coronary artery bypass grafting.[196] Polymorphism of the glycoprotein IIIa constituent of the platelet integrin receptor has also been correlated with postoperative cognitive decline.

Summary

The risks related to anesthesia have dramatically decreased over the past several decades. It is clear that death totally attributable to anesthesia is rare. Patient disease and the type and perhaps the location of surgical procedures have a greater effect on overall outcome. With these changes in risk, the anesthesiologist must now focus on nonmorbid outcomes, and there must be continued vigilance to maintain the high standards of hospital-based anesthesia in nonhospital settings. Finally, anesthesiologists should play a role in systems-based thinking to improve all aspects of care.

References

1. Fleisher LA, Pasternak LR, Herbert R, Anderson GF: Inpatient hospital admission and death after outpatient surgery in elderly patients: Importance of patient and system characteristics and location of care. Arch Surg 139:67-72, 2004.
2. Kim LJ, Martinez EA, Faraday N, et al: Cardiac troponin I predicts short-term mortality in vascular surgery patients. Circulation 106:2366-2371, 2002.
3. Mangano DT, Browner WS, Hollenberg M, et al: Long-term cardiac prognosis following noncardiac surgery. The Study of Perioperative Ischemia Research Group. JAMA 268:233-239, 1992.
4. Christopherson R, Beattie C, Frank SM, et al: Perioperative morbidity in patients randomized to epidural or general anesthesia for lower extremity vascular surgery. Perioperative Ischemia Randomized Anesthesia Trial Study Group. Anesthesiology 79:422-434, 1993.
5. Tuman KJ, McCarthy RJ, March RJ, et al: Effects of epidural anesthesia and analgesia on coagulation and outcome after major vascular surgery. Anesth Analg 73:696-704, 1991.
6. Goldman L, Caldera DL, Nussbaum SR, et al: Multifactorial index of cardiac risk in noncardiac surgical procedures. N Engl J Med 297:845-850, 1977.
7. Frank SM, Beattie C, Christopherson R, et al: Unintentional hypothermia is associated with postoperative myocardial ischemia. The Perioperative Ischemia Randomized Anesthesia Trial Study Group. Anesthesiology 78:468-476, 1993.
8. Frank SM, Fleisher LA, Breslow MJ, et al: Perioperative maintenance of normothermia reduces the incidence of morbid cardiac events. A randomized clinical trial. JAMA 277:1127-1134, 1997.
9. Lagasse RS: Anesthesia safety: Model or myth? A review of the published literature and analysis of current original data. Anesthesiology 97:1609-1617, 2002.
10. Beecher HK, Todd DP: A study of deaths associated with anesthesia and surgery. Ann Surg 140:2-34, 1954.
11. Buck N, Devlin HB, Lunn JL: Report of a Confidential Enquiry into Perioperative Deaths. London, The King's Fund Publishing House, 1987.
12. Cheney FW, Posner K, Caplan RA, Ward RJ: Standard of care and anesthesia liability. JAMA 261:1599-1603, 1989.
13. Mangano DT: Aspirin and mortality from coronary bypass surgery. N Engl J Med 347:1309-1317, 2002.
14. Mathew JP, Parks R, Savino JS, et al: Atrial fibrillation following coronary artery bypass graft surgery: Predictors, outcomes, and resource utilization. MultiCenter Study of Perioperative Ischemia Research Group. JAMA 276:300-306, 1996.
15. Clark RE: The development of The Society of Thoracic Surgeons voluntary national database system: Genesis, issues, growth, and status. Best Pract Benchmarking Healthc 1:62-69, 1996.
16. Grover FL, Shroyer AL, Edwards FH, et al: Data quality review program: The Society of Thoracic Surgeons Adult Cardiac National Database. Ann Thorac Surg 62:1229-1231, 1996.
17. Grover FL, Shroyer AL, Hammermeister KE: Calculating risk and outcome: The Veterans Affairs database. Ann Thorac Surg 62:S6-S11, 1996.
18. Nugent WC: Clinical applications of risk-assessment protocols in the management of individual patients. Ann Thorac Surg 64:S68-S72, discussion S80-S82, 1997.
19. Todd CJ, Freeman CJ, Camilleri-Ferrante C, et al: Differences in mortality after fracture of hip: The East Anglian audit. BMJ 310:904-908, 1995.
20. Pronovost PJ, Angus DC, Dorman T, et al: Physician staffing patterns and clinical outcomes in critically ill patients: A systematic review. JAMA 288:2151-2162, 2002.
21. Marx GF, Mateo CV, Orkin LR: Computer analysis of postanesthetic deaths. Anesthesiology 39:54-58, 1973.
22. Reich DL, Bodian CA, Krol M, et al: Intraoperative hemodynamic predictors of mortality, stroke, and myocardial infarction after coronary artery bypass surgery. Anesth Analg 89:814-822, 1999.
23. Ghali WA, Ash AS, Hall RE, Moskowitz MA: Statewide quality improvement initiatives and mortality after cardiac surgery. JAMA 277:379-382, 1997.
24. Hannan EL, Racz MJ, Jollis JG, Peterson ED: Using Medicare claims data to assess provider quality for CABG surgery: Does it work well enough? Health Serv Res 31:659-678, 1997.
25. Mukamel DB, Mushlin AI: Quality of care information makes a difference: An analysis of market share and price changes after publication of the New York State Cardiac Surgery Mortality Reports. Med Care 36:945-954, 1998.
26. Silber JH, Williams SV, Krakauer H, Schwartz JS: Hospital and patient characteristics associated with death after surgery. A study of adverse occurrence and failure to rescue. Med Care 30:615-627, 1992.
27. Beecher HK: The first anesthesia death with some remarks suggested by it on the fields of the laboratory and clinic in the appraisal of new anesthetic agents. Anesthesiology 2:443, 1941.
28. Snow J: On chloroform and other anesthetics. London, John Churchill, 1858.
29. Ruth HS: Anesthesia study commissions. JAMA 127:514, 1945.
30. Macintosh RR: Deaths under anaesthetics. Br J Anaesth 21:107-136, 1948.
31. Dornette WHL, Orth OS: Death in the operating room. Anesth Analg 35:545-569, 1956.
32. Dripps RD, Lamont A, Eckenhoff JE: The role of anesthesia in surgical mortality. JAMA 178:261-266, 1961.
33. Gebbie D: Anaesthesia and death. Can Anaesth Soc J 13:390-396, 1966.
34. Phillips OC, Frazier TM, Graff TD, DeKornfeld TJ: The Baltimore anesthesia study committee; review of 1,024 postoperative deaths. JAMA 174:2015-2019, 1960.
35. Schapira M, Kepes ER, Hurwitt ES: An analysis of deaths in the operating room and within 24 hours of surgery. Anesth Analg 39:149-157, 1960.
36. Clifton BS, Hotten WIT: Deaths associated with anaesthesia. Br J Anaesth 35:250-259, 1963.
37. Dinnick OP: Deaths associated with anaesthesia. Anaesthesia 19:536-556, 1964.
38. Bodlander FMS: Deaths associated with anaesthesia. Br J Anaesth 47:36-40, 1975.
39. Cohen MM, Duncan PG, Pope WDB, Wolkenstein C: A survey of 112,000 anesthetics at one teaching hospital (1975-1983). Can Anaesth Soc J 33:22-31, 1986.
40. Farrow SC, Fowkes FG, Lunn JN, et al: Epidemiology in anaesthesia: A method for predicting hospital mortality. Eur J Anaesthesiol 1:77-84, 1984.
41. Farrow SC, Fowkes FGR, Lunn JN, et al: Epidemiology in anaesthesia II: Factors affecting mortality in hospital. Br J Anaesth 54:811-817, 1982.
42. Harrison GG: Death attributable to anaesthesia: A 10-year survey (1967-1976). Br J Anaesth 50:1041-1046, 1978.
43. Holland R: Anaesthetic mortality in New South Wales. Br J Anaesth 59:834-841, 1987.
44. Warden JC, Horan BF: Deaths attributed to anaesthesia in New South Wales, 1984-1990. Anaesth Intensive Care 24:66-73, 1996.
45. Tiret L, Desmonts JM, Hatton F, Vourc'h G: Complications associated with anaesthesia—a prospective survey in France. Can Anaesth Soc 33:336-344, 1986.
46. Tikkanen J, Hovi-Viander M: Death associated with anaesthesia and surgery in Finland in 1986 compared to 1975. Acta Anaesthesiol Scand 39:262-267, 1995.
47. Lunn JN: The study on anaesthetic-related mortality. Anaesthesia 35:617, 1980.
48. Lunn JN, Devlin HB: Lessons from the Confidential Enquiry into Perioperative Deaths in three NHS regions. Lancet 2:1384-1386, 1987.
49. Lunn JN, Hunter AR, Scott DB: Anaesthesia-related surgical mortality. Anaesthesia 38:1090-1096, 1983.
50. Lunn JN, Mushin WW: Mortality associated with anesthesia. Anaesthesia 37:856, 1982.
51. Pedersen T, Eliasen K, Henriksen E: A prospective study of mortality associated with anaesthesia and surgery: Risk indicators of mortality in hospital. Acta Anaesthesiol Scand 34:176-182, 1990.
52. Charuluxananan S, Chinachoti T, Pulnitiporn A, et al: The Thai Anesthesia Incidents Study (THAI Study) of perioperative death: Analysis of risk factors. J Med Assoc Thai 88(Suppl 7):S30-S40, 2005.
53. Keenan RL, Boyan CP: Cardiac arrest due to anesthesia. JAMA 253:2373-2377, 1985.
54. Olsson GL, Hallen B: Cardiac arrest during anaesthesia. A computer-aided study in 250,543 anaesthetics. Acta Anaesthesiol Scand 32:653-664, 1988.
55. Biboulet P, Aubas P, Dubourdieu J, et al: Fatal and non fatal cardiac arrests related to anesthesia. Can J Anaesth 48:326-332, 2001.
56. Newland MC, Ellis SJ, Lydiatt CA, et al: Anesthetic-related cardiac arrest and its mortality: A report covering 72,959 anesthetics over 10 years from a US teaching hospital. Anesthesiology 97:108-115, 2002.
57. Kawashima Y, Takahashi S, Suzuki M, et al: Anesthesia-related mortality and morbidity over a 5-year period in 2,363,038 patients in Japan. Acta Anaesthesiol Scand 47:809-817, 2003.
58. Sprung J, Warner ME, Contreras MG, et al: Predictors of survival following cardiac arrest in patients undergoing noncardiac surgery: A study of 518,294 patients at a tertiary referral center. Anesthesiology 99:259-269, 2003.
59. Braz LG, Modolo NS, do Nascimento P Jr, et al: Perioperative cardiac arrest: A study of 53,718 anaesthetics over 9 yr from a Brazilian teaching hospital. Br J Anaesth 96:569-575, 2006.
60. Chiang TM, Sukis AE, Ross DE: Tonsillectomy performed on an out-patient basis: Report of a series of 40,000 cases without a death. Arch Otolaryngol 88:307-310, 1968.
61. Raymond CA: Study questions safety, economic benefits of outpatient tonsil/adenoid surgery. JAMA 256:311-312, 1986.

62. Carithers JS, Gebhart DE, Williams JA: Postoperative risks of pediatric tonsilloadenoidectomy. Laryngoscope 97:422-429, 1987.
63. Brigger MT, Brietzke SE: Outpatient tonsillectomy in children: A systematic review. Otolaryngol Head Neck Surg 135:1-7, 2006.
64. Gabalski EC, Mattucci KF, Setzen M, Moleski P: Ambulatory tonsillectomy and adenoidectomy. Laryngoscope 106:77-80, 1996.
65. Mitchell RB, Pereira KD, Friedman NR, Lazar RH: Outpatient adenotonsillectomy. Is it safe in children younger than 3 years? Arch Otolaryngol Head Neck Surg 123:681-683, 1997.
66. Schloss MD, Tan AK, Schloss B, Tewfik TL: Outpatient tonsillectomy and adenoidectomy: Complications and recommendations. Int J Pediatr Otorhinolaryngol 30:115-122, 1994.
67. Warren JL, Riley GF, Potosky AL, et al: Trends and outcomes of outpatient mastectomy in elderly women. J Natl Cancer Inst 90:833-840, 1998.
68. Warner MA, Shields SE, Chute CG: Major morbidity and mortality within 1 month of ambulatory surgery and anesthesia. JAMA 270:1437-1441, 1993.
69. Fleisher LA, Pasternak LR, Lyles A: A novel index of elevated risk of inpatient hospital admission immediately following outpatient surgery. Arch Surg 142:263-268, 2007.
70. Chukmaitov AS, Menachemi N, Brown LS, et al: A Comparative Study of Quality Outcomes in Freestanding Ambulatory Surgery Centers and Hospital-Based Outpatient Departments: 1997. Health Services Research, 43:1485-1504, 2008.
71. Morello DC, Colon GA, Fredricks S, et al: Patient safety in accredited office surgical facilities. Plast Reconstr Surg 99:1496-1500, 1997.
72. Vila H Jr, Soto R, Cantor AB, Mackey D: Comparative outcomes analysis of procedures performed in physician offices and ambulatory surgery centers. Arch Surg 138:991-995, 2003.
73. Coldiron B, Shreve E, Balkrishnan R: Patient injuries from surgical procedures performed in medical offices: Three years of Florida data. Dermatol Surg 30:1435-1443, discussion 1443, 2004.
74. Coldiron BM, Healy C, Bene NI: Office surgery incidents: What seven years of Florida data show us. Dermatol Surg 34:285-291, discussion 291-292, 2008.
75. Clayman MA, Seagle BM: Office surgery safety: The myths and truths behind the Florida moratoria—six years of Florida data. Plast Reconstr Surg 118:777-785, discussion 786-787, 2006.
76. Sanborn KV, Castro J, Kuroda M, Thys DM: Detection of intraoperative incidents by electronic scanning of computerized anesthesia records. Comparison with voluntary reporting. Anesthesiology 85:977-987, 1996.
77. Kheterpal S, Han R, Tremper KK, et al: Incidence and predictors of difficult and impossible mask ventilation. Anesthesiology 105:885-891, 2006.
78. Kheterpal S, Tremper KK, Englesbe MJ, et al: Predictors of postoperative acute renal failure after noncardiac surgery in patients with previously normal renal function. Anesthesiology 107:892-902, 2007.
79. Caplan RA, Ward RJ, Posner K, Cheney FW: Unexpected cardiac arrest during spinal anesthesia: A closed claims analysis of predisposing factors. Anesthesiology 68:5-11, 1988.
80. Tinker JH, Dull DL, Caplan RA, et al: Role of monitoring devices in prevention of anesthetic mishaps: A closed claims analysis. Anesthesiology 71:541-546, 1989.
81. Caplan RA, Posner KL, Ward RJ, Cheney FW: Adverse respiratory events in anesthesia: A closed claims analysis. Anesthesiology 72:828-833, 1990.
82. Bhananker SM, Posner KL, Cheney FW, et al: Injury and liability associated with monitored anesthesia care: A closed claims analysis. Anesthesiology 104:228-234, 2006.
83. Hove LD, Steinmetz J, Christoffersen JK, et al: Analysis of deaths related to anesthesia in the period 1996-2004 from closed claims registered by the Danish Patient Insurance Association. Anesthesiology 106:675-680, 2007.
84. Cooper JB: Toward prevention of anesthetic mishaps. Int Anesthesiol Clin 22:167-183, 1984.
85. Cooper JB, Newbower RS, Kitz RJ: An analysis of major errors and equipment failures in anesthesia management: Considerations for prevention and detection. Anesthesiology 60:34-42, 1984.
86. Cooper JB, Newbower RS, Long CD, McPeek B: Preventable anesthesia mishaps: A study of human factors. Anesthesiology 49:399-406, 1978.
87. Singleton RJ, Webb RK, Ludbrook GL, Fox MA: The Australian Incident Monitoring Study. Problems associated with vascular access: An analysis of 2000 incident reports. Anaesth Intensive Care 21:664-669, 1993.
88. Van der Walt JH, Webb RK, Osborne GA, et al: The Australian Incident Monitoring Study. Recovery room incidents in the first 2000 incident reports. Anaesth Intensive Care 21:650-652, 1993.
89. Russell WJ, Webb RK, Van der Walt JH, Runciman WB: The Australian Incident Monitoring Study. Problems with ventilation: An analysis of 2000 incident reports. Anaesth Intensive Care 21:617-620, 1993.
90. Buffington CW, Ramanathan S, Turndorf H: Detection of anesthesia machine faults. Anesth Analg 63:79-82, 1984.
91. Lopez-Jimenez F, Goldman L, Sacks DB, et al: Prognostic value of cardiac troponin T after noncardiac surgery: 6-month follow-up data. J Am Coll Cardiol 29:1241-1245, 1997.
92. Yeager RA, Moneta GL, Edwards JM, et al: Late survival after perioperative myocardial infarction complicating vascular surgery. J Vasc Surg 20:598-606, 1994.
93. Mangano DT, Layug EL, Wallace A, Tateo I: Effect of atenolol on mortality and cardiovascular morbidity after noncardiac surgery. Multicenter Study of Perioperative Ischemia Research Group. N Engl J Med 335:1713-1720, 1996.
94. Wallace A, Layug B, Tateo I, et al: Prophylactic atenolol reduces postoperative myocardial ischemia. McSPI Research Group. Anesthesiology 88:7-17, 1998.
95. Monk TG, Saini V, Weldon BC, Sigl JC: Anesthetic management and one-year mortality after noncardiac surgery. Anesth Analg 100:4-10, 2005.
96. Saklad M: Grading of patients for surgical procedures. Anesthesiology 62:206, 1941.
97. Keats AS: The ASA classification of physical status—a recapitulation. Anesthesiology 49:233, 1978.
98. Vacanti CJ, VanHouten RJ, Hill RC: A statistical analysis of the relationship of physical status to postoperative mortality in 68,388 cases. Anesth Analg 49:564-566, 1970.
99. Cohen MM, Duncan PG, Tate RB: Does anesthesia contribute to operative mortality? JAMA 260:2859-2863, 1988.
100. Owens WD, Felts JA, Spitznagel J, et al: ASA physical status classifications. Anesthesiology 49:239-243, 1978.
101. Zeldin RA: Assessing cardiac risk in patients who undergo noncardiac surgical procedures. Can J Surg 27:402, 1984.
102. Larsen SF, Olesen KH, Jacobsen E, et al: Prediction of cardiac risk in non-cardiac surgery. Eur Heart J 8:179-185, 1987.
103. Domaingue CM, Davies MJ, Cronin KD: Cardiovascular risk factors in patients for vascular surgery. Anaesth Intensive Care 10:324-327, 1982.
104. Jeffrey CC, Kunsman J, Cullen DJ, Brewster DC: A prospective evaluation of cardiac risk index. Anesthesiology 58:462-464, 1983.
105. White GH, Advani SM, Williams RA, Wilson SE: Cardiac risk index as a predictor of long-term survival after repair of abdominal aortic aneurysm. Am J Surg 156:103-107, 1988.
106. Lette J, Waters D, Lassonde J, et al: Postoperative myocardial infarction and cardiac death. Predictive value of dipyridamole-thallium imaging and five clinical scoring systems based on multifactorial analysis. Ann Surg 211:84-90, 1990.
107. McEnroe CS, O'Donnell TF, Yeager A, et al: Comparison of ejection fraction and Goldman risk factor analysis to dipyridamole-thallium imaging 201 studies in the evaluation of cardiac morbidity after aortic aneurysm surgery. J Vasc Surg 11:497-504, 1990.
108. Prause G, Ratzenhofer-Comenda B, Pierer G, et al: Can ASA grade or Goldman's cardiac risk index predict peri-operative mortality? A study of 16,227 patients. Anaesthesia 52:203-206, 1997.
109. Detsky A, Abrams H, McLaughlin J, et al: Predicting cardiac complications in patients undergoing non-cardiac surgery. J Gen Intern Med 1:211-219, 1986.
110. Palda VA, Detsky AS: Perioperative assessment and management of risk from coronary artery disease. Ann Intern Med 127:313-328, 1997.
111. Lee TH, Marcantonio ER, Mangione CM, et al: Derivation and prospective validation of a simple index for prediction of cardiac risk of major noncardiac surgery. Circulation 100:1043-1049, 1999.
112. Hannan EL, Kilburn H Jr, O'Donnell JF, et al: Adult open heart surgery in New York State. An analysis of risk factors and hospital mortality rates. JAMA 264:2768-2774, 1990.
113. Hannan EL, Kumar D, Racz M, et al: New York State's Cardiac Surgery Reporting System: Four years later. Ann Thorac Surg 58:1852-1857, 1994.
114. Hannan EL, Stone CC, Biddle TL, DeBuono BA: Public release of cardiac surgery outcomes data in New York: What do New York state cardiologists think of it? [corrected and republished article originally printed in Am Heart J 1997 Jul;134(1):55-61]. Am Heart J 134:1120-1128, 1997.
115. Vanzetto G, Machecourt J, Blendea D, et al: Additive value of thallium single-photon emission computed tomography myocardial imaging for prediction of perioperative events in clinically selected high cardiac risk patients having abdominal aortic surgery. Am J Cardiol 77:143-148, 1996.
116. Goldman L, Caldera DL: Risks of general anesthesia and elective operation in the hypertensive patient. Anesthesiology 50:285-292, 1979.
117. Hollenberg M, Mangano DT, Browner WS, et al: Predictors of postoperative myocardial ischemia in patients undergoing noncardiac surgery. The Study of Perioperative Ischemia Research. JAMA 268:205-209, 1992.
118. Fleisher LA, Beckman JA, Brown KA, et al: ACC/AHA 2007 Guidelines on perioperative cardiovascular evaluation and care for noncardiac surgery: Executive summary. A report of the American College of Cardiology/American Heart Association

Task Force on Practice Guidelines (Writing Committee to Revise the 2002 Guidelines on Perioperative Cardiovascular Evaluation for Noncardiac Surgery). Circulation 116:1971-1996, 2007.

119. Kaunitz AM, Hughes JM, Grimes DA, et al: Causes of maternal mortality in the United States. Obstet Gynecol 65:605-612, 1985.

120. Endler GC, Mariona FG, Sokol RJ, Stevenson LB: Anesthesia-related maternal mortality in Michigan, 1972 to 1984. Am J Obstet Gynecol 159:187-193, 1988.

121. Rochat RW, Koonin LM, Atrash HK, Jewett JF: Maternal mortality in the United States: Report from the Maternal Mortality Collaborative. Obstet Gynecol 72:91-97, 1988.

122. Morgan M: Anaesthetic contribution to maternal mortality. Br J Anaesth 59:842-855, 1987.

123. Chadwick HS, Posner K, Caplan RA, et al: A comparison of obstetric and nonobstetric anesthesia malpractice claims. Anesthesiology 74:242-249, 1991.

124. Hawkins JL, Koonin LM, Palmer SK, Gibbs CP: Anesthesia-related deaths during obstetric delivery in the United States, 1979-1990. Anesthesiology 86:277-284, 1997.

125. Panchal S, Arria AM, Labhsetwar SA: Maternal mortality during hospital admission for delivery: A retrospective analysis using a state-maintained database. Anesth Analg 93:134-141, 2001.

126. Gibbs CP, Krischer J, Peckham BM, et al: Obstetric anesthesia: A national survey. Anesthesiology 65:298-306, 1986.

127. Hawkins JL, Gibbs CP, Orleans M, et al: Obstetric anesthesia work force survey, 1981 versus 1992. Anesthesiology 87:135-143, 1997.

128. Mhyre JM, Riesner MN, Polley LS, Naughton NN: A series of anesthesia-related maternal deaths in Michigan, 1985-2003. Anesthesiology 106:1096-1104, 2007.

129. Bloom SL, Spong CY, Weiner SJ, et al: Complications of anesthesia for cesarean delivery. Obstet Gynecol 106:281-287, 2005.

130. Graff TD, Phillips OC, Benson DW, Kelley G: Baltimore Anesthesia Study Committee: Factors in pediatric anesthesia mortality. Anesth Analg 43:407, 1964.

131. Tiret L, Nivoche Y, Hatton F, et al: Complications related to anaesthesia in infants and children. A prospective survey of 40240 anaesthetics. Br J Anaesth 61:263-269, 1988.

132. Cohen MM, Cameron CB, Duncan PG: Pediatric anesthesia morbidity and mortality in the perioperative period. Anesth Analg 70:160-167, 1990.

132a. Flick RP, Sprung J, Harrison TE, et al: Perioperative cardiac arrests in children between 1988 and 2005 at a tertiary referral center: A study of 92,881 patients. Anesthesiology 106:226-237, 2007.

133. Odegard KC, DiNardo JA, Kussman BD, et al: The frequency of anesthesia-related cardiac arrests in patients with congenital heart disease undergoing cardiac surgery. Anesth Analg 105:335-343, 2007.

134. Morray JP, Geiduschek JM, Ramamoorthy C, et al: Anesthesia-related cardiac arrest in children: Initial findings of the Pediatric Perioperative Cardiac Arrest (POCA) Registry. Anesthesiology 93:6-14, 2000.

135. Bhananker SM, Ramamoorthy C, Geiduschek JM, et al: Anesthesia-related cardiac arrest in children: Update from the Pediatric Perioperative Cardiac Arrest Registry. Anesth Analg 105:344-350, 2007.

136. Denney JL, Denson JS: Risk of surgery in patients over 90. Geriatrics 27:115-118, 1972.

137. Djokovic JL, Hedley-Whyte J: Prediction of outcome of surgery and anesthesia in patients over 80. JAMA 242:2301-2306, 1979.

138. Del Guercio LR, Cohn JD: Monitoring operative risk in the elderly. JAMA 243:1350-1355, 1980.

139. Subcommittee of the National Halothane Study of the Committee on Anesthesia, National Academy of Sciences, National Research Council: Summary of the National Halothane Study: Possible association between halothane anesthesia and postoperative hepatic necrosis. JAMA 197:775, 1966.

140. Aach R: Halothane and liver failure. JAMA 211:2145-2147, 1970.

141. DeBacker LJ, Longnecker DS: Prospective and retrospective searches for liver necrosis following halothane anesthesia. Serum enzyme study and case report. JAMA 195:157-160, 1966.

142. Levine MF, Sarner J, Lerman J, et al: Plasma inorganic fluoride concentrations after sevoflurane anesthesia in children. Anesthesiology 84:348-353, 1996.

143. Nishiyama T, Aibiki M, Hanaoka K: Inorganic fluoride kinetics and renal tubular function after sevoflurane anesthesia in chronic renal failure patients receiving hemodialysis. Anesth Analg 83:574-577, 1996.

144. Conzen PF, Nuscheler M, Melotte A, et al: Renal function and serum fluoride concentrations in patients with stable renal insufficiency after anesthesia with sevoflurane or enflurane. Anesth Analg 81:569-575, 1995.

145. Rooke GA, Ebert T, Muzi M, Kharasch ED: The hemodynamic and renal effects of sevoflurane and isoflurane in patients with coronary artery disease and chronic hypertension. Sevoflurane Ischemia Study Group. Anesth Analg 82:1159-1165, 1996.

146. Becker LC: Is isoflurane dangerous for the patient with coronary artery disease? [editorial]. Anesthesiology 66:259-261, 1987.

147. Buffington CW, Romson JL, Levine A, et al: Isoflurane induces coronary steal in a canine model of chronic coronary occlusion. Anesthesiology 66:280-292, 1987.

148. Leung JM, Goehner P, O'Kelly BF, et al: Isoflurane anesthesia and myocardial ischemia: Comparative risk versus sufentanil anesthesia in patients undergoing coronary artery bypass graft surgery. The SPI (Study of Perioperative Ischemia) Research Group. Anesthesiology 74:838-847, 1991.

149. Leung JM, Hollenberg M, O'Kelly BF, et al: Effects of steal-prone anatomy on intraoperative myocardial ischemia. The SPI Research Group. J Am Coll Cardiol 20:1205-1212, 1992.

150. Slogoff S, Keats AS: Randomized trial of primary anesthetic agents on outcome of coronary artery bypass operations. Anesthesiology 70:179-188, 1989.

151. Slogoff S, Keats AS, Dear WE, et al: Steal-prone coronary anatomy and myocardial ischemia associated with four primary anesthetic agents in humans. Anesth Analg 72:22-27, 1991.

152. Rodgers A, Walker N, Schug S, et al: Reduction of postoperative mortality and morbidity with epidural or spinal anaesthesia: Results from overview of randomised trials. BMJ 321:1493, 2000.

153. Bode RH Jr, Lewis KP, Zarich SW, et al: Cardiac outcome after peripheral vascular surgery. Comparison of general and regional anesthesia. Anesthesiology 84:3-13, 1996.

154. Tuman KJ, McCarthy FJ, Spiess BD: Epidural anaesthesia and analgesia decreases postoperative hypercoagulability in high-risk vascular patients. Anesth Analg 70:S414, 1990.

155. Krupski WC, Layug EL, Reilly LM, et al: Comparison of cardiac morbidity between aortic and infrainguinal operations. Study of Perioperative Ischemia (SPI) Research Group. J Vasc Surg 15:354-363, 1992.

156. L'Italien GL, Cambria RP, Cutler BS, et al: Comparative early and late cardiac morbidity among patients requiring different vascular surgery procedures. J Vasc Surg 21:935-944, 1995.

157. Ashton CM, Petersen NJ, Wray NP, et al: The incidence of perioperative myocardial infarction in men undergoing noncardiac surgery. Ann Intern Med 118:504-510, 1993.

158. Ashton CM, Lahart CJ, Wray NP: The incidence of perioperative myocardial infarction with transurethral resection of the prostate. J Am Geriatr Soc 37:614-618, 1989.

159. Backer CL, Tinker JH, Robertson DM, Vlietstra RE: Myocardial reinfarction following local anesthesia for ophthalmic surgery. Anesth Analg 59:257-262, 1980.

160. Schein OD, Katz J, Bass EB, et al: The value of routine preoperative medical testing before cataract surgery. Study of Medical Testing for Cataract Surgery. N Engl J Med 342:168-175, 2000.

161. Warner MA, Shields SE, Chute CG: Major morbidity and mortality within 1 month of ambulatory surgery and anesthesia. JAMA 270:1437-1441, 1993.

162. Eagle KA, Rihal CS, Mickel MC, et al: Cardiac risk of noncardiac surgery: Influence of coronary disease and type of surgery in 3368 operations. CASS Investigators and University of Michigan Heart Care Program. Coronary Artery Surgery Study. Circulation 96:1882-1887, 1997.

163. Fleisher LA, Beckman JA, Brown KA, et al: ACC/AHA 2007 guidelines on perioperative cardiovascular evaluation and care for noncardiac surgery: A report of the American College of Cardiology/American Heart Association Task Force on Practice Guidelines (Writing Committee to Revise the 2002 Guidelines on Perioperative Cardiovascular Evaluation for Noncardiac Surgery) developed in collaboration with the American Society of Echocardiography, American Society of Nuclear Cardiology, Heart Rhythm Society, Society of Cardiovascular Anesthesiologists, Society for Cardiovascular Angiography and Interventions, Society for Vascular Medicine and Biology, and Society for Vascular Surgery. J Am Coll Cardiol 50:e159-e241, 2007.

164. Birkmeyer JD, Siewers AE, Finlayson EV, et al: Hospital volume and surgical mortality in the United States. N Engl J Med 346:1128-1137, 2002.

165. Kantonen I, Lepantalo M, Salenius JP, et al: Mortality in abdominal aortic aneurysm surgery—the effect of hospital volume, patient mix and surgeon's case load. Eur J Vasc Endovasc Surg 14:375-379, 1997.

166. Slogoff S, Keats AS: Does perioperative myocardial ischemia lead to postoperative myocardial infarction? Anesthesiology 62:107-114, 1985.

167. Birkmeyer JD, Stukel TA, Siewers AE, et al: Surgeon volume and operative mortality in the United States. N Engl J Med 349:2117-2127, 2003.

168. Arbous MS, Meursing AE, van Kleef JW, et al: Impact of anesthesia management characteristics on severe morbidity and mortality. Anesthesiology 102:257-268 quiz 491-492, 2005.

169. Bechtoldt AA: Committee on anesthesia study. Anesthetic-related deaths: 1969-1976. N C Med J 42:253-259, 1981.

170. Forrest WH: Outcome—the effect of the provider. *In* Hirsh RA, Forrest WH (eds): Health Care Delivery in Anesthesia. Philadelphia, George F Stickley, 1980, pp 137-142.

171. Silber JH: Anesthesiologist direction and patient outcomes. LDI Issue Brief 6:1-4, 2000.

172. Fleisher LA, Barash PG: Governmental databases, hospital information systems, and clinical outcomes: Big brother or big help? [editorial]. Anesth Analg 89:811-813, 1999.
173. Silber JH, Kennedy SK, Even-Shoshan O, et al: Anesthesiologist board certification and patient outcomes. Anesthesiology 96:1044-1052, 2002.
174. Pine M, Holt KD, Lou YB: Surgical mortality and type of anesthesia provider. AANA J 71:109-116, 2003.
175. Smith AF, Kane M, Milne R: Comparative effectiveness and safety of physician and nurse anaesthetists: A narrative systematic review. Br J Anaesth 93:540-545, 2004.
176. Brown RH, Schauble JF, Hamilton RG: Prevalence of latex allergy among anesthesiologists: Identification of sensitized but asymptomatic individuals. Anesthesiology 89:292-299, 1998.
177. Berry AJ, Greene ES: The risk of needlestick injuries and needlestick-transmitted diseases in the practice of anesthesiology. Anesthesiology 77:1007-1021, 1992.
178. Berry AJ, Isaacson IJ, Hunt D, Kane MA: The prevalence of hepatitis B viral markers in anesthesia personnel. Anesthesiology 60:6-9, 1984.
179. Berry AJ, Isaacson IJ, Kane MA, et al: A multicenter study of the prevalence of hepatitis B viral serologic markers in anesthesia personnel. Anesth Analg 63:738-742, 1984.
180. Denes AE, Smith JL, Maynard JE, et al: Hepatitis B infection in physicians. Results of a nationwide seroepidemiologic survey. JAMA 239:210-212, 1978.
181. Henderson DK: HIV-1 in the health care setting. *In* Mandell GL, Douglas RG, Bennett JE (eds): Principles and Practice of Infectious Disease, 3rd ed. New York, Churchill Livingstone, 1990, pp 2221-2236.
182. Kiyosawa K, Sodeyama T, Tanaka E, et al: Hepatitis C in hospital employees with needlestick injuries. Ann Intern Med 115:367-369, 1991.
183. Marcus R: CDC Cooperative Needlestick Surveillance Group: Surveillance on health care workers exposed to blood from patients infected with the human immunodeficiency virus. N Engl J Med 319:1118-1123, 1988.
184. Busby J: Through the valley of many shadows: HIV infected physicians. Tex Med 87:36-46, 1991.
185. Greene ES, Berry AJ, Arnold WP 3rd, Jagger J: Percutaneous injuries in anesthesia personnel. Anesth Analg 83:273-278, 1996.
186. Buergler JM, Kim R, Thisted RA, et al: Risk of human immunodeficiency virus in surgeons, anesthesiologists, and medical students. Anesth Analg 75:118-124, 1992.
187. Practice guidelines for management of the difficult airway: An updated report by the American Society of Anesthesiologists Task Force on Management of the Difficult Airway. Anesthesiology 98:1269-1277, 2003.
188. Practice guidelines for pulmonary artery catheterization: An updated report by the American Society of Anesthesiologists Task Force on Pulmonary Artery Catheterization. Anesthesiology 99:988-1014, 2003.
189. Practice guidelines for perioperative blood transfusion and adjuvant therapies: An updated report by the American Society of Anesthesiologists Task Force on Perioperative Blood Transfusion and Adjuvant Therapies. Anesthesiology 105:198-208, 2006.
190. Gaba DM, Maxwell M, DeAnda A: Anesthetic mishaps: Breaking the chain of accident evolution. Anesthesiology 66:670-676, 1987.
191. Holzman RS, Cooper JB, Gaba DM, et al: Anesthesia crisis resource management: Real-life simulation training in operating room crises. J Clin Anesth 7:675-687, 1995.
192. Howard SK, Gaba DM, Fish KJ, et al: Anesthesia crisis resource management training: Teaching anesthesiologists to handle critical incidents. Aviat Space Environ Med 63:763-770, 1992.
193. Popp HJ, Schecke T, Rau G, et al: An interactive computer simulator of the circulation for knowledge acquisition in cardio-anesthesia. Int J Clin Monit Comput 8:151-158, 1991.
194. Schwid HA, O'Donnell D: Anesthesiologists' management of simulated critical incidents. Anesthesiology 76:495-501, 1992.
195. Hopkins PM: Malignant hyperthermia: Advances in clinical management and diagnosis. Br J Anaesth 85:118-128, 2000.
196. Tardiff BE, Newman MF, Saunders AM, et al: Preliminary report of a genetic basis for cognitive decline after cardiac operations. The Neurologic Outcome Research Group of the Duke Heart Center. Ann Thorac Surg 64:715-720, 1997.

Stephen P. Fischer, Angela M. Bader, and BobbieJean Sweitzer

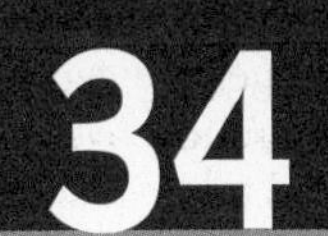

34 Preoperative Evaluation

Key Points

1. The anesthesia preoperative evaluation is the clinical foundation and framework of perioperative patient management and can potentially reduce operative morbidity and enhance patient outcomes.
2. The fundamental purpose of preoperative evaluation is to obtain pertinent information regarding the patient's current and past medical history and to formulate an assessment of the patient's intraoperative risk and requisite clinical optimization.
3. Basic and complex medical diseases and syndromes that can potentially affect anesthesia perioperative management require the anesthesiologist to be clinically knowledgeable and current in many aspects of internal medicine.
4. Patients require preoperative diagnostic and laboratory studies that are consistent with their medical history, the proposed surgical procedure, and the potential for intraoperative blood loss. Routine preoperative testing cannot be justified and is costly and clinically inappropriate.
5. Preoperative patient education and individual discussion can significantly reduce patient anxiety and fears of the perioperative anesthesia process.
6. Under the clinical directorship of an anesthesiologist, the anesthesia preoperative evaluation clinic can enhance operating room efficiency, decrease day-of-surgery cancellations and delays, reduce hospital costs, and enhance the quality of patient care.
7. New and updated preoperative evaluation consensus and evidence-based guidelines published by multiple medical specialties have led to evaluation protocols for preparing patients for anesthesia and surgery.
8. Increasing regulatory and reporting requirements involving preoperative issues by agencies such as the Joint Commission on Accreditation of Healthcare Organizations require awareness and compliance by anesthesiologists.
9. Information technology and decision support systems in preoperative evaluation can enhance the quality of patient care and clinical management through electronic integration and standardization of patient data.
10. The anesthesiologist is the perioperative medical specialist and the only preoperative evaluation physician who can truly evaluate the risks associated with anesthesia, discuss these risks with the patient, and manage them intraoperatively.

Virtually every practicing anesthesiologist has experienced and contributed to the evolution of anesthesia's involvement in perioperative care. Furthermore, the rapid transformation from admission of the patient to the hospital the night before surgery to the morning of surgery has necessitated that preoperative evaluation be conducted in a different manner. Although the historical basic concept of preoperative evaluation and an anesthesia clinic is not new to anesthesia, what has occurred in this specialty is unique, remarkable, and revolutionary. Many anesthesiologists have essentially taken back from multiple medical specialties the primary responsibility, coordination, and recognition for assessment and optimization of preoperative risk in patients being prepared for surgery.

Some anesthesiologists have evolved into perioperative medical specialists by demonstrating their unique qualification of focused knowledge and experience to evaluate and successfully manage medical complexities related to anesthesia and surgery.[1,2] Anesthesia care is no longer limited to the operating room. Many departments of anesthesiology have even changed their official departmental titles to include anesthesia and "perioperative care."

This chapter on preoperative evaluation is intended to provide the reader with a comprehensive discussion of the basics and fundamental practice of preoperative assessment, as well as provide a review of new concepts, regulatory requirements, consensus guidelines, medical-legal responsibilities, and clinical options.

The Evolution in Preoperative Evaluation

Preoperative evaluation of a surgical patient for anesthesia increases the practitioner's awareness of the patient's medical condition and becomes the foundation of the individual patient's perioperative management plan. The fundamental purpose in preoperative evaluation is to obtain pertinent information regarding the patient's current and past medical history and to formulate an assessment of the patient's intraoperative risk.

Anesthesiologists preoperatively perform focused clinical examinations, develop a plan of medical intervention and optimization, reduce the patient's (and family's) anxiety and fears through education, discuss perioperative care and options for postoperative pain control, determine the appropriate laboratory tests and diagnostic studies to perform, discuss anesthesia risks, and obtain informed consent. The anesthesia preoperative evaluation can decrease surgical morbidity, minimize expensive delays and cancellations on the day of surgery, and increase perioperative efficiency. The practice of preoperative evaluation for anesthesia has changed. Fewer patients are admitted to the hospital before surgery unless their medical condition is unstable and requires optimization. Currently, approximately 80% of surgeries in the United States are performed on an outpatient or same-day admission basis, even including major neurosurgical, cardiac, and radical cancer procedures. The previous process of admitting the majority of patients to the hospital at least the day before is no longer financially supported or justified.

Although patients are still assessed for the first time by the anesthesiologist just before surgery, the trend toward preparing and evaluating patients in a preoperative program or "clinic" before the surgical date has increased. This has been especially important in patients with multiple medical risks and comorbid conditions. In other settings, the preoperative evaluation is completed for many patients by the surgeon (or designee) or primary care physician, and only patients at highest risk are referred for consultation by an anesthesiologist. In such circumstances, the anesthesia department must interact with the surgical departments to establish general protocols for acquiring the information needed to safely perform anesthesia or there could be a potential for an increased incidence of delays or cancellations at the time of surgery to obtain additional information or evaluation.

A change in the procedure and manner of preoperative evaluation requires the anesthesiologist to achieve a high level of efficiency and accuracy in assessment of the patient's history, physical examination, differential diagnosis, and planning of management. It presents the anesthesiologist with a formidable challenge from both an organizational and a clinical perspective because of a decreased amount of time available to evaluate often medically complex patients. Providing consistent quality and cost-effective preoperative preparation of patients is an important issue in perioperative patient management.

Both The Joint Commission (TJC) and the American Society of Anesthesiologists (ASA) have developed standards and requirements for preoperative anesthesia evaluation.[3] Recent and updated preoperative evaluation guidelines published by multiple medical specialties have led to protocols for evaluation in preparing patients for anesthesia and surgery. Several of the current practice guidelines challenge the historical manner of practicing anesthesia.

These guidelines require objective review, reasonable consideration, and possibly changes in the manner of customary anesthesia practice.[4] For example, the routine "nothing by mouth" (NPO) after midnight or 6 hours before surgery has been redefined by the ASA Task Force on Preoperative Fasting.[5] The American College of Cardiologists/American Heart Association (ACC/AHA) preoperative evaluation guidelines, recently updated in 2007, recommend proceeding with elective surgery in certain patients who have experienced a myocardial infarction (MI) in terms of weeks rather than months. Both these and other changes and challenges in anesthesia practice are reviewed and the implications discussed in this chapter.

If anesthesia and surgery were not associated with perioperative risk or adverse patient outcome, anesthesia preoperative evaluation and management would not be required. Although the incidence of patient morbidity and mortality has decreased in the past decades, many patients still have an abundance of fear and anxiety regarding anesthesia risk. We begin this preoperative chapter with a current review and identification of the concepts, evaluation, and goals in assessment of patient risk.

Preoperative Risk Assessment

The current ASA risk classification system was developed in 1941 by Meyer Saklad at the request of the ASA (Table 34-1). This classification was the first attempt to quantify the risk associated with anesthesia and surgery. Neither the type of anesthesia nor the location of the procedure or operation was considered in the development or as components of this risk classification. The system attempts to give a subjective and relative risk based only on the patient's preoperative medical history (i.e., no consideration of diagnostic studies). ASA physical status (ASA-PS) 2

Table 34-1 American Society of Anesthesiologists Physical Status Classification

ASA 1	Healthy patient without organic, biochemical, or psychiatric disease
ASA 2	A patient with mild systemic disease, e.g., mild asthma or well-controlled hypertension. No significant impact on daily activity. Unlikely to have an impact on anesthesia and surgery
ASA 3	Significant or severe systemic disease that limits normal activity, e.g., renal failure on dialysis or class 2 congestive heart failure. Significant impact on daily activity. Probable impact on anesthesia and surgery
ASA 4	Severe disease that is a constant threat to life or requires intensive therapy, e.g., acute myocardial infarction, respiratory failure requiring mechanical ventilation. Serious limitation of daily activity. Major impact on anesthesia and surgery
ASA 5	Moribund patient who is equally likely to die in the next 24 hours with or without surgery
ASA 6	Brain-dead organ donor

"E" added to the classification indicates emergency surgery.
Available from www.asahq.org.

patients are at higher risk than ASA-PS 1 patients, but only if undergoing the *same* operation. Most importantly, there is no attempt to *quantify* the risk, which hampers the ability to use this risk assessment tool for communicating meaningful expectations to patients and other caregivers.

Despite these limitations, some studies have corroborated an association of mortality and morbidity with ASA-PS scores. Studies have also shown a correlation between ASA-PS and unanticipated intensive care unit admissions, longer hospital stays for some procedures, and adverse cardiopulmonary outcomes. No correlation has been shown between ASA-PS class and cancellations, cost, unplanned admissions, and other perioperative complications, and traditionally, surgical risk has been considered more important than anesthetic risk. However, few studies have evaluated the effect of combining the risk inherent in the surgical procedure and the ASA-PS score. Among the first was the Johns Hopkins Risk Classification System, but this system focuses only on surgical risk. As surgery has evolved with innovations in minimally invasive and endoscopic techniques, a general anesthetic requiring instrumentation of the airway with associated significant physiologic perturbations may pose a significant and greater risk than the surgery itself to some extremely fragile individuals.

Even the location of the procedure may alter the risk. A study of ambulatory surgery in Medicare beneficiaries older than 65 years found no deaths on the day of surgery when the procedure was performed in a physician's office; 2.3 deaths per 100,000 performed in a freestanding ambulatory surgical center; and 2.5 deaths per 100,000 performed at an outpatient hospital. The 7-day mortality was 35 per 100,000, 25 per 100,000, and 50 per 100,000, respectively. Age older than 85 years, significant comorbidity, and the type of procedure predicted adverse events.[6]

Other specialties have developed risk assessment tools for patients undergoing anesthesia and surgery. One of the first was Goldman, who further advanced risk assessment by identifying risk factors and cardiac complications in patients undergoing noncardiac surgery. Several studies followed, culminating in one of the most widely used guidelines for assessment of the common, significant perioperative complication of cardiac morbidity and mortality associated with noncardiac surgery. The joint ACC/AHA guideline was first published in 1996 and updated in 2007.[7] This guideline combines patient and surgical risk but is specific only for cardiac complications. There is no comprehensive risk assessment tool available at the time of this writing.

The concept of risk associated with anesthesia (see Chapter 33) is unique in that rarely does the anesthetic itself offer benefit but merely allows others to do things that potentially offer benefit. The goals in assessing risk are to inform patients so that they can weigh their options and to identify opportunities to alter that risk. Analysis of the Australian Incident Monitoring Study (AIMS) database showed that 11.6% of reports identified inadequate or incorrect preoperative *assessment* (478 of 6271) or preoperative *preparation* (248/6271).[8] Of adverse events, 3.1% (197) were indisputably related to inadequate or incorrect preoperative assessment or preparation. Of these 197 patients, major morbidity occurred in 23, and 7 patients died. The investigators concluded that patient factors contributed only 1% of the time. More than half of the incidents were preventable; an additional 21% were possibly preventable. Unpreventable events accounted for just 5% of cases. Almost a quarter of the time, communication failure was cited as the most significant factor. Analysis of the first 2000 reports submitted to AIMS found a sixfold increase in mortality in patients who were inadequately assessed preoperatively.[9] In a different study of anesthetic-related perioperative deaths, 53 of 135 deaths involved inadequate preoperative assessment and management.

Many anesthesiologists perform preoperative evaluations, review diagnostic studies (chosen and ordered by someone else), discuss anesthetic risks, and obtain informed consent moments before patients undergo major, potentially life-threatening or disfiguring procedures. This choice offers little opportunity to optimize comorbid conditions or alter risk. The effects of extensive disclosure are stressful for patients and families at a time when they may be ill prepared to consider the implications rationally. An increase in preoperative anxiety probably affects postoperative outcomes because increased anxiety correlates with increased postoperative analgesic requirements and prolonged recovery and hospital stay. Anxiety impairs retention of information, with attendant medicolegal implications because of inadequate communication or discussion of the risks associated with anesthesia.

Some assessment of risk is important to prepare for anesthesia and the surgical procedure. Patients have a right to be informed during the consent process of possible complications and, if possible, be given some estimate of the chance of complications occurring. Identified modifiable risk factors such as poorly controlled hypertension or unstable ischemic heart disease should be addressed. Risk assessment is useful to compare outcomes, control costs, allocate compensation, postpone surgery until interventions improve risk, or assist in the difficult decision of canceling or recommending that a procedure not be done when the risks are too high. The need for special techniques, postoperative care in the intensive care unit, and special monitoring must be considered and planned for. Yet risk assessment, at its best, is hampered by individual patient variability.

Detecting Disease in Preoperative Evaluation

Several studies have proved the utility of the history and physical examination in determining diagnoses. A study of general medical clinic patients found that 56% of correct diagnoses were made with the history alone, which increased to 73% with the addition of physical examination. In patients with cardiovascular disease, the history establishes the diagnosis two thirds of the time, and physical examination contributes to a quarter of diagnoses. Diagnostic tests such as chest radiographs and electrocardiograms (ECGs) helped with only 3% of diagnoses, and special tests (e.g., exercise ECG) assisted with 6%. In patients with respiratory, urinary, and neurologic conditions, the history has also been shown to be the most important diagnostic method. The skill of performing a clinical examination derives from pattern recognition learned by listening to and seeing patients and assimilating the stories and outcomes of their illnesses. The diagnostic acumen of the physician is a result of the ability to integrate and develop an overall impression rather than just reviewing a compilation of facts.

Importance of the Preoperative Medical History

The variability of the medical history and the words that both patients and physicians use to describe symptoms is a common problem. Using lay language and recording symptoms in ordinary words leads to greater interobserver agreement between practitioners and can lessen communication errors, which are common obstacles in medical care. Common errors occur when diagnostic labels such as "angina" are written in the record when the patient actually complained of "chest pain." Conversely, true angina or cardiac ischemia/infarction is rarely described by a patient as chest *pain*. More likely, the patient will have complaints of tightness or squeezing, often in the upper part of the abdomen, shoulder, or neck. Therefore, medical interviewers should not be surprised that patients may deny ever having chest *pain* if this is the only noun used when inquiring about symptoms to elicit a history, thus missing a history of angina. Obtaining the patient's history is not simply asking questions but asking the right questions, frequently in a variety of ways, and interpreting and carefully recording the answers. Complete and thorough histories assist in planning appropriate and safe anesthesia care and are more accurate and cost-effective in establishing diagnoses than screening laboratory tests are.

Components of the Preoperative Medical History

The important components of the anesthesia history are shown in Figure 34-1. The form can be completed by the patient in person (paper or electronic version), via Web-based programs, through a telephone interview, or by anesthesia staff.

The classic "history of present illness, or HPI," as it relates to evaluation for anesthesia starts with the reason that the patient is having surgery and the planned procedure. Often one needs to inquire further about how the surgical condition developed and any previous therapies related to this problem. Current and past medical problems, previous surgeries and types of anesthesia, and any anesthesia-related complications need to be noted. Rarely is simply a notation of diseases or symptoms such as hypertension, diabetes mellitus, coronary artery disease (CAD), shortness of breath, or chest pain sufficient. Equally important in identifying the presence of a disease is to establish the severity, current or recent exacerbations, the stability, and previous treatment of the condition or planned interventions. The extent, degree of control, and activity-limiting nature of the problems are equally important. The patient's medical problems, previous surgeries, and response to questions will elicit further inquiry to establish a complete history.

Prescription and over-the-counter medications, including supplements and herbals, should be carefully recorded, along with dosages and schedules. Any recent but currently interrupted medications should be included because this may lead to recognition of important issues. It is necessary to inquire about allergies to drugs and substances such as latex or radiographic dye, with special emphasis on the specifics of the patient's response to the exposure. Frequently, patients claim an allergy to a substance when in reality the reaction was a common, expected side effect (e.g., nausea or vomiting with narcotics). Use of tobacco, alcohol, or illicit drugs should be documented. Quantitatively documenting tobacco exposure by pack-years (number of packs of cigarettes smoked per day times the number of years of smoking) is best. For example, if one has smoked two packs of cigarettes daily for the last 10 years, this is recorded as 20 pack/years of tobacco use.

A history of malignant hyperthermia (MH) or a suggestion of it (hyperthermia or rigidity during anesthesia) in either a patient or family member should be clearly documented to allow appropriate arrangements to be made before the day of surgery. A personal or family history of pseudocholinesterase deficiency should be identified preoperatively. Records from previous anesthesia may clarify an uncertain history.

A screening review of systems is especially useful to uncover symptoms that may lead to the establishment of previously undiagnosed conditions. During the review of systems for anesthesia purposes, special emphasis needs to be placed on airway abnormalities; a personal or family history of adverse events related to anesthesia; and cardiovascular, pulmonary, hepatic, renal, endocrine, or neurologic symptoms. Questioning the patient about snoring and daytime somnolence may suggest undiagnosed sleep apnea, which has implications for anesthesia management (see the section "Preoperative Evaluation of Patients with Obstructive Sleep Apnea" and Chapter 64). The presence of any two of the following increases the chance that a patient has sleep apnea:

- Snoring
- Daytime sleepiness
- Hypertension
- Obesity

A significant history of heartburn, especially with associated reflux or after a period of fasting comparable to what will occur preoperatively, is important. Women of childbearing age need to be prompted to recall their last normal menstrual period and their likelihood of being pregnant. This history is more reliable if the woman, especially if a minor child, is questioned in privacy.

Determination of the patient's cardiorespiratory fitness or functional capacity is useful in guiding additional preanesthetic evaluation and predicting outcome and perioperative complications.[7,10] Exercise or work activity can be quantified in metabolic equivalents of the task (METs), which refers to a measure of the volume of oxygen consumed during an activity (Table 34-2). One's ability to exercise is two-pronged in that better fitness decreases mortality through improved lipid and glucose profiles and reductions in blood pressure (BP) and obesity. Lack of exercise increases the risk for development of cardiac disease. Conversely, an inability to exercise may be the result of cardiopulmonary disease. Patients with peripheral vascular disease (PVD) will be limited by claudication, and those with ischemic heart disease may complain of shortness of breath or chest discomfort with exertion. Patients may not volunteer this information until asked why they cannot walk more than a certain distance or climb stairs. Several studies have shown that inability to perform average levels of exercise (4 to 5 METs) identifies patients at risk for perioperative complications (see Table 34-2).[7]

One should inquire about chest discomfort (pain, pressure, tightness), duration of the discomfort, precipitating factors, associated symptoms, and methods of relief. One should note diagnoses, diagnostic tests, therapies, and names of treating physicians.

Shortness of breath with exertion or when lying flat (orthopnea) or peripheral edema is important to note. Patients are asked about a history of heart murmurs and what diagnostic studies have been performed to evaluate a murmur. The cardinal symptoms of severe aortic stenosis are angina, heart failure, and syncope, although patients are much more likely to complain of a decrease in exercise tolerance and exertional dyspnea.

A general examination of all organ systems needs to be performed. For example, asking patients whether they have ever had problems with their heart, lungs, kidneys, liver, or nervous system, whether they have had cancer, anemia, or bleeding problems, or whether thay have ever been hospitalized for any reason will often prompt recall of medical problems. Similarly, obtaining a complete listing of previous surgeries can help complete the medical history. Finally, a review of records from primary care physicians, specialists, or the hospital can reveal issues that the patient may not recall.

The Preoperative Physical Examination

At a minimum, the preanesthetic examination should include vital signs (e.g., BP, heart rate [HR], respiratory rate, oxygen saturation), height, and weight. Body mass index (BMI) is calculated from height and weight and is more accurate than weight in establishing obesity. Online BMI calculators can be found at

Patient's name________ Age____ Sex____ Date of surgery____

Planned operation ________ Surgeon________

Primary care doctor/phone #________ Other physicians/phone #s________

1. Please list **all operations** (and approximate dates)

a. ____ d. ____
b. ____ e. ____
c. ____ f. ____

2. Please list any **allergies** to medicines, latex or other (and your reactions to them)

a. ____ c. ____
b. ____ d. ____

3. Please list **all medications** you have taken in the last month (include over-the-counter drugs, inhalers, herbals, dietary supplements and aspirin)

	Name of Drug	Dose and How Often		Name of Drug	Dose and How Often
a.			f.		
b.			g.		
c.			h.		
d.			i.		
e.			j.		

(Please check YES or NO and circle specific problems)

	YES	NO
4. Have you taken steroids (prednisone or cortisone) in the last year?	☐	☐
5. Have you *ever* smoked? (Quantify in ____ packs/day for ____ years)	☐	☐
Do you still smoke?	☐	☐
Do you drink alcohol? (If so, how much?) ____	☐	☐
Do you use or have you ever used any illegal drugs? (we need to know for your safety)	☐	☐
6. Can you walk up one flight of stairs without stopping?	☐	☐
7. Have you had any problems with your heart? **(circle)** (chest pain or pressure, heart attack, abnormal ECG, skipped beats, heart murmur, palpitation, heart failure [fluid in the lungs], require antibiotics before routine dental care)	☐	☐
8. Do you have high blood pressure?	☐	☐
9. Have you had any problems with your lungs or your chest? **(circle)** (shortness of breath, emphysema, bronchitis, asthma, TB, abnormal chest x-ray)	☐	☐
10. Are you ill now or were you recently ill with a cold, fever, chills, flu or productive cough? Describe recent changes ____	☐	☐

Figure 34-1 Sample patient preoperative history form.

Continued

(Please check YES or NO and circle specific problems)	YES	NO
11. Have you or anyone in your family had serious bleeding problems? **(circle)** (prolonged bleeding from nosebleed, gums, tooth extractions, or surgery)	☐	☐
12. Have you had any problems with your blood (anemia, leukemia, sickle cell disease, blood clots, transfusions)?	☐	☐
13. Have you ever had problems with your: **(circle)**		
Liver (cirrhosis, hepatitis, jaundice)?	☐	☐
Kidney (stones, failure, dialysis)?	☐	☐
Digestive system (frequent heartburn, hiatus hernia, stomach ulcer)?	☐	☐
Back, neck or jaws (TMJ, rheumatoid arthritis)?	☐	☐
Thyroid gland (underactive or overactive)?	☐	☐
14. Have you ever had: **(circle)**		
Seizures, epilepsy, or fits?	☐	☐
Stroke, facial, leg or arm weakness, difficulty speaking?	☐	☐
Cramping pain in your legs with walking?	☐	☐
Problems with hearing, vision or memory?	☐	☐
15. Have you ever been treated for cancer with chemotherapy or radiation therapy? **(circle)**	☐	☐
16. Women: Could you be pregnant? Last menstrual period began: __________	☐	☐
17. Have you ever had problems with anesthesia or surgery? **(circle)** (severe nausea or vomiting, malignant hyperthermia (in blood relatives or self), prolonged drowsiness, anxiety, breathing difficulties, or problems during placement of a breathing tube)	☐	☐
18. Do you have any chipped or loose teeth, dentures, caps, bridgework, braces, problems opening your mouth, swallowing or choking? **(circle)**	☐	☐
19. Do your physical abilities limit your daily activities?	☐	☐
20. Do you snore?	☐	☐
21. Please list any medical illnesses not noted above:		
22. Additional comments or questions for nurse or anesthesiologist?		

Figure 34-1, cont'd

http://www.cdc.gov/nccdphp/dnpa/bmi/index.htm or http://www.nhlbisupport.com/bmi/. Formulas for calculating BMI are as follows:

English formula:

$$\text{BMI} = \left(\frac{\text{Weight in pounds}}{(\text{Height in inches}) \times (\text{Height in inches})}\right) \times 703$$

Metric formula:

$$\text{BMI} = \frac{\text{Weight in kilograms}}{(\text{Height in meters}) \times (\text{Height in meters})}$$

or

$$\text{BMI} = \left(\frac{\text{Weight in kilograms}}{(\text{Height in centimeters}) \times (\text{Height in centimeters})}\right) \times 10{,}000$$

A BMI of 40 or greater defines extreme obesity, obesity is defined as a BMI of 30 to 39.9, and an overweight person has a BMI of 25 to 29.9. An increased BMI is predictive of airway difficulties in some studies and one of many factors associated with the development of chronic diseases such as heart disease, cancer, and diabetes.[11]

Table 34-2 Metabolic Equivalents of Functional Capacity

MET	Functional Levels of Exercise
1	Eating, working at a computer, dressing
2	Walking down stairs or in your house, cooking
3	Walking 1-2 blocks
4	Raking leaves, gardening
5	Climbing 1 flight of stairs, dancing, bicycling
6	Playing golf, carrying clubs
7	Playing singles tennis
8	Rapidly climbing stairs, jogging slowly
9	Jumping rope slowly, moderate cycling
10	Swimming quickly, running or jogging briskly
11	Skiing cross country, playing full-court basketball
12	Running rapidly for moderate to long distances

From Jette M, Sidney K, Blumchen G: Metabolic equivalents (METs) in exercise testing, exercise prescription, and evaluation of functional capacity. Clin Cardiol 13:555-565, 1990.
MET, metabolic equivalent of the task. 1 MET = consumption of 3.5 mL O_2/min/kg of body weight.

Not infrequently, patients will have increased BP during the preoperative visit, even without a history of hypertension. This may be due to anxiety or missing doses of drugs because patients often do not take their medications before an appointment or procedure. This reading is probably not reflective of their usual control. Repeating the BP measurement, especially after the administration of anxiolytics if this is planned, obtaining previous readings from either medical records or asking patients what their "usual" BP measurements are, can be informative.

Inspection of the airway may be the single most important component of the physical examination from an anesthesiologist's perspective. Without specialized training in airway evaluation and management, including advanced techniques such as fiberoptic intubation, it is unlikely that nonanesthesiologists will be capable of performing an adequate assessment. See Box 34-1 for components of the airway examination.

All patients should have thorough documentation of an airway examination, whether in a preoperative evaluation clinic or immediately before surgery (see Chapter 50). The Mallampati classification is performed by having patients open the mouth widely and protruding the tongue completely forward. A tongue depressor is not used. In class I, the soft palate, fauces, entire uvula, and pillars are visualized; in class II, the soft palate, fauces, and a portion of the uvula; in class III, the soft palate and base of the uvula; and in class IV, the hard palate only. The evaluation should also document the status of teeth, range of motion of the neck, neck circumference (increasing size predicts difficulty with laryngoscopy), thyromental distance, body habitus, and pertinent deformities.[12] Because of the relatively high incidence of dental injuries during anesthesia, thorough documentation of preexisting tooth abnormalities is useful. A good time to discuss with patients variant options of airway management or techniques other than general anesthesia when applicable and prepare patients for possible awake fiberoptic intubation is after examination of the airway. When challenging airways are identified, advance planning ensures that the necessary equipment and skilled personnel are available.

Evaluation of the heart, lungs, and skin is necessary, as well as further focus on the organ systems involved with disease as reported by the patient. Auscultation of the heart and, when indicated, inspection of the pulses and peripheral and central veins and assessment for the presence of edema in the extremities may aid in developing a perioperative plan. One should auscultate for murmurs, rhythm disturbances, and signs of volume overload. Physical findings should focus on examination for third or fourth heart sounds, rales, jugular venous distention, ascites, hepatomegaly, and edema.

Observing whether the patient can walk up one to two flights of stairs can predict a variety of postoperative complications, including pulmonary and cardiac events and mortality, and aid in decisions regarding the need for further specialized testing such as pulmonary function tests (PFTs) or noninvasive cardiac stress testing.[13] This is frequently not practical, and a report by the patient is often sufficient.

The pulmonary examination should include auscultation for wheezing and decreased or abnormal breath sounds and notation of cyanosis or clubbing, use of accessory muscles, and effort of breathing.

A basic neurologic examination to document deficits in mental status, speech, cranial nerves, gait, and motor and sensory function may be indicated, depending on the surgical procedure and patient's history. For selective patients (e.g., those with deficits or disease or undergoing neurosurgery), a more extensive or focused neurologic examination is necessary to document specific preexisting abnormalities that may aid in diagnosis or interfere with positioning. Establishing a baseline allows comparison postoperatively for evaluation of new deficits and can aid in defense of potential malpractice claims of adverse events.

Obesity, hypertension, and large neck circumference (>17 inches in men, >16 inches in women, or >60 cm in anyone) predict an increased incidence of obstructive sleep apnea (OSA).[14] These same neck measurements also predict difficulty with mask ventilation and intubation. Intravenous access sites should be

Box 34-1 Components of the Airway Examination

- Length of the upper incisors
- Condition of the teeth
- Relationship of the upper (maxillary) incisors to the lower (mandibular) incisors
- Ability to protrude or advance the lower (mandibular) incisors in front of the upper (maxillary) incisors
- Interincisor or intergum (if edentulous) distance
- Tongue size
- Visibility of the uvula
- Presence of heavy facial hair
- Compliance of the mandibular space
- Thyromental distance with the head in maximum extension
- Length of the neck
- Thickness or circumference of the neck
- Range of motion of the head and neck

noted. If this is limited, one should discuss possible central line placement with the patient or arrange for assistance from interventional radiology. Auscultation for bruits is important in patients with a history of head and neck irradiation, stroke, or transient ischemic attack.

Preoperative Evaluation of Patients with Coexisting Disease

Many of these concerns and conditions, including intraoperative and postoperative anesthesia management, are discussed in greater detail in other chapters of this text. This section briefly reviews specific medical conditions that are commonly seen in preoperative evaluation and for which preoperative assessment and intervention are important. Identification of patients with these comorbid conditions often presents an opportunity for the anesthesiologist to intervene to lower risk. The following conditions are best managed before the day of surgery, which allows ample time for thoughtful evaluation, consultation, and planning of anesthesia care.

Cardiovascular Disease

Cardiovascular complications are the most common serious perioperative adverse event (see Chapter 33). It is estimated that cardiac morbidity will occur in 1% to 5% of unselected patients undergoing noncardiac surgery. In specific circumstances, perioperative interventions have been shown to modify cardiovascular morbidity and mortality.[7,15-17]

Hypertension

Hypertension, defined as two or more BP readings greater than 140/90 mm Hg, affects 1 billion individuals worldwide and increases with age. In the United States, 25% of adults and 70% of patients older than 70 years have hypertension, less than 30% are adequately treated, and 30% are undiagnosed. The degree of end-organ damage and morbidity and mortality correlate with the duration and severity of hypertension. Ischemic heart disease is the most common type of organ damage associated with hypertension. Each 20–mm Hg incremental elevation in systolic BP or 10–mm Hg incremental elevation in diastolic BP above 115/75 doubles the lifetime risk for cardiovascular disease in individuals 40 to 70 years of age. The odds ratio for an association between hypertension and perioperative cardiac risk is 1.31.[7,18] However, there is little evidence of an association between a preoperative BP reading of less than 180/110 mm Hg and perioperative cardiac risk. Heart failure, renal insufficiency, and cerebrovascular disease are common in hypertensive patients.

Preoperative evaluation identifies causes of hypertension, other cardiovascular risk factors, end-organ damage, and therapy. Paroxysmal hypertension or hypertension in young individuals should prompt a search for causes such as coarctation, hyperthyroidism, pheochromocytoma, or even illicit drug use such as cocaine, amphetamines, or anabolic steroids. (See the section "Pheochromocytoma" for further evaluation guidelines.) Physical examination focuses on the cardiovascular system, pulses, vital signs (BP needs to be repeated and previous records obtained to establish long-term values), the thyroid gland, and signs of volume overload. Asking about episodic tachycardia, palpitations, and syncope, measuring BP in both arms, listening for bruits, and assessing the pulses in both the upper and lower extremities are necessary if there is concern the patient may have more than essential hypertension. Testing should be determined by the history and physical examination. Patients with long-standing, severe (often based on the number and dosages of prescribed antihypertensive medications), or poorly controlled hypertension need an ECG and determination of blood urea nitrogen (BUN) and creatinine, depending on the surgical procedure. Those taking diuretics should have an evaluation of electrolytes. Patients with significant left ventricular hypertrophy (LVH), especially those with a strain pattern on the ECG, which is indicative of chronic ischemia, should have a careful assessment of symptoms and other risk factors for CAD. In the presence of heart failure or dyspnea of unknown origina, an echocardiogram may provide additional information that will modify management. LVH independently increases the risk for perioperative cardiac morbidity. Patients suspected of having hyperthyroidism require thyroid function tests.

It is generally recommended that elective surgery be delayed for severe hypertension (diastolic BP >115 mm Hg, systolic BP >200 mm Hg) until BP is less than 180/110 mm Hg. If severe end-organ damage is present, the goal should be to normalize BP *as much as possible* before surgery.[18] A careful history and physical examination to determine cardiac, neurologic, or renal disease is important (see appropriate sections of this chapter). Effective lowering of risk may require 6 to 8 weeks of therapy to allow regression of vascular and endothelial changes, but too rapid or extreme lowering of BP may increase cerebral and coronary ischemia; therefore, the benefits of delaying surgery for treatment must be weighed against the risks. The Antihypertensive and Lipid Lowering Treatment to Prevent a Heart Attack Trial (ALLHAT) showed that effective treatment of hypertension is not simply a matter of decreasing BP.[19] Thus, if surgery cannot be postponed, the goal is to not decrease chronically increased BP too rapidly. Severely elevated BP should be lowered over a period of several weeks. Studies suggest that hypotension intraoperatively is far more dangerous than hypertension.[18] For a BP lower than 180/110 mm Hg, there is no evidence to justify cancellation of surgery, although interventions preoperatively are appropriate. It is important to identify patients who have undiagnosed hypertension (although typically three separate occasions of increased BP in nonstressful situations are required to diagnosis true hypertension) and differentiate those who have poorly controlled hypertension from those who have episodic increased BP because of pain, anxiety, or stress.

Because the perioperative period is an excellent opportunity to alter the long- and short-term consequences of diseases, appropriate referral for future management is vital. Guidelines suggest that cardioselective β-blocker therapy is the best treatment preoperatively because of a favorable profile in lowering cardiovascular risk, although the Perioperative Ischemia Evaluation (POISE) trial has recently questioned the safety of starting these agents acutely.[7] The optimal time to start β-blocker therapy to achieve its benefit while minimizing risk is unknown. Even though diuretics are first-line therapies in most circumstances, starting them in the preoperative period is not generally a good idea because of the alterations in potassium (both hypokalemia and hyperkalemia) that may occur and the need for close monitoring and replacement. Calcium channel blockers (e.g., amlodipine, 5 to 10 mg daily) can be very effective. Frequently, anxiety increases BP, and therefore antianxiolytics can be used as adjunctive therapy. BP should not be lowered too rapidly. Continuation of antihypertensive treatment preoperatively is critical.

Ischemic Heart Disease

The goals of preoperative evaluation are to

- Identify the risk for heart disease based on risk factors (Fig. 34-2, Box 34-2)
- Identify the presence and severity of heart disease from symptoms, physical findings, or diagnostic tests
- Determine the need for preoperative interventions
- Modify the risk for perioperative adverse events

The basis of cardiac assessment is the history, physical examination, and ECG. Risk factors for CAD are as important or more important than symptoms of ischemia because CAD is not diagnosed in 40% of men and 65% of women before an acute coronary syndrome (unstable angina, acute MI, or sudden death) occurs. The traditional risk factors for CAD, such as smoking, hypertension, age, male gender, hypercholesterolemia, and family history, are not the same risk factors that are associated with an increased incidence of perioperative cardiac events (see Fig. 34-2 and Box 34-2). However, traditional risk factors are important in assessing the significance of chest pain, dyspnea, or an abnormal ECG. The Revised Cardiac Risk Index (RCRI; Box 34-2) has been validated in several studies as the best scoring system to predict

Box 34-2 Revised Cardiac Risk Index

High-risk surgery (intraperitoneal, intrathoracic, or suprainguinal vascular procedures)*
Ischemic heart disease (by any diagnostic criteria)
History of congestive heart failure
History of cerebrovascular disease
Diabetes mellitus requiring insulin†
Creatinine >2.0 mg/dL

*This risk factor is not considered a clinical predictor in the ACC/AHA 2007 guidelines for perioperative cardiac evaluation for noncardiac surgery.[7]
†This risk factor has been changed to simply diabetes mellitus in the ACC/AHA 2007 guidelines for perioperative cardiac evaluation for noncardiac surgery.[7]
From Lee TH, Marcantonio ER, Mangione CM, et al: Derivation and prospective validation of a simple index for prediction of cardiac risk of major noncardiac surgery. Circulation 100:1043-1049, 1999.

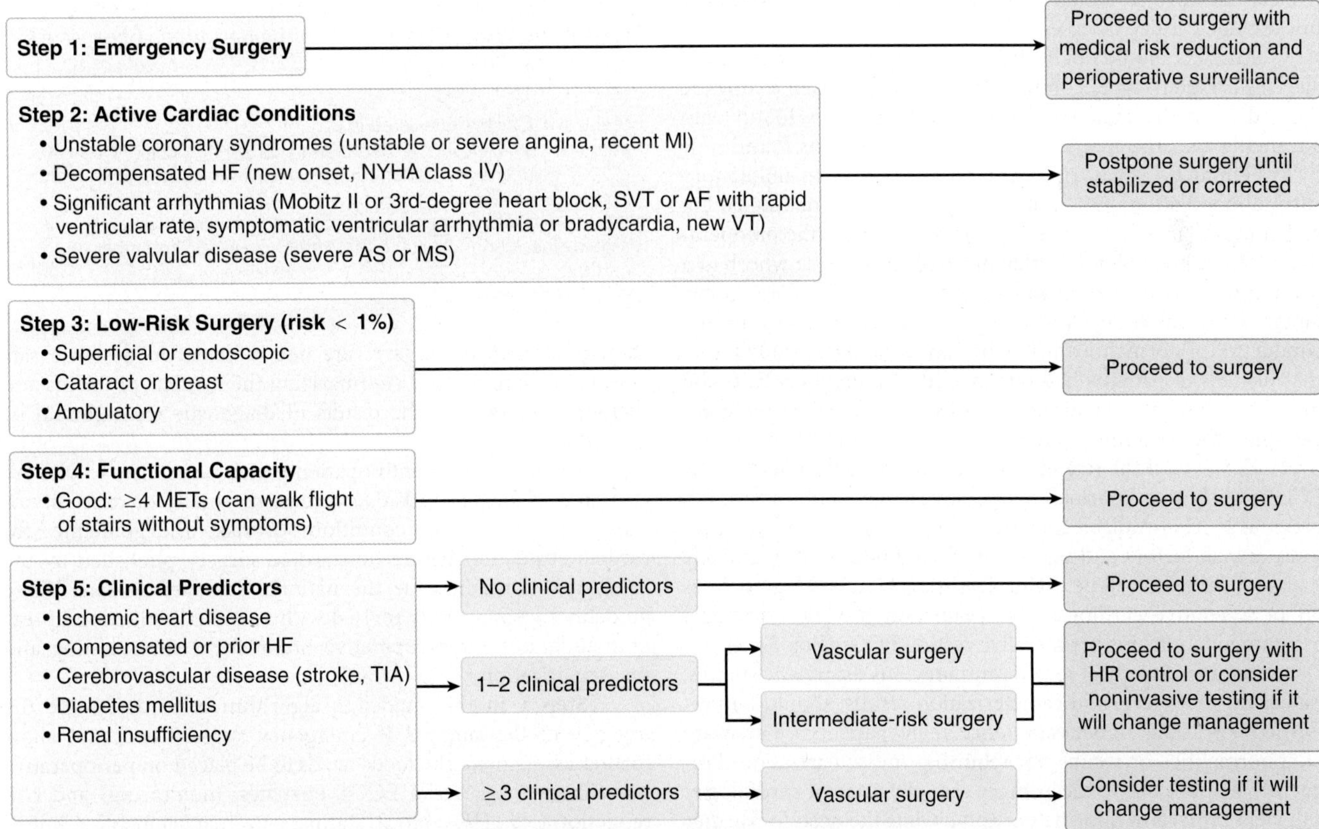

Figure 34-2 Simplified cardiac evaluation for noncardiac surgery. AF, atrial fibrillation; AS, aortic stenosis; HF, heart failure; HR, heart rate; METs, metabolic equivalents of the task; MI, myocardial infarction; MS, mitral stenosis; NYHA, New York Heart Association; SVT, supraventricular tachycardia; TIA, transient ischemic attack; VT, ventricular tachycardia. *(From Fleisher LA, Beckman JA, Brown KA, et al: ACC/AHA 2007 guidelines on perioperative cardiovascular evaluation and care for noncardiac surgery. J Am Coll Cardiol 50:e159-e241, 2007. Available at http://www.acc.org/qualityandscience/clinical/guidelines/Periop_/ Accessed September 28, 2007.)*

perioperative cardiac risk in patients undergoing noncardiac surgery.[20] The most important risk factors for adverse events are a history of ischemic heart disease, heart failure, diabetes, cerebrovascular disease, and renal insufficiency; advanced age; and high-risk surgery, especially open vascular procedures.

One should inquire about chest discomfort (pain, pressure, tightness), the duration of the discomfort, precipitating factors, associated symptoms, and methods of relief. Regardless of symptoms, the most important prognostic indicators of heart disease and perioperative adverse events are risk factors. Shortness of breath with exertion is a common angina-equivalent. Dyspnea is nonspecific and can be a result of deconditioning, pulmonary disease, or heart failure. Dyspnea in patients with risk factors for CAD (see Fig. 34-2 and Box 34-2) may necessitate an investigation for ischemic heart disease. Women are particularly likely to have atypical symptoms of ischemic heart disease. One should note diagnoses, diagnostic tests, therapies, and names of treating physicians.

Patients with risk factors for CAD or symptoms suggestive of ischemia, including atypical ones such as dyspnea, need an ECG. Tait and colleagues suggested that routine preoperative ECGs are not indicated in patients without a history of cardiovascular disease and no significant risk factors.[21] An abnormal ECG is found in 62% of patients with known cardiac disease, in 44% of those with strong risk factors, but in only 7% of individuals younger than 50 years with no risk factors. Additionally, the specificity of an abnormality on the ECG in predicting postoperative cardiac adverse events is only 26%, and a normal ECG does not exclude cardiac disease.[22]

An ECG should not be ordered simply because of advanced age (see Chapter 71). Recommendations for age-based testing are derived from the high incidence of abnormalities found with advancing age. The frequency of Q-wave infarctions found only by ECG in men 75 years or older is about 0.5%. In an ambulatory surgical population, 43% of patients had an abnormal ECG, but only 1.6% had an adverse perioperative event and the preoperative ECG was of potential value in just half of those who had a complication. Only certain abnormalities on the ECG are important in preoperative assessment (e.g., Q waves, especially if recent; conduction abnormalities and arrhythmias), and one study found that just 2% of patients had one or both if a previous ECG did not show these abnormalities. Establishing a baseline for comparison is the most important reason to obtain an ECG preoperatively. However, if the rate of probable events is infrequent or the ECG is likely to be normal preoperatively, the yield lessens. If a previous ECG is available and there has been no change in symptoms or risk factors and no new physical findings, it is unlikely that a repeat ECG will be useful. The 2007 ACC/AHA guidelines on perioperative cardiovascular evaluation provide additional recommendations for preoperative resting ECGs (Box 34-3).[7]

Review of medical records and previous diagnostic studies, especially stress tests and catheterization results, should be performed if possible. In our experience, many patients are unaware of abnormalities or results not requiring revascularization. Frequently, a phone call to the primary care physician or cardiologist will yield important information and obviate the need for further testing or consultation. Consultation initiated by the preoperative physician should seek specific advice regarding diagnosis and status of the patient's condition. Asking specific questions such as "*Does this patient have CAD?*" or "*Is this patient optimized for planned radical nephrectomy?*" is the first step. Letters or notes stating "*cleared for surgery*" are not sufficient to design a safe anesthetic plan. A letter summarizing the medical problems and therapies, along with the results of diagnostic tests, should be requested.

Box 34-3 Recommendations for Preoperative Resting 12-Lead Electrocardiogram

Class I

A preoperative resting 12-lead ECG is recommended for patients with at least one clinical risk factor* who are undergoing vascular surgical procedures

A preoperative resting 12-lead ECG is recommended for patients with known congestive heart failure, peripheral arterial disease, or cerebrovascular disease who are undergoing intermediate-risk surgical procedures

Class IIa

A preoperative resting 12-lead ECG is reasonable in persons with no clinical risk factors who are undergoing vascular surgical procedures

Class IIb

A preoperative resting 12-lead ECG may be reasonable in patients with at least one clinical risk factor who are undergoing intermediate-risk operative procedures

Class III

Preoperative and postoperative resting 12-lead ECGs are not indicated for asymptomatic persons undergoing low-risk surgical procedures

Class I recommendations: the procedure *should* be performed; class IIa: it is reasonable to perform the preocedure; class IIb: the procedure may be considered; class III: the procedure should *not* be performed because it is not helpful.

*Clinical risk factors are listed in Box 34-2.

Adapted from Fleisher LA, Beckman JA, Brown KA, et al: ACC/AHA 2007 guidelines on perioperative cardiovascular evaluation and care for noncardiac surgery. J Am Coll Cardiol 50:e159-e241, 2007. Available at http://www.acc.org/qualityandscience/clinical/guidelines/Periop_Fulltext_2007.pdf/ Accessed September 28, 2007.

The goal is to identify patients with heart disease who are at high risk for perioperative cardiac morbidity or mortality or those with modifiable conditions or risk. The guidelines for cardiac evaluation before noncardiac surgery published by the ACC/AHA have become the national standard of care. These guidelines were recently revised with a marked reduction in recommendations for preoperative noninvasive stress testing and revascularization.[7]

Step 1 in this guideline algorithm is to determine the urgency of the surgery. If emergency surgery does not allow further assessment, the focus needs to be placed on perioperative surveillance (e.g., serial ECGs, enzymes, monitoring) and risk reduction (e.g., HR control, statins, pain management). Clinical predictors, functional or exercise capacity, and level of surgical risk guide further diagnostic and therapeutic interventions.

Step 2 is to determine whether the patient has an active cardiac condition, such as acute MI, unstable or severe angina, decompensated heart failure, severe valvular disease (e.g., severe aortic stenosis), or significant arrhythmias (e.g., ventricular tachycardia or atrial fibrillation with a rapid rate), that warrants postponement of all except lifesaving emergency procedures (e.g., ruptured aneurysms). After evaluating and treating these conditions according to the AHA/ACC guidelines, surgery may be considered if the benefits outweigh the risks. Traditionally, patients who experienced an MI within 3 to 6 months were considered high risk and surgery was delayed. More recent evidence and the ACC/AHA guidelines suggest that *acute* MI, defined as occurring within the past 7 days, should still be considered high risk and elective surgeries postponed. A *recent* MI, defined as occurring within the past 30 days (but more than 7 days) *with evidence of myocardium at risk* (generally based on persistent symptoms or results of stress testing), is also a high-risk condition. However, a recent (8 to 30 days previously) MI *without evidence of myocardium at risk* is considered an active cardiac condition and equivalent to any history of CAD.

Step 3 involves determination of the surgical risk or severity. Patients without active cardiac conditions who are undergoing low-risk surgery (reported cardiac risk generally <1%; endoscopic or superficial procedures, cataract, breast, or ambulatory surgeries) can proceed to surgery without further cardiac testing other than an ECG within 3 months.

Step 4 assesses the patient's functional capacity (see Table 34-2). Asymptomatic patients who are highly functional can proceed to surgery. The 2007 ACC/AHA guidelines use the RCRI (see Box 34-2) derived from a cohort study showing an incidence of major cardiac events of 0.4%, 0.9%, 7%, and 11% in patients with zero, one, two, or three risk predictors, respectively.[20] The RCRI medical conditions have been confirmed in independent studies as valid predictors of risk.[15]

Step 5 is the last and most complicated determination for patients with poor or indeterminate functional capacity. The presence and number of clinical predictors as shown in Box 34-2 drive the recommendations for and probable benefit of further cardiac testing. Patients with no clinical predictors proceed to surgery. Those undergoing vascular surgery with three or more clinical risk factors are the group most likely to benefit from further testing, but the ACC/AHA guidelines recommend further testing only "if it will change management." Patients with one or more clinical predictors undergoing intermediate-risk surgery (1% to 5% risk for cardiac complications, including orthopedic, intra-abdominal, and intrathoracic procedures) or those with one or two risk factors undergoing vascular surgery can either proceed to surgery with HR control or undergo noninvasive testing if it will change management.

Chronic inflammatory conditions (e.g., rheumatoid arthritis, systemic lupus erythematosus [SLE]), chronic steroid use, and chest irradiation) increase the risk for CAD but have not been shown to be significant predictors of perioperative cardiac complications.[23,24] The substantial pullback of ACC/AHA recommendations advocating noninvasive stress testing and coronary revascularization before noncardiac surgery is due to the general lack of definitive benefit and risk reduction with this approach. The only randomized prospective study of revascularization (coronary artery bypass grafting [CABG] or percutaneous coronary intervention [PCI] with stenting) versus medical management failed to show a difference in outcome. This study was performed in intermediate- to high-risk patients with known CAD undergoing major vascular surgery.[25] Numerous retrospective and observational studies have failed to show a benefit of coronary revascularization before noncardiac surgery. Noncardiac surgery soon after revascularization (CABG or PCI with or without stents) is associated with high rates of perioperative cardiac morbidity and mortality.[26] Factors to consider are the urgency of the noncardiac surgery (e.g., patients with cancer) and the potential long-term benefits of revascularization. Patients who need noncardiac surgery within the next year are not good candidates for implantation of drug-eluting stents, and if revascularization is absolutely necessary, these patients need to be considered for either CABG or PCI without stenting or with a bare metal stent.[27] See the section on recent coronary stents and antiplatelet agents.

Stress testing identifies CAD and its severity, but the positive predictive value for perioperative cardiac complications is generally only 5% to 25%.[28] The negative predictive value of noninvasive tests for predicting perioperative events generally approaches 100%, so these tests are typically more informative about a patient who will *not* have an event than one who will. However, studies of the predictive value of noninvasive testing predated the era of drug-eluting stents and the risk of perioperative acute thrombosis with these stents. Cardiac catheterization, which some consider the gold standard for evaluation of coronary lesions, does not absolutely risk-stratify patients.[29] This lack of prognostic value is partly due to the approximately 50% incidence of plaque rupture (with intermediate-sized plaque of 40% to 70% being most vulnerable to rupture) as the causative event during the perioperative period combined with the hypercoagulable state and the typical withdrawal of antiplatelet agents.

Exercise treadmill testing can be ordered for patients with normal ECGs who can exercise and are likely to achieve an adequate HR response (68% to 81% sensitivity and 66% to 77% specificity for finding ischemia).[7] Prognostic information such as functional capacity and the workload at which ischemia occurs predict outcome. The test result is adequate when the patient can exercise to at least greater than 85% of the target HR (the target HR is defined as 220 − age). The individual's ability to exercise and symptoms that limit activity, such as dyspnea, have long-term prognostic implications, even in those without evidence of ischemia.

Pharmacologic tests such as dobutamine echocardiography or nuclear perfusion imaging are necessary for patients unable to exercise, those with pacemakers or significant bradycardia, or those taking high-dose β-adrenergic blockers.[7]

A combination of exercise and imaging can be used in patients able to exercise who have significant abnormalities on the ECG that may interfere with the interpretation of ischemia via the ECG (e.g., LVH with a strain pattern, ST-T wave changes, or left bundle branch block [LBBB]). Exercise combined with perfusion imaging in patients with LBBB results in a high incidence of false-positive tests because of septal perfusion defects not caused by CAD.[7] For most patients, the choice of which pharmacologic test is immaterial. Dobutamine uncovers ischemia by increasing contractility, HR, and BP and may therefore not be the best test in patients with pacemakers, significant bradycardia, aortic or cerebral aneurysms, or poorly controlled hypertension. Adenosine radionucleotide imaging (one of the most common methods of nuclear stress testing) uses the vasodilatory properties of adenosine (stenotic vessels are maximally vasodilated at rest) and uptake of the radioisotope by viable myocardium. This type of test is not dependent on the HR response but may exacerbate bronchospasm in patients taking theophylline or reduce preload, which may be dangerous in patients with severe aortic stenosis, hypertrophic cardiomyopathy (HCM), or carotid stenosis.

Echocardiography, combined with exercise or a pharmacologic agent, is used to look for wall motion abnormalities. Abnormalities present at rest (baseline) indicate scar tissue from previous infarction. Areas of myocardium that are normal at rest but show abnormalities with increased isotropy and chronotropy are consistent with stenotic lesions and limited blood flow. Similarly, nuclear imaging perfusion abnormalities at rest are consistent with infarction. Normal coronary arteries vasodilate with adenosine or exercise, and uptake of isotope is normal. Myocardium with limited blood flow will be normal at rest but show decreased uptake of isotope with exercise or administration of adenosine. Perioperative cardiac risk increases with increasing amounts of at-risk myocardium. If a patient has undergone a specific test in the past, it is most useful to obtain the same test for comparison.

Patients with ischemic heart disease require a complete blood count (CBC), and transfusion for anemia should be considered. In nonoperative settings but in populations with critical illness or chronic disease states associated with known CAD or risk factors for CAD, hemoglobin levels higher than 13.5 g/dL are associated with adverse outcomes.[30] A recent study suggests that even mild preoperative anemia increases postoperative mortality and cardiac morbidity in men but not in women.[31] Individuals with preoperative hematocrits between 39% and 51% had the lowest risk of adverse outcomes in this Veteran's Administration surgical population.

A thorough discussion of the optimal perioperative medical treatment of patients with ischemic heart disease can be found in Chapter 35. In brief, patients already taking statins and β-blockers need to have these drugs continued without interruption throughout the perioperative period. Those already taking β-blockers need their dosages adjusted to achieve an HR lower than 70 beats/min if at all possible. The optimal use of β-blockers in patients who are at significant risk for perioperative cardiac events and are currently not taking them in accord with national guidelines is controversial and discussed more fully in Chapter 35. Strong consideration should be given to continuing aspirin perioperatively or discontinuing for the shortest duration possible if used for secondary prevention of vascular events (Fig. 34-3).

By applying the ACC/AHA recommendations or using the predictive value of the RCRI and developing practice guidelines as shown in Figure 34-2, anesthesiologists in preanesthetic clinics are well positioned to risk-stratify patients, thus obviating the need for cardiac consultation. The preoperative period is an opportunity to identify patients with CAD who will benefit from long-term risk modification with statins, aspirin, exercise, and diet adjustment. Patients with symptoms consistent with ischemia (but without a diagnosis of CAD) or significant risk factors

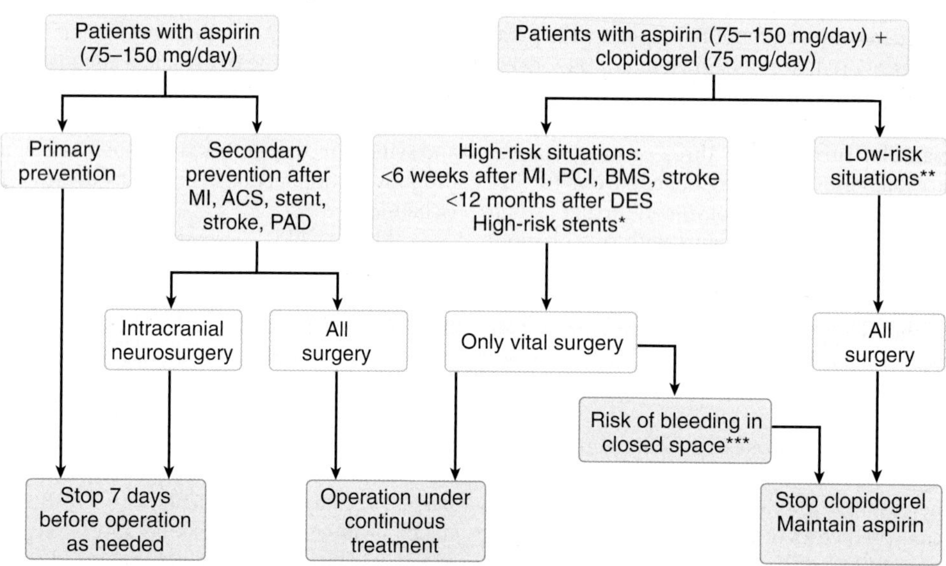

*High-risk stents: long (>36 mm), proximal, overlapping, or multiple stent implantation, stents for chronic total occlusions, stents in small vessels or bifurcated lesions.
**Examples of low-risk situations: >3 months after BMS, stroke, uncomplicated MI, PCI without stenting.
***Risk of bleeding in closed space: intracranial neurosurgery, intra-medullary canal surgery, posterior eye chamber ophthalmic surgery. In these situations, the risk/benefit ratio of upholding vs withdrawing aspirin must be evaluated for each case individually; in case of aspirin upholding, early postoperative re-institution is important.

Figure 34-3 Algorithm for preoperative management of patients receiving antiplatelet therapy. ACS, acute coronary syndrome; BMS, bare metal stent; DES, drug-eluting stent; MI, myocardial infarction; PAD, peripheral arterial disease; PCI, percutaneous coronary intervention. *(From Chassot P-G, Delabays A, Spahn DR: Perioperative antiplatelet therapy: The case for continuing therapy in patients at risk of myocardial infarction. Br J Anaesth 99:316-328, 2007. Available at http://bja.oxfordjournals.org.)*

without medical management such as statins and aspirin may benefit from evaluation by a cardiologist regardless of whether they are having surgery. Preoperative evaluation should not simply focus on perioperative risk.

Heart Failure

Heart failure affects 4 to 5 million people (2% of the population) in the United States and is a significant risk factor for postoperative adverse events (see Chapter 60).[32] One in 100 individuals between 50 and 59 years of age has a 5% to 7% risk of perioperative cardiac complications, but those with decompensated failure have a 20% to 30% incidence. Heart failure may be due to systolic dysfunction (decreased ejection fraction because of abnormal contractility), diastolic dysfunction (elevated filling pressure because of abnormal relaxation but normal contractility and ejection fraction), or a combination. Diastolic failure accounts for almost half of all cases, but there is little science to guide perioperative care of these individuals. Hypertension is a cause of diastolic dysfunction, and LVH on an ECG should raise suspicion. Ischemic heart disease is the most common cause of systolic dysfunction in the United States (50% to 75% of cases). Cardiomyopathies occur from a variety of causes, including infectious causes (human immunodeficiency virus [HIV], coxsackievirus, influenza virus, adenovirus, Chagas' or Lyme disease), ischemia, stress, toxins, alcohol, the peripartum period, drugs (doxorubicin [Adriamycin], cocaine), muscular dystrophies, and idiopathic causes, which can be familial and inherited in an autosomal dominant or X-linked autosomal recessive pattern.

The preoperative evaluation history and physical examination focus on identifying and minimizing the effects of heart failure. Recent weight gain, complaints of shortness of breath, fatigue, orthopnea, paroxysmal nocturnal dyspnea, nocturnal cough, peripheral edema, hospitalizations, and recent changes in management are all significant. Patients with decompensated heart failure feel as though they are "suffocating" or have "air hunger."[33] Angina or a history of CAD may indicate heart failure.

The physical examination focuses on finding third or fourth heart sounds, tachycardia, a laterally displaced apical pulse, rales, jugular venous distention, ascites, hepatomegaly, or peripheral edema. Classifying the patient's medical status according to the New York Heart Association (NYHA) categories is useful.[34]

NYHA Classification

Class I: no limitation of physical activity; ordinary activity does not cause fatigue, palpitations, or syncope

Class II: slight limitation of physical activity; ordinary activity results in fatigue, palpitations, or syncope

Class III: marked limitation of physical activity; less than ordinary activity results in fatigue, palpitations, or syncope; comfortable at rest

Class IV: inability to perform any physical activity without discomfort; symptoms at rest

Decompensated heart failure is considered a high-risk cardiac condition, and elective surgery should be postponed (see Fig. 34-2).[7] Brain naturetic peptide (BNP), which is released from the ventricles of the heart, can be useful in evaluating patients suspected of having decompensated heart failure.[35] In an emergency room study of patients with dyspnea, a plasma BNP level higher than 100 pg/mL diagnosed heart failure with a sensitivity, specificity, and predictive accuracy of 90%, 76%, and 83%, respectively. The plasma concentration of BNP correlated with NYHA functional class, with BNP levels ranging from 244 to 817 pg/mL corresponding to classes I to IV.[36] In patients undergoing noncardiac surgery, preoperative BNP levels predict cardiac complications and death.[37] An N-terminal pro-BNP level elevated to greater than 450 pg/mL in patients younger than 50 years and to greater than 900 pg/mL in patients 50 years or older is highly sensitive and specific for the diagnosis of acute failure. An N-terminal pro-BNP level less than 300 pg/mL has a 99% negative predictive value for acute heart failure. A study of patients undergoing vascular surgery showed that preoperatively elevated levels of N-terminal pro-BNP predicted cardiac events and mortality.[38]

A preoperative ECG plus determination of electrolytes, BUN, creatinine, and possibly BNP is indicated in all patients with or suspected of having heart failure. Digoxin levels should not be routinely measured unless toxicity under treatment or noncompliance is suspected. One should determine *trough* levels of digoxin, which is not always possible in a preoperative evaluation setting. Paroxysmal atrial tachycardia with a 2 : 1 atrioventricular (AV) block is pathognomonic of digoxin toxicity. Junctional tachycardia, ventricular ectopic beats, bigeminy, second-degree AV block, nausea, lethargy, altered color perception, and mental status changes or agitation are symptoms of digoxin toxicity. Chest radiography is useful in those suspected of pulmonary edema or decompensation. An objective measure of the left ventricular ejection fraction (LVEF), ventricular performance, and diastolic function with echocardiography is helpful if not previously performed, especially in patients with NYHA class III or IV heart failure. Normal LVEF is greater than 50%, mildly diminished is 41% to 49%, moderately diminished is 26% to 40%, and severely diminished is less than 25%. In patients with class III or IV heart failure, cardiology consultation would be useful before the patient undergoes general anesthesia or any intermediate- or high-risk procedure. Minor procedures under monitored anesthesia care may proceed as long as the patient's condition is stable.

Medical therapy, including β-blockers, hydralazine, nitrates, and digoxin, needs to be optimized and continued preoperatively. Angiotension-converting enzyme inhibitors (ACEIs), angiotensin receptor blockers (ARBs), diuretics (including aldosterone antagonists such as spironolactone), and anticoagulants may be beneficial, even on the day of surgery. Selectively continuing or discontinuing these drugs depends on the volume and hemodynamic status of the patient, the degree of cardiac dysfunction, and the anticipated surgery and volume challenges. Continuing all medications for patients with severe dysfunction who are scheduled for minor procedures is probably best. The other extreme occurs when patients with well-compensated NYHA class I failure are scheduled for lengthy high-risk procedures with projected significant blood loss or fluid requirements; in this case it is best to discontinue potent diuretics on the morning of surgery. Short-acting calcium channel antagonists depress left ventricular function, worsen symptoms, and increase the risk for death. Some patients will have pacemakers or implantable cardiac defibrillators, which have special considerations perioperatively (see the section on devices for management of cardiac rhythm for recommendations and Chapter 43).

Unless truly an emergency and life preserving, surgery should be postponed in patients with decompensated or untreated heart failure. There is no consensus on how long after an acute exacerbation patients remain at risk. Severely affected individuals or those with decompensation are best managed in concert with a heart failure specialist and may benefit from preoperative hospitalization for interventions designed to improve function.

Murmurs and Valvular Abnormalities

The quandary in the preoperative clinic is to determine the cause of cardiac murmurs and to distinguish between significant murmurs and clinically unimportant ones (see Chapter 60).[39] Functional murmurs occur as a result of turbulent flow across the aortic or pulmonic outflow tracts. These benign murmurs occur with high-outflow states such as hyperthyroidism, pregnancy, or anemia. However, noncardiologists or even cardiologists often cannot distinguish benign from pathologic murmurs. In elderly patients and those with risk factors for heart disease, other abnormal heart sounds, a history of rheumatic fever or anorectic drug use, evidence of volume overload, pulmonary disease, cardiomegaly, or an abnormal ECG, echocardiography should be considered (Box 34-4).[40] Although echocardiography may be useful in the diagnosis of many of these murmurs, the evaluation may not be required preoperatively if the information will not change management.

Diastolic murmurs are always pathologic and require further evaluation. Regurgitant disease is tolerated perioperatively much better than stenotic disease is. Heart failure in concert with any valvular disease is associated with a 20% risk of decompensation in the perioperative period. Murmurs are graded according to loudness: grade I, a faint murmur that can be heard with difficulty; grade II, faint but easily heard; grade III, moderately loud without a thrill; grade IV, loud with a palpable thrill; grade V, very loud but still needs a stethoscope (thrill present); and grade VI, murmur heard without a stethoscope. However, the usefulness of this distinction is debatable because severe lesions can be associated with soft murmurs and vice versa. The location of the murmur and changes in intensity with maneuvers guide diagnosis (Table 34-3). A Valsalva maneuver decreases filling of the right and left heart chambers and reduces the intensity of most murmurs, except those associated with mitral valve prolapse (MVP) and HCM. Standing will also increase the intensity of murmurs of MVP and HCM. Squatting increases venous return and afterload and therefore increases most murmurs, except those related to MVP and HCM. Asking the patient to repeatedly perform a handgrip will increase HR and afterload (increases BP) and will augment murmurs of mitral regurgitation and stenosis and aortic insufficiency but decrease aortic stenosis and HCM murmurs. All patients with murmurs require an ECG. In patients with significant abnormalities found by history, physical examination, or ECG, further evaluation by echocardiography or by a cardiologist should be considered (see Box 34-4).

Box 34-4 ACC/AHA Guideline Summary—Echocardiography in Asymptomatic Patients with Cardiac Murmurs*

Class I—There is evidence or general agreement (or both) that echocardiography is useful in asymptomatic patients with the following cardiac murmurs:

- Diastolic murmurs
- Continuous murmurs
- Late systolic murmurs
- Murmurs associated with ejection clicks
- Murmurs that radiate to the neck or back
- Grade 3 or louder systolic murmurs

Class IIa—The weight of evidence or opinion is in favor of the usefulness of echocardiography in asymptomatic patients with the following cardiac murmurs:

- Murmurs associated with other abnormal physical findings on cardiac examination
- Murmurs associated with an abnormal electrocardiogram or chest radiograph

Class III—There is evidence or general agreement (or both) that echocardiography is not useful in asymptomatic patients with the following murmurs:

- Grade 2 or softer midsystolic murmurs considered innocent or functional by an experienced observer

*These are indications for general evaluation but do not necessarily need to be performed preoperatively.

From Bonow, RO, Carabello, BA, Chatterjee, K, et al: ACC/AHA 2006 guidelines for the management of patients with valvular heart disease. A report of the American College of Cardiology/American Heart Association Task Force on Practice Guidelines (Writing Committee to Revise the 1998 Guidelines for the Management of Patients with Valvular Heart Disease). J Am Coll Cardiol 48:e1, 2006.

Table 34-3 Descriptions of Murmurs Associated with Cardiac Abnormalities

Lesion	Location	Timing	Description
Aortic stenosis	Second parasternal interspaces	Midsystolic	Crescendo-decrescendo, radiates to the carotids; ± S_3, S_4; Valsalva and sustained handgrip exercise decrease intensity
Aortic insufficiency	Third and fourth parasternal interspaces	Holodiastolic	Decrescendo, blowing, high pitched, radiates to the carotids; Austin-Flint rumble at the apex; squatting, handgrip exercise, and leaning forward increase intensity
Mitral stenosis	Apex	Mid-diastolic	Opening snap; low-pitched rumble radiates to the axilla; squatting and handgrip exercise increase intensity
Mitral regurgitation	Apex	Holosystolic	High pitched, blowing, radiates to the axilla; loud S_3; standing decreases intensity; squatting and handgrip exercise increase intensity
Mitral valve prolapse	Apex	Late systolic	Crescendo, midsystolic click; Valsalva and standing increase intensity; squatting decreases intensity
Hypertrophic cardiomyopathy	Apex, lower left sternal border	Midsystolic	S_4, single S_2; Valsalva and standing increase intensity; squatting, passive leg raising, and handgrip exercise decrease intensity

Aortic Stenosis

Aortic stenosis, the most common valvular lesion in the United States, affects 2% to 4% of adults older than 65 years; severe stenosis is associated with high risk for perioperative complications.[7] Once considered a degenerative lesion associated with age or a congenital bicuspid valve, aortic stenosis is now thought to have much in common with ischemic heart disease and is an independent marker of CAD.[41] In patients with bicuspid valves, stenosis typically develops at a younger age (fourth and fifth decades of life); those with stenosis of the tricuspid valves are usually older than 60 years, but there is overlap.

Aortic *sclerosis*, which also causes a systolic ejection murmur similar to that of aortic stenosis, is present in 25% of people 65 to 74 years of age and in almost half of those older than 84 years.[41] Aortic sclerosis is associated with a 40% increase in risk for MI and a 50% increase in risk for cardiovascular death in patients without a history of CAD.[42] There is no hemodynamic compromise with aortic sclerosis.

The cardinal symptoms of severe aortic stenosis are angina, heart failure, and syncope, although patients are much more likely to complain of a decrease in exercise tolerance and exertional dyspnea. Aortic stenosis causes a systolic ejection murmur, best heard in the right upper sternal border and often radiating to the neck. There is delayed carotid upstroke and a paradoxically split S_2, and exercise will increase HR and decrease an aortic stenosis murmur. Patients with a previously undiagnosed murmur need an ECG, and an echocardiogram should be considered in patients with an abnormality on the ECG (see Box 34-4). Such abnormalities may consist of LVH, often with a strain pattern (ST-T wave changes), left axis deviation, or LBBB.

Aortic stenosis severity is based on the mean transvalvular pressure gradient and valve area (Table 34-4). The pressure gradient falls if the left ventricle begins to fail. Current guidelines recommend echocardiography annually for patients with severe aortic stenosis, every 2 years for moderate stenosis, and every 5 years for mild stenosis.[40] Patients with aortic stenosis are at risk for sudden death from arrhythmias, heart failure, and myocardial ischemia and infarction from concomitant CAD (high incidence) or a supply-demand mismatch. Patients with aortic sclerosis or stenosis need evaluation for CAD regardless of other risk factors. Those with severe or critical stenosis should not undergo noncardiac surgery (unless emergency and lifesaving) without a cardiology evaluation and careful consideration of risks or until valve replacement. Patients with moderate to severe aortic stenosis have an increased risk of bleeding (especially from gastrointestinal angiodysplasia). The cause appears to be an acquired von Willebrand syndrome resulting from mechanical disruption of von Willebrand multimers during turbulent blood flow through a narrowed valve. See the section "von Willebrand's Disease" for more details. An activated partial thromboplastin time (aPTT) is indicated. Prophylaxis for infective endocarditis in patients with aortic stenosis is no longer recommended.[43]

Table 34-4 Severity of Aortic Stenosis

Grade	Velocity of Aortic Jet (m/sec)	Mean Pressure Gradient (mm Hg)	Valve Area (cm^2)
Mild	<3	<25	≥1.5
Moderate	3-4	25-40	1.0-1.5
Severe	4-4.5	40-50	0.7-1.0
Critical	>4.5	>50	<0.7

Aortic Insufficiency

Insufficiency of the aortic valve occurs with true valvular disease affecting the leaflets, from aortic root dilation, or as a result of both. Rheumatic heart disease, a bicuspid valve, collagen vascular diseases, and endocarditis can all lead to valvular disease. Aortic root dilation can complicate ankylosing spondylitis, osteogenesis imperfecta, syphilis, hypertension, age-related degeneration, Marfan's syndrome, and collagen vascular diseases. Acute insufficiency with pulmonary edema and hypertension can occur with trauma, infection, or aortic dissection and is an emergency. The murmur of aortic insufficiency is described in Table 34-3. The intensity of the murmur does not correlate with the severity of regurgitation.[44] Patients typically have a widened pulse pressure (normal or elevated systolic BP and low diastolic BP) manifested as Corrigan's or water-hammer pulses (bounding carotid pulse with a rapid downstroke). de Musset's sign is a head bob with each heartbeat, Duroziez's sign is a systolic and diastolic bruit heard over the femoral artery when it is partially compressed, Quincke's pulses are capillary pulsations in the fingertips or lips, and Müller's sign is systolic pulsations of the uvula.

An ECG is needed and an echocardiogram should be considered if finding could change management (see Box 34-4); a chest radiograph may be useful. LVH with ST- and T-wave changes as a result of volume overload or underlying chronic ischemia may be present. Left atrial hypertrophy and left axis deviation along with premature atrial and ventricular contractions are not uncommon. Generally, chronic insufficiency is well tolerated in the perioperative period. Patients with good functional status and preserved left ventricular systolic function have a low risk of complications with anesthesia. Prophylaxis for infective endocarditis is no longer recommended.[43]

Mitral Stenosis

Mitral stenosis is much less common than aortic stenosis and is usually associated with a history of rheumatic heart disease. It can occur with aortic valvular disease or mitral regurgitation. A normal mitral valve has an area of 4 to 6 cm^2; stenosis is mild when the mitral valve area is 1.5 to 2.5 cm^2, moderate with an area of 1.1 to 1.5 cm^2, and critical when the area is 0.6 to 1.0 cm^2. A resting mean transvalvular gradient greater than 10 mm Hg also denotes severe stenosis. Symptoms typically occur 10 to 20 years after acute rheumatic fever and are often precipitated by pregnancy or illness. Unrecognized mitral stenosis is included in the differential diagnosis of pulmonary edema.

Preoperative evaluation includes determining whether the patient has a history of dyspnea, fatigue, orthopnea, pulmonary edema, and hemoptysis. These findings result from elevated left atrial pressure and decreased cardiac output. Atrial fibrillation can be due to a dilated left atrium, which can acutely precipitate failure and chronically cause thrombosis. Patients with atrial fibrillation require anticoagulation to avoid a left atrial thrombus. Tachycardia decreases cardiac output. Pulmonary hypertension and right heart failure may occur with significant stenosis. A loud S_2 suggests pulmonary hypertension. The characteristics of the murmur are described in Table 34-3. Sustained handgrip exercise increases HR and BP and may increase the murmur. Examination should look for rales and signs of right heart failure such as jugular venous distention, peripheral edema, hepatomegaly, right ventricular heave, and ascites.

A preoperative ECG is necessary and an echocardiogram should be considered if it will change management (see Box 34-4). A chest radiograph should also be considered. β-Blockers are used to control HR, and antiarrhythmics prevent or control atrial fibrillation. These medications have to be continued preoperatively because HR needs to be controlled before surgery. Anticoagulation is managed in conjunction with the treating cardiologist and surgeon. Prophylaxis for infective endocarditis is no longer recommended.[43]

Mitral Regurgitation

Mitral regurgitation can be acute in the setting of ischemia or infarction or can be chronic and associated with mitral stenosis, mitral valve prolapse, collagen vascular diseases, or cardiomyopathies. The course is typically very gradual, and symptoms develop late and only after the development of left ventricular dysfunction. Preoperative symptoms are vague and often attributed to other causes. Fatigue, dyspnea, and atrial fibrillation can be present. Description of murmurs is presented in Table 34-3. A loud murmur associated with a thrill (grade ≥4) has a specificity of 91% for severe regurgitation but a sensitivity of 24%.[44] Severe regurgitation is rarely present with a grade 1 to 2 murmur; however, there is a wide range of severity with a grade 3 murmur. Chronic mitral regurgitation is generally well tolerated perioperatively unless other valvular lesions (e.g., mitral or aortic stenosis) or left ventricular dysfunction coexist. Prophylaxis for infective endocarditis is no longer recommended.[43]

Mitral Valve Prolapse

Also known as click-murmur or floppy valve syndrome, mitral valve prolapse is commonly diagnosed in young women during evaluation for atypical chest pain, palpitations, or syncope. Whether these symptoms are truly related is questionable. Interestingly, men older than 55 years with mitral valve prolapse are more likely to have regurgitation complications and are at greatest risk for infective endocarditis. The important issue preoperatively is to differentiate patients with clinically significant mitral valve degeneration and regurgitation from those with an incidental finding of prolapse or a click, which does not warrant further evaluation or change in management. Patients taking β-blockers for control of palpitations or atypical chest pain continue these medications perioperatively. Prophylaxis for infective endocarditis is no longer recommended.[43]

Tricuspid Regurgitation

Tricuspid regurgitation is a relatively common abnormality, but because it is usually asymptomatic and not audible on physical examination, it is most commonly noted by echocardiography performed for other reasons. A small degree of tricuspid regurgitation is present in approximately 70% of normal adults. Tricuspid regurgitation is most commonly caused by dilatation of the right ventricle and the tricuspid annulus. Right ventricular dilatation is caused by conditions that directly involve the right ventricle (ischemia, cardiomyopathy) or is due to pulmonary hypertension and elevated right ventricular systolic pressure. Tricuspid and mitral regurgitation often occurs together. Tricuspid regurgitation is less often due to processes that directly affect the tricuspid valve, such as Ebstein's anomaly (a congenital malformation), infective endocarditis, rheumatic fever, carcinoid syndrome, connective tissue disorders (Marfan's syndrome), myxomatous degeneration or prolapse (occurs in as many as 40% of patients with mitral valve prolapse), or injury from a pacemaker, central line, or implantable cardioverter-defibrillator (ICD) lead. Drugs such as the anorectics fenfluramine and phentermine and the dopamine agonist pergolide may cause tricuspid regurgitation by a mechanism similar to that seen with carcinoid syndrome. The aforementioned drugs are no longer available in the United States.

Tricuspid regurgitation is classically associated with a holosystolic murmur that is best heard at the right or left midsternal border or at the subxiphoid area. When the right ventricle is very enlarged, the murmur may even be appreciated at the apex. There is usually little radiation of the murmur, and a thrill is not palpable. However, the murmur of tricuspid insufficiency is often soft or absent, even when regurgitation is severe. Interventions that result in an increase in venous return (leg raising, exercise, hepatic compression) will augment the murmur of tricuspid regurgitation. The murmur may also become louder after a premature beat and prolonged diastole. In contrast, reducing venous return (by standing or with amyl nitrate) will diminish the intensity of the murmur. In patients with pulmonary hypertension, the intensity of the murmur may change with alterations in pulmonary artery pressure and therefore the right ventricle. Patients with (or suspected of having) pulmonary hypertension need to be managed in conjunction with a pulmonary hypertension specialist (see the section "Pulmonary Hypertension"). Prophylaxis for infective endocarditis is no longer recommended.[43] An echocardiogram should be considered if it will change management.

Hypertrophic Cardiomyopathy

Previously known as hypertrophic obstructive cardiomyopathy and before that as idiopathic hypertrophic subaortic stenosis, HCM can be familial. Patients with hypertrophic obstructive cardiomyopathy are often young and male and may be asymptomatic without murmurs. An ECG and echocardiogram should be considered if there is a personal or family history of syncope with exertion or sudden death or when a murmur consistent with this disorder is detected. Characteristics of the murmur are described in Table 34-3. A maneuver that decreases diastolic volume or increases contractility increases the intensity of the murmur. Passive leg raising and squatting decrease the intensity, and a Valsalva maneuver increases it. In an otherwise healthy nonhypertensive patient with LVH and ST-segment and T-wave abnormalities on an ECG, an echocardiogram should be considered.

Patients are at risk for sudden cardiac death probably from arrhythmias (see Box 34-4). Holter monitoring may be useful in some patients. Many patients are treated with β-blockers to decrease contractility; these medications are continued perioperatively. ICDs may be in place to prevent sudden death; see discussion in the appropriate section of this chapter. Prophylaxis for infective endocarditis is no longer recommended.[43]

Prosthetic Heart Valves

In patients with prosthetic valves, the most important issues preoperatively are determination of the underlying condition requiring replacement, the type of prosthesis, the need for anticoagulation, and the planned management of such patients in the perioperative period. Occasionally, patients will have valve-related hemolysis. The risk for thrombosis is greatest with multiple prosthetic valves, followed by valves in the mitral position and then aortic valve replacements. Caged-ball valves (Starr-Edwards) have the highest risk, single tilting-disk valves (Björk-Shiley, Medtronic-Hall, Omnicarbon) have an intermediate risk, and the lowest risk is seen with bileaflet tilting-disk prostheses (St. Jude, CarboMedics, Edwards Duromedics). Bioprosthetic valves such as Carpentier-Edwards (porcine heterograft or pericardial) or Hancock (porcine) brands generally do not require long-term anticoagulation. The decision to stop anticoagulants, the duration off anticoagulants, and the need to "bridge" with a shorter-acting drug and the type of bridging agent (intravenous heparin or low-molecular-weight heparin [LMWH]) need to be made in conjunction with the treating cardiologist and surgeon. See the section on anticoagulation for a discussion of bridging.

Rhythm Disturbances and Electrocardiographic Abnormalities

Arrhythmias and conduction disturbances are common in the perioperative period (see also Chapter 42). Supraventricular and ventricular arrhythmias are associated with a greater risk of perioperative adverse events because of the arrhythmia itself and because they are markers for cardiopulmonary disease. Uncontrolled atrial fibrillation and ventricular tachycardia are high-risk clinical predictors, and elective surgery should be postponed until evaluation and stabilization are complete.[7] New-onset atrial fibrillation, symptomatic bradycardia, or high-grade heart block (second or third degree) identified in the preoperative clinic warrant consideration of postponement of elective procedurest and referral to cardiology for further evaluation. First-degree AV block is defined as a PR interval longer than 0.20 msec with an HR of 50 to 100 beats/min and is generally benign. Second-degree heart block occurs when the PR interval is prolonged greater than 0.20 msec, and eventually the atrial beat is blocked, which results in a dropped or missing QRS complex after a P wave. Two types of second-degree block exist. A Mobitz type I or Wenckebach block is more benign, rarely progresses to complete heart block, and responds to atropine. It is characterized by a progressive lengthening of the PR interval until the dropped beat occurs and is usually due to AV nodal delay. Mobitz type II results from an infranodal block, can progress to complete heart block, and is generally treated with a pacemaker unless secondary to a reversible cause such as ischemia or drugs. It is characterized by a fixed, prolonged PR interval that does not change before the dropped QRS complex. Third-degree or complete heart block is complete dissociation between the atrial and ventricular beats (P waves and QRS complexes) and requires a pacemaker unless a reversible source is identified. The ventricular beats in a patient with complete heart block are independent of the atria and should not be depressed. Two general factors are considered when determining the need for a pacemaker: an arrhythmia associated with symptoms and the location of the conduction abnormality. Syncope or near syncope associated with bradycardia or conduction delays is generally an indication for placement of a pacemaker. Disease below the AV node, in the His-Purkinje system, is more ominous and is suggested by a normal or minimally prolonged PR interval, a Mobitz type II block, and QRS abnormalities (bundle branch block, fascicular block, or both). Because disease in the His-Purkinje system is generally less stable, permanent pacemaker placement is likely to be beneficial. The indications for a pacemaker perioperatively are the same as those in nonsurgical patients (Box 34-5).[45]

Box 34-5 Indications for a Pacemaker

Class I Indications

- Sinus bradycardia with symptoms clearly related to the bradycardia (usually with a heart rate <40 beats/min or frequent sinus pauses)
- Symptomatic chronotropic incompetence
- Complete (third-degree) AV block*
- Advanced second-degree AV block (block of ≥2 consecutive P waves)
- Symptomatic Mobitz I or II second-degree AV block
- Mobitz II second-degree AV block with a widened QRS or chronic bifascicular block, regardless of symptoms

Class II Indications

- Sinus bradycardia (heart rate <40 beats/min) with symptoms suggestive of bradycardia but without a clear association between bradycardia and symptoms
- Sinus node dysfunction with unexplained syncope
- Chronic heart rates <30 beats/min in an awake patient

Class I conditions are those in which permanent pacing is definitely beneficial and effective, provided that the condition is not due to a transient cause. Class II conditions are those in which permanent pacing may be indicated but there is conflicting evidence or divergence of opinion (or both).

*Controversy exists concerning complete atrioventricular (AV) block without symptoms. The current ACC/AHA guidelines classify asymptomatic third-degree AV block with average awake ventricular rates of 40 beats/min or greater as a class IIa indication, although others recommend definite pacemaker placement.

From Gregoratos, G, Abrams, J, Epstein, AE, et al: ACC/AHA/NASPE 2002 guideline update for implantation of cardiac pacemakers and antiarrhythmia devices: Summary article. A report of the American College of Cardiology/American Heart Association Task Force on Practice Guidelines (ACC/AHA/NASPE Committee to Update the 1998 Pacemaker Guidelines). Circulation 106:2145-2161, 2002.

Bundle branch blocks are complete or incomplete and either right (RBBB) or left (LBBB). They result from aging or fibrosis of the conducting system, ischemia, pulmonary disease, radiation, or cardiomyopathies or can be normal variants. Traditionally, LBBB has been considered more ominous and has been shown to be associated with CAD and heart failure.[46,47] LBBB is strongly associated with CAD, and in a patient with a recent onset or no previous evaluation of LBBB, stress testing or cardiology consultation may be warranted. Obtaining a previous ECG for comparison can establish the stability. RBBB is likely to be congenital, a result of calcification and degeneration of the conduction system or secondary to pulmonary disease. Brugada's syndrome is a congenital disease characterized by RBBB with ST-segment elevation in the right precordial leads and is associated with a risk for sudden death and lethal arrhythmias. If the history and physical examination do not suggest significant pulmonary, congenital, or ischemic heart disease or Brugada's syndrome, no further evaluation is warranted because of an isolated RBBB. An RBBB in a patient with pulmonary symptoms (including pulmonary hypertension) may be suggestive of severe respiratory or vascular compromise and may warrant pulmonary evaluation and echocardiography if intermediate- or high-risk surgery is planned. If congenital heart disease, pulmonary hypertension (see the appropriate section in this chapter), or Brugada's syndrome is suspected, cardiology consultation is indicated. LVH and ST-segment depression on a preoperative ECG are associated with a greater risk for MI and cardiac death perioperatively.[48] LVH may be associated with diastolic dysfunction and poorly controlled hypertension. Prolonged QT intervals should prompt an evaluation of electrolytes, magnesium, and calcium and a search for potentiating drugs. In a patient with a prolonged QT interval and syncope, near syncope, or a family history of sudden death, further evaluation should be considered.

Atrial Fibrillation

Atrial fibrillation occurs in elderly patients and those with thyrotoxicosis, valvular disease, and ischemic heart disease. It can be intermittent (paroxysmal), persistent (able to be cardioverted), or permanent (unable to be converted). Evidence suggests that rate control is more important than rhythm control. Patients with rapid ventricular rates (>100 beats/min) require control before elective surgery.[7] Patients with slow ventricular rates not caused by rate-controlling medications are at risk for sick sinus syndrome, need a careful history to uncover syncopal or near-syncopal episodes, and may need a Holter monitor. Most patients with atrial fibrillation will require long-term anticoagulation, which becomes an issue in the perioperative period. If they are being treated with only prophylactic therapy (no history of emboli or left atrial thrombi), bridging perioperatively is not cost-effective. Patients with atrial or ventricular thrombi or a previous history of thromboembolic events are at higher risk, and anticoagulant therapy is managed on a case-by-case basis in concert with the treating physician. β-Blockers, digoxin, and calcium channel blockers taken chronically to control rate or rhythm need to be continued perioperatively.

Supraventricular Arrhythmias

Supraventricular tachycardias result from rapidly firing ectopic atrial foci with rapid conduction via the AV node or from a reentry mechanism via accessory pathways. With a reentry mechanism the cycle self-perpetuates because conduction occurs down one pathway and up the other, with both the AV node–Purkinje system and the accessory pathway or pathways being involved. Various degrees of AV block may slow the ventricular rate. Wolff-Parkinson-White (WPW) syndrome is a classic supraventricular tachycardia with an accessory pathway but unique in that impulses can travel both retrograde and antegrade. Antegrade conduction over the accessory pathway results in a short PR interval (<0.12 msec) and slurring of the upstroke of the QRS, termed a delta wave. AV nodal–blocking drugs such as β-blockers, calcium channel blockers, and digoxin can paradoxically increase conduction over the accessory pathway and cause ventricular fibrillation. Lidocaine and procainamide are the preferred drugs to slow the tachycardia in patients with WPW syndrome. Certain patients may require ablation for long-term management of WPW syndrome, and this should be performed before elective surgery.

Ventricular Arrhythmias

Ventricular ectopics can be differentiated from atrial ectopics by a widen QRS (>0.12 msec) and lack of a P wave. The traditional grading system of Lown, organized by morphology (unifocal or multifocal), frequency (less than or greater than 30 beats/min), and other characteristics (couplets, R on T phenomenon), is limited in its ability to stratify risk. Classifying ventricular arrhythmias according to the type of rhythm disturbance and the presence of coexisting heart disease better predicts the risk for sudden death.

- Benign: isolated ventricular premature beats (VPBs) without heart disease
  - No need for further evaluation
  - No risk of sudden cardiac arrest
- Potentially lethal: greater than 30 VPBs/hr or nonsustained ventricular tachycardia with underlying heart disease
  - Requires cardiology evaluation with possible echocardiography, stress testing, catheterization, or electrophysiologic testing
  - Moderately high risk of sudden cardiac arrest; may benefit from an ICD
- Lethal: sustained ventricular tachycardia, ventricular fibrillation), syncope, or hemodynamic compromise associated with VPBs with underlying heart disease and often depressed cardiac function
  - Requires cardiology evaluation with possible stress testing, echocardiography, catheterization, or electrophysiologic testing
  - High risk of sudden cardiac arrest; likely to benefit from an ICD

Preoperative evaluation focuses on reversible causes such as hypokalemia, ischemia, acidosis, hypomagnesemia, drug toxicity, and endocrine dysfunction, which should be further evaluated and treated. Patients taking amiodarone are at risk for hypothyroidism and require thyroid function tests before surgery. Antiarrythmics should be continued perioperatively.

Cardiac Rhythm Management Devices: Pacemakers and Implantable Cardioverter-Defibrillators

More than 100,000 new cardiac rhythm management devices are implanted yearly in the United States. A complete discussion of the perioperative management of these devices can be found in Chapter 43.

Peripheral Vascular Disease

Also called peripheral arterial disease, PVD refers to aneurysmal or occlusive arterial disease of the extremities, visceral organs, head, neck, and brain. Many of these patients have disease secondary to tobacco abuse, diabetes, hyperlipidemia and hypertension, or combinations of these causes. Patients with Marfan's or Ehlers-Danlos syndrome may have aneurysmal disease without other risk factors. Renal insufficiency and cerebrovascular disease are frequent in this cohort of patients. Up to 75% of patients with PVD have CAD. In a study of 1000 consecutive patients scheduled for major vascular surgery, almost 60% had critical stenosis in at least one major coronary vessel. In addition, undiagnosed PVD (e.g., patients who smoke, are of increased age, have diabetes, or have cerebrovascular disease) should be considered when assessing patients scheduled for major surgery. Because claudication often limits functional capacity, symptoms of ischemic heart disease are often not apparent.

Determination of BP in both upper extremities and the presence or absence of peripheral pulses is important. Listening for bruits over the abdomen and femoral arteries or palpating for abdominal masses is part of the vascular examination but is rarely necessary preoperatively. BUN and creatinine should be determined before procedures involving injection of radiocontrast dye (see the section "Contrast-Induced Nephropathy" for management to reduce risk). Many patients take aspirin or dipyridamole, a vasodilator with some antiplatelet effects that are reversible on discontinuation; its elimination half-life is approximately 10 hours. Therefore, stopping this drug 48 hours before surgery eliminates the antiplatelet effect. However, because dypyridamole is often combined with aspirin (Aggrenox), this drug must be stopped 5 to 7 days before surgery if complete reversal of its antiplatelet effects is desired, although the risks related to stopping antiplatelet medications must also be considered.

Pulmonary Disorders (See Chapter 59)

Asthma

Asthma is a chronic inflammatory disease characterized by obstruction of the airways that is partially or completely reversible with treatment or spontaneously.[49] Bronchoconstriction is precipitated by irritants (smoke), allergens, infections, medications, or instrumentation of the larynx, trachea, or bronchi. Asthma is classified as intermittent (mild) or persistent (mild, moderate, or severe) based on how frequently symptoms occur and whether they are sporadic or constant. Patients with mild, well-controlled asthma have no greater risk associated with anesthesia and surgery than normal individuals do.

Reporting of asthma should prompt further questioning about shortness of breath, chest tightness, coughing (especially nocturnal), recent exacerbations, therapy (especially the use of steroids, particularly within the previous year) or oxygen use, hospitalizations, and intubations. The patient's best exercise level is important information for assessment of risk. A history of previous exacerbations with anesthesia should be elicited. Patients with asthma are quite good at estimating their current status and breathing capacity when asked about what percentage they are presently at (100% being normal). Adequate and appropriate medical therapy must be determined. The quality of breath sounds, quantity of air movement, and degree of wheezing are important. The degree of wheezing does not always correlate with the severity of bronchoconstriction. With severe obstruction, airflow is dangerously restricted and wheezing diminishes. Observing the degree of accessory muscle use often gauges the severity of the bronchoconstriction. Determination of oxygen saturation by pulse oximetry is useful. Arterial blood gas analysis is not generally necessary unless the patient is having a severe acute exacerbation. Patients taking oral steroids need blood glucose checked and may require perioperative steroid supplementation.

Wheezing is a common symptom in asthmatics but is not specific for this disease. Patients with chronic obstructive pulmonary disease (COPD), gastroesophageal reflux disease, vocal cord dysfunction, tracheal or bronchial stenosis, cystic fibrosis, allergic bronchopulmonary aspergillosis, and heart failure may wheeze. Spirometry is the preferred diagnostic test, but a normal result does not exclude asthma. A methacholine challenge test or a trial of bronchodilator therapy is indicated if spirometry is normal but there is still a strong suspicion of asthma. PFTs have no perioperative predictive value but in rare instances may be useful to gauge the severity of disease or the adequacy of therapy. Typical findings on PFTs are reduced forced expiratory volume in 1 second (FEV_1) and normal to increased functional residual capacity (FVC).

A preoperative chest radiograph is necessary only for evaluation of infections or pneumothorax. Bronchodilators, inhaled and oral steroids, and antibiotics (if taken) need to be continued on the day of surgery. β-Agonists are the most useful prophylactic intervention to lower the risk for bronchospasm on induction of anesthesia. A short course of steroids (20 to 60 mg of prednisone daily for 3 to 5 days) preoperatively may be useful in any patient who is not at baseline and surgery must proceed.

Chronic Obstructive Pulmonary Disease

COPD includes chronic bronchitis and emphysema and is characterized by obstruction to airflow that is not fully reversible. It is often due to exposure to pollutants such as cigarette smoke or substances in the environment (air pollution, allergens, grain, dust, and coal), α_1-antitrypsin deficiency, chronic infections, and long-standing asthma. Chronic bronchitis is the presence of symptoms on most days for at least 3 months for 2 successive years or recurrent excessive sputum that severely impairs expiratory airflow. Dyspnea, coughing, wheezing, and sputum production are common features. An acute exacerbation is defined as an increase in symptoms that requires a change in management.

The preoperative history and physical examination for patients with COPD are similar to that for patients with asthma, but with additional emphasis on the change in amount of sputum, color, or other signs of infection. A barrel chest and pursed-lip breathing suggest advanced disease. Typically, FEV_1 is reduced because of obstructed airflow, but FVC is increased because of reduced airflow, loss of elasticity, and overexpansion. Diffusing capacity (DLCO) is typically decreased, and its severity often correlates with the degree of hypoxia and hypercapnia, which in turn can predict the presence of pulmonary hypertension. However, PFTs have not been shown to predict perioperative outcome. Determination of oxygen saturation by pulse oximetry is appropriate to establish a baseline. Patients found to be hypoxic or using oxygen may benefit from further testing, including arterial blood gas determination. A chest radiograph is useful only when infection is suspected. An ECG may demonstrate right axis deviation, RBBB, or peaked P waves, which suggest pulmonary hypertension and possibly right ventricular changes in response to the chronic lung disease (see the section "Pulmonary Hypertension").

Restrictive Pulmonary Disorders

Restrictive lung disease is distinguished by a reduction in total lung capacity. Both pulmonary and extrapulmonary conditions cause restrictive disease. Pulmonary conditions include idiopathic interstitial pneumonia, interstitial lung disease related to connective tissue disease, lung resection, and pulmonary fibrosis. Extrapulmonary disorders are caused by chest wall limitations (kyphoscoliosis, obesity, ankylosing spondylitis), muscle dysfunction (muscular dystrophies, myasthenia gravis, paralyzed diaphragm), or pleural disease (mesothelioma, effusion, pneumothorax).

The preoperative medical history of associated diseases or symptoms prompts the directed evaluation. A chest radiograph and PFTs may be indicated to establish a diagnosis or evaluate acute or progressive worsening but are not routinely necessary preoperatively. FEV_1 and FVC are reduced proportionally, so the ratio is normal. These patients are at risk for pulmonary hypertension, which may not be diagnosed or communicated to caregivers because of overlapping symptoms with restrictive lung disease. See the section "Pulmonary Hypertension" for more details.

Dyspnea

Dyspnea is a subjective experience of breathing discomfort. It is a symptom of deconditioning, obesity, and disorders of ventilation, cardiac function, perfusion, and oxygen delivery. Dyspnea is associated with cardiac, pulmonary, hematologic, and neuromuscular diseases.

Patients with an insidious onset may not seek attention until quite late, and frequently they and their caregivers assume that the dyspnea is due to being "out of shape," although this should be a diagnosis of exclusion. The majority of patients with chronic dyspnea of unclear etiology have one of four diagnoses: asthma, COPD, interstitial lung disease, or cardiac dysfunction.

The important facts to determine are the onset, progression, precipitating factors, type and level of provocative activity, associated symptoms (chest pain, leg edema, syncope or near syncope, fatigue), other conditions (arthritis, connective tissue disease, cardiac disease, smoking), and drug or toxin exposure. Asking about the quality of dyspnea can differentiate causes. Dyspnea secondary to deconditioning is usually described as "heavy breathing," and one can often determine that the patient is actually describing fatigue more than true dyspnea. The bronchoconstriction in exacerbations of asthma is more commonly described as "tightness" or "air hunger," whereas patients with COPD complain of "not being able to take a deep breath" or "an increased effort to breathe." Patients with heart failure feel as though they are "suffocating" or have "air hunger."[33] Orthopnea (dyspnea while recumbent) suggests heart failure or sleep apnea. Coughing can be a symptom of heart failure, asthma, or COPD. Angina or a history of CAD may indicate heart failure. Anorexic drugs can cause pulmonary hypertension or valvular abnormalities. Connective tissue disease is associated with interstitial lung disease. On physical examination one should look for pallor, cyanosis, a "barrel" chest, rales, wheezing, crackles, murmurs, abnormal heart sounds or rhythms, an enlarged heart, tachycardia, jugular venous distention, joint involvement, clubbing, fibrotic skin changes, and edema. Patients with severe airflow obstruction may have pursed lips and a slow deep breathing pattern, and those with interstitial fibrosis or kyphoscoliosis typically have rapid shallow breathing.

The preoperative history and physical examination lead to accurate diagnoses in two thirds of cases. Initial testing may include an ECG, hematocrit (to exclude anemia), arterial blood gas analysis, thyroid function tests, a chest radiograph, spirometry, and oximetry at rest and while walking several feet. BNP levels may be useful. Most dyspnea patients with heart failure have BNP values higher than 400 pg/mL, whereas left ventricular dysfunction without exacerbation, pulmonary embolism, and cor pulmonale should be considered in dyspnea patients with plasma BNP concentrations between 100 and 400 pg/mL. Other testing depends on findings on these tests and is directed by the history and physical examination. Computed tomography scans and cardiopulmonary exercise testing are rarely necessary but can be useful if the aforementioned tests are not diagnostic.

Patients with Risk Factors for Postoperative Pulmonary Complications

Postoperative pulmonary complications develop in 5% to 10% of patients undergoing nonthoracic surgery and in 22% of high-risk patients. As many as one in four deaths occurring within a week of surgery are related to pulmonary complications, thus making it the second most common serious morbidity after cardiovascular adverse events.[50,51]

Established risk factors for an increased risk for pulmonary complications include the following[52]:

- History of cigarette use (current or >40 pack-years)
- ASA-PS scores higher than 2
- Age >70 years
- COPD
- Neck, thoracic, upper abdominal, aortic, or neurologic surgery
- Anticipated prolonged procedures (>2 hours)
- Planned general anesthesia (especially with endotracheal intubation)
- Albumin less than 3 g/dL
- Exercise capacity of less than two blocks or one flight of stairs
- BMI greater than 30

Surprisingly absent predictors in this list are asthma and results from arterial blood gas analysis or PFTs. The risk for complications is surprisingly low in patients with well-controlled asthma or those treated preoperatively with corticosteroids.[53] The risk is greater in asthmatics with recent exacerbations or a history of postoperative pulmonary complications or recent hospitalization or intubation for asthma. Arterial blood gas analysis is useful in predicting pulmonary function after lung resection surgery but does not predict risk for complications. The degree of airway obstruction, measured by FEV_1, is not predictive of pulmonary complications.[54] PFTs, arterial blood gas analysis, or chest radiographs should not be used routinely to predict the risk for postoperative pulmonary complications. PFTs may be indicated to diagnose disease (dyspnea caused by lung disease or heart failure?) or to assess management (can dyspnea or wheezing be improved further?) but should *not* be used as a risk assessment tool or to deny a beneficial procedure.[54]

Laboratory results and patient- and procedure-related determinants of risk for perioperative pulmonary complications have recently been reviewed in the literature.[55] Some of these factors can be modified to alter risk. The pulmonary status of patients with recent exacerbations or infections should be improved whenever possible. Prescriptions for antibiotics, bronchodilators, and steroids, referral to pulmonologists or internists, and postponing surgery are important in patients at high risk. Training patients preoperatively in lung expansion maneuvers, such as deep-breathing exercises and incentive spirometry, reduces pulmonary complications more than training postoperatively does. Additionally, a change in perioperative management, including altering the planned surgical procedure if possible, discussing alternatives to general anesthesia, especially when peripheral nerve blocks are an option, and educating the patient about the benefits of epidural pain management, may provide effective measures to decrease pulmonary complications.[56]

Patients Scheduled for Lung Resection

Most patients scheduled for lung resection surgery have underlying lung disease, and PFTs may be useful in predicting risk or excluding patients who may not have adequate pulmonary reserve after resection. This topic is covered more fully in Chapter 59.

Pulmonary Hypertension

Pulmonary hypertension may occur in isolation or with associated medical conditions and is classified into five groups (Box 34-6) according to the World Health Organization. Idiopathic

Box 34-6 Classification of Pulmonary Hypertension

Pulmonary Arterial Hypertension
Primary pulmonary hypertension
- Sporadic
- Familial

Associated with
- Collagen vascular disease
- Congenital shunts
- Portal hypertension
- Human immunodeficiency virus infection
- Drugs/toxins
- Persistent pulmonary hypertension of the newborn

Pulmonary Venous Hypertension
Left-sided heart disease
Extrinsic compression of central pulmonary veins
Pulmonary veno-occlusive disease

Pulmonary Hypertension Related to Lung Disease or Hypoxemia
Chronic obstructive pulmonary disease
Interstitial lung disease
Sleep-disordered breathing
Neonatal lung disease
Chronic exposure to high altitude

Pulmonary Hypertension Caused by Chronic Thromboembolic Disease
Pulmonary thrombosis or embolism
Sickle cell disease

Pulmonary Hypertension from Disorders Directly Affecting the Pulmonary Vasculature
Schistosomiasis
Sarcoidosis

Available from http://www.who.int/ncd/cvd/pph.html.

pulmonary arterial hypertension, formerly called primary pulmonary hypertension, is rare, but other forms are more common and occur with a variety of diseases, including cardiac, pulmonary, liver, thromboembolic, and collagen vascular disease. Pulmonary hypertension is associated with HIV infection, exposure to anorexics such as fenfluramine, chronic liver disease, especially if portal hypertension is present, and collagen vascular diseases, including scleroderma, SLE, and rheumatoid arthritis. Pulmonary hypertension is defined as a persistent elevation in mean pulmonary artery pressure greater than 25 mm Hg with a pulmonary artery occlusion pressure of less than 15 mm Hg. Occult pulmonary hypertension is more problematic than fully recognized disease because symptoms may be attributed to other diseases and perioperative decompensation may occur unexpectedly.

The manifestation of pulmonary hypertension is usually nonspecific, insidious, and associated with delayed diagnosis. Dyspnea is the initial symptom in 60% of patients but is present in 98% by the time of diagnosis. Dyspnea is nonspecific and associated with a multitude of conditions (see the section "Dyspnea"). Near syncope or syncopal episodes suggest severe disease. Hypoxia, hypercapnia, vasoconstrictors, and increased sympathetic tone (even from anxiety) increase pulmonary vascular resistance and lead to acute decompensation with right heart failure.

Patients with pulmonary arterial hypertension have a high rate of perioperative morbidity and mortality.[57] Mild pulmonary hypertension rarely affects anesthetic management, but moderate to severe disease increases the risk for right heart failure. Signs and symptoms of disease severity include[58]

- Dyspnea at rest
- Metabolic acidosis
- Hypoxemia
- Right heart failure (peripheral edema, hepatomegaly, jugular venous distention)
- History of syncope

Physical examination may reveal a split S_2 with a loud second component, right ventricular heave, a murmur of tricuspid regurgitation, ascites, hepatomegaly, jugular venous distention, and peripheral edema.

An echocardiogram is the screening test of choice and can used to estimate pulmonary artery pressure, assess right ventricular function, and identify left heart failure and valvular or congenital heart disease.[59] Patients with significant findings may require right and left heart catheterization, although the need for catheterization preoperatively depends on the surgical procedure. An ECG, chest radiograph, and echocardiogram are useful in patients with more than mild disease. Findings on the ECG include right axis deviation, RBBB, right ventricular hypertrophy, and tall R waves in leads V_1 and V_2. Right atrial hypertrophy and "P pulmonale" may be present in severe pulmonary hypertension, with peaked P waves most apparent in leads II, III, aVF, and V_1. Enlargement of the main pulmonary artery and a globular heart shape with loss of the retrosternal air space as a result of right ventricular dilation can be seen on the chest radiograph. Evaluators should inquire about a history of OSA, which can also be the cause of pulmonary hypertension.[60] A CBC with platelets, electrolytes, BUN, creatinine, and liver function tests (LFTs; may be elevated as a result of congestion or the use of bosentan) are needed.

Preoperatively, patients may be treated with diuretics, anticoagulants, calcium channel blockers, supplemental oxygen, sildenafil (a phosphodiesterase inhibitor), endothelin receptor antagonists (bosentan), and prostanoids (iloprost, epoprostenol). Some of these agents are given by continuous intravenous infusion, and even momentary interruption of therapy can be catastrophic. All drugs need to be continued preoperatively. Management of these patients in conjunction with a pulmonary hypertension specialist is advised.

Smokers and Those Exposed to Second-Hand Smoke

Exposure to tobacco, directly or through "second-hand" smoke, increases the risk for many perioperative complications. Smokers are more likely to experience wound infections, respiratory or airway complications (including oxygen desaturation), and severe coughing.[61] Smoking decreases macrophage function, negatively affects coronary flow reserve, and causes vascular endothelial dysfunction, hypertension, and ischemia. Smokers require longer hospital stays than nonsmokers do and often need postoperative intensive care admission.

The greatest benefit of smoking abstinence is probably realized only after several months of cessation. In studies reporting greater perioperative risk in recent quitters than in smokers, selection bias may have contributed to the results. Patients who were motivated to stop or advised to quit smoking may have been at greater risk because of health status. Soon after a patient quits smoking, carbon monoxide levels decrease, which improves oxygen delivery and utilization. Cyanide levels decrease, which benefits mitochondrial oxidative metabolism. Lower nicotine levels improve vasodilation, and many toxic substances that impair wound healing decrease. Patients without a history of ischemic heart disease who smoked shortly before surgery had significantly more episodes of rate-pressure product–related ST-segment depression than did nonsmokers, former smokers, or chronic smokers who did not smoke in the immediate preoperative period.[62]

A preoperative smoking cessation intervention in patients who underwent knee and hip replacement decreased rates of surgical site infection (SSI) from 23% in the conventional group to 4% in those who stopped smoking. The U.S. Public Health Service recommends that "*all* physicians should strongly advise every patient who smokes to quit because evidence shows that physician advice to quit smoking increases abstinence rates."[63] Nearly 70% of smokers want to quit.

Effective interventions include medical advice and pharmacotherapy, such as nicotine replacement therapy, which is safe in the perioperative period (see Chapter 35). Nicotine patches, gum, and lozenges are available without a prescription; nasal spray and buproprion (Wellbutrin) require prescriptions. Clonidine is also effective. Buproprion or clonidine should be started 1 to 2 weeks before an attempt at quitting; nicotine replacement therapy is effective immediately.[64] Individual and group counseling may increase rates of long-term abstinence. Many hospitals, insurance companies, and communities offer smoking cessation programs. Excellent resources are available on the Internet and from the U.S. government. Advice and guidelines are available at http://www.surgeongeneral.gov/tobacco/default.htm. Tobacco intervention training during medical school and residency can significantly improve the quality of physician counseling and rates of abstinence.

Endocrine Disorders (See also Chapter 35)

Diabetes Mellitus

Type 1 diabetes is an autoimmune disease that results in destruction of pancreatic insulin-producing (beta) cells; patients have an absolute deficiency of insulin but normal sensitivity to insulin, are at risk for ketoacidosis, and generally have an onset of disease at a younger age. Because of the often-difficult nature of control and the long duration of disease, by the time that these individuals reach adulthood, they are at increased risk for premature vascular disease, especially myocardial ischemia, even in the second decade of life. Type 2 diabetes is initially a result of insulin resistance, which with time can result in pancreatic "burnout," and is usually found in older, overweight adults. Using terms such as insulin dependent, non–insulin dependent, or adult onset is confusing and not recommended.

In the United States, approximately 20 million persons have diabetes, with 1 million new cases diagnosed each year. In as many as a third of patients, the disease is diagnosed only after significant diabetes-related complications develop. Unfortunately, the symptoms of diabetes are nonspecific, so the history, other than a family history of the disease, is not reliable in screening for the disease. However, patients who are overweight, have excessive abdominal fat (even if their BMI is normal), take steroids, or have polycystic ovarian syndrome are at increased risk. Certain ethnic groups (Native American, non-Hispanic black, Hispanic, and Asian American) have a higher incidence. Diabetes develops in females twice as commonly as in males.

Diabetics are at risk for multiorgan dysfunction, with renal insufficiency, stroke, peripheral neuropathy, autonomic dysfunction, and cardiovascular disease being most prevalent. Delayed gastric emptying, retinopathy, and reduced joint mobility occur in these patients. Diabetes is considered a CAD equivalent and an intermediate risk factor for perioperative cardiac complications, on a par with angina or a previous MI.[7] Diabetic patients without known coronary stenosis or angina have the same risk of myocardial ischemia or cardiac death as a nondiabetic with a previous MI.[65] Autonomic neuropathy is the best predictor of silent ischemia. Erectile dysfunction has been shown to be a strong predictor as well. Poorly controlled blood glucose and longer duration of disease also correlate with cardiac risk. See the section "Ischemic Heart Disease" and Figure 34-2 for further guidance on this topic.

Heart failure is twice as common in men and five times as common in women with diabetes as in those without diabetes. Poor glycemic control is associated with an increased risk for heart failure, and both systolic and diastolic dysfunction may be present. Diabetics are at increased risk for renal failure perioperatively and for postoperative infections. Recent studies suggest that tighter perioperative control may be warranted. Patients with poor preoperative management of glucose are likely to be more out of control intraoperatively and postoperatively. Aggressive management of hyperglycemia decreases postoperative complications.

Chronic kidney disease is usually asymptomatic until quite advanced. Diabetes is responsible for almost half of the patients requiring dialysis in the United States. The combination of hypertension, diabetes, and age older than 55 years accounts for more than 90% of patients with renal insufficiency. "Screening" for kidney disease is accepted practice in patients with diabetes. Patients with poorly controlled diabetes are at risk for the development of stiff joint syndrome with reduced cervical mobility, which may influence airway management.

The preoperative evaluation should focus on assessing organ damage and control of blood sugar. Cardiovascular, renal, and neurologic systems need close evaluation. Ischemic heart disease is often asymptomatic in diabetics. Inquiring about early satiety, erectile dysfunction, numbness in the hands and feet, and postprandial vomiting is important. Documenting pulses, skin breakdown, a sensory examination, and orthostatic vital signs (BP and HR both lying and standing) are important in most diabetics, especially those with long-standing disease or poor control. Patients with autonomic dysfunction or hypovolemia will have greater than a 20–mm Hg drop in systolic or greater than a 10–mm Hg decrease in diastolic BP pressure when assuming an upright position from recumbency.

A preoperative ECG plus determination of electrolytes, BUN, creatinine, and blood glucose is recommended for all diabetic patients. Frequently, patients are not fasting when evaluated in a preoperative clinic, and relying on reported glucose values is problematic. If patients bring a diary of multiple glucose values at varying times of the day (preprandial and postprandial), one can estimate the adequacy of therapy. However, patients often will only randomly check AM fasting blood glucose, which is likely to be lower because of an overnight fast than glucose values obtained later in the day. The glycosolated hemoglobin (HbA_{1c}) level is not influenced by fasting and, if available, can identify those with poor control. The American Diabetes Association recommends a target HbA_{1c} of less than 7%. Suggestions for hypoglycemic medication management on the day of surgery are discussed in Chapter 35. The goals of perioperative diabetic management include avoidance of hypoglycemia and marked hyperglycemia. The American College of Endocrinologists position statement recommends a target fasting glucose level of less than 110 mg/dL in noncritically ill hospitalized patients.[66]

Thyroid Disease

Thyroid hormones are important for metabolism and its regulation. Mild to moderate dysfunction probably has minimal impact perioperatively. Significant hyperthyroidism or hypothyroidism appears to increase perioperative risk. Hyperthyroid patients may have tachycardia, arrhythmias, palpitations, tremors, weight loss, and diarrhea. Hypothyroid patients may be hypotensive, bradycardic, and lethargic and exhibit weight gain, depressed cardiac function, pericardial effusions, and an impaired ventilatory response to hypoxia and hypercapnia. Symptoms and findings of both hypothyroidism and hyperthyroidism can be subtle and nonspecific, especially in the elderly. Patients may have goiters with related symptoms such as dysphagia, dyspnea, wheezing, and orthopnea. Grave's ophthalmopathy or proptosis is more common in smokers. Patients taking amiodarone are at risk for hypothyroidism and require evaluation of thyroid function before surgery.

Determination of medical therapy is important. Patients with a history of chronic thyroid disease need thyroid function tests before surgery. If symptomatology and therapy have not changed, tests within the 6 month before surgery are generally adequate. Thyroid-stimulating hormone (TSH) assays are best to evaluate for hypothyroidism. Measuring both *free* triiodothyronine (T_3) and thyroxine (T_4) and TSH is useful in hyperthyroid patients and avoids the confusion of protein-binding effects seen with total hormone levels. Elective surgery should be postponed until patients are euthyroid. Surgery, stress, or illness can precipitate myxedema or thyroid storm in patients with untreated or severe thyroid dysfunction. Preoperative consultation with an endocrinologist should be considered if surgery is urgent in patients with clinical thyroid dysfunction. Hyperthryoid patients should be treated with β-blockers, antithyroid medications, and steroids if surgery is urgent. Chest radiography or computed tomography is useful to evaluate tracheal or mediastinal involvement by a goiter. Continuation of medications (thyroid replacement and antithyroid drugs such as propylthiouracil) on the day of surgery is important.

Parathyroid Disease

Parathyroid hormone regulates calcium, and most cases of hyperparathyroidism are discovered when an elevated calcium level is found incidentally during diagnostic testing. Primary hyperparathyroidism is caused by a primary disorder of the parathyroid glands (adenomas or hyperplasia). Secondary hyperparathyroidism is hyperplasia of the parathyroid gland caused by hyperphosphatemia and hypocalcemia from chronic renal failure. Tertiary hyperparathyroidism occurs when the parathyroid hyperplasia in secondary hyperparathyroidism functions autonomously and results in hypercalcemia. Hypercalcemia from parathyroid disease is associated with osteoporosis and bone loss. Rarely, the parathyroid glands can become so enlarged that they compromise the airway. Hypoparathyroidism is rare but can result from total parathyroidectomy. Hypercalcemia and hypocalcemia are discussed in the section on calcium disorders.

Hypothalamic-Pituitary-Adrenal Disorders

Corticotropin-releasing hormone is released by the hypothalamus and regulates adrenocorticotropic hormone (ACTH) from the anterior pituitary gland, which in turn regulates cortisol from the adrenal cortex. A key component is the negative-feedback suppression by endogenous or exogenous glucocorticoids. Cortisol secretion varies with the circadian rhythm, being highest in the morning and with stress, fever, hypoglycemia, and surgery. Surgery is one of the most potent activators of the hypothalamic-pituitary-adrenal (HPA) axis. ACTH concentrations increase with incision and during surgery, but the greatest secretion of ACTH occurs during reversal of anesthesia, during extubation, and in the immediate postoperative period.

Excess adrenal hormone results from glucocorticoid treatment of disorders such as asthma or inflammatory diseases or from pituitary or adrenal tumors. Cushing's disease denotes the constellation of findings associated with a pituitary tumor; Cushing's syndrome refers to the same findings resulting from either an adrenal tumor or hyperplasia, ectopic ACTH from neoplasms, or exogenous steroids.

Preoperative findings on evaluation include significant hypertension, weight gain, myopathy, diabetes, moon facies, and a buffalo hump, which can influence airway management. Striae, virilization in females, and easy bruising are common. Exogenous steroids will suppress the adrenals, and the normal hypersecretion expected from stress or surgery will be blunted. Therefore, patients at risk will need "steroid coverage," which is discussed in Chapter 35. An ECG and electrolyte and glucose levels should be obtained preoperatively for most surgical procedures. Despite bruising easily, patients have normal coagulation profiles.

Adrenal insufficiency results from destruction of the pituitary or adrenal glands or from long-term administration of exogenous glucocorticoid. Tuberculosis and HIV infection can cause primary hypoadrenalism. Prednisone or its equivalent in doses of greater 20 mg/day for longer than 3 weeks suppresses the HPA axis. The HPA axis is not suppressed with doses of less than 5 mg/day of prednisone or its equivalent. Intermediate doses of steroids taken for longer than 3 weeks have equivocal effects on the HPA axis. The risk remains for up to 1 year after cessation of steroids. Patients with adrenal insufficiency exhibit weakness, weight loss, hypotension, orthostasis, hypovolemia, hyperpigmentation, and electrolyte abnormalities. Electrolytes and orthostatic vital signs should be evaluated.

Serum cortisol and plasma ACTH can establish the diagnosis and cause of adrenal insufficiency in most cases. If the serum cortisol concentration is inappropriately low and a simultaneous plasma ACTH concentration is very high, primary adrenal insufficiency (primary adrenal disease) is the cause. Secondary (pituitary disease) or tertiary (hypothalamic disease) insufficiency is the diagnosis if both the serum cortisol and plasma ACTH concentrations are inappropriately low. However, in more urgent situations one may not be able to wait for the ACTH results, so an ACTH stimulation test can be performed unless the diagnosis has been ruled out by a basal serum cortisol value in the upper end of the reference range or higher.[67] Cosyntropin is synthetic ACTH and can be administered in either a high-dose or a low-dose test. The time of day is not important because in patients with adrenal insufficiency, the response to cosyntropin is the same in the morning and afternoon. A normal response to the high-dose (250 μg as an intravenous bolus) ACTH stimulation test is a rise in serum cortisol concentration, measured after 30 to 60 minutes, to a peak of 18 to 20 μg/dL or greater. Low-dose (1-μg intravenous bolus) ACTH causes a rise in cortisol of 17 to 22.5 μg/dL or greater after 20 to 30 minutes. For both tests, a subnormal response confirms the diagnosis of adrenal insufficiency, but further studies are necessary to establish the type and cause.

Preoperative electrolytes should be evaluated and an ECG obtained if appropriate. Patients continue steroids on the day of surgery and may need supplementation with additional doses (see the section on medication).

Aldosterone, which is produced by the adrenal cortex, regulates volume and electrolytes (absorption of sodium and chloride, secretion of potassium and hydrogen ions) and is controlled by renin-angiotensin, not the HPA axis.

Multiple Endocrine Neoplasia Syndromes

The multiple endocrine neoplasia (MEN) syndromes are rare, but recognition is important both for treatment and for evaluation of family members.[68] MEN type II (MEN II) is subclassified into three distinct syndromes: MEN IIA, MEN IIB, and familial medullary thyroid cancer. Inheritance of MEN I and II is autosomal dominant.

Hyperparathyroidism is the most common manifestation of MEN I, with almost 100% penetrance by 40 to 50 years of age. Hypersecretion of gastrin in MEN I in association with Zollinger-Ellison syndrome is often manifested as multiple peptic ulcers. The *MEN1* gene has been identified, and therefore testing for *MEN1* mutations is possible. There is little evidence that early, presymptomatic detection reduces morbidity or mortality in MEN I. Screening of asymptomatic family members can also be done by measurement of serum calcium because of the high penetrance of hyperparathyroidism in MEN I.

An undiagnosed pheochromocytoma can cause substantial morbidity or even death during surgery. It is important to consider this preoperative diagnosis as a component of possible MEN II and, if present, remove the tumor before eliminating other endocrine tumors. Extra-adrenal pheochromocytoma is rare in MEN II, but bilateral adrenal disease is common. It is unusual for pheochromocytoma to precede the development of medullary thyroid carcinoma or be the initial manifestation of MEN II.

Hyperparathyroidism in MEN IIA is often clinically occult. DNA testing is the optimal test in MEN II syndromes. In contrast to MEN I, in which the long-term benefit of early diagnosis by genetic screening is not well established, early diagnosis by screening of at-risk family members in MEN II kindreds is essential because medullary thyroid carcinoma is a life-threatening disease that can be cured or prevented by early thyroidectomy.

Please refer to the appropriate sections in this chapter for discussion of the preoperative evaluation of patients with thyroid, hyperparathyroid, and pituitary diseases and pheochromocytomas.

Pheochromocytoma

Tumors that arise from chromaffin cells of the adrenal medulla and sympathetic ganglia and secrete catecholamines are referred to as pheochromocytomas and extra-adrenal catecholamine-secreting paragangliomas (extra-adrenal pheochromocytomas), respectively.[69] The term "pheochromocytoma" is often used for both types of tumors because of similar clinical findings and therapies. Pheochromocytomas are discovered when patients have symptoms, a family history, or discovery of an incidental adrenal mass. Approximately 3% to 10% of adrenal incidentalomas prove to be pheochromocytomas. The classic triad of symptoms is episodic headache, sweating, and tachycardia. Paroxysmal hypertension occurs in half of the patients. Many of the rest have what appears to be essential hypertension. Approximately 5% to 15% of patients have normal BP.

Preoperative evaluation may demonstrate paroxysmal hypertension, which is a classic sign of pheochromocytoma; however, patients with this finding rarely have the disorder. Headache, which is variable in severity and duration, occurs in up to 90% of symptomatic patients. Sweating occurs in up to 60% to 70% of patients. Other symptoms include palpitations, dyspnea, weakness, and panic attacks (particularly with pheochromocytomas that produce an increase in epinephrine). Pallor, orthostatic hypotension, blurred vision, weight loss, polyuria, polydipsia, hyperglycemia, psychiatric disorders, cardiopulmonary dysfunction (especially with the initiation of β-adrenergic blockers), and dilated cardiomyopathy are due to excess catecholamines. Marked hypertension has also been reported.

Pheochromocytoma should be suspected in patients who have one or more of the following:

- Hyperadrenergic spells (nonexertional palpitations, diaphoresis, headache, tremor, pallor)
- Difficult-to-control hypertension
- A familial syndrome that includes catecholamine-secreting tumors (MEN II, neurofibromatosis 1, von Hippel-Lindau disease), often with bilateral disease
- A family history of pheochromocytoma
- An incidentally discovered adrenal mass
- Unusual BP response during anesthesia, surgery, or angiography
- Hypertension at a young age (e.g., <20 years old)
- Idiopathic dilated cardiomyopathy
- A history of gastric stromal tumor or pulmonary chondromas (Carney's triad)

Preoperative measurements of urinary and plasma fractionated metanephrines and catecholamines generally establishes the diagnosis. The history and physical examination focus on the cardiovascular system and evaluation of vital signs, orthostatic BP, and findings of heart failure. An ECG and determination of electrolytes, BUN, creatinine, and glucose should be performed in all patients. Computed tomography, echocardiography, and cardiac consultation may be useful. A complete discussion of the anesthetic implications can be found in Chapter 35.

Renal Disease

The type and degree of impairment are important. Patients with renal dysfunction have many associated comorbid conditions that are generally related to the accompanying vasculopathy (see Chapters 18 and 45). Hypertension, cardiovascular disease, and electrolyte disturbances are most common. Chronic kidney disease (CKD) is defined as a decreased glomular filtration rate (GFR <60 mL/min/1.73 m^2) for at least 3 months or significant proteinuria. Chronic renal failure is defined as a GFR of less than 15 mL/min/1.73 m^2; acute renal failure (ARF) is a sudden decrease in renal function with a urine output of less than 0.5 mL/kg/hr. End-stage renal disease (ESRD) is loss of renal function for 3 or more months. Diabetes accounts for almost half of all cases of ESRD, hypertension for more than a quarter, and the combination of these plus age older than 55 years predicts more than 90% of cases. Polycystic kidney disease (autosomal dominant 90% of the time) is the causative factor in 10% of cases of ESRD and can be associated with intracranial aneurysms and mitral valve prolapse.

ARF may be reversible if precipitating factors are identified and corrected. Dividing ARF into prerenal, renal, and postrenal categories allows a systematic approach. Prerenal causes can often be differentiated by calculating the BUN-creatinine ratio. A ratio of 20 or greater suggests a prerenal cause, with hypovolemia or hypotension being most common. Fractional excretion of sodium (FE_{Na}) of less than 1% also suggests prerenal azotemia and can be calculated by the following formula:

$$FE_{Na} = \frac{P_{Cr}/U_{Cr}}{P_{Na}/U_{Na}}$$

Obstruction will result in dilated ureters and enlarged kidneys and is always in the differential diagnosis of ARF. Prompt identification with ultrasound leads to attempts to decompress the outflow tract. Rhabdomyolysis can cause ARF and is treatable.

GFR decreases with age, and the renal reserve of a normal 80-year-old is less than half that of a 40-year-old. The creatinine level is often not an accurate indicator of renal function, especially in elderly individuals. A doubling of serum creatinine from 0.8 to 1.6 mg/dL represents a halving of the GFR. The GFR can be reduced 50% or more without a rise in creatinine. Creatinine does not exceed the normal limits until the GFR has fallen below 50 mL/min. The Cockcroft-Gault formula can be used to estimate GFR:

$$\text{Creatinine clearance} = \frac{(140 - \text{Age}) \times \text{Weight (kg)} \times (0.85 \text{ if female})}{72 \times \text{Serum creatinine (mg/dL)}}$$

Online calculators to estimate renal function are available at www.nephron.com. Calculation of an eGFR can be done in elderly patients, those with an elevated serum creatinine, or individuals with other risk factors for CKD.

Chronic renal disease is a significant risk factor for cardiovascular morbidity and mortality and is an ACC/AHA intermediate cardiac risk factor considered to be equal to angina, MI, or a history of known CAD. The annual incidence of death from CAD in patients with both diabetes and ESRD who require hemodialysis is 8.2%. A creatinine concentration of 2.0 mg/dL or higher should trigger an assessment of cardiac risk under the ACC/AHA guidelines, simplified in Figure 34-2.[7] See the section "Ischemic Heart Disease" for a more detailed discussion of these guidelines. Pericarditis, pericardial effusions, and diastolic and systolic dysfunction can be present. Valvular heart disease is common in patients undergoing maintenance dialysis. Abnormalities include valvular and annular thickening and, most significantly, calcification of the heart valves resulting in regurgitation or stenosis (or both).[70] Mitral and aortic valve calcifications (40% and 55% of patients, respectively) and stenosis (11% to 13%) occur. Valvular calcifications progress to stenosis at an accelerated rate in dialysis patients.[71] Systemic hypertension is almost ubiquitous but is generally easier to manage with initiation of dialysis. Pulmonary hypertension and increased cardiac output occur in many patients with an arteriovenous fistula.

Renal failure results in anemia from lack of erythropoietin production by the kidneys, but in the present era of aggressive erythropoietin replacement, many of these patients have normal or high hematocrits, which actually increases morbidity and vascular events.[30] Patients with CKD can have platelet dysfunction and increased bleeding despite a normal platelet count, prothrombin time (PT), and aPTT. Once on dialysis, patients are more prone to hypercoagulable states. Chronic metabolic acidosis is common but usually mild and compensated for by chronic hyperventilation. Patients may exhibit electrolyte and calcium abnormalities, pulmonary and peripheral edema, anemia, hypercholesterolemia, and hypoalbuminemia. Hyperkalemia is the most serious electrolyte disturbance. Hypocalcemia is common with dialysis, and eventually secondary and tertiary hyperparathyroidism develops. Chronically elevated troponin and creatine kinase levels are common in patients maintained on dialysis. Worsening renal function should be suspected in diabetics who have improved glycemic control or unexpected hypoglycemia because insulin is metabolized by the kidneys and has a prolonged duration of action with progressive renal dysfunction. Autonomic and peripheral (sensory and motor) neuropathies can occur.

Patients at risk for perioperative renal failure include those with preexisting renal insufficiency (the single strongest predictor) or diabetes, especially in combination, and those undergoing procedures with the administration of contrast medium. If all three conditions are present, the risk of renal failure may be as high as 12% to 50%. Preoperative identification of at-risk patients alters management, such as hydration, administration of sodium bicarbonate, a change in the type of contrast medium, and avoidance of hypovolemia (see Chapter 65). This may require admission preoperatively. Nonsteroidal anti-inflammatory drugs (NSAIDs) and cyclooxygenase (COX-2) inhibitors interfere with autoregulation of renal perfusion and should be avoided or discontinued in patients with or at risk for renal insufficiency. Cyclosporine and aminoglycoside antibiotics can cause renal insufficiency. ACEIs and ARBs prevent deterioration in patients with diabetes or renal insufficiency but may worsen function during hypoperfusion states.

Many drugs are metabolized or cleared by the kidneys. Drugs with particular implications for anesthesia and surgery are the LMWHs because there is no easy method of monitoring their anticoagulation effects. All the LMWHs available in the United States are cleared by the kidneys and are not removed during dialysis. Therefore, LMWH has a prolonged duration of action in patients with CKD. The risk of significant bleeding or hematomas with centroneuraxial anesthesia may be increased.

Preoperative evaluation of patients with renal insufficiency or failure should focus on the cardiovascular and cerebrovascular systems, fluid volume, and electrolyte status. The early stages of

CKD typically cause no symptoms. Inquiring about the cardiovascular systems (chest pain, orthopnea, paroxysmal nocturnal dyspnea), urine output, associated comorbid conditions, medications, and dialysis schedules is vital. Understanding changes in patient weight is one method of assessing volume status.

In patients with or at risk for renal disease (especially those with two of the following: diabetes, poorly controlled hypertension, advanced age), an ECG and determination of electrolytes, calcium, glucose, albumin, BUN, and creatinine should be performed if the results will have an impact on management. LVH (from hypertension), peaked T waves (hypokalemia), flattened T waves, and prolonged PR and QT intervals (hypokalemia) prompt further evaluation. A chest radiograph (infection or volume overload), echocardiogram (for murmurs or heart failure), and stress testing (see ACC/AHA guidelines) may be indicated in certain patients. Many of these patients will benefit from cardiology evaluation based on these tests as discussed earlier. Venous access or blood draws from the brachial, cephalic (antecubital), and central veins in the nondominant upper extremity should be avoided in patients who may need fistulas for dialysis in the future.

Preoperative renal replacement therapy (dialysis) schedules should be determined, with scheduling of surgery ideally within 24 hours after dialysis. In elective cases, dialysis is best performed within 24 hours of surgery but not immediately before because of acute volume depletion and electrolyte alterations. Dialysis is associated with fluid and electrolyte (sodium, potassium, magnesium, phosphate) imbalance and shifting of electrolytes between the intracellular and extracellular compartments. Dialysis should be performed to correct volume overload, hyperkalemia, and acidosis. Coordinating the scheduling of dialysis and elective surgery is an important aspect of preoperative care.

Contrast-Induced Nephropathy

Contrast-induced nephropathy is defined as a 25% rise in creatinine above baseline after the administration of a radiocontrast agent (see Chapter 79). Patients with diabetes and CKD are at greatest risk, although radiocontrast media causes a transient decrease in the GFR in most individuals. Renal failure requiring dialysis after contrast-induced nephropathy is associated with less than a 20% 2-year survival rate, and a third of patients die during the initial hospitalization.

Hepatic Disorders

Liver disease can affect hepatocytes, the biliary system, or both (see Chapters 17 and 66). Liver disease affects protein synthesis, including coagulation factors and albumin, drug and toxin metabolism, and bile regulation. Hepatocellular diseases, including viral, alcoholic, and autoimmune hepatitis or hepatocellular carcinoma, affect hepatocytes and synthetic function of the liver. Obstructive disorders, including choledocholithiasis and bile duct tumors (extrahepatic), primary biliary cirrhosis (intrahepatic), or primary sclerosing cholangitis (extrahepatic and intrahepatic), cause bile stasis. Most drug-induced liver disease and some forms of viral hepatitis affect both hepatocytes and the biliary system.

Hepatitis

Hepatitis is a term used to describe inflammation of hepatocytes and can be caused by drugs, alcohol, viruses (hepatitis A, B, C, D, and E), or autoimmune diseases. All of these conditions have acute and chronic phases that can progress to cirrhosis, which is irreversible fibrosis of the liver. Risk factors for hepatitis are alcohol use, sexual activity (multiple partners, sex industry workers, sex with sex industry workers, or men who have sex with men), intravenous drug use, blood transfusions before 1992, travel to underdeveloped countries, obesity, tattoos, and body piercing. Hepatitis A is caused by contaminated food or water or contact with an infected person and rarely progresses beyond the acute illness. A remote history of hepatitis A has no significance perioperatively. Hepatitis B is transmitted by sexual activity or contact with blood (rarely from transfusions since screening was implemented in 1986). It varies in severity but is much less common since the widespread use of vaccination against this virus. Hepatitis C is caused primarily by blood exposure (blood has been screened since 1992), most often in intravenous drug users. Many patients are unaware of infection because the acute phase is frequently asymptomatic but can advance to cirrhosis. Hepatitis D occurs only with hepatitis B, and hepatitis E is rare in developed countries. Alcoholic hepatitis generally occurs after at least 10 years of daily moderate to heavy alcohol intake (>3 drinks/day for women; >5/day for men) and may progress to cirrhosis. Autoimmune hepatitis primarily affects young women and has no known cause. Virtually any drug, as well as herbals and over-the-counter preparations, can cause hepatitis, including statins, isoniazid, and acetaminophen.

Obstructive Jaundice

Extrahepatic bile duct obstruction is caused by gallstones, tumors (pancreatic, gallbladder, bile duct, ampulla of Vater), or scarring. Patients may have jaundice, pruritus, and abdominal pain. Predictors of surgical mortality are a preoperative hemocrit of less than 30%, bilirubin concentration greater than 11 mg/dL, and malignancy, and death may occur in as many as 60% if all three are present.[72] Renal failure develops in up to 8% of these patients postoperatively, which may be lessened with administration of bile salts or lactulose.[73]

Miscellaneous Liver Diseases

Wilson's disease, hemochromatosis, and α_1-antitrypsin deficiency are less common than hepatitis, are hereditary, and commonly occur in members of the same family. Obesity can result in nonalcoholic steatohepatitis, also known as "fatty liver," which causes abnormal LFT results and can progress to fibrosis. Primary biliary cirrhosis is an autoimmune disorder that results in intrahepatic biliary obstruction; it occurs most frequently in middle-aged women and is associated with antimitochondrial antibodies. Primary sclerosing cholangitis destroys bile ducts, is most frequent in young males, is associated with inflammatory bowel disease but can be idiopathic, and may progress to cirrhosis. Acute illnesses such as sepsis, surgery, and anesthesia can cause hepatic dysfunction. Gilbert's syndrome is a benign familial disorder with mildly elevated bilirubin and has no perioperative significance.

Remote History of "Hepatitis"

Patients may recount a history of "having hepatitis" many years before but little other information is known. One must take a careful preoperative history to determine circumstances surrounding the onset (e.g., transfusions, travel, exposure to risky situations) and whether any sequelae of chronic liver disease are present. It is important to clarify whether the episode occurred during or soon after surgery. Although halothane is rarely used in adults in the United States today, those who previously had halothane hepatitis may be at risk for cross-sensitivity to other fluorinated volatile agents with trifluoroacetyl metabolites (enflurane, isoflurane, desflurane).

Cirrhosis

Cirrhosis is the end result of most hepatotoxic conditions. Portal hypertension with splenomegaly, varices, ascites, and pleural effusions occur. The liver fails to synthesize proteins and clotting factors or clear toxins and drugs. Patients may have encephalopathy, bleeding, thrombocytopenia, and a prolonged PT and are at risk for renal insufficiency or failure. Pulmonary shunting may cause hypoxemia and pulmonary hypertension. Hepatorenal syndrome is the occurance of renal insufficiency in patients with hepatic disease in the absence of primary renal disease and may be related to hypoperfusion. Jaundiced patients are at particular risk for hepatorenal syndrome. Spontaneous bacterial peritonitis may develop in patients with ascites and increases perioperative mortality.

The Child-Turcotte-Pugh classification (Table 34-5) can predict perioperative morbidity and mortality. The Model for End-Stage Liver Disease (MELD) formula, which factors bilirubin, the international normalized ratio (INR), creatinine, and the cause of the liver disease, is used to select patients for transplantation, may be useful to predict risk for other surgery, and may do so better than the Child class.[74] Online calculators to determine MELD can be found at www.unos.org. Higher scores indicate more severe disease. One study showed that a MELD score lower than 14 predicted 77% of patients with poor outcomes.[74] Anemia increases postoperative mortality in patients with obstructive jaundice. One study did show that a serum albumin concentration of less than 2.1 mg/dL was a strong predictor of mortality in veterans undergoing major noncardiac surgery.[75]

Unexpected Increased Liver Function Test Values

Elevated alanine aminotransferase (ALT) and aspartate aminotransferase (AST) reflect damage to hepatocytes, bilirubin measures the liver's ability to conjugate or excrete bile (or both), alkaline phosphatase rises with degradation of hepatic excretion (also from bone turnover and thus nonspecific for liver disease), and albumin and PT measure synthetic function of the liver. Only 1 in 700 preoperative patients is unexpectedly found to have liver disease, and the vast majority are not severe disorders. However, if abnormal LFT values are unexpectedly found, further testing or referral may be warranted. In patients with elevations in ALT or AST, screening for hepatitis with hepatitis A IgM antibody, hepatitis B surface and core antigens, hepatitis B surface antibody, and hepatitis C antibody can help in establishing a diagnosis. Elevated alkaline phosphatase or bilirubin with normal or mildly to moderately increased transaminases suggests obstruction of the biliary system, and abdominal ultrasound, computed tomography, and endoscopic retrograde cholangiopancreatography can establish a diagnosis.

Table 34-5 Child-Turcotte-Pugh Classification

	Points (For Each with a Maximum of 15)		
Parameter	**1**	**2**	**3**
Ascites	Absent	Slight	Moderate
Bilirubin (mg/dL)	<2	2-3	>3
Albumin (g/dL)	>3.5	2.8-3.5	<2.8
Prothrombin time (seconds over control)	<4	4-6	>6
Encephalopathy	None	Grade 1-2	Grade 3-4

Class A: <7 points; Class B: 7-9 points; Class C: >9 points.

All Forms of Liver Disease

The preoperative history often uncovers the cause of the liver disease, therapies, and associated complications. Important issues to explore include the cause and degree of hepatic dysfunction. Patients with liver disease may be asymptomatic or complain of fatigue, weight loss, dark urine, pale stools, pruritus, right upper quadrant pain, bloating, and jaundice. Weight and vital signs, including oxygen saturation, are needed. Physical examination may reveal jaundice, bruising, ascites, pleural effusions, peripheral edema, or hypoxia. The presence of encephalopathy, coagulopathy, ascites, volume overload, and infectivity needs to be determined and explored preoperatively. The bilirubin level is generally higher than 2.5 mg/dL before icterus can be seen in mucous membranes and sclerae. Examination may reveal hepatomegaly, splenomegaly, and altered mental status. New-onset or worsening encephalopathy prompts an evaluation for precipitating factors such as worsening liver disease, infection, drug effects, bleeding, or electrolyte disturbances.

In selected patients, preoperative evaluation may warrant further testing consisting of an ECG, CBC with platelet count, electrolytes, BUN, creatinine, LFTs, albumin, and PT. An ammonia level may be helpful in patients with encephalopathy. A chest radiograph may identify effusions. Coagulopathy can be a result of vitamin K deficiency caused by an inability to secrete bile (cholestatic disorders), deficiency of coagulation factors because of loss of synthetic function as a result of cirrhosis, or thrombocytopenia secondary to splenomegaly and portal hypertension.

Therapy to correct coagulopathy is directed at the cause. Vitamin K, fresh frozen plasma, or platelets are used to correct deficiencies. Vitamin K, 1 to 5 mg orally or subcutaneously daily for 1 to 3 days, may correct a prolonged PT and carries minimal risk. However, the coagulopathy in patients with synthetic failure will probably not correct with such measures, and performing a type and screen will prepare the patient for platelet and fresh frozen plasma transfusions with the goal of achieving a platelet count higher than 50,000/mm^3 and an INR less than 1.5, respectively. Correction of anemia is controversial but may limit renal dysfunction. Lactulose (30 mL orally every 6 hours for 3 days before surgery with the last dose given within 12 hours of surgery) or oral bile salts with intravenous hydration beginning the night before surgery may reduce perioperative progression of renal disease in patients at risk.[76] Reduction of ascites preoperatively may decrease the risk of wound dehiscence and improve pulmonary function. Sodium restriction (in diet and intravenous solutions), diuretics (especially spironolactone, which inhibits aldosterone), and even paracentesis are useful. If fluid is aspirated, it is important to analyze it for infection. Encephalopathy is frequently caused by an acute insult such as infection, gastrointestinal bleeding, hypovolemia, or sedatives. It is important to determine reversible factors and treat accordingly. Lactulose, 30 mL every 6 hours orally, is first-line therapy. Addressing nutritional deficiencies with enteral or parenteral supplementation may have benefit, especially in alcoholic patients. Patients who abuse alcohol are at risk for neurologic deterioration if thiamine, folate, and vitamin B_{12} supplements are not provided, particularly when nutrition or glucose is given. These patients are also at risk for alcohol withdrawal syndromes (see the appropriate section).

Delaying elective surgery until after an acute episode of hepatitis or an exacerbation of chronic disease has resolved or until a diagnosis is established if hepatic dysfunction is newly detected is appropriate.[74] Elective surgery is contraindicated in patients with acute or fulminant liver disease, including alcoholic (mortality >55%), viral (mortality >10%), or undefined hepatitis. Perioperative risk in patients with chronic hepatitis or cirrhosis is predicted by its histologic severity (bridging or multilobular necrosis on biopsy), impairment of the synthetic and excretory functions of the liver, and portal hypertension (ascites, varices, bleeding).

Patients with severe liver disease have increased perioperative morbidity and mortality.[77] Perioperative management is discussed in Chapter 66. The most common adverse events are bleeding, infection, liver failure, and hepatorenal syndrome (renal failure in patients with portal hypertension but otherwise normal kidneys).

Hematologic Disorders

Anemia

Anemia may be a known problem or a suspected possibility based on a patient's history of underlying medical conditions or the reason for surgery. It is useful to determine the etiology, duration, and stability of the anemia, related symptoms, and therapy (especially transfusions), although the evaluation needs to consider the extent and type of surgery, the anticipated blood loss, and the patient's comorbid conditions that may influence oxygenation or be affected by hypoxia, such as pulmonary, cerebrovascular, or cardiovascular disease. Inquiring about a personal or family history of anemia is important.

The World Health Organization defines anemia as a hemoglobin level lower than 13 g/dL in adult men and less than 12 g/dL in adult women. The consequences of moderate levels of anemia and hemoglobin levels of 6.0 g/dL or higher in patients without CAD are minimal. The ASA Task Force on Blood Component Therapy concluded that red blood cells should not be transfused solely because of a hemoglobin level but rather because of risk for complications from inadequate oxygenation (see Chapter 55).[78] A recent Veteran's Affairs study suggests that even mild preoperative anemia increases postoperative mortality and cardiac morbidity, but only in men.[31] This study found that individuals with hematocrits between 39% and 51% had the lowest risk for adverse outcomes.

Preoperative patients at risk for anemia include those with a history of colon cancer, gastrointestinal or genitourinary bleeding, metrorrhagia, chronic infections, inflammatory diseases, nutritional deficiencies (including gastric bypass recipients), and a host of other conditions. Anemia is the most common preoperative hematologic disorder. An important component of the history and physical examination includes asking about palpitations, fatigue, chest pain, black or bloody stools, weight loss, pallor, murmurs, hepatospenomegaly, or lymphadenopathy.

Preoperative evaluation of patients with anemia or suspected anemia will benefit from a CBC. Generally, further evaluation should be done by a primary care physician or hematologist, but initial studies include a peripheral smear, determination of mean corpuscular volume (MCV), a reticulocyte count, and further testing such as iron studies, vitamin B_{12}, or folate levels, depending on the findings on the smear and the MCV. MCV, iron, and ferritin are low and total iron-binding capacity (TIBC) is high in iron deficiency anemia. MCV and TIBC are low or normal and iron and ferritin are normal or high in anemia associated with chronic disease. MCV is high and vitamin B_{12} or folate levels are low in macrocytic anemia associated with these deficiencies. Type and screening and preoperative transfusion may be necessary, depending on the level of anemia and anticipated surgical blood loss.

In special circumstances, such as a patient's refusal of perioperative blood transfusion or elective procedures with expected significant blood loss in anemic patients, postponement of surgery to treat with recombinant human erythropoietin and iron may be warranted.

Sickle Cell Disease

Sickle cell disease, a hereditary hemoglobinopathy with vaso-occlusion, is responsible for most of the associated complications. Patients homozygous for hemoglobin S (HbS) have disease and are at risk for major morbidity and a shortened life expectancy. Patients with SC disease have both HbS and HbC and a much less severe clinical course with moderate anemia. Heterozygous patients (HbS and HbA) have sickle cell trait and rarely have any consequences related to this condition. Preoperative assessment should focus on identification of organ dysfunction and acute exacerbations.[80] Patients may have renal insufficiency, splenomegaly, pulmonary hypertension and infarction, cerebrovascular accidents, and heart failure. They are at increased risk for infection because of splenic infarction. Frequent hospitalizations or a recent increase in hospitalizations, advanced age, preexisting infections, and pulmonary disease are predictive of perioperative vaso-occlusive complications.[79]

The preoperative history and physical examination should focus on the frequency, severity, and pattern of vaso-occlusive crises and the degree of pulmonary, cardiac, renal, and central nervous system damage. Pulse oximetry, hematocrit, measurement of BUN and creatinine, an ECG, and a chest radiograph should be considered. Additional testing (e.g., echocardiogram, arterial blood gases) may be needed in rare instances. Prophylactic transfusion may be beneficial, especially before intermediate- to high-risk cases. Preoperative prophylactic transfusion is controversial, and the decision to transfuse should be made in concert with a hematologist familiar with the disease. The Cooperative Study of Sickle Cell Disease concluded that preoperative transfusion was beneficial, although patients undergoing low-risk surgery had few complications even without transfusion.[80] Another study showed that a conservative transfusion regimen (decreasing HbS to <60% and hemoglobin to 10 g/dL) was as effective as a more traditional approach (transfusing to decrease HbS to <30% and hemoglobin to 10 g/dL). Additional benefits included fewer transfusion-related complications.[81]

Glucose-6-Phosphate Dehydrogenase Deficiency

Glucose-6-phosphate dehydrogenase deficiency is an X-linked hereditary Coombs-positive hemolytic anemia. Hemolysis occurs with exposure to drugs (antipyretics, nitrates, sulfonamides), infections, hypoxia, hypothermia, blood products, or stress. The severity of the hemolysis varies among patients and the offending agent or condition. Steroids are usually effective. The preoperative history focuses on previous episodes of hemolysis, identification of predisposing factors, and determination of the current hematocrit.

Coagulopathies

Hypocoagulable states are either inherited disorders such as the hemophilias and thrombocytopenia or are acquired disorders secondary to liver disease, malnutrition, or drug exposure. To determine the diagnosis and risk of bleeding, one inquires about known diagnoses, tests, treatments, previous bleeding episodes, and family history. Asking about excessive bruising, prolonged bleeding after cuts, heavy menstrual cycles, and bleeding gums is sensitive but not specific. A *change* in one of these factors is more meaningful than a chronic history becauses what one individual considers excessive may actually be normal.

The preoperative evaluation inquires into excessive bleeding after previous procedures or childbirth, especially if transfusions were unexpectedly required; such bleeding is more definitive but not diagnostic. Petechiae, multiple bruises, hematomas, jaundice, and frank bleeding are important findings. Diagnostic testing may include a platelet count, CBC, PT, and aPTT. *Routine* screening for coagulopathies with a PT, aPTT, or a bleeding time without an indication is not indicated. If specific causes of bleeding are suspected or known, such as liver disease or malnutrition, targeted testing with liver enzyme, protein, and albumin levels and a PT is needed.

In the case of a prolonged PT without a history of warfarin use, the most common cause is laboratory error, liver disease, or malnutrition. One should first repeat the test. If the test is abnormal again, referral to a hematologist or the primary care physician or evaluation of liver enzymes and a hepatitis panel may be warranted, depending on the surgery. A trial of vitamin K (1 to 5 mg orally once a day for 3 days) can be initiated. A prolonged aPTT can result from both hypocoagulable and hypercoagulable conditions. The first step is to repeat the test and ascertain exposure to heparin. Even small amounts of heparin present in indwelling catheters, especially if the blood is drawn from that site, can prolong the aPTT. The most common cause of a prolonged aPTT other than heparin exposure is von Willebrand's disease (vWD), but other hemophilias discussed later can prolong the aPTT. Factor V Leiden, anticardiolipin antibody, and lupus anticoagulants, which result in increased clotting, cause prolongation of the aPTT. Further testing for a prolonged aPTT includes a repeat aPTT; an aPTT mixing study; lupus anticoagulant; evaluation of coagulation factors VII, IX, XI, and XII; and checking von Willebrand factor (vWF) antigen and ristocetin cofactor levels. A mixing study, in which normal blood is mixed with the subject's blood, will detect factor deficiencies (the aPTT will correct with this test) or inhibitors (the aPTT will not correct).

Hemophilias

Hemophilia A (factor VIII deficiency) and hemophilia B (or Christmas disease) are X-linked recessively inherited disorders that occur almost exclusively in males. Hemophiliacs have a prolonged aPTT and normal PT. The severity of bleeding varies among individuals but tends to be similar in relatives and is directly related to the degree of factor deficiency. Even mild trauma can result in significant hemorrhage. Orthopedic procedures account for 50% of operations in hemophiliacs because recurrent bleeding destroys joints. Hemophilia A accounts for 85% of all cases of hemophilia.

A hematologist should be involved in the perioperative care of these patients. A detailed plan to monitor and replace deficient factors is paramount. Typically, factors VIII and IX are maintained at 75% to 100% in the immediate perioperative period and then at 50% until any risk of bleeding is past. Each unit of recombinant or purified factor concentrate raises the factor level by 2% per kilogram. Intramuscular injections are to be avoided.

Von Willebrand's Disease

vWD is an inherited disorder of factor VIII and vWF that affects both genders. It is the most common congenital coagulopathy and is estimated to occur in 1% of individuals.[82] Several types (1, 2A, 2B, 2M, and 2N) are autosomal dominant, and type 3 is recessive. Factor VIII and vWF circulate as a complex, and vWD results from both quantitative and qualitative deficiencies. Most patients have a prolonged aPTT, but those with mild disease may have a normal aPTT. The most common cause of a prolonged aPTT in patients not taking heparin is vWD. vWD is diagnosed by measuring ristocetin cofactor (a functional assay for vWF that causes platelet aggregation in the presence of ristocetin), vWF antigen, and factor VIII. vWF is an acute-phase reactant that increases with certain conditions such as stress or surgery, which sometimes makes the diagnosis difficult. Most patients with vWD will have a history of bleeding, but in some the diagnosis will not be made until a second challenge to coagulation occurs, including major surgery or exposure to drugs such as aspirin or NSAIDs.

Involvement of a hematologist in the care of these patients is beneficial. Desmospressin (1-desamino-8-D-arginine vasopressin [DDAVP]) increases release of factor VIII, vWF, and plasminogen activator from endothelial cells. An intravenous dose of 0.3 μg/kg (given over a period of 15 to 30 minutes to avoid hypotension, flushing, and tachycardia) typically raises vWF threefold to fourfold. However, there is considerable variation among individuals, so vWF and factor VIII levels must be monitored. Desmopressin is available as a nasal spray and should not be given more frequently than every 48 hours to avoid depletion of endothelial stores. To avoid release of plasminogen activator by desmopressin, ε-aminocaproic acid or tranexamic acid is given. Desmopressin is contraindicated in patients with type 2B because it increases abnormal vWF and may result in thrombocytopenia. Cryoprecipitate or factor VIII concentrates containing vWF will replace abnormal vWF.

Thrombocytopenia

Thrombocytopenia is a platelet count lower than 150,000/mm^3 and results from decreased production, increased destruction, or sequestration. Malignancies, drugs, autoimmune disorders, preeclampsia, hereditary disease, and disseminated intravascular coagulation can cause thrombocytopenia. In patients found to have low platelet counts unexpectedly, first repeat the test, examine the peripheral smear, and collect blood for a platelet count in a tube without ethylenediaminetetraacetic acid (EDTA). EDTA is a chelating agent added to tubes commonly used for determination of the CBC because it prevents clotting. However, in some patients it causes clumping of platelets resulting in pseudothrombocytopenia.

Recent exposure to heparin raises the issue of heparin-induced thrombocytopenia (HIT), which generally occurs within

5 to 10 days after exposure to heparin.[83] HIT is an immune-mediated disorder with antibodies directed against platelets and can result in arterial or venous thrombosis, stroke, amputations, and death in up to 30% of patients. Immediate discontinuation of heparin and testing for heparin-induced platelet antibodies are indicated. LMWH is less likely than unfractionated heparin to cause HIT but is contraindicated in patients with HIT. Alternative anticoagulants are danaparoid sodium, lepirudin, and argatroban. Idiopathic thrombocytopenic purpura is a chronic autoimmune disorder with autoantibodies against platelets that results in increased destruction. Patients are treated with corticosteroids and splenectomy (to eliminate the major site of platelet removal). Patients often have minimal bleeding at even very low platelet levels, probably because of increased turnover and a predominance of young platelets.

Surgery can be performed safely in patients with platelet counts higher than 50,000/mm^3. The risk of bleeding is inversely related to platelet counts lower than 50,000/mm^3. Anemia, fever, infections, and drugs that affect platelet function increase bleeding at any platelet level. Centroneuraxial anesthesia is safe with platelet counts higher than 100,000/mm^3.[84] Patients with newly discovered thrombocytopenia may benefit from hematology consultation before elective surgery. One unit of platelets transfused typically raises the count by 10,000/mm^3.

Thrombocytosis

Thrombocytosis is a platelet count greater than 500,000/mm^3 and may be physiologic (exercise, pregnancy), primary (myeloproliferative disorder), or secondary (iron deficiency, neoplasm, surgery, chronic inflammation). Platelet counts greater than 1,000,000/mm^3 place patients at risk for thrombotic events such as stroke, MI, pulmonary and mesenteric emboli, and peripheral arterial and venous clots. Patients with primary thrombocytosis (essential thrombocythemia) have a bleeding tendency that is worsened by exposure to drugs such as aspirin. Older patients and those with a previous history of bleeding or thrombosis may be at increased risk. Hydroxyurea, anagrelide (these drugs decrease production, so 7 to 10 days is needed), or plasmapheresis (removes platelets, so the effect is immediate) may be used to lower the platelet count. Treatment of the underlying disorder of secondary causes of thrombocytosis usually results in normalization of the platelet count.

Polycythemia

Polycythemia is a hematocrit greater than 54% and can be primary (polycythemia vera) or secondary to chronic hypoxia (COPD, high altitude, congenital heart disease). A steep increase in blood viscosity, which is thrombogenic, occurs with hematocrits higher than 50%. High hematocrits are associated with increased atherosclerosis (carotid stenosis, stroke) and cardiovascular disease (heart failure, MI). There are contradictory reports on whether polycythemia increases perioperative risk. A recent study showed an increase in postoperative mortality in men but not women with hematocrits higher than 51%.[31] However, an earlier report found no increased perioperative complications in patients with secondary polycythemia.

The preoperative evaluation (history and physical examination) focuses on the pulmonary and cardiovascular systems. Examination for cyanosis, clubbing, wheezing, and murmurs is necessary. Oxygen saturation, an ECG, and possibly arterial blood gas analysis and a chest radiograph are needed in patients with polycythemia. An unexpected preoperative finding of polycythemia should prompt an investigation to find the cause and, if not readily apparent, the possibility of polycythemia vera.

Risk of Thromboembolism or Pulmonary Emboli

Fatal pulmonary embolism occurs in 0.1% to 0.8% of patients undergoing elective general surgery, 2% to 3% of patients having elective hip replacement, and 4% to 7% of patients undergoing repair of a fractured hip who do not receive prophylaxis. The risk for venous thrombosis is increased in patients with previous venous thromboembolism, obesity, varicose veins, diabetes, cancer, heart failure, pregnancy, paralysis, the presence of an inhibitor deficiency state, or age younger than 50 years.[85] Factor V Leiden is the most common cause of inherited thrombophilia (40% to 50% of cases). The prothrombin gene mutation and deficiencies in protein S, protein C, and antithrombin account for most of the remaining cases. The risk of perioperative venous thromboembolism depends on the surgical procedure (e.g., degree of invasiveness, trauma, and immobilization) and patient-related variables (e.g., inflammatory bowel disease, acute illness, smoking, malignancy, obesity, increasing age, previous thromboembolism, estrogen use, hypercoagulable state).[86] Primary thromboembolic prophylaxis is beyond the scope of this chapter, but it is important to risk-stratify patients preoperatively so that appropriate measures can be implemented on the day of surgery. Because of the high risk of thromboembolism in patients undergoing elective lower extremity joint replacement, these patients are often given a dose of warfarin the night before surgery. American Society of Regional Anesthesiologists guidelines specifically state that if a single dose of warfarin has been administered within the previous 24 hours, it is safe to perform neuraxial anesthesia.[87]

Recent arterial or deep venous thromboembolism (DVT) requires perioperative interventions or postponement of nonlifesaving procedures. Without anticoagulation, the risk for recurrent DVT within 3 months of a proximal DVT is approximately 50%. A month of warfarin treatment reduces the risk to 10%, and 3 months reduces it to 5%. Patients with a hereditary hypercoagulable state (e.g., antithrombin III or protein C or S deficiency, prothrombin gene mutation, Factor V Leiden), cancer, or multiple episodes of DVT are at higher risk indefinitely. Patients with nonvalvular atrial fibrillation who have had a previous cerebral embolism are also at higher risk. Patients with mechanical heart valves, especially multiple valves, are at risk for embolism. Risk is greater with mitral than with aortic valves. Surgery increases the risk for DVT, but there is no such evidence that surgery increases the risk for arterial embolism in patients with atrial fibrillation or mechanical valves.[84]

Preoperative evaluation determines whether "bridging" with either unfractionated heparin intravenously or LMWH subcutaneously as an outpatient (or not to bridge) is warranted for patients with mechanical heart valves or previous episodes of thromboembolism secondary to atrial fibrillation. The decision needs to be made in concert with the treating physician or a cardiologist.

The authors believe that elective surgery should be postponed in the first month after an episode of venous or arterial thromboembolism. If postponement is not possible, the patient should receive preoperative heparin while the INR is below 2.0.[84] Ideally, 3 months of anticoagulation is recommended before elective surgery. Typically, withholding warfarin for 5 days will allow the PT/INR to fall to normal if the INR is chronically maintained between 2.0 and 3.0, the usual therapeutic targets. It may be necessary to withhold more doses if the INR is more prolonged or fewer doses if subtherapeutic. Therefore, it is necessary to check the INR during the preoperative visit to guide cessation of therapy. During the time without warfarin, patients may be at risk for recurrent thromboembolism, but the risk is relatively small in all but the highest-risk patients. It is controversial whether patients require "bridging" or heparin during this period. Previously, the only option was hospital admission for intravenous heparin therapy, which is costly. However, with the availability of LMWH, patients can receive subcutaneous (usually self-administered) LMWH at home without the need for monitoring.

Neurologic Disease

In patients with neurologic disease, a detailed history is required with a focus on recent events, exacerbations, or evidence of poor control of the medical condition. Information about previous investigations or therapy is important. A basic preoperative neurologic examination documenting deficits in mental status, speech, cranial nerves, gait, and motor and sensory function is important. This baseline determination allows comparison of new deficits postoperatively.

Cerebrovascular Disease

If a stroke or transient neurologic deficit has not been fully evaluated or has occurred recently, elective surgery should be considered pending complete evaluation because a history of stroke or symptoms of cerebrovascular insufficiency are strong predictors of perioperative stroke.[88] High-quality data are lacking on how soon after an event anesthesia and surgery are safe. The etiology and treatment guide further perioperative management. An embolic stroke from a patent foramen ovale (PFO) may require correction of the PFO or strict attention to avoidance of air emboli. A left atrial or ventricular thrombus or an embolic stroke secondary to atrial fibrillation or mechanical heart valves requires a minimum of 1 month and preferably 3 months of anticoagulation and possible bridging with short-acting anticoagulants for elective surgery.[84] Atrial fibrillation (either chronic or new onset) is a common cause of perioperative stroke, especially those occurring postoperatively, the most common time for stroke.[89]

Asymptomatic Bruit

A newly discovered carotid bruit requires a careful searching for symptoms of cerebral ischemia or transient ischemic attack, especially if the procedure is likely to involve manipulation of the neck or the patient has a potentially difficult airway. Frequently, patients will not have volunteered pertinent symptoms until specifically probed, especially if they were transient. Patients with risk factors for carotid atherosclerosis, including those who have undergone head and neck irradiation, especially at a younger age, need to be questioned specifically about amaurosis fugax, dysphagia, dysarthria, and other symptoms of cerebovascular insufficiency. One of the authors met a college professor in the preoperative clinic who was scheduled for an abdominal procedure and had a history of Hodgkin's lymphoma as a teenager. After a carotid bruit was ausculated, the patient confirmed receiving mantle irradiation for her lymphoma, but it took much probing to elicit a history of two transient episodes of slurred speech within the previous month. The patient was found to have 99% occlusion of her left internal carotid artery.

In patients who have truly asymptomatic bruits, significant carotid lesions are present 40% to 60% of the time, the risk of stroke in this group is 1% to 2% per year, and most strokes are preceded by transient symptoms.[90] A significant prospective, randomized multicenter trial found that patients with asymptomatic carotid stenosis of 60% or greater benefited from revascularization if they were considered good risk and the surgeon had a 3% or lower perioperative morbidity and mortality rate.[91] However, after reviewing the published data, a more recent Symposium on Cerebrovascular Diseases concluded that because progression rates are extremely slow and patients with carotid stenosis are at substantial risk for MI and vascular death, revascularization should be contemplated only in centers with low complication rates for medically stable patients, those expected to live at least 5 years with 80% or greater stenosis.[90] There is no evidence that truly asymptomatic bruits increase the risk for perioperative stroke. Carotid Doppler ultrasound studies are simple effective tools to evaluate at-risk patients who might benefit from further evaluation. Significant abnormalities on Doppler studies should prompt referral to a vascular surgeon or neurologist.

Seizure Disorder

The type and frequency of seizures (e.g., grand mal or absence) and the specifics of symptoms such as staring or focal findings are important to ascertain and document. Absence (previously petit mal) seizures may be particularly difficult to recognize because they lack generalized motor signs. More typical symptoms such as staring and obtundation may be misinterpreted as residual anesthetic effects in the postoperative period. Brain tumors, aneurysms, arteriovenous malformations (AVMs), classic epilepsy, drug toxicity, electrolyte disorders, infections, and vascular disease from arteriosclerosis, stroke, sickle cell disease, or SLE can all cause seizures.

Preoperative evaluation and documentation of anticonvulsants and the adequacy of seizure control are necessary. Routinely ordering tests for serum drug levels of anticonvulsant medications is not indicated unless toxicity is a concern or the patient is having breakthrough seizures. Patients with good control of seizures may have levels outside the therapeutic range, and the results may be confounded if the timing of administration of the drugs in relation to when the blood is drawn is not considered. Generally, trough levels are necessary for accurate interpretation. Medications to control seizures have multiple side effects (bone marrow suppression, macrocytic anemia, leukopenia, hyponatremia), and testing should be directed at suspected abnormalities. A CBC with a platelet count and electrolyte levels are most commonly obtained. Poorly controlled or new-onset seizures require consultation with a neurologist before proceeding with anything other than emergency surgery. Continuation of anticonvulsants in the perioperative period is necessary.

Multiple Sclerosis

Multiple sclerosis is thought to be an inflammatory immune disorder with two general patterns of disability: exacerbating-remitting and chronic progressive.[92] Symptomatology can include ataxia, motor weakness, sensory deficits, autonomic dysfunction, emotional lability, bladder or bowel dysfunction, and visual disturbances. Exacerbations can be triggered by stress, infections, the peripartum, and elevated temperatures. Varieties of treatments have been evaluated, including steroids, immunosuppressants, monoclonal antibodies, plasmapheresis, benzodiazepines, and baclofen. Preoperatively, it is important to document the history and pattern of disease, including symptoms and physical deficits, with special emphasis on respiratory compromise. Medications and previous triggers are important. There has been no documented association with the type of anesthetic or particular anesthetic agents and exacerbation of disease. Regional anesthesia may offer advantages for patients with respiratory compromise or cognitive dysfunction. Detailed documentation of preexisting neurologic deficits is important. Determination of oxygen saturation is needed. Testing is directed toward possible medication effects (e.g., azathioprine can suppress bone marrow and affect liver function, cyclophosphamide may cause electrolyte abnormalities, and steroids can cause hyperglycemia) and associated disturbances (e.g., chest radiography and white blood cell count if pulmonary infection is suspected). Patients with minor, stable disease require no special testing. Medications are continued on the day of surgery.

Aneurysms and Arteriovenous Malformations

Cerebral and spinal vascular lesions consist of aneurysms and AVMs, which may be intact or ruptured, symptomatic, or an incidental finding (see Chapter 63). Patients with polycystic kidney disease, fibromuscular dysplasia, type IV Ehlers-Danlos syndrome, or a family history of aneurysms are at increased risk for aneurysms. An AVM may be large enough to cause a mass effect. Pregnancy increases the risk for aneurysmal and possibly AVM bleeding. Before rupture, most patients will have minimal symptoms other than headache or seizures, but it is important to document complaints in all patients. With rupture, altered mental status, syncope, increased intracranial pressure with the typical signs and symptoms, inappropriate secretion of antidiuretic hormone, and hemodynamic perturbations are common. Bradycardia, tachycardia, ectopic beats, and ST-T wave changes, often mimicking those seen with ischemia, are common. Significant cardiac dysfunction with depressed contractility and wall motion abnormalities can be present on echocardiography. Preoperatively, concomitant CAD or preexisting cardiomyopathy should be considered and it not be assumed that these changes are related only to the bleeding. A preoperative ECG with determination of electrolytes, glucose, BUN, and creatinine is necessary. Chest radiography and echocardiography may also be helpful.

Parkinson's Disease

Parkinson's disease is a degenerative disorder of the basal ganglia in which failure of dopamine secretion results in diminished inhibition of the extrapyramidal motor system.[93] Preoperative patients typically have diminution of spontaneous movements, rigidity (cogwheel rigidity is classic), resting tremor, masked facies, difficulty speaking and walking, and frequently depression and dementia. Autonomic dysfunction with orthostatic hypotension, excessive salivation, and difficulty regulating temperature also occurs.

Patients are at risk for pulmonary complications because of difficulty swallowing and altered mental status and have an increased risk of aspiration and dysfunction of ventilatory muscles. Replacement of dopamine with levodopa, often combined with carbidopa, anticholinergic agents, bromocriptine, amantadine, and selegiline, is standard treatment. Levodopa can cause dyskinesias (dystonic and myoclonic involuntary movements). Pergolide, a dopamine receptor agonist, was recalled in early 2007 because of an increased risk for mitral and aortic regurgitation.[94] Patients exposed to this drug need a careful examination for murmurs and, if present, require an ECG and may require an echocardiogram. Selegiline is a monoamine oxidase inhibitor that inhibits dopamine degradation. Metoclopramine, phenothiazines, and butyrophenones may exacerbate symptoms by interfering with dopamine.

Preoperative evaluation focuses on the pulmonary system and degree of disability, especially dysphagia and dyspnea. Determination of room-air saturation and orthostatic BP and HR is important. Significant pulmonary symptoms, especially symptoms of infection or if worsening, may require a chest radiograph, pulmonary consultation, and delay of the procedure for improvement. Patients who have taken pergolide need auscultation for murmurs and, if present, may benefit from an ECG and echocardiogram. Deep brain stimulators need to be deactivated before procedures in which electrocautery will be used. All parkinsonian medications are continued. Abrupt withdrawal of levodopa may exacerbate symptoms, epecially dysphagia and chest wall rigidity, or result in neuroleptic malignant syndrome (NMS). NMS is characterized by autonomic instability, altered mental status, rigidity, and fever.

Neuromuscular Junction Disorders

Myasthenia gravis is an autoimmune disorder of skeletal muscle neuromuscular junctions that is due to antibodies against nicotinic acetylcholine receptors.[95] It is characterized by muscle weakness that worsens with activity and improves with rest.

Preoperative evaluation determines whether the patient has clinical or progressive weakness that can be exacerbated by stress, infections, hypokalemia, medications (aminoglycoside antibiotics, propranolol, ciprofloxacin, clindamycin), and surgery. Cardiac and smooth muscles are unaffected. Thymic hyperplasia and tumors may be present. The thymus is located in the anterior mediastinum and, when enlarged, has implications related to anesthesia (see "Mediastinal Masses"). Cranial nerve and bulbar involvement is common with pharyngeal and laryngeal muscle weakness, which increases the risk for aspiration. Ocular symptoms (diplopia, ptosis) are usually present and are frequently the initial or only complaints. Ventilatory function can be compromised. Preoperative PFTs are indicated for severely affected individuals and may be useful in predicting who may require postoperative ventilation.[96] PFTs may be particularly helpful if patients are being considered for ambulatory surgery, especially in freestanding surgical centers. Other autoimmune diseases such as rheumatoid arthritis, polymyositis, and thyroid disorders are common in myasthenics. See the appropriate sections of this chapter for discussion of these topics.

Patients are treated by thymectomy and with anticholinesterase and immunosuppressant medications. Worsening symptoms may be due to deteriorating disease (a myasthenic crisis) or excessive anticholinesterase treatment (a cholinergic crisis). By using a short-acting anticholinesterase (edrophonium), the two can be distinguished; only a myasthenic crisis will improve with more anticholinesterase. Plasmapheresis and intravenous immunoglobulins have been used to treat myasthenic crises or prepare patients for surgery but require several days to weeks for improvement.

Preoperative patients taking azathioprine require a CBC and LFTs because of the bone marrow suppression and liver dysfunction associated with this drug. Patients treated with steroids need an ECG and glucose determination and may require higher doses in the perioperative period. Even though anticholinesterases may cause bradycardia (necessitating a preoperative ECG) and salivation and alter the effects of neuromuscular blocking and reversal agents, they need to be continued to prevent a myasthenic crisis. Documentation of dosages and schedules and continuation of these medications up until the time of surgery are paramount. Avoidance of drugs that can exacerbate myasthenic symptoms is necessary. Management with a neurologist is important.

Lambert-Eaton syndrome is similar to myasthenia gravis and consists of muscle weakness, including oculobulbar involvement, and dysautonomia. It is caused by antibodies against voltage-gated calcium channels, which results in a decrease in acetylcholine. It is not associated with thymic abnormalities but is most common with malignancies; small cell lung cancer is the most frequent cause, but it also occurs with gastrointestinal tumors. The other distinguishing feature is that the muscle weakness classically improves with activity and is worse after inactivity. Therapies similar to that used for myasthenia, along with 3,4-diaminopyridine, a selective potassium channel blocker, are used and continued perioperatively. Preoperative evaluation and management are similar to that for myasthenia gravis.

Muscular Dystrophies and Myopathies

Muscular dystrophies and myopathies are inherited disorders of the neuromuscular junction (see Chapter 14). They share many similarities but have a few differences. Progressive skeletal muscle weakness commonly leading to respiratory failure and no effective therapy are the hallmarks of these disorders. Many have associated cardiomyopathies and possibly an association with MH. Duchenne's and Becker's muscular dystrophies are X-linked recessive disorders that occur in males. Patients have elevated creatine phosphokinase levels, often detected before the onset of symptoms. Males with a family history of Duchenne's or Becker's muscular dystrophy who have not been tested are considered at risk and require similar precautions as those with diagnosed disease. Cardiomyopathy and respiratory failure are common causes of death. Otherwise, normal female carriers may have dilated cardiomyopathy.

Preoperative evaluation for symptoms such as palpitations, dyspnea, chest pain, syncope, orthopnea, edema, aspiration, and pneumonia is important. Physical examination focuses on the cardiopulmonary system. An ECG, PFTs, and echocardiography are important in the preoperative evaluation.

Fascioscapulohumeral dystrophy is autosomal dominant, affects both genders, and causes a slowly progressive weakness of muscles of the shoulders and face. Cardiomyopathy is much less frequent than in the other dystrophies, but arrhythmias have been reported. Limb-girdle dystrophies have a variable inheritance and primarily affect the muscles of the shoulders and pelvis. Conduction abnormalities are present in some patients, although frank cardiomyopathies are less frequent. Inquiring about palpitations, syncope, and cardiac symptoms, examining patients as noted earlier for Duchenne's muscular dystrophy, and obtaining an ECG preoperatively are important.

Myotonic Dystrophies

Myotonia is prolonged contraction and delay of relaxation of muscles. It is a common symptom of several dystrophies, including classic myotonic dystrophy, congenital myotonic dystrophy, myotonia congenita, and central core disease. Myotonic dystrophy is the most common of these conditions and is an autosomal dominant inherited disorder that affects both genders. Congenital myotonic dystrophy is a severe form of this disease that is noted in infancy, often in the offspring of mothers with myotonic dystrophy.

Preoperative classic findings are severe muscle wasting, typically involving the face, hands, diaphragm, and pharyngeal, laryngeal, and pretibial muscles. Cold can trigger myotonia. The severity of disease is variable and it may not be apparent until the second to third decades of life, so a family history is important. Cardiomyopathies, arrhythmias, and conduction abnormalities are common, and some patients have cardiac valvular abnormalities. Cardiac involvement may not correlate with skeletal muscle atrophy or weakness. Patients require pacemakers once any evidence of second- or third-degree AV block develops, even if the patient is asymptomatic, because there may be unpredictably rapid progression of AV conduction disease. As a result of this potential for rapid progression, pacemaker placement is considered in these patients even with a first-degree AV block, regardless of symptoms. Aspiration with pneumonia and respiratory or cardiac failure are common. An increased risk for pulmonary complications postoperatively has been reported.[97]

Central core disease is a rare disorder consisting of a deficiency of mitochondrial enzymes. The name derives from the pathology of muscle biopsy specimens in which "cores" of abnormalities are apparent. Patients have proximal muscle weakness and scoliosis and may have cardiomyopathies. They are at risk for respiratory failure and aspiration, much like patients with myotonic dystrophy. Myotonia congenita is a hereditary disorder involving only skeletal muscles, is less severe, and does not cause cardiac abnormalities.

Patients with myotonia may be at increased risk for MH, although this is controversial. They may have similar findings as those with MH as a result of uncontrolled myotonic contraction with elevated metabolism and rhabdomyolysis.

Steroids, quinine, and procainamide may relieve myotonic contractions, but there is no cure for these diseases. These medications need to be continued perioperatively. The history and physical examination focus on the cardiopulmonary systems with special emphasis on findings of pulmonary infection, heart failure, palpitations, syncope, and conduction and valvular abnormalities. Preoperative testing includes an ECG and echocardiogram (except for patients with myotonia congenita), as well as a chest radiograph if acute symptoms of pulmonary disease are present. Any conduction abnormality on the ECG may benefit from cardiology consultation.

Central Nervous System Tumors

Pituitary tumors may be functioning (associated with endocrine abnormalities) or nonfunctioning and benign (adenomas are the most common pituitary lesion) or malignant (see Chapter 63).

Preoperative evaluation determines whether symptoms related to a mass effect of the tumor are present (e.g., headaches, visual field defects) or symptoms related to elevations in intracranial pressure are present (e.g., gait disturbances, vomiting, cranial nerve deficits, or bladder or bowel incontinence). Symptoms may be related to pituitary insufficiency (hypoadrenalism, hypothyroidism, or infertility being most common) or overactivity (Cushing's syndrome from tumors secreting ACTH; acromegaly from growth hormone secretion; hyperthyroidism from TSH production; gynecomastia, lactation, and sex hormone–

related changes from secretion of prolactin and gonadotropin [follicle-stimulating and luteinizing hormone]). These hormones are all produced by the anterior lobe of the pituitary and controlled via a feedback loop by the hypothalamus. The posterior pituitary stores and secretes vasopressin and oxytocin, which are synthesized in the hypothalamus. Cushing's syndrome results from excess cortisol production by the adrenals (stimulated by ACTH from the pituitary) and is discussed in the metabolic section of this chapter.

Acromegaly is caused by excess growth hormone and results in enlargement of connective tissue, bone, and visceral organs. On the preoperative physical examination, patients classically have an enlarged jaw (macrognathia), nose, feet, hands, and pharyngeal and laryngeal tissues, including the epiglottis and tongue (macroglossia). Patients have an increased incidence of both central sleep apnea and OSA, neuropathies from nerve entrapment, hypertension, LVH, diastolic dysfunction, and valvular abnormalities. CAD, heart failure, diabetes, hypothyroidism, and difficulty with mask ventilation, laryngoscopy, and intubation occur.

Preoperative solicitation and documentation of symptoms such as chest pain, dyspnea, snoring, numbness, polydipsia, headaches, and visual disturbances are important. Physical examination focuses on BP, airway features, murmurs, neurologic findings, and edema. Planning for difficult airway management plus discussion with the patient of possible awake fiberoptic intubation is necessary. An ECG, echocardiogram, electrolyte and glucose determination, and thyroid function tests are usually obtained.

TSH increases production of thyroid hormones (T_3 and T_4) by the thyroid gland. See the section "Thyroid Disease."

Posterior pituitary tumors result in failure to secrete vasopressin, also known as antidiuretic hormone, which regulates excretion of water by the kidneys. Deficiency of antidiuretic hormone results in excessive urine output from failure to reabsorb water and causes diabetes insipidus. These patients need estimation of volume status with orthostatic BP and HR measurement and electrolyte, BUN, and creatinine determination. Patients may have hypernatremia and volume depletion unless maintained on DDAVP.

Prolactin- and gonadotropin-secreting tumors have little impact on anesthetic management, but associated symptoms may alert clinicians to an undiagnosed pituitary tumor.

Patients with tumors or postpartum hemorrhage that cause pituitary insufficiency or those who have undergone resection of a pituitary tumor may require hormonal replacement such as steroids, thyroid medications, or DDAVP. It is important that these medications not be interrupted during the perioperative period. The preoperative history and physical examination should determine whether patients are adequately treated. Determining electrolyte, BUN, and creatinine levels and performing thyroid function tests and an ECG are necessary.

Intracranial tumors include gliomas (45% of tumors), such as glioblastoma multiforme, astrocytoma, ependymoma, medulloblastoma, and oligodendrocytoma, which are malignant and highly lethal. Benign meningiomas (15%) arise from the dura or meninges. Metastatic lesions (6%) are associated with virtually all types of malignancies. Schwannomas, craniophyaryngiomas, and dermoid tumors also occur. Most intracranial tumors are detected when symptoms related to a mass effect develop, patients have seizures, or they are found incidentally. Symptoms include headaches, stroke-like symptoms, vomiting, visual disturbances, altered cognitive function, and ataxia. If intracranial pressure becomes elevated, hypertension, bradycardia, arrhythmias, ECG abnormalities, and risk of brainstem herniation develop.

Careful questioning and documentation of neurologic deficits and symptomatology are important. For patients with metastatic lesions, issues pertaining to the primary malignancy or previous treatment need to be clarified. Continuation of steroids to decrease brain edema and anticonvulsant medications is essential.

Preoperative Evaluation of Patients with Psychiatric Disorders

Key issues in the preoperative assessment of patients with psychiatric disorders include assessing cognitive capacity, obtaining an accurate psychiatric history, evaluating the patient's capacity to give informed consent, and assessing the impact of psychotropic medications.[98]

Cognition is usually unimpaired in patients suffering from illnesses such as depression or schizophrenia and impaired in those suffering from disorders such as delirium, dementia, and autism. Orientation and memory should be assessed by the preoperative clinician to ensure that cognition is sufficient to obtain an accurate history and consent. Basic orientation to person, place, and time can be determined during the preoperative conversation or by looking at the way the patient has answered questions on forms. Mild cognitive impairment is frequently associated with mild dementia in elderly patients, who are at risk for postoperative delirium. More severe cognitive impairment raises issues regarding the reliability of the history and ability to obtain informed consent. Family members can aid by providing the history and countersigning consent forms.

Musculoskeletal and Connective Tissue Diseases

Deformities and chronic inflammation are key components of many of these disorders. The deformities need to be determined because of potential challenges in airway and regional anesthesia management. Chronic inflammation and associated vasculopathy with diseases such as rheumatoid arthritis, SLE, and scleroderma or systemic sclerosis often result in multiorgan dysfunction. The cardiovascular, pulmonary, renal, hematologic, integumentary, gastrointestinal, central, and peripheral nervous systems can all be involved.

Rheumatoid Arthritis

Rheumatoid arthritis affects up to 1% of the population (females more than males) and is a chronic autoimmune disorder primarily affecting the joints but often multiple systems.[99] Both large and small joints become inflamed, and severe deformity is possible, although the disease course varies dramatically. The temporomandibular joints and cricoarytenoid cartilage can be involved and result in limited mouth opening and hoarseness. Atlantodens subluxation and cervical spine instability can occur.

Subluxation is caused by laxity of the ligaments, not joint disease, and may be present in as many as 46% of patients.[100] Cervical spine diseases can occur without symptoms. Vasculitis or entrapment results in peripheral neuropathy. CAD, pericardial effusion, aortic regurgitation, and conduction abnormalities are frequently present.[101] The often severely limited functional status in these patients masks ischemic symptoms. Dyspnea, which can be an anginal equivalent, especially in women, may be confused with pulmonary symptomatology. Restrictive lung disease from decreased thoracic mobility, interstitial fibrosis, and pleural effusions may occur. Patients have an increased incidence of renal dysfunction from both vasculitis and chronic use of NSAIDs. Anemia, leukocytosis, and both thrombocytosis (from chronic inflammation) and thrombocytopenia (from splenomegaly) can be found. Rheumatoid nodules occur subcutaneously, usually over extensor joints, or in the lungs.

The preoperative history and physical examination are performed to document symptoms related to the many organ systems affected by rheumatoid arthritis (refer to appropriate sections of this chapter). Special detail needs to be given to the airway and to the neurologic, pulmonary, and cardiovascular systems. A careful history may elicit neurologic deficits, neck and upper extremity pain, and a crunching sound with neck movement. Patients who have neurologic deficits or symptoms or long-standing, severely deforming disease or who are scheduled to undergo procedures requiring manipulation of the cervical spine or special positioning, such as turning prone, require anteroposterior and lateral cervical spine radiographs with special flexion, extension, and open-mouth odontoid views.[100] Significant abnormalities (anterior atlas-dens interval >9 mm or posterior interval <14 mm) may benefit from consultation with a neurologist or neurosurgeon. However, the duration, severity, or symptoms of the disease do not correlate with cervical spine subluxation.

Preoperative documentation of deformities and neurologic deficits is important to establish a baseline level of function. For patients with significant hoarseness, referral to an otolaryngologist to assess mobility of the vocal cords and the degree of cricoarytenoid arthritis may be of benefit.[102] Acute or worsening pulmonary symptoms may trigger a need for pulse oximetry, chest radiographs, PFTs, or a pulmonary consultation (see the section "Pulmonary Disorders"). An ECG is always indicated, and abnormalities may prompt further testing or referral to a cardiologist, or both. Muffled heart sounds, pericardial rubs, and an enlarged heart detected by examination or on a chest radiograph together with low voltage on an ECG suggest a pericardial effusion, which can be evaluated with an echocardiogram. Many murmurs, especially if new, would benefit from further investigation (see Table 34-4 and Box 34-4). A CBC with a platelet count and determination of BUN and creatinine are indicated, except for the most minor of procedures.

Advanced planning for the management of identified or potential difficult airways is important. Discussion of regional anesthetic options and awake fiberoptic intubation is necessary. Continuation of steroids and chronic pain medications is optimal, but drugs with antiplatelet effects are generally discontinued and immunosuppressants may have to be temporarily stopped to allow normalization of blood counts. Patients with complex regimens and severe disease are best managed in concert with their rheumatologist or primary physician.

Ankylosing Spondylitis

Ankylosing spondylitis is a progressive inflammatory arthropathy that affects mainly the spine and sacroiliac joints.[103] It occurs primarily in males and can be accompanied by uveitis, peripheral arthritis, and vasculitis causing aortitis and aortic insufficiency. Restrictive lung disease can result from pulmonary fibrosis or poor chest wall movement secondary to joint fixation and kyphosis. Kyphosis can be so extreme that patients cannot face forward and are extremely difficult to intubate or even mask ventilate.

Preoperative evaluation by history and physical examination focuses on the skeletal and cardiopulmonary systems. A murmur warrants an ECG and may benefit from an echocardiogram. If ventilatory compromise is suspected or present, room-air pulse oximetry and a chest radiograph are necessary, as well as PFTs when appropriate. Acute processes must be managed preoperatively.

Patients taking NSAIDs require determination of BUN and creatinine levels, and a CBC with a platelet count and LFTs are indicated for those treated with leflunomide. Planning for airway management and discussion with the patient about the possibility of awake fiberoptic intubation are important. Peripheral nerve blocks are options, but centroneuraxial anesthesia is often unsuccessful because of severe spinal involvement.

Systemic Lupus Erythematosus

SLE is a systemic autoimmune disease predominately caused by vasculitis; it has a variable course, often with remissions punctuated by flares.[104] SLE affects mainly females and is typically more severe in African Americans than in other groups.

Preoperative evaluation determines whether the patient has chronic fatigue, weakness, respiratory compromise, fevers, and migratory arthritis affecting primarily the small joints of the hands and feet, which is common. Fevers may be a result of the disease itself or the frequent infections that develop because of the immune dysfunction and immunosuppressants used to treat the disease. Many patients have dermatologic conditions, including alopecia, the typical "butterfly rash" across the cheeks and nose, and photosensitivity. Vasospasm of the digits, dubbed Raynaud's phenomenon or disease, often with atrophy of the nails and fingernails, makes it difficult to obtain pulse oximetry readings.

Preoperative evaluation for interstitial lung disease, pleural effusions, frequent infections, and pulmonary hypertension is important and presents a significant concern. Pulmonary hypertension can result from interstitial lung disease, recurrent pulmonary emboli, or cardiomyopathy and carries a high risk of perioperative complications (see "Pulmonary Hypertension"). Cardiac involvement includes premature coronary artery arterosclerosis, pericarditis, myocarditis, aseptic endocarditis, and pleural effusions.

Coronary vasculitis and cardiomyopathy may occur. Hypertension, frequently difficult to control, is almost ubiquitous. Neuropsychiatric manifestations consisting of cerebral vasculitis, stroke, cognitive dysfunction, seizures, peripheral neuropathy, headache, affective disorders, and carotid artery disease are common. Lupus nephritis is a common morbidity with a poor prognosis that frequently results in renal failure. Patients with SLE often have anemia and may have leukopenia and thrombocytopenia.

Antiphospholipid antibodies occur frequently and can result in a coagulopathy with recurrent episodes of venous and arterial thrombosis, including pulmonary emboli and stroke. Typically, the aPTT is prolonged in these patients. Antinuclear antibodies are present in most cases and can help establish a diagnosis, especially with atypical manifestations.

The preoperative history and physical examination must evaluate all major organ systems and identify medications. Patients with severe disease, exacerbations, or infections are best managed along with the physicians primarily responsible for their care or a rheumatologist. Detailed questioning regarding neurologic symptoms, coughing, dyspnea, chest pain, orthopnea, fever, the course of disease, and medications is paramount. Any history of thromboembolic events is important, but recent events regarding precipitating factors, type and duration of treatment, and severity of the event (e.g., pulmonary embolus or DVT) must be detailed so that one can plan discontinuation of anticoagulants and need for bridging. Because of the significant incidence of both cerebrovascular and coronary artery lesions in these patients, careful questioning about exercise capacity, atypical symptoms of ischemia, and any previous diagnostic studies such as computed tomography, magnetic resonance imaging, echocardiography, or stress testing may be revealing.

Systemic Sclerosis

Systemic sclerosis, previously known as scleroderma, is an autoimmune disease characterized by excessive fibrosis that occurs more commonly in females.[105] Raynaud's phenomenon is the most common occurrence besides skin thickening. Localized scleroderma involves just the skin without involvement of other organs. Limited cutaneous systemic sclerosis is "limited" to the skin of the face and upper extremities as the cutaneous manifestation, but with systemic involvement, the gastrointestinal tract (dysphagia, reflux) and lungs (interstitial lung disease, pulmonary hypertension) can be affected. Pulmonary hypertension is associated with a poor prognosis and increases perioperative risk (see "Pulmonary Hypertension").[106] Diffuse cutaneous systemic sclerosis causes generalized skin thickening and multiple end-organ damage. Myocardial fibrosis, pericarditis, heart failure, and coronary artery fibrosis or spasm can occur. Patients often have severe hypertension, renal failure, dysphagia, fatigue, weight loss, reflux, and right heart failure.

The preoperative history and physical examination focus on the organ systems as outlined in the section "Systemic Lupus Erythematosus," with special attention paid to signs or symptoms of pulmonary hypertension (see "Pulmonary Hypertension"). A careful history to elicit symptoms of pulmonary disease (cough, dyspnea) or cardiac disease (dyspnea, orthopnea, chest pain) is vital. A murmur of tricuspid regurgitation and a split second heart sound are suggestive of pulmonary hypertension. Because of the thickened and fibrosed skin, microstomia, limited neck mobility, poor dentition, and oropharyngeal lesions, airway examination and planning for management are essential. Dermal thickening, scarring, edema, and contractures make venous access and regional anesthesia challenging. Discussing central venous access, even arranging for interventional radiology to place intravenous lines, and explaining the possibility for awake fiberoptic intubation will help on the day of surgery.

Preoperatively, patients with systemic sclerosis need an ECG and determination of BUN and creatinine levels. A CBC with a platelet count is indicated in those taking immunosuppressants. A chest radiograph and PFTs can be useful when evaluating patients with symptoms (cough, dyspnea) or signs (rales, hypoxemia) of possible interstitial lung disease or pulmonary fibrosis. Echocardiography is useful to screen for pulmonary hypertension in patients suspected of having this significant end-organ complication. Calcium channel blockers to treat Raynaud's phenomenon, antihypertensive agents, and immunosuppressants need to be continued preoperatively.

Inherited Connective Tissue Disorders

Ehlers-Danlos syndrome, a disorder of collagen synthesis, consists of several subtypes that have various manifestations, but almost all are characterized by joint hypermobility. Type IV is one of the most serious because those affected may have vascular and skin fragility and are at risk for vascular and visceral rupture and pneumothorax. Patients with type VI Ehlers-Danlos syndrome have muscle weakness, scoliosis, ocular and skin fragility, and osteopenia.

Marfan's syndrome is characterized by tall stature, arachnodactyly (long digits), scoliosis, pectus excavatum, ascending aortic dilatation and even dissection, valvular disease (aortic insufficiency, mitral valve prolapse, mitral regurgitation), and arrhythmias. Ocular (ectopia lentis, strabismus, glaucoma) and pulmonary (blebs, spontaneous pneumothorax) complications can occur.[107] Patients may have retrognathia and high arched palates. Careful auscultation for the diastolic murmur of aortic insufficiency is important (see Table 34-3). An ECG, echocardiogram, and chest radiograph should be obtained if a murmur is detected and management will be changed.

The most distinguishing feature of osteogenesis imperfecta is the propensity of patients for fractures from extremely fragile bones. Patients may have blue sclerae, short stature, scoliosis, joint hypermobility, hearing loss, pulmonary complications, muscle weakness, mitral valve prolapse, aortic insufficiency, and platelet dysfunction. An ECG and echocardiogram are necessary if a murmur is detected.

Epidermolysis bullosa is distinguished by blistering, skin fragility, and scarring because of abnormal epidermal-dermal anchoring. Even obtaining a BP reading may cause skin blistering and breakdown.

Kyphoscoliosis

Kyphoscoliosis is a curvature of the spine both laterally and anteriorly and may involve the thoracic or lumbar regions, or both. It occurs alone as as a manifestation of other diseases, including collagen vascular disorders, Marfan's syndrome, neurofibromatosis, muscular dystrophies, and cerebral palsy, among others. Therefore, the preoperative evaluation is aimed at identifying coexisting abnormalities. Pulmonary and cardiac compromise can occur with severe thoracic deformity. Restrictive lung disease, pulmonary hypertension, tracheobronchial and cardiac compression, and heart failure are possible.

The preoperative history focuses on functional capacity and cardiopulmonary symptoms. The ability of the patient to lie supine and allow airway access and management needs to be determined. Vital signs and performance of pulse oximetry are important. Auscultation for rales, decreased air entry, murmurs, and additional heart sounds and examination for edema and jugular venous distention are crucial. An ECG and chest radiograph are needed, and if patients are scheduled for spine correction surgery, a CBC and type and screen are required. An echocardiogram may be indicated if symptoms or signs of heart failure are present. Reversible lung disease or heart failure needs to be addressed and optimized before surgery.

Raynaud's Phenomenon

Raynaud's phenomenon or disease is an exaggerated vascular response to cold or emotional stress (thought to be due to stimulation of the sympathetic nervous system) that results in color changes of the digits.[108] It can be primary (idiopathic without a known cause) or secondary (associated with connective tissue diseases, autoimmune disorders, drugs, use of vibrating tools). It is estimated that more than 95% of patients with systemic sclerosis have Raynaud's phenomenon; 20% to 30% of patients with Sjögren's syndrome or SLE have it, but less than 5% of patients with rheumatoid arthritis. Raynaud's phenomenon most often affects the hands and typically results in a sudden onset of cold digits (fingers more common than toes) with sharply demarcated pallor or cyanosis. Cutaneous vasospasm is common in other sites such as the face and ears and can cause pain and numbness. Criteria for the diagnosis of primary disease include symmetric episodic attacks, no PVD, no tissue injury or gangrene, normal nail fold capillary examination, normal erythrocyte sedimentation rate, and a negative antinuclear antibody test. Primary Raynaud's phenomenon requires no special preoperative evaluation. Secondary disease should direct the assessment for associated disease states as outlined elsewhere in this chapter. It is important to distinguish Raynaud's phenomenon from PVD because of the difference in associated comorbid conditions. Calcium channel blockers are useful in many patients and need to be continued in the perioperative period.

Cancer/Tumors in Preoperative Patients

Cancer Patients

Patients with a history of cancer may have complications related to the disease or the treatment. Typically, patients will be aware of the side effects of treatment that they have experienced or are at risk of having. Asking them if any "unexpected complications" occurred or if chemotherapy or radiotherapy had to be interrupted because of adverse effects is important. A hypercoagulable state is common in patients with cancer, particularly those with advanced disease and primary brain tumors, ovarian adenocarcinoma, and pancreatic, colon, stomach, lung, prostate, and kidney cancer. Patients with cancer have a sixfold increased risk for thromboembolic events, and active cancer accounts for 20% of new episodes of thromboembolism (see "Risk of Thromboembolism or Pulmonary Emboli").

Preoperative evaluation should focus on evaluation of the heart, lungs, and neurologic and hematologic systems. Previous head and neck irradiation may cause carotid artery disease, hypothyroidism, or difficulty with airway management.[109] In these patients, auscultation for bruits, thyroid function tests, and carotid Doppler studies are recommended.

Mediastinal, chest wall, or left breast irradiation can cause pericarditis, conduction abnormalities, cardiomyopathy, valvular abnormalities, and premature CAD, even without traditional risk factors.[110] Therefore, younger patients who might not otherwise be expected to be at risk for heart disease but who have a history of radiation therapy for cancer should be assessed for symptoms of cardiac disease as part of the preoperative history and should have a preoperative ECG.

Cardiovascular disease is the second most common cause of mortality in survivors of Hodgkin's disease. One study found that 88% of patients had echocardiographic abnormalities 5 to 20 years after treatment, most of them asymptomatic. Treatment at a younger age increases the risk. Radiation exposure is not considered in the ACC/AHA guidelines for cardiac evaluation for noncardiac surgery but can be an important predictor of CAD.[110] A preoperative ECG, echocardiography, and stress testing may be indicated. Radiation pneumonitis can occur in those who have received irradiation of the lungs, breast, or mediastinum. A chest radiograph and oxygen saturation with pulse oximetry are indicated. PFTs may be needed.

Chemotherapy with doxorubicin can cause cardiomyopathy, bleomycin can produce pulmonary toxicity, vincristine and cisplatin may cause peripheral neuropathy, and cyclophosphamide may trigger hemorrhagic cystitis. Many agents cause renal and hepatic toxicity or suppress bone marrow, which may result in pancytopenia. Anemia is most common. A chest radiograph, CBC with platelets, determination of electrolytes, BUN, and creatinine, and LFTs may be indicated based on the type of chemotherapy.

Patients with hepatocellular cancer have a high incidence of chronic liver disease (see the appropriate section). One study found that almost 25% of patients with Child's class C disease (see Table 34-5) undergoing liver resection died in the hospital and almost 20% more died within the first month after discharge.[111] A CBC with platelets, electrolyte, BUN, creatinine, and albumin levels, LFTs, and PT are needed.

Intracranial neoplasms can be primary or metastatic and can be complicated by seizures, increased intracranial pressure with mental status changes, nausea, vomiting, gait disturbances, and hemodynamic alterations or neurologic deficits. Previous therapies, including radiation, steroids, and anticonvulsants, need to be determined. If the tumor is metastatic, the primary tumor site, the course of the illness, and complications of therapy are important. Cancers that typically metastasize to the brain include breast, colorectal, and lung cancer.

Preoperative neuroimaging, an ECG, and electrolytes and glucose levels are reviewed or obtained. Steroids and anticonvulsants are continued. Breast, colorectal, lung, head, and neck tumors commonly metastasize to bone and the liver. Bone lesions can result in hypercalcemia or pancytopenia. Pancytopenia, with anemia being most common, occurs with many cancers or with treatment of these cancers. Head and neck tumors or therapy for them (surgery, radiation) may cause difficulty with airway management and thyroid dysfunction. Lung cancer can compromise pulmonary function and cause airway problems or mediastinal masses (discussed later). Computed tomography scans of the head, neck, or chest may be indicated. Paraneoplastic syndromes can complicate almost any malignancy but are commonly associated with lung cancer. Hypercalcemia, inappropriate secretion of antidiuretic hormone, Lambert-Eaton or Cushing's syndrome (discussed in this chapter), and neuropathies may occur.

Preoperative patients who are chronically receiving opioids for cancer pain are likely to require greater than usual doses of medication for postoperative pain control. They should take their usual pain therapies the day of surgery with the exception of antiplatelet agents. Patients at risk for adrenal insufficiency should be assessed with a corticotropin (ACTH) stimulation test (see "Hypothalamic-Pituitary-Adrenal Disorders") or should be considered for additional perioperative steroids. A preoperative ECG is indicated for patients who have received mediastinal, breast, or lung irradiation or doxorubicin. All patients with cancer require a preoperative CBC with platelets and determination of electrolytes, BUN, creatinine, and calcium. Patients who are significantly malnourished benefit from 7 to 10 days of enteral or parenteral nutrition before major surgery. Surgery is delayed to allow neutropenia and thrombocytopenia to resolve if possible. Type and screening and planning blood component replacement can avoid delays on the day of surgery.

Mediastinal Masses

Lymphomas, thymomas, teratomas, metastatic disease, and goiters can occur in the anterior mediastinal space. Anterior mediastinal masses can cause obstruction of the great vessels, including the aorta, pulmonary arteries and veins, and superior vena cava, as well as the heart, trachea, and bronchi. Evaluation of patients with a mediastinal mass can be found in Chapter 59.

Von Hippel-Lindau Disease

von Hippel-Lindau disease is an inherited, autosomal dominant syndrome manifested by a variety of benign and malignant tumors. The spectrum of associated tumors includes hemangioblastoma, retinal angioma, clear cell renal cell carcinoma, pheochromocytoma, and neuroendocrine tumors of the pancreas. Preoperative evaluation of these patients focuses on evaluation of renal function and determination of symptoms or diagnoses compatible with pheochromocytomas or neuroendocrine tumors (see the section "Pheochromocytoma"). A careful history and physical examination with vital signs, an ECG, and determination of electrolytes, BUN, creatinine, and glucose is necessary in all patients. Further testing is guided by the history and laboratory findings.

Carcinoid Tumors

Carcinoid tumors are rare neuroendocrine tumors that release mediators and typically occur in the gastrointestinal tract; they are the most common neoplasm of the appendix but are also found in the pancreas and bronchi.

Preoperatively, patients with carcinoid syndrome complain of flushing, tachycardia, arrhythmias, diarrhea, malnutrition, bronchospasm, and carcinoid heart disease caused by vasoactive amines (serotonin, norepinephrine, histamine, dopamine), polypeptides (bradykinin, somatostatin, vasoactive intestinal peptide, glucagon), and prostaglandins released by the tumors. The majority of patients are asymptomatic. The liver inactivates the bioactive products of carcinoid tumors, which is why patients with gastrointestinal tumors have manifestations of carcinoid syndrome only if they have hepatic metastases. Heart disease can involve endocardial fibrosis of the pulmonic and tricuspid valves and cause stenosis and regurgitation, respectively. Right heart failure with peripheral edema and hepatomegaly can occur. Carcinoid tumors occur in MEN I.

Preoperative diagnostic tests are guided by the history and physical findings such as dyspnea, orthopnea, wheezing, edema, arrhythmias, and murmurs. Patients with diarrhea need determination of orthostatic BP, electrolytes, BUN, and creatinine. Patients with cardiac involvement need an ECG, electrolye assay, and echocardiography. Malnourished patients need orthostatic BP determination, an ECG, and electrolyte and albumin levels. Elevated urinary 5-hydroxyindoleacetic acid levels and carcinoid heart disease increase perioperative adverse events.[112] H_1 and H_2 histamine receptor blockers, ketanserin (a serotonin receptor antagonist), and octreotide may be useful to block release or the effects of mediators.

Special Issues in Preoperative Evaluation

Patients with Upper Respiratory Infections

Analysis of the literature available on patients with upper respiratory infections and anesthesia provides guidelines to help ensure patient safety while minimizing unnecessary cancellations. Although children with active and recent upper respiratory infections have been shown to be at increased risk for postoperative respiratory complications, these complications are generally manageable and have not been associated with long-term sequelae. Tait and Malviya summarized the literature on patients with upper respiratory infections and have provided a useful practice algorithm.[113] According to this algorithm, afebrile patients with symptoms of an uncomplicated upper respiratory infection, including clear secretions, should be able to undergo surgery.

The preoperative evaluation distinguishes patients with more severe symptoms, including purulent secretions, productive cough, temperature higher than 38°C, or signs of pulmonary involvement, and elective surgery should be postponed for about 4 weeks. This period was suggested because airway hyperreactivity persists for several weeks after an upper respiratory infection and patients recovering from one have been shown to have a rate of complications similar to those who have acute symptoms. Additional risk factors that should be considered include a history of asthma, need for intubation, surgery on the airway, smoking history, and a history of prematurity in pediatric patients. In patients with severe symptoms, especially those with underlying conditions (e.g., significant asthma, heart disease, and immunosuppression) that may further compromise safe anesthesia, elective surgery should be postponed for at least 4 weeks as well.[113] Preoperative laboratory testing and chest films may not be helpful in the decision; patients with viral infections may not have elevated white blood cell counts, and chest film findings typically lag behind clinical symptoms in patients with lower respiratory infections.

The risk-benefit ratio in each individual case needs to be assessed. Most would agree that surgery in patients with mild uncomplicated upper respiratory infections should not be canceled and surgery in those with more severe symptoms should be postponed for 4 weeks. Management should include awareness and prevention of potential complications.

Preoperative Evaluation of Patients with a Transplanted Organ

The number of patients with transplanted organs requiring nontransplant surgery increases yearly. These patients present special issues for preoperative evaluation because of concerns about transplant function, allograft denervation, immunosuppression, and post-transplant physiologic and pharmacologic issues (see Chapter 67). Close interaction with the transplant team is considered one of the most important steps in the perioperative care of these patients, and clinicians performing the preoperative assessment should ensure that the transplant care providers are aware of the upcoming procedure and be given an opportunity to make recommendations.

During the preoperative evaluation, the dosage regimen of all agents should be noted and patients should be instructed to continue taking all of these medications. However, these drugs can modify the pharmacology of many agents administered during the perioperative period. Impact on agents administered during anesthesia is discussed elsewhere and has been summarized in the literature.[114,115]

There are some general preoperative considerations in all transplant patients, as well as concerns specific to the type of organ transplanted.[116] In all transplant patients, the level of function of the transplanted organ and the presence of rejection should be evaluated. Immunosuppressant therapy results in hyperglycemia and adrenal suppression (steroids); risk of infection, hypertension, and renal insufficiency (steroids, cyclosporine, tacrolimus); and myelosuppresion with anemia, thrombocytopenia, and leukopenia (azathioprine, sirolimus). Because these patients are chronically immunosuppressed, the potential for infection should be considered in any preoperative evaluation. Although these patients are at higher risk for the development of infectious complications, there is no evidence suggesting that heightened antibiotic prophylaxis has any added benefit, and the usual preoperative recommendations should be followed. The need for "stress dose" supplementation in patients taking low-dose corticosteroids is controversial, although because of the low risks involved with this therapy, it is used frequently.

Careful cardiac evaluation is important in all transplant patients because the incidence of cardiovascular disease is increased. This is due to a variety of factors, including the association of organ failure with a number of cardiovascular risk factors, as well as the role of drug regimens, transplantation, and rejection episodes in creating new and worsened cardiovascular risk factors. Patients with heart transplants periodically undergo evaluation for CAD (stress testing or catheterization) and function (echocardiogram or multiple gated acquisition [MUGA]).

Renal function should be assessed preoperatively because chronic renal insufficiency is becoming a significant problem in recipients of other solid organs secondary to long-term use of immunosuppressive regimens. Although the effects of transplantation and immunosuppressive regimens on intravascular coagulation are controversial, DVT prophylaxis should be considered in all transplant patients.

Kidney transplant recipients present some specific issues. Despite the presence of a normal creatinine level, the average GFR is generally decreased. This predisposes patients to electrolyte abnormalities and altered drug metabolism, as reviewed in the articles referenced earlier. The risk for cardiovascular disease in renal transplant recipients is approximately twice that in the general population, and careful presurgical cardiac evaluation is essential. Nephrotoxic drugs, NSAIDs, and COX-2 inhibitors should be avoided in renal transplant recipients.

Liver transplant patients require careful evaluation of pulmonary function. Hepatopulmonary syndrome, which consists of intrapulmonary shunting caused by intrapulmonary vascular dilatation, can result in hypoxemia. These patients can also have ventilation-perfusion mismatching as a result of effusion, ascites, and diaphragmatic dysfunction. Diffusion abnormalities can result from interstitial pneumonitis and impaired hypoxic pulmonary vasoconstriction. In some cases, pretransplant pulmonary disturbances do not completely resolve after transplantation.

Lung transplant patients may require months to achieve peak pulmonary functional capacity. Because of exposure to the external environment, the transplanted lung is susceptible to infection and rejection. Lung transplant patients have a high rate of pulmonary infection, and the airway anastomosis is subject to risk of injury with intubation. Loss of the cough reflex and airway hyperresponsiveness may be present. These patients are also at increased risk for pulmonary edema. Preoperative pulmonary function testing can be extremely helpful.

Most of the issues relating to heart transplant patients evolve from the absence of autonomic innervation; specific drug effects are described in detail in the items referenced. The preoperative ECG may show two P waves, one from the native atria, which is not conducted, as well as one from the donor atria. The heart transplant lacks innervation, and thus ischemia is silent and autonomic reflexes are absent (lack of chronotropic response to exercise, anemia, or hypovolemia). Conduction abnormalities are common. Permanent pacemakers are required in a significant number of patients, and their function should be confirmed during preoperative assessment.

Preoperative Evaluation of Patients with Allergies

The patient's history of allergies and adverse drug reactions should be carefully documented in the preoperative record. True anaphylactic reactions should be distinguished from adverse side effects. The patient's definition of allergy may be very different from the true clinical definition, and patients may incorrectly think that previous perioperative difficulties are due to "allergies" to anesthetic or pain medications.

The incidence of true anaphylactic and anaphylactoid reactions during anesthesia is in the range of 1 in 6000; muscle relaxants account for 69% of these reactions, followed by latex (12%) and antibiotics (8%).[117] A careful history will allow avoidance of precipitating agents; premedication with histamine blockers and steroids is not generally recommended.

Anaphylactic reactions to amide local anesthetics are extremely rare. Allergies to preservatives such as para-aminobenzoic acid used with esters are more common. Patients may perceive, especially with dental procedures, adverse side effects from epinephrine in local anesthetic solutions as allergies, and this needs to be carefully distinguished. Similarly, true allergies to opioids are rare, and opioid side effects, such as nausea and emesis, may be misinterpreted as allergies. Skin testing can be used to determine the presence of a true allergy. Allergies to muscle relaxants are more common; there are no reports of anaphylaxis to volatile anesthetics.

Penicillin is the most common cause of anaphylaxis; however, of all who report an allergy, only about 10% to 20% actually have a true allergy. There is a small risk of cross reactivity with cephalosporins, but most of these reported reactions involve rashes and not anaphylaxis. Anaphylactic reactions to solutions such as bacitracin or providone-iodine have only rarely been reported; contact dermatitis in association with these agents is a more common reaction.

The rate of latex sensitization continues to increase; however, as better ways of identifying at-risk patients are developed, the incidence of latex-induced anaphylaxis is decreasing.[118] Diagnosis of a latex allergy during preoperative evaluation is based on a careful history. Patients at risk for latex allergy include those with a history of multiple surgical procedures, health care workers, and those with atopic histories. When latex allergy is identified during the preoperative visit, the operative team should be notified in advance to ensure that all appropriate equipment is available. The ASA task force outlines in detail intraoperative considerations for these patients.[119]

The scientific status of multiple chemical sensitivity disorder is controversial. Patients with this disorder report chronic, diffuse, nonspecific symptoms with low levels of multiple chemical substances. Symptoms involve multiple organ systems and include fatigue, headache, memory loss, palpitations, and gastrointestinal symptomatology. The symptoms are not generally accompanied by biologic test abnormalities or changes on physical examination. This disorder is frequently associated with chronic fatigue syndrome and fibromyalgia.[120] Performing a preoperative evaluation on these patients can be extremely difficult because patients have significant concerns about the multiple exposures involved during the perioperative period and the impact on their symptomatology. Cultural, historical, and behavioral issues, possibly in combination with some as yet undetermined physiologic abnormalities, may be responsible for the genesis of this disorder. There are no specific treatments and no current recommendations regarding perioperative care of these patients.

Preoperative Evaluation of Morbidly Obese Patients

A morbidly obese patient presents a special set of preoperative risks (see Chapter 64). Obesity is associated with an increased incidence of risk factors, including diabetes and cardiovascular disease. These patients have a higher incidence of difficult tracheal intubation, decreased arterial oxygenation, increased gastric volume, decreased gastric pH, postoperative wound infection, pulmonary embolism, and sudden death.[121]

Obesity is an independent risk factor for heart disease. Hypertension, stroke, hyperlipidemia, osteoarthritis, diabetes mellitus, cancer, and obstructive sleep apnea (OSA) are more common in obese people. Obese individuals have increased oxygen consumption and work of breathing but decreased lung volume and capacity. They have LVH and often decreased functional capacity. They frequently complain of dyspnea, which may be related to cardiac or pulmonary insufficiency or deconditioning. They are at risk for nonalcoholic steatohepatitis, also known as "fatty liver," which results in elevated LFT values and can progress to fibrosis.

Preoperative evaluation should be directed toward coexisting diseases. Patients with extreme obesity are at risk for heart failure and pulmonary hypertension. Obesity-hypoventilation syndrome (OHS), also known as pickwickian syndrome, is distinct from OSA. OHS is associated with awake, chronic hypoxemia (Pa_{O_2} <65 mm Hg) without a diagnosis of COPD or primary lung disease. These patients have impaired central ventilatory drive. Drugs or methods of weight reduction (purging, diuretics, laxatives, gastric bypass procedures) may result in electrolyte abnormalities, vitamin deficiencies, malnutrition, anemia, and cardiopulmonary disorders. Fenfluramine and dexfenfluramine, unavailable since 1997, caused mainly regurgitant valvular lesions and pulmonary hypertension. It is recommended that anyone ever exposed to these drugs undergo a cardiovascular evaluation. An ECG and echocardiogram (frequently done in the past) are recommended for those suspected of having dysfunction.

The preoperative history and physical examination focus on the airway, a history of snoring or daytime sleepiness, the cardiopulmonary system, and vital signs, including pulse oximetry. The BP cuff needs to have a width of approximately two thirds that of the arm and a length to adequately encircle the extremity. Neck circumference predicts difficulty with intubation. Depending on the history and physical findings, additional testing may be indicated.

These patients also have an increased incidence of OSA, which can be associated with pulmonary and systemic hypertension, left and right ventricular hypertrophy, and an increased incidence of arrhythmias, MI, and stroke.[122]

Preoperative Evaluation of Patients with Obstructive Sleep Apnea

Sleep-disordered breathing affects up to 9% of middle-aged women and 24% of middle-aged men; less than 15% of these cases have been diagnosed. Asking patients whether they snore, about the intensity of their snoring and whether it bothers others, about observed awakenings or choking, about daytime sleepiness and whether it interferes with activities, and about falling asleep while driving can identify those with probable sleep apnea. OSA, the most common serious manifestation of sleep-disordered breathing, is caused by intermittent airway obstruction. OSA is characterized by total collapse of the airway with complete obstruction for more than 10 seconds. Obstructive hypopnea is partial collapse (30% to 99%) associated with at least 4% arterial oxygen desaturation. The severity of OSA is measured with the apnea-hypoxia index, or the number of apneic and hypopneic episodes per hour of sleep. Patients with severe OSA have more than 30 episodes per hour.

Cardiovascular disease is common in patients with OSA. These patients have an increased incidence of hypertension, atrial fibrillation, bradyarrhythmias, ventricular ectopy, endothelial damage, stroke, heart failure, pulmonary hypertension, dilated cardiomyopathy, and atherosclerotic CAD.[60] Mask ventilation, direct laryngoscopy, endotracheal intubation, and even fiberoptic visualization of the airway are more difficult in patients with OSA than in healthy patients (see Chapters 50 and 64). Patients with OSA are more sensitive to the respiratory depressant effects of opioids than individuals without OSA are.

Preoperative evaluation should focus on identifying patients at risk for OSA and improving associated comorbid conditions in those with OSA. Echocardiography may be indicated if heart failure or pulmonary hypertension is suspected. Many of these patients are obese, and even if not, many of the same issues that apply to obese patients affect those with OSA. Patients should be instructed to bring their continuous positive airway pressure devices to the hospital on the day of surgery. Postoperative pain management and monitoring are critical.

Human Immunodeficiency Virus and Acquired Immunodeficiency Syndrome

The HIV pandemic has spread to every country in the world. Acute infection with the virus causes a mononucleosis-like illness that progresses to chronic lymphadenopathy (lasting 3 to 5 years) and culminates in a cell-mediated immune deficiency characterized by opportunistic infections, malignancies such as Kaposi's sarcoma and non-Hodgkin's lymphoma, and death, usually secondary to infections, wasting, or cancer. Risk factors for HIV infection include sexual contact with an infected individual, blood-borne contamination, men who have sex with men, sexual workers, and those having contact with sexual workers. Most infection transmitted by blood exposure occurs in intravenous drug users, and infection via transfusion in the United States is rare (1 per 1.5 to 2 million blood transfusions). Mothers can transmit the disease to their infants, usually during breastfeeding or delivery.[123] Minority populations are at increased risk for HIV infection. Many patients infected with HIV are unaware of their status.

HIV can affect all organs and cause multiple complications. Myocarditis, dilated cardiomyopathy, valvular disease, pulmonary hypertension, pericardial effusions, and tamponade are possible. Antiretroviral-induced lipodystrophy causes CAD. Pulmonary infections with *Pneumocystis jiroveci*, *Mycobacterium avium* or *tuberculosis*, cytomegalovirus, and *Cryptococcus* are common and often drug resistant. Central nervous system tumors, infections, aseptic meningitis, and acquired immunodeficiency syndrome (AIDS)-related dementia occur, as well as lymphomas, Kaposi's sarcoma, cervical cancer, and lymphoid interstitial pneumonitis. Supraglottic or intraoral Kaposi's sarcoma may interfere with ventilation and intubation; non-Hodgkin's lymphoma can cause mediastinal masses. Dysphagia, diarrhea, esophagitis, and renal dysfunction can lead to malnutrition, dehydration, and electrolyte imbalance (hyponatremia and hyperkalemia are the two major electrolyte disorders). Acute tubular necrosis, glomerulonephritis, renovascular disease, and HIV-associated nephropathy with nephritic syndrome can be present. The nucleoside reverse transcriptase inhibitors (i.e., zidovudine, didanosine, stavudine, lamivudine, abacavir, emtricitabine) may cause lactic acidosis, electrolyte abnormalities, neuropathy, autonomic dysfunction, gastrointestinal upset, renal or hepatic dysfunction, and pancreatitis. Zidovudine can cause pancytopenia.

The preoperative evaluation may illicit a history of thrush, fever of unknown origin, chronic diarrhea, lymphadenopathy, or herpes zoster in more than one dermatome. In a relatively young, otherwise healthy individual, this should raise concern of HIV infection. The enzyme-linked immunosorbent assay (ELISA) is the primary screening test and is greater than 99% sensitive but has a high number of false-positive results. The Western blot technique is used to confirm ELISA results. Patients with known HIV infection will frequently require further evaluation, including an ECG, CBC with platelets, determination of electrolytes, BUN, and creatinine, LFTs, and a chest radiograph, depending on the surgical procedure. If malnourished or evidence of nephritic syndrome is present, measurement of albumin, total protein, and magnesium levels may be beneficial. Determining the $CD4^+$ lymphocyte cell count and viral load, which reflects the patient's immunologic status during the previous 3 months, can have prognostic value. A 13% mortality rate within 6 months of surgery has been reported when the $CD4^+$ count is less than 50/mm^3 and a 0.8% mortality rate with $CD4^+$ counts greater than 200/mm^3.[109] Antiretroviral therapy is continued perioperatively.

Evaluation of Patients with a History of Substance Abuse

A patient with a history of current or previous alcohol or drug addiction presents special challenges for the perioperative team (see Chapter 101). Although the prevalence of these addictions is significant (14% and 7%, respectively), there is limited information based on prospective clinical trials to guide perioperative management.[124]

The preoperative evaluation allows an opportunity to obtain a detailed history of addiction and recovery. Addictive disease is considered permanent, even in patients who have had long periods of abstinence. If a patient is in recovery, knowledge of the dosages and effects of medications used for maintenance of recovery is essential. Verification of all medication doses is vital. In a recovering patient, anxiety may be heightened as a result of concern about the possibility of both relapse into addiction and inadequate pain treatment because of the history of addiction. The patient should be assured during the preoperative interview that anxiety and pain will be adequately treated. Clinicians may have prejudicial attitudes and may lack the educational background to formulate appropriate plans for pain management. Pain medication may be inadequate and restricted because of concern about provoking a relapse. Identifying these at-risk patients during the preoperative evaluation and involving the acute pain service to assist in management may be helpful.

Patients who are actively abusing cocaine and amphetamines are at significant risk during anesthesia because of intraoperative hemodynamic instability. Urine testing (especially on the day of surgery) is appropriate to ensure the absence of abused substances in patients about to undergo procedures. Patients who are currently substance abusers have a variety of clinical manifestations, depending on the drug abused. Jage and Heid suggest classifying the substances into three categories: central nervous system depressors (e.g., heroin, alcohol, sedatives, hypnotics), stimulants (e.g., cocaine, amphetamines), and other psychotropic substances (e.g., cannabis).[125] The preoperative period should be used to plan for appropriate management. Heroin addicts may require substitution with methadone, and those addicted to alcohol, sedatives, or hypnotics may require stabilization with benzodiazepines. Discussion of regional techniques, avoidance of inadequate analgesia, and optimization of analgesia with non-opioids is essential. Inadequate analgesia can potentially activate addiction. All information and potential management plans should be clearly transmitted to members of the operative team.

Many addicts are polysubstance abusers, and psychiatric disorders are common comorbid conditions. Addicts may be at risk for a myriad of perioperative complications, including withdrawal, acute intoxication, altered tolerance of anesthetic and opioid medications, infections, and end-organ damage.[126] Intravenous drug use should prompt an evaluation for cardiovascular, pulmonary, neurologic, and infectious complications such as endocarditis, abscesses, osteomyelitis, hepatitis, and HIV infection or AIDS. Alcohol abusers are specifically at risk for potentially life-threatening withdrawal with autonomic instability and hyperpyrexia. Cocaine and amphetamine addicts can have cerebrovascular accidents, cardiomyopathy, and arrhythmias. Additionally, cocaine and amphetamine inhibit the uptake of sympathomimetic neurotransmitters, increase BP, raise HR, and can cause paranoia, anxiety, seizures, angina, and MI (even in patients without CAD).[127] Long-term use causes ventricular hypertrophy, myocardial necrosis, and nasal septal perforation. Solvents can cause cardiac dysrhythmias, pulmonary and cerebral edema, diffuse cortical atrophy, and hepatic failure. Hallucinogens, including lysergic acid diethylamide (LSD), can cause autonomic dysregulation and paranoia. 3,4-Methylenedioxymethamphetamine (MDMA), commonly known as *ecstasy*, can cause excessive thirst, resulting in hyponatremia and pulmonary or cerebral edema.

Alcoholics are at risk for alcoholic hepatitis, cirrhosis, portal hypertension, cardiomyopathy, arrhythmias, seizures, neuropathies, dementia, Wernicke-Korsakoff syndrome (ataxia, cognitive dysfunction), and macrocytic anemia from vitamin deficiencies, delirium tremens, pneumonia, gastrointestinal bleeding, and coagulopathies secondary to either hepatic dysfunction or vitamin K deficiency. Marijuana can affect the cardiovascular and autonomic nervous systems and result in tachycardia, dysrhythmias, ECG abnormalities (T-wave and ST-segment changes), and increased cardiac output.

Patients who smoke marijuana are at the same risk as patients who smoke tobacco. Opioid (including heroin) users will have a tolerance to narcotics. It is important to document dosages of opioids taken, as well as any drugs to treat addiction such as methadone, clonidine, or buprenorphine (Suboxone or Subutex; with and without naloxone, respectively), a partial μ-agonist. Patients who are receiving opioid substitution therapy will experience normal pain responses to nociceptive stimuli and will require additional analgesia for control of postprocedure pain.[128]

Patients who use alcohol or prescription opioids to excess or illicit drugs may not give a reliable history. Vital signs, including temperature, are needed. Cocaine and amphetamines may raise BP and HR. Acute opioid use can slow the respiratory rate and cause lethargy and pinpoint pupils. Alcohol can often be detected by smell. Examination of venous access sites for signs of abscesses and skin and soft tissue infections is important. Auscultation for murmurs in intravenous drug users is essential. Symptoms and signs of heart failure or arrhythmias may be present in cocaine or alcohol abusers. Long-term use of alcohol causes liver dysfunction (see the appropriate section).

Preoperative testing depends on symptoms and findings from the history and physical examination. An ECG may be warranted in patients taking methadone because this drug can cause prolongation of the QT interval. It is important to ascertain whether and for how long patients can stop consuming alcohol or addictive drugs. In addition, more importantly, what happens when they do interrupt use? Does delirium tremens develop; do they have seizures or other signs of withdrawal? Ideally, patients with drug or alcohol dependence should be drug free well before elective surgery. Acute preoperative abstinence in alcoholics, however, has been associated with a poorer outcome postoperatively than if drinking is continued.[129] Preanesthesia clinic staff should be prepared to refer patients to addiction specialists or programs or prescribe medications to prevent withdrawal in the preoperative period if patients agree to abstinence.

Benzodiazepines are useful in preventing or treating alcohol withdrawal symptoms. Patients with a history of alcohol abuse who are taking disulfiram may have an altered response to sympathomimetic drugs; Hernandez and coworkers suggest that this agent be discontinued 10 days before surgery. If disulfram is continued, users can be sensitive to small amounts of alcohol (even from skin preparations or medications) and can experience flushing, nausea, and tachycardia. These authors also suggest that patients taking naltrexone for a history of alcohol or opioid abuse discontinue the drug 3 days before surgery. Patients taking SSRIs or methadone should continue maintenance doses. Marijuana users should be advised to avoid use at least 7 days before surgery because of its long half-life.[124]

Patients on methadone maintenance regimens continue the drug through the day of surgery. Because it may be difficult to overcome the analgesic agonist effect of Suboxone, it should be stopped 3 days before surgery. Patients may require substitution to avoid relapse of addiction during this period. Preoperative consultation with pain or addiction specialists (or both) may be useful for opioid abusers or patients taking methadone to combat addiction if the planned procedure will result in significant postoperative pain.

Preoperative Nutritional Evaluation

Patients who need surgery may be malnourished, either because of a chronic disease process (e.g., cancer or difficulty swallowing after a stroke) or because of a medical condition such as intermittent bowel obstruction (see Chapter 95). Malnutrition is associated with postoperative complications ranging from a prolonged hospital stay for patients undergoing total hip replacement to more major morbidity, such as wound breakdown, abscesses, infections, anastomotic breakdown, respiratory failure, and death.[130,131]

There is clear evidence that preoperative nutrition therapy in appropriate patients can reduce postoperative complications. TJC emphasizes the importance of preoperative nutritional evaluation and planning by requiring that nutritional screening be performed within 24 hours of admission, with full nutritional assessment in at-risk patients. Organizations must establish guidelines for nutrition screening and assessment that will identify patient characteristics known to be associated with nutrition problems and appropriately refer for planning. Reasonable agreement exists about predictive indicators of poor nutritional status: weight loss greater than 10% in the 6 months before surgery, change in dietary intake relative to normal, gastrointestinal symptoms that persist for longer than 2 weeks, decreased functional capacity (from lethargic to bedridden), and other physical factors such as loss of subcutaneous fat, muscle wasting, ankle edema, sacral edema, and ascites. Detsky and colleagues have incorporated these factors into the Subjective Global Assessment Scale.[132] The physical factors are rated as normal (0), mild (1+), moderate (2+), or severe (3+). Because of the high incidence of elective procedures that occur without previous admission, screening and assessment by TJC guidelines can be done either during the preoperative visit or during the first 24 hours of admission. This makes it extremely difficult to implement preoperative nutrition support in patients who may benefit. Kudsk reported that in a group of patients undergoing gastrointestinal procedures, TJC-required assessments were performed in the vast majority of cases between 12 and 25 hours after surgery.[133] As a result, although the TJC mandate was met, the clinical team did not have the opportunity to provide preoperative nutrition support if indicated. Proper identification of at-risk patients would best be accomplished at the time of preoperative assessment and in an outpatient setting to allow time for implementation of preoperative nutrition plans.

The best places to look for loss of subcutaneous fat are the triceps region of the arms, the midaxillary line at the costal margin, the interosseous and palmar areas of the hand, and the deltoid region of the shoulder. Muscle wasting is best assessed in the quadriceps femoris and deltoid region. The nutritional status of patients can be classified A (well nourished), B (moderately malnourished; weight loss of 5% to 10% without stabilization or weight gain, poor dietary intake, and mild loss of subcutaneous tissue), or C (severely malnourished; ongoing weight loss of >10%, severe subcutaneous tissue loss, muscle wasting, and edema).

A serum albumin level of less than 3.5 g/dL in the general surgical population or less than 3.9 g/dL in patients who need total hip replacement is an accurate predictor of malnutrition.[130,131] Serum albumin less than 2.1 mg/dL was a strong predictor of mortality in veterans undergoing major noncardiac surgery.[75] The combination of history plus physical examination and serum albumin level provides slightly improved accuracy in predicting malnutrition than either indicator alone does.

When possible, nutritional status should be improved preoperatively in severely malnourished patients. Enteral nutrition is the preferred means, but if the gut cannot be used, total parenteral nutrition (TPN), though not without its own risks, is acceptable. In a Veterans Affairs study, severely malnourished patients who received TPN had fewer noninfectious complications than controls did (5% versus 43%), with no concomitant increase in infectious complications.[80]

Breastfeeding Patients

There is little science to guide recommendations for the safety of anesthetics and medications in the babies of mothers who breastfeed and receive these agents. For elective cases, women need to be advised to pump and store milk preoperatively, which can be used in the first 24 hours after administration of an anesthetic or for the duration of breast milk exposure to potentially harmful agents. The mother should discard milk produced within the first 24 hours after anesthesia and generally resume breastfeeding after this period. Very young or premature babies, especially those at risk for apnea, may have complications if the mother continues to take opioid or sedating drugs. Mothers should be advised to discuss with their child's pediatrician the safety of breastfeeding while taking medications.

Patients with Do-Not-Resuscitate Orders

Some patients scheduled for procedures will have advance directives or a do-not-resuscitate (DNR) status (see Chapter 97). In 1993 the ASA adopted guidelines for the care of these patients and updated them in 2001 (Box 34-7).[134] Frequently, in circumstances with DNR orders, care providers are focused on a procedure-directed approach (i.e., do not intubate, no resuscitative drugs), which is problematic in the perioperative period when much of anesthesia care involves this approach. It has been suggested that a better tactic would be to discuss DNR status in the context of anesthesia in a goal-directed approach (i.e., from the perspective of the patient's values and objectives, such as "quality-of-life" concerns).[135] The ideal time to discuss this emotional, complex issue is during the preoperative evaluation. It has been shown that short discussions in a preoperative clinic can foster dialogue among patients, their proxies, and physicians regarding advance directives concerning end-of-life care. A durable power of attorney was completed by 27% of intervention patients versus 10% of controls, and 87% of the intervention group discussed end-of-life care with the appropriate individuals versus 66% of the control group.[136]

Box 34-7 Do-Not-Resuscitate Orders in the Perioperative Period

Policies automatically suspending DNR orders or other directives that limit treatment before procedures involving anesthetic care may not sufficiently address a patient's rights to self-determination in a responsible and ethical manner. Such policies, if they exist, should be reviewed and revised, as necessary, to reflect the content of these guidelines.

1. Full Attempt at Resuscitation: The patient or designated surrogate may request full suspension of existing directives during anesthesia and the immediate postoperative period, thereby consenting to the use of any resuscitation procedures that may be appropriate to treat clinical events that occur during this time.
2. Limited Attempt at Resuscitation Defined with Regard to Specific Procedures: The patient or designated surrogate may elect to continue to refuse certain specific resuscitation procedures (e.g., chest compressions, defibrillation, or tracheal intubation). The anesthesiologist should inform the patient or designated surrogate about which procedures are (1) essential to the success of anesthesia and the proposed procedure and (2) which procedures are not essential and may be refused.
3. Limited Attempt at Resuscitation Defined with Regard to the Patient's Goals and Values: The patient or designated surrogate may allow the anesthesiologist and surgical team to use clinical judgment in determining which resuscitation procedures are appropriate in the context of the situation and the patient's stated goals and values. For example, some patients may want full resuscitation procedures to be used to manage adverse clinical events that are believed to be quickly and easily reversible but to refrain from treatment of conditions that are likely to result in permanent sequelae, such as neurologic impairment or unwanted dependence on life-sustaining technology.

From Committee on Ethics, American Society of Anesthesiologists: Ethical guidelines for the anesthesia care of patients with do not resuscitate orders, 2001. Available at http://www.asahq.org/publicationsAndServices/standards/09.html.

Pseudocholinesterase Deficiency

A personal or family history of pseudocholinesterase (specifically, butyrylcholinesterase) deficiency should be identified preoperatively (see Chapter 29). When patients report an "allergy to succinylcholine," one should suspect this disorder or MH. Inquiring whether the patient had to remain intubated postoperatively, was gravely ill, or required intensive care may help differentiate these disorders. Pseudocholinesterase activity may be reduced permanently because of abnormal genotypes or transiently altered because of disease, drug effects, parturition, or infancy. Patients should be educated that this enzyme also metabolizes ester-linked local anesthetics.

Preoperative records from previous anesthesia may clarify an uncertain history. A dibucaine number and plasma pseudocholinesterase, chloride, and fluoride levels should be obtained. The *dibucaine number* is a measure of the qualitative activity of pseudocholinesterase and is the percentage of inhibition of the enzyme by the local anesthetic dibucaine. Normal individuals are homozygous for the wild type, and their dibucaine number is 80 because their plasma cholinesterase is 80% inhibited by dibucaine. Those who are homozygous for the atypical genes have a dibucaine number of 20 because of 20% inhibition. Heterozygous individuals have a dibucaine number of 60 because of approximately 60% inhibition. The plasma cholinesterase level is a quantitative measure of this enzyme. Plasma cholinesterase should not be confused with cholinesterase activity, which is an assessment of erythrocyte or red blood cell cholinesterase. The combination of dibucaine number and plasma cholinesterase can differentiate genetic from nongenetic causes of prolonged apnea after the administration of succinylcholine. A transient decrease in pseudocholinesterase activity as a result of drug interactions or other identified reasons has been observed soon after episodes of suspected pseudocholinesterase deficiency, so diagnostic testing should be delayed at least 24 hours. Patients with known or suspected pseudocholinesterase deficiency should be urged to obtain proper identification (Web search for "medical alert identification").

Malignant Hyperthermia

A history of MH or a suggestion of it (hyperthermia or rigidity during anesthesia) in either a patient or family member should be clearly documented so that special arrangements can made before the day of surgery (see Chapter 37). Individuals are genetically predisposed to MH and are asymptomatic until exposed to triggering agents. Certain neuromuscular diseases are associated with a risk for MH, including Duchenne's, Becker's, and myotonic muscular dystrophies, King-Denborough syndrome, central core disease, periodic paralysis, osteogenesis imperfecta, myelomeningocele, and strabismus.

Residency Training in Preoperative Evaluation

The evolution of preoperative evaluation, as well as the anesthesiologist's role in this area, challenges training programs to educate practitioners who can function well in roles both inside and outside the operating room. Optimal preoperative assessment, as well as continued improvement, will rely on properly educating anesthesiologists in the skills of physical diagnosis and patient assessment, personnel and business management, and conducting and understanding outcome-based research in this area. It is unrealistic to expect the next generation of anesthesiologists to successfully manage administrative and clinical roles in perioperative medicine without adequate exposure during residency training. A survey of training programs published in 2001 revealed that although almost all program directors agreed that competency in preoperative evaluation was an important skill, less than half had a formal curriculum in this area, nearly 50% did not teach patient interview skills, and 39% of programs did not expose their residents to a preoperative clinic experience.[137] The American College of Graduate Medical Education (ACGME) has recognized the importance of adequate training in this area during anesthesia residency. Requirements have been amended and became effective in July 2008; requirements in preoperative education have been increased and more specifically defined.[138] During the 3 clinical anesthesia training years, 1 month must be spent in a preoperative evaluation clinic. This may occur in divided rotations not less than 1 week in length. Successive experiences must reflect increased responsibility and learning opportunities. Program objectives must include adequate training not only in the clinical aspect of preoperative assessment but also in interpersonal skills, effective communication, and business practices. Practice management, operating room management, and systems-based practice issues should be included in the curriculum.

Assessment of skills in this area requires a definition of objectives. Instruments for assessing resident performance in this area should be developed. A "Preanesthesia Consultation Scoring Checklist" has been developed that contains 37 items grouped into the domains of physician-patient relationship, medical history, physical examination, patient education, and preanesthesia records.[139] This instrument was shown to have high construct validity, moderate internal consistency, and high probability of inter-rater agreement. Analysis of the scores could reliably assess resident performance at the defined criteria. The development of similar instruments in conjunction with the institution of a specific curriculum in preoperative evaluation will be of great help in assessing resident performance, as well as in meeting ACGME requirements.

Meeting Regulatory and Reporting Requirements

Appropriate and safe clinical assessment includes elements that are considered standard of care medically, in addition to elements that are requirements mandated by outside agencies. These outside agencies may be those mandating practice for quality accreditation, such as the TJC. Agencies may mandate practice for payment, such as the Center for Medicare and Medicaid Services (CMS) or other agencies that provide payment based on practice or performance. A detailed discussion of the use of technology in the preoperative clinic to meet requirements will follow in a later section. Regulatory requirements may exist internally as well. Institutions generally develop practice guidelines or standards, and it is incumbent on all practicing clinicians to abide by the standards of their respective institutions. A number of these standards involve preoperative care issues, and a number of requirements for accreditation by TJC involve preoperative issues. These requirements are described in detail in the TJC manual referenced and are available through the TJC website (www.jointcommission.org).

As far as the timing of preoperative assessment is concerned, TJC requires that the history and physical examination be completed within 30 days before the procedure and that a reassessment be done within the 24-hour period immediately preceding the surgery. No other TJC requirements exist regarding the timing of assessments, consents, or laboratory testing. It should be realized, however, that insurance payers might have specific requirements regarding the timing of assessments in relation to the surgical procedure and payment; providers may obtain information from their respective institutional compliance departments about the timing of assessments and payment by carrier. Hospital policies must ensure that patients have the right to refuse care, treatment, and services in accordance with the law. When the patient is not legally responsible, the surrogate decision-maker has the right to refuse care on the patient's behalf. To this end, the hospital must have a framework for ensuring that such advance directives are completed. TJC requires that the hospital document and have available to clinicians the patient's decision regarding such advance directives. The preoperative visit is an opportunity to supply the patient with information regarding advance directives, as well as to document the patient's wishes regarding such directives. TJC also requires that patients with special needs be assessed and these needs addressed. Such patients may be victims of abuse or neglect, alcohol or substance abusers, patients with significant emotional or behavioral disorders, and patients with specific nutritional needs. These assessments can be performed and documented at the time of the preoperative evaluation.

Many of these elements are documented as portions of the patient's nursing assessment, which TJC mandates be performed on each patient by a registered nurse. The preoperative history and physical examination may be performed by any licensed practitioner who is credentialed to do so. The anesthesia assessment may be performed by a physician or advanced practice nurse (nurse practitioner or certified registered nurse anesthetist) with appropriate training. TJC mandates that pain be assessed in all patients. A comprehensive pain assessment can be performed as part of the preoperative nursing or physician assessments. Establishing a baseline for the pattern of pain existing preoperatively is extremely important in formulating a postoperative care plan.

Patients who are taking significant amounts of narcotics and other pain relievers preoperatively can be identified and appropriate postoperative care plans formulated and communicated to the perioperative care team. TJC also supports a number of National Patient Safety Goals (NPSGs).[140] How an appropriate preoperative process can advance achievement of the 2007 NPSGs is illustrated in Table 34-6.

Table 34-6 Role of the Preoperative Clinic in Achieving National Patient Safety Goals

2007 National Patient Safety Goal	Preoperative Clinic Role
Improve the accuracy of patient identification	Use two patient identifiers when doing evaluation or testing; verify that all information on the operating room chart is correctly labeled
Improve the effectiveness of communication among caregivers	Communicate patient issues among multidisciplinary perioperative care providers Use a standardized list of abbreviations in the preoperative chart; eliminate the use of acronyms
Reduce the risk of health care–associated infection	Identify and transfer information to the operating room and postoperative areas regarding patients colonized with antibiotic-resistant organisms
Accurately and completely reconcile medications across the continuum of care	Begin a single accurate list of prescription and nonprescription medications and dosages that can follow the patient throughout the perioperative experience
Encourage patients' active involvement in their own care as a patient safety strategy	Perform patient and family education related to the upcoming procedure
Identify safety risks inherent in its patient population	Establish and implement a universal protocol to prevent wrong-sided procedures; verify sidedness at the time of preoperative assessment and correct errors

Preoperative Medical-Legal Issues

In a malpractice action involving preoperative professional negligence, the burden is on the plaintiff to show the generally recognized standard of medical care, deviation from that standard by the defendant, and that the deviation was the proximate cause of the patient's alleged injuries (see Chapter 10). Expert testimony is generally used to demonstrate the standard of care, as well as deviation from such standards. The ultimate decision of whether practice deviated from the standard of care should be a matter of fact, not opinion. However, in the preoperative area, many clinical "standards" are in actuality only guidelines based on general consensus or expert opinion, not on outcome data from large population-based studies. Compliance with the specific institutional guidelines, as well as with guidelines and standards set forth by credible groups such as the TJC and ASA, is heavily considered. The court generally accepts statements from these groups regarding definitions of standard of care. For example, there are a number of cases in which performance of preoperative assessment as defined by the TJC or guidelines for preoperative assessment as defined by the ASA have been placed into evidence as defining standard of care. Understanding the components of proper informed consent and establishing an effective system for obtaining consent are critical elements of the preoperative process. A review of legal decisions in this area by Raab has attempted to define appropriate parameters.[141] The absence of appropriate informed consent can result in consideration of the tort of battery. Lack of adequate informed consent has also been found to constitute the main cause of negligence, even when malpractice or substandard care cannot be proved. Courts apply either of two standards for adequate disclosure; one refers to what a reasonable clinician would consider important to the patient's decision (reasonable practitioner standard), and the other is whether the clinician has disclosed what a prudent patient would need to know in order to make an intelligent decision (prudent patient standard). These are different legal concepts that are applied on a state-by-state basis. The law requires that nontrivial risks be disclosed; extremely rare complications need not be disclosed. As far as disclosure regarding risks associated with anesthesia is concerned, Raab believes that the risk of anesthesia-related death or severe injury in a patient whose health is otherwise reasonably good would be in the range of a rare consequence; however, most reasonable patients would still want to be aware of this. The signed consent form is documentation that such discussions have occurred. Raab thinks that the dilemma regarding informing patients of rare probabilities of anesthesia complications remains unsolved. With regard to surgical informed consent, a closed claims analysis has revealed that documentation of discussion in the surgeon's office notes was a significant factor in reducing indemnity risk, regardless of whether the actual consent form was signed by the surgeon, resident, or nurse practitioner.[142]

Clinicians may be concerned about liability in overordering or underordering preoperative testing. In general, clinicians are not held liable for errors in judgment; liability holds only when the testing rendered would be considered to fall below accepted standards of practice.[143] It is extremely difficult to decide what is standard of practice for routine preoperative laboratory testing because of numerous articles demonstrating lack of impact of routine preoperative screening tests on management. However, failure to order appropriate laboratory testing that would diagnose an important presurgical comorbidity would imply that the clinician had performed a substandard assessment. This emphasizes the importance of a complete and well-documented preoperative history and physical examination with testing geared toward comorbid diseases revealed by this evaluation. Routine screening batteries in the setting of inadequate evaluation would seem to put the clinician at a much greater risk of missing an important preoperative condition. A review of more than 400 diagnostic malpractice claims in the outpatient setting would support this view.[144] These investigators reported that the most common breakdowns in the diagnostic process were failure to obtain an adequate history or perform an adequate physical examination, failure to order a specific diagnostic test, failure to follow up on rest results, and incorrect interpretation of test results.

A clinician who has informed discussions with the presurgical patient and documents a proper history, physical examination, and anesthesia and nursing assessment in the chart would minimize medical-legal risk. Additionally, the clinician must provide chart evidence of discussions regarding consent, risks, and alternatives; orders of preoperative testing geared to the results of the patient's particular assessment, along with appropriate follow-up of the abnormalities documented; and notes that all the patient's questions were answered.

Information Technology and Decision Support Systems in Preoperative Evaluation

Decision support algorithms can suggest appropriate clinical management and preoperative testing based on factors documented in the patient's history and physical examination (see Chapter 4). These algorithms can be generated by clinical leadership and distributed as part of the educational and orientation process for the preoperative clinic providers. Appropriate use of clinical and testing algorithms by clinicians, even in the absence of computer-based prompts, has been demonstrated to decrease laboratory costs as a result of unnecessary or unreimbursed testing and consultations.[145]

Algorithms can be built into computer-based programs; integration with patient data stored as part of the hospital's electronic medical record would be particularly valuable. Because institutions frequently store data in programs using different platforms, there is often difficulty in attempting to integrate multiple data storage programs within a single institution and even greater difficulty in considering complete integration of patient data with commercially available systems.

Despite the potential benefits, there are a number of barriers to implementation of electronic preoperative systems. The lack of uniformity in coding medical conditions presents significant impediments to computer-based preoperative assessment systems. Coding of physician data is extremely complex, in contrast to computer recording of laboratory data. Most of the commercially available systems involve pull-down menus, which may or may not be consistent with the physician's thought processes. Pull-down menus may result in information being recorded where it "best fits" and therefore may not be completely accurate. The use of free text results in loss of the ability to generate a plan based on decision support and also prevents the use of aggregate data for reporting.

Coding needs to be recorded in such a way that the data can be used for individual patient billing, as well as in aggregate for reporting of quality performance measures. It will be difficult to demonstrate an impact of quality reporting programs on clinical outcomes until adequate physician coding through information technology can be achieved. Because of lack of this focus in coding, regulatory quality reporting programs have been shown to influence hospital improvement activities but have not been shown to have a positive impact on outcomes.[146]

Confidentiality issues in protecting computer-based data from interception are of great concern. Unlike paper-based records, computer-stored data have the potential for security risks as a result of inappropriate access to information on large numbers of patients. Proper policies and education of staff regarding privacy issues are essential. The Health Insurance Portability and Accountability Act (HIPAA) is legislation regarding the privacy of health care information and related transactions. HIPAA requirements from the Department of Health and Human Services are outlined in their website (www.hhs.gov/ocr/hipaa). Business partners of health care institutions, such as billing agencies and insurance companies, must comply with these regulations as well.

There is some concern that a change from manual to computer-based data entry during the patient visit would decrease the efficiency of established workflow patterns. The effect on the patient interview needs to be considered as well. Clinicians will need to ensure that the quality of the interview does not suffer as they divide their time between the computer terminal and the patient. The resource savings may not be demonstrated if information is merely being typed instead of written, thus again emphasizing the need for integration among platforms and reduction of requirements for free text entry. There is no evidence-based literature demonstrating truly successful implementation, quality outcomes, and resource management with either commercially based or internally developed systems that address all of the necessary elements.

Groups such as Leapfrog and the National Surgical Quality Improvement Program have encouraged the development and use of such systems to record and report quality indicators and develop technologies to improve patient safety (www.leapfroggroup.org and www.acsnsqip.org). Because of the difficulties described with development and implementation of technology, adaption has been slow.[147] No "off-the-shelf" products are available, and no standards have been developed between vendors and institutions. Regulatory groups promote the ability of such systems to decrease errors and improve standardization and safety. Physicians are concerned about cost and the impact on workflow. The use of such systems may actually increase physician workload; one study estimated that computerized order entry would require 5% of a resident's weekly work hours.[148] Again, the ability of integration to allow medications already known in primary care and specialist's offices to be automatically entered into preoperative and order entry systems would vastly increase their appeal and efficiency.

Appropriate technology can address the TJC mandate regarding medicine reconciliation. According to this mandate, providers must enter an accurate single list of all prescription and nonprescription medications and dosages that starts at the time of entrance into the hospital for services. Development of such preoperative systems and incorporation into automated electronic perioperative information systems will aid in achieving efficient assessment before surgery. Acceptance of such systems and adequate patient and clinician use will require instruction, encouragement, and delineation of potential impact for improvement of the perioperative process.

Preoperative Involvement in Prevention of Surgical Site Infections

The preoperative visit provides an opportunity to intervene in the prevention of surgical site infections (SSIs). The Centers for Disease Control and Prevention (CDC) has used the National Nosocomial Infections Surveillance system to monitor nosocomial infections in acute care hospitals in the United States since 1970. Detailed information on this topic can be found on the CDC website (http://www.cdc.gov). In addition to considerable morbidity and mortality, SSIs significantly increase health care costs.[149] The CDC has developed standardized criteria for defining SSIs so that surveillance and comparisons can be done. Many institutions monitor the incidence of SSIs among various surgical services and procedures as a quality indicator. An analysis of one's own institutional performance and comparison with CDC benchmarks can yield extremely useful information. SSIs occurring after what would be defined by the CDC as clean surgery are probably due to certain factors, many of which can be identified during the preoperative visit (Box 34-8). The CDC recommends preoperative antiseptic showering. Preoperative showering with an antiseptic skin wash product is a well-accepted procedure for reducing skin bacteria, and showering on successive days with a skin antiseptic reduces counts progressively. However, there are no clear studies showing a direct independent relationship between preoperative antiseptic showering and a lower incidence of SSIs. Nevertheless, because of the CDC recommendation, many institutions instruct preoperative patients to perform these showers. At Brigham and Women's Hospital in Boston, patients undergoing non–mucous membrane surgery are given a skin antiseptic at the time of their preoperative clinic visit and instructed to take an antiseptic shower on each of the 2 days before the procedure. The preoperative visit can also provide an opportunity to ensure that appropriate SSI prophylaxis is ordered. If an institution establishes suggested guidelines, these algorithms can be followed and antibiotic orders written and available in the chart when the patient arrives for surgery, which would allow ample time for administration as indicated in the recommendations.

Box 34-8 Factors Influencing Surgical Site Infection after Clean Surgery

Patient Risk Factors
Age
Nutritional status
Diabetes
Obesity

Factors Associated with Preoperative Preparation
Preoperative antiseptic showering
Preoperative hair removal
Preoperative antibiotic prophylaxis

Factors Associated with the Procedure
Preoperative hand and arm antisepsis
Length of the procedure
Surgical technique

Infective Endocarditis Prophylaxis

The preoperative evaluation can also be used to identify patients in need of antibiotic prophylaxis to prevent subacute bacterial endocarditis. The recommendations by the AHA that were last published in 1997 were updated in 2006 and have included significant changes from the previous version. In this update the committee concludes that administration of antibiotics solely to prevent endocarditis is not recommended for patients undergoing a procedure on the genitourinary or gastrointestinal tract. Prophylaxis for dental procedures is recommended only for patients with underlying cardiac conditions associated with the highest risk of an adverse outcome from infective endocarditis. Infectious endocarditis is thought to be more likely to develop from frequent exposure to bacteremia associated with daily activities than from bacteremia associated with a dental, gastrointestinal, or gastrourinary procedure. The risk of antibiotic-associated adverse events and the cost-effectiveness of prophylactic therapy are such that the benefits are outweighed. Under these revised guidelines, many fewer patients will be candidates for prophylaxis.

The committee defined cardiac conditions associated with the highest risk for an adverse outcome from endocarditis. Such conditions include patients with prosthetic heart valves, unrepaired cyanotic congenital heart disease, congenital heart disease repaired with prosthetic devices for 6 months after the procedure (at which time endothelialization should have occurred), repaired congenital heart disease with residual defects, and cardiac transplantation with valvuloplasty. These are also the conditions for which prophylaxis during oral/dental procedures involving gingival manipulation or perforation of the oral mucosa are recommended, although the efficacy of such prophylaxis is unknown. Prophylaxis is recommended for the patients listed who are to undergo respiratory procedures that involve incision or biopsy of the mucosa. Prophylaxis for bronchoscopy is not recommended unless the procedure involves incision of the respiratory mucosa. Administration of prophylactic antibiotics solely to prevent endocarditis is not recommended for patients who undergo genitourinary or gastrointestinal procedures. Treatment is recommended if patients have an established infection or urinary tract colonization with enterococci. Antibiotics solely for the prevention of endocarditis are not recommended for patients with other cardiac conditions, including those with previous bypass surgeries or stents.

Prophylaxis for patients after total joint replacement was reviewed and an advisory statement issued in 2003. According to this advisory, patients with joint replacement who are undergoing high-risk procedures may need preventive antibiotics. This includes all patients during the first 2 years after joint replacement, immunocompromised/immunosuppressed patients, patients with inflammatory arthropathies such as rheumatoid arthritis and SLE, and patients with comorbid conditions, including previous prosthetic joint infections, malnourishment, hemophilia, HIV infection, insulin-dependent diabetes, and malignancy. The statements conclude that prophylaxis is not indicated for patients with pins, plates, or screws. The preoperative clinic visit can be an opportunity to identify those with joint replacements requiring prophylaxis and to ensure that appropriate orders are available at the time that the patient arrives for the procedure so that optimal timing of antibiotic administration can occur.

Recommended prophylaxis is amoxicillin, 2 g orally in adults and 50 mg/kg orally in children given 30 to 60 minutes before the procedure. This dose can be administered intravenously or intramuscularly if necessary. In patients allergic to penicillin, clindamycin (600 mg orally, intramuscularly, or intravenously in adults or 20 mg/kg orally, intramuscularly, or intravenously in children) can be used. Cephalexin (2 g orally in adults and 50 mg/kg orally in children) or cefazolin (1 g intramuscularly or intravenously in adults and 50 mg/kg intramuscularly and intravenously in children) can be used unless the patient has a history of anaphylaxis, angioedema, or urticaria with penicillin.

Preoperative Planning for Postoperative Pain Management

The preoperative evaluation provides an important opportunity to discuss and plan for the management of acute postoperative pain (see Chapter 87). Patients may be extremely concerned about this issue. Patients with chronic pain conditions need to have a plan for the management of acute pain in the setting of the chronic situation. In institutions that have an acute pain service, patients with particularly difficult management issues, patients taking large doses of analgesics, or patients with histories of analgesic abuse can be referred for consultation and appropriate perioperative managment. Patients can also be evaluated by the acute pain service postoperatively for management recommendations. In the absence of an acute pain service, the surgical service will generally be responsible for postoperative pain management.

TJC is particularly concerned that patients with pain issues be appropriately assessed and treated. A baseline pain assessment is an important part of any preoperative evaluation and is generally performed as part of the nursing assessment.[150] The preoperative pain standards in this regard state that patients have the right to appropriate assessment and management of pain and that pain must be assessed in all patients preoperatively.

Standardization of pain measurement is difficult because of the subjective nature of the variable. Scales used fall into the categories of single-dimension scales, such as visual analog and numerical rating scales, and multidimensional scales, such as the McGill pain questionnaire.[151] Figure 34-4 shows one example used for pain assessment in a preoperative evaluation. The location of the pain is noted on the figure; the character, duration, and frequency are documented, and intensity is recorded with a numerical rating scale from 1 to 10, with 1 being no pain and 10 being the worst pain imaginable. If a numerical scale cannot be used, a scale using faces can be substituted. Use of these scales readily allows comparison when reassessments are performed postoperatively.

As part of the preoperative pain assessment, any information regarding previous and ongoing pain issues should be documented, including pain control methods that have worked or not worked in the past. Some understanding of patients' attitude toward pain medication (e.g., fear of addiction) is helpful. The exact dose of their current analgesic medications is essential. If patients take them as needed, how many are being used on average per day should be recorded.

Patients with chronic pain conditions present a special management problem. There is no reason to wean patients from pain medicine before surgery. If the patient's analgesic is an NSAID or COX-2 inhibitor, the patient may be told to discontinue use before surgery. If so, the patient may need to be given a different analgesic for pain control before the procedure. Patients should be told to take their usual morning doses of pain medicine. If the patient wears a fentanyl transdermal patch, it can be left on. It is important to inform the patient that care providers will do everything possible to maintain comfort postoperatively, but the expectation of having no pain should not be given. It should be expected that a chronic pain patient's requirement for pain medication will be increased postoperatively and should be managed accordingly. There are no useful algorithms for treatment of acute pain in chronic pain patients, and care needs to be individualized. A pain service consultation may be very useful in this situation, especially when the surgical staff is not familiar with complicated chronic pain regimens and alternative options.

Preoperative Use of Alternative and Complementary Therapies

A significant number of patients have been reported to use alternative and complementary therapies in the preoperative period (see Chapter 32). A survey of preoperative clinic patients demon-

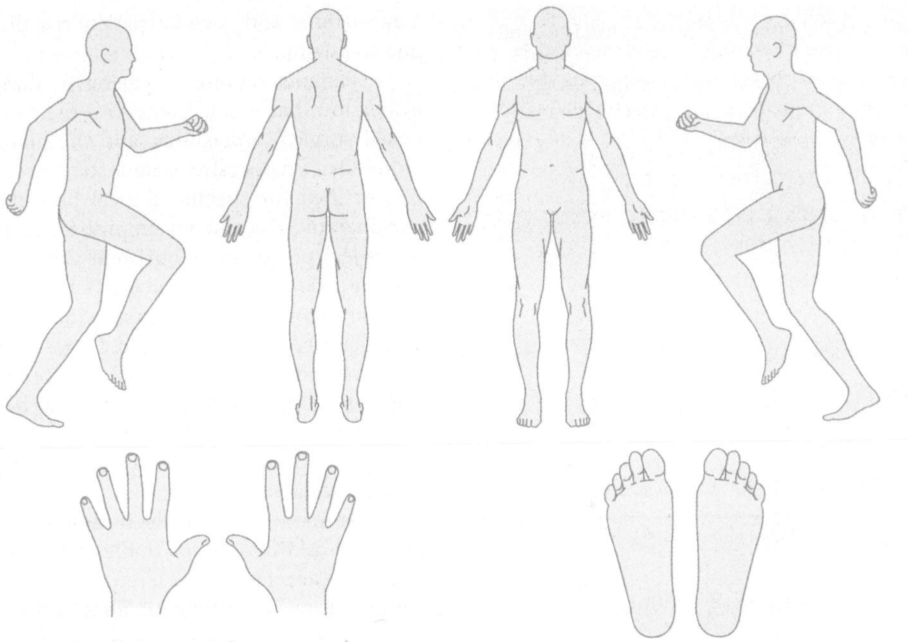

Do you currently have pain?

☐ Yes ☐ No If Yes, location: ____________________

Character: ☐ sharp ☐ throbbing ☐ dull ☐ burning

Duration: ____________________

Frequency: ____________________

Intensity scale: ____________________

☐ Numeric

☐ Faces

What makes the pain better? ____________________

What makes the pain worse? ____________________

What is an acceptable pain level to you? ____________________

Figure 34-4 Pain/status/history form.

strated that 22% reported the use of herbal medications and 51% used vitamins.[152] Women and patients in the age range of 40 to 60 years were more likely to use herbal medicine. The most commonly used compounds, from highest to lowest, included echinacea, *Ginkgo biloba*, St. John's wort, garlic, and ginseng. The pediatric population has a significant amount of use as well, which varies with ethnic subgroup.[153] Use of nonprescribed dietary supplements was significantly higher in Hispanic than in white children (33% versus 9%).

Of concern is that unless specifically questioned, patients may not report the use of these nonprescription agents. In a group of patients awaiting cardiac surgery, 56% did not inform the anesthesiologists before surgery regarding the use of these products.[154] Because patients may fail to disclose the use of alternative therapies unless specifically questioned, it is difficult to make specific associations between potential drug and herb interactions. In addition, the U.S. Food and Drug Administration (FDA) does not have regulatory oversight of purity and other standards of these nonprescription medications. Many of the herbs sold are ineligible to be approved as a drug, and the FDA can take action only when a substance is determined to be unsafe.

The ASA has published two documents on dietary supplements, one for patients and one for providers.[155] Both these pamphlets are available through the ASA website. The ASA recommends discontinuation of all alternative therapies 2 weeks before elective procedures, although there are no definite data supporting this recommendation.

The impact of alternative therapies on perioperative outcome is unclear. In a Hong Kong cohort study, 80% of presurgical patients took self-prescribed traditional Chinese herbal medicines (TCHMs).[156] Despite the high use of alternative therapies in this group, there was no significant association between any type of TCHM and the occurrence of either intraoperative or postoperative events when adjusted for covariates. Patients who used TCHMs were more likely to have a preoperative event, including a prolonged aPTT and hypokalemia.

The most common potential adverse effects of herbal medicines in the perioperative period include impaired coagulation, cardiovascular side effects, electrolyte disturbances, and prolongation of the effects of anesthetic agents.[157] There is little information available about the epidemiology of perioperative events related to alternative therapies, and there is no agency currently

Box 34-9 Potential Adverse Effects of Alternative Therapies

Cardiovascular instability, including high blood pressure, tachycardia, angina, and atrial arrhythmias: saw palmetto, ginseng, black cohosh, St. John's wort

Thromboembolic events: saw palmetto, ginseng

Enhanced potential for bleeding: black cohosh, ginkgo, garlic, ginseng, ginger, chamomile, vitamin E

Prolongation of anesthesia: St. John's wort

Hypothyroidism: soy

Hyperthyroidism: triiodoacetic acid

Hepatotoxicity: echinacea, kava

Decreased effectiveness of HIV protease inhibitors: St. John's wort

Seizures: black cohosh

Enhanced effect of opioid analgesics: valerian, kava, chamomile

Inhibited effect of opioid analgesics: ginseng

responsible for overseeing manufacturing and safety, regulating sales, and reporting adverse events. Starting in 2005, TJC required that alternative therapies be considered like any other drug when documentation of patient medications is performed. Potential adverse effects of the more commonly used agents are summarized in Box 34-9. However, much of these data is based on anecdotal evidence, theoretical proposals, and case reports—not from good epidemiologic studies with large databases.[158,159] Further in vitro data, animal studies, and clinical epidemiologic studies are needed to assess the significance of these potential interactions.

A significant number of patients also report the use of nonherbal alternative therapies. The most common complementary and alternative therapies reported in a survey of preoperative patients were massage therapy (15%), herbal therapy (10%), relaxation (8%) and acupuncture (7%).[160]

Preoperative Laboratory and Diagnostic Studies

The value and outcome of preoperative diagnostic studies and testing have become a central issue in evaluating cost-effective health care in presurgical patients. It is estimated that up to $4.0 billion is spent annually in the United States on preoperative diagnostic and laboratory evaluation. The value of obtaining preoperative studies as a screening tool to detect disease and evaluate the stability of the patient's medical condition for anesthesia and surgery has been extensively published in the academic literature.[161] The concept of standardized testing in all presurgical patients regardless of age or medical condition is no longer considered medically appropriate. Unnecessary testing is inefficient and expensive, and it requires additional technical resources. Inappropriate studies may lead to costly evaluation of borderline or false-positive laboratory and diagnostic test abnormalities. This may result in unnecessary operating room delays, cancellations, and potential patient risk through additional testing and follow-up.

Patients require preoperative diagnostic and laboratory evaluation that is consistent with their medical history, the proposed surgical procedures, and the potential for intraoperative blood loss. Preoperative diagnostic and laboratory testing should be obtained for specific clinical indications that may increase perioperative risk and not simply because the patient is to undergo a surgical procedure. Consistent accuracy of diagnostic testing and the problems associated with false positives are reason enough to limit preoperative tests to specific indications. The sensitivity, specificity, reproducibility, and clinical predictive value of preoperative diagnostic studies have been comprehensively reviewed in previous editions of this chapter. It has been well documented in academic studies that routine preoperative screening tests in an asymptomatic healthy patient have no beneficial effect on surgical or anesthesia outcomes.

At many hospitals, the tradition has been that all preoperative tests and diagnostic studies be ordered by the surgeon or primary care physician. Frequently, these tests are obtained without a specific diagnostic focus other than a speculation that the anesthesiologist may "require them" to proceed with surgery and thus avoid delays and cancellations. Other reasons include routine screening for disease states, establishment of a diagnostic baseline, personal habit (using a "standard" checklist for all patients), physician reassurance, and a perceived medicolegal necessity "not to miss anything." This historical method of ordering preoperative laboratory tests as screening devices and to avoid cancellations and delays cannot be justified and is clinically inappropriate.

Nonselective laboratory testing and diagnostic studies result in significant cost to the hospital and expense for the patient.[162,163] Routine presurgical screening tests are no longer supported or reimbursed by Medicare and most private insurance carriers without specific indications. Implementation of changes is necessary to reduce these costs and enhance patient care. Anesthesiologists are the perioperative medicine experts and are best qualified to establish appropriate and necessary preoperative laboratory and diagnostic tests for intraoperative anesthesia management. Providing specific guidelines and education to physician colleagues and surgical services for recommended preoperative testing reduces costs, expedites patient care, and enhances the anesthesiologist's recognition as the perioperative physician specialist.

Several academic studies have demonstrated reductions in hospital cost for preoperative diagnostic evaluation when diagnostic testing is coordinated through the anesthesia preoperative evaluation clinic.[164,165] Preoperative diagnosis-based guidelines (Table 34-7) provide basic recommendations for perioperative management of patients with medical conditions that increase operative risk. These disease-specific guidelines are not intended as absolute or standard requirements. There are no consistent recommendations or protocols in anesthesia texts or the literature or by medical/anesthesia society consensus of what constitutes recommended laboratory and diagnostic studies in an asymptomatic healthy patient at any age. After 6 years of extensive discussion, The ASA Task Force on Preanesthesia Evaluation published recommendations in 2002 that testing and consultation be done on the basis of a reasonable expectation that the patient may have an abnormal value and that such a value will have an effect on the decision whether and how to provide care during perioperative

Table 34-7 Diagnosis-Based Preoperative Testing

Preoperative Diagnosis	ECG	CXR	Hct/Hb	CBC	Lytes	Renal	Glucose	Coag	LFTs	Drug Levels	Ca
Cardiac disease											
MI history	X				±						
Stable angina	X				±						
CHF	X	±									
HTN	X	±			X*	X					
Chronic atrial fibrillation	X									X†	
PVD	X										
Valvular heart disease	X	±									
Pulmonary disease											
Emphysema	X	±								X‡	
Asthma	(PFTs only if symptomatic; otherwise no tests required)										
Chronic bronchitis	X	±		X							
Diabetes	X				±	X	X				
Hepatic disease											
Infectious hepatitis								X	X		
Alcohol/drug induced								X	X		
Tumor infiltration								X	X		
Renal disease			X		X	X					
Hematologic disorders				X							
Coagulopathies				X				X			
CNS disorders											
Stroke	X			X	X		X			X	
Seizures	X			X	X		X			X	
Tumor	X			X							
Vascular/aneurysms	X		X								
Malignancy				X							
Hyperthyroidism	X		X		X						X
Hypothyroidism	X		X		X						
Cushing's disease				X	X		X				
Addison's disease				X	X		X				
Hyperparathyroidism	X		X		X						X
Hypoparathyroidism	X				X						X
Morbid obesity	X	±					X				
Malabsorption/poor nutrition	X			X	X	X	X				
Select drug therapies											
Digoxin (digitalis)	X				±					X	
Anticoagulants			X					X			
Dilantin										X	
Phenobarbital										X	
Diuretics					X	X					
Steroids				X			X				
Chemotherapy				X							
Aspirin/NSAID (no tests)											
Theophylline										X	

*Patients taking diuretics.
†Patients taking digoxin.
‡Patients taking theophylline.
X, obtain; ±, consider.
Ca, calcium; CBC, complete blood count; CHF, congestive heart failure; Coag, coagulation; CXR, chest x-ray; ECG, electrocardiogram; Hb, hemoglobin; Hct, hematocrit; HTN, hypertension; LFTs, liver function tests; Lytes, electrolytes; MI, myocardial infarction; NSAID, nonsteroidal anti-inflammatory drug; PFTs, pulmonary function tests; PVD, peripheral vascular disease.

management.[3] Specific preoperative laboratory testing will be reviewed as follows, with an emphasis on diagnosis-based/clinical indications.

Complete Blood Count, Hemoglobin, and Hematocrit

The proposed surgical procedure and potential blood loss, together with individualized clinical indications, should determine the requirement for a blood count preoperatively. Primary clinical indications include a history of increased bleeding, hematologic disorders, renal disease, chemotherapy or radiation treatment, steroid or anticoagulant therapy, poor nutrition/malabsorption status, surgical procedures with anticipated high blood loss, and trauma.

Liver Function Testing

There is no routine preoperative anesthesia requirement for liver function testing. It should be based on a history of hepatic injury and physical examination findings. Primary clinical indications include a history of viral, alcohol, or drug-induced hepatitis, jaundice, cirrhosis, portal hypertension, biliary or gallbladder disease, hepatotoxic drug exposure, infiltration of tumor, certain immunologic disorders, and bleeding disorders.

Renal Function Testing

Tests of renal function measure the degree of renal tubular dysfunction and glomerular filtration. Primary clinical indications include patients with diabetes; hypertension; cardiac disease; dehydration; nausea and vomiting; anorexia; bulimia; increase fluid overload, such as in congestive heart failure, peripheral edema, or ascites; renal, hepatic, or cardiac impairment; hematuria; nocturia; polyuria; oliguria; anuria; and a history of renal transplantation.

Coagulation Testing

Clotting studies are not indicated as a routine preoperative evaluation, even in patients undergoing regional procedures, unless there is specific indication of a known or suspected coagulopathy. A careful history that includes drug therapies and physical examination will provide guidance if coagulation testing is indicated. Primary clinical indications include a history of a bleeding disorder or previous excessive intraoperative surgical bleeding, hepatic disease, poor nutritional status, and use of anticoagulants or other drugs that affect coagulation.

Urinalysis

There is no indication during preoperative anesthesia evaluation for routine urinalysis. Primary clinical indications could include a suspected urinary tract infection or unexplained fever or chills.

Pregnancy Test

Pregnancy testing is often determined by individual group practice protocols and can be based on the history and specific questions. Clinical indications can include the date of the last menstrual period, sexual activity, type or absence of birth control method, and patient or physician intuition.

The Electrocardiogram

The ECG is used to determine a previous history of MI, conduction/rhythm disturbances, ischemia, chamber hypertrophy, and metabolic/electrolyte disorders. Primary clinical indications preoperatively include a history of CAD or MI, hypertension, diabetes, congestive heart failure, chest pain, palpitations, abnormal valvular murmurs, peripheral edema, syncope, dizziness, dyspnea on exertion, shortness of breath, paroxysmal nocturnal dyspnea, and cerebrovascular disease. The ACC/AHA 2007 guidelines on perioperative cardiovascular evaluation provide additional recommendations for preoperative resting ECGs (see Box 34-3).[7]

The Chest Radiograph

There is no routine indication to obtain a chest radiograph in preoperative evaluation. The chest radiograph should be used to assess concerned abnormalities that are present by history or physical examination. Primary clinical indications for a preoperative chest radiograph include auscultation of rales or rhonchi, advanced COPD and blebs, pulmonary edema, suspected pneumonia, pulmonary or mediastinal masses, tracheal deviation, aortic aneurysm, atelectasis, cardiomegaly, pulmonary hypertension, or dextrocardia.

Preoperative Pulmonary Function Assessment

PFTs are not considered routine for patients with a history of asthma, emphysema, or COPD. Patients with pulmonary diseases have often undergone pulmonary function testing through their primary care physician, obtainable as needed. Clinical examination and a careful history will indicate the patient's current respiratory status and the potential for anesthesia/surgical pulmonary compromise.

Preoperative PFTs can assess potential respiratory complications in patients undergoing surgical resection of the lung. PFTs determine the patient's pulmonary reserve and whether the patient may require postoperative chronic ventilation support. The specifics of preoperative pulmonary function testing in patients undergoing lung resection are reviewed in another section of this chapter.

The Preoperative Evaluation Clinic

Many anesthesia groups and major medical centers have developed preoperative evaluation programs and clinics with the goal of enhancing operating room efficiency and the quality of patient care.[166,167] There are many variations in the staffing, structure, financial support, and daily operations of preoperative programs; however, all have a common goal of avoiding cancellations, delays, and adverse patient outcomes that could have been addressed before the day of surgery.

The development and implementation of a preoperative evaluation clinic depend on the daily volume of patients, the predominant medical patient acuity, the availability of facilities, the demographics of distance of the patient from the hospital, and a perioperative staff, hospital administrative, and anesthesia departmental commitment that supports changes.

It is essential that the anesthesiologist develop the leadership and management position in the preoperative evaluation program. When internal medicine departments and other medical specialties develop preoperative programs within hospitals, the anesthesiologist's role and expertise in perioperative patient management often become secondary. This can result in significant interdepartmental conflict and disagreement concerning a patient's evaluation, risk stratification, and optimal stability to proceed with anesthesia.

When patients are "cleared for surgery" by other specialties, this is often considered by the surgeon as evidence that the patient is appropriate and suitable for anesthesia. Unfortunately, this clearance is frequently provided with limited knowledge of current anesthesia practice and intraoperative patient management. The preoperative history, physical examination, and assessment by a medical specialist may not address specific anesthesia concerns of risk assessment[168,169] and patient optimization, thus providing the framework for potential surgical delays and cancellations. Additionally, patients may have had medications preoperatively withdrawn, changed, or added to their treatment in preparation for surgery, which further complicates intraoperative anesthesia management.

When cases are delayed or canceled by the assigned anesthesiologist on the day of surgery, it often creates significant frustration in the surgeon and patient. The anesthesiologist is the only specialist who can make the final determination of whether the patient is appropriate for anesthesia and whether the patient is stable to proceed. It is advantageous to accentuate this fact to hospital administrators and those who plan the development of a preoperative clinical program but remain uncertain regarding which speciality to support. Clinical studies have demonstrated that the anesthesiologist's leadership and direct clinical responsibility in a preoperative program will reduce hospital costs by decreasing operating room delays, cancellations,[164,170] and potential adverse intraoperative patient events.

Good outcomes depend strongly on awareness and planning. Anesthesia groups with a predominantly healthy outpatient and to-be-admitted population and hospital facilities with limited resources and staffing may be unable to evaluate all patients preoperatively before the day of surgery. This requires a means of screening patients and triaging them from the preoperative program in a manner that ensures a high level of accuracy in determining the patient's current health status. Accurate triaging results in time savings and avoidance of costly cancellation and delays on the day of surgery without compromising patient quality of care and outcomes.

One process of triaging involves having an anesthesia questionnaire (see Fig. 34-1) available in the surgeon's office, which could be filled out by the patient during the initial assessment by the surgeon. The questionare would be faxed to the group's anesthesia location before the surgical date. Reviewing the patient's medical history before the day of surgery, even by paper, reduces unresolved or unexpected medical concerns. A decision could then be made of whether the patient requires a formal preoperative consultation or could be evaluated on the day of surgery. A phone call by an anesthesiologist to a patient with a questionable medical history could clarify issues of concern. Another method of triaging patients to reduce the impact of unnecessary clinic evaluations would be to provide patients at the initial surgical visit with an anesthesia department Internet address where patients could fill out their medical questionnaire online for review.

Anesthesia groups with a larger number of medically complex presurgical patients may benefit from a more formal preoperative facility with multiple examination rooms, dedicated staffing, and a full-time operational system. The following sections describe the development and implementation of an anesthesia preoperative evaluation clinic with a focus on the necessary protocols, policies, and requirements for recognition, accomplishment, and success. Not every aspect of what is described becomes necessary. Various modifications and adaptations for individual practices, facility expansion, and financial support are expected.

Establishment of a successful anesthesia preoperative evaluation clinic requires interdepartmental commitment, collaboration, and financial support of several hospital disciplines.[164,171] The departments of anesthesia, surgery, nursing, and hospital administration must agree that a centralized preoperative clinic has value for the hospital, and each discipline must firmly support the necessary changes and operational goals of a preoperative evaluation clinic (Box 34-10).

Collaboration, Commitment, and Teamwork

The preoperative evaluation clinic is a visible partnership and collaboration between the departments of anesthesia, surgery, nursing, and hospital administration in achieving common goals as illustrated in Figure 34-5. It conveys the important concept that the development of this new clinical program is an integrated enterprise and requires obligation, sharing of endeavor, and financial responsibility.

Initially, surgeons may be reluctant to send patients to a newly developed anesthesia preoperative evaluation clinic. This hesitation stems from an unclear understanding of the supportive process, significance, and enhanced outcomes of a medical evaluation by an anesthesiologist. A surgeon's hesitation to send patients to the preoperative evaluation clinic can be reduced by identifying the clinical advantages of the preoperative program.

For example, informal assurances should be given to the surgical services that if a patient is evaluated in the preoperative program, the case will proceed to surgery without cancellation or delay by the assigned anesthesiologist, the only exception being illness or an adverse medical event between the time of evaluation and the time of the planned surgery. Cancellations and delays on the day of surgery can be a prominent source of aggravation and even antagonism for surgeons and patients and results in loss of revenue. Additionally, patients are often billed for hospital services although their actual surgical procedure was not performed.

Box 34-10 Operational Goals for a Preoperative Evaluation Clinic

Improve the client's perception of the preoperative evaluation experience by increasing personalized patient care, comfort, and convenience.

Provide a centralized site for preoperative evaluation.

Institute an anesthesia scheduling system for timely patient access and flow.

Ensure the presence of an anesthesiologist on site when patients are present.

Appoint a medical director to coordinate all activities.

Ensure the availability of medical records and surgical notes at the time of preoperative evaluation.

Decrease logistic shuffling of patients to multiple hospital service areas.

Integrate and coordinate services through on-site facilities for admission/registration, insurance authorization, laboratory tests, and electrocardiographic studies.

Improve the education of patients and families about the elements of their surgical procedure and the proposed anesthesia care, including postoperative pain control options.

Educate patients about what to expect regarding postoperative feeding and discharge needs.

Ensure and coordinate cost-effective ordering of preoperative laboratory and diagnostic studies.

Provide an anesthesia medical consultation service for evaluation of medically complex inpatients and outpatients.

Decrease the number of cancellations and delays in operative procedures on the day of surgery.

Enlist the skills of a nurse practitioner to assist in preoperative evaluation and patient/family education.

Develop protocols, policies, and clinical pathways.

Perform quality assurance reviews.

Maximize efficiency in operating room function and turnover time by coordinating all preoperative information at one location in the anesthesia preoperative evaluation clinic.

Enhance patient and surgeon satisfaction.

It is of paramount importance that anesthesia departmental practitioners discuss and agree on individual practice variations. Differences, such as at what fasting blood glucose level a surgical case would be canceled or what degree of preoperative hypertension is acceptable, require departmental clarification and agreement. If half the anesthesiologists would perform a particular surgical case with increased patient risk and the other half would cancel the case, the inconsistency demonstrated to the surgeon would foster a lack of support and reluctance to have patients evaluated, and essentially the clinic would be unsuccessful.

The anesthesia preoperative evaluation clinic can become a valued perioperative and hospital asset by providing consistent quality patient management and cost-effective outcomes that decrease surgical delays and cancellations. If a special medical concern related to anesthesia is identified before surgery, the preoperative program coordinates collecting the medical data, managing any additional workup or consultations, and discussing the case with the surgeon and the assigned anesthesiologist before the date.

Financial Concerns in Developing a Preoperative Clinic

Health care reforms have resulted in closer evaluation of the cost-benefit ratio and operational efficiency of many hospital programs.[172,173] Economic changes have decreased reimbursement and reduced the patient's length of stay in the hospital. At the same time there has been rapid advancement in outpatient services, especially in ambulatory surgery. The percentage of surgical patients entering the hospital as outpatients or admitted on the same day as surgery continues to increase and challenge perioperative personnel, especially the anesthesiologist.

Physicians are the primary decision-makers concerning the utilization of health care services. In preparing a patient for surgery, physicians are directly responsible for ordering virtually all of the patient's evaluations, including preoperative diagnostic testing and referral to specialists. Although health care continues to be in an active state of reform, it is frequently difficult for an individual physician or group to change the manner or routine of clinical practice patterns. There is increasing demand from hospitals and insurance carriers that providers demonstrate veri-

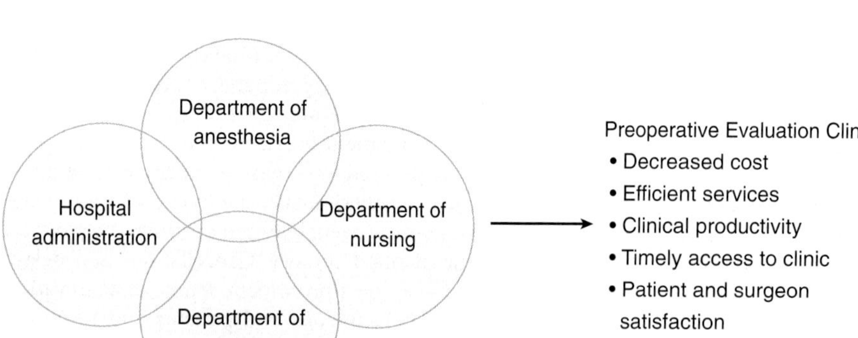

Figure 34-5 The anesthesia preoperative evaluation clinic is a constructive partnership toward common goals. Sharing of resources and budgetary costs is apportioned.

fiable evidence of decreasing costs while maintaining productivity and a high level of quality patient care.

Hospital support and financial contribution for a preoperative evaluation clinic will focus on price, quality, and value. Economic analysis of a proposed preoperative evaluation clinic is imperative to align administrative, operational, and financial support. It requires a documented comparison between the current preoperative resource utilization, costs, and outcomes (operating room delays, cancellations) with the projected preoperative evaluation clinic and anticipated operational improvements (decreased operating room delays, cancellations, enhanced operating room efficiency, etc.)

This document must be comprehensive and focused on opportunities for improvement. It is presented for hospital financial analysis in a business plan (Box 34-11) linked with academic publications demonstrating cost-effectiveness and outcomes in the preoperative clinic model. A preoperative clinic that offers no improvement and an increase in cost is unsuitable and economically detrimental to the hospital. Financial support for the anesthesia medical director is derived from both the department of anesthesia and hospital administration because the preoperative evaluation clinic is a hospital improvement–based program and can reduce hospital costs.

Facility Restructuring and Modernization

Focusing all preoperative clinical services into one hospital location establishes a center of visibility, competitiveness, and efficiency. The preoperative clinic should be regarded as a long-term investment for the hospital, physicians, and patients.

Facilities that have been developed at Stanford University Hospital are listed in Box 34-12 and are provided as an example of an extensive facility already in need of expansion because of increasing patient volume. However, not all hospital centers have the facilities or funding to construct a formal preoperative evaluation clinic. A compromise of sharing the preoperative clinic space with another medical specialty clinic could be beneficial in terms of staffing and reducing costs. The simplest of preoperative evaluation areas might be a private space in the presurgical holding area or the postanesthesia care unit as patient census decreases later in the day. Cross-trained staff from available resources such as the operating room or recovery room can assist in the preoperative evaluation program during downtime/low patient volume to process preliminary paperwork, obtain medical and outside records, record vital signs, collect laboratory specimens, and perform ECGs, for example.

The predominant costs of operating a preoperative evaluation clinic are essentially the number of staff per diem. Facility renovation can be costly or nominal. Material and supplies are usually minimal. A preoperative facility with a comfortable, low-stress patient waiting area is a positive investment in patient relationships. Patients often express their primary complaint with hospital services as waiting for excessive periods. A thoughtfully designed clinic facility enhances the patient's anesthesia experience.

Hospital administrators, surgeons, and other physicians will monitor performance of the preoperative evaluation clinic in terms of outcome measurements, personal observations, and value analysis. Achievement and success are often linked to renewed or additional financial support.

Quality assurance measurements and clinical benchmark indicators for the preoperative clinic should be entered into a database, which can then be used to determine performance standards and areas in need of improvement.[174,175] This information could measure, for example, operating room cancellation and delays, the specific causes, cost, and resource time loss. It provides the basis for operational changes and improvements in hospital service. Figure 34-6 is an example of a quality and service indicator form for a preoperative evaluation clinic.

Preoperative Standardization and Accuracy of Documentation

Standardization of the preoperative process is essential for both clinical and administrative reasons. Important reasons to encourage standardization in process and documentation are listed in Box 34-13.

Standardization maximizes reimbursement by ensuring accurate coding for the diagnosis-related group (DRG) and for preoperative testing. In many institutions, nonclinical personnel are used to review the preoperative history and physical assessment, from which comorbid conditions are coded to define the appropriate reimbursement level based on the surgical diagnosis and procedure. In some cases, a variety of clinicians in outside offices may be submitting preoperative history and physical assessments in nonstandard ways, thus making coding difficult. These assessments may focus on the surgical diagnosis and may not appropriately list all existing comorbid conditions. If an institution does not have a standardized process for preoperative recording of the history and physical examination, appropriate reimbursement for these issues may not be attained. This can be a major source of institutional revenue loss. In addition, a standardized process allows the clinician to accurately code for preoperative laboratory testing by diagnoses that can be reimbursed, as opposed to screening laboratory tests, which are no longer reimbursed by the CMS.

Standardization maximizes reimbursement by standardizing coding and data collection regarding pay-for-performance measures. Numerous strategies, including pay-for-performance measures, are being instituted across the country in an attempt to improve quality. Standardizing preoperative processes will allow the development and implementation of protocols so that the measures are met and appropriately documented. This is particularly important if implementation of these protocols is required before the day of the procedure. Presently, this could include implementing some of the national Surgical Care Improvement Project measures (e.g., appropriate perioperative β-blocker therapy).

Standardization allows the implementation of clinical algorithms based on best practice, which will optimize preoperative medical management and potentially reduce complications and ensure the best possible outcomes. Preoperative risk factors have been shown to be effective predictors of hospital cost.[176] Therefore, preoperative intervention to reduce risk could lead to significant cost savings. For example, despite the existing evidence, a significant number of patients who would be candidates for perioperative β-blockade are not receiving it at the time of the preoperative visit. There is inconsistent application of these guidelines by surgeons and referring physicians, thus again leading to

Box 34-11 Outline of a Business Plan for an Anesthesia Preoperative Evaluation Clinic (APEC)

The business plan provides or describes the following items:

I. An Executive Summary

One-paragraph summary of the proposed APEC program

II. Description of the APEC

Objective or mission of the APEC

Names of the proposed APEC medical director, department chair

Location within the hospital designated for the APEC (define an area, even if currently occupied)

Development stage (is there an existing preoperative program?)

Services of the APEC (see operational goals, Box 34-10)

Anesthesiology specialty information (i.e., anesthesiologists are the experts in operating room medicine and preoperative evaluation)

III. Analysis of General Factors Affecting Viability of the APEC

Volume and medical condition of preoperative patients (present a graph for past years)

Anticipated growth trends

Vulnerability to economic factors (e.g., fee-for-service payment is decreasing, managed care is increasing, hospitals need to decrease cost)

Technologic factors (e.g., anesthesia and surgical procedures are increasingly becoming more complex)

Regulatory issues (the APEC conforms to all local, state, and federal policies)

Financial considerations

IV. Definition of Target Markets

All outpatient and same-day admissions (i.e., increased smooth flow of a healthy patient through the health care system and educational processes, often starting in the surgical office)

Medically complex patient undergoing anesthesia and surgery

V. Discussion of Factors Relating to Competition

Competitive position of the APEC (the anesthesiologist is the operating room and preoperative medicine expert)

Barriers to entry (primary care physicians/consultants believe that they have sufficient specialty knowledge to clear patients for anesthesia and surgery)

Future competition

VI. Description of Effective Marketing Strategies

Increased visibility, which increases viability of the APEC

Use of hospital/health system news media to explain who anesthesiologists are and what they do

Formation of strategic partnerships with the departments of nursing and surgery and with the hospital/health system administration

Informal assurance that cases will be facilitated by anesthesia if seen in the APEC

Presentations at surgical, medical, gynecologic, pediatric, and administrative grand rounds (as well as others) and conferences

VII. Description of Operational Aspects of the APEC

Facilities (e.g., examination rooms, phlebotomy/electrocardiography room)

Equipment and supplies

Variable labor requirements (e.g., nurse practitioner, anesthesiologist)

Daily anticipated operations and flow

Quality assurance and utilization review

Management information systems

VIII. Description of Management and Organization of the APEC

Clinical and administrative director

Inclusion of the department of nursing and hospital administration

Organization management (presented in a flow chart)

IX. Description of the Developmental Goals of the APEC

Short-term goals (changes in clinical practice)

Long-term goals (e.g., renovation of facilities)

A time line (demonstrates a developmental plan)

The growth strategy (projection of 6-month, 1-year, and 5-year goals)

Evaluation of risk

X. Discussion of Financial Matters

Income statement (consider a facility fee, anesthesia medical consultation charge, projected hospital/health system cost savings, and market share enrichment)

Variable expenditures (e.g., APEC personnel and resources, facility housekeeping and supplies)

Balance sheet

Box 34-12 Facilities of the Anesthesia Preoperative Evaluation Clinic at Stanford University Hospital

Five combination office and examination rooms

A patient and family education room (preoperative teaching)

A patient-centered media and video room

A phlebotomy and electrocardiography room

An on-site office for the medical director

A registration and reception area

On-site restroom facilities

A large, comfortable patient lounge

An area for admitting and financial services

Approximately 2200 square feet for facilities

Conference room and shared chart and computer support room

the question of accountability for the preoperative process. An anesthesia preoperative clinic can develop and standardize clinical presurgical evaluation policies and guidelines to coordinate the process of implementing appropriate protocols before the day of surgery. This could result in decreased cost for prolonged hospitalizations caused, for example, by perioperative cardiac complications. Providing algorithms for clinical practice in areas where outcome-based data are unavailable may result in the use of arbitrary parameters based on consensus opinion. An algorithm provided to clinical staff performing preoperative assessment is provided in Box 34-14.

A second example in which implementation of a preoperative protocol may reduce postoperative complications is protocols that address reduction of SSIs. A standardized preoperative process provides a means for instruction in this regard; for example, at the time of the preoperative visit, patients can be given antiseptic agents to shower with before surgery.

Standardized processes allow more accurate data collection for quality reporting. Hospitals may be contributing data on their operational results to organizations such as TJC, the National Surgical Quality Improvement Program, or the Institution for Health Care Improvement. In addition, state law may mandate reporting requirements. For example, in the state of Massachusetts, information on the preoperative, operative, and postoperative factors and outcomes of cardiac surgical patients must be collected in a standardized fashion and reported to the state.

Standardized processes help minimize complications caused by communication errors. Recent work shows that serious communication breakdowns occur throughout the continuum of surgical care.[177] In a review of surgical malpractice claims, 81 communication breakdowns occurred in a total of 444 cases. Of these breakdowns, 38% involved problems with communication of preoperative information. Ambiguity about responsibility was a commonly associated factor. Standardization of documentation would improve transfer of care from preoperative clinicians to the operative team. Responsibility for dealing with abnormalities identified during the preoperative assessment could be clearly delineated.

Information Management and Centralization

For a patient's surgery to proceed without delay, all required paperwork and information must be present. At many hospitals, the surgeon's history and physical examination, operation consent form, laboratory test results, nursing operating room admission form, and anesthesia preoperative notes must be present in the patient's chart before entering the operating room.

The preoperative evaluation clinic can coordinate, process, and centralize all patient presurgical information in the medical chart. A simple checklist of required content can reduce delays and increase operating room efficiency by correcting problems before the day of surgery.

Because patients from out of the local area may be staying in hotels or with family or friends, it is important that a "day before surgery" local/cellular phone number be recorded in the presurgical chart so that the patient can be contacted before surgery. The preoperative staff telephones patients on the evening before surgery to ensure compliance with arrival time, to reinforce instructions, and to answer any questions. This contact by telephone avoids day-of-surgery delays and potential cancellations.

Accuracy of preoperative records is imperative, with multiple health care professionals, regulatory agencies, and occasionally the legal profession reading and reviewing medical entries. Preoperative issues that result in misinterpretation of intended documentation or physician orders can be a factor in adverse patient outcome and potential legal responsibility. Box 34-15 reviews preoperative evaluation documentation fundamentals and concerns.

Box 34-13 Importance of Preoperative Process Standardization

Standardization maximizes reimbursement by diagnosis-related group and for preoperative testing by standardization and accuracy of documentation in the preoperative assessment.

Standardization maximizes reimbursement by standardizing coding and data collection regarding pay-for-performance measures.

Standardization allows the implementation of clinical algorithms based on best practice, which will optimize preoperative medical management and potentially reduce complications and ensure the best possible outcomes.

Standardized care protocols and optimization of clinical care with a potential impact on reduction of complications can reduce the cost of admission and length of stay.

Standardized processes allow more accurate data collection for quality reporting.

Standardized processes help minimize complications caused by communication errors.

(Addressograph)

Preop Program
Quality & Service Indicator Form

Today's date: ____________

Date of surgery: ____________

• Anesthesia evaluator: ____________ Referring clinic: ____________

• Scheduled appointment: ☐ Yes ☐ No
• Arrived ± 30 minutes of appt. time: ☐ Yes ☐ No
• Patient triaged out: ☐ Yes ☐ No
• Patient chart available: ☐ Yes ☐ No ☐ Ordered
• Time first seen in preop clinic: ____________ (military time)
• Time in preop program < 90 minutes: ☐ Yes ☐ No

If No, cause of delay in preop program:

☐ No chart
☐ Outside records/tests did not arrive with patient
Time to find old/recent: ☐ ECG ☐ Chest X-ray ☐ MUGA ☐ PFTs
☐ ECHO ☐ Stress test ☐ Lab work
☐ Complex history, No H&P, start from the beginning for history
☐ Lab order problems/changes ☐ Call resident
☐ Wait to clear patient's ECG
☐ Consult with medical director
☐ Medical director not available, find appropriate person
☐ Contact outside source for additional information
☐ Patient arrived after 5:00 P.M.
☐ Patient had surgery recently, chart not available, start all over with information
☐ Clinical complication that could postpone or cancel surgery
☐ Language barrier w/interpreter ☐ Language barrier w/NO interpreter
☐ Physical disabilities
☐ Teaching
☐ Nursing assessment forms
☐ Solved problems unrelated to anesthesia; explain: ____________
☐ Cardiac surgical team not available

Evaluator
(Military Time)

Time in: ____________
Time out: ____________
Pt. Level: ____________
Teach: Yes ( ) No ( )
TOTAL
Visit time in: ____________
Visit time out: ____________

Comments: ____________

Figure 34-6 Preoperative program quality and service indicator form. ECG, electrocardiogram; ECHO, echocardiography.

Structure and Activities of the Preoperative Evaluation Clinic

The daily operations of an anesthesia preoperative clinic will vary according to patient volume, acuity of the patient's medical conditions, availability of facilities, and employee resources. However, a generalized operational structure can be suggested by examining several preoperative clinic models currently in practice.

Centers with a large volume of patients should have their patients formally scheduled in the clinic before the day of evaluation so that medical records and appropriate outside information would be available. The surgeon's office should schedule the anesthesia clinic appointment at the same time that the operating room case is booked. Flexibility in scheduling appointments is needed in the clinic to accommodate patients with urgent surgical requirements and those residing outside the local hospital area.

The anesthesia evaluator interviews and examines the patient, obtains historical medical information and outside records (via facsimile and phone as needed), and determines the appropriate diagnostic, laboratory, ECG, and other evaluation requirements. Phlebotomy, ECG, and hospital admitting/insurance registration are available in the preoperative clinic. Such centralization of multiservices provides a significant convenience to patients, who no longer must search for multiple hospital locations to complete preoperative requirements. It also centralizes all

Box 34-14 Algorithm for Preoperative Clinical Assessment

A. Assess Surgical Risk:

High risk (>5%)

- Aortic surgery
- Major vascular surgery
- Peripheral vascular surgery
- Prolonged procedures with fluid shifts*

Moderate risk (1% to 5%)

- Head and neck surgery
- Intraperitoneal and intrathoracic surgery
- Carotid endarterectomy
- Orthopedic surgery
- Prostate surgery

Low risk (1%)

- Superficial procedures
- Cataract surgery
- Breast surgery

B. Assess Functional Status

Low functional status: METs less than 4, unable to climb two flights of stairs, or inability to assess functional status

Acceptable functional status: METs greater than 4 or able to climb two flights of stairs without symptoms

C. Assess Stability

1. Does the patient have shortness of breath that is not due to pulmonary disease?
2. Does the patient have a history of syncope that has not been investigated?
3. Does the patient have a change in the pattern of chest pain or a history of chest pain that has not been investigated?
4. Does the patient have an increase in leg swelling, rales on lung examination, or new leg swelling that has not been investigated?
5. Does the patient have a history of paroxysmal nocturnal dyspnea or orthopnea that has not been investigated or has worsened?

D. Decision for Referral Based on A, B, C:

With a "yes" answer to any of the questions in C, consider referral to the PCP or cardiology regardless of functional status or surgical risk

If the answer to questions 1 to 5 is "no" and functional status is low, consider referral to cardiology only if the surgery is very high risk

If the answer to questions 1 to 5 is "no" and functional status is adequate, the patient does not warrant referral based on stability

Consider Cardiology Evaluation:

- Pacemaker not checked within 6 months
- Automatic implanted cardioverter-defibrillator not checked within 3 months
- History of positive exercise tolerance test without follow-up (Bruce <6 minutes, >4 segments with perfusion abnormalities)
- New left bundle branch block
- Atrial fibrillation (new or old) with a ventricular rate greater than 120 beats/min
- New T-wave inversions or new ST elevations or depressions greater than 2 mm
- New atrial fibrillation
- Second-degree atrioventricular block with a wide QRS complex (not investigated)
- New pathologic Q waves consistent with myocardial infarction
- Prolonged QT (>520 msec)

Consider Primary Care Evaluation

- New anemia (hematocrit less than 30% with unknown cause)
- Diastolic blood pressure greater than 110 mm Hg
- Glycohemoglobin greater than 8.5
- Wheezing on physical examination
- Potassium less than 3.2
- Platelet count less than 100,000, cause unknown or not investigated
- New hyperthyroidism
- Abnormal urinalysis suggestive of urinary tract infection
- Unexplained coagulation abnormalities
- New murmur

*Mastectomy with reconstruction, major bowel resection with colectomy, major lung resection procedures, hip revision, major back surgery, pelvic debulking.

METs, metabolic equivalents of the task; PCP, primary care provider.

hospital data into one chart, which remains in the preoperative evaluation clinic area until the time of surgery.

The patient's ECG is assessed during the clinic visit, and laboratory test results are evaluated at the end of each clinic day, with follow-up of abnormal findings as needed. In this manner, significant abnormalities can be addressed immediately, and if needed, cancellation of a surgical case would occur before the day of surgery.

One of the fundamental goals of the preoperative evaluation clinic is patient perioperative education to increase awareness and comfort by decreasing anxiety and fear. A nurse educator specifically trained in perioperative teaching discusses in detail the forthcoming surgical/hospital process with each patient and family member.

Enhanced Operating Room Efficiency and Outcomes

Appropriate utilization of perioperative services yields net benefits to the hospital and achieves a cost-benefit framework. Unnecessary surgical delays result in increased cost to the hospital and reduce operating room efficiency. The preoperative evaluation

Box 34-15 Preoperative Documentation and Concerns

Legibility of records. Poor handwriting results in misinterpretation or failure to implement important orders preoperatively.

Entries that are not signed or the signature is illegible. Print your last name and beeper/contact number.

All preoperative evaluation entries must be dated and timed in the document.

Do not black-out, obliterate, or white-out an error. Place one line through the entry, initial, and write "error."

Document all phone calls, time, and date to consulting physicians with their name and specifically what was discussed.

Note HIPAA* guidelines regarding unapproved abbreviations, which can result in patient medication and treatment errors.

If the patient has an abnormal diagnostic test result, document it and indicate what follow-up is planned. If you order a laboratory test, chest radiograph, electrocardiogram, or any test, you are responsible for knowing the results, follow-up, or referral if needed. Document it in the chart.

*Health Insurance Portability and Accountability Act.

program focuses on patient management and preparation for a smooth transition to surgery.

In one study on start times of the first case of the day, 91% of patients evaluated in the preoperative evaluation clinic entered the operating room by 6:50 AM for 7:30 AM start times. Delays were considered the exception rather than the customary occurrence. The operating room day ends earlier with decreased cost and overtime staffing when delays and problems are minimized. The preoperative evaluation clinic can establish a standard of efficient clinical services, including a contribution to on-time starts, decreased delays, and increased patient and surgeon satisfaction.

Although there are defined costs in developing and maintaining a preoperative evaluation clinic, a comparison with previous outcomes clearly demonstrates the clinic's utility, performance, and an improvement in operating room efficiency in terms of energy, time, and money.

Patient Education and Patient Satisfaction

The benefits of an effective preoperative evaluation process on efficiency have been well documented; however, there is limited information on the benefit of these clinics to the patient's experience. The use of patient satisfaction has been advocated as a unique clinical end point and as an indicator of the quality of the health care provided. Fung and Cohen believed that this outcome could be more insightful than the use of rare major outcomes such as death or common minor outcomes such as pain and nausea, which can be influenced by many other factors. Patient education and patient satisfaction with the preoperative process are closely linked. In work using an internally generated patient satisfaction questionnaire to assess satisfaction with all elements of the preoperative evaluation, the subscale that involved information and communication had the highest correlation with the overall satisfaction subscale.[178] Providing good patient education may facilitate patients' involvement in their care, give them a sense of control over the process, and contribute to increased patient satisfaction. Consumerism and transparency in quality measures, with patient satisfaction being one of these quality measures, are becoming ever more important issues in health care. Measuring patient satisfaction with the various elements of the preoperative process is essential to evaluate success and plan process improvement. Although health care leaders realize the importance of feedback systems, they often do not use the information they receive to pinpoint opportunities for change and correction.[166,179] Gail Scott provides tools and techniques that would allow feedback on the preoperative process to drive improvement.[179] These techniques are summarized in Box 34-16.

Most currently available surveys used by hospitals, such as the commonly used Press Ganey survey, reflect the overall perioperative experience. These standard questions are not effective at discerning patient satisfaction with particular elements of the preoperative process. For this reason, studies have developed internal questionnaires to measure this. Studies using this questionnaire (Box 34-17) show successful evaluation of preoperative process improvement. As noted, in this study the subscale that involved information and communication had the highest correlation with the overall satisfaction subscale. The authors conclude that the clinical and functional aspects of the preoperative evaluation visit have a significant impact on patient satisfaction, with information and communication versus the total amount of time

Box 34-16 Using Feedback to Drive Preoperative Process Improvement

Raise awareness; make sure that everyone in the organization understands the focus of process improvement.

Create measurable targets and goals (e.g., decreasing wait time).

Set service expectations and standards of behavior.

Allow direct service providers (frontline staff) access to hear feedback and input into problem solving.

Develop skills. Teach staff members customer service skills such as interviewing, dealing with difficult people, and conflict management.

Identify and remove barriers. Policies that do not make sense need to be eliminated.

Develop and support teams and relationships.

Listen to your customers: surveys, interviews, comments, shadowing.

Do not forget internal customers; obtain feedback from other teams and departments in the organization.

Share feedback in ways that teach. Eliminate an environment of blame.

Box 34-17 Sample Preoperative Satisfaction Questionnaire

Your feedback is important to us in assessing our services and helping us make changes. Please rate the quality of the services you received during your visit to the Pre-Admitting Test Center. To indicate your answer, just fill in the circle. *Please do not "check" or "X" circles.*

What Type of Surgery Are You Having?		Use these ratings:
O Orthopedic	O Neurosurgery	*Poor*
O Thoracic	O Ear, nose, throat/ophthalmology	*Fair*
O Cardiac	O Gynecology	*Good*
O General surgery	O Urology	*Very Good*
O Plastic	O Other/Don't know	*Excellent*

Please rate the following about your visit to the Weiner Center for Preoperative Evaluation (CPE):

1. Explanation of the CPE process by your surgeon's office ______________.
2. Ease of locating the CPE in the hospital ______________.
3. How clearly the CPE receptionist explained what would happen during your visit ______________.
4. Courtesy and efficiency of the CPE receptionist ______________.
5. Length of time you spent waiting to be seen ______________.
6. If you called the CPE, how promptly and efficiently were your questions answered ______________.

Visit with the Anesthesia Care Provider

1. Courtesy and respect you were given by your anesthesia provider ______________.
2. Explanation of your options and plan for anesthesia ______________.
3. Amount of time spent with the anesthesia provider ______________.

Visit with a Nurse or Nurse Practitioner

1. Courtesy and respect you were given by your nurse/nurse practitioner______________.
2. Explanation of your planned operation ______________.
3. Amount of time spent with the nurse/nurse practitioner ______________.
4. Explanation of how you should prepare for your surgery ______________.

Visit with Laboratory/X-Ray Technicians

1. Courtesy and respect you were given by the lab and x-ray technicians ______________.
2. Skill of the lab and x-ray technicians ______________.

Other

1. Overall, how would you rate the care and service you received in the CPE?______________.
2. To what degree were your questions answered clearly and completely? ______________.
3. After your CPE visit, how prepared do you feel for your surgery? ______________.
4. If you submitted information to the CPE over the Internet, such as medical history, how would you rate the service?

______________.

spent being the most positive and negative components, respectively. Of note is that after the preoperative visit, the vast majority of patients felt appropriately prepared for their upcoming procedure regarding education and communication of information (Box 34-17).

It is the role of the preoperative staff to educate the patient about issues regarding anesthesia, surgery, and the perioperative experience and to address specific patient anxieties about the procedure. A variety of ways to provide this have been evaluated, including direct communication, written information, videos, and websites. When comparing a face-to-face interview with an interview plus a brochure or a video, patients in the group receiving an interview plus a video had the highest scores in patient satisfaction and information gain.[167] An Internet tool may be a viable way for patients to receive information about their particular upcoming procedure, as well as to express concerns and formulate questions without the pressure of a rushed preoperative visit. Past studies have shown that patients may in fact be more likely to provide more information and reveal more problems, especially social and psychiatric issues, at a computer interface instead of to a health care provider.[180] By being aware of patient concerns, the visit can be tailored to better meet the needs of the patient. Time that would otherwise be spent trying to extract information from the patient can be used instead to answer patient questions more comprehensively, build rapport, and decrease stress.

How best can education be provided and patient concerns addressed? To answer this requires some understanding of what concerns patients have regarding their anesthetic and surgical experience. A number of studies have been reviewed to understand this information. Failure to wake up from an anesthetic has consistently been shown to be a major concern. Younger patients and women tend to express more anxiety regarding their anesthesia. Some practitioners believe that informing patients of all possible risks in detail will serve only to increase anxiety. Several studies have shown that more information does not necessarily decrease anxiety. It may be more important to identify subgroups of patients and focus the information toward the patient's coping style. A British study showed that although there was no correlation between the level of information provided preoperatively and patient anxiety, there was a strong correlation between patients' satisfaction with the amount of information provided and decreased anxiety. Identifying patient subgroups that may benefit from specific educational methodologies and providing this education to these subgroups in a cost-effective manner remain a challenge. In addition, optimal skills in the practitioner providing the patient education must be ensured. Diverse levels of educator experience can result in inconsistent patient information. Skill levels and core competencies in providing patient education must be established.

Preoperative patient education has been demonstrated to be a factor in reducing postoperative pain. Egbert found reduced narcotic requirements and reduced length of stay in patients who had intensive preoperative instruction about pain. Reduction in length of stay and postoperative medication was also shown in patients undergoing spinal surgery for back pain who received teaching sessions before surgery. In patients undergoing CABG, the group receiving information plus coping preparations had a lower incidence of postoperative hypertension, although this study did not show a decrease in length of stay or postoperative narcotic requirements.

In addition, patients who are taught to use a pain scale during the preoperative visit can more effectively self-report pain postoperatively.[181] Preoperative education can also provide an opportunity for intervention to improve patient lifestyle, such as an introduction to smoking cessation programs.

Optimal preoperative patient education can influence a number of factors that affect overall operating room efficiency. For example, appropriate preoperative fasting and medication orders can be given, thereby preventing delays and cancellations. An adequate discussion of informed consent during the clinic visit prevents delays in the preoperative holding area to address these issues. The preoperative visit can ensure that the patient receives adequate bowel preparation and stoma care instructions, and patients undergoing day surgery can be educated regarding the requirement for transportation home.

Preoperative Fasting Status

Preoperative fasting recommendations have been made to reduce the occurrence of pulmonary aspiration. The ASA has published practice guidelines for preoperative fasting based on the evidence available.[5] The task force supports a fasting period of 2 hours for clear liquids in all patients. The volume of liquid ingested is less important than the type of liquid ingested. A fasting period of 4 hours for neonates and infants receiving breast milk and 6 hours for those receiving formula and solids is recommended. For non-infants, a fasting period of 6 hours after a light meal and 8 hours after a meal that includes fried or fatty foods is recommended. These guidelines recommend that the preoperative evaluation include assessment of factors that may increase the risk for aspiration, including gastrointestinal motility disorders, the potential for difficult airway management, and diabetes mellitus. Separate fasting guidelines are not provided for patients with these and other conditions that may increase the risk of regurgitation and pulmonary aspiration. There is great diversity among institutions in the current practice patterns for preoperative fasting, with many being more conservative than the ASA guidelines would suggest.[182]

There is agreement among most institutions in this study that ingestion of clear fluids up to 2 to 3 hours before anesthesia is acceptable. There is diversity regarding solids, with many institutions still restricting intake of solids after midnight.

Role of the Medical Consultant in Preoperative Evaluation

The use of medical consultation for preoperative patients will vary by institution, depending on the level of expertise in perioperative medicine of the clinicians performing preoperative assessments. The comfort level of the preoperative staff in interpreting ECGs and in ordering and interpreting stress testing and echocardiograms will have a major influence on the amount of consultation requested, as demonstrated by Tsen and colleagues. Park has summarized the recommendations for preoperative cardiology consultation in a 2003 review.[183] This analysis suggests that anesthesiologists need consultation for a significant number of patients with cardiac disease who are undergoing noncardiac surgery.[184] However, as Kleinman states in the accompanying editorial, the level of expertise of the cardiology consultant over and beyond that of the requesting anesthesiologist is related to the immediate management of acute coronary syndromes.

As a perioperative physician, the anesthesiologist should have adequate expertise to quantify and manage perioperative risk. For example, in the one generally accepted effective intervention of perioperative β-blockade, a cardiologist is not needed to provide this therapy. In Kleinman's opinion, the cardiologist's major role is in the perioperative management of acute coronary syndromes and in long-term management of chronic medical conditions. There seems to be little agreement among cardiologists, anesthesiologists, and surgeons regarding the purposes and utility of consultation; a review of 55 consecutive cardiology consultations suggests that most give little advice that truly affects management.[169] When requesting a cardiology or any specialty consultation, the anesthesiologist should ask specific questions regarding the information desired to increase the value of the consultation and perioperative management.

The anesthesiologist is the final physician who questions and determines the patient's appropriateness and stability for surgery. There can be considerable frustration and tension in the presurgical holding area when a patient's surgery is delayed or canceled just before entering the operating room. Essential diagnostic studies such as a cardiac stress test or specific laboratory tests may not have been obtained. A perioperative risk concern may not have been evaluated by the specialty consultation. To avoid day-of-surgery delays and cancellations by the anesthesiologist, some surgeons have developed a pattern of obtaining more medical specialty consultations than are necessary or appropriate. When the anesthesiologist is involved in the determination of whether a medical consultation is needed, overall numbers of specialty consultations decrease—a substantial savings in cost and time.[164]

Role of the Preoperative Clinic in Guiding Intraoperative Management Choices

The role of preoperative evaluation is to provide data and guidance so that the team managing the case on the day of the procedure can make appropriate choices. It is inappropriate for clinic providers or any preoperative consultant to make ultimate decisions regarding a specific type of anesthesia to be provided. Possible options that depend on the type of procedure, patient comorbid conditions, and patient preference should be discussed. Documentation in the final anesthesia assessment should include a statement that the options have been discussed with the patient and any patient preference noted. The patient should be informed that the final decision regarding the anesthetic plan would be made by the team managing the case. The preoperative clinician should provide ample opportunity for the patient to have any questions or concerns regarding anesthetic options addressed. Patients are often concerned that they are not speaking with the anesthesia clinician who will be providing their care. They should be reassured that all information obtained in the clinic is transferred and reviewed by the team and that they will have a chance to speak with their actual care providers on the day of surgery if additional questions arise.

Additionally, should a high-risk case warrant the skills of a specialty anesthesiologist, this assessment and request can be facilitated through the preoperative evaluation clinic before the day of surgery. A personal discussion the day before surgery between the preoperative evaluator and anesthesiologist assigned a difficult case or airway enhances the perioperative management plan and avoids operating room delays, cancellations, and potential adverse outcomes.

Summary

The practice of anesthesiology has changed.[185,186] The expanding role of the anesthesiologist outside the operating room has redefined our specialty in the hospital and with our physician colleagues with regard to our clinical expertise, effectiveness, and contribution to quality patient care.

Anesthesiologists have noticeably evolved from a specialty practicing only inside the operating rooms to an acknowledged position as perioperative medicine specialists who comprehensively evaluate and manage patients preoperatively, intraoperatively, and through their postoperative pain requirements. Frequently this occurs in formalized hospital service programs or anesthesia preoperative/pain management clinics. The anesthesiologist's visibility and leadership position in perioperative patient management has enhanced hospital opportunities, leadership recognition, and the viability of our specialty.

Anesthesiologists need to be clinically knowledgeable and skilled in assessing patients in the preoperative period, whether it be in an evaluation clinic setting before the day of surgery or at the bedside immediately before induction of anesthesia. Preparation for anesthesia and surgery can be straightforward or complex and difficult. Medicine is increasingly fragmented and extremely specialized. Patients are getting older and living longer with chronic diseases. Surgical technologies, procedures, and settings where anesthesia is administered, as well as regulatory requirements, are constantly changing and requiring anesthesiologists to accept expanding perioperative responsibilities.

Guidelines and evidence-based medicine practices are being developed and updated frequently. Virtually all disease states have an impact on perioperative patients and their care. Anesthesiologists can collaborate with primary care providers, physician extenders, and specialists, but none can truly evaluate the risks associated with anesthesia, discuss these risks with patients, or manage them perioperatively other than a physician trained in anesthesiology.

Although health care changes, regulatory issues, consensus guidelines, and medical developments will occur, the primary purpose of preoperative evaluation will never change. The anesthesia preoperative evaluation is the clinical foundation and framework of perioperative patient management and can potentially reduce operative morbidity and enhance patient outcome.

References

1. Saidman LJ: The 33rd Rovenstine Lecture. What I have learned from 9 years and 9,000 papers. Anesthesiology 83:191-197, 1995.
2. Longnecker D: Planning the future of anesthesiology. Anesthesiology 84:495-497, 1996.
3. Practice advisory for preoperative evaluation: A report by the American Society of Anesthesiologists Task Force on Preanesthetic Evaluation. Anesthesiology 96:485-496, 2002.
4. Ginsburg WH Jr: When does a guideline become a standard? The new American Society of Anesthesiologists guidelines give us a clue. Ann Emerg Med 22:1891-1896, 1993.
5. American Society of Anesthesiologists Task Force on Preoperative Fasting.: Practice guidelines for preoperative fasting and the use of pharmacologic agents to reduce the risk of pulmonary aspiration: Application to healthy patients undergoing elective procedures. Anesthesiology 20:896-905, 1999.
6. Fleisher LA, Pasternak LR, Herbert R, et al: Inpatient hospital admission and death after outpatient surgery in elderly patients. Arch Surg 139:67-72, 2004.
7. Fleisher LA, Beckman JA, Brown KA, et al: ACC/AHA 2007 guidelines on perioperative cardiovascular evaluation and care for noncardiac surgery. J Am Coll Cardiol 50:e159-e241, 2007. Available at http://www.acc.org/qualityandscience/clinical/guidelines/Periop_/ Accessed September 28, 2007.
8. Kluger MT, Tham EJ, Coleman NA, et al: Inadequate pre-operative evaluation and preparation: A review of 197 reports from the Australian incident monitoring study. Anaesthesia 55:1173-1178, 2000.
9. Runciman WB, Webb RK: Anaesthesia related mortality in Australia, 1994–1995. Aust Soc Anaesth Newsl 94:15-17, 1994.
10. Hlatky MA, Boineau RE, Higginbotham MB, et al: A brief self-administered questionnaire to determine functional capacity (the Duke Activity Status Index). Am J Cardiol 64:651-654, 1989.
11. Calle EE, Rodriquez C, Walker-Thurmond K, et al: Overweight, obesity, and mortality from cancer in a prospectively studied cohort of U.S. adults. N Engl J Med 348:1625-1638, 2003.
12. Mallampati SR, Gatt SP, Gugino LD, et al: A clinical sign to predict difficult tracheal intubation: A prospective study. Can Anaesth Soc J 32:429-434, 1985.

13. Girish M, Trayner E, Dammann O, et al: Symptom-limited stair climbing as a predictor of postoperative complications after high-risk surgery. Chest 120:1147-1151, 2001.
14. Katz I, Stradling J, Slutsjy AS, et al: Do patients with obstructive sleep apnea have thick necks? Am Rev Respir Dis 141:1228-1231, 1990.
15. Poldermans D, Boersma E, Bax JJ, et al: The effect of bisoprolol on perioperative mortality and myocardial infarction in high-risk patients undergoing vascular surgery. N Engl J Med 341:1789-1794, 1999.
16. Fleisher LA, Beckman JA, Brown KA, et al: ACC/AHA 2006 guideline update on perioperative cardiovascular evaluation for noncardiac surgery: Focused update on perioperative beta-blocker therapy: A report of the American College of Cardiology/American Heart Association Task Force on Practice Guidelines. Circulation 113:2662-2674, 2006.
17. Feringa HH, Bax JJ, Boersma E, et al: High-dose beta-blockers and tight heart rate control reduce myocardial ischemia and troponin T release in vascular surgery patients. Circulation 114(1 Suppl):I344-I349, 2006.
18. Howell SJ, Sear JW, Foex P: Hypertension, hypertensive heart disease and perioperative cardiac risk. Br J Anaesth 92:570-583, 2004.
19. Furberg CD, Psaty BM, Pahor M, et al: Clinical implications of recent findings from the Antihypertensive and Lipid-Lowering Treatment To Prevent Heart Attack Trial (ALLHAT) and other studies of hypertension. Ann Intern Med 135:1074-1078, 2001.
20. Lee TH, Marcantonio ER, Mangione CM, et al: Derivation and prospective validation of a simple index for prediction of cardiac risk of major noncardiac surgery. Circulation 100:1043-1049, 1999.
21. Tait AR, Parr HG, Tremper KK: Evaluation of the efficacy of routine preoperative electrocardiograms. J Cardiothorac Vasc Anesth 11:752-755, 1997.
22. Liu LL, Dzankic S, Leung JM: Preoperative electrocardiogram abnormalities do not predict postoperative cardiac complications in geriatric surgical patients. J Am Geriatr Soc 50:1186-1191, 2002.
23. Wei L, MacDonald TM, Walker BR: Taking glucocorticoids by prescription is associated with subsequent cardiovascular disease. Ann Intern Med 141:764-770, 2004.
24. Asanuma Y, Oeser A, Shintani AK, et al: Premature coronary-artery atherosclerosis in systemic lupus erythematosus. N Engl J Med 349:2407-2415, 2003.
25. McFalls EO, Ward HB, Mortiz TE, et al: Coronary-artery revascularization before elective major vascular surgery. N Engl J Med 351:2795-2804, 2004.
26. Breen P, Wee JW, Pomposelli F, et al: Timing of high-risk vascular surgery following coronary artery bypass surgery: A 10-year experience from an academic medical centre. Anaesthesia 59:422-427, 2004.
27. Grines CL, Bonow RO, Casey DE, et al: Prevention of premature discontinuation of dual antiplatelet therapy in patients with coronary artery stents. J Am Coll Cardiol 49:734-739, 2007.
28. Grayburn PA, Hillis LD: Cardiac events in patients undergoing noncardiac surgery: Shifting the paradigm from noninvasive risk stratification to therapy. Ann Intern Med 138:506-511, 2003.
29. Topol EJ, Nissen SE: Our preoccupation with coronary luminology: The dissociation between clinical and angiographic findings in ischemic heart disease. Circulation 92:2333-2342, 1995.
30. Singh AK, Szczech L, Tang KL, et al: Correction of anemia with epoetin alfa in chronic kidney disease. N Engl J Med 355:2085-2098, 2006.
31. Wu W-C, Schifftner TI, Henderson WG, et al: Preoperative hematocrit levels and postoperative outcomes in older patients undergoing noncardiac surgery. JAMA 297:2481-2488, 2007.
32. Thom T, Haase N, Rosamond W, et al: Heart disease and stroke statistics—2006 update: A report from the American Heart Association Statistics Committee and Stroke Statistics Subcommittee. Circulation 113:e85-e151, 2006.
33. Mahler DA, Harver A, Lentine T, et al: Descriptors of breathlessness in cardiorespiratory diseases. Am J Respir Crit Care Med 154:1357-1363, 1996.
34. Criteria Committee of the New York Heart Association: Nomenclature and Criteria for Diagnosis of Disease of the Heart and Great Vessels, 9th ed. Boston, Little, Brown, 1994.
35. Januzzi JL Jr, Camargo CA, Anwaruddin S, et al: The N-terminal Pro-BNP investigation of Dyspnea in the Emergency Department (PRIDE) study. Am J Cardiol 95:948-954, 2005.
36. Maisel AS, Krishnaswamy P, Nowak RM, et al: Rapid measurement of B-type natriuretic peptide in the emergency diagnosis of heart failure. N Engl J Med 347:161-167, 2002.
37. Dernellis J, Panaretou M: Assessment of cardiac risk before non-cardiac surgery: Brain natriuretic peptide in 1590 patients. Heart 92:1645-1650, 2006.
38. Feringa HH, Schouten O, Dunkelgrun M, et al: Plasma N-terminal pro–B-type natriuretic peptide as long-term prognostic marker after major vascular surgery. Heart 93:226-231, 2007.
39. Carabello BA, Crawford FA: Valvular heart disease. N Engl J Med 337:32-41, 1997.
40. Bonow RO, Carabello B, de Leon AC Jr, et al: ACC/AHA guidelines for the management of patients with valvular heart disease. J Am Coll Cardiol 32:1486-1588, 1998. Available at http://www.acc.org/ Accessed July 5, 2007.
41. Otto CM, Lind BK, Kitzman DW, et al: Association of aortic-valve sclerosis with cardiovascular mortality and morbidity in the elderly. N Engl J Med 341:142-147, 1999.
42. Aronow WS, Ahn C, Shirani J, et al: Comparison of frequency of new coronary events in older subjects with and without valvular aortic sclerosis. Am J Cardiol 83:599-600, 1999.
43. Wilson W, Taubert K, Gewitz M, et al: Prevention of infective endocarditis. Guidelines from the American Heart Association. Circulation 116:1736-1754, 2007.
44. Desjardins VA, Enriquez-Sarano M, Tajik AJ, et al: Intensity of murmurs correlates with severity of valvular regurgitation. Am J Med 100:149-156, 1996.
45. Gregoratos G, Abrams J, Epstein AE, et al: ACC/AHA/NASPE 2002 guideline update for implantation of cardiac pacemakers and antiarrhythmia devices: Summary article. A report of the American College of Cardiology/American Heart Association Task Force on Practice Guidelines (ACC/AHA/NASPE Committee to Update the 1998 Pacemaker Guidelines). Circulation 106:2145-2161, 2002.
46. Eriksson P, Wilhelmsen L, Rosengren A: Bundle-branch block in middle-aged men: Risk of complications and death over 28 years. The Primary Prevention Study in Goteborg, Sweden. Eur Heart J 26:2300-2306, 2005.
47. Dhingra R, Pencina MJ, Wang TJ, et al: Electrocardiographic QRS duration and the risk of congestive heart failure: The Framingham Heart Study. Hypertension 47:861-867, 2006.
48. Landesberg G, Einav S, Christopherson R, et al: Perioperative ischemia and cardiac complications in major vascular surgery: Importance of the preoperative twelve-lead electrocardiogram. J Vasc Surg 26:570-578, 1997.
49. National Asthma Education and Prevention Program. Expert Panel Report: Guidelines for the diagnosis and management of asthma update on selected topics—2002. J Allergy Clin Immunol 110:S141-S219, 2002.
50. Wong DH, Weber EC, Schell MJ, et al: Factors associated with postoperative pulmonary complications in patients with severe chronic obstructive pulmonary disease. Anesth Analg 80:276-284, 1995.
51. McAlister FA, Bertsch K, Man J, et al: Incidence of and risk factors for pulmonary complications after nonthoracic surgery. Am J Respir Crit Care Med 171:514-517, 2005.
52. Arozullah AM, Daley J, Henderson WG, et al: Multifactorial risk index for predicting postoperative respiratory failure in men after major noncardiac surgery. Ann Surg 232:242-253, 2000.
53. Warner DO, Warner MA, Barnes RD, et al: Perioperative respiratory complications in patients with asthma. Anesthesiology 85:460-467, 1996.
54. De Nino LA, Lawrence VA, Averyt EC, et al: Preoperative spirometry and laparotomy: Blowing away dollars. Chest 111:1536-1541, 1997.
55. Smetana GW, Lawrence VA, Cornell JE, American College of Physicians: Preoperative pulmonary risk stratification for noncardiothoracic surgery. Ann Intern Med 144:581-595, 2006.
56. Ballantyne JC, Carr DB, deFerranti S, et al: The comparative effects of postoperative analgesic therapies on pulmonary outcome: Cumulative meta-analyses of randomized, controlled trials. Anesth Analg 86:598-612, 1998.
57. Ramakrishna G, Sprung J, Ravi BS, et al: Impact of pulmonary hypertension on the outcomes of noncardiac surgery: Predictors of perioperative morbidity and mortality. J Am Coll Cardiol 45:1691-1699, 2005.
58. Blaise G, Langleben D, Hurbert B: Pulmonary arterial hypertension: Pathophysiology and anesthetic approach. Anesthesiology 99:1415-1432, 2003.
59. McGoon M, Gutterman D, Steen V, et al: Screening, early detection, and diagnosis of pulmonary artery hypertension. Chest 126(Suppl):14-34, 2004.
60. Bradley TD, Floras JS: Sleep apnea and heart failure: Part I. Obstructive sleep apnea. Circulation 107:1671-1678, 2003.
61. Myles PS, Iacono GA, Hunt JO, et al: Risk of respiratory complications and wound infection in patients undergoing ambulatory surgery: Smokers versus nonsmokers. Anesthesiology 97:842-847, 2002.
62. Woehlck HJ, Connolly LA, Cinquegrani MP, et al: Acute smoking increases ST depression in humans during general anesthesia. Anesth Analg 89:856-860, 1999.
63. A clinical practice guideline for treating tobacco use and dependence. JAMA 283:3244-3254, 2000.
64. Warner DO: Helping surgical patients quit smoking: Why, when and how? Anesth Analg 101:481-487, 2005.
65. Haffner SM, Lehto S, Ronnemaa T, et al: Mortality from coronary heart disease in subjects with type 2 diabetes and in nondiabetic subjects with and without prior myocardial infarction. N Engl J Med 339:229-234, 1998.
66. Garber AJ, Moghissi ES, Bransome ED Jr, et al: American College of Endocrinology position state-

ment on inpatient diabetes and metabolic control. Endocr Pract 10:77-82, 2004.

67. Dickstein G, Shechner C, Nicholson WE, et al: Adrenocorticotropin stimulation test: Effects of basal cortisol level, time of day, and suggested new sensitive low dose test. J Clin Endocrinol Metab 72:773-778, 1991.
68. Brandi ML, Gagel RF, Angeli A, et al: Guidelines for diagnosis and therapy of MEN type 1 and type 2. J Clin Endocrinol Metab 86:5658-5671, 2001.
69. Kinney MAO, Narr BJ, Warner MA: Perioperative management of pheochromocytoma. J Cardiothorac Vasc Anesth 16:359-369, 2002.
70. Straumann E, Meyer B, Misteli M, et al: Aortic and mitral valve disease in patients with end stage renal failure on long-term haemodialysis. Br Heart J 67:236-239, 1992.
71. Umana E, Ahmed W, Alpert MA: Valvular and perivalvular abnormalities in end-stage renal disease. Am J Med Sci 325:237-242, 2003.
72. Hirakata RG, Alphorns N, Joshi RM, et al: Palliative surgery in malignant obstructive jaundice: Prognostic indicators of early mortality. J R Coll Surg Edinb 42:238-243, 1997.
73. Fogarty BJ, Parks RW, Rowlands BJ, et al: Renal dysfunction in obstructive jaundice. Br J Surg 82:877-884, 1995.
74. Befeler AS, Palmer DE, Hoffman M, et al: The safety of intra-abdominal surgery in patients with cirrhosis: Model for End-Stage Liver Disease score is superior to Child-Turcotte-Pugh classification in predicting outcome. Arch Surg 140:650-654, 2005.
75. Gibbs J, Cull W, Henderson W, et al: Preoperative serum albumin level as a predictor of operative mortality and morbidity. Arch Surg 134:36-42, 1999.
76. Pain JA, Cahill CJ, Gilbert JM, et al: Prevention of postoperative renal dysfunction in patients with obstructive jaundice: A multicentre study of bile salts and lactulose. Br J Surg 78:467-469, 1991.
77. Rizvon MK, Chou CL: Surgery in the patient with liver disease. Med Clin North Am 87:211-227, 2003.
78. Practice guidelines for blood component therapy: A report by the American Society of Anesthesiologists Task Force on Blood Component Therapy. Anesthesiology 84:732-747, 1996. Available at http://www.asahq.org/ Accessed July 5, 2007.
79. Firth PG, Head CA: Sickle cell disease and anesthesia. Anesthesiology 101:766-785, 2004.
80. Koshy M, Weiner SJ, Miller ST, et al: Surgery and anesthesia in sickle cell disease. Cooperative Study of Sickle Cell Diseases. Blood 86:3676-3684, 1995.
81. Vichinsky EP, Haberkern CM, Neumayr L, et al: A comparison of conservative and aggressive transfusion regimens in the perioperative management of sickle cell disease. N Engl J Med 333:206-213, 1995.
82. Michiels JJ, Gadisseur A, Budde U, et al: Characterization, classification, and treatment of von Willebrand diseases: A critical appraisal of the literature and personal experiences. Semin Thromb Hemost 31:577-601, 2005.
83. Warkentin TE, Kelton JG: Temporal aspects of heparin-induced thrombocytopenia. N Engl J Med 344:1286-1292, 2001.
84. Kearon C, Hirsh J: Management of anticoagulation before and after elective surgery. N Engl J Med 336:1506-1511, 1997.
85. Zurawska U, Parasuraman S, Goldhaber SZ: Prevention of pulmonary embolism in general surgery patients. Circulation 115:e302-e307, 2007.
86. Geerts WH, Pineo GF, Heit JA, et al: Prevention of venous thromboembolism. The Seventh ACCP Conference on Antithrombotic and Thrombolytic Therapy. Chest 126:338S-400S, 2004.
87. Horlocker TT, Wedel DJ, Benzon H, et al: Regional anesthesia in the anticoagulated patient: Defining the risks (the Second ASRA Consensus Conference on Neuraxial Anesthesia and Anticoagulation). Reg Anesth Pain Med 28:172-197, 2003.
88. Selim M: Perioperative stroke. N Engl J Med 356:706-713, 2007.
89. Hart R, Hindman B: Mechanisms of perioperative cerebral infarction. Stroke 13:766-773, 1982.
90. Dodick DW, Meissner I, Meyer FB, et al: Evaluation and management of asymptomatic carotid artery stenosis. Mayo Clin Proc 79:937-944, 2004.
91. Endarterectomy for asymptomatic carotid artery stenosis. Executive Committee for the Asymptomatic Carotid Atherosclerosis Study. JAMA 273:1421-1428, 1995.
92. Weiner HL: Multiple sclerosis is an inflammatory T-cell–mediated autoimmune disease. Arch Neurol 61:1613-1615, 2004.
93. Olanow CW, Watts RL, Koller WC: An algorithm (decision tree) for the management of Parkinson's disease (2001); treatment guidelines. Neurology 56:S1-S88, 2001.
94. www.fda.gov/cder/drug/advisory/pergolide.htm/ Accessed July 15, 2007.
95. O'Neill GN: Acquired disorders of the neuromuscular junction. Int Anesthesiol Clin 44:107-121, 2006.
96. Naguib M, el Dawlatly A, Ashour M, et al: Multivariate determinants of the need for postoperative ventilation in myasthenia gravis. Can J Anaesth 43:1006-1013, 1996.
97. Mathicu J, Allard P, Gobeil G, et al: Anesthetic and surgical complications in 219 cases of myotonic dystrophy. Neurology 49:1646-1650, 1997.
98. Desan PH, Powsner S: Assessment and management of patients with psychiatric disorders. Crit Care Med 32(Suppl):S166-S173, 2004.
99. Lee DM, Weinblatt ME: Rheumatoid arthritis. Lancet 358:903-911, 2001.
100. Tokunaga D, Hase H, Mikami Y, et al: Atlantoaxial subluxation in different intraoperative head positions in patients with rheumatoid arthritis. Anesthesiology 104:675-679, 2006.
101. Manzi S, Wasko MCM: Inflammation-mediated rheumatic diseases and atherosclerosis. Ann Rheum Dis 59:321-325, 2000.
102. Miyanohara T, Igarashi T, Suzuki H, et al: Aggravation of laryngeal rheumatoid arthritis after use of a laryngeal mask airway. J Clin Rheumatol 12:142-144, 2006.
103. Clegg DO: Treatment of ankylosing spondylitis. J Rheumatol Suppl 78:24-31, 2006.
104. Mills JA: Systemic lupus erythematosus. N Engl J Med 330:1871-1879, 1994.
105. Charles C, Clements P, Furst DE: Systemic sclerosis: Hypothesis-driven treatment strategies. Lancet 367:1683-1691, 2006.
106. Racz H, Mehta S: Dyspnea due to pulmonary hypertension and interstitial lung disease in scleroderma: Room for improvement in diagnosis and management. J Rheumatol 33:1723-1725, 2006.
107. Ho NC, Tran JR, Bektas A: Marfan's syndrome. Lancet 366:1978-1981, 2005.
108. Wigley FM: Clinical practice. Raynaud's phenomenon. N Engl J Med 347:1001-1008, 2002.
109. Cameron EH, Lipshultz SE, Tarbell NJ, et al: Cardiovascular disease in long-term survivors of pediatric Hodgkin's disease. Circulation 8:139-144, 1998.
110. Adams MJ, Hardenbergh PH, Constine LS, Lipshultz SE: Radiation-associated cardiovascular disease. Crit Rev Oncol Hematol 45:55-75, 2003.
111. Nagasue N, Kohno H, Tachibana M, et al: Prognostic factors after hepatic resection for hepatocellular carcinoma associated with Child-Turcotte class B and C cirrhosis. Ann Surg 229:84-90, 1999.
112. Kinney MA, Warner ME, Nagorney DM, et al: Perianesthetic risks and outcomes of abdominal surgery for metastatic carcinoid tumours. Br J Anaesth 87:447-452, 2001.
113. Tait AR, Malviya S: Anesthesia for the child with an upper respiratory tract infection: Still a dilemma? Anesth Analg 100:59-65, 2005.
114. Kostopanagiotou G, Smyrniotis V, Arkadopoulos N, et al: Anesthetic and perioperative management of adult transplant patients in nontransplant surgery. Anesth Analg 89:613-622, 1999.
115. Kostopanagiotou G, Smyrniotis V, Arkadopoulos N, et al: Anesthetic and perioperative management of paediatric organ recipients in nontransplant surgery. Paediatr Anaesth 13:754-763, 2003.
116. Gohh RY, Warren G: The preoperative evaluation of the transplanted patient for nontransplant surgery. Surg Clin North Am 86:1147-1166, 2006.
117. Hepner DL, Castells MC: Anaphylaxis during the perioperative period. Anesth Analg 97:1381-1395, 2003.
118. Hepner DL, Castells MC: Latex allergy: An update. Anesth Analg 96:1219-1229, 2003.
119. Berry AJ, Katz JD, Brown RH, et al: Natural Rubber Latex Allergy: Considerations for Anesthesiologists. Park Ridge, IL, American Society of Anesthesiologists, 1999, pp 1-34.
120. Ziem G, McTamney J: Profile of patients with chemical injury and sensitivity. Environ Health Perspect 105(Suppl 2):417-436, 1997.
121. Hood DD, Dewan DM: Anesthetic and obstetric outcome in morbidly obese parturients. Anesthesiology 79:1210-1218, 1993.
122. Strollo PJ, Rogers RM: Obstructive sleep apnea. N Engl J Med 334:99-104, 1996.
123. Evron S, Glezerman M, Harow E, et al: Human immunodeficiency virus: Anesthetic and obstetric considerations. Anesth Analg 98:503-511, 2004.
124. May JA, White HC, Leonard-White A, et al: The patient recovering from alcohol or drug addiction: Special issues for the anesthesiologist. Anesth Analg 92:1601-1608, 2001.
125. Jage J, Heid F: Anesthesia and analgesia in addicts: Basis for establishing a standard operating procedure. Anaesthesist 55:611-628, 2006.
126. Kennedy JM, van Rij AM, Spears GF, et al: Polypharmacy in a general surgical unit and consequences of drug withdrawal. Br J Clin Pharmacol 49:353-362, 2000.
127. Hill GE, Ogunnaike BO, Johnson ER: General anaesthesia for the cocaine abusing patient. Is it safe? Br J Anaesth 97:654-657, 2006.
128. Savage SR: Addiction in the treatment of pain: Significance, recognition, and management. J Pain Symptom Manage 8:265-278, 1993.
129. Hernandez M, Birnbach DJ, Van Zundert AAJ: Anesthetic management of the illicit-substance–using patient. Curr Opin Anaesthesiol 18:315-324, 2005.
130. Del Savio GC, Zelicof SB, Wexler LM, et al: Preoperative nutritional status and outcome of elective total hip replacement. Clin Orthop Relat Res 326:153-161, 1996.
131. The Veterans Affairs Total Parenteral Nutrition Cooperative Study Group: Perioperative total parenteral nutrition in surgical patients. N Engl J Med 325:525-532, 1991.
132. Detsky AS, Smalley PS, Chang J: Is this patient malnourished? JAMA 271:54-58, 1994.

133. Kudsk K: Joint Commission for Accreditation of Health Care Organizations guidelines; too late to intervene for nutritionally at-risk surgical patients. JPEN J Parenter Enteral Nutr 27:288-290, 2003.
134. Committee on Ethics, American Society of Anesthesiologists: Ethical guidelines for the anesthesia care of patients with do not resuscitate orders, 2001. Available at http://www.asahq.org/publicationsAndServices/standards/09.html.
135. Truog RD, Waisel DB, Burns JP: DNR in the OR. A goal-directed approach. Anesthesiology 90:3-6, 1999.
136. Grimaldo DA, Wiener-Kronish JP, Jurson T, et al: A randomized controlled trial of advance care planning discussions during preoperative evaluations. Anesthesiology 95:43-50, 2001.
137. Tsen L, Segal S, Pothier M, Bader A: Survey of residency training in preoperative evaluation. Anesthesiology 93:1134-1137, 2000.
138. ACGME website. Available at http://www.acgme.org/acWebsite/downloads/RRC_progReq/040pr07012008_TCC.pdf.
139. de Oliveira Filho GR, Schonhorst L: The development and application of an instrument for assessing resident competence during pre anesthesia. Anesth Analg 99:62-69, 2004.
140. Joint Commission on Accreditation of Healthcare Organizations: Comprehensive Accreditation Manual for Hospitals: Official Handbook. 2007. Available at http://www.jointcommission.org.
141. Raab EL: The parameters of informed consent. Trans Am Opthalmol Soc 102:225-232, 2004.
142. Bhattacharyya T, Yeon H, Harris M: The medical-legal aspects of informed consent in orthopaedic surgery. J Bone Joint Surg Am 87:2395-2400, 2005.
143. Szalados J: Legal issues in the practice of critical care medicine: A practical approach. Crit Care Med 35(Suppl):S44-S58, 2007.
144. Gandhi TK, Kachalia A, Thomas E, et al: Missed and delayed diagnosis in the ambulatory setting: A study of closed malpractice claims. Ann Intern Med 145:488-496, 2006.
145. Tsen LC, Segal S, Pothier M, et al: The effect of alterations in a preoperative assessment clinic on reducing the number and improving the yield of cardiology consultations. Anesth Analg 95:1563-1568, 2002.
146. Pham HH, Coughlan J, O'Malley AS: The impact of quality reporting programs on hospital operations. Health Affairs 25:1412-1422, 2006.
147. Berger RG, Kichak JP: Computerized physician order entry: Helpful or harmful? J Am Med Inform Assoc 11:100-103, 2004.
148. Perkins NA, Murphy JE, Malone DC, et al: Performance of drug-drug interaction software for personal digital assistants. Ann Pharmacother 40:850-855, 2006.
149. Mangram AJ, Horan TC, Pearson ML, et al: Guideline for prevention of surgical site infection, 1999. Hospital Infection Control Practice Advisory Committee. Infect Control Hosp Epidemiol 20:250-278, 1999.
150. Correll DJ: The measurement of pain: Objectifying the subjective. *In* Waldman SD (ed): Pain Management. Philadelphia, Elsevier, 2007, pp 197-211.
151. Melzack R: The McGill pain questionnaire: Major properties and scoring methods. Pain 1:277-299, 1975.
152. Tsen L, Segal S, Pothier M, et al: Alternative medicine use in presurgical patients. Anesthesiology 93:148-151, 2000.
153. Guenther E, Mendoza J, Crouch BI, et al: Differences in herbal and dietary supplement use in the hispanic and nonhispanic pediatric populations. Pediatr Emerg Care 21:507-514, 2005.
154. Leung JM, Dzankic S, Manku K, Yuan S: The prevalence and predictors of the use of alternative medicine in presurgical patints in five California hospitals. Anesth Analg 93:1062-1068, 2001.
155. American Society of Anesthesiologists: What You Should Know about Herbal Use and Anesthesia, 1st ed, 1999; 2nd ed, 2003. Park Ridge, IL, American Society of Anesthesiologists.
156. Lee A, Chui PT, Aun CS, et al: Incidence and risk of adverse perioperative events among surgical patients taking traditional Chinese herbal medicines. Anesthesiology 105:454-461, 2006.
157. Hodges PJ, Kam PC: The perioperative implications of herbal medicines. Anaesthesia 57:889-899, 2002.
158. Alexander JA: The potential hazards of used and abused perioperative drugs, herbs and dietary supplements. ASA Refresher Courses Anesthesiol 34:1-19, 2006.
159. Abebe W: Herbal medication: Potential for adverse interactions with analgesic drugs. J Clin Pharm Ther 27:391-401, 2002.
160. Wang SM, Peloquin C, Kain ZN: Attitudes of patients undergoing surgery toward alternative medical treatment. J Altern Complement Med 8:351-356, 2002.
161. Johnson RK, Mortimer AJ: Routine pre-operative blood testing: Is it necessary? Anaesthesia 57:914-917, 2002.
162. Imasogie N, Wong DT, Luk K, et al: Elimination of routine testing in patients undergoing cataract surgery allows substantial savings in laboratory costs. A brief report. Can J Anaesth 50:246-248, 2003.
163. Finegan BA, Rashiq S, McAlister FA, O'Connor P: Selective ordering of preoperative investigations by anesthesiologists reduces the number and cost of tests. Can J Anaesth 52:575-580, 2005.
164. Fischer SP: Development and effectiveness of an anesthesia preoperative evaluation clinic in a teaching hospital. Anesthesiology 85:196-206, 1996.
165. Starsnic MA, Guarnieri DM, Norris MC: Efficacy and financial benefit of an anesthesiologist-directed university preadmission evaluation center. J Clin Anesth 9:299-305, 1997.
166. Scott G: The voice of the customer: Is anyone listening? J Healthc Manage 46:221-223, 2001.
167. Snyder-Ramos SA, Seintsch H, Bottinger BW, et al: Patient satisfaction and information gain after the preanesthetic visit: A comparison of face-to-face interview, brochure, and video. Anesth Analg 100:1753-1758, 2005.
168. Minai FN, Kamal RS: Evaluation of cardiology consultations sought from the anaesthesia clinic. J Coll Physicians Surg Pak 14:199-201, 2004.
169. Katz RI, Barnhart JM, Ho G, et al: A survey on the intended purposes and perceived utility of preoperative cardiology consultations. Anesth Analg 87:830-836, 1998.
170. Ferschl MB, Tung A, Sweitzer B, et al: Preoperative clinic visits reduce operating room cancellations and delays. Anesthesiology 103:855-859, 2005.
171. Schmiesing CA, Brodsky JB: The preoperative anesthesia evaluation. Thorac Surg Clin 15:305-315, 2005.
172. Macario A: Are your hospital operating rooms "efficient"? A scoring system with eight performance indicators. Anesthesiology 105:237-240, 2006.
173. Macario A, Vitez TS, Dunn B, et al: Where are the costs in preoperative care? Analysis of hospital costs and charges for inpatient surgical care. Anesthesiology 83:1138-1144, 1995.
174. Archer T, Schmiesing CA, Macario A: What is quality improvement in the preoperative period? Int Anesthesiol Clin 40(2):1-16, 2002.
175. Ausset S, Bouaziz H, Brosseau M, et al: Improvement of information gained from the pre-anaesthetic visit through a quality-assurance programme. Br J Anaesth 88:280-283, 2002.
176. Davenport DL, Henderson WG, Khuri SF, et al: Preoperative risk factors and surgical complexity are more predictive of costs than postoperative complications: A case study using the National Surgical Quality Improvement Program (NSQIP) database. Ann Surg 242:463-471, 2005.
177. Greenberg CC, Regenbogen SE, Studdert DM, et al: Patterns of communication breakdowns resulting in injury to surgical patients. J Am Coll Surg 204:533-540, 2007.
178. Hepner DL, Bader AM, Hurwitz S, et al: Patient satisfaction with preoperative assessment in a preoperative assessment testing clinic. Anesth Analg 98:1099-1105, 2004.
179. Scott G: Customer satisfaction: Six strategies for continuous improvement. J Healthc Manage 46(2):82-85, 2001.
180. Bachman JW: The patient-computer interview: A neglected tool that can aid the clinician. Mayo Clin Proc 78:67-78, 2003.
181. Bond LM, Flickinger D, Aytes L, et al: Effects of preoperative teaching of the use of a pain scale with patients in the PACU. J Perianesth Nurs 20:333-340, 2005.
182. Ferrari LR, Rooney FM, Rockoff MA: Preoperative fasting practice in pediatrics. Anesthesiology 90:978-980, 1999.
183. Park K: Preoperative cardiology consultation. Anesthesiology 98:754-762, 2003.
184. Kleinman B: Preoperative cardiology consultation: How helpful is it? Anesthesiology 99:1240-1241, 2003.
185. Deutschman CS, Traber K: Evoultion of anesthesiology. Anesthesiology 85:1-3, 1996.
186. Wiklund RA, Rosenbaum SH: Medical progress: Anesthesiology (first of two parts). N Engl J Med 337:1132-1141, 1997.

Michael F. Roizen and Lee A. Fleisher

35 Anesthetic Implications of Concurrent Diseases

Key Points

1. The history and physical examination most accurately predict the risks and the likelihood of changes in monitoring or therapy.
2. For diabetic patients, end-organ dysfunction and the degree of glucose control in the perioperative and periprocedural periods are the critical issues with regard to risk.
3. The key to managing blood glucose levels in diabetic patients perioperatively is to set clear goals and then monitor blood glucose levels frequently enough to adjust therapy to achieve these goals.
4. Obesity is associated with multiple comorbid conditions, including diabetes, hyperlipidemia, and chololithiasis, but the primary concern is derangements of the cardiopulmonary system.
5. Obstructive sleep apnea is important to recognize because of the increased sensitivity to and the consequence of depressing the effects of hypnotics and opioids on airway muscle tone and respiration, as well as the difficulty with laryngoscopy and mask ventilation.
6. Although no controlled, randomized prospective clinical studies have been performed to evaluate the use of adrenergic receptor blocking drugs in patients undergoing resection of pheochromocytoma, the preoperative use of such drugs is generally recommended.
7. For patients with hypertension, we recommend the routine administration of all drugs preoperatively except angiotensin-converting enzyme inhibitors and angiotensin II antagonists.
8. Evaluation of a patient with cardiovascular disease depends on clinical risk factors, the extent of surgery, and exercise tolerance.
9. In patients with pulmonary disease, the following should be assessed: dyspnea, coughing and the production of sputum, recent respiratory infection, hemoptysis, wheezing, previous pulmonary complications, smoking history, and physical findings.
10. In patients with pulmonary disease, several strategies have been suggested, including cessation of smoking 8 weeks or more before surgery.
11. Risk factors for perioperative renal dysfunction include advanced age, congestive heart failure, previous myocardial revascularization, diabetes, and elevated baseline creatinine.
12. The main concern for a patient with renal disease is making it worse and thereby increasing the chance for renal failure, coma, and death.
13. Mild perioperative anemia may be significant only in patients with ischemic heart disease.
14. Careful management of chronic drug administration can include questions about the effects and side effects of alternative as well as prescription drugs.

This chapter reviews many conditions requiring special preoperative and preprocedure evaluation, intraoperative or intraprocedure management, or postprocedure care with particular focus on preprocedure care for those with increased waist size (see Chapter 64). Patients undergoing surgery move through a continuum of medical care to which a primary care physician, an internist or pediatrician, an anesthesiologist, and a surgeon, radiologist, or obstetrician-gynecologist contribute to ensure the best outcome possible. No aspect of medical care requires greater cooperation among physicians than does performance of a surgical operation or complex procedure involving multiple specialists and the perioperative care of a patient. Moreover, nowhere else can counseling make so huge a difference in so many lives. Because over 40% of medical costs are occasioned by tobacco use, physical inactivity, and poor food choices, the anesthesiologist has an important role in initiating change while assessing and ameliorating risk. We spend twice as much as developed Europe on medical care, largely because we in the United States have twice the incidence of chronic disease.[1] However, costs in the United States and the world will increase dramatically if we and other physicians do not use preoperative and other similar situations to influence patient lifestyle choices. The importance of integrating physicians' expertise is even greater within the context of the increasing life span of our population.[2] As the number of the elderly and the very old (those >85 years) grows, so does the need of surgical patients for preoperative consultation to help plan for comorbidity and multiple drug regimens, knowledge of which is crucial to successful patient management (also see Chapter 71). At a time when medical information is encyclopedic, it is difficult, if not impossible for even the most conscientious anesthesiologist to keep abreast of the medical issues relevant to every aspect of perioperative or periprocedure patient management. This chapter reviews such issues with primary emphasis on the anesthesiologist providing preoperative evaluation and care rather than transferring these responsibilities to other providers.

As with "healthy" patients (also see Chapter 34), it is the history and physical examination that most accurately predict not only the associated risks but also the likelihood that a monitoring technique or change in therapy will be beneficial or necessary for survival. This chapter emphasizes instances in which specific information should be sought in history taking, physical examination, or laboratory evaluation. Although controlled studies designed to confirm that optimizing a patient's preoperative or preprocedure physical condition would result in lower morbidity have not been performed for most diseases, it is logical to assume that such is the case. Studies showing the benefits of optimizing specific preprocedure conditions are highlighted. The fact that such preventive measures would cost less than treating the morbidity that would otherwise occur is an important consideration in a cost-conscious and soon cost-restricted environment.

Minimally invasive procedures such as cataract extraction, magnetic resonance imaging (MRI), or diagnostic arthroscopy, performed in conjunction with the best current anesthetic practices, may pose no greater risk than daily living does and thus might not be considered an opportunity for special evaluation. Nonetheless, preanesthetic and preprocedure evaluations have provided information that has led to changes in health care plans for more than 15% of all American Society of Anesthesiologists (ASA) class I and II patients (and for >20% of all patients in general) at the University of Florida (Gibby GL, et al., personal communication). Although these changes in care plans were attributable to data found by history taking and observation (the most common being gastric reflux, diabetes mellitus requiring insulin, asthma, and suspected difficult endotracheal intubation), no data show that patient outcome was improved by such changes. Nevertheless, logic caused practitioners to alter plans for such patients in ways that would optimize operating room schedules and decrease costs. Examples would be administering a β-adrenergic blocking drug, aspirin, or a statin (or any combination) the night before rather than delaying surgery to do so on the morning of surgery; administering a histamine type 2 (H_2) antagonist 1 to 2 hours before and an oral antacid immediately before entry into the operating room; ensuring the availability of equipment to measure blood glucose levels; obtaining a history of the patient's diabetic course and treatment from the primary care doctor, as well as from the patient; and performing a fiberoptic laryngoscopic examination or procuring additional skilled attention. Counseling to begin walking even 5 days in advance of surgery anecdotally reduces perioperative complications and speeds return to typical behavior. Thus, even if preoperative and preprocedure evaluation might not alter the outcome in an important way, its ability to decrease cost by reducing unwarranted laboratory testing and delays in obtaining treatment and equipment perceived to be beneficial (and medicolegally required) would be substantial and would warrant its use.

The following conditions are discussed in this chapter:

1. Diseases involving the endocrine system and disorders of nutrition (we have put this first because of its increasing importance to care)
2. Diseases involving the cardiovascular system
3. Disorders of the respiratory and immune system (including a tobacco cessation counseling plan—Breathe Free)
4. Diseases of the central nervous system (CNS), neuromuscular diseases, and mental disorders
5. Diseases involving the kidney, infectious diseases, and disorders of electrolytes
6. Diseases involving the gastrointestinal (GI) tract or the liver
7. Diseases involving hematopoiesis and various forms of cancer
8. Diseases of aging or those that occur more commonly in the aged, as well as chronic and acute medical conditions requiring drug therapy (also see Chapter 71).

Role of the Primary Care Physician or Consultant

The role of the primary care physician or consultant is not to select or suggest anesthetic or surgical methods but rather to optimize the patient's preoperative and preprocedure status regarding conditions that increase the morbidity and mortality associated with surgery and to alert the anesthesia care team about these conditions.

Quotations and a box in a Medical Knowledge Self-Assessment Program published by the leading organization representing internists, the American College of Physicians, highlight this role for the consultant[2]:

> *Effective interaction with colleagues in other specialties requires a thorough grounding in the language and science of these other disciplines as well as an awareness of basic guidelines for consultation [Box 35-1]. The consulting internists' role in perioperative care is focused on the elucidation of medical factors that may increase the risks of anesthesia and surgery. Selecting the anesthetic technique for a given patient, procedure, surgeon, and anesthetist is highly individualized and remains the responsibility of the anesthesiologist rather than the internist.*

Optimizing a patient's preoperative and preprocedure condition and counseling a patient about needed future lifestyle changes such as walking, food choices, and tobacco cessation are cooperative ventures between the anesthesiologist and the internist, pediatrician, surgeon, or family physician. If the primary care physician cannot affirm that the patient is in the very best physical state attainable (for that patient), the anesthesiologist and physician should do what is necessary to optimize that condition. Failure to consult with the primary care physician preoperatively

Box 35-1 Guidelines for Consultation Practice

Complete a prompt, thorough, generalist-oriented evaluation.

Respond specifically to the question or questions posed.

Indicate clearly the perioperative importance of any observations and recommendations outside the area of initial concern.

Provide focused, detailed, and precise diagnostic and therapeutic guidance.

Emphasize verbal communication with the anesthesiologist and surgeon, particularly to resolve complex issues.

Avoid chart notations that unnecessarily create or exacerbate regulatory or medicolegal risk.

Use frequent follow-up visits in difficult cases to monitor clinical status and compliance with recommendations.

From American College of Physicians: Medical consultation. *In* Medical Knowledge Self-Assessment Program IX, Part C, Book 4. Philadelphia, American College of Physicians, 1992, p 939.

or before a complex procedure is as risky as not checking the oxygen in the spare tanks. In fact, statements that describe the preoperative and preprocedure physical condition of the patient (e.g., "This patient is in optimum shape" and "I believe the mitral stenosis is more severe than the slight degree of mitral insufficiency") are much more useful to the anesthesiologist than statements that suggest overall clearance ("cleared for surgery") or perioperative procedures ("prevent hypoxia and hypotension"). Knowing the patient's waist size and exercise capacity is much more important than learning that his T waves did not flip by the time he completed his stress test (knowing his maximum metabolic equivalents of the task [METs] and heart rate recovery from a stress test are very useful).

Primary care physicians can prepare and treat a patient to provide optimal conditions for daily life. However, they do not have the depth of understanding of the anesthesiologist regarding the physiologic changes brought on by surgery and the manipulations in function that must be made to facilitate surgery and procedures and optimize perioperative and periprocedure outcomes. One example would be the induction of some degree of prerenal azotemia in a patient with congestive heart failure (CHF) by the primary care physician. The intravascular volume depletion associated with prerenal azotemia may make a cardiac patient more comfortable in daily life but would predispose that patient to hypovolemic problems during and after surgery and complex procedures. Thus, even though it would be desirable for the primary care physician to start the process of preparing the patient for the needs of surgery or complex procedures, this activity would not be compatible with the current state of knowledge or functioning of the vast majority of primary care physicians. Although such education is more readily available and of better quality than in previous decades[3-5] and although Fleisher, Goldman, Charlson, and their coworkers and even cardiologic organizations have provided considerable data regarding the importance of this aspect of care,[6-8] the training, knowledge, and ability of primary care physicians are still very deficient in this aspect of consultation. Without understanding the physiologic changes that occur perioperatively, it is difficult to prescribe the appropriate therapy. It is therefore part of the anesthesiologist's job to instruct the patient's consultants about the type of information needed from the preoperative and preprocedure consultation.

Diseases Involving the Endocrine System and Disorders of Nutrition

Pancreatic Disorders

Preoperative and Preprocedure Diabetes Mellitus

This section makes nine major points regarding diabetes:

1. The number of people known to be diabetic has more than tripled in 17 years in the United States to 25 million and is increasing substantially in the world. This growth has been fueled by the rise in type 2 diabetes caused by waist gain in the adult and now pediatric population (also see Chapter 82).
2. Diabetes itself may not be as important to perioperative outcome as its end-organ effects are (see point 4 for exceptions). Although the presence of diabetes has long been assumed to increase perioperative risk, results from epidemiologic studies may not support this assumption in patients not requiring management in the intensive care unit (ICU). These studies segregated the effects of diabetes per se on the organ system from the effects of the complications of diabetes (e.g., cardiac, nervous system, renal, and vascular disease) and the effects of old age and the accelerated aging that diabetes causes. Even in patients requiring ICU management, long-standing diabetes does not appear to be as important an issue as the end-organ dysfunction that exists and the degree of glucose control in the perioperative/periprocedure and ICU periods.[9-14]
3. Because diabetes represents at least two disease processes, its perioperative management may differ between these processes.
4. The Diabetes Control and Complication Trial for type 1 diabetics, the U.K. Prospective Diabetes Study for type 2 diabetics, The Advance Studies, and the Kumamoto studies all show that chronic tight control of blood sugar and blood pressure (BP), along with physical activity, results in a major delay in microvascular complications and perhaps indefinite postponement in type 2 diabetic patients.[15,16] However, current debate centers on the benefit associated with tight control in the perioperative period and on the benefit-risk ratio. Evidence indicates that tight control of blood glucose might be of benefit for pregnant diabetics (and their future offspring) (also see Chapter 69), for diabetics undergoing cardiopulmonary bypass (also see Chapter 60), for those with (global) CNS ischemia (also see Chapters 13 and 63), and for patients requiring postoperative or postprocedure care in an ICU. Little evidence indicates that perioperative tight control is of substantial benefit to any other group; moreover, the benefit-risk ratio of tight control has not been examined for any other group of patients.[9-14]

5. Different regimens permit almost any degree of perioperative control of blood glucose levels, but the tighter the control desired, the more frequently blood glucose levels must be monitored. Three treatment regimens are outlined later.
6. The major risk factors for diabetics undergoing surgery are the end-organ diseases associated with diabetes: cardiovascular dysfunction, renal insufficiency, joint collagen tissue abnormalities (limitation in neck extension,[17] poor wound healing), inadequate granulocyte production, and neuropathies.[9-19] Thus, a major focus of the anesthesiologist should be the preoperative and preprocedure evaluation and treatment of these diseases to ensure optimal preoperative and preprocedure conditions.
7. Regional anesthesia may be indicated to facilitate some procedures (also see Chapter 52). The following considerations should be kept in mind regarding the use of regional anesthesia for diabetic patients. Local anesthetic requirements are lower and the risk of nerve injury is higher in diabetic patients.[20] In addition, combining local anesthetics with epinephrine may pose an even greater risk for ischemic or edematous nerve injury (or both) in diabetics.
8. Nosocomial infection rates are probably decreased with outpatient surgery; the frequency of complications may be decreased in diabetics most at risk by either tight control of blood glucose or intense postoperative care, or both.
9. Both forms of diabetes cause accelerated aging (also see Chapter 71). Thus, the risks involved in caring for someone with diabetes are similar to those for someone much older, that is, someone who has a much higher physiologic age (or "RealAge").[21-23]

Non–insulin-dependent (type 2) diabetics account for more than 95% of the over 25 million diabetics in the United States. At the current rate of growth, there will be 300 million diabetics in the world in 2010. These individuals tend to be overweight, relatively resistant to ketoacidosis, and susceptible to the development of a hyperglycemic-hyperosmolar nonketotic state. The diagnosis of diabetes is made with a fasting blood glucose level greater than 110 mg/dL (6.1 mmol/L), and impaired glucose tolerance is diagnosed if the fasting level is less than 110 mg/dL (6.1 mmol/L) but greater than 100 (5.5). Plasma insulin levels are normal or increased in type 2 diabetics but are relatively low for the level of blood glucose. This hyperinsulinemia by itself is postulated to cause accelerated cardiovascular disease.

Diabetes mellitus is a heterogeneous group of disorders that have the common feature of a relative or absolute lack of insulin. The disease is characterized by a multitude of hormone-induced metabolic abnormalities, by diffuse microvascular lesions, and by long-term end-organ complications. Diabetes can be divided into two very different diseases that share these end-organ abnormalities. Type 1 diabetes is associated with autoimmune diseases and has a concordance rate of 40% to 50% (i.e., if one of a pair of monozygotic twins had diabetes, the likelihood that the other twin would have diabetes is 40% to 50%). In type 1 diabetes, the patient is insulin deficient and susceptible to ketoacidosis if insulin is withheld. In type 2, the concordance rate is 100% (i.e., genetic material is both necessary and sufficient for the development of type 2 diabetes). How markedly the aging and end-organ effects of these genes are expressed is based on lifestyle choices of food and physical activity. These patients are not susceptible to the development of ketoacidosis in the absence of insulin, and they have peripheral insulin resistance. Gestational diabetes develops in more than 3% of all pregnancies and increases the risk for type 2 diabetes to 17% to 63% within 15 years.

Type 1 and type 2 diabetes differ in other ways as well. Contrary to long-standing belief, patient age does not allow a firm distinction between type 1 and type 2 diabetes; type 1 diabetes can develop in an older person, and clearly, type 2 diabetes can develop in overnourished children. A diabetes-producing variant of Coxsackie B4 virus has been isolated from the pancreas of a patient who died of diabetic ketoacidosis (type 1 diabetes). This virus was also recovered from mice bred to be diabetes prone after inoculation of the virus had produced hyperglycemia and pancreatic beta cell necrosis coincident with rising antibody titers. Thus, the intrinsic genetic "vulnerability" in insulin-dependent type 1 diabetes mellitus may consist of a diminished capacity of beta cells to survive exposure to potentially damaging extrinsic agents. Type 1 diabetes is associated with a 15% prevalence of other autoimmune diseases, including Graves' disease, Hashimoto's thyroiditis, Addison's disease, and myasthenia gravis.

The common orally administered drugs can be classified into six groups in the sulfonylurea class of antidiabetic medications: tolazamide (Tolinase), tolbutamide (Orinase), and the newer sulfonylureas glyburide (Micronase), glipizide (Glucotrol), gliclazide (Diamicron), and glimepiride (Amaryl). Some of these medications have a longer blood glucose–lowering effect that persists for 24 hours or more and fewer drug-drug interactions. Oral hypoglycemic drugs may produce hypoglycemia for as long as 50 hours after intake (chlorpropamide [Diabinese] has the longest half-life). Other drugs and drug classes that fit into the category of hypoglycemic agents include the biguanide metformin, which decreases hepatic glucose output and may increase peripheral responsiveness to glucose (and is associated with lactic acidosis if the patient becomes dehydrated); the α-glucosidase inhibitors acarbose and miglitol, which decrease glucose absorption; the thiazolidinediones (such as pioglitazone), which increase peripheral responsiveness to insulin; and meglitinides and other noninsulin secretagogues such as repaglinide (Prandin), nateglinide (Starlix), and sitagliptin (Januvia). Recent experience with rosiglitazone (Avandia) for control of blood sugar makes one question whether examination of the mechanism or end-organ effects may lead to the best outcome for patients. Nevertheless, physicians advocating tight control of blood sugar levels usually give insulin to "maturity-onset" insulin-dependent diabetic patients twice a day or even more frequently.

Insulin-dependent diabetics tend to be young, nonobese, and susceptible to the development of ketoacidosis. Plasma insulin levels are low or nonmeasurable, and therapy requires insulin replacement. Patients with insulin-dependent diabetes experience an increase in their insulin requirements in the post-midnight hours, which may result in early-morning hyperglycemia (dawn phenomenon). This accelerated glucose production and impaired glucose utilization are due to nocturnal surges in secretion of growth hormone (GH). Normal patients and diabetics taking insulin have steady-state levels of insulin in their blood. (Unfortunately, traditional values for insulin pharmacokinetics are derived from studies designed as though the diabetic received only one shot of insulin in a lifetime.) Absorption of insulin is highly variable and dependent on the type and species of insulin, the site of administration, and subcutaneous blood flow. Nevertheless, attainment of a steady state is dependent on periodic administration of the preparations received by the patient. Thus, it seems logical to perioperatively continue the combinations of preparations that the patient had been receiving chronically after examining the patient's blood glucose monitoring logbook for the degree of control. (In our clinical experience, erratic control can foreshadow perioperative hypoglycemia.)

Acute complications in diabetic patients include hypoglycemia and diabetic ketoacidosis, as well as hyperglycemic, hyperosmolar, nonketotic coma. Diabetic patients are also subject to a series of long-term complications that lead to considerable morbidity and premature mortality, including cataracts, neuropathies, retinopathy, and angiopathy involving peripheral and myocardial vessels. The leading cause of the blindness associated with renal failure in the United States is diabetes. Many of these complications will bring the diabetic patient to surgery. The evidence that hyperglycemia itself accelerates these complications or that tight control of blood sugar levels decreases the rapidity of progression of microangiopathic disease is becoming more definitive.[24]

Glucose itself may be toxic because high levels can promote nonenzymatic glycosylation reactions leading to the formation of abnormal proteins that may decrease elastance and wound-healing tensile strength. The decrease in elastance is responsible for the stiff joint syndrome and for the fixation of the atlanto-occipital joint that makes intubation difficult. Furthermore, elevations in glucose may increase the production of macroglobulins by the liver, thereby increasing blood viscosity, and may promote intracellular swelling by favoring the production of nondiffusible, large molecules (e.g., sorbitol). Newer drug therapies (e.g., aldose reductase inhibitors) aim to decrease intracellular swelling by inhibiting the formation of such large molecules.

Studies on the long-term outcome of type 1 and type 2 diabetics indicate that tight control of blood glucose and blood sugar substantially prevents such complications (Table 35-1).[15,16]

Perioperative management of a diabetic patient may affect the surgical outcome. Physicians advocating tight control of blood

Table 35-1 Tight Control of Blood Glucose Levels Reduces Chronic Complications in Type 1 Diabetic Patients

	Type 1 Diabetic Patients	
Measure and Results	**Group Undergoing Intensive Control of Blood Glucose**	**Control Group**
Measurement of blood glucose levels	≥4/day	1/day
Insulin injections	≥3/day or an insulin pump was used	1-2/day
Diet	Special diet	Usual diabetic diet
Physician office visits	1-4/mo	Once every 3 mo
Results after 6 yr		
Diabetic retinopathy	70% less than control	
Treatment needed for retinopathy	50% less than control	
Significant nephropathy	50% less than control	
Neuropathy	60% less than control	

Modified from Reichard P, Nilsson BY, Rosenqvist U: The effect of long-term intensified insulin treatment on the development of microvascular complications of diabetes mellitus. N Engl J Med 329:304-309, 1993.

glucose levels point to the evidence of increased wound-healing tensile strength and decreased wound infections in animal models of diabetes (type 1) under tight control and the development of infections, renal failure, other serious complications, and death in patients requiring intensive care.[9-14]

Infections account for two thirds of postoperative complications and about 20% of perioperative deaths in diabetic patients. Experimental data suggest that many factors can make a diabetic patient vulnerable to infection. Many alterations in leukocyte function have been demonstrated in hyperglycemic diabetics, including decreased chemotaxis and impaired phagocytic activity of granulocytes, as well as reduced intracellular killing of pneumococci and staphylococci.[25] Keeping glucose levels in the vicinity of 150 mg/dL appears to maintain the ability of immunoglobins to form complexes. When diabetic patients are treated aggressively and blood glucose levels are kept below 270 mg/dL, the phagocytic function of granulocytes is improved and intracellular killing of bacteria is restored to nearly normal levels.[25]

Diabetic patients experience more infections in clean wounds than nondiabetics do. In a review of 23,649 surgical patients, the rate of wound infection in clean incisions was 10.7% for diabetics versus 1.8% for nondiabetics.[26] In addition, hyperglycemia may worsen the neurologic outcome after intraoperative cerebral ischemia.

Blood glucose levels may affect neurologic recovery after a global ischemic event. In a study of 430 consecutive patients resuscitated after out-of-hospital cardiac arrest, mean blood glucose levels were higher in patients who never awakened (341 ± 13 mg/dL) than in those who did awaken (262 ± 7 mg/dL).[27] Among patients who awakened, those with persistent neurologic deficits had higher mean glucose levels (286 ± 15 mg/dL) than those without deficits did (251 ± 7 mg/dL). These results are consistent with the finding that hyperglycemia during a stroke is associated with poorer short- and long-term neurologic outcomes. Although several questions remain, the likelihood that blood glucose is a determinant of brain damage after global ischemia is supported by the vast majority of animal studies after global CNS ischemia and by most, but not all studies after focal CNS ischemia. The preponderance of data after CNS ischemia indicates that levels of glucose higher than 150 or 250 mg/dL have an adverse effect on CNS recovery. Until better data are available, many will argue that a diabetic patient about to undergo surgery in which hypotension or reduced cerebral blood flow may occur should have a blood glucose level below 200 mg/dL during a period of cerebral ischemia. Some special situations may also influence how tightly one should manage a patient's glucose level, such as surgery requiring cardiopulmonary bypass, surgery in pregnant patients, and emergency surgery in patients with diabetic ketoacidosis or hyperosmolar nonketotic coma.

Diabetics undergoing coronary artery bypass grafting (CABG) in 1980 had a perioperative mortality rate of 5% versus 1.5% for nondiabetics.[28] In this study and in most other studies of diabetic patients undergoing CABG, important additional risk factors or confounding variables were not considered, including the incidence and extent of hypertension, ventricular dysfunction, and CHF or the severity of coronary artery disease.

The aforementioned study of 340 diabetics and 2522 nondiabetics undergoing CABG in 1980 demonstrated only a moderate increase in operative mortality for diabetics (1.8% versus 0.6%).[28] In the postbypass phase, patients with diabetes were found to require inotropic therapy and intra-aortic balloon pump support five times more frequently than nondiabetics did. This increased need for therapy in diabetics is due to several possible factors. Diabetics with angina have more extensive coronary artery disease than nondiabetic patients do. They are also more likely to have hypertension, cardiomegaly, diffuse hypokinesis, and previous myocardial infarction (MI). Insulin-dependent diabetics with coronary artery disease, impaired stress responses, and autonomic nerve dysfunction appear to have stiffer ventricles with a large increase in left ventricular end-diastolic pressure than matched nondiabetic controls do.[29] During cardiopulmonary bypass, hypothermia and stress reactions decrease the response to insulin and result in marked hyperglycemia (even when the perfusate and intravenous solutions do not contain glucose) (also see Chapter 60). Administration of washed cells has been advocated for small individuals because acid citrate dextrose– or adenine-supplemented blood can result in significant hyperglycemia. These changes are exaggerated in diabetic patients, and administration of insulin may have little effect until rewarming is achieved. Inotropic drugs are ineffective in maintaining cardiac contractility, although filling pressures, sinus rhythm, serum electrolytes, and arterial blood gases were adequate. Blood sugar levels were elevated in each case. After intravenous infusion of insulin, effective myocardial contractions returned and allowed easy and rapid weaning from bypass. The effect of glucose levels on neurologic outcome during cardiopulmonary bypass is both unclear and controversial.

Many diabetics requiring emergency surgery for trauma or infection have significant metabolic decompensation, including ketoacidosis. Frequently, little time is available for stabilization of the patient, but even a few hours may be sufficient for correction of any fluid and electrolyte disturbances that are potentially life threatening. It is futile to delay surgery in an attempt to eliminate ketoacidosis completely if the underlying surgical condition will lead to further metabolic deterioration. The likelihood of intraoperative cardiac arrhythmias and hypotension resulting from ketoacidosis will be reduced if intravascular volume depletion and hypokalemia are at least partially treated.

Insulin therapy is initiated with a 10-unit intravenous bolus of regular insulin, followed by continuous insulin infusion. The rate of infusion is determined most easily if one divides the last serum glucose value by 150 (or 100 if the patient is receiving steroids, has an infection, or is considerably overweight [body mass index ≥35]). The actual amount of insulin administered is less important than regular monitoring of glucose, potassium, and pH. Because the number of insulin binding sites is limited, the maximum rate of decline in glucose is fairly constant and averages 75 to 100 mg/dL/hr, regardless of the dose of insulin.[30] During the first 1 to 2 hours of fluid resuscitation, the glucose level may fall more precipitously. When serum glucose reaches 250 mg/dL, the intravenous fluid should include 5% dextrose.

The volume of fluid required for therapy varies with the overall deficit; it ranges from 3 to 5 L and may be as high as 10 L. Despite losses of water in excess of losses of solute, sodium levels are generally normal or reduced. Factitious hyponatremia caused by hyperglycemia or hypertriglyceridemia may result in this seeming contradiction. The plasma sodium concentration decreases by about 1.6 mEq/L for every 100-mg/dL increase in plasma glucose above normal. Initially, normal saline is infused at a rate of 250 to 1000 mL/hr, depending on the degree of volume depletion and cardiac status. Some measure of left ventricular volume should be monitored in diabetics who have a history of myocardial dysfunction. About a third of the estimated fluid deficit is corrected during the first 6 to 8 hours and the remaining two thirds over the next 24 hours.

The degree of acidosis is determined by measurement of arterial blood gases and detection of an increased anion gap (also see Chapter 49):

$$Na^+ - (Cl^- + HCO_3^-)$$

Acidosis with an increased anion gap (≥16 mEq/L) in an acutely ill diabetic may be caused by ketones in ketoacidosis, lactic acid in lactic acidosis, increased organic acids from renal insufficiency, or all three problems. In ketoacidosis, plasma levels of acetoacetate, β-hydroxybutyrate, and acetone are increased. Plasma and urinary ketones are measured semiquantitatively with Ketostix and Acetest tablets. The role of bicarbonate therapy in diabetic ketoacidosis is controversial. Myocardial function and respiration are known to be depressed at a blood pH below 7.0 to 7.10, yet rapid correction of acidosis with bicarbonate therapy may result in alterations in CNS function and structure. These alterations may be caused by (1) paradoxical development of cerebrospinal fluid and CNS acidosis from rapid conversion of bicarbonate to carbon dioxide and diffusion of the acid across the blood-brain barrier, (2) altered CNS oxygenation with decreased cerebral blood flow, and (3) the development of unfavorable osmotic gradients. After treatment with fluids and insulin, β-hydroxybutyrate levels decrease rapidly, whereas acetoacetate levels may remain stable or even increase before declining. Plasma acetone levels remain elevated for 24 to 42 hours, long after blood glucose, β-hydroxybutyrate, and acetoacetate levels have returned to normal; the result is continuing ketonuria.[30] Persistent ketosis with a serum bicarbonate level less than 20 mEq/L in the presence of a normal glucose concentration is an indication of the continued need for intracellular glucose and insulin for reversal of lipolysis.

The most important electrolyte disturbance in diabetic ketoacidosis is depletion of total-body potassium. Deficits range from 3 to 10 mEq/kg body weight. Serum potassium levels decline rapidly and reach a nadir within 2 to 4 hours after the start of intravenous insulin administration. Aggressive replacement therapy is required. The potassium administered moves into the intracellular space with insulin as the acidosis is corrected. Potassium is also excreted in urine because of the increased delivery of sodium to the distal renal tubules that accompanies volume expansion. Phosphorus deficiency in ketoacidosis as a result of tissue catabolism, impaired cellular uptake, and increased urinary losses may give rise to significant muscular weakness and organ dysfunction. The average phosphorus deficit is approximately 1 mmol/kg body weight. Replacement is needed if the plasma concentration decreases below 1.0 mg/dL.[30]

Glucotoxicity

Chronic tight control of blood glucose has been motivated by a theoretical concern about four potential glucotoxicities, plus the results from three major randomized outcome studies involving diabetic patients.[9-17]

1. Glucose itself may be toxic because high levels can promote nonenzymatic glycosylation reactions that lead to the formation of abnormal proteins. These proteins may weaken endothelial junctions and decrease elastance, which is responsible for the stiff joint syndrome (and difficult intu-

bation secondary to fixation of the atlanto-occipital joint), as well as decrease wound-healing tensile strength.

2. Furthermore, elevations in glucose may increase macroglobulin production by the liver (which would increase blood viscosity) and promote intracellular swelling by favoring the production of nondiffusible, large molecules (such as sorbitol). Some drug therapies (e.g., aldose reductase inhibitors) endeavor to decrease intracellular swelling by inhibiting the formation of such large molecules.
3. Glycemia also disrupts autoregulation. Glucose-induced vasodilation prevents target organs from protecting against increases in systemic BP. A glycosylated hemoglobin level of 8.1% is the threshold at which the risk for microalbuminuria increases logarithmically. A person with type 1 diabetes who has microalbuminuria of greater than 29 mg/day has an 80% chance of experiencing renal insufficiency. The threshold for glycemic toxicity differs for various vascular beds. For example, the threshold for retinopathy is a glycosylated hemoglobin value of 8.5% to 9.0% (12.5 mmol/L or 225 mg/dL), and that for cardiovascular disease is an average blood glucose value of 5.4 mmol/L (96 mg/dL). Thus, different degrees of hyperglycemia may be required before different vascular beds are damaged, or certain degrees of glycemia are associated with other risk factors for vascular disease. Another view is that perhaps severe hyperglycemia and microalbuminuria are simply concomitant effects of a common underlying cause. For instance, diabetics in whom microalbuminuria develops are more resistant to insulin, insulin resistance is associated with microalbuminuria in first-degree relatives of type 2 diabetics, and persons who are normoglycemic but subsequently have clinical diabetes are at risk for atherogenesis before the onset of disease.

Tight control retards all these glucotoxicities and may have other benefits in retarding the severity of diabetes itself.[9-17,31]

Thus, management of intraoperative glucose might be influenced by specific situations, such as the type of operation, pregnancy,[32] and the expected global CNS insult; the bias of the patient's primary care physician; or the type of diabetes. Type 1 diabetic patients definitely need insulin and might be considered candidates for tight control of blood glucose levels. Type 2 diabetic patients have insulin, and current data indicate that they do not benefit from tight perioperative control unless they need intensive care.[9-14]

The key to managing blood glucose levels perioperatively in diabetic patients is to set clear goals and then monitor blood glucose levels frequently enough to adjust therapy to achieve these goals. Three regimens that afford various degrees of perioperative control of blood glucose levels are discussed in the following sections.

Classic "Non–Tight Control" Regimen

Aim: To prevent hypoglycemia, ketoacidosis, and hyperosmolar states.

Protocol:

1. On the day before surgery, the patient should be given nothing by mouth (NPO) after midnight; a 13-oz glass of clear orange juice should be at the bedside or in the car for emergency use.
2. At 6 AM on the day of surgery, infuse a solution of intravenous fluids containing 5% dextrose through plastic cannulas at a rate of 125 mL/hr/70 kg body weight.
3. After starting the intravenous infusion, give half the usual morning insulin dose (and the usual type of insulin) subcutaneously.
4. Continue 5% dextrose solutions through the operative period and give at least 125 mL/hr/70 kg body weight.
5. In the recovery room, monitor blood glucose concentrations and treat on a sliding scale.

Such a regimen has been found to meet its goals.

"Tight Control" Regimen 1

Aim: To keep plasma glucose levels at 79 to 120 mg/dL. Maintenance of such levels may improve wound healing and prevent wound infections, improve neurologic outcome after global or focal CNS ischemic insults, or improve weaning from cardiopulmonary bypass.

Protocol:

1. On the evening before surgery, determine the preprandial blood glucose level.
2. Through a plastic cannula, begin an intravenous infusion of 5% dextrose in water at a rate of 50 mL/hr/70 kg body weight.
3. "Piggyback" an infusion of regular insulin (50 units in 250 mL or 0.9% sodium chloride) to the dextrose infusion with an infusion pump (Fig. 35-1). Before attaching this piggyback line to the dextrose infusion, flush the line with 60 mL of infusion mixture and discard the flushing solution. This approach saturates insulin binding sites on the tubing.

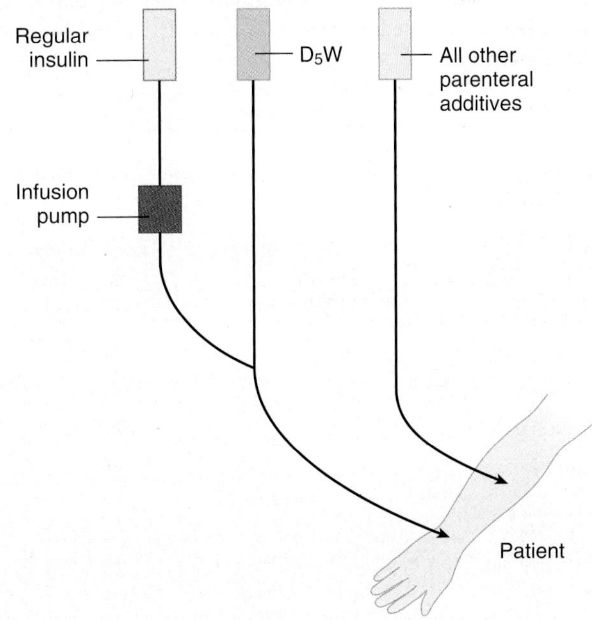

Figure 35-1 Arrangement of intravenous lines for infusion of regular insulin in a regimen tightly controlling blood glucose levels in diabetic patients undergoing surgery. D_5W, 5% dextrose in water.

4. Set the infusion rate by using the following equation: Insulin (U/hr) = plasma glucose (mg/dL)/150. (*Note*: The denominator should be 100 if the patient is taking corticosteroids, e.g., 10 mg of prednisolone a day or its equivalent, not to include inhaled steroids, or has a body mass index of ≥35.)
5. Repeat blood glucose measurements every 4 hours as needed, and adjust insulin appropriately to obtain blood glucose levels of 100 to 200 mg/dL.
6. On the day of surgery, intraoperative fluids and electrolytes are managed by continued administration of non–dextrose-containing solutions, as described in steps 3 and 4.
7. Determine the plasma glucose level at the start of surgery and every 1 to 2 hours for the rest of the 24-hour period. Adjust the insulin dosage appropriately.

Although we have not found it necessary to treat hypoglycemia (i.e., blood glucose levels <50 mg/dL), we have been prepared to do so with 15 mL of 50% dextrose in water. In such circumstances, the insulin infusion would be terminated. This regimen has been found to accomplish its objectives, with the exception of such tight goals for blood glucose, even in very "brittle" diabetics (i.e., those extremely resistant to treatment) given high doses of steroids.

"Tight Control" Regimen 2

Aim: Same as for Tight Control Regimen 1.

Protocol:

1. Obtain a "feedback mechanical pancreas" and set the controls for the desired plasma glucose regimen.
2. Institute two appropriate intravenous lines.

This last regimen may well supersede all others if the cost of a mechanical pancreas can be reduced and if control of hyperglycemia is shown to make a meaningful difference perioperatively; it has superseded all others in many ICUs and for good reason (Table 35-2).[11-13]

Table 35-2 Therapy for 1548 Postsurgical Diabetics in the Leuven Intensive Care Unit Study*

	Intensive Glucose Therapy (80-110 mg/dL)	Conventional Glucose Therapy (180-200 mg/dL)
Death in the ICU	4.6%	8.0%
After 5 days in the ICU	10.6%	20.2%
First 5 ICU days	1.7%	1.8%
All deaths	7.2%	10.9%
>14 days in the ICU	11.4%	15.7%
>14 days ventilated	7.5%	11.9%
Rx dialysis	4.8%	8.2%
Polyneuropathy	28.7%	51.9%

*Decreased complication rates and improved survival were observed in the group treated by tight control.

Diabetes and Accelerated Physiologic Aging

Adverse perioperative outcomes have repeatedly and substantially correlated with the age of the patient,[6,7,21-23,33] and diabetes does cause physiologic aging. When one translates the results of the Diabetes Control and Complications Trials into age-induced physiologic changes, a type 1 diabetic who has poor control of blood sugar ages approximately 1.75 years physiologically for every chronologic year of the disease and 1.25 years if blood sugar has been controlled tightly.[21-23] A type 2 diabetic ages about 1.5 years for every chronologic year of the disease and about 1.06 years with tight control of blood sugar and BP.[16,21-23,34] Thus, when providing care for a diabetic patient, one must consider the associated risks to be those of a person who is much older physiologically. That is, a diabetic's physiologic age ("RealAge") is considerably higher than that person's calendar age just by virtue of having the disease.[2]

The increased prevalence of obesity and lack of physical exercise seem to be major contributors to the increased prevalence of type 2 diabetes. As with type 1 diabetes, tight control of blood sugar, increased physical activity, and reduction in weight appear to reduce the accelerated aging associated with type 2 diabetes and even to substantially delay appearance of the disease and aging from it (Box 35-2).[21-23,34] Although such a reduction in aging should reduce the perioperative risk for diabetic patients, no controlled trials have confirmed this theory.

Other Conditions Associated with Diabetes

Diabetes is associated with microangiopathy (in retinal and renal vessels), peripheral neuropathy, autonomic dysfunction, and infection. Diabetics are often treated with angiotensin-converting enzyme (ACE) inhibitors, even in the absence of gross hypertension, in an effort to prevent the effects of disordered autoregulation, including renal failure.[15,16,35]

Before surgery, assessment and optimization of treatment of the potential and potent end-organ effects of diabetes are at least as important as assessment of the diabetic's current overall metabolic status. The preoperative evaluation of diabetics is also discussed in Chapter 34.

If one is to believe the few studies we have, the presence of autonomic neuropathy makes the operative period more hazardous and the postoperative period crucial to survival. Evidence of autonomic neuropathy might be routinely sought before surgery. Patients with diabetic autonomic neuropathy are at increased risk for gastroparesis (and consequent aspiration) and for intraoperative and postoperative cardiorespiratory arrest. Data indicate that diabetics who exhibit signs of autonomic neuropathy, such as early satiety, lack of sweating, lack of pulse rate change with inspiration or orthostatic maneuvers, and impotence, have a very high incidence of painless myocardial ischemia[19,36] and gastroparesis. Some investigators have successfully used 10 mg of metoclopramide preoperatively to facilitate gastric emptying of solids (Fig. 35-2). Interference with respiration or sinus automaticity by pneumonia or by anesthetics, pain medications, or sedative drugs appears to be the precipitating cause in most cases of sudden cardiorespiratory arrest. Measuring the degree of sinus arrhythmia or beat-to-beat variability provides a simple, accurate test for significant autonomic neuropathy. The difference between the maximum and minimum heart rate on deep inspiration is normally 15 beats/min but is 5 beats/min or less in all patients who sustained cardiorespiratory arrest.[19,36]

Box 35-2 The YOU Docs Plan for Reversing the Aging from Type 2 Diabetes and Metabolic Syndrome*

We or you have told us of tests and measurements that indicate you have type 2 diabetes or metabolic syndrome. Don't be alarmed; you can control the genes that predispose you to such so that this syndrome will not be as much problem to you in the future. BUT YOU HAVE TO DO IT—it is not your docs or your mother, IT IS UP TO YOU TO CONTROL YOUR GENES.

Because you have been diagnosed with type 2 diabetes or these syndromes, you can begin getting healthier by reducing your weight. Without a doubt, diabetes can be as damaging to your health as an annoyed anaconda. However, if you can hit these goals and even gradually decrease your waist size and your weight (aim for 2 pounds a week for the first 4 weeks, then 1 pound a week for 4 weeks, then 1 pound every month—after all you didn't get this big all at once), you'll decrease the aging effects of diabetes or metabolic syndrome by 80%, perhaps even more. Here's what has worked for our typical patient with your physique and tests and how to lose the weight and waist:

1. Avoid all white food—we're talking icing and white bread, not cauliflower.
2. Walk 30 minutes a day, no matter what.
3. Get a buddy and a plan for making YOU-turns: If you can walk 30 minutes every day and call (or e-mail) a support person each day after you've walked, you can lose the weight and have the waist you want, at least that's what review of weight and waist loss from over 190,000 buddy pairs tells us. So get a buddy you tell you walked daily and who will call you to check up if you do not call her within 15 minutes of your usual time (her's work better as buddies than him's). Have a plan for when you slip up—because you will. Here's a three-step approach for getting back on the right path:
   - Relax and say something positive to steer yourself back on course. Be confident that you can overcome the slip.
   - Do something physical right away—for instance, take a brisk walk or do a yoga pose. I recommend the downward-facing dog posture. This will help you refocus, take a deep breath, and remind yourself of your goals.
   - Eat something nutritious. Certain foods—such as carrots and apples—can help counteract stress, probably because they're crunchy and a touch sweet. You could choose a crisp vegetable, too. Whatever it is, make this the nutritious food "YOU-turn" to whenever you're stressed.
4. Once you have walked 30 minutes a day for 30 consecutive days, learn to lift weights and then integrate a resistance training program for 20 minutes three times a week into your weekly routine (you can download one for free at www.realage.com/youdocs); start with the beginner level no matter what your age.
5. Measure your waist around your belly button every Sunday. Suck in (you will anyway). Aim to lose an inch a month.
6. Get a blood pressure monitor and take it every Sunday. Your goal is 115/75.
7. Avoid the five aging foods: all added sugars and syrups, including all high-fructose corn syrup; saturated fats (four-legged plus palm or coconut oil) and *trans*-fats (blends or partially hydrogenated fats); and any grain except 100% whole grain, especially if it's one of the first five ingredients listed on a label.
8. Have as much fruit—whole, not fruit mixes or canned—and veggies as you want. By the way, Fruit Loops doesn't cut it.
9. Eat half an ounce of nuts—6 walnut halves, 12 almonds, or 20 peanuts—8 minutes before each meal, followed by a glass of water 4 minutes later.
10. Make eating automatic. I know I've said this before, but if you can train yourself—over 2 weeks or longer—to eat the right foods and make the right activity choices, you'll reprogram your body so that gradually eating right and exercising becomes a habit, one you'll do automatically. One tip for making your eating automatic is to have the same foods every day for two meals, say breakfast and lunch, and vary only one meal, such as dinner. Perhaps you're thinking "No one could do that." In fact, I practice what I preach by eating steel cut oatmeal for breakfast everyday. You can even prepare a week's worth of oats in advance to save time.
11. Inform and work with your primary care doctor. Keep taking your antidiabetic medications (and all others such as anti–high blood pressure medications), but follow your blood sugar and blood pressure closely. Our typical patients have to reduce antidiabetic medications and insulin after about 2 weeks and gets rid of them by the time they have lost 15% to 20% of the excess waist and weight they have gained since age 18 (women) or age 21 (men). Moreover, that reduction in medications occurs for their anti–high blood pressure medications too.

*The Type II Diabetes Disease Reversal plan is copywritten by the YOU Docs in *YOU On a Diet: The Owner's Manual for Waist Management* (Free Press, 2006 in the United States), reprinted here by permission of the copyright owner and offered to all who want to use it—feel free to copy and hand to patients (as long as credit is given).

Other characteristics of patients with autonomic neuropathy include postural hypotension with a decrease in BP of more than 30 mm Hg, resting tachycardia, nocturnal diarrhea, and dense peripheral neuropathy. Diabetics with significant autonomic neuropathy may have impaired respiratory responses to hypoxia and are particularly susceptible to the action of drugs that have depressant effects. These patients may warrant very close, continuous cardiac and respiratory monitoring for 24 to 72 hours postoperatively, although such logical treatment has not been tested in a rigorous, controlled trial.[19] In the absence of autonomic neuropathy, we would favor outpatient surgery for a diabetic (Table 35-3).

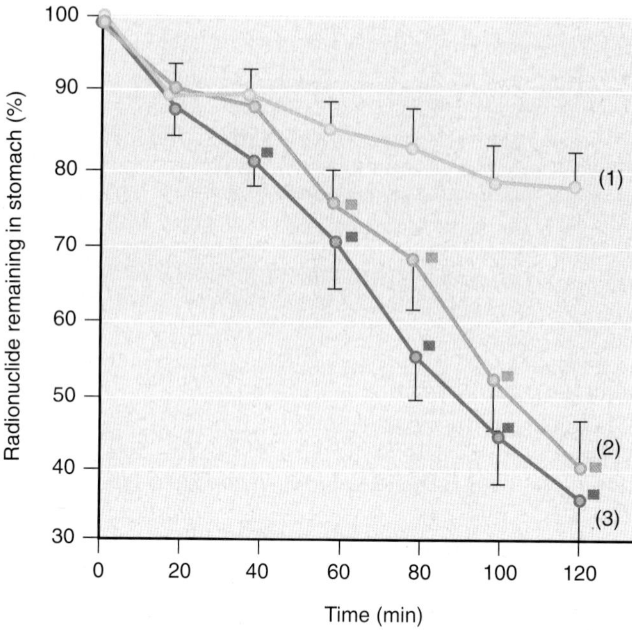

Figure 35-2 Gastric emptying time (mean ± SD) of a solid test meal in three groups of patients: diabetics (line 1), diabetics given metoclopramide (10 mg intravenously) 1.5 hours before the test meal (line 2), and nondiabetics (line 3). *(From Wright RA, Clemente R, Wathen R: Diabetic gastroparesis: An abnormality of gastric emptying of solids. Am J Med Sci 289:240, 1985.)*

Anticipated Newer Treatments of Diabetes

At least three major changes in the care of diabetic patients have made it to the clinical trial stage:

- Implanted (like a pacemaker) glucose analyzer with electronic transmission to a surface (watch) monitor
- New islet transplantation medication that makes islet cell transplants much more successful and rejection medication less hazardous
- Medications such as INGAP (islet neogenesis–associated protein) peptide, which may cause regrowth of normally functioning islet cells (without needing transplantation)

One can imagine how some of these treatments may radically change the therapies used in the perioperative period. If regrowth of islets becomes common, type 1 diabetes could all but disappear; if implanted minute-to-minute glucose reading is possible, tight control may be much easier and more expected.

Insulinoma and Other Causes of Hypoglycemia

Hypoglycemia in persons not treated for diabetes is rare. Hypoglycemia in nondiabetics can be caused by such diverse entities as pancreatic islet cell adenoma or carcinoma, large hepatoma, large sarcoma, alcohol ingestion, use of β-adrenergic receptor blocking drugs, haloperidol therapy, hypopituitarism, adrenal insufficiency, altered physiology after gastric or gastric bypass surgery, hereditary fructose intolerance, ingestion of antidiabetic drugs, galactosemia, or autoimmune hypoglycemia.[37] The last four entities cause postprandial reactive hypoglycemia. Because restriction of oral intake prevents severe hypoglycemia, the practice of keeping the patient NPO and infusing small amounts of a solution containing 5% dextrose greatly lessens the possibility of perioperative postprandial reactive hypoglycemia. The other causes of hypoglycemia can cause serious problems during the perioperative period.[37]

Symptoms of hypoglycemia fall into two groups: adrenergic excess (tachycardia, palpitations, tremulousness, or diaphoresis) and neuroglycopenia (headache, confusion, mental sluggishness, seizures, or coma). All these symptoms may be masked by anesthesia, so blood glucose levels should be determined frequently in such patients to ensure that hypoglycemia is not present. Because manipulation of an insulinoma can result in massive insulin release, this tumor should probably be operated on only at centers equipped with a mechanical pancreas. Perioperative use of the somatostatin analog octreotide, which suppresses insulin release from such tumors, appears to make the perioperative period a logarithm safer in anecdotal experience.

Disorders of Nutrition, Including Obesity

Hyperlipoproteinemia, Hyperlipidemia, and Hypolipidemia

Hyperlipidemia may result from obesity, estrogen or corticoid therapy, uremia, diabetes, hypothyroidism, acromegaly, alcohol ingestion, liver disease, inborn errors of metabolism, or pregnancy. Hyperlipidemia may cause premature coronary or peripheral vascular disease or pancreatitis.

Data showing that coronary events can be reduced by treating individuals with even normal levels of low-density cholesterol (LDL) cholesterol with the "statins"—drugs that raise high-density cholesterol (HDL) and lower LDL cholesterol levels—resulted from a decade of rapid progress in preventing reinfarction in high-risk patients.[38-40] Secondary prevention efforts were successful when these high-risk patients stopped smoking, reduced their BP, controlled stress, increased physical activity, and used aspirin, folate, β-blocking drugs, angiotensin inhibitors, diet, and other drugs to reduce their levels of LDL and increase their levels of HDL.

Table 35-3 Should a Diabetic Be an Outpatient or a Morning Admittance Patient?

Outpatient If	Morning Admittance Patient If
Can evaluate the history in advance	Cannot evaluate the history
End-organ disease does not require monitoring	End-organ disease requires invasive monitoring
Prehydration is available	Needs careful prehydration or is unnecessary
No CNS ischemia or planned cardiopulmonary bypass	CNS ischemia is present or cardiopulmonary bypass is planned
Not pregnant	Pregnant
Patient or vested home "mate" can determine blood glucose level	Patient cannot determine blood glucose level
Has vested home "mate"	No vested individual
Can take temperature or look for "red" wound	Cannot take temperature or look for "red" wound
Plan higher admission rate (no data)	Social care network is unsuitable

Although controlling the diet remains a major treatment modality for all types of hyperlipidemia, the drugs fenofibrate and gemfibrozil, which are used to treat hypertriglyceridemia, can cause myopathy, especially in patients with hepatic or renal disease; clofibrate is also associated with an increased incidence of gallstones. Cholestyramine binds bile acids, as well as oral anticoagulants, digitalis drugs, and thyroid hormones. Nicotinic acid causes peripheral vasodilation and should probably not be continued through the morning of surgery. Probucol (Lorelco) decreases the synthesis of apoprotein A-I; its use is associated on rare occasion with fetid perspiration or prolongation of the QT interval (or both) and sudden death in animals.

The West of Scotland Coronary Prevention Study and its congeners produced convincing evidence that drugs in the "statin" class (3-hydroxy-3-methylglutaryl–coenzyme A [HMG-CoA] reductase inhibitors) prevent the morbidity and mortality related to arterial aging and vascular disease, as well as their consequences, such as coronary artery disease, stroke, and peripheral vascular insufficiency.[39] Thus, the statins—lovastatin (Mevacor), pravastatin (Pravachol), simvastatin, fluvastatin, atorvastatin (Lipitor), and rosuvastatin (Crestor)—are mainstays of therapy.

However, the report of Downs and coworkers[39] from the Air Force/Texas Coronary Atherosclerosis Prevention Study went further. It showed a 37% reduction in the risk for first acute major coronary events in patients who had no risk factors and normal (average) LDL cholesterol levels. In this study lovastatin did not alter mortality rates, but that had been true for many early short-term trials with the statins. Although much of the effect of the statins has been attributed to their lipid-lowering effects, at least 40% of the effect of statins is modification by them of endothelial function, inflammatory responses, plaque stability, and thrombogenicity (Steven Nissen, MD, personal communcation). The report of Downs and colleagues broadened the use of statins, and they remain mainstays of therapy for hyperlipidemia. Statins are drugs that block HMG-CoA reductase, the rate-limiting enzyme of cholesterol synthesis. Their use is occasionally accompanied by liver dysfunction, CNS dysfunction, and severe depression not related to the high cost of each drug and its cogeners. Other drugs that reduce LDL and increase HDL cholesterol and decrease triglycerides are docosahexaenoic acid (DHA, an ω-3 fatty acid) and niacin. Recent data indicate that statins also provide the substantial benefit of reversing inflammation in arteries, as evidenced by their ability to decrease highly specific C-reactive protein and pull cholesterol from plaque.[41]

Hypolipidemic conditions are rare diseases often associated with neuropathy, anemia, and renal failure. Although anesthetic experience with hypolipidemic conditions has been limited, some specific recommendations can be made: continuation of caloric intake and intravenous administration of protein hydrolysates and glucose throughout the perioperative period.

Obesity

Although many conditions associated with obesity (diabetes, hyperlipidemia, cholelithiasis, gastroesophageal reflux disease, cirrhosis, degenerative joint and disk disease, venous stasis and thrombotic/embolic disease, sleep disorders, and emotional and altered body image disorders) contribute to chronic morbidity in the obese, the main concerns for the anesthesiologist have been the same for more than 4 decades—derangements of the cardiopulmonary system (also see Chapter 64).

Morbid obesity with minimal or no coexisting pulmonary conditions (e.g., no obesity-hypoventilation syndrome or chronic obstructive pulmonary disease [COPD]) will be referred to as "simple" obesity. In simple obesity, the pathophysiology of mild alterations in daytime gas exchange and pulmonary function may also result from compression and restriction of the chest wall and diaphragm by excess adipose tissue.[42] Typically, in the obese, the expiratory reserve volume and functional residual capacity are most affected and reduced to 60% and 80% of normal, respectively. Morbid obesity and its perioperative implications are also discussed in Chapters 34 and 64.

Other Eating Disorders: Anorexia Nervosa, Bulimia, and Starvation

Many endocrine and metabolic abnormalities occur in patients with anorexia nervosa, a condition characterized by starvation to the point of 40% loss of normal weight, hyperactivity, and a psychiatrically distorted body image. Many anorectic patients exhibit impulsive behavior, including suicide attempts, and intravenous drug use is much more common than in the general population. Acidosis, hypokalemia, hypocalcemia, hypomagnesemia, hypothermia, diabetes insipidus, and severe endocrine abnormalities mimicking panhypopituitarism need attention before anesthesia and surgery. Similar problems occur in bulimia (bulimorexia), a condition that may affect as many as 50% of female college students[43] and is even unintentionally present in many elderly.[44] As in severe protein deficiency (kwashiorkor), anorexia nervosa and bulimia may be accompanied by alterations on the electrocardiogram (ECG), including a prolonged QT interval, atrioventricular (AV) block, and other arrhythmias; sensitivity to epinephrine; and cardiomyopathy.[43] Total depletion of body potassium makes the addition of potassium to glucose solutions useful; however, fluid administration can precipitate pulmonary edema in these patients. Esophagitis, pancreatitis, and aspiration pneumonia are more frequent in these patients, as is delayed gastric emptying. Thus, invasive monitoring (radial artery and pulmonary artery catheterization) may be indicated for anorectic, bulimic, and malnurtured patients requiring emergency surgery. Elective surgery should probably be delayed until the abnormalities are treated.

Hyperalimentation (Total Parenteral or Enteral Nutrition)

Hyperalimentation (i.e., total parenteral nutrition [TPN]) consists of concentrating hypertonic glucose calories in the normal daily fluid requirements (also see Chapter 95). The solutions contain protein hydrolysates, soybean emulsions (i.e., Intralipid), or synthetic amino acids (or any combination of these ingredients). The major benefits of TPN or enteral nutrition have been fewer complications postoperatively and shorter hospital stays for patients scheduled to have no oral feeding for 7 days or who were malnourished preoperatively.[45,46] Starker and colleagues[47] found that the response to TPN, as monitored by serum albumin levels, predicted the postoperative outcome. The group demonstrating a rise in serum albumin with TPN had diuresis, weight loss, and fewer complications (1 of 15 patients) than did the group that gained weight and had a decrease in serum albumin (8 of 16 patients had 15 complications) (Fig. 35-3). These data are echoed by those in the Veterans Administration (VA) studies, which

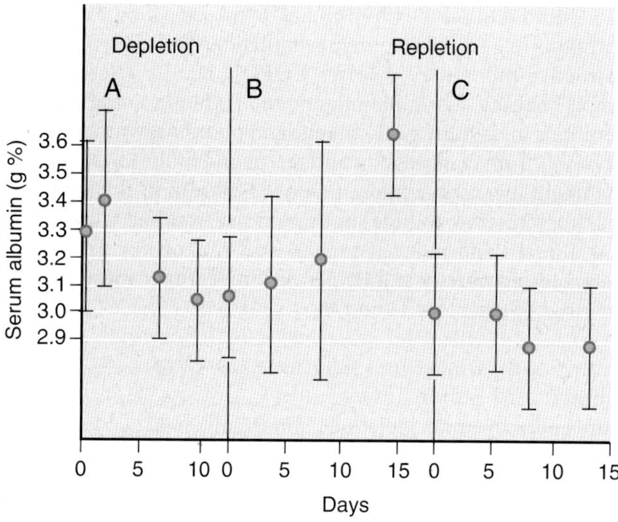

Figure 35-3 The response to hyperalimentation A, (repletion), as measured by variation in serum albumin levels, predicted the outcome of surgery. Patients who responded (B) to nutritional support with increased albumin levels had a significantly better outcome than did those whose albumin level did not increase (C). See the text for a more complete explanation. *(Adapted from Starker PM, Group FE, Askanazi J, et al: Serum albumin levels as an index of nutritional support. Surgery 91:194, 1982.)*

reported that the serum albumin level was one of the most powerful predictors of perioperative outcome.[45]

The major complications of hyperalimentation are sepsis and metabolic abnormalities. The central lines used for TPN require application with an absolutely aseptic technique and should not be used routinely as an intravenous route for drug administration. Major metabolic complications of TPN relate to deficiencies and the development of hyperosmolar states. Complications of hypertonic dextrose can develop if the patient has insufficient insulin (diabetes mellitus) to metabolize the sugar or if insulin resistance occurs (e.g., because of uremia, burns, or sepsis).

A gradual decrease in the infusion rate of TPN prevents the hypoglycemia that can occur on abrupt discontinuance. Thus, the infusion rate of TPN should be decreased the night before anesthesia and surgery or be continued throughout the operation at its current rate. The main reason for slowing or discontinuing TPN before anesthesia is to avoid intraoperative hyperosmolarity secondary to accidental rapid infusion of the solution or hypoglycemia if the infusion is discontinued because of high levels of endogenous insulin and lower levels of glucose present in the usual crystalloid solutions.[45] Hypophosphatemia is a particularly serious complication that results from the administration of phosphate-free or phosphate-depleted solutions for hyperalimentation. The low serum phosphate level causes a shift of the oxygen dissociation curve to the left. The resulting low 2,3-diphosphoglycerate and adenosine triphosphatase levels mean that cardiac output must increase for oxygen delivery to remain the same. Hypophosphatemia of less than 1.0 mg/dL of blood may cause hemolytic anemia, cardiac failure, tachypnea, neurologic symptoms, seizures, and death. In addition, long-term TPN is associated with deficiencies in trace metals such as copper (refractory anemia), zinc (impaired wound healing), and magnesium.

For these reasons, one author (M.F.R.) has adopted the following practices. Infusion of TPN or enteral nutrition is reduced beginning the night before surgery, and a 5% or 10% dextrose solution is substituted preoperatively. If serum glucose, phosphate, and potassium concentrations (measured preoperatively) are abnormal, they are restored to within normal limits. Strict asepsis is maintained. Conversely, one should continue infusing the TPN solution by using a pump system or enteral nutrition while strictly maintaining its normal rate and asepsis, administering all fluids through a different intravenous site, and performing a rapid-sequence induction of anesthesia (for those who received enteral nutrition).

Adrenocortical Malfunction

Three major classes of hormones—androgens, glucocorticoids, and mineralocorticoids—are secreted by the adrenal cortex. For each class, an excess or a deficiency of hormone produces a characteristic clinical syndrome. The widespread use of steroids can also make the adrenal cortex unable to respond normally to the demands placed on it by surgical trauma and subsequent healing. The increase in unindicated (scanning) computed tomography (CT) abdominal imaging procedures has meant that many adrenal masses have unfortunately been discovered only incidentally. These adrenal "incidentalomas," as they are termed because they were initially thought a nuisance discovered by unindicated body scans, have proved more serious. As many as 30% are hormonally active; in one recent review of 2000 such masses, 82% were not hormonally active, 5.3% proved to be cortisone-secreting adenomas, 5.1% were pheochromocytomas, 4.7% were adrenal carcinomas, 2.5% were unsuspected metastatic disease, and 1% were aldosterone-secreting adenomas. Incidentalomas may therefore require serious pursuit. Several points relative to adrenal cortical management deserve attention.

Controlled comparisons of the perioperative management of patients who have disorders of adrenal function are lacking, although we use steroids more and more commonly, with the results of some controlled trials available for specific uses. However, a review of the possible pathophysiologic changes in the adrenal cortex and techniques for their management should enable us to improve the perioperative care of patients with adrenal abnormalities.

Physiologic Properties of Adrenocortical Hormones

Androgens

Androstenedione and dehydroepiandrosterone, weak androgens arising from the adrenal cortex, constitute major sources of androgen in women (and have gained prominence for their use or abuse by baseball players seeking to hit more home runs). Excess secretion of androgen causes masculinization, pseudopuberty, or female pseudohermaphroditism. With some tumors, androgen is converted to an estrogenic substance, in which case feminization results. No special anesthetic evaluation is needed for such patients. Some congenital enzyme defects that cause androgen abnormalities also result in glucocorticoid and mineralocorticoid abnormalities that should be evaluated before surgery. Most of these patients are treated with exogenous glucocorticoids and mineralocorticoids and consequently require supplementation of these hormones perioperatively (see later).

Glucocorticoids

The principal glucocorticoid, cortisol, is an essential regulator of carbohydrate, protein, lipid, and nucleic acid metabolism. Cortisol exerts its biologic effects through a sequence of steps initiated by binding of hormone to stereospecific intracellular cytoplasmic receptors. This bound complex stimulates nuclear transcription of specific mRNA molecules. These molecules are then translated to give rise to proteins that mediate the ultimate effects of hormones.

Most cortisol is bound to corticosterone-binding globulin (CBG, transcortin). It is the relatively small amounts of unbound cortisol that enter cells to induce actions or to be metabolized. Conditions that induce changes in the amount of CBG include liver disease and nephrotic syndrome, both of which result in decreased circulating levels of CBG, and estrogen administration and pregnancy, which result in increased CBG production. Total serum cortisol levels may become elevated or depressed under conditions that alter the amount of bound cortisol, and yet the unbound, active form of cortisol is present in normal amounts. The most accurate measure of cortisol activity is the level of urinary cortisol—that is, the amount of unbound, active cortisol filtered by the kidney.

The serum half-life of cortisol is 80 to 110 minutes. However, because cortisol acts through intracellular receptors, pharmacokinetic data based on serum levels are not good indicators of cortisol activity. After a single dose of glucocorticoid, serum glucose is elevated for 12 to 24 hours; improvement in pulmonary function in patients with bronchial asthma can still be measured 24 hours after glucocorticoid administration. Treatment schedules for glucocorticoid replacement are therefore based not on the measured serum half-life but on the well-documented prolonged end-organ effect of these steroids. Hospitalized patients requiring chronic glucocorticoid replacement therapy are usually treated twice daily, with a slightly higher dose given in the morning than in the evening to simulate the normal diurnal variation in cortisol levels. For patients who require parenteral "steroid coverage" during and after surgery (see later paragraphs), administration of glucocorticoid every 12 hours is appropriate.[48] The relative potencies of glucocorticoids are listed in Table 35-4. Cortisol is inactivated primarily in the liver and is excreted as 17-hydroxycorticosteroid. Cortisol is also filtered and excreted unchanged into urine.

The synthetic glucocorticoids vary in their binding specificity in a dose-related manner. When given in supraphysiologic doses (>30 mg/day), cortisol and cortisone bind to mineralocorticoid receptor sites and cause salt and water retention and loss of potassium and hydrogen ions. When these steroids are administered in maintenance doses of 30 mg/day or less, patients require a specific mineralocorticoid for electrolyte and volume homeostasis. Many other steroids do not bind to mineralocorticoid receptors, even at high doses, and have no mineralocorticoid effect (see Table 35-4).

Secretion of glucocorticoids is regulated by pituitary adrenocorticotropic hormone (ACTH). ACTH is synthesized from a precursor molecule (pro-opiomelanocortin) that is metabolized to form an endorphin (β-lipotropin) and ACTH. Episodic secretion of ACTH has a diurnal rhythm that is normally greatest during the early morning hours in men, later in women, and is regulated at least in part by light-dark cycles. Its secretion is stimulated by release of corticotropin-releasing factor (CRF) from the hypothalamus. (An abnormality in the diurnal rhythm of corticoid secretion has been implicated as a cause of so-called jet lag.) Cortisol and other glucocorticoids exert negative feedback at both the pituitary and hypothalamic levels to inhibit the secretion of ACTH and CRF. If the CRF- or ACTH-producing cells are destroyed, the adrenal gland takes more than 30 days to atrophy to the point where acute administration of exogenous ACTH will cause almost no adrenal responsiveness.

Table 35-4 Relative Potencies and Equivalent Doses for Commonly Used Glucocorticoids

Steroids	Relative Glucocorticoid Potency	Equivalent Glucocorticoid Dose (mg)
Short Acting		
Cortisol (hydrocortisone)	1.0	20.0
Cortisone	0.8	25.0
Prednisone	4.0	5.0
Prednisolone	4.0	5.0
Methylprednisolone	5.0	4.0
Intermediate Acting		
Triamcinolone	5.0	4.0
Long Acting		
Betamethasone	25.0	0.60
Dexamethasone	30.0	0.75

Data from Axelrod L: Glucocorticoid therapy. Medicine (Baltimore) 55:39, 1976.

Mineralocorticoids

Aldosterone, the major mineralocorticoid secreted in humans, comes from the zona glomerulosa of the adrenal cortex and causes reabsorption of sodium and secretion of potassium and hydrogen ions, thereby contributing to electrolyte and volume homeostasis. This action is most prominent in the distal renal tubule but also occurs in the salivary and sweat glands. The major regulator of aldosterone secretion is the renin-angiotensin system. Juxtaglomerular cells in the cuff of renal arterioles are sensitive to decreased renal perfusion pressure or volume and, consequently, secrete renin. Renin splits the precursor angiotensinogen (from the liver) into angiotensin I, which is further converted by a converting enzyme, primarily in the lung, to angiotensin II. Angiotensin II binds to specific receptors to increase mineralocorticoid secretion, which is also stimulated by an increased potassium concentration and, to a lesser degree, by ACTH.

Adrenocortical Hormone Excess

Glucocorticoid Excess

Glucocorticoid excess (Cushing's syndrome) resulting from either endogenous oversecretion or chronic treatment with glucocorticoids at higher than physiologic doses produces a moon-faced plethoric individual with a centripetal distribution of fat (truncal obesity and skinny extremities), thin skin, easy bruising, and striae. Muscle wasting is common, but the heart and diaphragm are usually spared. A test for this syndrome is to ask the patient

Table 35-5 Clinical Features of Hyperadrenalism (Cushing's Syndrome) and Hypoadrenalism

Cushing's Syndrome	Hypoadrenalism
Central obesity	Weight loss
Proximal muscle weakness	Weakness, fatigue, lethargy
Osteopenia at a young age	Muscle and joint pain and back pain
Hypertension	Postural hypotension and dizziness
Headache	Headache
Psychiatric disorders	Anorexia, nausea, abdominal pain, constipation, diarrhea
Purple striae	
Spontaneous ecchymoses	
Plethoric facies	
Hyperpigmentation	Hyperpigmentation
Hirsutism	
Acne	
Hypokalemic alkalosis	Hyperkalemia, hyponatremia
Glucose intolerance	Occasional hypoglycemia
Kidney stones	Hypercalcemia
Polyuria	Prerenal azotemia
Menstrual disorders	
Increased leukocyte count	

to get up from a chair without using the hands. An inability to do so indicates proximal muscle weakness consistent with Cushing's syndrome. These patients often have osteopenia as a result of decreased formation of bone matrix and impaired absorption of calcium. Fluid retention and hypertension (because of increases in renin substrate and vascular reactivity caused by glucocorticoid) are common. Such patients may also have hyperglycemia and even diabetes mellitus from inhibition of peripheral use of glucose, as well as anti-insulin action and concomitant stimulation of gluconeogenesis (Table 35-5).

The most common cause of Cushing's syndrome is the administration of glucocorticoids for such conditions as arthritis, asthma, and allergies.[49] In these conditions, the adrenal glands atrophy and cannot respond to stressful situations (e.g., the preoperative and preprocedure period) by secreting more steroid. Thus, additional glucocorticoids may be required perioperatively (see the later section "Patients Taking Steroids for Other Reasons"). Spontaneous Cushing's syndrome may be caused by pituitary production of ACTH (65% to 75% of all spontaneous cases), which is usually associated with pituitary microadenoma, or by nonendocrine ectopic ACTH production (principally by tumors of the lung, pancreas, or thymus).[50] Ten percent to 20% of cases of spontaneous Cushing's syndrome are caused by an ACTH-independent process, either an adrenal adenoma or carcinoma.

Special preoperative and preprocedure considerations for patients with Cushing's syndrome include regulating diabetes and hypertension and ensuring that intravascular fluid volume and electrolyte concentrations are normal. Ectopic ACTH production may cause marked hypokalemic alkalosis. Treatment with the aldosterone antagonist spironolactone will stop the potassium loss and help mobilize excess fluid. Because of the high incidence of severe osteopenia and the risk of fractures, meticulous attention must be paid to positioning of the patient. In addition, glucocorticoids are lympholytic and immunosuppressive and thus increase the patient's susceptibility to infection. The tensile strength of healing wounds decreases in the presence of glucocorticoids, an effect that is at least partially reversed by the topical administration of vitamin A.

Specific considerations pertain to the surgical approach for each cause of Cushing's syndrome. For example, nearly three fourths of cases of spontaneous Cushing's disease result from a pituitary adenoma that secretes ACTH. One author's (M.F.R.) perioperative treatment of patients who have Cushing's disease and a pituitary microadenoma differs from that of patients who have a pituitary adenoma associated with amenorrhea and galactorrhea. A patient with Cushing's disease is inclined to bleed more easily and (on the basis of anecdotal evidence) tends to have higher central venous pressure (CVP). Thus, during transsphenoidal tumor resection in such patients, the practice is to routinely monitor CVP and maintain it at the low end of the normal range. In other cases of transsphenoidal resection of microadenoma, such monitoring is needed only infrequently.

Ten percent to 15% of patients with Cushing's syndrome exhibit adrenal overproduction of glucocorticoids from an adrenal adenoma or carcinoma. If either unilateral or bilateral adrenal resection is planned, we normally begin administering glucocorticoids at the start of resectioning of the tumor. Despite the absence of definitive studies, we normally give 100 mg of hydrocortisone hemisuccinate or hydrocortisone phosphate every 24 hours intravenously. We reduce this amount over a period of 3 to 6 days until a maintenance dose is reached. Beginning on day 3, the surgeons that we have worked with most also give a mineralocorticoid, 9α-fluorocortisol (0.05 to 0.1 mg/day). In certain patients, both steroids may require several adjustments. This therapy continues if the patient has undergone bilateral resection. For a patient who has undergone unilateral adrenal resection, therapy is individualized according to the status of the remaining adrenal gland. The incidence of pneumothorax in open adrenal resection approaches 20%; the diagnosis of pneumothorax is sought and treatment is begun before the wound is closed. This problem has almost vanished with use of the laparoscopic technique, which means that patients who need open resection merit even closer postoperative scrutiny.

Bilateral adrenalectomy in patients with Cushing's syndrome is associated with a high incidence of postoperative complications and a perioperative mortality rate (greater than that of even cardiac surgery) of 5% to 10%; it often results in permanent mineralocorticoid and glucocorticoid deficiency. Ten percent of patients with Cushing's syndrome who undergo adrenalectomy have an undiagnosed pituitary tumor. After reduction of high levels of cortisol by adrenalectomy, the pituitary tumor enlarges. These pituitary tumors are potentially invasive and may produce large amounts of ACTH and melanocyte-stimulating hormone, thereby increasing pigmentation.

Adrenal tumors are at least 85% incidentalomas—that is, discovered incidentally during screening (and largely unindicated) CT scans. Nonfunctioning adrenal adenomas are found in patients on autopsy, ranging from 1% to 32% in different series. Functioning adenomas are generally treated surgically; often, the contralateral gland resumes functioning after several months. Frequently, however, the effects of carcinomas are not cured by surgery. In such cases, administration of inhibitors of steroid synthesis, such as metyrapone or mitotane (*o,p′*-DDD[2,2-bis(2-chlorophenyl4-chlorophenyl)-1,1-dichloroethane]), may ameliorate some symptoms but may not improve survival. These drugs and specific aldosterone antagonists may aid in reducing symptoms in the case of ectopic ACTH secretion if the primary tumor proves unresectable. Patients given these adrenal suppressants are also prescribed chronic glucocorticoid replacement therapy (i.e., the goal of therapy is complete adrenal suppression). These patients should be considered to have suppressed adrenal function, and glucocorticoid replacement should be increased perioperatively.

Mineralocorticoid Excess

Excess mineralocorticoid activity (common with glucocorticoid excess because most glucocorticoids have some mineralocorticoid properties) leads to potassium depletion, sodium retention, muscle weakness, hypertension, tetany, polyuria, inability to concentrate urine, and hypokalemic alkalosis. These symptoms constitute primary hyperaldosteronism, or Conn's syndrome (a cause of low-renin hypertension because renin secretion is inhibited by the effects of the high levels of aldosterone).

Primary hyperaldosteronism is present in 0.5% to 1% of hypertensive patients who have no other known cause of hypertension. Primary hyperaldosteronism most often results from unilateral adenoma, although 25% to 40% of patients have been found to have bilateral adrenal hyperplasia. Intravascular fluid volume, electrolyte concentrations, and renal function should be restored to within normal limits preoperatively by administering the aldosterone antagonist spironolactone. The effects of spironolactone are slow in onset and increase for 1 to 2 weeks. A patient who has a serum potassium level of 2.9 mEq/L may have a total-body potassium deficit of as little as 40 mEq or as much as 400 mEq. Frequently, at least 24 hours is required to restore potassium equilibrium. A normal serum potassium level does not necessarily imply correction of a total-body deficit of potassium. In addition, patients with Conn's syndrome have a high incidence of hypertension and ischemic heart disease; hemodynamic monitoring should be appropriate for the degree of cardiovascular impairment.

A retrospective anecdotal study indicated that intraoperative hemodynamic status was more stable when BP and electrolytes were controlled preoperatively with spironolactone than when other antihypertensive drugs were used. However, the efficacy of optimizing the perioperative status of patients who have disorders of glucocorticoid or mineralocorticoid secretion has not been clearly established. We have assumed that gradual restoration of a normal condition is good medicine and that it would decrease perioperative morbidity and mortality.

Adrenocortical Hormone Deficiency

Glucocorticoid Deficiency

Withdrawal of steroids or suppression of synthesis by steroid therapy is the leading cause of underproduction of corticosteroids. Management of this type of glucocorticoid deficiency is discussed in the later section "Patients Taking Steroids for Other Reasons." Other causes of adrenocortical insufficiency include defects in ACTH secretion and destruction of the adrenal gland by autoimmune disease, tuberculosis, hemorrhage, or cancer; some forms of congenital adrenal hyperplasia (see previous discussion); and administration of cytotoxic drugs.

Primary adrenal insufficiency (Addison's disease) is associated with local destruction of all zones of the adrenal cortex and results in both glucocorticoid and mineralocorticoid deficiency if the insufficiency is bilateral; common symptoms and signs are listed in Table 35-5. Autoimmune disease is the most common cause of primary (nonexogenous) bilateral ACTH deficiency in the United States, whereas tuberculosis is the most common cause worldwide. Tuberculosis is associated with decreased adrenal function but large adrenal glands, as is also common in sarcoidosis, histoplasmosis, amyloidosis, metastatic malignancy, and adrenal hemorrhage. Destruction or partial destruction by trauma and by human immunodeficiency virus (HIV) and other infections, such as cytomegalovirus, mycobacteria, and fungi, is being recognized more frequently.

An increasingly common cause of adrenal insufficiency associated with large adrenal glands is heparin-induced thrombocytopenia, which might be considered in every patient who has received heparin and has hypotension.

Autoimmune destruction of the adrenals may be associated with other autoimmune disorders, such as some forms of type 1 diabetes and Hashimoto's thyroiditis. Enzymatic defects in cortisol synthesis also cause glucocorticoid insufficiency, compensatory elevations in ACTH, and congenital adrenal hyperplasia. Because adrenal insufficiency usually develops slowly, such patients are subject to marked pigmentation (from excess ACTH trying to stimulate an unproductive adrenal gland) and cardiopenia (apparently secondary to chronic hypotension).

Secondary adrenal insufficiency occurs when ACTH secretion is deficient, often because of a pituitary or hypothalamic tumor. Treatment of pituitary tumors by surgery or radiation therapy may result in hypopituitarism and subsequent adrenal failure.

If unstressed, glucocorticoid-deficient patients usually have no perioperative problems. However, acute adrenal crisis (addisonian crisis) can occur when even a minor stress is present (e.g., upper respiratory infection). Preparation of such a patient for anesthesia and surgery should include treatment of hypovolemia, hyperkalemia, and hyponatremia. Because these patients cannot respond to stressful situations, it was traditionally recommended that they be given a stress dose of glucocorticoids (about 200 mg hydrocortisone/70 kg body weight/day) perioperatively. However, Symreng and colleagues[51] gave 25 mg of hydrocortisone phosphate intravenously to adults at the start of the operative procedure, followed by 100 mg intravenously over the next 24 hours. Because using the minimum drug dose that would produce an appropriate effect is desirable, this latter regimen seems attractive. Such a regimen has proved to be as successful as a regimen using maximum doses (about 300 mg hydrocortisone per 70 kg body weight per day—see the later section "Patients Taking Steroids for Other Reasons"). Thus, we now recommend giving 100 mg of hydrocortisone phosphate intravenously every 24 hours.

Mineralocorticoid Deficiency

Hypoaldosteronism, a less common condition, can be congenital or can occur after unilateral adrenalectomy or prolonged administration of heparin. In addition, it can also be a consequence of long-standing diabetes and renal failure. Nonsteroidal inhibitors of prostaglandin synthesis may also inhibit renin release and exacerbate this condition in patients with renal insufficiency.

Plasma renin activity is below normal and fails to increase appropriately in response to sodium restriction or diuretic drugs. Most symptoms are caused by hyperkalemic acidosis rather than hypovolemia; in fact, some patients are hypertensive. These patients can have severe hyperkalemia, hyponatremia, and myocardial conduction defects. These defects can be treated successfully by administering mineralocorticoids (9α-fluorocortisol, 0.05 to 0.1 mg/day) preoperatively. Doses must be carefully titrated and monitored to avoid an increase in hypertension.

Patients Taking Steroids for Other Reasons

Perioperative Stress and the Need for Corticoid Supplementation

Many experimental studies and other reports (mostly anecdotal) concerning the adrenal responses of normal patients to the perioperative period, as well as the responses of patients taking steroids for other diseases, indicate the following:

1. Perioperative stress is related to the degree of trauma and the depth of anesthesia. Deep general or regional anesthesia causes the usual intraoperative glucocorticoid surge to be postponed to the postoperative period.
2. A few patients with suppressed adrenal function will have perioperative cardiovascular problems if they do not receive supplemental steroids perioperatively.
3. Although on occasion a patient who chronically takes steroids becomes hypotensive perioperatively, only rarely has this event been documented sufficiently to implicate glucocorticoid or mineralocorticoid deficiency as the cause.
4. Acute adrenal insufficiency occurs only rarely but can be life-threatening.
5. There is little risk in giving these patients steroid coverage equivalent to 100 mg of hydrocortisone hemisuccinate perioperatively.

In a well-controlled study of glucocorticoid replacement in primates, the investigators clearly defined the life-threatening events that can be associated with inadequate perioperative corticosteroid replacement.[48] This study further defined the physiologic and hemodynamic consequences of inadequate cortisol replacement; an alternative dose regimen is suggested that has stood the test of a decade and has altered management methods to possibly improve patient safety. In this study, adrenalectomized primates and sham-operated controls were maintained on physiologic doses of steroids for 4 months. The animals were then randomly allocated to groups that received subphysiologic (a 10th of the normal cortisol production), physiologic, or supraphysiologic (10 times the normal cortisol production) doses of cortisol for 4 days preceding abdominal surgery (cholecystectomy). Hemodynamic variables were measured by means of arterial and pulmonary artery catheters. The animals were maintained on their randomized dosage schedules during and after surgery. The group given subphysiologic doses of steroid perioperatively had a significant increase in postoperative mortality. Death rates for the physiologic and supraphysiologic replacement groups were the same and did not differ from the rate for sham-operated controls. Death in the subphysiologic replacement group was related to severe hypotension associated with a significant decrease in systemic vascular resistance and a reduced left ventricular stroke work index. Filling pressures of the heart were unchanged when compared with those in control animals. There was no evidence of hypovolemia or severe CHF. Despite the low systemic vascular resistance, the animals did not become tachycardic. All these responses are compatible with the previously documented interaction of glucocorticoids and catecholamines and thus suggest that glucocorticoids mediate catecholamine-induced increases in cardiac contractility and maintenance of vascular tone.

The investigators used a sensitive measure of wound healing involving accumulation of hydroxyproline. All treatment groups, including the group given supraphysiologic doses of glucocorticoids, had the same capacity for wound healing. Furthermore, perioperative administration of supraphysiologic doses of corticosteroids produced no adverse metabolic consequences.

This well-conducted study confirms several long-standing intuitive impressions concerning patients who have inadequate adrenal function as a result of either underlying disease or administration of exogenous steroids. Inadequate replacement of corticosteroids perioperatively can lead to addisonian crisis and death. Administration of supraphysiologic doses of steroids for a short time perioperatively caused no discernible complications. However, at least theoretical negative consequences can occur when large doses of steroids are given (see later). It is clear that inadequate corticosteroid coverage can cause death. What is not so clear is what dose of steroid should be recommended for replacement therapy. The authors of the previously discussed study on monkeys were reluctant to recommend simple physiologic steroid replacement doses for human patients perioperatively.[48] We never supplement perioperatively with a dose lower than what the patient has already been receiving.

Which patients definitely need supplementation? If in doubt, how can a patient's need for glucocorticoid supplementation be determined? Because the risk is low, we normally provide supplementation for any patient who has received steroids within a year.[48,51] Data indicate that topical application of steroids (even without the use of occlusive dressings) can suppress normal adrenal responses for as long as 9 months to 1 year (Table 35-6).

How can one determine when adrenal responsiveness has returned to normal? The morning plasma cortisol level does not reveal whether the adrenal cortex has recovered sufficiently to ensure that cortisol secretion will increase adequately to meet the demands of stress. Inducing hypoglycemia with insulin has been advocated as a sensitive test of pituitary-adrenal competence but is impractical and probably a more dangerous practice than simply administering glucocorticoids. If the plasma cortisol concentration is measured during acute stress, a value of greater than 25 μg/dL assuredly (and a value >15 μg/dL probably) indicates normal pituitary-adrenal responsiveness. In another test of pituitary-adrenal sufficiency, the baseline plasma cortisol level is determined. Then, 250 μg of synthetic ACTH (cosyntropin) is given, and plasma cortisol is measured 30 to 60 minutes later. An increase in plasma cortisol of 6 to 20 μg/dL or more is normal.[52,53] A normal response indicates recovery of pituitary-adrenal axis function. A lesser response usually indicates pituitary-adrenal insufficiency, possibly requiring perioperative supplementation with steroids.

It is unusual for laboratory data defining pituitary-adrenal adequacy to be available before surgery. Rather than delay surgery or test most patients, we assume that any patient who has taken steroids at any time during the preceding year has sup-

Table 35-6 Recovery of Hypothalamic-Pituitary-Adrenal Function after Withdrawal of Steroids

Recovery Time (mo)	Plasma 17-Hydroxycorticoid Values	Plasma ACTH Values	Adrenal Response to Exogenous ACTH	Response to Metyrapone
1	Low*	Low	Low	Low
2-5	Low	High†	Low	Low
6-9	Normal	Normal	Low	Low
>9	Normal	Normal	Normal	Normal

*Various subjective manifestations of mild adrenal insufficiency occur during this stage.
†The diurnal rhythm of plasma concentrations is qualitatively normal during this stage.
ACTH, adrenocorticotropic hormone.
Data from Graber AL, Ney RI, Nicholson WE, et al: Natural history of pituitary-adrenal recovery following long-term suppression with corticosteroids. J Clin Endocrinol Metab 25:11, 1965.

pressed pituitary-adrenal function and will require perioperative supplementation.

Under perioperative conditions, the adrenal glands secrete 116 to 185 mg of cortisol daily. Under maximum stress, they may secrete 200 to 500 mg/day. Good correlation exists between the severity and duration of the operation and the response of the adrenal gland. "Major surgery" would be represented by procedures such as laparoscopic colectomy and "minor surgery" by procedures such as herniorrhaphy. In one study of 20 patients during major surgery, the mean maximal concentration of cortisol in plasma was 47 μg/dL (range, 22 to 75 μg/dL). Values remained above 26 μg/dL for a maximum of 72 hours after surgery. During minor surgery, the mean maximal concentration of cortisol in plasma was 28 μg/dL (range, 10 to 44 μg/dL).

Although the precise amount required has not been established, we usually intravenously administer the maximum amount of glucocorticoid that the body manufactures in response to maximal stress (i.e., approximately 200 mg/day of hydrocortisone phosphate per 70 kg body weight). For minor surgical procedures, we usually give hydrocortisone phosphate intravenously, 100 mg/day per 70 kg body weight. Unless infection or some other perioperative complication develops, we decrease this dose by approximately 25% per day until oral intake can be resumed. At this point, the usual maintenance dose of glucocorticoids can be administered.

Risks of Supplementation

Rare complications of perioperative steroid supplementation include aggravation of hypertension, fluid retention, inducement of stress ulcers, and psychiatric disturbances. Although data are not available to assess the incidence of the following risks, two common complications of short-term perioperative supplementation with glucocorticoids are described in the literature: abnormal wound healing and an increased rate of infections. This evidence is inconclusive, however, because it relates to acute glucocorticoid administration and not to chronic administration of glucocorticoids with increased doses at times of stress. In contrast to some studies that suggest a deleterious effect of perioperative glucocorticoid administration on wound healing in rats, a study involving primates suggests that high doses of glucocorticoids, administered perioperatively, do not impair sensitive measures of wound healing.[48] Other data are not conclusive regarding a short-term increase in supplementation. However, an overall assessment of these results suggests that short-term perioperative supplementation with steroids has a small, but definite deleterious effect on wound healing that is perhaps partially reversed by topical administration of vitamin A.

Information regarding the risk of infection from perioperative glucocorticoid supplementation is also unclear. In many studies of chronic patient use and supplementation, no increased risk of serious infections was reported with chronic use alone. Data indicate that the risk of infection in a patient chronically taking steroids is real, but these data are inadequate to conclude that perioperative supplementation with steroids increases that risk.

Adrenal Cortex Function in the Elderly

Production of androgens by the adrenal gland progressively decreases with age (also see Chapter 71). This decrease in androgen activity has no known implications for anesthesia. Plasma levels of cortisol are unaffected by increasing age. Levels of CBG are also unaffected by age, which suggests that a normal fraction of free cortisol (1% to 5%) is present in elderly patients. Several investigators have noted a progressively impaired ability of aged patients to metabolize and excrete glucocorticoids. In normal individuals, the quantity of 17-hydroxycorticosteroids excreted is reduced by half by the seventh decade. This decreased excretion undoubtedly reflects the reduced renal function that occurs with aging. When excretion of cortisol metabolites is expressed as a function of creatinine clearance, the age difference disappears. Further reductions in cortisol clearance may be due to impaired hepatic metabolism of circulating cortisol.

The rate of secretion of cortisol is 30% lower in the elderly. This reduced secretion may be an appropriate compensatory mechanism for maintaining a normal cortisol level in the face of decreased hepatic and renal clearance of cortisol. It is important to the anesthesiologist that the reduced cortisol production can be overcome during periods of stress and that even the very elderly (those older than 100 years) display an entirely normal adrenal response to the administration of ACTH and to stresses such as hypoglycemia.

Both underproduction and overproduction of glucocorticoids are generally considered diseases of younger individuals. The highest incidence of Cushing's disease of either pituitary or adrenal origin occurs during the third decade of life. The most common cause of spontaneous Cushing's disease is benign pituitary adenoma. However, in patients older than 60 years in whom Cushing's disease develops, the most likely cause is adrenal carcinoma or ectopic ACTH production from tumors usually located in the lung, pancreas, or thymus.

Adrenal Medullary Sympathetic Hormone Excess: Pheochromocytoma

Less than 0.1% of all cases of hypertension are caused by pheochromocytomas, or catecholamine-producing tumors derived from chromaffin tissue.[54] Nevertheless, these tumors are clearly important to the anesthetist inasmuch as 25% to 50% of hospital deaths in patients with pheochromocytoma occur during induction of anesthesia or during operative procedures for other causes.[55] Though usually found in the adrenal medulla, these vascular tumors can occur anywhere, such as in the right atrium, the spleen, the broad ligament of the ovary, or the organs of Zuckerkandl at the bifurcation of the aorta. Malignant spread, which occurs in less than 15% of pheochromocytomas, usually proceeds to venous and lymphatic channels with a predisposition for the liver. This tumor is occasionally familial or part of the pluriglandular-neoplastic syndrome known as multiple endocrine adenoma type IIa or type IIb and is manifested as an autosomal dominant trait. Type IIa consists of medullary carcinoma of the thyroid, parathyroid adenoma or hyperplasia, and pheochromocytoma. What used to be called type IIb is now often called pheochromocytoma in association with phakomatoses such as von Recklinghausen's neurofibromatosis and von Hippel-Lindau disease with cerebellar hemangioblastoma. Frequently, bilateral tumors are found in the familial form. Localization of tumors can be achieved by MRI or CT, metaiodobenzylguanidine (MIBG) nuclear scanning, ultrasonography, or intravenous pyelography (in decreasing order of combined sensitivity and specificity).

Symptoms and signs that may be solicited before surgery or procedures and are suggestive of pheochromocytoma are excessive sweating; headache; hypertension; orthostatic hypotension; previous hypertensive or arrhythmic response to induction of anesthesia or to abdominal examination; paroxysmal attacks of sweating, headache, tachycardia, and hypertension; glucose intolerance; polycythemia; weight loss; and psychological abnormalities. In fact, the occurrence of combined symptoms of paroxysmal headache, sweating, and hypertension is probably a more sensitive and specific indicator than any one biochemical test for pheochromocytoma (Table 35-7). Despite more than 2000 articles in the literature about pheochromocytoma, little is known about what factors in care affect perioperative morbidity.[56,57]

Although no controlled, randomized, prospective clinical studies have investigated the value of preoperative and preprocedure use of adrenergic receptor blocking drugs, the use of such drugs is generally recommended before surgery. These drugs probably reduce the complications of hypertensive crisis, the wide BP fluctuations during manipulation of the tumor (especially until venous drainage is obliterated), and the myocardial dysfunction that occurs perioperatively. A reduction in mortality associated with resection of pheochromocytoma (from 40% to 60% to the current 0% to 6%) occurred when α-adrenergic receptor blockade was introduced as preoperative and preprocedure preparatory therapy for such patients.[56-60]

α-Adrenergic receptor blockade with prazosin or phenoxybenzamine restores plasma volume by counteracting the vasoconstrictive effects of high levels of catecholamines. This re-expansion of fluid volume is often followed by a decrease in hematocrit. Because some patients may be very sensitive to the effects of phenoxybenzamine, it should initially be given in doses of 20 to 30 mg/70 kg orally once or twice a day. Most patients usually require 60 to 250 mg/day. The efficacy of therapy should be judged by the reduction in symptoms (especially sweating) and stabilization of BP. For patients who have carbohydrate intolerance because of inhibition of insulin release mediated by α-adrenergic receptor stimulation, α-adrenergic receptor blockade may reduce fasting blood sugar levels. For patients who exhibit ST-T changes on the ECG, long-term preoperative and preprocedure α-adrenergic receptor blockade (1 to 6 months) has produced ECG and clinical resolution of catecholamine-induced myocarditis.[56,57,59-63]

β-Adrenergic receptor blockade with propranolol is suggested for patients who have persistent arrhythmias or tachycardia[56,57,59-63] because these conditions can be precipitated or aggravated by α-adrenergic receptor blockade. β-Adrenergic receptor blockade should not be used without concomitant α-adrenergic receptor blockade lest the vasoconstrictive effects of the latter go unopposed and thereby increase the risk for dangerous hypertension.

The optimal duration of preoperative therapy with phenoxybenzamine has not been studied. Most patients require 10 to 14 days, as judged by the time needed to stabilize BP and ameliorate symptoms. On the basis of our experience, this is a minimal period.[59,60,63] Because the tumor spreads slowly, little is lost by waiting until medical therapy has optimized the patient's preop-

Table 35-7 Characteristics of Tests for Pheochromocytoma

			Likelihood Ratio	
Test/Symptoms	**Sensitivity (%)**	**Specificity (%)**	**Positive Result***	**Negative Result†**
Vanillylmandelic acid excretion	81	97	27.0	0.20
Catecholamine excretion	82	95	16.4	0.19
Metanephrine excretion	83	95	16.6	0.18
Abdominal computed tomography	92	80	4.6	0.10
Concurrent paroxysmal hypertension, headache, sweating, and tachycardia‡	90	95	18.0	0.10

*The ratio representing the likelihood of a positive result is obtained by dividing the sensitivity by 1 and then subtracting the specificity.
†The ratio representing the likelihood of a negative result is obtained by subtracting the sensitivity from 1 and then dividing by the specificity.
‡Data for concurrent paroxysmal symptoms are best estimates from available data.
Modified from Pauker SG, Kopelman RI: Interpreting hoofbeats: Can Bayes help clear the haze? N Engl J Med 327:1009, 1992.

erative condition. Accordingly, we recommend using the following criteria:

1. No in-hospital BP reading higher than 165/90 mm Hg should be evident for 48 hours before surgery. We often measure arterial BP every minute for 1 hour in a stressful environment (our postanesthesia care unit). If no BP reading is greater than 165/90, this criterion is considered satisfied.
2. Orthostatic hypotension should be present, but BP on standing should not be lower than 80/45 mm Hg.
3. The ECG should be free of ST-T changes that are not permanent.
4. No more than one premature ventricular contraction (PVC) should occur every 5 minutes.

Other drugs, including prazosin, calcium channel blocking drugs, clonidine, dexmedetomidine, and magnesium, have also been used to achieve suitable degrees of α-adrenergic blockade before surgery.

Although specific anesthetic drugs have been recommended, we believe that optimal preoperative preparation, gentle induction of anesthesia, and good communication between the surgeon and anesthesiologist are most important. Virtually all anesthetic drugs and techniques (including isoflurane, sevoflurane, sufentanil, remifentanil, fentanyl, and regional anesthesia) have been used with success. In fact, all drugs studied are associated with a high rate of transient intraoperative arrhythmias.[59] One author (M.F.R.) has avoided desflurane because it may precipitate non-neurogenic catecholamine release. No good data indicate that these biases are appropriate.

Because of ease of use, there is a preference to give phenylephrine hydrochloride (Neo-Synephrine) or dopamine for hypotension and nitroprusside for hypertension. Phentolamine (Regitine) has too long an onset and duration of action. Occasionally (five times in >80 pheochromocytoma resections), we have used a β-adrenergic blocking agent (esmolol is now the preferred agent) for severe tachycardia without hypertension or volume depletion. Painful or stressful events such as intubation often cause an exaggerated stress response in less than perfectly anesthetized patients who have pheochromocytoma. This response is caused by release of catecholamines from nerve endings that are "loaded" by the reuptake process. Such stresses may result in catecholamine levels of 200 to 2000 pg/mL in normal patients. For a patient with pheochromocytoma, even simple stress can lead to blood catecholamine levels of 2000 to 20,000 pg/mL. However, infarction of a tumor, with release of products onto peritoneal surfaces, or surgical pressure causing release of products can result in blood levels of 200,000 to 1,000,000 pg/mL—a situation that should be anticipated and avoided (ask for a temporary stay of surgery, if at all possible, while the rate of nitroprusside infusion is increased). Once the venous supply is secured and if intravascular volume is normal (as measured by pulmonary wedge pressure or echocardiography), normal BP usually results. However, some patients become hypotensive and occasionally require massive infusions of catecholamines. On rare occasion, patients remain hypertensive intraoperatively. Postoperatively, about 50% remain hypertensive for 1 to 3 days—and initially have markedly elevated but declining plasma catecholamine levels—at which time all but 25% become normotensive. It is important to interview other family members and perhaps advise them to inform their future anesthetist about the potential for such familial disease.

Hypofunction or Aberration in Function of the Sympathetic Nervous System (Dysautonomia)

Disorders of the sympathetic nervous system include Shy-Drager syndrome, Riley-Day syndrome, Lesch-Nyhan syndrome, Gill's familial dysautonomia, diabetic dysautonomia, and the dysautonomia of spinal cord transection.

Although individuals can function well without an adrenal medulla, a deficient peripheral sympathetic nervous system occurring late in life poses major problems for many facets of life; nevertheless, perioperative sympathectomy or its equivalent has been recommended by some.[64-70] A primary function of the sympathetic nervous system appears to be regulation of BP and intravascular fluid volume during changing of body position. Common features of all the syndromes of hypofunctioning of the sympathetic nervous system are orthostatic hypotension and decreased beat-to-beat variability in heart rate. These conditions can be caused by deficient intravascular volume, deficient baroreceptor function (as also occurs in carotid artery disease[71]), abnormalities in CNS function (as in Wernicke or Shy-Drager syndrome), deficient neuronal stores of norepinephrine (as in idiopathic orthostatic hypotension[72] and diabetes), or deficient release of norepinephrine (as in traumatic spinal cord injury[73]). These patients may have an increased number of available adrenergic receptors (a compensatory response) and an exaggerated response to sympathomimetic drugs. In addition to other abnormalities, such as retention of urine or feces and deficient heat exchange, hypofunctioning of the sympathetic nervous system is often accompanied by renal amyloidosis. Thus, electrolyte and intravascular fluid volume status should be evaluated preoperatively. Because many of these patients have cardiac abnormalities, intravascular fluid volume might be assessed preoperatively with a Swan-Ganz catheter or intraoperatively via transesophageal echocardiography rather than measurement of CVP.

Inasmuch as functioning of the sympathetic nervous system is not predictable in these patients, we generally use slow, gentle induction of anesthesia and treat sympathetic excess or deficiency by infusing, with careful titration, drugs that directly constrict (phenylephrine) or dilate (nitroprusside) blood vessels or that stimulate (isoproterenol) or depress (esmolol) the heart rate. We prefer these drugs to agonists or antagonists, which may indirectly release catecholamines. A 20% perioperative mortality rate for 2600 patients after spinal cord transection has been reported, thus indicating that such patients are difficult to manage and deserve particularly close attention.

After reviewing 300 patients with spinal cord injuries, Kendrick and coworkers[74] concluded that autonomic hyperreflexia syndrome does not develop if the lesion is below spinal dermatome T7. If the lesion is above that level (splanchnic outflow), 60% to 70% of patients experience extreme vascular instability. The trigger to this instability, or a mass reflex involving noradrenergic and motor hypertonus,[75] can be a cutaneous, proprioceptive, or visceral stimulus (a full bladder is a common initiator). The sensation enters the spinal cord and causes a spinal reflex, which in normal persons is inhibited from above. Sudden increases in

Table 35-8 Biochemical Measurements of Thyroid Function That Account for Variation in Production of Thyroid-Binding Globulin

	Examples of Normal Thyroid Status						
	FT_4E	=	T_4	×	THBR	TSH
Normal	0.19 (0.12-0.25)	=	0.6 (0.4-0.9)	×	31% (25%-35%)	0.2 (0.2-0.8)
During use of oral contraceptives	0.19	=	1.3	×	15%	0.3
During use of corticosteroids	0.18	=	0.3	×	60%	0.3

FT_4E is the free T_4 (thyroxine) estimate. It is usually obtained by multiplying the total T_4 concentration (the free amount and the amount bound to protein) by the thyroid hormone–binding ratio (THBR, formerly called the resin T_3 uptake). THBR is a measure of the bound thyroid hormone–binding protein. TSH is the thyroid-stimulating hormone secreted by the pituitary in the negative feedback loop. (TSH increases when FT_4E is low in hypothyroidism.)

BP are sensed in the pressure receptors of the aorta and carotid sinus. The resulting vagal hyperactivity produces bradycardia, ventricular ectopia, or various degrees of heart block. Reflex vasodilation may occur above the level of the lesion and result in flushing of the head and neck. Two new techniques to help reduce acute injury or aid in repair (high-dose DHA and acute cooling) may also have anesthetic implications, but reports of these effects, if any, have not been published.

Depending on the length of time since spinal cord transection, other abnormalities may occur. Acutely (i.e., <3 weeks from the time of spinal injury), retention of urine and feces is common and, by elevating the diaphragm, may impair respiration. Disimpaction of the intestine alleviates this respiratory problem. Hyperesthesia is present above the lesion; reflexes and flaccid paralysis are present below the lesion. The intermediate period (3 days to 6 months) is marked by a hyperkalemic response to depolarizing drugs.[76] The chronic phase is characterized by return of muscle tone, a Babinski sign, and frequently, the occurrence of hyperreflexia syndromes (e.g., mass reflex, see earlier).

Thus, in addition to meticulous attention to perioperative intravascular volume and electrolyte status, the anesthesiologist should know—by history taking, physical examination, and laboratory data—the status of the patient's myocardial conduction (as revealed by the ECG), the status of renal functioning (by noting the ratio of creatinine to blood urea nitrogen [BUN]), and the condition of the respiratory muscles (by determining the ratio of forced expiratory volume in 1 second [FEV_1] to forced vital capacity [FVC]) (also see Chapter 44). The anesthesiologist may also obtain a chest radiograph if atelectasis or pneumonia is suspected on the basis of history taking or the physical examination. Temperature control, the presence of bone fractures or decubitus ulcers, and normal functioning of the urination and defecation systems must be assessed. Confirmation of the latter prevents postoperative pneumonia or atelectasis caused by high positioning of the diaphragm.

Thyroid Dysfunction

The major thyroid hormones are thyroxine (T_4), a prohormone product of the thyroid gland, and the more potent 3,5,3-triiodothyronine (T_3), a product of both the thyroid and extrathyroidal enzymatic deiodination of T_4. Under normal circumstances, approximately 85% of T_3 is produced outside the thyroid gland. Production of thyroid secretions is maintained by secretion of thyroid-stimulating hormone (TSH) in the pituitary, which in turn is regulated by secretion of thyrotropin-releasing hormone (TRH) in the hypothalamus. Secretion of TSH and TRH appears to be negatively regulated by T_4 and T_3. Many believe that all effects of thyroid hormones are mediated by T_3 and that T_4 functions only as a prohormone.

Because T_3 has greater biologic effect than T_4 does, one would expect the diagnosis of thyroid disorders to be based on levels of T_3. However, this is not usually the case. The diagnosis of thyroid disease is confirmed by one of several biochemical measurements: levels of free T_4 or total serum concentrations of T_4 and the "free T_4 estimate." This estimate is obtained by multiplying total T_4 (free and bound) by the thyroid-binding ratio (formerly called resin T_3 uptake) (Table 35-8). Free T_4 can be accurately measured by many laboratories. Direct measurement of free T_4 obviates the need to account for changes in binding protein synthesis and affinity caused by other conditions. The T_3-binding ratio measures the extra quantity of serum protein-binding sites. This measurement is necessary because thyroxine-binding globulin (TBG) is abnormally high during pregnancy, hepatic disease, and estrogen therapy (all of which would elevate the total T_4 level) (Box 35-3). Reliable interpretation of measurements of the total hormone concentration in serum necessitates

Box 35-3 Factors Influencing Serum Levels of Thyroxine-Binding Globulin

Conditions Increasing Serum Levels

Use of oral contraceptives
Pregnancy
Use of estrogen
Infectious hepatitis
Chronic active hepatitis
Neonatal state
Acute intermittent porphyria
Inherited conditions

Conditions Decreasing Serum Levels

Testosterone
Use of corticosteroids
Severe illness
Cirrhosis
Nephrotic syndrome
Inherited conditions

data on the percentage of bound hormone. The thyroid hormone–binding ratio test provides this information. In this test, I-labeled T_3 is added to a patient's serum and allowed to reach an equilibrium binding state. A resin is then added that binds the remaining radioactive T_3. Resin uptake is greater if the patient has fewer TBG-binding sites. In normal patients, resin T_3 uptake (the thyroid hormone–binding ratio) is 25% to 35%. When serum TBG is elevated, the thyroid hormone–binding ratio is diminished (see Table 35-8). When serum TBG is diminished, as in nephrotic syndrome, in conditions in which glucocorticoids are increased, or in chronic liver disease, the thyroid hormone–binding ratio is increased.

The free T_4 estimate and the free T_3 estimate are frequently used as measures of a patient's serum T_4 and T_3 hormone concentration. To obtain these estimates, the concentration of total serum T_4 or total serum T_3 is multiplied by the measured thyroid hormone–binding ratio. Values of these two indices are normal in the event of a primary alteration in binding but not with an alteration in secretion of thyroid hormone.

Hyperthyroidism can be diagnosed by measuring levels of TSH after the administration of TRH. Although administering TRH normally increases TSH levels in blood, even a small increase in the T_4 or T_3 level in blood abolishes this response. Thus, a subnormal or absent serum TSH response to TRH is a very sensitive indicator of hyperthyroidism. In one group of disorders involving hyperthyroidism, serum TSH levels are elevated in the presence of elevated levels of free thyroid hormone.

Measurement of the α-subunit of TSH has been helpful in identifying the rare patients who have a pituitary neoplasm and who usually have increased α-subunit concentrations. Some patients are clinically euthyroid in the presence of elevated levels of total T_4 in serum. Certain drugs, notably gallbladder dyes, propranolol, glucocorticoids, and amiodarone, block the conversion of T_4 to T_3, thereby elevating T_4 levels. Severe illness also slows this conversion. Levels of TSH are often high in situations in which the rate of conversion is decreased. In hyperthyroidism, cardiac function and responses to stress are abnormal; return of normal cardiac function parallels the return of TSH levels to normal.

Hyperthyroidism

Although hyperthyroidism is usually caused by the multinodular diffuse enlargement in Graves' disease (also associated with disorders of the skin or eyes, or both), it can also occur with pregnancy, thyroiditis (with or without neck pain), thyroid adenoma, choriocarcinoma, or TSH-secreting pituitary adenoma. Five percent of women have thyrotoxic effects 3 to 6 months postpartum and tend to have recurrences with subsequent pregnancies. Major manifestations of hyperthyroidism are weight loss, diarrhea, warm moist skin, weakness of large muscle groups, menstrual abnormalities, osteopenia, nervousness, jitteriness, intolerance to heat, tachycardia, cardiac arrhythmias, mitral valve prolapse, and heart failure. When the thyroid is functioning abnormally, the entity most threatened is the cardiovascular system. When diarrhea is severe, dehydration should be corrected preoperatively. Mild anemia, thrombocytopenia, increased serum alkaline phosphatase, hypercalcemia, muscle wasting, and bone loss frequently occur in hyperthyroidism. Muscle disease usually involves the proximal muscle groups; it has not been reported to cause respiratory muscle paralysis. In the apathetic form of hyperthyroidism (seen most commonly in persons older than 60 years), cardiac effects dominate the clinical picture. Signs and symptoms include weight loss, anorexia, and cardiac effects such as tachycardia, irregular heart rhythm, atrial fibrillation (in 10%), heart failure, and occasionally, papillary muscle dysfunction.

Although β-adrenergic receptor blockade can control the heart rate, its use is fraught with hazard in a patient already experiencing CHF. However, a decreasing heart rate may improve heart-pumping function. Thus, hyperthyroid patients who have fast ventricular rates, who are in CHF, and who require emergency surgery are given esmolol guided by changes in pulmonary artery wedge pressure and their condition. If slowing the heart rate with a small dose of esmolol (50 μg/kg) does not aggravate the heart failure, we administer more esmolol. We believe that we should aim to avoid imposing surgery on any patient whose thyroid function is clinically abnormal. Therefore, we believe that only "life or death" emergency surgery should preclude making the patient pharmacologically euthyroid, a process that can take 2 to 6 weeks. Evaluation of hyperthyroidism is also covered in Chapter 34. Antithyroid medications include propylthiouracil and methimazole, both of which decrease the synthesis of T_4 and may enhance remission by reducing TSH receptor antibody levels (the primary pathologic mechanism in Grave's disease). Propylthiouracil also decreases the conversion of T_4 to the more potent T_3. However, the literature indicates a trend toward preoperative preparation with propranolol and iodides alone.[77] This approach is quicker (i.e., 7 to 14 days versus 2 to 6 weeks); it shrinks the thyroid gland, as does the more traditional approach; it decreases conversion of the prohormone T_4 into the more potent T_3; and it treats symptoms but may not correct abnormalities in left ventricular function. Regardless of the approach, antithyroid drugs should be administered chronically and on the morning of surgery. If emergency surgery is necessary before the euthyroid state is achieved, if subclinical hyperthyroidism progresses without adequate treatment, or if hyperthyroidism gets out of control during surgery, intravenous administration of esmolol, 50 to 500 μg/kg, could be titrated to restore a normal heart rate (assuming the absence of CHF) (see earlier). In addition, intravascular fluid volume and electrolyte balance should be restored. However, administering propranolol or esmolol does not invariably prevent "thyroid storm."

No controlled study has demonstrated clinical advantages of any anesthetic drug over another for surgical patients who are hyperthyroid. A review of cases performed at the University of California, San Francisco, from 1968 to 1982 revealed that virtually all anesthetic drugs and techniques[78] have been used without adverse effects even remotely being attributable to the drug or technique. Furthermore, although some investigators have recommended that anticholinergic drugs (especially atropine) be avoided inasmuch as they interfere with the sweating mechanism and cause tachycardia, atropine has been given as a test for the adequacy of antithyroid treatment. Because patients are now subjected to operative procedures only (or almost only) when euthyroid, the traditional "steal" of a heavily premedicated hyperthyroid patient (so commonly found in the iodine-deficient locales surrounding the Lahey, Mayo, and Cleveland clinics) in the operating room has vanished.

A patient with a large goiter and an obstructed airway can be handled in the same way as any other patient with problematic airway management. Preoperative medication should avoid excessive sedation, and an airway should be established, often with the patient awake. A firm armored endotracheal tube is preferable and should be passed beyond the point of extrinsic compression. It is most useful to examine CT scans of the neck preoperatively to determine the extent of compression. Maintenance of anesthesia usually presents little difficulty. Postoperatively, extubation should be performed under optimal circumstances for reintubation in the event that the tracheal rings have been weakened and the trachea collapses.

Of the many possible postoperative complications (nerve injury, bleeding, and metabolic abnormalities), "thyroid storm" (discussed later), bilateral recurrent nerve trauma, and hypocalcemic tetany are the most feared. Bilateral recurrent laryngeal nerve injury (secondary to trauma or edema) causes stridor and laryngeal obstruction as a result of unopposed adduction of the vocal cords and closure of the glottic aperture. Immediate endotracheal intubation is required, usually followed by tracheostomy to ensure an adequate airway. This rare complication occurred only once in more than 30,000 thyroid operations at the Lahey Clinic. Unilateral recurrent nerve injury often goes unnoticed because of compensatory overadduction of the uninvolved cord. However, we often test vocal cord function before and after this surgery by asking the patient to say "e" or "moon." Unilateral nerve injury is characterized by hoarseness and bilateral nerve injury by aphonia. Selective injury to the adductor fibers of both recurrent laryngeal nerves leaves the abductor muscles relatively unopposed, and pulmonary aspiration is a risk. Selective injury to the abductor fibers leaves the adductor muscles relatively unopposed, and airway obstruction can occur. Bullous glottic edema, an additional cause of postoperative respiratory compromise, has no specific cause or known preventive measure.

The intimate involvement of the parathyroid gland with the thyroid gland can result in inadvertent hypocalcemia during surgery for thyroid disease. Complications related to hypocalcemia are discussed in the later section "Hypocalcemia."

Because postoperative hematoma can compromise the airway, neck and wound dressings are placed in a crossing fashion (rather than vertically or horizontally) and should be examined for evidence of bleeding before a patient is discharged from the recovery room.

Thyroid Storm

"Thyroid storm" is the name for the clinical diagnosis of a life-threatening illness in a patient whose hyperthyroidism has been severely exacerbated by illness or surgery. Thyroid storm is characterized by hyperpyrexia, tachycardia, and striking alterations in consciousness. It can thus be manifested very similarly to malignant hyperthermia, pheochromocytoma, or neuroleptic malignant syndrome. No laboratory tests are diagnostic of thyroid storm, and the precipitating (nonthyroidal) cause is the major determinant of survival. Therapy can include blocking the synthesis of thyroid hormones by administering antithyroid drugs, blocking the release of preformed hormone with iodine, meticulous attention to hydration and supportive therapy, and correcting the precipitating cause. Blocking the sympathetic nervous system with reserpine, α- and β-receptor antagonists, or α_2-agents may be exceedingly hazardous and requires skillful management and constant monitoring of the critically ill patient.

Thyroid dysfunction, either hyperthyroidism or hypothyroidism, develops in more than 10% of patients treated with the antiarrhythmic agent amiodarone.[79] Approximately 35% of the drug's weight is iodine, and a 200-mg tablet releases about 20 times the optimal daily dose of iodine. This iodine can lead to reduced synthesis of T_4 or increased synthesis. In addition, amiodarone inhibits the conversion of T_4 to the more potent T_3.

Patients receiving amiodarone might be considered to be in need of special attention preoperatively and may even require special attention to anesthesia, not just because of the arrhythmia that led to such therapy but also to ensure that no perioperative dysfunction or surprises occur because of unsuspected thyroid hyperfunction or hypofunction.[80] Many patients with amiodarone-induced thyrotoxicosis receive steroids for a period, another area of questioning that might be triggered by the use of amiodarone in a preoperative patient.

Hypothyroidism

Hypothyroidism is a common disease that has been detected in 5% of a large population in Great Britain, in 3% to 6% of a healthy older population in Massachusetts, and in 4.5% of a medical clinic population in Switzerland. The apathy and lethargy that often accompany hypothyroidism frequently delay its diagnosis, so the perioperative period may be the first opportunity to spot many such hypothyroid patients. However, hypothyroidism is usually subclinical, serum concentrations of thyroid hormones are in the normal range, and only serum TSH levels are elevated. The normal range of TSH is 0.3 to 4.5 mU/L, and TSH values of 5 to 15 mU/L are characteristic of this entity. In such cases, hypothyroidism may have little or no perioperative significance. However, a retrospective study of 59 mildly hypothyroid patients found that more hypothyroid patients than control subjects required prolonged postoperative intubation (9 of 59 versus 4 of 59) and had significant electrolyte imbalances (3 of 59 versus 1 of 59) and bleeding complications (4 of 59 versus 0 of 59).[81] Because only a small number of charts were examined, these differences did not reach statistical significance. In another study, overt hypothyroidism later developed in a high percentage of patients with a history of subclinical hypothyroidism.[82,83] Thus, a previous history of subclinical hypothyroidism may indicate the need to search for and be concerned about the possibility of overt hypothyroidism.

In the less frequent occurrences of overt hypothyroidism, the relative lack of thyroid hormone results in slow mental functioning, slow movement, dry skin, arthralgias, carpal tunnel syndrome, periorbital edema, intolerance to cold, depression of the ventilatory responses to hypoxia and hypercapnia, impaired clearance of free water with or without hyponatremia, "hung-up reflexes," slow gastric emptying, sleep apnea,[84] and bradycardia. In extreme cases, cardiomegaly, heart failure, and pericardial pleural effusions are manifested as fatigue, dyspnea, and orthopnea. Hypothyroidism is often associated with amyloidosis, which may produce an enlarged tongue, abnormalities of the cardiac conduction system, and renal disease. Hypothyroidism decreases the anesthetic requirement slightly. The tongue may be enlarged in a hypothyroid patient even in the absence of amyloidosis, and such enlargement may hamper endotracheal intubation.

A rising TSH level is the most sensitive indicator of failing thyroid function. Ideal preoperative and preprocedure management of hypothyroidism consists of restoring normal thyroid status: we routinely administer the normal dose of levothyroxine the morning of surgery, even though these drugs have long half-lives (1.4 to 10 days). (Levothyroxin is the preferred therapy because it allows the controlling enzyme systems to regulate TSH secretion, as well as conversion to T_3.) Reduced GI absorption of levothyroxine may occur with the coadministration of cholestyramine or aluminum hydroxide, iron, a high-bran meal, or sucralfate or colestipol. For patients in myxedema coma requiring emergency surgery, liothyronine can be given intravenously (with fear of precipitating myocardial ischemia, however) while supportive therapy is undertaken to restore normal intravascular fluid volume, body temperature, cardiac function, respiratory function, and electrolyte balance.

Treating hypothyroid patients with symptomatic coronary artery disease poses special problems and may require compromises in the general practice of preoperatively restoring euthyroidism with drugs. Although both levothyroxine and esmolol may be given, adequate amelioration of both ischemic heart disease and hypothyroidism may be difficult to achieve. The need for thyroid therapy must be balanced against the risk of aggravating the anginal symptoms. One review suggested early consideration of coronary artery revascularization.[85] It advocated initiating thyroid replacement therapy in the ICU soon after the patient's arrival from the operating room and myocardial revascularization surgery. However, several deaths from arrhythmia and CHF, as well as cardiogenic shock with infarction, have occurred while patients who were not given thyroid therapy were awaiting surgery. Thus, true emergency coronary artery revascularization should be considered in patients with both severe coronary artery disease and significant hypothyroidism.

In hypothyroidism, respiratory control mechanisms do not function normally. However, the response to hypoxia and hypercapnia and clearance of free water become normal with thyroid replacement therapy. Drug metabolism is anecdotally reported to be slowed, and awakening times from sedatives are reported to be prolonged during hypothyroidism. However, few formal studies and none in humans of the pharmacokinetics and pharmacodynamics of sedatives or anesthetic drugs have been published. These concerns disappear when thyroid function is normalized preoperatively. Addison's disease (with its relative steroid deficiency) is more common in hypothyroidism, and some endocrinologists routinely treat noniatrogenic hypothyroid patients with stress doses of steroids perioperatively because both conditions are commonly caused by autoimmune responses. The possibility that this steroid deficiency exists should be considered if the patient becomes hypotensive perioperatively. Body heat mechanisms are inadequate in hypothyroid patients, so temperature should be monitored and maintained, especially in patients requiring emergency surgery. Because of an increased incidence of myasthenia gravis in hypothyroid patients, it may be advisable to use a peripheral nerve stimulator to guide administration of muscle relaxants (see Chapter 29).

Thyroid Nodules and Carcinoma

More than 90% of thyroid nodules are benign, yet identifying malignancy in a solitary thyroid nodule is a difficult and important procedure. Male patients and patients with previous radiation therapy to the head and neck have an increased likelihood of malignant disease in their nodules. Often, needle biopsy and scanning are sufficient for the diagnosis, but occasionally, excisional biopsy is needed. Papillary carcinoma accounts for more than 70% of all thyroid carcinomas. Simple excision of lymph node metastases appears to be as efficacious for patient survival as radical neck procedures. Follicular carcinoma accounts for about 15% of thyroid carcinomas, is more aggressive, and has a less favorable prognosis.

Medullary carcinoma, the most aggressive form of thyroid carcinoma, is associated with a familial occurrence of pheochromocytoma, as are parathyroid adenomas. For this reason, a history might be obtained from patients who have a surgical scar in the thyroid region so that the possibility of occult pheochromocytoma can be ruled out.

Disorders of Calcium Metabolism

The three substances that regulate serum concentrations of calcium, phosphorus, and magnesium—parathyroid hormone (parathyrin, PTH), calcitonin, and vitamin D—act on bone, kidney, gut, and their own receptors (the last has led to an important advance in treatment in the last few years). Calcium excess in blood is due to either malignancy or hyperparathyroidism in more than 90% of patients.[86] PTH stimulates bone resorption, inhibits renal excretion of calcium, and increases conversion to active vitamin D, three conditions that lead to hypercalcemia. Calcitonin can be considered an antagonist to PTH. Through its metabolites, vitamin D aids in the absorption of calcium, phosphate, and magnesium from the gut and facilitates the bone resorptive effects of PTH. Secretion of PTH is modulated through the calcium-sensing receptor on the cell surface of parathyroid cells. An increase in ionized calcium stimulates this receptor, which causes a decrease in PTH secretion. Recognition of this effect has led to re-evaluation of the therapy for hyperparathyroidism inasmuch as a drug upregulating this receptor's sensitivity reduces PTH levels and the presence of increased calcium in over 60% of people who have elevated calcium levels from this cause.[87]

Hyperparathyroidism and Hypercalcemia

Primary hyperparathyroidism occurs in about 0.1% of the population, most commonly begins in the third to fifth decades of life, and occurs two to three times more frequently in women than men. Primary hyperparathyroidism usually results from enlargement of a single gland, commonly an adenoma and very rarely a carcinoma. Hypercalcemia almost always develops.

Calcium is the chief mineral component of the body; it provides structure to the skeleton and performs key roles in neural transmission, intracellular signaling, blood coagulation, and neuromuscular functioning. Ninety-nine percent of the 1000 g of calcium present in the average human body is stored in the bone mineral reservoir. The normal total serum calcium level is 8.6 to 10.4 mg/dL, as measured in most laboratories. Fifty percent to 60% is bound to plasma proteins or is complexed with phosphate or citrate. The value is dependent on the albumin level, with a decline of 0.8 mg/dL for each 1-g/dL drop in albumin. Binding of calcium to albumin is dependent on pH: binding decreases with acidic pH and increases with alkaline pH. It should be noted that serum calcium and not ionized calcium decreases with decreases in albumin levels. Although ionized calcium is the clinically significant fraction, the cost and technical difficulties of stabilizing the electrodes used for measurement have limited the available assays. Nevertheless, PTH and vitamin D_3 work to keep the level stable within 0.1 mg/dL in any individual.

Many of the prominent symptoms of hyperparathyroidism are a result of the hypercalcemia that accompanies it. Regardless of the cause, hypercalcemia can produce any of a number of symptoms, the most prominent of which involve the renal, skeletal, neuromuscular, and GI systems—anorexia, vomiting, constipation, polyuria, polydipsia, lethargy, confusion, formation of renal calculi, pancreatitis, bone pain, and psychiatric abnormalities. Free intracellular calcium initiates or regulates muscle contraction, release of neurotransmitters, secretion of hormones, enzyme action, and energy metabolism.

Nephrolithiasis occurs in 60% to 70% of patients with hyperparathyroidism. Sustained hypercalcemia can result in tubular and glomerular disorders, including proximal (type II) renal tubular acidosis. Polyuria and polydipsia are common complaints.

Skeletal disorders related to hyperparathyroidism are osteitis fibrosa cystica, simple diffuse osteopenia, and osteoporosis. The rate of bone turnover is five times higher in patients with hyperparathyroidism than in normal controls. Patients may have a history of frequent fractures or complain of bone pain, the latter especially in the anterior margin of the tibia.

Because free intracellular calcium initiates or regulates muscle contraction, neurotransmitter signaling, hormone secretion, enzyme action, and energy metabolism, abnormalities in these end organs are often symptoms of hyperparathyroidism. Patients may experience profound muscle weakness, especially in proximal muscle groups, as well as muscle atrophy. Depression, psychomotor retardation, and memory impairment may occur. Lethargy and confusion are frequent complaints.

Peptic ulcer disease is more common in these patients than in the rest of the population. Production of gastrin and gastric acid is increased. Anorexia, vomiting, and constipation may also be present.

Approximately a third of all hypercalcemic patients are hypertensive, but the hypertension usually resolves with successful treatment of the primary disease. Neither hypertension nor minimally invasive surgery seems to alter the perioperative risk associated with surgery in such patients in comparison to the usual hypertensives.[88,89] Even octogenarians with asymptomatic hyperparathyroidism can be operated on without mortality and with morbidity no different from that in younger individuals, thus encouraging the use of parathyroidectomy as preventive therapy.[89,90] Long-standing hypercalcemia can lead to calcifications in the myocardium, blood vessels, brain, and kidneys. Cerebral calcifications may cause seizures, whereas renal calcifications lead to polyuria that is unresponsive to vasopressin.

The most useful confirmatory test for hyperparathyroidism is a radioimmunoassay for PTH. In fact, two recent changes have radically reduced anesthesia involvement in the care of patients with primary hyperparathyroidism. One, the drug class that modulates the calcium-sensitive PTH cell receptor and thereby decreases calcium levels, the calcimimetics, has been discussed (earlier) and its use emphasized in older individuals (see later). The other is to use minimally invasive approaches after imaging procedures with just local anesthesia or a cervical plexus block—as with thyroidectomy.[91,92] Most surgeons now performing minimally invasive parathyroid removal monitor PTH levels intraoperatively to determine whether they have resected the causative adenoma. In hyperparathyroid patients, hormone levels are abnormal for a given level of calcium. The level of inorganic phosphorus in serum is usually low, but it may be within normal limits. Alkaline phosphatase is elevated if considerable skeletal involvement is present.

Glucocorticoid administration reduces the level of calcium in blood in many other conditions that cause hypercalcemia, but not usually in primary hyperparathyroidism. In sarcoidosis, multiple myeloma, vitamin D intoxication, and some malignant diseases, all of which can cause hypercalcemia, administration of glucocorticoids may lower serum calcium levels through an effect on GI absorption. This effect occurs to a lesser degree in primary hyperparathyroidism.

Hypercalcemia may also occur as a consequence of secondary hyperparathyroidism in patients who have chronic renal disease. When phosphate excretion decreases as a result of lower nephron mass, serum calcium levels fall because of deposition of calcium and phosphate in bone. Secretion of PTH subsequently increases, which causes the fraction of phosphate excreted by each nephron to increase. Eventually, the chronic intermittent hypocalcemia of chronic renal failure leads to chronically high levels of serum PTH and hyperplasia of the parathyroid glands—one of the entities termed secondary hyperparathyroidism.

What should be done for asymptomatic patients with primary hyperparathyroidism or even ones with secondary hyperparathyroidism? This question has become the subject of a major controversy, for which no definitive answer exists. Symptomatic primary hyperparathyroidism in those younger than 50 years or with serum calcium levels more than 1 mg/dL above the upper limit of normal, a 30% or greater reduction in the glomerular filtration rate (GFR), or severe bone demineralization is usually treated surgically. If the patient refuses surgery or if other illnesses make surgery inadvisable, medical management with the new calcimimetic cinacalcet has made management much more feasible. The difficulty with such management is that the hyperfunctioning parathyroid glands secrete more hormone as the serum calcium concentration is lowered—as though the calcium set point for feedback regulation of PTH secretion had been raised.

Patients with moderate hypercalcemia who have normal renal and cardiovascular function present no special preoperative and preprocedure problems. The ECG can be examined preoperatively and intraoperatively for shortened PR or QT intervals (Fig. 35-4). Because severe hypercalcemia can result in hypovolemia, normal intravascular volume and electrolyte status should be restored before commencement of anesthesia and surgery.

Management of hypercalcemia preoperatively should include (even in urgent or emergency situations) treatment of the underlying cause—a frequent strategy in malignancy-associated hypercalemic patients coming to surgery. Antitumor therapy preoperatively for both malignant and nonmalignant causes of hypercalcium can include hydration and diuresis to increase urinary calcium excretion. Restoration of intravascular volume, augmentation and excretion of urinary sodium (with saline infusion), and administration of diuretics (furosemide is commonly used) generally increase urinary calcium excretion substantially. Infusion rates of 200 to 400 mL/hr preoperatively are commonly used, but monitoring is needed to avoid fluid overload, especially since many patients have compromised cardiac pumping ability. Other complications of these interventions include hypomagnesemia and hypokalemia.

In emergency situations, vigorous expansion of intravascular volume usually reduces serum calcium to a safe level (<14 mg/dL); administration of furosemide is also often helpful in these situations. Phosphate should be given to correct hypophosphatemia because it decreases calcium uptake into bone, increases calcium excretion, and stimulates breakdown of bone. Hydration and diuresis, accompanied by phosphate repletion, suffice in the management of most hypercalcemic patients. Other measures to decrease reabsorption of bone include the bisphosphonates pamidronate sodium (90 mg intravenously) and zoledronate

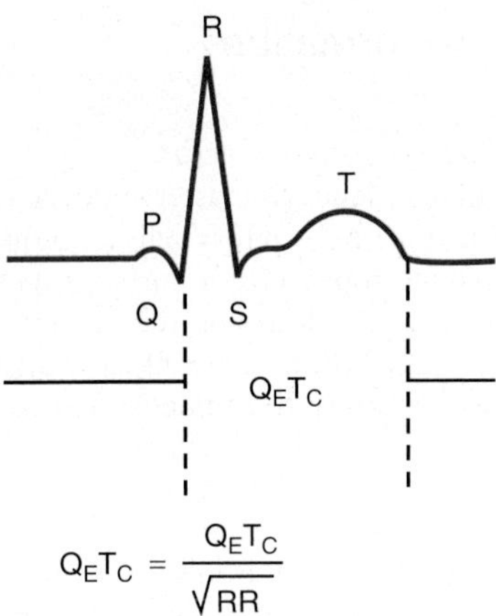

Figure 35-4 Measurement of the QTc interval (properly termed Q_ET_C to indicate that it begins with the start of the Q wave, lasts throughout the QT interval, ends with the end of the T wave, and is corrected for heart rate). RR is the RR interval in seconds. *(From Hensel P, Roizen MF: Patients with disorders of parathyroid function. Anesthesiol Clin North Am 5:287, 1987.)*

(4 mg intravenously), salmon calcitonin (100 to 400 units every 12 hours), and plicamycin (15 to 25 µg/kg intravenously).

Calcitonin lowers serum calcium levels through direct inhibition of bone resorption. It can decrease serum calcium levels within minutes after intravenous administration. Side effects include urticaria and nausea. It is so rapid acting that it can be used to reduce calcium levels while waiting for hydration and a bisphosphonate to take effect. Dialysis can also be used when appropriate.

It is especially important to know whether the hypercalcemia has been chronic because serious cardiac, renal, or CNS abnormalities may have resulted.

Hypocalcemia

Hypocalcemia (caused by hypoalbuminemia, hypoparathyroidism, hypomagnesemia, hypovitaminosis D, hungry bones after correction of hyperparathyroidism, anticonvulsant therapy, citrate infusion, or chronic renal disease) is not usually accompanied by a clinically evident cardiovascular disorder. The most common cause of hypocalcemia is hypoalbuminemia. In true hypocalcemia (i.e., when the free calcium concentration is low), myocardial contractility is affected. That is, myocardial contractility varies directly with levels of blood ionized calcium, although contractility decreased only 20% when ionized calcium levels changed from 1.68 to 1.34 mmol/L. The clinical signs of hypocalcemia are clumsiness; convulsions; laryngeal stridor; depression; muscle stiffness; paresthesia (oral and perioral); parkinsonism; tetany; Chvostek's sign; dry scaly skin, brittle nails, and coarse hair; low serum concentrations of calcium; prolonged QT intervals; soft tissue calcifications; and Trousseau's sign.

Hypocalcemia delays ventricular repolarization, hence increasing the QTc interval (normal, 0.35 to 0.44 second). With electrical systole prolonged, the ventricles may fail to respond to the next electrical impulse from the sinoatrial node, and a 2:1 heart block results. Prolongation of the QT interval is a moderately reliable ECG sign of hypocalcemia, not for the population as a whole, but for the individual patient.[93] Thus, monitoring the QT interval as corrected for the heart rate (see Fig. 35-4) is a useful, but not always accurate means of monitoring hypocalcemia in any individual patient. CHF may also occur with hypocalcemia, but this is rare. Because CHF in patients with coexisting heart disease is reduced in severity when calcium and magnesium ion levels are restored to normal, these levels may be normalized before surgery in a patient with impaired exercise tolerance or signs of cardiovascular dysfunction; normalization can be achieved intravenously over a 15-minute period if absolutely necessary.[94,95] Sudden decreases in blood levels of ionized calcium (as with chelation therapy) can result in severe hypotension.

Patients with hypocalcemia may have seizures. They may be focal, jacksonian, petit mal, or grand mal in appearance, indistinguishable from such seizures in the absence of hypocalcemia. Patients may also have a type of seizure called cerebral tetany, which consists of generalized tetany followed by tonic spasms. Therapy with standard anticonvulsants is ineffective and may even exacerbate these seizures (by an anti–vitamin D effect). In long-standing hypoparathyroidism, calcifications may appear above the sella; these calcifications represent deposits of calcium in and around small blood vessels of the basal ganglia. They may be associated with a variety of extrapyramidal syndromes.

The most common cause of acquired hypoparathyroidism is surgery on the thyroid or parathyroid glands. Other causes include autoimmune disorders, therapy with iodine 131, hemosiderosis or hemochromotosis, neoplasia, and granulomatous disease. Idiopathic hypoparathyroidism has been divided into three categories: an isolated persistent neonatal form, branchial dysembryogenesis, and autoimmune candidiasis related to multiple endocrine deficiency.

Pseudohypoparathyroidism and pseudopseudohypoparathyroidism are rare hereditary disorders characterized by short stature, obesity, rounded face, and shortened metacarpals. Patients with pseudohypoparathyroidism have hypocalcemia and hyperphosphatemia despite high serum levels of PTH. These patients have a deficient end-organ response to PTH as a result of abnormalities in G-protein function.

Because treatment of hypoparathyroidism is not surgical, hypoparathyroid patients who come to the operating room are those who require surgery for an unrelated condition. Their calcium, phosphate, and magnesium levels should be measured both preoperatively and postoperatively. Patients with symptomatic hypocalcemia might be treated with intravenous calcium gluconate before surgery. Initially, 10 to 20 mL of 10% calcium gluconate may be given at a rate of 5 mL/min. The effect on serum calcium levels is of short duration, but a continuous infusion with 10 mL/min of 10% calcium gluconate in 500 mL of solution over a period of 6 hours helps keep serum calcium at adequate levels. Magnesium and phosphate levels may require normalization as well to normalize cardiovascular and nervous system function.

The objective of therapy is to bring the symptoms under control before surgery and anesthesia. For patients with chronic hypoparathyroidism, the objective is to keep the serum calcium level in the lower half of the normal range. A preoperative and preprocedure ECG is useful for maintaining the QTc interval. The preoperative and preprocedure QTc value may be used as a guide to the serum calcium level if rapid laboratory assessment is not possible. Changes in the calcium level may alter the duration of muscle relaxation, so such alterations might be monitored by using a twitch monitor in these (as well as all other) patients.

The intimate involvement of the parathyroid gland with the thyroid gland can result in unintentional hypocalcemia during surgery for diseases of either organ. Because of the affinity of their bones for calcium, this relationship is crucial in patients with advanced osteitis. Internal redistribution of magnesium, calcium, or both ions may occur (into "hungry bones") after parathyroidectomy and cause hypomagnesemia, hypocalcemia, or both conditions. Because the tendency to tetany increases with alkalosis, hyperventilation is usually assiduously avoided. The most prominent manifestations of acute hypocalcemia are distal paresthesias and muscle spasm (tetany). Potentially fatal complications of severe hypocalcemia include laryngeal spasm and hypocalcemic seizures. The clinical sequelae of magnesium deficiency include cardiac arrhythmias (principally ventricular tachyarrhythmias), hypocalcemic tetany, and neuromuscular irritability independent of hypocalcemia (tremors, twitching, asterixis, and seizures).

In addition to monitoring total serum calcium or ionized calcium postoperatively, one can test for the Chvostek and Trousseau signs. (Note that serum calcium and not ionized calcium is dependent on the albumin level, with a decline of about 0.8 mg/dL for each 1-g/dL drop in serum albumin level.) Because the Chvostek sign can be elicited in 10% to 15% of patients who are not hypocalcemic, an attempt should be made to elicit it preoperatively to ensure that its appearance is meaningful. The Chvostek sign is a contracture of the facial muscles produced by tapping the ipsilateral facial nerves at the angle of the jaw. The Trousseau sign is elicited by applying a BP cuff at a level slightly above the systolic level for a few minutes. The resulting carpopedal spasm, with contraction of the fingers and inability to open the hand, stems from the increased muscle irritability in hypocalcemic states, aggravated by ischemia produced by the BP cuff.

Osteoporosis

Fifty percent of women older than 65 years sustain an osteoporotic fracture. (Because men are living longer, osteoporosis has become an increasing problem for them too, and recent reports indicate a 15% per decade hip fracture rate for men older than 65 years).[93] Men with COPD (even without steroid treatment) are at high risk for vertebral fractures and thus might be allowed to position and move themselves onto and off surgical tables. Furthermore, in either gender, each vertebral fracture is associated with a 10% decrease in lung capacity. Diagnosis and treatment of these conditions have increased with routine use of dual-energy x-ray absorptiometry (DEXA) or quantitative ultrasonography. Because "T" and "Z" scores were developed to relate changes in white postmenopausal women to those at age 21, care must be used in interpreting the results. Known risk factors include age, relative lifetime estrogen deficiency (late menarche, amenorrhea, early menopause, nulliparity), deficiency of dietary calcium, tobacco use, increased aerobic exercise in combination with decreased weight-bearing exercise, decreased weight-bearing exercise by itself, use of soft drinks, and Asian or white ancestry. Although therapy for osteoporosis (use of biphosphates, bone mineral depositors, weight-bearing exercises, calcium, vitamin D, estrogen, and now designer estrogens that may be useful for men such as Evista) does not have major known implications for anesthesia care,[96-98] bone fractures in such patients have occurred on movement to and from an operating table. Recombinant PTH and calcitonin are also used, but again, no reports of perioperative interactions have been prominent. Thus, the precautions mentioned earlier for hyperparathyroid patients relative to self-positioning and careful positioning may be useful.

Pituitary Abnormalities

Anterior Pituitary Hypersecretion

The anterior pituitary gland (or master endocrine gland) consists of five identifiable types of secretory cells (and the hormones that they secrete): somatotrophs (GH), corticotrophs (ACTH), lactotrophs (prolactin), gonadotrophs (luteinizing hormone [LH] and follicle-stimulating hormone [FSH]), and thyrotrophs (TSH). Secretion of these pituitary hormones is largely regulated by a negative-feedback loop by hypothalamic regulatory hormones and by signals that originate from the target site of pituitary action. Six hypothalamic hormones have been characterized: dopamine, the prolactin-inhibiting hormone; somatostatin, the GH release– inhibiting hormone; GH-releasing hormone (GHRH); corticotropin-releasing hormone (CRH); gonadotropin-releasing hormone (GnRH or LHRH); and TRH. Most pituitary tumors (>60%) are hypersecretory and are classified according to the excess production of a specific anterior pituitary hormone.

The three most common disorders of pituitary hypersecretion are those related to excesses of prolactin (amenorrhea, galactorrhea, and infertility), ACTH (Cushing's syndrome), or GH (acromegaly). In addition to knowing the pathophysiologic processes of the disease involved, the anesthesiologist must determine whether the patient recently underwent air pneumoencephalography (almost obsolete, but still used rarely). If so, nitrous oxide should not be used to lessen the risk of intracranial hypertension from gas collection. CT or MRI of the sella has largely replaced neuroencephalography, but as stated, the latter is still performed.

Preoperative evaluation of patients with acromegaly is found in Chapter 34. More than 99% of cases of acromegaly are attributable to pituitary adenoma (or use of recombinant GH for unapproved aging prevention, which it does not do as of current data). Thus, the primary treatment of acromegaly is transsphenoidal surgery (or withdrawal of drug) and symptomatic treatment of the carpal tunnel or other syndromes provoked. If the pituitary tumor is not totally removed, patients are often offered external pituitary irradiation. In the case of suprasellar extension, conventional transfrontal hypophysectomy is often performed. The dopaminergic agonist bromocriptine can lower GH levels, but the long-term follow-up with this drug is not favorable. Octreotide, a long-acting analog of somatostatin, now given in depot form about once a month, produces effective palliation in 50% of patients. Other medical therapies such as pegvisomant or somatostatin analogs are also medications that have been tried before surgery.

Difficulty with endotracheal intubation should be anticipated in an acromegalic patient; lateral neck films or CT scans of the neck and direct or indirect visualization can identify patients with subglottic stenosis or an enlarged tongue, mandibles, epiglottis, or vocal cords. If placement of an arterial line is necessary, a brachial or femoral site may be preferable to a radial site.[99]

Anterior Pituitary Hypofunction

Anterior pituitary hypofunction results in deficiency of one or more of the following hormones: GH, TSH, ACTH, prolactin, or gonadotropin. Preoperative and preprocedure preparation of patients who are chronically deficient in ACTH and TSH is discussed in Chapter 34. No special preoperative and preprocedure preparation is required for a patient deficient in prolactin or gonadotropin; deficiency in GH, however, can result in atrophy of cardiac muscle, a condition that may necessitate preoperative and preprocedure cardiac evaluation. Nonetheless, anesthetic problems have not been documented in patients with isolated GH deficiency. Acute deficiencies are another matter.

Acute pituitary deficiency is often caused by bleeding into a pituitary tumor. In surgical specimens of resected adenomas, as many as 25% show evidence of hemorrhage. These patients often have acute headache, visual loss, nausea or vomiting, ocular palsy, disturbances of consciousness, fever, vertigo, or hemiparesis. In such patients, rapid transsphenoidal decompression should be accompanied by consideration of replacement therapy, including glucocorticoids, and treatment of increased intracranial pressure.

Obstetric anesthesiologists are often aware of these pituitary failure problems (also see Chapter 69); Sheehan's syndrome is the clinical manifestation of pituitary infarction associated with hypotension after or during obstetric hemorrhage. Conditions that strongly suggest this diagnosis are failure to start postpartum lactation, increasing fatigue, cold intolerance, and especially hypotension unresponsive to volume replacement and pressors.

Posterior Pituitary Hormone Excess and Deficiency

Secretion of vasopressin or antidiuretic hormone (ADH) is enhanced by increased serum osmolality or the presence of hypotension. Inappropriate secretion of vasopressin, without relation to serum osmolality, results in hyponatremia and fluid retention. This inappropriate secretion can result from a variety of CNS lesions; from drugs such as nicotine, narcotics, chlorpropamide, clofibrate, vincristine, vinblastine, and cyclophosphamide; and from pulmonary infections, hypothyroidism, adrenal insufficiency, and ectopic production from tumors. Preoperative and preprocedure management of a surgical patient with inappropriate secretion of vasopressin includes appropriate treatment of the causative disorders and restriction of water. Occasionally, drugs that inhibit the renal response to ADH (e.g., lithium or demeclocycline) should be administered preoperatively to restore normal intravascular volume and electrolyte status.

Most of the clinical features associated with the syndrome of inappropriate secretion of antidiuretic hormone (SIADH) are related to hyponatremia and the resulting brain edema; such features include weight gain, weakness, lethargy, mental confusion, obtundation, and disordered reflexes and may culminate in convulsions and coma. This form of edema rarely leads to hypertension.

Recently, it has been recognized that 10% to 20% of long-distance and marathon runners have SIADH with increased vasopressin secretion. Because such people not infrequently undergo surgical treatment of injuries, SIADH symptoms and laboratory evaluation might be routine for that group as well.

SIADH should be suspected in any patient with hyponatremia who excretes urine that is hypertonic relative to plasma. The following laboratory findings further support the diagnosis:

1. Urinary sodium >20 mEq/L
2. Low serum levels of BUN, creatinine, uric acid, and albumin
3. Serum sodium <130 mEq/L
4. Plasma osmolality <270 mOsm/L
5. Urine hypertonic relative to plasma

Noting the response to water loading is a useful way of evaluating patients with hyponatremia. Patients with SIADH are unable to excrete dilute urine even after water loading. Assay of ADH in blood can confirm the diagnosis. Too vigorous treatment of chronic hyponatremia can result in disabling demyelination.[100,101] The increase in serum sodium should not be greater than 1 mEq/L/hr[100,101] (see discussion of hyponatremia in the later section "Electrolyte Disorders").

Patients with mild to moderate symptoms of water intoxication (and worse outcomes are seen in children, those with hypoxic episodes, and menstruant women) can be treated with restriction of fluid intake to about 500 to 1000 mL/day. Patients with severe water intoxication and CNS symptoms may need vigorous treatment consisting of intravenous administration of 200 to 300 mL of a 5% saline solution over a period of several hours, followed by fluid restriction.

Treatment should be directed at the underlying problem. If SIADH is drug induced, use of the drug should be withdrawn. Inflammation should be treated with appropriate measures, and neoplasms should be managed by surgical resection, irradiation, or chemotherapy, whichever is indicated.

No drugs are available that can suppress release of ADH from the neurohypophysis or from a tumor. Phenytoin (Dilantin) and narcotic antagonists such as naloxone and butorphanol have some inhibiting effect on physiologic ADH release but are clinically ineffective in patients with SIADH. Drugs that block the effect of ADH on renal tubules include lithium, which is rarely used because its toxicity often outweighs its benefits, and demethylchlortetracycline in doses of 900 to 1200 mg/day. The latter drug interferes with the ability of the renal tubules to concentrate urine, thereby causing excretion of isotonic or hypotonic urine and lessening the hyponatremia. Demethylchlortetracycline can be used in ambulatory patients with SIADH when it is difficult to restrict fluids.

When a patient with SIADH comes to the operating room for any surgical procedure, fluids are managed by measuring central volume status by CVP, pulmonary artery lines, or the cross-sectional left ventricular area at end-diastole on transesophageal echocardiography and by frequent assays of urine osmolarity, plasma osmolarity, and serum sodium, including the period immediately after surgery. Despite the common impression that SIADH is frequently seen in elderly patients in the postoperative period, studies have shown that the patient's age and the type of anesthetic used have no bearing on the postoperative development of SIADH. It is not unusual to see several patients in the neurosurgical ICU suffering from this syndrome. The diagnosis is usually one of exclusion. Patients with SIADH generally require only fluid restriction; very rarely is hypertonic saline needed.

Lack of ADH, which results in diabetes insipidus, is caused by pituitary disease, brain tumors, infiltrative diseases such as sarcoidosis, head trauma (including trauma after neurosurgery), or lack of a renal response to ADH. The last can occur as a result of such diverse causes as hypokalemia, hypercalcemia, sickle cell anemia, obstructive uropathy, and renal insufficiency. Preoperative or preprocedure treatment of diabetes insipidus consists of restoring normal intravascular volume by replacing urinary losses, administering desmopressin nasally, and giving daily fluid requirements intravenously.

Perioperative management of patients with diabetes insipidus is based on the extent of the ADH deficiency. Management of a patient with complete diabetes insipidus and a total lack of ADH does not usually present any major problem as long as the side effects of the drug are avoided and the presence of the condition is known before surgery. Just before surgery, the patient is given the usual dose of DDAVP (desmopressin acetate) intranasally or an intravenous bolus of 100 mU of aqueous vasopressin, followed by a constant infusion of 100 to 200 mU/hr.[2] The dose is usually adjusted to permit the daily breakthrough polyuria that avoids the iatrogenic syndrome of SIADH. We have found it useful to continue that dosing regimen perioperatively in all ambulatory patients who can take fluid orally in the postoperative period. All the intravenous fluids given intraoperatively should be isotonic to reduce the risk of water depletion and hypernatremia. Plasma osmolality should be measured every hour, both intraoperatively and immediately after surgery. If plasma osmolality rises well above 290 mOsm/L, hypotonic fluids can be administered; the rate of the intraoperative vasopressin infusion can be increased to greater than 200 mU/hr.

For patients who have a partial deficiency of ADH, it is not necessary to use aqueous vasopressin perioperatively unless plasma osmolality rises above 290 mOsm/L. Nonosmotic stimuli (e.g., volume depletion) and the stress of surgery usually cause the release of large quantities of ADH perioperatively. Consequently, these patients require only frequent monitoring of plasma osmolality during this period.

Because of side effects, the dose of vasopressin should be limited to that necessary for control of diuresis. The oxytoxic and coronary artery–constricting properties of vasopressin make this limit especially applicable to patients who are pregnant or have coronary artery disease.

Another problem for anesthesiologists is the care of patients who come to the operating room with a vasopressin drip for the treatment of bleeding from esophageal varices. This treatment is less common since the advent of laser therapy for varices. However, when vasopressin is given, the vasoconstrictive effect of vasopressin on the splanchnic vasculature is used to decrease bleeding. Such patients are often volume depleted and may have concomitant coronary artery disease. Because vasopressin has been shown to markedly decrease oxygen availability, primarily as a result of decreased stroke volume and heart rate, monitoring of tissue oxygen delivery may be useful. In patients with a history of angina pectoris who received a combination of cimetidine and vasopressin for esophageal varices, bradyarrhythmias and AV block have occurred. This effect indicates that the combination of cimetidine and vasopressin could be deleterious to the heart because of the combined negative inotropic and arrhythmogenic effects of the two drugs.

Diseases Involving the Cardiovascular System

Hypertension

Analysis of the perioperative treatment of hypertension is important because of the prevalence of the condition (30% of the general population in the United States), the great risk in perioperative care of a hypertensive patient, and the high cost of unnecessary delays in surgery (also see Chapter 34). The controversy centers around two issues. Does inadequate control of hypertension result in complications that could be prevented with some control? How much control of BP is needed and for how long? That is, does overzealous control just create unnecessary postponements of elective surgery or, worse, predispose the patient to exaggerated adverse drug reactions and greater hemodynamic instability than not so zealous control does?

Because of the controversy regarding the appropriateness of preoperative treatment of hypertension, the original articles that stimulated this controversy have been evaluated fully in previous editions.

Several schools of thought exist, the two oldest represented by studies conducted by Prys-Roberts and colleagues[102] in 1971 and by Goldman and Caldera[103] in 1979. Several other studies (Bedford and Feinstein,[104] Asiddao et al.,[105] Stone et al.,[106] Flacke et al.,[107] Ghignone et al.,[108] Tuman et al.,[109] Ellis et al.,[110] Mangano et al.,[111] Pasternack et al.[112]) have also been cited. Weksler and colleagues[113] studied 989 chronically treated hypertensive patients who underwent noncardiac surgery with diastolic BP between 110 and 130 mm Hg and no previous MI, unstable or severe angina pectoris, renal failure, pregnancy-induced hypertension, left ventricular hypertrophy, previous coronary revascularization, aortic stenosis, preoperative dysrhythmias, conduction defects, or stroke.[113] The control group had their surgery postponed and remained in the hospital for control of BP, and the study patients received 10 mg of nifedipine intranasally. No statistically significant differences in postoperative complications were observed, thus suggesting that this subset of patients without significant cardiovascular comorbid conditions can proceed with surgery despite elevated BP the day of surgery.

Only one study has directly assessed the relationship between cardiovascular disease and preoperative isolated systolic hypertension. In a multicenter study of patients undergoing CABG, the presence of isolated systolic hypertension has been associated with a 30% increased incidence of perioperative cardiovascular complications when compared with normotensive individuals, but no study has addressed the importance of isolated systolic hypertension in noncardiac surgery.[114] Unfortunately, each of these studies has deficiencies that prevent the establishment of a definitive answer to this question.

Recommendations

Although preoperative systolic BP is a significant predictor of postoperative morbidity, no data definitively establish whether preoperative treatment of hypertension reduces perioperative risk. Until a definitive study is performed (and that would unfortunately be extremely difficult to do), we recommend letting the weight of evidence guide preoperative treatment of a patient with hypertension. Such treatment would be based on three general beliefs: (1) the patient should be educated regarding the importance of lifelong treatment of hypertension, even isolated systolic hypertension; (2) perioperative hemodynamic fluctuations occur less frequently in treated than in untreated hypertensive patients (as demonstrated by Prys-Roberts and colleagues[102] and confirmed by Goldman and Caldera[103] and Mangano and associates,[111]); and (3) hemodynamic fluctuations have some relationship to morbidity. The data of Pasternack and colleagues[112] and Weksler and associates[113] imply that rapid correction of BP or prevention of increases in heart rate may be all that is needed. However, data from animals that had declining renal function with acute reductions in arterial BP accentuate the risks of such reductions.[115] Even though other epidemiologic data confirm these risks,[116,117] the hazards of BP fluctuations and acute hypertension may be serious in an untreated hypertensive subject.[118] Modern drug therapy for hypertension appears to reduce these risks but does so for many with a decrement in quality of life that causes many patients to avoid such medications.[119] Specific racial differences need to be considered before treatment (African Americans respond less well to β-adrenergic receptor blocking drugs and ACE inhibitors but as well to calcium channel antagonists as whites do).[120]

We use preoperative data to determine the individualized range of values that we consider tolerable by a particular patient during and after surgery. That is, if BP is 180/100 mm Hg and the heart rate is 96 beats/min on admission with no signs or symptoms of myocardial ischemia, we feel confident that the patient can tolerate these levels during surgery. If during the night BP decreases to 80/50 mm Hg and the heart rate to 48 beats/min and the patient does not wake with signs of a new cerebral deficit, we believe that the patient can safely tolerate such levels during anesthesia. Therefore, on the basis of preoperative data, we derive an individualized set of values for each patient. We then try to keep cardiovascular variables within that range and, in fact, plan before induction what therapies to use to accomplish that goal (e.g., administration of more/less anesthesia, nitroglycerin or nitroprusside/dopamine, dobutamine, phenylephrine, propranolol/isoproterenol, or atropine). We believe that this type of planning is especially important for a patient with suspected cardiovascular disease and relatively unimportant for a totally healthy patient. We do not know for certain that keeping cardiovascular variables within an individualized range of acceptable values improves the surgical outcome, but we do believe that such a plan reduces morbidity. For example, the POISE study demonstrated that acute β-blocker administration resulted in an increased incidence of stroke and death that was associated with an increased rate of hypotension.[121]

Preoperative Administration of All Antihypertensive Drugs

We routinely administer all antihypertensive drugs preoperatively, except ACE inhibitors or angiotensin II antagonists (AIIAs), which we tailor to the individual patient. Coriat and colleagues[122] found that ACE inhibitors were associated with hypotension in 100% of patients during induction versus about 20% in whom ACE inhibitors were withheld on the morning of surgery. Bertrand and coworkers performed a prospective randomized study in which it was demonstrated that more severe hypotensive episodes requiring vasoconstrictor treatment occur after induction of general anesthesia in patients chronically treated with an AIIA and receiving the drug on the morning before surgery than in those in whom AIIAs were discontinued on the day before surgery.[123] Kheterpal and colleagues performed a propensity-matched analysis of 12,381 noncardiac surgery cases.[124] Patients with chronic ACE inhibitor/angiotensin receptor blocker and diuretic therapy showed more periods with a mean arterial BP lower than 70 mm Hg, periods with a 40% decrease in systolic BP, periods with a 50% decrease in systolic BP, and vasopressor boluses than patients receiving diuretic therapy alone did. If these drugs are continued, vasopressin is the drug of choice for refractory hypotension. Although the long-term adverse effects of withholding therapy on the morning of surgery were not assessed, we withhold therapy until either oral fluid is able to be consumed (ambulatory patients) or we can convert to intravenously or nasogastrically administered alternatives (patients who remain NPO postoperatively). We even administer the patient's chronic diuretics on the morning of surgery because the major effect of diuretics after 1 week of therapy is arteriolar vasodilation and assessment of urine output may be inaccurate if the diuretic is abruptly discontinued on the morning of surgery.

Ischemic Heart Disease

Preoperative evaluation of a patient with ischemic heart disease (also see Chapter 60) and a discussion of the American Heart Association/American College of Cardiology (AHA/ACC) guidelines can be found in Chapter 34.[125]

Role of Coronary Artery Bypass Graft or Percutaneous Coronary Interventions before Noncardiac Surgery

Coronary revascularization has been suggested as a means of reducing perioperative risk before noncardiac surgery. Previous retrospective evidence has shown that prior successful preoperative revascularization may decrease postoperative cardiac risk twofold to fourfold in patients undergoing elective vascular surgery.[126,127] The strongest retrospective evidence comes from the Coronary Artery Surgery Study (CASS) registry, which enrolled patients from 1978 to 1981. Operative mortality in patients with CABG performed before noncardiac surgery was 0.9% but was significantly higher at 2.4% in patients without previous CABG. However, there was a 1.4% mortality rate associated with the CABG procedure itself. Eagle and colleagues reported on a long-term analysis of patients entered into CASS.[128] They studied patients assigned to medical or surgical therapy for coronary artery disease for over 10 years who subsequently underwent 3368 noncardiac operations in the years after assignment of coronary treatment. Intermediate-risk surgery such as abdominal, thoracic, or carotid endarterectomy was associated with a combined morbidity and mortality rate of 1% to 5% and a small but significant improvement in outcome in patients who had previously undergone revascularization. The most significant improvement in outcome occurred in patients who underwent major vascular surgery such as abdominal or lower extremity revascularization. However, this observational study did not randomize patients and was undertaken in the 1970s and 1980s, before significant advances in medical, surgical, and percutaneous coronary strategies.[128] Landesberg and coauthors retrospectively reviewed long-term outcomes in 578 major vascular procedures.[129] By multivariate analysis, age, type of vascular surgery, presence of diabetes, previous MI, and moderate to severe ischemia on preoperative thallium scanning (PTS) independently predicted mortality, and preoperative coronary revascularizaton predicted improved survival. Long-term survival after major vascular surgery was significantly improved if patients with moderate to severe ischemia on PTS underwent selective coronary revascularization.

The benefit of percutaneous coronary intervention (PCI) before noncardiac surgery has also been examined in several cohort studies. Posner and colleagues used an administrative data set of patients who underwent PCI and noncardiac surgery in Washington State.[130] They matched patients with coronary disease who were undergoing noncardiac surgery with and without previous PCI and looked at cardiac complications. In this nonrandomized design, they noted a significantly lower rate of 30-day cardiac complications in patients who underwent PCI at least 90 days before the noncardiac surgery. Importantly, however, PCI within 90 days of noncardiac surgery did not improve outcome. Although the explanation for these results is unknown, they may support the notion that PCI performed "to get the patient through surgery" may not improve perioperative outcome because cardiac complications may not occur in patients with stable or asymptomatic coronary stenosis. PCI may actually destabilize coronary plaque, which becomes manifest in the days or weeks after noncardiac surgery. Godet and associates studied a cohort of 1152 patients after abdominal aortic surgery in which 78 patients underwent PCI.[131] In the PCI group, the observed percentages of patients with a severe postoperative coronary event (9.0%; 95% confidence interval [CI], 4.4 to 17.4) or death (5.1% [95% CI, 2.0 to 12.5]) were not significantly different from the expected percentages (8.2% and 6.9%, respectively), which was confirmed by propensity analysis. PCI did not seem to significantly limit cardiac risk or death after aortic surgery.

Several randomized trials have now addressed the value of testing and CABG or PCI (or both) in a subset of patients. McFalls and colleagues reported the results of a multicenter randomized trail in the VA Health System in which patients with documented coronary artery disease on coronary angiography, excluding those with left main disease or a severely depressed ejection fraction (<20%), were randomized to CABG (59%) or percutaneous transluminal coronary angioplasty (PTCA) (41%) versus routine medical therapy.[132] At 2.7 years after randomization, mortality in the revascularization group was not significantly different (22%) from that in the no-revascularization group (23%) (Fig. 35-5). Within 30 days after the vascular operation, postoperative MI, defined by elevated troponin levels, occurred in 12% of the revascularization group and 14% of the no-revascularization group (P = .37). The authors suggested that coronary revascularization is

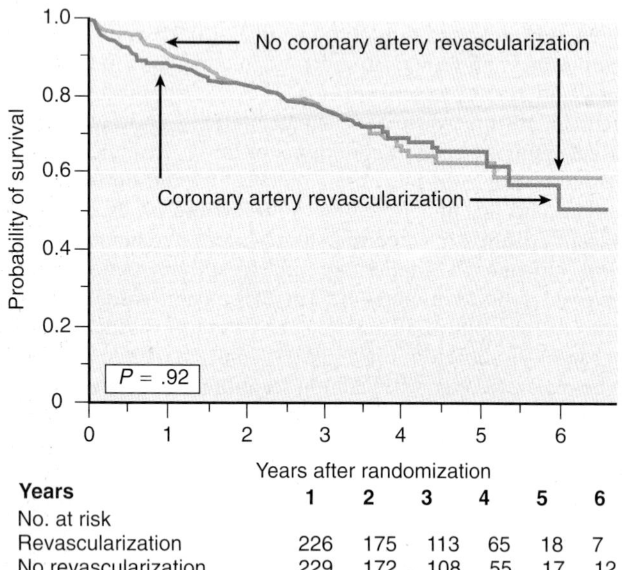

Years	1	2	3	4	5	6
No. at risk						
Revascularization	226	175	113	65	18	7
No revascularization	229	172	108	55	17	12

Figure 35-5 Long-term survival in patients randomized to coronary revascularization or routine care in patients with coronary artery disease on angiography and undergoing major vascular surgery in the Coronary Artery Revascularization Prophylaxis trial. *(Reproduced with permission from McFalls EO, Ward HB, Moritz TE, et al: Coronary-artery revascularization before elective major vascular surgery. N Engl J Med 351:2795-2804, 2004.)*

not indicated in patients with stable coronary artery disease, and their results further support the lack of efficacy of PCI or CABG for single- or double-vessel disease before noncardiac surgery. However, in a follow-up analysis, Ward and coauthors reported improved outcome in the subset who underwent CABG versus PCI.[133] Poldermans and colleagues randomized 770 patients about to undergo major vascular surgery and considered to have intermediate cardiac risk, defined as the presence of one or two cardiac risk factors, to either undergo further risk stratification with stress imaging or proceed directly to surgery.[134] All patients received bisoprolol with a targeted heart rate of 60 to 65 beats/min initiated before and continued after surgery. The 30-day incidence of cardiac death and nonfatal MI was similar in both groups (1.8% in the no-testing group versus 2.3% in the tested group). The conclusion of the authors was that further risk stratification in this group of patients considered to be at intermediate risk based on clinical history alone was unnecessary as long as perioperative β-blockers were used and that testing only delayed necessary vascular surgery. In a pilot study, Poldermans and associates tested patients with more than three risk factors; 101 (23%) showed extensive ischemia and were randomly assigned to revascularization (n = 49) or no revascularization.[135] Revascularization did not improve 30-day outcome; the incidence of the composite end point was 43% versus 33% (odds ratio [OR], 1.4; 95% CI, 0.7 to 2.8; P = .30). In addition, no benefit during 1-year follow-up was observed after coronary revascularization (49% versus 44%; OR, 1.2; 95% CI, 0.7 to 2.3; P = .48).

One issue in interpreting the results is that the length of time between coronary revascularization and noncardiac surgery most likely has an impact on its protective effect and potential risks. Back and coworkers studied 425 consecutive patients undergoing 481 elective major vascular operations at an academic VA Medical Center.[136] Coronary revascularization was classified as recent (CABG <1 year; PTCA <6 months) in 35 cases (7%), prior (CABG >1 year and ≤5 years; PTCA >6 months and ≤2 years) in 45 cases (9%), and remote (CABG ≥5 years; PTCA ≥2 years) in 48 cases (10%). Outcomes in patients with previous PTCA were similar to those after CABG (P = .7). Significant differences in adverse cardiac events and mortality were found between patients with CABG performed within 5 years or PTCA within 2 years (6.3%, 1.3%, respectively), individuals with remote revascularization (10.4%, 6.3%), and nonrevascularized patients stratified at high risk (13.3%, 3.3%) or intermediate/low risk (2.8%, 0.9%). The authors concluded that previous coronary revascularization (CABG <5 years; PTCA <2 years) may provide only modest protection against adverse cardiac events and mortality after major arterial reconstruction.

PCI using coronary stenting poses several special issues. Kaluza and associates reported on the outcome of 40 patients who underwent prophylactic coronary stent placement less than 6 weeks before major noncardiac surgery requiring general anesthesia.[137] There were seven MIs, 11 major bleeding episodes, and 8 deaths. All deaths and MIs, as well as 8 of the 11 bleeding episodes, occurred in patients subjected to surgery less than 14 days after stenting. Four patients expired after undergoing surgery 1 day after stenting. Wilson and colleagues reported on 207 patients who underwent noncardiac surgery within 2 months of stent placement.[5] Eight patients died or suffered an MI, all of whom were among the 168 patients who had surgery 6 weeks after stent placement. Vincenzi and coworkers studied 103 patients and reported that the risk of suffering a perioperative cardiac event

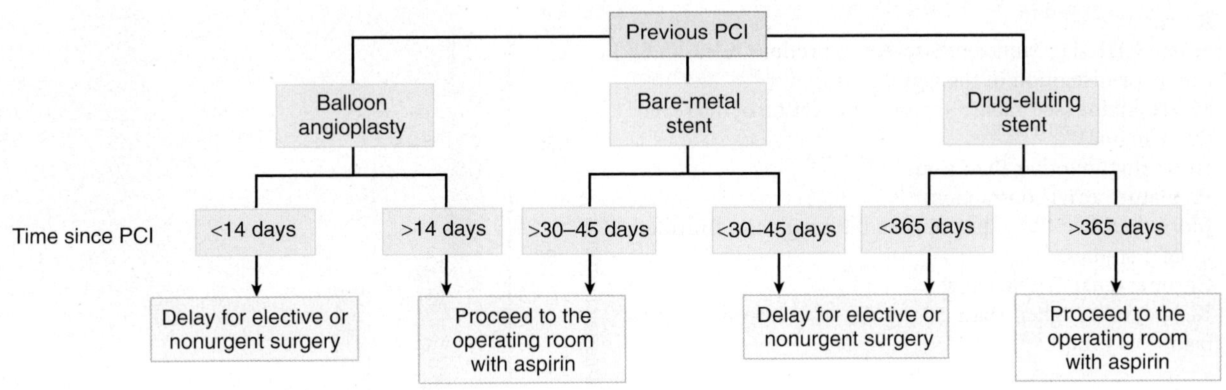

Figure 35-6 Recommendation for management of a patient with a previous percutaneous coronary intervention (PCI) from the American Heart Association/American College of Cardiology. *(Reproduced with permission from Fleisher LA, Beckman JA, Brown KA, et al: ACC/AHA 2007 guidelines on perioperative cardiovascular evaluation and care for noncardiac surgery: A report of the American College of Cardiology/American Heart Association Task Force on Practice Guidelines (Writing Committee to Revise the 2002 Guidelines on Perioperative Cardiovascular Evaluation for Noncardiac Surgery): Developed in collaboration with the American Society of Echocardiography, American Society of Nuclear Cardiology, Heart Rhythm Society, Society of Cardiovascular Anesthesiologists, Society for Cardiovascular Angiography and Interventions, Society for Vascular Medicine and Biology, and Society for Vascular Surgery. Circulation 116(17): e418-e499, 2007.)*

was 2.11-fold greater in patients with recent stents (<35 days before surgery) than in those who underwent PCI more than 90 days before surgery.[138] Leibowitz and associates studied a total of 216 consecutive patients who underwent PCI within 3 months of noncardiac surgery (PTCA, 122; stent, 94).[139] A total of 26 patients (12%) died, 13 in the stent group (14%) and 13 in the PTCA group (11%), a nonsignificant difference. The incidence of acute MI and death within 6 months was not significantly different (7% and 14% in the stent group and 6% and 11% in the PTCA group, respectively). Significantly more events occurred in the two groups when noncardiac surgery was performed within 2 weeks of PCI. Based on the accumulating data, elective noncardiac surgery after PCI, with or without stent placement, should be delayed for 4 to 6 weeks.

Drug-eluting stents may represent an even greater problem during the perioperative period based on case reports. Nasser and coauthors described two patients with in-stent thrombosis occurring 4 and 21 months after the implantation of sirolimus-eluting stents.[140] Several reports suggest that drug-eluting stents may represent an additional risk over a prolonged period (up to 12 months), particularly if antiplatelet agents are discontinued.[141] The new guidelines suggest continuing aspirin therapy in all patients with a coronary stent and discontinuing clopidogrel for as short an interval as possible for patients with bare-metal stents in place for less than 30 days or drug-eluting stents for less than 1 year (Fig. 35-6).

Summary of Preoperative and Intraoperative Factors That Correlate with Perioperative Morbidity

Summarizing a large number of studies, we list the following preoperative findings as conditions that correlate with perioperative morbidity and that can be corrected before surgery:

Table 35-9 Cardiovascular Disease Classification Chart

Class	New York Heart Association Functional Classification	Canadian Cardiovascular Society Functional Classification
I	Patients have cardiac disease but without the resulting limitations of physical activity. Ordinary physical activity does not cause undue fatigue, palpitation, dyspnea, or anginal pain.	Ordinary physical activity such as walking or climbing stairs does not cause angina. Angina with strenuous or rapid prolonged exertion at work or recreation
II	Patients have cardiac disease resulting in slight limitation of physical activity. They are comfortable at rest. Ordinary physical activity results in fatigue, palpitation, dyspnea, or anginal pain.	Slight limitation of ordinary activity. Ordinary walking or climbing stairs rapidly, walking uphill, and walking or stair climbing after meals or in the cold, in wind, under emotional stress, or only for a few hours after awakening. Walking more than two blocks on a level surface or up more than one flight of stairs at a normal pace and under normal conditions
III	Patients have cardiac disease resulting in marked limitation of physical activity. They are comfortable at rest. Less than ordinary physical activity causes fatigue, palpitation, dyspnea, or anginal pain.	Marked limitation of ordinary physical activity. Walking one or two blocks on a level surface and climbing more than one flight of stairs under normal conditions
IV	Patients have cardiac disease resulting in inability to carry on any physical activity without discomfort. Symptoms of cardiac insufficiency or of the anginal syndrome may be present even at rest. If any physical activity is undertaken, discomfort is increased.	Inability to carry out physical activity without discomfort—anginal syndrome *may* be present at rest

Modified from Wong DH, Weber EC, Schell MJ, et al: Factors associated with postoperative pulmonary complications in patients with severe COPD. Anesth Analg, 80: 276, 1995.

1. Recent MI[91,119,142-144]
2. Severe CHF (i.e., sufficiently severe to produce rales, an S_3 gallop, or distention of the jugular vein)[91,111,130,137,142,145-164]
3. Severe angina (see Table 35-9 for classification of the severity of angina)[137,142,145-152]
4. Heart rhythm other than sinus[142,145,153,154]
5. Premature atrial contractions[142]
6. More than five PVCs per minute (although unconfirmed in later studies)[142]
7. Chronic renal insufficiency
8. BUN levels higher than 50 mg/dL or potassium levels below 3.0 mEq/L[142,148,149,155]

Preoperative factors that correlate with perioperative risk but cannot be altered include (1) old physiologic or chronologic age (perioperative risk increases with age),* (2) significant aortic stenosis,[142,155,169] (3) emergency surgery,[91,142,145,147,153-155,165] (4) cardiomegaly,[142,145,147,153-156] (5) history of CHF,[91,142,145-147,153-158,160-163,170,171] (6) angina (or a history of angina or ischemia) on the ECG,[91,111,142,145-147,153,154,157-162,170,172] (7) abnormal ST-segment or inverted or flat T waves on the ECG,[8,142,145,154] or abnormal QRS complex on the ECG,[142] and (8) a significant mitral regurgitant murmur.[142,155]

Significant intraoperative factors that correlate with perioperative risk and that may be avoided or altered are (1) unnecessary use of vasopressors,[173,174] (2) unintentional hypotension[120,142,175] (this point is controversial, however, because some investigators have found that unintentional hypotension does not correlate with perioperative morbidity[174]), (3) hypothermia,[176] (4) too low or too high a hematocrit,[177,178] and (5) lengthy operations.[142]

Significant intraoperative factors that correlate with perioperative morbidity and probably cannot be avoided are (1) emergency surgery and (2) thoracic or intraperitoneal surgery or above-the-knee amputations.[142,145-147,153-155,157-159,161,162,168,170,171]

Although the evidence for these factors is fairly substantial, virtually no data are derived from prospective randomized studies indicating that treatment of the aforementioned conditions reduces perioperative risk in patients with ischemic heart disease. Nevertheless, all logic dictates that such treatment does reduce risk. Thus, the goal in giving anesthesia to patients with ischemic heart disease is to achieve the best preoperative condition obtainable by treating conditions that correlate with perioperative risk. The next step is to intraoperatively monitor for conditions that correlate with perioperative risk and, by careful attention to detail, avoid circumstances that lead to perioperative risk. Although local anesthesia may reduce perioperative risk, epidemiologic studies do not indicate any significant differences in perioperative morbidity in patients with ischemic heart disease who are given local anesthesia as opposed to general anesthesia.

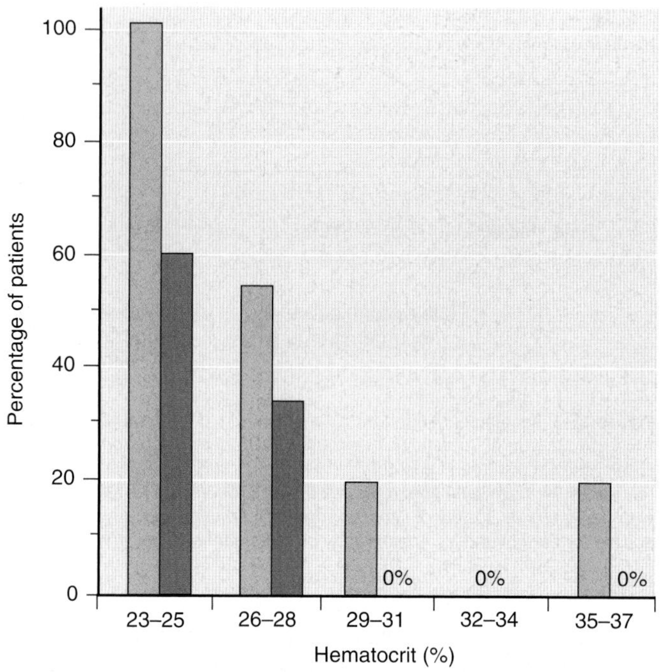

Figure 35-7 Relationship of postoperative myocardial ischemia (*yellow bars*) and morbid cardiac events (*blue bars*) to hematocrit for 27 high-risk patients undergoing infrainguinal arterial bypass. *(Data from Nelson AH, Fleisher LA, Rosenbaum SH: The relationship between postoperative anemia and cardiac morbidity in high risk vascular patients in the ICU. Crit Care Med 21:860, 1993.)*

Preoperative and Preprocedure Therapy

The only way known to increase oxygen supply to the myocardium of patients with coronary artery stenosis is to maintain diastolic BP, hemoglobin concentration (Fig. 35-7), and oxygen saturation. The main goal of anesthesia practice for these patients has been to decrease the determinants of myocardial oxygen demand, heart rate, ventricular wall tension, and contractile performance and improve plaque stabilization. Thus, medical management designed to preserve all viable myocardial tissue may include the following:

1. Continuation of β-adrenergic receptor blocking drugs (propranolol, atenolol, esmolol, or metoprolol) to avoid β-blocker withdrawl leading to increased contractility and heart rate. Multiple studies have demonstrated improved outcome in patients given perioperative β-blockers, especially if the heart rate is controlled.[179,180] However, newer studies have demonstrated that β-blockers may not be effective if the heart rate is not well controlled or in lower-risk patients.[181-183] Recently, the POISE trial was published in which 8351 high-risk β-blocker–naive patients were randomized to high-dose continuous-release metoprolol versus placebo.[121] There was a significant reduction in the primary outcome of cardiovascular events along with a 30% reduction in the MI rate, but a significantly increased rate of 30-day all-cause mortality and stroke. The current ACC/AHA guidelines on perioperative β-blockade advocate that perioperative β-blockade is a class I indication and should be used in patients previously taking β-blockers and those with a positive stress test undergoing major vascular surgery, although acute administration without titration may be associated with harm (Table 35-10).
2. Vasodilation (with nitroglycerin or its "long-acting" analogs nitroprusside, hydralazine, or prazosin) to decrease ventricular wall tension may be beneficial, although there are currently no randomized trials that support the prophylactic use of these agents.[110-112] The use of Swan-Ganz catheters[159,184] and transesophageal echocardiography for this type of patient is described in Chapters 40 and 41, and the

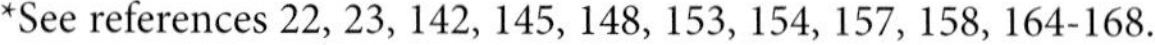

*See references 22, 23, 142, 145, 148, 153, 154, 157, 158, 164-168.

Table 35-10 Recommendations for Perioperative β-Blocker Therapy Based on Published Randomized Clinical Trials

Surgery	No Clinical Risk Factors	One or More Clinical Risk Factors	CHD or High Cardiac Risk	Patients Currently Taking β-Blockers
Vascular	Class IIb; level of evidence: B	Class IIa; level of evidence: B	Patients found to have myocardial ischemia on preoperative testing: class I; level of evidence: B* Patients without ischemia or no previous test: class IIa; level of evidence: B	Class I; level of evidence: B
Intermediate risk	...	Class IIb; level of evidence: C	Class IIa; level of evidence: B	Class I; level of evidence: C
Low risk	...	...	...	Class I; level of evidence: C

Ellipses (...) indicate that data were insufficient to determine a class of recommendation or level of evidence.
*Applies to patients found to have coronary ischemia on preoperative testing.
CHD, coronary heart disease.
Reproduced with permission from Fleisher LA, Beckman JA, Brown KA, et al: ACC/AHA 2007 guidelines on perioperative cardiovascular evaluation and care for noncardiac surgery: A report of the American College of Cardiology/American Heart Association Task Force on Practice Guidelines (Writing Committee to Revise the 2002 Guidelines on Perioperative Cardiovascular Evaluation for Noncardiac Surgery): Developed in collaboration with the American Society of Echocardiography, American Society of Nuclear Cardiology, Heart Rhythm Society, Society of Cardiovascular Anesthesiologists, Society for Cardiovascular Angiography and Interventions, Society for Vascular Medicine and Biology, and Society for Vascular Surgery." Circulation 116(17):e418-e499, 2007.

intraoperative management of patients with ischemic heart disease is discussed in further detail in Chapters 60 and 62 and in recent guidelines.[125]

3. Aspirin, statins, exercise, and diet. These choices seem to be indicated in many patients. Briefly, we believe that drugs given chronically (e.g., antihypertensive medications and some ACE inhibitors) should be continued through the morning of surgery (see earlier). The topic of chronic drug therapy is discussed in more detail in the last section of this chapter.

Valvular Heart Disease

Major alterations in the preoperative management of patients with valvular heart disease have been made regarding the use of anticoagulant therapy and are now based on the causes of the disease. Preoperative and intraoperative management of patients with valvular heart disease is discussed in Chapters 34 and 60.

The prognosis and, presumably, the perioperative risk for patients with valvular heart disease depend on the stage of the disease. Although stenotic lesions progress faster than regurgitant lesions do, regurgitant lesions secondary to infective endocarditis, rupture of the chordae tendineae, or ischemic heart disease can be rapidly fatal. Left ventricular dysfunction is common in the late stage of valvular heart disease.

Preoperative maintenance of drug therapy can be crucial; for example, a patient with aortic stenosis can deteriorate rapidly with the onset of atrial fibrillation or flutter because the atrial contribution to left ventricular filling can be critical in maintaining cardiac output. One of the most serious complications of valvular heart surgery and valvular heart disease before surgery is cardiac arrhythmia. Conduction disorders and chronic therapy with antiarrhythmic and inotropic drugs are discussed elsewhere in this chapter. The reader is referred elsewhere in this book (Chapter 83) or to other sources[185] for discussion of the management of a child with congenital heart disease who is undergoing noncardiac surgery.

Preoperative Antibiotic Prophylaxis for Endocarditis

Patients who have any form of valvular heart disease, as well as those with intracardiac (ventricular septal or atrial septal defects) or intravascular shunts, should be protected against endocarditis at the time of a known bacteremic event. Endocarditis has occurred in a sufficiently significant number of patients with hypertrophic cardiomyopathy (subvalvular aortic stenosis, asymmetric septal hypertrophy) and mitral valve prolapse to warrant the inclusion of these two conditions in the prophylaxis regimen.

Is endotracheal intubation associated with bacteremia? Bacteremia occurs after the following events: dental extraction, 30% to 80%; brushing of teeth, 20% to 24%; use of oral irrigation devices, 20% to 24%; barium enema, 11%; transurethral resection of the prostate (TURP), 10% to 57%; upper GI endoscopy, 8%; nasotracheal intubation, 16% (4 of 25 patients); and orotracheal intubation, 0% (0 of 25 patients). There are new guidelines from the AHA that are substantially different from those published in 2006.[186] There is also an update in 2008 from the AHA/ACC on endocarditis in patients with valvular heart disease, with changes from the 2006 document shown in Table 35-11.[187]

Cardiac Valve Prostheses and Anticoagulant Therapy and Prophylaxis for Deep Venous Thrombosis

In patients with prosthetic valves, the risk of increased bleeding during a procedure in a patient receiving antithrombotic therapy has to be weighed against the increased risk of thromboembolism caused by stopping the therapy. Common practice in patients undergoing noncardiac surgery with a mechanical prosthetic valve in place is cessation of anticoagulant therapy 3 days before surgery. This timeframe allows the international normalized ratio to fall to less than 1.5 times normal. The oral anticoagulants can then be resumed on postoperative day 1. Using a similar protocol, Katholi and colleagues found no perioperative episodes of thromboembolism or hemorrhage in 25 patients.[188] An alternative approach in patients at high risk for thromboembolism is conversion to heparin during the perioperative period. The heparin can then be discontinued 4 to 6 hours before surgery and resumed shortly thereafter. Current prosthetic valves may have a lower

Table 35-11 Changes Related to Endocarditis Prophylaxis: AHA/ACC Guidelines on Valvular Heart Disease

2006 VHD Guideline Recommendations	2008 VHD Focused Update Recommendations	Comments
Class I	**Class IIa**	
1. Prophylaxis against infective endocarditis is recommended for the following patients: • Patients with prosthetic heart valves and patients with a history of infective endocarditis (*level of evidence: C*) • Patients who have complex cyanotic congenital heart disease (e.g., single-ventricle states, transposition of the great arteries, tetralogy of Fallot) (*level of evidence: C*) • Patients with surgically constructed systemic pulmonary shunts or conduits (*level of evidence: C*) • Patients with congenital cardiac valve malformations, particularly those with bicuspid aortic valves, and patients with acquired valvular dysfunction (e.g., rheumatic heart disease) (*level of evidence: C*) • Patients who have undergone valve repair (*level of evidence: C*) • Patients who have hypertrophic cardiomyopathy when there is latent or resting obstruction (*level of evidence: C*) • Patients with MVP and auscultatory evidence of valvular regurgitation and/or thickened leaflets on echocardiography* (*level of evidence: C*)	1. Prophylaxis against infective endocarditis is reasonable for the following patients at highest risk for adverse outcomes from infective endocarditis who undergo dental procedures that involve manipulation of either gingival tissue or the periapical region of teeth or perforation of the oral mucosa: • Patients with prosthetic cardiac valves or prosthetic material used for cardiac valve repair (*level of evidence: B*) • Patients with previous infective endocarditis (*level of evidence: B*) • Patients with CHD (*level of evidence: B*) • Unrepaired cyanotic CHD, including palliative shunts and conduits (*level of evidence: B*) • Completely repaired congenital heart defect repaired with prosthetic material or device, whether placed by surgery or by catheter intervention, during the first 6 months after the procedure (*level of evidence: B*) • Repaired CHD with residual defects at the site or adjacent to the site of a prosthetic patch or prosthetic device (both of which inhibit endothelialization) (*level of evidence: B*) • Cardiac transplant recipients with valve regurgitation as a result of a structurally abnormal valve (*level of evidence: C*)	Modified recommendation (changed class of recommendation from I to IIa, changed text). There are no class I recommendations for infective endocarditis prophylaxis
Class III		
1. Prophylaxis against infective endocarditis is not recommended for the following patients: • Patients with isolated secundum atrial septal defect (*level of evidence: C*) • Patients 6 or more months after successful surgical or percutaneous repair of atrial septal defect, ventricular septal defect, or patent ductus arteriosus (*level of evidence: C*) • Patients with MVP without MR or thickened leaflets on echocardiography* (*level of evidence: C*) • Patients with physiologic, functional, or innocent heart murmurs, including patients with aortic valve sclerosis as defined by focal areas of increased echogenicity and thickening of the leaflets without restriction of motion and a peak velocity of less than 2.0 m/sec (*level of evidence: C*) • Patients with echocardiographic evidence of physiologic MR in the absence of a murmur and with structurally normal valves (*level of evidence: C*) • Patients with echocardiographic evidence of physiologic TR and/or pulmonary regurgitation in the absence of a murmur and with structurally normal valves (*level of evidence: C*)	1. Prophylaxis against infective endocarditis is not recommended for nondental procedures (such as transesophageal echocardiography, esophagogastroduodenoscopy, or colonoscopy) in the absence of active infection (*level of evidence: B*)	Modified recommendation (changed text)

*This footnote is obsolete. Please see 2006 VHD Guideline (3) for footnote text.
CHD, congestive heart disease; MR, mitral regurgitation; MVP, mitral valve prolapse; TR, tricuspid regurgitation; VHD, valvular heart disease.
From Nishimura RA, Carabello BA, Faxon DP, et al: ACC/AHA 2008 guideline update on valvular heart disease: Focused update on infective endocarditis: A report of the American College of Cardiology/American Heart Association Task Force on Practice Guidelines: Endorsed by the Society of Cardiovascular Anesthesiologists, Society for Cardiovascular Angiography and Interventions, and Society of Thoracic Surgeons. Circulation 118:887-896, 2008.

incidence, and the risk associated with heparin may outweigh its benefit in the perioperative setting. According to the AHA/ACC guidelines, heparin can usually be reserved for those who have had a recent thrombus or embolus (arbitrarily within 1 year), those with demonstrated thrombotic problems when previously off therapy, those with a Björk-Shiley valve, and those with more than three risk factors (atrial fibrillation, previous thromboembolism, hypercoagulable condition, and mechanical prosthesis).[189] A lower threshold for recommending heparin should be considered in patients with mechanical valves in the mitral position, in whom a single risk factor would be sufficient evidence of high risk. Subcutaneous low-molecular-weight heparin offers an alternative outpatient approach.[190] It is appropriate for the surgeon and cardiologist to discuss the optimal perioperative management for such a patient, including a review of the most recent guidelines.[191]

Regional anesthetic techniques might be avoided, although this issue is controversial.[192] Many practitioners do not hesitate to use regional anesthesia in the face of prophylaxis for deep venous thrombosis.[193-195] However, epidural hematoma has been associated with anticoagulant therapy in many reports. Large retrospective reviews of outcome after epidural or spinal anesthesia, or both, during or shortly before initiation of anticoagulant therapy with heparin have not reported neurologic dysfunction related to hematoma formation in any patient.[196,197] This paucity of damaging epidemiologic evidence, though reassuring, does not reduce the need for frequent evaluation of neurologic function and a search for back pain in the perioperative period after regional anesthesia in any patient receiving any clotting function inhibitor, including aspirin.[192,198-200] The risk of regional anesthesia concurrent with prophylaxis for deep venous thrombosis with heparin is greater with the use of low-molecular-weight heparin. (Heparin-induced thrombocytopenia has been treated successfully with intravenous immunoglobulin.[194]) The American Society of Regional Anesthesia and Pain Management has issued a consensus statement on the use of regional anesthesia in anticoagulated patients.[201] They suggest that the decision to perform spinal or epidural anesthesia/analgesia and the timing of catheter removal in a patient receiving antithrombotic therapy should be made on an individual basis, with the small though definite risk of spinal hematoma weighed against the benefits of regional anesthesia for a specific patient.

Deep venous thrombosis is so common in postoperative patients that almost 1% of postsurgical patients die of fatal pulmonary embolism (Table 35-12).[202] Because of this high mortality risk, prophylaxis against deep venous thrombosis has attained widespread acceptance; thus, prophylaxis often begins with 5000 units of heparin given subcutaneously 2 hours before surgery.[202-204] Other trials have shown equal effect with external pneumatic compression.[203,205] Persuading surgeons to use this technique may provide greater assurance in using regional anesthesia. Such an option, however, is not available for patients

Table 35-12 Incidence of Deep Venous Thrombosis and Fatal Pulmonary Embolism

	Incidence of		
Type of Surgery	**Deep Venous Thrombosis (%)**	**Proximal Deep Venous Thrombosis (%)**	**Fatal Pulmonary Embolism (%)**
General			
Age >40 yr	10	<1	0.1
Age >60 yr	10-40	3-15	0.8
Malignancy	50-60		
Thoracic	30		
Vascular			
Aortic repair	26		
Peripheral	12		
Urologic			
Open prostatectomy	40		
TURP	10		
Other urologic	30-40		
Major gynecologic			
With malignancy	40		
Without malignancy	10-20		
Neurosurgery			
Craniotomy	20-80		
Laminectomy	4-25		1.5-3.0
Orthopedic			
Total-hip replacement	40-80	10-20	1.0-5.0
Hip fracture	48-75		1.0-5.0
Tibial fracture	45		
Total knee	60-70	20	1.0-5.0
Head, neck, chest wall	11		
Medical			
Acute myocardial infarction	30	6	
Stroke	60-75		
Acute spine injury	60-100		
Other bed bound	26		

TURP, transurethral resection of the prostate.

with a prosthetic valve. New recommendations are available from the American College of Chest Physicians for prophylaxis against venous thromboembolism.[235a]

Another problem that can arise is managing a pregnant patient with a prosthetic valve during delivery. It is recommended that warfarin be replaced by subcutaneous heparin during the peripartum period. During labor and delivery, elective induction is advocated with discontinuance of all anticoagulant therapy, as indicated for the particular valve prosthesis (discussed earlier).[206]

Auscultation of the prosthetic valve should be performed preoperatively to verify normal functioning (Fig. 35-8).[207] Abnormalities in such sounds warrant preoperative consultation and verification of functioning.

Cardiac Conduction Disturbances: Cardiac Arrhythmias

Bradyarrhythmias, especially if profound or associated with dizziness or syncope, are generally managed with pacemakers (also see Chapters 34, 43, and 61). However, chronic bifascicular block (right bundle branch block with a left anterior or posterior hemiblock or a left bundle branch block with combined left anterior and posterior hemiblocks), even when only a first-degree heart block is present, can progress to complete heart block and sudden perioperative death on rare occasion. In six studies, less than 2% of the approximately 266 patients with bifascicular block progressed to complete heart block perioperatively.[208] On the other hand, these patients have a high 5-year mortality rate (160 of 554 patients, or 29%). Most of the deaths were related to tachyarrhythmias or MI—events not usually preventable by traditional pacemakers.[209] Thus, the presence of a bifascicular block on the ECG should make the anesthesiologist more worried about associated coronary artery disease or left ventricular dysfunction. Nevertheless, these patients rarely have complete heart block perioperatively. Therefore, prophylactic preoperative insertion of temporary pacing wires for bifascicular block does not seem warranted. However, a central route can be established in advance in the event that a temporary pacemaker needs to be inserted (most operating rooms do not rely on transthoracic pacing, although such might be attempted if available).[210] The actual pacemaker equipment and appropriate personnel should be immediately available and tested regularly because symptomatic heart block does occur perioperatively in more than 1% of patients. One study appears to have confirmed this rate of at least 1% for patients undergoing cardiac surgery.[211] One percent of patients in whom a pacing pulmonary artery catheter was not inserted preoperatively subsequently required pacing before cardiopulmonary bypass. By contrast, 19% of patients who had such a catheter in place underwent cardiac pacing before cardiopulmonary bypass. Predictors of the need for pacing included previous symptomatic bradyarrhythmia, a history of transient complete AV block, and aortic valve disease.

More than five PVCs per minute on preoperative examination correlates with perioperative cardiac morbidity.[142,147,153,154] To the classic criteria for treating PVCs (the presence of R-on-T couplets, the occurrence of more than three PVCs per minute,

Prosthesis Type	Mitral Prosthesis	Acoustic Characteristics	Aortic Prosthesis	Acoustic Characteristics
Ball valves	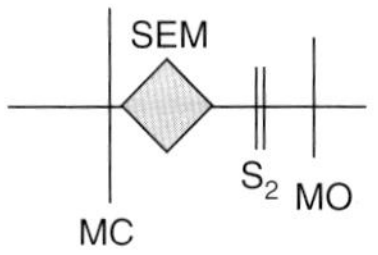 SEM S_2 MO MC	1) A_2–MO Interval 0.07–0.11 sec. 2) MV > MC 3) II-III/VI Systolic ejection murmur (SEM) 4) No diastolic murmur	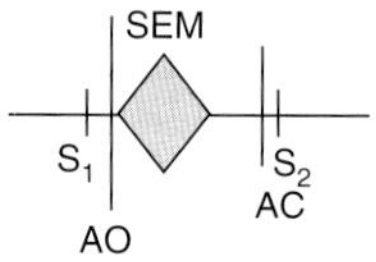 SEM S_1 S_2 AC AO	1) S_1–AO Interval 0.07 sec. 2) AO > AC 3) II/VI harsh SEM 4) No diastolic murmur
Disk valves	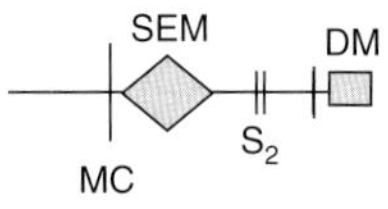 SEM DM S_2 MC	1) A_2–MO Interval 0.05–0.09 sec. 2) MO is rarely heard 3) II/VI is usually heard 4) II-III/VI diastolic rumble is usually heard	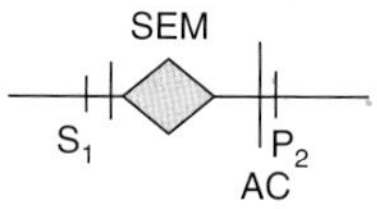 SEM S_1 P_2 AC	1) S_1–AO Interval 0.04 sec. 2) AO is uncommonly heard AC is usually heard 3) II/VI SEM is usually heard 4) Occasional diastolic murmur
Porcine valves	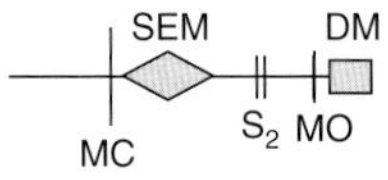 SEM DM S_2 MO MC	1) A_2–MO Interval 0.01 sec. 2) MO is audible 50% 3) I-II/VI apical SEM 50% 4) Diastolic rumble 1/2–2/3	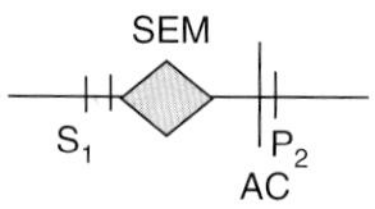 SEM S_1 P_2 AC	1) S_1–AO Interval 0.03–0.08 sec. 2) AO is uncommonly heard AC is usually heard 3) II/VI SEM in most 4) No diastolic murmur
Bileaflet valve (St. Jude)			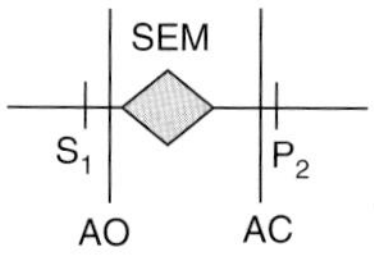 SEM S_1 P_2 AO AC	1) AO and AC commonly heard 2) A soft SEM is common

Figure 35-8 Summary of the normal acoustic characteristics of valve prostheses according to type and location. A_2, aortic second sound; AC, aortic valve closure sound; AO, aortic valve opening sound; DM, diastolic murmur; MC, mitral valve closure sound; MO, mitral valve opening sound; MV, mitral valve; P_2, pulmonary second sound; S_1, first heart sound; S_2, second heart sound; SEM, systolic ejection murmur. *(Redrawn from Smith ND, Raizada V, Abrams J: Auscultation of the normally functioning prosthetic valve. Ann Intern Med 95:594, 1981.)*

and multifocality of PVCs) must be added frequent (>10/hr over a 24-hour period) and repetitive ventricular beats. Electrophysiologic and programmed ventricular stimulation studies are being used to indicate and guide treatment of patients with ischemic heart disease or recurrent arrhythmias and survivors of out-of-hospital cardiac arrest. Although such patients are often treated with antiarrhythmic therapy, attention to their underlying condition should be a focus of our preoperative management. Chronic antiarrhythmic therapy is discussed in the last section of this chapter. Torsades de pointes is an arrhythmia characterized by episodes of alternating electrical polarity such that the major vector of the QRS complex seems to alternate around an isoelectric line. The hallmark enabling differential diagnosis from ventricular tachycardia is the unusual response of this arrhythmia to commonly used antiarrhythmic drugs. That is, the use of drugs that prolong the QT interval (e.g., quinidine, procainamide, disopyramide, some of the antihistamines, and the antipsychotic phenothiazines) may well make the arrhythmia more frequent or of longer duration. Reports of the sudden occurrence of torsades de pointes during surgery have been rare in the anesthesia literature. Immediate therapy consists of the administration of magnesium or electrical cardioversion, followed by overdrive cardiac pacing or the administration of β-adrenergic agonists and discontinuation of drugs that prolong the QT interval.

Premature atrial contractions and cardiac rhythm other than sinus also correlate with perioperative cardiac morbidity.[142,153] These arrhythmias may be more a marker of poor cardiovascular reserve than a specific cause of perioperative cardiac complications.

Pre-excitation syndrome is the name for supraventricular tachycardias associated with AV bypass tracts.[212] Successful treatment, which is predicated on an understanding of the clinical and electrophysiologic manifestations of the syndrome, consists of either catheter ablation techniques[209] or surgery using preoperative and intraoperative techniques that avoid release of sympathetic and other vasoactive substances and therefore tachyarrhythmias.[213,214] Anesthesia for electrophysiologic procedures is discussed in Chapter 61.

Disorders of the Respiratory and Immune Systems

General Preoperative and Preprocedure Considerations

Pulmonary complications after procedures requiring anesthesia are as common as cardiovascular complications—even more common if deep venous thrombosis is included. Moreover, pulmonary complications are equally or more important to the patient and health system in terms of morbidity, mortality, length-of-stay extension, and cost.

Although little may seem to have changed in the preoperative preparation of patients with respiratory disease, this impression is not true. Major changes in drug therapy have occurred, and appreciation of the effects of smoking and sleep apnea on perioperative and chronic care has increased.[215-232] (Preoperative and preprocedure identification and perioperative care of patients with sleep apnea are discussed in the earlier section on obesity and in Chapter 64.)

The main purpose of preoperative testing is to identify patients at risk for perioperative complications so that appropriate perioperative therapy can be instituted to foster return to functional status. Preoperative assessment can also establish baseline function and the feasibility of surgical intervention. Whereas numerous investigators have used pulmonary function tests to define inoperability or high-risk versus low-risk groups for pulmonary complications, few have been able to demonstrate that the performance of any specific preoperative or intraoperative measure, save perhaps smoking cessation and physical activity such as a walking program, reliably decreases perioperative pulmonary morbidity or mortality. Because routine preoperative pulmonary testing and care are discussed extensively in Chapters 44 and 59, the current discussion is limited to an assessment of the effectiveness of this type of care.

In fact, few randomized prospective studies indicate an outcome benefit of preoperative preparation, and we do not even have such for smoking cessation or walking—only epidemiologic data; a larger cohort has implied a benefit of intraoperative and postoperative pain therapy techniques (usually planned preoperatively).[227-232] Stein and Cassara[228] randomly allocated 48 patients to undergo preoperative therapy (cessation of smoking, administration of antibiotics for purulent sputum, and use of bronchodilating drugs, postural drainage, chest physiotherapy, and ultrasonic nebulizer) or no preoperative therapy. The no-treatment group had a mortality of 16% and morbidity of 60%, as opposed to 0% and 20%, respectively, for the treatment group. In addition, the treatment group spent an average of 12 postoperative days in the hospital as compared with 24 days for the 21 survivors in the no-treatment group.

Collins and colleagues[233] prospectively examined the benefits of preoperative antibiotics, perioperative chest physiotherapy and therapy with bronchodilating drugs, and routine postoperative analgesia (morphine) on postoperative respiratory complications in patients with COPD. Of these therapies, only preoperative treatment with antibiotics had a beneficial effect.

Warner and coworkers[234] collected data retrospectively about smoking history and prospectively (concurrently) about pulmonary complications for 200 patients undergoing CABG. These investigators documented that 8 weeks or more of smoking cessation was associated with a 66% reduction in postoperative pulmonary complications. Smokers who stopped for less than 8 weeks actually had an increase (from 33% for current smokers to 57.1% for recent quitters) in the rate of one or more of the six complications surveyed: purulent sputum with pyrexia; need for respiratory therapy care; bronchospasm requiring therapy; pleural effusion or pneumothorax (or both) necessitating drainage; segmental pulmonary collapse, as confirmed by radiography; or pneumonia necessitating antibiotic therapy. Others have found that both shorter and longer periods of cessation of smoking were needed before achieving cardiovascular[235] and hematologic benefit.[236] Of note, Bluman and associates[237] performed a retrospective chart review of 410 patients undergoing noncardiac surgery at a VA hospital. Current smoking was associated with a nearly sixfold increase in risk for a postoperative pulmonary complication. Reduction in smoking within 1 month of surgery was not associated with a decreased risk for postoperative pulmonary complications. Nakagawa and coauthors also reported higher pulmonary complication rates in patients undergoing pulmonary surgery who quit within 4 weeks of surgery than in current smokers or those who had stopped smoking for more than 4 weeks.[238] The fact that anesthesiologists rarely see their patients 4 weeks or more before surgery presents a dilemma: if one is unable to advise the patient to stop smoking 8 weeks or more before surgery, is it preferable for the patient to continue smoking? Perhaps these data will further support the implementation of preoperative and preprocedure assessment clinics in which anesthesiologists are able to advise and counsel patients about risk reduction.

At the Cleveland Clinic we have embarked on an active campaign motivated by several articles[239,240] and the ASA's efforts to use the preprocedure time of heightened awareness of health to try to motivate each patient who smokes to quit smoking as soon as recovery from surgery has begun. In the first 7 months we referred more than 1000 patients (of about 5000 admitted smokers) to a "breath free" clinic that follows a low-cost Web-based doctor-supervised process (Box 35-4) and succeeded in helping over 50% of those who kept their initial appointment successfully quit. Although that rate is lower than rates in patients self-referred and self-reported to websites that use the same protocol (Oprah.com and Real Age.com—where we have more than 120,000 self-reported successful quitters), we consider the effort worthwhile. Many fewer patients (about 100) have decided to quit before surgery (L. Skolaris and I. Hasan, personal communication).

When Skolnick and coworkers[226] studied 602 children prospectively, exposure to passive smoking (as measured by urinary cotinine, the major metabolite of nicotine) correlated directly with airway complications. Children with the least exposure to passive smoke had the fewest complications. Second-hand smoke may be a model for particulate air pollution with PM 2.5 particles, which have immediate and long-term effects in increasing lung dysfunction and inflammatory stimuli throughout the body.[241,242] In this sense, reducing particulate and diesel exhaust exposure in the 2 weeks before surgery might make sense, but such a hypothesis has not been tested (and outpatient surgery centers off busy freeways might prove to make such subtle inhibition of healing secondary to diesel particles an appropriate site to study).

As for things to do, Celli and associates[243] performed a randomized prospective controlled trial of intermittent positive-pressure breathing (IPPB) versus incentive spirometry and deep-breathing exercises in 81 patients undergoing abdominal surgery. The groups exposed to a respiratory therapist (regardless of the treatment given) had more than a 50% lower incidence of clinical complications (30% to 33% versus 88%) and shorter hospital stays than the control group did. Thus, this third prospective study indicates that outcome improves when there is any concern about

Box 35-4 You Tool: Breathe Free Program

Smoking Cessation Plan*

One of the most powerful addictions isn't bridal reality shops; it's cigarette smoking. Here, in our Breathe Free Program, developed with Daniel Seidman, MD, and the Cleveland Clinic team, we're going to teach you how to stop the addiction so that you can gain back the 8 to 13 years you've taken off your life (half in length and half in disability and illness) through those nasty sticks. Yes, you get a do-over here too and can make yourself younger even if you've burned your fingers with 20 cigarettes every day.

Step 1: Assess Yourself

Answer the following questions to see if you've lost control of your smoking behavior and it's turned into a full-fledged dependence.

1. **Have you smoked every day for at least the past several weeks?**
2. **Do you experience any of the following withdrawal symptoms after you stop or reduce your amount of smoking ("withdrawal symptoms can begin within a few hours of cessation")?**
   - Depressed mood
   - Insomnia
   - Irritability, frustration, or anger
   - Anxiety
   - Difficulty concentrating
   - Restlessness
   - Decreased heart rate
   - Increased appetite or weight gain
3. **Do you experience significant distress because of the symptoms in Question 2? Do you avoid social or work obligations—or leave in the middle of these obligations—because of significant distress or discomfort from not smoking?**

   If you answer "yes" to Question 1, "yes" to at least four of the symptoms in Question 2, and/or "yes" to Question 3, then you have a problem and may even meet the psychiatric definition for nicotine withdrawal. Knowing this can help build your commitment to change and to learning to breathe free.
4. **In the past year, was there a day you didn't smoke at all—not even a puff?**

   If you answered "yes," think about how you did it and how you then went back to smoking. Try to learn from what worked and what didn't.

   If you answered "no," don't despair. The movie in your head about how impossible breaking free from smoking will be probably is greatly exaggerated. With proper use of medicines and a good behavioral plan, it's possible to break free of smoking. We know, we helped over 700 people individually and over 80,000 using our Web-based programs (see oprah.com or realage.com). If you follow our plan and have a buddy to help, we believe your chance of success is over 60% each time you try—so three tries will get you to over a 90% chance of success.

*The Breath Free plan is copywritten by the YOU Docs in *YOU Being Beautiful: The Owner's Manual to Outer and Inner Beauty* (Free Press, 2008, United States), reprinted here by permission of the copyright owner and offered to all who want to use it—feel free to copy and hand to patients (as long as credit is given).

Box 35-4 You Tool: Breathe Free Program—cont'd

5. **Do you continue to smoke despite having a tobacco-caused medical problem such as bronchitis or COPD (chronic obstructive pulmonary disease)?**

   If you answered "yes," consider that almost all smokers are well aware of the medical problems associated with smoking. After all, they are listed on every pack you smoke. Even when told it is a matter of life and death, many continue to smoke after having a heart attack, lung surgery, or oral cancer removed. This behavior mystifies your loved ones and even leaves you, the smoker, bewildered, yet this is a hallmark of addiction and distinguishes it from "bad habits," which also involve automatic behavior. The difference is that bad habits predictably don't cause real and serious life consequences—a 20-can-a-day diet cola habit doesn't invariably result in troubles, nor does picking your nose.
6. **Do you get less of an effect—of pleasure or satisfaction—from the same number of cigarettes each day?**
7. **Do you continue to smoke, even though you enjoy only 10% to 20% of the cigarettes you light up?**

   If you answered "yes" to Questions 6 and 7, know that many people get sick of their addiction over time, especially after age 40. What was social and fun becomes rote habit with less pleasure than advertised. Keeping this in mind can motivate you to move forward with breathing free.
8. **Do you still enjoy smoking most or all of the time?**

   If you answered "yes," ask yourself if it would be nice to shed the burden of guilt and shame you carry from smoking? Remember, this is your body, and there is only one available for each customer. So even with all the new replacement parts available, you still can't protect your body from all the pollution in the cigarette smoke.
9. **Do you feel anxious and nervous, and has this continued every day for the past 2 weeks?**

   If you answered "yes," you may have more anxiety about getting through your breathe-free day—the day you go completely tobacco free. In that case, you may need to pay extra attention to the next step—working on preparation, confidence building, and motivation.
10. **Do you feel sad and blue, and has this continued every day for the past 2 weeks?**

    If you answered "yes," you may have more emotional discomfort after getting through your breathe-free day. You may also need to carefully review with your doctor nicotine withdrawal symptoms and the use of successful strategies to learn to live well without tobacco.

Step 2: Do the Prep Work

You're about to make a big change, one that requires some planning. Give yourself a month (31 days) to do all the prep work.

- **Promise yourself**: Make a personal pact with yourself to quit.
- **Set a quit date:** Make it at least a month from today
- **Take the Breathe Free Pledge:** See below.

As of ______________________, my official "Quit Date," I pledge to commit to breathing free!

My reasons for quitting smoking: ________________________ ____________.

I have found a buddy I will call daily: ____________________ __________.

I recognize that this may be one of the greatest challenges of my life, but I also know that breathing free is the best decision I can make to protect and improve my health. Upon signing this contract, I make a commitment to myself to breathe free and free myself from the limitations placed on me by my addiction.

I don't know what will happen or how difficult it will be, but I can get help from __________________________________ __________, and I have decided to (check one):

___ 1. Walk for 30 days and try nicotine patches (21 or 22 mg if I smoke a pack a day or so) and bupropion (100 mg twice a day—a reduced dose of Zyban) plus my buddy

___ 2. Use nicotine patches (or nicotine gum or nicotine oral inhaler) alone (plus my buddy)

___ 3. Use varenicline (Chantix) alone (plus my buddy)

I also know that staying smoke free (not having "just one") after the initial breathe-free period is important, and I have asked my friends and family to support me and not smoke around me. I will also continue to talk daily to my buddy for at least 6 months, and then I'll become a buddy to others.

By committing to a life of breathing free, I will ensure a healthier future for myself, and I will protect the well-being of my loved ones and everyone around me who will no longer be exposed to the dangers of second-hand smoke. I know that I am not only motivated but also committed and willing to make the effort to become a nonsmoker.

I deserve to give myself the healthiest life possible and breathe free!

- **Think of the three biggest reasons why you're quitting**: Write them on a card that you can carry with you and look at several times each day.
- **Be restrictive**: Eliminate smoking in two or three situations that usually prompt you to smoke.
- **Cut back**: Reduce the number of cigarettes you smoke to one pack a day or less.
- **Go cheap**: Change to a less desirable brand of cigarettes.
- **Need a light**: Discard your lighter and matches.
- **Misplace your cigarettes:** Carry them in a different place than you usually do.
- **Role-play**: Spend a little time each day imagining yourself in stressful situations in which you are not smoking.

(Continued)

Box 35-4 You Tool: Breathe Free Program—cont'd

Do the following four things, which will make quitting easier and could be the keys to your success.

- **Start walking 30 minutes a day—every day.**

Before you actually stop smoking, you have to establish another behavior—walking 30 minutes a day, every day—in its place. No excuses—you miss a day, you reset the clock to day 0. That is because another behavior takes at least 30 days to form. However, after a month of walking, you'll have two of the things you need to stick with our plan: more physical stamina and greater mental discipline.

- **Find a quitting buddy**.

Don't quit alone. We know from experience that everyone needs to be encouraged by someone—and your buddy is that someone. However, you shouldn't be the only one relying on other people; try to find a support partner who needs you as much as you need him or her.

- **See if you're covered**.

More and more insurance plans are offering some level of coverage for quit-smoking efforts. Ask your insurance company about its coverage. If your aren't insured, ask your HR department—many cover the cost (about $600 for 6 months—it really is cheaper than a pack a day, but we know dollars spent for medical expenses and smoking are usually segregated in smokers' minds and hearts).

- **Schedule a checkup.**

Quitting smoking is physically and mentally stressful, and you want to be sure you have no conditions that might interfere with the tools, techniques, and medications suggested in this program. So talk to your doctor about the following prescriptions to help you stop smoking:

1. Bupropion (Zyban or Wellbutrin) in 100-milligram tablets—one twice a day. Bupropion is an anticraving drug (it's also an antidepressant at higher doses) that can help you make the transition from smoker to quitter. It can interact with other medications, so make sure your doctor's aware of any drugs you're taking, particularly for high blood pressure or seizure disorders.
2. Nicotine patches. Talk with your doctor to figure out what strength would be best for you—for a one-pack-a-day habit it's usually 22 milligrams.

Quitting day is almost here—it's time to start getting your body ready to fight future cravings.

- **Start taking bupropion.** On day 30, 2 days before you'll actually stop smoking, take one tablet in the morning.
- **Keep taking bupropion**. On day 31, take one bupropion tablet in the morning.

Step 3: Break the Habit

Today's the day you stop smoking. If you've done the prep work, you're ready.

- **On day 32, QUIT**: Throw away all your cigarettes, and get rid of all ashtrays and any other smoking-related objects.
- **Put on a nicotine patch**. Place one on your arm, chest, or thigh (you'll be doing this daily for a while).
- **Take your bupropion**: One in the morning and one at night.

Here are your daily to-do's for days 33 through 61.

- **Take two**: Increase your bupropion to two tablets a day—one in the morning and another in the evening.
- **Patch up**: Put on a new one every day (and don't forget to take the old one off).
- **Keep walking**: Every day for 30 minutes.
- **Reach out**: Check in with your buddy.
- **Drink up**: Have as much coffee or water as you wish.

Step 4: Enjoy Life as an Ex-Smoker

Making it through a month without smoking is a huge accomplishment. It's time to celebrate the new YOU! Here are some to-do's for day 62 and beyond.

- **Breathe in**: Enjoy how quitting has made your lungs happier.
- **Push yourself**: Use your newfound vitality to start a strength-building routine. But take it slow; don't increase your physical activity by more than 10% a week.
- **Love life without the patch**: Every 2 months, decrease the dose of your nicotine patch by a third. Your goal is to be patch free after 6 months.
- **Say bye-bye bupropion**: But make it a slow goodbye. At 5 months, decrease your bupropion to one tablet in the evening, and aim to be off it entirely by your 8-month anniversary. Tip: Just in case you feel a craving, for the rest of your life carry one bupropion tablet with you at all times so that you can take it if you need to.

lung function on the part of someone knowledgeable in maneuvers designed to clear lung secretions.

Bartlett and coworkers[244] randomly assigned 150 patients undergoing extensive laparotomy to one of two groups. One group received preoperative instruction in and postoperative use of incentive spirometry (10 times per hour). The other group received similar medical care but no incentive spirometry. Only 7 of 75 patients using incentive spirometry had postoperative pulmonary complications, as opposed to 19 of 75 in the control group. However, other studies have not shown a benefit for specific treatments or have been too contaminated with bias to have a clear result emerge. Lyager and colleagues[245] randomly assigned 103 patients undergoing biliary or gastric surgery to receive either incentive spirometry with preoperative and postoperative chest physiotherapy or only preoperative and postoperative chest physiotherapy. No difference in the postoperative course or pulmonary complications was found between the two groups. Other studies have shown a specific benefit (i.e., above that provided by routine care) for chest physiotherapy and IPPB. These studies are usually poorly controlled, not randomized, or retrospective in design (or any combination of the three); these deficiencies probably substantially bias the results toward finding a benefit in

Table 35-13 Grade of Dyspnea Caused by Respiratory Problems (Assessed In Terms of Walking on a Level Surface at a Normal Pace)

Category	Description
0	No dyspnea while walking on a level surface at a normal pace
I	"I am able to walk as far as I like, provided I take my time"
II	Specific (street) block limitation ("I have to stop for a while after one or two blocks")
III	Dyspnea on mild exertion ("I have to stop and rest while going from the kitchen to the bathroom")
IV	Dyspnea at rest

Modified from Boushy SF, Billing DM, North LB, et al: Clinical course related to preoperative pulmonary function in patients with bronchogenic carcinoma. Chest 59:383, 1971.

reducing postoperative pulmonary complications. Although randomized prospective studies showed no benefit or actual harm from chest physiotherapy and IPPB on the resolution of pneumonia or postoperative pulmonary complications, the four studies cited earlier[228,233,243,244] and numerous retrospective studies strongly suggest that preoperative evaluation and treatment of patients with pulmonary disease actually decrease perioperative respiratory complications, even if only by causing a change in anesthetic techniques.

Recent meta-analyses have suggested a benefit of anesthetic and pain management with respect to respiratory outcomes. Rodgers and associates reviewed 141 trials involving 9559 patients who had been randomized to receive neuraxial blockade or general anesthesia. Overall mortality was significantly lower in the neuraxial blockade group (2.1% versus 3.1%). The relative risk of pneumonia in the neuraxial group was 0.61 (CI, 0.48 to 0.81), and the relative risk of respiratory depression was 0.41 (CI, 0.23 to 0.73).[227]

Not all studies demonstrate beneficial effects of pretreatment. In afebrile outpatient ASA class I and II children with no lung disease or findings who underwent noncavitary, nonairway surgery lasting less than 3 hours, neither albuterol nor ipratropium premedication decreased adverse events.[246]

Evaluation of dyspnea is especially useful and thus warrants discussion here (for a review of specific pulmonary function tests that identify high-risk groups, see Chapter 44). Boushy and coworkers[247] found that grades of preoperative dyspnea correlated with postoperative survival. (Grades of respiratory dyspnea are provided in Table 35-13.) Mittman[248] demonstrated an increased risk of death after thoracic surgery, from 8% in patients without dyspnea to 56% in patients who were dyspneic. Similarly, Reichel[249] found that no patients died after pneumonectomy if they were able to complete a preoperative treadmill test for 4 minutes at the rate of 2 mph on level ground. Other studies have found that the history and physical examination of an asthmatic subject can also predict the need for hospitalization.[217] Wong and colleagues[250] found that the risk index (Table 35-14) correlated with postoperative pulmonary complications. Other than dyspnea, what preoperative conditions make postoperative respiratory complications more likely? (See also Chapter 34.)

Arozullah and associates developed the first validated multifactorial risk index for postoperative respiratory failure, defined as mechanical ventilation for more than 48 hours after surgery or reintubation and mechanical ventilation after postoperative extubation.[251] In a prospective cohort study of 181,000 male veterans as part of the National Veterans Administration Surgical Quality Improvement Program, seven factors independently predicted risk (Table 35-15). With increasing numbers of risk factors present, the rate of complications increased from 0.5% (class 1) to 26.6% (class 4). Arozullah and colleagues subsequently developed a risk index for postoperative pneumonia by using data on 160,805 patients undergoing major noncardiac surgery and validated the index by using data on an additional 155,266 patients.[252] Patients were divided into five risk classes by using risk index scores (Table 35-16). Pneumonia rates were 0.2% in those with 0 to 15 risk points, 1.2% in those with 16 to 25 risk points, 4.0% in those with 26 to 40 risk points, 9.4% in those with 41 to 55 risk points, and 15.3% in those with more than 55 risk points.

Preoperative evaluation of patients with pulmonary disease can be found in Chapters 34 and 44. Despite the lack of definitive data establishing the efficacy of preoperative pulmonary testing and therapy, we recommend the following approach:

1. Eradicate acute infections and suppress chronic infections by using appropriate diagnostic measures and antibiotic treatment.
2. Relieve bronchospasm by using inhaled corticosteroids and bronchodilating drugs and document such relief with measurements of FEV_1 (also see Chapter 44).

Table 35-14 Classification of Risk of Pulmonary Complications for Thoracic and Abdominal Procedures

Category	Points*
I. Expiratory spirogram	
A. Normal (% FVC + [% FEV_1/FVC] > 150)	0
B. % FVC + (% FEV_1/FVC) = 100-150	1
C. % FVC + (% FEV_1/FVC) < 100	2
D. Preoperative FVC > 20 mL/kg	3
E. Postbronchodilator FEV_1/FVC < 50%	3
II. Cardiovascular system	
A. Normal	0
B. Controlled hypertension, myocardial infarction without sequelae for more than 2 yr	0
C. Dyspnea on exertion, orthopnea, paroxysmal nocturnal dyspnea, dependent edema, congestive heart failure, angina	1
III. Nervous system	
A. Normal	0
B. Confusion, obtundation, agitation, spasticity, discoordination, bulbar malfunction	1
C. Significant muscular weakness	1
IV. Arterial blood gases	
A. Acceptable	0
B. $Paco_2$ >50 mm Hg or Pao_2 <60 mm Hg on room air	1
C. Metabolic pH abnormality >7.50 or <7.30	1
V. Postoperative ambulation	
A. Expected ambulation (minimum, sitting at bedside) within 36 hr	0
B. Expected complete bed confinement for ≥36 hr	1

Modified from Wong DH, Weber EC, Schell MJ, et al: Factors associated with postoperative pulmonary complications in patients with severe COPD. Anesth Analg 80:276, 1995.

Table 35-15 Preoperative Predictors of Postoperative Respiratory Failure

Variable	Odds Ratio (95% Confidence Interval)
Type of surgery	
Abdominal aortic aneurysm	14.3 (12.0-16.9)
Thoracic	8.14 (7.17-9.25)
Neurosurgery, upper abdominal, or peripheral vascular	4.21 (3.80-4.67)
Neck	3.10 (2.40-4.01)
Other surgery*	1.00 (reference)
Emergency surgery	3.12 (2.83-3.43)
Albumin <0.30 g/L	2.53 (2.28-2.80)
Blood urea nitrogen >0.30 mg/dL	2.29 (2.04-2.56)
Partially or fully dependent status	1.92 (1.74-2.11)
History of COPD	1.81 (1.66-1.98)
Age (yr)	
≥70	1.91 (1.71-2.13)
60-69	1.51 (1.36-1.69)
<60	1.00 (reference)

*Other surgeries include ophthalmologic, ear, nose, mouth, lower abdominal, extremity, dermatologic, spine, and back surgery.
COPD, chronic obstructive pulmonary disease.
From Arozullah AM, Daley J, Henderson WG, et al: Multifactorial risk index for predicting postoperative respiratory failure in men after major noncardiac surgery. The National Veterans Administration Surgical Quality Improvement Program. Ann Surg 232:242-253, 2000, with permission.

3. In patients with bronchial asthma, consider the administration of corticosteroids beginning at least 48 hours before surgery in patients with a significant history of bronchospastic disease to achieve the maximal effect at the time of surgery. No randomized data support such an approach, but studies have not shown an increase in the risk for respiratory infection or wound complications.[253]
4. Institute measures to improve sputum clearance and familiarize the patient with respiratory therapy equipment (incentive spirometry) and postural drainage maneuvers. Initiate practice coughing and deep-breathing exercises.
5. Treat uncompensated right ventricular heart failure and heart rate with digoxin, diuretics, oxygen, and drugs that decrease pulmonary vascular resistance (e.g., hydralazine).[254]
6. The use of low-dose heparin prophylactically to decrease the incidence of venous thrombosis (and pulmonary emboli) has been the standard.[255,256] More recently, the use of low-molecular-weight heparin and intermittent compression stockings has become the standard for high-risk patients.[235a,255,256]
7. Identify and treat suspected or diagnosed sleep apnea with continuous positive airway pressure (CPAP), biphasic positive airway pressure (BiPAP), or other measures as indicated earlier (in the section "Disorders of Nutrition, Including Obesity").
8. Encourage reduction or cessation of smoking at least 4 weeks and preferably 8 weeks or more before surgery.[234,239,240]

Specific Diseases

Pulmonary Vascular Diseases

Pulmonary vascular diseases include pulmonary hypertension secondary to heart disease (postcapillary disorders), parenchymal lung disease (pulmonary precapillary disorders), pulmonary embolism, and cor pulmonale from COPD.[257] Optimal preoperative management of these conditions requires treatment of the underlying disease.[257-259] Because pulmonary embolism can be particularly difficult to diagnose, it is crucial to be especially alert to the possibility of this disease. The clinical findings of pulmonary emboli are not always present or specific for the diagnosis. The history may include tachypnea, dyspnea, palpitations, syncope, chest pain, or hemoptysis. Physical examination can reveal a pleural rub, wheezing, rales, a fixed and split second heart sound, right ventricular lift, or evidence of venous thrombosis, none of which are present in most patients. If the ECG shows an

Table 35-16 Postoperative Pneumonia Risk Index

Preoperative Risk Factor	Point Value
Type of surgery	
Abdominal aortic aneurysm repair	15
Thoracic	14
Upper abdominal	10
Neck	8
Neurosurgery	8
Vascular	3
Age	
80 yr	17
70-79 yr	13
60-69 yr	9
50-59 yr	4
Functional status	
Totally dependent	10
Partially dependent	6
Weight loss >10% in past 6 mo	7
History of chronic obstructive pulmonary disease	5
General anesthesia	4
Impaired sensorium	4
History of cerebrovascular accident	4
Blood urea nitrogen level	
<2.86 mmol/L (0.8 mg/dL)	4
7.85-10.7 mmol/L (22-30 mg/dL)	2
≥10.7 mmol/L (≥30 mg/dL)	3
Transfusion >4 U	3
Emergency surgery	3
Steroid use for chronic condition	3
Current smoker within 1 yr	3
Alcohol intake >2 drinks/day in past 2 wk	2

From Arozullah AM, Khuri SF, Henderson WG, et al: Development and validation of a multifactorial risk index for predicting postoperative pneumonia after major noncardiac surgery. Ann Intern Med 135:847-857, 2001, with permission.

S_1Q_3 pattern, spiral CT or lung perfusion scans can be obtained to rule out the diagnosis of pulmonary emboli. A high degree of suspicion is necessary to warrant angiography and anticoagulation or fibrinolytic therapy. If possible, the reactivity of the pulmonary vasculature should be determined, for it may be enhanced or decreased by such drugs as nifedipine, hydralazine, nitroglycerin, prazosin, tolazoline, phentolamine, sildenafil citrate, and nitric oxide. Monitoring of pulmonary artery pressure is often required; preoperative measures should be undertaken to ensure that the patient is not exposed to conditions that elevate pulmonary vascular resistance (e.g., hypoxia, hypercapnia, acidosis, lung hyperinflation, hypothermia)[260] or that decrease blood volume (prolonged restriction of fluid intake) or systemic vascular resistance.

Infectious Diseases of the Lung

Preoperative evaluation and treatment should follow the basic guidelines outlined in the introduction to this section and Chapter 34; treatment of the underlying disease should be completed before all but emergency surgery is performed.

Even though elective surgery should be postponed whenever infectious diseases of the lung are present, patients undergoing emergency surgery often have nosocomial infections and immunocompromised systems. The predominant pathogens for nosocomial pneumonia are gram-negative bacilli, *Staphylococcus aureus*, *Haemophilus influenzae*, anaerobes, and pneumococci. Furthermore, tuberculosis increased rapidly in the late 1980s and in the 1990s, probably because of reactivation in patients infected with HIV. Increased funding and directly observed antituberculosis therapy have more than offset immigrant and travel risk to cause it to decrease recently. Tuberculosis leads to chronic pulmonary and systemic symptoms. Affected patients may have malaise, headache, fever, hemoptysis, and extrapulmonary diseases affecting the skin, cervical lymph nodes, kidneys, pericardium, and meninges. Active disease is treated with four-drug therapy: isoniazid, pyrazinamide, ethambutol or streptomycin, and rifampin for 9 months. Therapy should probably be started before surgery. Management of these emergency patients (many of whom have adult respiratory distress syndrome) before they are brought to the operating room might include initiation of anti-infective therapy, optimization of fluid status and gas exchange, and therapy for the underlying pathophysiologic process.

Chronic Diseases of the Lung

Treatment of COPD (reactive airways) may include the use of β-adrenergic drugs, parasympatholytic agents (especially for exercise-induced asthma), systemic or inhaled corticosteroids, and leukotriene antagonists. An estimated 5% of the population has bronchospasm. Some investigators recommend using inhaled bronchodilators as first-line drugs and reducing the dose of inhaled steroids, such as beclomethasone dipropionate, budesonide, mometasone, or fluticasone, which are inactivated after absorption. However, in large doses, these "inhaled" steroids can suppress adrenal function, and supplemental systemic corticosteroids may be needed at times of stress (see earlier discussion under the section "Adrenocortical Malfunction"). Preoperative assessment must include gaining knowledge of drug regimens and their effects and education of the patient regarding proper use of an inhaler (Box 35-5) because these drugs can interact dangerously with anesthetics (see the last section of this chapter) or can be used inappropriately and therefore produce side effects without maximum benefit.[215-225] No known interaction between the inhaled anticholinergic ipratropium bromide and muscle relaxants has been reported. Patients can feel fine at rest but must be tested by exercise or spirometry to document the degree of current bronchospasm. Furthermore, a symptomatic response to bronchodilators in an asymptomatic patient may not predict whether the patient responds to bronchodilator therapy. An estimated 10% of asthmatic patients exhibit sensitivity to aspirin and may react not only to compounds containing aspirin but also to tartrazine, yellow dye No. 5, indomethacin, other nonsteroidal anti-inflammatory drugs, and aminopyrine.[261]

Box 35-5 Procedures for Correct Use of a Metered-Dose Inhaler

Remove the cap and hold the inhaler upright.

Shake the inhaler.

Tilt the head back slightly and exhale steadily to functional residual capacity.

Position the inhaler by using a spacer between the actuator and the mouth.

Press down on the inhaler while taking a slow, deep breath (3 to 5 seconds).

Hold the full inspiration for at least 5 and up to 10 seconds, if possible, to allow the medication to reach deeply into the lungs.

Repeat inhalations as directed. Waiting 1 minute after inhalation of the bronchodilator may permit subsequent inhalations to penetrate more deeply into the lungs and is necessary to ensure proper delivery of the dose. Rinse your mouth and expectorate after using the inhaler.

Cystic fibrosis is characterized by dilatation and hypertrophy of the bronchial glands, mucous plugging of the peripheral airways, and frequently, bronchitis, bronchiectasis, and bronchiolectasis. For all these conditions, the measures recommended earlier in this section, as well as appropriate hydration to allow mobilization of secretions, constitute optimal preprocedure therapy.

Surgical resection is the primary therapy for non–small cell carcinomas (e.g., adenocarcinoma, squamous cell carcinoma, and large cell carcinoma). These carcinomas account for 75% of all lung carcinomas, 12% of all malignant tumors, and 20% of all cancer deaths in the United States.[262] Success of surgery can be predicted by the stage of the tumor.

The combination of chemotherapy and radiation therapy is the current treatment of choice for small cell carcinomas of the lung.[263] Oat cell (small cell) carcinoma of the lung and bronchial adenomas are known for their secretion of endocrinologically active substances, such as ACTH-like hormones. Squamous cell cancers in the superior pulmonary sulcus produce Horner's syndrome, as well as characteristic pain in areas served by the eighth cervical nerves and first and second thoracic nerves. These tumors are now treated with preoperative radiation; surgical resection leads to an almost 30% "cure" rate.

Anaphylaxis, Anaphylactoid Responses, and Allergic Disorders Other Than Those Related to Lung Diseases and Asthma

Anaphylactic and Anaphylactoid Reactions

Anaphylaxis is a severe life-threatening allergic reaction. *Allergic* applies to immunologically mediated reactions, as opposed to those caused by pharmacologic idiosyncrasy, by direct toxicity or drug overdosage, or by drug interaction.[264-266] Anaphylaxis is the typical immediate hypersensitivity reaction (type I). Such reactions are produced by immunoglobulin E (IgE)-mediated release of pharmacologically active substances. These mediators in turn produce specific end-organ responses in the skin (urticaria), the respiratory system (bronchospasm and upper airway edema), and the cardiovascular system (vasodilation, changes in inotropy, and increased capillary permeability). Vasodilation occurs at the level of the capillary and postcapillary venule and leads to erythema, edema, and smooth muscle contraction. This clinical syndrome is called *anaphylaxis*. By contrast, *anaphylactoid reaction* denotes an identical or very similar clinical response that is not mediated by IgE or (usually) an antigen-antibody process.[265,266]

In anaphylactic reactions, an injected or inhaled (or injested) substance—usually drugs, food, or insect venom—can serve as the allergen itself. Low-molecular-weight agents are believed to act as haptens that form immunologic conjugates with host proteins. The offending substance, regardless of whether it is a hapten, may be the parent compound, a nonenzymatically generated product, or a metabolic product formed in the patient's body. When an allergen binds immunospecific IgE antibodies on the surface of mast cells and basophils, histamine and eosinophilic chemotactic factors of anaphylaxis are released from storage granules in a calcium- and energy-dependent process.[265,266] Other chemical mediators are rapidly synthesized and subsequently released in response to cellular activation. These mediators include slow-reacting substance of anaphylaxis, which is a combination of three leukotrienes; other leukotrienes[265,266]; kinins; platelet-activating factors; adenosine; chemotactic factors; heparin; tryptase; chymase; and prostaglandins, including the potent bronchoconstrictor prostaglandin D_2, eosinophil growth and activating factors, mast cell growth factors, and proinflammatory and other factors that contribute to the IgE isotype switch.

The end-organ effects of the mediators produce the clinical syndrome of anaphylaxis. Usually, a first wave of symptoms, including those caused by vasodilation and a feeling of impending doom, is quickly followed by a second wave as the cascade of mediators amplifies the reactions. In a sensitized patient, onset of the signs and symptoms caused by these mediators is usually immediate but may be delayed 2 to 15 minutes or, in rare instances, as long as 2.5 hours after the parenteral injection of antigen.[267,268] After oral administration, manifestations may occur at unpredictable times.

Mast cell proliferation, together with severe progressive inflammation, contributes to the worsening of symptoms that occurs even after an allergen load is no longer present. The antigen present in cells and lymphocytes, as well as activated mast cells, starts to induce the production of cytokines. These proinflammatory cytokines recruit more inflammatory cells, which leads to tissue edema and mediates a second wave of mast cell degranulation. This second wave can promote the recurrence of severe symptoms 6 to 8 hours later and necessitates, some believe, at least 8 hours of continued ICU-like observation.

In addition, there are multiple effector processes by which biologically active mediators can be generated to produce an anaphylactoid reaction. Activation of the blood coagulation and fibrinolytic systems, the kinin-generating sequence, or the complement cascade can produce the same inflammatory substances that result in an anaphylactic reaction. The two mechanisms known to activate the complement system are called classical and alternative. The classical pathway can be initiated through IgG or IgM (transfusion reactions) or plasmin. The alternative pathway can be activated by lipopolysaccharides (endotoxin), drugs (Althesin), radiographic contrast media,[269] membranes (nylon tricot membranes for bubble oxygenators), cellophane membranes of dialyzers, vascular graft material,[270] latex or latex-containing products,[271,272] and perfluorocarbon artificial blood. The most common agents responsible for intraoperative anaphylaxis are muscle relaxants.[272] However, latex accounts for a significant number of these reactions, and the incidence of intraoperative anaphylaxis caused by latex is increasing. It is now probably the second most important cause of intraoperative anaphylaxis. In addition, histamine can be liberated independent of immunologic reactions.[273] Mast cells and basophils release histamine in response to chemicals or drugs. Most narcotics can release histamine[273] and produce an anaphylactoid reaction, as can radiographic contrast media,[269] *d*-tubocurarine, and thiopental. What makes some patients susceptible to release of histamine in response to drugs is unknown, but hereditary and environmental factors may play a role.

Intravenous contrast material is probably the most frequently used agent that causes anaphylactoid reactions. Because diagnostic (skin and other) tests are helpful only in IgE-mediated reactions, pretesting is not useful for contrast reactions. Pretreatment with diphenhydramine, cimetidine (or ranitidine), and corticosteroids has been reported to be useful in preventing or ameliorating anaphylactoid reactions to intravenous contrast material[269,274] and perhaps to narcotics. Unfortunately, very large doses of steroids (1 g of methylprednisolone intravenously) may be necessary to obtain a beneficial effect.[275] The efficacy of large-dose steroid therapy has not been confirmed. Other common substances associated with anaphylactic or anaphylactoid reactions that might merit preoperative therapy include antibiotics, volume expanders, and blood products (Table 35-17).[265] The anesthesiologist should be prepared preoperatively to treat an anaphylactic or anaphylactoid response.

In some cases, a patient with a history of an anaphylactic or anaphylactoid reaction must receive a substance suspected of producing such a reaction (e.g., iodinated contrast material). In addition, some patients have a higher than average likelihood of having a reaction, thus warranting well-planned pretreatment and therapy for possible anaphylactic and anaphylactoid reactions.[269]

Minimizing Risks Preoperatively

Although virtually all evidence on this subject is merely anecdotal, enough consistent thought recurs through the literature to justify proposing an optimal approach to these problems. First, predisposing factors should be sought; patients with a history of atopy or allergic rhinitis should be suspected of being at risk. Because anaphylactic and anaphylactoid reactions to contrast media occur 5 to 10 times more frequently in patients with a previously suspected reaction, consideration should be given to the administration of low-osmotic agents and both H_1 and H_2 receptor antagonists for 16 to 24 hours before exposing these

Table 35-17 Incidence of Anaphylactic or Anaphylactoid Reactions to Some Common Agents

Agent	Incidence
Plasma protein	
Plasma protein derivative	0.019
Human serum albumin	0.011
Dextran 60/75	0.069
Dextran 40	0.007
Hydroxyethyl starch	0.085
Penicillin	0.002*
Chymopapain	0.3-1.5

*Fatal reactions.
Data modified from Levy JH, Roizen MF, Morris JM: Anaphylactic and anaphylactoid reactions: A review. Spine 11:282, 1986; and Moss J, McDermott DJ, Thisted RA, et al: Anaphylactic/anaphylactoid reactions in response to Chymodiactin (chymopapain). Anesth Analg 63:253, 1984.

patients to a suspected allergen. H_1 receptor antagonists appear to require this much time to act on the receptor. Volume status can be optimized,[265] and perhaps large doses of steroids (1 g of hydrocortisone) should also be administered before exposing patients to agents associated with a high incidence of anaphylactic or anaphylactoid reactions.[275] Older patients and patients taking β-adrenergic blocking drugs present special problems; they are at higher risk of having complications from both pretreatment (especially vigorous hydration) and therapy for anaphylactic reactions (glucagon is useful here) and are less responsive to treatment regimens.[276] One approach is to avoid drugs likely to trigger anaphylactic or anaphylactoid reactions or alter the treatment protocol for this group. Drawing blood for later analysis, especially of tryptase, can be useful in clarifying the diagnosis.[277]

With the increasing incidence of latex hypersensitivity, attempts have been made to make much of the operating room environment latex free; however, costs and preferences have resulted in the continued use of latex-containing gloves in many hospitals. Nonetheless, more hospitals are totally latex free. In allergic patients, care should be taken to ensure that no latex-containing products are present in the operating room.

Primary Immunodeficiency Diseases

Primary immunodeficiency diseases are usually manifested early in life as recurrent infections. Along with survival achieved with antibiotic and antibody treatment have come new prominent features: cancer and allergic and autoimmune disorders. Hereditary angioneurotic edema is an autosomal dominant genetic disease characterized by episodes of angioneurotic edema involving the subcutaneous tissues and submucosa of the GI tract and airway and often manifested as abdominal pain. These patients have a functionally impotent inhibitor or deficiency of an inhibitor to complement component C1. Treatment of an acute attack is supportive because epinephrine, antihistamines, and corticosteroids often fail to work. Plasma transfusions have been reported to resolve attacks or make them worse (theoretically by supplying either C1 esterase inhibitor or previously depleted complement components). The severity of attacks can be prevented or decreased by drugs that are either plasmin inhibitors (e.g., ε-aminocaproic acid [EACA] and tranexamic acid) or androgens (e.g., danazol). Because trauma can precipitate acute attacks, prophylactic therapy with danazol, intravenous EACA, plasma, or all three is recommended before elective surgery. Reports have also described the successful use of a partially purified C1 esterase inhibitor in two patients.

Most of the 1 in 700 persons who have selective IgA deficiency (i.e., <5 mg/dL) have repeated serious infections or connective tissue disorders. These infections commonly involve the respiratory tract (e.g., sinusitis, otitis) or GI tract (manifested as diarrhea, malabsorption, or both). If the patient has rheumatoid arthritis, Sjögren's syndrome, or systemic lupus erythematosus, the anesthetist should consider the possibility of isolated IgA deficiency. However, patients with this disorder can be otherwise healthy. Because antibodies to IgA may develop in these patients if previously exposed to IgA (as might occur from a previous blood transfusion), subsequent blood transfusions can cause anaphylaxis, even when they contain washed erythrocytes. Transfusions should therefore consist of blood donated by another IgA-deficient patient.

Many immunomodulators are now being given to augment cancer treatments[278]; no interactions between these modulators, no effects on the incidence of immune reactions during anesthesia, and no interactions with anesthetic effects have been reported except those regarding immune-suppressing drugs (see the last section of this chapter).

Immunonutrition[271] is increasingly being used preprocedurally by patients and prescribed by providers to decrease inflammatory responses. Whereas excellent data on the benefits of probiotics in changing the intestinal mileau to decrease inflammation can be found, limited data are available on their effects on periprocedural recovery or outcomes.

Diseases of the Central Nervous System, Neuromuscular Diseases, and Psychiatric Disorders

Evaluation of a patient with neurologic or psychiatric disease can be found in Chapter 34. Information gathered from the history that would warrant further investigation includes a previous need for postoperative ventilation in a patient without inordinate lung disease, which would indicate the possibility of metabolic neurologic disorders such as porphyria, alcoholic myopathy, other myopathies, neuropathies, and neuromuscular disorders such as myasthenia gravis. Other historical information warranting further investigation would be the use of drugs such as steroids; guanidine; anticonvulsant, anticoagulant, and antiplatelet drugs; lithium; tricyclic antidepressants; phenothiazines; and butyrophenones.

Although preoperative treatment of most neurologic disorders has not been reported to lessen perioperative morbidity, knowledge of the pathophysiologic characteristics of these disorders is important in planning intraoperative and postoperative management. Thus, preoperative knowledge about these disorders and their associated conditions (e.g., cardiac arrhythmias with Duchenne's muscular dystrophy or respiratory and cardiac muscle weakness with dermatomyositis) may reduce perioperative morbidity. A primary goal of neurologic evaluation is to determine the site of the lesion in the nervous system. Such localization to one of four levels (supratentorial compartment, posterior fossa, spinal cord, peripheral nervous system) is essential for accurate diagnosis and appropriate management. (Disorders accompanied by increased intracranial pressure and cerebrovascular disorders are discussed in Chapters 13 and 63.)

Coma

Little is known about specific anesthetic or perioperative or periprocedural choices that alter outcome for a comatose patient, but as for all other conditions, it is imperative to know the cause of the coma so that drugs can be avoided that might worsen the condition or that might not be metabolized because of organ dysfunction. First, the patient should be observed. Yawning, swallowing, or licking of the lips implies a "light" coma with major brainstem function intact. If consciousness is depressed but respiration, pupillary reactivity to light, and eye movements are normal and no focal motor signs are present, metabolic depression is likely. Abnormal pupillary responses may indicate hypoxia, hypothermia, local eye disease, or drug intoxication with belladonna alkaloids, narcotics, benzodiazepines, or glutethimide; pupillary responses may also be abnormal, however, after the use of eye drops. Other metabolic causes of coma include uremia, hypoglycemia, hepatic coma, alcohol ingestion, hypophosphatemia, myxedema, and hyperosmolar nonketotic coma. Except in extreme emergencies, such as uncontrolled bleeding or a perforated viscus, care should be taken to render the patient as metabolically normal as possible before surgery. This practice and documenting the findings on the chart preoperatively lessen any confusion regarding the cause of intraoperative and postoperative problems. However, too rapid correction of uremia or hyperosmolar nonketotic coma can lead to cerebral edema, a shift of water into the brain as a result of a reverse osmotic effect caused by dysequilibrium of the urea concentration.

The physical examination can be extremely helpful preoperatively in assessing the prognosis. Arms flexed at the elbow (i.e., decorticate posture) imply bilateral hemisphere dysfunction but an intact brainstem, whereas extension of the legs and arms (bilateral decerebrate posture) implies bilateral damage to structures at the upper brainstem or deep hemisphere level. Seizures are often seen in patients with uremia and other metabolic encephalopathies. Hyperreflexia and upward-pointing toes suggest a structural CNS lesion or uremia, hypoglycemia, or hepatic coma; hyporeflexia and downward-pointing toes with no hemiplegia generally indicate no structural CNS lesion.

Epileptic Seizures

Epileptic seizures result from paroxysmal neuronal discharges of abnormally excitable neurons. Six percent to 10% of individuals younger than 70 years will experience a seizure at some time during their lifetime. Fifty percent to 70% of patients with one seizure will never have another. However, 70% of people with two seizures will have an epileptic focus, be candidates for antiseizure medications, and be subject to withdrawal seizures after anesthesia if such medications are not continued.[279] A seizure is the term for the clinical event defined as a paroxysmal alteration in neurologic function caused by a synchronous, rhythmic depolarization of brain cortical neurons. Epilepsy is the condition manifested by recurrent, unprovoked seizures. Sometimes syncopal episodes can be mistaken for seizures, especially when interviews are compressed in the short timeframe of a preoperative visit. We believe that each patient who gives a history of recent undiagnosed syncope or seizure should be seen by a specialist in this field before proceeding with anesthesia because anesthesia can provoke these conditions (see later).[280] Twenty-five percent of patients with a seizure have a normal electroencephalogram (EEG) when interictal. Thus, a negative EEG does not indicate that someone with a seizure will not have a withdrawal seizure when emerging from anesthesia. Seizures can be generalized (arising from deep midline structures in the brainstem or thalamus, usually without an aura or focal features during the seizure), partial focal motor, or sensory (the initial discharge comes from a focal unilateral area of the brain, often preceded by an aura). As with cerebrovascular accidents and coma, knowing the origin may be crucial to understanding the pathophysiologic processes of the disease and to managing the intraoperative and postoperative course.

Epileptic seizures can arise from discontinuation of sedative-hypnotic drugs or alcohol, use of narcotics, uremia, traumatic injury, neoplasms, infection, congenital malformation, birth injury, drug use (e.g., amphetamines, cocaine), hypercalcemia or hypocalcemia, blood in the ventricle or hypoxia, and vascular disease and vascular accidents. Thirty percent of epileptic seizures have no known cause. Most partial seizures are caused by structural brain abnormalities (secondary to tumor, trauma, stroke, infection, and other causes).

An epileptic patient requires no special anesthetic management other than that for the underlying disease. Most authorities believe that anticonvulsant medications should be given in the therapeutic range[279-281] and continued through the morning of surgery, even in pregnant women; they should also be given postoperatively, even in mothers who plan to breast-feed, according to guidelines published by the American Academy of Neurology. Many of the epileptic drugs, including phenytoin, carbamazepine, and phenobarbiturate, alter the hepatic metabolism of many drugs and induce cytochrome P450 enzyme activity. Drug-drug interactions are much less problematic with the newer epileptic drugs such as gabapentin and topirimate.[279] Appropriate treatment of status epilepticus may include general anesthesia.[281] In one controlled trial, phenobarbital was more rapidly effective in controlling status epilepticus than was diazepam followed by phenytoin.[281] The frequency of side effects and required tracheal intubation was similar for both regimens. High concentrations of enflurane (especially with hyperventilation) can be associated with EEG evidence of epileptic activity and tonic-clonic movements. These seizures, however, do not appear to have serious sequelae. Enflurane anesthesia does not seem to increase seizure activity in patients with a history of convulsive disorders, and it even suppresses seizures induced by electroshock, pentylenetetrazole, strychnine, picrotoxin, or bemegride. Thus, other than the use of current drug therapy and heeding precautions taken for the underlying disease, no known changes in perioperative management seem to be indicated.

Infectious Diseases of the Central Nervous System, Degenerative Disorders of the Central Nervous System, and Headache

Many degenerative CNS disorders have been traced to slowly developing viral diseases or even the presence of certain proteins or viral particles ("prions"). No special perioperative anesthetic considerations appear to apply for infectious disorders of the CNS other than those for increased intracranial pressure and avoidance of occupational exposure and transmission of disease to health care workers (also see Chapter 101). The appropriate prophylactic measures to take if one comes in contact with meningococcal disease or other infectious CNS diseases are still not well established. The use of *H. influenzae* type b vaccine has made meningitis an adult disease.[282]

Parkinson's disease is a degenerative disorder of the CNS that may or may not be caused by a virus. Clinically, Parkinson's disease, chronic manganese intoxication, phenothiazine or butyrophenone toxicity, Wilson's disease, Huntington's chorea, traumatic boxing injury, the effects of street drug toxins such as methylphenyltetrahydropyridine (MPTP), and carbon monoxide encephalopathy all have similar initial features: bradykinesia, muscular rigidity, and tremor.

Newer therapies have been developed to arrest or even reverse the progression of Parkinson's disease. Therapy is directed at (1) increasing the neuronal release of dopamine or the receptor's response to dopamine, (2) stimulating the receptor directly with bromocriptine and lergotrile, (3) implanting dopaminergic tissue, or (4) decreasing cholinergic activity. New therapies using the monoamine oxidase inhibitor (MAOI) deprenyl or adrenal medullary transplants to slow the progression of disease appear promising,[283,284] and even treatment with high-dose coenzyme Q10 seems to be strikingly beneficial.[22] Experience with deprenyl in the perioperative milieu is insufficient to make proscriptions about its use. Anticholinergic agents have been the initial drugs of choice because they decrease tremor more than muscle rigidity. Dopamine does not pass the blood-brain barrier, so its precursor L-dopa (levodopa) is used. Unfortunately, L-dopa is decarboxylated to dopamine in the periphery and can cause nausea, vomiting, and arrhythmia. These side effects are diminished by the administration of α-methylhydrazine (carbidopa), a decarboxylase inhibitor that does not pass the blood-brain barrier. Refractoriness to L-dopa develops, and it is now debated whether the drug should be used only when symptoms cannot be controlled with other anticholinergic medications. "Drug holidays" have been suggested as one means of restoring the effectiveness of these compounds, but cessation of such therapy may result in a marked deterioration of function and need for hospitalization. Therapy for Parkinson's disease should be initiated before surgery and be continued through the morning of surgery; such treatment seems to decrease drooling, the potential for aspiration, and ventilatory weakness.[285,286] Reinstituting therapy promptly after surgery is crucial,[280,283-287] as is avoiding drugs such as the phenothiazines and butyrophenones (droperidol), which inhibit the release of dopamine (and perhaps alfentanil) or compete with dopamine at the receptor.[285] Carbidopa/levodopa in low doses (20 to 200 mg nightly versus the usual 60 to 600 mg/day for Parkinson's disease) is commonly used in the nonparkinsonian restless leg syndrome of the elderly (present in 2% to 5% of individuals older than 60 years). This drug too should be given the night before and the night immediately after surgery. Clozapine (a benzodiazepine) does not appear to worsen the movement disorders of Parkinson's disease and has been used postoperatively to stop levodopa-induced hallucinations.

Dementia, a progressive decline in intellectual function, can be caused by treatable infections (e.g., syphilis, cryptococcosis, coccidioidomycosis, Lyme disease, tuberculosis), depression (a trial of antidepressants is indicated in most patients), side effects of medications (digitalis has slowed brain function more than the heart rate), myxedema, vitamin B_{12} deficiency, chronic drug or alcohol intoxication, metabolic causes (liver and renal failure), neoplasms, partially treatable infections (HIV), untreatable infections (Creutzfeldt-Jakob syndrome), or decreased acetylcholine in the cerebral cortex (Alzheimer's disease). This last condition occurs in more than 0.5% of Americans.[288-291] Although these patients are often given cholinergic agonists, controlled trials of these drugs have not as yet shown major significant benefit.[289,290,292] Gingko has been advocated and has improved subjective symptoms in 37% of patients versus 23% of those given placebo. Although later controlled trials have failed to confirm its benefit in early Alzheimer's disease or in healthy elderly individuals, gingko is still popular. However, the prevalence of Alzheimer's disease and the desperation of the patients and their families have now widened such therapies. Cholinergic medications have been shown to improve functioning in patients with Alzheimer's disease.[293] These families often desire surgery, but the interactions of these drugs and therapies with perioperative analgesic and anesthetic drug therapies are not well established. There is one case report of intraoperative bradycardia in such patients with two cholinergic drugs.[294] Based on basic science research, there is some concern about a link between Alzheimer's disease, postoperative cognitive dysfunction, and inhaled agents.[295] Several investigators have demonstrated β-amyloid deposition in animals exposed to inhaled anesthetics.[296-298] Further research is required to determine whether this link is clinically relevant in humans. Most reversible dementias are either drug-induced delirium or depression.[289,290,299] At present, early results with stimulation at "threshold testing" are promising and seem to stimulate dendritic regrowth and may reverse some or much of the cognitive decline. Such computer programs and games are in early testing. Creutzfeldt-Jakob disease has been transmitted inadvertently by surgical instruments and corneal transplants; the causative virus or protein particle is not inactivated by heat, disinfectants, or formaldehyde.

More than 90% of patients with chronic recurring headaches are categorized as having migraine, tension, or cluster headaches. The mechanism of tension or cluster headaches may not differ qualitatively from that for migraine headaches; all may be manifestations of labile vasomotor regulation.[300] A headache is said to be migraine if it is characterized by four of the following five "POUNDing" conditions: if it is Pulsating, if it lasts One day or more, if it is Unilateral, if there is Nausea, and if it Disturbs daily activities.[301]

Treatment of cluster and migraine headaches centers on the use of serotonin drugs such as sumatriptan or ergotamine and its derivatives.[300-302] Other drugs that may be effective are propranolol, calcium channel inhibitors, cyproheptadine, prednisone, antihistamines, tricyclic antidepressants, phenytoin, and diuretic drugs, as well as biofeedback. Giant cell arteritis, glaucoma, and all the meningitides, including Lyme disease, are other causes of headache that might benefit from treatment before surgery.[303] No other special treatment is indicated preoperatively for a patient who has a well-delineated cause for the headaches. Acute migraine attacks can sometimes be terminated by ergotamine tartrate aerosol or by injection of sumatriptan or dihydroergotamine mesylate intravenously; general anesthesia has also been used. We normally continue all prophylactic headache medicine, although the decision to continue aspirin through the morning of surgery is usually left to the surgeon.

Back Pain, Neck Pain, and Spinal Canal Syndromes

Acute spinal cord injury is discussed earlier in the section on autonomic dysfunction. Although it is a common problem, little is written about the anesthetic management of syndromes related to herniated disks, spondylosis (usually of advancing age), and the congenital narrowing of the cervical and lumbar canal that gives rise to symptoms of nerve root compression. One report stresses the importance of the vascular component in the mechanism of damage to the spinal cord and, hence, the theoretical desirability of slight hypertension perioperatively.[304] Another report suggests the use of awake intubation, a fiberoptic bronchoscope, and monitoring of evoked potentials.[305] Other than the commonsense approach of seeking neurologic consultation or, if necessary, using awake positioning of patients in a comfortable position before emergency root decompression procedures, no special procedures appear to be necessary.

Demyelinating Diseases

Demyelinating diseases constitute a diffuse group of diseases ranging from those with uncertain cause (e.g., multiple sclerosis, where genetic, epidemiologic, and immunologic factors are probably all involved and interferon beta appears to be a promising treatment[306]) to those that follow infection, vaccination (e.g., Guillain-Barré syndrome), or antimetabolite treatment of cancer. Therefore, demyelinating diseases can have very diverse symptoms. Apparently, there is a risk of relapse of these diseases immediately after surgery. Because relapse may occur as a result of rapid electrolyte changes in the perioperative period, such changes might be avoided. In addition, perioperative administration of steroids has been advocated as a protective measure.[99] Although there are concerns about the use of neuraxial anesthesia in these patients, epidural anesthesia has been administered without problems.[307] Multiple sclerosis and demyelinating diseases in general are the most common cause of nontraumatic disability in young adults. The age-adjusted survival rate is 80% of that of unaffected individuals, or put another way, the average patient with multiple sclerosis ages 1.2 years for every year with the disease. However, the variability of the disease makes this average rate of aging almost meaningless. Thus far, no mode of treatment has been shown to alter most of these disease processes, although ACTH, steroids, interferon beta, glatiramer acetate (Copaxone), and plasmapheresis may ameliorate or abbreviate a relapse, even alter disease progression, especially progression of multiple sclerosis and (if started within 2 weeks of onset) Guillain-Barré syndrome.[308] Such an effect is consonant with the hypothesis of an immunologic disorder being the cause of these diseases. Care should be taken to avoid succinylcholine in these patients because of the risk of hyperkalemia

Sleep apnea may be considered a demyelinating or degenerative CNS disease or a peripheral disease of obesity, depending on its etiology. Both types (central and peripheral causes) appear to be increasingly common and are present in more than 5% of elderly African Americans. Preprocedure and preoperative identification of patients and therapy for sleep apnea are discussed in Chapter 64.

Metabolic Diseases

Included in the category of metabolic diseases is nervous system dysfunction secondary to porphyrias, alcoholism, uremia, hepatic failure, and vitamin B_{12} deficiency. The periodic paralysis that can accompany thyroid disease is discussed under "Neuromuscular Disorders" (see later).

Alcoholism or heavy alcohol intake is associated with acute alcoholic hepatitis (also see Chapter 66), the activity of which declines as alcohol is withdrawn; with myopathy and cardiomyopathy, which can be severe; and with withdrawal syndromes. Within 6 to 8 hours of withdrawal, the patient may become tremulous, a state that usually subsides within days or weeks. Alcoholic hallucinosis and withdrawal seizures generally occur within 24 to 36 hours. These seizures are generalized grand mal attacks; when focal seizures occur, other causes should be sought. Delirium tremens usually appears within 72 hours of withdrawal and is often preceded by tremulousness, hallucinations, or seizures. These three symptoms, combined with perceptual distortions, insomnia, psychomotor disturbances, autonomic hyperactivity, and in a large percentage of cases, another potentially fatal illness (e.g., bowel infarction or subdural hematoma), are components of delirium tremens. This syndrome is now treated with benzodiazepines. Nutritional disorders of alcoholism include alcoholic hypoglycemia and hypothermia, alcoholic polyneuropathy, Wernicke-Korsakoff syndrome, and cerebellar degeneration. In alcoholic patients (i.e., those who drink at least two six packs of beer or 1 pint of whiskey per day or the equivalent), emergency surgery and anesthesia (despite alcoholic hepatitis) are not associated with worsening abnormalities in liver enzymes. In addition, about 20% of alcoholic patients also have COPD. A patient who has a history of alcohol abuse therefore warrants careful examination of many systems for quantification of preoperative physical status.

Although hepatic failure can lead to coma with high-output cardiac failure, unlike uremia, it does not lead to chronic polyneuropathy. Uremic polyneuropathy is a distal symmetric sensorimotor polyneuropathy that may be improved by dialysis. The use of depolarizing muscle relaxants in patients with polyneuropathies has been questioned (also see Chapter 29). We believe that patients who have a neuropathy associated with uremia should not be given succinylcholine because of a possible exaggerated hyperkalemic response.

Pernicious anemia caused by vitamin B_{12} deficiency may result in subacute combined degeneration of the spinal cord; the signs are similar to those of chronic nitrous oxide toxicity. Both pernicious anemia and nitrous oxide toxicity are associated with peripheral neuropathy and disorders of the pyramidal tract and posterior column (which governs fine motor skills and the sense of body position). Combined-system disease can also occur without anemia, as can nitrous oxide toxicity in dentists and nitrous oxide abusers. Patients with vitamin B_{12} deficiency and anemia, if treated with folate, improve hematologically but progress to dementia and severe neuropathy. It may thus be prudent to give an intramuscular injection of 100 μg of vitamin B_{12} or 800 μg orally before giving folate to a patient who has signs of combined-system degeneration.[309]

The porphyrias are a constellation of metabolic diseases that result from an autosomally inherited lack of functional enzymes active in the synthesis of hemoglobin. Figure 35-9 schematically depicts the abnormalities that result from these enzyme deficits. It is important to note that type 1, 3, and 4 porphyrias can cause life-threatening neurologic abnormalities. These conditions are characterized by the presence of aminolevulinic acid (ALA) or porphobilinogen (or both) in urine; these substances do not occur in porphyria cutanea tarda, a disease that does not incur neurologic sequelae.[310] In acute intermittent porphyria, the typical pattern consists of acute attacks of colicky pain, nausea, vomiting, severe constipation, psychiatric disorders, and lesions of the lower motor neuron that can progress to bulbar paralysis. Certain drugs can induce the enzyme ALA synthetase and thereby exacerbate the disease process.[311-313] Such sensitizing drugs include barbiturates, meprobamate, chlordiazepoxide, glutethimide, diazepam, hydroxydione, phenytoin, imipramine, pentazocine, birth control pills, ethyl alcohol, sulfonamides, griseofulvin, and ergotamine preparations. Patients often have attacks during infection, fasting, or menstruation. Administration of glucose suppresses ALA synthetase activity and prevents or ablates acute attacks. Drugs used in anesthetic management that are reported to be safe for patients with porphyria include neostigmine (Prostigmin), atropine, gallamine, succinylcholine, *d*-tubocurarine, pancuronium, nitrous oxide, procaine, propofol, propanidid, etomidate, meperidine, fentanyl, morphine, droperidol, promazine, promethazine, and chlorpromazine.[311-313] Although ketamine has been used, postoperative psychoses attributable to the disease may be difficult to distinguish from those possibly caused by ketamine. In addition, although ketamine and etomidate are reported to be safe in humans, they seem to be porphyrinogenic in rats. Propofol has been used without provoking porphyria in at least two susceptible patients.[311,312]

Neuromuscular Disorders

Neuromuscular disorders consist of conditions affecting any major component of the motor unit: motor neuron, peripheral nerve, neuromuscular junction, and muscle. Neuropathies may involve all components of the nerve, thereby producing sensory, motor, and autonomic dysfunction, or only one component. Myopathies may involve only the proximal or distal muscles, or both.

Myasthenia gravis (also see Chapter 34) is a disorder of the muscular system caused by partial blockade or destruction of nicotinic acetylcholine receptors by IgG antibodies. The severity of the disease correlates with the ability of antibodies to decrease the number of available acetylcholine receptors.[314] Treatment of myasthenia is usually begun with anticholinesterase drugs, but in moderate and severe disease, treatment progresses to steroids and thymectomy.[314,315] Immunosuppressive drugs and plasmapheresis are initiated if the more conservative measures fail, and intravenous immunoglobulin, a rapid-onset therapy, is reserved for acute exacerbations and myasthenic crises.[314,315]

One major problem for the anesthesiologist involves the use of muscle relaxants and their reversal.[316] Because much of the care of myasthenia gravis patients involves tailoring the amount

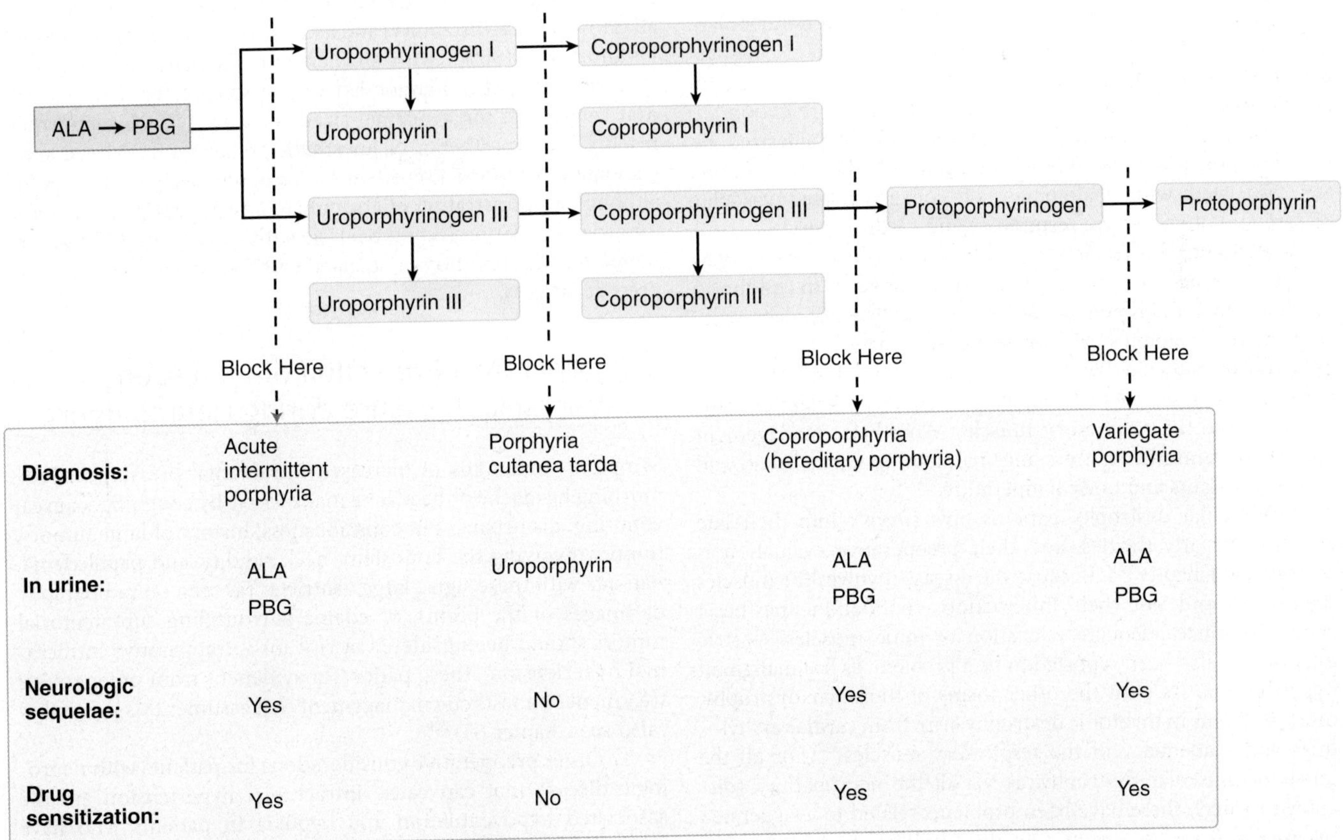

Figure 35-9 Schematic depiction of the functional enzyme deficits that occur in some of the porphyrias. ALA, aminolevulinic acid; PBG, porphobilinogen.

of anticholinesterase medication to the maximal muscle strength of the patient, derangement of the course of the patient during surgery could necessitate reassessment of the drug dosage. For that reason, several researchers recommend withholding all anticholinergic drugs for 6 hours before surgery and reinstituting medication postoperatively with extreme caution because the sensitivity of these patients to such drugs may have changed. In addition, there has been some concern that anticholinergic drugs may lead to a high incidence of bowel anastomotic leaks in patients who have undergone bowel anastomosis. Small doses of succinylcholine can be used to facilitate endotracheal intubation; tiny doses of nondepolarizing drugs can be used for intraoperative relaxation not achieved by regional anesthesia or volatile anesthetics. Controlled ventilation is frequently required for at least 24 to 48 hours postoperatively, although immediate extubation has become more common.[315-317] Postoperative ventilation is especially important in cases involving myasthenia gravis of more than 6 years' duration, COPD, a daily pyridostigmine requirement of 750 mg in association with significant bulbar weakness, and vital capacity of less than 40 mL/kg.[317]

Lambert-Eaton syndrome (myasthenic syndrome) is characterized by proximal limb muscle weakness and is associated with antibodies directed against the voltage-gated calcium channels in presynaptic nerve terminals. Strength or reflexes may increase with repetitive effort. Affected patients exhibit decreased release of acetylcholine at the neuromuscular junction. Guanidine therapy enhances the release of acetylcholine from nerve terminals and improves strength. Men with this syndrome generally have small cell carcinoma of the lung or other malignancy, whereas women often have malignancy, sarcoidosis, thyroiditis, or a collagen-related vascular disease. In addition, these patients have increased sensitivity to both depolarizing and nondepolarizing muscle relaxants.[318] Lambert-Eaton syndrome is also associated with an autonomic nervous system defect manifested by gastroparesis, orthostatic hypotension, and urinary retention.

Dermatomyositis and polymyositis are characterized by proximal limb muscle weakness with dysphagia. These conditions are associated with malignancy or collagen-related vascular disease and often involve respiratory and cardiac muscle.

Periodic paralysis is another disease in which sensitivity to muscle relaxants increases. Periodic weakness starts in childhood or adolescence and is precipitated by rest after exercise, sleep, cold, surgery, or pregnancy. Hypokalemic and hyperkalemic forms exist and are associated with cardiac arrhythmias. Like thyrotoxic periodic paralysis, these hypokalemic and hyperkalemic forms usually spare the respiratory muscles. Anesthetic management consists of minimizing stress and maintaining normal fluid and electrolyte status and body temperature.[318-321]

Muscular dystrophy patients now survive into their late twenties or early thirties, and their preoperative evaluation is reviewed in Chapter 34. Because the disease involves the muscles themselves and not their innervation, conduction anesthesia cannot produce adequate relaxation of tonic muscles. Gastric dilation has also been reported to be a problem, as has malignant hyperthermia. As with the other forms of muscular dystrophy, most problems in myotonic dystrophy arise from cardiac arrhythmias and inadequacy of the respiratory muscles.[322] For all the forms of muscular dystrophy, as for all the neuropathies (discussed earlier), there have been problems related to exaggerated release of serum potassium after the administration of depolarizing muscle relaxants (also see Chapter 29).

Malignant hyperthermia (also see Chapter 37) in the patient or in a relative of the patient merits careful history taking and at least consideration of performing a test for susceptibility to the condition. Prophylaxis with intravenous dantrolene sodium (Dantrium) may also be warranted. In some cases, malignant hyperthermia has been associated with recognizable musculoskeletal abnormalities such as strabismus, ptosis, myotonic dystrophy, hernias, kyphoscoliosis, muscular dystrophy, central core disease, and marfanoid syndrome. Appropriate preparation for a patient with previous masseter spasm, or trismus, is a matter of considerable debate. We prepare for malignant hyperthermia (i.e., we ensure a contaminant-free machine, use nontriggering agents, and have a malignant hyperthermia cart in the room) but do not routinely perform muscle biopsy or prescribe dantrolene prophylaxis.[323,324] Malignant hyperthermia occurs most frequently in children and adolescents, the incidence being 1 in 14,000 administrations of anesthetic. The incidence increases to 1 in 2500 patients requiring squint surgery.

Down Syndrome

Down syndrome (trisomy 21) occurs once in 1000 live births. It is associated with congenital cardiac lesions such as endocardial cushion defects (40%), ventricular septal defects (27%), patent ductus arteriosus (12%), and tetralogy of Fallot (8%), and prophylactic antibiotics should be used before predictable bacteremic events. Down syndrome is also associated with upper respiratory infections, with atlanto-occipital instability (in about 15% of patients,[325-328] in whom it is asymptomatic in most cases, but it is recommended that all patients be treated as though they have atlanto-occipital instability) and laxity of other joints, with thyroid hypofunction (50%), with an increased incidence of subglottic stenosis, and with enlargement of the tongue (or a decreased oral cavity size for a normal-sized tongue).[327,329] No abnormal responses to anesthetics or anesthetic adjuvants have been substantiated. A reported sensitivity to atropine has been disproved, although administration of atropine to any patient given digoxin for atrial fibrillation should be done with extreme care.[329] Examination for the conditions associated with Down syndrome should precede surgery.

Preoperative Prediction of Increased Intracranial Pressure during Neurosurgery

Symptoms and signs of increased intracranial pressure include morning headache or headache made worse by coughing, nausea, vomiting, disturbances in consciousness, history of large tumors, tumors involving the brainstem, neck rigidity, and papilledema. Patients with these signs, large ventricles (as seen on radiography or images of the brain), or edema surrounding supratentorial tumors should be considered at risk for intraoperative intracranial hypertension. These patients may benefit from preoperative treatment or anesthetic management that assumes this possibility (also see Chapter 63).[330]

Other preoperative considerations for patients with neurologic disease that can cause intracranial hypertension are the associated hypoventilation and hypoxia in patients who have severe hemiplegia and the presence of subarachnoid bleeding or other forms of intracranial hemorrhage (especially likely in women given heparin who have two or more cerebral infarcts noted on CT). Many strokes or transient ischemic attacks have a possible cardiac origin (59 of 184 patients).[331,332] The drugs used to prevent cerebral arterial spasm—calcium channel blockers—are discussed in the last section of this chapter.

Mental Disorders

Perhaps the most important preoperative consideration for patients with mental disorders, in addition to developing rapport, is understanding their specific drug therapy and its effects and side effects. More than 15% of all adult patients undergoing surgery are taking one of these therapies or have recently been taking one of these therapies. Lithium, tricyclic antidepressants, selective serotonin reuptake inhibitors (SSRIs), other antidepressants that defy classification such as bupropion, phenothiazines, butyrophenones, and MAOIs are used in these patients.[333] These drugs have potent effects and side effects that are discussed in the last section of this chapter.

Renal Disease, Infectious Diseases, and Electrolyte Disorders

One may ask why preoperative preparation of a patient with renal disease is discussed in the same section as preoperative preparation of a patient with an infectious disease. Although it is commonly recommended that no surgery except emergency or curative (e.g., drainage of an abscess) operations be performed in patients with infectious disease, it has become evident that renal insufficiency can be caused by antimicrobial drugs[334] and that sepsis, not shock, is probably the leading cause of acute postoperative renal failure. The anesthesiologist has an important role to play in preventing the onset and consequences of renal failure and its initiators. The linking of renal failure to electrolyte disorders is more obvious: the kidney is the primary organ for regulating body osmolality and fluid volume and has a major role in excretion of the end products of metabolism. In performing these functions, the kidney becomes intimately involved in the excretion of electrolytes.

A patient with renal insufficiency whose own kidneys are still functioning is distinct not only from a patient with end-stage renal disease whose renal functions are provided by dialysis but also from a patient who has a transplanted kidney. These three groups of patients require very different preoperative preparation. In addition, acute changes in renal function present quite a different problem than do chronic alterations in function. Certain renal diseases require different preoperative preparation than others, but generally, renal disease of any origin presents the same preoperative problems (also see Chapters 18, 34, and 45).

Renal Disease

Causes and Systemic Effects of Renal Disorders

Nephrotic syndrome may develop in patients with glomerular diseases without disturbing tubular function. The soundness of tubular function is an important consideration because tubular dysfunction with attendant uremia presents quite different problems than glomerular disease with only nephrotic syndrome does. This is not to minimize the adverse effects of glomerular disease; nephrotic syndrome consists of massive proteinuria and consequent hypoalbuminemia. The resulting reduction in plasma oncotic pressure diminishes plasma volume and calls forth compensatory mechanisms that result in retention of sodium and water. As a result, a common clinical finding in nephrotic syndrome is edema. Thus, patients with nephrotic syndrome may have excess total-body water and decreased intravascular volume. In addition, diuretics are often given in an attempt to decrease edema. Although serum creatinine and creatinine clearance estimations have limitations as indices of the GFR (inulin clearance is still the gold standard), these measurements are, for now, the most readily available to the anesthesiologist. Plasma creatinine levels reflect endogenous muscle catabolism and dietary intake, as well as urinary excretion. Urinary excretion depends on both filtration and secretion by the kidney. Drugs that are commonly used in the preoperative and perioperative periods can distort this measure of glomerular filtration: cimetidine and trimethoprim interfere with secretion by increasing plasma creatinine and decreasing creatinine clearance without altering filtration. It should also be remembered that the commonly used methods for measuring creatinine have a 95% confidence limit of greater than 20% for a GFR higher than 30 mL/min. Thus, a normal creatinine level of 1.3 mg/dL might give a measured value ranging from 1.0 to 1.5 mg/dL.

Furthermore, in patients with nephrotic syndrome in whom renal tubular function has been preserved, hypovolemia appears to be a significant cause of deteriorating tubular renal function.[335-337] Consequently, we advocate the same intense preoperative, intraoperative, and postoperative fluid management for patients with nephrotic syndrome as we do for patients with diminished tubular function. Admittedly, no randomized study has shown that close control of intravascular volume status in these groups of patients preserves renal tubular function (or any other measure of perioperative morbidity) to a greater degree than less rigid control does.

Uremia, the end result of renal tubular failure (i.e., failure of the concentrating, diluting, acidifying, and filtering functions) is manifested in many ways. Changes occur in the cardiovascular, immunologic, hematologic, neuromuscular, pulmonary, and endocrine systems, as well as in bone. These alterations are ascribed either to the toxic end products of protein metabolism or to an imbalance in functioning of the kidney. As the number of functioning nephrons diminishes, the still-functioning nephrons attempt to increase some solute and body composition preservation functions at the expense of other functions, such as excretion of phosphate. The accumulation of phosphate increases PTH levels, which in turn produces osteodystrophy. Osteodystrophy can be managed by (1) restriction of dietary phosphate, (2) the use of gels (e.g., aluminum hydroxide or carbonate) that bind with intestinal phosphate, (3) calcium supplementation, or (4) parathyroidectomy.

Certain alterations in patients with uremia, such as neuropathy, are most logically attributed to an accumulation of toxic metabolites. Peripheral neuropathy is most often sensory and involves the lower extremities, but it may also be motor; peripheral neuropathies are frequently improved with hemodialysis and can be dramatically reversed with transplantation. The use of depolarizing muscle relaxants in patients with peripheral neuropathy is controversial and is discussed in the section on neuropathies. Tubular function is commonly assessed by acidifying and concentrating capabilities.[338] Although such tests are crude, these capabilities are usually readily assessed by measuring urine pH and specific gravity. Better assessment of renal blood flow, for the purpose of improving renal blood flow and its distribution, is promised by the use of contrast-enhanced ultrasound in the operating room.[339] Along with the altered volume status and cardiac complications in uremic patients, autonomic neuropathy may contribute to hypotension during anesthesia. Atherosclerosis is often accelerated in uremic patients; hypertension, with its attendant consequences, is very common.

Cardiac failure (especially episodic failure) frequently occurs in uremic patients because of the presence of many adverse conditions: anemia with increasing myocardial work, hypertension, atherosclerosis, and altered volume status. Pericarditis can be manifested by pericardial rub alone or by pain (with or without hemorrhage). Cardiac tamponade should be ruled out on the basis of clinical features and by echocardiography if this diagnosis is seriously suspected preoperatively. In addition, cardiac tamponade should be treated or planned for preoperatively.

If anemia is present, its severity generally parallels the degree of uremia; chronically uremic patients seem to adapt well to anemia. No hard data have substantiated the need to give a preoperative blood transfusion to a chronically uremic patient, even when the preoperative hematocrit is as low as 16 or 18 vol%. Even in nonuremic patients in an ICU, a randomized trial was unable to demonstrate improved outcome with a liberal transfusion strategy,[340] and transfusions increase the risk for immune system compromise (also see Chapter 55).[341] Thus, one of the major historical reasons for not transfusing blood in patients with end-stage renal disease has been disproved by this finding: data show that the more blood transfusions a transplant recipient receives before transplantation, the greater the chance that the transplant will function successfully.[342] This immunosuppressive effect of transfusions is now routinely used in transplantation. However, the development of recombinant human erythropoietin has obviated the need for transfusions in chronically uremic patients. Balancing of the immunosuppressive use of blood transfusions versus the benefits of erythropoietin and the risks of transfusion remains to be determined. In uremic patients, coagulation and platelet adhesiveness may be abnormal and factor III activity decreased. Even uremic patients not given corticosteroids or immunosuppressive drugs may demonstrate abnormal immunity, perhaps warranting increased attention regarding procedures that lessen patient cross-contamination.

Uremic patients exhibit a wide variety of metabolic and endocrinologic disorders in addition to hyperparathyroidism, including impaired carbohydrate tolerance, insulin resistance, type IV hyperlipoproteinemia, autonomic insufficiency, hyperkalemia, and anion-gap acidosis (caused by an inability of the kidneys to reabsorb filtered bicarbonate and excrete sufficient ammonium into urine). Furthermore, the excretion and pharmacokinetics of drugs are different in uremic patients than in normal patients. In addition, complications of hemodialysis include nutritional deficiencies, electrolyte and fluid imbalances, and mental disorders. Because these conditions can lead to serious perioperative morbidity, they should be evaluated before surgery. No data, however, have substantiated the hypothesis that preoperative optimization of these metabolic and endocrinologic disorders reduces perioperative risk in uremic patients.

As with uremic patients, preoperative optimization of volume status is paramount in patients with kidney stones, and both are affected by carbohydrate intolerance.[343,344] Seventy-five percent of all kidney stones are composed of calcium oxalate. Patients with these stones frequently take diuretic drugs, consume calcium- and citrate-rich foods, and restrict salt intake. Prevention of dehydration by institution of intravenous fluid therapy along with restricted oral intake of protein may be as important for these patients as it is for those with struvite or uric acid stones. Struvite stones often result from urinary infection. Uric acid stones can be prevented by treatment with allopurinol, by preoperative hydration, or by alkalization of urine. Acidosis may contribute to stone formation. Again, optimal intravascular volume status is important in preventing stones and preserving renal function. More thorough discussion of renal function and physiology is provided in Chapter 18. Chapter 65 deals with the complexities of managing patients for renal surgery and other urologic procedures.

Creatinine clearance in conjunction with free water clearance appears to be the most accurate way of quantifying, for pharmacokinetic purposes, the degree of decreased renal function (also see Chapter 18).[344] For a patient with stable renal function, creatinine clearance, which is a rough estimate of GFR, can be approximated by noting the serum creatinine level: a doubling of the creatinine level represents a halving of the GFR. Thus, a patient with a stable serum creatinine level of 2 mg/dL would have a GFR of approximately 60 mL/min. A stable serum creatinine level of 4 mg/dL would accompany a GFR of approximately 30 mL/min, and a stable serum creatinine level of 8 mg/dL would accompany a GFR of 15 mL/min or less. When pregnancy and considerable edema are not present and the serum creatinine level is stable, the following formulas can be used to estimate creatinine clearance and free water clearance.[344-346]

$$\text{Creatinine clearance} = \frac{(140 - \text{Age}[\text{yr}]) \times \text{Body weight (kg)}}{72 \times \text{Serum creatinine (mg/dL)}}$$

$$\text{Free water clearance} = \text{Urine flow (mL/hr)} - \frac{\text{Urine osmolality (mOsm/L)} \times \text{Urine flow (mL/hr)}}{\text{Plasma osmolality (mOsm/L)}}$$

Note that renal function must be stable. Unstable renal function is often associated with changes in serum creatinine levels that lag by several days. Although knowing the serum creatinine level is more useful than knowing the BUN level, the latter provides some information, as discussed in the next section.

Free water clearance is a measure of renal concentrating ability and is normally −25 to +100 mL/hr; it becomes more positive in renal insufficiency states. It may also become more positive in patients who have a head injury or high blood alcohol levels or in those undergoing aggressive fluid infusion or administration of diuretics.[345]

Patients with Insufficient but Functioning Kidneys

One of the greatest challenges for the anesthesiologist is presented by patients with insufficient renal function whose renal function must be preserved during surgery. Additionally, the presence of chronic renal failure is associated with higher rates of perioperative cardiac morbidity, which may warrant further evaluation for the presence of occult coronary artery disease.[346] The many uremic symptoms and great perioperative morbidity associated with uremia can probably be avoided by attention to detail in the preoperative and perioperative management of patients with insufficient, but still functioning kidneys.[335-337]

First, studies demonstrate that acute postoperative renal failure is associated with an extremely high mortality rate.[347] There are multiple risk factors for the development of perioperative renal dysfunction, the most important of which include preexisting renal disease, heart surgery involving cardiopulmonary bypass or aortic surgery involving cross-clamping of the thoracic or abdominal aorta, and ongoing sepsis. In a systematic review of 28 studies by Novis and colleagues, preoperative renal risk factors such as increased serum creatinine, increased BUN, and preoperative renal dysfunction were repeatedly found to predict postoperative renal dysfunction.[345] Mangano and coworkers performed a prospective cohort study of 2222 patients with or without concurrent vascular surgery.[347] They identified five independent preoperative predictors of renal dysfunction: age 70 to 79 years (relative risk [RR], 1.6; 95% CI, 1.1 to 2.3) or age 80 to 95 years (RR, 3.5; CI, 1.9 to 6.3), CHF (RR, 1.8; CI, 1.3 to 2.6), previous myocardial revascularization (RR, 1.8; CI, 1.2 to 2.7), type 1 diabetes mellitus (RR, 1.8; CI, 1.1 to 3.0) or preoperative serum glucose levels exceeding 16.6 mmol/L (RR, 3.7; CI, 1.7 to 7.8), and preoperative serum creatinine levels of 124 to 177 μmol/L (RR, 2.3; CI, 1.6 to 3.4).

Moreover, acute perioperative renal failure is most likely to occur in patients who have renal insufficiency before surgery, are older than 60 years, and have preoperative left ventricular dysfunction.[345,347] Proper hydration before surgery probably decreases the mortality after acute renal failure induced by radiocontrast agents.[337] Clues regarding the presence of hypovolemia or hypervolemia should be sought from the history and physical examination (e.g., weight loss or gain, thirst, edema, orthostatic hypotension and tachycardia, flat neck veins, dry mucous membranes, decreased skin turgor). In seriously ill patients, insertion of a pulmonary artery catheter will permit more precise monitoring of intravascular fluid volume. Other causes of deterioration in function in chronic renal insufficiency are low cardiac output or low renal blood flow (in prerenal azotemia, whether because of cardiac failure or fluid depletion from diuretic drugs, BUN often increases disproportionately to increases in creatinine), urinary tract infection, use of nephrotoxic drugs, hypercalcemia, and hyperuricemia. These conditions and drugs should be avoided; if any of these conditions exist, they should be treated preoperatively.

To preserve normal renal function, infusion of saline, mannitol, furosemide, or low-dose dopamine has been recommended.[348-350] However, these therapies should be initiated with caution because saline infusions and mannitol can lead to fluid overload and myocardial damage; in addition, diuretic drugs given intraoperatively can produce postoperative hypovolemia, which worsens renal function. Very high concentrations of mannitol may also cause acute renal failure.[351] A meta-analysis of 58 trials involving the use of dopamine for renal protection/treatment, only 17 of which were randomized, was unable to demonstrate any benefit from the use of low-dose dopamine.[352] Maintenance of normal intravascular fluid volume can be guided by pulmonary capillary wedge pressure and has prevented impairment of renal function after open abdominal aortic reconstruction, even when urinary volumes were low.[353] Fenoldopam is a dopamine analog that causes natriuresis and increases renal blood flow and urine output. Several small studies have reported renoprotective effects of fenoldopam in patients undergoing cardiopulmonary bypass and infrarenal aortic aneurysm repair.[354-356]

Anesthetic drugs have been studied in patients with renal insufficiency. In a randomized trial, general anesthesia with desflurane or isoflurane did not exacerbate renal insufficiency.[357] Despite concern that sevoflurane leads to the production of compound A, which impairs renal functioning, a randomized trial of low-flow sevoflurane versus low-flow isoflurane anesthesia in patients with stable renal insufficiency did not demonstrate any difference in any measured renal function parameter.[358]

Patients Undergoing Dialysis

Patients with chronic (and at times acute) renal failure require renal replacement therapy, including conventional intermittent hemodialysis, peritoneal dialysis, and continuous renal replacement therapy (CRRT). CRRT includes a wide variety of techniques whose perioperative management has recently been reviewed (Table 35-18).[359] Although the primary indication for CRRT is acute renal failure, it can also be used for fluid clearance, correction of electrolyte abnormalities, and management of metabolic acidosis. It can be used in surgical patients without significant hemodynamic abnormalities. These patients may return to the operating room and their assessment and management may be complicated by the underlying disease and the use of systemic anticoagulation to prevent filter and circuit clotting. In patients undergoing intermittent treatment with hemodialysis or peritoneal dialysis, the procedure is discontinued before entering the operating room. For CRRT, the anesthesiologist must determine the appropriateness of discontinuing the therapy. With short procedures, the therapy can almost always be stopped and the arterial and venous ends of the circuit connected and run in the bypass mode. CRRT can also be used to manage fluids during surgery by changing the dialysate. If CRRT is continued, its effect on drug dosing must be recognized. In addition to effects on renal elimination of drugs, there are effects from changes in protein binding and volume of distribution, as well as drug removal effects from membrane permeability, membrane surface area, the ultrafiltration rate, and the dialysate flow rate.

Because a patient undergoing dialysis has already lost natural renal functioning, the emphasis in preoperative assessment shifts toward protecting other organ systems and optimally maintaining vascular access sites for cannulation. Usually, this does not require invasive monitoring. Emphasis is placed on intravascular fluid volume and electrolyte status, which can be ascertained by knowing when the patient last underwent dialysis, how much weight was normally gained or lost with dialysis, whether the fluid loss was peritoneal or intravascular, and what electrolyte composition the blood was dialyzed against. Although preoperative dialysis may benefit patients who have hyperkalemia, hypercalcemia, acidosis, neuropathy, and fluid overload, the resulting dysequilibrium between fluid and electrolytes can cause problems. Because hypovolemia induced by dialysis can lead to intraoperative hypotension, we try to avoid weight and fluid

Table 35-18 Characteristics of Renal Replacement Therapy

Renal Replacement Therapy	Blood Pump	Replacement Fluid (RF)/Dialysate (D)	Intraoperative Use
Conventional intermittent hemodialysis	Yes	D	No
Peritoneal dialysis	No	D	No
Slow continuous ultrafiltration	Yes/no	None	Yes
Continuous arteriovenous hemodialysis	No	D	No
Continuous arteriovenous hemodiafiltration	No	RF/D	No
Continuous venovenous hemofiltration	Yes	RF	Yes
Continuous venovenous hemodialysis	Yes	D	Yes
Continuous venovenous hemodiafiltration	Yes	RF/D	Yes

From Petroni KC, Cohen NH: Continuous renal replacement therapy: Anesthetic implications. Anesth Analg 94:1288-1297, 2002, with permission.

reduction in patients undergoing preoperative dialysis. In addition, hypopnea has been found to occur during and after dialysis when the dialysate contained acetate. Avoiding an acetate bathing solution may prevent this cause of hypoventilation.

Patients Who Have Received a Renal Transplant

More than 175,000 patients have received renal transplants (versus 300,000 currently undergoing dialysis in the United States). Approximately 50% are still alive, although a third must undergo dialysis (approximately 60,000 patients are now awaiting transplantation).[360] When these patients have subsequent surgery, the status of their renal function must be determined (i.e., whether they have normal renal function, insufficient but still functioning kidneys, or end-stage renal disease requiring hemodialysis). Descriptions of side effects from immunosuppressive drugs should also be sought. The drugs used preoperatively and intraoperatively to prevent acute rejection themselves have serious side effects that encourage close monitoring of blood glucose and cardiovascular function.[342,361] Because renal transplantation greatly increases the risk of infection, it is very important to avoid invasive monitoring and prevent patient cross-contamination.

Drugs in Patients with Renal Failure

Patients with renal azotemia have a threefold or higher risk of having an adverse drug reaction than those with normal renal function do.[362-364] The risk is increased by two conditions. (1) Excessive pharmacologic effects result from high levels of a drug or its metabolite (e.g., the metabolite of meperidine) in blood because of physiologic changes in target tissues induced by the uremic state. An example would be excessive sedation in a uremic patient with standard blood levels of sedative-hypnotic drugs. (2) Excessive administration of electrolytes with drugs also increases the risk of having an adverse drug reaction. For example, penicillin standardly has 1.7 mEq of potassium per 1 million units.[362-364] Administration of standard doses of drugs that depend on renal excretion for their elimination can result in drug accumulation and enhanced pharmacologic effect. Bennett and associates[362] have provided dosing guidelines for many drugs used by anesthesiologists for patients with and without renal failure. For example, patients with end-stage renal disease required significantly higher propofol doses to achieve the clinical end point of hypnosis than patients with normal renal function did.[364]

Infectious Disease

Because it is commonly recommended that no surgery except emergency or essential surgery (e.g., drainage of an abscess) be performed when an acute infectious disease is present and because renal insufficiency can be caused by antimicrobial drugs,[334,336,337] renal function and organ damage from renal insufficiency should be assessed preoperatively when infectious disease is present. Prophylactic administration of antibiotics (see Table 35-11) helps prevent sepsis from bacteremic interventions.[365] If therapeutic levels of an antibiotic are achieved and a reduction in fever occurs (presumably because of decreased levels of interleukin-2 released), spinal anesthesia might be considered by the anesthesiologist (using benefit-risk judgments) when an acute infectious disease is present.[366]

Sepsis is a leading cause of postoperative morbidity,[334,337] probably through a decrease in systemic vascular resistance related to activation of the complement system and other mediators. Thus, attention to the effects of antibiotic drugs must be supplemented by attention to intravascular volume status.[334-337,367,368] The degree of impairment of the infected organ and its effect on anesthesia should be assessed. For instance, endocarditis merits examination of volume status; antibiotic and other drug therapy and side effects[369]; myocardial function; and renal, pulmonary, neurologic, and hepatic function—organ systems that can be affected by endocarditis.

Although all surgery except emergency or essential operations is proscribed when an acute infectious disease is present (also see the section on upper respiratory infections in the pulmonary section of this chapter), many such diseases (e.g., influenza and pneumococcal pneumonia) and even inflammatory conditions are becoming less frequent because of successful immunization recommendations and programs.[370] Furthermore, even though acute infections are less common, surgery in patients with chronic viral diseases such as hepatitis and HIV infection is more frequent. Many of these patients may also harbor opportunistic infections such as tuberculosis or may have other systemic problems. Whether anesthesia or surgery, or both, exacerbates these infections or their systemic manifestations is not clear.

At least two other considerations merit preoperative consideration: patient isolation to prevent contamination of the patient and health care providers. Both concerns are real and are the focus of at least several published volumes. Nosocomial infection is a major source of postsurgical morbidity and has been radically reduced by consistent practices such as hand washing.[371,372] Acquired immunodeficiency syndrome (AIDS) and many forms of hepatitis (A, B, and C) appear to be due to viral infections but require direct contact with blood or body fluids. Screening for specific viruses or for the chronic end-organ effects of these viruses[373] is now being done to reduce the risk of infection to both recipients and health care personnel during blood transfusions. The usual precautions appear to be largely effective, but the risk is considerable if these precautions are not followed meticulously.[374]

Electrolyte Disorders

Disorders of calcium, magnesium, and phosphate balance were discussed in the section on diseases involving the endocrine system and disorders of nutrition (also see Chapters 34 and 49).

Hyponatremia and Hypernatremia

Electrolyte disorders are usually detected by determining the levels of electrolytes in serum. These concentrations reflect the balance between water and electrolytes. The osmolality of all body fluids is normally maintained within the narrow physiologic range of 285 to 290 mOsm/kg H_2O by integration of three key processes: thirst, release of ADH, and responsiveness of the medullary collecting ducts to ADH. Because of the permeability of biologic membranes, intracellular osmolality and extracellular osmolality are almost always equal and can be estimated by the following formula:

$$2[\mathrm{NA}^+](\mathrm{mEq/L}) + \frac{[\mathrm{Glucose}](\mathrm{mg/dL})}{18} + \frac{[\mathrm{BUN}](\mathrm{mg/dL})}{2.8} = \mathrm{mOsm/kg}$$

This formula will become easier to calculate when we convert fully to the Système International d'Unités (metric system) because millimoles (mmol) can be substituted for mg/(factor) in the above formula to read

$$2[\mathrm{Na}^{2+}] + [\mathrm{Glucose}] + [\mathrm{BUN}] = \mathrm{mOsm/kg}$$

with concentrations expressed in millimoles per liter (mmol/L). Although secretion of ADH is tightly controlled by osmotic stimuli at 285 to 290 mOsm/kg, the osmotic threshold for thirst is high (300 mOsm/kg), thus making this sign an important guide to volume deficiency.

Hyponatremia is perhaps the third most common fluid electrolyte abnormality in hospitalized patients. (Magnesium deficiency occurs in as many as 25% [see Chapter 54] and potassium deficiency, discussed later in this section, in as many as 10%.) Hyponatremia can occur in isotonic, hypertonic, or hypotonic forms. For example, isotonic hyponatremia can develop in protein or liquid accumulation states such as myeloma. Hypertonic hyponatremia can be present with hyperglycemia or with infusions of glycine (as in the TURP syndrome[375]). Hypotonic hyponatremia is the largest classification and is subdivided according to the status of the extracellular fluid into hypovolemic, isovolumic, or hypervolemic hypotonic hyponatremia. All three types require that excretion of renal water be impaired despite continued intake of dilute fluid. Common causes of hypovolemic hypotonic hyponatremia (Box 35-6) are GI losses[376] (vomiting, diarrhea), third-space losses (diuretics or salt-wasting nephropathy), or adrenal insufficiency. Hypervolemic hypotonic hyponatremic states complicate severe cardiac failure,[377] cirrhosis, nephrotic syndrome, or renal failure and are characterized by retention of sodium with disproportionately larger amounts of water.

The more common isovolumic hypotonic hyponatremia is caused by retention of water without sodium. Because edema is not usually clinically apparent, such patients appear isovolumic. Edema is most often caused by SIADH, which in turn may be caused by CNS or pulmonary tumors or dysfunction. Secretion of ADH increases with age, thus rendering the elderly more prone to hyponatremia. Drugs that potentiate the secretion of ADH (tricyclic antidepressants and vincristine) or its effects on the medullary collecting duct system in the kidney (nonsteroidal anti-inflammatory drugs and chlorpropamide) or that have similar effects (oxytocin) may be more likely to cause hyponatremia in the elderly. To establish the diagnosis of SIADH, the physician should determine that the patient is free of renal and cardiac dysfunction, has normal adrenal and thyroid function, and is normovolemic. Urine osmolality would then be found to exceed 100 mOsm/kg, serum osmolality would be low, and urine sodium excretion would be higher than 20 mEq/L (20 mOsm/L).

Disturbances in serum sodium therefore reflect alterations in glucose metabolism, renal function, or accumulation of body water. The last can be affected by disturbances in thirst, release of ADH, and renal function. Thus, hyponatremia reflects a relative excess of free water and can occur when total-body sodium

Box 35-6 Types and Causes of Hypotonic Hyponatremia*

Hypovolemic
Gastrointestinal losses
- Vomiting
- Diarrhea

Skin losses
Third-space losses
Lung losses
Renal losses
- Diuretics
- Renal damage
- Urinary tract obstruction

Adrenal insufficiency

Isovolemic
Syndrome of inappropriate secretion of antidiuretic hormone
Renal failure
Water intoxication
Hypokalemia
Dysfunctional osmostat

Hypervolemic
Congestive heart failure
Nephrosis
Liver dysfunction

*Serum osmolality less than 280 mOsm/L.

increases (as in edematous disorders), when total-body sodium is normal (as in excess of free water because of SIADH), or when total-body sodium decreases (as occurs with too aggressive use of diuretic drugs). Definition of the cause defines the treatment. For instance, water restriction is the mainstay of therapy for SIADH. Administration of demeclocycline is another option that corrects SIADH by inducing a reversible nephrogenic diabetes insipidus. The anesthesiologist is faced with the question of what levels of electrolytes require treatment before anesthesia. Although slowly developing hyponatremia usually produces few symptoms, the patient may be lethargic and apathetic. Chronic hyponatremia is better tolerated than acute hyponatremia because of mechanisms regulating intracellular fluid volume that alleviate brain edema; the loss of other solutes from cells decreases the osmotic movement of water into cells. Nonetheless, severe chronic hyponatremia (i.e., serum sodium levels <123 mEq/L) can cause brain edema.

By contrast, acute hyponatremia may be manifested by severe symptoms requiring emergency treatment: profound cerebral edema with obtundation, coma, convulsions, and disordered reflexes and thermoregulatory control.[99,100,378] Depending on the cause and relative total sodium and water content, treatment can range from the administration of hypertonic saline or mannitol (with or without diuretic drugs) to restriction of fluids or administration of other drugs.[99,100,378] Because neurologic damage may develop if the serum sodium concentration is increased too rapidly, the rate of increase should not exceed 1 mEq/L/hr.[99,100,378] After the serum sodium concentration has reached 125 mEq/L, therapy may consist of water restriction; more rapid correction may result in CNS demyelination.[99,100,378] In hyponatremic patients who have excess total-body water secondary to SIADH, serum levels can be corrected by giving furosemide, 1 mg/kg, and hypertonic saline to replace the loss of electrolytes in urine.[99,100,378] The diagnosis of SIADH is discussed earlier in this chapter (see the section "Pituitary Abnormalities").

Neither acute nor chronic hyponatremia necessitates restoration of serum sodium to normal levels; brain swelling usually disappears at a serum sodium level of 130 mEq/L. This leaves us with the question of what levels of serum sodium make anesthesia more risky. Because no data exist to answer this question, to allow for some error in caring for patients, we have arbitrarily chosen a flexible concentration of 131 mEq/L as the lower sodium limit for elective surgery.

Hypernatremia occurs much less commonly than hyponatremia. It is often iatrogenic in origin (e.g., it can be caused by failure to provide sufficient free water to a patient who is unconscious or who has had a recent stroke-induced deficit of the thirst mechanism) and can occur in the presence of low, normal, or excess total-body sodium. The primary symptoms of hypernatremia relate to brain cell shrinkage. Because too rapid correction of hypernatremia can lead to cerebral edema and convulsions, correction should be made gradually. Again, with no data to support this stance, we believe that all patients undergoing surgery should have serum sodium concentrations of less than 150 mEq/L before anesthesia.

Hypokalemia and Hyperkalemia

Hypokalemia and hyperkalemia are also discussed in Chapters 34 and 54. The relationship between the measured potassium concentration in serum and total-body potassium stores can best be described with a scattergram. Only 2% of total-body potassium is stored in plasma (4200 mEq in cells and 60 mEq in extracellular fluid). In normal persons, 75% of the 50 to 60 mEq/L of total-body potassium is stored in skeletal muscle, 6% in red blood cells, and 5% in the liver. Thus, a 20% to 25% change in potassium levels in plasma could represent a change in total-body potassium of 1000 mEq or more if the change were chronic or as little as 10 to 20 mEq if the change were acute.

As with serum sodium levels,[99,100,378] acute changes in serum potassium levels appear to be less well tolerated than chronic changes. Chronic changes are relatively well tolerated because of the equilibration of serum and intracellular stores that takes place over time to return the resting membrane potential of excitable cells to nearly normal levels.

Hyperkalemia can result from factitious elevation of potassium (as in red blood cell hemolysis); excessive exogenous potassium from sources such as salt substitutes or, in large amounts, bananas; cellular shifts in potassium (as a result of metabolic acidosis, tissue and muscle damage after burns, use of depolarizing muscle relaxants, or intense catabolism of protein); and decreased renal excretion (as occurs in renal failure, renal insufficiency with trauma, and therapy with potassium-sparing diuretic drugs, especially when combined with ACE inhibitors or mineralocorticoid deficiency).[379-381] Factitious hyperkalemia can occur when a tourniquet is left on too long or even by simple fist clenching.[382]

The major danger in anesthetizing patients who have disorders in potassium balance appears to be abnormal cardiac function—that is, both electrical disturbance[379] and poor cardiac contractility. Hyperkalemia lowers the resting membrane potential of excitable cardiac cells and decreases the duration of the myocardial action potential and upstroke velocity. This decreased rate of ventricular depolarization, plus the beginning of repolarization in some areas of the myocardium while other areas are still undergoing depolarization, produces a progressively widening QRS complex that merges with the T wave into a sine wave on the ECG.

Above a potassium level of 6.7 mEq/L, the degree of hyperkalemia and the duration of the QRS complex correlate well.[379] This correlation is even better than the correlation between the serum potassium level and T-wave changes. Nevertheless, the earliest manifestations of hyperkalemia are narrowing and peaking of the T wave. Though not diagnostic of hyperkalemia, T waves are almost invariably peaked and narrow when serum potassium levels are 7 to 9 mEq/L. When serum potassium levels exceed 7 mEq/L, atrial conduction disturbances appear, as manifested by a decrease in P-wave amplitude and an increase in the PR interval. Supraventricular tachycardia, atrial fibrillation, PVCs, ventricular tachycardia, ventricular fibrillation, or sinus arrest may all occur.

The ECG and cardiac alterations associated with hyperkalemia are potentiated by low serum levels of calcium and sodium. Intravenous administration of saline, bicarbonate, glucose with insulin (1 U/2 g glucose), and calcium can reverse these changes by shifting some extracellular potassium into the cell.

β-Adrenergic stimuli also cause redistribution of potassium into the cell. Indeed, the plasma potassium concentration measured in samples immediately before surgery is usually 0.2 to 0.8 mEq/L lower than that measured during the less stressful period 1 to 3 days before surgery.[383] β-Adrenergic receptor blocking drugs such as propranolol can be used to prevent such an effect preoperatively. A β-adrenergic receptor stimulating agent (20 mg of nebulized albuterol for a 70-kg patient) can be used to treat hyperkalemia when it occurs; it decreases potassium levels 1.0 mEq/L within 30 minutes, and its effect lasts 2 hours.[384] Although nebulized β_2-agonists effectively lower plasma potassium concentrations by stimulating sodium- and potassium-dependent adenosine triphosphatase, this therapy should be used as an adjunct to rather than a substitute for more established measures. Kayexalate (sodium polystyrene sulfonate) enemas can be given to bind potassium in the gut in exchange for sodium. Dialysis against a hypokalemic solution will also decrease serum potassium levels. However, in a hyperkalemic patient, hypoventilation can be dangerous during anesthesia because each 0.1 change in pH can produce a 0.4- to 1.5-mEq/L change in serum potassium levels in the opposite direction. For example, if pH decreases from 7.4 to 7.3, serum potassium levels could increase from 5.5 to 6.5 mEq/L.

Hypokalemia can be caused by inadequate intake of potassium, excessive GI loss (through diarrhea, vomiting, nasopharyngeal suctioning, chronic use of laxatives, or ingestion of cation exchange resins, as in certain wines), excessive renal loss (because of the use of diuretic drugs, renal tubular acidosis, chronic chloride deficiency, metabolic alkalosis, mineralocorticoid excess, excessive ingestion of licorice, use of antibiotics, ureterosigmoidostomy, and diabetic ketoacidosis), and shifts of potassium from extracellular to intracellular compartments (as occurs in alkalosis, insulin administration, administration of a β-adrenergic agonist or stress, barium poisoning, and periodic paralysis). As with hyperkalemia, knowledge of the cause of the potassium deficiency and appropriate preoperative evaluation and treatment of that cause may be as important as treatment of the deficiency itself. Also like hyperkalemia, hypokalemia may reflect small or vast changes in total-body potassium. Acute hypokalemia may be much less well tolerated than chronic hypokalemia. The major worrisome manifestations of hypokalemia pertain to the circulatory system, both the cardiac and peripheral components. In addition, chronic hypokalemia results in muscle weakness, hypoperistalsis, and nephropathy.

Cardiovascular manifestations of hypokalemia include autonomic neuropathy, which results in orthostatic hypotension and decreased sympathetic reserve; impaired myocardial contractility; and electrical conduction abnormalities, which can result in sinus tachycardia, atrial and ventricular arrhythmias, and disturbances in intraventricular conduction that can progress to ventricular fibrillation. In addition to arrhythmias, the ECG shows widening of the QRS complex, ST-segment abnormalities, progressive diminution of the T-wave amplitude, and a progressive increase in the U-wave amplitude. Surawicz[379] found these changes to be invariably present when serum potassium levels decreased to below 2.3 mEq/L. Although U waves are not specific for hypokalemia, they are sensitive indicators of the condition. Replenishing the total-body potassium deficit for a depletion reflected by a serum deficit of 1 mEq/L (e.g., from 3.3 to 4.3 mEq/L) may require 1000 mEq of potassium. Even if this amount could be given instantaneously (and it should not be replenished at a rate exceeding 250 mEq/day), it would take 24 to 48 hours to equilibrate in all tissues. Potassium-depleted myocardium is unusually sensitive to digoxin, calcium, and most important, potassium. Rapid potassium infusion in a hypokalemic patient can produce arrhythmias as severe as those produced by hypokalemia itself.[385] One potential strategy to prevent hypokalemia from anxiety and stress includes premedication with clonidine.[386]

Thus, the decision to proceed with surgery and anesthesia in the face of acute or chronic depletions or excesses of potassium depends on many factors.[387-392] It is essential to know the cause and treatment of the underlying condition creating the electrolyte imbalance and the effect of that imbalance on perioperative risk and physiologic processes. The urgency of the operation, the degree of electrolyte abnormality, the medications given, the acid-base balance, and the suddenness or persistence of the electrolyte disturbance are all considerations. For example, one small study of patients undergoing vascular access procedures with preoperative potassium levels of greater than 6 mmol/L demonstrated no adverse outcomes.[390] Similarly, in a cohort study in which 38 patients had a preoperative potassium level higher than 5.5 mEq/L, there were no dysrhythmias or major morbidity associated with the use of succinylcholine.[391]

Retrospective epidemiologic studies attribute significant risk to the administration of potassium (even chronic oral administration).[387] In one study, 1910 of 16,048 consecutive hospitalized patients were given oral potassium supplements. Of these 1910 patients, hyperkalemia contributed to death in 7, and the incidence of complications of potassium therapy was 1 in 250. Armed with such data, many internists do not prescribe oral potassium therapy for patients given diuretic drugs. Yet these patients frequently become moderately hypokalemic.[393] Modest hypokalemia occurs in 10% to 50% of patients given diuretic drugs. Should surgery be delayed to subject such patients to the risks of potassium therapy?

Three studies investigated whether modest hypokalemia was a problem by prospectively seeking arrhythmias on the ECGs of patients who had various preoperative levels of potassium.[388,389,392] No difference in the incidence of arrhythmias occurred in 25 normokalemic ($K > 3.4$ mEq/L) patients, 25 moderately hypokalemic ($K = 3$ to 3.4 mEq/L) patients, and 10 severely hypokalemic ($K < 2.9$ mEq/L) patients.[388] Wahr and coauthors studied 2402 patients undergoing elective CABG and reported that a serum potassium level less than 3.5 mmol/L was a predictor of serious perioperative arrhythmia (OR, 2.2; 95% CI, 1.2 to 4.0), intraoperative arrhythmia (OR, 2.0; 95% CI, 1.0 to 3.6), and postoperative atrial fibrillation/flutter (OR, 1.7; 95% CI, 1.0 to 2.7).[392] The inability of the eye to pick up these changes—or even the inability of Holter recordings for short periods (which seem not to have been used in this study)—points to the need for confirming studies.

Other studies indicate that modest hypokalemia can have severe consequences.[393,394] Holland and coworkers[394] treated 21 patients with 50 mg of hydrochlorothiazide twice a day for 4 weeks. These patients had a history of becoming hypokalemic during diuretic therapy; none of them had cardiac disease or was taking other medications. Before and after diuretic therapy, 24-hour ambulatory ECGs were recorded. This study is also subject to the limitations of Holter monitoring. Ventricular ectopy, including complex ventricular ectopy (multifocal PVCs, ventricular couplets, ventricular tachycardia), developed in 7 of the 21 patients (33%). Potassium repletion decreased the number of ectopic ventricular beats per patient from 71.2 to 5.4/hr. Apparently, some patients are sensitive to even minor potassium depletion. In the Multiple Risk Factor Intervention Trial involving 361,662 patients, more than 2000 of whom were treated for hypertension with diuretics, the reduction in serum potassium after diuretic therapy was greater in those with PVCs.[393] Although we recommend that hypokalemic patients be given potassium supplements, the merit of this practice is unclear.

Our personal criteria for preoperative potassium therapy are as follows. As a rule, all patients undergoing elective surgery should have normal serum potassium levels. However, we do not recommend delaying surgery if the serum potassium level is above 2.8 mEq/L or below 5.9 mEq/L, if the cause of the potassium imbalance is known, and if the patient is in otherwise optimal condition. This range of safe potassium levels is arbitrary and has changed from 3.3 in 1979, to 3.1 in 1986, to 2.9 in 1990 on the lower side and from 5.6 in 1979, to 5.7 in 1986, to 5.9 in 1990 on the upper side as more data have become available on the safety of preoperative hypokalemia and the dangers of replacing potassium in a hospital environment.[387] We subject all patients with end-stage renal failure to dialysis (using the same arbitrary safe range) before all surgical procedures except truly emergency ones (as in instances of imminent exsanguination). In studies on dogs in 1978, Tanifuji and Eger[395] determined the relationships between electrolyte status and anesthetic requirements that may require intraoperative consideration: hyponatremia and hypo-osmolality decreased the minimum alveolar concentration (MAC), hypernatremia increased MAC, and hyperkalemia did not affect the anesthetic requirement.

Gastrointestinal and Liver Diseases

Gastrointestinal Disease

Preoperative Search for Diverse Associated Disorders in Gastrointestinal Disease

Although preoperative preparation of the GI tract is usually the responsibility of the surgeon and although the GI tract frequently does not need to be extensively evaluated by the anesthesiologist, GI disease can and often does cause derangements in many or all other systems. Such disturbances can affect the safety of anesthesia for the patient. Thus, the anesthesiologist may need to not only optimize the patient's condition through extensive preoperative preparation but also have knowledge of disease processes and their effects to guide the patient smoothly through the perioperative period. The major advances of correcting fluid and electrolyte disorders and optimizing nutritional status before surgery now allow surgery to be performed in patients with GI disease previously deemed to be at too great a risk and may have lessened the risk for others.[45-47,396] Still, in patients with GI disease, thorough assessment of intravascular fluid volume, electrolyte concentrations, and nutrition is essential, including an evaluation of the supervening side effects of these therapies (e.g., hypophosphatemia from parenteral nutrition, hyperkalemia or cardiac arrhythmias from too vigorous treatment of hypokalemia, and CHF from too rapid or too vigorous treatment of hypovolemia).

In addition to the vast alterations in fluids, electrolytes, and nutrition that can occur with such diverse GI diseases as neoplasms and pancreatitis, patients with GI disorders can have gastroesophageal reflux disease,[397] bowel obstruction, vomiting, or hypersecretion of acid. These effects may merit rapid induction of anesthesia with the application of cricoid pressure or awake endotracheal intubation, preoperative nasogastric suctioning, or preoperative use of histamine receptor blocking agents. Clotting abnormalities may need to be corrected because fat-soluble vitamin K (often malabsorbed) is necessary for the synthesis of factors V, VII, IX, and X in the liver (also see Chapter 56). Liver disease is often associated with GI disease and, if severe enough, can also result in a deficiency of clotting factors synthesized by the liver.

Other factors should be remembered in the perioperative management of any patient with GI disease. First, closed spaces containing gas expand by absorbing nitrous oxide. Such expansion can lead to ischemic injury, rupture of GI viscera, or both. Second, GI surgery predisposes the patient to sepsis; sepsis and decreased peripheral vascular resistance can lead to massive fluid requirements, cardiac failure, and renal insufficiency. Recently, the surgical site infection rate has been declining. This decrease may be attributable to the use of better technique, more appropriate prophylactic timing and use of antibiotics, better nutrition, less invasive (laparoscopic and endoscopic) surgery, maintenance of normothermia, or surgical resection of even solid tumors.[398-402] Third, patients with GI disease may have many other associated disorders not directly related to the GI tract. For example, they may be anemic from deficiencies in iron, intrinsic factor, folate, or vitamin B_{12}. They may also manifest neurologic changes from combined-system disease. Respiration may be impaired because of heavy cigarette smoking, peritonitis, abscess, pulmonary obstruction, previous incisions, aspiration, or pulmonary embolism (as occurs with ulcerative colitis or with thrombophlebitis in the bedridden). These patients may also have hepatitis, cholangitis, side effects from antibiotic drugs or other medications, massive bleeding with anemia and shock, or psychological derangements.

Because GI disease can be accompanied by so many diverse associated disorders, the clinician must clearly search for involvement of other systems and preoperatively assess and treat such disorders appropriately. Discussion of two specific diseases, ulcerative colitis and carcinoid tumor, will highlight the importance of involvement of other systems in GI disease.

Ulcerative Colitis and Carcinoid Tumors as Examples of Gastrointestinal Disease Affecting Other Systems

Patients with ulcerative colitis often have psychological problems. They may also have phlebitis; deficiencies in iron, folate, or vitamin B_{12}; anemia; or clotting disorders caused by malabsorption. They may be malnourished or dehydrated or have electrolyte abnormalities. In addition, ulcerative colitis can be accompanied by massive bleeding, bowel obstruction or perforation or toxic megacolon causing respiratory compromise, hepatitis, arthritis, iritis, spondylitis, or diabetes secondary to pancreatitis.

The site of origin of carcinoid tumors in more than 75% of patients is the GI tract. Within the GI tract, carcinoid tumors have been documented to occur from the esophagus to the rectum. The most frequent site is the appendix, but carcinoids in this location rarely, if ever metastasize or produce carcinoid syndrome. Tumors arising in the ileocecal region have the highest incidence of metastases. Carcinoid tumors originating from sites other than the GI tract, such as the head and neck, lung, gonads, thymus, breast, and urinary tract, have also been reported. Cardiac involvement, though frequently reported, is usually limited to right-sided valvular and myocardial plaque formation.[403]

Not all patients with carcinoid tumors have symptoms attributable to secretion of hormone by the tumor. Some can, however, and unexpected carcinoid can be manifested during surgery by hypersecretion of gastric fluid. The most comprehensive series in the literature indicates that only 7% of patients have carcinoid syndrome, which typically consists of flushing, diarrhea, and valvular heart disease. Of those with the syndrome, approximately 74% have cutaneous flushing; 68%, intestinal hypermotility; 41%, cardiac symptoms; and 18%, wheezing. Factors influencing symptoms include the location of the tumor and the specific hormones produced and secreted. Although it is generally believed that if patients do not exhibit carcinoid syndrome, the tumors are not producing serotonin (5-hydroxytryptamine [5-HT]), but such may not be the case. Approximately 50% of patients with carcinoid tumors of the GI tract demonstrate evidence of 5-HT production as manifested by elevated urinary levels of 5-hydroxyindoleacetic acid (5-HIAA), a metabolic product of 5-HT. Carcinoid syndrome is usually associated with ileal carcinoid tumors that have metastasized to the liver. Presumably, the liver clears mediators released from the tumor. Impairment of this clearing ability by the metastatic tumor results in carcinoid syndrome.

Most patients with carcinoid tumors and increased urinary 5-HIAA have typical carcinoid tumors originating from the midgut (ileum or jejunum). These patients excrete only small amounts of 5-hydroxytryptophan (5-HTP). Patients with atypical carcinoid tumors that originate in the foregut (bronchus, stomach, and pancreas) excrete large amounts of 5-HT and 5-HTP, as well as moderately higher amounts of 5-HIAA.

Although it is generally agreed that 5-HT is responsible for the diarrhea experienced by patients with carcinoid tumors, other neurohumoral agents may contribute to the flushing and hypotension, including dopamine, histamine, and some of the neuropeptides such as substance P, neurotensin, vasoactive intestinal peptide, and somatostatin.

The net physiologic effect of circulating 5-HT represents a composite of both direct action (mediated by 5-HT receptors) and indirect action (mediated through modulation of adrenergic neurotransmission). The existence of several subtypes of 5-HT receptors may account for the different effects of 5-HT on various serotonin-sensitive tissue beds. Indirect actions are effected through alterations in catecholamine release and depend on the level of circulating 5-HT.

5-HT has little if any direct effect on the heart. With elevated levels, however, positive chronotropic and inotropic myocardial effects may occur, mediated by the release of noradrenaline (norepinephrine). Effects of serotonin on the vasculature include both vasoconstriction and vasodilation.

Alterations in GI function attributed to 5-HT include increased motility and net intestinal secretion of water, sodium chloride, and potassium. 5-HT reportedly causes bronchoconstriction in many animals, but rarely in humans. Asthmatics are a possible exception. Carcinoid tumors are frequently manifested as diarrhea with fluid and electrolyte abnormalities. Because these tumors secrete vasoactive substances, patients can exhibit hypotension or hypertension along with the flush associated with release of vasoactive substances. Vasoactive substances can be released from the tumor by any number of substances, including catecholamines. Until the 1990s, management of patients with this tumor was a real challenge for the anesthesiologist. Thus, anesthesiologists of that era had to tread a fine line between avoiding substances known to release 5-HT (e.g., *d*-tubocurarine and morphine) and inducing anesthesia so light that painful stimuli activate a sympathetic stress response.[404] The anesthesiologist also needed to be ready and able to treat hypotension, decreased peripheral vascular resistance, bronchospasm, and hypertension. α-Adrenergic receptor blockade with the phenothiazines, butyrophenones, or phenoxybenzamine and β-adrenergic receptor blockade with propranolol have been advocated to prevent catecholamine-mediated release of vasoactive substances. These practices, however, can lead to hypotension. Nevertheless, the difficulty in managing carcinoid syndrome seemed to change with the availability of a somatostatin analog. In fact, somatostatin is now such a powerful inhibitor of the release of peptides from carcinoid tumors and an inhibitor of the peptic effects on receptor cells that it is the therapy of choice for preoperative, intraoperative, and postoperative management of carcinoid symptoms and crises.[404,405] In cardiac surgical patients there has been a reduction in mortality over time, and vasopressors were shown to be safe in conjunction with octreotide.[406] However, the ease of management of most patients[404,405,407-410] should not lull the anesthesiologist into being unprepared—in fact, somatostatin has caused problems of its own and has failed to prevent severe hypotension and bronchospasm.[411,412]

In patients with severe hypotension that is not treatable with somatostatin, the drug of choice is either angiotensin or vasopressin. (Angiotensin is not commercially available in the United States.) However, the vasoactive substances released by carcinoid tumors cause fibrosis of the heart valves that often results in pulmonic stenosis or tricuspid insufficiency. To increase cardiac output in a patient with tricuspid insufficiency, the anesthesiologist should avoid drugs or situations that increase pulmonary vascular resistance (e.g., angiotensin, vasopressin, acidosis, hypercapnia, hypothermia). In addition, the production of large amounts of 5-HT (equal to 200 mg/day of 5-HIAA) can lead to the development of niacin deficiency with pellagra (as occurs with diarrhea, dermatitis, and dementia).

Acute elevation of plasma kinin activity in carcinoid patients has been postulated for many years as the explanation for the symptoms of carcinoid syndrome. The physiologic effects of kinins are known to include vasodilation of smaller resistance vessels and stimulation of the release of histamine from mast cells. The latter action potentiates their own vasodilating properties and further reduces systolic and diastolic BP. In addition, increases in vascular permeability may lead to edema. Kinins are not known to affect the myocardium directly.

Steroids have been effective in treating the symptoms of bronchial carcinoid tumors. Although prophylactic preoperative administration and intraoperative therapeutic use have been described, controlled studies of beneficial effects are lacking. Aprotinin, like steroids, inhibits the kallikrein cascade. This drug is capable of blocking the proteinase activity of kallikrein, and some reports have described a dramatic clinical response.

A subset of patients with symptoms of carcinoid syndrome excrete histamine at increased levels in their urine. Histamine causes vasodilation of small blood vessels, which leads to flushing and decreased total peripheral resistance. Histamine is known to cause bronchoconstriction, particularly in patients with bronchial asthma and other pulmonary diseases. Its role in carcinoid bronchospasm, if any, is uncertain. Histamine receptor blocking drugs have been used with some success in alleviating the flushing associated with carcinoid syndrome. H_2 antagonism alone was found to be just as effective as combination therapy in preventing symptoms; pure H_1 antagonism, however, was ineffective. These therapies have been relegated to a second-line defense since the use of somatostatin.

Catecholamines aggravate the symptoms of carcinoid syndrome, presumably by stimulating release of hormone by the tumor. The mechanism by which this release occurs remains obscure. Adrenergic receptors have not been demonstrated in carcinoid tumors, nor do these tumors usually have neural innervation. Perhaps adrenergic stimuli work through their mechanical effects on the gut and vessels to stimulate the release of tumor products. Treatment of patients with carcinoid tumors by means of α- and β-adrenergic antagonists has been beneficial in ameliorating flushing in some instances but ineffective in others.

The results of prospective studies on somatostatin to ameliorate the symptoms of carcinoid syndrome have been dramatic. Somatostatin appears to be a major advancement in the treatment of carcinoid syndrome.

It might logically be concluded that preoperative preparation of a patient with carcinoid syndrome would be similar to that for a patient with pheochromocytoma: titration of adrenergic, histaminic, and serotonergic receptor blocking drugs to maximum effect while monitoring intravascular volume status and adding somatostatin before surgery. Although this approach is logical, preoperative symptoms do not correlate with perioperative symptoms, and only the last two therapeutic options (optimization of intravascular fluid status and administration of somatostatin) are most effective.

Bronchospasm with or without flushing also develops in many patients when vasoactive substances are released. Thus, a patient with carcinoid tumor may be well or may be severely incapacitated by pulmonary, neurologic, nutritional, fluid, electrolytic, or cardiovascular disturbances. Therefore, although the GI system in itself may not require extensive preoperative preparation, GI disease can cause disturbances in any or all other systems that require extensive preoperative preparation to optimize the patient's condition plus preoperative knowledge of physiology and the effects of diseases to guide patients through the perioperative period smoothly. In addition, the anesthesiologist's understanding of the nature of the surgery probably aids in determining the system involvement caused by the GI disorder.

Another perioperative consideration is that patients with GI diseases (perhaps even more so than those with other diseases) have had to endure the psychosocial trauma of having to live with their disease for long periods or the necessity of facing such a prospect.[413] They need emotional support and holistic kindnesses as much as, if not more than others, without sacrificing scientific rigor in the treatment of their condition. Obtaining relevant psychological data while gathering medical information, sitting (not standing) while taking the history, and empathizing with the patient about how difficult it must be to accomplish tasks with this disease (stressing accomplishments, we have found) legitimize the physician's interests in and support of the patient's pain and other psychosocial issues. The time spent sitting and talking with the patient also allows the anesthesiologist to discuss options for pain therapy with the patient, why systemic morphine might be avoided in a patient with a fresh bowel anastomosis,[414] and other issues that show the anesthesiologist to be both a competent physician and particularly concerned with that patient's well-being. In addition to an appreciation of the organic effects of their disease, attention to emotional support of these patients perioperatively presents opportunities to use one's full skills as a physician to bring about healing.

Liver Disease

What are the risks of giving anesthesia to patients with acute liver disease who require emergency surgery? What are the risks of giving anesthesia to patients with chronic impairment of liver function? What can be done to minimize these risks? Although one might think that the experiences gained from providing anesthesia for liver transplantation would answer many of these questions, there is a substantial difference between optimizing cardiovascular function to meet the needs of a new liver (e.g., supply of nutrients) and maintaining liver function in a diseased liver. Because hepatic function and physiology are discussed in Chapter 17 and the preoperative evaluation is reviewed in Chapter 34, we will mention only that the liver performs many functions: it synthesizes substances (e.g., proteins, clotting factors), detoxifies the body of both drugs and the products of normal human metabolism, excretes waste products, and stores and supplies energy.

Hematologic Disorders and Oncologic Disease

Hematologic Disorders

Anemia and Polycythemia

Chapters 55 and 57 discuss the evidence that normovolemic anemia or polycythemia increases perioperative morbidity. The results indicate that knowledge and pretreatment of polycythemia might decrease perioperative morbidity and mortality.

Except for patients with ischemic heart disease (see later), no such evidence exists for normovolemic anemia.[415] Thus, there are no specific preoperative routines for anemia itself, except regarding patients who have or are likely to have ischemic heart disease (as determined by risk factors).[416-418] For these patients, hematocrits above or below 29% to 34% were found in two separate studies to be associated with increased episodes of myocardial ischemia after vascular surgery (Fig. 35-10).[178] For patients at risk for current ischemic heart disease, data indicate that transfusion to a hematocrit level of 29% to 34% may be appropriate (also, see the earlier section on cardiovascular diseases).[419,420] It should be remembered that anemia is a reduction in circulatory erythrocyte mass below the range of values considered normal for persons of the same sex at the same location (age older than 6 months, race, and ethnic background do not explain anemia). Each erythrocyte lives for approximately 120 days; therefore, replacement of 15 to 20 mL of senescent cells needs to be accomplished in the absence of diseases that destroy or cause loss of blood cells. Moreover, the symptoms of anemia—headache, weakness, exertional dyspnea, and loss of endurance—do not provide much information about the severity, rapidity of onset, and cardiorespiratory effects of the underlying cause of the anemia.

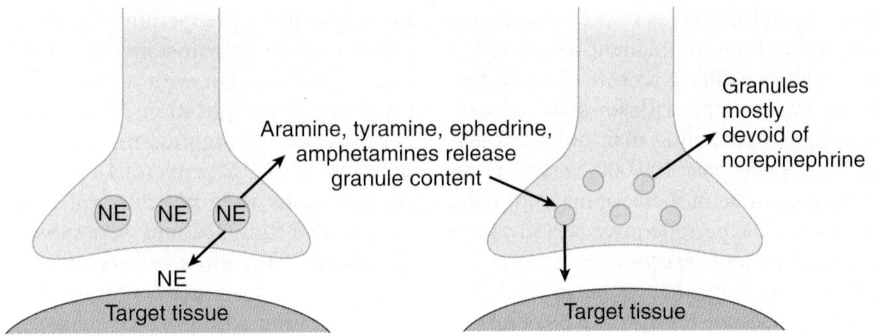

Figure 35-10 Antihypotensive drugs such as metaraminol (Aramine), tyramine, and ephedrine create their effect by releasing catecholamines from granules of the nerve terminal. Therefore, when treatment with drugs such as methyldopa, reserpine, or guanethidine depletes store of norepinephrine (NE) in the granules, little NE remains for release, and the antihypotensive drugs have been rendered ineffective.

Furthermore, because anemia can be a hallmark of many other diseases possibly affecting perioperative anesthetic management, the preoperative presence of anemia requires a search for and treatment of the underlying cause. For instance, anemia could indicate renal insufficiency or a drug reaction, both of which could alter anesthetic management. For this reason, the cause of the anemia should be known preoperatively. Similarly, polycythemia can be a primary disease (e.g., polycythemia vera), or it can be secondary to smoking, the use of diuretic drugs, chronic use of androgens, hypoxia, or other forms of chronic lung/heart disease. Phlebotomies are quite effective for patients with mild polycythemia. Cerebral blood flow improves when the hematocrit is kept below 45%. No prospective controlled study has been performed on humans regarding a possible decrease in perioperative morbidity or wound healing[178,416-418] as a result of perioperative treatment of anemia or polycythemia, although a National Institutes of Health–sponsored trial in hip fracture patients is ongoing. The time of most danger to the patient may be the early recovery room period, during which time oxygen delivery to the lungs is perhaps at its worst.[178] Options for alternatives to blood therapy are discussed in Chapters 55 and 57.

Erythropoietin is one of the substances necessary for normal production of red blood cells. Production and secretion of erythropoietin from the peritubular cells of the kidney are stimulated by tissue hypoxia. Signal transduction of this hypoxic stimulus depends on a heme-containing oxygen-sensing protein that mediates changes in the stability of messenger RNA from chromosome 7 in erythropoietin-producing cells. Erythropoietin triggers quiescent, early erythroid progenitor cells into cycle by acting like a mitogen and facilitating differentiation into late committed erythroid progenitor cells. In normoxic individuals, synthesis of erythropoietin is not stimulated until the concentration of hemoglobin falls below 10.5 g/dL. In severe anemia, erythropoietin levels can increase more than 1000-fold. Iron, folic acid, and vitamin B_{12} are also needed for normal maturation of erythrocytes. Several forms of anemia present special situations, such as sickle cell anemia, hereditary spherocytosis, and the autoimmune hemolytic anemias.

Sickle Cell Anemia and Related Hemoglobinopathies

The sickle cell syndromes constitute a family of hemoglobinopathies caused by abnormal genetic transformation of amino acids in the heme portion of the hemoglobin molecule. The sickle cell syndromes arise from a mutation in the β-globin gene that changes the sixth amino acid from valine to glutamic acid. A major pathologic feature of sickle cell disease is the aggregation of irreversibly sickled cells in blood vessels. The molecular basis of sickling is the aggregation of deoxygenated hemoglobin B molecules along their longitudinal axis.[421] This abnormal aggregation distorts the cell membrane and thereby produces a sickle shape. Irreversibly sickled cells become dehydrated and rigid and can cause tissue infarcts by impeding blood flow and oxygen to tissues.[421-424] Some have challenged this hypothesis, with several studies showing enhanced adhesion of sickled erythrocytes to vascular endothelium.[425] Some other abnormal hemoglobins interact with hemoglobin S to various degrees and give rise to symptomatic disease in patients heterozygous for hemoglobin S and one of the other hemoglobins such as the hemoglobin of thalassemia (hemoglobin C).

Three tenths of 1% of the African American population in the United States have sickle cell–thalassemia disease (hemoglobin SC); these patients also have end-organ disease and symptoms suggestive of organ infarction. For these patients, perioperative considerations should be similar to those for patients with sickle cell disease (hemoglobin SS), discussed later.

Whereas 8% to 10% of African Americans have the sickle cell trait (hemoglobin AS), 0.2% are homozygous for sickle cell hemoglobin and have sickle cell anemia. Sickle cell trait is a heterozygous condition in which the individual has one βS globin gene and one βA globin gene, which results in the production of both hemoglobin S and hemoglobin A, with a predominance of hemoglobin A. Sickle cell trait should not be considered a disease because hemoglobin AS cells begin to sickle only when the oxygen saturation of hemoglobin is below 20%. No difference has been found between normal persons (those with hemoglobin AA) and those with hemoglobin AS regarding survival rates or the incidence of severe disease, with one exception: patients with hemoglobin AS have a 50% increase in pulmonary infarction. However, single case reports of a perioperative death and a perioperative brain infarct in two patients with hemoglobin AS disease do exist, and a report of death believed to be due to aortocaval compression during general anesthesia that resulted in a sickling crisis does exist.[426] The need for exchange transfusion before cardiac surgery has been debated.[427,428] Frequent measurement of oxygen saturation (pulse oximetry) in multiple areas of the body is recommended, including the ear and toe in pregnant patients.[426] A retrospective review of exercise in military recruits showed that soldiers with sickle cell trait had a higher risk for sudden death after extreme exertion during basic training than did black soldiers with only hemoglobin A—32 per 100,000 versus 1 per 1,000,000.[429] Although this magnitude of increase may not seem great, the vasoactive responses of the perioperative period can be similar to those of moderate to extreme exertion.

The pathologic end-organ damage that occurs in sickle cell states is attributable to three processes: the sickling or adhesion (or both) of cells in blood vessels, which causes infarcts and subsequent tissue destruction secondary to tissue ischemia; hemolytic crisis secondary to hemolysis; and aplastic crises that occur with bone marrow exhaustion, which can rapidly result in severe anemia. Logic dictates that patients currently in crisis not undergo surgery except for extreme emergencies, and then only after an exchange transfusion.[423,425-429]

Because sickling is increased with lowered oxygen tensions, acidosis, hypothermia, and the presence of more desaturated hemoglobin S, current therapy includes keeping the patient warm and well hydrated, giving supplemental oxygen, maintaining high cardiac output, and not creating areas of stasis with pressure or tourniquets. Meticulous attention to these practices in periods when we do not usually pay most careful attention (i.e., waiting in the preinduction area) or when gas exchange may be most unmatched to the cardiovascular-metabolic demands (early postoperative period) may be important in lessening morbidity. Even following these measures routinely, with no special emphasis placed on the periods described, succeeded in reducing mortality to 1% in several series of patients with sickle cell syndromes.[426,429,430] Retrospective review of patient charts led the authors of those studies to conclude that at most, a 0.5% mortality rate could be attributed to the interaction between sickle cell anemia and anesthetics.

Can this rate be decreased?[422,430] Several investigators have advocated using partial exchange transfusions perioperatively. In children with sickle cell anemia and acute lung syndromes, partial exchange transfusion improved clinical symptoms and blood oxygenation. In addition, serum bilirubin levels decreased in patients with acute liver injury. Clinical improvement of pneumococcal meningitis and cessation of hematuria in papillary necrosis also accompanied exchange transfusion.[422] The goal of exchange transfusion is to increase the concentration of hemoglobin A to 40% and the hematocrit to 35%. The 40% figure is an arbitrary one because no controlled studies have established a threshold ratio of hemoglobin A to hemoglobin S that would render blood unable to sickle in vivo. To achieve the 40% ratio in a 70-kg adult, about 4 units of washed erythrocytes would have to be exchanged; the system is inexpensive but efficient.

The possible decrease in preoperative morbidity after partial exchange transfusion has not been compared with the risks of exchange, except in two studies,[424,431] in which the risks of exchange were found to exceed the benefits. In the first study, a retrospective review of 82 surgical procedures performed between 1978 and 1986 in 60 patients, no advantage was noted for preoperative exchange transfusion, as measured by a decrease in postoperative complications.[431] (However, only the sickest may have received exchange transfusions because patients were not randomly allocated to exchange or nonexchange groups.) A slight increase in postoperative atelectasis requiring treatment was seen in patients given preoperative transfusions. More than 50% of the patients given transfusions had a postoperative complication. Patients who began with a hematocrit higher than 36% had a lower rate of complications.[431] In the second study, a randomized comparison of aggressive versus conservative transfusion practices in 551 patients (604 operations), perioperative sickling complications were not different between groups, and transfusion-related complications were substantially less in the conservative group.[424] Therefore, our recommendation is to pay meticulous attention to preventing conditions that increase sickling or that cause infection and to limit exchange transfusion to crisis situations. Perhaps giving higher concentrations of enriched oxygen to patients undergoing laparoscopic procedures should also become routine. Induction of hyponatremia has been shown to abort acute sickle cell crisis; however, this treatment has not gained widespread acceptance. Other conditions are common in sickle cell syndromes: pulmonary dysfunction with increased shunting, renal insufficiency, gallstones, small MIs, priapism, stroke, aseptic necrosis of bones and joints, ischemic ulcers, retinal detachment as a result of neovascularization, and complications of repeated transfusions.

In thalassemia, globin structures are normal, but because of gene deletion, the rate of synthesis of either the α- or β-chains of hemoglobin (α- and β-thalassemia, respectively) decreases.[432-434] Two copies of the gene that codes for the α-globin chain are located on chromosome 16. Deletion of all four of these genes causes cell death in utero, and three deletions cause severe chronic hemolysis and a shortened life span. "α-Thalassemia-1 (trait)" occurs when two genes have been deleted and mild anemia results; "α-thalassemia-2 (silent)" occurs when the two genes have been deleted but no mild anemia or microcytosis results. In α-thalassemia trait, the hemoglobin A_2 level is normal. β-Thalassemia is associated with an excess of α-chains, which denature developing erythrocytes, thereby leading to their premature death in marrow or to shortened survival in the circulation. An elevated hemoglobin A_2 level is the hallmark of β-thalassemia trait, a common cause of mild anemia and microcytosis. Bone marrow transplantation and pharmacologic manipulation of hemoglobin F synthesis are being tried in these hemoglobinopathies, as is direct gene replacement therapy. These therapies seem to be promising in even reversing liver failure from previous iron overload.[435] These syndromes are common in Southeast Asia, India, and the Middle East and in people of African descent.

In thalassemia, facial deformity from erythropoietin-stimulated ineffective erythropoiesis (ineffective because of a genetic inability to produce useful hemoglobin) has been reported to make endotracheal intubation difficult.[432,433] This one case report[433] has not been amplified, and there are no reports of this complication in patients with sickle cell anemia. However, the anemia associated with these syndromes often produces a compensatory hyperplasia of the erythroid marrow, which in turn is associated with severe skeletal abnormalities.[432-434]

Cytoskeletal Anemias (Hereditary Spherocytosis and Elliptocytosis), Enzyme-Deficient Anemias, and Autoimmune Hemolytic Anemias

Congenital abnormalities of the erythrocyte membrane are becoming better understood. In elliptocytosis and hereditary spherocytosis, the membrane is more permeable to cations and more susceptible to lipid loss when cell energy is depleted than is the membrane of a normal red blood cell. Both hereditary spherocytosis (present in 1 in 5000 people) and hereditary elliptocytosis are inherited as autosomal dominant traits. In both disorders, defects in the membrane are thought to result from a mutation of spectrin, a structural protein of the membrane cytoskeleton.[436] Although the therapeutic role of splenectomy in these diseases is not fully defined, in severe disease, splenectomy is known to improve the shortened life span of the red blood cell 100% (from 20 to 30 days to 40 to 70 days). Because splenectomy predisposes the patient to gram-positive septicemia (particularly pneumococcal), perhaps patients should be given pneumococcal vaccine preoperatively before predictable bacteremic events. No specific problems related to anesthesia have been reported for these disorders.

Glucose-6-phosphate dehydrogenase (G6PD) deficiency (a gender-linked recessive trait) is also reported to occur in approximately 8% of African American men.[437] Young cells have normal activity, but older cells are grossly deficient when compared with normal cells. A deficiency in G6PD results in hemolysis of the erythrocyte and the formation of Heinz bodies. Red cell hemolysis can also occur with intercurrent infections or after the administration of drugs that produce substances requiring G6PD for detoxification (e.g., methemoglobin, glutathione, and hydrogen peroxide). Drugs to be avoided are sulfa drugs, quinidine, prilocaine, lidocaine, antimalarial drugs, antipyretic drugs, nonnarcotic analgesics, vitamin K analogs, and perhaps sodium nitroprusside.

The autoimmune hemolytic anemias include cold antibody anemia, warm antibody anemia (idiopathic), and drug-induced anemia.[438-440] Cold antibody hemolytic anemias are mediated by IgM or IgG antibodies, which at room temperature and below cause red blood cells to clump. When these patients are given blood transfusions, the cells and all fluid infusions must be warm, and body temperature must be meticulously maintained at 37°C if hemolysis is to be prevented. Warm antibody (or "idiopathic") hemolytic anemia is a difficult management problem characterized by chronic anemia, the presence of antibodies active against red blood cells, a positive Coombs test, and difficulty crossmatching blood. For patients undergoing elective surgery, autologous transfusions, predeposit of blood with or without erythropoietin stimulation,[441] and blood from rare Rh-negative red blood cell donors or the patient's first-degree relatives (or both) can be used. In emergency situations, the possibility of autotransfusion, splenectomy, or corticosteroid treatment should be discussed with a hematologist knowledgeable in this area.

Drug-induced anemias have three mechanisms. In receptor-type hemolysis, a drug (e.g., penicillin) binds to the membrane of the red blood cell, and the complex stimulates the formation of an antibody against the complex. In "innocent bystander" hemolysis, a drug (e.g., quinidine, sulfonamide) binds to a plasma protein, thereby stimulating an antibody (IgM) that cross-reacts with an erythrocyte. In autoimmune hemolysis, the drug stimulates the production of an antibody (IgG) that cross-reacts with the erythrocyte. Drug-induced hemolytic anemias generally cease when therapy with the drug ends. In emergency situations, the least incompatible cells available should be used for blood transfusion.

Granulocytopenia

Granulocyte mechanisms have undergone experimental elaboration in the last decade, partly because of the molecular biologic revolution: in addition to erythropoietin (discussed earlier), more than 14 hemolymphopoietic growth factors or cytokines have been characterized biochemically and cloned genetically. These growth factors interact with cell-surface receptors to produce their major actions (Table 35-19).[442] Use of the colony-stimulating factors has permitted more intense oncologic treatment. The few reports related to their perioperative effects detail the unfavorable adverse consequences that such therapies can have on gas exchange when adverse immunologic effects occur.[443]

In patients who have fewer than 500 granulocytes per milliliter of blood and established sepsis, the use of growth factor and granulocyte transfusion has been shown to prolong life.[444-446] Although bone marrow transplantation is being used increasingly, complications usually occur after transplantation, not on harvesting of cells (at which time the anesthesiologist who is not involved in critical care is most frequently involved). Abnormal results on pulmonary function testing before bone marrow transplantation seem to predict complications after transplantation, but not so strongly as to preclude transplantation.[447]

Platelet Disorders

Although inherited platelet disorders are rare, acquired disorders are quite common and affect at least 20% of all patients in medical and surgical ICUs, with infections and drug therapies being the leading causes (also see Chapter 55).[448] Both acquired and inherited platelet conditions cause skin and mucosal bleeding, whereas defects in plasma coagulation produce deep tissue bleeding or delayed bleeding. Perioperative treatment of inherited platelet disorders (e.g., Glanzmann's thrombasthenia, Bernard-Soulier syndrome, Hermansky-Pudlak syndrome) consists of platelet transfusions. EACA has recently been used successfully (experimentally, 1 g/70 kg four times daily) to decrease perioperative bleeding in thrombocytopenic patients. The much more common acquired disorders may respond to one of several therapies (see Chapter 55). Immune thrombocytopenias, such as those associated with lupus erythematosus, idiopathic thrombocytopenic purpura, uremia, hemolytic-uremic syndrome, platelet transfusions, heparin, and thrombocytosis, may respond to steroids, splenectomy, plateletpheresis, eradication of *Helicobacter pylori*, or alkylating agents or may require platelet transfusions, plasma exchange, whole blood exchange, or transfusion; sometimes these disorders do not respond to anything.[194,449,450] Traditionally, splenectomy is performed when steroid therapy fails or reaches a dosage that poses unacceptable risks of toxicity. Newer agents such as anti-D immune globulin and rituximab may induce desirable remissions in idiopathic thrombocytopenic purpura without splenectomy.

Thrombotic thrombocytopenic purpura is a rare disorder of unknown cause. Despite various therapies, this disorder carries a very high mortality rate. However, the introduction of plasmapheresis has improved response rates dramatically in patients with this disease. One uncontrolled study implies that the benefit lies not only in improvement of the hematologic picture but also in prevention of adult respiratory distress syndrome, a leading cause of death in these patients.[450] In that study, early institution of plasmapheresis improved oxygenation.

By far the largest number of platelet abnormalities consists of drug-related defects in the aggregation and release of platelets. Aspirin irreversibly acetylates platelet cyclooxygenase, the enzyme that converts arachidonic acid to prostaglandin endoperoxidases. Because cyclooxygenase is not regenerated in the circulation within the life span of the platelet and because this enzyme is

Table 35-19 Major Effects of Hemolymphopoietic Growth Factors/Cytokines

Cytokine	Other Names	Biologic Effects
Erythropoietin		Erythrocyte production
Interleukin-3 (IL-3)	Multicolony-stimulating factor Stem cell–activating factor Persisting cell-stimulating factor Hemopoietin-2	Stimulates proliferation and differentiation of granulocyte, macrophage, eosinophil, mast cell, megakaryocyte, and T- and B-cell lineage and early myeloid stem cells. Interacts with erythropoietin to stimulate erythroid colony formation, stimulates proliferation of AML blasts, and stimulates histamine release by mast cells
Granulocyte colony-stimulating factor (G-CSF)	Differentiation factor MGI-2	Stimulates granulocyte lineage proliferation and differentiation. Acts on early myeloid stem cells, especially in association with other factors; synergizes with IL-3 to stimulate megakaryocyte colony formation. Increases neutrophil phagocytes and antibody-dependent cell-mediated cytotoxicity. Releases neutrophils from bone marrow and is chemotactic for neutrophils and monocytes. Enhances phagocytosis and antibody dependent cell-mediated cytotoxicity and oxidative metabolism of neutrophils. Stimulates monocyte killing of *Mycobacterium avium-intracellulare* and *Candida* species, tumoricidal activity of monocytes, antibody-dependent cell-mediated cytotoxicity, and expression of cell-surface proteins
Granulocyte-macrophage colony-stimulating factor (GM-CSF)		Stimulates granulocyte, macrophage, and megakaryocyte proliferation and differentiation, early myeloid stem cells, and—in the presence of erythropoietin—erythropoiesis. Enhances the cytotoxic and phagocytic colony-stimulating factor activity of neutrophils against bacteria, yeast, parasites, and antibody-coated tumor cells. Increases surface expression of neutrophil adhesion proteins and enhances eosinophil cytotoxicity, macrophage phagocytosis, and basophil histamine release. Amplifies IL-2–stimulated T-cell proliferation and stimulates B-cell lines to proliferate
Colony-stimulating factor-1	Macrophage colony-stimulating factor	Stimulates predominantly macrophage-monocyte proliferation and differentiation with lesser effects on granulocytes. Acts synergistically with other factors on earlier myeloid stem cells. Stimulates macrophage phagocytosis, killing, migration, antitumor activity, and metabolism. Stimulates secretion of plasminogen activator, G-CSF, interferon, IL-3, or tumor necrosis factor by peritoneal macrophages
Interleukin-1 (α and β)	Endogenous pyrogen Hemopoietin-1 Osteoclast-activating factor Lymphocyte-activating factor	Induces synthesis of acute-phase proteins by hepatocytes. Activates resting T cells, cofactor for T- and B-cell proliferation. Chemotactic for monocytes and neutrophils. Induces production of growth factors, including G-CSF, GM-CSF, IL-6, CSF-1, IL-3, and interferon by many cells. Radioprotective in mice
Interleukin-2	T-cell growth factor	Growth factor for T cells, activates cytotoxic T lymphocytes, promotes synthesis of other cytokines, enhances natural killer cell function
Interleukin-4	B-cell–stimulating factor-1 B-cell differentiation factor (BCDF) IgG induction factor	Enhances antibody production (IgG and IgE) and upregulates class II MHC molecules and Fc receptors on B cells. Costimulant with anti-IgM antibodies for induction of DNA synthesis in resting B cells. Stimulates growth of activated T cells. In the presence of IL-3, enhances mast cell growth; with G-CSF, enhances granulocytes of GM colony formation; and with erythropoietin and/or IL-1, stimulates erythroid and megakaryocyte colony formation
Interleukin-5	Eosinophil differentiation factor (EDF) T-cell–replacing factor (TRF) B-cell growth factor-II (BCGF-II) B-cell differentiation factor (BCDF)	Enhances antibody production (IgA). Promotes proliferation and IgG secretion by B-cell lines and induces hapten-specific IgG secretion in vitro by in vivo–primed B cells. Promotes differentiation by normal B cells. Stimulates eosinophil production and differentiation (GM-CSF and IL-3 act synergistically with IL-5 to stimulate eosinophil proliferation and differentiation). Enhances synthesis of IL-2 receptors
Interleukin-6	B-cell–stimulating factor-2 (BSF-2) Interferon-β_2 T-cell activation factor Hybridoma growth factor	B-cell differentiation and IgG secretion. T cells activated to cytotoxicity. Synergizes with IL-3 on early marrow myeloid stem cells and stimulates proliferation and differentiation of granulocytes, macrophages, eosinophils, mast cells, and megakaryocytes, as well as platelet production (may be a thrombopoietin)
Interleukin-7	Lymphopoietin-1	Stimulates pre–B-cell production. Stimulates T-cell proliferation
Interleukin-8*	Neutrophil-activating factor T-cell chemotactic factor	Inflammatory mediator; stimulates activation of neutrophils
Interleukin-9		Stimulates erythroid colony formation and proliferation of a megakaryocyte cell line
Interleukin-10	Cytokine synthesis– inhibiting factor	Inhibits cytokine production by T_H1 cells
Interleukin-11		Stimulates B-cell, megakaryocyte, and mast cell lineages
C-kit ligand	Mast cell factor Stem cell factor Hemolymphopoietic growth factor-1	Acts on relatively early stem cells synergistically with other cytokines. Stimulates pre-B cells

*Not considered a true growth factor but included here for completeness.

AML, acute myeloblastic leukemia; MHC, major histocompatibility complex; T_H1, first of the thymus-derived cells.

Modified from Quesenberg PJ, Schafer AI, Schreiber AD, et al: Hematology. *In* American College of Physicians: Medical Knowledge Self-Assessment. Philadelphia, American College of Physicians, 1991, p 374.

essential for the aggregation of platelets, one aspirin tablet may affect platelet function for a week. All other drugs that inhibit platelet function (e.g., vitamin E, indomethacin, sulfinpyrazone, dipyridamole, tricyclic antidepressant drugs, phenothiazines, furosemide, steroids) do not inhibit cyclooxygenase function irreversibly; these drugs disturb platelet function for only 24 to 48 hours. If emergency surgery is needed before the customary 8-day period for platelet regeneration after aspirin therapy or if the 2-day period for other drugs has not elapsed, administration of 2 to 5 units of platelet concentrates will return platelet function in a 70-kg adult to an adequate level and platelet-induced clotting dysfunction to normal. Only 30,000 to 50,000 normally functioning platelets per milliliter is needed for normal clotting. Because low-dose aspirin therapy (<650 mg/day) allows aspirin to be gone from the body 24 hours after the last dose and because the body makes 70,000 platelets/mL blood per day, a 48-hour period after the last aspirin in minidose therapy should be sufficient time for platelet aggregation to become normal. This may be the period that must pass to avoid platelet transfusions and their associated risks. One platelet transfusion will increase the platelet count from 4000 to 20,000/mL blood; the platelet half-life is about 8 hours.

Heparin-induced thrombocytopenia can develop within hours on re-exposure to heparin in a previously sensitized patient. Lepirudin and argatroban are direct thrombin inhibitors effective as therapy for heparin-induced thrombocytopenia.[451]

Major risk factors for thrombosis include factor V Leiden and prothrombin 20210A mutations, elevated plasma homocysteine, and the antiphosphoid antibody syndrome.[452,453] Clinicians facing these challenging patients might seek expert local consultation for help with management. This issue is discussed more fully in Chapter 56.

Hemophilia and Related Clotting Disorders

Abnormalities in blood coagulation as a result of defects in plasma coagulation factor are either inherited or acquired. Inherited disorders include X-linked hemophilia A (a defect in factor VIII activity), von Willebrand's diseases (defect in the von Willebrand component of factor VIII), hemophilia B (a sex-linked deficiency of factor IX activity), and other less common disorders. The sex-linked origin of some of these disorders means that hemophilia occurs almost exclusively in the male offspring of female carriers; men do not transmit the disease to their male offspring.

In elective surgery, levels of the deficient coagulation factor should be assayed 48 hours before surgery and the level restored to 40% of normal before surgery. One unit of factor concentrate per kilogram of body weight normally increases the factor concentration by 2%. Thus, in an individual essentially devoid of activity, administration of 20 U/kg body weight would be required as an initial dose. Because the half-life is 6 to 10 hours for factor VIII and 8 to 16 hours for factor IX, approximately 1.5 U/hr/kg of factor VIII or 1.5 U/2 hr/kg of factor IX should be given. Additional administration of factors VIII and IX should be guided by the activity of the clotting factors for about 6 to 10 days postoperatively.[454-456]

These factors are available in various preparations; the newer genetically engineered von Willebrand factor, cryoprecipitate, which contains 20 U/mL, is obtained from regular donors (the risk of hepatitis being 1 in 200 for 5-mL lots) or from fresh frozen plasma (which contains 1 U/mL). Some risk of transmitting hepatitis and AIDS accompanies transfusion but, with better testing, much less than formerly.[457-460] Current screening of blood for aspartate or alanine aminotransferase levels is believed to result in a much lower risk of hepatitis C and even AIDS from transfusion. Theoretically, antigenic testing for HIV should further decrease the risk of transmission by blood products. Heat treatment is also reported to reduce the risk substantially. Factor IX, but not factor VIII is contained in prothrombin complex concentrates; however, these concentrates may contain activated clotting factors, which can lead to disseminated intravascular coagulation (DIC) and a high risk for hepatitis. In addition, although EACA or tranexamic acid is sometimes administered as a fibrinolytic inhibitor, these substances carry with them a significant risk for DIC. Additional hazards of modern therapy include acute and chronic hepatitis, AIDS, hypersensitivity reactions, psychic trauma, chronic pain with narcotic addiction, and inhibition of factors, especially VIII.

An antibody that inactivates factor VIII or IX (fresh frozen plasma fails to increase clotting factor activity after incubation with the patient's plasma) develops in approximately 10% of patients with either hemophilia A or B. These acquired anticoagulants are usually composed of IgG, are poorly removed by plasmapheresis, and are variably responsive to immunosuppressive drugs. The use of prothrombin complex concentrates can be lifesaving but carries the risk of DIC and hepatitis.

Vitamin K deficiency is discussed in the section on liver disease. To review, vitamin K–dependent clotting factors (II, VII, IX, and X) require vitamin K for the postsynthetic addition of γ-carboxyl groups to glutamate residues; administration of vitamin K or fresh frozen plasma can correct these deficiencies.

Patients who come to the operating room after having received many units of blood (as in massive GI bleeding) may have deficient clotting. This impaired clotting is initially caused by depletion of platelets, which occurs after approximately 10 to 15 units of blood has been given, and later, by depletion of coagulation factors (see Chapter 56). Treatment of these deficiencies can be corrected with platelet concentrates—each concentrate is normally suspended in 50 mL of fresh plasma; thus, coagulation factors are also replaced.

Urokinase, streptokinase, and tissue plasminogen activator (t-PA) have been used to treat pulmonary embolism, deep venous thrombosis, stroke, and arterial occlusive disease. These drugs accelerate the lysis of thrombi and emboli, in contrast to heparin, which may prevent, but not dissolve a thrombus. Bleeding complications associated with these fibrinolytic agents are the result of dissolution of hemostatic plugs and can be quickly reversed by discontinuing the medication and replenishing plasma fibrinogen with cryoprecipitate or plasma. However, cryoprecipitate and plasma are seldom needed preoperatively because the fibrinolytic activity of urokinase and streptokinase usually dissipates within 1 hour of discontinuing their administration. Nonetheless, insufficient data have accumulated to prescribe the ideal preoperative preparation and intraoperative management of hemostasis in patients recently treated with urokinase, streptokinase, or t-PA. Postponing surgery for three half-lives of the drug (increases in plasmin activity in blood can be assayed for ≥4 to 8 hours) may not be possible, and meticulous observation of the operative field for hemostasis may not suffice.[461,462] The process may be even more complex in a vascular or cardiac patient who requires heparin administration intraoperatively. To correct the fibrinogen deficiency in these patients, some clinicians administer fibrinogen before surgery and EACA at heparin administration. We usually delay or avoid giving EACA until heparin is administered in an effort to minimize the risk for thrombosis.

Desmopressin is now being tried in operations associated with high blood loss as a routine measure to decrease bleeding and transfusion requirements. Desmopressin therapy began as treatment of platelet dysfunction in von Willebrand's disease but has since expanded to routine use in patients undergoing cardiovascular surgery and frequent use in other high–blood loss operations. This increased use was prompted by the finding that desmopressin decreases bleeding and transfusion requirements.[463] Whether the side effects of desmopressin exceed its benefits remains to be determined and will probably influence how routine its administration becomes.

The problem of patients taking oral anticoagulants is discussed in the cardiovascular section of this chapter.[193-200,202-205] Regional anesthetic techniques might be avoided in patients given anticoagulant drugs.[193-200,202-205] Whether these regional techniques should also be avoided in patients treated prophylactically with low-dose subcutaneous heparin has not been studied. The effects of heparin sulfate can be reversed by titrating protamine, with the activated clotting time used as a guide.

Pharmacologic research is searching for specific molecular subtypes of heparin that have different anticoagulant potencies, binding affinities for antithrombin III, antithrombotic effects, and platelet-aggregating effects (see the pulmonary section in this chapter on prophylaxis for deep venous thrombosis). The search is on for a "new" heparin preparation that will block thrombosis without causing clinical bleeding (see earlier). Such a development might change our ways of monitoring clotting function. As of now, the new heparins appear to increase the risk for epidural hematoma. Determining the bleeding time, platelet count, partial thromboplastin time, and prothrombin time will identify almost all problems in patients with a suspected clotting or bleeding disorder (also see Chapter 56). As explained in Chapter 34, these screening tests should probably not be obtained for asymptomatic patients.

Oncologic Disease

Patients with malignant tumors may be otherwise healthy or may be desperately ill with nutritional, neurologic, metabolic, endocrinologic, electrolyte, cardiac, pulmonary, renal, hepatic, hematologic, or pharmacologic disabilities. Thus, determining the other disabilities accompanying malignant tumors requires evaluation of all systems. Abnormalities frequently accompanying such tumors include hypercalcemia either by direct bone invasion or by ectopic elaboration of PTH or other bone-dissolving substance, uric acid nephropathy, hyponatremia (especially with small cell, or oat cell, carcinoma of the lung), nausea, vomiting, anorexia and cachexia, fever, tumor-induced hypoglycemia, intracranial metastases (10% to 20% of all cancers), peripheral nerve or spinal cord disorders, meningeal carcinomatosis, toxic neuropathies secondary to anticancer therapy, and paraneoplastic neurologic syndromes (dermatomyositis, Eaton-Lambert syndrome, myopathies, and distal neuropathies).

Many patients with malignant tumors are given large doses of analgesics and should be kept comfortable during the perioperative period. Avoiding drug dependence is of no practical importance in terminally ill patients.[464] Marijuana (tetrahydrocannabinol) depresses the CNS vomiting center and may be more effective than the phenothiazines or butyrophenones in suppressing the nausea associated with cancer and its therapy; marijuana decreases anesthetic requirements 15% to 30%. Immunomodulators, stimulating factors or cytokines, gene identification,[465,466] and drugs for treating side effects (e.g., midazolam or ondansetron) have given new hope for safer, more effective therapy with fewer limiting side effects. The effect of ondansetron in preventing vomiting and the effect of midazolam in preventing "memory-stimulated vomiting" have been important additions. The NK-1 antagonists have also been approved for treatment in oncologic patients."

The toxicity of cancer chemotherapy is related to the drugs used and the dose. For radiation therapy, damage occurs when the following doses are exceeded: lungs, 1500 rad; kidneys, 2400 rad; heart, 3000 rad; spinal cord, 4000 rad; intestine, 5500 rad; brain, 6000 rad; and bone, 7500 rad. The toxicities of biologic and immunomodulating therapies are related to the change in immune function that they cause. Alkylating agents cause bone marrow depression, including thrombocytopenia, as well as alopecia, hemorrhagic cystitis, nausea, and vomiting. The alkylating agents, including cyclophosphamide and mechlorethamine, can act as an anticholinesterase and prolong neuromuscular blockade.[467] The antineoplastic alkaloid vincristine produces peripheral neuropathy and SIADH, and vinblastine produces myelotoxicity. Cisplatin is also associated with peripheral neuropathy and severe nausea. Nitrosoureas can produce severe hepatic and renal damage, as well as bone marrow toxicity, myalgia, and paresthesia. Folic acid analogs such as methotrexate have been linked to bone marrow depression, ulcerative stomatitis, pulmonary interstitial infiltrates, GI toxicity, and occasionally, severe liver dysfunction. Fluorouracil and floxuridine, both pyrimidine analogs, cause bone marrow toxicity, megaloblastic anemia, nervous system dysfunction, and hepatic and GI alterations. Purine analogs (mercaptopurine, thioguanine) have bone marrow depression as their primary toxic effect. Anthracycline antibiotics (doxorubicin, daunorubicin, mithramycin, mitomycin C, bleomycin) can all cause pulmonary infiltrates; cardiomyopathy (especially doxorubicin and daunorubicin); myelotoxicity; and GI, hepatic, and renal disturbances.

The wisdom of anesthetizing patients given bleomycin has been questioned. A retrospective study by Goldiner and coauthors[468] reported postoperative deaths in five consecutive patients given bleomycin. All five patients died of postoperative respiratory failure. Using the same anesthetic technique, Goldiner and coworkers[468] then anesthetized 12 patients, limited the inspired oxygen concentration to 22% to 25% perioperatively, and replaced much of the blood loss with colloids rather than crystalloids. None of the 12 patients died. These investigators postulated that bleomycin caused epithelial cell edema that progressed to necrosis of type I alveolar cells, leakage of fluid into the alveolar space, and the formation of "hyaline membranes" similar to that associated with oxygen toxicity. Goldiner and colleagues[468] believe that this pathophysiologic similarity indicates a possible synergistic relationship between oxygen and bleomycin. However, LaMantia and coworkers[469] retrospectively analyzed the changes in 16 patients undergoing surgery after bleomycin therapy. Thirteen patients were given oxygen at inspired concentrations of 37% to 45%. No instances of postoperative respiratory failure occurred. Animal data do not support this effect of bleomycin in altering the toxicity of hyperoxia.[470] Thus, data are currently available to support all practices regarding administration of oxygen to patients given bleomycin. We prefer to keep inspired oxygen concentrations at the lowest level that provides adequate tissue oxygenation. When in doubt about side effects in patients undergoing cancer chemotherapy, our practice is to seek advice from two experts.

Patients Given Drug Therapy for Chronic and Acute Medical Conditions

A steadily increasing number of potent drugs are being used to treat disease, and the average hospitalized patient receives more than 10 drugs. Many drugs have side effects that might make anesthesia more risky or patient management more difficult. Knowing the pharmacologic properties and potential side effects of commonly used drugs helps the anesthesiologist avoid pitfalls during anesthesia and surgery.

The first step in avoiding these pitfalls is to obtain a drug history from the patient, including vitamins, herbs, and supplements.[21-23,471,472] Then, for every drug, medicine, and over-the-counter preparation that the patient is using, the anesthesiologist should know the name, classification of drug, diseases and conditions for which it is prescribed, and common side effects. Having this knowledge before surgery helps the anesthesiologist avoid making mistakes that might turn minor side effects into life-threatening situations. If necessary, the anesthesiologist should return to the patient's bedside (or telephone outpatients) to search for signs or symptoms of these effects. Unnecessary drugs should be discontinued for at least three and preferably five half-lives of the drugs. This period should be longer if metabolites of the drug have activity and longer half-lives. For essential or beneficial drugs, the optimal dose should be determined in consultation with the treating physician; the optimal dose is that maximizing the ratio of therapeutic value to the risk of drug toxicity. Side effects should be sought and either corrected preoperatively or at least planned for in anesthetic management. For instance, if a patient is made hypokalemic with diuretic drugs, hypokalemia might be corrected before surgery; an additional tactic would be to avoid hyperventilation during surgery (see the earlier section on hypokalemia). This line of reasoning and planning is best done at least 1 week before surgery. Ideally, the surgeon, internist, primary care practitioner, and anesthesiologist should communicate regarding these topics well in advance of surgery. Understanding the side effects of chronic drug therapy that affect the sympathetic nervous system requires some knowledge of the basic pharmacologic characteristics of the sympathetic nervous system (see Chapter 12).

Pharmacologic Processes in the Sympathetic Nervous System

It is important to remember several points related to the pharmacology of the sympathetic nervous system when considering chronic drug therapy.

Norepinephrine, dopamine, and epinephrine exert their physiologic effect by interacting with an appropriate receptor at the target tissue. The primary receptor acts through intermediary messenger systems (including cyclic 3′,5′-adenosine monophosphate [cAMP] or G-stimulatory or G-inhibitory proteins, or both) or can change the conformation (and hence the affinity for ligands) of bordering or neighboring receptors. These bordering or neighboring receptor effects may account for many of the multitude of effects associated with catecholamines.

The action of sympathomimetic substances is terminated through an unusual process: the nerve ending uses an active reuptake system to recapture most of the norepinephrine from the target tissue (see Chapter 12). Obviously, blockage of this system permits more norepinephrine to remain free to produce physiologic effects. In addition to this reuptake system, two enzymes transform catecholamines metabolically: monoamine oxidase (MAO) and catechol-*O*-methyltransferase (COMT).

Antihypertensive Drugs

Many antihypertensive drugs and almost all mind-altering drugs affect sympathetic neuronal storage, uptake, metabolism, or release of neurotransmitters. For instance, the antihypertensive drug reserpine depletes the granules of norepinephrine, epinephrine, and dopamine in both the brainstem and periphery. Depletion of transmitters in sympathetic nerve endings renders drugs such as ephedrine and metaraminol ineffective because these drugs act primarily by releasing catecholamines (see Fig. 35-10). Guanethidine and guanadrel deplete granular norepinephrine and affect only the peripheral sympathetic system. In amounts used clinically, reserpine decreases MAC by 20% to 30%, whereas guanethidine has no effect on anesthetic requirements. In addition to causing a lack of response to indirect-acting vasopressors, reserpine can cause denervation supersensitivity and hyperresponsiveness (with hypertension or tachycardia, or both) to the usual doses of direct-acting sympathetic amines such as phenylephrine (Neo-Synephrine), isoproterenol, norepinephrine, epinephrine, and dopamine.[471,472] Thus, in patients who have been treated with drugs that alter sympathetic neurotransmitter release, uptake, metabolism, or receptor function, some problems may occur: hypotension, hypertension, and bradycardia should be treated by titrating doses of direct-acting vasoconstrictors such as phenylephrine, vasodilators such as nitroprusside, or chronotropic drugs such as atropine, isoproterenol, or dopamine.

Another group of antihypertensive drugs consists of "false neurotransmitters." False neurotransmitters replace norepinephrine in the granules at the nerve ending. α-Methyldopa (Aldomet) becomes α-methyldopamine, which is further metabolized to α-methylnorepinephrine (Fig. 35-11). In some nerve endings and for some receptors, α-methyldopamine or α-methylnorepinephrine is more potent than dopamine or norepinephrine as dopaminergic or α-adrenergic receptor stimulants. However, at most nerve endings, the false neurotransmitters are less potent stimulants; this lower degree of stimulation is one means by which their antihypertensive action is produced. Alternatively, α-methyldopa may act by stimulating the brainstem sympathetic nervous system. When this system antagonizes the peripheral sympathetic nervous system, the activity of the latter decreases and BP is reduced. Through its central effect, α-methyldopa decreases anesthetic requirements 20% to 40%.

In addition to altering the response to exogenously administered vasopressors, these neurotransmitter-depleting drugs can

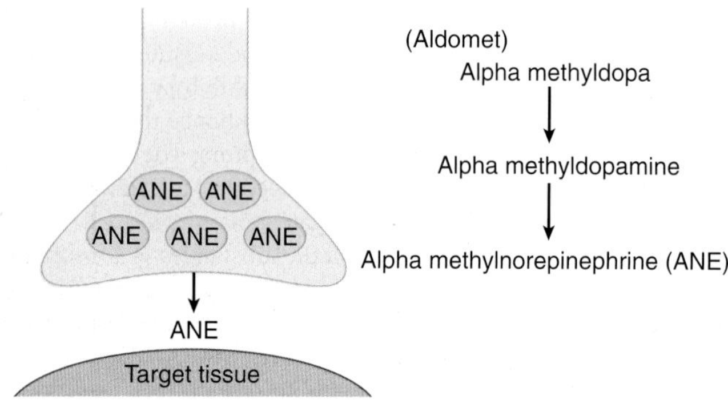

Figure 35-11 In the granules of the nerve terminal, α-methyldopa (Aldomet) is converted enzymatically to α-methyldopamine by the same enzyme that converts dopa to dopamine. α-Methyldopamine is converted to α-methylnorepinephrine by the same enzyme that converts dopamine to norepinephrine.

also produce side effects: psychic depression, nightmares, drowsiness, nasal stuffiness, diarrhea, bradycardia, and orthostatic hypotension with impotence (reserpine).[473-475] Guanethidine and guanadrel can cause orthostatic hypotension, bradycardia, asthma, diarrhea, and inhibition of ejaculation. α-Methyldopa is associated with drowsiness, orthostatic hypotension, bradycardia, diarrhea, acute or chronic hepatitis, cirrhosis, and autoimmune hemolytic anemia (i.e., a positive Coombs test result).[472] Because of these side effects, ACE inhibitors (captopril, enalapril, lisinopril, enalaprilat, and ramipril) and angiotensin II receptor blockers are being used increasingly as first-line drugs and appear to improve the quality of life of patients taking antihypertensive drugs. One of the angiotensin II receptor blockers—valsartan—when combined with a diuretic, actually increases libido in both men and women while decreasing BP. However, ACE inhibitors and angiotensin II receptor blockers may be associated with more peripheral vasodilation and hypotension on induction of anesthesia than sympatholytics are. Added to this group are the ACE receptor blocking agents. These last two classes of drugs are associated with such severe hypotension with standard anesthetic induction that we discontinue or at least consider discontinuing the use of these drugs preoperatively (see earlier).

Catecholamine or sympathetic receptor blocking drugs affect the three major types of catecholamine receptors: α-adrenergic, β-adrenergic, and dopaminergic. The existence of subdivisions (e.g., β_1 and β_2) suggested the possibility that some drugs would be found to affect only one set of receptors. For example, terbutaline is used more frequently than isoproterenol because terbutaline is said to exert a preferential effect on α_2-receptors (i.e., dilation of bronchial smooth muscle), thereby avoiding the cardiac stimulation produced by drugs that stimulate β_1-receptors. In fact, the selectivity is dose related. At a certain dose, a direct β_2-receptor stimulating drug will affect only those receptors but, at a higher dose, will stimulate both β_1- and β_2-receptors. The effect of a given dose varies with each patient. A certain dose may stimulate β_1- and β_2-receptors in one patient but neither receptor in another patient. More and more selective blocking drugs are being developed in hope of widening the margin between β_1- and β_2- and α-adrenergic effects. Ultimately, however, even more selectivity is desired. It would be advantageous to be able to decrease the heart rate without changing myocardial contractility or to increase contractility without changing the heart rate. Such is the goal of much drug research and the development of dobutamine and fenoldopam. However, to date, all such selectivity appears to be dose related, even for dobutamine.

Metoprolol (Lopressor) and atenolol (Tenormin) (both β_1-adrenergic receptor blocking drugs) and propranolol, betaxolol, timolol, esmolol, pindolol, oxprenolol, acebutolol, carteolol, penbutolol, and nadolol are widely available β-adrenergic receptor blocking drugs used for chronic therapy in the United States. Because nadolol has poor lipid solubility, it has a long elimination half-life (17 to 24 hours) and does not cross the blood-brain barrier readily. Although selective β-adrenergic receptor blocking drugs should be more appropriate in patients with increased airway resistance or diabetes, this advantage is apparent only when low doses are used. The use of β-adrenergic receptor blocking drugs has become widespread because these drugs treat everything from angina and hypertension to priapism and stage fright. These drugs appear to decrease morbidity and mortality in patients who have initially survived MI[476,477] and may increase perioperative survival in selected patients (see the earlier section on cardiovascular disease).

Smulyan and colleagues[478] studied the problems of long-term propranolol hydrochloride therapy in adult patients who must undergo abdominal surgery. Because these patients cannot take oral medications postoperatively for many days, they must be protected against perioperative sympathetic stimulation and the propranolol withdrawal syndrome. It is therefore common to develop intravenous β-blocker protocols for patients chronically taking these agents, although it is important to recognize the risk of β-blockers. The hypotensive and bradycardic effects of propranolol and general anesthesia appear to be additive. Because of its shorter half-life (3 to 10 minutes), esmolol has replaced propranolol in critical care (including anesthesia) settings because errors in therapy or side effects, such as increased airway resistance, vanish much more quickly than if propranolol were administered.[479] Propranolol does not affect anesthetic requirements, and one would expect the same lack of effect from other "pure" β-adrenergic receptor blocking drugs.

α-Adrenergic receptor blocking drugs include phentolamine, prazosin, terazosin, doxazosin, phenoxybenzamine, the phenothiazines, and the butyrophenones (e.g., droperidol). Dopaminergic receptor antagonists include the antischizophrenic drugs (phenothiazines and butyrophenones) and metoclopramide. The receptor blocking drugs inhibit the action of sympathomimetic drugs at the receptor in a dose-related fashion. Thus, propranolol lowers BP by blocking the tendency of norepinephrine and epinephrine to increase the rate and force of contractions of the heart (and perhaps their tendency to increase the secretion of renin as well). To overcome this blockade, one need only provide more β-receptor stimulating drug. Thus, high doses of vasopressors may be needed to increase BP in a patient given large doses of propranolol.

When administration of β-adrenergic receptor blocking drugs is terminated, sympathetic stimulation often increases, as though the body had responded to the presence of these drugs by increasing sympathetic neuron activity. Thus, propranolol and nadolol (to name just two) withdrawal can be accompanied by a hyper–β-adrenergic condition that increases myocardial oxygen demands. Administering propranolol or metoprolol can cause bradycardia, CHF, fatigue, dizziness, depression, psychoses, bronchospasm, and Peyronie's disease. The POISE study emphasizes the concerns that inadequate titration of these agents can lead to stroke or increased mortality.[121] Side effects of dopaminergic receptor blocking drugs are discussed later in this chapter. Prazosin (Minipress), terazosin, and oxazocin are α_1-adrenergic receptor blocking drugs used to treat hypertension, ischemic cardiomyopathy, receding hairlines, and benign prostatic hypertrophy because they dilate both veins and arteries and reduce sphincter tone. These drugs are associated with vertigo, palpitations, depression, dizziness, weakness, and anticholinergic effects.

Some sympathomimetic drugs stimulate α-adrenergic receptors in the brainstem. Clonidine (Catapres), a drug with a half-life of 12 to 24 hours, guanabenz, and guanfacine (Tenex) are α_2-adrenergic receptor stimulants. Presumably, α_2-adrenergic agonists, including clonidine, guanabenz, and guanfacine, chronically lower BP through the central brainstem adrenergic stimulation referred to previously. They may also be used chronically to treat opiate, cocaine, food, and tobacco withdrawal. Occasionally, withdrawal from clonidine can precipitate a sudden hypertensive crisis, analogous to that occurring on withdrawal from propranolol, and cause a hyper–β-adrenergic condition. The degree of hypertensive crisis after clonidine withdrawal is now being debated. (Although intravenous clonidine is not available in the United States, a skin patch of clonidine is being used preoperatively to ablate sympathomimetic responses perioperatively.) Tricyclic antidepressant drugs and presumably phenothiazines and the butyrophenones interfere with the action of clonidine. Although administration of a butyrophenone (e.g., droperidol) to a patient taking clonidine, guanabenz, or guanfacine chronically could theoretically precipitate a hypertensive crisis, none has been reported. Clonidine administration can be accompanied by drowsiness, dry mouth, orthostatic hypotension, bradycardia, and impotence. Acute clonidine or dexmedetomidine administration decreases anesthetic requirements by at least 40% to 60%; chronic administration decreases requirements by 10% to 20%.[480,481] Because of the relative safety of these drugs and their ability to decrease anesthetic requirements, block narcotic-induced muscle rigidity, and provide pain relief, their popularity preoperatively, introperatively, and in ICU sedation is increasing dramatically.[480-484]

Three other classes of antihypertensive drugs affect the sympathetic nervous system indirectly: diuretics, arteriolar dilators, and slow (calcium) channel blocking agents. Thiazide diuretic drugs are associated with hypochloremic alkalosis, hypokalemia, hyperglycemia, hyperuricemia, and hypercalcemia. The potassium-sparing diuretic drug spironolactone is associated with hyperkalemia, hyponatremia, gynecomastia, and impotence. All diuretic drugs can cause dehydration. The thiazide diuretics and furosemide appear to prolong neuromuscular blockade. The arteriolar dilator hydralazine can cause a lupus-like condition (usually with renal involvement), nasal congestion, headache, dizziness, CHF, angina, and GI disturbances. Such a syndrome is nonexistent with the other direct vasodilator on the U.S. market, minoxidil.

The slow-channel calcium ion antagonists ("calcium channel blocking drugs") inhibit the transmembrane influx of calcium ions into cardiac and vascular smooth muscle. Such inhibition reduces the heart rate (negative chronotropy); depresses contractility (negative inotropy); decreases conduction velocity (negative dromotropy); and dilates coronary, cerebral, and systemic arterioles (Fig. 35-12).[485] Verapamil, diltiazem, and nifed-

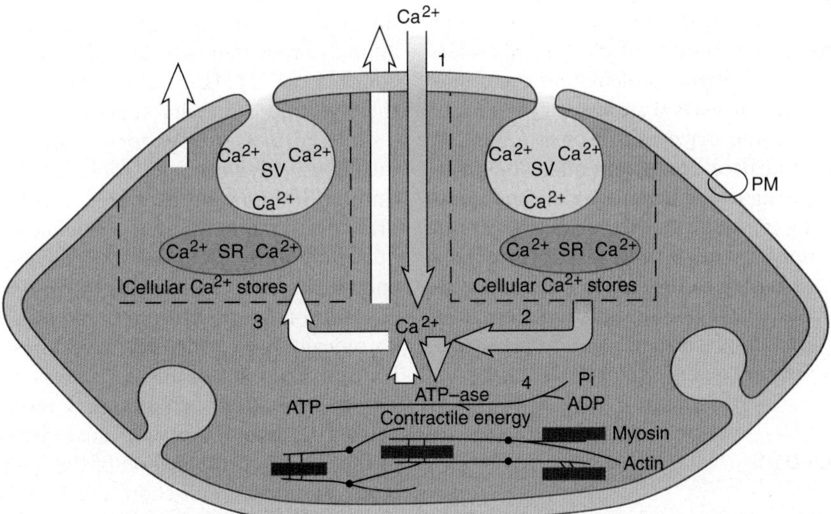

Figure 35-12 Schematic drawing of a smooth muscle cell showing calcium flux and possible sites of interference by halothane and nifedipine. The concentration of calcium (Ca^{2+}) in the cytoplasm increases (*green arrows*) because of entry through the plasma membrane (PM) and release from surface vesicles (SV) or the sacroplasmic reticulum (SR). When the concentration of cytoplasmic Ca^{2+} is sufficiently high, adenosine triphosphate (ATP) is activated. Splitting of ATP by adenosine triphosphatase (ATPase) into phosphatidylinositol (Pi) and adenosine diphosphate (ADP) provides the interaction and contraction of actin filaments and myosin particles constituting muscle fibers. The concentration of cytoplasmic Ca^{2+} decreases (*white arrows*) with the return of Ca^{2+} to cellular stores and the extracellular transport of Ca.[2+] Both halothane and nifedipine probably (1) inhibit the entry of Ca^{2+} and (2) may also interfere with cytoplasmic Ca^{2+} flux by reducing the release of Ca^{2+} by the SR, by (3) reducing storage and reuptake, or by (4) blocking ATPase or the contractile mechanism (or both). *(Redrawn from Tosone SR, Reves JG, Kissin I, et al: Hemodynamic responses to nifedipine in dogs anesthetized with halothane. Anesth Analg 62:903, 1983.)*

ipine all produce such effects, but to varying degrees and apparently by similar, but different mechanisms. These mechanisms relate to the three different classes of calcium channel antagonists that they represent: the phenylalkyl amines, the benzothiazepines, and the dihydropyridines, respectively. Nifedipine is the most potent of the three as a smooth muscle dilator, whereas verapamil and diltiazem have negative dromotropic and inotropic effects and vasodilating properties. Diltiazem has weak vasodilating properties when compared with nifedipine and has less of an AV conduction effect than verapamil does. Thus, verapamil and diltiazem can increase the PR interval and produce AV block. In fact, reflex activation of the sympathetic nervous system may be necessary during the administration of diltiazem, and especially during verapamil therapy, to maintain normal conduction. Clearly, verapamil and diltiazem must be titrated very carefully when a patient is already taking a β-adrenergic receptor blocking drug or when adding β-blocking drugs to a patient already taking verapamil or diltiazem.

The use of calcium channel blocking drugs has several important implications for anesthetic management.[485-487] First, the effects of inhaled and narcotic anesthetics and nifedipine in decreasing systemic vascular resistance, BP, and contractility may be additive. Similarly, verapamil and anesthetics (inhaled anesthetics, nitrous oxide, and narcotics) increase AV conduction times and additively decrease BP, systemic vascular resistance, and contractility. Second, verapamil and presumably the other calcium channel blocking drugs have been found to decrease anesthetic requirements by 25%. These drugs can produce neuromuscular blockade, potentiate both depolarizing and nondepolarizing neuromuscular blocking drugs, and in at least one type of myopathy (Duchenne's muscular dystrophy), even precipitate respiratory failure. Finally, because slow-channel activation of calcium is necessary to cause spasms of cerebral and coronary vessels, bronchoconstriction, and normal platelet aggregation, these drugs may have a role in treating ischemia of the nervous system, bronchoconstriction, and unwanted clotting disorders perioperatively. All three drugs are highly protein bound and may displace or be displaced by other drugs that are also highly protein bound (e.g., lidocaine, bupivacaine, diazepam, disopyramide, and propranolol). Adverse consequences can be minimized by titrating the inhaled or narcotic drug to the hemodynamic and anesthetic effects. By monitoring for side effects, the anesthetist can prevent them from becoming serious (S. Slogoff and coworkers, personal communication). Hemodynamic, but not electrophysiologic changes can usually be reversed by administering calcium. Reversal of the electrophysiologic effects may occur if "industrial" doses of β-adrenergic agonists are given.

Mood-Altering Drugs

Mood-altering drugs are the most frequently prescribed medications in the United States.[474,475] They include MAOIs, SSRIs, phenothiazines, tricyclic antidepressant drugs, other antidepressants that fail previous drug category classification such as bupropion, and drugs of abuse such as cocaine. MAOIs, which include isocarboxazid (Marplan), phenelzine (Nardil), pargyline (Eutonyl), tranylcypromine (Parnate), and deprenyl, bind irreversibly to the enzyme MAO, thereby increasing intraneuronal levels of amine neurotransmitters (serotonin, norepinephrine, dopamine, epinephrine, octopamine). This increase is associated with an antidepressant effect, an antihypertensive effect, an antinarcoleptic effect, elevation of liver enzymes, and delayed onset of Parkinson's disease (deprenyl). Because two forms of the enzyme (MAO-A and MAO-B) are selective in vitro for substrate (MAO-A is selective for serotonin, dopamine, and norepinephrine; MAO-B for tyramine and phenylethylamine), presumably MAOIs selective for MAO-A or MAO-B would have different effects.[488] This is not known for certain inasmuch as deprenyl (selegiline [Eldepryl]), an MAO-B–selective drug, improves a dopamine deficiency state, parkinsonism.

Interactions between MAOIs and a variety of foods and drugs containing indirect-acting sympathomimetic substances such as ephedrine or tyramine (found especially in aged cheeses) can occur for as long as 2 weeks after the last dose of MAOI is given. The most serious effects of this interaction are convulsions and hyperpyrexic coma (particularly after narcotics).

Anesthetic management of a patient given an MAOI can be chaotic; for this reason it is widely accepted practice to discontinue MAOIs at least 2 to 3 weeks before any planned operation.[474,475,488-492] An alternative point of view has been expressed regarding severely psychotic patients or emergency surgery.[488,493-495] Clearly, the risk of discontinuing MAOIs must be weighed against the risk of suicidal tendencies in some patients deprived of MAOIs. There are no reported experiences of interactions between narcotics and deprenyl, so judgments about possible worsening of Parkinson's disease and continuing MAOIs have no basis in data. It should be noted that severe reactions have occurred when too short an interval existed between the administration of MAOIs and tricyclic antidepressants. Emergency surgery on patients given MAOIs can be punctuated by hemodynamic instability. A regional block can be attempted as treatment of postoperative pain to avoid having to give narcotics. Cases of hyperpyrexic coma after the administration of most narcotics have been reported in humans, and animal studies document a 10% to 50% incidence of hyperpyrexic coma in animals pretreated with MAOIs and then given a variety of narcotics.[474,475,488-492] These reactions appear to be treated best by therapy supporting vital functions.

Alternative drugs for the treatment of severe depression include the tricyclic antidepressant drugs: amitriptyline (Elavil, Endep), imipramine (Tofranil, Presamine), desipramine (Norpramin), doxepin (Adapin, Sinequan), nortriptyline (Aventyl), fluoxetine (Prozac), trazodone (Desyrel), bupropion (Wellbutrin), and others.[474,475] Tricyclic antidepressant drugs also block the reuptake of neurotransmitters and cause their acute release. Given chronically, these drugs decrease stores of noradrenergic catecholamines. Tricyclic antidepressant drugs also produce side effects similar to those of atropine (dry mouth, tachycardia, delirium, urinary retention) and can cause changes on the ECG (changes in the T wave, prolongation of the QRS complex, bundle branch block or other conduction abnormalities, or PVCs). Although arrhythmias induced by tricyclic antidepressants have been treated successfully with physostigmine, bradycardia has sometimes occurred.[474,475] Drug interactions with tricyclic antidepressants include those related to blockade of the reuptake of norepinephrine (such as interference with the action of guanethidine) and fatal arrhythmias after halothane and pancuronium.[496,497] Such interactions, though predictable for a population of patients, may not alter a patient's threshold for arrhythmias. The newer antidepressants (the SSRIs) can also have serious side effects. Fluoxetine, a tricyclic that also has an SSRI effect, causes nausea, vomiting, headaches, nervousness, and possibly paranoia and ideas of suicide more commonly than the other tricyclics do[474,475]; however, it is less likely to cause anticholinergic effects or orthostatic hypotension. Bupropion may cause nausea, vomiting, seizures, agitation, tremor, excitement, and increased motor activity, but it only rarely causes anticholinergic effects or orthostatic hypotension. Discontinuing drugs can cause withdrawal symptoms or precipitate recurrence of psychiatric illness. Switching between drugs for depression can cause hyperpyrexia and coma. Thus, switching before surgery should not be requested casually.[474,475]

The effectiveness of phenothiazines and butyrophenones in schizophrenia suggests a dopamine receptor blocking action. In addition, these drugs possess varying degrees of parasympathetic stimulation and ability to block α-adrenergic receptors. The phenothiazines include chlorpromazine (Thorazine, Chlor-PZ), promazine (Sparine), triflupromazine (Vesprin), fluphenazine (Prolixin), trifluoperazine, prochlorperazine (Compazine), and many others. The butyrophenones include droperidol and haloperidol (Haldol). Both the phenothiazines and butyrophenones produce sedation, depression, and antihistaminic, antiemetic, and hypothermic responses. They are also associated with cholestatic jaundice, impotence, dystonia, and photosensitivity. Other side effects associated with phenothiazines include orthostatic hypotension (partly as a result of α-adrenergic blockade) and abnormalities on the ECG such as prolongation of the QT or PR intervals, blunting of T waves, depression of the ST segment, and on rare occasion, PVCs and torsades de pointes.[474,475,496,497] Although few data are available on the antidepressant drugs selective for serotonin (the SSRIs), occasional case reports of severe hypotension and cardiac arrest with severe bradycardia have been presented in abstract form.

Several important drug interactions are noteworthy for the phenothiazine derivatives. The effects of CNS depressants (especially narcotics and barbiturates) are enhanced by the concomitant administration of phenothiazines. In addition, the CNS seizure threshold is lowered by the administration of phenothiazines, which should be avoided in patients who are epileptic or withdrawing from any drug that depresses the CNS. The antihypertensive effects of guanethidine and guanadrel are blocked by tricyclic antidepressant drugs and the phenothiazines.[472] Lithium carbonate is used to treat manic depression, but it is more effective in preventing mania than relieving depression. In excitable cells, lithium mimics sodium and decreases the release of neurotransmitters both centrally and peripherally. Lithium prolongs neuromuscular blockade and may decrease anesthetic requirements because it blocks brainstem release of norepinephrine, epinephrine, and dopamine.

Psychoactive drugs such as the amphetamines (including methamphetamines and their smokable derivative in crystal form known as "ice") and cocaine acutely release norepinephrine, epinephrine, and dopamine and block their reuptake. Taken chronically, they deplete nerve endings of these neurotransmitters.

Drugs that appear to increase central α-adrenergic release increase anesthetic requirements, whereas drugs that appear to decrease central α-adrenergic release decrease anesthetic requirements. (This may not be the mechanism by which they alter anesthetic requirements, but it is a convenient way of remembering the alteration.) Drugs that affect only the β-adrenergic receptors do not alter anesthetic requirements.

Sympathomimetic Drugs

Many antiasthmatic drugs (bronchodilators) such as terbutaline, aminophylline, and theophylline are sympathomimetic drugs that can interact with volatile anesthetics to cause cardiac arrhythmias (also see Chapter 16). Halothane (and to some degree most other volatile anesthetics) sensitizes the myocardium to exogenous catecholamines.[498,499] Sensitization means that the minimum dose of exogenous epinephrine administered intravenously that is needed to produce PVCs would be lower in patients anesthetized with halothane than in awake patients.

How much epinephrine is safe to give when halothane is the anesthetic? Katz and Bigger[498] reported that the administration of 0.15 mL/kg of a 1 : 100,000 epinephrine solution per 10-minute period (not to exceed 0.45 mL/kg of a 1 : 100,000 solution per hour) was safe. Several studies have shown that lidocaine given with epinephrine affords extra protection and that enflurane and isoflurane are less sensitizing than halothane. Xanthines are effective bronchodilators because they produce β-adrenergic stimulation in two ways: they cause the release of norepinephrine[500,501] and also inhibit the breakdown of cAMP,[502] the mediator of many of the actions of β-adrenergic receptor agonists. Phosphodiesterase catalyzes the breakdown of cAMP. Thus, inhibition of phosphodiesterase by theophylline increases the concentration of cAMP. Marcus and associates[500] and Westfall and Flemming[501] showed that at least 40% of the inotropic effects of aminophylline are due to its ability to release norepinephrine directly.

Plasma theophylline levels of 5 mg/L are needed to reduce abnormally high airway resistance. No further beneficial effects are obtained when levels exceed 20 mg/L; instead, toxic effects appear. Theophylline (aminophylline is a combination of 85% theophylline and 15% ethylenediamine) is metabolized largely by the liver, with less than 10% being excreted unchanged in urine. The average half-life is 4.4 ± 1.15 hours in adults, and clearance is 1.2 mL/min/kg. Significant liver disease or pulmonary edema can decrease clearance of the drug by half and by a third, respectively.

An interaction between aminophylline and halothane appears to be a frequent, predictable occurrence: of 16 dogs anesthetized with 1% halothane and given high-dose bolus injections of aminophylline, 12 had ventricular arrhythmias and 8 had ventricular tachycardia or fibrillation. Thus, it is advisable to wait three drug half-lives after the last dose of aminophylline is given (i.e., approximately 13 hours in normal individuals) before using halothane to anesthetize an asthmatic patient. Using another anesthetic that is a bronchodilator but is less likely to predispose the patient to catecholamine-induced arrhythmias (e.g., enflurane, isoflurane, or sevoflurane) or using inhaled or systemic steroids started several days in advance might be alternatives in patients requiring aminophylline or other exogenous sympathomimetic drugs before or during surgery.

Other Drugs

Drugs other than those discussed earlier in this chapter have implications for anesthetic management. The therapies that have been discussed include anticoagulants and fibrinolytics (in the hematologic section), endocrinologic preparations excluding birth control pills but including corticosteroids (in the section on endocrinologic disease), antihypertensive drugs (earlier in this section and in the section on cardiovascular diseases), anticonvulsant drugs (in the section on neurologic disorders), and cancer chemotherapeutic agents (in the section on oncology).

Antiarrhythmic Drugs

Antiarrhythmic drugs include local anesthetics (lidocaine, procaine), anticonvulsant (phenytoin) or antihypertensive (propranolol) drugs, calcium channel blocking drugs, or primary antiarrhythmic drugs. These drugs are classified into five major categories: local anesthetics that alter phase 0 and phase 4 depolarization (quinidine, procainamide, and flecainide), local anesthetics that affect only phase 4 depolarization (lidocaine, tocainide, phenytoin, encainide), β-adrenergic receptor antagonists, antiadrenergic drugs (bretylium, disopyramide, amiodarone), and calcium entry blockers. These drugs are discussed elsewhere in this chapter. A useful reference with suggestions about drug therapy for cardiac arrhythmias and monitoring of side effects was published by the *Medical Letter on Drugs and Therapeutics*.[503] A lack of adverse reports does not indicate that all these drugs should be continued through the time of surgery; pharmacokinetic studies have not yet determined whether anesthesia (or anesthesia with specific agents) alters the volume of distribution or clearance of these drugs to an extent sufficient to warrant changing the dosage or dosage schedule in the perioperative period. The dearth of reports on this subject may be due to a lack of significant drug interaction or to a lack of awareness that untoward events could be caused by such an interaction.

The pharmacologic characteristics of the various antiarrhythmic drugs can affect anesthetic management. Disopyramide is similar to quinidine and procainamide in its antiarrhythmic effectiveness. Disopyramide is excreted mainly by the kidneys, but hepatic disease increases its half-life. This drug often produces anticholinergic effects, including tachycardia, urinary retention, and psychosis. Hepatitis has also been reported to have occurred after its use.[503] Little is known of the interaction of bretylium with anesthetics. Because bretylium blocks the release of catecholamines, chronic therapy with this drug has been associated with hypersensitivity to vasopressors.[503] Quinidine is dependent on the kidneys for excretion, can produce vagolytic effects that can decrease AV block, and is associated with blood dyscrasias and GI disturbances.[503] Most of the antiarrhythmic drugs enhance nondepolarizing neuromuscular blockade. Reports have confirmed this enhancement for quinidine, phenytoin, lidocaine, procainamide, and propranolol.[504-512] Amiodarone, an antiadrenergic drug used to treat recurrent supraventricular and ventricular tachycardia, causes thyroid dysfunction as a result of the large amount of iodine in its structure (see the section on thyroid disorders earlier in this chapter), as well as peripheral neuropathy, and has been associated with hypertension, bradyarrhythmias, and reduced cardiac output during anesthesia.[513] The drug has a half-life of 29 days, and its pharmacologic effects persist for over 45 days after discontinuance.[514] No data document such an effect for depolarizing muscle relaxants.

Antibiotics

Many antibacterial agents are nephrotoxic or neurotoxic (or both), and many prolong neuromuscular blockade (also see Chapter 29).[506-512] The only antibiotics devoid of neuromuscular effects appear to be penicillin G and the cephalosporins.[511] Most enzyme-inducing drugs do not increase the metabolism of enflurane or isoflurane. However, isoniazid appears to induce the microsomal enzymes responsible for the metabolism of at least enflurane, thereby increasing the possibility of fluorine-associated renal damage after enflurane.[515] Appropriate antibiotic prophylaxis for surgery requires a knowledge of the probability of infection for that type of surgical procedure and, if the incidence of infection warrants, the use of a drug regimen directed against the most likely infecting organisms.[516]

Digitalis

Digitalis preparations have a limited margin of safety, and the risk of toxicity increases with hypokalemia.[517] Although there is good rationale for administering digoxin prophylactically before surgery,[518] we generally avoid doing so because potassium concentrations can fluctuate widely during anesthesia as a result of fluid shifts, ventilatory acid-base derangements, and adjuvant treatments and because intraoperative arrhythmias caused by digitalis toxicity may be difficult to differentiate from those having other sources. Digitalis intoxication can be manifested by such diverse cardiac arrhythmias as junctional escape rhythm, PVCs, ventricular bigeminy or trigeminy, junctional tachycardia, paroxysmal atrial tachycardia with or without block, sinus arrest, sinus exit block, Mobitz type I or II block, or ventricular tachycardia.[517] However, anesthetics appear to protect against digitalis toxicity, at least in animal studies.[519-522] A titrated cardioversion technique using at first 10- and then 20-, 30-, 40-, 50-, 75-, 100-, 150-, and 200-J doses resulted in safe cardioversion in the presence of digitalis and propofol or midazolam hypnosis.[523] For patients in atrial fibrillation, the ventricular response should guide the choice of dose of digitalis.

Medications for Glaucoma

Medications for glaucoma include two organophosphates: echothiophate and isoflurophate (also see Chapter 75). These drugs inhibit serum cholinesterase, which is responsible for the hydrolysis and inactivation of succinylcholine and ester-type local anesthetics such as procaine, chloroprocaine, and tetracaine.[524,525] These ester-type local anesthetics should be avoided in patients treated with eye drops containing organophosphate. Table 35-20 lists other medications related to anesthesia and their side effects (from the National Registry for Drug-Induced Ocular Side Effects, Oregon Health Sciences University, 3181 SW Sam Jackson Park Road, Portland, OR 97201; 503-279-8456).

Magnesium, Cimetidine, and Oral Contraceptives

Although information on drugs long used in therapy is old, it is still pertinent and useful to review for these old "standby" drugs. Magnesium is given to treat eclampsia; it can cause neuromuscular blockade by itself and potentiates neuromuscular blockade by both nondepolarizing and depolarizing muscle relaxants. Cimetidine reduces hepatic blood flow and inhibits enzymatic degradation of drugs by the liver. Thus, higher blood levels and prolonged elimination half-lives may result when drugs that are metabolized by the liver (e.g., lidocaine, procaine, some narcotics, and propranolol) are given to patients taking cimetidine chronically or acutely.[526,527] The risk of postoperative venous thrombosis increases when oral contraceptives are used preoperatively. Although some authorities recommend changing from oral con-

Table 35-20 Common Ophthalmologic Drugs and Their Anesthetically Important Interactions

Drug (Trade Name)	Toxicities and Specific Treatments
Glaucoma: Primary goal is to reduce IOP by Miotics and epinephrine: increase outflow of aqueous humor β-Blockade and carbonic anhydrase inhibitors: reduce production of aqueous humor Osmotic drugs: transiently decrease volume	
Miotics Parasympathomimetics Pilocarpine (Adsorbocarpine, Isopto Carpine, Pilocar, Pilocel) Carbachol	
Acetylcholinesterase inhibitors Physostigmine Demecarium Isoflurophate (Floropryl) Echothiophate (Echodide, Phospholine)	Tox: Hypersalivation, sweating, N/V, bradycardia, hypotension, bronchospasm, CNS effects, coma, respiratory arrest, death Rx: Atropine, pralidoxime (Protopam) Ix: Succinylcholine—prolonged apnea (drugs must be discontinued 4 wk before)
Epinephrine (Epitrate, Murocoll, Mytrate, Epifrin, Glaucon, Epinal, Eppy)	Tox: (rare) Tachycardia, PVCs, HTN, headache, tremors Ix: Avoid drugs that sensitize to catecholamines, e.g., halothane
β-Blockers Timolol (Timoptic) Betaxolol (Betoptic) Levobunolol (Betagan)	Tox: J-blockade with bradycardia, exacerbation of asthma, CNS depression, lethargy, confusion Synergy noted with systemic drugs
Carbonic anhydrase inhibitors Acetazolamide (Diamox) Dichlorphenamide (Daranide, Oratrol) Ethoxzolamide (Cardrase, Ethamide) Methazolamide (Neptazane)	Tox: Anorexia, GI disturbances, "general miserable feeling" and malaise, paresthesias, diuresis, hypokalemia (transient), renal colic and calculi, hyperuricemia, thrombocytopenia, aplastic anemia, acute respiratory failure in patients with COPD
Osmotic drugs Glycerin (Glyrol, Osmoglyn) Isosorbide (Ismotic) Urea (Urevert, Ureaphil) Mannitol (Osmitrol)	Tox: Dehydration, hyperglycemia, nonketotic hyperosmolar coma (rare). Fatalities with mannitol secondary to CHF or intracranial bleeding Urea may cause thrombosis
Intraocular acetylcholine (Miochol)	Tox: Hypotension, bradycardia Rx: Atropine
Mydriatics and cycloplegics: Provide pupillary dilatation and paralysis of accommodation Anticholinergics block muscarinic receptors; paralyzing in iris α-Adrenergics contract the dilator of the iris	
Anticholinergics Atropine (Atropisol, Bufopto, Isopto Atropine) Cyclopentolate, alone (Cyclogyl) or with phenylephrine-homatropine (Cyclomydril) Scopolamine tropicamide (Homatrocel, Isopto Homatropine, Isopto Hyoscine, Murocoll #19, Mydriacyl)	Tox: Dry mouth, flushing, thirst, tachycardia, seizure, hyperactivity, transient psychosis, rare coma, and death Rx: Physostigmine
α-Adrenergics Phenylephrine (Efricel, Mydfrin, Neo-Synephrine) Hydroxyamphetamine (Paredrine)	Tox: Tachycardia, HTN, PVCs, myocardial ischemia, agitation

CHF, congestive heart failure; CNS, central nervous system; COPD, chronic obstructive pulmonary disease; GI, gastrointestinal; HTN, hypertension; IOP, intraocular pressure; Ix, interaction; N/V, nausea and vomiting; PVCs, premature ventricular contractions; Rx, treatment; Tox, toxicity.

traceptives to topical methods of birth control 2 to 4 weeks before surgery, no controlled study has determined whether birth control pills should be discontinued before surgery or the resulting incidence of pregnancy. Moreover, year-long pellets make discontinuation impractical for some. Other authorities recommend preventing venous thromboembolism by using low-dose heparin, guided by a determination of efficacy and cost-effectiveness. In addition, estrogens with micronized progestins are effective at reducing all-cause mortality for at least the first 10 years after menopause.[22,23,528] Thus, the uncertainty surrounding prophylaxis for heart disease (created by the dilemma of long-term benefit versus the short-term risk of thromboembolism) needs better data for resolution.

Interrupting a Drug Regimen before Surgery

If a drug is needed for treatment preoperatively, it should be continued through surgery. One of us (M.F.R.) provides patients and other professionals with a detailed list (Box 35-7) that we supply through our preanesthesia and preprocedure assessment clinic. It must often be specifically requested because many patients and nurses perceive the NPO directive to include drugs.[529,530] The only exception to this general rule of not altering preoperative drug therapy might pertain to (1) MAOIs, (2) anticoagulants and fibrinolytic drugs (e.g., clopidogrel [Plavix]) if surgical hemostasis is needed, (3) nicotinic acid, (4) dosage adjustments for insulin and corticosteroids, (5) ACE inhibitors and receptor antagonists (angiotensin II receptor blocking drugs), and (6) drugs for erectile dysfunction (i.e., sildenafil [Viagra], vardenafil [Levitra], tadalafil [Cialis], or similar drugs). These recommendations require that the anesthesiologist be aware of the pharmacologic characteristics, interactions, and anesthetic implications of drugs described earlier in this chapter.

When in doubt about a disease or a drug, we consult the following textbooks: *Harrison's Principles of Internal Medicine*; *Anesthesia and Uncommon Diseases: Pathophysiologic and Clinical Correlations*; *Anesthesia and Co-Existing Disease*; *Essence of Anesthesia Practice*; *Anesthetic Implications of Congenital Anomalies in Children*; *Pharmacology and Physiology in Anesthetic Practice*; and *Goodman and Gilman's The Pharmacologic Basis of Therapeutics*. It is then wise to consult two experts on the drug or disease and determine who is best able to care for the patient. The

Box 35-7 Preoperative and Preprocedure Medication Instruction Guidelines (PPAC Form 5)

Instruct patients to take the following medications with a small sip of water EVEN IF OTHERWISE NPO:

Antihypertensive medications—Continue on the day of the operation or procedure

Diuretics—Continue on the day of the operation or procedure

Cardiac medications (e.g., digoxin)—Continue on the day of the procedure

Antidepressant, antianxiety, and psychiatric medications—Continue on the day of the operation or procedure

Thyroid medications—Continue on the day of the operation or procedure

Birth control pills—Continue on the day of the operation or procedure

Eye drops—Continue on the day of the operation or procedure

Heartburn or reflux medications (e.g., Prilosec, Zantac)—Continue on the day of the operation or procedure

Narcotic pain medications—Continue on the day of the operation or procedure

Antiseizure medications—Continue on the day of the operation or procedure

Asthma medications—Continue on the day of the operation or procedure

Steroids (oral and inhaled)—Continue on the day of the operation or procedure

Statins (e.g., Zocor, Lipitor)—Continue on the day of the operation or procedure

Aspirin—Usually continue; discontinue 7 days before plastic surgery and surgery on the retina

COX-2 inhibitors—Continue on the day of the operation or procedure unless the surgeon specifies (usually concerned about bone healing)

NSAIDs—Usually continue; discontinue 48 hours before plastic surgery and surgery on the retina

Vitamins, iron, Premarin—Discontinue on the day of the operation or procedure

Topical medications (e.g., creams and ointments)—Discontinue on the day of the operation or procedure

Oral hypoglycemic drugs—Discontinue on the day of the operation or procedure

Insulin—For all patients, discontinue all regular or combination (70/30 preparations) insulin on the day of the operation or procedure. Type 2 diabetics should discontinue all insulins of any type. Type 1 diabetics should take a small amount (usually a third) of their usual AM long-acting insulin (e.g., Lente or NPH) on the day of the operation or procedure. Type 1 diabetics should not take any short-acting insulin, such as regular insulin, on the day of the procedure. Patients with an insulin pump should continue their basal rate only.

Viagra, Levitra, Cialis, or similar drugs—Discontinue 36 hours before surgery

Warfarin (Coumadin)—Discontinue 4 days before surgery except for patients undergoing cataract surgery without a bulbar block

Plavix (clopidogrel)—Discontinue 7 days before surgery except for vascular patients or those undergoing cataract surgery

Herbals and nonvitamin supplements—Discontinue 7 days before surgery

MAOIs—Patients taking these antidepressant medications need an anesthesia consultation before surgery (preferably 3 weeks before surgery)

COX, cyclooxygenase; MAOIs, monoamine oxidase inhibitors; NPO, nothing by mouth; NSAIDs, nonsteroidal anti-inflammatory drugs.

expert who is best qualified should be observed while attending to the patient, not only preoperatively and intraoperatively but also postoperatively. It is important to remember that few prospective controlled studies have shown that any preoperative technique, treatment, or management decreases perioperative risk. However, common sense and foreknowledge of potential pitfalls, as well as diligence in avoiding these pitfalls, should reduce avoidable perioperative complications.

References

1. Thorpe KE, Howard DH, Galactionova K: Differences in disease prevalence as a source of the U.S.-European health care spending gap. Health Affairs 26:w678-w686, 2007.
2. Wei JY: Age and the cardiovascular system. N Engl J Med 327:1735, 1992.
3. Perioperative medicine. *In* Medical Knowledge Self-Assessment Program 14, General Internal Medicine. Philadelphia, American College of Physicians, 2006, p 128.
4. Roizen M: The preoperative cardiology consult: What the cardiologist should know about anesthesia. *In* Parmley W, Chatterjee K (eds): Cardiology. Philadelphia, JB Lippincott, 1993, p 1.
5. Wilson SH, Fasseas P, Orford JL, et al: Clinical outcome of patients undergoing non-cardiac surgery in the two months following coronary stenting. J Am Coll Cardiol 42:234-240, 2003.
6. Fleisher LA, Eagle KA: Clinical practice. Lowering cardiac risk in noncardiac surgery. N Engl J Med 345:1677, 2001.
7. Goldman L, Caldera DL, Nussbaum SR, et al: Multifactorial index of cardiac risk in noncardiac surgical procedures. N Engl J Med 297:845, 1977.
8. Fleisher LA, Beckman JA, Brown KA, et al: ACC/AHA 2007 guidelines on perioperative cardiovascular evaluation and care for noncardiac surgery—a report of the American College of Cardiology/American Heart Association Task Force on Practice Guidelines (Writing Committee to Revise the 2002 Guidelines on Perioperative Cardiovascular Evaluation for Noncardiac Surgery). J Am Coll Cardiol 50:159-211, 2007.
9. Krinsley JS: Effect of an intensive glucose management protocol on the mortality of critically ill adult patients. Mayo Clin Proc 79:992-1000, 2004.
10. Advance Collaborative Group: Intensive broad glucose control and vascular outcomes in patients with type 2 diabetes. N Engl J Med 358:2560-2572, 2008.
11. Van den Berghe G, Wouters P, Weekers F, et al: Intensive insulin therapy in critically ill patients. N Engl J Med 345:1359-1367, 2001.
12. Ingels C, Debaveye Y, Milants I, et al: Strict blood glucose control with insulin after cardiac surgery: Impact on 4-year survival, depending on medical care, and quality of life. Eur Heart J 27:2716-2724, 2006.
13. Finney SJ, Zekveld C, Elia A, Evans TW: Glucose control and mortality in critically ill patients. JAMA 290:2041-2047, 2003.
14. Krinsley JS: Association between hyperglycemia and increased hospital mortality in a heterogeneous population of critically ill patients. Mayo Clin Proc 78:1471-1478, 2003.
15. The Diabetes Control and Complications Trial (DCCT)/Epidemiology of Diabetes Interventions and Complications Research Group: Retinopathy and nephropathy in patients with type I diabetes four years after a trial of intensive therapy. N Engl J Med 342:381-389, 2000.
16. UK Prospective Diabetes Study Group: Tight blood pressure control and risk of macrovascular and microvascular complications in type II diabetes. BMJ 317:703-713, 1998.
17. Albacker T, Carvalho G, Schricker T, et al: High-dose insulin therapy attenuates systemic inflammation response in coronary artery bypass grafting patients. Ann Thorac Surg 86:20-27, 2008.
18. Freeman R: Autonomic peripheral neuropathy. Lancet 365:1259-1270, 2005.
19. Charlson ME, MacKenzie CR, Gold JP: Preoperative autonomic function abnormalities in patients with diabetes mellitus and patients with hypertension. J Am Coll Surg 179:1, 1994.
20. Kalichman MW, Calcutt NA: Local anesthetic–induced conduction block and nerve fiber injury in streptozotocin-diabetic rats. Anesthesiology 77:941, 1992.
21. Roizen MF: RealAge: Are You As Young As You Can Be? New York, HarperCollins, 1999.
22. Roizen MF: The RealAge Makeover: Take Years Off Your Looks and Add Them to Your Life! New York, HarperCollins, 2004.
23. Roizen MF, Oz MC: YOU: The Owner's Manual. New York, HarperCollins, 2005.
24. Dormandy JA, Charbonnel B, Ecklund DJ, et al: Secondary prevention of mascrovascular events in patients with type 2 diabetes in the PROactive Study (PROspective pioglitAzone Clinical Trial In macro Vascular Events): A randomized controlled trial. Lancet 366:1279-1289, 2005.
25. Nolan CM, Beaty HN, Bagdade JD: Further characterization of the impaired bactericidal function of granulocytes in patients with poorly controlled diabetes. Diabetes 27:889, 1978.
26. Cruse PJ, Foord R: A 5-year prospective study of 23,649 surgical wounds. Arch Surg 107:206, 1973.
27. Longstreth WT, Inui TS: High blood glucose level on hospital admission and poor neurological recovery after cardiac arrest. Ann Neurol 15:59, 1984.
28. Johnson WD, Pedraza PM, Kayser KL: Coronary artery surgery in diabetics: 261 consecutive patients followed four to seven years. Am Heart J 104:823-827, 1982.
29. Borow KM, Jaspan JB, Williams KA, et al: Myocardial mechanics in young adult patients with diabetes mellitus: Effects of altered load, inotropic state and dynamic exercise. J Am Coll Cardiol 15:1508, 1990.
30. Chiasson JL, Aris-Jilwan N, Belanger R, et al: Diagnosis and treatment of diabetic ketoacidosis and the hyperglycemic hyperosmolar state. CMAJ 168:859-866, 2003.
31. The Diabetes Control and Complications Trial Research Group: Effect of intensive therapy on residual β-cell function in patients with type 1 diabetes in the Diabetes Control and Complications Trial. A randomized, controlled trial. Ann Intern Med 128:517, 1998.
32. Ramanathan S, Khoo P, Arismendy J: Perioperative maternal and neonatal acid-base status and glucose metabolism in patients with insulin-dependent diabetes mellitus. Anesth Analg 73:105, 1991.
33. Khuri SF, Daley J, Henderson W, et al: Risk adjustment of the postoperative mortality rate for the comparative assessment of the quality of surgical care: Results of the National Veterans Affairs Surgical Risk Study. J Am Coll Surg 185:315, 1997.
34. Tuomilehto J, Lindstrom J, Eriksson JG, et al: Finnish Diabetes Prevention Study Group. Prevention of type 2 diabetes mellitus by changes in lifestyle among subjects with impaired glucose tolerance. N Engl J Med 344:1343-1350, 2001.
35. Ravid M, Brosh D, Levi Z, et al: Use of enalapril to attenuate decline in renal function in normotensive, normoalbuminuric patients with type 2 diabetes mellitus. A randomized, controlled trial. Ann Intern Med 128:982, 1998.
36. Page MM, Watkins PJ: Cardiorespiratory arrest and diabetic autonomic neuropathy. Lancet 1:14, 1978.
37. Pasternak JJ, McGregor DG, Schroeder DR, et al: Hypoglycemia in patients undergoing cerebral aneurysm surgery: Its association with long-term gross neurologic and neuropsychological function. Mayo Clin Proc 83:406-417, 2008.
38. Larsen ML, Illingworth DR: Drug treatment of dyslipoproteinemia. Med Clin North Am 78:225, 1994.
39. Downs JR, Clearfield M, Weis S, et al: Primary prevention of acute coronary events with lovastatin in men and women with average cholesterol levels. Results of AFCAPS/TexCAPS. JAMA 279:1615, 1998.
40. Fowkes FGR, Price JF, Leng GC: Targeting subclinical atherosclerosis. BMJ 316:1764, 1998.
41. Nissen SE, Tazcu EM, Schoenhagen P, et al: Effect of intensive compared with moderate lipid-lowering therapy on progression of coronary atherosclerosis. A randomized clinical trial. JAMA 291:1071-1080, 2004.
42. Pelosi P, Croci M, Ravagnan I, et al: Respiratory system mechanics in sedated, paralyzed, morbidly obese patients. J Appl Physiol 82:811-818, 1997.
43. Daniels L: Good nutrition for good surgery: Clinical and quality of life outcomes. Australian Prescriber 26:136-140, 2003.
44. Donini LM, Savina C, Cannella C: Eating habits and appetite control in the elderly: The anorexia of aging. Int Psychogeriatr 15:73-87, 2003.
45. Veterans Administration Total Parenteral Nutrition Cooperative Study Group: Perioperative total parenteral nutrition in surgical patients. N Engl J Med 325:525, 1991.
46. Nicholas JM, Cornelius MW, Tchorz KM, et al: A two institution experience with 226 endoscopically placed jejunal feeding tubes in critically ill surgical patients. Am J Surg 186:583-590, 2003.
47. Starker PM, La Sala PA, Askanazi J, et al: The responses to TPN, a form of nutritional assessment. Ann Surg 198:720, 1983.
48. Udelsman R, Ramp J, Gallucci WT, et al: Adaptation during surgical stress: A reevaluation of the role of glucocorticoids. J Clin Invest 77:1377, 1986.

49. Lampe GH, Roizen MF: Anesthesia for patients with abnormal function of the adrenal cortex. Anesthesiol Clin North Am 5:245, 1987.
50. Ezzat S, Asa SL, Couldwell WT, et al: The prevalence of pituitary adenomas: A systematic review. Cancer 101:613-619, 2004.
51. Symreng T, Karlberg BE, Kågedal B, et al: Physiological cortisol substitution of long-term steroid-treated patients undergoing major surgery. Br J Anaesth 53:949, 1981.
52. Nieman LK, Oldfield EH, Wesley R, et al: A simplified morning corticotrophin-releasing hormone stimulation test for the differential diagnosis of adrenocorticotrophin-dependent Cushing's syndrome. J Clin Endocrinol Metab 77:1308, 1993.
53. Dorin RI, Qualls CR, Crapo LM: Diagnosis of adrenal insufficiency. Ann Intern Med 139:194-204, 2003.
54. Bravo EL: Evolving concepts in the pathophysiology, diagnosis and treatment of pheochromocytoma. Endocr Rev 15:356, 1994.
55. St John Sutton MG, Sheps SG, Lie JT: Prevalence of clinically unsuspected pheochromocytoma: Review of a 50-year autopsy series. Mayo Clin Proc 56:354, 1981.
56. Prys-Roberts C: Phaeochromocytoma—recent progress in its management. Br J Anaesth 85:44-57, 2000.
57. Witteles RM, Kaplan EL, Roizen MF: Safe and cost-effective preoperative preparation of patients with pheochromocytoma. Anesth Analg 91:302-304, 2000.
58. Lucon AM, Pereira MAA, Mendonça BB, et al: Pheochromocytoma: Study of 50 cases. J Urol 157:1208, 1997.
59. Roizen MF, Horrigan RW, Koike M, et al: A prospective randomized trial of four anesthetic techniques for resection of pheochromocytoma [abstract]. Anesthesiology 57:A43, 1982.
60. Roizen MF, Hunt TK, Beaupre PN, et al: The effect of alpha-adrenergic blockade on cardiac performance and tissue oxygen delivery during excision of pheochromocytoma. Surgery 94:941, 1983.
61. Allen GC, Rosenberg H: Pheochromocytoma presenting as acute malignant hyperthermia—a diagnostic challenge. Can J Anaesth 37:593, 1990.
62. Zakowski M, Kaufman B, Berguson P, et al: Esmolol use during resection of pheochromocytoma: Report of three cases. Anesthesiology 70:875, 1989.
63. Roizen MF, Schreider BD, Hassan SZ: Anesthetic for patients with pheochromocytoma. Anesthesiol Clin North Am 5:269, 1987.
64. Roizen MF: Should we all have a sympathectomy at birth? Or at least preoperatively? Anesthesiology 68:482, 1988.
65. Stone JG, Foëx P, Sear JW, et al: Myocardial ischemia in untreated hypertensive patients. Effect of a single small oral dose of a beta-adrenergic blocking agent. Anesthesiology 68:495, 1988.
66. Mangano DT, Layug EL, Wallace A, et al: Effect of atenolol on mortality and cardiovascular morbidity after noncardiac surgery. N Engl J Med 335:1713, 1996.
67. Flacke JW, Bloor BC, Flacke WE, et al: Reduced narcotic requirement by clonidine with improved hemodynamic and adrenergic stability in patients undergoing coronary bypass surgery. Anesthesiology 67:11, 1987.
68. Yeager MP, Glass DD, Neff RK, Brinck-Johnsen T: Epidural anesthesia and analgesia in high-risk surgical patients. Anesthesiology 66:729, 1987.
69. Fleisher LA, Rosenbaum SH, Nelson AH, Barash PG: The predictive value of preoperative silent ischemia for postoperative ischemic cardiac events in vascular and nonvascular surgery patients. Am Heart J 122:980, 1991.
70. Levine JD, Dardick SJ, Roizen MF, et al: The contribution of sensory afferents and sympathetic efferents to joint injury in experimental arthritis. J Neurosci 6:3423, 1986.
71. Wade JG, Larson CP, Hickey RF, et al: Carotid endarterectomy and carotid chemoreceptor and baroreceptor function in man. N Engl J Med 282:823, 1970.
72. Ziegler MG, Lake CR, Kopin IJ: The sympathetic nervous system defect in primary orthostatic hypotension. N Engl J Med 296:293, 1977.
73. Goldstein DS, Holmes C, Cannon RO III, et al: Sympathetic cardioneuropathy in dysautonomias. N Engl J Med 336:696, 1997.
74. Kendrick WW, Scott JW, Jousse AT, et al: Reflex sweating and hypertension in traumatic transverse myelitis. Treat Serv Bull (Ottawa) 8:437, 1953.
75. Naftchi NE, Wooten GF, Lowman EW, et al: Relationship between serum dopamine-β-hydroxylase activity, catecholamine metabolism, and hemodynamic changes during paroxysmal hypertension in quadriplegia. Circ Res 35:850, 1974.
76. Gronert GA, Theye RA: Pathophysiology of hyperkalemia induced by succinylcholine. Anesthesiology 43:89, 1975.
77. Feek CM, Sawers JSA, Irvine WJ, et al: Combination of potassium iodide and propranolol in preparation of patients with Graves' disease for thyroid surgery. N Engl J Med 302:883, 1980.
78. Roizen MF, Becker CE: Thyroid storm: A review of cases at University of California, San Francisco. Calif Med 115:5, 1971.
79. Loh KC: Amiodarone-induced thyroid disorders: A clinical review. Postgrad Med J 76:133-140, 2000.
80. Williams M, Lo Gerfo P: Thyroidectomy using local anesthesia in critically ill patients with amiodarone-induced thyrotoxicosis: A review and description of the technique. Thyroid 12:523-525, 2002.
81. Weinberg AD, Brennan MD, Gorman CA, et al: Outcome of anesthesia and surgery in hypothyroid patients. Arch Intern Med 143:893, 1983.
82. Surks MI, Ortiz E, Daniels GH, et al: Subclinical thyroid disease: Scientific review and guidelines for diagnosis and management. JAMA 291:228-238, 2004.
83. Vanderpump MPJ, Tunbridge WMG, French JM, et al: The incidence of thyroid disorders in the community: A twenty-year follow-up of the Wickham Survey. Clin Endocrinol 43:55, 1995.
84. Hattori H, Hattori C, Yonekura A, Nishimura T: Two cases of sleep apnea syndrome caused by primary hypothyroidism. Acta Otolaryngol Suppl 550:59-64, 2003.
85. Levine HD: Compromise therapy in the patient with angina pectoris and hypothyroidism: A clinical assessment. Am J Med 69:411, 1980.
86. Stewart AF: Clinical practice. Hypercalcemia associated with cancer. N Engl J Med 352:373-379, 2005.
87. Peacock M, Bilezikian JP, Klassen PS, et al: Cinacalcet hydrochloride maintains long-term normocalcemia in patients with primary hyperparathyroidism. J Clin Endocrinol Metab 90:135-141, 2005.
88. Lind L, Ljunghall S: Blood pressure reaction during the intraoperative and early postoperative periods in patients with primary hyperparathyroidism. Exp Clin Endocrinol 102:409-413, 1994.
89. Kebebew E, Duh QY, Clark OH: Parathyroidectomy for primary hyperparathyroidism in octogenarians and nonagenarians: A plea for early surgical referral. Arch Surg 138:867-871, 2003.
90. Boonen S, Vanderschueren D, Pelemans W, Bouillon R: Primary hyperparathyroidism: Diagnosis and management in the older individual. Eur J Endocrinol 151:297-304, 2004.
91. Carling T, Donovan P, Rinder C, Udelsman R: Minimally invasive parathyroidectomy using cervical block—reasons for conversion to general anesthesia. Arch Surg 141:401-404, 2006.
92. Allain TJ, Dhesi J: Hypovitaminosis D in older adults. Gerontology 49:273-278, 2003.
93. Rumancik WM, Denlinger JK, Nahrwold ML, et al: The QT interval and serum ionized calcium. JAMA 240:366, 1978.
94. Hensel P, Roizen MF: Patients with disorders of parathyroid function. Anesthesiol Clin North Am 5:287, 1987.
95. Lang RM, Fellner SK, Neumann A, et al: Left ventricular contractility varies directly with blood ionized calcium. Ann Intern Med 108:524, 1988.
96. Moyad MA: Preventing male osteoporosis: Prevalence, risks, diagnosis and imaging tests. Urol Clin North Am 31:321-330, 2004.
97. Cauley JA, Robbins J, Chen Z, et al: Effects of estrogen plus progestin on risk of fracture and bone mineral density: The Women's Health Initiative randomized trial. JAMA 290:1729-1738, 2003.
98. Keller MI: Treating osteoporosis in post-menopausal women: A case approach. Cleve Clin J Med 71:829-837, 2004.
99. Rojiani AM, Prineas JW, Cho ES: Protective effect of steroids on electrolyte-induced demyelination. J Neuropathol Exp Neurol 46:495, 1987.
100. Ayus JC, Wheeler JM, Arieff AI: Postoperative hyponatremic encephalopathy in menstruant women. Ann Intern Med 117:891-897, 1992.
101. Robertson GL: Diabetes insipidus. Endocrinol Metab Clin North Am 24:549, 1995.
102. Prys-Roberts C, Meloche R, Foëx P: Studies of anesthesia in relation to hypertension. I: Cardiovascular responses of treated and untreated patients. Br J Anaesth 43:122, 1971.
103. Goldman L, Caldera DL: Risks of general anesthesia and elective operation in the hypertensive patient. Anesthesiology 50:285, 1979.
104. Bedford RF, Feinstein B: Hospital admission blood pressure: A predictor for hypertension following endotracheal intubation. Anesth Analg 59:367, 1980.
105. Asiddao CB, Donegan JH, Whitesell RC, et al: Factors associated with perioperative complications during carotid endarterectomy. Anesth Analg 61:631, 1982.
106. Stone JG, Foëx P, Sear JW, et al: Risk of myocardial ischemia during anesthesia in treated and untreated hypertensive patients. Br J Anaesth 61:675, 1988.
107. Flacke JW, Bloor BC, Flacke WE, et al: Reduced narcotic requirement by clonidine with improved hemodynamic and adrenergic stability in patients undergoing coronary bypass surgery. Anesthesiology 67:11, 1987.
108. Ghignone M, Calvillo O, Quintin L: Anesthesia and hypertension: The effect of clonidine on perioperative hemodynamics and isoflurane requirements. Anesthesiology 67:3, 1987.
109. Tuman KJ, McCarthy RJ, Spiess BD, et al: Effect of pulmonary artery catheterization on outcome in patients undergoing coronary artery surgery. Anesthesiology 70:199, 1989.
110. Ellis JE, Drijvers G, Shah MN, et al: Topical clonidine fails to reduce postoperative stress response after noncardiac surgery. Anesth Analg 74:S85, 1992.
111. Mangano DT, Browner WS, Hollenberg M, et al: Association of perioperative myocardial ischemia

with cardiac morbidity and mortality in men undergoing noncardiac surgery. N Engl J Med 323:1781, 1990.
112. Pasternack PF, Grossi EA, Baumann FG, et al: Beta blockade to decrease silent myocardial ischemia during peripheral vascular surgery. Am J Surg 158:113, 1989.
113. Weksler N, Klein M, Szendro G, et al: The dilemma of immediate preoperative hypertension: To treat and operate, or to postpone surgery? J Clin Anesth 15:179-183, 2003.
114. Aronson S, Boisvert D, Lapp W: Isolated systolic hypertension is associated with adverse outcomes from coronary artery bypass grafting surgery. Anesth Analg 94:1079-1084, 2002.
115. Okuda S, Onoyama K, Motomura K, et al: Effect of acute reduction in blood pressure on renal function of rats with diseased kidneys. Nephron 45:311, 1987.
116. Farnett L, Mulrow CD, Linn WD, et al: The J-curve phenomenon and the treatment of hypertension. Is there a point beyond which pressure reduction is dangerous? JAMA 265:489, 1991.
117. Hasebe N, Kido S, Ido A, et al: Reverse J-curve relation between diastolic blood pressure and severity of coronary artery lesion in hypertensive patients with angina pectoris. Hypertens Res 25:381-387, 2002.
118. Mayhan WG, Faraci FM, Heistad DD: Disruption of the blood-brain barrier in cerebrum and brain stem during acute hypertension. Am J Physiol 251:H1171, 1986.
119. Croog SH, Levine S, Testa MA, et al: The effects of antihypertensive therapy on the quality of life. N Engl J Med 314:1657, 1986.
120. Materson BJ, Reda DJ, Cushman WC, et al: Single-drug therapy for hypertension in men. A comparison of six antihypertensive agents with placebo. N Engl J Med 328:914, 1993.
121. POISE Study Group, Devereaux PJ, Yang H, Yusuf S, et al: Effects of extended-release metoprolol succinate in patients undergoing non-cardiac surgery (POISE trial): A randomised controlled trial. Lancet 371:1839-1847, 2008.
122. Coriat P, Richer C, Douraki T, et al: Influence of chronic angiotensin-converting enzyme inhibition in anesthetic induction. Anesthesiology 81:299, 1994.
123. Bertrand M, Godet G, Meersschaert K, et al: Should the angiotensin II antagonists be discontinued before surgery? Anesth Analg 92:26-30, 2001.
124. Kheterpal S, Khodaparast O, Shanks A, et al: Chronic angiotensin-converting enzyme inhibitor or angiotensin receptor blocker therapy combined with diuretic therapy is associated with increased episodes of hypotension in noncardiac surgery. J Cardiothorac Vasc Anesth 22:180-186, 2008.
125. Fleisher LA, Beckman JA, Brown KA, et al: ACC/AHA 2007 guidelines on perioperative cardiovascular evaluation and care for noncardiac surgery: A report of the American College of Cardiology/American Heart Association Task Force on Practice Guidelines (Writing Committee to Revise the 2002 Guidelines on Perioperative Cardiovascular Evaluation for Noncardiac Surgery): Developed in collaboration with the American Society of Echocardiography, American Society of Nuclear Cardiology, Heart Rhythm Society, Society of Cardiovascular Anesthesiologists, Society for Cardiovascular Angiography and Interventions, Society for Vascular Medicine and Biology, and Society for Vascular Surgery. Circulation 116(17):e418-e499, 2007.
126. Hertzer NR, Young JR, Beven EG, et al: Late results of coronary bypass in patients with peripheral vascular disease: I. Five-year survival according to age and clinical cardiac status. Cleve Clin Q 53:133-143, 1986.
127. Hertzer NR, Young JR, Beven EG, et al: Late results of coronary bypass in patients with peripheral vascular disease. II. Five-year survival according to sex, hypertension, and diabetes. Cleve Clin Q 54:15-23, 1987.
128. Eagle KA, Rihal CS, Mickel MC, et al: Cardiac risk of noncardiac surgery: Influence of coronary disease and type of surgery in 3368 operations. CASS Investigators and University of Michigan Heart Care Program. Coronary Artery Surgery Study. Circulation 96:1882-1887, 1997.
129. Landesberg G, Mosseri M, Wolf YG, et al: Preoperative thallium scanning, selective coronary revascularization, and long-term survival after major vascular surgery. Circulation 108:177-183, 2003.
130. Posner KL, Van Norman GA, Chan V: Adverse cardiac outcomes after noncardiac surgery in patients with prior percutaneous transluminal coronary angioplasty. Anesth Analg 89:553-560, 1999.
131. Godet G, Riou B, Bertrand M, et al: Does preoperative coronary angioplasty improve perioperative cardiac outcome? Anesthesiology 102:739-746, 2005.
132. McFalls EO, Ward HB, Moritz TE, et al: Coronary-artery revascularization before elective major vascular surgery. N Engl J Med 351:2795-2804, 2004.
133. Ward HB, Kelly RF, Thottapurathu L, et al: Coronary artery bypass grafting is superior to percutaneous coronary intervention in prevention of perioperative myocardial infarctions during subsequent vascular surgery. Ann Thorac Surg 82:795-800, discussion 800-801, 2006.
134. Poldermans D, Bax JJ, Schouten O, et al: Should major vascular surgery be delayed because of preoperative cardiac testing in intermediate-risk patients receiving beta-blocker therapy with tight heart rate control? J Am Coll Cardiol 48:964-969, 2006.
135. Poldermans D, Schouten O, Vidakovic R, et al: A clinical randomized trial to evaluate the safety of a noninvasive approach in high-risk patients undergoing major vascular surgery: The DECREASE-V Pilot Study. J Am Coll Cardiol 49:1763-1769, 2007.
136. Back MR, Stordahl N, Cuthbertson D, et al: Limitations in the cardiac risk reduction provided by coronary revascularization prior to elective vascular surgery. J Vasc Surg 36:526-533, 2002.
137. Kaluza GL, Joseph J, Lee JR, et al: Catastrophic outcomes of noncardiac surgery soon after coronary stenting. J Am Coll Cardiol 35:1288-1294, 2000.
138. Vicenzi MN, Meislitzer T, Heitzinger B, et al: Coronary artery stenting and non-cardiac surgery—a prospective outcome study. Br J Anaesth 96:686-693, 2006.
139. Leibowitz D, Cohen M, Planer D, et al: Comparison of cardiovascular risk of noncardiac surgery following coronary angioplasty with versus without stenting. Am J Cardiol 97:1188-1191, 2006.
140. Nasser M, Kapeliovich M, Markiewicz W: Late thrombosis of sirolimus-eluting stents following noncardiac surgery. Catheter Cardiovasc Interv 65:516-519, 2005.
141. Schouten O, van Domburg RT, Bax JJ, et al: Noncardiac surgery after coronary stenting: Early surgery and interruption of antiplatelet therapy are associated with an increase in major adverse cardiac events. J Am Coll Cardiol 49:122-124, 2007.
142. Goldman L, Caldera DL, Southwick FS, et al: Cardiac risk factors and complications in noncardiac surgery. Medicine (Baltimore) 57:357, 1978.
143. Schoeppel SL, Wilkinson C, Waters J, et al: Effects of myocardial infarction on perioperative cardiac complications. Anesth Analg 62:493, 1983.
144. Shah KB, Kleinman BS, Sami H, et al: Reevaluation of perioperative myocardial infarction in patients with prior myocardial infarction undergoing noncardiac operations. Anesth Analg 71:231, 1990.
145. Eagle KA, Boucher CA: Cardiac risk of noncardiac surgery. N Engl J Med 321:1330, 1989.
146. Lette J, Waters D, Lapointe J, et al: Usefulness of the severity and extent of reversible perfusion defects during thallium-dipyridamole imaging for cardiac risk assessment before noncardiac surgery. Am J Cardiol 64:276, 1989.
147. Kennedy JW, Kaiser GC, Fisher LD, et al: Clinical and angiographic predictors of operative mortality from the Collaborative Study in Coronary Artery Surgery (CASS). Circulation 63:793, 1981.
148. Poldermans D, Arnese M, Fioretti PM, et al: Improved cardiac risk stratification in major vascular surgery with dobutamine-atropine stress echocardiography. J Am Coll Cardiol 26:648-653, 1995.
149. Lee TH, Marcantonio ER, Mangione CM, et al: Derivation and prospective validation of a simple index for prediction of cardiac risk of major noncardiac surgery. Circulation 100:1043-1049, 1999.
150. Fleisher LA, Skolnick ED, Halroyd KJ, Lehmann HP: Coronary artery revascularization before abdominal aortic aneurysm surgery: A decision analytic approach. Anesth Analg 79:661-669, 1994.
151. Mason JJ, Owens DK, Harris RA, et al: The role of coronary angiography and coronary revascularization before noncardiac surgery. JAMA 273:1919-1925, 1995.
152. Glance LG: Selective preoperative cardiac screening improves five-year survival in patients undergoing major vascular surgery: A cost-effectiveness analysis. J Cardiothorac Vasc Anesth 13:265-271, 1999.
153. Detsky AS, Abrams HB, McLaughlin JR, et al: Predicting cardiac complications in patients undergoing non-cardiac surgery. J Gen Intern Med 1:211, 1986.
154. Gerson MC, Hurst JM, Hertzberg VS, et al: Cardiac prognosis in noncardiac surgery. Ann Intern Med 103:832, 1985.
155. Higgins TL, Estafanous FG, Loop FD, et al: Stratification of morbidity and mortality outcome by preoperative risk factors in coronary artery bypass patients. A clinical severity score. JAMA 267:2344, 1992.
156. Charlson ME, MacKenzie CR, Gold JP, et al: Risk for postoperative congestive heart failure. Surg Gynecol Obstet 172:95, 1991.
157. Rivers SP, Scher LA, Gupta SK, Veith FJ: Safety of peripheral vascular surgery after recent acute myocardial infarction. J Vasc Surg 11:70-75, discussion 76, 1990.
158. Berlauk JF, Abrams JH, Gilmour IJ, et al: Preoperative optimization of cardiovascular hemodynamics improves outcome in peripheral vascular surgery: A prospective, randomized clinical trial. Ann Surg 214:289, 1991.
159. American Society of Anesthesiologists Task Force on Pulmonary Artery Catheterization: Practice guidelines for pulmonary catheterization. A report by the American Society of Anesthesiologists Task Force on Pulmonary Artery Catheterization. Anesthesiology 78:380, 1993.
160. Roizen MF: Anesthesia goals for surgery to relieve or prevent visceral ischemia. *In* Roizen MF (ed):

Anesthesia for Vascular Surgery. New York, Churchill Livingstone, 1990, p 171.
161. Eagle KA, Coley CM, Newell JB, et al: Combining clinical and thallium data optimizes preoperative assessment of cardiac risk before major vascular surgery. Ann Intern Med 110:859, 1989.
162. Boucher CA, Brewster DC, Darling RC, et al: Determination of cardiac risk by dipyridamole-thallium imaging before peripheral vascular surgery. N Engl J Med 312:389, 1985.
163. Charlson ME, MacKenzie R, Gold JP, et al: Postoperative renal dysfunction can be predicted. Surg Gynecol Obstet 169:303, 1989.
164. Eagle KA, Rihal CS, Mickel MC, et al: Cardiac risk of noncardiac surgery: Influence of coronary disease and type of surgery in 3368 operations. CASS Investigators and University of Michigan Heart Care Program. Coronary Artery Surgery Study. Circulation 96:1882-1887, 1997.
165. Cohen MM, Duncan PG: Physical Status Score and trends in anesthetic complications. J Clin Epidemiol 41:83, 1988.
166. Mantha S, Roizen MF, Barnard J, et al: Relative effectiveness of preoperative noninvasive cardiac evaluation tests on predicting adverse cardiac outcomes following vascular surgery: A meta-analysis. Anesth Analg 79:422, 1994.
167. Froehlich JB, Karavite D, Russman PL, et al: American College of Cardiology/American Heart Association preoperative assessment guidelines reduce resource utilization before aortic surgery. J Vasc Surg 36:758-763, 2002.
168. Santos AL, Gelperin A: Surgical mortality in the elderly. J Am Geriatr Soc 23:42, 1975.
169. O'Keefe JH, Shub C, Rettke SR: Risk of noncardiac surgical procedures in patients with aortic stenosis. Mayo Clin Proc 64:400, 1989.
170. Raby KE, Goldman L, Creager MA, et al: Correlation between preoperative ischemia and major cardiac events after peripheral vascular surgery. N Engl J Med 321:1296, 1989.
171. Fletcher JP, Antico VF, Gruenwald S, Kershaw LZ: Dipyridamole-thallium scan for screening of coronary artery disease prior to vascular surgery. J Cardiovasc Surg 29:666, 1988.
172. Goldschlager N: Use of the treadmill test in the diagnosis of coronary artery disease in patients with chest pain. Ann Intern Med 97:383, 1982.
173. Smith JS, Roizen MF, Cahalan MK, Benefiel DJ: Does anesthetic technique make a difference? Augmentation of systolic blood pressure during carotid endarterectomy: Effects of phenylephrine versus light anesthesia and of isoflurane versus halothane on the incidence of myocardial ischemia. Anesthesiology 69:846, 1988.
174. Riles TS, Kopelman I, Imparato AM: Myocardial infarction following carotid endarterectomy: A review of 683 operations. Surgery 85:249, 1979.
175. Charlson ME, MacKenzie CR, Gold JP, et al: Preoperative characteristics predicting intraoperative hypotension and hypertension among hypertensives and diabetics undergoing noncardiac surgery. Ann Surg 212:66, 1990.
176. Frank SM, Fleisher LA, Breslow MJ, et al: Perioperative maintenance of normothermia reduces the incidence of morbid cardiac events: A randomized clinical trial. JAMA 277:1127, 1997.
177. Erikssen G, Thaulow E, Sandvik L, et al: Haematocrit: A predictor of cardiovascular mortality? J Intern Med 234:493, 1993.
178. Nelson AH, Fleisher LA, Rosenbaum SH: Relationship between postoperative anemia and cardiac morbidity in high-risk vascular patients in the intensive care unit. Crit Care Med 21:860, 1993.
179. Mangano DT, Layug EL, Wallace A, Tateo I: Effect of atenolol on mortality and cardiovascular morbidity after noncardiac surgery. Multicenter Study of Perioperative Ischemia Research Group. N Engl J Med 335:1713-1720, 1996.
180. Poldermans D, Boersma E, Bax JJ, et al: The effect of bisoprolol on perioperative mortality and myocardial infarction in high-risk patients undergoing vascular surgery. Dutch Echocardiographic Cardiac Risk Evaluation Applying Stress Echocardiography Study Group. N Engl J Med 341:1789-1794, 1999.
181. Lindenauer PK, Pekow P, Wang K, et al: Perioperative beta-blocker therapy and mortality after major noncardiac surgery. N Engl J Med 353:349-361, 2005.
182. Juul AB, Wetterslev J, Gluud C, et al: Effect of perioperative beta blockade in patients with diabetes undergoing major non-cardiac surgery: Randomised placebo controlled, blinded multicentre trial. BMJ 332:1482, 2006.
183. Yang H, Raymer K, Butler R, et al: The effects of perioperative beta-blockade: Results of the Metoprolol after Vascular Surgery (MaVS) study, a randomized controlled trial. Am Heart J 152:983-990, 2006.
184. Naylor CD, Sibbald WJ, Sprung CL, et al: Pulmonary artery catheterization: Can there be an integrated strategy for guideline development and research promotion? JAMA 269:2407, 1993.
185. Hollinger I: Diseases of the cardiovascular system. *In* Katz R, Steward D (eds): Anesthesia and Uncommon Pediatric Diseases. Philadelphia, WB Saunders, 1993, p 93.
186. Wilson W, Taubert KA, Gewitz M, et al: Prevention of infective endocarditis: Guidelines from the American Heart Association: A guideline from the American Heart Association Rheumatic Fever, Endocarditis, and Kawasaki Disease Committee, Council on Cardiovascular Disease in the Young, and the Council on Clinical Cardiology, Council on Cardiovascular Surgery and Anesthesia, and the Quality of Care and Outcomes Research Interdisciplinary Working Group. Circulation 116:1736-1754, 2007.
187. Nishimura RA, Carabello BA, Faxon DP, et al: ACC/AHA 2008 guideline update on valvular heart disease: Focused update on infective endocarditis: A report of the American College of Cardiology/American Heart Association Task Force on Practice Guidelines: Endorsed by the Society of Cardiovascular Anesthesiologists, Society for Cardiovascular Angiography and Interventions, and Society of Thoracic Surgeons. Circulation 118:887-889, 2008.
188. Katholi RE, Nolan SP, McGuire LB: Living with prosthetic heart valves. Subsequent noncardiac operations and the risk of thromboembolism or hemorrhage. Am Heart J 92:162-167, 1976.
189. Bonow RO, Carabello B, de Leon AC Jr, et al: Guidelines for the management of patients with valvular heart disease: Executive summary. A report of the American College of Cardiology/American Heart Association Task Force on Practice Guidelines (Committee on Management of Patients with Valvular Heart Disease). Circulation 98:1949-1984, 1998.
190. Ezekowitz MD: Anticoagulation management of valve replacement patients. J Heart Valve Dis 11(Suppl 1):S56-S60, 2002.
191. Bonow RO, Carabello BA, Kanu C, et al: ACC/AHA 2006 guidelines for the management of patients with valvular heart disease: A report of the American College of Cardiology/American Heart Association Task Force on Practice Guidelines (Writing Committee to Revise the 1998 Guidelines for the Management of Patients with Valvular Heart Disease): Developed in collaboration with the Society of Cardiovascular Anesthesiologists: Endorsed by the Society for Cardiovascular Angiography and Interventions and the Society of Thoracic Surgeons. Circulation 114(5):e84-e231, 2006.
192. Vandermeulen EP, Van Aken H, Vermylen J: Anticoagulants and spinal-epidural anesthesia. Anesth Analg 79:1165, 1994.
193. Rao TLK, El-Etr AA: Anticoagulation following placement of epidural and subarachnoid catheters: An evaluation of neurologic sequelae. Anesthesiology 55:618, 1981.
194. Frame JN, Mulvey KP, Phares JC, Anderson MJ: Correction of severe heparin-associated thrombocytopenia with intravenous immunoglobulin. Ann Intern Med 111:946, 1989.
195. Waldman SD, Feldstein GS, Waldman HJ, et al: Caudal administration of morphine sulphate in anticoagulated and thrombocytopenic patients. Anesth Analg 66:267, 1987.
196. Bargon HC, LaRaja RD, Rossi G, Atkinson D: Continuous epidural analgesia in the heparinized vascular surgical patient: A retrospective review of 912 patients. J Vasc Surg 6:144, 1987.
197. Onishchuk JL, Carlsson C: Epidural hematoma associated with epidural anesthesia: Complications of anticoagulant therapy. Anesthesiology 77:1221, 1992.
198. Horlocker TT, Wedel DJ, Offord KP: Does preoperative antiplatelet therapy increase the risk of hemorrhagic complications associated with regional anesthesia? Anesth Analg 70:631, 1990.
199. Macdonald R: Aspirin and extradural blocks. Br J Anaesth 66:1, 1991.
200. Amrein PC, Ellman L, Harris WH: Aspirin-induced prolongation of bleeding and perioperative blood loss. JAMA 245:1825, 1981.
201. Horlocker TT, Wedel DJ, Benzon H, et al: Regional anesthesia in the anticoagulated patient: Defining the risks (the second ASRA Consensus Conference on Neuraxial Anesthesia and Anticoagulation). Reg Anesth Pain Med 28:172-197, 2003.
202. International Multicentre Trial: Prevention of fatal postoperative pulmonary embolism by low doses of heparin. Lancet 2:45, 1975.
203. Consensus Conference: Prevention of venous thrombosis and pulmonary embolism. JAMA 256:744, 1988.
204. Collins R, Scrimgeour A, Yusuf S, Peto R: Reduction in fatal pulmonary embolism and venous thrombosis by perioperative administration of subcutaneous heparin. N Engl J Med 318:1162, 1988.
205. Gallus A, Raman K, Darby T: Venous thrombosis after elective hip replacement—the influence of preventive intermittent calf compression and on surgical technique. Br J Surg 70:17, 1983.
206. Lutz DJ, Noller KL, Spittell JA Jr, et al: Pregnancy and its complications following cardiac valve prostheses. Am J Obstet Gynecol 131:460, 1978.
207. Smith ND, Raizada V, Abrams J: Auscultation of the normally functioning prosthetic valve. Ann Intern Med 95:594, 1981.
208. Gauss A, Hübner C, Radermacher P, et al: Perioperative risk of bradyarrhythmias in patients with asymptomatic chronic bifascicular block or left bundle branch block. Does an additional first-degree atrioventricular block make any difference? Anesthesiology 88:679, 1998.
209. Ruskin JN: Catheter ablation for supraventricular tachycardia. N Engl J Med 324:1660, 1991.

210. Kelly JS, Royster RL: Noninvasive transcutaneous cardiac pacing. Anesth Analg 69:229, 1989.
211. Risk SC, Brandon D, D'Ambra MN, et al: Indications for the use of pacing pulmonary artery catheters in cardiac surgery. J Cardiothorac Vasc Anesth 6:275, 1992.
212. Prystowsky EN: Diagnosis and management of the pre-excitation syndromes. Curr Probl Cardiol 13:225, 1988.
213. McAnulty JH, Rahimtoola SH, Murphy E, et al: Natural history of "high-risk" bundle-branch block. Final report of a prospective study. N Engl J Med 307:137, 1982.
214. Rose MR, Koski G: Anesthesia in patients with Wolff-Parkinson-White syndrome [abstract]. Anesthesiology 69:A146, 1988.
215. Anthonisen NR, Connet JE, Kiley JP, et al: Effect of smoking intervention and the use of an inhaled anticholinergic bronchodilator on the rate of decline of FEV_1. The Lung Health Study. JAMA 272:1497, 1994.
216. European Respiratory Society: Optimal assessment and management of chronic obstructive pulmonary disease (COPD). Eur Respir J 8:1398, 1995.
217. Holleman DR Jr, Simel DL: Does the clinical examination predict airflow limitation? JAMA 273:313, 1995.
218. Lacasse Y, Guyatt GH, Goldstein RS: The components of a respiratory rehabilitation program: A systematic overview. Chest 111:1077, 1997.
219. Saint S, Bent S, Vittinghoff E, Grady D: Antibiotics in chronic obstructive pulmonary disease exacerbations. A meta-analysis. JAMA 273:957, 1995.
220. Thompson WH, Nielson CP, Carvalho P, et al: Controlled trial of oral prednisone in outpatients with acute COPD exacerbations. Am J Respir Crit Care Med 154:407, 1996.
221. NAEP Expert Panel Report 2: Guidelines for the diagnosis and management of asthma. Public Health Service. US Department of Health and Human Services Publication No. 97-4051A, May 1997. Available at http://www.nhlbi.nih.gov/nhlbi/nhlbi.htm.
222. Sin DD, Man J, Sharpe H, et al: Pharmacological management to reduce exacerbations in adults with asthma: A systematic review and meta-analysis. JAMA 292:367-376, 2004.
223. Tilles SA: Differential diagnosis of adult asthma. Med Clin North Am 90:61-76, 2006.
224. Dompeling E, van Schayck CP, van Grunsven PM, et al: Slowing the deterioration of asthma and chronic obstructive pulmonary disease observed during bronchodilator therapy by adding inhaled corticosteroids. A 4-year prospective study. Ann Intern Med 118:770, 1993.
225. Calligaro KD, Azurin DJ, Dougherty MJ, et al: Pulmonary risk factors of elective abdominal aortic surgery. J Vasc Surg 18:914, 1993.
226. Skolnick ET, Vomvolakis MA, Buck KA, et al: Exposure to environmental tobacco smoke and the risk of adverse respiratory events in children receiving general anesthesia. Anesthesiology 88:1144, 1998.
227. Rodgers A, Walker N, Schug S, et al: Reduction of postoperative mortality and morbidity with epidural or spinal anaesthesia: Results from overview of randomised trials. BMJ 321:1493, 2000.
228. Stein M, Cassara EL: Preoperative pulmonary evaluation and therapy for surgery patients. JAMA 211:787, 1970.
229. Khan MA, Hussain SF: Review article—pre-operative pulmonary evaluation. J Ayub Med Coll Abbottabad 17(4):82-86, 2005.
230. Rock P, Passannante A: Preoperative assessment: Pulmonary. Anesthesiol Clin North Am 22:77-91, 2004.
231. Qaseem A, Snow V, Fitterman N, et al: Risk assessment for and strategies to reduce perioperative pulmonary complications for patients undergoing noncardiothoracic surgery: A guideline from the American College of Physicians. Ann Intern Med 144:575-580, 2006.
232. Smetana GW, Lawrence VA, Cornell JE: Preoperative pulmonary risk stratification for noncardiothoracic surery: Systematic review for the American College of Physicians. Ann Intern Med 144:581-595, 2006.
233. Collins CD, Darke CS, Knowelden J: Chest complications after upper abdominal surgery: Their anticipation and prevention. BMJ 1:401, 1968.
234. Warner MA, Offerd KP, Warner ME, et al: Role of preoperative cessation of smoking and other factors in postoperative pulmonary complications: A blinded prospective study of coronary artery bypass patients. Mayo Clin Proc 64:609, 1989.
235. Robinson K, Conroy RM, Mulcahy R: When does the risk of acute coronary heart disease in ex-smokers fall to that in non-smokers? A retrospective study of patients admitted to hospital with a first episode of myocardial infarction or unstable angina. Br Heart J 62:16, 1989.
235a. Geerts WH, Bergqvist D, Pineo GF, et al: Prevention of venous thromboembolism: American College of Chest Physicians Evidence-Based Clinical Practice Guidelines (8th Edition). Chest 133(6Suppl):381S-453S, 2008.
236. Ernst E, Matrai A: Abstention from chronic cigarette smoking normalizes blood rheology. Atherosclerosis 64:75, 1987.
237. Bluman LG, Mosca L, Newman N, Simon DG: Preoperative smoking habits and postoperative pulmonary complications. Chest 113:883-889, 1998.
238. Nakagawa M, Tanaka H, Tsukuma H, Kishi Y: Relationship between the duration of the preoperative smoke-free period and the incidence of postoperative pulmonary complications after pulmonary surgery. Chest 120:705-710, 2001.
239. Warner DO: Perioperative abstinence from cigarettes: Physiologic and clinical consequences. Anesthesiology 104:356-367, 2006.
240. Quraishi SA Orkin FK, Roizen MF: The anesthesia preoperative assessment: An opportunity for smoking cessation intervention. J Clin Anesth 18:635-640, 2006.
241. McCreanor J, Cullinan P, Nieuwenhuijsen MJ, et al: Respiratory effects of exposure to diesel traffic in persons with asthma. N Engl J Med 357:2348-2358, 2007.
242. Downs SH, Schindler C, Liu LJS, et al: Reduced exposure to PM10 and attenuated age-related decline in lung function. N Engl J Med 357:2338-2347, 2007.
243. Celli BR, Rodriguez KS, Snider GL: A controlled trial of intermittent positive pressure breathing, incentive spirometry, and deep breathing exercises in preventing pulmonary complications after abdominal surgery. Am Rev Respir Dis 130:12, 1984.
244. Bartlett RH, Brennan ML, Gazzaniga AB, et al: Studies on the pathogenesis and prevention of postoperative pulmonary complications. Surg Gynecol Obstet 137:925, 1973.
245. Lyager S, Wernberg M, Rajani N, et al: Can postoperative pulmonary conditions be improved by treatment with the Bartlett-Edwards incentive spirometer after upper abdominal surgery? Acta Anaesthesiol Scand 23:312, 1979.
246. Elwood T, Morris W, Martin LD, et al: Bronchodilator premedication does not decrease respiratory adverse events in pediatric general anesthesia. Can J Anaesth 50:277-284, 2003.
247. Boushy SF, Billing DM, North LB, et al: Clinical course related to preoperative pulmonary function in patients with bronchogenic carcinoma. Chest 59:383, 1971.
248. Mittman C: Assessment of operative risk in thoracic surgery. Am Rev Respir Dis 84:197, 1961.
249. Reichel J: Assessment of operative risk of pneumonectomy. Chest 62:570, 1972.
250. Wong DH, Weber EC, Schell MJ, et al: Factors associated with postoperative pulmonary complications in patients with severe COPD. Anesth Analg 80:276, 1995.
251. Arozullah AM, Daley J, Henderson WG, Khuri SF: Multifactorial risk index for predicting postoperative respiratory failure in men after major noncardiac surgery. The National Veterans Administration Surgical Quality Improvement Program. Ann Surg 232:242-253, 2000.
252. Arozullah AM, Khuri SF, Henderson WG, et al: Development and validation of a multifactorial risk index for predicting postoperative pneumonia after major noncardiac surgery. Ann Intern Med 135:847-857, 2001.
253. Kabalin CS, Yarnold PR, Grammer LC: Low complication rate of corticosteroid-treated asthmatics undergoing surgical procedures. Arch Intern Med 155:1379-1384, 1995.
254. Selzer A, Walter RM: Adequacy of preoperative digitalis therapy in controlling ventricular rate in postoperative atrial fibrillation. Circulation 34:119, 1966.
255. Geerts WH, Heit JA, Clagett GP, et al: Prevention of venous thromboembolism. Chest 119(1 Suppl):132S-175S, 2001.
256. O'Donnell M, Weitz JI: Thromboprophylaxis in surgical patients. Can J Surg 46:129-135, 2003.
257 Matthay RA, Niederman MS, Wiedemann HP: Cardiovascular pulmonary interaction in chronic obstructive pulmonary disease with special reference to pathogenesis and management of cor pulmonale. Med Clin North Am 74:571, 1990.
258. Fedullo PF, Auger WR, Kerr KM, Rubin LJ: Chronic thromboembolic pulmonary hypertension. N Engl J Med 345:1465-1472, 2001.
259. Galie N, Ghofrani HA, Torbicki A, et al: Sildenafil citrate therapy for pulmonary arterial hypertension. N Engl J Med 353:2148-2157, 2005.
260. Domino KB, Wetstein L, Glasser SA, et al: Influence of mixed venous oxygen tension ($P\bar{v}O_2$) on blood flow to atelectatic lung. Anesthesiology 59:428, 1983.
261. Settipane GA, Dudupakkam RK: Aspirin intolerance. III: Subtypes, familial occurrence and cross reactivity with tartrazine. J Allergy Clin Immunol 56:215, 1975.
262. Cancer Statistics for the United States. Available at www.cdc.gov/nchs/products/pubs/pubd/hus/trendtables.htm 200.
263. Aisner J: Extensive-disease small-cell lung cancer: The thrill of victory the agony of defeat. J Clin Oncol 14:658, 1996.
264. Cooper JAD (ed): Drug-induced pulmonary disease. Clin Chest Med 11:1, 1990.
265. Levy JH, Roizen MF, Morris JM: Anaphylactic and anaphylactoid reactions: A review. Spine 11:282, 1986.
266. Kemp SF, Lockey RF: Anaphylaxis: A review of causes and mechanisms. J Allergy Clin Immunol 110:341-348, 2002.

267. Smith PL, Kagey-Sobotka A, Bleecker ER, et al: Physiologic manifestations of human anaphylaxis. J Clin Invest 66:1072, 1980.
268. Delage C, Irey NS: Anaphylactic deaths: A clinicopathologic study of 43 cases. J Forensic Sci 17:525, 1972.
269. Bettman MA: Radiographic contrast agents—a perspective. N Engl J Med 317:891, 1987.
270. Roizen MF, Rodgers GM, Valone FH, et al: Anaphylactoid reactions to vascular graft material presenting with vasodilation and subsequent disseminated intravascular coagulation. Anesthesiology 71:331, 1989.
271. Mertes PM, Laxenaire MC: Allergic reactions occurring during anaesthesia. Eur J Anaesthesiol 19:240-262, 2002.
272. Lieberman P: Anaphylactic reactions during surgical and medical procedures. J Allergy Clin Immunol 110(2 Suppl):S64-S69, 2002.
273. Rosow CE, Moss J, Philbin DM, et al: Histamine release during morphine and fentanyl anesthesia. Anesthesiology 56:93, 1982.
274. Millbern SM, Bell SD: Prevention of anaphylaxis to contrast media. Anesthesiology 50:56, 1979.
275. Halevy S, Altura BT, Altura BM: Pathophysiological basis for the use of steroids in the treatment of shock and trauma. Klin Wochenschr 60:1021, 1982.
276. Toogood JH: Risk of anaphylaxis in patients receiving beta-blocker drugs. J Allergy Clin Immunol 81:1, 1988.
277. Van Arsdel PP Jr, Larson EB: Diagnostic tests for patients with suspected allergic disease. Ann Intern Med 110:304, 1989.
278. Heyland DK, Novak F, Drover JW, et al: Should immunonutrition become routine in critically ill patients? A systematic review of the evidence. JAMA 286:944-953, 2001.
279. Drugs for epilepsy. Med Lett Drugs Ther 45:57-64, 2003.
280. Roberts R: Differential diagnosis of sleep disorders, non-epileptic attacks and epileptic attacks. Curr Opin Neurol 11:135-139, 1998.
281. Shaner DM, McCurdy SA, Herring MO, et al: Treatment of status epilepticus: A prospective comparison of diazepam and phenytoin versus phenobarbital and optional phenytoin. Neurology 38:202, 1988.
282. Schuchat A, Robinson K, Wenger JD, et al: Bacterial meningitis in the United States in 1995. N Engl J Med 337:970, 1997.
283. Parkinson Study Group: Impact of deprenyl and tocopherol treatment on Parkinson's disease in DATA TOP patients requiring levodopa. Ann Neurol 39:37, 1996.
284. Goetz CG, Olanow CW, Koller WC, et al: Multicenter study of autologous adrenal medullary transplantation to the corpus striatum in patients with advanced Parkinson's disease. N Engl J Med 320:337, 1989.
285. Mets B: Acute dystonia after alfentanil in untreated Parkinson's disease. Anesth Analg 72:557, 1991.
286. Muzzi DA, Black S, Cucchiara RF: The lack of effect of succinylcholine on serum potassium in patients with Parkinson's disease. Anesthesiology 71:322, 1989.
287. Wiklund RA, Ngai SH: Rigidity and pulmonary edema after Innovar in a patient on levodopa therapy: Report of a case. Anesthesiology 35:545-547, 1971.
288. Barry PP, Moskowitz MA: The diagnosis of reversible dementia in the elderly, a critical review. Arch Intern Med 148:1914, 1988.
289. Skoog I, Nilsson J, Palmertz B, et al: A population-based study of dementia in 85-year-olds. N Engl J Med 328:153, 1993.
290. Petersen RC, Smith GE, Waring SC, et al: Mild cognitive impairment: Clinical characterization and outcome. Arch Neurol 56:303-308, 1999.
291. Ross GW, Abbott RD, Petrovitch H, et al: Frequency and characteristics of silent dementia among elderly Japanese-American men. The Honolulu-Asia Aging Study. JAMA 277:800, 1997.
292. Snowdon DA, Greiner LH, Mortimer JA, et al: Brain infarction and the clinical expression of Alzheimer disease. The Nun Study. JAMA 277:813, 1997.
293. Drugs for Alzheimer's disease. Med Lett Drugs Ther 43:53, 2001.
294. Jones PM, Soderman RM: Intra-operative bradycardia in a patient with Alzheimer's disease treated with two cholinesterase inhibitors. Anaesthesia 62:201, 2007.
295. Xie Z, Tanzi RE: Alzheimer's disease and post-operative cognitive dysfunction. Exp Gerontol 41:346-359, 2006.
296. Eckenhoff RG, Johansson JS, Wei H, et al: Inhaled anesthetic enhancement of amyloid-beta oligomerization and cytotoxicity. Anesthesiology 101:703-709, 2004.
297. Wei H, Liang G, Wang Q, et al: The common inhalational anesthetic isoflurane induces apoptosis via activation of inositol 1,4,5-trisphosphate receptors. Anesthesiology 108:251-260, 2008.
298. Zhang B, Dong Y, Zhang G, et al: The inhalation anesthetic desflurane induces caspase activation and increases amyloid beta-protein levels under hypoxic conditions. J Biol Chem 283:11866-11875, 2008.
299. Hemmelgarn B, Suissa S, Huang A, et al: Benzodiazepine use and the risk of motor vehicle crash in the elderly. JAMA 278:27, 1997.
300. Mozkowitz MA: Basic mechanisms in vascular headache. Neurol Clin 8:801, 1990.
301. Michel P, Henry P, Letenneur L, et al: Diagnostic screen for assessment of IHS criteria for migraine by general practitioners. Cephalagia 12:54, 1993.
302. MacIntyre PD, Bhargava B, Hogg KJ, et al: Effect of subcutaneous sumatriptan, a selective 5HT-1 agonist, on the systemic, pulmonary, and coronary circulation. Circulation 87:401, 1993.
303. Shadick NA, Phillips CB, Logigian EL, et al: The long-term clinical outcomes of Lyme disease. A population-based retrospective cohort study. Ann Intern Med 121:560, 1994.
304. Ferguson RJ, Caplan LR: Cervical spondylitic myelopathy. Neurol Clin 3:373, 1985.
305. Ovassapian A, Land P, Schafer MF, et al: Anesthetic management for surgical corrections of severe flexion deformity of the cervical spine. Anesthesiology 58:370, 1983.
306. Rudick RA, Cohen JA, Weinstock-Guttman B, et al: Management of multiple sclerosis. N Engl J Med 337:1604, 1997.
307. Kocabas S, Karaman S, Firat V, Bademkiran E: Anesthetic management of Guillain-Barré syndrome in pregnancy. J Clin Anesth 19:299-302, 2007.
308. McKhann GM, Griffin JW, Cornblath DR, et al: Plasmapheresis and Guillain-Barré syndrome: Analysis of prognostic factors and the effect of plasmapheresis. Ann Neurol 23:347, 1988.
309. Toh B-H, van Driel IR, Gleeson PA: Pernicious anemia. N Engl J Med 337:1441, 1997.
310. Jensen NF, Fiddler DS, Striepe V: Anesthetic considerations in porphyrias. Anesth Analg 80:591, 1995.
311. Kantor G, Rolbin SH: Acute intermittent porphyria and caesarean delivery. Can J Anaesth 39:282, 1992.
312. Meissner PN, Harrison GG, Hift RJ: Propofol as an I.V. anaesthetic induction agent in variegate porphyria. Br J Anaesth 66:60, 1991.
313. McNeill MJ, Bennet A: Use of regional anaesthesia in a patient with acute porphyria. Br J Anaesth 64:371, 1990.
314. Massey JM: Treatment of acquired myasthenia gravis. Neurology 48:S46-S51, 1997.
315. d'Empaire G, Hoaglin DC, Perlo VP, et al: Effect of prethymectomy plasma exchange on postoperative respiratory function in myasthenia gravis. J Thorac Cardiovasc Surg 89:592, 1985.
316. Eisenkraft JB, Book WJ, Mann SM, et al: Resistance to succinylcholine in myasthenia gravis: A dose response study. Anesthesiology 69:760, 1988.
317. Eisenkraft JB, Papatestas AE, Kahn CH, et al: Predicting the need for postoperative mechanical ventilation in myasthenia gravis. Anesthesiology 65:79, 1986.
318. Small S, Ali HH, Lennon VA, et al: Anesthesia for unsuspected Lambert-Eaton myasthenic syndrome with autoantibodies and occult small cell lung carcinoma. Anesthesiology 76:142, 1992.
319. Lema G, Urzua J, Moran S, Canessa R: Successful anesthetic management of a patient with hypokalemic familial periodic paralysis undergoing cardiac surgery. Anesthesiology 74:373, 1991.
320. Ashwood EM, Russell WJ, Burrow DD: Hyperkalaemic periodic paralysis. Anaesthesia 47:579, 1992.
321. Gutmann DH, Fischbeck KH: Molecular biology of Duchenne and Becker's muscular dystrophy: Clinical applications. Ann Neurol 26:189, 1989.
322. Smith CL, Bush GH: Anesthesia and progressive muscular dystrophy. Br J Anaesth 57:1113, 1985.
323. Schwartz L, Rockoff MA, Koka BV: Masseter spasm with anesthesia: Incidence and implications. Anesthesiology 61:772, 1984.
324. Rosenberg H: Trismus is not trivial [editorial]. Anesthesiology 67:453, 1987.
325. Pueschel SM, Scola FH: Atlantoaxial instability in individuals with Down syndrome: Epidemiologic, radiographic, and clinical studies. Pediatrics 80:55, 1987.
326. Morray JP, MacGillivray R, Duker G: Increased perioperative risk following repair of congenital heart disease in Down's syndrome. Anesthesiology 65:221, 1986.
327. Roizen NJ, Patterson D: Down's syndrome Lancet 361:1281-1289, 2003.
328. Freeman SB, Taft LF, Dopoley KJ, et al: Population-based study of congenital heart defects in Down syndrome. Am J Med Genet 80:213-217, 1998.
329. Kobel M, Creighton RE, Steward DJ: Anaesthetic considerations in Down's syndrome: Experience with 100 patients and a review of the literature. Can J Anaesth 29:593, 1982.
330. Bedford RF, Morris L, Jane JA: Intracranial hypertension during surgery for supratentorial tumor: Correlation with preoperative computed tomography scans. Anesth Analg 61:430, 1982.
331. Ramirez-Lassepas M, Quinones MR: Heparin therapy for stroke: Hemorrhagic complications and risk factors for intracerebral hemorrhage. Neurology 34:114, 1984.
332. Rem JA, Hachinski VC, Boughner DR, Barnett HJ: Value of cardiac monitoring and echocardiography in TIA and stroke patients. Stroke 16:950, 1985.
333. Drugs for psychiatric disorders. Treatment guideline. Med Lett Drugs Ther 11:69-76, 2003.
334. Appel GB, Neu HC: The nephrotoxicity of antimicrobial agents. N Engl J Med 296:663, 722, 784, 1977.

335. Byrick RJ, Rose DK: Pathophysiology and prevention of acute renal failure: The role of the anaesthetist. Can J Anaesth 37:457, 1990.
336. Berns AS: Nephrotoxicity of contrast media. Kidney Int 36:730, 1989.
337. Myers BD, Moran SM: Hemodynamically mediated acute renal failure. N Engl J Med 314:97, 1986.
338. Thadhani R, Pascual M, Bonventre JV: Acute renal failure. N Engl J Med 334:1448, 1996.
339. Aronson S, Thisthelwaite RJ, Walker R, et al: Safety and feasibility of renal blood flow determination during surgery with perfusion ultrasonography. Anesth Analg 80:353, 1995.
340. Hebert PC, Wells G, Blajchman MA, et al: A multicenter, randomized, controlled clinical trial of transfusion requirements in critical care. Transfusion Requirements in Critical Care Investigators, Canadian Critical Care Trials Group. N Engl J Med 340:409-417, 1999.
341. Koch CG, Khandwala F, Li L, et al: Persistant effect of red cell transfusion on health-related quality of life after cardiac surgery. Ann Thorac Surg 82:13-20, 2006.
342. Rao KV, Anderson RC, O'Brien TJ: Factors contributing for improved graft survival in recipients of kidney transplants. Kidney Int 24:210, 1983.
343. Coe FL, Parks JH, Asplin JR: The pathogenesis and treatment of kidney stones. N Engl J Med 327:1141, 1992.
344. Kellen M, Aronson S, Roizen MF, et al: Predictive and diagnostic tests of renal failure: A review. Anesth Analg 78:134, 1994.
345. Novis BK, Roizen MF, Aronson S, Thisted RA: Association of preoperative risk factors with postoperative acute renal failure. Anesth Analg 78:143, 1994.
346. Lee TH, Marcantonio ER, Mangione CM, et al: Derivation and prospective validation of a simple index for prediction of cardiac risk of major noncardiac surgery. Circulation 100:1043-1049, 1999.
347. Mangano CM, Diamondstone LS, Ramsay JG, et al: Renal dysfunction after myocardial revascularization: Risk factors, adverse outcomes, and hospital resource utilization. The Multicenter Study of Perioperative Ischemia Research Group. Ann Intern Med 128:194-203, 1998.
348. Flancbaum L, Choban PS, Dasta JF: Quantitative effects of low-dose dopamine on urine output in oliguric surgical intensive care unit patients. Crit Care Med 22:61, 1994.
349. Paul MD, Mazer CD, Byrick RJ, et al: Influence of mannitol and dopamine on renal function during elective infrarenal aortic clamping in man. Am J Nephrol 6:427, 1986.
350. Crowley K, Clarkson K, Hannon V, et al: Diuretics after transurethral prostatectomy: A double-blind controlled trial comparing furosemide and mannitol. Br J Anaesth 65:337, 1990.
351. Dorman, HR, Sondheimer JH, Cadnapaphornchai P: Mannitol-induced acute renal failure. Medicine (Baltimore) 69:153-159, 1990.
352. Kellum JA, Decker J: Use of dopamine in acute renal failure: A meta-analysis. Crit Care Med 29:1526-1531, 2001.
353. Alpert RA, Roizen MF, Hamilton WK, et al: Intraoperative urinary output does not predict postoperative renal function in patients undergoing abdominal aortic revascularization. Surgery 95:707, 1984.
354. Halpenny M, Lakshmi S, O'Donnell A, et al: The effects of fenoldopam on coronary conduit blood flow after coronary artery bypass graft surgery. J Cardiothorac Vasc Anesth 15:72-76, 2001.
355. Halpenny M, Rushe C, Breen P, et al: The effects of fenoldopam on renal function in patients undergoing elective aortic surgery. Eur J Anaesthesiol 19:32-39, 2002.
356. Caimmi PP, Pagani L, Micalizzi E, et al: Fenoldopam for renal protection in patients undergoing cardiopulmonary bypass. J Cardiothorac Vasc Anesth 17:491-494, 2003.
357. Litz RJ, Hubler M, Lorenz W, et al: Renal responses to desflurane and isoflurane in patients with renal insufficiency. Anesthesiology 97:1133-1136, 2002.
358. Conzen PF, Kharasch ED, Czerner SF, et al: Low-flow sevoflurane compared with low-flow isoflurane anesthesia in patients with stable renal insufficiency. Anesthesiology 97:578-584, 2002.
359. Petroni KC, Cohen NH: Continuous renal replacement therapy: Anesthetic implications. Anesth Analg 94:1288-1297, 2002.
360. Renal Data System: USRDS 2001 Annual Data Report: Atlas of End Stage Renal Disease in the United States. Bethesda, MD, National Institute of Diabetes and Digestive and Kidney Diseases, 2001.
361. Myers BD, Sibley R, Newton L, et al: The long-term course of cyclosporine-associated chronic nephropathy. Kidney Int 33:590, 1988.
362. Bennett WM, Aronoff GR, Morrison G, et al: Drug prescribing in renal failure: Dosing guidelines for adults. Am J Kidney Dis 3:155, 1983.
363. Bennett WM, Aronoff GR, Golper TA, et al: Drug Prescribing in Renal Failure. Dosing Guidelines for Adults. 2nd ed. Philadelphia, American College of Physicians, 1991.
364. Goyal P, Puri GD, Pandey CK, Srivastva S: Evaluation of induction doses of propofol: Comparison between endstage renal disease and normal renal function patients. Anaesth Intensive Care 30:584-587, 2002.
365. Platt R, Zaleznik DF, Hopkins CC, et al: Perioperative antibiotic prophylaxis for herniorrhaphy and breast surgery. N Engl J Med 322:153, 1990.
366. Chestnut DH: Spinal anesthesia in the febrile patient. Anesthesiology 76:667, 1992.
367. Rackow EC, Astiz ME: Pathophysiology and treatment of septic shock. JAMA 266:548, 1991.
368. Knaus WA, Wagner DP: Multiple systems organ failure: Epidemiology and prognosis. Crit Care Clin 5:522, 1989.
369. The choice of antibacterial drugs. Med Lett Drugs Ther 46:13, 2004.
370. Nichol KL, Nordin JD, Nelson DB, et al: Effectiveness of influenza vaccine in the community-dwelling elderly. N Engl J Med 357:1373-1381, 2007.
371. Maki DG, Botticelli JT, Le Roy ML, Thielke TS: Prospective study of replacing administration sets for intravenous therapy at 48- vs 72-hour intervals: 72 hours is safe and cost-effective. JAMA 258:1771, 1987.
372. Maki DG, Ringer M: Evaluation of dressing regimens for prevention of infection with peripheral intravenous catheters: Gauze, a transparent polyurethane dressing, and an iodophor-transparent dressing. JAMA 258:2396, 1987.
373. Dodd RY: The risk of transfusion-transmitted infection. N Engl J Med 327:419, 1992.
374. Buergler JM, Kim R, Thisted RA, et al: The risk of human immunodeficiency virus in surgeons, anesthesiologists, and medical students. Anesth Analg 75:118, 1992.
375. Jensen V: The TURP syndrome. Can J Anaesth 38:90, 1991.
376. Ostia JR: The binge-purge syndrome: A common albeit unappreciated cause of acid-base and fluid electrolyte disturbances. South Med J 80:58, 1987.
377. Schrier RW: Pathogenesis of sodium and water retention in high-output and low-output cardiac failure, nephrotic syndrome, cirrhosis, and pregnancy (Pts 1 and 2). N Engl J Med 319:1065, 1127, 1988.
378. Sterns RH: Severe symptomatic hyponatremia: Treatment and outcome. Ann Intern Med 107:656, 1987.
379. Surawicz B: Relationship between electrocardiogram and electrolytes. Am Heart J 73:814, 1967.
380. Rimmer JM, Horn JF, Gennari FJ: Hyperkalemia as a complication of drug therapy. Arch Intern Med 147:867, 1987.
381. Busch EH, Ventura HO, Lavie CJ: Heparin-induced hyperkalemia. South Med J 80:1450, 1987.
382. Don BR, Sebastian A, Cheitlin M, et al: Pseudohyperkalemia caused by fist clenching during phlebotomy. N Engl J Med 322:1290, 1990.
383. Kharasch ED, Bowdle TA: Hypokalemia before induction of anesthesia and prevention by β_2 adrenoceptor antagonism. Anesth Analg 72:216, 1991.
384. Allon M, Dunlay R, Copkney C: Nebulised albuterol for acute hyperkalemia in patients on hemodialysis. Ann Intern Med 110:426, 1989.
385. Wong KC, Kawamura R, Hodges MR, et al: Acute intravenous administration of potassium chloride to furosemide pretreated dogs. Can J Anaesth 24:203, 1977.
386. Hahm TS, Cho HS, Lee KH, et al: Clonidine premedication prevents preoperative hypokalemia. J Clin Anesth 14:6-9, 2002.
387. Lawson DH: Adverse reactions to potassium chloride. Q J Med 43:433, 1974.
388. Vitez TS, Soper LE, Wong KC, Soper P: Chronic hypokalemia and intraoperative dysrhythmias. Anesthesiology 63:130, 1985.
389. Hirsch IA, Tomlinson DL, Slogoff S, Keats AS: The overstated risk of preoperative hypokalemia. Anesth Analg 67:131, 1988.
390. Olson RP, Schow AJ, McCann R, et al: Absence of adverse outcomes in hyperkalemic patients undergoing vascular access surgery. Can J Anaesth 50:553-557, 2003.
391. Schow AJ, Lubarsky DA, Olson RP, Gan TJ: Can succinylcholine be used safely in hyperkalemic patients? Anesth Analg 95:19-122, 2002.
392. Wahr JA, Parks R, Boisvert D, et al: Preoperative serum potassium levels and perioperative outcomes in cardiac surgery patients. Multicenter Study of Perioperative Ischemia Research Group. JAMA 281:2203-2210, 1999.
393. Cohen JD, Neaton JD, Prineas RJ, Daniels KA: Diuretics, serum potassium and ventricular arrhythmias in the multiple risk factor intervention. Am J Cardiol 60:548, 1987.
394. Holland OB, Nixon JV, Kuhnert L: Diuretic-induced ventricular ectopic activity. Am J Med 70:762, 1981.
395. Tanifuji Y, Eger EI II: Brain sodium, potassium and osmolality: Effect on anesthetic requirement. Anesth Analg 57:404, 1978.
396. Kornbluth A, Sachar DB: Ulcerative colitis practice guidelines in adults. American College of Gastroenterology, Practice Parameters Committee. Am J Gastroenterol 92:204, 1997.
397. Kahrilas PJ: Gastroesophageal reflux disease. JAMA 276:983, 1996.
398. Kurz A, Sessler DI, Lenhardt R: Perioperative normothermia to reduce the incidence of surgical-wound infection and shorten hospitalization. Study of Wound Infection and Temperature Group. N Engl J Med 334:1209-1215, 1996.
399. Antimicrobial prophylaxis. Med Lett Drugs Ther 43:92-97, 2001.

400. Jain NK, Larson DE, Schroeder KW, et al: Antibiotic prophylaxis for percutaneous endoscopic gastrostomy. Ann Intern Med 107:824, 1987.
401. Gorbach SL: Antimicrobial prophylaxis for appendectomy and colorectal surgery. Rev Infect Dis 13(Suppl 10):S815, 1991.
402. Peterson WJ: Peptic ulcer—an infectious disease? West J Med 152:167, 1990.
403. Botero M, Fuchs R, Paulus DA, Lind DS: Carcinoid heart disease: A case report and literature review. J Clin Anesth 14:57-63, 2002.
404. Veall GRQ, Peacock JE, Bax NDS, Reilly CS: Review of the anaesthetic management of 21 patients undergoing laparotomy for carcinoid syndrome. Br J Anaesth 72:335, 1994.
405. Longnecker M, Roizen MF: Patients with carcinoid syndrome. Anesthesiol Clin North Am 5:313, 1987.
406. Weingarten TN, Abel MD, Connolly HM, et al: Intraoperative management of patients with carcinoid heart disease having valvular surgery: A review of one hundred consecutive cases. Anesth Analg 105:1192-1199, 2007.
407. Marsh HM, Martin JK Jr, Kvols LK, et al: Carcinoid crisis during anesthesia: Successful treatment with a somatostatin analogue. Anesthesiology 66:89, 1987.
408. Watson JT, Badner NH, Ali MJ: The prophylactic use of octreotide in a patient with ovarian carcinoid and valvular heart disease. Can J Anaesth 37:798, 1990.
409. McCrirrick A, Hickman J: Octreotide for carcinoid syndrome. Can J Anaesth 38:339, 1991.
410. Quinlivan JK, Roberts WA: Intraoperative octreotide for refractory carcinoid-induced bronchospasm. Anesth Analg 78:400, 1994.
411. Dilger JA, Rho EH, Que FG, Sprung J: Octreotide-induced bradycardia and heart block during surgical resection of a carcinoid tumor. Anesth Analg 98:318-320, 2004.
412. Zimmer C, Kienbaum P, Wiesemes R, Peters J: Somatostatin does not prevent serotonin release and flushing during chemoembolization of carcinoid liver metastases. Anesthesiology 98:1007-1011, 2003.
413. Drossman DA, McKee DC, Sandler RS, et al: Psychosocial factors in the irritable bowel syndrome. A multivariate study of patients and non-patients with irritable bowel syndrome. Gastroenterology 95:701, 1988.
414. Aitkenhead AR, Robinson S: Influence of morphine and pethidine on the incidence of anastomotic dehiscence after colonic surgery. Br J Anaesth 63:230P, 1989.
415. Green J, Beyar R, Sideman S, et al: The "jaundiced heart": A possible explanation for postoperative shock in obstructive jaundice. Surgery 100:14, 1986.
416. Audet A-M, Goodnough LT: Practice strategies for elective red blood cell transfusion. American College of Physicians. Ann Intern Med 116:403, 1992.
417. Welch HG, Meehan KR, Goodnough LT: Prudent strategies for elective red blood cell transfusion. Ann Intern Med 116:393, 1992.
418. Crystal GJ, Rooney MW, Salem MR: Myocardial blood flow and oxygen consumption during isovolumic hemodilution alone and in combination with adenosine-induced controlled hypotension. Anesth Analg 67:539, 1988.
419. Nelson AH, Fleisher LA, Rosenbaum SH: Relationship between postoperative anemia and cardiac morbidity in high-risk vascular patients in the intensive care unit. Crit Care Med 21:860-866, 1993.
420. Wu WC, Schifftner TL, Henderson WG, et al: Preoperative hematocrit levels and postoperative outcomes in older patients undergoing noncardiac surgery. JAMA 297:2481-2488, 2007.
421. Bunn HF: Pathogenesis and treatment of a sickle cell disease. N Engl J Med 337:762, 1997.
422. Adams RJ, McKie VC, Hsu L, et al: Prevention of a first stroke by transfusions in children with sickle cell anemia and abnormal results on transcranial Doppler ultrasonography. N Engl J Med 339:5, 1998.
423. Platt OS, Thorington BD, Brambella DJ, et al: Pain in sickle cell disease: Rates and risk factors. N Engl J Med 325:11, 1991.
424. Vichinsky EP, Haberkern CM, Neumayr L, et al: A comparison of conservative and aggressive transfusion regimens in the perioperative management of sickle cell disease. N Engl J Med 333:206, 1995.
425. Turhan A, Weiss LA, Mohandas N, et al: Primary role for adherent leukocytes in sickle cell vascular occlusion: A new paradigm. Proc Natl Acad Sci U S A 99:3047-3051, 2002.
426. Dunn A, Davies A, Eckert G, et al: Intraoperative death during caesarean section in a patient with sickle-cell trait. Can J Anaesth 34:67, 1987.
427. Hemming AE: Pro: Exchange transfusion is required for sickle cell trait patients undergoing cardiopulmonary bypass. J Cardiothorac Vasc Anesth 18:663-665, 2004.
428. Messent M: Con: Exchange transfusion is not required for sickle cell trait patients undergoing cardiopulmonary bypass. J Cardiothorac Vasc Anesth 18:666-667, 2004.
429. Kark JA, Posey DM, Schumaeker HR, Ruehle CJ: Sickle cell trait as a risk factor for sudden death in physical training. N Engl J Med 317:781, 1987.
430. Bischoff RJ, Williamson A III, Dalali MJ, et al: Assessment of the use of transfusion therapy perioperatively in patients with sickle cell hemoglobinopathies. Ann Surg 207:434, 1988.
431. Tuck SM, James CE, Brewster EM, et al: Prophylactic blood transfusion in maternal sickle cell syndromes. Br J Obstet Gynaecol 94:121, 1987.
432. Beutler E: The common anemias. JAMA 259:2433, 1988.
433. Orr D: Difficult intubation: A hazard in thalassemia. A case report. Br J Anaesth 39:585, 1967.
434. Pootrakul P, Hungsprenges S, Fucharoen S, et al: Relation between erythropoiesis and bone metabolism in thalassemia. N Engl J Med 304:1470-1473, 1981.
435. Muretto P, Angelucci E, Lucarelli G: Reversibility of cirrhosis in patients cured of thalassemia by bone marrow transplantation. Ann Intern Med 136:667-672, 2002.
436. Lux SE, Wolfe LC: Inherited disorders of the red cell membrane skeleton. Pediatr Clin North Am 27:463, 1980.
437. Beutler E: Glucose-6-phosphate dehydrogenase deficiency. N Engl J Med 324:169, 1991.
438. Engelfriet CP, Overbeeke MA, van der Berne AE: Autoimmune hemolytic anemia. Semin Hematol 29:3, 1992.
439. Schilling RF: Is nitrous oxide a dangerous anesthetic for vitamin B_{12}-deficient subjects? JAMA 255:1605, 1986.
440. Beebe DS, Bergen L, Palahniuk RJ: Anesthesia utilizing plasmapheresis and forced air warming in a patient with severe cold agglutinin hemolytic anemia. Anesth Analg 76:1144, 1993.
441. Goodnough LT, Rudnick S, Price TH, et al: Increased preoperative collection of autologous blood with recombinant human erythropoietin therapy. N Engl J Med 321:1163, 1989.
442. Quesenberg PJ, Schafer AI, Schreiber AD, et al: Hematology. *In* American College of Physicians: Medical Knowledge Self-Assessment. Philadelphia, American College of Physicians, 1991, p 374.
443. Tobias JD, Furman WL: Anesthetic considerations in patients receiving colony-stimulating factors (G-CSF and GM-CSF). Anesthesiology 75:536, 1991.
444. Alavi JB, Root RK, Djerassi I, et al: A randomized clinical trial of granulocyte transfusion for infection in acute leukemia. N Engl J Med 296:706, 1977.
445. Gabrilove JL, Jakubowski A, Scher H, et al: Effect of granulocyte colony stimulating factor on neutropenia and associated morbidity due to chemotherapy for transitional-cell carcinoma of the urothelium. N Engl J Med 318:1414, 1988.
446. Quie PG: The white cells: Use of granulocyte transfusions. Rev Infect Dis 9:189, 1987.
447. Crawford SW, Fisher L: Predictive value of pulmonary function tests before marrow transplantation. Chest 101:1257, 1992.
448. McCrae KR, Bussel JB, Mannucci PM, et al: Platelets: An update on diagnosis and management of thrombocytopenic disorders. Hematology (Am Soc Hematol Educ Program) 282-305, 2001.
449. Kelton JG: Management of the pregnant patient with idiopathic thrombocytopenic purpura. Ann Intern Med 99:796, 1983.
450. Douzinas EE, Markakis K, Karabinis A, et al: Early plasmapheresis in patients with thrombotic thrombocytopenic purpura. Crit Care Med 20:57, 1992.
451. Lewis BE, Wallis DE, Berkowitz MD, et al: Argatroban anticoagulant therapy in patients with heparin-induced thrombocytopenia. Circulation 103:1838-1843, 2001.
452. Bauer KA: The thrombophilias: Well-defined risk factors with uncertain therapeutic implications. Ann Intern Med 135:367-373, 2001.
453. Levine JS, Branch DW, Rauch J: The antiphospholipid syndrome. N Engl J Med 346:752-763, 2002.
454. Evans BE: Dental treatment for hemophiliacs: Evaluation of dental program (1975-1976) at the Mount Sinai Hospital International Hemophilia Training Center. Mt Sinai J Med 44:409, 1977.
455. Zauber NP, Levin J: Factor IX levels in patients with hemophilia B (Christmas disease) following transfusion with concentrates of factor IX or fresh frozen plasma (FFP). Medicine (Baltimore) 56:213, 1977.
456. Brettler DB, Levine PH: Factor concentrates for treatment of hemophilia: Which one to choose? Blood 73:2067, 1989.
457. Centers for Disease Control and Prevention (CDC): Safety of therapeutic products used for hemophilia patients. MMWR Morb Mortal Wkly Rep 37(29):441, 449-450, 1988.
458. Briere RO: Serum ALT levels: Effect of sex, race, and obesity on unit rejection rate. Transfusion 28:392, 1988.
459. Sloand EM, Pitt E, Klein HG: Safety of the blood supply. JAMA 274:1368, 1995.
460. Preparation of von Willebrand's factor. Med Lett Drugs Ther 35:51, 1993.
461. Lee KF, Manchell J, Rankin JS, et al: Immediate versus delayed coronary grafting after streptokinase treatment: Postoperative blood loss and clinical results. J Thorac Cardiovasc Surg 95:216, 1988.
462. Dickman CA, Shedd SA, Spetzler RF, et al: Spinal epidural hematoma associated with epidural anesthesia: Complications of systemic heparinization in patients receiving peripheral vascular thrombolytic therapy. Anesthesiology 72:947, 1990.
463. Czer LS, Bateman TM, Gary RJ, et al: Treatment of severe platelet dysfunction and hemorrhage after

cardiopulmonary bypass: Reduction in blood product usage with desmopressin. J Am Coll Cardiol 9:1139, 1987.
464. Brigden ML, Barnett JB: A practical approach to improving pain control in cancer patients. West J Med 146:580, 1987.
465. Drugs of choice for cancer chemotherapy. Med Lett Drugs Ther 39:21, 1997.
466. Bishop JM: Molecular themes in oncogenesis. Cell 64:235, 1991.
467. Chung F: Cancer, chemotherapy, and anesthesia. Can J Anaesth 29:364, 1982.
468. Goldiner P, Carlon GC, Cvitkovic E, et al: Factors influencing postoperative morbidity and mortality in patients treated with bleomycin. BMJ 1:1664, 1978.
469. LaMantia KR, Glick JH, Marshall BE: Supplemental oxygen does not cause respiratory failure in bleomycin-treated surgical patients. Anesthesiology 60:65, 1984.
470. Matalon S, Harper WV, Nickerson PA, Olszowka J: Intravenous bleomycin does not alter the toxic effects of hyperoxia in rabbits. Anesthesiology 64:614, 1986.
471. Roizen MF: Is a patient's history of food supplement use simply supplementary? J Clin Anesth 10:89, 1998.
472. How herbal products increase surgical risks. Nursing Sept:24-25, 2007.
473. Drugs for hypertension. Med Lett Drugs Ther 37:45, 1995.
474. Drugs that cause psychiatric symptoms. Med Lett Drugs Ther 35:65, 1993.
475. Huyse FJ, Touw DJ, van Schijndel RS, et al. Psychotropic drugs and the perioperative period: A proposal for a guideline in elective surgery. Psychosomatics 47:8-22, 2006.
476. The Norwegian Multicenter Study Group: Timolol-induced reduction in mortality and reinfarction in patients surviving acute myocardial infarction. N Engl J Med 304:801, 1981.
477. Frishman WH, Furberg CD, Friedewald WT: Beta-adrenergic blockade for survivors of acute myocardial infarction. N Engl J Med 310:830, 1984.
478. Smulyan H, Weinberg SE, Howanitz PJ: Continuous propranolol infusion following abdominal surgery. JAMA 247:2539, 1982.
479. Gold MR, Dec GW, Cocca-Spofford DC, Thompson BT: Esmolol and ventilatory function in cardiac patients with COPD. Chest 100:1215, 1991.
480. Bloor BC, Flacke WE: Reduction in halothane anesthetic requirement by clonidine, an alpha-adrenergic agonist. Anesth Analg 61:741, 1982.
481. Weinger MB, Segal IS, Maze M: Dexmedetomidine, acting through central alpha-2 adrenoceptors, prevents opiate-induced muscle rigidity in the rat. Anesthesiology 71:242, 1989.
482. Maze M, Tranquilli W: Alpha-2 adrenoreceptor agonists: Defining the role in clinical anesthesia. Anesthesiology 74:581, 1991.
483. Segal IS, Jarvis DJ, Duncan SR, et al: Clinical efficacy of oral-transdermal clonidine combinations during the perioperative period. Anesthesiology 74:220, 1991.
484. Pandharipande PP, Pon BT, Herr DL, et al: Effect of sedation with dexmedetanidine vs. lorazepam on acute brain dysfunction in mechanically ventilated patients: The MENDS randomized controlled trial. JAMA 298:2644-2653, 2007.
485. Katz AM: Cardiac ion channels. N Engl J Med 328:1244, 1993.
486. Merin RG, Chelly JE, Hysing ES, et al: Cardiovascular effects of and interaction between calcium blocking drugs and anesthetics in chronically instrumented dogs. IV: Chronically administered oral verapamil and halothane, enflurane, and isoflurane. Anesthesiology 66:140, 1987.
487. Kapur PA, Matarazzo DA, Fung DM, Sullivan KB: The cardiovascular and adrenergic actions of verapamil or diltiazem in combination with propranolol during halothane anesthesia in the dog. Anesthesiology 66:122, 1987.
488. Michaels I, Serrins M, Shier NQ, Barash PG: Anesthesia for cardiac surgery in patients receiving monoamine oxidase inhibitors. Anesth Analg 63:1014, 1984.
489. Evans-Prosser CDG: The use of pethidine and morphine in the presence of monamine oxidase inhibitors. Br J Anaesth 40:279, 1968.
490. Roizen MF: Monoamine oxidase inhibitors: Are we condemned to relive history, or is history no longer relevant? J Clin Anesth 2:293, 1990.
491. Noble WH, Baker A: MAO inhibitors and coronary artery surgery: A patient death. Can J Anaesth 39:1061, 1992.
492. Hirshman CA, Linderman KS: Anesthesia and monoamine oxidase inhibitors. JAMA 261:3407, 1989.
493. El-Ganzouri AR, Ivankovich AD, Braverman B, McCarthy R: Monoamine oxidase inhibitors: Should they be discontinued preoperatively? Anesth Analg 64:592, 1985.
494. Ebrahim ZY, O'Hara JF, Borden L, Tetzlaff J: Monoamine oxidase inhibitors and elective surgery. Cleve Clin J Med 60:129, 1993.
495. Clarke AG: MAOI's and anaesthesia. Can J Anaesth 43:641, 1996.
496. Veith RC, Raskind MA, Caldwell JH, et al: Cardiovascular effects of tricyclic antidepressants in depressed patients with chronic heart disease. N Engl J Med 306:954, 1982.
497. Richelson E, El-Fakahany E: Changes in the sensitivity of receptors for neurotransmitters and the actions of some psychotherapeutic drugs. Mayo Clin Proc 57:576, 1982.
498. Katz RL, Bigger JT: Cardiac arrhythmias during anesthesia and operation. Anesthesiology 33:193, 1970.
499. Horrigan RW, Eger EI II, Wilson CB: Epinephrine-induced arrhythmias during enflurane anesthesia in man: A nonlinear dose-response relationship and dose-dependent protection from lidocaine. Anesth Analg 57:547, 1978.
500. Marcus ML, Skelton CL, Graver LE, et al: Effects of theophylline on myocardial mechanics. Am J Physiol 222:1361, 1972.
501. Westfall DP, Flemming WW: Sensitivity changes in the dog heart to norepinephrine, calcium and aminophylline resulting from pretreatment with reserpine. J Pharmacol Exp Ther 159:98, 1968.
502. Rall TW, West TC: The potentiation of cardiac inotropic responses to norepinephrine by theophylline. J Pharmacol Exp Ther 139:269, 1963.
503. Drugs for cardiac arrhythmias. Med Lett Drugs Ther 38:75, 1996.
504. Harrah MD, Way WL, Katzung BG: The interaction of *d*-tubocurarine with antiarrhythmic drugs. Anesthesiology 33:406, 1970.
505. Telivuo L, Katz RL: The effects of modern intravenous local anesthetics on respiration during partial neuromuscular block in man. Anaesthesia 25:30, 1970.
506. Miller RD, Way WL, Katzung BG: The potentiation of neuromuscular blocking agents by quinid Anesthesiology 28:1036, 1967.
507. Pittinger CB, Eryasa Y, Adamson R: A induced paralysis. Anesth Analg 49:487
508. Singh YN, Harvey AL, Marshall IG: Antibiotic-induced paralysis of the mouse phrenic nerve–hemidiaphragm preparation, and reversibility by calcium and by neostigmine. Anesthesiology 48:418, 1978.
509. Pittinger CB, Adamson R: Antibiotic blockade of neuromuscular function. Annu Rev Pharmacol 12:169, 1972.
510. Becker LD, Miller RD: Clindamycin enhances a non-depolarizing neuromuscular blockade. Anesthesiology 45:84, 1976.
511. Snavely SR, Hodges GR: The neurotoxicity of antibacterial agents. Ann Intern Med 101:92, 1984.
512. McIndewar IC, Marshall RJ: Interactions between the neuromuscular blocking drug Org NC45 and some anaesthetic, analgesic and antimicrobial agents. Br J Anaesth 53:785, 1981.
513. Navalgund AA, Alifimoff JK, Jakymec AJ, Bleyaert AL: Amiodarone-induced sinus arrest successfully treated with ephedrine and isoproterenol. Anesth Analg 65:414, 1986.
514. Kannan R, Nademane K, Hendrickson JA, et al: Amiodarone kinetics after oral doses. Clin Pharmacol Ther 31:438, 1982.
515. Rice SA, Sbordone L, Mazzo RI: Metabolism by rat hepatic microsomes of fluorinated ether anesthetics following isoniazid administration. Anesthesiology 53:489, 1980.
516. Antimicrobial prophylaxis in surgery. Med Lett Drugs Ther Guidelines 20:27, 2004.
517. Beller GA, Smith TW, Abelmann WH, et al: Digitalis intoxication. N Engl J Med 284:989, 1971.
518. Ritchie AJ, Danton M, Gibbons JRP: Prophylactic digitalisation in pulmonary surgery. Thorax 47:41, 1992.
519. Morrow DH: Anesthesia and digitalis toxicity. VI. Effect of barbiturates and halothane on digoxin toxicity. Anesth Analg 49:305, 1970.
520. Pratila MG, Pratilas V: Anesthetic agents and cardiac electromechanical activity. Anesthesiology 49:338, 1978.
521. Logic JR, Morrow DH: The effect of halothane on ventricular automaticity. Anesthesiology 36:107, 1972.
522. Ivankovich AD, Miletich DJ, Grossman RK, et al: The effect of enflurane, isoflurane, fluroxene, methoxyflurane and diethyl ether on ouabain tolerance in the dog. Anesth Analg 55:360, 1976.
523. Ali N, Dais K, Banks T, Sheikh M: Titrated electrical cardioversion in patients on digoxin Clin Cardiol 5:417, 1982.
524. Adverse systemic effects from orthalmic drugs. Med Lett Drugs Ther 24:53, 198
525. The Medical Letter Handbo of Adverse Drug Interactions, 2003.
526. Feely J, Wilkinson G McAllister CB, et al: Increased toxicity an educed clearance of lidocaine by cimetidi Ann Intern Med 96:592, 1982.
527. Lam AM, Pa JA: Cimetidine and prolonged post-operat omnolence. Can J Anaesth 28:450, 1981.
528. Derry Update on hormones, menopause, and ase: Evaluating the professional response hea Woman's Health Initiative. Health Care ten Int 29:720-737, 2008.
52 ld R, Nimmo WS: Do patients fasting before and after surgery receive their prescribed drug treatment? BMJ 296:744, 1988.
. Lesar TS, Briceland LL, Delcoure K, et al: Medication prescribing errors in a teaching hospital. JAMA 263:2329, 1990.

Lydia Cassorla and Jae-Woo Lee

36 Patient Positioning and Anesthesia

Key Points

1. Patient positioning is a major responsibility that is shared by the entire operating room team. A balance between optimal surgical positioning and patient well-being is sometimes required.
2. Many patient positions that are used for surgery result in undesirable physiologic consequences, including significant cardiovascular and respiratory compromise. Anesthetics blunt natural compensatory mechanisms, rendering surgical patients vulnerable to positional changes.
3. Peripheral nerve injury, although rare, accounted for 18% of cases in the 1990-1994 American Society of Anesthesiologists (ASA) Closed Claims Database, second only to death. Peripheral nerve injury is often a result of patient positioning. The mechanisms of injury are stretching, compression, and ischemia.
4. Ulnar neuropathy is the most common postoperative nerve injury, followed by injury to the brachial plexus, lumbosacral nerve roots, and spinal cord.
5. Not all postoperative neuropathies, including ulnar neuropathy, are currently explainable and may not be entirely preventable. Many postoperative ulnar nerve deficits do not seem to be related to intraoperative patient position because they appear days after surgery.
6. The ASA issued a Practice Advisory in 2000 for the prevention of perioperative peripheral neuropathies. Only 6 of 509 studies reviewed met the standard, however, for a scientifically proven relationship between intervention and outcome.
7. Postoperative visual loss is a rare but devastating complication that is associated with the prone position. The causes are multifactorial and incompletely understood.
8. Anesthetics administered outside classic operating rooms present special challenges with regard to patient positioning because of equipment limitations and differences in the work environment and culture.

Anesthesiologists share a critical responsibility for the proper positioning of patients in the operating room. Positions deemed optimal for surgery often result in undesirable physiologic changes, such as hypotension from impaired venous return to the heart or oxygen desaturation owing to ventilation-perfusion mismatching. In addition, peripheral nerve injuries during surgery remain a significant source of perioperative morbidity.[1-3]

Proper positioning requires the cooperation of anesthesiologists, surgeons, and nurses to ensure patient well-being and safety while providing surgical exposure. During anesthesia care, whenever possible, patients should be placed in a position that they would tolerate when awake. Jewelry and hair ornaments are removed. Padded surfaces, lumbar support, and natural joint position are optimal. The head should remain midline without substantial extension or flexion whenever possible. At no time should pressure on the eyes occur. Because surgeons wish to have optimal exposure, and positions may be maintained for long periods, prevention of complications often requires compromise and judgment. The duration of more extreme positions, if such are necessary, should be limited as much as possible. Expected tilting of the operating room table during surgery should be anticipated before draping, and the patient should be secured accordingly. Use of safety straps and prevention of a patient fall are fundamental.

Cardiovascular Concerns

Complex arterial, venous, and cardiac physiologic responses have evolved to blunt the effects of positional changes on arterial blood pressure and maintain perfusion to vital organs. Central, regional, and local mechanisms are involved. This is particularly important for humans who maintain an upright posture, owing to the vertical distance from the heart to the brain and its need for constant perfusion.

Normally, as an individual reclines from an erect to a supine position, venous return to the heart increases as pooled blood from the lower extremities redistributes toward the heart. Preload, stroke volume, and cardiac output are augmented. The resultant increase in arterial blood pressure activates afferent baroreceptors from the aorta (via the vagus nerve) and within the walls of the carotid sinuses (via the glossopharyngeal nerve) to decrease sympathetic outflow and increase parasympathetic impulses to the sinoatrial node and myocardium. The result is a compensatory decrease in heart rate, stroke volume, and cardiac output. Mechanoreceptors from the atria and ventricle also are activated to decrease sympathetic outflow to muscle and splanchnic vascular beds. Lastly, atrial reflexes are activated to regulate renal sympathetic nerve activity, plasma renin, atrial natriuretic peptide, and arginine vasopressin levels.[4] As a result, systemic arterial blood pressure is maintained within a narrow range during postural changes in the unanesthetized setting.

General anesthesia, muscle relaxation, positive-pressure ventilation, and neuraxial blockade interfere with venous return to the heart, arterial tone, and autoregulatory mechanisms, rendering patients under anesthesia especially vulnerable to relatively uncompensated circulatory effects of changes in position. The use of spinal or epidural anesthesia causes a significant sympathectomy across all affected dermatomes, independent of the presence of general anesthesia, reducing preload and potentially blunting cardiac response if the sympathetic output to the heart is affected (see Chapter 51). Positive-pressure ventilation increases mean intrathoracic pressure, diminishing the venous pressure gradient from peripheral capillaries to the right atrium. Because small pressure gradients are active in the venous circulation, this may significantly affect cardiac filling and consequently cardiac output. Positive end-expiratory pressure increases mean intrathoracic pressure further, as do conditions associated with low lung compliance, such as airways disease, obesity, ascites, and light anesthesia. Venous return and cardiac output may be compromised further.[5]

For these reasons, arterial blood pressure is often particularly labile immediately after the initiation of anesthesia and during patient positioning. It is crucial for the anesthesiologist to anticipate, monitor, and treat these effects, and to assess the safety of positional changes for each patient. Blood pressure should be measured frequently after induction of anesthesia or initiation of neuraxial blockade. It is often necessary to increase intravenous fluid administration, adjust the level of anesthesia, or administer vasopressors during this hemodynamic transition. Temporary use of head-down positions may be helpful. Sometimes a delay in repositioning of the patient for surgery may be necessary until systemic blood pressure reaches an acceptable level of homeostasis. Interruptions in monitoring to facilitate positioning or turning of the operating room table must be minimized during this dynamic period. Patient positioning is always secondary to patient safety.

Pulmonary Concerns

Anesthetized patients who are breathing spontaneously have a reduced tidal volume and functional residual capacity and an increased closing volume compared with the nonanesthetized state. Positive-pressure ventilation with muscle relaxation may ameliorate ventilation-perfusion mismatches under general anesthesia by maintaining adequate minute ventilation and limiting atelectasis. The diaphragm assumes an abnormal shape, however, owing to the loss of muscle tone, and is displaced less in the dependent portions of the lung.[6] This decreases ventilation-perfusion matching and consequently arterial Po_2. Patients undergoing neuraxial anesthesia lose abdominal and thoracic muscle function in affected dermatomes, but diaphragmatic function is retained if general anesthesia and muscle relaxation are not concurrently administered. In addition to these effects of anesthesia, patient position has distinct effects on pulmonary function. In particular, any position that limits movement of the diaphragm, chest wall, or abdomen may increase atelectasis and intrapulmonary shunt.

Spontaneous ventilation results from small negative intrathoracic pressure shifts during inspiration owing to diaphragmatic displacement and chest wall expansion. This pressure decrease also promotes venous return to the thorax by reducing the pressure in the great veins and right atrium compared with the periphery. Normal distribution of ventilation is determined by the excursion of the diaphragm, movement of the chest wall, and compliance of the lung. When an individual shifts from standing to supine, functional residual capacity decreases owing to cephalad displacement of the diaphragm. The relative contribution to ventilation of the chest wall compared with the diaphragm decreases from 30% to 10%. With spontaneous ventilation in either position, diaphragmatic movement is greatest adjacent to the most dependent portions of the lung, helping to bring new ventilation to the zones of the lung that are preferentially perfused. The preferential perfusion of the dependent portions is dominated by gravity; however, other factors, such as pulmonary vascular length, also may be important. Perfusion seems to follow a central-to-peripheral spectrum in each lobe that is maintained with changes in cardiac output.[7-9]

The prone position has been used to improve respiratory function in patients with adult respiratory distress syndrome.[10] In anesthetized patients, the prone position has advantages over the supine position with regard to lung volumes and oxygenation without adverse effects on mechanics,[11,12] including obese[13] and pediatric patients (see Chapter 82).[14] When patients are prone, weight should be distributed to the thoracic cage and bony pelvis, allowing the abdomen to move with respiration, as outlined subsequently.

Specific Positions

Supine

The most common position for surgery is the supine, or dorsal decubitus position (Fig. 36-1). Because the entire body is close to the level of the heart, hemodynamic reserve is best maintained. Because compensatory mechanisms are blunted by anesthesia, however, even a few degrees of head-down (Trendelenburg) position or head-up (reverse Trendelenburg) position are sufficient to cause significant cardiovascular changes.

Associated Arm Position

In a supine patient, one or both arms may be abducted out to the side or adducted (tucked) alongside the body. It is recommended that upper extremity abduction be limited to less than 90 degrees to minimize the likelihood of brachial plexus injury by caudad pressure in the axilla from the head of the humerus.[15] The hand

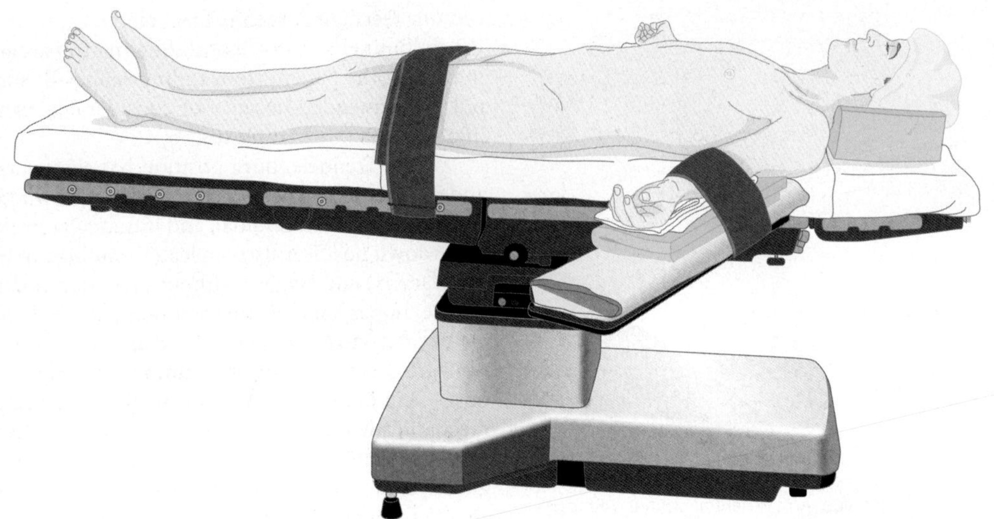

Figure 36-1 Supine position. Note the asymmetry of the base of the table, placing the patient's center of gravity over the base if positioned in the usual direction.

and forearm are either supinated or kept in a neutral position with the palm toward the body to reduce external pressure on the spiral groove of the humerus and the ulnar nerve (Fig. 36-2).[16-18] When the arms are adducted, they are usually held alongside the body with a "draw sheet" that passes under the body and over the arm, and is then tucked directly under the torso (not the mattress) to ensure that the arm remains properly placed next to the body. Alternatively, in surgeries in which access to the chest or abdomen is not necessary, curved arm cradles may be used. In all cases, the arms are placed in a neutral position.[16] The elbows and any protruding objects, such as intravenous fluid lines and stopcocks, are padded (Fig. 36-3).

Variations of the Supine Position

Several variations of the supine position are frequently used. The *lawn chair position,* in which the hips and knees are slightly flexed (Fig. 36-4), reduces stress on the back, hips, and knees, and is better tolerated by patients who are awake or undergoing monitored anesthesia care. In addition, because the legs are slightly above the heart, venous drainage from the lower extremity is facilitated. Also, the xiphoid to pubic distance is decreased, reducing the tension on the ventral abdominal musculature and easing closure of laparotomy incisions. Proper positioning of the patient's hips on the operating room table and several modifications to the table are required to achieve this position. Typically, the back of

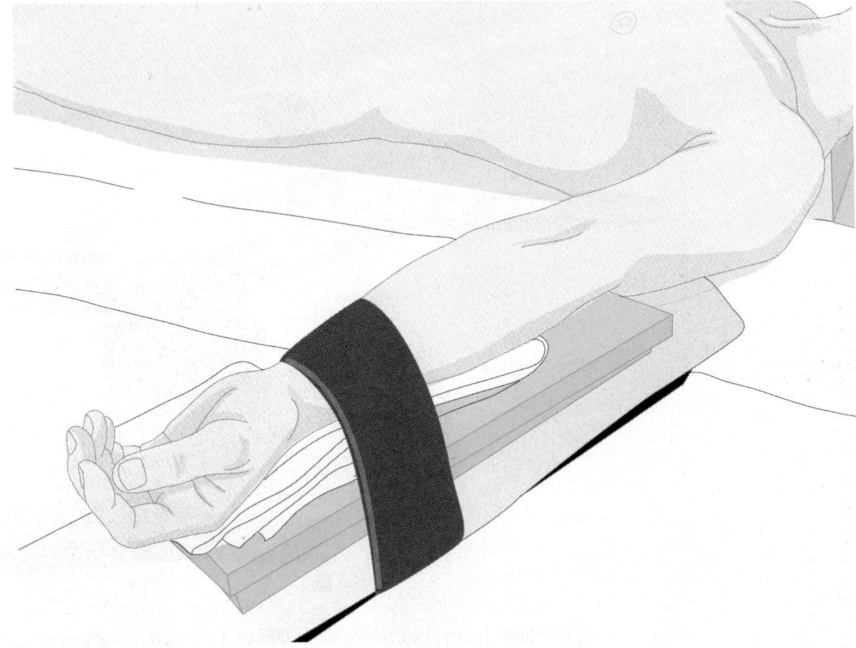

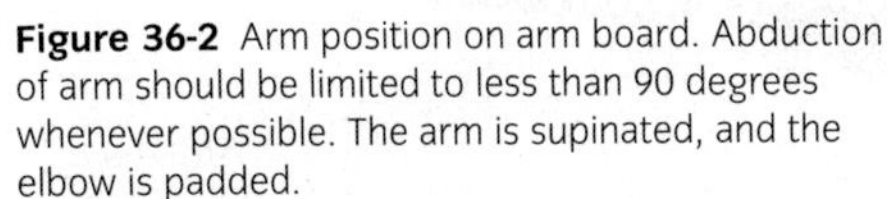

Figure 36-2 Arm position on arm board. Abduction of arm should be limited to less than 90 degrees whenever possible. The arm is supinated, and the elbow is padded.

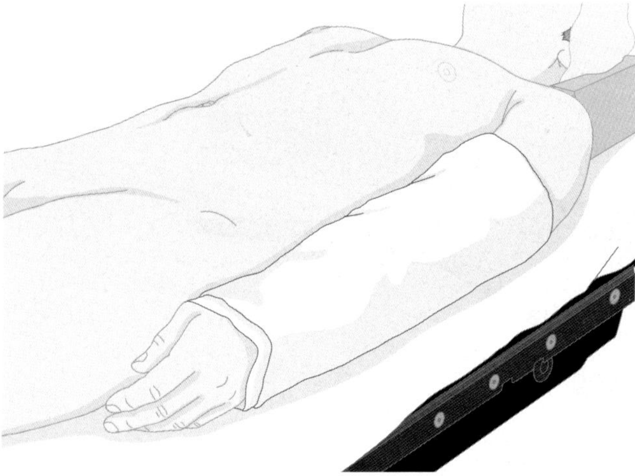

Figure 36-3 Arm tucked at patient's side. Arm in neutral position with palm to hip. The elbow is padded, and one needs to ensure that the arm is supported.

the bed is raised, the legs below the knees are lowered to an equivalent angle, and a slight Trendelenburg tilt is used to level the hips with the shoulders, if desired. These modifications reduce venous pooling in the legs and permit an arm board or table to be parallel with the floor if desired for upper extremity surgery.

The *frog-leg position,* in which the hips and knees are flexed, and the hips are externally rotated with the soles of the feet facing each other, allows access to the perineum, medial thighs, genitalia, and rectum. Care must be taken to minimize stress and postoperative pain in the hips and prevent dislocation by supporting the knees appropriately.

Tilting a supine patient head down, the *Trendelenburg position* (Fig. 36-5), is often used to increase venous return during hypotension, to improve exposure during abdominal and laparoscopic surgery, and to prevent air emboli and facilitate cannulation during central line placement. It is linked by name to a 19th century German surgeon, Trendelenburg, who described its use for abdominal surgery. Nonsliding mattresses are recommended to prevent the patient from sliding cephalad. Shoulder braces are not recommended because of considerable risk of compression injury to the brachial plexus.

The Trendelenburg position has significant cardiovascular and respiratory consequences. The head-down position increases central venous, intracranial, and intraocular pressures. Prolonged head-down position also can lead to swelling of the face, conjunctiva, larynx, and tongue with an increased potential for postoperative upper airway obstruction. The cephalic movement of abdominal viscera against the diaphragm also decreases functional residual capacity and pulmonary compliance. In spontaneously ventilating patients, the work of breathing increases. In mechanically ventilated patients, airway pressures must be higher to ensure adequate ventilation. The stomach also lies above the glottis. Endotracheal intubation is often preferred to protect the airway from pulmonary aspiration related to reflux and to reduce atelectasis. Because of the risk of edema to the trachea and mucosa surrounding the airway during surgeries in which patients have been in the Trendelenburg position for prolonged periods, it may be prudent to verify an air leak around the endotracheal tube or visualize the larynx before extubation.

Reverse Trendelenburg position (head-up tilt) (see Fig. 36-5) is often employed to facilitate upper abdominal surgery by shifting the abdominal contents caudad. This position is increasingly popular because of the growing number of laparoscopic surgeries. Caution is advised to prevent patients from slipping on the table, and more frequent monitoring of arterial blood pressure may be prudent to detect hypotension owing to decreased venous return. In addition, the position of the head above the heart reduces perfusion pressure to the brain and should be taken into consideration when determining optimal blood pressure.

In all positions in which the head is at a different level than the heart, the effect of the hydrostatic gradient on cerebral arterial and venous pressures should be carefully considered in terms of cerebral perfusion pressure. Careful documentation of any potential arterial pressure gradients is especially prudent.

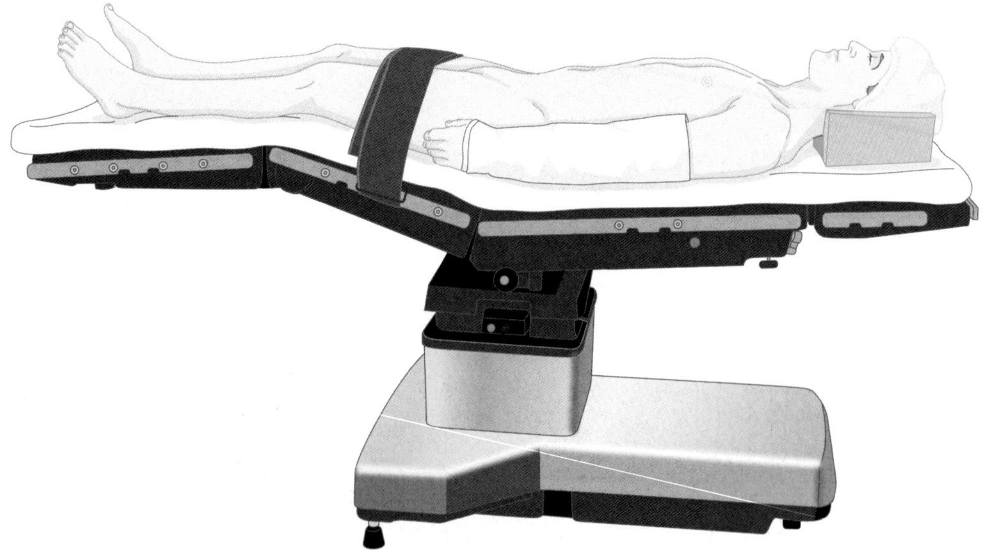

Figure 36-4 Lawn chair position. Flexion of the hips and knees decreases tension on the back.

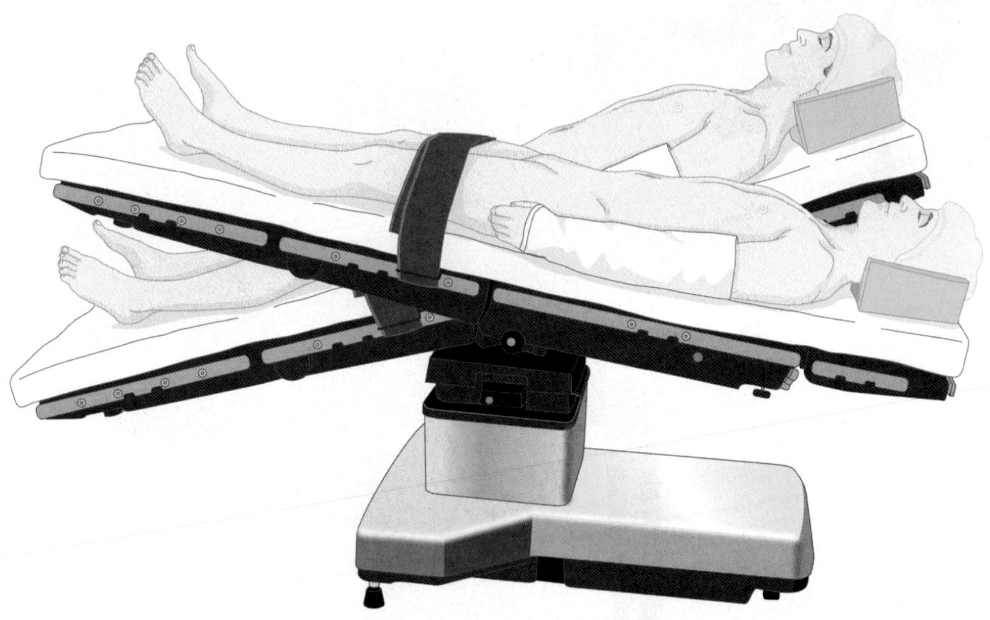

Figure 36-5 Trendelenburg position and reverse Trendelenburg position. Shoulder braces should be avoided to prevent brachial plexus compression injuries.

Complications

Pressure alopecia resulting from ischemic hair follicles is related to prolonged immobilization of the head with its full weight falling on a limited area, usually the occiput. Lumps, such as those caused by monitoring cable connectors, should not be placed under head padding because they may create focal areas of pressure. Hypothermia and hypotension during surgery, such as during cardiopulmonary bypass, may increase the incidence of this complication. Consequently, it is prudent to cushion the head well, and if possible during prolonged surgery, periodic rotation of the head to redistribute the weight may be considered.

Backache may occur in the supine position as the normal lumbar lordotic curvature, particularly the tone of the paraspinous musculature, is lost during general anesthesia with muscle relaxation or a neuraxial block. Consequently, patients with extensive kyphosis, scoliosis, or a previous history of back pain may require extra padding of the spine or slight flexion at the hip and knee. Tissues overlying all bony prominences, such as the heels and sacrum, must be padded to prevent soft tissue ischemia owing to pressure, especially during prolonged surgery.[19]

Peripheral nerve injury (discussed in detail subsequently) is a complex phenomenon with a multifactorial etiology. The American Society of Anesthesiologists (ASA) published a practice advisory in 2000 to help prevent perioperative neuropathies.[16] Ulnar neuropathy is the most common lesion. Although there is no direct evidence that positioning or padding alone can prevent perioperative ulnar neuropathies, the committee has recommended, as mentioned earlier, to limit arm abduction in a supine patient to less than 90 degrees at the shoulder with the hand and forearm either supinated or kept in a neutral position. Regardless of the position of the upper extremities, maintaining the head in a relatively midline position can help minimize the risk of stretch injury to the brachial plexus.[20]

When patients are very heavy, caution is advised when placing them in reverse axis on the operating room table (see Chapter 64). The base of the operating room table is asymmetric, with the torso over the foot of the table. Patients are often positioned with the torso over the open side of the table, however, to improve surgical access or to permit use of equipment such as C-arm x-ray devices. This positioning places the heaviest part of the body and the patient's center of gravity opposite the weighted foot of the table, with substantial leverage. The operating room table can tilt and tip over if sufficient weight is placed away from the base, particularly if extensions are used, or the bed is tilted in the Trendelenburg position. Operating room table weight limits differ substantially with regard to normal and reverse positioning and should be strictly observed.

Lithotomy

The classic lithotomy position is frequently used during gynecologic, rectal, and urologic surgeries. The hips are flexed 80 to 100 degrees from the trunk, and the legs are abducted 30 to 45 degrees from the midline. The knees are flexed until the lower legs are parallel to the torso, and the legs are held by supports or stirrups, usually "candy cane," knee crutch, or calf support style (Figs. 36-6, 36-7, and 36-8). The foot section of the operating room table is lowered. If the arms are on the operating table alongside the patient, the hands and fingers may lie near the open edge of the lowered section of the table. When raising the foot of the table at the end of surgery, strict attention to the position of the hand must be paid to avoid a potentially disastrous crush injury to the fingers (Fig. 36-9). For this reason, positioning the arms on armrests far from the table hinge point is recommended at all times when patients are in the lithotomy position.

Initiation of the lithotomy position requires coordinated positioning of the lower extremities by two assistants to avoid torsion of the lumbar spine. Both legs should be raised together, flexing the hips and knees simultaneously. The lower extremities should be padded to prevent compression against the stirrups. After the surgery, the patient must be returned to the supine posi-

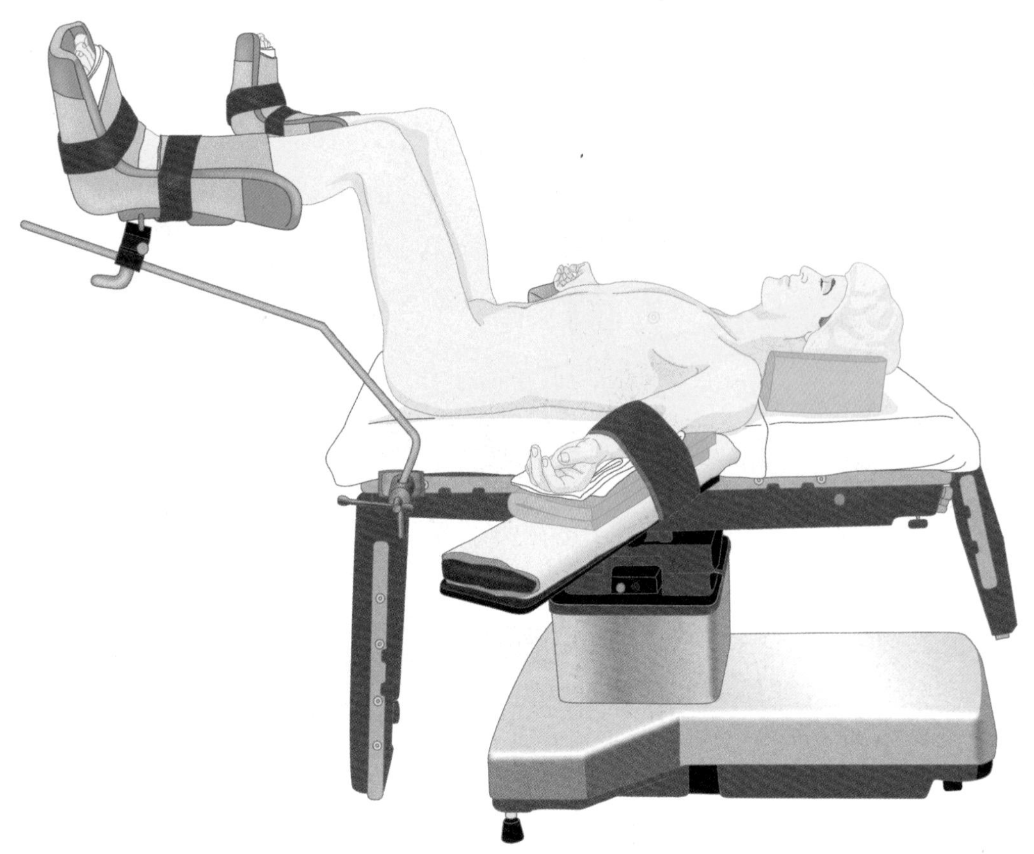

Figure 36-6 Lithotomy position. Hips are flexed 80 to 100 degrees with lower leg parallel to body. Arms are on armrests away from hinge point of foot section.

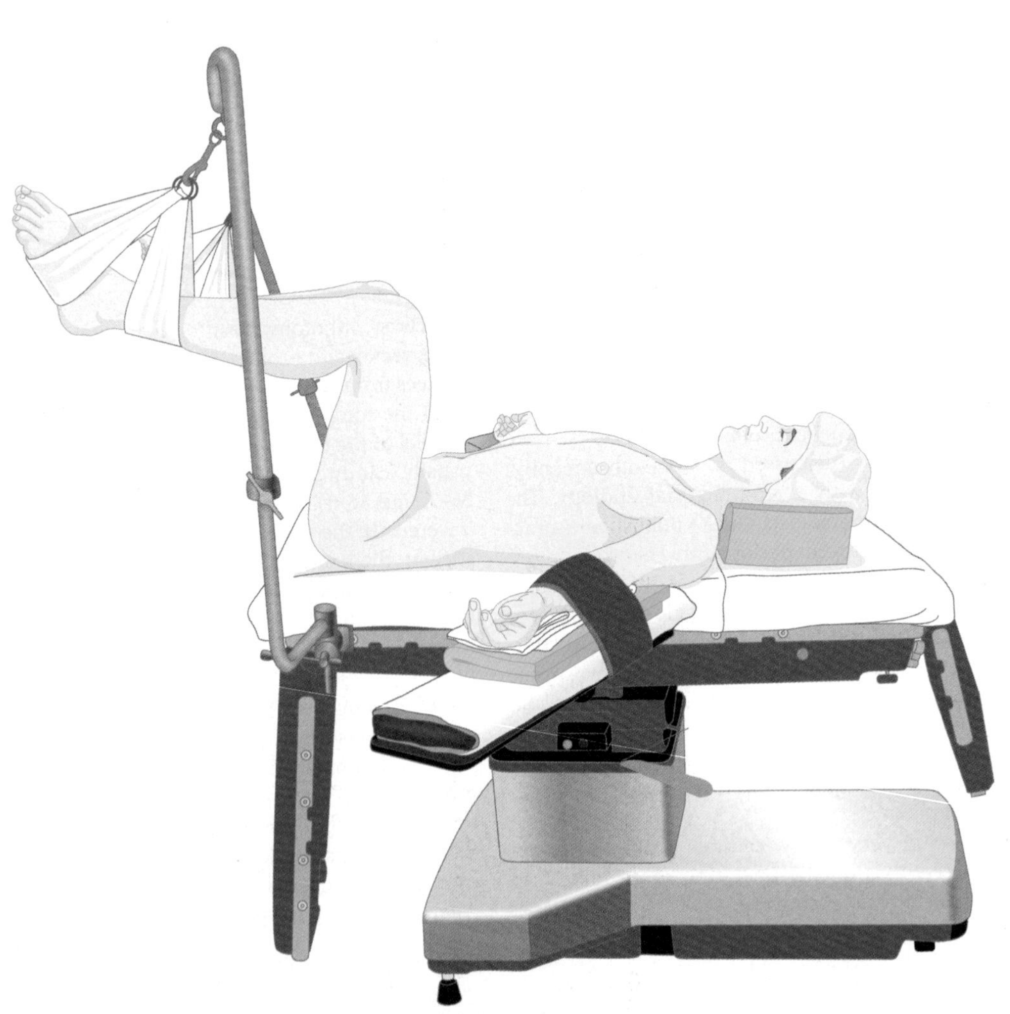

Figure 36-7 Lithotomy position with "candy cane" supports.

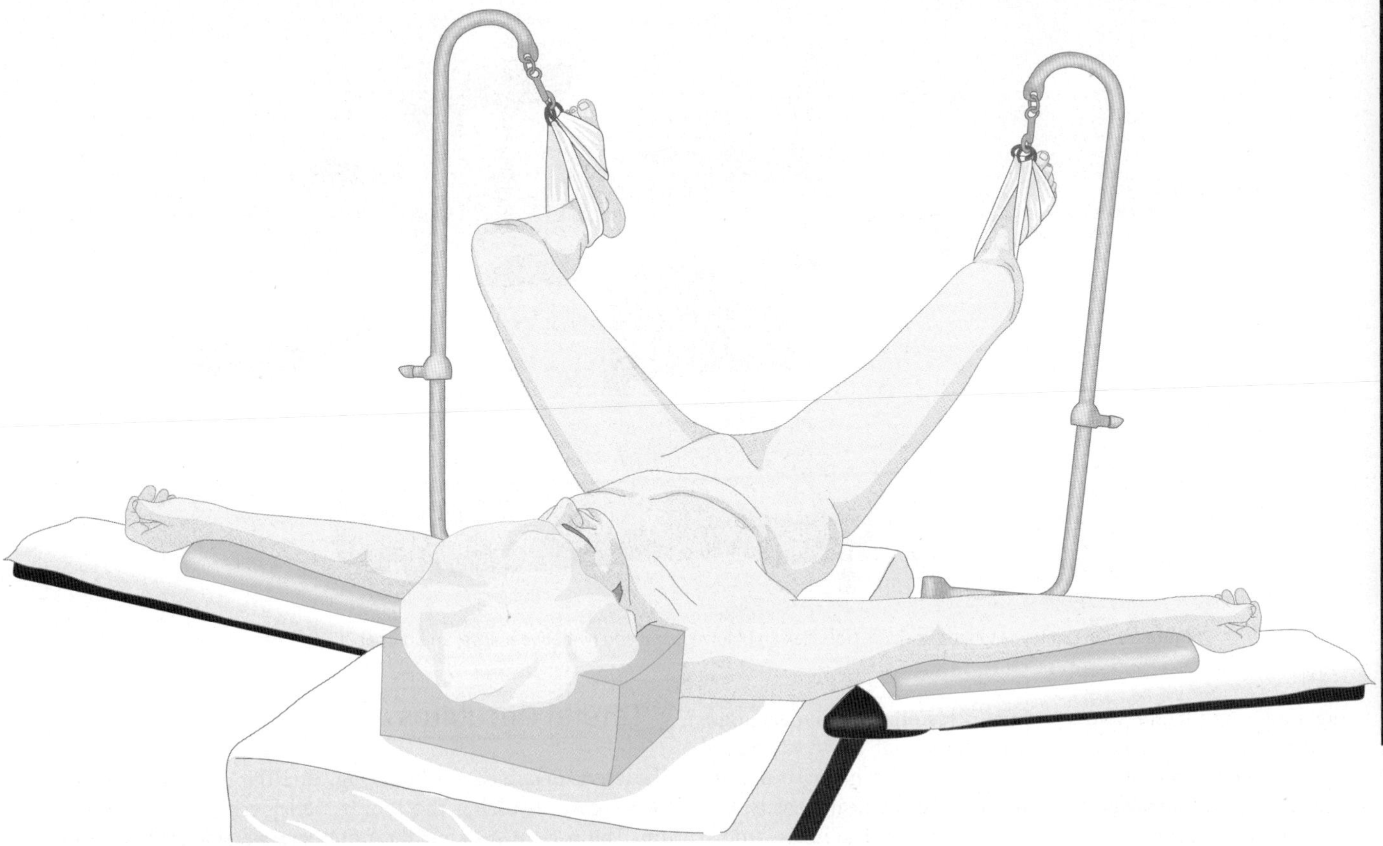

Figure 36-8 Lithotomy position with correct position of "candy cane" stirrups well away from lateral fibular head.

tion in a coordinated manner. As mentioned, the hands should be positioned to prevent entrapment in any moving or articulating sections of the operating room table. The legs should be removed from the holders simultaneously, knees brought together in the midline, and the legs slowly straightened and lowered onto the operating room table.

The lithotomy position also may cause significant physiologic changes. When the legs are elevated, preload increases, causing a transient increase in cardiac output and, to a lesser extent, cerebral venous and intracranial pressure in otherwise healthy patients. In addition, the lithotomy position causes the abdominal viscera to displace the diaphragm cephalad, reduc-

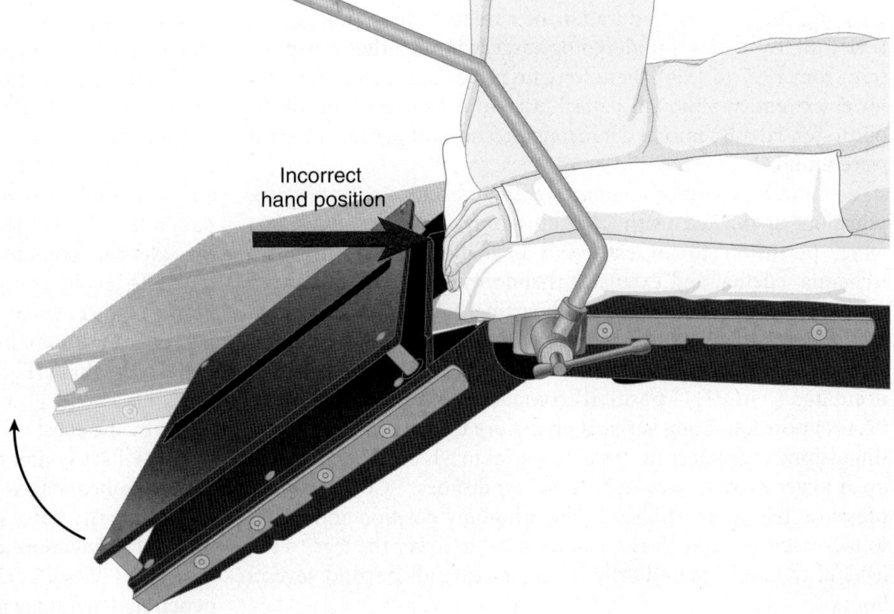

Figure 36-9 Improper position of arms in lithotomy position with fingers at risk for compression when the lower section of the bed is raised.

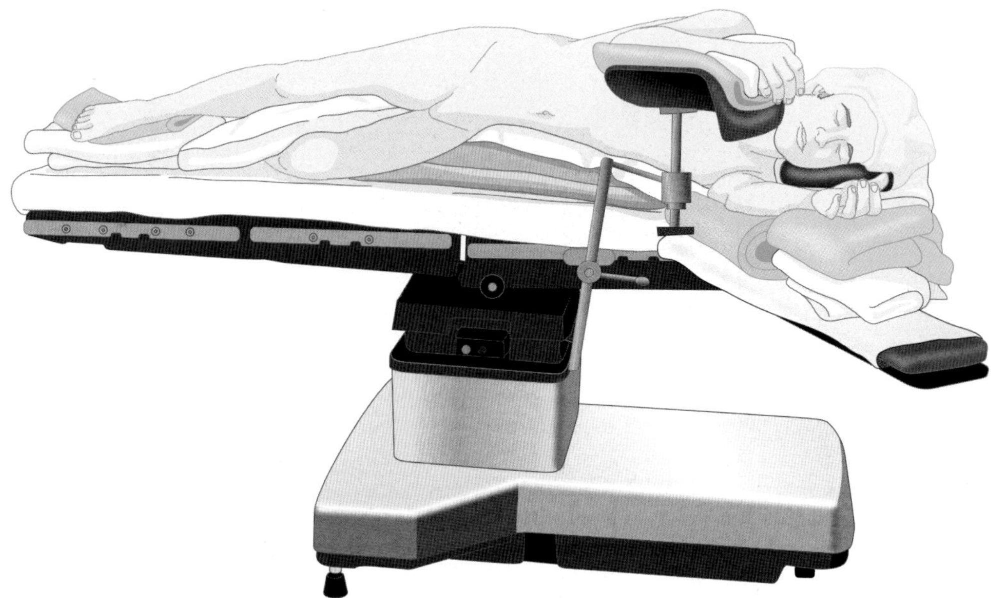

Figure 36-10 Lateral decubitus position. Note flexion of lower leg, padding between legs, and proper support of both arms.

ing lung compliance and potentially resulting in a decreased tidal volume. If obesity or a large abdominal mass is present (tumor, gravid uterus), abdominal pressure may increase significantly enough to obstruct venous return to the heart. Lastly, the normal lordotic curvature of the lumbar spine is lost in the lithotomy position, potentially aggravating any previous lower back pain.[21]

In a retrospective review of 198,461 patients undergoing surgery in the lithotomy position from 1957 to 1991, injury to the common peroneal nerve was the most common lower extremity motor neuropathy, representing 78% of nerve injuries. A potential cause of the injury was the compression of the nerve between the lateral head of the fibula and the bar holding the legs. When the candy cane stirrups are used, special attention must be paid to avoid compression (see Fig. 36-8). The injury was more common with patients who had low body mass index, recent cigarette smoking, or prolonged duration of surgery.[22] In a prospective review of 991 patients undergoing surgery in the lithotomy position from 1997 to 1998, there were no motor neuropathies in the lower extremity, although paresthesias in the distribution of the obturator, lateral femoral cutaneous, sciatic, and peroneal nerves were found.[23]

Lower extremity compartment syndrome is a rare complication associated with the lithotomy position. It occurs when perfusion to an extremity is inadequate, resulting in ischemia, edema, and extensive rhabdomyolysis from increased tissue pressure within a fascial compartment. In a large retrospective review of 572,498 surgeries, the incidence of compartment syndromes was higher in the lithotomy (1 in 8720) and lateral decubitus (1 in 9711) positions compared with the supine (1 in 92,441) position. Long surgical procedure time was the only distinguishing characteristic of the surgeries in which patients developed lower extremity compartment syndromes.[24] Compartment pressures have been studied in the lithotomy position and found to increase over time. It is recommended to lower the legs to the level of the body periodically if surgery extends beyond several hours.[25-27]

Lateral Decubitus

The lateral decubitus position (Fig. 36-10) is used most frequently for surgery involving the thorax, retroperitoneal structures, or hip. The patient rests on the nonoperative side and is balanced with anterior and posterior support, such as bedding rolls or a deflatable beanbag, and a flexed dependent leg. The arms usually are positioned in front of the patient. The dependent arm rests on a padded arm board perpendicular to the torso. The nondependent arm is often supported over folded bedding or suspended with an armrest or foam cradle. If possible, the arm should not be abducted more than 90 degrees. For some high thoracotomies, the nondependent arm may need to be elevated above the shoulder plane for exposure; however, vigilance is warranted to prevent neurovascular compromise.

The act of positioning a patient in the lateral decubitus position requires the cooperation of the entire operating room staff to prevent potential injuries. The patient's head must be kept in a neutral position to prevent excessive lateral rotation of the neck and stretch injuries to the brachial plexus. Additional head support may be required (Fig. 36-11). The dependent ear should be checked to avoid folding and undue pressure. It is advised to verify that the eyes are securely taped before repositioning if the patient is asleep. The dependent eye must be checked frequently for external compression.

To avoid compression injury to the dependent brachial plexus or vascular compression, an "axillary roll" (generally a liter bag of intravenous fluid) is frequently placed just caudal to the dependent axilla (Fig. 36-12). This roll should never be placed *in* the axilla. Its purpose is to ensure that the weight of the thorax is borne by the chest wall caudal to the axilla and avoid compression of the axillary contents. Many practitioners do not use a roll if the deflatable beanbag is used to cradle the torso. Regardless of the technique, the pulse should be monitored in the dependent arm for early detection of compression to axillary neurovascular structures. Vascular compression and venous engorgement in the dependent arm may affect the pulse oximetry reading, and a low

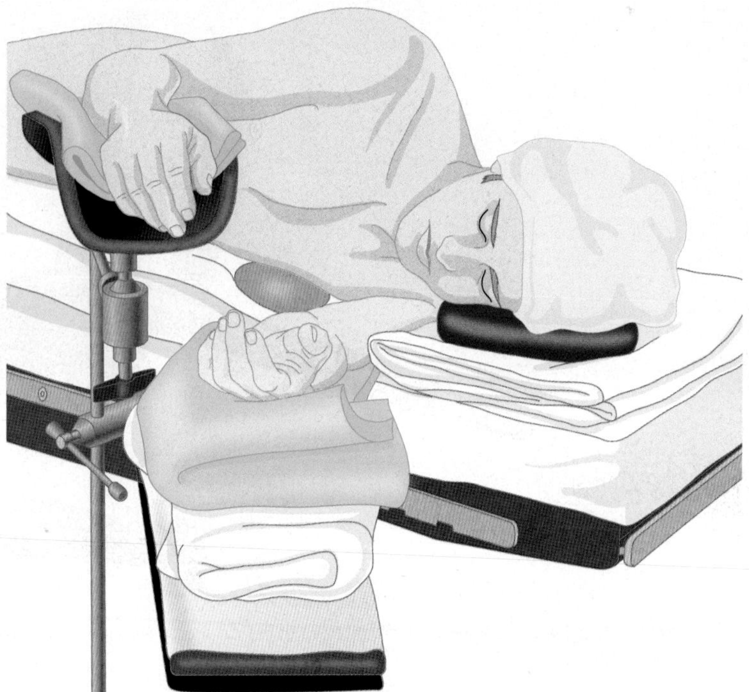

Figure 36-11 Lateral decubitus position showing placement of arms and head. Note additional padding under headrest to ensure alignment of head with spine. Headrest should be kept away from dependent eye.

saturation reading may be an early warning of compromised circulation. Hypotension measured in the dependent arm may be due to axillary arterial compression, so it is useful to retain the ability to measure blood pressure in both arms. When a kidney rest is used, it must be properly placed under the dependent iliac crest to prevent inadvertent compression of the inferior vena cava. Finally, a pillow or other padding is generally placed between the knees with the dependent leg flexed to minimize excessive pressure on bony prominences and stretch of low extremity nerves.

The lateral decubitus position also is associated with pulmonary compromise.[28] In a patient who is mechanically ventilated, the combination of the lateral weight of the mediastinum and disproportionate cephalad pressure of abdominal contents on the dependent lung favors overventilation of the nondependent lung. At the same time, pulmonary blood flow to the underventilated, dependent lung increases owing to the effect of gravity. Consequently, ventilation-perfusion matching worsens, potentially affecting gas exchange and ventilation.

The lateral decubitus position is preferred during pulmonary surgery and one-lung ventilation. The minute ventilation of the dependent lung is usually increased when the nondependent lung is collapsed. The increase in minute ventilation combined with decreased compliance owing to positioning may exacerbate further the airway pressure required to achieve adequate ventilation. Head-down tilt in the lateral position

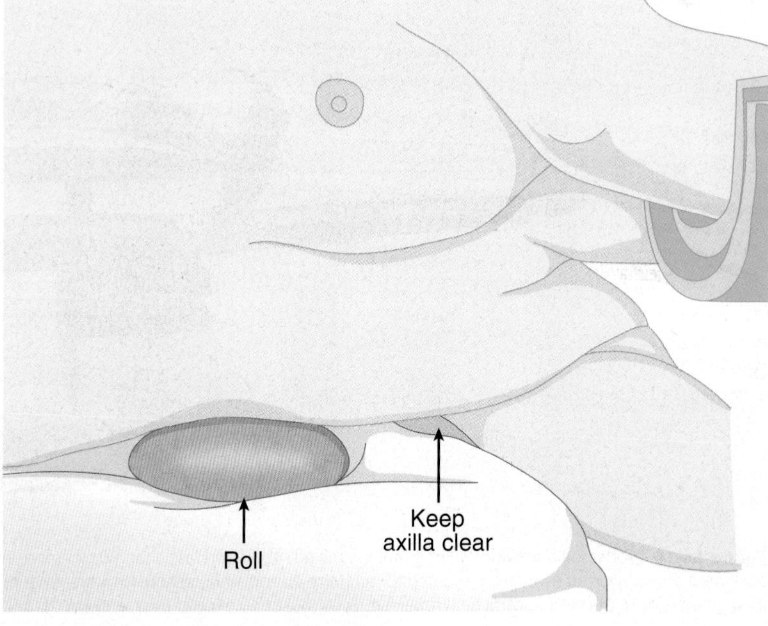

Figure 36-12 Use of axillary roll in lateral decubitus position. Roll, in this case a bag of intravenous fluid, is placed well away from axilla to prevent compression of the axillary artery and brachial plexus.

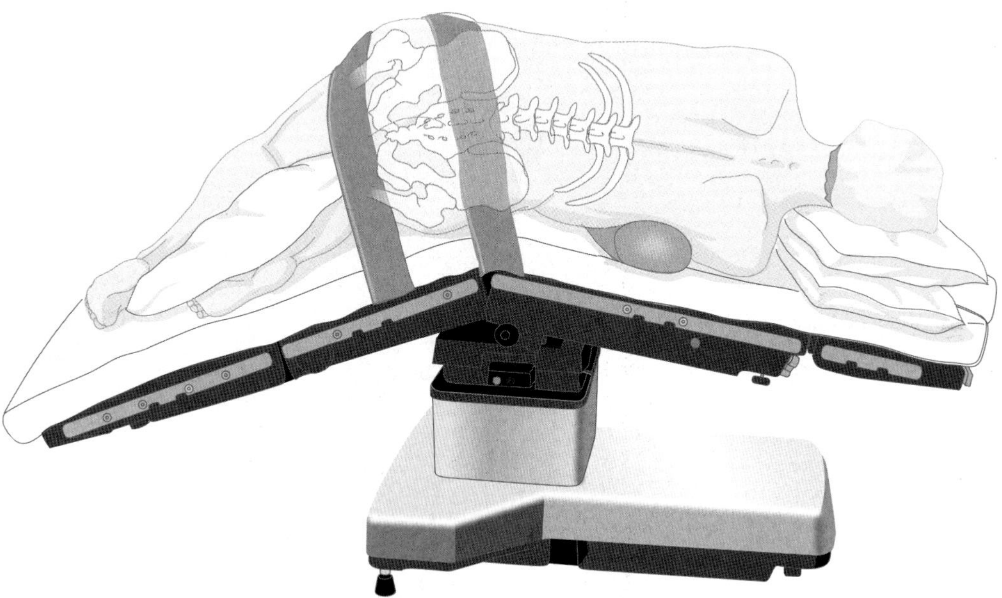

Figure 36-13 Flexed lateral decubitus position. Point of flexion should lie under iliac crest, rather than the flank or lower ribs, to optimize ventilation of the dependent lung.

worsens pulmonary function still further, increasing shunt fraction.[29]

Patients may be flexed while in the lateral position to spread the ribs during thoracotomies or improve exposure of the retroperitoneum for renal surgeries. The point of flexion, and the kidney rest if raised, should lie under the iliac crest rather than the flank or ribcage to minimize compression of the dependent lung (Fig. 36-13). This position is often accompanied by a component of reverse Trendelenburg positioning, creating the potential for venous pooling in the lower body. For these reasons, use of the flexed, lateral position is discouraged when not actively needed for surgical exposure.

Prone

The prone or ventral decubitus position (Fig. 36-14) is used primarily for surgical access to the posterior fossa of the skull, the posterior spine, the buttocks and perirectal area, and the lower extremities. As with the supine position, if the legs are in plane with the torso, hemodynamic reserve is maintained; however, if there is any significant lowering of the legs or tilt of the entire table, venous return may be decreased or augmented accordingly. Pulmonary function may be superior to the supine or lateral decubitus positions if there is no significant abdominal pressure, and the patient is properly positioned.[30,31] The legs should be

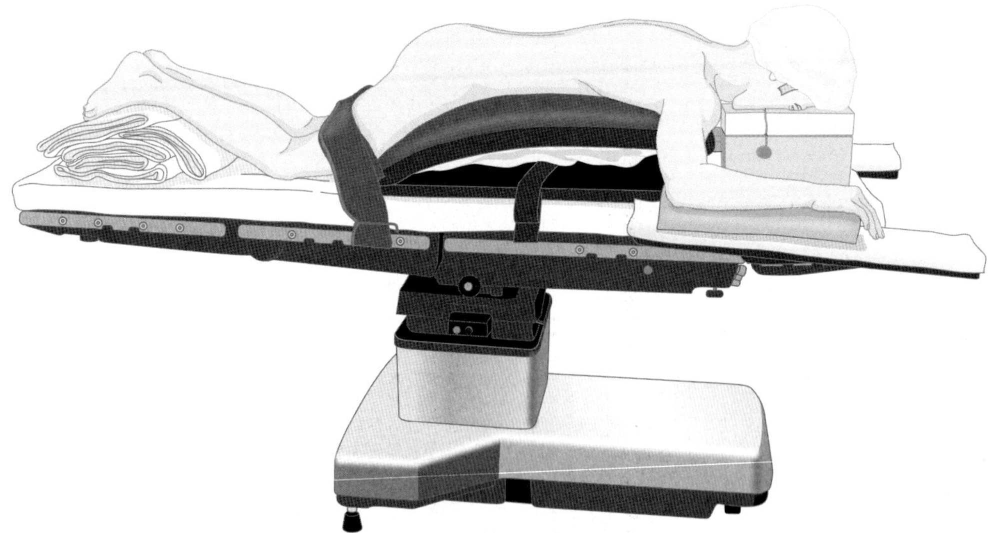

Figure 36-14 Prone position with Wilson frame. Arms are abducted less than 90 degrees whenever possible. Pressure points are padded, and chest and abdomen are supported away from the bed to minimize abdominal pressure and preserve pulmonary compliance. Soft head pillow has cutouts for eyes and nose and a slot to permit endotracheal tube exit. Eyes must be checked frequently.

padded and flexed slightly at the knees and hips. The head may be supported face-down with its weight borne by the bony structures or turned to the side.

Both arms may be positioned to the patient's sides and tucked in the neutral position as described for a supine patient, or placed next to the patient's head on arm boards—sometimes called the prone "superman" position. Extra padding under the elbow is needed to prevent compression of the ulnar nerve. The arms should not be abducted greater than 90 degrees to prevent excessive stretching of the brachial plexus, especially in patients with the head turned. Finally, elastic stockings and active compression devices are needed for the lower extremities to minimize pooling of the blood, especially with any flexion of the body.

When general anesthesia is planned, the patient is first intubated on the stretcher, and all intravascular access is obtained as needed. The endotracheal tube is well secured to prevent dislodgment and loosening of tape owing to drainage of saliva when prone. With the coordination of the entire operating room staff, the patient is turned prone onto the operating room table, keeping the neck in line with the spine during the move. The anesthesiologist is primarily responsible for coordinating the move and for repositioning of the head. An exception might be cases in which rigid pin fixation is used, and the surgeon holds the pin frame. It is recommended to disconnect blood pressure cuffs and arterial and venous lines that are on the side that rotates furthest to avoid dislodgment, although some clinicians prefer to disconnect all lines and monitors before moving. Pulse oximetry usually can be maintained if applied to the "inside" arm, and full monitoring should be reinstituted as rapidly as possible. Endotracheal tube position and adequate ventilation are reassessed immediately after the move.

Head position is crucial. The patient's head may be turned to the side when prone if neck mobility is adequate. As in the lateral decubitus position, the dependent eye must be checked frequently for external compression. In addition, in patients with cervical arthritis or cerebrovascular disease, lateral rotation of the neck may compromise carotid or vertebral arterial blood flow or jugular venous drainage. In most cases, the head is kept in a neutral position using a surgical pillow, horseshoe headrest, or Mayfield head pins. Numerous commercially available pillows are specially designed for the prone position. Most, including disposable foam versions, support the forehead, malar regions, and the chin, with a cutout for the eyes, nose, and mouth (see Fig. 36-14). The face is not always visible, however, making eye checks more difficult. Mirror systems are available to facilitate intermittent visual confirmation that the eyes are unimpinged, although direct visualization or tactile confirmation of at least the initial appearance is prudent (Fig. 36-15).

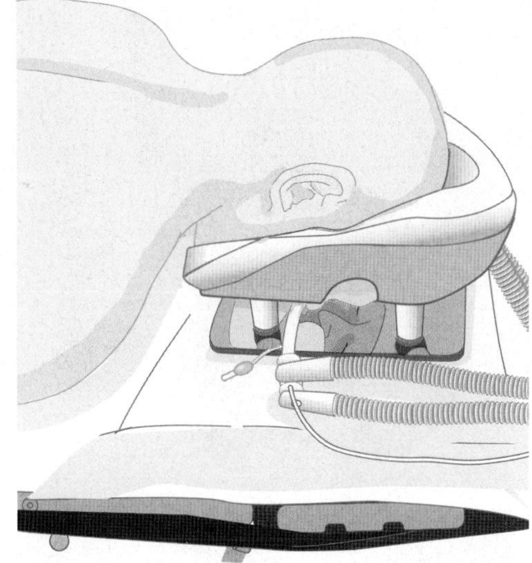

Figure 36-15 Mirror system for prone position. Bony structures of head and face are supported, and monitoring of eyes and airway is facilitated with a plastic mirror.

The horseshoe headrest supports only the forehead and malar regions and allows excellent access to the airway, but it is more rigid and potentially dangerous if the head moves (Figs. 36-16 and 36-17). Mayfield rigid pins support the head without any direct pressure on the face, allow access to the airway, and hold the head firmly in one position that can be finely adjusted for optimal neurosurgical exposure (Fig. 36-18). Rigid pin fixation is rarely used outside cranial or cervical spine surgeries. When properly applied, the pins cause significant periosteal stimulation. A high degree of vigilance also is necessary to prevent patient movement when the head is held in rigid pins; skidding out of pins can result in scalp lacerations or cervical spine injury. Because horseshoe and pin headrests attach to adjustable articu-

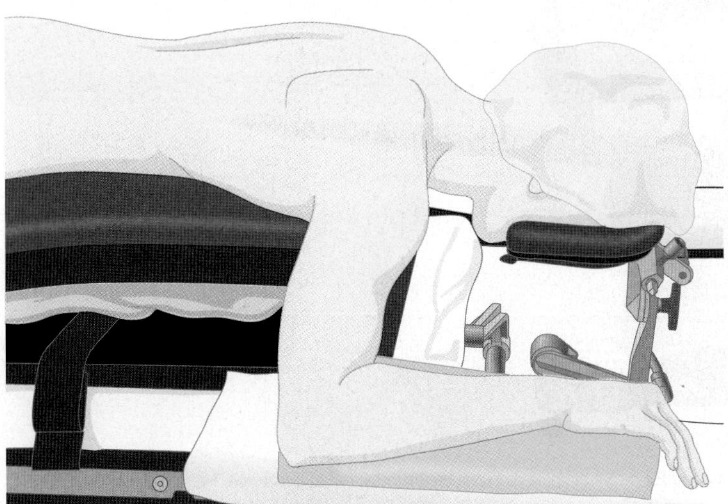

Figure 36-16 Prone position with horseshoe adapter. Head height is adjusted to position neck in a natural position.

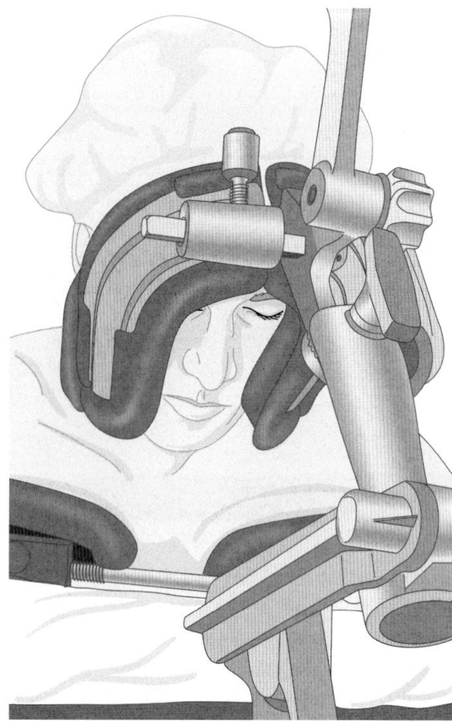

Figure 36-17 Prone position, face seen from below. Horseshoe adapter permits superior access to airway and visualization of eyes. Width may be adjusted to ensure proper support by facial bones.

lating supports, any slippage or failure of this bracketing device may lead to complications if the head suddenly drops.

Regardless of the technique employed to support the head, the eyes, face, and airway must be checked periodically to ensure that the weight is borne only by the bony structures, and that there is no pressure on the eyes. Proper position is verified frequently and noted in the anesthetic record. The face should be rechecked if any patient motion occurs during surgery, or if the table is significantly repositioned. The prone position is a risk factor for perioperative visual loss, which is discussed in detail subsequently.

Because the abdominal wall is easily displaced, external pressure on the abdomen may elevate intra-abdominal pressure in the prone position. This elevated pressure compromises respiration and transmits elevated venous pressures to the abdominal and spine vessels, including the epidural veins. During spinal surgery, low venous pressure is desirable to minimize bleeding and facilitate surgical exposure. External pressure on the abdomen may push the diaphragm cephalad, decreasing functional residual capacity and pulmonary compliance, and increasing peak airway pressure. Abdominal pressure also may impede venous return through compression of the inferior vena cava. For these reasons, careful attention must be paid to the ability of the abdomen to hang free and to move with respiration.

The thorax is generally supported by firm rolls or bolsters placed along each side from the clavicle to the iliac crest. Multiple commercial rolls and bolsters are available, including the Wilson frame (see Fig. 36-14), Jackson table, Relton frame, and the Mouradian/Simmons modification of the Relton frame. All devices serve to minimize abdominal compression by the operating room table and maintain normal pulmonary compliance. To prevent tissue injury, pendulous structures (e.g., male genitalia and female breasts) should be clear of compression; the breasts should be placed medial to the bolsters. The lower portion of each roll or bolster must be placed under its respective iliac crest to prevent pressure injury to the genitalia and the femoral vasculature.[32] The prone position presents special risks for morbidly obese patients, whose respiration is already compromised, and who may be difficult to reposition quickly. Sometimes it may be necessary to discuss alternative positioning options with the surgeon to ensure patient safety.

Sitting

The sitting position, although infrequently used because of the perception of risk from venous and paradoxical air embolism, offers advantages to the surgeon in approaching the posterior

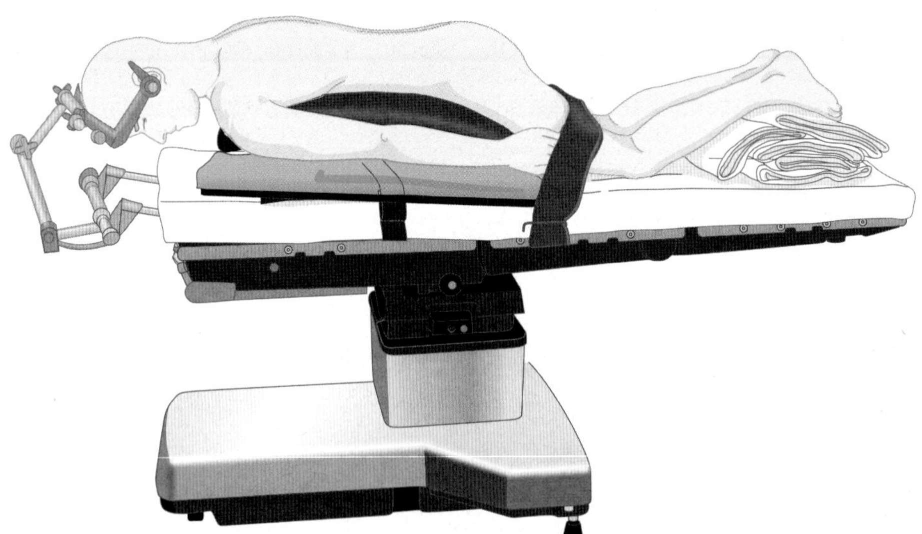

Figure 36-18 Prone position with Mayfield head pins. Rigid fixation is provided for cervical spine and posterior intracranial surgeries. Head position may include neck torsion or flexion that affects endotracheal tube position.

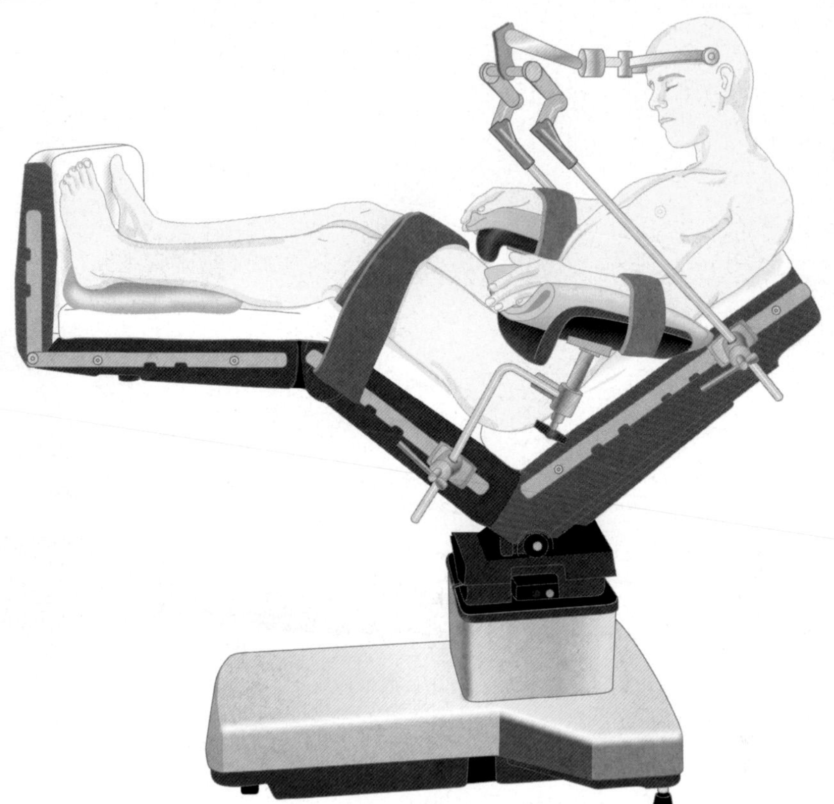

Figure 36-19 "Sitting" position with Mayfield head pins. This is actually a modified recumbent position as the legs are kept as high as possible to promote venous return. Arms must be supported to prevent shoulder traction. In a commonly used variation they are padded and rest on the abdomen, as illustrated in Figure 63-8. Note that the head holder support is preferably attached to the back section of the table so that the patient's back may be adjusted or lowered emergently without first detaching the head holder. If the head holder is connected to the thigh section of the table this cannot be done.

cervical spine and the posterior fossa (Fig. 36-19). The main advantages of the sitting position over the prone position for neurosurgical and cervical spine surgeries are excellent surgical exposure, decreased blood in the operative field, and, possibly, reduced perioperative blood loss.[33] The main advantages to the anesthesiologist are superior access to the airway, reduced facial swelling, and improved ventilation, particularly in obese patients. A variation of the sitting position, the beach chair position is increasingly used for shoulder surgeries, including arthroscopic procedures (Fig. 36-20). Its attraction to the surgeon is superior access to the shoulder from the anterior and posterior aspect, and potential for great mobility of the arm at the shoulder joint.

The head may be fixed in pins for neurosurgery or taped in place with adequate support for other surgeries. Because gravity is pulling the arms caudad, they must be supported to the point of slight elevation of the shoulders to avoid traction on the shoulder muscles and potential stretching of upper extremity neurovascular structures. The knees are usually slightly flexed for balance and to reduce stretching of the sciatic nerve, and the feet are supported and padded.[34]

The hemodynamic effects of placing a supine patient in the sitting position are dramatic. Because of the pooling of blood into the lower body under general anesthesia (see earlier), patients are particularly prone to hypotensive episodes. Incremental positioning and the use of intravenous fluids, vasopressors, and appropriate adjustments of anesthetic depth can reduce the degree and duration of hypotension. Elastic stockings and active leg compression devices can help maintain venous return.

Head and neck position has been associated with complications during surgery to the posterior spine or skull in the sitting position. Excessive cervical flexion has numerous adverse consequences. It can impede arterial and venous blood flow, causing hypoperfusion or venous congestion of the brain. It may impede normal respiratory excursion. Excessive flexion also can obstruct the endotracheal tube and place significant pressure on the tongue, leading to macroglossia. Generally, maintaining at least two fingers' distance between the mandible and the sternum is recommended for a normal-sized adult, and patients should not be positioned at the extreme of their range of motion.[35] Extra caution with neck flexion is advised if transesophageal echocardiography (TEE) is used for air embolism monitoring because the esophageal probe lies between the flexed spine and the airway and endotracheal tube, adding potential for compression of laryngeal structures and the tongue.

Because of the elevation of the surgical field above the heart, and the inability of the dural venous sinuses to collapse because of their bony attachments, the risk of venous air embolism is a constant concern. Arrhythmia, desaturation, pulmonary hypertension, circulatory compromise, or cardiac arrest may occur if sufficient quantities are entrained. If the foramen ovale is patent, even small amounts of venous air may result in a stroke or myocardial infarction owing to paradoxical embolism. TEE has shown some degree of venous air in most patients studied during neurosurgery in the sitting position (≤100%).[36,37] Because of the risk of paradoxical embolus, screening contrast echocardiography to investigate the patency of the interatrial septum is

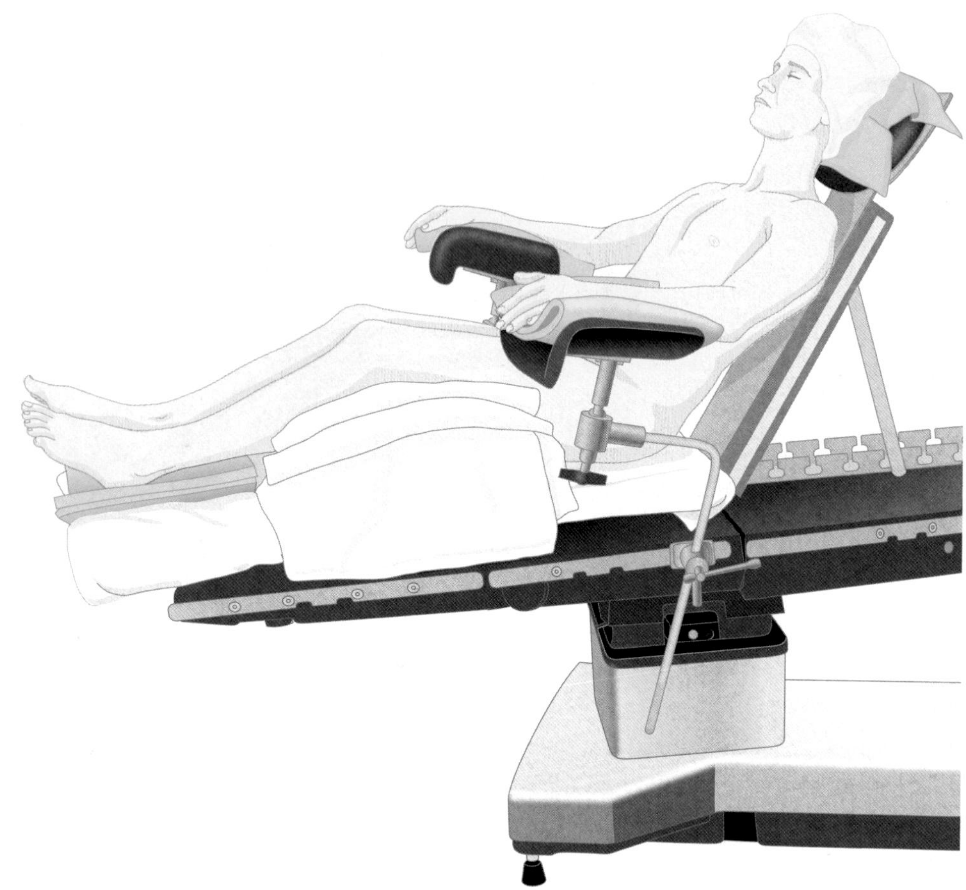

Figure 36-20 Sitting position adapted for shoulder surgery. This is sometimes called the "beach chair position". Arms must be supported to prevent stretching of the brachial plexus.

often performed before sitting position intracranial or cervical spine surgery. Septal patency may not always be detected, however. Adequate hydration and early detection of entrained air with the use of TEE or precordial Doppler ultrasound may decrease the incidence and severity of venous air embolism.[36]

Peripheral Nerve Injury

Peripheral nerve injury remains a serious perioperative complication and a significant source of professional liability despite the low incidence (approximately 0.11% of 81,000 anesthetic procedures reviewed from 1987 to 1993).[38] Injuries occur when peripheral nerves are subjected to stretch, ischemia, or compression during surgery.[39] Because sensation is blocked by unconsciousness or regional anesthesia, early warning symptoms of pain and the normal spontaneous repositioning are absent. In 1984, the ASA developed a Closed Claims Project to evaluate adverse anesthetic outcomes from the closed claims files of 35 U.S. liability insurance companies. Since the initial report in 1990, the incidence of nerve injury has remained essentially constant, representing 18% of all claims during 1990 through 1994, second only to death (22%).[1-3] Among the total 670 claims filed, ulnar neuropathy remained the most frequent site of injury (28%), followed by the brachial plexus (20%), lumbosacral nerve root (16%), and spinal cord (13%) (Table 36-1).

The distribution of nerve injuries has changed significantly over time. Ulnar neuropathy decreased from 37% in 1980-1984 to 17% in the 1990s, and spinal cord injury increased from 8% in 1980-1984 to 27% in 1990s. Spinal cord injury and lumbosacral nerve root neuropathy were predominantly associated with regional anesthesia. Epidural hematoma and chemical injury represented 29% of the known mechanisms of injury among the claims filed. The injuries probably were related to the use of neuraxial block in anticoagulated patients and the increased usage of blocks for chronic pain management (Table 36-2).[3,40,41]

With the exception of spinal cord injury, the mechanism of nerve injury remains largely unknown. Most injuries, particularly injuries to nerves of the upper extremity, such as the ulnar nerve and brachial plexus, occurred in the presence of adequate positioning and padding. Because of the significant morbidity associated with peripheral nerve injury, in 2000 the ASA published a practice advisory for the prevention of peripheral neuropathies.[16] The advisory was not based on scientific evidence, but the consensus of a consultant expert group. Only 6 of 509 positioning studies reviewed "... exhibited sufficiently acceptable methods and analyses that provided a clear indication of the relationships between interventions and outcomes of interest" (Table 36-3).

Because of the paucity of clear data on the causes and the prevention of peripheral injuries, individual practices vary with regard to specific padding and positional details. Prolonged duration is a risk factor. Good sense would avoid positions that permit stretching of the nerves and pressure to anatomic locations known

Table 36-1 Nerve Injury Claims in the American Society of Anesthesiologists Closed Claims Database

Nerve	No. Claims in Current Database (*N* = 4183)	% of Total (*N* = 670)	No. Claims since 1990 Report	% of Total since 1990 (*N* = 445)
Ulnar	190	28	113	25
Brachial plexus	137	20	83	19
Lumbosacral nerve root	105	16	67	15
Spinal cord	84	13	73	16
Sciatic*	34	5	23	5
Median	28	4	19	4
Radial	18	3	13	3
Femoral	15	2	9	2
Other single nerves	43	6	35	8
Multiple nerves	16	2	10	2
Total	*670*	*100*	*445*	*100*

*Includes peroneal nerve.
From Cheney FW, Domino KB, Caplan RA, et al: Nerve injury associated with anesthesia. Anesthesiology 90:1064, 1999.

to carry nerves prone to injury, such as the ulnar cubital tunnel and the peroneal nerve coursing over the fibular head. Whenever possible, the patient's position should appear as natural as possible. Padding and support should distribute weight over as wide an area as possible; however, no padding material has been shown to be superior. It also is important to anticipate the additional effects of anesthesia and muscle relaxation.

In a retrospective study of 1000 consecutive spine surgeries that used somatosensory evoked potential (SSEP) monitoring, five arm positions were compared with regard to SSEP changes in the upper extremities. A modification of arm position reversed 92% of upper extremity SSEP changes. The incidence of position-related upper extremity SSEP changes was significantly higher in the prone superman (7%) and lateral decubitus (7.5%) positions compared with the supine arms out, supine arms tucked, and prone arms tucked positions (1.8% to 3.2%). Reversible SSEP changes were not associated with postoperative deficits (see Chapter 46).[42]

Ulnar Nerve

The etiology of perioperative ulnar neuropathy is complex and incompletely understood. The ulnar nerve lies in a superficial

Table 36-2 Most Common Nerve Injuries in American Society of Anesthesiologists Closed Claims Database after 1990

Injury	Recommendations for Prevention
Ulnar nerve (25%)	Avoid excessive pressure on postcondylar groove of humerus Keep hand and forearm either supinated or in neutral position
Brachial plexus (19%)	Avoid the use of shoulder braces in patients in Trendelenburg position (use nonsliding mattresses) Avoid excessive lateral rotation of head either in supine or prone position Limit abduction of the arm to <90 degrees in supine position Avoid placement of high axillary roll in decubitus position—keep roll out of axilla Use ultrasound to find internal jugular vein for central line placement
Spinal cord (16%) and lumbosacral nerve root (15%)	Be aware that the fraction of spinal cord injuries is increasing, probably in relation to use of epidural catheters for pain management Follow current guidelines for regional anesthesia in anticoagulated patients*
Sciatic and peroneal (5%)	Minimize time of surgery in lithotomy position Use two assistants to coordinate simultaneous movement of both legs to and from lithotomy position Avoid excessive flexion of hips, extension of knees, or torsion of lumbar spine Avoid excessive pressure on peroneal nerve at the fibular head
Median (4%) and radial (3%)	Be aware that 25% of injuries to the median and radial nerves were associated with axillary block, and 25% of injuries were associated with traumatic insertion or infiltration of an intravenous line

*Horlocker TT, Wedel DJ, Benzon H, et al: Regional anesthesia in the anticoagulated patient: Defining the risks (The Second ASRA Consensus Conference on Neuraxial Anesthesia and Anticoagulation). Reg Anesth Pain Med 28:172-197, 2003.
Data from references 1-3.

Table 36-3 Summary of American Society of Anesthesiologists Task Force Consensus Findings on Prevention of Perioperative Peripheral Neuropathies

Preoperative Assessment
When judged appropriate, it is helpful to ascertain that patients can comfortably tolerate anticipated operative position
Upper Extremity Positioning
Arm abduction should be limited to 90 degrees in supine patients; patients who are positioned prone may comfortably tolerate arm abduction >90 degrees
Arms should be positioned to decrease pressure on the postcondylar groove of the humerus (ulnar groove). When arms are tucked at the side, a neutral forearm position is recommended. When arms are abducted on armboards, either supination or a neutral forearm position is acceptable
Prolonged pressure on radial nerve in spiral groove of humerus should be avoided
Extension of elbow beyond a comfortable range may stretch median nerve
Lower Extremity Positioning
Lithotomy positions that stretch hamstring muscle group beyond a comfortable range may stretch sciatic nerve
Prolonged pressure on peroneal nerve at fibular head should be avoided
Neither extension nor flexion of hip increases risk of femoral neuropathy
Protective Padding
Padded armboards may decrease risk of upper extremity neuropathy
Use of chest rolls in laterally positioned patients may decrease risk of upper extremity neuropathies
Padding at elbow and at fibular head may decrease risk of upper and lower extremity neuropathies
Equipment
Properly functioning automated blood pressure cuffs on upper arms do not affect risk of upper extremity neuropathies
Shoulder braces in steep head-down positions may increase risk of brachial plexus neuropathies
Postoperative Assessment
Simple postoperative assessment of extremity nerve function may lead to early recognition of peripheral neuropathies
Documentation
Charting specific positioning actions during care of patients may result in improvements of care by (1) helping practitioners focus attention on relevant aspects of patient positioning, and (2) providing information that continuous improvement processes can use to effect refinements in patient care

From ASA Task Force on Prevention of Perioperative Peripheral Neuropathies: Practice advisory for the prevention of perioperative peripheral neuropathies. Anesthesiology 92:1168-1182, 2000.

position at the elbow. Although the incidence is low, the morbidity associated with ulnar neuropathy can be severe. In a prospective study among 1502 patients undergoing noncardiac surgery, 7 patients developed perioperative ulnar neuropathy, of which 3 patients had residual symptoms after 2 years.[43] The neuropathy, if permanent, results in the inability to abduct or oppose the fifth finger, diminished sensation in the fourth and fifth fingers, and eventual atrophy of the intrinsic muscle of the hands creating a claw-like hand.

Previously, injury was thought to be associated with hyperflexion of the elbow and compression by the operating room table of the nerve at the condylar groove and the cubital tunnel against the posterior aspect of the medial epicondyle of the humerus. The current consensus is that the etiology of ulnar nerve palsy is multifactorial and not always preventable. In a large retrospective review of perioperative ulnar neuropathy lasting longer than 3 months, the onset of symptoms occurred more than 24 hours postoperatively in 57% of patients, 70% were male, and 9% experienced bilateral symptoms. Very thin or obese patients were at increased risk, as were patients on prolonged postoperative bed rest. There was no association with intraoperative patient position or anesthetic technique.[44]

The Closed Claims Project also showed that perioperative ulnar neuropathy occurred predominantly in men, in an older population, and with a delayed onset (median of 3 days).[3] Although most ulnar damage claims were associated with general anesthesia, payment also was made for claims where the patient had been awake or sedated during regional anesthesia involving the lower extremity. In a prospective study of medical patients who did not undergo surgical procedures, 2 of 986 patients developed ulnar neuropathy.[45] The large predominance of ulnar injury in men may be explained by anatomic differences. Men have a more developed and thickened flexor retinaculum with less protective adipose tissue and a larger (1.5 ×) tubercle of the coronoid process that can predispose to nerve compression in the cubital tunnel.[46,47] Other risk factors, including diabetes mellitus, vitamin deficiency, alcoholism, cigarette smoking, and cancer, need further studies to be substantiated. In the ASA Closed Claims Project, only 9% of ulnar injury claims had an explicit mechanism of injury, and, in 27% of claims, the padding of the elbows was explicitly stated.[3] It has become accepted that postoperative ulnar nerve palsy can occur without any apparent cause, even when padding and positioning of the patient's arm were done carefully and documented in the anesthetic record.[18]

Brachial Plexus

The brachial plexus is susceptible to injury from stretching or compression because of its long superficial course in the axilla between two points of fixation, the vertebra and the axillary fascia, in association with the mobile clavicle and humerus (Fig. 36-21). The patient often complains of sensory deficit in the distribution of the ulnar nerve. Injury is most commonly associated with arm abduction greater than 90 degrees, lateral rotation of the head, asymmetric retraction of the sternum for internal mammary artery dissection during cardiac surgery, and direct trauma. To avoid brachial plexus injury, patients ideally should be positioned with the head midline, arms kept at the sides, the elbow mildly flexed, and the forearm supinated.

In cardiac surgery patients requiring median sternotomy, brachial plexus injury has been specifically associated with the C8-T1 nerve roots. In a prospective study in which the incidence of injury was 4.9%, the authors found that 73% of the injuries occurred on the same side as the internal jugular vein cannulation.[48] Among noncardiac surgery patients, the incidence is reported to be 0.02%.[49] In the ASA Closed Claims Project, 16% of brachial plexus injuries occurred during a regional block, particularly the axillary block.[3]

Brachial plexus injury also is associated with direct compression, particularly with the use of shoulder braces in patients undergoing surgery in the Trendelenburg position. The nerves are vulnerable to compression as they pass between the clavicle and

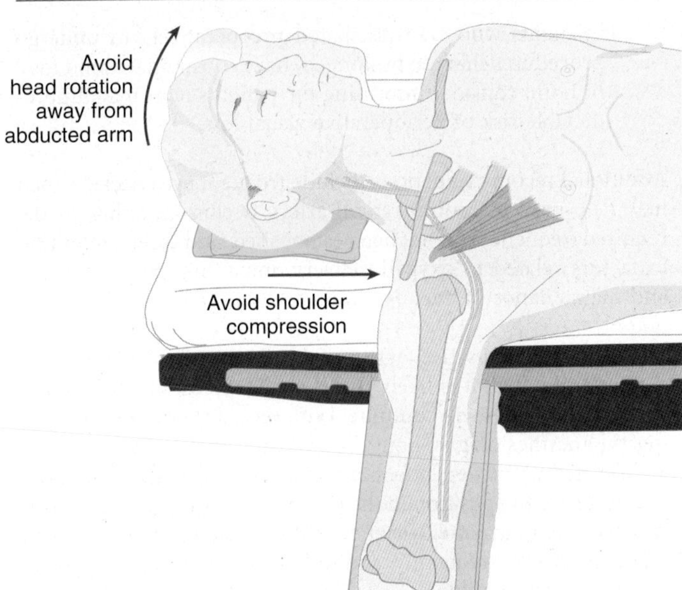

Figure 36-21 The brachial plexus is vulnerable to stretch and compression. Arm abduction is limited to less than 90 degrees whenever possible. Excessive head rotation, especially away from an abducted arm, should be avoided. Shoulder braces should be avoided because they may cause direct compression of the plexus medially between the clavicle and first rib, or laterally below the head of the humerus.

the first rib. Medial placement of the braces can compress the proximal roots, and lateral placement of the braces can stretch the plexus by displacing the shoulders (see Fig. 36-21). The patient with injury often complains of painless motor deficit in the distribution of the radial and median nerves. In the ASA Closed Claims Project, 10% of brachial plexus injuries were directly attributed to patient positioning. Of those, one half involved the use of shoulder braces in patients in the Trendelenburg position.[3] Consequently, nonsliding mattresses should be used in place of shoulder braces.

Other Upper Extremity Nerves

Although quite rare, the radial nerve can be injured from direct pressure as it traverses the spiral groove of the humerus in the lower third of the arm. The injury often manifests as a wrist drop with an inability to abduct the thumb or extend the metacarpophalangeal joints. Isolated median nerve injury most often occurs during the insertion of an intravenous needle into the antecubital fossa in an anesthetized patient where the nerve is adjacent to the medial cubital and basilic veins. Patients with this injury are unable to oppose the first and fifth digits and have decreased sensation over the palmar surface of the lateral three and a half fingers. In an evaluation of the ASA Closed Claims database from 1970 to 2001, Liau[50] found that peripheral intravenous and arterial line insertion accounted for 2.1% of all claims filed, particularly among patients undergoing cardiac surgery where the arms are tucked and the lines are not visible for inspection. Nerve injury accounted for 17% of intravenous line complications second only to skin slough or necrosis (28%) and swelling, inflammation, and infection (17%).

Lower Extremity Nerves

Injuries to the sciatic and common peroneal nerves occur most often in the lithotomy position. Because of its fixation between the sciatic notch and the neck of the fibula, the sciatic nerve can be stretched with external rotation of the leg. Hyperflexion of the hips or extension of the knees also can aggravate nerve stretch in this position. The common peroneal nerve, a branch of the sciatic nerve, can be damaged from the compression of the nerve between the head of the fibula and the frame of the leg support. Most often, patients who sustain injury complain of a foot drop and the inability to extend the toes in a dorsal direction or evert the foot.

In a prospective study of 991 patients undergoing surgery under general anesthesia in the lithotomy position, the incidence of lower extremity neuropathies was 1.5%, with injuries to the sciatic and peroneal nerves representing 40% of the cases. Symptoms were predominantly paresthesia with onset within 4 hours of surgery and resolution generally within 6 months. No motor deficits were noted, but in a previous retrospective study, the same authors found the incidence of severe motor disability in patients undergoing surgery in the lithotomy position to be 1 in 3608.[22,23]

Injury to the femoral or obturator nerves generally occurs during lower abdominal surgical procedures with excessive retraction. The obturator nerve also can be injured during a difficult forceps delivery or by excessive flexion of the thigh to the groin. A femoral neuropathy manifests with decreased flexion of the hip, decreased extension of the knee, or a loss of sensation over the superior aspect of the thigh and medial/anteromedial side of the leg. An obturator neuropathy manifests with inability to adduct the leg with decreased sensation over the medial side of the thigh.

Perioperative Eye Injury and Visual Loss

Although quite rare (incidence of 0.056% in one retrospective review),[51] perioperative eye injuries are a source of significant morbidity and liability (see Chapter 90). In the ASA Closed Claims database, eye complications constituted 3% of all claims and were associated with greater monetary settlements compared with nonocular injuries.[3]

Corneal abrasion is the most common type of perioperative eye injury and is associated with direct trauma to the cornea from facemasks, surgical drapes, or other foreign objects. Corneal abrasion also can be associated with decreased basal tear production or swelling of the dependent eye in patients in the prone position. Patients complain of pain associated with a foreign body sensation in the eye on awakening from surgery. This injury also can occur from a dried section of cornea. Symptoms are generally transient, and treatment comprises supportive care and antibiotic ointment to prevent bacterial infection.

In a prospective study of 671 patients undergoing nonocular surgery, 4.2% of patients reported a new onset of blurred vision lasting at least 3 days after surgery. For most patients, the symptoms resolved within 2 months without complication; 1% required visits to eye care providers.[52] Precautionary measures to reduce the incidence of corneal abrasion include early and careful taping of the eyelids after induction of anesthesia, care regarding dangling objects when leaning over patients, and close observation as patients awaken. Before they are completely awake, patients often try to rub their eye or nose with pulse oximeter probes, armboards, and intravenous lines attached, inadvertently endangering their eyes.

Postoperative visual loss is a devastating complication that has been associated with specific surgeries and patient risk factors (see Chapter 90). Risk varies with type of surgery. The incidence varies from a range of 1 in 60,965 to 1 in 125,234 for patients undergoing noncardiac, nonocular surgeries[51,53] to 0.06% to 0.113% for patients undergoing cardiac surgery with cardiopulmonary bypass,[54,55] and 0.09% for patients undergoing spine surgery in the prone position.[56] Ischemic optic neuropathy (ION) and, to a lesser extent, central retinal arterial occlusion from direct retinal pressure are the conditions most sited as potential causes. Perioperative factors associated with an increased risk of ION include prolonged hypotension, long duration of surgery especially in the prone position, large blood loss, large crystalloid use, anemia or hemodilution, and increased intraocular or venous pressure from the prone position.[57,58] Intraocular pressure increases in the dependent eye in the lateral decubitus position as well.[59] Patient risk factors associated with ION include hypertension, diabetes, atherosclerosis, morbid obesity, and tobacco use. With the exception of obvious external compression of the eyes, however, the cause of perioperative visual loss seems to be multifactorial in nature with no consistent underlying mechanism.

In 1999, the ASA Committee on Professional Liability established the ASA Postoperative Visual Loss Registry to understand the complication better. By 2005, 131 cases were reported to the registry, of which 73% of reported cases involved patients undergoing spine surgeries, and 9% involved cardiac surgery.[60-62] Of 93 patients with postoperative visual loss after prone spine surgery, Lee and colleagues[62] reported that 89% were diagnosed with ION, predominantly posterior, and 11% were diagnosed with central retinal artery occlusion. In patients who were diagnosed with ION, 66% had documented bilateral involvement, of which 42% had eventual improvement in vision, although often clinically insignificant. Compared with central retinal artery occlusion, patients with ION had significantly higher anesthetic duration (9.8 ± 3.1 hours versus 6.5 ± 2.2 hours), estimated blood loss (median 2 L versus 0.75 L), and crystalloid infusion (9.7 ± 4.7 L versus 4.6 ± 1.7 L). Patients with ION also were relatively healthy (64% ASA class I and II), and 73% were men.[62]

In 2006, the ASA issued a practice advisory for perioperative visual loss associated with spine surgery. No definite recommendations were made concerning the issue of induced hypotension, use of vasopressors, or transfusion threshold owing to the multifactorial nature and the low incidence of the injury. Despite a lack of direct evidence, several suggestions were made for "high risk" patients undergoing complex spine surgery, as follows:[63]

Discuss the possibility of staging the spine surgery in consultation with the surgeon.

Avoid excessive increase in intraocular pressure from head position below the body and external compression of the abdomen or chest. Keep the head neutral.

Use colloids along with crystalloids to maintain intravascular volume. Consider placement of a central venous line for monitoring preload.

For patients who are anticipated preoperatively to undergo procedures that are prolonged, have substantial blood loss, or both, consider informing the patients of a small, unpredictable risk of perioperative visual loss.

Additional recommendations include frequent eye checks, which may help prevent central retinal artery occlusion, although the required frequency has not been established, and careful attention to factors related to oxygen delivery, including oxygen tension and maintenance of adequate intravascular volume and cardiac output.[64]

Until the causative factors of this devastating type of injury are better defined, it is likely that debate regarding patient management strategies will continue. With regard to patient positioning, the anesthesiologist should be aware that intraocular pressures are elevated in the dependent eye in the lateral position and both eyes in the prone position in the absence of any external pressure. It is sensible to avoid external eye pressure at all times, to document eye checks frequently, and to limit time in the prone position whenever possible.

Evaluation and Treatment of Perioperative Neuropathies

When a nerve injury becomes apparent postoperatively, it is essential to perform and document a directed physical examination to correlate the extent of sensory or motor deficits with the preoperative examination and any intraoperative events. Whether or not an etiology is suspected, it is prudent to seek neurologic consultation to define the neurogenic basis, localize the site of the lesion, and determine the severity of injury for guiding prognostication.[65,66] With proper diagnosis and management, most injuries resolve; however, months to years may be required.[39]

For motor neuropathy, an electromyogram can be performed to determine the exact location of the injury. An electromyogram involves recording the electrical activity of muscle from a needle electrode inserted within it. If present, abnormalities may point to the affected component within the motor unit, which consists of the anterior horn cell, its axon and neuromuscular junctions, and the muscle fibers that it innervates. Certain findings are suggestive of denervation, including the presence of abnormal spontaneous activity in the resting muscle (fibrillation potentials and positive sharp waves, which result from muscle irritability) and increased insertion activity. Insertion activity increases within a few days of muscle denervation, whereas abnormal spontaneous activity takes 1 to 4 weeks to develop, depending on the distance from the nerve lesion to the muscle. From a medicolegal standpoint, the presence of abnormal spontaneous activity in the acute setting may suggest the nerve injury was present preoperatively. In addition, depending on the pattern of abnormalities, an electromyogram may distinguish between radiculopathies, plexopathies, and neuropathies.

For anesthesiologists, nerve conduction studies may be more useful to evaluate potential peripheral nerve injuries, such as ulnar neuropathy. Nerve conduction studies permit the assessment of motor and sensory nerves. To evaluate motor integrity, the nerve is stimulated supramaximally at two points along its course, and a recording is made of the electrical response of one of the muscles that it innervates. The size of the muscle action potential provides an estimate of the number of motor axons and muscle fibers that are activated by the stimulus. For sensory conduction studies, the nerve fiber is stimulated supramaximally at one point, and the sensory nerve action potential is recorded from another point. The latency of the response can be interpreted as a reflection of the number of functioning sensory axons. Nerve conduction studies are useful for several reasons because they may reveal the presence of a subclinical polyneuropathy that made the individual nerves more susceptible to injury, and help distinguish between axon loss and demyelination, which has significant implications regarding course and overall prognosis.

Most sensory neuropathies are generally transient and require only reassurance to the patient with follow-up, whereas most motor neuropathies include demyelination of peripheral fibers of a nerve trunk (neurapraxia) and generally take 4 to 6 weeks for recovery. Injury to the axon within an intact nerve sheath (axonotmesis) or complete nerve disruption (neurotmesis) can cause severe pain and disability. When reversible, recovery often takes 3 to 12 months. Interim physical therapy is recommended to prevent contractures and muscle atrophy.[65,66]

If a new sensory or motor deficit is found postoperatively, electrophysiologic evaluation by a neurologist within the first week may provide useful information concerning the characteristic and temporal pattern of the injury. Another examination after 4 weeks, when enough time has elapsed for the electrophysiologic changes to evolve, provides more definitive information about the site, nature, and severity of the nerve injury. Regardless, electrophysiologic testing must be interpreted within the clinical content for which it was obtained. No single test can define the etiology of injury.

Anesthesia outside the Operating Room

Anesthesia care providers are increasingly involved with procedures performed for gastrointestinal endoscopy, cardiac catheterization, interventional radiology, neuroradiology, and magnetic resonance imaging/computed tomography, and for office-based procedures (see Chapter 79).[67] Anesthesia care may be requested specifically because a patient is not expected to tolerate the position required for the procedure owing to comorbidities, such as congestive heart failure, pulmonary disease, or morbid obesity. Additionally, positions that are generally safe for patients who are awake may pose serious risks to patients under anesthesia.

Vigilance is particularly important outside the operating room to maintain patient safety because of the less familiar environment, lack of positioning equipment, and variability in staff and nursing training with regard to patient positioning. Many locations do not routinely have safety straps or arm supports available. Diagnostic tables may not lend themselves to established intraoperative solutions to patient positioning challenges. The ability to institute Trendelenburg positioning to augment venous return and cardiac output rapidly is often lacking. In some settings, such as magnetic resonance imaging, the anesthesiologist is not in direct proximity to the patient, and vigilance is more difficult.

Currently, the number of claims in the ASA Closed Claims database for injury during anesthesia care outside the operating room is very small (33 versus 4291 claims for intraoperative surgical anesthesia). Of these claims, 54% were associated with death; 63% were associated with substandard care (predominantly owing to inadequate monitoring); and 58% involved monitored anesthesia care among patients who were ASA class III to V, most of whom were at the extremes of age.[68] In such an environment, where practice patterns have often evolved in the context of nonanesthetized patients, the anesthesiologist is primarily responsible for verifying the safety of each patient's position, and for implementing guidelines for patients under anesthesia.

Summary

The positioning of patients under anesthesia care is a major responsibility requiring great attention to detail and constant vigilance. Rapid positioning and optimal surgical exposure are virtues that may be appreciated instantly, but the potential for lasting harm to patients from improper positioning and physiologic compromise must be kept in mind. Each position has significant physiologic effects on ventilation and circulation. In addition, despite increased awareness, position-related complications, including peripheral nerve injuries, remain a significant source of patient morbidity. Anesthesiologists, surgeons, and nurses must work together when positioning patients to ensure their comfort and safety in addition to the desired surgical exposure. Ideally, the final position should appear natural: a position that the patient would comfortably tolerate if awake and unsedated for the anticipated duration of the procedure.

References

1. Cheney FW: The American Society of Anesthesiologists Closed Claims Project: What have we learned, how has it affected practice, and how will it affect practice in the future. Anesthesiology 91:552-556, 1999.
2. Kroll DA, Caplan RA, Posner K, et al: Nerve injury associated with anesthesia. Anesthesiology 73:202-207, 1990.
3. Cheney FW, Domino KB, Caplan R, Posner KL: Nerve injury associated with anesthesia: A closed claim analysis. Anesthesiology 90:1062-1069, 1999.
4. O'Brien TJ, Ebert TJ: Physiologic changes associated with the supine position. *In* Martin JT, Warner MA (eds): Positioning in Anesthesia and Surgery, 3rd ed. Philadelphia, WB Saunders, 1997.
5. Luecke T, Pelosi P: Positive end-expiratory pressure and cardiac output. Crit Care 9:607-621, 2005.
6. Froese AB: Gravity, the belly, and the diaphragm: You can't ignore physics. Anesthesiology 104:193-196, 2006.
7. Hakim TS, Lisbona R, Dean GW: Gravity-independent inequality in pulmonary blood flow in humans. J Appl Physiol 63:1114-1121, 1987.
8. Burrowes KS, Tawhai MH: Computational predictions of pulmonary blood flow gradients: Gravity versus structure. Respir Physiol Neurobiol 154:515-523, 2006.
9. Galvin I, Drummond GB, Nirmalan M: Distribution of blood flow and ventilation in the lung: Gravity is not the only factor. Br J Anaesth 98:420-428, 2007.
10. Girard TD, Bernard GR: Mechanical ventilation in ARDS: A state-of-the-art review. Chest 131:921-929, 2007.
11. Pelosi P, Croci M, Calappi E, et al: The prone positioning during general anesthesia minimally affects

respiratory mechanics while improving functional residual capacity and increasing oxygen tension. Anesth Analg 80:955-960, 1995.
12. Soro M, García-Pérez ML, Belda FJ, et al: Effects of prone position on alveolar dead space and gas exchange during general anaesthesia in surgery of long duration. Eur J Anaesthesiol 24:431-437, 2007.
13. Pelosi P, Croci M, Calappi E, et al: Prone positioning improves pulmonary function in obese patients during general anesthesia. Anesth Analg 83:578-583, 1996.
14. von Ungern-Sternberg BS, Hammer J, Frei FJ, et al: Prone equals prone? Impact of positioning techniques on respiratory function in anesthetized and paralyzed healthy children. Intensive Care Med 33:1771-1777, 2007.
15. Britt BA, Gordon RA: Peripheral nerve injuries associated with anaesthesia. Can Anaesth Soc J 11:514-536, 1964.
16. ASA Task Force on Prevention of Perioperative Peripheral Neuropathies: Practice advisory for the prevention of perioperative peripheral neuropathies. Anesthesiology 92:1168-1182, 2000.
17. Prielipp RC, Morell RC, Walker FO, et al: Ulnar nerve pressure: Influence of arm position and relationship to somatosensory evoked potentials. Anesthesiology 91:345-354, 1999.
18. Stewart JD, Shantz SH: Perioperative ulnar neuropathies: A medicolegal review. Can J Neurol Sci 30:15-19, 2003.
19. Warner MA: Supine positions. *In* Martin JT, Warner MA (eds): Positioning in Anesthesia and Surgery, 3rd ed. Philadelphia, WB Saunders, 1997.
20. Coppieters MW, Van De Velde M, Stappaerts KH: Positioning in anesthesiology: Toward a better understanding of stretch-induced perioperative neuropathies. Anesthesiology 97:75-81, 2002.
21. Martin JT: Lithotomy. *In* Martin JT, Warner MA (eds): Positioning in Anesthesia and Surgery, 3rd ed. Philadelphia, WB Saunders, 1997.
22. Warner MA, Martin JT, Schroeder DR, et al: Lower-extremity motor neuropathy associated with surgery performed on patients in a lithotomy position. Anesthesiology 81:6-12, 1994.
23. Warner MA, Warner DO, Harper CM, et al: Lower extremity neuropathies associated with lithotomy positions. Anesthesiology 93:938-942, 2000.
24. Warner ME, LaMaster, LM, Thoeming AK, et al: Compartment syndrome in surgical patients. Anesthesiology 94:705-708, 2001.
25. Chase J, Harford F, Pinzur MS, Zussman M: Intraoperative lower extremity compartment pressures in lithotomy-positioned patients. Dis Colon Rectum 43:678-680, 2000.
26. Wassenaar EB, van den Brand JG, van der Werken C: Compartment syndrome of the lower leg after surgery in the modified lithotomy position: Report of seven cases. Dis Colon Rectum 49:1449-1453, 2006.
27. Turnbull D, Farid A, Hutchinson S, et al: Calf compartment pressures in the Lloyd-Davies position: A cause for concern? Anaesthesia 57:905-908, 2002.
28. Dunn PF: Physiology of the lateral decubitus position and one-lung ventilation. Int Anesthesiol Clin 38:25-53, 2000.
29. Choi YS, Bang SO, Shim JK, et al: Effects of head-down tilt on intrapulmonary shunt fraction and oxygenation during one-lung ventilation in the lateral decubitus position. J Thorac Cardiovasc Surg 134:613-618, 2007.
30. Douglas WW, Rehder K, Beynen FM, et al: Improved oxygenation in patients with acute respiratory failure: The prone position. Am Rev Respir Dis 115:559-566, 1977.
31. Lumb AB, Nunn JF: Respiratory function and ribcage contribution to ventilation in body positions commonly used during anesthesia. Anesth Analg 73:422-426, 1991.
32. Martin JT: The ventral decubitus (prone) positions. *In* Martin JT, Warner MA (eds): Positioning in Anesthesia and Surgery, 3rd ed. Philadelphia, WB Saunders, 1997.
33. Black S, Ockert DB, Oliver WC Jr, Cucchiara RF: Outcome following posterior fossa craniectomy in patients in the sitting or horizontal positions. Anesthesiology 69:49-56, 1988.
34. Newberg Milde L: The head-elevated positions. *In* Martin JT, Warner MA (eds): Positioning in Anesthesia and Surgery, 3rd ed. Philadelphia, WB Saunders, 1997.
35. Warner MA: Positioning of the head and neck. *In* Martin JT, Warner MA (eds): Positioning in Anesthesia and Surgery, 3rd ed. Philadelphia, WB Saunders, 1997.
36. Mammoto T, Hayashi Y, Ohnishi Y, Kuro M: Incidence of venous and paradoxical air embolism in neurosurgical patients in the sitting position: Detection by transesophageal echocardiography. Acta Anaesthesiol Scand 42:643-647, 1998.
37. Papadopoulos G, Kuhly P, Brock M, et al: Venous and paradoxical air embolism in the sitting position: A prospective study with transoesophageal echocardiography. Acta Neurochir 126:140-143, 1994.
38. Blitt CD, Kaufer-Bratt C, Ashby J, Caillet JR: QA program reveals safety issues, promotes development of guidelines. Anesthesia Patient Safety Found Newsl 9:17, 1994.
39. Winfree CJ, Kline DG: Intraoperative positioning nerve injuries. Surg Neurol 63:5-18, 2005.
40. Lee LA, Posner KL, Domino KB, et al: Injuries associated with regional anesthesia in the 1980s and 1990s: A closed claim analysis. Anesthesiology 101:143-152, 2004.
41. Fitzgibbon DR, Posner KL, Domino KB, et al: Chronic pain management. American Society of Anesthesiologists Closed Claims Project. Anesthesiology 100:98-105, 2004.
42. Kamel IR, Drum ET, Koch SA, et al: The use of somatosensory evoked potentials to determine the relationship between patient positioning and impending upper extremity nerve injury during spine surgery: A retrospective analysis. Anesth Analg 102:1538-1542, 2006.
43. Warner MA, Warner DO, Matsumoto JY, et al: Ulnar neuropathy in surgical patients. Anesthesiology 90:54-59, 1999.
44. Warner MA, Warner ME, Martin JT: Ulnar neuropathy: Incidence, outcome, and risk factors in sedated or anesthetized patients. Anesthesiology 81:1332-1340, 1994.
45. Warner MA, Warner DO, Harper CM, et al: Ulnar neuropathy in medical patients. Anesthesiology 92:614-615, 2000.
46. Contreras MG, Warner MA, Charboneau WJ, Cahill DR: Anatomy of the ulnar nerve at the elbow: Potential relationship of acute ulnar neuropathy to gender differences. Clin Anat 11:372-378, 1998.
47. Morell RC, Prielipp RC, Harwood TN, et al: Men are more susceptible than women to direct pressure on unmyelinated ulnar nerve fibers. Anesth Analg 97:1183-1188, 2003.
48. Hanson MR, Breuer AC, Furlan AJ, et al: Mechanism and frequency of brachial plexus injury in open-heart surgery: A prospective analysis. Ann Thorac Surg 36:675-679, 1983.
49. Cooper DE, Jenkins RS, Bready L, Rockwood CA Jr: The prevention of injuries to the brachial plexus secondary to malposition of the patient during surgery. Clin Orthop 228:33, 1988.
50. Liau DW: Injuries and liability related to peripheral catheters: A closed claim analysis. ASA Newsletter 70:11-13, 2006.
51. Roth S, Thisted RA, Erickson JP, et al: Eye injuries after nonocular surgery: A study of 60,965 anesthetics from 1988 to 1992. Anesthesiology 85:1020-1027, 1996.
52. Warner ME, Fronapfel PJ, Hebl JR, et al: Perioperative visual changes. Anesthesiology 96:855-859, 2002.
53. Warner ME, Warner MA, Garrity JA, et al: The frequency of perioperative vision loss. Anesth Analg 93:1417-1421, 2001.
54. Kalyani SD, Miller NR, Dong LM, et al: Incidence of and risk factors for perioperative optic neuropathy after cardiac surgery. Ann Thorac Surg 78:34-37, 2004.
55. Nuttall GA, Garrity JA, Dearnani JA, et al: Risk factors for ischemic optic neuropathy after cardiopulmonary bypass: A matched case/control study. Anesth Analg 93:1410-1416, 2001.
56. Roth S, Barach P: Postoperative visual loss: Still no answers-yet. Anesthesiology 95:575-577, 2001.
57. Hunt K, Bajekal R, Calder I, et al: Changes in intraocular pressure in anesthetized prone patients. J Neurosurg Anesthesiol 16:287-290, 2004.
58. Cheng MA, Todorov A, Tempelhoff R, et al: The effect of prone positioning on intraocular pressure in anesthetized patients. Anesthesiology 95:1351-1355, 2001.
59. Hwang JW, Jeon YT, Kim JH, et al: The effect of the lateral decubitus position on the intraocular pressure in anesthetized patients undergoing lung surgery. Acta Anaesthesiol Scand 50:988-992, 2006.
60. Lee LA: ASA Postoperative Visual Loss Registry. Preliminary analysis of factors associated with spine operations. ASA Newsletter 67:7-8, 2003.
61. Ho V, Newman NJ, Song S, et al: Ischemic optic neuropathy following spine surgery. J Neurosurg Anesthesiol 17:38-44, 2005.
62. Lee LA, Roth S, Posner L, et al: The American Society of Anesthesiologists Postoperative Visual Loss Registry. Analysis of 93 spine cases with postoperative visual loss. Anesthesiology 105:652-659, 2006.
63. Practice advisory for perioperative visual loss associated with spine surgery: A report by the American Society of Anesthesiologists Task Force on Perioperative Blindness. Anesthesiology 104:1319-1328, 2006.
64. Weiskopf RB, Feiner J, Lieberman J, Hu SS: Visual loss after spinal surgery. Anesthesiology 106:1250-1251, 2007.
65. Aminoff MJ: Electrophysiologic testing for the diagnosis of peripheral nerve injuries. Anesthesiology 100:1298-1303, 2004.
66. Dylewsky W, McAlpine FS: Peripheral nervous system. *In* Martin JT, Warner MA (eds): Positioning in Anesthesia and Surgery, 3rd ed. Philadelphia, WB Saunders, 1997.
67. Lalwani K: Demographics and trends in nonoperating-room anesthesia. Curr Opin Anaesthesiol 19:430-435, 2006.
68. Robbertze R, Posner KL, Domino KB. Closed claims review of anesthesia for procedures outside the operating room. Curr Opin Anaesthesiol 19:436-442, 2006.

Jie Zhou, Paul D. Allen, Isaac N. Pessah, and Mohamed Naguib

37 Neuromuscular Disorders and Malignant Hyperthermia

Key Points

1. Dystrophin, along with dystrophin-associated glycoproteins, is involved in sarcolemmal stability. Its defects are responsible for Duchenne's muscular dystrophy (DMD) and Becker's muscular dystrophy (BMD).
2. Whereas the risk for a malignant hyperthermia (MH) mutation in DMD/BMD patients is similar to that in the general population, the incidence of MH-like anesthetic events has been reported to be 0.002 with DMD and 0.00036 with BMD.
3. Succinylcholine is contraindicated in DMD/BMD patients because of the risk of rhabdomyolysis and hyperkalemia as a result of their unstable sarcolemmal membrane.
4. The majority of complications in patients with myotonic dystrophy (MD) were found to be pulmonary related. Pulmonary complications of MD are the result of hypotonia, chronic aspiration, and central and peripheral hypoventilation.
5. Although patients with sodium channel pathology have often been considered to be susceptible to MH, there is no increased risk for MH in these patients.
6. MH is an anesthetic-related disorder of increased skeletal muscle metabolism. It is an inherited condition and it occurs in swine and humans.
7. Skeletal muscle accounts for approximately 40% of body weight; its increased metabolism therefore has a profound effect on whole-body metabolism.
8. Signs of MH, including tachycardia, increased expired CO_2, muscle rigidity, and increased temperature, are related to the increased metabolism.
9. The abnormal function of the ryanodine receptor of skeletal muscle in MH causes barely controlled concentration of calcium within the cell when it is not exposed to triggering agents.
10. The added loss of control of intracellular calcium on exposure to triggering agents or heat stress leads to marked metabolic stimulation within the cell to provide extra adenosine triphosphate to drive the calcium pumps that restore calcium to its reservoirs (e.g., sarcoplasmic reticulum, mitochondria, extracellular fluid).
11. Dantrolene markedly attenuates myoplasmic Ca^{2+} concentrations and thereby restores metabolism to normal, with reversal of the signs of metabolic stimulation.
12. MH is inherited; one mutation accounts for all porcine MH, whereas more than 130 mutations account for human MH.
13. Evaluation of persons susceptible to MH includes contracture of a skeletal muscle biopsy specimen with halothane and caffeine and evaluation of DNA to identify mutations. Only DNA testing is needed to evaluate swine MH.
14. Future MH goals include advancement of genetic evaluations in North American and European medical programs and stronger finances to support genetic studies, identification of the mode of action of dantrolene, determination of the immediate cause of triggering of MH, and the development of effective, nondestructive tests for MH susceptibility.

Neuromuscular disorders, although rarely encountered in routine anesthetic practice, are a group of disorders that challenges both perioperative management and intensive care.

In this chapter, diseases that affect the normal function of peripheral nerves, the neuromuscular junction, and muscles are described. Although such diseases are thought to be rare, the number of patients that a clinician may encounter is increasing annually because of better medical care, increasing longevity, and possibly other yet unidentified factors. As a rule, neuromuscular disorders have significant potential to interact with an improper anesthetic plan, and all affected patients require special perioperative attention for anesthetic management. In this area, the armamentarium of invasive and noninvasive diagnostic tools is being developed, especially in genetics. Also covered in this chapter is malignant hyperthermia (MH). This fulminant syndrome is elicited by the administration of triggering anesthetic agents, such as a volatile anesthetic or a depolarizing neuromuscular blocking agent. MH has been and continues to be a life-threatening complication of anesthesia if the diagnosis is not made promptly and treatment is not begun in a timely fashion. Unlike other disorders described in this chapter, MH has virtually no characteristic phenotype before exposure to the triggering agent and is truly an example of the interaction of genes and environment.

Multiple Sclerosis

Multiple sclerosis (MS) is an autoimmune disorder characterized by T-cell–mediated autoantibodies against myelin and a subsequent inflammatory response within the central nervous system (CNS: brain and spinal cord). Thus, MS is a disorder of the myelinated part of the axon that leads to secondary nerve conduction failure. The disease affects mainly women, primarily between 20 and 40 or 45 and 60 years of age. Although the etiology is unknown, it has been speculated that MS is caused by environmental factors combined with a genetic predisposition. Naturally, researchers have focused on identifying key events and the genetic origin of the disorder to provide diagnostic and possibly also therapeutic tools for the management of MS patients.

Patients with MS frequently report paresthesias, muscle weakness, and sensory disturbances. Typically, there is a localized or, late in the course of disease, generalized muscle weakness with the legs affected more than the arms. In severe cases, respiration may be involved with the development of hypoxemia. Diplopia and other cranial nerve–dependent impairments are early and frequent signs, along with sensory abnormalities and sometimes disturbed bowel and bladder function. As a rule, symptoms are closely related to the site affected within the CNS, and the amount of symptoms is related to the extent of sclerosing CNS plaque. Notably, MS can be associated with impaired autonomic function, which may lead to adverse reactions to sympathomimetic drugs.[1]

Diagnosis of MS is currently based on a combination of clinical and laboratory tests, including cerebrospinal fluid (CSF) antibody analysis and radiology (detection of CNS plaque by magnetic resonance imaging). Medication consists of various combinations of immunosuppression modalities.

Anesthetic Considerations. It has been speculated that general anesthesia and surgery may increase the risk for aggravation of MS.[2] At present, there is no general consensus on this matter, and patients should therefore be informed of the potential for aggravated symptoms in the postoperative period. In general, preoperative chronic immunosuppressive medication should be continued during the perioperative period. Patients with MS are sensitive to physical (pain, fever, infection) and emotional stress, which makes it more likely that symptoms will be intensified in the perioperative period. Great care must be exercised to minimize changes in body temperature, fluid homeostasis, and central hemodynamics (preload, afterload) and to maintain respiration. Although intravenous induction agents and volatile anesthetics have been used safely, it is wise to avoid administering depolarizing neuromuscular blocking drugs to MS patients. MS-induced denervation or misuse myopathy may lead to a risk for succinylcholine-induced hyperkalemia, which can result in fatal cardiac arrhythmias (see also Chapter 29). Use of nondepolarizing neuromuscular blockers appears to be safe. Regional anesthesia, including epidural application of low concentrations of local anesthetics, has been used in MS patients. Spinal anesthesia exacerbates symptoms in MS and is therefore not recommended for MS patients by most authorities. Notably, postpartum worsening of MS symptoms is noted in 20% of females (also see Chapter 69). The need for postoperative care is dependent on the preoperative symptoms, type of surgery, and status of the patient at the end of the surgical procedure. In this context, MS patients with severe weakness and respiratory distress, including pharyngeal dysfunction, may need extended postoperative care, such as noninvasive respiratory support and intense physiotherapy, to avoid further impairment of their pulmonary function.

Motor Neuron Disorders

Motor neuron disorders involve either the upper or the lower motor neurons of the cerebral cortex, brainstem, and spinal cord. Some forms are mixed, whereas others have predominately upper or lower motor neuron involvement. Amyotrophic lateral sclerosis (ALS) is the most common disease within this group and involves both upper and lower motor neurons. Other examples of motor neuron disease are Kennedy's disease (spinobulbar muscular atrophy), Friedreich's ataxia (mixed upper and lower motor neurons), and spinal muscular atrophy (lower motor neurons).

ALS (Lou Gehrig's disease) is characterized by progressive and variable loss of motor neurons within the cerebral cortex, medullary nuclei of cranial nerves, and nuclei of the ventral horn in the spinal cord. Degenerative loss of these neurons leads to progressive muscle weakness, muscle atrophy, and loss of neuronal mass in these locations. Sensory functions, including intellectual capacity and cognition, as well as bowel and bladder function, are not usually affected in ALS.

ALS has an incidence of about 2 in 100,000, and onset of the disease usually takes place around 40 to 50 years of age, with males more often affected than females. Most cases are sporadic, but rare familial forms (autosomal dominant and recessive forms) do exist. The underlying mechanism or mechanisms for this selective and progressive motor neuronal death are thus far unclear, but it has recently been suggested that superoxide dismutase mutations may have a key role in the increased formation of free radicals seen in subsets of patients. The diagnosis is made by electrophysiology (electromyography [EMG] and electroneurography) and by neurologic examination, which demonstrates early spastic weakness of the upper and lower extremities, typical subcutaneous muscle fasciculations, and bulbar involvement affecting pharyngeal function, speech, and the facial muscles. No curative treatment is currently available, and patients are therefore treated symptomatically.

Anesthetic Considerations. Bulbar involvement in combination with respiratory muscle weakness leads to a risk for aspiration and pulmonary complications. Notably, these patients may have increased sensitivity to the respiratory depressant effects of sedatives and hypnotics. There are reports of sympathetic hyperreactivity and autonomic failure.[3] Succinylcholine should be avoided because of the risk for hyperkalemia as a result of denervation and immobilization. Nondepolarizing neuromuscular blocking agents may cause prolonged and pronounced neuromuscular blockade and hence should be used with great caution.[4] General anesthesia combined with epidural anesthesia has been used without complications.

Guillain-Barré Syndrome

Guillain-Barré syndrome (GBS) is an acute inflammatory polyneuritis caused by an immunologic reaction. Although the etiology is unknown, in many cases a timely association with a viral (influenza-like) or bacterial infection or even lymphomatous disease can be demonstrated.[5] Symmetric peripheral flaccid muscle weakness and sensory loss develop. The lower extremities are affected first, after which the disease progresses to the upper extremities and cranial nerve–innervated muscles in some cases. Importantly, patients may also have autonomic involvement that could lead to sudden fatal cardiac and circulatory collapse. The diagnosis is made after careful neurologic examination, clinical electrophysiology, and CSF analysis. CSF analysis may show a typical increase in CSF protein in combination with a normal cell count, which is a classic sign of the disease. Treatment focuses on respiratory support, nutritional support, and early initiation of plasmapheresis.

Anesthetic Considerations. Succinylcholine should not be used because of the risk of hyperkalemia. Nondepolarizing muscle relaxants are not contraindicated but should be avoided as a result of the increased sensitivity and risk for prolonged muscle weakness in the postoperative period. The risk for autonomic dysfunction, respiratory failure, and aspiration may require assisted or mechanical ventilation, even in the postoperative period. Great care should be taken to maintain circulatory stability, including adequate cardiac preload and afterload. Careful hemodynamic monitoring is therefore essential in these patients. General anesthesia can be used; however, the combination of general anesthesia and epidural anesthesia is more controversial.[6] Although regional anesthesia is not contraindicated, there are reports of an association between GBS and epidural anesthesia.[7]

Hereditary Motor-Sensory Neuropathies, including Charcot-Marie-Tooth Disease

Hereditary motor-sensory neuropathies include a spectrum of peripheral neurologic disorders, among which Charcot-Marie-Tooth (CMT) disease is often listed. They are caused by a specific mutation in one of several myelin genes that results in defects in myelin structure, maintenance, and formation. Hereditary motor-sensory neuropathies have been classified into seven types and multiple subtypes according to the age at onset, mode of inheritance, predominately involved muscle groups, and genotypes.[8,9] CMT types 1 and 2 are the most common hereditary peripheral neuropathies, with an estimated prevalence of 40 per 100,000.[9] Patients with CMT disease typically experience slow and progressive distal muscle weakness and wasting. Damage to sensory axons may also lead to sensory loss resulting in frequent tripping and falls. Neuropathic pain may develop in some patients. CMT patients usually have normal life expectancy. CMT type 3, also known as Dejerine-Sottas disease, is a very severe condition with an early onset of hypotonia during infancy. Nerve conduction velocity is typically significantly reduced to less than 10 msec.[9] The genetic inheritance pattern for CMT disease is heterogeneous.

Anesthetic Considerations. The anesthesia experience in patients with CMT disease is limited because of the small number of cases. Major considerations include the use of hypnotic agents, muscle relaxants, volatile agents, and neuraxial techniques. CMT type 1 patients have been reported to have significantly increased sensitivity to thiopental at induction that correlates with the severity of both motor and sensory defects. However, total intravenous anesthesia (TIVA) has been performed successfully in a number of cases without any reported problems.[10-12]

Because of the reduced number of acetylcholine receptors, sensitivity to nondepolarizing muscle relaxants is elevated and the response to succinylcholine is also reduced.[13] Although succinylcholine has been used without adverse effect,[14,15] the risk of an exaggerated hyperkalemic response may be sufficient to preclude it from being used in patients with suspected muscular denervation.[15] Prolonged neuromuscular blockade with vecuronium has been reported.[16] As a result of the large variety of disabilities in this patient group, careful baseline assessment of neuromuscular status should be conducted before the use of nondepolarizing neuromuscular relaxants. Normal response to atracurium and mivacurium has been demonstrated.[17,18] Both TIVA and volatile anesthetics have been used safely in CMT patients in a series of cases.[14] Neuraxial techniques for obstetric procedures have been reported to generally be successful in CMT patients.[19-22] However, the use of regional anesthesia can be controversial given that the possible complications may exacerbate the neurologic symptoms.[23] Similar medicolegal concerns may apply to the surgical and anesthesia positioning of CMT patients because of the sensory deficits and limb deformities.

Duchenne's Muscular Dystrophy and Becker's Muscular Dystrophy

Duchenne's muscular dystrophy (DMD) is the most common and severe type of muscular dystrophy, with an incidence of 1 per 3500 live male births[24] and a total male prevalence of about 50 to 60×10^{-6}.[25] Becker's muscular dystrophy (BMD) is relatively rare and has an incidence of about 1 in 18,000 live male births and a prevalence of 23.8×10^{-6}.[25] Both DMD and BMD are X-linked recessive diseases. The defect is located on the short arm of the X chromosome at the Xp21 region, which contains the gene for the large protein Dp427, also known as dystrophin. The dystrophin gene is 2500 kilobases long with more than 70 exons.[25] Dystrophin is distributed not only in skeletal, cardiac, and smooth muscle but also in the brain.[26] Because of the large size of the dystrophin gene, spontaneous new mutations are common and account for a third of new cases.[27]

The most common form of mutation is a deletion within the gene (65% to 70% of cases of DMD and >80% of BMD). Duplication and point mutations are responsible for the rest. It

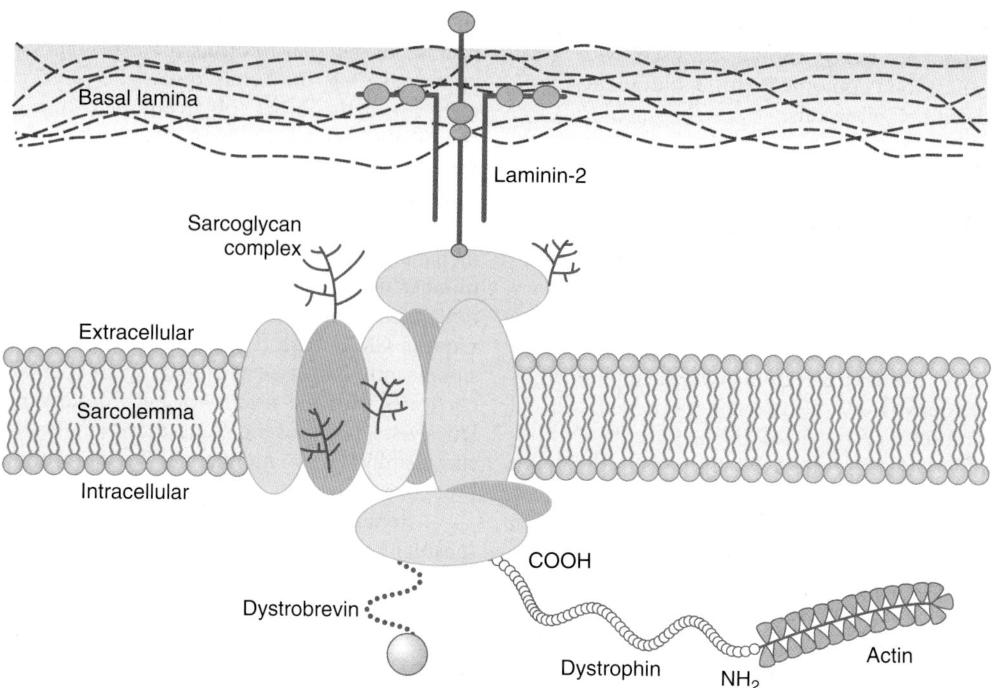

Figure 37-1 Diagram of the cell-surface and cytoskeleton protein complex.

also appears that there are "hot spots" within the first 20 exons and in the central region of the gene (exons 45 to 55) where deletion and duplication are likely to occur.[25] Female cases of DMD have been reported with the 45,X and 46,XX karyotypes. The disease mechanism for the female 46,XX karyotype was thought to be preferential loss of the paternal X chromosome by postzygotic nondisjunction and manifestation of the DMD gene from the maternal X chromosome in muscle cells.[28] BMD is usually milder in severity than DMD because disruption of the translation process occurs in the relatively distal part of the gene, which leads to a reduced amount of truncated dystrophin protein.[25,29]

Dystrophin, along with dystrophin-associated glycoproteins (DAGs), is involved in sarcolemmal stability. Dystrophin is responsible for maintenance of muscle membrane integrity despite the fact that it accounts for only approximately 0.002% of the protein in striated muscle.[30] Dystrophin aggregates and links to actin (at its N terminus) and the DAG complex (at its C terminus) to form a stable structure that interacts with laminin in the extracellular matrix (Fig. 37-1). Lack or dysfunction of dystrophin leads to cellular and membrane instability, with progressive leakage of intracellular components and elevation of creatine phosphokinase (CPK) levels. Eventually, damaged muscle cell units are invaded by macrophages and destroyed. Current study suggests that cytotoxic T cells are probably the culprit. Consequently, clinical pseudohypertrophy of the muscle occurs when the dead muscle shells are replaced by fibrofatty infiltrates. Loss of muscle units accounts for the weakness and contracture.[26]

Both DMD and BMD are characterized by progressive weakness and wasting of predominantly the proximal musculature. Pseudohypertrophy of the calves and other muscle groups is common. As the more severe of the two diseases, DMD tends to be symptomatic early in life. Seventy-four percent of children with DMD were found to manifest the disease by 4 years of age.[24] DMD patients do not usually begin to walk until they are about 18 month of age or later. The initial clinical findings include a waddling gait, frequent falling, and difficulty climbing stairs because of proximal muscle weakness in the pelvic girdle. The classic Gower maneuver describes rising from a sitting to a standing position with the help of both arms. Patients may also show weakness in the shoulder girdle and trunk erectors that leads to thoracolumbar scoliosis. The earlier the onset of disease, the more rapid the disease course. In most cases, children with DMD are unable to walk by the age of 9 to 11. Proximal deep tendon reflexes in the upper extremities and patella may also disappear despite the lack of denervation.[29] Nevertheless, the tendo Achillis reflex remains intact even in later stages of the disease. Sixty percent of patients will have pseudohypertrophy of the calves, and 30% will have macroglossia. Some may also suffer from pain in the calves with activity. The intellectual impairment that can be associated with the disease was thought to be related to limitation of educational opportunities. However, with equalization of educational opportunities, psychometric studies have revealed a significantly lower average intelligence quotient in DMD patients than in healthy groups.[31] This implies a possible effect of dysfunctional dystrophin in the brain on learning. Death in patients with DMD is commonly due to cardiopulmonary compromise in their 30s.[24] BMD is a mild form of DMD. The mutation that causes BMD produces dystrophin that retains partial function. The onset of symptoms occurs in the second or third decade of life. As a result, the life span of BMD patients can reach the early 40s. Pneumonia is the most common cause of death (Fig. 37-2).[29]

The heart is also affected to various degrees, depending on the stage of the disease and the type of mutation. Cardiac degeneration is due to replacement of myocardium by connective tissue or fat, which leads to dilated cardiomyopathy.[32] Cardiac involvement starts early in the course of the disease, although clinical

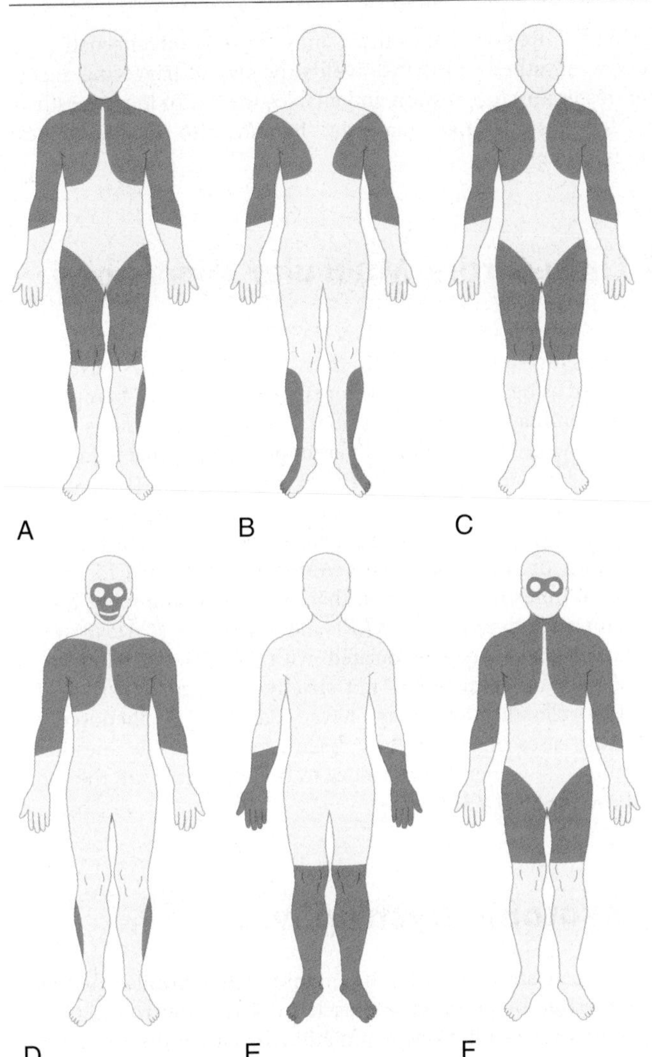

Figure 37-2 Distribution of predominant muscle weakness in different types of dystrophy: **A,** Duchenne type and Becker type; **B,** Emery-Dreifuss; **C,** limb girdle; **D,** facioscapulohumeral; **E,** distal; and **F,** oculopharyngeal. *(Redrawn from Emery AE: The muscular dystrophies. BMJ 317:991-995, 1998.)*

signs are not usually obvious in the early stage. No correlation has been established between the severity of cardiac disease and the severity of skeletal disease. Studies at necropsy have shown that the cardiomyopathy in DMD involves the posterobasal and contiguous lateral left ventricular walls as initial and primary sites of myocardial dystrophy in the absence of small vessel coronary artery disease in these areas.[33] Typical initial manifestations on the electrocardiogram (ECG) in DMD and BMD are sinus tachycardia, tall R waves in the right precordial leads, prominent left precordial Q waves, increased QT dispersion, and inverted T waves from scarring of the posterobasal portion of the left ventricle. Initially, echocardiography is normal or shows regional wall motion abnormalities in areas of fibrosis. With the spreading of fibrosis, left ventricular dysfunction can be seen and ventricular arrhythmias frequently occur as well. In the final stages of the disease, systolic dysfunction may lead to heart failure and sudden death. Subclinical or clinical cardiac involvement is present in about 90% of DMD/BMD patients, but it is the cause of death in only 20% of DMD and 50% of BMD patients. Angiotensin-converting enzyme inhibitors are recommended in early stages of the disease, and β-blockers may be an additional option if indicated.[32]

Pulmonary insufficiency is a leading cause of morbidity and mortality in DMD.[34] Usually, expiratory muscle function is affected first because of the early onset of abdominal muscle weakness. By contrast, inspiratory muscle function is relatively preserved in the first decade, implying sparing of the diaphragm.[35] Vital capacity (VC) increases in the first decade because of overall body growth, plateaus in early adolescence, and then declines dramatically as the diaphragmatic weakness progresses.[35] Other measured lung volumes such as inspiratory reserve volume and total lung capacity (TLC) follow the same pattern. A disproportionate loss of VC and TLC relative to the respiratory muscle dysfunction results in part from additional factors, such as altered chest wall and lung mechanics, modifications in the distribution of surfactant, micro-atelectasis, and local fibrosis secondary to recurrent pneumonia.[35] Scoliosis further impairs pulmonary function. On average, for each 10 degrees of thoracic scoliosis curvature, forced vital capacity (FVC) decreases by 4%.[30] In 90% of patients, a curvature of greater than 20 degrees develops 3 to 4 years after they are wheelchair bound. Respiratory failure inevitably occurs in the second decade of life and is the most common cause of death.[36]

Diagnosis and Differential Diagnosis. Chronic elevation of the serum CPK level is a general indication of muscle disease. Three serum tests showing elevated CPK levels obtained 1 month apart is diagnostic of muscular dystrophy. CPK represents leakage of enzyme from muscle cells and does not correlate with severity of the disease. CPK could reach 50 to 300 times the normal value in early stages of the disease. The level tends to decrease with the loss of muscle mass. Elevation of the MB fraction of creatine kinase (CK) precludes its use as a marker for cardiac injury.[29] EMG can be supportive of the diagnosis; however, it can be very difficult to perform on children. Muscle biopsy, followed by immunostaining or Western blot analysis for dystrophin, is recommended for diagnostic testing. Multiple polymerase chain reaction is also useful in detecting more than 98% of the existing deletions.[26] The result is usually available within 24 hours, which may render muscle biopsy, the old "gold standard," obsolete.

Anesthetic Considerations. Patients with DMD and BMD may require anesthesia for muscle biopsy, correction of scoliosis, release of contractures, and exploratory laparotomy for ileus,[29] as well as for dental[37] and obstetric[38] procedures. As the natural course of the disease progresses, the risk of surgery increases concomitant with the increased comorbid conditions associated with the later phase of the disease. However, perioperative complications are not proportional to the severity of the disease. They occur even in mildly affected patients. Consequently, patients should undergo careful preoperative consultation and evaluation.

Fifty percent to 70% of patients with muscular dystrophy demonstrate some cardiac abnormality, although it is clinically significant in only 10%.[29] Preoperative cardiology assessment with an ECG and echocardiography is essential. Continuous cardiac Holter monitoring is necessary if an arrhythmia is captured on the ECG or the patient describes symptoms that can be related to cardiac arrhythmias. Echocardiography will demonstrate mitral valve prolapse in 10% to 25% of patients. It may also show posterobasilar hypokinesis in a thin-walled ventricle and a slow relaxation phase with normal contraction characterizing the cardiomyopathy seen in DMD.[29] However, echocardiography may not always reflect the ability of the diseased myocardium to respond to perioperative stress. Stress echocardiography using angiotensin to detect latent heart failure and identify inducible contraction abnormalities has been advocated.[39]

An estimated 30% of deaths in individuals with DMD are due to respiratory causes.[40] Therefore, careful preoperative pulmonary assessment is important. Webster demonstrated that the manual muscle strength test has a strong statistical correlation with all of the timed functional tests. Peak expiratory flow was not only easy to perform but also correlated statistically with all timed functional tests.[41] The correlation was not significant for VC or forced expiratory volume in 1 second (FEV_1).

Intraoperatively, in terms of airway management, patients with DMD and BMD may have decreased laryngeal reflexes and prolonged gastric emptying time, which increases the risk for aspiration.[42] Decreased ability to cough up the accumulation of oral secretions predisposes muscular dystrophy patients to postoperative respiratory tract infections.[29] Masseter spasm is also a possible complication during induction of anesthesia in these patients.[43] Preparedness for a difficult airway is necessary, especially in patients with potential airway problems.

Postoperatively, DMD patients are at an increased risk for respiratory compromise.[44] Retrospective reviews have indicated that the incidence of prolonged postoperative ventilation (>36 hours) was greatest in DMD patients who had a preoperative FVC of less than 40% of the predicted value.[45,46] Preoperative pulmonary function studies are valuable in determining the postoperative course. Patients with a VC of greater than 30% of the predicted value can usually be extubated immediately after surgery.[29] Sleep apnea may also compound the condition and contribute to the development of pulmonary hypertension. Continuous positive airway pressure and bilevel positive airway pressure have been demonstrated to be effective in the management of postoperative respiratory depression. Delayed pulmonary insufficiency may occur up to 36 hours postoperatively despite the apparent recovery of skeletal muscle strength.[47]

Reports have suggested a relationship between DMD/BMD and MH, but this association is not based on good rational grounds. Whereas the risk for an MH mutation in DMD/BMD patients is similar to that of the general population, the incidence of MH-like anesthetic events has been reported to be 0.002 with DMD and 0.00036 with BMD.[48] Unexplained cardiac arrest[43,49] and acute heart failure[50] have been reported in DMD/BMD patients. Succinylcholine is contraindicated in these patients because of the potential for rhabdomyolysis and hyperkalemia as a result of their unstable sarcolemmal membrane. Succinylcholine-induced hyperkalemia during acute rhabdomyolysis is more likely to result in cardiac arrest and unsuccessful resuscitation than is the potassium efflux resulting from upregulation of acetylcholine receptors in burn patients.[47] The use of nondepolarizing muscle relaxants is usually accompanied by an increase in both maximal effect and duration of action.[51] Narcotics can be used, but small incremental dosing and short-acting medications are recommended given the respiratory depression associated with these medications. Because of reports of inadvertent reactions to volatile anesthetics,[29] TIVA has become more popular.[52] However, consideration needs to be given to the myocardial status of the patient when propofol or barbiturates are used because they may lead to profound hypotension and reduced organ perfusion.[29,53] Regional anesthesia may be a good alternative to general anesthesia in that it avoids the risk of triggering agents and respiratory depression and enables the use of local anesthetics for postoperative analgesia. It may also facilitate chest physiotherapy.[54]

Limb-Girdle Muscular Dystrophy

Limb-girdle muscular dystrophy (LGMD) is a group of disorders with heterogeneous causes. To date, at least 18 genes have been identified as being responsible for this disease, with 7 being autosomal dominant and 11 autosomal recessive.[55] Mutations within the same gene may result in different phenotypes that sometimes are not consistent with LGMD. Proximal muscle (shoulder or pelvic) girdle weakness is the characteristic feature of this group of diseases. Given the marked genetic heterogeneity, clinical manifestations of the disease vary. Autosomal recessive forms are about 10 times more common than autosomal dominant forms. Fukutin-related protein (*FKRP*) and calpain 3 (*CAPN3*) gene mutations have been associated with LGMD. In addition, a number of other disorders not strictly included under LGMD in this classification may have LGMD-like phenotypes.[55] Sporadic cases of LGMD have been reported in the anesthesia literature.[56-58] General approaches to these patients are the same as those for DMD/BMD.

Myotonic Dystrophy

Myotonic dystrophy (MD) is an inherited muscular disorder characterized by progressive muscle weakness and wasting. Two types of MD result from a mutation in either the dystrophia myotonica–protein kinase (*DMPK*) gene, located on chromosome 19q13.3 (MD1, also known as Steinert's disease), or the CysCysHisCys (CCHC)-type zinc finger, nucleic acid binding protein (*CNBP*) gene, located on chromosome 3q21 (MD2).[59] The incidence of MD is 1 in 8000. MD1 is by far the most common of the two types and accounts for about 98% of all cases. MD1 is caused by expansion of a CTG trinucleotide repeat in the *DMPK* gene and is inherited in an autosomal dominant manner.[60] Typical signs and symptoms include muscle weakness and wasting (most prominent in the cranial and distal limb musculature), periodic myotonia, progressive myopathy, insulin resistance, defects in cardiac conduction, neuropsychiatric impairment, cataracts, testicular atrophy, and frontal balding in males. The typical cranial muscle weakness and wasting are manifested not only in the facial, temporalis, masseter, and sternocleidomastoid muscles but also in the vocal cord apparatus. Mitral valve prolapse is found in 20% of patients.[47] The severity of the disease is related to the number of extra trinucleotide repeats.[61] MD1 patients may also have mildly elevated CK levels. Myotonic discharges can be identified on EMG, as well as an inability to relax from a handgrip. During pregnancy, the symptoms may be exacerbated. Uterine atony and retained placenta may also complicate vaginal delivery. First-degree atrioventricular heart block is a common finding on the ECG before the onset of symptoms.[47]

MD2 is also called proximal myotonic myopathy. Intron 1 of the *CNBP* gene contains a complex repeat motif,

(TG)n(TCTG)n(CCTG)n, and expansion of the CCTG repeat was determined as the cause of MD2. Patients with MD2 suffer from myotonia (90% of those affected), muscle dysfunction (82% weakness, pain, and stiffness), and less commonly, cardiac conduction defects, iridescent posterior subcapsular cataracts, insulin-insensitive type 2 diabetes mellitus, and testicular failure.[62]

Anesthetic Considerations. General considerations for MD are similar to those for other muscular dystrophies. Mathieu and coworkers conducted a retrospective study on the anesthetic and surgical complications of MD. The majority of complications were found to be pulmonary related and significantly more frequent in patients undergoing upper abdominal operations and those with severe disability, as assessed by the presence of proximal limb weakness.[63] The pulmonary complications of MD are the result of hypotonia, chronic aspiration, and central and peripheral hypoventilation.[29] Smooth muscle atrophy, which leads to poor gastric motility, when coupled with a diminished cough reflex, promotes aspiration. Succinylcholine will produce contractions lasting for several minutes, thus making intubation and ventilation a challenge. These contractions are not antagonized by nondepolarizing muscle relaxants. Other agents, including methohexital, etomidate, propofol, and even neostigmine, may also induce myotonic reactions. Short-acting nondepolarizing muscle relaxants or avoidance of relaxation is therefore advised.[29] Triggering factors, such as hypothermia, shivering, and mechanical or electrical stimulation, may cause a myotonic reaction.[64] The reaction can be treated with phenytoin (4 to 6 mg/kg/day) or quinine (0.3 to 1.5 g/day).[29] Furthermore, MD patients can be very sensitive to anesthetic agents, with hypersomnolence and CO_2 retention sometimes being observed. Careful titration with relatively short-acting anesthetic agents may be beneficial. Close cardiac monitoring is required for MD patients. Pacing equipments should be readily available because a third of first-degree atrioventricular blocks may not respond to atropine.[29] All patients should be treated as though they have both cardiomyopathy and conduction defects.

Myotonia Congenita

Myotonia congenita (MC) is a congenital form of muscular dystrophy characterized by uncontrolled temporary skeleton muscle excitability as a result of mutations in the muscle chloride channel gene (*CLCN1*). There are two forms of MC, one with autosomal dominant and the other with recessive inheritance. The former is also known as Thomsen's disease and the later as Becker's myotonia. The myotonia in MC patients is usually initiated by a forceful muscle contraction, particularly after rest for at least 10 minutes. The myotonic muscle stiffness then becomes increasingly obvious after a second and third short, but forceful contraction. Further contractions usually dampen the myotonia.[65]

Thomsen's disease was the first myotonic disease to be described. Patients may have a hypertrophic and athletic appearance. The sign of percussion myotonia is described as an indenting-appearing myotonia triggered by tapping the muscle. Lid lag is common and muscle stretch reflexes are normal.[65] Myotonia symptoms in Becker's myotonia usually start at 10 to 14 years of age or even later and are more severe than those of Thomsen's disease. Becker's myotonia may be associated with severe generalized stiffness resulting in falling. It can frequently be misdiagnosed as epilepsy. Antiepileptic medications do improve the symptoms, however.[65]

Anesthetic Considerations. As with many muscle diseases, there have been reports that MC patients are predisposed to MH, but as is the case for almost all of them, there are no data to support this hypothesis.[66-68] However, depolarizing muscle relaxant can lead to severe masseter spasm in MC patients. Generalized spasm involving the respiratory and skeletal muscles has been reported.[66] The findings resemble those of MH, so dantrolene is sometimes administered.[65] Because dantrolene is an inhibitor of calcium release from the sarcoplasmic reticulum (SR), it can usually abolish the myotonia effectively.[66,67] Some believe that local anesthetics and class Ib antiarrhythmic drugs such as lidocaine should be used for myotonic reactions rather than dantrolene.[69] Because shivering in the operating room can trigger the myotonic reaction, MC patients should be kept normothermic during surgery.[65]

Myotubular Myopathy

Myotubular myopathy (MTM) is pathologically defined by the presence of centrally placed nuclei in the majority of extrafusal muscle fibers, an appearance resembling fetal myotubes during normal muscle development. Consequently, MTM is also called centronuclear myopathy (CNM).[70] However, MTM now mostly refers to the X-linked form of the disease, whereas CNM is used for the autosomal form.[70]

MTM and CNM are rare. The estimated incidence of MTM is 1 in 50,000 newborn males.[70] MTM has been linked to the myotubularin (*MTM1*) gene on Xq28. Pregnancy is often complicated by polyhydramnios and reduced fetal movements. Affected males typically have severe floppiness and weakness and respiratory distress at birth. Cardiac muscles are not generally involved. The patient usually has a normal response to pain, but tendon reflexes are absent. The long-term prognosis for MTM is extremely poor.[70] In patients who survive the first year of life, most are either completely or partially ventilator dependent.[71] These patients often have abnormal liver function.[71] Both autosomal recessive and autosomal dominant forms have been observed in CNM patients. Its clinical features include respiratory distress, hypotonia, bulbar weakness, ophthalmoplegia, ptosis, and facial diplegia. Although the exact genetic mechanism is not fully understood, the *MTM1*, myotubularin-related protein (*MTMR2*), and myotubularin-related phosphatase (*MTMR3*) genes have been implicated.[70] Pathologically, MTM and CNM share a similar characteristic histologic feature: predominantly type 1 fiber with centrally placed nuclei seen on hematoxylin-eosin staining of formalin-fixed, paraffin-embedded tissue.[70]

Anesthetic Considerations. Reports of anesthesia for patients with MTM are sparse.[72-77] Nontriggering general anesthesia has been used because of the unfounded concern of possible susceptibility to MH. Agents such as propofol, fentanyl, remifentanil, and nitrous oxide have been used successfully without adverse effects.[72-77] The possibility of a prolonged effect of nondepolarizing muscle relaxants has been suggested with mechanomyography.[72-77] However, in reality, intubation of such patients may not require any muscle relaxant because of their hypotonic state. Costi and van der Walt suspected that the defect in MTM is distal to the neuromuscular junction,[73] whereas Dorchies and coworkers suggested that muscle in MTM might be intrinsically normal, with myotubularin-deficient motor neurons involved in development of the disease.[78]

Metabolic Myopathies

Two major energy sources for muscle exist: glycogen and fatty acid. Glycogen serves as a dynamic, but limited reservoir of glucose, mainly stored in skeletal muscle and liver. Glycogen storage disorders (GSDs) are a group of metabolism disorders caused by enzyme deficiency or dysfunction. They reduce effective glucose storage by interfering with normal glycogen synthesis and degradation. Synthetic errors cause decreased normal glycogen, whereas degradation errors tend to block the breakdown of glycogen. Subsequently, hypoglycemia and accumulation of glycogen in tissues could occur as a result of substrate use. There are more than 12 types of GSD that are assigned Roman numerals based on the enzyme deficiencies. Types I and II are discussed here.

Glycogen Storage Disease Type I

The incidence of GSD I is approximately 1 in 100,000 live newborns.[79] The incidence in non-Ashkenazi Jews from North Africa may be as high as 1 in 5420 people.[79] The defective enzyme causing the disease is glucose-6-phosphatase, which is the enzyme that converts glucose 6-phosphate (G6P) to glucose in the liver. Type Ia (von Gierke's disease) is due to a deficiency in G6P hydrolase (catalytic subunit) activity and accounts for more than 80% of cases. Types Ib (G6P transporter deficiency), Ic, and Id represent allelic defects in the translocase associated with G6P. Their inheritance is autosomal recessive. The G6P gene (*G6PC*) encoding the hydrolase resides at 17q21, with the gene encoding G6P translocase (*G6PT*) located at 11q23. Mutations responsible for GSD I have been described in both type Ia and Ib patients.[79]

Impaired glycogenolysis results in accumulation of glycogen and G6P in the liver, kidney, intestine, skeletal muscle, and heart and is manifested as hepatomegaly, renomegaly, proximal tubular dysfunction, and diarrhea.[80] Fasting hypoglycemia is the initial manifestation of the disease. As a result, upregulation of the synthesis and transport of counter-regulatory hormones, such as glucagon, cortisol, catecholamines, and growth hormone, becomes obvious and leads to the release of pyruvate, lactate, and free fatty acid. Lipid deposition in lean tissues such as the liver, skeletal muscle, cardiac muscle, and pancreas results in lipotoxicity and organ failure, including pulmonary hypertension, steatohepatitis, end-stage renal disease, insulin resistance, cardiac contractile dysfunction, and pancreatic beta cell failure.[79] For type Ib disease, specific problems such as neutropenia and neutrophil dysfunction are prominent. Patients may have recurrent infections and inflammatory bowel disease.[81]

Anesthesia Considerations. Anesthesia case reports for GSD I patients are rare.[82,83] Patients with GSD I diseases should be given intravenous glucose-containing fluid preoperatively when they have fasted. Lactate-containing solutions should be avoided because these patients are not able to convert the lactic acid to glycogen.[29] Patients need to be monitored frequently to avoid hypoglycemia.

Glycogen Storage Disease Type II (Acid Maltase Deficiency)

The incidence of acid maltase deficiency (AMD) is estimated to be 1 in every 14,000 to 40,000 births. Its inheritance is autosomal recessive with a few exceptions.[84,85] Mutations of the acid maltase gene on chromosome 17q25 cause deficiency of lysosomal acid maltase (acid α-1,4-glucosidase).[85] Cases of AMD have been arbitrarily classified into three groups—infantile, childhood, and adult—according to the age at onset or death, rate of progression, and tissue-organ involvement.[85]

Acid maltase is a lysosomal enzyme that catalyzes the one-way hydrogenation of glycogen to G6P and is found in all tissues, including skeletal and cardiac muscle.[86] Consequently, glycogen accumulates within the muscle tissues of maltase-deficient patients. Infantile AMD, also known as Pompe's disease, is usually manifested within the first few months of life as rapidly progressive weakness and hypotonia and enlargement of the tongue, heart, and liver. Massive amounts of glycogen (8% to 15% of the wet weight of the tissue) accumulate in the heart, liver, and skeletal muscle, with relatively smaller deposits in smooth muscle, eyes, kidneys, endothelial cells, lymphocytes, brain, and spinal cord. Accumulation of glycogen in cardiac muscle leads to cardiac failure in the infantile form.[85] Echocardiography demonstrates marked thickening of the interventricular septum and posterior left ventricular wall, left ventricular outflow obstruction, and trabecular hypertrophy.[85] Ventricular wall thickness may be increased to up to 25 mm.[87] Wolff-Parkinson-White syndrome has been reported.[88] The signs and symptoms of infantile AMD may resemble those of DMD. Death usually results from cardiorespiratory decompensation within several years of disease progression.[89]

Childhood AMD occurs in infancy to early childhood and is manifested by clinical signs of myopathy. Respiratory muscles tend to be selectively affected. Calf enlargement can also occur. The disease progresses relatively slowly in this form, with a few patients surviving beyond the second decade of life.[85] Tongue, heart, and liver enlargement occur infrequently.[90] However, involvement of vascular smooth muscle is more severe than in the infantile form. There has been a report of extensive glycogen deposition in the arterial wall causing basilar aneurysms.[90]

Adult AMD usually occurs after age 20 and is characterized by slow progressive myopathy or symptoms of respiratory failure.[85] The weakness in proximal muscles is more prominent than the weakness in distal muscles. A third of adult AMD patients suffer from respiratory failure with a restrictive pattern. Weakness in the diaphragm causes extensive atelectasis. VC may be significantly reduced.[85]

Anesthetic Considerations. Anesthesia reports in AMD patients are rare.[91-94] Isolated intraoperative cardiac arrest during halothane anesthesia in infantile AMD has been documented.[94] Despite the problem noted with halothane, enflurane[92] and sevoflurane[93] have been used without complications. Theoretically, total intravenous general anesthesia with propofol may cause a reduction in afterload leading to an increased risk for myocardial ischemia. This may become significant when the patient is tachycardic.[93]

Subendocardial ischemia may occur in patients with a thickened ventricular wall and result in higher left ventricular end-diastolic pressure at lower ventricular volume.[93,95] Close cardiac monitoring is therefore necessary. A central venous or pulmonary artery catheter is not essential in patients who are normovolemic without preexisting heart failure.[93] Adequate filling pressure and normal to high systemic vascular resistance (SVR) are required to ensure effective coronary perfusion.[93] Ketamine has been used successfully in a number of cases because of its ability to maintain SVR and contractility. Respiratory failure and muscle weakness are the other concerns for anesthesiologists. A spectrum of uses of muscle relaxants from none[92] to atracurium[91] to rocuronium[93] have been attempted. Low-dose rocuronium, 0.5 mg/kg, with close monitoring of neuromuscular function and adequate use of reversal agents, has been sufficient to prevent prolonged postoperative weakness.[93] Depolarizing agents should be avoided because of the potential risk of hyperkalemia and rhabdomyolysis.[93,94]

Mitochondrial Myopathies

Mitochondrial diseases refer to defects in the five main steps of mitochondrial metabolism: substrate transport, substrate utilization, the Krebs cycle, the electron transport chain, and oxidation-phosphorylation coupling.[96] However, the term *mitochondrial myopathy* has been reserved for disorders caused by defects in the respiratory chain.[96] The respiratory chain is composed of five multimeric complexes (I to V) embedded in the inner mitochondrial membrane, plus two small mobile electron carriers, coenzyme Q_{10} (CoQ_{10}) and cytochrome *c*, for a total of more than 80 proteins,[96] among which 13 are encoded by mitochondrial DNA (mtDNA) and all others by nuclear DNA (nDNA). mtDNA is different from nDNA in several aspects: (1) mtDNA is circular and contains no intron, (2) it has larger numbers of copies than nDNA does and a much higher spontaneous mutation rate, and (3) its inheritance is maternal. Diagnosis of mitochondrial diseases is difficult because of their clinical heterogeneity.

Primary mtDNA mutations may include point mutations in polypeptide, tRNA, or rRNA encoding regions and large-scale rearrangements, duplications, or deletions.[97] Some of the common conditions caused by point mutations include myoclonic epilepsy with ragged-red fibers (MERRF); mitochondrial encephalopathy, lactic acidosis, and stroke-like episodes (MELAS); neuropathy, ataxia, and retinitis pigmentosa (NARP); maternally inherited Leigh's syndrome; and Leber's hereditary optic neuropathy (LHON).[96] Sporadic large-scale mutations may lead to Kearns-Sayre syndrome, progressive external ophthalmoplegia, and Pearson's syndrome.[96] nDNA mutations can cause deficiencies in complexes I to IV and CoQ_{10} of the electron transport chain.[96]

Mitochondrial myopathy is estimated to have an incidence of 1 in 4000.[98] Among all the mitochondrial functions, abnormalities in electron transport and oxidative phosphorylation are the most common causes of mitochondrial myopathies.[99] Mitochondrial myopathies are characterized by proximal muscle weakness with increased lactic acid and positive muscle biopsy for mitochondrial cytopathy.[100] The hallmark of mitochondrial myopathies is the "ragged red fiber" when muscle biopsy specimens are stained with modified Gomori trichrome stain,[101] and specific defects in the activity of these enzymes have been demonstrated in patients with mitochondrial disease.[102] Fatigue and poor stamina are prominent clinical features. Movement disorders such as ataxia, dystonia, myoclonus, chorea, athetosis, and tremors have also been described as being due to mitochondrial abnormalities.[102]

Anesthetic Considerations

Preoperative Evaluation. Given the heterogeneous types of mitochondrial disease, patients with mitochondrial disease will need a comprehensive preoperative evaluation with a particular focus on neurologic, cardiac, respiratory, musculoskeletal, endocrinopathic, and metabolic compromise (also see Chapters 34 and 35). An ECG and echocardiogram should be considered in patients with signs and symptoms of cardiomyopathy or conduction defects (or both). Although normal lactate and glucose levels cannot rule out mitochondrial diseases, laboratory studies consisting of glucose, electrolytes with anion gap, complete blood count, blood urea nitrogen, lactate, pyruvate, ammonia, CK, biotinidase, acyl carnitines, and blood and urine amino and organic acids could be used as initial investigation for suspected mitochondrial disorders.[103] Further workup should include an erythrocyte sedimentation rate, glycosylated hemoglobin (HbA_{1C}), liver and renal profiles, thyroid function tests, arterial blood gas, and urinalysis.[98,102] Multidisciplinary consultation with special laboratory and imaging studies may be required.[102]

Induction and Maintenance of Anesthesia. Anesthesia has a significant impact on mitochondrial function. Both barbiturates and propofol inhibit complex I of the electron transport chain.[103] Local anesthetics have been demonstrated to disrupt oxidative phosphorylation and decrease the bioenergetic capacity of mitochondria.[103] Sensitivity to intravenous barbiturates and etomidate has been reported.[104,105] However, midazolam,[106] thiopental,[107] propofol,[108,109] remifentanil,[110] and ketamine[109] have all been used safely. Premedication should avoid respiratory depression caused by impaired respiratory responses to hypoxemia. Volatile agents such as halothane, isoflurane, and sevoflurane have been shown to inhibit complex I.[103] This direct inhibition of mitochondrial electron transport system enzymes and altered mitochondrial bioenergetics in the heart were thought to be the mechanism of cardiac preconditioning by volatile anesthetics.[111,112] Inhaled sevoflurane has been widely used for induction because of its low pungency.[100] In some cases, halothane[106] and isoflurane[106,113] have also been used. Isoflurane has been recommended as the agent of choice in patients with Kearns-Sayre syndrome because rhythm disturbances have been reported with halothane in such patients.[106,113] In addition, artificial pacing capability is recommended when dealing with this specific subset of patients.[100] With use of the bispectral index, higher sensitivity to volatile agents has been suggested in children with mitochondrial diseases, especially with dysfunction of complex I.[114] However, its methodology has been criticized.[115] A decreased minimum alveolar concentration of halothane in patients with mental retardation has also been reported.[116]

Despite no real evidence and the fact that volatile anesthetics are frequently the anesthetic of choice when muscle relaxants are considered, several papers have expressed concern that these myopathies are associated with increased sensitivity to MH. This conclusion is not supported by any data. Increased sensitivity to nondepolarizing muscle relaxants has been documented for mivacurium,[117] atracurium,[118] and rocuronium.[118,119] In contrast, normal responses to depolarizing and nondepolarizing neuromuscular blockers such as pancuronium,[120] vecuronium,[121] and atracurium[108,122] are also reported. Although muscle relaxants are not absolutely contraindicated based on current literature and research, it is necessary for anesthesia practitioners to administer depolarizing or nondepolarizing neuromuscular blockers with caution to patients with mitochondrial diseases and to use neuromuscular monitoring (see Chapter 47).[98]

Nonsteroidal anti-inflammatory drugs[100] and regional techniques consisting of local,[100,123] spinal,[124] and epidural administration have been reported. However, it is suggested that regional anesthesia be performed when neurologic abnormalities of the spinal cord and peripheral nerves have definitely been ruled out.[124] Importantly, coagulation function should be assessed because of the possibility of hepatic dysfunction.[100]

Opioids should be used with caution because of the increased risk for respiratory depression and their potential to induce respiratory acidosis in addition to the underlying metabolic acidosis.[100] Because patients with mitochondrial diseases have dysfunctional aerobic metabolism, any increase in the basic metabolic rate should be prevented.[102] Shivering, hypoxia, fasting, and hypotension in such patients may exacerbate the lactic acidosis and should therefore be avoided.[125] Finally, the increased postoperative infection rate in patients with mitochondrial diseases may be due to low hepatic mitochondrial activity, phagocytosis by Kupffer cells, and decreased activity of the reticuloendothelial system.[126]

Myasthenia Gravis

Myasthenia gravis (MG) is an autoimmune disorder of the neuromuscular junction. Autoantibodies against the α-subunit of the muscle-type nicotinic acetylcholine receptor destroy acetylcholine receptors of the neuromuscular junction and cause classic transmission failure with muscle weakness and fatigue. Sparing of other α-subunits of neuronal-type nicotinic acetylcholine receptors provides an explanation for the lack of autonomic or CNS involvement of the disease. The incidence of MG varies between geographic regions, being 1.2 per million in Japan and about 14 per 100,000 in some areas of the United States.[127,128] In younger age groups, females are affected more often than males are, whereas in elderly age groups (>60 years), males are more frequently affected.

There is a striking association between MG and hyperplasia of the thymus, with more than 70% of MG patients having thymus hyperplasia and 10% having thymomas.[128] MG may also be seen as a part of a paraneoplastic syndrome.[128]

Typically, patients first report bulbar symptoms consisting of diplopia and ptosis. The bulbar symptoms are often followed by unevenly distributed muscle weakness and fatigue of the extremities and face. Speech and chewing may be affected, as well as pharyngeal function and coordination of swallowing, with a subsequent increased frequency of aspiration of oral contents. The muscle weakness is often exacerbated during exercise and throughout the course of the day. Apart from the patchy distribution of muscle weakness, symptoms may also vary from day to day, and there may be periods of remission of varying duration.

The diagnosis of MG is made by neurologic examination and testing of the tendency to fatigue and exhibit increased weakness during exercise or repeated contractions. The diagnosis can be confirmed by the Tensilon test (administration of an anticholinesterase, e.g., edrophonium). Improvement is usually seen within 5 minutes after administration of the drug and lasts for about 10 minutes. In addition, electrophysiologic evaluation is often performed and shows a classic decrement in the compound muscle action potential after repetitive nerve stimulation.

Anesthetic Considerations. Ideally, careful neurologic consultation in addition to preoperative evaluation should be performed on MG patients with the aim of optimizing drug therapy and preparing for postoperative care. Pulmonary function tests may be indicated to determine the need for mechanical ventilation postoperatively.[117] As a general rule, patients should keep taking their anticholinesterase medication and be informed about the possibility of postoperative ventilator support. Succinylcholine can be used if needed for rapid tracheal intubation. However, patients with MG might need larger than normal doses (1.5 to 2.0 mg/kg body weight) because of the decreased number of functional acetylcholine receptors.[129] On the other hand, as a result of the decrease in cholinesterase activity achieved by anticholinesterase treatment, neuromuscular blocks with succinylcholine or mivacurium are frequently prolonged.[130,131] Nondepolarizing neuromuscular blockers can be used in patients with MG but should be given with caution because their effects are highly unpredictable and the distribution of muscle weakness is often uneven. Consequently, monitoring of neuromuscular function with a peripheral nerve stimulator is not always reliable in MG patients, and dosing of any nondepolarizing muscle relaxant should be increased in small increments corresponding to 0.1 to 0.2 times the 95% effective dose (ED_{95}) until the desired neuromuscular blocking effect is achieved. Perioperative anticholinesterase treatment will modify the response to reversal agents because of the already existing acetylcholinesterase block, and in some cases, recovery of neuromuscular function after the administration of a reversal agent has been reported to be prolonged.[132]

Potent volatile anesthetics have been used successfully in MG patients. Because of the impaired margin of safety at the neuromuscular junction, a volatile anesthetic usually provides adequate muscular paralysis to allow most surgical procedures to be performed without the need for a neuromuscular blocking agent. Epidural and spinal anesthesia can be used in MG patients, provided that muscle function and ventilation are carefully monitored perioperatively, as for general anesthesia. For a more detailed review, see Baraka[133] and Abel and Eisenkraft.[134]

Eaton-Lambert Myasthenic Syndrome

Eaton-Lambert myasthenic syndrome (ELMS) is an immune-mediated channelopathy caused by decreased release of acetylcholine as a result of autoantibodies against presynaptic voltage-gated calcium channels and other presynaptic elements.[135] Patients with ELMS have muscle weakness and fatigability, generally of the proximal limb muscles, with the lower extremities affected more often than the extraocular and bulbar muscle groups. The syndrome is frequently part of a paraneoplastic phenomenon, usually combined with small cell lung carcinoma. Unlike MG, patients with ELMS are usually worse in the morning with gradual improvement throughout the day. Improvement of muscle function with exercise is due to the accumulation of presynaptic calcium and subsequent improved release of acetylcholine.[136] A minority of patients exhibit autonomic dysfunction. The diagnosis of ELMS is made by careful physical examination combined with clinical electrophysiology showing the typical facilitation of motor action potential with high-frequency nerve stimulation (30 to 50 Hz). Anticholinesterase treatment has little effect on patients with ELMS. Plasmapheresis, immunoglobulin therapy, and 3,4-diaminopyridine (DAP) result in transient improvement.

Anesthetic Considerations. As in patients with MG, those with ELMS should be carefully evaluated for the risk of postoperative respiratory failure and the need for prolonged respiratory monitoring in the postoperative period. Sensitivity to depolarizing and nondepolarizing neuromuscular blocking agents is usually increased. In patients treated with DAP or an anticholinesterase agent, reversal of neuromuscular blockade may be ineffective.

Periodic Paralysis (Hyperkalemic and Hypokalemic)

Hyperkalemic periodic paralysis (HyperPP) is an autosomal dominant disorder first described by Tyler and associates in 1951.[65] It is characterized by attacks of flaccid weakness associated with increased serum potassium.[137] A potassium-rich meal or rest after strenuous exercise may precipitate an attack. Stressful situations may also provoke the onset of paralysis. The paralysis may last for 15 minutes to an hour, with decreased tendon reflexes. In the interictal state, HyperPP is usually associated with mild myotonia that does not impede voluntary movements.[65]

The pathogenesis of HyperPP involves mutations in the voltage-gated sodium channel NaV1.4 of mature muscle fibers; such mutations lead to pathologically increased sodium current and an increased tendency of the muscle fiber to become depolarized.[65,137] Influx of sodium into the muscle is accompanied by simultaneous efflux of potassium and hyperkalemia. Mutant channels exhibit sustained sodium currents that lead to prolonged membrane depolarization, causing myotonia followed by membrane desensitization (or inactivation) and resulting in paralysis. In HyperPP patients, serum CK can be elevated, sometimes 5 to 10 times above the normal limit, whereas serum sodium and potassium levels are normal in the interictal state.[65]

Hypokalemic periodic paralysis (HypoPP) is characterized by a decrease in potassium levels in blood. Attacks of HypoPP can be triggered by rigorous exercise, stress, high-carbohydrate or high-salt meals, pregnancy, menstruation, hypothermia, or drugs such as insulin.[138,139] EMG does not usually show myotonia.[137] The severity of attacks is usually greater than those occurring in patients with HyperPP. HypoPP is an autosomal dominant disease with higher penetration in males. The disease is due to loss of function of one of the two different ion channel types: CaV1.1 and NaV1.4.[137] The most common muscle groups affected are those in the arms and legs; however, the disorder can also affect swallowing and respiratory muscles, which can be fatal in severe cases.[140] The diagnosis of HypoPP is made by laboratory testing demonstrating hypokalemia during attacks and normokalemia between attacks.

Anesthetic Considerations. Potassium, cholinesterase inhibitors, and depolarizing muscle relaxants will aggravate the myotonia in HyperPP patients.[65] Prolonged muscle weakness has been reported when succinylcholine is used.[141] Although one third of patients had no signs of myotonia,[142] masseter spasm and respiratory and skeletal muscles stiffness could still occur during intubation and ventilation.[65] Therefore, neostigmine and succinylcholine should be contraindicated in HyperPP patients. Ideally, all patients with HyperPP need to be admitted preoperatively so that proper preoperative fasting can be accompanied by the administration of dextrose-containing potassium-free maintenance fluid.[143] Postoperatively, HyperPP patients may remain paralyzed for up to several hours. Preventive measures such as maintaining normal body temperature and low serum potassium levels and avoiding hypoglycemia are helpful in limiting such paralysis.[144] Although patients with sodium channel pathology have often been considered to be susceptible to MH, there is no increased risk for MH in these patients.[145] General anesthesia with and without nondepolarizing muscle relaxants has been shown to have satisfactory outcomes.[141,143,144,146] Regional techniques may also be appropriate for this patient group.[142,146] Abortion of the hyperkalemic attack may be accomplished by administering glucose, insulin, epinephrine, and calcium supplements, or alternatively, glucagon may be used. β-Adrenergic treatment with metaproterenol has also been shown to prevent attacks and facilitate recovery.[143]

Management of HypoPP patients should focus on avoiding triggers and medications causing shift of potassium. General anesthesia, postoperative stress, glucose-containing intravenous solutions, and long-acting neuromuscular blockers are associated with postoperative paralytic events.[138] Epidural analgesia has been shown to reduce both pain-related hyperventilation and serum catecholamines, thereby minimizing changes in serum potassium levels.[138] The sympathomimetic effect of epinephrine-containing local anesthetics may also precipitate hypokalemia.[138]

Malignant Hyperthermia

MH is a pharmacogenetic clinical syndrome that in its classic form occurs during anesthesia with a volatile halogenated alkane such as halothane and the depolarizing muscle relaxant succinylcholine. Clinical MH produces rapidly increasing body temperature (by as much as 1°C/5 min) and extreme acidosis as a result of acute loss of control of intracellular calcium levels and compensatory uncontrolled increases in skeletal muscle metabolism that may proceed to severe rhabdomyolysis. Although MH was initially associated with a mortality rate of 70%, earlier diagnosis and the use of dantrolene have reduced the mortality to less than 5%. Current cases of MH are restricted in severity because of diagnostic awareness, early detection through end-expired carbon dioxide, use of less potent anesthetic triggers, and administration of drugs that attenuate its progression. Wilson and colleagues[147] first used the term *malignant hyperthermia* in print in 1966. A Danish survey[148] reported an incidence of fulminant MH of one case per 62,000 anesthetics administered when triggering agents were not used, but the number of suspected cases was one per 4500 anesthetics administered when triggering agents were administered. Public education and communication in the United States are provided by a layman's organization, Malignant Hyperthermia Association of the United States (MHAUS, 11 E. State Street, P.O. Box 1069, Sherburne, NY 13460-1069; telephone: 1-607-674-7901; fax: 1-607-674-7910; e-mail: info@mhaus.org; website: www.mhaus.org), and by emergency consultation with the MH Hotline (1-800-MHHYPER, or 1-800-644-9737). The North American MH Registry, a professional subsidiary of MHAUS, collates findings from muscle biopsy centers in Canada and the United States and provides access to specific patient data through the hotline or its director Dr. Barbara Brandom (North American MH Registry of MHAUS, Room 7449, Department of Anesthesiology, Children's Hospital, University of Pittsburgh, 3705 Fifth Avenue at DeSoto St., Pittsburgh, PA, 15213-2583; telephone: 1-888-274-7899; fax: 1-412-692-8658; e-mail: bwb@pitt.edu).

Between 50% and 80% of genotyped patients who have had a clinical MH syndrome and a positive muscle biopsy have had their disease linked to 1 of more than 110 mutations in the type 1 ryanodine receptor (RyR1; SR Ca^{2+} release channel) gene and 2 mutations in the L-type Ca^{2+} channel CaV1.1.[149] The genetics of MH and the related abnormal function of RyR1, the dihydropyridine receptor (DHPR), and associated proteins are being investigated at the molecular biologic level, with a porcine model and several new mouse models providing intricate details about the etiology of the disorder. Parallel studies in humans are limited by scarce material for scientific study and are complicated by the fact that phenotypes within a genotype vary as a result of genetic, epigenetic, and environmental modifiers. In vitro muscle biopsy testing remains the only "approved" stand-alone screening test currently available in the United States and elsewhere.

History

Between 1915 and 1925, one family experienced three anesthetic-induced MH deaths with rigidity and hyperthermia and was puzzled for decades regarding the cause of these deaths. MH susceptibility (MHS) was eventually confirmed in three descendants by in vitro muscle biopsy tests.[150] In 1929, Ombrédanne[151] described anesthesia-induced postoperative hyperthermia and pallor in children accompanied by significant mortality but did not detect any familial relationships. Critical worldwide attention to MH began in 1960, when Denborough and Lovell[152] reported a 21-year-old Australian with an open leg fracture who was more anxious about anesthesia than about surgery because 10 of his relatives had died during or after anesthesia. Lovell initially anesthetized him with the then-new agent halothane, halted it when signs of MH appeared, successfully treated the symptoms and aborted the syndrome, and subsequently used spinal anesthesia. Further evaluations by George Locher in Wausau, Wisconsin, and Beverly Britt in Toronto, Canada, led to the discovery that MH risk was indeed familial.[153] It was also found that the cause of the syndrome was the result of skeletal muscle involvement rather than central loss of temperature control by the recognition of increased muscle metabolism or muscle rigidity early in the syndrome, low-threshold contracture responses, and elevated CK values.[154]

Interestingly, a similar syndrome was discovered in swine inbred with breeding patterns designed to produce a rapid growth rate and superior muscle development (e.g., Landrace, Pietrain, Duroc, Poland, China). *Porcine stress syndrome*,[155] which is associated with increased metabolism, acidosis, rigidity, fever, and death from rapid deterioration of muscle and results in pale, soft, exudative pork,[156] can be triggered by any stress, such as separation, shipping conditions, weaning, fighting, coitus, or preparation for slaughter, and had become a significant problem for meat production. In 1966, Hall and coworkers[157] reported that a syndrome that appeared to be identical to MH could be induced in stress-susceptible swine by the administration of halothane and succinylcholine. The cause of this syndrome in pigs was discovered to be a single missense mutation in *RYR1*, and all susceptible swine have the same Arg615Cys mutation in the SR calcium release channel RyR1.[158]

In 1975, Harrison[159] described the efficacy of dantrolene in preventing and treating porcine MH, which was rapidly confirmed in humans by a multihospital evaluation of dantrolene used to treat anesthetic-induced episodes.[160] Today, dantrolene still remains the primary basis for successful MH therapy.

Physiology and Pathophysiology of Excitation-Contraction Coupling and Malignant Hyperthermia

MH is a syndrome caused by dysregulation of excitation-contraction (EC) coupling in skeletal muscle. Normal muscle contraction is initiated by nerve impulses arriving at the neuromuscular junction (i.e., the motor end plate) that trigger the release of acetylcholine from the nerve terminal. Acetylcholine activates cation channels on the muscle membrane essential for initiating action potentials that propagate rapidly along the surface membrane of the muscle. Invaginations of the surface membrane (transverse or T tubules) act as conduits to rapidly and uniformly direct action potentials deep within the myofibrils, where they are transduced by a "voltage sensor," the slow voltage-gated Ca^{2+} channels (DHPRs). In response to membrane depolarization, the voltage sensor then undergoes a conformational change that is mechanically transmitted to the Ca^{2+} release channels (RyR1) concentrated in the junctional face of the SR. The mechanical coupling of DHPRs and RyR1 channels that occurs at specialized junctions (*triadic junctions*) is essential for initiating release of Ca^{2+} stored within the SR. Release of SR Ca^{2+} causes the free, intracellular Ca^{2+} concentration to increase from 10^{-7} to about 10^{-5} M. The Ca^{2+} binds to proteins (troponin C and tropomyosin) in the thin filament to expose the myosin binding sites on actin that activate the thick filament (myosin) and cause muscle contraction. The whole process is called EC coupling. Intracellular Ca^{2+} pumps (i.e., sarcoplasmic/endoplasmic reticulum Ca^{2+}-adenosine triphosphatase [ATPase], or SERCA pumps) rapidly propel Ca^{2+} actively back into the SR, and muscle relaxation begins when the Ca^{2+} concentration falls below 10^{-6} M and ends when the resting myoplasmic Ca^{2+} concentration is restored to 10^{-7} M. Because both contraction and relaxation are energy-related processes that consume adenosine triphosphate (ATP), knowing the molecular events contributing to EC coupling and the associated relaxation is essential to understanding the cause of MH (Fig. 37-3). Clinical and laboratory data from swine and

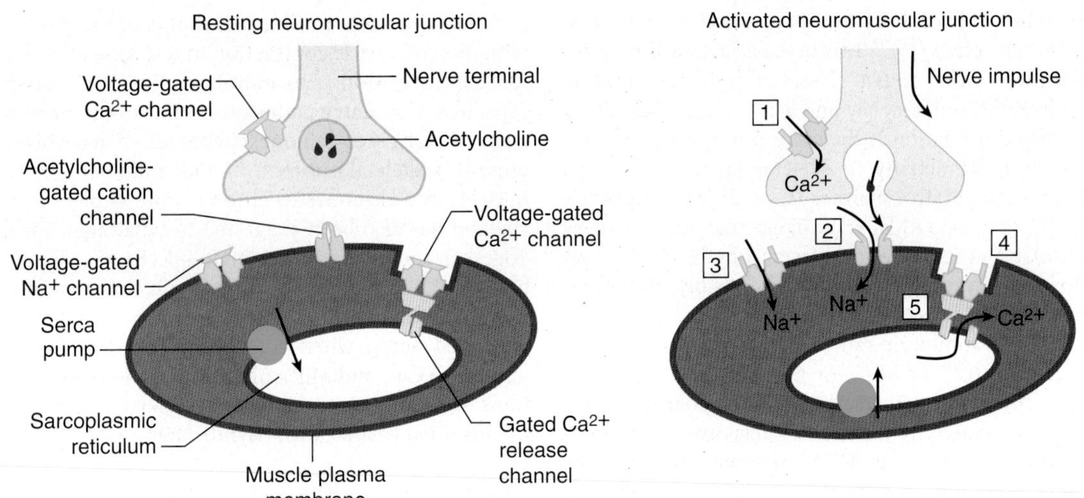

Figure 37-3 Key ion channels involved in neuromuscular transmission and excitation-contraction coupling. Nerve impulses arriving at the nerve terminal activate voltage-gated Ca^{2+} channels (1). The resulting increase in cytoplasmic Ca^{2+} concentration is essential for the exocytosis of acetylcholine. Binding of acetylcholine to postsynaptic nicotinic cholinergic receptors activates an integral nonselective cation channel that depolarizes the sarcolemmal membrane (2). Depolarizing the sarcolemma to threshold activates voltage-gated Na^+ channels (3), which propagate action potential impulses deep into the muscle through the transverse tubule system. Within the transverse tubule system, L-type voltage-gated Ca^{2+} channels sense membrane depolarization and undergo a conformational change (4). A physical link between the α_1-subunit and the ryanodine receptor is thought to be the means by which the signal is transferred to the sarcoplasmic reticulum to induce the release of stored Ca^{2+} (5). *(Adapted from Alberts B, Bray D, Lewis J, et al: Molecular Biology of the Cell, 3rd ed. New York, Garland Press, 1994.)*

humans indicate that the fulminant MH syndrome is associated with a persistent increase in intracellular Ca^{2+}.[161-164] The increased activity of pumps and exchangers trying to correct the increase in Ca^{2+} causes a need for ATP, which in turn produces heat. Thus, the end result is hyperthermia. The rigidity that is frequently seen during a fulminant MH episode is the result of the inability of the Ca^{2+} pumps and transporters to reduce the unbound myoplasmic Ca^{2+} below the contractile threshold. Dantrolene is therapeutic because it reduces the concentration of myoplasmic Ca^{2+}. However, the pathway by which dantrolene lowers myoplasmic Ca^{2+} is complex and still not fully understood.

Malignant Hyperthermia Is the Result of Abnormal Function of Muscle Calcium Release Units

Ryanodine receptors (RyRs), which in muscle are synonymous with the junctional foot protein/SR calcium release channel, are so named because they specifically bind the toxic plant alkaloid ryanodine.[165,166] There are three RyR isoforms encoded by three genes located on human chromosomes 19q13.1, 1q42.1-q43, and 15q14-q15, the "skeletal" (RyR1), "cardiac" (RyR2), and "brain" (RyR3) isoforms, respectively. Each functional RyR consists of four identical subunits (≈5000 amino acids each), and each subunit binds with an accessory protein, calstabin 1 (FK506 12-kd binding protein [FKBP12]). The total mass of the tetramer exceeds 2 megadaltons. Thus, it is one of the largest known proteins and the largest known channel in mammalian species. Evidence of direct coupling of CaV1.1 and RyR1 has been demonstrated by expressing chimeric CaV1.1/CaV1.2 cDNA dysgenic myotubes that lack constitutive expression of either Ca^{2+} channel protein.[167,168] Such studies have provided compelling evidence that the cytoplasmic region between repeats II and III (i.e., cytosolic II-III loop) contains a stretch of 46 amino acids (L720 to Q765) that are essential for engaging bidirectional signaling with RyR1.[169]

In the last 5 years our understanding of EC coupling has increased significantly by identifying protein-protein interactions that regulate both the release and sequestration of Ca^{2+} within skeletal muscle. The elemental unit of function has been named the Ca^{2+} release unit (CRU), and it is localized within junctional regions of T-tubule and SR membranes.[170] The CRU is a macromolecular assembly of interacting proteins that participate in tightly regulating EC coupling. RyR1 is a high-conductance channel that regulates release of SR Ca^{2+} and is the central component of the CRU. The functional RyR1 physically interacts with tetrads composed of four voltage-activated CaV1.1 subunits within the T-tubule membrane to engage bidirectional signaling. Proteins localized within the triad junction that interact with either or both RyR1 and CaV1.1 include Homer 1, which physically binds and functionally couples target proteins, calstabin 1, triadin, junctin, Mg29, junctophilin 1 and 2, calsequestrin, calmodulin, the catalytic and regulatory subunits of protein kinase A, and protein phosphatase 1 (for review see elsewhere[171-174]), and it is likely that this list is not complete. There is experimental support that mutations found in RyR1 ($_{MH}$RyR) alter protein-protein interactions in the CRU.[175-177]

In the presence of certain chemical substances, MH mutations in RyR1 or DHPR cause severe dysregulation of RyR1 channel function. This can be seen in vitro as heightened sensitivity to volatile anesthetics, 4-chloro-*m*-cresol, caffeine, ryanodine, and potassium depolarization.[178-180] Chemically induced dysfunction of the RyR1 complex appears to be the principal cause of triggering uncontrolled skeletal muscle metabolic acidosis (aerobic and glycolytic), rigidity, and hyperkalemia, but the mechanisms governing the syndrome are unclear.

Two essential cations greatly shape the kinetics and magnitude of Ca^{2+} release in response to depolarizing triggers: Ca^{2+} itself and Mg^{2+}. The normal RyR1 complex responds to Ca^{2+} in a biphasic manner. First, Ca^{2+} activates the channel in a graded manner between 100 nM and 100 μM, whereas higher concentrations inhibit channel activity.[181,182] This biphasic action is thought to occur via binding of Ca^{2+} to two classes of regulatory sites on RyR1, a high-affinity stimulatory site and a low-affinity inhibitory site.[173] Mg^{2+}-induced inhibition is the second important physiologic regulator of RyR1 activity in skeletal muscle.[183,184] Mg^{2+} inhibits RyR1 in a cooperative manner ($n_H \approx 2$; 50% inhibitory concentration [IC_{50}] ≈ 650 μM). It is likely that Mg^{2+} acts by competing with Ca^{2+} at its activator sites and by binding to yet unidentified low-affinity inhibitory sites.[185,186] Possibly, MH mutations introduce allosteric instability into the RyR1 complex that leads to a reduction of inhibition rather than directly altering the binding properties of Ca^{2+} or Mg^{2+}, or both, at the activator or inhibitor sites. Therefore, hypersensitivity to pharmacologic agents is likely to be closely tied to altered responses to physiologic ligands. However, whether MHS channels are primarily hyposensitive to inhibition by Mg^{2+} [187,188] or Ca^{2+} (or both), are hypersensitive to activation by Ca^{2+}, or exhibit altered sensitivities in both directions to both ions remains controversial. Recent studies have also pursued the "leaky channel" hypothesis by examining SR preparations from homozygous R615C MHS pigs and heterozygous R163C and C512S mice; they observed a significantly lower Ca^{2+} loading capacity (38%, 23%, and 22% lower than matched wild type mice, respectively) primarily mediated by the presence of leaky channels that remain active even with 100-nM extravesicular Ca^{2+}.[189,190] These direct measures of MHS RyR1 channel dysfunction are consistent with intracellular calcium measurements made in MHS muscles, myotubes, and myoball preparations and in dyspedic myotubes expressing $_{MH}$RyR1s, all of which have been shown to have chronically elevated resting cytoplasmic $[Ca^{2+}]_i$.[177,179,191] Dirksen and coworkers demonstrated that cells expressing the CaV1.1 R1086H MHS mutation have enhanced RyR1 sensitivity to activation by endogenous (voltage sensor) and exogenous (caffeine) activators.[192-196]

Some experimental evidence suggests that long-range interdomain interactions between regions of RyR1 are involved in channel regulation by stabilizing protein conformations critical for normal channel transitions.[197]

Factors Other Than Ryanodine Receptor Abnormalities

Other cellular processes can affect MH episodes. It has been demonstrated that concurrent administration of nondepolarizing neuromuscular blocking drugs at the same time as triggering agents can delay or prevent the onset of clinical MH syndrome. Pretreatment of MH-susceptible pigs with sufficient nondepolarizing neuromuscular blocking agent to completely abolish muscle twitch elicited by electrical stimulation of the nerve prevented halothane from triggering the clinical syndrome for 90 minutes, the longest time point tested.[198] However, in the continued presence of halothane, when function of the neuromuscular junction was restored by administration of the cholinesterase inhibitor neostigmine, clinical MH was triggered immediately. This suggested a close relationship between functional neuromuscular junctions or depolarization of the sarcolemma (or both) and the clinical syndrome.

Recently, it has been shown that sarcolemmal excitation-coupled Ca^{2+} entry (ECCE) is sensitive to the conformation of the RyR1 and is enhanced by several mutations in RyR1, including MH mutations.[171,176,199] This enhancement is responsible for the observation that MHS muscles are more sensitive to depolarization with KCl. Although the sarcolemmal channel responsible for ECCE has not yet been identified, it is one target for dantrolene's reduction of muscle contraction in response to both electrical and KCl depolarization.[175] In addition to ECCE, classic store-operated capacitive Ca^{2+} entry pathways similar to the store-operated Ca^{2+} entry (SOCE) seen in nonexcitable cells[200] have been shown to be present in skeletal muscle[201-203] and could be more active in MHS muscles as a response to chronic store depletion. Such a SOCE channel has also been suggested to be a target for dantrolene.[204] Together, these data suggest that $_{MH}$RyRs or $_{MH}$CaV1.1 and possibly $_{MH}$Csq1 or another $_{MH}$CRU protein could assume a conformation that enhances Ca^{2+} entry via ECCE or SOCE (or both). This enhanced entry, when combined with decreased sensitivity of $_{MH}$RyRs to Ca^{2+} and Mg^{2+} inhibition, could provide cellular conditions that heighten sensitivity to triggering agents and perpetuate the fulminant clinical MH syndrome.

Dantrolene

Dantrolene is the only drug that has been shown to be effective in reversing the symptoms of MH. Preadministration of dantrolene will also prevent the development of fulminant MH in homozygous pigs or heterozygous MH mice when exposed to a triggering stimulus. Dantrolene sodium is a hydantoin derivative (1-[5-(4-nitrophenyl)-2-furanyl]methylene]imino]-2,4-imidazolidinedione) that does not block neuromuscular transmission but causes muscle weakness by direct muscular action. The properties of dantrolene have been closely correlated with its ability to reduce efflux of Ca^{2+} from the SR in vitro. Dantrolene (20 μM) counteracts the effect of reduced Mg^{2+} inhibition in MH-affected muscle.[61] Dantrolene (20 μM) can inhibit the enhanced sensitivity to caffeine seen in MH muscles, and both dantrolene and its water-soluble analog azumolene (150 μM) have been shown to reduce depolarization-induced release of Ca^{2+}, both in muscle and in triadic vesicles.[205] The idea that dantrolene suppresses SR Ca^{2+} release as a result of direct interactions with RyR1 is somewhat controversial. Paul-Pletzer and associates[206] demonstrated that [^{3}H]azidodantrolene specifically labels the amino terminus of RYR1 defined by the 1400–amino acid residue N-terminal calpain digestion fragment of RYR1. More detailed analysis further localized the [^{3}H]azidodantrolene binding site to a single domain containing the core sequence corresponding to amino acid residues 590 through 609 of RyR1.[206] However, to date we lack evidence of a direct action of dantrolene on single RyR1 channels studied in lipid bilayers, even in the presence of calstabin 1, ATP, and activating concentrations of Ca^{2+}, suggesting that dantrolene's main action is to alter key protein-protein interactions.

Genetics

RYR1 mutations have been found in 50% to 80% of patients and relatives who are labeled MH susceptible by positive contracture tests and in almost all families with central core disease (CCD) and King-Denborough syndrome. More than 143 missense mutations and 8 deletions associated with MH have thus far been detected. Another 29 missense mutations are associated with CCD and multiminicore disease in patients with unknown MH testing status.[149] Interestingly, 40% of missense *RYR1* mutations occur at CpG dinucleotide sequences. Five other loci (17q21-24, 1q32, 3q13, 7q21-24, and 5p) have been linked to families with positive contracture tests and an unusual response to anesthesia and have been designated MHS loci 2 through 6, respectively. However, of these five, the only gene that has been shown to be associated with MH is *CACNL1A3*,[207] which codes for CaV1.1 (the α_{1S}-subunit of DHPR), in the MHS3 locus. Two causative mutations in this gene are linked to less than 1% of MHS families worldwide. In some of the other loci, all genes within the locus have been ruled out as causing susceptibility to MH. Hence for practical reasons, the *RYR1* gene remains the primary target for current clinical genetic analysis.

Distribution of *RYR1* Mutations

The missense mutations associated with MHS, CCD, or in some cases both, are dispersed throughout the coding region of the *RYR1* gene, and all allow transcription of a protein that is putatively functional.[149,208] Until recently, it was thought that most *RYR1* mutations were clustered in three "hot spots": between amino acid residues 35 and 614 (MH/CCD region 1), between amino acid residues 2163 and 2458 (MH/CCD region 2) in the myoplasmic foot region of the protein, and between amino acids 4643 and 4898 in the carboxyl-terminal transmembrane loop or pore region (MHS/CCD region 3)[209] (Fig. 37-4). It appears that the supposition that there were "hot spots" was simply due to bias in sample analysis inasmuch as the missense mutations associated with MH or CCD (or both) are scattered over 54 of the 107 exons of *RYR1*. Approximately 41% of reported MH mutations are found in multiple families. CCD mutations are predominantly found in the C-terminal region of the gene (exons 85 to 103), and only 10 mutations (17%) have been described in more than one family: R4861H ($n = 14$), V4849I ($n = 9$), I4898T ($n = 7$), L4824P ($n = 4$), A4940T ($n = 4$), G4638D ($n = 3$), R4893W ($n = 3$), R4861C ($n = 2$), R4893Q ($n = 2$), and G4899E ($n = 2$).

MH and CCD have been reported in Western populations predominantly, but more likely than not this is incorrect and the result of the manner and frequency in which cases are reported. The true ethnic distribution of MH and CCD is difficult to ascertain. It does appear that the associated mutations are clustered in a given region of the world, but the distribution and frequency appear to be somewhat population specific. In the United Kingdom, 69 *RYR1* mutations have been discovered, 25 of which are found in only a single family. G2434R is found in approximately 40% of the 434 mutation-positive MH families investigated in the United Kingdom, with the next most common mutations being T2206M (10%) and G341R (8%). In Switzerland, V2168M and I2336H are the predominant mutations,[210] and in Germany, R163C (MH and CCD), R614C (MH), T2206M (MH), G2434R (MH), and R2454H (MH) have each been detected in five or more independent cases.[211,212] G341R and R614C are common in France,[213] and R614C has also been found in several MH families from Italy[213] and Canada.[214] G341R has been found frequently in Belgium.[213] The mutation common to Europe and North America is G2434R, which occurs in 4% to 7% of European and 5.5% of North American families.[215] Single-family mutations are the most common mutations reported in Japanese, Chinese, Taiwanese, Australian, and New Zealand MH families,[216-218] but it is likely that this may reflect the small number of cases investigated there. Because genetic screening in European and North American studies has predominantly targeted only regions 1 and 2 of the original hot spots in the gene, the absence of *RYR1* mutations in some of the screened population could be explained by

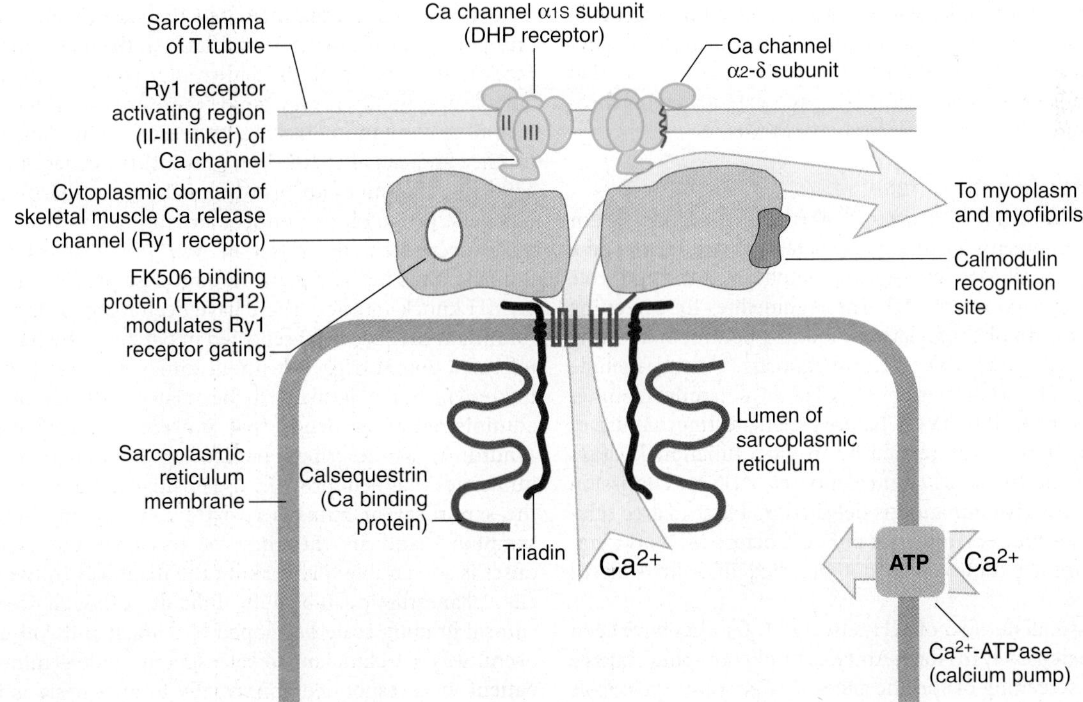

Figure 37-4 Schematic representation of the triad junction of skeletal muscle shows the junctional foot protein (ryanodine [Ry1] receptor) and its associated proteins. In skeletal muscle, the α_{1S}-subunit of the dihydropyridine receptor (DHPR) participates in excitation-contraction coupling. These physical links transmit essential signals across the narrow gap of the triadic junction that activate the Ry1 receptor and release Ca^{2+} from the sarcoplasmic reticulum. *(Adapted from Pessah IN, Lynch C III, Gronert GA: Complex pharmacology of malignant hyperthermia. Anesthesiology 84:1275, 1996.)*

RYR1 mutations located outside these two regions or by involvement of other genes.

Inheritance and Penetrance of Malignant Hyperthermia

Inheritance of human MH can no longer be considered to be solely autosomal dominant with variable penetrance because more than one MH-linked mutation has been identified in some probands and families. Six nonconsanguineous families harbor at least two *RYR1* mutations that have both been linked to MHS, and in two families one is an *RYR1* mutation and the second is a *CaV1.1* mutation.[219] Although MHS homozygotes are common in affected pigs, they are rare in human and transgenic mouse populations. The known MHS homozygous humans appear clinically normal but exhibit stronger responses to IVCT and caffeine/halothane contracture tests (CHCTs) than heterozygous individuals do.[220-223] Homozygosity of two MH mutations in "hot spot" 1 leads to perinatal lethality in mice.[189,190] Double heterozygous individuals do not appear to show any additive effect of the second mutation on IVCT.[219]

Discordance between Genetic and IVCT/CHCT Malignant Hyperthermia Testing

Discordance has confounded linkage analysis worldwide. Examples include MHN patients carrying an *RYR1* mutation associated with MH and MHS patients who do not carry the familial *RYR1* mutation. Several explanations are possible, the most likely being that IVCT/CHCT is not clinically precise and that the thresholds for IVCT or CHCT are inexact. This would lead to errors in determining whether a patient was MHN or MHS. A second possibility is variable penetrance with possible allelic silencing,[224] and a third is that individuals with discordance have mutations in other unknown genes or modifier genes that affect the function of RyR1 and its phenotypic penetrance. The rarity of large kindreds with MH makes linkage analysis and understanding variability in clinical manifestations difficult. Robinson and associates demonstrated by the transmission disequilibrium test (TDT) that loci on chromosomes 5 and 7 and, to a lesser extent, loci on chromosomes 1 and 7 influence susceptibility to MH.[213]

Guidelines for Genetic Screening

In 2000, the European MH group[225] formulated guidelines for *RYR1* mutation screening with linkage data to other loci for some MH families, but all MH investigators emphasized the vital role of IVCT in the diagnosis of MH. These guidelines for screening have reduced the number of relatives requiring contracture testing without increasing the risk of misdiagnosis[226,227] and include the following: (1) confirmation of MHS in a family member (preferably a proband) by IVCT before genetic testing; (2) use of 15 *RYR1* mutations characterized by in vitro functional assays for the genetic protocol; (3) confirmation of MHS and omission of IVCT if a causative mutation is detected in a first-degree relative; and (4) need for performance of IVCT before MHN is diagnosed if a familial mutation is not detected in a first-degree relative.

Only a small number of MH-susceptible families have been investigated extensively in North America by phenotyping, linkage analysis, and screening of specific genes. Collaborative protocols over the past several years between MH biopsy centers and molecular biologists have screened 209 unrelated MHS subjects for mutations in the *RYR1* gene (see "Distribution of *RYR1* Mutations").

A recent consensus meeting agreed to the following: (1) limitations of genetic testing include low sensitivity because of the diversity of mutations and genes; (2) the *RYR1* gene is the primary focus for genetic testing, but further studies are required for more complete understanding of the relationship between mutations and susceptibility; (3) guidelines for referral and education are needed to establish clinical testing in a Clinical Laboratories Improvement Act (CLIA)—certified laboratory; and (4) a North American MH *RYR1* Mutation Panel was not changed from the original panel set out in 2002 (Table 37-1).

Fulminant Malignant Hyperthermia

Fulminant MH is rare. Acute episodes of MH depend on four variables: a genetic (perhaps rarely acquired) predisposition, the absence of inhibiting factors, the presence of an anesthetic or nonanesthetic trigger, and the presence of environmental factors that could potentiate the action of one or more of the other three variables.

Anesthetic Triggering

Anesthetic drugs that trigger MH include ether, halothane, enflurane, isoflurane, desflurane, sevoflurane, and depolarizing muscle relaxants, the only currently used of which is succinylcholine. Desflurane and sevoflurane appear to be less potent triggers than halothane and produce a more gradual onset of MH.[228,229] The onset may be explosive if succinylcholine is used. MH-susceptible swine were traditionally screened by induction with a volatile anesthetic, which led to pronounced hind limb rigidity within 5 minutes, frequently sooner.[230] Prior exercise even an hour before induction of anesthesia increased the severity and hastened the onset of rigidity in swine.[230] Similarly, in the new knock-in mouse models, the onset of limb rigidity after commencing exposure to volatile anesthetics is very rapid. There are also several modifying factors that are more likely to be present in humans than in pigs or mice and can alter (or even prevent) the onset of clinical MH. Mild hypothermia and preadministration of barbiturates, tranquilizers, propofol, or nondepolarizing neuromuscular blockers delay or prevent the onset of MH[163,230-232] in MH-susceptible humans, thus making them respond less predictably than swine or MH knock-in mice. There have been many instances in which fulminant MH has been reported in patients who have previously tolerated potent triggers without difficulty.[233] Why this occurs is unknown, but it is likely to be related to prior or concurrent administration of drugs that prevent or delay onset of the syndrome, as described earlier, or unknown environmental influences that help provoke the positive incident. Thus, onset of the syndrome in humans is extremely variable both in initial symptoms and in the time of onset of the syndrome. Its onset is so variable that making the diagnosis in the setting of a clinical anesthetic can be quite difficult. Although not perfect, the clinical grading scale developed by Larach and colleagues[234] is a useful way for clinicians to retrospectively determine whether a patient who responded abnormally to anesthesia is in any way likely to actually have had a clinical MH episode. However, MH is most easily diagnosed prospectively by vigilance, recognizing its signs and symptoms, and knowing how to treat the syndrome.

Table 37-1 Findings of the North American Malignant Hyperthermia Mutation Panel, 2002

Exon	Mutation*	RyR1 Amino Acid Change	No. of Families in North America†	Estimated Incidence in Europe (%)	Phenotype
6	C487T	R163C	2	2-7	MHS, CCD
9	G742A	G248R	2 (11)	2	MHS
11	G1021A	G341R	1	6-17	MHS
17	C1840T	R614C	6 (42)	4-45	MHS
39	C6487T	R2163C	2	4	MHS
39	G6488A	R2163H	0	1	MHS, CCD
39	G6502A	V2168M	1	8	MHS, CCD
40	C6617T	T2206M	2	One family	MHS
44	Deletion	ΔG2347	2	0	MHS
44	G7048A	A2350T	1	0	MHS
45	G7303A	G2434R	9 (54)	4-10	MHS
45	G7307T	R2435H	1	2.5	MHS, CCD
46	G7361A	R2454H	4	One family	MHS
46	C7372	R2458C	0	4	MHS
46	G7373A	R2458H	0	4	MHS
101	G14582A	A4861H	0	Multiple families	CCD
102	T14693C	I4898T	0	Multiple families	MHS, CCD

*Criteria for the 17 mutations: (1) they occur in more than one family in North America or Europe, and (2) previous testing of a sequence variant shows that it is not a polymorphism.
†Data collaboration of the Uniformed Services University of the Health Sciences, Thomas Jefferson University, Wake Forest University, University of California, Davis, and Barrow Neurological Institute indicates those also found in Canada (e.g., for exon 45, four families with the mutation G2434R were found in Canada).
CCD, central core disease; MHS, malignant hyperthermia susceptibility; RyR1, ryanodine receptor type 1.

The two classic clinical manifestations of fulminant MH syndrome may start in one of the following two scenarios.

1. Rigidity after induction with thiopental and succinylcholine but successful intubation, followed rapidly by the symptoms listed after scenario 2
2. Normal response to induction of anesthesia and uneventful anesthetic course until onset of the following symptoms:
   - Unexplained sinus tachycardia or ventricular arrhythmias, or both
   - Tachypnea if spontaneous ventilation is present
   - Unexplained decrease in O_2 saturation (because of a decrease in venous O_2 saturation)
   - Increased in end-tidal P_{CO_2} with adequate ventilation (and in most cases unchanged ventilation)
   - Unexpected metabolic and respiratory acidosis
   - Central venous desaturation
   - Increase in body temperature above 38.8°C with no obvious cause

The usually muted onset of MH (scenario 2) is in most cases detected quickly by the development of tachycardia, increased levels of expired carbon dioxide, and muscle rigidity. It can be delayed for several reasons and may not be overt until the patient is in the recovery room. Once initiated, the course of MH can be rapid. When clinical signs such as increased expired carbon dioxide, muscle rigidity, tachycardia, and fever suggest MH, more than one abnormal sign must be observed before making the diagnosis because according to a meta-analysis of many reported cases, a single adverse sign does not usually indicate MH.[234] The mechanism by which anesthetics and depolarizing muscle relaxants trigger MH is unsolved, *but* it cannot be ignored that they are etiologic agents and that early diagnosis is critical for successful treatment.

During a fulminant MH episode, triggering agents cause affected subjects to undergo a very large increase in aerobic and anaerobic metabolism that results in intense production of heat, carbon dioxide, and lactate and an associated respiratory and metabolic acidosis.[230,235] These reactions markedly alter whole-body acid-base balance and temperature and are magnified as temperature increases because skeletal muscle makes up 40% of the body mass. Whole-body rigidity occurs in almost all susceptible pigs and mice, as well as in most humans. Temperature may exceed 43°C (109.4°F), Pa_{CO_2} may exceed 100 mm Hg, and arterial pH (pH_a) may decrease well below 7.00. The increased permeability of skeletal muscle results in increased serum levels of potassium, ionized calcium, CK (although MH-related changes in serum CK do not differ overall from changes in CK observed during surgery[236]), myoglobin, and serum sodium.[230] Sympathetic hyperactivity is responsible for the cardinal sign of MH—tachycardia—which occurs early as an indication of increased metabolism. With metabolic exhaustion, cellular permeability increases along with whole-body edema, including acute cerebral edema. As MH progresses untreated, disseminated intravascular coagulation and cardiac or renal failure may develop. It is important to note that MH is a disorder of increased muscle metabolism and, despite its name, need not involve increased temperature! For example, if heat loss is greater than production or if cardiac output plummets early, central temperature will not increase.

Awake Triggering: Exercise and Heat

Whether MH can be triggered in humans in the absence of a triggering agent is controversial. Porcine environmental stress such as exercise, heat, anoxia, apprehension, and excitement triggers fulminant MH (see "History").[230,235] These responses are related to muscle movement or to increased temperature. Increased ambient temperature triggers fulminant MH in two strains of MH mice.[190,191] Epidemiologic studies have shown that exercise-induced symptoms, including rhabdomyolysis, occur more frequently in MHS patients[237]; an Arg401Cys *RYR1* mutation was present in three cases of exercise-induced rhabdomyolysis.[216] Other reports are largely anecdotal and relate heat stroke, sudden and unexpected death, unusual stress and fatigue, or myalgias to possible awake MH episodes. Stresses associated with these episodes include exercise and environmental exposure to volatile nonanesthetic vapors.[238-240]

Malignant Hyperthermia–Associated Syndromes

MASSETER SPASM ("THIOPENTAL-SUCCINYLCHOLINE OR HALOTHANE-SUCCINYLCHOLINE RIGIDITY"). Masseter spasm is defined as jaw muscle rigidity in association with limb muscle flaccidity after the administration of succinylcholine. The masseter and lateral pterygoid muscles contain slow tonic fibers that can respond to depolarizing neuromuscular blockers with a contracture.[241,242] This is manifested clinically on exposure to succinylcholine as an increase in jaw muscle tone, well defined by van der Spek and associates.[243] There is a spectrum of responses: a tight jaw that becomes a rigid jaw and then a very rigid jaw (Fig. 37-5). This jaw rigidity may occur even after pretreatment with a "defasciculating" dose of a nondepolarizing relaxant. If there is rigidity of other muscles in addition to trismus, the association with MH is absolute; anesthesia should be halted as soon as possible and treatment of MH begun. However, in more than 80% of patients with trismus but no rigidity of other muscles, it is a variant found in normal patients. If trismus occurs, proper monitoring should include end-expired CO_2, examination for pigmenturia, and arterial or venous blood sampling for CK, acid-base status, and electrolyte levels, particularly potassium. Although scientifically unproven, it is thought that the initial tightness of the jaw and its duration may predict the gravity of the response. For patients with "jaws of steel," the procedure should be halted, especially if the condition persists for more than several minutes. If the jaw is slightly resistant to opening, the anesthesiologist may continue anesthesia with proper monitoring. If the jaw is moderately tight and distinctly a problem, there are two choices: halt the procedure or continue with nontriggering agents. Any suggestion of MH should prompt MH therapy, including administration of dantrolene.

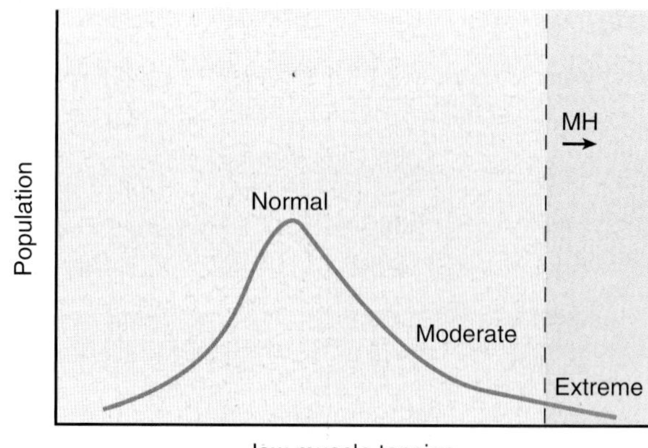

Figure 37-5 Succinylcholine usually increases jaw muscle tone slightly. In some patients this increase is moderate, and in very few, the effect is extreme (i.e., "jaws of steel"). As many as 50% of this latter group may be susceptible to malignant hyperthermia (MH). Somewhere in the area of the declining curve is the boundary for the MH population.

Diagnosis in the Operating Room and Postanesthesia Care Unit

As stated earlier, fulminant MH is rare, and early signs of clinical MH may be subtle. These signs must be distinguished from other disorders with similar signs (Box 37-1). When the diagnosis is obvious (i.e., fulminant MH or succinylcholine-induced rigidity with rapid metabolic changes), marked hypermetabolism and heat production occur, and there may be little time left for specific therapy to prevent death or irreversible morbidity. If the syndrome begins with slowly increasing end-tidal CO_2 (defined earlier), specific therapy can await a complete clinical workup before treatment. In general, MH is not expected to occur when no triggers are administered (see "Anesthesia for Susceptible Patients"). When volatile anesthetics or succinylcholine is used, MH should be suspected whenever there is an unexpected increase in end-expired CO_2, undue tachycardia, tachypnea, arrhythmias, mottling of the skin, cyanosis, increased temperature, muscle rigidity, sweating, or unstable blood pressure. If any of these occur, signs of increased metabolism, acidosis, or hyperkalemia must be sought. Analysis of arterial blood gases demonstrates metabolic acidosis and may show respiratory acidosis if the patient is unable to increase ventilation as metabolism increases. O_2 and CO_2 change more markedly in the central venous compartment than in arterial blood; therefore, end-expired or venous CO_2 levels more accurately reflect whole-body stores. Venous carbon dioxide, unless the blood drains an area of increased metabolic activity, should have PCO_2 levels of only about 5 mm Hg greater than that of expected or measured $PaCO_2$. In small children, particularly those without oral food or fluid for a prolonged period, the base deficit may be 5 mEq/L because of their smaller energy stores. Any patient suspected of having an MH episode should be reported to the North American Registry via the rare disease protocol (American Medical Record Association [AMRA]), available from the MHAUS website at http://www.mhaus.org/.

Box 37-1 Mimics of Malignant Hyperthermia Disorder

Alcohol therapy for limb arteriovenous malformation
Contrast dye
Cystinosis
Diabetic coma
Drug toxicity or abuse
Environmental heat gain more than loss
Equipment malfunction with increased carbon dioxide
Exercise hyperthermia
Freeman-Sheldon syndrome
Heat stroke
Hyperthyroidism
Hypokalemic periodic paralysis
Intracranial free blood
Muscular dystrophies (Duchenne's, Becker's)
Myotonias
Neuroleptic malignant syndrome
Osteogenesis imperfecta
Pheochromocytoma
Prader-Willi syndrome
Rhabdomyolysis
Sepsis
Ventilation problems
Wolf-Hirschhorn syndrome

Treatment

Acute therapy for MH can be summarized as follows: (1) Discontinue all anesthetic agents and hyperventilate with 100% oxygen. Normal ventilation is that required to remove metabolic carbon dioxide. With increased aerobic metabolism, normal ventilation must increase. However, carbon dioxide production is also increased because of neutralization of fixed acid by bicarbonate; hyperventilation removes this additional CO_2. (2) Administer dantrolene (2.5 mg/kg intravenously [IV] to a total dose of 10 mg/kg IV) every 5 to 10 minutes until symptoms subside. (3) Administer bicarbonate (2 to 4 mEq/kg IV) to correct the metabolic acidosis with frequent monitoring of blood gases and pH. (4) Control fever by administering iced fluids, cooling the body surface, cooling body cavities with sterile iced fluids, and if necessary, using a heat exchanger with a pump oxygenator. Cooling should be halted at 38°C to 39°C to prevent inadvertent hypothermia. (5) Monitor urinary output and establish diuresis to protect the kidney from probable myoglobinuria. (6) Further therapy is guided by blood gases, electrolytes, temperature, arrhythmia, muscle tone, and urinary output. Treatment of hyperkalemia with glucose and insulin should be slow. The most effective way to lower serum potassium is reversal of MH by effective doses of dantrolene. (7) Analyze coagulation studies (e.g., international normalized ratio, platelet count, prothrombin time, fibrinogen, fibrin split or degradation products).

Discontinuation of the trigger may be adequate therapy for acute MH if the onset is slow or if exposure was brief. Dantrolene is packaged in 20-mg bottles with sodium hydroxide for a pH of 9 to 10 (otherwise it will not dissolve) and with mannitol (converts the hypotonic solution to isotonic). The initial dose should be 2.5 mg/kg dantrolene reconstituted in sterile water and administered intravenously. Dantrolene *must* be reconstituted in sterile water rather than salt solutions or it will precipitate. Dantrolene has a half-life of at least 10 hours in children and adults.[244,245] At therapeutic concentrations, dantrolene may prolong the need for intubation and assisted ventilation. Aside from cholestasis during long-term (>3 weeks) therapy, dantrolene has no serious side effects.

The clinical course will determine further therapy and studies. Dantrolene should probably be repeated at least every 10 to 15 hours (its half-life) for at least one and possibly several doses. Recrudescence of MH can approach 50%, usually within 6.5 hours.[246,247] When indicated, calcium and cardiac glycosides may be used safely. They can be lifesaving during persistent hyperkalemia. Permanent neurologic sequelae, such as coma or paralysis, may occur in advanced cases, probably because of inadequate cerebral oxygenation and perfusion for the increased metabolism and because of the fever, acidosis, hypo-osmolality with fluid shifts, and potassium release. Slow voltage-gated calcium channel blockers do not increase porcine survival.[248,249] If uncertain at any time, the physician should contact the MH Hotline to verify treatment and report the case with an AMRA form.

Anesthesia for Susceptible Patients

Safe anesthetics consist of nitrous oxide, barbiturates, etomidate, propofol, opiates, tranquilizers, and nondepolarizing muscle relaxants. Potent volatile anesthetics and succinylcholine must be avoided, even in the presence of dantrolene. There are anecdotal reports that some human patients have experienced a hypermetabolic state despite these precautions, but they have always responded favorably to the administration of intravenous dantrolene. Preoperative dantrolene is never needed because the use of nontriggering agents is almost always associated with uneventful anesthesia. Regional anesthesia is safe and may be preferred. Amide anesthetics such as lidocaine were once considered dangerous in susceptible patients because they were thought to induce or worsen muscle contractures in vitro as a result of their effect of increasing calcium efflux from the SR. Porcine and human studies have consistently demonstrated the lack of danger of amide anesthetics. Before use for MH-susceptible patients, anesthetic machines may be "cleansed" of potent volatile agents by removal or sealing of the vaporizers, changing the soda lime, perhaps replacing the fresh gas outlet hose, and using a disposable circle with a flow of 10 L/min for 5 minutes.[250,251]

The anesthesiologist should confidently discuss anesthetic care with MH-susceptible patients and assure them that all will be done to avoid difficulties with MH and that the appropriate drugs, knowledge, and skills are immediately at hand if any problems occur. Many of these patients have undergone procedures uneventfully, such as dental analgesia and obstetric anesthesia, before the diagnosis of susceptibility was made. The patient can enter the therapeutic environment in a reassured, relaxed, and comfortable state. Outpatient procedures are feasible in most environments; the time of discharge depends on the usual outpatient criteria.

Any facility using MH triggers on an inpatient or outpatient basis should have dantrolene available immediately.

Evaluation of Susceptibility

Evaluation of susceptibility includes a history and physical examination to detect any subclinical abnormality. A genealogy with specific information about anesthetic exposure and agents can estimate the likelihood of exposure to triggering agents. Blood CK values, when determined in a resting, fasting state without recent trauma, reflect muscle membrane stability. When the CK level is elevated in a close relative of a person with known MHS, the relative may be considered to have MHS without contracture testing. If the CK level is normal on several occasions, there is no predictive value, and contracture studies are necessary. The patient must travel to the test center for surgical biopsy to ensure viability and accurate results. Muscle biopsy contracture studies, performed at about 30 centers around the world, involve exposure to halothane, caffeine, halothane plus caffeine, and ryanodine.[225] 4-Chloro-*m*-cresol may add to precision.[176] It is also important to note that contracture responses are sometimes positive in patients with myopathies that bear no direct relationship to MH and therefore may not indicate susceptibility. Dantrolene must be avoided before biopsy because it masks the response to contracture-producing drugs. After a patient is diagnosed as being MH susceptible, DNA testing for mutations should follow. When a mutation is detected, other relatives with that mutation should be considered to be MH susceptible without the need for an invasive contracture test, and they need not travel to a testing center (see "Genetics").

Advice should be given to susceptible patients. Precautions are necessary in regard to general anesthesia, and triggers include all potent volatile agents and succinylcholine. Awake episodes are uncommon, and if not experienced before diagnosis, they are an unlikely problem. The true predictive value (i.e., percentage of positive results that are true positives) or efficiency (i.e., percentage of all results that are true, whether positive or negative) of contracture testing in determining susceptibility in the general population cannot be estimated because of the selection process that has been used to date for testing (i.e., limited to those with anesthesia reactions who do not have any other muscle disease pathology). False-positive results from cautious interpretation or decreased specificity are masked because the patient will never be exposed to triggering agents. A promising innovative in vivo human application involves physiologically based microdialysis infusion of caffeine or halothane into muscle of MH-susceptible patients to trigger exaggerated localized changes in acid-base balance.[252-256] White blood cells express MH mutations and provide a substrate for genetic analysis.[257-261] Nuclear magnetic resonance has promise,[262,263] but it is difficult to standardize a stress, such as forearm ischemia, that can differentiate susceptible from normal tissue.

Summary

MH is a subclinical myopathy featuring an eerie and erratic metabolic mayhem that is unmasked on exposure to potent volatile anesthetics or succinylcholine. Skeletal muscle acutely and unexpectedly increases its myoplasmic Ca^{2+} concentration, thereby leading to increased oxygen consumption and lactate production and resulting in greater heat production, respiratory and metabolic acidosis, muscle rigidity, sympathetic stimulation, and increased cellular permeability. MH-susceptible skeletal muscle differs from normal muscle in that it is always closer to loss of control of Ca^{2+} concentration within the muscle fiber, and it can involve a generalized alteration in cellular or subcellular membrane permeability. This is an EC coupling defect resulting from an alteration in protein-protein interaction in the CRU. It is a homozygous, single point mutation of *RYR1* in swine and a heterozygous disorder in humans, in whom there may also be a modification of RyR1 protein function by interacting structures, membranes, or enzymes. Diagnosis rests on acute awareness of the signs and symptoms of this syndrome, of which hyperthermia is a late sign. Specific treatment is administration of dantrolene to lower muscle Ca^{2+} levels; symptomatic treatment consists of reversal of the acid-base and temperature changes. Evaluation of affected families is guided by analysis of drug-induced muscle contractures (by European IVCT and North American CHCT protocols) and genetic testing of DNA samples. General or regional anesthesia is safe for patients susceptible to MH, provided that care is taken to specially prepare the anesthesia machine and avoid all potent volatile anesthetics and succinylcholine if a general anesthesia technique is chosen. Research on MH has yielded insight into the physiology of metabolism and into the molecular biology of genetic muscle disorders. Challenges remaining include identification of all genetic mutations responsible for human MH, elucidation of the mechanism that links exposure to subsequent loss of control of Ca^{2+}, development of noninvasive and nondestructive testing for susceptibility, and determination of the mode of action of dantrolene.

References

1. Bannister R, Davies B, Holly E, et al: Defective cardiovascular reflexes and supersensitivity to sympathomimetic drugs in autonomic failure. Brain 102:163-176, 1979.
2. Bader AM, Hunt CO, Datta S, et al: Anesthesia for the obstetric patient with multiple sclerosis. J Clin Anesth 1:21-24, 1988.
3. Shimizu T, Kawata A, Kato S, et al: Autonomic failure in ALS with a novel *SOD1* gene mutation. Neurology 54:1534-1537, 2000.
4. Rosenbaum KJ, Neigh JL, Strobel GE: Sensitivity to nondepolarizing muscle relaxants in amyotrophic lateral sclerosis: Report of two cases. Anesthesiology 35:638-641, 1971.
5. Jacobs BC, Rothbarth PH, van der Meche FG, et al: The spectrum of antecedent infections in Guillain-Barré syndrome: A case control study. Neurology 51:1110-1111, 1998.
6. Brooks H, Christian AS, May AE: Pregnancy, anaesthesia and Guillain Barré syndrome. Anaesthesia 55:894-898, 2000.

7. Steiner I, Argov Z, Cahan C, Abramsky O: Guillain-Barré syndrome after epidural anesthesia: Direct nerve root damage may trigger disease. Neurology 35:1473-1475, 1985.
8. Rudnik-Schneborn S, De Visser M, Zerres K: Spinal muscular atrophies. *In* Engel A, Franzini-Armstrong C (eds): Myology. New York, McGraw-Hill, 2004, pp 1845-1864.
9. Cruse R: Hereditary primary motor sensory neuropathies, including Charcot-Marie-Tooth disease. April 29, 2007. Available from: http://www.uptodate.com/ Accessed July 2007.
10. Ginz HF, Ummenhofer WC, Erb T, Urwyler A: [The hereditary motor-sensory neuropathy Charcot-Marie-Tooth disease: Anesthesiologic management —case report with literature review.] Anaesthesist 50:767-771, 2001.
11. Gratarola A, Mameli MC, Pelosi G: Total intravenous anaesthesia in Charcot-Marie-Tooth disease. Case report. Minerva Anestesiol 64:357-360, 1998.
12. Sugino S, Yamazaki Y, Nawa Y, et al: [Anesthetic management of a patient with Charcot-Marie-Tooth disease using propofol and nitrous oxide.] Masui 51:1016-1019, 2002.
13. Baur CP, Schara U, Schlecht R, et al: [Anesthesia in neuromuscular disorders. Part 2: Specific disorders.] Anasthesiol Intensivmed Notfallmed Schmerzther 37:125-137, 2002.
14. Antognini JF: Anaesthesia for Charcot-Marie-Tooth disease: A review of 86 cases. Can J Anaesth 39:398-400, 1992.
15. Baranov D, Kelton T, McClung H, et al: Neurological diseases. *In* Fleisher L (ed): Anesthesia and Uncommon Diseases. Philadelphia, Saunders Elsevier, 2006.
16. Pogson D, Telfer J, Wimbush S: Prolonged vecuronium neuromuscular blockade associated with Charcot Marie Tooth neuropathy. Br J Anaesth 85:914-917, 2000.
17. Naguib M, Samarkandi AH: Response to atracurium and mivacurium in a patient with Charcot-Marie-Tooth disease. Can J Anaesth 45:56-59, 1998.
18. Schmitt HJ, Munster T: Mivacurium-induced neuromuscular block in adult patients suffering from Charcot-Marie-Tooth disease. Can J Anaesth 53:984-988, 2006.
19. Reah G, Lyons GR, Wilson RC: Anaesthesia for caesarean section in a patient with Charcot-Marie-Tooth disease. Anaesthesia 53:586-588, 1998.
20. Scull T, Weeks S: Epidural analgesia for labour in a patient with Charcot-Marie-Tooth disease. Can J Anaesth 43:1150-1152, 1996.
21. Sugai K, Sugai Y: [Epidural anesthesia for a patient with Charcot-Marie-Tooth disease, bronchial asthma and hypothyroidism.] Masui 38:688-691, 1989.
22. Tanaka S, Tsuchida H, Namiki A: [Epidural anesthesia for a patient with Charcot-Marie-Tooth disease, mitral valve prolapse syndrome and second degree AV block.] Masui 43:931-933, 1994.
23. Schmitt HJ, Muenster T, Schmidt J: Central neural blockade in Charcot-Marie-Tooth disease. Can J Anaesth 51:1049-1050, 2004.
24. Dubowitz V: Muscle Disorders in Childhood, 2nd ed. Philadelphia, WB Saunders, 1995, pp 34-132.
25. Dalakas M, Palace J, Rose M: The muscular dystrophies. *In* Barnes P, Hilton-Jones D (eds): Myopathies in Clinical Practice. London, Martin Dunitz, 2003, pp 59-83.
26. Do T: Muscular Dystrophy. Available from http://www.imedicine.com/printtopic.asp?bookid=9&topic=418/ Accessed March 30, 2007.
27. Emery A: Population frequencies of inherited neuromuscular diseases—a world survey. Neuromuscul Disord 1:19-29, 1991.
28. Sano M, Saito F, Yamamoto K, et al: Duchenne muscular dystrophy in a female with 45,X/46,XX chromosome constitution. Jinrui Idengaku Zasshi 32:257-262, 1987.
29. Urban M, Lahlou S: Muscle diseases. *In* Fleisher L (ed): Anesthesia and Uncommon Diseases. Philadelphia, Saunders Elsevier, 2006, pp 303-325.
30. Hoffman E: Dystrophin: The protein product of the Duchenne muscular dystrophy locus. Cell 51:919-928, 1987.
31. Leibowitz D, Dubowitz V: Intellect and behaviour in Duchenne muscular dystrophy. Dev Med Child Neurol 23:577-590, 1981.
32. Finsterer J, Stollberger C: The heart in human dystrophinopathies. Cardiology 99:1-19, 2003.
33. Perloff JK, Henze E, Schelbert HR: Alterations in regional myocardial metabolism, perfusion, and wall motion in Duchenne muscular dystrophy studied by radionuclide imaging. Circulation 69:33-42, 1984.
34. Morris P: Duchenne muscular dystrophy: A challenge for the anaesthetist. Paediatr Anaesth 7:1-4, 1997.
35. Hahn A, Bach JR, Delaubier A, et al: Clinical implications of maximal respiratory pressure determinations for individuals with Duchenne muscular dystrophy. Arch Phys Med Rehabil 78:1-6, 1997.
36. Ames WA, Hayes JA, Crawford MW: The role of corticosteroids in Duchenne muscular dystrophy: A review for the anesthetist. Paediatr Anaesth 15:3-8, 2005.
37. Kawaai H, Tanaka K, Yamazaki S: Continuous infusion propofol general anesthesia for dental treatment in patients with progressive muscular dystrophy. Anesth Prog 52:12-16, 2005.
38. Molyneux MK: Anaesthetic management during labour of a manifesting carrier of Duchenne muscular dystrophy. Int J Obstet Anesth 14:58-61, 2005.
39. Angermann C, Spes C, Pongratz D: [Cardiac manifestation of progressive muscular dystrophy of the Duchenne type.] Z Kardiol 75:542-551, 1986.
40. Smith CL, Bush GH: Anaesthesia and progressive muscular dystrophy. Br J Anaesth 57:1113-1118, 1985.
41. Webster R: Respiratory function as a measure of muscle strength in young boys with Duchenne muscular dystrophy. *In* Neurology. University of N.S.W., School of Women and Children's Health, 2003.
42. Stevens RD: Neuromuscular disorders and anesthesia. Curr Opin Anaesthesiol 14:693-698, 2001.
43. Breucking E, Reimnitz P, Schara U, Mortier W: [Anesthetic complications. The incidence of severe anesthetic complications in patients and families with progressive muscular dystrophy of the Duchenne and Becker types.] Anaesthesist 49:187-195, 2000.
44. Benson ER, Thompson JD, Smith BG, Banta JV: Results and morbidity in a consecutive series of patients undergoing spinal fusion for neuromuscular scoliosis. Spine 23:2308-2317, discussion 2318, 1998.
45. Miller F, Moseley CF, Koreska J: Spinal fusion in Duchenne muscular dystrophy. Dev Med Child Neurol 34:775-786, 1992.
46. Jenkins JG, Bohn D, Edmonds JF, et al: Evaluation of pulmonary function in muscular dystrophy patients requiring spinal surgery. Crit Care Med 10:645-649, 1982.
47. Stoelting R, Dierdorf S: Anesthesia and Co-existing Disease. Philadelphia, Churchill Livingstone, 2002, pp 505-549.
48. Brandom B, Apuya J: Epidemiological challenges in malignant hyperthermia. Available from http://www.publichealth.pitt.edu/supercourse/SupercoursePPT/4011-5001/4881.ppt/ Accessed July 2007.
49. Farell P: Anesthesia-induced rhabdomyolysis causing cardiac arrest: Case report and review of anesthesia and the dystrophinopathies. Anesth Intensive Care 22:597-601, 1994.
50. Schummer W, Schummer C: Acute heart failure during spinal surgery in a boy with Duchenne muscular dystrophy. Br J Anaesth 92:149, author reply 149-150, 2004.
51. Ririe DG, Shapiro F, Sethna NF: The response of patients with Duchenne's muscular dystrophy to neuromuscular blockade with vecuronium. Anesthesiology 88:351-354, 1998.
52. Yemen TA, McClain C: Muscular dystrophy, anesthesia and the safety of inhalational agents revisited; again. Paediatr Anaesth 16:105-108, 2006.
53. Fairfield MC: Increased propofol requirements in a child with Duchenne muscular dystrophy. Anaesthesia 48:1013, 1993.
54. Murat I, Esteve KC, Montay G, et al: Pharmacokinetics and cardiovascular effects of bupivacaine during epidural anesthesia in children with Duchenne muscular dystrophy. Anesthesiology 67:249-252, 1987.
55. Kirschner J, Bonnemann CG: The congenital and limb-girdle muscular dystrophies: Sharpening the focus, blurring the boundaries. Arch Neurol 61:189-199, 2004.
56. Moro C, Dangelser G, Veyckemans F: [Anesthetic management of a child with delta sarcoglycanopathy.] Ann Fr Anesth Reanim 26:359-362, 2007.
57. Egi M, Tokioka H, Chikai T, et al: [Propofol anesthesia for a patient with progressive muscular dystrophy.] Masui 51:196-198, 2002.
58. Pash MP, Balaton J, Eagle C: Anaesthetic management of a parturient with severe muscular dystrophy, lumbar lordosis and a difficult airway. Can J Anaesth 43:959-963, 1996.
59. Myotonic Dystrophy, November 2006. Available from http://ghr.nlm.nih.gov/condition=myotonic-dystrophy/ Accessed July 2007.
60. Bird T: Myotonic Dystrophy Type 1, 2005. Available from http://www.genetests.org/query?dz=myotonic-d/ Accessed July 2007.
61. Krivickas LS, Ansved T, Suh D, Frontera WR: Contractile properties of single muscle fibers in myotonic dystrophy. Muscle Nerve 23:529-537, 2000.
62. Dalton J, Ranum L, Day J: Myotonic dystrophy type 2. *In* GeneReviews 2007. Available at http://www.geneclinics.org/profiles/myotonic-d2.
63. Mathieu J, Allard P, Gobeil M, et al: Anesthetic and surgical complications in 219 cases of myotonic dystrophy. Neurology 49:1646-1650, 1997.
64. Catena V, Del Monte DD, Rubini A, et al: Anesthesia and myotonic dystrophy (Steinert's syndrome). The role of total intravenous anesthesia with propofol, cisatracurium and remifentanyl. Case report. Minerva Anestesiol 73:475-479, 2007.
65. Lehmann-Horn F, Reinhardt R, Jurkat-Rott K: Altered excitability of the cell membrane. *In* Engel A, Franzini-Armstrong C (eds): Myology. New York, McGraw-Hill, 2004, pp 1257-1300.
66. Farbu E, Softeland E, Bindoff LA: Anaesthetic complications associated with myotonia congenita: Case study and comparison with other myotonic disorders. Acta Anaesthesiol Scand 47:630-634, 2003.

67. Newberg LA, Lambert EH, Gronert GA: Failure to induce malignant hyperthermia in myotonic goats. Br J Anaesth 55:57-60, 1983.
68. Beck CL, Fahlke C, George AL Jr: Molecular basis for decreased muscle chloride conductance in the myotonic goat. Proc Natl Acad Sci U S A 93:11248-11252, 1996.
69. Rosenbaum HK, Miller JD: Malignant hyperthermia and myotonic disorders. Anesthesiol Clin North Am 20:623-664, 2002.
70. North K: Congenital myopathies. *In* Engel A, Franzini-Armstrong C (eds): Myology. New York, McGraw-Hill, 2004, pp 1473-1533.
71. Herman GE, Finegold M, Zhao W, et al: Medical complications in long-term survivors with X-linked myotubular myopathy. J Pediatr 134:206-214, 1999.
72. Breslin D, Reid J, Hayes A, Mirakhur RK: Anaesthesia in myotubular (centronuclear) myopathy. Anaesthesia 55:471-474, 2000.
73. Costi D, van der Walt JH: General anesthesia in an infant with X-linked myotubular myopathy. Paediatr Anaesth 14:964-968, 2004.
74. García-Aguado R, Núñez M, Tommasi Rosso M, et al: [Myotubular myopathy (centronuclear) and expected difficult intubation. Anesthetic management.] Rev Esp Anestesiol Reanim 41:302-303, 1994.
75. Gottschalk A, Heiman-Patterson T, deQuevedo R 2nd, Quinn PD: General anesthesia for a patient with centronuclear (myotubular) myopathy. Anesthesiology 89:1018-1020, 1998.
76. Schmid E, Johr M, Berger TM: X-linked myotubular myopathy: Anesthetic management for muscle biopsy. Paediatr Anaesth 16:218-220, 2006.
77. Tokarz A, Gaszynski T, Gaszynski W, Arkuszewski P: General anaesthesia with remifentanil and propofol for a patient with centronuclear (myotubular) myopathy. Eur J Anaesthesiol 19:842-844, 2002.
78. Dorchies OM, Laporte J, Wagner S, et al: Normal innervation and differentiation of X-linked myotubular myopathy muscle cells in a nerve-muscle coculture system. Neuromuscul Disord 11:736-746, 2001.
79. Raghavan V: Glucose-6-phosphatase deficiency. 2007. Available from http://www.emedicine.com/med/byname/Glucose-6-Phosphatase-Deficiency.htm/ Accessed July 2007.
80. Rake JP, Visser G, Labrune P, et al: Guidelines for management of glycogen storage disease type I—European Study on Glycogen Storage Disease Type I (ESGSD I). Eur J Pediatr 161(Suppl 1):S112-S119, 2002.
81. Visser G, Rake JP, Labrune P, et al: Consensus guidelines for management of glycogen storage disease type 1b—European Study on Glycogen Storage Disease Type 1. Eur J Pediatr 161(Suppl 1):S120-S123, 2002.
82. Kakinohana M, Tokumine J, Shimabukoro T, et al: [Patient-controlled sedation using propofol for a patient with von Gierke disease.] Masui 47:1104-1108, 1998.
83. Kawai T: [Anesthetic management for an emergency operation in a patient with von Gierke disease.] Masui 54:924-925, 2005.
84. Loonen MC, Busch HF, Koster JF, et al: A family with different clinical forms of acid maltase deficiency (glycogenosis type II): Biochemical and genetic studies. Neurology 31:1209-1216, 1981.
85. Engel A, Hirschhorn R, Huie M: Acid maltase deficiency. *In* Engel A, Franzini-Armstrong C (eds): Myology. New York, McGraw-Hill, 2004, pp 1559-1586.
86. Anderson W: Glycogen Storage Disease, Type II. Jan 18, 2006. Available from http://www.emedicine.com/med/topic908.htm/ Accessed July 2007.
87. Ehlers KH, Hagstrom JW, Lukas DS, et al: Glycogen-storage disease of the myocardium with obstruction to left ventricular outflow. Circulation 25:96-109, 1962.
88. Bulkley BH, Hutchins GM: Pompe's disease presenting as hypertrophic myocardiopathy with Wolff-Parkinson-White syndrome. Am Heart J 96:246-252, 1978.
89. Weinik M, King F: Acid Maltase Deficiency Myopathy. eMedicine, 2006.
90. Makos MM, McComb RD, Hart MN, Bennett DR: Alpha-glucosidase deficiency and basilar artery aneurysm: Report of a sibship. Ann Neurol 22:629-633, 1987.
91. Gitlin MC, Jahr JS, Margolis MA, McCain J: Is mivacurium chloride effective in electroconvulsive therapy? A report of four cases, including a patient with myasthenia gravis. Anesth Analg 77:392-394, 1993.
92. Kotani N, Hirota K, Anzawa N, et al: Motor and sensory disability has a strong relationship to induction dose of thiopental in patients with the hypertropic variety of Charcot-Marie-Tooth syndrome. Anesth Analg 82:182-186, 1996.
93. Ing RJ, Cook DR, Bengur RA, et al: Anaesthetic management of infants with glycogen storage disease type II: A physiological approach. Paediatr Anaesth 14:514-519, 2004.
94. McFarlane HJ, Soni N: Pompe's disease and anaesthesia. Anaesthesia 41:1219-1224, 1986.
95. Mohiddin SA, Fananapazir L: Systolic compression of epicardial coronary and intramural arteries in children with hypertrophic cardiomyopathy. Tex Heart Inst J 29:290-298, 2002.
96. DiMauro S, Bonilla E: Mitochondrial encephalomyopathies. *In* Engel A, Franzini-Armstrong C (eds): Myology. New York, McGraw-Hill, 2004, pp 1623-1662.
97. Siciliano G, Volpi L, Piazza S, et al: Functional diagnostics in mitochondrial diseases. Biosci Rep 27:53-67, 2007.
98. Wisely NA, Cook PR: General anaesthesia in a man with mitochondrial myopathy undergoing eye surgery. Eur J Anaesthesiol 18:333-335, 2001.
99. Mehndiratta MM, Agarwal P, Tatke M, Krishmamurthy M: Neurological mitochondrial cytopathies. Neurol India 50:162-167, 2002.
100. Wallace JJ, Perndt H, Skinner M: Anaesthesia and mitochondrial disease. Paediatr Anaesth 8:249-254, 1998.
101. Swash M, Schwartz MS, Sargeant MK: The significance of ragged-red fibres in neuromuscular disease. J Neurol Sci 38:347-355, 1978.
102. Shipton EA, Prosser DO: Mitochondrial myopathies and anaesthesia. Eur J Anaesthesiol 21:173-178, 2004.
103. Levy E, Muravchick S: Mitochondrial diseases. *In* Fleisher L (ed): Anesthesia and Uncommon Diseases. Philadelphia, Saunders Elsevier, 2006, pp 455-467.
104. James RH: Thiopentone and ophthalmoplegia plus. Anaesthesia 40:88, 1985.
105. James RH: Induction agent sensitivity and ophthalmoplegia plus. Anaesthesia 41:216, 1986.
106. Driessen J, Willems S, Dercksen S, et al: Anesthesia-related morbidity and mortality after surgery for muscle biopsy in children with mitochondrial defects. Paediatr Anaesth 17:16-21, 2007.
107. Burns AM, Shelly MP: Anaesthesia for patients with mitochondrial myopathy. Anaesthesia 44:975-977, 1989.
108. Kelly A, O'Connor M: Mitochondrial myopathy and anaesthesia. Anaesthesia 45:596, 1990.
109. Ramchandra DS, Anisya V, Gourie-Devi M: Ketamine monoanaesthesia for diagnostic muscle biopsy in neuromuscular disorders in infancy and childhood: Floppy infant syndrome. Can J Anaesth 37:474-476, 1990.
110. Guasch E, Civantos B, Aguilar JM, et al: Progressive external ophthalmoplegia and ambulatory remifentanil-propofol based anaesthesia. Anaesthesia 58:607-608, 2003.
111. Stowe DF, Kevin LG: Cardiac preconditioning by volatile anesthetic agents: A defining role for altered mitochondrial bioenergetics. Antioxid Redox Signal 6:439-448, 2004.
112. Stadnicka A, Marinovic L, Ljubkovic M, et al: Volatile anesthetic–induced cardiac preconditioning. J Anesth 21:212-219, 2007.
113. Lauwers MH, Van Lersberghe C, Camu F: Inhalation anaesthesia and the Kearns-Sayre syndrome. Anaesthesia 49:876-878, 1994.
114. Morgan PG, Hoppel CL, Sedensky MM: Mitochondrial defects and anesthetic sensitivity. Anesthesiology 96:1268-1270, 2002.
115. Allen GC: Bispectral index and mitochondrial myopathies. Anesthesiology 98:282, author reply 283, 2003.
116. Frei FJ, Haemmerle MH, Brunner R, Kern C: Minimum alveolar concentration for halothane in children with cerebral palsy and severe mental retardation. Anaesthesia 52:1056-1060, 1997.
117. Naguib M, el Dawlatly AA, Ashour M, al-Bunyan M: Sensitivity to mivacurium in a patient with mitochondrial myopathy. Anesthesiology 84:1506-1509, 1996.
118. Finsterer J, Stratil U, Bittner R, Sporn P: Increased sensitivity to rocuronium and atracurium in mitochondrial myopathy. Can J Anaesth 45:781-784, 1998.
119. Sharma AD, Erb T, Schulman SR, et al: Anaesthetic considerations for a child with combined Prader-Willi syndrome and mitochondrial myopathy. Paediatr Anaesth 11:488-490, 2001.
120. D'Ambra MN, Dedrick D, Savarese JJ: Kearns-Sayre syndrome and pancuronium-succinylcholine–induced neuromuscular blockade. Anesthesiology 51:343-345, 1979.
121. Wiesel S, Bevan JC, Samuel J, Donati F: Vecuronium neuromuscular blockade in a child with mitochondrial myopathy. Anesth Analg 72:696-699, 1991.
122. Rowe RW, Helander E: Anesthetic management of a patient with systemic carnitine deficiency. Anesth Analg 71:295-297, 1990.
123. Rosaeg OP, Morrison S, MacLeod JP: Anaesthetic management of labour and delivery in the parturient with mitochondrial myopathy. Can J Anaesth 43:403-407, 1996.
124. Hsiao PN, Cheng YJ, Tseng HC, et al: Spinal anesthesia in MELAS syndrome: A case with mitochondrial myopathy, encephalopathy, lactic acidosis and stroke-like episodes. Acta Anaesthesiol Sin 38:107-110, 2000.
125. Sasano N, Fujita Y, So M, et al: Anesthetic management of a patient with mitochondrial myopathy, encephalopathy, lactic acidosis, and stroke-like episodes (MELAS) during laparotomy. J Anesth 21:72-75, 2007.
126. Farag E, Argalious M, Narouze S, et al: The anesthetic management of ventricular septal defect (VSD) repair in a child with mitochondrial cytopathy. Can J Anaesth 49:958-962, 2002.
127. Vincent A, Palace J, Hilton-Jones D: Myasthenia gravis. Lancet 357:2122-2128, 2001.
128. Lindstrom JM: Acetylcholine receptors and myasthenia. Muscle Nerve 23:453-477, 2000.
129. Eisenkraft JB, Book WJ, Mann SM, et al: Resistance to succinylcholine in myasthenia gravis: A dose-response study. Anesthesiology 69:760-763, 1988.

130. Baraka A: Suxamethonium block in the myasthenic patient. Correlation with plasma cholinesterase. Anaesthesia 47:217-219, 1992.
131. Seigne RD, Scott RP: Mivacurium chloride and myasthenia gravis. Br J Anaesth 72:468-469, 1994.
132. Kim JM, Mangold J: Sensitivity to both vecuronium and neostigmine in a sero-negative myasthenic patient. Br J Anaesth 63:497-500, 1989.
133. Baraka A: Onset of neuromuscular block in myasthenic patients. Br J Anaesth 69:227-228, 1992.
134. Abel M, Eisenkraft JB: Anesthetic implications of myasthenia gravis. Mt Sinai J Med 69:31-37, 2002.
135. Takamori M, Maruta T, Komai K: Lambert-Eaton myasthenic syndrome as an autoimmune calcium-channelopathy. Neurosci Res 36:183-191, 2000.
136. Hewett SJ, Atchison WD: Serum and plasma from patients with Lambert-Eaton myasthenic syndrome reduce depolarization-dependent uptake of $^{45}Ca^{2+}$ into rat cortical synaptosomes. Brain Res 566:320-324, 1991.
137. Jurkat-Rott K, Lehmann-Horn F: Paroxysmal muscle weakness: The familial periodic paralyses. J Neurol 253:1391-1398, 2006.
138. Viscomi CM, Ptacek LJ, Dudley D: Anesthetic management of familial hypokalemic periodic paralysis during parturition. Anesth Analg 88:1081-1082, 1999.
139. Robinson JE, Morin VI, Douglas MJ, Wilson RD: Familial hypokalemic periodic paralysis and Wolff-Parkinson-White syndrome in pregnancy. Can J Anaesth 47:160-164, 2000.
140. Periodic Paralyses. 2007. Available from http://www.clevelandclinic.org/health/health-info/docs/2400/2452.asp?index=9499/ Accessed December 2007.
141. Depoix JP, Julliard JM, Aubry P: Propofol-remifentanil target-controlled anesthesia in a patient with hyperkalemic familial periodic paralysis. Anesth Analg 99:302, 2004.
142. Aouad R, Atanassoff PG: Epidural anesthesia in a patient with hyperkalemic periodic paralysis undergoing orthopedic surgery. Can J Anaesth 51:92, 2004.
143. Aarons JJ, Moon RE, Camporesi EM: General anesthesia and hyperkalemic periodic paralysis. Anesthesiology 71:303-304, 1989.
144. Ashwood EM, Russell WJ, Burrow DD: Hyperkalaemic periodic paralysis and anaesthesia. Anaesthesia 47:579-584, 1992.
145. Lehmann-Horn F, Iaizzo PA: Are myotonias and periodic paralyses associated with susceptibility to malignant hyperthermia? Br J Anaesth 65:692-697, 1990.
146. Weller JF, Elliott RA, Pronovost PJ: Spinal anesthesia for a patient with familial hyperkalemic periodic paralysis. Anesthesiology 97:259-260, 2002.
147. Wilson RD, Nichols RJ, Dent TE: Disturbances of the oxidative-phosphorylation mechanism as a possible etiological factor in sudden unexplained hyperthermia occurring during anesthesia. Anesthesiology 27:231, 1996.
148. Ording H: Investigation of malignant hyperthermia susceptibility in Denmark. Dan Med Bull 43:111-125, 1996.
149. Robinson R, Carpenter D, Shaw MA, et al: Mutations in *RYR1* in malignant hyperthermia and central core disease. Hum Mutat 27:977-989, 2006.
150. Harrison GG, Isaacs H: Malignant hyperthermia. An historical vignette. Anaesthesia 47:54-56, 1992.
151. Ombrédanne L: De l'influence de l'anesthésique employé dans la ganèse des accidents post-opératoires de pâleurhyperthermie observés chez les nourrissons. Rev Med Française 10:617, 1929.
152. Denborough MA, Lovell R: Anaesthetic deaths in a family. Lancet 2:45, 1960.
153. Kalow W, Britt BA, Terreau ME, Haist C: Metabolic error of muscle metabolism after recovery from malignant hyperthermia. Lancet 296:895-898, 1970.
154. Britt BA, Locher WG, Kalow W: Hereditary aspects of malignant hyperthermia. Can Anaesth Soc J 16:89-98, 1969.
155. Ball RA, Annis CL, Topel DG, Christian LL: Clinical and laboratory diagnosis of porcine stress syndrome. Vet Med Small Anim Clin 68:1156-1159, 1973.
156. Briskey EJ: Etiological status and associated studies of pale, soft, exudative porcine musculature. Adv Food Res 13:89-178, 1964.
157. Hall LW, Woolf N, Bradley JW, Jolly DW: Unusual reaction to suxamethonium chloride. BMJ 2:1305, 1966.
158. Fujii J, Otsu K, Zorzoto F, et al: Identification of a mutation in porcine ryanodine receptor associated with malignant hyperthermia. Science 253:448-451, 1991.
159. Harrison GG: Control of the malignant hyperpyrexic syndrome in MHS swine by dantrolene sodium. Br J Anaesth 47:62-65, 1975.
160. Kolb ME, Horne ML, Martz R: Dantrolene in human malignant hyperthermia. Anesthesiology 56:254-262, 1982.
161. López JR, Alamo LA, Jones D, et al: [Determination of intracellular free calcium concentration, in vivo, in swine susceptible to malignant hyperthermia syndrome.] Acta Cient Venez 36:102-104, 1985.
162. López JR, Alamo LA, Jones D, et al: $[Ca^{2+}]_i$ in muscles of malignant hyperthermia susceptible pigs determined in vivo with Ca^{2+} selective microelectrodes. Muscle Nerve 9:85-86, 1986.
163. López JR, Allen PD, Alamo LA, et al: Myoplasmic free $[Ca^{2+}]$ during a malignant hyperthermia episode in swine. Muscle Nerve 11:82-88, 1988.
164. López JR, Gerardi A, López MJ, Allen PD: Effects of dantrolene on myoplasmic free $[Ca^{2+}]$ measured in vivo in patients susceptible to malignant hyperthermia. Anesthesiology 76:711-719, 1992.
165. Pessah IN, Waterhouse AL, Casida JE: The calcium-ryanodine receptor complex of skeletal and cardiac muscle. Biochem Biophys Res Commune 128:449-456, 1985.
166. Pessah IN, Anderson KW, Casida JE: Solubilization and separation of Ca^{2+}-ATPase from the Ca^{2+}-ryanodine receptor complex. Biochem Biophys Res Commune 139:235-243, 1986.
167. Beam KG, Tanabe T, Numa S: Structure, function, and regulation of the skeletal muscle dihydropyridine receptor. Ann N Y Acad Sci 560:127-137, 1989.
168. Tanabe T, Beam KG, Adams BA, et al: Regions of the skeletal muscle dihydropyridine receptor critical for excitation-contraction coupling. Nature 346:567-569, 1990.
169. Nakai J, Tanabe T, Konno T, et al: Localization in the II-III loop of the dihydropyridine receptor of a sequence critical for excitation-contraction coupling. J Biol Chem 273:24983-24986, 1998.
170. Flucher BE, Franzini-Armstrong C: Formation of junctions involved in excitation-contraction coupling in skeletal and cardiac muscle. Proc Natl Acad Sci U S A 93:8101-8106, 1996.
171. Cherednichenko G, Hurme AM, Fessenden JD, et al: Conformational activation of Ca^{2+} entry by depolarization of skeletal myotubes. Proc Natl Acad Sci U S A 101:15793-15798, 2004.
172. Gaburjakova M, Gaburjakova J, Reiken S, et al: FKBP12 binding modulates ryanodine receptor channel gating. J Biol Chem 276:16931-16935, 2001.
173. Meissner G: Regulation of mammalian ryanodine receptors. Front Biosci 7:d2072-d2080, 2002.
174. Ward CW, Feng W, Tu J, et al: Homer protein increases activation of Ca^{2+} sparks in permeabilized skeletal muscle. J Biol Chem 279:5781-5787, 2004.
175. Cherednichenko G, Ward CW, Feng W, et al: Enhanced excitation-coupled calcium entry (ECCE) in myotubes expressing malignant hyperthermia mutation R163C is attenuated by dantrolene. Mol Pharmacol 73:1203-1212, 2008.
176. Yang T, Allen PD, Pessah IN, Lopez JR: Enhanced excitation-coupled calcium entry in myotubes is associated with expression of *RYR1* malignant hyperthermia mutations. J Biol Chem 282:37471-37478, 2007.
177. Yang T, Esteve E, Pessah IN, et al: Elevated resting $[Ca^{2+}](i)$ in myotubes expressing malignant hyperthermia RyR1 cDNAs is partially restored by modulation of passive calcium leak from the SR. Am J Physiol Cell Physiol 292:C1591-C1598, 2007.
178. Wappler F, Anetseder M, Baur CP, et al: Multicentre evaluation of in vitro contracture testing with bolus administration of 4-chloro-*m*-cresol for diagnosis of malignant hyperthermia susceptibility. Eur J Anaesthesiol 20:528-536, 2003.
179. Yang T, Ta TA, Pessah IN, Allen PD: Functional defects in six ryanodine receptor isoform-1 (RyR1) mutations associated with malignant hyperthermia and their impact on skeletal excitation-contraction coupling. J Biol Chem 278:25722-25730, 2003.
180. Reuter DA, Anetseder M, Müller R, et al: The ryanodine contracture test may help diagnose susceptibility to malignant hyperthermia. Can J Anaesth 50:643-648, 2003.
181. Pessah IN, Stambuk RA, Casida JE: Ca^{2+}-activated ryanodine binding: Mechanisms of sensitivity and intensity modulation by Mg^{2+}, caffeine, and adenine nucleotides. Mol Pharmacol 31:232-238, 1987.
182. Zimanyi I, Pessah IN: Pharmacological characterization of the specific binding of $[^3H]$ryanodine to rat brain microsomal membranes. Brain Res 561:181-191, 1991.
183. Jona I, Szegedi C, Sárközi S, et al: Altered inhibition of the rat skeletal ryanodine receptor/calcium release channel by magnesium in the presence of ATP. Pflugers Arch 441:729-738, 2001.
184. Laver D: The power of single channel recording and analysis: Its application to ryanodine receptors in lipid bilayers. Clin Exp Pharmacol Physiol 28:675-686, 2001.
185. Laver DR, Baynes TM, Dulhunty AF: Magnesium inhibition of ryanodine-receptor calcium channels: Evidence for two independent mechanisms. J Membr Biol 156:213-229, 1997.
186. Voss AA, Allen PD, Pessah IN, Perez CF: Allosterically coupled calcium and magnesium binding sites are unmasked by ryanodine receptor chimeras. Biochem Biophys Res Commun 366:988-993, 2008.
187. Lamb GD: Ca^{2+} inactivation, Mg^{2+} inhibition and malignant hyperthermia. J Muscle Res Cell Motil 14:554-556, 1993.
188. Laver DR, Owen VJ, Juankar PR, et al: Reduced inhibitory effect of Mg^{2+} on ryanodine receptor-Ca^{2+} release channels in malignant hyperthermia. Biophys J 73:1913-1924, 1997.
189. Chelu MG, Goonasekera SA, Durham WJ, et al: Heat- and anesthesia-induced malignant hyperthermia in an RyR1 knock-in mouse. FASEB J 20:329-330, 2006.
190. Yang T, Riehl J, Esteve E, et al: Pharmacologic and functional characterization of malignant hyperthermia in the R163C RyR1 knock-in mouse. Anesthesiology 105:1164-1175, 2006.

191. López JR, Linares N, Pessah IN, Allen PD: Enhanced response to caffeine and 4-chloro-*m*-cresol in malignant hyperthermia–susceptible muscle is related in part to chronically elevated resting $[Ca^{2+}]_i$. Am J Physiol Cell Physiol 288:C606-C612, 2005.
192. Avila G, Dirksen RT: Functional effects of central core disease mutations in the cytoplasmic region of the skeletal muscle ryanodine receptor. J Gen Physiol 118:277-290, 2001.
193. Avila G, O'Brien JJ, Dirksen RT: Excitation-contraction uncoupling by a human central core disease mutation in the ryanodine receptor. Proc Natl Acad Sci U S A 98:4215-4220, 2001.
194. Avila G, O'Connell KM, Dirksen RT: The pore region of the skeletal muscle ryanodine receptor is a primary locus for excitation-contraction uncoupling in central core disease. J Gen Physiol 121:277-286, 2003.
195. Dirksen RT, Avila G: Altered ryanodine receptor function in central core disease: Leaky or uncoupled Ca^{2+} release channels? Trends Cardiovasc Med 12:189-197, 2002.
196. Weiss RG, O'Connell KM, Flucher BE, et al: Functional analysis of the R1086H malignant hyperthermia mutation in the DHPR reveals an unexpected influence of the III-IV loop on skeletal muscle EC coupling. Am J Physiol Cell Physiol 287:C1094-C1102, 2004.
197. Ikemoto N, Yamamoto T: Regulation of calcium release by interdomain interaction within ryanodine receptors. Front Biosci 7:d671-d683, 2002.
198. Jones DE, Ryan JF, Taylor B, et al: Pancuronium in large doses protects susceptible swine from halothane induced malignant hyperthermia. Anesthesiology 63:A344, 1985.
199. Hurne AM, O'Brien JJ, Wingrove D, et al: Ryanodine receptor type 1 (RyR1) mutations C4958S and C4961S reveal excitation-coupled calcium entry (ECCE) is independent of sarcoplasmic reticulum store depletion. J Biol Chem 280:36994-37004, 2005.
200. Putney JW Jr, Broad LM, Braun FJ, et al: Mechanisms of capacitative calcium entry. J Cell Sci 114:2223-2229, 2001.
201. Kurebayashi N, Ogawa Y: Depletion of Ca^{2+} in the sarcoplasmic reticulum stimulates Ca^{2+} entry into mouse skeletal muscle fibres. J Physiol 533:185-199, 2001.
202. Ma J, Pan Z: Junctional membrane structure and store operated calcium entry in muscle cells. Front Biosci 8:d242-d255, 2003.
203. Pan Z, Yang D, Nagaraj RY, et al: Dysfunction of store-operated calcium channel in muscle cells lacking mg29. Nat Cell Biol 4:379-383, 2002.
204. Zhao X, Weisleder N, Han X, et al: Azumolene inhibits a component of store-operated calcium entry coupled to the skeletal muscle ryanodine receptor. J Biol Chem 281:33477-33486, 2006.
205. Yamaguchi N, Igami K, Kasai M: Kinetics of depolarization-induced calcium release from skeletal muscle triads in vitro. J Biochem (Tokyo) 121:432-439, 1997.
206. Paul-Pletzer K, Yamamoto T, Bhat MB, et al: Identification of a dantrolene-binding sequence on the skeletal muscle ryanodine receptor. J Biol Chem 277:34918-34923, 2002.
207. Monnier N, Procaccio V, Stieglitz P, Lunardi J: Malignant-hyperthermia susceptibility is associated with a mutation of the alpha 1-subunit of the human dihydropyridine-sensitive L-type voltage-dependent calcium-channel receptor in skeletal muscle. Am J Hum Genet 60:1316-1325, 1997.
208. Sambuughin N, Sei Y, Gallagher KL, et al: North American malignant hyperthermia population: Screening of the ryanodine receptor gene and identification of novel mutations. Anesthesiology 95:594-599, 2001.
209. Brown RL, Pollack AN, Couchman KG, et al: A novel ryanodine receptor mutation and genotype-phenotype correlation in a large malignant hyperthermia New Zealand Maori pedigree. Hum Mol Genet 9:1515-1524, 2000.
210. Girard T, Urwyler A, Censier K, et al: Genotype-phenotype comparison of the Swiss malignant hyperthermia population. Hum Mutat 18:357-358, 2001.
211. Brandt A, Schleithoff L, Jurkat-Rott K, et al: Screening of the ryanodine receptor gene in 105 malignant hyperthermia families: Novel mutations and concordance with the in vitro contracture test. Hum Mol Genet 8:2055-2062, 1999.
212. Rueffert H, Olthoff D, Deutrich C, et al: A new mutation in the skeletal ryanodine receptor gene (*RYR1*) is potentially causative of malignant hyperthermia, central core disease, and severe skeletal malformation. Am J Med Genet A 124:248-254, 2004.
213. Robinson R, Hopkins P, Carsana A, et al: Several interacting genes influence the malignant hyperthermia phenotype. Hum Genet 112:217-218, 2003.
214. Gillard EF, Otsu K, Fujii J, et al: A substitution of cysteine for arginine 614 in the ryanodine receptor is potentially causative of human malignant hyperthermia. Genomics 11:751-755, 1991.
215. Sei Y, Sambuughin NN, Davis EJ, et al: Malignant hyperthermia in North America: Genetic screening of the three hot spots in the type I ryanodine receptor gene. Anesthesiology 101:824-830, 2004.
216. Davis M, Brown R, Dickson A, et al: Malignant hyperthermia associated with exercise-induced rhabdomyolysis or congenital abnormalities and a novel *RYR1* mutation in New Zealand and Australian pedigrees. Br J Anaesth 88:508-515, 2002.
217. Oyamada H, Oguchi K, Sitoh N, et al: Novel mutations in C-terminal channel region of the ryanodine receptor in malignant hyperthermia patients. Jpn J Pharmacol 88:159-166, 2002.
218. Yeh HM, Tsai MC, Su YN, et al: Denaturing high performance liquid chromatography screening of ryanodine receptor type 1 gene in patients with malignant hyperthermia in Taiwan and identification of a novel mutation (Y522C). Anesth Analg 101:1401-1406, 2005.
219. Monnier N, Krivasic-Horber R, Payen JF, et al: Presence of two different genetic traits in malignant hyperthermia families: Implication for genetic analysis, diagnosis, and incidence of malignant hyperthermia susceptibility. Anesthesiology 97:1067-1074, 2002.
220. Fletcher JE, Tripolitis L, Hubert M, et al: Genotype and phenotype relationships for mutations in the ryanodine receptor in patients referred for diagnosis of malignant hyperthermia. Br J Anaesth 75:307-310, 1995.
221. Lynch PJ, Krivasic-Horber R, Reyford H, et al: Identification of heterozygous and homozygous individuals with the novel *RYR1* mutation Cys35Arg in a large kindred. Anesthesiology 86:620-626, 1997.
222. Monnier N, Ferreiro A, Marty I, et al: A homozygous splicing mutation causing a depletion of skeletal muscle RYR1 is associated with multi-minicore disease congenital myopathy with ophthalmoplegia. Hum Mol Genet 12:1171-1178, 2003.
223. Rueffert H, Olthoff, Deutrich C, et al: Homozygous and heterozygous Arg614Cys mutations (1840C→T) in the ryanodine receptor gene co-segregate with malignant hyperthermia susceptibility in a German family. Br J Anaesth 87:240-245, 2001.
224. Zhou H, Brockington M, Jungbluth H, et al: Epigenetic allele silencing unveils recessive *RYR1* mutations in core myopathies. Am J Hum Genet 79:859-868, 2006.
225. Urwyler A, Deufel T, McCarthy T, et al: Guidelines for molecular genetic detection of susceptibility to malignant hyperthermia. Br J Anaesth 86:283-287, 2001.
226. Robinson RL, Brooks C, Brown SL, et al: *RYR1* mutations causing central core disease are associated with more severe malignant hyperthermia in vitro contracture test phenotypes. Hum Mutat 20:88-97, 2002.
227. Rueffert H, Othoff D, Deutrich C, et al: Mutation screening in the ryanodine receptor 1 gene (*RYR1*) in patients susceptible to malignant hyperthermia who show definite IVCT results: Identification of three novel mutations. Acta Anaesthesiol Scand 46:692-698, 2002.
228. Allen GC, Brubaker CL: Human malignant hyperthermia associated with desflurane anesthesia. Anesth Analg 86:1328-1331, 1998.
229. Shulman M, Braverman B, Ivankovich AD, Gronert G: Sevoflurane triggers malignant hyperthermia in swine. Anesthesiology 54:259-260, 1981.
230. Gronert GA: Malignant hyperthermia. Anesthesiology 53:395-423, 1980.
231. Hall GM, Lucke JN, Lister D: Proceedings: Neuromuscular blocking drugs in porcine malignant hyperthermia. Br J Anaesth 48:270-271, 1976.
232. Denborough M, Hopkinson KC: Propofol and malignant hyperpyrexia. Lancet 1:191, 1988.
233. Bendixen D, Skovgaard LT, Ording H: Analysis of anaesthesia in patients suspected to be susceptible to malignant hyperthermia before diagnostic in vitro contracture test. Acta Anaesthesiol Scand 41:480-484, 1997.
234. Larach MG, Localio AR, Allen GC, et al: A clinical grading scale to predict malignant hyperthermia susceptibility. Anesthesiology 80:771-779, 1994.
235. Rosenberg H, Davis M, James D, et al: Malignant hyperthermia. Orphanet J Rare Dis 2:21, 2007.
236. Antognini JF: Creatine kinase alterations after acute malignant hyperthermia episodes and common surgical procedures. Anesth Analg 81:1039-1042, 1995.
237. Wappler F, Fiege M, Steinfath M, et al: Evidence for susceptibility to malignant hyperthermia in patients with exercise-induced rhabdomyolysis. Anesthesiology 94:95-100, 2001.
238. Anetseder M, Hartung E, Klepper S, Reichmann H: Gasoline vapors induce severe rhabdomyolysis. Neurology 44:2393-2395, 1994.
239. Denborough MA, Hopkinson KC, Banney DG: Firefighting and malignant hyperthermia. BMJ (Clin Res Ed) 296:1442-1443, 1988.
240. Ryan JF, Tedeschi LG: Sudden unexplained death in a patient with a family history of malignant hyperthermia. J Clin Anesth 9:66-68, 1997.
241. Butler-Browne GS, Eriksson PO, Laurent C, Thornell LE: Adult human masseter muscle fibers express myosin isozymes characteristic of development. Muscle Nerve 11:610-620, 1988.
242. Morgan DL, Proske U: Vertebrate slow muscle: Its structure, pattern of innervation, and mechanical properties. Physiol Rev 64:103-169, 1984.
243. van der Spek AF, Reynolds PI, Fang WB, et al: Changes in resistance to mouth opening induced by depolarizing and non-depolarizing neuromuscular relaxants. Br J Anaesth 64:21-27, 1990.
244. Flewellen EH, Nelson TE, Jones WP, et al: Dantrolene dose response in awake man: Implications for management of malignant hyperthermia. Anesthesiology 59:275-280, 1983.

245. Lerman J, McLeod ME, Strong HA: Pharmacokinetics of intravenous dantrolene in children. Anesthesiology 70:625-629, 1989.
246. Burkman JM, Posner KL, Domino KB: Analysis of the clinical variables associated with recrudescence after malignant hyperthermia reactions. Anesthesiology 106:901-906, quiz 1077-1078, 2007.
247. Hopkins PM: Recrudescence of malignant hyperthermia. Anesthesiology 106:893-894, 2007.
248. Gallant EM, Foldes FF, Rempel WE, Gronert GA: Verapamil is not a therapeutic adjunct to dantrolene in porcine malignant hyperthermia. Anesth Analg 64:601-606, 1985.
249. Harrison GG, Wright IG, Morrell DF: The effects of calcium channel blocking drugs on halothane initiation of malignant hyperthermia in MHS swine and on the established syndrome. Anaesth Intensive Care 16:197-201, 1988.
250. McGraw TT, Keon TP: Malignant hyperthermia and the clean machine. Can J Anaesth 36:530-532, 1989.
251. Schonell LH, Sims C, Bulsara M: Preparing a new generation anaesthetic machine for patients susceptible to malignant hyperthermia. Anaesth Intensive Care 31:58-62, 2003.
252. Anetseder M, Hager M, Müller-Reible C, Roewer N: Regional lactate and carbon dioxide concentrations in a metabolic test for malignant hyperthermia. Lancet 362:494, discussion 494-495, 2003.
253. Bina S, Cowan G, Karaian J, et al: Effects of caffeine, halothane, and 4-chloro-*m*-cresol on skeletal muscle lactate and pyruvate in malignant hyperthermia–susceptible and normal swine as assessed by microdialysis. Anesthesiology 104:90-100, 2006.
254. Bina S, Muldoon S, Bunger R: Effects of ryanodine on skeletal muscle lactate and pyruvate in malignant hyperthermia–susceptible and normal swine as assessed by microdialysis. Eur J Anaesthesiol 25:48-57, 2008.
255. Schuster F, Metterlein T, Kranke P, et al: Intramuscular injection of sevoflurane detects malignant hyperthermia predisposition in susceptible pigs. Anesthesiology 107:616-620, 2007.
256. Schuster F, Schöll H, Hager M, et al: The dose-response relationship and regional distribution of lactate after intramuscular injection of halothane and caffeine in malignant hyperthermia–susceptible pigs. Anesth Analg 102:468-472, 2006.
257. Girard T, Cavagna D, Padovan E, et al: B-lymphocytes from malignant hyperthermia–susceptible patients have an increased sensitivity to skeletal muscle ryanodine receptor activators. J Biol Chem 276:48077-48082, 2001.
258. Litman RS, Rosenberg H: Malignant hyperthermia: Update on susceptibility testing. JAMA 293:2918-2924, 2005.
259. McKinney LC, Butler T, Mullen SP, Klein SG: Characterization of ryanodine receptor–mediated calcium release in human B cells: Relevance to diagnostic testing for malignant hyperthermia. Anesthesiology 104:1191-1201, 2006.
260. Ording H, Foder B, Scharff O: Cytosolic free calcium concentrations in lymphocytes from malignant hyperthermia susceptible patients. Br J Anaesth 64:341-345, 1990.
261. Sei Y, Brandom BW, Bina S, et al: Patients with malignant hyperthermia demonstrate an altered calcium control mechanism in B lymphocytes. Anesthesiology 97:1052-1058, 2002.
262. Gareau PJ, Janzen EG, Towner RA, Stewart WA: In vivo ^{31}P NMR spectroscopy studies of halothane induced porcine stress syndrome. No effect of C-phenyl N-tert-butyl nitrone (PBN). Free Radic Res Commun 19:43-50, 1993.
263. Payen JF, Bosson JL, Bourdon L, et al: Improved noninvasive diagnostic testing for malignant hyperthermia susceptibility from a combination of metabolites determined in vivo with ^{31}P-magnetic resonance spectroscopy. Anesthesiology 78:848-855, 1993.

38 Fundamental Principles of Monitoring Instrumentation

Key Points

1. Accuracy and precision are different. Accuracy is how close a value is to the true value. Precision is how repeatable the measurements are. An inaccurate, but precise monitor can be recalibrated to be accurate, but an imprecise monitor cannot be improved.
2. Filtering can improve the signal display, but it also can result in smoothing and loss of information.
3. A signal can be extracted from noise by repeated measurements because the noise is random over time, but the signal is not.
4. Electrical signals can be converted from analog to digital. Conversion can introduce some artifacts, but can allow for greater storage and analysis capabilities.
5. Invasive pressure monitors are affected by damping and resonance. Damping leads to distortion, signal loss, and reduction of peak values. Resonance can lead to amplification and overestimation of the peak value.
6. Pulse oximetry combines analysis of optical plethysmography and absorption analysis with empirical data to produce an estimate of Sao_2.
7. Wavelength and frequency are related to the speed of the wave by the following formula: speed = wavelength × frequency. Shorter wavelengths improve the resolution of light and ultrasound measurements.
8. Flow measurements are among the most difficult to obtain and usually involve indirect measures. (For example, a temperature change or pressure decrease is measured, and a flow value is derived. A small error in the initial measurement leads to a much larger error in the derived flow value.)

Why Fundamental Principles Are Important

Patient monitoring has been a key aspect of anesthesiology since its beginnings as a medical specialty. As anesthesiology has grown more sophisticated and complex, so have the monitors and the data that they produce. The anesthesiologist's senses of sight, hearing, and touch, at first expanded with the stethoscope, sphygmomanometer, and electrocardiograph, are now supplemented by the pulse oximeter, expired gas analyzer, evoked potential monitor, and transesophageal echocardiograph, to name a few. The complexity of some of these devices can be intimidating, and the anesthesiologist may be tempted to regard them as incomprehensible "black boxes" that provide clinical data. To do so, however, would be to shirk an important part of the anesthesiologist's clinical responsibility. Anesthesiologists must be able not only to understand and interpret the data from the monitors, but also to anticipate and recognize errors associated with their use. Anesthesiologists cannot accomplish this goal without understanding how these devices work.

This chapter provides an understanding of the scientific principles underlying the design and function of the most commonly used monitors. Some concepts of basic physics are defined first, followed by more detailed descriptions of the principles and their monitoring applications. The text and figures explain these principles predominantly in a qualitative manner. For readers desiring a more quantitative explanation, the relevant physics and equations are provided in the appendices to this chapter.

Basic Principles

Nature of Physics and Measurement

Physics is the science of matter and energy and interactions between the two—that is, it is the study of everything in the physical universe. Physics encompasses everything from the motions and inner workings of the atom to those of galaxies. Physics is quantitative, and mathematics is the language of physics. Newton and Leibnitz invented "the calculus" as a mathematical tool for

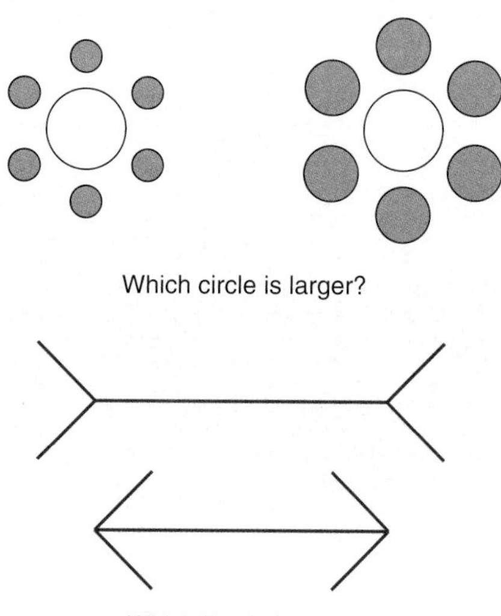

Figure 38-1 Optical illusions. We perceive the circles to be different sizes because we infer the size by relative dimension. The closeness of the smaller circles makes the inner circle appear smaller, and vice versa. The lines appear to be different sizes because we use straight-line perspective to estimate size and distance. This illusion reportedly does not work in cultures where straight lines are not used. Our internal perceptions lead us to err in estimating size and length. In the same way, the internal programming of our monitors can lead us to misinterpret results.

expressing and studying the laws of physics. Our monitors are also quantitative. Before we can discuss and understand the complexity of modern anesthetic monitors, we must quantitatively define what we are attempting to measure and understand the limitations of measurement.

We measure and monitor mass and energy: how much of a substance is present and in what energy state. Much of what we desire to monitor is outside the range of human physical senses. We must make measurements in this insensible realm with devices that enhance or extend our senses. Just as the senses have limitations and can be "fooled" under certain circumstances (Fig. 38-1), our physiologic monitors are limited by their design and can be fooled under some conditions. Intelligent users of these devices must understand their basic design assumptions to predict when they are likely to produce erroneous data.

Accuracy and Precision of Measurements

All measurements have errors. Error is usually determined by the comparison of a measurement with a "gold standard" of that measure. All measurements, even the so-called gold standards, are subject to errors with respect to reproducibility. From a clinician's perspective, a physiologic measurement is dependable only if it is accurate to the degree required for clinical decision making.

Systemic blood pressure can be measured in several ways. We can listen to Korotkoff sounds by the use of a sphygmomanometer cuff and stethoscope; we can rely on an oscillometric automated noninvasive blood pressure device, or if we need continuous measurement, we may place an intra-arterial cannula.[1] Each of these techniques provides slightly different arterial blood pressure values, and each has different sources of error. Our choice of method may be determined by accuracy or by our needs for the frequency of the data and the ease of retrieving these data. An automatic oscillometric device is usually chosen over manual auscultatory measurements for ease of acquisition and reproducibility. Two individuals taking auscultatory blood pressure measurements may hear the Korotkoff sounds at slightly different points and record different blood pressures. The required accuracy of a clinical monitor is determined by the smallest change in the measured variable that could affect a clinical decision. The requirements for "absolute accuracy" (is the measured value correct?) may be different from the requirements for "relative accuracy" (does the measured value follow trends?).

A pulse oximeter estimates arterial hemoglobin oxygen saturation by measuring light absorbance. The pulse oximeter saturation estimate, Spo_2, is compared with the hemoglobin oxygen saturation determined from analysis of an arterial blood sample by a laboratory carbon monoxide oximeter, Sao_2. Some errors are associated with arterial blood sampling and in vitro analysis of the sample by the carbon monoxide oximeter. Nevertheless, the carbon monoxide oximeter is considered to be the gold standard in this comparison of methods.

The pulse oximeter's saturation value can be compared with that of the carbon monoxide oximeter by the determination of bias and precision, as recommended by Bland and Altman (Fig. 38-2).[2] Bias is the average difference between simultaneous values from the two methods, or the systematic error. If a pulse oximeter reads an average of 5% higher than the carbon monoxide oximeter, it has a bias of 5%, and we can adjust for that systematic error by recalibrating the device. Precision is the standard deviation of the difference between the two measurements, and it quantifies the random error, or "scatter." A higher value for precision indicates a larger random error. (This statistic may be more appropriately called "imprecision.") If the random error is too large, the device may not be clinically useful. We can adjust for systematic error (bias) by recalibration, but there is no way to adjust for random error.

Measurement of Mass

Measurement is the determination of a physical quantity. A "dimension" is a specific category or type of physical quantity, such as mass, length, time, energy, or any of their derivatives. Units are specific ways of measuring a given dimension. Examples of units are the meter (length), second (time), kilogram (mass), ampere (current), and degree Kelvin (temperature). Describing a measurement without defining the unit is meaningless. A 30° day in Fahrenheit is literally freezing; a 30° day in Celsius is hot. Units can be base units or derived units. There are seven base units (meter, kilogram, second, ampere, degree-Kelvin, mole, and candela) in the SI (*Système International* [International System of Units]) system used in science, from which multiple other units can be derived.

When we "weigh" a patient, we are determining the force of gravity acting on the patient's mass. We generally mean this to be on the earth's surface, but the concept of weight is applicable to other locations. (On the surface of Jupiter, a 70-kg man would weigh 12 times his Earth weight, but his mass would still be 70 kg.) Because force = mass × acceleration due to gravity (Newton's second law), we *balance* the force on the patient with a known mass to determine the patient's "weight" (the SI units of force or weight are "Newtons") and mass (kg) (Fig. 38-3). The concept of balancing forces applies to multiple other monitoring

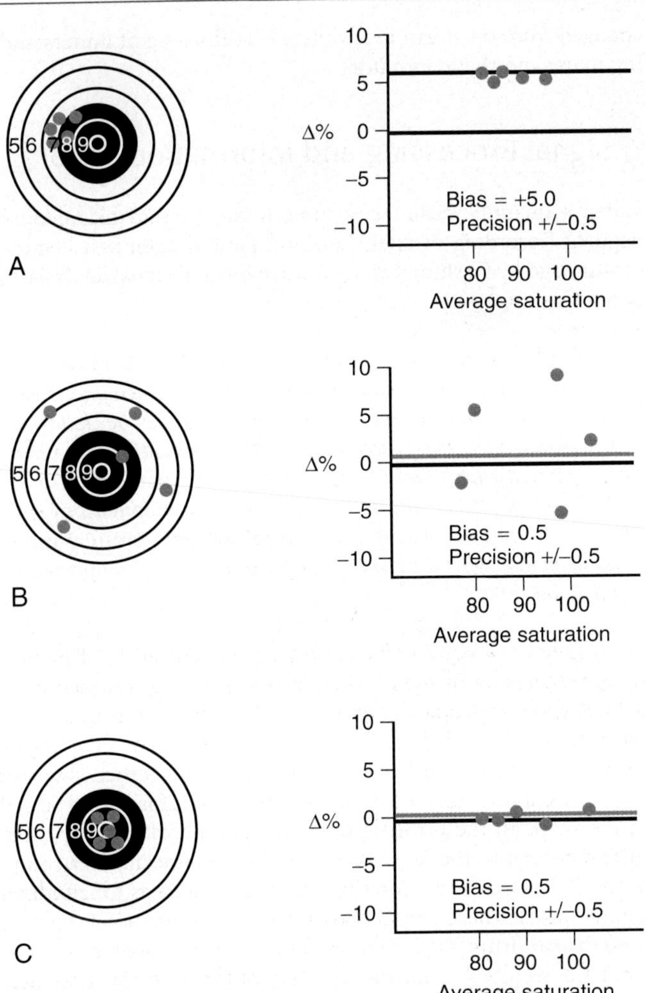

Figure 38-2 Accuracy and precision. The bias plot is a way to compare two different methods of measuring the same variable. **A-C,** Examples are plotted above on the right for saturation values, blood analysis versus pulse oximetry. It is a plot of the difference between the two measurements being compared versus the average of those two measurements. **A,** If one method constantly measures slightly higher than the other by a consistent value, it has a positive bias. If it has only slight variation around that bias, it is said to have very low random error (or precision, which equals the standard deviation of the differences). **B,** The values are randomly scattered, such that the average difference is near zero, but the precision value is very large. This large random error makes the device unusable because calibration would not improve this random error. **C,** The optimal device has a bias near zero and a very small precision (standard deviation of the differences). No amount of calibrating or "sighting in" could cause the device in **B** to become more accurate because the error is randomly scattered.

modalities. When we measure the central venous pressure using a simple manometer, we are observing the balance of forces between the patient's venous pressure and the force of gravity acting on a fluid column (Fig. 38-4). When the same pressure is measured electronically, we are "balancing" a Wheatstone bridge (a system of resistors used to determine an unknown resistance) (Fig. 38-5).

Measurement of Energy

Energy can exist in many different forms. Even matter is related to energy, mathematically defined by Einstein's famous $E = mc^2$

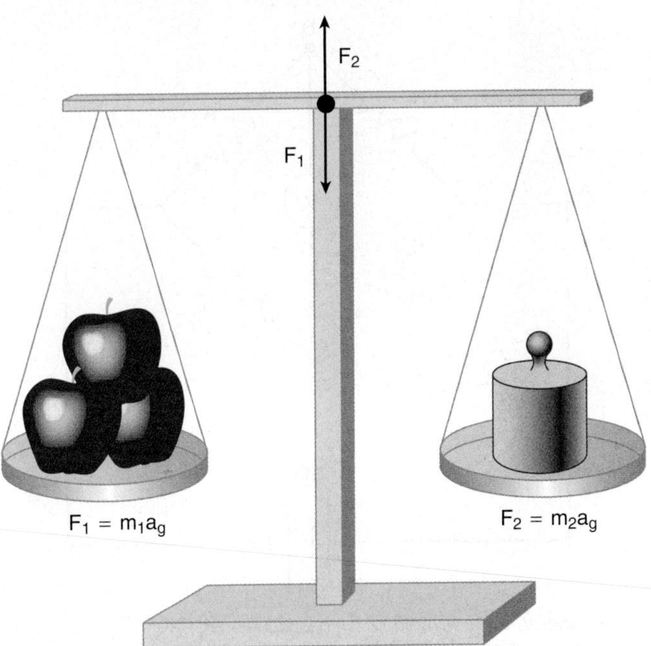

Figure 38-3 Balance. A scale is in balance when the forces are equal and in opposite directions. The force of gravity on the unknown mass of fruit is balanced by the known standard masses on the opposite side of the balance. $F_1 = F_2$, hence $m_1\ a_g = m_2\ a_g$; because $a_g = a_g$, $m_1 = m_2$ (a_g = acceleration due to gravity).

equation; that is to say, matter and energy are different forms of the same "stuff." In the absolute sense, usually reserved for thermonuclear weapons, atomic reactors, and the sun, matter can be converted into energy, and vice versa. If a 1-kg mass were completely converted to energy by means of $E = mc^2$, it would yield 8.987×10^{16} J (Table 38-1).The energy of motion is described as kinetic energy (KE = ½ mv^2). Temperature is a form of kinetic

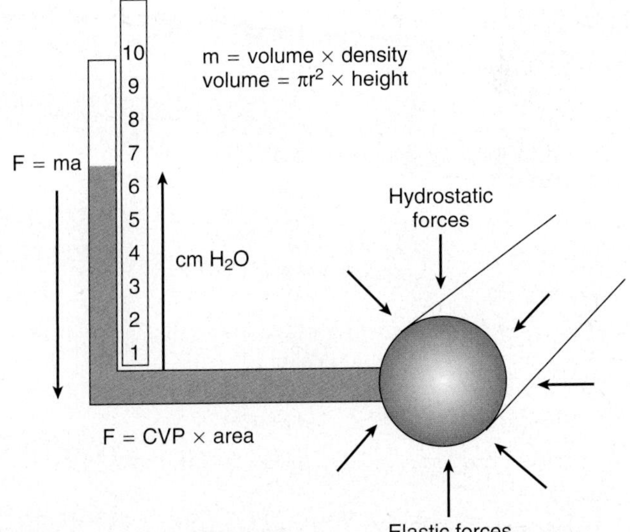

Figure 38-4 Manometer. A water manometer uses a balance of forces. In this case, the downward pressure of the fluid, as determined by its density and height, balances the upward pressure of the central venous system, caused by hydrostatic and elastic recoil forces. CVP, central venous pressure; F, force.

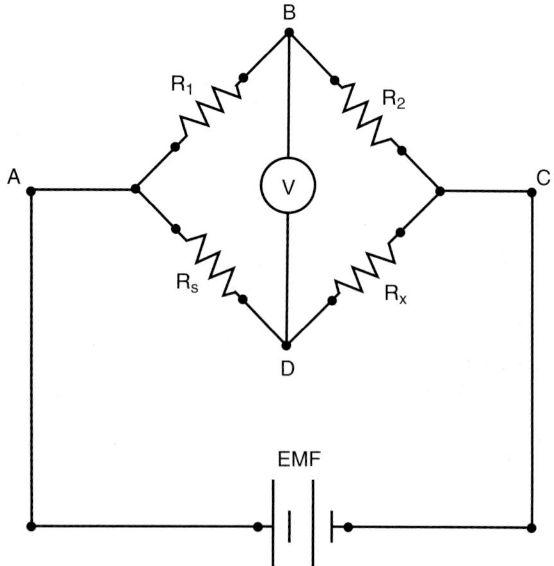

Figure 38-5 Wheatstone bridge. A Wheatstone bridge is an electronic circuit designed so that an unknown resistance can be calculated by knowing two sets of variables: (1) the voltage drop across the bridge and (2) the other resistances in the circuit (see Appendix 3).

energy at the molecular level. Acoustic energy (sound) is a wave of pressure energy transmitted through matter. Light is a form of electromagnetic energy. Potential energy is stored energy and can be of many forms, including gravitational, chemical, pressure, and electromagnetic. The fundamental law of conservation of energy (energy and matter can neither be created nor destroyed, only changed from one form to another) is at the core of understanding many anesthetic monitors.

Table 38-1 Comparison of Energy Levels of Common and Uncommon Events

Event	Energy
1-kg mass falling 1 m on Earth	9.8 J
Heart beat	10 J (at rest, 60 beats/min, 10 W)
Internal defibrillation for ventricular fibrillation	30 J
Maximum output of surface defibrillator	360 J
1 kcal	4186 J
Car battery	1.8 mJ = 1.8×10^6 J
1 kg of fat	3.8×10^7 J
Ton of TNT	4.2×10^9 J
Atomic bomb (Hiroshima)	15 kilotons = $15 \times 10^3 \times 4.2 \times 10^9$ J = 6.3×10^{14} J
Hydrogen bomb	1 megaton = 4.2×10^{15} J
1 kg converted completely to energy	8.987×10^{16} J
The sun (4.2×10^9 kg matter/sec)	3.8×10^{26} J/sec

Modified from Hecht E: Physics: Algebra/Trig. Pacific Grove, CA, Brooks/Cole, 1994.

Signal Processing and Information Theory

When a quantity varies over time, it can be said to contain a "signal." Recording of vital signs and patient data, first begun a century ago by Cushing,[3] is a primitive form of signal analysis. To quote Cushing[4]:

> *In all serious or questionable cases the patient's pulse and blood-pressure, their usual rate and level having been previously taken under normal ward conditions, should be followed throughout the entire procedure, and the observations recorded on a plotted chart. Only in this way can we gain any idea of physiological disturbances—whether given manipulations are leading to shock, whether there is a fall of blood-pressure from loss of blood, whether the slowed pulse is due to compression, and so on.*

Often the signals (the energy or concentration of matter) we are interested in monitoring are too small for our senses to define changes adequately. We must either concentrate or amplify the signal. Often, this information is "transduced" or changed from one form to another for amplification and processing. An old-style gramophone is a good example: The information stored in the shape of the record groove moves a needle attached to a mica diaphragm (the reproducer), which is connected to a sound horn. The mechanical vibrations are reproduced as longitudinal sound waves. These sound waves enter the human ear, contact onto the ear drum, causing it to vibrate, which moves the ossicular chain, resulting in an amplification of the pressure at the oval window, transmitted through the fluid of the inner ear where the appropriate hair cell resonates and generates a neural signal (transduction) (Fig. 38-6). This process is analogous to the process by which our arterial pressure transducers work (Fig. 38-7).

Data Processing

When an analog signal (e.g., voltage versus time) is amplified, the background noise and the desired signal are amplified (Fig. 38-8). Various techniques can be used to enhance the signal-to-noise ratio. Most pulse oximeters assume that a patient's pulse rate is between 30 and 300 beats/min. The instrument filters out any pulsations that occur at frequencies less than 30 or greater than 300 (see the section on alternating current, capacitors, and impedance and Fig. 38-25). Filtering can remove the noise that is outside of this frequency range, improving our ability to discern the signal of interest. Improper filtering can destroy the true signal. In some cases, a desired periodic signal can be repeated and summated, and the accompanying random noise becomes a smaller fraction of the signal. Evoked potentials are an excellent example of this process of "ensemble averaging." The evoked response signal for a single stimulus is actually much smaller than the random noise, but this signal is nearly identical after each stimulus. By summing the potentials after many stimuli, we reinforce the evoked response signal, but not the noise (Fig. 38-9).

Finally, the waveform of any periodic signal can be represented by a summation of sinusoidal waves, called a "Fourier

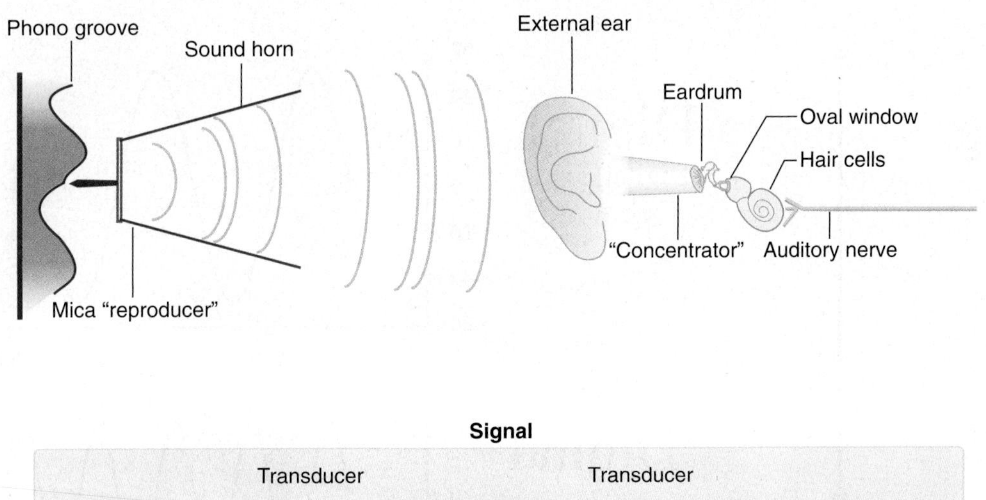

Figure 38-6 Transduction in mechanical and biologic systems. Mechanical energy of the winding mechanism causes the cylinder of the phonograph to rotate. The bumps and curves in the cylinder then move the needle, converting that energy into acoustic energy (a longitudinal wave). The mechanical vibrations are reproduced as longitudinal sound waves. These sound waves enter the human ear, contact the ear drum, causing it to vibrate, which moves the ossicular chain, resulting in an amplification of the pressure at the oval window, transmitted through the fluid of the inner ear where the appropriate hair cell resonates and generates a neural signal (transduction). Loss of hair cells leads to deafness, most commonly in the higher frequency range as one ages. This is analogous to a monitor lacking sensitivity in the desired range.

series" (Fig. 38-10).[5] The component sine waves can be described by their frequency and amplitude (or power, which is proportional to the square of the amplitude). A waveform originally expressed as amplitude versus time is transformed into a plot of power versus frequency (Fig. 38-11). The resulting plot, called the "power spectrum," is a common form for displaying and interpreting some types of waveform data, such as the electroencephalogram (see Chapter 39).

Errors in Signal Analysis

We have all seen movies where car wheels appear to be rotating backward while the car is moving forward. This is the result of a specific type of error, called "aliasing," which occurs when the sampling frequency is too slow to capture the rapid variations of the true signal (Fig. 38-12). Aliasing also can happen with ultrasound, where the display may show echoes from objects that do not actually exist.

In mechanical systems, such as the conventional liquid-filled tubing and pressure transducer for measuring arterial blood pressure, frictional forces can dampen the signal. The signal also can be distorted by resonant amplification, where the energy of the signal is temporarily stored in the compliance of the tubing, and then released (see Appendix 4) (Fig. 38-13). If the display rate is too fast, we also can miss important signals. The systolic pressure variation (alteration in systolic blood pressure with positive-pressure ventilation)[6,7] has been used to determine volume

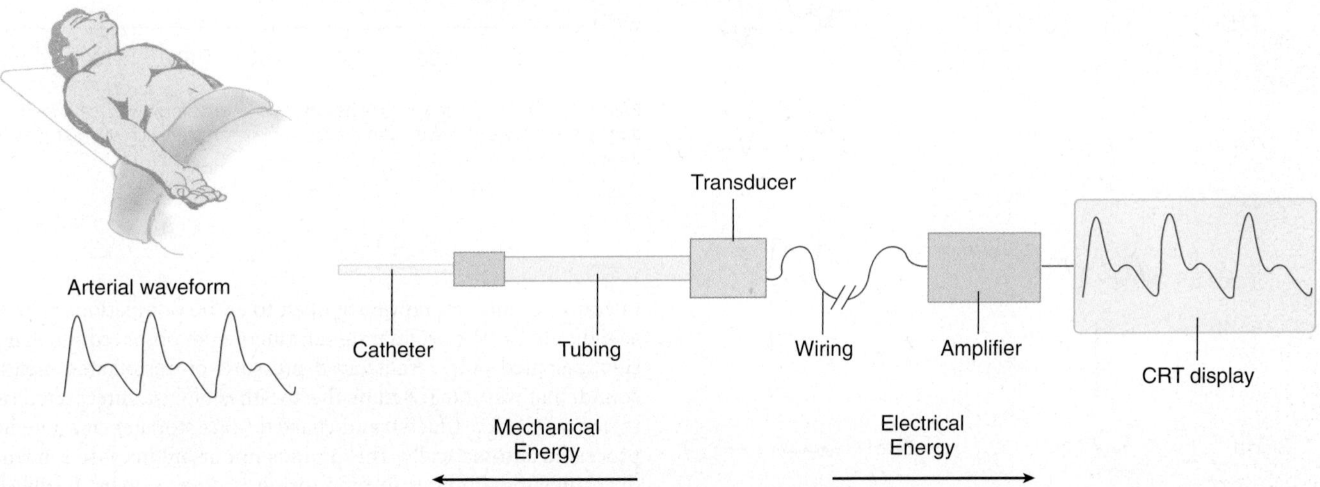

Figure 38-7 Transducer. A transducer changes a signal from one form of energy to another. A common transducer in anesthesia changes mechanical energy (e.g., an arterial pulse) into electrical energy, which is then displayed as time versus amplitude on an LCD or CRT display. Microphones and speakers are also examples of transducers.

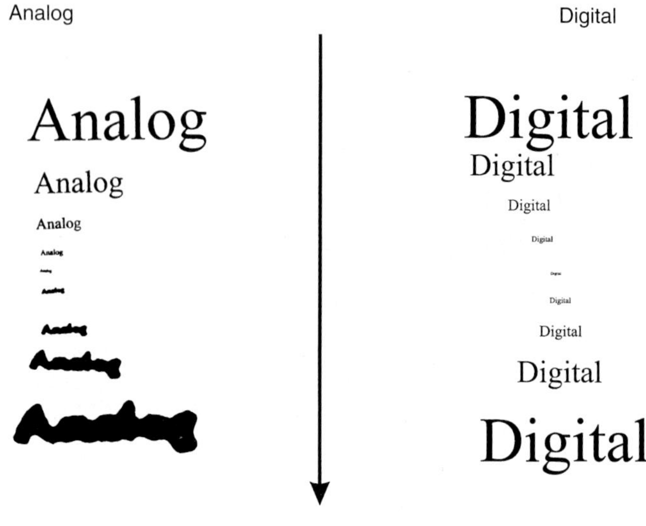

Figure 38-8 Digital and analog signal processing. The analog signal shows distortion and loss of fidelity as it is reduced and then amplified. The digital signal shows no such loss. To create the analog example, a copy machine was used to shrink the text and then enlarge it. For the digital signal, the font size was reduced, the text copied, and the process reversed.

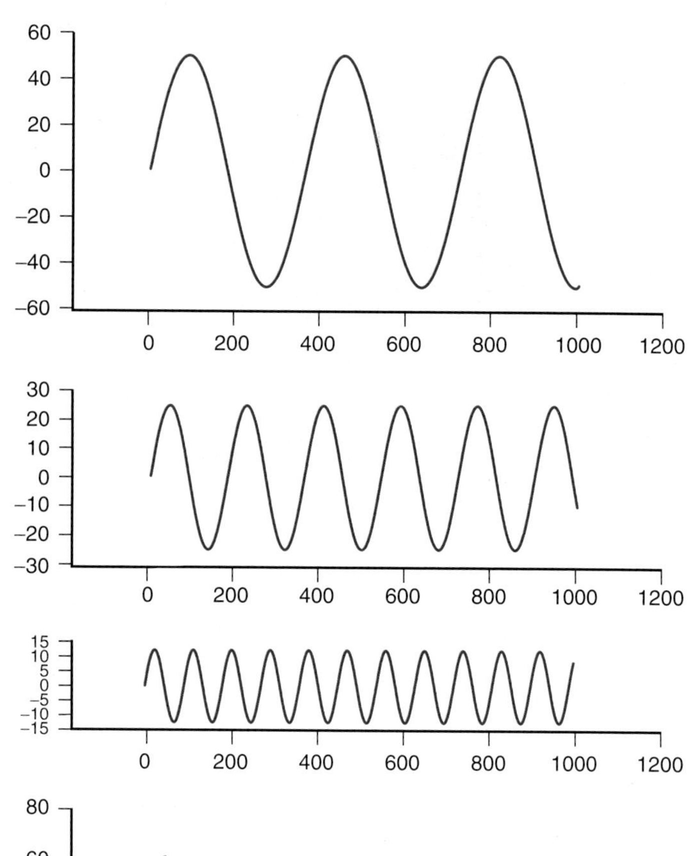

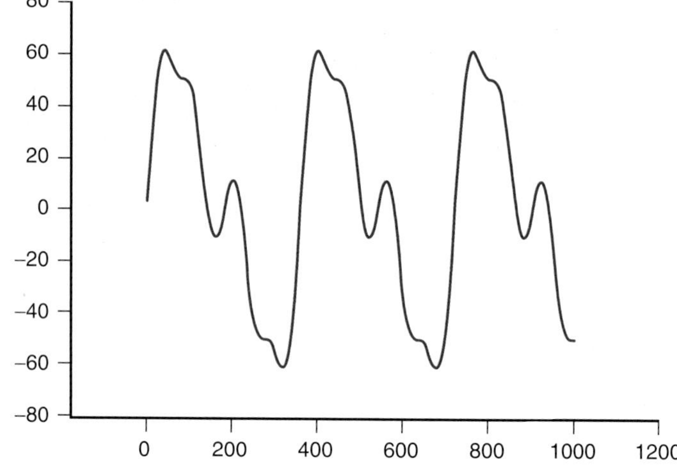

Figure 38-10 Fourier series. This pseudoarterial waveform was generated by adding the three sine waves with the following characteristics, y = 50 sinx, y = 25 sin2x, y = 12 sin4x.

responsiveness in hypotension. Because this change happens much more slowly than the heart rate, and because many displays employ "auto-gain"—that is, they control the size of the display to maintain a constant waveform amplitude (e.g., the plethysmograph display of most pulse oximeters)—the systolic pressure variation has been clinically neglected for many years.

With modern data recording and storage, Cushing's original rationale of correlating changes in patient physiology to intraoperative events can now be applied to entire populations as well as individuals. The original signal, whether an observed pupillary sign, palpated pulse, transduced pressure, or auscultated breath sound, that was integrated by the anesthesiologist, interpreted (is this real or is it artifact?), and charted (data storage) can now be processed automatically. This point is important because it introduces new possibilities in monitoring (trends, signals, feedback to user) and new pitfalls. Imagine an anesthesia record that would alert you to future potential physiologic issues from currently monitored data and predictive algorithms, that is, an intelligent

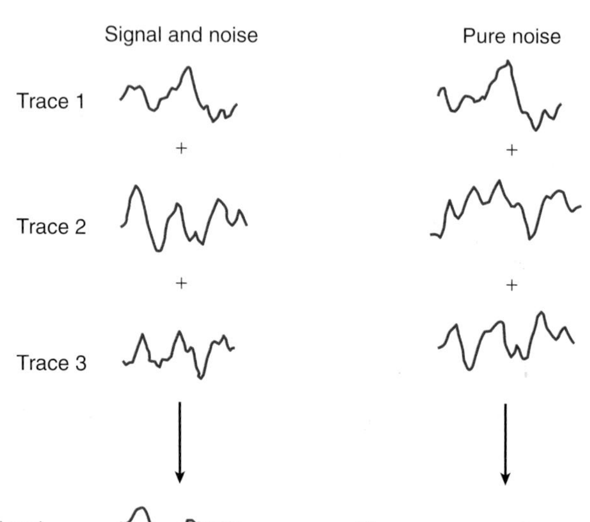

Figure 38-9 Somatosensory evoked potentials. A background signal can be separated from random noise by repeatedly adding the signals. The noise (random) is equally likely to be positive or negative; adding positive and negative yields zero with multiple summations.

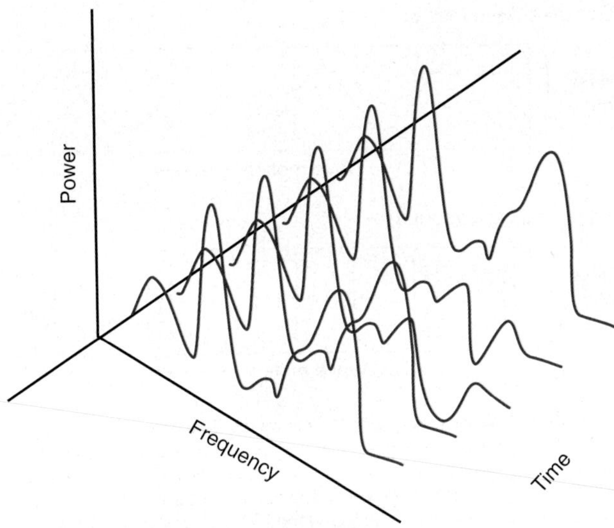

Figure 38-11 Spectral arrays. A compressed spectral array can display the frequency on the *x* axis and power on the *y* axis. A number of these can be aligned with time as a third axis, giving an indication of changes in power over time.

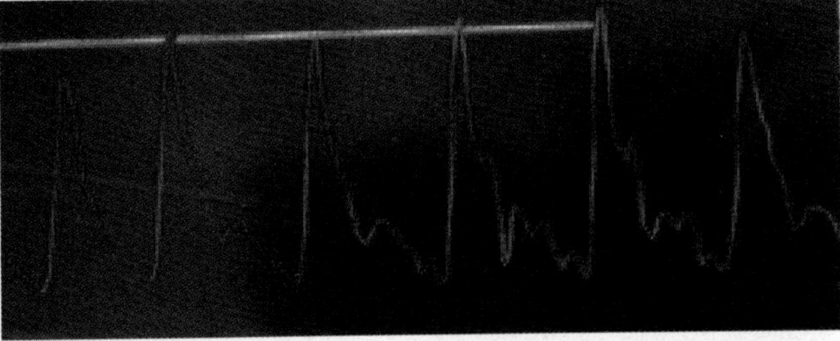

A

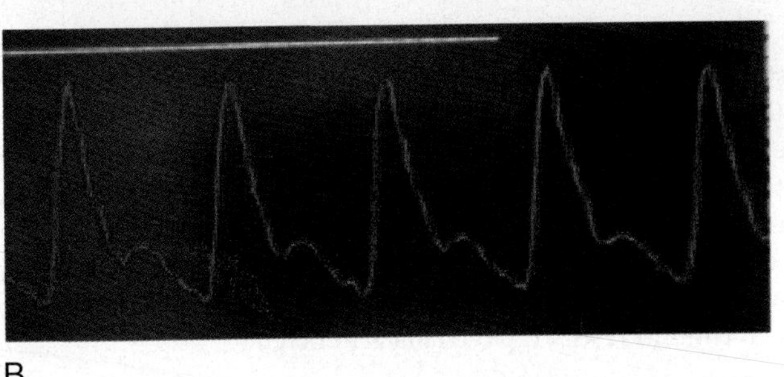

B

Figure 38-13 Arterial waveform resonance. **A,** A peaked arterial waveform indicating some resonance with overestimation of the systolic blood pressure. **B,** The same patient when damping is added to the system.

anesthesia record. New problems are introduced by such technology, including security, potential loss of data (loss of not only a single chart or data point, but of all the charts), and erroneous signal processing (imagine a faulty algorithm denying you the very information Cushing sought to use to improve patient care).

Pressure Measurement

Principles of Pressure Measurement

With some of the basics of measurement behind us, we can now work through an example of clinical measurement. As part of a clinical examination, we can note the distention of the jugular vein. What are we really doing? We are visualizing the reflection of light off of the patient's skin changing as the underlying structure (the jugular vein) fills and collapses. But what are the physics of this distention? If we were to insert a clear tube into the vein and hold the tube vertical with respect to gravity, we would observe the mass of blood in the tube raised a certain distance (centimeters) against the force of gravity by the central venous pressure until a balance point is reached. Energy is lost in the work done in raising the fluid column, distending the tubing, and frictional losses. The actual venous pressure is slightly greater than we can reasonably measure. Despite these limitations, a liquid manometer is a simple and effective way to determine central venous pressure.

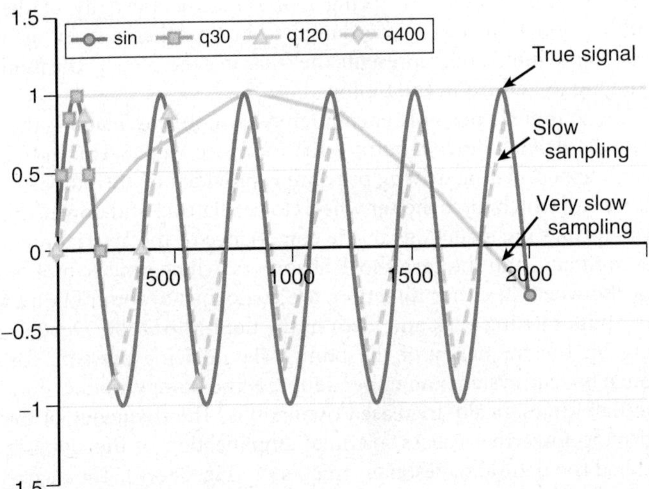

Figure 38-12 Aliasing. Improper sampling leads to an erroneous waveform. A slower sampling rate results in a change in the amplitude and wavelength.

The units of pressure measurement can tell us something about how the measurement is made. We commonly define pressure in terms of millimeters of mercury (mm Hg), centimeters of water (cm H_2O), pounds per square inch (psi), or atmospheres (atm). What we have measured in our clear manometer tube is a pressure in centimeters of blood. Given that the content of blood in the tube can vary, we need to have more standard units than centimeters of patient blood. To do so, we must understand the physics of the manometer. The density of a fluid is its mass per unit volume, which has SI units of kilograms per cubic meter (kg/m^3) or, more commonly, grams per milliliter (g/mL). The pressure exerted by a liquid column of height z and density ρ is simply ρgz (see Appendix 2 for derivation). If the manometer liquid is mercury, which has a density of 13,600 kg/m^3 (13.6 g/mL), the manometer pressure in pascals (the SI unit of pressure) is:

$$P\,(\text{Pa}) = 13{,}600 \times 9.8 \times z\,(\text{m}) = 1.333 \times 105 \times z\,(\text{m})$$

Because these large numbers are awkward, we often express P in kilopascals (kPa) and z in mm Hg:

$$P\,(\text{kPa}) = 0.1333z\,(\text{mm Hg})$$

A useful reference for the various pressure units in use today is the pressure of the earth's atmosphere at sea level, called "1 atmosphere" or 1 atm:

$$\begin{aligned} 1\,\text{atm} &= 101.3\,\text{kPa} \\ &= 760\,\text{mm Hg} = 29.92\,\text{inches-Hg} \\ &= 14.7\,\text{psi} \\ &= 988\,\text{cm}\,H_2O \end{aligned}$$

If a fluid-filled catheter is connected to the circulatory system of a patient, the height of the fluid in the manometer determines the mean pressure at the tip of the catheter. If the pressure measured is central venous pressure, we can use these data to infer right ventricular preload. For slowly changing pressures, a water or mercury manometer is simple and dependable (see Fig. 38-4). The manometer cannot respond quickly to rapid changes in pressure because of its inertia; that is, the mass of the liquid column resists rapid changes in height.

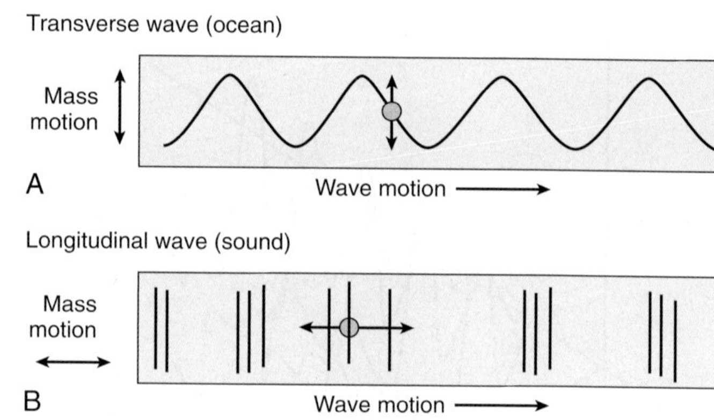

Figure 38-15 Transverse and longitudinal waves. **A,** In transverse waves (e.g., ocean waves), the particles move perpendicular to the motion of the wave. **B,** In longitudinal waves (e.g., sound waves), the particles move back and forth in the direction of the wave. The actual matter in either wave does not move much. The energy transfers without mass transfer. In arterial systems, this can clarify the fact that pressure does not equal flow.

Dynamic Pressure Measurement (Transducer)

Accurate measurement of a rapidly changing pressure signal, such as arterial blood pressure, is more difficult and complex. There are many characteristics of the arterial pressure versus time waveform (Fig. 38-14) that we might wish to determine. Systolic, diastolic, and mean arterial pressures are given by the maximum, minimum, and average pressure values during the cardiac cycle. In addition, we can measure the maximum upward slope of the waveform during systole, which is related to the speed of ventricular ejection. An abnormally rapid downslope after aortic valve closure (indicated by the dicrotic notch) suggests possible aortic insufficiency. The details of the pressure-time waveform and its maxima and minima are important to the clinician. Despite our display of the waveform on a vertical axis, it is important to remember that the arterial pressure is not a transverse wave (similar to a wave on the ocean), but a longitudinal wave (similar to a sound wave or a pulse transmitted through a coiled spring) (Fig. 38-15).

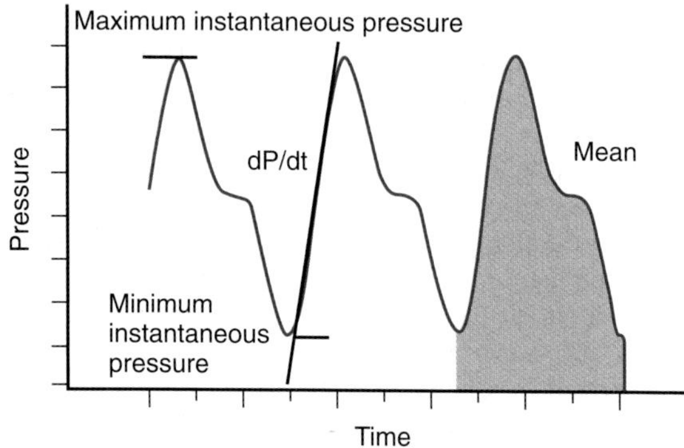

Figure 38-14 Arterial waveform. Systolic pressure is defined as the instantaneous maximal pressure; diastolic, the instantaneous minimum pressure; and mean, the average pressure over a cycle. dP/dT refers to the upstroke of the arterial pressure (i.e., the rate of pressure generation). The mean pressure is estimated as the diastolic plus ⅓ the pulse pressure (systolic-diastolic) when only the systolic and diastolic pressures are known.

A modern pressure transducer is a device that changes either electric resistance or capacitance in response to changes in pressure on a solid-state device. The variable transducer electric resistance is placed in a circuit involving three known resistances (Wheatstone bridge [see Fig. 38-5]; see Appendix 3), and the change in resistance is converted into electric voltage. The moving part of the transducer itself is very small and has little mass. It is not clinically or commercially practical to place the transducer in direct contact with arterial blood (although one manufacturer has done exactly this), so we use a liquid-filled tube to connect the intra-arterial catheter to the external pressure transducer. This system of a fluctuating driving pressure (i.e., the arterial pressure being measured), a liquid-filled tube, and a pressure transducer is mechanically equivalent to the mass-spring harmonic oscillator shown in Figure 38-16. The mass (m) represents the mass of the fluid in the tubing. The spring represents the elasticity of the tubing and transducer. The damper, shown schematically as a piston moving in oil, represents the friction generated by the fluid moving to and fro in the tubing.

A more commonly encountered harmonic oscillator is that of a car driving down a bumpy dirt road (see Fig. 38-16). In this case, the oscillating driving pressure is provided by the bumps in the road, which force the car wheels to oscillate up and down. The car springs are analogous to the compliance of the arterial pressure tubing, and the car's shock absorbers, which oppose motion of the wheel in either direction, are analogous to the friction of the fluid moving back and forth in the fluid-filled tube. Depending on the frequency of the bumps (i.e., driving pressure frequency), the system can either suppress the bumpy road or may initiate dramatically increased oscillations. The frequency of the driving force that causes maximal amplification of the signal is called the natural or resonant frequency (Fig. 38-17). The degree of amplification is directly related to the mass and inversely related to the amount of friction present; for large amounts of

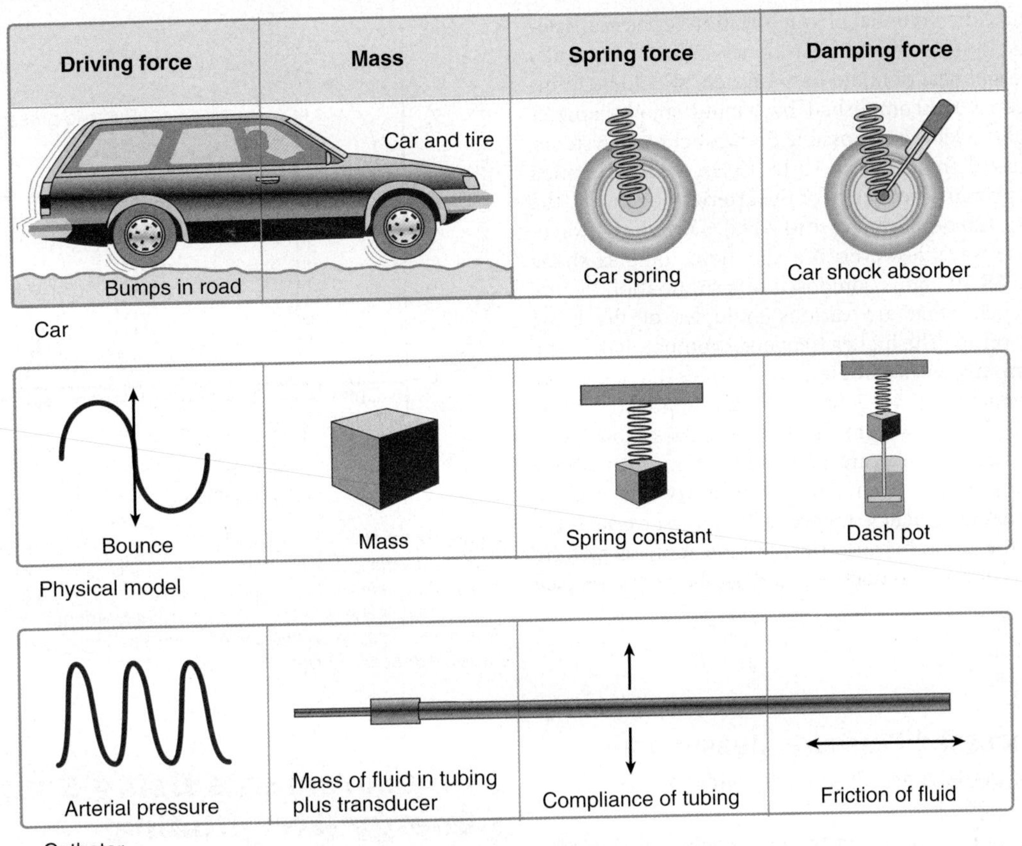

Figure 38-16 Damping and resonance. Pressure measured in an invasive arterial catheter can overshoot or amplify the actual blood pressure. This phenomenon is referred to as the dynamic frequency response of the fluid-filled arterial line and transducer system. This phenomenon has a physical model, which can generate an equation to predict the output pressure response, depending on the frequency of the input pressure and several physical parameters of the system. In the physical model, the driving pressure (the arterial blood pressure) acts on a mass (the fluid within the arterial pressure tubing), pushing it up and down against a spring, which stores energy (the compliant pressure tubing), and a dash pot, which opposes motion in either direction (the resistance of the fluid as it moves to and fro within the pressure tubing). Depending on the input frequency, the output may go through an amplification as it reaches a specific frequency, known as the resonant frequency of the system. There is a common phenomenon noted when a car drives along a bumpy dirt road. In this situation, the driving force is the bumps in the road, which act on the tire. The car spring is equivalent to the compliance to the pressure tubing, and the shock absorber corresponds to the resistance of fluid moving back and forth in the arterial line. The mass of the fluid is analogous to the mass of the front of the car. You may have experienced the phenomenon in which you reach a certain speed as you are driving along a bumpy road when the front of the car starts to oscillate with increasing amplitude. If you speed up or slow down, this phenomenon disappears. The car bounces highest when you have reached the resonant frequency of this harmonic oscillator. (See Appendix 4 for a detailed mathematical description of this process.)

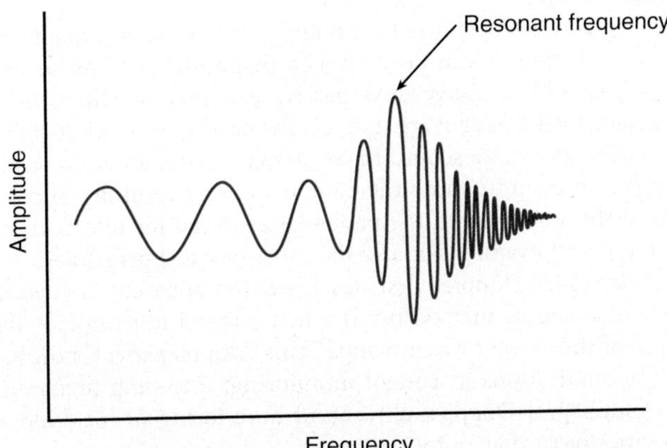

Figure 38-17 Amplitude and frequency. As the frequency increases, the amplification can increase to a maximum, and then the signal becomes attenuated. *(Adapted from Sykes MK, Vickers MD, Hull CJ: Principles of Measurement and Monitoring in Anesthesia and Intensive Care, 3rd ed. Oxford, Blackwell, 1991.)*

friction, attenuation rather than amplification occurs (see Appendix 4).

To visualize this concept intuitively, hang a weight on the end of a rubber band while holding the upper end of the band in your hand. If you move your hand up and down slowly, the weight follows your hand movements almost exactly. As you increase the frequency of your hand oscillations, the weight begins to "lag" behind your hand, and the amplitude of the weight movement begins to increase. As you approach the natural frequency of this simple system, you will observe the phenomenon of "resonance," when the amplitude of the weight motion becomes very large. If you try different rubber bands and weights, you will find that stiffer bands or smaller weights yield higher natural frequencies. The same is true of our fluid-coupled pressure transducer system. Stiffer (i.e., less compliant) tubing or a shorter length of tubing (less mass) produces higher natural frequencies in this system; that is, it requires a much higher pulse rate before amplification.

To minimize the potential of amplification of the real arterial pressure, the system should have noncompliant (i.e., stiff) tubing, and the total mass of liquid in the system should be minimized, which can be accomplished by having small-diameter tubing and as short a length as possible. In most clinical systems, the natural resonant frequency is 10 to 15 Hz, which is much higher than the primary frequency of the arterial waveform (the heart rate is 60 to 120 beats/min or 1 to 2 Hz). The arterial waveform is not a sine wave, however; it is the more complex shape shown in Figure 38-10 and is composed of a summation of sine waves of frequencies that are various multiples of the heart rates—a Fourier series. The higher frequency components of the arterial waveform (higher harmonics) are the ones that are closer to the natural frequency of the system and are amplified. This is why we see a "whip" in the waveform when the peak systolic pressure and the initial upstroke are amplified significantly above the true systolic pressure, even though the heart rate itself is not near the resonant frequency. Theoretically, mean arterial pressure should be the same because this amplification of systolic pressure also produces a reduction in diastolic pressure (see Appendix 4).

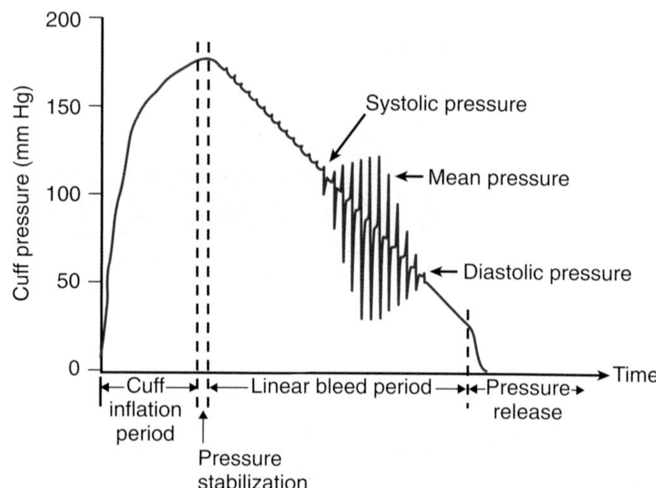

Figure 38-18 Noninvasive blood pressure measurement. Using the signal from the arterial pulse, oscillometric blood pressure measurements are obtained by determining the point at which the signal is first detected, its maximal amplitude, and the signal decay rate. *(Adapted from Ehrenwerth J, Eisenkraft J: Anesthesia Equipment: Principles and Applications. St. Louis, Mosby-Year Book, 1993.)*

Signal-Processed Pressure Measurement (Noninvasive Blood Pressure Monitor)

Systolic pressure can be estimated by noting return of the flow pulse after occlusion of the brachial artery by a cuff. The return of flow can be detected by (1) simple palpation of the radial artery, (2) recording with a Doppler device over the radial artery, or (3) the use of a pulse oximeter. Most anesthesiologists are familiar with the loss of pulse oximeter signal when the noninvasive blood pressure monitor is cycling.

Automated noninvasive blood pressure monitoring devices used in operating rooms employ a more sophisticated application of this principle. These devices monitor the oscillating signal generated in the cuff by the arterial pressure changes. The cuff first inflates to above systolic pressure, at which point the signal and oscillations are abolished. Then the cuff slowly deflates in a stepwise fashion. The pressure at which the oscillating pressure signal first appears is interpreted as the systolic pressure. The signal increases in amplitude as the cuff pressure decreases. The point at which the signal is at maximal amplitude is interpreted as mean arterial pressure. As cuff pressure decreases further, the oscillations drop off rapidly. Diastolic pressure is mathematically inferred from the systolic and mean values (Fig. 38-18).[8]

Errors can be introduced in the same manner as for manual auscultation of Korotkoff sounds: Too small or too large a cuff requires a higher or a lower pressure to occlude arterial flow, and stiff atherosclerotic arteries are resistant to compression. External compression caused by patient motion or the surgeon leaning on the blood pressure cuff can cause pressure oscillations that are not related to arterial pressure and may result in an erroneous reading, most commonly a higher diastolic pressure. Mercury sphygmomanometers are being phased out of use in some countries and hospitals, which leads to questions regarding the accuracy and precision of alternative devices, such as the aforementioned automated noninvasive blood pressure monitors and aneroid sphygmomanometers.[9,10]

Measurements Using Sound Energy (Longitudinal Pressure Wave)

Principles of Sound

Sound waves are small fluctuations in pressure, density, and velocity that can propagate through matter of any form: solid, liquid, or gas (see Fig. 38-15). In contrast to electromagnetic waves such as light (see the section on light), sound cannot propagate in a vacuum. The commonly used unit of sound, the decibel (dB), is not an SI unit, but a logarithmic ratio of the sound energy referenced to 20 μPa (or 0.0002 millibar), the threshold of normal human hearing.

Sound has been used for many years in medical diagnosis and monitoring. It can be used as a diagnostic method in two ways: passive and active. In a passive examination, the sounds generated by the patient are studied. The basic examination of this type uses the stethoscope. In an active examination, acoustic energy is transmitted into the patient, and the resulting interaction of this energy with the patient is analyzed for information. Both types of examination use the same physical principles.

In 1842, Doppler first described the apparent change in pitch of a sound that occurred when either the source of the sound or the listener was moving.[11] This "Doppler effect" now has several applications in patient monitoring, including precordial and esophageal Doppler ultrasound monitoring of local blood velocities or cardiac output.

When a sound source is moving toward the listener, the apparent pitch increases, and vice versa. The exact amount of frequency shift depends on whether the listener or the sound source is moving (Fig. 38-19; see Appendix 7). Because changes in the frequency of sine waves can be measured precisely, the Doppler principle provides a very accurate method of measuring

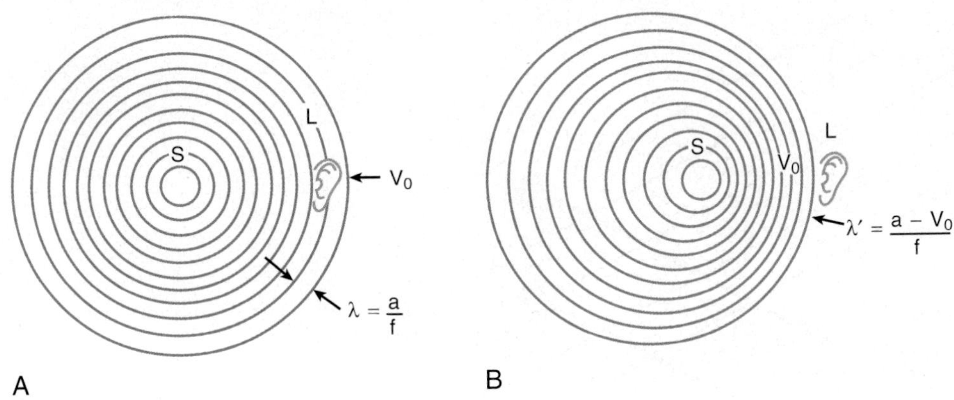

Figure 38-19 Doppler effect. **A,** When a listener is moving toward a stationary sound source, the frequency increases because the listener transverses more waves per unit time than a stationary listener. **B,** When a sound source is moving toward a stationary listener, the wave fronts "stack up," causing an apparent increased frequency.

the velocities of moving sound reflectors. At the high frequencies often used (>5 MHz), objects as small as red corpuscles can scatter enough sound for detection.

Passive Sound Examination (Stethoscope)

Vibrations, such as those caused by the closing and opening of heart valves or air moving through the respiratory passages, travel through the body as sound waves. Sound is conducted better and more rapidly in liquids than in gases. Bronchial breath sounds are heard better when the bronchi are surrounded by lung consolidation. When sound waves reach a sudden change in density (e.g., a liquid-gas interface), some of the energy is reflected.

Some simple facts about sound waves can facilitate an understanding of the reflection and scattering process in the body. First, all sound waves can be represented as a summation of sinusoidal waves of various frequencies and amplitudes. This process of Fourier or power spectral analysis was discussed earlier in this chapter. A note from a musical instrument consists of a sine wave at the "fundamental frequency" plus many "harmonics" at multiples of this frequency. The fundamental frequency describes the pitch of the tone: middle C is standardized at 256 Hz, for example.

All of these many frequencies propagate at the same speed, the speed of sound (called "a"). For ideal gases, the speed of sound is proportional to the square root of temperature. The speed of sound in air at room temperature is 344 msec, or 1129 ft/sec or 770 miles/hr (mph). At an altitude of 13,000 m (40,000 ft), where the standard air temperature is −57°C, the speed of sound is only 295 msec, or 661 mph. The speed of sound is much higher in liquids than in gases. The speed of sound through water at 15°C is 1450 m/sec. This value also approximates the speed of sound through most of the solid parts of the human body. In other solids, the speed of sound varies greatly, with a range of 54 m/sec in rubber to 6000 m/sec in granite. Reflection of sound occurs at interfaces where the product of the density and the speed of sound ($\rho \times a$) changes suddenly. Larger changes in this "acoustic impedance" result in greater reflection and less transmission. In the human body, the largest changes in acoustic impedance occur at gas-tissue boundaries: the lungs and the gastrointestinal tract. Reflection of sound by the lungs makes it difficult to auscultate heart tones through an air-filled, emphysematous chest. For the same reason, a transthoracic echocardiograph provides less detail than the transesophageal technique; in the former case, the lungs are in the way.

The first attempts to gather information about the inside of the patient by using sound involved placing one's ear directly on the patient. Although this procedure had many limitations, it led to the development of the modern stethoscope, which is based on the physical principles of sound transmission. The stethoscope uses a large diaphragm to transmit and concentrate the sound energy. The bell acts as an amplifier and a low-pass filter to transmit low-frequency diastolic rumbles. The physics of stethoscopy were described in depth by Rappaport and Sprague.[12]

In a simple stethoscopic examination, errors are introduced by "signal processing," that is, lack of experience or appropriate knowledge on the part of the listener. Because it is a nonpowered, nontechnologic device (the energy levels come from the phenomena themselves), an esophageal or precordial stethoscope has unique value in being a continuous monitor during power outages. Physical limits to the technique include airspace disease (in itself an informational finding), inability to place the monitor appropriately, and lack of quantifiable data.

Active Sound Examination (Percussion, Echo, Doppler)

The earliest "active" acoustic diagnostic technique was percussion of the chest wall. A skilled clinician can use this method to detect consolidation of the lungs, pleural effusion, and a few other chest pathologies. Although based on transmission and reflection of sound, percussion is purely qualitative and is unable to localize pathologic changes accurately. Modern ultrasound improves on percussion by using shorter wavelength sound waves and quantitative detection of their reflections (echoes). The spatial resolution of an examination is limited by the wavelength of the sound used (Fig. 38-20). Using ultrasound at frequencies in the megahertz (10^6 cycles/sec) range allows resolution of much smaller objects. The wavelength of 1-MHz sound waves in solid tissue is about 1.5 mm, whereas the wavelength of a 256-Hz tone (middle C) in tissue is 5.7 m.

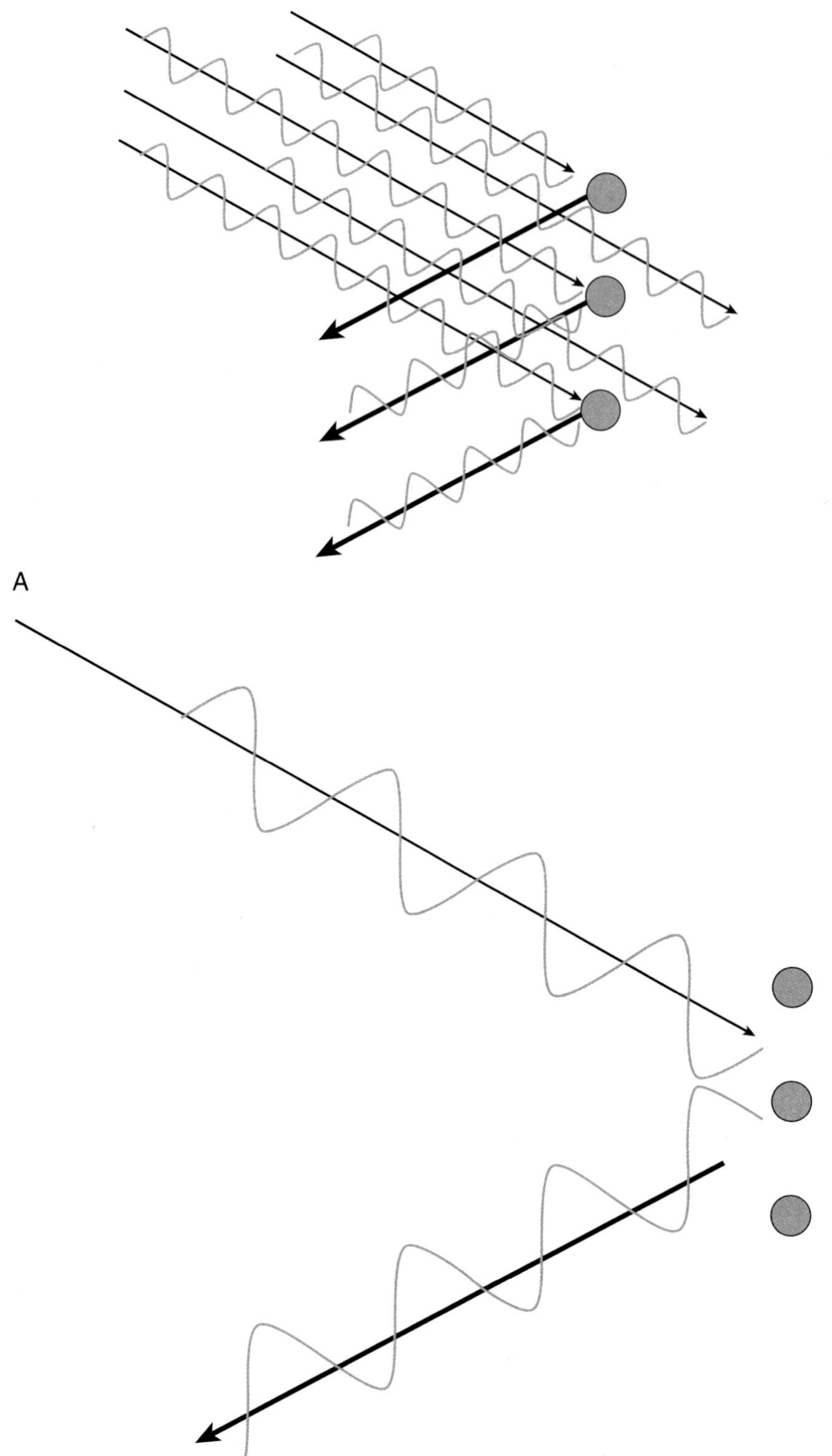

Figure 38-20 Wave size and resolution. Wave reflection depends on the relative size of waves and objects. For small objects, small waves are needed for good reflection and resolution. **A,** The object size is large relative to the wave size, resulting in good spatial resolution. **B,** The object size is small relative to the wavelength, leading to poor resolution of the objects. This principle also applies to light waves. Electron microscopes can resolve smaller objects than light microscopes because the wavelengths used are smaller. Imagine running an unsharpened pencil over a fine (1-mm grid) or coarse (1-cm grid) screen. The pencil sticks in the larger holes, while passing over the smaller ones. Sharpening the pencil to a point improves the resolution.

With the use of esophageal transducers, echocardiography has become a popular intraoperative monitoring technique.[13,14] Sound waves in the 2- to 10-MHz range are transmitted toward the heart in short bursts or pulses. After each pulse, the transducer passively listens to the reflected echoes from various tissues. The ability to place the transducer in the esophagus is advantageous because sound does not have to pass through airspaces or bone on its way to and from the heart. The speed of sound through the heart and surrounding soft tissues is a nearly constant 1540 msec. Exact measurement of the elapsed time between transmission of the pulse and receipt of the echo provides the distance to the reflecting structure. The sound beam from the transducer is projected in a narrow "searchlight" pattern, so the exact direction of reflecting structures also is known.

The Doppler effect is used in echocardiography to determine the presence and degree of valvular regurgitation by converting the Doppler shift of sound waves reflected from erythrocytes into a color display (see Appendix 7; also see Chapter 41). Cardiac output also can be estimated from descending thoracic aortic blood velocity by using a Doppler technique. These devices estimate the blood flow in the descending aorta and ignore flow to the head and arms. They calibrate descending aortic flow to cardiac output by assuming a constant proportional relationship between the two flows.[15]

Measurements Using Electric Energy (Transverse Wave) (see also Chapter 100)

Principles of Electricity

Most monitors and other anesthesiology apparatus use the basic principles of electricity and magnetism. Nearly all transducers use some form of electric energy as their output, and the subsequent data processing and display are entirely electric. We review some basic electromagnetic principles in this section by using examples from medical equipment. Electromagnetic waves, including light, are transverse waves, meaning that the electric and magnetic field vectors are oriented perpendicular to the direction of wave propagation. In contrast to sound, these waves require no media in which to propagate.

Static Electricity

Electricity is a manifestation of a property called "charge" that is inherent in matter. The charge can be negative, positive, or neutral. Static electricity involves charges at rest: Like charges repel one another, whereas opposite charges attract. What we usually mean by the word "electricity" involves the flow of charges, or electric current. Current flows in one direction in direct-current (DC) electronic devices and alternates back and forth in alternating-current (AC) devices.

The SI unit of charge is the coulomb, and the smallest quantum of charge is the charge of an electron (1.6×10^{-19} Coulomb), which is equal but opposite to the charge of a proton. (More recently discovered subatomic particles called "quarks" actually have smaller charges, but this is beyond the scope of this chapter and not relevant to medicine.) An electrostatic force is exerted between two charged objects and is directly proportional to the product of the two charges and inversely proportional to the square of the distance between them:

$$F = k \times q_1 \times q_2 / r^2 \text{—Coulomb's law} \quad (1)$$

This force is attractive when the charges are of opposite sign, and repulsive when they are of the same sign. In a Nobel Prize–winning experiment, Millikan determined the charge of an electron by suspending charged oil drops between two horizontal charged plates such that the electrostatic force balanced the gravitational force, and the drops were held in midair (Fig. 38-21). Approximately 20 years later in 1940, Millikan's son developed one of the earliest infrared ear oximeters, the forerunner of the pulse oximeter (see the section on the pulse oximeter).

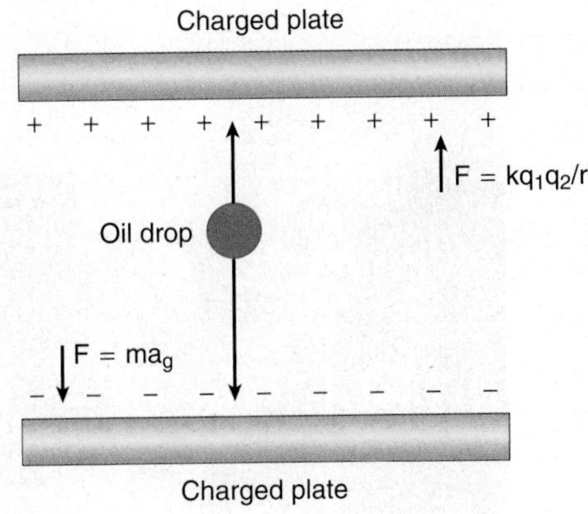

Figure 38-21 Electric force. The quantity of charge on an electron was determined by balancing the electric force on an oil drop against the gravitational force on the same drop. $F_1 = kq_1\, q_2/r^2 = F_2 = m_1\, a_g$.

Direct Current

Just as mechanical energy may be stored as potential energy, electric energy can be stored as a "potential difference." A common analogy is to compare electric potential difference with water pressure (Fig. 38-22 and Table 38-2). The potential difference (V) between points *A* and *B* is defined as the work required to move a unit charge from *A* to *B*. The SI unit of potential difference is the volt; the term *voltage* is often used for potential difference. Charges can move easily through conductors, but they do not move well through insulators, also called "dielectrics." If a potential difference (V) exists between *A* and *B*, and these two points are connected by a conductor, charges will flow between them and produce an electric current (I).

The SI unit of current is the coulomb per second, called the "ampere." If points *A* and *B* are separated by an insulator, no current will flow until the potential difference becomes so great that a breakdown of the insulator occurs. If *A* and *B* are separated by dry air, no current will flow until the potential difference reaches 3000 V/mm. At this very large potential gradient, air ionizes and becomes a conductor, and a current flows in the form of a visible (and audible) spark. To generate a spark between two electrodes 1 cm apart, one must create a potential difference of 30,000 V. The spark plugs in a car have an electrode gap of about 0.8 mm, requiring at least 2400 V from the ignition coil to generate a spark. Lightning is a larger manifestation of the same phenomenon.

A battery is a chemical cell that produces a nearly constant potential difference between two electrodes, which is called "electromotive force (EMF)". The battery can provide a continuous source of electrons, or current, to flow through any conducting circuit connected between its electrodes. Flow of electricity is opposed by resistance, analogous to resistance in water pipes. In most materials, resistance (R) is related to voltage (V) and current flow (I) in the following manner:

$$V = IR \quad (2)$$

This relationship is called Ohm's law, and materials that follow this behavior are called "ohmic" materials. This example is analogous to hemodynamic flow, in which the pressure decrease across the systemic vasculature (mean arterial pressure—central

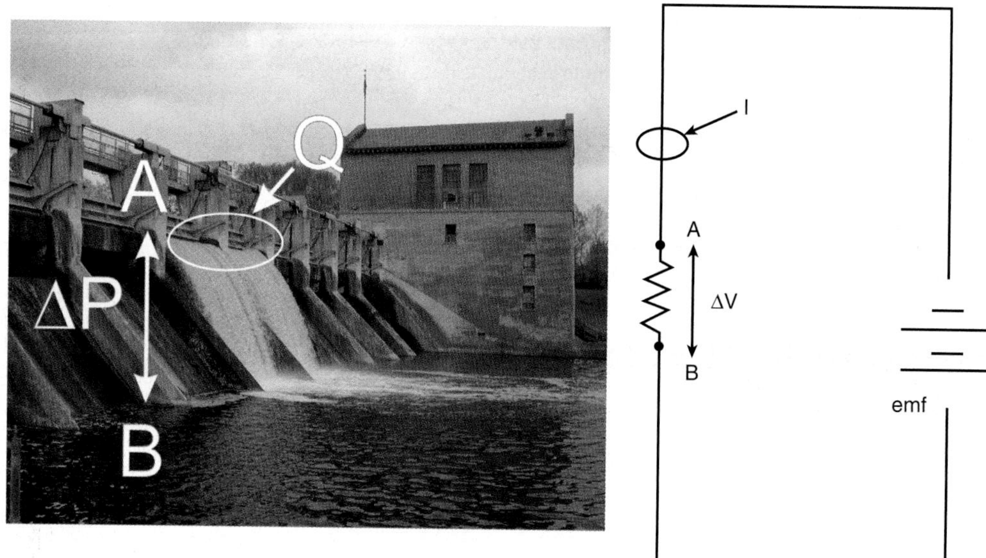

Figure 38-22 Water and electricity. The pressure drop over the dam (*A* to *B*) is analogous to the voltage drop over the resistance (*A* to *B*) (e.g., light bulb). The amount of flow (width of water) (*Q*) is analogous to the current (*I*). Both falling water and electric potential can do work, as evidenced by the use of dams to generate electricity and electricity to pump water.

venous pressure) equals cardiac output times systemic vascular resistance:

$$\Delta P = CO \times SVR \quad (3)$$

The power (i.e., rate of work; see discussion earlier in this chapter) required to produce an electric current is the product of voltage and current: P = VI. By combining this formula with Ohm's law (V = IR), we have $P = I^2R = V^2/R$. If we double the current through a fixed resistance (R), we use four times the original power. This power loss in resistors is dissipated as heat, which is the reason why nearly all electric devices become warm during use. The filament in an incandescent light bulb is merely a resistor that becomes so hot from ohmic heating that it glows, or radiates light.

A capacitor is a device that stores charge (Q) in direct proportion to the potential difference (V) between its two electrodes: Q = CV. The proportionality constant (C) is called "capacitance," which is measured in SI units of farads (1 farad = 1 coulomb/volt). When a capacitor is connected to a battery, current flows until the capacitor is charged to the point that the potential across the capacitor equals the EMF of the battery: V = Q/C = EMF (Fig. 38-23). When we push the "charge" button of a cardiac defibrillator, this kind of circuit is activated to charge a capacitor to the desired level. As shown in Figure 38-23B, time is required to charge a capacitor. For a large capacitor, more time is required. It takes longer to charge a defibrillator to 200 J than to 50 J.

Table 38-2 Comparison of Hydrodynamic and Electrical Energy Commonly Encountered

Water	Electricity	Energy
Squirt gun	Static electric spark	High pressure, low flow, low energy
Garden hose	House current	Moderate pressure, moderate flow, moderate energy
	Car battery	Low pressure, moderate flow, moderate energy
River flood		Low pressure, huge flow, huge energy
Fire hose	High tension wires	High pressure, high flows
	Lightning	High pressure, high flow

Alternating Current

In an AC circuit, the current and the voltage fluctuate rapidly (Fig. 38-24). There are many important differences between AC and DC power. The voltage in common AC "house power" fluctuates sinusoidally at a frequency of 60 Hz (50 Hz in Europe). We characterize the amplitude of such a fluctuating voltage by its root mean square (RMS), that is, the square root of the time average of V^2. For AC house power, V_{RMS} = 115 V (230 V in Europe). Current in an AC system also is constantly changing and is likewise measured as an RMS value.

AC circuits have three forms of impedance: resistance (R), capacitance (C), and inductance (L). An inductor is a circuit element whose impedance, called "inductive reactance," increases with the frequency (f) of the current fluctuations ($R_L = 2\pi fL$). Conversely, the impedance of a capacitor, called "capacitive reactance," decreases with increasing frequency ($R_C = ½\,\pi fC$). Inductors tend to block high frequencies, whereas capacitors tend to block low frequencies (Fig. 38-25). This principle is used in stereo systems to direct the signal to either the "woofer" (low-frequency speaker) or the "tweeter" (high-frequency speaker). In medical instruments, inductance and capacitance circuits can be used to "filter" the signal (e.g., decreasing the amount of 60-Hz interference from AC wiring).

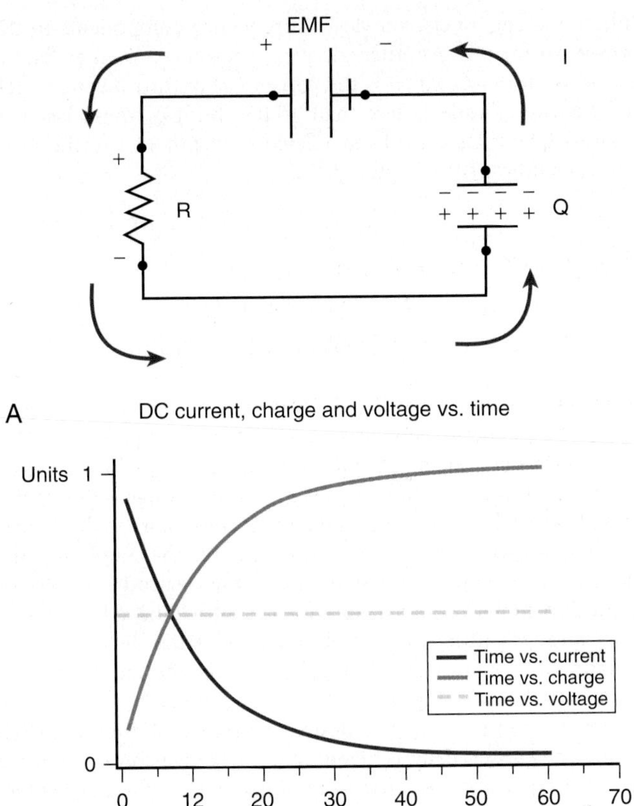

Figure 38-23 Resistance and capacitance in a direct-current circuit. **A,** Under direct current, the resistance impedes flow, resulting in a voltage decrease across the resistance. The capacitor allows current to flow until the charge builds on the capacitor. **B,** Under direct current, the voltage is constant over time, and the current flow decreases as the charge on the capacitor increases. This type of circuit is used to charge a defibrillator.

Passive Electric Examination (Electrocardiograph, Electroencephalograph)

Now that some of the basics of electricity have been described, we can discuss the electrocardiograph (ECG) and the electroencephalograph (EEG), where the sources of EMF are the heart and the brain (see Chapters 40 and 42). Electric potentials on biologic surfaces are too small to observe directly and must be amplified and processed before display. ECG potentials on the skin are in the 1-mV range, and EEG potentials are near 0.1 mV.

Figure 38-26 illustrates why electric potentials on biologic surfaces are so small. The heart generates an electric signal as a result of the synchronous depolarization and repolarization of multiple cells. The electric potentials generated by the heart are measured between two skin electrodes, *A* and *B*. As the figure shows, there are multiple effective resistances and capacitances in the tissues between the EMF source and the measuring electrodes. These impedances reduce the magnitude of the voltage signal at the skin. The "shunt" resistors R_3, R_4, and R_5 combined with the "series" resistors R_1, R_2, and R_3 form what is called a "voltage divider network." Lower values of shunt resistance or higher values of series resistance result in smaller voltages at the skin. The capacitance of the skin (C_s) also acts to attenuate the low-frequency components and distort the waveform. Skin resistance, which may be a megaohm (10^6 ohms) for dry skin, can be reduced to a few hundred ohms by conductive gels.

If a DC voltage is applied between two body surface electrodes, current flows through the tissues between them. Although the electric current in metals consists entirely of electron flow, in tissues, positive and negative ions migrate. Negative ions tend to accumulate at the positive electrode (the anode), and positive ions accumulate at the negative electrode (the cathode). This collection of anions and cations near each electrode creates its own EMF, which opposes the EMF that set up the original current. The current decreases, so the effective impedance between the electrodes increases. This phenomenon, called "polarization of electrodes," has two harmful effects. First, the increased impedance from polarization can attenuate the ECG signal for several seconds after defibrillation or DC cardioversion. Such attenuation could be misinterpreted as a lack of electric activity and result in inappropriate administration of a second shock. The second consequence of prolonged application of DC voltage is accumulation of a local concentration of toxic ions near electrode sites, a condition that can cause burns or tissue necrosis.

A partial solution to the problem is the use of a nonpolarizable electrode, such as a silver and silver chloride combination.

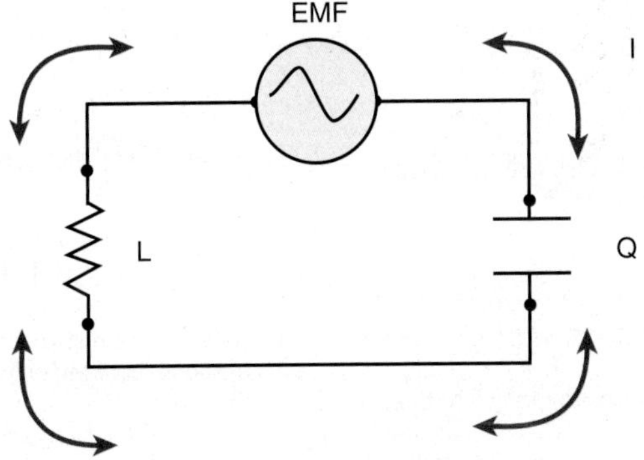

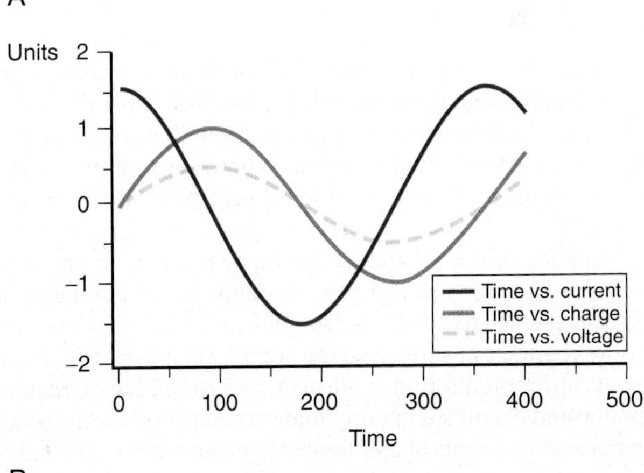

Figure 38-24 Resistance and capacitance in an alternating-current (AC) circuit. **A,** In an AC circuit, in contrast to a direct-current circuit, the capacitor does not block current flow. **B,** The capacitor and resistance act to shift the phase of the AC current. Current changes lag behind voltage changes. EMF, electromotive force.

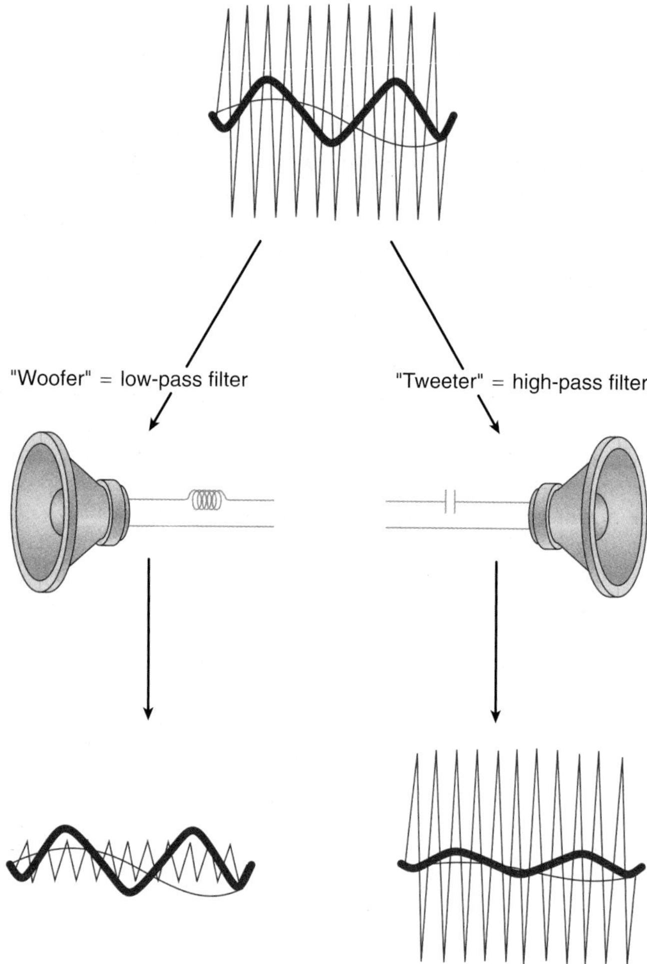

Figure 38-25 Woofer and tweeter. Stereo speakers use resistors to act as an impedance to high-frequency components of sound, allowing only the bass frequencies to pass on to the woofer speaker. Capacitors are used as a high-pass filter to allow only the high frequencies to get to the tweeter. By a similar process, 60-Hz interference from electrical appliances can be decreased. *(From Hecht E: Physics: Algebra/Trig. Pacific Grove, CA, Brooks/Cole, 1994.)*

This electrode can act as a source of, or "sink," for anions and cations, minimizing the accumulation of ions. Most disposable ECG electrodes now use such materials. Even these electrodes are nonpolarizable for only a limited time, however, and the application of prolonged DC voltage between any tissue electrodes must be avoided.

Similar problems complicate measurements of the EEG, but in this case, the raw signal is one tenth the amplitude of the ECG: 100 μV versus 1 mV. The spontaneous EEG provides eight or more channels of surface voltage versus time data, which is of limited use for monitoring in the operating room. For rapid interpretation and diagnosis, the amplitude versus time data are usually transformed into plots of amplitude (or power) versus frequency. This process of power spectral analysis was discussed in the section on signal processing. The EEG power spectrum facilitates rapid diagnosis of hemisphere asymmetries and changes in frequency content that accompany either deep anesthesia or cerebral hypoxia. "Bispectral density" is another method of analyzing the raw EEG that determines levels of correlation (or degree of "phase-locking") between various frequency components in the power spectrum. Another derived parameter is the "burst-suppression ratio," which is the percentage of time during which the EEG amplitude is less than +5 μV. Both of these last two derived quantities have been related to depth of anesthesia in clinical studies (see Chapter 39).

Active Electric Examination (Neuromuscular Block Monitor, Somatosensory Evoked Potentials)

A muscle twitch can be elicited by generating a 0.2- to 0.3-msec pulse of current to depolarize a peripheral motor nerve. This motor nerve conducts the impulse to the muscle, where a twitch is generated. We can understand the "in-use" failings of this device by following the path of the signal. We must start with an adequate power source (no power = no twitch). If the coupling of the electrodes to the patient is poor (i.e., if the electrodes are dry or good skin contact is not made), the circuit will have high resistance, and very little current will flow (see earlier discussion and equation 8), resulting in a diminished twitch. The simplest way to be certain that this monitor is functioning properly is to perform a positive control (see the desired response of thumb twitch before the chosen drug is given) and a negative control (see the twitch disappear in response to administered drug) (see Chapters 46 and 47).

Evoked potential (evoked response) monitors can determine the status of multiple parts of the sensory nervous system by measuring the central nervous system response to a discrete sensory stimulus. The stimulus can be auditory, optical, or peripheral somatosensory. The amplitude of the evoked response measured at the skin can be very small—less than 1 μV in the case of acoustic cortical potentials. This very small signal is in a "sea" of spontaneous EEG (>100-μV amplitude) signals. We resort to a signal enhancement technique called "ensemble averaging." Rather than trying to measure the small response to a single stimulus, we average the responses from hundreds (or thousands) of stimuli. Because the evoked responses that we seek occur consistently at the same time after the known stimulus, this averaging process

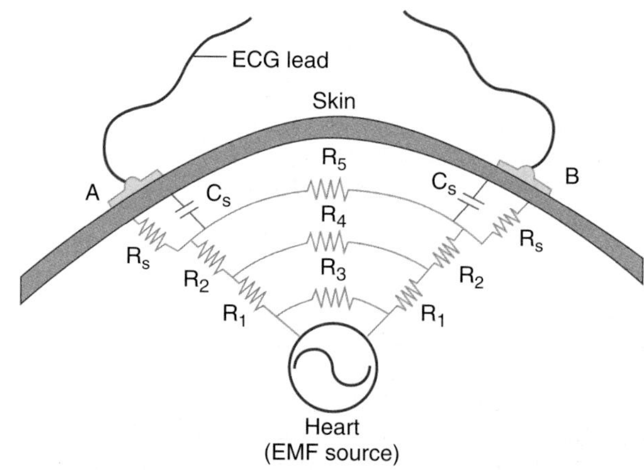

Figure 38-26 Why the electrocardiograph (ECG) is so small. Multiple resistances and capacitances in the body decrease the potential and distort the waveform before the electromotive force (EMF) reaches the surface.

reinforces the signal from the evoked response, and the random "noise" tends to cancel itself. In this way, we commonly measure signals whose amplitude is roughly 1% the amplitude of the background noise (see Fig. 38-9).

Whenever charged particles are moving, a magnetic field is generated in a direction perpendicular to the motion. Paramagnetism is a form of magnetism exhibited only in specific substances in the presence of an external magnetic field. Oxygen is a paramagnetic gas. This property is used to measure inspired and expired oxygen concentrations—chemical methods such as fuel cell amperometric sensors and polarographic electrodes are too slow to respond. In a fast responding paramagnetic oxygen sensor, 100% oxygen can exert a pressure of 3 Pa in a 2.4-T magnetic field.

Measurement Using Light Energy

Principles of Light

What we commonly refer to as light is electromagnetic radiation in the visible range of wavelengths. Every substance with a temperature greater than absolute zero emits electromagnetic radiation, called "black body radiation." This radiation is characterized by a frequency and wavelength that are related by the speed of light: frequency = speed of light ÷ wavelength (c = speed of light = 3×10^8 m/sec or 186,400 miles/sec or 7.5 times around the earth's circumference in 1 second, in a vacuum). High energies or temperatures are associated with high frequencies and short wavelengths, such as those of gamma rays and x-rays. As wavelength increases to the micron range, ultraviolet radiation proceeds to visible light (approximately 0.5 to 0.8 μ), and at larger wavelengths, infrared is followed by microwaves and radio waves with wavelengths in the kilometer range.

Electromagnetic waves and sound waves have some important differences. The particles in motion in sound waves are in the same direction as the propagation (longitudinal waves), whereas in electromagnetic waves, the electric and magnetic fields are perpendicular to the direction of propagation (transverse waves). Sound waves can propagate only through matter, whereas electromagnetic waves propagate through a vacuum without attenuation. The speed of light is about 1 million times faster than the speed of sound in sea-level air. If an observer is moving relative to a sound source, measurement of the speed of sound depends on the observer's own motion, but the speed of light is the same to any observer in any frame of reference. This last statement is the basic premise of Einstein's special theory of relativity. In the high-frequency range of the electromagnetic spectrum are two forms of ionizing radiation: x-rays and gamma rays. These high-frequency waves are capable of knocking electrons out of their orbits and can cause cell injury and death or ontogenesis. Gamma rays are commonly emitted by decaying radioactive nuclei.

Visible light and infrared light have several properties common to all electromagnetic radiation. Light represents a form of energy that, when passing through matter, may be reflected, transmitted, or absorbed. Although light itself cannot be stored, it can be converted into some other form of energy, such as electricity, chemical energy, and heat. In addition, light can be generated from other forms of energy, including heat (incandescent), electric (gas discharge), and chemical (photoluminescent) energy.

Light as a Multifunctional Tool: Beer-Lambert Law

When light passes through matter, it is transmitted, absorbed, or reflected. The relative absorption or reflection of light at different wavelengths is used in several monitoring devices to estimate the concentrations of dissolved substances (e.g., carbon dioxide in respiratory gas and hemoglobin in plasma). This type of measurement is called spectrophotometry and is based on the Beer-Lambert law of absorption, which states that if a known intensity of light illuminates a chamber of known dimensions, the concentration of a dissolved substance can be determined if the incident and transmitted light intensity is measured:

$$I_t = I_i e^{-dC\alpha} \qquad (4)$$

Solved for C:

$$C = (1/d\alpha)\ln\left[I_i/I_t\right] \qquad (5)$$

where C is the concentration of the dissolved substance, d is the path length of the light *a*, and α is an absorption constant for the dissolved substance at the light wavelength used. I_i and I_t are the incident and transmitted light intensity. The unknown C is inversely proportional to d and directly proportional to the log of the ratio of I_i to I_t (Fig. 38-27). Red and infrared light (wavelength 0.6 to 1 μ) are generally used because the constituents of interest to anesthesiologists (anesthetic agents, carbon dioxide, hemoglobin) absorb light within that range. Red and infrared light can penetrate soft tissues and may be used to measure the concentrations of hemoglobin species in vivo (see the section on pulse oximeters). Infrared light is absorbed by small molecules only if they have bonds and are asymmetric; in other words, their molecules have a dipole moment. Nitrogen, oxygen, and helium cannot be measured by infrared light. Another limitation of infrared light is that it is absorbed by ordinary glass; the measurement chambers for these devices must be made of sapphire or other infrared-permeable materials.

Simple Absorbance Monitors (Capnometer, Anesthetic Analyzer)

Capnometers, capnographs, and anesthetic gas analyzers all use the Beer-Lambert law to analyze constituents of the respiratory gas stream (see Chapter 25). A capnometer measures and displays only discrete values of partial pressure of carbon dioxide ($P{CO_2}$), such as the end-tidal value. A capnograph provides a continuous plot of $P{CO_2}$ in the airway versus time. The physical design of capnometers is divided into two categories: mainstream and sidestream. In mainstream capnometers, the light absorption chamber is placed directly in the airway, and the light source shines through the chamber, with carbon dioxide being measured during inspiration and expiration directly. Advantages of this technique are a very fast response time and no problems with clogging of the sampling tubes, which is a disadvantage of sidestream capnometers. Disadvantages of the mainstream geometry include the

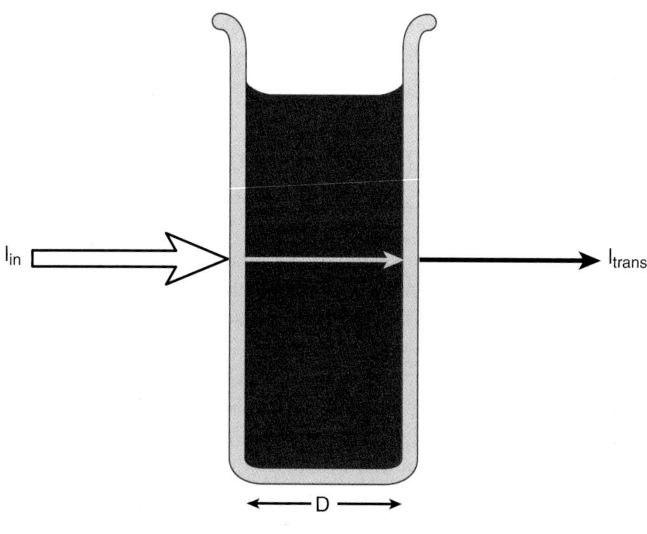

Figure 38-27 Cuvette. Light entering the cuvette is reflected and absorbed. The concentration of substances absorbing and reflecting light can be determined by measuring the amount of light entering and exiting the system.

necessity of having a potentially heavy, expensive infrared measurement device placed directly in the airway at the endotracheal tube, and the unavailability of devices that can measure anesthetic agents and carbon dioxide.

The most commonly used devices in the operating room are sidestream capnometers. A thin sampling tube is attached to the airway near the endotracheal tube, and samples are aspirated at 200 to 400 mL/min into the measurement chamber, which is located within the monitor itself. The advantages of this method are the opposite of the disadvantages of the mainstream capnometers; the sampling tube is lightweight, and the device can be used to measure carbon dioxide and anesthetic agents. Disadvantages of sidestream capnometers relate mostly to the delayed response time and potential clogging of the aspiration tubing.[16]

Anesthetic agent analyzers and capnographs function by the same physical principles, but with different wavelengths of light being used (Fig. 38-28). The light absorbances of a mixture of gases can interfere with each other, so compensations are built into current devices.

Processed Absorbance Monitors (Pulse Oximeter)

Oximeters are devices that use light absorbance measurements to determine the concentration of various species of hemoglobin. One of the first in vivo oximeters was a noninvasive monitor used in aviation research during World War II. This device transilluminated tissue (the earlobe) with light of two wavelengths. One wavelength was sensitive to changes in oxyhemoglobin, and the other was not. In effect, the earlobe acted as a test tube containing the suspended hemoglobin. For a review of the development of pulse oximetry, the reader is referred to the excellent article by Severinghaus and Astrup.[17]

Before specific engineering problems are discussed, we need to define what we wish to measure. Adult blood usually contains four species of hemoglobin: oxyhemoglobin (HbO_2), reduced hemoglobin (Hb), methemoglobin (metHb), and carboxyhemoglobin (COHb). The latter two are abnormal hemoglobins (called "dyshemoglobins"), and are normally present in only small amounts. Each of these hemoglobin species has a different light absorption profile. Figure 38-29 illustrates the different absorption constants for each hemoglobin species light from red to infrared light. Fractional hemoglobin saturation ($O_2Hb\%$) is defined as the ratio of HbO_2 to total hemoglobin:

$$O_2Hb\% = HbO_2/(HbO_2 + Hb + metHb + COHb)$$

Measuring this quantity in the presence of metHb and COHb requires at least four wavelengths of light, which yield four simultaneous Beer-Lambert equations to solve for the four hemoglobin species. Because metHb and COHb do not contribute to oxygen transport, functional saturation is defined as the ratio of HbO_2 to HbO_2 plus reduced hemoglobin:

$$Sa{O_2} = HbO_2/(HbO_2 + Hb)$$

Although functional saturation depends explicitly on only HbO_2 and Hb, four light wavelengths are still required to measure it in the presence of significant concentrations of COHb and metHb.[18,19] If the concentrations of metHb and COHb are zero, $O_2Hb\%$ and SaO_2 become identical.

The pulse oximeter performs substantial signal processing of optically transduced physiologic data. Although the physical

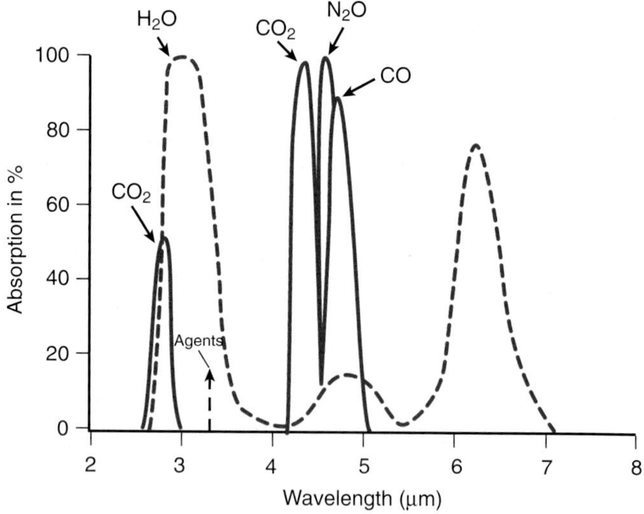

Figure 38-28 Absorption spectra of some gases and materials important to anesthesia. The absorption is not constant over wavelengths. It is important to choose the proper wavelength to measure. Also, when multiple substances are present, it is still possible to measure their concentrations, provided that enough wavelengths are available. (The solution becomes one of multiple equations with multiple unknowns.) *(From Gravenstein JS, Paulus DA, Hayes TJ: Capnography in Clinical Practice. Boston, Butterworths, 1989.)*

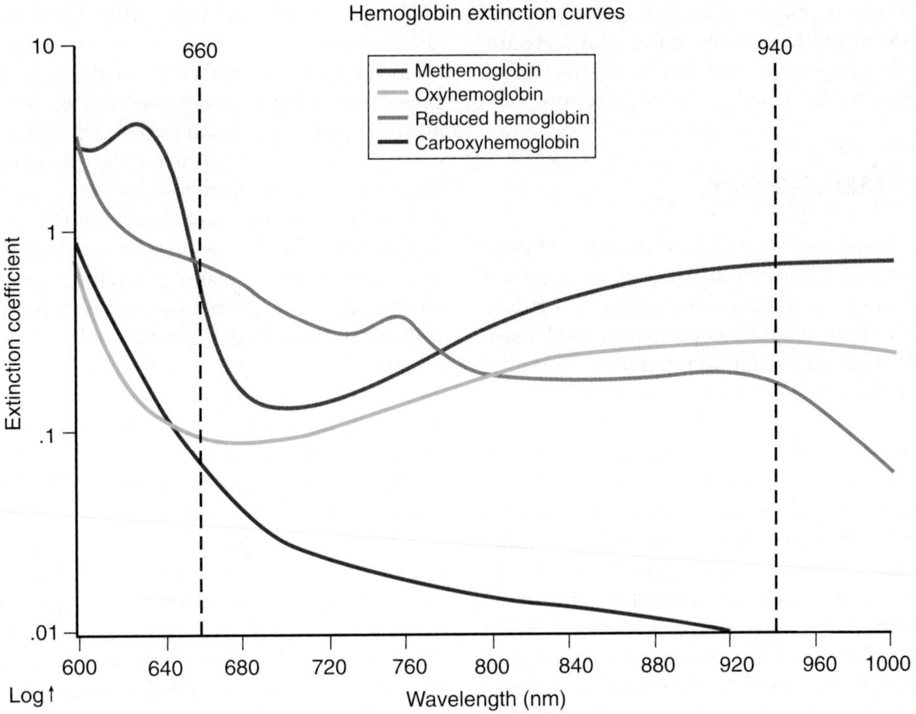

Figure 38-29 Hemoglobin extinction curves. Pulse oximetry uses the wavelengths of 660 nm and 940 nm because these are available in solid state emitters (not all wavelengths are able to be emitted from diodes). Carboxyhemoglobin and oxyhemoglobin absorb equally at 660 nm, and so both read as Sao_2 to a conventional pulse oximeter. In addition, methemoglobin and reduced hemoglobin share absorption at 660 nm and interfere with correct Sao_2 measurement. *(Courtesy of Susan Manson, Biox/Ohmeda, Boulder, CO, 1986.)*

principle governing pulse oximetry is straightforward, application of this principle to produce a clinically useful device involves significant engineering problems.[18,20] The remainder of this section describes the physical and physiologic problems of pulse oximeter design and the engineering solutions to these problems. The discussion is divided into basic design and management of signal artifacts.

Basic Design of Pulse Oximeters

Noninvasive in vivo oximeters measure red and infrared light transmitted through and reflected by a tissue bed. Accurate estimation of Sao_2 by this method entails several technical problems. There are many light absorbers in the transmitted light path other than arterial hemoglobin (e.g., skin, soft tissue, and venous and capillary blood). The pulse oximeter accounts for the effects of absorption of light by tissue and venous blood by assuming that only arterial blood pulsates. Figure 38-30 schematically illustrates the series of absorbers in a typical sample of living tissue. At the top of the figure is the AC component, which represents absorption of light by the pulsating arterial blood. The DC (baseline) component represents absorption of light by the tissue bed, including venous, capillary, and nonpulsatile arterial blood. Pulsatile expansion of the arteriolar bed increases the light path length (see equations 4 and 5), increasing absorbency. Conventional pulse oximeters (including all commercial pulse oximeters until 2005) use only two wavelengths of light, typically 660 nm (red light) and 940 nm (near-infrared light). The pulse oximeter first determines the fluctuating or "AC" component of absorbance at each wavelength and then divides this value by the nonfluctuating or "DC" component to obtain the "pulse-added absorbance," which is independent of the incident light intensity. The oximeter then calculates the ratio (R) of the two pulse-added absorbances (one for each wavelength)[18]:

$$R = \left(AC\,660/DC\,660\right)/\left(AC\,940/DC\,940\right) \qquad (6)$$

Finally, the value of R (often called the "ratio of ratios") is related to the displayed saturation estimate Spo_2 by a "look-up table" programmed into the oximeter's software. The tables used in all commercial pulse oximeters are based on experimental studies in healthy human volunteers. Although each manufactur-

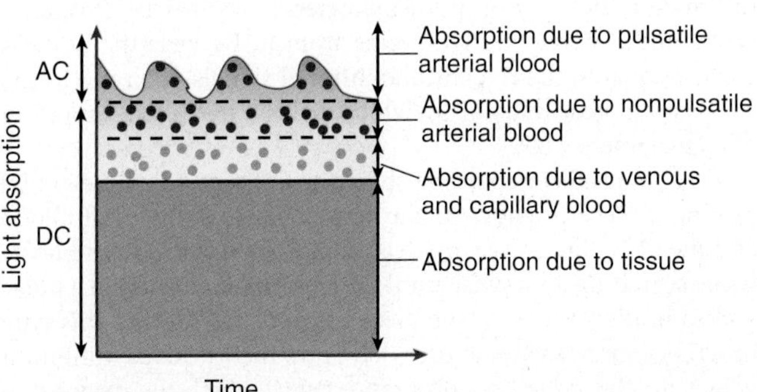

Figure 38-30 Pulse oximetry signals. A primary difficulty with pulse oximetry is that the pulsatile signal is small compared with the total absorbance of the ear or finger being examined. Pulsatile flow is needed to determine the Sao_2. AC, alternating current; DC, direct current. *(Adapted from Ohmeda Pulse Oximeter model 3700 Service Manual.)*

er's exact calibration curve is proprietary, these curves are very similar. When the ratio of red-to-infrared pulse-added absorbance is 1.0, the displayed Spo_2 is approximately 85%. This fact has clinical implications that are discussed in the next section.

Signal Artifact Management

One of the most difficult engineering problems in pulse oximetry is identification of the fluctuating absorbance pattern of arterial blood in a sea of electromagnetic and other artifacts. Artifacts have four major sources: ambient light, low perfusion (weak pulse, low AC-to-DC signal ratio), venous blood pulsations (caused by patient motion, among other things) and additional light absorbers in the blood (e.g., dyshemoglobins, intravenous dyes). All these sources of artifacts produce a low signal-to-noise ratio, resulting in either erroneous Spo_2 values or no value at all.

The photodiodes used in the sensor to detect light cannot differentiate one wavelength of light from another. The detector does not know whether the light received originates from the red (660 nm) light-emitting diode (LED), the infrared (940 nm) LED, or the room lights. This problem is solved in most pulse oximeters by alternating the red and infrared LED sources. The red LED is turned on first, and the photodiode detector produces a current resulting from the red LED plus the room lights. Next, the red LED is turned off, and the infrared LED is turned on. The photodiode signal then represents the infrared LED plus the room lights. Finally, both LEDs are turned off, and the photodiode generates a signal from the room lights alone. This sequence is repeated hundreds of times per second. In this way, the oximeter attempts to eliminate light interference even in a quickly changing background of room light.[18] Some sources of fluctuating light can cause problems despite this clever design. Artifact from ambient light can be minimized simply by covering the sensor with an opaque shield.

Another engineering problem is that of a low AC-to-DC signal ratio, or low perfusion. When a small pulsatile absorbance signal is detected, the conventional pulse oximeter amplifies the signal and estimates saturation from the ratio of the amplified absorbances. In this way, the pulse oximeter can estimate saturation values of Spo_2 for a wide range of patients who generate different amplitudes for pulsatile absorbance. As with a radio receiver, when a weak signal is amplified, the background noise, or "static," also is amplified. At the highest amplifications (which can be up to 1 million times), some pulse oximeters may "analyze" this noise signal and generate an Spo_2 value from it. Because the noise is usually equal in the red and the infrared signals, the ratio of the two is often near unity (1.0), which yields a displayed saturation of approximately 85%.

This problem could be shown in early pulse oximeters by placing a piece of paper in the sensor between the photodiode and the LED. Some early models amplified the background noise while searching for a pulse until they eventually displayed a pulse and saturation value for the piece of paper. To prevent this type of artifact, many manufacturers have now incorporated minimum values for the signal-to-noise ratio, below which the device displays no value for Spo_2. Some oximeters also display a low signal strength error message; in addition, many display a plethysmographic wave for visual identification of noise.

Patient motion, causing venous pulsations with a high AC-to-DC signal ratio, may be the most difficult artifact to eliminate. Engineers have tried several approaches to this problem, beginning with simply increasing the signal averaging time. If the device averages its measurements over a longer period, the effect of an intermittent artifact is usually less. This longer averaging period also slows the response time to an acute change in Sao_2, however, and it may result in "frozen" Spo_2 values being displayed when the true saturation is rapidly changing. Most pulse oximeters now allow the user to select one of several time-averaging modes. In addition, some manufacturers use more sophisticated algorithms to identify and reject spurious signals.

One innovation aimed at reducing motion artifact is based on the premise that motion causes pulsations of venous blood within the tissue bed. Conventional pulse oximetry cannot distinguish venous pulsations from those of arterial blood; large low-reading errors or loss of signal can result. In the newer signal-processing algorithm developed by Masimo, Inc. (Irvine, CA), the oximeter computes a venous "noise reference signal," which is common to both light wavelengths. The noise reference is subtracted from the total signal, and a "true" arterial signal is left. This is one of five "parallel engine" algorithms that Masimo SET (Signal Extraction Technology) uses simultaneously to find the most reliable Spo_2 value for the current signal conditions. Tests in human volunteers and preliminary clinical studies indicate that this new technology represents an improvement in pulse oximeter performance in low signal-to-noise ratio situations.[21,22]

More recently, Masimo has brought to market the first multiwavelength pulse oximeter: the Rainbow Rad-57 Pulse CO-oximeter. This device employs eight light wavelengths rather than the usual two, making it capable of measuring COHb and MetHb, in addition to the conventional Spo_2 value and pulse rate. The first human volunteer study of this instrument shows that it can measure COHb with an uncertainty of ±2%, and MetHb with an uncertainty of ±0.5%.[23]

Other in vivo oximeters have been developed to measure light reflected by living tissue in an attempt to determine hemoglobin saturation in specific organs. Using reflected rather than transmitted light adds complexity because the path lengths of the light through the tissue may be varied and tortuous, making calibration difficult. Nevertheless, a signal reflected from living tissue may produce useful information regarding the average saturation of the hemoglobin within that tissue.[24] A cerebral oximeter may be able to measure mean brain hemoglobin saturation, which reflects the intracerebral balance among venous, arterial, and capillary blood, and the oxygenation of all three.

Measurement of Temperature

Principles of Temperature

Moving matter contains energy. Even stationary objects are moving at the atomic level. This kinetic energy of molecules and atoms is described as temperature. When all molecular motion (translational, vibrational, and rotational) ceases, the substance is said to be at a temperature of absolute zero—the lowest possible temperature. This temperature is equivalent to −273°C, and is defined as 0°K. This state provides a reference point for all temperature measurements, which in all thermodynamic calculations must be expressed in degrees Kelvin.

Heat is a form of internal kinetic energy that can flow between two contacting bodies that are at different temperatures.

The amount of heat required to increase the temperature of 1 g of a given substance by 1°C is called the specific heat of that substance. The calorie, a common heat unit, is the amount of heat required to increase the temperature of 1 g of water from 14.5°C to 15.5°C. One calorie is equivalent to 4.184 J of energy. When we refer to calories in terms of the calories in the food that we eat or the calories that we expend while exercising, we are actually referring to kilocalories, or thousands of calories (also called "kitchen calories"). The total amount of heat energy in an object depends on its specific heat, its temperature, and its mass. Although a cup of 60°C coffee is much "hotter" than a 30°C swimming pool, the coffee contains much less total thermal energy than the pool does. The same is true for potential energy stored as pressure potential or electric potential. A small container at high pressure may have less potential energy than a larger container at lower pressure (see Chapter 48).

Temperature Monitors (Thermometer, Thermistor, Thermopile, Liquid Crystal)

Three techniques are commonly used for measuring temperature: based on expansion of a material as its temperature increases, based on changes in electric properties with temperature, and based on optical properties of a material. As heat is added to most substances (gases, liquids, or solids), motion of the molecules increases, and the volume of the material increases at constant pressure. Depending on the material, this expansion can be calibrated directly to changes in temperature. Liquids are most commonly used, such as mercury because its effective range extends from its freezing point of −39°C to approximately 250°C.[25] Mercury thermometers have two disadvantages. First, they require 2 to 3 minutes for complete thermal equilibration (mercury is a liquid metal with a high specific heat). Second, they are enclosed in a glass tube, which may break and cause injuries.[26] Thermometers based on the expansion of gas (Bourdon tube) or metal (bimetallic strip) are frequently used in thermostats because they also respond slowly to transient changes in temperature.

Electric techniques for measuring temperature can be subdivided into three categories: resistance thermometers, thermistors, and thermocouples. Resistance thermometers operate on the principle that the electric resistance of metals increases with temperature. These devices most frequently use a platinum wire as the temperature-sensitive resistor, a battery, and a galvanometer to measure current, which can be calibrated to temperature. The platinum wire is incorporated into a Wheatstone bridge circuit, which accurately measures very small changes in resistance (see Fig. 38-5).

Compared with a platinum thermometer, a thermistor is a semiconductor that displays the opposite behavior with regard to electric resistance. As the thermistor is heated, its resistance decreases. Thermistors, being solid-state devices, can be manufactured in extremely small sizes and have a fast response to change in temperature (i.e., little heat is needed to increase their temperature). Most of the temperature probes used in anesthesia, from the ones at the end of pulmonary artery catheters to esophageal probes, are thermistors. Physical problems with thermistors are few: Cracked or broken wires lead to high resistance and incorrect temperature readings. More common problems are poor probe placement and misinterpretation of the resulting value (e.g., placing an esophageal probe in the oropharynx and measuring airway temperature rather than core temperature). Thermocouples are conductors that generate a voltage in response to a temperature gradient.

The optical properties of materials can be used to measure temperature in two ways: (1) the infrared "black body" emissions of an object can be measured by using a device known as a thermopile, and the emission can be converted to temperature, and (2) a liquid crystal "matrix" can be placed in direct contact with the desired zone, and an optical change can be observed (a change in color). The most commonly encountered example of infrared temperature measurement involves the tympanic membrane temperature monitor used in recovery rooms, pediatrics, and hospital wards.[27] The infrared detector produces an electric signal that is proportional to the fourth power of the difference in absolute temperatures of the objects. The following formula describes this phenomenon: $Q_{1,2} = K(T_1^4 - T_2^4)$, where $Q_{1,2}$ is net heat transfer (W/cm^2), K is the Stefan-Boltzmann constant, and T_1 and T_2 are the absolute temperatures of the two objects (°K).

In theory, this method of measuring the core temperature should be accurate. In practice, improper placement and lack of calibration, but not ear canal cerumen, contribute to real-world errors.[28-30] Additionally, the probe is large for intraoperative use.

Liquid crystal measures of temperature (found in "mood rings") are often used for skin temperature monitoring. Just as the molecules in a liquid crystal watch display change their optical properties with a small electric current, becoming polarized and dark, the molecules in a liquid crystal temperature device change their optical properties with temperature, resulting in a rainbow of colors. The crystal matrix is sensitive to pressure and temperature. (By touching an LCD display panel, one can note the visual rainbow of changing colors.) The reported clinical accuracy of liquid crystal devices varies.[31,32]

Measurement of Flow

Principles of Flow

Although conceptually one of the easier measurements to understand as volume or mass movement over time, flow is actually not easy to measure. We must clearly distinguish between fluid flow and fluid velocity, which are often confused. Flow (Q) refers to the volume of fluid passing a particular surface area per unit of time; its SI units are cubic meters per second (m^3/sec), but in medicine, it is more commonly measured in mL/sec or L/min. Fluid velocity (U) is simply the speed of the fluid at a particular point in space, measured in msec. By analogy, imagine a multilane freeway: the speed (velocity) of individual cars may vary depending on the lane; the flow is the number of cars passing a point per minute.

Mass and Volume Flow Meters (Urometer, Volumeter)

Flow can be measured directly, by diverting the flow into a measuring chamber. We can measure the mass or volume of fluid flowing per unit time by catching the fluid in a container and either weighing it or measuring its volume. The common urometer for measuring urine volume is an example. The volumeter used in North American Drager anesthesia machines also measures aliquots of volume integrated over time to measure tidal and minute volume (Fig. 38-31).[33]

Dilutional Flow Meters (Thermodilution, Fick Principle)

Volume and mass flow also can be measured by dilutional techniques. If some measurable indicator (a bolus of dye, a thermal pulse, oxygen consumption, carbon dioxide production) is injected into a flow, and its concentration is measured as a function of time at a point downstream, the volume flow (Q) can be calculated by integration. The most common medical application is determination of cardiac output by the pulmonary artery thermodilution method (see Appendix 6). Errors associated with these methods involve using the wrong injectate volume (too small a volume resulting in an overestimate of flow) or an error in temperature measurement (see the section on temperature).

"Continuous" thermodilution cardiac output using an electric heating coil to warm the pulmonary artery blood removes errors associated with fluid injectate techniques but introduces the need to average the smaller signal over a longer time interval. Additionally, there is an upper limit to warming the blood without cellular damage, so signal quality is reduced in febrile patients.[34] A slightly different approach is to measure the electric current required to maintain a constant temperature at the catheter tip. This is the principle of a constant temperature hot wire anemometer (used to measure gas flows in wind tunnels and in some anesthesia machines) applied to cardiac output.

The rate of carbon dioxide production or oxygen consumption can be used to measure cardiac output by modifications of the Fick equation (see Appendix 6). When using these variables, a change in metabolic rate can lead to errors in cardiac output measurement.

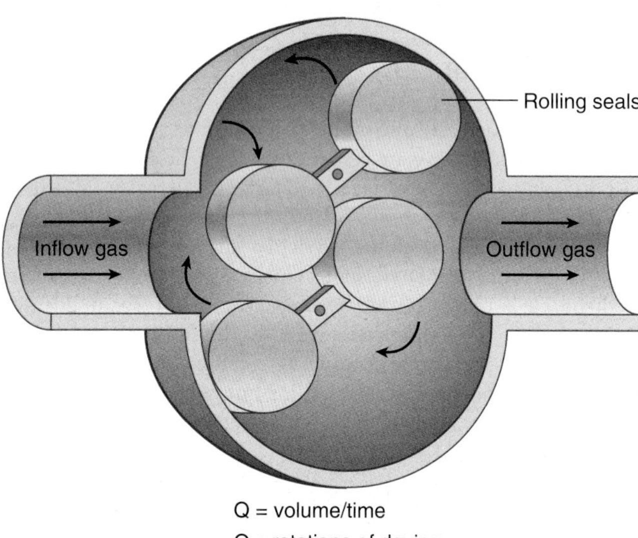

Figure 38-31 Volumeter. Flow can be described as volume over time. This design of flow meter allows gas to pass in only small aliquots, each of which turns a counter to measure the amount flowing past. When divided by time, this results in a flow measurement. *(Adapted from Ehrenwerth J, Eisenkraft J: Anesthesia Equipment: Principles and Application. St. Louis, Mosby-Year Book, 1993.)*

Velocity and Pressure Flow Meters (Venturi, Pitot)

Flowing fluids in tubes generate velocity and pressure, which can be used to measure the flow indirectly. Pressure in fluids can be thought of as a form of potential energy, as described earlier. Kinetic energy in fluids is expressed in terms of flow, the bulk movement of fluid with a given direction and magnitude. The potential energy of pressure can be converted into the kinetic energy of flow; for example, the hydrostatic pressure generated by gravity acting on a vertical column of liquid can be transformed into flow by opening a valve at the bottom of the column. Pressure and flow also can change independently. With the human circulatory system used as an example, a healthy young trauma patient in hypovolemic shock can have normal blood pressure, but low blood flow with high systemic vascular resistance. A septic patient can have very low blood pressure accompanied by high blood flow and low systemic vascular resistance (high-output septic shock). The total mechanical energy of a moving fluid is the sum of the kinetic (flow) energy and the potential (pressure) energy (see Table 38-2).

A pressure gradient (changing pressure in a particular spatial direction) exerts a force on the fluid, and the fluid tends to accelerate in the direction of decreasing pressure. Pressure gradient is only one of the forces that commonly act on fluids; other forces include gravity (discussed earlier) and viscous force or friction. If these other forces are negligible, and the fluid is incompressible (i.e., a liquid with constant density), the equation of motion (F = ma) can be integrated to yield:

$$P + \tfrac{1}{2}\rho U^2 = P_0 \qquad (7)$$

where P is pressure, ρ is fluid density, U is the magnitude of the fluid velocity, and P_0 is a constant called the "stagnation pressure" (see Appendix 5). This form of the Bernoulli equation tells us that pressure decreases as velocity increases in a frictionless flow, and vice versa. This equation dispells the common misconception that pressure always decreases in the direction of flow. In the flow inside a tube (a pipe or a large vein) of gradually increasing diameter, fluid velocity (U) decreases in the downstream direction as the diameter and cross-sectional area of the tube increase. As U decreases, equation 5 tells us that P increases in the direction of flow. This example shows the relationship of potential and kinetic energy in fluids: As the kinetic energy of this tube flow decreases (U^2 falls) in the flow direction, the potential energy increases (P rises) by an equal amount. The total energy remains constant because we have assumed no friction.

Flow can be determined by measuring the average velocity of the fluid across the tube. In laminar tube flow (Fig. 38-32A), the velocity profile has a parabolic shape, with the highest velocity at the center line and the fluid at the walls being stationary. In turbulent tube flow, the velocity profile is "flattened" as shown in Figure 38-32B.

The Bernoulli equation applies to a specific subset of frictionless flows, as described earlier. Many flows important to anesthesiologists do not follow the Bernoulli equation. Most com-

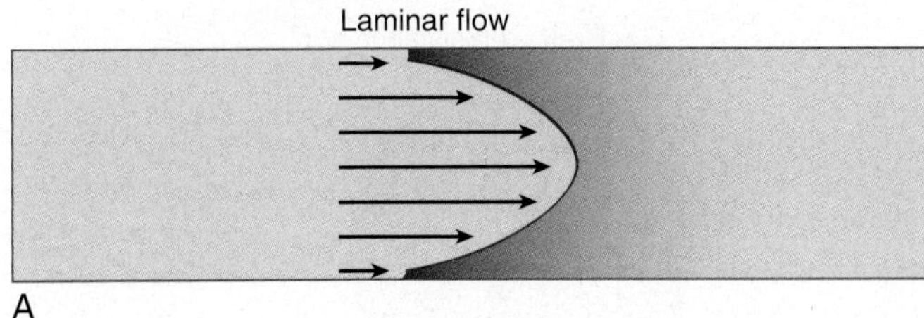

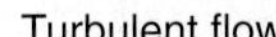

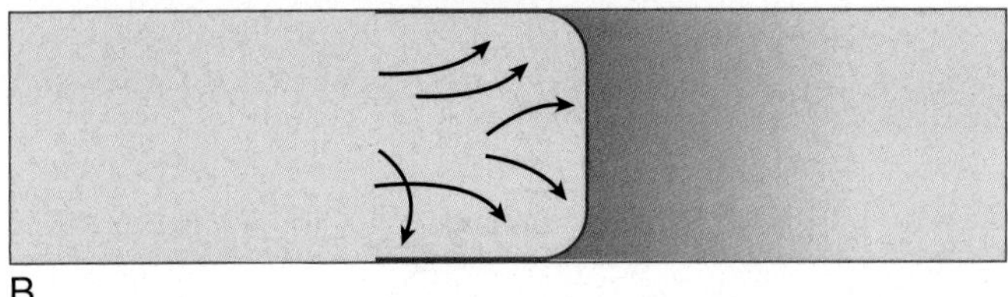

Figure 38-32 Laminar and turbulent flow. **A,** In a smooth-walled tube at low flow rates (i.e., small pressure gradients), the flow rate is laminar; that is, flow moves smoothly in concentric circles, with the centermost area having the greatest flow velocity and the area nearest the wall of the tube being virtually stationary. **B,** As flow rate (and pressure gradient) increases, the flow transitions from laminar to turbulent. Instead of a neatly ordered flow, the velocities are more randomly distributed, energy is dissipated as heat, and the energy needed for a given flow rate increases. Many factors govern this transition, including size of the tube, viscosity of the fluid, flow rate, and pressure gradient. These factors are combined in the determination of the Reynolds number (see Appendix 5).

monly, the flow that we desire to measure is not laminar, but turbulent. The transition from laminar to turbulent flow depends on the type of fluid, the speed of the flow, and the shape of the flow. The fluid factors are combined in a dimensionless ratio called the "Reynolds number (Re)":

$$Re = \rho UL/\mu \tag{8}$$

where ρ is the density of the fluid, U is the mean flow velocity, L is a characteristic dimension (length) of the flow, and μ is the viscosity of the fluid. For a given flow geometry (e.g., flow through a tube of circular cross-section), transition from laminar to turbulent flow occurs at a critical value of Re. In straight, smooth, circular tubes, transition from laminar to turbulent flow occurs at Re of approximately 2100 (see Appendix 5).

A Venturi tube is a circular tube with a gradual contraction and expansion in diameter, in contrast to the sudden contraction-expansion of an orifice flow meter (Fig. 38-33). Because the contraction is smooth and gradual, the Bernoulli equation (equation 7) applies to this geometry. For conservation of mass and energy to apply, as we restrict the flow by narrowing the tube, the speed *increases*; the pressure on the walls *decreases* to keep the total energy (the "stagnation pressure" of the Bernoulli equation) constant. The total mass flow on both sides of the contraction must be equal (we have not created or lost any matter). If we measure the pressure difference between the widest and the narrowest parts of the Venturi tube, we can solve the Bernoulli equation for velocity (see Appendix 5). The Venturi tube derives fluid velocity (U) from the pressure difference, not volume flow (Q). The Venturi tube is used in many industrial applications and is used on some aircraft to measure speed.

To have a measurable pressure gradient, there must be some resistance in the fluid path. The lower the rate of flow, the

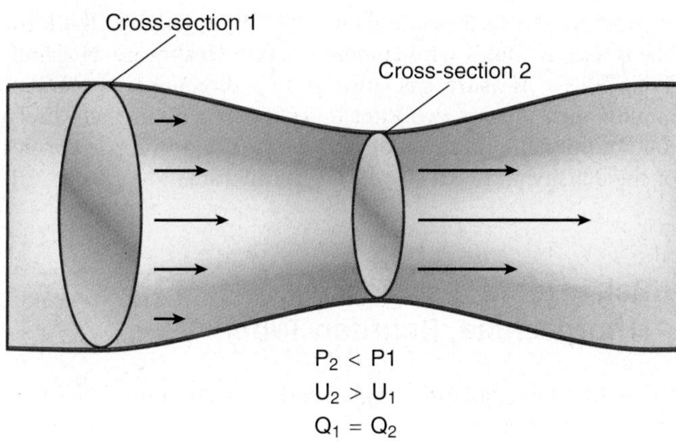

Figure 38-33 Venturi tube. By measuring the pressure difference between two points in a laminar flow, the average flow velocity can be determined because the mass flow and total energy (minus frictional losses) must be the same (see Appendix 5).

greater the resistance must be to generate the same pressure gradient. In respiratory applications, pediatric flow meters have too much resistance (owing to lower flows) to use in adults, and adult flow meters do not generate enough resistance to give an adequate signal (pressure change) in pediatric patients. A variable resistance flow meter has been devised (Ohmeda 7900/Aisys (GE Healthcare, Madison, WI) wherein the orifice is a flap that moves as the flow increases. No simple equation or relationship exists between the pressure above and below the restriction; this flow meter must be empirically calibrated, and the calibration curve for each sensor must be stored electronically.

A Pitot tube is a cylindric tube whose open end is pointed directly into the flow, that is, "upstream" (Fig. 38-34). The pressure measured in the Pitot tube approximates the stagnation pressure, given earlier by equation 7. If we independently measure the static pressure p (the p_1 side port in the Fig. 38-34) at the same location, and we know the fluid density ρ, we can easily solve equation 7 for the fluid velocity U. The Pitot tube derives velocity U, not volume flow Q. The Pitot tube is simple and reliable, and is used

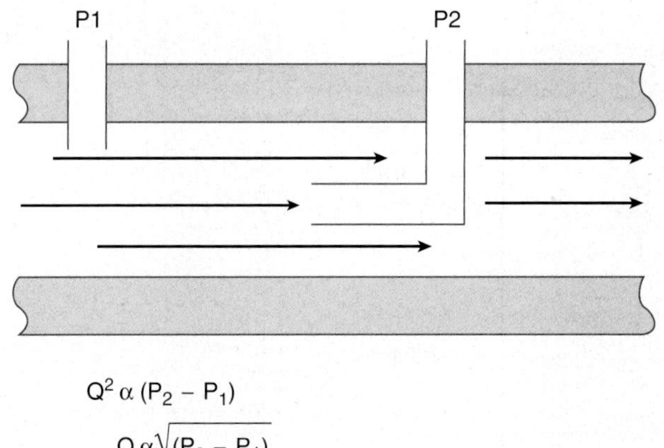

Figure 38-34 Pitot tube. As flows increase, wall pressure decreases as a result of the Bernoulli principle. The Pitot tube measures the difference in pressure from the middle of the flow to the wall and converts this to a flow measurement (see Appendix 5). *(Adapted from Ehrenwerth J, Eisenkraft J: Anesthesia Equipment: Principles and Applications. St. Louis, Mosby-Year Book, 1993.)*

on most aircraft to measure their speed. In anesthesia, the Pitot tube is used in Datex Ultima monitors (GE Healthcare, Helsinki, Finland). To measure gas flow in two directions, the Datex monitor incorporates two Pitot tubes, one facing in each direction. Additionally, the monitor samples gas composition to correct for the density and viscosity of the gas mixture.

Balance-of-Pressure Flow Meters (Thorpe Tube, Bourdon Tube)

If flow in a tube passes through a sudden restriction such as an orifice, the volume flow Q is proportional to the area of the orifice and the square root of the pressure drop through the orifice. (The Bernoulli equation does not apply to this flow geometry.) This is the principle of all orifice flow meters, including the rotameter of an anesthesia machine (see Appendix 5).

The most common flow meter seen by anesthesiologists is the floating bobbin rotameter on the anesthesia machine, the Thorpe tube (Fig. 38-35). This variable-orifice flow meter uses a balance of forces to determine pressure change and measure flow. When the flow meter valve is opened, the flow of gases through the annular orifice between the bobbin and the tapered glass tube provides a force to raise the bobbin. As the bobbin rises, the area of the annular gap between the bobbin and the tube increases as a result of the taper of the tube. As the area of this gap (orifice) increases, the pressure change across the bobbin decreases because the pressure change across an orifice is inversely proportional to the square of the orifice area. The bobbin ceases its upward motion at an equilibrium point when the downward force of gravity (weight of the bobbin) is balanced by the upward pressure force. The height of the bobbin in the tube is directly related to the gas flow. Although this flow meter is simple in principle, its application becomes more complex when the flow in the tube changes from laminar to turbulent as velocity and diameter increase. For mathematical derivations, see Appendix 5.

Another flow meter, the Bourdon tube (Fig. 38-36), keeps the orifice constant and allows the pressure to vary. As flow Q increases, the gradient of P_1 to P_2 increases and causes the flattened metal tube to uncoil and move the pointer.

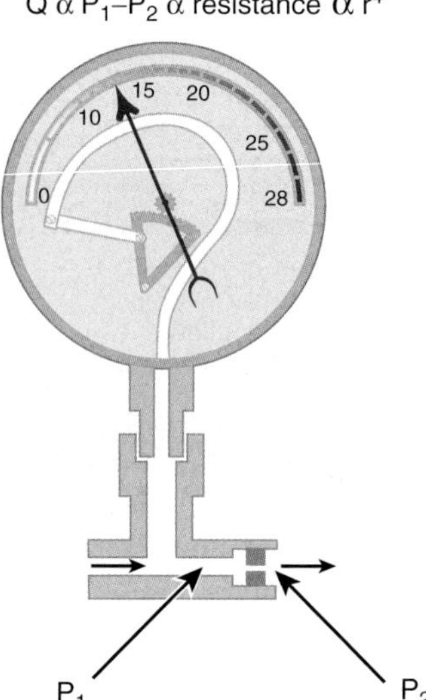

Figure 38-36 Bourdon tube flow meter. In contrast to the Thorpe tube, which has a constant pressure, but a variable orifice, the Bourdon tube has a constant orifice, but a variable pressure. The tube uncoils under the high back pressure. This drawback makes it unsuitable for use in low-pressure respiratory systems. It receives much use in portable oxygen tanks, however. If the orifice is increased in radius, the flow meter will under-read actual flow. If the orifice is dirty (i.e., decreased radius), the flow will be overestimated. *(From Mushin WW, Jones PL: Physics for the Anaesthetist, 4th ed. Oxford, Blackwell, 1987.)*

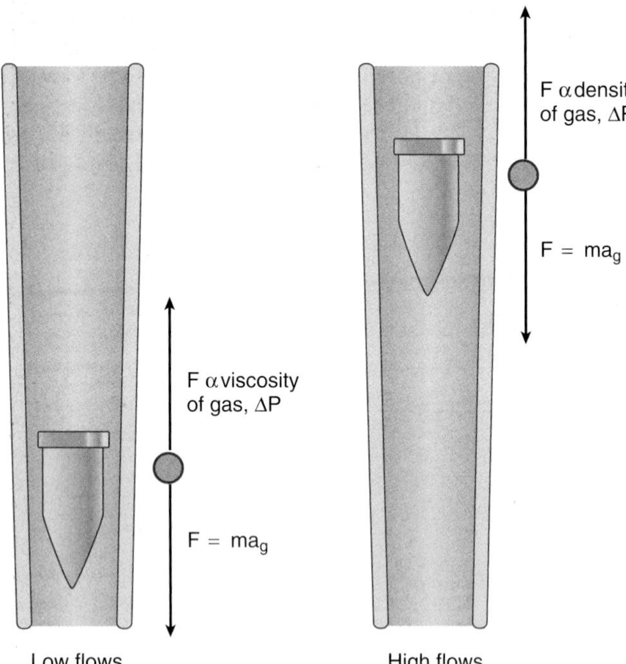

Figure 38-35 Thorpe tube flow meter. At low flows, viscosity of gas predominates, and the flows balance when the gravitational attraction equals the pressure gradient across the equivalent orifice. At higher flows, density takes over, and the balance is the same except for the formula determining pressure (acts like an orifice) (see Appendix 5).

Kinetic Energy Flow Meters (Wright Spirometer)

Vanes or propellers placed in a confined flow turn at a rate proportional to the volume flow if there is no friction in the propeller bearings. Various vane spirometers (Fig. 38-37) (e.g., Wright spirometer) work by this principle. These devices tend to be less accurate at very high and low flow rates because of frictional forces.

Summary of Flow Measurement

Every method of measuring flow has its particular limitations and uncertainties. Because gases are not always pure with a known, constant density, flow meters based on the Bernoulli equation (equation 7) are subject to errors. Any device inserted into a fluid flow can disturb the flow by its presence. A rotating vane spirom-

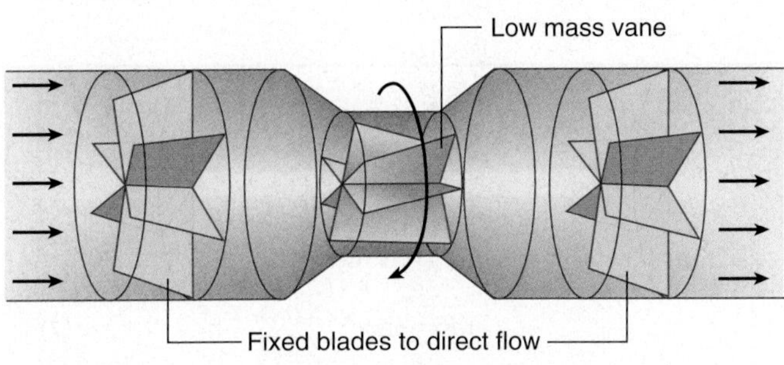

Figure 38-37 Vane spirometer. Moving gases contain kinetic energy. This can be sampled by a rotating "windmill" in the gas stream. *(Adapted from Ehrenwerth J, Eisenkraft J: Anesthesia Equipment: Principles and Applications. St. Louis, Mosby-Year Book, 1993.)*

eter may reduce the gas flow at high flow rates because of internal friction. Several methods of flow or fluid velocity measurement depend on a pressure measurement (Pitot tube, Venturi tube, orifice flow meter); the flow measurement is no more accurate than the pressure measurement.

Conclusion

New monitors are being developed almost continuously, but new physical principles are revealed only rarely. The science of physics is a constant effort to understand, simplify, and predict the behavior of the universe in quantitative terms. The terms and principles outlined here will be referred to multiple times in subsequent chapters.

References

1. DeGowin EL, DeGowin RL: Bedside Diagnostic Examination, 5th ed. New York, Macmillan, 1987.
2. Bland JM, Altman DG: Statistical methods for assessing agreement between two methods of clinical measurement. Lancet 1:307-310, 1986.
3. Beecher HK: The first anesthetic record (Cushing and Codman). Surg Gynecol Obstet 71:689-692, 1940.
4. Cushing H: Technical methods of performing certain operations. Surg Gynecol Obstet 6:237-246, 1908.
5. Sykes MK, Vickers MD, Hull CJ: Principles of Measurement and Monitoring in Anaesthesia and Intensive Care, 3rd ed. Boston, Blackwell, 1991.
6. Dorje P, Tremper K: Systolic pressure variation: A dynamic measure of the adequacy of intravascular volume. Semin Anesth Periop Med Pain 24:147-153, 2005.
7. Michard F: Changes in arterial pressure during mechanical ventilation. Anesthesiology 103:419-428, 2005.
8. Quill TJ: Blood pressure monitoring. *In* Ehrenqerth J (ed): Anesthesia Equipment Principles and Applications. St. Louis, Mosby-Year Book, 1993.
9. O'Brien E: Has conventional sphygmomanometry ended with the banning of mercury? Blood Press Monit 7:37-40, 2002.
10. Ireland J: In praise of mercury sphygmomanometers: Electronic readings of blood pressure seem to be higher than readings obtained with mercury sphygmomanometers. BMJ 322:1249, 2001.
11. Resnick R, Halliday D: Physics for Students of Science and Engineering. New York, John Wiley & Sons, 1960.
12. Rappaport MB, Sprague H: Physiologic and physical laws that govern auscultation, and their clinical applications. Am Heart J 21:257-318, 1941.
13. Cahalan MK, Litt L, Botvinick EH, Schiller NB: Advances in noninvasive cardiovascular imaging: Implications for the anesthesiologist. Anesthesiology 66:356-372, 1987.
14. Clements FM, de Bruijn NP: Perioperative evaluation of regional wall motion by transesophageal two-dimensional echocardiography. Anesth Analg 66:249-261, 1987.
15. Wong D, Tremper K, Stemmer E, et al: Noninvasive cardiac output: Simultaneous comparison of different methods with thermodilution. Anesthesiology 72:784-792, 1990.
16. Gravenstein JS, Paulus JS, Hayes TJ: Capnography in Clinical Practice. Boston, Butterworths, 1989.
17. Severinghaus JW, Astrup PB: History of blood gas analysis. Int Anesthesiol Clin 25:1-224, 1987.
18. Tremper KK, Barker SJ: Pulse oximetry. Anesthesiology 70:98-108, 1989.
19. Barker SJ, Tremper KK, Hyatt J: Effects of methemoglobinemia on pulse oximetry and mixed venous oximetry. Anesthesiology 70:112-117, 1989.
20. Pologe JA: Pulse oximetry: Technical aspects of machine design. Int Anesthesiol Clin 25:137-153, 1987.
21. Dumas C, Wahr JA, Tremper KK: Clinical evaluation of a prototype motion artifact resistant pulse oximeter in the recovery room. Anesth Analg 83:269-272, 1996.
22. Barker SJ, Shah NK: The effects of motion on the performance of pulse oximeters in volunteers (revised publication). Anesthesiology 86:101-108, 1997.
23. Barker S, Curry J, Redord D, Morgan S: Measurement of COHb and MetHb by pulse oximetry: A human volunteer study. Anesthesiology 892-897, 2006.
24. Wahr JA, Tremper KK, Samra S, Delpy DT: Near-infrared spectroscopy: Theory and applications. J Cardiothorac Vasc Anesth 10:406-418, 1996.
25. Budavari S, O'Neil MJ, Smith A, Heckelman P: The Merck Index, 11th ed. Rahway, NJ, Merck, 1989.
26. Moxham JP, Lee PK: Broken glass mercury thermometer: A difficult airway foreign body. Otolaryngol Head Neck Surg 127:339-341, 2002.
27. Shinozaki T, Deane R, Perkins FM: Infrared tympanic thermometer: Evaluation of a new clinical thermometer. Crit Care Med 16:148-150, 1988.
28. Pransky SM: The impact of technique and conditions of the tympanic membrane upon infrared tympanic thermometry. Clin Pediatr (Phila) 30:50-52, 1991.
29. Terndrup TE, Rajk J: Impact of operator technique and device on infrared emission detection tympanic thermometry. J Emerg Med 10:683-687, 1992.
30. Chamberlain JM, Terndrup TE: New light on ear thermometer readings. Contemp Pediatr 11:66-76, 1994.
31. Vaughn MS, Cork RC, Vaughn RW: Inaccuracy of liquid crystal thermometry to identify core temperature trends in postoperative adults. Anesth Analg 61(3):284-287, 1982.
32. Ikeda T, Sessler DI, Marder D, Xiong J: Influence of thermoregulatory vasomotion and ambient temperature variation on the accuracy of core-temperature estimates by cutaneous liquid-crystal thermometers. Anesthesiology 86:603-612, 1997.
33. Cicman JH, Gotzon J, Himmelwright C, et al: Operating Principles of Narkomed Anesthesia Systems, 2nd ed. Telford, PA, WE Andrews, 1998.
34. Q2 CCO/SvO2 Monitoring System Operating Manual [computer program]. North Chicago, Abbott Laboratories, 1998.

Appendix 1

Distance versus Time under Constant Acceleration: Equivalence of Potential and Kinetic Energy

Velocity (v) is the rate at which distance is changing; that is, it is the time derivative of distance:

$$\mathbf{v} = dx/dt \quad (1)$$

The variable v is in boldface type to indicate that it is a vector: it has magnitude and direction. Distance **x** is a vector pointing from the origin to the present location of the particle or object; it is called the "position vector." Time (t) is a scalar; it has magnitude, but no direction and is in plain type.

Acceleration (**a**) is the time rate of change of velocity. It is the time derivative of the velocity vector, or the second derivative of distance with respect to time:

$$\mathbf{a} = dv/dt = (d/dt)(dx/dt) = d^2\mathbf{x}/dt^2 \quad (2)$$

If an object starts with zero velocity (**v** = 0) at time zero (t = 0) and then accelerates with constant acceleration (a), its velocity at time t will be simply **v** = at. To calculate the distance traveled by the object between time t = 0 and time t, we must divide the time interval 0 to t into a series of very small intervals, each of time length dt. The distance traveled during the interval dt is simply the velocity at that time multiplied by the time interval:

$$dx = vdt = (\mathbf{a}t)dt \quad (3)$$

In the second step, we have substituted the constant acceleration relationship **v** = **a**t from above. Now to compute the total distance traveled, we must sum the distance from all of the small dt time intervals that occur between 0 and t:

$$\mathbf{x} = \Sigma(\mathbf{a}t)dt \quad (4)$$

If we allow the length of the time interval dt to approach zero, the summation process becomes the integral with respect to time from time zero to time t:

$$\mathbf{x} = \int vdt = \int (\mathbf{a}t)dt = \frac{1}{2}\mathbf{a}t^2 \quad (5)$$

An object starting from rest at t = 0 and moving with constant acceleration (**a**) will move a distance ½ **a**t² in time t. If this is a falling object (in a vacuum, where there is no air resistance), a = g = 9.8 msec², and the distance formula becomes:

$$\mathbf{x} = \frac{1}{2}gt^2 = (4.9)t^2 \quad (6)$$

In the first second, the object falls 4.9 m; at the end of 2 seconds, it has fallen 19.6 m; after 3 seconds, 44.1 m; and so on.

The kinetic energy (KE) of a moving object is

$$KE = \frac{1}{2}mv^2 \quad (7)$$

where m is the mass of the object, and v is the magnitude of its velocity (also called speed). Note that v used in this sense is in plain type, not boldface. Consider again the falling object that started at position x = 0 at time t = 0 and falls a distance h:

$$h = \frac{1}{2}gt^2, \text{ or}$$

$$t = \sqrt{(2h/g)} \quad (8)$$

Because velocity v = at = gt, we have by substitution from equation 8:

$$V = gt = g\sqrt{(2h/g)} = \sqrt{(2gh)} \quad (9)$$

The kinetic energy is given by:

$$KE = \frac{1}{2}mv^2 = \frac{1}{2}m(2gh) = mgh \quad (10)$$

Now let us consider the work required to lift the fallen object back to its original height of h. Work is defined as the force exerted times the distance over which the force acts: W = Fd. The force of gravity acting on our object is F_g = mg, so the work required to lift it the distance (h) back to x = 0 is:

$$W = Fd = (mg)d = mgh \quad (11)$$

The work required to restore the object equals the kinetic energy possessed by the object at the bottom of its fall, KE = W = mgh. When we lift the object from x = h back to x = 0, we have increased its potential energy (PE) by the amount mgh. This potential energy can be converted to kinetic energy by allowing the object to fall the distance h. This type of potential energy, called gravitational potential, has a value that clearly depends on where we locate the origin of our coordinates, x = 0. It is the change in potential energy, however, and not its absolute value, that the potential energy/kinetic energy balances:

$$\Delta KE = -\Delta PE \quad (12)$$

The change in kinetic energy is equal to and of opposite sign to the change in potential energy.

Appendix 2

Physics of Hydrostatic Pressure

A liquid manometer is a simple and reliable means of monitoring pressures that do not change rapidly. It simply uses the weight of a measured vertical column of liquid to balance the pressure exerted against the bottom of the column. We have defined weight as the force exerted by gravity on a mass (m): F_g = mg. To determine the weight of a column of liquid of known dimensions (the manometer in Fig. 38-4), we must first know the density (mass per unit volume) of the liquid. Density has dimensions of m/L^3, and the SI units are kilograms per cubic meter (kg/m³). Because liquids are almost incompressible, their density is influenced little by pressure (but affected by temperature). The density of water at room temperature is 997.8 kg/m³, or 1 g/cm³.

The pressure (p) exerted by the bottom of the vertical column of liquid in a manometer (see Fig. 38-4) is determined as follows. If the cross-sectional area of the liquid cylinder is A, and the height of the cylinder is z, its volume is V = Az. If the liquid has a density of ρ, the mass of the column is:

$$m = \rho V = \rho Az \tag{1}$$

Its weight is:

$$W = mg = \rho Azg \tag{2}$$

The liquid column exerts a force equal to its weight on its base, whose surface area is A, creating the following pressure on the surface:

$$p = \text{force/area} = \rho Azg/A = \rho gz \tag{3}$$

The pressure exerted by the manometer is independent of its cross-sectional area (A); it depends on only the density of the working fluid and the vertical height of the column. If we know the liquid density, measurement of the column height (z) allows us to calculate the pressure (p). If the working fluid is mercury (e.g., sphygmomanometers), the density is 13,680 kg/m^3 (13.68 g/cm^3, or 13.68 times the density of water). The relationship of pressure to height of the column is:

$$\begin{aligned} p &= \rho gz = (13{,}600\ \text{kg/m}^3)(9.8\ \text{N/kg})(z) \\ p[\text{N/m}^2] &= 133{,}300(z) \end{aligned} \tag{4}$$

The unit of pressure newton/meter^2 (N/m^2) is called the pascal (Pa). Because a pascal is a small unit of pressure, we usually use kilopascals (10^3 Pa or kPa). If we express p in kPa and z in mm Hg (rather than meters), equation 4 becomes:

$$p[\text{kPa}] = 0.1333(z)[\text{mm}] \tag{5}$$

Appendix 3

Wheatstone Bridge

The Wheatstone bridge is a network of four resistors connected as shown in Figure 38-5, with a battery or direct-current voltage source (electromotive force) connected between *A* and *C* and a voltmeter (V) connected between *B* and *D*. The bridge is said to be "balanced" when the voltmeter reads zero potential difference between points *B* and *D*. From Ohm's law (V = IR), it is easy to show that balance occurs when $R_x = R_s \times (R_2/R_1)$. If R_s is an adjustable standard resistor, and R_1 and R_2 are fixed known resistors, the balanced bridge provides a very precise means of determining R_x, the unknown resistance. This principle has many applications in biomedical engineering, including strain gauge pressure transducer measurements. In this case, the transducer itself is the unknown resistance R_x.

Appendix 4

Amplification Artifact of a Fluid Tube/Transducer Pressure Wave

The amplification artifact of a fluid tube/transducer pressure waveform can be calculated if a few properties of the system are known. The most relevant part of this solution is the response amplitude, which is plotted against the driving frequency (f) in Figure 38-17. This figure shows some important properties of fluid-coupled transducers and other harmonic oscillators. One of these properties is the existence of a resonant frequency, f_0, which is defined as follows:

$$f_0 = \frac{1}{2}\pi\sqrt{k/m} \tag{1}$$

m is the mass of the system, and k is the elasticity, or spring constant.

As we increase the amount of damping (i.e., friction; c is the friction constant), we observe a decrease in the peak amplitude at resonance, and the frequency at which the peak occurs decreases slightly. The damping coefficient (z) is defined as follows:

$$z = c/\sqrt{2km} \tag{2}$$

Although the arterial pressure waveform is not actually sinusoidal, Figure 38-16 shows the most important characteristics of the pressure transducer response. Any combination of catheter, tubing, and transducer can be characterized by two quantities: a resonant frequency (f_0) and a damping coefficient (z). Gardner measured these quantities for many transducer and tubing systems and found that most systems have resonant frequencies of 10 to 20 cycles/sec or Hz and damping coefficients of 0.2 to 0.3. For clinical systems, the maximum amplification factor (ratio of transducer output to input waveform amplitude) at resonance is near 2.5.

If the resonant frequency is 10 Hz (600 cycles/min), one might conclude that amplification plays little role in the clinical range of pulse rates, which are 5 to 10 times smaller. The arterial pressure waveform is not a sine wave, however. It can be represented as a summation of sine waves (a Fourier series) with frequencies up to many times the pulse rate. These higher harmonic frequencies are amplified most and yield the spiked appearance of a poorly processed arterial waveform. Depending on the shape of the actual arterial pressure wave, this distortion can introduce a 20% to 40% "overshoot" error in systolic blood pressure readings. Even worse, this error depends on the pulse rate, so an error determined for a particular patient at the beginning of administration of an anesthetic may not remain constant.

From this discussion, we can easily predict how to optimize the performance of a pressure transducer system. First, the resonant frequency (f_0) should be as high as possible. The value for k in equation 1 should be large (i.e., the spring should be "stiff"), and the value for m should be small (i.e., the cannula and pressure tubing should be as stiff and inelastic as possible). To minimize the mass of the moving fluid, the tubing should be short in length and small in diameter. Judging from plots of amplitude versus frequency/resonant frequency at different damping coefficients, the optimal damping coefficient would be 0.4 to 0.5. One also should carefully eliminate air bubbles from the system because they add elasticity and friction, lowering the resonant frequency. In a clinical system, one can determine the approximate f_0 and z of a transducer system if graphic output is available. If the high-pressure flush is turned on and then quickly turned off at a high chart speed (50 mm/sec), the tracing oscillates through several cycles at a frequency near f_0. The damping coefficient can be found by determining the ratio of amplitudes of successive peaks on the tracing. This is a practical example of how fundamental principles of mechanics can be used to predict and optimize the performance of monitoring systems. These concepts of mechanics recur in other sections of this chapter.

Appendix 5

Flow Meters, Bernoulli's Principle, Laminar and Turbulent Flow

The equations governing the motion of fluids are expressions of Newton's second law, F = ma. Forces associated with fluids fall into three major categories: (1) gravity, (2) pressure, and (3) friction. In the example using manometers, the gravitational force per unit volume of fluid is simply ρg, acting in the vertical direction. Pressure forces are the result of differences in pressure from one point to another and are expressed mathematically as the negative of the pressure gradient. (A pressure gradient is a vector in the direction of the maximal rate of pressure increase, with magnitude equal to the pressure derivative in that direction.) Friction is proportional to viscosity, the physical property of a fluid that relates shear stress to rate of strain:

$$P_0 = p + \frac{1}{2}\rho U^2 + \rho g z \qquad (1)$$

Equation 1 shows the relationship between velocity and pressure of a fluid in a flow that meets the conditions described. For flows in tubes, the manometer technique provides an easy method of measuring mean pressure. The simplest flow meters apply a combination of these two principles to a tube of changing cross-sectional diameter. The Venturi flow meter shown in Figure 38-33 consists of a tube of varying cross-sectional area that has two ports for measurement of pressure. The Bernoulli equation for points 1 and 2 in the figure becomes:

$$P_1 + \frac{1}{2}\rho U_1^2 = P_2 + \frac{1}{2}\rho U_2^2 \qquad (2)$$

Here, the gravity terms have canceled out because the tube is horizontal, but these terms are usually negligible for gas flows in any direction.

The volume of the fluid flow (Q) (also called flux) at both locations must be the same because no fluid is entering or leaving through the tube walls. The dimensions and SI units for the volume of fluid flow are L^3/t and m^3/sec. This volume is determined at each cross-section of the tube by multiplying the average velocity (U) by the cross-sectional area (A):

$$Q = U_1 A_1 = U_2 A_2 \qquad (3)$$

Assuming that A_1, A_2, P_1, and P_2 are known, we now have two equations for the two unknowns U_1 and U_2. Solving these for the velocity U_1 produces:

$$U_1 = \sqrt{\left[2(P_1 - P_2)/\rho\left(1 - A_1^2 - A_2^2\right)\right]} \qquad (4)$$

To find the volume of the flow (Q), we multiply this result by A_1. Velocity is proportional to the square root of the pressure drop, or the pressure change varies as velocity is squared. For a given U_1, or the magnitude of flow velocity, the pressure drop varies as the square of the ratio of the areas, or the fourth power of the ratio of the diameters. If we choose an A_2 greater than A_1, equation 4 implies that P_2 is greater than P_1. In this case, the pressure increases in the direction of flow, a change that initially seems contrary to intuition.

The bobbin flow meters (also called variable-orifice flow meters) in anesthesia machines use a similar principle. These devices consist of a slightly tapered vertical tube and a bobbin or ball that fits inside the tube (see Fig. 38-35). The cross-sectional area of the ring-shaped gap between the bobbin and the tube wall is proportional to the height of the bobbin. Because changes in the cross-sectional area of flow are abrupt rather than gradual (as in Fig. 38-33), the Bernoulli equation does not accurately describe this type of flow. The flow above the bobbin (i.e., downstream) is highly turbulent, and turbulence is a condition that dissipates kinetic energy into heat. Introduction of the empirical constant C_d enables one to use the same formulation as in equation 4:

$$Q = C_d A\sqrt{\left[2(P_1 - P_2)\right]/\rho} \qquad (5)$$

and

$$P_1 - P_2 = \left(\frac{1}{2}\rho Q^2\right)/\left(C_d^2 A^2\right) \qquad (6)$$

where C_d is a dimensionless constant called the "discharge coefficient." This constant varies with the shape of the orifice and with the value for another dimensionless parameter, the Reynolds number (Re). Re, the overall ratio of inertial forces to viscous forces in a particular flow, is determined as follows:

$$Re = \rho U L/\mu \qquad (7)$$

where U is mean flow velocity, L is a characteristic length for the flow (in our flow meter, L is the diameter of the tube), and μ is the viscosity of the fluid. The dimension for viscosity is M/LT. The value for Re is important to any fluid flow because it determines some of the most important characteristics of the flow. The transition from laminar, or "smooth," flow to turbulent flow is determined by the shape of the flow and Re. Flow in a long, straight, smooth-walled tube becomes turbulent at an Re value of approximately 2100. Flow through an abrupt orifice, such as that of the flow meter in Figure 38-36, becomes turbulent at an Re value of less than 100.

Returning now to the function of the flow meter, one can see that as gas flows upward through the tapered tube, the bobbin begins to rise. As the bobbin rises, the cross-sectional area of the orifice (A) increases because of the taper of the tube; the drop in pressure ($P_1 - P_2$) decreases. The bobbin reaches an equilibrium position for a given volume of flow (Q) when the pressure lifting the bobbin is exactly equal to the weight of the bobbin. In this type of flow meter, the pressure difference is fixed by the bobbin weight, and the area of the orifice varies with the volume of the flow—hence the name "variable-orifice flow meter." Equations 5 and 6 show that calibration of these flow meters depends on the density and the viscosity of the gas: density (ρ) appears explicitly, and viscosity (μ) appears in the dependence of Cd on Re. If we use the wrong gas in a particular flow meter, equations 5 and 6 and the viscosity and density of the new gas enable us to predict the change in calibration.

Appendix 6

Measurement of Cardiac Output by Thermal Dilution and Mass Flow Technique

A commonly used method of measuring blood flow is dilutional calculation—dye or thermal dilution. These methods are simply mass or energy balances that determine the volume of fluid that has been diluted by adding a volume of dye or a given thermal energy. If you have a bucket of water at room temperature (25°C), and you want to determine the volume of water in the bucket, you could add a known volume of water at a known temperature. If 100 mL of water at 35°C is added to the bucket, and the final temperature is 27°C, the unknown volume can be calculated by balancing the heat energy associated with the dilutional process, assuming that no heat is lost to the environment. This dilutional process can be used to measure blood flow by completing this same heat balance measured over time. Thermodilution cardiac output measurements can have significant error as a result of the many assumptions associated with the technique, such as rapid injection of the thermodilution injectate; accurate temperature and volume of the injected fluid; constant known heat capacity of blood, which in reality is a function of the hematocrit value; and little heat loss to the lung.

Thermistor probes are most commonly used for clinical monitoring of patient temperature because they are inexpensive, small, and flexible. For these reasons, the thermistor probe also is used to measure cardiac output determined by the thermodilution technique. Computation of cardiac output performed in this manner is, in effect, a heat balance for the right side of the heart. (Heat balance is a method of accounting for all heat in a process or change involving transfer of heat.) The technique consists of quick injection of a known volume of a sterile solution (usually 10 mL of 5% dextrose in water) into the right side of the heart, while a sensor notes the temperature of the blood in the pulmonary artery. It is assumed that the cold injected solution equilibrates thermally with the blood as it perfuses the pulmonary artery, but that the solution does not acquire heat from other tissues. The following equation is the solution of this heat balance:

$$CO = \left[\rho i Ci Vi\left(T_b - T_i\right)(60Cr)\right] / \left[\left(\rho_b C_b \int_0^\infty T_b(t)dt\right)\right] \quad (1)$$

where CO is cardiac output (L/min), ρ_i and ρ_b are the densities of the injectate and blood, C_i and C_b are the heat capacities of the injectate and blood, V_i is the volume of the injectate, T_b and T_i are the temperature of the blood and the injectate, *Cr* is a computational constant that corrects for the increasing temperature of the injectate, and the integration is the area under the thermodilution curve. Because the injectate warms as it is injected through the catheter before mixing with the blood, the correction factor Cr is applied to the equation.

The same principle of balance used for temperature determination of cardiac output can be applied to oxygen or carbon dioxide (CO_2) balance as well. Classically, oxygen balance is used as described by Fick. Measurement of oxygen consumption and content is cumbersome, and a modification of the Fick equation using CO_2 production is used. NICO is a new partial rebreathing method using the following equation:

$$Q = \dot{V}_{CO_2} / \left(C\bar{V}_{CO_2} - Ca_{CO_2}\right) \quad (2)$$

Cardiac output (Q) is simply the expired CO_2 divided by the arterial-venous difference in CO_2. Assuming that Q does not change, the equations for CO_2 elimination must be the same with or without rebreathing, where *N* indicates normal breathing, and *R* indicates rebreathing. By rearranging the equations, cardiac output is the ratio of the change in elimination of CO_2 divided by the change in arterial CO_2 content. Arterial CO_2 content is derived from the slope of end-tidal pressure of CO_2 (P_{ETCO_2}):

$$Q = \dot{V}_{CO_2N} / \left(C\bar{V}_{CO_2N} - Ca_{CO_2N}\right) = \dot{V}_{CO_2R} / \left(C\bar{V}_{CO_2R} - Ca_{CO_2R}\right) = \frac{\Delta\dot{V}CO_2}{\Delta CaCO_2} \quad (3)$$

We can see that potential errors are induced by violations of the following assumptions: (1) change in Q during the measurement period, (2) change in metabolic rate and production of CO_2, and (3) change in ventilation. As a trend analysis, patients with chronic obstructive lung disease, in which the absolute value of Pa_{CO_2} is widely different from P_{ETCO_2}, may have an absolute error in Q determination by this method, but the relative changes should track.

Appendix 7

Ultrasound

The simplest sound wave to represent mathematically is a sinusoidal wave propagating in one dimension:

$$p' = p_0 \sin[(2\pi/\lambda)(x - at)] \quad (1)$$

where p' is the pressure fluctuation, λ is the wavelength (distance between waves), x is the coordinate in the direction of propagation, and *a* is the speed of propagation, or the speed of sound.

The amplitude of a sound wave is measured by the root mean square value of the pressure fluctuations. This value is called the sound pressure level (SPL). Because the range of SPL values is often very wide, a logarithmic scale is used:

$$SPL = 20\log(p^*/P_0) \quad (2)$$

where p^* is the root mean square pressure fluctuation, and P_0 is a reference pressure chosen as the lowest sound pressure detectable by the human ear. This pressure representing the threshold of hearing is 2×10^{-8} kPa at a sound frequency of 2 kHz (2000 cycles/sec). The units in this SPL scale are called decibels. A sound pressure of 2×10^{-8} kPa corresponds to an SPL of 0 dB, the lowest audible sound level [$(p^*/P_0 = 1$; $\log(1) = 0)$]. Quiet conversation has an SPL of approximately 40 to 50 dB, or a pressure 10 to 300 times that of the threshold of hearing.

When sound waves encounter a sudden change in the properties of the conducting medium, some of the sound is transmitted through the new medium, and some of it is reflected, or "scattered," in many directions. Although the mathematics of this process are complex, one conclusion is readily apparent: The greater the mismatch in density and compressibility between the two media, the more sound that is reflected. The quantity that best determines the degree of reflection at an interface between two media is the ratio (R) of the products of density (ρ) and the speed of sound (a) through the two media:

$$R = (\rho_1 a_1)/(\rho_2 a_2) \quad (3)$$

We can easily see that the greatest acoustic mismatch in the body occurs between solid tissues and the lungs. The density and the speed of sound are much lower in the air-filled lungs than in solid tissues. Ultrasonography cannot "look" through the lungs at tissues or organs on the other side. The second greatest mismatch occurs between soft tissues and bone, the latter having a much higher ρa than the former. In 1842, Doppler first described the apparent change in pitch of a sound that occurred when either the source of the sound or the listener was moving. This Doppler effect now has several applications in patient monitoring, including precordial and esophageal Doppler ultrasound devices that measure local blood velocities or cardiac output. If a sound source radiating a frequency (f) is stationary, and the listener is moving (see Fig. 38-19A), the wavelength of the waves can be determined by the equation:

$$\lambda = a/f \quad (4)$$

because the time between wave fronts is 1/f, and the waves are moving at the speed of sound (a). If the listener moves toward the source at speed V_0, the velocity of the listener relative to the moving wave fronts is $(a + V_0)$. The number of wave fronts that the listener encounters per unit time is:

$$f' = \text{velocity/distance between waves} = (a + V_0)/\lambda \quad (5)$$

Because the sound frequency for a stationary listener is $f = a/\lambda$ (equation 4), the frequency f' heard by the moving listener becomes:

$$f' = (a + V_0)/\lambda = f + (V_0/\lambda) = f + (V_0 f/a) = f[1 + (V_0/a)] \quad (6)$$

The apparent frequency of the listener is increased by the factor $[1 + (V_0/a)]$. A listener moving toward the source at half the speed of sound hears a frequency 1.5 times that of a stationary listener.

Now consider a stationary listener and a source moving at speed V_0, as shown in Figure 38-19B. The wave fronts are no longer concentric circles; they are more closely spaced in the direction that the source is moving. If the frequency of the sound emitted at the source is f, the source moves a distance V_0/f during each vibration. The wavelength in the direction of motion is shortened by V_0/f and becomes $l = (a - V_0)/f$. The waves themselves are traveling at speed a, so the frequency heard by the stationary listener is:

$$f' = a/\lambda' = af/(a - V_0) = f[1/(1 - V_0/a)] \quad (7)$$

If the source is moving at half the speed of sound toward the listener, the apparent frequency doubles. Compare this situation with the preceding one in which the listener is moving, and the apparent frequency increases by only 50%. Doppler ultrasound systems combine the two situations shown in Figure 38-19. The initial acoustic source is a stationary transducer, and the sound from this device is scattered from a moving target (e.g., red blood cells). The scattered sound returns to a stationary listener—the receiving transducer. In effect, the target is a moving listener hearing a stationary source; the target re-radiates the sound as a moving source toward a stationary listener. The frequency heard by the receiving transducer is obtained by combining equations 6 and 7:

$$f' = f\left[\frac{1 + V/a}{1 - V/a}\right] \quad (8)$$

In this example, we have assumed that the target is moving toward the ultrasound transducers at speed V. If the target is moving at half the speed of sound, the observed frequency is increased by a factor of 3. Because changes in the frequency of sine waves can be measured precisely, the Doppler principle provides an accurate method of measuring the velocity of moving sound reflectors. At the high frequencies often used (ε5 MHz), objects as small as red corpuscles can scatter enough sound for detection.

Ultrasound imaging is exceptionally complex. For simplicity's sake, recall the submarine movies wherein the sonar operator calls out "range 2000 yards, bearing 36 degrees." These two parameters are crucial in describing some of the math of ultrasound.

The first factor to consider is the maximal range of the ultrasound, which is described by the following relationship:

$$r_{max} = cT/2 \quad (9)$$

That is, the maximal range equals the speed of sound in tissue (≈1540 msec) multiplied by time T between pulses divided by 2. A further limitation is the fact that the energy dissipates in the tissue. (You need to tap harder when percussing to detect deeper structures). For deeper penetration into tissues, one requires higher energies and slower pulse rates. Wavelength and frequency are related in the following manner:

$$\lambda = c/f \tag{10}$$

where f is the frequency, λ is the wavelength, and c is the speed of sound.

Next, we need to consider the axial resolution (is the enemy destroyer 2000 yards distant, or 2005?) and the annular resolution (is the bearing 36 or 38 degrees?). Sound in tissue spreads out in a bandwidth around a fundamental frequency. To determine the necessary bandwidth for an axial resolution of 2 mm, the following rough approximation holds:

$$B = 2c/\Delta r \tag{11}$$

where Δr is the axial resolution. We need a bandwidth of 1.54 MHz to get an axial resolution of 2 mm.

For annular resolution (Δθ), the beam spreads out the farther it goes from the source. Without deriving the mathematics, two factors determine annular resolution—the frequency and the aperture. Aperture size is limited to a size that fits into or onto a human. A 1-degree error at a 1-cm range increases at a 10-cm range: circumference = 2πr: $\frac{1}{360} \times 2 \times \pi \times 1 = 0.17$ mm; at 10 cm, circumference = 1.7 mm.

39 Monitoring the Depth of Anesthesia

Key Points

1. The definition of "depth of anesthesia" has constantly evolved since the first demonstration of clinical anesthesia in the 1840s. The changing definitions have revolved around the available drugs used to provide anesthesia and the body of knowledge on their effects in humans.
2. Anesthesia is not a single pharmacologic process. It is a complex interaction of multiple stimuli, diverse responses, and the drug-induced probability of nonresponsiveness to the stimuli.
3. Anesthesia can be defined by hypnotic (unconsciousness) and analgesic (pain relief) components. The hypnotic component can be created by intravenous and inhaled anesthetics, whereas the analgesic component can be created by opioids and local anesthetics. Some drugs, such as ether, nitrous oxide, and ketamine, provide both hypnotic and analgesic components to some degree.
4. Hypnotics, when given alone, allow significant hemodynamic response to intense noxious stimuli. Opioids, when given alone, do not guarantee consistent unconsciousness or lack of movement response to intense noxious stimuli. The combination of the two can result in predictable unconsciousness and lack of hemodynamic response to intense noxious stimuli.
5. The interaction of the hypnotic and analgesic components can be characterized by a three-dimensional surface with hypnotic concentration on the *y* axis, analgesic concentration on the *x* axis, and the probability of nonresponse on the *z* axis.
6. Characterization of the three-dimensional surface requires precise stimuli to be applied and specific responses to be measured at defined effect-site concentrations of the hypnotic and analgesic.
7. The specific stimuli-response pairs used to define anesthetic depth range from easily suppressed responses to mild stimulation, such as the verbal response to a verbal command, to difficult-to-suppress responses to intense stimuli, such as the hemodynamic response to intubation.
8. The interaction of hypnotics and analgesics is generally synergistic.
9. Current clinical anesthesia involves the physician carefully observing the clinical response to defined stimuli and then adjusting the hypnotic or analgesic dosage (or both) by using the synergistic interaction to achieve the clinical goals of hemodynamic control, lack of awareness, and rapid, safe induction and emergence.
10. The hypnotic effects of the intravenous and inhaled anesthetics can be measured with empirically derived indices calculated from the electroencephalogram (EEG).
11. EEG-based indices of hypnotic drug effect correlate with hypnotic-induced sedation, amnesia, loss of consciousness, and reduced cerebral metabolic rate.
12. A consequence of inadequate anesthetic depth is intraoperative awareness. The incidence of awareness in healthy patients is approximately 0.1% and can increase to 1.0% to 1.5% in higher-risk patient populations.
13. There is emerging evidence that intraoperative monitoring of the hypnotic component of an anesthetic regimen may significantly decrease the risk of awareness associated with anesthesia. However, it does not totally eliminate the risk.
14. Maintenance of a high steady-state concentration of a volatile anesthetic may reduce the risk of awareness if the consequences of a high concentration can be tolerated by the patient.

A corollary to the aphorism "if you don't know where you are going, then any road will do" is that if you don't know what anesthesia is, any monitor of anesthetic depth will do. What is anesthesia? Anesthesiologists have multiple inconsistent definitions of the anesthetic state and hold strong opinions on how to measure it. Fortunately, an integrated, quantitative concept of the anesthetic state can now be built on the incremental knowledge developed since the introduction of anesthesia more than a century ago. As our understanding of the anesthetic state has advanced, so has our ability to control it pharmacologically and monitor it in real time.

The chapter is divided into four sections. The first reviews evolving definitions of depth of anesthesia. Anesthesia will be defined in terms of two fundamental pharmacologic components, the hypnotic effect and the analgesic effect, with clinical anesthesia requiring both components. The second section reviews memory and awareness, critical components of anesthetic depth. The third reviews basic pharmacologic concepts that are linked to depth of anesthesia. The last section discusses electrophysiologic approaches to assessing depth of anesthesia, including the influence of specific drugs on electrophysiologic approaches. The perspective of the authors is that anesthesia is a pharmacologically induced state that renders patients insensitive to surgery. Because pharmacology is inextricably linked to defining and measuring anesthetic depth, the pharmacology of hypnotics and opioids is discussed from different perspectives in each section. There is unavoidable overlap because monitoring the depth of anesthesia, the focus of this chapter, means monitoring the pharmacologic effects of the drugs used to render patients insensate.

Definitions of Anesthetic Depth

In a 1987 editorial, Prys-Roberts[1] examined clinical components truly relevant to the depth of anesthesia. He began by observing that depth of anesthesia is difficult to define because anesthetists have approached the issue in terms of the drugs available to them rather than the patient's needs during surgery. Prys-Roberts believed that the noxious stimulation of surgery induces a variety of reflex responses that may be independently modulated. One important observation was that pain is the conscious perception of noxious stimulation. Thus, he defined anesthesia as a state of drug-induced unconsciousness in which the patient neither perceives nor recalls noxious stimulation. The loss of consciousness is an all-or-none phenomenon. By this definition, there can be no variable depth of anesthesia. The patient is either conscious or unconscious.

Prys-Roberts defined noxious stimulation as a mechanical, chemical, thermal, or radiation-induced trespass causing potential or actual cell damage. Figure 39-1 shows the somatic and autonomic responses to noxious stimulation. Noxious stimulation arises from somatic or visceral tissue, and responses can be somatic or autonomic. Somatic responses include both sensory and motor activity. A sensory response is perception of pain. Low concentrations of inhaled or intravenously administered anesthetics can eliminate pain, particularly in combination with opioids, but they allow a motor response. The motor response to noxious stimuli is typically an all-or-none withdrawal of the stimulated part. This is the same concept that Eger and colleagues[2] used more than 4 decades earlier when they defined the minimum

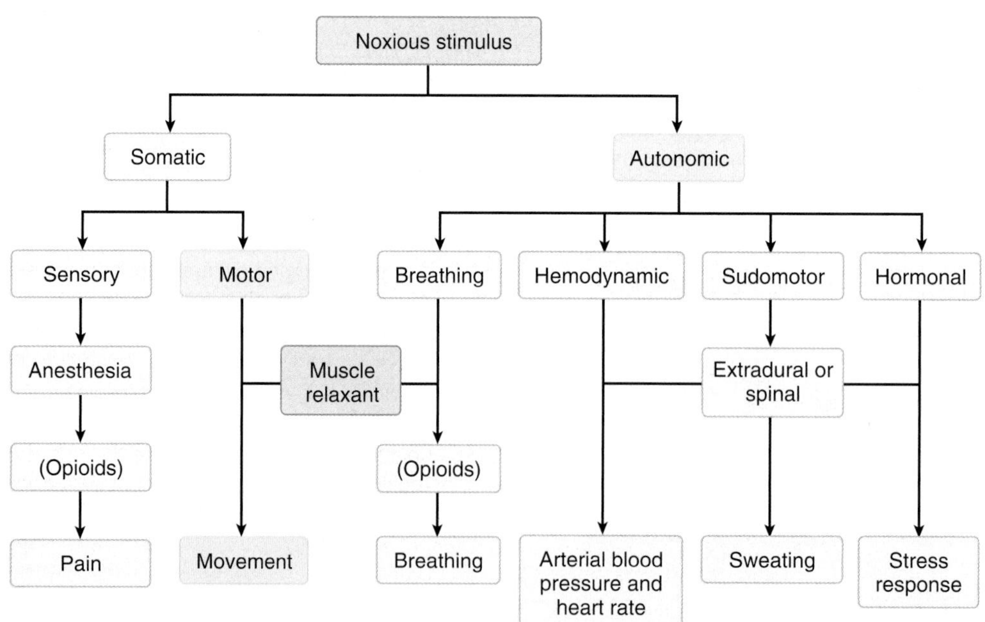

Figure 39-1 Depth of anesthesia can be defined by suppression of the clinically relevant responses to noxious stimuli, as proposed by Prys-Roberts. The figure is read from left to right and from top to bottom to see the order in which reflex responses are suppressed by anesthetic drugs. *(Modified from Prys-Roberts C: Anaesthesia: A practical or impossible construct? [editorial] Br J Anaesth 59:1341, 1987.)*

alveolar concentration (MAC) as the drug concentration that blocked movement in response to noxious stimulation.

Prys-Roberts divided autonomic responses into four categories: breathing, hemodynamic, sudomotor, and hormonal. The ventilatory response may occur even if there is no somatic motor response to surgical stimulation. A higher concentration is required to suppress the breathing response than is required to suppress the somatic response to noxious stimuli.

The hemodynamic response consists of autonomic responses to noxious stimuli, namely, increased sympathetic tone, which elevates arterial blood pressure and the heart rate. The sudomotor response consists of sweating, whereas the hormonal response consists of catecholamines and corticosteroids.

Prys-Roberts considered pain relief, muscle relaxation, and suppression of autonomic activity to be discrete pharmacologic effects. Some drugs can produce all these end points. Others produce only one or two. The only feature common to most anesthetics is suppression of sensory perception and production of unconsciousness. He considered the inclusion of muscle relaxation in the definition of the anesthetic state to be illogical and confusing. Although muscle relaxation is necessary for laryngoscopy and surgical access, it is neither a component of anesthesia nor an alternative to adequate anesthesia.

In a 1993 editorial, Kissin[3] expanded, refined, and further contributed to the definition of anesthesia. Similar to Prys-Roberts, Kissin began by indicating that a wide spectrum of pharmacologic actions via different drugs can be used to create the anesthetic state. Such pharmacologic actions include analgesia, anxiolysis, amnesia, unconsciousness, and suppression of somatic motor, cardiovascular, and hormonal responses to the stimulation of surgery. Kissin stated that the spectrum of effects that constitutes the state of general anesthesia should not be regarded as several components of anesthesia resulting from one anesthetic action but, rather, regarded as representing separate pharmacologic actions, even if the anesthesia is produced by one drug. Kissin then reviewed a series of investigative studies and concepts that supported his hypothesis:

1. Several groups of drugs (benzodiazepines, opioids, α_2-agonists) that induce anesthesia by acting on specific receptors can have their anesthetic effects reversed by the administration of a specific receptor antagonist.
2. There is growing understanding that the molecular mechanisms of general anesthesia are more specific than was suggested by the previous unitary hypothesis of anesthesia.
3. The rank order of effects for two important goals of anesthesia (hypnotic effect and blockade of somatic motor response to noxious stimuli) can be different for different classes of anesthetics. Opioids induce blockade of movement response to noxious stimulation before hypnosis occurs. For intravenous anesthetics, the opposite occurs.
4. When studies of anesthetic interactions are undertaken, the type of interaction (synergism, antagonism, summation) for one component of anesthesia may differ from that of another component.
5. Classic theories of anesthesia, based on the unitary nonspecific mechanisms of anesthetic action, suggest that one anesthetic may be freely replaceable by another and that the effects of anesthetic combinations should be additive. This appears to be true for inhaled anesthetics,[4] but most combinations of intravenous anesthetic drugs are synergistic for hypnotic effects, a finding that suggests diverse drug targets for drug-induced hypnosis.

If one understands general anesthesia as a spectrum of separate pharmacologic actions that vary according to the goals of anesthesia, certain conclusions can be made regarding the measurement of anesthetic potency and depth of anesthesia. Kissin stated that the "diversity of pharmacological actions that in combination provide anesthesia make[s] it almost impossible to determine the potency of different actions with one measure."[3]

A Modern Definition of the Anesthetic State

What is Anesthesia?

The sine qua non of the anesthetized state is unconsciousness or the lack of thought processing. The crux of the difficulty in defining "anesthetic depth" is that unconsciousness cannot be measured directly. What can be measured is response to stimulation. Does the patient respond to command? Does the response to incision suggest conscious perception? Does the heart rate or blood pressure go up in response to surgical manipulation? Does the patient remember events, conversations, or pain? As observed by Prys-Roberts, anesthesia is nonresponsiveness. The "depth" of anesthesia is determined by the stimulus applied, the response measured, and the drug concentration at the site of action that blunts responsiveness.

The state of consciousness can be assessed clinically with tools such as the Modified Observer Assessment of Alertness/Sedation (MOAA/S) scale (Table 39-1).[5] As defined later in this chapter, the state of consciousness can be inferred, although not directly measured, by analysis of information on the electroencephalogram (EEG). This can be done with either spectral techniques, such as the bispectral index (BIS) or with evoked potentials, such as auditory evoked potentials (AEPs). These indices do not directly measure unconsciousness or unresponsiveness. However, we know through extensive validation that these measures are predictive of the likelihood of response, provided that the anesthetic state has been induced with the drugs used to calibrate the electrophysiologic measure.

Nonresponsiveness can be induced by deep sleep or by 2% isoflurane. What distinguishes the nonresponsiveness of the anesthetic state from the nonresponsiveness of normal sleep is the stimulus intensity required to penetrate the state of nonrespon-

Table 39-1 Modified Observer's Assessment of Alertness/Sedation Scale

Score	Responsiveness
5	Responds readily to name spoken in a normal tone
4	Lethargic response to name spoken in a normal tone
3	Responds only after name is called loudly and/or repeatedly
2	Responds only after mild prodding or shaking
1	Responds only after painful trapezius squeeze
0	No response after painful trapezius squeeze

Box 39-1 Components Needed to Define Depth of Anesthesia

Afferent stimulus
Efferent response
Equilibrated concentrations of analgesic drugs
Equilibrated concentrations of hypnotic drugs
Equilibrated concentrations of other relevant drugs (e.g., β-blockers, muscle relaxants, local anesthetics)
Interaction surface relating the drug concentrations to the probability of the given response to the given stimulus

siveness and rouse the brain to conscious perception. The hypnotic drugs used in anesthesia (propofol, thiopental, inhaled anesthetics, ketamine) are each capable of producing such profound central nervous system (CNS) depression that even the most painful surgical stimulus cannot rouse the patient from a state of near-total nonresponsiveness. However, if the painful surgical stimulus can be attenuated before reaching the cortical level, the dose required to maintain the state of nonresponsiveness can be reduced.

Attenuation of surgical stimulation is the function of systemic analgesics (e.g., opioids) and local anesthetics. The interaction between analgesics and hypnotics is thus fundamental to understanding and defining anesthetic depth. Box 39-1 indicates the components of defining the depth of anesthesia used in the remainder of this chapter.

Extending ideas proposed by Glass in 1998,[6] consciousness can be perceived as the balance between depression and excitation within the cortex (Fig. 39-2, upper right). The cortex is primarily depressed by hypnotics, although opioids and nitrous oxide also have sedating properties that depress the cortex. Cortical depression promotes unconsciousness. These effects are opposed by ambient stimulation (e.g., loud music, a hard cold operating table) and the excitatory effects of pain projected on the cortex.

Figure 39-2 also shows the influence of opioids, nitrous oxide, and local anesthetics in preventing noxious stimulation from reaching the cortex. Systemic opioids act on the midbrain and thalamus,[7] although spinal actions are also critical for their analgesic effects.[8] Neuraxial opioids clearly act primarily on the spinal cord. Local anesthetics act either at the spinal cord (for neuraxial blocks) or on peripheral nerves (e.g., nerve blocks and local infiltration). Nitrous oxide exerts some of its analgesic effects through spinal mechanisms,[9,10] as well as the midbrain,[11] but for simplicity we will lump nitrous oxide with opioids at the midbrain. The net effect of analgesic and local anesthetics is to attenuate the transmission of painful sensation to the cortex, thereby reducing the amount of hypnotic required to obtain a state of nonresponsiveness.

Pharmacologic View of the Anesthetic State

Figure 39-3 reduces the model in Figure 39-2 to a highly simplified pharmacologic view.[12] The subcortical actions in Figure 39-2 have been compressed to a single site of action in the lower left of Figure 39-3, and all analgesics, including nitrous oxide, local anesthetics, and opioids, have been compressed to just "opioids." The simplification produces a mathematically tractable pharmacologic structure and may provide insight into the interaction between analgesics and hypnotics on consciousness and responsiveness.

In Figure 39-3, painful stimuli arrive in the lower left. Opioids (and all other analgesics) attenuate the painful stimulus.

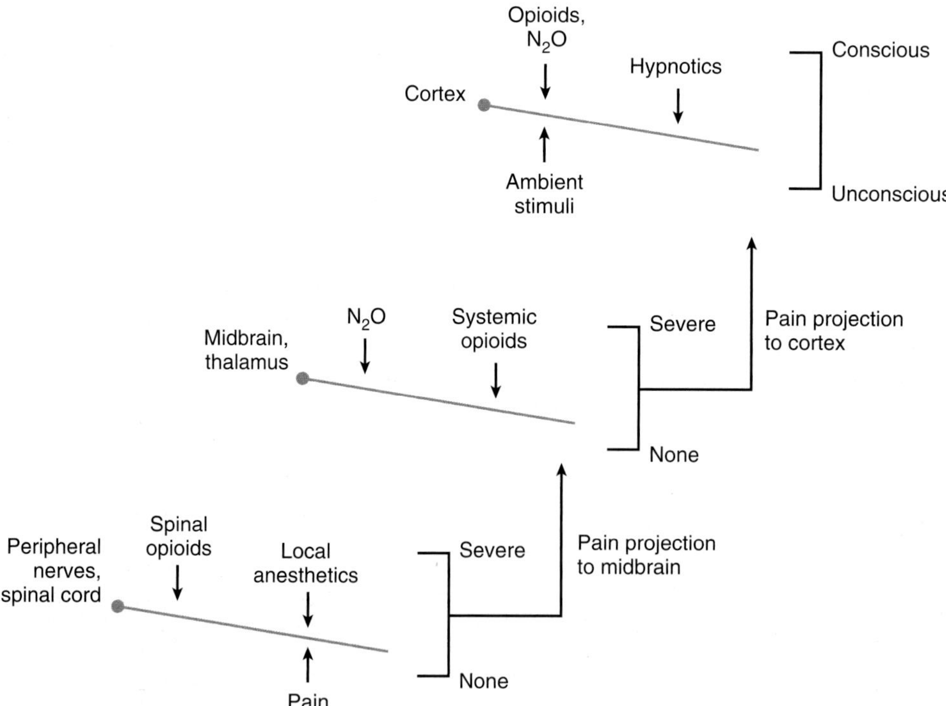

Figure 39-2 Stylized view of the interaction between hypnotics, which depress consciousness, and analgesics, which suppress noxious stimuli.

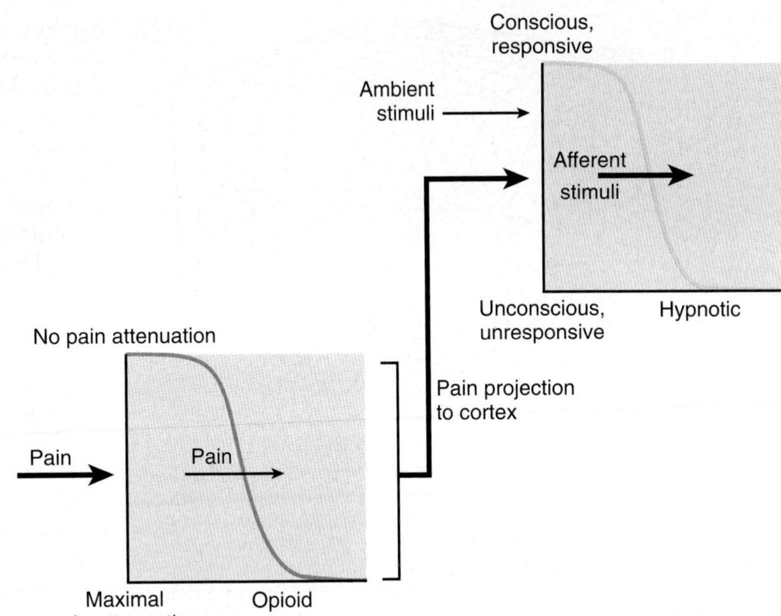

Figure 39-3 Pharmacologic interpretation of the interaction between hypnotics and analgesics. All measures of responsiveness appear in the upper right as "unconsciousness, unresponsive" which lumps the cortical and subcortical responses.

The magnitude of the stimulus affects both the magnitude of the output and the apparent potency of the opioids. Another way of saying this is that it takes more opioid to attenuate a powerfully painful stimulus than a moderately painful stimulus. This has repeatedly been demonstrated, as shown in Figure 39-4.[13] Pharmacologically, the effect of "opioids" on attenuating the pain signal can be expressed by using a standard sigmoid Emax pharmacodynamic equation:

$$\text{Pain out} = \text{Pain in} \cdot \left(1 - \frac{\text{Opioid}^{\gamma}}{\text{Opioid}^{\gamma} + \left[\text{Opioid}_{50} \cdot \text{Pain in}\right]^{\gamma}}\right)$$

in which "pain in" is the afferent painful stimulus, "pain out" is the efferent painful stimulus transmitted to the cortex, "opioid" is the steady-state opioid concentration, "opioid$_{50}$" is the equilibrated opioid concentration associated with 50% attenuation of the "pain in" for an afferent pain intensity of 1, and γ is the steepness of the opioid concentration-versus-response relationship. Opioid$_{50}$ is multiplied by "pain in" to reflect the decreased potency of opioids in attenuating severe pain, as shown in Figure 39-4.

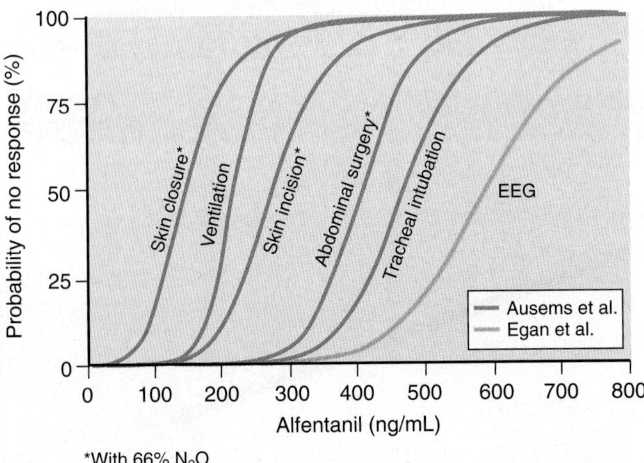

Figure 39-4 The effect of increasingly painful stimulation on the opioid concentration-versus-response relationship.[13] As pain intensity increases, the apparent potency of the opioids decreases. EEG, electroencephalogram.

In Figure 39-3 the output of the attenuated noxious stimulation is projected to the cortex, where the CNS-arousing characteristics of pain are balanced by the CNS-depressant effects of hypnotics. The pharmacologic expression of this would be

$$\text{Probability of responsiveness} = 1 - \frac{\text{Hypnotic}^{\eta}}{\text{Hypnotic}^{\eta} + \left[\text{Hypnotic}_{50} \cdot \text{Stimulus in}\right]^{\eta}}$$

where "stimulus in" is the "pain out" projecting from lower structures plus the ambient stimulation, "hypnotic" is the steady-state concentration of the sedative-hypnotic, "hypnotic$_{50}$" is the concentration associated with a 50% probability of nonresponsiveness when the "stimulus in" equals 1, and η is the steepness of the hypnotic concentration–versus–probability of nonresponsiveness relationship.

This cascading model of drug effect produces the response surface shown in Figure 39-5. The x and y axes in Figure 39-5 are the equilibrated concentrations of opioid and hypnotic, respectively, The z axis in Figure 39-5 is the probability of nonresponsiveness. This surface has the fundamental properties of the opioid-hypnotic relationship. Near the origin for drug concentrations, labeled "1" on the surface, there is no chance of nonresponsiveness, and the patient is probably wide awake. In fact, the floor of the figure indicates that there is a minimum amount of drug that must be given before the patient has any chance of nonresponsiveness. On the other side of the surface, labeled "2", there is enough opioid and hypnotic to ensure virtually no chance of response. The red line in the middle of the surface, labeled "5", is the 50% isobole. This line shows the opioid and hypnotic concentrations associated with a 50% probability of responsiveness. It extends from the curve for the hypnotic-versus-response relationship in the absence of opioids on the far left, labeled "3," to

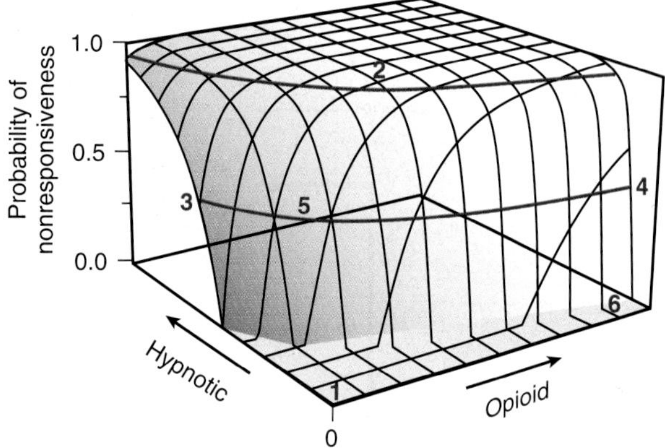

Figure 39-5 Relationship between opioid and hypnotic drug concentrations and the probability of nonresponsiveness. 1, No chance of nonresponsiveness; 2, no chance of response; 3, hypnotic-versus-response relationship in the absence of opioids; 4, hypnotic-versus-response relationship in the presence of large doses of opioids; 5, area of maximum synergy between opioids and hypnotics; 6, in the absence of opioids even profound levels of opioids cannot suppress response; *blue line* in the middle of the surface, the 50% isobole; *blue curve* at the top of the surface, 95% isobole.

the hypnotic-versus-response relationship in the presence of large quantities of opioids on the right, labeled "4." The relationship between hypnotics and opioids is highly synergistic in that when the drugs are used in combination (for example, at the point labeled "5"), it takes far less of either drug than would be the case were the opioids or hypnotics used alone. The model predicts that some hypnotic is required to achieve the anesthetized state. In the absence of a hypnotic, even profound levels of opioids are unable to produce a state of nonresponsiveness, as can be seen at point "6" on the surface.[14-17] However, a modest amount of opioid profoundly reduces the concentration of hypnotic necessary for nonresponsiveness, as seen at point "5." Beyond this, additional opioid has only modest effect in further reducing the hypnotic dose required for a drug effect. The corollary is that large doses of hypnotic are required in the absence of an opioid.[18-20] The blue curve at the top of the surface is the 95% isobole. This curve defines the opioid and hypnotic combinations associated with a 95% probability of nonresponsiveness. Because the surface is very steep, as soon as there is a modest probability of nonresponsiveness, a modest increase in drug concentration is all that is required to move from a 50% chance of nonresponsiveness to a 95% chance of nonresponsiveness.

Figure 39-5 shows that the model of the anesthetic state presented in Figure 39-2 generates a pharmacologic response surface that is very much like those seen in virtually all drug interaction trials.[21]

The ability of inhaled anesthetics to induce immobility in response to noxious stimulation is mediated by the spinal cord, not the cortex.[22,23] Experimentally, the interaction between inhaled anesthetics and opioids in preventing movement response to noxious stimulation[24] resembles Figure 39-5. As such, a pharmacologic model of the effect of opioids on MAC would resemble Figure 39-3 except that the response end point (movement) is mediated by the spinal cord rather than the cortex.

Experimental Characterization of the Anesthetic State

To quantify anesthetic depth, we must be rigorous about the definition of the *z* axis in Figure 39-5, the probability of nonresponsiveness. Consider the matrix of stimuli and responses shown in Figure 39-6. Stimuli can be roughly divided into benign and noxious. Benign stimuli are not physically painful. Thus, responses to benign stimuli are readily suppressed by hypnotics alone, with minimal need for analgesic drugs. Noxious stimuli are physically painful, and thus responses to noxious stimuli are more readily suppressed in the presence of analgesics. Skin incision appears somewhat in the middle of noxious stimuli, being more stimulating than electrical pain but much less stimulating than laryngoscopy and intubation. Figure 39-6 represents the noxious stimuli in approximately increasing order of intensity.

Figure 39-6 shows 10 responses in approximate rank order of difficulty to suppress and 14 stimuli of approximately increas-

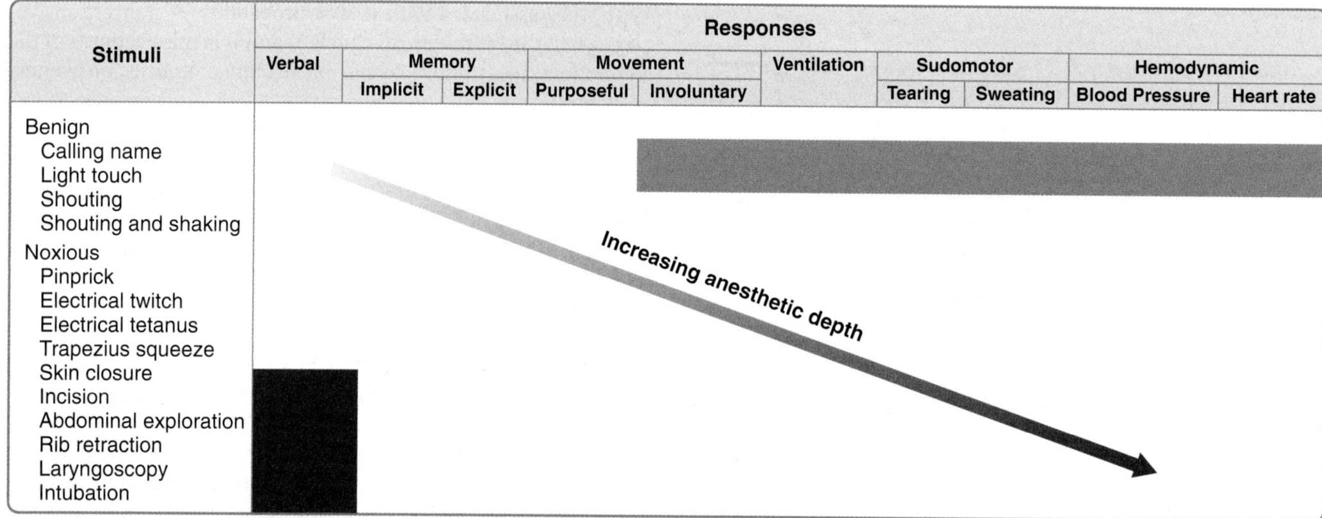

Figure 39-6 Matrix of relevant stimuli and responses. Stimuli are in approximately increasing order of noxiousness. Responses are in approximately increasing order of difficulty of suppression. As the cells progress from left to right and from top to bottom, increasingly larger doses of anesthetic drug are required to suppress the given response to the given stimulus.

ing intensity. The grayed-out cells have been removed as being clinically uninteresting, which leaves 122 cells to define anesthetic depth. If we wanted to fully characterize the ability of isoflurane and fentanyl to create a state of nonresponsiveness for each of the listed responses to any of the listed stimuli, we would need to characterize the response surface (i.e., Fig. 39-5) for each clinically relevant cell! With so many choices of stimuli and interactions, it is not surprising that anesthesiologists cannot agree on a simple definition of anesthetic depth.

Fortunately, it is not necessary to characterize the response to every stimulus. If we characterize the response to a benign stimulus, such as shaking and shouting, and several noxious stimuli, such as electrical tetanus, incision, laryngoscopy, and intubation, we will have captured the clinically relevant range of benign and noxious stimulation.

To our matrix of stimuli and responses we must add the matrix of hypnotics and opioids. Commonly used hypnotics include the anesthetic vapors halothane, isoflurane, sevoflurane, and desflurane and the intravenous hypnotics propofol, thiopental, etomidate, and midazolam. Commonly used opioids include fentanyl, alfentanil, sufentanil, remifentanil, morphine, meperidine, hydromorphone, methadone, tramadol, and piritramide. With 8 hypnotics and 10 opioids, there are 80 combinations. Eighty combinations times 122 interactions yields 9760 combinations of opioids, hypnotics, stimuli, and responses. To this we must then add the influence of age, disease, genetics, and other factors. Clearly, it is impossible to create response surfaces to characterize how opioids and hypnotics produce a state of nonresponsiveness for all possible combinations of drugs, patients, stimuli, and responses.

Fortunately, there are powerful generalizations that provide clinical insight and tractable experimental design. The most important is that for any stimulus-response pair, the depth of anesthesia is the probability of nonresponse. Specifically, *the depth of anesthesia is the drug-induced probability of nonresponse to stimulation, calibrated against the strength of the stimulus and the difficulty of suppressing the response.* Anesthetic depth ranges from fully awake (i.e., verbally responsive to a simple command) to a 100% probability of nonresponse for a difficult-to-suppress (e.g., tachycardia) to a profoundly noxious stimulation (e.g., intubation). Thus, a fully integrated view of anesthetic depth requires consideration of the components shown in Box 39-1.

Figure 39-7 shows an experimentally tractable and clinical useful distillation of the matrix of stimuli and responses from Figure 39-6. The matrix has been reduced to three stimuli, calling name, incision, and intubation, and three responses, verbal response, purposeful movement, and hemodynamic response. Within three of the cells are representative opioid-hypnotic interaction surfaces. As seen in the cells, verbal response to name calling is readily suppressed by hypnotics, with only modest effect from opioids. The middle surface shows that suppression of movement in response to incision requires more hypnotic and opioid to suppress than does a verbal response to a patient's name being called. Additionally, the vertical probability axis stretches for the more profound stimuli to indicate that a 100% chance of nonresponse to incision is a more profound level of drug effect than is a 100% chance of nonresponse to calling the patient's name. Suppressing the most refractory response, hypertension and tachycardia, to the most profound stimulus, intubation, requires yet more opioid and hypnotic. As demonstrated by Figure 39-7, anesthetic depth ranges from a 100% chance of a verbal response to a verbal command (wide awake, no drug) to enough opioid and hypnotic to provide a 100% chance of no hemodynamic response to intubation.

MAC creates a unifying principle of anesthetic depth for the inhaled anesthetics. Although each inhaled anesthetic has some pharmacologic peculiarities, in general they have parallel dose-response curves across drugs (e.g., isoflurane versus sevoflurane versus desflurane) and across stimuli-response pairs. Examples are the inhaled concentration associated with response to

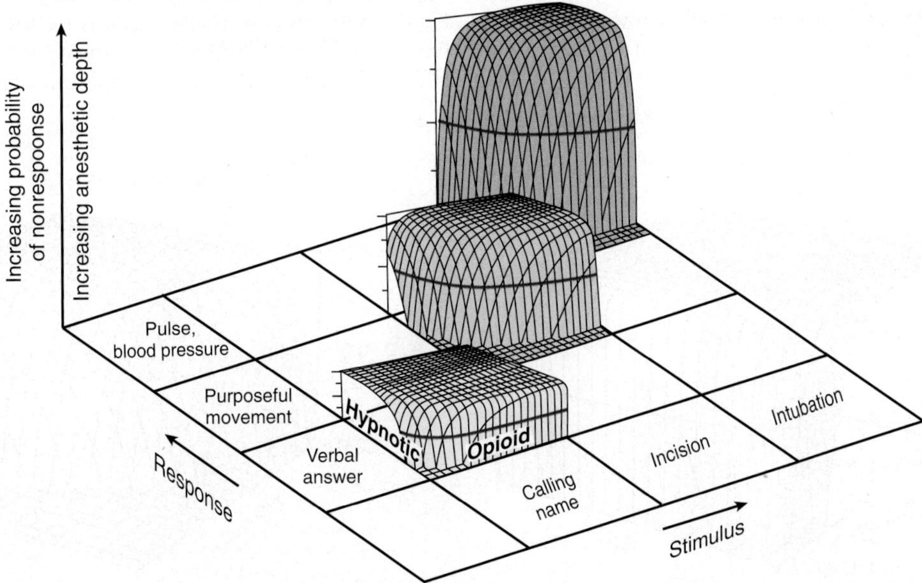

Figure 39-7 The role of opioid and hypnotics in the stimulus-response relationship for three stimuli of increasing intensity and three increasingly difficult responses to suppress. Each cell would have its own opioid-hypnotic interaction surface, and three are displayed. The vertical axis is the probability of nonresponse. Verbal nonresponsiveness to name calling is readily suppressed, even at light levels of anesthesia. In contrast, profound levels of anesthesia are required to suppress the hemodynamic response to intubation.

verbal stimulation (MAC-awake),[25] movement to incision (MAC), and hemodynamic response to incision (MAC-BAR).[26] Thus, by knowing the relative values of MAC, one can infer the relative values of the other stimulus-response relationships. There is less similarity among the intravenous hypnotics. Fortunately, the only intravenous drugs regularly used to maintain the anesthetic state are propofol and midazolam, which limits the number of clinically interesting intravenous anesthetic combinations.

Fentanyl, alfentanil, sufentanil, and remifentanil appear to differ mainly in potency and time course of drug effect, despite conflicting reports of pharmacologic idiosyncrasies for each member of the fentanyl series. Morphine, meperidine, hydromorphone, and methadone appear to differ in potency and intrinsic efficacy and have a slightly reduced maximum analgesic effect than the fentanyl series of opioids does. These latter four drugs also have their own pharmacologic quirks, particularly meperidine, which has only a limited role as an analgesic in contemporary practice.

Nitrous oxide is not only the oldest of the anesthetic drugs still in common use but also remains one of the least well understood. It has properties of hypnotics, with a MAC that slightly exceeds 1 atm,[27] as well as potent analgesic properties. Although the interaction of nitrous oxide with opioids,[28] inhaled anesthetics,[29] and propofol,[30] has been characterized, no studies have gathered enough data to generate the response surfaces needed to fully understand the interactions of this nearly ubiquitous anesthetic drug.

Fundamental Relationships That Characterize the Anesthetic State

Based on the simplifying assumptions just stated, we can comprehend anesthetic depth by understanding a limited number of prototypical drug combinations: isoflurane-fentanyl, isoflurane-nitrous oxide, nitrous oxide-fentanyl, propofol-fentanyl, propofol-nitrous oxide, midazolam-nitrous oxide, and midazolam-fentanyl. For each of these combinations, characterization of the response surface for a handful of stimuli and responses, as suggested in Figure 39-7, would allow understanding of current clinical practice and provide for definition of the full range of anesthetic depth:

1. Loss of response to shouting and shaking:
   a. Any response is considered, (i.e., "MAC-awake")
2. Loss of response to electrical tetanus:
   a. Verbal response or purposeful movement
   b. Any autonomic (hemodynamic or sudomotor) response
   c. Any memory response
3. Loss of response to an intermediate stimulus (incision, trapezius muscle squeeze):
   a. Purposeful movement (i.e., "MAC")
   b. Any autonomic (hemodynamic or sudomotor) response (i.e., "MAC-BAR")
   c. Any memory response
4. Loss of response to laryngoscopy/intubation:
   a. Purposeful movement
   b. Any autonomic (hemodynamic or sudomotor) response
   c. Any memory response
5. The concentration-versus-EEG response relationship in the absence of stimulation

We now have a matrix of just 11 stimuli-versus-response relationships. Multiplied by our seven prototypical drug combinations yields 77 response surfaces, from which we can infer the rest of the surfaces through scaling based on the MAC for inhaled drugs and C_{50} (concentration associated with a 50% probability of drug effect) for intravenous drugs and the relative rankings of stimuli and responses. Moreover, the combinations range from light anesthesia with modest stimulation and easily attenuated responses, found in the upper left corner of Figure 39-6, to deep anesthesia with profound stimuli and very difficult-to-ablate responses, found in the lower right corner of Figure 39-6.

Figure 39-8 shows examples of response surfaces for a modest and a profound stimulus. These interaction surfaces are based on the same model as the interaction surface shown in Figure 39-5, differing only in the intensity of the afferent painful signal. We find the same pattern when we examine real data. Figure 39-9 shows response surfaces for the potentiation of isoflurane by fentanyl (left)[16] and for the potentiation of propofol by alfentanil (right).[17] The shapes of these curves are not exactly like

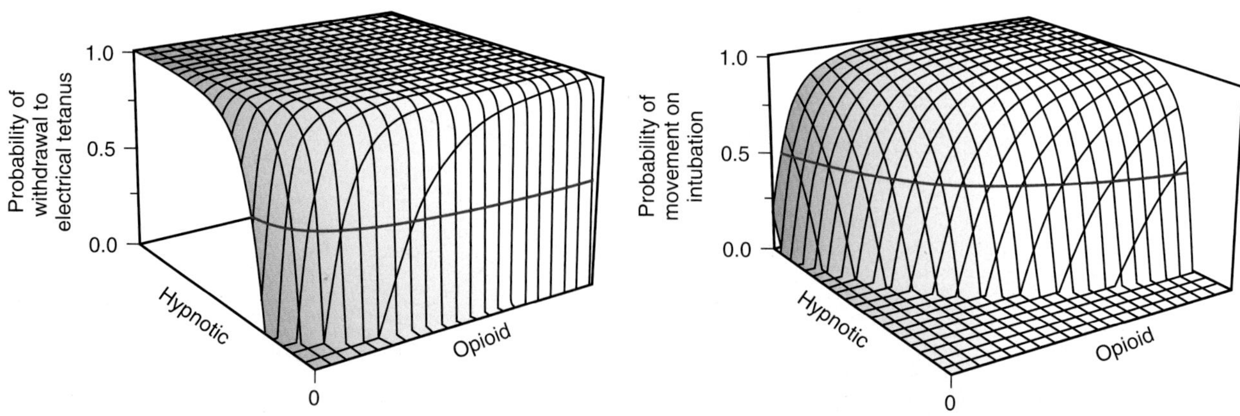

Figure 39-8 Examples of response surfaces for a modest stimulus on the *left* (withdrawal to electrical tetanus) and a profound stimulus on the *right* (movement response to intubation) based on the model shown in Figure 39-5 with differing intensity of the afferent painful signal. The figure on the *left* shows a relatively mild stimulus-response combination, whereas the figure on the *right* shows a profoundly noxious stimulus-response combination.

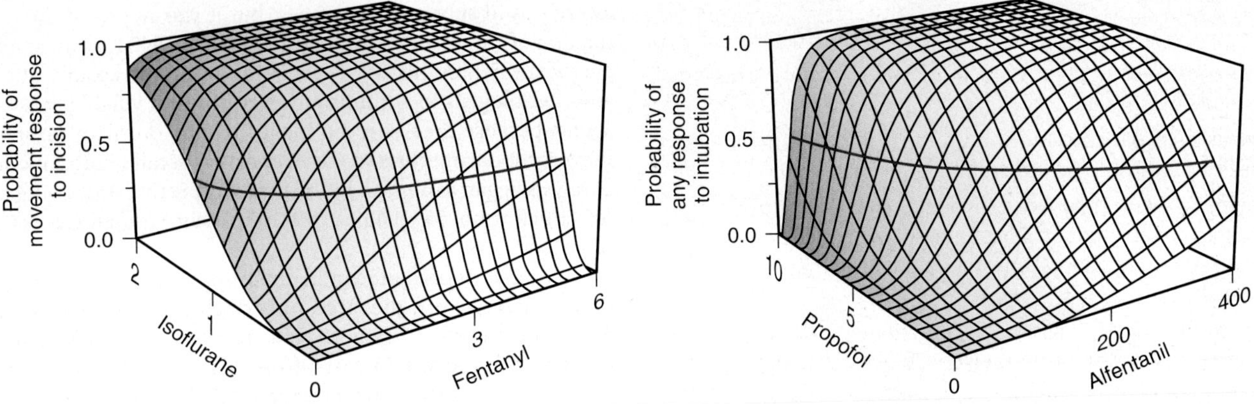

Figure 39-9 The *left* image shows the response surface for reduction in the minimum alveolar concentration of isoflurane by fentanyl.[16] The *right* image shows the interaction of propofol with alfentanil on blunting all responses to intubation.[17] Both figures demonstrate the intrinsic synergy between opioids and hypnotics in producing unresponsiveness.

the shapes derived from our hypnotic-opioid interaction model because (1) the investigators were interested only in characterizing the interaction at the 50% response level and thus did not gather enough data to characterize the upper and lower edges of either curve and (2) the mathematical function was logistic regression, which has several shortcomings as a model of drug interaction. Nevertheless, the figures demonstrate the intrinsic synergy between opioids and hypnotics in producing unresponsiveness, as well as the tendency for more profoundly noxious stimulation (e.g., intubation) to generate more synergy between the analgesic and hypnotic components of anesthesia.

Given our broad definition of anesthetic depth as providing nonresponsiveness to a wide range of stimuli-response pairs (see Fig. 39-6), one might wonder what drugs constitute "anesthetics"? Drugs are defined by their actions, and "anesthesia" is too nonspecific to characterize a drug effect. Because creation of a state of nonresponsiveness ("anesthesia") involves so many drug actions, the term "anesthetic" should not be used to suggest a particular drug class. In particular, "anesthetics" should not be used to describe drugs that suppress consciousness inasmuch as these drugs are more accurately termed "hypnotics." The one exception might be "inhaled anesthetics" because the drugs in this class (halothane, isoflurane, desflurane, and sevoflurane) suppress most of the responses to noxious stimuli.

Awareness and Memory

A spectrum of cognitive activity, including awareness, unconscious memory formation, and dreaming, has been reported during the administration of drugs that are intended to induce and maintain general anesthesia (Fig. 39-10). In addition, a range of physical and physiologic responses have been reported that may indicate perception of painful stimulation, whether conscious or unconscious. The nomenclature used to describe these phenomena has been varied and confusing. In this chapter we use the following widely accepted definitions (Box 39-2).

Awareness

Awareness during anesthesia is an important clinical problem that sometimes results in disabling psychological sequelae for the patient.[34] Although substantial improvements in prevention and treatment of awareness have been made in recent decades, further reductions are hopefully possible through improved training, continuing education, and perioperative care.

Incidence of Awareness

Measuring the Incidence of Awareness

No "cast-iron" method of measuring the incidence of awareness is available because awareness is a subjective cognitive experience that may not be completely understood by the patient or revealed by the patient to the interviewer.[35] Nevertheless, a consensus has developed about an acceptable form of questioning that is based on the questions first used by Brice, Hetherington, and Utting[36] published in 1970:

1. What was the last thing you remembered happening before you went to sleep?

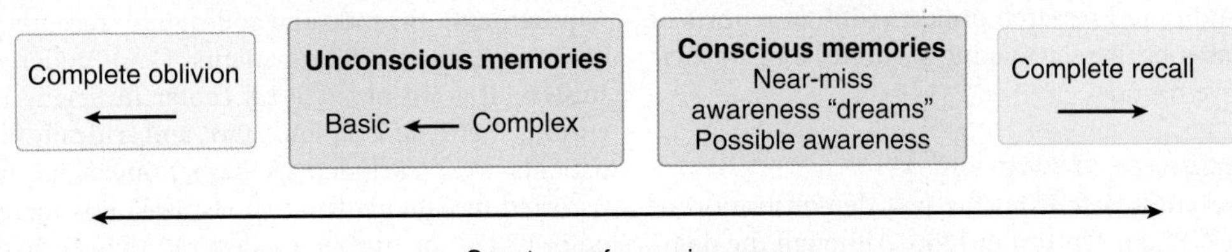

Figure 39-10 Spectrum of cognitive activity reflecting the pharmacologic activity of drugs that induce and maintain the anesthetized state, including awareness, unconscious memory formation, and dreaming.

Box 39-2 Definitions of Awareness and Memory

Awareness—Postoperative recall of events occurring during general anesthesia[31]

Amnesic wakefulness—Responsiveness during general anesthesia without postoperative recall[31]

Dreaming—Any experience (excluding awareness) that patients are able to recall postoperatively that they think occurred during general anesthesia and that they believe is dreaming[32]

Explicit memory—Conscious recollection of previous experiences ("awareness" is evidence of explicit memory)[33]

Implicit memory—Changes in performance or behavior that are produced by previous experiences but without any conscious recollection of those experiences ("unconscious memory formation" during general anesthesia)[33]

2. What is the first thing you remembered happening on waking?
3. Did you dream or have any other experiences while you were asleep?

Abouleish and Taylor[37] modified the Brice questionnaire to the form most commonly used in subsequent studies:

1. What was the last thing you remembered before going to sleep?
2. What was the first thing you remembered on waking?
3. Do you remember anything between going to sleep and waking?
4. While you were sleeping during the operation, did you dream?

An important feature of the modified questionnaire is that it includes a direct question about memory of intraoperative events without making any suggestion about what form these memories might take. A direct question is desirable inasmuch as previous research has suggested that patients may not volunteer information about their awareness episode.[38] In addition, patients should be questioned on more than one occasion postoperatively to maximize the likelihood of detecting all cases of awareness. Residual anesthetic effects, preoccupation with immediate postoperative problems such as pain, and memory suppression as a result of post-traumatic stress disorder[39] (PTSD) may inhibit patients from reporting their awareness experience at an early postoperative interview.

Clinicians should note that the modified Brice questionnaire has been administered to tens of thousands of patients in quality assurance audits and research projects without reports of undue distress to patients, thereby making it a useful tool for their routine postoperative rounds.

Studies of the Incidence of Awareness

Case reports of awareness date from the first demonstration of ether anesthesia by William Morton in 1846. Although the demonstration was deemed a success—because the patient was unresponsive during surgery—it was later revealed that the patient recalled part of the procedure. Patients continued to experience awareness in subsequent decades, but it was not until the introduction of curare into anesthetic practice in 1942 that the modern era of awareness began. The use of muscle relaxants allowed anesthesiologists to administer lower doses of volatile anesthetic agents because they were no longer relying on them to prevent movement during surgery. Case reports of recall of intraoperative paralysis began to appear. In the first prospective study, published by Hutchinson in 1960, a 1.2% incidence of awareness was reported.[40]

Many cohort studies and randomized trials have been published subsequently, the largest of which are presented in Table 39-2. This table reveals a 10-fold decrease in the incidence of awareness in the last 50 years, from about 1% to about 0.1%. In these recent studies, patients undergoing high-risk surgery were included in the mix and a substantial proportion received muscle relaxants. Most patients were attending tertiary referral centers where anesthesia was provided by qualified anesthesiologists and nurse anesthetists, as well as practitioners in training. Patients were asked a direct question about awareness and in two studies were interviewed more than once.

Several other recent studies have reported a substantially different incidence of awareness. Enlund and Hassan[52] did not identify any episode of awareness in 5216 patients undergoing minor surgery at a surgery center. A "high-dose" propofol-opioid protocol without muscle relaxants was administered to 93% of the patients. These patients were interviewed once at discharge from the postanesthesia care unit with the modified Brice questionnaire. The authors and others[62] questioned whether the patient mix, anesthesia protocol, and timing or number of interviews were responsible for the absence of awareness. Pollard and coauthors[33] also reported a low incidence of awareness in 87,361 patients undergoing all types of surgery (six cases [0.0068%]). Four of the aware patients were having cardiac surgery (incidence of 0.12% in cardiac surgery patients). This study was conducted in a tertiary referral hospital (56% of patients) and seven community hospitals and surgery centers (44% of patients). Anesthesia was administered by qualified nurse anesthetists and anesthesiologists using volatile anesthetic–based protocols. The authors and others[63,64] questioned whether the data collection method, which did not include a direct question about recall of events during surgery, the patient population, the absence of anesthesia providers in training, and the anesthetic protocols were responsible for the low incidence of awareness.

In contrast, several recent studies have reported higher rates of awareness. Chaiwat and colleagues[54] reported five cases of awareness in 802 American Society of Anesthesiologists (ASA) class 1 and 2 patients (0.62%) undergoing elective noncardiac, nonobstetric surgery in a Thai tertiary referral center. Volatile-based anaesthesia with muscle relaxants was administered. A cogent reason for each of the cases was present (i.e., inadequate anesthetic delivery, cardiovascular instability, increased anesthetic requirement). Errando and colleagues[61] recently reported 39 cases of awareness in 3921 patients (1%) undergoing noncardiac surgery at a tertiary referral center in Spain. The patients were enrolled between 1995 and 2001, and critically ill and traumatized patients were excluded. A higher incidence of awareness was reported in patients whose anesthesia was maintained with propofol (1.1%) or nitrous oxide (5%) than in patients maintained with a volatile anesthetic (0.59%).

Many studies have sought to determine the incidence of awareness in specific patient groups. These studies report an

Table 39-2 Prospective Cohort Studies of Awareness in Adult Patients

Year	Patients	N	Interviews	Incidence (%)	Type of anesthesia	Reference
1960	General surgery*	656	1	1.2	N_2O based and volatile based combined	Hutchinson[40]
1971	Obstetric surgery	880	1	3.3; 0.2	N_2O based versus volatile based	Crawford[41]
1975	General surgery	490	1	1	N_2O based and volatile based combined	Wilson[42]
1985	Cesarean section	777	1	6; 1	Low versus higher dose volatile based	Crawford[42a]
1991	General surgery	1000	1	0.2	Not stated	Liu[43]
1991	Cesarean section	3076	1	1.3; 0.4	Low- versus higher-dose thiopental/volatile	Lyons[44]
1993	Cardiac surgery	700	1	1.1	Volatile based	Phillips[45]
1993	Noncardiac surgery	1727	1	0.3	Propofol based	Sandin[46]
1997	General surgery	1000	3	0.2	Propofol based	Nordstrom[47]
1998	General surgery	2612	1	0.4	Volatile based and propofol based combined	Ranta[48]
1998	Cardiac surgery	617	1	0.3	Volatile based	Dowd[49]
2000	Noncardiac surgery	11,785	3	0.18; 0.10	Volatile based; muscle relaxant versus no muscle relaxant	Sandin[50]
2000	Nonobstetric surgery	10,811	1	0.11	Not stated	Myles[51]
2002	Minor general surgery	5216	1	0	Propofol based	Enlund[52]
2002	Cardiac surgery	929	1	0.5	Not stated	Ranta[53]
2002	General surgery	802	1	0.62	Volatile based	Chaiwat[54]
2004	High risk of awareness	2463	3	0.89; 0.16	Volatile based and propofol based; routine care or BIS guided	Myles[55]
2004	Nonobstetric surgery	19,575	2	0.13	Not stated	Sebel[56]
2004	General surgery	4945	3	0.04	Volatile based (all BIS monitored)	Ekman[57]
2005	All surgery	126,078	1	0.08	Volatile based	Rungreungvanich[58]
2007	All surgery	87,361	2	0.0068	Volatile-based	Pollard[33]
2007	Cesarean section	763	2	0.26	(33% BIS monitored)	Paech[59]
2008	High risk of awareness	1941	3	0.2; 0.2	Volatile based; end-tidal agent monitoring guided versus BIS guided	Avidan[60]
2008	Noncardiac surgery	3921	3	1.1; 0.59; 5	Propofol based, volatile based or N_2O based	Errando[61]

*General surgery corresponds to nonobstetric, noncardiac surgery.
BIS, bispectral index.

increased risk in patients undergoing cardiac surgery,[65] trauma surgery,[66,67] cesarean section,[44,59] airway endoscopic surgery,[68,69] and pediatric surgery[70,71] (although these incidences have also decreased over time). The reasons that these patients may be more at risk for awareness are discussed in the following paragraphs.

Risk Factors for Awareness

Awareness results from an imbalance between anesthetic requirement and anesthetic delivery. This imbalance may be summarized under three main headings:

Normal Requirement—Low Delivery

Inadequate delivery of anesthesia to patients with a normal anesthetic requirement is a common cause of awareness and one that exposes anesthesiologists to peer review, media attention, and litigation.[72,73]

Historically, anesthesia was commonly maintained with nitrous oxide supplemented by residual premedication and induction drugs—a technique associated with a greater than 1% incidence of awareness.[40] Appreciation of this fact resulted in increased use of volatile anesthetics and opioids and a decline in the incidence of awareness, particularly during cesarean section. Similarly, for cardiac surgery, high doses of opioids with or without an adjuvant hypnotic were favored because of stable patient hemodynamics. Unfortunately, however, responsiveness to noxious stimulation was ablated and a high risk of awareness was reported.[65,74] Influential commentary that questioned whether opioids were really capable of producing general anesthesia,[75] as well as a desire for rapid tracheal extubation ("fast tracking"), led to a change in practice and a reduced risk of awareness.[68]

Errors in knowledge, judgment, vigilance, or technical expertise can lead to inadequate anesthetic delivery during any type of general anesthesia.[76-78] However, inhaled and intravenous anesthetics each have their unique problems. During anesthesia with inhaled agents, awareness can result from vaporizer, anesthetic circuit, or end-tidal anesthetic gas monitor malfunctions that lead to inadequate delivery of nitrous oxide or volatile anesthetic agents (or both).[78] Interruptions in delivery of volatile anesthetics when moving patients from anesthetic induction rooms to operating rooms may also have contributed to the historical incidence of awareness, especially in children.[31,70,71] During intravenous anesthesia, problems in every part of the system from the syringe driver to the site of intravenous access have been reported.[76,79] However, despite early concern about an increased incidence of awareness during propofol-maintained anesthesia,[80] only the Errando study identified a risk,[61] with other studies failing to confirm this risk.[52]

Low Requirement—Very Low Delivery

Delivering adequate anesthesia to patients with a low anesthetic requirement or low cardiovascular reserve presents a particular challenge. For example, pregnant women have a lower anesthetic requirement than nonpregnant women do.[81,82] However, concern about uterine contractility, placental blood flow, and neonatal respiratory depression makes anesthesiologists cautious about anesthetic delivery during cesarean section. The incidence of awareness during cesarean section was particularly high when nitrous oxide–based anesthesia was the norm. Recently, however, the risk of awareness appears to have diminished because of supplementation with volatile anesthetics and possibly the advent of EEG-based monitors.

Patients with low perfusion states as a result of hypovolemia or cardiac failure have a lowered anesthetic requirement, but the anesthetic doses required for adequate anesthesia may still be greater than those that can be tolerated by the cardiovascular system. The result is a higher incidence of awareness in cardiac[65,77] and trauma surgery patients.[66,67] This issue applies particularly to young cardiac and trauma patients, in whom the discrepancy between the vigor of the brain and the cardiovascular system is greatest.

High Requirement—Normal Delivery

Anesthetic requirements may be higher than usual in patients who are tolerant of sedative or analgesic drugs, such as alcohol, benzodiazepines, and opioids (unless the patient is acutely intoxicated, in which case anesthetic requirements may be lower).[54] In addition, there is normal variability in the population with respect to anesthetic requirements. Some patients have multiple episodes of awareness or have family members who have suffered awareness, thus suggesting a genetic etiology.[38,54] Recent evidence also links increased anesthetic requirements to the phenotype of red hair[83] and to childhood.[71] Finally, women recover more rapidly from anesthesia than men do, which potentially increases their risk of awareness if anesthetic delivery becomes inadequate.[84,85]

Preventing Awareness

The incidence of awareness has decreased substantially over recent decades, possibly because of the recognition that awareness has significant consequences for patients and their anesthesiologists and that some anesthetic techniques are associated with increased risk. Nevertheless, further reductions are hopefully possible through further training, continuing education, and perioperative care (Fig. 39-11).

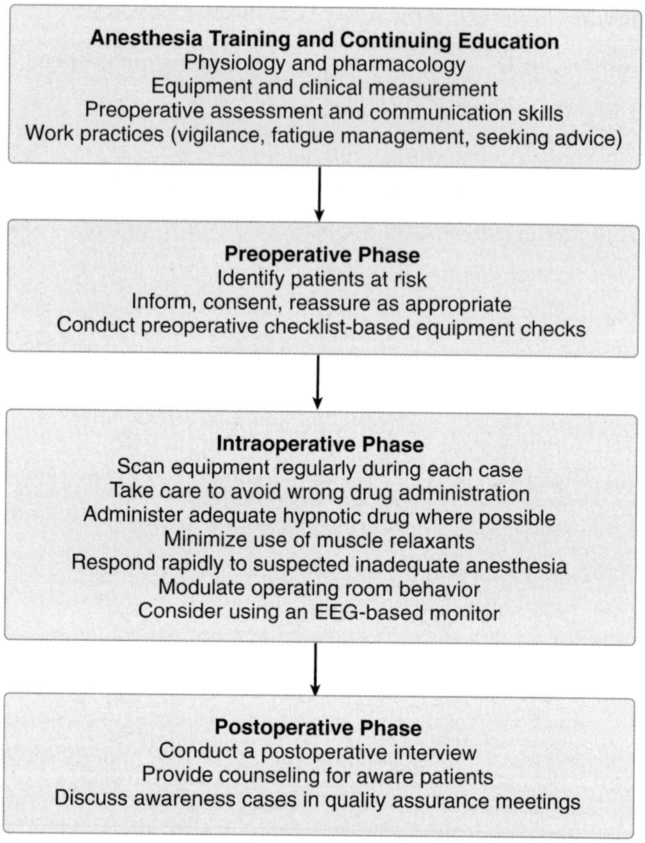

Identifying Patients at Risk

An ASA task force recently promulgated a Practice Advisory that combined an evidence-based approach with expert opinion and open forum commentary.[34] The consensus was that a preoperative interview may be useful in identifying patients at increased risk for awareness and that patients at increased risk should be informed of the possibility of awareness preoperatively.[61] To elicit a past history of awareness, direct questioning may be required.[86]

Anesthesia Training and Continuing Education
Physiology and pharmacology
Equipment and clinical measurement
Preoperative assessment and communication skills
Work practices (vigilance, fatigue management, seeking advice)

↓

Preoperative Phase
Identify patients at risk
Inform, consent, reassure as appropriate
Conduct preoperative checklist-based equipment checks

↓

Intraoperative Phase
Scan equipment regularly during each case
Take care to avoid wrong drug administration
Administer adequate hypnotic drug where possible
Minimize use of muscle relaxants
Respond rapidly to suspected inadequate anesthesia
Modulate operating room behavior
Consider using an EEG-based monitor

↓

Postoperative Phase
Conduct a postoperative interview
Provide counseling for aware patients
Discuss awareness cases in quality assurance meetings

Figure 39-11 Steps to reduce intraoperative awareness by integrating training with perioperative vigilance. EEG, electroencephalogram.

Reducing Intraoperative Risk

A thorough checklist-based evaluation of equipment should be adhered to preoperatively.[61] During anesthesia, anesthesiologists should develop the habit of scanning drug delivery systems regularly to specifically detect inadequate delivery (e.g., leakage of propofol or air entrainment). Special care should be taken to avoid incorrect drug administration (e.g., giving a muscle relaxant instead of midazolam before induction).[73] Sufficient hypnotic should be administered when possible, and muscle relaxants should be avoided unless required. There should be a rapid response to suspected inadequate anesthesia because memories can take some seconds or minutes to be encoded. This response may include increasing delivery of hypnotic drug, reducing nociception by halting surgery and administering analgesics, and speaking reassuringly to the patient.[86]

Awareness cannot be directly measured as it occurs because by definition, it relies on postoperative recall of intraoperative events.[33] Traditional clinical signs such as movement, tachycardia, hypertension, pupillary responses, and lacrimation are thought to be unreliable predictors of awareness, but they should still be monitored in every patient and treated on their merits.[35,37,54,55,61,86,87]

The utility of the BIS (Aspect Medical Systems, Inc.) in preventing awareness has been investigated in three large studies. Ekman and colleagues[88] conducted a prospective cohort study in Swedish patients undergoing noncardiac surgery under relaxant general anesthesia with routine BIS monitoring. Patients were interviewed three times with a modified Brice questionnaire. The incidence of awareness was significantly reduced in the BIS-monitored group in comparison to a historical control group without BIS monitoring (0.04% versus 0.18%; $P = .038$).

Myles and coworkers[55] conducted an international randomized controlled trial in 2463 patients at high risk of awareness who were undergoing all types of surgery under relaxant general anesthesia (the B-Aware Trial). Patients were randomized to receive BIS-guided anesthesia (BIS titrated to 40 to 60) or routine care and were interviewed three times with a modified Brice questionnaire. The overall incidence of awareness was 0.5%. There were two confirmed cases of awareness in the BIS-guided group and 11 confirmed cases in the control group (odds ratio, 0.18; 95% confidence interval, 0.02 to 0.84; $P = .022$). Awareness was not predicted from clinical signs in any case. The authors concluded that BIS monitoring is warranted in patients at high risk for awareness undergoing relaxant general anesthesia.

Recently, Avidan and coauthors[60] reported the results of a single-center randomized controlled trial in 1941 patients at higher risk for awareness who were undergoing all types of surgery under relaxant general anesthesia. Patients were randomized to receive BIS-guided anesthesia (BIS titrated to 40 to 60) or end-tidal anesthetic gas (ETAG) concentrations of 0.7 to 1.3 MAC and were interviewed three times with a modified Brice questionnaire. The overall incidence of awareness was 0.2%. There were two cases of awareness in each group (absolute difference, 0%; 95% confidence interval, −0.56% to 0.57%). The authors concluded that their results did not support routine BIS monitoring. Subsequently, it has been shown that the study was underpowered to confirm a difference inasmuch as the incidence of awareness was much lower than anticipated by the sample size calculation, the patients were at relatively low risk, and ETAG concentrations in the 0.7 to 1.3 MAC range are likely to prevent awareness (if the hemodynamic consequences can be tolerated by the patient).[89] In fact, adequate power to detect a difference between BIS and ETAG would have required a group size of more than 9000 patients.[90] Although it is not possible to draw a conclusion about the relative effectiveness of BIS and ETAG from this study, Avidan and coworkers have provoked a discussion about whether ETAG-guided anesthesia is a viable means of preventing awareness.[60] This hypothesis awaits confirmation by a suitably designed trial.

Overall, the current evidence indicates that BIS monitoring may reduce but not eliminate the risk of awareness.[91,92] Failure to respond adequately to changes in the index (i.e., allowing sustained BIS values above the recommended range),[55,60] failure to recognize the possibility of misleading values or artifact,[93,94] and the possibility that awareness may occur at BIS values within the recommended range[55,60] are all reasons why awareness may still occur in BIS-monitored patients. Furthermore, no specific data exist for the other available EEG-based monitors. On this basis, the ASA taskforce concluded that "the decision to use a brain function monitor should be made on a case-by-case basis by the individual practitioner for selected patients (e.g., light anesthesia)."[34] This analysis should also take into account the potential cost of using this technology to prevent a relatively rare complication of anesthesia.[55,60,95]

Consequences of Awareness

Earlier reports on the psychological consequences of awareness were based on retrospective study designs in which patients were identified by advertisement, referral, or analysis of closed claims.[35,72,96] These studies illustrated the distress that may result from an awareness episode but did not confirm the spectrum of symptoms or the incidence of PTSD. More recently, Lennmarken and colleagues[97] audited the incidence of psychological sequelae in 18 prospectively identified awareness cases. Three weeks after the episode, all patients appeared to be coping well and follow-up was discontinued. Two years later, two patients could not be contacted, one had died, and six refused to be interviewed. Of the nine interviewed patients, four were severely disabled by PTSD and another three reported more minor symptoms. These authors suggested that the incidence of PTSD could be greater than 50% inasmuch as avoidance of medical situations is one of the signs of PTSD. Subsequently, this group of researchers reported a contrasting result.[38] They asked 2681 consecutive patients whether they had been aware in the past and identified greater emotional stress in the few days after the episode than later (incidence of late psychological symptoms, 33%). They concluded that the study methodology may influence the result.

Risk factors for PTSD in the awareness setting have not been identified. Commentators have suggested that memory of the pain of surgery and an unsympathetic response from caregivers may contribute.[35,97] The psychological literature suggests that peritraumatic dissociation is a predictor of the severity of post-traumatic symptoms.[39] Further research is required in this area.

An episode of awareness may have consequences for the anesthesiologist as well. Most patients who suffer an awareness episode do not proceed to litigation or generate unwanted attention from the media or regulatory authorities. One could hope that good communication and patient support may prevent not only adverse patient sequelae but also lawsuits.[98] The ASA Closed Claims Project provides a valuable analysis of cases that have proceeded to litigation in the United States. In the period 1990 to 2001, 55 claims were made, substandard care was identified in 47% of cases, and 46% were settled with a patient payment (median payment, $41,210 [substantially lower than the median payment for other general anesthesia claims]).[98] It is difficult to say whether the recent attention paid to awareness[34] and the advent of EEG-based monitoring[55] will increase or decrease the liability for awareness in the future.

Unconscious Memory Formation During Anesthesia

Whether patients can form unconscious memories during anesthesia and whether these memories matter are interesting questions and ones that have occupied researchers for the last 40 years.[99] In the first systematic study of this subject, Levinson[100] staged a mock crisis during anesthesia and then hypnotized the patients to determine whether unconscious memories of the crisis had been retained. No patient had active recall of events occurring during anesthesia, but under hypnosis, 4 of the 10 patients could recount the crisis accurately. However, this study and subsequent ones[99] were confounded by the inability to discount inadequate anesthesia or reduce the influence of active recall when testing for unconscious memory.

Since the mid-1990s, investigators have more carefully controlled anesthetic depth by using EEG-based monitoring and have used perceptual priming tests that measure explicit and implicit memory in a single test involving the process dissociation paradigm.[101] These studies revealed that unconscious memories are retained if anesthesia is relatively light or variable in depth and word presentation occurs during surgery.[102-104] For example, Lubke and coworkers[102] investigated patients in whom general anesthesia was induced for trauma surgery by using the word stem completion test and process dissociation paradigm. The number of stem completions with words presented during surgery ("hits") increased with increasing BIS values, and implicit memory was demonstrated at BIS values of less than 60. Stonell and coauthors[103] reported successful priming at BIS values greater than 50, whereas Deeprose and colleagues[104] reported priming at mean BIS values of 42. In contrast, Kerssens and colleagues[105] targeted a similar BIS range but achieved a lot less fluctuation in BIS values (1% versus 8% to 11% in the previously mentioned studies[103,104]). They could not demonstrate any unconscious memory formation. This study emphasizes that excursions into light planes of anesthesia appear to be necessary for memory formation.

Finally, does unconscious memory formation during anesthesia have any consequences for the patient? In the psychological literature, priming has been reported to enhance existing tendencies—this is the foundation of subliminal advertising techniques. However, there is no evidence yet that unconscious memory formation has adverse or even therapeutic effects after general anesthesia. Nevertheless, we should avoid making comments during anesthesia that we do not want our patients to hear.[106]

Dreaming During Anesthesia

Dreaming during anesthesia is a commonly reported and fascinating phenomenon that nevertheless remains poorly understood. The incidence of dreaming during anesthesia varies according to the age and sex of the patients, the type of anesthesia, and the timing of the postoperative interview. Dreaming is more commonly reported by younger patients[107,108] and after propofol-based,[108] opioid-based,[36] or ketamine-based[109] anesthesia. If an interview is conducted at emergence from anesthesia, about 25% of patients will report that they have been dreaming.[108] However, if the interview is delayed until discharge from the postanesthesia care unit, the incidence falls to around 6%.[55]

Early reports of dreaming were often suggestive of near-miss awareness: (1) "A patient dreamed that he was at a fairground and someone was throwing darts at his stomach,"[110] (2) "A patient dreamt that the pages of a heavy book were being slowly turned over at regular intervals,"[40] and (3) "A patient dreamed of a party at a public house in which there was a generous supply of gin and the anaesthetist was the landlord!"[36] It was also reported that dreaming patients exhibited more signs of light anesthesia, were more likely to report awareness, and were less likely than non-dreaming patients to have been BIS monitored.[36,107,111]

Subsequent studies suggested, however, that most dreaming is not related to inadequate anesthesia and may occur during recovery. Leslie and coworkers[108] conducted a prospective cohort study of 300 young healthy patients undergoing relaxant general anesthesia for noncardiac surgery. No difference in median BIS values during surgery between dreamers and nondreamers was reported. The form and content of the dreams were suggestive of the dreams of sleep onset, and the authors postulated that dreaming was occurring during physiologic sleep (a hypothesis that awaits confirmation).

Almost all dreaming during anesthesia is harmless, unimportant, and quickly forgotten. Only dreams that worry the patient or that are suggestive of awareness should receive further attention. These patients should receive similar follow-up to patients with frank recall of intraoperative events.[108]

Hypnotics, Analgesics, and Anesthetic Depth

Inhaled Anesthetics

Movement Response and the MAC Concept

Purposeful movement of a body part in response to noxious stimuli has been extensively used as a clinical sign of anesthesia. Using this movement to quantitate anesthetic response induced by potent inhaled anesthetics, Eger, Merkel, and their colleagues[2,112] defined MAC as the minimum alveolar concentration of inhaled anesthetic required to prevent 50% of subjects from "gross purposeful movement" in response to a skin incision. As suggested by the definition, "minimum" is a slight misnomer, and "median" would probably have been a better descriptor. Readers are referred to the excellent review articles that document development of the MAC concept and its many applications in anesthesia.[113,114]

The MAC concept has three basic components: (1) an all-or-none (quantal) movement response must occur after applications of a "supramaximal" noxious stimulus; (2) end-tidal concentrations of anesthetic in the alveoli, considered an equilibrated sample site, are used as an indication of the concentration of anesthetic in the brain; and (3) MAC is a unifying concept of inhaled anesthetic potency.

For determination of MAC in humans, the standard noxious stimulus has been the initial surgical skin incision.[2] Skin incision represents a reproducible noxious stimulation. There has been no systematic examination of other perioperative surgical stimuli (e.g., peritoneal traction) representing more profound surgical manipulation than skin incision or endotracheal intubation. For determination of MAC in animals, the standard stimulus has been application of a surgical clamp to the base of the tail. After examining other noxious stimuli in dogs, Eger and colleagues[2] concluded that tail clamping represented the most noxious stimulation that was experimentally reproducible and not excessively traumatic.

A second component of the MAC concept involves use of the alveolar concentration of an anesthetic as an indication of drug concentration. The steady-state (i.e., equilibrated) partial pressures of inhaled anesthetics must be identical in all body tissues, such as alveoli, blood, and brain. Thus, the measured end-tidal partial pressure of an inhaled anesthetic (representative of the alveolar concentration) is in direct proportion to the underlying concentration in the brain at steady state. Because the brain is so well perfused relative to its mass, it is possible to achieve an equilibration among end-tidal, alveolar, arterial, and brain anesthetic partial pressures within 15 minutes of exposure to a constant end-tidal anesthetic concentration.[115]

A third component of MAC is that it has served as a unifying measure of inhaled anesthetic potency. This has resulted in the concept of MAC fractions or MAC multiples for end points other than movement response to skin incision. Stoelting and colleagues determined the MAC of an anesthetic that would allow opening of the eyes on verbal command during emergence from anesthesia ("MAC-awake").[116] This stimulation is less intense than surgical skin incision, and response occurs at lower concentrations of anesthetic than movement to skin incision does. Generally, the MAC-awake values are a third to a fourth of the MAC values for surgical incision. Yakaitis and coworkers[117] determined the MAC of an inhaled anesthetic that would inhibit movement and coughing during endotracheal intubation ("MAC-intubation"). Intubation is significantly more stimulating than skin incision, with higher concentrations of inhaled anesthetic required to eliminate movement response. Finally, Roizen and associates[118] investigated the MAC of anesthetics necessary to prevent an adrenergic response to skin incision ("MAC-BAR"), as measured by the concentration of catecholamine in venous blood. When one examines the values for (1) MAC-awake, (2) MAC–skin incision, (3) MAC-intubation, and (4) MAC-BAR, one sees a family of concentration-versus-response curves that characterize the hypnotic effects of inhaled anesthetics relative to defined clinical stimuli.

Zbinden and colleagues undertook a comprehensive examination of the effects of different noxious stimuli on the purposeful movement response with isoflurane.[119] Twenty-six healthy surgical patients were administered only isoflurane with adequate inspired/end-tidal equilibration. Multiple noxious stimuli were applied at varying end-tidal isoflurane concentrations. From the resulting data, the authors were able to define a family of concentration-versus-response curves for different noxious stimuli, as displayed in Figure 39-12. The percent end-tidal isoflurane concentrations that resulted in a 50% probability of no movement response for different stimuli were as follows: verbal responsiveness, 0.37%; trapezius muscle squeeze, 0.84%; laryngoscopy, 1.0%; 50-Hz electrical tetanus, 1.03%; skin incision, 1.16% (MAC, by definition); and laryngoscopy with intubation, 1.76%. This study demonstrates how varying clinical stimuli require different isoflurane concentrations to prevent a clinical response and can be used to define a concentration-versus-response relationship for the hypnotic effects of isoflurane. When different inhaled anesthetics are compared, the ratio of MAC–skin incision to MAC-intubation or MAC-awake is relatively constant.

Table 39-3 Factors that Affect Minimum Alveolar Concentration

Effect on MAC	Factors (Study Subjects)
Decrease	Hypothermia (animals) Severe hypotension (animals) Advanced age (humans) Opioids, ketamine (humans, animals) Chronic administration of amphetamine (animals) Reserpine, α-methyldopa (animals) Cholinesterase inhibitors (animals) Intravenous local anesthetics (humans, animals) Pregnancy (animals) Hypoxemia (Pa_{O_2} < 40 mm Hg) (animals) Anemia (animals) α_2-Agonists (animals, humans)
Increase	Hyperthermia (animals) Hyperthyroidism (animals) Alcoholism (humans) Acute administration of dextroamphetamine (animals) Young age (humans, animals)
No effect	Duration of anesthesia (humans, animals) Sex (human, animals) Metabolic acid-base status (animals) Hypercapnia and hypocapnia (humans, animals) Isovolemic anemia (animals) Hypertension (animals)

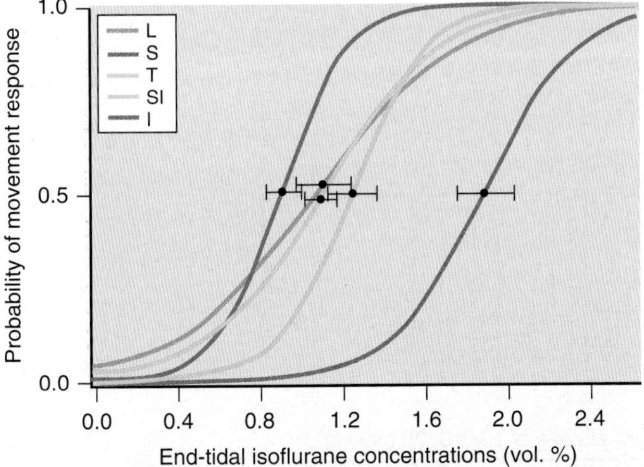

Figure 39-12 Logistic regression analysis of the end-tidal isoflurane concentration relative to the predicted probability of no movement response for different noxious stimuli. *Bars* indicate the 95% confidence intervals the end-tidal concentration with a 50% probability of response. I, laryngoscopy/intubation; L, laryngoscopy; S, trapezius muscle squeeze; SI, skin incision; T, tetanic nerve stimulation. *(Modified from Zbinden AM, Maggiorini M, Petersen-Felix S, et al: Anesthetic depth defined using multiple noxious stimuli during isoflurane/oxygen anesthesia. I. Motor reactions. Anesthesiology 80:253-260, 1994.)*

Other drugs used in anesthesia increase the apparent potency of inhaled anesthetics by decreasing the anesthetic requirement, as measured by a reduction in MAC. Numerous altered physiologic states (e.g., aging) also change the apparent potency of inhaled anesthetics. Several review articles have described the many studies applying the MAC concept to the clinical practice and science of anesthesia.[38] Table 39-3 summarizes the results of these studies regarding the factors that affect MAC.

Much of the previous research on MAC assumed that the lack of movement response from inhaled anesthetics was due to anesthetic effects on the central, cortical brain tissues. This assumption has been challenged. In 1993, Rampil and coworkers demonstrated in decorticate rats that the spinal cord was the primary site mediating immobility for inhaled anesthetics.[22] Antognini and Schwartz also drew the same conclusions from experiments in goats with isolated brain/body perfusion.[23] These investigators demonstrated that the MAC value for the goat was

Table 39-4 Hemodynamic Response to Defined Noxious Stimuli Under Isoflurane Anesthesia

Stimulus	End-Tidal Concentration That Suppresses Movement In 50% of Patients (ET_{50}) (Percent atm)	Change in Systolic Blood Pressure for Patients at ET_{50} (mm Hg)	Change in Heart Rate for Patients at ET_{50} (Beats/min)
Trapezius muscle squeeze	0.90	9	5
Electrical tetanus	1.10	15	15
Laryngoscopy	1.07	23	17
Skin incision	1.24	34	35
Laryngoscopy and intubation	1.87	53	36

ET, end-tidal concentration.

approximately twice as large when only the brain was exposed to isoflurane than when both the brain and spinal cord were exposed to the anesthetic.

Other Clinical Responses

Responses other than purposeful movement have been investigated as possible clinical measures of the depth of anesthesia: the rate and volume of ventilation in spontaneously breathing subjects, eye movement, the diameter and reactivity of pupils to light, heart rate, arterial blood pressure, and autonomic signs such as sweating. It has not been possible to use these clinical signs to generate uniform measures of the depth of anesthesia for inhaled anesthetics. Although some clinical signs do correlate with depth of anesthesia for certain inhaled anesthetics, the same cannot be said for other inhaled anesthetics.[120]

We have previously noted that the hemodynamic response is harder to suppress than movement. This was particularly well demonstrated by Zbinden and colleagues[121] in a systematic study of the hemodynamic response to different noxious stimuli at increasing isoflurane concentrations. In 26 healthy surgical patients receiving different equilibrated end-tidal concentrations of isoflurane, the following noxious stimuli were applied, several of them on multiple occasions: trapezius muscle squeeze, 50-Hz electrical tetanus, laryngoscopy, laryngoscopy with intubation, and skin incision. With continuous recording of intra-arterial hemodynamics, acute increases in heart rate and systolic blood pressure were recorded and related to the isoflurane concentration and presence or absence of purposeful movement. Table 39-4 presents the absolute increase in systolic blood pressure and heart rate at the isoflurane end-tidal concentration that had a 50% probability of no purposeful movement for that specific stimulus. As stated earlier, different noxious stimuli result in different degrees of hemodynamic response. There is a relative rank order of the degree of hemodynamic response, with laryngoscopy and intubation being the most intense stimuli. Multiple regression analysis demonstrated that the type of stimulation had the most influence on the increase in blood pressure, with the isoflurane concentration being the least important. Figure 39-13 presents the baseline systolic blood pressure and subsequent increase in systolic pressure at a measured isoflurane concentration for subjects receiving a skin incision. Increasing isoflurane concentration did not prevent the increase in systolic blood pressure, even at very high end-tidal concentrations. Rather, increasing isoflurane concentration only decreased the prestimulation systolic

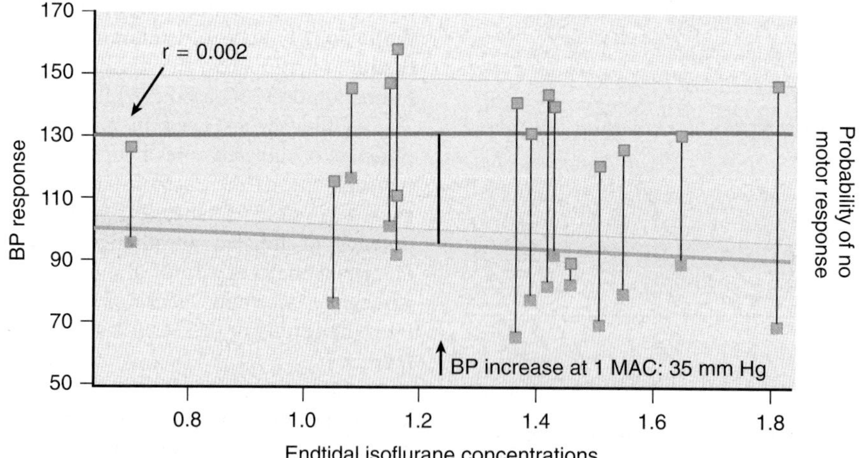

Figure 39-13 Response of systolic blood pressure (BP, in mm Hg) to skin incision as a function of end-tidal isoflurane concentration. Yellow squares, systolic blood pressure before stimulation; Blue squares, systolic blood pressure after stimulation; *lower oblique line*, regression line to systolic BP before stimulation (r = −0.46); *upper line*, regression line to systolic BP after skin incision (r = 0.0002); *shaded area*, 95% confidence interval for regression lines; *vertical arrow*, median effective isoflurane concentration for the motor response of the stimulation pattern. The *shaded areas* represent the linear regression relationship of isoflurane concentration versus prestimulus and poststimulus systolic BP. MAC, minimul alveolar concentration. *(From Zbinden AM, Maggiorini M, Petersen-Felix S, et al: Anesthetic depth defined using multiple noxious stimuli during isoflurane/oxygen anesthesia. I. Motor reactions. Anesthesiology 80:253-260, 1994.)*

pressure such that the noxious stimuli returned systolic pressure closer to the normal, awake values.

The clinical implications of these data relative to judging anesthetic depth from the hemodynamic response for inhaled anesthetics are significant. When used as a sole agent, even in high concentrations, isoflurane is unable to suppress hemodynamic responses to noxious stimuli. Rather, the hemodynamic control seen with high isoflurane concentrations occurs as a result of a decrease in the prestimulation hemodynamic baseline. Thus, although hemodynamic responses are the most commonly used clinical measures to judge inhaled anesthetic depth of anesthesia, the scientific basis for such application is tenuous.

Zbinden's work is important evidence that isoflurane provides hypnotic effects with minimal analgesic effect, as judged by the profound hemodynamic response to noxious stimuli in the presence of 1.8 MAC isoflurane. In clinical practice, additional drugs are commonly used with inhaled anesthetics. Daniel and colleagues[26] examined how fentanyl (0 to 3 μg/kg) and 60% nitrous oxide alter the heart rate, mean arterial blood pressure, and catecholamine response (components of MAC-BAR) during desflurane and isoflurane anesthesia. Fentanyl, 1.5 μg/kg, reduced MAC-BAR for desflurane from 1.3 to 0.4 MAC and for isoflurane from 1.3 to 0.55 MAC. Increasing the fentanyl dose to 3 μg/kg did not cause further change in MAC-BAR values for both inhaled anesthetics. Figure 39-14 shows an interaction surface for fentanyl and isoflurane based on modifying the model reported by McEwan to increase C_{50} in the absence of fentanyl by 1.3 and adjusting the isoflurane C_{50} in the presence of an effect-site fentanyl concentration of 1.36 ng/mL (corresponding to a 1.5-μg/kg bolus) to 0.4 MAC. The red arrow shows the reduction in MAC-BAR demonstrated by Daniel and coworkers.[26] It is clear from the figure that additional opioid would not be expected to yield further significant reductions in MAC-BAR. This study suggests that the addition of analgesic components, such as nitrous oxide and fentanyl, can prevent the sympathetic stimulation and hemodynamic responses seen with noxious surgical stimuli when inhaled anesthetics are used.

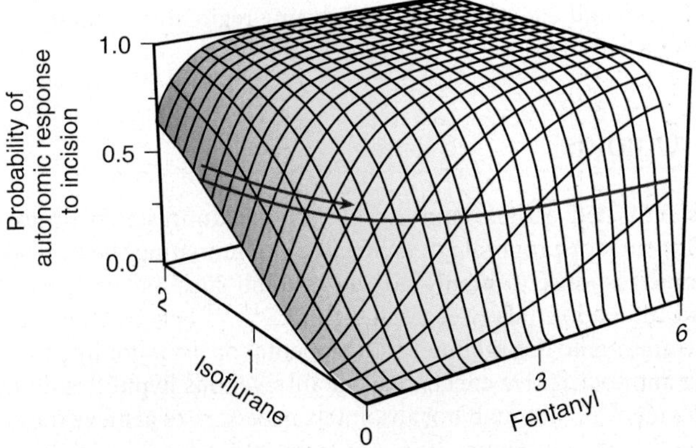

Figure 39-14 Interaction surface for fentanyl and isoflurane reflecting suppression of the autonomic response. The surface is based on the isoflurane interaction reported by McEwan and colleagues,[16] but modified to increase the C_{50} of isoflurane in the absence of fentanyl by 1.3 minimum alveolar concentration (MAC) and adjusting the isoflurane C_{50} in the presence of an effect-site fentanyl concentration of 1.36 (corresponding to a 1.5-μg/kg bolus) to 0.4 MAC, as reported by Daniel and coauthors.[26] The *red arrow* shows the reduction in MAC-BAR demonstrated by Daniel and coworkers.[26]

Intravenously Administered Hypnotics

Traditionally, intravenous hypnotics were used for induction of anesthesia as a single intravenous bolus. The introduction of propofol allowed these drugs to be infused for maintenance of anesthesia, where assessment of depth of anesthesia becomes more relevant.

Assessing Depth During Induction of Anesthesia

Induction of anesthesia often consists of a rapid intravenous bolus injection of an intravenous hypnotic (e.g., propofol, thiopental, etomidate). Plasma concentrations peak within a half to 1 minute and decline rapidly on redistribution of the drug. The rapidly changing plasma concentrations cause a corresponding fluctuation in the degree of CNS depression. Depth of anesthesia increases rapidly (causing loss of consciousness), peaks, and then decreases as plasma concentrations decline. CNS depression lags behind plasma concentrations and is manifested as hysteresis on curves plotting effect against plasma concentration. All the concepts discussed earlier regarding non–steady-state conditions produced by rapid administration of a drug make assessment of the relationship of plasma concentration and depth of anesthesia difficult, if not impossible, during bolus intravenous administration.

Clinical end points useful in assessing depth of anesthesia during induction include loss of verbal responsiveness, loss of eyelid reflex, and loss of corneal reflex. Typical stimulation occurring during induction of anesthesia includes laryngoscopy and intubation, which are profoundly noxious stimuli. Frequently, response to these two procedures cannot be eliminated completely with just the intravenously administered hypnotic. In one study, administration of thiopental (6 mg/kg) was followed by an average increase in systolic blood pressure of 53 mm Hg on laryngoscopy and intubation.[122] In another study, administration of thiamylal (4 mg/kg) was followed by an increase in mean arterial blood pressure from 92 mm Hg (control) to 136 mm Hg on laryngoscopy.[123] Because most intravenous hypnotics do not provide significant analgesia, the hemodynamic response to major noxious stimuli is great, even when large doses are given. Thus, assessment of depth of anesthesia with clinically relevant noxious stimuli such as laryngoscopy and intubation requires the concurrent administration of other analgesic drugs (opioids or nitrous oxide) to provide reasonable and clinically acceptable hemodynamic control.

Assessing Depth During Maintenance of Anesthesia

Becker[124] presented one of the first studies that quantified the relationship between plasma concentrations of an intravenous anesthetic (in this case, thiopental) and clinical measures of depth of anesthesia.

Hung and coauthors[125] proposed a conceptual approach that used clinical measures to examine intravenous anesthetic pharmacodynamics. A target controlled infusion of thiopental rapidly achieved and then maintained a low (10 to 40 μg/mL) and then high (40 to 90 μg/mL) thiopental concentration in 26 surgical patients. After allowing 5 minutes for blood-brain equilibration, increasingly noxious stimuli (verbal command, 50-Hz electrical tetanus, trapezius muscle squeeze, laryngoscopy, and intubation) were applied at 1-minute intervals until the patient responded verbally or moved purposefully. The approach separated the increasing levels of thiopental required to block increasingly noxious stimulation.

Kazama and colleagues[19] examined the pharmacodynamics of propofol alone and then of propofol with fentanyl by using the defined noxious stimuli/movement responses that Hung and coworkers[125] used for thiopental and the hemodynamic methodology developed by Zbinden and associates[121] for isoflurane. These results are shown in Figure 39-15. Verbal response was easily suppressed by propofol, whereas the response to intubation was the most difficult to suppress. Tetanus, incision, and laryngoscopy were similarly noxious in this paradigm. Kazama and colleagues also found that addition of a steady-state fentanyl concentration of 1 or 3 ng/mL minimally decreased the amount of propofol required to suppress verbal response but profoundly decreased the amount of propofol required to suppress the response to tetanus, laryngoscopy, skin incision, and intubation.[19] Similar to what Zbinden and associates[121] described for isoflurane, the addition of fentanyl to propofol attenuated the increases in systolic blood pressure in a dose-dependent manner. The conceptual methodology used by Kazama and coworkers allows characterization of anesthetic depth by using multiple, defined noxious stimuli, as discussed previously in this chapter, and supports the intellectual framework for anesthetic depth shown in Figure 39-7.

Quantitation of clinical depth of anesthesia for the combination of an opioid and intravenous anesthetic was reported by Vuyk and coauthors.[126] Using the pharmacodynamic methodology developed by Ausems and colleagues,[28] the interaction of a constant plasma concentration of propofol (in place of nitrous oxide) was examined as the alfentanil was titrated to clinical responses. Propofol exhibited a significant interaction with alfentanil, thus decreasing the total dose of alfentanil and the alfentanil plasma concentrations needed for adequate anesthesia. Table 39-5 indicates how the total dose of alfentanil needed decreased from 22.8 mg with 66% nitrous oxide to 10.3 mg with a steady-state propofol plasma concentration of 4 μg/mL. The mechanism of this decreased dose requirement was marked potentiation of alfentanil such that the alfentanil plasma concentrations needed to achieve the same degree of pharmacologic effect were two to four times lower with propofol.

Table 39-5 Interaction of Propofol and Nitrous Oxide with Alfentanil in Lower Abdominal Surgery

Event	Alfentanil Cp_{50} (ng/mL) in Conjunction with	
	Propofol	**Nitrous Oxide**
Steady-state propofol or nitrous oxide concentration	4.0 ± 0.6 μg/mL (range, 3.2 to 4.9)	66%
Intubation	92 ± 20*	429 ± 42*
Skin incision	55 ± 16*	101 ± 16*
Intra-abdominal dissection	66 ± 38†	206 ± 65†
Total alfentanil dose (mg)	10.3 ± 6.1†	22.8 ± 6.4†

*± standard error.

†± standard deviation.

Modified from Vuyk J, Lim T, Engbers FH, et al: Pharmacodynamics of alfentanil as a supplement to propofol or nitrous oxide for lower abdominal surgery in female patients. Anesthesiology 78:1036-1045, 1993.

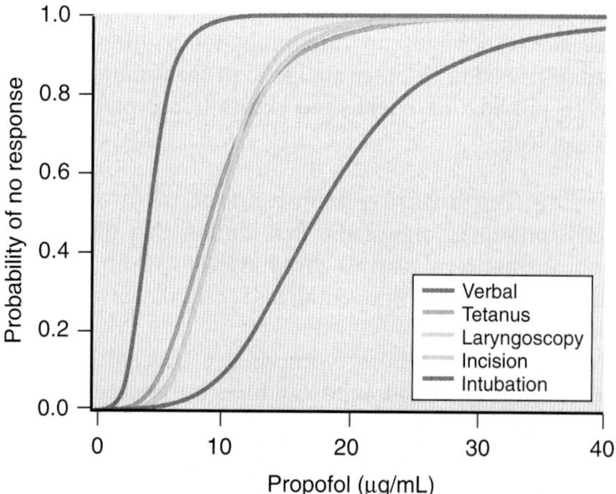

Figure 39-15 Propofol concentration-versus-response relationship for five clinically relevant stimuli: verbal, electrical tetanus, laryngoscopy, incision, and intubation. *(From Kazama T, Ikeda K, Morita K: Reduction by fentanyl of the Cp_{50} values of propofol and hemodynamic responses to various noxious stimuli. Anesthesiology 87:213-227, 1997.)*

In a subsequent study, Vuyk and colleagues used this same methodology, but they randomized the surgical subjects to a range of constant propofol blood concentrations.[17] With blood propofol concentrations increasing from 2 to 10 μg/mL, the alfentanil Cp_{50} decreased from 170 to 25 ng/mL for laryngoscopy, from 280 to 23 ng/mL for intubation, from 259 to 9 ng/mL for opening of the peritoneum, and from 209 to 16 ng/mL for the intra-abdominal surgical stimulus. With plasma alfentanil concentrations increasing from 10 to 150 ng/mL, the propofol Cp_{50} for regaining of consciousness decreased from 3.8 to 0.8 μg/mL. This study confirms the profound, synergistic interaction of propofol with alfentanil. Vuyk and colleagues used computer simulations of their gathered data to suggest that the optimal blood propofol and plasma alfentanil concentrations that allow the most rapid recovery from intraoperative anesthesia occur at 3.5 and 85 ng/mL, respectively. An editorial[127] comment on this study provided more general guidelines for using the quantitative interaction of propofol and alfentanil to design dosing regimens for total intravenous anesthesia.

Opioids

As indicated earlier, large intravenously administered doses of thiopental or propofol are ineffective at eliminating the hemodynamic response to highly noxious stimuli such as laryngoscopy and intubation (also see Chapter 27).[19,122,123] Fentanyl decreases the anesthetic requirement for thiopental or propofol by providing antinociceptive effects that the intravenous hypnotics do not provide.[19,128] Although not absolutely necessary to achieve the end points shown in Figure 39-6, as Figure 39-7 suggests, opioids are typically combined with hypnotic drugs to create the state of nonresponsiveness we recognize as anesthesia.

Opioids as Complete Anesthetics

In 1947, Neff and associates[129] used meperidine as an intravenous supplement to nitrous oxide/oxygen anesthesia. The later use of opioids without the concurrent use of hypnotics coincided with the development of cardiac surgery and intensive care during the 1970s. Providing anesthesia for patients with severe valvular or congenital heart disease without causing cardiovascular collapse was difficult before the introduction of high-dose opioid anesthesia. These early cardiac surgery patients were extremely ill and had little or no circulatory reserve. During the late 1960s, Lowenstein and coauthors[130] noted the hemodynamic stability of patients undergoing mechanical ventilation who were given frequent large doses of intravenous morphine to suppress respiration in the intensive care units. This observation encouraged Lowenstein and coworkers to become the first to administer morphine (0.5 to 3.0 mg/kg) as the only "anesthetic" drug. The resulting cardiovascular stability in acutely ill patients with acquired valvular heart disease was impressive. As cardiac surgery advanced in methodology, patients with ischemic heart disease began to undergo surgical anesthesia. Unfortunately, morphine anesthesia was less satisfactory for these patients, in whom hypertension, tachycardia, and awareness developed during surgery.[130]

In 1978, Stanley and Webster[131] introduced the use of high-dose fentanyl for cardiac anesthesia. This technique minimized the undesirable effects of morphine on induction (hypotension) and provided better hemodynamic stability in patients with good ventricular function and ischemic heart disease. As clinical experience with fentanyl increased, however, investigators found that even enormous doses of fentanyl could not reliably produce the anesthetic state, as defined in Figure 39-7, for the most potent stimuli and difficult-to-suppress responses.[132] This discovery demonstrated that opioids are not "anesthetics," but only potent analgesics and weak hypnotics, as suggested by Figure 39-2.

Many studies confirm this finding. Wynands and colleagues[14] used moderate to large doses of fentanyl (50 to 150 µg/mL) only, with no other anesthetic drugs (no hypnotic component), and measured plasma concentrations at defined surgical stimuli (intubation, skin incision, sternotomy, aortic root dissection) in patients undergoing coronary surgery with good ventricular function. In approximately 20% of patients, extremely high plasma concentrations of fentanyl (15 ng/mL) did not eliminate hemodynamic responses, defined as a 20% increase in systolic blood pressure. These results have been confirmed by Hynynen and colleagues[133] and Philbin and associates.[134]

Murphy and Hug[135] measured the ability of fentanyl to decrease enflurane MAC in dogs. They first anesthetized the dogs with enflurane and determined MAC. Fentanyl was then infused at progressively higher rates to obtain a constant steady-state plasma concentration of fentanyl in each animal. After each increase in infusion rate, enflurane MAC was determined again. Murphy and Hug found that even very high plasma concentrations of fentanyl (20 ng/mL) did not decrease enflurane MAC beyond 60% to 70% of its initial value (Fig. 39-16). That is, there was a ceiling to the enflurane-sparing effect. Morphine, sufentanil, and alfentanil also decrease enflurane MAC and have a similar ceiling effect in dogs.[136-138]

McEwan and colleagues undertook similar studies in humans and characterized the decrease in isoflurane MAC with varying constant fentanyl plasma concentrations achieved with a computer-driven infusion pump.[16] Movement response to initial skin incision was examined relative to end-tidal isoflurane concentrations. McEwan and coworkers[16] found the results in humans to be very similar to those observed by Hug and colleagues in dogs. Isoflurane MAC decreased 39% at a steady-state fentanyl plasma concentration of 1 ng/mL and 63% at a fentanyl plasma

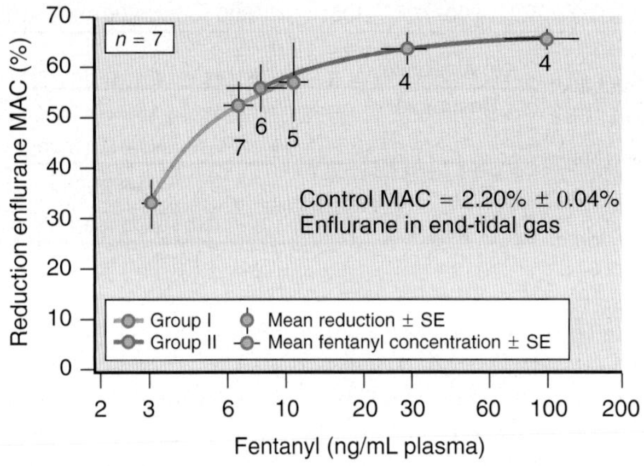

Figure 39-16 Percent reduction in enflurane minimum alveolar concentration (MAC) as a function of the plasma concentrations of fentanyl. Each point represents the mean concentration (± SEM) for fentanyl in plasma and the average percent (± SEM) reduction in enflurane MAC. Numbers of dogs below the vertical standard error bars indicate the numbers per data point. SE, standard error. *(From Murphy MR, Hug CC Jr: The anesthetic potency of fentanyl in terms of its reduction of enflurane MAC. Anesthesiology 57:485-488, 1982.)*

concentration of 3 ng/mL. Increasing fentanyl plasma concentrations to more than 3 ng/mL produced a minimal further reduction in isoflurane MAC. The maximal reduction in MAC was 82% at a steady-state fentanyl plasma concentration of 10.6 ng/mL. Similar MAC reduction results have been obtained with other inhaled anesthetics (desflurane, sevoflurane) and other opioids (alfentanil, sufentanil, remifentanil).[6,139]

Similar results are found when other end points of inhaled anesthetics and opioid interactions are examined, including MAC-awake and MAC-BAR[118,140,141]: a ceiling effect of the opioid occurs at defined steady-state plasma concentrations.

Clinical Signs of Inadequate Anesthesia and Plasma Concentration of Opioids

Ausems and colleagues[142] used pharmacodynamic modeling concepts to relate clinical signs of inadequate opioid anesthesia to plasma concentrations of the drug. In their study paradigm, patients were premedicated with a benzodiazepine, anesthesia was induced with alfentanil (150 µg/kg), and the trachea was intubated with the aid of succinylcholine. Anesthesia was maintained with 70% nitrous oxide and a variable-rate infusion of alfentanil. The infusion was titrated to the following clinical end points: (1) systemic arterial blood pressure increased to greater than 15 mm Hg higher than the patient's normal value; (2) heart rate exceeding 90 beats/min in the absence of hypovolemia; (3) somatic responses, such as body movements (minimal muscle paralysis allowed physical movement), swallowing, coughing, grimacing, or opening of the eyes; and (4) autonomic signs of inadequate anesthesia (e.g., lacrimation, flushing, or sweating). If any clinical signs occurred, the infusion rate was increased 25 to 50 µg/kg/hr, and a small bolus dose (7 µg/kg) was given. Good hemodynamic control was possible in all subjects. If no clinical signs occurred, however, the infusion rate was decreased at regular 15-minute intervals.

Figure 39-17A shows the relationship between the plasma concentration of alfentanil and response/no response for three clinical end points: intubation, skin incision, and skin closure. Figure 39-17B shows the individual subject curves for the proba-

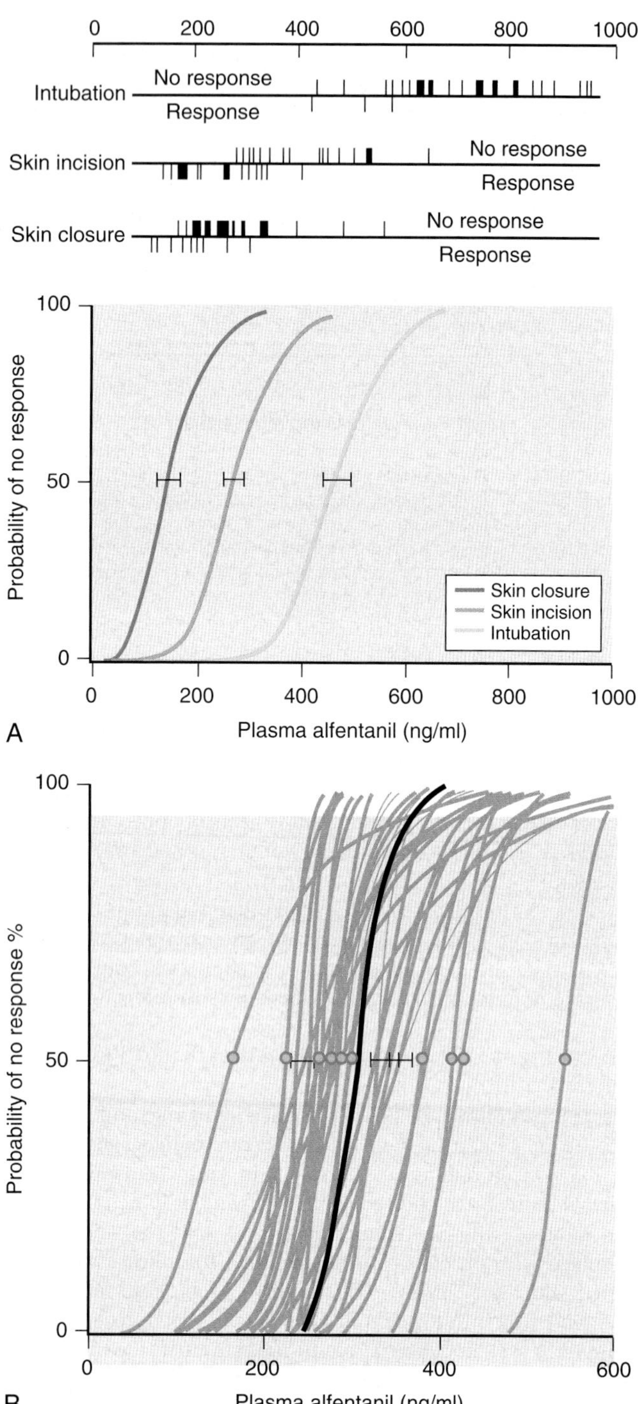

Figure 39-17 A, Relationship between the plasma concentration of alfentanil and response/no response at three specific events of short duration. The quantal data are characterized by logistic regression in the lower panel, ± standard error for Cp_{50}, which is the alfentanil plasma concentration associated with a 50% probability of no response. **B,** Plasma concentration of alfentanil versus the probability of no response for each of 34 patients during the intra-abdominal phase of lower abdominal surgery. *Circles* represent the Cp_{50} values, and the *black line* represents the average response of the 34 patients. *(**A,** From Ausems ME, Hug CC Jr, Stanski DR, Burm AG: Plasma concentrations of alfentanil required to supplement nitrous oxide anesthesia for general surgery. Anesthesiology 65:362-373, 1986; **B,** from Ausems ME, Vuyk J, Hug CC Jr, Stanski DR: Comparison of computer-assisted infusion versus intermittent bolus administration of alfentanil as a supplement to nitrous oxide for lower abdominal surgery. Anesthesiology 68:851-861, 1988.)*

bility of no response during surgery. Attenuating the response to intubation required significantly higher plasma concentrations of alfentanil than attenuating the response to skin incision did. Cp_{50} values for these clinical responses are shown in Table 39-6.

Remifentanil is the newest opioid in the fentanyl family and has a unique ester bond that is susceptible to hydrolysis by nonspecific blood and tissue esterases, which results in very rapid metabolism. Minto and colleagues[143,144] quantitated the population pharmacokinetics and dynamics of this opioid by using simulation techniques to develop dosing guidelines. Drover and Lemmens[145] applied the opioid anesthetic depth concepts developed by Ausems and coworkers[28] to define therapeutic plasma concentrations of remifentanil in surgical patients.

The approach to opioid administration presented by Ausems and colleagues[28] provides useful insight into the clinical assessment of depth of anesthesia. Overdosage with opioids cannot be judged intraoperatively in a paralyzed patient. Only at the end of anesthesia, when spontaneous ventilation should occur, does one know whether administration of opioids has been excessive. To prevent overdosage, Ausems and coworkers[28] proposed titrating the alfentanil infusion rate to clinical effect to find the lowest possible effective rate of opioid administration. Once the infusion rate associated with hemodynamic responsiveness (i.e., "light anesthesia") has been determined, one increases the rate slightly to provide an adequate analgesic component to achieve a nonresponsive state. Intermittent intravenous bolus administration of opioids is not as efficient as variable-rate infusion when titrating plasma concentrations of opioids to clinical effect.[142] The steep slope of the concentration-versus-response curve for alfentanil (Fig. 39-17B) demonstrates that a small increase in the plasma concentration of the drug rapidly converts an inadequate anesthetic state (100% probability of response to stimuli) to an adequate anesthetic state. Because of moderate variability in the pharmacokinetics of alfentanil, this process of titrating the infusion rate against clinical effect and pharmacodynamics is necessary for each patient. Egan and Shafer have referred to this concept as "surfing" the concentration-versus-response curve.[146] This concept is nearly ideal for remifentanil because of the rapid and

Table 39-6 Cp_{50} Values for Perioperative Events and Intraoperative Manipulation Associated with Three Types of Surgical Procedures During Alfentanil Anesthesia

Event	Cp_{50} (ng/mL)
Single events	
Intubation	475 ± 28*
Skin incision	279 ± 20
Skin closure	150 ± 23
Spontaneous ventilation	233 ± 13
Intraoperative manipulation	
Breast surgery (*n* = 12)	270 ± 63†
Lower abdominal (*n* = 14)	309 ± 44
Upper abdominal (*n* =11)	412 ± 135

*Standard error of the estimated value for the parameter.
†Values are presented as means ± SD.
Cp_{50}, plasma concentration of a drug producing a 50% chance of suppressing response to the given stimulus.
From Ausems ME, Vuyk J, Hug CC Jr, Stanski DR: Comparison of computer-assisted infusion versus intermittent bolus administration of alfentanil as a supplement to nitrous oxide for lower abdominal surgery. Anesthesiology 68:851-861, 1988.

predictable pharmacokinetic profile along with rapid blood-brain equilibration.[143]

Electrophysiologic Monitoring

(see also Chapter 46)

Spontaneous Electroencephalogram

The realization that anesthetic drugs alter the EEG dates back to the discovery that the brain produces electrical activity. In 1875, Caton used chloroform to convince himself that the electrical oscillations from the brain were indeed biologic in origin.[147] During the 1920s and 1930s, when electronic amplifiers allowed recording of these small voltages through the skull, Berger measured the influence of chloroform on the EEG.[148] In 1937, Gibbs and coauthors reported that anesthetics changed EEG activity from low-voltage fast waves to high-voltage slow waves and postulated that the EEG could be used to measure the effects of anesthesia.[149] In 1952, Faulconer demonstrated with ether that the depth of anesthesia, based on recognition of EEG patterns, correlated with the arterial concentration of ether.[150] He also demonstrated that the presence of nitrous oxide lowered the arterial concentration of ether necessary to produce a given effect on the EEG.

Hypnotic general anesthetics produce a biphasic EEG effect that was first described by Martin and colleagues.[151] With light anesthesia, there is EEG desynchronization and increased frequency associated with the excitement phase. This is followed by progressive synchronization, slowing, and an initial increased amplitude eventually leading to burst suppression with lengthening periods of EEG silence. With induction of anesthesia the topographic distribution also changes from occipital dominance to frontal dominance. Loss of spatial localization may occur with arousal.

The EEG can be considered a measure of the depth of anesthesia for several reasons:

1. It represents cortical electrical activity derived from summated excitatory and inhibitory postsynaptic activity, which in turn is the result of subcortical events, including those that pass through subcortical thalamic nuclei.
2. Cerebral blood flow and cerebral metabolism are related to the degree of EEG activity.[152]
3. Anesthetic drugs affect cerebral blood flow, metabolism, and EEG patterns.
4. Surgical stimulation affects cerebral blood flow, metabolism, and the EEG.

The EEG is thus a continuous, responsive, noninvasive indicator of cerebral function even when the patient is unconscious and unresponsive.

Noxious stimulation during inadequate anesthesia generally causes EEG activation. Peripheral noxious stimuli reach the brain through afferent systems that pass through the ascending reticular activating systems of the brainstem. These systems regulate cerebral function and thus affect the underlying EEG pattern. Noxious stimuli can cause three types of changes in the EEG:

1. Desynchronization with the appearance of 20- to 60-Hz fast rhythms (EEG activation)
2. The appearance of 6- to 10-Hz spindles
3. Bursts of 1- to 3-Hz slow waves[153]

These EEG patterns vary with individual anesthetics and with the nature of the stimulation, and there is a distinct drug plasma concentration that blocks responses to noxious stimulation.[154,155]

Early studies concluded that the EEG was not a meaningful measure of the depth of anesthesia. Galla and colleagues examined raw EEG signals for 43 patients and correlated EEG patterns with clinical signs of anesthesia.[156] A discrepancy seemed to exist between the clinical signs and EEG patterns, especially during induction and emergence. During induction, clinical signs indicated that the patients were more lightly anesthetized than the EEG patterns suggested, whereas on emergence, clinical signs indicated greater anesthetic depth.

Although recording of raw EEG signals involves accumulating a large amount of information and EEG tracings, current computer analysis techniques can summarize and distill the EEG into a condensed, descriptive format (the "processed" EEG).[157,158] Levy investigated processed EEG signals during induction and before cardiopulmonary bypass.[159] He examined a series of univariate descriptors, including median frequency (the frequency below which 50% of the EEG power is located) and spectral edge (the frequency below which 95% of the EEG power is located). He concluded that the multimodal EEG activity observed in 64% of cases precluded the use of single univariate parameters to describe the anesthetic state.

Clinical assessment of the depth of anesthesia did not correlate well with EEG patterns but suggested that some patterns may be useful trend monitors. Drummond and colleagues examined five numeric descriptors derived from the processed EEG during imminent arousal (spontaneous movement, coughing, or eye opening) from isoflurane/nitrous oxide anesthesia.[160] These authors determined the threshold value for each parameter that best predicted imminent arousal. Although several parameters (median frequency, spectral edge 90% frequency, total power, and frequency band ratio) predicted imminent arousal with a sensitivity of 90% and specificities of 82% to 90%, none of the EEG descriptors could serve as a completely reliable, sole predictor of imminent arousal. Long and coworkers undertook a similar analysis using either isoflurane or fentanyl anesthesia.[161] For isoflurane anesthesia, these investigators found that awakening was always presaged by an abrupt overall decrease in power in the 1- to 4-Hz frequency range (decrease in delta power). During emergence from fentanyl/nitrous oxide anesthesia, obvious change in the overall EEG power spectrum was not noted; however, the same numeric EEG descriptors that were predictive of awakening from isoflurane also occurred during emergence from fentanyl. These two studies concluded that consistent trends in the EEG can be expected to occur with changing depth of anesthesia, with the available EEG descriptors providing potentially useful trend information regarding the changing depth of anesthesia. However, the sensitivity and specificity of the available parameters are such that no one parameter can serve as the sole indicator of anesthetic depth.

Dwyer and colleagues examined the power spectrum of the EEG in surgical patients receiving 0.6 to 1.4 MAC isoflurane-only anesthesia with skin incision.[162] A second group of volunteers received 0.15 to 0.45 MAC isoflurane with memory testing. Different time-dependent EEG frequency parameters (e.g., spectral edge, median frequency) were examined relative to the clinical measures. The authors found that isoflurane caused some decrease in EEG activity. However, no difference in EEG parameters was found between subjects who moved and those who did not move with skin incision. In volunteers receiving low-dose isoflurane, memory of the information presented did not correlate with values of any EEG parameter. The authors concluded that the EEG parameters examined did not predict depth of anesthesia as defined by response to surgical skin incision, response to verbal command, or development of memory.

The previously described clinical research attempting to relate EEG effects to clinical anesthetic depth resulted in inconclusive findings. When single anesthetic drugs are examined under defined conditions, it has been possible to demonstrate unambiguous relationships between EEG parameters and anesthetic drug concentrations and to use pharmacokinetic and pharmacodynamic modeling concepts to link drug concentrations to EEG drug effects.[163] Application of the EEG to measure clinical depth of anesthesia failed previously for several reasons:

1. A lack of understanding of the effects of interactions of several concurrently administered anesthetic drugs on the EEG
2. No standard approach to choosing an optimal EEG parameter
3. No clear definition of a "gold standard" for measurement and assessment of the clinical depth of anesthesia

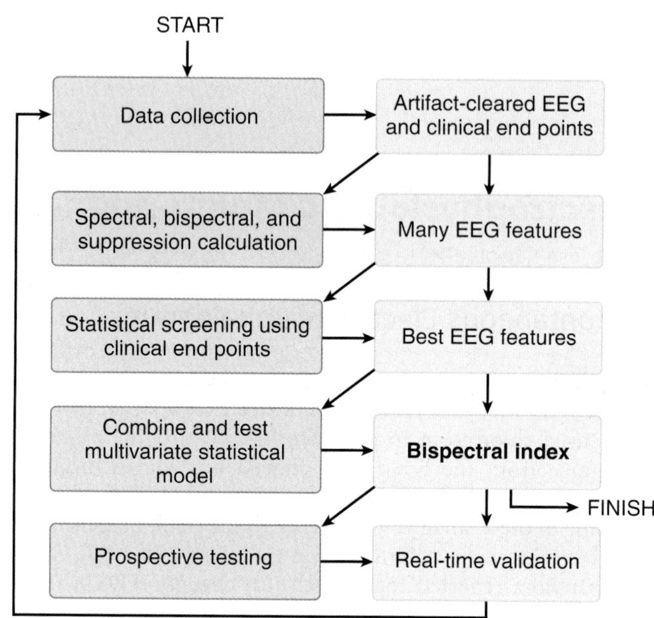

Figure 39-18 Key steps used during development of the bispectral index algorithm. Statistical modeling was used to identify the best features of the electroencephalogram (EEG) for recognition of clinical end points. The circular path notes that the process was iterative. *(From Kelley SD: Monitoring Level of Consciousness during Anesthesia and Sedation. Aspect Medical Systems, 2003.)*

Multiparameter Electroencephalographic Monitoring

In the 1990s, Aspect Medical Systems undertook an integrated research effort to develop the EEG as a measure of anesthetic depth. The Aspect EEG monitor, or the BIS, quantitates anesthetic effects on the brain, specifically, the hypnotic component of anesthesia. Other devices have followed this example but have used somewhat different approaches to EEG analysis (see later). Manufacturers differ in their willingness to disclose all the details of the algorithms, but they typically follow principles similar to those used by Aspect. In terms of clinical evaluation, the volume of literature on the BIS far exceeds that of any other device.

The common principles are shown in Figure 39-18:

1. The devices present a continuous EEG parameter, the specific index, that ranges from an awake, no-drug-effect value of 95 to 100 to 0 with no detectable EEG activity.
2. Multiple EEG signal–processing approaches that capture incremental information not captured with traditional approaches based on a single signal-processing approach, such as fast Fourier transformation, are used simultaneously.
3. Multiple clinically relevant measures (movement, hemodynamics, lash reflex, response to verbal command, recall, and drug concentration) were gathered in volunteers and patients with concurrent EEG data as part of the validation process.
4. Advanced multivariate statistical data analysis was used to correlate the components of the multiple EEG signal–processing approaches with the clinical data to create the univariate parameter.
5. Prospective clinical evaluation of the index is performed at multiple institutions under varying anesthetic and surgical conditions.
6. The indices measure the hypnotic components of the anesthetic and are relatively insensitive to the analgesic (e.g., opioid) components of an anesthetic.
7. Prospective clinical trials demonstrate that the monitors can improve the outcome of an anesthetic regimen.
8. Simple hardware and sensors were developed and are commercially available to facilitate capture of high-quality signals despite the noisy electrical environment of the operating room.

Electroencephalographic Signal Processing

Most EEG signal processing has previously involved a form of spectral analysis that examines the EEG signal during a small slice of time (epoch) as a function of frequency. The frequency analysis decomposes the EEG signal into a series of sine waves by Fourier analysis. Because the signal is digitally sampled, Fourier analysis is performed by a mathematical transformation called the discrete Fourier transformation. The discrete Fourier transformation calculates the phase and amplitude of discrete sine waves at frequencies ranging from 0 to half the sampling frequency in increments of 1/x (x is the number of seconds in each "epoch" or segment of the EEG signal). The frequency of each sine wave is the number of cycles per second, although the mathematics of the discrete Fourier transformation necessarily calculate only uniformly spaced frequencies. The amplitude is half the peak-to-peak voltage. The phase angle describes the time offset of the sine wave relative to the start of the epoch.

The conventional output of the discrete Fourier analysis is a spectral histogram showing the frequency and amplitudes of the sine waves in the underlying EEG signal. The phase information is typically ignored. Fourier analysis assumes that the signal pattern is constant during the epoch. Thus, it poorly handles signals that abruptly change during an epoch, such as burst suppression.

In "bispectral" analysis, the phase information is not ignored, and a more complex algorithm incorporates the phase information to look for evidence of phase coupling among frequency bands, such as bicoherence. Bispectral analysis was originally developed by the statistician John Tukey[164] and found one of its first applications in submarine warfare.[165] The anatomic, electrophysiologic, and clinical meaning of EEG phase relationships is unknown. However, the general notion is that an awake brain has multiple signal generators working independently and hence displays little synchronization. With progressive drug-induced loss of consciousness, fewer independent signal generators are active, and thus the resulting EEG is more likely to reflect coupling between signal generators. In addition, several useful techniques that promote noise suppression beyond what is possible with conventional spectral analysis are used.[166] Thus, the analyses provide additional information about the EEG signal than is captured by traditional spectral analysis approaches in which only frequency and amplitude are considered.

The Bispectral Index

Bispectral EEG signal processing has been reviewed by Rampil[166] and by Sigl and Chamoun.[167] Johansen and Sebel reviewed the clinical development of BIS monitoring.[168] Its development and validation are described here in some detail because it has the largest literature describing its development and it serves to illustrate the path that other devices would have to follow.

The BIS is a complex, proprietary EEG parameter developed by Aspect Medical Systems. In 1996, the U.S. Food and Drug Administration approved the commercially available version as a monitor of anesthetic effect on the brain. Figure 39-18 displays the conceptual process whereby Aspect took EEG and clinical data from approximately 1500 subjects and 5000 hours of EEG signal gathered under a broad range of anesthetic regimens. The EEG was processed by first removing high- and low-frequency artifacts, electrocardiographic signals, pacemaker spikes, eye blinks, wandering baseline, and interference by alternating current. The EEG data were then analyzed by three different approaches: Fourier spectral analysis, bispectral analysis, and time domain analysis (Fig. 39-19). Time domain analysis was used to characterize burst suppression (seen at a BIS value of less than 40) and isoelectricity. The EEG was smoothed across the power spectrum and bispectrum by using a moving average. The analysis then examined the degree of beta or high frequency (14 to 30 Hz), the amount of low-frequency synchronization, and the

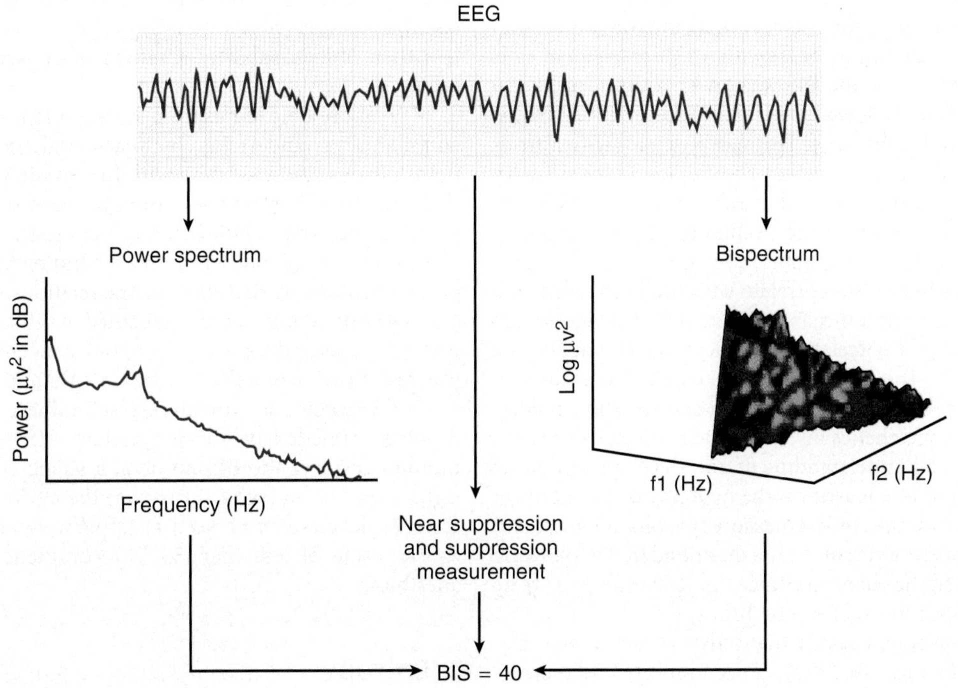

Figure 39-19 Schematic diagram of signal processing paths integral to generating a single bispectral index (BIS) value. After digitization and artifact rejection, original electroencephalographic (EEG) epochs undergo three primary paths of analysis: power spectral analysis, bispectral analysis, and time-based analysis for suppression/near suppression to look for key EEG features. The BIS algorithm, based on statistical modeling, combines the contributions of each of the identified features to generate the scaled BIS. *(From Kelley SD: Monitoring Level of Consciousness during Anesthesia and Sedation. Aspect Medical Systems, 2003.)*

presence of fully or nearly suppressed periods (i.e., isoelectric signal). The algorithm to determine the relative weighting in the final calculation of the BIS value (0 to 100) involved performing a multivariate statistical analysis, similar to semilinear canonic correlation, on the aforementioned EEG data relative to a clinical database that was gathered from multiple different clinical studies over the past 15 years.[169] As prototype versions of the BIS were developed over a period of several years, subsequent clinical testing was used to improve and refine the algorithms and components of the EEG parameter. The BIS algorithm was adapted to handle burst suppression EEG, to minimize the initial activation of the EEG seen with some anesthetic drugs, and to optimally use the components of Fourier analysis and bispectrum analysis. Thus, the BIS is a complex parameter composed of a combination of time domain, frequency domain, and higher-order spectral components derived from clinical data that measure the hypnotic component of an anesthetic.[166] Over the past decade, the BIS parameter has been modified on the basis of new data about the EEG response to novel anesthetic drugs and drug combinations, as well as to incorporate new signal collection and noise rejection technology. This is important to bear in mind as one reviews studies performed years apart.

The initial studies with early versions of the BIS algorithm in the early 1990s attempted to correlate the BIS to predict movement in response to skin incision with the use of isoflurane/oxygen,[167] propofol/nitrous oxide,[170] or propofol/alfentanil anesthesia.[171] In the first major clinical evaluation of the BIS technology, a large, multicenter study by Sebel and colleagues randomized 300 patients into two groups.[172] Both groups received an anesthetic regimen designed so that approximately half of all patients would move at skin incision. In the control group, the BIS was passively recorded and not used for titration. In the BIS-titrated group, drug concentrations were increased to produce a BIS value of less than 60. In the control group, the BIS was a mean of 66 ± 19 (standard deviation [SD]) with a 43% movement rate. In the BIS-adjusted group, the BIS was lower, a mean of 51 ± 9 (SD) with a significantly lower movement rate of 13%. In this multicenter trial, some centers used primarily opioids with nitrous oxide, whereas others used propofol or isoflurane as the primary anesthetic. The study also found that reliability of the BIS was strongly influenced by anesthetic technique. When hypnotic drugs such as propofol or isoflurane are used as the primary anesthetic, changes in the BIS correlate with the probability of a movement response to skin incision. When opioid analgesics are used at higher doses, the correlation to patient movement became much less significant. This information, when linked to the understanding that purposeful movement upon skin incision reflects the spinal action of anesthetics instead of their cortical effects,[22,23] provided fundamental understanding of how development of the BIS algorithm had to be focused on the hypnotic components of anesthesia, specifically, the clinical measures of consciousness and memory. A subsequent series of studies described in the following paragraphs provided the data and clinical understanding to create the current algorithm to calculate the BIS.

Glass and coworkers designed a study to examine the relationship among BIS, measured drug concentrations, and increasing levels of sedation when the anesthetic drugs propofol, midazolam, isoflurane, and alfentanil were given to volunteers in a controlled manner.[173] Data from this study were used to further optimize the BIS algorithm. Seventy-two volunteers received a single drug at four or five defined, increasing target plasma concentrations that ultimately created an unconscious subject. The BIS, arterial drug or end-tidal concentrations, and subjective sedation and memory scores were measured. The BIS was significantly correlated to measured drug concentrations, as well as clinical measures of sedation. None of the alfentanil patients lost consciousness and had minimal change in the BIS, a finding confirming that the BIS is not sensitive to low concentrations of opioid analgesics. Fifty percent and 95% of the volunteers were unconscious at BIS values of 67 and 50, respectively.

Liu and colleagues demonstrated in 26 surgical subjects that the BIS accurately tracked the degree of clinical sedation with intermediate (4 mg) to large (20 mg) doses of midazolam given during regional anesthesia.[174] Response to a loud voice corresponded to a BIS of 87 ± 6 (SD) and a 40% probability of recall. A deeper end point, lack of response to mild prodding, corresponded to a BIS value of 81 ± 8 (SD) and resulted in complete lack of recall. When midazolam created an unresponsive subject, the mean BIS value was 69.2 ± 13.9 (SD). Similar results were found by these investigators for propofol when given under regional anesthesia[175] and were reported by Katoh and coworkers with low, sedating doses of sevoflurane and also with higher, anesthetic concentrations in 69 surgical patients.[176] Both the BIS and end-tidal sevoflurane concentrations were correlated to clinical sedation scores of the patients. The BIS decreased almost linearly from a median value of 95 to 45 with an end-tidal sevoflurane concentration increasing from 0.2% to 1.4%. Sevoflurane concentrations greater than 1.4% produced a limited further reduction in the BIS.

Flaishon and colleagues examined the behavior of the BIS when surgical patients were given a single intravenous bolus of propofol, 2 mg/kg, or thiopental, 4 mg/kg, with concurrent muscle relaxants.[177] The isolated arm technique was used to identify loss and then return of consciousness. No patient with a BIS value of less than 58 was conscious; a BIS value of less than 65 signified a less than 5% probability of return of consciousness within 50 seconds.

A more detailed examination of memory and response to command was undertaken by Kearse and associates during propofol/nitrous oxide sedation with BIS monitoring.[178] These investigators found a strong association between the BIS and response to command, whether the command consisted simply of a uniform voice asking a volunteer to move a hand or foot or incorporated graded and then varied stimuli. The relationship between the BIS and responsiveness scores remained consistent over time and with increases or decreases in propofol concentrations. No subject was responsive when the BIS was less than 57.

Clinically, a unilateral self-adhesive frontotemporal montage provided by the proprietary BIS sensor is used. The monitor displays the BIS number, a single channel of raw EEG signals, and an index of activity on the electromyogram (EMG). Current devices can be seen at http://www.aspectmedical.com/. A BIS value of less than 55 is recommended during general anesthesia.

Entropy

Because the EEG displays chaotic or nonlinear behavior, it seems reasonable to apply methods from the theories of nonlinear dynamics. Entropy is used in chemistry to describe the microstates of gases and liquids and the ability of atoms to move in multiple directions (i.e., the amount of disorder). As a substance changes from a solid to a liquid to a gas, the mobility and potential for interaction among atoms increases and entropy also increases. The converse applies in going from a gas to a solid.

In 1948, Claude Shannon applied these concepts to information theory such that entropy described the complexity, irregularity, or unpredictability of a signal.[179] A pure sinusoidal wave would have an entropy of zero because it is regular and predictable, whereas a wave containing hugely variable frequencies (e.g., noise) would have very high entropy. Unfortunately, as originally described by Shannon, entropy is not normalized to the total power, so there is great interindividual variation. This limits clinical use because one wants the same index value to indicate a similar depth of anesthesia among patients.

There are multiple entropy algorithms, but only spectral entropy has been used in a commercially available device, the GE Healthcare Entropy Module (formerly Datex-Ohmeda M-Entropy), which was commercially released in 2003. The exact algorithm was published in 2004 and is in the public domain.[180,181] The algorithm uses the time domain (i.e., burst suppression) and frequency domain from Fourier analysis and then also applies the Shannon function to the frequency data. This approach has been termed "time-frequency balanced spectral entropy."

The facial EMG has a frequency range (approximately >20 Hz) that overlaps with the "traditional" EEG (0.8 to 32 Hz), thereby confounding analysis of cortical activity. The facial EMG changes with level of consciousness and the use of neuromuscular blocking drugs. EMG analysis was briefly and unsuccessfully tried as a depth-of-anesthesia monitor.[182,183] Some authorities have the impression that the EMG may be more related to analgesia requirements. Datex-Ohmeda tried to exploit this by creating two indices, State Entropy (SE) and Response Entropy (RE). SE is computed from the EEG in the 0.8- to 32-Hz range and should encompass mainly the hypnotic elements of the EEG, whereas RE is computed from 0.8 to 47 Hz, which includes a significant amount of the facial EMG.[180] Thus when EMG activity is low, SE and RE should be the same, but with arousal and an increase in facial EMG, RE should increase. The initial clinical studies with this device showed that it produced results comparable to those of the BIS when tested with intravenous and inhaled hypnotic anesthetics.[184-186]

The GE Entropy Module uses the same unilateral self-adhesive frontotemporal sensor as the BIS but specifically made for the GE product (i.e., they are not interchangeable). The module works only with GE monitoring systems with the appropriate software loaded. The SE, RE, and a single channel of the raw EEG are displayed on the same screen as the other monitored variables. The displayed SE range is 0 (isoelectric EEG) to 91 (fully awake), and the RE range is 0 to 100. The anesthetic range is 40 to 60, and the manufacturer recommends that SE outside this range may require a change in hypnotic dosing, whereas if the SE is in this range but the RE is more than 10 above the SE, more analgesic may be required. Good substantiation of this recommendation is lacking.

Patient State Index

The Patient State Index (PSI) from Physiometrix, Inc., also incorporates a proprietary algorithm. In addition to using time, frequency, and phase information, the PSI also uses spatial information as EEG dominance changes with induction of anesthesia from occipital to frontal and with arousal.[187,188] A self-adhesive five-lead bilateral frontotemporal montage is used that provides greater spatial analysis than can be achieved with a unilateral montage. Development of the algorithm involved extensive use of EEG databases[189] and is illustrated in Figure 39-20. Development of the PSI has recently been reviewed.[190] Figure 39-21 shows the complexity of analyses continuously performed in the process of updating the PSI. Similar complexity occurs with most such monitors. Initial studies show it to be comparable to the BIS in tracking sedation levels.[191,192]

The portable monitor displays the PSI, with 25 to 50 being the anesthetic range. The index is shown as the current number, as well as the trend, which is color-coded to indicate whether it is in the anesthetic range, too light, or too deep. In addition, there are qualitative indicators of the EMG, artifacts, and burst suppres-

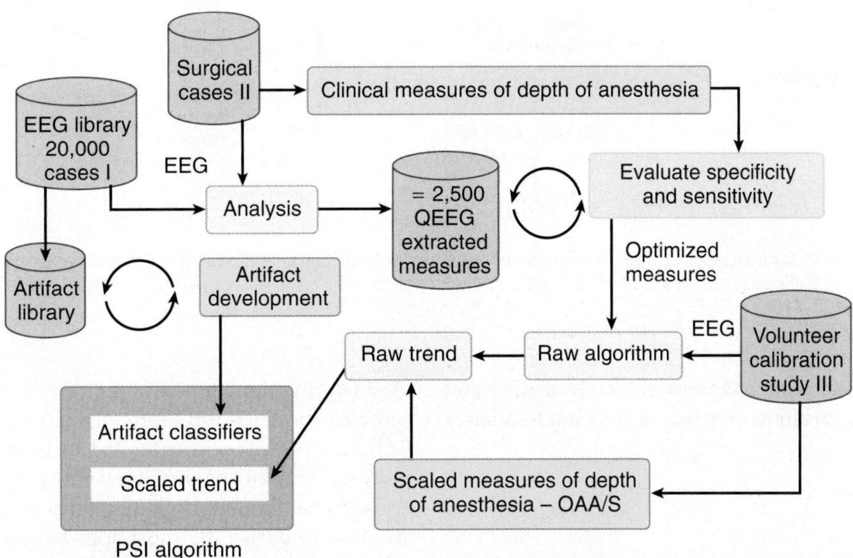

Figure 39-20 Algorithm used to develop the Patient State Index (PSI). EEG, electroencephalogram; OAA/S, Observer Assessment of Alertness/Sedation scale; QEEG, quantitative EEG. *(From Drover DR, Ortega R: Patient State Index. Best Pract Res Clin Anaesthesiol 20:121-128, 2006.)*

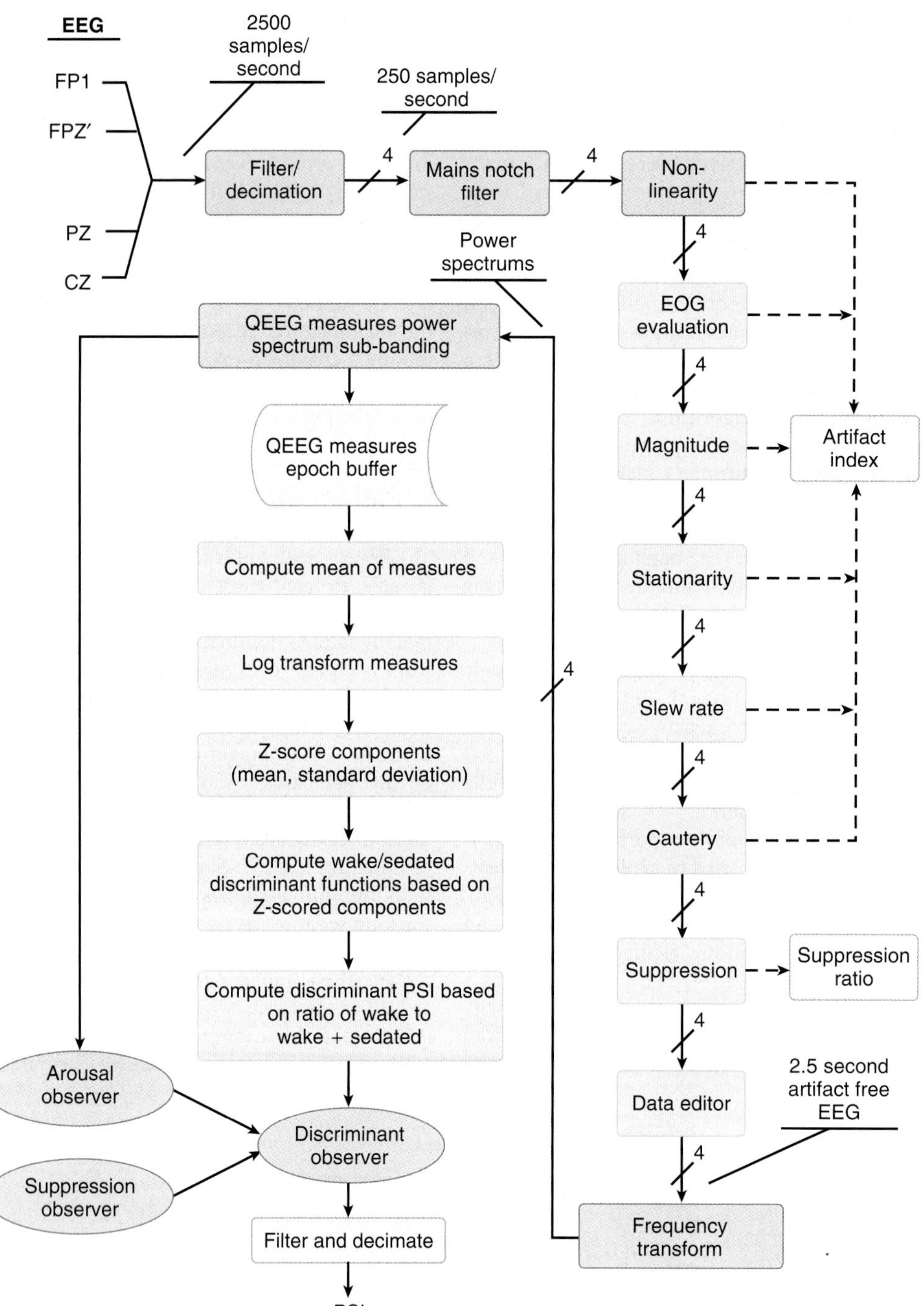

Figure 39-21 The Patient State Index (PSI) involves a series of steps that consider both the linear and nonlinear spectral components of the electroencephalogram (EEG). EOG, electro-oculogram; QEEG, quantitative electroencephalogram. *(From Drover DR, Ortega R: Patient State Index. Best Pract Res Clin Anaesthesiol 20:121-128, 2006.)*

sion. Other optional displays include four channels of EEG and the digital spectral array, an alternative way of showing frequency data.

Narcotrend

The Narcotrend monitor takes a somewhat different approach to EEG analysis by using a categorization system initially developed for analyzing the sleep EEG. In 1937, Loomis and coworkers categorized the sleep EEG into characteristic patterns labeled A to E.[193] This pattern was extended to include substages and made more appropriate for anesthesia with stages labeled A to F.[194] After artifact rejection, multiple time and frequency domain analyses are used to derive the most appropriate anesthetic stage. Initial validation also involved testing a large data set of EEGs during anesthesia. Early clinical studies found the Narcotrend to be similar to the BIS.[195-197]

This monitor uses standard electrocardiography electrodes rather than a proprietary electrode strip. The monitor displays a single channel of raw EEG, the Narcotrend stage indicated by a capital letter and a numerical subscript (e.g., D_2), the power spectrum, and the trend of the stages.

Other EEG-Based Devices

There is a steady increase in the number of devices emerging on the market. Although they differ in display format, size, electrodes, and other features, they are to a greater or lesser extent similar in principle to the devices described earlier. Examples include the SNAP Index (Viasys Healthcare, Madison, WI) and Cerebral State Monitor (Danmeter, Odense, Denmark).

Evoked Responses as Monitors of the Depth of Anesthesia

Sensory, including auditory, stimulation produces a low-amplitude signal, or evoked response, within the CNS. This evoked response can be separated by means of computer signal-averaging techniques from the underlying, spontaneous EEG. The ability to evoke a response is a measure of the functional integrity of the pathways between the sensory receptor and the neural generator of peaks in the evoked response waveform. Because evoked responses are sensitive to anesthetic drugs, they have been investigated as possible measures of anesthetic drug effect and depth of anesthesia.[198]

Recording of evoked responses involves recording EEG epochs synchronized to the repetitive sensory stimuli. Computer techniques extract the evoked potential from the underlying EEG. Typically, the algorithm requires 100 to 1000 stimuli to confidently extract the evoked potential from the underlying EEG signal. Therefore, the evoked response represents a time-versus-voltage relationship that can be quantitated by measuring the poststimulus latency and interpeak amplitudes in the waveform. Evoked response methodology has been reviewed in detail.[199]

Many investigations have been performed with evoked potentials, with special emphasis on midlatency auditory evoked potentials (MLAEPs).[198,200-203] MLAEPs have been shown to be significantly affected by anesthetic hypnotic drugs in a graded, reversible, and nonspecific manner. Specifically, the amplitudes (microvolts) and the latency (milliseconds) of the waves Pa and Nb have been examined. Hypnotic anesthetic drugs decrease the amplitudes and increase the latencies of these two waves. Opioids in clinically relevant concentrations produce minimal changes in MLAEPs.[204]

Measuring MLAEPs can be inconvenient, and this may have limited their clinical use to date. Limitations include the following:

1. Considerable time needed to produce a response, 0.5 to 5 minutes
2. Complex setup, with MLAEPs typically requiring more than 5 minutes of patient preparation
3. Need for intact hearing
4. Lack of a univariate parameter calibrated to the anesthetic state

Kenny and colleagues addressed some of these limitations by introducing a new MLAEP parameter, the AEP index, based on a proprietary algorithm.[205,206] The AEP index simplifies interpretation of the MLAEP waveforms, but it still requires significant time for the signal-averaging process. Jensen and coworkers developed a new adaptive method for extracting the MLAEP from the EEG signal that involves an autoregressive model with an exogenous input (ARX) to allow extraction of the AEP signal within 15 to 25 sweeps of 110-msec duration; the process results in only a 6-second delay.[207] This concept has been incorporated into a commercial device that calculates the A-Line ARX Index (AAI) from the fast-extracted MLAEP waveform analysis (A-Line Monitor, Danmeter A/S, Odense, Denmark). The AAI, like the BIS, ranges from 100 (awake) to 0 (deep hypnotic effect), and the recommended surgical anesthesia range is 15 to 25. The software has recently been updated and the current iteration, the AEP monitor/2, also uses EEG-derived data to supplement the AEP data.[208]

In clinical studies the A-Line performed comparably to the BIS and other EEG-based monitors but did not demonstrate advantages that would outweigh the nuisance of ear plugs and continuous high-frequency clicking sounds in patients' ears.[209-211]

Clinical Interpretation and Effects of Drugs on Electrophysiologic Monitors

All of the currently available devices have adopted a scale of 0 to 100, where 0 represents an isoelectric EEG and 100 represents an awake patient. The documentation for these monitors recommends specific ranges for wakefulness, sedation, light anesthesia, deep anesthesia, and excessive anesthesia. The clinical ranges are not identical across devices, so care is required when using or comparing different devices. For example, the BIS "anesthesia" range is 40 to 60, whereas the PSI "anesthesia" range is 25 to 50. Figure 39-22 displays the numerical value of the BIS from 0 to 100 relative to clinical end points and the underlying EEG signal.

After administration of a hypnotic drug, the index decreases from awake values of 80 to 100 as the patient's level of consciousness undergoes a series of transitions. At a device's threshold index of anesthesia, the probability of consciousness is low. The "anesthesia" range reflects adequate hypnotic effect for loss of consciousness with reasonably rapid recovery to consciousness. Like all electrophysiologic measures, in each patient one must correlate the clinical state to the reported value to adjust for variability between patients. Figure 39-23 displays the relationship between the BIS value and the probability of response to voice or the probability of explicit memory recall during propofol anesthesia.[212] Response to verbal command is preserved at lower BIS values than explicit recall is.

A limited number of studies examined the relationship of the BIS to direct measures of brain function. Alkire[213] studied the correlation between the cerebral metabolic rate, as measured by positron emission tomography, and the BIS during propofol and isoflurane anesthesia. Volunteers served as their own controls. After baseline measurements, volunteers received increasing amounts of propofol or isoflurane until they were unconscious (BIS values of 30 to 50). This study demonstrated a linear relation-

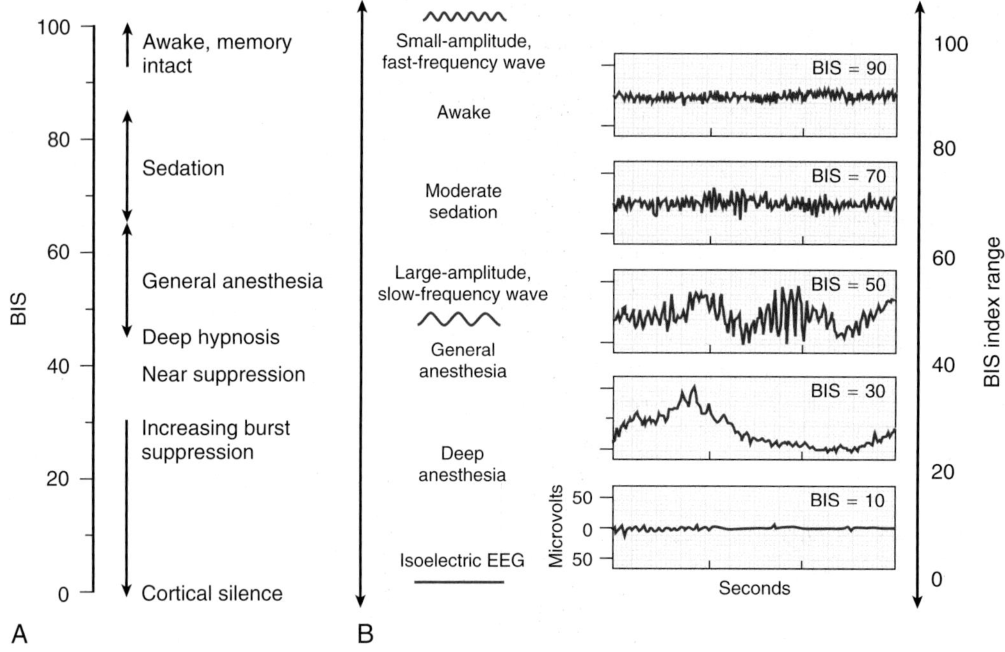

Figure 39-22 **A,** Clinical correlations of the bispectral index (BIS). Maintaining the BIS value of 45 to 60 during general anesthesia appears to ensure unconsciousness with a hypnotic/opioid anesthetic technique while providing for rapid emergence. **B,** Changes on the electroencephalogram (EEG) observed with increasing depth of anesthesia. *(**A,** Adapted from Johansen JW, Sebel PS: Development and clinical application of electroencephalographic bispectrum monitoring. Anesthesiology 93:1336-1344, 2000; **B,** from Kelley SD: Monitoring Level of Consciousness during Anesthesia and Sedation. Aspect Medical Systems, 2003.)*

ship between decreasing BIS and a reduction in cerebral metabolic rate (r = −0.81), indicating a physiologic link between the EEG and the cerebral metabolic response to hypnotic drugs.

Ludbrook and colleagues examined the relationship between propofol brain concentrations, as estimated by simultaneous arterial/jugular bulb venous blood sampling during propofol induction of anesthesia, cerebral blood flow, and BIS measurements.[214] Although significant intersubject variability

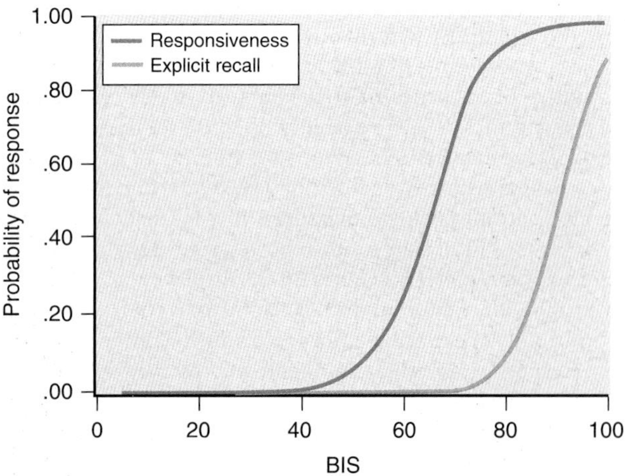

Figure 39-23 Reduction in verbal responsiveness to command (*blue line*) and memory (*yellow line*) with decreased bispectral index (BIS) values during propofol anesthesia. BIS values less than 60 are associated with 0 probability of awareness. *(Iselin-Chaves IA, Flaishon R, Sebel PS, et al: The effect of the interaction of propofol and alfentanil on recall, loss of consciousness, and the bispectral index. Anesth Analg 87:949-955, 1998.)*

was seen, calculated propofol brain concentrations and BIS values correlated closely. Similar results have been found by using the estimated propofol or sevoflurane effect-site concentration. There is high correlation in the prediction probability of BIS, entropy, and effect-site propofol concentration, but differences between the devices are not of clinical significance.[185,186]

Hypnotics

The relationship between depth-of-anesthesia indices and commonly used hypnotics such as midazolam, propofol, isoflurane, sevoflurane, and desflurane has been assessed in both patients and volunteers. The approach is to use stepwise increases in drug concentration and correlate this with a clinical sedation grading scale such as MOAA/S (see Table 39-1).[5] The MOAA/S scale requires stimulating the subject, which may change the depth-of-anesthesia index. Whether the index is recorded before or after stimulation is not always reported.

Studies of all currently available devices show a good relationship with the MOAA/S scale for commonly used hypnotics.[173-176,190,209,210,215-220] Indeed, such a relationship is a requirement for regulatory approval and integral for development of the software (see earlier). The relationship between sedation and the derived electrophysiologic index does not seem to be influenced by age in adults.[221] Although the average index tracks the sedation scale well at steady state, there is huge interindividual variation, particularly during non–steady-state conditions such as induction and emergence.[222] While awake, the index may range from 70 to 100, but once anesthetized, the index might be in the range of 25 to 65. Schnider and colleagues reported an extreme example in a patient with genetically determined low-voltage EEG.[223] This otherwise unremarkable volunteer had a baseline BIS of 40, which paradoxically increased with the administration of xenon. Thus, intersubject variability in the EEG requires assessment of awake values before titration of hypnotic to a given target EEG index.

Opioids

Early studies demonstrated that low concentrations of opioids did not change the BIS response during propofol or inhaled anesthesia.[172,173] Iselin-Chaves and coworkers performed a volunteer study that examined sedation score and the presence/absence of recall during stepped increases in propofol and propofol with alfentanil (50 or 100 ng/mL).[212] The BIS, sedation, and memory function were highly correlated, and the BIS value was not affected by the low alfentanil concentration.

A similar limited interaction has also been found with remifentanil[224] and sufentanil.[225] In contrast, Koitabashi and associates found that the addition of increasing doses of remifentanil reduced BIS for the same propofol dose.[226] Struys and colleagues examined the propofol estimated effect-compartment concentration needed to prevent response to verbal stimulation, eye lash reflex, and tetanic stimulation in patient volunteers given one of three remifentanil target concentrations: 0, 2, or 4 ng/mL.[215] BIS and the AAI were monitored as well. The indices decreased monotonically as propofol was increased. For both indices, the value at loss of response was higher with each successive dose of remifentanil; specifically, with remifentanil the volunteers were "asleep" with less propofol and at higher BIS or AAI. This relates to the definition of anesthetic depth at the beginning of the chapter. Struys and colleagues required a stimulus to assess anesthetic depth, and interpretation of the index from the processed EEG requires consideration of the opioid and hypnotic component together.

Ferenets and coworkers used a similar paradigm to study entropy and complexity measures, including spectral entropy, approximate entropy, Higuchi fractal dimension, Lempel-Ziv complexity, relative [beta] ratio, and the SyncFastSlow measure.[227] They found that the effect of remifentanil was critically dependent on the frequency range used for the calculations, which may further explain the conflicting literature on opioids and depth-of-anesthesia devices.

Bouillon and colleagues used response surface modeling to assess the likelihood of response, BIS, and approximate entropy.[12] Figure 39-24 shows the synergy between propofol and remifentanil on the probability of response to laryngoscopy (A) and the additive effects of propofol and remifentanil effect on the BIS (B). Most critically, the trajectory lines on figure B show the trajectory of equipotent combinations of propofol and remifentanil for probabilities of no response to laryngoscopy ranging from 5% to 95%. Because the interaction on the BIS has a different shape from the interaction on the probability of nonresponse to noxious stimulation, the "right" BIS value for any desired probability of nonresponse is a function of the relative amounts of propofol and remifentanil. If the drugs are used at the point of maximum interaction, the "right" BIS value associated with nonresponse will be higher than if the drugs are not well balanced and synergy is reduced.

Most commercially available monitors have been calibrated for the combination of opioids and hypnotics, as suggested by Figure 39-24. The commercially available indices are therefore most accurate when used with anesthesia consisting of a low or moderate dose of opioid and a hypnotic drug (volatile inhaled anesthetic, intravenous anesthetic) titrated to the average anesthetic range of the monitored index. When using high doses of opioids it is important to provide an adequate dose of hypnotic to guarantee lack of awareness.[228]

Nitrous Oxide

Most studies suggest that nitrous oxide given in concentrations of up to 70% has minimal effect on the BIS. Rampil and coworkers demonstrated in volunteers that nitrous oxide concentrations of up to 50% alter the spectral content of the EEG with surprisingly little change in the BIS.[229] However the subjects did not exhibit CNS depression at these concentrations. In a different study, 70% nitrous oxide produced unconsciousness but still did not alter the BIS.[230] The addition of nitrous oxide to a hypnotic, even up to 70%, may reduce the BIS, have no effect, or increase it.[231-233] The effect of nitrous oxide appears to be dependent on the monitor used. Soto and colleagues found that neither BIS nor PSI demon-

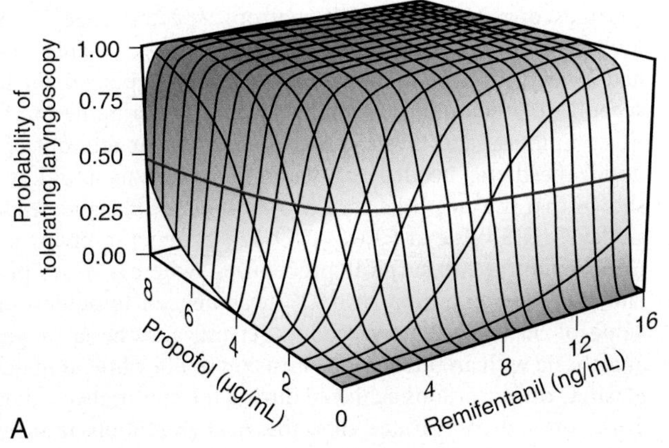

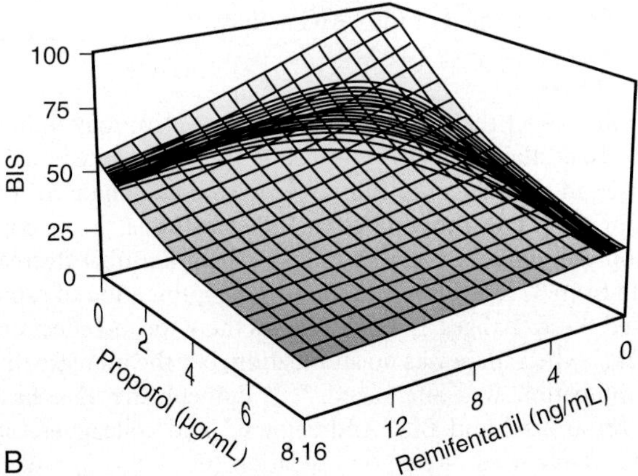

Figure 39-24 A, Interaction between propofol and remifentanil for a decreased probability of response to laryngoscopy based on the model shown in Figure 39-3. **B,** Interaction between propofol and remifentanil for their effects on the bispectral index (BIS); additivity is demonstrated. The trajectory lines show the BIS values at equipotent combinations of propofol and remifentanil for 5% to 95% probabilities of no response to laryngoscopy based on **A.** *(From Bouillon TW, Bruhn J, Radulescu L, et al: Pharmacodynamic interaction between propofol and remifentanil regarding hypnosis, tolerance of laryngoscopy, bispectral index, and electroencephalographic approximate entropy. Anesthesiology 100:1353-1372, 2004.)*

strated a change in index but SE did when nitrous oxide was added or removed.[234]

Ketamine

The dissociative anesthetic ketamine produces excitatory effects on the EEG. Ketamine doses that create unresponsiveness (0.25 to 0.5 mg/kg) did not change the BIS.[235]

When ketamine is used with propofol, an additive anesthetic interaction occurs[24] that is not reflected in the BIS,[236] and the response to ketamine may differ by device used.[237] Thus, the addition of ketamine to an anesthetic complicates interpretation of the processed EEG, again emphasizing the need to consider the clinical circumstance and drugs used when interpreting a "depth-of-anesthesia" index.

Interaction with Muscle Relaxants

The algorithms used in the currently available devices all, to a greater or lesser extent, include some EMG activity inasmuch as EMG and EEG frequencies overlap at values greater than 30 Hz. Indeed, the GE Entropy device deliberately includes EMG in the belief that it may be an index of need for analgesia (see earlier). Muscle relaxants may confound the accuracy of devices in relation to the depth of anesthesia (also see Chapter 29). Ekman and coworkers[238] recently found that BIS and AAI responses to noxious stimulation were affected by the degree of neuromuscular block and that the block did not affect the indices in the absence of noxious stimulation.

Fluctuating muscle tension and tonic input from muscle spindles contribute to CNS arousal. As a result, muscle relaxants may deepen anesthesia by reducing neural traffic.[239] Multiple studies have demonstrated an effect of muscle relaxants in appearing to deepen anesthesia.[240-242] The most bizarre was the study by Messner and associates, in which awake volunteers (the investigators themselves) received succinylcholine with no hypnotic (!) and the BIS decreased to as low as 33.[243] Reversal of muscle relaxation can also change the amount of EMG activity and influence the monitor.[244]

Not all studies have demonstrated an effect of muscle relaxants.[245] The differences among studies probably reflect the algorithm being used,[246] which may change among iterations of the same device. Additionally, deep anesthesia at baseline may already have eliminated much of the EMG activity.[247]

Other Drugs

Drugs that affect the sympathetic nervous system may influence depth-of-anesthesia devices. Infusion of a β-blocker such as esmolol can also alter the BIS in some studies. Johansen found that during stable propofol/alfentanil anesthesia, a 30-minute infusion of esmolol (1-mg/kg bolus, 250 μg/kg/min) decreased the BIS from 37 ± 6 (SD) to 22 ± 6.[248] Discontinuation of esmolol reversed these changes. In other studies there was no effect of the β-blocker when there was no stimulation, but the increase in BIS with intubation was attenuated.[249,250] Epinephrine also has an effect on arousal and BIS. Andrzejowski and colleagues established a stable level of propofol sedation (OAA/S = 2) and then gave a bolus of 15 μg of epinephrine.[251] The sedation level increased (OAA/S = 4) and the BIS rose on average by 13. These studies indicate that there is a complex interaction among β-receptors, level of arousal, and BIS during anesthesia. β-Adrenoreceptor blockade can alter the EEG arousal response to noxious stimuli even when inadequate analgesia is present and can decrease the BIS during adequate clinical anesthesia. The effect of dexmedetomidine on depth-of-anesthesia monitors has not yet been well studied. Initial studies indicate that the BIS performs appropriately, whereas auditory responses do not change substantially.[252,253]

Response to Noxious Stimulation

Guignard and associates examined the response of the BIS to laryngoscopy and tracheal intubation during propofol administration with and without remifentanil.[254] Hemodynamics, movement response, and BIS were measured. With propofol at a target effect-site concentration of 4 μg/mL, the BIS decreased to a mean of approximately 45. Intubation increased the BIS to a mean of 70. When computer-controlled infusion of remifentanil was added to achieve target effect-site concentrations of 2 to 16 ng/mL, the interaction of remifentanil on BIS values was obvious. Before intubation, these remifentanil concentrations did not change the BIS values during propofol hypnosis. Progressively increasing concentrations of remifentanil blunted the increase in BIS after intubation. Remifentanil target effect-site concentrations of 8 and 16 ng/mL resulted in a minimal increase in the BIS, hemodynamic stability, and no purposeful movement. This study demonstrated that significant noxious stimuli given with only a hypnotic present (e.g., propofol, inhaled anesthetics) will result in a significant hemodynamic response with an increase in BIS values. The addition of adequate opioid analgesia results in hemodynamic control and less or no change in the BIS value. Ropcke and colleagues demonstrated similar EEG activation and an increase in BIS values when desflurane only (no opioids) was given to surgical patients during intra-abdominal surgery.[255] They demonstrated that in unstimulated patients before the initiation of surgery, a desflurane end-tidal concentration of 2.2% was needed to achieve a mean BIS value of 50. The desflurane end-tidal concentration needed to achieve a BIS value of 50 increased to 6.8% during intra-abdominal noxious surgical stimulation. The authors did not examine whether opioid analgesia would change the response observed with desflurane. A study in volunteers subjected to different combinations of propofol and remifentanil and progressively increasing stimulation (shouting, shaking, laryngoscopy) found that BIS, entropy, spectral edge 95, measured drug concentrations, and predicted drug concentrations all had a very good prediction probability for hypnosis but barely acceptable prediction probability for airway manipulation.[216]

Epidural anesthesia can also decrease the amount of hypnotic anesthetic needed for sedation. Hodgson and Liu have shown that the end-tidal concentration of sevoflurane needed to achieve a BIS value of 50 was 0.59% in patients receiving a lidocaine epidural for surgical procedures, whereas a sevoflurane end-tidal concentration of 0.92% was needed to achieve a BIS value of 50 in patients receiving general anesthesia or general anesthesia with an intravenous infusion of lidocaine to match the plasma concentrations achieved during the epidural anesthetic.[256] This study demonstrates that the deafferentation induced by regional anesthesia results in supraspinal effects that change hypnotic anesthetic requirements.

Studies such as these show that EEG activation is dependent on the amount of neural traffic. Processed EEG indices are good indicators of hypnosis at a given amount of stimulation but may not accurately predict the changes that will occur when stimulation changes. The behavioral, hemodynamic, and EEG response to painful stimuli can be prevented by adequate analgesia.

Clinical Utility of Depth-of-Anesthesia Devices

Drug Titration

Depth-of-anesthesia devices primarily measure the effects of hypnotics on the EEG. The synergistic interaction of opioids on clinical end points (hemodynamics, movement responses) is more profound than reflected by the EEG. As a result, these devices are most accurate when used with anesthesia consisting of a low or moderate dose of opioid analgesic and a hypnotic drug (volatile inhaled anesthetic, intravenous anesthetic).

Clinical use involves separating the hypnotic and analgesic components of an anesthetic regimen. The concept entails titration of the hypnotic component to the anesthetic range that is associated with a high probability of unconsciousness. A small to moderate amount of analgesic (opioid) decreases the noxious input to the CNS, thus providing hemodynamic stability and decreasing the probability of response.

The anesthesiologist must continuously evaluate the clinical and monitored responses to the surgical stimulation. During intense surgical stimulation, if the index increases or the patient exhibits movement and hemodynamic responses (or both), the anesthesiologist should respond by increasing the hypnotic component to lower the index if it is elevated. Incremental opioid should be given to increase the analgesic component until movement and hemodynamics are controlled. As the end of the anesthetic regimen approaches, the hypnotic component should be decreased to allow the index to increase. These devices therefore add another monitored parameter but in no way relieve the anesthesiologist of the need to use clinical judgment and to be vigilant at all times to ensure that patients are adequately anesthetized.

Drug Consumption, Costs, and Recovery

Several studies have examined the clinical and economic outcome benefits of BIS monitoring in routine surgery. Gan and colleagues[257] studied 302 subjects receiving a propofol/alfentanil/nitrous oxide anesthetic regimen in four different institutions. Half the subjects were randomized to "standard practice" whereby the propofol and alfentanil were titrated to provide stable anesthesia with the fastest possible recovery. The BIS was recorded in this group but not displayed to the practitioner. The remaining subjects received "standard practice plus BIS monitoring." In this group, propofol infusions were titrated to achieve a target BIS value between 45 and 60 during surgery and 60 to 75 during the final 15 minutes of anesthesia. Patients in the BIS group required significantly lower normalized propofol infusion rates (134 versus 116 μg/kg/min), were extubated significantly sooner (11.2 versus 7.3 minutes), had a higher percentage of patients oriented on arrival in the recovery room (43% versus 23%), and had more rapid discharge from the recovery room. This study demonstrated that titrating propofol with BIS monitoring during balanced anesthesia decreased propofol use and significantly improved recovery with no difference in intraoperative conditions.

Song and colleagues[258] presented similar findings with inhaled anesthetics. Sixty surgical patients were randomized to receive desflurane or sevoflurane with 65% nitrous oxide and low doses of fentanyl. Half the patients were randomized to standard practice in which the inhaled anesthetic was titrated according to clinical end points and judgment. The second group had the volatile anesthetic titrated to a BIS value of 60. During the maintenance period, BIS values were significantly lower in the standard-treatment group (mean of 42), a finding suggesting deeper anesthesia than in the BIS-titrated group with a mean of 60. Volatile anesthetic use in the BIS-titrated group was 30% to 38% lower than in the control group. Similarly, times to verbal responsiveness were 30% to 55% shorter in the BIS-titrated group. This study demonstrated that titrating desflurane and sevoflurane with the use of BIS monitoring decreased utilization of the drugs and contributed to faster emergence from anesthesia.

A meta-analysis of 11 trials involving 1380 patients found that BIS monitoring reduced drug consumption by 19%, nausea and vomiting by 6%, and recovery room time by 4 minutes.[259] The cost saving from drugs was offset by the cost of the monitoring electrodes, so the actual cost was 5.55 U.S. dollars higher in the monitored group. A recent review for the Cochrane Database of 20 studies with 4056 patients found that BIS monitoring reduced drug consumption and shortened recovery times by 2 to 8 minutes.[260] Similar results have been found with other devices.[261,262] Although it seems the devices can save on drug costs and time in the early recovery period, the overall benefit from a cost and time perspective is probably modest.

Outcome

The relationship of anesthetic management to patient morbidity and mortality has generally focused on the immediate perioperative period. Information on the effects of anesthetic management on long-term postoperative mortality rates is limited. Monk and coworkers monitored the BIS in 1064 patients undergoing general anesthesia for major elective surgery (excluding cardiac and intracranial procedures) lasting at least 2 hours.[263] The anesthetic technique was not controlled, and the anesthesiologist was blind to the BIS values. The authors examined the incidence of death at 1 year. Independent predictors of mortality were comorbid conditions (relative risk [RR] of 16), cumulative deep hypnotic time with a BIS value less than 45 (RR of 1.24), and systolic hypotension (RR of 1.03). There are many concerns with this study, including the fact that it has not been replicated nor has the outcome parameter "cumulative deep hypnotic time" been validated.

Lindholm and colleagues looked at mortality within 2 years of surgery in 4087 surgical patients monitored with the BIS.[264] They found that the duration of a BIS value less than 45 was statistically associated with increased 1- and 2-year postoperative mortality (hazard ratio, 1.13 and 1.18, respectively) if preexisting malignancy was not included among the covariates. Importantly, when preexisting malignancy was included among the covariates, the hazard ratio was reduced to 1.08 and did not reach statistical significance. They concluded that the linkage of a BIS value lower than 45 to postoperative mortality is "very weak in comparison with co-morbidity as assessed by ASA physical score, the preexisting malignancy status at surgery, and age," and a causal relationship, if any, can only be assessed in a prospective randomized trial.

Conclusions

Anesthetic depth can be defined as the drug-induced probability of nonresponse to stimulation, calibrated against the strength of the stimulus and the difficulty of suppressing the response. This definition requires that multiple different stimuli and responses are measured at precisely defined drug concentrations to permit estimation of the full drug-versus–probability of nonresponse surface for clinically important stimuli. There is no one stimulus and response measurement that will capture depth of anesthesia in a clinically or scientifically meaningful manner. The anesthesiologist must understand a complex matrix of stimuli, responses, and "anesthetic" drugs, including their pharmacodynamic (and generally synergistic) interactions. This definition captures the nature of routine clinical care whereby anesthesiologists observe a series of stimuli ranging from talking to the patient preoperatively to intubation to skin incision. They also observe a range of responses ranging from verbal response to movement to tachycardia and hypertension, and they calibrate these observations of stimuli and responses against the drugs used to reduce the probability of response by constantly adjusting the administered dose to achieve the desired anesthetic depth.

Our definition of "depth of anesthesia" identifies two critical components to maintain the anesthetic state: hypnosis from drugs such as propofol or the inhaled anesthetics and analgesia from opioids or nitrous oxide. We demonstrate the scientific evidence that profound degrees of hypnosis in the absence of analgesia will not prevent the hemodynamic responses to profoundly noxious stimuli and that profound degrees of analgesia do not guarantee unconsciousness. However, the combination of hypnosis and analgesia suppresses the hemodynamic response to noxious stimuli and guarantees unconsciousness. The synergy between hypnotics and analgesics is used every day by every anesthesiologist in clinical practice. We also demonstrate that this concept can be captured with a three-dimensional interaction surface (hypnotic concentration on the y axis, analgesic concentration on the x axis, probability of nonresponsiveness for defined stimuli on the z axis) that can be accurately estimated with available clinical data for currently used anesthetic drugs.

Awareness during anesthesia is an important clinical problem that sometimes results in prolonged disabling psychological sequelae for the patient. Comprehensive understanding of the sciences underpinning anesthesia, thorough preoperative evaluation and preparation, careful intraoperative observation, and postoperative debriefing may help reduce the incidence of awareness and the severity of its consequences. Unconscious memory formation and dreaming remain fascinating but probably harmless phenomena.

There are now many electrophysiologic monitors that can be used to assess the magnitude of the drug-induced changes in the EEG and evoked responses and help guide titration of anesthetics. Of these, the BIS is the most extensively validated. These monitors correlate well with the effects of hypnotics (particularly propofol, thiopental, and inhaled anesthetics) on memory, sedation, and consciousness but should always be used in conjunction with clinical assessment of the patient, the stimulus, and the drugs used. Titration guided by the BIS decreases the incidence of intraoperative awareness. An electrophysiologic measure of analgesia is not currently available.

There is considerable room for the development of additional technology and pharmacologic insight into measures of the depth of anesthesia. The opioid/hypnotic concentration-versus-response surface has not been characterized for many stimulus-response pairs. There are many additional drug interactions that might be profitably characterized (e.g., opioids versus α_2-adrenergic agonists), as well as higher-dimensional drug interactions (e.g., three-drug interaction surfaces). There are cells in the stimulus-response matrix for which only poor EEG predictors exist (e.g., movement with opioid/nitrous oxide anesthesia, ketamine). There are important responses that are poorly understood (e.g., inflammatory, humeral, neurophysiologic, and psychological responses). Our definition of anesthetic depth, as well as measurement of anesthetic depth, will expand as the matrix of stimuli, responses, and drugs that influence the probability of nonresponse expands with new research and new knowledge.

References

1. Prys-Roberts C: Anaesthesia: A practical or impossible construct? [editorial] Br J Anaesth 59:1341, 1987.
2. Eger EL II, Saidman LJ, Brandstater B: Minimum alveolar anesthetic concentration: A standard of anesthetic potency. Anesthesiology 26:756-763, 1965.
3. Kissin I: General anesthetic action: An obsolete notion? [editorial] Anesth Analg 76:215-218, 1993.
4. Eger EI II, Tang M, Liao M, et al: Inhaled anesthetics do not combine to produce synergistic effects regarding MAC in rats. Anesth Analg 107:479-485, 2008.
5. Chernik DA, Gillings D, Laine H, et al: Validity and reliability of the Observer's Assessment of Alertness/Sedation Scale: Study with intravenous midazolam. J Clin Psychopharmacol 10:244-251, 1990.
6. Glass PS: Anesthetic drug interactions: An insight into general anesthesia—its mechanism and dosing strategies. Anesthesiology 88:5-6, 1998.
7. Bencherif B, Fuchs PN, Sheth R, et al: Pain activation of human supraspinal opioid pathways as demonstrated by [^{11}C]-carfentanil and positron emission tomography (PET). Pain 99:589-598, 2002.
8. Chen SR, Pan HL: Blocking mu opioid receptors in the spinal cord prevents the analgesic action by subsequent systemic opioids. Brain Res 1081:119-125, 2006.
9. Fukuhara N, Ishikawa T, Kinoshita H, et al: Central noradrenergic mediation of nitrous oxide–induced analgesia in rats. Can J Anaesth 45:1123-1129, 1998.
10. Quock RM, Best JA, Chen DC, et al: Mediation of nitrous oxide analgesia in mice by spinal and supraspinal kappa-opioid receptors. Eur J Pharmacol 175:97-100, 1990.
11. Fang F, Guo TZ, Davies MF, Maze M: Opiate receptors in the periaqueductal gray mediate analgesic effect of nitrous oxide in rats. Eur J Pharmacol 336:137-141, 1997.
12. Bouillon TW, Bruhn J, Radulescu L, et al: Pharmacodynamic interaction between propofol and remifentanil regarding hypnosis, tolerance of laryngoscopy, bispectral index, and electroencephalographic approximate entropy. Anesthesiology 100:1353-1372, 2004.
13. Egan TD, Muir KT, Hermann DJ, et al: The electroencephalogram (EEG) and clinical measure of opioid potency: Defining the EEG–clinical potency relationship ("fingerprint") with application to remifentanil. Int J Pharm Med 15:1-9, 2001.
14. Wynands JE, Wong P, Townsend GE, et al: Narcotic requirements for intravenous anesthesia. Anesth Analg 63:101-105, 1984.
15. Sebel PS, Glass PS, Fletcher JE, et al: Reduction of the MAC of desflurane with fentanyl. Anesthesiology 6:52-59, 1992.
16. McEwan AI, Smith C, Dyar O, et al: Isoflurane minimum alveolar concentration reduction by fentanyl. Anesthesiology 78:864-869, 1993.
17. Vuyk J, Lim T, Engbers FH, et al: The pharmacodynamic interaction of propofol and alfentanil during lower abdominal surgery in women. Anesthesiology 83:8-22, 1995.
18. Smith C, McEwan AI, Jhaveri R, et al: The interaction of fentanyl on the Cp_{50} of propofol for loss of

consciousness and skin incision. Anesthesiology 81:820-828, 1994.

19. Kazama T, Ikeda K, Morita K: Reduction by fentanyl of the Cp_{50} values of propofol and hemodynamic responses to various noxious stimuli. Anesthesiology 87:213-227, 1997.
20. Kazama T, Ikeda K, Morita K, et al: Propofol concentration required for endotracheal intubation with a laryngoscope or fiberscope and its interaction with fentanyl. Anesth Analg 86:872-879, 1998.
21. Minto CF, Schnider TW, Short TG, et al: Response surface model for anesthetic drug interactions. Anesthesiology 92:1603-1816, 2000.
22. Rampil IJ, Mason P, Singh H: Anesthetic potency (MAC) is independent of forebrain structures in the rat. Anesthesiology 78:707-712, 1993.
23. Antognini JF, Schwartz K: Exaggerated anesthetic requirements in the preferentially anesthetized brain. Anesthesiology 79:1244-1249, 1993.
24. Hendrickx JFA, Eger EI II, Sonner JM, Shafer SL: Is synergy the rule? A review of anesthetic interactions producing hypnosis and immobility. Anesth Analg 107:494-506, 2008.
25. Eger EI II: Age, minimum alveolar anesthetic concentration, and minimum alveolar anesthetic concentration–awake. Anesth Analg 93:947-953, 2001.
26. Daniel M, Weiskopf RB, Noorani M, Eger EI II: Fentanyl augments the blockade of the sympathetic response to incision (MAC-BAR) produced by desflurane and isoflurane: Desflurane and isoflurane MAC-BAR without and with fentanyl. Anesthesiology 88:43-49, 1998.
27. Hornbein TF, Eger EI II, Winter PM, et al: The minimum alveolar concentration of nitrous oxide in man. Anesth Analg 61:553-556, 1982.
28. Ausems ME, Hug CC Jr, Stanski DR, Burm AG: Plasma concentrations of alfentanil required to supplement nitrous oxide anesthesia for general surgery. Anesthesiology 65:362-373, 1986.
29. Ghouri AF, White PF: Effect of fentanyl and nitrous oxide on the desflurane anesthetic requirement. Anesth Analg 72:377-381, 1991.
30. Stuart PC, Stott SM, Millar A, et al: Cp_{50} of propofol with and without nitrous oxide 67%. Br J Anaesth 4:638-639, 2000.
31. Hobbs A, Bush G, Downham D: Perioperative dreaming and awareness in children. Anaesthesia 43:560-562, 1988.
32. Ghoneim M: Awareness during Anesthesia. Oxford, Butterworth-Heinemann, 2001, pp 1-22.
33. Pollard R, Coyle J, Gilbert R, Beck J: Intraoperative awareness in a regional medical system. A review of 3 years' data. Anesthesiology 106:269-274, 2007.
34. ASA Advisory Committee: Practice advisory for intraoperative awareness and brain function monitoring: A report by the American Society of Anesthesiologists Task Force on Intraoperative Awareness. Anesthesiology 104:847-864, 2006.
35. Moerman N, Bonke B, Oosting J: Awareness and recall during general anesthesia. Facts and feelings. Anesthesiology 79:454-464, 1993.
36. Brice D, Hetherington R, Utting J: A simple study of awareness and dreaming during anaesthesia. Br J Anaesth 42:535-542, 1970.
37. Abouleish E, Taylor FH: Effect of morphine-diazepam on signs of anesthesia, awareness and dreams of patients under N_2O for cesarian section. Anesth Analg 55:702-706, 1976.
38. Samuelsson P, Brudin L, Sandin R: Late psychological symptoms after awareness among consecutively included surgical patients. Anesthesiology 106:26-32, 2007.
39. Shalev A, Peri T, Canetti L, Schreiber S: Predictors of PTSD in injured trauma survivors: A prospective study. Am J Psychiatry 153:219-225, 1996.
40. Hutchinson R: Awareness during surgery. Br J Anaesth 33:463-469, 1960.
41. Crawford J: Awareness during operative obstetrics under general anaesthesia. Br J Anaesth 43:179-182, 1971.
42. Wilson S, Vaughan R, Stephen C: Awareness, dreams, and hallucinations associated with general anesthesia. Anesth Analg 54:609-617, 1975.

42a. Crawford JS, Lewis M, Davies P: Maternal and neonatal responses related to the volatile agent used to maintain anaesthesia at caesarean section. Br J Anaesth 57:482-487, 1985.

43. Liu WH, Thorp TA, Graham SG, Aitkenhead AR: Incidence of awareness with recall during general anaesthesia. Anaesthesia 46:435-437, 1991.
44. Lyons G, Macdonald R: Awareness during caesarean section. Anaesthesia 46:62-64, 1991.
45. Phillips A, McLean R, Devitt J, et al: Recall of intraoperative events after general anaesthesia and cardiopulmonary bypass. Can J Anaesth 40:922-926, 1993.
46. Sandin R, Nordstrom O: Awareness during total iv anaesthesia. Br J Anaesth 71:782-787, 1993.
47. Nordstrom O, Engstrom A, Persson S, Sandin R: Incidence of awareness in total i.v. anaesthesia based on propofol, alfentanil and neuromuscular blockade. Acta Anaesthesiol Scand 41:978-984, 1997.
48. Ranta S, Laurila R, Saario J, et al: Awareness with recall during general anesthesia: Incidence and risk factors. Anesth Analg 86:1084-1089, 1998.
49. Dowd M, Cheng D, Karski J, et al: Intraoperative awareness in fast-track cardiac anaesthesia. Anesthesiology 89:1068-1073, 1998.
50. Sandin R, Enlund G, Samuelsson P, Lennmarken C: Awareness during anaesthesia: A prospective case study. Lancet 355:707-711, 2000.
51. Myles P, Williams D, Hendrata M, et al: Patient satisfaction after anaesthesia and surgery: Results of a prospective survey of patients. Br J Anaesth 84:6-10, 2000.
52. Enlund M, Hassan H: Intraoperative awareness: Detected by the structured Brice interview. Acta Anaesthesiol Scand 46:345-349, 2002.
53. Ranta S, Herranen P, Hynynen M: Patients' conscious recollections from cardiac anesthesia. J Cardiothorac Vasc Anesth 16:426-430, 2002.
54. Chaiwat O, Vacharaksa K, Prakanrattana U: Awareness under general anesthesia. J Med Assoc Thai 85(Suppl 3):S948-S955, 2002.
55. Myles P, Leslie K, McNeil J, et al: A randomised controlled trial of BIS monitoring to prevent awareness during anaesthesia: The B-Aware Trial. Lancet 363:1757-1763, 2004.
56. Sebel P, Bowdle T, Ghoneim M, et al: The incidence of awareness during anesthesia: A multicenter United States study. Anesth Analg 99:833-839, 2004.
57. Ekman A, Lindholm M, Lennmarken C, Sandin R: Reduction in the incidence of awareness using BIS monitoring. Acta Anaesthesiol Scand 48:20-26, 2004.
58. Rungreungvanich M, Lekprasert V, Sirinan C, et al: An analysis of intraoperative awareness in Thai Anesthesia Incidence Study. Anesthesiology 103:A1283, 2005.
59. Paech M, Clavisi O, Scott K, et al: The Australasian Obstetric General Anaesthesia for Caesarean Section Survey. Paper presented at the ANZCA 2007Annual Scientific Meeting, Melbourne, Australia.
60. Avidan M, Zhang L, Burnside B, et al: Anesthesia awareness and the bispectral index. N Engl J Med 358:1097-1108, 2008.
61. Errando CL, Sigl JC, Robles M, et al: Awareness with recall during general anaesthesia: A prospective observational evaluation of 4001 patients. Br J Anaesth 10:178-185, 2008.
62. Sandin R: Relax, be aware, and know what you are doing. Acta Anaesthesiol Scand 46:343-344, 2002.
63. Sebel P, Bowdle T, Rampil I, et al: Don't ask, don't tell. Anesthesiology 107:672-673, 2007.
64. Leslie K: Awareness in a community-based practice. Anesthesiology 107:671-672, 2007.
65. Goldmann L, Shah M, Hebden M: Memory of cardiac anaesthesia. Anaesthesia 42:596-603, 1987.
66. Bogetz M, Katz J: Recall of surgery for major trauma. Anesthesiology 61:6-9, 1984.
67. Lubke G, Sebel P: Awareness and different forms of memory in trauma anaesthesia. Curr Opin Anaesthesiol 13:161-165, 2000.
68. Moore J: Awareness during bronchoscopy. Ann R Coll Surg Engl 69:45-47, 1987.
69. Kelly JS, Roy RC: Intraoperative awareness with propofol-oxygen total intravenous anesthesia for microlaryngeal surgery. Anesthesiology 77:207-209, 1992.
70. McKie B, Thorpe E: Awareness and dreaming during anaesthesia in a paediatric hospital. Anaesth Intensive Care 1:407-414, 1973.
71. Davidson A, Huang G, Czarnecki C, et al: Awareness during anesthesia in children: A prospective cohort study. Anesth Analg 100:653-661, 2005.
72. Domino K, Posner K, Caplan R, Cheney F: Awareness during anesthesia: A closed claims analysis. Anesthesiology 90:1053-1061, 1999.
73. Bergman I, Kluger M, Short T: Awareness during general anaesthesia: A review of 81 cases from the Anaesthetic Incident Monitoring Study. Anaesthesia 57:549-556, 2002.
74. Hilgenberg J: Intraoperative awareness during high-dose fentanyl–oxygen anesthesia. Anesthesiology 54:341-343, 1981.
75. Hug CC: Does opioid anesthesia exist? Anesthesiology 73:1-4, 1990.
76. Luginbuhl M, Schnider T: Detection of awareness with the bispectral index: Two case reports. Anesthesiology 96:241-243, 2002.
77. Moerman A, Herregods L, Foubert L, et al: Awareness during anaesthesia for implantable cardioverter defibrillator implantation. Anaesthesia 50:733-735, 1995.
78. Caplan R, Vistica M, Posner K, Cheney F: Adverse anesthetic outcomes arising from gas delivery equipment: A closed claims analysis. Anesthesiology 87:741-748, 1997.
79. Rowan K: Awareness under TIVA: A doctor's personal experience. Anaesth Intensive Care 30:505-506, 2002.
80. Tong D, Chung F: Recall after total intravenous anaesthesia due to an equipment misuse. Can J Anaesth 44:73-77, 1997.
81. Gin T, Chan M: Decreased minimum alveolar concentration of isoflurane in pregnant humans. Anesthesiology 81:829-832, 1994.
82. Gin T, Mainland P, Chan M, Short T: Decreased thiopental requirements in early pregnancy. Anesthesiology 86:73-78, 1997.
83. Liem E, Lin C-M, Suleman M, et al: Anesthetic requirement is increased in redheads. Anesthesiology 101:279-283, 2004.
84. Gan T, Glass P, Sigl J, et al: Women emerge from general anesthesia with propofol/alfentanil/nitrous oxide faster than men. Anesthesiology 90:1283-1287, 1999.

85. Buchanan F, Myles P, Leslie K, et al: Gender and recovery after general anesthesia combined with neuromuscular blocking drugs. Anesth Analg 102:291-297, 2006.
86. Myles PS: Prevention of awareness during anaesthesia. Best Pract Res Clin Anaesthesiol 21:345-355, 2007.
87. Nordström O, Sandin R: Recall during intermittent propofol anaesthesia. Br J Anaesth 76:699-701, 1996.
88. Ekman A, Lindholm M, Lennmarken C, Sandin R: Reduction in the incidence of awareness using BIS monitoring. Acta Anaesthesiol Scand 48:20-26, 2004.
89. Myles P, Leslie K, Forbes A: Anesthesia awareness and the bispectral index. Letter to the editor. N Engl J Med 359:428-429, 2008.
90. Kelley SD, Manberg PJ, Sigl JC: Anesthesia awareness and the bispectral index. N Engl J Med 359:427-428, 2008.
91. Sneyd JR, Mathews DM: Memory and awareness during anaesthesia. Br J Anaesth 100:742-744, 2008.
92. Divan, AY, Mathews DM: The Impact of anesthesia awareness risk reduction strategies: A literature review. ASA abstract, 2008.
93. Dahaba A: Different conditions that could result in the bispectral index indicating an incorrect hypnotic state. Anesth Analg 101:765-773, 2005.
94. Voss L, Sleigh J: Monitoring consciousness: The current status of EEG-based depth of anaesthesia monitors. Best Pract Res Clin Anaesthesiol 21:313-325, 2007.
95. O'Connor M, Daves S, Tung A, et al: BIS monitoring to prevent awareness during general anesthesia. Anesthesiology 94:520-522, 2001.
96. Osterman J, Hopper J, Heran W, et al: Awareness during anesthesia and the development of post-traumatic stress disorder. Gen Hosp Psychiatry 23:198-204, 2001.
97. Lennmarken C, Bildfors K, Enlund G, et al: Victims of awareness. Acta Anaesthesiol Scand 46:229-231, 2002.
98. Kent C, Domino K: Awareness: Practice, standards and the law. Best Pract Res Clin Anaesthesiol 21:369-383, 2007.
99. Ghoneim M, Block R: Learning and memory during general anesthesia. An update. Anesthesiology 87:387-410, 1997.
100. Levinson B: States of awareness during general anaesthesia. Br J Anaesth 37:544-546, 1965.
101. Jacoby L: A process dissociation framework: Separating automatic from intentional uses of memory. J Mem Lang 30:513-541, 1991.
102. Lubke G, Kerssens C, Phaf H, Sebel P: Dependence of explicit and implicit memory on hypnotic state in trauma patients. Anesthesiology 90:70-80, 1999.
103. Stonell C, Leslie K, He C, Lee L: No sex differences in memory formation during general anesthesia. Anesthesiology 105:920-926, 2006.
104. Deeprose C, Andrade J, Harrison D, Edwards N: Unconscious auditory priming during surgery with propofol and nitrous oxide anaesthesia: A replication. Br J Anaesth 94:57-62, 2005.
105. Kerssens C, Ouchi T, Sebel P: No evidence of memory formation during anesthesia with propofol or isoflurane with close control of hypnotic state. Anesthesiology 102:57-62, 2005.
106. Andrade J, Deeprose C: Unconscious memory formation during anaesthesia. Best Pract Res Clin Anaesthesiol 21:385-401, 2007.
107. Leslie K, Myles P, Forbes A, et al: Dreaming during anaesthesia in patients at high risk of awareness. Anaesthesia 60:239-244, 2005.
108. Leslie K, Skrzypek H, Paech M, et al: Dreaming during anesthesia and anesthetic depth in elective surgery patients: A prospective cohort study. Anesthesiology 106:33-42, 2007.
109. Grace R: The effect of variable-dose diazepam on dreaming and emergence phenomena in 400 cases of ketamine-fentanyl anaesthesia. Anaesthesia 58:904-910, 2003.
110. Harris T, Brice D, Hetherington R, Utting J: Dreaming associated with anaesthesia: The influence of morphine premedication and two volatile adjuvants. Br J Anaesth 43:172-178, 1971.
111. Huang G, Davidson A, Stargatt R: Dreaming during anaesthesia in children: Incidence, nature and associations. Anaesthesia 60:854-861, 2005.
112. Merkel G, Eger EI II: A comparative study of halothane and halopropane anesthesia: Including the method for determining equipotency. Anesthesiology 24:346-357, 1963.
113. Quasha AL, Eger EI II, Tinker JH: Determination and applications of MAC. Anesthesiology 53:315-334, 1980.
114. Cullen DJ: Drugs and anesthetic depth. *In* Smith NT, Miller RD, Corbascio AN (eds): Drug Interactions in Anesthesia. Philadelphia, Lea & Febiger, 1981, p 287.
115. Eger EI II, Bahlman SH: Is the end-tidal anesthetic partial pressure an accurate measure of the arterial anesthetic partial pressure? Anesthesiology 35:301-303, 1971.
116. Stoelting RK, Longnecker DE, Eger EI II: Minimum alveolar concentrations in man on awakening from methoxyflurane, halothane, ether and fluroxene anesthesia: MAC awake. Anesthesiology 33:5-9, 1970.
117. Yakaitis RW, Blitt CD, Angiulo JP: End-tidal halothane concentration for endotracheal intubation. Anesthesiology 47:386-388, 1977.
118. Roizen MF, Horrigan RW, Frazer BM: Anesthetic doses blocking adrenergic (stress) and cardiovascular responses to incision—MAC BAR. Anesthesiology 54:390-398, 1981.
119. Zbinden AM, Maggiorini M, Petersen-Felix S, et al: Anesthetic depth defined using multiple noxious stimuli during isoflurane/oxygen anesthesia. I. Motor reactions. Anesthesiology 80:253-260, 1994.
120. Cullen DJ, Eger EI II, Stevens WC, et al: Clinical signs of anesthesia. Anesthesiology 36:21-36, 1972.
121. Zbinden AM, Petersen-Felix S, Thomson DA: Anesthetic depth defined using multiple noxious stimuli during isoflurane/oxygen anesthesia. II. Hemodynamic responses. Anesthesiology 80:261-267, 1994.
122. King BD, Harris LC Jr, Greifenstein FF, et al: Reflex circulatory responses to direct laryngoscopy and tracheal intubation performed during general anesthesia. Anesthesiology 12:556-566, 1951.
123. Stoelting RK: Circulatory changes during direct laryngoscopy and tracheal intubation: Influence of duration of laryngoscopy with or without prior lidocaine. Anesthesiology 47:381-384, 1977.
124. Becker KE Jr: Plasma levels of thiopental necessary for anesthesia. Anesthesiology 49:192-196, 1978.
125. Hung OR, Varvel JR, Shafer SL, Stanski DR: Thiopental pharmacodynamics. II. Quantitation of clinical and electroencephalographic depth of anesthesia. Anesthesiology 77:237-244, 1992.
126. Vuyk J, Lim T, Engbers FH, et al: Pharmacodynamics of alfentanil as a supplement to propofol or nitrous oxide for lower abdominal surgery in female patients. Anesthesiology 78:1036-1045, 1993.
127. Stanski DR, Shafer SL: Quantifying anesthetic drug interaction: Implications for drug dosing [editorial]. Anesthesiology 83:1, 1995.
128. Tammisto T, Aromaa U, Korttila K: The role of thiopental and fentanyl in the production of balanced anaesthesia. Acta Anaesthesiol Scand 24:31-35, 1980.
129. Neff W, Mayer EC, de la Luz Percales M: Nitrous oxide and oxygen anesthesia with curare relaxation. Calif Med 66:67-69, 1947.
130. Lowenstein E, Hallowell P, Levine FH, et al: Cardiovascular response to large doses of intravenous morphine in man. N Engl J Med 281:1389-1393, 1969.
131. Stanley TH, Webster LR: Anesthetic requirements and cardiovascular effects of fentanyl-oxygen and fentanyl-diazepam-oxygen anesthesia in man. Anesth Analg 57:411-416, 1978.
132. Waller JL, Hug CC Jr, Nagle DM, Craver JM: Hemodynamic changes during fentanyl-oxygen anesthesia for aortocoronary bypass operation. Anesthesiology 55:212-217, 1981.
133. Hynynen M, Lehtinen AM, Salmenperä M, et al: Continuous infusion of fentanyl or alfentanil for coronary artery surgery. Effects on plasma cortisol concentration, beta-endorphin immunoreactivity and arginine vasopressin. Br J Anaesth 58:1260-1266, 1986.
134. Philbin DM, Rosow CE, Schneider RC, et al: Fentanyl and sufentanil anesthesia revisited: How much is enough? Anesthesiology 73:5-11, 1990.
135. Murphy MR, Hug CC Jr: The anesthetic potency of fentanyl in terms of its reduction of enflurane MAC. Anesthesiology 57:485-488, 1982.
136. Hall RI, Murphy MR, Hug CC Jr: The enflurane sparing effect of sufentanil in dogs. Anesthesiology 67:518-525, 1987.
137. Hall RI, Szlam F, Hug CC Jr: The enflurane-sparing effect of alfentanil in dogs. Anesth Analg 66:1287-1291, 1987.
138. Murphy MR, Hug CC Jr: The enflurane sparing effect of morphine, butorphanol, and nalbuphine. Anesthesiology 57:489-492, 1982.
139. Glass PS, Gan TJ, Howell S, Ginsberg B: Drug interactions: Volatile anesthetics and opioids. J Clin Anesth 9:18S-22S, 1997.
140. Katoh T, Kobayashi S, Suzuki A, et al: The effect of fentanyl on sevoflurane requirements for somatic and sympathetic responses to surgical incision. Anesthesiology 90:398-405, 1999.
141. Katoh T, Ikeda K: The effect of fentanyl on sevoflurane requirements for loss of consciousness and skin incision. Anesthesiology 88:18-24, 1998.
142. Ausems ME, Vuyk J, Hug CC Jr, Stanski DR: Comparison of computer-assisted infusion versus intermittent bolus administration of alfentanil as a supplement to nitrous oxide for lower abdominal surgery. Anesthesiology 68:851-861, 1988.
143. Minto CF, Schnider TW, Egan TD, et al: Influence of age and gender on the pharmacokinetics and pharmacodynamics of remifentanil. I. Model development. Anesthesiology 86:10-23, 1997.
144. Minto CF, Schnider TW, Shafer SL: Pharmacokinetics and pharmacodynamics of remifentanil. II. Model development. Anesthesiology 86:24-33, 1997.
145. Drover DR, Lemmens HJM: Population pharmacodynamics and pharmacokinetics of remifentanil as a supplement to nitrous oxide anesthesia for elective abdominal surgery. Anesthesiology 89:869-877, 1998.
146. Egan TD, Shafer SL: Target-controlled infusions for intravenous anesthetics: Surfing USA not! Anesthesiology 99:1039-1041, 2003.
147. Caton R: The electrical currents of the brain [abstract]. BMJ 2:278, 1875.

148. Berger H: Uber das Elektrenkaphalogramm des Menschen. Arch Psychiatry 101:452, 1933.
149. Gibbs FA, Gibbs EL, Lennox WG: Effect on the electro-encephalogram of certain drugs which influence nervous activity. Arch Intern Med 60:154, 1937.
150. Faulconer A Jr: Correlation of concentrations of ether in arterial blood with electro-encephalographic patterns occurring during ether-oxygen and during nitrous oxide, oxygen and ether anesthesia of human surgical patients. Anesthesiology 13:361-369, 1952.
151. Martin JT, Faulconer A Jr, Bickford RG: Electroencephalography in anesthesiology. Anesthesiology 20:359-376, 1959.
152. Kuramoto T, Oshita S, Takeshita H, Ishikawa T: Modification of the relationship between cerebral metabolism, blood flow, and electroencephalogram by stimulation during anesthesia in the dog. Anesthesiology 51:211-217, 1979.
153. Prior PF: The EEG and detection of responsiveness during anaesthesia and coma. *In* Rosen M, Lunn JN (eds): Consciousness, Awareness, and Pain in General Anesthesia. London, Butterworths, 1987, p 34.
154. Bimar J, Bellville JW: Arousal reactions during anesthesia in man. Anesthesiology 47:449-454, 1977.
155. Miyauchi Y, Sakabe T, Maekawa T, et al: Responses of EEG, cerebral oxygen consumption and blood flow to peripheral nerve stimulation during thiopentone anaesthesia in the dog. Can Anaesth Soc J 32:491-498, 1985.
156. Galla SJ, Rocco AG, Vandam LD: Evaluation of the traditional signs and stages of anesthesia: An electroencephalographic and clinical study. Anesthesiology 19:328-338, 1958.
157. Levy WJ, Shapiro HM, Maruchak G, Meathe E: Automated EEG processing for intraoperative monitoring: A comparison of techniques. Anesthesiology 53:223-236, 1980.
158. Rampil IJ: What every neuroanesthesiologist should know about electroencephalograms and computerized monitors. Anesthesiol Clin North Am 10:683-718, 1992.
159. Levy WJ: Intraoperative EEG patterns: Implications for EEG monitoring. Anesthesiology 60:430-434, 1984.
160. Drummond JC, Brann CA, Perkins DE, Wolfe DE: A comparison of median frequency, spectral edge frequency, a frequency band power ratio, total power and dominance shift in the determination of depth of anesthesia. Acta Anaesthesiol Scand 35:693-699, 1991.
161. Long CW, Shah NK, Lounghlin C, et al: A comparison of EEG determinants of near awakening from isoflurane and fentanyl anesthesia. Anesth Analg 69:169-173, 1989.
162. Dwyer RC, Rampil IJ, Eger EI II, Bennett HL: The electroencephalogram does not predict depth of isoflurane anesthesia. Anesthesiology 81:403-409, 1994.
163. Stanski DR: Pharmacodynamic modeling of anesthetic EEG drug effects. Annu Rev Pharmacol Toxicol 32:423-447, 1992.
164. Blackman RB, Tukey JW: The Measurement of Power Spectra. New York, Dover, 1958.
165. Abarbanel H, Davis R, MacDonald GJ, Munk W: Bispectra. Defense Technical Information Center, Document ADA150870, 1984.
166. Rampil IJ: A primer for EEG signal processing in anesthesia. Anesthesiology 89:980-1002, 1998.
167. Sigl JC, Chamoun NG: An introduction to bispectral analysis for the electroencephalogram. J Clin Monit 10:392-404, 1994.
168. Johansen JW, Sebel PS: Development and clinical application of electroencephalographic bispectrum monitoring. Anesthesiology 93:1336-1344, 2000.
169. Gregg K, Varvel JR, Shafer SL: Application of semilinear canonical correlation to the measurement of opioid drug effect. J Pharmacokinet Biopharm 20:611-635, 1992.
170. Kearse LA Jr, Manberg P, Chamoun N, et al: Bispectral analysis of the electroencephalogram correlates with patient movement to skin incision during propofol/nitrous oxide anesthesia. Anesthesiology 81:1365-1370, 1994.
171. Vernon JM, Lang E, Sebel PS, Manberg P: Prediction of movement using bi-spectral EEG during propofol/alfentanil or isoflurane/alfentanil anesthesia. Anesth Analg 80:780-785, 1995.
172. Sebel PS, Lang E, Rampil IJ, et al: A multicenter study of bispectral electroencephalogram analysis for monitoring anesthetic effect. Anesth Analg 84:891-899, 1997.
173. Glass PS, Bloom M, Kearse L, et al: Bispectral analysis measures sedation and memory effects of propofol, midazolam, isoflurane and alfentanil in healthy volunteers. Anesthesiology 86:836-847, 1997.
174. Liu J, Singh H, White PF: Electroencephalogram bispectral analysis predicts the depth of midazolam-induced sedation. Anesthesiology 84:64-69, 1996.
175. Liu J, Singh H, White PF: Electroencephalographic bispectral index correlates with intraoperative recall and depth of propofol-induced sedation. Anesth Analg 84:185-189, 1997.
176. Katoh T, Suzuki A, Ikeda K: Electroencephalographic derivatives as a tool for predicting the depth of sedation and anesthesia induced by sevoflurane. Anesthesiology 88:642-650, 1998.
177. Flaishon R, Windsor A, Sigl J, Sebel PS: Recovery of consciousness after thiopental or propofol: Bispectral index and the isolated forearm technique. Anesthesiology 86:613-619, 1997.
178. Kearse LA, Rosow C, Zaslavsky A, et al: Bispectral analysis of the electroencephalogram predicts conscious processing of information during propofol sedation and hypnosis. Anesthesiology 88:25-34, 1998.
179. Shannon CE: A mathematical theory of communication. Bell Syst Tech J 27:379-423, 623A-656A, 1948.
180. Viertiö-Oja H, Maja V, Särkelä M, et al: Description of the Entropy algorithm as applied in the Datex-Ohmeda S/5 Entropy Module. Acta Anaesthesiol Scand 48:154-161, 2004.
181. Jäntti V, Alahuhta S: Spectral entropy—what has it to do with anaesthesia, and the EEG? Br J Anaesth 93:150-151, 2004.
182. Chang T, Dworsky WA, White PF: Continuous electromyography for monitoring depth of anesthesia. Anesth Analg 67:521-525, 1988.
183. Dutton RC, Smith WD, Bennett HL, et al: Craniofacial electromyogram activation response: Another indicator of anesthetic depth. J Clin Monit Comput 14:5-17, 1998.
184. Vakkuri A, Yli-Hankala A, Talja P, et al: Time-frequency balanced spectral entropy as a measure of anesthetic drug effect in central nervous system during sevoflurane, propofol, and thiopental anesthesia. Acta Anaesthesiol Scand 48:145-153, 2004.
185. Ellerkmann RK, Soehle M, Alves TM, et al: Spectral entropy and bispectral index as measures of the electroencephalographic effects of propofol. Anesth Analg 102:1456-1462, 2006.
186. Ellerkmann RK, Liermann VM, Alves TM, et al: Spectral entropy and bispectral index as measures of the electroencephalographic effects of sevoflurane. Anesthesiology 101:1275-1282, 2004.
187. Tinker JH, Sharbrough FW, Michenfelder JD: Anterior shift of the dominant EEG rhythm during anesthesia in the Java monkey: Correlation with anesthetic potency. Anesthesiology 46:252-259, 1977.
188. Kochs E, Bischoff P, Pichlmeier U, Schulte am Esch J: Surgical stimulation induces changes in brain electrical activity during isoflurane/nitrous oxide anesthesia. A topographic electroencephalographic analysis. Anesthesiology 80:1026-1034, 1994.
189. Drover DR, Lemmens HJ, Pierce ET, et al: Patient State Index: Titration of delivery and recovery from propofol, alfentanil, and nitrous oxide anesthesia. Anesthesiology 97:82-89, 2002.
190. Drover DR, Ortega R: Patient State Index. Best Pract Res Clin Anaesthesiol 20:121-128, 2006.
191. Chen X, Tang J, White PF, et al: A comparison of Patient State Index and bispectral index values during the perioperative period. Anesth Analg 95:1669-1674, 2002.
192. White PF, Tang J, Ma H, et al: Is the patient state analyzer with the PSArray2 a cost-effective alternative to the bispectral index monitor during the perioperative period? Anesth Analg 99:1429-1435, 2004.
193. Loomis AL, Harvey EN, Hobart CA: Cerebral states during sleep as studied by human brain potentials. J Exp Psychol 21:127-144, 1937.
194. Schultz B, Schultz A, Grouven U: Sleeping stage based systems (Narcotrend). *In* Bruck HP, Koeckerling F, Bouchard F, Schug-Pass C (eds): New Aspects of High Technology in Medicine 2000. Bolognia, Italy, Monduzzi Editore, 2000, pp 285-291.
195. Kreuer S, Biedler A, Larsen R, et al: The Narcotrend—a new EEG monitor designed to measure the depth of anaesthesia. A comparison with bispectral index monitoring during propofol-remifentanil-anaesthesia. Anaesthesist 50:921-925, 2001.
196. Schmidt GN, Bischoff P, Standl T, et al: Narcotrend and bispectral index monitor are superior to classic electroencephalographic parameters for the assessment of anesthetic states during propofol-remifentanil anesthesia. Anesthesiology 99:1072-1077, 2003.
197. Kreuer S, Wilhelm W, Grundmann U, et al: Narcotrend index versus bispectral index as electroencephalogram measures of anesthetic drug effect during propofol anesthesia. Anesth Analg 98:692-697, 2004.
198. Thornton C, Barrowcliffe MP, Konieczko KM, et al: The auditory evoked response as an indicator of awareness. Br J Anaesth 63:113-115, 1989.
199. Freye E: Cerebral monitoring in the operating room and the intensive care unit—an introductory for the clinician and a guide for the novice wanting to open a window to the brain. Part II: Sensory-evoked potentials (SSEP, AEP, VEP). J Clin Monit Comput 19:77-168, 2005.
200. Thornton C, Heneghan CPH, Navaratnarajah M, et al: Effect of etomidate on the auditory evoked response in man. Br J Anaesth 57:554-561, 1985.
201. Heneghan CPH, Thornton C, Navaratnarajah M, Jones JG: Effect of isoflurane on the auditory evoked response in man. Br J Anaesth 59:277-282, 1987.
202. Thornton C, Konieczko K, Jones JG, et al: Effect of surgical stimulation on the auditory evoked response. Br J Anaesth 60:372-378, 1988.

203. Newton DEF, Thornton C, Konieczko K, et al: Auditory evoked response and awareness: A study in volunteers at sub-MAC concentrations of isoflurane. Br J Anaesth 69:122-129, 1992.
204. Schwender D, Rimkus T, Haessler R, et al: Effect of increasing doses of alfentanil, fentanyl and morphine on mid-latency auditory evoked potentials. Br J Anaesth 71:622-628, 1993.
205. Mantzaridis H, Kenny GN: Auditory evoked potential index: A quantitative measure of changes in auditory evoked potentials during general anesthesia. Anaesthesia 52:1030-1036, 1997.
206. Kurita T, Doi M, Katoh T, et al: Auditory evoked potential index predicts the depth of sedation and movement in response to skin incision during sevoflurane anesthesia. Anesthesiology 95:364-370, 2001.
207. Jensen EW, Nygaard M, Hennenberg SW: On-line analysis of middle latency auditory evoked potentials (MLAEP) for monitoring depth of anesthesia in laboratory rats. Med Eng Phys 20:722-728, 1998.
208. Vereecke HE, Vasquez PM, Jensen EW, et al: New composite index based on midlatency auditory evoked potential and electroencephalographic parameters to optimize correlation with propofol effect site concentration: Comparison with bispectral index and solitary used fast extracting auditory evoked potential index. Anesthesiology 103:500-507, 2005.
209. Iselin-Chaves IA, El Moalem HE, Gan TJ, et al: Changes in the auditory evoked potentials and the bispectral index following propofol or propofol and alfentanil. Anesthesiology 92:1300-1310, 2000.
210. Struys MMRF, Jensen EW, Smith W, et al: Performance of the ARX-derived auditory evoked potential index as an indicator of anesthetic depth. Anesthesiology 96:803-816, 2002.
211. Schmidt GN, Bischoff P, Standl T, et al: ARX-derived auditory evoked potential index and bispectral index during the induction of anesthesia with propofol and remifentanil. Anesth Analg 97:139-144, 2003.
212. Iselin-Chaves IA, Flaishon R, Sebel PS, et al: The effect of the interaction of propofol and alfentanil on recall, loss of consciousness, and the bispectral index. Anesth Analg 87:949-955, 1998.
213. Alkire MT: Quantitative EEG correlations with brain glucose metabolic rate during anesthesia in volunteers. Anesthesiology 89:323-333, 1998.
214. Ludbrook GL, Visco E, Lam AM: Propofol: Relation between brain concentrations, electroencephalogram, middle cerebral blood flow velocity and cerebral oxygen extraction during induction of anesthesia. Anesthesiology 97:1363-1370, 2002.
215. Struys MM, Vereecke H, Moerman A, et al: Ability of the bispectral index, autoregressive modelling with exogenous input–derived auditory evoked potentials, and predicted propofol concentrations to measure patient responsiveness during anesthesia with propofol and remifentanil. Anesthesiology 99:802-812, 2003.
216. Bruhn J, Bouillon TW, Radulescu L, et al: Correlation of approximate entropy, bispectral index, and spectral edge frequency 95 (SEF95) with clinical signs of "anesthetic depth" during coadministration of propofol and remifentanil. Anesthesiology 98:621-627, 2003.
217. Bonhomme V, Plourde G, Meuret P, et al: Auditory steady-state response and bispectral index for assessing level of consciousness during propofol sedation and hypnosis. Anesth Analg 91:1398-1403, 2000.
218. Schmidt GN, Bischoff P, Standl T, et al: Comparative evaluation of the Datex-Ohmeda S/5 Entropy Module and the bispectral index monitor during propofol-remifentanil anesthesia. Anesthesiology 101:1283-1290, 2004.
219. Jensen EW, Litvan H, Revuelta M, et al: Cerebral state index during propofol anesthesia: A comparison with the bispectral index and the A-line ARX index. Anesthesiology 105:28-36, 2006.
220. Schmidt GN, Bischoff P, Standl T, et al: Comparative evaluation of Narcotrend, bispectral index, and classical electroencephalographic variables during induction, maintenance, and emergence of a propofol/remifentanil anesthesia. Anesth Analg 98:1346-1353, 2004.
221. Katoh T, Bito H, Sato S: Influence of age on hypnotic requirement, bispectral index, and 95% spectral edge frequency associated with sedation by sevoflurane. Anesthesiology 92:55-61, 2000.
222. Anderson RE, Barr G, Assareh H, Jakobsson J: The AAI index, the BIS index and end-tidal concentration during wash in and wash out of sevoflurane. Anaesthesia 58:531-535, 2003.
223. Schnider TW, Luginbühl M, Petersen-Felix S, Mathis J: Unreasonably low bispectral index values in a volunteer with genetically determined low-voltage electroencephalographic signal. Anesthesiology 89:1607-1608, 1998.
224. Wang LP, McLoughlin P, Paech MJ, et al: Low and moderate remifentanil infusion rates do not alter target-controlled infusion propofol concentrations necessary to maintain anesthesia as assessed by bispectral index monitoring. Anesth Analg 104:325-331, 2007.
225. Hans P, Brichant JF, Dewandre PY, et al: Effects of two calculated plasma sufentanil concentrations on the hemodynamic and bispectral index responses to Mayfield head holder application. J Neurosurg Anesthesiol 11:81-85, 1999.
226. Koitabashi T, Johansen JW, Sebel PS: Remifentanil dose/electroencephalogram bispectral response during combined propofol/regional anesthesia. Anesth Analg 94:1530-1533, 2002.
227. Ferenets R, Vanluchene A, Lipping T, et al: Behavior of entropy/complexity measures of the electroencephalogram during propofol-induced sedation: Dose-dependent effects of remifentanil. Anesthesiology 106:696-706, 2007.
228. Yli-Hankala A: Awareness despite low spectral entropy values. Anesth Analg 106:1585, author reply 1586, 2008.
229. Rampil IJ, Kim JS, Lenhardt R, et al: Bispectral EEG index during nitrous oxide administration. Anesthesiology 89:671-677, 1998.
230. Barr G, Jakobsson JG, Owall A, Anderson RE: Nitrous oxide does not alter bispectral index: Study with nitrous oxide as sole agent and as an adjunct to i.v. anaesthesia. Br J Anaesth 82:827-830, 1999.
231. Coste C, Guignard B, Menigaux C, Chauvin M: Nitrous oxide prevents movement during orotracheal intubation without affecting BIS value. Anesth Analg 91:130-135, 2000.
232. Oda Y, Tanaka K, Matsuura T, et al: Nitrous oxide induces paradoxical electroencephalographic changes after tracheal intubation during isoflurane and sevoflurane anesthesia. Anesth Analg 102:1094-1102, 2006.
233. Karalapillai D, Leslie K, Umranikar A, Bjorksten AR: Nitrous oxide and anesthetic requirement for loss of response to command during propofol anesthesia. Anesth Analg 102:1088-1093, 2006.
234. Soto RG, Smith RA, Zaccaria AL, Miguel RV: The effect of addition of nitrous oxide to a sevoflurane anesthetic on BIS, PSI, and entropy. J Clin Monit Comput 20:145-150, 2006.
235. Suzuki M, Edmonds HL Jr, Tsueda K, et al: Effect of ketamine on bispectral index and levels of sedation. J Clin Monit Comput 14:373, 1998.
236. Sakai T, Singh H, Mi WD, et al: The effect of ketamine on clinical endpoints of hypnosis and EEG variables during propofol infusion. Acta Anaesthiol Scand 43:212-216, 1999.
237. Vereecke HE, Vanluchene AL, Mortier EP, et al: The effects of ketamine and rocuronium on the A-Line auditory evoked potential index, bispectral index, and spectral entropy monitor during steady state propofol and remifentanil anesthesia. Anesthesiology 105:1122-1134, 2006.
238. Ekman A, Stålberg E, Sundman E, et al: The effect of neuromuscular block and noxious stimulation on hypnosis monitoring during sevoflurane anesthesia. Anesth Analg 105:688-695, 2007.
239. Forbes AR, Cohen NH, Eger EI II: Pancuronium reduces halothane requirement in man. Anesth Analg 58:497-499, 1979.
240. Bruhn J, Bouillon TW, Shafer SL: Electromyographic activity falsely elevates the bispectral index. Anesthesiology 92:1485-1487, 2000.
241. Vivien B, Di Maria S, Ouattara A, et al: Overestimation of bispectral index in sedated intensive care unit patients revealed by administration of muscle relaxants. Anesthesiology 99:9-17, 2003.
242. Liu N, Chazot T, Huybrechts I, et al: The influence of a muscle relaxant bolus on bispectral and Datex-Ohmeda Entropy values during propofol-remifentanil induced loss of consciousness. Anesth Analg 101:1713-1718, 2005.
243. Messner M, Beese U, Romstöck J, et al: The bispectral index declines during neuromuscular block in fully awake persons. Anesth Analg 97:488-491, 2003.
244. Vasella FC, Frascarolo P, Spahn DR, Magnusson L: Antagonism of neuromuscular blockade but not muscle relaxation affects depth of anaesthesia. Br J Anaesth 94:742-747, 2005.
245. Greif R, Greenwald S, Schweitzer E, et al: Muscle relaxation does not alter hypnotic level during propofol anesthesia. Anesth Analg 94:604-608, 2002.
246. Dahaba AA, Mattweber M, Fuchs A, et al: The effect of different stages of neuromuscular block on the bispectral index and the bispectral index-XP under remifentanil/propofol anesthesia. Anesth Analg 99:781-787, 2004.
247. Inoue S, Kawaguchi M, Sasaoka N, et al: Effects of neuromuscular block on systemic and cerebral hemodynamics and bispectral index during moderate or deep sedation in critically ill patients. Intensive Care Med 32:391-397, 2006.
248. Johansen JW: Esmolol promotes electroencephalographic burst suppression during propofol/alfentanil anesthesia. Anesth Analg 93:1526-1531, 2001.
249. Menigaux C, Guignard B, Adam F, et al: Esmolol prevents movement and attenuates the BIS response to orotracheal intubation. Br J Anaesth 89:857-862, 2002.
250. Oda Y, Nishikawa K, Hase I, Asada A: The short-acting beta1-adrenoceptor antagonists esmolol and landiolol suppress the bispectral index response to tracheal intubation during sevoflurane anesthesia. Anesth Analg 100:733-737, 2005.
251. Andrzejowski J, Sleigh JW, Johnson IA, Sikiotis L: The effect of intravenous epinephrine on the bispectral index and sedation. Anaesthesia 55:761-763, 2000.
252. Triltsch AE, Welte M, von Homeyer P, et al: Bispectral index–guided sedation with dexmedetomidine

in intensive care: A prospective, randomized, double blind, placebo-controlled phase II study. Crit Care Med 30:1007-1014, 2002.
253. Haenggi M, Ypparila H, Hauser K, et al: The effects of dexmedetomidine/remifentanil and midazolam/remifentanil on auditory-evoked potentials and electroencephalogram at light-to-moderate sedation levels in healthy subjects. Anesth Analg 103:1163-1169, 2006.
254. Guignard B, Menigaux C, Dupont X, et al: The effect of remifentanil on the bispectral index change and hemodynamic response after orotracheal intubation. Anesth Analg 90:161-167, 2000.
255. Ropcke H, Rehberg B, Koennen-Bergmann M, et al: Surgical stimulation shifts EEG concentration-response relationship with desflurane. Anesthesiology 94:390-399, discussion 5A, 2001.
256. Hodgson PS, Liu SS: Epidural lidocaine decreases sevoflurane requirement for adequate depth of anesthesia as measured by the bispectral index monitor. Anesthesiology 94:799-803, 2001.
257. Gan TJ, Glass PS, Windsor A, et al: Bispectral index monitoring allows faster emergence and improved recovery from propofol, alfentanil and nitrous oxide anesthesia. Anesthesiology 87:808-815, 1997.
258. Song D, Joshi GP, White PF: Titration of volatile anesthetics using bi-spectral index facilitates recovery after ambulatory anesthesia. Anesthesiology 87:842-848, 1997.
259. Liu SS: Effects of bispectral index monitoring on ambulatory anesthesia: A meta-analysis of randomized controlled trials and a cost analysis. Anesthesiology 101:311-315, 2004.
260. Punjasawadwong Y, Boonjeungmonkol N, Phongchiewboon A: Bispectral index for improving anaesthetic delivery and postoperative recovery. Cochrane Database Syst Rev 4:CD003843, 2007.
261. Vakkuri A, Yli-Hankala A, Sandin R, et al: Spectral entropy monitoring is associated with reduced propofol use and faster emergence in propofol–nitrous oxide–alfentanil anesthesia. Anesthesiology 103:274-279, 2005.
262. Kreuer S, Biedler A, Larsen R, et al: Narcotrend monitoring allows faster emergence and a reduction of drug consumption in propofol-remifentanil anesthesia. Anesthesiology 99:34-41, 2003.
263. Monk TG, Saini V, Weldon BC, et al: Anesthetic management and one-year mortality after noncardiac surgery. Anesth Analg 100:4-10, 2005.
264. Lindholm ML, Träff S, Granath F, et al: Mortality within two years after surgery in relation to low intraoperative BIS values and preexisting malignant disease. Anesth Analg (in press).

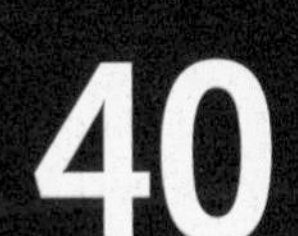

Rebecca A. Schroeder, Atilio Barbeito, Shahar Bar-Yosef, and Jonathan B. Mark

40 Cardiovascular Monitoring

Key Points

1. Although a stethoscope should be present in every anesthetizing location, continuous stethoscopy is an insensitive method for early detection of untoward hemodynamic events.
2. Most automated noninvasive blood pressure measuring devices use an oscillometric measurement technique and rarely cause complications. Caution should be exercised in patients who cannot complain of arm pain, those with irregular rhythms that force repeated cuff inflation, and individuals receiving anticoagulant therapy.
3. Direct arterial pressure monitoring should be widely used in operative patients with severe cardiovascular diseases or those undergoing major surgical procedures that involve significant blood loss or fluid shifts.
4. The Allen test for palmar arch collateral arterial flow is not a reliable method to predict complications from radial artery cannulation. Despite the absence of anatomic collateral flow at the elbow, brachial artery catheterization for perioperative blood pressure monitoring is a safe alternative to radial or femoral arterial catheterization.
5. The accuracy of a directly recorded arterial pressure waveform is determined by the natural frequency and damping coefficient of the pressure monitoring system. Optimal dynamic response of the system will be achieved when the natural frequency is high, thereby allowing accurate pressure recording across a wide range of damping coefficients.
6. Rather than the common placement at the midaxillary line, the preferred position for alignment (or "leveling") of external pressure transducers is approximately 5 cm posterior to the sternomanubrial junction. When using external transducers and fluid-filled monitoring systems, this transducer location will eliminate confounding hydrostatic pressure measurement artifacts.
7. Because of wave reflection and other physical phenomena, arterial blood pressure recorded from peripheral sites has a wider pulse pressure than central aortic pressure does.
8. Dynamic measures of cardiac preload, such as systolic pressure variation and pulse pressure variation, are better predictors of volume responsiveness than static indicators such as central venous pressure (CVP) or pulmonary capillary wedge pressure.
9. Selecting the best site, catheter, and method for safe and effective central venous cannulation requires that the physician consider the purpose of the catheterization, the patient's underlying medical condition, the intended operation, and the skill and experience of the physician performing the procedure. Right internal jugular vein cannulation is favored by most anesthesiologists because of its consistent, predictable anatomic location and its relative ease of access intraoperatively.
10. Methods to reduce mechanical complications from central venous catheters include the use of ultrasound vessel localization, venous pressure measurement before insertion of large catheters, and radiographic confirmation that the catheter tip rests outside the pericardium and parallel to the walls of the superior vena cava.
11. When using CVP as a measure of intravascular volume, the influences of ventricular compliance and intrathoracic pressure must be taken into consideration. In general, a trend in CVP values or its change with therapeutic maneuvers is more reliable than a single measurement. Important pathophysiologic information can be obtained by careful assessment of the CVP waveform morphology.
12. Of the many complications of central venous and pulmonary artery catheters, catheter misuse and data misinterpretation are among the most common.
13. Pulmonary artery wedge pressure is a delayed and damped reflection of left atrial pressure. The wedge pressure provides a close estimate of pulmonary capillary pressure in many cases but may underestimate capillary pressure when postcapillary pulmonary vascular resistance is increased, as in patients with sepsis.

14. Use of central venous, pulmonary artery diastolic, or pulmonary artery wedge pressure as an estimate of left ventricular preload is subject to many confounding factors, including changes in diastolic ventricular compliance and juxtacardiac pressure.
15. Most randomized prospective clinical trials have failed to show that pulmonary artery catheter monitoring results in improved patient outcome. Reasons cited for these results include misinterpretation of catheter-derived data and failure of hemodynamic therapies that are guided by specific hemodynamic indices.
16. Thermodilution cardiac output monitoring, the most widely used clinical technique, is subject to measurement errors introduced by rapid intravenous fluid administration, intracardiac shunts, and tricuspid valve regurgitation.
17. Mixed venous hemoglobin oxygen saturation is a measure of the adequacy of cardiac output relative to body oxygen requirements. It is also dependent on arterial hemoglobin oxygen saturation and hemoglobin concentration.
18. Newer methods of cardiac output monitoring, including esophageal Doppler and pulse contour analysis, allow beat-to-beat estimation of left ventricular stroke volume and measurement of other cardiovascular variables.

Introduction to Cardiovascular Monitoring: Focused Physical Examination

Although cardiovascular monitors receive prime emphasis, the fundamental basis for circulatory monitoring remains in the eyes, hands, and ears of the anesthesiologist. In many ways, the clinician's senses capture more information than even the most sophisticated electronic monitors do. Combined with knowledge, experience, and sound clinical judgment, the clinician's senses offer an integrated, panoramic view of the patient's condition, made even more valuable by an understanding of the clinical context present. Whereas electronic instruments accurately and monotonously collect huge volumes of quantitative data, the clinician plays a vital role in patient monitoring by integrating, evaluating, and interpreting these data.[1] Just as inspection, palpation, and auscultation are the cornerstones of physical examination of the cardiovascular system, these same clinical procedures are fundamental elements of perioperative cardiovascular monitoring. However, they must be adapted and focused on the unique requirements of surgical and critically ill patients, and their limitations must be recognized.

Many standard physical means of assessing the circulation are used throughout an operation. For many healthy patients undergoing minor procedures, these physical signs provide a considerable fraction of the total cardiovascular monitoring. For higher-risk patients and longer, more complicated operations, the extent of supplemental electronic monitoring grows accordingly. However, careful physical assessment still provides the clinician with an all-important backup system to confirm or refute information derived from other monitoring devices. The most obvious, perhaps trivial, example is a patient whose electrocardiogram (ECG) shows asystole. Detection of a normal pulse by direct palpation focuses the anesthesiologist on correcting the monitoring artifact rather than initiating cardiopulmonary resuscitation.

Early advances in cardiovascular assessment beyond basic physical examination were not readily accepted into medical practice. Around 1900, the introduction of sphygmomanometry to measure blood pressure was criticized because it would weaken clinical acuity by blunting the senses and acute perceptions of the clinician. Even stethoscopy had its critics, simply on the basis that it placed the physician at greater distance from the patient.

Palpation of the pulse and its rate and character should not be forgotten in the perioperative setting. Environmental constraints in the operating room may dictate which pulses are accessible for monitoring, but they also provide unique opportunities for pulse monitoring during surgery. For example, during cardiac surgery the beating heart may be observed directly, and palpation of the ascending aorta by the surgeon provides a useful estimate of aortic blood pressure. In fact, the surgeon's evaluation of any arterial pulse within the surgical field should be considered whenever severe hemodynamic instability develops.

Clinical evaluation of venous pressure during anesthesia is technically difficult because of unusual patient positions, positive-pressure mechanical ventilation, and lack of access to observe the neck veins. However, early recognition of venous obstruction in an extremity or in the head and neck may have important clinical consequences. Not only might this observation herald hemodynamic problems for the patient, but communicating these observations to the operating surgeon should also allow timely correction of contributing surgical factors.

Given that the cardiovascular system is responsible for the transport of substrates and by-products to and from all organ systems, monitoring end-organ function can be used to assess the adequacy of cardiovascular performance. Inspection of mucous membranes, skin color, and skin turgor can reveal pertinent clues about hydration, oxygenation, and perfusion. Additional simple clinical techniques include empirical estimation of fluid deficits and blood loss, measurement of urine output, and detection of altered mental status. Unfortunately, interpretation of these clinical signs and symptoms is often confounded by preexisting organ dysfunction and the direct effects of anesthetic drugs on organs. As a result, use of these clinical assessment tools is of limited value in many anesthetized or critically ill patients. Frequently, additional cardiovascular monitoring techniques are required.

Stethoscopy

Although Laennec is credited with introducing the stethoscope into general medical practice in 1818, nearly a century elapsed before Harvey Cushing proposed in 1908 that the stethoscope be used as a routine cardiopulmonary monitoring device during surgery.[2] For many years thereafter, intraoperative monitoring with either a precordial or an esophageal stethoscope became the most common simple method for monitoring ventilation and circulation in anesthetized patients.

Stethoscopy provides a simple and reliable means of listening to heart and breath sounds continuously throughout an operation. The most common equipment used for precordial stethoscopy consists of a heavy metal bell or accumulator attached to a length of rubber or plastic extension tubing and a custom-molded monaural plastic earpiece. Electronically amplified stethoscopes have been designed to improve the quality and clarity of heart and breath sounds but have not supplanted standard inexpensive mechanical devices in everyday practice.[3] Though minimally invasive and practical only for patients receiving general endotracheal anesthesia, the esophageal stethoscope provides monitoring benefits not available with its precordial cousin. Clear breath sounds and distinct heart sounds are audible in most patients when the tip of the stethoscope is positioned 28 to 30 cm from the incisors, and esophageal temperature can be measured with an incorporated thermistor.[4] Although use of the esophageal stethoscope is generally without significant risk, rare complications include hypoxemia from unintended tracheobronchial placement or compression of the membranous posterior portion of the trachea in small infants, loss down the esophagus, detachment of the acoustic cuff, and distortion of surgical anatomy in the neck. Placement of the esophageal stethoscope may also cause pharyngeal or esophageal trauma and interfere with nasogastric tube positioning or transesophageal echocardiography.

Despite the purported value of the precordial or esophageal stethoscope for basic monitoring of patient safety, its widespread application in clinical practice has diminished in recent years.[5,6] This decline may be driven by the routine use of pulse oximetry, capnography, and other electronic monitors that have become ubiquitous.[7] As a practical matter, clinicians may not recognize changing heart or breath sounds as readily as might be expected because of reliance on more modern electronic devices, distraction, or operating room noise. These practice patterns appear to be borne out by the 1993 Australian Incident Monitoring Study, which noted that a stethoscope was used in only 5% of the 1256 critical incidents reported and was the first monitor to detect the morbid incident—cardiac arrest—in only one instance.[5] As a result, the current role of intraoperative stethoscopy as a continuous monitor has become limited to special applications (e.g., pediatric anesthesia) and to institutions with insufficient resources to purchase electronic monitors.

Heart Rate Monitoring

The simplest and least invasive form of cardiac monitoring remains measurement of the heart rate. Under most circumstances in modern anesthesia practice, electronic devices are used to continuously monitor this vital sign and provide an important guide to the influence of anesthetics and surgical stimuli on the patient's condition. The ability to estimate the heart rate quickly with a "finger on the pulse" is a skill as important as this expression is common.

Although any monitor that measures the period of the cardiac cycle can be used to determine the heart rate, the ECG is the most common method used in the operating room (see Chapter 42). Measurement of the heart rate by ECG begins with accurate detection of the R wave and measurement of the R-R interval. The digital value displayed for the heart rate is generated from an algorithm designed to count and average a certain number of beats and then display a number that is updated every 5 to 15 seconds.[8] As a result, transient dysrhythmias may have little impact on the displayed digital heart rate value (Fig. 40-1).

Occasionally, the clinician must check electrode attachment, increase signal gain on the ECG, or select alternative ECG leads to improve the accuracy of heart rate monitoring. Most monitors allow manual adjustment of the threshold or sensitivity for R-wave detection and recognition of electronic pacing spikes. In the operating room, ECG artifacts are common, particularly those caused by the electrosurgical unit. The ECG trace should always be inspected visually to confirm the numeric value for the heart rate displayed on the monitor. In addition, the arterial pressure waveform or the pulse oximeter plethysmograph should be used to confirm the pulse rate in these instances.

Electrical interference in the ECG trace may arise from sources other than the electrosurgical unit. Power line noise appears as a 60-Hz artifact and may be eliminated by selecting narrower-bandpass ECG filters, including a 60-Hz notch filter. Other artifacts result from muscle twitching and fasciculations, as well as from various medical devices, including lithotripsy machines, cardiopulmonary bypass equipment, and fluid warmers.[9] Paced rhythms can produce problems with measurement of the heart rate on the ECG. When tall pacing spikes are present, the monitor may misinterpret these high-amplitude signals as R waves and miscalculate the heart rate. Tall T waves may produce the same artifact when the monitor mistakenly

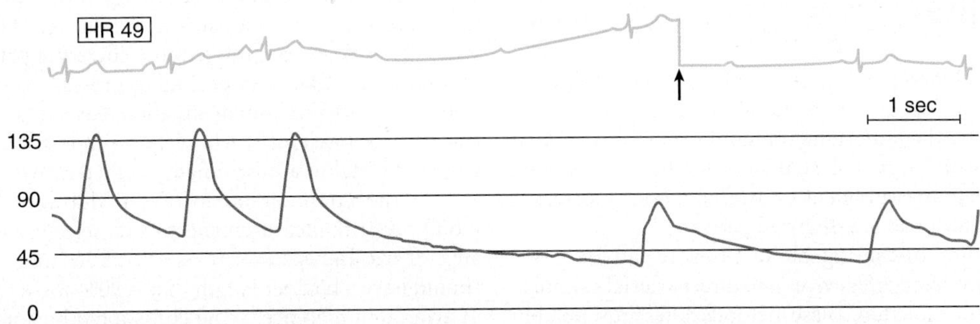

Figure 40-1 Digital heart rate (HR) displays may fail to warn of dangerous bradyarrhythmias. Direct observation of the electrocardiogram (ECG) and the arterial blood pressure traces reveals a complete heart block and a 4-second period of asystole, whereas the digital display reports an HR of 49 beats/min. Note that the ECG filter (*arrow*) corrects the baseline drift so that the trace remains on the recording screen. *(From Mark JB: Atlas of Cardiovascular Monitoring. New York, Churchill Livingstone, 1998, Fig. 13-2.)*

counts these T waves as R waves. These problems may be ameliorated by decreasing ECG gain, adjusting the sensitivity for detection of R waves, changing the ECG lead to one with a smaller pacing spike or T-wave amplitude, or selecting pacing detection modes that distinguish pacing spikes from other ECG features.

Pulse Rate Monitoring

The distinction between heart rate and pulse rate centers on whether a given electrical depolarization and systolic contraction of the heart (heart rate) generate a palpable, peripheral arterial pulsation (pulse rate). Pulse deficit describes the extent to which the pulse rate is less than the heart rate. Such deficit is typically seen in patients with atrial fibrillation, in which short R-R intervals compromise cardiac filling during diastole and result in reduced stroke volume and an imperceptible arterial pulse. The most extreme example of a pulse deficit is electrical-mechanical dissociation, or pulseless electrical activity, seen in patients with cardiac tamponade, extreme hypovolemia, and other conditions in which cardiac contraction does not generate a palpable peripheral pulse.

Most monitors report heart rate and pulse rate separately. The former is measured from the ECG trace and the latter is determined from a selectable pulse source. The pulse oximeter plethysmograph trace is the most common source for measurement of the pulse rate, but it may be of poor quality in patients with severe arterial occlusive disease or marked peripheral vasoconstriction. In addition to indicating the pulse rate, this waveform may also provide supplementary diagnostic clues to cardiovascular function[10,11] (see systolic pressure variation in the later section "Arterial Pressure Monitoring for Prediction of Volume Responsiveness"). Other pulse rate sources include the directly measured arterial pressure waveform and automatic noninvasive blood pressure (NIBP) monitors, which determine the pulse rate from the pressure oscillations detected by the surrounding cuff. Pulse rate monitoring and heart rate monitoring complement one another. Although monitoring both may seem redundant, such redundancy is intentional and being applied to modern computerized monitoring algorithms to reduce measurement errors and false alarms.[12]

Arterial Blood Pressure Monitoring

Like the heart rate, blood pressure is a fundamental cardiovascular vital sign and a critical part of monitoring anesthetized or seriously ill patients. The importance of monitoring this vital sign is underscored by the fact that standards for basic anesthetic monitoring mandate measurement of arterial blood pressure at least every 5 minutes in all anesthetized patients.[13]

Techniques for measuring blood pressure fall into two major categories: indirect cuff devices and direct arterial cannulation and pressure transduction. These methods differ most notably in terms of the physical signal being monitored and their level of invasiveness. Although direct arterial blood pressure measurement is the reference standard against which other methods are compared, even this technique can yield spurious results. Consequently, blood pressure measured in clinical practice with different techniques often yields significantly different values.[14]

Indirect Measurement of Arterial Blood Pressure

Manual Intermittent Techniques

Most indirect methods of measuring blood pressure rely on a sphygmomanometer similar to the one first described by Riva-Rocci in 1896.[15] This apparatus included an arm-encircling inflatable elastic cuff, a rubber bulb to inflate the cuff, and a mercury manometer to measure cuff pressure. Riva-Rocci described the measurement of systolic arterial blood pressure by determining the pressure at which the palpated radial arterial pulse disappeared as the cuff was inflated.

A commonly used variation of the Riva-Rocci method, termed the "return-to-flow technique," records the pressure during cuff deflation at which the pulse reappears and is detected by palpation. When the patient has a finger pulse oximeter or an indwelling arterial catheter in the ipsilateral arm, return to flow can be detected by reappearance of the plethysmographic or arterial pressure waveforms. Return-to-flow methods provide a simple, rapid estimation of systolic blood pressure during urgent situations but do not allow measurement of diastolic blood pressure.

To measure both systolic and diastolic arterial pressure, the most widely used intermittent manual method is the auscultatory technique, originally described by Korotkoff in 1905.[16] Using a sphygmomanometer, cuff, and stethoscope, Korotkoff measured blood pressure by auscultating sounds generated by arterial blood flow. These sounds are a complex series of audible frequencies produced by turbulent flow beyond the partially occluding cuff. The pressure at which the first Korotkoff sound is heard is generally accepted as systolic pressure (phase I). The character of the sound progressively changes (phases II and III), becomes muffled (phase IV), and is finally absent (phase V). Diastolic pressure is recorded at phase IV or V. However, phase V may never occur in certain pathophysiologic states such as aortic regurgitation.[17]

A fundamental shortcoming of the auscultatory method of blood pressure measurement is its reliance on blood flow to generate Korotkoff sounds. Pathologic or iatrogenic causes of decreased peripheral blood flow, such as cardiogenic shock or high-dose vasopressor infusion, can attenuate or obliterate the generation of sound and result in significant underestimation of blood pressure.[18] In contrast, low compliance of the tissues underlying the cuff, as encountered in a shivering patient, will require an excessively high cuff-occluding pressure and produce "pseudohypertension." A similar situation exists in patients with severe calcific arteriosclerosis, whose noncompressible arteries may be palpated distal to a fully inflated cuff (positive Osler sign).[17]

Other common sources of error during intermittent manual blood pressure measurement include selection of an inappropriate cuff size and excessively rapid cuff deflation. The optimal cuff should have a bladder length that is 80% and a width at least 40% of arm circumference.[17] The cuff should be applied snugly, with the bladder centered over the artery and any residual air squeezed out. Although too large a cuff will generally work well and produce little error, use of cuffs that are too small will result in overestimation of blood pressure.[17] The cuff deflation rate is another important variable that influences manual blood pressure measurement. The decrease in cuff pressure should proceed slowly enough for the Korotkoff sounds to be detected and properly assigned to the current pressure in the cuff. Failure to identify the initial Korotkoff sounds will result in a falsely low measurement of blood pressure.

Automated Intermittent Techniques

Many limitations of manual intermittent blood pressure measurement have been overcome by automated NIBP devices, which are now used widely. In addition, automated NIBP devices provide audible alarms and can transfer data to a computerized information system. However, the greatest advantage of automated NIBP devices over manual methods of blood pressure measurement is that they provide frequent, regular blood pressure measurements and free the operator to perform other vital clinical duties.

Most automated NIBP devices are based on oscillometry, a technique first described by Marey in 1876.[17] In this method, variations in cuff pressure resulting from arterial pulsations during cuff deflation are sensed by the monitor and used to determine arterial blood pressure values. The pressure at which the peak amplitude of arterial pulsations occurs corresponds closely to directly measured mean arterial pressure (MAP), and values of systolic and diastolic pressure are derived from proprietary formulas that examine the rate of change of the pressure pulsations.[19,20] Consequently, systolic and diastolic values are less reliable than MAP values.[17] Systolic pressure is typically identified as the pressure at which pulsations are increasing and are at 25% to 50% of maximum. Diastolic pressure is the most unreliable oscillometric measurement and is commonly recorded when the pulse amplitude has declined to a small fraction of its peak value (Fig. 40-2).

Although oscillometry is used primarily in automated NIBP measurement, the same principles may be applied to determine blood pressure manually with a standard cuff and aneroid manometer. If the cuff is deflated slowly until the needle on the aneroid gauge begins to flicker or oscillate, the corresponding pressure value provides a close estimate of systolic blood pressure. Like the return-to-flow technique, "manual oscillometry" can be performed quickly, with only one hand on the inflation bulb and pressure relief valve and observing the aneroid gauge needle for the onset of oscillation.

In clinical practice, oscillometric automated NIBP measurement has focused largely on pressure measured from the upper part of the arm. If a patient's surgical procedure or medical condition requires that the cuff be applied to the calf, ankle, or thigh, an appropriately sized cuff must be used.

Other methods using a variety of sensing techniques, including Doppler, photo-oscillometry, and motion of the arterial wall, have also been described for automated intermittent NIBP measurement.[21] Although these methods have been found to measure blood pressure with reasonable accuracy under limited clinical circumstances, they all require additional sensing transducers, their accuracy in critically ill patients is uncertain, and consequently, none has supplanted the standard oscillometric technique.

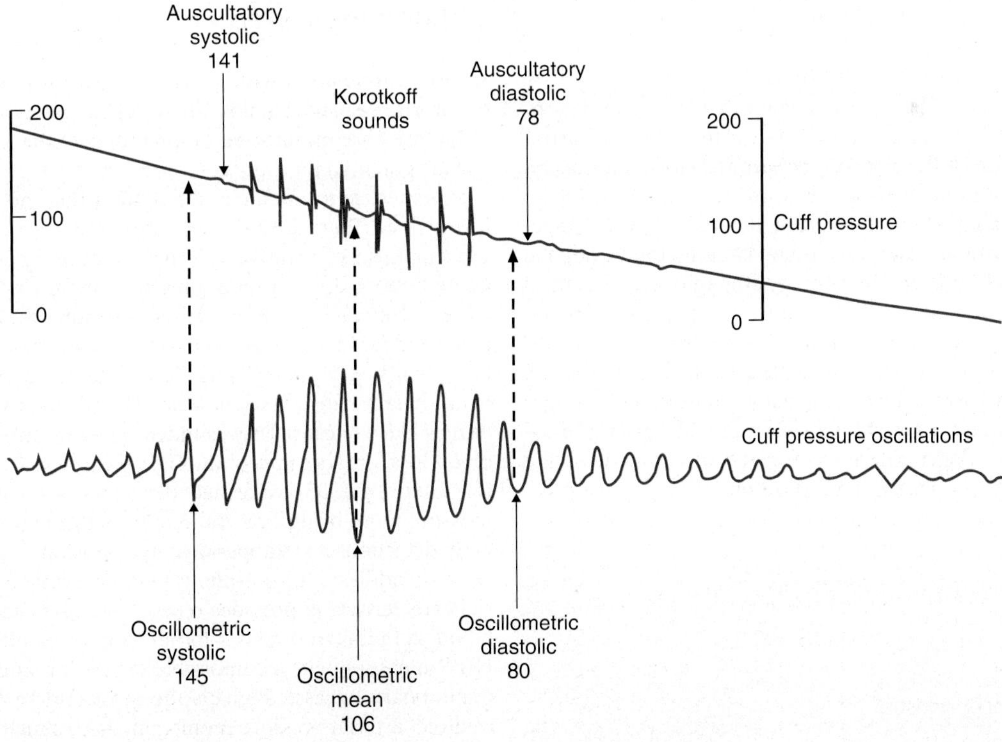

Figure 40-2 Comparison of blood pressure measurements via Korotkoff sounds and oscillometry. Oscillometric systolic blood pressure is recorded at the point where cuff pressure oscillations begin to increase, mean pressure corresponds to the point of maximal oscillations, and diastolic pressure is measured at the point where the oscillations become attenuated. Note the correspondence between these measurements and the Korotkoff sounds that determine auscultatory systolic and diastolic pressure. *(From Geddes LA: Cardiovascular Devices and Their Applications. New York, John Wiley, 1984, Fig. 34-2. Reprinted by permission of John Wiley & Sons, Inc.)*

Even though automated NIBP measurements have been shown to closely approximate directly measured arterial pressure in controlled clinical settings, numerous investigations underscore the disagreement that often exists when direct and indirect pressure measurements are compared, particularly when techniques are compared under changing hemodynamic conditions.[14,17] Standards for performance of automated NIBP devices have been advanced by the Association for the Advancement of Medical Instrumentation, the British Hypertension Society, and other organizations. These standards generally require accuracy within 5 mm Hg with respect to reference methods.[17,21] However, the clinical performance of an NIBP monitor should be evaluated by other criteria, including the number of outlier values, duration of discrepancies, magnitude of individual errors, and performance under variable clinical conditions.[21]

Complications of Noninvasive Blood Pressure Measurement

Although automated blood pressure measurement techniques are considered noninvasive and relatively safe, complications have been reported, including rare severe events such as compartment syndrome (Box 40-1).[22] These morbid events occur more often after prolonged periods of excessively frequent cycles of cuff inflation/deflation and are due to trauma or impaired distal limb perfusion. Other factors that may contribute include cuff misplacement across a joint or repeated attempts to determine blood pressure in the presence of an artifact-producing condition such as involuntary muscle tremors. Caution should be exercised when using these monitors in patients with depressed consciousness, preexisting peripheral neuropathies, arterial or venous insufficiency, or irregular cardiac rhythms, as well as in those receiving anticoagulant or thrombolytic therapy.

Automated Continuous Techniques

Advances in microprocessor and servomechanical control technology have enabled noninvasive techniques to provide a reasonable representation of the arterial pressure waveform and nearly continuous assessment of blood pressure without resorting to direct arterial cannulation. One such device measures finger blood pressure with an arterial volume-clamp method designed and first reported by Penaz in 1973.[23] Although several clinical investigators have demonstrated reasonable accuracy of finger blood pressure as a surrogate for intra-arterial pressure measurements, a number of factors have precluded more widespread application of this technology.[24] In many circumstances, finger blood pressure monitoring will not reflect brachial arterial pressure. In addition, finger arteries are prone to spasm with the potential for distal ischemia, hand position will influence pressure values, and blood sampling cannot be performed without indwelling catheters.

Other automatic continuous noninvasive techniques have been used to measure blood pressure by applying technologies based on arterial wall displacement, pulse transit time, arterial tonometry, and other methods. All techniques have limitations, including the need for calibration, sensitivity to motion artifact, and limited applicability in critically ill patients.[17,21,25] It remains unclear whether any noninvasive technique will reduce the need for direct arterial pressure monitoring or whether these methods will replace automated intermittent oscillometry as the standard NIBP monitoring method in anesthesia and critical care.

Box 40-1 Complications of Noninvasive Blood Pressure Measurement

- Pain
- Petechiae and ecchymoses
- Limb edema
- Venous stasis and thrombophlebitis
- Peripheral neuropathy
- Compartment syndrome

Box 40-2 Indications for Arterial Cannulation

- Continuous, real-time blood pressure monitoring
- Planned pharmacologic or mechanical cardiovascular manipulation
- Repeated blood sampling
- Failure of indirect arterial blood pressure measurement
- Supplementary diagnostic information from the arterial waveform
- Determination of volume responsiveness from systolic pressure or pulse pressure variation

Direct Measurement of Arterial Blood Pressure

Arterial cannulation with continuous pressure transduction and waveform display remains the accepted reference standard for blood pressure monitoring despite the fact that it is more costly, has the potential for more complications, and requires more technical expertise to initiate and maintain than noninvasive monitoring does. There are a number of reasons why clinicians should use this form of invasive pressure monitoring (Box 40-2). First and foremost, direct arterial pressure monitoring should be used when moment-to-moment blood pressure changes are anticipated and rapid detection is vital. These conditions typically apply to patients with preexisting severe cardiovascular disease or hemodynamic instability or when the planned operative procedure is likely to cause large, sudden cardiovascular changes, rapid blood loss, or large fluid shifts. The Australian Incident Monitoring Study of 1993 confirmed the superiority of direct arterial pressure monitoring over indirect monitoring techniques for the early detection of intraoperative hypotension.[26]

In addition to continuous blood pressure monitoring, arterial catheterization provides reliable vascular access for frequent blood sampling and allows monitoring of blood pressure when NIBP measurement is impossible (as during nonpulsatile cardiopulmonary bypass). Perhaps the most underemphasized value of direct arterial pressure monitoring is that analysis of the arterial pressure waveform may provide many important diagnostic clues to the patient's condition. More than a half-century ago, Eather and colleagues emphasized these diagnostic insights in a paper that first introduced and advocated direct monitoring of "arterial pressure and pressure pulse contours" in anesthetized patients.[27] Some of these diagnostic insights are readily apparent and commonly sought, such as identification of the arterial dicrotic notch to guide proper timing for intra-aortic balloon counterpulsation, whereas others are more subtle, such as recognition of excessive variation in systolic blood pressure as a sign of hypovolemia.[28]

Percutaneous Radial Artery Cannulation

The radial artery is the most common site for invasive blood pressure monitoring in anesthesia and critical care because it is technically easy to cannulate and complications are uncommon, in part because of the good collateral circulation of the hand.[29] Slogoff and coauthors described the results of radial artery cannulation in 1700 cardiovascular surgical patients who underwent the procedure without ischemic complications despite evidence of radial artery occlusion after decannulation in more than 25% of the patients.[30]

Before attempting radial artery cannulation, many clinicians assess the adequacy of collateral flow to the hand by performing a modified Allen test. This bedside examination, originally described by E. V. Allen in 1929, provided a technique to assess arterial stenosis in the hands of patients with thromboangiitis obliterans.[31] To perform the Allen test, the examiner compresses the radial and ulnar arteries and asks the patient to make a tight fist to exsanguinate the palm. The patient then opens the fist while avoiding hyperextension of the wrist or fingers, and as occlusion of the ulnar artery is released, the color of the open palm is observed. Normally, the palm will show a striking flush in several seconds; severely reduced ulnar collateral flow is present when the palm remains pale for more than 10 seconds.

Although the Allen test is often used to identify patients at high risk for ischemic complications from radial artery catheterization, the predictive value of this test is uncertain. Numerous reports of permanent ischemic sequelae note that a normal Allen test result was present before catheterization.[32] In contrast, there are many descriptions of uncomplicated radial artery catheterization despite the presence of an abnormal Allen test result before the procedure.[30] In recent years, the radial artery has been used safely as an access site for coronary stenting or excised and used as a graft for coronary bypass surgery, even in individuals with abnormal Allen test results.[33,34] Although most patients show radial artery dominance with respect to overall hand perfusion, total radial artery occlusion does not appear to compromise distal perfusion, perhaps because of collateral recruitment.[34] Furthermore, Allen test results bear little relation to distal blood flow, as measured by fluorescein dye injection or photoplethysmography. Although it is obviously of great importance that the clinician minimize the chance of significant distal ischemia from arterial pressure monitoring, the Allen test cannot be relied on to avoid this adverse outcome.

Consistent, successful radial artery cannulation should be easily achievable with attention to a number of procedural details. The wrist and hand are immobilized in mild dorsiflexion and secured with the wrist resting across a soft pad. Excessive dorsiflexion of the wrist should be avoided because of the possibility of attenuating the pulse. The course of the radial artery proximal to the wrist is identified by gentle palpation, the skin is prepared with an antiseptic, and a local anesthetic is injected intradermally and subcutaneously alongside the artery. Arterial catheterization can then be performed with a standard intravenous catheter or an integrated guidewire-catheter assembly designed for this purpose. A recent educational video provides greater detail about this standard procedure.[35]

Once the catheter is fully advanced into the vessel lumen, the radial artery is occluded by applying proximal pressure, the needle is removed, the monitoring system pressure tubing is fastened to the catheter, an appropriate sterile dressing is applied, and the apparatus is taped and secured to the wrist. Although a soft armboard can be used to maintain the wrist in an anatomically neutral position during arterial pressure monitoring, extreme wrist dorsiflexion should always be avoided because it may lead to median nerve injury.[36,37]

Some clinicians choose the "transfixion" technique for arterial cannulation, in which the front and back walls of the artery are punctured intentionally, the needle is removed from the catheter, and the catheter is withdrawn into the vessel lumen. Although it is unnecessary to place an additional hole in the back wall of the radial artery for successful cannulation, the technique per se does not appear to influence the success rate or incidence of postcannulation complications.

Other aids to arterial cannulation include the use of ultrasound imaging to guide catheter insertion.[38] This may be particularly helpful when standard placement attempts by palpation have failed. Although some authors have suggested that ultrasound or guidewire-based techniques will improve success rates of arterial cannulation, it appears that this is more a function of operator experience and personal preference.[39]

Alternative Arterial Pressure Monitoring Sites

If the radial arteries are unsuitable for monitoring pressure, several alternative cannulation sites are available. The *ulnar artery* is cannulated with a technique much like that described for the radial artery.[40] Even in circumstances in which previous attempts to cannulate the ipsilateral radial artery have failed, the ulnar artery may be cannulated safely.[30]

Although in theory the *brachial artery* does not have the anatomic benefit of the collateral circulation present in the hand, clinical trials have confirmed the safety of this cannulation site. Bazaral and coauthors reported the use of more than 3000 brachial artery catheters in patients undergoing cardiac surgery over a 3-year period, with only one patient requiring postoperative thrombectomy and no untoward sequelae.[41] A slightly longer catheter is preferred for the brachial site because of the need for the catheter to traverse the elbow joint. Other peripheral arteries occasionally chosen for monitoring pressure include the *dorsalis pedis*, *posterior tibial*, and *superficial temporal arteries*. The dorsalis pedis and posterior tibial arteries are generally reserved for pediatric applications.

The *axillary artery* provides another site for long-term pressure monitoring. Advantages include patient comfort, mobility, and access to a central arterial pressure waveform. Complications appear to be infrequent and similar in incidence to radial and femoral artery catheterization.[42] If the axillary approach is chosen, the left side is preferred over the right because the axillary catheter tip will lie distal to the aortic arch and great vessels. Clinicians should be aware, however, that the risk of cerebral embolization is increased whenever more centrally located arterial catheters are used.

The *femoral artery* is the largest artery commonly selected for monitoring blood pressure, and it appears to have a safety record comparable to that of other sites.[42] As with axillary artery pressure monitoring, the femoral artery waveform more closely resembles aortic pressure than do waveforms recorded from peripheral sites. When compared with radial artery catheterization, the risk of distal ischemia after femoral artery cannulation may be reduced because of the large diameter of the artery, but atherosclerotic plaque embolization is more likely during initial guidewire and catheter placement. Catheterization of the femoral artery is best achieved with a guidewire technique. The operator must be careful to puncture the femoral artery below the inguinal ligament, thereby limiting the risk of arterial injury causing uncontained hemorrhage into the pelvis or peritoneum, a potentially catastrophic complication.[43]

Complications of Direct Arterial Pressure Monitoring

Widespread application of invasive arterial pressure monitoring in anesthesia and intensive care is related, no doubt, to the extremely good safety record of this technique. Large clinical investigations confirm the low incidence of long-term complications after radial artery cannulation, in particular, the small risk of distal ischemia, which is probably less than 0.1%.[29,30,42] Although vascular complications from radial artery cannulation are uncommon, factors that may increase risk include vasospastic arterial disease, previous arterial injury, thrombocytosis, protracted shock, high-dose vasopressor administration, prolonged cannulation, and infection.[44,45]

Additional rare, but serious complications have been reported after arterial cannulation (Box 40-3). In most cases there were technical problems during catheter placement or confounding medical problems such as shock or coagulopathy. The Australian Incident Monitoring Study provides some noteworthy observational data on the incidence and types of complications of blood pressure monitoring.[26,46] Of 2000 untoward clinical events reported in this investigation, only 13 were related to peripheral arterial cannulation, less than the number associated with central venous or peripheral venous cannulation (18 and 33 incidents, respectively). Five of these 13 cases involved equipment faults or misassembly, in 3 cases the arterial line was mistaken for an intravenous line and used for injection of drugs, in 3 cases the arterial line was either disrupted or kinked, in 1 case a fragment of guidewire broke off inside the patient, and in only 1 instance did transient vasospasm follow radial artery cannulation. A second report from this study noted that direct pressure monitoring failed or gave misleading results in 10 instances, including 5 in which there was either incorrect calibration, incorrect interpretation of the pressure display, or unrecognized subclavian artery stenosis. These data suggest that most complications of direct arterial pressure monitoring can be attributed to equipment misuse. This serves to highlight the importance of having a backup system readily available for manual measurement of blood pressure.

Box 40-3 Complications of Direct Arterial Pressure Monitoring

- Distal ischemia, pseudoaneurysm, arteriovenous fistula
- Hemorrhage, hematoma
- Arterial embolization
- Local infection, sepsis
- Peripheral neuropathy
- Misinterpretation of data
- Misuse of equipment

Technical Aspects of Direct Blood Pressure Measurement

Direct measurement of arterial blood pressure requires that the pressure waveform from the cannulated artery be reproduced accurately on the bedside monitor. Not surprisingly, the displayed pressure signal is influenced significantly by the measuring system, including the arterial catheter, extension tubing, stopcocks, flush devices, transducer, amplifier, and recorder.[47]

Blood pressure monitoring systems used in the operating room and intensive care units are described as underdamped, second-order dynamic systems.[47-49] These fluid-filled systems may be modeled after mass-spring systems that demonstrate simple harmonic motion and exhibit similar behavior that depends on the physical properties of elasticity, mass, and friction. These three properties determine the system's operating characteristics, termed the *frequency response* or *dynamic response*, which in turn are characterized by two important system parameters, *natural frequency* (f_n, ω) and *damping coefficient* (ζ, Z, α, D). The natural frequency of the monitoring system quantifies how rapidly the system oscillates, and the damping coefficient quantifies the frictional forces that act on the system and determine how rapidly it comes to rest. Both parameters may be estimated or measured at the bedside, and they dramatically influence the appearance of the recorded pressure waveform.

Natural Frequency, Damping Coefficient, and Dynamic Response of Pressure Monitoring Systems

The arterial blood pressure waveform is a periodic complex wave that can be reproduced by Fourier analysis, which recreates the original complex pressure wave by summing a series of simpler sine waves of different amplitudes and frequencies.[50,51] The original pressure wave has a characteristic periodicity termed the *fundamental frequency*, which is equal to the pulse rate. Although the pulse rate is reported in beats per minute, fundamental frequency is reported in cycles per second or hertz (Hz).

The sine waves that sum to produce the complex wave have frequencies that are multiples or harmonics of the fundamental frequency. A crude arterial waveform that displays a systolic upstroke, systolic peak, dicrotic notch, and so forth can be reconstructed with reasonable accuracy from two sine waves, the fundamental frequency, and the second harmonic (Fig. 40-3). If the original arterial pressure waveform contains high-frequency components such as a steep systolic upstroke, higher-frequency sine waves (and more harmonics) are needed to provide faithful reconstruction of the original pressure waveform. As a general rule, 6 to 10 harmonics are required to provide distortion-free reproduction of most arterial pressure waveforms.[50,52] Hence, accurate blood pressure measurement in a patient with a pulse rate of 120 beats/min (2 cycles/sec or 2 Hz) requires a monitoring system dynamic response of 12 to 20 Hz. The faster the heart rate and the steeper the systolic pressure upstroke, the greater the dynamic response demands on the monitoring system.

If the monitoring system has a natural frequency that is too low, frequencies in the monitored pressure waveform will overlap the natural frequency of the measurement system. As a result, the system will resonate and pressure waveforms recorded on the monitor will be exaggerated or amplified versions of true intra-arterial pressure (Fig. 40-4). This phenomenon is the familiar

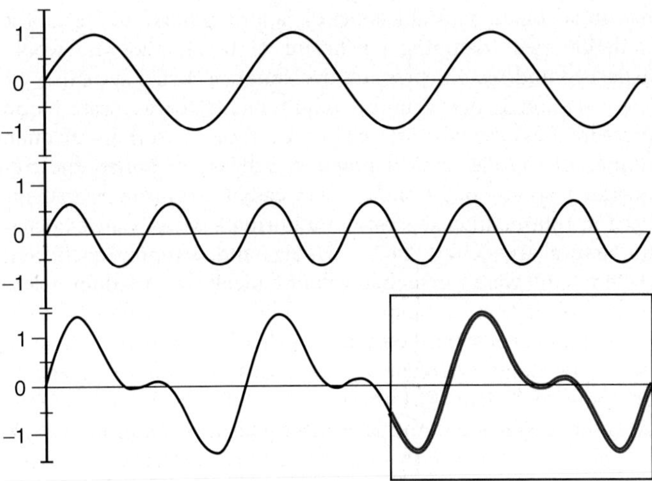

Figure 40-3 Arterial blood pressure waveform produced by summation of sine waves. The fundamental wave (*top*) added to 63% of the second harmonic wave (*middle*) results in a pressure wave (*bottom*) that resembles an arterial blood pressure waveform (*box*). *(From Mark JB: Atlas of Cardiovascular Monitoring. New York, Churchill Livingstone, 1998, Fig. 9-1.)*

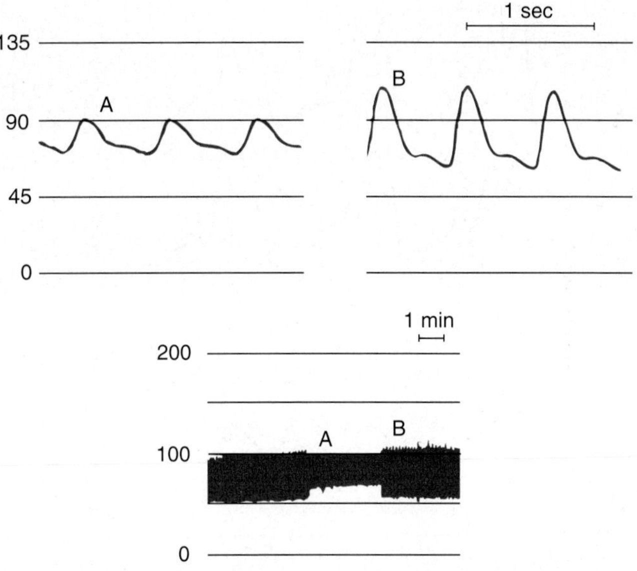

Figure 40-5 Overdamped arterial pressure waveform. The overdamped pressure waveform (A) shows a diminished pulse pressure when compared with the normal waveform (B). The slow-speed recording below demonstrates a 3-minute period of damped arterial pressure. Despite the damped pressure waveform, mean arterial pressure remains unchanged during this period. *(From Mark JB: Atlas of Cardiovascular Monitoring. New York, Churchill Livingstone, 1998, Fig. 9-3.)*

arterial pressure waveform that displays overshoot, ringing, or resonance. In these instances, the recorded systolic blood pressure overestimates true intra-arterial pressure.

In addition to a sufficiently high natural frequency, the bedside monitoring system must also have an appropriate damping coefficient. An overdamped arterial pressure waveform is recognized by its slurred upstroke, absent dicrotic notch, and loss of fine detail. Severely overdamped pressure waves display a falsely narrowed pulse pressure, although MAP may remain reasonably accurate (Fig. 40-5). In contrast, underdamped pressure waveforms display systolic pressure overshoot and contain additional artifacts produced by the measurement system that are not part of the original intravascular pressure wave (see Fig. 40-4). It is a mistake to attach physiologic significance to these small artifactual waves produced by an underdamped monitoring system that continues to ring or oscillate abnormally in response to the input pressure signal.

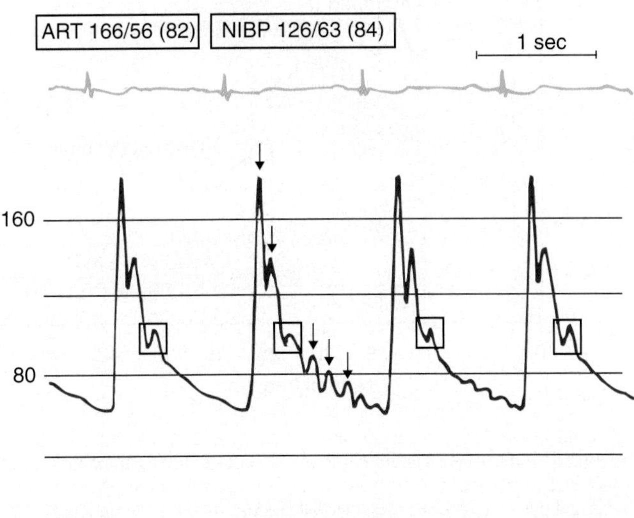

Figure 40-4 Underdamped arterial pressure waveform. Systolic pressure overshoot and additional small, nonphysiologic pressure waves (*arrows*) distort the waveform and make it hard to discern the dicrotic notch (*boxes*). Digital values displayed for direct arterial blood pressure (ART, 166/56; mean, 82 mm Hg) and noninvasive blood pressure (NIBP, 126/63; mean, 84 mm Hg) show the differences in pressure measurement that arise because of an underdamped arterial pressure waveform. *(From Mark JB: Atlas of Cardiovascular Monitoring. New York, Churchill Livingstone, 1998, Fig 9-4.)*

Most catheter-transducer systems are underdamped but have an acceptable natural frequency that exceeds 12 Hz. If the system's natural frequency is lower than 7.5 Hz, the pressure waveform is often distorted, and no amount of damping adjustment can restore the monitored waveform to adequately resemble the original waveform.[47] If, on the other hand, the natural frequency can be increased sufficiently (e.g., 24 Hz), damping will have minimal effect on the monitored waveform, and faithful reproduction of intravascular pressure is achieved more easily (Figs. 40-6 and 40-7). In other words, the lower the natural frequency of the monitoring system, the more narrow the range of damping coefficients that can be tolerated to ensure faithful reproduction of the pressure wave. For example, if the monitoring system's natural frequency is 10 Hz, the damping coefficient must be between 0.45 and 0.6 for accurate monitoring of the pressure waveform. If the damping coefficient is too low, the monitoring system will be underdamped, resonate, and display factitiously elevated systolic blood pressure; if the damping coefficient is too high, the system will be overdamped, systolic pressure will be falsely decreased, and fine detail in the pressure trace will be lost.

From these considerations it follows that a pressure monitoring system will have optimal dynamic response if its natural frequency is as high as possible.[51] In theory, this is best achieved by using short lengths of stiff pressure tubing and limiting the

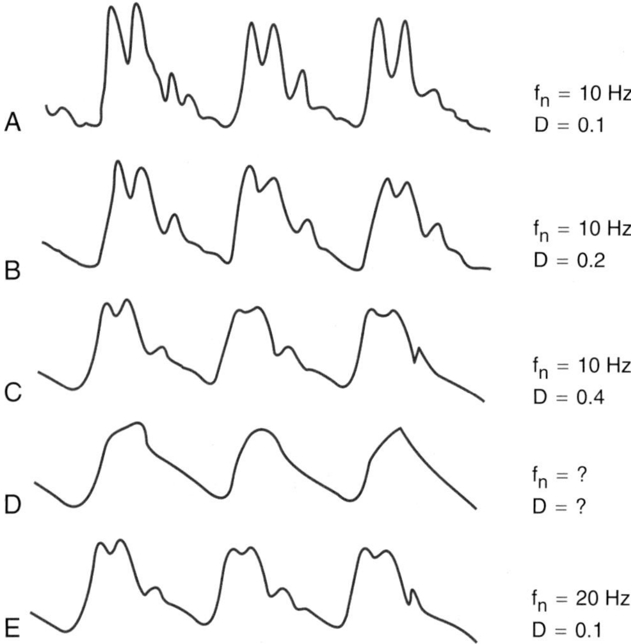

Figure 40-6 Interaction between damping coefficient (D) and natural frequency (f_n) in pressure waveform recordings. **A,** An underdamped pressure waveform (f_n = 10 Hz; D = 0.1) displays small artifactual waves and systolic pressure overshoot. **B,** A small increase in D (0.2) diminishes these artifacts. **C,** Critical damping (D = 0.4) provides an accurate pressure waveform even though f_n remains low. **D,** Overdamping results in loss of fine detail and precludes determination of f_n or D. **E,** Increased f_n (20 Hz) allows a low D (0.1) to have minimal impact on waveform morphology. Notice the similarities between waveforms **C** and **E**. *(From Mark JB: Atlas of Cardiovascular Monitoring. New York, Churchill Livingstone, 1998, Fig. 9-7.)*

number of stopcocks and other monitoring system appliances. Blood clots and air bubbles trapped and concealed in stopcocks and other connection points will have similar adverse influences on the system's dynamic response. As a general rule, adding air bubbles to monitoring systems will not improve their dynamic response because any increase in system damping is always accompanied by a decrease in natural frequency. Somewhat paradoxically, monitoring system resonance may increase and cause even greater systolic pressure overshoot (Fig. 40-8).

To assess the amount of distortion existing in a pressure monitoring system, the fast-flush test provides a convenient bedside method for determining the system's dynamic response.[47,49,51] To perform this test, the fast-flush valve is opened briefly, and the resulting flush artifact is examined. Natural frequency is inversely proportional to the time between adjacent oscillation peaks. It can be calculated as 1 cycle/1.7 mm × 25 mm/sec = 14.7 cycles/sec (14.7 Hz) (Fig. 40-9). Monitoring systems with shorter oscillation cycles will have higher natural frequencies.[51]

The damping coefficient is related to the amplitudes of successive oscillation peaks. The amplitude ratio thus derived indicates how quickly the measuring system comes to rest. The damping coefficient can be calculated mathematically, but it is usually determined graphically from the amplitude ratio.[47,51] For example, if the amplitudes of two successive oscillation cycles are 24 and 17 mm, the amplitude ratio is 17/24, or 0.71. This corresponds to a damping coefficient of 0.11 based on the graphic solution (Fig. 40-9). Note that the monitoring system illustrated has an adequate natural frequency (approximately 15 Hz) but is underdamped (damping coefficient of 0.11), and one would expect to find systolic pressure overshoot in such a system.

Although the technical requirements for accurate blood pressure measurement are well known, these conditions are often unmet in routine clinical practice. Schwid examined the frequency response of 30 radial artery catheter-transducer systems used in routine intensive care monitoring.[53] Mean values (± SD) for natural frequency (14.7 ± 3.7 Hz) and damping coefficient (0.24 ± 0.07) were worse than values typically reported for measurements made under laboratory conditions, instead falling in the underdamped response region reported by Gardner.[47] Furthermore, the range of frequency responses (10.2 to 25.3 Hz) and damping coefficients (0.15 to 0.44) measured in this setting suggests that distortion of the arterial waveform is common in clinical practice, particularly systolic arterial pressure overshoot resulting from an underdamped system (see Fig. 40-7).

Components of Pressure Monitoring Systems

Arterial pressure monitoring systems have a number of components, beginning with the intra-arterial catheter and including extension tubing, stopcocks, in-line blood sampling set, pressure transducer, continuous-flush device, and electronic cable connecting the bedside monitor and waveform display screen. The stopcocks in the system provide sites for blood sampling and allow the transducer to be exposed to atmospheric pressure to establish a zero reference value. Needleless blood sampling ports and in-line aspiration systems permit drawing of blood without the use of sharp needles and allow aspirated waste blood to be

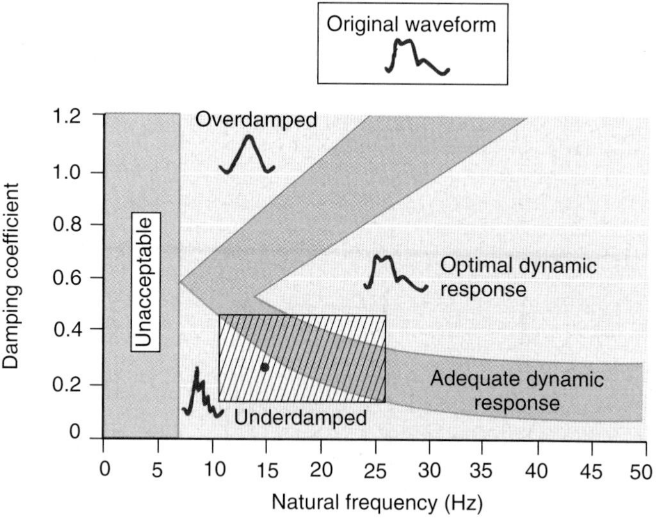

Figure 40-7 Interaction between damping coefficient and natural frequency. Depending on these two system parameters, catheter tubing-transducer systems fall into one of five different dynamic response ranges. Systems with an optimal dynamic response will faithfully record the most demanding pressure waveforms, whereas those with an adequate dynamic response will accurately record most pressure waveforms seen in clinical practice. Overdamped and underdamped systems introduce artifacts characteristic of these technical limitations. Systems with a natural frequency of less than 7 Hz are considered unacceptable. The *rectangular crosshatched box* indicates the ranges of damping coefficients and natural frequencies commonly encountered in clinical pressure measurement systems. The point within the box shows the mean values of 30 such systems recorded by Schwid.[53] *(From Mark JB: Atlas of Cardiovascular Monitoring. New York, Churchill Livingstone, 1998, Figs.9-6, 9-8, and 9-11.)*

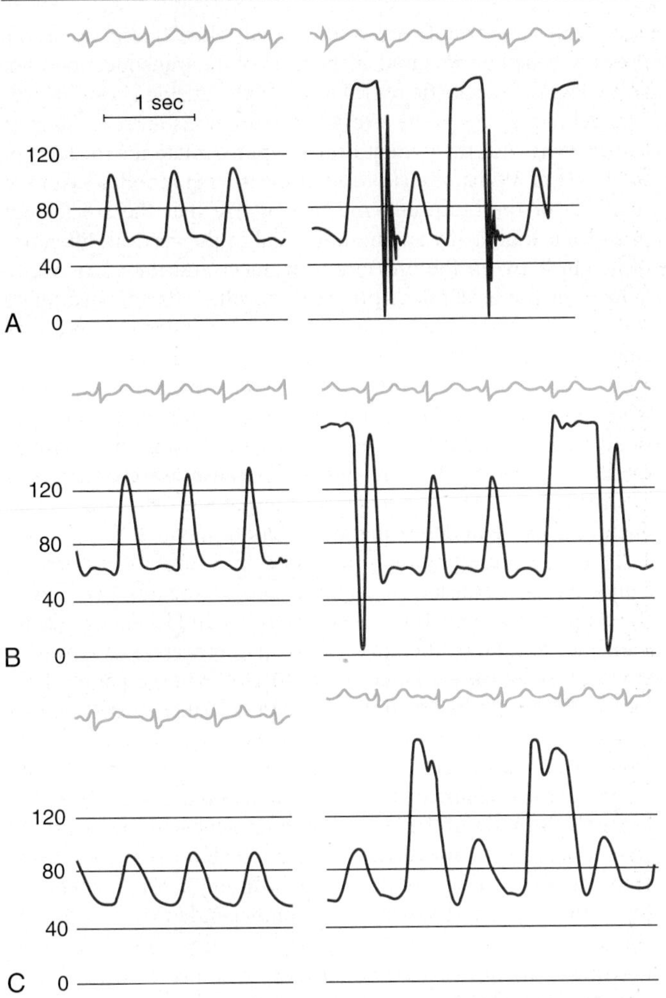

Figure 40-8 Effect of small air bubbles within arterial pressure monitoring systems. Arterial pressure waveforms are displayed, along with superimposed fast-flush square-wave artifacts. **A,** The original monitoring system has an adequate dynamic response (natural frequency, 17 Hz; damping coefficient, 0.2). **B,** A small 0.1-mL air bubble added to the monitoring system produces a paradoxical increase in arterial blood pressure. Note the decreased natural frequency of the system. **C,** A larger 0.5-mL air bubble further degrades the dynamic response and produces spurious arterial hypotension. *(From Mark JB: Atlas of Cardiovascular Monitoring. New York, Churchill Livingstone, 1998, Fig. 9-14.)*

returned to the patient within a convenient closed system. Modifications such as these are intended to reduce the incidence of needle injury and decrease waste of the patient's blood during sampling. However, these additional features may degrade the dynamic response of the monitoring system and further exacerbate systolic arterial pressure overshoot.

The flush device provides a continuous, slow (1 to 3 mL/hr) infusion of saline to purge the monitoring system and prevent thrombus formation within the arterial catheter. Dextrose solutions should not be used because flush contamination of sampled blood may cause serious errors in blood glucose measurement.[54] A dilute concentration of heparin (1 to 2 units heparin/mL saline) has been added to the flush solution to further reduce the incidence of catheter thrombosis, but this practice increases the risk for heparin-induced thrombocytopenia and should be avoided. The flush device not only ensures continuous slow flushing of the line and catheter but also includes a spring-loaded valve for periodic, high-pressure flushing. This rapid flushing is used to purge the extension line of blood after an arterial sample has been taken or to restore the dynamic response characteristics of the pressure monitoring system, which will otherwise slowly deteriorate over time.[55]

Transducer Setup: Zeroing and Leveling

Before initiating patient monitoring, the pressure transducer must be zeroed, calibrated, and leveled to the appropriate position on the patient. The initial step in this process is to expose the transducer to atmospheric pressure by opening the adjacent stopcock to air, pressing the zero pressure button on the monitor, and

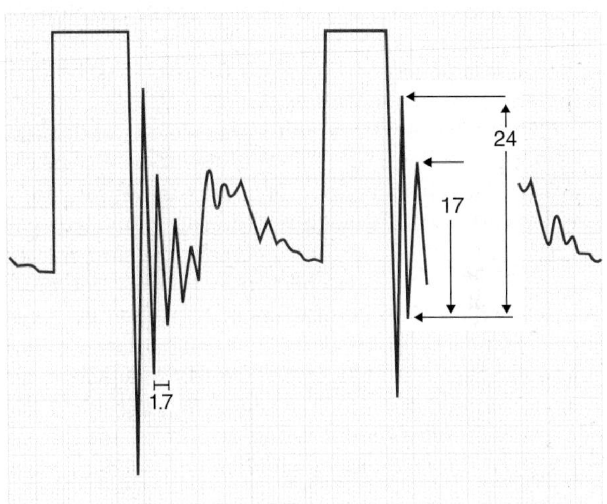

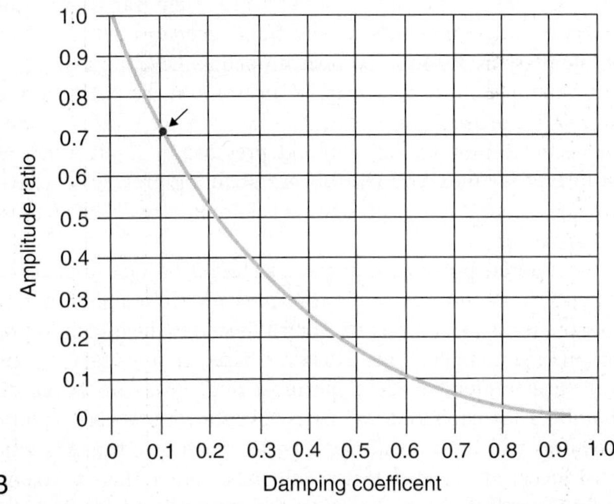

Figure 40-9 Clinical measurement of natural frequency and damping coefficient. **A,** Two square-wave fast-flush artifacts interrupt an arterial pressure waveform recorded on standard 1-mm grid paper at a speed of 25 mm/sec. Natural frequency is determined by measuring the period of one cycle of adjacent oscillation peaks (1.7 mm). The damping coefficient is determined by measuring the heights of adjacent oscillation peaks (17 and 24 mm). From these measurements a natural frequency of 14.7 Hz and an amplitude ratio of 0.71 may be calculated. See text for greater detail. **B,** Relationship between amplitude ratio and damping coefficient. The amplitude ratio determined in the fast-flush test in **A** corresponds to a damping coefficient of 0.11. *(From Mark JB: Atlas of Cardiovascular Monitoring. New York, Churchill Livingstone, 1998, Figs.9-9 and 9-10.)*

thereby establishing the zero pressure reference value. The transducer now has a reference—ambient atmospheric pressure—against which all intravascular pressures are measured. This process underscores the fact that all pressures displayed on the monitor are referenced to atmospheric pressure outside the body. Although clinicians generally refer to "zeroing the transducer," the transducer is actually exposed to atmospheric pressure through an open stopcock affixed to the transducer. To be precise, it is this air-fluid interface at the level of the stopcock that is the zero pressure locus. This point must be aligned with a specific position on the patient to ensure the correct transducer level.

When a significant change in pressure occurs, the zero reference value can be rechecked quickly by opening the stopcock and noting that the pressure value on the bedside monitor is still zero.[52] Occasionally, a faulty transducer, cable, or monitor will cause the zero baseline to drift. Though uncommon with modern monitoring components, this zero drift artifact must be identified to avoid important diagnostic errors.[56,57]

Historically, calibration of the transducer was the next step after zeroing. Calibration is an adjustment in system gain to ensure accurate transducer measurement relative to a known reference pressure value. Though traditionally calibrated against a mercury manometer, current disposable pressure transducers meet accuracy standards established by the Association for the Advancement of Medical Instrumentation and the American National Standards Institute.[56] As a result, bedside calibration of the transducer is no longer performed. Nonetheless, on rare occasion, despite successful transducer zeroing, the measured blood pressure values seem erroneous, and a malfunctioning pressure transducer, cable, or monitor must be suspected and replaced.[57]

The final step in transducer setup is to adjust the pressure monitoring zero point to the appropriate level relative to the patient. Note that transducer zeroing and leveling are two distinct procedures. Zeroing exposes the transducer to ambient atmospheric pressure through an open stopcock. Leveling assigns this zero reference point to a specific position on the patient's body. Although precise location of the zero reference level is essential for accurate monitoring of blood pressure, it is also critically important for measurement of cardiac filling pressures, where a small absolute error in pressure measurement will cause a large relative error.

Arterial pressure transducers should be placed at a level that will best estimate aortic root pressure. In a supine patient, pressure transducer levels are often adjusted to the midchest position in the midaxillary line. However, based on physical principles and measurement of the uppermost fluid levels in the cardiac chambers, Courtois and associates have shown that cardiac filling pressures will be overestimated by as much as 7 mm Hg when transducers are leveled to the midchest rather than a position approximately 5 cm posterior to the sternal border.[58] This preferred (more anterior) transducer location obviates the confounding effect of hydrostatic pressure on cardiac filling pressure measurements. Inasmuch as this transducer location will provide the most accurate measurement of left ventricular pressure, the same transducer level is optimal for arterial blood pressure measurement. Other investigators have confirmed that leveling of pressure transducers to the midchest position will cause overestimation of cardiac filling pressure and presumably aortic root pressure.[59]

In some circumstances, the clinician may choose to adjust the arterial transducer level to a different position on the body. It is critically important to recognize that when this is done, the pressure is being measured at the level of the transducer and not at the level of the aortic root. For example, during sitting neurosurgical operations, if the arterial pressure transducer is raised to a level even with the patient's ear to approximate the location of the circle of Willis, the clinician is measuring blood pressure at the level of the brain and must recognize that the aortic root pressure is higher (by an amount equal to the vertical difference in height between the pressure transducer and the aortic root). Whenever the level of the pressure transducer is adjusted, there is no need to rezero the transducer because atmospheric pressure changes little over the few inches of height adjustment.

Common errors in blood pressure measurement occur when pressure transducers are fixed to an intravenous pole and the height of the patient's bed is adjusted. Raising the height of the bed relative to the transducer will cause overestimation of blood pressure, whereas lowering the patient below the transducer will cause underestimation of blood pressure.

Proper interpretation of blood pressure measurements from a patient in the lateral decubitus position requires an understanding of the distinction between zeroing and leveling pressure transducers and the differences between noninvasive and invasive blood pressure measurement (Fig. 40-10). When a patient is in the lateral decubitus position, one arm is higher than the heart (and aortic root) and the other arm is lower. Regardless of whether direct arterial pressure is measured from the right or the left arm, as long as the pressure transducer remains fixed at the level of the heart, the location of the arms has no influence on the measured arterial pressure. However, noninvasive cuff blood pressure measurements will be different in the two arms, higher in the dependent (down) arm and lower in the nondependent (up) arm (see Fig. 40-10). Note that if the arterial pressure transducers were attached to the arms rather than fixed at the level of the heart, pressures recorded from the right and left radial artery catheters would equal those recorded by the ipsilateral noninvasive cuffs and would be higher in the dependent arm than in the nondependent arm.

Normal Arterial Pressure Waveforms

Direct arterial pressure monitoring in anesthetized patients began nearly 60 years ago.[27] In that early era, arterial pulse waveform analysis was noted to provide useful diagnostic information, but somewhat surprisingly, modern physicians pay little attention to the morphology and detail of the arterial pressure waveform. O'Rourke and Gallagher attribute this change in practice to the reliance on cuff sphygmomanometry, which provides "numbers which came to be linked in a simplistic way to cardiac strength (systolic pressure) and arteriolar tone (diastolic pressure). Pseudoscience had arrived with (these) numbers. … Even when monitored directly in operating theatres and critical care areas, anesthetists and intensivists show little interest in the waveform and base their judgments on values of systolic, diastolic and mean pressure."[60]

Because clinicians today benefit from the widespread availability of high-resolution, multicolored monitor displays, renewed interest in waveform analysis should expand clinical monitoring capabilities.[28] Appreciation of the diagnostic clues provided by the direct arterial pressure waveform requires full understanding of normal waveform components, their relationship to the cardiac cycle, and differences in waveforms recorded from different sites in the body.

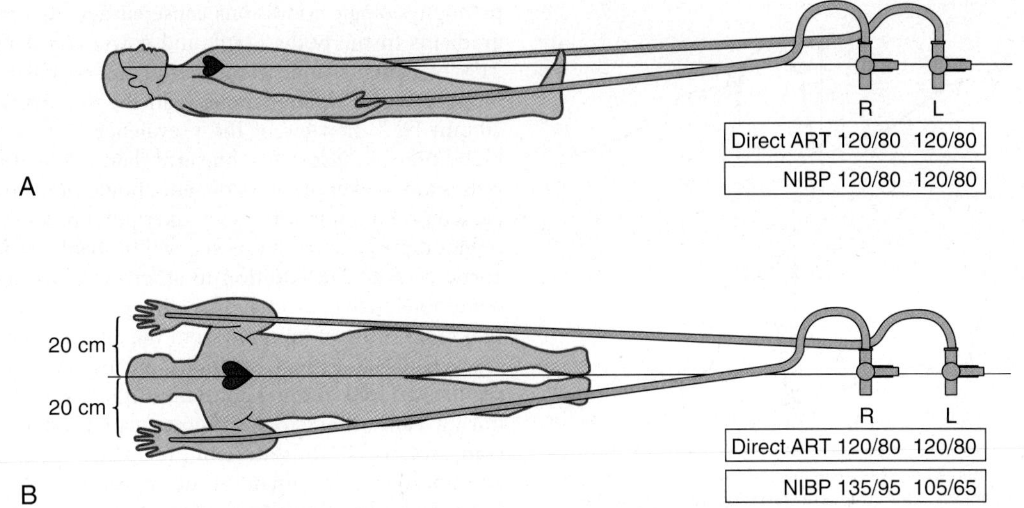

Figure 40-10 Effect of patient position on the relationship between direct arterial blood pressure (ART) and indirect noninvasive blood pressure (NIBP) measurements. **A,** In a supine patient, pressures measured from the right (R) or left (L) arms by either technique will be the same. **B,** In the right lateral decubitus position, ART recorded directly from the right and left radial arteries will remain unchanged as long as the respective pressure transducers remain at heart level. However, NIBP will be higher in the dependent right arm and lower in the nondependent left arm. Differences in NIBP are determined by the positions of the arms above and below the level of the heart and are equal to the hydrostatic pressure differences between the level of the heart and the respective arm. A 20-cm difference in height produces a 15–mm Hg difference in pressure. *(From Mark JB: Atlas of Cardiovascular Monitoring. New York, Churchill Livingstone, 1998, Fig. 9-22.)*

The systemic arterial pressure waveform results from ejection of blood from the left ventricle into the aorta during systole, followed by peripheral arterial runoff of this stroke volume during diastole (Fig. 40-11). The systolic components follow the ECG R wave and consist of a steep pressure upstroke, peak, and decline and correspond to the period of left ventricular systolic ejection. The downslope of the arterial pressure waveform is interrupted by the dicrotic notch, then continues its decline during diastole after the ECG T wave, and reaches its nadir at end-diastole. The dicrotic notch recorded directly from the central aorta is termed the *incisura* (from the Latin, "a cutting into"). The incisura is sharply defined and is undoubtedly related to closure of the aortic valve.[61] In contrast, the peripheral arterial waveform generally displays a later, smoother dicrotic notch that only approximates the timing of aortic valve closure and depends more on properties of the arterial wall. Note that the systolic upstroke of the radial artery pressure trace does not appear for 120 to 180 msec after inscription of the ECG R wave (see Fig. 40-11). This interval reflects the sum of times required for spread of electrical depolarization through the ventricular myocardium, isovolumic left ventricular contraction, opening of the aortic valve, left ventricular ejection, transmission of the aortic pressure wave to the radial artery, and finally, transmission of the pressure signal from the arterial catheter to the pressure transducer.

The bedside monitor displays numeric values for the systolic peak and end-diastolic nadir pressures. Measurement of mean pressure is more complicated and depends on the algorithm used by the monitor. In simplest terms, MAP is equal to the area beneath the arterial pressure curve divided by the beat period and averaged over a series of consecutive heartbeats. Although MAP is often estimated as diastolic pressure plus one third times pulse pressure, this estimate is valid only at slower heart rates because the proportion of the cardiac cycle spent in diastole decreases during tachycardia.[62]

One of the most important features of the arterial pressure waveform is the phenomenon of distal pulse amplification. Pressure waveforms recorded simultaneously from different arterial sites will have different morphologies because of the physical characteristics of the vascular tree, namely, impedance and harmonic resonance[21,60] (Fig. 40-12). As the arterial pressure wave travels from the central aorta to the periphery, the arterial upstroke

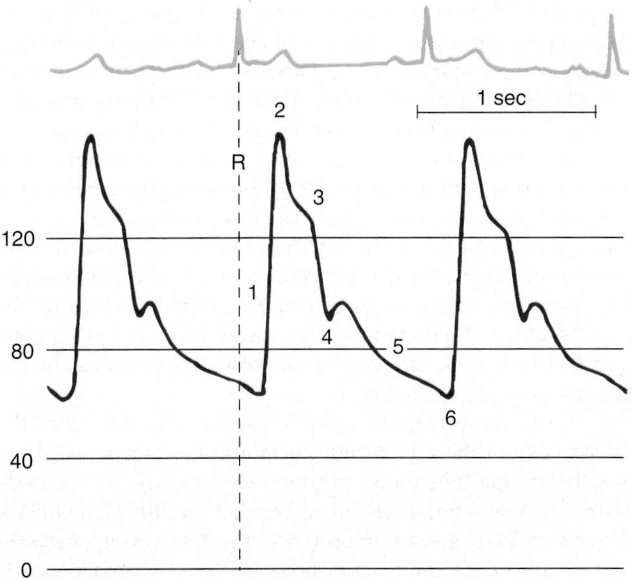

Figure 40-11 Normal arterial blood pressure waveform and its relationship to the electrocardiographic R wave. 1, Systolic upstroke; 2, systolic peak pressure; 3, systolic decline; 4, dicrotic notch; 5, diastolic runoff; 6, end-diastolic pressure. *(From Mark JB: Atlas of Cardiovascular Monitoring. New York, Churchill Livingstone, 1998, Fig. 8-1.)*

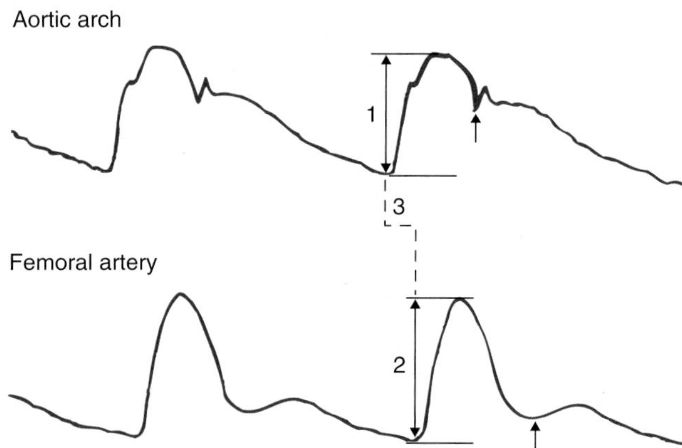

Figure 40-12 Distal pulse wave amplification of the arterial pressure waveform. When compared with pressure in the aortic arch, the more peripherally recorded femoral artery pressure waveform demonstrates a wider pulse pressure (compare 1 and 2); a delayed upstroke (3); a delayed, slurred dicrotic notch (compare *arrows*); and a more prominent diastolic wave. *(From Mark JB: Atlas of Cardiovascular Monitoring. New York, Churchill Livingstone, 1998, Fig. 8-4.)*

becomes steeper, the systolic peak becomes higher, the dicrotic notch appears later, the diastolic wave becomes more prominent, and end-diastolic pressure becomes lower. Thus, when compared with central aortic pressure, peripheral arterial waveforms have higher systolic pressure, lower diastolic pressure, and wider pulse pressure. Furthermore, there is a delay in arrival of the pressure pulse at peripheral sites, so the systolic pressure upstroke begins approximately 60 msec later in the radial artery than in the aorta. Despite morphologic and temporal differences between peripheral and central arterial waveforms, MAP in the aorta is just slightly greater than MAP in the radial artery.

Pressure wave reflection is the predominant factor that influences the shape of the arterial pressure waveform as it travels peripherally.[60] As blood flows from the aorta to the radial artery, mean pressure decreases only slightly because of little resistance to flow in the major conducting arteries. At the arteriolar level, mean blood pressure falls markedly as a result of the dramatic increase in vascular resistance at this site. This high resistance to flow diminishes pressure pulsations in small downstream vessels but acts to augment upstream arterial pressure pulses because of pressure wave reflection.[63] These intrinsic vascular phenomena determine the shape of the arterial pulse wave recorded from different sites in the body, in both health and disease. For example, elderly patients have reduced arterial distensibility, which results in early return of reflected pressure waves, increased pulse pressure, a late systolic pressure peak, and disappearance of the diastolic pressure wave (Fig. 40-13).

From these considerations it becomes evident that the morphology of the arterial waveform and the precise values of systolic and diastolic blood pressure vary throughout the body under normal conditions in otherwise healthy individuals. Perhaps of even greater importance, the relationship between central and peripheral arterial pressure varies with age and is altered by various physiologic changes, pathologic conditions, and pharmacologic interventions.

Arterial Blood Pressure Gradients

In addition to the normal physiologic phenomena that exert subtle influences on the arterial pressure waveform, a number of pathophysiologic conditions cause exaggerated arterial pressure gradients in the body. Frank and coworkers demonstrated that 21% of patients undergoing peripheral vascular surgery had a blood pressure difference between the two arms that exceeded 20 mm Hg.[64] In view of the prevalence of this problem, when blood pressure is lower in one arm than in the other or when the pulses are weaker on one side, one should never insert an arterial catheter on the side with the weaker pulse because determination of blood pressure from this site will probably underestimate true aortic pressure. In addition to atherosclerosis, other pathologic conditions such as arterial dissection or embolism preclude accurate monitoring of pressure from the affected sites.

Unusual patient positions during surgery may produce regional arterial compression, and surgical retraction, particularly during cardiothoracic operations, can produce local vascular compression.[65,66] The nature of the operative procedure is always an important determinant of the appropriate site for monitoring arterial pressure. Operations requiring placement of a descending thoracic aortic cross-clamp may interrupt arterial flow to the left subclavian artery and its tributaries in the left arm, as well as branches of the aorta beyond the clamp. In these cases, blood pressure monitored from the right arm best estimates aortic root pressure and carotid arterial pressure and is used to guide anesthetic management. In addition, pressure may be monitored simultaneously from a femoral artery in an attempt to estimate perfusion pressure to vital organs distal to the aortic cross-clamp.

Various pathophysiologic disturbances may produce generalized arterial pressure gradients in the body and should be considered when choosing a site for monitoring arterial pressure. Large differences in peripheral and central arterial pressure may be seen in patients in shock. Femoral artery systolic pressure may exceed radial artery systolic pressure by more than 50 mm Hg in septic patients who require vasopressor infusions, an observation that has significant therapeutic implications for the management of critically ill patients.[67] Other vasoactive drugs, anesthetics (particularly neuraxial blockade), and changes in patient temperature produce pressure gradients that alter the relationship between central and peripheral arterial pressure measurements.[21] During hypothermia, thermoregulatory vasoconstriction causes radial

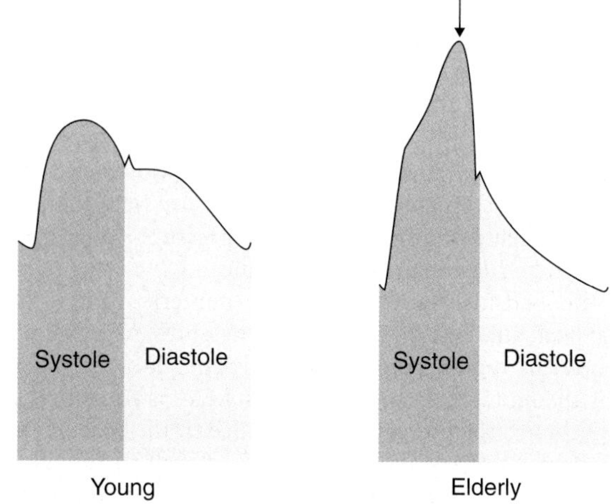

Figure 40-13 Impact of pressure wave reflection on arterial pressure waveforms. In elderly individuals with reduced arterial distensibility, early return of reflected waves increases pulse pressure, produces a late systolic pressure peak (*arrow*), and attenuates the diastolic pressure wave.

artery systolic pressure to exceed femoral artery systolic pressure, whereas during rewarming, vasodilation reverses this gradient and causes radial artery pressure to underestimate femoral artery pressure.[68]

Large differences between central and peripheral arterial blood pressure have also been described in cardiac surgical patients undergoing cardiopulmonary bypass (Fig. 40-14). Shortly after initiation of cardiopulmonary bypass, mean radial artery pressure is lower than mean femoral artery pressure, and this difference seems to persist during the bypass procedure.[69] Furthermore, in the initial minutes after bypass, radial arterial pressure continues to be lower than central aortic pressure, often by more than 20 mm Hg.[70] In most patients, these pressure differences persist after bypass for only several minutes and resolve within an hour, but occasionally these pressure gradients are still present during the postoperative period.

Abnormal Arterial Pressure Waveforms

Detailed examination of the morphologic features of individual arterial pressure waveforms can provide important diagnostic clues to a variety of pathologic conditions (Table 40-1). *Aortic stenosis* produces a fixed obstruction to left ventricular ejection that results in reduced stroke volume and an arterial pressure waveform that rises slowly (*pulsus tardus*), peaks late in systole, and is small in amplitude (*pulsus parvus*) (Fig. 40-15A and B). A distinct shoulder, termed the *anacrotic notch*, often distorts the pressure upstroke, and the dicrotic notch may not be discernible. These features make the arterial pressure waveform appear overdamped.

In *aortic regurgitation*, the arterial pressure wave displays a sharp rise, wide pulse pressure, and low diastolic pressure as a result of runoff of blood into the left ventricle and the periphery during diastole. Because of the large stroke volume ejected from the left ventricle in this condition, the arterial pressure pulse may have two systolic peaks (*bisferiens pulse*) (see Fig. 40-15C). These peaks represent separate percussion and tidal waves, the former resulting from left ventricular ejection and the latter arising from the periphery as a reflected wave. In *hypertrophic cardiomyopathy*, the arterial pressure waveform assumes a peculiar bifid shape termed a "spike-and-dome" configuration. After an initial sharp pressure upstroke that results from rapid left ventricular ejection in early systole, arterial pressure falls rapidly as dynamic left ventricular outflow obstruction develops during midsystole and is followed by a late systolic reflected wave, thereby creating the characteristic double-peaked waveform (see Fig. 40-15D).

Observation of arterial waveform patterns over consecutive heartbeats provides an additional set of diagnostic clues. *Pulsus alternans* is recognized by the alternating beats of larger

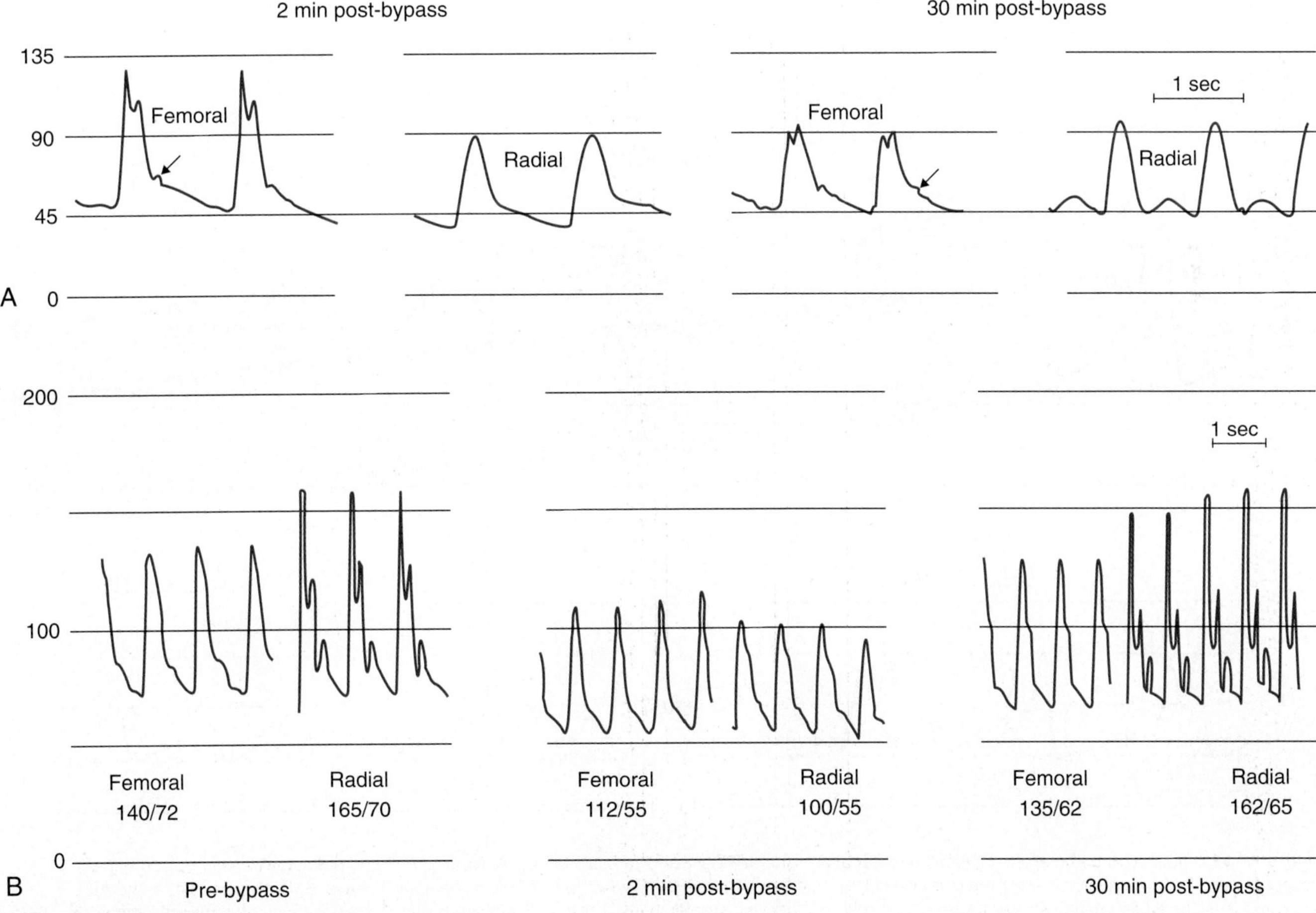

Figure 40-14 Arterial pressure gradients after cardiopulmonary bypass. **A,** Femoral and radial artery pressure traces recorded 2 minutes after bypass, when radial artery pressure underestimates the more centrally measured femoral artery pressure, and 30 minutes later, when radial and femoral arterial pressure has been equalized and radial pressure has assumed a more typical morphology. Note that the dicrotic notch (*arrows*) is visible in the femoral pressure trace after bypass but not initially in the radial pressure trace. **B,** Femoral and radial artery pressure traces recorded before cardiopulmonary bypass, 2 minutes after bypass, and 30 minutes after bypass. Note the changing relationship between femoral and radial artery pressure measurements (in mm Hg) at these different times.

Table 40-1 Arterial Blood Pressure Waveform Abnormalities

Condition	Characteristics
Aortic stenosis	Pulsus parvus (narrow pulse pressure) Pulsus tardus (delayed upstroke)
Aortic regurgitation	Bisferiens pulse (double peak) Wide pulse pressure
Hypertrophic cardiomyopathy	Spike-and-dome pattern (midsystolic obstruction)
Systolic left ventricular failure	Pulsus alternans (alternating pulse pressure amplitude)
Cardiac tamponade	Pulsus paradoxus (exaggerated decrease in systolic blood pressure during spontaneous inspiration)

and smaller pulse pressures (Fig. 40-16A). In general, it is considered to be a sign of severe left ventricular systolic dysfunction, often noted in patients with advanced aortic stenosis. Pulsus alternans should be distinguished from the bigeminal pulse that arises from a bigeminal rhythm, usually ventricular bigeminy. Both abnormalities create an alternating pulse pressure in the arterial pressure waveform, but the rhythm is regular in pulsus alternans.

Pulsus paradoxus is an exaggerated inspiratory fall in systolic arterial pressure that exceeds 10 to 12 mm Hg during quiet breathing (see Fig. 40-16B).[71,72] The term is confusing because a small inspiratory reduction in blood pressure is a normal phenomenon and pulsus paradoxus is not truly paradoxical, but rather an exaggeration of the normal inspiratory decline in blood pressure. Pulsus paradoxus is a characteristic, almost universal finding in cardiac tamponade that occurs in many patients with pericardial constriction. It is said to occur in patients with airway obstruction, bronchospasm, dyspnea, or any condition characterized by large swings in intrathoracic pressure. However, in cardiac tamponade, pulse pressure and left ventricular stroke volume decrease during inspiration, in contrast to the blood pressure changes observed in patients with forced breathing patterns and exaggerated changes in intrathoracic pressure, in whom pulse pressure is relatively unchanged.[73]

The arterial pressure waveform provides diagnostic clues in other unusual physiologic states, such as for proper timing of intra-aortic balloon counterpulsation (Fig. 40-17A). During nonpulsatile cardiopulmonary bypass, minor variations in blood pressure created by the arterial roller head allow calculation and confirmation of the adequacy of systemic blood flow[28] (see Fig. 40-17B).

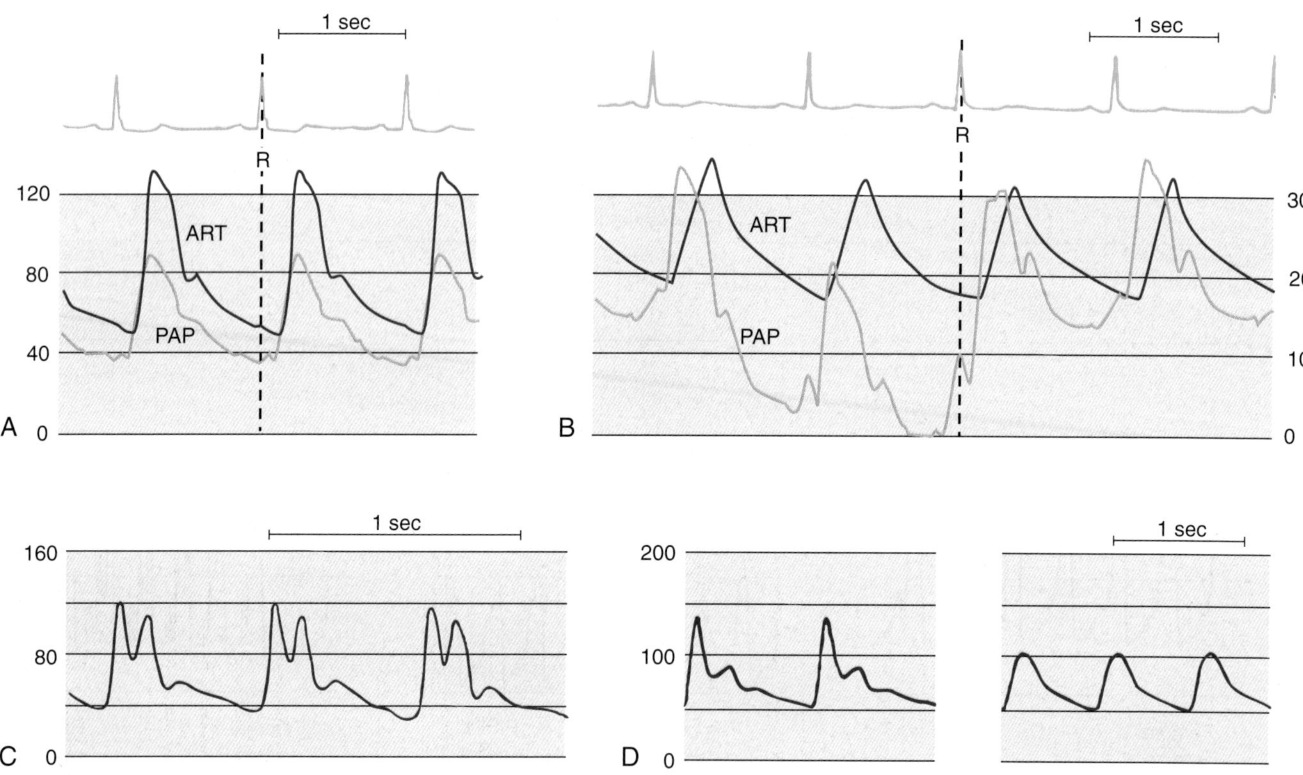

Figure 40-15 Influence of pathologic conditions on arterial pressure (ART) waveform morphology. **A,** *Normal* ART and pulmonary artery pressure (PAP) waveform morphologies demonstrating the similar timing of these waveforms relative to the electrocardiographic R wave. **B,** In *aortic stenosis*, the ART waveform is distorted and demonstrates a slurred upstroke and delayed systolic peak. These changes are particularly striking in comparison to the normal PAP waveform. Note the beat-to-beat respiratory variation in the PAP waveform. See text for greater detail. For **A** and **B,** the ART scale is on the *left* and the PAP scale is on the *right*. **C,** *Aortic regurgitation* produces a bisferiens pulse and a wide pulse pressure. See text for greater detail. **D,** The arterial pressure waveform in *hypertrophic cardiomyopathy* shows a peculiar "spike-and-dome" configuration. The pressure waveform assumes a more normal morphology after surgical correction of this condition. *(From Mark JB: Atlas of Cardiovascular Monitoring. New York, Churchill Livingstone, 1998, Figs.3-3, 17-21, and 17-24.)*

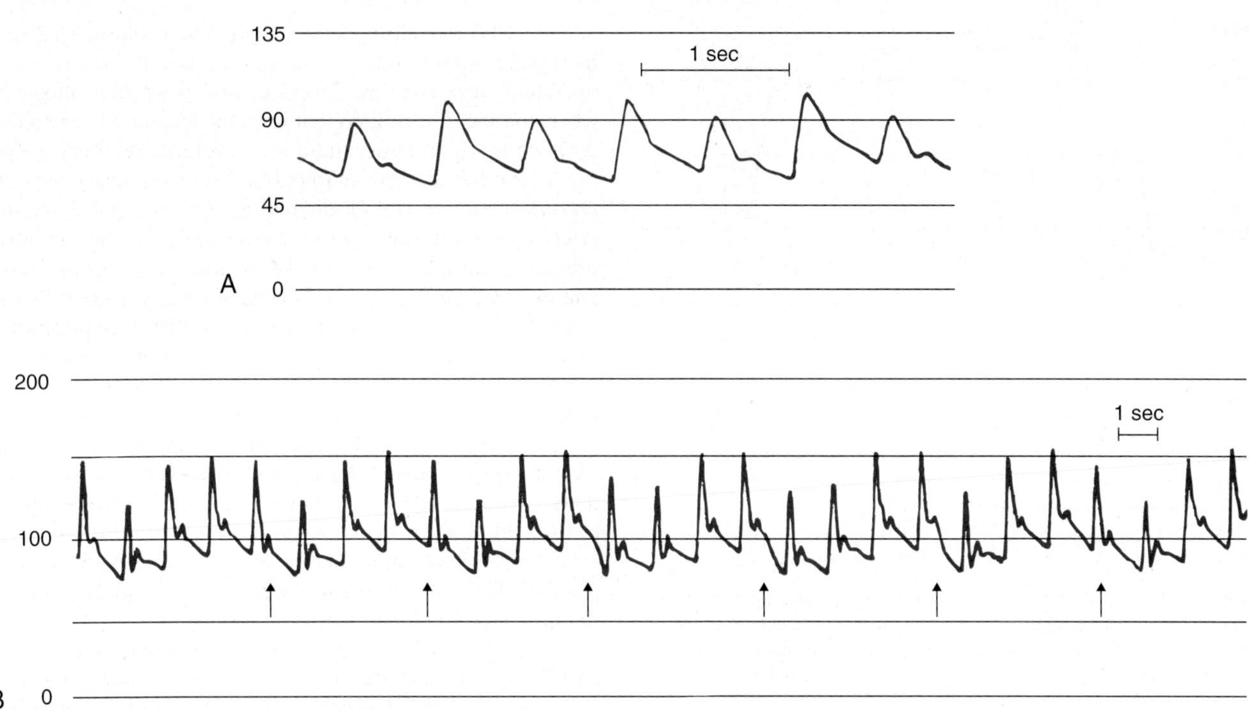

Figure 40-16 Beat-to-beat variability in arterial pressure waveform morphologies. **A,** *Pulsus alternans*. **B,** *Pulsus paradoxus*. The marked decline in systolic arterial pressure and pulse pressure during spontaneous inspiration (*arrows*) is characteristic of cardiac tamponade. *(From Mark JB: Atlas of Cardiovascular Monitoring. New York, Churchill Livingstone, 1998, Fig. 18-10.)*

Arterial Pressure Monitoring for Prediction of Volume Responsiveness

The starting point for hemodynamic resuscitation begins with optimizing cardiac preload. The limitations of static indicators of preload, such as central venous pressure (CVP), have been increasingly recognized because of the many factors that confound their interpretation.[74] Newer dynamic markers of volume responsiveness have been described that provide more useful information for determining appropriate end points for fluid resuscitation. Variations in arterial blood pressure observed during positive-pressure mechanical ventilation are the most widely studied of these dynamic indicators. These changes in blood pressure are readily observed on the bedside monitor in patients who are receiving direct arterial blood pressure monitoring, and they result from the changes in intrathoracic pressure and lung volume that occur during the respiratory cycle.

During positive-pressure inspiration, increasing lung volume compresses and displaces the pulmonary venous reservoir and propels blood into the left heart chambers, thereby increasing left ventricular preload. Simultaneously, the increase in intrathoracic pressure reduces left ventricular afterload. The increase in left ventricular preload and decrease in afterload produce an increase in left ventricular stroke volume and an increase in systemic arterial pressure. In most patients the preload effects are more important, but in patients with severe left ventricular systolic failure, the reduction in afterload plays an important role in increasing left ventricular ejection. At the same time that left heart filling is increasing during early inspiration, the rising intrathoracic pressure causes a decrease in systemic venous return and right ventricular preload. The increased lung volume may also increase pulmonary vascular resistance (PVR) slightly and thereby increase right ventricular afterload. These effects combine to reduce right ventricular ejection during inspiration. During early expiration, the reduced right ventricular stroke volume that occurred during inspiration crosses the pulmonary vascular bed and leads to reduced left ventricular filling. As a result, left ventricular stroke volume falls and systemic arterial blood pressure decreases. This cyclic variation in systemic arterial pressure may be measured and quantified as the *systolic pressure variation* (SPV).

SPV is often subdivided into inspiratory and expiratory components by measuring the increase (Δ Up) and decrease (Δ Down) in systolic pressure in relation to the end-expiratory, apneic baseline pressure (Fig. 40-18). In a mechanically ventilated patient, normal SPV is 7 to 10 mm Hg, with Δ Up being 2 to 4 mm Hg and Δ Down being 5 to 6 mm Hg.[75] The greatest clinical use of SPV has been for the early diagnosis of hypovolemia.[76] In both experimental animals and patients, hypovolemia causes a dramatic increase in SPV, particularly the Δ Down component. An increase in SPV, particularly in Δ Down, may herald hypovolemia, even in patients in whom arterial blood pressure is maintained near normal levels by compensatory arterial vasoconstriction.

In a heterogeneous group of intensive care patients, Marik demonstrated that a large SPV (>15 mm Hg) was highly predictive of low pulmonary artery wedge pressure (PAWP) (<10 mm Hg).[77] Using echocardiography to measure the left ventricular cross-sectional area as a surrogate for preload, Coriat and colleagues found Δ Down to be better than wedge pressure as a predictor of preload.[78] Other uses of SPV focus on changes in the Δ Up portion of the arterial pressure trace. Just as Δ Down may

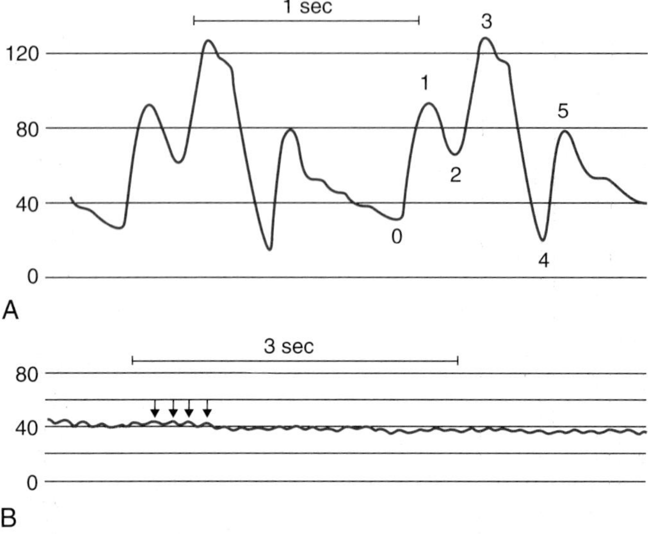

Figure 40-17 Unusual arterial pressure waveforms. **A,** *Intra-aortic balloon counterpulsation* with a 1:2 balloon-assist ratio produces a characteristic change in the arterial pressure waveform. Four cardiac cycles are shown, two with balloon assistance and two without. 0, Unassisted end-diastolic pressure; 1, unassisted systolic pressure; 2, dicrotic notch; 3, assisted or augmented diastolic pressure; 4, end-diastolic or presystolic dip; 5, assisted systolic pressure. Effective afterload reduction by the intra-aortic balloon is evidenced by the presystolic dip pressure (4) lower than the unassisted end-diastolic pressure (0) and the assisted systolic pressure peak (5) lower than the unassisted systolic pressure peak (1). **B,** Arterial pressure waveform during *cardiopulmonary bypass*. Small phasic pressure variations (*arrows*) result from the mechanical action of the bypass roller pump. The bypass pump flow rate may be estimated by measuring these pulsations. Nineteen pulsations are recorded in a 3-second time interval. In this case, the pump configured with ⅜-in tubing has an effective stroke volume of 27 mL. The pump flow rate may be calculated as follows: (19 pulsations/3 sec) × (1 pump revolution/two pulsations) × (27 mL/revolution) × (60 sec/min) = 5130 mL/min. This calculated pump flow rate should equal the flow rate displayed on the pump console (i.e., 5.2 L/min). *(From Mark JB: Atlas of Cardiovascular Monitoring. New York, Churchill Livingstone, 1998, Figs.20-3 and 19-8.)*

reveal changes in cardiac preload, the Δ Up portion of the arterial pressure trace may provide clues to the afterload dependence of the left ventricle.

As a dynamic indicator of cardiac preload, SPV and Δ Down provide valuable clinical information beyond that provided by static preload indicators such as CVP or PAWP. It appears that the magnitude of blood pressure variation accurately predicts patients who will subsequently respond to a volume challenge by increasing stroke volume and cardiac output. Using receiver-operator curve analysis, Tavernier and coworkers showed that when compared with PAWP or left ventricular end-diastolic area, Δ Down was a far better indicator of volume responsiveness.[79]

Another dynamic marker of volume responsiveness is *pulse pressure variation* (PPV), defined as the maximal difference in arterial pulse pressure measured over the course of the positive-pressure respiratory cycle divided by the average of the maximal and minimal pulse pressure[80,81] (Fig. 40-19). Normal PPV should not exceed 13%.[82] In addition to SPV and PPV, new pulse contour methods for measurement of cardiac output (see later) allow online measurement of variations in left ventricular stroke volume, so-called *stroke volume variation* (SVV). Like the other related dynamic indicators of volume responsiveness, normal SVV is approximately 10%, and greater variability accurately predicts a positive response to a fluid challenge.[83] Another approach to assessing fluid responsiveness has focused on the respiratory cycle–induced variation in the pulse plethysmogram, but this physiologic signal is even more subject to confounding influences than the arterial blood pressure waveform is.[82,84]

Despite rapidly accumulating evidence of the value of SPV and PPV and their related measures as accurate predictors of cardiac preload, they have not found widespread clinical adoption for a number of reasons. The original description of this method required transient interruption of mechanical ventilation to identify an apneic baseline for measurement of Δ Down and Δ Up.[75] Newer monitors use computerized algorithms to measure and display SPV or PPV continuously, but these automated measures are not yet routinely available in standard bedside monitors.[85,86]

A number of additional factors have precluded the wider application of SPV and PPV for monitoring volume responsiveness. The magnitude of blood pressure variation observed in any patient will be influenced by positive-pressure ventilation parameters, including tidal volume and peak inspiratory pressure. SPV and PPV cannot be used reliably in patients with cardiac arrhythmias or significant changes in chest wall or lung compliance. As noted earlier, respiratory cycle–induced variations in arterial pressure are not solely related to changes in left ventricular preload but depend in part on afterload influences. Although it is clear that the magnitude of SPV and PPV predict fluid responsiveness, precise threshold values remain uncertain, and the variety of techniques described have not been standardized.[83] Perhaps most important, all these measures have been validated only in mechanically ventilated patients and are not applicable to

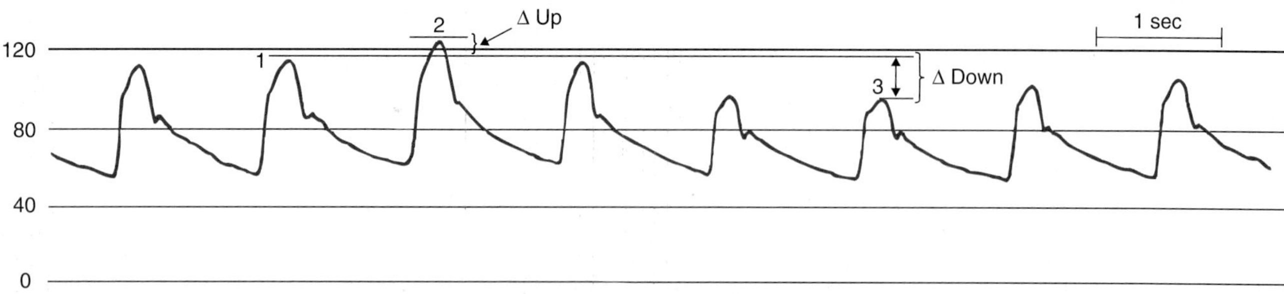

Figure 40-18 Systolic pressure variation. When compared with the systolic blood pressure recorded at alpha (1), a small increase occurs during positive-pressure inspiration (2, Δ Up), followed by a decrease (3, Δ Down). Normally, total systolic pressure variation does not exceed 10 mm Hg. In this instance, the large Δ Down indicates hypovolemia even though systolic arterial pressure and the heart rate are relatively normal. *(From Mark JB: Atlas of Cardiovascular Monitoring. New York, Churchill Livingstone, 1998, Fig. 16-16.)*

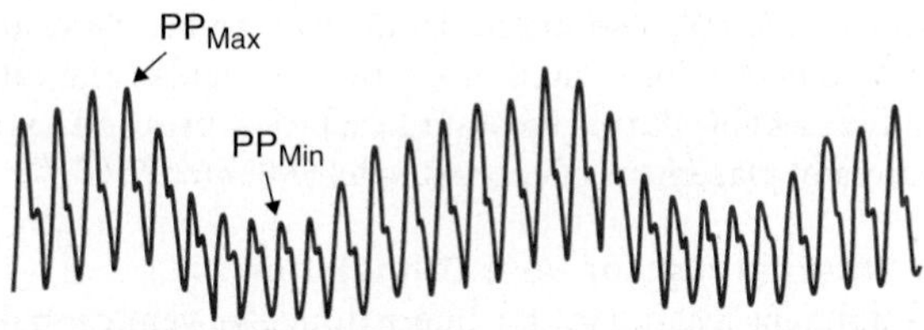

Note: The arterial blood pressure tracing is not drawn to scale

$PP_{Max} = 150 - 70 = 80$
$PP_{Min} = 120 - 60 = 60$
$PPV = (PP_{Max} - PP_{Min})/([PP_{Max} + PP_{Min}]/2)$
$PPV = 80 - 60/([80 + 60]/2) = 29\%$

Figure 40-19 Pulse pressure variation. Pulse pressure variation (PPV) is calculated as the difference between the maximal (PP_{Max}) and minimal (PP_{Min}) pulse pressure values during one mechanical respiratory cycle, divided by the average of these two values. (Note that the arterial blood pressure trace is drawn for illustrative purposes and not to scale.)

spontaneously breathing subjects, thereby precluding their use in many anesthetized and critically ill patients.

Central Venous Pressure Monitoring

Indirect assessment of CVP through physical examination of the neck veins is a fundamental aspect of cardiovascular assessment, but one that has many shortcomings. The jugular veins may be impossible to identify in up to 20% of patients, and the bedside diagnosis of low, normal, or high CVP is often inaccurate, particularly in critically ill patients.[87,88] This problem is compounded in the perioperative period, when visualization of the neck veins is further obscured and abrupt changes, sometimes of great magnitude, are not uncommon. As a result, direct measurement of CVP is frequently necessary in hemodynamically unstable patients and those undergoing major operations.

Central Venous Cannulation

Cannulation of a large central vein is the standard clinical method for monitoring CVP and is also performed for a number of additional therapeutic interventions, such as providing secure vascular access for the administration of vasoactive drugs or to initiate rapid fluid resuscitation. Frequently, the central venous location is the only site available for intravenous access of any kind. Patients at risk for venous air emboli may have central venous catheters placed for aspiration of entrained air. In addition, central venous access is required to initiate transvenous cardiac pacing, temporary hemodialysis, or pulmonary artery catheterization for more comprehensive cardiac monitoring (Box 40-4).

The decision to perform central venous cannulation before or after induction of anesthesia is guided most often by individual patient and physician preferences or institutional practice. One should consider abandoning attempts at preoperative central venous cannulation in any patient who becomes overly sedated or uncooperative during the procedure and proceed with inducing anesthesia and obtaining secure control of the airway. At that point, further attempts at gaining central vascular access are appropriate.

Choosing the Catheter, Site, and Method of Central Venous Cannulation

Central venous catheters come in a variety of lengths, gauges, composition, and lumen number.[89,90] These characteristics vary according to the purpose of the catheterization, whether for CVP monitoring or other therapeutic indications and whether intended for short- or long-term use. This makes it critical for the physician to choose the best catheter for any given application. Seven-French, 20-cm multiport catheters that allow monitoring of CVP and infusion of drugs and fluids simultaneously are the most common.[91] It should be noted that rapid fluid resuscitation is more efficient with short, large-bore intravenous catheters inserted peripherally because the smaller diameter of each individual lumen and the overall catheter length increase resistance to flow significantly. For example, according to the manufacturer's product specifications, the maximal flow rate of the 16-gauge lumen of a standard 7-Fr, 20-cm central venous catheter is a quarter that of a 16-gauge, 3-cm intravenous catheter in a large peripheral vein.

A popular alternative method for multilumen central venous access uses a large introducer sheath with an integrated T-connector sidearm for multiple drug infusions combined with a single-lumen catheter inserted through the hemostasis valve for continuous CVP monitoring. Although use of these larger introducer sheaths is not free of complications, they do allow rapid placement of a pacing wire or pulmonary artery catheter (PAC) for more intensive monitoring should the need arise.

Selecting the best site for safe and effective central venous cannulation ultimately requires consideration of the indication for catheterization (pressure monitoring versus drug or fluid administration), the patient's underlying medical condition, the clinical setting, and the skill and experience of the physician performing the procedure. In patients with severe bleeding diatheses, it is best to choose a puncture site at which bleeding from the vein or adjacent artery is easily detected and controlled with

Box 40-4 Indications for Central Venous Cannulation

- Central venous pressure monitoring
- Pulmonary artery catheterization and monitoring
- Transvenous cardiac pacing
- Temporary hemodialysis
- Drug administration
  - Concentrated vasoactive drugs
  - Hyperalimentation
  - Chemotherapy
  - Agents irritating to peripheral veins
  - Prolonged antibiotic therapy (e.g., endocarditis)
- Rapid infusion of fluids (via large cannulas)
  - Trauma
  - Major surgery
- Aspiration of air emboli
- Inadequate peripheral intravenous access
- Sampling site for repeated blood testing

local compression. In such a patient, an internal or external jugular approach would be preferable to a subclavian site. Likewise, patients with severe emphysema or others who would be severely compromised by pneumothorax would be better candidates for internal jugular than subclavian cannulation because of the higher risk with the latter approach. If transvenous cardiac pacing is required in an emergency situation, catheterization of the right internal jugular vein is recommended because it provides the most direct route to the right ventricle. Trauma patients with their necks immobilized in a hard cervical collar are best resuscitated via a femoral or subclavian approach; the latter may be used even more safely if the risk of pneumothorax is obviated by prior placement of a thoracostomy tube. The physician must recognize that the length of catheter inserted to position the catheter tip properly in the superior vena cava will vary according to puncture site, being slightly (3 to 5 cm) greater when the left internal or external jugular veins are chosen versus the right internal jugular vein.[92] Finally, a physician's personal experience undoubtedly plays a significant role in determining the safest site for central venous cannulation, particularly when the procedure is performed under urgent or emergency circumstances.

Since its introduction into clinical practice in the late 1960s, percutaneous puncture of the right internal jugular vein has been the method preferred by anesthesiologists for central venous cannulation.[93-95] Reasons for this preference include consistent, predictable anatomic location of the internal jugular vein, readily identifiable and palpable surface landmarks, and a short, straight course to the superior vena cava. An internal jugular vein catheter is highly accessible during most surgical procedures and has a rate of successful placement of approximately 90% to 99%.[94,96]

Right Internal Jugular Vein Cannulation

Many different techniques for internal jugular vein cannulation have been described, although the "central" approach described by Daily and colleagues is among the most popular and is described with minor modifications here.[97] Careful positioning will make the patient comfortable, improve identification of surface landmarks, and increase the likelihood of success. The patient is placed in the supine position with the head turned slightly to the left to expose the right side of the neck and keep the chin from interfering with the procedure. Pillows that cause the neck to be flexed should be removed, but forceful neck extension or extreme leftward rotation of the head should be avoided because this alters cervical vascular anatomy and may cause the internal jugular vein to overlie the carotid artery, thereby increasing the risk for carotid arterial puncture.[98] Anatomic landmarks, including the sternal notch, clavicle, and sternocleidomastoid muscle, should be identified before skin preparation and draping for the sterile procedure because these landmarks are more easily appreciated before they are covered by the sterile drape (Fig. 40-20). The patient should be calm, sedated, receiving supplemental oxygen if necessary, and monitored with an ECG, blood pres-

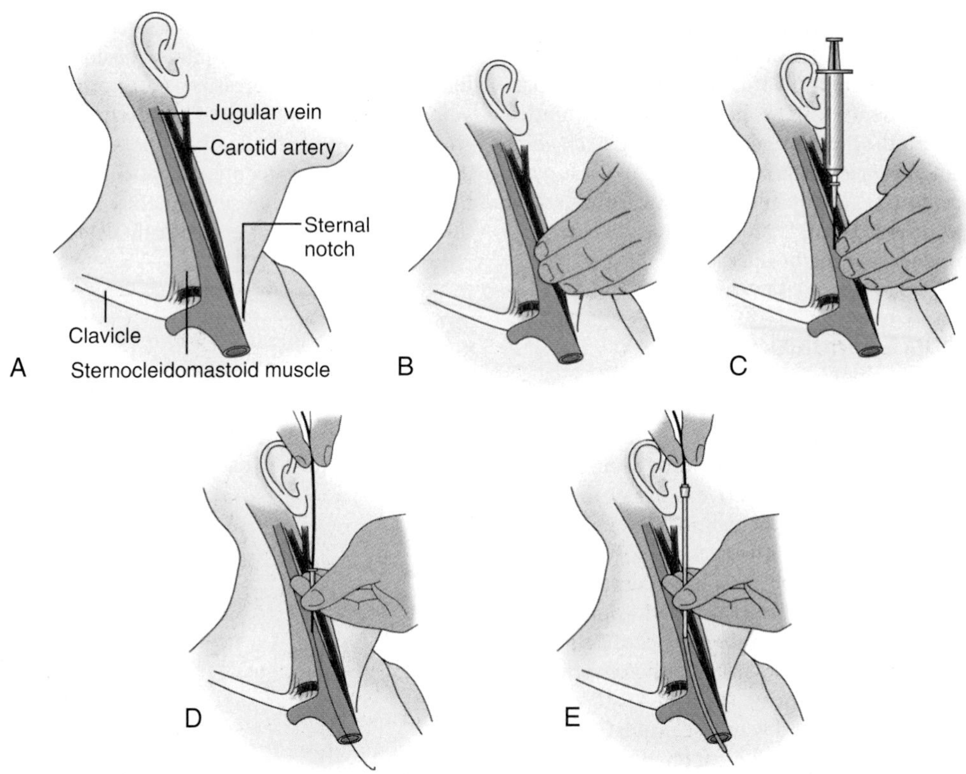

Figure 40-20 Technique for central venous cannulation of the right internal jugular vein. **A,** Important surface landmarks are identified. **B,** The course of the internal carotid artery is palpated. **C,** The internal jugular vein is punctured at the apex of the triangle formed by the two heads of the sternocleidomastoid muscle, with the needle tip directed toward the ipsilateral nipple. **D,** A guidewire is introduced through the thin-walled needle into the vein. **E,** The central venous cannula is inserted over the guidewire while making sure that the proximal end of the guidewire protrudes beyond the catheter and is controlled by the operator.

sure monitor, and pulse oximeter. Because of the frequency and serious morbidity of infectious complications from central venous catheterization, strict aseptic technique is required. Formal guidelines to reduce these complications have been published by the Centers for Disease Control and Prevention and provide prudent recommendations that should be followed during all catheterizations.[99]

Good aseptic technique begins with hand washing before the procedure. A mask, cap, sterile gloves, and gown should always be used, regardless of the procedural setting. The skin is cleaned widely from earlobe to clavicle to sternal notch, preferably with 2% chlorhexidine, an agent that has been shown to be superior to the more traditional 10% povidone-iodine.[99,100] Aseptic preparation is completed with the application of a large sterile drape that provides maximal barrier precautions, preferably a full-body drape.

Under these sterile conditions, the relevant anatomy is again identified, particularly the course of the carotid artery in the neck. The internal jugular vein lies in the groove between the sternal and clavicular heads of the sternocleidomastoid muscle, lateral and slightly anterior to the carotid artery in most cases. In many patients, venous pulsations from the internal jugular vein are observed directly within this groove and further identify the approximate site for skin puncture. An assistant then places the patient in a slight head-down (Trendelenburg) position to increase jugular vein diameter in the neck. This step may be omitted in a hypervolemic, dyspneic patient. The intended skin is anesthetized by subcutaneous infiltration of a local anesthetic solution (typically 1% lidocaine) with a 25-gauge needle if the patient is awake. Venipuncture then proceeds with a 22-gauge, 1½-inch (3.8-cm) finder needle mounted on a 5-mL syringe (see Fig. 40-20). The needle is inserted at the apex of the triangle formed by the two heads of the sternocleidomastoid muscle, at an angle of approximately 30 degrees from the plane of the skin, and directed toward the ipsilateral nipple. Gentle aspiration will identify the jugular vein when dark venous blood enters the syringe. Although use of the small finder needle is an extra step in this procedure, it presumably increases the margin of safety because unintentional puncture of the carotid artery with this small needle is less likely to result in significant bleeding and hematoma formation.[101] If blood is not aspirated as the finder needle is advanced and then withdrawn, additional needle passes may locate the internal jugular vein by fanning laterally in a small arc from the point where the needle enters the skin. If the vein is not located after several needle passes, the finder needle is withdrawn completely and checked for patency, the anatomy is reassessed, and the puncture may then proceed with the needle entering the skin several millimeters closer to the palpated carotid pulse but still directed in a sagittal or slightly lateral direction. One should resist the temptation to explore with a medial or leftward direction of the finder needle when this technique is being used because such exploration will increase the likelihood of unintentional puncture of the carotid artery.

After the internal jugular vein is located with the finder needle, the needle is gently withdrawn while the skin and surface anatomy remain fixed by the left hand. The vein is then punctured with an 18-gauge, 2½-inch (6.4-cm), thin-walled needle attached to a 5-mL syringe along the same track used with the finder needle while keeping in mind the three-dimensional location and depth of the identified internal jugular vein. It is not uncommon for the lumen of the jugular vein to be compressed as this larger thin-walled needle is advanced and both the front and back walls pierced almost simultaneously.[102,103] Consequently, the thin-walled needle should be inserted only slightly beyond the expected depth of the vein and then slowly withdrawn while maintaining gentle aspiration on the syringe. As such, venous entry of the needle is recognized during needle withdrawal by the sudden return of free-flowing venous blood.

Many individuals choose to substitute a 2-inch, 18-gauge intravenous catheter for the 18-gauge thin-walled needle for venipuncture. In this method, the catheter is advanced over the needle and into the vein immediately after blood is seen returning into the barrel of the syringe. Although this catheter can be advanced completely into the vein, it may be kinked or occluded, thereby making it more difficult to differentiate pulsatile arterial blood flow from unintentional arterial puncture. It is vital to confirm the intravenous location of this catheter. The color of the aspirated blood is examined, and it may be compared with a simultaneously obtained arterial sample, although this technique is not completely reliable.[104] A safer method is to manually transduce the pressure by attaching sterile intravenous extension tubing to the catheter and observing the fluid column.[104,105] When using this technique, it is important to allow the blood to fill more than 30 cm of the tubing and then raise it vertically and observe a fall in the column of blood. This excludes the possibility of a kinked catheter or the catheter tip abutting the arterial wall, either of which may mask an arterial puncture. Continuous pressure transduction of the thin-walled needle has been advocated as an even better method of detecting arterial puncture and preventing arterial cannulation.[96,106] Although none of these measures are foolproof, they may provide a greater margin of safety and reduce the rate of serious complications resulting from unintentional cannulation of the carotid artery with a large-bore catheter.

Once successful venipuncture is confirmed, the hub of the thin-walled needle or catheter is fixed with the fingers of the left hand, the syringe is detached, and venous blood should be observed to drip from the needle hub. A guidewire (usually 0.032 or 0.035 inch) with either a J-shaped tip or a soft, flexible straight end is inserted through the needle. The wire should advance easily into the vein with little resistance. The ECG is monitored continuously to detect arrhythmias, which are common if the wire tip is inserted too far and contacts the wall of the right atrium or ventricle.[107] From this point in the procedure, it is critical that the clinician maintain control over the guidewire and monitor its depth of insertion and continued sterility.

The puncture site is enlarged with a No. 11 scalpel blade to accommodate the greater size required for the intended catheter. A firm, tapered-tip vessel dilator may be inserted to dilate the subcutaneous tissues around the guidewire and allow a larger catheter to pass smoothly without damage to the tip of the catheter. (When an introducer sheath is to be used, the dilator and sheath form a single unit, and this separate dilation step is usually omitted.) The vessel dilator is removed, and the central venous catheter is inserted over the guidewire while countertraction on the skin is maintained. Again, the clinician must be attentive to the guidewire and ensure that a sufficient length protrudes from the catheter hub before advancing the catheter into the vein so that the wire may be extracted easily. The catheter is inserted to an appropriate depth that will place the tip in the superior vena cava, above its junction with the right atrium. This depth is typically 15 to 18 cm if the catheter is placed via the technique described. The guidewire is then withdrawn, the catheter is attached by a Luer-Lok connector to monitoring or infusion tubing and secured in place, and sterile dressing is applied. Antibiotic ointment should not be applied to the insertion site because it may increase the risk of catheter colonization with multidrug-resistant bacteria or *Candida*.[108,109]

In patients at risk for major intraoperative blood loss and hemodynamic instability, two central venous catheters may frequently be required. Some physicians advocate double cannulation of the same central vein (usually the right internal jugular) with two catheters in close proximity. With this technique, a guidewire is introduced into the internal jugular vein by the standard method. Then, before catheter placement, a second jugular venipuncture is performed, approximately 1 to 2 cm cephalad or caudad, and a second guidewire is introduced into the vein. Placing appropriate catheters over each guidewire and securing them at the skin in the normal fashion complete the procedure. Although limited evidence suggests that the incidence of major complications with this double-cannulation technique is no greater than with single central venous catheterization, it is not clear whether this approach is safer than central venous cannulation in two separate central veins.[110] Serious complications of the double-cannulation technique include facial vein avulsion, catheter entanglement, and catheter fracture.[111,112] Double central venous cannulation must be reserved for patients whose needs for venous access and hemodynamic monitoring cannot be met through single cannulation.

Alternative Central Venous Cannulation Sites

Left Internal Jugular Vein

Cannulation of the left internal jugular vein may be accomplished with a technique similar to the one described earlier, although several anatomic details make the left side less attractive than the right. The cupola of the pleura is higher on the left, thereby theoretically increasing the risk for pneumothorax. The thoracic duct may be injured during the procedure as it enters the venous system at the junction of the left internal jugular and subclavian veins.[113] The left internal jugular vein is often smaller than the right and demonstrates a greater degree of overlap of the adjacent carotid artery during head rotation.[114] Catheters inserted from the left side of the patient must traverse the innominate (i.e., left brachiocephalic) vein and enter the superior vena cava perpendicularly, and their distal tips may impinge on the right lateral wall of the superior vena cava and thereby increase the potential for vascular injury. (This anatomic disadvantage pertains to all left-sided catheterization sites and highlights the need for radiographic confirmation of proper catheter location.) Furthermore, there is less familiarity with the technique simply because clinicians cannulate the left internal jugular vein much less often, a situation that results in more adverse events and morbidity.[98,115]

Subclavian Vein

The subclavian vein is an important site for central venous cannulation and is particularly popular among surgeons and other physicians who place central venous catheters for emergency volume resuscitation and long-term intravenous therapy or dialysis rather than for shorter-term monitoring purposes.[116,117] Advantages of subclavian venous cannulation include a lower risk of infection than with internal jugular or femoral sites, ease of insertion in trauma patients who may be immobilized in a cervical collar, and increased patient comfort, especially for long-term intravenous therapy such as hyperalimentation and chemotherapy.[99,118]

For subclavian central access, the patient is placed in a slight head-down position with the arms fully adducted and the head turned slightly away. A small roll is placed between the shoulder blades to expose the infraclavicular area fully. The skin is punctured 2 to 3 cm caudad to the midpoint of the clavicle, far enough from its inferior edge to avoid downward angulation of the needle as it is inserted just beneath the posterior surface of the clavicle. The needle tip is directed toward the suprasternal notch, which may be constantly identified by the fingers of the operator's other hand. Again, the needle is always advanced with gentle negative pressure exerted against the plunger of the syringe. If the subclavian vein is not entered in the first pass, the needle may be withdrawn and a second pass attempted in a slightly more cephalad direction while ensuring that the needle continues to hug the undersurface of the clavicle as it is advanced and avoiding the tendency to increase the downward angulation of the needle. Once the subclavian vein is punctured, catheterization proceeds in a manner similar to that described for jugular vein catheterization.

Several important technical details must be followed to ensure successful subclavian vein cannulation and avoid complications, particularly pneumothorax. Venipuncture generally proceeds without first identifying the vein with a smaller-gauge finder needle because the depth of the subclavian vein is often beyond the reach of the standard 1½-inch, 22-gauge finder needle. A thin-walled needle is preferred over an 18-gauge catheter/needle assembly because the catheter would be very easily kinked as it courses under the clavicle, thereby precluding both confirmation of venous puncture and passage of the guidewire. Of greatest importance, however, the clinician should resist the temptation to make multiple needle passes if the subclavian vein is not punctured on the second or third attempt. It is clear that complications from this procedure, particularly the incidence of pneumothorax and subclavian artery puncture, are directly related to the number of attempts.[117,119] Bilateral attempts at subclavian venipuncture are highly discouraged because of the serious morbidity of bilateral pneumothorax and the difficulty detecting and treating injury to the subclavian artery. Perhaps to an even greater degree than with internal jugular vein cannulation, the safety of subclavian venous line placement rests in the experience of the operator. In more practiced hands, the incidence of complications should be low, with pneumothorax developing in less than 2% and arterial puncture in less than 5% of cases.[117,119]

External Jugular Vein

Both the right and left external jugular veins provide a safe, albeit somewhat problematic alternative to internal jugular or subclavian vein cannulation. Because the external jugular veins are superficial, they allow central venous cannulation with essentially no risk of pneumothorax or unintended arterial puncture. In most instances, it is best to use an 18-gauge catheter rather than the thin-walled needle to introduce the guidewire because of the tortuous course of the external jugular vein and the frequent need to manipulate the guidewire repeatedly to guide it into the superior vena cava. A J-tipped guidewire should always be used because it may be advanced under the clavicle and into the central circulation more successfully than a straight-tipped wire.[120,121] When the guidewire does not advance as desired and appears to be moving peripherally into the subclavian vein, abducting the ipsilateral shoulder beyond 90 degrees before advancing the wire may facilitate central venous passage. Alternatively, the patient's ipsilateral arm is placed at the side and an assistant applies mild caudad traction on the shoulder to straighten the course of the external jugular vein while the wire is advanced. Essentially the only factors that preclude use of the external jugular veins for CVP monitoring are an inability to visualize and cannulate the vessel in the neck and to advance a catheter into the central circulation. Care should be taken to not use excessive force when advancing catheters and stiff dilators into the external jugular vein because the sharp angle that this vein makes with the subclavian vein may increase the risk for venous injury. Unfortunately, problems with successful placement occur in approximately 20% of patients, thus limiting more widespread application of this technique.[104,122]

Femoral Vein

Femoral vein cannulation provides a useful site for CVP monitoring when the more common jugular and subclavian sites are not accessible, as is commonly the case in patients with burns or trauma, during surgical procedures that involve the head, neck, and upper part of the thorax, or during cardiopulmonary resuscitation. Use of the femoral vein obviates many of the common complications of central venous catheterization, specifically pneumothorax, but it does carry the risk of femoral artery and, more rarely, femoral nerve injury. Femoral venipuncture is performed below the inguinal ligament just medial to the palpated femoral arterial pulse in a manner similar to that used for femoral artery cannulation. Either a long (40 to 70 cm) catheter is positioned, under ECG or fluoroscopic guidance, in the inferior vena cava close to the cavoatrial junction or a shorter (15 to 20 cm) catheter is inserted from the femoral vein into the common iliac vein.[123,124] Both techniques provide intra-abdominal venous pressure measurements that appear to agree closely with pressures measured in the superior vena cava in mechanically ventilated, critically ill adults.[123,124] It is not clear whether this correlation remains valid in patients who are breathing spontaneously, those with elevated intra-abdominal or intrathoracic pressure, or those not in the supine position. Disadvantages of the femoral venous route include an increased risk of thromboembolic and infectious complications, as well as vascular injury, which may lead to intra-abdominal or retroperitoneal hemorrhage.[125] Moreover, catheters inserted at the femoral site generally preclude ambulation during recovery.

Axillary and Other Peripheral Veins

In patients with extensive, severe burn injuries, the axillary region is often spared and provides a useful site for either arterial or venous pressure monitoring.[126] Standard 20-cm CVP catheters placed in the axillary veins, approximately 1 cm medial to the palpated axillary artery, allow measurement of pressure from the superior vena cava. Even more distal pressures measured from peripheral veins in the hand and forearm may provide a reasonably accurate estimate of CVP in selected surgical patients.[127] Modified volumetric infusion pumps can even measure in-line peripheral venous pressure without the need for additional transducers and monitoring equipment.[128] Although this method of measuring CVP incurs no risk beyond that associated with placing any standard peripheral intravenous catheter, it has not been validated widely and cannot replace central venous cannulation in most circumstances.

Peripherally inserted central venous catheters (*PICCs*) have become a popular alternative to centrally inserted catheters in patients requiring long-term intravenous therapy. Advantages of a PICC include bedside placement under local anesthesia, an extremely low risk of major insertion-related complications, and safe placement by nonphysicians (i.e., registered nurses and physician assistants). This technique may be particularly cost-effective because it eliminates the need for a minor operative procedure in patients who require a Hickman or Broviac central venous catheter.[129] Venous access for a PICC is obtained through an antecubital vein, preferably the basilic vein, which is generally more successfully catheterized than the cephalic vein because of its more linear course. Early reports described only modest success positioning PICCs in an appropriate central location, as well as considerable risk for venous thrombosis, but improvements in catheter design and insertion technique now result in successful placement and few complications in most patients.[129-131] Most PICCs are placed for long-term therapeutic indications (chemotherapy or parenteral nutrition) and use very flexible, nonthrombogenic silicone catheters. Less commonly, a standard polyurethane 40-cm intravenous catheter is inserted peripherally and advanced to a central location for short-term infusion of vasoactive drugs or monitoring of CVP or pulmonary artery pressure (PAP). CVP recorded via PICCs is slightly higher than the pressure measured with centrally inserted catheters, but this difference is clinically insignificant.[132] When these standard long venous catheters are inserted from an antecubital vein, the catheter tip may advance into the heart as the arm is abducted, thereby increasing the risk for cardiac perforation or arrhythmias.[133,134] Whenever a PICC line is in place, the clinician should exercise caution when placing any additional central venous catheters because of the risk of shearing the PICC line within the central venous circulation.

Ultrasound-Guided Central Venous Cannulation

First described in 1984, ultrasound-guided placement of central venous catheters has proved beneficial in most settings, including the intensive care unit and the operating room.[135,136] Available evidence suggests that fewer needle passes are required for successful venous cannulation when two-dimensional ultrasound guidance is used. In addition, most investigators have shown that ultrasound guidance reduces the time required for catheterization, increases overall success rates, and results in fewer complications.[137,138] The benefit is most evident when the internal jugular vein rather than the subclavian or femoral vein is cannulated, when inexperienced rather than experienced operators perform the procedure, and for adult rather than pediatric patients. Based on this evidence, the Agency for Healthcare Research and Quality has listed the use of real-time ultrasound guidance for central venous catheterization as 1 of 11 practices to improve health care.[139] Nonetheless, the use of ultrasound for placement of central venous catheters continues to be low. Recent surveys show that both house staff physicians at one academic tertiary care center and a group of practicing American anesthesiologists routinely use ultrasound for central venous cannulation less than 15% of the time.[93,140] Some aspects of the use of ultrasound for placement of all central venous access remain controversial. It is still largely unknown whether the additional equipment and manipulation associated with real-time ultrasound guidance may increase the rate of catheter-related infections or whether the increased dependence on this technology by trainees will prove detrimental in clinical settings in which it may be unavailable.

Ultrasound guidance can be used in several different ways during central venous catheterization. For example, Doppler ultrasound transforms the sound waves reflected from the moving red blood cells into an amplified audio signal that can be used to locate the artery and vein before or during cannulation.[135] Two-dimensional ultrasound can be used to confirm vessel location and patency and mark the skin, and then the catheterization can proceed in the usual fashion. Alternatively, the technology can be incorporated into the procedure itself to give real-time visualization of vessel cannulation, a method that is coming to replace the more limited, "one-look" technique.[141]

Real-time, two-dimensional ultrasound guidance for internal jugular vein cannulation requires a 7.5- to 10-MHz transducer protected by a sterile sheath. The operator holds the ultrasound probe in the nondominant hand to obtain a view of the target vessel. The vein and artery appear as two circular black structures on the ultrasound image. The vein is identified by anatomic location and by its compressibility. The artery appears mildly pulsatile (Fig. 40-21). When using ultrasound guidance, either transverse (short axis) or longitudinal (long axis) views are adequate. In general, the transverse view is easier to learn and allows simultaneous identification of the artery and vein, whereas the longitudinal view allows visualization of the needle tip at all times, which may reduce perforation of the posterior wall of the vein.[142] After positioning the vein in the center of the ultrasound screen, the vessel is punctured under direct vision with the 18-gauge needle of choice. The technique then proceeds as in the standard landmark technique described earlier, but with confirmation of the intravenous location of the guidewire with a longitudinal view before proceeding with dilation of the vessel.

Ultrasound imaging of the subclavian vessels is more difficult and often hampered by the patient's body habitus and probe configuration. When using ultrasound to guide cannulation of the subclavian vein, the transducer is placed in the infraclavicular groove at the level of the middle or lateral third of the clavicle, and the axillary vein and artery are imaged as they exit the bony canal formed by the clavicle and the first rib.[143] The artery is most commonly cephalad to the vein and noncompressible, and it does not vary in size with respiration. Either a transverse or longitudinal view can be obtained and used to guide needle insertion.[144] Another approach has been described in children in which the probe is placed in the supraclavicular space to obtain a longitudinal view of the subclavian vein while cannulation is performed via the usual infraclavicular route.[145]

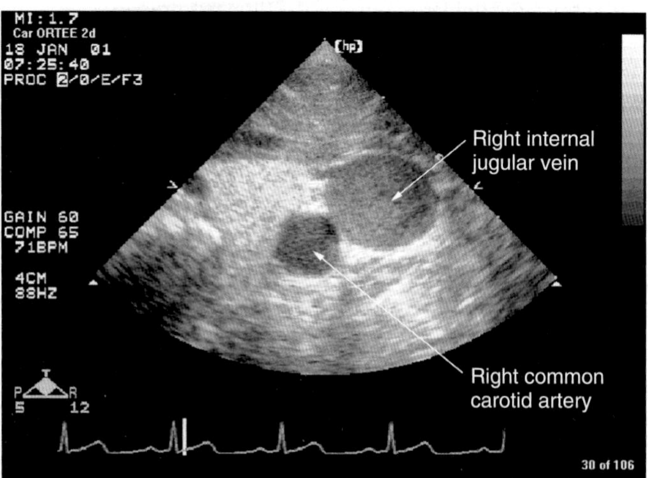

Figure 40-21 Transverse-plane ultrasound image showing the right internal jugular vein and its typical anatomic position anterior and lateral to the right common carotid artery.

Confirming Catheter Position

Central venous catheters placed in the operating room are commonly used for the duration of the surgical procedure without radiologic confirmation of the location of the catheter tip. Before monitoring or infusion commences, aspiration of blood should confirm the intravenous location of each lumen of a multilumen catheter and remove any residual air from the catheter-tubing system. After surgery, however, the position of the catheter tip must be confirmed radiographically. Catheter tips located within the heart or below the pericardial reflection of the superior vena cava increase the risk for cardiac perforation and fatal cardiac tamponade. Ideally, the catheter tip should lie within the superior vena cava, parallel to the vessel walls, and be positioned *below* the inferior border of the clavicles and *above* the level of the third rib, the T4 to T5 interspace, the azygos vein, the tracheal carina, or the takeoff of the right mainstem bronchus.[146,147] Using fresh human cadavers, Albrecht and colleagues recently confirmed that the tracheal carina was always above the pericardial reflection on the superior vena cava, thus suggesting that catheter tip should always be located superior to this radiographic landmark.[148]

Complications of Central Venous Pressure Monitoring

Complications of central venous cannulation are increasingly being recognized as major sources of morbidity, with more than 15% of patients experiencing some sort of related adverse event.[125] Although serious immediate complications are infrequent when these procedures are performed by well-trained, experienced clinicians, infectious complications are common, and the use of CVP catheters continues to result in significant morbidity and mortality. Complications are often divided into mechanical, thromboembolic, and infectious causes (Box 40-5).

Mechanical Complications of Central Venous Catheterization

The incidence of complications depends on a number of factors, including the catheter insertion site and the patient's medical condition. Large retrospective and observational studies provide the best estimates of the incidence and frequency of complications. In general, *unintended arterial puncture* is the most common acute mechanical complication, with an incidence ranging from 1.9% to 15%.[149] Many of these injuries result in localized hematoma formation, but on rare occasion even small-gauge needle punctures may lead to serious complications such as arterial thromboembolism.[150]

If arterial puncture with a small needle occurs during central venous cannulation, the needle should be removed and external pressure applied for several minutes to prevent hematoma formation. When unintentional carotid artery cannulation occurs, it can usually be managed conservatively by removing the catheter, applying local compression to the puncture site, and monitor-

Box 40-5 Complications of Central Venous Pressure Monitoring

Mechanical
- Vascular injury
  - Arterial
  - Venous
  - Hemothorax
  - Cardiac tamponade
- Respiratory compromise
  - Airway compression from hematoma
  - Tracheal, laryngeal injury
  - Pneumothorax
- Nerve injury
- Arrhythmias
- Subcutaneous/mediastinal emphysema

Thromboembolic
- Venous thrombosis
- Pulmonary embolism
- Arterial thrombosis and embolism (air, clot)
- Catheter or guidewire embolism

Infectious
- Insertion site infection
- Catheter infection
- Bloodstream infection
- Endocarditis

Misinterpretation of data

Misuse of equipment

ing the patient's airway and neurologic status. A vascular surgeon should be consulted promptly to help manage the complication. Only under exceptional circumstances should the catheter be allowed to remain in the vessel because of a high risk for arteritis, thrombus formation, and cerebral embolization.[151]

Vascular injuries from central venous catheterization have a range of clinical consequences. The most common minor complications are localized hematoma or injury to the venous valves.[152] More serious complications include perforation into the pleural space or mediastinum resulting in hydrothorax, hemothorax, hydromediastinum, hemomediastinum, chylothorax, or any combination of these sequelae.[113,153-156] Other catastrophic and thankfully rare vascular injuries have been reported, including aortic perforation and avulsion of the facial vein.[111,157] Delayed vascular complications after central venous catheterization are uncommon but should be considered consequences of this procedure. A number of these delayed complications have been described in the literature, including aortoatrial fistula, venobronchial fistula, carotid artery–internal jugular vein fistula, and pseudoaneurysm formation.[158-161]

The most important life-threatening vascular complication of central venous catheterization is *cardiac tamponade* resulting from perforation of the intrapericardial superior vena cava, right atrium, or right ventricle and subsequent hemopericardium or unintentional pericardial instillation of intravenous fluid.[162] This injury was the second most common complication related to central venous catheters in an analysis of the American Society of Anesthesiologists Closed Claims Project in 2004.[163] Cardiac tamponade resulted in death in 81% of cases in this report and often had a delayed manifestation (1 to 5 days), thus indicating that this complication is related to catheter maintenance and use more often than to the vascular access procedure itself. Most reports document the avoidable nature of this catastrophic event and highlight that patients are predisposed to this complication when central venous catheter tips are malpositioned within the heart chambers or abutting the wall of the superior vena cava at a steep angle. This latter position can be recognized radiographically as a gentle curvature of the catheter tip within the superior vena cava.[164] These observations emphasize that objective confirmation of proper catheter tip location is mandatory, regardless of whether the catheter is inserted from a central or peripheral site. In fact, many early reports of catheter-related cardiovascular perforation suggested that peripheral catheters may be associated with an unusually high risk for this complication because arm abduction may cause the catheter tip to advance into a dangerous location within the heart.[133,165] When cardiac tamponade is caused by catheter-induced cardiac perforation, symptoms develop suddenly, so a high index of suspicion is required if severe hypotension occurs in any patient with a central venous catheter in place. Cardiac arrhythmias may provide an early clue to intracardiac location of the catheter tip.[134] Occasionally, both posteroanterior and lateral chest radiographs, as well as injection of radiopaque contrast material, are required to locate the catheter tip precisely.[166]

Pneumothorax is often cited as the most common complication of subclavian vein cannulation, although it appears that unintended arterial puncture is actually more frequent.[46,119] Mansfield and coauthors reported a 1.5% incidence of pneumothorax and a 3.7% incidence of arterial puncture in 821 patients who underwent attempted subclavian vein cannulation.[119] Pneumothorax is even less frequent with the internal jugular approach. Shah and coworkers reported a 0.5% incidence of pneumothorax in their series of nearly 6000 internal jugular catheterizations.[149] This estimate is most likely high because these patients had undergone sternotomy for cardiac surgery, a procedure that may have been responsible for the pneumothorax in many cases. Small pneumothoraces may be managed conservatively, whereas tube thoracostomy is the best treatment for larger air collections or pneumothorax in patients receiving positive-pressure mechanical ventilation or scheduled for major surgery. The physician must always be prepared for the possibility of tension pneumothorax and its adverse hemodynamic sequelae. In addition to pneumothorax, other respiratory tract injuries have been reported after central venous catheterization, including subcutaneous and mediastinal emphysema, tracheal perforation, and rupture of an endotracheal tube cuff.[167]

Nerve injury is another potential complication of central venous cannulation. Damage may occur to the brachial plexus, stellate ganglion, phrenic nerve, or vocal cords.[168,169] In addition, chronic pain syndromes have been attributed to this procedure.[170]

Thromboembolic Complications of Central Venous Catheterization

Catheter-related thrombosis varies according to the site of central venous catheterization and occurs in as many as 21.5% of patients with femoral vein catheters and 1.9% of those with subclavian vein catheters.[118] Catheters that are positioned low in the right atrium may be more prone to thrombus formation, possibly because of mechanical irritation of the right atrial endocardium by the catheter.[171] Thrombi that form at the catheter tip or adhere to the endocardium have the potential to become a nidus for infection, cause superior vena cava syndrome, or embolize into the pulmonary circulation.[172,173] Occasionally, surgical removal is required.[174]

In addition to thromboembolism, other reported embolic complications of central venous catheterization include embolism of portions of the catheter or guidewire and air embolism.[175,176] Almost invariably, these problems are the result of misuse of equipment, thus highlighting the need for proper education and training of nurses and physicians responsible for the use of these devices.

Infectious Complications of Central Venous Catheterization

By far the most common major late complication of central venous cannulation is *infection*. Bloodstream infections occur in approximately 5% of patients with standard central venous catheters and thus lead to an estimated 150,000 to 250,000 cases of catheter-related bacteremia or fungemia annually.[99,177] Given that the crude mortality of patients with nosocomial bloodstream infections is approximately 35% and the cost of these infections can exceed $50,000 per episode, even basic strategies to reduce this complication appear to be both cost-effective and lifesaving.[177,178]

As previously noted, the starting point for prevention of infection is meticulous attention to aseptic technique.[179] When more long-term central venous access is anticipated, the subclavian site is preferred because use of the jugular or femoral veins carries a higher risk for infection.[118,180] Multilumen catheters may carry a higher risk for infection than single-lumen catheters, although the added clinical functionality of such catheters often mandates their use.[99,125] Catheters are made from materials such as silicone, polyvinyl chloride, Teflon, and polyurethane. Furthermore, catheters of the same material may be manufactured differently, which influences their surfaces and the frequency of bacterial adherence to the surface.[181] Heparin-bonded central venous catheters have been shown to reduce the incidence of catheter-related thrombosis and infection in children and adults.[182] Incorporation of antimicrobial treatments onto the catheter surface, such as combinations of chlorhexidine and silver sulfadiazine or monocycline and rifampin, have been shown to reduce rates of catheter colonization and bloodstream infection.[177,183] The added expense has prevented more widespread adoption of these catheters, although an analysis has suggested their cost-effectiveness in settings in which the rate of catheter-related infection remains high (>3.3 per 1000 catheter-days).[184] The use of catheters with a silver-impregnated subcutaneous cuff has not been shown to be beneficial.[185] A chlorhexidine gluconate–impregnated sponge dressing has been shown to reduce catheter colonization in infants and children but does not reduce the rate of catheter-associated bloodstream infections.[186,187] Current guidelines from the Centers for Disease Control and Prevention do not support routine catheter site changes or scheduled changes over a guidewire and instead provide other detailed recommendations for catheter management to reduce the risk for infectious complications.[99]

Other Complications of Central Venous Catheterization

Miscellaneous other adverse sequelae of central venous cannulation have been reported (see Box 40-5), and although their incidence is not clearly known, most appear to be uncommon. All physicians performing these procedures should be familiar with them, particularly since many of these complications are related to *operator error*.[46,188]

Use of *guidewires, vessel dilators,* and *large-bore catheters* carries certain additional risks that mandate meticulous attention to technique. The proximal tip of the guidewire must remain under the physician's control at all times to avoid inserting the wire too far into the heart and thus causing arrhythmias or potentially losing the guidewire within the circulation.[175,189] By design, vessel dilators are stiffer than the catheters and may cause significant trauma if inserted forcefully or farther than necessary to dilate the subcutaneous tissue tract from skin to vein.[190] Large-bore introducer sheaths and multilumen catheters have become popular because of their clinical utility, yet their size may increase the risk for cannulation-associated trauma, hemorrhage from unrecognized line disconnections, and major venous air embolism. Not only may air be entrained during initial cannulation, but improperly connected large-bore cannulas may pose an additional risk because of the large site for entry of air directly into the central venous circulation.[176,191]

Although many complications of CVP monitoring relate to equipment misuse, the frequency of complications caused by misinterpretation of data remains unknown. It is extremely likely, however, that clinicians misinterpret CVP measurements and have suboptimal understanding of CVP monitoring, just as has been demonstrated repeatedly for PAP monitoring (see discussion later). Safe and effective use of CVP monitoring requires a detailed understanding of cardiovascular physiology, normal CVP waveforms, and common pathologic abnormalities in these measurements.

Physiologic Considerations for Central Venous Pressure Monitoring: Diastolic Pressure-Volume Relationships and Transmural Pressure

Cardiac filling pressures are monitored to estimate cardiac filling volumes, which in turn determine the stroke output of the left and right ventricles. According to the Frank-Starling principle, the force of cardiac contraction is directly proportional to end-diastolic muscle fiber length at any given level of intrinsic contractility or inotropy. This muscle fiber length or preload is proportional to end-diastolic chamber volume. Even though it would be ideal to monitor cardiac chamber volumes continuously in critically ill patients, this goal remains elusive in clinical practice.

When a cardiac filling pressure is measured as a surrogate for estimating cardiac volume, one must not assume that these two variables always change in direct proportion or even in the same direction. In fact, the diastolic pressure-volume relationship in cardiac muscle is not linear, but rather curvilinear, with a progressively steeper slope at higher volumes (Fig. 40-22).[192,193] This diastolic pressure-volume relationship is one limb of a pressure-volume loop that describes the relationship between pressure and volume for the left or right ventricle during an entire cardiac cycle. When a ventricle is operating along the flat portion of its diastolic filling curve, a significant increase in filling volume or preload results in a small increase in filling pressure. In contrast,

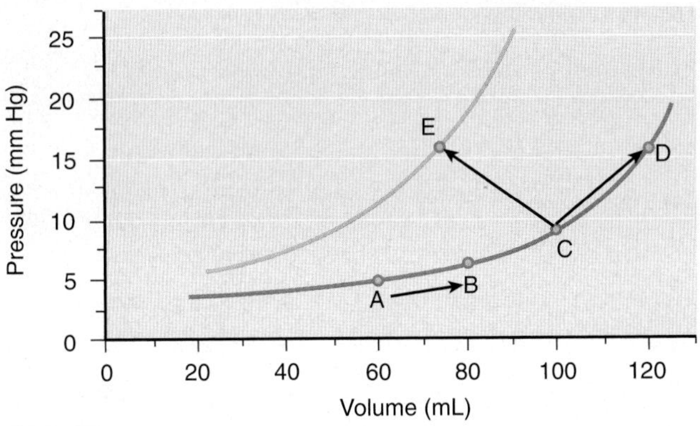

Figure 40-22 Ventricular diastolic pressure-volume relationship. Along the flat portion of the curve, a 20-mL increase in ventricular volume causes a small increase in ventricular pressure (A to B). In contrast, the same increase in volume along the steep portion of the ventricular filling curve causes a marked increase in filling pressure (C to D). Another problem associated with the use of filling pressure as a surrogate for filling volume arises when shifts in the pressure-volume relationship occur. At point C, ventricular volume is 100 mL and ventricular pressure is 8 mm Hg. An increase in filling pressure to 15 mm Hg may accompany either an increased volume (D) or decreased volume (E). The latter occurs when ventricular compliance changes and shifts the ventricular diastolic pressure-volume relationship up and to the left. *(From Mark JB: Atlas of Cardiovascular Monitoring. New York, Churchill Livingstone, 1998, Fig. 15-2.)*

the same increase in filling volume causes a significant increase in filling pressure when the ventricle is operating on the steep portion of its curve.[194] An even more confusing situation arises when the diastolic pressure-volume relationship of the ventricle changes, for example, with the onset of myocardial ischemia. Rather than moving along the same diastolic pressure-volume curve, the ventricle now shifts to a different, steeper curve, where somewhat paradoxically, an increase in filling pressure may accompany a decrease in filling volume.[195] As in this example, not only can one not assume that a given measured change in cardiac filling pressure reflects a proportional change in ventricular preload, it cannot even be assumed that diastolic pressure and volume change in a similar direction.[195]

The relationship between ventricular volume and filling pressure depends on the portion of the pressure-volume curve over which the patient's heart is operating and the shape or slope of the curve. Commonly termed ventricular compliance, this change in pressure for a given change in volume ($\Delta P/\Delta V$) is actually the reciprocal of compliance and is more accurately termed ventricular elastance, distensibility, or stiffness.[196] A patient with an abnormally stiff ventricle will have a greater change in end-diastolic pressure for any given change in end-diastolic volume, and the converse is true for a patient with an abnormally compliant ventricle. By definition, diastolic dysfunction is present when changes in ventricular pressure are abnormally elevated for any given change in ventricular volume.

The ventricular diastolic pressure-volume relationship is influenced by the intrinsic properties of the ventricle, such as the passive mechanical characteristics of cardiac muscle, chamber geometry, and relaxation. In addition, external forces exerted by the pericardium, the adjacent ventricle, the coronary vasculature, and pleural pressure will further influence ventricular pressure-volume relationships.[197,198] One should not equate cardiac filling pressures with filling volumes when patients are functioning over wide ranges of their diastolic pressure-volume curve or under conditions in which diastolic stiffness is abnormal or changing rapidly.

In general, all intravascular pressures measured in clinical practice are referenced to ambient atmospheric pressure. Indeed, the first step in pressure transducer setup is to zero the transducer by exposing it to atmospheric pressure and assigning this pressure a value of zero by pressing the zero pressure button on the monitor (see "Technical Aspects of Direct Blood Pressure Measurement"). Thus, a cardiac filling pressure of 10 mm Hg is 10 mm Hg higher than ambient atmospheric pressure. Does this pressure value accurately represent the distending force across the cardiac chamber wall at end-diastole?

To answer this question, one needs to consider transmural pressure. The cardiac chambers are all contained within the pericardium and thorax. Changes in pressure in the structures surrounding the heart will influence pressures recorded within the heart. Transmural pressure is the difference between chamber pressure and juxtacardiac or pericardial pressure. This transmural pressure determines ventricular preload, end-diastolic volume, or fiber length. The same measured filling pressure, referenced to atmospheric pressure, can be associated with markedly different transmural pressures and chamber volumes, depending on whether juxtacardiac pressure is high or low. Although juxtacardiac pressure can be ignored under some circumstances, marked alterations in pleural and pericardial pressure occur commonly and must be considered when any cardiac filling pressure is interpreted. Transmural pressure is always the pressure of physiologic interest. Because juxtacardiac pressure is not measured routinely, one must always consider that the measured central venous pressure, referenced to ambient atmosphere, may be a poor estimate of transmural pressure.[194,199]

Cardiac filling pressures are measured directly from a number of sites in the vascular system. CVP monitoring is the least invasive method, followed by monitoring of PAP and left atrial pressure (LAP). Proper interpretation of all cardiac filling pressures requires knowledge of normal values for these pressures, as well as pressures in the cardiac chambers, the great vessels, and other measured and derived hemodynamic variables (Table 40-2).

Normal Central Venous Pressure Waveforms

Strictly speaking, CVP is the pressure measured at the junction of the venae cavae and the right atrium and reflects the driving force for filling the right atrium and ventricle. Because the large veins of the thorax, abdomen, and proximal extremities form a compliant reservoir for a sizable percentage of total blood volume, CVP is highly dependent on intravascular blood volume and the intrinsic vascular tone of these capacitance vessels. In other words, CVP or right atrial pressure in part reflects the relationship of blood volume to the capacity of the venous system.[200] In addition, CVP also reflects the functional capacity of the right ventricle. Based on the Frank-Starling mechanism, higher right heart filling pressures are required to maintain ventricular stroke output when ventricular contractility is impaired. Thus, in clinical practice, CVP monitoring is used for assessment of blood volume and right heart function.[201] Normal CVP in an awake, spontaneously breathing patient ranges between 1 and 7 mm Hg.

Table 40-2 Normal Cardiovascular Pressures

Pressure	Average (mm Hg)	Range (mm Hg)
Right Atrium		
a wave	6	2-7
v wave	5	2-7
Mean	3	1-5
Right Ventricle		
Peak systolic	25	15-30
End-diastolic	6	1-7
Pulmonary Artery		
Peak systolic	25	15-30
End-diastolic	9	4-12
Mean	15	9-19
Pulmonary Artery Wedge		
Mean	9	4-12
Left Atrium		
a wave	10	4-16
v wave	12	6-21
Mean	8	2-12
Left Ventricle		
Peak systolic	130	90-140
End-diastolic	8	5-12
Central Aorta		
Peak systolic	130	90-140
End-diastolic	70	60-90
Mean	90	70-105

Mechanical events during the cardiac cycle are responsible for the sequence of waves seen in a typical CVP trace. The CVP waveform consists of five phasic events, three peaks (a, c, v) and two descents (x, y) (Table 40-3, Fig. 40-23).[202,203] The most prominent wave is the *a wave* of atrial contraction, which occurs at end-diastole after the ECG P wave. Atrial contraction increases atrial pressure and provides the "atrial kick" to fill the right ventricle through the open tricuspid valve. Atrial pressure decreases after the a wave as the atrium relaxes. This smooth decline in pressure is interrupted by the *c wave*. This wave is a transient increase in atrial pressure produced by isovolumic ventricular contraction, which closes the tricuspid valve and displaces it toward the atrium. The c wave always follows the ECG R wave because it is generated during the onset of ventricular systole. (Note that the c wave observed in a jugular venous pressure trace might have a slightly more complex origin. This wave has been attributed to early systolic pressure transmission from the adjacent carotid artery and may be termed a carotid impact wave.[204] Because jugular venous pressure also reflects right atrial pressure, however, this c wave probably represents both arterial [carotid impact] and venous [tricuspid motion] origins.) Atrial pressure continues its decline during ventricular systole because of continued atrial relaxation and changes in atrial geometry produced by ventricular contraction and ejection. This is the *x descent*, or systolic collapse in atrial pressure. The *x* descent can be divided into two portions, x and x′, corresponding to segments before and after the c wave. The last atrial pressure peak is the *v wave*, which is caused by venous filling of the atrium during late systole while the tricuspid valve remains closed. The v wave usually peaks just after the ECG T wave. Atrial pressure then decreases, thereby inscribing the *y descent*, or diastolic collapse, as the tricuspid valve opens and blood flows from atrium to ventricle. (A final compo-

Table 40-3 Central Venous Pressure Waveform Components

Waveform Component	Phase of Cardiac Cycle	Mechanical Event
a wave	End diastole	Atrial contraction
c wave	Early systole	Isovolumic ventricular contraction, tricuspid motion toward the right atrium
v wave	Late systole	Systolic filling of the atrium
h wave	Mid to late diastole	Diastolic plateau
x descent	Mid systole	Atrial relaxation, descent of the base, systolic collapse
y descent	Early diastole	Early ventricular filling, diastolic collapse

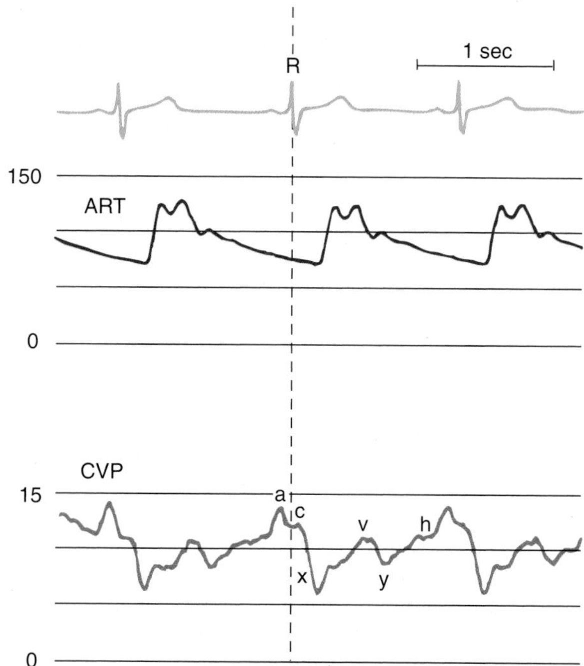

Figure 40-23 Normal central venous pressure (CVP) waveform. The diastolic components (y descent, end-diastolic a wave) and the systolic components (c wave, x descent, end-systolic v wave) are all clearly delineated. A mid-diastolic plateau wave, the h wave, is also seen because the heart rate is slow. Identification of the waveform is aided by timing the relationship between individual waveform components and the electrocardiographic R wave. Waveform timing using the arterial (ART) pressure trace is more confusing because of the relative delay in systolic arterial pressure upstroke. *(From Mark JB: Atlas of Cardiovascular Monitoring. New York, Churchill Livingstone, 1998, Fig. 2-5.)*

nent of the CVP waveform, the *h wave*, occasionally appears as a pressure plateau in mid to late diastole. The h wave is not normally seen unless the heart rate is slow and venous pressure is elevated.[204,205]) In summary, the normal venous waveform components may be remembered as follows: the a wave results from atrial contraction; the c wave results from closure of the tricuspid valve and isovolumic right ventricular contraction; the x descent is the systolic decrease in atrial pressure caused by atrial relaxation; the v wave results from ventricular ejection, which drives venous filling of the atrium; and the y descent is the diastolic decrease in atrial pressure caused by flow across the open tricuspid valve.

In relation to the cardiac cycle and ventricular mechanical actions, the CVP waveform can be considered to have three systolic components (c wave, x descent, v wave) and two diastolic components (y descent, a wave). By recalling the mechanical actions that generate the pressure peaks and troughs, it is easy to identify these waveform components properly by aligning the CVP waveform and the ECG trace and using the ECG R wave to mark end-diastole and the onset of systole. When the radial artery pressure trace is used for timing of the CVP waveform instead of the ECG, confusion may arise because the arterial pressure upstroke occurs nearly 200 msec after the ECG R wave (see Fig. 40-23). This normal physiologic delay reflects the times required for spread of electrical depolarization through the ventricle (~60 msec), isovolumic left ventricular contraction (~60 msec), transmission of the rise in aortic pressure to the radial artery (~50 msec), and transmission of the rise in radial artery pressure through fluid-filled tubing to the transducer (~10 msec).[61,206]

The normal CVP peaks are designated systolic (c, v) or diastolic (a) according to the phase of the cardiac cycle in which the wave begins. However, one generally identifies these waves not by their onset or upstroke but rather by the location of their peaks. For instance, the a wave generally begins and peaks in end-diastole, but the peak may appear delayed to coincide with the ECG R wave, especially in a patient with a short PR interval. In this instance the a and c waves merge, and this composite wave is termed an a-c wave. Designation of the CVP v wave as a systolic event may be even more confusing. Although ascent of the v wave begins during late systole, the peak of the v wave occurs during isovolumic ventricular relaxation, immediately before opening of the atrioventricular valve and the y descent. Consequently, the most precise description would be that the v wave begins in late systole but peaks during isovolumic ventricular relaxation, the earliest portion of diastole. For clinical purposes, it is simplest to consider the v wave to be a systolic wave.

Although three distinct CVP peaks (a, c, v) and two troughs (x, y) are discernible in the normal venous pressure trace, heart rate changes and conduction abnormalities alter this pattern. A short ECG PR interval causes fusion of the a and c waves, and tachycardia reduces the length of diastole and the duration of the y descent, which causes the v and a waves to merge. In contrast, bradycardia causes each wave to become more distinct, with separate x and x′ descents visible and a more prominent h wave. Although there are circumstances in which other pathologic waves may be evident in the CVP trace, one should resist the temptation to assign physiologic significance to each small pressure peak because many will arise as artifacts of fluid-filled tubing-transducer monitoring systems. It is more useful to search for the expected waveform components, including those characteristic of the pathologic conditions suspected.

Abnormal Central Venous Pressure Waveforms

Various pathophysiologic conditions may be diagnosed or confirmed by examination of the CVP waveform (Table 40-4). One of the most common applications is rapid diagnosis of cardiac arrhythmias.[207] In *atrial fibrillation*, the a wave disappears and the c wave becomes more prominent because atrial volume is greater at end-diastole and the onset of systole as a result of the absence of effective atrial contraction (Fig. 40-24A). Occasionally, atrial fibrillation or flutter waves may be seen in the CVP trace when the ventricular rate is slow. Isorhythmic *atrioventricular dissociation* or *junctional (nodal) rhythm* (see Fig. 40-24B) alters the normal sequence of atrial contraction before ventricular contraction. Instead, atrial contraction now occurs during ventricular systole when the tricuspid valve is closed, thereby inscribing a tall "cannon" a wave in the CVP waveform. Absence of normal atrioventricular synchrony during ventricular pacing (see Fig. 40-24C) can be identified in a similar fashion by searching for cannon waves in the venous pressure trace. In these instances, the CVP waveform helps diagnose the cause of the arterial hypotension; loss of the normal end-diastolic atrial kick may not be as evident in the ECG trace as it is in the CVP waveform.

Right-sided valvular heart diseases alter the CVP waveform in different ways.[208] *Tricuspid regurgitation* produces abnormal systolic filling of the right atrium through the incompetent valve (Fig. 40-25A). A broad, tall systolic c-v wave results, beginning in early systole and obliterating the systolic x descent in atrial pressure. The CVP trace is said to be ventricularized and resembles right ventricular pressure. Note that this regurgitant wave differs in onset, duration, and magnitude from a normal v wave caused by end-systolic atrial filling from the venae cavae. In patients with tricuspid regurgitation, right ventricular end-diastolic pressure is

Table 40-4 Central Venous Pressure Waveform Abnormalities

Condition	Characteristics
Atrial fibrillation	Loss of a wave Prominent c wave
Atrioventricular dissociation	Cannon a wave
Tricuspid regurgitation	Tall systolic c-v wave Loss of x descent
Tricuspid stenosis	Tall a wave Attenuation of y descent
Right ventricular ischemia	Tall a and v waves Steep x and y descents M or W configuration
Pericardial constriction	Tall a and v waves Steep x and y descents M or W configuration
Cardiac tamponade	Dominant x descent Attenuated y descent
Respiratory variation during spontaneous or positive-pressure ventilation	Measure pressures at end-expiration

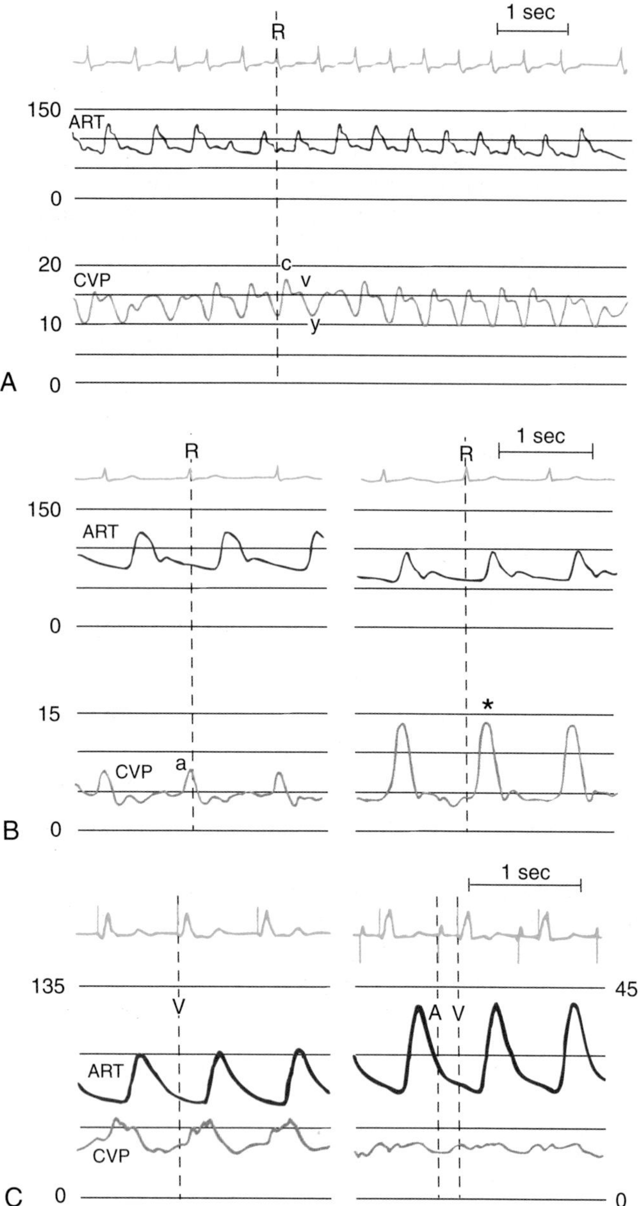

Figure 40-24 Changes in central venous pressure (CVP) caused by cardiac arrhythmias. **A,** Atrial fibrillation. Note the absence of the a wave, a prominent c wave, and a preserved v wave and y descent. This arrhythmia also causes variation in the electrocardiographic (ECG) R-R interval and left ventricular stroke volume, which can be seen in the ECG and arterial pressure (ART) traces. **B,** Isorhythmic atrioventricular dissociation. In contrast to the normal end-diastolic a wave in the CVP trace *(left panel)*, an early systolic cannon wave is inscribed (*, *right panel*). Reduced ventricular filling accompanying this arrhythmia causes decreased arterial blood pressure. **C,** Ventricular pacing. Systolic cannon waves are evident in the CVP trace during ventricular pacing *(left panel)*. Atrioventricular sequential pacing restores the normal venous waveform and increases arterial blood pressure *(right panel)*. The ART scale is shown on the *left*; the CVP scale is on the *right*. *(From Mark JB: Atlas of Cardiovascular Monitoring. New York, Churchill Livingstone, 1998, Figs.14-1, 14-5, and 14-6.)*

overestimated by the numeric display on the bedside monitor, which reports a single mean value for CVP. Instead, right ventricular end-diastolic pressure is best estimated by measuring CVP at the time of the ECG R wave, before the regurgitant systolic wave (see Fig. 40-25A). Unlike tricuspid regurgitation, *tricuspid stenosis* produces a diastolic defect in atrial emptying and ventricular filling (see Fig. 40-25B). Mean CVP is elevated, and a pressure gradient exists throughout diastole between the right atrium and ventricle. The a wave is unusually prominent and the y descent is attenuated as a result of the impaired diastolic egress of blood from the atrium. Other conditions that reduce right ventricular compliance, such as right ventricular ischemia, pulmonary hypertension, or pulmonic valve stenosis, may produce a prominent end-diastolic a wave in the CVP trace but do not attenuate the early diastolic y descent. CVP waveform morphology changes in other characteristic ways in the presence of pericardial disease and right ventricular infarction. These patterns are

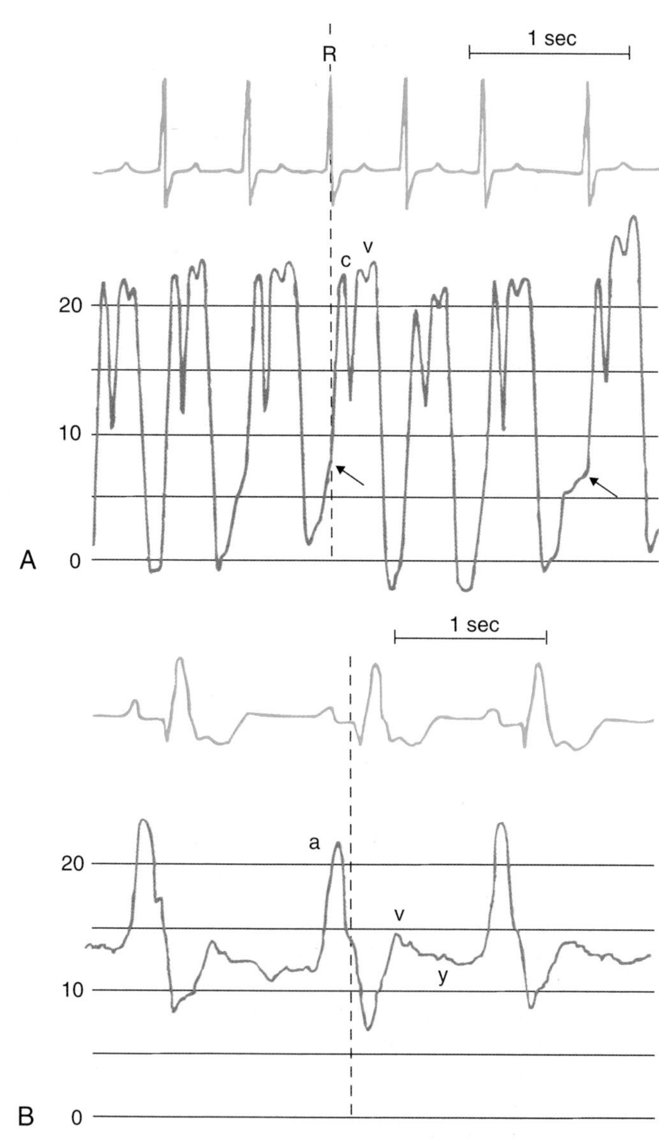

Figure 40-25 Changes in central venous pressure (CVP) in tricuspid valve disease. **A,** Tricuspid regurgitation increases mean CVP, and the waveform displays a tall systolic c-v wave that obliterates the x descent. In this example the a wave is not seen because of atrial fibrillation. Right ventricular end-diastolic pressure is estimated best at the time of the electrocardiographic R wave *(arrows)* and is lower than mean CVP. **B,** Tricuspid stenosis increases mean CVP, the diastolic y descent is attenuated, and the end-diastolic a wave is prominent. *(From Mark JB: Atlas of Cardiovascular Monitoring. New York, Churchill Livingstone, 1998, Figs. 17-3 and 17-15.)*

best interpreted in conjunction with monitoring of PAP, which is discussed later.

Perhaps the most important application of CVP monitoring is to provide an estimate of the adequacy of circulating blood volume and right ventricular preload. As noted earlier, transmural CVP is the pressure of physiologic interest, although in clinical practice we measure and record pressures referenced to ambient atmospheric pressure. Consequently, accurate interpretation of CVP requires the physician to consider the alterations in intrathoracic or juxtacardiac pressure that occur during the respiratory cycle.[194,199] During spontaneous breathing, inspiration causes a decrease in pleural and juxtacardiac pressure, which is transmitted, in part, to the right atrium and lowers CVP (Fig. 40-26A). This same decrease in pleural pressure will influence other measured central vascular pressures in similar fashion. Note a subtle, but critically important observation about the measurement of central vascular pressures. Although CVP measured relative to atmospheric pressure decreases during the inspiratory phase of spontaneous ventilation, transmural CVP, the difference between right atrial pressure and juxtacardiac pressure, may actually increase slightly as more blood is drawn into the right atrium. The opposite pattern is observed during positive-pressure ventilation, in which inspiration increases intrathoracic pressure while raising the measured CVP but decreases transmural CVP because the elevated intrathoracic pressure reduces venous return (see Fig. 40-26B). As mentioned earlier, transmural pressures are rarely measured in clinical practice because of difficulty assessing juxtacardiac or intrathoracic pressure. Instead, end-expiratory values for cardiac filling pressures should be recorded in all patients to provide the best estimate of transmural pressure. At the end of expiration, intrathoracic and juxtacardiac pressures approach atmospheric pressure regardless of ventilatory status, and the CVP values will coincide (see Fig. 40-26). Proper pressure values can also be determined by visual inspection of the CVP waveform on a calibrated monitor screen or paper recording. This facilitates comparison of CVP values (and other cardiac filling pressures) obtained from the same patient under varying patterns of ventilation, a common situation in anesthesia and critical care.

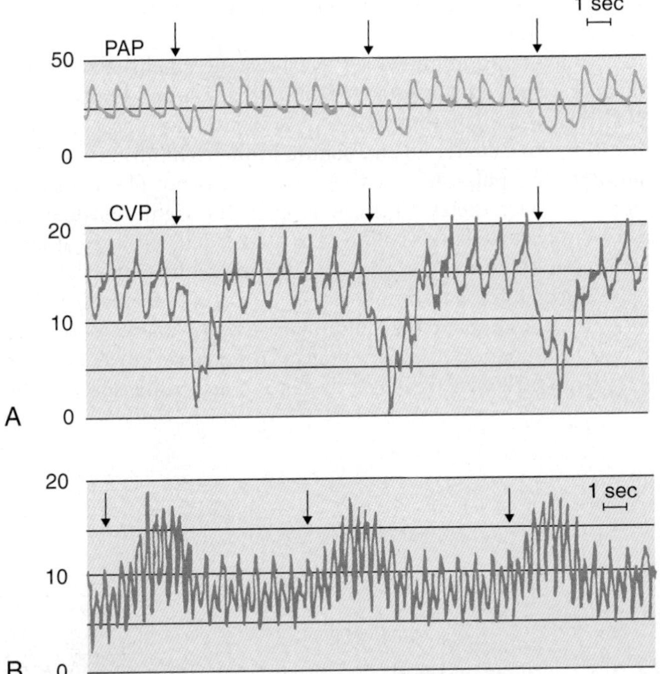

Figure 40-26 Respiratory influences on the measurement of central venous pressure (CVP). **A,** During spontaneous ventilation, the onset of inspiration (*arrows*) causes a reduction in intrathoracic pressure, which is transmitted to both the CVP and pulmonary artery pressure (PAP) waveforms. CVP should be recorded at end-expiration (mean CVP, 14 mm Hg). **B,** During positive-pressure ventilation, the onset of inspiration (*arrows*) causes an increase in intrathoracic pressure. CVP is still recorded at end-expiration (mean CVP, 8 mm Hg). *(From Mark JB: Atlas of Cardiovascular Monitoring. New York, Churchill Livingstone, 1998, Figs. 16-1 and 16-2.)*

Not only can individual CVP waveforms provide unique diagnostic clues about the circulation, but trends in CVP over time may also be useful in estimating fluid or blood loss and guiding replacement therapy. It is important to remember that there is a significant range of normal values and that a small change in CVP may reflect a significant alteration in circulating blood volume and right ventricular preload. Additional useful information may be derived from examining how a fluid bolus simultaneously alters CVP and other variables of clinical interest, such as blood pressure, urine output, and so forth.

Pulmonary Artery Catheter Monitoring

In 1970, Swan, Ganz, and colleagues introduced pulmonary artery catheterization into clinical practice for hemodynamic assessment of patients with acute myocardial infarction.[209,210] These catheters allowed accurate measurement of important cardiovascular physiologic variables at the bedside, and their popularity soared. By the mid-1990s, estimated annual PAC sales in the United States approached 2 million catheters, with an estimated cost associated with their use in excess of $2 billion each year.[211]

The PAC provides measurements of several hemodynamic variables that many clinicians, including experts in intensive care, cannot predict accurately from standard clinical signs and symptoms.[212] However, it remains uncertain whether PAC monitoring leads to improved patient outcome.[213]

Pulmonary Artery Catheterization

PACs can be placed from any of the central venous cannulation sites described earlier, but the right internal jugular vein is preferred because it provides the most direct route to the right heart chambers. The procedure is conducted in a manner similar to that for central venous cannulation. However, before PAC insertion, a slightly larger skin nick is made to accommodate a large-bore introducer sheath with a hemostasis valve at its outer end and a side-arm extension for intravenous access. A tapered-tip, stiff dilator stylet is placed inside an introducer sheath to facilitate passage into the vein. Utmost care must be exercised when introducing this large dilator-cannula assembly by advancing it only to the depth required to enter the vein and then threading the introducer into the vein. Finally, the guidewire and dilator are removed, and the introducer sheath is sutured in place.

The standard PAC has a 7.0- to 9.0-Fr circumference, is 110 cm in length marked at 10-cm intervals, and contains four internal lumens. The distal port at the catheter tip is used for monitoring of PAP, whereas the second is 30 cm more proximal and is used for monitoring of CVP. The third lumen leads to a balloon near the tip, and the fourth houses wires for a temperature thermistor, the end of which lies just proximal to the balloon.

The steps in placing a PAC require the aid of a skilled assistant. Before insertion, the PAC is passed through a sterile sheath that attaches to the hub of the introducer and allows sterile manipulation of PAC position during use. The assistant attaches the distal and proximal port hubs to pressure transducers and flushes them to ensure proper function and exclude air from the system. The balloon is tested by filling it completely with 1.5 mL of air from a volume-limited syringe to ensure symmetry of expansion and patency. The air-filled balloon at the tip of the catheter serves to "float" the catheter forward with blood flow through the right heart chambers and into its proper position in the pulmonary artery.

It is important to check the assembly for proper function. When the tip of the PAC is held near heart level, the recorded pressure should be 0 mm Hg, thus confirming that the transducer was correctly adjusted at the beginning of the procedure. The catheter tip is then raised up straight to create a 30-cm-tall vertical fluid column, which should produce a pressure of 22 mm Hg (equivalent to 30 cm H_2O) on the bedside monitor.

The PAC is then inserted through the hemostasis valve of the introducer to a depth of 20 cm or approximately 5 cm beyond the tip of the introducer sheath. A characteristic CVP waveform should be visible. The gentle curvature of the PAC should be oriented to point just leftward of the sagittal plane (the 11-o'clock position as viewed from the patient's head) to facilitate passage through the anteromedially located tricuspid valve. The balloon is inflated and the catheter is advanced into the right atrium; through the tricuspid valve, right ventricle, and pulmonic valve; into the pulmonary artery; and finally into the wedge position. Characteristic waveforms from each of these locations confirm proper catheter passage and placement (Fig. 40-27).

After PAWP is measured, the balloon is deflated and the PAP waveform should reappear. Wedge pressure may be obtained as needed by reinflating the balloon and allowing the catheter to float distally until pulmonary artery occlusion occurs again. The clinician must recognize that the tip of the PAC advances to a smaller pulmonary artery each time that the balloon is inflated to measure wedge pressure. In some patients the PAC may migrate distally even without balloon inflation. This problem is more common during cardiopulmonary bypass because of the repeated cardiac manipulations and temperature changes, which alter the stiffness of the catheter.[214] Consequently, proper catheter position must be ensured throughout the monitoring period by frequent observation of the pressure waveform. If a PAWP trace appears without balloon inflation or with only partial balloon inflation, the balloon should be deflated and the catheter withdrawn several centimeters to reduce the risk of pulmonary vascular injury. Although the external protective sleeve covering the PAC is intended to maintain sterility during these minor adjustments, the sleeve does not preclude contamination. Therefore, PACs should be manipulated only as necessary to maintain a proper safe location.[215]

Additional Guidelines for Placement of Pulmonary Artery Catheters

From a right internal jugular vein puncture site, the right atrium should be reached when the PAC is inserted 20 to 25 cm, the right ventricle at 30 to 35 cm, the pulmonary artery at 40 to 45 cm, and the wedge position at 45 to 55 cm. When other sites are chosen for catheter placement, additional distance is required, typically an extra 5 to 10 cm from the left internal jugular and left and right external jugular veins, 15 cm from the femoral veins, and 30 to 35 cm from the antecubital veins.[216] These distances serve only as a rough guide, and waveform morphology must always be verified and catheter position confirmed with a chest radiograph as soon as practical. The tip of the PAC should be within 2 cm of the cardiac silhouette on a standard anteroposterior chest film.[217]

Keeping in mind these typical distances helps avoid complications caused by unintended catheter loops and knots within the heart. If a right ventricular waveform is not observed after inserting the catheter 40 cm, coiling in the right atrium is likely. Similarly, if a pulmonary artery waveform is not observed after inserting the catheter 50 cm, coiling in the right ventricle has probably occurred. The balloon should be deflated, the catheter withdrawn to 20 cm, and the PAC floating sequence repeated.

Although the right internal jugular vein is the primary site for catheterization of the pulmonary artery, failure to achieve venous cannulation or other medical and surgical considerations may require the use of alternative sites. For cardiac surgery, the

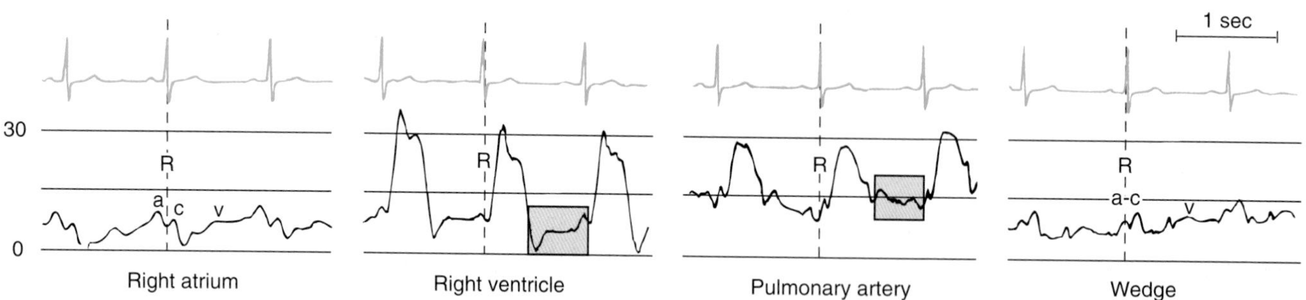

Figure 40-27 Characteristic waveforms recorded during passage of the pulmonary artery catheter. Right atrial pressure resembles a central venous pressure waveform and displays a, c, and v waves. Right ventricular pressure shows higher systolic pressure than seen in the right atrium, although the end-diastolic pressures are equal in these two chambers. Pulmonary artery pressure shows a diastolic step-up when compared with ventricular pressure. Note also that right ventricular pressure increases during diastole whereas pulmonary artery pressure decreases during diastole (*shaded boxes*). Pulmonary artery wedge pressure has a similar morphology to right atrial pressure, although the a-c and v waves appear later in the cardiac cycle relative to the electrocardiogram. *(From Mark JB: Atlas of Cardiovascular Monitoring. New York, Churchill Livingstone, 1998, Fig. 3-1.)*

left internal jugular vein is often the second choice because a PAC inserted by the subclavian route may be compressed and kinked under the clavicle, thus making it extremely difficult to withdraw or advance after sternotomy.[219]

Regardless of the intended surgical procedure, whenever one plans to insert a PAC through the left internal jugular, subclavian, and particularly the external jugular veins, the more tortuous course of these vessels may make it difficult to advance the large-bore introducer sheath fully into the vessel. This is not a problem as long as the introducer cannula is withdrawn slightly to maintain a position in the vein that allows unimpeded intravenous infusion and free aspiration of venous blood. Frequently, the introducer cannula needs to remain in this partially inserted position while the PAC is introduced through its hemostasis valve. Because the tip of the PAC is more flexible and smaller than the tip of the introducer, the PAC might advance easily and completely into the central vein and right atrium. The PAC balloon may then be inflated and the procedure completed in the normal fashion with the PAC serving as the de facto guidewire. Occasionally, the introducer sheath must remain partially or completely withdrawn to avoid acute angulation and kinking of the PAC as it leaves the sheath and enters the central vein.[218,219]

After successful venous cannulation, if attempts to advance the PAC to the right ventricle prove difficult, the physician should consider whether this difficulty might result from abnormal venous anatomy. The most common abnormality of the systemic veins is persistence of the left superior vena cava, which is present in approximately 0.1% to 0.2% of the general population and 2% to 9% of patients with other forms of congenital heart disease.[220,221] A persistent left superior vena cava descends along the left mediastinum and empties into a dilated coronary sinus. As a result of its benign nature, virtually all cases are asymptomatic and discovered incidentally at the time of failed central venous or pulmonary artery catheterization. Because a normal right superior vena cava is present in most of these patients, the anomaly is recognized only when attempted PAC placement proceeds from a left-sided vein. More rarely, difficult PAC placement is encountered during attempted right-sided venous cannulation because the right superior vena cava is absent as well. In these cases, the right internal jugular vein joins the persistent left superior vena cava by a bridging innominate vein. A rare form of atrial septal defect, termed *unroofed coronary sinus*, may also be encountered in these patients and provide coronary sinus–left atrial communication and the potential for a PAC to enter the left atrium and systemic circulation.[221] With any of these venous anomalies, advancement of the PAC into the coronary sinus may disclose an unexpected pressure waveform, coronary sinus pressure. This waveform has characteristics of both the downstream right atrial pressure and an indirectly transmitted, dampened left ventricular pressure waveform.

A few additional points might aid successful positioning of the PAC. The air-filled balloon tends to float to nondependent regions as it passes through the heart into the pulmonary vasculature. Consequently, positioning a patient head down will aid flotation past the tricuspid valve, and tilting the patient onto the right side and placing the head up will encourage flotation out of the right ventricle.[222] Deep inspiration during spontaneous ventilation will increase venous return and right ventricular output transiently and may facilitate catheter flotation in a patient with low cardiac output. On occasion, a catheter may be floated to proper position when stiffened by injecting 10 to 20 mL of an iced solution through the distal lumen. Finally, a catheter that is initially difficult to place may be positioned easily when hemodynamic conditions change, as commonly occurs after induction of general anesthesia and initiation of positive-pressure ventilation.

Complications of Pulmonary Artery Catheter Monitoring

Complications of PAC use may be divided into several groups: those resulting from catheter placement, those associated with the in vivo presence of the catheter, and those resulting from catheter use and misuse. For the most part, problems encountered during catheter placement are the same for both PAP and CVP monitoring (see Box 40-5). However, catheterization of the right ventricle and pulmonary artery causes complications uniquely associated with PACs (Box 40-6).

When all adverse effects from PAC use are considered, including self-limited arrhythmias observed during catheter insertion, it appears that minor complications occur in more than 50% of catheterized patients.[211] However, major morbidity specifically attributable to PAC use is uncommon.[223] In both an initial exhaustive review of the literature and in its 2003 update, the American Society of Anesthesiologists Task Force on Pulmonary Artery Catheterization emphasized that the reported incidence of complications from PAC monitoring varies widely, although it seems that serious complications occur in 0.1% to 0.5% of PAC-monitored surgical patients.[211] In 1984, Shah and coworkers reported the use of PACs in 6245 patients undergoing cardiac and noncardiac operations.[149] Quite remarkably, only 10 patients (0.16%) had serious complications resulting in morbidity and only 1 patient (0.016%) died as a result of pulmonary artery catheterization. Furthermore, a 1998 European report of PAC use in 5306 patients undergoing cardiac surgery confirmed this low incidence of major morbidity, with injury to the right ventricle or pulmonary artery occurring in only 4 patients (0.07%).[224] Finally, only 1 of 2000 adverse events reported in the Australian Incident Monitoring Study of 1993 involved the use of a PAC, in contrast to 64 adverse events involving access to the arterial or venous

Box 40-6 Complications of Pulmonary Artery Catheter Monitoring

Catheterization
- Arrhythmias, ventricular fibrillation
- Right bundle branch block, complete heart block

Catheter residence
- Mechanical, catheter knots
- Thromboembolism
- Pulmonary infarction
- Infection, endocarditis
- Endocardial damage, cardiac valve injury
- Pulmonary artery rupture
- Pulmonary artery pseudoaneurysm

Misinterpretation of data

Misuse of equipment

systems.[46] However, it is important to acknowledge that although these large studies indicate a low incidence of serious complications attributable to the use of PACs, the frequency of complications in a particular clinical setting or patient group remains unknown.

Arrhythmias are the primary complication observed during pulmonary artery catheterization. In fact, self-limited atrial or ventricular arrhythmias are so common during PAC passage through the heart that most clinicians do not consider them complications, but instead confirmation that the PAC is traversing the cardiac chambers appropriately. Shah and associates observed transient premature ventricular contractions in 68% and atrial dysrhythmias in 1.3% of their catheterized patients.[149] Of greater clinical significance, persistent ventricular dysrhythmias requiring treatment occurred in only 3.1% of patients, none of whom suffered prolonged hemodynamic instability. Although the balloon-tipped PAC is less arrhythmogenic when it strikes the endocardium than a standard intravenous catheter or transvenous pacing wire is, PACs have been reported to induce sustained atrial fibrillation, ventricular tachycardia, and even ventricular fibrillation.[222,224,225]

Prophylactic use of intravenous lidocaine before pulmonary artery catheterization is not effective in reducing ventricular ectopy.[226] When such problems arise, the balloon should be deflated and the catheter withdrawn to the right atrium. When hemodynamically significant dysrhythmias develop hours or even days after placement, it is unlikely that the PAC is responsible. However, the position of the catheter tip should always be checked by observation of the pressure waveform and chest radiograph to identify catheters that have migrated back into the right ventricle.

As the PAC passes through the right ventricle and strikes the interventricular septum, transient right bundle branch block occurs in up to 5% of patients.[227,228] This is of no clinical significance except in patients with preexisting left bundle branch block. In these patients, complete heart block may be precipitated, although this is rare. Shah and coworkers catheterized 113 patients with preexisting left bundle branch block, and complete heart block developed in only 1 patient (0.9%).[149] In a different population of 47 high-risk patients with left bundle branch block, many of whom had acute myocardial infarction or heart failure, Morris and colleagues inserted 82 PACs without a single episode of complete heart block for the initial 24-hour period.[227] However, transcutaneous pacing equipment, an external pulse generator, and a temporary transvenous pacing wire or pacing PAC should be readily available as a precaution, especially since the onset of heart block in this setting may be delayed.

A dizzying array of mechanical problems have been reported with PACs or introducer sheaths since their introduction into clinical use. In the setting of cardiac surgery, PACs may be damaged by surgical instruments or become entrapped in sutures or bypass cannulas.[149,229-231] Whenever right heart structures are involved, it is prudent to ensure free movement of the PAC before chest closure. Sternal retraction during cardiac surgery may pose other problems, particularly when the PAC is inserted via the external jugular or subclavian route. The PAC may kink as it exits the introducer sheath and makes an acute angle between the sheath and vessel wall.[218,219] These mechanical difficulties should be suspected whenever there is a damped appearance of the monitored pressure trace or difficulty infusing fluids or withdrawing blood through one of the catheter lumens.

Although gross structural defects in the catheter itself should be recognized by inspection of the catheter before insertion, more subtle manufacturing problems may escape detection. Some, such as communications between the PAP, CVP, and balloon inflation lumens, may be suspected only when the data are contradictory or inconsistent.[232,233]

PACs may dislodge temporary transvenous pacing wires, become entangled with other cardiac catheters, or form knots within the heart.[234,235] Arnaout and coauthors reported a PAC knot around the tricuspid valve chordae tendineae that resulted in severe tricuspid valve regurgitation after catheter removal.[234] Catheter knots should be suspected when there is difficulty withdrawing a PAC, and the diagnosis may be confirmed by chest radiography. Knots may be untied by radiologists with the use of intravascular snares and fluoroscopic guidance.[236] If the knot has already been drawn tight, surgical exploration and removal are usually required.

Although the incidence of thromboembolic complications is increased in patients who require PAC monitoring for longer periods, thrombi have been detected on PACs within hours of placement.[237] When drugs such as aprotinin and ε-aminocaproic acid are used to reduce perioperative bleeding, the risk of thrombus formation on the PAC may be increased.[238,239] Although heparin bonding to the external surface has unquestionably reduced the thrombogenicity of PACs, it does not entirely eliminate the possibility.[237,240] Fortunately, major pulmonary embolism is a rare occurrence.[241]

The incidence of PAC-related infection increases after 3 days of continuous monitoring and in patients with preexisting sepsis.[242] The most catastrophic of these infections is endocarditis, most often of the right-sided valves.[243,244] Using sophisticated microbiologic techniques in 297 critically ill patients, Mermel and associates demonstrated a 22% incidence of local infection of the introducer sheath but only a 0.7% incidence of bacteremia related to the PAC.[245] In view of these findings, it is not surprising that scheduled PACs changes do not reduce the risk for bloodstream infection, particularly when the catheter is changed over a guidewire.[246] However, cannulation at a new site carries a significant risk of vascular complications. The specific risks and benefits must be weighed in each patient.

In addition to infectious injury, mechanical injury may also result from PAC use.[243,244] In a series of 55 autopsies of patients who had been monitored with a PAC, Rowley and colleagues identified right-sided endocardial lesions in 53%.[243] Even though both severe tricuspid regurgitation and severe pulmonic regurgitation have been reported, these complications of PAC use are rare.[234,244,247] Using color flow Doppler echocardiography, Sherman and coworkers demonstrated that placement of a PAC caused a slight increase in the magnitude of tricuspid regurgitation, but in no instances did the PAC lead to severe right-sided valvular insufficiency.[248]

Pulmonary artery rupture, the most deadly but also the most preventable of complications, occurs in approximately 0.02% to 0.2% of catheterized patients and appears to carry a mortality rate of 50%.[149,249] Several factors appear to increase the risk for this catastrophic event, including hypothermia, anticoagulation, and advanced age, although many reported cases involve heart transplant procedures.[249-251] Pulmonary hypertension may also possibly predispose patients to arterial injury during balloon inflation because of the increased gradient between proximal arterial and distal wedge pressure or because pulmonary hypertension distends the pulmonary vasculature and causes the PAC to wedge in a distal, less compliant vessel.[252]

Several mechanisms of pulmonary artery injury have been proposed and investigated, including forceful inflation of the PAC balloon and chronic erosion by the catheter tip abutting the vessel wall or eccentric balloon inflation forcing the uncushioned catheter tip through the vessel wall.[251,253] Regardless of the precise mechanism by which pulmonary arterial injury occurs, case reports highlight that this complication often results from suboptimal catheter insertion and management techniques. Procedural errors include unnecessary catheter manipulation, excessive insertion depth, unrecognized persistent wedge pressure, prolonged balloon inflation, or improper balloon inflation with liquid rather than air.[252-254] It is critical that the clinician recognize artifactual "overwedged" pressure recordings that indicate peripheral location of the PAC tip or impaction against the vessel wall and correct this problem immediately by withdrawing the catheter into the proximal pulmonary artery (see later).

The hallmark of catheter-induced pulmonary artery rupture is hemoptysis, which may cause life-threatening exsanguination or hypoxemia. Less commonly, occult hypotension or respiratory compromise may develop. If the visceral pleura fails to contain the bleeding, free rupture into the pleural space produces a large hemothorax. When time allows, a chest radiograph helps make the diagnosis by revealing the hemothorax or a new infiltrate near the tip of a distally positioned PAC. Although its initial appearance may be confused with catheter-related pulmonary infarction, its pattern of resolution and clinical course differentiate these diagnoses. In confusing cases the diagnosis may be made by performing a wedge angiogram, in which radiopaque dye injected through the wedged PAC will extravasate into the pulmonary parenchyma and thus identify the site of arterial disruption.[250]

Treatment of pulmonary artery rupture focuses on resuscitation and immediate control of the hemorrhage. Specific therapeutic steps are highly individualized, depending on the setting. The first priority is ensuring adequate oxygenation and ventilation, which may require endobronchial intubation with either a single- or double-lumen endotracheal tube to selectively ventilate and protect the unaffected lung. In addition, positive end-expiratory pressure (PEEP) applied to the affected lung may help control hemorrhage.[255] Any anticoagulation should be reversed unless the patient must remain on cardiopulmonary bypass and bronchoscopy is performed to localize and control the site of bleeding. A bronchial blocker may be guided into the involved bronchus to tamponade the bleeding and prevent contamination of the uninvolved lung.[256] Management of the PAC itself is more controversial. Some experts recommend removing the catheter, but others suggest leaving the PAC in place to monitor PAP and guide antihypertensive therapy targeted at lowering this pressure and reducing bleeding.[257,258] Others have suggested that the PAC balloon may be carefully reinflated and the catheter floated into the involved pulmonary artery to occlude the bleeding arterial segment as a temporizing measure.[256] Although these techniques may be effective in some cases, many patients will require definitive surgical therapy, such as oversewing the involved pulmonary artery or resecting the involved segment, lobe, or lung.[250,256] In addition, some authors have recommended distant follow-up with angiography to rule out pseudoaneurysm formation in those managed conservatively because of the high morbidity associated with secondary hemorrhage.[249,256,259,260]

A more insidious but possibly more common complication of PAC use is misinterpretation of data.[261,262] Although the magnitude of the problem is not clear, there is reason to believe that there are widespread knowledge deficits among practitioners who use PACs. In 1990, Iberti and coauthors reported the results of a 31-question multiple-choice examination taken by 496 resident and staff physicians in the medicine, surgery, and anesthesiology departments in 13 North American medical centers. The authors found a poor overall level of knowledge of PACs, as evidenced by a mean score of only 67% correct answers. Although higher scores were demonstrated by individuals with more training and more experience inserting and using catheter-derived information, none of these factors ensured a high level of knowledge.[263] These results have been duplicated in a variety of other specialty care groups.[264] It is especially concerning that PAWP measurement was performed incorrectly by 30% to 50% of the clinicians in these studies and that educational programs failed to improve performance.[265,266] Taken together, these observations highlight the fact that effective use of PACs requires a great deal of expertise and clinical experience and that even measuring the most fundamental PAC-derived variable, namely, wedge pressure, is a complicated endeavor.[267]

Physiologic Considerations for Pulmonary Artery Catheter Monitoring: Prediction of Left Ventricular Filling Pressure

Pulmonary artery catheterization allows measurement of a variety of hemodynamic variables, including cardiac output, mixed venous oxygen saturation, and most important, pulmonary artery diastolic and wedge pressure. These values, in turn, are used to estimate left ventricular filling pressure and, in combination with other clinical information, help guide administration of fluid and vasoactive drugs.

When a PAC floats to the wedge position, the inflated balloon isolates the distal pressure-monitoring orifice from upstream PAP. A continuous static column of blood now connects the wedged PAC tip to the junction of the pulmonary veins and left atrium. Thus, wedging the PAC, in effect, extends the catheter tip to measure the pressure at the point at which blood flow resumes on the venous side of the pulmonary circuit. Because resistance in the large pulmonary veins is negligible, PAWP provides an accurate, indirect measurement of both pulmonary venous pressure and LAP.[50,268]

Pulmonary artery diastolic pressure (PADP) is often used as an alternative to PAWP to estimate left ventricular filling pressure. This is acceptable in normal circumstances because when pulmonary venous resistance is low, the pressure in the pulmonary artery at the end of diastole will equilibrate with downstream pressure in the pulmonary veins and left atrium.[269,270] From a monitoring standpoint, PADP has the added advantage of being available for continuous monitoring, whereas PAWP is measured only intermittently.

For PADP or PAWP to be valid estimates of left ventricular filling pressure, the column of blood connecting the tip of the wedged catheter and the draining pulmonary vein must be continuous and static. At the microcirculatory level, this channel consists of pulmonary capillaries that are subject to external compression by surrounding alveoli. West and colleagues described a three-zone model of the pulmonary vasculature based on the gravitationally determined relationships between relative pressure in the pulmonary arteries, the pulmonary veins, and the surrounding alveoli.[271] This model provides useful insight into conditions when PAC measurements are erroneous.

In West zone 1, alveolar pressure exceeds that in both the pulmonary artery and the pulmonary veins, whereas in zone 2, it is intermediate between these two pressures (Fig. 40-28). A PAC positioned in both zone 1 and 2 will be highly susceptible to alveolar pressure, and measurements will reflect alveolar or airway pressure rather than left ventricular filling pressure. As such, the tip of the PAC must lie in zone 3 for PAWP measurements to be accurate. In most clinical settings, a supine position of the patient favors zone 3 conditions, a finding that has been confirmed by radiographic studies.[272] However, when patients are placed in the lateral or semi-upright position, zone 2 may expand significantly. In general, zones 1 and 2 become more extensive when LAP is low, when the PAC tip is located vertically above the left atrium, or when alveolar pressure is high. Clues to an incorrectly positioned catheter include absence of normal PAWP a and v waves, marked respiratory variation in PAWP, and a PADP that exceeds the PAWP measurement without excessively tall a or v waves visible on the trace.[49]

Normal Pulmonary Artery and Wedge Pressure Waveforms

As the balloon-tipped PAC is floated to its proper position in the pulmonary artery, characteristic pressure waveforms are recorded (see Fig. 40-27). In the superior vena cava or right atrium, a CVP waveform should be observed, with its a, c, and v waves and low mean pressure. At this point the PAC balloon is inflated and the catheter advanced until it crosses the tricuspid valve to record right ventricular pressure, which is characterized by a rapid systolic upstroke, a wide pulse pressure, and low diastolic pressure. The PAC next enters the right ventricular outflow tract and floats past the pulmonic valve into the main pulmonary artery. Premature ventricular beats are common during this period as the balloon-tipped catheter strikes the right ventricular infundibular wall. Entry into the pulmonary artery is heralded by a step-up in diastolic pressure and a change in waveform morphology.

On occasion it may be difficult to distinguish right ventricular pressure from PAP, particularly if only the numeric values for these pressures are examined. However, careful observation of the pressure waveform by focusing on the diastolic pressure contours allows differentiation. During diastole, PAP will fall because of interruption of flow during pulmonic valve closure, while simultaneously, pressure in the right ventricle will increase because of filling from the right atrium (see Fig. 40-27).[216]

Under normal conditions, the PAP upstroke slightly precedes the radial artery pressure upstroke because of the longer duration of left ventricular isovolumic contraction, as well as the time required for propagation of the pressure wave to a distal monitoring site. As a practical matter, though, the pulmonary and systemic arterial pressure waveforms appear to overlap on the bedside monitor (Fig. 40-29). Understanding these temporal relationships is critically important for proper interpretation of abnormal pulmonary artery and wedge pressure waveforms, particularly when tall v waves are present (see later).

As noted previously, wedge pressure is an indirect measurement of pulmonary venous pressure and LAP and should therefore resemble these venous waveforms, with characteristic a and v waves and x and y descents. However, because of interposition of the pulmonary vascular bed between the PAC tip and left atrium, wedge pressure is a delayed representation of LAP.[268] On average, 160 msec is required for the LAP pulse to traverse the pulmonary veins, capillaries, arterioles, and arteries. As a consequence of this delay, the wedge pressure a wave appears to follow the ECG R wave in early ventricular systole even though the a wave is an end-diastolic event (see Fig. 40-29).

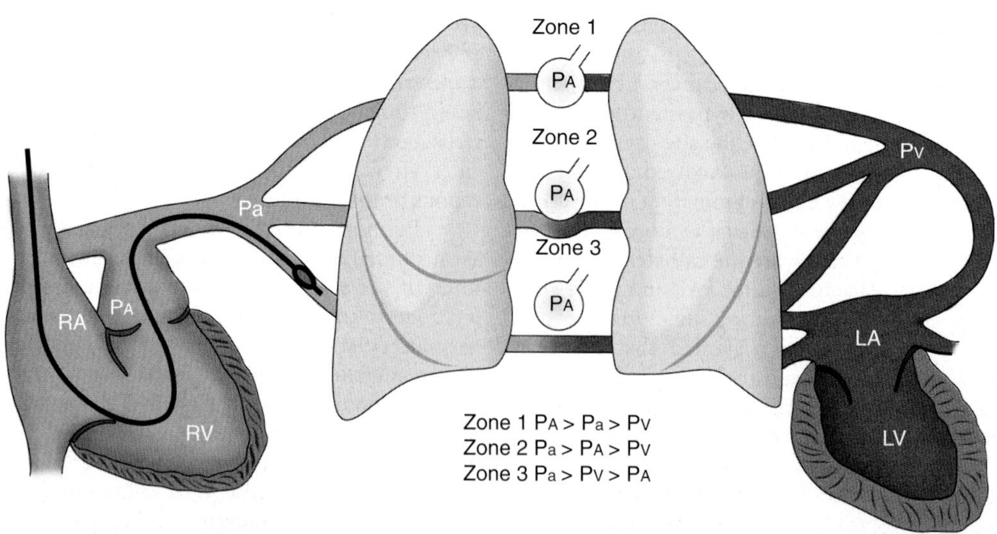

Figure 40-28 The tip of the pulmonary artery catheter must be wedged in lung zone 3 to provide an accurate measure of pulmonary venous (Pv) or left atrial (LA) pressure. When alveolar pressure (PA) rises above Pv in lung zone 2 or above pulmonary arterial pressure (Pa) in lung zone 1, wedge pressure will reflect alveolar pressure rather than intravascular pressure. LV, left ventricle; PA, pulmonary artery; RA, right atrium; RV, right ventricle. *(From Mark JB: Atlas of Cardiovascular Monitoring. New York, Churchill Livingstone, 1998, Fig. 6-10.)*

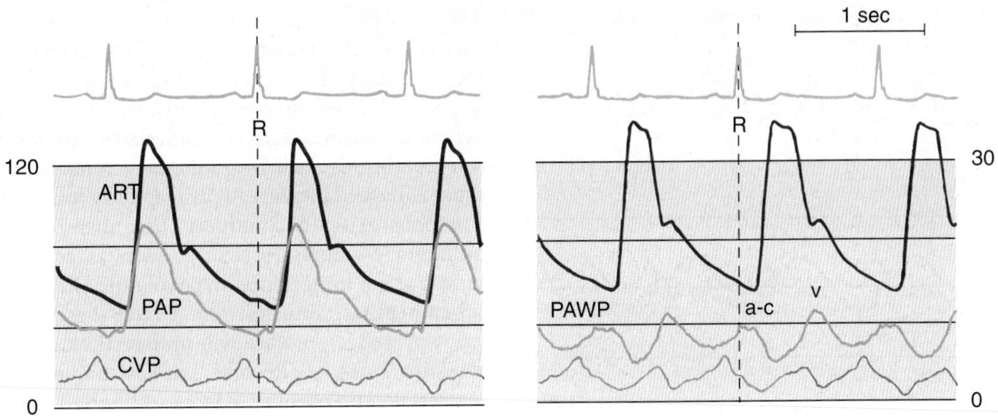

Figure 40-29 Temporal relationships between normal systemic arterial pressure (ART), pulmonary artery pressure (PAP), central venous pressure (CVP), and pulmonary artery wedge pressure (PAWP). Note that the PAWP a-c and v waves appear to occur later in the cardiac cycle than their counterparts on the right side of the heart seen in the CVP trace. The ART scale is on the *left*; the PAP, CVP, and PAWP pressure scales are on the *right*. *(From Mark JB: Atlas of Cardiovascular Monitoring. New York, Churchill Livingstone, 1998, Fig. 3-3.)*

To recognize prominent a or v waves in the wedge pressure trace, it is not always necessary to inflate the PAC balloon. Because the PCWP trace reflects pressure waves transmitted in retrograde fashion from the left atrium, these waves will not normally be visible within the antegrade PAP waves produced by right ventricular ejection. In the setting of prominent a or v waves, the PAP trace becomes a composite wave that reflects both retrograde and antegrade components. Tall left atrial a or v waves will distort the normal PAP waveform appearance, with the a wave inscribed at the onset of the systolic upstroke and the v wave distorting the dicrotic notch (Fig. 40-30).[268,273] Once these waves are identified by wedging the PAC and comparing the PAP and PAWP traces, it is wise to "follow" the "wedge pressure" a and v waves in the unwedged PAP trace rather than repeatedly inflating the balloon.

In summary, PAWP measured with a balloon-tipped PAC provides a delayed, damped estimate of LAP by measuring the pressure near the junction of the pulmonary veins and the left atrium. Mean wedge pressure should be lower than mean PAP; otherwise, blood would not flow in an antegrade direction. The PAWP waveform should display small but visible a and v waves if the pressure trace is displayed with sufficient gain and resolution on the monitor screen.

Left Atrial Pressure, Pulmonary Artery Wedge Pressure, and Pulmonary Capillary Pressure

The most common technique for monitoring LAP during cardiac surgery involves catheterization of the left atrium with a thin catheter introduced through the right superior pulmonary vein and secured with a purse-string suture. The catheter is brought out through the skin beneath the xiphoid process and attached to a closed pressure monitoring system. Because LAP monitoring is discontinued simply by withdrawing the left atrial catheter through the skin, transseptal methods for LAP monitoring during surgery have been proposed to reduce the risk of bleeding after catheter removal.[274]

Today, direct LAP monitoring has largely been supplanted by PAC monitoring, no doubt because the latter provides a wider array of hemodynamic data. Furthermore, PAWP generally provides an excellent estimate of LAP after cardiac surgery.[275,276] On the other hand, there are a host of pathophysiologic conditions that alter the relationships between PADP, PAWP, and LAP and lead to erroneous measurements and potential clinical errors (see later).

Direct LAP monitoring continues to be particularly useful in pediatric patients undergoing complex congenital heart surgery, in part because of technical difficulties in this patient population. Gold and coauthors reported complications from left-sided monitoring occurring in only 0.68% of 2393 catheters.[277] However, direct access to the left heart chambers carries the grave risk of air and particulate embolization to the systemic circulation, especially during routine flushing of the lines.

Catheter removal may result in bleeding, the most common complication from LAP catheters. Consequently, these lines must be removed before the mediastinal chest drains, and if attempted withdrawal is met with resistance, surgical re-exploration is required. More unusual complications include catheter entrapment in mechanical aortic or mitral valve prostheses, fistulas between the right superior pulmonary vein and the right mainstem bronchus, and embolization of catheter fragments.[277-279]

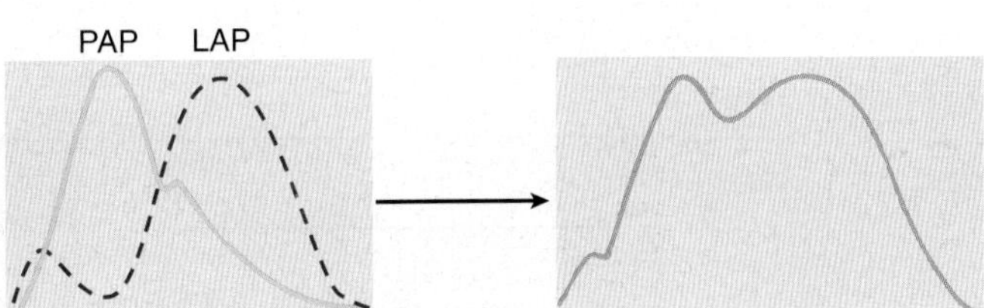

Figure 40-30 Tall left atrial pressure (LAP) a and v waves transmitted in a retrograde direction through the pulmonary vasculature distort the antegrade pulmonary artery pressure (PAP) waveform. The LAP a wave distorts the systolic upstroke, and the v wave distorts the dicrotic notch. *(From Mark JB: Atlas of Cardiovascular Monitoring. New York, Churchill Livingstone, 1998, Fig. 4-10.)*

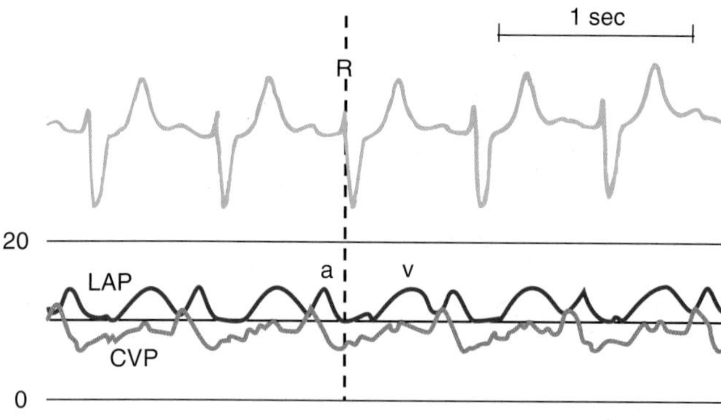

Figure 40-31 Normal temporal relationships between the electrocardiographic, central venous pressure (CVP), and left atrial pressure (LAP) traces. The LAP and CVP waveforms have nearly identical morphologies, although the CVP a wave slightly precedes the LAP a wave. *(From Mark JB: Atlas of Cardiovascular Monitoring. New York, Churchill Livingstone, 1998, Fig. 2-9.)*

Normal LAP waveforms resemble those from CVP catheters, although there are a few subtle morphologic distinctions. Because atrial depolarization originates in the sinoatrial node located at the junction of the superior vena cava and the right atrium, the right-sided a wave appears slightly earlier than the left-sided a wave (Fig. 40-31). Although the a wave is the most prominent pressure peak in a normal CVP trace, the v wave is often taller than the a wave in a normal LAP waveform, thus suggesting that atrial contraction is stronger on the right than the left and that the left atrium is less distensible than the right.[61] Finally, the interval between atrial and ventricular contraction is approximately 40 msec longer on the right than on the left.[61] Consequently, a and c waves are seen as separate waves in a right atrial pressure trace, whereas on the left they merge into a composite a-c wave. In the PAWP waveform, the c wave is obscured even further by the damping effect of the lung vasculature.

The terms *pulmonary artery wedge pressure* and *pulmonary artery occlusion pressure* are used interchangeably and refer to the same measurement obtained from the tip of a PAC after balloon inflation and flotation to the wedged position. However, pulmonary capillary pressure must not be confused with wedge pressure or LAP, nor should the term *pulmonary capillary wedge pressure* be used at all. The hydrostatic pressure in the pulmonary capillaries that causes edema formation according to the Starling equation is different from LAP. This is the pressure that must exceed LAP to maintain antegrade blood flow through the lungs. Although the magnitude of the difference between pulmonary capillary pressure and wedge pressure is generally small, it can increase markedly when resistance to flow in the pulmonary veins is elevated.[280] In most situations, the major component of PVR occurs at the precapillary, pulmonary arteriolar level. However, rare conditions such as pulmonary veno-occlusive disease may cause a marked increase in postcapillary resistance to flow. Similar situations arise in conditions that disproportionately increase pulmonary venous resistance, such as central nervous system injury, acute lung injury, hypovolemic shock, endotoxemia, and norepinephrine infusion.[273,274] Under these conditions, measurement of wedge pressure will underestimate pulmonary capillary pressure substantially and thereby underestimate the risk of hydrostatic pulmonary edema. Although pulmonary capillary pressure may be measured at the bedside by analyzing the decay in the PAP trace after PAC balloon inflation, these techniques have not been adopted widely in clinical practice.[281,282] To avoid confusion, the phrase "pulmonary capillary wedge pressure" should be abandoned because it is imprecise and misleading.

Abnormal Pulmonary Artery and Wedge Pressure Waveforms

PAC monitoring is subject to the same technical artifacts inherent in all invasive pressure monitoring techniques, as well as some additional problems unique to this method.[253,283,284] Because the PAC is longer and passes through the cardiac chambers, it is more prone to distortions from clot or air bubbles, and motion-related artifacts are more problematic. Artifactual pressure spikes may be distinguished from the underlying physiologic pressure waveform by their unique morphology and timing.

At the onset of systole, tricuspid valve closure accompanied by right ventricular contraction and ejection resulting in excessive catheter motion are responsible for the most common PAC trace artifact.[283,285] Note that this pressure artifact occurs simultaneous with the CVP c wave and may produce either an artificially low pressure or a pressure peak. If the monitor detects this inappropriate pressure nadir, it may erroneously be designated as PADP (Fig. 40-32). Repositioning the PAC often solves the problem.

Another common artifact in PAC pressure measurement occurs when the balloon is overinflated and occludes the lumen orifice. This phenomenon is termed *overwedging* and is usually caused by distal catheter migration and eccentric balloon infla-

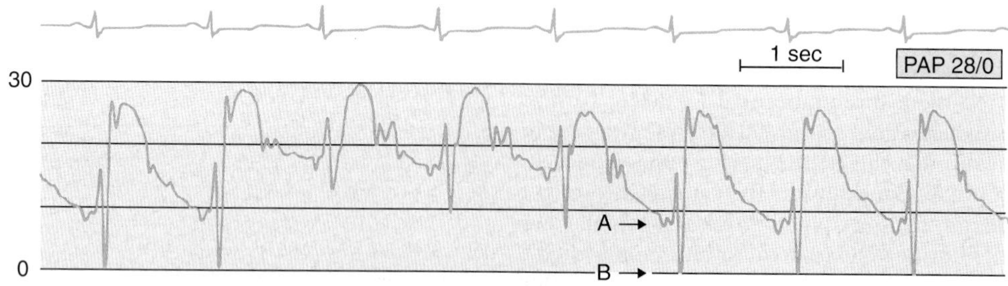

Figure 40-32 Artifactual pressure peaks and troughs in the pulmonary artery pressure (PAP) waveform caused by catheter motion. The correct value for pulmonary artery end-diastolic pressure is 8 mm Hg (A), although the monitor digital display erroneously reports the PAP as 28/0 mm Hg (B). *(From Mark JB: Atlas of Cardiovascular Monitoring. New York, Churchill Livingstone, 1998, Fig. 5-6.)*

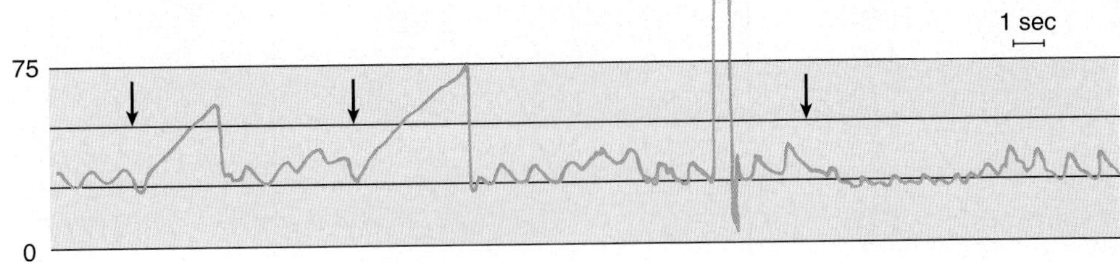

Figure 40-33 Overwedging of the pulmonary artery (PA) catheter causes artifactual waveform recordings. The first two attempts to inflate the PA catheter balloon (first *two arrows*) produce a nonpulsatile increasing pressure caused by an occluded catheter tip. After the catheter is withdrawn slightly, balloon inflation allows proper wedge pressure measurement (*third arrow*). Before the third attempt at balloon inflation, the PA pressure lumen is flushed, which restores the appropriate pulsatile pressure detailed to the PA and wedge pressure waveforms on the right side of the trace. *(From Mark JB: Atlas of Cardiovascular Monitoring. New York, Churchill Livingstone, 1998, Fig. 5-7.)*

tion, which forces the catheter tip against the vessel wall. The catheter now records a gradually rising pressure produced by the continuous flush system and builds up pressure against the obstructed distal opening (Fig. 40-33). For a catheter that has migrated to a more distal position, it is possible for overwedging to occur without balloon inflation. Note that the overwedged pressure is devoid of pulsatility, is higher than expected, and rises continuously to the flush pressure. Such a pattern should arouse suspicion and prompt corrective action.

As emphasized earlier, with each PAC balloon inflation and wedge measurement, the catheter tip migrates distally. When a wedge pressure tracing appears during partial balloon inflation, it suggests that the PAC is inappropriately located in a smaller, distal branch of the pulmonary artery. The catheter should be withdrawn before overwedging results in vascular injury or pulmonary infarction.

Pathophysiologic conditions involving the left-sided cardiac chambers or valves produce characteristic changes in the pulmonary artery and wedge pressure waveforms. One of the characteristics of these waveforms is the tall v wave of mitral regurgitation. Unlike a normal wedge pressure v wave produced by late systolic pulmonary venous inflow, the prominent v wave of mitral regurgitation begins in early systole. Mitral regurgitation causes fusion of the c and v waves and obliteration of the systolic x descent because the isovolumic phase of left ventricular systole is eliminated as a result of retrograde ejection of blood into the left atrium.[208] Because the prominent v wave of mitral regurgitation is generated during ventricular systole, mean wedge pressure overestimates left ventricular filling pressure. Consequently, in cases of severe disease, left ventricular end-diastolic pressure is best estimated by measuring wedge pressure before onset of the regurgitant v wave (Fig. 40-34). Although mean wedge pressure exceeds left ventricular end-diastolic pressure in patients with severe mitral regurgitation, mean wedge pressure remains a good approximation for mean LAP. Retrograde pressure reflected by the regurgitant v wave contributes to left atrial hypertension and the subsequent risk of hydrostatic pulmonary edema.

When large v waves are present in the wedge pressure trace, it is critically important to recognize them and be able to distinguish the wedged from the unwedged pressure waveform. At first glance, a wedge trace with a tall systolic v wave resembles a typical unwedged PAP trace, but closer observation reveals a number of discriminating details. The PAP upstroke is steeper and slightly precedes the systemic arterial pressure upstroke, whereas a wedge tracing with a prominent v wave has a more gradual upstroke that begins after the radial artery pressure upstroke. Furthermore, the wedge pressure v wave reaches its peak later in the cardiac cycle, after the ECG T wave, as opposed to the simultaneous systemic and pulmonary arterial peaks (see Fig. 40-34).[208,286] Another distinguishing feature in patients with severe mitral regurgitation is the unusual morphology of the pulmonary artery waveform itself. The larger the v wave, the more the regurgitant v wave distorts the pulmonary artery waveform by giving it a bifid appearance and obscuring the normal end-systolic dicrotic notch (see Fig. 40-34).[273] Through recognition of these subtle but important diagnostic details, a clinician may assess the wedge pressure v wave by observing the unwedged PAP trace. This would eliminate the need for repeated balloon inflation and avoid the potential for catastrophic arterial rupture.

A close look at left atrial pressure-volume relationships helps explain the apparently paradoxical coexistence of severe mitral regurgitation and a normal PAWP trace.[287,288] Three factors determine whether mitral regurgitation produces a prominent v wave in the left atrial or wedge pressure traces: left atrial volume (often termed the patient's "volume status"), left atrial compliance, and regurgitant volume (Fig. 40-35). Given that the left atrial

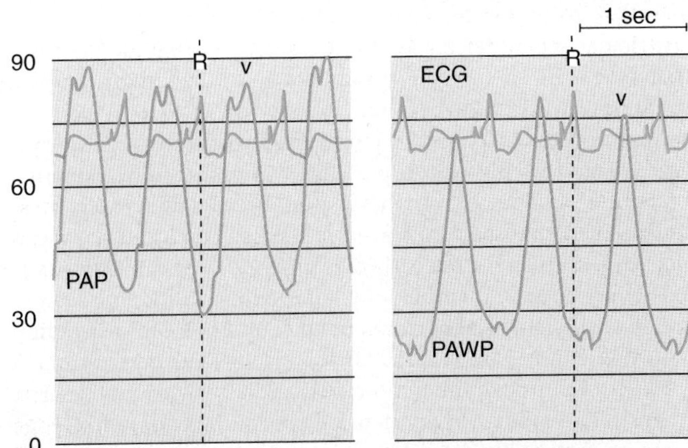

Figure 40-34 Severe mitral regurgitation. A tall systolic v wave is inscribed in the pulmonary artery wedge pressure (PAWP) trace and also distorts the pulmonary artery pressure (PAP) trace, thereby giving it a bifid appearance. The electrocardiogram (ECG) is abnormal because of ventricular pacing. Left ventricular end-diastolic pressure is estimated best by measuring PAWP at the time of the electrocardiographic R wave, before onset of the regurgitant v wave. Note that mean PAWP exceeds left ventricular end-diastolic pressure in this condition. *(From Mark JB: Atlas of Cardiovascular Monitoring. New York, Churchill Livingstone, 1998, Fig. 17-11.)*

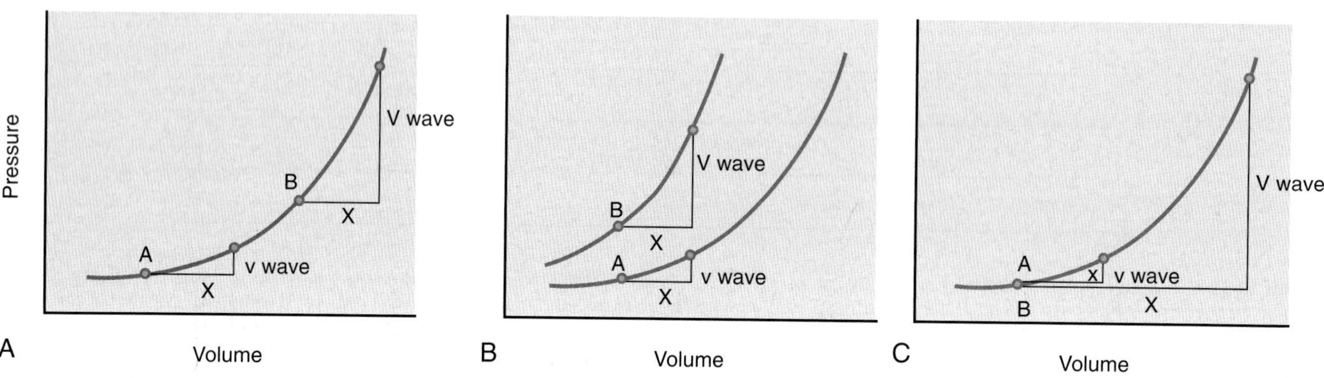

Figure 40-35 V wave height as an indicator of the severity of mitral regurgitation. Left atrial pressure-volume curves describe the three factors that determine v wave height. **A,** Influence of left atrial volume. For the same regurgitant volume (x), the left atrial v wave will be taller if baseline atrial volume is greater (point B versus point A). **B,** Influence of left atrial compliance. For the same regurgitant volume (x), the left atrial v wave will be taller if baseline atrial compliance is reduced (point B versus point A). **C,** Influence of regurgitant volume. Beginning at the same baseline left atrial volume (points A and B), if regurgitant volume increases (X versus x), the left atrial pressure v wave will increase (V versus v). *(From Mark JB: Atlas of Cardiovascular Monitoring. New York, Churchill Livingstone, 1998, Fig. 17-13.)*

pressure-volume relationship is not linear, the same volume of regurgitation will result in a variable increment in systolic pressure, depending on the preexisting atrial volume at the onset of systole. Furthermore, the nature of that relationship is dependent on the compliance (i.e., stiffness) of the left atrium. Although the total regurgitant volume of blood entering the left atrium will influence the height of the v wave, this clearly is not the only determinant of v wave magnitude. This may explain why patients with acute mitral regurgitation tend to have tall wedge pressure v waves—they have smaller, stiffer left atria with poorer compliance than patients with long-standing disease do. It is not surprising that wedge pressure v waves are neither sensitive nor specific indicators of the severity of mitral regurgitation, and the height of these waves should not be used in such a manner.[287] Prominent wedge pressure v waves may exist in the absence of mitral regurgitation when LAP is high, as might occur when the left atrium is compressed.[289] Tall v waves are also seen commonly in patients with hypervolemia, congestive heart failure, and ventricular septal defects.[287] Note that the giant v waves observed in patients with ventricular septal defects are not caused by retrograde flow, but rather excessive antegrade systolic flow into the left atrium as a result of the intracardiac shunt.[290]

In contrast to mitral regurgitation, which distorts the systolic portion of the wedge pressure waveform, mitral stenosis alters its diastolic aspect. In this condition, the holodiastolic pressure gradient across the mitral valve results in an increased mean wedge pressure, a slurred early diastolic y descent, and a tall end-diastolic a wave. Similar hemodynamic abnormalities are seen in patients with left atrial myxoma or whenever there is obstruction to mitral flow. Diseases that increase left ventricular stiffness (e.g., left ventricular infarction, pericardial constriction, aortic stenosis, and systemic hypertension) produce changes in wedge pressure that partly resemble those seen in mitral stenosis. In these conditions, mean wedge pressure is increased and the trace displays a prominent a wave, but the y descent remains steep because there is no obstruction to flow across the mitral valve during diastole. Because patients with advanced mitral stenosis often have coexisting atrial fibrillation, the a wave will not be present in many of these cases (Fig. 40-36).[208]

Myocardial ischemia may be detected with the PAC in several ways. Ischemia itself impairs left ventricular relaxation and thus results in diastolic dysfunction, a pattern particularly characteristic of demand ischemia associated with tachycardia or induced by rapid atrial pacing.[195,291,292] Impaired ventricular relaxation results in a stiffer, less compliant left ventricle, which leads to increased left ventricular end-diastolic pressure. Not only does this in turn increase left atrial and wedge pressure, but the morphology of these waveforms changes as well, with the phasic a and v wave components becoming more prominent as diastolic filling pressure increases.[293-295] Although myocardial ischemia will often be detectable as a rise in pulmonary artery diastolic, mean, or systolic pressure, these changes are generally less striking than the accompanying change in wedge pressure and the new appearance of tall a and v waves (Fig. 40-37). In patients with left ventricular ischemia, the tall wedge pressure a wave is produced by end-diastolic atrial contraction into a stiff, incompletely relaxed left ventricle.[296] Although the diastolic dysfunction accompanying myocardial ischemia leads to an increase in left ventricular end-diastolic pressure, this elevation in pressure often coexists with decreased left ventricular end-diastolic volume or preload.[195] The dissociation between filling pressure and filling volume in this condition must be appreciated to avoid diagnostic and therapeutic errors.

Myocardial ischemia also produces a characteristic pattern of left ventricular systolic dysfunction. Systolic dysfunction is the hallmark of supply ischemia, which is caused by a sudden reduction or cessation of coronary blood flow to a region of the myocardium.[292,297] With severe systolic dysfunction, changes in global left ventricular contractile performance may be detected by hemodynamic monitoring. As the ejection fraction falls significantly, left ventricular end-diastolic volume and pressure rise, and systemic arterial hypotension and elevated pulmonary diastolic and wedge pressure develop.[298] A more common hemodynamic manifestation of myocardial ischemia occurs when left ventricular geometry is distorted or when the region of ischemic myocardium underlies a papillary muscle and results in acute mitral regurgitation.[299] This form of mitral regurgitation is often termed "papillary muscle ischemia" or "functional mitral regurgitation." As noted earlier, PAC monitoring is particularly well suited to detect this event by revealing the onset of new regurgitant v waves in the pulmonary artery or wedge pressure traces (see Fig. 40-34).

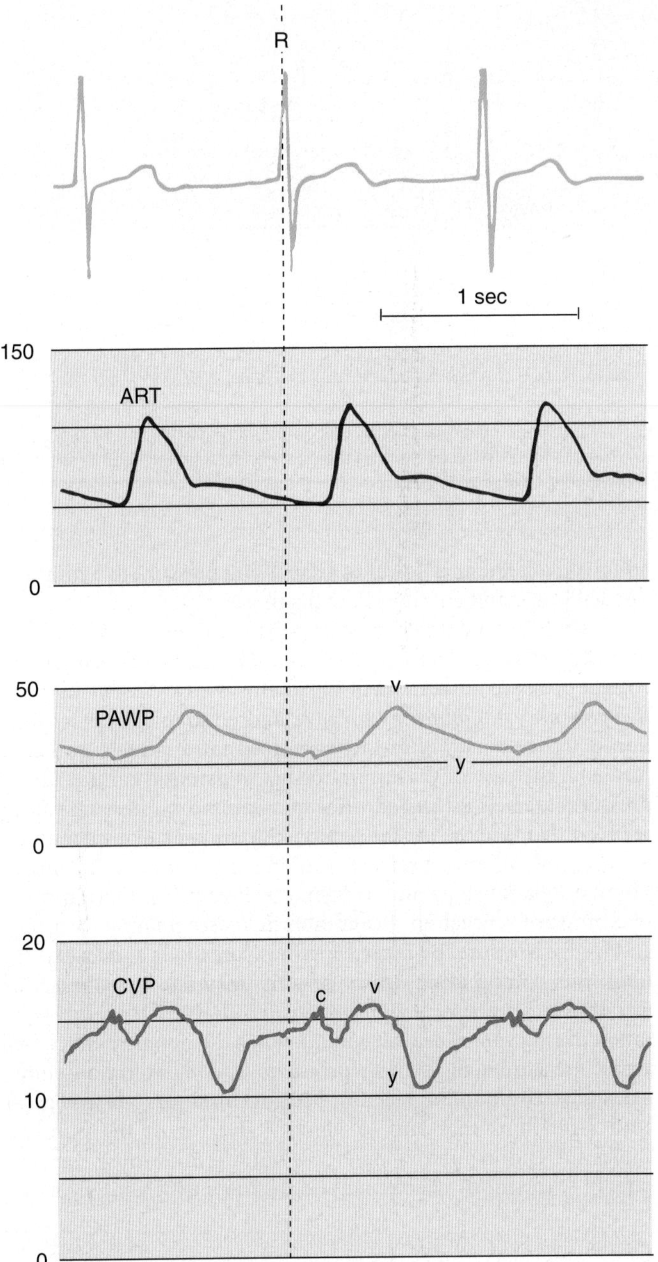

Figure 40-36 Mitral stenosis. Mean pulmonary artery wedge pressure (PAWP) is increased (35 mm Hg) and the diastolic y descent is markedly attenuated. Compare the slope of the y descent in the PAWP trace with the y descent in the central venous pressure (CVP) trace. In addition, compare this PAWP y descent with the PAWP y descent in mitral regurgitation (see Fig 40-34). A waves are not seen in the PAWP or CVP traces because of atrial fibrillation. ART, arterial blood pressure. *(From Mark JB: Atlas of Cardiovascular Monitoring. New York, Churchill Livingstone, 1998,: Fig. 17-19.)*

Whether the PAC should be used in high-risk patients as a supplemental monitor for detection of myocardial ischemia remains controversial.[295,300-302] None of the current methods for detecting perioperative myocardial ischemia are perfectly sensitive or specific. Although patients with left ventricular ischemia are likely to have higher mean wedge pressure than those without ischemia, these differences are small and may be difficult to detect clinically.[295] Furthermore, clear quantitative threshold values for mean wedge pressure or a and v wave peak pressures that are diagnostic of ischemia have not been identified, perhaps because of the wide variations found in normal patients. Consequently, when a PAC is used to diagnose myocardial ischemia, the best approach is to integrate the PAC data with other clinical data.[303]

Right ventricular ischemia produces characteristic PAC trace patterns that may be helpful in diagnosis and management. Just as left ventricular ischemia increases PAWP, right ventricular ischemia increases CVP. In fact, this is one of the few situations in which CVP may be higher than wedge pressure. In addition, CVP waveforms may display a prominent a wave resulting from right ventricular diastolic dysfunction and a prominent v wave resulting from ischemia-induced tricuspid regurgitation.[304,305] This particular CVP waveform is described as having an M or W configuration, which refers to the tall a and v waves and interposed steep x and y descents. Severe pulmonary artery hypertension may also result in right ventricular ischemia and dysfunction and increases in CVP, but this can be distinguished from primary right ventricular dysfunction in that the PAP and calculated PVR are normal in primary ventricular failure.

The CVP waveform in right ventricular infarction is similar to that in restrictive cardiomyopathy or pericardial constriction, including elevated mean pressure, prominent a and v waves, and steep x and y descents.[306] The cardinal feature common to these conditions is impaired right ventricular diastolic compliance, often termed "restrictive physiology." In restrictive cardiomyopathy and right ventricular infarction, diastolic dysfunction impairs ventricular relaxation and decreases wall compliance, whereas in pericardial constriction, also termed constrictive pericarditis or pericardial restriction, cardiac filling is limited by the rigid, often calcified pericardial shell. Impaired venous return decreases end-diastolic volume, stroke volume, and cardiac output. Despite reduced cardiac volumes, cardiac filling pressures are markedly elevated and equal in all four chambers of the heart at end-diastole (Fig. 40-38). Although PAC monitoring reveals this pressure equalization, the characteristic M or W configuration is more apparent in the CVP trace, most likely because of the damping effect of the pulmonary vasculature on left-sided filling pressures.[307-309]

Another hallmark of pericardial constriction is observed in the right and left ventricular pressure traces. These traces demonstrate rapid, but short-lived early diastolic ventricular filling, which produces a diastolic "dip-and-plateau" pattern or "square root sign."[72,310] In some cases, particularly when the heart rate is slow, a similar waveform pattern may be noted in the CVP trace: a steep y descent (the diastolic dip) produced by rapid early diastolic flow from the atrium to the ventricle, followed by a mid-diastolic h wave (the plateau) from the interruption in flow imposed by the restrictive pericardial shell (see Fig. 40-38).

Like pericardial constriction, cardiac tamponade impairs cardiac filling, but in the case of tamponade, a compressive pericardial fluid collection produces this effect. This fluid collection results in a marked increase in CVP and reduced diastolic volume, stroke volume, and cardiac output. Despite many similar hemodynamic features, tamponade and constriction may be distinguished by the different CVP waveforms seen in these two conditions. In tamponade, the venous pressure waveform appears more monophasic and is dominated by the systolic x pressure descent. The diastolic y pressure descent is attenuated or absent because early diastolic flow from the right atrium to the right ventricle is impaired by the surrounding compressive pericardial

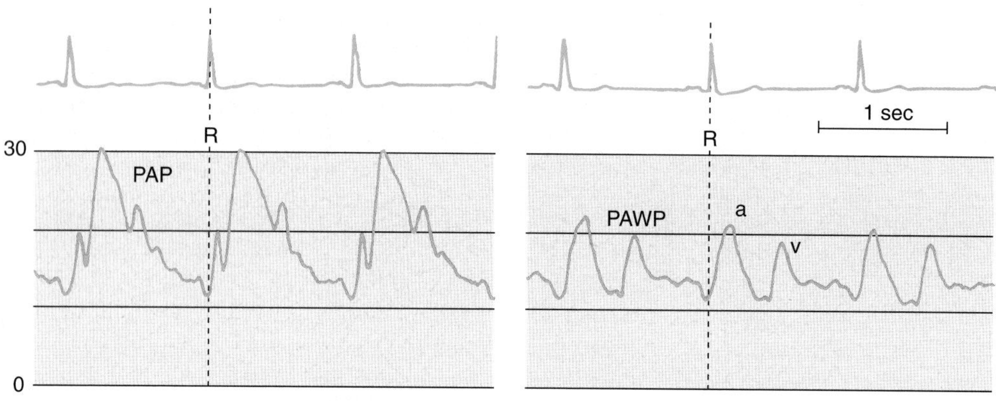

Figure 40-37 Myocardial ischemia. Pulmonary artery pressure (PAP) is relatively normal and mean pulmonary artery wedge pressure (PAWP) is only slightly elevated (15 mm Hg). However, PAWP morphology is markedly abnormal, with tall a waves (21 mm Hg) resulting from the diastolic dysfunction seen in this condition. *(From Mark JB: Atlas of Cardiovascular Monitoring. New York, Churchill Livingstone, 1998, Fig. 12-4.)*

fluid collection (Fig. 40-39).[307,311,312] Clearly, other clinical and hemodynamic clues help identify these diagnoses, such as the presence of *pulsus paradoxus*, an almost invariable finding in cardiac tamponade (see Fig. 40-16).[313] Coexisting abnormalities such as tachycardia, arrhythmias, and atrial contractile failure may complicate interpretation of these waveforms. On occasion, localized pericardial constriction may simulate valvular stenosis, and hypovolemia may lower cardiac filling pressure to within the normal range and confound the diagnosis.

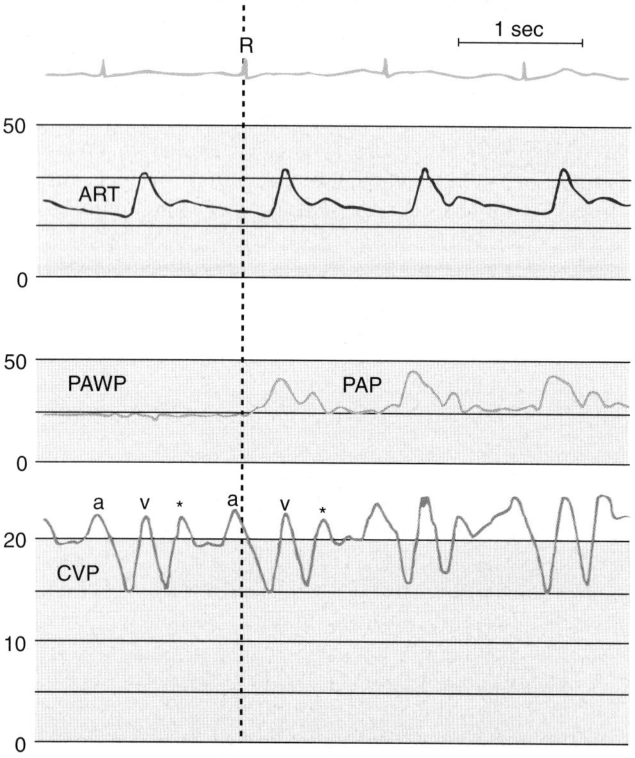

Figure 40-38 Pericardial constriction. This condition causes elevation and equalization of diastolic filling pressure in the pulmonary artery pressure (PAP), pulmonary artery wedge pressure (PAWP), and central venous pressure (CVP) traces. The CVP waveform reveals tall a and v waves with steep x and y descents and a mid-diastolic plateau wave (*) or h wave. *(From Mark JB: Atlas of Cardiovascular Monitoring. New York, Churchill Livingstone, 1998, Fig. 18-1.)*

Probably the single most important waveform abnormality or interpretive problem in PAC monitoring is discerning the correct pressure measurement in patients who are receiving *positive-pressure ventilation* or who have labored spontaneous respiration or other causes of greatly increased intrathoracic pressure. Just as in the case of CVP monitoring, transmural cardiac filling pressures are best estimated when end-expiratory pressure values are recorded (see the earlier section "Physiologic Considerations for Central Venous Pressure Monitoring: Diastolic Pressure-Volume Relationships and Transmural Pressure"). During positive-pressure ventilation, inspiration increases pulmonary artery and wedge pressure. By measuring these pressures at end-expiration, the confounding effect of this inspiratory increase in intrathoracic pressure is minimized (Fig. 40-40).[199] Forceful inspiration during spontaneous ventilation has the opposite effect, but again, measurement of these pressures at end-expiration eliminates this confounding factor. Bedside monitors are designed with algorithms that aim to identify and report the numeric values for end-expiratory pressures but are notoriously inaccurate.[314,315] The most reliable method for measuring central vascu-

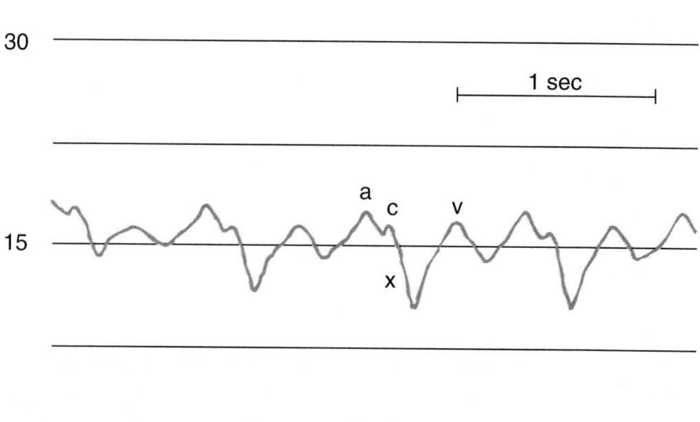

Figure 40-39 Cardiac tamponade. The central venous pressure waveform shows increased mean pressure (16 mm Hg) and attenuation of the y descent. Compare with Figure 40-38. *(From Mark JB: Atlas of Cardiovascular Monitoring. New York, Churchill Livingstone, 1998, Fig. 18-5.)*

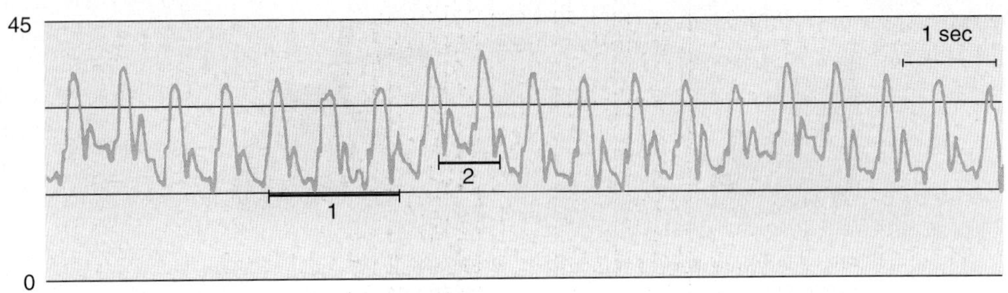

Figure 40-40 Influence of positive-pressure mechanical ventilation on pulmonary artery pressure. Pulmonary artery pressure should be measured at end-expiration #1, 15 mm Hg) to obviate the artifact caused by positive pressure inspiration (#2, 22 mm Hg). Compare with Figure 40-26. *(From Mark JB: Atlas of Cardiovascular Monitoring. New York, Churchill Livingstone, 1998, Fig. 16-3.)*

lar pressures at end-expiration is examination of the waveforms on a calibrated monitor screen or paper recording.[315,316]

Use of Central Vascular Pressures to Estimate Left Ventricular Preload

A detailed understanding of the relationship between left ventricular filling pressure and preload is important for clinically meaningful interpretation of PAC-derived data. Although surrogates such as PADP and PAWP are used as measures of left ventricular filling, many factors influence the relationship between filling pressure and chamber volume. For example, a PAWP of 20 mm Hg is somewhat higher than normal, but depending on its interpretation and the clinical setting, different treatments would be indicated. Proper interpretation of this filling pressure depends on juxtacardiac pressure and ventricular compliance. Most commonly, a wedge pressure of 20 mm Hg is assumed to mean that juxtacardiac pressure and ventricular compliance are normal and the diagnosis is hypervolemia, with increased left ventricular end-diastolic volume causing the increased PAWP. However, different conclusions are reached if juxtacardiac pressure is increased by certain condition, including tamponade, constriction, or positive-pressure ventilation. Furthermore, a wedge pressure of 20 mm Hg may mean that ventricular compliance is decreased, such as might occur with diastolic dysfunction secondary to myocardial ischemia, hypertrophy, or cardiomyopathy (Fig. 40-41).

Determining an ideal central vascular pressure is often a clinical challenge. At the extremes of high and low, the appropriate intervention is more obvious. Unfortunately, things are rarely so clear-cut in critically ill patients, and the optimal wedge pressure must often be chosen empirically. A fluid challenge may be useful in determining the optimal pressure by comparison with the baseline hemodynamics of the particular patient. An intravenous bolus of crystalloid or colloid solution (250 to 500 mL) is given over a period of 15 minutes, and the change in wedge pressure is measured. Small increases in wedge pressure after the fluid challenge (e.g., <3 mm Hg) suggest that the ventricle is operating on the flat portion of its diastolic filling curve, whereas large increases in wedge pressure (e.g., ≥7 mm Hg) suggest that the steep portion of the curve has been reached and that little further increase in stroke volume and cardiac output can be achieved without a substantial risk of producing hydrostatic pulmonary edema.[50,315]

Clinicians have recognized for years that CVP is a poor indicator of volume status for a variety of reasons.[317,318] The diastolic pressure-volume curves for the left and right ventricles are different even in healthy individuals, with the left ventricle being less compliant. Although investigators have shown that CVP, PADP, and PAWP all vary in the same direction, the more important question is whether small changes in CVP are clinically meaningful or even reliably detectable.[319,320]

The shared septum of the left and right ventricles, as well as the presence of the pericardium, leads to further interpretive problems in the use of CVP for assessing ventricular preload. Ventricular interdependence and pericardial constraint couple changes in right and left ventricular function such that a primary change in right ventricular filling may produce a secondary change in left ventricular filling by altering its diastolic pressure-volume relationship.[198,321] For example, acute pulmonary artery hypertension increases right ventricular end-diastolic volume and pressure, shifts the ventricular septum leftward, and increases left ventricular end-diastolic pressure while simultaneously decreasing left ventricular end-diastolic volume because of a shift

Transduced PAWP	20	20	20
Transmural PAWP	25	10	25
LV compliance	Normal	Normal	Stiff
LV volume	Increased	Normal (or reduced)	Normal (or reduced)

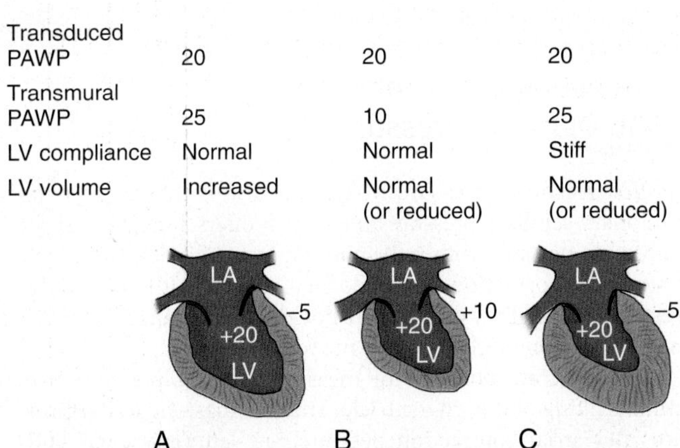

Figure 40-41 Influence of juxtacardiac pressure and ventricular compliance on left ventricular (LV) preload. There are three interpretations of increased transduced pulmonary artery wedge pressure (PAWP, 20 mm Hg). **A,** Juxtacardiac pressure (–5 mm Hg) and LV compliance are normal, transmural PAWP is increased (25 mm Hg), and LV volume is increased. **B,** Juxtacardiac pressure is increased (+10 mm Hg), LV compliance is normal, transmural PAWP is decreased (10 mm Hg), and LV volume is normal or decreased. **C,** Juxtacardiac pressure is normal, LV compliance is decreased, transmural PAWP is increased (25 mm Hg), and LV volume is normal or decreased. *(From Mark JB: Atlas of Cardiovascular Monitoring. New York, Churchill Livingstone, 1998, Fig. 15-8.)*

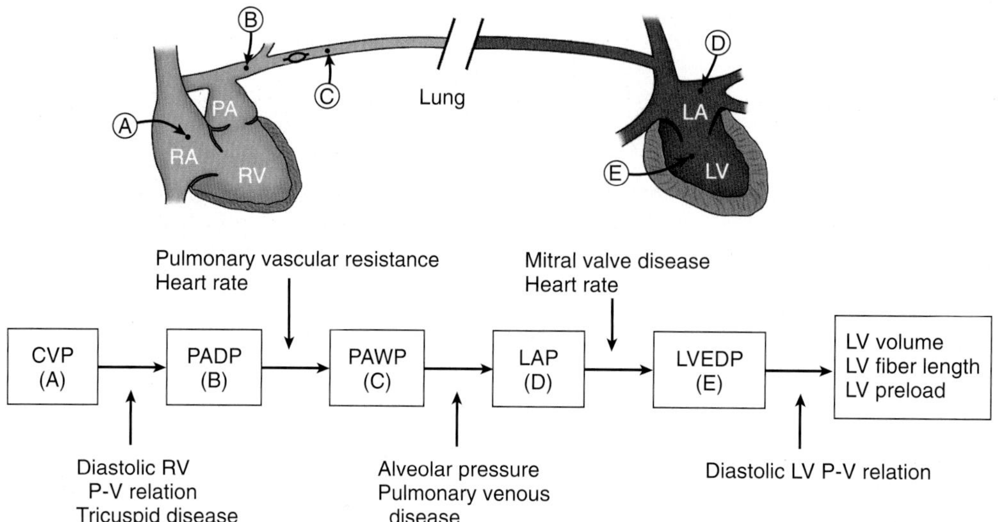

Figure 40-42 Anatomic and physiologic factors that influence the relationships between various measures of left ventricular (LV) filling and true LV preload. The further upstream filling pressure is measured, the more confounding factors may influence the relationship between this measurement and LV preload. CVP, central venous pressure; LA, left atrium; LAP, left atrial pressure; LVEDP, left ventricular end-diastolic pressure; PA, pulmonary artery; PADP, pulmonary artery diastolic pressure; PAWP, pulmonary artery wedge pressure; P-V, pressure-volume; RA, right atrium, RV, right ventricle. *(From Mark JB: Atlas of Cardiovascular Monitoring. New York, Churchill Livingstone, 1998, Fig. 15-5.)*

in the left ventricular pressure-volume relationship to a steeper, stiffer curve. Conversely, primary changes on the left side can adversely affect the right heart structures in similar ways.

Finally, numerous additional factors may alter the relationship between CVP and left ventricular preload (Fig. 40-42).[194] The further upstream from the left ventricle one records the "filling pressure," the greater the multitude of factors that conspire to nullify the relationship between the monitored pressure and left ventricular preload. In view of these considerations, it should be no surprise that reliance on CVP to estimate left ventricular preload in critically ill patients is poorly placed.

Predicting Left Ventricular End-Diastolic Pressure

The first reason to measure wedge pressure is that it estimates pulmonary capillary pressure and as such offers a measure of the hydrostatic pressure within the pulmonary capillaries that largely controls the formation of pulmonary edema. Although wedge pressure and capillary pressure are not identical, changes in PAWP and capillary pressure generally mirror each other.

The second purpose for measuring wedge pressure is to estimate filling of the left ventricle. The end-diastolic wedge pressure after atrial contraction best predicts left ventricular end-diastolic filling pressure or preload.[315] Left ventricular end-diastolic pressure is measured at the Z-point (the point at which the slope of the left ventricular pressure upstroke changes, approximately 50 msec after the ECG Q wave and generally coinciding with the ECG R wave) (Fig. 40-43).[61]

PAC Underestimation of Left Ventricular End-Diastolic Pressure

When a PAC is used to estimate left ventricular filling pressure, there are a number of situations in which this pressure is either underestimated or overestimated (Tables 40-5 and 40-6, respectively). Left ventricular diastolic dysfunction leading to decreased ventricular compliance is the most common cause of underestimation of left ventricular end-diastolic pressure.[322] The atrial contribution to left ventricular end-diastolic volume and pressure is normally less than 20%, but with diastolic dysfunction, it may approach 50%.[296] Under these conditions, the wedge pressure a wave will be unusually prominent and will provide a close estimate of left ventricular end-diastolic pressure, but the mean wedge pressure will underestimate left ventricular filling (see Fig. 40-37).[269] In patients with aortic regurgitation, abnormal diastolic left ventricular filling from the aorta occurs as soon as left ventricular pressure falls below aortic pressure and continues after left atrial contraction and closure of the mitral valve. Left ventricular diastolic pressure continues to rise until end-diastolic pressure is reached at the onset of mechanical systole. Because mitral valve closure occurs before end-diastole, mean PAWP and the wedge pressure a wave both underestimate left ventricular end-diastolic pressure.[269]

In the presence of pulmonic regurgitation, diastolic flow from the proximal pulmonary artery becomes bidirectional, moving both antegrade into the left atrium and retrograde into the right ventricle. When right ventricular diastolic pressure is lower than LAP, pulmonary artery diastolic flow seeks the lower-pressure pathway toward the right ventricle, and PADP will underestimate PAWP, LAP, and left ventricular end-diastolic pressure.[323]

When PVR is normal, there is no pressure gradient across the pulmonary vascular bed at the end of diastole, and PADP equilibrates with the downstream LAP. However, when right ventricular systole is delayed because of right bundle branch block, PAP continues to fall with the x or systolic descent in LAP. In such circumstances, PADP may underestimate left ventricular end-diastolic pressure by as much as 7 mm Hg.[324]

Under normal conditions, inflation of the PAC balloon to measure wedge pressure interrupts antegrade blood flow through

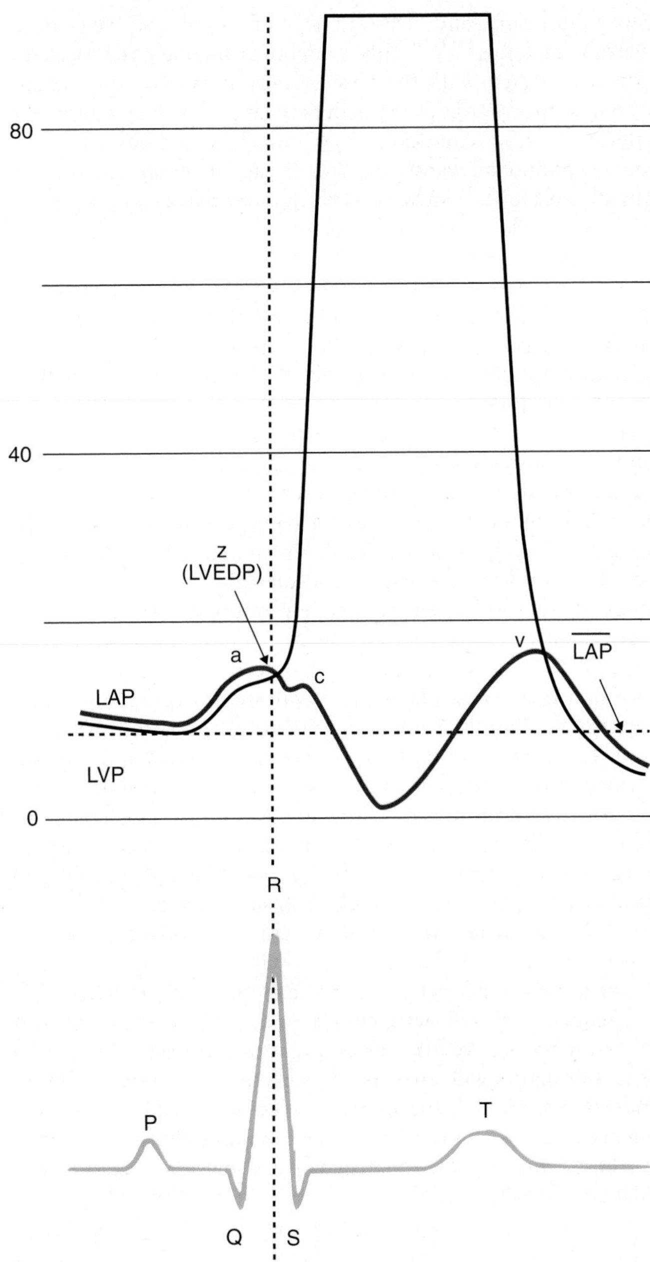

Figure 40-43 Relationship between left atrial pressure (LAP) and left ventricular end-diastolic pressure (LVEDP). LVEDP is measured at the Z-point on the left ventricular pressure (LVP) trace at the time of the electrocardiographic R wave. Mean LAP (9 mm Hg) underestimates LVEDP (15 mm Hg), but the LAP a wave pressure peak closely estimates LVEDP. *(From Mark JB: Atlas of Cardiovascular Monitoring. New York, Churchill Livingstone, 1998, Fig. 6-1.)*

a small section of the lung and has no measurable effect on total pulmonary blood flow or left heart filling. However, after pneumonectomy and in other rare conditions that markedly decrease the pulmonary vascular bed, balloon inflation may occlude a significant portion of the remaining pulmonary vascular cross-sectional area. Mechanical obstruction of pulmonary blood flow ensues and causes increased CVP, as well as decreased LAP, cardiac output, and systemic blood pressure.[325] Therefore, because inflation of the PAC balloon for measurement of wedge pressure leads to obstruction of pulmonary blood flow, the measured wedge pressure underestimates the left atrial and left ventricular end-diastolic pressures that existed before balloon inflation.

Table 40-5 Underestimation of Left Ventricular End-Diastolic Pressure

Condition	Site of Discrepancy	Cause of Discrepancy
Diastolic dysfunction	Mean LAP < LVEDP	Increased end-diastolic a wave
Aortic regurgitation	LAP a wave < LVEDP	Mitral valve closure before end-diastole
Pulmonic regurgitation	PADP < LVEDP	Bidirectional runoff for pulmonary artery flow
Right bundle branch block	PADP < LVEDP	Delayed pulmonic valve opening
After pneumonectomy	PAWP < LAP or LVEDP	Obstruction of pulmonary blood flow

LAP, left atrial pressure; LVEDP, left ventricular end-diastolic pressure; PADP, pulmonary artery diastolic pressure; PAWP, pulmonary artery wedge pressure. Modified from Mark JB: Predicting left ventricular end-diastolic pressure. *In* Mark JB (ed): Atlas of Cardiovascular Monitoring. New York, Churchill Livingstone, 1998, p 59.

PAC Overestimation of Left Ventricular End-Diastolic Pressure

Respiratory influences on the pulmonary artery and wedge pressure traces are the most common cause of overestimation of left ventricular end-diastolic pressure (see Table 40-6). Mechanical ventilation with PEEP poses a particular problem inasmuch as it may expand zone 1 or zone 2 lung conditions and allow PAWP to be influenced by alveolar pressure. In general, mechanical ventilation with PEEP increases wedge pressure by an amount less

Table 40-6 Overestimation of Left Ventricular End-Diastolic Pressure

Condition	Site of Discrepancy	Cause of Discrepancy
Positive end-expiratory pressure	Mean PAWP > mean LAP	Creation of lung zone 1 or 2 or pericardial pressure changes
Pulmonary arterial hypertension	PADP > mean PAWP	Increased pulmonary vascular resistance
Pulmonary veno-occlusive disease	Mean PAWP > mean LAP	Obstruction to flow in large pulmonary veins
Mitral stenosis	Mean LAP > LVEDP	Obstruction to flow across the mitral valve
Mitral regurgitation	Mean LAP > LVEDP	Retrograde systolic v wave raises mean atrial pressure
Ventricular septal defect	Mean LAP > LVEDP	Antegrade systolic v wave raises mean atrial pressure
Tachycardia	PADP > mean LAP > LVEDP	Short diastole creates pulmonary vascular and mitral valve gradients

LAP, left atrial pressure; LVEDP, left ventricular end-diastolic pressure; PADP, pulmonary artery diastolic pressure; PAWP, pulmonary artery wedge pressure. Modified from Mark JB: Predicting left ventricular end-diastolic pressure. *In* Mark JB (ed): Atlas of Cardiovascular Monitoring. New York, Churchill Livingstone, 1998, p 59.

than half the value of PEEP applied (i.e., 10 cm H_2O PEEP will raise wedge pressure less than 5 cm H_2O or 4 mm Hg).[50,326] However, the ratio of chest wall compliance to lung compliance has a significant impact on the relationship between PEEP and its effect on PAWP, and simple mathematical methods to adjust for this effect are not adequate.[50,321,327] Alternative methods to correct for PEEP, such as measuring pleural pressure, are cumbersome and not generally used. Prolonged discontinuation of PEEP before measuring wedge pressure is to be discouraged. Not only might circulatory dynamics change dramatically as a result of rebound central hypervolemia caused by translocation of blood into the core, but respiratory gas exchange may also deteriorate and be slow to recover.[50] As an alternative, Pinsky and coworkers found that transient airway disconnection for 2 to 3 seconds in patients receiving mechanical ventilation with PEEP allowed measurement of nadir wedge pressure, which proved to be a better and safer way to estimate left ventricular filling pressure at higher levels of PEEP.[327] When wedge pressure measurement did not change after abrupt airway disconnection, the on-PEEP wedge pressure measurement accurately reflected left ventricular filling pressure. However, when wedge pressure decreased after airway disconnection, the nadir wedge pressure reached within 3 seconds provided a more accurate measurement. Studying patients with adult respiratory distress syndrome, Teboul and colleagues found that PAWP closely estimates left ventricular end-diastolic pressure at all levels of PEEP up to 20 cm H_2O.[328] This relative microvascular "protection" from the effects of PEEP presumably occurred because of the marked increase in lung stiffness seen in these patients.

When the pulmonary vasculature is normal, pulmonary blood flow ceases at end-diastole, and PADP equals LAP. However, if PVR increases, PAP equilibration with downstream pressure does not occur. Under these conditions, the pulmonary vascular bed begins to resemble the systemic vasculature, where a large pressure gradient between systemic arterial pressure and right atrial pressure persists at end-diastole. Therefore, in the presence of pulmonary arterial hypertension, PADP overestimates PAWP, LAP, and left ventricular end-diastolic pressure.[329]

In contrast to the precapillary pulmonary vasoconstriction that exists in patients with pulmonary arterial hypertension, post-capillary obstruction to flow in the pulmonary veins may occur in the rare condition pulmonary veno-occlusive disease. Patients with this condition have normal LAP, but some disagreement exists about whether these patients have normal or elevated PAC-derived wedge pressure measurements.[50,330,331] In part, these different observations may relate to whether the PAC has been wedged successfully because the wedge position may be difficult to obtain in these patients or in some instances the measured wedge pressure may be recorded from a totally occluded vascular channel. The most important factor, however, is whether the patient has predominantly small-vein occlusion or large-vein occlusion. Obstruction to flow in the small pulmonary veins narrows the static column of blood connecting the wedged PAC tip with the flowing column in the larger pulmonary veins. Given that the partial obstruction involves only the static column, wedge pressure will measure normal left atrial and pulmonary venous pressure because there is no pressure drop across this partially obstructed vascular segment in the absence of flow. Conversely, large-vein obstruction creates a pressure gradient across the large veins as blood flows in these vessels toward the left atrium. In this instance, wedge pressure will detect an increased pulmonary venous pressure and overestimate left atrial and ventricular diastolic pressure.[50,330,331] This model of pulmonary vein obstruction is consistent with the observations of Zidulka and Hakim, who measured wedge pressure in both large and small pulmonary arteries.[332] Other conditions may mimic the hemodynamic features of pulmonary veno-occlusive disease, including mediastinal fibrosis and intrathoracic or atrial tumors that obstruct pulmonary venous flow near the left atrium.

Mitral stenosis obstructs blood flow between the left atrium and left ventricle, and consequently LAP will exceed left ventricular pressure throughout diastole. Furthermore, all upstream pressures recorded by the PAC will overestimate left ventricular end-diastolic pressure as a result of the valvular obstruction. Because the pressure gradient across the mitral valve is directly related to flow, PADP and PAWP will overestimate left ventricular filling pressure even more when transmitral flow is increased by tachycardia or elevated cardiac output.[333]

LAP is increased in mitral regurgitation because of the abnormal leakage of blood across the incompetent valve during systole, and left ventricular end-diastolic pressure is better approximated by measuring wedge pressure before onset of the regurgitant c-v wave (see Fig. 40-34).[334] In contrast to patients with mitral stenosis, in whom LAP exceeds left ventricular pressure throughout diastole, patients with mitral regurgitation have appropriate diastolic equilibration of atrial and ventricular pressure. The problem in mitral regurgitation is choosing the appropriate end-diastolic, pre–v wave pressure to use as an estimate for left ventricular end-diastolic pressure. Mean PAWP will overestimate left ventricular end-diastolic pressure in any patient whose wedge pressure displays tall systolic v waves, including those with ventricular septal defect and left ventricular failure.[287,290]

When tachycardia develops, the duration of diastole is shortened. At both the mitral and pulmonary vascular levels, pressure gradients develop as diastole progressively shortens.[335,336] Consequently, PADP overestimates mean PAWP, which in turn overestimates left ventricular end-diastolic pressure. Patients in atrial fibrillation will have more complete equilibration of PADP and left ventricular end-diastolic pressure during longer R-R intervals. Consequently, these beats should be chosen to provide the best estimate of left ventricular end-diastolic pressure and preload.

Additional Features of Pulmonary Artery Catheters

The popularity of PACs is largely due to the fact that they are multipurpose and provide a wide range of supplementary features for therapeutic and diagnostic applications. Some catheters have a third lumen, which is often used as an additional venous infusion line that opens either 20 or 30 cm from the catheter tip. Others have specific modifications designed for monitoring continuous cardiac output, right heart function, or mixed venous oximetry, thereby vastly expanding the types of physiologic information available to those caring for critically ill patients. Specialized PACs also allow temporary endocardial pacing or intracardiac ECG recording and may even have combinations of electrodes permanently implanted along its length to allow bipolar ventricular, atrial, or atrioventricular pacing.[337] Other models have a special lumen that opens in the right ventricle, through which a thin bipolar wire may be introduced for endocardial ventricular pacing, or have separate atrial and ventricular lumens for passage of two pacing wires for bichamber sequential pacing.[338]

Pulmonary Artery Catheterization and Outcome Controversies

Pulmonary artery catheterization has stimulated a great deal of vigorous controversy. It is an expensive, invasive technique that is widely used but still not proven to improve patient outcome. The PAC controversy has been fueled in part by strongly worded editorials written by prominent physicians debating whether PAC use should be suspended pending scientific proof of its efficacy.[339-341] Although similar controversies have surrounded the use of other widely adopted, highly technical clinical monitoring techniques such as electronic fetal monitoring, physicians who use PACs should especially appreciate the uncertainties surrounding PAC monitoring and be fully informed of the evidence that must guide patient selection.[342,343]

In 2003, the American Society of Anesthesiologists published an updated practice guideline for pulmonary artery catheterization that included a current exhaustive review of the scientific evidence for the clinical effectiveness of PAC monitoring.[211] The inconsistent findings of the many studies in the literature were striking, with evidence both supporting and refuting the benefits of this technique.[213,301,344-346] A great amount of the published literature concerning the use of PACs had been plagued by problems in study design (lack of randomization, small sample size), lack of standardization, and heterogeneity of both patients and clinical settings (medical versus surgical, cardiac surgery patients versus patients with acute congestive heart failure). Furthermore, even within a given clinical setting there is little consensus on which hemodynamic parameters are the most relevant to obtain from use of the PAC and no agreement on appropriate therapeutic interventions in response to specific findings.

Perhaps the most provocative of the early studies was published by Connors and colleagues, who examined the association between PAC use during the first 24 hours of intensive care and subsequent survival.[347] This prospective cohort study included 5735 patients in five teaching hospitals as part of a larger 9000 patient cohort.[348,349] Entry into the study required predicted 6-month mortality in excess of 50%. Patients who were in the PAC-monitored group were judged to be sicker by every measurement recorded, although to the extent statistically possible, the authors used case-matching analyses and applied a propensity score to adjust for these confounding medical covariates. These patients had increased mortality, increased length of hospital stay, and increased cost. Moreover, there was no subgroup of patients who appeared to benefit from PAC monitoring. Publication of this study was accompanied by a strongly worded editorial calling for a moratorium on PAC use or initiation of a randomized controlled trial to define its efficacy.[339]

In the intervening years, a great deal of work and energy have been devoted to determining whether patients are being helped or harmed by the use of PACs. Fortunately, a series of large, randomized, adequately powered studies have been published that specifically address this issue. Three trials enrolling a total of 3468 patients showed no effect on mortality or on hospital or intensive care unit length of stay despite a higher incidence of adverse events.[213,350,351] These complications were most commonly infection or "insertion-related" events. These trials included medical and surgical patients, elderly and high-risk patients, and those with severe heart failure. These findings were confirmed by two meta-analyses of 11 and 13 published randomized, controlled trials involving PAC use.[352,353]

Some investigators have even been able to show a treatment benefit from PAC use in selective populations, a finding that helps guide future use and research. A review of 53,312 patients from the National Trauma Data Bank showed no mortality benefit in those treated with PACs in the group as a whole. However, in patients with an injury severity scale score greater than 25, those who arrived at the hospital in severe shock, or those older than 60 years, mortality was decreased significantly.[354] In a mixed medical and surgical population, patients with Acute Physiology and Chronic Health Evaluation (APACHE) scores less than 25 showed increased mortality when treated with PACs, whereas those with scores higher than 31 showed significant benefit.[355]

Indications for Pulmonary Artery Catheterization

The most recent recommendations governing the use of PACs are the American Society of Anesthesiologists practice guideline published in 2003.[211] The task force considered PAC monitoring to be appropriate in surgical patients undergoing procedures associated with a high risk of complications from hemodynamic changes (e.g., cardiac surgery) or patients with advanced cardiopulmonary diseases that would place them at increased risk for adverse perioperative events. Furthermore, the specific practice setting, as well as the proficiency and experience of clinicians, should be considered.

PAC use must be tailored to the degree of risk for the patient and the risk posed by the procedure itself. For example, a patient with advanced ischemic cardiomyopathy who needs lower extremity amputation under regional anesthesia would not warrant PAC monitoring, whereas a patient with stable ischemic heart disease scheduled for extensive abdominal cancer resection may benefit from perioperative use. Furthermore, the individual practice setting must be considered.[211] Keats has termed this feature "the role of environment in the outcome of operation," by which he means important unmeasurable aspects of the clinical setting, including, but not limited to technical skill and experience.[356] Clearly, all physicians and nurses using a PAC must have the requisite knowledge and skills to use it safely and effectively. Unfortunately, this is a goal that eludes objective definition and remains unattained by current postgraduate training programs.[266]

Several important points should be kept in mind when indications for PAC monitoring are being considered. First, uses of the catheter are different in different patient populations. For example, whereas acute titration of fluids and inotropic agents is most relevant in the perioperative period, in the heart failure population, fine management of oral medications or delineation of drug combinations may be most important. Use of the catheter should be timely; that is, it should not be withheld until irreversible injury has occurred and therapies would be futile. Patients arriving in shock may benefit from immediate PAC placement, whereas others may warrant "watchful waiting." In addition, no catheter should be placed unless the data will be used. Finally, it is of the utmost importance to consider the clinical expertise and experience of those manipulating the catheter and interpreting the data.

It seems a reasonable conclusion from the bulk of published research that PAC use should be limited, although a moratorium on use is ill advised. Use should be reserved to centers with significant experience and expertise. Moreover, PACs should generally be used to monitor and guide therapy in patients at high risk for hemodynamic instability, those who are judged more critically ill by a variety of clinical means, and those who are in shock, especially if older than 60 years.

There remains a great deal of uncertainty and controversy surrounding PAC use. Among the many measurements and calculations possible from a PAC, there is little consensus on which is the most meaningful and useful. Furthermore, therapies based on these findings have not been systematically studied or validated. Indeed, the variations in PAC design have moved so far beyond simple wedge pressure measurement that the PAC is becoming as much a physiologic monitor as it is a hemodynamic one. A PAC itself has no capacity to benefit and only limited risk. However, the potential for adverse outcomes from therapies based on PAC measurements is tremendous. This is the direction that future research needs to take.

Table 40-7 Normal Hemodynamic Values

	Average	Range
Cardiac output (L/min)	5.0	4.0-6.5
Stroke volume (mL)	75	60-90
Systemic vascular resistance		
Wood units	15	10-20
Dynes•sec/cm^5	1200	800-1600
Pulmonary vascular resistance		
Wood units	1	0.5-3
Dynes•sec/cm^5	80	40-180
Arterial oxygen content (mL/dL)	18	16-20
Mixed venous oxygen content (mL/dL)	14	13-15
Mixed venous oxygen saturation (%)	75	70-80
Arteriovenous oxygen difference (mL/dL)	4	3-5
Oxygen consumption (mL/min)	225	200-250

Cardiac Output Monitoring

Aside from its pressure monitoring capabilities, one of the more important features of the PAC is its ability to measure cardiac output via the thermodilution method. Cardiac output is the total blood flow generated by the heart, and in a normal adult at rest it ranges from 4.0 to 6.5 L/min. Measurement of cardiac output provides a global assessment of the circulation, and when combined with other hemodynamic measurements (heart rate, arterial blood pressure, CVP, PAP, and PAWP), it allows calculation of additional important circulatory variables such as systemic vascular resistance (SVR), PVR, and ventricular stroke work (Table 40-7).

Three factors have driven efforts to measure cardiac output in clinical practice. The first is the recognition that in many critically ill patients, low cardiac output leads to significant morbidity and mortality.[357] In addition, clinical assessment of cardiac output is often inaccurate; for example, seriously ill patients with decreased cardiac output might have normal systemic arterial blood pressure.[358] Finally, newer techniques for measurement of cardiac output are less invasive than PAC monitoring and thus might provide benefit to many patients without the attendant risks associated with invasive monitoring.[358-360] The advantages and disadvantages of each technique must be appreciated for proper clinical application.

Thermodilution Cardiac Output Monitoring

The thermodilution technique has become the de facto clinical standard for measuring cardiac output because of its ease of implementation and extensive clinical experience with its use in various settings. It is a variant of the *indicator dilution* method, in which a known amount of a tracer substance is injected into the bloodstream and its change in concentration measured over time at a downstream site (see Chapter 38 for more details). For thermodilution, (negative) heat is injected, and change in temperature downstream is measured.

In practical terms, a fixed volume of iced or room-temperature fluid is injected as a bolus into the proximal (right atrial) lumen of the PAC, and the resulting change in pulmonary artery blood temperature is recorded by a thermistor at the catheter tip. As in all other forms of cardiovascular monitoring, it is important to have a real-time display of the thermodilution curve resulting from each cardiac output measurement.[361] This allows the clinician to discern artifacts that would invalidate the cardiac output measurement, such as unstable blood temperature, recirculation, or incomplete indicator injection. Usually, a series of three cardiac output measurements performed in rapid succession are averaged to provide a more reliable result. When only a single injection was used to determine cardiac output, a difference between sequential cardiac output measurements of 22% was required to suggest a clinically significant change. In contrast, when three injections were averaged to determine the thermodilution measurement, a change greater than 13% indicated a clinically significant change in cardiac output.[362]

Even when carefully performed, some studies have found that thermodilution cardiac output measurements may not agree with other reference methods.[363,364] However, few complications are directly attributable to the technique itself, and monitoring the trend in cardiac output is probably more clinically useful than emphasizing any absolute value.

Sources of Error in Thermodilution Cardiac Output Monitoring

Several important technical issues and potential sources of error must be considered to interpret thermodilution cardiac output measurements properly (Box 40-7).[361] The thermodilution technique measures right ventricular output. In the face of an *intracardiac shunt*, right ventricular and left ventricular output will not be equal. In patients with left-to-right shunts, early recirculation of the thermal indicator can be seen to distort the downward slope of the thermodilution curve, and in patients with right-to-

Box 40-7 Factors Influencing the Accuracy of Thermodilution Cardiac Output Measurement

Intracardiac shunts
Tricuspid or pulmonic valve regurgitation
Inadequate delivery of thermal indicator
- Central venous injection site within the catheter introducer sheath
- Warming of iced injectate

Thermistor malfunction from fibrin or a clot
Pulmonary artery blood temperature fluctuations
- Post–cardiopulmonary bypass status
- Rapid intravenous fluid administration

Respiratory cycle influences

left shunt, some of the injected indicator will bypass the thermistor and result in overestimation of left ventricular cardiac output.

Patients with *tricuspid* or *pulmonic valve regurgitation* pose additional problems for thermodilution cardiac output measurement because of recirculation of the indicator across the incompetent valve. In patients with severe tricuspid regurgitation, the thermodilution curves have an abnormally prolonged decay time, and the measured cardiac output may be inaccurate. Unfortunately, there is no simple method to correct for this problem. In the presence of significant tricuspid regurgitation, thermodilution cardiac output techniques are simply unreliable, either underestimated or overestimated, depending on the severity of valvular regurgitation and the magnitude of the cardiac output.[361,365]

Other technical problems with thermodilution cardiac output measurement are caused by *inadequate delivery of the thermal indicator*. Mishandling of an iced injectate syringe can warm the solution and reduce the signal of the thermal indicator administered. In addition, fibrin or blood clot on the PAC tip may lead to *thermistor malfunction* and result in spurious cardiac output values.

Unrecognized *fluctuation in blood temperature* may also influence cardiac output measurement. In most patients, pulmonary artery blood temperature falls rapidly in the initial minutes *after cardiopulmonary bypass* when the rewarmed body core redistributes the heat gained at the end of bypass. Because of this progressive decline in central core and pulmonary artery blood temperature, the thermal baseline is unstable. Thermodilution cardiac output measurements made in the minutes after bypass are notoriously unreliable, most often leading to marked underestimation of true cardiac output.[366] Other inaccuracies in thermodilution cardiac output measurement occur when pulmonary artery blood temperature changes because of *rapid fluid infusion*.[367] Either overestimation or underestimation of cardiac output occurs, depending on the timing of the additional fluid bolus.

The choice of iced (0°C) or room-temperature injectate has been examined in detail to determine the preferred method for accurate measurement of cardiac output. Although the size of the thermal bolus (and hence the signal-to-noise ratio) is increased when an iced injectate is used, this indicator is more time-consuming, expensive, and cumbersome to prepare than a room-temperature injectate is. Because several groups have demonstrated equivalent accuracy in cardiac output determinations when iced and room-temperature injectates are compared, it appears that room-temperature injectate is preferred for almost all clinical applications.[368] In adults, an injectate volume of 10 mL should be used, whereas in children, an injectate volume of 0.15 mL/kg is recommended.[361]

One of the more controversial issues in standard bolus thermodilution cardiac output monitoring is the proper timing of measurement in relation to the *respiratory cycle*, particularly in patients receiving positive-pressure mechanical ventilation. Because the stroke output of the right ventricle varies as much as 50% during the respiratory cycle, the limited "sampling" of right ventricular stroke volumes measured with the bolus thermodilution technique may lead to widely variable measurements of cardiac output, depending on the point during the respiratory cycle when the measurements are performed.[369] Although reproducibility of consecutive measurements improves markedly when the bolus injections are synchronized to the same phase of the respiratory cycle, accurate measurement of average cardiac output is achieved more reliably by making multiple injections during the different phases of the respiratory cycle and then averaging the results.[361,369]

Continuous Thermodilution Cardiac Output Monitoring

Newer technologies applied to PAC monitoring allow nearly continuous cardiac output (CCO) monitoring with a warm thermal indicator.[370,371] In brief, small quantities of heat are released from a 10-cm thermal filament incorporated into the right ventricular portion of a PAC, approximately 15 to 25 cm from the catheter tip, and the resulting thermal signal is measured by the thermistor at the tip of the catheter in the pulmonary artery. The heating filament is cycled on and off in a pseudorandom binary sequence, and cardiac output is derived from cross-correlation of the measured pulmonary artery temperature with the known sequence of heating filament activation.[371] Typically, the value displayed for cardiac output is updated every 30 to 60 seconds and represents the average value for the cardiac output measured over the previous 3 to 6 minutes. In a laboratory investigation examining how CCO measurements responded to unstable hemodynamic conditions, such as hemorrhage and fluid resuscitation, Siegel and colleagues showed that changes in CCO were markedly slower than changes detected by ultrasonic flow probe, blood pressure, or mixed venous oxygen saturation.[372] In view of these inherent time delays, the PAC CCO method should be considered a continual rather than a continuous real-time monitor.

In general, the CCO method appears to have good agreement with standard bolus thermodilution cardiac output measurements or electromagnetic flow probe techniques.[370,373] In a small, multicenter study, Mihm and associates found that CCO provided a clinically reliable measurement in a group of 47 intensive care unit patients.[370] The device performed well in patients with a wide range of cardiac output (1.6 to 10.6 L/min) and core temperature (33.2°C to 39.8°C), and the method showed no deterioration in performance over the 72-hour monitoring period. Reproducibility and precision appear to be better with the CCO method than with the standard bolus thermodilution techniques, probably because of the fact that the continuous method displays a time-weighted average cardiac output value as opposed to a single instantaneous measurement.[374,375]

The CCO PAC has been widely accepted into clinical use for a number of practical reasons. Although these catheters are more expensive than standard PACs, obviating the need for bolus injections reduces nursing workload and the potential risk of fluid overload or infection. Furthermore, because the CCO PAC provides a cardiac output value that is an average derived over the previous several minutes, the beat-to-beat variations in stroke volume that occur during a single respiratory cycle are all equally represented. As a result, cardiac output measured by the CCO method may provide a more accurate measurement of global cardiac output in patients receiving positive-pressure mechanical ventilation.

However, like cold bolus thermodilution techniques, warm thermal CCO has certain methodologic pitfalls that must be recognized and avoided. The CCO computer and catheter require a significant amount of time to warm up and may work poorly in an environment with a great deal of thermal noise, such as the cardiac operating room. As already emphasized, CCO monitors have an inherent 5- to 15-minute delay in responding to abrupt changes in cardiac output, and the magnitude of this delay depends on the type of physiologic perturbation, as well as the CCO computer monitor algorithm.[372] Although modifications of CCO algorithms provide a "STAT Mode" rapid response time, acute changes in cardiac output are still detected more slowly by CCO monitoring than by other methods, such as direct arterial pressure or mixed venous oximetry. In effect, the CCO technique involves a fundamental tradeoff between rapid response time and overall accuracy of measurement. Standards for these performance characteristics have not been defined but must balance the response time against the stability of the displayed value and its immunity from thermal noise.[374]

Mixed Venous Oximetry Pulmonary Artery Catheter

Although the formal Fick cardiac output method is not widely applied in clinical practice, the physiologic relationships described by the Fick equation form the basis for another PAC-based monitoring technique termed *continuous mixed venous oximetry*. Rearrangement of the Fick equation reveals the four determinants of mixed venous hemoglobin saturation:

$$S\overline{v}O_2 = SaO_2 - \frac{\dot{V}O_2}{\dot{Q} \times 1.36 \times Hb} \quad (1)$$

where $S\overline{v}O_2$ = mixed venous hemoglobin saturation (%)
SaO_2 = arterial hemoglobin saturation (%)
$\dot{V}O_2$ = oxygen consumption (mL O_2/min)
$\dot{Q}$ = cardiac output (L/min)
Hb = hemoglobin concentration (g/dL)

To the extent that arterial hemoglobin saturation, oxygen consumption, and hemoglobin concentration remain stable, mixed venous hemoglobin saturation may be used as an indirect indicator of cardiac output. For example, when cardiac output falls, tissue oxygen extraction increases and the mixed venous blood will have a lower oxygen content and lower hemoglobin oxygen saturation. However, as noted in this equation, mixed venous hemoglobin saturation also varies directly with arterial hemoglobin concentration and saturation and inversely with oxygen consumption. When any of these other variables change significantly, one cannot assume that a change in mixed venous hemoglobin saturation results solely from a change in cardiac output. Although these considerations may confound the use of mixed venous hemoglobin saturation as an indicator of cardiac output, monitoring this variable provides more comprehensive information about the balance of oxygen delivery and consumption by the body—not just the raw cardiac output, but also the adequacy of that cardiac output.[376]

Although mixed venous hemoglobin saturation may be determined by intermittent blood sampling from the pulmonary artery, a specially designed PAC can provide this information reliably and continuously. Fiberoptic bundles incorporated into the PAC determine the hemoglobin saturation in pulmonary artery blood based on the principles of reflectance oximetry using either a two- or three-wavelength system. A special computer connected to this PAC displays the mixed venous hemoglobin saturation continuously. The technology is typically incorporated into the standard PAC or the CCO PAC, in the latter case providing both CCO and venous oximetry data.

Technical problems with continuous mixed venous oximetry are generally limited to improper positioning of the PAC tip against the vessel wall or inaccurate calibration.[377] Multi-wavelength fiberoptic technology and reflection intensity algorithms help reduce wall artifacts caused by spurious reflections from a PAC thrombus or the pulmonary arterial walls. These catheters are calibrated at the bedside before use but may also be calibrated in vivo from a pulmonary artery blood gas sample if the mixed venous saturation values are questionable. Most clinical trials comparing PAC-derived continuous venous oximetry values with laboratory analysis of pulmonary artery blood samples have shown good agreement between techniques.[378] It is important to remember that mixed venous oxygenation is a global, whole-body measurement. Therefore, regionally inadequate blood flow and tissue oxygen delivery (such as limb or intestinal ischemia) can coexist with a normal or a high mixed venous oximetry value.

The continuous mixed venous oximetry PAC may be used to measure thermodilution cardiac output and arterial and mixed venous oxygen content values and thereby calculate oxygen consumption by rearrangement of the Fick equation. However, values for oxygen consumption derived from these measurements generally underestimate direct oxygen consumption measured by mass spectrometry, metabolic cart, or water-sealed spirometry.[379]

Oxygen delivery may also be calculated as shown in Equation 2:

$$\dot{D}O_2 = \dot{Q} \times CaO_2 \quad (2)$$

where $\dot{D}O_2$ = oxygen delivery (mL/min)
$\dot{Q}$ = cardiac output (dL/min)
CaO_2 = oxygen content of arterial blood (mL O_2/dL blood)

Many physicians have used these derived measures of oxygen consumption and oxygen delivery to guide the treatment of critically ill patients, although the success of this "goal-oriented therapy" in improving patient outcomes is still inconclusive. However, a recent randomized study in patients undergoing cardiac surgery has shown better outcome in patients randomized to protocol-driven interventions aimed at achieving mixed venous oxygen saturation higher than 70% (and blood lactate <2 mg/dL).[380] Similarly, optimizing central venous oxygen saturation (measured in superior vena cava blood) has been shown to improve outcome in patients with early sepsis[381] and in high-risk surgical patients.[382]

It is important to note that these studies have used strict protocol-driven therapeutic interventions. A large Veterans Affairs observational trial of 3265 cardiac surgical patients noted that 49% of patients received continuous mixed venous oximetry PACs and that use of this catheter was associated with increased cost but no better outcome than achieved in the standard PAC group.[383] In this study, however, no protocol was used to guide therapeutic interventions based on monitoring results.

Right Ventricular Ejection Fraction Pulmonary Artery Catheters

Although cardiovascular monitoring has focused predominantly on left ventricular performance, in some instances, right ventricular dysfunction may be the more important factor limiting circulation. Patient populations at increased risk for right ventricular dysfunction include those with chronic obstructive pulmonary disease, adult respiratory distress syndrome, pulmonary hypertension, and right ventricular ischemia and infarction.[384] Standard techniques are available for monitoring right ventricular performance in patients with acute myocardial infarction involving the right ventricle. PAC monitoring in patients with right ventricular infarction often reveals the characteristic hemodynamic patterns described earlier. However, accurate evaluation of right ventricular performance has proved more complicated. In patients with severe respiratory failure, for example, the confounding effects of mechanical ventilation with high levels of PEEP have made interpretation of cardiac filling pressures difficult and, in some cases, misleading.[385]

Measurement of right ventricular ejection fraction (RVEF) with a specially designed PAC offers another method for evaluating right ventricular function. This method uses a standard PAC equipped with a rapid-response thermistor that detects and quantifies the small changes in pulmonary artery blood temperature that occur with each heartbeat, in a manner somewhat analogous to a standard CCO PAC. The cardiac output computer measures the residual fraction of thermal signal after each heartbeat and derives RVEF.[386] Clearly, all factors that confound standard thermodilution cardiac output measurement will also interfere with accurate determination of RVEF. In addition, because the temperature changes measured by the RVEF PAC are small beat-to-beat changes, the method will not work if the ECG R waves cannot be detected accurately, the R-R interval is short because of tachycardia, or the cardiac rhythm is irregular.[377] Comparison of PAC-based RVEF measurements with angiographic or nuclear techniques has yielded mixed results in terms of accuracy, but this may reflect, in part, the absence of a widely accepted reference standard for this measurement.[386,387] Intraoperative use of the RVEF PAC has focused primarily on detection of right ventricular dysfunction in patients with coronary artery disease undergoing surgical revascularization. Reduced RVEF has been noted after cardiopulmonary bypass, particularly in patients with preexisting right coronary artery obstruction.[388] However, RVEF is an extremely load-dependent measurement of right ventricular performance, and the clinician must keep this fact in mind to interpret this measurement properly.[377,389] Clinical use of the RVEF PAC appears to have found its greatest application to date in critically ill patients, especially those with respiratory failure.[389,390] In these applications, the measurement of greatest interest has been right ventricular end-diastolic volume, which is derived mathematically from RVEF:

$$\text{RVEDV} = \frac{\text{SV}}{\text{RVEF}} \tag{3}$$

where RVEDV = right ventricular end-diastolic volume (mL)
SV = stroke volume (mL)
RVEF = right ventricular ejection fraction

Right ventricular end-diastolic volume appears to correlate better with cardiac output than standard preload measurements such as CVP or PAWP do.[390,391] These findings are not surprising given all the interpretive problems associated with monitoring cardiac filling pressure previously discussed. It should be kept in mind, however, that the better correlation between right ventricular end-diastolic volume and cardiac output may result from the mathematical coupling of measurements because both are derivatives of stroke volume determined with the PAC. Furthermore, as in the case of standard PAC monitoring, the benefit of RVEF PAC monitoring in terms of patient outcome remains unproven.[392]

Pulmonary Artery Catheter–Derived Hemodynamic Variables

The cardiovascular system is often modeled as an electrical circuit, with the relationship between cardiac output, blood pressure, and resistance to flow related in a manner similar to Ohm's law:

$$\begin{aligned} \text{SVR} &= \frac{\text{MAP} - \text{CVP}}{\text{CO}} \times 80 \\ \text{PVR} &= \frac{\text{MPAP} - \text{PAWP}}{\text{CO}} \times 80 \end{aligned} \tag{4}$$

where SVR = systemic vascular resistance (dyne·sec·cm^{-5})
PVR = pulmonary vascular resistance (dyne·sec·cm^{-5})
MAP = mean arterial pressure (mm Hg)
CVP = central venous pressure (mm Hg)
MPAP = mean pulmonary artery pressure (mm Hg)
PAWP = pulmonary artery wedge pressure (mm Hg)
CO = cardiac output (L/min)

Normal values for SVR and PVR are given in Table 40-7. Note that these calculations of SVR and PVR are based on a hydraulic fluid model that assumes continuous laminar flow through a series of rigid pipes.[393] These calculations also use atrial pressure as the downstream pressure for systemic or pulmonary flow, with CVP used for right atrial pressure in the SVR calculation and PAWP used for LAP in the PVR calculation. Alternative methods to calculate resistance ignore the effect of these downstream pressures. For the systemic circulation, total resistance may be calculated from MAP and cardiac output alone, and for the pulmonary circulation, total pulmonary resistance describes the ratio of mean PAP and cardiac output.

All these resistance formulas oversimplify the behavior of the cardiovascular system to a tremendous degree. A more physiologic model of the systemic circulation considers the vasculature to be a series of collapsible vessels with intrinsic tone. This model, also called the *vascular waterfall*, describes a critical closing pressure in the downstream end of the circuit that exceeds right atrial pressure and serves to limit flow—an effective downstream pressure that is higher than the right atrial pressure used in the SVR formula. Detailed consideration of these issues is beyond the scope of this discussion and is available from other sources.[394,395] The important point for clinicians, though, is that therapy focused on fine adjustment of SVR may be very misleading and should be avoided.

Additional problems arise in considering the pulmonary vasculature and using the formulas just presented as a measure of resistance to flow through the lung. The pulmonary vasculature is more compliant than the systemic vasculature, and marked increases in pulmonary blood flow may not produce any significant increase in PAP. In addition, flow usually ceases at end-diastole in the low-resistance pulmonary circuit.[396] Thus, changes in PVR may result from intrinsic alterations in pulmonary vascular tone (constriction or dilation) or vascular recruitment or from rheologic changes. For the pulmonary circuit, a better approach to evaluating changes in PVR may be to examine the end-diastolic gradient between PADP and PAWP (Fig. 40-44).[397]

Another set of common calculations derived from standard hemodynamic variables adjusts these measurements for the patient's body surface area (BSA) in an attempt to normalize these measurements for patients of different size. BSA is generally determined from a standard nomogram based on height and weight. The most commonly indexed variables are the cardiac index (cardiac index = cardiac output/BSA) and stroke volume index (stroke volume index = stroke volume/BSA). On occasion, SVR and PVR are indexed as well (SVR index = SVR × BSA; PVR index = PVR × BSA). In theory, normalizing hemodynamic values through "indexing" should help clinicians determine appropriate normal physiologic ranges to help guide therapy. Unfortunately, there is little evidence that these additional calculations provide valid normalizing adjustments. BSA is a biometric measurement with an obscure relationship to blood flow, and it does not adjust for variations between individuals based on age, sex, body habitus, or metabolic rate.[398] Although it is important to be aware of a patient's size and medical history when interpreting and treating changes in any of the measured or calculated hemodynamic variables, it is not appropriate to target therapy solely at achieving normal indexed values.

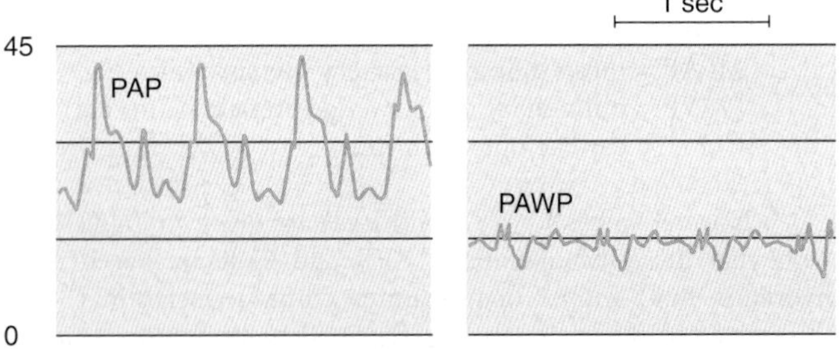

Figure 40-44 Pulmonary hypertension. The increased gradient across the pulmonary vasculature causes pulmonary artery diastolic pressure to exceed pulmonary artery wedge pressure (PAWP). PAP, pulmonary artery pressure. *(From Mark JB: Atlas of Cardiovascular Monitoring. New York, Churchill Livingstone, 1998, Fig. 6-11.)*

Other Methods for Monitoring Cardiac Output and Perfusion

Ultrasound-Based Methods for Monitoring Cardiac Output

All of the ultrasound-based methods for monitoring cardiac output use the Doppler principle. When ultrasound waves strike moving objects, these waves are reflected back to their source at a different frequency, termed the *Doppler shift frequency*, which is directly related to the velocity of the moving objects and the angle at which the ultrasound beam strikes these objects. For measurement of blood flow, the red blood cells flowing through a major artery serve as the moving objects targeted by the ultrasound beam. To measure blood flow velocity, the Doppler equation is rearranged to solve for velocity:

$$v = \frac{f \times c}{2f_0 \times \cos\theta} \quad (5)$$

where v = velocity of red blood cell targets
f = Doppler shift frequency
f_0 = transmitted ultrasound beam frequency
θ = angle between the ultrasound beam and the vector of red blood cell flow
c = velocity of ultrasound in blood (approximately 1570 m/sec)

In general, determining blood flow velocity requires just a single measurement, the Doppler shift frequency, because the velocity of ultrasound in blood and the transmitted ultrasound frequency are known and cos θ is assumed to equal 1 as long as the angle of insonation is small. This assumption requires that the ultrasound beam be oriented as much as possible in a direction that is parallel to the flow of blood. For example, for angles of less than 20 degrees, cos θ will be greater than 0.94, thereby introducing an error of less than 6% in calculation of cardiac output. Once the Doppler shift frequency is measured and blood flow velocity is calculated, stroke volume can be determined from Equation 6:

$$SV = v \times ET \times CSA \quad (6)$$

where SV = stroke volume (mL)
v = spatial average velocity of blood flow (cm/sec)
ET = systolic ejection time (sec)
CSA = cross-sectional area of the vessel (cm^2)

Several different ultrasound-based methods can be used to measure cardiac output, each using slightly different equipment and measuring blood flow from a different site in the body.

Suprasternal Doppler Cardiac Output Monitoring

This method was developed to measure blood flow velocity in the distal aortic arch with an ultrasound transducer applied to the suprasternal notch.[399] Although the suprasternal Doppler cardiac output technique showed reasonable agreement with the thermodilution method, it is relatively labor intensive, requires a fair degree of experience and expertise, and cannot be accomplished in a significant number of critically ill medical and surgical patients.[399,400] Because it provides only an intermittent measurement at best, clinical acceptance of this method was limited.

Esophageal Doppler Cardiac Output Monitoring

The evolution of Doppler techniques into practical clinical monitoring tools required an ultrasound transducer that could be positioned and left in place for continuous monitoring without the need for repeated adjustments or time-consuming measurements by the physician or ultrasonographer. Such a transducer was incorporated into the tip of a standard esophageal stethoscope to allow continuous monitoring of cardiac output by interrogating the blood flow profile in the descending thoracic aorta. In brief, the Doppler probe is inserted into the esophagus to a depth of approximately 35 cm from the incisors. Probe position is adjusted to optimize the audible Doppler flow sound from the descending aorta. In most patients, optimal probe tip position is at the T5-T6 vertebral interspace or the third sternocostal junction because the esophagus and the descending aorta lie in close proximity and run essentially parallel to one another at this location.[401] The ultrasound transducer is mounted at a fixed angle that is anatomically defined and known by the cardiac output computer. This angle is then used to correct the resulting Doppler shift frequency to provide an accurate velocity measurement.

Several limitations of the esophageal Doppler technique must be appreciated by the physician to avoid pitfalls in interpretation of data. This monitoring method interrogates blood flow in the descending thoracic aorta and therefore measures only a fraction of total cardiac output. To report total cardiac output, either the esophageal Doppler measurement must be "calibrated" by some alternative method or an empirically determined correction constant of 1.4 must be used.[402] This constant is accurate for most patients but does not apply universally, especially in the presence of conditions that redistribute blood flow, such as pregnancy, aortic cross-clamping, and post–cardiopulmonary bypass status.[401,403] In addition, the diameter of the descending aorta is either measured by using A-mode ultrasound or calculated on the basis of the patient's age, sex, height, and weight via a nomogram.[404] When calculated, it is assumed that the diameter of the descending aorta does not change throughout the cardiac cycle.[405] Moreover, the technique is likely to be inaccurate in the presence of aortic valve stenosis or regurgitation or in patients with thoracic aortic disease, it is not easily applied in nonintubated patients, and it cannot be used in individuals with esophageal pathology. Finally, like all ultrasound techniques, the acoustic window needed to acquire the Doppler signal may not be adequate in some individuals, thereby precluding use of this method.

Advantages of the esophageal Doppler monitoring technique include its ease of use, minimal invasiveness, and inherent safety. It appears that limited experience is needed for clinical success—as few as 10 to 12 cases for accurate application of the technique.[401] In a recent review describing 25 clinical trials in which esophageal Doppler cardiac output measurement was compared with PAC thermodilution measurements, it was noted that the Doppler cardiac output values correlated well with the thermodilution measurements and showed minimal overall bias and good tracking of directional changes in thermodilution cardiac output with low intraobserver and interobserver measurement variability.[401]

The esophageal Doppler method has enjoyed renewed popularity.[402,406] Current devices provide a clear visual display of the spectral Doppler waveform, but they also calculate and display additional hemodynamic variables, including peak blood flow velocity, flow acceleration, and heart rate–corrected flow time (Fig. 40-45). Some studies have shown that these additional measures provide useful information about left ventricular preload, contractility, and SVR.[402,407] One of the more important values of the monitor may be focusing clinical attention on optimizing stroke volume rather than total cardiac output. Indeed, in critically ill patients, complications may be better predicted by low stroke volume than by low cardiac output.[408] Several studies have shown that volume resuscitation guided by maximizing esophageal Doppler–measured stroke volume in moderate-risk surgical patients reduces perioperative morbidity and shortens hospital stay.[409-411]

Bioimpedance Cardiac Output Monitoring

The technique of bioimpedance cardiac output monitoring was first described by Kubicek and colleagues and is based on changes in electrical impedance of the thoracic cavity occurring with ejection of blood during cardiac systole.[412] Their original formula relates these bioimpedance measurements to stroke volume:

$$SV = \frac{\rho L^2}{Zo^2} \times VET \times \max \frac{dZ}{dt} \qquad (7)$$

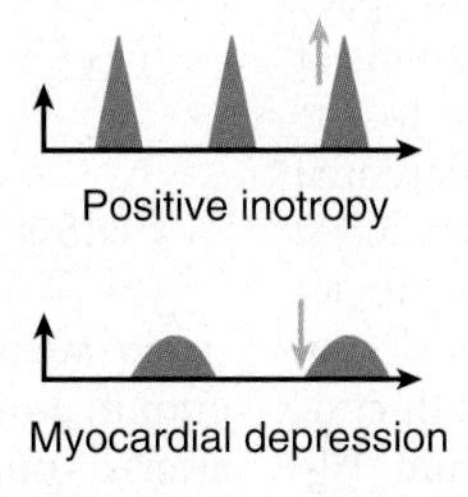

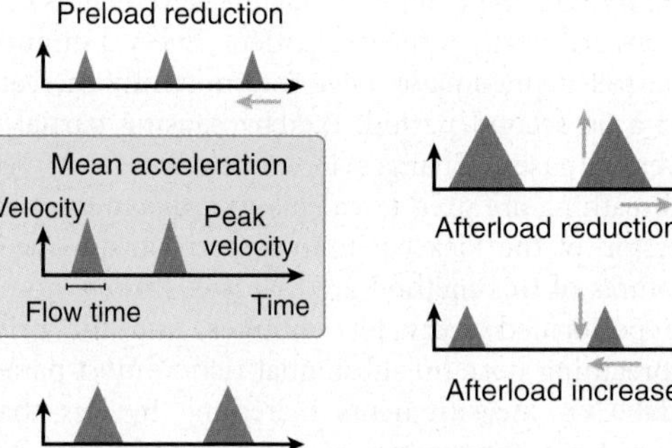

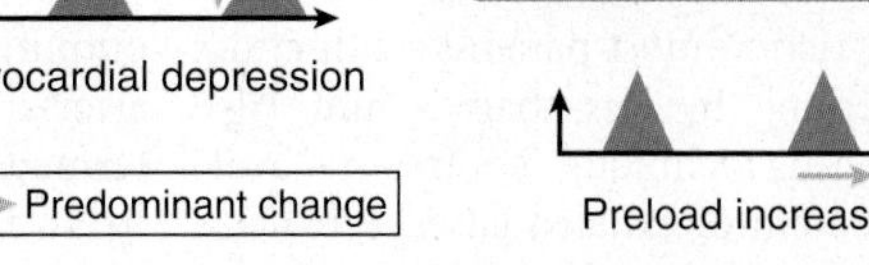

Figure 40-45 Spectral Doppler tracings of aortic blood flow recorded with esophageal Doppler cardiac output monitoring. The velocity-time waveform shape reflects alterations in contractility (mainly affecting peak velocity and mean acceleration), preload (mainly affecting systolic flow time corrected for heart rate [FTc]), and afterload (which affects FTc, mean acceleration, and peak flow velocity). *(Modified with permission from Singer M: Esophageal Doppler monitoring of aortic blood flow: Beat-by-beat cardiac output monitoring. Int Anesthesiol Clin 31:99-125, 1993.)*

where SV = stroke volume
ρ = specific resistivity of blood
L = thoracic length
Zo = basal thoracic impedance
VET = ventricular ejection time
$\max \frac{dZ}{dt}$ = maximum rate of impedance change during systolic upstroke

For performing the measurements, disposable electrodes are applied to the skin surface along the sides of the neck and lateral aspect of the lower part of the thorax, and a continuous small electrical current is applied across the chest. Patient height, weight, and gender are used to calculate the volume of the thoracic cavity. Bioimpedance cardiac output is computed for each cardiac cycle and continuously displayed as an average value over several heartbeats.

Although many studies suggest that the bioimpedance method is accurate in healthy volunteers, its reliability deteriorates in critically ill patients, including those with sepsis, increased lung water, aortic regurgitation, and electronic cardiac pacing.[413-415] More recent changes in signal processing techniques have improved the accuracy of thoracic bioimpedance measurements and might increase its clinical acceptance.[416]

Partial CO_2 Rebreathing Cardiac Output Monitoring

Another method of monitoring cardiac output that does not require pulmonary artery catheterization is the partial CO_2 rebreathing technique.[417,418] Because of the difficulty encountered in the standard Fick method involving measuring oxygen consumption and mixed venous hemoglobin saturation, this new technique is based on a restatement of the Fick equation for carbon dioxide elimination rather than oxygen uptake:

$$\dot{Q} = \frac{\dot{V}CO_2}{C\bar{v}CO_2 - CaCO_2} \quad (8)$$

where $\dot{Q}$ = cardiac output
$\dot{V}CO_2$ = rate of carbon dioxide elimination
$C\bar{v}CO_2$ = carbon dioxide content of mixed venous blood
$CaCO_2$ = carbon dioxide content of arterial blood

This method uses the change in CO_2 production and end-tidal CO_2 concentration in response to a brief, sudden change in minute ventilation. With a specially designed breathing system and monitoring computer, this measurement is easily performed in any tracheally intubated patient. Every 3 minutes a computer-controlled pneumatic valve intermittently increases dead space for a 50-second period, thereby causing partial rebreathing of exhaled gases. Changes in end-tidal CO_2 in response to the rebreathing are used to calculate cardiac output by a differential version of the Fick equation for carbon dioxide. The attractive features of this method are that it is entirely noninvasive, it can be performed every few minutes, and the brief episodes of rebreathing pose no substantial risk to most patients, with end-tidal CO_2 measurements increasing by less than 3 mm Hg. However, as currently designed, this technique requires tracheal intubation for accurate measurement of exhaled gases. Furthermore, changing patterns of ventilation may have an unpredictable influence on the measurement. As with all Fick-based techniques, the partial CO_2 rebreathing method measures pulmonary capillary blood flow as an indicator of total cardiac output and thus requires correction for pulmonary shunt.

The initial clinical trials suggested reasonably good agreement between the partial rebreathing CO_2 cardiac output method and other techniques such as thermodilution. However, as with most of these newer monitoring methods, the clinical trials are small and mainly focused on specific patient groups, particularly coronary artery bypass patients.[419] At present, the clinical role of this technique is primarily focused on short-term intraoperative applications or mechanically ventilated postoperative patients.

Lithium Dilution Cardiac Output Monitoring

The lithium dilution technique is another cardiac output monitoring method that derives its fundamental basis from indicator dilution principles.[420] In brief, after an intravenous bolus injection of a small dose of lithium chloride, an ion-selective electrode attached to a peripheral arterial catheter measures the lithium dilution curve, from which cardiac output is derived. Preliminary investigations suggest that this technique is accurate when compared with standard thermodilution methods or electromagnetic flowmetry.[421,422] As originally described, the technique required a central venous catheter for injection of lithium, but recent studies indicate comparable accuracy with peripheral intravenous bolus administration of the lithium indicator.[423] Thus, the technique seems to provide a method for accurate cardiac output measurement in a wide variety of critically ill patients who only have peripheral intravenous and arterial catheters.

Transpulmonary Thermodilution Cardiac Output

For transpulmonary thermodilution measurement, ice-cold saline is injected into a central line and the change in temperature is measured in a large peripheral artery (femoral, axillary, or brachial artery) via a special arterial catheter equipped with a thermistor.[424] Several studies have shown adequate correspondence to standard thermodilution cardiac output.[425,426] Because the measurement lasts over several cardiac cycles, respiratory effects on stroke volume are averaged and eliminated, in contrast to standard thermodilution.[427] Mathematical derivation from the thermodilution curve can produce two additional clinically useful indices: extravascular lung water, which is a measure of pulmonary edema,[428,429] and intrathoracic blood volume, which is a measure of preload. Several studies have found this index to be a better measure of cardiac preload than traditional measurements such as CVP or PAWP.[430,431]

Pulse Contour Cardiac Output Monitoring

In an attempt to provide continuous measurement of cardiac output, a number of techniques have focused on analysis of the arterial pulse pressure waveform. These methods, generally termed *pulse contour cardiac output*, determine the cardiac output from computerized analysis of the arterial pressure waveform recorded from an arterial catheter or even a noninvasive finger blood pressure waveform.[432,433] Pulse contour methods offer the potential for continuous, beat-to-beat monitoring of cardiac output. In addition, the change in stroke volume from beat to beat can be used to evaluate volume status in ventilated patients.[434]

However, several disadvantages exist.[435] First, baseline calibration with a known cardiac output is required to account for individual differences in vascular resistance, impedance, and wave reflectance. Additionally, recalibration is required every 8 to 12 hours to account for changes in vasculature characteristics over time. A reasonably well-defined arterial pressure waveform is needed for accurate identification of systole and diastole, a condition that might not exist in patients with severe tachycardia or dysrhythmia.

Although early studies comparing these techniques showed fairly poor agreement with other cardiac output measurements, more recent clinical trials in surgical patients have shown that the pulse contour methods provide an acceptable level of accuracy.[433,436,437]

Gastric Tonometry

Gastric tonometry aims at monitoring gastric circulation as an early indication of splanchnic hypoperfusion.[438] A balloon-tipped tube is inserted into the stomach, and the saline or air in the balloon is allowed to equilibrate with the CO_2 in the gastric lumen. Intermittently, the saline or air is aspirated and the CO_2 level is measured. With the development of gastric hypoperfusion, clearance of CO_2 from the gastric mucosa decreases while CO_2 production increases from titration of acid released by anaerobic metabolism. The CO_2 from the mucosa diffuses freely to the gastric lumen and is detected by the tonometry.

Several studies have shown that gastric mucosal CO_2 and pH are a predictor of post-trauma or perioperative complications or death.[439-441] Furthermore, several studies have shown that therapy guided by gastric tonometry can improve clinical outcome in critically ill or perioperative patients.[442,443]

References

1. Gravenstein JS: Monitoring with our good senses. J Clin Monit Comput 14:451-453, 1998.
2. McIntyre JWR: Stethoscopy during anaesthesia. Can J Anaesth 44:535-542, 1997.
3. Biro P: Electrically amplified precordial stethoscope. J Clin Monit 10:410-412, 1994.
4. Manecke GR, Poppers PJ: Esophageal stethoscope placement depth: Its effect on heart and lung sound monitoring during general anesthesia. Anesth Analg 86:1276-1279, 1998.
5. Klepper ID, Webb RK, Van Der Walt JH, et al: The stethoscope: Applications and limitations—an analysis of 2000 incident reports. Anaesth Intensive Care 21:575-578, 1993.
6. Prielipp RC, Kelly JS, Roy RC: Use of esophageal or precordial stethoscopes by anesthesia providers: Are we listening to our patients? J Clin Anesth 7:367-372, 1995.
7. Watson MO, Sanderson P: Designing for attention with sound: Challenges and extensions to ecological interface design. Hum Factors 49:331-346, 2007.
8. Block FE: What is heart rate, anyway? J Clin Monit 10:366-370, 1994.
9. Mark JB: Monitoring heart rate. *In* Mark JB (ed): Atlas of Cardiovascular Monitoring. New York, Churchill Livingstone, 1998, pp 205-217.
10. Murray WB, Foster PA: The peripheral pulse wave: Information overlooked. J Clin Monit 12:365-377, 1996.
11. Reisner A, Shaltis PA, McCombie D, Asada HH: Utility of the photoplethysmogram in circulatory monitoring. Anesthesiology 108:950-958, 2008.
12. Zong W, Moody GB, Mark RG: Reduction of false arterial blood pressure alarms using signal quality assessment and relationships between the electrocardiogram and arterial blood pressure. Med Biol Eng Comput 42:698-706, 2004.
13. American Society of Anesthesiologists: Standards for Basic Anesthetic Monitoring. 2005. Available at http://www.asahq.org/publicationsAndServices/standards/02.pdf/ Accessed May 5, 2008.
14. Bruner JMR, Krenis LJ, Kunsman JM, Sherman AP: Comparison of direct and indirect methods of measuring arterial blood pressure. Med Instrum 15:11-21, 97-101, 182-188, 1981.
15. Riva-Rocci S: Un nuovo sfigmomanometro. Gaz Med Torino 47:981, 1896.
16. Korotkoff NS: On the subject of methods of determining blood pressure. Bull Imp Med Acad St Petersburg 11:365, 1905.
17. Pickering TG, Hall JE, Appel LJ, et al: Recommendations for blood pressure measurement in humans and experimental animals: Part 1: Blood pressure measurement in humans: A statement for professionals from the Subcommittee of Professional and Public Education of the American Heart Association Council on High Blood Pressure Research. Hypertension 45:142-161, 2005.
18. Cohn JN: Blood pressure measurement in shock. Mechanism of inaccuracy in auscultatory and palpatory methods. JAMA 199:972-976, 1967.
19. Posey JA, Geddes LA, Williams H, Moore AG: The meaning of the point of maximum oscillations in cuff pressure in the indirect measurement of blood pressure. Part 1. Cardiovasc Res Center Bull 8:15-25, 1969.
20. Yelderman M, Ream AK: Indirect measurement of mean blood pressure in the anesthetized patient. Anesthesiology 50:253-256, 1979.
21. Weiss BM, Pasch T: Measurement of systemic arterial pressure. Curr Opin Anaesthesiol 10:459-466, 1997.
22. Alford JW, Palumbo MA, Barnum MJ: Compartment syndrome of the arm: A complication of noninvasive blood pressure monitoring during thrombolytic therapy for myocardial infarction. J Clin Monit Comput 17:163-166, 2002.
23. Penaz J: Photoelectric measurement of blood pressure, volume, and flow in the finger. Paper presented at the 10th International Conference on Medical and Biological Engineering, 1973, p 104.
24. Bos WJW, van Goudoever J, van Montfrans GA, et al: Reconstruction of brachial artery pressure from noninvasive finger pressure measurements. Circulation 94:1870-1875, 1996.
25. Belani K, Ozaki M, Hynson J, et al: A new noninvasive method to measure blood pressure: Results of a multicenter trial. Anesthesiology 91:686-692, 1999.
26. Cockings JGL, Webb RK, Klepper ID, et al: Blood pressure monitoring—applications and limitations: An analysis of 2000 incident reports. Anaesth Intensive Care 21:565-569, 1993.
27. Eather KF, Peterson LH, Dripps RD: Studies of the circulation of anesthetized patients by a new method for recording arterial pressure and pressure pulse contours. Anesthesiology 10:125-132, 1949.
28. Mark JB: Atlas of Cardiovascular Monitoring. New York, Churchill Livingstone, 1998.
29. Mandel MA, Dauchot PJ: Radial artery cannulation in 1000 patients. Precautions and complications. J Hand Surg 2:482-485, 1977.
30. Slogoff S, Keats AS, Arlund C: On the safety of radial artery cannulation. Anesthesiology 59:42-47, 1983.
31. Allen EV: Thromboangiitis obliterans: Methods of diagnosis of chronic obstructive lesions distal to the wrist with illustrative cases. Am J Med Sci 178:237, 1929.
32. Wilkins RG: Radial artery cannulation and ischaemic damage: A review. Anaesthesia 40:896-899, 1985.
33. Abu-Omar Y, Mussa S, Anastasiadis K, et al: Duplex ultrasonography predicts safety of radial artery harvest in the presence of an abnormal Allen test. Ann Thorac Surg 77:116-119, 2004.
34. Barbeau GR, Arsenault F, Dugas L, et al: Evaluation of the ulnopalmar arterial arches with pulse oximetry and plethysmography: Comparison with the Allen's test in 1010 patients. Am Heart J 147:489-493, 2004.
35. Tegtmeyer K, Brady G, Lai S, et al: Videos in clinical medicine. Placement of an arterial line. N Engl J Med 354:e13, 2006.
36. Chowet AL, Lopez JR, Brock-Utne JG, Jaffe RA: Wrist hyperextension leads to median nerve conduction block: Implications for intra-arterial catheter placement. Anesthesiology 100:287-291, 2004.
37. Kuo MH, Leong CP, Chang YF, Chang HW: Static wrist position associated with least median nerve compression: Sonographic evaluation. Am J Phys Med Rehabil 80:256-260, 2001.
38. Levin PD, Sheinin O, Gozal Y: Use of ultrasound guidance in the insertion of radial artery catheters. Crit Care Med 31:481-484, 2003.

39. Gerber DR, Zeifman WE, Khouli HI, et al: Comparison of wire-guided and nonwire-guided radial artery catheters. Chest 109:761-764, 1996.
40. Karacalar S, Ture H, Baris S, et al: Ulnar artery versus radial artery approach for arterial cannulation: A prospective, comparative study. J Clin Anesth 19:209-213, 2007.
41. Bazaral MG, Welch M, Golding LAR, Badhwar K: Comparison of brachial and radial arterial pressure monitoring in patients undergoing coronary artery bypass surgery. Anesthesiology 73:38-45, 1990.
42. Scheer B, Perel A, Pfeiffer UJ: Clinical review: Complications and risk factors of peripheral arterial catheters used for haemodynamic monitoring in anaesthesia and intensive care medicine. Crit Care 6:199-204, 2002.
43. Muralidhar K: Complication of femoral artery pressure monitoring. J Cardiothorac Vasc Anesth 12:128-129, 1998.
44. Rehfeldt KH, Sanders MS: Digital gangrene after radial artery catheterization in a patient with thrombocytosis. Anesth Analg 90:45-46, 2000.
45. Rose SH: Ischemic complications of radial artery cannulation: An association with a calcinosis, Raynaud's phenomenon, esophageal dysmotility, sclerodactyly, and telangiectasia variant of scleroderma. Anesthesiology 78:587-589, 1993.
46. Singleton RJ, Webb RK, Ludbrook GL, Fox AL: Problems associated with vascular access: An analysis of 2000 incident reports. Anaesth Intensive Care 21:664-669, 1993.
47. Gardner RM: Direct blood pressure measurement—dynamic response requirements. Anesthesiology 54:227-236, 1981.
48. Kleinman B: Understanding natural frequency and damping and how they relate to the measurement of blood pressure. J Clin Monit 5:137-147, 1989.
49. Kleinman B, Powell S, Kumar P, Gardner RM: The fast flush test measures the dynamic response of the entire blood pressure monitoring system. Anesthesiology 77:1215-1222, 1992.
50. O'Quin R, Marini JJ: Pulmonary artery occlusion pressure: Clinical physiology, measurement, and interpretation. Am Rev Respir Dis 128:319-326, 1983.
51. Mark JB: Technical requirements for direct blood pressure measurement. *In* Mark JB (ed): Atlas of Cardiovascular Monitoring. New York, Churchill Livingstone, 1998, pp 99-126.
52. Geddes LA: Handbook of Blood Pressure Measurement. Clifton, NJ, Humana Press, 1991.
53. Schwid HA: Frequency response evaluation of radial artery catheter-manometer systems: Sinusoidal frequency analysis versus flush method. J Clin Monit 4:181-185, 1988.
54. Sinha S, Jayaram R, Hargreaves CG: Fatal neuroglycopaenia after accidental use of a glucose 5% solution in a peripheral arterial cannula flush system. Anaesthesia 62:615-620, 2007.
55. Promonet C, Anglade D, Menaouar A, et al: Time-dependent pressure distortion in a catheter-transducer system. Anesthesiology 92:208-218, 2000.
56. Gardner RM: Accuracy and reliability of disposable pressure transducers coupled with modern pressure monitors. Crit Care Med 24:879-882, 1996.
57. Skidmore K, Chen J, Litt L: Arterial catheter pressure cable corrosion leading to artifactual diagnosis of hypotension. Anesth Analg 95:1192-1195, 2002.
58. Courtois M, Fattal PG, Kovacs SJ, et al: Anatomically and physiologically based reference level for measurement of intracardiac pressures. Circulation 92:1994-2000, 1995.
59. Seo JH, Jung CW, Bahk JH: Uppermost blood levels of the right and left atria in the supine position: Implication for measuring central venous pressure and pulmonary artery wedge pressure. Anesthesiology 107:260-263, 2007.
60. O'Rourke MF, Gallagher DE: Pulse wave analysis. J Hypertens 14:S147-S157, 1996.
61. Braunwald E, Fishman AP, Cournand A: Time relationship of dynamic events in the cardiac chambers, pulmonary artery and aorta in man. Circ Res 4:100-107, 1956.
62. Stouffer G: Arterial pressure. *In* Stouffer G (ed): Cardiovascular Hemodynamics for the Clinician. Malden, MA, Blackwell Futura, 2008, pp 57-66.
63. Franklin SS, Weber MA: Measuring hypertensive cardiovascular risk: The vascular overload concept. Am Heart J 128:793-803, 1994.
64. Frank SM, Norris EJ, Christopherson R, Beattie C: Right- and left-arm blood pressure discrepancies in vascular surgery patients. Anesthesiology 75:457-463, 1991.
65. Kinzer JB, Lichtentrhal PR, Wade LD: Loss of radial artery pressure trace during internal mammary artery dissection for coronary artery bypass graft surgery. Anesth Analg 64:1134-1136, 1985.
66. Mark JB: Arterial blood pressure. Direct vs. indirect measurement. *In* Mark JB (ed): Atlas of Cardiovascular Monitoring. New York, Churchill Livingstone, 1998, pp 81-89.
67. Dorman T, Breslow MJ, Lipsett PA, et al: Radial artery pressure monitoring underestimates central arterial pressure during vasopressor therapy in critically ill surgical patients. Crit Care Med 26:1646-1649, 1998.
68. Urzua J, Sessler D, Meneses G, et al: Thermoregulatory vasoconstriction increases the difference between femoral and radial arterial pressures. J Clin Monit 10:229-236, 1994.
69. Chauhan S, Saxena N, Mehrotra S, et al: Femoral artery pressures are more reliable than radial artery pressures on initiation of cardiopulmonary bypass. J Cardiothorac Vasc Anesth 14:274-276, 2000.
70. Hynson JM, Katz JA, Mangano DT: On the accuracy of intra-arterial pressure measurement: The pressure gradient effect. Crit Care Med 26:1623-1624, 1998.
71. McGregor M: Pulsus paradoxus. N Engl J Med 301:480-482, 1979.
72. Shabetai R, Fowler NO, Guntheroth WG: The hemodynamics of cardiac tamponade and constrictive pericarditis. Am J Cardiol 26:480-489, 1970.
73. Mark JB: Pericardial constriction and cardiac tamponade *In* Mark JB (ed): Atlas of Cardiovascular Monitoring. New York, Churchill Livingstone, 1998, pp 313-326.
74. Gelman S: Venous function and central venous pressure: A physiologic story. Anesthesiology 108:735-748, 2008.
75. Perel A: Assessing fluid responsiveness by the systolic pressure variation in mechanically ventilated patients. Anesthesiology 89:1309-1310, 1998.
76. Rooke GA: Systolic pressure variation as an indicator of hypovolemia. Curr Opin Anaesthesiol 8:511-515, 1995.
77. Marik PE: The systolic blood pressure variation as an indicator of pulmonary capillary wedge pressure in ventilated patients. Anaesth Intensive Care 21:405-408, 1993.
78. Coriat P, Vrillon M, Perel A, et al: A comparison of systolic blood pressure variations and echocardiographic estimates of end-diastolic left ventricular size in patients after aortic surgery. Anesth Analg 78:46-53, 1994.
79. Tavernier B, Makhotine O, Lebuffe G, et al: Systolic pressure variation as a guide to fluid therapy in patients with sepsis-induced hypotension. Anesthesiology 89:1313-1321, 1998.
80. Gunn SR, Pinsky MR: Implications of arterial pressure variation in patients in the intensive care unit. Curr Opin Crit Care 7:212-217, 2001.
81. Preisman S, Kogan S, Berkenstadt H, Perel H: Predicting fluid responsiveness in patients undergoing cardiac surgery: Functional haemodynamic parameters including the Respiratory Systolic Variation Test and static preload indicators. Br J Anaesth 95:746-755, 2005.
82. Perel A: Automated assessment of fluid responsiveness in mechanically ventilated patients. Anesth Analg 106:1031-1033, 2008.
83. Berkenstadt H, Margalit N, Hanani M, et al: Stroke volume variation as a predictor of fluid responsiveness in patients undergoing brain surgery. Anesth Analg 92:984-989, 2001.
84. Cannesson M, Delannoy B, Morand A, et al: Does the Pleth variability index indicate the respiratory-induced variation in the plethysmogram and arterial pressure waveforms? Anesth Analg 106:1189-1194, 2008.
85. Cannesson M, Slieker J, Desebbe O, et al: The ability of a novel algorithm for automatic estimation of the respiratory variations in arterial pulse pressure to monitor fluid responsiveness in the operating room. Anesth Analg 106:1195-1200, 2008.
86. Auler JO Jr, Galas F, Hajjar L, et al: Online monitoring of pulse pressure variation to guide fluid therapy after cardiac surgery. Anesth Analg 106:1031-1033, 2008.
87. McGee SR: Physical examination of venous pressure: A critical review. Am Heart J 136:10-18, 1998.
88. Cook DJ: Clinical assessment of central venous pressure in the critically ill. Am J Med Sci 299:175-178, 1990.
89. Gravenstein N, Blackshear RH: In vitro evaluation of relative perforating potential of central venous catheters: Comparison of materials, selected models, number of lumens, and angles of incidence to simulated membrane. J Clin Monit 7:1-6, 1991.
90. Fisher KL, Leung AN: Radiographic appearance of central venous catheters. AJR Am J Roentgenol 166:329-337, 1996.
91. Graham AS, Ozment C, Tegtmeyer K, et al: Videos in clinical medicine. Central venous catheterization. N Engl J Med 356(21):e21, 2007.
92. Peres PW: Positioning central venous catheters—a prospective study. Anaesth Intensive Care 18:536-539, 1990.
93. Bailey PL, Glance LG, Eaton MP, et al: A survey of the use of ultrasound during central venous catheterization. Anesth Analg 104:491-497, 2007.
94. Sanford TJ: Internal jugular vein cannulation versus subclavian vein cannulation. An anesthesiologist's view: The right internal jugular vein. J Clin Monit 1:58-61, 1985.
95. English IC, Frew RM, Pigott JF, Zaki M: Percutaneous catheterisation of the internal jugular vein 1969 (classical article). Anaesthesia 50:1071-1076, 1995.
96. Oliver WC Jr, Nuttall GA, Beynen FM, et al: The incidence of artery puncture with central venous cannulation using a modified technique for detection and prevention of arterial cannulation. J Cardiothorac Vasc Anesth 11:851-855, 1997.
97. Daily PO, Griepp RB, Shumway NE: Percutaneous internal jugular vein cannulation. Arch Surg 101:534-536, 1970.
98. Sulek CA, Gravenstein N, Blackshear RH, Weiss L: Head rotation during internal jugular vein cannulaton and the risk of carotid artery puncture. Anesth Analg 82:125-128, 1996.

99. O'Grady NP, Alexander M, Dellionger EP, et al: Guidelines for prevention of intravascular catheter–related infections. Centers for Disease Control and Prevention. MMWR Recomm Rep 51(RR-10):1-29, 2002.
100. Chaiyakunapruk N, Veenstra DL, Lipsky BA, Saint S: Chlorhexidine compared with povidone-iodine solution for vascular catheter-site care: A meta-analysis. Ann Intern Med 136:792-801, 2002.
101. Civetta JM, Gabel JC, Gemer M: Internal-jugular-vein puncture with a margin of safety. Anesthesiology 36:622-623, 1972.
102. Ellison N, Jobes DR, Troianos CA: Internal jugular vein cannulation. Anesth Analg 78:198, 1994.
103. Mangar D, Turnage WS, Mohamed SA: Is the internal jugular vein cannulated during insertion or withdrawal of the needle during central venous cannulation. Anesth Analg 76:1375, 1993.
104. Jobes DR, Schwartz AJ, Greenhow DE, et al: Safer jugular vein cannulation: Recognition of arterial puncture and preferential use of the external jugular route. Anesthesiology 59:353-355, 1983.
105. Fabian JA, Jesudian MC: A simple method of improving the safety of percutaneous cannulation of the internal jugular vein. Anesth Analg 64:1032-1033, 1985.
106. Alexander R: Using continuous pressure monitoring to aid central vein cannulation. Can J Anaesth 44:99-100, 1997.
107. Royster RL, Johnston WE, Gravelee GP: Arrhythmias during venous cannulation prior to pulmonary artery catheter insertion. Anesth Analg 64:1214-1216, 1985.
108. Flowers RH 3rd, Schwenzer KJ, Kopel RF, et al: Efficacy of an attachable subcutaneous cuff for the prevention of intravascular catheter–related infection. A randomized, controlled trial. JAMA 261:878-883, 1989.
109. Zakrzewska-Bode A, Muytjens HL, Liem KD, Hoogkamp-Korstanje JA: Mupirocin resistance in coagulase-negative staphylococci, after topical prophylaxis for the reduction of colonization of central venous catheters. J Hosp Infect 31:189-193, 1995.
110. Reeves ST, Roy RC, Dorman BH, et al: The incidence of complications after the double-catheter technique for cannulation of the right internal jugular vein in a university teaching hospital. Anesth Analg 81:1073-1076, 1995.
111. Reeves ST, Baliga P, Conroy JM, et al: Avulsion of the right facial vein during double cannulation of the internal jugular vein. J Cardiothorac Vasc Anesth 9:429-430, 1995.
112. Inoue S, Ohnishi Y, Kuro M: Accidental penetration of an indwelling retrograde introducer sheath by an introducer needle during right internal jugular vein cannulation. J Cardiothorac Vasc Anesth 12:67-68, 1998.
113. Khalil KG, Parker FB, Mukherjee N, Webb WR: Thoracic duct injury. A complication of jugular vein catheterization. JAMA 221:908-909, 1972.
114. Parry G: Trendelenburg position, head elevation and a midline position optimize right internal jugular vein diameter. Can J Anaesth 51:379-381, 2004.
115. Lobato EB, Myers JA, Sulek CA, Blas ML: A randomized study of right versus left internal jugular venous cannulation in adults. Anesthesiology 89(3A):A1189, 1998.
116. Haire WD, Lieberman RP: Defining the risks of subclavian-vein catheterization. N Engl J Med 331:1769-1770, 1994.
117. Hoyt DB: Internal jugular vein cannulation versus subclavian vein cannulation. A surgeon's view: The subclavian vein. J Clin Monit 1:61-63, 1985.
118. Merrer J, De Jonghe B, Golliot R, et al: Complications of femoral and subcalvian venous catheterization in critically ill patients. A randomized controlled trial. JAMA 286:700-707, 2001.
119. Mansfield PF, Hohn DC, Fornage BD, et al: Complications and failures of subclavian-vein catheterization. N Engl J Med 331:1735-1738, 1994.
120. Blitt CD, Wright WA, Petty WC, Webster TA: Central venous catheterization via the external jugular vein: A technique employing the J-wire. JAMA 229:817-818, 1974.
121. Blitt CD, Carlson GL, Wright WA: J-wire versus straight wire for central venous system cannulation via the external jugular vein. Anesth Analg 61:536-537, 1982.
122. Schwartz AJ, Jobes DR, Levy WJ, et al: Intrathoracic vascular catheterization via the external jugular vein. Anesthesiology 56:400-402, 1982.
123. Joynt GM, Comersall CD, Buckley TA, et al: Comparison of intrathoracic and intra-abdominal measurements of central venous pressure. Lancet 347:1155-1157, 1996.
124. Ho KM, Joynt GM, Tan P: A comparison of central venous pressure and common iliac venous pressure in critically ill mechanically ventilated patients. Crit Care Med 26:461-464, 1998.
125. McGee DC, Gould MK: Preventing complications of central venous catheterization. N Engl J Med 348:1123-1133, 2003.
126. Andel H, Koller R, Andel D, et al: Central venous approach via vena axillaris in critically burned patients. Anesthesiology 89(9):B26, 1998.
127. Amar D, Melendez JA, Zhang H, et al: Correlation of peripheral venous pressure and central venous pressure in surgical patients. J Cardiothorac Vasc Anesth 15:40-43, 2001.
128. Philip JH, Philip BK: Hydrostatic and central venous pressure measurement by the IVAC 560 Infusion Pump. Med Instrum 19:232-235, 1985.
129. Ng PK, Ault MJ, Ellrodt AG, Maldonado L: Peripherally inserted central catheters in general medicine. Mayo Clin Proc 72:225-233, 1997.
130. Kellner GA, Smart JF: Percutaneous placement of catheters to monitor "central venous pressure." Anesthesiology 36:515-516, 1972.
131. Webre DR, Arens JF: Use of cephalic and basilic veins for introduction of central venous catheters. Anesthesiology 38:389-392, 1973.
132. Black IH, Blosser SA, Murray WB: Central venous pressure measurements: Peripherally inserted catheters versus centrally inserted catheters. Crit Care Med 28:3833-3836, 2000.
133. Kuiper DH: Cardiac tamponade and death in a patient receiving total parenteral nutrition. JAMA 230:877, 1974.
134. Kasten GW, Owens E, Kennedy D: Ventricular tachycardia resulting from central venous catheter tip migration due to arm position changes: Report of two cases. Anesthesiology 62:185-187, 1985.
135. Legler D, Nugent M: Doppler localization of the internal jugular vein facilitates central venous cannulation. Anesthesiology 60:481-482, 1984.
136. Wigmore TJ, Smythe JF, Hacking MB, et al: Effect of the implementation of NICE guidelines for ultrasound guidance on the complication rates associated with central venous catheter placement in patients presenting for routine surgery in a tertiary referral centre. Br J Anaesth 99:662-665, 2007.
137. Randolph AG, Cook DJ, Gonzales CA, Pribble CG: Ultrasound guidance for placement of central venous catheters: A meta-analysis of the literature. Crit Care Med 24:2053-2058, 1996.
138. Hind D, Calvert N, McWilliams R, et al: Ultrasonic locating devices for central venous cannulation: Meta-analysis. BMJ 327:361, 2003.
139. Rothschild JM: Ultrasound guidance of central vein catheterization. Evidence Report/Technology Assessment No. 43. Making Health Care Safer. A Critical Analysis of Patient Safety Practices. Agency for Healthcare Research and Quality, 2001, pp 245-253.
140. Girard TD, Schectman JM: Ultrasound guidance during central venous catheterization: A survey of use by house staff physicians. J Crit Care 20:224-229, 2005.
141. Milling TJ Jr, Rose J, Briggs WM, et al: Randomized, controlled clinical trial of point-of-care limited ultrasonography assistance of central venous cannulation: The Third Sonography Outcomes Assessment Program (SOAP-3) Trial. Crit Care Med 33:1764-1769, 2005.
142. Feller-Kopman D: Ultrasound-guided internal jugular access: A proposed standardized approach and implications for training and practice. Chest 132:302-309, 2007.
143. Gualtieri E, Deppe S, Sipperly ME, Thompson DR: Subclavian venous catheterization: Greater success rate for less experienced operators using ultrasound guidance. Crit Care Med 23:692-697, 1995.
144. Brooks AJ, Alfredson M, Pettigrew B, Morris DL: Ultrasound-guided insertion of subclavian venous access ports. Ann R Coll Surg Engl 87:25-27, 2005.
145. Pirotte T, Veyckemans F: Ultrasound-guided subclavian vein cannulation in infants and children: A novel approach. Br J Anaesth 98:509-514, 2007.
146. Caruso LJ, Gravenstein N, Layon AJ, et al: A better landmark for positioning a central venous catheter. J Clin Monit Comput 17:331-334, 2002.
147. Kapadia CB, Heard SO, Yeston NS: Delayed recognition of vascular complications caused by central venous catheters. J Clin Monit 4:267-271, 1988.
148. Albrecht K, Nave H, Breitmeier D, et al: Applied anatomy of the superior vena cava—the carina as a landmark to guide central venous catheter placement. Br J Anaesth 92:75-77, 2004.
149. Shah KB, Rao TLK, Laughlin S, El-Etr AA: A review of pulmonary artery catheterization in 6,245 patients. Anesthesiology 61:271-275, 1984.
150. Heath KJ, Woulfe J, Lownie S, et al: A devastating complication of inadvertent carotid artery puncture. Anesthesiology 89:1273-1275, 1998.
151. Brown CQ: Inadvertent prolonged cannulation of the carotid artery. Anesth Analg 61:150-152, 1982.
152. Imai M, Hanaoka Y, Kemmotsu O: Valve injury: A new complication of internal jugular vein cannulation. Anesth Analg 78:1041-1046, 1994.
153. Beilin Y, Bronheim D, Mandelbaum C: Hemothorax and subclavian artery laceration during "J" wire change of a right internal jugular vein catheter. Anesthesiology 88:1399-1400, 1998.
154. Bernard RW, Stahl WM: Mediastinal hematoma: Complication of subclavian vein catheterization. NY State J Med 74:83-86, 1974.
155. Naguib M, Farag H, Joshi RN: Bilateral hydrothorax and hydromediastinum after a subclavian line insertion. Can Anaesth Soc J 32:412-414, 1985.
156. Rudge CJ, Bewick M, McColl I: Hydrothorax after central venous catheterization. BMJ 3:23-25, 1973.
157. Fangio P, Mourgeon E, Romelaer A, et al: Aortic injury and cardiac tamponade as a complication of subclavian venous catheterization. Anesthesiology 96:1520-1522, 2002.
158. Ezri T, Szmuk P, Cohen Y, et al: Carotid artery–internal jugular vein fistula: A complication of internal jugular vein catheterization. J Cardiothorac Vasc Anesth 15:231-232, 2001.

has revolutionized the storage and processing of TEE images. Secure digital servers have replaced videotape libraries of clinical studies, thereby resulting in vastly faster access to and fidelity of stored images, and after decades of work on real-time three-dimensional (3D) imaging, it is finally a reality. Its impact on clinical practice remains to be determined, but we predict that it will simplify and speed mastery of the assessment of valvular anatomy and pathology.[4]

Practice Guidelines for Transesophageal Echocardiography

In 1992, the American Society of Echocardiography (ASE) Committee for Physician Training in Echocardiography published its guidelines for training in TEE.[5] They are based on previous recommendations for training in transthoracic echocardiography (TTE) and are directed at training for TEE in both operative and nonoperative applications. These guidelines require the trainee to attain at least an intermediate level of training in echocardiography and perform and interpret no less than 50 supervised TEE examinations. In 1996, a joint task force of the American Society of Anesthesiologists and the Society of Cardiovascular Anesthesiologists (SCA) published guidelines for perioperative TEE that defined two levels of practice: basic and advanced.[6] Anesthesiologists with basic training in perioperative TEE "should be able to use TEE for indications that lie within the customary practice of anesthesiology" and "must be able to recognize their limitations in this setting and request assistance, in a timely manner, from a physician with advanced training." Anesthesiologists with advanced training in perioperative TEE "should, in addition to the above, be able to exploit the full diagnostic potential of TEE in the perioperative period." These guidelines broadly defined the general principles for training in perioperative TEE, including cognitive and technical objectives. In addition, the guidelines delineated three categories of evidence-based indications for TEE, including category I indications, in which TEE was judged to frequently be useful in improving clinical outcomes in patients with hemodynamic instability, valvular pathology, cardiac source of emboli, and aortic pathology (Box 41-1). These indications were based on available data in 1995 when the task force wrote the guidelines. In 2007, the task force was reconvened to update the guidelines. Publication of their recommendations is expected in 2009. Based on the information available today, we anticipate a recommendation that TEE be used in all patients undergoing cardiac or thoracic aortic surgery and in other surgical patients in whom known or suspected cardiovascular pathology might result in significant hemodynamic, pulmonary, or neurologic compromise.

In 1999, a joint task force of the ASE and SCA published recommendations for a comprehensive TEE examination.[7] These recommendations described in detail the 20 TEE cross sections included in the comprehensive examination. In 2002, a joint task force of the ASE and SCA used the principles and recommendations published in the aforementioned guidelines to formulate guidelines for training in perioperative TEE, including the prerequisite medical knowledge and training, echocardiographic knowledge and skills, training components and duration, training environment and supervision, and equivalence requirements for postgraduate physicians already in practice.[8] A minimum number of cases are delineated; however, these numbers are less important than the depth and diversity of the clinical experience and the quality of training. Like previous published guidelines, these guidelines provide training recommendations for a basic and an advanced level of perioperative echocardiography. Unlike previous guidelines, these guidelines do not specify the duration of training. Instead, they emphasize the goals of training and the number and diversity of cases required to meet these goals (Table 41-1). The time required for perioperative training will vary markedly depending on the volume and diversity of the affiliated cardiac surgical program.

The American Heart Association (AHA), American College of Cardiology (ACC), ASE, and other professional organizations have issued other guidelines that involve TEE. In 2003, the AHA, ACC, and ASE published practice guidelines for the clinical use of echocardiography, including intraoperative and critical care TEE applications.[9] Their class I indications are essentially the

Box 41-1 Indications for Perioperative Transesophageal Echocardiography

Category I indications: Supported by the strongest evidence or expert opinion; TEE is frequently useful in improving clinical outcomes in these settings and is often indicated, depending on individual circumstances, for the following:

Intraoperative evaluation of acute, persistent, and life-threatening hemodynamic disturbances in which ventricular function and its determinants are uncertain and have not responded to treatment

Intraoperative use in valve repair

Intraoperative use in congenital heart surgery for most lesions requiring cardiopulmonary bypass

Intraoperative use in repair of hypertrophic obstructive cardiomyopathy

Intraoperative use for endocarditis when preoperative testing was inadequate or extension of infection to perivalvular tissue is suspected

Preoperative use in unstable patients with suspected thoracic aortic aneurysms, dissection, or disruption who need to be evaluated quickly

Intraoperative assessment of aortic valve function during repair of aortic dissections with possible aortic valve involvement

Intraoperative evaluation of pericardial window procedures

Use in the intensive care unit for unstable patients with unexplained hemodynamic disturbances, suspected valve disease, or thromboembolic problems (if other tests or monitoring techniques have not confirmed the diagnosis or patients are too unstable to undergo other tests)

Adapted with permission from Practice guidelines for perioperative transesophageal echocardiography. A report by the American Society of Anesthesiologists and the Society of Cardiovascular Anesthesiologists Task Force on Transesophageal Echocardiography. Anesthesiology 84:986-1006, 1996.

Table 41-1 Recommendations for Basic and Advanced Perioperative Echocardiography

	Basic*	Advanced*
Minimum number of examinations†	150	300
Minimum number personally performed‡	50	150
Program director qualifications	Advanced perioperative echocardiography training	Advanced perioperative echocardiography training plus at least 150 additional perioperative TEE examinations
Program qualifications	Wide variety of perioperative applications of echocardiography	Full spectrum of perioperative applications of echocardiography

*Totals for basic training may be counted toward advanced training provided that the basic training was completed in an advanced training environment.
†Complete echocardiographic examinations interpreted and reported by the trainee under appropriate supervision; may include transthoracic studies recorded by qualified individuals other than the trainee.
‡Comprehensive intraoperative transesophageal echocardiographic examinations personally performed, interpreted, and reported by the trainee under appropriate supervision.
Adapted from Cahalan MK, Abel M, Goldman M, et al: American Society of Echocardiography and Society of Cardiovascular Anesthesiologists task force guidelines for training in perioperative echocardiography. Anesth Analg 94:1384-1388, 2002.

same as those listed in Box 41-1. In 2005, the ASE published its recommendations for indications and performance guidelines for pediatric TEE, including intraoperative applications,[10] and in 2007, the ACC, ASE, and multiple other societies issued their appropriateness criteria (i.e., summary of proven indications) for TTE and TEE. However, in this publication, intraoperative applications were explicitly excluded.

Properties of Ultrasound

To noninvasively visualize structures inside the body, ultrasound machines generate an imperceptible vibration within a transducer that, when put next to tissue surfaces, vibrates the surrounding tissue (muscle, blood, fat, or bone). During vibration, particles within the tissue compress and then spread apart. This dual process is called *compression* and *rarefaction*. The sequence of compression and rarefaction is described by sine waves and is characterized in terms of wavelength, frequency, amplitude, and propagation velocity (Fig. 41-1).

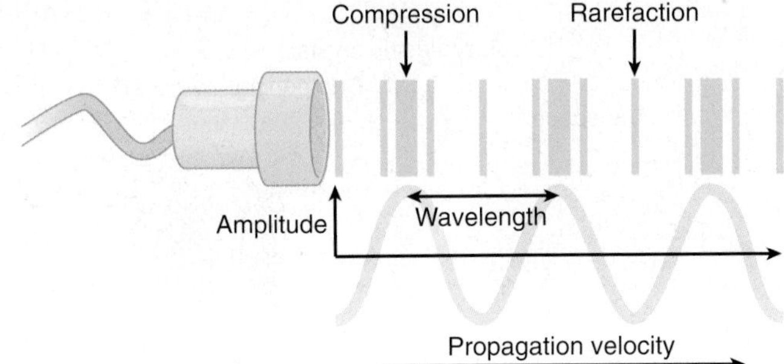

Figure 41-1 Illustration of terms used to describe transmission of ultrasound energy from a transducer into adjacent tissue. As ultrasound vibrations enter surrounding tissue, particles within the tissue compress and then spread apart (compression and rarefaction). Sine waves are used to characterize the sequence of compression and rarefaction, wavelength is the distance between two peaks of the sine wave, amplitude is a measure of tissue compression, and propagation velocity is the speed of the ultrasound wave within tissue.

Wavelength is the distance between two peaks of the sine wave. Wavelengths used in ultrasound are measured in millimeters. *Frequency* is the number of cycles that occur in 1 second. One cycle per second is defined as 1 hertz (abbreviated Hz). Ultrasound is sound with frequencies higher than the audible range for humans, or greater than 20,000 cycles per second (20 kHz). Frequencies typically used for sonographic imaging are 2 to 10 mega hertz (MHz). Wavelength is inversely related to frequency.

Amplitude is a measure of tissue compression. Amplitude represents the *loudness* of an ultrasound wave. Amplitude can vary over a large range and is described by decibels (dB). Decibels is a logarithmic transformation that allows large amplitudes to be presented next to small amplitudes (i.e., 1000 and 0.001) on the same display. A rule of thumb is that a 6-dB change is equivalent to doubling or halving of the amplitude.

Propagation velocity describes the speed of an ultrasound wave traveling through tissue. In blood it is 1540 m/sec. The relationship between propagation velocity, frequency, and wavelength is described by Equation 1:

$$\text{Propagation velocity} = \text{Frequency} \times \text{Wavelength} \quad (1)$$

Assuming that propagation velocity is constant, the wavelength for any frequency can be calculated (Table 41-2).

Transducers, typically made of quartz or titanate ceramic, use crystals that exhibit the piezoelectric effect. With electricity,

Table 41-2 Relationship Among Frequency, Wavelength, and Depth of Penetration

Frequency	Wavelength	Depth of Penetration (200-400 × Wavelength)	Approximate Resolution (2 × Wavelength)
3.5 MHz	0.44 mm	9-18 cm	0.9 mm
5.0 MHz	0.31 mm	6-12 cm	0.6 mm
6.0 MHz	0.26 mm	5-10 cm	0.5 mm
7.5 MHz	0.21 mm	4-8 cm	0.4 mm

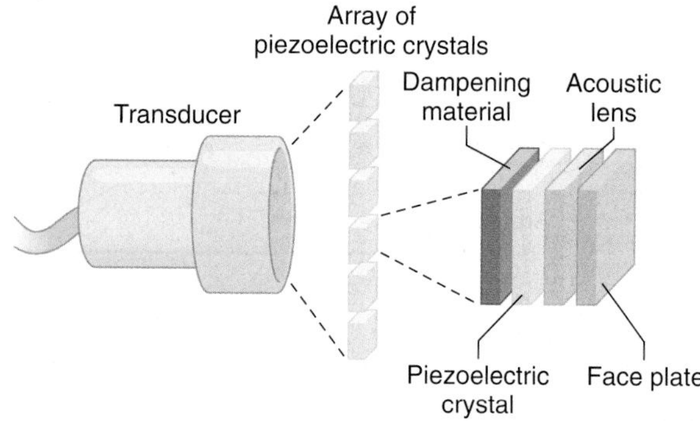

Figure 41-2 Illustration of an array of piezoelectric crystals contained within an ultrasound transducer. When pulsed with alternating current, piezoelectric crystals "ring" much like a bell. The crystal continues to vibrate after an electrical pulse has ended. To achieve a crisper pulse, a backing material is applied to the crystal to *dampen* the ring after the pulse has ended. To optimize transmission from the crystal into tissue, an *acoustic lens* focuses the ultrasound beam and an *impedance-matching face plate* improves conductance of ultrasound from the transducer into tissue.

the crystal vibrates and emits ultrasound. The reverse also holds: When ultrasound waves strike a piezoelectric crystal and make it vibrate, the crystal generates electricity. Thus, the same crystals can serve as emitters and receivers of ultrasound. The *frequency* of vibration is determined by the thickness of the piezoelectric crystal. To refine and control the emitted ultrasound beam, several layers of material are placed adjacent to the crystal (Fig. 41-2).

Transducer Frequency, Image Resolution, and Depth of Penetration

Echocardiography uses ultrasound waves with frequencies of 2.5 to 7.5 million cycles/sec (MHz). Important relationships between transducer frequency, depth, and resolution include (1) the slower the frequency, the greater the depth of penetration at the expense of resolution, and (2) the faster the frequency, the greater the resolution at the expense of depth of penetration (Table 41-3). Frequencies greater than 7.5 MHz are not used because they produce wavelengths too short for adequate penetration into tissue (an exception would be epiaortic scanning). Penetration is limited to about 200 to 400 times the wavelength. Resolution is limited to about twice the wavelength.

Image resolution is characterized in terms of axial, elevational, lateral, and temporal resolution. Axial resolution is resolution along the length of an ultrasound beam. It is a function of transducer frequency and pulse width. Long wavelengths (slow frequency) have deeper tissue penetration but are unable to resolve objects that are close together along the ultrasound beam scan line. Short wavelengths (fast frequency) do the opposite. Similarly, short-duration pulses improve and long pulses worsen axial resolution. Elevational resolution refers to the thickness of the ultrasound image: typically 8 to 10 mm.

Lateral resolution is a function of ultrasound beam formation. The initial segment (near field) of an ultrasound beam is columnar, and the length is dependent on transducer width and wavelength. Beyond the near field, the beam diverges (far field). Divergence is also a function of transducer frequency. As the frequency rises, the near field gets longer and the divergence angle decreases. For example, for transducer frequencies of 3.5 and 7 MHz, the divergence angles are 26 and 12 degrees, respectively. As the transducer width gets smaller, the angle of divergence gets larger. The lack of lateral resolution at greater depths accounts for blurring of the image in the far field (Fig. 41-3A and B).

Another descriptor of lateral resolution is the grating lobe. A grating lobe is a diverging ultrasound beam that emerges from the transducer along with the main ultrasound beam. The angle of the diverging grating lobe is determined by the spacing between the crystals in a transducer array. At angles at which the path length of an ultrasound wave between the two adjacent transducer crystals differs by one wavelength, a grating lobe is formed (Fig. 41-4).

An example of a grating lobe artifact is a properly positioned pulmonary artery catheter that appears to go through the aorta. The artifact appears as an echo-dense archlike object that traverses structures within the heart and is at equal distance from the transducer throughout the image. In this example, a diverging ultrasound beam from a grating lobe is reflected back to the transducer. The ultrasound machine cannot differentiate between reflected ultrasound from the main beam and the grating lobe beam.

Temporal resolution is the ability to accurately locate moving structures at a particular instant in time. The more images displayed per second (frame rate), the better the temporal resolution. A typical frame has 128 lines in a 90-degree 2D image. If the depth is set to 20 cm, the time required for sampling one line is 260 μsec. To scan all 128 lines requires 33 msec. In 1 second, the sector is scanned 30 times. To image moving structures inside the heart, a frame rate of at least 30 frames/sec is required. Decreasing

Table 41-3 Clinical Features of Pulsed Wave, Continuous Wave, and Color Flow Doppler

Doppler Technique	Advantages	Disadvantages	Clinical Uses
Pulsed wave	Measures blood flow velocities at selected areas of interest 3-5 mm wide along the ultrasound scan line	Cannot measure fast blood flow velocities (>1 m/sec) because of aliasing	To measure blood flow velocities through the pulmonary veins and mitral valve and in low-flow areas within the heart
Continuous wave	Detects blood flow velocities up to 7 m/sec (not subject to the Nyquist limit)	Cannot identify location of the peak velocity along the ultrasound scan line	To measure blood flow velocities through the aorta, aortic valve, stenotic valve lesions, and regurgitant valvular jets
Color flow	Presents the spatial relationships between structure and blood flow	Like pulsed wave Doppler, cannot measure fast blood flow velocities because of aliasing	To enhance recognition of valvular abnormalities, aortic dissections, and intracardiac shunts

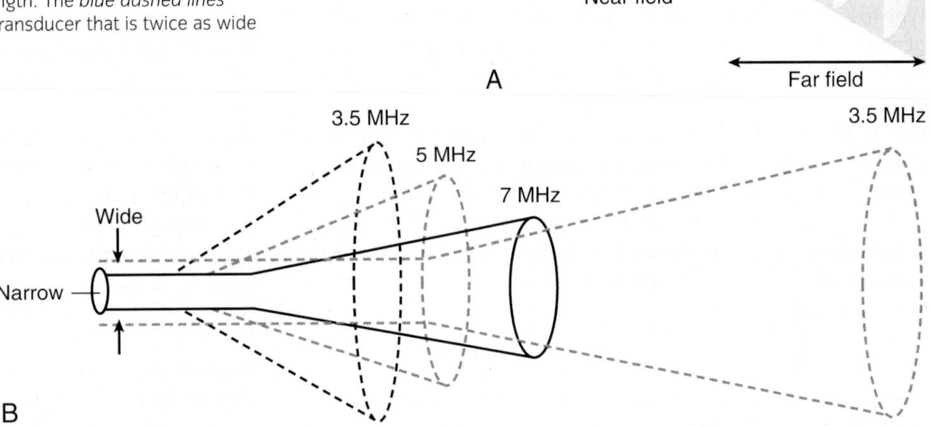

Figure 41-3 **A,** Near- and far-field beam formation. The near field is the columnar portion of the beam and the far field is the diverging segment of the beam. Theta (Θ) represents the angle of divergence. Structures within the near field (target 1) are imaged with crisp lateral resolution, whereas structures in the far field (target 2) are imaged with blurred lateral resolution. **B,** Relationship between near-field length and transducer frequency and width. The length of the near field is a function of transducer width and frequency. As frequency increases, the near field lengthens. The angle of divergence is also a function of transducer frequency. With increasing transducer frequency, the angle of divergence decreases. The *black dashed*, *dotted*, and *solid lines* represent beam divergence for a 3.5-, 5.0-, and 7.0-MHz transducer, respectively. With wider transducers, the near field increases in length. The *blue dashed lines* represent the near and far fields for a 3.5-MHz transducer that is twice as wide as the narrow transducer.

image depth will improve temporal resolution. Ultrasound machines allow the operator to zoom in on a region of interest within the 2D display. This function redistributes the number of scan lines used to generate a full 2D image into a smaller region of interest and thereby improve temporal resolution.

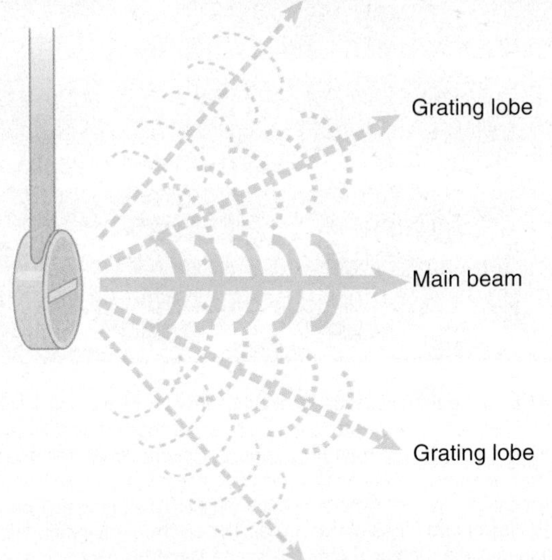

Figure 41-4 The main ultrasound beam (*solid line*) emitted from a transducer is accompanied by a series of grating lobes (*dotted lines*). The grating lobes are a phenomenon of beam formation that is a function of the array of piezoelectric crystals within the transducer. At certain angles from the main beam, the ultrasound wave from each crystal within the array is exactly one wavelength behind the wavelength from the adjacent crystal. This generates a grating lobe. The clinical implications of grating lobes are that highly echogenic objects such as a Swan-Ganz catheter or a mitral valve prosthesis can "appear" to be locations within the heart (i.e., the aorta) that are incorrect.

As ultrasound waves penetrate tissue, signal strength is attenuated. *Attenuation* is a function of tissue *absorption* (ultrasound energy converted to heat), *divergence* of ultrasound energy as it moves away from the transducer, *reflection*, and *scattering* (Fig. 41-5). Absorption is dependent on tissue type. For example, air absorbs more ultrasound energy than bone does, but bone absorbs more than blood or water does. A term used to describe absorption is half-power distance, which is the distance required

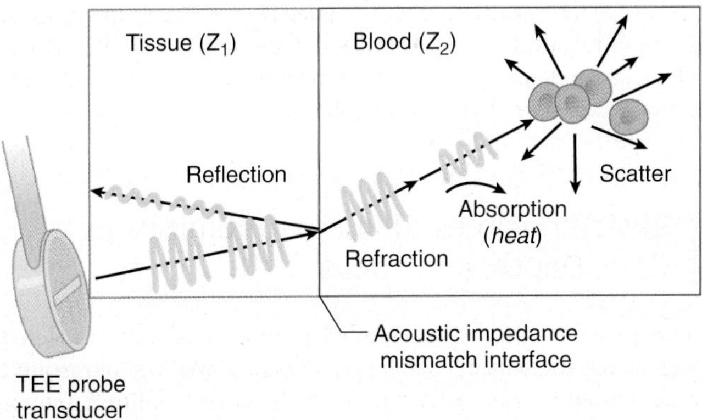

Figure 41-5 Diagram of specular reflection, refraction, absorption, scatter, and acoustic impedance. As ultrasound waves strike an interface between two different tissue types, some of it is reflected and the remainder passes through. The reflected ultrasound wave has a trajectory angle equal to the incident angle. Refraction refers to deflection of the ultrasound beam as it travels from one tissue type to another. Scattering occurs when an ultrasound wave strikes a structure that is less than one wavelength in lateral dimension (a red blood cell). Absorption represents the amount of ultrasound energy that dissipates as heat. Acoustic impedance refers to the resistance that an ultrasound wave meets when traveling though tissue. Acoustic impedance (Z) is defined as the product of tissue density and propagation velocity.

to decrease the ultrasound energy by 50%. The half-power distances for air, bone, blood, and water are 0.08, 0.8, 15, and 380 cm, respectively.

As ultrasound waves strike an interface between two different tissue types, some of it is reflected and the remainder passes through. Just as light is reflected from a mirror, the reflected ultrasound wave has a trajectory angle equal to the incident angle. The amplitude of reflected ultrasound waves is decreased by 40 to 60 dB (100- to 1000-fold). Ultrasound waves that pass through to adjacent tissue are subject to *refraction*. Refraction refers to deflection of the ultrasound beam as it travels from one tissue type to another. An example of refraction is distortion of an image of an object when partially submerged in a fish tank or swimming pool. Refraction can bend ultrasound beams and thus make objects appear in locations where they do not exist. Scattering occurs when an ultrasound wave strikes a structure that is less than one wavelength in lateral dimension (a red blood cell). The scattered ultrasound energy is radiated in all directions.

Acoustic impedance refers to the resistance that an ultrasound wave meets when traveling though tissue. It is a function of tissue density and is defined by Equation 2:

$$\text{Acoustic impedance (Z)} = \text{Tissue density} \times \text{Propagation velocity} \quad (2)$$

The greater the tissue density, the faster the ultrasound beam moves through the tissue. For example, ultrasound waves are much slower in air (330 m/sec), faster in blood (1540 m/sec), and very fast in bone (4080 m/sec). The extent of ultrasound beam reflection is a function of the difference in acoustic impedance between two adjacent tissues. The larger the difference in acoustic impedance, the more ultrasound energy will be reflected. Bone–soft tissue and air–soft tissue interfaces reflect most of the ultrasound beam. Imaging structures deep to these interfaces is difficult.

Mismatches in acoustic impedance and attenuation are important to consider in imaging the heart with TEE. For example, the upper aortic arch is difficult to visualize from the esophagus because of interposition of the air-filled trachea. In addition, most of the ultrasound energy that does make it to the trachea-tissue interface is reflected as a result of the large difference in acoustic impedance between air and tissue.

Basic Principles of Image Optimization: Gain, Depth, and Focus

Gain is used to amplify low-amplitude ultrasound waves reflected back to the transducer. Gain represents how well the ultrasound system *listens*. It can be used to offset the large-amplitude signals returned from proximal structures from the low-amplitude signals returned from distant structures. Many ultrasound machines have a series of sliding controls called *time gain compensation* controls that allow the operator to adjust the gain at a given depth. One temptation when structures are not readily visualized in the brightly lit operating room is to turn up the gain. Although gain increases structure brightness, it comes at the cost of amplifying background noise. A better approach is to brighten the display screen settings and keep gain at normal settings.

In echocardiography, the crystals emit very short pulses of ultrasound (0.5 to 3 μsec containing two wavelengths) and receive or "listen" for the reflected ultrasound for 250 to 500 μsec. The *pulse repetition frequency* (PRF) is the number of pulses that leave and return to the transducer in a single second. As image depth is increased, the time required to reach the target depth and return increases. Thus, the number of cycles that can be completed within 1 second is reduced. The opposite also holds: as imaging depth decreases, PRF increases. PRF is also described in hertz; it is audible and ranges from 1 to 10 kHz.

Early echocardiography displays used this principle to map out the depth of structures within the heart. The first echocardiograms, "motion" or "M-mode" studies, were one-dimensional views of cardiac structures produced by single-crystal transducers with the results traced on moving photosensitive paper. Today, M-mode echocardiography is used principally to view rapidly moving structures, such as valve leaflets, because M-mode transducers can produce up to 1800 images/sec (Fig. 41-6). However, M-mode images reveal only a small portion of the heart at one time, thus making orientation and interpretation of spatial relationships difficult.

To generate 2D images, ultrasound machines were configured to sequentially redirect the beam over an area (sector) of interest. Transducers contain a row of piezoelectric crystals (a linear array). By introducing a small delay in the firing of adjacent crystals in the array (a phased array), the ultrasound machine is able to steer the resultant ultrasound beam. Hence, by varying the time delay between crystals, ultrasound machines are able to steer

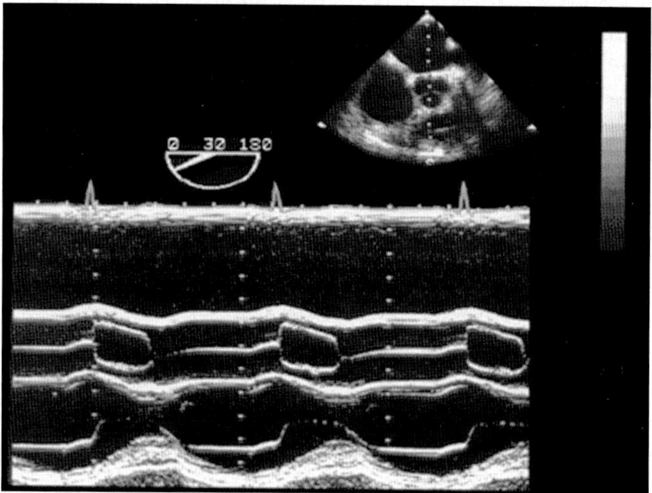

Figure 41-6 M-mode transesophageal echocardiogram of a normal aortic valve. For reference, a single frame (stop action) of the two-dimensional cross section is shown at the top right of the figure. The *dotted vertical line* through the two-dimensional echocardiogram depicts the single line of sampling provided by the M-mode echocardiogram over time (the horizontal axis for the lower two thirds of the figure). The electrocardiogram defines systole and diastole. Note in the middle of the M-mode image the three tilted *rectangles* connected by the slightly *undulating line*. These rectangles and lines are formed by the motion of the leaflets of the aortic valve as they open and close during the cardiac cycles shown. From top to bottom in this M-mode echocardiogram, the structures indicated by the *white lines* are the posterior wall of the left atrium (just under the electrocardiogram), the posterior wall of the aortic annulus, the aortic valve (as described above), the anterior wall of the aortic annulus, a pulmonary artery catheter, and the myocardium of the right ventricular outflow tract. *(Reproduced with permission from Cahalan MK: Intraoperative Transesophageal Echocardiography. An Interactive Text and Atlas. New York, Churchill Livingstone, 1997.)*

the beam through a sector of interest (typically a 90-degree sector). Although 2D techniques produce only about 30 images/sec, definition in two dimensions provides an enormous advantage in recognizing anatomic and pathologic landmarks (Fig. 41-7). Images are displayed in "real time" on a monitor screen and digitally recorded for later review. In a similar fashion to steering the ultrasound beam, the *focal depth* of an ultrasound beam can be adjusted by triggering the piezoelectric crystals to concentrate the ultrasound beam at a desired depth (Fig. 41-8). The focal depth is typically set at or just below the structure of interest in a 2D image.

The advance from 2D to real-time 3D echocardiography has proved difficult. The time needed to acquire the requisite 2D images, the computing challenge of collating them into 3D images, and the display challenge of depicting 3D images on a 2D video screen all contributed to the difficulty. Matrix-array transducers solved the image acquisition problem. Typically, they contain over 3000 imaging elements and electronically rotate the 2D ultrasound beam through 180 degrees in milliseconds to acquire the requisite 2D images in a fraction of the time possible with mechanically rotated multiplane transducers. Computing power and commercially patented display algorithms solved the other problems (Fig. 41-9).[11]

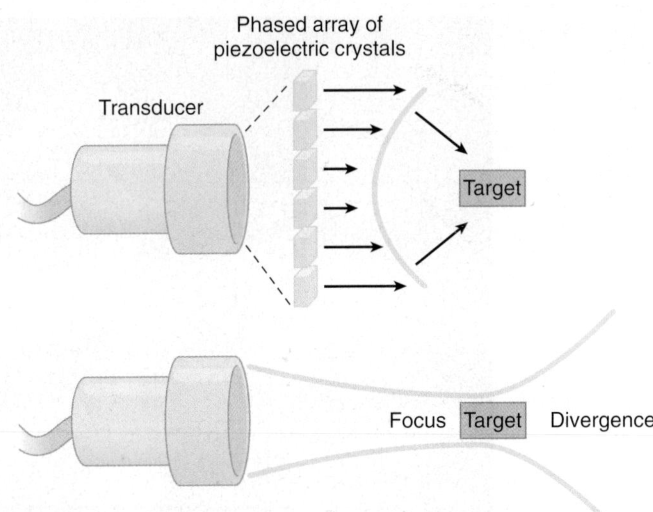

Figure 41-8 Schematic illustration of phasing the start of an array of piezoelectric crystals to focus an ultrasound beam. Crystals are sequentially fired from the outer edge to the middle of the array. The resultant concave wave converges at a point some distance from the transducer. The focal distance from the transducer is a function of the time delay between firing crystals from the edge to the middle of the array.

Integration of Flow and Structure

Christian Doppler, a physicist, studied a band playing a specific pitch on a moving train. He observed a change in pitch as the train passed by. In this experiment he characterized the relationship between train velocity and frequency (pitch), known as the Doppler shift. When applied to echocardiography, Doppler shift provides a significant enhancement to 2D imaging. With Doppler, blood flow velocity can be measured as blood flows through structures inside the heart. The ultrasound that bounces off moving red blood cells is reflected back to the transducer at a slightly different frequency than that emitted from the transducer. The shift in frequency allows the ultrasound machine to estimate blood flow velocity and direction of flow. Blood flow toward a transducer increases the frequency and vice versa with blood flowing away from the transducer. Doppler shifts are between 20 and 2000 Hz (within the audible range). Many ultrasound machines allow the user, if interested, to listen to the Doppler shift.

One important feature of assessing Doppler shift is the intercept angle (i.e., θ). To get the most accurate estimate of red blood cell speed, Doppler shift should be measured with an ultrasound beam that travels in the direction of blood flow. As the intercept angle deviates from zero degrees, blood flow will be underestimated. To compensate for this, the cosine of θ is used to account for the sampling angle. Most ultrasound machines

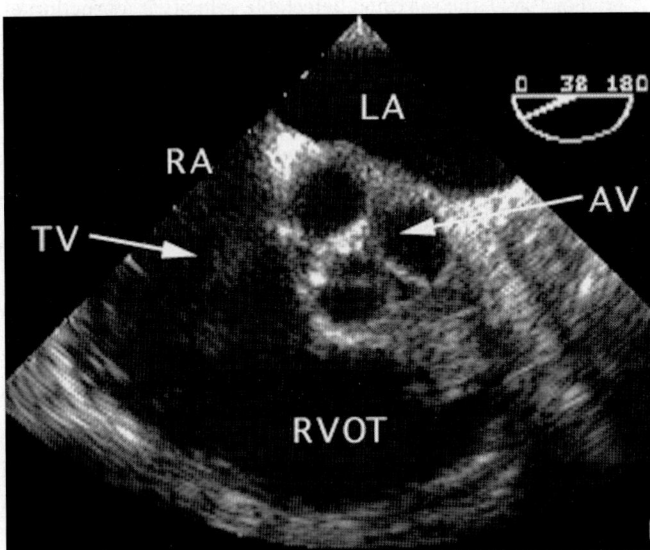

Figure 41-7 Stop-action short-axis two-dimensional cross section of a normal aortic valve (AV). This midesophageal view of the AV reveals the morphology of the three cusps of this normal valve. LA, left atrium; RA, right atrium; RVOT, right ventricular outflow tract; TV, tricuspid valve. *(Reproduced with permission from Cahalan MK: Intraoperative Transesophageal Echocardiography. An Interactive Text and Atlas. New York, Churchill Livingstone, 1997.)*

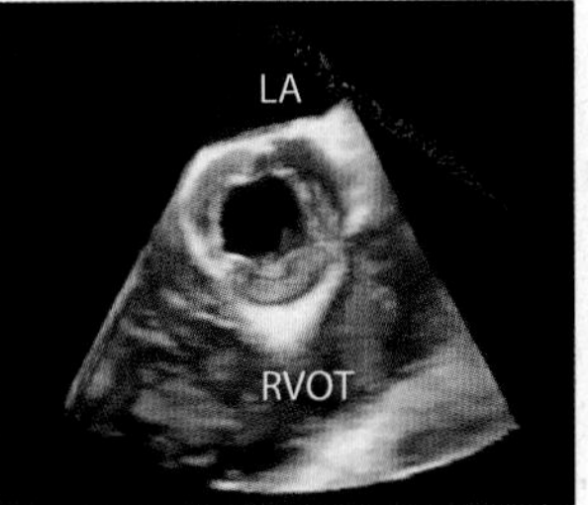

Figure 41-9 Stop-action image of a short-axis three-dimensional cross section of a normal aortic valve during systole. The partially open leaflets of aortic valve are seen in the center of the figure. Shadowing and color variation are used to depict the actual three-dimensional contours and shape of the valve and surrounding structures. In stop-action mode, these techniques are not as effective as when the real-time images are displayed. LA, left atrium; RVOT, right ventricular outflow tract.

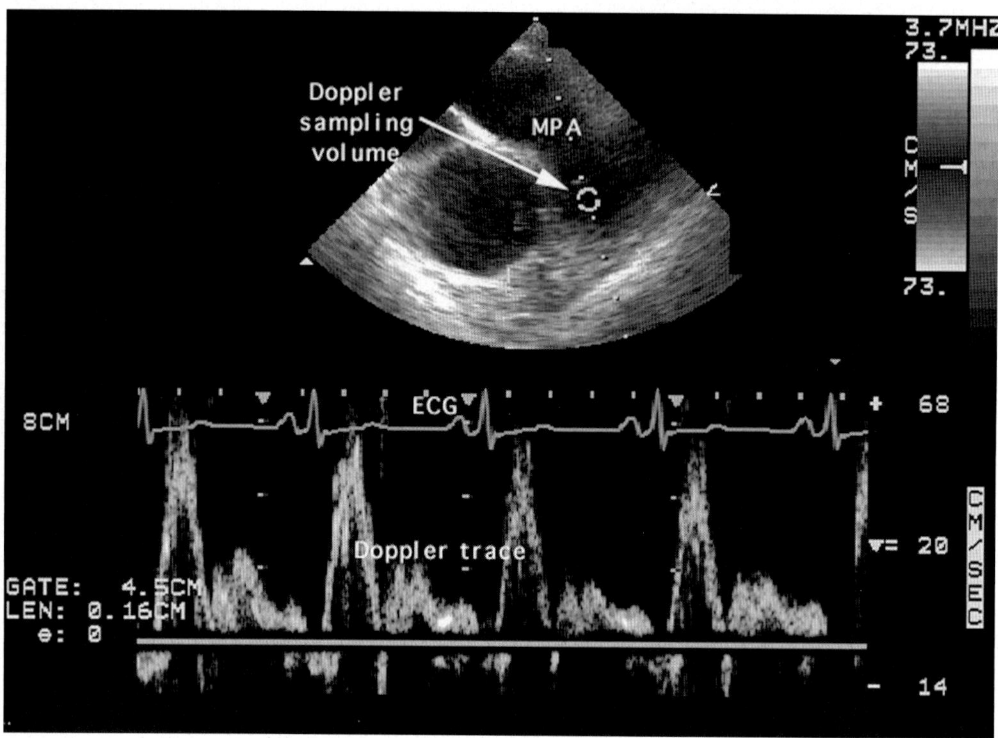

Figure 41-10 Pulsed wave Doppler echocardiogram of the main pulmonary artery (MPA). At the top of the echocardiogram is a still-frame image of the two-dimensional cross section used to position the Doppler sampling volume (*broken circle* at point of *white arrow*). On the bottom two thirds of the echocardiogram is the display in white of the instantaneous blood flow velocities (vertical axis) versus time (horizontal axis) occurring in that sample volume. The electrocardiogram (ECG) provides timing, and the *bold horizontal line* is the baseline (zero flow) for the flow velocities. Flow velocities above this line are positive (i.e., toward the transducer) to a maximum of 68 cm/sec. Flow below this line is negative (i.e., away from the transducer) to a maximum of –14 cm/sec. *(Reproduced with permission from Cahalan MK: Intraoperative Transesophageal Echocardiography. An Interactive Text and Atlas. New York, Churchill Livingstone, 1997.)*

ignore the cosine term (assume that $\theta = 0$ and cosine $\theta = 1$). At angles of 20, 30, and 60 degrees, Doppler shift will underestimate the velocity by 6%, 13%, and 50%, respectively. An intercept angle of up to 30 degrees is usually acceptable.

Doppler shifts are presented in three ways: pulsed wave Doppler (PWD), continuous wave Doppler (CWD), and color flow Doppler (CFD). The clinical features of each are presented in Table 41-3. With PWD, a small sampling volume (cursor) is placed in an area of interest within a 2D image. The transducer generates a pulse of ultrasound and then switches to the receive mode and awaits the arrival of a reflected portion of the ultrasound pulse from the sampling area (Fig. 41-10). The ultrasound machine then measures the frequency shift (or Doppler shift) to estimate the speed of blood cells in the sample volume.

One limitation of PWD is that it may be too slow to capture the velocity of fast-moving blood cells. This phenomenon is known as *aliasing*. An example of aliasing is when one watches the spokes on a wagon wheel in a western movie. As velocity increases, the movie camera detects an increase in rotational velocity of the wheel up to a point, and then the wheel appears to start spinning backward. As rotational velocity increases beyond the movie camera's sample rate, the wheel appears to be slowing down even though in reality it is speeding up.

The limit at which the sampling rate fails to accurately capture the true velocity is called the *Nyquist limit*. The sampling frequency, in this example the movie camera's sampling rate, must be at least twice the speed of the rotational velocity of the wagon wheel. With PWD, if the velocity of blood flow exceeds the Nyquist limit for the PRF (defined as PRF/2), blood flow will appear to reverse direction (Fig. 41-11).

For PWD, the maximal detectable velocity is a function of depth and transducer frequency. For depth, the farther the ultrasound pulse has to travel, the slower the maximal detectable velocity. For transducer frequency, the faster the frequency, the slower the maximal detectable velocity. To minimize aliasing with PWD, the slowest transducer setting is used. Aliasing of PWD occurs at blood flow velocities greater than 0.8 to 1.0 m/sec. Normal flow within the heart may reach 1.4 m/sec and pathologic flow up to 6 m/sec. To measure such velocities, CWD is needed.

CWD uses two sets of separate crystals: one to continuously emit ultrasound and one to continuously receive it. CWD has an infinite PRF, which eliminates the problem of aliasing (Fig. 41-12). However, this infinite pulse repetition rate allows insufficient time for the first pulse to return to the transducer before the next is emitted. Consequently, the ultrasound machine cannot precisely define the location of the moving blood cells.

CFD is based on PWD and uses multiple sample volumes along a scan line. The operator selects an area of interest ("color sector"). Scan lines are sequentially scanned through this sector. Blood flow velocity measurements are taken at several points along each scan line. A color code is used to depict flow toward (red) and away (blue) from the transducer; lighter and darker shades of red and blue, respectively, denote relatively faster and slower velocities. Continuous color maps of flow are superimposed on gray-scale cross-sectional echocardiograms. CFD has the same limitations as described previously for PWD. The

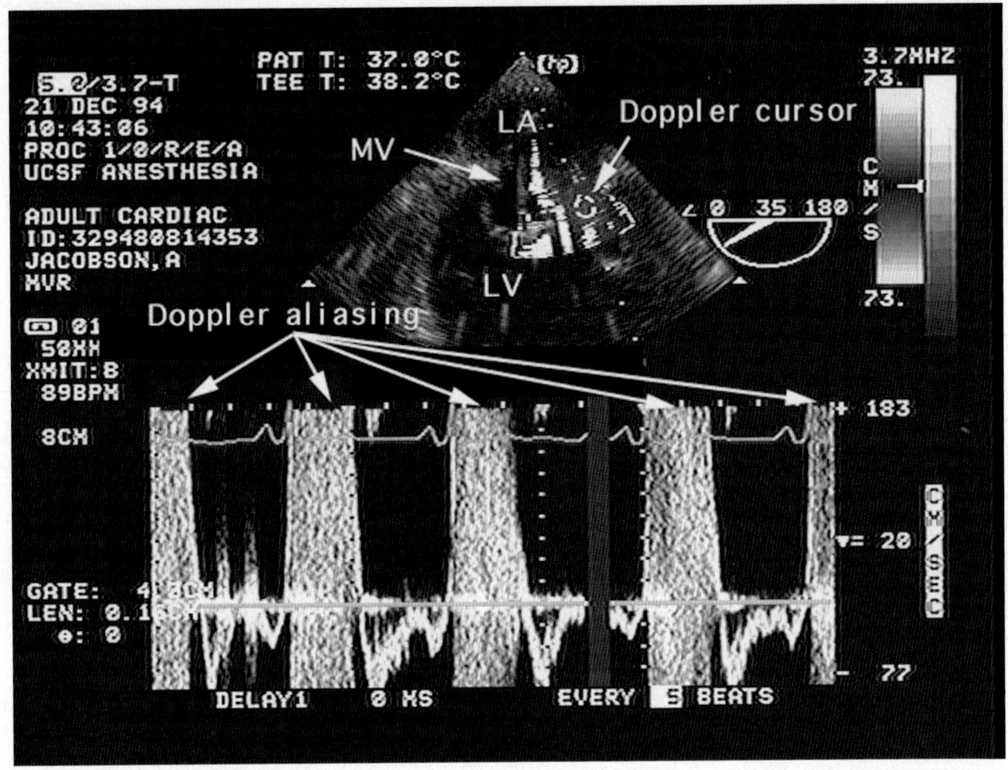

Figure 41-11 Pulsed wave Doppler (PWD) echocardiogram with aliasing at high velocities. PWD measurement of blood flow velocities in a mitral valve (MV) orifice during four cardiac cycles is shown. At the top of the figure is a still-frame image of the two-dimensional cross section used to position the Doppler sampling volume (indicated by the Doppler cursor–labeled *arrow*). On the bottom two thirds of the figure is the display in white of the instantaneous blood flow velocities (vertical axis) versus time (horizontal axis) occurring in that sample volume. The electrocardiogram provides timing, and the *bold horizontal line* is the baseline (zero flow) for the flow velocities. Flow velocities above this line are positive (i.e., toward the transducer) to a maximum of 183 cm/sec. Flow velocities below this line are negative (i.e., away from the transducer) to a maximum of −77 cm/sec. This tracing documents significant mitral regurgitation (the positive systolic velocities) but does not measure the peak velocity of regurgitant flow because it is beyond the Nyquist limit—the systolic velocities off the top of the scale are said to alias; that is, they go off scale and wrap around into the domain of negative velocities. LA, left atrium; LV, left ventricle. *(Reproduced with permission from Cahalan MK: Intraoperative Transesophageal Echocardiography. An Interactive Text and Atlas. New York, Churchill Livingstone, 1997.)*

maximal blood velocity that can be detected with CFD is a function of sector depth and PRF. PRF is considerably longer with CFD because of the numerous series of samples taken throughout the sector of interest, so the Nyquist limit is typically lower than with PWD.

Two aliasing patterns are easily recognized. The first is "normal" aliasing, in which the area of apparent flow reversal forms one or more broad, relatively homogeneous color surfaces (Fig. 41-13). Blood flow velocities within a normal heart often produce this type of aliasing because they exceed the Nyquist limit for color Doppler (0.6 to 0.8 m/sec). The second type of aliasing results from disturbed or turbulent flow within the heart (e.g., mitral regurgitation) and is never normal (Fig. 41-14). When the ultrasound machine detects two different velocities within the same small sample volume (as a result of disturbed flow), it displays a mixture, or mosaic, of colors. In most cardiovascular abnormalities these mosaics form jetlike configurations and are called "color jets." Minimizing the color sector area or reducing the distance between the transducer and the sector (or both) increases the overall PRF and thus allows an increase in the maximal measurable flow velocity before aliasing occurs. When evaluating color jets caused by valvular regurgitation, jet size is affected markedly by the Nyquist limit and gain settings. To facilitate consistent interpretation, the ASE recommends using a Nyquist limit (aliasing velocity) of 50 to 60 cm/sec and a color gain that just eliminates random color speckle from nonmoving regions.[12]

Tissue Doppler

Tissue Doppler imaging is a relatively new use of PWD technology adapted to measure myocardial velocity instead of blood flow velocity.[13] During normal LV contraction, the mitral annulus descends toward the apex of the heart. Tissue Doppler imaging measures the velocity of this descent (S_m), and S_m correlates with traditional measures of LV function, including ejection fraction and the rate of rise in LV systolic pressure (dP/dt).[14,15] In addition, S_m decreases in the presence of myocardial ischemia and responds as expected with changes in inotropy.[16,17] The four-chamber cross-sectional view is best for measuring S_m; the sampling volume is placed at the lateral insertion point of the mitral valve into the left ventricle and the cross section is aligned so that the sampling cursor is directly parallel to the motion of the annulus. S_m is an easy and reproducible measurement. However, like fractional area change and fractional shortening, it should be interpreted with caution when preload changes. Ama and associates tested its load dependence in 42 hemodynamically stable patients with normal

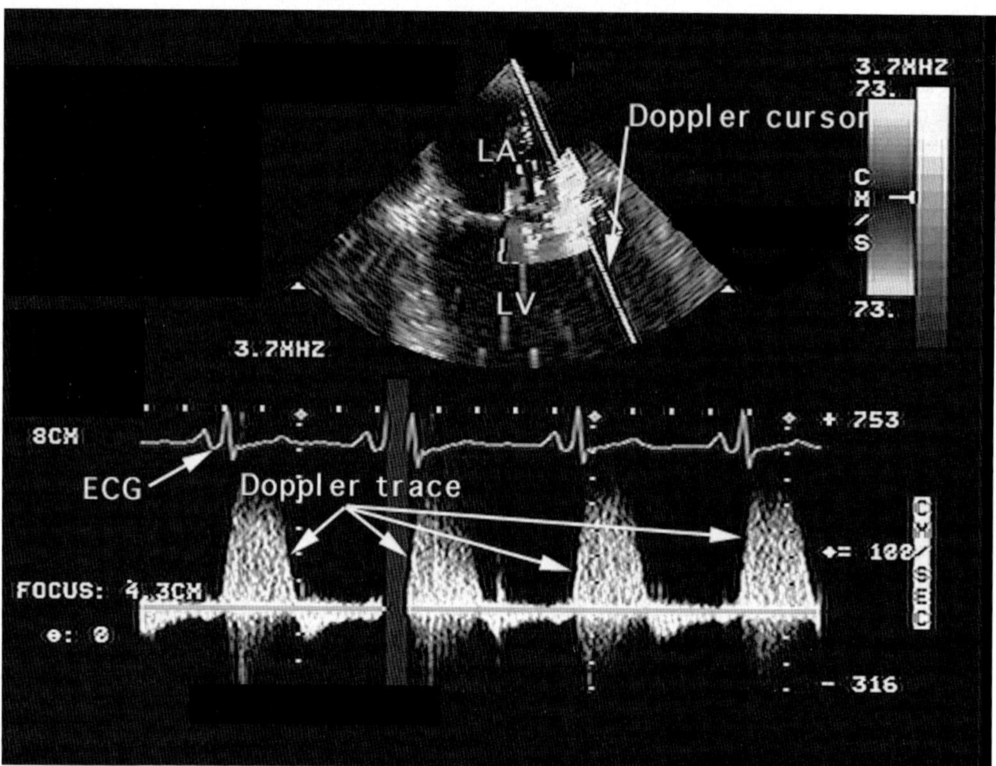

Figure 41-12 Continuous wave Doppler (CWD) measures high-velocity flow without aliasing. CWD measurement of blood flow velocities in a mitral valve orifice during four cardiac cycles is shown. At the top of the figure is a still-frame image of the two-dimensional cross section used to position the Doppler sampling cursor (the *diagonal white line*). On the bottom two thirds of the figure is the display in white of all the instantaneous blood flow velocities (vertical axis) versus time (horizontal axis) occurring anywhere along that cursor. The electrocardiogram (ECG) provides timing, and the *bold horizontal line* is the baseline (zero flow) for the flow velocities. Flow velocities above this line are positive (i.e., toward the transducer) to a maximum of 753 cm/sec. Flow velocities below this line are negative (i.e., away from the transducer) to a maximum of –316 cm/sec. This tracing documents significant mitral regurgitation (the positive systolic velocities) with a peak blood flow velocity of approximately 5 m/sec (each *white dot* on the vertical axis equals 100 cm/sec or 1 m/sec). LA, left atrium; LV, left ventricle. *(Reproduced with permission from Cahalan MK: Intraoperative Transesophageal Echocardiography. An Interactive Text and Atlas. New York, Churchill Livingstone, 1997.)*

segmental LV function after coronary surgery. S_m did not change significantly in response to a 20% increase or decrease in mean arterial pressure induced by phenylephrine or nitroglycerin. However, it increased significantly when preload was augmented by rapid infusion of colloid.[18] In summary, S_m is less dependent on afterload than fractional area change and fractional shortening are but, like these other two measures, remains critically dependent on preload. The few measures of LV function that appear to be independent of both preload and afterload (e.g., preload-recruitable stroke work) are not practical for clinical use.

Equipment Design and Operation

TEE probes are a marvel of engineering: a miniaturized echocardiographic transducer (about 40 mm long, 13 mm wide, and 11 mm thick) mounted on the tip of a gastroscope. Typically, the transducer is a phased-array configuration with 64 piezoelectric elements operating at 3.7 to 7.5 MHz. With sequential firing of the elements and an acoustic lens in the transducer housing, the ultrasound waves are formed into a 90-degree beam approximately 2 to 10 mm in thickness that emanates at right angles to the transducer. Like standard gastroscopes, two rotary knobs ("wheels") control movement of the tip of the scope. One wheel anteflexes and retroflexes the transducer (i.e., moves the transducer toward and away from the heart). The other wheel flexes the transducer rightward and leftward (Fig. 41-15).

Currently, most multiplane transducers use the same transducer technology but mount the transducer on a rotating device that allows it to spin on its axis from 0 to 180 degrees within the tip of the gastroscope (transducer housing). Because cardiac structures and blood flow are not precisely aligned relative to the transducer, this design has significantly refined imaging capability. Matrix transducers accomplish the same rotation of the beam but do so electronically (i.e., without mechanically moving the transducer). The size of the probes has been decreased for pediatric application by reducing the number of crystals, and probes are now small enough for use in infants and neonates.

Ultrasonographs contain high-powered computers capable of initiating the ultrasound beam and processing the returning data. A series of electronic transforms (some guarded commercial secrets) produce the real-time images displayed on the video screen. All ultrasonographs share common technical aspects, including gain, depth, and Doppler controls. However, the differences in technical aspects between manufacturers and even between models from the same manufacturer are sufficiently great to prevent formulation of any universal operating instruc-

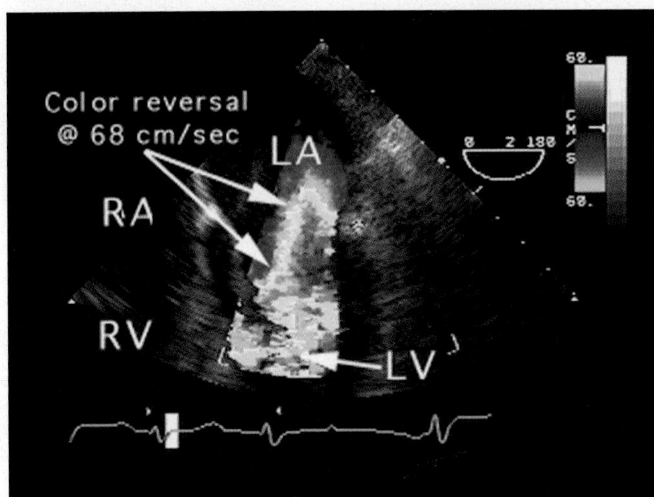

Figure 41-13 "Normal" color Doppler aliasing. In this echocardiogram, "normal" color Doppler aliasing is seen because laminar flow of blood through the mitral valve and into the left ventricle (LV) exceeds the Nyquist limit (68 cm/sec in this example—see the color reference icon at the upper right of the figure), thereby resulting in reversal of the color coding of flow direction. Notice that this color reversal occurs across fairly broad, regular areas and not in a random or point-by-point fashion as occurs with turbulent flow (always abnormal). In this example, follow the blue flow from high in the left atrium (LA) as it accelerates into the mitral orifice, and notice how color Doppler depicts the increasing flow velocities: the blue color becomes lighter and lighter until the Nyquist limit is reached. Color reversal then occurs, with light blue becoming yellow. Just at that reversal point, the velocity equals the Nyquist limit, in this example 68 cm/sec. Subsequent reversals may occur at that limit or multiples of that limit. RA, right atrium; RV, right ventricle. *(Reproduced with permission from Cahalan MK: Intraoperative Transesophageal Echocardiography. An Interactive Text and Atlas. New York, Churchill Livingstone, 1997.)*

tions. Fortunately, detailed instructions for each model are available in the operator's manual supplied with each ultrasonograph. Alternatively, cardiac sonographers are often excellent sources of instruction in the operation of these machines.

Basic Transesophageal Examination

Before performing TEE, the operator must determine that the benefits of TEE outweigh the risks. Except in the presence of esophageal disease or injury, the risk is quite low. Absolute contraindications include previous esophagectomy, severe esophageal obstruction, esophageal perforation, and ongoing esophageal hemorrhage. Relative contraindications include an esophageal diverticulum, varices, fistula, and previous esophageal surgery, as well as a history of gastric surgery, mediastinal irradiation, unexplained swallowing difficulties, and other conditions that might be worsened by placement and manipulation of the TEE probe.

In some studies, TEE is associated with a low incidence of oral and pharyngeal injuries (0.1% to 0.3%), but in other studies, the incidence of postoperative gastrointestinal complaints did not differ significantly from that in comparable patients who had not undergone TEE.[19,20] Uncontrolled studies have reported a 0.1% to 12% incidence of transient hoarseness after TEE. Serious pharyngeal or esophageal injury after TEE has been reported but is rare.[21] Two case reports indicate the possibility of TEE-associated splenic injury.[22,23] Among 10,218 patients (European multicenter study) undergoing TEE (primarily outpatients), esophageal perforation occurred in 1, who subsequently died; autopsy revealed a malignant tumor invading the esophagus.[24] Although bacteremia during TEE is uncommon, endocarditis has been reported in outpatients.[25,26] Endocarditis from intraoperative TEE has not been reported, and the risk is probably near zero because antibiotics are usually administered for prevention of surgical wound infection. In infants, TEE has a low complication rate, but even an appropriately sized TEE probe may obstruct the airway distal to the endotracheal tube or compress the descending aorta.[27]

Once the patient is anesthetized and the trachea securely intubated, the contents of the stomach are suctioned. Gentle massage of the left upper quadrant of the abdomen during suctioning may help remove air, which can otherwise degrade the imaging. The patient's neck is then extended and the well-lubricated TEE probe is introduced into the midline of the hypopharynx with the transducer side facing anteriorly. Usually, with minimal force the probe will pass blindly into the esophagus, especially if the neck is extended. If the probe does not pass blindly, a laryngoscope is used to lift the larynx anteriorly and the probe is placed into the esophagus under direct vision. During insertion or withdrawal of the transducer, the controls of the gastroscope must be in the neutral or relaxed position to allow the transducer to follow the natural course of the esophagus, thereby potentially minimizing the chance for injury.

Because of time constraints and relatively narrow diagnostic goals, anesthesiologists often perform a more limited intraoperative examination than described in the ASE/SCA's task force recommendation for a comprehensive TEE examination (see the

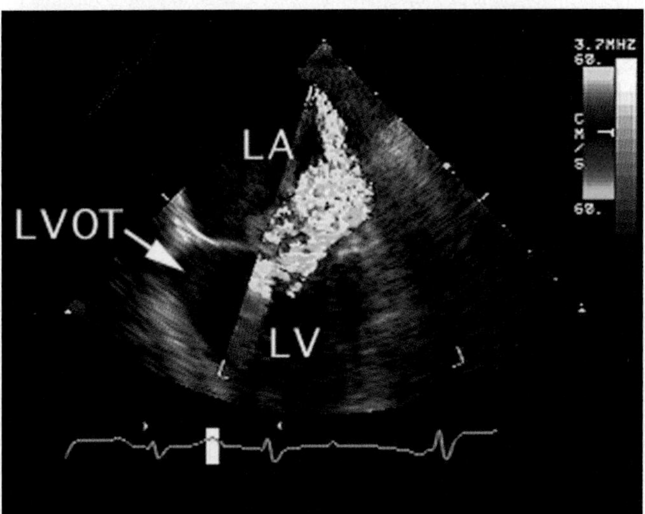

Figure 41-14 Color Doppler aliasing depicting turbulent flow. In this echocardiogram, color Doppler reveals aliasing caused by severe mitral regurgitation: a broad-based systolic color jet emanating from the mitral valve and extending far into the left atrium (LA). This jet is composed of a mosaic of colors mixed in a seemingly random, point-by-point fashion because the jet results from the turbulent flow of mitral regurgitation. Turbulence is never normal in the heart, and thus mosaic jets such as the one shown here are highly valuable diagnostic signs of underlying pathology. LV, left ventricle; LVOT, left ventricular outflow tract. *(Reproduced with permission from Cahalan MK: Intraoperative Transesophageal Echocardiography. An Interactive Text and Atlas. New York, Churchill Livingstone, 1997.)*

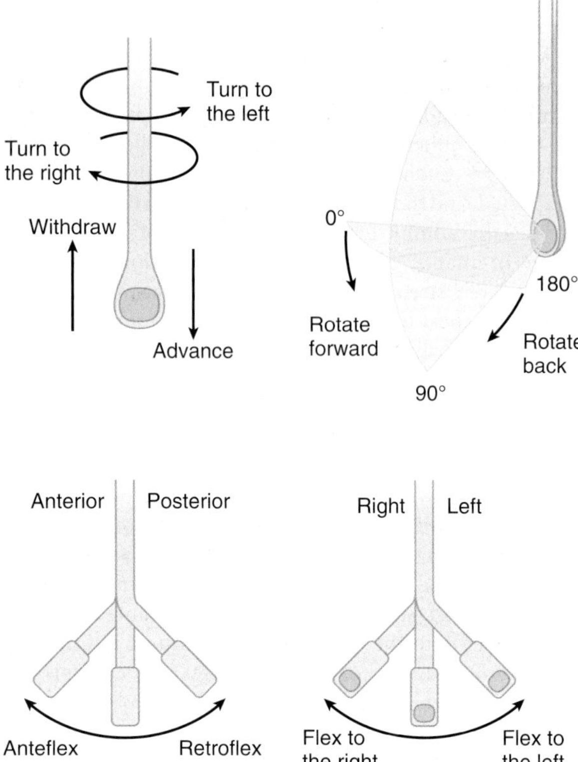

Figure 41-15 Terminology used to describe transesophageal echocardiography probe movements. *(Reproduced with permission from Shanewise JS, Cheung AT, Aronson S, et al: ASE/SCA guidelines for performing a comprehensive intraoperative multiplane transesophageal echocardiography examination: Recommendations of the American Society of Echocardiography Council for Intraoperative Echocardiography and the Society of Cardiovascular Anesthesiologists Task Force for Certification in Perioperative Transesophageal Echocardiography. Anesth Analg 89:870-884, 1999.)*

subsequent section).[7,28] However, even when time is critical, the examination performed should allow at least the basic applications of TEE as outlined in the 1996 guidelines for perioperative TEE: detection of markedly abnormal ventricular filling or function, extensive myocardial ischemia or infarction, large air embolism, severe valvular dysfunction, large cardiac masses or thrombi, large pericardial effusions, and major lesions of the great vessels.[6] A minimum of eight different cross sections drawn from the 20 cross sections delineated in the comprehensive examination are required to meet these diagnostic goals. Four of the cross sections are imaged in both 2D and color Doppler to assess valvular function. The next paragraph describes the probe manipulations required to achieve these cross sections. The reader should review Figure 41-15 to understand the terms used in this description.

After the TEE probe is introduced safely into the esophagus, it is advanced to the midesophageal (ME) level (28 to 32 cm measured at the upper incisors), and the aortic valve (AV) is imaged in the short axis (SAX) by turning the probe, adjusting its depth in the esophagus, and rotating the multiplane transducer 25 to 45 degrees until the three cusps of the valve are seen as being approximately equal in size and shape (Fig. 41-16H). Image depth is set at 10 to 12 cm as required to position the AV in the center of the video screen. This cross section is ideal for detection of aortic stenosis. This and all subsequent cross sections are digitally recorded. Next, the probe is turned slightly to position the AV in the center of the video screen, and then the multiplane angle is rotated forward to 110 to 130 degrees to bring the long axis (LAX) of the AV in view (see Fig. 41-16I). This cross section is best for detection of ascending aortic abnormalities, including type I aortic dissection. Color Doppler is used for assessment of AV competence. For detection of valvular stenosis and regurgitation, the Nyquist limit is set to 50 to 60 cm/sec.[12] Next, Doppler is discontinued and the probe is turned rightward until the ME bicaval cross section comes into view (see Fig. 41-16L). This cross section is usually seen best at a multiplane angle between 90 and 110 degrees and is ideal for assessing caval abnormalities, as well as compression of the right atrium from anteriorly located masses or effusions and compression of the left atrium from posteriorly located masses or effusions. In addition, the bicaval cross section may reveal collections of air located anteriorly in the left or right atrium, as well as the structure of the interatrial septum, including the foramen ovale. Next, the multiplane angle is rotated back to 60 to 80 degrees and the probe is turned leftward just past the AV to bring the ME right ventricular (RV) inflow and outflow cross section into view (see Fig. 41-16M). Usually, an image depth of 12 to 14 cm is required to position the RV outflow tract in the center of the video screen. This cross section reveals RV contractile function, the outflow tract, and pulmonary valve function with the application of color Doppler. Next, the transducer is rotated back to 0 degrees and the probe advanced 4 to 6 mm into the esophagus and gently retroflexed until all four cardiac chambers are visualized (ME four-chamber cross section) (see Fig. 41-16A). Rotating the transducer 10 to 15 degrees will often enhance the view of the tricuspid annulus. Usually, an image depth of 14 to 16 cm is required to include the LV apex in the sector scan. In 2D imaging, the free wall of the right ventricle and the lateral and septal LV wall segments are evaluated for contractile function. With color Doppler, both the mitral and tricuspid valves are assessed. Stenotic and regurgitant lesions can be diagnosed accurately. During this assessment, image depth is decreased to 10 to 12 cm to afford a magnified view of the valves and color Doppler flow patterns. Next, color Doppler is discontinued, the left ventricle is positioned in the center of the screen, and the multiplane angle is rotated forward to 90 degrees to bring into view the ME two-chamber cross section (see Fig. 41-16B). Image depth is returned to 14 to 16 cm. This cross section is best for revealing the function of the basal and apical segments of the anterior and inferior LV walls, as well as anterior and inferior pericardial collections. When air emboli collect in the left ventricle, they can generally best be seen in this view as very echogenic areas located along the anterior apical endocardial surface. The transducer is then rotated forward to 135 degrees to reveal the ME LAX cross section, which is best for assessment of the anteroseptal and posterior wall segments for contractile LV function (see Fig. 41-16C). Together, the ME four-chamber, two-chamber, and LAX cross sections reveal all 16 segments of the left ventricle (Fig. 41-17). However, the next and last of the basic cross sections provides a second look at the midventricular segments, as well as other benefits. To achieve this cross section, the transducer is rotated back to 0 degrees, the left ventricle is centered in the screen, and the probe is advanced 4 to 6 cm into the stomach. It is then gently flexed anteriorly to reveal the transgastric (TG) SAX cross section (see Fig. 41-16D). This cross section is ideal for monitoring LV filling and contractile function. All major coronary arteries supplying the myocardium are viewed in this cross section. Moreover, changes in preload cause greater changes

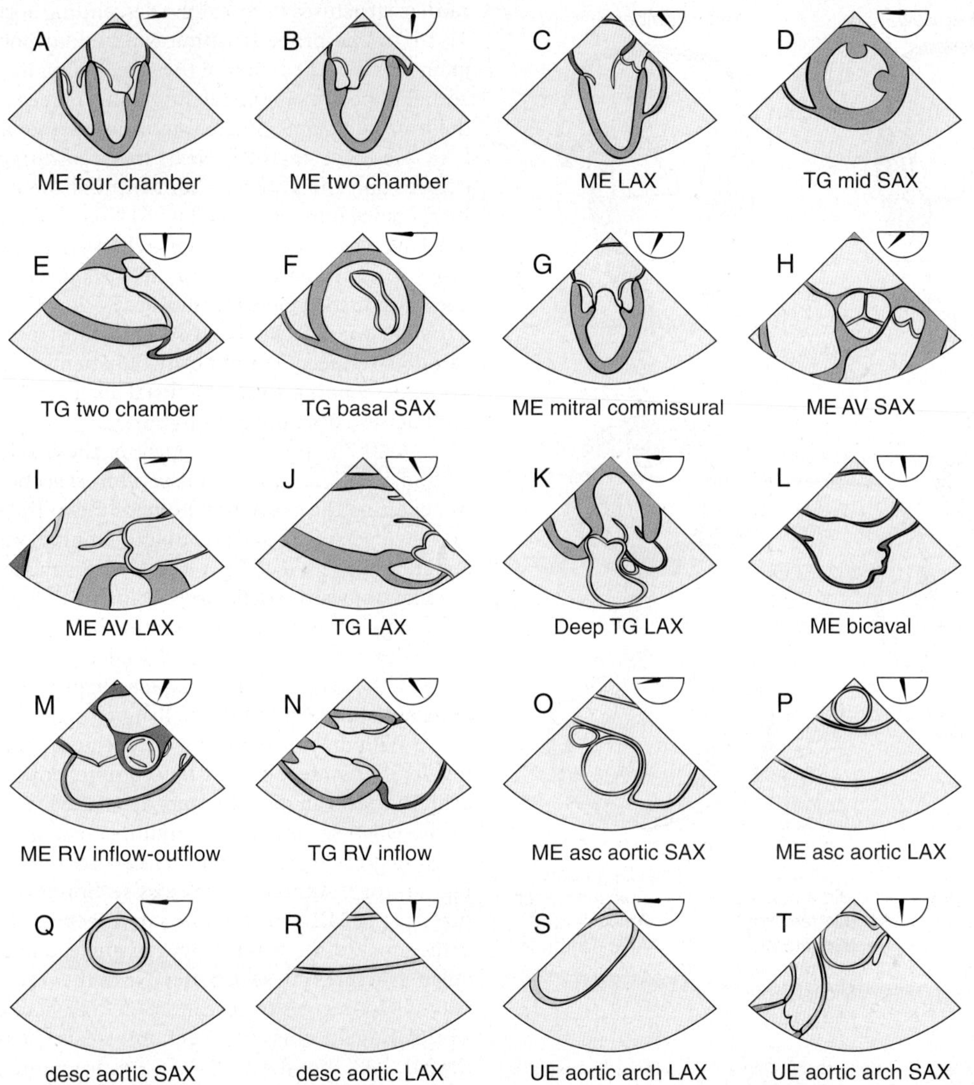

Figure 41-16 Transesophageal echocardiography cross sections in a comprehensive examination. Twenty standard cross sections and their abbreviated names are depicted by the line drawings. The text describes the probe manipulations required to produce each of these cross sections. *(Reproduced with permission from Shanewise JS, Cheung AT, Aronson S, et al: ASE/SCA guidelines for performing a comprehensive intraoperative multiplane transesophageal echocardiography examination: Recommendations of the American Society of Echocardiography Council for Intraoperative Echocardiography and the Society of Cardiovascular Anesthesiologists Task Force for Certification in Perioperative Transesophageal Echocardiography. Anesth Analg 89:870-884, 1999.)*

in the LV SAX than in the LAX dimension, and movement of the probe from this cross section is readily apparent inasmuch as the papillary muscles provide prominent landmarks. Because this cross section is used to judge filling and ejection, image depth is consistently set to 12 cm so that the size and function of the heart can easily be judged relative to previously examined hearts.

Comprehensive Transesophageal Examination

In addition to the 8 cross sections described in the preceding paragraph, 12 other cross sections are required to complete the comprehensive perioperative TEE examination delineated in the 1999 ASE/SCA task force recommendations.[7] When time permits or the diagnostic questions require, the comprehensive examination can be completed in any order deemed most appropriate by the operator. Shanewise and colleagues described an examination sequence based on anatomic structures, and the reader is referred to this very detailed reference for one excellent approach.[7] However, when a single individual is responsible for anesthetic care and the TEE examination, the comprehensive examination is completed as time permits after the basic examination has been recorded. When such is the case, the operator can use 3 of the 8 basic cross sections as takeoff points for the other 12 cross sections, thus making completion of the comprehensive examination a relatively easy sequence to remember and quick to perform.

With the probe positioned for the AV SAX cross section, the other six cross sections of the aorta are easily achieved. First, the probe is withdrawn slowly 1 to 3 cm while keeping the aorta in the center of the video screen to view the ascending aorta in SAX (see Fig. 41-16O). As the probe is withdrawn, the operator progressively views more superior SAX cross sections of the aorta beginning with the sinotubular junction until the image is lost

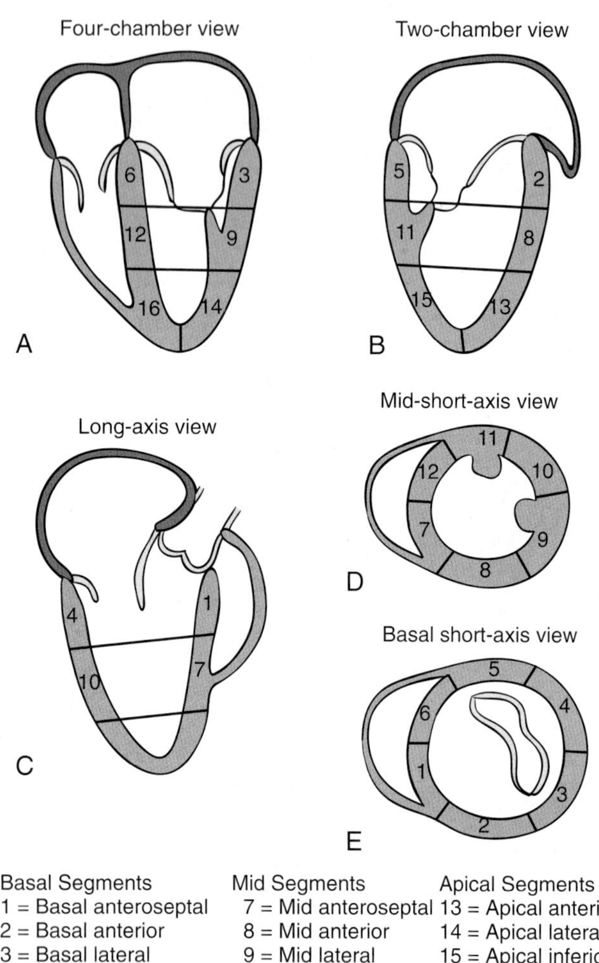

Figure 41-17 Five transesophageal echocardiography cross sections with myocardial segments identified. A total of 16 myocardial segments are identified and named according to standards adopted by the American Society of Echocardiography and the Society of Cardiovascular Anesthesiologists. *(Reproduced with permission from Shanewise JS, Cheung AT, Aronson S, et al: ASE/SCA guidelines for performing a comprehensive intraoperative multiplane transesophageal echocardiography examination: Recommendations of the American Society of Echocardiography Council for Intraoperative Echocardiography and the Society of Cardiovascular Anesthesiologists Task Force for Certification in Perioperative Transesophageal Echocardiography. Anesth Analg 89:870-884, 1999.)*

because of interposition of the trachea between the esophagus and aorta. Next, the multiplane angle is rotated forward to 100 to 120 degrees and advanced slowly 1 to 3 cm while keeping the aorta in the center of the video screen to view the ascending aorta in LAX (see Fig. 41-16P). These two cross sections are ideal for assessment of pathology of the ascending aorta, such as type I aortic dissection and aortic atheromas. However, the most superior aspect of the aorta is rarely seen, including the takeoff of the innominate artery, because of the aforementioned tracheal interposition. Next, the transducer is returned to 0 degrees, the image depth decreased to 6 cm, and the probe turned leftward past the cardiac structures to reveal the descending aorta in SAX (see Fig. 41-16Q). The probe is withdrawn and advanced with the aorta maintained in the center of the screen until the entire descending aorta has been examined in SAX. This maneuver is repeated with the transducer at 90 degrees to examine the descending aorta in LAX (see Fig. 41-16R). Next, the transducer is returned to 0 degrees and the probe withdrawn until the distal aortic arch in LAX comes into view (see Fig. 41-16S). Rotating the transducer to 90 degrees reveals the distal arch in SAX (see Fig. 41-16T). The probe is turned leftward until the aorta just disappears from view and then turned slowly rightward to identify the takeoff of the left subclavian artery (well seen in most patients) and the left carotid (well seen in a minority of patients). These cross sections of the descending aorta and distal aortic arch reliably reveal dissections and atheromatous disease.

With the probe positioned for the ME four-chamber cross section, the ME mitral commissural cross section is easily achieved by centering the coaptation point of the mitral valve in the center of the video screen and rotating the multiplane angle forward to about 60 degrees (see Fig. 41-16G). This maneuver positions the ultrasound beam parallel to the closure line of the mitral leaflets and completes the LAX examination of the mitral valve. Although a detailed discussion of mitral leaflet structure and function is beyond the scope of this chapter, Figure 41-18 summarizes an excellent approach to this challenging task.[29]

With the probe positioned for the TG mid SAX, the remaining five cross sections of the comprehensive examination are achieved easily in most patients. First, the left ventricle is centered in the video screen and the multiplane angle is rotated forward to 90 degrees to reveal the TG two-chamber cross section (see Fig. 41-16E). Although this cross section reveals the same structures as the ME two-chamber cross section, the viewing angle is orthogonal to the former viewing angle, and as a result, subvalvular structures are seen better. Next, the transducer is rotated to 100 to 120 degrees to reveal the TG LAX cross section (see Fig. 41-16J). Again, this cross section reveals the same structures as the ME LAX, but the TG LAX permits a more parallel alignment of the ultrasound beam with blood flow through the LV outflow track and AV. Next, the TG RV inflow cross section is achieved by returning the probe to the TG mid SAX position, turning it rightward until the right ventricle is centered in the video screen, and then rotating the multiplane angle to 100 to 120 degrees to bring the RV apex into view (see Fig. 41-16N). This cross section is ideal for viewing the RV inferior free wall. Next, the TG basal SAX is achieved by returning the probe to the TG mid SAX, releasing the flexion of the probe, withdrawing 1 to 2 cm, and then flexing the probe gently until the orifice of the mitral valve is seen in SAX (Fig. 41-16F). This cross section can prove vital in determining the precise location of mitral regurgitation.[29] Finally, the TG deep LAX cross section is achieved by returning the probe to the TG mid SAX position, releasing the flexion of the probe, advancing it 6 to 8 cm into the stomach, fully flexing it once in the stomach, gently withdrawing it until minimal resistance is met at the gastroesophageal junction, and then slightly turning it leftward or rightward to reveal the LV outflow tract and AV (Fig. 41-16K). Usually, this cross section does not resolve structures as well as the ME LAX does, but it provides optimal beam alignment for Doppler interrogation of the LV outflow tract and AV. Frequently, this cross section is the most difficult of the cross sections to visualize. If a few gentle attempts fail to accomplish it, it should be abandoned.

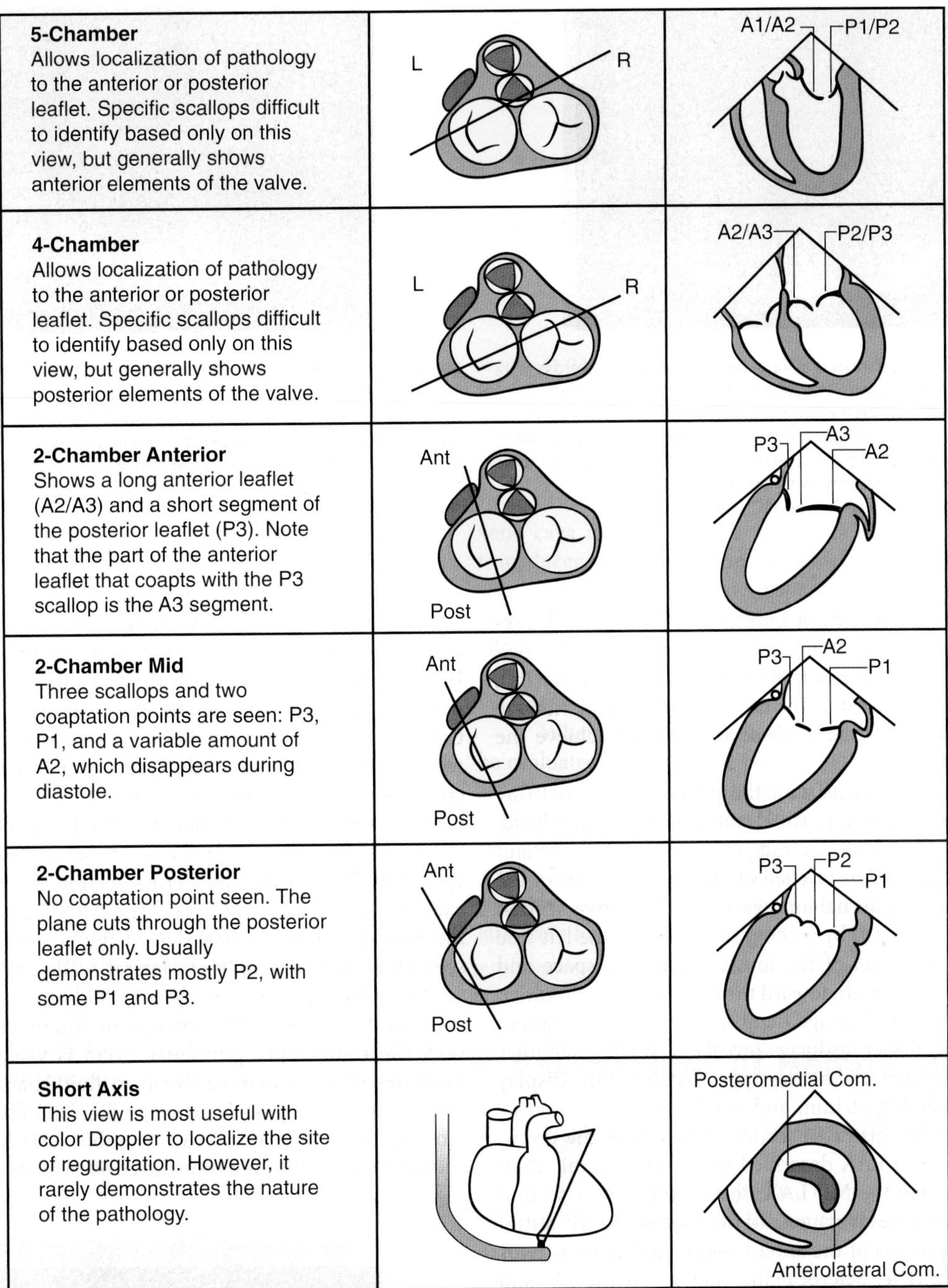

Figure 41-18 A systematic examination of the mitral valve is depicted. In this examination, the mitral valve is viewed in multiple cross sections to delineate the leaflet anatomy. The five-chamber cross section is accomplished by withdrawing the probe slightly from the standard four-chamber cross section until the left ventricular outflow track is in view. The *center column* shows the planes of the different cross sections as viewed from directly above the base of the heart. The two-chamber anterior, mid, and posterior cross sections are variations on the standard two-chamber cross section that are accomplished by turning the probe from the patient's right to left. P1, P2, and P3 refer to the three scallops of the posterior mitral leaflet, and A1, A2, and A3 refer to the juxtaposed segments of the anterior mitral leaflet. The *right column* shows the leaflet segments seen in the corresponding cross section. *(Reproduced with permission from Lambert AS, Miller JP, Foster E, et al: Improved evaluation of the location and mechanism of mitral valve regurgitation with a systematic transesophageal echocardiography examination. Anesth Analg 88:1205-1212, 1999.)*

Basic Transthoracic Examination

In patients with an unsecured airway, TTE is easier to perform than TEE because TTE is entirely noninvasive. TTE uses frequencies lower (1 to 3 MHz) than TEE does to penetrate the greater distances inherent in the transthoracic technique, but all previously discussed modalities (M-mode, spectral Doppler, color Doppler, and tissue Doppler) can be performed with TTE. Transthoracic cardiac probes are significantly different from the linear probes used to identify superficial vascular structures and nerve bundles. Thus, the probes used for ultrasound-guided nerve

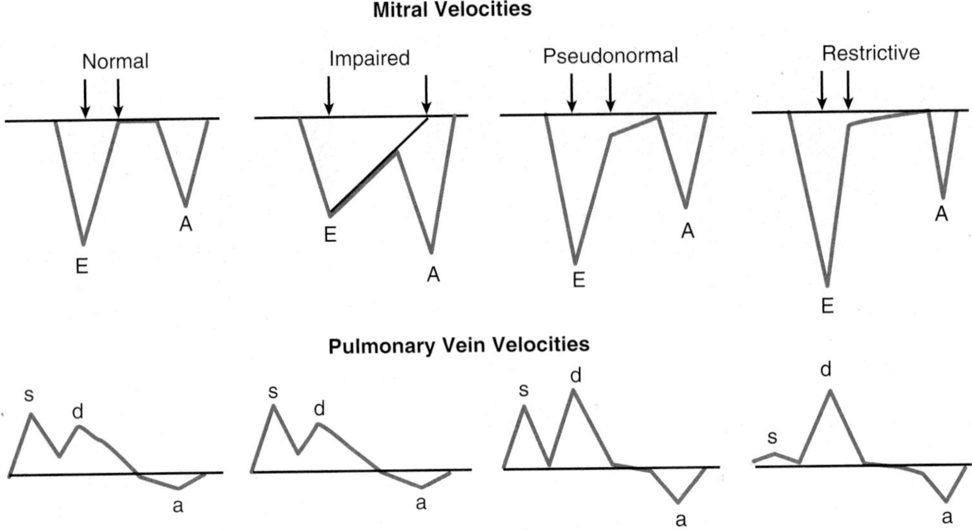

Figure 41-28 Line drawings representing simultaneous transesophageal pulsed wave Doppler recordings from the mitral annulus and right upper pulmonary vein are shown for normal, impaired, pseudonormal, and restrictive left ventricular diastolic function. The *solid black line* represents the slope of the E-wave velocity. From the start of the line at the inflection point of the E wave until its intercept at the base line is the deceleration time. This time is depicted in each of the mitral velocity drawings by *black arrows*. Please see text for further details. *(Adapted From Zile MR, Brutsaert DL: New concepts in diastolic dysfunction and diastolic heart failure: Part I: Diagnosis, prognosis and measurements of diastolic function. Circulation 105:1387-1393, 2002.© 2002 American Heart Association, Inc.)*

impaired relaxation, left atrial pressure is normal, and therefore so is the pattern of pulmonary venous flow: the S wave is greater than the D wave. The second and more severe degree of diastolic dysfunction is termed "pseudonormal" and is characterized by return of the normal E-to-A ratio because of a pathologic increase in left atrial pressure that results in abnormal pulmonary venous flow: the D wave is greater than the S wave. One simple way to confirm that the mitral flow pattern is pseudonormal and not normal is to transiently reduce left atrial filling with a Valsalva maneuver. If diastolic function is pseudonormal, the E-to-A ratio will transiently reverse, with A being greater than E. If diastolic function is normal, the normal ratio of E greater than A will persist and both waves will decrease in size. The third and most severe degree of diastolic dysfunction is termed "restrictive" and is characterized by very high E-wave velocity, a short deceleration time, and low A-wave velocity. In restrictive diastolic function, left atrial pressure is very high and results in a very small S wave and large D wave in the pulmonary veins. Patients with this pattern have a poor prognosis and suffer symptoms of congestive heart failure regardless of their systolic function.[41]

Transesophageal Echocardiography During Life-Threatening Hypotension

Ultimately, hypotension has only two possible causes: inadequate cardiac output or inappropriately low systemic vascular resistance. TEE is remarkably well suited for addressing this differential diagnosis. During severe hypotension, qualitative TEE estimates of ventricular filling and function serve as practical guides for the administration of fluids, inotropes, and vasopressors. An experienced observer can differentiate severe ventricular dysfunction from other life-threatening causes of hypotension. In severe LV failure, ventricular filling (as assessed by end-diastolic area) is increased and ejection is decreased, whereas in inappropriately low systemic vascular resistance, ventricular filling is usually normal or slightly decreased and ejection is markedly increased. Hypovolemia is easily recognized as a marked decrease in ventricular filling and a marked increase in ejection. Although inappropriately low systemic vascular resistance, severe aortic regurgitation, severe mitral regurgitation, and ventricular septal defects can manifest the same LV filling and ejection pattern on the TG SAX cross section, distinguishing these causes of hypotension is not difficult with the use of other cross sections and color Doppler. A dramatic example of the use of TEE in hypotensive patients is provided by a study of 60 consecutive patients with severe, persistent hypotension after cardiac surgery despite intensive therapy guided by invasive monitors.[42] TEE confirmed the presumed etiology of the hypotension in only 30 of these patients. In two patients, TEE revealed unsuspected cardiac tamponade and in six others unsuspected hypovolemia. In five patients, TEE prevented unnecessary reoperations by proving that tamponade was not present despite hemodynamic data suggesting that it was. In another study, unstable cardiac surgical patients in the operating room ($n = 57$) or intensive care unit ($n = 83$) underwent emergency TEE.[43] Based on TEE findings alone, 22 of these patients underwent urgent surgical interventions. The average time to diagnosis was 11 minutes. In still another study involving critically ill surgical patients, TEE proved to be more cost-effective than TTE because the latter so often fails to reveal diagnostic images.[44] Moreover, TEE has prognostic value in hypotensive, critically ill patients: when it reveals nonventricular causes of hypotension (e.g., valvular or pericardial), patients are twice as likely to survive as those with other causes of hypotension.[45] Even in the setting of prolonged cardiopulmonary resuscitation, TEE may reveal crucial diagnostic information.[46]

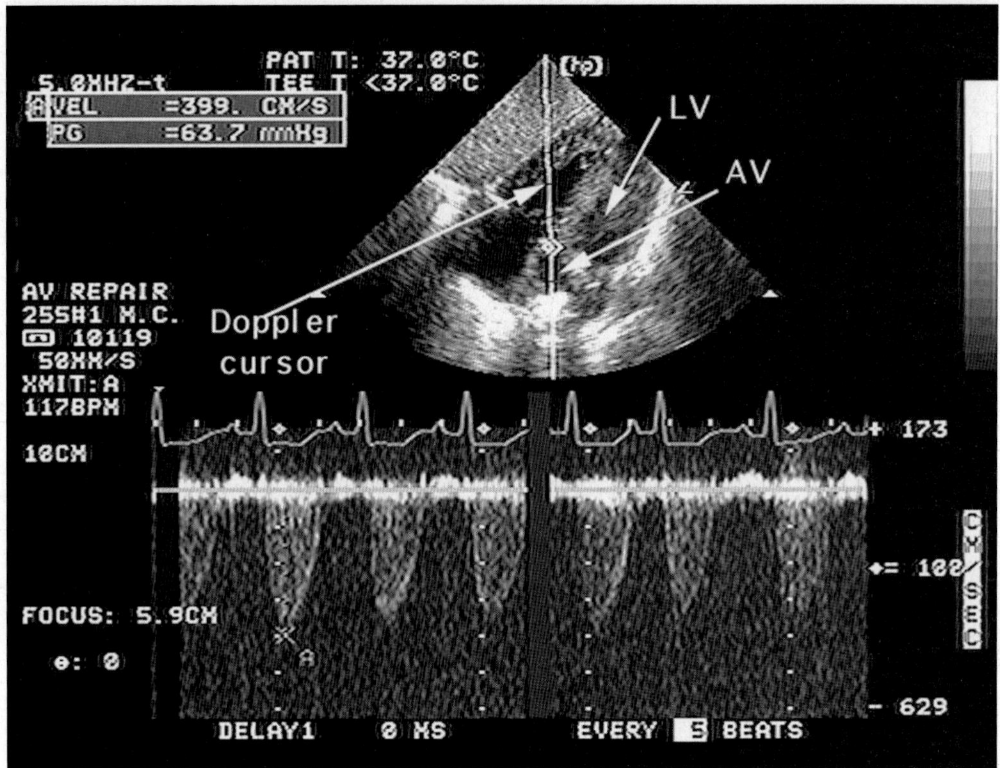

Figure 41-29 Continuous wave Doppler measurement of blood flow velocities immediately above the aortic valve (AV) during seven cardiac cycles. At the top of the figure is a still-frame image of the two-dimensional cross section used to position the Doppler sampling cursor (the *diagonal white line*). On the bottom two thirds of the figure is the display in white of the instantaneous blood flow velocities (vertical axis) versus time (horizontal axis) occurring anywhere along that cursor. The electrocardiogram provides timing, and the *bold horizontal line* is the baseline (zero flow) for the flow velocities. With this Doppler alignment, all flow velocities are negative (i.e., away from the transducer). The Doppler scale has been set to a maximum of −629 cm/sec, and this tracing documents significant aortic stenosis: a peak blood flow velocity of approximately 4 m/sec (each *white dot* on the vertical axis equals 100 cm/sec or 1 m/sec), corresponding to a peak gradient across the AV of 64 mm Hg. LV, left ventricle. *(Reproduced with permission from Cahalan MK: Intraoperative Transesophageal Echocardiography. An Interactive Text and Atlas. New York, Churchill Livingstone, 1997.)*

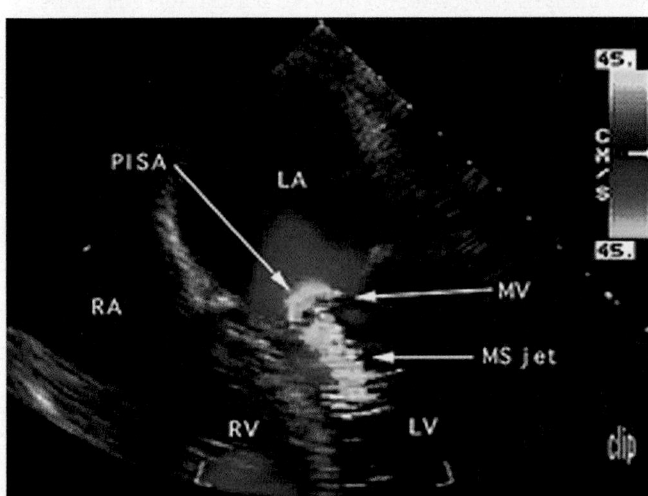

Figure 41-30 This four-chamber echocardiogram reveals a thickened and narrowed mitral valve (MV) indicative of mitral stenosis (MS). Color Doppler demonstrates (1) acceleration of blood flow into the stenotic valve (a light blue semicircular area immediately above the valve [PISA (proximal isovelocity surface area)]), (2) a narrow color jet across the valve itself, and (3) a 1- by 4-cm color jet extending from the undersurface of the valve into the left ventricle (LV). LA, left atrium; RA, right atrium; RV, right ventricle. *(Reproduced with permission from Cahalan MK: Intraoperative Transesophageal Echocardiography. An Interactive Text and Atlas. New York, Churchill Livingstone, 1997.)*

contrast agents but to aggregation of red cells in areas of low flow. Whenever left atrial enlargement and spontaneous contrast are noted, thrombus in the left atrium and, in particular, the left atrial appendage should be suspected and investigated carefully.

The presence and severity of mitral regurgitation are evaluated from the same cross sections used for evaluation of mitral stenosis and with the same grading strategy used for aortic regurgitation (Table 41-5). Mild regurgitation is characterized by a narrow-based, systolic color jet (<2 mm at its origin in the valve) that occupies less than 25% of the left atrial cross-sectional area and extends less than half the distance to the posterior wall of the left atrium. Moderate regurgitation is a broader-based, systolic color jet (3 to 5 mm at its origin in the valve) occupying less than 50% of the left atrial cross-sectional area and extending 50% to 90% of the distance to the posterior wall of the left atrium. Severe regurgitation is a broad-based, systolic color jet (>5 mm) occupying most of the left atrium and extending into the pulmonary veins and left atrial appendage (Fig. 41-32). Eccentrically directed jets of mitral regurgitation that hug the wall of the atrium are generally associated with more severe valvular regurgitation than their cross-sectional area might suggest (see Fig. 41-32). Moreover, eccentrically directed jets usually point away from the defective leaflet (i.e., laterally directed jets are typically associated with anterior leaflet defects and medially directed jets with posterior leaflet defects), provided that the mechanism of regurgitation is leaflet prolapse or flail.[78] Severe mitral regurgitation is invariably

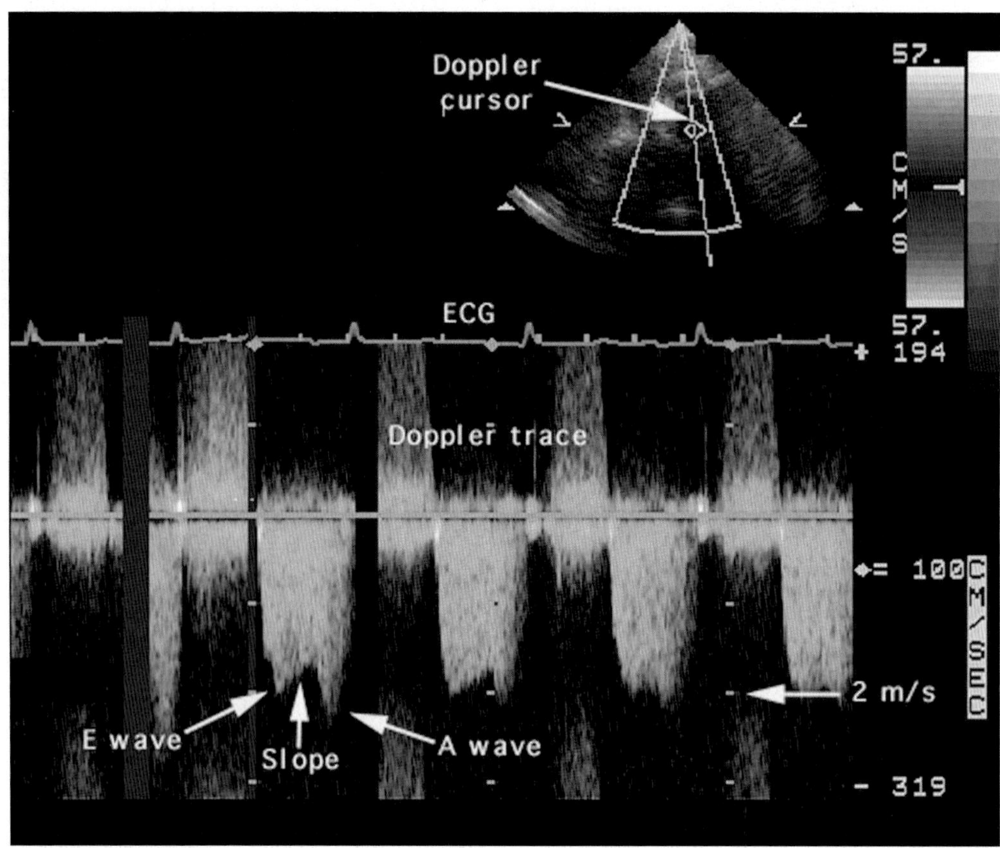

Figure 41-31 Continuous wave Doppler measurement of blood flow velocities through a stenotic mitral valve. At the top of the figure is a still-frame image of the four-chamber cross section used to position the Doppler cursor. On the bottom two thirds of the figure is the display in white of the instantaneous blood flow velocities (vertical axis) versus time (horizontal axis) occurring anywhere along that cursor. The electrocardiogram (ECG) is shown for timing purposes, and the *bold horizontal line* running through the Doppler tracing is the baseline (zero flow) for the flow velocities. Velocities displayed above the baseline are positive and represent flow toward the transducer. These velocities are due to mitral regurgitation and are so high they exceed the scale used in this example. Velocities displayed below the baseline are negative and represent flow away from the transducer. These velocities are due to severe mitral stenosis and average about 2 m/sec, indicative of a 16 mm Hg gradient across the mitral valve. Also note how slowly flow velocity decreases after the peak of the E wave (i.e., the Slope). The pressure half-time can be calculated from this slope and is markedly increased in the presence of severe mitral stenosis. *(Reproduced with permission from Cahalan MK: Intraoperative Transesophageal Echocardiography. An Interactive Text and Atlas. New York, Churchill Livingstone, 1997.)*

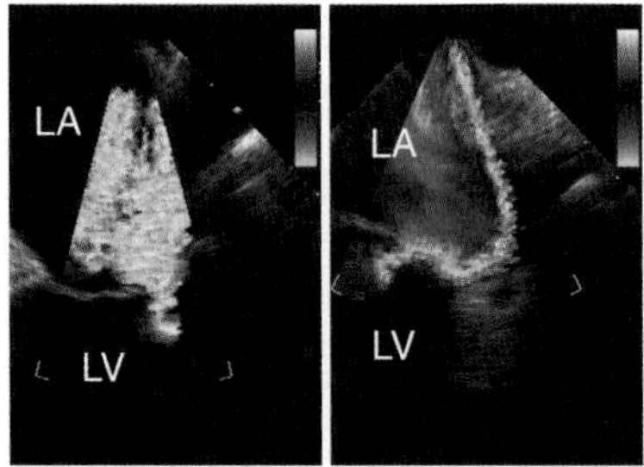

Figure 41-32 Two honed-down stop-action four-chamber transesophageal echocardiograms demonstrating severe mitral regurgitation. The one on the *left* reveals a large color jet depicting turbulent flow emanating from the center of the mitral valve at its coaptation point. The mechanism of the regurgitation in this patient is annular dilatation. Notice the broad base of the jet at the level of the valve leaflet and the extent of the jet's penetration into the left atrium (LA). The stop-action echocardiogram on the *right* reveals another broad-based jet with eccentric direction indicative of prolapse of the anterior leaflet of the mitral valve. Wall-hugging jets such as this one have a small cross-sectional area because much of their energy is absorbed by the wall of the atrium. LV, left ventricle.

associated with systolic reversal of pulmonary venous inflow (Fig. 41-33).[79] The general guidelines listed earlier are widely used, but many more criteria have been described for assessment of mitral regurgitation.[12] Of most importance, the degree of regurgitation is exquisitely dependent on LV loading conditions. For practical purposes, quantitative measures of regurgitation, such as the regurgitant orifice area based on the theory of proximal isovelocity surface area, are less often used in operating rooms because of time restriction.

Pulmonary and tricuspid valve pathology is assessed in a fashion analogous to that described previously for the aortic and mitral valves.

Coronary Disease

In a study of 82 high-risk patients undergoing coronary artery surgery, the investigators used staged blinding of the cardiac surgeons and anesthesiologists at critical points during surgery to document the clinical impact of TEE. After these clinicians docu-

Table 41-5 Simplified Grading for Mitral Regurgitation*

	Jet Width at Origin (mm)	Jet Area (% LA_a)	Jet Depth (% LA_d)
Mild	>2	<25	<50
Moderate	3-5	25-50	50-90
Severe	>5	<50	>100

*Systolic jet width is assessed with color Doppler in the five- or four-chamber view at the closure point of the mitral valve (the origin of the regurgitant jet). The transducer should be repositioned until the origin of the jet is clearly imaged. Failure to image the origin of the jet may lead to overestimation of its severity. Systolic jet area is assessed with color Doppler in the five- or four-chamber view. % LA_a is the percentage of the LA_a occupied by the plume of the color jet (the area of turbulent flow depicted by the mosaic of color pixels). This parameter is markedly affected by left ventricular systolic pressure. Failure to adjust color or two-dimensional gains correctly may lead to underestimation or overestimation of the severity of the regurgitation. Color gain should be set just below the level that results in random color sparkle, and two-dimensional gains should be set at the minimum levels allowing adequate visualization of cardiac structures. Systolic jet depth is assessed with color Doppler in the five- or four-chamber view. % LA_d is the depth of penetration of the jet into the left atrium expressed as a percentage of the distance from the mitral annulus to the posterior wall of the left atrium. This parameter is also markedly affected by left ventricular systolic pressure. In severe mitral regurgitation, the regurgitant jet may extend into one or more pulmonary veins and cause transient reversal of pulmonary venous blood flow.
From Cahalan MK: Intraoperative Transesophageal Echocardiography: An Interactive Text and Atlas. New York, Churchill Livingstone, 1996.

mented their planned management at each stage, the TEE results were revealed and led to at least one significant change in anesthetic management in 51% of patients and surgical management in 33% of patients, including additional unplanned or revised grafts (15%) and unplanned valve procedures (20%).[80] These high-risk patients had postoperative infarction and mortality rates below predicted (1% versus 3% predicted, difference not statistically significant). In the study noted in the section earlier involving 457 consecutive patients undergoing coronary artery surgery, TEE identified 71 new findings in 13% of patients. The new finding resulted in a change in surgical management in 6% of patients. After bypass, surgical management, including graft evaluation or revision and mitral repair, was initiated in 10 patients.

Congenital Heart Surgery

Pediatric TEE probes are used in infants as small as 3 kg (also see Chapter 83). Stevenson and coauthors reported that intraoperative TEE reliably detected residual cardiac defects in 17 (7.4%) of 230 consecutive patients undergoing congenital heart surgery.[81] These patients were reoperated on immediately for revision of the residual defects. However, a subsequent publication from the same center reported that the number of residual defects missed

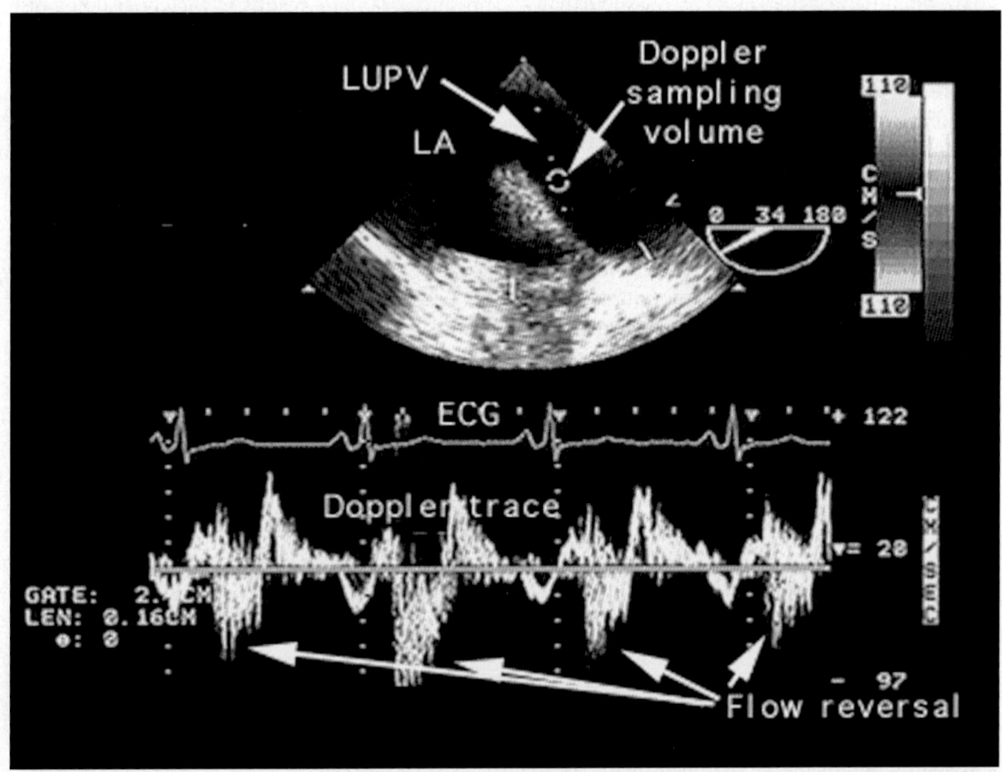

Figure 41-33 Pulsed wave Doppler measurement of blood flow velocities in the left upper pulmonary vein (LUPV). At the top of the figure is a still-frame image of the two-dimensional cross section used to position the Doppler sampling cursor (*broken circle* at point of *arrow*). On the bottom two thirds of the figure is a display of the instantaneous blood flow velocities (vertical axis) versus time (horizontal axis) occurring in the LUPV. The electrocardiogram (ECG) is shown for timing purposes, and the *bold horizontal line* running through the Doppler tracing is the baseline (zero flow) for the flow velocities. Velocities displayed above the baseline are positive and represent flow toward the transducer (in this case, into the left atrium [LA]). Velocities displayed below the baseline are negative and represent flow away from the transducer (in this case, into the LUPV). This Doppler tracing documents systolic flow reversal (normally it is positive, that is, toward the LA in systole) and confirms the presence of severe mitral regurgitation. *(Reproduced with permission from Cahalan MK: Intraoperative Transesophageal Echocardiography. An Interactive Text and Atlas. New York, Churchill Livingstone, 1997.)*

by intraoperative TEE increased from 2% to 13% when the attending anesthesiologist and not a separate echocardiographer performed TEE.[82] This study generated considerable controversy. Although it does not resolve the issue of whether a separate echocardiographer is required to perform TEE adequately in patients undergoing congenital heart repair, it does amply demonstrate that patients can suffer severe consequences when intraoperative TEE is not expertly performed, interpreted, and acted on. In this study, the deaths of seven patients may have been related to the delayed recognition of residual defects. With progress in pediatric congenital heart surgery, more and more children with palliated congenital heart disease will survive to adulthood and undergo cardiac and other kinds of surgery. For an excellent update on TEE in adult congenital heart disease, please see the recent review by Russell and associates.[83]

Other Cardiac Diseases and Applications

In addition to use in valve repair, congenital heart surgery, and thoracic aortic surgery and in hemodynamically unstable patients, the 1996 ASA/SCA guidelines identify intraoperative use of TEE during surgery for hypertrophic cardiomyopathy, endocarditis, and pericardial window procedures as category I indications.[6] Subsequent publications have documented the critical role that TEE may provide in minimally invasive cardiac surgery and in placement of cardiac support devices.[84,85] Thousands of other published reports have documented that TEE can reveal virtually any significant morphologic or functional pathology of the heart. TEE is particularly sensitive for abnormalities involving the left atrium and mitral valve, including masses, thrombi, and emboli, because of the proximity of the left atrium and mitral valve to the TEE transducer. In contrast, pathologies of the RV and LV apex are less reliably detected. TEE is exquisitely sensitive to air embolism, and as a result, even insignificant amounts of air in the circulation give rise to impressive densities on the video display. Currently, accurate estimation of the amount of air in the circulation is impossible with TEE. However, large amounts typically opacify the involved chambers until collections (very bright densities) are formed in the most superiorly positioned parts of the chambers (e.g., the anterior endocardial surface of the left ventricle in a supine patient). Pulmonary emboli may be seen with TEE if they lodge proximal to the bifurcation of the main pulmonary artery.

Transesophageal Echocardiography in Noncardiac Surgery and Critical Care

TEE has many of the same applications in noncardiac surgical patients and critically ill patients as in cardiac surgical patients (also see Chapter 91). Numerous case reports and case series have documented the impact that it can have on patient management and outcome. In our practice, the leading indications are hemodynamic instability and massive blood loss, where TEE has a vital role in determining the etiology of the instability (see the previous section on this topic) and in guiding volume resuscitation.[86,87] In the intensive care unit, TEE has similar applications, and these have been reviewed recently.[88,89]

Data Storage, Documentation, and Quality Assurance

Traditionally, echocardiograms were stored on videotape and written reports of the results were placed in the patient's medical record. Currently, digital recording of individual cardiac cycles or multiple cycles is the standard. The resulting "loops" are transported via hospital networks or the Internet to secure servers, where the studies can be retrieved rapidly. The SCA has published guidelines for TEE reporting (http://www.scahq.org/sca3/peri_op_report4-02.rtf) and a recommended report form (http://www.scahq.org/sca3/TEEREPORfin4-02.rtf).

The ASE and SCA have published guidelines for continuous quality improvement (CQI) in perioperative echocardiography.[90] However, even relatively simple CQI interventions may produce dramatic results in the consistency of image acquisition and storage.[28] Periodic expert review of TEE interpretations is essential if practitioners are to reach and maintain their diagnostic potential. Collaboration between the departments of anesthesiology and cardiology is one approach to this review process that minimizes the duplication inherent in the formation of independent CQI programs.

Certification

The SCA and ASE formed the National Board of Echocardiography (www.echoboards.org). This new board offers a written examination and certification in perioperative echocardiography. The written examination is open to all licensed physicians. Certification requires additional documented experience for physicians who completed their training before 2009. For physicians completing their training after 2009, certification will require fellowship training in perioperative echocardiography (http://www.echoboards.org/certification/pte/reqs.html).

References

1. Frazin L, Talano JV, Stephanides L, et al: Esophageal echocardiography. Circulation 54:102-108, 1976.
2. Matsumoto M, Oka Y, Strom J, et al: Application of transesophageal echocardiography to continuous intraoperative monitoring of left ventricular performance. Am J Cardiol 46:95-105, 1980.
3. Schluter M, Langenstein BA, Polster J, et al: Transoesophageal cross-sectional echocardiography with a phased array transducer system. Technique and initial clinical results. Br Heart J 48:67-72, 1982.
4. Sharma R, Mann J, Drummond L, et al: The evaluation of real-time 3-dimensional transthoracic echocardiography for the preoperative functional assessment of patients with mitral valve prolapse: A comparison with 2-dimensional transesophageal echocardiography. J Am Soc Echocardiogr 20:934-940, 2007.
5. Pearlman AS, Gardin JM, Martin RP, et al: Guidelines for physician training in transesophageal echocardiography: Recommendations of the American Society of Echocardiography Committee for Physician Training in Echocardiography. J Am Soc Echocardiogr 5:187-194, 1992.
6. Practice guidelines for perioperative transesophageal echocardiography. A report by the American Society of Anesthesiologists and the Society of Cardiovascular Anesthesiologists Task Force on Transesophageal Echocardiography. Anesthesiology 84:986-1006, 1996.
7. Shanewise JS, Cheung AT, Aronson S, et al: ASE/SCA guidelines for performing a comprehensive intraoperative multiplane transesophageal echocardiography examination: Recommendations of the American Society of Echocardiography Council for Intraoperative Echocardiography and the Society of Cardiovascular Anesthesiologists Task Force for Certification in Perioperative Transesophageal Echocardiography. Anesth Analg 89:870-884, 1999.
8. Cahalan MK, Abel M, Goldman M, et al: American Society of Echocardiography and Society of Cardiovascular Anesthesiologists task force guidelines for training in perioperative echocardiography. Anesth Analg 94:1384-1388, 2002.
9. Cheitlin MD, Armstrong WF, Aurigemma GP, et al: ACC/AHA/ASE 2003 Guideline update for the clinical application of echocardiography: Summary article. A report of the American College of Cardiology/American Heart Association Task Force on Practice Guidelines (ACC/AHA/ASE Committee to Update the 1997 Guidelines for the Clinical Application of Echocardiography). J Am Soc Echocardiogr 16:1091-1110, 2003.
10. Ayres NA, Miller-Hance W, Fyfe DA, et al: Indications and guidelines for performance of transesophageal echocardiography in the patient with pediatric acquired or congenital heart disease: Report from the task force of the Pediatric Council of the American Society of Echocardiography. J Am Soc Echocardiogr 18:91-98, 2005.
11. Hung J, Lang R, Flachskampf F, et al: 3-D echocardiography: A review of the current status and future directions. J Am Soc Echocardiogr 20:213-233, 2007.
12. Zoghbi WA, Enriquez-Sarano M, Foster E, et al: Recommendations for evaluation of the severity of native valvular regurgitation with two-dimensional and Doppler echocardiography. J Am Soc Echocardiogr 16:777-802, 2003.
13. Pai RG, Bodenheimer MM, Pai SM, et al: Usefulness of systolic excursion of the mitral anulus as an index of left ventricular systolic function. Am J Cardiol 67:222-224, 1991.
14. Mishiro Y, Oki T, Yamada H, et al: Evaluation of left ventricular contraction abnormalities in patients with dilated cardiomyopathy with the use of pulsed tissue Doppler imaging. J Am Soc Echocardiogr 12:913-920, 1999.
15. Yamada H, Oki T, Mishiro Y, et al: Effect of aging on diastolic left ventricular myocardial velocities measured by pulsed tissue Doppler imaging in healthy subjects. J Am Soc Echocardiogr 12:574-581, 1999.
16. Gorcsan J 3rd, Strum DP, Mandarino WA, et al: Quantitative assessment of alterations in regional left ventricular contractility with color-coded tissue Doppler echocardiography. Comparison with sonomicrometry and pressure-volume relations. Circulation 95:2423-2433, 1997.
17. Alam M, Wardell J, Andersson E, et al: Effects of first myocardial infarction on left ventricular systolic and diastolic function with the use of mitral annular velocity determined by pulsed wave Doppler tissue imaging. J Am Soc Echocardiogr 13:343-352, 2000.
18. Ama R, Segers P, Roosens C, et al: The effects of load on systolic mitral annular velocity by tissue Doppler imaging. Anesth Analg 99:332-338, 2004.
19. Hulyalkar AR, Ayd JD: Low risk of gastroesophageal injury associated with transesophageal echocardiography during cardiac surgery. J Cardiothorac Vasc Anesth 7:175-177, 1993.
20. Rousou JA, Tighe DA, Garb JL, et al: Risk of dysphagia after transesophageal echocardiography during cardiac operations. Ann Thorac Surg 69:486-489, 2000.
21. Huang CH, Lu CW, Lin TY, et al: Complications of intraoperative transesophageal echocardiography in adult cardiac surgical patients—experience of two institutions in Taiwan. J Formos Med Assoc 106:92-95, 2007.
22. Olenchock SA Jr, Lukaszczyk JJ, Reed J 3rd, Theman TE: Splenic injury after intraoperative transesophageal echocardiography. Ann Thorac Surg 72:2141-2143, 2001.
23. Chow MS, Taylor MA, Hanson CW 3rd: Splenic laceration associated with transesophageal echocardiography. J Cardiothorac Vasc Anesth 12:314-316, 1998.
24. Daniel WG, Erbel R, Kasper W, et al: Safety of transesophageal echocardiography. A multicenter survey of 10,419 examinations. Circulation 83:817-821, 1991.
25. Mentec H, Vignon P, Terre S, et al: Frequency of bacteremia associated with transesophageal echocardiography in intensive care unit patients: A prospective study of 139 patients. Crit Care Med 23:1194-1199, 1995.
26. Read RC, Finch RG, Donald FE, et al: Infective endocarditis after transesophageal echocardiography. Circulation 87:1426, 1993.
27. Stevenson JG: Incidence of complications in pediatric transesophageal echocardiography: Experience in 1650 cases. J Am Soc Echocardiogr 12:527-532, 1999.
28. Miller JP, Lambert AS, Shapiro WA, et al: The adequacy of basic intraoperative transesophageal echocardiography performed by experienced anesthesiologists. Anesth Analg 92:1103-1110, 2001.
29. Lambert AS, Miller JP, Merrick SH, et al: Improved evaluation of the location and mechanism of mitral valve regurgitation with a systematic transesophageal echocardiography examination. Anesth Analg 88:1205-1212, 1999.
30. Kircher BJ, Himelman RB, Schiller NB: Noninvasive estimation of right atrial pressure from the inspiratory collapse of the inferior vena cava. Am J Cardiol 66:493-496, 1990.
31. Cheung AT, Savino JS, Weiss SJ, et al: Echocardiographic and hemodynamic indexes of left ventricular preload in patients with normal and abnormal ventricular function. Anesthesiology 81:376-387, 1994.
32. Tousignant CP, Walsh F, Mazer CD: The use of transesophageal echocardiography for preload assessment in critically ill patients. Anesth Analg 90:351-355, 2000.
33. Swenson JD, Bull D, Stringham J: Subjective assessment of left ventricular preload using transesophageal echocardiography: Corresponding pulmonary artery occlusion pressures. J Cardiothorac Vasc Anesth 15:580-583, 2001.
34. Kuecherer HF, Muhiudeen IA, Kusumoto FM, et al: Estimation of mean left atrial pressure from transesophageal pulsed Doppler echocardiography of pulmonary venous flow. Circulation 82:1127-1139, 1990.
35. Kusumoto FM, Muhiudeen IA, Kuecherer HF, et al: Response of the interatrial septum to transatrial pressure gradients and its potential for predicting pulmonary capillary wedge pressure: An intraoperative study using transesophageal echocardiography in patients during mechanical ventilation. J Am Coll Cardiol 21:721-728, 1993.
36. Nomura M, Hillel Z, Shih H, et al: The association between Doppler transmitral flow variables measured by transesophageal echocardiography and pulmonary capillary wedge pressure. Anesth Analg 84:491-496, 1997.
37. Balik M, Pachl J, Hendl J, et al: Effect of the degree of tricuspid regurgitation on cardiac output measurements by thermodilution. Intensive Care Med 28:1117-1121, 2002.
38. Darmon PL, Hillel Z, Mogtader A, et al: Cardiac output by transesophageal echocardiography using continuous-wave Doppler across the aortic valve. Anesthesiology 80:796-805, 1994.
39. Hoit BD: Left ventricular diastolic function. Crit Care Med 35:S340-S347, 2007.
40. Aurigemma GP, Gaasch WH: Clinical practice. Diastolic heart failure. N Engl J Med 351:1097-1105, 2004.
41. Oh JK, Hatle L, Tajik AJ, Little WC: Diastolic heart failure can be diagnosed by comprehensive two-dimensional and Doppler echocardiography. J Am Coll Cardiol 47:500-506, 2006.
42. Reichert CL, Visser CA, Koolen JJ, et al: Transesophageal echocardiography in hypotensive patients after cardiac operations. Comparison with hemodynamic parameters. J Thorac Cardiovasc Surg 104:321-326, 1992.
43. Cicek S, Demirilic U, Kuralay E, et al: Transesophageal echocardiography in cardiac surgical emergencies. J Card Surg 10:236-244, 1995.
44. Cook CH, Praba AC, Beery PR, Martin LC: Transthoracic echocardiography is not cost-effective in critically ill surgical patients. J Trauma 52:280-284, 2002.
45. Heidenreich PA, Stainback RF, Redberg RF, et al: Transesophageal echocardiography predicts mortality in critically ill patients with unexplained hypotension. J Am Coll Cardiol 26:152-158, 1995.
46. van der Wouw PA, Koster RW, Delemarre BJ, et al: Diagnostic accuracy of transesophageal echocardiography during cardiopulmonary resuscitation. J Am Coll Cardiol 30:780-783, 1997.
47. Smith JS, Cahalan MK, Benefiel DJ, et al: Intraoperative detection of myocardial ischemia in high-risk patients: Electrocardiography versus two-

dimensional transesophageal echocardiography. Circulation 72:1015-1021, 1985.
48. van Daele ME, Sutherland GR, Mitchell MM, et al: Do changes in pulmonary capillary wedge pressure adequately reflect myocardial ischemia during anesthesia? A correlative preoperative hemodynamic, electrocardiographic, and transesophageal echocardiographic study. Circulation 81:865-871, 1990.
49. Rouine-Rapp K, Ionescu P, Balea M, et al: Detection of intraoperative segmental wall-motion abnormalities by transesophageal echocardiography: The incremental value of additional cross sections in the transverse and longitudinal planes. Anesth Analg 83:1141-1148, 1996.
50. Cwajg JM, Cwajg E, Nagueh SF, et al: End-diastolic wall thickness as a predictor of recovery of function in myocardial hibernation: Relation to rest-redistribution T1-201 tomography and dobutamine stress echocardiography. J Am Coll Cardiol 35:1152-1161, 2000.
51. Afridi I, Kleiman NS, Raizner AE, Zoghbi WA: Dobutamine echocardiography in myocardial hibernation. Optimal dose and accuracy in predicting recovery of ventricular function after coronary angioplasty. Circulation 91:663-670, 1995.
52. Seeberger MD, Cahalan MK, Rouine-Rapp K, et al: Acute hypovolemia may cause segmental wall motion abnormalities in the absence of myocardial ischemia. Anesth Analg 85:1252-1257, 1997.
53. Qaddoura FE, Abel MD, Mecklenburg KL, et al: Role of intraoperative transesophageal echocardiography in patients having coronary artery bypass graft surgery. Ann Thorac Surg 78:1586-1590, 2004.
54. Click RL, Abel MD, Schaff HV: Intraoperative transesophageal echocardiography: 5-year prospective review of impact on surgical management. Mayo Clin Proc 75:241-247, 2000.
55. Mishra M, Chauhan R, Sharma KK, et al: Real-time intraoperative transesophageal echocardiography—how useful? Experience of 5,016 cases. J Cardiothorac Vasc Anesth 12:625-632, 1998.
56. Mihalatos DG, Gopal AS, Kates R, et al: Intraoperative assessment of mitral regurgitation: Role of phenylephrine challenge. J Am Soc Echocardiogr 19:1158-1164, 2006.
57. Schroder JN, Williams ML, Hata JA, et al: Impact of mitral valve regurgitation evaluated by intraoperative transesophageal echocardiography on long-term outcomes after coronary artery bypass grafting. Circulation 112:I293-I298, 2005.
58. Buckmaster MJ, Kearney PA, Johnson SB, et al: Further experience with transesophageal echocardiography in the evaluation of thoracic aortic injury. J Trauma 37:989-995, 1994.
59. Vignon P, Gueret P, Vedrinne JM, et al: Role of transesophageal echocardiography in the diagnosis and management of traumatic aortic disruption. Circulation 92:2959-2968, 1995.
60. Erbel R, Engberding R, Daniel W, et al: Echocardiography in diagnosis of aortic dissection. Lancet 1:457-461, 1989.
61. Torossov M, Singh A, Fein SA: Clinical presentation, diagnosis, and hospital outcome of patients with documented aortic dissection: The Albany Medical Center experience, 1986 to 1996. Am Heart J 137:154-161, 1999.
62. Nienaber CA, von Kodolitsch Y, Nicolas V, et al: The diagnosis of thoracic aortic dissection by noninvasive imaging procedures. N Engl J Med 328:1-9, 1993.
63. Movsowitz HD, Levine RA, Hilgenberg AD, Isselbacher EM: Transesophageal echocardiographic description of the mechanisms of aortic regurgitation in acute type A aortic dissection: Implications for aortic valve repair. J Am Coll Cardiol 36:884-890, 2000.
64. Katz ES, Tunick PA, Rusinek H, et al: Protruding aortic atheromas predict stroke in elderly patients undergoing cardiopulmonary bypass: Experience with intraoperative transesophageal echocardiography. J Am Coll Cardiol 20:70-77, 1992.
65. Gold JP, Torres KE, Maldarelli W, et al: Improving outcomes in coronary surgery: The impact of echo-directed aortic cannulation and perioperative hemodynamic management in 500 patients. Ann Thorac Surg 78:1579-1585, 2004.
66. Hartman GS, Yao FS, Bruefach MR, et al: Severity of aortic atheromatous disease diagnosed by transesophageal echocardiography predicts stroke and other outcomes associated with coronary artery surgery: A prospective study. Anesth Analg 83:701-708, 1996.
67. Konstadt SN, Reich DL, Kahn R, Viggiani RF: Transesophageal echocardiography can be used to screen for ascending aortic atherosclerosis. Anesth Analg 81:25-28, 1995.
68. Trehan N, Mishra M, Kasliwal RR, Mishra A: Reduced neurological injury during CABG in patients with mobile aortic atheromas: A five-year follow-up study. Ann Thorac Surg 70:1558-1564, 2000.
69. Mishra M, Malhotra R, Karlekar A, et al: Propensity case-matched analysis of off-pump versus on-pump coronary artery bypass grafting in patients with atheromatous aorta. Ann Thorac Surg 82:608-614, 2006.
70. Agricola E, Oppizzi M, Maisano F, et al: Detection of mechanisms of immediate failure by transesophageal echocardiography in quadrangular resection mitral valve repair technique for severe mitral regurgitation. Am J Cardiol 91:175-179, 2003.
71. Shin HJ, Lee YJ, Choo SJ, et al: Analysis of recurrent mitral regurgitation after mitral valve repair. Asian Cardiovasc Thorac Ann 13:261-266, 2005.
72. Brown ML, Abel MD, Click RL, et al: Systolic anterior motion after mitral valve repair: Is surgical intervention necessary? J Thorac Cardiovasc Surg 133:136-143, 2007.
73. Shapira Y, Vaturi M, Weisenberg DE, et al: Impact of intraoperative transesophageal echocardiography in patients undergoing valve replacement. Ann Thorac Surg 78:579-583, 2004.
74. Hoffmann R, Flachskampf FA, Hanrath P: Planimetry of orifice area in aortic stenosis using multiplane transesophageal echocardiography. J Am Coll Cardiol 22:529-534, 1993.
75. Blumberg FC, Pfeifer M, Holmer SR, et al: Transgastric Doppler echocardiographic assessment of the severity of aortic stenosis using multiplane transesophageal echocardiography. Am J Cardiol 79:1273-1275, 1997.
76. Moisa RB, Zeldis SM, Alper SA, Scott WC: Aortic regurgitation in coronary artery bypass grafting: Implications for cardioplegia administration. Ann Thorac Surg 60:665-668, 1995.
77. Stoddard MF, Prince CR, Tuman WL, Wagner SG: Angle of incidence does not affect accuracy of mitral stenosis area calculation by pressure half-time: Application to Doppler transesophageal echocardiography. Am Heart J 127:1562-1572, 1994.
78. Himelman RB, Kusumoto F, Oken K, et al: The flail mitral valve: Echocardiographic findings by precordial and transesophageal imaging and Doppler color flow mapping. J Am Coll Cardiol 17:272-279, 1991.
79. Klein AL, Obarski TP, Stewart WJ, et al: Transesophageal Doppler echocardiography of pulmonary venous flow: A new marker of mitral regurgitation severity. J Am Coll Cardiol 18:518-526, 1991.
80. Savage RM, Lytle BW, Aronson S, et al: Intraoperative echocardiography is indicated in high risk coronary bypass surgery. Ann Thorac Surg 64:368-373, 1997.
81. Stevenson JG, Sorensen GK, Gartman DM, et al: Transesophageal echocardiography during repair of congenital cardiac defects: Identification of residual problems necessitating reoperation. J Am Soc Echocardiogr 6:356-365, 1993.
82. Stevenson JG: Adherence to physician training guidelines for pediatric transesophageal echocardiography affects the outcome of patients undergoing repair of congenital cardiac defects. J Am Soc Echocardiogr 12:165-172, 1999.
83. Russell IA, Rouine-Rapp K, Stratmann G, Miller-Hance WC: Congenital heart disease in the adult: A review with Internet-accessible transesophageal echocardiographic images. Anesth Analg 102:694-723, 2006.
84. Chumnanvej S, Wood MJ, MacGillivray TE, Melo MF: Perioperative echocardiographic examination for ventricular assist device implantation. Anesth Analg 105:583-601, 2007.
85. Shanewise JS, Zaffer R, Martin RP: Intraoperative echocardiography and minimally invasive cardiac surgery. Echocardiography 19:579-582, 2002.
86. Schulmeyer MC, Santelices E, Vega R, Schmied S: Impact of intraoperative transesophageal echocardiography during noncardiac surgery. J Cardiothorac Vasc Anesth 20:768-771, 2006.
87. Burns JM, Sing RF, Mostafa G, et al: The role of transesophageal echocardiography in optimizing resuscitation in acutely injured patients. J Trauma 59:36-40, discussion 40-42, 2005.
88. Denault AY, Couture P, McKenty S, et al: Perioperative use of transesophageal echocardiography by anesthesiologists: Impact in noncardiac surgery and in the intensive care unit. Can J Anaesth 49:287-293, 2002.
89. Porembka DT: Importance of transesophageal echocardiography in the critically ill and injured patient. Crit Care Med 35:S414-S430, 2007.
90. Mathew JP, Glas K, Troianos CA, et al: ASE/SCA recommendations and guidelines for continuous quality improvement in perioperative echocardiography. Anesth Analg 103:1416-1425, 2006.

Zak Hillel and Giora Landesberg

42 Electrocardiography

Key Points

1. Electrocardiographic monitoring is mandatory and a standard of care.
2. Electrocardiography permits detection of electrical disturbances that may influence the mechanical function of the heart.
3. With carefully selected lead combinations, most arrhythmias and myocardial ischemic events can be detected in the perioperative setting.
4. Appropriate diagnosis of arrhythmias and ischemia will allow proper and effective treatment.

The electrocardiogram (ECG) was first invented by William Einthoven in 1901, who used a string galvanogram for his recordings. This time-honored and relatively simple tool remains, even today, a mainstay in clinical cardiac diagnosis and therapy. In the perioperative setting, electrocardiography serves two main functions: diagnosis and monitoring. In the preoperative period, the standard 12-lead ECG is performed mainly for risk assessment. It is used to provide information on the patient's baseline (chronic) cardiac status with regard to myocardial ischemia and conduction or rhythm abnormalities as part of the whole preoperative clinical assessment. Occasionally, the preoperative ECG may reveal acute or new abnormalities, especially when dealing with urgent or emergency operations, and in such cases comparing current with previous ECGs is of extreme importance. During and after surgery the ECG is used mainly for monitoring to detect changes in rate and rhythm or myocardial ischemia. With many patients undergoing surgery with pacemakers or implantable cardiac defibrillators in place, the ECG enables the anesthesiologist to monitor the proper function of these devices during the surgical procedure. Perioperative management of these devices is described in Chapter 43. During cardiac surgery, both myocardial ischemia and different types of arrhythmia are common, especially after separation from cardiopulmonary bypass. Proper diagnosis and management of intraoperative ischemia and arrhythmias are part of the expertise of the anesthesiologist. A postoperative 12-lead ECG is often obtained in patients at high cardiac risk when new ischemic or rhythm changes are suspected. In all these scenarios, a good understanding of the principles of interpretation of the ECG is vital for the clinical anesthesiologist. This chapter is intended to cover most aspects of interpretation of the ECG, with special emphasis on issues relevant to anesthesia and perioperative care.

Electrocardiographic Lead Systems

Standard Recording Electrodes and Leads

The small electric currents produced by the electrical activity of cardiac muscle spread an electrical field throughout the body that behaves as a volume conductor, which allows it to be recorded at various sites on the surface of the body as electrocardiographic signals. The electrical potentials reaching the skin are recorded by electrodes (leads) placed at specific locations, and the output of these leads is amplified, filtered, and displayed on various electronic devices. There are two types of electrocardiographic leads: *bipolar* and *unipolar*. A bipolar lead consists of two electrodes placed at different sites to measure the difference in potential between them. Unipolar leads measure the "absolute" electrical potential at one site in relation to a *reference*, or *remote site*, at which the potential is deemed to be zero. The standard clinical ECG includes recordings from 12 leads. These 12 leads include three *bipolar* (leads I, II, and III), six *unipolar precordial* (leads V_1 through V_6), and three *modified unipolar limb leads* (the augmented limb leads aVR, aVL, and aVF) (Table 42-1).

Standard Electrocardiographic Recordings

The ECG is normally recorded on special paper consisting of grids of horizontal and vertical lines. Distances between vertical lines represent time intervals, whereas distances between hori-

Table 42-1 Location of electrodes and lead connections for the standard 12-lead electrocardiogram and additional leads

Lead Type	Positive Input	Negative (Reference) Input
Bipolar Limb Leads		
Lead I	Left arm	Right arm
Lead II	Left leg	Right arm
Lead III	Left leg	Left arm
Augmented Unipolar Limb Leads		
aVR	Right arm	Left arm plus left leg
aVL	Left arm	Right arm plus left leg
aVF	Left leg	Left arm plus left arm
Precordial Leads		
V_1	Right sternal margin, 4th intercostals space	Wilson central terminal
V_2	Left sternal margin, 4th intercostal space	Wilson central terminal
V_3	Midway between V_2 and V_4	Wilson central terminal
V_4	Left midclavicular line, 5th intercostal space	Wilson central terminal
V_5	Left anterior axillary line	Wilson central terminal
V_6	Left midaxillary line	Wilson central terminal

Adapted from Zipes DP, Libby P, Bonow R, Braunwald E: Braunwald's Heart Disease: A Textbook of Cardiovascular Medicine, 7th ed. Philadelphia, WB Saunders, 2005.

zontal lines represent voltage. The lines are 1 mm apart, with every fifth line intensified. The speed of the paper is standardized to 25 mm/sec. On the horizontal axis, 1 mm represents 0.04 second, and 0.5 cm represents 0.20 second. On the vertical axis, 10 mm represents 1 mV. On every recording, a 1-cm (1-mV) calibration mark should indicate that the ECG is appropriately calibrated.

Normal Electrical Activity

P Wave

Under normal circumstances, the sinoatrial (SA) node has the most rapid spontaneous depolarization rate and is therefore the dominant cardiac pacemaker. From the SA node, the impulse normally spreads to the atrioventricular (AV) node through one left-sided and two right-sided pathways. The P wave is the result of normal depolarization of the atria, and identification of this wave is important for determination of normal sinus rhythm. The anatomically anterior right atrium is activated earlier, and only later does the signal shift posteriorly as activation proceeds over the left atrium. Therefore, the P wave in the right precordial leads (V_1 and, occasionally, V_2) is commonly biphasic, a positive deflection followed by a negative one, whereas in the lateral leads, the P wave is upright and reflects right-to-left spread of the activation front.

PR Interval

The PR interval is the temporal bridge between atrial and ventricular activation, during which the AV node, the bundle of His, the bundle branches, and the intraventricular conduction systems are activated (Fig. 42-1). Most of the conduction delay during this segment is due to slow conduction within the AV node. The normal PR interval is 120 to 200 msec in duration.

Myocardial Activation—The QRS Complex

The QRS complex is the manifestation of left and right ventricular muscle depolarization. Its pattern in each electrocardiographic lead represents the sum of all electrical forces emanating from the wavefront propagation of ventricular electrical excitation aimed in the direction of that lead. Ventricular excitation spreads within several milliseconds from the bundle branches to the His-Purkinje fibers, which are dispersed broadly throughout the entire endocardial surfaces of both ventricles. Excitation of the Purkinje–ventricular muscle junctions in the endocardium then proceeds by conduction from muscle cell to muscle cell to activate the entire ventricle thickness toward the epicardium. The normal pattern of activation of the ventricles starts in the interventricular septum with a vector oriented from left to right in the frontal plane and anteriorly in the horizontal plane (as determined by the anatomic position of the septum within the chest). This produces an initial small positive R wave in the right-sided leads (aVR and V_1) and small negative waves (septal q waves—less than 30 to 40 msec) in the left-sided leads (I, aVL, V_5, and V_6). Subsequent QRS complex elements reflect activation of the free walls of the left and right ventricles. Because the right ventricular muscle mass is considerably smaller than that of the left ventricle, the QRS primarily represents left ventricular (LV) activity with its main vector proceeding from right to left in the axial plane and anterior followed by posterior vectors in the horizontal plane (R wave followed by a small S wave in the left-sided leads). The

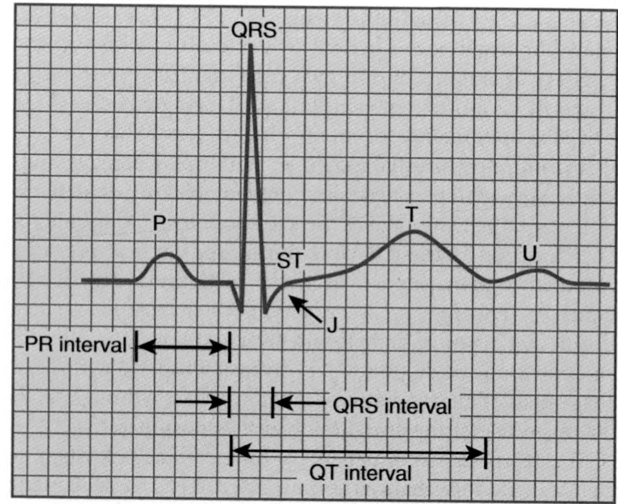

Figure 42-1 Waves and intervals of a normal electrocardiogram. *(From Goldberger AL: Clinical Electrocardiography: A Simplified Approach, 6th ed. St Louis, CV Mosby, 1999; and Zipes DP, Libby P, Bonow R, Braunwald E: Braunwald's Heart Disease: A Textbook of Cardiovascular Medicine, 7th ed. Philadelphia, WB Saunders, 2005.)*

main vector of the QRS complex in the frontal plane serves to calculate the electrical axis of the heart, which is normally between −30 and +90 degrees. An axis more negative than −30 degrees is called *left axis deviation*, and an axis higher than +90 degrees is termed *right axis deviation*. The duration of the normal QRS complex is less than 120 msec.

ST Segment and T Wave

Repolarization of the ventricles generates the ST segment and T wave. Repolarization, like activation, occurs in a characteristic geometric pattern. Because the endocardial action potential lasts longer than that of its overlying epicardium, repolarization of the epicardium often starts earlier than in the endocardium. However, under normal conditions, there are regional differences in electrical recovery properties of the ventricles, and the transmural gradients predominantly determine the ST patterns.

Normally, there is concordance between the orientation of the QRS complex and the T wave, with both deflecting in the same direction. The junction of the QRS and the ST segment is called the J junction. The QT interval—the duration from the Q wave to the end of the T wave—is highly dependent on heart rate, and formulas have been developed to calculate the corrected QT interval (QTc), which if prolonged may be associated with serious ventricular arrhythmias. The T wave is sometimes followed by a small U wave, which may be associated with hypokalemia or hypomagnesemia (see Fig. 42-1). An example of a normal 12-lead electrocardiogram is shown in Figure 42-2.

The Abnormal Electrocardiogram

Atrial Abnormality

Initiation of atrial electrical activation from a site other than the SA node occurs in one of two ways: either as an escape rhythm if the normal SA nodal pacemaker slows or fails or as an accelerated atrial ectopic rhythm if the automaticity of the ectopic site is associated with a rate higher than the SA node. Ectopic atrial activation is often manifested by an abnormal morphology of the P wave (different from the native P). Most commonly, negative P waves are seen in the leads where the P wave is normally upright (leads I, II, aVF, and V_4 through V_6), with or without shortening of the PR interval. The exact site of an ectopic atrial pacemaker is usually of little clinical significance except that left-sided atrial ectopy is seen more often in association with LV or left heart valvular abnormalities, whereas right-sided ectopy is more common in patients with chronic obstructive lung disease or other causes of right heart dysfunction.

Ventricular Hypertrophy and Enlargement

Left ventricular hypertrophy (LVH) or enlargement produces changes throughout the QRST complex. The most characteristic change is increased voltage of the QRS complex: tall R waves in the left-sided leads (I, aVL, V_5, and V_6) and deep S waves in the right-sided leads (V_1 and V_2). ST-segment and T-wave amplitudes can be normal or increased. ST-segment depression with downsloping from a depressed J point and inverted asymmetric T waves are common in long-standing and severe LVH. Similarly, a QRS duration prolonged beyond 110 msec reflects the longer duration of activation of the thickened ventricular wall. Many sets of diagnostic electrocardiographic criteria for LVH have been developed, although their diagnostic importance in the era of echocardiography has obviously diminished. For example, Sokolow and Lyon found the following voltage criteria to correlate best with postmortem pathologic findings of LVH: SV_1 + (RV_5 or RV_6) > 3.5 mV or RaVL > 1.1 mV (or both) (Fig. 42-3).

Right ventricular hypertrophy is manifested on the ECG by abnormally tall R waves in the rightward-directed leads (aVR, V_1, and V_2), reversal of normal R-wave progression in the precordial leads, deep S waves with abnormally small R waves in the left-sided leads (I, aVL, V_5, and V_6), and marked right axis deviation (>110 degrees). Chronic obstructive pulmonary disease can lead to right ventricular hypertrophy, changes in the position of the heart within the chest, and hyperinflation of the lungs. Acute right ventricular pressure overload, such as that caused by pulmonary embolism, can produce a characteristic pattern on the ECG: a QR or qR pattern in the right-sided leads, an $S_1Q_3T_3$ pattern, and an acute incomplete or complete right bundle branch block (RBBB). However, even the classic $S_1Q_3T_3$ pattern occurs in only about 10% of cases of acute pulmonary embolism (Fig. 42-4).

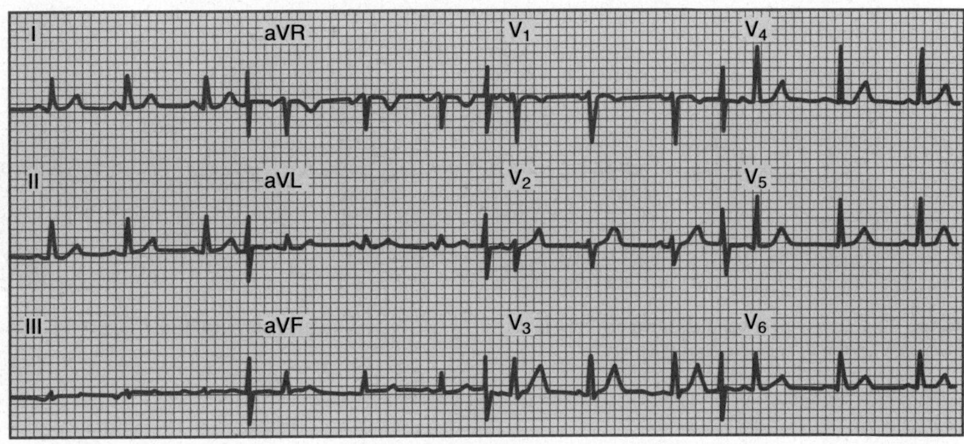

Figure 42-2 Example of a normal 12-lead electrocardiogram. *(From Zipes DP, Libby P, Bonow R, Braunwald E: Braunwald's Heart Disease: A Textbook of Cardiovascular Medicine, 7th ed. Philadelphia, WB Saunders, 2005.)*

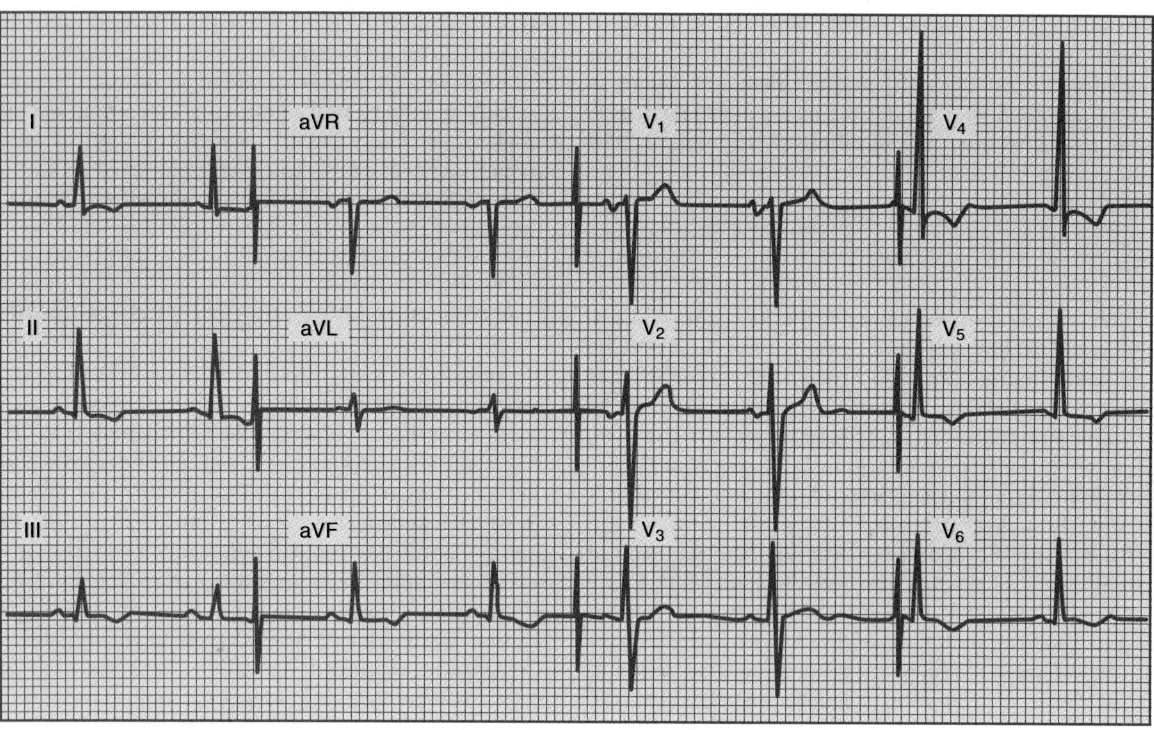

Figure 42-3 Left ventricular hypertrophy on electrocardiography. Tall R waves on the left-sided leads and deep S waves on the right-sided ones, down-sloping ST-segment depression and T-wave inversion opposite the main R-wave axis, and a biphasic p wave signify left atrial abnormality. *(From Zipes DP, Libby P, Bonow R, Braunwald E: Braunwald's Heart Disease: A Textbook of Cardiovascular Medicine, 7th ed. Philadelphia, WB Saunders, 2005.)*

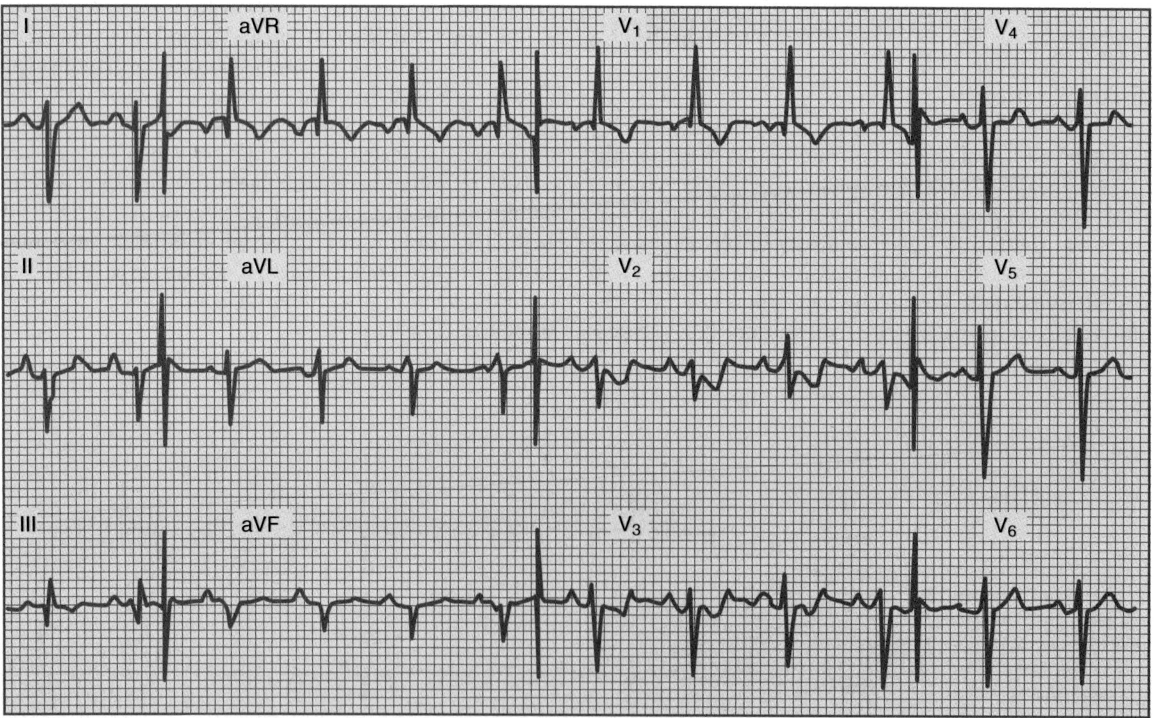

Figure 42-4 Severe right ventricular hypertrophy indicated by tall R waves on the right-sided leads, deep S waves on the left-sided leads, and T-wave inversions on the right-sided leads ($S_1Q_3T_3$).

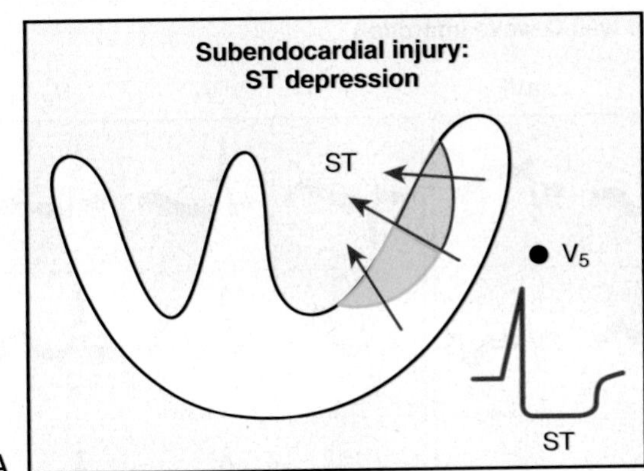

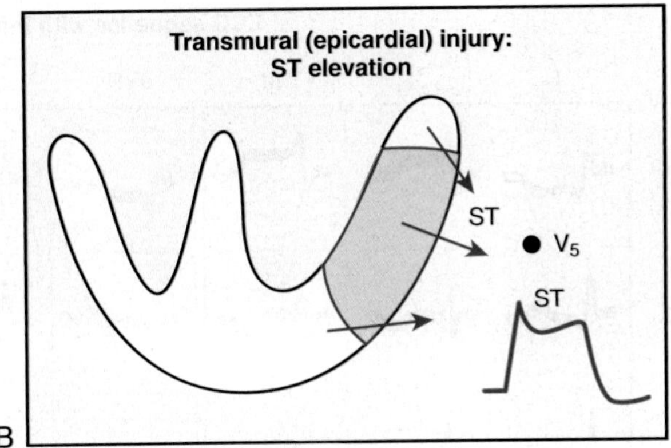

Figure 42-5 Patterns of injury currents. **A,** Acute subendocardial, ST-depression type. **B,** Transmural, ST-elevation type (ischemia). *(From Zipes: Braunwald's Heart Disease: A Textbook of Cardiovascular Medicine, 7th ed.)*

Myocardial Ischemia

The ST-T segment, representing myocardial repolarization, is the component of the ECG most sensitive to acute myocardial ischemia. ST elevation, which may be accompanied by tall positive (hyperacute) T waves, indicates transmural ischemia and is most often the result of acute coronary artery occlusion caused by either coronary thrombosis or vasospasm (Prinzmetal's variant angina). Reciprocal ST depression may appear in the contralateral leads. Ischemia confined to the subendocardial area is usually denoted by ST-segment depression. Subendocardial, ST depression–type ischemia typically occurs during episodes of symptomatic or asymptomatic ("silent") stable angina pectoris. It is characteristic of ischemia occurring during exercise, tachycardia, or a pharmacologic stress test in patients with significant but stable coronary artery disease (CAD) (Fig. 42-5).

Myocardial Infarction

With prolonged ischemia, there is a risk of developing myocardial necrosis or myocardial infarction (MI). The electrocardiographic manifestation of MI includes decreased R-wave amplitude and pathologic Q waves (>1 mm in depth and >40 msec in duration), which may develop as a result of loss of electromotive forces in the infarcted area. Transmural infarctions are more likely to culminate in pathologic Q waves, whereas subendocardial (nontransmural) infarcts are less likely to produce Q waves. However, pathologic studies have shown such a wide overlap between the two entities and their electrocardiographic expression that "Q-wave" or "non–Q-wave" infarction is not synonymous with transmural or nontransmural infarction. Pathologic Q waves usually develop days after the onset of acute MI, and once they develop, they infrequently disappear and serve as an indicator of the location of the infarction. Persistent T-wave inversion may also be the only sign of chronic ischemia and recent or old MI. Pathologic Q waves with ST elevation that persists for weeks or longer after MI correlate strongly with severe myocardial mechanical dysfunction, akinesis, or ventricular aneurysm.

Electrocardiographic leads demonstrating ST-T changes or Q waves may help define the location and the coronary artery responsible for the ischemia or MI. For example, precordial leads V_1 to V_3 correspond to the anteroseptal or apical walls of the left ventricle; leads V_4 to V_6 to the apical or lateral LV walls (Fig. 42-6); leads II, III, and aVF to the inferior LV wall (Fig. 42-7); and the

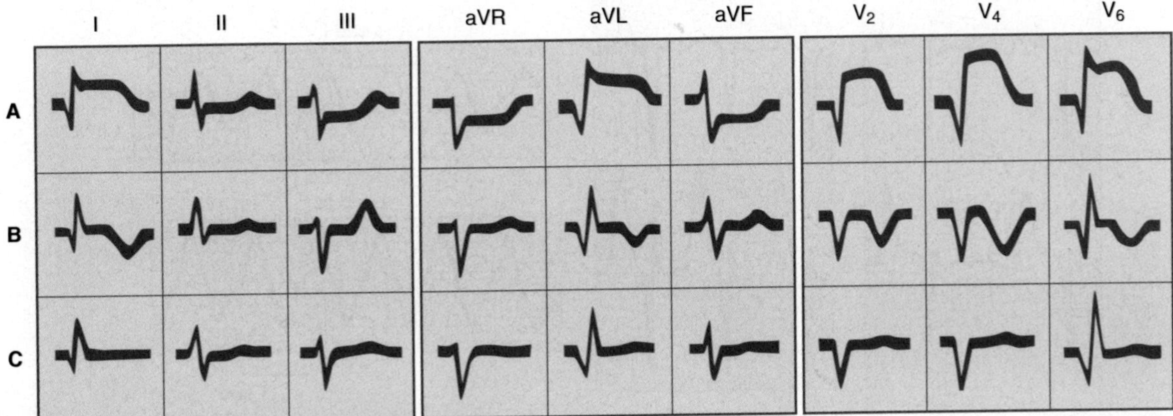

Figure 42-6 Acute, ST-elevation–type anterior wall myocardial infarction. **A,** Acute phase: ST elevations and new Q waves. **B,** Evolving phase: deep T-wave inversions. **C,** Resolving phase: partial or complete regression of the ST-T changes (and sometimes Q waves). Notice the reciprocal ST-T changes in the inferior leads (II, III, and aVF). *(From Goldberger AL: Clinical Electrocardiography: A Simplified Approach, 7th ed. St Louis, CV Mosby, 2006.)*

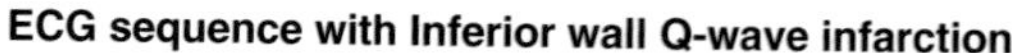

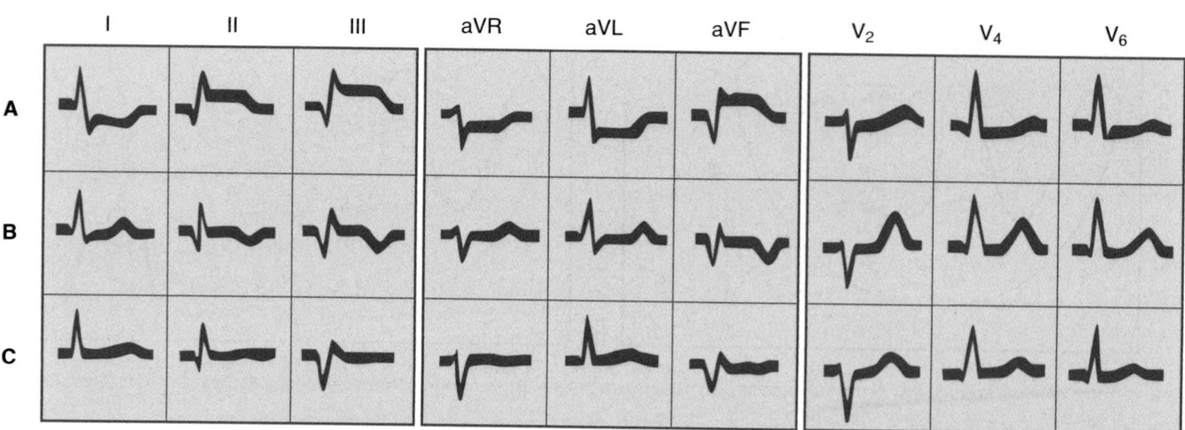

Figure 42-7 Inferior wall myocardial infarction. **A,** Acute phase: ST elevations and new Q waves. **B,** Evolving phase: deep T-wave inversions. **C,** Resolving phase: partial or complete regression of the ST-T changes (and sometimes Q waves). Notice the reciprocal ST-T changes in the anterior leads (I, aVL, and V_2). *(From Goldberger AL: Clinical Electrocardiography: A Simplified Approach, 7th ed. St Louis, CV Mosby, 2006.)*

right-sided leads to the right ventricle. Posterior wall infarction induces ST elevation or Q waves in leads placed over the left side and back (V_7 to V_9), and reciprocal ST depression or tall R′ waves may develop in leads V_1 to V_3.

Electrolyte Abnormalities

The ECG is affected not only by structural or functional myocardial abnormalities but also by numerous metabolic and electrolyte aberrations (see Chapter 54).

CALCIUM. Hypercalcemia shortens and hypocalcemia prolongs phase 2 of the action potential duration, thus leading to abbreviation or prolongation of the QT interval, respectively. Severe hypercalcemia (e.g., total serum Ca^{2+} >15 mg/dL) causes a decrease in T-wave amplitude or T-wave inversion, and hypercalcemia may produce a high-takeoff ST segment in leads V_1 and V_2 simulating acute ischemia.

POTASSIUM. Hyperkalemia leads to a distinctive sequence of changes on the ECG, starting with narrowing and peaking of the T wave and shortening of the QT interval. Progressive hyperkalemia causes widening of the QRS complex, a low P-wave amplitude, and prolongation of the PR interval with the possibility of a second- to third-degree AV block (Fig. 42-8). Severe hyperkalemia results in sine-wave ventricular flutter and eventually asystole. Hypokalemia, in contrast, may cause ST depression, flattened T waves, and a prominent U wave that may sometimes exceed the amplitude of T waves. Hypokalemia prolongs repolarization and leads to long QT(U) syndrome, which predisposes to a torsades de pointes–type ventricular fibrillation.

MAGNESIUM. Mild to moderate hypermagnesemia or hypomagnesemia is not associated with specific changes on the ECG. Yet severe hypermagnesemia can cause AV and intraventricular conduction disturbances, including complete heart block and cardiac arrest (Mg^{2+} >15 mEq/L). Hypomagnesemia is often associated with hypocalcemia or hypokalemia

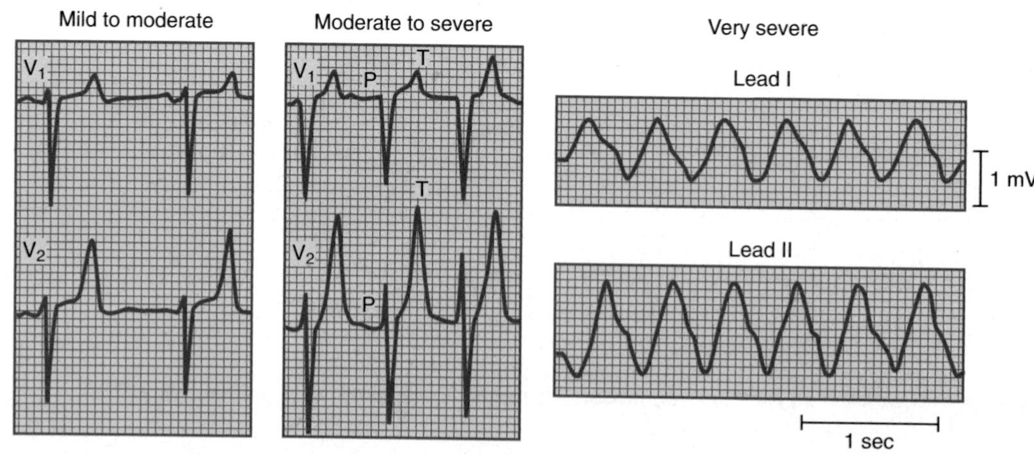

Figure 42-8 Electrocardiographic signs of hyperkalemia. The earliest change with hyperkalemia is peaking ("tenting") of the T waves. With progressive increases in the serum potassium concentration, the QRS complexes widen, the P waves decrease in amplitude and may disappear, and finally a sine-wave pattern leads to asystole unless emergency therapy is initiated. *(From Goldberger AL: Clinical Electrocardiography: A Simplified Approach, 7th ed. St Louis, CV Mosby, 2006.)*

and may predispose to long QT(U) syndrome and torsades de pointes.

Electrocardiographic Monitoring Systems

Noise Filtering

Low-Frequency Filtering. All electrocardiographic monitors use filters to narrow the signal bandwidth in an attempt to reduce environmental artifacts and improve signal quality. Low-frequency noise, such as that produced by respiration or any other patient motion, causes the tracing to wander above and below the baseline. Therefore, low-frequency filters are used in electrocardiographic monitoring. The heart rate in beats per minute forms a rough lower bound for the frequency content in hertz (Hz, cycles per second). Because heart rates below 40 beats/min (0.67 Hz) are uncommon, traditional low-frequency analog filters are used to cut signals off at frequencies below 0.5 Hz. However, such filters introduce considerable distortion on the ECG, particularly with respect to the level of the ST segment. It results in phase nonlinearities in areas of the electrocardiographic signal where frequency content and wave amplitude change abruptly, as occurs where the end of the QRS complex meets the ST segment. The 1975 American Heart Association (AHA) recommendations included a 0.05-Hz low-frequency cutoff for diagnostic electrocardiography. This recommendation preserves the fidelity of repolarization, but it does not eliminate the problem of baseline drift. Current modern digital filtering provides more sophisticated methods to achieve a higher cutoff for low-frequency filtration without the phase distortions seen with analog filtering. Thus, current AHA recommendations[1] to reduce artifactual distortion of the ST segment are that the low-frequency cutoff should be (1) 0.05 Hz for monitors with analog filters and (2) 0.67 Hz or lower for monitors and electrocardiographic recording devices with linear digital filters and zero phase distortion.

High-Frequency Filtering. High-frequency filters are needed to reduce distortions from muscle fasciculations, tremors, and electromagnetic interference from other electrical equipment. Older monitors used a 40-Hz filter to reduce the interference from electrical current. However, the higher the frequencies contained in the filtered signal, the more accurate the measurement of rapid upstroke velocity, peak amplitude, and waves of short duration. A high-frequency cutoff of 100 Hz was considered adequate by the AHA in 1975 to maintain diagnostic accuracy during visual inspection of the ECG, even though it has long been recognized that higher-frequency components of the QRS complex may have clinical significance in patients with various forms of heart disease. According to current AHA recommendations, an upper frequency cutoff of at least 150 Hz is required to accurately measure routine duration and amplitudes in adults, adolescents, and children, and an upper frequency cutoff of 250 Hz is more appropriate for infants.

Most modern electrocardiographic monitors allow the operator a choice of several bandwidths. The actual filter frequencies tend to vary among manufacturers. One manufacturer allows a choice of three different filtering modes: (1) a diagnostic mode with a bandwidth of 0.05 to 130 Hz for adults and 0.5 to 130 Hz for neonates, (2) a monitoring mode with a bandwidth of 0.5 to 40 Hz for adults and 0.5 to 60 Hz for neonates, and (3) a filter mode with a bandwidth of 0.5 to 20 Hz. The importance of bandwidth selection for detection of perioperative myocardial ischemia was evaluated by Slogoff and coworkers, who showed that the position of the ST segment was similar in all systems using the lower filter limit (0.05 Hz) recommended by the AHA.[2]

Three-Electrode Electrocardiographic Monitoring

In contrast to the standard 12-lead ECG, in which the four limb electrodes are placed on the wrists and ankles, electrode placement for continuous cardiac monitoring is on the torso to reduce artifacts from limb movement, as well as to avoid tethering the patient. Therefore, the right and left arm (RA/LA) electrodes are placed in the infraclavicular fossae close to the right and left shoulders, respectively, and the left leg (LL) electrode is placed below the rib cage on the left side of the abdomen. The ground or reference electrode (RL), if present, can be positioned anywhere, but it is usually placed on the right side of the abdomen.

The three-electrode system is the simplest and most common mode of electrocardiographic monitoring in operating rooms and intensive care units (ICUs). It allows monitoring of three bipolar leads by recording the potential difference between each of three pairs of electrodes: lead I (positive electrode, LA; negative electrode, RA), lead II (positive electrode, LL; negative electrode, RA), lead III (positive electrode, LL; negative electrode, LA), or other modified chest leads.[3] Three-electrode monitoring is usually good enough to track the heart rate, detect R waves for synchronized direct-current (DC) shock in cardioversion, and detect ventricular fibrillation. However, it is inadequate for diagnosing more complex arrhythmias, such as distinguishing between RBBB and left bundle-branch block (LBBB) or between ventricular tachycardia (VT) and supraventricular tachycardia (SVT) with aberrant ventricular conduction, for which a "true" V_1 lead is necessary. The three-electrode system is also inadequate for ST-segment monitoring because it does not provide multilead monitoring or precordial leads, which are frequently the most sensitive for detecting ischemia. The older literature[4] suggested that modified chest leads such as CS_5 (RA electrode placed under the right clavicle and LA electrode placed in the V_5 position) or CB_5 (RA electrode over the center of the right scapula and LA electrode in the V_5 position) may be suitable for detection of anterior wall myocardial ischemia; however, these leads are currently considered not accurate enough and are not recommended for monitoring myocardial ischemia.

Five-Electrode Electrocardiographic Monitoring

In the five-electrode monitoring system, the four limb electrodes, LA, RA, LL, and RL placed at their corresponding monitoring locations, allow any of the six limb leads to be obtained (leads I, II, III, aVR, aVL, and aVF), and a fifth chest electrode can be placed in any of the standard V_1 through V_6 locations (Fig. 42-9).

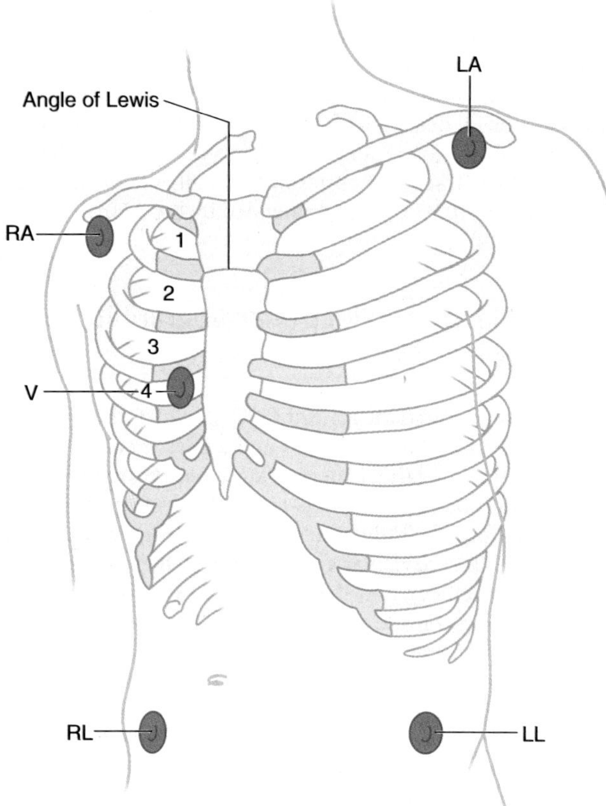

Figure 42-9 Commonly used five-electrode lead system that allows recording any of the six limb leads plus one precordial (V) lead. Shown here is lead placement for recording V_1. A limitation of this system is that only one precordial lead can be recorded. *(From Drew BJ, Califf RM, Funk M, et al: Practice standards for electrocardiographic monitoring in hospital settings: An American Heart Association Scientific Statement from the Councils on Cardiovascular Nursing, Clinical Cardiology, and Cardiovascular Disease in the Young. Circulation 110:2721-2746, 2004.)*

V_1 is the preferred lead for special arrhythmia monitoring, whereas the other precordial leads, especially V_3 to V_5, are the preferred leads for ischemia monitoring. The five-electrode monitoring system is currently the standard for monitoring patients with suspected perioperative myocardial ischemia. Differences in sensitivity and specificity among the different electrocardiographic leads in detecting myocardial ischemia are discussed later.

Ten-Electrode, Twelve-Lead Electrocardiographic Monitoring

Mason and Likar in 1966 introduced a variation on positioning the standard limb electrodes of the 12-lead ECG during exercise stress testing to minimize artifacts in the limb leads caused by movement.[5] In this design, the RA and LA electrodes were attached to the right and left infraclavicular fossae, and the LL electrode was attached to the left iliac fossa. The RL electrode could be placed anywhere but was usually placed on the right iliac fossa for symmetry. Studies have shown that although the limb lead QRS complexes are slightly different in amplitude and axis and the precordial leads may also vary slightly from the standard 12-lead recording, the ST-segment measurements during exercise stress testing were only incidentally affected when the Mason and Likar 12-lead electrocardiographic system was used as compared with the standard 12-lead ECG.[6] A major advantage of cardiac monitors using the Mason-Likar 12-lead system is that ST-segment monitoring software has been developed to analyze all 12 leads and to sound an alarm for ST-segment changes, regardless of whether multiple leads are being displayed on the bedside or central monitor. Therefore, if lead II is being displayed but the patient has a transient ischemic event involving lead V_5, an ST alarm would be triggered. Not all manufacturers who offer the Mason-Likar lead system perform full 12-lead ST-segment analysis, nor do they store all 12 leads for printing at a later time. Another advantage of the Mason-Likar lead system is that more than one precordial lead can be displayed at the same time. The disadvantage of the system for cardiac monitoring is that 10 electrodes are required and the 6 precordial electrodes often interfere with diagnostic (e.g., echocardiography, chest radiography) and emergency (defibrillation sites) procedures. In addition, the precordial sites are difficult to maintain on patients with large breasts or hirsute chests (Fig. 42-10).

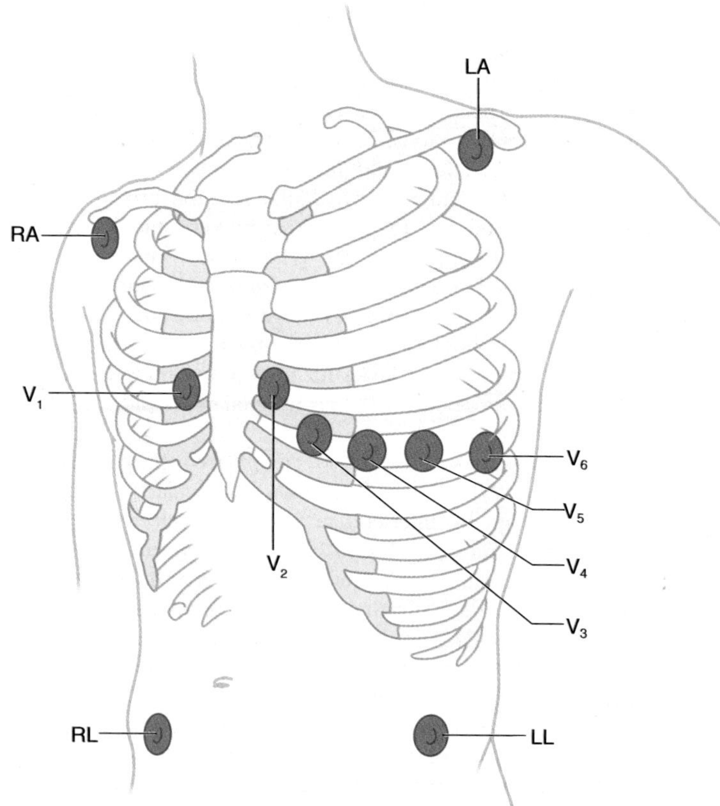

Figure 42-10 Mason-Likar 12-lead electrocardiographic (ECG) system. Anatomic locations for precordial leads are the same as for recording a standard 12-lead electrocardiogram, except that the limb leads are relocated from standard 12-lead ECG positions on the wrists and ankles to the torso. *(From Drew BJ, Califf RM, Funk M, et al: Practice standards for electrocardiographic monitoring in hospital settings: An American Heart Association Scientific Statement from the Councils on Cardiovascular Nursing, Clinical Cardiology, and Cardiovascular Disease in the Young. Circulation 110:2721-2746, 2004.)*

Holter Monitoring

Holter monitoring, originally a cardiologist's tool, has been used by a number of anesthesiologists to document the perioperative incidence of arrhythmias or ischemia. In Holter monitoring, electrocardiographic information from two or three bipolar leads is recorded by a miniature recorder. Up to 48 hours of electrocardiographic signals can be collected. Subsequently, the data are processed via a playback system, and the electrocardiographic signals are analyzed. On most modern systems, the playback unit includes a dedicated computer for rapid analysis and automatic recognition of arrhythmias and ischemia.

A significant early obstacle to the widespread use of conventional Holter monitoring in the perioperative period was the delayed, retrospective analysis and interpretation. This limitation was to some extent overcome by real-time Holter monitors, which both record specific electrocardiographic segments for later playback and also analyze the rhythm and ST segment in real time to alert the user to an acute event.[7,8] Despite significant technical progress, Holter monitoring devices continue to be limited primarily to clinical investigations.

Interpretation and Management of Arrhythmias

There is little doubt that during prolonged visual electrocardiographic monitoring on a video display, arrhythmias may go undetected. It has been demonstrated long ago that coronary care unit staff failed to detect serious ventricular arrhythmias in 84% of their patients.[9] Subsequently, computerized monitors have been designed for the automatic detection of arrhythmias in an attempt to increase the rate of detection of abnormal, potentially dangerous rhythms. These monitors use proprietary sophisticated algorithms such as pattern recognition, measurements of QRS width, onset, offset, and amplitude, and calculations of area to classify complexes into morphologic families.[10,11] Most monitors are capable of detecting potentially fatal arrhythmias such as severe bradycardia or asystole and dangerous tachyarrhythmias such as VT or ventricular fibrillation. Yet no published study has evaluated the accuracy, sensitivity, and specificity of these automated, real-time arrhythmia detection monitors. It has been shown, though, that detection of clinically important arrhythmias in the cardiac ICU improves significantly if a nurse watches the monitor and pays attention to the alarms.[12] Thus, today's computerized monitoring systems still have not achieved the level of accuracy sufficient to eliminate the need for human surveillance; the alarms must be recognized and the ECG interpreted and acted on by a knowledgeable person in a timely fashion.

Diagnosis of Arrhythmias

Arrhythmias are common during and after surgery and have numerous causes. Postoperative dysrhythmias are most likely to occur in patients with structural heart disease. The initiating factor for an arrhythmia after surgery is usually a transient insult such as hypoxemia, cardiac ischemia, catecholamine excess, or electrolyte abnormality.[13] Using perioperative Holter recordings, Mahla and colleagues[14] evaluated how anesthesia and surgery affect the course of ventricular dysrhythmias (premature ventricular beats and repetitive forms of ventricular beats: couplets and nonsustained VT) noted preoperatively in patients with structural heart disease undergoing noncardiac surgery. They concluded that the frequency of ventricular dysrhythmias was not associated with adverse cardiac outcomes. The incidence of perioperative dysrhythmia in patients with an adverse outcome (8%) did not differ from the incidence in those with a good outcome. Patients undergoing cardiac surgery obviously have a higher incidence of cardiac dysrhythmias. The incidence of new-onset atrial fibrillation after cardiac surgery approaches 33%, such arrhythmias are associated with a worse outcome.[15] Several major factors contribute to the development of perioperative arrhythmias:

1. *General anesthetics*: Volatile anesthetics, such as halothane or enflurane, produce arrhythmias, probably by a reentrant mechanism.[16] Halothane also sensitizes the myocardium to endogenous and exogenous catecholamines. Drugs that block the reuptake of norepinephrine, such as cocaine and ketamine, can facilitate the development of epinephrine-induced arrhythmias (see Chapter 23). In contrast, volatile anesthetics may have an antifibrillatory effect in response to acute coronary occlusion and reperfusion, at least in a canine model.[17] Sevoflurane may cause severe bradycardia and nodal rhythm when used in high concentrations during induction in infants,[18] and desflurane may prolong the QTc within the first minute of anesthesia in patients with a normal heart.[19]
2. *Local anesthetics*: Regional anesthesia by central neuraxial blockade, the goal of spinal or epidural anesthesia, may be associated with profound, albeit transient pharmacologic sympathectomy. This phenomenon may cause parasympathetic nervous system dominance leading to mild to very severe bradyarrhythmias, especially when the blockade extends to very high thoracic levels (see Chapter 51). Inadvertent intravascular injection of a large dose of local anesthetic may lead to asystole and cardiac arrest, which are very difficult to treat.[20] One proposed treatment is the administration of 20% Intralipid.[21,22]
3. *Abnormal arterial blood gases or electrolyte levels*: Excessive hyperventilation, particularly in the presence of low serum potassium levels, may precipitate severe cardiac arrhythmias.[23] Alterations in blood gases or electrolytes may lead to arrhythmias by producing reentrant mechanisms or by altering the phase 4 depolarization of conduction fibers. Electrolyte disturbances associated with cardiopulmonary bypass can also result in intraoperative arrhythmias (see Chapters 54 and 60).
4. *Endotracheal intubation*: This maneuver may be the most common cause of arrhythmias during surgery and is frequently associated with hemodynamic disturbances by eliciting autonomic reflexes (see also Chapter 50).
5. *Autonomic reflexes*: Vagal stimulation may produce sinus bradycardia and allow ventricular escape mechanisms to occur. It may also produce AV block or even asystole. These reflexes may be related to traction on the peritoneum or direct pressure on the vagus nerve during carotid surgery (see Chapter 62). During jugular vein cannula-

tion, stimulation of the carotid sinus by palpation of the neck can lead to bradyarrhythmias. Specific reflexes, such as the oculocardiac reflex, can also produce severe bradycardia or asystole.

6. *Central nervous system stimulation and dysfunction of the autonomic nervous system*: Many electrocardiographic abnormalities can occur in patients with intracranial disease, especially subarachnoid hemorrhage. These abnormalities are most commonly ST-T wave changes and may easily mimic myocardial ischemia and infarction (see Chapter 63).[24] The mechanism of these arrhythmias appears to be related to changes in autonomic nervous system tone.
7. *Preexisting cardiac disease*: This is probably the most common background for arrhythmias during anesthesia and surgery.[25] Patients with a preexisting tendency for atrial or ventricular arrhythmias are more likely to exhibit them during or after surgery in response to perioperative stress or secondary to acute withdrawal of oral antiarrhythmic medications, most commonly β-blockers.
8. *Central venous cannulation*: Insertion of catheters or wires into the central circulation frequently leads to arrhythmias (see Chapter 40).
9. *Surgical manipulation of cardiac structures*: Arrhythmias are frequently observed during insertion of atrial sutures or placement of venous cannulas for cardiopulmonary bypass during cardiac surgery (see Chapters 60 and 83). They are usually self-limited and cease at the end of manipulation.
10. *Location of surgery*: Dental surgery is often associated with arrhythmias because profound stimulation of the sympathetic and parasympathetic nervous systems frequently occurs.[26] Junctional rhythms are often seen and may be caused by stimulation of the autonomic nervous system by the fifth cranial nerve. The oculocardiac reflex leads to severe bradycardia in response to traction on the rectus muscles of the orbit. This reflex, which is mediated by the trigeminal nerve as the afferent limb and the vagus nerve as the efferent limb, is especially sensitive in *neonates* and children and common during strabismus operations.

After an arrhythmia is recognized, does it produce a hemodynamic disturbance, what type of treatment is required, and how urgently should therapy be instituted? Treatment should be initiated promptly if the arrhythmia results in marked hemodynamic impairment. Prompt treatment should also be instituted if the arrhythmia is a precursor for a more severe arrhythmia (e.g., frequent multifocal ventricular premature beats [VPBs] with an R-on-T phenomenon can lead to ventricular fibrillation). Immediate attention is required for arrhythmias in a patient with underlying cardiac disease (e.g., any tachycardia in a patient with mitral valve stenosis, aortic valve stenosis, or ischemic heart disease). Arrhythmias can be classified by heart rate or by anatomic origin within the heart. By heart rate criteria, arrhythmias can be broken down into three categories: bradyarrhythmias (heart rate <60 beats/min), tachyarrhythmias (heart rate >100 beats/min), and conduction blocks (at any heart rate). The anatomic origin of an arrhythmia can be ventricular, supraventricular, junctional, or elsewhere. Diagnosis and treatment of arrhythmias can be simplified by using the following checklist when looking at an electrocardiographic display:

1. What is the heart rate?
2. Is the rhythm regular?
3. Is there one P wave for each QRS complex?
4. Is the QRS complex normal?
5. Is the rhythm dangerous?
6. Does the rhythm require treatment?

The following is analysis of some common intraoperative arrhythmias.

Sinus Bradycardia

Sinus bradycardia is diagnosed when the pacemaker site is in the sinus node but the rate is slower than normal. Etiologic factors include drug effects, acute inferior MI, hypoxia, vagal stimulation, and high sympathetic blockade. Sinus bradycardia accounts for roughly 11% of intraoperative arrhythmias.

1. *Heart rate*: Slower than 60 beats/min. In patients maintained on chronic β-blocker therapy, it is defined as a heart rate of less than 50 beats/min.
2. *Rhythm*: Regular, except for occasional escape beats from other pacemaker sites.
3. *P/QRS*: Ratio of 1 : 1.
4. *QRS complex*: Normal morphology.
5. *Significance*: Heart rates lower than 40 beats/min are poorly tolerated, even in healthy patients, and should be evaluated on the basis of their effect on cardiac output. Treatment is recommended if hypotension, ventricular arrhythmias, or signs of poor peripheral perfusion are observed. Sinus bradycardia may be part of the sick sinus syndrome in which sinus node dysfunction can precipitate bradycardia, heart block, tachyarrhythmia, or alternating bradyarrhythmia and tachyarrhythmia.[27]
6. *Treatment*: Usually none is necessary. When treatment is deemed necessary, the following approach may be considered: (1) atropine, 0.5 to 1.0 mg by intravenous bolus repeated every 3 to 5 minutes, up to 0.04 mg/kg or approximately a 3.0-mg total dose for the average 75-kg male patient; (2) ephedrine, 5 to 25 mg by intravenous bolus; (3) dopamine or dobutamine (if blood pressure is adequate), 5 to 20 μg/kg/min by intravenous infusion; (4) epinephrine, 2 to 10 μg/min by intravenous infusion; (5) isoproterenol, 2 to 10 μg/min by intravenous infusion. Temporary transcutaneous or transvenous pacing may be necessary for severe, drug-refractory sinus bradycardia. Immediate institution of transcutaneous pacing is especially important in symptomatic patients.

Sinus Tachycardia

The pacemaker site in patients with sinus tachycardia is in the sinus node, and the rate is faster than normal. Sinus tachycardia is the most common arrhythmia in the perioperative period. It occurs with such frequency that it is not included in most studies of the incidence of arrhythmias. Common causes include pain, inadequate anesthesia, hypovolemia, fever, hypoxia, hypercapnia, heart failure, and drug effects.

1. *Heart rate*: Faster than 100 beats/min in adult patients and may be as high as 170 beats/min. Patients with significant CAD may not tolerate heart rates even as low as 70 to 80 beats/min, and subendocardial ischemia can develop. Similarly, patients with severe mitral or aortic stenosis may be sensitive to even moderate increases in heart rate.
2. *Rhythm*: Regular.
3. *P/QRS*: Ratio of 1:1.
4. *QRS complex*: Normal but there may be associated ST-segment depression with severe increases in heart rate and resulting myocardial ischemia.
5. *Significance*: Prolonged tachycardia in patients with underlying heart disease can precipitate MI and congestive heart failure (CHF) as a result of the increased myocardial work required and decreased myocardial oxygen supply because of decreased diastolic coronary perfusion time. A major diagnostic problem is encountered when the heart rate is 150 beats/min because this is a common rate for sinus tachycardia, paroxysmal atrial tachycardia, or atrial flutter with a 2:1 block. These three arrhythmias can sometimes be distinguished by the use of carotid sinus massage or intravenous administration of edrophonium or adenosine phosphate.
6. *Treatment*: The underlying disorder should be treated. Hypovolemia and light anesthesia are the most common causes. In patients with ischemic heart disease in whom tachycardia develops, β-adrenergic blockers should be used judiciously to prevent myocardial ischemia regardless of whether ST-segment changes are present. Hypovolemia or other causes should also be addressed in these patients.

Sinus Arrhythmia

In sinus arrhythmia, the impulses arise from the SA node, and the rhythm is characterized by a variable rate. The PR interval is normal, as is the QRS complex. Most commonly, but not invariably, the rate increases with inspiration and decreases with expiration. This arrhythmia occurs more often in children than in adults. The heart rate is 60 to 100 beats/min, the rhythm is irregular, the P/QRS ratio is 1:1, and the QRS complex has normal morphology. Sinus arrhythmia has little clinical significance, is considered a normal finding, and requires no treatment.

Atrial Premature Beats

An ectopic pacemaker site in the left or right atrium initiates an atrial premature beat (APB). The shape of the P wave is different from the usual SA node P wave and may be inverted. The PR interval may be shorter or longer than normal, depending on the site of the ectopic focus and the refractoriness of the AV nodal pathway. The APB spreads through the AV node and ventricular conduction system and, in retrograde fashion, reaches the SA node and resets the sinus pacemaker. The interval from the APB to the next sinus beat is therefore a normal sinus cycle (i.e., no compensatory pause). The absence of a compensatory pause is an important distinguishing feature between APBs and VPBs. Occasionally, APBs may find part of the ventricular conduction system refractory, in which case they travel down an aberrant pathway and create an abnormal QRS complex. They are then called APBs with aberrant ventricular conduction and can easily be confused with VPBs. Because the recovery period of the right ventricular conduction system is longer than that of the left, the most common form of aberration appears as an RBBB. Helpful points in differentiating APBs with aberrant ventricular conduction from VPBs include (1) the presence of a preceding P wave, usually abnormally shaped; (2) an RBBB configuration of the QRS complex; (3) the presence of an rsR′ ventricular complex in V_1; and (4) the finding that the initial vector forces are identical to the preceding beat, which is usually the opposite with a VPB. Other characteristics of APBs are as follows:

1. *Heart rate*: Variable, depending on the frequency of the APBs.
2. *Rhythm*: Irregular.
3. *P/QRS*: Usually 1:1. The P waves have various shapes and may even be lost in the QRS or T waves. Occasionally, the P wave is so early that it finds the ventricle refractory, and a nonconducted beat occurs.
4. *QRS complex*: Usually normal unless ventricular aberration is present.
5. *Significance*: In one study, APBs represented 10% of all intraoperative arrhythmias. They have little clinical significance, but frequent APBs may lead to other, more serious supraventricular arrhythmias or may be a sign of digitalis intoxication.
6. *Treatment*: Rarely necessary.

Paroxysmal Supraventricular Tachycardia

Paroxysmal SVT (PSVT) is characterized by a rapid regular rhythm, generally with a narrow QRS complex and lacking the normal SA node P wave. Inclusion of tachycardias involving the AV node (Fig. 42-11) allows a useful classification of tachycardias as being caused by reentry in the AV node, by apparent or concealed accessory AV pathways, or less often, by SA node reentry. Ectopic atrial or ectopic nodal tachycardias are among the less frequent SVTs. Inappropriate or persistent sinus tachycardia is another variant. PSVT rhythms are usually abrupt in onset and termination. PSVT is easily distinguished from rapid atrial fibrillation, which is an irregular rhythm, and from rapid atrial flutter, which has flutter waves.

1. Heart rate: 130 to 270 beats/min.
2. *Rhythm*: Usually regular unless the impulse originates from multiple atrial foci.
3. *P/QRS*: 1:1 relationship, although the P wave may often be hidden in the QRS complex or T wave.
4. *QRS complex*: Generally normal, but ST-T changes indicative of ischemia may be observed. Aberration of ventricular conduction may occur and complicate the differential diagnosis with VT. SVT may also be confused with sinus tachycardia, atrial flutter, and atrial fibrillation. In differentiating these rhythms, carotid sinus massage or edrophonium (5 to 10 mg given intravenously) was traditionally used. More recently, adenosine (6 to 12 mg by intravenous bolus) has been used to slow the rate by transiently enhancing the normal degree of AV block or to terminate the arrhythmia.[28] Esophageal electrocardiographic leads may also be helpful to better define atrial activity.[29]

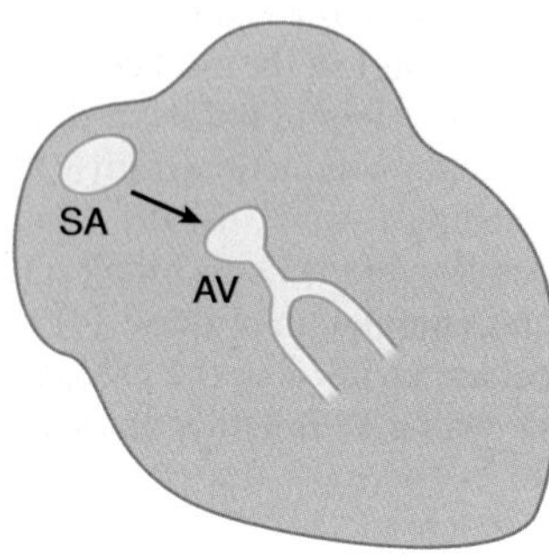

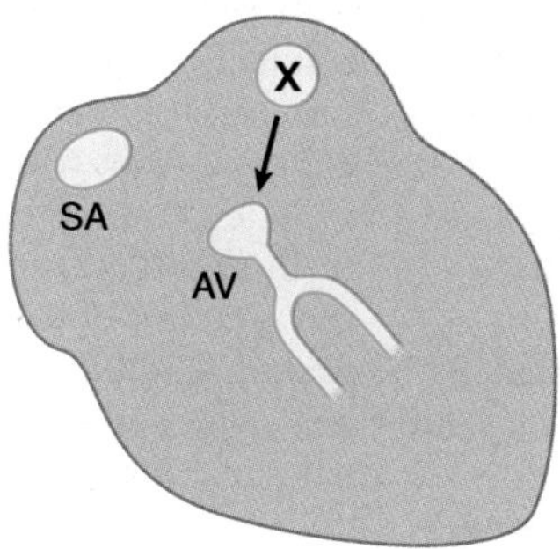

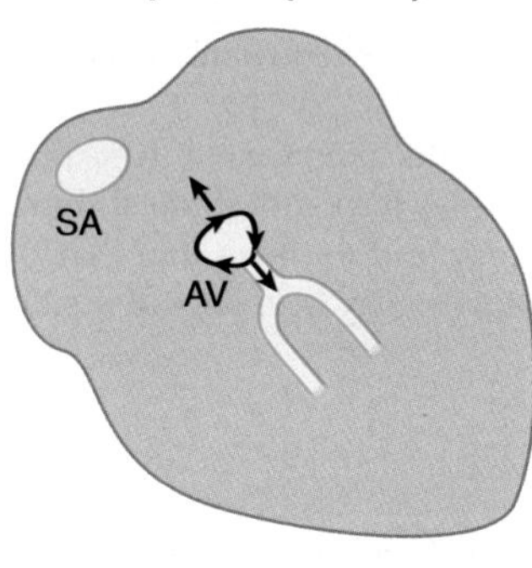

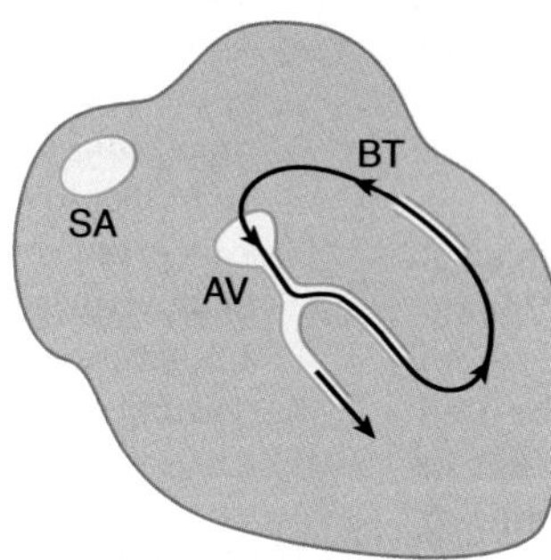

Figure 42-11 Major types of paroxysmal supraventricular tachycardia. **A,** Normal sinus rhythm. **B,** Atrial tachycardia. A focus (X) outside the sinoatrial (SA) node fires off automatically at a rapid rate. **C,** Atrioventricular (AV) nodal reentrant tachycardia. The cardiac stimulus originates as a wave of excitation that spins around the AV nodal (junctional) area. As a result, retrograde P waves may be buried in the QRS or appear immediately before or just after the QRS complex (*arrows*) because of nearly simultaneous activation of the atria and ventricles. **D,** A similar type of reentrant (circus-movement) mechanism may occur with a bypass tract (BT) of the type found in Wolff-Parkinson-White syndrome. This mechanism is referred to as atrioventricular reentrant tachycardia (AVRT). Note the negative P wave (*arrow*) in lead II, somewhat after the QRS complex. (With AVRT, the P wave in lead II may be negative or isoelectric.) *(From Goldberger AL: Clinical Electrocardiography: A Simplified Approach, 7th ed. St Louis, CV Mosby, 2006.)*

5. *Significance*: PSVT can be seen in 5% of normal young adults and in patients with Wolff-Parkinson-White syndrome or other pre-excitation syndromes. During anesthesia, PSVT accounts for up to 2.5% of all arrhythmias. This arrhythmia has no association with any intrinsic heart disease or systemic illness. When a patient is anesthetized, PSVT can be precipitated by changes in autonomic nervous system tone, by drug effects, or by intravascular volume shifts and can produce severe hemodynamic deterioration. Sometimes the PSVT may be associated with AV block because of the fast atrial rate and slow AV conduction. PSVT with a 2:1 block represents digitalis intoxication in many patients.
6. *Treatment*: Even though this arrhythmia is not usually associated with hemodynamic deterioration, the following can be undertaken to treat it:
   a. Vagal maneuvers such as carotid sinus massage should be applied only to one side.[30]
   b. Adenosine, which is the drug of choice, is given by 6-mg rapid (2 seconds) intravenous bolus, preferably through an antecubital or central vein. If no response is elicited, second and third doses of 12 to 18 mg of adenosine may be administered by rapid intravenous bolus.[31]
   c. Verapamil (2.5 to 10 mg given intravenously) terminates AV nodal reentry successfully in about 90% of cases.[32] Unlike adenosine, verapamil has the advantage of providing long-term relief.
   d. Amiodarone (150-mg infusion over a 10-minute period for the loading dose) is a recent addition.[33]
   e. Esmolol (1 mg/kg by bolus and 50 to 200 mg/kg/min by infusion) has been shown to be effective.[34]
   f. Edrophonium or neostigmine can be given by intravenous bolus.[35]
   g. Phenylephrine (100 μg by intravenous bolus) is administered if the patient is hypotensive.[36]
   h. Intravenous digitalization is performed with one of the short-acting digitalis preparations: ouabain (0.25 to 0.5 mg given intravenously) or digoxin (0.5 to 1.0 mg given intravenously).[36]

i. Rapid overdrive pacing may be done in an effort to capture the ectopic focus.[37]

j. Synchronized cardioversion may be performed with incremental doses of energy of 100, 200, 300, and 360 J, preferably after light sedative premedication.[38] Electrode catheter ablation with radiofrequency energy has evolved as the definitive, long-term treatment of most persistent AV reentrant or focal atrial SVTs.[39]

Atrial Flutter

Atrial flutter most commonly represents a macro-reentrant arrhythmia that circulates in a specific manner in the right atrium (i.e., counterclockwise rotation as viewed in the angiographic left anterior oblique view). Because it is associated with very fast heart rates, it is generally accompanied by AV block. Classic sawtooth flutter waves (F waves) are usually present (Fig. 42-12). The characteristics of atrial flutter are as follows:

1. *Heart rate*: The atrial heart rate is 250 to 350 beats/min with a ventricular rate of about 150 beats/min (2 : 1 or varying AV conduction block).
2. *Rhythm*: The atrial rhythm is regular. The ventricular rhythm may be regular if a fixed AV block is present or irregular if a variable block exists.
3. *P/QRS*: Usually there is a 2 : 1 block with an atrial rate of 300 beats/min and a ventricular rate of 150 beats/min, but it may vary between 2 : 1 and 8 : 1. F waves are best seen in leads V_1 and II and the esophageal lead.
4. *QRS complex*: Normal. T waves are lost in the f waves.
5. *Significance*: Atrial flutter does not always indicate severe heart disease. It can be seen in patients with CAD, mitral valve disease, pulmonary embolism, hyperthyroidism, cardiac trauma, cancer of the heart, and myocarditis.
6. *Treatment*: Pharmacologic or synchronized DC cardioversion, when indicated, should be performed only after careful consideration or evaluation of a possible thromboembolic event. Initial treatment should consist of control of the ventricular response rate with drugs that slow AV node conduction:

a. β-Blockers such as esmolol (1 mg/kg by intravenous bolus) or propranolol.

b. Calcium channel blockers such as verapamil (5 to 10 mg given intravenously) or diltiazem.[40] β-Blockers and calcium channel blockers are also effective as pharmacoprophylaxis for the prevention of postoperative atrial tachyarrhythmias after thoracic and cardiac surgery.[41]

If the ventricular response is excessively rapid or hemodynamic instability is present, or both, the following guidelines should be used:

c. Synchronized DC cardioversion starting at a relatively high energy of 100 J and gradually increasing to 360 J is indicated.

d. The class III antiarrhythmic agent ibutilide (Corvert, 1 mg in 10 mL saline or 5% dextrose in water [D_5W] infused slowly intravenously over a 10-minute period) has been documented to convert atrial flutter to sinus rhythm in most patients with relatively new-onset atrial flutter.[42] This may be repeated once, and although it is highly effective, life-threatening torsades de pointes (discussed later) may occur hours after ibutilide administration, thus making 4- to 8-hour monitoring after treatment highly desirable.

e. Procainamide (5 to 10 mg/kg for the intravenous loading dose, infused no faster than 0.5 mg/kg/min) may rarely be used in an attempt to restore sinus rhythm after the ventricular response has been adequately controlled.[43]

f. Amiodarone (150-mg intravenous loading dose infused over a 10-minute period, followed by 1 mg/min intravenously for 6 hours, a 0.5-mg/min intravenous infusion for 18 hours, and then a reduced intravenous dose or switching to an oral dose) has recently been shown to be effective.

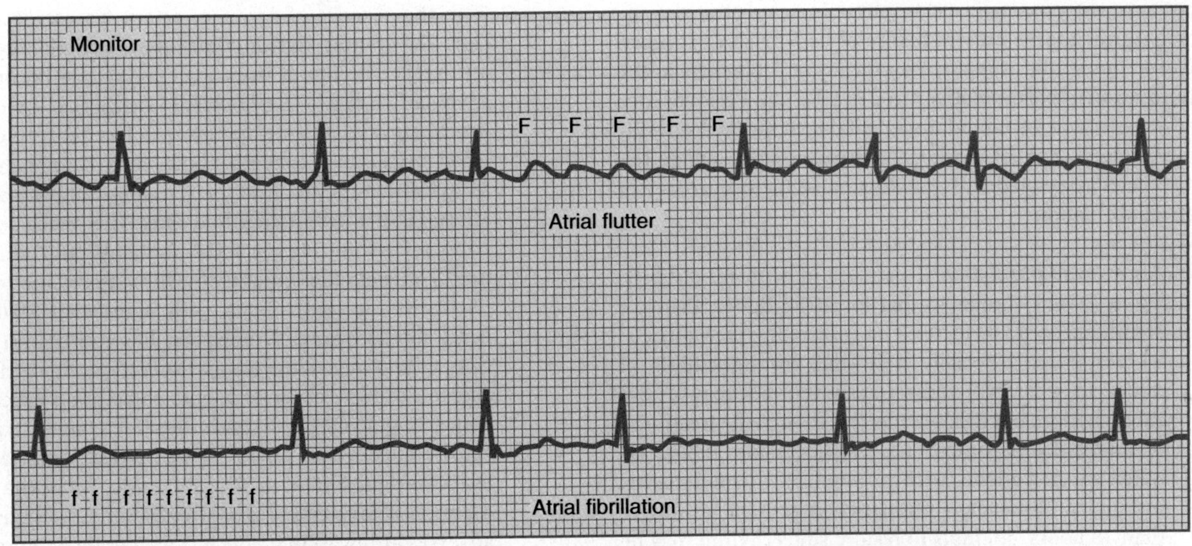

Figure 42-12 Atrial flutter and fibrillation. Notice the "sawtooth" waves (F waves) with atrial flutter and the irregular fibrillatory waves (f waves) with atrial fibrillation. *(From Goldberger AL: Clinical Electrocardiography: A Simplified Approach, 7th ed. St Louis, CV Mosby, 2006.)*

Atrial Fibrillation

Atrial fibrillation is an excessively rapid and irregular atrial focus with no P waves appearing on the ECG; instead, fine fibrillatory activity is seen (f waves, see Fig. 42-12). This is the most commonly encountered irregular rhythm. It is often described as irregularly irregular and may be associated with a pulse deficit. Its characteristics are as follows:

1. *Heart rate*: The atrial rate is 350 to 500 beats/min, and the ventricular rate is 60 to 170 beats/min.
2. *Rhythm*: Irregularly irregular.
3. *P:QRS*: The P wave is absent and replaced by f waves or no obvious atrial activity at all.
4. *QRS complex*: Normal.
5. *Significance*: The causes of atrial fibrillation are similar to those of atrial flutter. This rhythm is often associated with significant cardiac disease; however, idiopathic, paroxysmal atrial fibrillation has become increasingly recognized. The clinical significance and treatment of atrial fibrillation are similar to that for atrial flutter, except for two important considerations. The loss of atrial "kick" from inefficient contraction of the atria may reduce ventricular filling and significantly compromise cardiac output. After 24 to 48 hours, atrial fibrillation may be associated with the development of atrial thrombi, possibly resulting in pulmonary or systemic embolization.

   Atrial fibrillation is the most common postoperative arrhythmia and has significant consequences on patient health. Postoperative atrial fibrillation complicates up to 8% of all noncardiac surgeries, between 3% and 30% of noncardiac thoracic surgeries, and between 16% and 46% of cardiac surgeries. It has been associated with increased morbidity, mortality, and longer, more costly hospital stays. The risk of atrial fibrillation after cardiac and noncardiac surgery may be affected by several epidemiologic and intraoperative factors, as well as by the presence of preexisting cardiovascular and pulmonary disorders. It is typically a transient, reversible phenomenon that may develop in patients who possess an electrophysiologic substrate for the arrhythmia that is present before or as a result of surgery. Numerous studies support the efficacy of β-blockers in the prevention of postoperative atrial fibrillation. Perioperative administration of amiodarone, sotalol, nondihydropyridine calcium channel blockers, and magnesium sulfate has also been associated with a reduction in the occurrence of atrial fibrillation.[44]
6. *Treatment*:
   a. *Acute atrial fibrillation*: Treatment of acute atrial fibrillation is very similar to that for atrial flutter. Primary attention should be focused on controlling the ventricular response, especially with the administration of diltiazem or esmolol intravenously. Ibutilide may restore sinus rhythm, but it is less effective than in the treatment of flutter. Synchronized DC cardioversion should be relied on in patients with pronounced hemodynamic instability. However, if fibrillation is present for longer than 48 hours, attempts to restore sinus rhythm may be associated with a heightened risk for thromboembolism. In a patient with a normal coagulation profile, adequate anticoagulation for 3 to 4 weeks should be considered before attempting to restore sinus rhythm. Alternatively, transesophageal echocardiographic examination to rule out atrial thrombi may be substituted. New developments in electrophysiologic techniques for ventricular defibrillation consisting of biphasic current shocks have shown superiority to the conventional monophasic current techniques (discussed later). However, data regarding the efficacy of biphasic shocks for conversion of atrial fibrillation are still emerging. A randomized, double-blind, multicenter trial by the BiCard investigators[45] demonstrated that for the cardioversion of atrial fibrillation, a biphasic shock waveform has greater efficacy, requires fewer shocks and lower delivered energy, and results in less dermal injury than a monophasic shock waveform does. These results mirror those seen in the ventricular fibrillation trials.

   b. *Long-term therapy*: Long-term therapy for atrial fibrillation varies and depends on factors such as whether the arrhythmia is constant or paroxysmal, the nature of the underlying heart disease, and the state of ventricular function or hemodynamic stability or reserve. In an older individual or in the setting of specific risk factors (e.g., hypertension, diabetes mellitus, severe LV systolic dysfunction), anticoagulation with warfarin (Coumadin) should be strongly considered. When control of ventricular response is difficult with standard agents (e.g., β-blockers, calcium channel blockers, digitalis), electrode catheter ablation of the AV junction and permanent pacemaker insertion have seen increased use. This method is not a curative, merely a rate-controlling procedure. It also produces a regular ventricular contraction rhythm. For patients who are in and out of atrial fibrillation, implanted atrial defibrillators that function much like their ventricular counterparts (see Chapter 43) were considered a therapeutic option. Today, these devices see very limited application. The current "curative" electrophysiologic procedure is transseptal pulmonary vein isolation via radiofrequency catheter ablation (see Chapter 61).[46]

   In the absence of coronary artery disease or significant LV systolic dysfunction, class Ic antiarrhythmic agents (i.e., flecainide or propafenone) have become the agents of choice.[47] Use of class Ia drugs (i.e., quinidine, procainamide, and disopyramide) has sharply diminished because of concern about their significant proarrhythmic function and their systemic and organ side effects. Use of antiarrhythmic drugs that block repolarizing potassium currents (i.e., sotalol[48] and amiodarone[49]) has gained popularity for the suppression of atrial fibrillation in individuals with significant structural heart disease. Sotalol, however, has much lower efficiency in converting atrial fibrillation than class Ic agents do. New class III agents show good efficacy in converting atrial fibrillation. Ibutilide converts rapidly, can be effective in up to 50% of cases,[50] and is more effective than sotalol or procainamide. All of the drugs mentioned for treating atrial fibrillation have significant adverse cardiovascular effects, torsades de pointes (ventricular fibrillation), CHF, bradycardia, and hypotension being the most prominent.[51]

Junctional Rhythms

The AV node itself and sites just above and below it can act as pacemakers. It makes sense to consider this ectopic activity as arrhythmias of the AV junction. The resultant P wave is abnormal and, depending on the position of the ectopic pacemaker, may be very close to, buried in, or after the QRS complex. Depending on the rate of fire of the ectopic pacemaker, the resultant rhythm is nodal premature; nodal quadrigeminy, trigeminy, or bigeminy; nodal rhythm; or nodal tachycardia.

1. *Heart rate*: Variable, 40 to 180 beats/min (i.e., nodal bradycardia to junctional tachycardia).
2. *Rhythm*: Regular.
3. *P/QRS*: 1 : 1, but there are three varieties:
   a. *High nodal rhythm*: The impulse reaches the atrium before the ventricle; the P wave therefore precedes the QRS but has a shortened PR interval (0.1 second).
   b. *Mid nodal rhythm*: The impulse reaches the atrium and the ventricle at the same time. The P wave is lost in the QRS.
   c. *Low nodal rhythm*: The impulse reaches the ventricle first and then the atrium, so the P wave follows the QRS complex.
4. *QRS complex*: Normal, unless altered by the P wave.
5. *Significance*: Junctional rhythms are common in patients under anesthesia (about 20%), especially with halogenated anesthetic agents. Junctional rhythms frequently decrease blood pressure and cardiac output by about 15%, but they can decrease it up to 30% in patients with heart disease.[52]
6. *Treatment*: Usually, no treatment is required, and the rhythm reverts spontaneously. If hypotension and poor perfusion are associated with the rhythm, treatment is indicated. Atropine, ephedrine, or isoproterenol can be used in an effort to increase the activity of the SA node so that it will take over as the pacemaker. Dual-chamber electrical pacing at a rate faster than a slow nodal rhythm is another option.

Ventricular Premature Beats

VPBs result from ectopic pacemaker activity arising below the AV junction. The VPB originates in and spreads through the myocardium or ventricular conducting system, thereby resulting in a wide (>0.12-second), bizarre QRS complex. The ST segment usually slopes in the direction opposite the main deflection of the QRS complex. There is no P wave associated with a VPB, but retrograde depolarization of the atria or blocked sinus beats may obscure the diagnosis.

The most important entity in the differential diagnosis is APB with aberrant ventricular conduction. The distinction should be made whenever possible.

Although an APB normally reaches the SA node and resets the sinus rhythm, such an occurrence is rare when the ectopic pacemaker is in the ventricle. A VPB often blocks the next depolarization from the SA node, but the following sinus beat occurs on time. The result is a fully compensatory pause consisting of the interval from the VPB to the expected normal QRS, which is blocked at the AV node, plus a normal sinus interval.

VPBs are common during anesthesia, where they account for 15% of observed arrhythmias. They are much more common in anesthetized patients with preexisting cardiac disease. Other than heart disease, known etiologic factors include electrolyte and blood gas abnormalities, drug interactions, brainstem stimulation, and trauma to the heart.

1. *Heart rate*: Depends on the underlying sinus rate and frequency of the VPBs.
2. *Rhythm*: Irregular.
3. *P/QRS*: No P wave with the VPB.
4. *QRS complex*: Wide and bizarre, with a width of more than 0.12 second. If it is of an RBBB nature, prominent R forces are present in V_1. If it is an LBBB in appearance, notching of the S wave and less acute downward sloping of the ST segment are common.
5. *Significance*: The new onset of VPBs must be considered a potentially serious event because in certain clinical situations, the arrhythmia may progress to VT or ventricular fibrillation. Such situations include coronary artery insufficiency, MI, digitalis toxicity with hypokalemia, and hypoxemia. VPBs are more likely to precede ventricular fibrillation if they are multiple, multifocal, or bigeminal; occur near the vulnerable period of the preceding ventricular repolarization (i.e., R-on-T phenomenon)[53]; or appear in short-long-short coupling sequences. VPBs are markers, not the cause of more severe arrhythmias.
6. *Treatment*: In most patients, VPBs (occurring as single, bigeminy, or trigeminy but excluding nonsustained VT) do not need to be treated, particularly if the patient does not have an acute coronary syndrome, and treatment is generally dictated by the presence of symptoms attributable to the VPBs. The first step in treatment is to correct any underlying abnormalities such as decreased serum potassium or low arterial oxygen tension. If the arrhythmia is of hemodynamic significance or if it is believed to be a harbinger of worse arrhythmias, lidocaine is the treatment of choice, with an initial bolus dose of 1.5 mg/kg. Recurrent VPBs can be treated with a lidocaine infusion at 1 to 4 mg/min; additional therapy includes esmolol, propranolol, procainamide, quinidine, disopyramide, atropine, verapamil, or overdrive pacing.

Ventricular Tachycardia

The presence of three or more sequential VPBs defines VT. Diagnostic criteria include the presence of fusion beats, capture beats, and AV dissociation. The specific morphologic appearance of the QRS complex may also be helpful in distinguishing VT from other arrhythmias. VT is classified by its duration and morphology. In duration, nonsustained VT lasts three beats and up to 30 seconds, and sustained VT lasts 30 seconds or longer. With monomorphic morphology, all complexes have the same pattern, and with polymorphic morphology, complexes constantly change patterns. Polymorphic VT with a long QTc is also called "torsades de pointes."

The characteristics of VT are as follows:

1. *Heart rate*: 100 to 200 beats/min.
2. *Rhythm*: Generally regular, but may be irregular if the VT is paroxysmal.

3. *P/QRS*: Usually there is no fixed relationship because VT is a form of AV dissociation in which the P waves can be seen marching through the QRS complex.
4. *QRS complex*: Wide, more than 0.12 second in width, with similar morphologic criteria in lead V_1 as for VPB.
5. *Significance*: Acute onset is life threatening and requires immediate treatment.
6. *Treatment*: If the patient is hemodynamically stable, amiodarone administered as one or more intravenous doses of 150 mg in 100 mL saline or D_5W over a period of 10 minutes, followed by an intravenous infusion of 1 mg/min for 6 hours and 0.5 mg/min thereafter, is the recommended current treatment (maximum intravenous dose, 2.2 g/24 hr). Although amiodarone is associated with substantially less hypotension than bretylium is, hypotension and bradycardia are its main side effects. Amiodarone's pharmacologic effects persist for more than 45 days. Lidocaine and procainamide have been used in the past with varying degrees of success to treat VT. Synchronized cardioversion is the indicated nonpharmacologic intervention in any wide-complex tachycardia, whether monomorphic VT or a wide-complex SVT. Polymorphic VT with a normal QT interval is treated with amiodarone and cardioversion. Metabolic abnormalities and drug toxicity must be considered and treated. Polymorphic VT with a prolonged QT interval is a more serious rhythm disturbance, and the recommended current treatment is an intravenous infusion of 1 g of magnesium administered over a 2- to 3-minute period. Precipitating metabolic or toxic causes should be treated. Overdrive pacing may also be helpful in this setting (Fig. 42-13).

Ventricular Fibrillation

Ventricular fibrillation is an irregular rhythm that results from a rapid discharge of impulses from one or more ventricular foci or from multiple wandering reentrant circuits in the ventricles. The ventricular contractions are erratic and are represented on the ECG by bizarre patterns of various size and configuration. P waves are not seen. Important causes of ventricular fibrillation include myocardial ischemia, hypoxia, hypothermia, electric shock, electrolyte imbalance, and drug effects (Fig. 42-14).

Its characteristics are as follows:

1. *Heart rate*: Rapid and grossly disorganized.
2. *Rhythm*: Totally irregular.
3. *P/QRS*: None seen.
4. *QRS complex*: Not present.

Paroxysmal nonsustained ventricular tachycardia

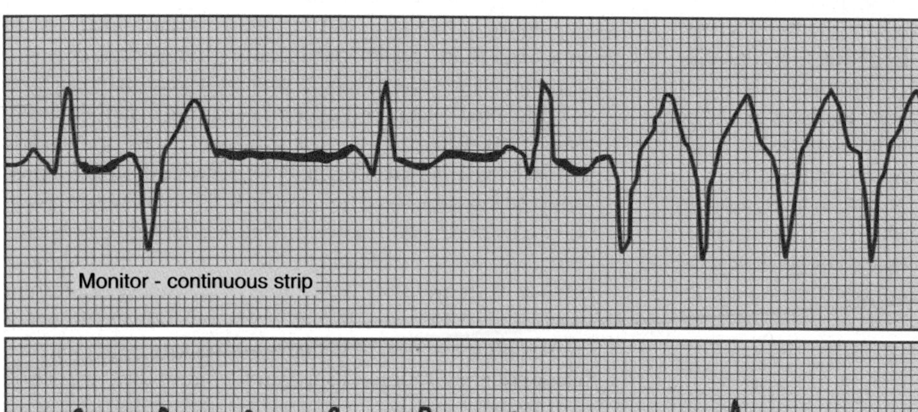

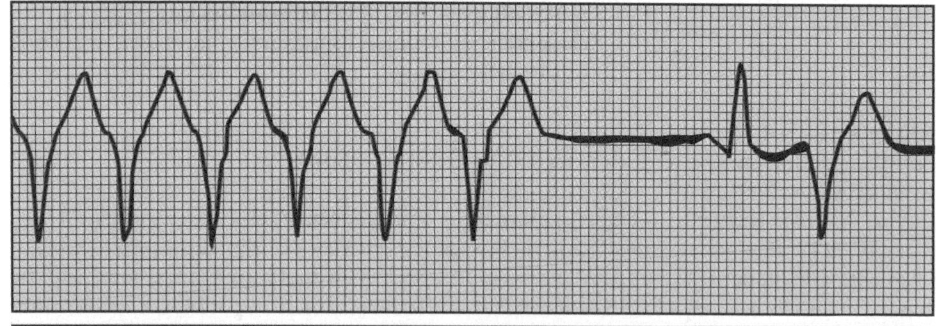

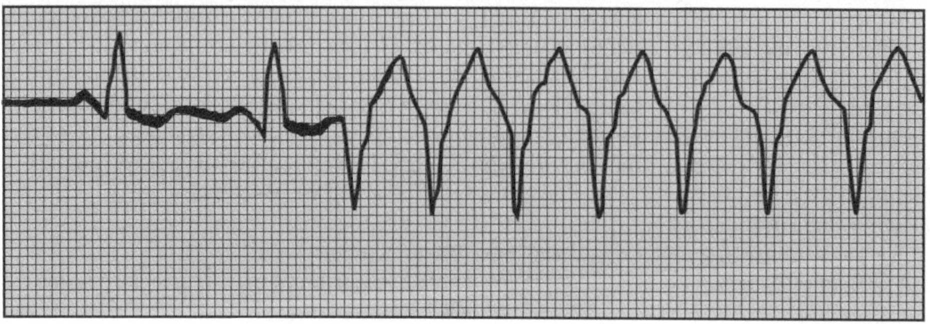

Figure 42-13 Short bursts of ventricular tachycardia. *(From Goldberger AL: Clinical Electrocardiography: A Simplified Approach, 7th ed. St Louis, CV Mosby, 2006.)*

Ventricular fibrillation

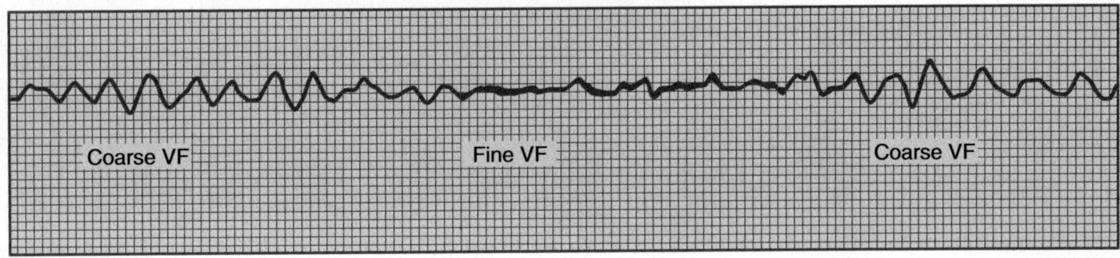

Figure 42-14 Ventricular fibrillation (VF) in the form of coarse and fine waves. *(From Goldberger AL: Clinical Electrocardiography: A Simplified Approach, 7th ed. St Louis, CV Mosby, 2006.)*

5. *Significance*: There is no effective cardiac output, and life must be sustained by artificial means, such as external cardiac massage.
6. *Treatment*:
   a. Cardiopulmonary resuscitation must be initiated immediately, and then defibrillation must be performed as rapidly as possible. Asynchronous external defibrillation should be performed with a DC defibrillator using incremental energies in the range of 200 to 360 J. The introduction of biphasic (and rectilinear) transthoracic shocks has reduced the energy levels required and increased the efficacy of ventricular defibrillation. In a prospective, randomized, multicenter trial conducted by the ZOLL investigators,[54,55] 120 J of biphasic current was superior to 200 J of monophasic current, especially in patients with increased chest wall impedance.
   b. Early administration of 1 g of magnesium sulfate may facilitate defibrillation. In some instances, epinephrine has been used for coarsening the fibrillation to facilitate defibrillation. Vasopressin has been added as a drug for the treatment of ventricular fibrillation. The vasopressin dose is a single 40-unit intravenous bolus. Subsequent administration of epinephrine should be delayed for at least 5 minutes after vasopressin. Supportive pharmacologic therapy may include lidocaine, amiodarone, bretylium, procainamide, phenytoin, or esmolol.
   c. Torsades de pointes, which may mimic ventricular fibrillation or VT, is a life-threatening arrhythmia that occurs in the presence of disturbed repolarization (hence its association with prolonged QT intervals).[56] Discontinuation of drugs that predispose to prolongation of the QT interval and correction of electrolyte abnormalities are essential in the treatment of torsades de pointes. Acute therapy may include defibrillation, 1 to 2 g of intravenous magnesium sulfate, intravenous isoproterenol, and overdrive pacing.[57]

Conduction Defects

Conduction defects are most often chronic, are present on the baseline preoperative ECG, and represent the underlying disease state of the myocardium or conduction system. However, conduction defects may be observed for the first time during surgery and anesthesia. They can occur as a result of simple manipulation, such as passage of a pulmonary artery catheter through the right ventricle, but they can also be a manifestation of myocardial ischemia. Because high-grade (second- and third-degree AV blocks) conduction defects often have deleterious effects on hemodynamic performance, intraoperative recognition is important.

Three types of conduction system blocks are possible: SA block, AV heart block, and intraventricular conduction block. The His bundle ECG used by cardiologists has greatly improved the understanding of conduction through the heart. In an SA block, the block occurs at the sinus node. Because atrial excitation is not initiated, P waves are not found on the ECG. The next beat can be a normal sinus beat, a nodal escape beat, or a ventricular escape beat.

The second type of heart block is an AV heart block, or AV block, which may be incomplete or complete. First- and second-degree AV blocks are generally considered incomplete, whereas a third-degree AV block is considered to be a complete heart block. First-degree AV block is often found in healthy hearts, but it is also associated with CAD or digitalis administration. It is characterized by a PR interval longer than 0.21 second. All atrial impulses progress through the AV node to the Purkinje system. This form of heart block ordinarily requires no treatment. Second-degree AV block is associated with the conduction of some of the atrial impulses to the AV node and into the Purkinje system. It is further subdivided into two specific types. A Mobitz type I block, or a Wenckebach block, is characterized by progressive lengthening of the PR interval until an impulse is not conducted and the beat is dropped (Fig. 42-15). This form of block is relatively benign and often reversible, and it does not require a pacemaker. It may be caused by digitalis toxicity or MI and is usually transient. A Mobitz type I block reflects disease of the AV node.

The other form of second-degree heart block is a Mobitz type II block, which may reflect disease of the bundle of His and Purkinje tissues, especially when the QRS complex is broad. In this, the less common and more serious form of second-degree heart block, dropped beats occur without any progressive lengthening of the PR interval (Fig. 42-16). This type of block has a serious prognosis because it frequently progresses to a complete heart block and may require pacemaker insertion before major surgical procedures.

Third-degree AV block, also called a complete heart block, occurs when all electrical activity from the atria fails to progress into the Purkinje system. The atrial and ventricular contractions have no relationship with each other, although each chamber

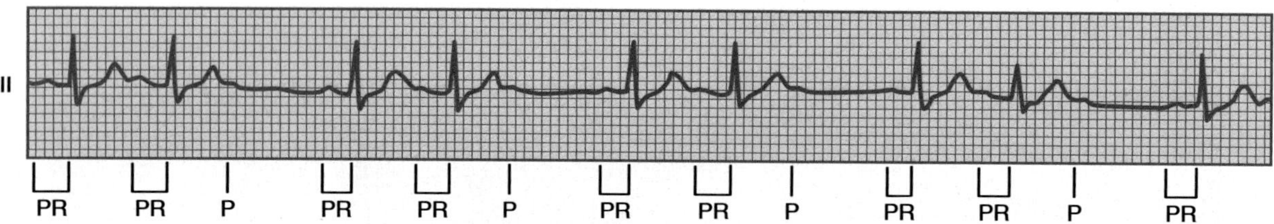

Figure 42-15 A Mobitz type I (Wenckebach) block produces a characteristically syncopated rhythm with grouping of the QRS complexes (group beating). Notice the progressive increase in PR intervals, with the third sinus P wave in each sequence not followed by a QRS complex. AV, atrioventricular. *(From Goldberger AL: Clinical Electrocardiography: A Simplified Approach, 7th ed. St Louis, CV Mosby, 2006.)*

contracts regularly. The ventricular rate is approximately 40 beats/min. The QRS complex may be normal if the pacemaker site is in the AV node, but it is usually widened to longer than 0.12 second when the pacemaker site is located in the ventricle (Fig. 42-17). The heart rate is usually too slow to maintain adequate cardiac output, and syncope or Adams-Stokes syndrome may occur, as well as heart failure. These patients generally require insertion of a transvenous endocardial or epicardial pacemaker to increase their heart rate and cardiac output.

Intraventricular blocks

Under normal conditions, activation of the left ventricle spreads simultaneously through both the left anterior and left posterior fascicles. Blockage or even a modest delay in conduction in one of these fascicles results in sequential rather than simultaneous activation of the corresponding sites and produces characteristic abnormal patterns on the ECG.

Left Anterior Fascicular Block. The left bundle branch of the bundle of His itself bifurcates distally into two fascicles, the anterior and posterior fascicles. A left anterior fascicular block (LAFB) is relatively common because of the delicate structure of the left fascicle. It causes delayed activation of the anterosuperior LV wall and is characterized by marked (−45- to −90-degree) left axis deviation. LAFB may occur in persons without overt cardiac disease but is it found mainly in patients with a wide range of diseases of the myocardial and conduction system, such as CAD or LVH. It has minimal to no independent prognostic significance.

Left Posterior Fascicular Block. A left posterior fascicular block (LPFB) is considerably less common than an anterior fascicular block because of the thicker structure of the right fascicle. It is also at a less vulnerable location near the LV inflow tract. LPFB results in delayed activation of the inferoposterior aspect of the left ventricle, and the electrocardiographic features of LPFB are marked right axis deviation (>120 degrees). LPFB can occur in patients with almost any cardiac disease but is unusual in otherwise healthy people. As in the case of LAFB, the overall QRS duration remains normal (<120 msec) (Fig. 42-18).

Left Bundle Branch Block. Caused by a serious delay or block of the main left bundle branch or both of its two fascicles, an LBBB results in a prolonged QRS duration, abnormal QRS complex, and ST-T wave abnormalities. A basic requirement is a QRS duration of 120 msec or longer. There is also a broad, sometimes notched R wave in the left-sided leads (I, aVL, V_5, V_6) with deep S waves in the right precordial leads and absent septal Q waves. The QRS axis is highly variable. It can be normal or devi-

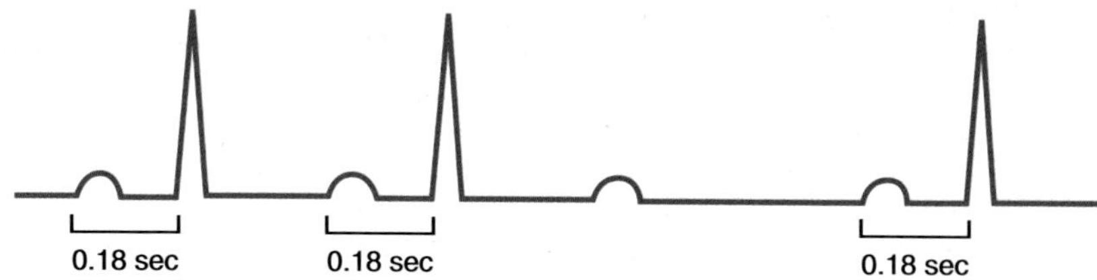

Figure 42-16 Mobitz type II atrioventricular block. Notice that the PR intervals remain constant as long as the QRS is not dropped, as in Mobitz type I. *(From Goldberger AL: Clinical Electrocardiography: A Simplified Approach, 7th ed. St Louis, CV Mosby.)*

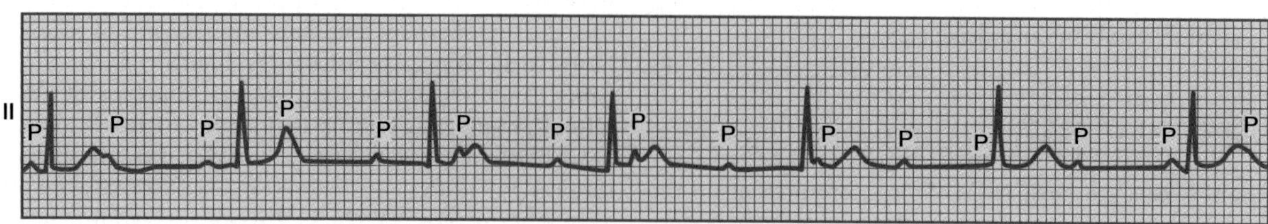

Figure 42-17 A complete heart block with underlying sinus rhythm is characterized by independent atrial (P) and ventricular (QRS complex) activity. The atrial rate is almost always faster than the ventricular rate. The PR intervals are completely variable. AV, atrioventricular. *(From Goldberger AL: Clinical Electrocardiography: A Simplified Approach, 7th ed. St Louis, CV Mosby, 2006.)*

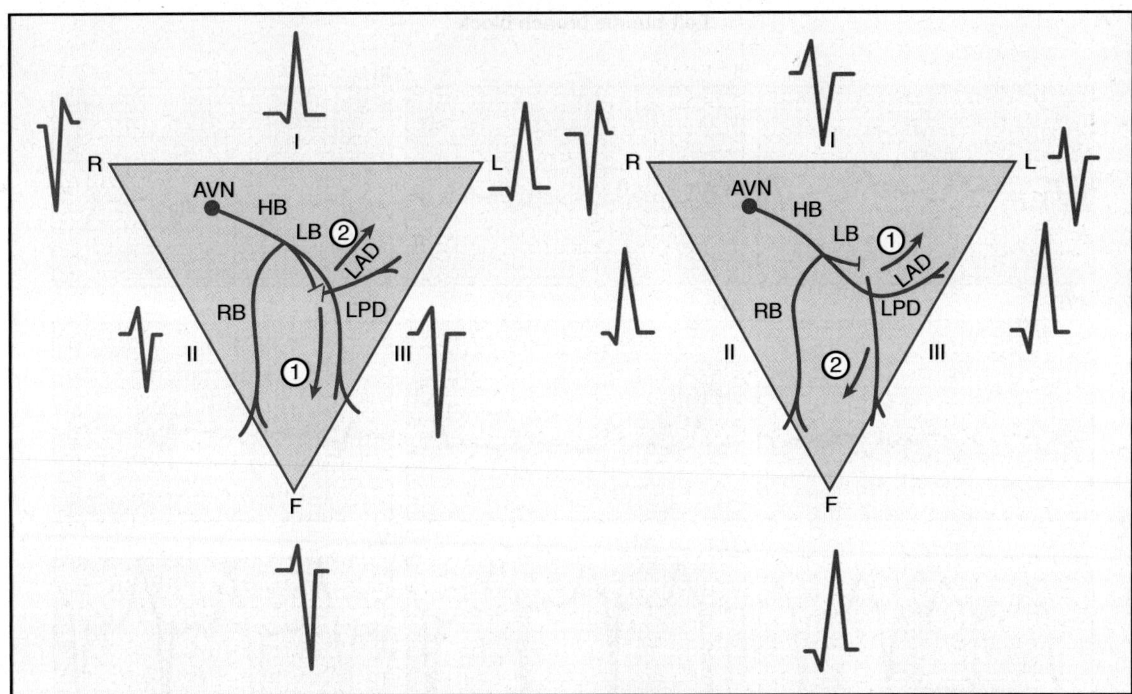

Figure 42-18 Diagrammatic representation of fascicular blocks in the left ventricle. Interruption of the left anterior fascicle (*left*) results in an initial inferior (1) followed by a dominant superior (2) direction of activation (negative in lead II and positive in leads I and aVL). Interruption of the left posterior fascicle (*right*) results in an initial superior (1) followed by a dominant inferior (2) direction of activation (negative in lead I and positive in leads II and III). AVN, atrioventricular node; HB, His bundle; LAD, left anterior descending artery; LB, left bundle; LPD, left posterior descending artery; RB, right bundle. *(Courtesy of C. Fisch, M.D.; From Zipes DP, Libby P, Bonow R, Braunwald E: Braunwald's Heart Disease: A Textbook of Cardiovascular Medicine, 7th ed. Philadelphia, WB Saunders, 2005.)*

ated to the left or even the right. The ST-T waves are usually discordant with the direction of the QRS complex. LBBB is an ominous prognostic sign and has associated survival rates as low as 50%, probably reflecting the severity of the underlying cardiac disease. The QRS duration correlates inversely with the LV ejection fraction and is one of the criteria for current ventricular resynchronization therapy (biventricular pacing).

LBBB obscures or simulates other patterns on the ECG. In the presence of LBBB, the diagnosis of LVH, acute ischemia, or MI may be difficult or impossible (Fig. 42-19).

Right Bundle Branch Block. An RBBB is caused by a conduction delay anywhere in the right-sided intraventricular conduction system. The high prevalence of RBBB corresponds to the relative fragility of the right bundle branch, as suggested by the development of RBBB after minor trauma produced by right ventricular catheterization. The electrocardiographic manifestation of RBBB consists of prominent and notched R waves with rsr′, rsR′, or rSR′ on the right-sided leads and wide S waves on the left-sided leads, along with QRS prolongation (≥120 msec). If the QRS duration is not prolonged, it is termed an incomplete RBBB. As with LBBB, the ST-T waves are discordant with the QRS complex.

RBBB is common in the general healthy population without clinical evidence of structural heart disease and has no prognostic significance in this group. However, in patients with organic heart disease, new onset of RBBB does predict a higher rate of CAD, CHF, and mortality (Fig. 42-20).

Trifascicular blocks usually consist of one of the foregoing bilateral bundle branch blocks (i.e., RBBB plus LAFB or LPFB), in addition to a prolonged PR interval. Bundle of His ECGs are necessary to determine whether the AV conduction disturbance is localized in the AV node or whether it is distal and possibly represents an incomplete fascicular block in the last remaining fascicle.

Electrocardiographic Criteria for Acute Myocardial Ischemia

ST Depression–Type Ischemia

The criteria most accepted for detecting myocardial ischemia on continuous electrocardiographic monitoring are those established and validated during exercise stress testing.[58] During stress testing and with acute subendocardial ischemia, the electrical forces responsible for the ST segment are deviated toward the inner layer of the heart, thereby causing depression of the ST segment. With acute transmural (epicardial) ischemia, the electrical forces in the ischemic area are deviated toward the outer layer of the heart, thereby causing ST-segment elevation in the overlying leads (see Fig. 42-5). As the heart rate increases, the J point, or junctional up-sloping depression, occurs normally. In patients with myocardial ischemia, however, the ST segment typically becomes horizontal (flattens) as the severity of ischemia increases. With progressive exercise or tachycardia during ischemia, the ST-segment depression may worsen, the ST segment may become down sloping, even causing T-wave inversion in more than one lead, and angina may develop. In about 10% of patients, especially asymptomatic ones, ischemia may appear only in the recovery phase after exercise.

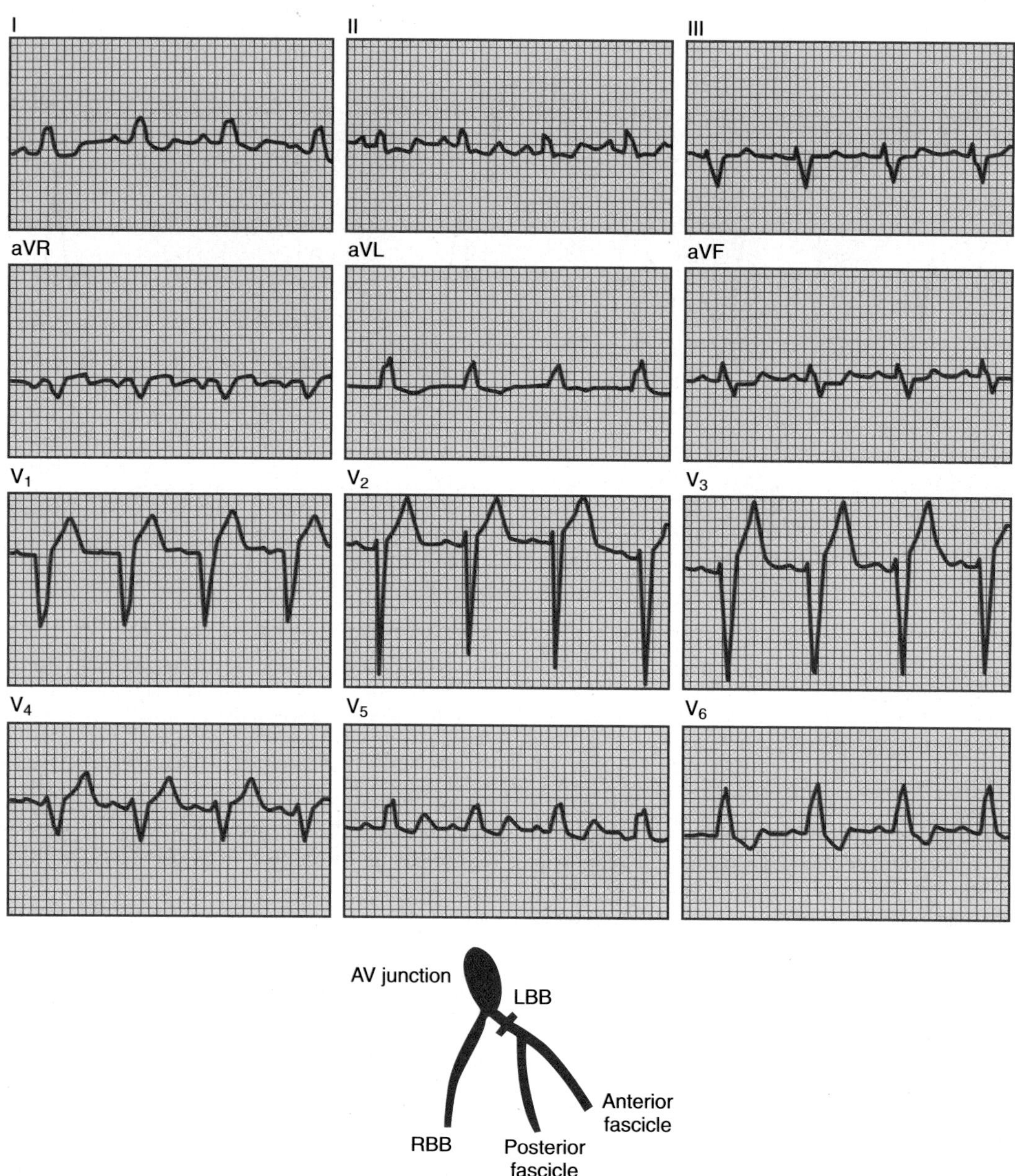

Figure 42-19 Left bundle branch (LBB) block with a characteristic wide QS complex in lead V_1 and a wide R wave in lead V_6 with slight notching at the peak. The inverted T waves in leads V_5 and V_6 (secondary T-wave inversions) are also characteristic of an LBB block. AV, atrioventricular; RBB, right bundle branch. *(From Goldberger AL: Clinical Electrocardiography: A Simplified Approach, 7th ed. St Louis, CV Mosby, 2006.)*

The criteria established for stress-induced ischemia are 1 mm (0.1 mV) or more of horizontal or down-sloping ST-segment depression measured 60 to 80 msec after the J point in at least three consecutive beats with a stable baseline. The ST depression may be accompanied by T-wave flattening or inversion. Junctional or J-point depression is normal during exercise. In addition, a *rapidly up-sloping* ST segment (>1 mV/sec) that is also *depressed less than 0.15 mV* (1.5 mm) is considered normal. In patients with *slowly up-sloping* ST-segment depression in which the ST segment is *depressed 0.15 mV (1.5 mm) or more* at J+80 msec, the slowly up-sloping ST depression may signify CAD (Figs. 42-21 and 42-22).

Some patients have preexisting ST-segment abnormalities from previous MI, bundle branch blocks, or LVH that make ST-segment interpretation more difficult. In these patients, additional horizontal or down-sloping ST-segment depression of 1 mm or greater from baseline is required to be considered myocardial ischemia. Causes of ST-segment changes other than myocardial ischemia include drugs (most notably digitalis), temperature changes, hyperventilation, and positional changes. The distribution of ST depression–type ischemia correlates poorly with the specific location of CAD.

ST Elevation–Type Ischemia

ST-segment elevation in a non–Q-wave lead is very uncommon during stress testing; it occurs in approximately 1% of patients

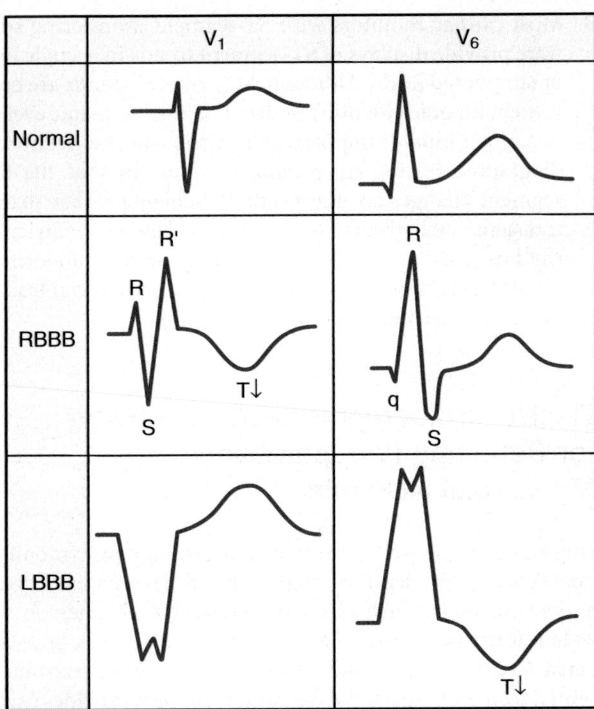

Figure 42-20 Comparison of QRST changes in left bundle branch block (LBBB) versus right bundle branch block (RBBB). *(From Zipes: Braunwald's Heart Disease: A Textbook of Cardiovascular Medicine, 7th ed; and Goldberger AL: Clinical Electrocardiography: A Simplified Approach. 6th ed. St Louis, CV Mosby, 1999.)*

with CAD and suggests transmural myocardial ischemia caused by coronary vasospasm or high-grade coronary narrowing. The electrocardiographic site of ST-segment elevation is relatively specific for the myocardial territory involved, in contrast to ST depression–type ischemia. ST elevation occurring during exercise testing in electrocardiographic leads with pathologic Q waves does not indicate myocardial ischemia but does correlate with reduced LV function and a worse prognosis.

T-Wave Changes

T-wave morphology is largely influenced by body position, respiration, hyperventilation, and drug therapy, as well as by myocardial ischemia/necrosis. Therefore, T-wave changes not accompanied by significant ST-segment displacement rarely signify myocardial ischemia. Pseudonormalization of T waves (inverted at rest, becoming upright during exercise) may in rare instances also be a marker for myocardial ischemia. In a meta-analysis that included 147 reports of patients who underwent both angiography and exercise testing, the sensitivity and specificity of the exercise electrocardiographic stress test for detection of CAD were 68% and 77%, respectively.[59]

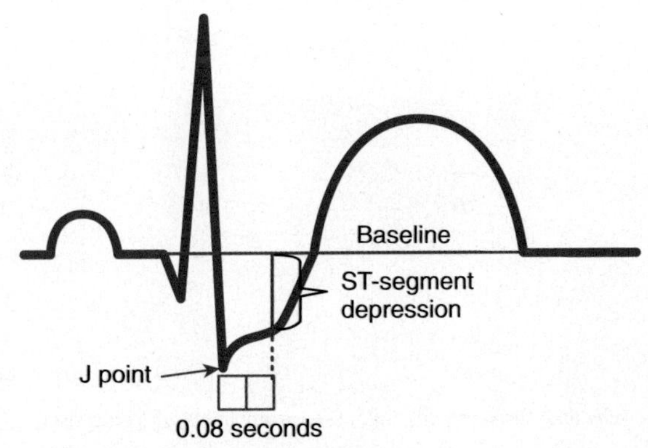

Figure 42-21 Illustration demonstrating how the ST-segment deviation is measured at 80 msec after the J point (J+80 msec).

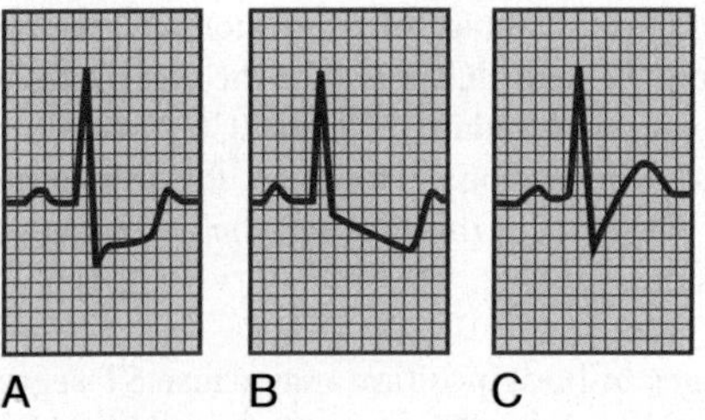

Figure 42-22 Horizontal ST depression (**A**) and down-sloping (**B**) ST depression—indicative of myocardial ischemia. Up-sloping ST depression (**C**) may be a normal finding.

Real-Time Myocardial Ischemia Monitoring

Real-time ST-segment analysis first appeared in cardiac monitoring in the mid-1980s, and currently this feature is standard in most electrocardiographic monitors. On some monitors, ST-segment analysis is automatic when a five-electrode system is used. However, the five-electrode monitoring system with automatic ST-segment analysis is primarily used by anesthesiologists in the operating room but widely underused postoperatively in the postanesthesia care unit or ICU. A recent study has shown that even among coronary care units, fewer than than 50% of clinicians routinely use ST-segment monitoring for the detection of myocardial ischemia in patients admitted with acute coronary syndromes.[60] Chief among the reasons for underuse of ST analysis are (1) a high number of false alarms, (2) lack of education on how to use the technology, and (3) what to do in response to ST alarms. In addition, there are no published randomized clinical trials to determine whether the addition of computerized ST-segment ischemia monitoring improves outcomes in patients with acute coronary syndromes or in postsurgical patients.[12]

The algorithm for ST-segment analysis is relatively simple. In each electrocardiographic lead, the computer determines the voltage of the ST segment at 60 or 80 msec after the J point (termed J+60 or J+80 msec) and compares it with the isoelectric point measured normally during the PR interval. One millimeter of ST-segment deviation is equivalent to a 100-mV difference. The changes in ST-segment level over time in each lead are displayed as ST-segment trends. To overcome problems of noise and artifacts, most monitors use filters to exclude erroneous or abnormal beats on the ECG. Averaging processes are used to calculate the mean ST-segment level over a period of 8 to 15 beats. Current monitors automatically detect the J point and calculate the J+60 msec ST-segment level. However, they also allow the operator to manually adjust the J point and the ST-segment measurement point in patients with abnormal patterns on the ECG.

One major advantage of continuous ST-segment monitoring over serial 12-lead ECGs is that the electrodes stay in place and do not vary as standard 12-lead ECGs may do between different measuring sessions. However, for improved diagnostic accuracy of ST-segment monitoring, the following points should be recognized:

1. Changes in body position may cause ST-segment changes and lead to false ST-segment deviations. However, these positional ST-segment changes are almost always accompanied by changes in QRS and therefore can easily be distinguished from true ST-segment deviations. In addition, returning the patient to the supine position may help distinguish true from positional ST-segment deviation. Changes in position of the heart in the mediastinum were also shown to affect the ST segment. Mark and coworkers[61] observed that placement of a Canadian sternal retractor during cardiac surgery was associated with a reduction in V_5 R-wave amplitude from 15 ± 1 to 10 ± 1 mm. Simultaneously, V_5 S-wave amplitude and absolute ST-segment deviation were reduced from 3.5 ± 0.4 to 1.7 ± 0.3 mm and from 0.50 ± 0.04 to 0.39 ± 0.05 mm, respectively (Table 42-2). These investigators concluded that inclusion of an R-wave gain factor may improve perioperative electrocardiographic ischemia monitoring.
2. Many patients with CAD do not have perfectly isoelectric ST segments. Early repolarization (a normal variant), intraventricular conduction delays, ventricular hypertrophy, digitalis, and nonspecific ST-T wave abnormalities may cause baseline ST-segment abnormalities. It is therefore important to tailor the ST alarm trending to the patient's baseline ST level. Many current cardiac monitors with ST-segment monitoring software allow clinicians to set alarm parameters manually. If alarm parameters are set 1 to 2 mm around the isoelectric (0 μV) line rather than at the patient's baseline ST level, frequent false alarms will occur. It is recommended that alarm parameters be set 1 mm above and below the baseline ST level in patients at high risk for ischemia. It should also be remembered that underlying electrocardiographic abnormalities may hinder ST analysis in about 10% of patients. Such abnormalities include hypokalemia, digitalis, LBBB, Wolff-Parkinson-White syndrome, LVH with strain, and acute pericarditis. In these patients, other modalities for diagnosis of myocardial ischemia should be considered, such as transesophageal echocardiography.
3. Most cardiac monitors with ST-segment monitoring software provide displays of ST-segment trends in a single lead or summated leads. Although such graphic trends are convenient for quick identification of potential ischemic events, it is of paramount importance to also print the electrocardiographic tracing in question to confirm that the ST-segment changes are the result of ischemia rather than a transient arrhythmia (e.g., an accelerated ventricular rhythm or a new bundle branch block) or other abnormality of the electrocardiographic complex, which can lead to inaccurate calculation.

Electrocardiographic Lead Sensitivity for Detecting Perioperative Myocardial Ischemia

During the perioperative period, electrocardiographic monitoring most commonly identifies stress-induced, ST-segment depression–type ischemia. Such electrocardiographic changes do not provide information about the location of the ischemic myocardial area. In contrast, ST-segment elevation indicating transmural ischemia, seen particularly during cardiac surgery, provides useful information about the myocardial segment and coronary perfusion territory responsible for the ischemic episode. Because the majority of modern patient-monitoring systems do not monitor all 12 electrocardiographic leads simultaneously, selecting which chest leads to monitor is of great importance, particularly in noncardiac surgery. During exercise stress testing, investigators have identified leads V_4 and V_5 as the most sensitive leads to detect exercise-induced ischemia (90% to 100% sensitivity).[62] London and colleagues[63] studied high-risk patients undergoing noncardiac surgery and showed that the greatest sensitivity for ischemia was obtained with lead V_5 (75%), followed by lead V_4 (61%). Combining leads V_4 and V_5 increased the sensitivity to 90%, whereas with the standard lead II and V_5 combination, the sensitivity was only 80%. They also suggested that if three leads (II, V_4, and V_5) could be examined simultaneously, the sensitivity would rise to 98%. More recently, Landesberg and associates[64] monitored continuous 12-lead ST-segment changes greater than 0.2 mV from baseline in a single lead, or greater than 0.1 mV in two contiguous leads at J+60 msec, lasting longer than 10 minutes in patients undergoing major vascular surgery. Troponins were used as markers for MI. They showed that in fact leads V_3 and V_4 were more sensitive than V_5 in detecting perioperative ischemia

Table 42-2 Electrocardiographic Changes during Sternal Retractor Placement in 83 Patients

Variable	Period	Mean ± SEM	*n* Increase	*n* Decrease	χ^2	P
V_5 RWA	Baseline	15.1 ± 0.8	—	—	—	—
	Retractor	9.9 ± 0.7	9	69	44.6	.001
V_5 SWA	Baseline	3.5 ± 0.4	—	—	—	—
	Retractor	1.7 ± 0.3	3	59	48.8	.001
V_5 ST-ABS	Baseline	0.05 ± 0.04	—	—	—	—
	Retractor	0.40 ± 0.05	20	51	12.68	.001

n, number of patients showing the indicated change; RWA, R-wave amplitude; ST-ABS, absolute value of ST displacement; SWA, S-wave amplitude; χ^2, comparison between *n* increase and *n* decrease.

Adapted from Mark JB, Chein GL, Steinbrook RA, et al: Electrocardiographic R-wave changes during cardiac surgery. Anesth Analg 74:26, 1992.

(87%, 79%, and 66%, respectively). Among the patients who experienced MI, V_4 was the most sensitive for ischemia (83.3%), followed by V_3 and V_5 (75% each). Combined monitoring of two of these leads (e.g., V_3 and V_5) increased the sensitivity to about 97%.[62] It was also demonstrated that on average, the baseline, preanesthesia ST segment was above the isoelectric point in V_1 through V_3 and below isoelectric in V_5 through V_6. Lead V_4 was closest to the isoelectric level on the baseline ECG, thus rendering it most suitable for detection of ischemia. Lead V_4 also detects ischemia earlier and shows a greater ST-segment deviation. These main findings were corroborated by Martinez and colleagues,[65] who also used the same method to monitor postoperative ischemia in ICU patients after major vascular surgery.

For patients with acute coronary syndromes (e.g., those with atherosclerotic plaque disruption), the recommendation is to monitor limb lead III and leads V_3 and V_5 as the most sensitive combination for detection of ischemia.[66] Monitoring of a right-sided precordial lead (V_4R) may be of benefit in patients with occlusive disease of the right coronary artery,[67] as might inspection of posterior leads (V_7 to V_9) in patients with suspected posterior ischemia.

It is commonly believed that monitoring for intraoperative myocardial ischemia is unnecessary in neonates. Whereas electrocardiographic lead systems for adults are concerned with detection of ischemia and arrhythmias, neonatal electrocardiographic monitoring has focused on recognition of arrhythmias alone. The results of some studies, however, suggest that the neonatal heart is more susceptible to ischemia than the adult heart is.[68] These studies have demonstrated the importance of calibrated electrocardiographic monitoring in neonates with congenital heart disease (see Chapter 83).

Perioperative Myocardial Ischemia and Infarction

Perioperative monitoring for myocardial ischemia in patients undergoing cardiac or noncardiac surgery started about 30 years ago. In 1980, Tinker[69] noted the importance of intraoperative ST-segment monitoring via lead V_5 and that large fluctuations in systolic blood pressure, heart rate, or hypothermia with postoperative shivering are associated with ischemia. Coriat and colleagues,[70] pioneers in using Holter monitoring in patients undergoing major vascular surgery, showed that the presence of intraoperative ischemia on Holter monitoring was strongly associated with the severity of preoperative angina pectoris. Slogoff and Keats[71] first demonstrated in 1985 an association between intraoperative ischemia and postoperative MI. They demonstrated that MI detected before induction of anesthesia or before the onset of cardiopulmonary bypass during coronary artery bypass graft surgery is strongly associated with ischemia on Holter monitoring. Several studies using perioperative (preoperative, intraoperative, and postoperative) Holter monitoring in patients undergoing major vascular surgery showed that early postoperative tachycardia-induced silent myocardial ischemia was frequent after vascular surgery and significantly associated with postoperative clinical ischemic events.[72-74] Mangano and coworkers[75] (1990) demonstrated that postoperative Holter-detected ischemia was common (41%) and predictive of adverse postoperative cardiac events, with a ninefold increase in the odds of postoperative cardiac morbidity and mortality when compared with intraoperative or preoperative ischemia.

Table 42-3 summarizes all the studies that were published in the English literature on perioperative ischemia and postoperative cardiac morbidity after major noncardiac surgery.[76-90] Altogether, these studies included more than 2400 patients. The majority of the studies involved major vascular surgery and Holter monitoring for detection of perioperative ischemia (except for the studies by Landesberg and colleagues, which used continuous on-line 12-lead electrocardiographic monitoring). The data revealed that perioperative ischemia was common in high-risk patients, with an incidence between 24% and 63%, and was almost exclusively ST depression consistent with ischemia (97% to 100%). The average postoperative MI rate in these studies was 3.9% (range, 0.6% to 15%), the majority of which were non–Q-wave infarctions (66% to 100%). The incidence of all ischemic postoperative cardiac events was 7.3% (range, 3% to 37%), and the average mortality was 1.04% (range, 0% to 2.8%). Another important observation was that the duration of postoperative ischemia was strongly associated with postoperative ischemic cardiac events. Patients with prolonged, often long hours of postoperative ST depression–type ischemia were likely to experience postoperative MI and elevated serum troponin levels, whereas short episodes of ischemia (<30 minutes) were unlikely to culminate in MI.[87] Additional studies have shown that perioperative ischemia is associated not only with early but also with long-term (5 years) postoperative morbidity and mortality.[88,91]

Examples of Perioperative Ischemia and Infarction

EXAMPLE 1. Frank and coauthors[76] published one of the first and most detailed cases of postoperative cardiac mortality related to heart rate–induced prolonged postoperative ST depression–type ischemia detected on Holter monitoring. A patient who underwent lower extremity arterial bypass surgery was monitored with a Holter monitor before, during, and after the operation. His records show that he had heart rate–related silent myocardial ischemia preoperatively that subsided intraoperatively, immediately after anesthesia was instituted, only to recur as soon as the patient woke up from surgery. Figure 42-23 shows the ischemia worsening progressively after surgery until the patient died suddenly 10 hours after the operation. The ST depression–type ischemia of this patient occurred at a relatively low heart rate of 80 to 85 beats/min and in the absence of significant alterations in blood pressure. Two snapshots of electrocardiographic disclosure are presented at around 12 midnight: one at a heart rate of approximately 90 beats/min, which showed deep ST-segment depression, and the other a short while later with temporary slowing of the heart rate to around 60 beats/min, which showed almost complete but transient resolution of the ST depression. Although cardiac markers were not measured and no data were provided on myocardial function by echocardiography, it is very suggestive that the patient died as a result of prolonged, silent, heart rate–related ST depression–ischemia, which was at least temporarily reversible by slowing his heart rate (Fig. 42-23).

EXAMPLE 2. A 70-year-old patient with a history of CAD (treated by coronary artery bypass grafting 7 years earlier), reduced LV function, insulin-dependent diabetes mellitus, and

Table 42-3 (Part 1) Studies Published in the English Literature on Perioperative Ischemia and Postoperative Cardiac Morbidity after Major Noncardiac Surgery

					Postoperative Ischemic Cardiac Events in Patients with Ischemia on Continuous Electrocardiographic Monitoring				
Publication	***N***	**Type of Surgery**	**Patients with Ischemia (%)**	**Patients with Any Ischemic Event (%)**	**Sensitivity (%)**	**Specificity (%)**	**Positive Predictive Value (%)**	**Negative Predictive Value (%)**	**Relative Risk (%)**
McCann and Clements,[72] J Vasc Surg, 1989	50	Vascular	38	8	100	62	21	100	Indefinite
Ouyang et al.,[73] Am J Cardiol, 1989	24	Vascular	63	37.5	89	37.5	53	89	4.8
Pasternack et al.,[74] J Vasc Surg, 1989	200	Vascular	50.5	4.5	100	36.5	7.1	100	Indefinite
Frank et al.,[75] J Clin Anesth, 1990	1	Vascular							
Mangano et al., N Engl J Med, 1990,[76] J Am Coll Cardiol, 1991[77]	474	Major noncardiac	41	3.2	85.7	82	13.9	99	8.6
Pasternack et al.,[78] J Vasc Surg, 1992	385	Vascular	46	4.9	84.2	68.8	13.3	98.8	11.7
Raby et al.,[79] JAMA, 1992	115	Vascular	30.4	13.9	87.5	69.5	40	97.5	16
Marsch et al.,[80] Anesthesiology, 1992	52	Hip arthroplasty	31	6 (11.5)	50	69.2	18.7	91.6	2.25
Landesberg et al.,[81] Lancet, 1993	151	Vascular	48	8.6	84.6	52.3	15.3	97.4	6
Andrews et al.,[82] J Vasc Med Biol, 1994	145	Vascular	24.8	4.1	100	75.2	16.7	100	Indefinite
Ganz et al.,[83] Am Heart J, 1994	1	Vascular							
Fleisher et al.,[84] J Clin Anesth, 1995	145	Major noncardiac	26	6.2	77.8	74.5	18.9	98.1	10.2
Wallace et al.,[85] Anesthesiology, 1998	101	Major noncardiac	34	11.0	?				
Groves et al.,[86] Br J Anaesth, 1999	82	Thoracotomy	24	10.9	55.5	75.6	25	93.5	3.8
Rapp et al.,[87] Acta Anaesthesiol Scand, 1999	20	Vascular	40	15	100	60	37.5	100	Indefinite
Gauss et al.,[88] Anesthesiology, 2001	204	Major noncardiac	1.5 with ischemia >30 min	8.6	18.75	96.3	100	83.5	6.1
Landesberg et al.,[89,90] J Am Coll Cardiol, 2001, 2003	447	Major Vascular	14.7 with ischemia >10 min	9.2	92.7	85.2	57.6	99.2	73

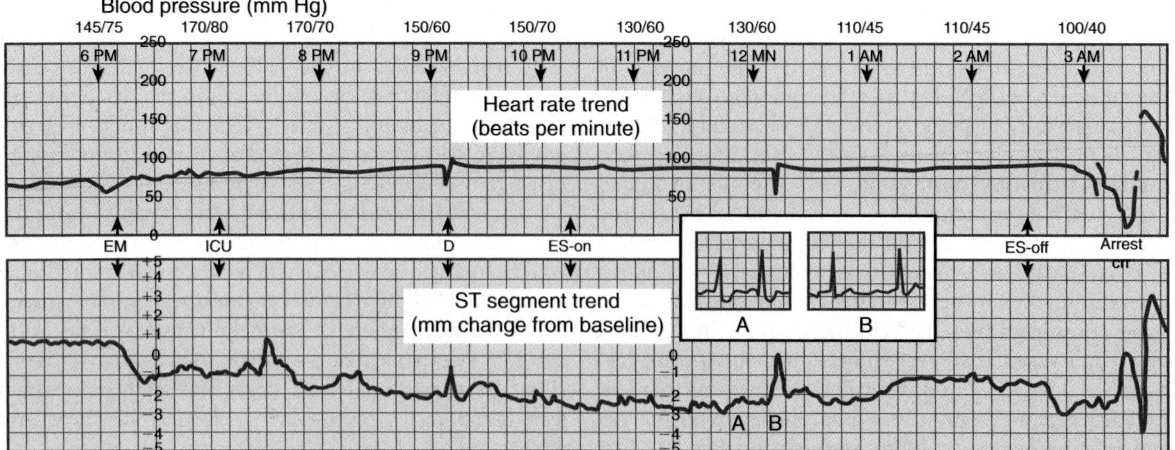

Figure 42-23 Heart rate and ST trends from emergence of anesthesia (EM) to cardiac arrest. CPR, cardiopulmonary resuscitation; D, brief decrease in heart rate; ES-on/off, start/end of esmolol infusion; ICU, intensive care unit admission. *(From Frank SM, Beattie C, Christopherson R, et al: Perioperative rate-related silent myocardial ischemia and postoperative death. J Clin Anesth 2:326-331, 1990.)*

Table 42-3 (Part 2)

Publication	% with ST Depression	Postoperative Ischemia Duration (hr)		Postoperative MI		Cardiac Mortality (%)	Electrocardiographic Leads Monitored
		Patients without MI	Patients with MI	%	% with non-Q MI		
McCann and Clements,[72] J Vasc Surg, 1989	Not specified			4	Not specified	4	Modified V_5
Ouyang et al.,[73] Am J Cardiol, 1989	100	Median = 1.05 (0.08-9.0) min		8.3	Not specified	0	2 inferior + 2 anterior
Pasternack et al.,[74] J Vasc Surg, 1989	Only ST depression was studied	2.9 ± 8.3	11.5 ± 13.1	4.5	Not specified	0.5	Single MC_5
Frank et al.,[75] J Clin Anesth, 1990	ST depression		>10 hr			100	L_2, V_5
Mangano et al., N Engl J Med, 1990,[76] J Am Coll Cardiol 1991[77]	98	1.3 ± 3.3		2.5	Not specified	1.3	CC_5 and MC_5
Pasternack et al.,[78] J Vasc Surg, 1992	Only ST-depression was studied	2.98 ± 8.76	8.1 ± 10.1	4.9	Not specified	1.3	Single CM_5
Raby et al.,[79] JAMA, 1992	Only ST-depression was studied	0.36 (0.02-4.7)		7.8	Not specified	2.6	Not specified
Marsch et al.,[80] Anesthesiology, 1992	100	Not specified		0.5	Not specified	0	CM_3, CM_5, aVF
Landesberg et al.,[81] Lancet, 1993	97	0.56 ± 0.36	8.44 ± 7.84 (>2 hr)	4.0	84	0	Modified V_4, V_5, aVF
Andrews et al.,[82] J Vasc Med Biol, 1994	Only ST-depression was studied		All were >2 hr	0.68	Not specified		Inferior and lateral leads
Ganz et al.,[83] Am Heart J, 1994	ST depression		> 12 hr			100	
Fleisher et al.,[84] J Clin Anesth, 1995	99.3		All were >30 min	6.2	100	0.68	Modified V_3, V_5
Wallace et al.,[85] Anesthesiology, 1998	100	4.7 ± 6.0		2	Not specified	2	CC_5, CM_5, ML
Groves et al.,[86] Br J Anaesth, 1999	Not specified	Not specified		4.8		2.4	V_2, V_5
Rapp et al.,[87] Acta Anaesthesiol Scand, 1999	100	4.3 ± 3.8	28.8 ± 26.9; >5.8 hr	15 (by cTn)	100	0	CC_5, CM_5
Gauss et al.,[88] Anesthesiology, 2001	100	Not reported	>30 min	3 (by cTn)	66	0	V_4, V_5
Landesberg et al.,[89,90] J Am Coll Cardiol, 2001, 2003	99	0.85 ± 0.81	6.26 ± 6.1	3.6 (by cTn)	100	0.4	12-lead ECG

cTn, cardiac troponin; ECG, electrocardiogram; MI, myocardial ischemia.

peripheral vascular disease exhibited prolonged myocardial ischemia and infarction immediately after carotid endarterectomy. On arrival at the operating room the patient was connected to a continuous, 12-lead electrocardiographic monitor with online ST-segment analysis. During surgery no ischemia was observed (Fig. 42-24). Immediately after surgery and on emergence from anesthesia, significant ST depression occurred in association with a moderate increase in heart rate to a maximum of 102 beats/min, in accordance with vague pain in his jaw. The ischemic ST-segment changes lasted 193 minutes, after which the ECG reverted completely to its baseline. Nevertheless, an increase in troponin I to 10.2 ng/mL was measured 6 hours after surgery and up to 32.1 ng/mL on the morning after surgery (see Fig. 42-24).[90] The figure insert depicts all 12-lead electrocardiographic complexes during peak ischemia superimposed on their baseline, preoperative pattern. Significant ST depression occurred in all the

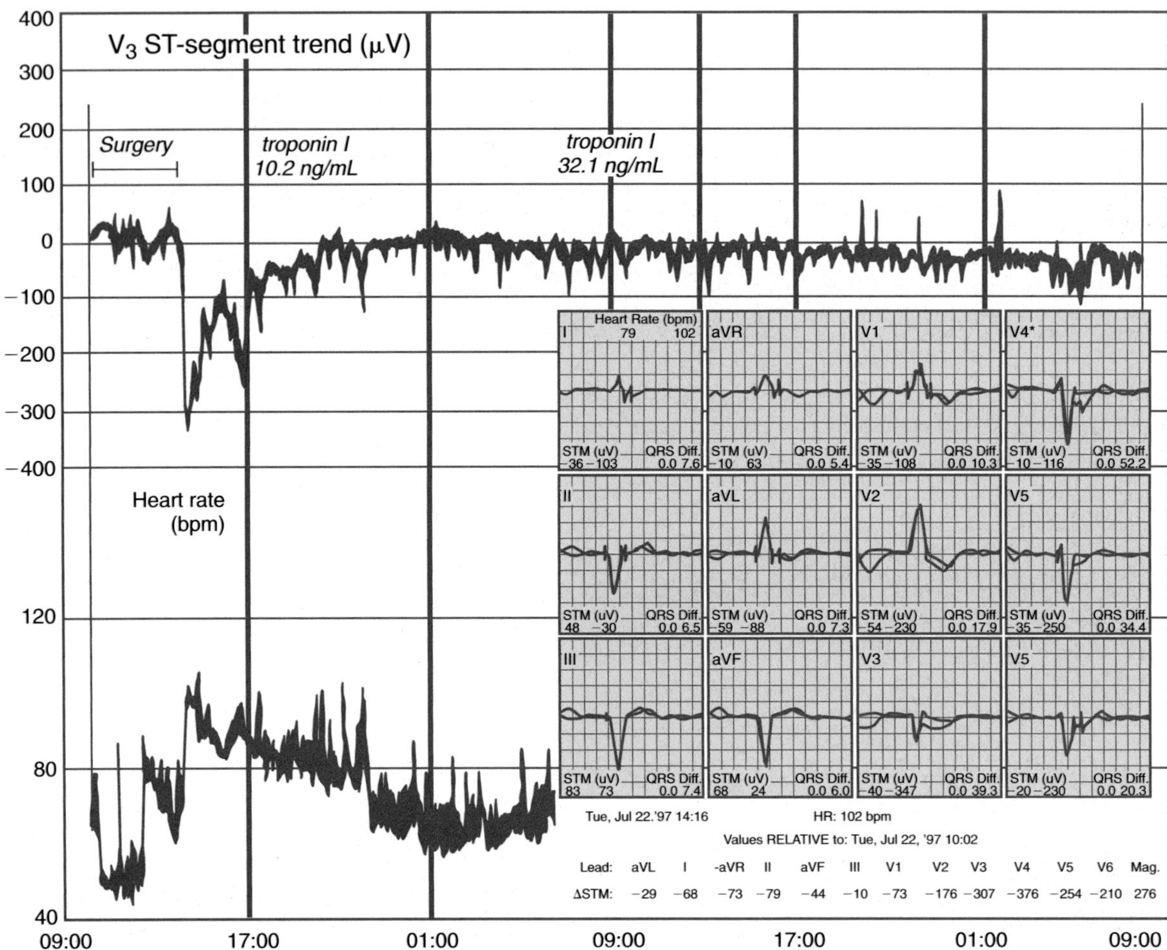

Figure 42-24 Lead V_3 ST-segment and heart rate trends in a patient with prolonged (193 minutes) postoperative ST-segment depression and troponin elevation. The *insert* shows the 12-lead electrocardiographic complexes at peak ischemia superimposed on their baseline patterns.

chest leads and was deepest in lead V_4 (−3.7 mm at peak ischemia). It is interesting to notice the marked abnormality of this patient's baseline ECG (LVH, RBBB, left anterior hemiblock, and baseline ST-T changes). Despite these baseline abnormalities on the ECG, the continuous ST trend monitoring in 12 leads combined with the marked troponin I elevation strongly suggests that the patient had prolonged (>3 hours) ischemia that culminated in elevation of troponin and MI.

Example 3. A 65-year-old patient was admitted for surgery because of an asymptomatic abdominal aortic aneurysm (7 cm) and exhibited prolonged postoperative ischemia and infarction with chronic total occlusion of a coronary artery. His past medical history was significant for hypertension, mild obesity (85 kg), and smoking until 12 years before admission. He had no clinical history of ischemic heart disease, but because of shortness of breath on climbing stairs, a preoperative thallium scan was performed (Fig. 42-25) and demonstrated a moderate to severe, large reversible defect in the entire LV anterior wall.

On echocardiography, the size and function of both ventricles were normal with moderate mitral regurgitation. In light of the thallium scan findings, the patient underwent preoperative coronary angiography (Fig. 42-26), which showed total ostial occlusion of the left anterior descending artery with retrograde filling through a large collateral from the right coronary artery.

Based on these findings, a decision was made to proceed to surgery without coronary revascularization. The patient was given bisoprolol (β_1-selective blocker), 50 mg daily for a month, before he returned for surgery (aortobifemoral bypass).

As in the previous example, this patient was monitored during and after surgery by continuous 12-lead electrocardiography with on-line ST-segment monitoring. Intraoperatively, the heart rate was 50 to 70 beats/min, and no significant ST-segment changes were observed. However, immediately at the end of surgery and extubation, significant ST-depression consistent with ischemia developed in association with an increase in heart rate to a maximum of 98 beats/min (Fig. 42-27) and blood pressure of 155/86. Intravenous esmolol and labetalol were administered immediately, and the ischemia subsided within 15 minutes. The patient was transferred extubated and comfortable to the ICU under continuous infusion of esmolol. In the ICU, the doses of esmolol had to be escalated gradually because of a persistent increase in heart rate. Postoperative pain was managed with the epidural catheter. Nevertheless, 5 hours after the end of surgery, severe ST depression recurred in the entire anterior wall. The ischemia lasted longer than 5 hours and responded poorly to β-adrenergic blocking agents (see Fig. 42-27). The patient became delirious and shortness of breath developed. Treatment included intravenous diuretics and a slow

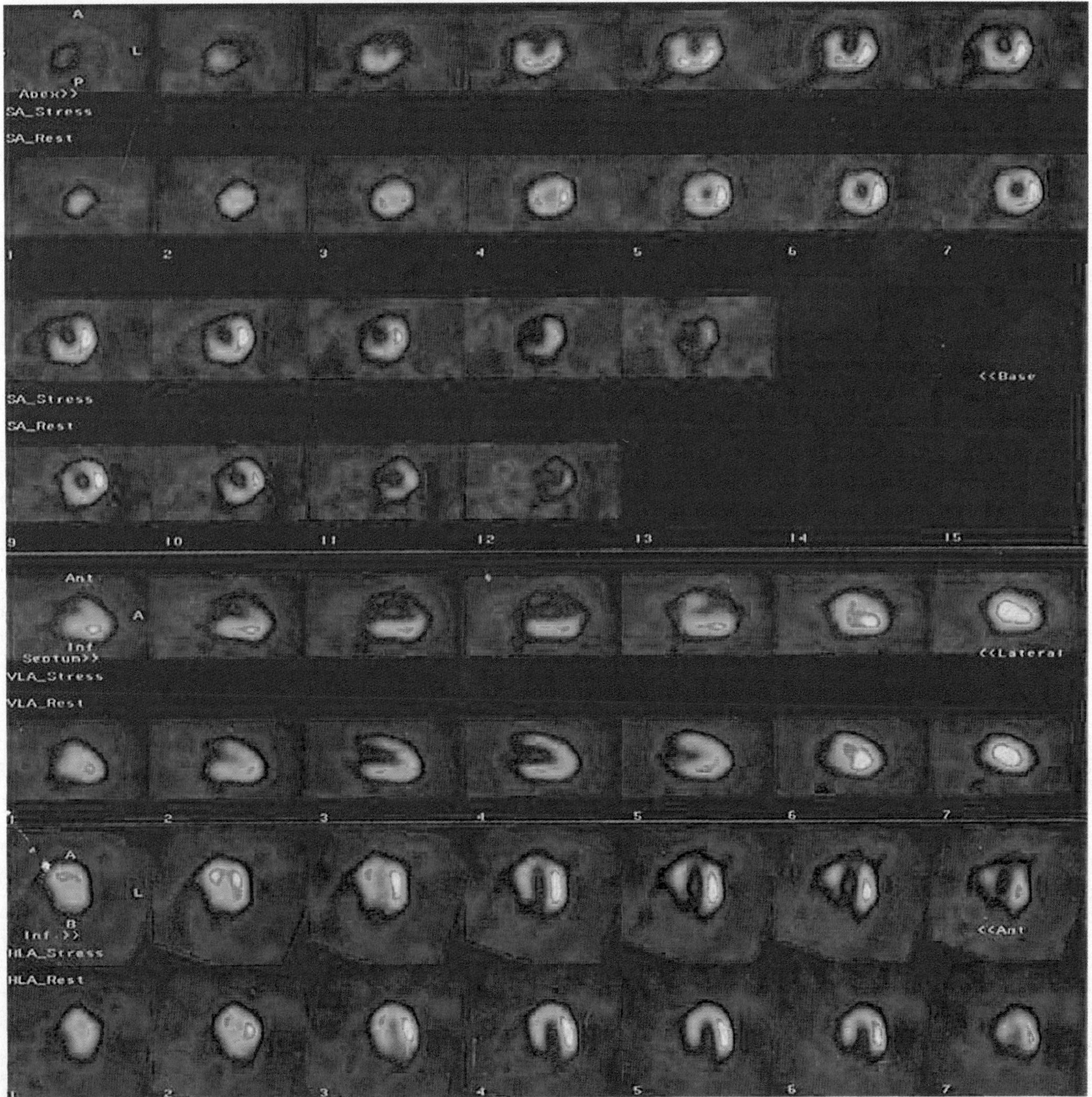

Figure 42-25 Preoperative dipyridamole-thallium single photon emission computed tomography scan of a patient scheduled for abdominal aortic surgery. A moderate to severe reversible defect is present in the entire anterior wall.

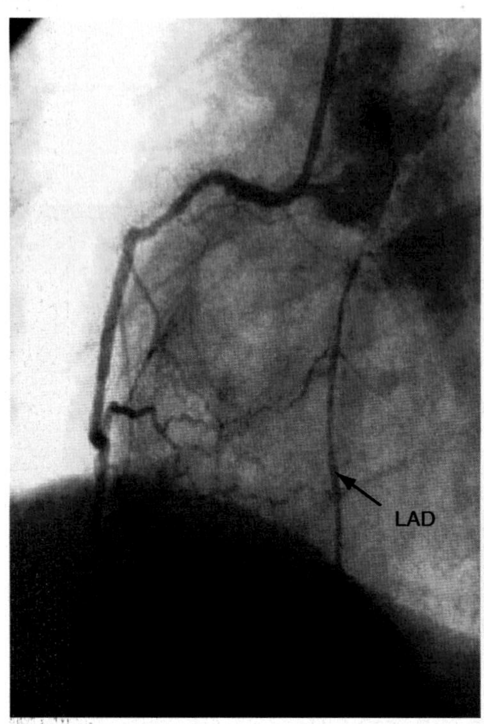

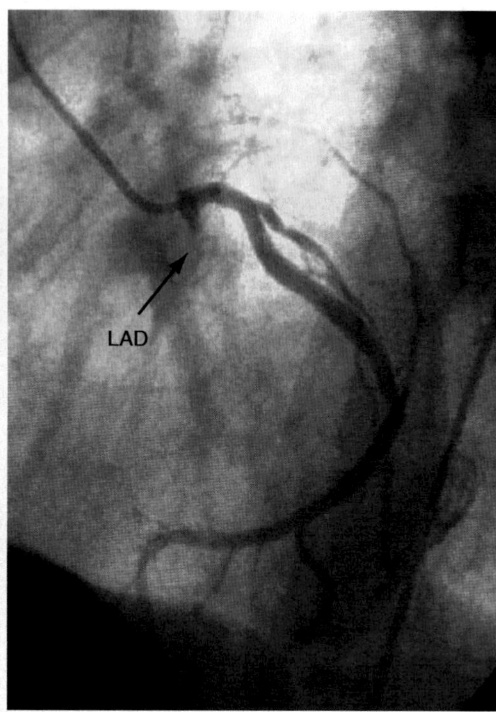

Figure 42-26 Coronary angiogram of the patient in Figure 42-25 showing chronic total ostial occlusion of the left anterior descending (LAD) artery with excellent filling of the distal LAD artery by a collateral from the right coronary artery. A possible mild stenosis is also noted in the first marginal coronary artery.

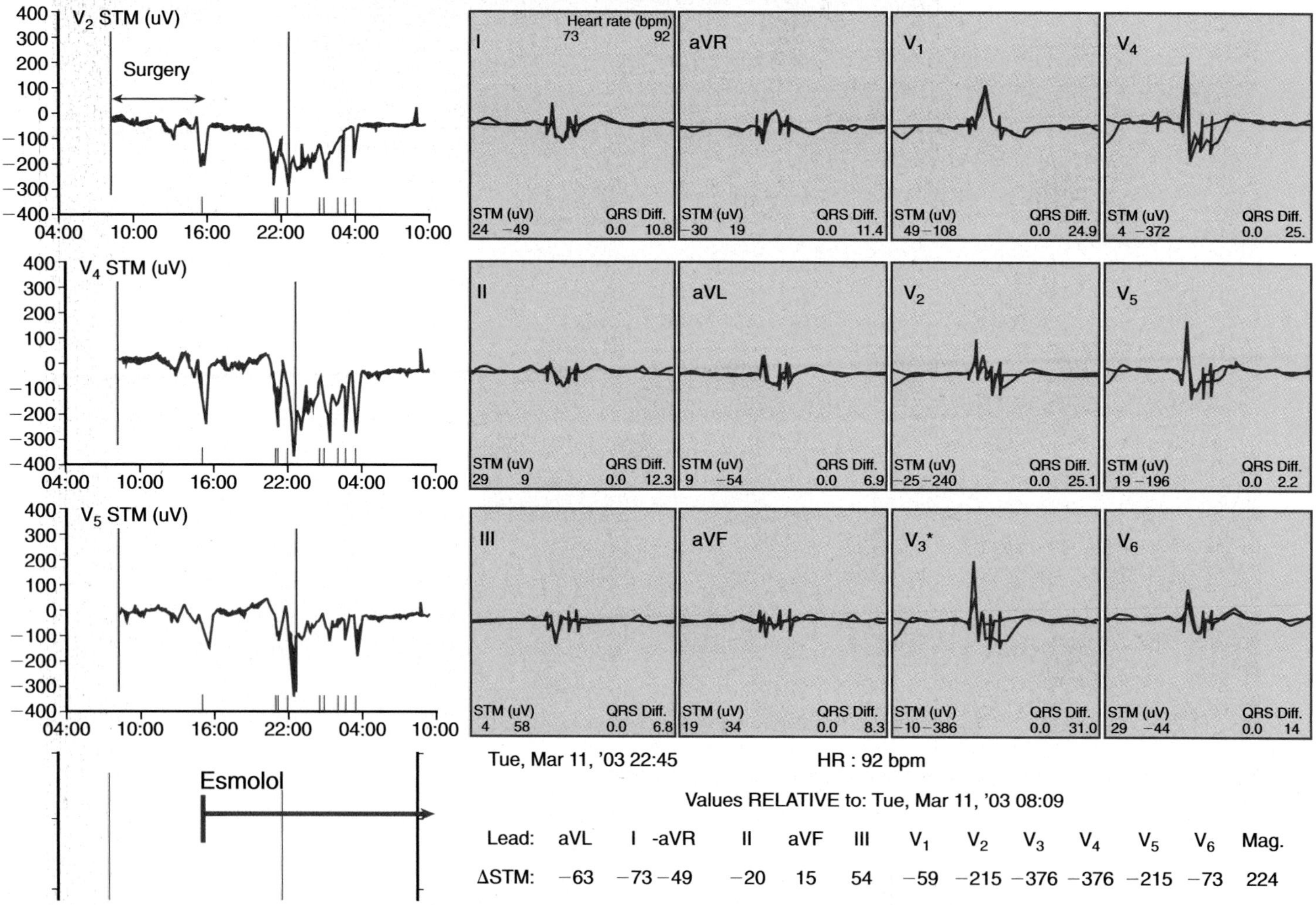

V$_2$ STM (uV)

Surgery

V$_4$ STM (uV)

V$_5$ STM (uV)

Esmolol

Heart rate (bpm) 73 92

	STM (uV)	QRS Diff.
I	24 −49	0.0 10.8
aVR	−30 19	0.0 11.4
V$_1$	49 −108	0.0 24.9
V$_4$	4 −372	0.0 25.
II	29 9	0.0 12.3
aVL	9 −54	0.0 6.9
V$_2$	−25 −240	0.0 25.1
V$_5$	19 −196	0.0 2.2
III	4 58	0.0 6.8
aVF	19 34	0.0 8.3
V$_3$*	−10 −386	0.0 31.0
V$_6$	29 −44	0.0 14

Tue, Mar 11, '03 22:45 HR : 92 bpm

Values RELATIVE to: Tue, Mar 11, '03 08:09

Lead:	aVL	I	−aVR	II	aVF	III	V$_1$	V$_2$	V$_3$	V$_4$	V$_5$	V$_6$	Mag.
ΔSTM:	−63	−73	−49	−20	15	54	−59	−215	−376	−376	−215	−73	224

Figure 42-27 Perioperative ST-segment and heart rate trends are demonstrated in the *left panels*. All 12-lead electrocardiographic complexes during peak ischemia, superimposed over the corresponding baseline (preoperative) complexes, are demonstrated in the *right panels*. The ST-segment trends show two episodes of ST-depression–type ischemia: a short episode of 15 minutes immediately at the end of surgery, followed by a 5-hour period of no ischemia and then another long episode of ST depression lasting more than 5 hours. Ischemia is evident in all anterior leads but is maximal in V_3 and V_4.

infusion of packed red blood cells. Twenty-fours hours after the end of surgery, the ischemic electrocardiographic changes regressed almost completely to normal, yet serum troponin T levels increased to 0.64 ng/mL and remained elevated for another 5 days.

This unique case demonstrates that postoperative MI may occur as a result of prolonged stress-induced ST depression–type ischemia in the presence of stable CAD with chronic total coronary artery occlusion of one coronary artery and no rupture of coronary plaque.

References

1. Kligfield P, Gettes LS, Bailey JJ, et al: Recommendations for the standardization and interpretation of the electrocardiogram: part I: The electrocardiogram and its technology: A scientific statement from the American Heart Association Electrocardiography and Arrhythmias Committee, Council on Clinical Cardiology; the American College of Cardiology Foundation; and the Heart Rhythm Society: Endorsed by the International Society for Computerized Electrocardiology. Circulation 115:1306-1324, 2007.
2. Slogoff S, Keats AS, David Y, Igo SR: Incidence of perioperative myocardial ischemia detected by different electrocardiographic systems. Anesthesiology 74:1171-1172, 1991.
3. Thys DM, Kaplan JA: The ECG in Anesthesia and Critical Care. New York, Churchill Livingstone, 1987.
4. Bazaral MG, Norfleet EA: Comparison of CB_5 and V_5 leads for intraoperative electrocardiographic monitoring. Anesth Analg 60:849-853, 1981.
5. Mason RE, Likar I: A new system of multiple-lead exercise electrocardiography. Am Heart J 71:196-205, 1966.
6. Krucoff MW, Loeffler KA, Haisty WK Jr, et al: Simultaneous ST-segment measurements using standard and monitoring-compatible torso limb lead placements at rest and during coronary occlusion. Am J Cardiol 74:997-1001, 1994.
7. London MJ: Validation testing of the SEER real-time digital Holter monitor. J Cardiothorac Vasc Anesth 10:497-501, 1996.
8. Dodds TM, Delphin E, Stone G, et al: Detection of perioperative myocardial ischemia using Holter with real-time ST segment analysis. Anesth Analg 67:890-893, 1988.
9. Romhilt DW, Bloomfield SS, Chou TC, Fowler NO: Unreliability of conventional electrocardiographic monitoring of arrhythmia detection in coronary care units. Am J Cardiol 31:457-461, 1973.
10. Chiang CM, Jenkins JM, DiCarlo LA, et al: Real-time arrhythmia identification from automated analysis of intraatrial and intraventricular electrograms. Pacing Clin Electrophysiol 16:223-227, 1993.
11. Igel DA, Wilkoff BL: Automated ventricular tachyarrhythmia recognition: A combination of cycle length and nonlinear dynamics measurements. J Cardiovasc Electrophysiol 8:388-397, 1997.
12. Drew BJ, Califf RM, Funk M, et al: Practice standards for electrocardiographic monitoring in hospital settings: An American Heart Association Scientific Statement from the Councils on Cardiovascular Nursing, Clinical Cardiology, and Cardiovascular Disease in the Young. Circulation 110:2721-2746, 2004.
13. Heintz KM, Hollenberg SM: Perioperative cardiac issues: Postoperative arrhythmias. Surg Clin North Am 85:1103-1114, 2005.
14. Mahla E, Rotman B, Rehak P, et al: Perioperative ventricular dysrhythmias in patients with structural heart disease undergoing noncardiac surgery. Anesth Analg 86:16-21, 1998.
15. Mathew JP, Fontes ML, Tudor IC, et al: A multicenter risk index for atrial fibrillation after cardiac surgery. Investigators of the Ischemia Research and Education Foundation; Multicenter Study of Perioperative Ischemia Research Group. JAMA 291:1720-1729, 2004.
16. Atlee JL 3rd, Rusy BF: Ventricular conduction times and AV nodal conductivity during enflurane anesthesia in dogs. Anesthesiology 47:498-503, 1977.
17. Kroll DA, Knight PR: Antifibrillatory effects of volatile anesthetics in acute occlusion/reperfusion arrhythmias. Anesthesiology 61:657-661, 1984.
18. Green DH, Townsend P, Bagshaw O, Stokes MA: Nodal rhythm and bradycardia during inhalation induction with sevoflurane in infants: A comparison of incremental and high-concentration techniques. Br J Anaesth 85:368-370, 2000.
19. Owczuk R, Wujtewicz MA, Sawicka W, et al: The Influence of desflurane on QTc interval. Anesth Analg 101:419-422, 2005.
20. Reiz S, Nath S: Cardiotoxicity of local anesthetic agents. Br J Anaesth 58:736-746, 1986.
21. Rosenblatt MA, Abel M, Fischer GW, et al: Successful use of a 20% lipid emulsion to resuscitate a patient after a presumed bupivacaine-related cardiac arrest. Anesthesiology 105:217-218, 2006.
22. Weinberg G: Lipid infusion resuscitation for local anesthetic toxicity: Proof of clinical efficacy. Anesthesiology 105:7-8, 2006.
23. Edwards R, Winnie AP, Ramamurthy S: Acute hypocapneic hypokalemia: An iatrogenic anesthetic complication. Anesth Analg 56:786-792, 1977.
24. Samuel MA: The brain-heart connection. Circulation 116:77-84, 2007.
25. Angelini L, Feldman MI, Lufschonowski R, Leachman RD: Cardiac arrhythmias during and after heart surgery: Diagnosis and management. Prog Cardiovasc Dis 16:469-495, 1974.
26. Alexander JP: Dysrhythmia and oral surgery. Br J Anaesth 43:773-778, 1971.
27. Dobrzynski H, Boyett MR, Anderson RH: New insights into pacemaker activity: Promoting understanding of sick sinus syndrome. Circulation 115:1921-1932, 2007.
28. diMarco JP, Sellers TD, Lerman BB, et al: Diagnostic and therapeutic use of adenosine in patients with supraventricular tachyarrhythmias. J Am Coll Cardiol 6:417-425, 1985.
29. Bushman GA: Clinical correlates of dysrhythmias requiring an esophageal ECG for accurate diagnosis in patients with congenital heart disease. J Cardiothorac Anesth 3:290-294, 1989.
30. Lim SH, Anantharaman V, Teo WS, et al: Comparison of treatment of supraventricular tachycardia by Valsalva maneuver and carotid sinus massage. Ann Emerg Med 31:30-35, 1998.
31. Camm AJ, Garratt CJ: Adenosine and supraventricular tachycardia. N Engl J Med 325:1621-1629, 1991.
32. DiMarco JP, Miles W, Akhtar M, et al: Adenosine for paroxysmal supraventricular tachycardia: Dose ranging and comparison with verapamil. Assessment in placebo-controlled, multicenter trials: The Adenosine for PSVT Study Group. Ann Intern Med 113:104-110, 1990.
33. Balser JR: The rational use of intravenous amiodarone in the perioperative period. Anesthesiology 86:974-987, 1997.
34. Balser JR, Martinez EA, Winters BD, et al: Beta-adrenergic blockade accelerates conversion of postoperative supraventricular tachyarrhythmias. Anesthesiology 89:1052-1059, 1998.
35. Eldor J, Frankel DZ: Use of low-dose neostigmine intravenously in the treatment of supraventricular tachycardia: An immediate bradycardic effect. Resuscitation 18:103-110, 1989.
36. Basta M, Klein GJ, Yee R, et al: Current role of pharmacologic therapy for patients with paroxysmal supraventricular tachycardia. Cardiol Clin 15:587-597, 1997.
37. Altamura G, Bianconi L, Toscano S, et al: Transcutaneous cardiac pacing for termination of tachyarrhythmias. Pacing Clin Electrophysiol 13:2026-2030, 1990.
38. Hood RE, Shorofsky SR: Management of arrhythmias in the emergency department. Cardiol Clin 24:125-133, 2006.
39. Morady F: Catheter ablation of supraventricular arrhythmias: State of the art. J Cardiovasc Electrophysiol 15:124-139, 2004.
40. Niebauer MJ, Chung MK: Management of atrial flutter. Cardiol Rev 9:253-258, 2001.
41. Sedrakyan A, Treasure T, Browne J, et al: Pharmacologic prophylaxis for postoperative atrial tachyarrhythmia in general thoracic surgery: Evidence from randomized clinical trials. J Thorac Cardiovasc Surg 129:997-1005, 2005.
42. Ellenbogen KA, Stambler BS, Wood MA, et al: Efficacy of intravenous ibutilide for rapid termination of atrial fibrillation and atrial flutter: A dose-response study. J Am Coll Cardiol 28:130-136, 1996.
43. Chapman MJ, Moran JL, O'Fathartaigh MS, et al: Management of atrial tachyarrhythmias in the critically ill: A comparison of intravenous procainamide and amiodarone. Intensive Care Med 19:48-52, 1993.
44. Mayson SE, Greenspon AJ, Adams S, et al: The changing face of postoperative atrial fibrillation prevention: A review of current medical therapy. Cardiol Rev 15:231-241, 2007.
45. Page RL, Kerber RE, Russell JK, et al: Biphasic versus monophasic shock waveform for conversion of atrial fibrillation: The results of an international randomized, double-blind multicenter trial. J Am Coll Cardiol 39:1956-1963, 2002.
46. O'Neill MD, Jais P, Hocini M, et al: Catheter ablation for atrial fibrillation. Circulation 116:1515-1523, 2007.
47. Naccarelli GV, Dorian P, Hohnloser SH, et al: Prospective comparison of flecainide versus quinidine for the treatment of paroxysmal atrial fibrillation/flutter: The Flecainide Multicenter Atrial Fibrillation Study Group. Am J Cardiol 77:53A, 1996.

48. Gallik DM, Kim SG, Ferrick KJ, et al: Efficacy and safety of sotalol in patients with refractory atrial fibrillation or flutter. Am Heart J 134:155-160, 1997.
49. Opolski G, Stanislawska J, Górecki A, et al: Amiodarone in restoration and maintenance of sinus rhythm in patients with chronic atrial fibrillation after unsuccessful direct-current cardioversion. Clin Cardiol 20:337-340, 1997.
50. Stambler BS, Wood MA, Ellenbogen KA, et al: Efficacy and safety of repeated intravenous doses of ibutilide for rapid conversion of atrial flutter or fibrillation. Ibutilide Repeat Dose Study Investigators. Circulation 94:1613-1621, 1996.
51. Donahue TP, Conti JB: Atrial fibrillation: Rate control versus maintenance of sinus rhythm. Curr Opin Cardiol 6:46-53, 2001.
52. Haldemann G, Sehaer H: Haemodynamic effects of transient atrioventricular dissociation in general anesthesia. Br J Anaesth 44:159-162, 1972.
53. Oupadia P, Ramaswamy K: Images in clinical medicine. "R-on-T" phenomenon. N Engl J Med 338:1812, 1998.
54. Mittal S, Ayati S, Stein KM, et al: Comparison of a novel rectilinear biphasic waveform with a damped sine wave monophasic waveform for transthoracic ventricular defibrillation. ZOLL Investigators. J Am Coll Cardiol 34:1595-1601, 1999.
55. Hong MF, Dorian P: Update on advanced life support and resuscitation techniques. Curr Opin Cardiol 20:1-6, 2005.
56. Roden DM: Torsades de pointes. Clin Cardiol 16:683-686, 1993.
57. Roden DM: A practical approach to torsades de pointes. Clin Cardiol 20:285-290, 1997.
58. Stern S: State of the art in stress testing and ischaemia monitoring. Card Electrophysiol Rev 6:204-208, 2002.
59. Gianrossi R, Detrano R, Mulvihill D, et al: Exercise-induced ST depression in the diagnosis of coronary artery disease. A meta-analysis. Circulation 80:87-98, 1989.
60. Patton JA, Funk M: Survey of use of ST-segment monitoring in patients with acute coronary syndromes. Am J Crit Care 10:23-34, 2001.
61. Mark JB, Chien GL, Steinbrook RA, Fenton T: Electrocardiographic R-wave changes during cardiac surgery. Anesth Analg 74:26-31, 1992.
62. Miller TD, Desser KB, Lawson M: How many ECG leads are required for exercise treadmill tests? J Electrocardiol 20:131-137, 1987.
63. London MJ, Hollenberg M, Wong MG, et al: Intraoperative myocardial ischemia: Localization by continuous 12-lead electrocardiography. Anesthesiology 69:232-241, 1988.
64. Landesberg G, Mosseri M, Wolf Y, et al: Perioperative myocardial ischemia and infarction: identification by continuous 12-lead ECG with on-line ST-segment monitoring. Anesthesiology 96:264-270, 2002.
65. Martinez EA, Kim LJ, Faraday N, et al: Sensitivity of routine intensive care unit surveillance for detecting myocardial ischemia. Crit Care Med 31:2302-2308, 2003.
66. Drew BJ, Krucoff MW: Multilead ST-segment monitoring in patients with acute coronary syndromes: A consensus statement for healthcare professionals. ST-Segment Monitoring Practice Guideline International Working Group. Am J Crit Care 8:372-386, quiz 387-388, 1999.
67. De Hert SG, Moens MM, Vermeyen KM, et al: Use of the right-sided precordial lead V_4R in the detection of intraoperative myocardial ischemia. J Cardiothorac Vasc Anesth 7:659-667, 1993.
68. Bell C, Rimar S, Barash P: Intraoperative ST segment changes consistent with myocardial ischemia in the neonate: A report of three cases. Anesthesiology 71:601-604, 1989.
69. Tinker JH: Anesthesia for patients with ischemic heart disease. Contemp Anesth Pract 2:85-87, 1980.
70. Coriat P, Harari A, Daloz M, Viars P: Clinical predictors of intraoperative myocardial ischemia in patients with coronary artery disease undergoing non-cardiac surgery. Acta Anaesthesiol Scand 26:287-290, 1982.
71. Slogoff S, Keats AS: Does perioperative myocardial ischemia lead to postoperative myocardial infarction? Anesthesiology 62:107-114, 1985.
72. McCann RL, Clements FM: Silent myocardial ischemia in patients undergoing peripheral vascular surgery: Incidence and association with perioperative cardiac morbidity and mortality. J Vasc Surg 9:583-587, 1989.
73. Ouyang P, Gerstenblith G, Furman WR, et al: Frequency and significance of early postoperative silent myocardial ischemia in patients having peripheral vascular surgery. Am J Cardiol 64:1113-1116, 1989.
74. Pasternack PF, Grossi EA, Baumann FG, et al: The value of silent myocardial ischemia monitoring in the prediction of perioperative myocardial infarction in patients undergoing peripheral vascular surgery. J Vasc Surg 10:617-625, 1989.
75. Frank SM, Beattie C, Christopherson R, et al: Perioperative rate-related silent myocardial ischemia and postoperative death. J Clin Anesth 2:326-331, 1990.
76. Mangano DT, Browner WS, Hollenberg M, et al: Association of perioperative myocardial ischemia with cardiac morbidity and mortality in men undergoing noncardiac surgery. The Study of Perioperative Ischemia Research Group. N Engl J Med 323:1781-1788, 1990.
77. Mangano DT, Hollenberg M, Fegert G, et al: Perioperative myocardial ischemia in patients undergoing noncardiac surgery—I: Incidence and severity during the 4 day perioperative period. The Study of Perioperative Ischemia (SPI) Research Group. J Am Coll Cardiol 17:843-850, 1991.
78. Pasternack PF, Grossi EA, Baumann FG, et al: Silent myocardial ischemia monitoring predicts late as well as perioperative cardiac events in patients undergoing vascular surgery. J Vasc Surg 16:171-179, 1992.
79. Raby KE, Barry J, Creager MA, et al: Detection and significance of intraoperative and postoperative myocardial ischemia in peripheral vascular surgery. JAMA 268:222-227, 1992.
80. Marsch SC, Schaefer HG, Skarvan K, et al: Perioperative myocardial ischemia in patients undergoing elective hip arthroplasty during lumbar regional anesthesia. Anesthesiology 76:518-527, 1992.
81. Landesberg G, Luria MH, Cotev S, et al: Importance of long-duration postoperative ST-segment depression in cardiac morbidity after vascular surgery. Lancet 341:715-719, 1993.
82. Andrews TC, Goldman L, Creager MA, et al: Identification and treatment of myocardial ischemia in patients undergoing peripheral vascular surgery. J Vasc Med Biol 5:8-15, 1994.
83. Ganz LI, Andrews TC, Barry J, Raby KE: Silent ischemia preceding sudden cardiac death in a patient after vascular surgery. Am Heart J 127:1652-1654, 1994.
84. Fleisher LA, Nelson AH, Rosenbaum SH: Postoperative myocardial ischemia: Etiology of cardiac morbidity or manifestation of underlying disease? J Clin Anesth 7:97-102, 1995.
85. Wallace A, Layug B, Tateo I, et al: Prophylactic atenolol reduces postoperative myocardial ischemia. Anesthesiology 88:7-17, 1998.
86. Groves J, Edwards ND, Carr B, Sherry KM: Perioperative myocardial ischaemia, heart rate and arrhythmia in patients undergoing thoracotomy: An observational study. Br J Anaesth 83:850-854, 1999.
87. Rapp HJ, Rabethge S, Luiz T, et al: Perioperative ST-segment depression and troponin T release. Identification of patients with highest risk for myocardial damage. Acta Anaesthesiol Scand 43:124-129, 1999.
88. Gauss A, Rohn HJ, Schauffelen A, et al: Electrocardiographic exercise stress testing for cardiac risk assessment in patients undergoing noncardiac surgery. Anesthesiology 94:38-46, 2001.
89. Landesberg G, Mosseri M, Zahger D, et al: Myocardial infarction following vascular surgery: The role of prolonged, stress-induced, ST-depression–type ischemia. J Am Coll Cardiol 37:1839-1845, 2001.
90. Landesberg G, Shatz V, Akopnik I, et al: Association of cardiac troponin, CK-MB and postoperative myocardial ischemia with long-term survival following major vascular surgery. J Am Coll Cardiol 42:1547-1554, 2003.
91. Browner WS, Li J, Mangano DT: In-hospital and long-term mortality in male veterans following noncardiac surgery. The Study of Perioperative Ischemia Research Group. JAMA 268:228-232, 1992.

43 Implantable Cardiac Pulse Generators: Pacemakers and Cardioverter-Defibrillators

Key Points

Preoperatively

1. Identify the generator manufacturer and whether the generator is a pacemaker or defibrillator.
2. Have the pacemaker or defibrillator interrogated by a competent authority shortly before administration of the anesthetic.
3. Obtain a copy of this interrogation. Ensure that the device will pace the heart.
4. Consider replacing any device near its elective replacement period in a patient scheduled to undergo either major surgery or surgery within 25 cm of the generator.
5. Determine the patient's underlying rate and rhythm, which then determines the need for backup (external) pacing support.
6. Identify the magnet rate and rhythm, if any.
7. Program minute ventilation rate responsiveness off, if present.
8. Program all rate enhancements off.
9. Consider increasing the lower rate limit to optimize oxygen delivery to tissues for major cases.
10. Disable antitachycardia therapy if a defibrillator is present.

Intraoperatively

1. Monitor cardiac rhythm with pulse oximetry (plethysmography) or arterial waveform analysis.
2. Ask the surgeon to operate without the monopolar electrosurgical unit (ESU).
3. Use a bipolar ESU if possible; if not possible, a pure cut is better than "blend" or "coag."
4. Place the ESU return pad so that electricity is prevented from crossing the generator-heart circuit, even if the pad must be placed on the distal part of the forearm and the wire covered with sterile drape.
5. If the ESU causes ventricular oversensing and pacer quiescence, limit the period or periods of asystole.

Postoperatively

1. Have the device interrogated by a competent authority immediately postoperatively. Some rate enhancements can be reinitiated, and the optimum heart rate and pacing parameters should be determined. Note that any patient with disabled antitachycardia therapy must be monitored until the antitachycardia therapy is restored.

Adapted from the ASA Practice Advisory for Perioperative Management of Patients with a Pacemaker or Defibrillator.

Battery-operated pacing devices were introduced by C. W. Lillehei (a cardiothoracic surgeon) and Earl Bakken (an electrical technician) in 1958, just 4 years after invention of the transistor. In 1960, Wilson Greatbatch, an engineer in Buffalo, New York, created the first implantable battery-powered device in his barn.[1] The natural progression of pacemaker (PM) developments led to invention of the implantable cardioverter-defibrillator (ICD*) around 1980 by Michael Morchower (of Baltimore). First approved by the U.S. Food and Drug Administration (FDA) in 1985, implantation of ICDs required a thoracotomy, a significant operation in a patient with poor heart function. Advances in electronic miniaturization, as well as improvements in battery technology, have led to the development of very small (10-mL volume), but electronically complicated, programmable pacing devices.

Technologic advances (transvenous lead placement, antitachycardia* pacing [ATP] capability, miniaturization permitting

*Although many authors and references identify this device as an "automatic implantable cardioverter-defibrillator or AICD," the term "AICD" is a brand name originally owned by CPI-Cardiac Pacemakers, Inc., which was acquired by Guidant Medical Corporation and is now a part of Boston Scientific (Natick, MA). The term "PCD" (for "Programmable Cardioverter-Defibrillator") belongs to the Medtronic Corporation (Minneapolis, MN).

*The terms *antibradycardia* and *antitachycardia* will be used throughout this chapter. Antibradycardia refers to pacing to maintain a minimum rate. Thus, conventional PMs are antibradycardia devices. Antitachycardia refers to therapy delivered in the setting of tachycardia, and it is designed to reduce the underlying heart rate.

pectoral pocket placement, and multiple-chamber, rate-responsive antibradycardia pacing) and numerous survival benefits[2,3] have led to increases in the use of ICDs. These changes in ICD implantation and indications have two important results for health care providers. First, a pectoral (rather than abdominal) pocket ICD with pacing capability might be mistaken, by virtue of pacing "spikes" on the surface electrocardiogram, for a (non-ICD) PM. At many centers, electrocardiograms are obtained from patients who have "PMs" with use of a magnet. Because some ICDs from Boston Scientific/Guidant Medical/CPI can undergo permanent deactivation of antitachycardia therapy with magnet placement, this mistake could leave a patient unprotected[4] and possibly result in death.[5] Second, pacing functions in an ICD often respond to external stimuli (magnet placement, electromagnetic interference [EMI]) differently than a PM does. These issues are addressed later in this chapter. Additionally, all ICDs now perform permanent cardiac pacing, so the issues in the sections on pacing will apply to ICD care as well. Distinguishing a conventional PM from an ICD can be accomplished by examining the right ventricular (RV) lead system on a chest radiograph (Fig. 43-1). A chest radiograph can also be used to identify the generator manufacturer (Fig. 43-2).

Pacemaking and defibrillation systems have a remarkable record for reliability, but they can and do fail. Maisel and colleagues reviewed FDA records for PM and ICD failures (death or explantation because of malfunction other than battery depletion) for the period 1990 to 2002. Even though the nature of this reporting scheme promotes under-reporting of problems, for these 12 years, 2.25 million PMs were implanted, with 8,834 (0.4%) confirmed (and reported) malfunctions and 30 deaths. For ICDs, 415,780 were implanted, with 8,489 (2%) confirmed malfunctions and 31 deaths.[6] Thus, every patient with a cardiac generator should undergo regular in-office follow-up. For appropriately selected devices, telephone checks can be used to identify battery depletion (PM and ICD) or detection of tachycardia (ICD), but telephone checks cannot ensure adequacy of pacing capture and sense safety margins at this time. For PMs, nationally published guidelines recommend at least a telephone check every 1 to 3 months, depending on implant duration.[7] No such guidelines exist for ICD follow-up, although most ICD manufacturers recommend follow-up periods not to exceed 4 months.

Issues also develop and lead to "notices," "product advisories," or "recalls" from the various manufacturers, which might affect perioperative care. For example, Guidant has 46,000 ICDs with potentially defective magnet sensors that could prevent delivery of shock or ATP. Their recommended action was to permanently disable the magnet switch by programming. An ICD thus programmed will therefore deliver a shock even with a magnet in place (Fig. 43-3).[8] The Sprint Fidelis ICD lead series from Medtronic will report ventricular activity in the absence of true electrical systoles (oversensing), which can result in failure to pace or inappropriate delivery of shock,[9] and Guidant has one such lead with similar issues (Model 0156) (Fig. 43-4).

The complexity of PMs and ICDs, as well as the multitude of programmable parameters, limits the number of generalizations that can be made about the perioperative care of a patient with an implanted pulse generator. Population aging, continued enhancements in implantable technology, and new indications for implantation of cardiac devices continue to drive the growing number of implants. The American Society of Anesthesiologists has taken note of these issues and is developing a Perioperative Practice Advisory[10]; the "Key Points" reflect this advisory. Practice guidelines have been issued by the American College of Cardiology (ACC) (hereafter called the ACC guidelines),[11] the American Heart Association (AHA), and the Heart Rhythm Society (formerly the North American Society of Pacing and Electrophysiology [NASPE]).[12] Reviews can also be found in a number of journals.[13-15]

Patients with an implanted cardiac pulse generator often have significant comorbid disease in addition to their cardiac rhythm disturbance. Our ability to care for these patients requires attention to both their medical and psychological problems. We also need an understanding of their pulse generator, its function, and its probable idiosyncrasies in the operating or procedure room.

Finally, not all electronic generators implanted in the chest are cardiac devices, and devices resembling cardiac pulse generators are being implanted at increasing rates for indications unrelated to cardiac issues. When implanted in the pectoral position (the usual place for current cardiac generators), these noncardiac devices can be mistakenly identified as cardiac generators.[16] Pulse generator implantation has been approved by the FDA for pain control, thalamic stimulation to control Parkinson's disease, phrenic nerve stimulation to stimulate the diaphragm in paralyzed patients, and vagus nerve stimulation to control epilepsy and depression.[17] Vagus nerve stimulation is also under consideration for the treatment of heart failure[18] and perhaps obesity. Thus, when evaluating a patient with any pulse generator, one must now determine whether the pulse generator will be pacing the heart, stimulating the central nervous system, stimulating the spinal cord, or stimulating the vagus nerve.

Pacemakers

PM manufacturers report that more than 2,500 generators have been manufactured by more than 26 named entities over the past 40 years. Currently, more than 250,000 adults and children in the United States undergo new PM placement each year, and nearly 2 million patients have PMs today. Many factors lead to confusion regarding the behavior of a device and the perioperative care of a patient with a device, especially since case reports, textbooks, and literature reviews have not kept pace with technologic developments.

A pacemaking system consists of an impulse generator and a lead or leads to carry the electrical impulse to the patient's heart. Leads are connected to the heart's chambers through the vena cava (transvenous leads) or are directly sewn onto the surface of the heart (epicardial leads). Leads can be unipolar (one electrode per lead), bipolar (two electrodes per lead), or multipolar (multiple electrodes and wires contained within one lead with connections in multiple chambers) (see Fig. 43-1A). Because two electrodes are required to complete a circuit, the second electrode in a unipolar configuration will be the metal generator case. Use of the case as an electrode requires that the generator pocket be devoid of gas, and electrical continuity has reportedly been disrupted by the use of nitrous oxide.[19]

PMs with unipolar leads seem to be more sensitive to the effects of EMI, and these systems produce larger "spikes" on an analog-recorded electrocardiogram. Most PM systems (except many Autocapture devices from St. Jude Cardiac Rhythm Management, Sylmar, CA) pace in bipolar mode because bipolar

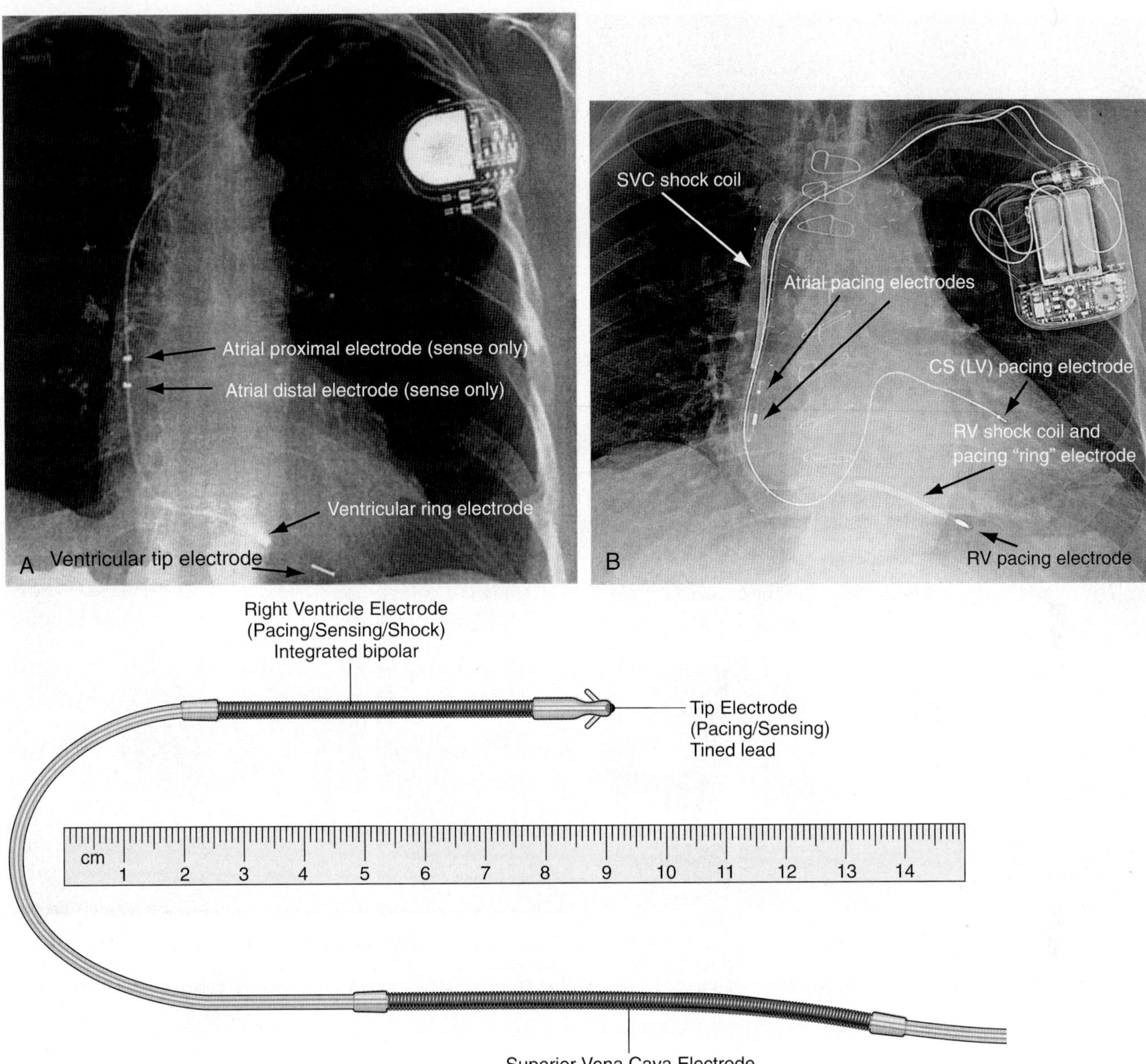

Figure 43-1 A conventional single lead pacemaker, an implantable cardioverter-defibrillator (ICD), and a right ventricular (RV) defibrillator lead are shown to assist in determination of the type of system on chest radiography. **A,** Conventional pacemaker with one quadripolar lead that provides atrial and ventricular sensing and ventricular pacing. This chest radiograph shows a number of features of a modern pacing system. The generator is located in the left pectoral region. The single lead enters the subclavian vein under the clavicle but superficial to the first rib (a common site for lead problems, although no problem is demonstrated here). This device has two electrodes positioned within the right atrium that can provide sensing to detect intrinsic atrial activity. The ventricular portion of the lead shows the classic bipolar pattern with a ring electrode just proximal to the tip electrode, and these electrodes can be used for sensing intrinsic ventricular activity, as well as depolarizing the ventricle. This particular system is a VDD pacemaking system, and this configuration is placed into patients with a functioning atrioventricular node. The system cannot be used to depolarize the atrium. Because the surface electrocardiogram will often demonstrate ventricular pacing that tracks the atrial activity, inspection of the surface electrocardiogram often produces an erroneous diagnosis of a dual-chamber (DDD) pacemaker. **B,** Defibrillator system with biventricular pacing capability. Note that three leads are placed: a conventional bipolar lead to the right atrium, a multipolar lead terminating in the right ventricle, and a unipolar lead to the coronary sinus (CS). The presence of a "shock" conductor in the right ventricle (called a "shock coil") distinguishes a defibrillation system from a conventional pacing system. Many ICDs have an additional shock coil in the superior vena cava (SVC). Typically, the SVC shock coil is electrically identical to the defibrillator case (called the "can"). When the defibrillation circuitry includes the ICD case, it is called "active can configuration." This particular system is designed to provide "resynchronization therapy" in the setting of dilated cardiomyopathy with a prolonged QRS interval (and frequently with a prolonged PR as well). The bipolar lead in the right atrium will perform both sensing and pacing function. Likewise, the tip electrode in the right ventricle along with the shock coil performs RV pacing and sensing function. When the second RV pacing electrode is merged with the shock coil, the lead is called "integrated bipolar" because unipolar RV pacing is not permitted in an ICD system. The lead in the CS depolarizes the left ventricle (LV). Failure to depolarize one of the ventricles might result in ventricular oversensing (and inappropriate antitachycardia therapy) in an ICD. **C,** Integrated bipolar RV defibrillator lead. The tip of this lead becomes enmeshed in the RV trabeculae (called a "tined" lead) rather than engaging the myocardial wall with a screw ("active fixation"). This particular lead has an SVC shock coil as well.

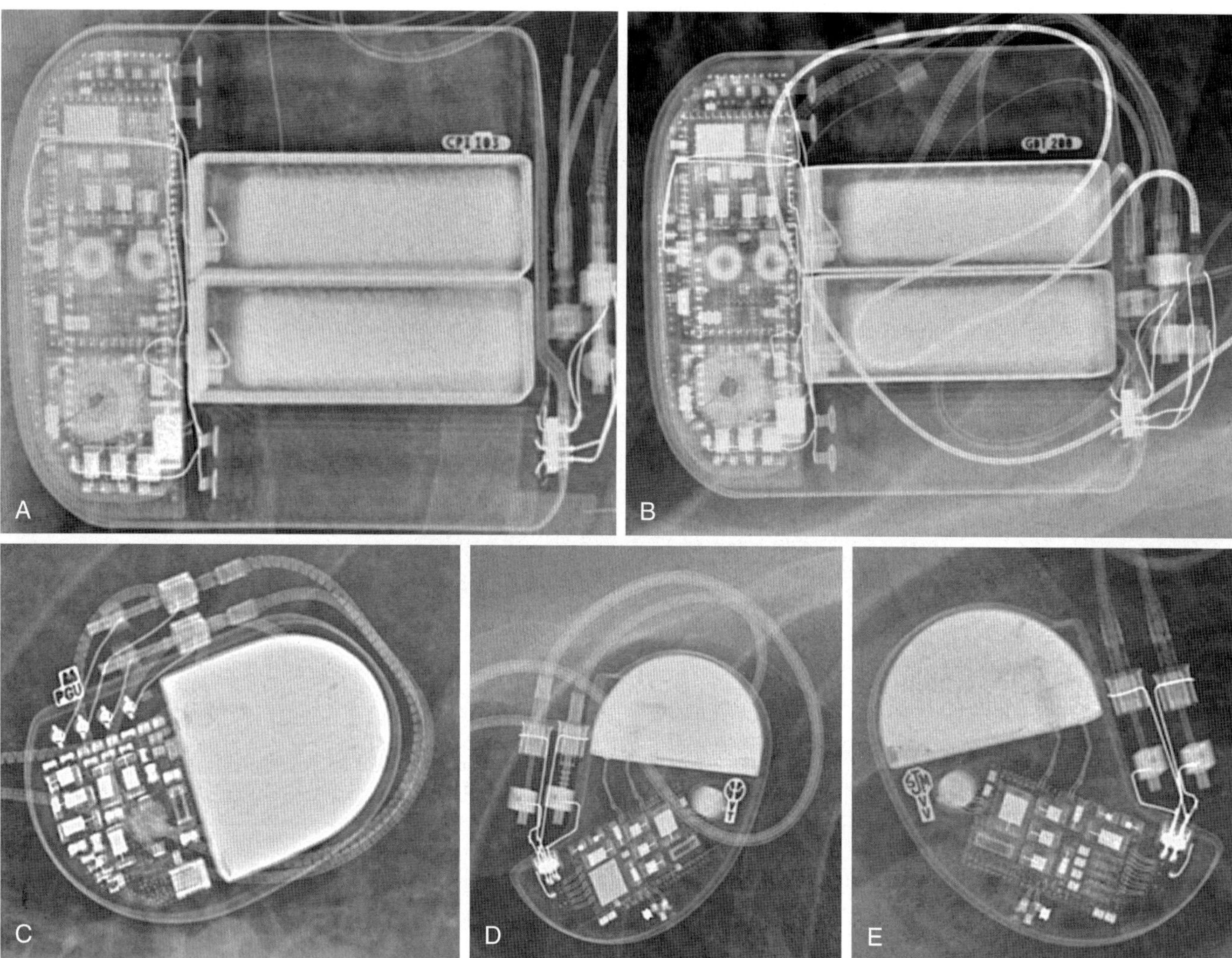

Figure 43-2 Radiographic identifiers for some generator manufacturers. Pacemaker and implantable cardioverter-defibrillator generators can be identified from operative dictations, patient cards, or some chest radiographs. Using digital x-ray equipment with postprocessing zoom capability, corporate x-ray logo identifiers from CPI (**A**), Guidant (**B**), Medtronic (**C**), Pacesetter (**D**), and St. Jude Medical (**E**) are shown. Not shown: BOS is the new Boston Scientific logo.

Setup

Magnet	INITIAL VALUE	PRESENT VALUE
*Enable magnet use		Off
*Change tachy mode with magnet		
Beeper		
Beep during capacitor charge		Off
Beep on sensed and paced ventricular events		Off
Beep when ERI is reached		On

Figure 43-3 Magnet mode setup from a Guidant Contak Renewal 3 HE model H179. This implantable cardioverter-defibrillator (ICD) is part of an "Urgent Medical Device Safety Information and Corrective Action" letter to physicians from the Guidant Corporation on June 23, 2005, in which a magnet switch problem was announced. The corrective action was designed to permanently disable the magnet switch by programming. As a result, this ICD will not disable shock therapy in response to magnet placement. According to the notice, approximately 46,000 Guidant ICDs were affected and should have their magnet switch permanently disabled. Note the line below the magnet switch report called "Change tachy mode with magnet." With magnet function operative in many Boston Scientific/Guidant Medical/CPI ICDs, enabling this setting allows permanent deactivation of ICD function with the application of a magnet for more than 30 seconds (see text).

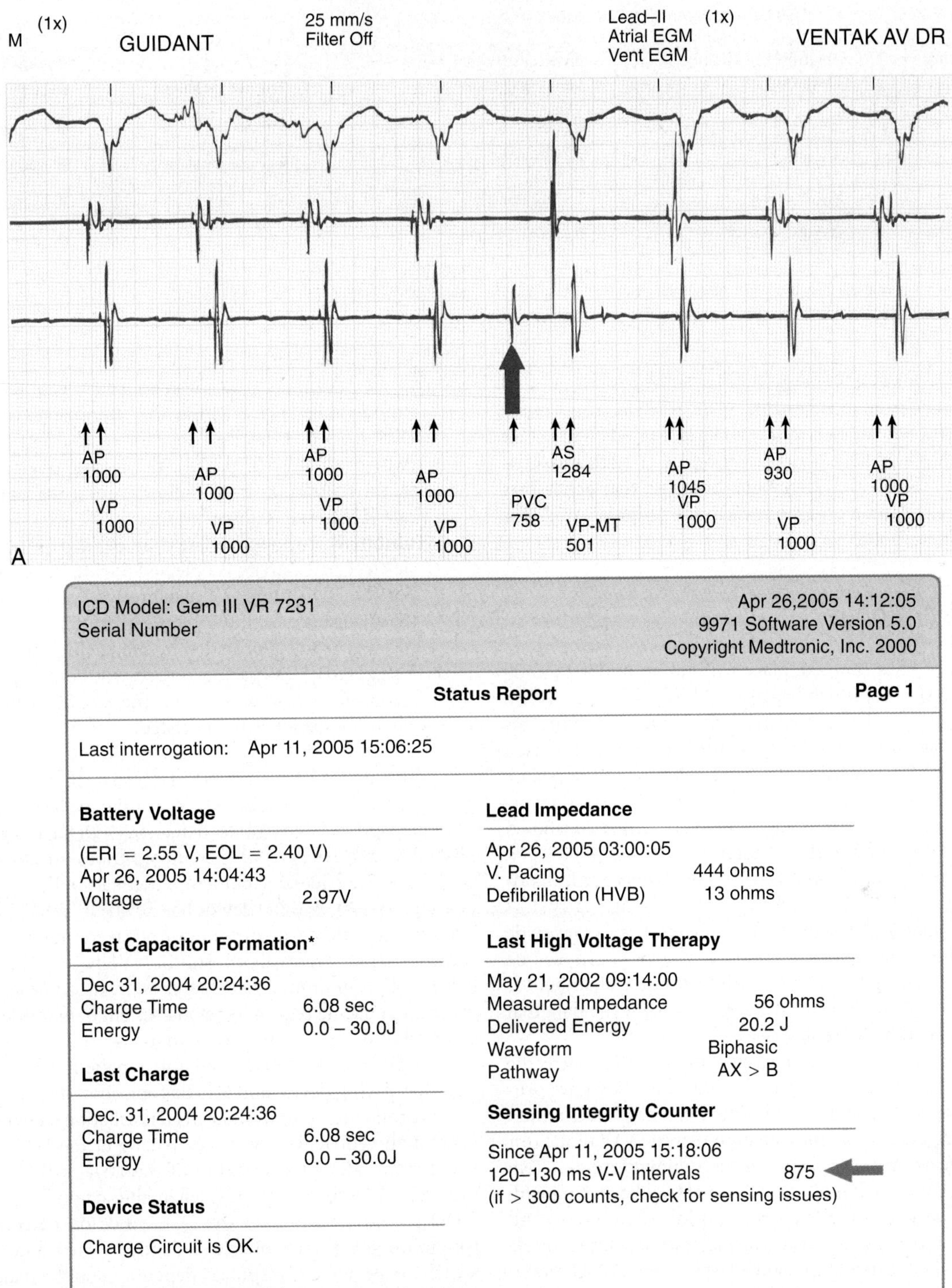

ICD Model: Gem III VR 7231
Serial Number

Apr 26,2005 14:12:05
9971 Software Version 5.0
Copyright Medtronic, Inc. 2000

Status Report **Page 1**

Last interrogation: Apr 11, 2005 15:06:25

Battery Voltage

(ERI = 2.55 V, EOL = 2.40 V)
Apr 26, 2005 14:04:43
Voltage 2.97V

Last Capacitor Formation*

Dec 31, 2004 20:24:36
Charge Time 6.08 sec
Energy 0.0 – 30.0J

Last Charge

Dec. 31, 2004 20:24:36
Charge Time 6.08 sec
Energy 0.0 – 30.0J

Device Status

Charge Circuit is OK.

Lead Impedance

Apr 26, 2005 03:00:05
V. Pacing 444 ohms
Defibrillation (HVB) 13 ohms

Last High Voltage Therapy

May 21, 2002 09:14:00
Measured Impedance 56 ohms
Delivered Energy 20.2 J
Waveform Biphasic
Pathway AX > B

Sensing Integrity Counter

Since Apr 11, 2005 15:18:06
120–130 ms V-V intervals 875
(if > 300 counts, check for sensing issues)

*Minimum Auto Cap Formation interval is 4 months

Figure 43-4 Ventricular oversensing from damaged leads. **A,** A real-time telemetry recording from a Guidant implantable cardioverter-defibrillator (ICD) with a Guidant 0156 right ventricular (RV) defibrillation lead reports a spontaneous ventricular (*arrow*) event that was not present on the surface electrocardiogram (ECG), termed ventricular oversensing. In this ICD, the pacing function was DDD (lower rate, 60 beats/min; atrioventricular delay, 180 msec), and this patient was dependent on the ICD pacing function for his ventricular systoles. The top tracing is the surface ECG, the second tracing is the intracardiac atrial electrogram (EGM), and the third tracing is the intracardiac ventricular EGM. Along the bottom is the "marker channel," which shows the pacemaker's interpretation of events—AP is atrial pace, AS is atrial sense, VP is ventricular pace, and the inappropriate ventricular sensed event is labeled "PVC" because it occurs after a ventricular event without an intervening atrial event. Note that this oversensing has prolonged the RR interval between the fourth and fifth ventricular systoles because this patient is dependent on the pacing function for his ventricular systoles. In a pacing-dependent patient, this type of oversensing can lead to asystole. It can also provoke inappropriate antitachycardia therapy (i.e., shock) in a patient with native ventricular activity because these oversensed events can increase the apparent heart rate count to the ICD. **B,** A patient with a single-chamber Medtronic ICD and a Medtronic Sprint Fidelis RV defibrillation lead was found to have a significant ventricular oversensing issue at interrogation 4/26/05 before his head and neck surgery. In this case the ICD is reporting 875 "short RR intervals" (note the *arrow*) since the previous interrogation 15 days earlier (4/11/05). These data are consistent with a lead fracture causing intermittent "make-break" contacts. In this case, new counts began accumulating 12 minutes after the previous interrogation was complete. More than 100 counts per month is considered a problem; indications to replace the lead include ventricular oversensing in a pacing-dependent patient or high rate detection triggered by this inappropriate oversensing.

Table 43-1 NASPE/BPEG Revised (2002) Generic Pacemaker Code (NBG)

Position I: Pacing Chamber(s)	Position II: Sensing Chamber(s)	Position III: Response(s) to Sensing	Position IV: Programmability	Position V: Multisite Pacing
O = none	**O** = none	**O** = none	**O** = none	**O** = none
A = atrium	**A** = atrium	**I** = inhibited	**R** = rate modulation	**A** = atrium
V = ventricle	**V** = ventricle	**T** = triggered		**V** = ventricle
D = dual (A + V)	**D** = dual (A + V)	**D** = dual (T + I)		**D** = dual (A + V)

The generic pacemaker code.[20] This code, initially published in 1983, was last revised in 2002 in an effort to keep current with technologic developments in the pacing field. The NBG code is a joint project by the North American Society of Pacing and Electrophysiology (NASPE) (the "N") and the British Pacing and Electrophysiology Group (BPEG) (the "B"). The "G" stands for generic.

pacing usually requires less energy. Bipolar sensing is more resistant to interference from muscle artifacts or stray electromagnetic fields. Frequently, bipolar electrodes can be identified on the chest film because they will have a ring electrode 1 to 3 cm proximal to the lead tip (see Fig. 43-1A). Note, however, that generators with bipolar leads can be programmed to the unipolar mode for pacing, sensing, or both.

Pacemaker Codes

No discussion of PMs can take place without an understanding of the generic PM code, which has been published by the NASPE and British Pacing and Electrophysiology Group (BPEG). This code (NBG*) was initially published in 1983 and was last revised in February 2002.[20] It describes the basic behavior of the pacing device (Table 43-1). PMs also come with a variety of terms generally unfamiliar to the anesthesiologist, many of which are shown in the glossary at the end of this chapter.

The first two positions of this code (chambers paced, chambers sensed) seem relatively straightforward. Although early PMs provided only ventricular support, current models can provide pacing in the atria and ventricles, and these devices can also be programmed to determine intrinsic activity in these chambers as well. The code does not describe the array of diagnostic data that can be accumulated by these devices.

Probably the most confusing aspect of the NBG code is the third position (response to the sensed event). Most PMs are programmed either to the DDD mode (dual-chamber pacing and sensing, both triggered and inhibited mode) or the VVI mode (for single-chamber, ventricular pacing in the inhibited mode). Two other modes frequently found are VDD (ventricular pacing with dual-chamber pacing in the triggered and inhibited mode) and DDI (dual-chamber pacing and sensing, but inhibited mode only). In the United States, atrial-only PM placement (AAI mode) is unusual, but these devices are implanted in patients with sinus node disease in other countries. This third position describes the following behavior:

D (Dual): DDD pacing provides atrioventricular (AV) synchrony. In the DDD setting, atrial pacing will take place in the "inhibited" mode; that is, the pacing device will emit an atrial pulse if no sensed atrial event (or intervening ventricular event because any ventricular event will reset atrial timing) takes place within the appropriate timeframe. In DDD or VDD devices, once an atrial event has occurred (whether native or paced), the pacing device will ensure that a ventricular event follows (up to the upper tracking rate [UTR, see "Glossary"]).

I (Inhibited): The appropriate chamber is paced unless intrinsic electrical activity is detected during the pacing interval. For the DDI mode, AV synchrony is provided only when the atrium is paced. If intrinsic atrial activity is present, no AV synchrony is provided by the pacing function.

T (Triggered): The pacing device will emit a pulse only in response to a sensed event. The triggered mode is used when the device is being tested.

The modes VDD and DDI deserve further comment. VDD pacing is used for a patient with AV nodal dysfunction but intact and appropriate sinus node behavior. VDD pacing is accomplished with a single lead that incorporates atrial sensing electrodes and ventricular conductors that can both pace and sense (see Fig. 43-1A). A VDD device has no atrial pacing capability. As a result, in a patient who depends on atrial contraction to augment cardiac output, events that result in VVI pacing (e.g., sinus rate below the programmed rate, battery depletion) or asynchronous ventricular pacing (e.g., magnet placement in many devices, EMI) can lead to deteriorating hemodynamics.[21,22]

DDI pacing is indicated for a patient who has a dual-chamber pacing device and also has episodes of paroxysmal atrial dysrhythmia (e.g., paroxysmal atrial fibrillation). DDI pacing prevents high ventricular rates (i.e., pacing at the UTR) that could result from attempted tracking of the atrial arrhythmia, and it provides AV synchrony only when the atrium is paced. Many DDD programs will enter the DDI mode on detection of high (programmable) atrial rates (called mode switch, automatic mode switch, or atrial tachy response, depending on the manufacturer). When the mode switches to DDI, perturbations (such as very high [>400/min] atrial rates, EMI from the electrosurgical unit [ESU], or magnet placement and removal) might revert the PM back to DDD pacing, with the resultant appearance of AV pacing or ventricular pacing at the UTR (see "Pacemaker Magnets").

Rate modulation (the fourth position) also remains a poorly understood concept. Because some patients cannot increase their heart rate in response to increased oxygen demand (chronotropic incompetence), PM manufacturers have devised a number of mechanisms to detect "patient exercise," such as sensors that detect vibration, respiration, and pressure (Box 43-1). As the sensor detects "exercise," it increases the pacing rate

*The NBG code is a joint project from the NASPE (the "N") and the BPEG (the "B"). The "G" stands for generic. NASPE reorganized as the Heart Rhythm Society (HRS) in 2004.

Box 43-1 Rate Modulation (Activity) Sensors Available or Under Investigation

Currently Approved in the United States

- Vibration sensor
- Motion sensor
- Minute ventilation (bioimpedance sensor)
- QT interval (Vitatron only)
- Right ventricular pressure (Biotronik only)

Under Investigation

- Right ventricular stroke volume
- Blood pH
- Blood temperature
- Mixed venous oxygen sensor
- Systolic time intervals
- Evoked response
- Intracardiac Impedance

Of the types of sensors used to detect exercise in a patient with a cardiac pacemaker, five are currently approved in the United States, although many others are under investigation. Some devices have two sensors and can be programmed for cross-checking to prevent increases in heart rate from spurious causes. Minute ventilation sensors are very sensitive to stray electromagnetic interference, and patients have been inappropriately treated for pacemaker-driven tachycardias as a result. There is very little perioperative experience with right ventricular pressure sensors at this time. Most pacemaker experts recommend that rate modulation be programmed to "OFF" in the perioperative period to prevent confusion between an intrinsic tachycardia versus a pacemaker-induced tachycardia (for example, see Schwartzenburg and colleagues[23]).

(termed "sensor-indicated rate"). As the exercise tapers, this sensor-indicated rate returns to the programmed lower rate. The sensitivity of these sensors to their exercise signals and the rates of change in pacing are programmable features in current generators. Activation of rate response algorithms resulting in an increased pacing rate in the operating room, whether from vigorous chest wall skin preparation, pressure on the generator, or EMI in a minute ventilation device, has led to inappropriate treatment and patient harm.[24,25]

With the 2002 revision of the NBG, the fifth column describes multisite pacing functionality (it had been used to describe antitachycardia functions, but this scheme has been abandoned and a generic defibrillator code has been established). Atrial multisite pacing might prevent atrial fibrillation,[26] and ventricular multisite pacing is an acceptable means of pacing patients with dilated cardiomyopathy (DCM).[27-29]

Pacemaker Indications

Indications for permanent pacing are shown in Box 43-2 and are reviewed in detail elsewhere.[30] Classically, antibradycardia pacing treats patients with sinus node disease (improper impulse formation) and AV node disease (improper impulse conduction). Pacing can be used to reduce the outflow tract obstruction in hypertrophic obstructive cardiomyopathy (HOCM) in both adults and children because paced ventricular conduction takes place in a left bundle branch pattern (the left ventricular [LV] septum depolarizes after the other segments rather than as an early systolic event).[31] Finally, in August 2001, devices were approved by the FDA for three-chamber pacing (right atrium, both ventricles) to treat DCM.[32] This pacing modality can also be called cardiac resynchronization therapy (CRT) or biventricular (BiV) pacing. To accomplish LV pacing, a pacing lead is placed into the coronary sinus (see Fig. 43-1B) or sewn onto the LV free wall. In patients with a significant RV-to-LV activation time, loss of capture in a ventricle can lead to ventricular overcounting with resultant inappropriate antitachycardia therapy in those with a DCM-pacing defibrillator.[33,34]

Pacing for HOCM and DCM requires careful attention to pacer programming. To be effective in these patients, the PM must provide the stimulus for ventricular depolarization, and AV synchrony must be preserved.[35] PM inhibition or loss of pacing (e.g., from native conduction, atrial irregularity, ventricular irregularity, development of junctional rhythm, or EMI) can lead to deteriorating hemodynamics in these patients.

BiV pacing might cause inappropriate lengthening of the QT interval in susceptible patients, and this lengthening has been reported to be associated with torsades de pointes.[36] As a result of this report, prudent anesthesiologists should ensure adequate access to rapid defibrillation for patients with BiV pacing accomplished without an ICD.

Pacemaker Magnets

Despite oft-repeated folklore, most PM manufacturers warn that magnets were never intended to treat PM emergencies or prevent the effects of EMI. Rather, magnet-activated switches were incorporated to produce pacing behavior that demonstrates remaining battery life and, sometimes, pacing threshold safety factors.

Placement of a magnet over a generator might produce no change in pacing because *not all pacemakers switch to a continuous asynchronous mode when a magnet is applied.* Moreover, not all models from a given company behave the same way. Possible effects of magnet placement are shown in Table 43-2.[37-39] In some devices magnet behavior can be altered by programming, whereas in others, magnet behavior can be completely eliminated by programming.

Box 43-2 Pacemaker Indications

- Symptomatic diseases of impulse formation (sinus node disease)
- Symptomatic diseases of impulse conduction (disease of the atrioventricular node)
- Long QT syndrome
- Hypertrophic obstructive cardiomyopathy*
- Dilated cardiomyopathy*

Indications for permanent pacing are listed. Most patients with pacemakers currently fall into the first two categories (sinus or atrioventricular nodal disease).

*Requires 100% ventricular pacing to be effective. Thus, short atrioventricular delays (around 120 to 150 msec) are programmed.

Table 43-2 Pacemaker Magnet Behavior

Pacemaker Company		Magnet Mode Designation	Explanation
Biotronik (except INOS and DROMOS)		AUTO	If battery okay, 10 asynchronous events at 90 beats/min, then returns to original programmed mode, without rate responsiveness. Pacing is at the lowest available rate (LRL, sleep rate, or hysteresis rate). If battery at ERI, 10 asynchronous events at 80 beats/min in the VOO mode, then either VDD (dual-chamber) or VVI (single-chamber) pacing at 11% lower than the lowest available rate. For any dual-chamber mode (DDD, DDI, or VDD), the AV delay shortens to 100 msec while the magnet is in place
		ASYNCH	Asynchronous pacing at 90 beats/min if battery okay. At ERI, 80 beats/min (single-step change) in the VOO mode regardless of original programming. For any dual-chamber mode (DDD, DDI, or VDD), the AV delay shortens to 100 msec while the magnet is in place
		SYNCH	If battery okay, pacing in original programmed mode, without rate responsiveness. Pacing is at the lowest available rate (LRL, sleep rate, or hysteresis rate). If battery at ERI, either VDD (dual-chamber) or VVI (single-chamber) pacing at 11% lower than the lowest available rate. For any dual-chamber mode (DDD, DDI, or VDD), the AV delay shortens to 100 msec while the magnet is in place
Boston Scientific/Guidant Medical/CPI		ASYNCH	Asynchronous pacing at 100 beats/min if okay, 85 beats/min at ERI (single-step change). The Insignia model has an intermediate step at 90 beats/min at IFI. For Triumph and Prelude models, see Medtronic pacemakers, below
		OFF	No change, magnet is ignored. OFF is the magnet mode after a "power on reset," which can occur secondary to EMI
		EGM mode	No change in pacing. Magnet application initiates data collection
Medtronic			Asynchronous pacing at 85 beats/min if okay, SSI at 65 beats/min regardless of original programming if ERI detected (single-step change). Most Medtronic pacemakers emit one or more ventricular pulses during the first 3-7 asynchronous events (which might be at a rate of 100 beats/min) at a reduced pulse width or voltage to demonstrate the adequacy of ventricular pacing output. Also, Medtronic pacemakers default to SSI pacing at 65 beats/min, without rate responsiveness, on detection of ERI, regardless of whether a magnet is present
St. Jude Medical (not including Telectronics)	"SJM" x-ray logo	Battery Test	Asynchronous pacing at 98.6 beats/min gradually decreasing to <86.3 beats/min at ERI
		OFF	No magnet response
		Event snapshots	No change in pacing. Magnet application causes pacemaker to collect data. Identity and Entity models lack this feature
		Event snapshots + Battery Test	For a magnet placed 2 seconds, pacing mode and rate are unchanged and the device stores an EGM. If the magnet is placed ≥5 seconds, the Battery Test mode (see above) is activated. Identity and Entity models lack this feature
	Pacesetter x-ray logo (ψ)	Battery Test	Asynchronous pacing, with rate depending on the specific model. In general, a pacing rate of less than 90 beats/min should prompt further evaluation
		OFF	No magnet response
		VARIO mode (present in some models)	VARIO results in a series of 32 asynchronous pacing events. The rate of the first 16 paces reflects battery voltage, which gradually declines from 100 to 85 beats/min at ERI. The next 15 paces are used to document the ventricular pacing capture safety margin. The rate will be 119 beats/min with gradually declining pacing voltage. The 16th pace of this group is at no output. The next pace restarts the 32-event sequence. The 32-event sequence repeats as long as the magnet remains in place

The effect or effects of appropriately placing a magnet over a pacemaker are shown. Column 1 shows the pacemaker manufacturer. If the magnet response is programmable, column 2 shows the various programmable modes available. The first mode shown for a company is the default mode. Column 3 shows the effect on pacing therapy for the magnet mode shown in column 2. Unless otherwise specified, asynchronous pacing takes place, without rate responsiveness, in the chambers originally programmed. Thus, a dual-chamber program would result in DOO pacing, and a single-chamber program would result in VOO pacing (unless an atrial device is used, which would be AOO), and a biventricular, dual-chamber device would be DOOOV.

AV, atrioventricular; EGM, electrogram; EMI, electromagnetic interference; EOL, end of life—the device should be replaced immediately; ERI, elective replacement indicator—the device should be replaced promptly; IFI, intensified follow-up interval—the device needs monthly battery checks; LRL, lower rate limit—the programmed lower rate, or set point, of the pacemaker; SSI, single-chamber, inhibited mode—if implanted for ventricular pacing, SSI = VVI; for an atrial pacemaker, SSI = AAI.

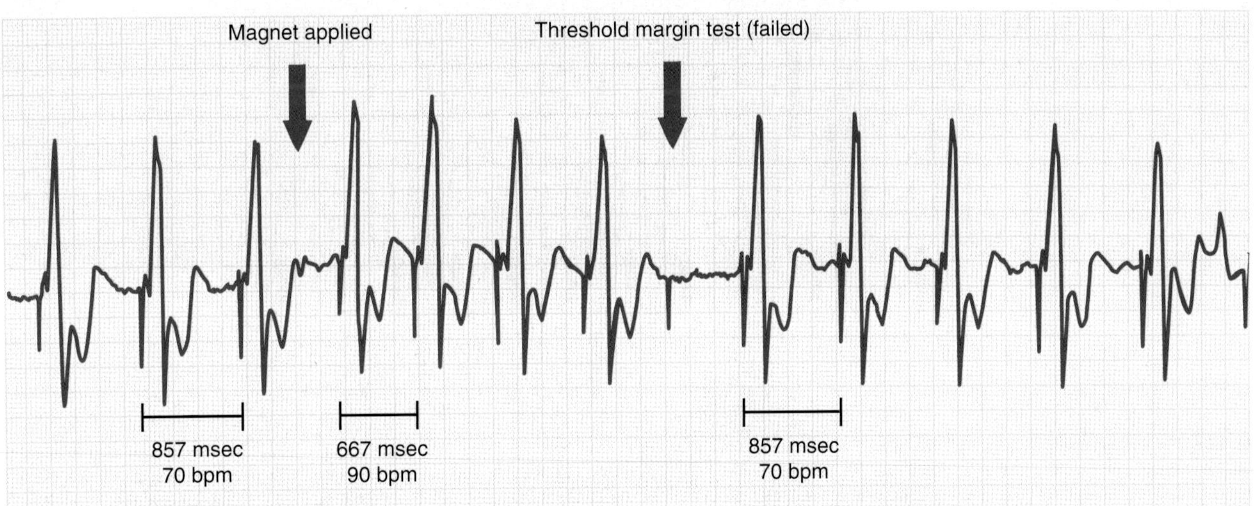

Figure 43-5 Threshold margin test (TMT) demonstrating an inadequate safety margin for pacing. Application of a magnet to some pacemakers will produce asynchronous pacing in which one or more pacing stimuli are emitted with reduced ventricular pacing voltage, pulse width, or both. This sequence is used to determine, without formal pacemaker interrogation, the adequacy of pacing energy settings. In this electrocardiographic strip from an Intermedics device, the patient was being paced in the VVI mode at a rate of 70/min (equal to 857-msec intervals). On application of the magnet, this pacemaker produced four intervals (five pacing stimuli) of asynchronous pacing at a rate of 90/min (667-msec intervals), thus demonstrating adequate battery voltage for this device (pacemaker response to magnet placement is dependent on the manufacturer and sometimes the programming). At the fifth pacing stimulus after magnet application, the pacemaker performs a TMT by reducing the stimulus pulse width to 50% of the programmed value (equal to 50% of programmed energy). Failure of this stimulus to produce ventricular systole (i.e., failure to capture) demonstrates a dangerously low safety margin for ventricular pacing because pacing pulse width should be at least three and generally four times the threshold for capture. After these five initial stimuli, Intermedics pacemakers then pace asynchronously at the programmed lower rate (70 in this case) for 60 additional cycles. On completion of these 64 cycles (65 stimuli), Intermedics pacemakers return to programmed values and ignore the magnet.

For all generators, calling the manufacturer remains the most reliable method of determining magnet response and using this response to predict remaining battery life (phone numbers for device manufacturers are shown in Appendix 2). As battery voltage falls, the magnet response can be used to detect the following:

IFI (Intensified follow-up required)—the device must be checked frequently (approximately every 4 weeks for most models).

ERI (Elective replacement indicator)—the device is nearing the end of its useful life and should be electively replaced.

EOL (End of life)—the device has insufficient battery power remaining and should be replaced immediately.

Upon application of a magnet, some devices perform a "threshold margin test" (TMT). In this test, one or more of the PM pulses are reduced in amplitude, pulse width, or both in an attempt to gauge the safety margin for pacing voltage. Loss of capture on these TMT pulses indicates an inadequate safety margin for pacing (Fig. 43-5). Some devices from St. Jude Medical (formerly Pacesetter) with the Siemens "Vario" feature will reduce the ventricular pacing energy over 16 cycles to demonstrate the pacing threshold. As a result, many pacing cycles can take place at insufficient energy for ventricular capture, which can produce periods of asystole while the magnet is applied.[40]

Occasionally, PM-mediated tachycardia (PMT) can ensue on removal of the magnet from a dual-chamber PM (Fig. 43-6). These PMTs result from retrogradely conducted P waves during asynchronous ventricular pacing, most commonly when the magnet rate is lower than the patient's intrinsic rate. These retrograde P waves are then "tracked" by a dual-chamber device (DDD, VDD modes only), which results in pacing at the UTR. Each paced ventricular cycle results in another retrograde P wave, thereby producing tachycardia. Should this behavior be observed, it can be subverted by reapplication and then removal of the magnet. Some devices can be programmed to recognize these PMTs and will periodically omit one ventricular pacing pulse or lengthen one AV delay cycle during UTR pacing.

In addition, as noted earlier, a patient with a dual-chamber device that has detected a rapid atrial rate and has "mode-switched" to prevent UTR pacing could have the mode switch reset upon application and removal of the magnet. These patients will then undergo UTR pacing until criteria are met to return to the mode-switch function. Distinguishing PMT caused by retrograde P waves from UTR pacing caused by rapid atrial rates (before mode-switch entry) can be very difficult. In general, though, mode switch secondary to rapid atrial rates will take place within 10 to 15 seconds, and PMT from retrograde P waves is quite persistent.

For generators with programmable magnet behavior (Boston Scientific/Guidant Medical/CPI, Pacesetter, St. Jude Medical, Telectronics, Biotronik), only interrogation with a programmer can reveal the current settings. Many manufacturers publish a generator reference guide, although not all of these guides list all magnet idiosyncrasies.

Preanesthetic Evaluation and Pacemaker Reprogramming

Preanesthetic management of a patient with a PM includes evaluation and optimization of coexisting disease (also see Chapter 34).

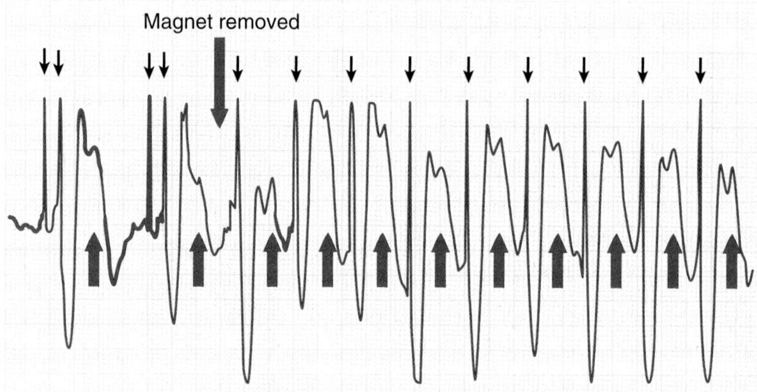

Figure 43-6 Pacemaker-mediated tachycardia (PMT) after removal of the magnet from a pacemaker. This patient had a dual-chamber pacemaker implanted for atrioventricular (AV) nodal disease, and she was pacemaker dependent for ventricular activity. She had a sinus rate of 75/min before application of the magnet with appropriate ventricular pacing (strip not shown). Her programmed AV delay is 200 msec. With magnet application, her pacemaker produced asynchronous AV sequential pacing (DOO mode) at a rate of 60/min. This strip is from an electrocardiographic recorder that enhances the pacemaker artifact with *black, downward arrows*. Because the asynchronous "magnet" rate of this device is lower than her intrinsic atrial rate, many of the atrial pacing stimuli were applied during an atrial refractory period (called functional noncapture). A consequence of atrial noncapture can be retrograde AV nodal conduction with depolarization of the atria after depolarization of the ventricle or ventricles. The retrograde P waves are shown with the *red upward arrows*. While the magnet is applied, this retrograde depolarization of the atria is ignored. Shortly after the magnet was removed (shown), there was a paced ventricular event, followed by retrograde AV nodal conduction. With the ensuing depolarization of the atria from this retrograde conduction, the pacemaker sensed an atrial event and responded by pacing the ventricle 200 msec later. Yet another retrograde P wave appears, and each pace in response to a retrograde P wave created yet another ventricular pace. The result is a PMT at the upper tracking rate (programmed here to 130/min) of the pacemaker. PMT from retrograde AV nodal conduction can occur in any DDD or VDD device with magnet removal, a premature ventricular contraction, or a noncaptured atrial pace. Treatment of this PMT should be reapplication of the magnet. Some pacemakers can be programmed to eventually delay one AV cycle when pacing at the upper tracking limit to "break" PMT.

ACC guidelines suggest that cardiac testing (stress tests, echocardiograms) be dictated by the patient's underlying disease, medications, symptomatology, interval from last testing, and planned intervention.[11]

No special laboratory tests or radiographs are needed for patients with a conventional PM. Chest films rarely depict lead problems, not all devices have radiographic markings, and a standard chest radiograph can exclude the generator or its markings. However, a patient with a BiV PM or ICD might need a chest film to document the position of the coronary sinus lead, especially if central line placement is planned. Currently, there are no data or guidelines regarding placement of a central line in the setting of a coronary sinus lead, and because these leads have no fixation, they might be more easily dislodged than a standard PM or ICD lead. In fact, in early studies, spontaneous dislodgement of the coronary sinus lead was detected in more than 11% of patients.[41,42]

Important features of preanesthetic device evaluation are shown in Appendix 1. Current NASPE and Medicare guidelines include telephone evaluation every 4 to 12 weeks (depending on device type and age) and at least one direct evaluation (i.e., device interrogation with a programmer) at least once per year.[7] In abstract form, Rozner and coauthors reported significant noncompliance with these guidelines in 161 consecutive patients, as well as the need to replace 5% of PMs preoperatively for battery depletion.[43] Telephone evaluation provides some assurance of battery longevity, but it does not provide rigorous evaluation of the pacemaking system. ACC guidelines recommend timely, preoperative interrogation of every PM.[11]

For current PMs, interrogation with a programmer remains the most reliable method for evaluating battery voltage, battery impedance, lead performance, and adequacy of the current settings. Special attention should be paid to patients from countries where PMs might be reused[44] because battery life (typically 5 to 7 years) might not be related to length of implantation in the current patient. For any PM with battery voltage less than 2.6 V or battery impedance (where available) greater than 3000 Ω, the company should be consulted about the possible need for elective replacement of the device before surgery.

Appropriate reprogramming (Box 43-3) is the safest way to avoid intraoperative problems, especially if monopolar "Bovie" electrosurgery will be used. Many PM manufacturers stand ready to assist with this task (see Appendix 2 for company telephone numbers). However, interrogation of any generator with or without reprogramming requires a medical prescription and supervision by an appropriately trained physician.[52] Hospital guidelines and policy should reflect the need for a competent physician to review and validate any care delivered by a company representative.

Reprogramming a PM to asynchronous pacing at a rate more rapid than the patient's underlying rate usually ensures that no oversensing during EMI will take place, thus protecting the patient. However, there is one case report involving a Telectronics device that would open its output circuitry (i.e., no pacing stimuli would be delivered) in the presence of high-voltage EMI.[53] Furthermore, at our institution we have observed two PMs in DOO mode decrease their rate during use of an ESU for monopolar coagulation, presumably because of high battery current drain.

Reprogramming a device *will not* protect the device from internal damage or reset caused by EMI. Additionally, setting a device to asynchronous mode causes the PM to ignore premature atrial or ventricular systoles, which could have the potential to create a malignant rhythm in a patient with significant structural compromise of the myocardium.[54]

In general, rate responsiveness and other "enhancements" ("afib" suppression [formerly dynamic atrial overdrive], hysteresis, managed ventricular pacing, sleep rate, AV search, and so on) should be disabled by programming to prevent misinterpretation of the cardiac rhythm.[46,55] Note that for many Guidant and CPI devices, Guidant Medical recommends increasing the pacing voltage to "5 V or higher" in any case in which an ESU will be used. Few cardiologists follow this recommendation, but there are reports of pacing threshold changes during both intrathoracic[56] and nonchest surgery,[57] as well as in patients with significant noncardiac acute disease.[58]

Special attention must be given to any device with a minute ventilation (bioimpedance) sensor (Box 43-4) because inappropriate tachycardia has been observed secondary to mechanical ventilation,[25,47] monopolar "Bovie" electrosurgery,[47,61,62] and connection to an electrocardiographic monitor with respiratory rate monitoring.[48-50,59,60,63] Sometimes this PMT has led to inappropriate, unsuccessful pharmacologic treatment of the tachycardia[25] with subsequent patient injury.[24]

Intraoperative (or Procedure) Management of Pacemakers

Although no special monitoring or anesthetic technique is required for a patient with a cardiac generator, attention must be given to a number of concerns (also see Chapters 40 and 60). First, electrocardiographic monitoring of a patient must include the ability to detect pacing discharges. Currently, most electrocardiographic monitors in both the operating room and the intensive care unit perform digital acquisition and analysis of electrocardiographic signals, and they are subject to considerable interference from a variety of sources.[64] In their default settings, these monitors often filter the pacing artifacts, and no pacing "spikes" will be shown. This filtering must be disabled so that the monitor will "paint" pacing spikes onto the display. Even with the filtering disabled, however, pacing artifacts do not always appear. Atrial signals are weak, and current monitors do a poor job detecting them. Moreover, because many digital monitors analyze only one lead for these signals (and then "paint on" artifacts on every lead), placement of the electrocardiographic leads can markedly affect the detection axis.* In practice, when a patient with known pacing is monitored, sometimes changing the "analysis" lead on the monitor will result in the appearance of pacing signals. Unfortunately, when the PM artifact filter is disabled, EMI, especially from use of a monopolar ESU, can lead to inappropriate "painting" of pacing artifacts on the monitor (Fig. 43-7).[65]

Second, patient monitoring must include the ability to ensure that paced electrical activity is converted to mechanical

Box 43-4 Pacemakers with Minute Ventilation (Bioimpedance) Sensors

ELA Medical
- Brio (212, 220, 222)
- Chorus RM (7034, 7134)
- Opus RM (4534)
- Rhapsody (2530)
- Symphony (2250, 2550)
- Talent (130, 213, 223)

Boston Scientific/Guidant Medical/CPI
- Pulsar (1172, 1272)
- Pulsar Max (1170, 1171, 1270)
- Pulsar Max II (1180, 1181, 1280)
- Insignia Plus (1194, 1297, 1298)

Medtronic
- Kappa 400 series (KDR401, KDR403, KSR401, KSR403)

Telectronics/St. Jude
- Meta (1202, 1204, 1206, 1230, 1250, 1254, 1256)
- Tempo (1102, 1902, 2102, 2902)

Pacemakers with minute ventilation (bioimpedance) sensors frequently respond to electromagnetic interference (EMI) with pacing at the upper sensor rate.[48,49] These tachycardias can also be produced by connection to an operating room electrocardiographic monitor because many of these devices inject electrical signals through the electrocardiographic leads to determine the respiratory rate or lead disconnection.[59,60] In 1998, the U.S. Center for Devices and Radiologic Health issued a safety alert calling for the deactivation of any minute ventilation (bioimpedance) sensor before exposing a patient to a potential source of EMI or connection to medical devices.[50]

Box 43-3 Situations Probably Requiring Pacemaker Reprogramming

- Any rate-responsive device—see text (problems are well known[23,45] and have been misinterpreted with the potential for patient injury[46-49]; the Food and Drug Administration has issued an alert regarding devices with minute ventilation sensors[50]—see Box 43-4)
- Special pacing indication (hypertrophic obstructive cardiomyopathy, dilated cardiomyopathy, pediatric patients)
- Pacemaker-dependent patients
- Major procedure in the chest or abdomen
- Rate enhancements present that should be disabled
- Special procedures (see text)
- Lithotripsy
- Transurethral resection
- Hysteroscopy
- Electroconvulsive therapy
- Succinylcholine use
- Magnetic resonance imaging (generally contraindicated by device manufacturers)[51]

In some situations and for certain patients, a pacemaker should be reprogrammed either to avoid potential patient injury or to prevent a pacemaker rhythm that could be confused with pacemaker malfunction.

*Most monitors manufactured since 2005 have much improved capability to detect and display pacing artifacts, although they still filter these high-frequency signals in their default setup mode.

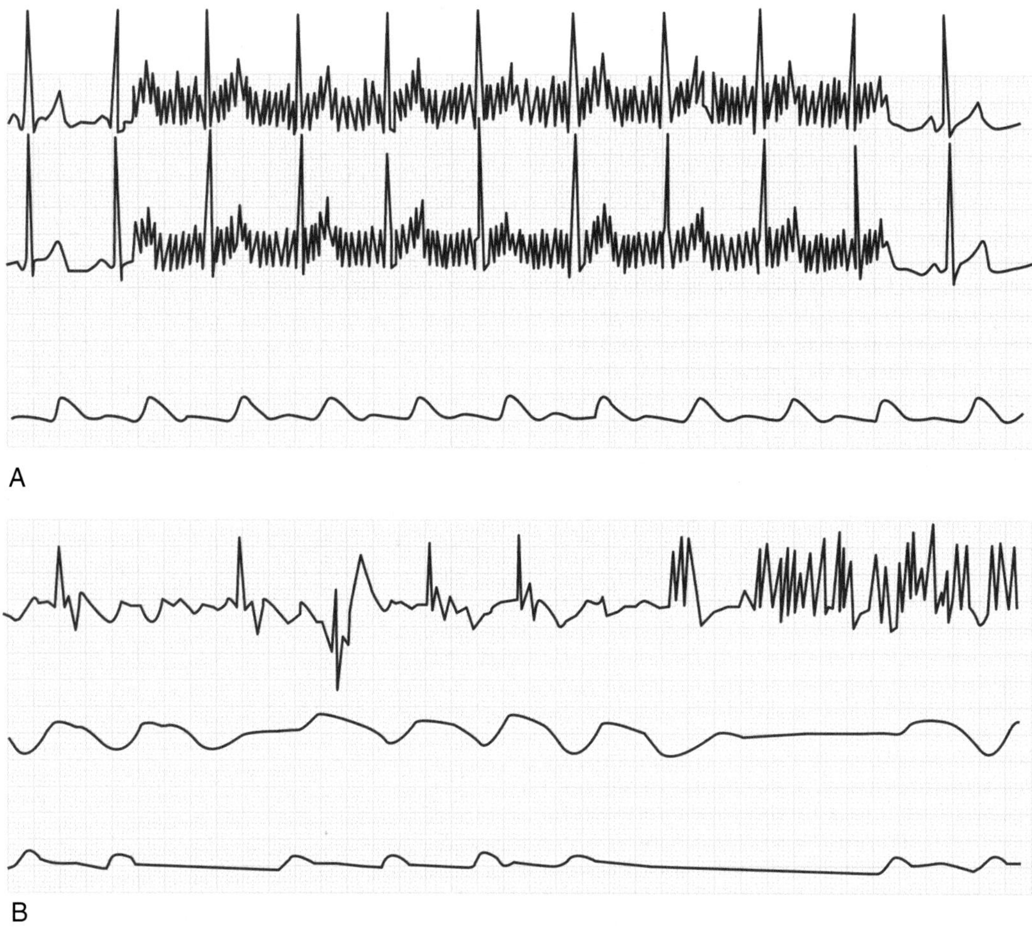

Figure 43-7 Disabling the pacemaker artifact filter on a digitally processed electrocardiographic monitor results in the "painting" of environmental noise (EMI) as pacemaker artifacts. **A,** Effects of "Cut" monopolar electrosurgical unit (ESU) application. Here, the patient's underlying rate exceeded the pacemaker's programmed lower rate limit, and no pacing took place. However, activation of the ESU in the "Cut" mode produced sufficient electromagnetic noise that the monitor began "painting" pacemaker artifacts at a rate of about 20 Hz. The *top tracing* is the electrocardiographic (ECG) lead II, the *middle tracing* is ECG lead V_5, and the *bottom tracing* is the invasive arterial pressure waveform. **B,** The effects of "Coagulation" ESU application produced ventricular oversensing with pacemaker inhibition and left this patient with compromised cardiac output. There is also evidence of inappropriate monitor "painting" of pacemaker artifacts from the EMI. The *top tracing* is ECG lead II, the *middle tracing* is the pulse oximeter plethysmogram, and the *bottom tracing* is the invasive arterial pressure waveform. *(From Rozner MA: Review of electrical interference in implanted cardiac devices. Pacing Clin Electrophysiol 26:923-925, 2003. Used by permission.)*

systole. Mechanical systole is best evaluated by pulse oximetry plethysmography, or arterial pressure waveform display.

Third, there remains limited published perioperative experience with intraoperative BiV pacing at this time. These patients often have ejection fractions of less than 30%, and they depend on pacing in both ventricles to improve their cardiac output. Loss of ventricular pacing from any cause (AV dyssynchrony [atrial fibrillation, atrial flutter, appearance of junctional rhythm], myocardial ischemia, acid-base disturbance, change in pacing threshold, ESU interference, etc.) can cause an immediate decrease in cardiac output. With the exception of transesophageal echocardiography, no beat-to-beat monitoring of cardiac output has demonstrated any utility in detecting loss of BiV pacing behavior. Patients with HOCM pacing can be dependent on ventricular pacing to limit LV outflow tract obstruction.

Fourth, some patients might need an increased pacing rate during the perioperative period to meet an increased oxygen demand. This subject is often not addressed. PM patients reportedly experience postoperative morbidity and mortality frequently,[66] and failure to address tissue oxygen demands and cardiac output needs might contribute to this problem.

Fifth, appropriate equipment must be on hand to provide backup pacing or defibrillation (or both) if needed. Cardiac generators, although hardy, occasionally perform some untoward maneuver or fail, even in the absence of EMI.[67] Acceptable, but inappropriate behavior of a PM or ICD can create an inhospitable situation. Even a properly working, dual-chamber PM can produce R-on-T pacing, especially in the setting of junctional rhythm or premature ventricular contractions (Fig. 43-8).

The medical team caring for a patient with an implanted cardiac pulse generator must understand that the patient has been deemed needy of this device by a physician who is an expert in the diagnosis and management of cardiac rhythm issues. Few anesthesiologists are qualified to contradict this diagnosis, yet some persist in providing an anesthetic without appropriate backup pacing and defibrillation equipment on hand.

Monopolar "Bovie" ESU use remains the principal intraoperative issue for patients with a PM. Between 1984 and 1997, the

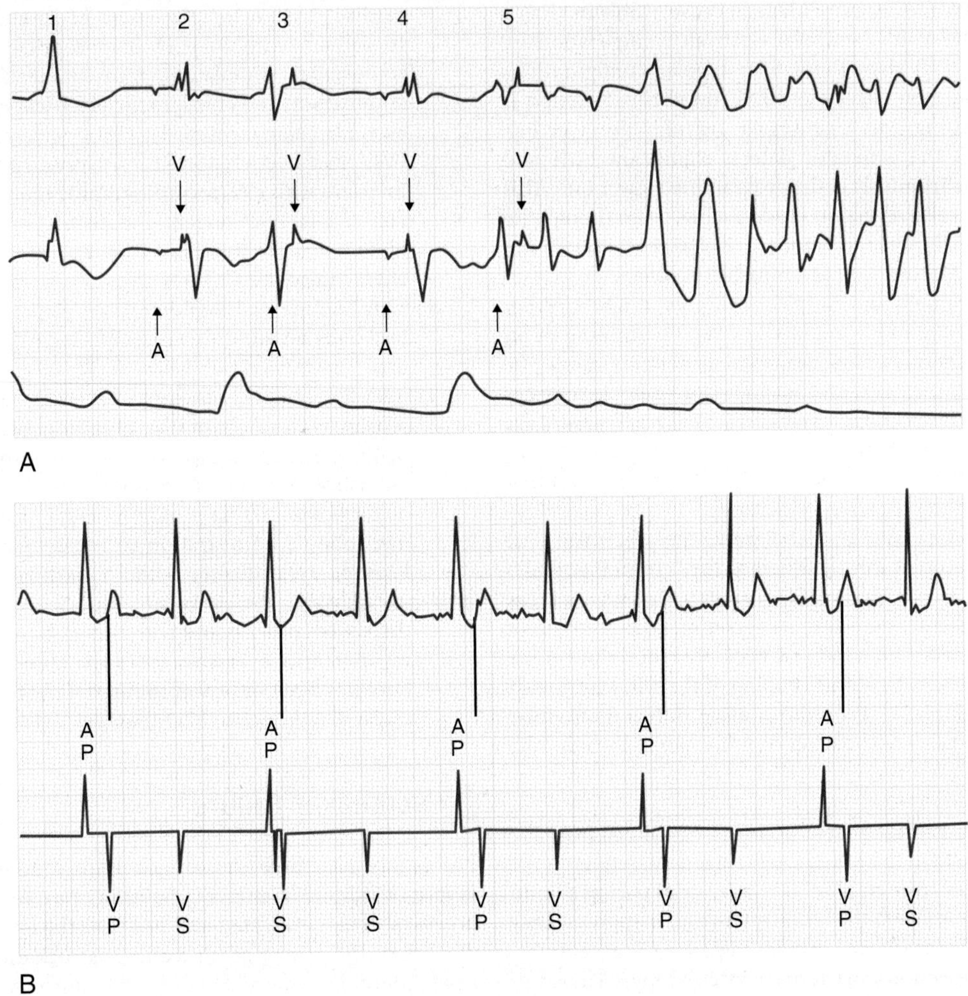

Figure 43-8 Normal dual-chamber pacemaker timing can produce R-on-T pacing. **A,** This strip demonstrates functional ventricular undersensing of a premature ventricular contraction (PVC) with resultant R-on-T pace leading to torsades de pointes. This patient had a dual-chamber pacemaker in the DDD mode with a programmed lower rate of 70/min (R-R interval of 857 msec) and atrioventricular (AV) delay of 200 msec. With these parameters, the pacemaker will pace the atrium 657 msec after any previous ventricular event. Atrial pacing is labeled "A" and ventricular pacing is labeled "V." The *top tracing* is electrocardiographic (ECG) lead II, the *middle tracing* is ECG lead V_5, and the *bottom tracing* is the invasive arterial blood pressure waveform. Approximately 660 msec after the first QRS (1) on the strip (which was adequately sensed by the pacemaker), an atrial stimulus is emitted. At 200 msec after this atrial pace, a ventricular stimulus is emitted and appears to depolarize the ventricle (2). About 660 msec later (3), the patient experienced a PVC. Because the pacemaker was preparing to emit the atrial stimulus, it had disabled its ventricular sensing element and failed to sense this PVC (termed *functional undersensing*). At 200 msec after the atrial stimulus, no ventricular event had been sensed, so the pacemaker emitted a ventricular stimulus on the T wave. Because the ventricle was in a refractory period from the PVC, there was no depolarization of the ventricle (called *functional noncapture*). At 660 msec from this attempted V-pace, the pacemaker again paces the atrium (4), and it appears that the next V-pace captures the ventricle. At point 5 there is a repeat of the events at point 3; that is, the pacemaker disabled its sensing elements in preparation to pace the atrium and failed to detect the PVC. This time, however, the V-pace on the T wave produced torsades de pointes. **B,** This strip was obtained from a Medtronic programmer during interrogation of a Kappa 700 dual-chamber pacemaker. The *top tracing* is ECG lead II, and the *bottom tracing* is the "marker channel," which shows the pacemaker's interpretation of events. This pacemaker was programmed to the DDD mode with a lower rate of 60/min. The AV delay was 200 msec. As a result, after any ventricular event, the pacemaker will emit an atrial pulse at 800 msec if no intervening atrial or ventricular event takes place. This patient had a junctional rhythm at 75/min (corresponding to an R-R interval of 800 msec), so the pacemaker emitted an atrial pulse just as the junctional event occurred. Because the pacemaker disables its ventricular sensing element when emitting the atrial pulse, it failed to detect the ventricular event and emitted the ventricular pulse 200 msec later, on the T wave. This inappropriate pacing takes place every other cycle because every other junctional event is sensed around 600 msec after the previous ventricular pace. Decreasing the AV delay will decrease the likelihood of pacing during the vulnerable period of the ventricle. AP is an atrial pace, VP is a ventricular pace, and VS is a ventricular sensed event. The third complex deserves comment. The pacemaker sensed this ventricular event as it re-enabled its sensing element, and the pacemaker cannot tell whether the sensed event is a true ventricular depolarization or an "echo" of the atrial pace. When a signal from the ventricle is sensed within 30 to 90 msec after an atrial pace, many pacemakers immediately emit a ventricular pacing stimulus. Called a "ventricular safety pace," this pacing stimulus is designed to protect the patient from inappropriate sensing of the atrial signal by the ventricular channel, which would then inhibit the ventricular output. The safety pace is emitted at 110 msec to prevent R-on-T pacing. This feature is also called "nonphysiologic AV delay" by some manufacturers. R-on-T pacing can be appropriate (but not ideal) behavior of a DDD or DDI pacemaker in the setting of PVCs, as well as a junctional rhythm. It can also be seen with atrial or ventricular undersensing.

FDA was notified of 456 adverse events with pulse generators, 255 from electrosurgery, and a "significant number" of device failures.[68] A monopolar ESU is more likely to cause problems than a bipolar ESU, and PMs with a unipolar electrode configuration are more sensitive to EMI than those with bipolar configurations are.[69] The most common effect of an ESU on pacing function is ventricular oversensing, which causes pacing inhibition (see Fig. 43-7B). Sometimes the generator detects significant EMI and begins pacing asynchronously at the programmed lower rate. This behavior is called "noise reversion mode pacing," even though the PM does not actually change "modes." Noise reversion is not present in some ICDs and is programmable in others.

Magnet placement during electrosurgery might prevent aberrant PM behavior, and it might allow reprogramming of an older (pre-1990) generator. Note that some generators cannot be programmed in the presence of a magnet (for example, devices from Boston Scientific, Guidant, and CPI). Newer generators are believed to be relatively immune to spurious reprogramming as a result of EMI, although they can undergo a reset condition that will probably alter the programmed settings.[70]

If a monopolar ESU is to be used, the electrosurgical current-return pad (often misidentified as the "grounding pad") must be placed to ensure that the ESU current path does not cross the pacemaking system. Some authors recommend placement of this pad on the shoulder for head and neck procedures or on the distal part of the arm (with sterile draping of the wire) for breast and axillary procedures.[69,71] Procedures using only a monopolar ESU or with special EMI pacing ramifications include the following:

Lithotripsy—The cardiac generator must be excluded from the lithotripter field. If the lithotripter triggers its output on the sensed electrocardiographic "R" wave, atrial pacing should be disabled to prevent the lithotripter from inappropriately firing on the atrial pacing artifact (also see Chapter 65).

Transurethral Resection and Uterine Hysteroscopy—Transurethral resection of the bladder or prostate and hysteroscopic procedures generally use a monopolar ESU, and device reprogramming might be needed to prevent PM oversensing with resultant PM inhibition. A resectoscope that includes the current-return electrode on the shaft (the irrigation medium will be normal saline) might limit EMI to the generator but has not been carefully tested in this environment (also see Chapter 65).

Magnetic Resonance Imaging (MRI)—Without special care, MRI is contraindicated by most device manufacturers, and deaths have been reported. According to physicians' manuals from most manufacturers, MRI might lead to magnet switch closure (magnet mode activation), reprogramming, inappropriate high-rate pacing, generator damage, myocardial injury, or generator movement within the pocket causing pain, lead failure, or arrhythmia. Nevertheless, safe performance of MRI in qualified patients with PMs and ICDs has been reported[72,73] (also see Chapter 79).

Electroconvulsive Therapy—Electroconvulsive therapy might require a nonsensing (asynchronous) mode to prevent myopotential-induced oversensing with resultant PM inhibition.[74]

Nerve Stimulator Testing/Therapy—Nerve stimulators can cause PM oversensing with resultant PM inhibition[75] and cardiac arrest.[76] Nerve stimulators have been used intraoperatively to inhibit undesired cardiac pacing[23] or arrest the cardiac rhythm for placement of an endovascular stent.[77] In patients with an ICD, inappropriate detection of neuromuscular stimulators, transcutaneous electrical nerve stimulation, and chiropractic electrical muscle stimulation as ventricular tachycardia (VT) or ventricular fibrillation (VF) has been reported.[78,79] Nerve stimulators can also interfere with electrocardiographic monitoring of PM artifacts.[65] Like ESU current, the electrical path for nerve stimulator current should not cross the generator system or the chest[80] (also see Chapter 47).

Succinylcholine or Etomidate Use—Reports of myopotential problems on administration of succinylcholine[81] or etomidate[82] have been published. In the case of succinylcholine, muscle fasciculations might have caused ventricular oversensing with resultant PM inhibition, but this report is difficult to interpret. No electrocardiographic tracings were published, and the PM was damaged during a subsequent defibrillation. Using programmers, I have witnessed succinylcholine administration to more than 50 patients with PMs or defibrillators without finding any myopotential oversensing. The etomidate issue is also not clear because there were other issues with the particular PM.[83] However, myopotential oversensing (in the absence of succinylcholine) has been observed to interfere with PM function[84] or cause inappropriate ICD therapy[85] (also see Chapter 29).

Pacemaker Failure

PM failure has three causes: generator failure, lead failure, or failure of capture. Generator failure is rare in a device that has previously been evaluated and not near the end of useful battery life, unless the generator (or leads) is struck directly by the ESU. Lead failure, also unusual but reported during patient repositioning,[86] can result in undersensing (intrinsic activity is not detected), oversensing ("detection" of events unrelated to intrinsic activity), or failure to deliver sufficient energy to the myocardium to produce depolarization (termed loss of capture). Myocardial changes that lengthen the refractory period or increase the energy requirement for depolarization (failure to capture) can result from myocardial ischemia/infarction, acid-base disturbance, electrolyte abnormalities, or abnormal antiarrhythmic drug levels.

The response to PM failure depends on the clinical situation: a patient with a perfusing rhythm and stable vital signs can be observed while a plan is made to correct the problem. For a patient with inadequate perfusion, the following steps can be attempted (while cardiopulmonary resuscitation is in progress when appropriate):

1. A magnet can be applied if the PM is known to revert to an asynchronous mode, which will also eliminate sensing behavior in these devices. For many of the St. Jude Autocapture devices with magnet mode enabled, magnet application might increase pacing amplitude and restore capture. Devices from ELA Medical (Denver, CO) typically increase their pacing amplitude when a magnet is applied. Some PMs perform threshold margin testing upon magnet placement, which can further reduce pacing.[38]

2. Temporary pacing can be initiated, and it can be transthoracic (transcutaneous), transvenous, or transesophageal. Transesophageal (atrial) pacing requires a functional atrium and AV node for ventricular activation, so it is contraindicated in patients with atrial fibrillation or flutter. It is also generally contraindicated in the presence of a permanent PM (or ICD).

In the setting of external pacing, the electrocardiogram can be misinterpreted because the PM artifacts are large in comparison to the QRS complexes (Fig. 43-9A). Successful ventricular pacing has been reported with transesophageal PMs, but it remains unreliable[87] and produces inferior hemodynamics when compared with atrial pacing (Fig. 43-9B). Note that any external pacing might further

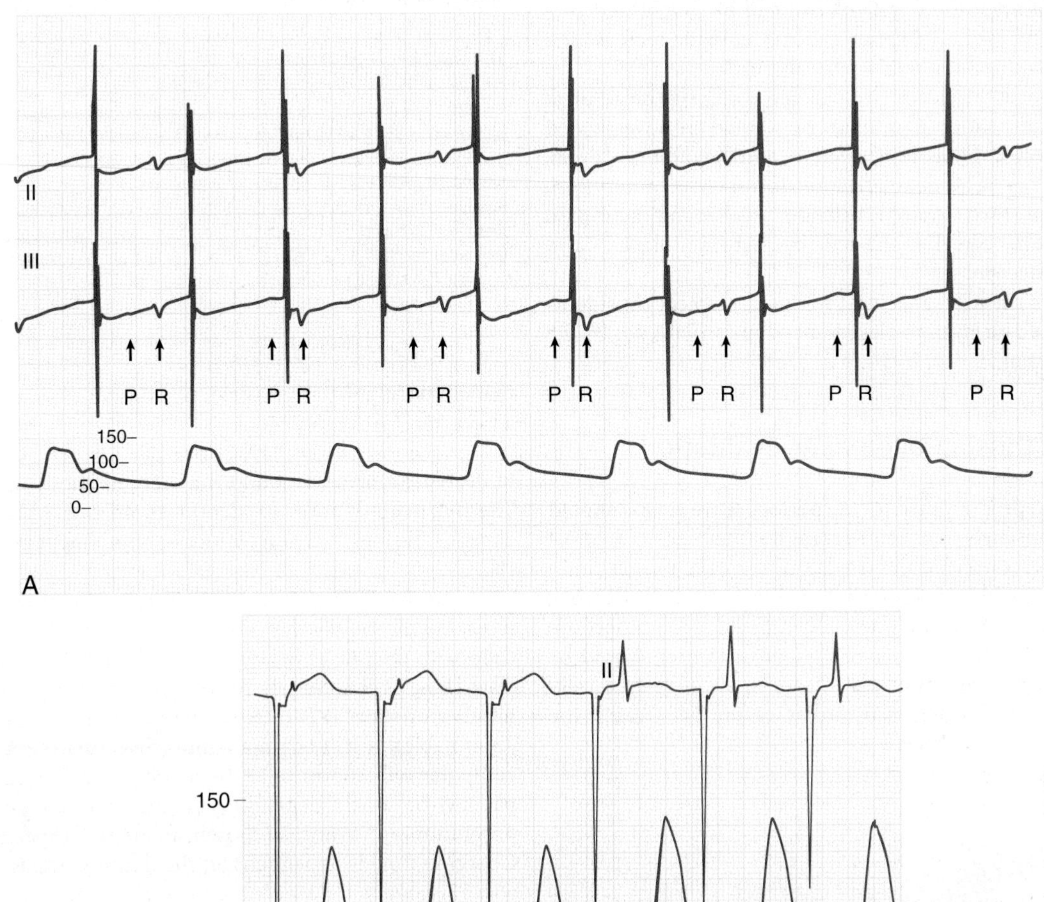

Figure 43-9 Issues with a transesophageal atrial pacemaker (TAP). **A,** Improper placement of a TAP demonstrating atrial noncapture. The *top recording* is electrocardiographic (ECG) lead II, the *middle recording* is ECG lead III, and the *bottom recording* is the invasive arterial pressure waveform. Sinus bradycardia with evidence of tissue underperfusion developed in this 72-year-old man. A TAP (CardioCommand, Tampa, FL) was placed, and the large ECG artifacts at 75/min were misinterpreted by personnel and the ECG monitor as ventricular systoles (capture). This patient has a sinus rate of 50/min with a first-degree atrioventricular block (PR interval of 280 msec). The patient's native atrial (P) and ventricular (R) depolarizations are noted. The arterial pressure waveform confirms pacing noncapture. **B,** Direct ventricular activation with a transesophageal pacemaker. The *top recording* is ECG lead II, and the *bottom recording* (enhanced vertical scale) is the invasive arterial pressure waveform. This strip is from an obese 61-year-old woman with diabetes and hypertension undergoing transsphenoidal hypophysectomy. Shortly after induction, sinus bradycardia at 37 beats/min and mild hypotension developed. A transesophageal pacemaker was placed but advanced too far into the esophagus. This strip was recorded during "pullback." The ventricle was directly activated in the first four events, with a resultant wide-complex QRS and average blood pressure of 135/75 mm Hg. On pullback, the atrium was activated, the QRS returned to a narrow complex, and blood pressure increased to 143/80 mm Hg. Except for the bradycardia, this patient had a normal heart and did not have a permanently placed generator.

inhibit PM output at energies that will not produce myocardial capture.[88]

3. Sympathomimetic drugs can decrease depolarization threshold or increase chronotropicity (or both). Epinephrine (0.5 to 1 μg/min) or dopamine (5 to 20 μg/kg/min) should be considered. Isoproterenol (0.5 μg/min) is often recommended but not widely available and is complicated by hypotension. Antimuscarinic drugs (atropine, glycopyrrolate) might be helpful.
4. Causes of myocardial ischemia should be sought and corrected. Myocardial ischemia can substantially increase the energy required for ventricular capture.[89]
5. Disturbances in electrolyte balance, antiarrhythmic drug levels, and acid-base equilibrium should be investigated and corrected. Potassium, calcium, and magnesium abnormalities can raise depolarization thresholds. In addition, potassium flux, ionized calcium levels, and acid-base equilibrium can be affected by hyperventilation and hypoventilation.
6. If none of the measures just presented succeed, consideration should be given to placement of epicardial leads by the surgical staff.

Postanesthesia Pacemaker Evaluation

A PM that was reprogrammed for the perioperative period should be reset appropriately. For non-reprogrammed devices, most manufacturers recommend interrogation to ensure proper functioning and acceptable remaining battery life if any electrosurgery was used. The ACC guidelines now recommend a postprocedure interrogation (also see Chapter 85).[11] Consideration should be given to increasing the lower paced rate in a chronotropically incompetent patient if increased cardiac output will benefit the patient during convalescence.

Implantable Cardioverter-Defibrillators

The development of an implantable, battery-powered device able to deliver sufficient energy to terminate VT or VF represents a major medical breakthrough for patients with a history of ventricular tachydysrhythmias. These devices reduce deaths in the setting of malignant ventricular tachydysrhythmias,[90,91] and they clearly remain superior to antiarrhythmic drug therapy.[92] Initially approved by the FDA in 1985, more than 60,000 devices will be implanted in the United States this year, and industry sources report that more than 250,000 patients have these devices today. Furthermore, results from the Sudden Cardiac Death–Heart Failure Trial (SCD-HeFT—showing that prophylactic placement of an ICD is superior to drug therapy in any patient with an ejection fraction less than 0.35 and *without* evidence of arrhythmic inducibility) have led to a significant increase in the number of patients for whom ICD therapy is indicated.[93]

A considerable number of technologic advances have been applied since the first ICD was placed, including substantial miniaturization (pectoral pocket placement with transvenous leads is the norm), as well as battery improvements that now permit permanent pacing with these devices. Thus, one could easily confuse a pectoral ICD for a PM.

Table 43-3 NASPE/BPEG Generic Defibrillator Code (NBD)

Position I: Shock Chambers(s)	Position II: Antitachycardia Pacing Chamber(s)	Position III: Tachycardia Detection	Position IV: Antibradycardia Pacing Chamber(s)*
O = none	**O** = none	**E** = electrogram	**O** = none
A = atrium	**A** = atrium	**H** = hemodynamic	**A** = atrium
V = ventricle	**V** = ventricle		**V** = ventricle
D = dual (A + V)	**D** = dual (A + V)		**D** = dual (A+V)

The NBD code is a joint project from the North American Society of Pacing and Electrophysiology (NASPE) (the "N") and the British Pacing and Electrophysiology Group (BPEG) (the "B").[94] The "D" stands for defibrillator.
*For robust identification, position IV is expanded into its complete NBG code. For example, a biventricular pacing-defibrillator with ventricular shock and antitachycardia pacing functionality would be identified as VVE-DDDRV, assuming that the pacing section was programmed DDDRV. Currently, no hemodynamic sensors have been approved for detection of tachycardia (position III).

Like PMs, ICDs have a four-place generic code (NBD*) to indicate lead placement and function, as shown in Table 43-3.[94] The most robust form of identification, called the "label form," expands the fourth character into its component generic PM code (NBG).

Newer ICDs (since 1993) have many programmable features, but essentially they measure each cardiac R-R interval and categorize the rate as normal, too fast (short R-R interval), or too slow (long R-R interval). When the device detects a sufficient number of short R-R intervals within a certain period (all programmable), it will begin an antitachycardia event. The internal computer will choose ATP (less energy use, better tolerated by patient) or shock, depending on the manifestation and device programming. If shock is chosen, an internal capacitor is charged. Charging time is dependent on the desired output, and it can be 6 to 15 seconds for a maximum shock. Charging time is lengthened by lower battery voltage, time from last charge,[†] and lower temperature.

Most ICDs can be programmed to "reconfirm" VT or VF after charging to prevent inappropriate shock therapy. Some ICDs can be programmed to begin ATP immediately on initiating a charge cycle. Typically, ICDs deliver 6 to 18 shocks per event. Once a shock is delivered, no further ATP will take place. Despite considerable improvement in detection of ventricular dysrhythmias, more than 10% of shocks are for rhythms other than VT or VF.[95,96] Supraventricular tachycardia (SVT) remains the most common etiology of inappropriate shock therapy,[97,98] and causes of inappropriate shock have been reviewed elsewhere.[99] Program-

*The NBD code is a joint project from the NASPE (the "N") and the BPEG (the "B"). The "D" stands for defibrillator.

†The capacitor in an ICD "deforms" during inactivity, which leads to increased time needed to charge the capacitor. To mitigate the effects of deformation, all ICDs perform nontherapeutic charging of their capacitor (called "reforming") at a programmable periodic interval (usually 1 to 6 months).

mable features in current ICDs to differentiate VT from a tachycardia of supraventricular origin (SVT) include the following[100]:

1. Onset criteria—in general, the onset of VT is abrupt, whereas the onset of SVT has a sequentially shortening R-R interval.
2. Stability criteria—in general, the R-R interval of VT is relatively constant, whereas the R-R interval of atrial fibrillation with rapid ventricular response is quite variable.
3. QRS width criteria—in general, the QRS width in SVT is narrow (<110 msec), whereas the QRS width in VT is wide (>120 msec).
4. "Intelligence" in dual-chamber devices attempting to associate atrial activity with ventricular activity.
5. Morphology waveform analysis with comparison to stored historical templates.

Note that once the R-R interval becomes sufficiently short for detection of VF, most ICDs will begin a shock sequence. As noted earlier, once the device delivers any shock therapy, no further ATP will take place.

An ICD with antibradycardia therapy capability will begin pacing when the R-R interval is too long. In July 1997, the FDA approved devices with sophisticated dual-chamber pacing modes and rate-responsive behavior for ICD patients who need permanent pacing (about 20% of ICD patients). Because of the DAVID study, which suggested that DDD pacing in a patient without a clear need for dual-chamber pacing decreases survival when compared with single-chamber device placement,[101] many electrophysiologists are programming long (>250 msec) AV delays in these patients to limit ventricular pacing. As noted previously, however, long AV delays can lead to R-on-T pacing (see Fig. 43-8A). In addition, many ICD manufacturers have designed algorithms to limit ventricular pacing. Some of these algorithms allow dropped QRS events, which can resemble a second-degree Mobitz II block or malfunction of the pacing system.

ICD Indications

Initially, ICDs were placed for hemodynamically significant VT or VF (Box 43-5). Newer indications associated with sudden death include patients awaiting heart transplantation[102] and those with long QT syndrome,[103] Brugada syndrome (right bundle branch block, ST-segment elevation in leads V_1 to V_3), and arrhythmogenic RV dysplasia.[104,105] Studies suggest that ICDs can be placed prophylactically (i.e., used for primary prevention) to prevent sudden death in young patients with hypertrophic cardiomyopathy,[106] as well as in post–myocardial infarction patients with an ejection fraction less than 30%,[93] but they are of no benefit after coronary artery bypass grafting. Three-chamber ICDs have been approved by the FDA for patients with DCM, and ICDs are in clinical trial for patients with HOCM who have experienced VT or VF.

ICD Magnets

Like PMs, magnet behavior in ICDs can be altered by programming. Most devices will suspend tachydysrhythmia detection (and therefore therapy) when a magnet is appropriately placed to

Box 43-5 Indications for Implantable Cardioverter-Defibrillators

Ventricular tachycardia

Ventricular fibrillation

Brugada syndrome (right bundle branch block, ST-segment elevation in V_1 to V_3)

Arrhythmogenic right ventricular dysplasia

Long Q-T syndrome

Hypertrophic cardiomyopathy

Prophylactic use in a patient who has a cardiomyopathy (CM) without electrophysiologic testing to justify placement: MADIT II (ejection fraction [EF] <30%, ischemic CM),[93] MUSTT (EF <40%, ischemic CM with unsustained ventricular tachycardia),[92] SCD-HeFT (EF <35% and causing CM).[3]

activate the magnet switch. Some devices from Angeion, Boston Scientific, CPI, Guidant, Pacesetter, St. Jude Medical, or Ventritex can be programmed to ignore magnet placement, and some Guidant ICDs have had their magnet function permanently disabled because of a magnet switch issue (e.g., see Fig. 43-3).[8]

Depending on programming, antitachycardia therapy in some Boston Scientific/Guidant Medical/CPI devices can be permanently disabled by magnet placement for 30 seconds, and as noted earlier, some patients have been discovered with their ICD antitachycardia therapy unintentionally disabled.[4,5] In Boston Scientific/Guidant Medical/CPI devices, if the magnet mode is enabled and the ICD is enabled for antitachycardia therapy, the ICD will emit beeps synchronized to R waves to signify adequate placement of the magnet and suspension of tachyarrhythmia detection (hence disabling therapy). If the ICD emits a constant tone, antitachycardia therapy has been programmed to "off," regardless of magnet placement. Depending on programming, ICDs from Boston Scientific/Guidant Medical/CPI can toggle between activated and inactivated states with 30 seconds of magnet application. Thus, to re-enable therapy, the magnet must be removed and then replaced until the constant tone reverts to beeps synchronized to R waves. Subsequent removal of the magnet then returns the antitachycardia therapy to the enabled state. Any Boston Scientific/Guidant Medical/CPI device that emits either beeps or constant tones while a magnet is placed will have its antitachycardia therapy disabled during the magnet session.

To ensure correct magnet placement on its devices, Medtronic marketed a device called the "Smart Magnet." Manufacturing ceased around 2005 because not many were sold. This battery-powered instrument contains a magnet and a radiofrequency (RF) receiver. All Medtronic generators broadcast RF destined for the programmer on magnet placement, and the Smart Magnet detects this RF transmission and illuminates the "found" light when an ICD is under the magnet. Medtronic recommends that the Smart Magnet be taped to the patient. Note that during the occurrence of EMI, transmission from the ICD to the Smart Magnet can be interrupted, and the ICD "found" light often turns off. In this setting, though, the ICD remains disabled because it is the physical presence of the magnet rather than the RF communication that disables the antitachycardia therapy.

In general, magnets will not affect ICD antibradycardia pacing mode or rate (except ELA [rate change] and Telectronics

Guardian 4202/4203 [disabled]). Intermedics devices transiently change the pacing rate (VVI mode) to reflect battery voltage. Interrogating the device and calling the manufacturer remain the most reliable method for determining magnet response.

The comments in the pacing section (including Appendix 1 and Box 43-3) apply here for any ICD with antibradycardia pacing. Many ICDs have no noise reversion behavior, so ESU-induced ventricular oversensing might lead to nonpacing in a patient who is dependent on the ICD for pacing.

Preanesthetic Evaluation and ICD Reprogramming

In addition to evaluating and optimizing any comorbid disease in ICD patients, I believe that every ICD should undergo preoperative interrogation. These devices store considerable data regarding the occurrence of dysrhythmias. Because ATP is well tolerated, most patients are not aware of this intervention. For any patient scheduled to undergo an elective procedure, the onset of new dysrhythmias probably warrants investigation of the problem before the procedure (Fig. 43-10).

Determination of the need for elective replacement of an ICD because of battery depletion is more complicated than with PMs. Because some ICDs can have multiple battery cells, predicting battery depletion based on battery voltage is difficult. In general, however, the manufacturer should be consulted for any device with a "charging time" in excess of 12 seconds.

Most ICDs should have their antitachycardia therapy disabled before the use of any device that causes EMI. Use of a monopolar ESU can produce inappropriate shocks. Casavant and associates found a stored electrogram sequence in an ICD suggesting that it had misinterpreted use of a monopolar ESU during dermatologic facial surgery as VF,[107] and Figure 43-11 shows VT detection that occurred during surgery. Additionally, there is one report of a central line guidewire interacting with the RV lead that led to a short-circuit shock and subsequent failure of the ICD.[108]

Intraoperative (or Procedure) Management of ICDs

At this time, no special monitoring (because of the ICD) is required for a patient with an ICD. Electrocardiographic monitoring and the ability to deliver external cardioversion or defibrillation must be present during the time of ICD disablement. Should cardioversion or defibrillation be needed, the defibrillator pads should be placed so that they avoid the pulse generator to the greatest extent possible. Nevertheless, one should remember that the patient, not the ICD, is being treated. The recommendations in the section "Intraoperative (or Procedure) Management of Pacemakers" apply here as well.

No special anesthetic techniques have been championed for patients with an ICD. Most of these patients will have severely depressed systolic function, dilated ventricular cavities, and significant valvular regurgitation. Thus, the choice of anesthetic technique should be dictated by the underlying physiologic derangements that are present. Conflicting data have been published regarding the choice of anesthetic agent or agents and changes in defibrillation threshold (DFT). In 1993, Gill and coworkers examined DFT in dogs and concluded that neither halothane nor isoflurane changed the DFT in open chest defibrillation when compared with pentobarbital infusion.[109] However, Weinbroum and associates evaluated DFTs in humans during ICD implantation and found that halothane, isoflurane, and fen-

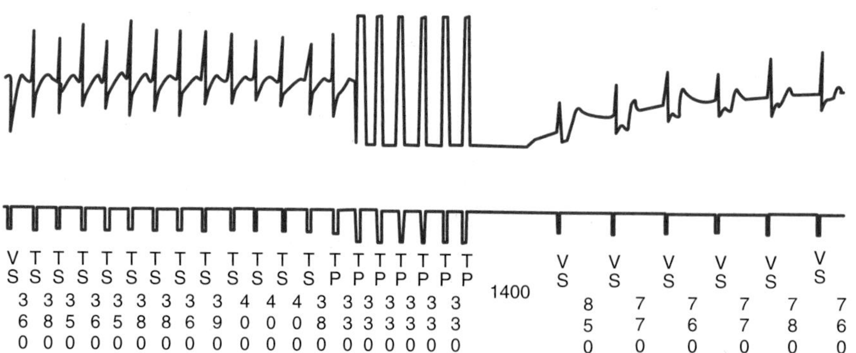

Figure 43-10 Unexpected ventricular tachycardia (VT) with antitachycardia pacing was found in this patient during her preoperative visit. A 65-year-old woman with a history of VT had undergone implantation of a Medtronic single-chamber defibrillator about 8 months previously. She had not had any dizziness or syncopal episodes since placement of an implantable cardioverter-defibrillator (ICD). Interrogation of her device in the preoperative center revealed VVE-VVI programming, along with an episode of tachycardia at 150 to 162 beats/min that was detected by the ICD as VT. The ICD delivered a six-beat burst of antitachycardia pacing at 182 beats/min, which converted the tachycardia back to sinus rhythm. No backup pacing was needed after the VT was terminated. The *upper tracing* is a digitized ventricular electrogram that was stored in the ICD during the tachycardic event. The *lower tracing* is the "marker channel," which reports the interpretation of each event by the ICD. The numbers below the marker channel represent the interval (in milliseconds). The rate is calculated by dividing the interval into 60,000 msec/min. TD marks the final event that starts therapy, TS represents an interval in the VT zone, TP is an antitachycardia pace event, and VS is an intrinsic ventricular depolarization with a rate that is neither too fast (short interval) nor too slow (long interval). This device was set to detect VT as 16 consecutive ventricular events with a rate between 146 and 200 per minute and to deliver antitachycardia pacing at 84% of the last R-R interval (the last interval was 400 msec, so antitachycardia pacing was delivered at a rate of 182/min (330 msec).

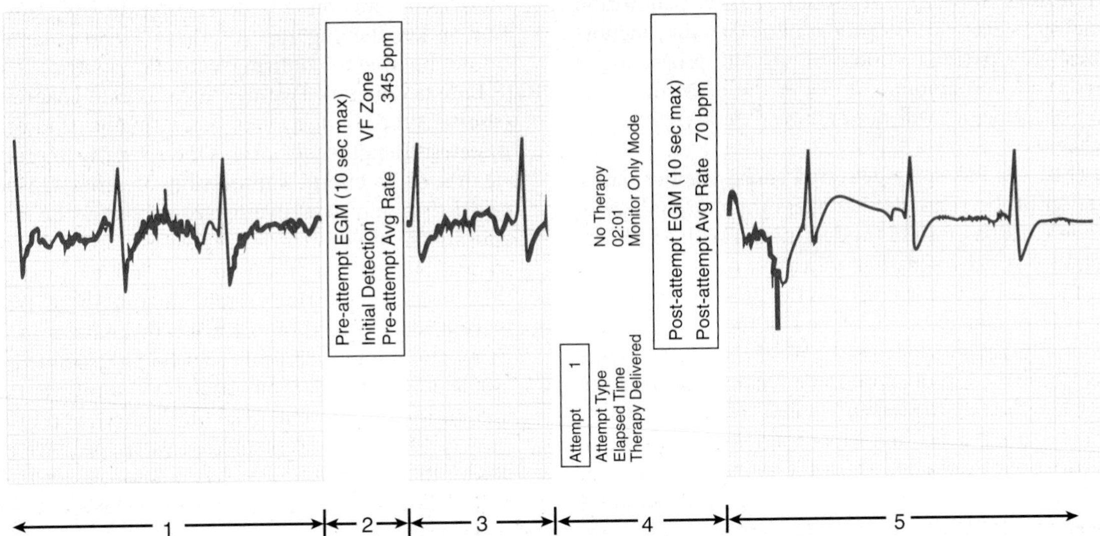

Figure 43-11 Electromagnetic interference (EMI) from the monopolar electrosurgery unit (ESU; "Bovie") caused an implantable cardioverter-defibrillator (ICD) to detect ventricular fibrillation (VF). This stored electrogram (EGM) was one of 73 found at the end of a 4-hour surgical procedure in which considerable monopolar electrosurgery was used. This patient had a Guidant Medical ICD in the VOE-VVI mode. The patient's ICD had been placed in a "monitor only" mode before surgery. As a result, the ICD recorded any instance of ventricular dysrhythmia that would have triggered therapy, but it could not actually deliver therapy. From left to right, (1) the EGM demonstrates a ventricular rate of 70/min, but with considerable noise on the baseline; (2) a VF event was declared for the detected heart rate of 345/min, and the ICD charged its capacitor; (3) the ICD was programmed to "reconfirm before shock," and the ventricular rate remains 70/min with noise on the baseline; (4) again, the noise caused the ICD to believe that the patient remained in VF, and the ICD would have delivered a shock, except that it was programmed to "monitor only"; and (5) because the noise is gone (the ESU had stopped), the ICD declares the event over after "successful" defibrillation.

tanyl increased the DFT.[110] Even with these increases, though, the increased DFTs were still substantially lower than the maximum energy generally available in ICDs, and these increases would not have been noted under the usual testing conditions.

Postanesthesia ICD Evaluation

The ICD must be reinterrogated and re-enabled, and deaths from failure to re-enable an ICD have been reported.[5] All recorded events should be reviewed and counters should be cleared. The pacing parameters must be checked and reprogrammed as necessary.

Summary

Electronic miniaturization has permitted the design and use of sophisticated electronics in patients who have need for artificial pacing or automated cardioversion/defibrillation of their heart. These devices are no longer confined to merely keeping the heart beating between a minimum rate (pacing function) and a maximum rate (ICD functions); they are now being used as therapy to improve a failing heart.

Both aging of the population and our ability to care for a patient with increasingly complex disease suggest that we will be caring for many more patients with these devices, and we must be prepared for this situation. Safe and efficient clinical management of these patients depends on our understanding of implantable systems, indications for their use, and the perioperative needs that they create.

Glossary

Afib Suppression (formerly Dynamic Atrial Overdrive)—A programmable rate enhancement for PMs that increases the pacing rate in response to the presence of intrinsic atrial activity. Afib suppression is designed to pace the atrium at a rate just above the intrinsic rate to prevent atrial fibrillation.[111] It should be disabled before an anesthetic to prevent high pacing rates.

Atrioventricular Delay—The time that a dual-chamber system waits after detecting (or initiating) an atrial event before pacing the ventricle. Some generators shorten this time as the heart rate increases (termed "rate-adaptive AV delay" or "dynamic AV delay"). Some generators can be programmed to extend the AV delay to search for intrinsic conduction ("search AV delay"). Some generators will prolong an AV delay after any atrial event when the last ventricular event was intrinsic ("AV delay hysteresis"). In a patient with a conducting AV node, the sensed AV delay will be slightly longer than the "PR" interval on the surface electrocardiogram (see Fusion Beat and Pseudofusion Beat) because the ventricular sensing element is attached to the apex of the right ventricle and the depolarization takes place only after RV activation (typically >60 msec after activation of the AV node).

Automatic Rate—see Lower Rate Limit.

Bipolar Lead—An electrode with two conductors. Bipolar pacing typically uses less energy than unipolar pacing does, and it will produce smaller artifacts on analog monitors. Bipolar sensing is more resistant to oversensing from muscle artifact or stray electromagnetic fields. Most pacing generators can be programmed to a unipolar mode (separate settings for pacing and sensing), even in the presence of bipolar electrodes.

Electrogram Storage Mode (EGM Mode)—Passive acquisition and internal storage of electrocardiographic data for diagnostic purposes while pacing (or monitoring) with programmed parameters. A PM programmed to enter the EGM mode on application of a magnet will not demonstrate asynchronous pacing behavior.

Fusion Beat (FB)—A PM spike delivered shortly before native depolarization of the ventricle that alters the morphology of the QRS, often misdiagnosed as undersensing. With an FB, the pacing stimulus is delivered after activation of the AV node, but before the sensing element detects the PM-induced depolarization. It is similar to pre-excitation of the ventricle seen in Lown-Ganong-Levine syndrome or Wolff-Parkinson-White syndrome. Confirmation of appropriate sensing behavior can be made by lengthening the sensing interval (i.e., lengthening the AV delay). Fusion beats suggest, but should not be used to confirm ventricular capture. See also Pseudofusion Beat.

Generator—Device with a power source and circuitry to produce an electrical impulse designed to be conducted to the heart. Typically, pacing generators are placed in a pectoral pocket, and leads are inserted into the right atrium, right ventricle, or both. Since 1995, however, ICDs have also been approved for pectoral pocket placement.

Hysteresis—If present, the amount by which the patient's intrinsic rate must fall below the programmed rate before the generator begins pacing. Some pacers periodically decrease the pacing rate to search for resumption of intrinsic activity (called "search hysteresis"). These functions, when present, can mimic PM malfunction.

Implantable Cardioverter-Defibrillator (ICD) Mode—Designation of chambers shocked, chambers paced for antitachycardia pacing, method of tachycardia detection, and chambers paced for antitachycardia therapy. Table 43-3 shows the NASPE/BPEG generic ICD code.

Lower Rate Limit (LRL, also **Automatic Rate** or **Programmed Rate)**—The lowest sustained regular rate at which the generator will pace. Typically, the device begins pacing when the patient's intrinsic rate falls below this value.

Oversensing—Detection of undesired signals that are interpreted as cardiac activity. Oversensing can lead to PM-driven tachycardia (pacing device, DDD mode with atrial oversensing and ventricular tracking), ventricular pause (pacing device with electrosurgically induced ventricular oversensing leading the pacer to "detect" ventricular activity), or inappropriate shock (defibrillator, event oversensing).

Pacing Mode—The designation of chambers paced, chambers sensed, sensing response, rate responsiveness, and antitachyarrhythmia function for a PM system. Table 43-1 shows the NASPE/BPEG generic PM code.

Programmed Rate—see Lower Rate Limit

Pseudofusion Beat (PFB)—A PM spike delivered shortly after native depolarization without alteration of the QRS morphology. PFBs are often misdiagnosed as undersensing, and they result from the position of the sensing electrode relative to the depolarizing wave front (see "Fusion Beat"). Confirmation of appropriate sensing behavior can be achieved by lengthening the sensing interval (i.e., decreasing the program rate [atrial FB] or lengthening the AV delay [ventricular PFB]). PFB cannot be used to confirm electronic capture.

Rate Enhancements—Features such as rate-adaptive AV delay (shortens the AV delay with increasing heart rate), AV search hysteresis (lengthens/shortens the AV delay to produce intrinsic AV conduction), suppression of atrial fibrillation (also called dynamic atrial overdrive—increases the lower rate on appearance of native atrial depolarization so that nearly constant atrial pacing is produced but at a rate only slightly higher than the patient's intrinsic rate), rate smoothing (limits changes in ventricular paced rates caused by changes in atrial rates; rising and falling rate limits can be programmed), sleep rate (see later), ventricular rate regulation (similar to rate smoothing but used to prevent atrial fibrillation), and hysteresis (see earlier). Each of these enhancements can produce pacing/nonpacing that can mimic PM dysfunction, and these enhancements should be programmed "OFF" before delivery of any anesthetic.

Rate Modulation—The ability of the generator to sense the need to increase the heart rate in response to patient activity. Mechanisms include (1) a mechanical sensor in the generator to detect motion or vibration, (2) electronic detection of the QT interval (shortens during exercise), (3) transthoracic impedance to measure changes in respiration, and (4) a sensor or sensors for central venous blood temperature or oxygen saturation (see Box 43-1). Some generators now incorporate multiple sensors. The pacing rate determined by the rate modulation algorithm is called the "Sensor Indicated Rate."

Sensor Indicated Rate—The pacing rate determined by the sensor in a PM programmed to a rate-responsive mode (the fourth character of NBG = "R").

Sleep Rate (also **Circadian Rate**)—The rate (lower than the Programmed Rate) at which the pacing generator will pace during programmed "nighttime" hours.

Undersensing—Failure to detect a desired event.

Unipolar Lead—An electrode with only one conductor. Some devices with bipolar leads are programmed to the unipolar lead mode. Systems with unipolar leads produce larger spikes on the electrocardiogram than bipolar leads do. Systems with unipolar leads use the generator case as the second conductor.

Upper Sensor Rate (**USR**, also **Upper Activity Rate** [**UAR**])—The maximum rate to which a rate-modulated PM can drive the heart. The USR is not affected by the UTR because when the USR becomes active, the PM is pacing the atrium.

Upper Tracking Rate (**UTR**, also called **Upper Rate Limit** [**URL**])—PMs programmed to the VDD or DDD mode cause the ventricles to track atrial activity. Should an atrial tachyarrhythmia develop, such as supraventricular tachycardia, atrial fibrillation, or atrial flutter, the generator acts to limit ventricular pacing. When the atrial rate exceeds the UTR, the generator can change mode (i.e., switch to DDI) or introduce a second-degree AV block. Second-degree blocks can be Mobitz type I (Wenckebach) or Mobitz type II, depending on a variety of programmed settings within the PM.

References

1. Chardack WM, Gage AA, Greatbatch W: A transistorized, self-contained, implantable pacemaker for the long-term correction of complete heart block. Surgery 48:643-654, 1960.
2. Saxon LA, Bristow MR, Boehmer J, et al: Predictors of sudden cardiac death and appropriate shock in the Comparison of Medical Therapy, Pacing, and Defibrillation in Heart Failure (COMPANION) Trial. Circulation 114:2766-2772, 2006.
3. Bardy GH, Lee KL, Mark DB, et al: Amiodarone or an implantable cardioverter-defibrillator for congestive heart failure. N Engl J Med 352:225-237, 2005.
4. Rasmussen MJ, Friedman PA, Hammill SC, Rea RF: Unintentional deactivation of implantable cardioverter-defibrillators in health care settings. Mayo Clin Proc 77:855-859, 2002.
5. Hauser RG, Kallinen L: Deaths associated with implantable cardioverter defibrillator failure and deactivation reported in the United States Food and Drug Administration Manufacturer and User Facility Device Experience Database. Heart Rhythm 1:399-405, 2004.
6. Maisel WH, Moynahan M, Zuckerman BD, et al: Pacemaker and ICD generator malfunctions: Analysis of Food and Drug Administration annual reports. JAMA 295:1901-1906, 2006.
7. Bernstein AD, Irwin ME, Parsonnet V, et al: Report of the NASPE Policy Conference on antibradycardia pacemaker follow-up: Effectiveness, needs, and resources. North American Society of Pacing and Electrophysiology. Pacing Clin Electrophysiol 17:1714-1729, 1994.
8. Guidant: Urgent medical device safety information and corrective action (Contak Renewal [3,4,RF] ICD [magnet switch]). Published June 23, 2005. Available at http://www.bostonscientific.com/templatedata/imports/HTML/PPR/ppr/support/current_advisories.pdf.
9. Medtronic: Urgent medical device information: Sprint Fidelis lead patient management recommendations. Published October 15, 2007. Available at http://www.medtronic.com/fidelis/physician-letter.html/ Accessed October 19, 2007.
10. Practice advisory for the perioperative management of patients with cardiac rhythm management devices: Pacemakers and implantable cardioverter-defibrillators: A report by the American Society of Anesthesiologists Task Force on Perioperative Management of Patients with Cardiac Rhythm Management Devices. Anesthesiology 103:186-198, 2005.
11. Fleisher LA, Beckman JA, Brown KA, et al: ACC/AHA 2007 guidelines on perioperative cardiovascular evaluation and care for noncardiac surgery. A report of the American College of Cardiology/American Heart Association Task Force on practice guidelines (Writing Committee to Revise the 2002 Guidelines on Perioperative Cardiovascular Evaluation for Noncardiac Surgery). Published September 27, 2007. Available at http://circ.ahajournals.org/cgi/content/abstract/CIRCULATIONAHA.107.185699v1/ Accessed November 16, 2007.
12. Goldschlager N, Epstein A, Friedman P, et al: Environmental and drug effects on patients with pacemakers and implantable cardioverter/defibrillators: A practical guide to patient treatment. Arch Intern Med 161:649-655, 2001.
13. Pinski SL, Trohman RG: Interference in implanted cardiac devices, part I. Pacing Clin Electrophysiol 25:1367-1381, 2002.
14. Pinski SL, Trohman RG: Interference in implanted cardiac devices, part II. Pacing Clin Electrophysiol 25:1496-1509, 2002.
15. Stone KR, McPherson CA: Assessment and management of patients with pacemakers and implantable cardioverter defibrillators. Crit Care Med 32:S155-S165, 2004.
16. Kazatsker M, Kusniek J, Hasdai D, et al: Two pacemakers in one patient: A stimulating case. J Cardiovasc Electrophysiol 13:522, 2002.
17. Marangell LB, Martinez M, Jurdi RA, Zboyan H: Neurostimulation therapies in depression: A review of new modalities. Acta Psychiatr Scand 116:174-181, 2007.
18. Zamotrinsky AV, Kondratiev B, de Jong JW: Vagal neurostimulation in patients with coronary artery disease. Auton Neurosci 88:109-116, 2001.
19. Lamas GA, Rebecca GS, Braunwald NS, Antman EM: Pacemaker malfunction after nitrous oxide anesthesia. Am J Cardiol 56:995, 1985.
20. Bernstein AD, Daubert JC, Fletcher RD, et al: The revised NASPE/BPEG generic code for antibradycardia, adaptive-rate, and multisite pacing. North American Society of Pacing and Electrophysiology/British Pacing and Electrophysiology Group. Pacing Clin Electrophysiol 25:260-264, 2002.
21. Forand JM, Schweiss JF: Pacemaker syndrome during anesthesia. Anesthesiology 60:588-590, 1984.
22. Ducey J, Fincher D, Baysinger C: Therapeutic suppression of a permanent ventricular pacemaker using a peripheral nerve stimulator. Anesthesiology 75:533-536, 1991.
23. Schwartzenburg CF, Wass CT, Strickland RA, Hayes DL: Rate-adaptive cardiac pacing: Implications of environmental noise during craniotomy. Anesthesiology 87:1252-1254, 1997.
24. Lau W, Corcoran SJ, Mond HG: Pacemaker tachycardia in a minute ventilation rate–adaptive pacemaker induced by electrocardiographic monitoring. Pacing Clin Electrophysiol 29:438-440, 2006.
25. von Knobelsdorff G, Goerig M, Nagele H, Scholz J: [Interaction of frequency-adaptive pacemakers and anesthetic management. Discussion of current literature and two case reports.] Anaesthesist 45:856-860, 1996.
26. Delfaut P, Saksena S: Electrophysiologic assessment in selecting patients for multisite atrial pacing. J Interv Card Electrophysiol 4(Suppl 1):81-85, 2000.
27. Peters RW, Gold MR: Pacing for patients with congestive heart failure and dilated cardiomyopathy. Cardiol Clin 18:55-66, 2000.
28. Abraham WT, Fisher WG, Smith AL, et al: Cardiac resynchronization in chronic heart failure. N Engl J Med 346:1845-1853, 2002.
29. Hare JM: Cardiac-resynchronization therapy for heart failure. N Engl J Med 346:1902-1905, 2002.
30. Atlee J, Bernstein A: Cardiac rhythm management devices part I. Anesthesiology 95:1265-1280, 2001.
31. Hayes DL: Evolving indications for permanent pacing. Am J Cardiol 83:161D-165D, 1999.
32. Auricchio A, Stellbrink C, Sack S, et al: The pacing therapies for congestive heart failure (PATH-CHF) study: Rationale, design, and endpoints of a prospective randomized multicenter study. Am J Cardiol 83:130D-135D, 1999.
33. Garcia-Moran E, Mont L, Brugada J: Inappropriate tachycardia detection by a biventricular implantable cardioverter defibrillator. Pacing Clin Electrophysiol 25:123-124, 2002.
34. Schreieck J, Zrenner B, Kolb C, et al: Inappropriate shock delivery due to ventricular double detection with a biventricular pacing implantable cardioverter defibrillator. Pacing Clin Electrophysiol 24:1154-1157, 2001.
35. Gras D, Mabo P, Tang T, et al: Multisite pacing as a supplemental treatment of congestive heart failure: Preliminary results of the Medtronic Inc. InSync Study. Pacing Clin Electrophysiol 21:2249-2255, 1998.
36. Medina-Ravell VA, Lankipalli RS, Yan GX, et al: Effect of epicardial or biventricular pacing to prolong QT interval and increase transmural dispersion of repolarization: Does resynchronization therapy pose a risk for patients predisposed to long QT or torsades de pointes? Circulation 107:740-746, 2003.
37. Rozner MA, Gursoy S, Monir G: Care of the patient with a pacemaker. *In* Stone DJ, Bogdanoff DL, Leisure GS, et al (eds): Perioperative Care: Anesthesia, Surgery and Medicine. Philadelphia, CV Mosby, 1997, pp 53-67.
38. Purday JP, Towey RM: Apparent pacemaker failure caused by activation of ventricular threshold test by a magnetic instrument mat during general anaesthesia. Br J Anaesth 69:645-646, 1992.
39. Bourke ME: The patient with a pacemaker or related device. Can J Anaesth 43:24-41, 1996.
40. Shapiro WA, Roizen MF, Singleton MA, et al: Intraoperative pacemaker complications. Anesthesiology 63:319-322, 1985.
41. Valls-Bertault V, Mansourati J, Gilard M, et al: Adverse events with transvenous left ventricular pacing in patients with severe heart failure: Early experience from a single centre. Europace 3:60-63, 2001.
42. Alonso C, Leclercq C, d'Allonnes FR, et al: Six year experience of transvenous left ventricular lead implantation for permanent biventricular pacing in patients with advanced heart failure: Technical aspects. Heart 86:405-410, 2001.
43. Rozner MA, Nguyen AD, Roberson JC: Inadequate pacemaker follow-up detected at the preanesthetic visit. Anesthesiology 96:A1071, 2002.
44. Panja M, Sarkar CN, Kumar S, et al: Reuse of pacemaker. Indian Heart J 48:677-680, 1996.
45. Aldrete JA, Brown C, Daily J, Buerke V: Pacemaker malfunction due to microcurrent injection from a bioimpedance noninvasive cardiac output monitor. J Clin Monit 11:131-133, 1995.
46. Levine PA: Response to "rate-adaptive cardiac pacing": Implications of environmental noise during craniotomy. Anesthesiology 87:1261, 1997.
47. Madsen GM, Andersen C: Pacemaker-induced tachycardia during general anaesthesia: A case report. Br J Anaesth 63:360-361, 1989.
48. Rozner MA, Nishman RJ: Pacemaker-driven tachycardia revisited. Anesth Analg 88:965, 1999.
49. Rozner MA, Nishman RJ: Electrocautery-induced pacemaker tachycardia: Why does this error continue? Anesthesiology 96:773-774, 2002.
50. Interaction between minute ventilation rate–adaptive pacemakers and cardiac monitoring and diagnostic equipment. Center for Devices and Radiologic Health. Published October 14, 1998. Available at http://www.fda.gov/cdrh/safety/minutevent.html/ Accessed January 1, 2007.
51. Martin ET, Coman JA, Shellock FG, et al: Magnetic resonance imaging and cardiac pacemaker safety at 1.5-Tesla. J Am Coll Cardiol 43:1315-1324, 2004.

52. Hayes JJ, Juknavorian R, Maloney JD: The role(s) of the industry employed allied professional. Pacing Clin Electrophysiol 24:398-399, 2001.
53. Kleinman B, Hamilton J, Hariman R, et al: Apparent failure of a precordial magnet and pacemaker programmer to convert a DDD pacemaker to VOO mode during the use of the electrosurgical unit. Anesthesiology 86:247-250, 1997.
54. Preisman S, Cheng DC: Life-threatening ventricular dysrhythmias with inadvertent asynchronous temporary pacing after cardiac surgery. Anesthesiology 91:880-883, 1999.
55. Andersen C, Madsen GM: Rate-responsive pacemakers and anaesthesia. A consideration of possible implications. Anaesthesia 45:472-476, 1990.
56. Levine PA, Balady GJ, Lazar HL, et al: Electrocautery and pacemakers: Management of the paced patient subject to electrocautery. Ann Thorac Surg 41:313-317, 1986.
57. Rozner MA, Nguyen AD: Unexpected pacing threshold changes during non-implant surgery. Anesthesiology 96:A1070, 2002.
58. Levine PA, Gauch P: Utilizacao clinica da autocaptura. Reblampa 16:31-41, 2003.
59. Chew EW, Troughear RH, Kuchar DL, Thorburn CW: Inappropriate rate change in minute ventilation rate responsive pacemakers due to interference by cardiac monitors. Pacing Clin Electrophysiol 20:276-282, 1997.
60. Walldén J, Gupta A, Carlsén HO: Supraventricular tachycardia induced by Datex patient monitoring system. Anesth Analg 86:1339, 1998.
61. Van Hemel NM, Hamerlijnck RP, Pronk KJ, Van der Veen EP: Upper limit ventricular stimulation in respiratory rate responsive pacing due to electrocautery. Pacing Clin Electrophysiol 12:1720-1723, 1989.
62. Wong DT, Middleton W: Electrocautery-induced tachycardia in a rate-responsive pacemaker. Anesthesiology 94:710-711, 2001.
63. Southorn PA, Kamath GS, Vasdev GM, Hayes DL: Monitoring equipment induced tachycardia in patients with minute ventilation rate–responsive pacemakers. Br J Anaesth 84:508-509, 2000.
64. Patel SI, Souter MJ: Equipment-related electrocardiographic artifacts: Causes, characteristics, consequences, and correction. Anesthesiology 108:138-148, 2008.
65. Rozner MA: Peripheral nerve stimulators can inhibit monitor display of pacemaker pulses. J Clin Anesth 16:117-120, 2004.
66. Samain E, Schauveliege F, Henry C, Marty J: Outcome in patients with a cardiac pacemaker undergoing noncardiac surgery. Anesthesiology 95:A142, 2001.
67. Samain E, Marty J, Souron V, et al: Intraoperative pacemaker malfunction during a shoulder arthroscopy. Anesthesiology 93:306-307, 2000.
68. Pressly N: Review of MDR reports reinforces concern about EMI. FDA User Facility Reporting #20. Published 1997. Available at http://www.fda.gov/cdrh/fuse20.pdf/ Accessed January 1, 2007.
69. Rozner MA: Review of electrical interference in implanted cardiac devices. Pacing Clin Electrophysiol 26:923-925, 2003.
70. Rozner MA, Burton AW, Kumar AJ: Pacemaker complication during MRI. J Am Coll Cardiol 45:161-162, 2005.
71. Trankina MF, Black S, Gibby G: Pacemakers: Perioperative evaluation, management and complications. Anesthesiology 93:A1193, 2000.
72. Gimbel JR, Johnson D, Levine PA, Wilkoff BL: Safe performance of magnetic resonance imaging on five patients with permanent cardiac pacemakers. Pacing Clin Electrophysiol 19:913-919, 1996.
73. Gimbel JR, Kanal E, Schwartz KM, Wilkoff BL: Outcome of magnetic resonance imaging (MRI) in selected patients with implantable cardioverter defibrillators (ICDs). Pacing Clin Electrophysiol 28:270-273, 2005.
74. Alexopoulos GS, Frances RJ: ECT and cardiac patients with pacemakers. Am J Psychiatry 137: 1111-1112, 1980.
75. Engelhardt L, Grosse J, Birnbaum J, Volk T: Inhibition of a pacemaker during nerve stimulation for regional anaesthesia. Anaesthesia 62:1071-1074, 2007.
76. O'Flaherty D, Wardill M, Adams AP: Inadvertent suppression of a fixed rate ventricular pacemaker using a peripheral nerve stimulator. Anaesthesia 48:687-689, 1993.
77. Moskowitz DM, Kahn RA, Camunas J, et al: External chest wall stimulation to suppress a permanent transvenous pacemaker in a patient during endovascular stent graft placement. Anesthesiology 89:531-533, 1998.
78. Philbin DM, Marieb MA, Aithal KH, Schoenfeld MH: Inappropriate shocks delivered by an ICD as a result of sensed potentials from a transcutaneous electronic nerve stimulation unit. Pacing Clin Electrophysiol 21:2010-2011, 1998.
79. Vlay SC: Electromagnetic interference and ICD discharge related to chiropractic treatment. Pacing Clin Electrophysiol 21:2009, 1998.
80. McKay RE, Rozner MA: Preventing pacemaker problems with nerve stimulators. Anaesthesia 63:554-556, author reply 556-557, 2008.
81. Finfer SR: Pacemaker failure on induction of anaesthesia. Br J Anaesth 66:509-512, 1991.
82. Altose M, Leon-Ruiz E: Etomidate-induced pacemaker-mediated ventricular tachycardia. Anesthesiology 106:1059-1060, 2007.
83. Rozner MA: Etomidate unlikely to have induced pacemaker-mediated tachycardia. Anesthesiology 107:1036, author reply 1037, 2007.
84. Bohm A, Kayser S, Pinter A, Preda I: Intermittent output failure of a VVI device due to the disintegration of the generator. Pacing Clin Electrophysiol 24:127-128, 2001.
85. Grimm W, Menz V, Hoffmann J, et al: Complications of third-generation implantable cardioverter defibrillator therapy. Pacing Clin Electrophysiol 22:206-211, 1999.
86. Rozner MA, Trankina MF: Intrathoracic gadgets: Update on pacemakers and implantable cardioverter defibrillators. ASA Refresher Course Anesthesiol 28:183-199, 2000.
87. Roth JV, Brody JD, Denham EJ: Positioning the pacing esophageal stethoscope for transesophageal atrial pacing without P-wave recording: Implications for transesophageal ventricular pacing. Anesth Analg 83:48-54, 1996.
88. Mychaskiw G, Eichhorn JH: Interaction of an implanted pacemaker with a transesophageal atrial pacemaker: Report of a case. J Clin Anesth 11:669-671, 1999.
89. Snow N: Acute myocardial ischemia during pacemaker implantation: Implication for threshold determinations and potential complications. Pacing Clin Electrophysiol 6:35-37, 1983.
90. Moss AJ, Hall WJ, Cannom DS, et al: Improved survival with an implanted defibrillator in patients with coronary disease at high risk for ventricular arrhythmia. Multicenter Automatic Defibrillator Implantation Trial Investigators. N Engl J Med 335:1933-1940, 1996.
91. A.V.I.D. Investigators: A comparison of antiarrhythmic-drug therapy with implantable defibrillators in patients resuscitated from near-fatal ventricular arrhythmias. The Antiarrhythmics versus Implantable Defibrillators (AVID) Investigators. N Engl J Med 337:1576-1583, 1997.
92. Buxton AE, Lee KL, Fisher JD, et al: A randomized study of the prevention of sudden death in patients with coronary artery disease. Multicenter Unsustained Tachycardia Trial Investigators. N Engl J Med 341:1882-1890, 1999.
93. Moss A, Zareba W, Hall W, et al: Prophylactic implantation of a defibrillator in patients with myocardial infarction and reduced ejection fraction. N Engl J Med 346:877-883, 2002.
94. Bernstein AD, Camm AJ, Fisher JD, et al: North American Society of Pacing and Electrophysiology policy statement. The NASPE/BPEG defibrillator code. Pacing Clin Electrophysiol 16:1776-1780, 1993.
95. Grimm W, Flores BF, Marchlinski FE: Electrocardiographically documented unnecessary, spontaneous shocks in 241 patients with implantable cardioverter defibrillators. Pacing Clin Electrophysiol 15:1667-1673, 1992.
96. Hurst TM, Krieglstein H, Tillmanns H, Waldecker B: Inappropriate management of self-terminating ventricular arrhythmias by implantable cardioverter defibrillators despite a specific reconfirmation algorithm: A report of two cases. Pacing Clin Electrophysiol 20:1328-1331, 1997.
97. Prasad K, Kishore AG, Anderson MH, et al: Inappropriate shocks in patients receiving internal cardioverter-defibrillators for malignant ventricular arrhythmias. Indian Heart J 49:403-407, 1997.
98. Schumacher B, Tebbenjohanns J, Jung W, et al: Radiofrequency catheter ablation of atrial flutter that elicits inappropriate implantable cardioverter defibrillator discharge. Pacing Clin Electrophysiol 20:125-127, 1997.
99. Rozner MA: The patient with an implantable cardioverter-defibrillator. Prog Anesthesiol 13:43-52, 1999.
100. Swerdlow CD: Supraventricular tachycardia–ventricular tachycardia discrimination algorithms in implantable cardioverter defibrillators: State-of-the-art review. J Cardiovasc Electrophysiol 12:606-612, 2001.
101. Wilkoff BL, Cook JR, Epstein AE, et al: Dual-chamber pacing or ventricular backup pacing in patients with an implantable defibrillator—The Dual Chamber and VVI Implantable Defibrillator (DAVID) Trial. JAMA 288:3115-3123, 2002.
102. Sandner SE, Wieselthaler G, Zuckermann A, et al: Survival benefit of the implantable cardioverter-defibrillator in patients on the waiting list for cardiac transplantation. Circulation 104:I171-I176, 2001.
103. Khan IA: Long QT syndrome: Diagnosis and management. Am Heart J 143:7-14, 2002.
104. McKenna WJ, Thiene G, Nava A, et al: Diagnosis of arrhythmogenic right ventricular dysplasia/cardiomyopathy. Task Force of the Working Group Myocardial and Pericardial Disease of the European Society of Cardiology and of the Scientific Council on Cardiomyopathies of the International Society and Federation of Cardiology. Br Heart J 71:215-218, 1994.
105. Brugada P, Geelen P: Some electrocardiographic patterns predicting sudden cardiac death that every doctor should recognize. Acta Cardiol 52:473-484, 1997.
106. Maron BJ, Shen WK, Link MS, et al: Efficacy of implantable cardioverter-defibrillators for the prevention of sudden death in patients with hypertrophic cardiomyopathy. N Engl J Med 342:365-373, 2000.
107. Casavant D, Haffajee C, Stevens S, Pacetti P: Aborted implantable cardioverter-defibrillator shock during

facial electrosurgery. Pacing Clin Electrophysiol 21:1325-1326, 1998.

108. Varma N, Cunningham D, Falk R: Central venous access resulting in selective failure of ICD defibrillation capacity. Pacing Clin Electrophysiol 24:394-395, 2001.

109. Gill RM, Sweeney RJ, Reid PR: The defibrillation threshold: A comparison of anesthetics and measurement methods. Pacing Clin Electrophysiol 16:708-714, 1993.

110. Weinbroum AA, Glick A, Copperman Y, et al: Halothane, isoflurane, and fentanyl increase the minimally effective defibrillation threshold of an implantable cardioverter defibrillator: First report in humans. Anesth Analg 95:1147-1153, 2002.

111. Carlson MD, Ip J, Messenger J, et al: A new pacemaker algorithm for the treatment of atrial fibrillation: Results of the Atrial Dynamic Overdrive Pacing Trial (ADOPT). J Am Coll Cardiol 42:627-633, 2003.

Appendix 1

Preanesthetic Pulse Generator (Pacemaker, Implantable Cardioverter-Defibrillator) Evaluation

Determining the indication for and date of initial device placement
Identifying the type of device (pacemaker, implantable cardioverter-defibrillator) and manufacturer
Determining the patient's underlying rhythm and rate (if any)
Identifying the number and types of leads
Determining the last generator test date and battery status
Obtaining a history of generator events (if any)
Obtaining the current program information (device interrogation), including mode, rate, and rate enhancements
Ensuring that generator discharges become mechanical systoles with adequate pacing safety margins
Ensuring adequate safety margin for sensing events (if intrinsic events are present)
Ensuring that magnet detection is enabled (magnet behavior and rate should be recorded)
Determining whether the pacemaker should be reprogrammed, depending on pacemaker dependency, surgery type and location, need for increased heart rate, and other factors

The preanesthetic pacemaker evaluation should consist of device interrogation. The above statements can be fashioned into a request to the cardiologist or pacemaker service. Note that for implantable cardioverter-defibrillators, the term "generator events" includes a history of antitachycardia therapy

Appendix 2

Pulse Generator Company Phone Numbers

AM Pacemaker Corp (Boston Scientific)	800-227-3422	Edwards Pacemaker Systems (Medtronic)	800-325-2518
Angeion	**800-264-2466**	**ELA Medical**	**800-352-6466**
Arco Medical (Boston Scientific)	800-227-3422	**Boston Scientific**	**800-227-3422**
Biotronik	**800-547-0394**	**Intermedics (Boston Scientific)**	**800-227-3422**
Boston Scientific	**800-227-3422**	**Medtronic**	**800-505-4636**
Cardiac Control Systems	Unavailable	**Pacesetter (St. Jude Medical)**	**800-722-3774**
Cardio Pace Medical, Inc. (Novacon)	Unavailable	Siemans—Elema (St. Jude Medical)	800-722-3774
Cardiac Pacemakers, Inc.—CPI (Boston Scientific)	**800-227-3422**	**Telectronics Pacing (St. Jude Medical)**	**800-722-3774**
Cook Pacemaker Corp.	800-245-4715	**Ventritex (St. Jude Medical)**	**800-722-3774**
Coratomic (Biocontrol Technology)	Unavailable	Vitatron (Medtronic)	800-328-2518
Cordis Corporation (St. Jude Medical)	800-722-3774		
Diag/Medcor (St Jude Medical)	800-722-3774		

Companies in bold text market implantable cardioverter-defibrillators.

44 Respiratory Monitoring

Key Points

1. Hypoxemia is caused by reduced P_{IO_2}, hypoventilation, increased ventilation-perfusion ($\dot{V}/\dot{Q}$) heterogeneity, increased shunt, and diffusion nonequilibrium. Hypercapnia is almost always due to hypoventilation.
2. During mechanical ventilation in the operative and intensive care settings, hypoxemia is most often due to increased $\dot{V}/\dot{Q}$ heterogeneity and shunt.
3. A clinically useful approximation to the alveolar gas equation for O_2 is given by $P_{AO_2} = (P_B - 47) \times F_{IO_2} - 1.2 \times P_{CO_2}$. Exchange of O_2 and CO_2 takes place independently in the lung.
4. The alveolar-arterial (A-a) gradient increases with age and supplemental O_2. The Pa_{O_2}/F_{IO_2} and A/a ratios typically do not change with increased age or inspired O_2.
5. When derangements in gas tensions are noted on arterial blood gas analysis, it is important to verify that the sample was obtained and analyzed in an appropriate and timely manner.
6. Refinements and further studies on continuous intravascular blood gas monitors may one day lead to widespread routine use of these devices.
7. Pulse oximetry is a rapid, reliable indicator of oxygenation status in surgical and critically ill patients. Newer oximeters feature reduced capability for errors attributable to motion artifact and hypoperfusion.
8. Multiwavelength pulse oximeters are commercially available and allow measurement of carboxyhemoglobin and methemoglobin. Pulse oximetry may one day prove to be a reliable noninvasive monitor of volume status and fluid responsiveness.
9. A sudden decrease in P_{ETCO_2} usually results from a circuit disconnection, airway obstruction, abrupt decrease in cardiac output, or pulmonary embolism. P_{ETCO_2} is not always a reliable approximation of Pa_{CO_2}, particularly during general anesthesia or in the critically ill.
10. Mapping of pressure-volume curves in patients with acute respiratory distress syndrome (ARDS) and acute lung injury (ALI) can provide valuable information about lung mechanics and help guide positive end-expiratory pressure (PEEP) and tidal volume settings. Sustained high airway pressure is needed to open collapsed alveoli, and PEEP stabilizes the recruited lung units.
11. Computed tomography has greatly increased our understanding of the complicated interaction between PEEP and lung recruitment in ARDS. Electrical impedance tomography may in the future emerge as a useful bedside monitor of lung recruitment, pulmonary edema, and respiratory mechanics.
12. Recruitment strategies and low–tidal volume ventilation have been shown to improve outcomes in ARDS and ALI. High-frequency ventilators are safe and effective in refractory ARDS and may some day prove to be the ideal mode of lung protective ventilation.

Gas Exchange

The realization that gas exchange takes place in the lung was made by the ancients. However, not until the 18th century, when oxygen was discovered by Joseph Priestley, did Lavoisier ascertain the true purpose of breathing: the biochemical combustion of carbon and oxygen to carbon dioxide, a process known as respiration.[1] More than 200 years later, the exact mechanisms by which the respiratory system takes up oxygen and eliminates carbon dioxide are still being debated.

Alveolar Gases

A practicable method for directly sampling and analyzing alveolar air was first described by Haldane and Priestly in 1905.[2] Because of the inaccuracies and technical difficulty involved in direct sampling, efforts to develop indirect methods of determining the composition of alveolar air ensued. Subsequently, many equations describing the concentration of alveolar gases have been derived, with a wide range of accuracy and complexity. All are based simply on the law of conservation of mass and derive from the universal alveolar air equation:

$$\text{Alveolar fraction of gas X} = (\text{Inspired fraction of X} \pm \text{Output or uptake of X}) / \text{Alveolar ventilation} \quad (\text{i.e., output for } CO_2\text{, uptake for } O_2) \tag{1}$$

The equation in this form is only approximate and requires corrections to account for differences in expired and inspired minute volume, discussed later. Moreover, because of the inhomogeneous nature of the lung, the partial pressures calculated should be interpreted as *averages* of various alveolar concentrations present in heterogeneous gas exchange units. Put simply, the gas concentrations in each alveolus are probably different, and values obtained from the equation represent the mean of all alveoli.

In the case of O_2, solving the universal equation for uptake $(\dot{V}O_2)$ yields a general Fick equation that can be solved for alveolar O_2:

$$\dot{V}O_2 = \dot{V}A(FIO_2 - FAO_2) \tag{2}$$

$$FAO_2 = (FIO_2 - \dot{V}O_2)/\dot{V}A \tag{3}$$

where FAO_2 is the alveolar O_2 fraction, FIO_2 is the inspired fraction, and $\dot{V}A$ is alveolar ventilation in volume per minute. In other words, the amount of O_2 in alveoli is equal to the difference between the amount inspired and the amount taken up by pulmonary capillaries (conservation of mass). Multiplying through by dry barometric pressure (PB_{dry}) to obtain partial pressures, Equation 3 becomes

$$PAO_2 = PB_{dry}(FIO_2 - \dot{V}O_2/\dot{V}A) \tag{4}$$

where PB_{dry} = barometric pressure − saturated water vapor pressure.

It is most clear in this form of the equation that PAO_2 is influenced only by four variables: barometric pressure, fraction of inspired O_2, uptake of O_2, and alveolar ventilation.[3]

The same manipulations of the universal equation yield a formula for determining alveolar CO_2:

$$PACO_2 = PB_{dry}(FICO_2 + \dot{V}CO_2/\dot{V}A) \tag{5}$$

Note that CO_2 output must be *added* to the inspired concentration to obtain $PACO_2$. However, because $FICO_2$ is usually zero and $\dot{V}CO_2$ is relatively constant, it is clear that $PACO_2$ is dependent mainly on one factor, alveolar ventilation, to which it is inversely proportional:

$$PACO_2 = c(1/\dot{V}A) \tag{6}$$

where c is a constant. This approximation becomes less accurate in clinical situations in which CO_2 output can be appreciably elevated, as with fever, sepsis, or shivering.[4]

Perhaps the simplest and most widely used approximation of the alveolar gas equation was derived by Riley and colleagues[5] and relates PAO_2 and $PACO_2$ in the following way:

$$PAO_2 = PIO_2 - PACO_2/R \tag{7}$$

where R is the respiratory exchange ratio defined as $\dot{V}CO_2/\dot{V}O_2$ and relates CO_2 output to O_2 uptake. Normally, the ratio is relatively constant at 0.8 (i.e., 0.8 mol CO_2 produced for every 1 mol O_2 consumed), and the equation becomes

$$PAO_2 = PIO_2 - 1.25 \times PACO_2 \tag{8}$$

Note that the term $PACO_2/R$ in Equation 7 replaces the term $(PB_{dry} \times \dot{V}O_2)/\dot{V}A$ from Equation 4. Because $PACO_2$ can be assumed to be equal to $PaCO_2$ based on the Enghoff modification and R relates O_2 uptake to CO_2 output, $PACO_2/R$ is essentially an indirect measure of O_2 uptake and is much easier to accurately calculate than $\dot{V}O_2/\dot{V}A$.[6]

A common misconception from the appearance of PCO_2 in Equations 7 and 8 is that PAO_2 is directly influenced by changes in $PACO_2$. Rather, exchange of O_2 and CO_2 takes place independently in the lung, and PAO_2 is influenced by only the four aforementioned factors. The apparent influence of $PACO_2$ on PAO_2 is actually reflective of a change in minute ventilation or O_2 consumption, more obvious in Equation 4. For example, as alveolar ventilation decreases, $PaCO_2$ rises and PAO_2 will decrease according to Equation 8 as a result of the reduced alveolar ventilation. There is no "displacement" or direct alteration of O_2 by CO_2.[6,7]

Despite being quite adequate for clinical use, the Riley equation does not account for small differences in expired and inspired gas volume because of (1) the respiratory exchange ratio (less CO_2 output than O_2 uptake at a ratio of 4:5) and (2) respired inert gases not being in equilibrium with blood (such as during nitrous oxide induction or washout). An equation proposed by Filley and coworkers[8] corrects for this difference and does not entail calculation of R, which can be higher than the normal 0.8 in certain clinical settings, such as with metabolic acidosis or overfeeding:

$$PAO_2 = PIO_2 - PACO_2[(PIO_2 - PEO_2)/PECO_2] \tag{9}$$

Though more accurate, it is more cumbersome than the Riley equation in that mixed expired gas concentrations must be measured. This equation should be used, for example, when calculating shunt fraction because precise PAO_2 values are imperative.[3]

Arterial Gases

Exchange of gases between alveoli and blood occurs at the pulmonary capillaries. Arterial blood is formed by mixture of this pulmonary capillary blood with the mixed venous shunt fraction. Thus, three major factors influence the efficiency of this exchange and the resultant arterial gas tensions: $\dot{V}/\dot{Q}$ matching, alveolar diffusion capacity, and shunt fraction. Along with hypoventilation and low PIO_2, derangements in any of these factors result in arterial hypoxemia (Box 44-1). Some determination of the cause of the hypoxemia can be made by evaluation of the A-a O_2 gradient; problems with gas exchange increase the gradient, whereas it is normal in hypoxemia because of low PIO_2 or hypoventilation. The A-a gradient is usually elevated in a patient breathing supplemental oxygen. Two other indices of oxygenation that remain unchanged with fluctuating FIO_2 are the PAO_2/FIO_2 and a/A ratios (normally 350 to 500 mm Hg and 0.8 to 0.85, respectively).

Box 44-1 Five Causes of Hypoxemia and the Associated Alveolar-to-Arterial (A-a) O_2 Gradient

Normal A-a O_2 Gradient
- Hypoventilation
- Reduced P_{IO_2}

Increased A-a O_2 Gradient
- Increased $\dot{V}/\dot{Q}$ heterogeneity
- Increased shunt
- Diffusion limitation

The extent to which these factors affect the makeup of arterial blood differs for CO_2 and O_2 because they have different arteriovenous gradients and diffusing capacities. CO_2 is estimated to have a diffusing capacity 20 to 30 times greater than that of O_2,[9] and its exchange is therefore minimally affected by derangements in alveolar membrane diffusion and $\dot{V}/\dot{Q}$ mismatching. The narrower arteriovenous gradient of CO_2 (≈6 mm) versus O_2 (~60 mm) leads to less profound effects of venous shunt on arterial P_{CO_2}. Except in extreme circumstances there is little evidence that impaired diffusion of O_2 or CO_2 across the alveolar membrane occurs to any clinically significant extent, so this is not discussed further in this chapter.

$\dot{V}/\dot{Q}$ Mismatch

In normal subjects, resting minute ventilation is roughly 4 L/m and pulmonary blood flow is 5 L/m, which results in a ventilation-to-perfusion ratio of roughly 0.8 for the entire lung.[10] This would represent the $\dot{V}/\dot{Q}$ ratio of each alveolus if ventilation and perfusion were uniformly distributed in the lung. In reality, distribution is not uniform, and ratios range anywhere from zero (shunt) to infinity (dead space ventilation). For example, alveoli in dependent lung regions are better perfused than those in the apices and therefore have lower $\dot{V}/\dot{Q}$ ratios.[11] Ventilation is usually more evenly distributed throughout the lung than blood flow is, so impaired oxygenation of arterial blood is most often due to derangements in perfusion.

$\dot{V}/\dot{Q}$ mismatching results in hypoxemia for two reasons. First, more blood tends to flow through alveoli with low $\dot{V}/\dot{Q}$, such as dependent lung.[9] Thus, when $\dot{V}/\dot{Q}$ scatter increases, flow through alveoli with low $\dot{V}/\dot{Q}$ (and therefore low P_{O_2}) is greater than flow through areas of high $\dot{V}/\dot{Q}$, which causes a disproportionately large effect from the areas of low $\dot{V}/\dot{Q}$ and hence a reduction in Pa_{O_2}. The second reason is due to the nature of oxyhemoglobin (HbO_2) dissociation. Alveoli with high $\dot{V}/\dot{Q}$ are on the plateau portion of the curve, where shifts in P_{AO_2} have little effect on O_2 content. These new areas of high (or higher) $\dot{V}/\dot{Q}$ introduced by scatter are unable to compensate for the new areas of low $\dot{V}/\dot{Q}$, which are on the steep portion of the curve and therefore more profoundly affected by changes in P_{AO_2} (Figs. 44-1 and 44-2).

Shunt

One extreme of $\dot{V}/\dot{Q}$ mismatch is a right-to-left shunt ($\dot{V}/\dot{Q}$ = 0), the other extreme being dead space ventilation ($\dot{V}/\dot{Q}$ = infinity). Normally, a small shunt fraction (<3% of cardiac output) exists because of drainage of bronchial and thebesian venous blood into the left heart.[7] However, as a result of the steep arterio-

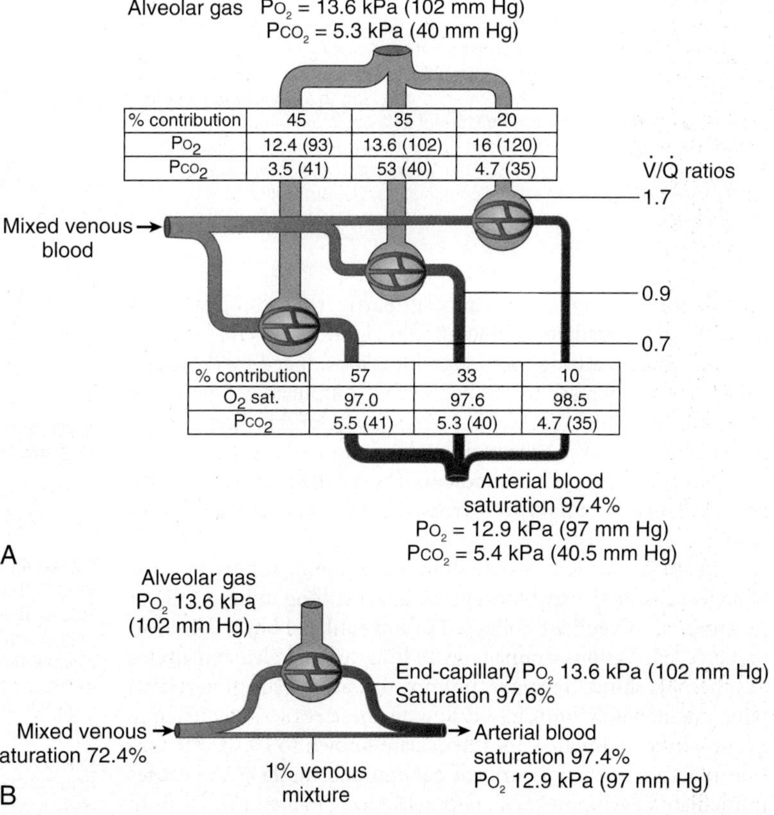

Figure 44-1 Alveolar-to-arterial P_{O_2} difference caused by scatter of $\dot{V}/\dot{Q}$ ratios and its representation by an equivalent degree of venous admixture. **A,** Scatter of $\dot{V}/\dot{Q}$ ratios corresponding roughly to the three zones of the lung in a normal upright subject. Mixed alveolar gas P_{O_2} is calculated with allowance for the contribution of gas volumes from the three zones. Arterial saturation is similarly determined and P_{O_2} derived. There is an alveolar-arterial P_{O_2} difference of 0.7 kPa (5 mm Hg). **B,** Theoretical situation that would account for the same alveolar-to-arterial P_{O_2} difference caused solely by venous admixture. This is a useful method of quantifying the functional effect of scattered $\dot{V}/\dot{Q}$ ratios but should be carefully distinguished from the actual situation. *(From Lumb AB: Nunn's Applied Respiratory Physiology, 6th ed. Philadelphia, Elsevier/Butterworth Heinemann, 2005.)*

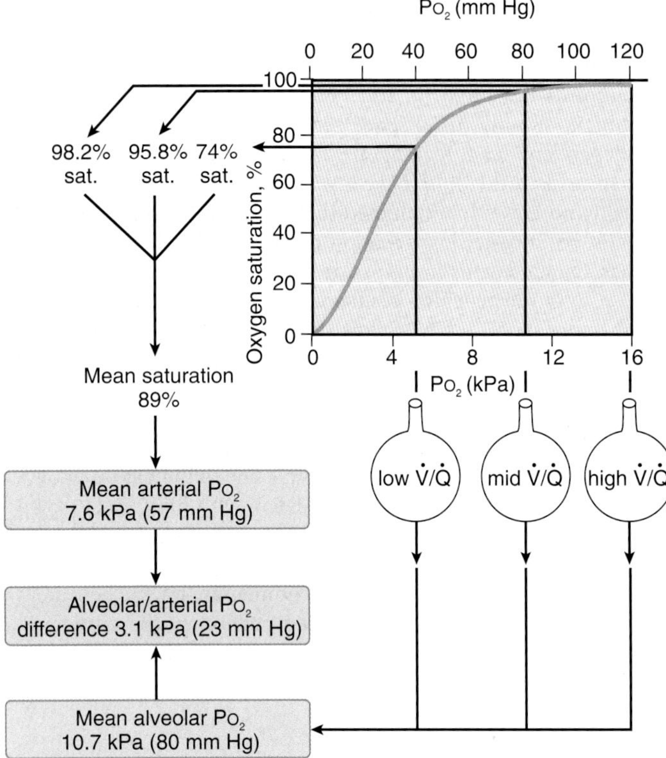

Figure 44-2 Alveolar-arterial Po_2 difference caused by scatter of $\dot{V}/\dot{Q}$ ratios resulting in oxygen tensions along the upper inflection of the oxygen dissociation curve. The diagram shows the effect of three groups of alveoli with Po_2 values of 5.3, 10.7, and 16.0 kPa (40, 80, and 120 mm Hg). Ignoring the effect of the different volumes of gas and blood contributed by the three groups, mean alveolar Po_2 is 10.7 kPa. However, because of the shape of the dissociation curve, the saturation of blood leaving the three groups is not proportional to their Po_2. The mean arterial saturation is in fact 89%, and Po_2 is therefore 7.6 kPa. The alveolar-arterial Po_2 difference is thus 3.1 kPa. The actual difference would be somewhat greater because gas with a high Po_2 would make a relatively greater contribution to alveolar gas and blood with a low Po_2 would make a relatively greater contribution to arterial blood. In this example, a calculated venous admixture of 27% would be required to account for the scatter of $\dot{V}/\dot{Q}$ ratios in terms of the measured alveolar-arterial Po_2 difference at an alveolar Po_2 of 10.7 kPa. *(From Lumb AB: Nunn's Applied Respiratory Physiology, 6th ed. Philadelphia, Elsevier/Butterworth Heinemann, 2005.)*

venous Po_2 gradient, this shunt is partly responsible for the normal A-a O_2 gradient of 5 to 10 mm Hg found in children and young adults breathing room air. Shunt introduced by these circulations can increase to 10% of cardiac output in the presence of severe bronchial disease and aortic coarctation.[9] The normal heterogeneity of $\dot{V}/\dot{Q}$ throughout the lung is the other contributor to the baseline A-a gradient. The gradient increases with age, probably secondary to increased closing capacity and $\dot{V}/\dot{Q}$ scatter.[7]

Pathologic right-to-left shunting of blood occurs in areas of atelectasis or airway blockage, as in acute lung injury (ALI) or pneumonia. Alveoli are collapsed or unventilated but continue to be perfused. Venous drainage from lung tumors also constitutes a pathologic shunt. If hypoxic pulmonary vasoconstriction (HPV) fails to adequately limit blood flow to these regions, hypoxemia occurs. Indeed, inhaled anesthetics are known to cause attenuation of HPV, and induction of general anesthesia (GA) causes immediate development of atelectasis (see Chapter 15).[12,13] Both phenomena are probably contributors to the 5% to 10% shunt found in patients undergoing GA with mechanical ventilation.[10]

Calculating Shunt Fraction and Dead Space

A simplified but useful three-compartment lung model aids in approximating what fraction of cardiac output $(\dot{Q}_T)$ constitutes shunt $(\dot{Q}_S)$ and what fraction of tidal volume (V_T) constitutes dead space ventilation $(\dot{V}_{DS})$. Commonly known as the Riley approach, the lung is considered as though it were made up of three compartments at the three extremes of $\dot{V}/\dot{Q}$ matching: (1) a shunt compartment with perfused but unventilated alveoli, (2) a dead space compartment with ventilated but unperfused alveoli, (3) and an ideal compartment with normally distributed ventilation and perfusion (Fig. 44-3).

As discussed earlier, the lung is actually composed of many compartments with a wide distribution of $\dot{V}/\dot{Q}$ ratios, and this as an oversimplified but clinically useful model.

The shunt fraction $(\dot{Q}_S/\dot{Q}_T)$ can be calculated by using the Berggren shunt equation to compare the O_2 content of mixed venous $(C\bar{v}O_2)$, pulmonary capillary $(Cc'O_2)$, and arterial (CaO_2) blood:

$$\dot{Q}_S/\dot{Q}_T = (Cc'O_2 - CaO_2)/(Cc'O_2 - C\bar{v}O_2) \qquad (10)$$

In a normal subject with capillary O_2 saturation close to 100%, the following approximation can be made

$$\dot{Q}_S/\dot{Q}_T = (1 - SaO_2)/(1 - S\bar{v}O_2) \qquad (11)$$

where $S\bar{v}O_2$ and SaO_2 are mixed venous and arterial O_2 saturation, respectively.

It is important to note that the fraction calculated in Equation 10 is not a *true* shunt (intrapulmonary shunt through alveoli

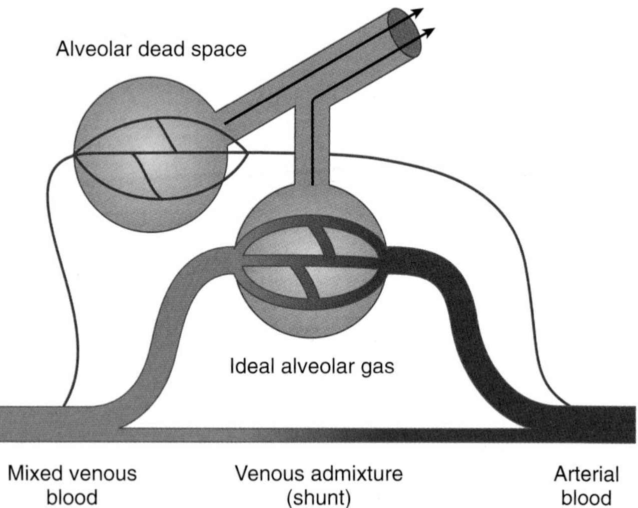

Figure 44-3 Three-compartment (Riley) model of gas exchange. The lung is imagined to consist of three functional units consisting of alveolar dead space, "ideal" alveoli, and venous admixture (shunt). Gas exchange occurs only in the "ideal" alveoli. The measured alveolar dead space consists of true alveolar dead space together with a component caused by $\dot{V}/\dot{Q}$ scatter. The measured venous admixture consists of true venous admixture (shunt) together with a component caused by $\dot{V}/\dot{Q}$ scatter. Note that "ideal" alveolar gas is exhaled contaminated with alveolar dead space gas, so it is not possible to sample "ideal" alveolar gas. *(From Lumb AB: Nunn's Applied Respiratory Physiology, 6th ed. Philadelphia, Elsevier/Butterworth Heinemann, 2005.)*

with zero $\dot{V}/\dot{Q}$) but should be thought of as a *total* shunt because it includes intracardiac and physiologic shunting and the contribution of areas with relatively low (shuntlike) but nonzero $\dot{V}/\dot{Q}$. Thus, the model is unable to predict how much each of these factors contributes to the calculated shunt because they all introduce undersaturated blood into the arterial circulation. It is though that breathing 100% O_2 eliminates the *shuntlike* contribution by fully saturating capillary blood in low- $\dot{V}/\dot{Q}$ alveoli, but it appears instead that these regions may progress via resorption atelectasis into areas of true shunt.[14] Making the distinction between true shunt and shuntlike regions caused by low $\dot{V}/\dot{Q}$ may be clinically important, particularly for anesthesiologists, in that reduced $\dot{V}/\dot{Q}$ has been shown to be more predictive of postoperative hypoxemia than increased shunt is.[10] Techniques allowing more accurate distinction between the components of calculated shunt and dead space have been developed and are described later.

A method has been derived to estimate shunt fraction without sampling arterial or mixed venous blood.[15] Arterial oxygen content is calculated from measured hemoglobin (Hb) and Spo_2, and Po_2 is obtained from the alveolar gas equation by using end-tidal Pco_2 as an estimate of $Paco_2$. Mixed venous O_2 content is estimated by assuming a fixed arterial–to–mixed venous O_2 gradient. Estimates of shunt fraction obtained by this method are expectedly somewhat imprecise (±16%) when compared with invasive measurements but are adequate for clinical use.

The dead space component in the three-compartment gas exchange model can be calculated with the Bohr equation:

$$V_{DS}/V_T = \left(Paco_2 - P_{ECO_2}\right)/Pao_2 \qquad (12)$$

where P_{EO_2} is the mixed expired Pco_2

The fraction calculated includes anatomic, alveolar, and apparatus (i.e., breathing circuit) dead space, which together represent *physiologic* dead space.

As with the shunt calculation described earlier, dead space determined by the equation is not *true* dead space because it includes an indeterminate contribution from relatively underperfused or *dead space–like* alveoli with high $\dot{V}/\dot{Q}$ (see Fig. 44-3). Another limitation of the model is that alterations in cardiac output or Hb concentration can lead to different calculated values of shunt fraction, even when actual $\dot{V}/\dot{Q}$ ratios have not changed. A substantial rise in cardiac output will increase $S\bar{v}o_2$ and cause a subsequent rise in the O_2 content of shunted blood and therefore arterial blood (Fig. 44-4). The calculated shunt fraction would decrease without an actual decrease in percent shunt by volume.

Distinguishing between Shunt and Altered $\dot{V}/\dot{Q}$ as the Cause of Impaired Oxygenation

In 1974, Wagner and coauthors described a technique known as multiple inert gas elimination (MIGET), which allows plotting of pulmonary ventilation and perfusion against the $\dot{V}/\dot{Q}$ ratio for a large number of lung compartments (rather than just three compartments as in the Riley approach), all with different $\dot{V}/\dot{Q}$ ratios.[14] Six inert tracer gases with widely varying blood solubility are infused intravenously and allowed to reach steady state. Arterial and mixed expired gas concentrations are measured, and the mixed venous concentration is calculated via the Fick principle. Retention-solubility and excretion-solubility curves are created and then translated into a continuous plot of perfusion against $\dot{V}/\dot{Q}$ and ventilation against $\dot{V}/\dot{Q}$, respectively, in relation to the heterogeneous spectrum of $\dot{V}/\dot{Q}$ ratios present throughout the lung. A host of other variables can be accurately measured, including intrapulmonary shunt and alveolar dead space. The technique is cumbersome and the numerical analyses rather complicated for routine use, but studies using the technique have been invaluable to our understanding of gas exchange in intensive care unit (ICU)[16] and surgical[17,18] settings. Figure 44-5 shows a typical plot in awake patients, with the development of shunt, increased dead space, and $\dot{V}/\dot{Q}$ scatter on induction of GA. Increasing shunt detected by multiple inert gas elimination (MIGET) has been correlated with increasing atelectasis noted on chest computed tomography (CT).[19] Distinguishing between true shunt and low $\dot{V}/\dot{Q}$ can also be performed noninvasively by simultaneously plotting Sao_2 versus P_{IO_2} (Fig. 44-6). Increasing shunt shifts the curve downward, whereas reducing $\dot{V}/\dot{Q}$ below the normal 0.8 shifts the curve rightward. The figure schematically shows the long-established observation that hypoxemia caused by true shunt is minimally responsive to increased P_{IO_2}, in contrast to hypoxemia caused by $\dot{V}/\dot{Q}$ mismatch. As mentioned, $\dot{V}/\dot{Q}$ reduction detected by a rightward shift of the curve intraoperatively has been shown to correlate with hypoxemia up to 30 hours postoperatively. The technique may help identify patients at risk for postoperative hypoxemia and in need of supplemental O_2 and closer monitoring. It can also be used in patients with chronic lung disease to determine whether additional O_2 may be needed during air travel or at altitude.[10]

Blood Gas Analysis

Measurement of Blood Gas Tensions

The basic design that modern blood gas analyzers still use today was introduced by Severinghaus and Bradley in 1958.[20] Designed by Leland Clark in 1953,[21] the Po_2 electrode is a platinum probe bathed in an electrolyte solution and separated from the sample (blood) by an O_2 permeable membrane. Oxygen molecules pass from blood through the membrane and are reduced to hydroxyl ions. Po_2 is proportional to the current generated by this reduction reaction. Similarly, the Stow/Severinghaus Pco_2 electrode is a pH-sensitive glass probe bathed in a bicarbonate solution and encased by a CO_2 permeable membrane. Pco_2 is proportional to the H^+ generated as CO_2 reacts with water to form H^+ and HCO_3^-. Severinghaus and Astrup have provided a detailed history of the development of blood gas analysis (BGA).[22,23]

Temperature Correction

Modern blood gas analyzers measure blood gas tensions at 37°C. Because patients rarely have a temperature of exactly 37°C, blood samples must be heated or cooled to 37°C for analysis. Heating a blood sample decreases pH, gas solubility, and Hb affinity for O_2 and CO_2. Thus, as the blood from a hypothermic patient (say 35°C) is heated and analyzed at 37°C, more gas becomes dissolved in solution and the measured Po_2 and Pco_2 will be higher than at 35°C. Raising the temperature also increases the H^+ concentration and would give a falsely low pH in a hypothermic patient. Modern analyzers use one of a number of algorithms to automatically correct pH and blood gas tensions for temperature, and Box 44-2 provides the formulas approved by the National Committee

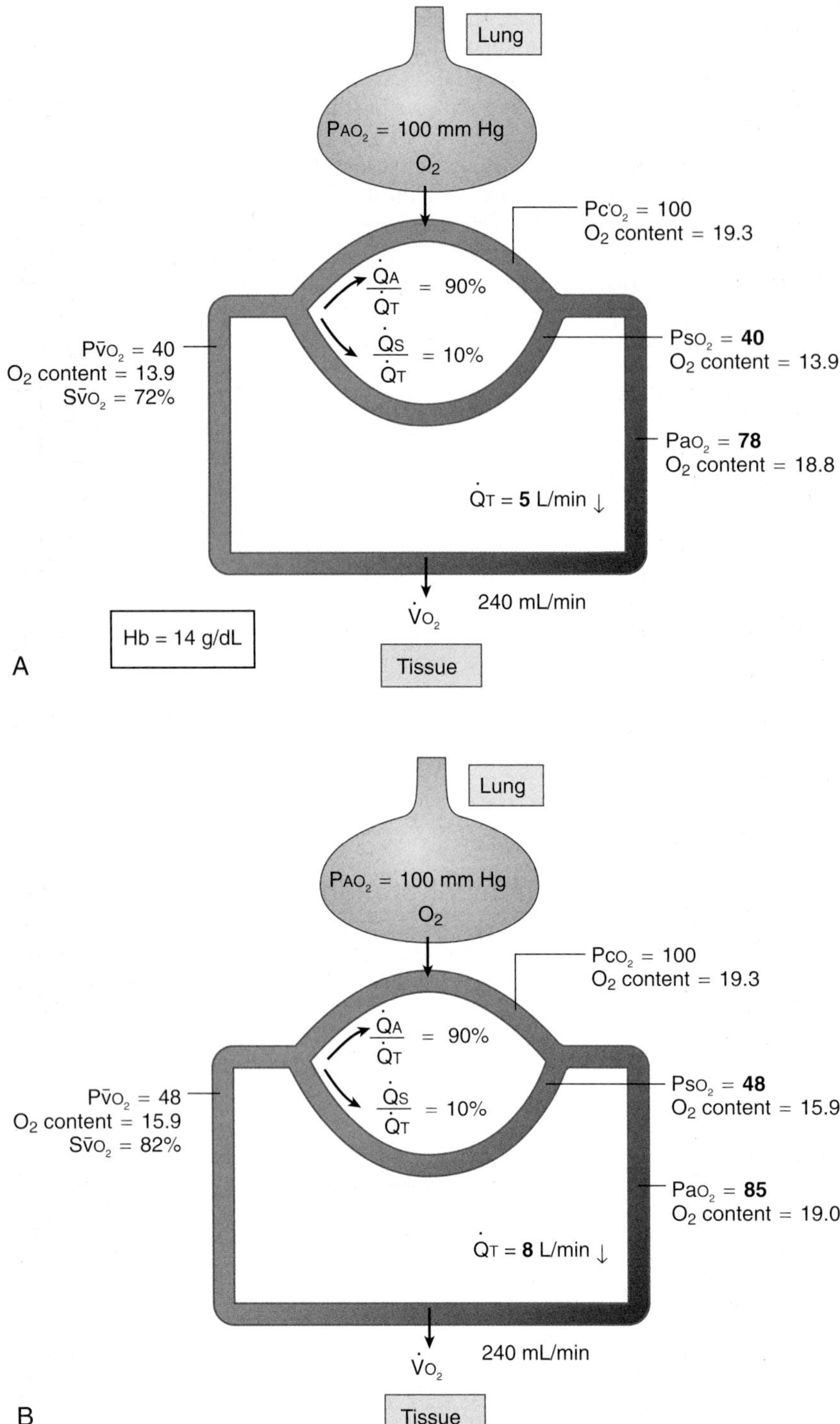

Figure 44-4 Effect of cardiac output on Po_2. **A,** Arterial and mixed venous O_2 tension and content are shown at a cardiac output of 5 L/min. **B,** Assuming constant $\dot{V}o_2$, an increase in cardiac output to 8 L/min increases Pao_2 from 78 to 85 mm Hg because $S\bar{v}o_2$ increases at higher cardiac output. The resulting increase in O_2 content of the shunted blood (here assumed to be 10% of cardiac output) then raises the arterial O_2 content and Pao_2. Po_2 values are in mm Hg, and O_2 content is in mL/dL.

for Clinical Laboratory Standards (NCCLS). The corrections are all rather slight, and there is little evidence to suggest that temperature-corrected values are clinically more useful than 37°C values. Two approaches, pH-stat and alpha-stat, have been used to manage pH in hypothermic patients undergoing cardiopulmonary bypass. The alpha-stat approach lets pH rise naturally into the alkalotic range as the patient is cooled, and pH-stat maintains normal pH and presumably cerebral perfusion by adding CO_2. Data favoring either approach are very limited.

Artifactual Changes in Arterial Blood Gas Values

Delay in analyzing a blood sample after it is drawn can artifactually change the measured pH and gas tensions. Storing a sample longer than 20 minutes can cause a significant elevation in Pco_2 and reduction in Po_2 and pH, probably secondary to cellular metabolism. Leukocytosis and thrombocytosis accelerate these

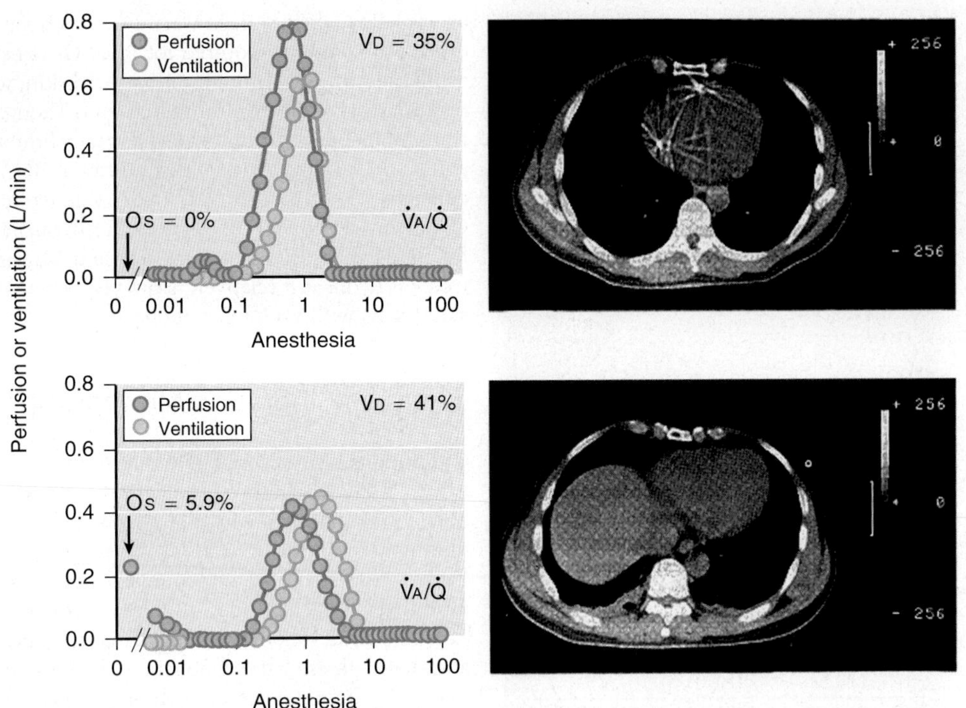

Figure 44-5 Ventilation-perfusion ($\dot{V}_A/\dot{Q}$) distribution and computed tomography in a supine subject. **Left,** $\dot{V}_A/\dot{Q}$ distribution in an awake (*top*) and anesthetized (*bottom*) subject. Note the appearance of a pulmonary shunt and an increase in $\dot{V}_A/\dot{Q}$ mismatch during general anesthesia with mechanical ventilation. **Right,** Computed tomography of the chest just above the top of the right diaphragm. Note the appearance of densities in the dependent lung regions during anesthesia. VD, volume of distribution. *(Redrawn from Gunnarsson L, Tokics L, Gustavsson H, et al: Influence of age on atelectasis formation and gas exchange impairment during general anesthesia. Br J Anaesth 66:423-432, 1991.)*

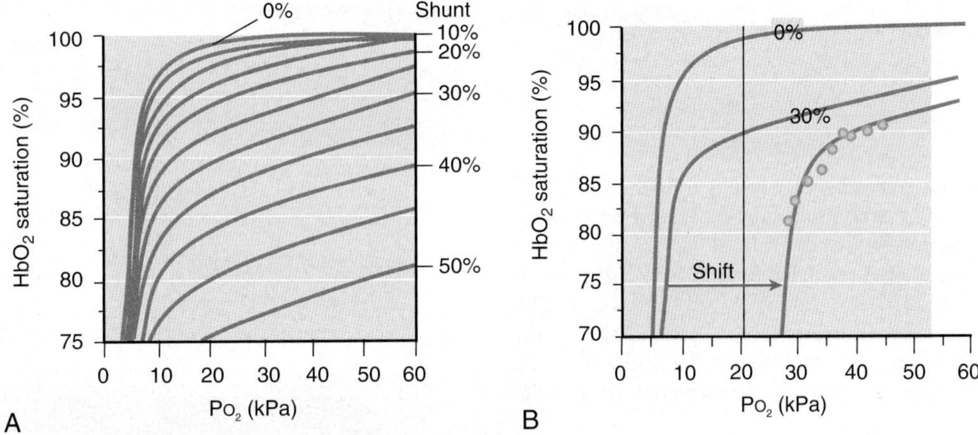

Figure 44-6 Hemoglobin-oxygen (HbO_2) saturation versus inspired partial pressure of oxygen (PO_2). The curves are plotted by changing inspired PO_2 in stepwise fashion. **A,** Series of theoretical curves obtained by calculating the effect of different degrees of right-to-left shunt. Increasing shunt displaces the curves downward. **B,** The curve on the *left* of the graph (0%) is from a normal subject. The *middle* curve (30%) represented a 30% right-to-left shunt from the 30% curve seen in **A**. The curve on the *right* of this graph is from a patient undergoing thoracotomy for esophageal surgery. The points cannot be fitted by any of the shunt curve, but the fit is quite good when the 30% curve is shifted to the right. This implies a combination of shunt and $\dot{V}_A/\dot{Q}$ mismatch. *(Adapted from Jones JG, Jones SE: Discriminating between the effect of shunt and reduced $\dot{V}_A/\dot{Q}$ on arterial oxygen saturation is particularly useful in clinical practice. J Clin Monit Comput 16:337, 2000.)*

Box 44-2 Algorithms for Correction to Body Temperature of Blood Gas Tensions Measured at 37°C

pH

$$\Delta pH/\Delta T = -0.0146 + 0.0065\ (7.4 - pH_m)$$

$$\Delta pH/\Delta T = -0.015$$

$$\Delta pH/\Delta T = -0.0147 + 0.0065\ (7.4 - pH_m)^*$$

$$\Delta pH/\Delta T = -0.0146$$

Pco_2

$$\Delta \log_{10} Pco_2/\Delta T = 0.019^*$$

$$\Delta \log_{10} Pco_2/\Delta T = 0.021$$

Po_2

$$\Delta \log_{10} Pco_2/\Delta T = \left(\frac{0.0252}{0.234(Po_2/100)^{3.88}+1}\right) + 0.00564$$

$$\Delta \log_{10} Pco_2/\Delta T = 0.0052 + 0.27\left[1 - 10^{-0.13(100 - SAo_2)}\right]$$

$$\Delta \log_{10} Pco_2/\Delta T = \frac{5.49\times10^{-11}\,Po_2^{3.88} + 0.071^*}{9.72\times10^{-9}\,Po_2^{3.88} + 2.3}$$

$$\Delta \log_{10} Pco_2/\Delta T = \frac{\begin{array}{c}0.012(Po_{2m}/714)+(So_2/100)\\(1-So_2/100)(Hb/0.6)+0.073\end{array}}{Po_{2m}/714+So_2/100(1-So_2/100)(Hb/0.6)}$$

$So_2 \le 95\%$: $\Delta \log_{10} Pco_2/\Delta T = 0.31$

$So_2 > 95\%$: $\Delta \log_{10} Pco_2/\Delta T = 0.032 - 0.0268e^{(0.3So_2 - 30)}$

*National Committee for Clinical Laboratory Standards (NCCLS)-approved standard.

Hb, blood hemoglobin concentration in g/dL; pH_m and Po_{2m}, pH and Po_2 values measured at an electrode temperature of 37°C; Po_2, partial pressure of oxygen in mm Hg; So_2, percent hemoglobin-oxygen (HbO_2) saturation; T, temperature in degrees centigrade (°C).

Data from Ashwood ER, Kost G, Kenny M: Temperature correction of blood-gas and pH measurements. Clin Chem 29:1877, 1983; and Siggaard-Andersen O, Wimberley PD, Gothgen I, Siggaard-Andersen M: A mathematical model of the hemoglobin-oxygen dissociation curve of human blood and of the oxygen partial pressure as a function of temperature. Clin Chem 30:1646, 1984.

changes.[24] Because red cells do not contain mitochondria, this phenomenon is not observed in polycythemia. However, anaerobic glycolysis can generate lactic acid and reduce pH. Placing the sample in ice immediately after it is obtained can maintain its stability, and addition of sodium fluoride or cyanide can inhibit cellular O_2 consumption.[24] The presence of air bubbles in the sample syringe can falsely elevate Po_2 but has little effect on pH and Pco_2. Syringes are usually heparinized to prevent coagulation.

Transcutaneous Blood Gas Monitoring

Although the turnaround time for obtaining Po_2 with traditional blood gas analyzers has drastically decreased since their inception, the ability to assess a patient's oxygenation status even more rapidly and easily has obvious advantages. One alternative is to measure gas tensions at the bedside transcutaneously. This technology relies on the tendency of capillary Po_2 to approximate arterial Po_2 when skin is warmed, which causes blood flow to exceed the amount required for local O_2 consumption. O_2 from capillaries diffuses through the warmed skin, where it is analyzed by a Clark-type electrode adhered to it. Though useful in infants, transcutaneous gas monitoring has many limitations despite good agreement of Po_2 values with traditional BGA.[25] Peripheral vascular disease or vasoconstriction can generate erroneous values. Cutaneous hypoxia caused by reduced cardiac output will give falsely decreased Po_2 readings. These devices must be calibrated frequently, have a relatively slow response time, and can cause skin burns with prolonged application.

In-Line Blood Gas Monitoring

Continuous intra-arterial pH measurement was accomplished as early as 1927 with antimony electrodes. Shortly after Clark developed his Po_2 electrode in 1956, the first continuous intravascular blood gas monitoring (CIBGM) devices were developed. Early devices consisted of electrochemical sensors and were essentially modified Clark electrodes. Problems with these devices included excessive drift, lack of reliability, large size, and interference from anesthetic gases. Later, Lubbers and Opitz, using a technology known as fluorescence quenching, created fiberoptic probes to continuously measure Po_2 and Pco_2, which they named *optodes*.[26] Absorbance-based fiberoptic sensors were also developed. Only two single-parameter devices became commercially available: the Continucath 1000 electrochemical Po_2 sensor for adults and the Neocath (Biomedical Sensors, High Wycomb, UK) O_2 sensor for neonatal umbilical artery placement.

Advances in the design of single-parameter systems inevitably led to the development of multiparameter devices capable of measuring pH, Pco_2, Po_2, and temperature. Most are pure optode systems, with the Paratrend 7 being the only hybrid optode-electrode system. The upgraded Paratrend 7+ replaced the Clark Po_2 electrode with an optode, thus making it a pure optode system (Fig. 44-7).

Agreement between sensor and traditional BGA measurements can be quantified by use of the Bland-Altman calculation

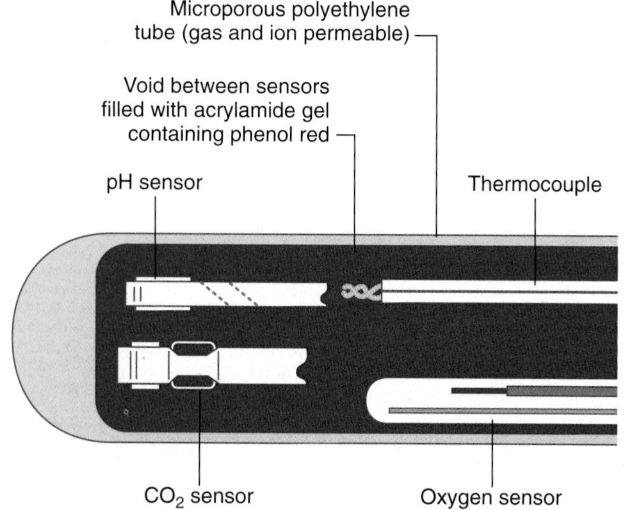

Figure 44-7 Cross section of the Paratrend 7 sensor tip. *(Courtesy of Biomedical Sensors, High Wycombe, UK.)*

of *bias* and *precision*.[27] Bias is the difference between mean values obtained by standard methods (BGA) and those obtained with the new device being tested. Precision is the standard deviation of these differences and measures reproducibility of the results.

Like their predecessors, newer probes remain fragile and continue to exhibit motion artifact, wall effect (decreased Po_2 readings because of contact with the arterial wall), and thrombogenicity. Their accuracy diminishes with insufficient blood flow to the cannulated artery. Moreover, despite encouraging in vitro and animal studies, results from clinical trials have not consistently been as favorable. Data for Pco_2 and pH measurements are impressive, but studies have found poor agreement of sensor Po_2 measurements with those obtained by BGA in elevated Po_2 ranges.[28,29] Weiss and colleagues found accurate results with minimal drift in all parameters up to 10 days after insertion in pediatric patients, but the O_2 sensor required frequent calibration.[30] Several published studies on the clinical performance of various CIABGM devices are summarized in Table 44-1.

Despite its limitations, CIABGM has many theoretical advantages over traditional BGA, although no outcome studies have proved these advantages (Box 44-3). Use of CIABGM in cardiac, thoracic, orthopedic, and transplant surgery may lead to earlier detection of severe blood gas and acid-base derangements.[35,36] Detection of Po_2 changes after cement implantation during hip replacement has been accomplished with this technology.[33] It has been validated for use in anesthesia and intensive care in pediatric patients.[32] Further technologic refinements, outcome studies, and data on cost-effectiveness are necessary for CIABGM to have widespread application in anesthesia and critical care.

Box 44-3 Advantages of a Continuous Intra-arterial Blood Gas Monitoring System over Intermittent Blood Gas Analysis

- Availability of continuous data
- Earlier detection of deleterious events
- Potential for trend analysis
- Decreased blood loss
- Decreased laboratory turnaround time
- Decreased exposure of staff to potentially infected blood

From Venkatesh B: In-line blood gas monitoring. *In* Papadakos PJ, Lachmann B (eds): Mechanical Ventilation: Clinical Applications and Pathophysiology. Philadelphia, Elsevier, 2008.

Oxygen Saturation

Although traditional BGA remains the standard modality for determining oxygen content, an alternative is to measure oxygen saturation (So_2). It can provide rapid and clinically useful information about oxygenation status.

Co-oximetry

The co-oximeter is a traditional blood gas analyzer that is also capable of measuring concentrations of HbO_2, reduced hemoglobin (HbR), carboxyhemoglobin (COHb), and methemoglobin (MetHb). Each of these species has unique absorption spectra, and corresponding wavelengths of light are used to analyze a small blood sample. It is currently the gold standard for measuring Sao_2. Results are usually obtained in less than 2 minutes.

Transcutaneous Oximetry

The principle of transcutaneous oximetry is similar to that of transcutaneous gas tension monitoring, but Sao_2 is measured instead of Po_2. Two wavelengths of light are used to measure quantities of oxygenated and deoxygenated blood to give an estimate of Sao_2, provided that the blood being analyzed is mostly arterial and other Hb species are absent. Two-wavelength ear oximeters were developed and used in practice more than 60 years ago.[37] Robert Shaw patented an eight-wavelength ear oximeter in 1972, and a device using this technology was marketed in the late 1970s by Hewlett Packard. Problems with size and reliability of data prevented its widespread use.

Pulse Oximetry

Some of the problems with transcutaneous oximetry were solved with the invention of pulse oximetry. Though first developed in Japan in the early 1970s, it was not until a decade later that its routine use began. Pulse oximetry works by analyzing the pulsatile arterial component of blood flow, thereby ensuring that arterial saturation (Spo_2) rather than venous saturation is being measured (Fig. 44-8). Two wavelengths of light are used, usually

Table 44-1 Results from Some Published Studies on Clinical Performance of Continuous Intra-arterial Blood Gas Monitoring

Investigator(s)	Device	Number of Patients	Clinical Setting and Insertion Site	pH Bias ± Precision (pH Units)	Pco_2 Bias ± Precision (mm Hg)	Po_2 Bias ± Precision (mm Hg)
Ganter[29]	Paratrend 7+	23	OR: thoracoscopic surgery (radial)	−0.01 ± 0.06	3 ± 9	−20 ± 86
Coule et al.[31]	Paratrend 7+	50 (Ped)	ICU (radial/femoral)	0.00 ± 0.04	0.38 ± 4.8	0.75 ± 25
Weiss et al.[30]	Paratrend 7	24 (Ped)	ICU (radial/femoral)	0.005 ± 0.03	−1.8 ± 6.3	1.2 ± 24
Venkatesh et al.[33]	Paratrend 7	10	OR: hip replacement (radial)	0.02 ± 0.03	0.53 ± 1.8	1.2 ± 20
Larson et al.[34]	PB 3300	29	OR/ICU (radial)	0.01 ± 0.04	1.2 ± 3.3	0.3 ± 9

ICU, intensive care unit; OR, operating room; Ped, pediatric.

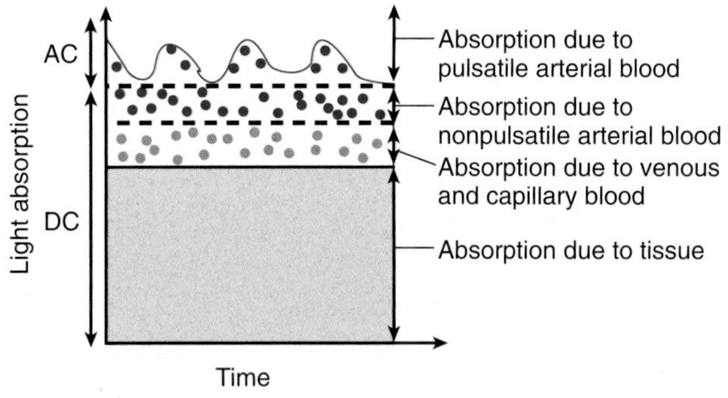

Figure 44-8 Principle of pulse oximetry. Light passing through tissue containing blood is absorbed by tissue and by arterial, capillary, and venous blood. Usually, only the arterial blood is pulsatile. Light absorption may therefore be split into a pulsatile component (AC) and a constant or nonpulsatile component (DC). Hemoglobin O_2 saturation may be obtained by application of Equation 19. *(Data from Tremper KK, Barker SJ: Pulse oximetry. Anesthesiology 70:98, 1989.)*

660 nm (red) and 940 nm (infrared), because oxygenated and deoxygenated blood each absorb light quite differently at these wavelengths. At 660 nm, HbO_2 absorbs less light than HbR does, whereas the opposite is observed with infrared light. Two diodes emitting light of each wavelength are placed on one side of the probe and a photo diode that senses the transmitted light on the opposite side. The amount of light absorbed at each wavelength by the pulsatile arterial component (AC) of blood flow can be distinguished from baseline absorbance of the nonpulsatile component and surrounding tissue (DC). The ratio R is calculated by the oximeter as follows and is empirically related to O_2 saturation:

$$R = \left(AC_{660}/DC_{660}\right)/\left(AC_{660}/DC_{660}\right) \qquad (13)$$

A calibration curve (Fig. 44-9) is derived from R and laboratory measurements of arterial oxygen saturation in healthy volunteers and the algorithm stored in the oximeter. Modern devices are calibrated against laboratory Sao_2 down to 70% saturation, and lower saturations are determined by extrapolation of the curve. Thus, pulse oximeters cannot be calibrated by the user, and their reliability is dependent on the quality of signal processing and the stored calibration curve.

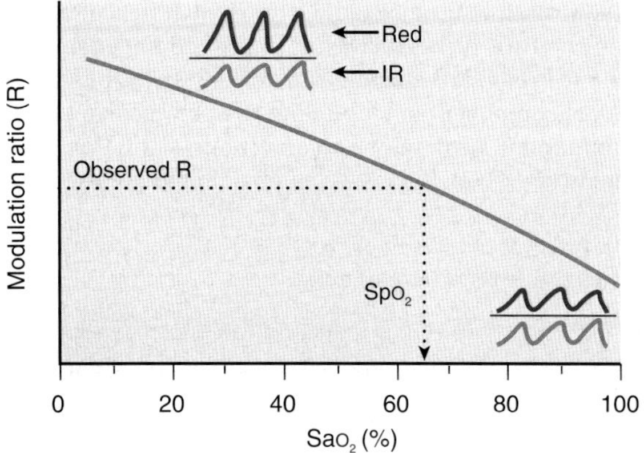

Figure 44-9 Red/infrared modulation ratio (R) versus oxygen saturation (Sao_2). At high Sao_2 (*right* side of the graph), the pulse amplitude (or modulation) of the red signal is less than that of the infrared signal, whereas the reverse is true at low Sao_2. Pulse oximeters measure R, the ratio of red to infrared pulse amplitudes (see Equation 13), and estimate Sao_2 by applying the calibration curve (*solid line*) as depicted by the *dashed line* and *arrow*. *(From Mannheimer PD: The light-tissue interaction of pulse oximetry. Anesth Analg 105(6 Suppl):S10-S17, 2007.)*

Accuracy of Pulse Oximetry

Because of its impressive accuracy, reliability, and convenience, pulse oximetry has become one of the most important technologic developments in clinical monitoring. Several studies comparing co-oximetry and pulse oximetry report substantial agreement between Spo_2 and Sao_2 over a wide range of Sao_2 values.[38,39]

Errors in Pulse Oximetry

Because Spo_2 measurements are averaged over a few seconds to provide readings, there is some degree of delay in response time. Hypothermia, low CO, and vasoconstriction secondary to drugs or peripheral hypoxia all increase bias, imprecision, and response time for hypoxic episodes (Table 44-2).[40] This appears to be more common with finger probes than with ear or forehead monitoring (Fig. 44-10).[41] Motion artifact and hypoperfusion are the most common causes of Spo_2 inaccuracy,[42,43] both of which are less problematic with newer oximeters. Caution is advised in using pulse oximetry to not make inferences about gas exchange. Spo_2 should not be used to assess the adequacy of ventilation because Sao_2 is only minimally affected by changes in Pco_2 (via the Bohr effect). In addition, when Po_2 is high, large decreases in oxygen tension produce only small changes (if any) in Sao_2 and may not be detected with pulse oximetry (see Fig. 44-2).

Anemia, with an Hb concentration as low as 2.3 g/dL, has little or no effect on Spo_2 readings when Sao_2 is normal,[44] but underestimation of Sao_2 has been observed during hypoxemia.[45] Because MetHb substantially absorbs both red and infrared light, falsely low Spo_2 readings are generated when actual Sao_2 is above 85%, and readings are falsely high when actual Sao_2 is below 85%. Spo_2 invariably reads 85% when very large amounts of MetHb are present.[46] Conversely, COHb absorbs very little infrared light, but it is very similar to HbO_2 in its red light absorbance. Oximeters using only two wavelengths therefore cannot distinguish between HbCO and HbO_2, and the presence of HbCO produces falsely elevated Spo_2 readings. Erroneous Spo_2 readings can be caused by structural hemoglobinopathies,[47,48] as well as by a host of other factors, many of which are summarized in Table 44-2.

Recent Advances in Pulse Oximetry

Error Correction. Motion sensitivity and signal loss secondary to hypoperfusion are two of the more common errors that occur with pulse oximetry. These inaccuracies have been reduced with the recent advances in signal analysis that have been incorporated into units from a number of manufacturers.[49] Several studies suggest that newer units can detect hypoxemic episodes more reliably than their predecessors can under these conditions.[50,51] Indeed, one study reported that during hypoperfusion or excessive motion, oximeters using this technology give accurate Sao_2 readings in 92% of cases in which older monitors failed.[52]

Multiwavelength Pulse Oximeters. Because only two wavelengths of light are used in traditional pulse oximeters, the presence of additional Hb species cannot be detected, which may result in erroneous readings. Using principles from both pulse

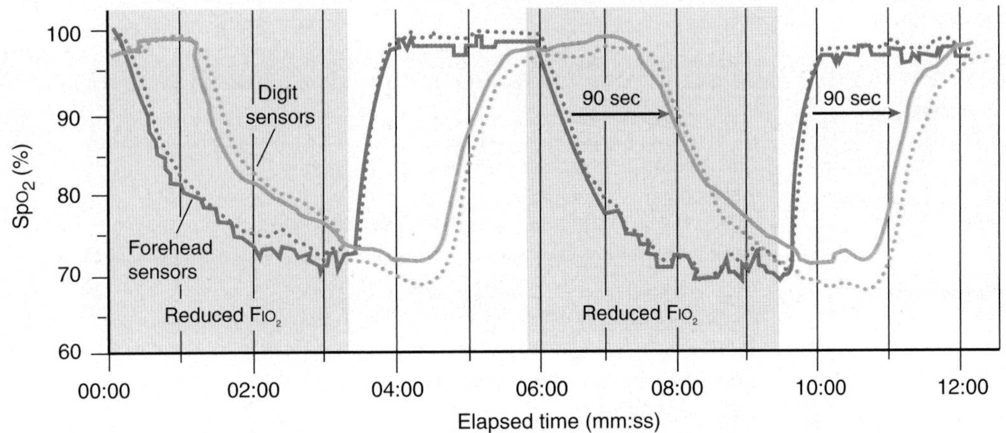

Figure 44-10 Effect of pulse oximeter probe replacement on delay from onset of hypoxemia to a drop in measured Spo_2. During cold-induced peripheral vasoconstriction in normal volunteers, the onset of hypoxemia was detected more quickly with an oximeter probe on the forehead than on the finger. Other studies have shown a similar advantage for pulse oximeter probes placed on the ear. *(From Bebout DE, Mannheimer PD, Wun C-C: Site-dependent differences in the time to detect changes in saturation during low perfusion. Crit Care Med 29:A115, 2002.)*

oximetry and co-oximetry, the first eight-wavelength pulse oximeter capable of measuring several species of Hb has become commercially available and may prove to be a major advance in oxygen monitoring. The Massimo Rad-57 (Massimo Corp, Irvine, CA) gained Food and Drug Administration (FDA) clearance in 2006 and boasts the ability to accurately measure MetHb and COHb, in addition to all the features of conventional pulse oximetry. Two large studies comparing measurements from the unit with conventional co-oximetry in emergency department patients have produced equivocal results, with one reporting a significant number of false-positive readings.[53,54] One smaller study in healthy volunteers reported good agreement between oximeter and laboratory measurements,[55] and other investigations to determine accuracy of the device are ongoing.

Reflectance Pulse Oximetry. The technology was developed to combat problems with signal transmission during hypoperfusion and for use when a transmission path is unavailable. Probes are commonly placed on the forehead, where motion artifact and hypoperfusion tend to be less of a problem than with other sites.[56] Forehead probes are commercially available and appear to detect hypoxemia more quickly than ear or finger probes do.[41] The light-emitting and light-sensing diodes are on the same side of the probe instead of opposite sides as in traditional pulse oximetry, and the reflected light from the tissue bed is analyzed. Indeed, reflectance oximetry has been used to monitor fetal oxygen saturation with scalp probes and been shown to decrease surgical intervention in the face of non-reassuring fetal status.[57] Esophageal probes have been designed and have shown success in measuring Spo_2 during cardiothoracic surgery when finger probes have failed.[58] The investigators reported minimal bias and narrow limits of agreement when compared with finger probes used in the study. Monitoring of gastric Spo_2 as an indicator of splanchnic perfusion has also shown promise.[59] Excessive edema, poor skin contact, and motion artifact are the most common sources of error in reflectance oximetry. Artifacts have also been shown to occur with probe placement directly over a pulsating superficial artery.[60]

Clinical Applications of Pulse Oximetry

Pulse oximetry is arguably most useful as an early warning sign of hypoxemia. Because this is of paramount importance in the surgical setting, pulse oximetry became a standard of care in anesthesia practice in 1986. In a large study comparing intraoperative pulse oximeter use with standard care, 80% of anesthesiologists felt more comfortable when using pulse oximetry.[61] It is interesting to note that despite its widely accepted value, there is little evidence that pulse oximetry affects outcomes in anesthesia,[62] and a study evaluating postsurgical patients did not demonstrate that routine Sao_2 monitoring reduces mortality, cost of hospitalization, or ICU transfer.[63]

Perioperative. In a randomized, controlled study of 200 surgical patients, Moller and colleagues found a reduced incidence of hypoxemia intraoperatively and in the postanesthesia care unit (PACU) when pulse oximetry was used. In the recovery room, patients in the oximeter group on average received higher Fio_2 and more naloxone, had a longer stay, and were discharged with supplemental O_2 more frequently.[64] The same group later conducted a study looking at postoperative complications with and without intraoperative pulse oximetry in 20,802 patients. No overall difference was found in complication rate, outcome, mean hospital stay, or in-hospital death between the groups, even though hypoxemia and hypoventilation were detected more frequently when pulse oximetry was used.[64] However, post hoc analysis of this trial suggests that pulse oximetry may have decreased the incidence of myocardial ischemia.[62] A number of studies report detection of hypoxemia several days postoperatively with pulse oximetry.[65,66] Intrapartum fetal pulse oximetry in the presence of a non-reassuring fetal heart rate is associated with a reduction in operative interventions.[57] The peak effects of analgesia may correlate with hypoxemia, so monitoring of patients receiving narcotics may be important to prevent adverse cardiac events.[67]

Critically Ill. The complicated pathophysiologic milieu of critical illness is such that many monitoring devices can produce inaccurate data in this patient population. Pulse oximetry, on the other hand, appears to maintain its reliability. Jubran and Tobin found that pulse oximeters accurately estimate Sao_2 in critically ill patients when Sao_2 is greater than 90% (bias, 1.7%; precision, ±1.2%) but are less accurate when Sao_2 falls below 90%.[68] An Spo_2 of 92% was indicative of adequate oxygenation when titrating O_2 in white patients. In black patients, however, significant hypoxemia was commonly present with an Spo_2 of

Table 44-2 Artifacts in Pulse Oximetry

Factor	Effect
Toxic Alterations in Hemoglobin	
Carboxyhemoglobin (COHb)	Slight reduction of the assessment of oxygen saturation (Sao_2) by pulse oximetry (Spo_2) (i.e., overestimates the fraction of hemoglobin available for O_2 transport)
Cyanmethemoglobin	Not reported
Methemoglobin (MetHb)	At high levels of MetHb, Spo_2 approaches 85%, independent of actual Sao_2
Sulfhemoglobin	Not reported (affects CO oximetry by producing a falsely high reading of MetHb)
Structural Hemoglobinopathies	
Hemoglobin F	No significant effect
Hemoglobin H	No significant effect (i.e., overestimates the fraction of hemoglobin available for O_2 transport)
Hemoglobin Köln	Artifactual reduction in Spo_2 of 8% to 10%
Hemoglobin S	No significant effect
Hemoglobin Replacement Solutions	
Diaspirin cross-linked hemoglobin	No significant effect
Bovine polymerized hemoglobin (oxygen carrier-201)	No significant effect
Dyes	
Fluorescein	No significant effect
Indigo carmine	Transient decrease
Indocyanine green	Transient decrease
Isosulfan blue (patent blue V)	No significant effect at low dose; prolonged reduction in Spo_2 at high dose
Methylene blue	Transient, marked decrease in Spo_2 lasting up to several minutes; possible secondary effects as a result of effects on hemodynamics
Hemoglobin Concentration	
Anemia	If Sao_2 is normal, no effect; during hypoxemia with Hb values less than 14.5 g/dL, progressive underestimation of actual Sao_2
Polycythemia	No significant effect
Other Factors	
Acrylic fingernails	No significant effect
Ambient light interference	Bright light, particularly if flicker frequency is close to a harmonic of the light-emitting diode switching frequency, can falsely elevate the Spo_2 reading
Arterial O_2 saturation	Depends on manufacturer; during hypoxemia, Spo_2 tends to be artifactually low
Blood flow	Reduced amplitude of pulsations can hinder obtaining a reading or cause a falsely low reading
Henna	Red henna, no effect; black henna, may block light sufficiently to preclude measurement
Jaundice	No effect; multiwavelength laboratory oximeters may register a falsely low Sao_2 and falsely high COHb and MetHb
Motion	Movement, especially shivering, may depress the Spo_2 reading
Nail polish	Slight decrease in Spo_2 reading, with greatest effect using blue nail polish, or no change
Sensor contact	"Optical shunting" of light from source to detector directly or by reflection from skin results in falsely low Spo_2 reading
Skin pigmentation	Small errors or no significant effect reported; deep pigmentation can result in reduced signal
Tape	Transparent tape between sensor and skin has little effect; falsely low Spo_2 has been reported when smeared adhesive is in the optical path
Vasodilatation	Slight decrease
Venous pulsation (e.g., tricuspid insufficiency)	Artifactual decrease in Spo_2

92%, and an Spo_2 of 95% was needed to ensure adequate oxygenation. After cardiac surgery, use of pulse oximetry has been shown to increase detection of hypoxemic episodes and decrease the number of arterial BGAs performed in the ICU.[69]

New and Future Applications

Analysis of the plethysmographic waveform generated by pulse oximeters has been advocated as a means of assessing volume status, fluid responsiveness, and a number of other clinical variables.[70,71] Respiratory variations in systolic pressure (dPs) and arterial pulse pressure (dPp) have been shown to be accurate indicators of volume status and fluid responsiveness in mechanically ventilated patients (Fig. 44-11).[72] Pulse pressure variation may predict fluid responsiveness more reliably than the use of dPs can. Such analyses require placement of an arterial catheter and are not always practical. Recently, variation in the pulse oximeter plethysmograph (dPOP) amplitude was shown to be a reliable noninvasive surrogate for dPp because both parameters are dependent on

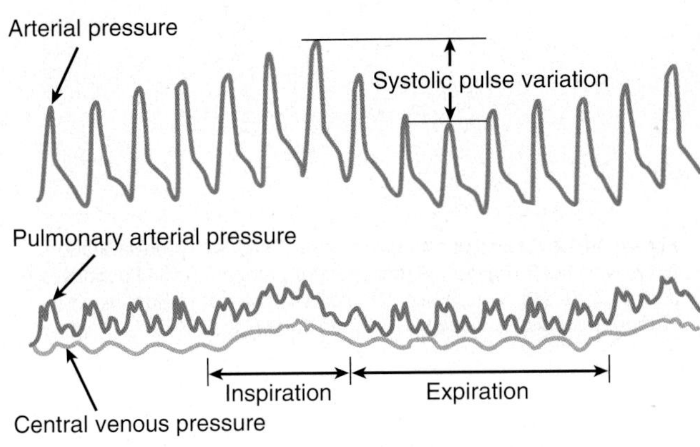

Figure 44-11 Cyclic variation of vascular pressures during positive-pressure ventilation. Inspiratory reduction in preload leads to reduced left ventricular volume after a lag phase of a few heartbeats because of pulmonary vascular transit time. The inspiratory decrease in left ventricular volume results in decreased stroke volume and systolic blood pressure during expiration. Similar variations in amplitude can be noted in pulse oximeter waveforms. *(From Nanchal R, Taylor RW. Hemodynamic monitoring. In Papadakos PJ, Lachmann B [eds]: Mechanical Ventilation: Clinical Applications and Pathophysiology. Philadelphia, Elsevier, 2008.)*

stroke volume.[73] In a study of patients under GA, Cannesson and colleagues found that baseline dPOP was correlated with percent change in cardiac index induced by volume expansion.[74] Similar results were obtained in a separate study on critically ill septic patients.[75] The authors of these trials concluded that dPOP can predict response to fluid administration and quantifies the effect of volume expansion on a number of hemodynamic parameters. To elucidate where the oximeter probe should be placed to best detect these variations, Shelley and colleagues analyzed plethysmographic waveforms from finger, ear, and forehead probes in patients undergoing positive-pressure ventilation during surgery, as well as in spontaneously breathing patients.[76] Their results suggest that the ear and forehead may be better monitoring sites than the finger for detection of variation in respiratory waveform. Because error and artifact correction in most commercial pulse oximeters can obscure the often subtle respiratory variations, unaltered plethysmographic waveforms are needed for such analyses.

Many other novel applications of pulse oximetry in anesthetic practice have been studied. Mowafi found that dPOP may be a better indicator of intravascular test dose injection during epidural placement than traditional hemodynamic markers are (i.e., heart rate and blood pressure).[77] A 10% decrease in POP indicated intravascular injection with 100% sensitivity, specificity, positive predictive value, and negative predictive value. Sensitivities using heart rate and blood pressure change as criteria were 85% to 95%. Changes in perfusion index (defined as AC_{940}/DC_{940}) have been used as confirmation of epidural placement and as an indicator of painful stimulus under anesthesia.[78,79] Many modern oximeters are programmed to measure perfusion index.

Mixed Venous Monitoring

Shock represents an imbalance between oxygen demand, delivery, and utilization at the tissue level. Monitoring of mixed venous oxygen saturation ($S\bar{v}O_2$) can give insight into the adequacy of this balance. It can be calculated by rearranging the Fick equation for O_2:

$$S\bar{v}O_2 = SaO_2 - \dot{V}O_2/(Hb \times 1.39 \times CO) \qquad (14)$$

From this equation, it is clear that decreased $S\bar{v}O_2$ can be caused by low SaO_2, low Hb, or low cardiac output, all of which decrease oxygen delivery (DO_2), or by increased O_2 consumption ($\dot{V}O_2$). These variables are related in the following way:

$$\dot{V}O_2 = DO_2 \times ERO_2 \qquad (15)$$

where ERO_2 is the extraction ratio (%) of O_2.

If oxygen delivery to tissue falls and consumption is to remain constant, oxygen extraction by tissues must increase. Blood returning to the right heart will therefore have a reduced O_2 content and $S\bar{v}O_2$. Thus, a reduced $S\bar{v}O_2$ is suggestive of global tissue hypoxia, which often precedes multiorgan failure and death.[80] Increased anaerobic metabolism as evidenced by increased lactate levels ensues and is associated with increased mortality.[81] These processes are usually under way as $S\bar{v}O_2$ approaches 40%. A pulmonary artery catheter is required to measure mixed venous saturation, and continuous monitoring can be performed with a catheter that incorporates a fiberoptic bundle. A superior vena cava sample obtained from a central venous catheter is often used as a surrogate for mixed venous saturation when a pulmonary artery catheter is impractical or unavailable.[82]

Shock of any etiology can cause the aforementioned turn of events, and a low $S\bar{v}O_2$ sheds no light on the cause of the global hypoxia. As mentioned, low $S\bar{v}O_2$ may not always be secondary to impaired delivery but may be due to increased oxygen consumption in the face of fever, thyrotoxicosis, and other conditions (Fig. 44-12). Moreover, a normal $S\bar{v}O_2$ is not necessarily indicative of adequate tissue oxygenation. Although cardiogenic and hypovolemic shock is very often associated with low $S\bar{v}O_2$, it can be normal or elevated in shock secondary to severe sepsis or hepatic failure because these conditions are frequently associated with microvascular dysfunction and impaired oxygen extraction by tissues. DO_2 is often elevated in these states.

In a novel application of continuous $S\bar{v}O_2$ measurement, pulse oximetry combined with $S\bar{v}O_2$ monitoring has been used in patients with acute respiratory failure to continuously monitor shunt fraction and adjust ventilator settings accordingly.[82] The authors of this study adjusted continuous positive airway pressure (CPAP) levels to obtain the lowest shunt fraction and showed that use of this method results in CPAP settings similar to those obtained by conventional means. Though somewhat invasive, the technique was found to be cost-effective and accurate in titrating CPAP in this subset of patients.

Tissue Oxygenation

The goal of optimizing pulmonary gas exchange is to ultimately optimize oxygenation at the cellular level. Analysis of alveolar, arterial, and venous gases is used in conjunction with clinical indices of tissue function (i.e., urine output, mental status) to make inferences about the state of affairs in cells. Oxygen is transported from alveoli with a PO_2 of around 100 mm Hg down a steep gradient, known as the oxygen cascade, to its final site of utilization, the mitochondrion, where PO_2 is estimated to be less

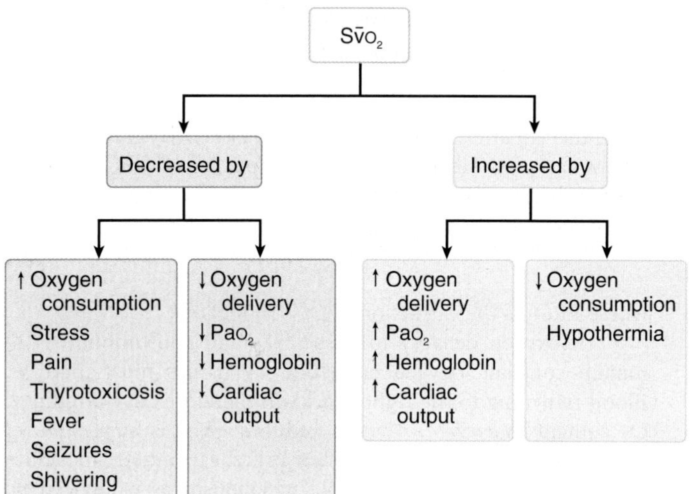

Figure 44-12 Causes of changes in mixed venous oxygen saturation. *(From Nanchal R, Taylor RW. Hemodynamic monitoring.* In *Papadakos PJ, Lachmann B [eds]: Mechanical Ventilation: Clinical Applications and Pathophysiology. Philadelphia, Elsevier, 2008.)*

than 1 mm Hg. Mitochondria from skeletal muscle appear to maintain their function with a Po_2 as low as 0.1 mm Hg.[83]

Unlike arterial Po_2 measurements, which should be nearly equal regardless of the artery sampled, Po_2 varies considerably within a particular organ or tissue bed because blood flow and O_2 consumption are not uniform but vary from point to point within the tissue. Because O_2 diffuses down a gradient from arterioles to mitochondria, measurements may also vary depending on where along this pathway a reading is obtained. Thus, it is generally thought that a distribution of Po_2 measurements across the tissue must be obtained to best describe its oxygenation status. Because of variable O_2 supply and demand, normal Po_2 levels and distributions differ from organ to organ.

A variety of methods have been devised to directly measure oxygen tensions and concentrations within tissues, and it has been an area of intense research for several decades. Most of the technologic advances have been made in the laboratory and have yet to be proved practical in the clinical setting.

Polarography is the current standard modality for measuring tissue oxygenation. It has the best resolution of all the available technology. Similar in principle to laboratory BGA, a Clark or needle-type electrode is inserted into tissue (rather than a blood sample), and Po_2 is proportional to the current generated as oxygen is reduced. Oxygen tension as low as 0.1 mm Hg can be resolved quite accurately. Though too invasive for routine clinical use, the technology is commercially available and has found application in neurosurgery and oncology.[84,85]

Near-infrared spectroscopy is a noninvasive system capable of measuring the oxygenation state of hemoglobin, myoglobin, and mitochondrial cytochromes.[86] The ability to monitor the oxygenation status of cytochromes along the electron transport chain will probably prove to be the best estimate of cellular oxygenation. Up to four wavelengths of light are applied to tissue, and the scattered light is returned via fiberoptic cables to the monitor for analysis. The technology has been incorporated into devices capable of measuring blood O_2 saturation in the brain, which have been commercially available for some 20 years.[87] Resolution is inferior to that of polarography, and problems with calibration and interference have limited its widespread use. Images can be obtained depicting changes in Hb concentration, but the resolution is poor.

A number of new systems for measuring tissue oxygenation are under laboratory investigation and have yet to reach commercial availability. Such systems include phosphorescence, fluorescence, electron paramagnetic resonance oximetry, and nuclear magnetic resonance spectroscopy. A number of reviews detailing all of these techniques have been compiled.[87]

Expired Gas Analysis

The ability to rapidly measure concentrations of inspired and expired gas is of paramount importance in anesthetic practice. Most anesthesia machines are equipped with oxygen sensors on the inspiratory limb of the circuit to help ensure that an adequate supply of oxygen is delivered to the patient at all times. Expired gas analysis is used to make inferences about blood concentrations and depth of anesthesia. Several systems are available for the measurement of gas tensions in exhaled air.

Mass Spectrometry

Mass spectrometry is a technique by which concentrations of gas particles in a sample can be determined according to their mass-charge ratio. A gas sample is passed through an ionizer and molecules become positively charged ions. Because all of the ions generated carry the same positive charge, this allows separation of particles based solely on mass. A detector then counts the number of ions of each mass, and the results are translated into concentrations. Measurements are quite reliable and can be obtained in fractions of a second.

Clinical use of mass spectrometry for expired gas analysis began in respiratory care units in the mid-1970s. They were introduced into operating rooms and anesthesia practice shortly thereafter. Because of their size and complexity, hospitals often connected many operating rooms to a single spectrometer and had the results relayed back to the anesthesiologist. The convenience plus low cost of infrared analyzers has largely phased mass spectrometry out of clinical use.

Infrared Absorption

Presently, most expired gas analyzers used in anesthesia involve infrared absorption. A gas sample is collected in a chamber through which infrared light is passed, and gas tensions are derived based on the intensity of the transmitted light. Today's infrared gas analyzers are capable of measuring all anesthetic agents currently in use, as well as CO_2 and N_2O. Oxygen does not absorb infrared light and therefore must be measured by other means, such as electrochemical or paramagnetic analysis.

Electrochemical Analysis

The same principles allowing electrochemical determination of oxygen in blood or tissue can be used to measure Po_2 in a mixture of gas. Polarographic (Clark type) electrodes, which require an applied voltage, or galvanic cells (most common) can be used for this purpose. In either arrangement, the amount of current generated as oxygen is reduced is proportional to the amount of oxygen present in the gas mixture, thus providing reliable estimates of Po_2 electrochemically. These sensor types are often used to measure inspired oxygen concentrations in anesthesia machines and conventional ventilators. Response time is somewhat slow and the method is rarely used for expired gas analysis.

Paramagnetic Analysis

Because the oxygen molecule has magnetic properties, its behavior in a magnetic field can be used to determine the concentration of oxygen in a gaseous mixture. Some newer anesthesia machines (e.g., Datex Ohmeda S/5) have incorporated paramagnetic oxygen analyzers capable of measuring oxygen in both the inspired and expired limbs of the circuit. Paramagnetic devices boast a longer life span and faster response time than electrochemical cells do.

Measurement of Nitric Oxide

Nitric oxide (NO) is a potent pulmonary vasodilator and has been used for a number of years to improve oxygenation in the face of acute respiratory distress syndrome (ARDS) and severe pulmonary hypertension (see also Chapter 31). It is produced endogenously and has multiple physiologic functions, including neurotransmission, regulation of vascular tone, and mediation of inflammation. Studies have identified NO as a marker of airway eosinophil activation, and exhaled levels are elevated in a number of inflammatory airway diseases such as asthma and chronic obstructive pulmonary disease (COPD).[88] Elevation of exhaled NO is greater than 90% specific for the diagnosis of asthma in both children and adults.[89,90] NO_2, the toxic oxidation product of NO, can accumulate with prolonged treatment or if stored NO is exposed to oxygen. Although accumulation of harmful levels is rare, NO_2 is known to cause pulmonary toxicity even at relatively low concentrations. Thus, an ideal NO analyzer would also have the ability to accurately measure NO_2 levels to avoid delivery or accumulation of toxic levels of this by-product. As the diagnostic and therapeutic use of NO has increased, methods to accurately quantify inhaled and exhaled concentrations of both NO and NO_2 have been sought.

Continuous measurement of inhaled NO has traditionally been accomplished with the use of electrochemical sensors. NO is oxidized to nitric acid, and its concentration is proportional to the current generated by the reaction. A number of electrochemical NO sensors have been independently evaluated and are reported to be quite accurate in measuring inhaled NO and NO_2.[91,92] The electrodes are sensitive to water vapor, and prolonged exposure can shorten the life span of the sensor and promote inaccurate readings. Accuracy also begins to wane at concentrations below 1 part per million (ppm), thus making them inappropriate for measurement of exhaled concentrations, which are typically in the parts-per-billion (ppb) range. Moreover, the slow response time of electrochemical sensors prevents their use for single-breath and exhaled NO analysis.

Because it is normally exhaled in very low concentrations, NO in expired air can be measured only with mass spectrometry or a process known as chemiluminescence. These analyzers, currently the most commonly used, have a shorter response time and can detect less than 1 ppb NO and NO_2. Wide variations in exhaled NO readings have been reported with chemiluminescence analyzers, and NO_2 levels may be underestimated in the presence of high oxygen concentrations.[93,94] Unstable instrument temperature, varying expiratory flow rate, and interference are some of the factors that may explain these variations.[95] Another study comparing four analyzers found that only the most rapid device provided accurate analysis in a continuous flow system and that the other three overestimated low levels and underestimated high levels.[96] A mid-infrared laser spectroscopy system has been developed that may eliminate some of the problems encountered with chemiluminescence analyzers by simultaneously measuring CO_2. It has shown promise in a small study comparing its results with typical exhaled NO levels.[95]

Waveform Analysis of Expired Respiratory Gases

Capnographs

Changes in the shape of the expired CO_2 waveform in an intubated patient can provide very useful monitoring information. Capnometry is the measurement of expired CO_2 and has become increasingly popular as a diagnostic tool in a number of settings. It is now the confirmation method of choice in anesthesia for proper placement of an endotracheal tube. CO_2 concentration is usually measured by infrared absorption with either a mainstream or sidestream capnometer. Measurements can then be plotted against time or exhaled volume to generate a *capnograph*. Capnography has found many useful clinical applications, and in 1998 it was adopted by the American Society of Anesthesiologists as standard care for all general anesthetics administered.

Mainstream versus Sidestream

The major difference between sidestream and mainstream capnometry is location of the sensor. However, this seemingly minor

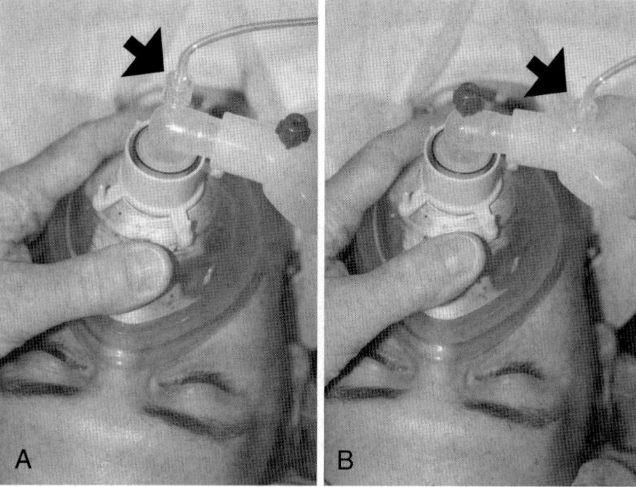

Figure 44-13 Sidestream sampling port placement. **A,** To minimize the effects of breathing circuit dead space, attachment of the sampling port should be as close to the patient as possible (*arrow*). **B,** Placement of the port as shown (*arrow*) can cause artifactual lowering of the end-tidal measurement.

difference plays a major role in the complexity, accuracy, and response time of each system.

SIDESTREAM. In sidestream capnometry, a fixed volume of gas is continuously sampled from the circuit. The sampled gas is aspirated through nylon or Teflon tubing into the measuring cell and then released into the atmosphere or returned to the circuit through a second tube (Fig. 44-13). Sampling should take place as close to the patient as possible to minimize the effects of circuit dead space, and the rate is usually adjusted to between 50 and 500 mL/min. It is imperative that the sampling rate be adjusted properly. Erroneous measurements will be obtained if the sampling rate exceeds the expiratory flow rate and causes inspired gas to be sampled. Hypoventilation may occur if the sampling flow exceeds fresh gas flow. Particular attention should be paid to this factor in the pediatric setting, in which expired and fresh gas flow can be quite low. Oxygen masks or nasal cannulas can be adapted to allow CO_2 monitoring (Fig. 44-14). The respiratory rate can be monitored adequately, but P_{ETCO_2} measurements may be falsely low unless the sample tubing is placed close to the nostril. Cannulas specifically designed to allow P_{ETCO_2} monitoring while administering O_2 have been developed and are commercially available.

There are several sources of potential error in sidestream capnometry. Water vapor condenses in the sample tubing and often accumulates in the measuring chamber. Liquids and particulate matter can also enter the measuring cell and produce erroneous readings. Most systems incorporate filters and water traps to help minimize these factors. Response time is delayed because gas samples must travel to the measuring cell through the sample tubing. Such delay can be minimized by using short tubing with a small lumen and high sample flow rates. The somewhat complicated sampling system and tubing connections provide multiple sites for damage or gas leakage. CO_2 can diffuse out of sample tubing and cause falsely low readings. Longer tubing and slower sampling rates increase this error, and nylon appears to be less permeable to CO_2 than other commonly used materials are.

MAINSTREAM. Mainstream capnometers incorporate the infrared sensor into the circuit very close to the endotracheal tube. Consequently, many of the problems with sidestream capnometry have been eliminated. CO_2 is measured directly in the circuit and no gas is subtracted, thus obviating the need for a complicated sampling system. The effects of breathing circuit and sample tubing dead space are minimized and the response time is therefore faster with mainstream systems. They are often used in the pediatric population, where circuit dead space can be more significant and response time is more critical. The measuring chamber must be warmed to about 40°C to prevent condensation of water vapor on the sensor window. Care must be taken to avoid skin contact with the chamber. It is somewhat heavy, and the

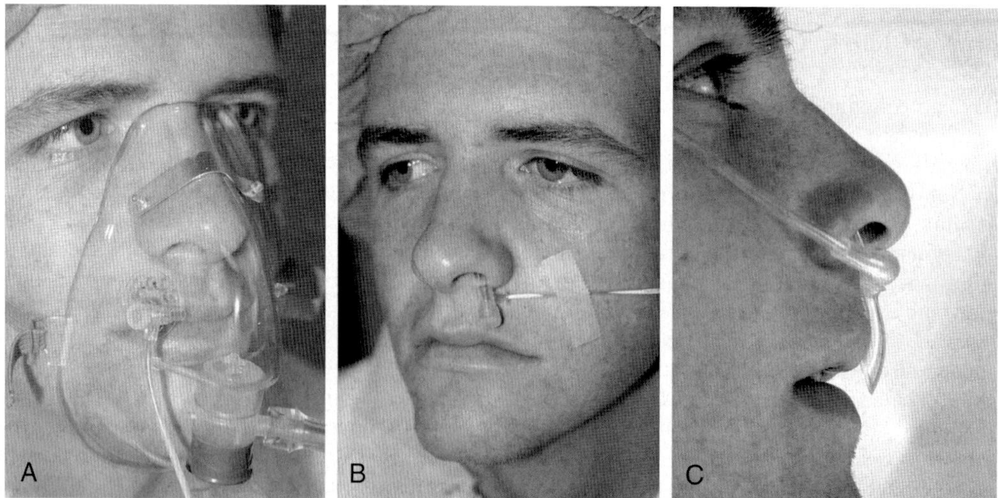

Figure 44-14 Monitoring a spontaneously breathing patient with a sidestream capnometer. **A,** Attachment of the sampling line to a non-rebreathing mask usually provides waveforms adequate for monitoring the respiratory rate, but end-tidal CO_2 tension (P_{ETCO_2}) is low because of mixing within the mask. **B,** Placement of a sample probe close to a nostril increases the accuracy of P_{ETCO_2} measurement. **C,** A specially designed probe (Oridion, Needham, MA) samples exhaled gas from the nose and mouth for assessing exhaled gas from mouth breathers. A second port in the same device can be used to administer supplemental oxygen.

circuit should be inspected frequently to avoid kinking of the endotracheal tube. Mainstream capnometers require frequent calibration, usually daily, and are prone to soiling with saliva or mucus because of their close proximity to the patient.

Time versus Volume Capnographs

TIME. The most commonly used type of capnograph plots P_{CO_2} versus time. The tracing is traditionally divided into an inspiratory phase and three (sometimes four) expiratory phases (Fig. 44-15):

Phase 0: inspiratory phase
Phase I: dead space and little or no CO_2
Phase II: mixture of alveolar and dead space gas
Phase III: alveolar plateau, with the peak representing end-expiratory (end-tidal) CO_2 (P_{ETCO_2}).

In patients with normal lung function, P_{ETCO_2} generally underestimates Pa_{CO_2} by 1 to 5 mm Hg because of the presence of a small amount of alveolar dead space.[7] Factors that increase alveolar dead space will widen this gradient and increase the slope of phase III. During anesthesia there is often increased alveolar dead space caused by reduced cardiac output and decreased perfusion of the lung apices.[97] It is therefore not surprising that studies under anesthesia have found the P_{ETCO_2}-Pa_{CO_2} gradient to be slightly elevated at 5 to 10 mm Hg.[98] An extreme example of acutely increased alveolar dead space is pulmonary embolism. Thus, an abruptly decreased P_{ETCO_2} with ventilation held constant is often indicative of a sudden decrease in cardiac output or pulmonary embolism. Other common causes of a widened gradient include obstructive lung disease, smoking, and advanced age. Examples of commonly encountered capnographic waveforms are shown in Figure 44-16.

The slope of the alveolar plateau (phase III) can also be increased in obstructive airway disease or during prolonged expiration. Two explanations for this phenomenon have generally been forwarded. First, obstructed (slow) lung units with low $\dot{V}/\dot{Q}$ and high P_{CO_2} empty slower and later than "fast" alveoli with normal $\dot{V}/\dot{Q}$ and low P_{CO_2}. This is manifested as a linear upsloping of phase III instead of the typical "plateau." Second, as lung volume decreases during exhalation and CO_2 excretion from capillaries remains constant, P_{CO_2} slowly rises throughout expiration and causes an upsloping plateau (Fig. 44-17).[99] Accordingly, even a person with completely normal lungs can have an upsloping plateau during prolonged expiration. End-tidal CO_2 therefore approximates *peak* alveolar CO_2, whereas Pa_{CO_2} can be thought of as average alveolar P_{CO_2}.

At the terminal end of the phase III plateau, a sharp rise in P_{CO_2} is sometimes observed and is referred to as phase IV. Although its exact cause is unknown, this rise is thought to occur when closing capacity is reached and small airways close, usually

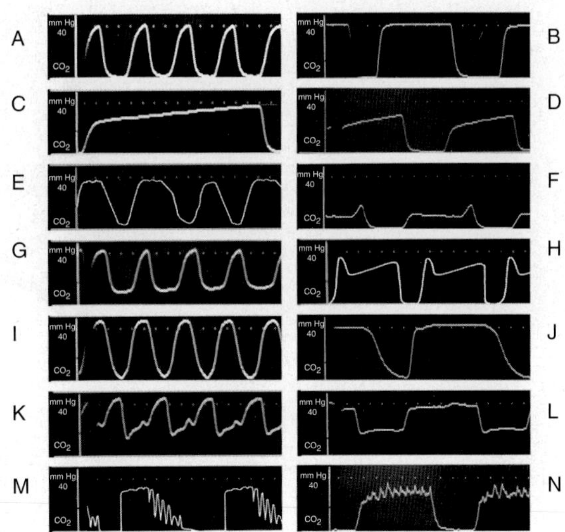

Figure 44-16 Examples of capnograph waves. **A,** Normal spontaneous breathing. **B,** Normal mechanical ventilation. **C,** Prolonged exhalation during spontaneous breathing. As CO_2 diffuses from mixed venous blood into alveoli, its concentration progressively rises (see Fig. 44-17). **D,** Increased slope of phase III in a mechanically ventilated patient with emphysema. **E,** Added dead space during spontaneous ventilation. **F,** Dual plateau (i.e., tails-up pattern) caused by a leak in the sample line. The alveolar plateau is artifactually low because of dilution of exhaled gas with air leaking inward. During each mechanical breath the leak is reduced because of higher pressure within the airway and tubing, thus explaining the rise in CO_2 concentration at the end of the alveolar plateau. This pattern is not seen during spontaneous ventilation because the required increase in airway pressure is absent. **G,** Exhausted CO_2 absorbent producing an inhaled CO_2 concentration greater than zero. **H,** Double peak in a patient with a single lung transplant. The first peak represents CO_2 from the transplanted (normal) lung. Exhalation of CO_2 from the remaining (obstructed) lung is delayed, thereby producing the second peak. **I,** Inspiratory valve stuck open during spontaneous breathing. Some backflow into the inspired limb of the circuit causes a rise in the level of inspired CO_2. **J,** Inspiratory valve stuck open during mechanical ventilation. The "slurred" downslope during inspiration represents a small amount of inspired CO_2 in the inspired limb of the circuit. **K** and **L,** Expiratory valve stuck open during spontaneous breathing and mechanical ventilation, respectively. Inhalation of exhaled gas causes an increase in inspired CO_2. **M,** Cardiogenic oscillations, when seen, usually occur on sidestream capnographs of spontaneously breathing patients at the end of each exhalation. Cardiac action causes to-and-fro movement of the interface between exhaled and fresh gas. The CO_2 concentration in gas entering the sampling line therefore alternates between high and low values. **N,** Electrical noise resulting from a malfunctioning component. The seemingly random nature of the signal perturbations (about three per second) implies a nonbiologic cause.

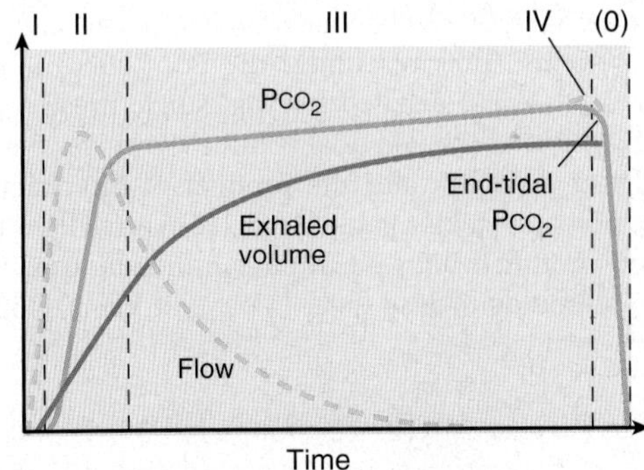

Figure 44-15 Time and volume capnographs. **A,** Expired P_{CO_2} versus time (i.e., standard time capnogram). The waveform is conventionally subdivided into phases. During phase I, exhaled gas from the large airways has a P_{CO_2} of 0. Phase II is the transition between airway and alveolar gas. Phase III (i.e., alveolar plateau) is normally flat, but in the presence of $\dot{V}_A/\dot{Q}$ mismatching, it has a positive slope. The downslope of the capnogram at the onset of inspiration is usually referred to as phase 0, but sometimes there is a terminal increase in the slope associated with the onset of airway closure (*dashed line* labeled IV). The P_{CO_2} value at the end of exhalation is referred to as the end-tidal P_{CO_2} (P_{ETCO_2}). Also shown are the exhaled gas flow rate and volume.

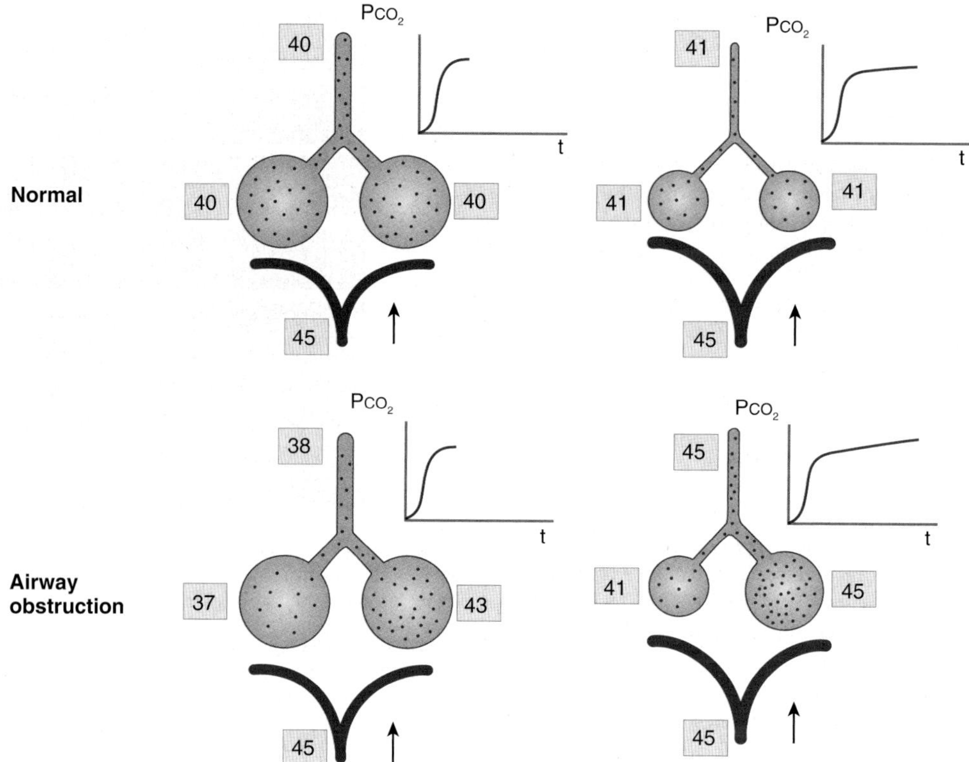

Figure 44-17 Mechanisms of airway obstruction producing an upsloping phase III capnogram. In a normal, healthy person (*upper panel*), there is a narrow range of $\dot{V}_A/\dot{Q}$ ratios with values close to 1. Gas exchange units therefore have similar Pco_2 and tend to empty synchronously, and the expired Pco_2 remains relatively constant. During the course of exhalation, alveolar Pco_2 slowly rises as CO_2 continuously diffuses from blood. This causes a slight increase in Pco_2 toward the end of expiration, and this increase can be pronounced if the exhalation is prolonged (see Fig. 44-16C). In a patient with diffuse airway obstruction (*lower panel*), the airway pathology is heterogeneous, with gas exchange units having a wide range of $\dot{V}_A/\dot{Q}$ ratios. Well-ventilated gas exchange units, with gas containing lower Pco_2, empty first; poorly ventilated units, with higher Pco_2, empty last. In addition to the continuous rise in Pco_2 mentioned previously, there is a progressive increase caused by asynchronous exhalation.

after prolonged expiration. These small airways may supply lung units with little CO_2 for various reasons, and their closure would therefore allow CO_2-rich gas from other lung units to abruptly reach the upper airway. Bhavani-Shankar and colleagues favor a different explanation and state that well-ventilated, open lung units have an upsloping increase in Pco_2 whereas Pco_2 in poorly ventilated, closure-prone units increases linearly. When poorly ventilated airways close, the pattern from well-ventilated units predominates and the slope of the plateau rises suddenly.[99] This concept is nicely cartooned at capnography.com in the phase IV section.

To summarize, any condition that increases alveolar dead space or $\dot{V}/\dot{Q}$ heterogeneity will increase the slope of phase III. This includes acute and chronic airway obstruction, and prolonged expiration in a normal subject can also generate this pattern. Sometimes this slope is so significant that the reported P_{ETCO_2} actually exceeds Pa_{CO_2}. This has been observed during anesthesia in obese patients and in 50% of both normal infants and pregnant women.[100] It is probably secondary to reduced thoracic compliance and functional residual capacity (FRC), increased cardiac output, and increased CO_2 production.[101] High mixed venous CO_2 tension and malignant hyperthermia have also been reported to cause a negative Pa_{CO_2}-P_{ETCO_2} gradient.[102] In such cases, P_{ETCO_2} is clearly not an accurate estimate of Pa_{CO_2}, and the average alveolar Pco_2 obtained from a volume capnograph may be more indicative of Pa_{CO_2}.[103]

VOLUME. A volume capnograph is obtained by plotting expired Pco_2 versus exhaled gas volume, usually obtained with a spirometer or pneumotachometer. There is no inspiratory phase in a volume capnograph, and the curve is divided into three expiratory phases. Several measurements that are not possible with time capnography can be made, such as partitioning of dead space components. The area under the Pco_2 curve is the total volume of CO_2 ($\dot{V}co_2$) exhaled for that single breath. Dividing this value by the total exhaled tidal volume (V_T) gives the fraction of expired CO_2 (F_{ECO_2}), and the product of this fraction and barometric pressure yields a value for mixed expired Pco_2 (P_{ECO_2}). The Enghoff-modified Bohr equation can then be used to determine total (physiologic) dead space (V_{DSphys} or V_{DStot}) (Figs. 44-18 and 44-19):

$$V_{DS_{tot}} = V_T\left[\left(Pa_{CO_2} - P_{ECO_2}\right)/Pa_{CO_2}\right] \quad (16)$$

Once $V_{DS_{tot}}$ has been determined, subtracting the anatomic dead space ($V_{DS_{anat}}$) derived from the capnograph (see Fig. 44-18) yields the alveolar dead space component ($V_{DS_{alv}}$):

$$V_{DS_{alv}} = V_{D_{tot}} - V_{DS_{anat}} \quad (17)$$

Alternatively, alveolar dead space can be calculated by replacing P_{ECO_2} in the Bohr equation with *average* alveolar Pco_2 ($P_{A'CO_2}$), which can be derived from the volume capnograph[104]:

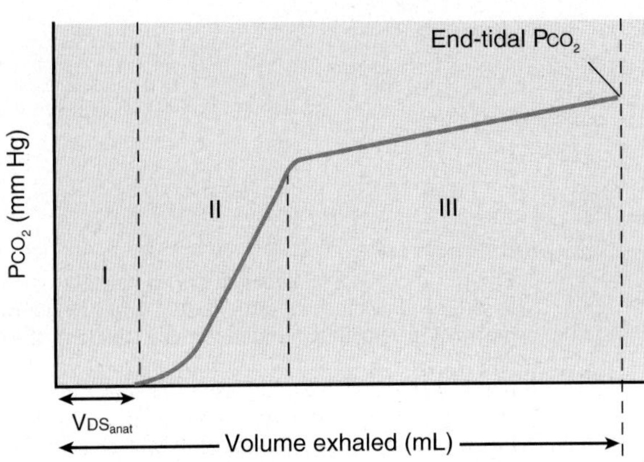

Figure 44-18 Volume capnograph: single-breath CO_2 ($SBCO_2$) curve. The horizontal axis of the graph represents expiratory/inspiratory tidal volume and is generally divided into three areas: I, the anatomic dead space volume (VDS_{anat}): II, the transitional phase II volume; and III, the phase III alveolar volume. The sum of these values is the tidal volume. The vertical axis represents the concentration of CO_2. PCO_2, partial pressure of carbon dioxide. *(From Pilbeam SP, Cairo JM: Mechanical Ventilation: Physiological and Clinical Applications, 4th ed. St. Louis, Elsevier, 2006.)*

$$V_{DS_{alv}} = (V_T - V_{DS_{anat}}) / \left[(Pa_{CO_2} - P_{A'CO_2}) / Pa_{CO_2} \right] \quad (18)$$

Capnography has been used to titrate positive end-expiratory pressure (PEEP) settings inasmuch as narrowing of the Pa_{CO_2}-P_{ETCO_2} gradient suggests reduced alveolar dead space and shunt fraction as a result of alveolar recruitment and improved $\dot{V}/\dot{Q}$ matching. These changes are often subtle or absent on a time capnograph and may be detectable only with volume capnography.[100] It has been suggested that an incompetent inspiratory valve and rebreathing during mechanical ventilation may require volume capnography to be detected reliably.[105] The technique may also be better than time capnography for the diagnosis of pulmonary embolism.[106]

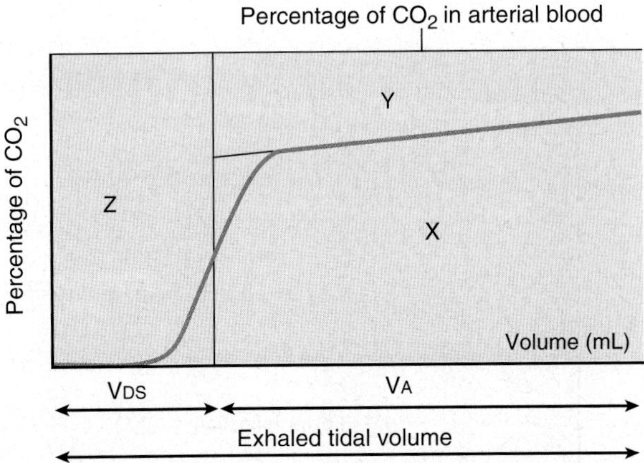

Figure 44-19 Volume capnograph: graph of the percentage of carbon dioxide ($\%CO_2$) (*y* axis) and volume (*x* axis). A *horizontal line* drawn at the top of the curve represents $\%CO_2$ in arterial blood. Three distinct regions are established. Area X represents the actual CO_2 exhaled in one breath (assuming that no CO_2 is rebreathed), area Y is the amount of CO_2 that is not eliminated because of alveolar dead space, and area Z is the amount of CO_2 not eliminated because of anatomic dead space. The ratios of these areas are the same as in the relationship seen in the Bohr equation: $(Pa_{CO_2} - P_{ECO_2})/Pa_{CO_2} = (Y + Z)/(X + Y + Z)$. P_{ECO_2}, mixed expired PCO_2; VA, alveolar volume; VDS, dead space volume.

Additional Clinical Applications of Capnography

In addition to those outlined in the preceding sections, capnography has a host of clinical applications. Monitoring of P_{ETCO_2} can be invaluable during mechanical ventilation in the operating room and ICU to make inferences about cardiovascular status, Pa_{CO_2} trends, and adequacy of ventilation. Disappearance of the capnograph waveform may warn of cardiovascular collapse or massive airway obstruction, but it is most often due to disconnection or a large leak in the circuit. Capnography has been used to assess the efficacy of chest compressions during cardiopulmonary resuscitation and even to verify proper placement of enteric feeding tubes.[107]

Errors

Various disease states discussed previously may cause overestimation or underestimation of Pa_{CO_2} with use of P_{ETCO_2}. Condensation of water vapor in the sample tubing and measuring cell can elevate the reported PCO_2 slightly. Warming these pieces of equipment plus avoiding the use of drying agents in the sample line reduces this error. Capnometers may underreport true P_{ETCO_2} at higher respiratory rates. Exhausted CO_2 absorbent increases inspired CO_2, and failure to recognize such depletion may lead to suspicion of rebreathing from other causes.

Pulmonary and Chest Wall Monitoring

Pressure-Volume Curve Analysis

Lung mechanics can be severely impaired in a number of respiratory disorders. Monitoring changes in mechanical function of the lung is vital in developing a safe and effective support strategy in the face of respiratory failure. In a mechanically ventilated patient, construction of pressure-volume (PV) curves can provide important information about mechanics and help guide ventilator management. A *dynamic* PV curve is one that is constructed during gas flow, whereas *static* curves are derived when flow is absent. Techniques for constructing static curves were introduced in the mid-1970s and soon thereafter were shown to be useful in determining the cause of acute respiratory distress (Fig. 44-20). In recent years, the PV relationship has been studied extensively as a means of determining optimal PEEP and tidal volume in ARDS and ALI.

Static Curve

A static curve is constructed by using the ventilator or a large syringe to deliver known tidal volumes, and patients must be sedated and paralyzed for an optimal study. The resultant plateau (P_{plat}) and peak inspiratory pressures (P_{pk}) are recorded after each breath to allow determination of both static (C_{stat}) and dynamic (C_{dyn}) compliance. Because C_{stat} is calculated by using plateau

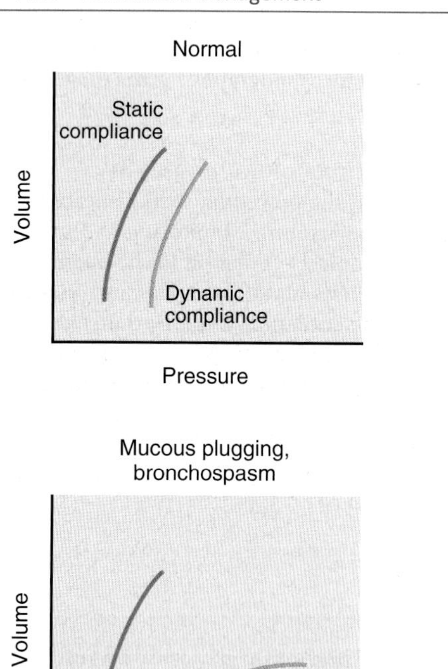

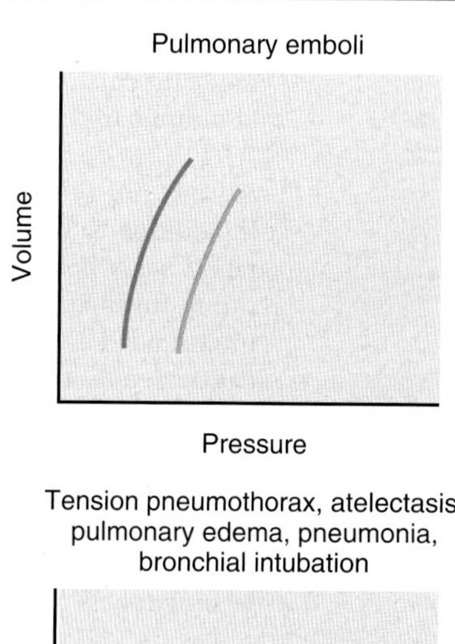

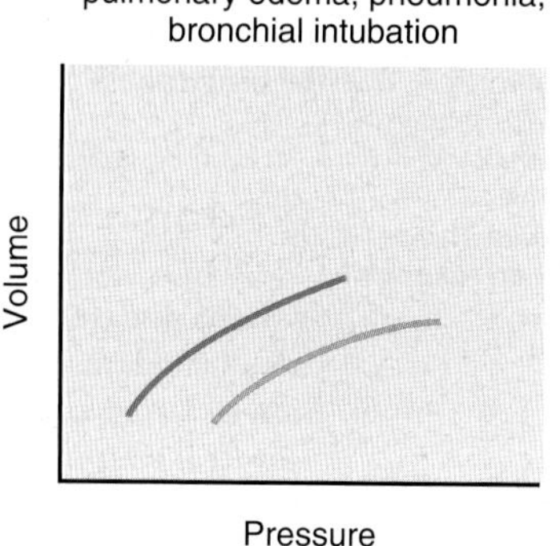

Figure 44-20 Pressure-volume curves reflecting changes in static and dynamic compliance (C_{stat} and C_{dyn}) during mechanical ventilation. Under normal conditions, the C_{stat} and C_{dyn} curves are similar. Because pulmonary emboli do not affect resistance or compliance, neither curve changes with this condition. With mucous plugging or bronchospasm, airway resistance (Raw) increases, the C_{dyn} curve shifts to the right and flattens (more pressure is required), and the C_{stat} curve remains unchanged. With conditions that reduce lung compliance (CL), both curves shift to the right and flatten. *(From Bone RC: Monitoring ventilatory mechanics in acute respiratory failure. Respir Care 28:597-604, 1983.)*

pressure, it is mainly influenced by chest wall and alveolar elastic recoil:

$$C_{stat} = V_T/(P_{plat} - PEEP) \quad (19)$$

C_{dyn} is derived by using P_{pk} and therefore takes airway and circuit resistance into account as well:

$$C_{dyn} = V_T/(P_{pk} - PEEP) \quad (20)$$

In patients with normal lung function, the static PV curve is usually linear, and C_{stat} ranges from 50 to 100 mL/cm H_2O (Fig. 44-21). In disorders such as ARDS and ALI, where compliance can be substantially decreased, the curve becomes sigmoidal or S shaped.[108,109] Upper (UIP) and lower (LIP) inflection points can often be identified. The LIP, sometimes called P_{flex}, signifies an abrupt increase in compliance and is thought to result from the sudden recruitment of a large number of alveoli. The plateau pressure at which the LIP occurs is often referred to as the *opening pressure* of the lung. Overdistention of alveoli begins to occur once a critical volume (or pressure) is reached, marked by the UIP. Maintaining airway pressures between the LIP and UIP is therefore believed by many to prevent derecruitment and overdistention of alveoli, both of which contribute to ventilator-induced lung injury.[108,109] Using this reasoning, PEEP would be set slightly above the LIP to keep recruited alveoli open.[110] Indeed, this approach has been shown to result in earlier weaning from the ventilator, less release of inflammatory cytokines, and a trend toward reduced mortality in ARDS patients.[108,111]

Despite positive results using the LIP and UIP to guide PEEP and VT settings, recent evidence suggests that the LIP does not correlate with the pressure at which recruited alveoli will begin to close, known as the *critical closing pressure*.[112,113] A probable explanation is that contrary to previous thought, recruitment has been shown to occur along the entire PV curve, independent of the LIP and UIP. Thus, setting PEEP above the LIP is not always beneficial and may instead increase the risk for overdistention and barotrauma.[114] Direct measures of appropriate response may be more suitable in determining the best PEEP level (see "Analysis of the Level of PEEP").

Once the lung has been fully recruited, a deflation curve can be drawn by stepwise deflation of the lung, similar to mapping of the inspiratory limb. As lung volume decreases, critical closing

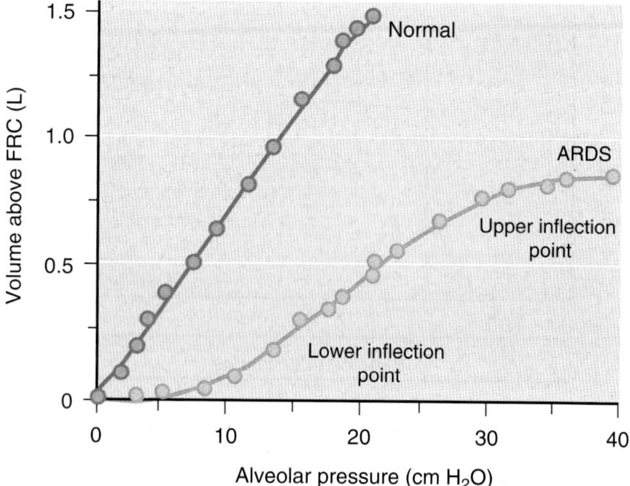

Figure 44-21 Example of a static, inspiratory pressure-volume curve of the respiratory system in a patient with acute respiratory distress syndrome (ARDS) versus a healthy subject. Upper (about 30 cm H_2O) and lower (about 10 cm H_2O) inflection points are present in the patient with ARDS. FRC, functional residual capacity. *(From Hess DR, Kacmarek RM: Essentials of Mechanical Ventilation, 2nd ed. New York, McGraw-Hill, 2002.)*

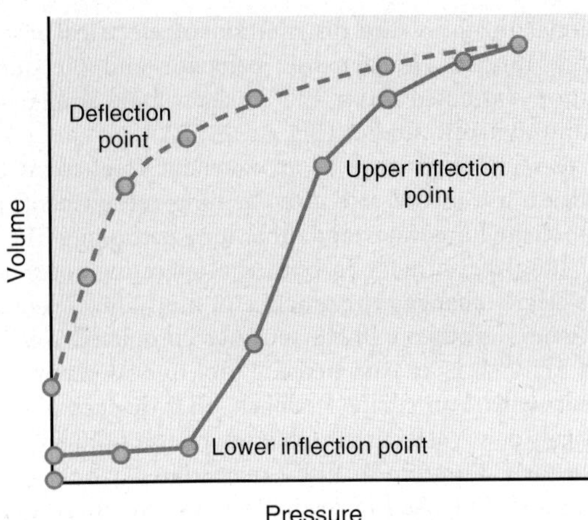

Figure 44-22 Pressure-volume relationship of the lung showing the inflation (*solid line*) and the deflation limb (*dashed line*). Note the clear difference in lung volume between both limbs at identical pressure (hysteresis). *(From van Kaam AHLC: Neonatal mechanical ventilation. In Papadakos PJ, Lachmann B [eds]: Mechanical Ventilation: Clinical Applications and Pathophysiology. Philadelphia, Elsevier, 2008.)*

pressure is reached, and a *deflection* point appears on the curve corresponding to a rapid decrease in compliance and closure of a large number of lung units (Fig. 44-22). Because compliance improves during inflation as lung units are recruited, higher volumes are observed at the same pressure during deflation than during inflation, a phenomenon referred to as *hysteresis*. Accordingly, critical closing pressure will be lower than opening pressure, and setting PEEP slightly above the deflection point rather than the LIP may provide superior alveolar stabilization with less risk of overdistention and ventilator-induced lung injury.[115,116] A number of recent studies suggest that the LIP does not reliably indicate the pressure at which maximal alveolar derecruitment occurs.[112,117] In addition, there is mounting evidence that using the deflation limb rather than the inflation limb of PV curves to guide ventilation may improve gas exchange and mechanics, often at lower mPaw and PEEP levels.[118,119] Therefore, although the presence of an LIP on the PV curve indicates a *need* for lung recruitment, the deflection point may be more valuable in determining the amount of PEEP required to prevent alveolar collapse. Evaluating deflation C_{stat} in this manner to determine closing pressure is at least as effective as monitoring $Pa{O_2}$ for selection of the optimum PEEP level.[115,116] Moreover, recruitment maneuvers have been shown to be quite safe and are less injurious than allowing shear stress damage associated with derecruitment to proceed unchecked.[120,121]

Static PV curves can also be obtained from a single breath delivered slowly (2 to 3 L/m) until a predetermined pressure is reached and are referred to as slow-flow or quasi-static PV loops. The curves derived are comparable to those obtained with typical static techniques, but the deflation limb is often difficult to acquire.[122,123] Several modern ventilators have incorporated this capability. The Hamilton Galileo ventilator allows selection of the desired flow rate for the PV study, and an interactive curve is then displayed on the monitor, usually within 30 seconds.

Dynamic Curve

A number of ventilators are capable of mapping dynamic PV curves during tidal breaths delivered with normal gas flow. Newer ventilators automatically display the curve with each tidal volume. Though useful in following general trends in compliance, identification of inflection points is more difficult on dynamic PV curves. Several factors can alter the loop from breath to breath, and using dynamic curves for determination of optimal V_T and PEEP is not generally recommended.[122]

Analysis of the Level of PEEP

Application of PEEP has long been known to improve lung mechanics and gas exchange in many forms of acute respiratory failure. Appropriate PEEP increases FRC, decreases pulmonary edema, and maintains the patency of airways and recruited alveoli. It is important to note that PEEP does not recruit the lung; rather, it is sustained high pressure that reopens closed alveoli and airways, and PEEP stabilizes these recruited lung units. A host of tools and parameters described in this chapter have been used by clinicians to evaluate PEEP settings, including capnography, titration to the best $Pa{O_2}/Sa{O_2}$ ratio, continuous $S\bar{v}{O_2}$ and shunt monitoring, PV curve analysis, and others. None have unequivocally been shown to result in superior outcome. Consequently, there is no consensus on a single method of titrating and evaluating clinical response to PEEP. More than 30 years ago it was noted that the PEEP level resulting in maximum O_2 delivery also produced optimal compliance while minimizing dead space and shunt fraction.[124] The authors coined the phrase "optimum" PEEP to refer to that producing the maximum improvement in pulmonary function with minimal hemodynamic compromise. Recent trials have shown that during a derecruitment study, measuring C_{stat} may be as useful and more cost-effective than measuring $Pa{O_2}$ in determining closing pressure and guiding PEEP selection.[115,116] Nowadays most clinicians use one of these two parameters to set PEEP after the recruitment maneuver. Inflection points on PV curves are not always easy to identify, and a decrease in $Pa{O_2}$ rather than C_{stat} should be used to identify closing pressure in such cases.

Patients under GA are prone to compression atelectasis in dependent lung regions (see Fig. 44-5).[125] Thus, it is tempting to apply PEEP to all patients undergoing surgery with mechanical ventilation to prevent this atelectasis. It has been shown that application of PEEP during GA can attenuate and reverse dependent atelectasis but does not improve gas exchange.[126] A study comparing normal and obese subjects also found that application of PEEP during GA did not alter gas exchange in normal patients, but some improvement was noted in the obese population.[127] Thus, there is no evidence to support routine use of PEEP during GA. However, these studies did not use recruitment maneuvers, and a trial by Tusman and colleagues showed that alveolar recruitment can improve oxygenation during GA (see also Chapter 15).[128] In addition, PEEP combined with recruitment maneuvers has been shown to provide a sustained increase in $Pa{O_2}$ and lung volume in mechanically ventilated postsurgical patients.[128,129]

Analysis of Lung Recruitment

The importance of early lung recruitment in respiratory failure and ARDS has been well documented.[130] Lung-protective ventilation in ARDS via frequent recruitment maneuvers results in improved 28-day survival, earlier weaning from mechanical ventilation, and less barotrauma than with conventional ventilation strategies.[111] Effective recruitment is performed by applying sustained high airway pressure, usually for 30 to 90 seconds. Many successful techniques, all using essentially these same principles, have been described.[131,132] Recruitment maneuvers are typically well tolerated, with no significant hemodynamic deterioration or inflammatory response.[133,134] Although improvements in pulmonary compliance and oxygenation are indicative of successful recruitment, direct methods of quantifying and monitoring lung recruitment are emerging.

Computed Tomography

Technologic advances in CT have made it a valuable tool for studying ARDS and lung recruitment. It has been used in numerous studies to evaluate the effects of a wide range of variables on alveolar recruitment and stabilization.[135] Recently, Gattinoni and colleagues performed a trial to examine whether measuring the amount of recruitable lung by CT could help predict how the lung would respond to PEEP after recruitment. They concluded that a higher amount of recruitable lung was correlated with a positive response to PEEP whereas PEEP was of little benefit and perhaps detrimental in patients with less recruitable lung measured by CT.[136] This conclusion was in line with previous studies showing that PEEP results in hyperinflation and increased stress in normal lung regions when the amount of recruitable lung is low.[137] Quantitative CT analysis of potentially recruitable lung may therefore be useful in determining the best PEEP level, but further studies are needed on the practicality of routine use. CT was instrumental in the discovery that lung recruitment occurs throughout inspiration and not solely around the LIP of the PV curve.[138]

Electrical Impedance Tomography

A new and exciting form of monitoring of pulmonary function may be electrical impedance tomography (EIT).[139,149] It is a noninvasive and radiation-free technique based on the measurement of electric potentials at the chest wall surface. Within a particular cross-sectional plane, harmless electrical currents are driven across the thorax in a rotating pattern to generate a potential gradient at the surface, which is then transformed into a two-dimensional image of the distribution of electrical impedance within the thorax. The dynamic behavior and the qualitative information extracted from EIT images look similar to that reported in dynamic studies (Fig. 44-23).[141,142]

This technology may be an excellent assessment tool for easy bedside use to evaluate alveolar lung recruitment, pulmonary embolism, lung water, and other lung pathology. The importance of lung recruitment in both the operating room and the ICU has clearly changed the practice of mechanical ventilation.

Amato's group in Brazil recently completed a validation study of EIT.[142] It is an easy bedside tool to evaluate mechanical ventilation with immediate feedback. EIT devices may, in the future, easily detect selective intubation, pneumothorax, and alveolar atelectasis. Titration of PEEP may someday be evaluated in real time, with EIT used instead of waiting for BGA, radiologic studies, and CT scans. This technology may one day be integrated into the bedside monitor or into closed-loop mechanical ventilators.

Inspiratory Pressure Monitoring

Impaired respiratory muscle function from fatigue or neuromuscular disorders can contribute to respiratory failure and difficulty weaning from mechanical ventilation. Measurement of maximum inspiratory pressure (MIP), also called negative inspiratory force, gives a useful bedside appraisal of respiratory muscle strength. It can be performed on intubated and nonintubated patients by attaching a pressure manometer to the endotracheal tube or a noninvasive mouthpiece. Alternatively, use of a one-way valve that allows exhalation only has been described, although it is quite uncomfortable for the patient.[143] Normal MIP is about −90 cm H_2O but can range between −50 and −120 cm H_2O. To obtain accurate measurements, MIP should be measured after maximal expiration because the diaphragm can generate the greatest pressure at residual volume. Studies have demonstrated that inability to generate MIP more negative than −20 cm results in tidal volumes that are insufficient for generating a strong cough. Moreover, this cutoff has been shown to result in weaning failure with

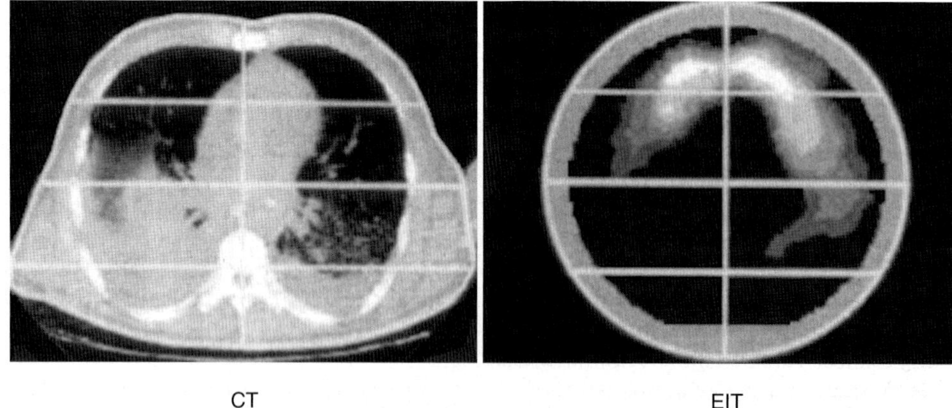

Figure 44-23 Comparison of a computed tomographic (CT) scan and an electrical impedance tomographic (EIT) image during mechanical ventilation of a patient with acute lung injury. The *gray* and *white* areas in the EIT image reflect areas with change in impedance (volume changes) and correlate with well-inflated areas on the CT scan. There is no impedance change on the EIT scan in the dorsal area, where atelectasis is present on the CT scan. *(From Wolf GK, Arnold JH: High-frequency oscillatory ventilation for adult acute respiratory distress syndrome: A decade of progress. Crit Care Med 33(Suppl):S163-S169, 2005.)*

a negative predictive value of 1.[144] Though not yet a firmly established predictor of weaning outcome, MIP is useful in determining whether patient weakness or neuromuscular dysfunction is playing a role in unsuccessful weaning trials.

Esophageal Monitoring

Transpulmonary pressure, rather than peak or plateau pressure, is the most important determinant of alveolar distention and is defined as alveolar pressure (PA) minus pleural pressure (Ppl).[145] Thus, true distending pressure of the lung cannot be measured without determination of Ppl. Direct measurement of Ppl is clinically impractical, but it can be estimated quite reliably in upright patients by measuring pressure in the distal third of the esophagus. The esophagus is a fairly passive structure and the third part is very close to the pleural space, thus allowing transmission of pleural pressure to an intraesophageal pressure monitor.[146] A balloon-tipped catheter is typically used, and this technique is considered the standard modality for evaluating inspiratory effort and work of breathing (WOB). In the supine position, this relationship is less predictable because gravitational forces cause compression of the esophagus and dependent lung, thereby skewing the measurements.

Placement of a second balloon catheter into the stomach allows simultaneous measurement of gastric pressure and provides a means of obtaining a host of useful information about respiratory mechanics. For example, transdiaphragmatic pressure monitoring can be performed to assess diaphragmatic contraction. As the diaphragm contracts and the domes descend, negative Ppl (or Pes) should coincide with positive abdominal pressure (or Pg) generating transdiaphragmatic pressure. Inability of the diaphragm to contract properly results in loss of transdiaphragmatic pressure and has been observed after uncomplicated upper abdominal surgery (Fig. 44-24). Diaphragmatic fatigue and phrenic nerve palsy elicit a similar pattern.[147] This can also be observed clinically inasmuch as impaired diaphragmatic activity is associated with paradoxical inward movement of the abdomen during inspiration.

Work of Breathing

The work involved in normal respiration, often referred to as *work of breathing (WOB)*, usually requires minimal energy expenditure. Work is defined as the force needed to move a mass times the distance moved: $W = F \times d$. In the respiratory system, it represents the pressure (or force) needed to inspire a certain volume of gas: $WOB = P \times V$. With respiratory compromise, WOB can be quite high, as much as 40% of total oxygen consumption (normally <5%). WOB can be estimated by measuring pressure and volume changes from a PV curve. Total work is the area enclosed by the curve (integral of pressure and volume). Thus, the larger the loop, the greater the WOB (Fig. 44-25). However, studies indicate that mechanical work calculated in this manner may underestimate true WOB and is weakly correlated with the $\dot{V}O_2$ of respiratory muscles. Alternatively, many clinicians believe that the *pressure-time product* (PTP) is the most accurate measure of work performed by the diaphragm during inspiration and better correlates with $\dot{V}O_2$[148] because the PTP takes isometric contraction of the diaphragm into account, which consumes additional O_2. Increases in PTP indicate stronger diaphragmatic contraction and vice versa. Calculation of PTP requires measurement of transdiaphragmatic pressure as outlined earlier and is not routinely performed. Occlusion pressures (P_{100}) measured with a dedicated valve system or conventional ventilator have also been shown to correlate with WOB.[148,149]

Closed-Loop Analysis

Closed-loop ventilation involves computer-based real-time interpretation of respiratory mechanics with continuous adjustment of the level of support delivered to the patient.[150] Any change in mechanics or patient effort is detected and a new breathing pattern is initiated by the ventilator. Ventilator dyssynchrony and WOB are minimized. Moreover, erroneous or unsafe settings could potentially be minimized with a system that continuously regulates ventilator support based on real-time assessment of the

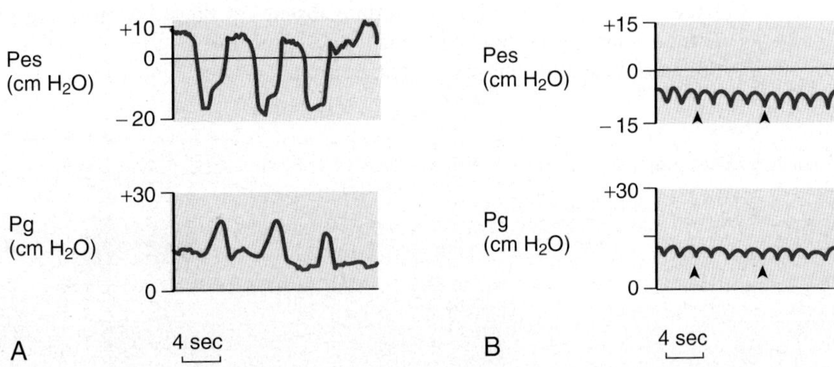

Figure 44-24 Examples of transdiaphragmatic pressure monitoring. **A,** Simultaneous esophageal (Pes) and gastric (Pg) pressure waveforms during tidal breathing in a normal individual. Negative esophageal (and therefore pleural) pressure swings are accompanied by positive gastric pressure waves indicative of the development of transdiaphragmatic pressure during inspiration. **B,** The same waveforms in a patient with phrenic nerve palsy (and therefore absent diaphragmatic contraction). Negative intrathoracic pressure swings (*arrowheads*) are accompanied by gastric pressure swings in the same direction. Intrathoracic pressure changes are directly transmitted through a passive diaphragm. These changes can also be observed in the early postoperative period in patients who have undergone upper abdominal surgery. *(From Brown KA, Hoffstein V, Byrick RJ: Bedside diagnosis of bilateral diaphragmatic paralysis in a ventilator-dependent patient after open-heart surgery. Anesth Analg 64:1208, 1985.)*

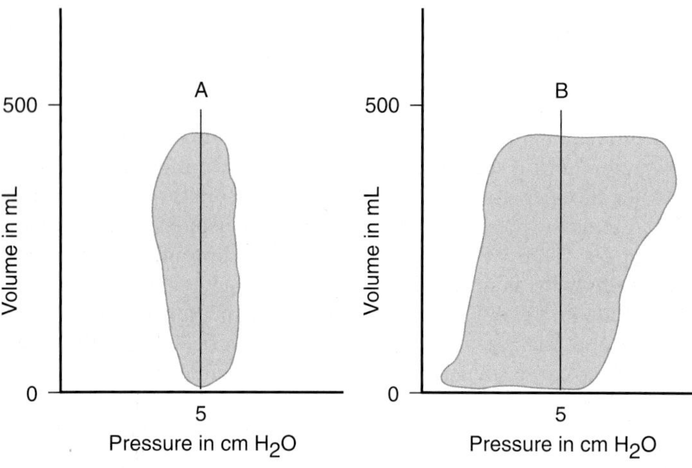

Figure 44-25 Work of breathing (WOB) during continuous positive airway pressure (CPAP). WOB in this figure is the integral of airway pressure and tidal volume. Loop A is an example of a freestanding CPAP system. Spontaneous breaths occur clockwise, inspiration to expiration. Loop B is CPAP through a ventilator demand valve system. Breathing occurs clockwise. *(Redrawn from Hirsch C, Kacmarek RM, Stanek K: Work of breathing during CPAP and PSV imposed by the new generation mechanical ventilators: A lung model study. Respir Care 36:815–828, 1991; and Kirby RR, Banner MJ, Downs JB: Clinical Applications of Ventilatory Support. New York, Churchill Livingstone, 1990.)*

patient. Table 44-3 summarizes the four commercially available closed-loop systems. A study was performed to compare ARDS and COPD patients ventilated with a closed-loop mode termed *adaptive support ventilation* (ASV) available on the Hamilton Galileo ventilator. The authors found that on average, ARDS patients received lower tidal volumes with a higher respiratory rate than COPD patients did.[151] This would be expected and desired based on current knowledge of mechanics and the importance of low–tidal volume ventilation in ARDS. Moreover, the results support the possibility that closed-loop ventilation with ASV can appropriately tailor ventilation based on respiratory mechanics. It is highly conceivable that closed-loop ventilator modes may one day prove to be safer and more convenient than traditional mechanical ventilation.

Apnea Monitoring

The postoperative period is often characterized by episodes of apnea and hypoxemia. Paradoxical breathing and other ventilatory disturbances can also occur frequently. Though more common with narcotic administration, residual effects of other anesthetic agents can play a role in the cause of these disturbances. They are often subtle and are more likely to be noticed with continuous respiratory monitoring as opposed to intermittent observation.[152] A wide variety of continuous apnea monitoring systems have been developed. Most methods detect changes in chest wall movement, gas exchange, or gas flow to make inferences about changes in respiratory pattern.

Movement of the chest wall is most commonly detected by transthoracic impedance. The technology is usually incorporated into the electrocardiographic (ECG) monitoring system. A small current is passed between two ECG leads, and chest wall movement is detected by a change in impedance to the current induced by the motion. Respiratory inductive plethysmography (RIP) is another method of apnea detection that monitors chest movement. The chest and abdomen are encircled by one or more coils that measure changes in their cross-sectional area occurring with respiration. Inductance of the bands depends on the area that they enclose and thereby allows detection of respiratory movements. A technique called photoplethysmography (PPG) also relies on detection of anatomic changes induced by breathing. Infrared PPG sensors placed near upper extremity veins can detect cyclic changes in venous blood flow occurring with respiration.[153] Respiratory muscle electromyography has also been used as a means of monitoring respiration. A limitation common to all these techniques is that respiratory efforts during episodes of obstructive apnea may be interpreted as normal respirations despite absent gas flow.[154] Monitoring of gas flow and exchange may therefore be a more reliable indicator of adequate respiration.

Table 44-3 Main Characteristics of Proportional Assist Ventilation (PAV), Neurally Adjusted Ventilatory Assist (NAVA), Knowledge-Based System (KBS), and Adaptive Support Ventilation (ASV)

	PAV	NAVA	KBS	ASV
Principle	P_{insp} proportional to $flow_{insp}$	P_{insp} proportional to EMG_{dia}	P_{insp} to maintain RR in comfort zone	P_{insp} and RR to minimize WOB
Breath type	Spontaneous	Spontaneous	PSV	PSV, PCV, P-SIMV
Sedated patients	No	No	No	Yes
Active patients	Yes	Yes	Yes	Yes
Automatic weaning	No	No	Yes	Yes

EMG_{dia}, diaphragmatic electromyographic activity; $Flow_{insp}$, inspiratory flow; PCV, pressure-controlled ventilation; P-SIMV, pressure-controlled intermittent mandatory ventilation; PSV, pressure-support ventilation; RR, respiratory rate; WOB, work of breathing.
From Wysocki M, Brunner JX: Closed-loop ventilation: An emerging standard of care? Crit Care Clin 23:223-240, 2007.

Apnea monitoring systems that rely on airflow detection may be a more sensitive alternative to monitors of patient movement. In a study comparing transthoracic impedance and a nasal-oral airflow system in the PACU, Wiklund and colleagues found that impedance monitoring failed to detect apneic episodes more frequently than flow detection did.[154] False alarm rates were similar between the two groups. Hök and associates studied an acoustic airflow monitoring system and reported that it was more sensitive in detecting episodes of apnea and hypoventilation than pulse oximetry was.[155] Another acoustic airflow sensor was compared with a thoracic impedance system by Werthammer and colleagues.[155a] Of 26 apneic episodes observed by direct observation, the airflow sensor detected all 26, whereas only 7 episodes were detected by the impedance monitor. Other airflow monitors detect respiration by measuring changes in humidity. Tatara and Tsuzaki studied a device called a rapid-response hygrometer that monitors changes in humidity at the nostril and can measure respiratory rates of up to 60 breaths per minute.[156] Respiratory phases could be identified almost 2 seconds faster than with capnography. The development of fiberoptic humidity-based systems has also been described.[157,158]

Because end-tidal CO_2 monitoring and pulse oximetry can rapidly detect derangements in gas exchange, they may prove to be the most dependable options for apnea monitoring. In a study of more than 4000 apneic episodes from overnight polysomnograms, detection of apnea by pulse oximetry was compared with manual detection, such as airflow or respiratory movement.[158a] Only 1.32% of apneic episodes were reportedly missed by pulse oximetry, whereas manual devices missed 7.9% of apnea events. Although end-tidal CO_2 monitoring can be performed easily and accurately on intubated patients, measurements from a mask or nasal cannula are often unreliable. However, the respiratory rate is usually reported accurately, and trends in P_{ETCO_2} can be monitored with these devices. As pulse oximetry and capnography systems become more portable and inexpensive, their use for apnea monitoring will probably continue to grow. Large outcome studies may be needed to demonstrate the possible superiority of one system over another.

Lung Water Analysis

Many disease states can cause abnormal accumulation of extravascular lung water (EVLW), commonly known as pulmonary edema. Clinicians have long been aware of the severe cardiac and respiratory insufficiency that pulmonary edema can cause, yet it remains unclear whether accurately quantifying it can guide management in a way that ultimately improves outcome. Nonetheless, investigators continue to seek simple and reliable methods for detecting and quantifying EVLW, and many advances have been made in recent years. Research in this field is complicated by the fact that gravimetry, which requires analysis of postmortem lung weight, remains the standard for EVLW measurement.[159,160] As a result, much of the data evaluating new techniques come from animal studies.

Radiographic Methods

The chest radiograph is the most widely used test to screen for pulmonary edema. Under ideal conditions, obtaining a chest film allows semiquantitative measures of EVLW, as well as determination of its distribution and possible etiology. Even under such conditions, sensitivity is rather poor; a 30% to 35% increase in EVLW is needed before radiographic changes consistent with pulmonary edema can be detected on the chest film.[161] In typical critical care settings, where image quality and acquisition technique can vary greatly, it is estimated that a 100% increase in EVLW may be needed to produce observable radiographic changes. Moreover, weak correlation of EVLW measurements between chest radiography and other established methods has been observed in the ICU environment.[159]

CT has been increasingly studied in recent years as a means of quantification of EVLW. In animal experiments, CT densitometry could detect an increase in EVLW by as little as 50%.[162] Using thin-section CT, Scillia and colleagues found that significant hypoxemia secondary to pulmonary edema may not develop until the increase in EVLW approaches the 200% to 300% range.[163] Lack of portability and high radiation exposure limit the use of CT for serial EVLW measurement. Research continues on a number of other imaging modalities, including ultrasonography,[164] positron emission tomography,[165] nuclear magnetic resonance,[166] and EIT,[167] but none have been incorporated into routine clinical use.

Indicator Dilution Methods

Quantification of EVLW via double indicator dilution curves was first described more than 50 years ago. More recently, a transpulmonary thermodilution technique that uses cold saline as a single indicator has been described. Although controversy exists over the accuracy of dilution techniques, many studies report excellent reproducibility and correlation with gravimetric methods.[159] One study using transpulmonary thermodilution reported that changes in EVLW of as little as 10% to 20% can be detected with high sensitivity.[168] Both techniques are somewhat invasive and require placement of arterial and central venous catheters. Although early devices were quite cumbersome, currently available systems are relatively safe and easy to implement and allow bedside measurements to be obtained.

Despite recent improvements in a number of the aforementioned modalities, chest radiography remains the only tool widely integrated into clinical practice. A probable explanation is that studies have suggested potential clinical utility in precise EVLW analysis, but none have shown that obtaining such measurements facilitates decision-making or improves patient outcome.

Monitoring High-Frequency Ventilation

Recent data on the benefits of low–tidal volume, high-PEEP ventilation in ARDS have prompted a search for the optimal lung protective mode of ventilation. First introduced in the late 1950s, high-frequency ventilation (HFV) offers an alternative to conventional ventilation in patients with ARDS and ALI. HFV is characterized by rapid delivery of small tidal volumes and maintenance of high mean airway pressure.[169] Whereas routine use in adults is a fairly recent trend, trials in preterm infants with neonatal respiratory distress syndrome began almost 20 years ago.[170] Clear evidence of outcome benefit with HFV versus conventional ventilation is lacking, but numerous studies have implied that HFV may reduce the risk for ventilator-induced lung injury,[171] improve oxygenation,[172] and be as safe as conventional ventilation in ARDS.[173] The FDA has defined HFV as any form of ventilation that delivers a respiratory rate greater than 150 breaths/min. Although several forms of HFV have evolved since its development, the most widely used method in both adults and pediatric patients is high-frequency oscillatory ventilation (HFOV). Other modes include high-frequency jet ventilation (HFJV), high-frequency flow interruption (HFFI), and high-frequency percussive ventilation (HFPV). Before the widespread availability of HFV modes, a conventional ventilator was used to deliver low tidal volumes with high frequency, a technique that became known as high-frequency positive-pressure ventilation (HFPPV).

Because mechanisms of gas exchange during HFV differ from those regulating conventional ventilation, standard monitoring equipment may not provide accurate data. Fortunately, the reliability of pulse oximetry in assessing oxygenation status with other modes of ventilation seems to extend to HFV. Early studies showed a correlation between airway pressure and gas exchange efficiency during HFJV, with higher peak and driving pressures resulting in lower $Pa{CO_2}$ and higher $Pa{O_2}$. Monitoring P_{ETCO_2} conventionally during HFV produces unreliable measurements for a number of reasons, but mainly because of difficulty obtaining undiluted, CO_2-rich gas samples.[174,175] Though useful in monitoring conventional ventilation, the concept of "end-tidal" CO_2 is altogether misguided in HFV because no inspiratory or expiratory phases are identifiable on capnographic waveforms.[176] Moreover, the likelihood that expired CO_2 tensions accurately reflect $Pa{CO_2}$ is low in patients requiring HFV inasmuch as alveolar dead space and intrapulmonary shunting can be extensive.[174]

Despite its limitations, studies have demonstrated the ability of capnometry to provide accurate $Pa{CO_2}$ estimates during HFV. A common technique is to interrupt or slow the ventilator down to deliver a normal breath. CO_2 tensions measured with intermittent capnography have been shown to agree well with simultaneously obtained $Pa{CO_2}$ values.[177] The accuracy of capnometric $P{CO_2}$ readings may also depend on where the sample is obtained. Gas sampled from the distal tip of the endotracheal tube seems to provide more valid approximations of $Pa{CO_2}$ than sampling proximally does.[176] However, these measurements must also be obtained intermittently. In an effort to eliminate this problem and others associated with expired gas analysis during HFV, Berkenbosch and Tobias studied the accuracy of continuous transcutaneous CO_2 monitoring in this setting. When compared with $Pa{CO_2}$ values from BGA obtained simultaneously, bias and precision were only 2.1 and 2.7 mm Hg, respectively.[174] Studies by these authors and other investigators have also demonstrated that transcutaneous CO_2 monitoring may approximate $Pa{CO_2}$ better than P_{ETCO_2} in both adults and children undergoing mechanical ventilation.[178,179] Although the technique has gained a footing in pediatric critical care, transcutaneous O_2 and CO_2 monitoring in adults will probably increase in popularity as refinements to this technology continue to be made.

As the potential benefits of HFV continue to be elucidated, investigators have sought practical techniques for bedside monitoring of lung mechanics, recruitment, and regional aeration. Portable chest radiography has been shown to be a poor tool for assessing lung morphology in ARDS.[179,180] CT has proved useful for such analyses but continues to be limited by portability issues. Recently, some investigators have focused on EIT and RIP as modalities that may be able to provide accurate lung volume measurements at the bedside during HFV.[181,182] RIP has been used experimentally to construct PV curves during HFV and thereby determine optimal lung volume and pressure settings.[183,184] In the first infant study of this kind, Tingay and colleagues used the open-lung concept to recruit lung and then map the deflation limb of the PV curve.[185,186] The authors concluded that RIP could be used during HFOV to construct satisfactory deflation curves. Ventilation along the deflation limb resulted in greater lung volume and oxygenation, often with lower distending pressure requirements, than did ventilation on the inflation limb (Fig. 44-26). This was in line with previous animal studies demonstrating improved mechanics and oxygenation with deflation limb ventilation after recruitment.[117] An earlier infant trial using single-occlusion compliance measurements failed to demonstrate the utility of PV curves in optimizing lung volume during HFV, but neither recruitment maneuvers nor deflation limb ventilation had been used.[187] EIT has the advantage of providing information about global and regional changes in lung volume, as well as continuous imaging of changes in impedance (and probably volume) occurring throughout the respiratory cycle. Bedside availability would potentially allow clinicians to detect aeration changes in real time and reverse them by adjusting ventilation parameters.[182]

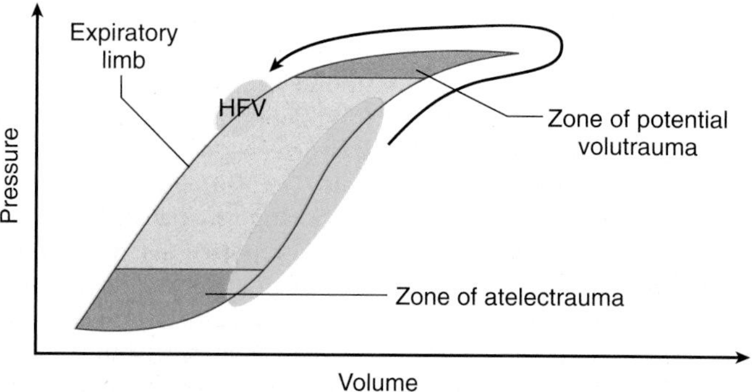

Figure 44-26 Pressure-volume curve depicting the "open lung" concept using high-frequency ventilation (HFV). Potential lung injury is reduced when ventilation of the lung is shifted onto the expiratory portion of the curve by aggressive lung recruitment. Lung volume is then maintained with high mean airway pressure and small tidal volumes. *(From Singh JM, Stewart TE: High-frequency ventilation.* In *Fink MP, Abraham E, Vincent JL, et al [eds]: Textbook of Critical Care, 5th ed. Philadelphia, Elsevier, 2005.)*

Estimation of pulmonary mechanics during HFV has most often been accomplished by the conventional passive techniques described earlier. This practice has raised concern among some authors, who argue that technical aspects of these strategies may exacerbate derecruitment and provide inadequate information about lung parenchyma.[187] In the study by Tingay and colleagues, passive deflation was not used for PV analysis, and derecruitment was further prevented by avoiding full deflation of the lung below closing pressure. Others suggest that the high frequencies and flow rates associated with HFV currently limit the feasibility of obtaining accurate dynamic measurements. Thus, efforts have been undertaken to identify safe alternatives for reliably assessing lung compliance and determining optimal airway pressure during

HFV. The oscillatory pressure ratio (OPR), defined as the ratio of pressure swings at the distal and proximal ends of the endotracheal tube, was shown to be inversely related to lung compliance in an animal model of ALI.[188] The mPaw setting resulting in the lowest OPR also generated the best lung compliance and oxygenation. Titrating mPaw to a minimal OPR may therefore prove to be a reliable, noninvasive means of optimizing lung mechanics and oxygenation during HFV. The low-frequency forced oscillation technique is another experimental monitor that allows partitioning of lung mechanics into airway and parenchymal components, as well as determination of chest wall impedance.[189] Monitoring chest vibration can provide a crude indicator of changes in compliance during HFOV. Oscillator power is often titrated to generate vibrations from the clavicle down to the mid-portion of the thigh, and a change in pattern may signal the development of an obstruction, pneumothorax, or worsening mechanics of any etiology.

Monitoring the Respiratory System in Transport

Intrahospital transport of critically ill and mechanically ventilated patients becomes necessary in a number of situations (see Chapter 79). The need for diagnostic or surgical procedures is among the most frequent reasons for patient transport. A number of studies have reported on the high number of transports that critically ill patients require.[190] Children and trauma victims seem to require more frequent transportation for diagnostic purposes than other critically ill patients do. Not surprisingly, intrahospital transport of this tenuous patient population can be fraught with problems ranging from simple equipment malfunction to major disasters such as anoxic brain injury and even death. Studies report a widely varying incidence of adverse events during transportation of critically ill patients. Complex and numerous pieces of equipment are often necessary to safely perform the transfer. One study looking at 125 transports from the ICU found a 34% incidence of equipment-related adverse events, the most common being ECG lead disconnection and monitor power failure.[190]

Lack of agreed-upon monitoring techniques and definitions of "adverse events" partly explains the wide discrepancy in reported incidence. Moreover, few outcome studies comparing monitoring strategies during transport have been performed. It has long been observed, however, that transport of critically ill patients may put them at increased risk for cardiovascular and respiratory compromise, both during and after transport.[191] A higher incidence of gas exchange deterioration and even pneumonia has been reported after intrahospital transport.[192,193] Arrhythmias, hypotensive episodes, and blood gas derangements are not uncommon. Studies in trauma patients have revealed widely variable heart rate and blood pressure during transportation for diagnostic procedures.[194] Thus, a continually displayed electrocardiogram and blood pressure must be available during transport of all critically ill patients. In addition, pulse oximetry should be used in light of its high reliability in forewarning of hypoxemia and deterioration in gas exchange. A good rule of thumb is to monitor critically ill patients at least as closely during transport as deemed necessary within the ICU before transport. Complications are reduced when personnel trained to deal with the intricacies of intrahospital transport are available.[195] Emergency cardiovascular drugs should be available for postoperative transport of all hemodynamically unstable and critically ill subjects. Preparation of equipment and medication checklists before transport can help ensure readiness for any untoward events. The receiving location should confirm before transport that it has the equipment and necessary staff in place to receive the patient.

Transport of a mechanically ventilated patient presents the inherent risks of airway loss and further derangements in gas exchange. Equipment and medications needed to establish and maintain a secure airway must accompany such patients during any transfer. The presence of adequate oxygen supply with properly functioning low-pressure alarms should be verified during pretransport preparation. Many authors advocate the use of a mechanical ventilator rather than manual ventilation devices for intrahospital transport because more variability in pH and CO_2 tension has been observed with the use of manual devices.[196] A higher incidence of significant PaO_2/FIO_2 deterioration may also be associated with manual versus mechanical ventilation (P = .056).[196] In a blinded study using capnography, Tobias and associates noted a high incidence of unintentional hyperventilation when using manual devices during the intrahospital transfer of intubated pediatric patients.[197] Similar findings have been noted in adults, and tighter control of $PaCO_2$ can be achieved if $PETCO_2$[198] or VT is monitored during manual ventilation. These findings have led many experts to recommend $PETCO_2$ monitoring in addition to standard monitoring for high-risk patients requiring a more optimal level of ventilation.

Obvious contraindications to the transport of critically ill patients include an inability to provide adequate oxygenation and ventilation during transport or at the receiving location. Unstable hemodynamics or an inability to adequately monitor cardiovascular status throughout the trip should prompt postponement or cancellation. The risk-benefit ratio should be considered before all transports to help determine whether a trip is truly warranted; performing such analyses may be the most effective way of avoiding adverse events during transportation. Indeck and coworkers found that 68% of patients transferred from a trauma unit for diagnostic testing experienced serious physiologic changes whereas only 24% of the transfers resulted in significant modification of patient management.[199] The development of increasingly sophisticated portable devices has provided a bedside alternative for many diagnostic and therapeutic procedures.

References

1. deMicheli A: [Regarding respiration and the so-called "animal heat." A historical sketch.] Rev Invest Clin 53:462-467, 2001.
2. Haldane JS, Priestley JG: The regulation of the lung-ventilation. J Physiol 32:225-266, 1905.
3. Nunn JF: Alveolar air equations. Anesthesiology 85:946, 1996.
4. Frank SM, Fleisher LA, Olson KF, et al: Multivariate determinants of early postoperative oxygen consumption in elderly patients. Effects of shivering, body temperature, and gender. Anesthesiology 83:241-249, 1995.
5. Riley RL, Lilienthal JL, Proemmel DO, Franke RE: On the determination of the physiologically effective pressures of oxygen and carbon dioxide. Am J Physiol 147:191-198, 1946.
6. Story DA: Alveolar oxygen partial pressure, alveolar carbon dioxide partial pressure, and the alveolar gas equation. Anesthesiology 84:1011, 1996.
7. Hlastala MP: Ventilation/perfusion: From the bench to the patient. Cardiologia 41:405-415, 1996.
8. Filley GF, MacIntosh DJ, Wright GW: Carbon monoxide uptake and pulmonary diffusing capacity in normal subjects at rest and during exercise. J Clin Invest 33:530-539, 1954.
9. Lumb AB: Nunn's Applied Respiratory Physiology, 6th ed. Elsevier, Butterworth Heinemann, 2005, pp 140, 125-126, 128-129.
10. Jones JG, Jones SE: Discriminating between the effect of shunt and reduced $\dot{V}A/\dot{Q}$ on arterial oxygen saturation is particularly useful in clinical practice. J Clin Monit Comput 16:337-350, 2000.
11. Hlastala MP, Glenny RW: Vascular structure determines pulmonary blood flow distribution. News Physiol Science 14:182-186, 1999.
12. Lundquist H, Hedenstierna G, Strandberg A, et al: CT-assessment of dependent lung densities in man during general anesthesia. Acta Radiol 36:626-632, 1995.
13. Warner DO, Warner MA, Ritman EL: Atelectasis and chest wall shape during halothane anesthesia. Anesthesiology 85:49-59, 1996.
14. Wagner PD, Laravuso RB, Uhl RR, West JB: Continuous distributions of ventilation-perfusion ratios in normal subjects breathing air and 100 per cent O_2. J Clin Invest 54:54-68, 1974.
15. Hope DA, Jenkins BJ, Willis N, et al: Non-invasive estimation of venous admixture: Validation of a new formula. Br J Anaesth 74:538-543, 1995.
16. Feihl F, Eckert P, Brimioulle S, et al: Permissive hypercapnia impairs pulmonary gas exchange in the acute respiratory distress syndrome. Am J Respir Crit Care Med 162:209-215, 2000.
17. Hachenberg T, Tenling A, Nyström SO, et al: Ventilation-perfusion inequality in patients undergoing cardiac surgery. Anesthesiology 80:509-529, 1994.
18. Andersson L, Lagerstrand L, Thörne A, et al: Effect of CO_2 pneumoperitoneum on ventilation-perfusion relationships during laparoscopic cholecystectomy. Acta Anaesthesiol Scand 46:552-560, 2002.
19. Tokics L, Hedenstierna G, Svensson L, et al: $\dot{V}/\dot{Q}$ distribution and correlation to atelectasis in anesthetized paralyzed humans. J Appl Physiol 81:1822-1833, 1996.
20. Severinghaus JW, Bradley AF: Electrodes of blood Po_2 and Pco_2 determination. J Appl Physiol 13:515-520, 1958.
21. Clark LC Jr, Wolf R, Granger D, Taylor Z: Continuous recording of blood oxygen tension by polarography. J Appl Physiol 6:189-193, 1953.
22. Severinghaus JW: First electrodes for blood Po_2 and Pco_2 determination. J Appl Physiol 97:1599-1600, 2004.
23. Severinghaus JW, Astrup P, Murray JF: Blood gas analysis and critical care medicine. Am J Respir Crit Care Med 157:S114-S122, 1998.
24. Schmidt C, Müller-Plathe O: Stability of Po_2, Pco_2 and pH in heparinized whole blood samples: Influence of storage temperature with regard to leukocyte count and syringe material. Eur J Clin Chem Clin Biochem 30:767-773, 1992.
25. Robertson PW, Hart BB: Assessment of tissue oxygenation. Respir Care Clin N Am 5:221-263, 1999.
26. Lubbers DW, Opitz N: The pco_2-/po_2-optode: A new probe for measurement of pco_2 or po_2 in fluids and gases (authors' transl). Z Naturforsch [C] 30:532-533, 1975.
27. Bland JM, Altman DG: Statistical methods for assessing agreement between two methods of clinical measurement. Lancet 1:307-310, 1986.
28. Ganter M, Zollinger A: Continuous intravascular blood gas monitoring: Development, current techniques, and clinical use of a commercial device. Br J Anaesth 91:397-407, 2003.
29. Ganter MT: Accuracy and performance of a modified continuous intravascular blood gas monitoring device during thoracoscopic surgery. J Cardiothorac Vasc Anesth 18:587-591, 2004.
30. Weiss IK, Fink S, Harrison R, et al: Clinical use of continuous arterial blood gas monitoring in the pediatric intensive care unit. Pediatrics 103:440-445, 1999.
31. Coule LW, Truemper EJ, Steinhart CM, Lutin WA: Accuracy and utility of a continuous intra-arterial blood gas monitoring system in pediatric patients. Crit Care Med 29:420-426, 2001.
32. Hatherill M, Tibby SM, Durward A, et al: Continuous intra-arterial blood-gas monitoring in infants and children with cyanotic heart disease. Br J Anaesth 79:665-667, 1997.
33. Venkatesh B, Pigott DW, Fernandez A, Hendry SP: Continuous measurement of arterial blood gas status during total hip replacement: A prospective study. Anaesth Intensive Care 24:334-341, 1996.
34. Larson CP Jr, Vender J, Seiver A: Multisite evaluation of a continuous intraarterial blood gas monitoring system. Anesthesiology 81:543-552, 1994.
35. Aschkenasy SV, Hofer CK, Zalunardo MP, et al: Patterns of changes in arterial Po_2 during one-lung ventilation: A comparison between patients with severe pulmonary emphysema and patients with preserved lung function. J Cardiothorac Vasc Anesth 19:479-484, 2005.
36. Pavlidis T, Papaziogas B, Vretzakis G, et al: Continuous monitoring of arterial blood gases and pH during laparoscopic cholecystectomy using a Paratrend sensor. Minerva Chir 57:17-22, 2002.
37. Severinghaus JW: Takuo Aoyagi: Discovery of pulse oximetry. Anesth Analg 105(6 Suppl):S1-S4, 2007.
38. Wouters PF, Gehring H, Meyfroid G, et al: Accuracy of pulse oximeters: The European multi-center trial. Anesth Analg 94:S13-S16, 2002.
39. Hannhart B, Haberer JP, Saunier C, Laxenaire MC: Accuracy and precision of fourteen pulse oximeters. Eur Respir J 4:115-122, 1991.
40. Tobin RM, Pologe JA, Batchelder PB: A characterization of motion affecting pulse oximetry in 350 patients. Anesth Analg 94:S54-S61, 2002.
41. Bebout DE, Mannheimer PD, Wun CC: Site-dependent differences in the time t o detect changes in saturation during low perfusion [abstract]. Crit Care Med 29:A115, 2001.
42. Welch JP, DeCesare R, Hess D: Pulse oximetry: Instrumentation and clinical application. Respir Care 35:584-601, 1990.
43. Salyer JW: Neonatal and pediatric pulse oximetry. Respir Care 48:386-396, 2003.
44. Jay GD, Hughes L, Renzi FP: Pulse oximetry is accurate in acute anemia from hemorrhage. Ann Emerg Med 24:32-35, 1994.
45. Severinghaus JW, Koh SO: Effect of anemia on pulse oximeter accuracy at low saturation. J Clin Monit 6:85-88, 1990.
46. Ralston AC, Webb RK, Runciman WB: Potential errors in pulse oximetry. III: Effects of interferences, dyes, dyshaemoglobins and other pigments. Anaesthesia 46:291-295, 1991.
47. Craft JA, Alessandrini E, Kenney LB, et al: Comparison of oxygenation measurements in pediatric patients during sickle cell crises. J Pediatr 124:93-95, 1994.
48. Katoh R, Miyake T, Arai T: Unexpectedly low pulse oximeter readings in a boy with unstable hemoglobin Köln. Anesthesiology 80:472-474, 1994.
49. Next-generation pulse oximetry. Health Devices 32:47-87, 2003.
50. Bohnhorst B, Poets CF: Major reduction in alarm frequency with a new pulse oximeter. Intensive Care Med 24:277-278, 1998.
51. Irita K, Kai Y, Akiyoshi K, et al: Performance evaluation of a new pulse oximeter during mild hypothermic cardiopulmonary bypass. Anesth Analg 96:11-14, 2003.
52. Durban CG, Rostow SK: Advantages of new technology pulse oximetry with adults in extremis. Anesth Analg 94:S81-S83, 2002.
53. O'Malley GF: Non-invasive carbon monoxide measurement is not accurate. Ann Emerg Med 48:477-478, 2006.
54. Suner S, Partridge R, Sucov A, et al: Non-invasive screening for carbon monoxide toxicity in the emergency department is valuable. Ann Emerg Med 49:718-719, author reply 719, 2007.
55. Barker SJ, Curry J, Redford D, Morgan S: Measurement of carboxyhemoglobin and methemoglobin by pulse oximetry: A human volunteer study. Anesthesiology 107:892-897, 2007.
56. Dassel ACM, Graaff R, Sikkema M, et al: Reflectance pulse oximetry at the forehead improves by pressure on the probe. J Clin Monit 11:237-244, 1995.
57. East CE, Brennecke SP, King JF, et al: The effect of intrapartum fetal pulse oximetry, in the presence of a nonreassuring fetal heart rate pattern, on operative delivery rates: A multicenter, randomized, controlled trial (the FOREMOST trial). Am J Obstet Gynecol 194:606.e1-606.e16, 2006.
58. Kyriacou PA, Powell SL, Jones DP, Langford RM: Evaluation of oesophageal pulse oximetry in patients undergoing cardiothoracic surgery. Anaesthesia 58:422-427, 2003.
59. Fournell A, Schwarte LA, Scheeren TW, et al: Assessment of microvascular oxygen saturation in gastric mucosa in volunteers breathing continuous positive airway pressure. Crit Care Med 31:1705-1710, 2003.
60. Nijland R, Jongsma HW, van den Berg PP, et al: The effects of pulsating arteries on reflectance pulse oximetry: Measurements in adults and neonates. J Clin Monit 11:118-122, 1995.
61. Moller JT, Pederson T, Rasmussen LS: Randomized evaluation of pulse oximetry in 20,802 patients: I.

Design, demography, pulse oximetry failure rate, and overall complication rate. Anesthesiology 78:436-444, 1993.
62. Young D, Griffiths J: Clinical trials of monitoring in anaesthesia, critical care and acute ward care: A review. Br J Anaesth 97:39-45, 2006.
63. Ochroch EA, Russell MW, Hanson WC 3rd et al: The impact of continuous pulse oximetry monitoring on intensive care unit admissions from a postsurgical care floor. Anesth Analg 102:868-875, 2006.
64. Moller JT, Johannessen NN, Espersen K, et al: Randomized evaluation of pulse oximetry in 20,802 patients: II. Perioperative events and postoperative complications. Anesthesiology 78:445-453, 1993.
65. Wheatley RG, Shepherd D, Jackson IJ, et al: Hypoxaemia and pain relief after upper abdominal surgery: Comparison of i.m. and patient-controlled analgesia. Br J Anaesth 69:558-561, 1992.
66. Rosenberg J, Oturai P, Erichsen CJ, et al: Effect of general anesthesia and major versus minor surgery on late postoperative episodic and constant hypoxemia. J Clin Anesth 6:212-216, 1994.
67. Gill NP, Wright B, Reilly CS: Relationship between hypoxaemic and cardiac ischaemic events in the perioperative period. Br J Anaesth 68:471-473, 1992.
68. Jubran A, Tobin MJ: Reliability of pulse oximetry in titrating supplemental oxygen therapy in ventilator-dependent patients. Chest 97:1420-1425, 1990.
69. Bierman MI, Stein KL, Snyder JV: Pulse oximetry in the postoperative care of cardiac surgical patients: A randomized controlled trial. Chest 102:1367-1370, 1992.
70. Shamir M, Eidelman LA, Floman Y, et al: Pulse oximetry plethysmographic waveform during changes in blood volume. Br J Anaesth 82:178-181, 1999.
71. Monnet X, Lamia B, Teboul JL: Pulse oximeter as a sensor of fluid responsiveness: Do we have our finger on the best solution? Crit Care 9:429-430, 2005.
72. Michard F, Boussat S, Chemla D, et al: Relation between respiratory changes in arterial pulse pressure and fluid responsiveness in septic patients with acute circulatory failure. Am J Respir Crit Care Med 162:134-138, 2000.
73. Cannesson M, Besnard C, Durand PG, et al: Relation between respiratory variations in pulse oximetry plethysmographic waveform amplitude and arterial pulse pressure in ventilated patients. Crit Care 9:R562-R568, 2005.
74. Cannesson M, Attof Y, Rosamel P, et al: Respiratory variations in pulse oximetry plethysmographic waveform amplitude to predict fluid responsiveness in the operating room. Anesthesiology 106:1105-1111, 2007.
75. Feissel M, Teboul JL, Merlani P, et al: Plethysmographic dynamic indices predict fluid responsiveness in septic ventilated patients. Intensive Care Med 33:993-999, 2007.
76. Shelley KH, Jablonka DH, Awad AA, et al: What is the best site for measuring the effect of ventilation on the pulse oximeter waveform? Anesth Analg 103:372-377, 2006.
77. Mowafi HA: The efficacy of plethysmographic pulse wave amplitude as an indicator for intravascular injection of epinephrine-containing epidural test dose in anesthetized adults. Anesth Analg 101:1506-1511, 2005.
78. Uemura A, Yagihara M, Miyabe M: Pulse oximeter perfusion index as a predictor for the effect of pediatric epidural block. Anesthesiology 105:A1354, 2006.
79. Hager H, Church S, Mandadi G, et al: The perfusion index measured by a pulse oximeter indicates pain stimuli in anesthetized volunteers. Anesthesiology 101:A514, 2004.
80. Beal AL, Cerra FB: Multiple organ failure syndrome in the 1990s: Systemic inflammatory response and organ dysfunction. JAMA 271:226-233, 1994.
81. Rivers E, Nguyen B, Havstad S, et al, for the Early Goal-Directed Therapy Collaborative Group: Early goal-directed therapy in the treatment of severe sepsis and septic shock. N Engl J Med 345:1368-1377, 2001.
82. Räsänen J, Downs JB, DeHaven B: Titration of continuous positive airway pressure by real-time dual oximetry. Chest 92:853-856, 1987.
83. Connett RJ, Honig CR, Gayeski TE, Brooks GA: Defining hypoxia: A systems view of Vo_2, glycolysis, energetics, and intracellular Po_2. J Appl Physiol 68:833-842, 1990.
84. Dings J, Meixensberger J, Jager A, Roosen K: Clinical experience with 118 brain tissue oxygen partial pressure catheter probes. Neurosurgery 43:1082-1095, 1998.
85. Hockel M, Knoop C, Schlenger K, et al: Intratumoral po_2 predicts survival in advanced cancer of the uterine cervix. Radiother Oncol 26:45-50, 1993.
86. McCormick PW, Stewart M, Goetting MG, et al: Noninvasive cerebral optical spectroscopy for monitoring cerebral oxygen delivery and hemodynamics. Crit Care Med 19:89-97, 1991.
87. Kavanagh MC, Tsang V, Chow S, et al: A comparison in individual murine tumors of techniques for measuring oxygen levels. Int J Radiat Oncol Biol Phys 44:1137-1146, 1999.
88. Barnes PJ, Liew FY: Nitric oxide and asthmatic inflammation. Immunol Today 16:128-130, 1995.
89. Gabriele C, Nieuwhof EM, Van Der Wiel EC, et al: Exhaled nitric oxide differentiates airway diseases in the first two years of life. Pediatr Res 60:461-465, 2006.
90. Dupont LJ, Demedts MG, Verleden GM: Prospective evaluation of the validity of exhaled nitric oxide for the diagnosis of asthma. Chest 123:751-756, 2003.
91. Purtz EP, Hess D, Kacmarek RM: Evaluation of electrochemical nitric oxide and nitrogen dioxide analyzers suitable for use during mechanical ventilation. J Clin Monit 13:25-34, 1997.
92. Strauss JM, Krohn S, Sümpelmann R, et al: Evaluation of two electrochemical monitors for measurement of inhaled nitric oxide. Anaesthesia 51:151-154, 1996.
93. Bernareggi M, Cremona G: Measurement of exhaled nitric oxide in humans and animals. Pulm Pharmacol Ther 12:331-352, 1999.
94. Etches PC, Harris ML, McKinley R, Finer NN: Clinical monitoring of inhaled nitric oxide: Comparison of chemiluminescent and electrochemical sensors. Biomed Instrum Technol 29:134-140, 1995.
95. Roller C, Namjou K, Jeffers J, et al: Simultaneous NO and CO_2 measurement in human breath with a single IV-VI mid-infrared laser. Opt Lett 27:107-109, 2002.
96. Nishimura M, Imanaka H, Uchiyama A, et al: Nitric oxide (NO) measurement accuracy. J Clin Monit 13:241-248, 1997.
97. Shibutani K, Muraoka M, Shirasaki S, et al: Do changes in end-tidal Pco_2 quantitatively reflect changes in cardiac output? Anesth Analg 79:829-833, 1994.
98. Tavernier B, Rey D, Thevenin D, et al: Can prolonged expiration manoeuvres improve the prediction of arterial Pco_2 from end-tidal Pco_2? Br J Anaesth 78:536-540, 1997.
99. Bhavani-Shankar K, Kumar AY, Moseley HS, Ahyee-Hallsworth R: Terminology and the current limitations of time capnography: A brief review. J Clin Monit 11:175-182, 1995.
100. Rich GF, Sconzo JM: Continuous end-tidal CO_2 sampling within the proximal endotracheal tube estimates arterial CO_2 tension in infants. Can J Anaesth 38:201-203, 1991.
101. Bhavani-Shankar K: Negative arterial to end-tidal CO_2 gradients in children. Can J Anaesth 41:1125-1126, 1994.
102. Kwetny I, Finucane BT: Negative arterial to end-tidal carbon dioxide gradient: An additional sign of malignant hyperthermia during desflurane anesthesia. Anesth Analg 102:815-817, 2006.
103. Breen PH, Mazumdar B, Skinner SC: Comparison of end-tidal Pco_2 and average alveolar expired Pco_2 during positive end-expiratory pressure. Anesth Analg 82:368-373, 1996.
104. Fletcher R: Relationship between alveolar deadspace and arterial oxygenation in children with congenital cardiac disease. Br J Anaesth 62:168-176, 1989.
105. Breen PH, Bradley PJ: Carbon dioxide spirogram (but not capnogram) detects leaking inspiratory valve in a circle circuit. Anesth Analg 85:1372-1376, 1997.
106. Verschuren F, Heinonen E, Clause D, et al: Volumetric capnography as a bedside monitoring of thrombolysis in major pulmonary embolism. Intensive Care Med 30:2129-2132, 2004.
107. Sanders AB: Capnometry in emergency medicine. Ann Emerg Med 18:1287-1290, 1989.
108. Ranieri VM, Suter PM, Tortorella C, et al: Effect of mechanical ventilation on inflammatory mediators in patients with acute respiratory distress syndrome: A randomized controlled trial. JAMA 282:54-61, 1999.
109. Ventilation with lower tidal volumes as compared with traditional tidal volumes for acute lung injury and the acute respiratory distress syndrome. The Acute Respiratory Distress Syndrome Network. N Engl J Med 342:1301-1308, 2000.
110. Muscedere JG, Mullen JB, Gan K, Slutsky AS: Tidal ventilation at low airway pressures can augment lung injury. Am J Respir Crit Care Med 149:1327-1334, 1994.
111. Amato MB, Barbas CS, Medeiros DM, et al: Effect of a protective-ventilation strategy on mortality in the acute respiratory distress syndrome. N Engl J Med 338:347-354, 1998.
112. Maggiore SM, Jonson B, Richard JC, et al: Alveolar derecruitment at decremental positive end-expiratory pressure levels in acute lung injury: Comparison with the lower inflection point, oxygenation, and compliance. Am J Respir Crit Care Med 164:795-801, 2001.
113. Rimmensberger PC, Pristine G, Mullen BM, et al: Lung recruitment during small tidal volume ventilation allows minimal positive end-expiratory pressure without augmenting lung injury. Crit Care Med 27:1940-1945, 1999.
114. Roupie E, Dambrosio M, Servillao G, et al: Titration of tidal volume and induced hypercapnia in acute respiratory distress syndrome. Am J Respir Crit Care Med 152:121-128, 1995.
115. Hickling KG: Best compliance during a decremental, but not incremental, positive end-expiratory pressure trial is related to open-lung positive end-expiratory pressure: A mathematical model of acute respiratory distress syndrome lungs. Am J Respir Crit Care Med 163:69-78, 2001.

116. Marini JJ, Gattinoni L: Ventilatory management of acute respiratory distress syndrome: A consensus of two. Crit Care Med 32:250-255, 2004.
117. Mergoni M, Volpi A, Bricchi C, Rossi A: Lower inflection point and recruitment with PEEP in ventilated patients with acute respiratory failure. J Appl Physiol 91:441-450, 2001.
118. van Genderingen HR, van Vught AJ, Duval EL, et al: Attenuation of pressure swings along the endotracheal tube is indicative of optimal distending pressure during high-frequency oscillatory ventilation in a model of acute lung injury. Pediatr Pulmonol 33:429-436, 2002.
119. Tingay DG, Mills JF, Morley CJ, et al: The deflation limb of the pressure-volume relationship in infants during high-frequency ventilation. Am J Respir Crit Care Med 173:414-420, 2006.
120. Suh GY, Koh Y, Chung MP, et al: Repeated derecruitments accentuate lung injury during mechanical ventilation. Crit Care Med 30:1848-1853, 2002.
121. Fujino Y, Goddon S, Dolhnikoff M, et al: Repetitive high-pressure recruitment maneuvers required to maximally recruit lung in a sheep model of acute respiratory distress syndrome. Crit Care Med 29:1579-1586, 2001.
122. Ranieri VM, Giuliani R, Fiore T, et al: Volume-pressure curve of the respiratory system predicts effects of PEEP in ARDS: "Occlusion" versus "constant flow" technique. Am J Respir Crit Care Med 149:19-27, 1994.
123. Albaiceta GM, Piacentini E, Villagrá A, et al: Application of continuous positive airway pressure to trace static pressure-volume curves of the respiratory system. Crit Care Med 31:2514-2519, 2003.
124. Suter PM, Fairley B, Isenberg MD: Optimum end-expiratory airway pressure in patients with acute pulmonary failure. N Engl J Med 292:284-289, 1975.
125. Gunnarsson L, Tokics L, Gustavsson H, Hedenstierna G: Influence of age on atelectasis formation and gas exchange impairment during general anaesthesia. Br J Anaesth 66:423-432, 1991.
126. Tokics L, Hedenstierna G, Strandberg A, et al: Lung collapse and gas exchange during general anesthesia: Effects of spontaneous breathing, muscle paralysis, and positive end-expiratory pressure. Anesthesiology 66:157-167, 1987.
127. Pelosi P, Ravagnan I, Giurati G, et al: Positive end-expiratory pressure improves respiratory function in obese but not in normal subjects during anesthesia and paralysis. Anesthesiology 91:1221-1231, 1999.
128. Tusman G, Böhm SH, Vazquez de Anda GF, et al: Alveolar recruitment strategy improves arterial oxygenation during general anaesthesia. Br J Anaesth 82:8-13, 1999.
129. Dyhr T, Laursen N, Larsson A: Effects of lung recruitment maneuver and positive end-expiratory pressure on lung volume, respiratory mechanics and alveolar gas mixing in patients ventilated after cardiac surgery. Acta Anaesthesiol Scand 46:717-725, 2002.
130. Papadakos PJ, Lachmann B: The open lung concept of alveolar recruitment can improve outcome in respiratory failure and ARDS. Mt Sinai J Med 69:73-77, 2002.
131. Grasso S, Mascia L, Del Turco M, et al: Effects of recruiting maneuvers in patients with acute respiratory distress syndrome ventilated with protective ventilatory strategy. Anesthesiology 96:795-802, 2002.
132. Schreiter D, Reske A, Stichert B, et al: Alveolar recruitment in combination with sufficient positive end-expiratory pressure increases oxygenation and lung aeration in patients with severe chest trauma. Crit Care Med 32:968-975, 2004.
133. Talmor D, Sarge T, Legedza A, et al: Cytokine release following recruitment maneuvers. Chest 132:1434-1439, 2007.
134. Reis Miranda D, Klompe L, Mekel J, et al: Open lung ventilation does not increase right ventricular outflow impedance: An echo-Doppler study. Crit Care Med 34:2555-2560, 2006.
135. Gattinoni L, Caironi P, Valenza F, Carlesso E: The role of CT-scan studies for the diagnosis and therapy of acute respiratory distress syndrome. Clin Chest Med 27:559-570, 2006.
136. Gattinoni L, Caironi P, Cressoni M, et al: Lung recruitment in patients with the acute respiratory distress syndrome. N Engl J Med 354:1775-1786, 2006.
137. Levy MM: PEEP in ARDS—how much is enough? N Engl J Med 351:389-391, 2004.
138. Gattinoni L, Caironi P, Pelosi P, Goodman LR: What has computed tomography taught us about the acute respiratory distress syndrome? Am J Respir Crit Care Med 164:1701-1711, 2001.
139. van Genderingen HR, van Vught AJ, Jansen JR: Estimation of regional volume changes by electrical impedance pressure tomography during a pressure-volume maneuver. Intensive Care Med 29:233-240, 2003.
140. Frerichs I, Dargaville PA, Dudykevych T, Rimensberger PC: Electrical impedance tomography: A method for monitoring regional lung aeration and tidal volume distribution. Intensive Care Med 29:2312-2316, 2003.
141. Gattinoni L, D'Andrea L, Pelosi P, et al: Regional effects and mechanism of positive end-expiratory pressure in early respiratory distress syndrome. JAMA 269:2122-2127, 1993.
142. Victorino JA, Borges JB, Okamato VN, et al: Imbalances in regional lung ventilation: A validation study on electrical impedance tomography. Am J Respir Crit Care Med 169:791-800, 2004.
143. Kacmarek RM, Cycyk-Chapman MC, Young-Palazzo PJ, Romagnoli DM: Comparison of two techniques for the determination of maximal inspiratory pressure (MIP) in mechanically ventilated patients. Respir Care 39:868-878, 1989.
144. Yang KL, Tobin MJ: A prospective study of indexes predicting the outcome of trials of weaning from mechanical ventilation. N Engl J Med 324:1445-1450, 1991.
145. Stewart TE: Establishing an approach to mechanical ventilation. Can Respir J 3:403-408, 1996.
146. Benditt JO: Esophageal and gastric pressure measurements. Respir Care 50:68-75, discussion 75-77, 2005.
147. Roussos C, Zakynthinos S: Fatigue of the respiratory muscles. Intensive Care Med 22:134-155, 1996.
148. Bellani G, Patroniti N, Weismann D, et al: Measurement of pressure-time product during spontaneous assisted breathing by rapid interrupter technique. Anesthesiology 106:484-490, 2007.
149. Pesenti A, Pelosi P, Foti G, et al: An interrupter technique for measuring respiratory mechanics and the pressure generated by respiratory muscles during partial ventilatory support. Chest 102:918-923, 1992.
150. Wysocki M, Brunner JX: Closed-loop ventilation: An emerging standard of care? Crit Care Clin 23:223-240, ix, 2007.
151. Arnal JM, Nafati C, Wysocki M, et al: Utilization of adaptive support ventilation (ASV) in a polyvalent intensive care unit [abstract]. Intensive Care Med 30:S84, 2004.
152. Catley DM, Thornton C, Jordan C, et al: Pronounced, episodic oxygen desaturation in the postoperative period: Its association with ventilatory pattern and analgesic regimen. Anesthesiology 63:20-28, 1985.
153. Nilsson L, Johansson A, Kalman S: Monitoring of respiratory rate in postoperative care using a new photoplethysmographic technique. J Clin Monit Comput 16:309-315, 2000.
154. Wiklund L, Hök B, Ståhl K, Jordeby-Jönsson A: Postanesthesia monitoring revisited: Frequency of true and false alarms from different monitoring devices. J Clin Anesth 6:182-188, 1994.
155. Hök B, Wiklund L, Henneberg S: A new respiratory rate monitor: Development and initial clinical experience. Int J Clin Monit Comput 10:101-107, 1993.
155a. Werthammer J, Krasner J, DiBenedetto J, Stark A: Apnea monitoring by acoustic detection of airflow. Pediatrics 71:53-55, 1983.
156. Tatara T, Tsuzaki K: An apnea monitor using a rapid-response hygrometer. J Clin Monit 13:5-9, 1997.
157. Folke M, Granstedt F, Hök B, Scheer H: Comparative provocation test of respiratory monitoring methods. J Clin Monit Comput 17:97-103, 2002.
158. Roback K, Nelson N, Johansson A, et al: A new fiberoptical respiratory rate monitor for the neonatal intensive care unit. Pediatr Pulmonol 39:120-126, 2005.
158a. George CF, Millar TW, Kryger MH: Identification and quantification of apneas by computer-based analysis of oxygen saturation. Am Rev Respiratory Disease 137:1238, 1988.
159. Lange NR, Schuster DP: The measurement of lung water. Crit Care 3:R19-R24, 1999.
160. Katzenelson R, Perel A, Berkenstadt H, et al: Accuracy of transpulmonary thermodilution versus gravimetric measurement of extravascular lung water. Crit Care Med 32:1550-1554, 2004.
161. Fernández-Mondéjar E, Guerrero-López F, Colmenero M: How important is the measurement of extravascular lung water? Curr Opin Crit Care 13:79-83, 2007.
162. Forster BB, Muller NL, Mayo JR, et al: High-resolution computed tomography of experimental hydrostatic pulmonary edema. Chest 101: 1434-1437, 1992.
163. Scillia P, Delcroix M, Lejeune P, et al: Hydrostatic pulmonary edema: Evaluation with thin-section CT in dogs. Radiology 211:161-168, 1999.
164. Agricola E, Bove T, Oppizzi M, et al: "Ultrasound comet-tail images": A marker of pulmonary edema: A comparative study with wedge pressure and extravascular lung water. Chest 127:1690-1695, 2005.
165. Serizawa S, Suzuki T, Niino H, et al: Using $H_2{}^{15}O$ and $C^{15}O$ in noninvasive pulmonary measurements. Chest 106:1145-1151, 1994.
166. Caruthers SD, Paschal CB, Pou NA, et al: Regional measurements of pulmonary edema by using magnetic resonance imaging. J Appl Physiol 84:2143-2153, 1998.
167. Freimark D, Arad M, Sokolover R, et al: Monitoring lung fluid content in CHF patients under intravenous diuretics treatment using bio-impedance measurements. Physiol Meas 28:S269-S277, 2007.
168. Fernandez-Mondejar E, Rivera-Ferna'ndez R, García-Delgado M, et al: Small increases in extravascular lung water are accurately detected by transpulmonary thermodilution. J Trauma 59:1420-1424, 2005.

169. Chan KP, Stewart TE, Mehta S: High-frequency oscillatory ventilation for adult patients with ARDS. Chest 131:1907-1916, 2007.
170. High-frequency oscillatory ventilation compared with conventional mechanical ventilation in the treatment of respiratory failure in preterm infants. The HIFI Study Group. N Engl J Med 320:88-93, 1989.
171. Bollen CW, Uiterwaal CS, van Vught AJ: Cumulative metaanalysis of high-frequency versus conventional ventilation in premature neonates. Am J Respir Crit Care Med 168:1150-1155, 2003.
172. Mehta S, Lapinsky SE, Hallett DC, et al: Prospective trial of high-frequency oscillation in adults with acute respiratory distress syndrome. Crit Care Med 29:1360-1369, 2001.
173. Derdak S, Mehta S, Stewart TE, et al: Multicenter Oscillatory Ventilation for Acute Respiratory Distress Syndrome Trial (MOAT) Study Investigators: High-frequency oscillatory ventilation for acute respiratory distress syndrome in adults: A randomized, controlled trial. Am J Respir Crit Care Med 166:801-808, 2002.
174. Berkenbosch JW, Tobias JD: Transcutaneous carbon dioxide monitoring during high-frequency oscillatory ventilation in infants and children. Crit Care Med 30:1024-1027, 2002.
175. Clark RH: High-frequency ventilation. J Pediatr 124:661-670, 1994.
176. Nishimura M, Imanaka H, Tashiro C, et al: Capnometry during high-frequency oscillatory ventilation. Chest 101:1681-1683, 1992.
177. Frietsch T, Krafft P, Becker HD, et al: Intermittent capnography during high-frequency jet ventilation for prolonged rigid bronchoscopy. Acta Anaesthesiol Scand 44:391-397, 2000.
178. Berkenbosch JW, Lam J, Burd RS, Tobias JD: Noninvasive monitoring of carbon dioxide during mechanical ventilation in older children: End-tidal versus transcutaneous techniques. Anesth Analg 92:1427-1431, 2001.
179. Rouby JJ, Puybasset L, Cluzel P, et al: Regional distribution of gas and tissue in acute respiratory distress syndrome. II. Physiological correlations and definition of an ARDS Severity Score. CT Scan ARDS Study Group. Intensive Care Med 26:1046-1056, 2000.
180. Puybasset L, Gusman P, Muller JC, et al: Regional distribution of gas and tissue in acute respiratory distress syndrome. III. Consequences for the effects of positive end-expiratory pressure. CT Scan ARDS Study Group. Intensive Care Med 26:1215-1227, 2000.
181. Brazelton TB III, Watson KF, Murphy M, et al: Identification of optimal lung volume during high-frequency oscillatory ventilation using respiratory inductive plethysmography. Crit Care Med 29:2349-2359, 2001.
182. Wolf G, Arnold J: Noninvasive assessment of lung volume: Respiratory inductance plethysmography and electrical impedance tomography. Crit Care Med 33(Suppl):S163-S169, 2005.
183. Gothberg S, Parker TA, Griebel J, et al: Lung volume recruitment in lambs during high-frequency oscillatory ventilation using respiratory inductive plethysmography. Pediatr Res 49:38-44, 2001.
184. Brazelton TB III, Watson KF, Murphy M, et al: Identification of optimal lung volume during high frequency oscillatory ventilation using respiratory inductive plethysmography. Crit Care Med 29:2349-2359, 2001.
185. Tingay DG, Mills JF, Morley CJ, et al: The deflation limb of the pressure-volume relationship in infants during high-frequency ventilation. Am J Respir Crit Care Med 173:414-420, 2006.
186. Lachmann B: Open up the lung and keep the lung open. Intensive Care Med 18:319-321, 1992.
187. Kalenga M, Battisti O, François A, et al: High-frequency oscillatory ventilation in neonatal RDS: Initial volume optimization and respiratory mechanics. J Appl Physiol 84:1174-1177, 1998.
188. Pillow JJ: High-frequency oscillatory ventilation: Mechanisms of gas exchange and lung mechanics. Crit Care Med 33(3 Suppl):S135-S141, 2005.
189. Pillow JJ, Sly PD, Hantos Z: Monitoring of lung volume recruitment and derecruitment using oscillatory mechanics during high-frequency oscillatory ventilation in the preterm lamb. Pediatr Crit Care Med 5:172-180, 2004.
190. Smith I, Fleming S, Cernaianu A: Mishaps during transport from the intensive care unit. Crit Care Med 18:278-281, 1990.
191. Waydhas C, Schneck G, Duswald KH: Deterioration of respiratory function after intrahospital transport of critically ill surgical patients. Intensive Care Med 21:784-789, 1995.
192. Kollef MH, Von Harz B, Prentice D, et al: Patient transport from intensive care increases the risk of developing ventilator-associated pneumonia. Chest 112:765-773, 1997.
193. Bercault N, Wolf M, Runge I, et al: Intrahospital transport of critically ill ventilated patients: A risk factor for ventilator-associated pneumonia—a matched cohort study. Crit Care Med 33:2471-2478, 2005.
194. Hurst JM, Davis K Jr, Johnson DJ, et al: Cost and complications during in-hospital transport of critically ill patients: A prospective cohort study. J Trauma 33:582-585, 1992.
195. Szem JW, Hydo LJ, Fischer E, et al: High-risk intrahospital transport of critically ill patients: Safety and outcome of the necessary "road trip." Crit Care Med 23:1660-1666, 1995.
196. Nakamura T, Fujino Y, Uchiyama A, et al: Intrahospital transport of critically ill patients using ventilator with patient-triggering function. Chest 123:159-164, 2003.
197. Tobias JD, Lynch A, Garrett J: Alterations of end-tidal carbon dioxide during the intrahospital transport of children. Pediatr Emerg Care 12:249-251, 1996.
198. Palmon SC, Liu M, Moore LE, Kirsch JR: Capnography facilitates tight control of ventilation during transport. Crit Care Med 24:608-611, 1996.
199. Indeck M, Peterson S, Smith J, Brotman S: Risk, cost, and benefit of transporting ICU patients for special studies. J Trauma 28:1020-1025, 1988.

Mark Stafford-Smith, Andrew Shaw, and Solomon Aronson

45 Renal Function Monitoring

Key Points

1. Perioperative acute renal failure (ARF), although uncommon, is associated with extremely high morbidity and mortality rates.
2. The mechanism for perioperative ARF is complex and most commonly involves multiple factors such as ischemia/reperfusion, inflammation, and toxins.
3. Repeated direct perioperative assessment of renal hemodynamics, tubular function, or pathogenesis of perioperative renal dysfunction is impractical; therefore, indirect assessments, such as serum creatinine trends, are the best practical currently available perioperative tool to assess renal function.
4. Intraoperative urine formation depends on a number of factors and is an insensitive and unreliable method for assessing postoperative risk of renal dysfunction.
5. Serum chemistries and urine indices such as blood urea nitrogen, creatinine, fractional excretion of sodium, and free water clearance are generally late indicators of renal function deterioration and do not enable the clinician to clearly delineate the cause of renal failure.
6. Creatinine clearance is the most sensitive and specific clinical method for determining renal function, but it is limited by time and measurement restrictions.
7. Early biochemical markers for renal function hold promise and are a current focus for research that may soon lead to new tests able to provide prompt clinical information.

Acute kidney injury (AKI) characterized by rapid decline in glomerular filtration and accumulation of nitrogenous waste products (blood urea nitrogen [BUN] and creatinine) is a common medical problem occurring in 5% and 30% of all hospital and intensive care unit (ICU) patients, respectively.[1] AKI is also a serious perioperative complication for patients undergoing major surgery (Fig. 45-1).[2-10] Disentangling the clinical effects of AKI from those of other conditions (e.g., sepsis) is difficult because renal impairment rarely presents in isolation in critically ill patients. However, a prevailing observation is that AKI itself portends poor prognosis, not only owing to the loss of renal function and potential for excessive volume and solutes but also from the ineffective clearance of "uremic toxins," such as inflammatory mediators,[11-13] and the numerous potentially life-threatening complications related to impaired renal function, including sepsis, respiratory failure, gastrointestinal hemorrhage, and central nervous system dysfunction. Acute renal failure (ARF) requiring dialysis develops in 1% to 7% of patients after cardiac or major vascular surgery (Fig. 45-2) and is strongly associated with morbidity and mortality (Fig. 45-3) (see Chapters 60 and 62).[14-17] The mortality rate of ARF was 91% during World War II, 68% in the Korean War, and 67% in the Vietnam War. Today, depending on associated comorbidities, postoperative renal failure is responsible for up to 60% mortality in the postoperative period.[3,4,7,8] ARF in the presence of no other comorbidities has a 10% to 40% mortality rate, whereas ARF in the ICU setting carries a 50% to 80% mortality rate (see Chapter 91).[18] Perioperative renal failure accounts for one half of all patients requiring acute dialysis.[18]

The overall reported frequency of ARF among all patients admitted to the hospital is 1%[19] and may increase to 2% to 5%[3,20] during hospitalization. The incidence of perioperative ARF requiring dialysis has remained largely unchanged since it was first described over 40 years ago[21,22]; however, recognition of this disorder is increasing[9] and reinvigorated efforts to reduce its occurrence are underway as medical populations shift toward older and more critically ill patients undergoing increasingly higher-risk procedures (see Chapter 71). An emerging strategy to reduce the incidence of perioperative renal failure involves improvement of renal function monitoring to allow prompt recognition of the onset of ARF in the operative and critical care setting.

Perioperative renal failure, for example, has long been defined as the need for postoperative dialysis; however, this is by no means the only tool that has been used as a marker to describe acute changes in kidney well-being. In one review of 28 studies,[23] no two definitions for perioperative ARF were the same. Because the implications of needing postoperative dialysis are quite

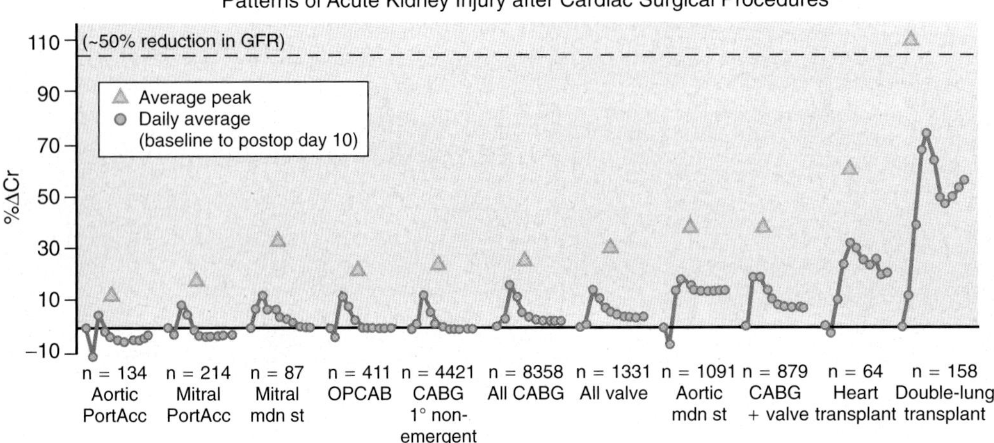

Figure 45-1 Average daily (*circles*) and unadjusted average peak (*triangles*) serum creatinine values for the first 10 days after several different cardiac surgery procedures, represented as change relative to preoperative serum creatinine.[118,334-340] The average peak value considerably exceeds the highest average daily value for each procedure because creatinine peaks on different days for different patients. % ΔCr, peak fractional serum creatinine rise; Aortic PortAcc, minimally invasive parasternotomy aortic valve replacement; Mitral PortAcc, port access mitral valve surgery; Mitral mdn st, median sternotomy mitral valve surgery; OPCAB, off-pump coronary artery bypass surgery; CABG, coronary artery bypass surgery 1° nonemergent; Aortic mdn st, median sternotomy aortic valve replacement. (*Used with permission from Stafford-Smith M, Patel U, Phillips-Bute B, et al: Acute kidney injury and chronic kidney disease after cardiac surgery. Adv Chronic Kidney Dis 15:157-177, 2008.*)

different for a patient starting with normal baseline function than one starting near the brink of filtration failure, even the usefulness of dialysis as a marker of outcome has been questioned.[24] Recent research efforts have been directed toward developing a universally accepted standard for describing AKI or renal failure.[25-32]

Although ischemic causes have long been believed to be primarily responsible for perioperative ARF,[33,34] lack of success with this paradigm in developing renoprotective strategies,[35] combined with accumulating evidence that postoperative renal dysfunction possesses characteristics of multiple types of AKI,[36,37] has resulted in a reevaluation of the pathophysiology of this disorder. Much can be learned from the many settings beyond ischemia-reperfusion where specific types of AKI occur; examples include contrast-associated nephropathy, pigment nephropathy (e.g., hemoglobin, myoglobin), cholesterol embolism (atheroembolism) nephropathy, aminoglycoside nephropathy, norepinephrine-induced nephropathy, and as part of the sepsis/systemic inflammatory response syndrome. In these examples, the disorder describes the renal pathophysiology and strategies to prevent or attenuate each condition are interventions directed specifically toward the cause. Animal studies of such "pure" nephropathies treated with logical renoprotective interventions often demonstrate success; unfortunately, this has rarely extended to equivalent renoprotection in human perioperative studies. However, it makes sense that a specific treatment for a "pure" nephropathy applied nonselectively to a mixture of nephropathies, variably expressed in different patients, would be unsuccessful. Protection from one perioperative nephropathy may even add

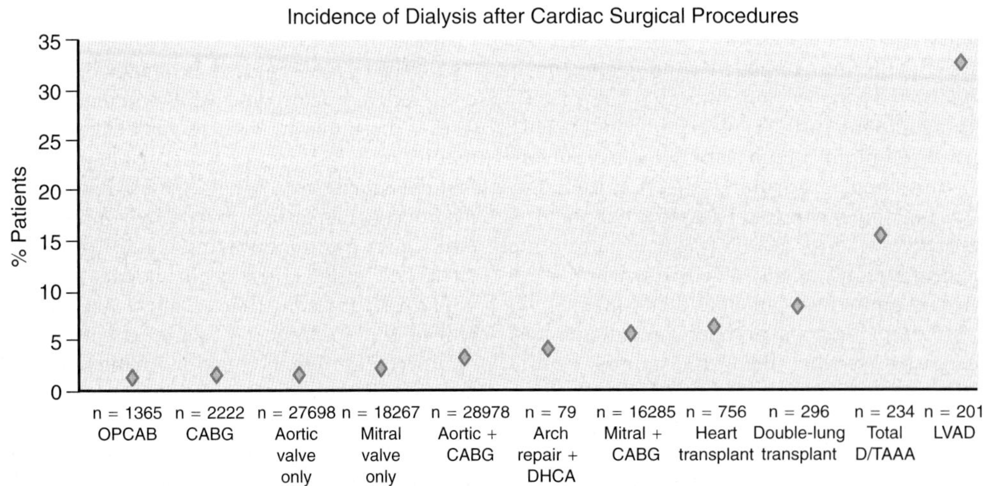

Figure 45-2 Rate of new-onset dialysis differs significantly for various surgical procedures.[4,341-348] OPCAB, off-pump coronary artery bypass surgery; CABG, coronary artery bypass surgery; DHCA, deep hypothermic circulatory arrest; D/TAAA, descending/thoracoabdominal aortic aneurysm; LVAD, left ventricular assist device. (*Used with permission from Stafford-Smith M, Patel U, Phillips-Bute B, et al: Acute kidney injury and chronic kidney disease after cardiac surgery. Adv Chronic Kidney Dis 15:157-177, 2008.*)

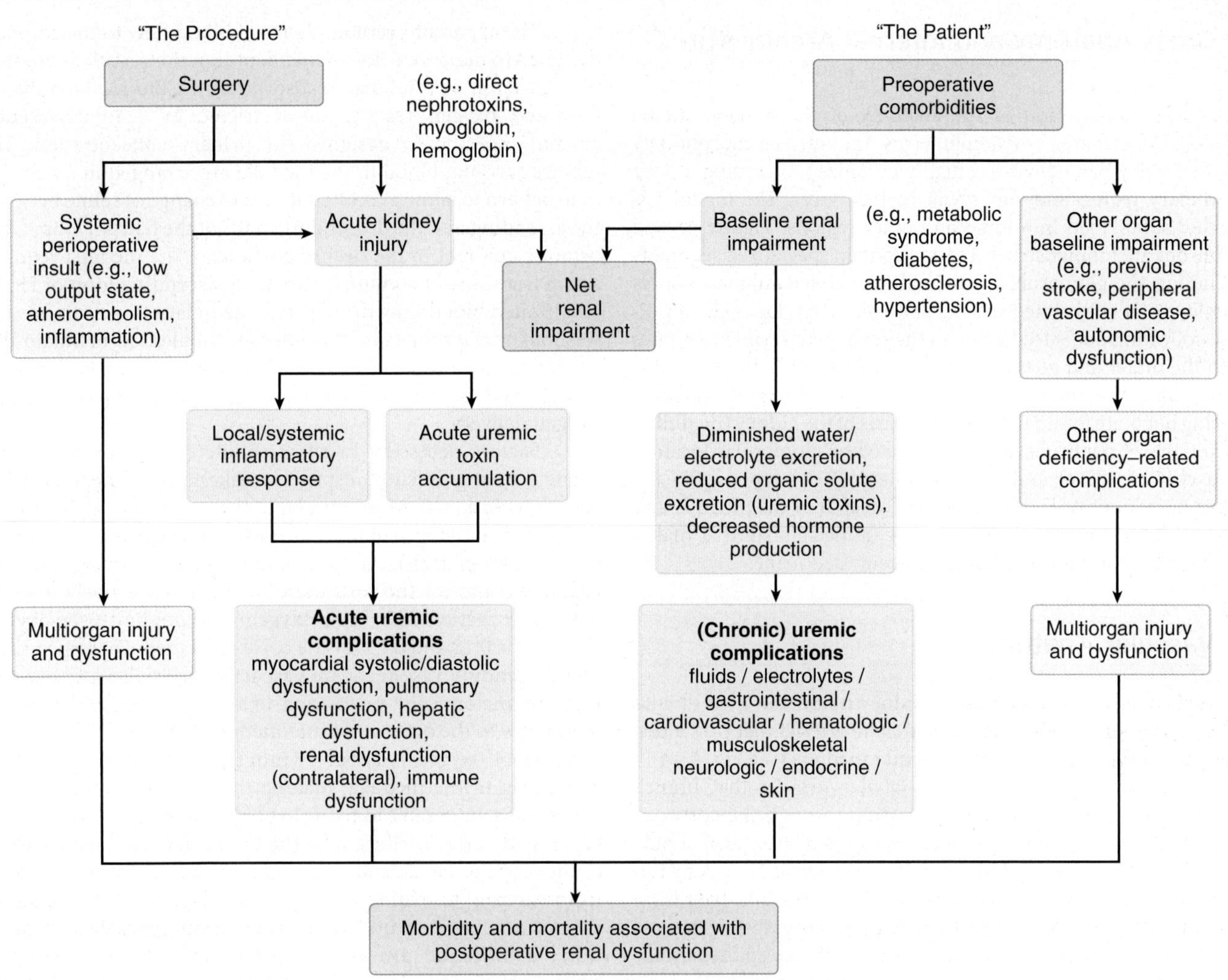

Figure 45-3 Procedural and patient factors related to surgery contributing to risk of perioperative acute kidney injury (AKI) and postoperative morbidity and mortality. Of note, although AKI contributes to this risk, a significant part of this association must also be attributed to other very serious conditions that can cause injury, such as sepsis, that themselves are major sources of adverse outcome. *(Modified with permission from Stafford-Smith M, Patel U, Phillips-Bute B, Shaw A, Swaminathan M: Acute kidney injury and chronic kidney disease after cardiac surgery. Adv Chr Kid Dis 15:157-177, 2008.)*

risk for another type; for example, augmenting renal blood flow (RBF) may attenuate ischemia-reperfusion injury while delivering more atheroemboli and inflammatory mediators. Evidence continues to grow supporting the idea that postoperative AKI is a mosaic of several "pure" nephropathies, each of varying importance for a particular patient and procedure, suggesting that only individualized renoprotection strategies, guided by timely point-of-care renal function monitoring, will be helpful in developing effective renoprotection strategies. Hence, advances in renal function monitoring are currently a major focus in the search for improved renal protection and risk stratification strategies for AKI (see Chapter 18).

Renal Physiology

The kidneys are mesoderm-derived, bean-shaped retroperitoneal organs and weigh approximately 150 g each. They are the most highly perfused major organs in the body, representing only 0.4% of body weight but receiving an impressive 25% of cardiac output; as a comparison, "at rest" blood flow to the kidneys is eightfold greater per gram of tissue than blood flow to muscle during heavy exercise. Notably, renal artery blood flow is not primarily linked to metabolic demand; it is this "excess" blood flow that allows filtration of plasma at rates as rapid as 125 to 140 mL/min in adults. However, autoregulatory reflexes do exist that regulate renal perfusion; these are myogenic and tubular-glomerular reflexes that exist to "protect" the glomeruli from damage due to pressure overload by restricting RBF at higher pressures (e.g., >80 mm Hg).[38,39] However, the kidneys may not receive a luxury supply of nutrients and oxygen, because marked regional differences in blood flow within the kidney paradoxically make some areas (i.e., the medulla) very vulnerable to ischemic injury. Cortical blood flow exceeds outer and inner medullary perfusion by 3- and 20-fold per gram of tissue, respectively.[40] Although there is strong evidence that paracrine regulation of oxygen delivery is important in the medulla, little is known about the specifics of this process.[41]

Gross Anatomy and Internal Architecture

A detailed description of the anatomy of the kidney can be obtained elsewhere.[42] In simple terms, the internal morphology of the kidney parenchyma is highly organized, including a deep medullary region and superficial cortical layer. The medulla is further subdivided into inner and outer regions. Tightly packed nephrons are tubular structures that contain specialized segments including the glomerulus, proximal convoluted tubule, loop of Henle, distal convoluted tubule, and collecting duct (Fig. 45-4). The collecting ducts feed urine to the renal pelvis, which empties into the ureter and goes on to the bladder. Each kidney contains approximately 1 million nephrons. The loops of Henle and collecting ducts are found in the deeper parts of the kidney (medulla). Two types of nephrons are differentiated by glomerular location into cortical (85%) and juxtamedullary (15%) types; only the latter have loops of Henle that course deep into the medulla and participate in *countercurrent exchange,* a mechanism that makes possible the formation of highly concentrated urine.

Vascular Anatomy

A single *renal artery* enters at the kidney hilum and then divides many times, ultimately producing *arcuate arteries* that pass along the boundary between cortex and outer medulla (see Fig. 45-4).[41] Arcuate arteries give rise to *interlobular arteries* that branch toward the outer kidney surface, passing through the cortex as they produce numerous *afferent arterioles,* which in turn supply a *capillary tuft* to each glomerulus. The glomerular capillary tuft is the barrier where plasma elements are filtered and pass from the vascular to tubular space. Specialized negatively charged fenestrated capillary endothelial cells and tubular epithelial cells (podocytes) separated by a basement membrane allow approximately 25% of plasma volume to pass into the glomerulus (Bowman's capsule); normally, only elements smaller than 60 to 70 kDa are small enough to be filtered. Many disease conditions cause abnormalities of this interface and allow much larger proteins and even red blood cells to pass through; this manifests as either nephrotic syndrome (proteinuria > 3.5 g/24 hr) or glomerulonephritis (proteinuria and hematuria). As the vascular tuft exits the glomerulus, capillaries merge and become the *efferent arteriole.* Subsequent branches of the afferent arterioles become *peritubular capillaries* to nourish the tubules. Peritubular capillaries receive reabsorbed fluids and solutes from tubular cells before rejoining to form *venules.* Peritubular vessels of juxtamedullary glomeruli are known as *vasa recta* and accompany the loops of Henle deep into the medulla. The venous system of the kidney runs parallel and close to the arterial vasculature, finally returning blood to the inferior vena cava through the *renal vein.* Vascular supply to the kidney is strictly segmental, and embolic arterial or venous obstruction affects renal tissue in a "pizza wedge" parenchymal distribution involving all cortical and medullary tubular elements of affected nephrons.

Medullary hypoxia is a key concept that refers to the low oxygen levels that exist in the renal medulla, even during normal resting conditions. Sodium and water reabsorption depend on the hypertonicity of the medullary interstitium. The countercurrent multiplier system in the loop of Henle is a critical component of the kidney's ability to excrete or conserve salt and water.

The apparent overabundance of blood flow to the cortex is designed to maximize flow-dependent functions, such as glomerular filtration and tubular reabsorption. In the medulla, blood flow and oxygen reserve are restricted by a tubulovascular anatomy specifically designed for urinary concentration. The tubules carrying blood to the medulla are arranged in a hairpin-loop pattern to allow a countercurrent exchange of solute between the ascending and the descending limbs of the hairpin loop.[43] The osmotic gradient in the deeper portions of the medulla requires active transport of sodium in the thick ascending loop of Henle and limited blood flow through the medullary vessels to prevent washout of the solutes in those deeper tubules. To maintain this concentration gradient in the thick ascending limb, high energy demand (i.e., active sodium transport) must be coupled with low oxygen delivery.

Factors necessary to allow countercurrent exchange and create a urea gradient conspire to make normal medullary Po_2 very low (e.g., 10 to 20 mm Hg); these include high oxygen demand from active solute transport and sluggish blood supply (5% to 10% of RBF). Average blood flow is 5.0 mL/g/min and 0.03 mL/g/min for the cortex and medulla, respectively, and the oxygen extraction ratio (i.e., oxygen consumption over oxygen delivery) is 0.18 and 0.79 for the cortex and medulla, respectively. The descending vasa recta are vasoactive arteriolar microvessels that are anatomically positioned to regulate total and regional blood flow to the outer and inner medulla.[43] Normally, the partial pressure of oxygen is about 50 mm Hg in the cortex and 8 to 15 mm Hg in the medulla, making the thick ascending loop of Henle most vulnerable to tissue hypoxia. Medullary oxygen delivery is made more inefficient by the unique hairpin loop anatomy of the loops of Henle and vasa recta that allows "oxygen escape" from entering to exiting capillaries (see Fig. 45-4).[44,45] This precarious arrangement underpins some of the specialized homeostatic abilities of the kidney, particularly the formation of concentrated urine, but also underlies the extreme vulnerability of the renal medulla to ischemic injury.[46]

The high metabolic requirement of the thick ascending loop of Henle in a hypoxic environment makes it especially vulnerable to injury associated with an imbalance in oxygen supply and demand.[47,48] Hypoxic perfusion of an isolated kidney preparation has demonstrated that the cells of the thick ascending limb of the loop of Henle in the medulla are extremely vulnerable to hypoxic damage.[48] Most recent available evidence suggests specific roles for prostaglandins (mediated by cyclooxygenase-2 receptors), angiotensin II, bradykinin, adenosine, nitric oxide (generated by nitric oxide synthase type 3), norepinephrine, and vasopressin in the paracrine autoregulation of medullary blood flow.[41] An adenosine receptor–mediated renal *ischemic preconditioning reflex* has been characterized, but the relevance of this to humans is unknown.[49-51]

Normal Function

The "resting" kidney continuously regulates body composition by processing plasma filtrate to keep fluid volume, osmolarity, acidity, and numerous electrolytes within narrow limits. Every 3 minutes a plasma volume equivalent to a 12-oz soft drink is filtered, and all but 1% (4 mL) is returned to circulation; the remnant is urine. Tightly regulated through tubular processing are extracellular solutes, including sodium, potassium, hydrogen ion, bicarbonate,

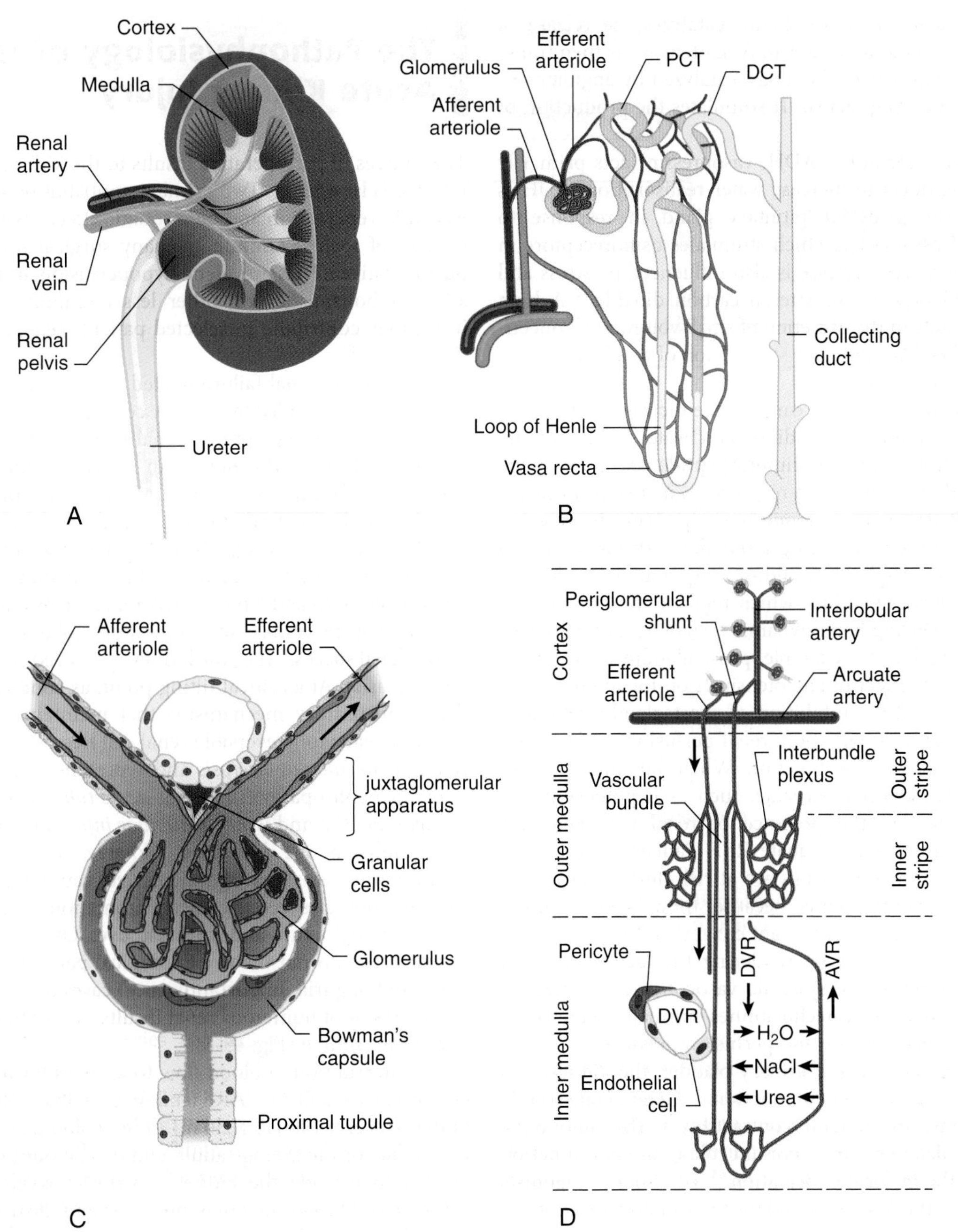

Figure 45-4 **A,** The internal structure of the kidney includes the vasculature, cortex and medulla regions, and urinary tract structures. **B,** The functional unit of the kidney is the nephron. **C,** The glomerulus is the site where plasma filtration occurs; approximately 20% of plasma entering the glomerulus will pass through the specialized capillary wall into Bowman's capsule and enter the tubule to be processed and generate urine. **D,** The vascular anatomy of the kidney is highly organized, and the medullary microcirculation is part of the mechanism that permits countercurrent exchange.[41] AVR, ascending vasa recta, DVR, descending vasa recta. PCT, proximal convoluted tubule; DCT, distal convoluted tubule. (***A*** *from http://www.nida.nih.gov/consequences/kidney/. Accessed February 17, 2008;* ***B*** *from http://www.pathology.vcu.edu/education/PathLab/pages/renalpath/rpsrhome.htm from Lecture 1. Accessed February 17, 2008;* ***C*** *from http://www.besthealth.com/besthealth/bodyguide/reftext/images/Nephron.jpg. Accessed February 17, 2008. Used with permission from Pallone TL, Zhang Z, Rhinehart K: Physiology of the renal medullary microcirculation. Am J Physiol Renal Physiol 284:F253-F266, 2003.)*

and glucose. The kidney also generates ammonia and eliminates metabolic and nitrogenous wastes, including creatinine, urea, and bilirubin, as well as toxins and many classes of drugs. Finally, the kidneys generate glucose and secrete circulating hormones that influence erythrocyte generation, systemic blood pressure, and calcium homeostasis.

High concentrations of aldosterone stimulate reabsorption of sodium and water, primarily in the distal tubule and the collecting ducts. Aldosterone is produced by the adrenal cortex in response to the feedback from the renin-angiotensin-aldosterone system, simplified as follows. Reduced delivery of sodium to the macula densa causes release of renin from the granular cells of

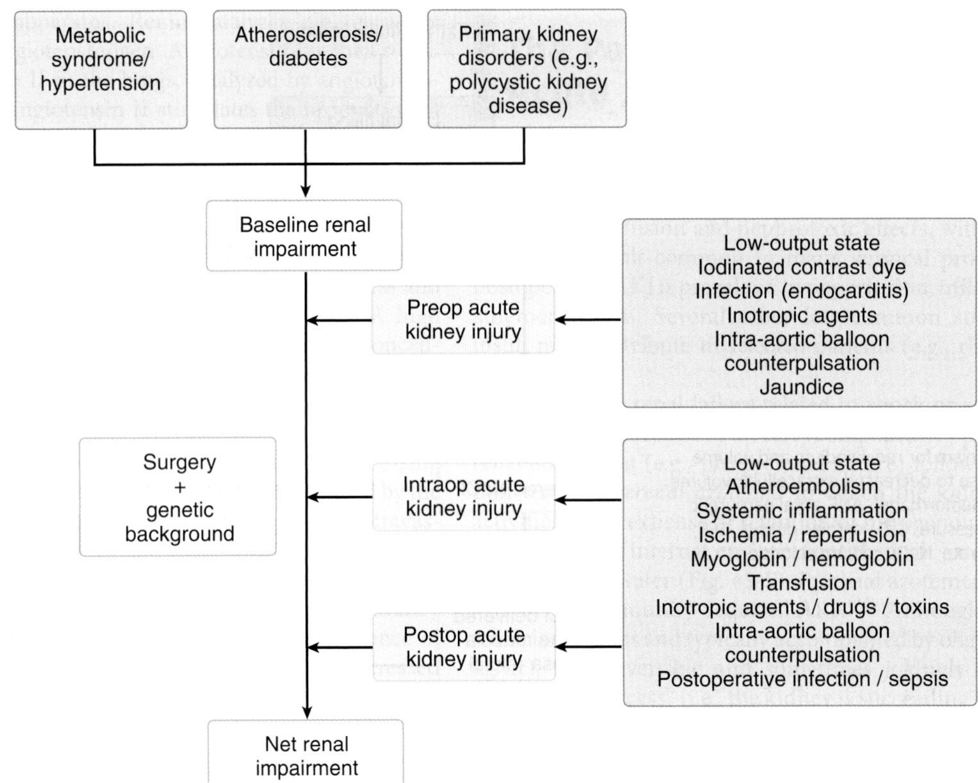

Figure 45-6 Perioperative clinical risk factors that predict risk of postoperative kidney injury and chronic kidney disease.

Surgical and anesthetic interventions may have autonomic consequences, such as increasing circulating catecholamines, that also reduce glomerular filtration by altering renal vascular resistance and decreasing RBF. The normal physiology of the kidney includes a role of adrenergic receptors in modulating vasoconstrictor (alpha 1) and vasodilating (alpha 2) effects, respectively. In animal models, infusion of norepinephrine is a well-described source of renal vasoconstriction and reduction in glomerular filtration[69,70]; this effect also appears to be relevant to human physiology.[71] The perioperative stress response to major surgery, particularly related to neurosurgical procedures, can further reduce urine output by increasing circulating ADH levels.[72,73]

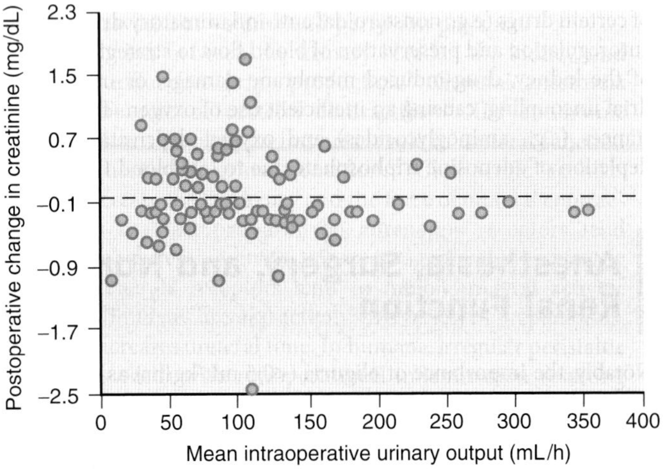

Figure 45-7 Low hourly urine flow (<0.5 mL/kg/hr) is a marker in some widely used criteria to diagnose AKI but is not a meaningful assessment to make this diagnosis in the immediate perioperative period. The lack of association of urine output with postoperative renal complications is exemplified by data in the figure comparing postoperative urine output and postoperative change in serum creatinine after aortic surgery. *(Used with permission from Alpert RA, Roizen MF, Hamilton WK, et al: Intraoperative urinary output does not predict postoperative renal function in patients undergoing abdominal aortic revascularization. Surgery 95:707-711, 1984.)*

Effects of Regional Anesthesia

Regional anesthetics and the kidneys interact in a complex manner that varies according to the underlying cardiovascular, renal, fluid, and electrolyte status of the patient (see Chapters 51 and 52).[74] Epidural and spinal anesthesia reduce systemic and renal vascular sympathetic tone.[75] Spinal cord segments T4 through L1 contribute to the sympathetic innervation of the renal vasculature, which is mediated by sympathetic fibers from the celiac and renal plexus.[76,77] Autonomic blockade above the fourth thoracic level also blocks cardioaccelerator sympathetic innervation to the heart. If neuraxial blockade reduces blood pressure and cardiac output, it will reduce RBF, with matching reductions in glomerular filtration and urine output. Suleiman and colleagues[78] demonstrated in healthy volunteers that RBF is unchanged during epidural anesthesia with a T6 sensory block. In their study, mean arterial pressure remained above 70 mm Hg and RBF never decreased below 6% of the baseline level.

The effect of neuraxial blockade varies not only on the level of sympathetic block but also the presence of underlying disease. In all perioperative settings, renal filtration and urine formation depend on the net sum of numerous endogenous effects, including circulating catecholamines, autonomic blockade, ADH, angiotensin, dopamine, vasopressin, prostaglandin, atrial natriuretic peptide, endothelin, and nitric oxide. Superimposed on endogenous factors are surgical and anesthetic interventions, such as aortic cross-clamping, cardiopulmonary bypass (CPB), diuretics, and vasoactive infusions (e.g., vasopressin, dopaminergic and adrenergic agonists).

Urine volume and free water clearance may decrease during spinal anesthesia as a result of increased ADH secretion. Increased renal sympathomimetic activity decreases RBF through α-adrenergic mediation and increases renin release through β-adrenergic innervation directly or by interaction with the renal tubular macula densa and the baroreceptor reflex mechanism.[79-82] Of note, thoracic epidural anesthesia has been shown to increase RBF and urine output in animal models of endotoxic shock.[83]

Two recent large reviews on epidural anesthesia have findings that relate to perioperative renal outcomes. Moraca and colleagues[81,82] conducted a meta-analysis and reported on the association of thoracic epidural anesthesia with improved surgical outcomes in part attributable to reduction of perioperative morbidity, including blunting of stress response, attenuating infections, reduced ileus, reduced blood loss, and reduction in ARF. Liu and Wu[80] reviewed 18 meta-analyses, 10 reviews, eight randomized controlled trials, and two observational studies on epidural analgesia and found that the data support the ability of epidural analgesia to reduce cardiovascular and pulmonary complications, including renal morbidity after major vascular surgery on high-risk patients.

Effects of Inhaled Anesthetics

There is a well-recognized nephrotoxic effect of the older volatile inhaled anesthetics that has been attributed to the liberation of inorganic fluoride when they are metabolized (see Chapter 24).[84] Methoxyflurane (no longer used clinically) and enflurane, when employed for prolonged periods (9.6 minimum alveolar concentration [MAC] hours), lead to significant generation of inorganic fluoride.[84-87] Increased serum levels of inorganic fluoride caused polyuric renal insufficiency.[84,85] Approximately 100 published cases of renal failure and 20 renal-related deaths attest to the significance of methoxyflurane-related nephrotoxicity.[84]

Because sevoflurane metabolism is similar to enflurane in regard to liberation of free fluoride ions,[84,88-91] (Fig. 45-8) concerns were raised during development that this agent may also impair the ability of the kidneys to concentrate urine.[89,92] Methoxyflurane studies indicated that AKI was likely to occur with circulating fluoride levels greater than 50 μM/L.[84,86] This presumed toxic threshold was extrapolated to the study of other halogenated anesthetic agents, including enflurane and sevoflurane (see Fig. 45-8). Notably, mean plasma fluoride levels in volunteers are approximately twice as high with sevoflurane as enflurane and 43% of volunteers receiving sevoflurane have plasma fluoride levels that exceed 50 μM/L. Healthy patients receiving 9 MAC hours of sevoflurane anesthesia have serum fluoride levels averaging 36.6 ± 4.3 μM/L.[88,93] However, relative to methoxyflurane, high fluoride levels with sevoflurane are short-lived, peaking 2 hours after the end of anesthesia and dropping by 50% within 8 hours. Despite high fluoride levels with sevoflurane, volunteers have no impairment in their ability to concentrate urine in

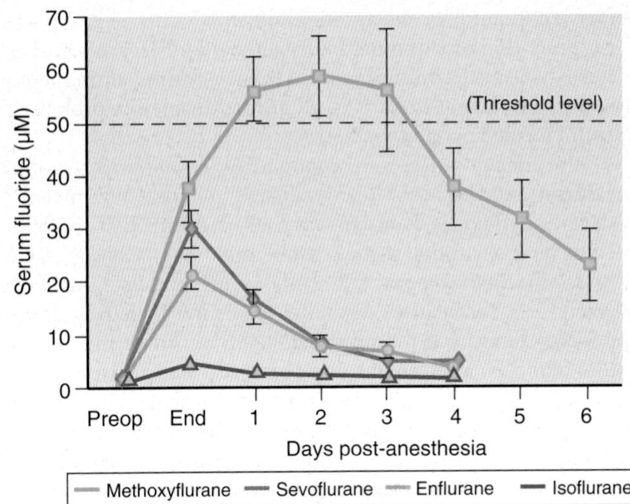

Figure 45-8 The nephrotoxic effect of the older volatile inhaled anesthetics are attributed to the liberation of inorganic fluoride when they are metabolized. Methoxyflurane-related AKI was related to threshold circulating fluoride levels greater than 50 μM/L. Levels of inorganic fluoride do not correlate as closely with the risk of AKI for modern volatile anesthetics such as sevoflurane. *(Used with permission from Mazze RI: Methoxyflurane revisited: tale of an anesthetic from cradle to grave. Anesthesiology 105:843-846, 2006.)*

response to desmopressin, whereas 20% of volunteers receiving enflurane have transient concentrating deficits on day 1 but not day 5 post exposure.[93] To interpret these findings, investigators postulate that intrarenal production of fluoride ion may be more important for nephrotoxicity than circulating plasma fluoride levels.[91] The intrarenal metabolism of methoxyflurane is fourfold greater than the intrarenal metabolism of sevoflurane.

Other explanations for differences in the renal effects of volatile agents were sought, including evaluation of variation in nephrotoxic compounds generated when an inhaled anesthetic agent interacts with carbon dioxide absorbents. In breathing circuit systems at high temperature and low flow rates, carbon dioxide absorbents degrade sevoflurane, creating fluoromethyl-2,2-difluoro-1-(trifluoroethyl) vinyl ether, also known as compound A. Metabolism of compound A includes conjugation in the liver with glutathione and then modification in the kidney by an enzyme (cysteineconjugate β-lyase). Some compound A metabolites can cause renal injury, characterized by diuresis, glycosuria, proteinuria, and elevated serum BUN and creatinine levels. AKI by this mechanism in experimental models is a function of the degree and duration of exposure to compound A,[94] with well-defined exposure thresholds in rats for injury (50-114 ppm for 3 hours) and death (331 for 3 hours, 203 for 6 hours, or 127 ppm for 12 hours).[95] However, a disparity exists between the results in rats and humans that may be due to differences in compound A processing; of the four recognized pathways for metabolism, three do not involve renal β-lyase nor result in kidney toxicity. Humans have 10- to 30-fold less renal β-lyase enzyme activity compared with rats, which may account for the absence of kidney injury from sevoflurane in humans. One study[96] compared the safety of low-flow sevoflurane and isoflurane anesthesia in patients having prolonged surgeries (>6 hr). The average MAC hours in both groups was similar, and the average compound A concentration in the sevoflurane group was 20 ± 7 ppm. Markers of renal injury, including BUN, creatinine, *N*-acetyl-β-D-glucosaminidase (NAG), and alanine aminopeptidase, were increased similarly in all groups during the prolonged exposure to the volatile anesthetics.

The concentrations of compound A possible with sevoflurane during anesthesia has been evaluated in human volunteers.[97] Fresh carbon dioxide absorbent was used, and 1.25 MAC sevoflurane was given (without nitrous oxide) for 8 hours. Compound A levels approached 50 ppm, and 24-hour urine collections were analyzed for 3 consecutive days after exposure. Urinary glutathione S-transferase (GST) and other highly sensitive markers of tubular damage after nephrotoxic and ischemic insults were measured.[98] The investigators reported transient elevations of urinary protein, albumin, glucose, α-GST, and π-GST in patients receiving sevoflurane. Interestingly, no such increases were observed after similar exposure to desflurane. A multicenter study[99] involving 73 elective surgical procedures lasting 2 to 8 hours compared the safety and efficacy of low flow (less than 2 L/min) sevoflurane to isoflurane. Fresh carbon dioxide absorbent was used for all cases, and nitrous oxide was not permitted. Sevoflurane use averaged 3.6 MAC hour, and compound A levels were as high as 223 ppm (mean 79 ± 54 ppm). No differences were found in urine albumin, glucose, protein, or osmolality between treatment groups. Moreover, within the sevoflurane group, there were no significant correlations between compound A levels and BUN, creatinine, or urinary excretion of protein, glucose, NAG, α-GST, or π-GST.[99]

Despite the fact that 7% to 15% of patients receiving sevoflurane may have (short-lived) circulating levels of fluoride in excess of 50 μM/L and/or significant exposure to compound A, adverse renal effects do not seem to occur.[84] While explanation for the apparent safety of sevoflurane in the presence of nephrotoxins is not completely understood, some have proposed that the source of methoxyflurane-related renal injury may even be some other metabolic "villain" than fluoride or compound A that is unique to methoxyflurane metabolism, such as dichloroacetic acid.[100] Potential benefits of sevoflurane to the kidney have been described. In patients undergoing cardiac surgery, preconditioning with sevoflurane has been reported to decrease biochemical markers for renal (as well as myocardial) dysfunction.[101] Seventy-two patients scheduled for coronary artery bypass graft surgery (CABG) were randomly assigned to preconditioning conditions (oxygen-air versus sevoflurane 4%) during the first 10 minutes of CPB. Sevoflurane preconditioning significantly decreased postoperative release of brain natriuretic peptide and plasma cystatin C concentrations compared with oxygen-air.

Perioperative Hemodynamic Instability and Renal Function

An early compensated phase of renal adaptation in response to decreased glomerular blood flow with oliguria is sometimes referred to as "pre-prerenal failure" or "acute renal success."[58] When compensatory mechanisms are overwhelmed, accumulation of nitrogenous waste ensues (e.g., blood urea nitrogen) and prerenal failure. Renal clearance is determined by the delivery of waste products to the kidney (i.e., RBF) and by the kidney's ability to extract them (i.e., glomerular filtration).

In animal models, RBF is interrupted mechanically or pharmacologically; flow reduction by more than 50% is followed by a timed episode of complete renal ischemia (e.g., 40 to 60 minutes); and the consequent functional and histologic lesion, laboratory, and pathologic features resemble significant AKI without the need for dialysis. A number of theories have been proposed to explain the pathogenesis of hemodynamically mediated AKI. Although an extreme reduction in RBF is clearly necessary,[34,102] the unpredictable degree of AKI after hypotension suggests that it is not always sufficient. Even with decreased glomerular perfusion, a series of compensatory mechanisms can still preserve renal filtration.[58] Salt and water retention can restore intravascular volume and fractional tubular reabsorption. At a given level of cardiac output, intrarenal factors affect the ratio of renal-to-systemic vascular resistance, thereby influencing the fraction of cardiac output received by the kidneys. At the glomerular capillary, plasma is separated into a protein-free ultrafiltrate and a nonfiltered portion. Normally, the filtration fraction (i.e., relationship of glomerular filtration to renal plasma flow) is about 0.2. Initially, the filtration fraction is maintained by efferent arteriolar constriction. Unabated, the mechanisms that influence efferent arteriolar vasoconstriction ultimately may influence afferent arteriolar vasoconstriction. The resulting decrease in filtration fraction is the hallmark of postischemic AKI.[58] Ischemic tubular damage may be exacerbated further by an imbalance between oxygen supply and demand. Most vulnerable to the imbalance are the thick ascending tubular cells of the loop of Henle in the medulla.[48,102-105]

Microsphere, xenon washout, and angiographic techniques have shown that outer cortical blood flow decreases in ischemic models of AKI.[106-108] Because 85% to 90% of RBF is normally distributed to cortical glomeruli, the finding of cortical pallor and RBF redistribution away from cortex suggests that redistribution may contribute to the functional lesions of AKI. In some cases, the return of perfusion to the cortex has correlated with a return of renal function.[107] The theory that intrarenal distribution of blood flow away from the outer cortex to the inner medulla decreases oxygen supply while increased tubular reabsorption of solute increases oxygen demand is further supported by studies of renal energetics during AKI.[109-111] A decrease in the glomerular filtration, and consequently in the energy requirement for tubular reabsorption, may be a mechanism by which the kidney reduces energy demands before energy supply is critically limited.

Other Perioperative Perturbations and Renal Function

Whereas aortic cross-clamping above the renal arteries has obvious influence on glomerular filtration, infrarenal aortic cross-clamping and declamping also has significant indirect effects on glomerular filtration and urine formation through changes in myocardial function, sympathetic activity, neuronal and hormonal activity (e.g., renin and angiotensin production), intravascular volume, and systemic vascular resistance.[112] During standard CPB, cardiorenal relationships are approximately as expected;

RBF falls to 12% to 13% of total pump flow and is predicted by flow rate and perfusion pressure; however, only mean pressure correlates with urine output.[65,66] The intactness of myogenic and tubular-glomerular autoregulatory feedback has not been evaluated during CPB.[38,39]

ARF after aortocoronary bypass surgery continues to be a devastating complication that is associated with multiorgan dysfunction, increased resource utilization, high cost, and increased mortality (see Chapters 60 and 62).[2-10] Annually, 1 million patients worldwide have coronary revascularization with use of CPB with approximately 77,000 patients a year developing postoperative AKI, among which approximately 14,000 require dialysis for the first time.[4] The mechanism of perioperative AKI during cardiac surgery appears to be multifactorial, involving preoperative and intraoperative risk factors, including preexisting renal dysfunction, diabetes, ventricular dysfunction, older age, hypertension, microembolic and macroembolic processes, inflammatory mediators, prolonged CPB time, sensitivity to sympathetic stimulation, perturbation in renovascular resistance and flow,[3,8,113] and hypertension subtype (namely, pulse pressure hypertension).[2]

The importance of CPB has been evaluated in numerous studies of postoperative AKI between patients undergoing off-pump and on-pump coronary revascularization surgeries[114-124] with no conclusive evidence that CPB directly contributes to postoperative AKI. In a recent multicenter study of patients undergoing cardiac surgery, independent and significant risk factors for AKI were age older than 75 years, preoperative congestive heart failure, prior history of myocardial infarction, preexisting renal disease, intraoperative use of multiple inotropes, intraoperative insertion of intra-aortic balloon pump, and extended duration of CPB (>2 hr). In addition, preoperative pulse pressure (systolic minus diastolic) greater than 40 mm Hg had an incremental and progressive relationship with renal risk, such that for every additional 20-mm Hg increment in pulse pressure there was an additive odds ratio of 1.49 (CI, 1.17 to 1.89; $P = .001$). In this large study, with a high incidence of AKI (4.8%) in both the derivation (n = 2381) and validation (n = 2402) cohorts, AKI was nearly two times and renal-related death three times more common in patients with a pulse pressure greater than 80 mm Hg.

Genetic variants are an established predictor of chronic kidney disease (e.g., renal transplant nephropathy) and explain twofold to threefold more variation in postoperative AKI than standard clinical risk factors alone.[125,126] A handful of candidate polymorphisms known to affect inflammation and vasoconstriction have been studied, and several demonstrate strong associations with postcardiac surgery AKI.[126,127] The most clinically relevant genetic findings to date identify co-possession of the IL-6 572C and angiotensinogen (AGT) 842C polymorphisms in whites (9% of patients) as a predictor of an approximately fourfold greater than average peak creatinine rise after coronary revascularization (121%) (Fig. 45-9) and may have potential as a preoperative screening tool if validated in other populations. In African Americans, a similar, but statistically less robust finding, co-possession of the endothelial nitric oxide synthase (eNOS) 894T and angiotensin-converting enzyme deletion polymorphisms, also predicts a large creatinine rise (162.5%) (see Fig. 45-9). This compelling evidence of a genetic basis for postoperative AKI has come from analysis of a relatively small number of candidate genetic variants.

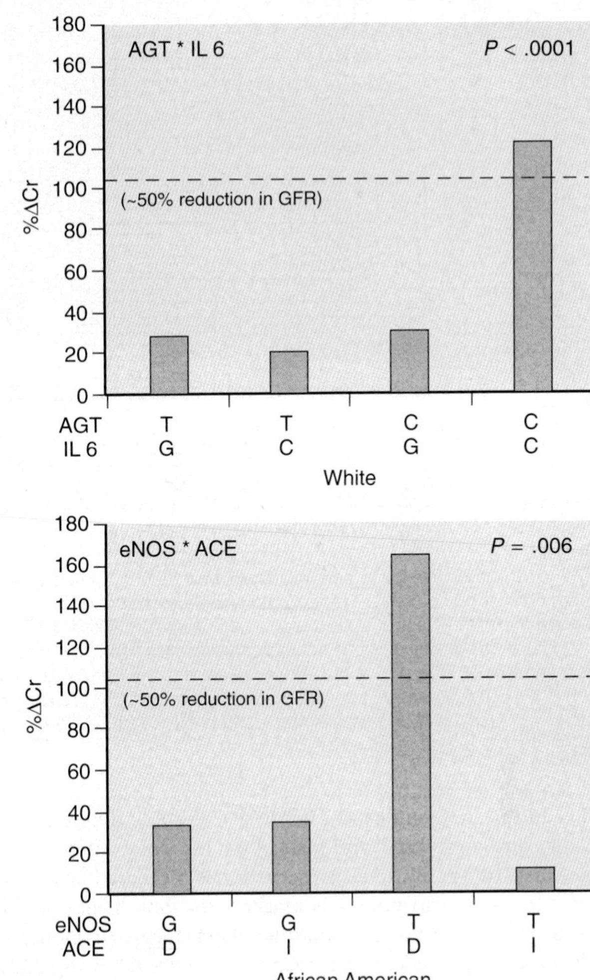

Figure 45-9 AKI after cardiac surgery is better predicted by knowledge of genetic variants than by standard clinical risk factors alone. Common gene polymorphism combinations predict increased risk; angiotensinogen (AGT) 842T→C and interleukin (IL) -6 572G→C in whites; endothelial nitric oxide synthase (eNOS) 894G→T and angiotensin-converting enzyme (ACE) insertion/deletion (I/D) in African Americans. % ΔCr, peak fractional serum creatinine rise; GFR, glomerular filtration rate. *(Used with permission from Stafford-Smith M, Podgoreanu M, Swaminathan M, et al: Association of genetic polymorphisms with risk of renal injury after coronary artery bypass graft surgery. Am J Kidney Dis 45:519-530, 2005.)*

Monitors of Renal Function

In patients with perioperative AKI, one of the major challenges to optimal perioperative management and early intervention has been the absence of tools for early recognition of subtle AKI. Traditional renal failure monitoring tools typically are insensitive until less than 40% of normal functioning nephrons remain (Fig. 45-10); this leaves only a small margin of renal function before uremic symptoms are apparent, when less than 5% of normal functioning nephrons remain.[58]

The highest standard for evidence of perioperative renal preservation is the avoidance of renal replacement therapy and reduced mortality. For example, optimal postoperative management of hyperglycemia in critically ill patients reduces the incidence of dialysis and improves survival.[128] Unfortunately, most

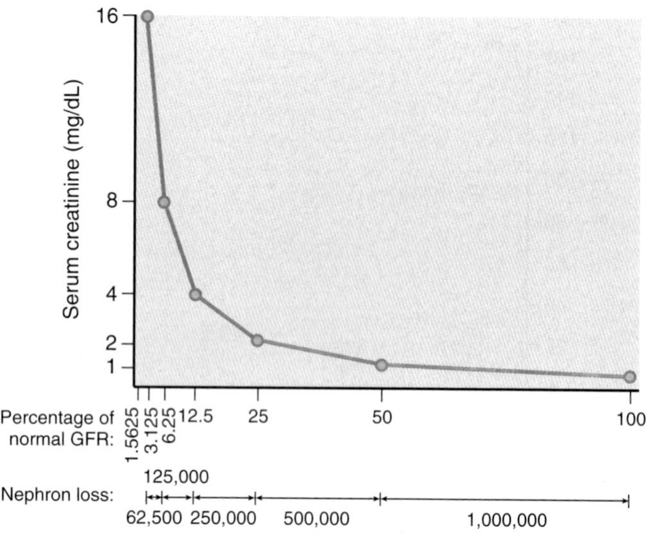

Figure 45-10 The inverse logarithmic relationship between serum creatinine concentration (*y* axis) and relative reductions in glomerular filtration rate (GFR) and approximate nephron loss (*x* axis). The nonlinear relationship means that serum creatinine level is not markedly increased until there is a 75% reduction in GFR (e.g., 120 to 30 mL/min). *(Modified from Faber MD, Kupin WL, Krishna G, Nairns RG: The differential diagnosis of ARF. In Lazarus JM, Brenner BM [eds]: ARF, 3rd ed. New York, Churchill Livingstone, 1993, p 133.)*

studies do not have sufficient sample size to show differences in mortality or dialysis rates and instead employ surrogates.

Most commonly, renal preservation is measured using secondary surrogate end points as markers for dialysis and death. Secondary measures most commonly reflect changes in glomerular filtration after surgery rather than renal failure requiring dialysis; peak filtration impairment is compared with a critical threshold or to renal function at baseline. Although most markers of renal filtration impairment based on serum creatinine have been validated through their association with postoperative mortality, there is little consensus on a standard assessment modality[129]; one review of 28 controlled perioperative studies found no two reports with the same AKI or ARF criteria.[23] Many studies present a variety of markers of AKI to describe an effect.[130]

Renal function is monitored indirectly. Among obstructive causes that may initiate ARF, an occluded or kinked urinary catheter must be eliminated as a source of oliguria. Toxic causes of ARF include antibiotics (e.g., aminoglycosides, amphotericin B) or radiocontrast agents. For example, with aminoglycosides, nephrotoxicity is poorly correlated with kidney tissue or plasma levels of the drug but is markedly augmented by concomitant volume depletion or liver cirrhosis.[20] In contrast, the likelihood of AKI correlates with baseline renal impairment and the amount of radiocontrast material injected, particularly when the contrast volume to creatinine clearance ratio is greater than 6.0.[131] The vigilance of the anesthesiologist is the first monitor required for preserving renal function.

The monitoring of renal function possible during the perioperative period is highly related to perioperative timing, postoperative disposition, and operative procedure. Unlike the postoperative/critical care setting where renal monitoring can involve periodic evaluation of kidney function under relatively stable conditions, intraoperative renal monitoring involves a briefer more unstable period, often involving significant blood loss, major fluid shifts, wide hemodynamic fluctuations, and even direct compromise to renal artery blood flow; all of these factors undermine the steady state so essential to most standard tests of renal function, such as creatinine clearance. The anesthesiologist often relies on indirect variables, such as urine volume, to assess renal perfusion. Unfortunately, urine output does not reliably reflect glomerular filtration and renal function under intraoperative conditions. Even knowledge of renal artery blood flow is not particularly informative, because increased flow mandates increased filtration and active transport demands, as well as increased oxygen delivery. As previously discussed, a monitor of balanced supply/demand of regional renal perfusion, particularly in the renal medulla, would be an ideal, although currently unavailable, direct monitoring tool. The best tools currently available intraoperatively are indirect hemodynamic monitors that can assist in optimizing conditions consistent with kidney wellbeing, such as ensuring adequate intravascular volume (i.e., preload), cardiac performance, and systemic perfusion. Serum chemistries and urinary indices may enable the assessment of adequate distribution of cardiac output to the kidneys themselves.

Indirect Markers of Optimal Renal Perfusion and Function

Nonoperative epidemiologic studies show a pattern for the development of renal failure that commonly involves the combination of severe dehydration with chronic renal conditions. For example, the combination of diabetes mellitus and volume depletion increases the chance of developing ARF by 100-fold.[20] The most practical preoperative methods to assess volume status are by standard preoperative history and physical examination and by evaluating changes in blood pressure in response to changing conditions. An awake patient normally does not have significant orthostatic changes in blood pressure unless he or she is dehydrated, whereas a similarly dehydrated anesthetized patient may demonstrate paradoxical arterial pulse changes with positive-pressure inspiration.[132]

Oxygen Delivery: Blood Gas, Acid-Base Balance, and Hematocrit

Severe arterial hypoxemia to a partial pressure of arterial oxygen ($Pa{O_2}$) value of less than 40 mm Hg is associated with decreased RBF and renal vasoconstriction.[133,134] It appears that systemic hypoxia can produce antidiuresis and antinatriuresis independent of renal nerve innervation.[135] Capnometry may be a useful monitor because hypercarbia has been associated with decreased RBF in patients requiring mechanical ventilation.[136] Animal studies indicate that oxygen supply demand inequalities are exaggerated and medullary hypoxia is extreme during CPB, effects that last well beyond separation from circulatory support.[137]

The effects of anemia on the kidney have been most studied in the context of CPB management. When crystalloid/colloid solutions are used to prime an extracorporeal circuit, initiation of CPB obligates an acute drop of approximately 30% in oxygen-carrying capacity. Animal studies endorse moderate hemodilution (hematocrit 20%-30%) as renoprotective during CPB through reduction of blood viscosity and improved regional blood flow.[138,139] However, although hematocrits less than 20% during CPB are commonly accepted clinically (extreme hemodilution), recent studies have linked very low hematocrit values with adverse outcome.[140-142] Several large retrospective studies identify lowest hematocrit during CPB as a predictor of postoperative AKI and renal failure.[130,143-145] Ironically, one alternative to tolerating extreme CPB hemodilution, transfusion, has also been considered risky for the kidney.[143,145]

Swaminathan and colleagues found an independent association of lowest CPB hematocrit (range, 22% to 24%) with postoperative AKI in a retrospective study of 1404 CABG surgery patients, a risk that was increased for obese patients.[143] These authors also observed a relationship between transfusion with renal impairment. In a similar study of AKI, Habib and colleagues[130] identified a near sigmoid-shaped detrimental CPB hematocrit "elbow" effect below 24%, even after adjustment for transfusion and extended CPB duration. Finally, Karkouti and colleagues evaluated the incidence of dialysis relative to lowest CPB hematocrit in 9080 cardiac surgery patients, noting a hematocrit less than 21% to be detrimental, compared with 21% to 25%, with a 2.3-fold increased risk of dialysis.[144] Interestingly, high hematocrits (>25%) were also associated with an increased risk for dialysis in this study. Although these studies endorse efforts to prevent extreme hemodilution during CPB, and guidelines for transfusion have been described,[146] support for transfusion as a treatment for all but the most extreme anemia (<15%)[147,148] is more controversial.[149]

Systemic Perfusion: Systolic Arterial and Pulse Pressure

Large multicenter epidemiologic studies have identified a relationship between markers of abnormal central aortic compliance, such as preoperative isolated systolic hypertension (>160 mm Hg) and wide pulse pressure hypertension (>40 mm Hg),[2,8,150] and postoperative AKI and dialysis. Preexisting systolic hypertension predicts a 40% greater risk, and wide pulse pressure also predicts postoperative AKI such that in cardiac surgery patients for every additional 20–mm Hg increment in pulse pressure greater than 40 mm Hg there is an OR of 1.49 (CI, 1.17 to 1.89; $P = .001$).

The systolic component of blood pressure is determined by stroke volume and the rate of ventricular ejection, whereas the pulsatile component of blood pressure is governed by the relationships among stroke volume, ventricular ejection, viscoelastic properties of large arteries, and peripheral vascular resistance. Pulse pressure is an index of the effects of large artery stiffness and the rate of pressure on propagation and reflection within the arterial tree. Early return of reflected arterial waves during late systolic rather than early diastolic pressure (from increased propagation velocity in stiff vessels) increases systolic blood pressure (i.e., afterload) and decreases diastolic blood pressure (i.e., perfusion pressure). It is likely that perfusion pressure and risk of perioperative renal dysfunction are linked by the preexisting capacity of the vasculature to compensate for low pressure as it determines flow. Those with a predisposition to low flow due to abnormal central aortic compliance may represent patients who require higher pressure to maintain adequate flow and minimize renal risk compared with normotensive patients.

RBF during CPB is not autoregulated and varies with pump flow rates and blood pressure.[65] However, CPB hypotension is not equivalent to hypotension with hemorrhagic shock or low cardiac output states, because low pressure during CPB is rarely associated with low flow. Fischer and colleagues retrospectively compared CPB flow rates and perfusion pressures in a case-control analysis of three groups of patients with normal baseline renal function who postoperatively either required dialysis (n = 44), sustained a renal injury without requiring dialysis (n = 51) or had no renal impairment (n = 48).[151] These authors noted that, on average, greater renal injury was associated with longer bypass durations, lower flows, and longer periods with CPB pressure less than 60 mm Hg. A serious limitation of this study is the potential for confounding CPB variables and known renal risk factors. In contrast, several large retrospective studies that accounted for known risk factors in evaluating perfusion management did not link low CPB blood pressure (with maintained flow) with postoperative AKI.[152-155]

RBF is affected by renal artery stenosis. In a retrospective study of 798 aortocoronary bypass patients whose cardiac catheterization procedures routinely included renal angiogram, Conlon and colleagues found that 18.7% of patients had at least 50% stenosis of one renal artery (9 patients had > 95% renal artery stenosis bilaterally).[156] However, in a multivariable logistic regression analysis there was no association of the presence or severity of renal artery stenosis with postoperative AKI.

Intravascular Volume Status: Central Venous Pressure, Pulmonary Capillary Wedge Pressure, Left Atrial Pressure, and Left Ventricular End-Diastolic Area

The decision to use any monitor should depend on the patient's functional cardiac reserve status and the extent of the proposed surgical insult. Although maintaining adequate cardiac output is necessary for maintaining adequate RBF, it may not guarantee adequate flow. Intravascular volume monitoring techniques must include caution to identify physiologic conditions that influence their validity as a reflection of preload in a particular patient (see Chapters 16, 18, 40, and 88). Monitoring central venous pressure to assess preload involves assumptions about normal left and right ventricular function, pulmonary vascular resistance, and mitral, pulmonary, and tricuspid valve function. Similarly, monitoring pulmonary artery pressure or pulmonary capillary wedge pressure assumes normal left ventricular compliance, mitral valve function, and normal airway pressure.

Direct measurements of left atrial pressure may offer insight into the kidney pressure-flow relationship because left atrial hypotension is a powerful stimulus for renal vasoconstriction.[85] Despite equivalent reductions in cardiac output and arterial blood pressure, RBF decreases much more when left atrial pressure is decreased (e.g., hemorrhagic shock) compared with when left atrial pressure is increased (e.g., cardiogenic shock).[157] Left atrial pressure receptors modulate renal vasoconstriction through release of atrial natriuretic peptide, a hormone secreted by the cardiac atria in response to intravascular volume expansion.[158] Atrial natriuretic hormone acts on the arterial and venous systems, the adrenals, and the kidneys to reduce intravascular volume and decrease blood pressure.[54] Within the kidney, the hormone increases hydraulic pressure in the glomerular capillaries through afferent arteriolar dilation and efferent arteriolar vasoconstriction. Atrial natriuretic peptide reduces blood pressure by relaxing smooth muscle and reducing sympathetic vascular stimulation and also inhibits renin and aldosterone secretion, causing renal vasodilation, natriuresis, and diuresis.[54]

Intraoperatively, one of the most direct ways to monitor intravascular volume may be by direct assessment of the left ventricular end-diastolic area with transesophageal echocardiography.[159,160] In addition, assessment of adequate cardiac function through pulse oximetry, acid-base assessment, cardiac output monitoring, and left ventricular fractional area of change as a surrogate for ejection fraction contribute to evidence of normovolemia and renal perfusion (see Chapters 16, 18, 40, and 88).[161] However, monitoring with invasive devices, such as pulmonary artery catheters, arterial cannulas, and transesophageal echocardiography, has never been demonstrated to reduce the incidence of ARF.

Blood Flow: Cardiac Output and Esophageal Doppler Ultrasonography–Guided "Fluid Optimization"

The electrocardiogram is essential to detect the depolarization-repolarization changes consistent with the electrolyte abnormalities of renal dysfunction and to monitor for normal rate and rhythm. The synchronized atrial kick preceding ventricular contraction may contribute significantly to cardiac output in the patient with a noncompliant left ventricle. Transesophageal echocardiography 2D and renal arterial Doppler waveform images, primarily of the left kidney, can be used to assess changes in pulsatility and resistive indices and qualitatively describe RBF changes over time.[162,163]

Many believe that dehydration, hypovolemia, and blood loss are major contributors to perioperative renal dysfunction.[164] An update to enhance traditional, somewhat unreliable guides to fluid administration (e.g., central venous pressure) is the concept of "guided fluid optimization." The principle behind fluid optimization is to maximize tissue-oxygen delivery by achieving a maximum stroke volume, typically achieved by esophageal Doppler ultrasonography–monitored fluid boluses.[165] Some randomized studies have evaluated fluid optimization, a strategy that leads to increased perioperative volume administration for almost all patients, and reported improved outcomes such as shorter hospital stays.[166] In contrast, other studies have studied restrictive fluid regimens and also reported improved outcomes without evidence of increased ARF, despite decreases in perioperative urine output.[167,168] A systematic review of over 80 perioperative fluid management randomized trials concluded that current evidence does not allow evidence-based recommendations of one type of fluid over another or on the optimal amount of fluid to be administered for fluid replacement in elective surgical procedures but recommended strict avoidance of fluid overload.[169] Others have described the disastrous and unpredictable occurrence of acute pulmonary edema related to postoperative fluid retention.[170] There is insufficient evidence on which to base judgments on the importance of fluid selection and management strategies on perioperative renal function.[165,169]

Autoregulation and Distribution of Cardiac Output to the Kidneys

Standard cardiorenal relationships identify cardiac output and perfusion pressure as major predictors of RBF, whereas pressure alone correlates with urine output.[65,66] As previously mentioned, renal artery autoregulatory reflexes are *not* influenced by metabolic need and serve to "protect" the glomeruli from overload by restricting blood flow at higher pressures (e.g., >80 mm Hg).[38,39] Renal reflexes guided by different stimuli are the afferent and efferent arteriolar myogenic and tubular-glomerular feedback reflexes and the paracrine reflexes of the medullary microcirculation.

The fraction of cardiac output perfusing the kidneys depends on the ratio of renal vascular resistance to systemic vascular resistance.[58] In general, the response to renal hypoperfusion involves three major regulatory mechanisms that support renal function: (1) afferent arteriolar dilation increases the proportion of cardiac output that perfuses the kidney; (2) efferent arteriolar resistance increases the filtration fraction; and (3) hormonal and neural responses improve renal perfusion by increasing intravascular volume, thereby indirectly increasing cardiac output. The afferent arterioles react to reductions in perfusion pressure by relaxing their smooth muscle elements to decrease renal vascular resistance. Decreased solute delivery to the macula densa in the cortical portion of the thick ascending loop of Henle results in relaxation of the juxtaposed afferent arteriolar smooth muscle cells, improving glomerular perfusion and filtration.

The kidney produces vasodilator prostaglandins to counteract the effects of systemic vasoconstrictor hormones such as angiotensin II.[171] In a state of low cardiac output when systemic blood pressure is preserved by the action of systemic vasopressors, RBF is not depressed because the effect of the vasopressors is blunted within the kidney.

A selective increase in efferent arteriolar resistance decreases glomerular plasma flow, thereby preserving GFR. Glomerular filtration is augmented because capillary pressure upstream from the site of vasoconstriction tends to rise. This mechanism enables the kidney to offer high organ vascular resistance to contribute to the maintenance of systemic blood pressure without compromising its function of filtration. Studies using specific inhibitors of angiotensin II have shown that efferent arteriolar resistance largely results from the action of angiotensin II.[172] At low concentrations, norepinephrine has a vasoconstricting effect on efferent arterioles, indicating that the adrenergic system may also be important for maintaining the renal compensatory response.[173]

Evidence supports the notion that reductions in cardiac output are accompanied by the release of vasopressin and by increased activity of the sympathetic nervous system and the renin-angiotensin-aldosterone system. These regulatory mechanisms to preserve RBF conserve salt and water. The control of blood delivery to the kidney, the fraction of plasma filtered, and the amount of volume returned to the systemic circulation are determined by regulatory mechanisms within the kidney that attempt to preserve filtration function during compromised circulation.

One study reported the normal response to hemorrhage in otherwise healthy patients, describing a 30% reduction in RBF with a decrease in mean perfusion pressure from 80 to 60 mm Hg.[174] Changes known to occur at the initiation of CPB include greater reduction in renal than systemic perfusion, loss of RBF autoregulation, and stress hormone and inflammatory responses known to be harmful to the kidney.[65,175,176] These effects may explain why the duration of CPB independently predicts post–cardiac surgery renal impairment.[3,4,177,178] Notably, during experimental CPB, medullary Po_2 drops from typically low levels to unmeasurable levels.[137]

Laboratory Tests of Serum and Urine as Markers of Renal Function

An ideal glomerular filtration monitor for perioperative AKI recognition would be accurate, point-of-care, simple, brief, and inexpensive and, in addition, should have confirmed links with AKI-related outcomes (e.g., mortality). Although no such test exists, trends in repeated serum creatinine determinations (relative or absolute changes), alone or integrated into estimates of GFR, are currently the most used clinical tool for this purpose.[179-181]

Although traditional tests are useful in identifying kidney failure, an inherent limitation of almost all currently available tools is the obligate delay between the *onset* of AKI and the *diagnosis* of AKI. One striking difference between management of AKI and acute myocardial infarction (AMI) is the lack of *early biomarkers* for AKI to guide prompt recognition and intervention when tissue is threatened (i.e., AMI—troponin, creatinine kinase-MB). Thus, one of the primary priorities of the largest current collaborative initiative, the AKI network (AKIN),[30] is to explore the existence and value of early AKI biomarkers. Therefore, the following discussion will be categorized into traditional diagnostic tools that provide only delayed recognition of AKI and the currently expanding field of early biomarkers for AKI.

Table 45-1 Biomarkers of Kidney Function*

Serum creatinine
Analysis tools
Baseline to peak postoperative fractional change
Peak in-hospital postoperative
Maximum change baseline-to-peak
ARF definitions
STS definition
AKIN criteria[30]
RIFLE criteria[31]
Modified contrast nephropathy
Creatinine clearance
Estimates
Cockroft-Gault equation[180]
MDRD equation[181]
Direct measures
24-hr urine collection
2-hr urine collection
Analysis tools
Nadir postoperative
Baseline-to-nadir postoperative
Baseline-to-nadir postoperative fractional change
Glomerular filtration rate
Inulin clearance
Iohexol clearance
Analysis tools
Nadir postoperative
Baseline-to-nadir postoperative
Baseline-to-nadir postoperative fractional change
Urine volume
Analysis tools
AKIN criteria[30]
RIFLE criteria[31]
Blood urea nitrogen
Urine specific gravity
Urine osmolality
Urine-to-plasma creatinine ratio
Urine-to-plasma urea ratio
Urinary sodium
Fractional excretion of sodium
Free water clearance
Renal blood flow

*Traditional biomarkers of kidney function primarily focus on measurements or estimates of function for comparison to expected normal values. With regard to diagnosis of prerenal azotemia and acute kidney injury, these tools typically provide information to confirm a diagnosis as long as 48 hours after the event.
STS, Society of Thoracic Surgeons; AKIN, AKI Network; MDRD, Modification of Diet in Renal Disease (study).

Traditional (Delayed) Biomarkers of Acute Kidney Injury

Biomarkers for renal failure and acute tubular necrosis, which are reviewed next, include urine volume, urine specific gravity, urine osmolality, serum creatinine level, serum blood urea nitrogen level, urine-to-plasma creatinine ratio, urine-to-plasma urea ratio, urine sodium level, fractional excretion of sodium (FE_{Na}), free water clearance, creatinine clearance, inulin clearance, and RBF (Table 45-1).

Urine Volume

Although recorded religiously, intraoperative urine output remains a controversial perioperative marker of renal function. Whereas the presence of urine (regardless of amount) confirms blood flow to the kidney, urine flow rate is an indirect parameter of renal function, and many nonrenal factors directly and profoundly influence urine production. Multiple studies have shown no correlation between urine volume and histologic evidence of acute tubular necrosis, GFR, creatinine clearance, or changes from preoperative to postoperative levels of BUN and creatinine levels in patients with burn injury,[182] trauma,[183,184] or shock status or in those undergoing cardiovascular surgery.[63,185,186] Alpert and colleagues observed oliguric aortic surgery patients (urine flow < 0.125 mL/kg/hr) given either additional crystalloid solution, intravenous mannitol, furosemide, or no intervention[63] and found no correlation between intraoperative mean or lowest hourly urine output and subsequent AKI (see Fig. 45-7).

In contrast to the intraoperative setting, significant prolonged preoperative or postoperative oliguria (<0.5 mL/kg/hr for >6 hr) is more predictive and even diagnostic of AKI; for example, oliguria has been incorporated into the AKIN and RIFLE AKI criteria.[30,31] The kidney concentrates the ultrafiltrate so that at maximal concentration, a minimum of 400 to 500 mL of urine is required to clear the daily obligatory nitrogenous wastes.[187] Among the factors that influence tubular excretion of solute and water are local and systemic levels of renin, aldosterone, and ADH. In the operating room, patients are often hemodynamically unstable; decreased blood volume or cardiac output, fluctuating hormone levels (e.g., aldosterone, renin, ADH), nervous system reflexes, and increased catecholamine concentrations, added to the effects of general anesthesia, can alter GFR. The data do not support oliguria as a reliable intraoperative sign of pending renal dysfunction.[63,182-187] Notably, the lack of correlation of immediate perioperative oliguria with AKI requires further incorporation into recent consensus statements developed primarily by nephrologists and critical care physicians as one of the criteria to diagnose AKI, such as the RIFLE and AKIN criteria.[30,31]

Urine Specific Gravity

Urine specific gravity reflects the mass of 1 mL of urine compared with 1 mL of distilled water. Normal values range between 1.001 and 1.035. In settings of poor perfusion or prerenal azotemia, urine specific gravity is high (e.g., 1.030), reflecting the kidney's ability to conserve sodium and water. With loss of concentrating ability due to acute tubular necrosis, urine specific gravity resembles plasma osmolarity (i.e., 1.010). Specific gravity is a surrogate for osmolarity (normal range, 50 to 1000 mOsm/kg). Unfortunately, when substances that raise specific gravity without significantly changing osmolarity are present in large amounts (e.g., glucose, protein, contrast dye) (Table 45-2), high urine specific gravity can provide misleading reassurance that renal concentrating ability is preserved.[188,189] The ability of the kidneys to concentrate urine after water deprivation is impaired in elderly patients, also making urine specific gravity an unreliable test.

Urine Osmolality

Osmolality is a measure of the number of osmotically active particles in solution in the solvent phase. It is one of the major forces that move fluid throughout the body, especially in the kidney. Theoretically, urine osmolality is physiologically superior to urine specific gravity as a test of renal function; however, the same substances and conditions that render urine specific gravity a nonspecific test can also affect the reliability of urine osmolality (see Table 45-2). A defective urinary concentrating mechanism tends to be one of the most consistent and lasting tubular defects of ARF.

Table 45-2 Substances and Conditions Affecting Urine Specific Gravity and Urine Osmolality

Proteins
Glucose
Mannitol
Dextran
Diuretics
Advanced age
Extremes of age
Radiographic contrast media
Antibiotics (e.g., carbenicillin)
Hydrometer calibration
Detergents
Temperature
Hormonal imbalances

The sensitivity and specificity of urine osmolality as a test for predicting or distinguishing acute tubular necrosis from prerenal azotemia are clinically inadequate.[186,190-195] With values greater than 500 mOsm, the positive predictive value for diagnosing prerenal azotemia ranges from 60% to 100%. With a value less than 350 mOsm, the positive predictive value for diagnosing acute tubular necrosis ranges from 69% to 95%.

Serum Creatinine Concentration

In spite of all its limitations, the serum creatinine concentration remains the most used clinical tool to assess renal function. However, due to its nonlinear relationship with changes in renal function (see Fig. 45-10), variability among individuals, and susceptibility to changes unrelated to changes in GFR (e.g., cimetidine, trimethoprim, acetylcysteine),[196,197] elevation of serum creatinine concentration is only somewhat reliable as a sign of renal dysfunction, and GFR may be reduced by as much as 75% before elevations reach abnormal levels.[198]

Creatinine, a cyclic anhydride of creatine, is a small molecule (113 daltons) that is continuously released during skeletal muscle protein catabolism. Muscle mass, which is smaller in women and declines with age, directly predicts creatinine release. Curiously, age- and gender-related differences in GFR are well matched with differences in creatinine release such that normal serum creatinine levels vary little with age or between genders (Fig. 45-11). Creatinine levels in body fluids (e.g., plasma, serum, urine) are also easy and inexpensive to measure. These properties have made serum creatinine a mainstay as a marker of steady-state changes in renal filtration.

Developing a consensus definition of AKI has been a recent focus. A consensus opinion from the Acute Kidney Injury Network asserts that the term *AKI* be used to represent the entire spectrum of ARF.[30] The AKIN definition, a 1.5-fold or 0.3 mg/dL (≥ 26.4 μmol/L) creatinine rise within a 48-hour period or more than 6 hours of oliguria (<0.5 mL/kg/hr), is a modification of its predecessor, the Acute Dialysis Quality Initiative (ADQI) Group so-called RIFLE criteria.[31] Specific to cardiac surgery is the Society of Thoracic Surgeons' definition of ARF as at least a twofold creatinine rise to a value exceeding 2.0 mg/dL or new dialysis or both.[25] Another commonly used AKI definition requires creatinine rise to exceed 25% or 0.5 mg/dL (44 μmol/L).[26,37]

Whereas creatinine has many advantages as a marker of changes in filtration function, its many drawbacks continue to fuel the search for a more ideal marker of renal filtration. In conditions such as the perioperative period where steady state is difficult to ascertain, serum creatinine may fail to accurately reflect the magnitude of nephron loss, and relative changes in serum creatinine may be more important than whether a value lies within or outside the normal range. Because creatinine production is proportional to muscle mass, many chronically ill, malnourished, elderly patients have serum creatinine values in the normal range, despite reduced renal concentrating ability and GFR. Conversely, many critically ill patients at risk for developing ARF may have high metabolic rates because of hyperalimentation, sepsis, or post-traumatic states. Higher metabolic rates mean higher nitrogenous waste production requiring greater than average RBF and urine flow rates to maintain normal serum creatinine concentration. Because creatinine is excreted by glomerular filtration and tubular secretion, as the GFR decreases the tubular secretion becomes a progressively more important fraction of creatinine excretion, such that creatinine clearance

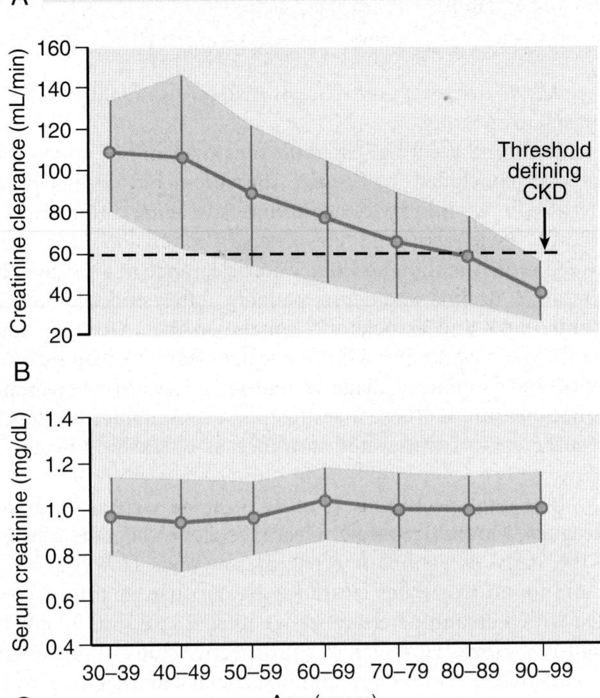

Figure 45-11 Several "rule of thumb" tools exist to estimate normal glomerular filtration rate (GFR) values based on age and gender (**A**). Creatinine clearance approximates but overestimates GFR due to creatinine secretion from the proximal renal tubule. Notably, owing to the similarity in rate of decline of GFR and creatinine release related to age (**B**), and based on gender, normal serum creatinine values remain remarkably similar throughout life (**C**). Notably, by the fifth decade some individuals, and by the ninth decade most individuals, with serum creatinine values in the normal range have GFR values reflecting chronic renal dysfunction (<60 mL/min). CKD, chronic kidney disease. (*Modified with permission from Davies DF, Shock NW: Age changes in glomerular filtration rate, effective renal plasma flow, and tubular excretory capacity in adult males. J Clin Invest 29:496-507, 1950.*)

overestimates the GFR by 50% to 100% if the true GFR is less than 15 mL/min.[198,199] Postoperative rise of serial serum creatinine measurements do not definitively identify AKI sometimes for several days after cardiac or noncardiac surgery.[32,200] Nonetheless, the serum creatinine concentration remains a useful, inexpensive, and, so far, unsurpassed clinical tool particularly to reflect *trends* of change in renal filtration function and predict outcome, even during the perioperative period.[179,201,202]

Blood Urea Nitrogen

BUN remains widely used to assess renal function but possesses few of the characteristics of an "ideal" substance. A product of protein metabolism, BUN level is increased by high protein intake, blood in the gastrointestinal tract, and accelerated catabolism (e.g., in traumatized or septic patients). The normal range is 8 to 20 mg/dL. Because urea is synthesized in the liver, hepatic dysfunction decreases urea production and, therefore, BUN concentration. BUN concentration fails in a key criterion as a reliable estimate of the GFR. Although urea is freely filtered at the glomerulus, it is reabsorbed to a large and variable extent. The reabsorption of urea is greater, approximately 60% of the filtered load, when urinary flow is low; only about 40% is reabsorbed when flow is high. In addition, perioperative hemodilution (e.g., CPB) may affect circulating BUN levels.

It was believed that combining BUN and serum creatinine levels would provide more reliable information than using either alone. If ratios of BUN to serum creatinine exceeded 20:1, for example, dehydration was suspected.

Urine-to-Plasma Creatinine Ratio

The urine-to-plasma creatinine index was first introduced in 1950 by Bull and colleagues[203] as a method of evaluating patients with acute tubular necrosis. It was determined retrospectively that patients whose urine-to-plasma creatinine levels rose above 10 after having been below 10 were no longer at serious risk for "uncontrolled mineral and water loss." This index was introduced primarily as a prognostic aid and not as a diagnostic test.

The sensitivity and specificity of the urine-to-plasma creatinine index are unfortunately clinically unreliable for diagnosing acute tubular necrosis and prerenal azotemia.[204] Miller and coworkers[191] concluded that the index was not useful, except in extreme situations, because of significant overlap between groups. Espinel and Gregory[192] prospectively studied 87 patients (61 with acute tubular necrosis or prerenal azotemia) and concluded that the urine-to-plasma creatinine ratio might be a useful indicator of acute tubular necrosis if the ratio was less than 10 and that it might be an indicator of prerenal azotemia if the ratio was less than 40. However, a significant overlap in values was found for 33% of patients.

Urine-to-Plasma Urea Ratio

In 1959, Perlmutter and colleagues[205] proposed that the ratio between urine and serum urea nitrogen levels could differentiate prerenal azotemia from acute tubular necrosis. These investigators thought that a ratio of greater than 14 was associated with transient oliguria and that a ratio of less than 10 was associated with acute tubular necrosis. In 1965, Eliahou and Bata[190] reported that the urine-to-blood urea ratio might not be useful for diagnosis in all cases. Subsequently, Chisholm and associates[206] confirmed that the urine-to-plasma urea ratio was often misleading in the diagnosis of uremia.

Urea production is not constant and is affected by many nonrenal variables.[207] Variables include sudden increases or decreases in protein intake, states of increased protein catabolism (i.e., trauma, infections, hyperthermia, or corticosteroid therapy), gastrointestinal bleeding, and liver dysfunction. Because urea levels can vary tremendously independent of renal function, it is not surprising that knowing the urine-to-plasma urea ratio does not make it possible to differentiate between prerenal azotemia and acute tubular necrosis.

Urinary Sodium Concentration

With decreasing perfusion, the normally functioning kidney conserves sodium and water. The factors affecting this phenomenon are numerous and include heterogenicity of nephrons, secretion of aldosterone, secretion of ADH, diuretic therapy, saline content of intravenous infusion solutions, sympathetic neural tone, and sodium-avid states (e.g., congestive heart failure, cirrhosis). It is traditionally accepted that a urinary sodium level of less than 20 mEq suggests prerenal azotemia and that a level of greater than 40 mEq indicates acute tubular necrosis.

The reported sensitivity and specificity of urinary sodium levels for diagnosis of acute tubular necrosis and prerenal azotemia suggest that the levels can be used for diagnosis of approximately one half of the patients with acute tubular necrosis.[186,191-193,203,208,209] Considering the complex physiology of sodium homeostasis, it is not surprising that levels of urinary sodium are unreliable indicators of prerenal azotemia or acute tubular necrosis. The test is nonspecific because a significant overlap exists between the diagnostic categories and because urinary sodium measurement tends to correlate more with volume and type of resuscitation fluid than with renal function.[184]

Fractional Excretion of Sodium

Failure of avid sodium reuptake by the kidney in the setting of dehydration manifests by increased urine sodium and is the principle underpinning the utility of FE_{Na} as a diagnostic tool. A sodium excretion value of less than 1% compared with greater than 1% often enables differentiation between prerenal azotemia and acute tubular necrosis, particularly in the presence of oliguria.[210] The FE_{Na} was first described by Espinel[208]; it represents the fraction of sodium excreted versus that filtered by the kidneys. Handa and Morrin[204] had previously described the "renal failure ratio," which is a derivative of the excreted fraction of filtered sodium. The only difference between the two is that in determining renal failure ratio the plasma sodium level is assumed to be constant. FE_{Na} is calculated as follows:

$$FE_{Na} = \frac{\text{Excreted Na}}{\text{Filtered Na} \times 100} = \frac{U_{Na}P_{Cr}}{\left(U_{Cr}P_{Na} \times 100\right)}$$

where P_{Cr} is the plasma creatinine level, P_{Na} is the plasma sodium level, U_{Cr} is the urinary creatinine level, and U_{Na} is the urinary sodium level.

At first, investigators reported that FE_{Na} permitted clear differentiation between prerenal azotemia and acute tubular necrosis.[191-193,208] However, subsequent case reports cast doubt on the sensitivity and specificity of FE_{Na} as a useful discriminator between these conditions.[208,209,211-213] Brown[211] suggested that the FE_{Na} was diagnostic of acute tubular necrosis but was of little or no value for the early prediction of renal failure. Brosius and Lau[212] showed that early determinations of the FE_{Na} were more likely to be misleading than later determinations, indicating that the measurement was unlikely to be helpful in the early diagnosis of acute tubular necrosis. Shin and colleagues[210] concluded that knowing the FE_{Na} was useful only when oliguria was already present. However, because this indicator is usually observed later in the course of renal disease than the changes in creatinine or free water clearance, the FE_{Na} is not a highly valuable tool for predicting imminent renal failure and is rarely used now for this purpose.[214,215]

Free Water Clearance

Water that contains no solutes is considered "free water." Thus, compared with normal isosmotic plasma, hyperosmotic urine can be considered to represent the clearance of a negative amount of free water (i.e., avid water retention). Normal free water clearance (C_{H2O}) in the setting of dehydration can be as high as −25 to −20 mL/hr, whereas free water clearance of −15 to +15 mL/hr reflects incipient renal dysfunction. Free water clearance is a measure of the kidney's ability to dilute or concentrate urine as necessary to maintain homeostasis and is determined using the following equation:

$$C_{H2O} = UV - \left(U_{Osm} \times UV/P_{Osm}\right)$$

where UV is urine volume, U_{Osm} is urinary osmolality, and P_{Osm} is plasma osmolality.

Jones and Weil[216] assessed the sensitivity of free water clearance and concluded that serial measurements predicted the patients who would experience progressive renal dysfunction.[186] However, Rosenberg and coworkers[184] found no correlation between renal function and free water clearance in a prospective study of 69 trauma and sepsis patients. After studying 38 ICU patients, Baek and associates[217] concluded that ARF was diagnosed 1 to 3 days sooner with free water clearance than by other clinical and laboratory diagnostic criteria (creatinine clearance was not measured). These investigators recommended sequential measurements of free water clearance as an early indicator of ARF.

In a retrospective study of 675 trauma victims, Shin and colleagues[183] found free water clearance alone was not sufficient for the early detection of renal dysfunction. However, these authors found free water clearance greater than 20 mL/hr combined with a creatinine clearance less than 25 mL/min identified a high-risk group. However, in a prospective study of postoperative patients,[210] these same authors concluded that free water clearance was not as sensitive as creatinine clearance for predicting ARF in trauma patients. The same substances and conditions that decrease the usefulness of urine osmolality for indicating renal failure can similarly decrease the usefulness of free water clearance (see Table 45-2).[218]

Creatinine Clearance

Substances used to assess GFR through their clearance from the circulation are presumed to have certain "ideal" properties, including a steady supply to the circulation, free glomerular filtration, and neither reabsorption or excretion by the tubules. As previously mentioned, creatinine partially fails these criteria, owing to its minimal secretion from the proximal tubule; however, because "gold standard" methodologies such as inulin, ^{51}Cr-EDTA, or ^{99m}Tc-DTPA clearance are expensive and cumbersome, creatinine clearance continues to be the most commonly used direct measurement of renal filtration function. Creatinine clearance is the volume of plasma that the kidneys can completely clear of creatinine per minute and is measured by calculating the amount of creatinine reaching the urine during a period of time (urine volume and urine creatinine concentration) and comparing it with the concentration of creatinine in the blood. Measurements of creatinine clearance are most useful to quantify renal reserve.

Precise measurements of creatinine clearance require collection of timed urine samples using the following formula:

$$GFR = UV/P$$

where U is the urinary concentration of creatinine (mg/dL), V is the volume of urine (mL/min), and P is the plasma concentration (mg/dL). The major limitation in the determination of creatinine clearance is the necessity of collecting urine accurately. Although

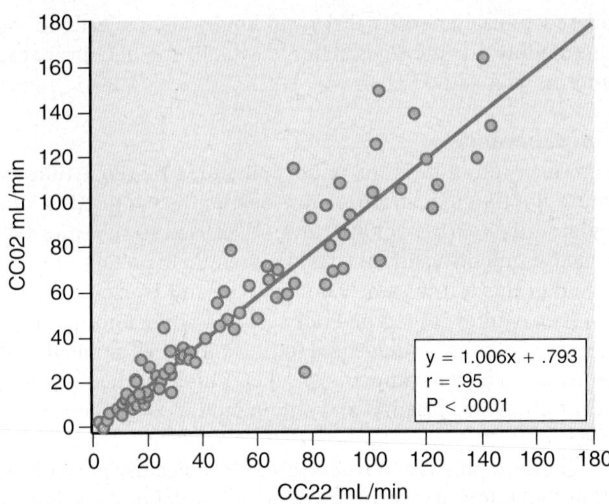

Figure 45-12 Correlation between the 2-hour creatinine clearance (CC02) and the 22-hour creatinine clearance (CC22). (*Adapted from Sladen RN, Endo E, Harrison T: Two-hour versus 22-hour creatinine clearance in critically ill patients. Anesthesiology 67:1013-1016, 1987.*)

reasonable correlation between 2-hour and 24-hour creatinine clearance (R = 0.85) has been reported for patients in ICUs (Fig. 45-12),[219,220] it remains true that the longer the urine collection period, the more accurate is the calculation of creatinine clearance. Changing hydration of the patient invalidates short-term determinations of the GFR, as does failure to record urine volume accurately. The error in calculation of creatinine clearance can vary from 10% to 27%, depending on the accuracy of urine collection,[221] body weight, surface area, and normal day-to-day variations. Another significant drawback is that for the patient with ARF a test that requires 24-hour urine collection is often impractical.

Perioperatively, creatinine clearance can be estimated by integrating serum creatinine values with other patient characteristics.[180] However, the dynamic changes in renal function and rapid fluid shifts typical of the surgical period often compromise precise measurement of renal glomerular filtration rate at this time. Until more precise validated perioperative markers are available, many believe that serum creatinine–derived markers are at least as accurate (and less expensive) than other more invasive tests.[179,201,202] A variety of algorithms have been developed to estimate creatinine clearance from a single steady-state serum creatinine value during conditions; these formulas are usually developed through modeling using data from large nonsurgical populations and require knowledge of factors that influence creatinine generation (gender, age, body weight). Of the many predictive tools that exist, the Cockcroft-Gault equation has been the most validated and durable.[180] The Cockcroft-Gault equation calculates estimated GFR (eGFR) based on patient gender, age (years), weight (kg), and serum creatinine (Cr) (mg/dL):

$$\text{Cockcroft-Gault eGFR}\left(\text{mL/min}\right) = \left(140-\text{age}\right)\times\text{weight}\left(\text{kg}\right)/\left(\text{Cr}\times 72\right)$$
$$\left(\times 0.85 \text{ for females}\right)$$

More recently, an estimating method from the Modification of Diet in Renal Disease (MDRD) study that adds knowledge of ethnicity (black versus nonblack) to standard components of the Cockcroft-Gault equation may improve accuracy.[181]

An abbreviated MDRD formula is available that can estimate GFR measured in mL/min/1.73 m^2

$$\text{GFR} = 186\times\left(\text{serum creatinine}\left[\text{mg/dL}\right]\right)^{-1.154}\times\left(\text{age}\right)^{-0.203}$$
$$\left(\times 0.742 \text{ for females}\right)$$
$$\left(\times 1.210 \text{ for blacks}\right)$$

However, even the most detailed MDRD eGFR equation under ideal conditions correlates poorly with GFR determined using "gold standard" tools, with a 30% or greater error in 10% patients and more than a 50% deviation in 2%.[181]

When Shin and associates[183] retrospectively reviewed the records of 26 patients who had acute tubular necrosis, they concluded that the diagnosis was likely to be made in patients who had a creatinine clearance of less than 25 mL/min and a free water clearance of greater than 15 mL/hr. In a follow-up study of 40 trauma patients who underwent surgery, these researchers[210] concluded that creatinine clearance of less than 25 mL/min alone permitted the early detection of renal dysfunction in patients with the potential for development of renal failure and that free water clearance was not as sensitive.

So-called Starling forces are important in understanding the factors that affect glomerular filtration. Glomerular filtration is governed by the following equation:

$$\text{GFR} = K_f \times (P_{GC} - P_{BC} - P_{PO})$$

where GFR is the glomerular filtration rate or the rate at which fluid is filtered through the glomerular capillaries into the Bowman capsule, K_f is the glomerular filtration coefficient or the factor that considers the permeability and surface area of the glomerular basement membrane, P_{GC} is the glomerular capillary pressure, P_{BC} is the pressure in the Bowman capsule, and P_{PO} is the plasma oncotic pressure.

Acute changes in GFR, and consequently in urine formation, are commonly caused by changes in glomerular capillary pressure. For example, events that reduce plasma flow rates reduce the hydraulic pressure of glomerular capillaries and favor decreased ultrafiltration whereas events that increase plasma flow rate have the opposite effect. Theoretically, varying concentrations of plasma proteins may influence urine formation and the GFR. As the concentration of proteins in plasma decreases, the oncotic pressure and the oncotic force opposing ultrafiltration also decrease. Conversely, an increase in oncotic pressure reduces the GFR. This effect is most likely offset by the oncotic force of plasma proteins (e.g., albumin), which enables adequate intravascular volume to be maintained. However, in one series,[222] patients resuscitated with albumin after massive transfusion had more renal dysfunction than those resuscitated with saline.

Intravenous fluid choices are associated with increased renal risk in some studies of postoperative AKI. When the impact of normal saline-based intravenous fluid replacement was evaluated and compared with lactated Ringer's solution (i.e., albumin 5% in normal saline, hetastarch in normal saline, or lactated Ringer's solution), renal function indices (i.e., creatinine clearance, serum creatinine, and urine output) were all inferior in the normal saline-based vehicle groups.[223] The patients receiving lactated Ringer's solution were more likely to exhibit a hypercoagulable state.[223] Outcome data, however, did not enable a distinction between albumin and normal saline as a fluid replacement option. Volume expansion using hydroxyethyl starch (HES) preparations is associated with AKI in critically ill and surgical patients in several retrospective reports.[224-227] In a randomized study of 129 patients with septic shock or severe sepsis that received either 3% gelatin or 6% HES, peak serum creatinine and the frequency of ARF and oliguria was higher in the HES group.[228] In the same study, a multivariable analysis also identified the use of HES as an independent predictor of ARF. In contrast, Boldt and colleagues found no evidence of increased renal risk in two small perioperative randomized studies of surgical patients receiving either gelatin or 6% HES.[229,230] Recent studies have focused on the contents of the solutions supporting the HES preparations and their potential to influence the development of metabolic hyperchloremic acidosis and variations in renal outcome.

Use of saline or saline-based colloid solutions in perioperative patients is commonly associated with the acid-base abnormality metabolic hyperchloremic acidosis. In a randomized, blinded trial, 47 elderly patients undergoing major surgery received 6% HES suspended in either 0.9% sodium chloride (HESPAN, B. Braun Medical, Inc., Irvine, CA) or a balanced salt solution (Hextend, BioTime, Inc., Berkeley, CA) (see Chapters 71 and 88). None of the patients receiving the balanced salt-based solution but two thirds of those receiving sodium chloride developed hyperchloremic metabolic acidosis ($P < .0001$).[231] In addition, in the saline group, gastric tonometry identified a larger increase in the CO_2 gap ($P = .04$), suggesting poorer splanchnic perfusion. Some have speculated that this metabolic abnormality may be a relevant modifier of perioperative renal vulnerability.[232] Increased chloride levels and acidosis can reduce RBF and GFR, increase afferent arteriolar tone, and alter renin release.[233,234] The avoidance of saline and the development of metabolic hyperchloremic acidosis may prove to be an important modifier of renal risk.

In general, the GFR is determined by the rate of glomerular plasma flow (as it influences ultrafiltration pressure), systemic oncotic pressure, glomerular hydraulic pressure differences, and an ultrafiltration coefficient. The ultrafiltration coefficient is the product of glomerular capillary hydraulic permeability and total surface area available for filtration. The filtration rate across a capillary bed is, therefore, the product of surface area, pressure gradients, and permeability. Hydrostatic pressures are normally maintained higher in glomerular capillaries than in other capillary beds by a delicate balance of preglomerular and postglomerular vascular tone in arterioles. The permeability of the glomerular capillary wall is equal for substances with molecular masses up to 5000 to 6000 daltons and decreases to almost zero at 60,000 to 70,000 daltons.[235] Metabolic wastes and essential nutrients are filtered freely, and larger proteins, such as albumin and immunoglobulin G, are filtered in trace amounts or not at all. The glomerulopathic process in diabetes,[236] for example, results from all of the factors that cause sustained increase in glomerular pressure and flow. Hyperglycemia induces a state of extracellular fluid volume expansion, structural hypertrophy of the kidney, and altered glucoregulatory and vasoregulatory hormone action. These hemodynamic consequences of hyperglycemia lead to renal vasodilation and increased plasma flow rate. The increase of plasma flow causes increased glomerular transcapillary flux of plasma proteins. The elevation in glomerular flow (i.e., pressure) also alters the permeability and selectivity of the glomerular basement membrane, resulting in increased protein filtration. The increased transglomerular flux of plasma proteins leads to their accumulation in the mesangium, which further propagates glomerulosclerosis.

Inulin Clearance

Glomerular filtration is an important index of renal function. Because the tubule reabsorbs most of the water filtered through the glomerulus, urine volume cannot be used to measure GFR. For measurement, a substance is required that is filtered through the glomerulus at the same rate as water and is excreted in the urine (i.e., neither reabsorbed nor secreted). The amount of such a substance filtered is then equal to the amount eliminated in the urine and can be determined from the product of the substances' concentration in plasma and the amount of plasma water filtered.

Inulin, a polymer of fructose with a molecular mass of 5200 daltons that is found in Jerusalem artichokes, dahlias, and chicory, has been used to measure GFR because it is filtered freely in the glomerulus, not reabsorbed or secreted, and is excreted in the urine. Purified inulin is expensive and difficult to measure. However, since its introduction in 1934, inulin clearance has been considered the standard for measurement of GFR.[237] To assess inulin clearance, the clinician administers a priming dose of inulin intravenously, followed by a continuous infusion calculated to maintain constant blood concentrations. After an equilibration period (usually 1 hour), clearance measurements are obtained. Urine is collected (typically with a Foley catheter), and venous blood samples are obtained at the midpoint of each clearance period. The longer the clearance period, the less likely is the introduction of error from incomplete voiding. The standard formula for calculation of clearance is as follows:

$$C_I = (U_I V)/P_I$$

where U_I and P_I are the urine and plasma concentrations of inulin, C_I is the rate of inulin clearance, and V is the urine flow rate.

Whereas inulin clearance is considered a "gold standard" tool to measure GFR in clinical practice, the endogenous substance creatinine is used to measure clearance. Creatinine is a smaller substance than inulin and is not an ideal substance for measuring clearance because a small amount is secreted under normal conditions. Although creatinine clearance may exceed inulin clearance, the clearance of endogenous creatinine approximates that of inulin and has proved to be a reasonable measure of GFR.[238] The creatinine-to-inulin clearance ratio is almost identical in healthy infants, children, and adults. In subjects with moderate to severe renal insufficiency, however, the creatinine-to-inulin clearance ratio is increased.[239] Increased secretion and clearance of creatinine in patients with renal insufficiency may, therefore, result in overestimates of true GFR.

Urea (molecular mass of 60 daltons) cannot be used to estimate GFR because, under normal conditions, it is filtered and reabsorbed. More importantly, urea clearance changes with the state of hydration; for example, under conditions of dehydration, urea clearance is significantly less than inulin clearance.

Renal Blood Flow

Although it is certainly true that an extended period of renal artery clamping (e.g., 30-40 min) sufficient to cause blood flow to cease is also sufficient to cause ischemic AKI, it is simplistic to assume that moderate increases and decreases in renal artery blood flow are good and bad for the kidney, respectively. Regional variations in perfusion result in a precarious balance between oxygen supply and demand in some renal tissues, particularly in the inner renal medulla. Notably, high levels of RBF also oblige high levels of oxygen demand to facilitate active transport of sodium and other solutes back into the circulation. Unfortunately, RBF is a very poor indicator of the adequacy of regional medullary perfusion and oxygen delivery. Despite an overwhelming number of clinical trials failing to demonstrate the value of the dopaminergic agonist effects of low dose intravenous dopamine (3-5 μg/kg/min) that include increased renal artery blood flow as renoprotective[240,241] and many editorials discouraging its use,[242,243] this strategy continues to be popular with some clinicians.[244,245]

Interest in RBF as a predictor of renal function was first stimulated in 1947 when Trueta and associates[246] introduced the concept of cortical ischemia and attributed the pathogenesis of ARF to increased blood flow through the medulla. Supporting evidence for this view has since been offered by many investigators who measured RBF distribution with various methods.[247-250] Perhaps nephrons in the outer cortex are "salt losers" and those in the inner cortex are "salt retainers." If this is true, salt-retaining states should occur with the selective reduction of RBF to the superficial cortex, and these states may or may not be accompanied by a rise in RBF to the deep cortex.[222,250]

It is essential to understand how hypovolemia affects distribution of RBF. Activation of the sympathetic nervous system and possibly the renin-angiotensin system reduces RBF and GFR. Despite well-maintained arterial blood pressure, blood flow may decrease to one third of its normal level but still significantly exceed the intrinsic oxygen needs of the kidney. Constriction of afferent arterioles becomes sufficient to reduce the hydrostatic pressure in glomerular capillaries to levels inadequate for maintenance of normal filtration. Only when hypovolemia or hemorrhage is extreme does this extend to adverse effects on the metabolic function of the kidney itself. As RBF decreases further, arteriolar vasoconstriction leads to ischemia and morphologic damage.

Renal arteriographic and xenon washout studies in patients with ARF have shown selected, profound reduction in RBF.[249] Arteriography reveals severe attenuation of the intrarenal arterial tree, inability to visualize cortical vessels, absence of a normal cortical nephrogram, and striking reduction in the velocity of contrast dye as it passed through the kidney. These same patients have no bleeding from the cortex during open renal biopsy. The xenon washout studies also show that the usual transit of xenon through the cortex (indicating cortical perfusion) that is usual in the normal kidney is absent in acute oliguria. Renal cortical perfusion at one third of its normal level, involving constriction of the afferent arterioles, appears sufficient to impair renal function.

The understanding that distribution of RBF is nonhomogeneous, the recognition of nephron structure and functional heterogenicity, and the suggestion that changes in the zonal distribution of RBF affect renal salt and water homeostasis have focused investigators on developing improved techniques to measure intrarenal blood flow.[250] Methods to measure distribution of RBF in humans include the clearance of para-aminohippurate, indicator dilution, renocortical tissue Po_2, radiolabeled tracers, Doppler ultrasonography, and external gas-washout techniques. Owing to the risks and limitations associated with these techniques their clinical use has been limited.

Any nontoxic substance cleared by the kidney and not metabolized may be used to measure RBF by application of the Fick principle, whereby renal plasma flow (RPF) is calculated as follows:

$$RPF = UV/(A - RV)$$

where U is urinary concentration, V is urine flow rate, A is arterial plasma concentration, and RV is renal venous plasma concentration. RBF is then calculated from the following formula:

$$RBF = RPF/(1 - \text{Hematocrit})$$

The volume of plasma from which the kidney can extract and excrete a specific substance in a given time is the renal clearance of the substance. An ideal substance for measuring renal plasma flow would be completely eliminated from the plasma in one pass through the renal circulation due to filtration at the glomerulus without any further tubular metabolism. Para-aminohippurate is a substance that almost meets these criteria. The practical advantage of measuring the extraction of para-aminohippurate is that its renal extraction is approximately 90% in humans after one passage. Measurement of RBF is based on the assumption that cortical extraction is 100% and that extraction in the medulla is 0%; therefore, it has been assumed that the nonextracted fraction (10%) should reflect the fraction of blood flowing through the medulla. However, experimental evidence shows that cortical extraction is not 100%,[251] casting doubt on the accuracy of intrarenal blood flow assessment with extraction techniques. Other limitations of the extraction technique include the requirement for a high rate of urine flow, a steady state for 15 to 30 minutes, and the sampling of systemic arterial and renal venous blood.

Indocyanine green, which is bound to albumin in plasma, has been used in the indicator dilution method with densitometry. The indicator dilution method necessitates catheterization of a renal artery and vein. Although attempts have been made to measure renocortical (fast) and medullar (slow) blood flows separately from dye dilution curves, no convincing results have been produced.[252] Measurement of RBF by a continuous thermodilution technique, which requires renal venous cannulation and continuous injection of normal saline, has been proposed.[253] Measurements have correlated with calculated RBFs derived from clearance techniques in patients after cardiac catheterization; however, only total RBF is measured with the thermodilution technique.

Tissue oxygen pressure is measured with a multiwire surface Po_2 electrode and temperature probe. This polarographic Clark-type electrode has multiple platinum microelectrodes arranged in an array in the center of the tissue contact area, with a polarographic silver anode positioned at its circumference. The probe is placed directly on the renal cortex and measures changes in local tissue Po_2, which is an indirect indicator of renal surface perfusion.[254-256] However, this device measures only outer cortical RBF changes. Because ischemic insults to the kidney are associated with a marked decrease in blood flow to the outer cortex, a redistribution of blood flow to the juxtamedullary glomeruli in the inner cortex and medulla is presumed.

Monitoring of urinary oxygen tension, as an indicator of medullary oxygen tension, has been examined as a method for assessing renal function.[257-260] Drops in urine Po_2 after CPB predict creatinine rise after cardiac surgery,[261] a finding possibly related to the strong correlation between medullary and urine oxygen levels observed in animal models.[137] Although urine Po_2 measured in the ureter provides a good "online" estimate of medullary Po_2 in a pig model of CPB, this technology has not been evaluated in humans.[137] Urine samples exposed to the atmosphere during collection from bladder catheters provide artificially high urine Po_2 values because samples are easily contaminated with oxygen from room air. Another problem with measuring urinary oxygen tension or saturation is that bladder wall oxygen tension differs considerably from urine measurements.

External krypton-85 and xenon-133 clearance are techniques that can estimate RBF per gram of tissue from gas clearance.[262] The gas-washout technique requires selective catheterization of the renal artery and is usually performed in conjunction with arteriography. Alternatively, the renal artery can be punctured intraoperatively for injection. After injection, the gas diffuses rapidly into the renal tissue, theoretically equilibrating in tissue and blood. The renal washout curve is then assessed by external counting. The reliability of washout methods in some circumstances has been questioned.[263]

Qualitative and semi-quantitative evaluation of renal perfusion can be obtained with a gamma camera recording of the transit of a radiopharmaceutical tracer through the kidney. Qualitative evaluation of renal perfusion consists of the visual assessment of the serial images and comparative assessment of the first transit of tracer from the aorta (or iliac-renal artery) to the kidney. Among the limitations associated with the renogram is movement of the radiopharmaceutical (injected intravenously as a bolus) before it reaches the kidney, necessitating that the pharmacokinetic model contain all the possible exchange compartments between the kidney and the plasma for accurate analysis of the tissue radioactivity curve. The presence of low urine flow rates, dilated pelvic caliceal cavities, or severely reduced renal function may also cause difficulties for test interpretation. In general, the information that can be derived from the renogram includes renal clearance (as a fraction of the radioisotope to blood volume) and blood flow of the two kidneys relative to each other.[264] Because the results obtained are comparative, lesions are revealed only when they have asymmetric distribution.

Intraoperative transesophageal echocardiography 2D and renal arterial Doppler waveform images, primarily of the left kidney, can be used to assess changes in pulsatility and resistive indices and qualitatively describe RBF changes over time.[162] Typically, an interlobar artery is selected for evaluation. The anatomic course and relationships of the vessel allow easy recognition on subsequent serial scans in the same patient; the vessel is large enough to assume laminar flow throughout its length; and the angle of the ultrasound beam can generally be minimized to assume maximum Doppler frequency shift. Renal vascular resistance can be assessed by the pulsatility index.[265] The lower the pulsatile index, the less resistance there is to flow. The value is derived by dividing the difference between systolic maximum height and diastolic minimum height of the waveform by its mean height. Change in flow velocity can be assessed from a change in the mean frequency shift. The frequency shift is proportional to the mean velocity of blood flow within the vessel multiplied by the cosine of the angle between the ultrasound beam and the direction of flow. The angle is assumed to be close to zero. With this method, only blood flow velocity in large interlobar arteries and resistance can be assessed. The duplex Doppler ultrasound technique may provide a unique opportunity to demonstrate the effects of drugs on the renal vasculature and to predict the onset of pending renal failure or transplanted kidney rejection. Overall, this technique should provide an opportunity for measuring relative changes in large vessel flow velocity but not in absolute RBF.

Contrast ultrasonography has been used to image RBF.[266-269] The microbubbles produced by ultrasonic cavitation (i.e., sonication) are smaller than red blood cells and, in passing with them through the microcapillary vascular bed, reflect an echo beam to permit direct ultrasonic imaging of tissue volume and flow. Sonicated microbubbles have been shown to exhibit intracavitary velocities comparable to those of red blood cells, as observed by Doppler ultrasound techniques. Modest correlations have been found between calculated RBF assessed by contrast ultrasonography and direct flow assessment.[269]

Although not evaluated in surgical patients, a novel approach to the recognition of AKI is scintigraphic functional magnetic resonance imaging that can characterize abnormal kidney physiology, including glomerular filtration rate, tubular concentration, transit, blood volume, perfusion, inflammation, and even hypoxia.[163]

Novel (Early) Biomarkers of Acute Kidney Injury

Disappointing progress in care for AKI has prompted a strategic reevaluation of research in this area and fueled a rebirth of interest in old early indicators and a search for new "early biomarkers."[270,271] While early biomarkers are as yet some of the least validated tools in clinical AKI management, a very large research initiative is underway.[270-280] A unifying theme is the goal of providing information to facilitate prompt intervention strategies to improve care of AKI. While a few of the new tools represent attempts to find a substitute "ideal" creatinine-like substance to use in estimates of renal filtration (e.g., cystatin C), most markers take advantage of one of the three early consequences of AKI: tubular cell damage, tubular cell dysfunction, and the adaptive stress response of the kidney. The hope is that prompt biomarker information will allow timely AKI risk identification, surveillance (i.e., recognition of "pre-AKI" states such as pre-renal azotemia), diagnosis, and prognosis. Strategic approaches to improve the usefulness of early biomarkers have included combining tests to create focused panels for specific AKI concerns. Test panels could address issues such as the timing of onset, grade of a problem, and even the type of AKI (e.g., ischemic versus inflammatory). For example, in children developing AKI after cardiac surgery, one early biomarker (neutrophil gelatinase-associated lipocalin) increases 25-fold within 2 hours of surgery, facilitating diagnosis of AKI 2 days sooner than by serum creatinine values,[281] whereas another biomarker (urinary IL-18) rises 4 to 6 hours postoperatively and persists for more than 48 hours (Fig. 45-13).[282] In septic AKI, elevated levels of urinary IL-18 and two other markers (platelet-activating factor and urinary sodium hydrogen exchanger isoform-3) precede overt kidney failure by as much as 48 hours.[271] Urinary IL-18 levels in this study also differentiated septic from nonseptic AKI. A collection of the most promising biomarkers are presented here, including classes reflecting impaired renal filtration, tubular cell damage (tubular enzymuria), tubular cell

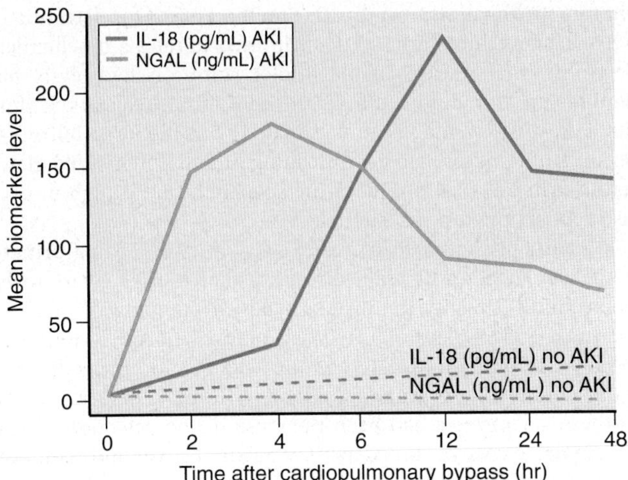

Figure 45-13 Pattern of early biomarkers urinary IL-18 and NGAL after CPB in 55 cardiac surgery patients with and without criteria for AKI diagnosed 48 to 72 hours postoperatively (defined as a peak rise in serum creatinine concentration greater than 50% of baseline). IL, interleukin; NGAL, neutrophil gelatinase-associated lipocalin. *(Used with permission from Parikh CR, Mishra J, Thiessen-Philbrook H, et al: Urinary IL-18 is an early predictive biomarker of acute kidney injury after cardiac surgery. Kidney Int 70:199-203, 2006.)*

dysfunction (tubular proteinuria), and adaptive responses of the kidney to stress (Table 45-3).

New Filtration-Based Markers of Renal Dysfunction

Examples of the search for a replacement for creatinine include cystatin C, proatrial natriuretic peptide(1-98) (proANP[1-98]), and tryptophan glycoconjugate. Cystatin C is a member of the cystatin "superfamily" of cysteine proteinase inhibitors and is produced by all nucleated cells at a constant rate. Cystatin C has been available clinically for more than 15 years and can be determined rapidly. Much like creatinine, cystatin C accumulates in the circulation with renal impairment and can be used as a marker of glomerular filtration. But cystatin C has theoretical advantages over creatinine, particularly as an indicator of mild chronic renal failure.[270,283,284] Equivalent to creatinine clearance, cystatin C clearance can be calculated using the Larsson equation.[285] Cystatin C outperformed creatinine in detecting AKI after cardiac and renal transplantation surgery in a small number of studies, although these studies have received valid criticism.[270,286] In one cardiac surgery study, serum creatinine peaked on day 3 while cystatin C peaked on day 2,[286] although another cardiac surgery study did not see such a clear-cut difference in timing.[287] Studies have linked rises in cystatin C with mortality in congestive heart failure and acute coronary syndrome patients,[288,289] validating cystatin C as a marker of important change in renal function, something notably lacking for many of the new early AKI biomarkers. However, there are concerns with the usefulness of cystatin C compared with creatinine.[290] Interindividual variability in steady-state cystatin C levels is much greater compared with creatinine (75% versus 7%). In addition, conditions such as malignancy, human immunodeficiency virus infection, corticosteroid, or thyroid hormone therapy are associated with increased serum levels without changes in renal function.[270] Finally, three studies in critically ill patients have questioned the prognostic ability of cystatin C in this setting.[270]

ProANP(1-98) is the remnant of the prohormone that remains when α-atrial natriuretic peptide is generated.[270] ProANP(1-98) disappears from the blood largely due to renal clearance and is, therefore, suitable to assess glomerular filtration. Although numerous studies of this substance have been performed in patients with chronic renal disease, understanding of this substance in AKI is limited to a single study.[291] In this investigation of 29 septic patients, proANP(1-98) was a better predictor for the occurrence of ARF than cystatin C. In addition, proANP(1-98) levels were four times higher in nonsurvivors.

Tryptophan glycoconjugate 2-(α-mannopyranosyl)-L-tryptophan is a novel circulating marker of glomerular filtration that is excreted independent of muscle mass and tubular secretion.[292] The behavior of this substance is very similar to that of inulin, making it an "ideal" substance to assess glomerular filtration; however, unfortunately measurement is currently prohibitively labor intensive and expensive.

Table 45-3 Early Biomarkers* of Acute Kidney Injury

Filtration-Based Markers of Renal Dysfunction
Cystatin C
Proatrial natriuretic peptide (1-98)
Tryptophan glycoconjugate
Biomarkers Reflecting Renal Tubular Cell Damage (Tubular Enzymuria)
α-Glutathione S-transferase
π-Glutathione S-transferase
β-*N*-Acetyl-β-D-glucosaminidase
γ-Glutamyl transpeptidase
Alkaline phosphatase
Lactate dehydrogenase
Ala-(Leu-Gly)-aminopeptidase
Proximal renal tubular epithelial antigen
Urinary sodium hydrogen exchanger isoform 3
Biomarkers Reflecting Renal Tubular Cell Dysfunction (Tubular Proteinuria)
α_1-Microglobulin
β_2-Microglobulin
Albumin
Adenosine deaminase binding protein
Renal tubular epithelial antigen-1
Retinol binding protein
Lysozyme
Ribonuclease
IgG
Transferrin
Ceruloplasmin
Lambda and kappa light chains
Urinary total protein
Biomarkers Reflecting the Renal Stress Response
Neutrophil gelatinase-associated lipocalin
Urinary interleukin-18
Platelet-activating factor
Kidney injury molecule-1
Cysteine-rich protein 61

*New early biomarkers are being developed to promptly provide information to improve risk stratification, surveillance, diagnosis, and prognostic information about acute kidney injury.

Biomarkers Reflecting Renal Tubular Cell Damage (Tubular Enzymuria)

Renal tubular cells contain enzyme proteins that are highly specific to their location within the kidney and even tubule region, making detected enzyme leakage from damaged tubular cells into urine an appealing target for early biomarker discovery. Many tubular enzyme tests have been available for years, but only recently has their clinical use been seriously considered. Segmental involvement and ultrastructural origin of AKI is known, for example, with α and π isomers of glutathione *S*-transferase (GST), which are cytosolic enzymes from proximal and distal tubular cells, respectively. *N*-acetyl-β-D-glucosaminidase (NAG) is a proximal tubular lysosomal enzyme. General brush border injury is reflected by other markers including γ-glutamyl transpeptidase (γ-GT), alkaline phosphatase, and Ala-(Leu-Gly)-aminopeptidase. The concentration of many of these substances measured soon after a renal stress, normalized relative to urine creatinine, appears able to differentiate AKI from other conditions. In a study of 26 critically ill patients, Westhuyzen and colleagues found that by testing for several tubular enzymes twice daily, detection of AKI was accelerated by 12 hours to 4 days compared with serum creatinine.[293] These authors speculated that low expense and easy automated assays for γ-GT and alkaline phosphatase made these enzyme tests appealing for identifying AKI in random urine samples. In a study of proximal renal tubular epithelial antigen (HRTE-1) urine levels from 36 normal subjects and 51 patients with renal conditions (acute tubular necrosis [ATN]), chronic nephropathies, prerenal azotemia), 79% of ATN patients had abnormal concentrations, whereas all other subjects had normal levels.[193] As a diagnostic test, HRTE-1 had 90% and 81% discrimination in differentiating ATN versus chronic nephropathies and ATN versus prerenal azotemia, respectively.

NAG is the most commonly used investigational urinary enzyme assay for assessment of renal disease and the detection of nephrotoxicity. Unlike a number of unstable enzymes excreted into the urine, NAG remains suitable for clinical diagnosis of renal disease. Increased NAG activity detected in urine is a sensitive test for renal tubular damage[294]; its molecular mass precludes filtration by the glomerulus, and it is neither absorbed nor secreted by the tubules. Any increase in urinary concentration of NAG may be considered a marker for tubular damage. The value of NAG as a diagnostic test is further enhanced by its presence in a number of isoenzyme forms. The relative amount of each isoenzyme varies at different stages of renal disease.

A number of analytical methods are available for the determination of urinary NAG, including fluorometric, colorimetric, spectrophotometric, and dipstick tests. Each of these methods is tedious, and this limits its clinical application. Low levels of NAG are excreted by normal individuals, and assay procedures must be sensitive enough to overcome the endogenous inhibitor urea.[295] Another factor to overcome is variation from urine collection that occurs over time. Factoring the enzyme activity with creatinine concentration over the same urine flow collection period is a reasonable approach for this problem.[296] In general, the sensitivity and reproducibility of the fluorometric method, when it is performed correctly, is excellent, but the equipment necessary is not commonly available in laboratories.

The colorimetric technique overcomes the limitations of the fluorometric technique by the incorporation of a calibrant for easy interlaboratory comparison and access in most clinical chemistry laboratories, with modification for use with spectrophotometric analysis.[297] A dipstick method exists for detection of NAG in the urine.[298] The NAG strip incorporates a biochemical derivative that releases a blue-violet color on hydrolysis but requires up to 30 minutes from the addition of reagents. Unfortunately, if the sample is contaminated with blood or bilirubin, results from this test can be misleading. Besides pigmented material in urine, a concentrated urine specimen that is high in urea also renders the test inaccurate.

Perhaps the most interesting discovery regarding urinary NAG for detection of renal disease is that there appears to be isoenzyme specificity for various types of pathology.[299] NAG is the most active lysosomal hydrolase and is normally found in tissues as two major forms: A and B. These major forms differ in their subunit composition. Traditionally, the main clinical interest in these isoenzymes had been their use in the detection of two autosomal recessive disorders: Tay-Sachs disease and Sandhoff disease. In 1970, Price and colleagues[300] reported that the B form increased in a urinary pattern of NAG after surgical trauma. Since that time it has been appreciated that the relative amount of the B form increased (i.e., the ratio of A to B forms decreased) compared with urine in the normal population. Automated methods for separation of NAG isoenzymes allow the pattern of excretion to be compared in various disease states. Of interest to the anesthesiologist is that evidence suggests that after major surgery the percentage of an intermediate isoenzyme (I) increases in the urine.[301] Smaller increases in the I form were also observed in rejection of renal transplants. Rejection was more strongly associated with a decrease in the A/B ratio in a cohort of renal transplant patients. No change in the isoenzyme profile was found in stable transplant patients, whereas reversible rejection was characterized by an increase in the I form and a decrease in the relative amount of the A form present. When a patient did not respond to treatment, the I and the B forms were elevated but levels of the A form decreased.[302]

Different nephrotoxic drugs or conditions appear to produce characteristic urinary NAG isoenzyme profiles. For example, the B and I forms are elevated after administration of aminoglycosides. Total urinary and serum NAG activity also has been reported to increase in diabetic patients. Overall, NAG activity in the urine reflects the activity of the disease or severity of the damage. Serial monitoring is, therefore, most useful because relative change over time is the most useful way to interpret the results. The NAG-to-creatinine ratio is a more sensitive and specific marker for renal tubular dysfunction. It is useful to express NAG as a ratio of urinary creatinine to minimize dilutional or concentration effects. The lack of sensitive, simple, inexpensive, and efficient methods is the limiting factor for widespread clinical use of NAG monitoring. Another urinary enzyme, clusterin, may prove to be more specific than NAG[303] for evaluating nephrotoxicity caused by aminoglycoside use while remaining equally sensitive.

Other urinary constituents can detect cytotoxic and abnormal processes in specific regions of the nephron. α-GST is found principally in the proximal convoluted tubules, and π-GST is found principally in the distal convoluted tubule. Ala-(Leu-Gly)-aminopeptidase and γ-GT excretion are specific markers for proximal tubular brush border injury. Of note, although enhanced urinary excretion of tubular enzymes can signal damaged tubular cells, it can also reflect an increased turnover of tubular cells or some other metabolic disturbance; thus, the signals of early, irreversible disease may not always be distinguished from the noise of biologic variability and use of these markers should be applied with appropriate caution. In addition, their validation compared to clinically important outcomes, such as dialysis or mortality, has received little attention.

Urinary sodium hydrogen exchanger isoform-3 (NHE-3) is the isoform of the Na^+/H^+ exchanger present in the apical membrane of proximal tubular cells and responsible for the majority of Na^+ uptake and H^+ excretion by the kidney.[304] NHE-3 is found in the urine with tubular injury, and levels can be estimated from semiquantitative immunoblots of the urine membrane fraction. In a study of 54 critically ill patients and 14 controls, NHE-3 was only seen with tubular injury and, when normalized to urinary creatinine, was six times higher with ATN than prerenal azotemia, without overlap.[305] In addition, urinary NHE-3 was not present with intrinsic ARF other than ATN, and the normalized level correlated with serum creatinine rise in patients with tubular injury.

Biomarkers Reflecting Renal Tubular Cell Dysfunction (Tubular Proteinuria)

When small proteins are filtered by the glomerulus, binding and endocytic reuptake in the proximal tubule normally returns these substances to the body through a megalin-mediated transport system. So-called tubular proteinuria results from functional impairment of this process and the escape of small proteins into the urine. Endogenous low-molecular-weight (LMW) proteins that are normally taken up in this way include β_2- and α_1-microglobulin, albumin, adenosine deaminase binding protein, renal tubular epithelial antigen-1, retinol binding protein, lysozyme, ribonuclease, IgG, transferrin, ceruloplasmin, lambda and kappa light chains, and urinary total protein. Appearance of any of these substances in the urine heralds abnormal proximal nephron function consistent with AKI. However, enthusiasm for LMW protein markers as perioperative tools to diagnose AKI has been reduced, particularly with cardiac surgery, by the confusion that can occur when an antifibrinolytic agent is used.[306] Lysine and its analog (e.g., ε-aminocaproic acid, tranexamic acid) specifically block renal binding sites, causing a profound but reversible inhibition of LMW protein reuptake (Fig. 45-14) [307]; the effect is transient and apparently benign but so potent that urine LMW protein measurement after a small dose of intravenous lysine has been proposed as a tool for estimating GFR.[307] The serine protease inhibitor antifibrinolytic drug aprotinin is a small protein and does not inhibit tubular reuptake but is itself metabolized by the same renal transport system as LMW proteins.[308] Although the influence of aprotinin on renal processing of LMW proteins has not been examined, α_1-microglobulinuria without change in serum creatinine has been reported in cardiac surgical patients after use of this agent.[309]

β_2-Microglobulin is a subunit of the class I antigen of the major histocompatibility complex and is structurally homologous to immunoglobulins.[310] Its mass is 11,600 daltons, it is freely filtered from plasma by the renal glomerulus, and more than 99.9% reabsorbed in the proximal tubule. β_2-Microglobulin is measured by radioimmunoassay and immunodiffusion techniques.[311] Specific limitations to its use include its unstable nature in urine of pH 5.5 or below, thereby precluding its use for patients with concomitant urinary tract infection or pyuria. Its degradation by proteolysis is affected by temperature, and its measurement requires a sophisticated laboratory that precludes widespread clinical use. α_1-Microglobulin is filtered at the glomerulus and is

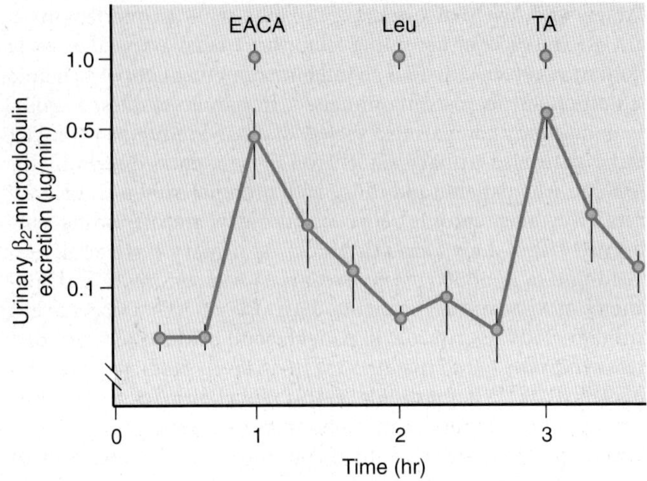

Figure 45-14 Spillage of low-molecular-weight proteins, such as β_2-microglobulin, into the urine, also known as tubular proteinuria, is a poor early biomarker of AKI when lysine analog antifibrinolytic agents are being used.[306] In volunteers, significant but transient increases in urinary β_2-microglobulin levels occur after injection with ε-aminocaproic acid (EACA) and tranexamic acid (TA), but not injection of an unrelated amino acid, leucine (Leu).[307] This potent but transient effect reflects inhibition of normal small protein reuptake by the proximal tubule transport system. (*Modified with permission from Mogensen CE, Solling K: Studies on renal tubular protein reabsorption: Partial and near complete inhibition by certain amino acids. Scand J Clin Lab Invest 37:477-486, 1977.*)

95% reabsorbed at the proximal tubule, thereby indicating proximal tubular dysfunction when present in the urine.[1,312,313]

Lysozymuria, an increase of the enzymatic protein lysozyme in urine, occurs if the serum level is elevated above the normal renal threshold (45 mg/mL) or when renal tubular function is impaired.[314] The normal urinary lysozyme level is less than 1.9 mg/mL, and a level greater than 5 mg/mL is regarded as evidence for significant renal tubular damage. Elevated serum levels of lysozyme may be a consequence of renal failure as well as a marker for it. Because white blood cells have a high concentration of lysozyme, urinary tract infections may also lead to elevated serum levels.

Biomarkers Reflecting the Renal Tubular Cell Response to Stress

Examples of markers that assess the response of the kidney to stress include neutrophil gelatinase–associated lipocalin (NGAL), urinary interleukin-18, platelet-activating factor, kidney injury molecule-1, and cysteine rich protein-61. NGAL is a small protease-resistant polypeptide. Although its role remains largely obscure, NGAL infusion in mice attenuates AKI after renal ischemia.[315] A transcriptome-wide interrogation for genes induced very early after renal ischemia identified NGAL as a protein generated by ischemic renal tubular cells.[316] NGAL appears in kidney parenchyma within 1 hour and in urine of cardiac surgery patients within 2 hours after injury (see Fig. 45-13), earlier than traditional markers,[282,317] and elevated levels are highly predictive of postoperative AKI.[281] Although NGAL demonstrates great promise as an early AKI biomarker, a notable limitation is the high variability among patients in baseline values. Like many early biomarkers, NGAL requires validation as a useful clinical tool in a wide variety of clinical settings and correlation with important outcomes.

Inflammation is a central aspect of the pathophysiology of AKI. Cytokines and adhesion molecules mediate injury in the kidney, and levels of urinary cytokines such as interleukin-18 (IL-18) and platelet-activating factor have been assessed as early biomarkers of AKI. IL-18 is an inflammatory mediator of ischemic acute tubular necrosis in animals.[318] In human studies, a cross-sectional study comparing a variety of renal conditions with AKI found increased urinary IL-18 level to be a good discriminator between AKI patients and those with prerenal azotemia, urinary tract infections, chronic renal insufficiency, and nephrotic syndrome.[319] This study found that a cut-off urinary IL-18-to-serum creatinine ratio of 500 pg/mg creatinine had sensitivity and specificity of 85% and 88% for the diagnosis of ATN, respectively. Another study in critically ill patients with adult respiratory distress syndrome found that urinary IL-18 levels predicted AKI and mortality risk.[318] Interestingly, in this report, urinary IL-18 levels were significantly higher in septic than nonseptic AKI patients, despite similar serum creatinine concentrations. In one study of cardiac surgery patients, increased urinary IL-18 levels within 6 hours postoperatively predicted subsequent diagnosis of AKI by traditional criteria (see Fig. 45-13).[282] Other plasma and urinary cytokines, such as IL-8, IL-10, IL-1 receptor antagonist, and tissue necrosis factor soluble receptor-2, are less studied but have been shown to correlate with proximal tubular dysfunction.[1]

Platelet-activating factor is a phospholipid mediator of inflammation also known to participate in the pathophysiology of AKI.[271] In a study of 12 critically ill patients with septic shock and AKI, blood and urinary concentrations of platelet-activating factor correlated with several standard clinical and laboratory parameters related to ARF.[320]

Kidney injury molecule-1 (KIM-1) is a transmembrane protein expressed at low levels in normal kidney that is markedly upregulated in proximal renal tubular cells in response to ischemic or nephrotoxic AKI.[271] Increases in rat urine KIM-1 levels correlate with increases in serum creatinine values.[321,322] In a study of humans with ARF, KIM-1 expression is markedly increased in renal biopsy samples with ATN and accompanied by elevated urine KIM-1 levels.[323] In this study, urine KIM-1 was also a better predictive tool than γ-GT and AP.[323] KIM-1 appears in urine within 12 hours of AKI and remains elevated; however, to date there are no published data to correlate the extent of damage with KIM-1 levels. KIM-1 also appears in the urine before a rise in serum creatinine level with cisplatin or high-dose folic acid nephrotoxicity.[270] Measurement of KIM-1 in urine requires Western blot analysis and quantification by enzyme-linked immunosorbent assay.

Cysteine-rich protein-61 (CYR61) is a heparin-binding protein that is secreted by injured tissues, including the kidney, and is involved in tissue growth and repair.[316] In an animal model, CYR61 was expressed in renal tissue within 1 hour and detected in urine 3 to 6 hours after ischemia, peaking in urine 6 to 9 hours after injury. The CYR61 gene is upregulated more than 10-fold after renal ischemic injury.[324] Notably, CYR61 does not appear in animals with prerenal azotemia.

Preoperative Evaluation of Renal Function

The greater the magnitude and duration of the surgical insult and the number of acute and chronic risk factors, the greater is the likelihood of perioperative renal compromise and the need for preoperative identification of renal function (see Chapters 34 and 35). In patients with inadequate blood flow, injury is commonly caused by the added risk of drugs, by abnormal hemodynamics, or by preexisting disease.[325] Studies have shown that 12% to 14% of patients who develop acute renal insufficiency during hospitalization do so after radiographic procedures requiring use of a contrast agent. If preexisting renal insufficiency exists, progressive deterioration in renal function occurs in 42% of cases, with a poor prognosis if dialysis is required.[326] Risk factors, such as volume depletion, aminoglycoside use, radiocontrast dye exposure, use of nonsteroidal anti-inflammatory drugs, septic shock, and pigmenturia all contribute to the development of ARF. It appears that the combined interaction of these multiple acute risk factors is central in the pathogenesis of ARF (see Fig. 45-6).[20] Patients with preexisting renal insufficiency, for example, are especially prone to develop ARF that requires dialysis as a result of cardiovascular surgery. Similarly, diabetic patients with renal insufficiency are especially vulnerable to radiocontrast agents. Of course, part of this association is due to the insensitivity of standard tools such as serum creatinine to loss of renal function (see Fig. 45-10), leaving limited reserve and only a small further loss in renal function required to push an individual to the brink of dialysis. Some key determinants of postoperative renal function are preoperative renal function, maintenance of appropriate intravascular volume, and normal myocardial function.[23]

The potential value of understanding the genetic makeup of patients has yet to be fully explored and is likely to be important (see earlier discussion). Genetic variants are an established predictor of chronic kidney disease (e.g., renal transplant nephropathy), and early perioperative studies in cardiac surgery patients have already identified genetic factors that explain twofold to threefold more variation in postoperative AKI compared with standard clinical risk factors alone.[125,126]

In addition to intrinsic renal disease, several extrinsic variables influence the outcome of renal function tests: intracellular and extracellular volume, cardiovascular function, and neuroendocrine factors.[327,328] Advanced age also markedly decreases renal function reserve. GFR, normally about 125 mL/min in a young adult, decreases to about 80 mL/min at 60 years of age and to 60 mL/min at 80 years (see Fig. 45-11). Although not necessarily the primary cause for end-stage renal disease, hypertension in up to 85% of patients with renal failure is a major risk factor for the high cardiovascular morbidity that occurs.[329] The role of metabolic syndrome in contributing to end-stage renal disease is also becoming more apparent.[330]

In addition to its contribution to renal failure in hypertensive nephrosclerosis resulting from essential hypertension and hyperfiltration in diabetic nephropathy, hypertension also contributes to the loss of renal function associated with aging. Preoperative isolated systolic blood pressure hypertension and wide pulse pressure (i.e., the difference between systolic and diastolic blood pressure) are strong independent predictors of postoperative renal dysfunction.[150,331] It appears that an increase in conduit vessel stiffness with inadequate flow during low-pressure states contributes to increased preoperative renal dysfunction and hemodialysis-dependent renal failure.

Urinalysis provides qualitative information that must be interpreted cautiously. Hematuria (i.e., more than one or two red blood cells per high-power field in a concentrated sediment) suggests glomerular disease or, in a trauma patient, injury to the kidneys or the lower urinary tract. A urine test result that is positive for blood in the absence of red blood cells suggests the presence of free hemoglobin or myoglobin in the urine. Pyuria (i.e., more than four white blood cells per high-power field) suggests urinary tract infection. Although urine may normally contain hyaline and granular casts, cellular casts represent a pathologic condition. Red blood cell casts suggest interstitial nephritis, including pyelonephritis. Urinary pH, although difficult to interpret on a spot urine sample, may assist in the diagnosis of some acid-base disturbances. The pH of urine tends to be more acidic when factors that initiate failure are prerenal rather than postrenal. The presence of proteinuria on a routine dipstick examination may be normal, or it may suggest severe renal disease. In a concentrated urine sample, trace or 1+ proteinuria is a nonspecific finding, whereas 3+ or 4+ proteinuria suggests glomerular disease. The existence of glucosuria without hyperglycemia indicates proximal tubular damage.

Serum creatinine levels offer rapid but inexact estimates of creatinine clearance. Acute elevations of serum creatinine levels occur in approximately 5% of all hospitalized patients and in up to 20% of patients in intensive care units.[32] The incidence increases directly with the severity of trauma and the degree of injury or disease. The incidence and severity of ARF usually are greater when the preoperative serum creatinine level is greater than 2 mg/dL[332]; however, an isolated serum creatinine measurement is an unreliable indicator of GFR when renal function is changing. There is an inverse logarithmic relationship between GFR and serum creatinine concentration (see Fig. 45-10). Decreasing the rate by one half results in twice the serum creatinine level. For example, a patient with a baseline serum creatinine level of 0.6 mg/dL who develops contrast nephropathy sufficient to reduce the number of glomeruli and filtration rate by one half would have a serum creatinine level of 1.2 mg/dL, still in the normal range. Thus, a trend in serum creatinine values is always more useful than a single serum creatinine measurement to evaluate renal function reserve, particularly when changes are anticipated. The measurement of creatinine clearance may constitute the best overall indicator of GFR, although this index also has limitations. In one study, more than one half of 131 critically ill patients had normal values for urine output, BUN, and serum creatinine but had reduced creatinine clearance. Creatinine clearance was the best predictor of mortality among these patients compared with the other measures of renal function.[333] Although serum creatinine level may be a more reliable measure of glomerular function than the BUN level, the simultaneous determination of BUN and serum creatinine levels offers a more complete evaluation of renal function than either determination alone. Ordinarily, the BUN-to-creatinine ratio is approximately 10, and if the BUN level is approximately 10 times as great as the serum creatinine level, the clinician may conclude that the measurements are probably correct. Conversely, if the ratio deviates significantly from 10, the clinician should consider the nonrenal factors influencing the BUN level or serum creatinine level or both. All three measurements (i.e., BUN, serum creatinine level, and creatinine clearance) require careful interpretation.

Summary

In patients with, or at risk for developing, AKI the perioperative management continues to be challenging. Numerous factors contribute to the heterogeneous condition referred to as perioperative AKI, but insults collectively combine through ischemic and toxic mechanisms. The recent revision of mission in the research community in regard to the investigation of AKI will likely lead to rapid developments in the field of renal function monitoring, including "early biomarker" tests or panels of tests that aid in risk prediction, identification of patients with conditions that precede AKI, such as prerenal azotemia, and the diagnosis and prognosis of AKI. The major hope is that improvements in monitoring will translate into better prevention, treatment, and outcome from AKI, something that has been disappointingly absent over the past half century since the problem of perioperative ARF was first described. As understanding of renal function and AKI evolves, traditional tests, such as serum creatinine, are being questioned as to allow sufficiently early intervention to improve the care of patients with AKI. The introduction of new "early biomarker" tests and even preoperative genetic testing may contribute significant advances to renal function monitoring. That this information will improve the prognosis of AKI is hoped for but not known. Meanwhile, serum creatinine continues to be the mainstay of most renal function monitoring strategies.

References

1. Flynn FV: Assessment of renal function: Selected developments. Clin Biochem 23:49-54, 1990.
2. Aronson S, Fontes ML, Miao Y, Mangano DT: Risk index for perioperative renal dysfunction/failure: Critical dependence on pulse pressure hypertension. Circulation 115:733-742, 2007.
3. Conlon PJ, Stafford-Smith M, White WD, et al: Acute renal failure following cardiac surgery. Nephrol Dial Transplant 14:1158-1162, 1999.
4. Mora-Mangano C, Diamondstone LS, Ramsay JG, et al: Renal dysfunction after myocardial revascularization: Risk factors, adverse outcomes, and hospital resource utilization. The Multicenter Study of Perioperative Ischemia Research Group. Ann Intern Med 128:194-203, 1998.
5. Wijeysundera DN, Karkouti K, Dupuis JY, et al: Derivation and validation of a simplified predictive index for renal replacement therapy after cardiac surgery. JAMA 297:1801-1809, 2007.
6. Ostermann ME, Taube D, Morgan CJ, Evans TW: Acute renal failure following cardiopulmonary bypass: A changing picture. Intensive Care Med 26:565-571, 2000.
7. Chertow GM, Levy EM, Hammermeister KE, et al: Independent association between acute renal failure and mortality following cardiac surgery. Am J Med 104:343-348, 1998.
8. Chertow GM, Lazarus JM, Christiansen CL, et al: Preoperative renal risk stratification. Circulation 95:878-884, 1997.
9. Swaminathan M, Shaw AD, Phillips-Bute BG, et al: Trends in acute renal failure associated with coronary artery bypass graft surgery in the United States. Crit Care Med 35:2286-2291, 2007.
10. Chukwuemeka A, Weisel A, Maganti M, et al: Renal dysfunction in high-risk patients after on-pump and off-pump coronary artery bypass surgery: A propensity score analysis. Ann Thorac Surg 80:2148-2153, 2005.
11. Vanholder R, Argiles A, Baurmeister U, et al: Uremic toxicity: Present state of the art. Int J Artif Organs 24:695-725, 2001.
12. Vanholder R, De Smet R, Glorieux G, et al: Review on uremic toxins: Classification, concentration, and interindividual variability. Kidney Int 63:1934-1943, 2003.
13. Vanholder R, Glorieux G, Lameire N: Uraemic toxins and cardiovascular disease. Nephrol Dial Transplant 18:463-466, 2003.
14. Chertow GM, Soroko SH, Paganini EP, et al: Mortality after acute renal failure: Models for prognostic

stratification and risk adjustment. Kidney Int 70:1120-1126, 2006.
15. Lin CY, Chen YC, Tsai FC, et al: RIFLE classification is predictive of short-term prognosis in critically ill patients with acute renal failure supported by extracorporeal membrane oxygenation. Nephrol Dial Transplant 21:2867-2873, 2006.
16. Shaheen IS, Watson AR, Harvey B: Acute renal failure in children: Etiology, treatment and outcome. Saudi J Kidney Dis Transpl 17:153-158, 2006.
17. Loef BG, Epema AH, Smilde TD, et al: Immediate postoperative renal function deterioration in cardiac surgical patients predicts in-hospital mortality and long-term survival. J Am Soc Nephrol 16:195-200, 2005.
18. Brivet FG, Kleinknecht DJ, Loirat P, Landais PJ: Acute renal failure in intensive care units—causes, outcome, and prognostic factors of hospital mortality; a prospective, multicenter study. French Study Group on Acute Renal Failure. Crit Care Med 24:192-198, 1996.
19. Kaufman J, Dhakal M, Patel B, Hamburger R: Community-acquired acute renal failure. Am J Kidney Dis 17:191-198, 1991.
20. Shusterman N, Strom BL, Murray TG, et al: Risk factors and outcome of hospital-acquired acute renal failure: Clinical epidemiologic study. Am J Med 83:65-71, 1987.
21. Doberneck RC, Reiser MP, Lillehei CW: Acute renal failure after open-heart surgery utilizing extracorporeal circulation and total body perfusion. J Thorac Cardiovasc Surg 43:441-452, 1962.
22. Thurlbeck W, Castleman B: Atheromatous emboli to the kidneys after aortic surgery. N Engl J Med 257:442-447, 1957.
23. Novis BK, Roizen MF, Aronson S, Thisted RA: Association of preoperative risk factors with postoperative acute renal failure. Anesth Analg 78:143-149, 1994.
24. Gaudino M, Luciani N, Giungi S, et al: Different profiles of patients who require dialysis after cardiac surgery. Ann Thorac Surg 79:825-829, 2005.
25. Ferguson TB Jr, Dziuban SW Jr, Edwards FH, et al: The STS National Database: Current changes and challenges for the new millennium. Committee to Establish a National Database in Cardiothoracic Surgery, The Society of Thoracic Surgeons. Ann Thorac Surg 69:680-691, 2000.
26. Barrett BJ, Parfrey PS: Prevention of nephrotoxicity induced by radiocontrast agents. N Engl J Med 331:1449-1450, 1994.
27. American Society of Nephrology Renal Research Report. J Am Soc Nephrol 16:1886-1903, 2005.
28. Eknoyan G, Lameire N, Barsoum R, et al: The burden of kidney disease: Improving global outcomes. Kidney Int 66:1310-1314, 2004.
29. Thompson BT, Cox PN, Antonelli M, et al: Challenges in end-of-life care in the ICU: Statement of the 5th International Consensus Conference in Critical Care: Brussels, Belgium, April 2003: executive summary. Crit Care Med 32:1781-1784, 2004.
30. Mehta RL, Kellum JA, Shah SV, et al: Acute Kidney Injury Network: Report of an initiative to improve outcomes in acute kidney injury. Crit Care 11:R31, 2007.
31. Bellomo R, Ronco C, Kellum JA, et al: Acute renal failure: Definition, outcome measures, animal models, fluid therapy and information technology needs. The Second International Consensus Conference of the Acute Dialysis Quality Initiative (ADQI) Group. Crit Care 8:R204-R212, 2004.
32. Charlson ME, MacKenzie CR, Gold JP, Shires GT: Postoperative changes in serum creatinine: When do they occur and how much is important? Ann Surg 209:328-333, 1989.
33. Myers BD, Miller DC, Mehigan JT, et al: Nature of the renal injury following total renal ischemia in man. J Clin Invest 73:329-341, 1984.
34. Myers B, Moran S: Hemodynamically mediated acute renal failure. N Engl J Med 314:97-105, 1986.
35. Friedrich JO, Adhikari N, Herridge MS, Beyene J: Meta-analysis: Low-dose dopamine increases urine output but does not prevent renal dysfunction or death. Ann Intern Med 142:510-524, 2005.
36. Myers BD, Hilberman M, Spencer RJ, Jamison RL: Glomerular and tubular function in non-oliguric acute renal failure. Am J Med 72:642-649, 1982.
37. Stafford-Smith M: Perioperative renal dysfunction: Implications and strategies for protection, *In* Newman MF (ed): Perioperative Organ Protection. Baltimore, Lippincott Williams & Wilkins, 2003, pp 89-124.
38. Loutzenhiser R, Griffin K, Williamson G, Bidani A: Renal autoregulation: New perspectives regarding the protective and regulatory roles of the underlying mechanisms. Am J Physiol Regul Integr Comp Physiol 290:R1153-R1167, 2006.
39. Arendshorst WJ, Brannstrom K, Ruan X: Actions of angiotensin II on the renal microvasculature. J Am Soc Nephrol 10(Suppl 11): S149-S161, 1999.
40. Geraghty JG, Nsubuga M, Angerson WJ, et al: A study of regional distribution of renal blood flow using quantitative autoradiography. Am J Physiol 263:F958-F962, 1992.
41. Pallone TL, Zhang Z, Rhinehart K: Physiology of the renal medullary microcirculation. Am J Physiol Renal Physiol 284:F253-F266, 2003.
42. Preuss HG: Basics of renal anatomy and physiology. Clin Lab Med 13:1-11, 1993.
43. Pallone TL, Turner MR, Edwards A, Jamison RL: Countercurrent exchange in the renal medulla. Am J Physiol Regul Integr Comp Physiol 284:R1153-R1175, 2003.
44. Leonhardt K, Landes R, McCauley R: Anatomy and physiology of intrarenal oxygen tension: Preliminary study of the effect of anesthetics. Anesthesiology 26:648-658, 1965.
45. Brezis M, Rosen S: Hypoxia of the renal medulla—its implications for disease. N Engl J Med 332:647-655, 1995.
46. Brezis M, Epstein FH: Cellular mechanisms of acute ischemic injury in the kidney. Annu Rev Med 44:27-37, 1993.
47. Brezis M, Rosen S, Silva P, Epstein FH: Selective anoxic injury to thick ascending limb: An anginal syndrome of the renal medulla? Adv Exp Med Biol 180:239-249, 1984.
48. Brezis M, Rosen S, Silva P, Epstein FH: Selective vulnerability of the medullary thick ascending limb to anoxia in the isolated perfused rat kidney. J Clin Invest 73:182-190, 1984.
49. Cochrane J, Williams BT, Banerjee A, et al: Ischemic preconditioning attenuates functional, metabolic, and morphologic injury from ischemic acute renal failure in the rat. Ren Fail 21:135-145, 1999.
50. Lee HT, Emala CW: Protective effects of renal ischemic preconditioning and adenosine pretreatment: Role of A(1) and A(3) receptors. Am J Physiol Renal Physiol 278:F380-F387, 2000.
51. Lee HT, Gallos G, Nasr SH, Emala CW: A_1 adenosine receptor activation inhibits inflammation, necrosis, and apoptosis after renal ischemia-reperfusion injury in mice. J Am Soc Nephrol 15:102-111, 2004.
52. Philbin DM, Baratz RA, Patterson RW: The effect of carbon dioxide on plasma antidiuretic hormone levels during intermittent positive-pressure breathing. Anesthesiology 33:345-349, 1970.
53. Brennan LA Jr, Malvin RL, Jochim KE, Roberts DE: Influence of right and left atrial receptors on plasma concentrations of ADH and renin. Am J Physiol 221:273-278, 1971.
54. Cogan MG: Renal effects of atrial natriuretic factor. Annu Rev Physiol 52:699-708, 1990.
55. Morita T, Wada I, Saeki H, et al: Ureteral urine transport: Changes in bolus volume, peristaltic frequency, intraluminal pressure and volume of flow resulting from autonomic drugs. J Urol 137:132-135, 1987.
56. Young CJ, Attele A, Toledano A, et al: Volatile anesthetics decrease peristalsis in the guinea pig ureter. Anesthesiology 81:452-458, 1994.
57. Makker SP, Tucker AS, Izant RJ Jr, Heymann W: Nonobstructive hydronephrosis and hydropureter associated with peritonitis. N Engl J Med 287:535-537, 1972.
58. Badr KF, Ichikawa I: Prerenal failure: A deleterious shift from renal compensation to decompensation. N Engl J Med 319:623-629, 1988.
59. Kellen M, Aronson S, Roizen MF, et al: Predictive and diagnostic tests of renal failure: A review [see comments]. Anesth Analg 78:134-142, 1994.
60. Barger A, Herd J: Renal vascular anatomy and distribution of blood flow. *In* Orlaff J, Berliner R (eds): Handbook of Physiology, section 8. Baltimore, Williams & Wilkins, 1973.
61. Schrier RW: Acute renal failure. JAMA 247:2518-2522, 2524, 1982.
62. Kreisberg J, Venkatachalam MA: Morphologic factors in acute renal failure. *In* Brenner B, Lazarus JM (eds): Acute Renal Failure, 2nd ed. New York, Churchill Livingstone, 1988.
63. Alpert RA, Roizen MF, Hamilton WK, et al: Intraoperative urinary output does not predict postoperative renal function in patients undergoing abdominal aortic revascularization. Surgery 95:707-711, 1984.
64. Mercatello A: Changes in renal function induced by anesthesia. Ann Fr Anesth Reanim 9:507-524, 1990.
65. Andersson LG, Bratteby LE, Ekroth R, et al: Renal function during cardiopulmonary bypass: Influence of pump flow and systemic blood pressure. Eur J Cardiothorac Surg 8:597-602, 1994.
66. Szabo G, Posch E, Rosivall L, et al: The effect of haemorrhage on renal blood flow and intrarenal flow distribution. Injury 9:146-150, 1977.
67. Everett GB, Allen GD, Kennedy WF Jr, et al: Renal hemodynamic effects of general anesthesia in outpatients. Anesth Analg 52:470-479, 1973.
68. Papper S, Papper EM: The effects of preanesthetic, anesthetic, and postoperative drugs on renal function. Clin Pharmacol Ther 5:205-215, 1964.
69. Taguma Y, Sasaki Y, Kyogoku Y, et al: Morphological changes in an early phase of norepinephrine-induced acute renal failure in unilaterally nephrectomized dogs. J Lab Clin Med 96:616-632, 1980.
70. Baehler RW, Williams RH, Work J, et al: Studies on the natural history of the norepinephrine model of acute renal failure in the dog. Nephron 26:266-273, 1980.
71. Hollenberg NK, Meyerovitz M, Harrington DP, Sandor T: Influence of norepinephrine and angiotensin II on vasomotion of renal blood supply in humans. Am J Physiol 252:H941-H944, 1987.
72. Amano J, Suzuki A, Sunamori M: Antidiuretic hormone and cardiovascular responses during and after coronary artery bypass surgery. Thorac Cardiovasc Surg 41:297-300, 1993.
73. Cregg N, Mannion D, Casey W: Oliguria during corrective spinal surgery for idiopathic scoliosis: The role of antidiuretic hormone. Paediatr Anaesth 9:505-514, 1999.
74. Mark JB, Steele SM: Cardiovascular effects of spinal anesthesia. Int Anesthesiol Clin 27:31-39, 1989.

75. Saada M, Duval AM, Bonnet F, et al: Abnormalities in myocardial segmental wall motion during lumbar epidural anesthesia. Anesthesiology 71:26-32, 1989.
76. Kennedy WF Jr, Sawyer TK, Gerbershagen HY, et al: Systemic cardiovascular and renal hemodynamic alterations during peridural anesthesia in normal man. Anesthesiology 31:414-421, 1969.
77. Kennedy WF Jr, Sawyer TK, Gerbershagen HU, et al: Simultaneous systemic cardiovascular and renal hemodynamic measurements during high spinal anaesthesia in normal man. Acta Anaesthesiol Scand Suppl 37:163-171, 1969.
78. Suleiman MY, Passannante AN, Onder RL, et al: Alteration of renal blood flow during epidural anesthesia in normal subjects. Anesth Analg 84:1076-1080, 1997.
79. Halperin BD, Feeley TW: The effect of anesthesia and surgery on renal function. Int Anesthesiol Clin 22:157-168, 1984.
80. Liu SS, Wu CL: Effect of postoperative analgesia on major postoperative complications: A systematic update of the evidence. Anesth Analg 104:689-702, 2007.
81. Moraca RJ, Sheldon DG, Thirlby RC: The role of epidural anesthesia and analgesia in surgical practice. Ann Surg 238:663-673, 2003.
82. Oremus K, Safaric Z: The role of epidural anesthesia and analgesia in surgical practice. Ann Surg 240: 561-562; author reply 562, 2004.
83. Daudel F, Bone HG, Traber DL, et al: Effects of thoracic epidural anesthesia on hemodynamics and global oxygen transport in ovine endotoxemia. Shock 26:615-619, 2006.
84. Mazze RI: Methoxyflurane revisited: Tale of an anesthetic from cradle to grave. Anesthesiology 105:843-846, 2006.
85. Mazze RI, Calverley RK, Smith NT: Inorganic fluoride nephrotoxicity: Prolonged enflurane and halothane anesthesia in volunteers. Anesthesiology 46:265-271, 1977.
86. Cousins MJ, Mazze RI: Methoxyflurane nephrotoxicity: A study of dose response in man. JAMA 225:1611-1616, 1973.
87. Mazze RI, Cousins MJ, Kosek JC: Dose-related methoxyflurane nephrotoxicity in rats: A biochemical and pathologic correlation. Anesthesiology 36:571-587, 1972.
88. Munday IT, Stoddart PA, Jones RM, et al: Serum fluoride concentration and urine osmolality after enflurane and sevoflurane anesthesia in male volunteers. Anesth Analg 81:353-359, 1995.
89. Kharasch ED, Armstrong AS, Gunn K, et al: Clinical sevoflurane metabolism and disposition: II. The role of cytochrome P450 2E1 in fluoride and hexafluoroisopropanol formation. Anesthesiology 82:1379-1388, 1995.
90. Conzen PF, Nuscheler M, Melotte A, et al: Renal function and serum fluoride concentrations in patients with stable renal insufficiency after anesthesia with sevoflurane or enflurane. Anesth Analg 81:569-575, 1995.
91. Kharasch ED, Hankins DC, Thummel KE: Human kidney methoxyflurane and sevoflurane metabolism: Intrarenal fluoride production as a possible mechanism of methoxyflurane nephrotoxicity. Anesthesiology 82:689-699, 1995.
92. Malan TP Jr: Sevoflurane and renal function. Anesth Analg 81:S39-S45, 1995.
93. Frink EJ Jr, Malan TP Jr, Isner RJ, et al: Renal concentrating function with prolonged sevoflurane or enflurane anesthesia in volunteers. Anesthesiology 80:1019-1025, 1994.
94. Morio M, Fujii K, Satoh N, et al: Reaction of sevoflurane and its degradation products with soda lime: Toxicity of the byproducts. Anesthesiology 77:1155-1164, 1992.
95. Gonsowski CT, Laster MJ, Eger EI 2nd, et al: Toxicity of compound A in rats: Effect of increasing duration of administration. Anesthesiology 80:566-573, 1994.
96. Bito H, Ikeuchi Y, Ikeda K: Effects of low-flow sevoflurane anesthesia on renal function: Comparison with high-flow sevoflurane anesthesia and low-flow isoflurane anesthesia. Anesthesiology 86:1231-1237, 1997.
97. Eger EI 2nd, Koblin DD, Bowland T, et al: Nephrotoxicity of sevoflurane versus desflurane anesthesia in volunteers. Anesth Analg 84:160-168, 1997.
98. Cressey G, Roberts DR, Snowden CP: Renal tubular injury after infrarenal aortic aneurysm repair. J Cardiothorac Vasc Anesth 16:290-293, 2002.
99. Kharasch ED, Frink EJ Jr, Zager R, et al: Assessment of low-flow sevoflurane and isoflurane effects on renal function using sensitive markers of tubular toxicity. Anesthesiology 86:1238-1253, 1997.
100. Kharasch ED, Schroeder JL, Liggitt HD, et al: New insights into the mechanism of methoxyflurane nephrotoxicity and implications for anesthetic development. Part 2. Identification of nephrotoxic metabolites. Anesthesiology 105:737-745, 2006.
101. Julier K, Da Silva R, Garcia C, et al: Preconditioning by sevoflurane decreases biochemical markers for myocardial and renal dysfunction in coronary artery bypass graft surgery: A double-blinded, placebo-controlled, multicenter study. Anesthesiology 98:1315-1327, 2003.
102. Brezis M, Rosen S, Silva P, Epstein FH: Renal ischemia: A new perspective. Kidney Int 26:375-383, 1984.
103. Byrick RJ, Rose DK: Pathophysiology and prevention of acute renal failure: The role of the anaesthetist. Can J Anaesth 37:457-467, 1990.
104. Zimmerhackl B, Robertson CR, Jamison RL: The microcirculation of the renal medulla. Circ Res 57:657-667, 1985.
105. Zimmerhackl BL, Robertson CR, Jamison RL: The medullary microcirculation. Kidney Int 31:641-647, 1987.
106. Flamenbaum W: Pathophysiology of acute renal failure. Arch Intern Med 131:911-928, 1973.
107. Chedru MF, Baethke R, Oken DE: Renal cortical blood flow and glomerular filtration in myohemoglobinuric acute renal failure. Kidney Int 1:232-239, 1972.
108. Knapp R, Hollenberg NK, Busch GJ, Abrams HL: Prolonged unilateral acute renal failure induced by intra-arterial norepinephrine infusion in the dog. Invest Radiol 7:164-173, 1972.
109. Ross B, Freeman D, Chan L: Contributions of nuclear magnetic resonance to renal biochemistry. Kidney Int 29:131-141, 1986.
110. Ratcliffe PJ, Moonen CT, Holloway PA, et al: Acute renal failure in hemorrhagic hypotension: Cellular energetics and renal function. Kidney Int 30:355-360, 1986.
111. Ratcliffe PJ, Moonen CT, Ledingham JG, Radda GK: Timing of the onset of changes in renal energetics in relation to blood pressure and glomerular filtration in haemorrhagic hypotension in the rat. Nephron 51:225-232, 1989.
112. Gamulin Z, Forster A, Morel D, et al: Effects of infrarenal aortic cross-clamping on renal hemodynamics in humans. Anesthesiology 61:394-399, 1984.
113. Page US, Washburn T: Using tracking data to find complications that physicians miss: The case of renal failure in cardiac surgery. Jt Comm J Qual Improv 23:511-520, 1997.
114. Ascione R, Nason G, Al-Ruzzeh S, et al: Coronary revascularization with or without cardiopulmonary bypass in patients with preoperative nondialysis-dependent renal insufficiency. Ann Thorac Surg 72:2020-2025, 2001.
115. Loef BG, Epema AH, Navis G, et al: Off-pump coronary revascularization attenuates transient renal damage compared with on-pump coronary revascularization. Chest 121:1190-1194, 2002.
116. Tang AT, Knott J, Nanson J, et al: A prospective randomized study to evaluate the renoprotective action of beating heart coronary surgery in low risk patients. Eur J Cardiothorac Surg 22:118-123, 2002.
117. Schwann NM, Horrow JC, Strong MD 3rd, et al: Does off-pump coronary artery bypass reduce the incidence of clinically evident renal dysfunction after multivessel myocardial revascularization? Anesth Analg 99:959-964, 2004.
118. Gamoso MG, Phillips-Bute B, Landolfo KP, et al: Off-pump versus on-pump coronary artery bypass surgery and postoperative renal dysfunction. Anesth Analg 91:1080-1084, 2000.
119. Hayashida N, Teshima H, Chihara S, et al: Does off-pump coronary artery bypass grafting really preserve renal function? Circ J 66:921-925, 2002.
120. Sabik JF, Gillinov AM, Blackstone EH, et al: Does off-pump coronary surgery reduce morbidity and mortality? J Thorac Cardiovasc Surg 124:698-707, 2002.
121. Karthik S, Musleh G, Grayson AD, et al: Effect of avoiding cardiopulmonary bypass in non-elective coronary artery bypass surgery: A propensity score analysis. Eur J Cardiothorac Surg 24:66-71, 2003.
122. Reston JT, Tregear SJ, Turkelson CM: Meta-analysis of short-term and mid-term outcomes following off-pump coronary artery bypass grafting. Ann Thorac Surg 76:1510-1515, 2003.
123. Al-Ruzzeh S, Ambler G, Asimakopoulos G, et al: Off-pump coronary artery bypass (OPCAB) surgery reduces risk-stratified morbidity and mortality: A United Kingdom multi-center comparative analysis of early clinical outcome. Circulation 108(Suppl 1): II1-II8, 2003.
124. Cheng DC, Bainbridge D, Martin JE, Novick RJ: Does off-pump coronary artery bypass reduce mortality, morbidity, and resource utilization when compared with conventional coronary artery bypass? A meta-analysis of randomized trials. Anesthesiology 102:188-203, 2005.
125. Yates RB, Stafford-Smith M: The genetic determinants of renal impairment following cardiac surgery. Semin Cardiothorac Vasc Anesth 10:314-326, 2006.
126. Stafford-Smith M, Podgoreanu M, Swaminathan M, et al: Association of genetic polymorphisms with risk of renal injury after coronary aftery bypass graft surgery. Am J Kidney Dis 45:519-530, 2005.
127. Chew ST, Newman MF, White WD, et al: Preliminary report on the association of apolipoprotein E polymorphisms, with postoperative peak serum creatinine concentrations in cardiac surgical patients. Anesthesiology 93:325-331, 2000.
128. van den Berghe G, Wouters P, Weekers F, et al: Intensive insulin therapy in the critically ill patients. N Engl J Med 345:1359-1367, 2001.
129. Stafford-Smith M, Reddan DN, Phillips-Bute B, et al: Association of perioperative creatinine-derived variables with mortality and other outcomes after coronary bypass surgery. Anesth Analg 92:SCA28, 2001.
130. Habib RH, Zacharias A, Schwann TA, et al: Role of hemodilutional anemia and transfusion during cardiopulmonary bypass in renal injury after coro-

nary revascularization: Implications on operative outcome. Crit Care Med 33:1749-1756, 2005.
131. Altmann D, Zwas D, Spartz AB, et al: Use of the contrast volume to estimated creatinine clearance ratio to predict renal failure after angiography. J Intervent Cardiol 10:113-119, 1997.
132. Perel A, Pizov R, Cotev S: Systolic blood pressure variation is a sensitive indicator of hypovolemia in ventilated dogs subjected to graded hemorrhage. Anesthesiology 67:498-502, 1987.
133. Kilburn KH, Dowell AR: Renal function in respiratory failure: Effects of hypoxia, hyperoxia, and hypercapnia. Arch Intern Med 127:754-762, 1971.
134. Pelletier CL, Shepherd JT: Effect of hypoxia on vascular responses to the carotid baroreflex. Am J Physiol 228:331-336, 1975.
135. Neylon M, Johns E, Marshall J: The renal response to systemic hypoxia in the anesthetized rat. J Physiol (Lond) 452:88P, 1992.
136. Sladen A, Laver MB, Pontoppidan H: Pulmonary complications and water retention in prolonged mechanical ventilation. N Engl J Med 279:448-453, 1968.
137. Stafford-Smith M, Grocott HP: Renal medullary hypoxia during experimental cardiopulmonary bypass: A pilot study. Perfusion 20:53-58, 2005.
138. Shah D, Corson J, Karmody A, Leather R: Effects of isovolemic hemodilution on abdominal aortic aneurysmectomy in high risk patients. Ann Vasc Surg 1:50-54, 1986.
139. Messmer K: Hemodilution. Surg Clin North Am 55:659-678, 1975.
140. DeFoe G, Ross C, Olmstead E, et al: Group NNECDS: Lowest hematocrit on bypass and adverse outcomes associated with coronary artery bypass grafting. Ann Thorac Surg 71:769-776, 2001.
141. Fang WC, Helm RE, Krieger KH, et al: Impact of minimum hematocrit during cardiopulmonary bypass on mortality in patients undergoing coronary artery surgery. Circulation 96:II-194-II-199, 1997.
142. Ranucci M, Pavesi M, Mazza E, et al: Risk factors for renal dysfunction after coronary surgery: The role of cardiopulmonary bypass technique. Perfusion 9:319-326, 1994.
143. Swaminathan M, Phillips-Bute BG, Conlon PJ, et al: The association of lowest hematocrit during cardiopulmonary bypass with acute renal injury after coronary bypass surgery. Ann Thorac Surg 76:784-791, 2003.
144. Karkouti K, Beattie WS, Wijeysundera DN, et al: Hemodilution during cardiopulmonary bypass is an independent risk factor for acute renal failure in adult cardiac surgery. J Thorac Cardiovasc Surg 129:391-400, 2005.
145. Kincaid EH, Ashburn DA, Hoyle JR, et al: Does the combination of aprotinin and angiotensin-converting enzyme inhibitor cause renal failure after cardiac surgery? Ann Thorac Surg 80:1388-1393, 2005.
146. Ferraris VA, Ferraris SP, Saha SP, et al: Perioperative blood transfusion and blood conservation in cardiac surgery: The Society of Thoracic Surgeons and the Society of Cardiovascular Anesthesiologists clinical practice guideline. Ann Thorac Surg 83:S27-S86, 2007.
147. Viele MK, Weiskopf RB: What can we learn about the need for transfusion from patients who refuse blood? The experience with Jehovah's Witnesses. Transfusion 34:396-401, 1994.
148. Carson JL, Duff A, Poses RM, et al: Effect of anaemia and cardiovascular disease on surgical mortality and morbidity. Lancet 348:1055-1060, 1996.
149. Spiess BD: Choose one: Damned if you do/damned if you don't! Crit Care Med 33:1871-1874, 2005.
150. Aronson S, Fontes ML, Mangano DT: Wide pulse pressure confers a blow to the kidneys [abstract]. Anesthesiology 2002.
151. Fischer UM, Weissenberger WK, Warters RD, et al: Impact of cardiopulmonary bypass management on postcardiac surgery renal function. Perfusion 17:401-406, 2002.
152. Abel RM, Buckley MJ, Austen WG, et al: Etiology, incidence, and prognosis of renal failure following cardiac operations: Results of a prospective analysis of 500 consecutive patients. J Thorac Cardiovasc Surg 71:323-333, 1976.
153. Bhat JG, Gluck MC, Lowenstein J, Baldwin DS: Renal failure after open heart surgery. Ann Intern Med 84:677-682, 1976.
154. Urzua J, Troncoso S, Bugedo G, et al: Renal function and cardiopulmonary bypass: Effect of perfusion pressure. J Cardiothorac Vasc Anesth 6:299-303, 1992.
155. Swaminathan M, Knauth K, Phillips-Bute B, et al: Lowest CPB hematocrit is inversely associated with creatinine rise after coronary bypass surgery. Anesth Analg 94:S70, 2002.
156. Conlon PJ, Crowley J, Stack R, et al: Renal artery stenosis is not associated with the development of acute renal failure following coronary artery bypass grafting. Ren Fail 27:81-86, 2005.
157. Gorfinkel HJ, Szidon JP, Hirsch LJ, Fishman AP: Renal performance in experimental cardiogenic shock. Am J Physiol 222:1260-1268, 1972.
158. Kahl FR, Flint JF, Szidon JP: Influence of left atrial distention on renal vasomotor tone. Am J Physiol 226:240-246, 1974.
159. Smith MD, MacPhail B, Harrison MR, et al: Value and limitations of transesophageal echocardiography in determination of left ventricular volumes and ejection fraction. J Am Coll Cardiol 19:1213-1222, 1992.
160. Helak JW, Reichek N: Quantitation of human left ventricular mass and volume by two-dimensional echocardiography: In vitro anatomic validation. Circulation 63:1398-1407, 1981.
161. Folland ED, Parisi AF, Moynihan PF, et al: Assessment of left ventricular ejection fraction and volumes by real-time, two-dimensional echocardiography: A comparison of cineangiographic and radionuclide techniques. Circulation 60:760-766, 1979.
162. Garwood S, Davis E, Harris SN: Intraoperative transesophageal ultrasonography can measure renal blood flow. J Cardiothorac Vasc Anesth 15:65-71, 2001.
163. Laissy JP, Idee JM, Fernandez P, et al: Magnetic resonance imaging in acute and chronic kidney diseases: Present status. Nephron Clin Pract 103:c50-c57, 2006.
164. Sear JW: Kidney dysfunction in the postoperative period. Br J Anaesth 95:20-32, 2005.
165. Jacob M, Chappell D, Rehm M: Clinical update: Perioperative fluid management. Lancet 369:1984-1986, 2007.
166. Price JD, Sear JW, Venn RM: Perioperative fluid volume optimization following proximal femoral fracture. Cochrane Database Syst Rev 1:CD003004, 2004.
167. Nisanevich V, Felsenstein I, Almogy G, et al: Effect of intraoperative fluid management on outcome after intraabdominal surgery. Anesthesiology 103: 25-32, 2005.
168. Brandstrup B, Tonnesen H, Beier-Holgersen R, et al: Effects of intravenous fluid restriction on postoperative complications: Comparison of two perioperative fluid regimens: A randomized assessor-blinded multicenter trial. Ann Surg 238:641-648, 2003.
169. Holte K, Kehlet H: Fluid therapy and surgical outcomes in elective surgery: A need for reassessment in fast-track surgery. J Am Coll Surg 202:971-989, 2006.
170. Arieff AI: Fatal postoperative pulmonary edema: Pathogenesis and literature review. Chest 115:1371-1377, 1999.
171. Makhoul RG, Gewertz BL: Renal prostaglandins. J Surg Res 40:181-192, 1986.
172. Packer M, Lee WH, Kessler PD: Preservation of glomerular filtration rate in human heart failure by activation of the renin-angiotensin system. Circulation 74:766-774, 1986.
173. Edwards RM: Segmental effects of norepinephrine and angiotensin II on isolated renal microvessels. Am J Physiol 244:F526-F534, 1983.
174. Stone AM, Stahl WM: Renal effects of hemorrhage in normal man. Ann Surg 172:825-836, 1970.
175. Reves JG, Karp RB, Buttner EE, et al: Neuronal and adrenomedullary catecholamine release in response to cardiopulmonary bypass in man. Circulation 66:49-55, 1982.
176. Laffey J, Boylan J, Cheng D: The systemic inflammatory response to cardiac surgery: Implications for the anesthesiologist. Anesthesiology 97:215-252, 2002.
177. Llopart T, Lombardi R, Forselledo M, Andrade R: Acute renal failure in open heart surgery. Ren Fail 19:319-323, 1997.
178. Hilberman M, Myers BD, Carrie BJ, et al: Acute renal failure following cardiac surgery. J Thorac Cardiovasc Surg 77:880-888, 1979.
179. Gowans EM, Fraser CG: Biological variation of serum and urine creatinine and creatinine clearance: Ramifications for interpretation of results and patient care. Ann Clin Biochem 25:259-263, 1988.
180. Cockcroft DW, Gault MH: Prediction of creatinine clearance from serum creatinine. Nephron 16:31-41, 1976.
181. Levey AS, Bosch JP, Lewis JB, et al: A more accurate method to estimate glomerular filtration rate from serum creatinine: A new prediction equation. Modification of Diet in Renal Disease Study Group. Ann Intern Med 130:461-470, 1999.
182. Vertel RM, Knochel JP: Nonoliguric acute renal failure. JAMA 200:598-602, 1967.
183. Shin B, Isenhower NN, McAslan TC, et al: Early recognition of renal insufficiency in post-anesthetic trauma victims. Anesthesiology 50:262-265, 1979.
184. Rosenberg IK, Gupta SL, Lucas CE, et al: Renal insufficiency after trauma and sepsis: A prospective functional and ultrastructural analysis. Arch Surg 103:175-183, 1971.
185. Knos GB, Berry AJ, Isaacson IJ, Weitz FI: Intraoperative urinary output and postoperative blood urea nitrogen and creatinine levels in patients undergoing aortic reconstructive surgery. J Clin Anesth 1:181-185, 1989.
186. Jones LW, Weil MH: Water, creatinine and sodium excretion following circulatory shock wtih renal failure. Am J Med 51:314-318, 1971.
187. Goldstein MB: Acute renal failure. Med Clin North Am 67:1325-1341, 1983.
188. Pru C, Kjellstrand C: Urinary indices and chemistries in the differential diagnosis of prerenal failure and acute tubular necrosis. Semin Nephrol 5:224-233, 1985.
189. Haskell LP, Tannenberg AM: Elevated urinary specific gravity in acute oliguric renal failure due to hetastarch administration. N Y State J Med 88:387-388, 1988.
190. Eliahou H, Bata A: The diagnosis of acute renal failure. Nephron 2:287, 1965.

191. Miller TR, Anderson RJ, Linas SL, et al: Urinary diagnostic indices in acute renal failure: A prospective study. Ann Intern Med 89:47-50, 1978.
192. Espinel CH, Gregory AW: Differential diagnosis of acute renal failure. Clin Nephrol 13:73-77, 1980.
193. Zager RA, Rubin NT, Ebert T, Maslov N: Rapid radioimmunoassay for diagnosing acute tubular necrosis. Nephron 26:7-12, 1980.
194. Miller PD, Krebs RA, Neal BJ, McIntyre DO: Polyuric prerenal failure. Arch Intern Med 140:907-909, 1980.
195. Heimann T, Brau S, Sakurai H, Peirce EC 2nd: Urinary osmolal changes in renal dysfunction following open-heart operations. Ann Thorac Surg 22:44-49, 1976.
196. Andreev E, Koopman M, Arisz L: A rise in plasma creatinine that is not a sign of renal failure: Which drugs can be responsible? J Intern Med 246:247-252, 1999.
197. Hoffmann U, Fischereder M, Kruger B, et al: The value of *N*-acetylcysteine in the prevention of radiocontrast agent-induced nephropathy seems questionable. J Am Soc Nephrol 15:407-410, 2004.
198. Shemesh O, Golbetz H, Kriss JP, Myers BD: Limitations of creatinine as a filtration marker in glomerulopathic patients. Kidney Int 28:830-838, 1985.
199. Moran SM, Myers BD: Course of acute renal failure studied by a model of creatinine kinetics. Kidney Int 27:928-937, 1985.
200. Doolan PD, Alpen EL, Theil GB: A clinical appraisal of the plasma concentration and endogenous clearance of creatinine. Am J Med 32:65-79, 1962.
201. Bloor GK, Welsh KR, Goodall S, Shah MV: Comparison of predicted with measured creatinine clearance in cardiac surgical patients. J Cardiothorac Vasc Anesth 10:899-902, 1996.
202. Morgan DB, Dillon S, Payne RB: The assessment of glomerular function: Creatinine clearance or plasma creatinine? Postgrad Med J 54:302-310, 1978.
203. Bull G, Joekes A, Lowe K: Renal function studies in acute tubular necrosis. Clin Sci 9:379, 1950.
204. Handa SP, Morrin PA: Diagnostic indices in acute renal failure. Can Med Assoc J 96:78-82, 1967.
205. Perlmutter M, Grossman SL, Rothenberg S, Dobkin G: Urine-serum urea nitrogen ratio; Simple test of renal function in acute azotemia and oliguria. JAMA 170:1533-1537, 1959.
206. Chisholm GD, Charlton CA, Orr WM: Urine-urea-blood-urea ratios in renal failure. Lancet 1:20-23, 1966.
207. Luke RG, Briggs JD, Allison ME, Kennedy AC: Factors determining response to mannitol in acute renal failure. Am J Med Sci 259:168-174, 1970.
208. Espinel CH: The FENa test: Use in the differential diagnosis of acute renal failure. JAMA 236:579-581, 1976.
209. Diamond JR, Yoburn DC: Nonoliguric acute renal failure associated with a low fractional excretion of sodium. Ann Intern Med 96:597-600, 1982.
210. Shin B, Mackenzie CF, Helrich M: Creatinine clearance of early detection of posttraumatic renal dysfunction. Anesthesiology 64:605-609, 1986.
211. Brown RS: Renal dysfunction in the surgical patient: Maintenance of high output state with furosemide. Crit Care Med 7:63-68, 1979.
212. Brosius FC, Lau K: Low fractional excretion of sodium in acute renal failure: Role of timing of the test and ischemia. Am J Nephrol 6:450-457, 1986.
213. Saha H, Mustonen J, Helin H, Pasternack A: Limited value of the fractional excretion of sodium test in the diagnosis of acute renal failure. Nephrol Dial Transplant 2:79-82, 1987.
214. Steiner RW: Interpreting the fractional excretion of sodium. Am J Med 77:699-702, 1984.
215. Zarich S, Fang LS, Diamond JR: Fractional excretion of sodium: Exceptions to its diagnostic value. Arch Intern Med 145:108-112, 1985.
216. Jones LW, Weil MH: Changes in urinary output and free water clearance in patients with acute circulatory failure (shock). J Urol 102:121-125, 1969.
217. Baek SM, Brown RS, Shoemaker WC: Early prediction of acute renal failure and recovery: I. Sequential measurements of free water clearance. Ann Surg 177:253-258, 1973.
218. Kosinski JP, Lucas CE, Ledgerwood AM: Meaning and value of free water clearance in injured patients. J Surg Res 33:184-188, 1982.
219. Sladen RN, Endo E, Harrison T: Two-hour versus 22-hour creatinine clearance in critically ill patients. Anesthesiology 67:1013-1016, 1987.
220. Wheeler LA, Sheiner LB: Clinical estimation of creatinine clearance. Am J Clin Pathol 72:27-32, 1979.
221. Greenblatt DJ, Ransil BJ, Harmatz JS, et al: Variability of 24-hour urinary creatinine excretion by normal subjects. J Clin Pharmacol 16:321-328, 1976.
222. Lucas CE, Weaver D, Higgins RF, et al: Effects of albumin versus non-albumin resuscitation on plasma volume and renal excretory function. J Trauma 18:564-570, 1978.
223. Bennett-Guerrero E, et al: Impact of normal saline based versus balanced salt intravenous fluid replacement on clinical outcomes: A randomized blinded clinical trial. Anesthesiology 94:A147, 2001.
224. Cittanova ML, Leblanc I, Legendre C, et al: Effect of hydroxyethylstarch in brain-dead kidney donors on renal function in kidney-transplant recipients. Lancet 348:1620-1622, 1996.
225. Peron S, Mouthon L, Guettier C, et al: Hydroxyethyl starch-induced renal insufficiency after plasma exchange in a patient with polymyositis and liver cirrhosis. Clin Nephrol 55:408-411, 2001.
226. Winkelmayer WC, Glynn RJ, Levin R, Avorn J: Hydroxyethyl starch and change in renal function in patients undergoing coronary artery bypass graft surgery. Kidney Int 64:1046-1049, 2003.
227. De Labarthe A, Jacobs F, Blot F, Glotz D: Acute renal failure secondary to hydroxyethylstarch administration in a surgical patient. Am J Med 111:417-418, 2001.
228. Schortgen F, Lacherade JC, Bruneel F, et al: Effects of hydroxyethylstarch and gelatin on renal function in severe sepsis: A multicentre randomised study. Lancet 357:911-916, 2001.
229. Boldt J, Brenner T, Lang J, et al: Kidney-specific proteins in elderly patients undergoing cardiac surgery with cardiopulmonary bypass. Anesth Analg 97:1582-1589, 2003.
230. Kumle B, Boldt J, Piper S, et al: The influence of different intravascular volume replacement regimens on renal function in the elderly. Anesth Analg 89:1124-1130, 1999.
231. Wilkes NJ, Woolf R, Mutch M, et al: The effects of balanced versus saline-based hetastarch and crystalloid solutions on acid-base and electrolyte status and gastric mucosal perfusion in elderly surgical patients. Anesth Analg 93:811-816, 2001.
232. Parekh N: Hyperchloremic acidosis. Anesth Analg 95:1821, 2002.
233. Wilcox C: Regulation of renal blood flow by plasma chloride. J Clin Invest 71:726-735, 1983.
234. Hansen PB, Jensen BL, Skott O: Chloride regulates afferent arteriolar contraction in response to depolarization. Hypertension 32:1066-1070, 1998.
235. Renkin EM, Robinson RR: Glomerular filtration. N Engl J Med 290:785-792, 1974.
236. Mauer SM, Steffes MW, Ellis EN, et al: Structural-functional relationships in diabetic nephropathy. J Clin Invest 74:1143-1155, 1984.
237. Richards A, Westfall B, Bott P: Renal excretion of inulin, creatinine, and xylose in normal dogs. Proc Soc Exp Biol Med 32:73, 1934.
238. Miller BF, Winkler AW: The renal excretion of endogenous creatinine in man. comparison with exogenous creatinine and inulin. J Clin Invest 17:31-40, 1938.
239. Skov PE: Glomerular filtration rate in patients with severe and very severe renal insufficiency: Determined by simultaneous inulin, creatinine and 125 iothalamate clearance. Acta Med Scand 187:419-428, 1970.
240. Carcoana OV, Hines RL: Is renal dose dopamine protective or therapeutic? Yes. Crit Care Clin 12:677-685, 1996.
241. Cottee DB, Saul WP: Is renal dose dopamine protective or therapeutic? No. Crit Care Clin 12:687-695, 1996.
242. Holmes CL, Walley KR: Bad medicine: Low-dose dopamine in the ICU. Chest 123:1266-1275, 2003.
243. Jones D, Bellomo R: Renal-dose dopamine: From hypothesis to paradigm to dogma to myth and, finally, superstition? J Intensive Care Med 20:199-211, 2005.
244. Prins I, Plotz FB, Uiterwaal CS, van Vught HJ: Low-dose dopamine in neonatal and pediatric intensive care: A systematic review. Intensive Care Med 27:206-210, 2001.
245. McHugh GJ: Current usage of dopamine in New Zealand intensive care units. Anaesth Intensive Care 29:623-626, 2001.
246. Trueta J, Barclay A, Daniel P, et al: Studies on the Renal Circulation. Oxford, Blackwell Scientific Publications, 1947.
247. Carriere S, Thorburn G, O'Morchoe C, et al: Intrarenal distribution of blood flow in dogs during hemorrhagic hypotension. Circ Res 19:167, 1966.
248. Barger AC, Herd JA: The renal circulation. N Engl J Med 284:482-490, 1971.
249. Rector JB, Stein JH, Bay WH, et al: Effect of hemorrhage and vasopressor agents on distribution of renal blood flow. Am J Physiol 222:1125-1131, 1972.
250. Aukland K: Intrarenal distribution of blood flow: Are reliable methods available for measurements in man? Scand J Clin Lab Invest 35:481-486, 1975.
251. Aukland K, Loyning EW: Intrarenal blood flow and para-aminohippurate (PAH) extraction. Acta Physiol Scand 79:95-108, 1970.
252. Reubi RC, Gossweiler N, Gurtler R: Renal circulation in man studied by means of a dye-dilution method. Circulation 33:426-442, 1966.
253. Haywood GA, Stewart JT, Counihan PJ, et al: Validation of bedside measurements of absolute human renal blood flow by a continuous thermodilution technique. Crit Care Med 20:659-664, 1992.
254. Muller M, Padberg W, Schindler E, et al: Renocortical tissue oxygen pressure measurements in patients undergoing living donor kidney transplantation. Anesth Analg 87:474-476, 1998.
255. Kram HB, Appel PL, Fleming AW, Shoemaker WC: Assessment of intestinal and renal perfusion using surface oximetry. Crit Care Med 14:707-713, 1986.
256. Schott G, Prom T: Intraoperative cortical Po_2 measurement in kidney transplantation: The effect of the calcium antagonist diltiazem. Urologe A 33:415-421, 1994.
257. Kainuma M, Kimura N, Shimada Y: Effect of acute changes in renal arterial blood flow on urine oxygen tension in dogs. Crit Care Med 18:309-312, 1990.
258. Rennie DW, Reeves RB, Pappenheimer JR: Oxygen pressure in urine and its relation to intrarenal blood flow. Am J Physiol 195:120-132, 1958.

259. Hong SK, Boylan JW, Tannenberg AM, Rahn H: Total and partial gas tensions of human bladder urine. J Appl Physiol 15:115-120, 1960.
260. Thorburn GD, Kopald HH, Herd JA, et al: Intrarenal distribution of nutrient blood flow determined with krypton 85 in the unanesthetized dog. Circ Res 13:290-307, 1963.
261. Kainuma M, Yamada M, Miyake T: Continuous urine oxygen tension monitoring in patients undergoing cardiac surgery. J Cardiothorac Vasc Anesth 10:603-608, 1996.
262. Hollenberg NK, Epstein M, Rosen SM, et al: Acute oliguric renal failure in man: Evidence for preferential renal cortical ischemia. Medicine (Baltimore) 47:455-474, 1968.
263. Grunfeld JP, Sabto J, Bankir L, Funck-Brentano JL: Methods for measurement of renal blood flow in man. Semin Nucl Med 4:39-50, 1974.
264. Farmelant MH, Burrows BA: The renogram: Physiologic basis and current clinical use. Semin Nucl Med 4:61-73, 1974.
265. Stevens PE, Gwyther SJ, Hanson ME, et al: Noninvasive monitoring of renal blood flow characteristics during acute renal failure in man. Intensive Care Med 16:153-158, 1990.
266. Aronson S, Thistlethwaite RJ, Walker R, et al: Safety and feasibility of renal blood flow determination during kidney transplant surgery with perfusion ultrasonography. Anesth Analg 80:353-359, 1995.
267. Aronson S, Wiencek JG, Feinstein SB, et al: Assessment of renal blood flow with contrast ultrasonography. Anesth Analg 76:964-970, 1993.
268. Wei K, Le E, Bin JP, et al: Quantification of renal blood flow with contrast-enhanced ultrasound. J Am Coll Cardiol 37:1135-1140, 2001.
269. Aronson S, Bilotta F, Wienceck J, et al: Assessment of renal blood flow distribution in dogs with contrast ultrasound following dopamine infusion. Anesth Analg 74:S11, 1992.
270. Trof RJ, Di Maggio F, Leemreis J, Groeneveld AB: Biomarkers of acute renal injury and renal failure. Shock 26:245-253, 2006.
271. Bagshaw SM, Langenberg C, Haase M, et al: Urinary biomarkers in septic acute kidney injury. Intensive Care Med 33:1285-1296, 2007.
272. Perco P, Pleban C, Kainz A, et al: Protein biomarkers associated with acute renal failure and chronic kidney disease. Eur J Clin Invest 36:753-763, 2006.
273. O'Riordan E, Goligorsky MS: Emerging studies of the urinary proteome: The end of the beginning? Curr Opin Nephrol Hypertens 14:579-585, 2005.
274. Parikh CR, Edelstein CL, Devarajan P, Cantley L: Biomarkers of acute kidney injury: Early diagnosis, pathogenesis, and recovery. J Invest Med 55:333-340, 2007.
275. Devarajan P: Proteomics for biomarker discovery in acute kidney injury. Semin Nephrol 27:637-651, 2007.
276. Han WK, Waikar SS, Johnson A, et al: Urinary biomarkers in the early diagnosis of acute kidney injury. Kidney Int 73:863-869, 2008.
277. Devarajan P: Emerging biomarkers of acute kidney injury. Contrib Nephrol 156:203-212, 2007.
278. Nguyen MT, Ross GF, Dent CL, Devarajan P: Early prediction of acute renal injury using urinary proteomics. Am J Nephrol 25:318-326, 2005.
279. Bonventre JV: Diagnosis of acute kidney injury: From classic parameters to new biomarkers. Contrib Nephrol 156:213-219, 2007.
280. Vaidya VS, Bonventre JV: Mechanistic biomarkers for cytotoxic acute kidney injury. Expert Opin Drug Metab Toxicol 2:697-713, 2006.
281. Mishra J, Dent C, Tarabishi R, et al: Neutrophil gelatinase-associated lipocalin (NGAL) as a biomarker for acute renal injury after cardiac surgery. Lancet 365:1231-1238, 2005.
282. Parikh CR, Mishra J, Thiessen-Philbrook H, et al: Urinary IL-18 is an early predictive biomarker of acute kidney injury after cardiac surgery. Kidney Int 70:199-203, 2006.
283. Levin A: Cystatin C, serum creatinine, and estimates of kidney function: Searching for better measures of kidney function and cardiovascular risk. Ann Intern Med 142:586-588, 2005.
284. Grubb A, Bjork J, Lindstrom V, et al: A cystatin C–based formula without anthropometric variables estimates glomerular filtration rate better than creatinine clearance using the Cockcroft-Gault formula. Scand J Clin Lab Invest 65:153-162, 2005.
285. Momeni M, Baele P, Jacquet L, et al: Cystatin C in cardiac surgery. Acta Anaesthesiol Belg 58:107-112, 2007.
286. Zhu J, Yin R, Wu H, et al: Cystatin C as a reliable marker of renal function following heart valve replacement surgery with cardiopulmonary bypass. Clin Chim Acta 374:116-121, 2006.
287. Abu-Omar Y, Mussa S, Naik MJ, et al: Evaluation of cystatin C as a marker of renal injury following on-pump and off-pump coronary surgery. Eur J Cardiothorac Surg 27:893-898, 2005.
288. Smith GL, Lichtman JH, Bracken MB, et al: Renal impairment and outcomes in heart failure: systematic review and meta-analysis. J Am Coll Cardiol 47:1987-1996, 2006.
289. Jernberg T, Lindahl B, James S, et al: Cystatin C: A novel predictor of outcome in suspected or confirmed non–ST-elevation acute coronary syndrome. Circulation 110:2342-2348, 2004.
290. Traynor J, Mactier R, Geddes CC, Fox JG: How to measure renal function in clinical practice. BMJ 333:733-737, 2006.
291. Mazul-Sunko B, Zarkovic N, Vrkic N, et al: Proatrial natriuretic peptide(1-98), but not cystatin C, is predictive for occurrence of acute renal insufficiency in critically ill septic patients. Nephron Clin Pract 97:c103-c107, 2004.
292. Takahira R, Yonemura K, Yonekawa O, et al: Tryptophan glycoconjugate as a novel marker of renal function. Am J Med 110:192-197, 2001.
293. Westhuyzen J, Endre ZH, Reece G, et al: Measurement of tubular enzymuria facilitates early detection of acute renal impairment in the intensive care unit. Nephrol Dial Transplant 18:543-551, 2003.
294. Price RG: Urinary enzymes, nephrotoxicity and renal disease. Toxicology 23:99-134, 1982.
295. Mueller PW, MacNeil ML, Steinberg KK: *N*-Acetyl-beta-D-glucosaminidase assay in urine: Urea inhibition. J Anal Toxicol 13:188-190, 1989.
296. Stolarek I, Howey JE, Fraser CG: Biological variation of urinary *N*-acetyl-beta-D-glucosaminidase: Practical and clinical implications. Clin Chem 35:560-563, 1989.
297. Yuen CT, Price RG, Chattagoon L, et al: Colorimetric assays for *N*-acetyl-beta-D-glucosaminidase and beta-D-galactosidase in human urine using newly-developed omega-nitrostyryl substrates. Clin Chim Acta 124:195-204, 1982.
298. Hofmann W, Guder WG: A diagnostic programme for quantitative analysis of proteinuria. J Clin Chem Clin Biochem 27:589-600, 1989.
299. Robinson D, Stirling JL: *N*-Acetyl-beta-glucosaminidases in human spleen. Biochem J 107:321-327, 1968.
300. Price RG, Dance N, Richards B, Cattell WR: The excretion of *N*-acetyl-beta-glucosaminidase and beta-galactosidase following surgery to the kidney. Clin Chim Acta 27:65-72, 1970.
301. Tucker SM, Pierce RJ, Price RG: Characterisation of human *N*-acetyl-beta-D-glucosaminidase isoenzymes as an indicator of tissue damage in disease. Clin Chim Acta 102:29-40, 1980.
302. Whiting PH, Petersen J, Power DA, et al: Diagnostic value of urinary N-acetyl-beta-D-glucosaminidase, its isoenzymes and the fractional excretion of sodium following renal transplantation. Clin Chim Acta 130:369-376, 1983.
303. Eti S, Cheng CY, Marshall A, Reidenberg MM: Urinary clusterin in chronic nephrotoxicity in the rat. Proc Soc Exp Biol Med 202:487-490, 1993.
304. Girardi AC, Degray BC, Nagy T, et al: Association of Na^+-H^+ exchanger isoform NHE3 and dipeptidyl peptidase IV in the renal proximal tubule. J Biol Chem 276:46671-46677, 2001.
305. du Cheyron D, Daubin C, Poggioli J, et al: Urinary measurement of Na^+/H^+ exchanger isoform 3 (NHE3) protein as new marker of tubule injury in critically ill patients with ARF. Am J Kidney Dis 42:497-506, 2003.
306. Stafford-Smith M: Antifibrinolytic agents make alpha1- and beta2-microglobulinuria poor markers of post cardiac surgery renal dysfunction. Anesthesiology 90:928-929, 1999.
307. Mogensen CE, Solling K: Studies on renal tubular protein reabsorption: Partial and near complete inhibition by certain amino acids. Scand J Clin Lab Invest 37:477-486, 1977.
308. Rustom R, Maltby P, Grime JS, et al: Effects of lysine infusion on the renal metabolism of aprotinin (Trasylol) in man. Clin Sci (Colch) 83:295-299, 1992.
309. Feindt PR, Walcher S, Volkmer I, et al: Effects of high-dose aprotinin on renal function in aortocoronary bypass grafting. Ann Thorac Surg 60:1076-1080, 1995.
310. Karlsson FA, Wibell L, Evrin PE: Beta 2-microglobulin in clinical medicine. Scand J Clin Lab Invest Suppl 154:27-37, 1980.
311. Norden AG, Flynn FV: Degradation of beta 2-microglobulin in infected urine by leukocyte elastase-like activity. Clin Chim Acta 134:167-176, 1983.
312. Dehne MG, Boldt J, Heise D, et al: Tamm-Horsfall protein, alpha-1- and beta-2-microglobulin as kidney function markers in heart surgery. Anaesthesist 44:545-551, 1995.
313. Gormley SM, McBride WT, Armstrong MA, et al: Plasma and urinary cytokine homeostasis and renal dysfunction during cardiac surgery. Anesthesiology 93:1210-1216, 2000.
314. Harrison JF, Parker RW, De Silva KL: Lysozymuria and acute disorders of renal function. J Clin Pathol 26:278-284, 1973.
315. Mishra J, Mori K, Ma Q, et al: Amelioration of ischemic acute renal injury by neutrophil gelatinase-associated lipocalin. J Am Soc Nephrol 15:3073-3082, 2004.
316. Mishra J, Ma Q, Prada A, et al: Identification of neutrophil gelatinase-associated lipocalin as a novel early urinary biomarker for ischemic renal injury. J Am Soc Nephrol 14:2534-2543, 2003.
317. Wagener G, Jan M, Kim M, et al: Association between increases in urinary neutrophil gelatinase-associated lipocalin and acute renal dysfunction after adult cardiac surgery. Anesthesiology 105:485-491, 2006.
318. Parikh CR, Abraham E, Ancukiewicz M, Edelstein CL: Urine IL-18 is an early diagnostic marker for acute kidney injury and predicts mortality in the intensive care unit. J Am Soc Nephrol 16:3046-3052, 2005.
319. Parikh CR, Jani A, Melnikov VY, et al: Urinary interleukin-18 is a marker of human acute tubular necrosis. Am J Kidney Dis 43:405-414, 2004.
320. Mariano F, Guida G, Donati D, et al: Production of platelet-activating factor in patients with sepsis-

associated acute renal failure. Nephrol Dial Transplant 14:1150-1157, 1999.

321. Ichimura T, Bonventre JV, Bailly V, et al: Kidney injury molecule-1 (KIM-1), a putative epithelial cell adhesion molecule containing a novel immunoglobulin domain, is up-regulated in renal cells after injury. J Biol Chem 273:4135-4142, 1998.
322. Ichimura T, Hung CC, Yang SA, et al: Kidney injury molecule-1: A tissue and urinary biomarker for nephrotoxicant-induced renal injury. Am J Physiol Renal Physiol 286:F552-F563, 2004.
323. Han WK, Bailly V, Abichandani R, et al: Kidney Injury Molecule-1 (KIM-1): A novel biomarker for human renal proximal tubule injury. Kidney Int 62:237-244, 2002.
324. Muramatsu Y, Tsujie M, Kohda Y, et al: Early detection of cysteine rich protein 61 (CYR61, CCN1) in urine following renal ischemic reperfusion injury. Kidney Int 62:1601-1610, 2002.
325. Davidman M, Olson P, Kohen J, et al: Iatrogenic renal disease. Arch Intern Med 151:1809-1812, 1991.
326. McCullough PA, Wolyn R, Rocher LL, et al: Acute renal failure after coronary intervention: Incidence, risk factors, and relationship to mortality. Am J Med 103:368-375, 1997.
327. Diehl JT, Cali RF, Hertzer NR, Beven EG: Complications of abdominal aortic reconstruction: An analysis of perioperative risk factors in 557 patients. Ann Surg 197:49-56, 1983.
328. Crawford ES, Crawford JL, Safi HJ, et al: Thoracoabdominal aortic aneurysms: Preoperative and intraoperative factors determining immediate and long-term results of operations in 605 patients. J Vasc Surg 3:389-404, 1986.
329. Luke RG: Can renal failure due to hypertension be prevented? Hypertension 18:I139-I142, 1991.
330. Kurella M, Lo JC, Chertow GM: Metabolic syndrome and the risk for chronic kidney disease among nondiabetic adults. J Am Soc Nephrol 16:2134-2140, 2005.
331. Aronson S, Boisvert D, Lapp W: Isolated systolic hypertension is associated with adverse outcomes from coronary artery bypass grafting surgery. Anesth Analg 94:1079-1084, 2002.
332. Hou SH, Bushinsky DA, Wish JB, et al: Hospital-acquired renal insufficiency: A prospective study. Am J Med 74:243-248, 1983.
333. Wilson RF, Soullier G, Antonenko D: Creatinine clearance in critically ill surgical patients. Arch Surg 114:461-467, 1979.
334. McCreath BJ, Swaminathan M, Booth JV, et al: Mitral valve surgery and acute renal injury: Port access versus median sternotomy. Ann Thorac Surg 75:812-819, 2003.
335. Fischer SS, Phillips-Bute B, Swaminathan M, et al: Symmetry aortic connector devices and acute renal injury: A comparison of renal dysfunction after three different aortocoronary bypass surgery techniques. Anesth Analg 102:25-31, 2006.
336. Stafford-Smith M, Swaminathan M, McCreath BJ, et al: Morbidity-related serum creatinine patterns after coronary bypass surgery. Anesth Analg 92: SCA123, 2001.
337. Swaminathan M, Knauth K, Phillips-Bute B, et al: Acute renal dysfunction after cardiac transplant surgery: A comparison with other forms of cardiac surgery. Anesth Analg 94:SCA102, 2002.
338. Morozowich S, Lin S, Phillips-Bute B, et al: Aprotinin use and allograft function after off-pump bilateral lung transplantation. Anesth Analg 102:SCA6, 2006.
339. Ten Clay S, Phillips-Bute B, Glower D, et al: Aortic valve replacement and acute kidney injury: Minimally invasive parasternotomy versus median sternotomy. Anesth Analg 106:SCA124, 2008.
340. Stafford-Smith M, Patel U, Phillips-Bute B, et al: Acute kidney injury and chronic kidney disease after cardiac surgery. Adv Chronic Kidney Dis 15:157-177, 2008.
341. Hix JK, Thakar CV, Katz EM, et al: Effect of off-pump coronary artery bypass graft surgery on postoperative acute kidney injury and mortality. Crit Care Med 34:2979-2983, 2006.
342. Mehta RH, Grab JD, O'Brien SM, et al: Bedside tool for predicting the risk of postoperative dialysis in patients undergoing cardiac surgery. Circulation 114:2208-2216; quiz 2208, 2006.
343. Appoo JJ, Augoustides JG, Pochettino A, et al: Perioperative outcome in adults undergoing elective deep hypothermic circulatory arrest with retrograde cerebral perfusion in proximal aortic arch repair: Evaluation of protocol-based care. J Cardiothorac Vasc Anesth 20:3-7, 2006.
344. Boyle JM, Moualla S, Arrigain S, et al: Risks and outcomes of acute kidney injury requiring dialysis after cardiac transplantation. Am J Kidney Dis 48:787-796, 2006.
345. Rocha PN, Rocha AT, Palmer SM, et al: Acute renal failure after lung transplantation: Incidence, predictors and impact on perioperative morbidity and mortality. Am J Transplant 5:1469-1476, 2005.
346. Safi HJ, Harlin SA, Miller CC, et al: Predictive factors for acute renal failure in thoracic and thoracoabdominal aortic aneurysm surgery [published erratum appears in J Vasc Surg 1997 Jan;25(1):93]. J Vasc Surg 24:338-344; discussion 344-345, 1996.
347. Topkara VK, Dang NC, Barili F, et al: Predictors and outcomes of continuous veno-venous hemodialysis use after implantation of a left ventricular assist device. J Heart Lung Transplant 25:404-408, 2006.
348. Lindeman RD, Tobin J, Shock NW: Longitudinal studies on the rate of decline in renal function with age. J Am Geriatr Soc 33:278-285, 1985.

Christoph N. Seubert and Michael E. Mahla

46 Neurologic Monitoring

Key Points

1. There are four key principles of intraoperative neurologic monitoring.
2. The pathway at risk during the surgical procedure must be amenable to monitoring.
3. If evidence of injury to the pathway is detected, there must be some intervention possible.
4. If changes in the neurologic monitor are detected, and no intervention is possible, although the monitor may be of prognostic value, it does not have the potential to provide direct benefit to the patient from early detection of impending neurologic injury.
5. The monitor must provide reliable and reproducible data.
6. There are few randomized prospective studies evaluating the efficacy of neurologic monitoring modalities.
7. Based on clinical experience and nonrandomized studies, practice patterns for use of neurologic monitoring have emerged.
8. There are procedures for which monitoring is recommended and used by most centers
9. There are procedures for which monitoring is used frequently in some centers, but not in others.
10. There are procedures for which there is no clear clinical experience or evidence indicating that monitoring is useful at all (experimental use).
11. There are procedures in which monitoring is used selectively for patients believed to be at higher-than-usual risk for intraoperative neurologic injury.

Neurologic monitoring in the context of anesthesia care for a patient spans a wide spectrum of techniques, diverse procedures, and various intraoperative or even postoperative settings. Techniques for monitoring fall into two broad categories: techniques to assess metabolic integrity of the nervous system, which typically entail either global or regional determinations of blood flow or oxygenation, or techniques to assess functional integrity, which likewise may be global or focused on specific anatomic components of the nervous system.

The procedures and settings in which neurologic monitoring is typically applied all share the characteristic that changes in the monitored parameters can be corrected or minimized by either modifying the surgical approach or manipulating parameters under the control of the anesthesiologist. Monitored procedures range from procedures where monitoring dictates the surgical approach, such as localization of the motor strip during tumor surgery or the neurologic examination during an "awake" craniotomy, to procedures that by their nature put parts of the nervous system at increased risk.

In many procedures that require neurologic monitoring, the surgical target overlaps with the site of action of drugs a patient receives. The anesthesiologist and the surgeon need to be aware not only of limitations inherent in individual monitoring techniques, but also of nonsurgical factors that influence the monitoring results. The monitoring approach ideally should anticipate nonsurgical factors by providing a degree of redundancy that helps distinguish a localized surgical trespass from a systemic event.

For some procedures, neurologic monitoring is a marker of the quality of care and is routinely employed because outcome data support its use. Examples include correction of scoliosis and resection of vestibular schwannomas. More frequently, the approach to monitoring is based on local conventions and surgical expectations. In this latter case, monitoring utility depends even more on a good understanding of the technique's capabilities and limitations by anesthesiologists and surgeons and on their mutual collaboration to allow corrective action in the face of changing signals or to prevent false alarms that disrupt surgery.

This chapter first discusses individual monitoring modalities in isolation so that the clinician can appreciate the inherent strengths and weaknesses of each. Subsequent sections apply this information by describing suitable approaches to various clinical settings that combine and integrate individual techniques to optimize neurologic outcome for patients. The chapter ends with a brief discussion of how neurologic monitoring is believed to be useful today, and where more work is needed to determine whether monitoring has a role in surgical patients in the future.

Monitoring Modalities

Monitors of Adequacy of Nervous System Blood Flow

Adequacy of cerebral blood flow (CBF) can be monitored by two principal methods. The first method assesses blood flow itself with the implicit assumption that "normal" flow provides adequately for the metabolic needs of the brain. The second approach assesses oxygen delivery either locally or globally with the implicit assumption that "normal" values at the site of measurement are reflective of adequate blood supply throughout the central nervous system (CNS). To illustrate the limitations imposed by such implicit assumptions, let us examine global or hemispheric CBF in the context of a patient's disease process.

In normal brain, values of hemispheric CBF of approximately 50 mL/100 g/min reflect adequate oxygen delivery for maintaining structural integrity and function. Values of less than 20 to 25 mL/100 g/min are associated first with failure of function and on further decrease with structural damage.[1] In neurosurgical patients, structural integrity and function may be altered by disease processes and anesthetics, which have an impact on the interpretation of measured CBF. A CBF of 40 mL/100 g/min in a patient in barbiturate coma after resection of an arteriovenous malformation may represent hyperemia (because metabolic demand is very low), whereas the same CBF in a patient with a mass lesion may reflect a modest decrease in cerebral perfusion pressure secondary to increasing intracranial pressure.

Global Blood Flow Monitoring Techniques (Noninvasive)

Intravascular Tracer Compounds. Direct measurement of CBF is possible by determining kinetics of washin or washout, or both, of an inert tracer compound, a method originally described by Kety and Schmidt.[2] The most widely used measurement technique involves administration of a radioactive isotope of xenon (^{133}Xe), followed by measurement of the radioactivity washout with gamma detectors placed over specific areas of the brain. Depending on the number of detectors, this method can provide a spatial resolution of 4 cm. In normal brain, flow at different depths may be inferred from the early washout, which should reflect high-perfusion cortical gray matter, and late washout from low-perfusion deeper white matter.

Drawbacks of the method are the patient's exposure to radioactive compounds and the need for externally placed and potentially cumbersome detector equipment, which may interfere with surgery itself in the case of intracranial surgery. Focal areas of hypoperfusion may be missed because of underlying or overlying adequate flow, a phenomenon described as "look-through."[3] Despite these shortcomings, ^{133}Xe washout has been used at a few major centers for intraoperative monitoring during operations such as carotid endarterectomy.[4-8] Modern variations of the same concept are mean transit time determinations of intravascular contrast agents during neuroimaging for determining locoregional blood flow[7,8] or a double-indicator technique for determining global CBF.[9] All these techniques share the limitation of providing a snapshot of CBF in time instead of continuous monitoring.

Transcranial Doppler Ultrasound. Transcranial Doppler (TCD) ultrasound is a technique that infers CBF from measurements of the blood flow velocity in the large conducting arteries of the brain. The TCD probe transmits pulses of sound waves through the thin temporal bone in a variation of the pulsed wave Doppler technique with which anesthesiologists may be familiar from echocardiography. When these sound waves are reflected off the red blood cells back toward the TCD probe, the velocity of the reflected sound waves is changed because the blood cells themselves are in motion toward or away from the probe. This phenomenon is known as the "Doppler shift," and is directly related to flow velocity and flow direction of the blood cells. Blood flow is faster during systole and in the center of a vessel and slower in diastole and near the vessel wall. TCD records a spectrum of flow velocities, whose outline resembles an arterial waveform tracing. These concepts are illustrated in Figure 46-1.

Intraoperatively, TCD measurements are most commonly and easily made by continuous monitoring of the middle cerebral artery for the purpose of detecting either significant changes in flow velocity or the presence of particulate emboli. As a diagnostic study, in addition to the middle cerebral artery, the anterior cerebral, anterior communicating, posterior cerebral, and posterior communicating arteries can be examined through the temporal bone window. The basilar, ophthalmic, and internal carotid arteries also can be insonated through the foramen magnum (TCD probe at the back of the flexed neck) (basilar artery), the closed eyelid (with reduced sound energy) (ophthalmic artery), and near the angle of the jaw (internal carotid artery). An important limitation of TCD results from the fact that most of the examination is done through the temporal bone, which may be thick enough to preclude an adequate examination in 10% to 20% of patients.[10,11]

Two assumptions that are intuitive and plausible, but ultimately unproven, must be made for TCD-measured blood flow velocity to have a direct relationship to CBF. First, blood flow velocity is directly related to blood flow only if the diameter of the artery where the flow velocity is measured and the measurement angle of the Doppler probe remain constant. In practical terms, the difficulty with this assumption lies in finding a means to affix the TCD probe in a way that prevents dislodgment or movement during monitoring. The second assumption requires that CBF in the basal arteries of the brain is directly related to cortical CBF. Because TCD monitoring is typically done mainly using the middle cerebral artery, this assumption may be invalid if collateral blood flow by leptomeningeal collaterals from anterior and posterior cerebral artery territories is adequate. Although these two assumptions constrain the utility of TCD as a stand-alone monitor of CBF, the changes in flow velocity seen in typical applications (discussed subsequently) are large enough to provide useful clinical information.

More importantly, TCD is the only continuous neurologic monitoring technique that provides early warning for hyperperfusion and for the number of emboli delivered to the brain during various phases of an operation. Because of their high echogenicity, emboli show up in the TCD spectrum as high-intensity transient signals (HITSs) (see Fig. 46-1) and are easily identified as brief beeps or chirps within the background of the Doppler sounds.

Jugular Bulb Venous Oxygen Saturation. The degree of oxygen extraction by an organ can be monitored by following the

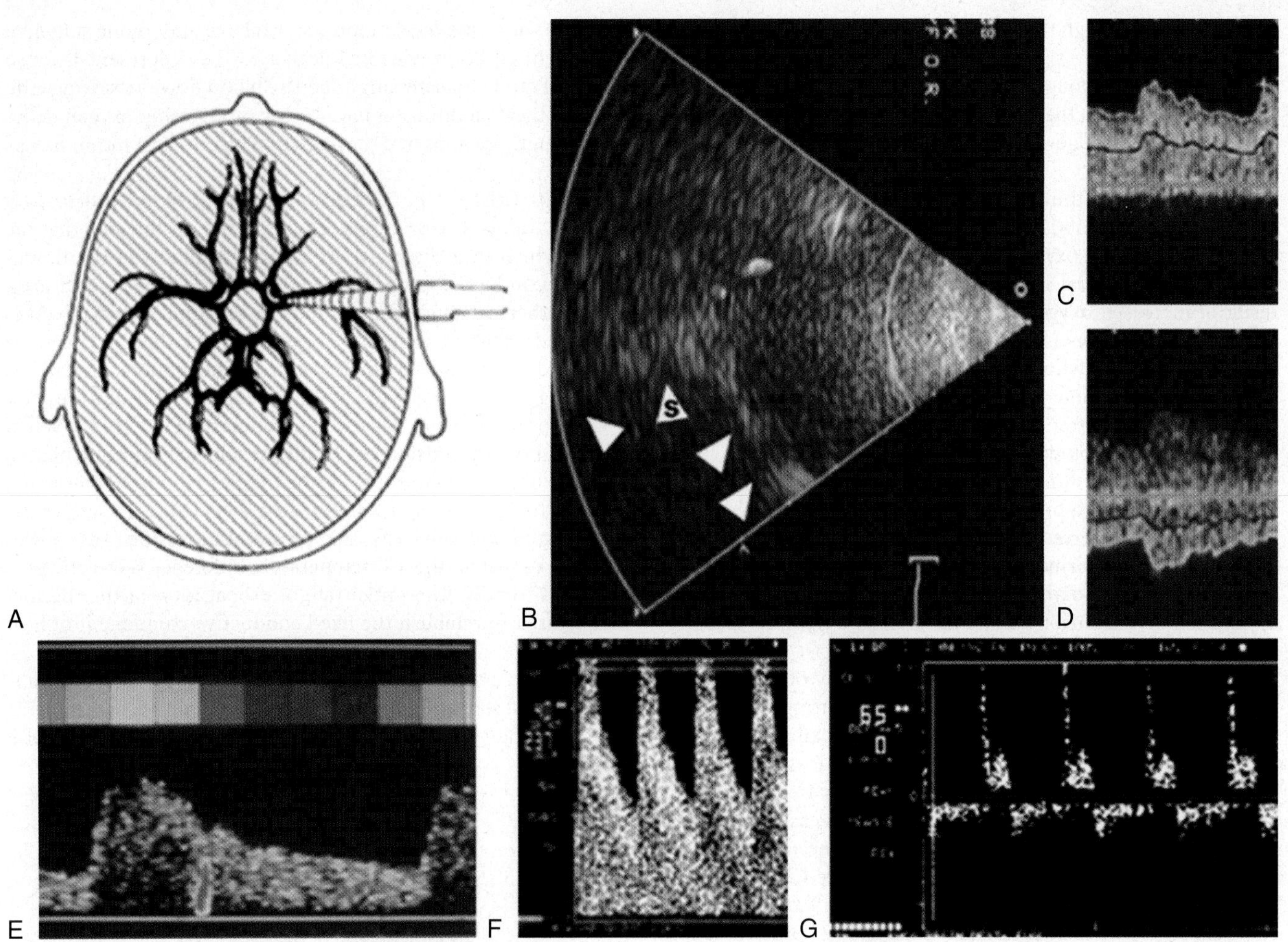

Figure 46-1 **A,** Transcranial Doppler monitoring is done by insonating the arteries at the base of the brain through a thin part of the temporal bone. **B,** If this is done with an imaging probe, some intracranial structures, such as the cerebral peduncles (*white triangles*) or the sella complex (*white triangle labeled* "S"), can be visualized. The Doppler signals originate from the right middle, right anterior, and left anterior cerebral arteries. **C,** Normal Doppler spectrum obtained from the middle cerebral artery. **D,** Doppler profile of the bifurcation of the terminal internal carotid artery as it branches into the middle cerebral artery (flowing toward the transducer) and the anterior cerebral artery (flowing away). This flow signal can be obtained if the transducer is focused as shown in **A. E-G,** Examples of three clinical applications of transcranial Doppler. **E,** Emboli are highly echogenic and show up as high-energy transient signals (HITS). On the audible output, these emboli are easily noticed as brief beeps or chirps. **F,** Doppler profile of a middle cerebral artery in a patient with severe vasospasm after an aneurysmal subarachnoid hemorrhage (compare with **C**). **G,** Transcranial Doppler examination consistent with intracranial circulatory arrest. There is a brief systolic inflow followed by retrograde flow during diastole.

oxygen saturation of the mixed venous blood that drains that organ. In the case of the brain, jugular bulb venous oxygen saturation ($Sjvo_2$) is believed to measure the degree of oxygen extraction and to represent the balance between cerebral oxygen supply and demand. To monitor $Sjvo_2$, a fiberoptic catheter is placed in a retrograde fashion into the jugular bulb through the internal jugular vein under fluoroscopic guidance. The fiberoptic bundle emits near-infrared light and records light reflected back to the catheter, a technique known as "reflectance oximetry." Because near-infrared light can travel several centimeters in tissue and is mostly absorbed by hemoglobin, it is possible to determine the oxygen saturation of the surrounding tissue (i.e., the jugular venous blood). Correct tip placement is crucial to minimize admixture of extracranial venous blood. To decrease the risk of complications, usually only one side is monitored.

Several theoretical limitations of the technique must be borne in mind to interpret $Sjvo_2$ values and trends properly. Although nearly all blood from the brain drains via the jugular veins, intracranial mixing of venous blood is incomplete and may result in differences between right-sided and left-sided measurements. The dominant jugular vein (i.e., the right for most patients) drains predominantly cortical venous blood, whereas the contralateral jugular vein drains more of the subcortical regions.[12] Despite such regional differences, $Sjvo_2$ must be considered a monitor of global cerebral oxygenation because inadequate perfusion to a focal brain region may not decrease $Sjvo_2$ values below the normal range of 55% to 75%. Because $Sjvo_2$ represents the balance between supply and demand, interpretation of the absolute value of $Sjvo_2$ must take the clinical circumstances into account.

Cerebral Oximetry. Cerebral oximetry is a noninvasive technique that, similar to $Sjvo_2$ monitoring, uses reflectance oximetry to measure the oxygen saturation of the tissues underneath the sensor. Typically, two sensors are applied to both sides of the forehead. The light passes not only through parts of the frontal brain, but also through the overlying skull and scalp. Contamination of the oximetry signal by extracranial blood sources is a serious concern, although the use of two sensing diodes with different distances from the light source within one sensor patch and adjustments of the algorithm of the oximeter may minimize this problem.[13,14]

Because two thirds to four fifths of the cerebral blood volume is venous blood, cerebral oximetry determines predominantly "local venous oxygen saturation."[15] It can be expected that in the face of cerebral ischemia, oximetry values decrease as a result of increased oxygen extraction, well before function fails, or permanent neuronal damage ensues. The simplicity of its use and the familiarity with the principles of treating decreases in systemic mixed venous oxygen saturation have made cerebral oximetry a popular trend monitor in operations that potentially cause decreases in blood flow to the vessels of the head. There are some significant limitations, however, of the use of cerebral oximetry during such procedures. First, adequacy of global cerebral perfusion is inferred from measurements over the frontopolar brain. Second, normative data on normal values or expected changes for cerebral oximetry are largely absent, but preoperative application of the sensors allows the start of a trend in conjunction with a neurologic baseline examination.

An example of how these limitations play out is provided by a study of the use of cerebral oximetry during 100 carotid endarterectomies in awake patients.[16] Cerebral oximetry was able to identify 97.4% of patients with adequate CBF as indicated by the absence of clinical symptoms. The monitor frequently indicated inadequate CBF, defined as a 20% decrease in cerebral oxygen saturation from the preclamp baseline, although the patient had no clinical symptoms of inadequate CBF. The false-positive rate of 66.7% may simply illustrate the fact that oxygen extraction increases before function fails. The real problem is that the lower limit for acceptable regional oxygen saturation is unknown in a large population of patients.[17] The value may be different from patient to patient, and addition of anesthetic drugs that influence cerebral metabolism may confuse the picture further.

Tissue-Level Blood Flow Monitoring Techniques (Invasive)

Tissue-level monitoring for the brain is by definition invasive. All monitors in current clinical or research use are implanted through a burr hole, extend either into the white matter or ventricular system, and typically use a bolt for stabilization. They all share a 1% to 2% risk of bleeding, infection, or ischemia owing to the implantation procedure.[18] A second shared feature is their limited spatial resolution (i.e., each monitoring probe monitors only a limited area of brain surrounding the probe). When these monitors were first developed, there was considerable debate regarding the optimal placement of the device given such limited spatial resolution. Based on today's appreciation for the impact of secondary neurologic insults on the ultimate outcome, there is growing agreement that tissue-level monitoring is best performed in morphologically and functionally normal tissue that is part of the penumbra or vulnerable zone of interest.[19-21] Placing a blood flow monitor into the brain tissue supplied by an aneurysm-carrying artery in the setting of a subarachnoid hemorrhage maximizes, but does not ensure, the chances of early detection of vasospasm.

Of the tissue-level monitors, two have undergone sufficient refinement to be in wider clinical use. They represent the two principal modes of assessing adequate blood flow—assessing CBF through thermal diffusion monitoring or assessing oxygen delivery through tissue partial pressure of oxygen (Po_2) monitoring.

Thermal Diffusion Cerebral Blood Flow Monitoring.

Thermal diffusion CBF monitoring is based on the idea that the rate at which heat dissipates in a tissue depends on the tissue's thermal conductive properties and the blood flow in that area. Because thermal conduction properties remain constant, changes in heat dissipation reflect changes in blood flow and can be expressed quantitatively in the conventional units of CBF as mL/100 g/min. In practice, the probe consists of a thin catheter with two thermistors placed 5 mm apart (Fig. 46-2). When inserted, both thermistors are located in subcortical white matter. The proximal or passive thermistor measures brain temperature, whereas the distal or active thermistor is heated to 2°C above the temperature measured by the passive thermistor. The power required to sustain the 2°C temperature difference is directly proportional to CBF. The initial rate of propagation of the thermal field is used to establish the fixed conductive component of heat transfer.

The acute performance of this technology has been validated against stable xenon computed tomography (CT) in patients with head injury and performed well across a wide range of CBF

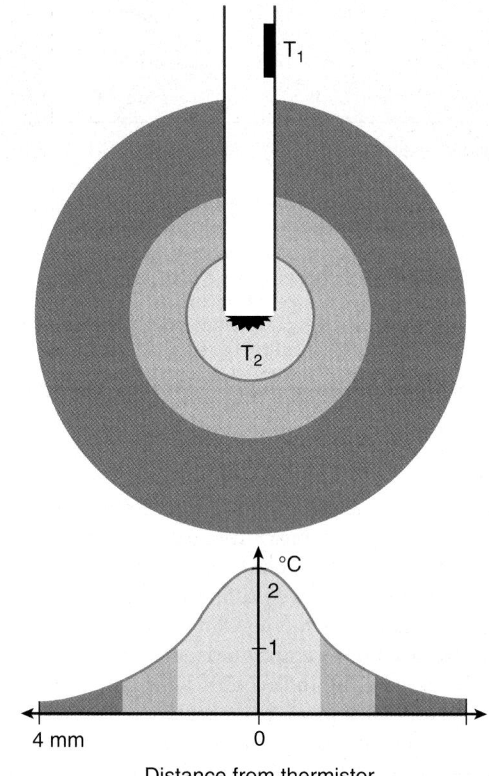

Figure 46-2 Thermal diffusion measurement of cerebral blood flow. The probe is placed in the subcortical white matter. It contains a passive thermistor (T_1) that measures brain temperature and is located outside of the area influenced by the active thermistor. The active thermistor (T_2) is heated to 2°C above brain temperature. The energy required to maintain that increase in temperature is proportional to cerebral blood flow.

values in a sheep model of hypercarbia, hyperventilation, and cardiac arrest.[22] In continuous clinical use, the probe shows some drift and recalibrates at regular intervals.[23] To avoid thermal tissue injury, measurement is automatically suspended if the passive thermistor measures a brain temperature of 39.1°C. Because fever is a frequent complication, particularly in patients with severe brain disease, the inability to monitor during a febrile episode may constitute a true limitation of the technique.

Tissue Partial Pressure of Oxygen Monitoring. Localized monitoring of tissue Po_2 is based on an oxygen-sensitive electrode originally described by Clark.[24] The diffusion of oxygen molecules through an oxygen-permeable membrane into an electrolyte solution causes an electric current that is proportional to Po_2. Currently available catheter-based electrodes provide stable recording conditions over long periods. Similar to regional CBF probes, they are placed into the subcortical white matter.

Most of the data on brain tissue oxygen levels ($P_{Br}O_2$) comes from studies in patients with head trauma. Comparison with stable xenon CT for assessment of CBF shows good correlation between $P_{Br}O_2$ and CBF.[25,26] Similarly, the time course of changes in $P_{Br}O_2$ after traumatic brain injury resembles that of CBF.[27,28] Critics of the technique argue that $P_{Br}O_2$ values are highly influenced by the partial pressure of arterial oxygen (Pao_2) and are merely an elaborate indicator of the quality of patient ventilation. This view is supported by the observation that increasing the fraction of inspired oxygen (Fio_2) increases $P_{Br}O_2$, but likely represents an oversimplification.[29] Concurrent microdialysis studies have shown that increasing Fio_2 not only increases $P_{Br}O_2$, but also decreases tissue lactate levels, suggesting a true improvement in the metabolic milieu of the brain tissue itself.[30,31]

Monitors of Nervous System Function

The most commonly used monitors of function are the electroencephalogram (EEG), sensory evoked responses (SERs), motor evoked responses, and the electromyogram (EMG). The EEG is a surface recording of the summation of excitatory and inhibitory postsynaptic potentials spontaneously generated by the pyramidal cells in the cerebral cortex. The signals are very small, and each recording electrode records only information generated directly beneath the electrode. Monitoring the EEG is usually directed toward one or more of four perioperative uses. First, the EEG is used to help identify inadequate blood flow to the cerebral cortex caused by either a surgically induced or anesthetic-induced reduction in blood flow or retraction on cerebral tissue. Second, the EEG may be used to guide an anesthetic-induced reduction of cerebral metabolism either in anticipation of a loss of CBF or in the treatment of high intracranial pressure, when a reduction in CBF and blood volume is desired. Third, the EEG may be used to predict neurologic outcome after a brain insult. Finally, the EEG may be used to gauge the depth of the hypnotic state of the patient under general anesthesia (see Chapter 39).

More than 50 years of experience monitoring the EEG has led to many known correlations of EEG patterns with clinical states of the normal and pathologic cerebral cortex. The electroencephalographer can accurately identify consciousness, unconsciousness, seizure activity, stages of sleep, and coma. In the absence of significant changes in anesthetic technique, the electroencephalographer also can accurately identify inadequate oxygen delivery to the brain (from either hypoxemia or ischemia). By using high-speed computerized EEG analysis and statistical methods, EEG patterns in the continuum from awake to deeply anesthetized are becoming, with few exceptions, much better understood. In addition, computer advances have made possible high-speed mathematic manipulation of the EEG signal to present the data in a manner more suitable to continuous trends for use during surgical or anesthetic monitoring.

Evoked potentials are electric activity generated in response to either a sensory or a motor stimulus. Measurements of evoked responses may be made at multiple points along an involved nervous system pathway. The evoked responses are generally smaller than other electric activity generated in nearby tissue (muscle or brain) and are readily obscured by these other biologic signals. In the case of SERs, repeated sampling and sophisticated electronic summation and averaging techniques are needed to extract the desired evoked potential signal from background biologic signals. Motor evoked responses are generally larger and commonly do not require averaging.

SERs are the most common type of evoked potentials monitored intraoperatively. During the last 2 decades, much research has been done on the use of intraoperative motor evoked potentials (MEPs). Although routine use of MEP monitoring is still not widespread, it is becoming more so. There are three basic types of sensory evoked responses: somatosensory evoked potentials (SSEPs), brainstem auditory evoked potentials (BAEPs), and visual evoked potentials (VEPs).

The SSEP is produced by electrically stimulating a peripheral (or rarely cranial) nerve. Responses may be recorded proximally over the stimulated nerve, the spinal cord, and the cerebral cortex. The recorded responses assess the function of the peripheral nerve, the posterior and lateral aspects of the spinal cord, a small portion of the brainstem, the ventral posterolateral nucleus of the thalamus, the thalamocortical radiation, and a portion of the sensory cortex. The BAEP is usually produced by a series of rapid, loud clicks applied directly to the external auditory canal. Responses are most commonly recorded from electrodes applied to the scalp, although more invasive direct recordings from auditory structures and nerves may also be made. BAEPs assess function of the auditory apparatus itself; cranial nerve VIII; the cochlear nucleus; and a small area of the rostral brainstem, the inferior colliculus, and the auditory cortex. The VEP is produced by flash stimulation of the retina. Recordings are made from cortically placed electrodes and assess visual pathways from the optic nerve to the occipital cortex.

MEP responses are generated most commonly by the application of a transcranial train of electric stimuli, and responses are recorded at various points along the spinal column, peripheral nerve, and innervated muscle. Electric stimuli to activate motor tracts also may be applied at the level of the spinal cord, but this method of stimulation is controversial (see later), with research suggesting that the response, as it is currently recorded, is at best a mixed response and at worst primarily a sensory response. Magnetic stimuli also may be applied transcranially or at the level of the spinal cord, but use of magnetic stimulation is much less common than electric stimulation, primarily for technical reasons involving fixation of the magnet to the patient to avoid shifts in magnetic field application, which would significantly alter responses. MEPs assess the integrity of the descending motor pathway through the internal capsule, the brainstem, the spinal cord, the peripheral nerve, and finally the muscle itself. The ability to record MEPs from some patients with cerebral palsy indicates that normal functional organization of the motor cortex cannot be inferred from MEPs.

Electroencephalogram

Basic Unprocessed Electroencephalogram Concepts. The EEG is produced by a summation of excitatory and inhibitory postsynaptic potentials produced in cortical gray matter. Because the EEG signal is generated only by postsynaptic potentials and is much smaller than action potentials recorded over nerves or from the heart, extreme care must be taken when placing electrodes to ensure proper placement and excellent contact with the skin to avoid significant signal loss. Alternatively, subdermal needle electrodes may be used, particularly when sterile application of an electrode close to a surgical field is necessary. When electrodes are applied directly to the surface of the brain, impedance is minimized by close electrode contact and saturation of the area with an electrolyte solution.

EEG electrodes generally are placed according to a mapping system that relates surface head anatomy to underlying brain cortical regions. The placement pattern of recording electrodes is called a montage. Use of a standard recording montage permits anatomic localization of signals produced by the brain and allows development of normative EEG patterns and comparison of EEG recordings made at different times. The standard EEG "map" is called the 10-20 system for EEG electrode placement (Fig. 46-3). This system is a symmetric array of scalp electrodes placed systematically based on the distance from the nasion to the inion and from the pretragal bony indentations associated with both temporomandibular joints. Based on 10% or 20% of these distances, recording electrodes are placed systematically over the frontal (F), parietal (P), temporal (T), and occipital (O) regions at increasing distances from the midline. Left-sided electrodes are given odd number subscripts, and right-sided electrodes are given even number subscripts. Increasing numbers indicate an increasing distance from the midline. Midline electrodes are designated with a "z" subscript. The standard diagnostic EEG uses at least 16 channels of information,[32] but intraoperative recordings have been reported using 1 to 32 discreet channels.

The intraoperative EEG is most commonly recorded from electrodes placed on the scalp. Recordings also may be made from electrodes placed on the surface of the brain (electrocorticography), or from microelectrodes placed transcortically to record from individual neurons (e.g., during surgery for Parkinson's disease).[33,34] The EEG signal is described using three basic parameters: amplitude, frequency, and time. Amplitude is the size, or voltage, of the recorded signal and ranges commonly from 5 to 500 μV (versus 1 to 2 mV for the electrocardiogram signal). Because neurons are irreversibly lost during the normal aging process, EEG amplitude decreases with age. Frequency can be thought of simply as the number of times per second the signal oscillates or crosses the zero voltage line. Time is the duration of the sampling of the signal; this is continuous and real time in the standard paper or digital EEG, but is a sampling epoch in the processed EEG (see later).

Normal Electroencephalogram. Normal patterns seen on the EEG vary among normal individuals, but are consistent enough to allow for accurate recognition of normal and pathologic patterns. The usual base frequency in an awake patient is the beta range (>13 Hz). This high-frequency and usually low-amplitude signal is common from an alert attentive brain and may be recorded from all regions. With eye closure, higher amplitude signals in the alpha frequency range (8 to 13 Hz) seen best in the occipital region appear (Fig. 46-4). This "eyes closed" resting pattern is the baseline awake pattern used when anesthetic effects on the EEG are described. When events that lead the brain to produce higher frequencies and larger amplitudes occur, the EEG is described as "activated," and when slower frequencies are produced (theta = 4 to 7 Hz, and delta = <4 Hz), the EEG is said to be "depressed." The EEG in a sleeping patient may contain all of these frequencies at various times. The slower frequencies occur during deep natural sleep with "sleep spindles" (Fig. 46-5), but during light sleep or rapid eye movement (REM) sleep, the EEG becomes activated, and the eye muscle EMG appears on the EEG.

In the normal EEG in awake and asleep patients, patterns recorded from corresponding electrodes on each hemisphere are symmetric in terms of frequency and amplitude, the patterns are predictable if clinical states are known, and spike (epileptic) waveforms are absent. In most cases, normal EEG patterns are associated with normal underlying brain function in awake and anesthetized patients.

Abnormal Electroencephalogram. General characteristics of the "abnormal" EEG include asymmetry with respect to frequency, amplitude, or both, recorded from corresponding electrodes on each hemisphere, and patterns of amplitude and

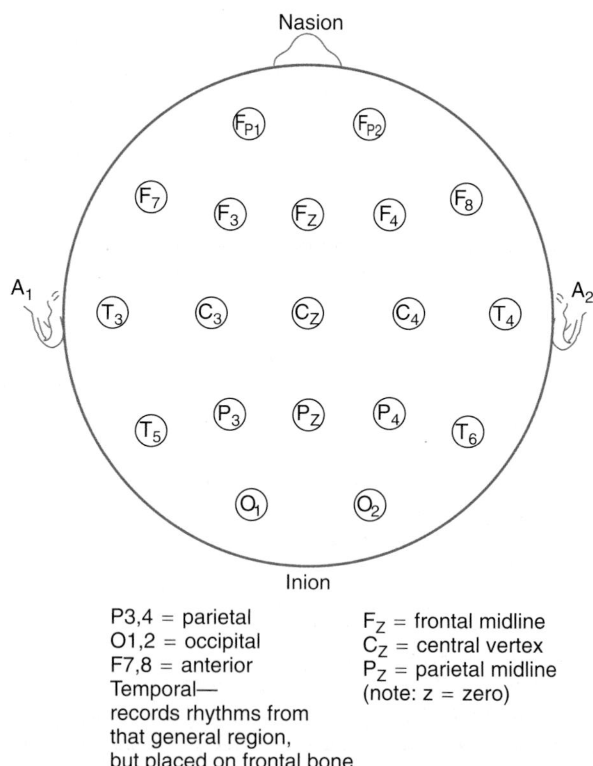

Figure 46-3 International 10-20 system of electrode placement for recording electroencephalogram and sensory evoked responses. *(From Hughes JR: EEG in Clinical Practice, 2nd ed. Newton, MA, Butterworth-Heinemann, 1994.)*

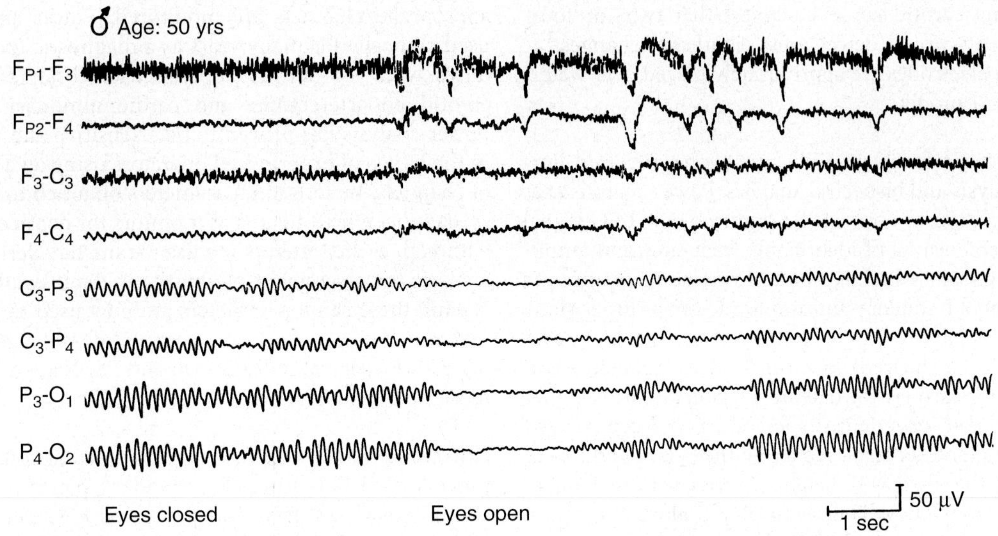

Figure 46-4 The loss and return of α activity as the eyes open and close can be seen. The large spikes are muscle artifact.

frequency that are unpredictable or unexpected in the normal recording. These abnormal patterns reflect either anatomic or metabolic alterations in the underlying brain. Regional asymmetry can be seen with tumors, epilepsy, and cerebral ischemia or infarction. Epilepsy may be recognized by high-voltage spike and slow waves, whereas cerebral ischemia manifests first with EEG slowing with preservation of voltage. Further slowing and loss of voltage occurs as ischemia becomes more severe. Factors affecting the entire brain may produce symmetric abnormalities of the signal. Identifying pathologic abnormal patterns in the global EEG signal is very important, although sometimes quite difficult, in the clinical situation. Many of the normal global pattern changes produced by anesthetic drugs are similar to pathologic patterns produced by ischemia or hypoxemia. Control of anesthetic technique is very important when the EEG is being used for clinical monitoring of the nervous system.

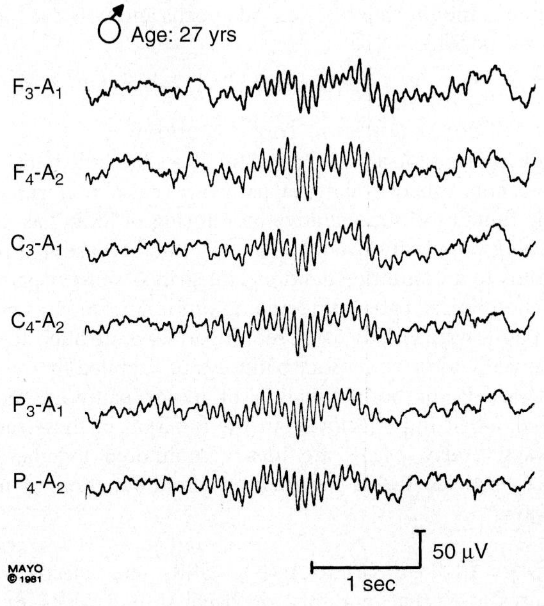

♂ Age: 27 yrs

F3-A1

F4-A2

C3-A1

C4-A2

P3-A1

P4-A2

50 μV

1 sec

MAYO ©1981

Figure 46-5 Characteristic sleep spindles in normal sleep are shown in the center.

Processed Electroencephalogram Concepts. Interpretation of the standard paper EEG tracing is a science and an art. Until the last quarter of the 20th century, the paper EEG was used during intraoperative monitoring with the technologist relying on memory of the baseline and on experience to determine when significant EEG changes occurred. This qualitative approach was used simply because the waveforms could not be described mathematically in a time frame that would make such information of any practical use. Computer hardware has dramatically improved in speed and size, and real-time signal processing is now possible and commonly used.

Numerous limitations are introduced when moving from the raw EEG domain to the processed EEG domain. First, artifact is processed in many cases along with desired signal leading to a perfectly believable processed EEG display that is materially incorrect. Second, the standard 16-channel EEG montage provides more information than can be practically analyzed or displayed by most processed EEG monitors and perhaps more than is needed for routine intraoperative use. Most available processed EEG devices used by anesthesiology personnel use four or fewer channels of information—translating to at most two channels per hemisphere. Processed EEG devices generally monitor less cerebral territory than a standard 16-channel EEG. Third, some intraoperative changes are unilateral (e.g., regional ischemia owing to carotid clamping), and some are bilateral (e.g., EEG depression by bolus administration of an anesthetic). Display of the activity of both hemispheres is necessary to delineate unilateral from bilateral changes. An appropriate number of leads over both hemispheres is needed. Most early studies validating intraoperative EEG monitoring used continuous visual inspection of a 16- to 32-channel analog EEG by an experienced electroencephalographer—such monitoring was considered the gold standard.[35,36] Adequate studies comparing the processed EEG with fewer channels with this gold standard across multiple uses and operations have not been done, although limited data using processed EEG monitoring during carotid surgery suggest that two- or four-channel instruments would detect most significant changes,[37,38] provided that the electrodes are appropriately placed over watershed areas of blood supply.

Devices. Two basic forms of EEG processing are used currently: power analysis and bispectral analysis. Power analysis uses Fourier transformation to convert the digitized raw EEG signal into component sine waves of identifiable frequency and amplitude. The raw EEG data, which is a plot of voltage versus time, is converted to a plot of frequency and amplitude versus time. Many commercially available processed EEG machines display power (voltage or amplitude squared) as a function of frequency and time. These monitors display the data in two general forms, either compressed spectral array or density spectral array. In compressed spectral array, frequency is displayed along the x axis, and power is displayed along the y axis with height of the waveform equal to the power at that frequency. Time is displayed along the z axis. Tracings overlap each other, with the most recent information in front (Fig. 46-6). Density spectral array also displays frequency along the x axis; time is displayed along the y axis, and power is reflected by the density of the dots at each frequency. Each display format provides the same data, and choice depends on the preference of the user.

Many changes that occur during anesthesia and surgery are reflected as changes in amplitude, frequency, or both. These changes can be clearly seen in these displays if adequate and appropriate channels are monitored. Power analysis has been used clinically for many years as a diagnostic tool during procedures with risk for intraoperative cerebral ischemia, such as carotid endarterectomy and cardiopulmonary bypass (CPB). Power analysis has proven to be a sensitive and reliable monitor in the hands of experienced operators using an adequate number of channels. In addition, parameters obtained from power analysis have been investigated as monitors for depth of anesthesia.[39-42] Although earlier attempts to use parameters derived from power analysis for assessment of anesthetic depth were largely unsuccessful, these same parameters are now used to varying degrees with much more success as a part of different algorithms (including BIS [Bispectral Index Score] and PSI [Patient State Index]) to measure hypnotic states.

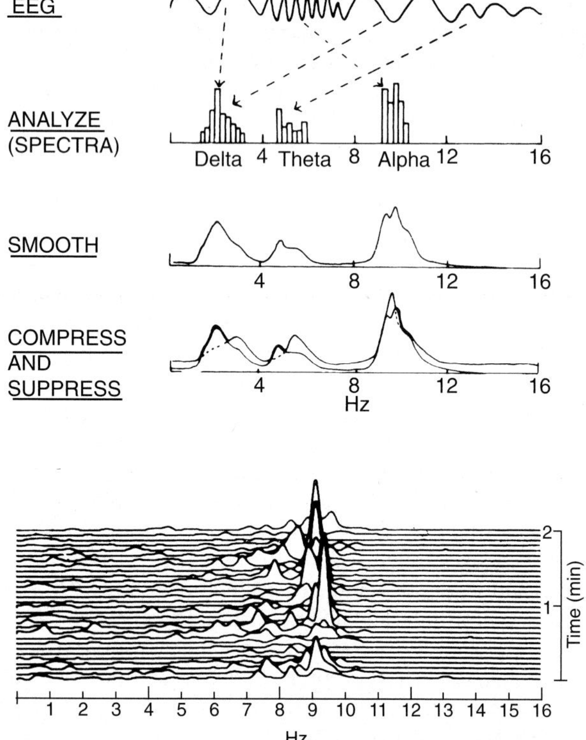

Figure 46-6 Diagram of technique used to generate compressed spectral array. Example at the bottom of the figure shows compressed spectra of the α rhythm from a normal subject. *(From Stockard JJ, Bickford RG: The neurophysiology of anaesthesia. In Gordon E [ed]: A Basis and Practice of Neuroanesthesia. New York, Elsevier, 1981, p 3.)*

Data Acquisition Period. An important consideration in the processed EEG is time. The standard paper or digital EEG is continuous in real time. The processed EEG samples data over a given time period (epoch), processes the data, and then displays information in various formats. There is a relationship between epoch length and spectral resolution. If a long epoch length is chosen, the waveform can be described precisely, but the time required for data processing is long and not real time. If a short length of data is sampled, analysis may be done in near real time, but the epoch chosen for analysis may not be representative of the overall waveform (i.e., the condition of the patient). There also may be insufficient data points for meaningful Fourier transformation. This issue, as related to the use of intraoperative EEG for analysis of anesthetic depth, has been studied by Levy.[43] A longer epoch may produce less epoch-to-epoch variability and allow more precise description of frequency and power; however, the longer epoch increases the delay before new information is processed and displayed, reducing the amount and timeliness of information available for clinical decision making. In studying EEG epochs of 2 to 32 seconds, Levy[43] concluded that 2-second epochs are appropriate during general anesthesia. Many commercially available devices have used 2-second epoch lengths, updated at varying user-selected intervals. With better and faster computers, continuous monitoring of 2-second epochs and now even longer epochs is possible.

Evoked Potentials

Basic Concepts Common to All Modalities. EEG signals provide information about cortical function, but little to no information about subcortical neural pathways crucial to normal neurologic function. Intraoperative monitoring of SERs has gained increasing popularity over the last 25 years because it provides the ability to monitor the functional integrity of sensory pathways in an anesthetized patient undergoing surgical procedures placing these pathways at risk. Because motor pathways are often adjacent anatomically to these sensory pathways or supplied by the same blood vessels, or both, function of motor pathways may be inferred, albeit imperfectly, from the function of these sensory pathways. Today, MEPs are ideally monitored together with SERs to provide direct information about function of motor pathways.

Sensory Evoked Responses. SERs are electric CNS responses to electric, auditory, or visual stimuli. SERs are produced by stimulating a sensory system and recording the resulting electric responses at various sites along the sensory pathway up to and including the cerebral cortex. Because of the very low amplitude of SERs (0.1 to 10 μV), it is often impossible to distinguish SERs from other background biologic signals, such as the EEG or EMG, which may be considered in this case undesirable "noise." To extract the SER from the background noise, the recorded signal is digitized, and signal averaging is applied. With this technique, signal recording is time-locked to the application of the sensory stimulus. During intraoperative median nerve SER monitoring, after nerve stimulation at the wrist, only signal information occurring less than 50 msec after the stimulus is recorded. The SER occurs at a constant time after the stimulus application; other electric activity, such as spontaneous EEG, occurs at random intervals after the sensory stimulus. The averaging technique improves the SER signal-to-noise ratio by eliminating random elements and enhancing the SER. This enhancing effect increases directly with the square root of the number of responses added into the averaged response.

SER recordings are of two general types determined by the distance of the recording electrode from the neural generator of the evoked response. SERs recorded from electrodes close to the neural generators (within approximately 3 to 4 cm in the average adult) are termed "near-field potentials."[44] Near-field potentials are recorded from electrodes placed very close to the actual signal generator site,[45] and the morphology is directly affected by electrode location.[44] Far-field potentials are recorded from electrodes located a greater distance from the neural generator and are conducted to the recording electrode through a volume conductor (brain, cerebrospinal fluid, and membranes). As a result, it is more difficult to locate the source of the recorded signal (the current spreads diffusely throughout the conducting medium), and the electrode position has little effect on the morphology of the recorded evoked potential.[44,45] As the distance between the recording electrode and the neural generator increases, the recorded SER becomes smaller. More responses have to be averaged to record far-field potentials (several thousand) than near-field potentials (50 to 100).[44,45]

SERs also may be described as cortical or subcortical in origin. Cortical SERs are generated by the arrival at the cortex of the volley of action potentials generated by stimulating the sensory system. Because they are recorded as a near-field potential, they are typically easy to identify by elapsed time, waveform morphology, and amplitude. Subcortical responses may arise from many different structures depending on the type of response, including peripheral nerves, spinal cord, brainstem, thalamus, cranial nerves, and others. Cortical SERs are usually recorded from scalp electrodes placed according to the standard 10-20 system for EEG recordings (see Fig. 46-3). Subcortical evoked responses also may be recorded as far-field potentials from scalp electrodes or, as appropriate, from electrodes placed over the spinal column or peripheral nerve.

Evoked potentials of all types (sensory or motor) are described in terms of latency and amplitude (Fig. 46-7). Latency is defined as the time measured from the application of the stimulus to the onset or peak (depending on convention used) of the response. The amplitude is simply the voltage of the recorded response. According to convention, deflections below the baseline are labeled "positive (P)," and deflections above the baseline are labeled "negative (N)." Because amplitude and latency change with recording circumstances, normal values must be established for each neurologic monitoring laboratory, and may differ from values recorded in other laboratories.

SERs used for intraoperative monitoring include SSEPs, BAEPs, and rarely VEPs. For all these techniques, cortical recording electrodes are placed on the scalp, using the same standard 10-20 system as for recording the EEG, whereas recordings for subcortical and peripheral signals are placed in various standardized anatomic locations. The surgical incision and the need for sterility may necessitate nonstandard electrode placements. Such deviations must be considered when interpreting baseline and subsequent SERs. In the case of MEPs, stimulating electrodes also are placed according to the 10-20 system of electrode placement, but over motor cortex instead. Recording electrodes may be

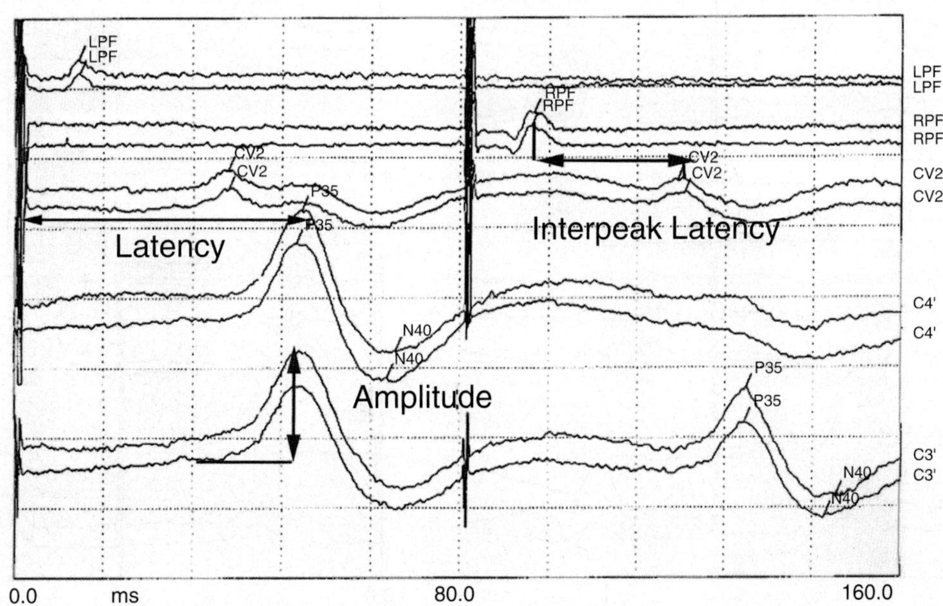

Figure 46-7 Sensory evoked responses are described in terms of latency and amplitude. Interpeak latency is the measured time between two peaks. Interpeak latency may be measured between two peaks in the same channel or between peaks in different channels (shown in figure). Note that the polarity of peaks is displayed contrary to standard convention (see text).

placed over the spinal column, peripheral nerve, and (most commonly) innervated muscle.

Intraoperative changes in evoked responses, such as decreased amplitude, increased latency, or complete loss of the waveform, may result from surgical trespass, such as retractor placement or ischemia, or they may reflect systemic changes, such as changes in anesthetic drug administration, temperature changes, or hypoperfusion. When these changes are detected and considered to be significant, the surgeon or anesthesiologist can make changes to relieve or lessen the insult to the monitored pathway (and presumably surrounding neural structures). Interventions by the anesthesiologist are directed at improving perfusion to the nervous tissue at risk and include increasing arterial blood pressure, especially if induced hypotension is used, or if the patient's pressure has decreased to below the preoperative level; transfusion, if significant anemia is present; volume expansion; augmentation of cardiac output; and normalization of arterial blood gas tensions if indicated. Changes in evoked potentials after retractor placement during a craniotomy or after compression of the blood supply to the spinal cord from spinal column distraction promptly allow the surgeon and the anesthesiologist to make appropriate changes to the operative procedure and anesthetic management that may prevent or minimize any postoperative neurologic deficit (Fig. 46-8).

Tolerance limits for degree of change in evoked response signals or duration of complete loss of waveform before permanent neurologic dysfunction occurs are not clearly defined, and this problem is especially true for transcranial MEPs. Such ambiguity is common among intraoperative monitors. Although we do know that increased frequency and duration of ST segment depression during coronary bypass surgery is associated with an increased risk of perioperative infarction, exact limits for degree and duration of ST segment depression for surgery do not exist, and likely vary significantly from patient to patient. The same problem may be exhibited with neurologic monitors.

Many centers using intraoperative SER monitoring define decreases in amplitude of 50% or more from baseline associated with a less than 10% prolongation in latency as clinically significant SER changes. Uncorrected, such changes are associated in clinical series and in case reports with onset of new postoperative neurologic deficits. As a result, such changes are immediately investigated. In practice, any SER changes directly associated with a surgical event are considered clinically significant, however, even if the magnitude of change is less than just described. Changes in SER that do not progress to complete loss of the waveform are less likely to be associated with a major new postoperative neurologic deficit. Complete loss of the SER waveform intraoperatively without recovery is highly likely to be associated with a major new deficit. If the SER recovers either spontaneously or after intraoperative interventions, the likelihood of neurologic injury depends on the procedure, the duration of the SER loss, and on whether the SER is mainly used to judge integrity of

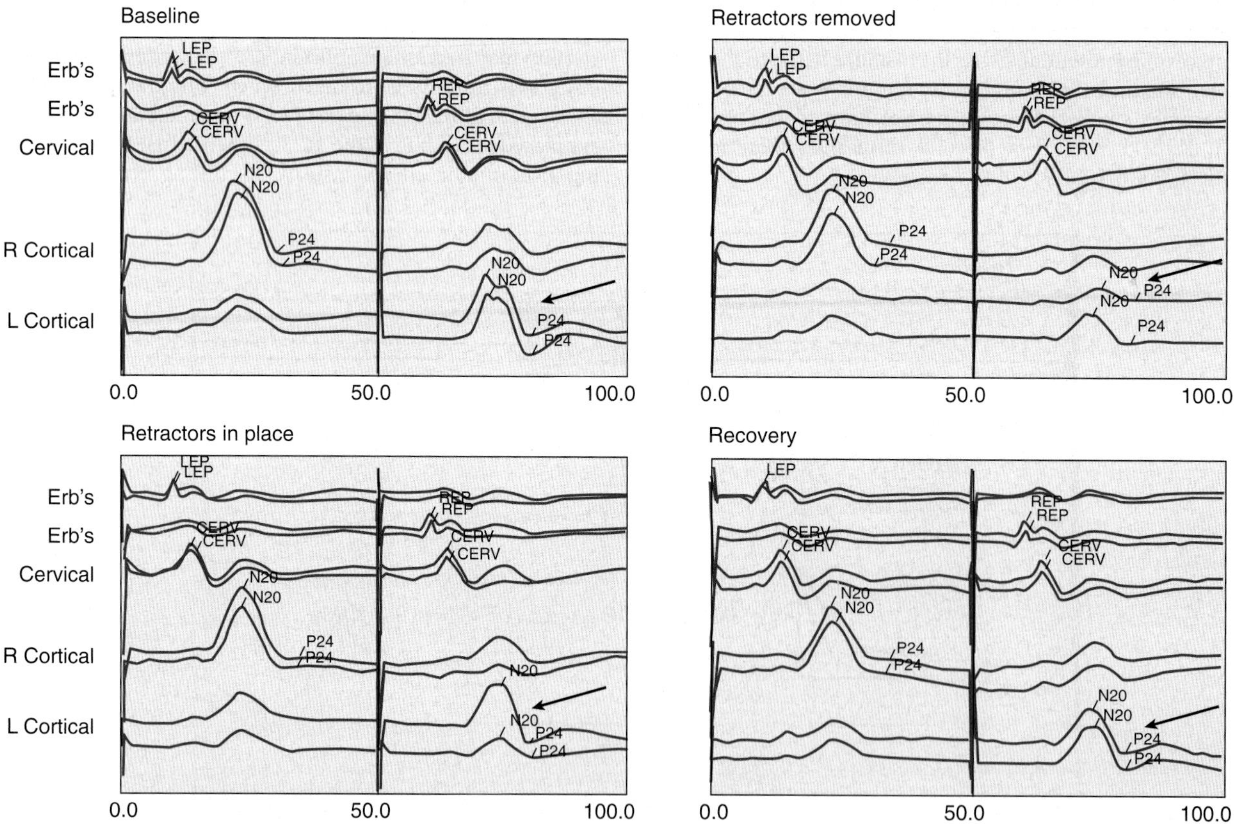

Figure 46-8 Somatosensory evoked potentials during an aneurysm clipping. Responses generated by the cortex at risk are indicated by *arrows*. Baseline, after retractor placement, after retractor removal, and recovery traces are shown. The initial evoked response change occurred 4 minutes after retractor placement. Note loss of voltage of cortical evoked response caused by inadvertent compression of the middle cerebral artery.

adjacent unmonitored structures. In one study of aortic vascular surgery in which SSEPs were monitored, loss of the SSEP waveform for less than 15 minutes was not associated with a new permanent neurologic deficit, whereas complete loss of the SSEP for longer periods was increasingly likely to reflect permanent neurologic injury, even if the response recovered completely to its intraoperative baseline during surgery.[46]

One of the most important principles of recording SERs intraoperatively is that reproducible, reliable tracings must be obtained at baseline before any intervention likely to cause changes in the evoked response. If good quality tracings with identifiable waveforms cannot be recorded and reproduced at baseline, evoked response monitoring would be of little use in monitoring the integrity of the CNS intraoperatively. If significant variability exists, or waveforms are difficult to identify, it would be impossible intraoperatively to distinguish SER changes that are clinically significant from a preexisting baseline variability of waveforms. When good, reproducible responses cannot be recorded at baseline, monitoring should not be used for clinical decision making.

Somatosensory Evoked Potentials. SSEPs are recorded after electric stimulation of a peripheral mixed nerve. Stimulation is provided most commonly with surface electrodes (e.g., electrocardiogram electrodes) placed on the skin above the nerve or with fine needle electrodes. A square wave stimulus of 50 to 250 μsec duration is delivered to the peripheral nerve, and the intensity is adjusted to produce a minimal muscle contraction. Increasing the stimulus intensity beyond the sum of the motor and sensory threshold does not influence the amplitude or latency of the recorded evoked potential. On a practical basis, however, many laboratories do not establish SSEP monitoring until after the patient is already anesthetized and paralyzed. In these cases, stimulus intensity is increased until no further increase in response size occurs at any recording site, typically constant current stimulation of 20 to 50 mA. For comparison, consider supramaximal stimulation used for the neuromuscular blockade monitor, commonly 80 mA. The rate of stimulation varies from 1 to 6 Hz. The common sites of stimulation include the median nerve at the wrist, the common peroneal nerve at the knee, and the posterior tibial nerve at the ankle.[47]

SSEP responses consist of short-latency and long-latency waveforms. Cortical short-latency SSEPs are most commonly recorded intraoperatively because they are less influenced by changes in anesthetic drug levels. The pathways involved in the generation of upper extremity short-latency SSEPs include large-fiber sensory nerves with their cell bodies in the dorsal root ganglia and central processes traveling rostrally in the ipsilateral posterior column of the spinal cord synapsing in the dorsal column nuclei at the cervicomedullary junction (first-order fibers), second-order fibers crossing and traveling to the contralateral thalamus via the medial lemniscus, and third-order fibers from the thalamus to the frontoparietal sensorimotor cortex. These primary cortical evoked responses, which are recordable with most anesthetic techniques, result from the earliest electric activity generated by the cortical neurons and are thought to arise from the postcentral sulcus parietal neurons. The longer latency secondary cortical waves are thought to arise in the association cortex. These responses have much greater variability in an awake patient,[45] habituate rapidly on repetitive stimulation,[44] and are only poorly reproducible during general anesthesia. Cortical SSEPs other than the primary cortical response are not monitored or interpreted intraoperatively because they are severely altered by general anesthesia.[44]

Although most evidence indicates that upper extremity evoked potentials are conducted rostrally in the spinal cord via dorsal column pathways, much data suggest that lower extremity SSEPs are conducted substantially by the lateral funiculus.[48] Stimulation of the posterior tibial nerve or common peroneal nerve at or above motor threshold activates group I fibers that synapse and travel rostrally through the dorsal spinocerebellar tract. After synapsing in nucleus Z at the spinomedullary junction, the pathway crosses and projects onto the ventral posterolateral thalamic nucleus.[49] Studies with dogs, cats, and monkeys support the concept that lower extremity SERs are conducted in all quadrants of the spinal cord, but primarily in the dorsal lateral funiculus.[50,51] This pathway difference is important because the dorsal lateral funiculus is supplied primarily by the anterior spinal artery, the artery that also supplies the descending motor pathway and neurons in the spinal cord. Manipulations, such as distraction of the spinal column to correct scoliosis, which may secondarily compress or distort radicular blood supply to the anterior spinal cord, should cause changes in the SSEP in the event blood supply is reduced to critical levels. This hypothesis is verified by the very low, but not zero, incidence of postoperative paraplegia on awakening without any intraoperative changes in SSEPs.

For SSEP recordings with median nerve stimulation, recording electrodes (usually electrocardiogram pads) are first placed at Erb's point, just above the midpoint of the clavicle. This point overlies the brachial plexus, and signals recorded here assure the clinician that the stimulus is actually being delivered properly to the patient. The next electrode (either an electrocardiogram pad or a gold cup electrode) is placed midline posteriorly over the neck at level of the second cervical vertebra, relatively near the dorsal column nuclei. Signals recorded here ensure proper transmission of the response from the peripheral nervous system into the spinal cord and rostral along the spinal cord to the lower medulla. The final electrodes (gold cup electrodes or needle electrodes) are placed on the scalp overlying the sensory (parietal) cortex contralateral to the stimulated limb. Signals recorded here ensure the integrity of the pathway through the brainstem, thalamus, and internal capsule, and may assess adequacy of CBF in this area of the cortex.[52-56]

To record SSEPs after posterior tibial nerve stimulation, electrodes (electrocardiogram pads) are placed first over the popliteal fossa to ensure proper stimulus delivery to the nervous system. Electrodes also may be placed over the lower lumbar spine to ensure proper transmission of the signal into the spinal cord itself, but this site is not commonly used because of the proximity of sterile surgical incisions. Cervical spine and scalp recording electrodes are placed in a similar fashion as described previously, although different locations may be used as required by the placement of the surgical incision. More invasive recording methods, such as epidural electrodes, also may be used intraoperatively.

Purported generators for short-latency SSEPs are listed in Table 46-1 and shown in Figure 46-9.[44,47] Induction of anesthesia and use of different recording electrode locations (montage), necessitated by the surgical incision, may significantly alter the appearance of the SSEP. In these cases, attribution of a particular generator to a given wave on the tracing may be quite difficult. During neurologic monitoring, such precision is not needed, and

Table 46-1 Generators of Somatosensory Evoked Potentials after Median Nerve Stimulation

Peak	Generators
N9 (EP)	Brachial plexus*
N11	Posterior columns or spinal roots
N13/P13	Dorsal column nuclei*
N14, 15	Brainstem or thalamus
N19/P22	Parietal sensory cortex*

*Indicates sites commonly recorded during surgery. All other waveforms indicated are not commonly monitored.

recorded waveforms are compared with tracings obtained at baseline and during earlier portions of the surgical procedure. After lower limb stimulation, absolute latencies are increased because of the greater distance the response to stimulation must travel along the peripheral sensory nerve and spinal cord. Interpeak latencies (see Fig. 46-7) also are evaluated to assess specific conduction times, such as N9 to N14 conduction time, reflecting transmission time from the brachial plexus to brainstem, or N14 to N19 conduction time, reflecting transmission time between the dorsal column nuclei and the primary sensory cortex.[57]

Brainstem Auditory Evoked Potentials. BAEPs are produced in the diagnostic laboratory by delivering repetitive clicks or tones via headphones. Headphones are not practical for surgical monitoring of neurosurgical procedures, and click stimuli are delivered using foam ear inserts attached to stimulus transducers (Fig. 46-10). Stimulus intensity is usually set at 60 to 70 dB above the patient's click-hearing threshold, although, practically speaking, many intraoperative laboratories establish monitoring after induction of anesthesia and instead begin with a stimulus intensity of 90 dB nHL (normal hearing level). The duration of the click is approximately 100 μsec, and the stimulus is given usually 10 to 15 times per second. Clicks are delivered using different "polarities"—that is, the click may cause initial movement of the tympanic membrane away from the transducer (rarefaction) or toward the transducer (condensation). Use of these two different methods commonly produces very different waveforms, amplitudes, and latencies in individual patients, and the method that produces the largest reproducible response is chosen. If stimulus artifact is a serious problem, clicks of alternating polarity may be used to decrease the artifact, but the waveforms produced are an average of those produced by either stimulating technique alone and may be more difficult to monitor.

Rate and intensity of stimulus delivery affect BAEPs.[44,58] Unilateral stimulation is used because responses from the other ear, which may remain normal during surgery, may obscure any abnormal responses from the monitored ear. Recording electrodes (usually gold cup electrodes) are placed on the lobe of the stimulated ear and on the top of the head (vertex).[58] White noise commonly may be delivered to the contralateral ear to prevent bone conduction from stimulation of the monitored ear from producing an evoked response from the contralateral ear. On average, 500 to 2000 repetitions are required because BAEPs recorded from the scalp are far-field potentials and extremely small (often <0.3 μV).[44,58]

Peaks in recordings of BAEPs are labeled I through VII; the purported neural generators for these peaks and the auditory pathway are shown in Figure 46-11. The anatomic auditory pathway would predict that BAEP monitoring would be most useful for surgical procedures in the posterior fossa that risk hearing or structures in the upper medulla, pons, and midbrain. As with other SERs, amplitude, absolute latencies, and interpeak latencies are evaluated to assess integrity of the auditory system,

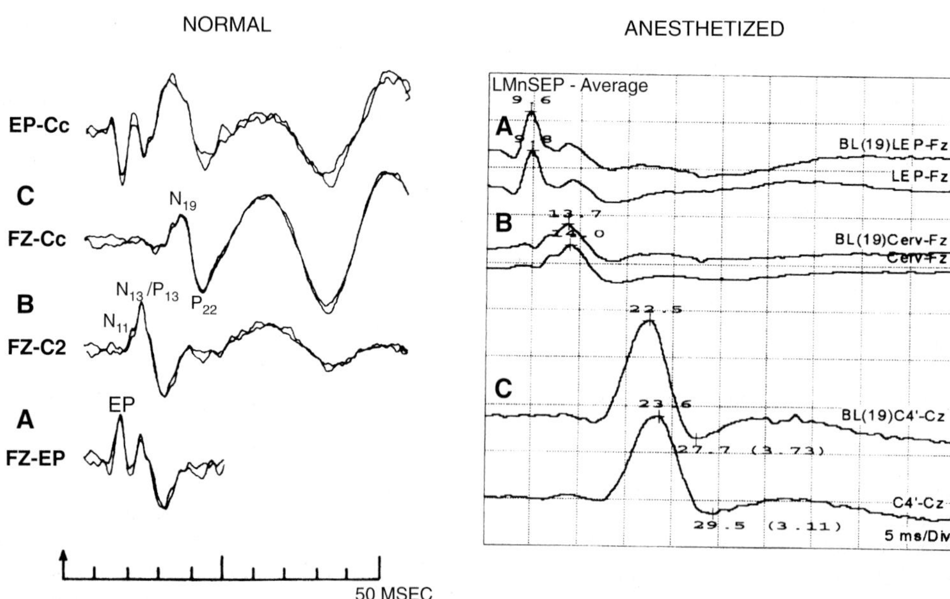

Figure 46-9 Short-latency somatosensory evoked potentials produced by stimulation of the median nerve at the wrist. The ability to identify each of the labeled peaks shown in the tracing from the awake patient is compromised by the anesthetic state and use of different recording electrode locations (**A** to **C**). Corresponding tracings are labeled with the same letter. *(From Chiappa KH, Ropper AH: Evoked potentials in clinical medicine. N Engl J Med 306:1205, 1982.)*

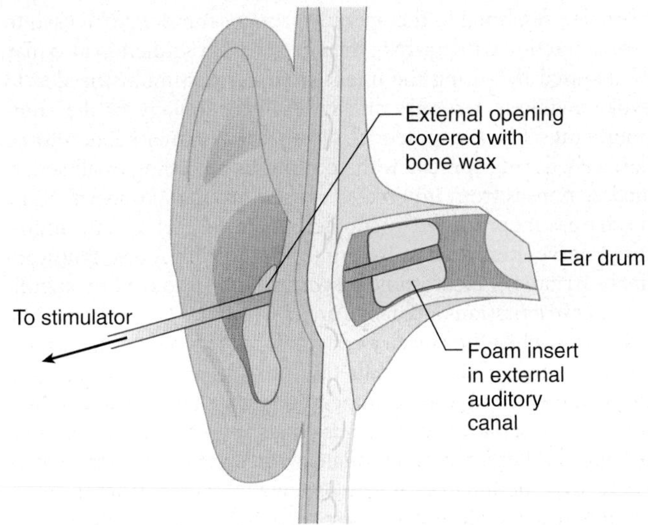

Figure 46-10 Schematic of brainstem auditory evoked potential stimulating apparatus. Loud click stimuli are delivered directly to the eardrum through the ear insert.

localize the functional defect when it occurs, and assess peripheral and central conduction times. Because waves VI and VII are inconsistent and variable, they are not routinely monitored,[58] and most articles reporting use of BAEP for surgical monitoring in the operating room monitor waves only up to wave V.[59-61]

Visual Evoked Potentials. VEPs are recorded after monocular stimulation with recording electrodes over the occipital, parietal, and central scalp.[60] Flash stimulation of the retina using light-emitting diodes embedded in soft plastic goggles through closed eyelids or as needed via contact lenses with built-in light-emitting diodes is provided. VEPs are cortical SERs, which vary with the type of stimulus, part of the retina stimulated, degree of pupil dilation, and patient's attention level.[44] Because some of these factors change commonly and even constantly during the course of every anesthetic, VEPs would be expected to be highly variable during surgery even when no surgical trespass on the visual system occurs. VEPs are the least commonly used evoked response monitoring technique intraoperatively.

Motor Evoked Potentials. MEPs are generated most commonly by the application of a transcranial train of electric stimuli, and responses are recorded at various points along the spinal column, peripheral nerve, and innervated muscle.

TRANSCRANIAL MOTOR EVOKED POTENTIALS. Monitoring of the integrity of the motor tracts within the spinal cord is a technique with great potential benefit, and even during the relative short history of MEP monitoring, there are reported cases of loss of MEPs with preservation of the SSEP.[62-67] This technique has potential applications in spinal surgery, in which transmission across the operative field can be assessed, and in aortic surgery, with the potential for impairment of the blood supply to the vulnerable anterior spinal cord. Relative to SER monitoring, MEP monitoring is quite invasive and, in the case of transcranial stimulation, uses much higher stimulus intensity (≥400 V).

Several variants of MEP monitoring exist. The first method involves transcranial stimulation, either electric or magnetic. During transcranial electric MEP monitoring, stimulating electrodes (usually small, metallic screw-type electrodes similar to those used in fetal monitoring) are placed into the scalp overlying the motor cortex, and a train of electric stimuli (usually around 400 to 500 V) is applied to the scalp. This stimulation definitely activates muscles of mastication, and bite-blocks must be placed to prevent serious damage to the tongue during stimulation. During magnetic stimulation, a powerful magnetic stimulator is placed on the scalp over the motor cortex. Magnetic stimulation is more difficult for two reasons. First, the magnetic stimulator must be fixed to the head to prevent movement because even a slight movement of the stimulator can substantially alter the

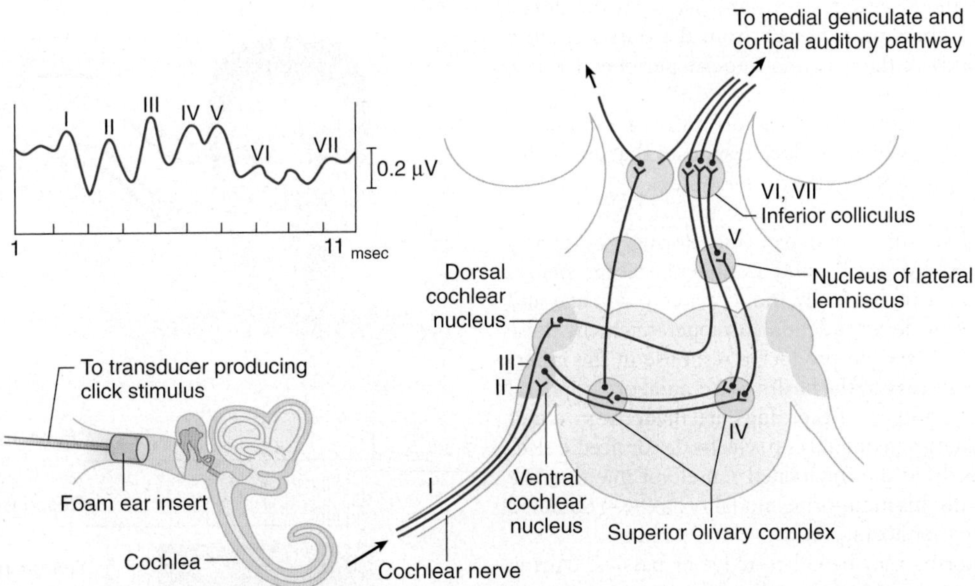

Figure 46-11 Schematic of auditory neural pathway. The brainstem auditory evoked potential is initiated by stimulation of the cochlea with a broadband click stimulus given via an ear insert in the external auditory canal. Neural generators of the brainstem auditory evoked potential peaks are shown.

stimulus applied to the motor cortex. Second, the stimulator is quite large and cannot practically be used intraoperatively if a craniotomy is performed. Brief repetitive applications of electric current or a strong magnetic field induce current in the motor cortex and produce an MEP.

These transcranial stimulating methods also may activate surrounding cortical structures and subcortical white matter pathways (sensory and motor). Distal antidromic propagation of the transcranially applied stimulus is blocked by synapses in all of the ascending sensory pathways. The stimulus is propagated easily orthodromically via descending motor pathways. The evoked responses may be recorded over the spinal cord, the peripheral nerve, and, most commonly, the muscle itself. To enhance the MEP, these responses may be averaged in the same manner as SERs, but averaging is almost always unnecessary.

Spinal Motor Evoked Potentials. Another method of producing the MEP involves electric stimulation of the spinal cord itself above the area of the cord at risk during surgery. Responses may be recorded over the distal spinal cord, peripheral nerve, and muscle.[68-70] Responses are recorded distally, usually over the peripheral nerve, and profound surgical muscle relaxation is used to prevent gross movement during surgery. This type of MEP is called a "neurogenic" MEP. Initially, investigators believed that this response, recorded over a peripheral nerve in the lower extremity (typically the tibial nerve in the popliteal fossa), was generated by stimulation of the descending motor tracts, activation of the anterior horn cells, and propagation of the nerve action potential via the peripheral nerve. Multiple clinical trials were conducted using this technique and comparing results of MEP monitoring with the SSEP with good results.[68-70] These responses also have the advantage that they do not show the same sensitivity to anesthetics that SSEPs do and may be recorded with any anesthetic technique.

Subsequent studies in animals and humans[71] have shown that neurogenic MEPs are, at best, mixed responses with a significant component of an antidromically conducted response along the sensory pathway. Stimulation of the dorsal column results in an antidromically conducted recordable signal peripherally because the somesthetic system does not synapse in the dorsal root ganglion, and fibers pass directly from the dorsal column through the cell body in the ganglion into the peripheral nerve. Because of this problem, use of neurogenic MEP monitoring has decreased significantly, replaced by the more invasive transcranial stimulation techniques, which produce responses that are exclusively produced by activation of the motor system.

Electromyography. Intraoperative monitoring of EMG responses generated by cranial and peripheral motor nerves allows early detection of surgically induced nerve damage and assessment of level of nerve function intraoperatively. In these cases, the ability of a nerve to produce a response in the innervated muscle is used to assess the health of a cranial or peripheral nerve at risk during surgery. Recordings are made from either surface (electrocardiogram or gold cup) electrodes or needle electrodes placed directly in the innervated muscle of interest. The most experience with this monitoring modality has been obtained during facial nerve monitoring.

EMG monitoring may be either active or passive. During active monitoring, a cranial or peripheral nerve is stimulated electrically, and the evoked EMG (compound muscle action potential) response from the muscle is recorded. Stimulation of the nerve proximal to the operative area or tumor can be used to assess functional integrity of the nerve.[72] Nerve function also may be assessed by noting the intensity of nerve stimulus needed to evoke a muscle response and by the morphology of the compound muscle action potential. Nerve function may be monitored passively during surgery with continuous recording of all generated responses from innervated muscle groups. "Popcorn" EMG discharges are produced by simple, benign contact with the monitored nerve. Response trains are produced with more significant nerve irritation. Neurotonic discharges are produced by significant nerve irritation or damage or both (Fig. 46-12).[72] These EMG responses, when they reach a certain voltage threshold, are usually converted into audible signals that provide immediate feedback to the surgeon and warn of impending nerve damage in real time. Real-time feedback is key because density and frequency of neurotonic discharges may correlate with degree of postoperative nerve dysfunction, as shown by data obtained from patients undergoing resection of acoustic tumors.[73]

Intraoperative monitoring of the motor component of other cranial nerves also has been successfully performed. EMG monitoring of the trigeminal nerve can be accomplished with electrodes placed over or in the temporalis or masseter muscles. Trigeminal nerve motor monitoring has been used during nerve section for tic douloureux to ensure preservation of the motor branch of the trigeminal nerve and in combination with facial nerve monitoring during resection of large posterior fossa lesions.[72] Using recording electrodes placed in or over the trapezius or sternocleidomastoid muscles, the spinal accessory nerve has been successfully monitored during resection of large meningiomas, glomus jugulare tumors, and neck carcinomas.[72] EMG monitoring of the hypoglossal nerve with needle electrodes placed in the tongue has been infrequently used for large posterior fossa lesions and clivus tumors.[72] Although EMG monitoring of the eye muscles can be performed using tiny hook wires for recording, it is rarely used.

Monitoring of peripheral motor nerves has been performed by placing needle electrodes in or over the muscles innervated by

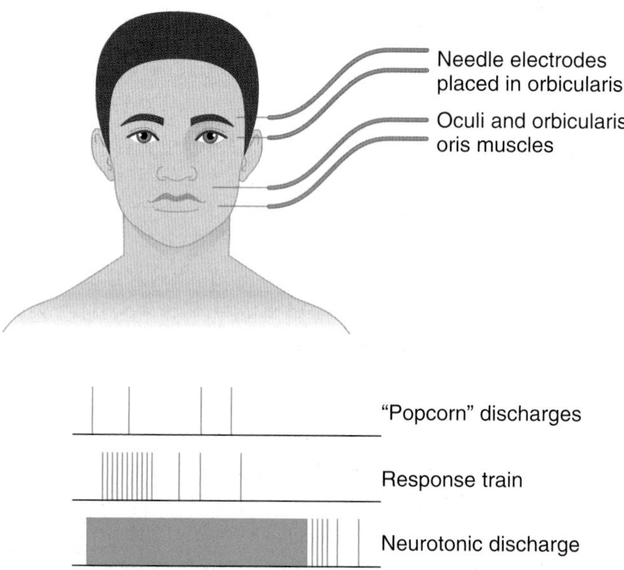

Figure 46-12 Schematic of facial nerve monitoring and typical responses seen during surgery.

nerves that traverse the operative area and are at risk from the planned surgical procedure. Auditory feedback from EMG monitoring can warn the surgeon of unexpected surgical trespass of the nerve, help locate a nerve within the field (e.g., during untethering of the spinal cord), and localize the level of any conduction block or delay. Because radiculopathies have been reported to occur after spine surgery, EMG monitoring of peripheral nerves has been used in patients undergoing spine surgery to decrease the risk of nerve root injury during the procedure.[72]

Clinical Applications of Neurologic Monitoring

Neurovascular Surgery (also see Chapter 63)

Extracranial Neurovascular Surgery: Carotid Vascular Surgery (Monitors: EEG, SSEPs, TCD, Cerebral Oximetry)

Electroencephalogram. The use of the EEG as a monitor of the adequacy of CBF during carotid endarterectomy has been established for many years. In a large series of patients undergoing carotid endarterectomy at the Mayo Clinic,[36] the EEG was compared with regional CBF using the ^{133}Xe washout method. This study validated the EEG as an indicator of the adequacy of regional CBF.

Normal CBF in gray and white matter averages 50 mL/100 g/min. With most anesthetic techniques, the EEG begins to become abnormal when CBF decreases to 20 mL/100 g/min. The threshold for EEG changes apparently is much lower (8 to 10 mL/100 g/min), however, when isoflurane is used.[74] Cellular survival is not threatened until CBF decreases to 12 mL/100 g/min (lower with isoflurane). The difference in blood flow between when the EEG becomes abnormal and the blood flow at which cellular damage begins to occur provides a rational basis for monitoring the EEG during carotid surgery. In many cases, prompt detection of EEG changes may allow intervention (e.g., shunting, increasing cerebral perfusion pressure) to restore CBF before onset of permanent neurologic damage. Standard hemodynamic monitoring provides no direct information about the adequacy of CBF. Blood pressure is not a specific indicator of the adequacy of CBF. Significant hypotension is not predictably associated with EEG evidence of cerebral ischemia. Severe anemia and decreases in oxygen saturation also decrease oxygen delivery. EEG activity becomes abnormal when increased blood flow cannot compensate for decreased arterial oxygen content.

Serious intraoperative reduction in cerebral oxygen supply may result from surgical factors (e.g., carotid cross-clamping) that are usually beyond the anesthesiologist's control, and from factors that the anesthesiologist can correct. Reduction in CBF produced by hyperventilation, hypotension, or temporary occlusion of major blood vessels may be corrected by reducing ventilation, by restoring normal blood pressure, or, in the case of temporary vessel occlusion, by increasing blood pressure above normal. Because the EEG may readily detect cerebral ischemia, continuous EEG monitoring may be used to evaluate the effectiveness of therapy instituted to correct ischemia.

If monitoring of the EEG could be proved scientifically to reduce the incidence of stroke during carotid vascular surgery, EEG monitoring would be established as a standard of care. Definitive data showing stroke reduction do not yet exist, however, and given the number of patients required to power a trial that would show a reduction in stroke rate from 2% to 1%, such studies are unlikely to be funded or forthcoming. What data are available do not provide a basis to recommend universal use of EEG monitoring during carotid surgery. In a large series of patients undergoing carotid endarterectomy with selective shunting who were monitored with 16-channel unprocessed EEG, no patient awakened with a new neurologic deficit that was not predicted by EEG.[75] Transient, correctable EEG changes were not associated with stroke. Persistent changes were associated with stroke. This study had no comparison group, however, analyzing stroke rate when EEG monitoring was not used during surgery.

In the North American Symptomatic Carotid Endarterectomy Trial and the European Carotid Surgery Trial, retrospective comparison of patients receiving EEG monitoring and patients not receiving EEG monitoring failed to show a significant difference in outcome.[76,77] Because the EEG detects reductions in CBF that would not otherwise be apparent in unmonitored patients, and permits intervention that may correct the problem (usually placing a shunt or increasing blood pressure), EEG monitoring should logically be useful in reducing the incidence of stroke when selective shunting is used. Data available from studies at this time bring us no closer to resolving this question, however, than we were 30 years ago. Advocates of monitoring and individuals who believe monitoring is of no value can cite multiple studies supporting each viewpoint.

Even more difficult to prove is that EEG monitoring is useful when all patients are shunted during carotid clamping. Such monitoring has detected correctable shunt malfunction, and investigators have described hypotension-related EEG changes in patients with critical stenoses and poor collateral circulation.[78] Advocates of selective shunting based on EEG (or other monitoring) criteria claim that inserting a shunt unnecessarily through a region of diseased vessel would surely increase embolization. A multicenter study of 1495 carotid endarterectomies provides some evidence that shunting of patients without evidence of decreased cerebral perfusion increases the incidence of stroke more than sixfold.[79] Although this study and other more recent studies[80-82] advocate that selective shunting using some form of monitoring of the adequacy of CBF should improve perioperative stroke rate, an analysis by the Cochrane Stroke Group[83] failed to show sufficient evidence to advocate for routine shunting, selective shunting, or even no shunting at all. Until compelling studies addressing this issue are done, it is unlikely that EEG monitoring during carotid vascular surgery would become a standard method.

Processed EEG also has been used during carotid vascular surgery. Two issues affect the efficacy and reliability of processed EEG as a monitor for cerebral ischemia. First, what is the minimum number of channels (or areas of the brain) to be monitored? The 16-channel unprocessed EEG is a reliable and sensitive monitor for intraoperative cerebral ischemia during carotid endarterectomy. In a series of more than 2000 patients monitored with 16-channel EEG at the Mayo Clinic, there were no false-negative EEGs[75]; in other words, no patient had undetected intraoperative cerebral injury. In operating rooms where carotid surgery is performed, however, 16-channel EEG monitored by a dedicated technician is unavailable. Processed EEG using less than 16 channels is used much more commonly. Clinical experience and clinical investigations suggest that four channels (two per side) are the minimum number of channels for adequate sensitivity and specificity.[37] When a limited number of channels were compared with 16-channel EEG monitoring, 100% sensitivity and specificity were obtained using 2 channels per hemisphere, provided that those channels monitored the middle cerebral artery territory. These results were obtained with a frontoparietal channel combined with a frontotemporal channel.[37]

The second issue is the experience level of the observer monitoring the processed EEG. Is a dedicated, experienced technician or electroencephalographer needed? In a study addressing this question, the 16-channel unprocessed EEG monitored by a dedicated technician was compared with a processed EEG reviewed by three anesthesiologists of differing levels of experience with processed EEG.[38] The three anesthesiologists interpreted the tracings without knowledge of the case. They were presented only with the written trace with an indication of the point at which the carotid artery was clamped. In these cases, the most important interpretation pitfall to avoid is the "false-negative" pattern. If the clinician interprets the EEG as showing adequate CBF when in fact it does not, the surgeon may fail to shunt an ischemic patient. A false-positive result may be less of a problem because that patient is not ischemic but is given a shunt anyway. In this case, only the risk of emboli from the "unnecessary" shunt is incurred. The positive predictive value of the anesthesiologist correctly interpreting the trace as unchanged after clamping was 91% to 98%, which indicates that the device can be used by novice interpreters with fair accuracy to determine the presence of cerebral ischemia at the time of carotid occlusion. In this study, the review by the anesthesiologist was not done during the course of the procedure, but rather "off line," and does not address the issue of whether an anesthesiologist providing the intraoperative anesthetic management of the patient can provide adequate monitoring of the processed EEG simultaneously.

EEG monitoring has limitations. Despite the data available from the Mayo Clinic, immediately evident postoperative strokes have been reported in patients without any evidence of EEG changes intraoperatively. In our experience, such strokes result from emboli via the lenticulostriate arteries to subcortical structures that do not generate or affect the EEG, but are critically involved in the descending motor pathway. Overall, such events are rare.

Should the patient undergoing carotid endarterectomy have EEG monitoring? That question cannot be answered based on any available data. EEG monitoring provides information about CBF that would not otherwise be available. The clinician has an opportunity to intervene to increase inadequate blood flow when it occurs. Anecdotally, many clinicians have found such monitoring useful and use it routinely. Population studies do not support routine use, and it is up to the clinician to decide whether to use it.

Somatosensory Evoked Potentials. SSEP monitoring also has been used to gauge adequacy of CBF to the cerebral cortex and subcortical pathways during carotid vascular surgery.[56,84,85] SSEPs have been found in the laboratory to have a similar but slightly lower threshold for failure compared with the EEG. SSEPs are generally intact until the cortical blood flow decreases to less than 15 mL/100 g/min.[54] In a few comparison studies with the EEG, a similar sensitivity and specificity for postoperative neurologic function was found. These studies involved few patients, however, and are inadequate to support the hypothesis that SSEP monitoring may substitute for EEG monitoring of the adequacy of CBF.[84-86] Logic also would suggest that changes in SSEP are unlikely, for example, with ischemia involving the anterior portions of either the frontal or temporal lobe, which could readily be detected by an appropriately placed EEG electrode. Finally, a more recent meta-analysis does not support the use of SSEPs during carotid vascular surgery as a sole monitor of neurologic function.[87] There is even less outcome evidence to support the use of SSEPs during carotid surgery than there is for the EEG, but the authors and others have found SSEPs to be useful as a simultaneous monitor with EEG to detect subcortical ischemia.

Transcranial Doppler. TCD monitoring during carotid vascular surgery is based on measurement of two primary parameters—blood flow velocity in major conducting arteries leading to the cerebral cortex (most commonly middle cerebral artery) and the number of emboli detected in the same artery. The hypothesis justifying the use of this monitoring during carotid vascular surgery has two components: blood flow velocity correlates with CBF, and increasing numbers of emboli increase the likelihood of emboli related cerebral ischemia or stroke. The first component has not been well tested and shows variable results. An early study in a small group of patients undergoing carotid surgery did not show good correlation between CBF and blood flow velocity.[88] Subsequent studies in patients with varying intracranial pathology have yielded mixed results.[89-92]

The correlation between CBF and TCD-measured blood flow velocity remains good over time only when the artery being insonated does not change diameter, and when cortical blood flow in the distribution of the measured artery does not have significant collateral sources of blood flow. The relationship between emboli count and stroke is better established with multiple studies conducted in the preoperative, intraoperative, and postoperative periods indicating that higher emboli counts are associated with higher stroke risk and warrant intervention.[93-99]

Intraoperative use of TCD has not been widely adopted for many reasons. As previously noted, good TCD signals cannot be obtained in many individuals who could benefit from monitoring. Also, TCD probe motion during surgery causes major problems with loss of signal or with angle of insonance–induced changes in the relationship between blood flow velocity and blood flow. Nonetheless, multiple series of carotid endarterectomies with TCD monitoring have been reported with good success, quoting a critical blood flow velocity reduction around 50% as indicative of inadequate CBF requiring intervention (shunt or increased blood pressure or both).[93-99] There are no good outcome data supporting TCD use intraoperatively, but data regarding emboli count and risk of stroke suggest that if technical issues with probe attachment to the patient can be overcome, TCD may be useful as a predictor of impending stroke in the preoperative, postoperative, and perhaps intraoperative periods.

Cerebral Oximetry (Near-Infrared Spectroscopy). Near-infrared spectroscopy (NIRS) is an attractive monitor because of its ease of application and lack of training required for interpretation. The hypothesis governing its use is very simple: As oxygen delivery to the brain decreases, oxygen extraction from arterial blood increases, and the oxygen saturation in cerebral venous blood decreases. NIRS applied to cerebral monitoring measures the oxygen saturation in the cerebral venous blood in the prefrontal cortex and promptly detects increases in oxygen extraction resulting from decreased oxygen delivery. Multiple case reports and series document the use of cerebral oximetry during neurovascular surgery, but several major questions surrounding use of NIRS during carotid surgery remain unanswered.

The first and most important question is what degree of decrease in oxygen saturation can be tolerated before intervention is necessary. Because most interventions involve some risk (e.g., shunt → emboli, increased BP → myocardial ischemia), the answer to this question is important. The answer does not yet exist, however, and may vary from patient to patient. Two more recent studies showed that in awake patients, the saturation value at which any patient would develop symptoms varied from patient to patient,[100,101] and an absolute value that required shunting could not be determined. Another study showed that cerebral oxygen saturation decreased before the EEG developed changes, and the authors used this observation to claim superiority for NIRS monitoring of the brain during carotid surgery.[102] This finding should not be surprising, however, because function of the brain (in this case, electric function) does not fail until increased extraction of oxygen no longer meets metabolic demands for the tissue. If metabolic demands are being met by increased extraction, it is unclear that intervention is needed.

Finally, a study by Friedell and colleagues[103] compared NIRS with EEG and SSEP monitoring during carotid surgery. In 24 of 323 patients, significant differences were observed between NIRS and monitors of electric function. Seventeen patients showed no changes in electric function with significant decreases in cerebral oxygen saturation. In seven patients, no change in cerebral oxygen saturation occurred despite significant change in the EEG and SSEP. These data in combination with the data from studies in awake patients suggest that use of NIRS alone during carotid vascular surgery may be inappropriate.

Intracranial Neurovascular Surgery (Monitors: SSEPs)

Somatosensory Evoked Potentials. SSEPs have been extensively studied during cerebral aneurysm surgery. During these procedures, the surgical incision and brain retraction precludes placement of scalp or brain surface electrodes that could detect cerebral ischemia in at-risk cortex. Recording electrodes placed on the surface of the brain have been used successfully, but they are commonly considered "in the way" by neurosurgeons. Scalp electrodes may be placed easily for SSEP monitoring, although the recording montage is frequently not the same as that used in an awake patient.

For aneurysms involving the anterior cerebral circulation, SSEP monitoring has an excellent, but not perfect, record for predicting postoperative neurologic function. Most patients without surgically induced SSEP changes during surgery awaken with an unchanged neurologic examination. Patients with significant SSEP changes that do not revert to normal awaken with a new neurologic deficit. Patients with SSEP changes that return to normal after a significant intraoperative change may show at least a transient postoperative deficit, with the severity and duration increasing as the duration of the SSEP change increases. Many authors have reported significant utility of SSEP monitoring in detecting improper aneurysm clip placement (see Fig. 46-8) and in guiding intraoperative blood pressure management, particularly in patients already showing or at significant risk for vasospasm after subarachnoid hemorrhage.[55,104-109] The same success cannot be reported, however, for posterior circulation aneurysms. In these cases, many areas of the cortex and subcortical structures are at risk for damage that cannot be monitored at all by somatosensory pathway function. A significant false-negative monitoring pattern exists for these patients, but changes can still be detected when a surgical insult is sufficiently severe to involve large portions of the brain.[110-113]

Supratentorial Intracranial Nonvascular Surgery (Monitors: Awake Patient, EEG, SSEPs)

During supratentorial procedures, neurologic monitoring can contribute to the precise localization of structures that need to be preserved or conversely supplement the anatomic information provided by imaging with functional data. Three techniques fall under this category: (1) Awake craniotomy can be a suitable approach for the resection of tumors and seizure foci. (2) Intraoperative electrocorticography (i.e., the recording from strategically placed subdural electrodes) is used to target more closely the resection of seizure foci. (3) Localization of the central sulcus and by extension the precentral motor cortex is sometimes helpful, if these structures have been displaced by a tumor.

The most comprehensive approach to the problem of functional localization of brain structures that need to be preserved to achieve a good outcome is to perform entire segments of a supratentorial craniotomy in an awake patient, who is undergoing repeated neurologic examinations targeted to assess the eloquent area at risk. Such procedures are typically divided into exposure, mapping, and resection phases, and can be done with the patient entirely awake or awake only during periods when the neurologic examination needs to be assessed.[114] Common to all these approaches is the need for meticulous locoregional anesthesia of the scalp at the craniotomy site and the pin sites of the head holder.[115] A second requirement is a patient who is well informed about the awake parts of the procedure and willing and able to cooperate. Dexmedetomidine, propofol, and remifentanil are the agents most frequently incorporated into the anesthetic regimens for awake craniotomy.[116] Complications of awake craniotomy include nausea and vomiting, respiratory problems, and "tight" brain, but are typically mild and occur in less than 10% of cases in experienced centers. Seizures triggered by cortical stimulation can be stopped by the application of iced saline to the exposed cortex or a small amount of barbiturate or propofol.

Seizure Focus Localization Surgery

Patients with epilepsy who have seizures that generalize from an anatomically distinct focus may benefit greatly from the surgical resection of that seizure focus.[117] Precise localization of a seizure focus is important for achieving the therapeutic objective of seizure control and for minimizing complications from the resection. With sensitive magnetic resonance tomography techniques, neuronavigation, and recordings of typical seizure activity in the awake patient after placement of subdural and depth electrodes, the anatomic location and the appropriate extent of the resection frequently can be determined preoperatively.[118] These developments have diminished the role of intraoperative recordings from the epileptogenic zone using electrocorticography.[119]

Neurologic monitoring during such a resection is performed using two different techniques. First, activity of the seizure focus can be recorded through electrocorticography. Second, eloquent brain areas next to the seizure focus can be monitored during an awake craniotomy as described in the previous section. Electrocorticography is done by placing a grid of subdural electrodes onto the exposed brain surface and recording spontaneous electric activity. Electrocorticography is constrained by several limitations. The time for such recordings is limited to a few minutes; recordings are limited to interictal discharges, which may not correlate with the epileptogenic focus; and recordings need to be obtained from a brain that is under the effects of general anesthetic agents, which alter the EEG.

To provide good conditions during the recording, the level of anesthesia is lightened (e.g., by use of a strict nitrous-narcotic technique or low concentrations of volatile agents). Provocative techniques, such as hyperventilation or administration of a small dose of methohexital, may be useful to activate the seizure focus. Intraoperative seizure mapping requires the involvement of an expert electroencephalographer familiar with this technique.

Motor Strip Localization

Electrophysiologic monitoring of the somatosensory system in anesthetized patients can provide a simple anatomic guide to the location of the rolandic fissure, which separates the parietal primary sensory and frontal primary motor cortex. The fissure is located by recording cortical SSEPs from a subdural strip electrode that is placed perpendicular to the presumed location of the fissure. The exact location of the fissure is characterized by a reversal in the polarity of the primary cortical response between the electrodes straddling the fissure, as illustrated in the clinical example in Figure 46-13.

Posterior Fossa Surgery (Monitors: BAEPs, Cranial Nerve Monitoring, SSEPs, MEPs)

Beside the cerebellum, the posterior fossa contains within the narrow space of the brainstem many crucial neural structures, including ascending and descending sensorimotor pathways; cranial nerve nuclei; cardiorespiratory centers; the reticular activating system; and the neural networks that underlie crucial protective reflexes, such as eye blink, swallowing, gag, and cough. Posterior fossa surgery is not undertaken lightly, and even small injuries can leave significant neurologic deficits. Although some of these neural structures, such as the sensory or auditory pathway, can be monitored consistently, intraoperative integrity of other neural structures is frequently only inferred from the well-being of neighboring structures amenable to monitoring.

Microvascular Decompression of Cranial Nerves V, VII, and IX

Microvascular decompression is done most frequently for trigeminal neuralgia (cranial nerve V) in patients who present acceptable medical risks for a posterior fossa craniotomy. More rarely, the same approach is used to treat hemifacial spasm or neurovascular compromise of lower cranial nerves. The surgery entails dissecting along the intracranial portion of the nerve, identifying offending blood vessels that encroach on the nerve, and placing an insulating Teflon pad between vessel and nerve. The surgery risks ischemic damage to perforating vessels coming off the offending arteries and cerebellar retraction–related damage to cranial nerves. The facial and vestibulocochlear nerves are at particular risk for stretch-induced injury caused by medial retraction of the cerebellum. Retraction-induced stretch produces a prolongation of the interpeak latency between peaks I and V of the BAEP waveform, ultimately leading to a complete loss of all waves beyond wave I (Fig. 46-14). Failure to release retraction in a timely manner results in postoperative hearing loss. Such monitoring increases the chances for preserved hearing after microvascular decompression.[120-124]

Vestibular Nerve Schwannoma

Vestibular nerve schwannomas are the most common tumors located in the cerebellopontine angle. Because of the common origin of the cochlear component of cranial nerve VIII and the essentially identical intracranial trajectory of the facial nerve, hearing loss and facial nerve palsy are concerns during surgical resection of these tumors. Size and preoperative auditory function are the best predictors of postoperative hearing.[125] For tumors up to about 2 to 3 cm in size, monitoring of BAEPs can increase the chances of preserving hearing.[126] In addition to BAEPs, the facial nerve is monitored through spontaneous and stimulated EMG. Prospective trials have shown a higher percentage of patients with a functional facial nerve 1 year after surgery if facial nerve monitoring was used as previously described. Tonic discharges warn of impending damage caused by stretch or heat (bovie). Sharp section of the nerve may elicit no discharge, and neuromuscular blockade may eliminate the ability to monitor. If the course of the nerve is displaced by the tumor, the surgeon can map its course with a hand-held stimulator and real-time auditory feedback.

Other Posterior Fossa Neoplasms

Monitoring for operations on other neoplasms located in the brainstem typically is individualized to each particular case or to the particular surgical approach. EMG may be recorded not only from the territory of the facial nerve, but also from the tongue to monitor the hypoglossal nerve, and from the glottis through electrodes embedded into a specialized endotracheal tube to monitor the vagus nerve. Such a setup can be used to map the floor of the fourth ventricle functionally, if it is distorted by a tumor.[127] Such monitoring may be insufficient to preserve vital reflexes because only the efferent limb of these reflexes is monitored by recording EMG from innervated muscle.

Use of neurologic monitoring for brainstem ischemia, although done in some centers, is not well documented or supported by clinical studies. Global well-being of the brainstem may be monitored by combining multiple modalities of evoked potentials, such as BAEPs, SSEPs, and MEPs. Each modality monitors a function whose integrity would be considered important in its own right for the functional outcome of an individual patient. As illustrated in Figure 46-15, the cross-section monitored by combining all these modalities still leaves out crucial areas. Given that perfusion occurs through perforating vessels, it is easy to see that monitoring may indicate that all is well or, more likely, that a therapeutic intervention was helpful in restoring function, when clinically the patient is still left with a significant deficit. This occurrence invalidates neither monitoring nor the therapeutic

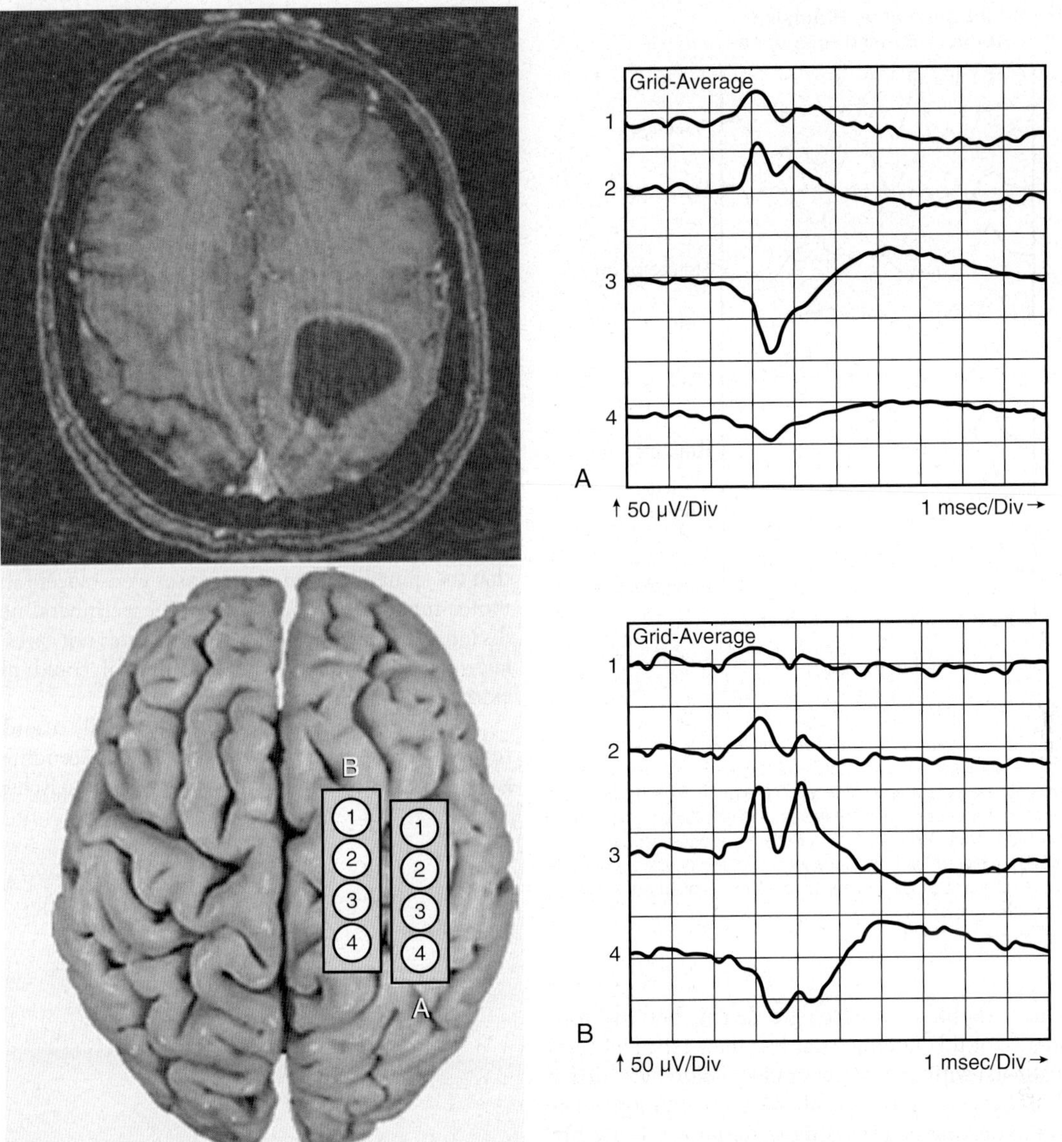

Figure 46-13 Intraoperative localization of the rolandic fissure separating the primary sensory and motor cortex. The clinical example is from a patient with a large parietal tumor shown in the scan. Two of the recordings made from a four-contact subdural electrode strip are shown. The relative positions of the strip electrode are labeled B and A. In recording A, the primary cortical response from the electrodes anterior to the rolandic fissure shows an upward deflection, whereas the response from electrodes posterior to the fissure shows a downward deflection. Moving the strip electrode anterior (recording B) moves this "phase reversal" between electrodes 3 and 4.

intervention, but indicates only that the monitored pathway was not located in an area at risk from the surgical procedure. Because of such obligatory "false-negatives," few studies address the utility of such monitoring. Because each individual monitoring modality comes with its own constraints, such an approach typically requires a dedicated neurophysiologist for interpretation and troubleshooting.

Spinal Column and Spinal Cord Surgery (Monitors: SSEPs, MEPs, EMG)

Intraoperative monitoring of SSEPs has been used most extensively in patients undergoing surgical procedures involving the spinal column or spinal cord, or both. Extensive experience has been gained in patients who have decompressive laminectomies or who have undergone corrective procedures for scoliosis. Intraoperative changes in SSEPs have been noted in 2.5% to 65% of patients undergoing surgical procedures on the spine or spinal cord.[128-131] When these changes are promptly reversed either spontaneously or with interventions by the surgeon or anesthesiologist (e.g., lessening the degree of spine straightening in scoliosis surgery or increasing arterial blood pressure), the patients most often have preserved neurologic function postoperatively. When these changes persisted, however, the patients most often awakened with worsened neurologic function.

False-negative (rare) and false-positive (common) results have been reported with SSEP monitoring during spine surgery. Patients with intact SSEPs throughout the procedure have awak-

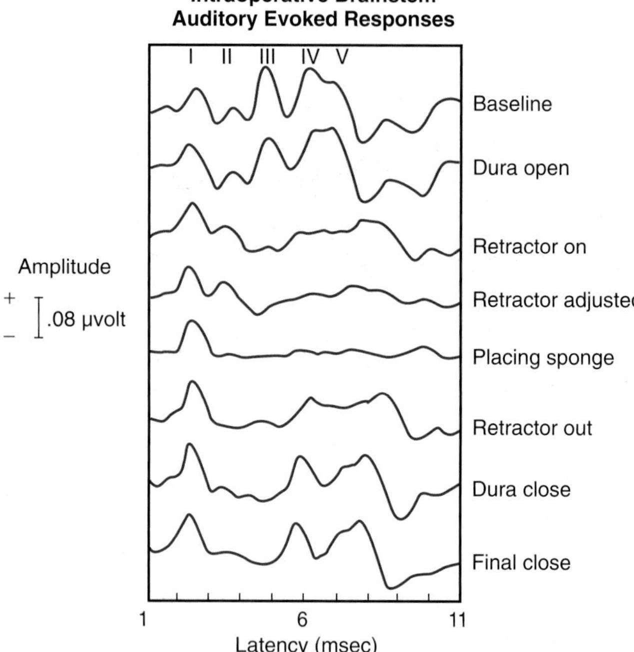

Figure 46-14 Intraoperative monitoring of brainstem auditory evoked responses during microvascular decompression. The baseline recording shows the typical five waves of the brainstem auditory evoked potential response. Intraoperative events are designated to the right of each trace. Placement of the retractor causes a severe increase in latency of wave V even after adjustment of retraction. During placement of the sponge, all waves subsequent to wave I, which originates in the inner ear, are nearly completely lost. Removal of the retractor causes brainstem auditory evoked potentials to revert toward baseline.

ened with a new significant neurologic deficit, but the total reported incidence of this finding is far less than 1% of all cases monitored. Patients with no postoperative neurologic deficit commonly experience significant changes in intraoperative SSEPs.[131] This monitoring pattern is most commonly caused by failure to control for other, nonpathologic factors that may alter the SSEP. Overall, the reliability of properly performed SSEP monitoring to predict the postoperative sensory and motor function has been reported to be excellent.[44,130,132] Motor tracts are not directly monitored by SSEPs, however. In addition, the blood supply to the dorsal columns of the spinal cord, which carries all of the upper extremity SSEPs and at least a portion of the lower extremity SSEPs, is derived primarily from the posterior spinal arteries. The blood supply to motor tracts and neurons is derived primarily from the anterior spinal artery. It is possible for a significant motor deficit to develop postoperatively in patients with intact SSEPs throughout the operative course. Such events have been reported.[133,134]

In operations on the spinal column and after acute spinal cord injury, the sensory and motor changes generally correlate well[44]; however, in patients with neurologic dysfunction after thoracic aortic vascular surgery, frequently posterior spinal cord function (proprioception, vibration, light touch) is left intact when motor and other sensory functions (pain, temperature) are impaired. This result occurred in 32% of patients with neurologic injury after aortic aneurysm repair in one series,[135] with similar results in many other series. Intraoperative SSEP monitoring in these patients carries a significant risk for false-negative results, and as a result, such monitoring is not widely used.

Multiple anecdotal reports and an increasing number of case series suggest that MEP monitoring during surgery on the spine or its blood supply is useful. Several series have reported significant changes in MEPs without changes in SSEPs. These series suggest that combined use of SSEP monitoring and MEP monitoring may eliminate false-negative monitoring patterns during spine surgery.[136-141] In the case of monitoring paraplegia risk during thoracoabdominal aneurysm surgery, the literature shows mixed but improving support for the use of MEP monitoring. Two earlier studies suggested that MEPs may not be as effective as hoped. The first study recorded MEPs from the lumbar spinal cord in dogs produced by transcranial electric stimulation.[135] Elmore and associates[142] found that these spinally recorded potentials did not accurately predict postoperative motor function. In a second study, Reuter and colleagues[143] recorded MEPs at the spinal cord and the peripheral nerve level in dogs produced by transcranial electric stimulation. They also found that the spinally recorded responses were inaccurate in predicting motor function postoperatively. The peripheral nerve responses disappeared in all animals and were not present 24 hours later regardless of whether the animal could move its lower extremities.

These studies suggest that the spinally recorded MEP likely represents a response generated by the descending corticospinal tract. This white matter pathway is resistant to ischemia compared

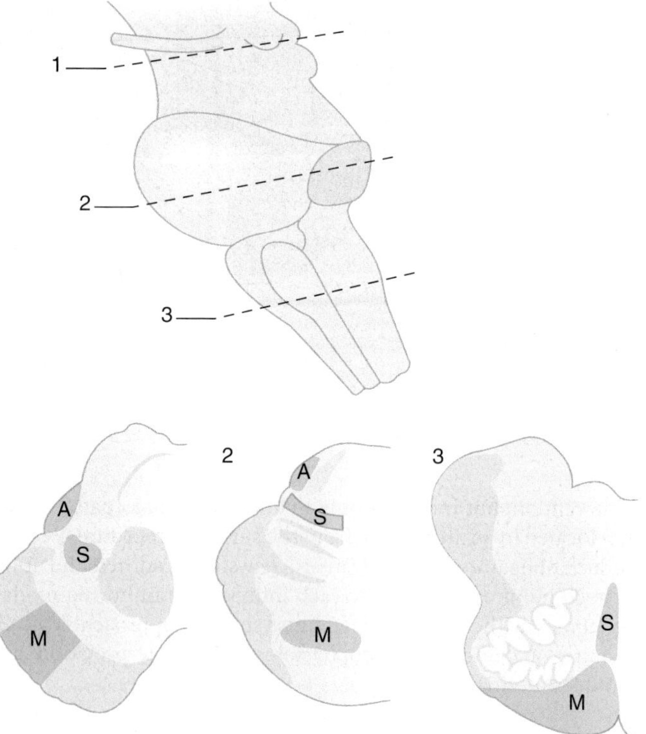

Figure 46-15 Monitoring of the brainstem with evoked potentials. Evoked potentials monitor specific tracts that encompass defined areas in the brainstem. This is shown in three transverse sections approximately at the levels indicated in the drawings. The areas directly monitored by a given modality are indicated in *blue* and labeled M (motor), S (somatosensory), and A (auditory). Conclusions about the well-being of the remainder of the brainstem are made by inference from the monitored areas.

with the more metabolically active anterior horn cells (gray matter). Recovery of this white matter–generated MEP response could occur after reperfusion of the cord, whereas the gray matter might not recover. Responses recorded from the peripheral nerve would reflect postsynaptic anterior horn cell function, but lower extremity ischemia occurring after aortic cross-clamping may preclude recording this or the response from muscles during surgery.

More recent clinical series have shown much greater success with MEP monitoring during aortic vascular surgery in correctly detecting inadequate spinal cord blood flow and in improving operative outcome. The technique has proven useful, particularly when operative strategies such as reimplantation of crucial intercostal vessels based on results of MEP monitoring, alteration of spinal cord perfusion pressure (blood pressure increase or cerebrospinal fluid drainage or both), spinal cord cooling, and other methods are used.[144-153] Although this monitoring technique holds promise in aortic surgery, much more clinical work is needed before MEP monitoring during aortic surgery becomes widely accepted and used.

Peripheral Nerve Surgery (Monitors: EMG, Nerve Action Potential)

Neurologic monitoring for surgeries involving peripheral nerves can be done in two different settings. In the first, the peripheral nerve is intact, but threatened by the surgery. Examples would be an intrinsic nerve tumor, such as a schwannoma or an extensive soft tissue tumor, particularly if it displaces the normal anatomic course of a nerve. Monitoring of spontaneous and stimulated muscle responses from muscle groups innervated by the nerve in question can be used to guide the resection. Spontaneous EMG discharges can be generated by stretch or compression of the nerve, by local heating from electrocautery, or from ischemia. Two caveats apply to the monitoring of spontaneous EMG. First, the neuromuscular junction is part of the monitored pathway, and muscle relaxation decreases/abolishes the sensitivity of monitoring in a dose-dependent manner. Second, sharp section of the nerve may not result in a noticeable discharge. To search out the course of the nerve intraoperatively, the surgeon may stimulate the wound area with a hand-held probe and listen for stimulated EMG or palpate for muscle contraction. The underlying concept should be familiar to anesthesiologists from the use of nerve stimulators in regional anesthesia.

A variation of this technique of monitoring that is gaining popularity is monitoring of pedicle screw placement during spinal instrumentation with the aim of avoiding nerve root injuries owing to malpositioned pedicle screws.[154,155] Typically, the shank of an implanted pedicle screw is stimulated repetitively with increasing current to determine the threshold for eliciting a dermatomal compound muscle potential. Because thresholds vary among cervical, thoracic, and lumbar spine, and between healthy and diseased nerve roots, this technique is currently not universally regarded as useful, but shows some promise.[156]

A second setting where monitoring of peripheral nerves is used is in patients with prolonged weakness and sensory loss after nerve injury undergoing nerve exploration.[157] The aim is to determine whether nerve reconstruction may improve outcome. The area of the lesion is determined by preoperative nerve conduction studies. Intraoperatively, the nerve is first stimulated proximal to the lesion, and a recording of the nerve action potential is made directly from the nerve distal to the lesion, as illustrated in Figure 46-16. If there is nerve conduction across the lesion, lysis of scar is performed, and the incision is closed. Natural recovery by means of axonal regrowth produces the best outcome. If conduction does not occur across the lesion, resection of the damaged nerve and nerve cable grafting is performed.[158-160]

Non-neurologic Surgery That Risks Damage to the Central Nervous System (Monitors: EEG, TCD, Cerebral Oximetry, $SjvO_2$)

Cardiopulmonary Bypass

Electroencephalogram. In humans, changes that occur with the institution of cardiopulmonary bypass (CPB) may alter the EEG via multiple different mechanisms. Plasma and brain levels of anesthetic drugs may be altered by CPB or by anesthetic drugs commonly given at the institution of CPB, alterations in arterial carbon dioxide tension and blood pressure may occur, and hemodilution with hypothermic perfusate nearly always occurs. These effects, all of which may produce EEG changes similar to pathologic changes seen with ischemia, make it difficult to interpret EEG changes occurring around the time of institution of CPB.

Levy and others[161,162] have tried to distinguish the normal effects of hypothermia from other events occurring at the institution of and conclusion of CPB. Initially, Levy concluded that only a qualitative relationship could be determined, but later, with the use of a much more sophisticated EEG analysis technique (approximate entropy), EEG changes associated with changes in temperature could be quantified.

Chabot and colleagues in Boston[163] and Edmonds and colleagues in Louisville[164] have attempted to use quantitative (processed, multiple-channel) EEG during CPB to detect cerebral hypoperfusion and relate these changes to postoperative neurologic function. In addition, some minimal work has been done with intervention after detection of cerebral hypoperfusion using quantitative EEG. Such monitoring techniques have not been widely adopted because although the data seem promising, only a few patients have been studied, and there are very few corroborating studies. In addition, this type of monitoring is extremely costly in time, personnel, and equipment costs, and given the lack of convincing outcome data, the cost-to-benefit ratio is unclear at best. Some other investigators failed to show any convincing relationship between intraoperative EEG parameters and postoperative neurologic function, especially in small infants and children.[165,166] Much work remains to be done studying use of the processed, quantitative EEG to provide information for clinical management of patients during CPB. None of the currently available studies and recommendations would support an evidence-based justification for their routine application.

Transcranial Doppler. TCD also has been used to monitor the cerebral circulation during CPB. Anecdotal reports and case series document the use of TCD for determining adequacy of CBF, detection of emboli, and detection of improper cannula placement.[167] Only very limited outcome data exist, and use of

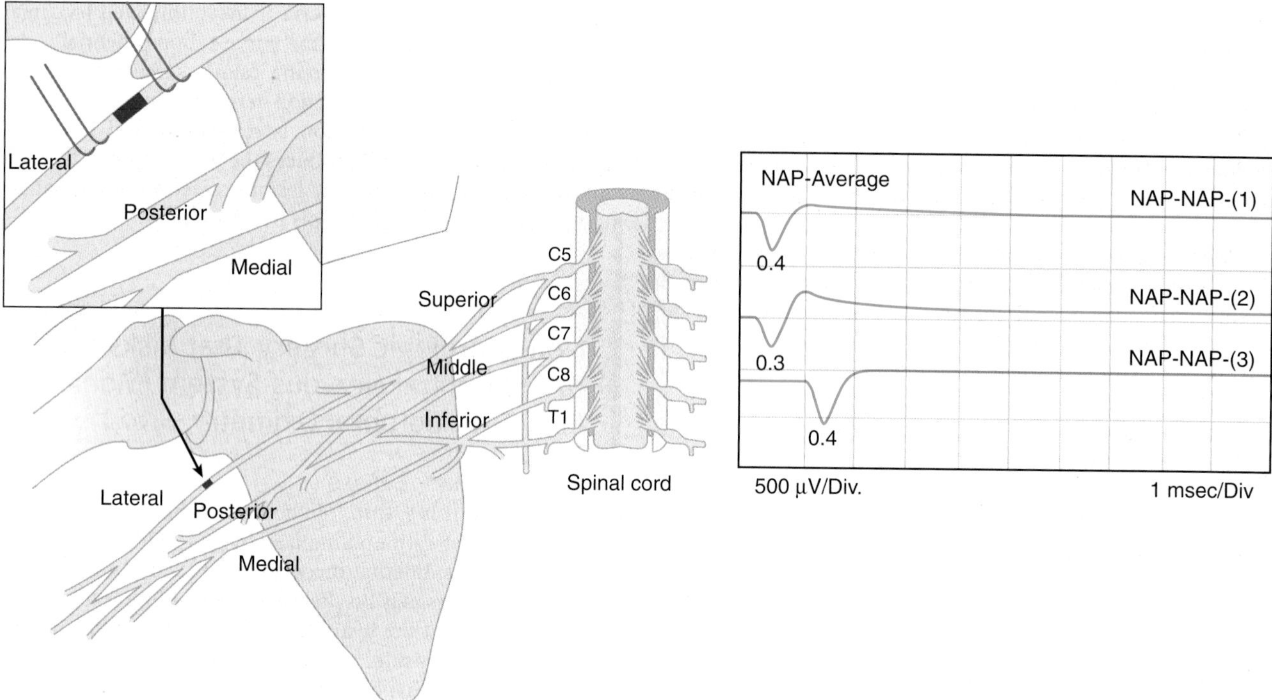

Figure 46-16 Recording a nerve action potential during a brachial plexus exploration. The site of the injury on the lateral fascicle is indicated in *red*. As shown in the *inset*, the surgeon places hook electrodes on either side of the exposed part of the nerve. If the injury is limited to an axonotmesis, proximal stimulation will result in a distal nerve action potential similar to the ones shown in the recording to the right. The delay in the response in the third tracing is simply due to a change in technical settings.

TCD during CPB does not stand up to evidence-based examination, primarily because of lack of information. Probe placement instability and inability to obtain signals in some patients also have limited the use of this monitor intraoperatively.

Cerebral Oximetry and Jugular Venous Oxygen Saturation. As is the case with EEG monitoring during CPB, there are multiple case reports and several series that advocate the use of NIRS or $Sjvo_2$ as indicators of adequate perfusion of the brain during CPB.[168,169] Incorrect placement of CPB cannulas has been detected clinically and in laboratory studies. One more recent series of patients undergoing CPB for coronary bypass surgery showed a higher incidence of major organ system dysfunction and longer hospital stays in patients with lower baseline and intraoperative cerebral oxygen saturation values.[170] The same questions exist for this application of NIRS, however, as do for the use of NIRS during carotid vascular surgery. Use of NIRS during CPB, although it provides information that would not otherwise be available, does not stand up to evidence-based examination, and much more work is needed before NIRS can be recommended as a standard of care during CPB.

$Sjvo_2$ is very invasive. Although data from case reports and studies suggest that $Sjvo_2$ may have utility in detecting inadequate CBF, lack of outcome data, lack of clearly defined critical values at different temperatures during CPB, and availability of more noninvasive modalities (EEG, cerebral oximetry) have resulted in only limited use of this monitoring method during CPB. Based on current information, no neurologic monitoring techniques either alone or in combination are clearly useful in improving outcome during surgery requiring CPB. Further research is needed before the cost in personnel and in equipment of neurologic monitoring during CPB can be justified.

Intensive Care Applications of Neurologic Monitoring (Monitors: EEG, Evoked Potentials, TCD, $Sjvo_2$)

Secondary injury to the CNS has been recognized in past decades as a major modifiable risk factor in patients with CNS disease. Aneurysmal subarachnoid hemorrhage, stroke, and traumatic brain injury are examples of CNS insults in which secondary injury has important implications for the ultimate functional outcome.[171-173] The same diseases frequently result in a primary insult to the CNS that severely constrains the utility of the clinical neurologic examination because of the need for mechanical ventilation and sedation. Many techniques of neurologic monitoring discussed earlier also have been used in the intensive care unit. Generally, however, techniques that require continued presence of skilled technologists, such as monitoring of evoked potentials, are prohibitively expensive and of less practical value than techniques that can be performed as a daily examination, or techniques that provide data easily integrated into the intensive care frame of mind. Along with monitoring, some of the techniques discussed previously also can provide important prognostic information in comatose patients and guide decision making.

Cerebral Ischemia

Cerebral ischemia is an important cause of secondary injury to the CNS. It can be difficult to detect in patients who are either comatose or sedated, but can occur even in the face of an adequate cerebral perfusion pressure.[174,175] Three techniques may provide intensivists with additional information about cerebral perfusion. None of the monitors is considered "standard of care." As with all monitors, the impact of the monitor on outcome depends on the quality of the therapeutic interventions that result from integration of the additional data into the clinical management of a given patient.

$Sjvo_2$ monitoring is used most extensively in the intensive care unit to monitor patients with traumatic brain injury. The data have been used to guide blood pressure and ventilatory management to optimize blood flow. $Sjvo_2$ monitoring has had a major effect on ventilatory management of head-injured patients and has significantly reduced the routine use of hyperventilation in neurosurgical patients.[176-180] $Sjvo_2$ values of less than 50% generally indicate cerebral ischemia. Increases in $Sjvo_2$ may occur in response to therapy, or may be an ominous sign if the increase is caused by falling demand because of neuronal death.

Similar to $Sjvo_2$ monitoring, monitoring of $P_{Br}O_2$ and blood flow is used most frequently in patients with traumatic brain injury. $P_{Br}O_2$ performs well in clinical practice. Decreases to less than 10 to 15 mm Hg are associated with worsening outcome,[27,180] whereas $P_{Br}O_2$-targeted treatment strategies may improve outcome.[181] The data for thermal diffusion CBF are not as comprehensive, perhaps reflecting the slightly less robust technology.[182] Nonetheless, in the setting of subarachnoid hemorrhage, thermal diffusion CBF less than 15 mL/100 g/min showed a sensitivity of 90% and a specificity of 75% for detecting symptomatic vasospasm.[19]

TCD is widely used in the intensive care unit to document the presence and severity of cerebral vasospasm after subarachnoid hemorrhage. As the major cerebral arteries narrow, flow velocity within the lumen must increase if blood flow is to be maintained. Such narrowing occurs 12 to 24 hours before the onset of clinical symptoms, allowing therapy to be initiated before the onset of clinical symptoms.[183-187] Mean flow velocities of more than 120 cm/sec seem to correlate well with angiographic vasospasm,[188,189] although intracranial pressure and concurrent therapy with hypertensive hypervolemic hemodilution modify the flow velocity. The latter two factors result in characteristic changes of the TCD waveform, however, preserving the utility of the examination.

Prognosis in Coma and Determination of Brain Death.

EEG monitoring may help to assess the clinical course and the prognosis of comatose patients. Assessment of prognosis must be separated from the insult that precipitated the coma by more than 24 hours. If not, the EEG may reflect predominantly the effect of the insult and may not predict prognosis. More than 24 hours after the insult, spontaneous sustained burst suppression correlates strongly with severe irreversible brain injury.[190] Absence of EEG variability portends a high likelihood of persistent vegetative state or death,[190,191] whereas spontaneous variability, reactivity to external stimuli, and typical sleep patterns are associated with more favorable outcomes.[192-194]

A specific indication for EEG monitoring is the therapeutic induction of a coma by barbiturate administration. Because neither blood nor cerebrospinal fluid concentrations of barbiturates reliably predict burst suppression and near-maximal reduction in cerebral metabolic rate of oxygen consumption,[195] and because barbiturate administration usually requires an increase in cardiovascular support, documentation of a burst suppression pattern on EEG allows the use of the minimal effective dose of barbiturate.

Similar to EEG, evoked potential studies have a place in predicting prognosis in comatose patients. The presence of normal SSEPs bilaterally is an excellent prognostic sign, whereas the absence of any SSEP cortical response is a poor prognostic indicator. The degree of bad outcome can be predicted by BAEPs. Intact and normal BAEPs with absent cortical SSEPs predict a best outcome of a chronic vegetative state. Outcome may be worse, however, because BAEPs commonly deteriorate later with rostral-to-caudal deterioration. Absent BAEP responses beyond wave I predict a high likelihood of brain death. Present but abnormal SSEPs are associated with outcomes intermediate between good/high function and a chronic vegetative state.[196-205]

TCD also has been used in the intensive care unit as an aid to the diagnosis of brain death. As intracranial pressure increases, the pulsatility of the TCD waveform increases, accentuating the systolic peak and diminishing flow during diastole. With further increases in intracranial pressure, a characteristic to-and-fro pattern of flow is established, which is consistent with clinical brain death.[206] TCD studies are easily performed at the bedside and can minimize the need for unnecessary transports of the patient for definitive radiologic studies.

Nonsurgical Factors Influencing Monitoring Results

Anesthesia and the Electroencephalogram

Anesthetic drugs affect the frequency and amplitude of EEG waveforms. Although each drug class and each specific drug has some specific, dose-related EEG effects (Table 46-2), some basic anesthesia-related EEG patterns may be described. Subanesthetic doses of intravenous and inhaled anesthetics usually produce an increase in frontal beta activity and abolish the alpha activity normally seen in the occipital leads in an awake, relaxed patient with the eyes closed. As the patient actually goes to sleep with general anesthesia, the brain waves become larger in amplitude and slower in frequency. In the frontal areas, small beta activity seen in an awake patient slows to the alpha range and increases in size. In combination with the loss of the occipital alpha activity, this phenomenon produces the appearance of a "shift" of the alpha activity from the posterior cortex to the anterior cortex. Further increases in the dose of the inhalation or intravenous agent produce further slowing of the EEG, and some agents have the capability to suppress EEG activity totally (see Table 46-2). Other agents never produce burst suppression or an isoelectric EEG, despite increasing dose, either because they are incapable of completely suppressing the EEG (e.g., opioids, benzodiazepines) or because cardiovascular toxicity of the drug (e.g., halothane) prevents administration of a large enough dose.

Intravenous Anesthetic Drugs

Barbiturates, Propofol, and Etomidate. Despite widely varying potencies and durations of action, barbiturates, propofol, and etomidate produce similar EEG patterns (Fig. 46-17 shows

Table 46-2 Anesthetic Drugs and Electroencephalogram (EEG)

Drug	Effect on EEG Frequency	Effect on EEG Amplitude	Burst Suppression?
Isoflurane			Yes, >1.5 MAC
Subanesthetic	Loss of alpha, ↑ frontal beta	↑	
Anesthetic	Frontal 4-13 Hz activity	↑	
Increasing dose >1.5 MAC	Diffuse theta and delta → burst suppression → silence	↑ → 0	
Desflurane	Similar to equi-MAC dose of isoflurane	Similar to equi-MAC dose of isoflurane	Yes, >1.5 MAC
Sevoflurane	Similar to equi-MAC dose of isoflurane	Similar to equi-MAC dose of isoflurane	Yes, >1.5 MAC
Nitrous oxide (alone)	Frontal fast oscillatory activity (>30 Hz)	↑, especially with inspired concentration >50%	No
Enflurane			Yes, >1.5 MAC
Subanesthetic	Loss of alpha, ↑ frontal beta	↑	
Anesthetic	↑ frontal 7-12 Hz activity	↑	
Increasing dose >1.5 MAC	Spikes/spike and slow waves → burst suppression; hypocapnia → seizures	↑↑ → 0	
Halothane			Not seen in clinically useful dosage range
Subanesthetic	↑ frontal 10-20 Hz activity	↑	
Anesthetic	↑ frontal 10-15 Hz activity	↑	
Increasing dose >1.5 MAC	Diffuse theta, slowing with increasing dose	↑	
Barbiturates			Yes, with high doses
Low dose	Fast frontal beta activity	Slight ↑	
Moderate dose	Frontal alpha frequency spindles	↑	
Increasing high dose	Diffuse delta → burst suppression → silence	↑↑↑ → 0	
Etomidate			Yes, with high doses
Low dose	Fast frontal beta activity	↑	
Moderate dose	Frontal alpha frequency spindles	↑	
Increasing high dose	Diffuse delta → burst suppression → silence	↑↑ → 0	
Propofol			Yes, with high doses
Low dose	Loss of alpha, ↑ frontal beta	↑	
Moderate dose	Frontal delta, waxing/waning alpha	↑	
Increasing high dose	Diffuse delta → burst suppression → silence	↑↑ → 0	
Ketamine			No
Low dose	Loss of alpha, ↑ variability	↑↓	
Moderate dose	Frontal rhythmic delta	↑	
High dose	Polymorphic delta, some beta	↑↑ (beta is low amplitude)	
Benzodiazepines			No
Low dose	Loss of alpha, increased frontal beta activity	↑	
High dose	Frontally dominant delta and theta	↑	
Opiates			No
Low dose	Loss of beta, alpha slows	↔ ↑	
Moderate dose	Diffuse theta, some delta	↑	
High dose	Delta, often synchronized	↑↑	
Dexmedetomidine	Moderate slowing, prominent spindles	↑↑	No

*delta = <4 Hz frequency; theta = 4-7 Hz frequency; alpha = 8-13 Hz frequency; beta = >13 Hz frequency.
MAC, minimum alveolar concentration.

EEG effects of thiopental). These drugs all follow the basic anesthesia-related EEG pattern described previously with initial EEG activation (see Fig. 46-17A), followed by dose-related depression. As the patient loses consciousness, characteristic frontal spindles are seen (see Fig. 46-17B), which are replaced by polymorphic 1- to 3-Hz activity (see Fig. 46-17C) as the drug dose is increased. Further increases in dose result in lengthening periods of suppression interspersed with periods of activity (burst suppression). With a very high dose, EEG silence results. All of these drugs have been reported to cause epileptiform activity in humans, but epi-

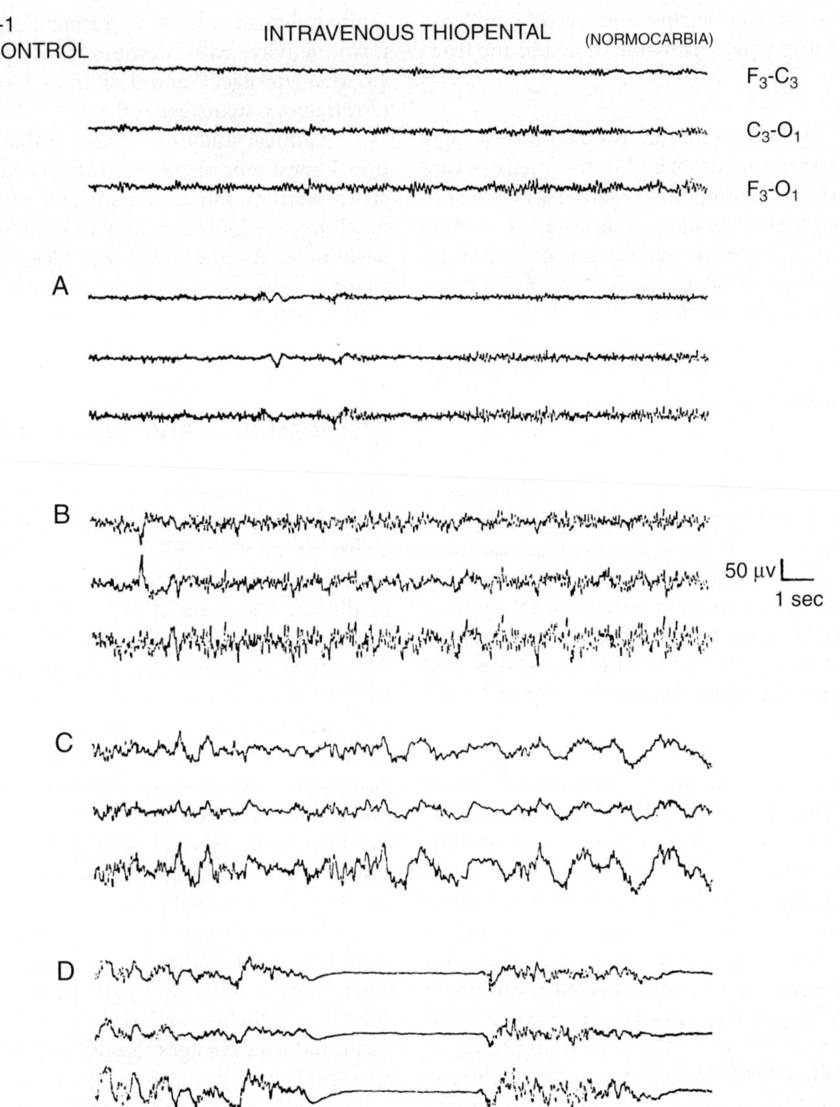

Figure 46-17 Electroencephalogram effects of intravenous administration of thiopental in humans. **A,** Rapid activity. **B,** Barbiturate spindles. **C,** Slow waves. **D,** Burst suppression. *(From Clark DL, Rosner BS: Neurophysiologic effects of general anesthetics. Anesthesiology 38:564, 1973.)*

leptiform activity is clinically significant only after methohexital and etomidate when given in subhypnotic doses.

Ketamine. Ketamine does not follow the basic anesthesia-related EEG pattern. Anesthesia with ketamine is characterized by frontally dominant rhythmic, high-amplitude theta activity. Increasing doses produce intermittent polymorphic delta activity of very large amplitude interspersed with low-amplitude beta activity.[207] Electrocortical silence cannot be produced with ketamine. EEG activity may be very disorganized and variable at all doses. This disorganization of the EEG with ketamine is responsible for the failure of the bispectral index to be useful in looking at the effect of ketamine on consciousness. Recovery of normal EEG activity even after a single bolus dose of ketamine is slow compared with barbiturates. There is no information available about the relationship between emergence reactions after ketamine and the EEG. Ketamine also has been associated with increased epileptiform activity.[207]

Benzodiazepines. Despite varying potencies and durations of action, benzodiazepines also follow the basic anesthesia-related EEG pattern. As a class, however, these drugs are incapable of producing burst suppression or an isoelectric EEG.

Opioids. As a class, opioids do not follow the basic anesthesia-related EEG pattern. Opioids generally produce a dose-related decrease in frequency and increase in amplitude of the EEG. If no further doses of opiates are given, alpha and beta activity return as drug redistribution occurs. The rapidity of return depends on the initial dose and on the drug. Remifentanil is associated with the most rapid return to normal.[208] Complete suppression of the EEG cannot be obtained with opioids. Epileptiform activity occurs in humans and in animals receiving large to supraclinical doses of opioids. Sharp wave activity is common after induction of anesthesia with fentanyl, with 20% of patients showing this phenomenon after 30 µg/kg; 60%, after 50 µg/kg; 58%, after 60 µg/kg; and 80%, after 70 µg/kg. Alfentanil bolus has been used clinically to activate seizure foci during epilepsy surgery.[209] This epileptiform activity is mainly noted in the frontotemporal region.[210]

Dexmedetomidine. Dexmedetomidine is being increasingly used for sedation in the operating room and in the intensive care unit. EEG studies of patients undergoing sedation with dexmedetomidine alone show patterns similar to those seen in normal human sleep with increased slow-wave activity and sleep spindles prominent.[211] Burst suppression or an isoelectric EEG pattern cannot be produced even with high doses of the drug. Level of sedation with dexmedetomidine can be effectively monitored using processed EEG parameters and has been reported using bispectral index and entropy techniques.[212]

Inhaled Anesthetics

Nitrous Oxide. Used alone, nitrous oxide causes a decrease in amplitude and frequency of the dominant occipital alpha rhythm. With the onset of analgesia and depressed consciousness, frontally dominant fast oscillatory activity (>30 Hz) is frequently seen.[213] This activity may persist to some extent for 50 minutes after discontinuation of nitrous oxide. When nitrous oxide is used in combination with other agents, it increases the effects that would be associated with the agent alone clinically and with respect to the EEG pattern seen.

Isoflurane, Sevoflurane, Enflurane, Halothane, and Desflurane. Potent inhaled anesthetics follow the basic anesthesia-related EEG pattern. Isoflurane initially causes an activation of the EEG followed by a slowing of the EEG activity that is more marked with increasing dose. Isoflurane begins to produce periods of EEG suppression at 1.5 minimum alveolar concentration (MAC), which become longer with increasing dose until electric silence is produced at 2 to 2.5 MAC. Isolated epileptiform patterns sometimes can be seen during intersuppression activity at 1.5 to 2 MAC isoflurane.[214] Sevoflurane causes similar dose-dependent EEG effects. Equi-MAC concentrations of sevoflurane and isoflurane cause similar EEG changes.[215] Epileptiform activity has been induced by administration of sevoflurane in patients without epilepsy, and seizure activity on EEG, but not clinical seizure activity, has been reported in pediatric patients with a history of epilepsy during induction of anesthesia with sevoflurane.[216,217] Despite these observations, sevoflurane, similar to other inhalation agents, is not suitable for use during electrocorticography for localization of seizure foci.[218] EEG patterns seen with enflurane are similar to the patterns seen with isoflurane except that epileptiform activity is considerably more prominent. At 2 to 3 MAC, burst suppression is seen, but virtually all intersuppression activity consists of large spike/wave pattern discharges. Hyperventilation with high concentrations of enflurane increases the length of suppression, decreases the duration of bursts, but increases the amplitude and main frequency component of the intersuppression epileptiform activity. Frank EEG seizures also may occur with enflurane that produce the same cerebral metabolic effects as pentylenetetrazol, a known convulsant.

Halothane also produces EEG patterns similar to those of isoflurane, but dosages of halothane that would produce burst suppression in the EEG (3 to 4 MAC) are associated with profound cardiovascular toxicity. Desflurane produces EEG changes similar in nature to equi-MAC concentrations of isoflurane. In limited clinical studies, there has been no evidence of epileptiform activity with desflurane, despite hyperventilation and 1.6 MAC dosage,[219] and desflurane has been used as a treatment of refractory status epilepticus.[220]

Clinical studies have shown that the EEG effects of inhalational anesthetic agents are influenced by age and baseline EEG characteristics. Older patients and patients with EEG slowing at baseline were more sensitive to the EEG effects of isoflurane and desflurane. As anesthesia was deepened, similar EEG pattern changes were noted, but these changes occurred at lower end-tidal anesthetic concentrations.[221]

Anesthesia and Sensory Evoked Responses

Volatile Anesthetics

Multiple drugs used in the perioperative period can influence the ability to monitor SERs accurately (Table 46-3). A more recent review provides the interested clinician with a detailed analysis of all drug effects on SERs,[222] which is beyond the scope of this chapter. Table 46-3 does not quantify drug effects, but rather lists whether an individual drug is capable of producing a change in any part of an evoked response that could be mistaken for a surgically induced change. A "no" designation in this table does not mean that there are no effects of a given drug on SERs. The "no" designation indicates that any effects that do occur would not be called clinically significant by *clinicians experienced in intraoperative monitoring*. Several general concepts (Table 46-4) help the clinician who is trying to determine the best choice of drugs for use during monitored cases.

The volatile anesthetics isoflurane, sevoflurane, desflurane, enflurane, and halothane have similar effects in differing degrees on all types of SERs. VEPs are the most sensitive to the effects of volatile anesthetics, and BAEPs are the most resistant to anesthetic-induced changes. Spinal and subcortical SSEP responses are significantly less affected than cortical potentials.[223-225]

SSEPs, because they are the most widely used intraoperative SER technique, are the most completely studied with respect to the effects of anesthetic drugs. The effects of the currently used volatile agents on cortical SSEPs are dose-dependent increases in latency and conduction times and a decrease in amplitude of cortically, but not subcortically recorded signals.[223-227] When comparing the different volatile agents, studies have reported conflicting results.[223,225] One study suggests that halothane has a greater impact on cortical SSEPs than either isoflurane or enflurane,[225] whereas another published report supports a greater effect produced by enflurane and isoflurane than halothane.[223] None of these differences are clinically important and may be ignored by the practicing clinician. With respect to the newer agents, desflurane and sevoflurane seem to have qualitatively and quantitatively similar effects on SERs as isoflurane.[228-232] In neurologically normal patients, 0.5 to 1 MAC of any of the potent inhaled agents in the presence of nitrous oxide is compatible with monitoring of cortical SSEPs (Figs. 46-18, 46-19, and 46-20).[223,227] Neurologically impaired patients may show a significantly greater sensitivity to inhaled agents, even to the point of not tolerating any recordable level of inhaled agent. Generally, better monitoring conditions are obtained, however, with narcotic-based anesthetics with less than 1 MAC total (nitrous oxide plus potent agent) end-tidal inhaled anesthetic concentration.

Table 46-3 Ability of an Individual Anesthetic Drug to Produce a Change in Sensory and Motor Evoked Potentials That Could Be Mistaken for a Surgically Induced Change

	SSEPs		BAEPs		VEPs		Transcranial MEPs	
Drug	**LAT**	**AMP**	**LAT**	**AMP**	**LAT**	**AMP**	**LAT**	**AMP**
Isoflurane	Yes	Yes	No	No	Yes	Yes	Yes	Yes
Enflurane	Yes	Yes	No	No	Yes	Yes	Yes	Yes
Halothane	Yes	Yes	No	No	Yes	Yes	Yes	Yes
Nitrous oxide*	Yes	Yes	No	No	Yes	Yes	Yes	Yes
Barbiturates	Yes	Yes	No	No	Yes	Yes	Yes	Yes
Etomidate	No	No	No	No	Yes	Yes	No	No
Propofol	Yes	Yes	No	No	Yes	Yes	Yes	Yes
Droperidol	No	No	No	No	—	—	Yes	Yes
Diazepam	Yes	Yes	No	No	Yes	Yes	Yes	Yes
Midazolam	Yes	Yes	No	No	Yes	Yes	Yes	Yes
Ketamine	No	No	No	No	Yes	Yes	No	No
Opiates	No	No	No	No	No	No	No	No
Dexmedetomidine	No	No	No	No	No	ND	ND	No

Note: This table is not quantitative in any way. "Yes" or "no" designations indicate whether an individual drug is capable of producing an effect on any portion of the evoked response that could be mistaken for a surgically induced change.
*Increases the effect of the agent(s) with which it is used.
(p): Use of this drug and any dose may render this type of monitoring impossible for a signifieant period of time.
AMP, amplitude; BAEPs, brainstem auditory evoked potentials; LAT, latency; MEPs, motor evoked potentials; ND, no data available from the literature; SSEPs, somatosensory evoked potentials; VEPs, visual evoked potentials.

The volatile anesthetics result in increases in latency of BAEPs without significantly affecting the amplitude.[227,233-235] Volatile anesthetics cause increases in latency and decreases in amplitude in the early (middle latency) cortical responses after auditory stimulation,[234] however, and these middle latency responses are now being used to monitor the hypnotic component of general anesthetics.[32] Adequate monitoring of BAEPs is possible with any clinically useful concentrations of inhaled agents (with or without nitrous oxide) (Figs. 46-21 and 46-22).[227,233-236]

Use of the volatile agents during monitoring of VEPs results in dose-dependent increases in latency with or without changes in amplitude.[227,237-240] Isoflurane results in dose-dependent increases in latency and decreases in amplitude up to 1.8% in 100% oxygen, at which time the waveform is lost.[227,237] Enflurane in the absence of hypocarbia also leads to decrease in amplitude.[237] Halothane causes increases in latency without changes in amplitude.[238,239] Although the data from these studies seem valid, the results are not clinically relevant because the variability of VEPs in anesthetized patients is so great that satisfactory monitoring, in the opinion of many experts, is impossible using any anesthetic technique.

Although volatile anesthetics cause significant changes in the SER waveforms, it is possible to provide adequate monitoring intraoperatively in the presence of anesthetic doses of volatile anesthetics. Doses of agents causing significant depression of the

Table 46-4 Guidelines for Choosing Anesthetic Techniques During Procedures in Which Sensory Evoked Responses Are Monitored

1. Intravenous agents have significantly less effect than "equipotent" doses of inhaled anesthetics
2. Combinations of drugs generally produce "additive" effects
3. Subcortical (spinal or brainstem) sensory evoked responses are very resistant to the effects of anesthetic drugs. If subcortical responses provide sufficient information for the surgical procedure, anesthetic technique is not important, and effects on cortically recorded responses may be ignored

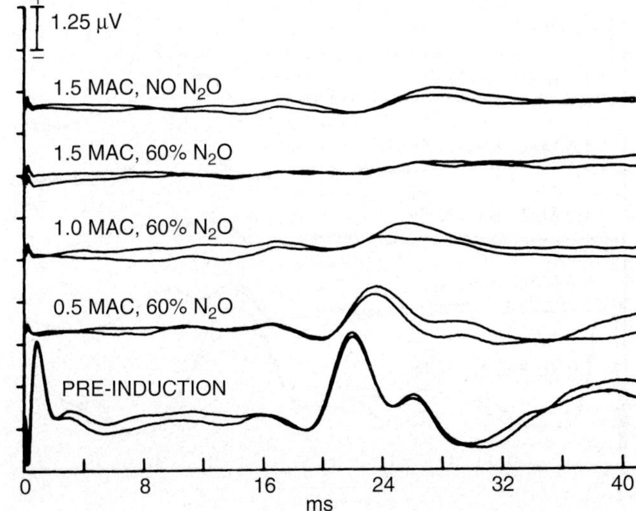

Figure 46-18 Representative somatosensory evoked potential cortical responses (C-3, C-4-FPz) at various minimum alveolar concentration (MAC) levels of isoflurane. *(From Peterson DO, Drummond JC, Todd MM: Effects of halothane, enflurane, isoflurane, and nitrous oxide on somatosensory evoked potentials in humans. Anesthesiology 65:35, 1986.)*

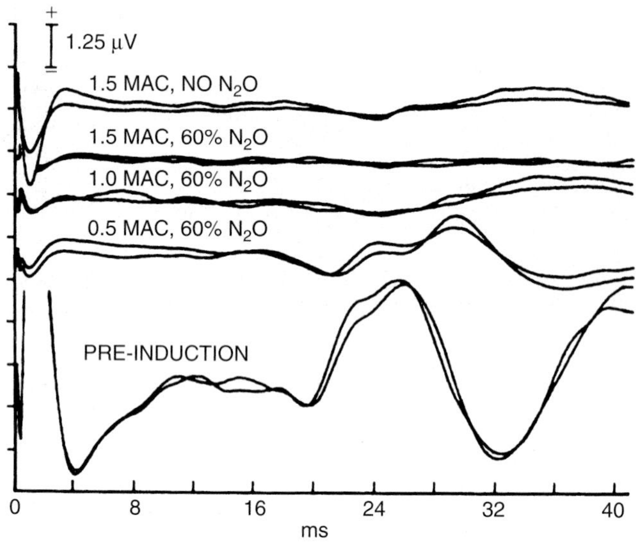

Figure 46-19 Representative somatosensory evoked potential cortical responses (C-3, or C-4-FPz) at various minimum alveolar concentration (MAC) levels of enflurane. *(From Peterson DO, Drummond JC, Todd MM: Effects of halothane, enflurane, isoflurane, and nitrous oxide on somatosensory evoked potentials in humans. Anesthesiology 65:35, 1986.)*

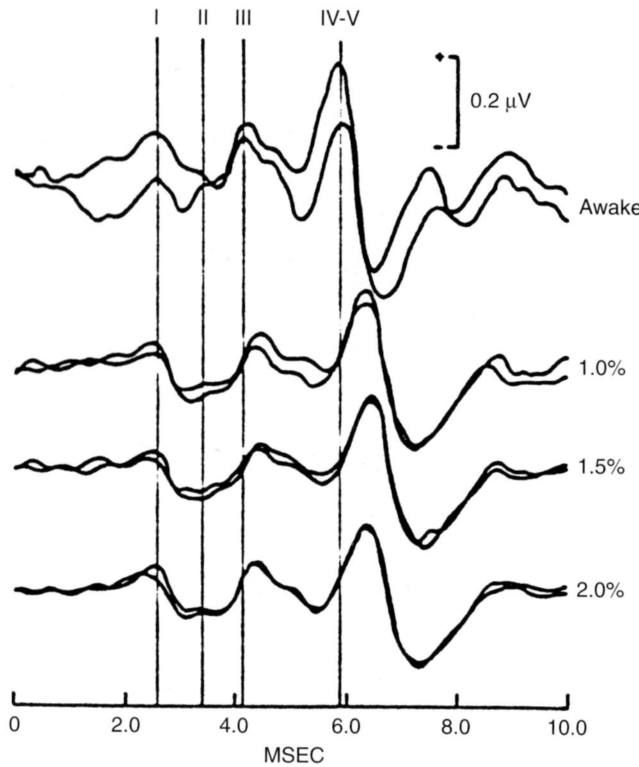

Figure 46-21 Influence of isoflurane alone on brainstem auditory evoked potential in a typical subject. Latency of peaks III and IV to V increased at 1.0%, but stabilized with increasing anesthetic depth. *(From Manninen PH, Lam AM, Nicholas JF: The effects of isoflurane–nitrous oxide anesthesia on brainstem auditory evoked potentials in humans. Anesth Analg 64:43, 1985.)*

response to be monitored must be prevented. In the authors' experience, end-tidal concentrations of inhaled agents totaling greater than 1.3 MAC have a dose-related, increasing probability of obliterating cortical SSEPs even in neurologically normal patients. Equally important, anesthetic concentration should not be changed during the critical periods of intraoperative monitoring. Critical periods are defined as periods in which surgical interventions are most likely to result in damage to neurologic tissue and changes in the SERs. Because the volatile anesthetic-induced changes in SERs are dose-dependent, increasing anesthetic dosage at a crucial point in the operative procedure can result in confusing changes in the SERs that potentially may be caused by the anesthetic, the surgical procedure, or both. The appropriate intervention is difficult to determine.

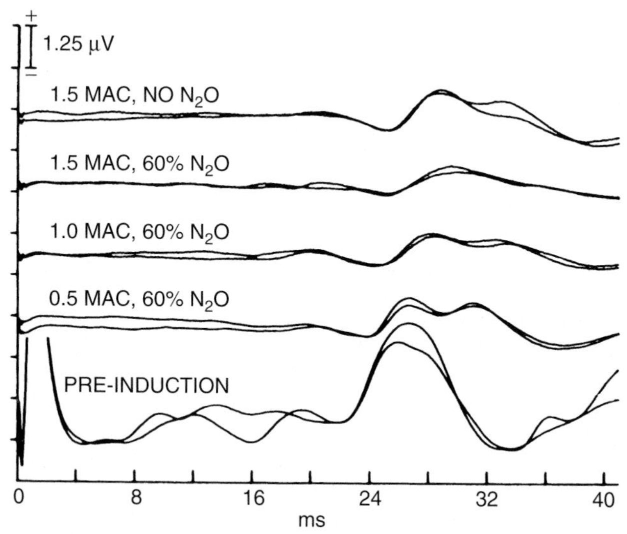

Figure 46-20 Representative somatosensory evoked potential cortical responses (C-3, C-4-FPz) at various minimum alveolar concentration (MAC) levels of halothane. *(From Peterson DO, Drummond JC, Todd MM: Effects of halothane, enflurane, isoflurane, and nitrous oxide on somatosensory evoked potentials in humans. Anesthesiology 65:35, 1986.)*

As with the volatile anesthetics, nitrous oxide causes differing effects on the SERs depending on the sensory system monitored. It causes decreases in amplitude without significant changes in latency in SSEPs when used alone or when added to a narcotic-based or volatile anesthetic.[223,224,241] The addition of nitrous oxide to a maintenance volatile anesthetic during the monitoring of BAEPs causes no further change.[233] Likewise, use of nitrous oxide alone causes no change in BAEPs, unless gas accumulates in the middle ear.[241] Use of nitrous oxide alone results in an increase in latency and a decrease in amplitude in VEPs, but when it is added to a volatile anesthetic technique, it causes no further changes in VEPs.[237,241]

Intravenous Agents

The effects of barbiturates on SERs have been studied in animal models and in humans. Increasing doses of thiopental in patients result in progressive dose-dependent increases in latency, decreases in amplitude of SSEPs, and progressive increases in latency of wave V in BAEPs. The changes in SSEPs are more pronounced than the changes in BAEPs, and waveforms beyond the initial primary cortical response are quickly obliterated. This finding is consistent with the theories that barbiturates affect synaptic transmission more than axonal conduction. Early wave-

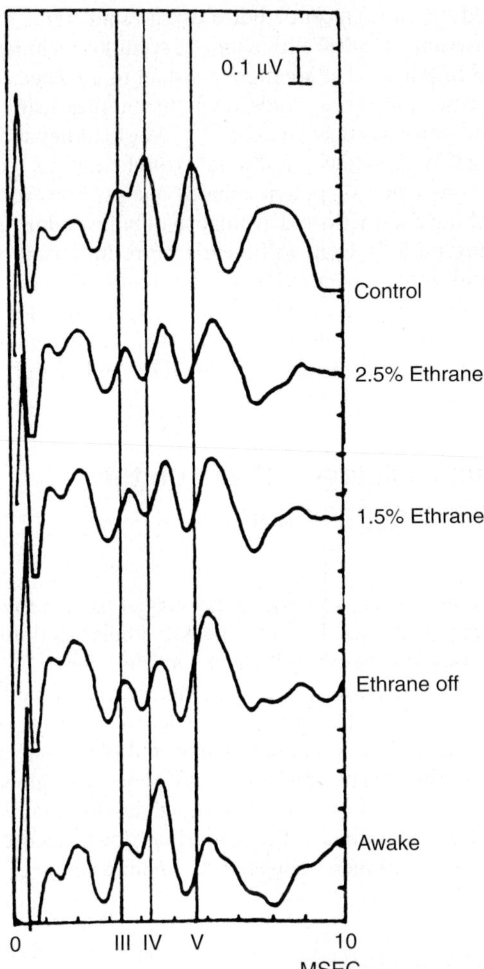

Figure 46-22 Brainstem auditory evoked potential recording obtained in one patient at different enflurane (Ethrane)-inspired concentrations. *(From Dubois MY, Sato S, Chassy J, et al: Effects of enflurane on brainstem auditory evoked responses in humans. Anesth Analg 61:898, 1982.)*

forms in SERs result primarily from axonal transmission, and later waves depend on multisynaptic pathways in addition to axonal transmission. At doses of thiopental far greater than doses producing an isoelectric EEG, adequate monitoring of early cortical and subcortical SSEPs and BAEPs was preserved.[242] Other barbiturate compounds show similar effects. Somatosensory and auditory SERs were never obliterated even at doses greater than those causing complete suppression of spontaneous EEG activity.[243] This observation is important, especially when attempting to monitor the adequacy of CBF during cerebrovascular surgery when the patient has been given large, "protective" doses of barbiturates. The EEG is isoelectric and not helpful for monitoring. The early cortical SSEP waveforms are still preserved, however, and may be very helpful in determining adequacy of CBF. Preserved ability to monitor SSEPs in head-injured patients receiving therapeutic thiopental infusions has been shown.[244] VEPs are much more sensitive to barbiturates. Low barbiturate doses obliterate all except the earliest waveforms. The early potentials persisted with increases in latency even to very high pentobarbital doses.[245] Except for VEPs, adequate perioperative monitoring of SERs is possible even in the presence of high-dose barbiturate therapy as long as the effects of the drug (increased latency with moderately decreased amplitude) are considered.

After bolus administration and intravenous infusions, etomidate causes increases in latency of all waves and prolongation of central conduction time in SSEPs. In contrast to virtually all other commonly used anesthetics, etomidate causes increases in amplitude of the cortical SSEP.[246,247] This effect may be due to an alteration in the balance of inhibitory and excitatory influences or an increase in the irritability of the CNS. This effect seems to be present in the cortex, but not in the spinal cord.[247] Etomidate infusions have been used to enhance SSEP recording in patients when it was impossible to obtain reproducible responses at the beginning of intraoperative monitoring because of the patients' pathology (Fig. 46-23). Following baseline responses that could not be monitored, the etomidate augmentation of the SSEP allowed adequate monitoring and detection of intraoperative

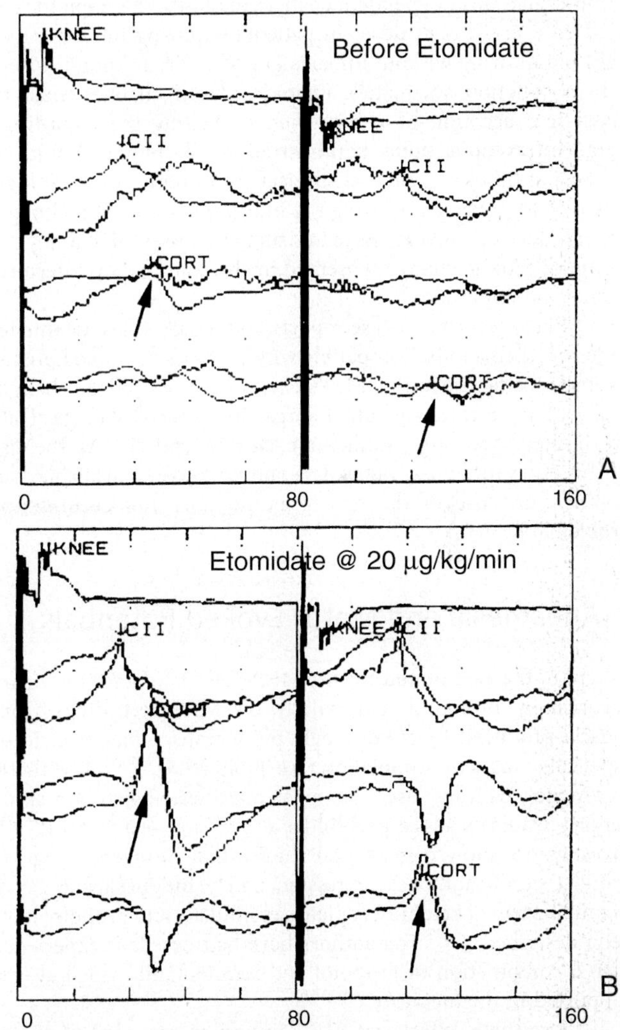

Figure 46-23 Effects of etomidate on somatosensory evoked potential. **A,** The *top tracings* were obtained from a mildly mentally impaired patient with severe kyphoscoliosis during the early maintenance phase of anesthesia using isoflurane and fentanyl. **B,** The *bottom tracings* were obtained after discontinuing isoflurane and instituting an etomidate infusion at 20 µg/kg/min. Note dramatically increased amplitude and clarity of the signal in the cortical channels (marked by *arrows*), which both are recorded with the same amplification scale.

events leading to compromise of the spinal cord.[247] The effects of etomidate on BAEPs are dose-dependent increases in latency and decreases in amplitude that are not clinically significant.[248]

Droperidol in premedicant doses has been shown to have varying effects on SSEPs. In most patients, decreases in amplitude and loss of late waves were noted. In a few patients, increases in amplitude were noted. In all patients, conduction time was prolonged.[249] Effects were not clinically significant. Benzodiazepines also can cause changes in SERs.[250,251] Diazepam causes increases in latency and decreases in amplitude of SSEPs, increases in latency in the cortical response after auditory stimulation, and no change in BAEPs.[250,251] Midazolam causes decreases in amplitude without changes in latency of SSEPs.[246]

Generally, opioids cause small dose-dependent increases in latency and decreases in amplitude of SSEPs. These changes are not clinically significant. Effects on amplitude are more variable than the latency increases.[252,253] Even at large doses of fentanyl (60 μg/kg), reproducible SSEPs can be recorded.[253] Other opiates cause similar dose-dependent changes in SSEPs.[252,254] Opioids can be used even in high doses in patients requiring intraoperative SSEP monitoring without impairment of ability to monitor neurologic function adequately. Opioid-induced changes must be taken into account, however, when evaluating the recordings. Large intravenous bolus administration of opioids should be avoided at times of potential surgical compromise to neurologic function to prevent confusing the interpretation of SEP changes if they develop. BAEPs were resistant to doses of fentanyl of 50 μg/kg with no changes observed in absolute latency, interpeak latency, or amplitude.[255]

Based on several case reports and small series, dexmedetomidine seems to be compatible with all types of evoked potential monitoring (including MEPs), and does not produce changes that would be mistaken for a surgically induced change. Data are limited, and large studies are lacking entirely. As the use of this drug increases, more data should become available, but at this time, use of dexmedetomidine does not seem to be problematic.

Anesthesia and Motor Evoked Potentials

Except in the case of neurogenic MEPs, effects of anesthetics are surprisingly profound, particularly on MEP recordings from muscle produced by either single pulse transcranial electric or especially magnetic stimulation (see Table 46-3).[256-261] Anesthetic techniques typically used by most anesthesiologists for spine surgery would produce prohibitive depression of the MEP.[262,263] Investigators showed in several studies that intravenous agents produce significantly less depression, and techniques using any of a combination of ketamine, opiates, etomidate, and propofol have been described.[264-270] The authors have had excellent experience with a combination of propofol and remifentanil, which also is supported in the literature.

Anesthetic effects on MEP responses recorded at spinal levels seem to be less serious. When responses are recorded from muscle, neuromuscular blocking agents should be monitored quantitatively, maintaining T1 twitch height at around 30% of control values to prevent excessive movement during the operation.[136,257] When responses are not recorded from muscle, profound relaxation is desirable because gross muscle movement produced by MEP stimulation is eliminated, facilitating the surgical procedure. More recent studies using rapid trains of stimuli with transcranial electric and magnetic stimulus techniques have produced responses that are more resistant to the effects of anesthetic agents, and more "traditional" techniques using inhaled agents and narcotics may be used.[271-273] Most studies support the use of total intravenous anesthesia as preferable to techniques using nitrous oxide or potent inhaled agents, however. Precise control of the anesthetic and avoidance of boluses during critical monitoring periods seem to be even more important than for SSEPs, and active cooperation of the anesthesia care team is essential for good, reproducible results. Figure 46-24 shows the dramatic effect of introduction of 0.3 MAC isoflurane to a total intravenous technique using propofol and remifentanil.

Pathophysiologic Effects on the Electroencephalogram

Hypoxia

Hypoxia may produce inadequate delivery of oxygen to the cerebral cortex generating EEG, and changes similar to those occurring with ischemia result. Initially, hypoxemia may not result in any EEG changes because the brain can increase blood flow to compensate. When the hypoxemia becomes severe enough, further increases in flow are impossible, and EEG changes occur. "Slowing" of the EEG during hypoxia is a nonspecific global effect. Fast frequencies are lost, and low frequencies dominate. Eventually, the EEG is abolished as the brain shuts down electric activity and diverts all oxygen delivered to maintenance of cellular integrity.

Hypotension

In a normal, awake patient, significant levels of hypotension seem to be needed to cause the earliest of CNS signs, as measured by discrimination tests such as the flicker-fusion test. This test examines the flicker rate at which the observer perceives the light to be continuous. In the early days of deliberate hypotension, this test was part of the preoperative evaluation to judge how far the pressure could be reduced during the operation. Clear signs of confusion and inability to concentrate or respond properly to simple commands generally represent very low levels of cerebral perfusion when caused by hypotension because the normal cerebral circulation has a large capacity to vasodilate and maintain normal flow in the face of significant hypotension.

The EEG changes associated with even this level of hypotension are not dramatic, although they are clear by comparison with a previously active recording. Herein lies the problem with using intraoperative EEG to determine whether a given level of hypotension has resulted in brain ischemia. EEG changes are not very pronounced and are bilateral. These changes also are nearly identical to the changes caused by increasing doses of many anesthetic drugs. EEG changes associated with hypotension can be detected, but when the hypotension is induced slowly and associated with changes in anesthetic drugs (e.g., use of isoflurane to reduce blood pressure), the changes are very difficult to interpret. EEG changes associated with acute, severe hypotension such as may be caused by sudden arrhythmias are easier to read. Many patients undergoing surgery do not have a normal cerebral circulation, however. In these individuals, even mild hypotension may result in significant cerebral ischemia. In these individuals, moni-

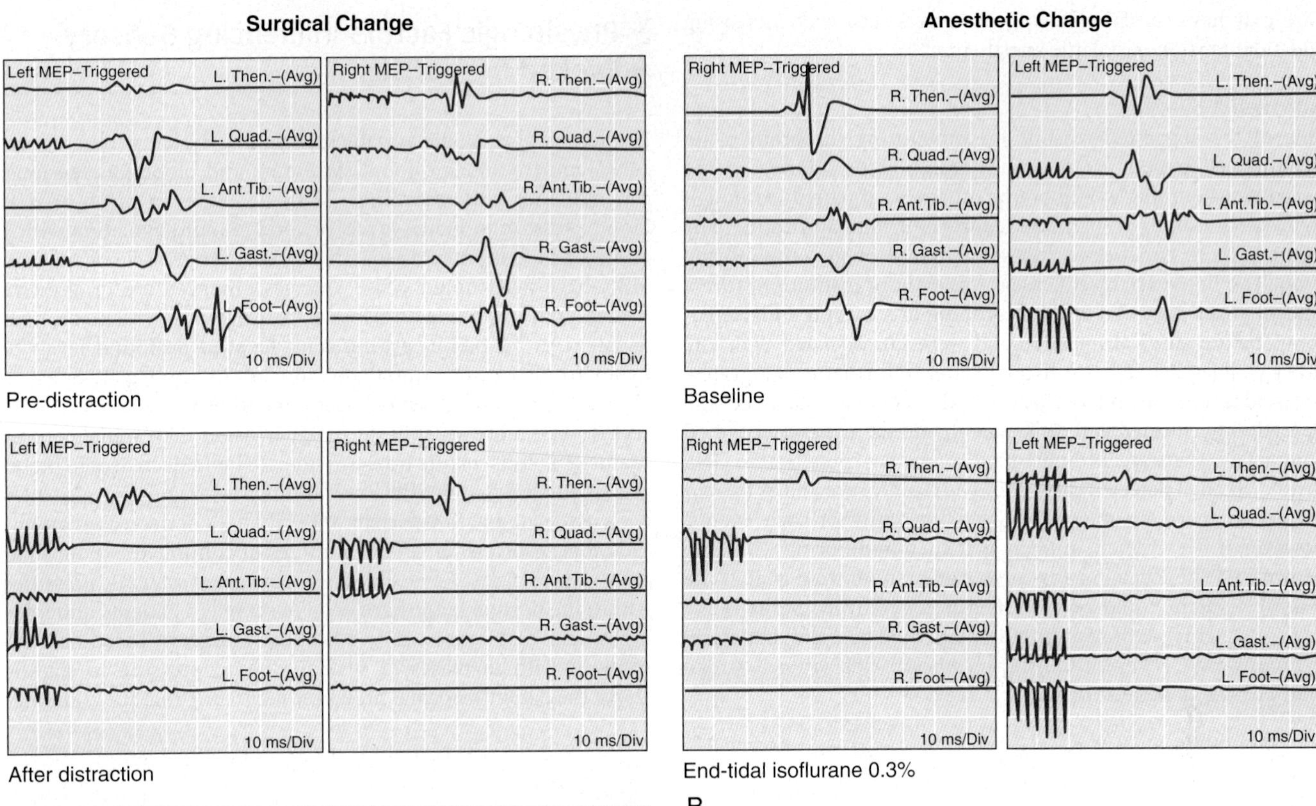

Figure 46-24 **A,** Transcranial electrical motor evoked potential recording showing surgically induced change during spine surgery (scoliosis repair). **B,** Motor evoked potential with an anesthetic-induced change. Note similarity of the change pattern except that in the anesthetic-induced change, the responses in the upper extremity also changed. Left-sided and right-sided responses are shown on the corresponding panel. A single upper extremity response is shown (*top tracing*) in each panel. Responses from four muscle groups in each lower extremity are shown directly below.

toring the EEG during planned hypotension may be helpful, provided that other causes of similar EEG changes may be carefully controlled. There remains little literature to support the use of EEG monitoring during hypotension, but in our opinion, when the EEG is being monitored (e.g., during carotid surgery), EEG changes secondary to hypotension really do represent cerebral ischemia of a significant degree and should be considered an important finding.

Hypothermia

During cooling on CPB, the total power and peak power frequency of the high-frequency band were highly correlated with temperature using Fourier analysis and spectral edge data; however, there was significant variability between subjects, especially during cooling.[274] Complete EEG suppression usually develops at 15°C to 18°C. Levy and colleagues[162] showed an improved ability to quantify the effects of hypothermia on the EEG using an EEG processing technique known as "approximate entropy."

Hypercarbia and Hypocarbia

Hypocapnia is known to activate excitable seizure foci, and in rare cases may produce EEG evidence of cerebral ischemia even in awake subjects.[275] Hypercapnia, unless severe and associated with hypoxemia, has only indirect effects secondary to increased CBF. In an anesthetized patient, hypercarbia-associated increases in

CBF may have similar effects to the effects seen with increasing end-tidal tension of volatile anesthetics.[276]

Untoward Events

One of the suggested reasons for monitoring the brain of an anesthetized patient is to enable detection of injuries to the nervous system that would not be otherwise apparent. Although there are hundreds of such case reports in the literature and many in the authors' experience, cost-effectiveness of such monitoring is unclear. In a more recent case at the authors' institution, severe EEG changes occurred at the beginning of a carotid endarterectomy, before surgical incision, and were unassociated with any other vital sign changes or hypotension. Immediate angiography revealed acute carotid occlusion and completely changed the operation performed with this patient, and the patient recovered completely. There are intraoperative events that could lead to CNS insult, which, if detected early, could be rapidly reversed or treated to prevent permanent injury. Given the rarity of such events, however, it is extremely unlikely that such monitoring would be shown to be beneficial in any foreseeable randomized trial. If the "at-risk" patient could be identified preoperatively, perhaps the EEG or other types of neuromonitoring could be useful in detecting untoward CNS events during anesthesia, such as a new stroke after elective general surgery.

Physiologic Factors Influencing Sensory Evoked Responses

Numerous physiologic variables, including systemic blood pressure, temperature (local and systemic), and blood gas tensions, can influence SEP recordings. With decreases in mean arterial blood pressure to below levels of cerebral autoregulation owing to either blood loss or vasoactive agents, progressive changes in SERs have been noted. SSEP changes observed are progressive decreases in amplitude until loss of the waveform with no changes in latency.[277,278] BAEPs are resistant to even profound levels of hypotension (mean arterial pressure of 20 mm Hg in dogs).[277] Cortical (synaptic) function necessary to produce cortical SERs seems to be more sensitive to hypoperfusion than spinal cord or brainstem, nonsynaptic transmission.[278] Rapid decreases in blood pressure to levels above the lower limit of autoregulation also have been associated with transient SSEP changes of decreased amplitude that resolve after several minutes of continued hypotension at the same level.[279] Reversible SSEP changes at systemic pressures within the normal range have been observed in patients undergoing spinal distraction during scoliosis surgery. These changes resolved with increases of systemic blood pressure to slightly above the patient's normal pressure, suggesting that the combina-

Table 46-5 Current Practices in Neurologic Monitoring

Procedure	Monitors	Current Practice
Carotid endarterectomy	Awake patient neurologic examination, EEG, SSEP, TCD	NIH recommends use of one of these four available monitors.
	CO	Threshold value not determined, inadequate normative population data
Scoliosis surgery	SSEP	Monitoring recommended, and may substitute for wake-up testing
	Wake-up test	Largely abandoned in centers using electrophysiologic monitoring. Monitoring is not continuous and false-negative monitoring patterns have been reported.
	MEP	Increased clinical use now that transcranial electrical stimulation is FDA approved. Useful in combination with SSEP
Acoustic neuroma	Facial nerve monitor	Facial nerve monitoring recommended
	BAEP	BAEP shows some clinical evidence of improved outcome in some procedures.
Intracranial aneurysm clipping	SSEP, EEG	Used routinely in some centers; limited clinical data on outcome, but appears clinically useful during anterior circulation procedures
Cranial nerve V decompression	BAEP	Used in some centers, reduces hearing loss
Cranial nerve VII decompression	BAEP	Data from small series show improved hearing preservation
Supratentorial mass lesions	SSEP	Used in some centers in selected high-risk procedures
Infratentorial mass lesions	BAEP/SSEP	BAEP to detect retractor-related cranial nerve VIII injury; SSEP in rare, high-risk lesions adjacent to ascending sensory pathways
Decompression of spinal stenosis	SSEP	Used in some centers in high-risk procedures (more often cervical)
Spinal cord trauma	SSEP/MEP	Used in some centers in high-risk procedures
Cardiopulmonary bypass	EEG, TCD, $Sjvo_2$, CO	Used routinely in some centers, actively studied, but no outcome data as of yet
Aortic coarctation	SSEP	Used routinely in a few centers, no widespread acceptance
Aortic aneurysm repair	SSEP	Used routinely in a few centers, no widespread acceptance
	MEP	Used routinely in a few centers, no widespread acceptance

BAEP, brainstem auditory evoked potential; CO, cerebral oximetry; EEG, electroencephalogram; FDA, U.S. Food and Drug Administration; MEP, motor evoked potential; NIH, National Institutes of Health; $Sjvo_2$, jugular bulb venous oxygen saturation; TCD, transcranial Doppler.

tion of surgical manipulation with levels of hypotension generally considered "safe" could result in spinal cord ischemia.[280]

Changes in temperature also affect SERs. Hypothermia causes increases in latency and decreases in amplitude of cortical and subcortical SERs after all types of stimulation.[281-283] Hyperthermia also alters SERs, with increases in temperature leading to decreases in amplitude in SSEPs and loss of SSEPs at 42°C during induced hyperthermia.[284]

Changes in arterial blood gas tensions have been reported to alter SERs, probably in relation to changes in blood flow or oxygen delivery to neural structures.[285,286] Hypoxia produces SSEP changes (decreased amplitude) similar to the changes seen with ischemia.[286] Decreased oxygen delivery associated with anemia during isovolemic hemodilution results in progressive increases in latency of SSEPs and VEPs that become significant at hematocrits less than 15%. Changes in amplitude were variable until very low hematocrits (approximately 7%) were reached, at which point the amplitude of all waveforms decreased.[287]

Summary

Regardless of the type of intraoperative neurologic monitor, several principles must be observed for neurologic monitoring to provide potential benefit to the patient. First, the pathway at risk during the surgical procedure must be amenable to monitoring. Second, if evidence of injury to the pathway is detected, there must be some intervention possible. If changes in the neurologic monitor are detected, and no intervention is possible, although the monitor may be of prognostic value, it does not have the potential to provide direct benefit to the patient from early detection of impending neurologic injury. Third, the monitor must provide reliable and reproducible data. If the data have a high degree of variability in the absence of clinical interventions, their utility for detecting clinically significant events is limited.

This chapter has reviewed the most common clinically used intraoperative neurologic monitors. Ideally, clinical studies would provide outcome data on the efficacy of a neurologic monitor in a given procedure to improve neurologic outcome. Although there is a wealth of clinical experience with many of these monitoring modalities, there is little in the way of randomized prospective studies evaluating the efficacy of neurologic monitoring. Based on clinical experience with neurologic monitoring and nonrandomized clinical studies in which neurologic monitoring is used and generally compared with historical controls, practice patterns for use of neurologic monitoring have developed. In certain procedures, neurologic monitoring is recommended and used by most centers; in other procedures, monitoring is used almost routinely in some centers, but not in others; and in some procedures, there is no clear clinical experience or evidence that would indicate that monitoring is useful at all (experimental use). Finally, there are procedures in which monitoring is used selectively for patients believed to be at higher-than-usual risk for intraoperative neurologic injury. Table 46-5 provides a summary of current clinical practice.

References

1. Martin NA, Doberstein C: Cerebral blood flow measurement in neurosurgical intensive care. Neurosurg Clin North Am 5:607-618, 1994.
2. Kety SS, Schmidt CF: The determination of cerebral blood flow in man by the use of nitrous oxide in low concentrations. Am J Physiol 143:53-66, 1945.
3. Skyhoj Olsen T, Larsen B, Bech Skriver E, et al: Focal cerebral ischemia measured by the intra-arterial ^{133}Xe method: Limitations of two-dimensional blood flow measurements. Stroke 12:736-744, 1981.
4. Messick JM Jr, Casement B, Sharbrough FW, et al: Correlation of regional cerebral blood flow (rCBF) with EEG changes during isoflurane anesthesia for carotid endarterectomy: Critical rCBF. Anesthesiology 66:344-349, 1987.
5. Sundt TM Jr, Sharbrough FW, Anderson RE, Michenfelder JD: Cerebral blood flow measurements and electroencephalograms during carotid endarterectomy. J Neurosurg 41:310-320, 1974.
6. Zampella E, Morawetz RB, McDowell HA, et al: The importance of cerebral ischemia during carotid endarterectomy. Neurosurgery 29:727-731, 1991.
7. Harrigan MR, Leonardo J, Gibbons KJ, et al: CT perfusion cerebral blood flow imaging in neurological critical care. Neurocrit Care 2:352-366, 2005.
8. Ostergaard L: Cerebral perfusion imaging by bolus tracking. Top Magn Reson Imaging 15:3-9, 2004.
9. Wietasch GJ, Mielck F, Scholz M, et al: Bedside assessment of cerebral blood flow by double-indicator dilution technique. Anesthesiology 92:367-375, 2000.
10. Bass A, Krupski WC, Schneider PA, et al: Intraoperative transcranial Doppler: Limitations of the method. J Vasc Surg 10:549-553, 1989.
11. Manno EM: Transcranial Doppler ultrasonography in the neurocritical care unit. Crit Care Clin 13:79-104, 1997.
12. White H, Baker A: Continuous jugular venous oximetry in the neurointensive care unit: A brief review. Can J Anaesth 49:623-629, 2002.
13. Hongo K, Kobayashi S, Okudera H, et al: Noninvasive cerebral optical spectroscopy: Depth-resolved measurements of cerebral haemodynamics using indocyanine green. Neurol Res 17:89-93, 1995.
14. Samra SK, Stanley JC, Zelenock GB, Dorje P: An assessment of contributions made by extracranial tissues during cerebral oximetry. J Neurosurg Anesthesiol 11:1-5, 1999.
15. Madsen PL, Secher NH: Near-infrared oximetry of the brain. Prog Neurobiol 58:541-560, 1999.
16. Samra SK, Dy EA, Welch K, et al: Evaluation of a cerebral oximeter as a monitor of cerebral ischemia during carotid endarterectomy. Anesthesiology 93:964-970, 2000.
17. Rigamonti A, Scandroglio M, Minicucci F, et al: A clinical evaluation of near-infrared cerebral oximetry in the awake patient to monitor cerebral perfusion during carotid endarterectomy. J Clin Anesth 17:426-430, 2005.
18. Haitsma IK, Maas AIR: Advanced monitoring in the intensive care unit: Brain tissue oxygen tension. Curr Opin Crit Care 8:115-120, 2002.
19. Vajkoczy P, Horn P, Thome C, et al: Regional cerebral blood flow monitoring in the diagnosis of delayed ischemia following aneurysmal subarachnoid hemorrhage. J Neurosurg 98:1227-1234, 2003.
20. Lang EW, Mulvey JM, Mudaliar Y, et al: Direct cerebral oxygenation monitoring: A systematic review of recent publications. Neurosurg Rev 30:99-107, 2007.
21. Vajkoczy P, Roth H, Horn P, et al: Continuous monitoring of regional cerebral blood flow: Experimental and clinical validation of a novel thermal diffusion microprobe. J Neurosurg 93:265-274, 2000.
22. Longhi L, Pagan F, Valeriani V, et al: Monitoring brain tissue oxygen tension in brain-injured patients reveals hypoxic episodes in normal-appearing and in peri-focal tissue. Intensive Care Med 33:2136-2142, 2007.
23. Jaeger M, Soehle M, Schuhmann MU, et al: Correlation of continuously monitored regional cerebral blood flow and brain tissue oxygen. Acta Neurochir (Wien) 147:51-56, 2005.
24. Clark LC: Monitor and control of blood and tissue oxygen tensions. Trans Am Soc Artif Int Org 2:41-45, 1956.
25. Siggaard-Andersen O, Fogh-Andersen N, Gothgen IH, Larsen VH: Oxygen status of arterial and mixed venous blood. Crit Care Med 23:1284-1293, 1995.
26. Gopinath SP, Valadka AB, Uzura M, Robertson CS: Comparison of jugular venous oxygen saturation and brain tissue PO_2 as monitors of cerebral ischemia after head injury. Crit Care Med 27:2337-2345, 1999.
27. Valadka AB, Gopinath SP, Contant CF, et al: Relation of brain tissue PO_2 to outcome after severe head injury. Crit Care Med 26:1576-1581, 1998.
28. Sarrafzadeh AS, Kiening KL, Bardt TF, et al: Cerebral oxygenation in contusioned vs. nonlesioned brain tissue: Monitoring of $PtiO_2$ with Licox and Paratrend. Acta Neurochir Suppl 71:186-189, 1998.

29. Rosenthal G, Hemphill JC 3rd, Sorani M, et al: Brain tissue oxygen tension is more indicative of oxygen diffusion than oxygen delivery and metabolism in patients with traumatic brain injury. Crit Care Med 36:1917-1924, 2008.
30. Menzel M, Doppenberg EM, Zauner A, et al: Increased inspired oxygen concentration as a factor in improved brain tissue oxygenation and tissue lactate levels after severe human head injury. J Neurosurg 91:1-10, 1999.
31. Menzel M, Doppenberg EM, Zauner A, et al: Cerebral oxygenation in patients after severe head injury: Monitoring and effects of arterial hyperoxia on cerebral blood flow, metabolism and intracranial pressure. J Neurosurg Anesthesiol 11:240-251, 1999.
32. Hughes JR: EEG in Clinical Practice, 2nd ed. Newton, MA, Butterworth-Heinemann, 1994.
33. Vitek JL, Bakay RAE, Hashimoto T, et al: Microelectrode-guided pallidotomy: Technical approach and its application in medically intractable Parkinson's disease. J Neurosurg 88:1027, 1998.
34. Garonzik IM, Hua SE, Ohara S, et al: Intraoperative microelectrode and semi-microelectrode recording during the physiological localization of the thalamic nucleus ventral intermediate. Movement Disorders 17:S135, 2002.
35. Martin JT, Faulconer A Jr, Bickford RG: Electroencephalography in anesthesiology. Anesthesiology 20:359, 1959.
36. Sharbrough FW, Messick JM Jr, Sundt TM: Correlation of continuous electroencephalograms with cerebral blood flow measurements during carotid endarterectomy. Stroke 4:674, 1973.
37. Craft RM, Losasso TJ, Perkins WJ, et al: EEG monitoring for cerebral ischemia during carotid endarterectomy (CEA): How much is enough? J Neurosurg Anesthesiol 6:301, 1994.
38. Spackman TN, Faust RJ, Cucchiara RF, et al: A comparison of a periodic analysis of the EEG with standard EEG and cerebral blood flow for detection of ischemia. Anesthesiology 66:229, 1987.
39. Billard V, Gambus PL, Chamoun N, et al: A comparison of spectral edge, delta power, and bispectral index as EEG measures of alfentanil, propofol, and midazolam drug effect. Clin Pharmacol Ther 61:45, 1997.
40. Schmidt GN, Bischoff P, Standl T, et al: Narcotrend and bispectral index monitor are superior to classic electroencephalographic parameters for the assessment of anesthetic states during propofol-remifentanil anesthesia. Anesthesiology 99:1072, 2003.
41. Willmann K, Springman S, Rusy D, et al: A preliminary evaluation of a new derived EEG index monitor in anesthetized patients. J Clin Monit Comput 17:345, 2002.
42. Drover DR, Lemmens HJ, Pierce ET, et al: Patient State Index: Titration of delivery and recovery from propofol, alfentanil, and nitrous oxide anesthesia. Anesthesiology 97:82, 2002.
43. Levy WJ: Effect of epoch length on power spectrum analysis of the EEG. Anesthesiology 66:489, 1987.
44. Grundy BL: Monitoring of sensory evoked potentials during neurosurgical operation: Methods and applications. Neurosurgery 11:556, 1982.
45. Greenberg RP, Ducker TB: Evoked potentials in the clinical neurosciences. J Neurosurg 56:1, 1982.
46. Freedman WA, Chadwick GM, Verhoeven JS, et al: Monitoring of somatosensory evoked potentials during surgery of middle cerebral artery aneurysms. Neurosurgery 29:98, 1991.
47. Chiappa KH, Ropper AH: Evoked potentials in clinical medicine. N Engl J Med 306:1205, 1982.
48. Cohen AR, Young W, Ransohoff J: Intraspinal localization of the somatosensory evoked potential. Neurosurgery 9:157, 1981.
49. York DH: Somatosensory evoked potentials in man: Differentiation of spinal pathways responsible for conduction from the forelimb vs. hindlimb. Progr Neurobiol 25:1, 1985.
50. Ealand-Snyder BG, Holliday TA: Pathways of ascending evoked spinal cord potentials of dogs. Electroencephalogr Clin Neurophysiol 58:140, 1984.
51. Gaines R, York DH, Watts C: Identification of spinal cord pathways responsible for the peroneal-evoked response in the dog. Spine 9:810, 1984.
52. Bundo M, Inao S, Nakamura A, et al: Changes of neural activity correlate with the severity of cortical ischemia in patients with unilateral major cerebral artery occlusion. Stroke 33:61, 2002.
53. Symon L: Flow thresholds in brain ischaemia and the effects of drugs. Br J Anaesth 57:34, 1985.
54. Brainston NM, Ladds A, Symon L, et al: Comparison of the effects of ischaemia on early components of the somatosensory evoked potential in brainstem, thalamus, and cerebral cortex. J Cereb Blood Flow Metab 4:68, 1984.
55. Lopez JR, Chang SD, Steinberg GK: The use of electrophysiological monitoring in the intraoperative management of intracranial aneurysms. J Neurol Neurosurg Psychiatry 66:189, 1999.
56. Guerit JM, Witdoeckt C, de Tourtchaninoff M, et al: Somatosensory evoked potential monitoring in carotid surgery, I: Relationships between qualitative SEP alterations and intraoperative events. Electroencephalogr Clin Neurophysiol 104:459, 1997.
57. Ganes T: A study of peripheral, cervical, and cortical evoked potentials and afferent conduction times in the somatosensory pathway. Electroencephalogr Clin Neurophysiol 49:446, 1980.
58. Chiappa KH, Ropper AH: Evoked potentials in clinical medicine. N Engl J Med 306:1140, 1982.
59. Grundy BL, Jannetta PJ, Procopio PT, et al: Intraoperative monitoring of brain-stem auditory evoked potentials. J Neurosurg 57:674, 1982.
60. Raudzens PA, Shetter AG: Intraoperative monitoring of brain-stem auditory evoked potentials. J Neurosurg 57:341, 1982.
61. Duncan PG, Sanders RA, McCollough DW: Preservation of auditory-evoked responses in anaesthetized children. Can Anaesth Soc J 26:492, 1979.
62. Levy WJ, York DH, McCaffrey M, et al: Motor evoked potentials from transcranial stimulation of the motor cortex in humans. Neurosurgery 15:287, 1984.
63. Legatt AD: Current practice of motor evoked potential monitoring: Results of a survey. J Clin Neurophysiol 19:454, 2002.
64. MacDonald DB, Al Zayed Z, Khoudeir I, et al: Monitoring scoliosis surgery with combined multiple pulse transcranial electric motor and cortical somatosensory-evoked potentials from the lower and upper extremities. Spine 28:194, 2003.
65. Szelenyi A, Bueno de Camargo A, Flamm E, et al: Neurophysiological criteria for intraoperative prediction of pure motor hemiplegia during aneurysm surgery: Case report. J Neurosurg 99:575, 2003.
66. Meylaerts S, Jacobs MJ, van Iterson V, et al: Comparison of transcranial motor evoked potentials and somatosensory evoked potentials during thoracoabdominal aortic aneurysm repair. Ann Surg 230:742, 1999.
67. Pelosi L, Lamb J, Grevitt M, et al: Combined monitoring of motor and somatosensory evoked potentials in orthopaedic spinal surgery. Clin Neurophysiol 113:1082, 2002.
68. Owen JH, Bridwell KH, Grubb R, et al: The clinical application of neurogenic motor evoked potentials to monitor spinal cord function during surgery. Spine 16(Suppl):S385, 1991.
69. Darden BV 2nd, Hatley MK, Owen JH: Neurogenic motor evoked-potential monitoring in anterior cervical surgery. J Spinal Disord 9:485, 1996.
70. Pereon Y, Bernard JM, Fayet G, et al: Usefulness of neurogenic motor evoked potentials for spinal cord monitoring: Findings in 112 consecutive patients undergoing surgery for spinal deformity. Electroencephalogr Clin Neurophysiol 108:17, 1998.
71. Toleikis JR, Skelly JP, Carlvin AO, et al: Spinally elicited peripheral nerve responses are sensory rather than motor. Clin Neurophysiol 111:736, 2000.
72. Harper CM, Daube RJ: Surgical monitoring with evoked potentials: The Mayo Clinic experience. *In* Desmedt JE (ed): Neuromonitoring in Surgery. New York, Elsevier Science, 1989, p 275.
73. Harner SG, Daube JR, Beatty CW: Improved preservation of facial nerve function with use of electrical monitoring during removal of acoustic neuromas. Mayo Clin Proc 62:92, 1987.
74. Michenfelder JD, Sundt TM, Fode N, et al: Isoflurane when compared to enflurane and halothane decreases the frequency of cerebral ischemia during carotid endarterectomy. Anesthesiology 67:336, 1987.
75. Sundt TW Jr, Sharbrough FW, Piepgras DG, et al: Correlation of cerebral blood flow and electroencephalographic changes during carotid endarterectomy: With results of surgery and hemodynamics of cerebral ischemia. Mayo Clin Proc 56:533, 1981.
76. Bond R, Warlow CP, Naylor AR, Rothwell PM: European Carotid Surgery Trialists' Collaborative Group. Variation in surgical and anesthetic technique and associations with operative risk in the European Carotid Surgery Trial: Implications for trials of ancillary techniques. Eur J Vasc Endovasc Surg 23:117-126, 2002.
77. Kalkman CJ: Con: Routine shunting is not the optimal management of the patient undergoing carotid endarterectomy, but neither is neuromonitoring. J Cardiothorac Vasc Anesth 18:381-383, 2004.
78. Plestis KA, Loubser P, Mizrahi EM, et al: Continuous electroencephalographic monitoring and selective shunting reduces neurologic morbidity rates in carotid endarterectomy. J Vasc Surg 25:620, 1997.
79. Darby JM, Stein K, Grenvik A, et al: Approach to management of the heart beating "brain dead" organ donor. JAMA 261:2222, 1989.
80. Roseborough GS: Pro: Shunting is the optimal management of the patient undergoing carotid endarterectomy. J Cardiothorac Vasc Anesth 18:375-380, 2004.
81. Schneider JR, Droste JS, Schindler N, et al: Carotid endarterectomy with routine electroencephalography and selective shunting: Influence of contralateral internal carotid artery occlusion and utility in prevention of postoperative strokes. J Vasc Surg 35:1114-1122, 2002.
82. Woodworth GF, McGirt MJ, Than KD, et al: Selective versus routine intraoperative shunting during carotid endarterectomy: A multivariate outcome analysis. Neurosurgery 61:1170-1177, 2007.
83. Bond R, Rerkasem K, Counsell C, et al: Routine or selective carotid artery shunting for carotid endarterectomy (and different methods of monitoring in selective shunting). Cochrane Database Syst Rev 2: CD000190, 2000.
84. Lam AM, Manninen PH, Ferguson GG, et al: Monitoring of electrophysiologic function during carotid endarterectomy: A comparison of somatosensory

evoked potentials and conventional electroencephalogram. Anesthesiology 75:15, 1991.

85. Ackerstaff RG, van de Vlasakker CJ: Monitoring of brain function during carotid endarterectomy: An analysis of contemporary methods. J Cardiothorac Vasc Anesth 12:341, 1998.

86. Kearse LA Jr, Brown EN, McPeck K: Somatosensory evoked potentials sensitivity relative to electroencephalography for cerebral ischemia during carotid endarterectomy. Stroke 23:498, 1992.

87. Wober C, Zeitlhofer J, Asenbaum S, et al: Monitoring of median nerve somatosensory evoked potentials in carotid surgery. J Clin Neurophysiol 15:429, 1998.

88. Halsey JH, McDowell HA, Gelman S: Transcranial Doppler and rCBF compared in carotid endarterectomy. Stroke 17:1206-1208, 1986.

89. Brauer P, Kochs E, Werner C, et al: Correlation of transcranial Doppler sonography mean flow velocity with cerebral blood flow in patients with intracranial pathology. J Neurosurg Anesthesiol 10:80-85, 1998.

90. Pindzola RR, Balzer JR, Nemoto EM, et al: Cerebrovascular reserve in patients with carotid occlusive disease assessed by stable xenon-enhanced CT cerebral blood flow and transcranial Doppler. Stroke 32:1811-1817, 2001.

91. Chieregato A, Sabia G, Tanfani A, et al: Xenon-CT and transcranial Doppler in poor-grade or complicated aneurysmatic subarachnoid hemorrhage patients undergoing aggressive management of intracranial hypertension. Intensive Care Med 32:1143-1150, 2006.

92. Poeppel TD, Terborg C, Hautzel H, et al: Cerebral haemodynamics during hypo- and hypercapnia: Determination with simultaneous ^{15}O-butanol-PET and transcranial Doppler sonography. Nuklearmedizin 46:93-100, 2007.

93. Ackerstaff RG, Moons KG, van de Vlasakker CJ, et al: Association of intraoperative transcranial Doppler monitoring variables with stroke from carotid endarterectomy. Stroke 31:1817-1823, 2000.

94. Ogasawara K, Suga Y, Sasaki M, et al: Intraoperative microemboli and low middle cerebral artery blood flow velocity are additive in predicting development of cerebral ischemic events after carotid endarterectomy. Stroke 39:3088-3091, 2008.

95. Mueller M, Behnke S, Walter P, et al: Microembolic signals and intraoperative stroke in carotid endarterectomy. Acta Neurol Scand 97:110-117, 1998.

96. Abbott AL, Levi CR, Stork J, et al: Timing of clinically significant microembolism after carotid endarterectomy. Cerebrovasc Dis 23:362-367, 2007.

97. Dunne VG, Besser M, Ma WJ: Transcranial Doppler in carotid endarterectomy. J Clin Neurosci 8:140-145, 2001.

98. Spencer MP: Transcranial Doppler monitoring and causes of stroke from carotid endarterectomy. Stroke 28:685-691, 1997.

99. Gaunte ME: Transcranial Doppler: Preventing stroke during carotid endarterectomy. Ann R Coll Surg Engl 80:377-387, 1998.

100. Rigamonti A, Scandroglio M, Minicucci F, et al: A clinical evaluation of near-infrared cerebral oximetry in the awake patient to monitor cerebral perfusion during carotid endarterectomy. J Clin Anesth 17:426-430, 2005.

101. Samra SK, Dy EA, Welch K, et al: Evaluation of a cerebral oximeter as a monitor of cerebral ischemia during carotid endarterectomy. Anesthesiology 93:964-970, 2000.

102. Calderon-Arnulphi M, Alaraj A, Amin-Janjani S, et al: Detection of cerebral ischemia in neurovascular surgery using quantitative frequency-domain near-infrared spectroscopy. J Neurosurg 106:283-290, 2007.

103. Friedell ML, Clark JM, Graham DA, et al: Cerebral oximetry does not correlate with electroencephalography and somatosensory evoked potentials in determining the need for shunting during carotid endarterectomy. J Vasc Surg 48:601-606, 2008.

104. Friedman WA, Chadwick GM, Verhoeven FJ, et al: Monitoring of somatosensory evoked potentials during surgery for middle cerebral artery aneurysms. Neurosurgery 29:83, 1991.

105. Mizoi K, Yoshimoto T: Intraoperative monitoring of the somatosensory evoked potentials and cerebral blood flow during aneurysm surgery—safety evaluation for temporary vascular occlusion. Neurol Med Chir (Tokyo) 31:318, 1991.

106. Misoi K, Yoshimoto T: Permissible temporary occlusion time in aneurysm surgery as evaluated by evoked potential monitoring. Neurosurgery 33:434, 1993.

107. Holland NR: Subcortical strokes from intracranial aneurysm surgery: Implications for intraoperative neuromonitoring. J Clin Neurophysiol 15:439, 1998.

108. Schramm J, Zentner J, Pechstein U: Intraoperative SEP monitoring in aneurysm surgery. Neurol Res 16:20, 1994.

109. Wiedemayer H, Fauser B, Sandalcioglu IE: The impact of neurophysiological intraoperative monitoring on surgical decisions: A critical analysis of 423 cases. J Neurosurg 96:255, 2002.

110. Manninen PH, Patterson S, Lam AM, et al: Evoked potential monitoring during posterior fossa aneurysm surgery: A comparison of two modalities. Can J Anaesth 41:92, 1994.

111. Manninen PH, Cuillerier DJ, Gelb AW, et al: Monitoring of brain stem function during posterior fossa surgery. Can J Anaesth 37(4 Pt 2):S23, 1990.

112. Friedman WA, Kaplan BL, Day AL: Evoked potential monitoring during aneurysm operation: Observations after fifty cases. Neurosurgery 20:678, 1987.

113. Little JR, Lesser RP, Luders H: Electrophysiological monitoring during basilar aneurysm operation. Neurosurgery 20:421, 1987.

114. Frost EA, Booij LH: Anesthesia in the patient for awake craniotomy. Curr Opin Anaesthesiol 20:331-335, 2007.

115. Costello TG, Cormack JR: Anaesthesia for awake craniotomy: A modern approach. J Clin Neurosci 11:16-19, 2004.

116. Erickson KM, Cole DJ: Anesthetic considerations for awake craniotomy for epilepsy. Anesthesiol Clin 25:535-555, 2007.

117. Beghi E, Tonini C: Surgery for epilepsy: Assessing evidence from observational studies. Epilepsy Res 70:97-102, 2006.

118. Kuzniecky R, Devinsky O: Surgery insight: Surgical management of epilepsy. Nat Clin Pract Neurol 3:673-681, 2007.

119. Quesney LF, Niedermeier E: Electrocorticography. *In* Niedermeier E, Lopes da Silva F (eds): Electroencephalography, 5th ed. Philadelphia, Lippincott Williams & Wilkins, 1994, pp 769-775.

120. Ramnarayan R, Mackenzie I: Brain-stem auditory evoked responses during microvascular decompression for trigeminal neuralgia: Predicting postoperative hearing loss. Neurol India 54:250-254, 2006.

121. Sindou MP: Microvascular decompression for primary hemifacial spasm: Importance of intraoperative neurophysiological monitoring. Acta Neurochir (Wien) 147:1019-1026, 2005.

122. Brock S, Scaioli V, Ferroli P, Broggi G: Neurovascular decompression in trigeminal neuralgia: Role of intraoperative neurophysiological monitoring in the learning period. Stereotact Funct Neurosurg 82:199-206, 2004.

123. Sindou M, Fobé JL, Ciriano D, Fischer C: Hearing prognosis and intraoperative guidance of brainstem auditory evoked potential in microvascular decompression. Laryngoscope 102:678-682, 1992.

124. Friedman WA, Kaplan BJ, Gravenstein D, Rhoton AL Jr: Intraoperative brain-stem auditory evoked potentials during posterior fossa microvascular decompression. J Neurosurg 62:552-557, 1985.

125. Khrais T, Sanna M: Hearing preservation surgery in vestibular schwannoma. J Laryngol Otol 120:366-370, 2006.

126. Bennett M, Haynes DS: Surgical approaches and complications in the removal of vestibular schwannomas. Otolaryngol Clin North Am 40:589-609, 2007.

127. Sala F, Manganotti P, Tramontano V, et al: Monitoring of motor pathways during brain stem surgery: What we have achieved and what we still miss? Clin Neurophysiol 37:399-406, 2007.

128. Maccabee PJ, Pinkhasov EI, Tsairis P, et al: Spinal and short latency scalp derived somatosensory evoked potentials during corrective spinal column surgery. Electroencephalogr Clin Neurophysiol 53:P32, 1982.

129. Luederes H, Gurd A, Hahn J, et al: A new technique for intraoperative monitoring of spinal cord function: Multichannel recording of spinal cord and subcortical evoked potentials. Spine 7:110, 1982.

130. Raudzens PA: Intraoperative monitoring of evoked potentials. Ann N Y Acad Sci 388:308, 1982.

131. McCallum JE, Bennett MH: Electrophysiologic monitoring of spinal cord function during intraspinal surgery. Surg Forum 26:469, 1975.

132. Grundy BL: Intraoperative monitoring of sensory evoked potentials. *In* Nodar RH, Barber C (eds): Evoked Potentials II. Boston, Butterworth, 1984, p 624.

133. Spielholz NI, Benjamin MV, Engler GL et al: Somatosensory evoked potentials during decompression and stabilization of the spine: Methods and findings. Spine 4:500, 1979.

134. Halliday AM, Wakefield GS: Cerebral evoked potentials in patients with dissociated sensory loss. J Neurol Neurosurg Psychiatry 26:211, 1963.

135. Szilagyi DE, Hageman JH, Smith RF, et al: Spinal cord damage in surgery of the abdominal aorta. Surgery 83:38, 1978.

136. Edmonds HL, Paloheimo MPJ, Backman MH, et al: Transcranial magnetic motor evoked potentials for functional monitoring of motor pathways during scoliosis surgery. Spine 14:683, 1989.

137. Boyd SG, Rothwell JC, Cowan JMA, et al: A method of monitoring function in corticospinal pathways during scoliosis surgery with a note on motor conduction velocities. J Neurol Neurosurg Psychiatry 49:251, 1986.

138. Sloan TB, Janik D, Jameson L: Multimodality monitoring of the central nervous system using motor-evoked potentials. Curr Opin Anesthesiol 21:560-564, 2008.

139. Padberg AM, Wilson-Holden TJ, Lenke LG, Bridwell KH: Somatosensory and motor evoked potential monitoring without a wake-up test during idiopathic scoliosis surgery: An accepted standard of care. Spine 23:1392-1400, 1998.

140. Schwartz DM, Auerbach JD, Dormans JP, et al: Neurophysiologic detection of impending spinal cord injury during scoliosis surgery. J Bone Joint Surg Am 89:2440-2449, 2007.

141. MacDonald DB, Al Zayed Z, Khoudeir I, Stigsby B: Monitoring scoliosis surgery with combined multiple pulse transcranial electric motor and cortical somatosensory-evoked potentials from the lower and upper extremities. Spine 28:194-203, 2003.
142. Elmore JR, Gloviczki P, Harper CM, et al: Failure of motor evoked potentials to predict neurologic outcome in experimental thoracic aortic occlusion. J Vasc Surg 14:131, 1991.
143. Reuter DG, Tacker WA, Badylak SF, et al: Correlation of motor-evoked potential response to ischemic spinal cord damage. J Thorac Cardiovasc Surg 104:262, 1992.
144. Dong CC, MacDonald DB, Janusz MT: Intraoperative spinal cord monitoring during descending thoracic and thoracoabdominal aneurysm surgery. Ann Thorac Surg 74:S1873, 2002.
145. Guerit JM, Dion RA: State-of-the-art of neuromonitoring for prevention of immediate and delayed paraplegia in thoracic and thoracoabdominal aorta surgery. Ann Thorac Surg 74:S1867, 2002.
146. Jacobs MJ, Elenbaas TW, Schurink GW, et al: Assessment of spinal cord integrity during thoracoabdominal aortic aneurysm repair. Ann Thorac Surg 74:S1864, 2002.
147. MacDonald DB, Janusz M: An approach to intraoperative neurophysiologic monitoring of thoracoabdominal aneurysm surgery. J Clin Neurophysiol 19:43, 2002.
148. Meylaerts SA, Jacobs MJ, van Iterson V, et al: Comparison of transcranial motor evoked potentials and somatosensory evoked potentials during thoracoabdominal aortic aneurysm repair. Ann Surg 230:742, 1999.
149. de Haan P, Kalkman CJ, Jacobs MJ: Spinal cord monitoring with myogenic motor evoked potentials: Early detection of spinal cord ischemia as an integral part of spinal cord protective strategies during thoracoabdominal aneurysm surgery. Semin Thorac Cardiovasc Surg 10:19, 1998.
150. Shine TS, Harrison BA, De Ruyter ML, et al: Motor and somatosensory evoked potentials: Their role in predicting spinal cord ischemia in patients undergoing thoracoabdominal aortic aneurysm repair with regional lumbar epidural cooling. Anesthesiology 108:580-587, 2008.
151. Lases EC, Schepens MA, Haas FJ, et al: Clinical prospective study of biochemical markers and evoked potentials for identifying adverse neurological outcome after thoracic and thoracoabdominal aortic aneurysm surgery. Br J Anaesth 95:651-661, 2005.
152. Weigang E, Hartert M, Siegenthaler MP, et al: Neurophysiological monitoring during thoracoabdominal aortic endovascular stent graft implantation. Eur J Cardiothorac Surg 29:392-396, 2006.
153. Jacobs MJ, Mess W, Mochtar B, et al: The value of motor evoked potentials in reducing paraplegia during thoracoabdominal aneurysm repair. J Vasc Surg 43:239-246, 2006.
154. Raynor BL, Lenke LG, Bridwell KH, et al: Correlation between low triggered electromyographic thresholds and lumbar pedicle screw malposition: Analysis of 4857 screws. Spine 32:2673-2678, 2007.
155. Shi YB, Binette M, Martin WH, et al: Electrical stimulation for intraoperative evaluation of thoracic pedicle screw placement. Spine 28:595-601, 2003.
156. Leppanen RE: Intraoperative monitoring of segmental spinal nerve root function with free-run and electrically-triggered electromyography and spinal cord function with reflexes and F-responses: A position statement by the American Society of Neurophysiological Monitoring. J Clin Monit Comput 19:437-461, 2005.
157. Shin AY, Spinner RJ, Steinmann SP, Bishop AT: Adult traumatic brachial plexus injuries. J Am Acad Orthop Surg 13:382-396, 2005.
158. Harper CM, Daube RJ: Surgical monitoring with evoked potentials: The Mayo Clinic experience. *In* Desmedt JE (ed): Neuromonitoring in Surgery. New York, Elsevier Science, 1989, p 275.
159. Kline DG, Kim D, Midha R, et al: Management and results of sciatic nerve injuries: A 24-year experience. J Neurosurg 89:13, 1998.
160. Kim DH, Cho YJ, Tiel RL, et al: Outcomes of surgery in 1019 brachial plexus lesions treated at Louisiana State University Health Sciences Center. J Neurosurg 98:1005, 2003.
161. Levy WJ: Quantitative analysis of EEG changes during hypothermia. Anesthesiology 60:291, 1984.
162. Levy WJ, Pantin E, Mehta S, et al: Hypothermia and the approximate entropy of the electroencephalogram. Anesthesiology 98:53, 2003.
163. Chabot RJ, Gugino LD, Aglio LS, et al: QEEG and neuropsychological profiles of patients after undergoing cardiopulmonary bypass surgical procedures. Clin Electroencephalogr 28:98, 1997.
164. Edmonds HL Jr, Griffiths LK, van der Laken J, et al: Quantitative electroencephalographic monitoring during myocardial revascularization predicts postoperative disorientation and improves outcome. J Thorac Cardiovasc Surg 103:555, 1992.
165. Miller G, Rodichok LD, Baylen BG: EEG changes during open heart surgery on infants aged 6 months or less: Relationship to early neurologic morbidity. Pediatr Neurol 10:124, 1994.
166. Williams GD, Ramamoorthy C: Brain monitoring and protection during pediatric cardiac surgery. Semin Cardiothorac Vasc Anesth 11:23-33, 2007.
167. Doblar DD: Intraoperative transcranial ultrasonic monitoring for cardiac and vascular surgery. Semin Cardiothorac Vasc Anesth 8:127-145, 2004.
168. Sakamoto T, Duebener LF, Laussen PC, Jonas RA: Cerebral ischemia caused by obstructed superior vena cava cannula is detected by near-infrared spectroscopy. J Cardiothorac Vasc Anesth 18:293-303, 2004.
169. Kussman BD, Wypij D, DiNardo JA, et al: An evaluation of bilateral monitoring of cerebral oxygen saturation during pediatric cardiac surgery. Anesth Analg 101:1294-1300, 2005.
170. Murkin JM, Adams SJ, Novick RJ, et al: Monitoring brain oxygen saturation during coronary bypass surgery: A randomized prospective study. Anesth Analg 104:51-58, 2007.
171. Gopinath SP, Robertson CS, Contant CF, et al: Jugular venous desaturation and outcome after head injury. J Neurol Neurosurg Psychiatry 57:717-723, 1994.
172. Fandino J, Stocker R, Prokop S, et al: Cerebral oxygenation and systemic trauma related factors determining neurological outcome after brain injury. J Clin Neurosci 7:226-233, 2000.
173. Cormio M, Valadka AB, Robertson CS: Elevated jugular venous oxygen saturation after severe head injury. J Neurosurg 90:9-15, 1999.
174. Cremer OL, van Dijk GW, van Wensen E, et al: Effect of intracranial pressure monitoring and targeted intensive care on functional outcome after severe head injury. Crit Care Med 33:2207-2213, 2005.
175. Stiefel MF, Udoetuk JD, Spiotta AM, et al: Conventional neurocritical care and cerebral oxygenation after traumatic brain injury. J Neurosurg 105:568-575, 2006.
176. Fortune JB, Feustel PJ, Graca L, et al: Effect of hyperventilation, mannitol, and ventriculostomy drainage on cerebral blood flow after head injury. J Trauma 39:1091, 1995.
177. Skippen P, Seear M, Poskitt K, et al: Effect of hyperventilation on regional cerebral blood flow in head-injured children. Crit Care Med 25:1402, 1997.
178. Imberti R, Bellinzona G, Langer M: Cerebral tissue PO_2 and $Sjvo_2$ changes during moderate hyperventilation in patients with severe traumatic brain injury. J Neurosurg 96:97, 2002.
179. Coles JP, Minhas PS, Fryer TD, et al: Effect of hyperventilation on cerebral blood flow in traumatic head injury: Clinical relevance and monitoring correlates. Crit Care Med 30:1950, 2002.
180. van den Brink WA, van Santbrink H, Steyerberg EW, et al: Brain oxygen tension in severe head injury. Neurosurgery 46:868-876, 2000.
181. Stiefel MF, Spiotta A, Gracias VH, et al: Reduced mortality rate in patients with severe traumatic brain injury treated with brain tissue oxygen monitoring. J Neurosurg 103:805-811, 2005.
182. Steiner LA, Andrews PJ: Monitoring the injured brain: ICP and CBF. Br J Anaesth 97:26-38, 2006.
183. Suarez JI, Qureshi AI, Yahia AB, et al: Symptomatic vasospasm diagnosis after subarachnoid hemorrhage: Evaluation of transcranial Doppler ultrasound and cerebral angiography as related to compromised vascular distribution. Crit Care Med 30:1348, 2002.
184. Topcuoglu MA, Pryor JC, Ogilvy CS, et al: Cerebral vasospasm following subarachnoid hemorrhage. Curr Treat Options Cardiovasc Med 4:3731, 2002.
185. Jarus-Dziedzic K, Juniewicz H, Wronski J, et al: The relation between cerebral blood flow velocities as measured by TCD and the incidence of delayed ischemic deficits: A prospective study after subarachnoid hemorrhage. Neurol Res 24:5822, 2002.
186. Aaslid R: Transcranial Doppler assessment of cerebral vasospasm. Eur J Ultrasound 16:3, 2002.
187. Mascia L, Fedorko L, ter Brugge K, et al: The accuracy of transcranial Doppler to detect vasospasm in patients with aneurysmal subarachnoid hemorrhage. Intensive Care Med 29:1088, 2003.
188. Sloan MA, Haley EC, Kassell NF, et al: Sensitivity and specificity of transcranial Doppler ultrasonography in the diagnosis of vasospasm following subarachnoid hemorrhage. Neurology 39:1514, 1989.
189. Sekhar LN, Wechsler LR, Yonas H, et al: Value of transcranial Doppler examination in the diagnosis of cerebral vasospasm after subarachnoid hemorrhage. Neurosurgery 22:813, 1988.
190. Vespa PM, Nenov V, Nuwer MR: Continuous EEG monitoring in the intensive care unit: Early findings and clinical efficacy. J Clin Neurophysiol 16:1-13, 1999.
191. Bricolo A, Turazzi S, Faccioli F, et al: Clinical application of compressed spectral array in long-term EEG monitoring of comatose patients. Electroencephalogr Clin Neurophysiol 45:211-225, 1978.
192. Gutling E, Gonser A, Imhof HG, Landis T: EEG reactivity in the prognosis of severe head injury. Neurology 45:915-918, 1995.
193. Alexandre A, Rubini L, Nertempi P, Farinello C: Sleep alterations during post-traumatic coma as a possible predictor of cognitive defects. Acta Neurochir Suppl (Wien) 28:188-192, 1979.
194. Bergamasco B, Bergamini L, Doriguzzi T, Fabiani D: EEG sleep patterns as a prognostic criterion in post-traumatic coma. Electroencephalogr Clin Neurophysiol 24:374-347, 1968.
195. Winer JW, Rosenwasser RH, Jimenez F: Electroencephalographic activity and serum and cerebrospi-

nal fluid pentobarbital levels in determining the therapeutic end point during barbiturate coma. Neurosurgery 29:739-741, 1991.

196. Facco E, Munari M, Baratto F, et al: Multimodality evoked potentials (auditory, somatosensory and motor) in coma. Neurophysiol Clin 23:237-258, 1993.

197. Pohlmann-Eden B, Dingethal K, Bender HJ, Koelfen W: How reliable is the predictive value of SEP (somatosensory evoked potentials) patterns in severe brain damage with special regard to the bilateral loss of cortical responses? Intensive Care Med 23:301-308, 1997.

198. Ruiz-Lopez MJ, Martinez de Azagra A, Serrano A, Casado-Flores J: Brain death and evoked potentials in pediatric patients. Crit Care Med 27:412-416, 1999.

199. Goodwin SR, Friedman WA, Bellefleur M: Is it time to use evoked potentials to predict outcome in comatose children and adults? Crit Care Med 19:518-524, 1991.

200. Morgalla MH, Bauer J, Ritz R, Tatagiba M: Coma: The prognostic value of evoked potentials in patients after traumatic brain injury. Anaesthesist 55:760-768, 2006.

201. Nuwer MR: Electroencephalograms and evoked potentials: Monitoring cerebral function in the neurosurgical intensive care unit. Neurosurg Clin North Am 5:647-659, 1994.

202. Lew HL, Poole JH, Castaneda A, et al: Prognostic value of evoked and event-related potentials in moderate to severe brain injury. J Head Trauma Rehabil 21:350-360, 2006.

203. Carter BG, Butt W: Review of the use of somatosensory evoked potentials in the prediction of outcome after severe brain injury. Crit Care Med 29:178-186, 2001.

204. Carter BG, Butt W: Are somatosensory evoked potentials the best predictor of outcome after severe brain injury? A systematic review. Intensive Care Med 31:765-775, 2005.

205. Fischer C, Luaute J: Evoked potentials for the prediction of vegetative state in the acute stage of coma. Neuropsychol Rehabil 15:372-380, 2005.

206. Petty GW, Mohr JP, Pedley T, et al: The role of transcranial Doppler in confirming brain death. Neurology 40:300, 1990.

207. Rosen I, Hagerdal M: Electroencephalographic study of children during ketamine anesthesia. Acta Anaesthesiol Scand 20:32, 1976.

208. La Marca S, Lozito RJ, Dunn RW: Cognitive and EEG recovery following bolus intravenous administration of anesthetic agents. Psychopharmacol (Berl) 120:426, 1995.

209. McGuire G, El-Beheiry H, Manninen P, et al: Activation of electrocorticographic activity with remifentanil and alfentanil during neurosurgical excision of epileptogenic focus. Br J Anaesth 91:651-655, 2003.

210. Sebel PS, Bovill JG, Wauquier A, et al: Effects of high dose fentanyl anesthesia on the electroencephalogram. Anesthesiology 55:203, 1981.

211. Hyypponen E, Maksimow A, Lapinlampi P, et al: Electroencephalogram spindle activity during dexmedetomidine sedation and physiological sleep. Acta Anaesthesiol Scand 52:289-294, 2008.

212. Maksimow A, Snapir A, Sarkela M, et al: Assessing the depth of dexmedetomidine-induced sedation with electroencephalogram (EEG)-based spectral entropy. Acta Anaesthesiol Scand 51:22-30, 2007.

213. Yamamura T, Fukuda M, Takeya H, et al: Fast oscillatory EEG activity induced by analgesic concentrations of nitrous oxide in man. Anesth Analg 60:283, 1981.

214. Clark DL, Hosick EC, Neigh JL: Neurophysiologic effects of isoflurane in man. Anesthesiology 39:261, 1973.

215. Artru AA, Lam AM, Johnson JO, et al: Intracranial pressure, middle cerebral artery flow velocity, and plasma inorganic fluoride concentrations in neurosurgical patients receiving sevoflurane or isoflurane. Anesth Analg 85:587, 1997.

216. Komatsu H, Taie S, Endo S, et al: Electrical seizures during sevoflurane anesthesia in two pediatric patients with epilepsy. Anesthesiology 81:1535, 1994.

217. Jaaskelainen SK, Kaisti K, Suni L, et al: Sevoflurane is epileptogenic in healthy subjects at surgical levels of anesthesia. Neurology 61:1073, 2003.

218. Endo T, Sato K, Shamoto H, et al: Effects of sevoflurane on electrocorticography in patients with intractable temporal lobe epilepsy. J Neurosurg Anesthesiol 14:59, 2002.

219. Rampil IJ, Lockhart SH, Eger EI, et al: The electroencephalographic effects of desflurane in humans. Anesthesiology 74:434, 1991.

220. Sharpe MD, Young GB, Mirsattari S, et al: Prolonged desflurane administration for refractory status epilepticus. Anesthesiology 97:261, 2002.

221. Hoffman WE, Edelman G: Comparison of isoflurane and desflurane anesthetic depth using burst suppression of the electroencephalogram in neurosurgical patients. Anesth Analg 81:811, 1995.

222. Banoub M, Tetzlaff JE, Schubert A: Pharmacologic and physiologic influences affecting sensory evoked potentials. Anesthesiology 99:716, 2003.

223. Peterson DO, Drummond JC, Todd MM: Effects of halothane, enflurane, isoflurane, and nitrous oxide on somatosensory evoked potentials in humans. Anesthesiology 65:35, 1986.

224. McPherson RW, Mahla M, Johnson R, et al: Effects of enflurane, isoflurane, and nitrous oxide on somatosensory evoked potentials during fentanyl anesthesia. Anesthesiology 62:626, 1985.

225. Pathak KS, Amaddio BS, Scoles PV, et al: Effects of halothane, enflurane, and isoflurane in nitrous oxide on multilevel somatosensory evoked potentials. Anesthesiology 70:207, 1989.

226. Samra SK, Vanderzant CW, Domer PA, et al: Differential effects of isoflurane on human median nerve somatosensory evoked potentials. Anesthesiology 66:29, 1987.

227. Sebel PS, Ingram DA, Flynn PJ: Evoked potentials during isoflurane anaesthesia. Br J Anaesth 58:580, 1986.

228. Scholz J, Bischoff P, Szafarczyk W, et al: Comparison of sevoflurane and isoflurane in ambulatory surgery: Results of a multicenter study. Anaesthetist 45:S63, 1996.

229. Haghighi SS, Sirintrapun SJ, Johnson JC, et al: Suppression of spinal and cortical somatosensory evoked potentials by desflurane anesthesia. J Neurosurg Anesthesiol 8:148, 1996.

230. Bernard JM, Pereon Y, Fayet G, et al: Effects of isoflurane and desflurane on neurogenic motor- and somatosensory-evoked potential monitoring for scoliosis surgery. Anesthesiology 85:1013, 1996.

231. Boisseau N, Madany M, Staccini P, et al: Comparison of the effects of sevoflurane and propofol on cortical somatosensory evoked potentials. Br J Anaesth 88:785, 2002.

232. Vaugha DJ, Thornton C, Wright DR, et al: Effects of different concentrations of sevoflurane and desflurane on subcortical somatosensory evoked responses in anaesthetized, non-stimulated patients. Br J Anaesth 86:59, 2001.

233. Manninen PH, Lam AM, Nicholas JF: The effects of isoflurane-nitrous oxide anesthesia on brainstem auditory evoked potentials in humans. Anesth Analg 64:43, 1985.

234. Thornton C, Catley DM, Jordan C, et al: Enflurane anaesthesia causes graded changes in the brainstem and early cortical auditory evoked response in man. Br J Anaesth 55:479, 1983.

235. Dubois MY, Sato S, Chassy J, et al: Effects of enflurane on brainstem auditory evoked responses in humans. Anesth Analg 61:898, 1982.

236. Cohen MS, Britt RH: Effects of sodium pentobarbital, ketamine, halothane, chloralose on brainstem auditory evoked responses. Anesth Analg 61:338, 1982.

237. Chi OZ, Field C: Effects of isoflurane on visual evoked potentials in humans. Anesthesiology 65:328, 1986.

238. Uhl RR, Squires KC, Bruce DL, et al: Effect of halothane anesthesia on the human cortical visual evoked response. Anesthesiology 53:273, 1980.

239. Domino EF, Corssen G, Sweet RB: Effects of various general anesthetics on the visually evoked response in man. Anesth Analg 42:735, 1963.

240. Burchiel KG, Stockard JJ, Myers RR, et al: Visual and auditory evoked responses during enflurane anesthesia in man and cats. Electroencephalogr Clin Neurophysiol 39:434P, 1973.

241. Sebel PS, Flynn PJ, Ingram DA: Effect of nitrous oxide on visual, auditory, and somatosensory evoked potentials. Br J Anaesth 56:1403, 1984.

242. Drummond JC, Todd MM, Sang H: The effect of high dose sodium thiopental on brain stem auditory and median nerve somatosensory evoked responses in humans. Anesthesiology 63:249, 1985.

243. Shimoji K, Kano T, Nakashima H, et al: The effects of thiamyl sodium on electrical activities of the central and peripheral nervous systems in man. Anesthesiology 40:234, 1974.

244. Ganes T, Lundar T: The effect of thiopentone on somatosensory evoked responses and EEGs in comatose patients. J Neurol Neurosurg Psychiatry 46:509, 1983

245. Sutton LN, Frewen T, Marsh R, et al: The effects of deep barbiturate coma on multimodality evoked potentials. J Neurosurg 57:178, 1982.

246. Koht A, Schutz W, Schmidt G, et al: Effects of etomidate, midazolam, and thiopental on median nerve somatosensory evoked potentials and the additive effects of fentanyl and nitrous oxide. Anesth Analg 67:435, 1988.

247. Sloan TB, Ronai AK, Toleikis JR, et al: Improvement of intraoperative somatosensory evoked potentials by etomidate. Anesth Analg 67:582, 1988.

248. Navaratnarajah M, Thornton C, Heneghan CPH, et al: Effect of etomidate on the auditory evoked response in man. Proc Anaesth Res Soc 55:1157P, 1983.

249. Grundy BL, Brown RH, Clifton PC: Effect of droperidol on somatosensory cortical evoked potentials. Electroencephalogr Clin Neurophysiol 50:158, 1980.

250. Doring WH, Daub D: Akustisch evozierte Hirstamm und Rindepotentiale bei sedierung mit diazepam. Arch Otorhinolaryngol 227:522, 1980.

251. Grundy BL, Brown RH, Greenbergh BA: Diazepam alters cortical potentials. Anesthesiology 51:538, 1979.

252. Pathak KS, Brown RH, Cascorbi HF, et al: Effects of fentanyl and morphine on intraoperative somatosensory cortical-evoked potentials. Anesth Analg 63:833, 1984.

253. Schubert A, Peterson DO, Drummond JC, et al: The effect of high-dose fentanyl on human median nerve somatosensory evoked responses. Anesth Analg 65:S136, 1986.

254. Grundy BL, Brown RH: Meperidine enhances somatosensory cortical evoked potentials. Electroencephalogr Clin Neurophysiol 50:177, 1980.
255. Samra SK, Lilly DJ, Rush NL, et al: Fentanyl anesthesia and human brain-stem auditory evoked potentials. Anesthesiology 61:261, 1984.
256. Zentner J, Kiss I, Ebner A: Influence of anesthetics—nitrous oxide in particular—on electromyographic response evoked by transcranial electrical stimulation of the cortex. Neurosurgery 24:253, 1989.
257. Jellinek D, Jewkes D, Symon L: Noninvasive intraoperative monitoring of motor evoked potentials under propofol anesthesia: Effects of spinal surgery on the amplitude and latency of motor evoked potentials. Neurosurgery 29:551, 1991.
258. Taniguchi M, Nadstawek J, Langenbach U, et al: Effects of four intravenous anesthetic agents on motor evoked potentials elicited by magnetic transcranial stimulation. Neurosurgery 33:407, 1993.
259. Ubags LH, Kalkman CJ, Been HD, et al: The use of ketamine or etomidate to supplement sufentanil/ N_2O anesthesia does not disrupt monitoring of myogenic transcranial motor evoked responses. J Neurosurg Anesthesiol 9:228, 1997.
260. Kalkman CJ, Drummond JC, Patel PM, et al: Effects of droperidol, pentobarbital and ketamine on myogenic motor evoked responses in humans. Neurosurgery 35:1066, 1994.
261. DeWitt LD, Wechsler LR: Transcranial Doppler. Stroke 19:915, 1988.
262. Sloan TB, Heyer EJ: Anesthesia for intraoperative neurophysiologic monitoring of the spinal cord. J Clin Neurophysiol 19:430, 2002.
263. Zentner J, Thees C, Pechstein U, et al: Influence of nitrous oxide on motor-evoked potentials. Spine 22:1002, 1997.
264. Nathan N, Tabaraud F, Lacroix F, et al: Influence of propofol concentrations on multipulse transcranial motor evoked potentials. Br J Anaesth 91:493, 2003.
265. Ghaly RF, Ham JH, Lee JJ: High-dose ketamine hydrochloride maintains somatosensory and magnetic motor evoked potentials in primates. Neurol Res 23:881, 2001.
266. Scheufler KM, Zentner J: Total intravenous anesthesia for intraoperative monitoring of the motor pathways: An integral view combining clinical and experimental data. J Neurosurg 96:571, 2002.
267. Taniguchi M, Nadstawek J, Langenbach U, et al: Effects of four intravenous anesthetic agents on motor evoked potentials elicited by magnetic transcranial stimulation. Neurosurgery 33:407, 1993.
268. Ubags LH, Kalkman CJ, Been HD, et al: The use of ketamine or etomidate to supplement sufentanil/ N_2O anesthesia does not disrupt monitoring of myogenic transcranial motor evoked responses. J Neurosurg Anesthesiol 9:228, 1997.
269. Yang LH, Lin SM, Lee WY, et al: Intraoperative transcranial electrical motor evoked potential monitoring during spinal surgery under intravenous ketamine or etomidate anesthesia. Acta Neurochir (Wien) 127:191, 1994.
270. Ubags LH, Kalkman CJ, Been HD, et al: A comparison of myogenic motor evoked responses to electrical and magnetic transcranial stimulation during nitrous oxide/opioid anesthesia. Anesth Analg 88:568, 1999.
271. Pechstein U, Nadstawek J, Zentner J, et al: Isoflurane plus nitrous oxide versus propofol for recording of motor evoked potentials after high frequency repetitive electrical stimulation. Electroencephalogr Clin Neurophysiol 108:175, 1998.
272. Pelosi L, Stevenson M, Hobbs GJ, et al: Intraoperative motor evoked potentials to transcranial electrical stimulation during two anaesthetic regimens. Clin Neurophysiol 112:1076, 2001.
273. Ubaga LH, Kalkman CJ, Been HD: Influence of isoflurane on myogenic motor evoked potentials to single and multiple transcranial stimuli during nitrous oxide/opioid anesthesia. Neurosurgery 43:90, 1998.
274. Stockard JJ, Bickford RG: The neurophysiology of anaesthesia. *In* Gordon E (ed): A Basis and Practice of Neuroanesthesia. New York, Elsevier, 1981, p 3.
275. Kraaier V, van Huffelen AC, Wieneke GH: Changes in quantitative EEG and blood flow velocity due to standardized hyperventilation: A model of transient ischaemia in young human subjects. Electroencephalogr Clin Neurophysiol 70:377, 1988.
276. Clowes GHA Jr, Kretchmer HE, McBurney RW, et al: The electroencephalogram in the evaluation of the effects of anesthetic agents and carbon dioxide accumulation during surgery. Ann Surg 138:558, 1953.
277. Eng DY, Dong WK, Bledsoe SW, et al: Electrical and pathological correlates of brain hypoxia during hypotension. Anesthesiology 53:S92, 1980.
278. Kobrine AI, Evans DE, Rizzoli HV: Relative vulnerability of the brain and spinal cord to ischemia. J Neurol Sci 45:65, 1980.
279. Bunegin L, Albin MS, Helsel P, et al: Evoked responses during trimethaphan hypotension. Anesthesiology 55:A232, 1981.
280. Grundy BL, Nash CL, Brown RH: Arterial pressure manipulation alters spinal cord function during correction of scoliosis. Anesthesiology 54:249, 1981.
281. Russ W, Kling D, Loesevitz A, et al: Effect of hypothermia on visual evoked potential (VEP) in humans. Anesthesiology 61:207, 1984.
282. Stockard JJ, Sharbrough FW, Tinker JA: Effects of hypothermia on the human brainstem auditory response. Ann Neurol 3:368, 1978.
283. Spetzler RF, Hadley MN, Rigamonti D, et al: Aneurysms of the basilar artery treated with circulatory arrest, hypothermia, and barbiturate cerebral protection. J Neurosurg 68:868, 1988.
284. Dubois M, Loppola R, Buchsbaum MS, et al: Somatosensory evoked potentials during whole body hyperthermia in humans. Electroencephalogr Clin Neurophysiol 52:157, 1981.
285. Nakagawa Y, Ohtsuka T, Tsura M, et al: Effects of mild hypercapnia on somatosensory evoked potentials in experimental cerebral ischemia. Stroke 25:275, 1984.
286. Grundy BL, Heros RC, Tung AS, et al: Intraoperative hypoxia detected by evoked potential monitoring. Anesth Analg 60:437, 1981.
287. Nagao S, Roccaforte P, Moody RA: The effects of isovolemic hemodilution and reinfusion of packed erythrocytes on somatosensory and visual evoked potentials. J Surg Res 25:S30, 1978.

Jørgen Viby-Mogensen

47 Neuromuscular Monitoring

Key Points

1. Residual postoperative neuromuscular blockade causes decreased chemoreceptor sensitivity to hypoxia, functional impairment of the pharyngeal and upper esophageal muscles, impaired ability to maintain the airway, and an increased risk for the development of postoperative pulmonary complications.
2. It is difficult and often impossible to exclude with certainty clinically significant residual curarization by clinical evaluation of recovery of neuromuscular function.
3. Absence of tactile fade in the response to train-of-four (TOF) stimulation, tetanic stimulation, and double-burst stimulation does not exclude significant residual blockade.
4. Adequate recovery of postoperative neuromuscular function cannot be guaranteed without objective neuromuscular monitoring.
5. Good evidence-based practice dictates that clinicians should always quantitate the extent of neuromuscular blockade by objective monitoring.
6. To exclude clinically significant residual neuromuscular blockade, the TOF ratio, when measured mechanically or by electromyography, must exceed 0.9.
7. Total twitch depression during surgery should be avoided. Whenever possible, one or two TOF responses should be maintained.
8. Antagonism of the neuromuscular block with a cholinesterase inhibitor should not be initiated before at least two or preferably three or four responses to TOF stimulation are observed.
9. If sufficient recovery (TOF ≥ 0.9) has not been documented objectively at the end of the surgical procedure, the neuromuscular block should be antagonized.

Quite often, the degree of neuromuscular blockade during and after anesthesia is evaluated with clinical criteria alone. However, clinically significant residual neuromuscular blockade (i.e., paralysis) may persist postoperatively.[1,2] Objective monitoring of the degree of neuromuscular block during and after anesthesia should reduce the problems of residual neuromuscular blockade.[3,4]

In awake patients, muscle power can be evaluated by tests of voluntary muscle strength, but during anesthesia and recovery from anesthesia this is not possible. Instead, the clinician uses clinical tests to assess muscle power directly and to estimate neuromuscular function indirectly (muscle tone; feel of the anesthesia bag as an indirect measure of pulmonary compliance, tidal volume, and inspiratory force). All these tests, however, are influenced by factors other than the degree of neuromuscular blockade. Therefore, whenever more precise information regarding the status of neuromuscular functioning is desired, the response of muscle to nerve stimulation should be assessed. This procedure also takes into account the considerable variation in individual response and sensitivity to muscle relaxants.

This chapter reviews the basic principles of peripheral nerve stimulation and the requirements for effective use of nerve stimulators. It also describes the response to nerve stimulation during depolarizing (phase I and phase II) and nondepolarizing neuromuscular blockade. Finally, methods of evaluating evoked neuromuscular responses with and without the availability of recording equipment are discussed.

Types of Peripheral Nerve Stimulation

Neuromuscular function is monitored by evaluating the muscular response to supramaximal stimulation of a peripheral motor nerve. Two types of stimulation can be used: electrical and magnetic. Electrical nerve stimulation is by far the most commonly used method in clinical practice and is described in detail in this chapter. In theory, magnetic nerve stimulation has several advantages over electrical nerve stimulation.[5,6] It is less painful and does not require physical contact with the body. However, the equipment required is bulky and heavy, it cannot be used for train-of-four (TOF) stimulation, and it is difficult to achieve supramaximal stimulation with this method. Therefore, magnetic nerve stimulation is very seldom used in clinical anesthesia.

Principles of Peripheral Nerve Stimulation

The reaction of a single muscle fiber to a stimulus follows an all-or-none pattern. In contrast, the response of the whole muscle depends on the number of muscle fibers activated. If a nerve is stimulated with sufficient intensity, all fibers supplied by the nerve will react, and the maximum response will be triggered. After administration of a neuromuscular blocking drug, the response of the muscle decreases in parallel with the number of fibers blocked. The reduction in response during constant stimulation reflects the degree of neuromuscular blockade.

For the preceding principles to be in effect, the stimulus must be truly maximal throughout the period of monitoring; therefore, the electrical stimulus applied is usually at least 20% to 25% above that necessary for a maximal response. For this reason the stimulus is said to be supramaximal; however, supramaximal electrical stimulation hurts, which is not a concern during anesthesia, but during recovery the patient may be awake enough to experience the discomfort of nerve stimulation. Therefore, some researchers advocate stimulation with submaximal current during recovery. Although several investigations indicate that testing of neuromuscular function can be reliably performed postoperatively with submaximal stimulation,[7,8] the accuracy of such monitoring is unacceptable with low current.[9]

Patterns of Nerve Stimulation

For evaluation of neuromuscular function, the most commonly used patterns of electrical nerve stimulation are single-twitch, TOF, tetanic, post-tetanic count (PTC), and double-burst stimulation (DBS).

Single-Twitch Stimulation

In the single-twitch mode of stimulation, single supramaximal electrical stimuli are applied to a peripheral motor nerve at frequencies ranging from 1.0 Hz (once every second) to 0.1 Hz (once every 10 seconds) (Fig. 47-1). The response to single-twitch stimulation depends on the frequency at which the individual stimuli are applied. If the rate of delivery is increased to greater than 0.15 Hz, the evoked response will gradually decrease and settle at a lower level. As a result, a frequency of 0.1 Hz is generally used. Because 1-Hz stimulation shortens the time necessary to determine supramaximal stimulation, this frequency is sometimes used during induction of anesthesia; however, the apparent time of onset and length of neuromuscular blockade depend on the pattern and duration of stimulation. Therefore, results obtained with 1-Hz single-twitch stimulation cannot be compared with results obtained by using, for instance, 0.1-Hz single-twitch stimulation or TOF stimulation.[10]

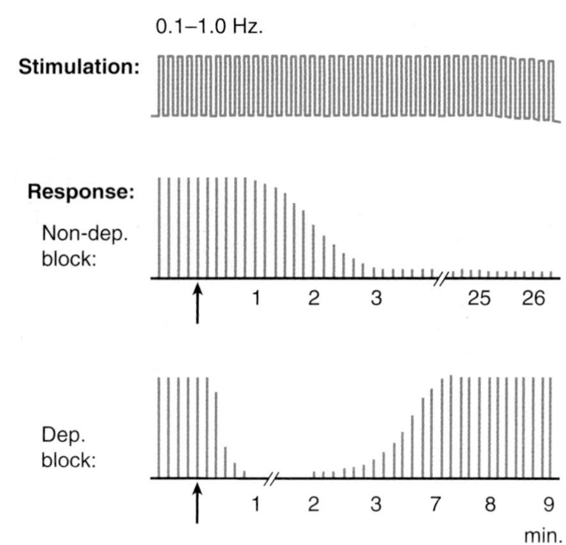

Figure 47-1 Pattern of electrical stimulation and evoked muscle responses to single-twitch nerve stimulation (at frequencies of 0.1 to 1.0 Hz) after injection of nondepolarizing (Non-dep.) and depolarizing (Dep.) neuromuscular blocking drugs (*arrows*). Note that except for the difference in time factors, no differences in the strength of the evoked responses exist between the two types of block.

Train-of-Four Stimulation

In TOF nerve stimulation, introduced by Ali and associates[11,12] during the early 1970s, four supramaximal stimuli are given every 0.5 second (2 Hz) (Fig. 47-2). When used continuously, each set (train) of stimuli is normally repeated every 10th to 20th second. Each stimulus in the train causes the muscle to contract, and "fade" in the response provides the basis for evaluation. That is, dividing the amplitude of the fourth response by the amplitude of the first response provides the TOF ratio. In the control response (the response obtained before the administration of a muscle relaxant), all four responses are ideally the same: the TOF

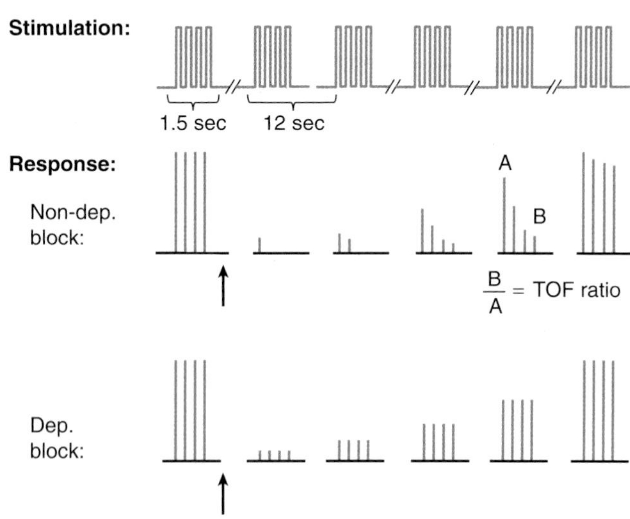

Figure 47-2 Pattern of electrical stimulation and evoked muscle responses to TOF nerve stimulation before and after injection of nondepolarizing (Non-dep.) and depolarizing (Dep.) neuromuscular blocking drugs (*arrows*).

ratio is 1.0. During a partial nondepolarizing block, the ratio decreases (fades) and is inversely proportional to the degree of blockade. During a partial depolarizing block, no fade occurs in the TOF response; ideally, the TOF ratio is approximately 1.0. Fade in the TOF response after injection of succinylcholine signifies the development of a phase II block (discussed later in the section on depolarizing neuromuscular blockade).

The advantages of TOF stimulation are greatest during nondepolarizing blockade because the degree of block can be read directly from the TOF response even though a preoperative value is lacking. In addition, TOF stimulation has some advantages over tetanic stimulation: it is less painful and, unlike tetanic stimulation, does not generally affect the degree of neuromuscular blockade.

Tetanic Stimulation

Tetanic stimulation consists of very rapid (e.g., 30-, 50-, or 100-Hz) delivery of electrical stimuli. The most commonly used pattern in clinical practice is 50-Hz stimulation given for 5 seconds, although some investigators have advocated the use of 50-, 100-, and even 200-Hz stimulation for 1 second. During normal neuromuscular transmission and a pure depolarizing block, the muscle response to 50-Hz tetanic stimulation for 5 seconds is sustained. During a nondepolarizing block and a phase II block after the injection of succinylcholine, the response will not be sustained (i.e., fade occurs) (Fig. 47-3).

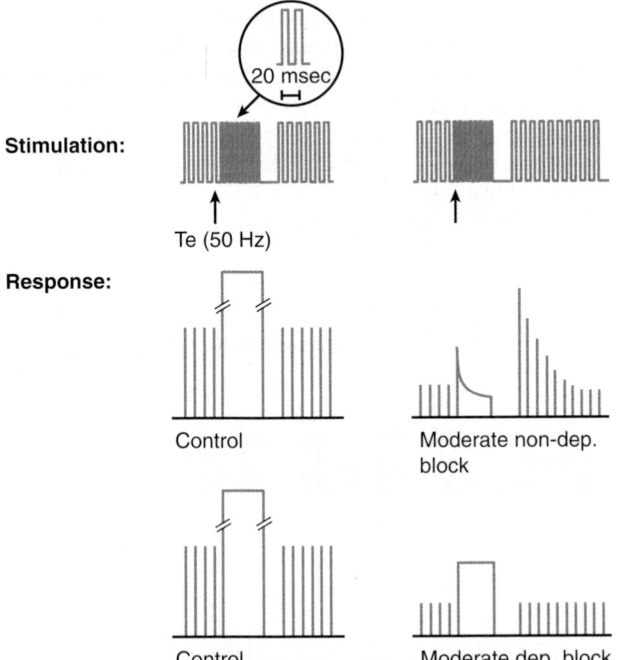

Figure 47-3 Pattern of stimulation and evoked muscle responses to tetanic (50-Hz) nerve stimulation for 5 seconds (Te) and post-tetanic twitch stimulation (1.0-Hz) (*arrows*). Stimulation was applied before the injection of neuromuscular blocking drugs and during moderate nondepolarizing (non-dep.) and depolarizing (dep.) blocks. Note the fade in the response to tetanic stimulation, plus the post-tetanic facilitation of transmission during nondepolarizing blockade. During depolarizing blockade, the tetanic response is well sustained, and no post-tetanic facilitation of transmission occurs.

Fade in response to tetanic stimulation is normally considered a presynaptic event; the traditional explanation is that at the start of tetanic stimulation, large amounts of acetylcholine are released from immediately available stores in the nerve terminal. As these stores become depleted, the rate of acetylcholine release decreases until equilibrium between mobilization and synthesis of acetylcholine is achieved. Despite this equilibrium, the muscle response caused by tetanic stimulation of the nerve at, for example, 50 Hz is maintained (given normal neuromuscular transmission) simply because the acetylcholine released is many times greater than the amount necessary to evoke a response. When the "margin of safety"[13] at the postsynaptic membrane (i.e., the number of free cholinergic receptors) is reduced by nondepolarizing neuromuscular blocking drugs, a typical reduction in twitch height is seen with a fade during, for instance, repetitive stimulation. In addition to this postsynaptic block, nondepolarizing neuromuscular blocking drugs may also block presynaptic neuronal-type acetylcholine receptors, thereby leading to impaired mobilization of acetylcholine within the nerve terminal.[14] This effect substantially contributes to fade in the response to tetanic (and TOF) stimulation. Although the degree of fade depends primarily on the degree of neuromuscular blockade, fade also depends on the frequency (Hz) and the length (seconds) of stimulation and on how often tetanic stimuli are applied. Unless these variables are kept constant, results from different studies using tetanic stimulation cannot be compared.

During partial nondepolarizing blockade, tetanic nerve stimulation is followed by a post-tetanic increase in twitch tension (i.e., post-tetanic facilitation of transmission) (see Fig. 47-3). This event occurs because the increase in mobilization and synthesis of acetylcholine caused by tetanic stimulation continues for some time after discontinuation of stimulation. The degree and duration of post-tetanic facilitation depend on the degree of neuromuscular blockade, with post-tetanic facilitation usually disappearing within 60 seconds of tetanic stimulation. Post-tetanic facilitation is evident in electromyographic, acceleromyographic, and mechanical recordings during partial nondepolarizing neuromuscular blockade. In contrast, post-tetanic twitch potentiation, which sometimes occurs in mechanical recordings before any neuromuscular blocking drug has been given, is a muscular phenomenon that is not accompanied by an increase in the compound muscle action potential.

Tetanic stimulation is very painful and therefore not normally acceptable to an unanesthetized patient. Furthermore, especially in the late phase of neuromuscular recovery, tetanic stimulation may produce lasting antagonism of neuromuscular blockade in the stimulated muscle such that the response of the tested site may no longer be representative of other muscle groups.[15]

Traditionally, tetanic stimulation has been used to evaluate residual neuromuscular blockade but is too painful to use in an unanesthetized patient. Except in connection with the technique of PTC (see later), tetanic stimulation has very little place in everyday clinical anesthesia. If the response to nerve stimulation is recorded, all the information required can be obtained from the response to TOF nerve stimulation. In contrast, if the response to nerve stimulation is evaluated only by tactile evaluation[16,17] or by eye (Viby-Mogensen and colleagues, unpublished observation), even experienced observers are unable to judge the response of tetanic stimulation with sufficient certainty to exclude residual neuromuscular blockade.

Post-Tetanic Count Stimulation

Injection of a nondepolarizing neuromuscular blocking drug in a dose sufficient to ensure smooth tracheal intubation causes intense neuromuscular blockade of the peripheral muscles. Because no response to TOF and single-twitch stimulation occurs under these conditions, these modes of stimulation cannot be used to determine the degree of blockade. It is possible, however, to quantify intense neuromuscular blockade of the peripheral muscles by applying tetanic stimulation (50 Hz for 5 seconds) and observing the post-tetanic response to single-twitch stimulation given at 1 Hz starting 3 seconds after the end of tetanic stimulation.[18] During intense blockade, there is no response to either tetanic or post-tetanic stimulation (Fig. 47-4). However, when the intense neuromuscular blockade dissipates and before the first response to TOF stimulation reappears, the first response to post-tetanic twitch stimulation occurs. As the intense block dissipates, more and more responses to post-tetanic twitch stimulation appear. For a given neuromuscular blocking drug, the time until return of the first response to TOF stimulation is related to the number of post-tetanic twitch responses present at a given time (i.e., the PTC) (Fig. 47-5).[18-22]

The PTC method is mainly used to assess the degree of neuromuscular blockade when there is no reaction to single-twitch or TOF nerve stimulation, as may be the case after injection of a large dose of a nondepolarizing neuromuscular blocking drug. However, PTC can also be used whenever sudden movements must be eliminated (e.g., during ophthalmic surgery). The necessary level of blockade of the adductor pollicis muscle to ensure paralysis of the diaphragm depends on the type of anesthesia and, in the intensive care unit, on the level of sedation. To ensure elimination of any bucking or coughing in response to tracheobronchial stimulation, neuromuscular blockade of the peripheral muscles must be so intense that no response to post-tetanic twitch stimulation can be elicited (PTC 0) (Fig. 47-6).[19-23]

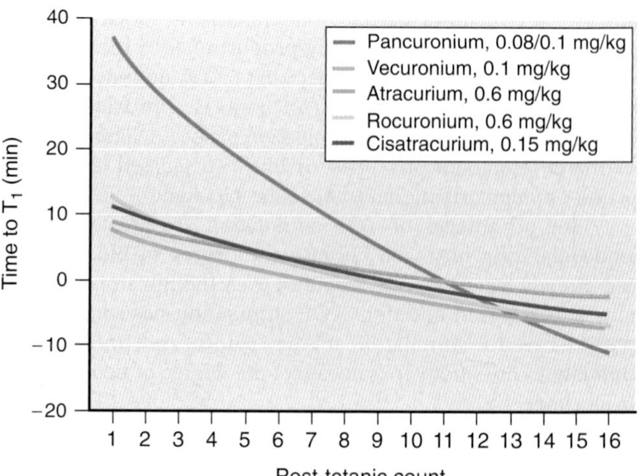

Figure 47-5 Relationship between the post-tetanic count and time when onset of train-of-four (T_1) is likely to be elicited for various neuromuscular blocking agents. *(From El-Orbany MI, Joseph JN, Salem MR: The relationship of post-tetanic count and train-of-four responses during recovery from intense cisatracurium-induced neuromuscular blockade. Anesth Analg 97:80, 2003.)*

The response to PTC stimulation depends primarily on the degree of neuromuscular blockade. It also depends on the frequency and duration of tetanic stimulation, the length of time between the end of tetanic stimulation and the first post-tetanic stimulus, the frequency of the single-twitch stimulation, and also (probably) the duration of single-twitch stimulation before tetanic stimulation. When the PTC method is used, these variables should be kept constant. In addition, because of possible antagonism of neuromuscular blockade in the hand, tetanic stimulation should not be performed more often than every 6 minutes.[18] If the hand muscles undergo antagonism of neuromuscular blockade while the rest of the body is still paralyzed, the hand muscles are no longer useful for monitoring.

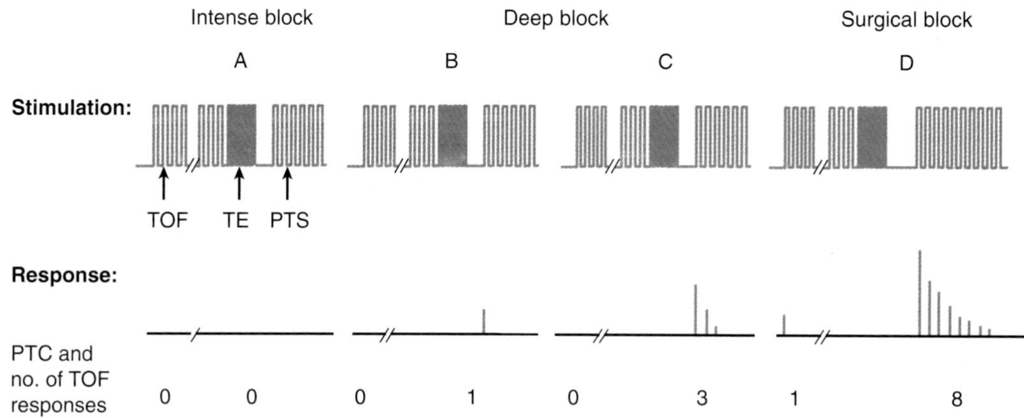

Figure 47-4 Pattern of electrical stimulation and evoked muscle responses to train-of-four (TOF) nerve stimulation, 50-Hz tetanic nerve stimulation for 5 seconds (TE), and 1.0-Hz post-tetanic twitch stimulation (PTS) during four different levels of nondepolarizing neuromuscular blockade. During intense blockade of peripheral muscles (**A**), no response to any of the forms of stimulation occurs. During less pronounced blockade (deep blockade, **B** and **C**), there is still no response to TOF stimulation, but post-tetanic facilitation of transmission is present. During surgical blockade (**D**), the first response to TOF appears and post-tetanic facilitation increases further. The post-tetanic count (see text) is 1 during very deep block (**B**), 3 during less deep block (**C**), and 8 during surgical (or moderate) block (**D**).

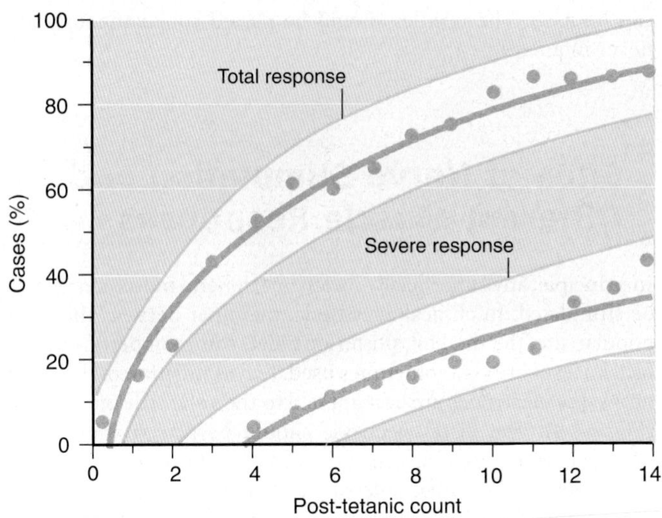

Figure 47-6 Relationship between the rate of muscle response to stimulation of the tracheal carina and the degree of neuromuscular blockade of peripheral muscles, as evaluated by post-tetanic count (PTC). The subjects were 25 patients anesthetized with thiopental, nitrous oxide, and fentanyl and given vecuronium (0.1 mg/kg) for tracheal intubation. For comparison, the first response to train-of-four stimulation usually occurs when the PTC is approximately 10 (range, 6 to 16). The carina was stimulated with a soft sterile rubber suction catheter introduced via the endotracheal tube. The total response consisted of mild responses plus severe responses. A mild response was said to occur if stimulation of the carina induced only slight bucking that did not interfere with surgery. A severe response was said to occur if stimulation elicited bucking that interfered with surgery and required intervention. Elimination of severe responses requires an intense neuromuscular blockade; PTC must be less than 2 to 3, and elimination of all reactions requires that PTC be 0. *(From Fernando PUE, Viby-Mogensen J, Bonsu AK, et al: Relationship between post-tetanic count and response to carinal stimulation during vecuronium-induced neuromuscular blockade. Acta Anaesthesiol Scand 31:593, 1987. Copyright 1987, Munksgaard International Publishers, Ltd. Copenhagen, Denmark.)*

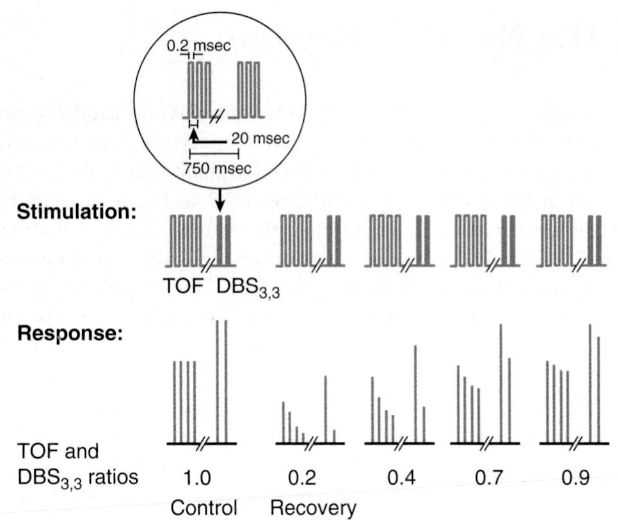

Figure 47-7 Pattern of electrical stimulation and evoked muscle responses to train-of-four (TOF) nerve stimulation and double-burst nerve stimulation (i.e., three impulses in each of two tetanic bursts, $DBS_{3,3}$) before injection of muscle relaxants (control) and during recovery from nondepolarizing neuromuscular blockade. The TOF ratio is the amplitude of the fourth response to TOF divided by the amplitude of the first response. The $DBS_{3,3}$ ratio is the amplitude of the second response to $DBS_{3,3}$ divided by the amplitude of the first response. (See text for further explanation.)

Double-Burst Stimulation

DBS consists of two short bursts of 50-Hz tetanic stimulation separated by 750 msec. The duration of each square wave impulse in the burst is 0.2 msec (Fig. 47-7). Although the number of impulses in each burst can vary, DBS with three impulses in each of the two tetanic bursts ($DBS_{3,3}$) is most commonly used.[24-26]

In nonparalyzed muscle, the response to $DBS_{3,3}$ is two short muscle contractions of equal strength. In a partly paralyzed muscle, the second response is weaker than the first (i.e., the response fades) (see Fig 47-7). Measured mechanically, the TOF ratio correlates closely with the $DBS_{3,3}$ ratio. DBS was developed with the specific aim of allowing manual (tactile) detection of small amounts of residual blockade under clinical conditions,[24] and during recovery and immediately after surgery, tactile evaluation of the response to $DBS_{3,3}$ is superior to tactile evaluation of the response to TOF stimulation.[26,27] However, as shown in Figure 47-8, absence of fade in the manually evaluated response to $DBS_{3,3}$ (and TOF) does not exclude residual neuromuscular blockade.[28]

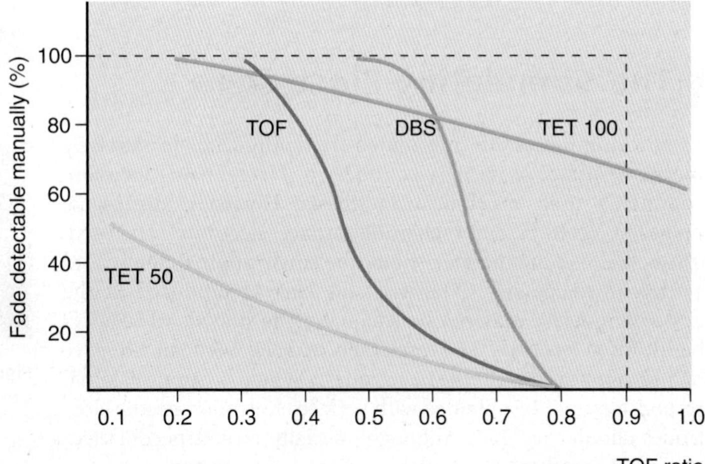

Figure 47-8 Fade detectable by feel in the response to train-of-four (TOF), double-burst stimulation ($DBS_{3,3}$), and 50- and 100-Hz tetanic stimulation (TET 50 and TET 100) in relation to the true TOF ratio, as measured mechanically. The axis indicates the percentage of instances in which fade can be felt at a given TOF ratio.[17,25,26] It appears that it is not possible to exclude residual neuromuscular block by any of the methods, regardless of whether a TOF ratio of 0.7 or 0.9 is taken to reflect adequate recovery of neuromuscular function. (See text for further explanation.)

The Nerve Stimulator

Although many nerve stimulators are commercially available, not all meet the basic requirements for clinical use. The stimulus should produce a monophasic and rectangular waveform, and the length of the pulse should not exceed 0.2 to 0.3 msec. A pulse exceeding 0.5 msec may stimulate the muscle directly or cause repetitive firing. Stimulation at a constant current is preferable to stimulation at a constant voltage because current is the determinant of nerve stimulation. Furthermore, for safety reasons, the nerve stimulator should be battery operated, include a battery check, and be able to generate 60 to 70 mA, but not higher than 80 mA. Many commercially available stimulators can deliver just 25 to 50 mA and provide a constant current only when skin resistance ranges from 0 to 2.5 kΩ. These limitations are a disadvantage; during cooling, skin resistance may increase to approximately 5 kΩ, which may cause the current delivered to the nerve to fall below the supramaximal level and lead to a decrease in the response to stimulation. As a result, the anesthesiologist may misjudge the degree of neuromuscular blockade. Ideally, the nerve stimulator should have a built-in warning system or a current level display that alerts the user when the current selected is not delivered to the nerve.

The ideal nerve stimulator should have other features as well. The polarity of the electrodes should be indicated, and the apparatus should be capable of delivering the following modes of stimulation: TOF (as both a single train and in a repetitive mode, with TOF stimulation being given every 10 to 20 seconds), single-twitch stimulation at 0.1 and 1.0 Hz, and tetanic stimulation at 50 Hz. In addition, the stimulator should have a built-in time constant system to facilitate PTC. The tetanic stimulus should last 5 seconds and be followed 3 seconds later by the first post-tetanic stimulus. If the nerve stimulator does not allow objective measurement of the response to TOF stimulation, at least one DBS mode should be available, preferably $DBS_{3,3}$. Single-twitch stimulation at 1 Hz is useful during initiation of monitoring because it shortens the time necessary to determine supramaximal stimulation. Most investigators agree that there is no need for tetanus at 100 or 200 Hz because 50-Hz tetanic stimulation stresses neuromuscular function to the same extent as maximal voluntary effort does. Furthermore, in contrast to 100- and 200-Hz stimulation, 50-Hz tetanic stimulation does not cause fatigue (fade) in nonparalyzed muscle.

The Stimulating Electrodes

Electrical impulses are transmitted from stimulator to nerve by means of surface or needle electrodes, the former being the more commonly used in clinical anesthesia. Normally, disposable pregelled silver or silver chloride surface electrodes are used. The actual conducting area should be small, approximately 7 to 11 mm in diameter.[29] Otherwise, the current produced in the underlying nerve may not be adequate. The skin should always be cleansed properly and preferably rubbed with an abrasive before application of the electrodes. When a supramaximal response cannot be obtained with surface electrodes, needle electrodes should be used. Although specially coated needle electrodes are commercially available, ordinary steel injection needles can be used. The needles should be placed subcutaneously but never in a nerve.

Sites of Nerve Stimulation and Different Muscle Responses

In principle, any superficially located peripheral motor nerve may be stimulated. In clinical anesthesia, the ulnar nerve is the most popular site; the median, posterior tibial, common peroneal, and facial nerves are also sometimes used. For stimulation of the ulnar nerve, the electrodes are best applied to the volar side of the wrist (Fig. 47-9). The distal electrode should be placed about 1 cm proximal to the point at which the proximal flexion crease of the wrist crosses the radial side of the tendon to the flexor carpi ulnaris muscle. The proximal electrode should preferably be placed so that the distance between the centers of the two electrodes is 3 to 6 cm (see Fig. 47-9). With this placement of the electrodes, electrical stimulation normally elicits only finger flexion and thumb adduction. If one electrode is placed over the ulnar groove at the elbow, thumb adduction is often pronounced because of stimulation of the flexor carpi ulnaris muscle. When this latter placement of electrodes (sometimes preferred in small children) is used, the active negative electrode should be at the wrist to ensure maximal response. Polarity of the electrodes is less crucial when both electrodes are close to each other at the volar side of the wrist; however, placement of the negative electrode distally normally elicits the greatest neuromuscular response.[30] When the temporal branch of the facial nerve is stimulated, the negative electrode should be placed over the nerve, and the positive electrode should be placed somewhere else over the forehead.

Because different muscle groups have different sensitivities to neuromuscular blocking agents, results obtained for one muscle cannot be automatically extrapolated to other muscles. The diaphragm is among the most resistant of all muscles to both depo-

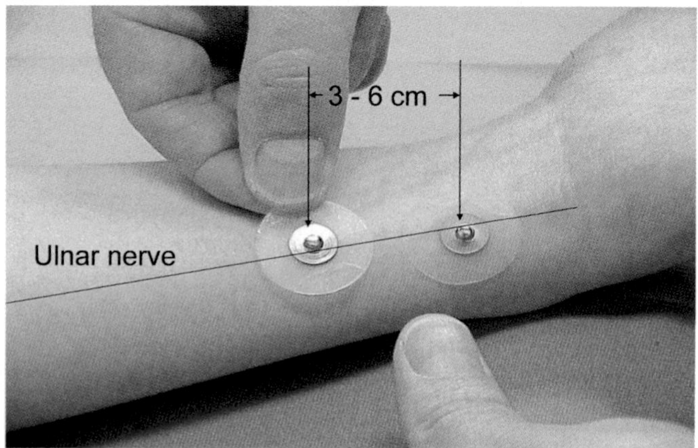

Figure 47-9 Stimulating electrodes with the appropriate contact area in the correct position over the ulnar nerve of the left forearm. *(From Fuchs-Buder T, Claudius C, Skovgaard LT, et al: Good clinical research practice in pharmacodynamic studies of neuromuscular blocking agents II: The Stockholm revision. Acta Anaesthesiol Scand 51:789, 2007.)*

larizing[31] and nondepolarizing neuromuscular blocking drugs.[32] In general, the diaphragm requires 1.4 to 2.0 times as much muscle relaxant as the adductor pollicis muscle for an identical degree of blockade (Fig. 47-10).[32] Also of clinical significance is that onset time is normally shorter for the diaphragm than for the adductor pollicis muscle and the diaphragm recovers from paralysis more quickly than the peripheral muscles do (Fig. 47-11).[33] The other respiratory muscles are less resistant than the diaphragm, as are the larynx and the corrugator supercilii muscles.[34-36] Most sensitive are the abdominal muscles, the orbicularis oculi muscle, the peripheral muscles of the limbs, and the geniohyoid, masseter, and upper airway muscles.[37-40] From a practical clinical point of view, it is worth noting that (1) the response of the corrugator supercilii to facial nerve stimulation reflects the extent of neuromuscular blockade of the laryngeal adductor muscles and abdominal muscles better than the response of the adductor pollicis to ulnar nerve stimulation does[34,41] and (2) the upper airway muscles seem to be more sensitive than the peripheral muscles.[37,38] Although three investigations using acceleromyography have indicated small differences in the response to TOF nerve stimulation in the arm (adductor pollicis muscle) and the leg (flexor hallucis brevis muscle), these differences are probably of little clinical significance.[42,43]

Even though the precise source of these differences is unknown, variations in acetylcholine receptor density, acetylcholine release, acetylcholinesterase activity, fiber composition, innervation ratio (number of neuromuscular junctions), blood flow, and muscle temperature may be possible explanations.

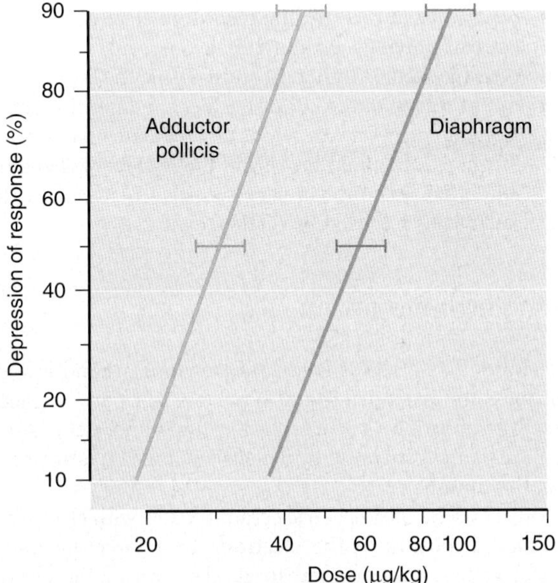

Figure 47-10 The mean cumulative dose-response curve for pancuronium in two muscles shows that the diaphragm requires approximately twice as much pancuronium as the adductor pollicis muscle for the same amount of neuromuscular blockade. The depression in muscle response to the first stimulus in train-of-four nerve stimulation (probit scale) was plotted against dose (log scale). The force of contraction of the adductor pollicis was measured on a force-displacement transducer; response of the diaphragm was measured electromyographically. *(From Donati F, Antzaka C, Bevan DR: Potency of pancuronium at the diaphragm and the adductor pollicis muscle in humans. Anesthesiology 65:1, 1986.)*

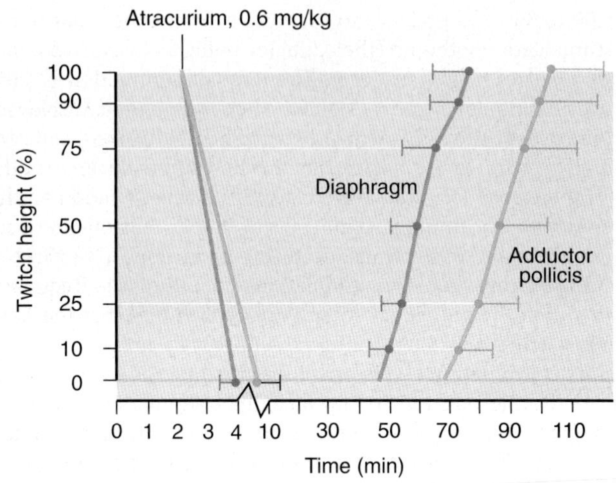

Figure 47-11 Evolution of twitch height (mean ± SD) of the diaphragm (*blue circles*) and the adductor pollicis muscle (*yellow circles*) in 10 anesthetized patients after the administration of atracurium, 0.6 mg/kg. *(From Pansard J-L, Chauvin M, Lebrault C, et al: Effect of an intubating dose of succinylcholine and atracurium on the diaphragm and the adductor pollicis muscle in humans. Anesthesiology 67:326, 1987.)*

In assessing neuromuscular function, use of a relatively sensitive muscle such as the adductor pollicis of the hand has both disadvantages and advantages. Obviously, during surgery it is a disadvantage that even total elimination of the response to single-twitch and TOF stimulation does not exclude the possibility of movement of the diaphragm, such as hiccupping and coughing. PTC stimulation, however, allows evaluation of the intense blockade necessary to ensure total paralysis of the diaphragm. On the positive side, the risk of overdosing the patient decreases if the response of a relatively sensitive muscle is used as a guide to the administration of muscle relaxants during surgery. In addition, during recovery, when the adductor pollicis has recovered sufficiently, it can be assumed that no residual neuromuscular blockade exists in the diaphragm or in other resistant muscles.

Recording of Evoked Responses

The choice of recording method is a practical decision. Five methods are available: measurement of the evoked mechanical response of the muscle (mechanomyography [MMG]), measurement of the evoked electrical response of the muscle (electromyography [EMG]), measurement of acceleration of the muscle response (acceleromyography [AMG]), measurement of the evoked electrical response in a piezoelectric film sensor attached to the muscle (piezoelectric neuromuscular monitor [P_ZEMG], and phonomyography [PMG]).

Mechanomyography

A requirement for correct and reproducible measurement of evoked tension is that the muscle contraction be isometric. In clinical anesthesia, this condition is most easily achieved by measuring thumb movement after the application of a resting tension of 200 to 300 g (a preload) to the thumb. When the ulnar nerve is stimulated, the thumb (the adductor pollicis muscle) acts on a force-displacement transducer. The force of contraction is then converted into an electrical signal, which is amplified, displayed, and recorded. The arm and hand should be rigidly fixed, and care should be taken to prevent overloading of the transducer. In addition, the transducer should be placed in correct relation to the thumb (i.e., the thumb should always apply tension precisely along the length of the transducer). It is important to remember that the response to nerve stimulation depends on the frequency with which the individual stimuli are applied and that the time used to achieve a stable control response may influence subsequent determination of the onset time and duration of blockade.[29] Generally, the reaction to supramaximal stimulation increases during the first 8 to 12 minutes after commencement of the stimulation. Therefore, in clinical studies, recording of the control response (before injection of muscle relaxant) should not be made until the response has stabilized for 8 to 12 minutes or a 2- or 5-second 50-Hz tetanic stimulation has been given.[44] Even then, twitch response often recovers to 110% to 150% of the control response after paralysis with succinylcholine. This increase in response, thought to be caused by a change in the contractile response of the muscle, normally disappears within 15 to 25 minutes.

Although numerous methods for mechanical recording of evoked mechanical responses exist, not all meet the criteria outlined.

Electromyography

Evoked EMG records the compound action potentials produced by stimulation of a peripheral nerve. The compound action potential is a high-speed event that for many years could be picked up only by means of a preamplifier and a storage oscilloscope. Modern neuromuscular transmission analyzers are able to make on-line electronic analyses and graphic presentations of the EMG response.

The evoked EMG response is most often obtained from muscles innervated by the ulnar or the median nerves. Stimulating electrodes are applied as in force measurements. Although both surface and needle electrodes may be used for recording, no advantage is obtained by using the latter. Most often, the evoked EMG response is obtained from the thenar or hypothenar eminence of the hand or from the first dorsal interosseous muscle of the hand, preferably with the active electrode over the motor point of the muscle (Fig. 47-12). The signal picked up by the analyzer is processed by an amplifier, a rectifier, and an electronic integrator. The results are displayed either as a percentage of control or as a TOF ratio.

Two new sites for recording the EMG response have been introduced: the larynx and the diaphragm.[45,46] By using a noninvasive disposable laryngeal electrode attached to the tracheal tube and placed between the vocal cords, it is possible to monitor the onset of neuromuscular blockade in the laryngeal muscles. Thus far, however, the method is mainly of interest in clinical research when investigating onset times of the laryngeal muscles. In paravertebral surface diaphragmatic EMG, the recording electrodes are placed on the right of vertebrae T12/L1 or L1/L2 for monitoring the response of the right diaphragmatic crux to transcutaneous stimulation of the right phrenic nerve at the neck.[45-47] As is the case with surface laryngeal EMG, surface diaphragmatic EMG is mainly of interest in clinical research because of difficulties connected with stimulation of the phrenic nerve transcutaneously at the neck.

Evoked electrical and mechanical responses represent different physiologic events. Evoked EMG records changes in the electrical activity of one or more muscles, whereas evoked MMG records changes associated with excitation-contraction coupling and contraction of the muscle as well. For these reasons, the results obtained with these methods may differ.[48,49] Although evoked EMG responses generally correlate well with evoked mechanical responses,[50] marked differences may occur, especially in the response to succinylcholine and in the TOF ratio during recovery from a nondepolarizing block.[48-50]

In theory, recording of evoked EMG responses has several advantages over recording of evoked mechanical responses. Equipment for measuring evoked EMG responses is easier to set up, the response reflects only factors influencing neuromuscular transmission, and the response can be obtained from muscles not accessible to mechanical recording. However, evoked EMG does entail some difficulties. Although high-quality recordings are possible in most patients, the results are not always reliable. For one thing, improper placement of electrodes may result in inadequate pickup of the compound EMG signal. If the neuromuscular transmission analyzer does not allow observation of the actual waveform of the compound EMG, determining optimal placement of the electrodes is difficult. Another source of unreliable results may be that fixation of the hand with a preload on the thumb might be more important than is generally appreciated[50] inasmuch as changes in the position of the electrodes in relation to the muscle may affect the EMG response. In addition, direct muscle stimulation sometimes occurs. If muscles close to the stimulating electrodes are stimulated directly, the recording electrodes may pick up an electrical signal even though neuromuscular transmission is completely blocked. Another difficulty is that the EMG response often does not return to the control value. Whether this situation is the result of technical problems, inadequate fixation of the hand, or changes in temperature is unknown (Fig. 47-13). Finally, the evoked EMG response is very sensitive to electrical interference, such as that caused by diathermy.

Acceleromyography

The technique of AMG is based on Newton's second law: force equals mass times acceleration.[51] If mass is constant, acceleration is directly proportional to force. Accordingly, after nerve stimulation, one can measure not only the evoked force but also acceleration of the thumb.

AMG uses a piezoelectric ceramic wafer with electrodes on both sides. Exposure of the electrode to a force generates an electrical voltage proportional to acceleration of the electrode. Consequently, when an accelerometer is fixed to the thumb and the ulnar nerve is stimulated, an electrical signal is produced whenever the thumb moves. This signal can be analyzed in a specially designed analyzer[52] or perhaps displayed on a recording system. At least one detached monitor based on measurement of acceleration is commercially available: the TOF-Watch (Organon, part of Schering-Plough Corp.) (Fig. 47-14).

AMG is a simple method of analyzing neuromuscular function, both in the operating room and in the intensive care

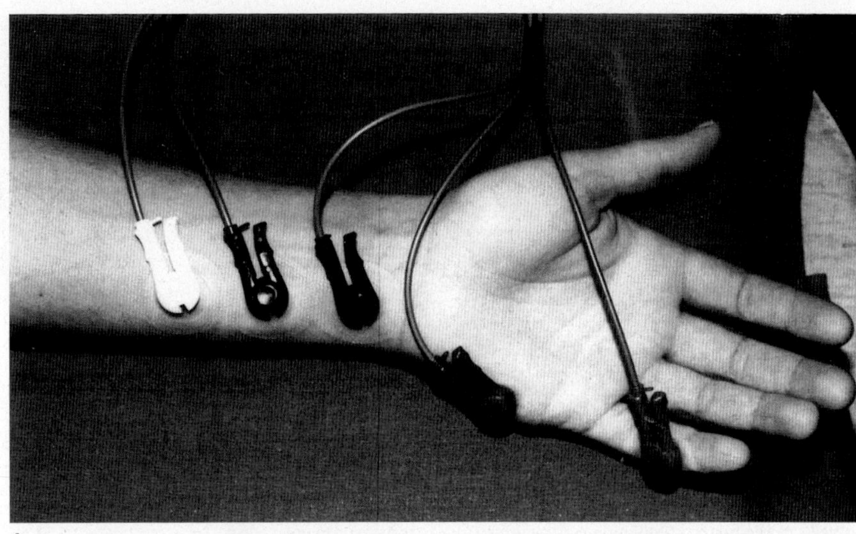

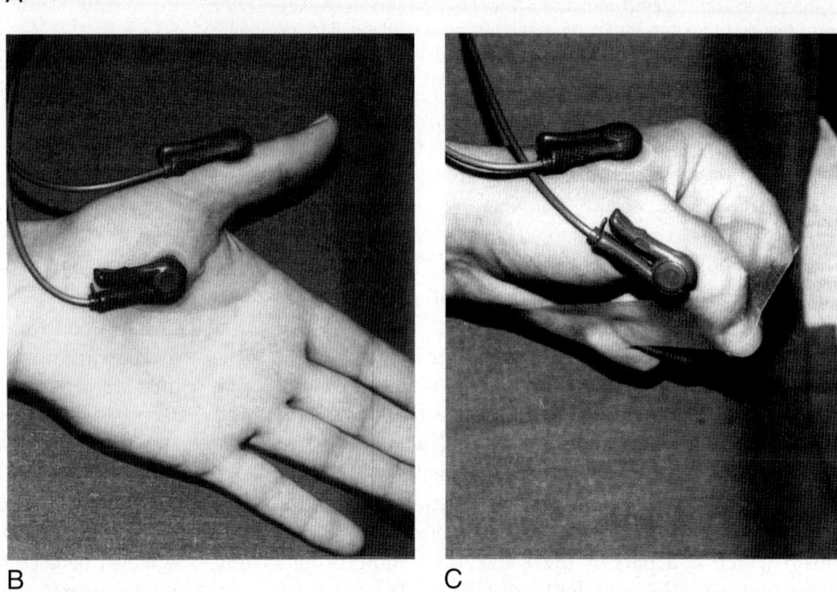

Figure 47-12 Electrode placement for stimulation of the ulnar nerve and for recording of the compound action potential from three sites of the hand. **A,** Abductor digiti minimi muscle (in the hypothenar eminence). **B,** Adductor pollicis muscle (in the thenar eminence). **C,** First dorsal interosseus muscle. *(Courtesy of Datex-Ohmeda, Helsinki, Finland.)*

unit. However, although good correlation exists between the TOF ratio measured by this method and the TOF ratio measured with a force-displacement transducer or EMG,[51,53,54] measurements made via AMG are not directly comparable with results obtained by the other two methods.[54-58] When AMG is used with a free-moving thumb, as originally suggested,[51] wide limits of agreements in twitch height (T1) and TOF ratio and differences in the onset and recovery course of blockade between AMG and MMG have been found. Moreover, the AMG control TOF ratio is consistently higher than when measured with a force-displacement transducer. In accordance with this, several studies have indicated that when using AMG, the TOF ratio indicative of sufficient postoperative neuromuscular recovery is 1.0 rather than 0.9 as when measured by MMG or EMG in the adductor pollicis muscle.[2,17,59,60]

One reason for the wide limits of agreement between AMG and MMG is probably and paradoxically connected with one of the originally claimed advantages of the method, that fixation of the hand could be reduced to a minimum as long as the thumb could move freely.[51] However, in daily clinical practice it is often not possible to ensure that the thumb can move freely and that the position of the hand does not change during a surgical procedure. The evoked response may therefore vary considerably. Several solutions have been proposed, and on-going clinical research indicates that the use of an elastic preload on the thumb may improve the agreement between results obtained with AMG and MMG (Fig. 47-15). Despite these reservations, it is my opinion that AMG at the thumb is a valuable clinical tool that when used with intelligence, may eliminate the problem of postoperative residual neuromuscular blockade.[61,62]

When the thumb is not available for monitoring during surgery, some clinicians prefer to monitor the AMG response of the orbicularis oculi or the corrugator supercilii in response to facial nerve stimulation.[41] However, neuromuscular monitoring of both these sites with AMG is subject to large uncertainty regarding the extent of paralysis, and it therefore cannot be recommended for routine monitoring. It provides only a rough estimate of the degree of block of the peripheral muscles.[63,64]

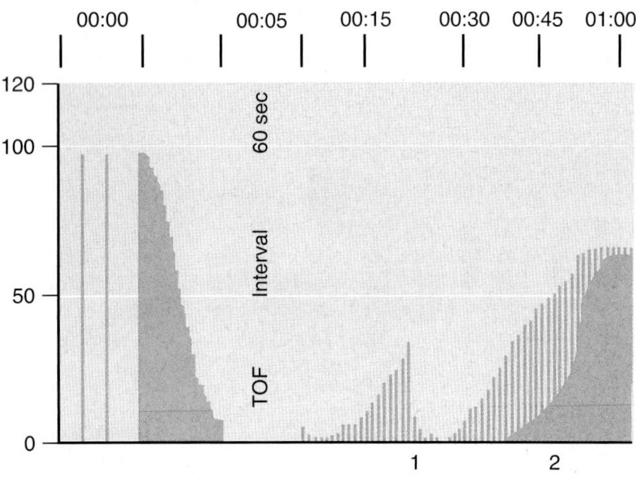

Figure 47-13 Evoked electromyographic printout from a Relaxograph. Initially, single-twitch stimulation was given at 0.1 Hz, and vecuronium (70 μg/kg) was administered intravenously for tracheal intubation. After approximately 5 minutes, the mode of stimulation was changed to train-of-four (TOF) stimulation every 60 seconds. At a twitch height (first twitch in the TOF response) of approximately 30% of control (marker 1), 1 mg of vecuronium was given intravenously. At marker 2, 1 mg of neostigmine was given intravenously, preceded by 2 mg of glycopyrrolate. The printout also illustrates the common problem of failure of the electromyographic response to return to the control level. *(Courtesy of Datex-Ohmeda, Helsinki, Finland.)*

Piezoelectric Neuromuscular Monitors

The technique of the piezoelectric monitor is based on the principle that stretching or bending a flexible piezoelectric film (e.g., one attached to the thumb) in response to nerve stimulation generates a voltage that is proportional to the amount of stretching or bending.[65,66] At least two devices based on this principle are available commercially: the ParaGraph Neuromuscular Blockade Monitor (Vital Signs, Totowa, NJ) and the M-NMT MechanoSensor, which is a part of the Datex AS/3 monitoring system (Datex-Ohmeda, Helsinki, Finland) (Fig. 47-16).

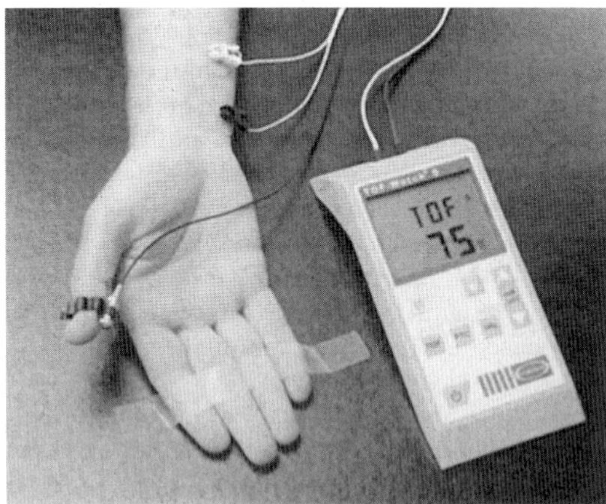

Figure 47-14 TOF-Watch (Organon, part of Schering-Plough, Corp.). This neuromuscular transmission monitor is based on measurement of acceleration with a piezoelectric transducer.[51,52] Note that the transducer is fastened to the thumb and the stimulating electrodes. On the display of the TOF-Watch, the train-of-four (TOF) ratio is given in percentage.

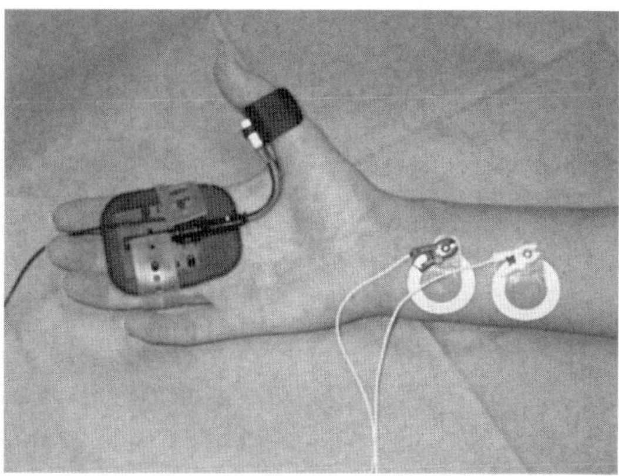

Figure 47-15 Hand adaptor (elastic preload) for the TOF-Watch transducer (Organon, part of Schering-Plough, Corp.).

Few studies have evaluated the function of these monitors.[65-67] The scarce data indicate a good relationship between results obtained with P_ZEMG, AMG, and MMG, but also wide limits of agreement between the methods. Therefore, although P_ZEMG may be a valuable clinical tool, the values obtained in an individual patient with this method may vary from those obtained with MMG or AMG.

Phonomyography

PMG (acoustic myography) is a relatively new method of monitoring neuromuscular function.[68-72] Contraction of skeletal muscles generates intrinsic low-frequency sounds, which can be recorded with special microphones. This method has been evaluated for clinical and research purposes. Several reports indicate good correlation between evoked acoustic responses and those obtained with more traditional methods of recording, such as MMG, EMG, and AMG. However, it is uncertain whether PMG will ever be used for monitoring neuromuscular blockade during routine anesthesia. What does make PMG interesting, however, is that in theory the method can be applied not only to the adductor pollicis muscle but also to other muscles of interest such as the diaphragm, larynx, and eye muscles. In addition, the ease of application is attractive.

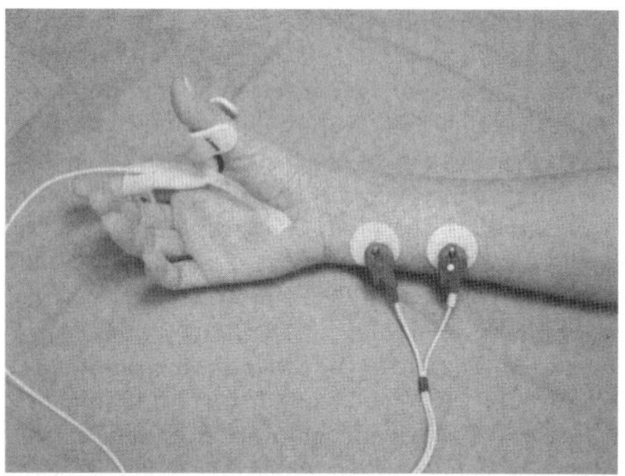

Figure 47-16 Datex-Engstrøm M-NMT MechanoSensor (a piezoelectric neuromuscular monitor).

For further information on recording evoked responses, the reader is referred to guidelines for good clinical research practice in pharmacodynamic studies of neuromuscular blocking drugs, published in *Acta Anaesthesiologica Scandinavica*.[29]

Evaluation of Recorded Evoked Responses

Nerve stimulation in clinical anesthesia is usually synonymous with TOF nerve stimulation. Therefore, the recorded response to this form of stimulation is used to explain how to evaluate the degree of neuromuscular blockade during clinical anesthesia.

Nondepolarizing Neuromuscular Blockade

After injection of a nondepolarizing neuromuscular blocking drug in a dose sufficient for smooth tracheal intubation, TOF recording demonstrates four phases or levels of neuromuscular blockade: intense blockade, deep blockade, moderate or surgical blockade, and recovery (Fig. 47-17).

Intense Neuromuscular Blockade

Intense neuromuscular blockade occurs within 3 to 6 minutes of injection of an intubating dose of a nondepolarizing muscle relaxant, depending on the drug and the dose given. This phase is also called the "period of no response" because no response to any pattern of nerve stimulation occurs. The length of this period varies, again depending primarily on the duration of action of the muscle relaxant and the dose given. The sensitivity of the patient to the drug also affects the period of no response.

Deep Neuromuscular Blockade

Intense neuromuscular blockade is followed by a period of deep block, characterized by absence of response to TOF stimulation, but presence of post-tetanic twitches (i.e., PTC ≥ 1; compare with Figure 47-4). Although it is not possible during this phase to determine exactly how long deep neuromuscular blockade will last, correlation does exist between PTC stimulation and the time until reappearance of the first response to TOF stimulation (see Fig. 47-5).

Moderate or Surgical Blockade

Moderate or surgical blockade begins when the first response to TOF stimulation appears. This phase is characterized by a gradual return of the four responses to TOF stimulation. Furthermore, good correlation exists between the degree of neuromuscular blockade and the number of responses to TOF stimulation. When only one response is detectable, the degree of neuromuscular blockade (the depression in twitch tension) is 90% to 95%. When the fourth response reappears, neuromuscular blockade is usually 60% to 85%.[73,74] The presence of one or two responses in the TOF pattern normally indicates sufficient relaxation for most surgical procedures. During light anesthesia, however, patients may move, buck, or cough. Therefore, when elimination of sudden movements is crucial, a deeper block (or a deeper level of anesthesia) may be necessary. The deep block can then be evaluated by PTC (see Fig. 47-6).

Antagonism of neuromuscular blockade with a cholinesterase inhibitor should not normally be attempted when the blockade is intense or deep because reversal will often be inadequate, regardless of the dose of antagonist administered.[75] Furthermore, after the administration of large doses of muscle relaxants, reversal of the block to clinically normal activity is not always possible if only one TOF response is present. In general, antagonism with cholinesterase inhibitors should not be initiated before at least two and preferably three or four responses are observed.

Recovery

Return of the fourth response in the TOF heralds the recovery phase. During neuromuscular recovery, a reasonably good correlation exists between the actual TOF ratio measured by MMG and clinical observation, but the relationship between the TOF ratio and signs and symptoms of residual blockade varies greatly

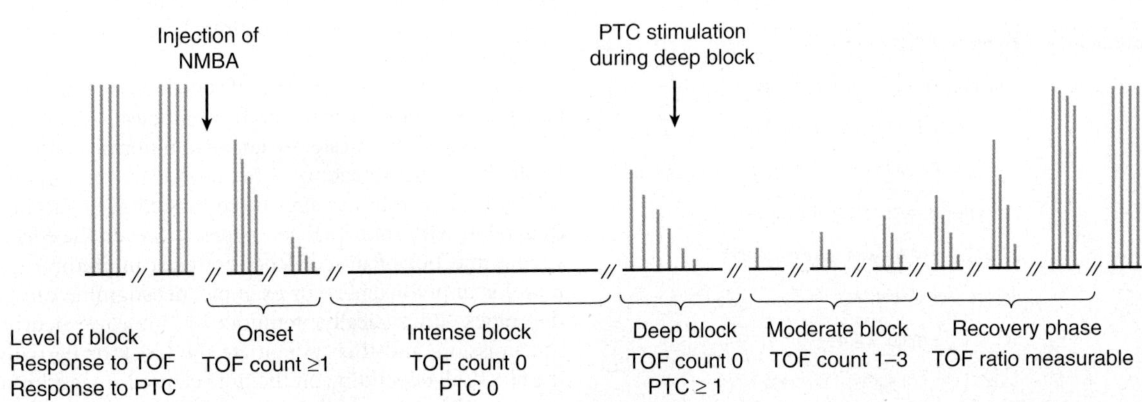

Figure 47-17 Levels of block after a normal intubating dose of a nondepolarizing neuromuscular blocking agent (NMBA) as classified by post-tetanic count (PTC) and train-of-four (TOF) stimulation. During intense (profound) block, there are no responses to either TOF or PTC stimulation. During deep block, there is response to PTC but not to TOF stimulation. Intense (profound) block and deep block together constitute the "period of no response to TOF stimulation." Reappearance of the response to TOF stimulation heralds the start of moderate block. Finally, when all four responses to TOF stimulation are present and a TOF ratio can be measured, the recovery period has started. *(From Fuchs-Buder T, Claudius C, Skovgaard LT, et al: Good clinical research practice in pharmacodynamic studies of neuromuscular blocking agents II: The Stockholm revision. Acta Anaesthesiol Scand 51:789, 2007.)*

among patients.[75] When the TOF ratio is 0.4 or less, the patient is generally unable to lift the head or arm. Tidal volume may be normal, but vital capacity and inspiratory force will be reduced. When the ratio is 0.6, most patients are able to lift their head for 3 seconds, open their eyes widely, and stick out their tongue, but vital capacity and inspiratory force are often still reduced. At a TOF ratio of 0.7 to 0.75, the patient can normally cough sufficiently and lift the head for at least 5 seconds, but grip strength may still be as low as about 60% of control.[76] When the ratio is 0.8 and higher, vital capacity and inspiratory force are normal.[12,77-79] The patient may, however, still have diplopia and facial weakness (Table 47-1).[75]

In clinical anesthesia, a TOF ratio of 0.70 to 0.75, or even 0.50, has been thought to reflect adequate recovery of neuromuscular function.[79] However, the TOF ratio, whether recorded mechanically or by EMG, must exceed 0.80 or even 0.90 to exclude clinically important residual neuromuscular blockade.[40,50,59,80-85] Moderate degrees of neuromuscular blockade decrease chemoreceptor sensitivity to hypoxia and thereby lead to insufficient response to a decrease in oxygen tension in blood.[80,81,83,85] Moreover, residual blockade (TOF < 0.90) is associated with functional impairment of the pharyngeal and upper esophageal muscles, which most probably predisposes to regurgitation and aspiration of gastric contents.[40] Recently, Eikerman and colleagues documented that partial neuromuscular blockade, even to a degree that does not evoke dyspnea or oxygen desaturation, may decrease inspiratory upper airway volume and can evoke partial inspiratory airway collapse.[86] Accordingly, residual blockade (TOF < 0.70) caused by the long-acting muscle relaxant pancuronium is a significant risk factor for the development of postoperative pulmonary complications (Table 47-2 and Fig. 47-18).[82] Even in volunteers without sedation or impaired consciousness, a TOF ratio of 0.9 or less may impair the ability to maintain the airway.[76] Adequate recovery of neuromuscular function requires return of an MMG or EMG TOF ratio to 0.90 or greater, which cannot be guaranteed without objective neuromuscular monitoring.[61,62,87-90]

Table 47-1 Clinical Signs and Symptoms of Residual Paralysis in Awake Volunteers After Mivacurium-Induced Neuromuscular Blockade

Train-of-Four Ratio	Signs and Symptoms
0.70-0.75	Diplopia and visual disturbances
	Decreased handgrip strength
	Inability to maintain apposition of the incisor teeth
	"Tongue depressor test" negative
	Inability to sit up without assistance
	Severe facial weakness
	Speaking a major effort
	Overall weakness and tiredness
0.85-0.90	Diplopia and visual disturbances
	Generalized fatigue

From Kopman AF, Yee PS, Neuman GG: Relationship of the train-of-four fade ratio to clinical signs and symptoms of residual paralysis in awake volunteers. Anesthesiology 86:765, 1997.

Table 47-2 Relationship between Train-of-Four Ratio at the First Postoperative Recording and Postoperative Pulmonary Complications*

	Pancuronium (*n* = 226)			Atracurium or Vecuronium (*n* = 450)		
		Patients with POPC			Patients with POPC	
	No. of Patients	*n*	%	No. of Patients	*n*	%
TOF ≥ 0.70	167	8	4.8	426	23	5.4
TOF < 0.70	59	10	16.9†	24	1	4.2

*Results from a prospective, randomized, and blinded study of postoperative pulmonary complications (POPC) in a total of 691 adult patients undergoing abdominal, gynecologic, or orthopedic surgery and receiving either pancuronium, atracurium, or vecuronium.[82] In 4 of the 46 patients with POPC (1 in the pancuronium group and 3 in the atracurium and vecuronium groups), the train-of-four (TOF) ratio was not available. Because there were no significant differences in the two groups of patients given the intermediate-acting muscle relaxants, the data from these groups are pooled.

†*P* < .02 versus patients in the same group with a TOF ratio of 0.70 or greater.

Depolarizing Neuromuscular Blockade (Phase I and II Blocks)

Patients with normal plasma cholinesterase activity who are given a moderate dose of succinylcholine (0.5 to 1.5 mg/kg) undergo a typical depolarizing neuromuscular block (phase I block; i.e., the response to TOF or tetanic stimulation does not fade, and no post-tetanic facilitation of transmission occurs). In contrast, some patients with genetically determined abnormal plasma cholinesterase activity who are given the same dose of succinylcholine undergo a nondepolarizing-like block characterized by fade in the response to TOF and tetanic stimulation and the occurrence of post-tetanic facilitation of transmission (Fig. 47-19). This type of block is called a phase II block (dual, mixed, or desensitizing block). In addition, phase II blocks sometimes occur in genetically normal patients after repetitive bolus doses or a prolonged infusion of succinylcholine.

From a therapeutic point of view, a phase II block in normal patients must be differentiated from a phase II block in patients with abnormal cholinesterase activity. In normal patients, a phase II block can be antagonized by administering a cholinesterase inhibitor a few minutes after discontinuation of succinylcholine. In patients with abnormal genotypes, however, the effect of intravenous injection of an acetylcholinesterase inhibitor (e.g., neostigmine) is unpredictable. For example, neostigmine can potentiate the block dramatically, temporarily improve neuromuscular transmission, and then potentiate the block or partially reverse the block, all depending on the time elapsed since administration of succinylcholine and the dose of neostigmine given. Therefore, unless the cholinesterase genotype is known to be normal, antagonism of a phase II block with a cholinesterase inhibitor should be undertaken with extreme caution. Even if neuromuscular function improves promptly, patient surveillance should continue for at least 1 hour.

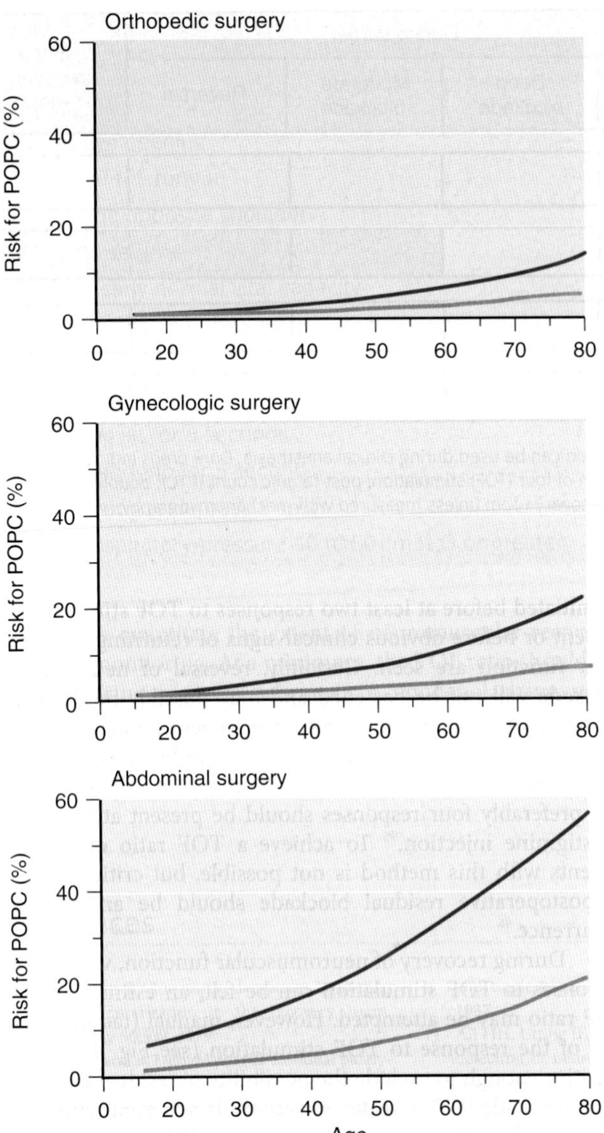

Figure 47-18 Predicted probabilities of a postoperative pulmonary complication (POPC) in different age groups in orthopedic, gynecologic, and major abdominal surgery with a duration of anesthesia of less than 200 minutes. The *red lines* represent patients with residual neuromuscular block (train-of-four [TOF] < 0.70) after the administration of pancuronium; the *blue lines* represent patients with a TOF of 0.70 or greater after the administration of pancuronium, as well as all patients after the administration of atracurium and vecuronium, independent of the TOF ratio at the end of anesthesia.[82]

Use of Nerve Stimulators Without Recording Equipment

Whenever a neuromuscular blocking drug is administered to a patient, tactile or visual evaluation of the evoked response is still the most common form of clinical neuromuscular monitoring. The following is a description of how this is best done.

First, for supramaximal stimulation, careful cleansing of the skin and proper placement and fixation of electrodes are essential. Second, every effort should be taken to prevent central cooling, as well as cooling of the extremity being evaluated. Both central and local surface cooling of the adductor pollicis muscle may reduce twitch tension and the TOF ratio.[91-93] Peripheral cooling may affect nerve conduction, decrease the rate of release of acetylcholine and muscle contractility, increase skin impedance, and reduce blood flow to muscles, thus decreasing the rate of removal of muscle relaxant from the neuromuscular junction. These factors may account for the occasional very pronounced difference in muscle response between a cold extremity and the contralateral warm extremity.[94] Third, when possible, the response to nerve stimulation should be evaluated by feel and not by eye, and the response of the thumb (rather than response of the fifth finger) should be evaluated. Direct stimulation of the muscle often causes subtle movement of the fifth finger when no response is present at the thumb. Finally, the different sensitivities of various muscle groups to neuromuscular blocking agents should always be kept in mind. Figure 47-20 shows which modes of nerve stimulation can be used at various perioperative times.

Use of a Peripheral Nerve Stimulator During Induction of Anesthesia

The nerve stimulator should be attached to the patient before induction of anesthesia but should not be turned on until after the patient is unconscious. Single-twitch stimulation at 1 Hz may be used initially when seeking supramaximal stimulation. However, after supramaximal stimulation has been ensured and before muscle relaxant is injected, the mode of stimulation should be changed to TOF (or 0.1-Hz twitch stimulation). Then, after the response to this stimulation has been observed (the control response), the neuromuscular blocking agent is injected. Although the trachea is often intubated when the response to TOF stimulation disappears, postponement of this procedure for 30 to 90

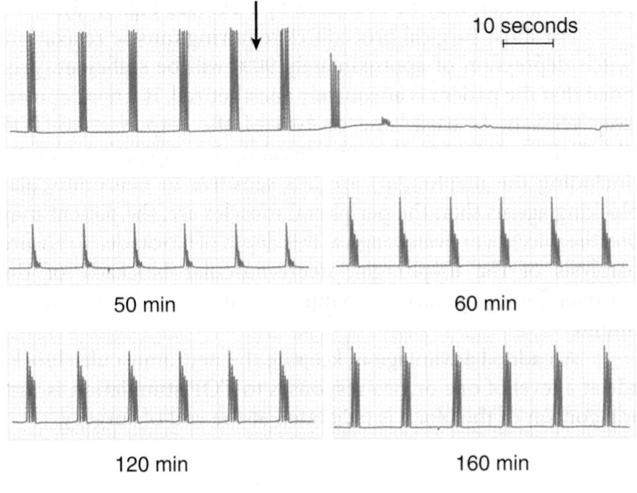

Figure 47-19 Typical recording of the mechanical response (Myograph 2000) to train-of-four ulnar nerve stimulation after injection of 1 mg/kg of succinylcholine (*arrow*) in a patient with genetically determined abnormal plasma cholinesterase activity. The prolonged duration of action and the pronounced fade in the response indicate a phase II block.

28. Fruergaard K, Viby-Mogensen J, Berg H, et al: Tactile evaluation of the response to double burst stimulation decreases, but does not eliminate the problem of postoperative residual paralysis. Acta Anaesthesiol Scand 42:1168, 1998.
29. Fuchs-Buder T, Claudius C, Skovgaard LT, et al: Good clinical research practice in pharmacodynamic studies of neuromuscular blocking agents II: The Stockholm revision. Acta Anaesthesiol Scand 51:789, 2007.
30. Brull SJ, Silverman DG: Pulse width, stimulus intensity, electrode placement, and polarity during assessment of neuromuscular block. Anesthesiology 83:702, 1995.
31. Smith CE, Donati F, Bevan DR: Potency of succinylcholine at the diaphragm and the adductor pollicis muscle. Anesth Analg 67:625, 1988.
32. Donati F, Antzaka C, Bevan DR: Potency of pancuronium at the diaphragm and the adductor pollicis muscle in humans. Anesthesiology 65:1, 1986.
33. Pansard J-L, Chauvin M, Lebrault C, et al: Effect of an intubating dose of succinylcholine and atracurium on the diaphragm and the adductor pollicis muscle in humans. Anesthesiology 67:326, 1987.
34. Plaud B, Debaene B, Donati F: The corrugator supercilii, not orbicularis oculi, reflects rocuronium neuromuscular blockade at the laryngeal adductor muscles. Anesthesiology 95:96, 2001.
35. Donati F, Meistelman C, Plaud B: Vecuronium neuromuscular blockade at the diaphragm, the orbicularis oculi, and adductor pollicis muscles. Anesthesiology 73:870, 1990.
36. Rimaniol JM, Dhonneur G, Sperry L, et al: A comparison of the neuromuscular blocking effects of atracurium, mivacurium, and vecuronium on the adductor pollicis and the orbicularis oculi muscle in humans. Anesth Analg 83:808, 1996.
37. Isono S, Ide T, Kochi T, et al: Effects of partial paralysis on the swallowing reflex in conscious humans. Anesthesiology 75:980, 1991.
38. Pavlin EG, Holle R, Schone R: Recovery of airway protection compared with ventilation in humans after paralysis with curare. Anesthesiology 70:381, 1989.
39. D'Honneur G, Guignard B, Slavov V, et al: Comparison of the neuromuscular blocking effect of atracurium and vecuronium on the adductor pollicis and the geniohyoid muscle in humans. Anesthesiology 82:649, 1995.
40. Eriksson LI, Sundman E, Olsson R, et al: Functional assessment of the pharynx at rest and during swallowing in partially paralyzed humans. Anesthesiology 87:1035, 1997.
41. Kirov K, Motamed C, Ndoko S-K, et al: TOF count at corrugator supercilii reflects abdominal muscles relaxation better than at adductor pollicis. Br J Anaesth 98:611, 2007.
42. Kern SE, Johnson JO, Orr JA, et al: Clinical analysis of the flexor hallucis brevis as an alternative site for monitoring neuromuscular block from mivacurium. J Clin Anesth 9:383, 1997.
43. Saitoh Y, Fujii Y, Takahashi K, et al: Recovery of post-tetanic count and train-of-four responses at the great toe and thumb. Anaesthesia 53:244, 1998.
44. Lee GC, Iyengar S, Szenohradszky J, et al: Improving the design of muscle relaxant studies. Anesthesiology 86:48, 1997.
45. Hemmerling TM, Schurr C, Walter S, et al: A new method of monitoring the effect of muscle relaxants on laryngeal muscle using surface laryngeal electromyography. Anesth Analg 90:494, 2000.
46. Hemmerling TM, Schmidt J, Wolf T, et al: Intramuscular versus surface electromyography of the diaphragm for determining neuromuscular blockade. Anesth Analg 92:106, 2001.
47. Hemmerling TM, Schmidt J, Hanusa C, et al: The lumbar paravertebral region provides a novel site to assess neuromuscular block at the diaphragm. Can J Anaesth 48:356, 2001.
48. Engbæk J, Skovgaard LT, Fries B, et al: Monitoring of neuromuscular transmission by electromyography (II). Evoked compound EMG area, amplitude and duration compared to mechanical twitch recording during onset and recovery of pancuronium-induced blockade in the cat. Acta Anaesthesiol Scand 37:788, 1993.
49. Kopman AF: The relationship of evoked electromyographic and mechanical responses following atracurium in humans. Anesthesiology 63:208, 1985.
50. Engbæk J, Østergaard D, Viby-Mogensen J: Clinical recovery and train-of-four ratio measured mechanically and electromyographically following atracurium. Anesthesiology 71:391, 1989.
51. Viby-Mogensen J, Jensen E, Werner M, et al: Measurement of acceleration: A new method of monitoring neuromuscular function. Acta Anaesthesiol Scand 32:45, 1988.
52. Jensen E, Viby-Mogensen J, Bang U: The accelerograph: A new neuromuscular transmission monitor. Acta Anaesthesiol Scand 32:49, 1988.
53. Werner MU, Kirkegaard Nielsen H, May O, Djernes M: Assessment of neuromuscular transmission by the evoked acceleration response. An evaluation of the accuracy of the acceleration transducer in comparison with a force displacement transducer. Acta Anaesthesiol Scand 32:395, 1988.
54. May O, Kirkegaard Nielsen H, Werner MU: The acceleration transducer—an assessment of its precision in comparison with a force displacement transducer. Acta Anaesthesiol Scand 32:239, 1988.
55. McCluskey A, Meakin G, Hopkinson JM, et al: A comparison of acceleromyography and mechanomyography for determination of the dose-response curve of rocuronium in children. Anaesthesia 52:345, 1997.
56. Kirkegaard-Nielsen H, Helbo-Hansen HS, Pedersen SH, et al: New equipment for neuromuscular transmission monitoring: A comparison of the TOF-Guard with the Myograph 2000. J Clin Monitor Comput 14:19, 1998.
57. Eikermann M, Groeben H, Husing J, et al: Predictive value of mechanomyography and accelerometry for pulmonary function in partially paralyzed volunteers. Acta Anaesthesiol Scand 48:365, 2004.
58. Samet A, Capron F, Alla F, et al: Single acceleromyographic train-of-four, 100-hertz tetanus or double-burst stimulation: Which test performs better to detect residual paralysis? Anesthesiology 102:51, 2005.
59. Eikermann M, Groeben H, Hüsing J, et al: Accelerometry of adductor pollicis muscle predicts recovery of respiratory function from neuromuscular blockade. Anesthesiology 98:1133, 2003.
60. Capron F, Alla F, Hottier C, et al: Can acceleromyography detect low levels of residual paralysis? A probability approach to detect a mechanomyographic train-of-four ratio of 0.9. Anesthesiology 100:1119, 2004.
61. Mortensen CR, Berg H, El-Mahdy A, et al: Perioperative monitoring of neuromuscular transmission using acceleromyography prevents residual neuromuscular block following pancuronium. Acta Anaesthesiol Scand 39:797, 1995.
62. Gätke MR, Viby-Mogensen J, Rosenstock C, et al: Postoperative muscle paralysis after rocuronium: Less residual block when acceleromyography is used. Acta Anaesthesiol Scand 46:207, 2002.
63. Gätke MR, Larsen PB, Engbæk J, et al: Acceleromyography of the orbicularis oculi muscle. I: Significance of the electrode position. Acta Anesthesiol Scand 46:1124, 2002.
64. Larsen PB, Gätke MR, Fredensborg BB, et al: Acceleromyography of the orbicularis oculi muscle. II: Comparing the orbicularis oculi and adductor pollicis muscles. Acta Anaesthesiol Scand 46:1131, 2002.
65. Kern SE, Johnson JO, Westenkow DR, et al: An effectiveness study of a new piezoelectric sensor for train-of-four measurement. Anesth Analg 78:978, 1994.
66. Pelgrims K, Vanacker B: Comparative study of the TOF-ratio measured by the ParaGraph versus the TOF-Guard, with and without thumb repositioning. Acta Anaesthesiol Belg 52:297, 2001.
67. Dahaba AA, von Klobucar F, Rehak PH, et al: The neuromuscular transmission module versus the relaxometer mechanomyograph for neuromuscular block monitoring. Anesth Analg 94:591, 2002.
68. Barry DT: Muscle sounds from evoked twitches in the hand. Arch Phys Med Rehabil 72:573, 1991.
69. Dascalu A, Geller E, Moalem Y, et al: Acoustic monitoring of intraoperative neuromuscular block. Br J Anaesth 83:405, 1999.
70. Hemmerling TM, Donati F, Beaulieu P, et al: Phonomyography of the corrugator supercilii muscle: Signal characteristics, best recording site and comparison with acceleromyography. Br J Anaesth 88:389, 2002.
71. Hemmerling TM, Babin D, Donati F: Phonomyography as a novel method to determine neuromuscular blockade at the laryngeal adductor muscles. Anesthesiology 98:359, 2003.
72. Trager G, Michaud G, Deschamps S, et al: Comparison of phonomyography, kinemyography and mechanomyography for neuromuscular monitoring. Can J Anaesth 53:103, 2006.
73. Gibson FM, Mirakhur RK, Clarke RSJ, et al: Quantification of train-of-four responses during recovery of block from non-depolarizing muscle relaxants. Acta Anaesthesiol Scand 31:655, 1987.
74. O'Hara DA, Fragen RJ, Shanks CA: Comparison of visual and measured train-of-four recovery after vecuronium-induced neuromuscular blockade using two anaesthetic techniques. Br J Anaesth 58:1300, 1986.
75. Engbæk J, Østergaard D, Theil Skovgaard L, et al: Reversal of intense neuromuscular blockade following infusion of atracurium. Anesthesiology 72:803, 1990.
76. Kopman AF, Yee PS, Neuman GG: Relationship of the train-of-four fade ratio to clinical signs and symptoms of residual paralysis in awake volunteers. Anesthesiology 86:765, 1997.
77. Ali HH, Wilson RS, Savarese JJ, et al: The effect of tubocurarine on indirectly elicited train-of-four muscle response and respiratory measurements in humans. Br J Anaesth 47:570, 1975.
78. Ali HH, Utting JE, Gray C: Quantitative assessment of residual antidepolarizing block (part I). Br J Anaesth 43:473, 1971.
79. Brand JB, Cullen DJ, Wilson NE, et al: Spontaneous recovery from non-depolarizing neuromuscular blockade: Correlation between clinical and evoked responses. Anesth Analg 56:55, 1977.
80. Eriksson LI, Lennmarken C, Wyon N, et al: Attenuated ventilatory response to hypoxaemia at vecuronium-induced partial neuromuscular block. Acta Anaesthesiol Scand 36:710, 1992.
81. Eriksson LI, Sato M, Severinghaus JW: Effect of a vecuronium-induced partial neuromuscular block on hypoxic ventilatory response. Anesthesiology 78:693, 1993.
82. Berg H, Viby-Mogensen J, Roed J, et al: Residual neuromuscular block is a risk factor for postoperative pulmonary complications. Acta Anaesthesiol Scand 41:1095, 1997.

83. Wyon N, Joensen H, Yamamoto Y, et al: Carotid body chemoreceptor function is impaired by vecuronium during hypoxia. Anesthesiology 89:1471, 1999.
84. Sundman E, Witt H, Olsson R, et al: The incidence and mechanism of pharyngeal and upper esophagus dysfunction in partially paralyzed humans. Anesthesiology 92:997, 2000.
85. Jonsson M, Kim C, Yamamoto Y, et al: Atracurium and vecuronium block nicotine-induced carotid body responses. Acta Anaesthesiol Scand 94:117, 2002.
86. Eikerman M, Vogt FM, Herbstreit F, et al: The predisposition to inspiratory upper airway collapse during partial neuromuscular blockade. Am J Respir Crit Care Med 175:9, 2007.
87. Shorten GD, Merk H: Perioperative train-of-four monitoring and residual curarization. Can J Anaesth 42:711, 1995.
88. Kopman AF, Ng J, Zank LM, et al: Residual postoperative paralysis. Pancuronium versus mivacurium, does it matter? Anesthesiology 85:1253, 1996.
89. Naguib M, Kopman AF, Ensor JE: Neuromuscular monitoring and postoperative curarization: A meta-analysis. Br J Anaesth 98:302, 2007.
90. Viby-Mogensen J, Claudius C, Eriksson LI: Neuromuscular monitoring and postoperative residual curarization. Br J Anaesth 99:297, 2007.
91. Heier T, Caldwell JE, Sessler DI, et al: The effect of local surface and central cooling on adductor pollicis twitch tension during nitrous oxide/isoflurane and nitrous oxide/fentanyl anesthesia in humans. Anesthesiology 72:807, 1990.
92. Eriksson LI, Lennmarken C, Jensen E, et al: Twitch tension and train-of-four ratio during prolonged neuromuscular monitoring at different peripheral temperatures. Acta Anaesthesiol Scand 35:247, 1991.
93. Heier T, Caldwell JE: Impact of hypothermia on the response to neuromuscular blocking drugs. Anesthesiology 104:1070, 2006.
94. Thornberry EA, Mazumdar B: The effect of changes in arm temperature on neuromuscular monitoring in the presence of atracurium blockade. Anaesthesia 43:447, 1988.
95. Kirkegaard H, Heier T, Caldwell JE: Efficacy of tactile-guided reversal from cisatracurium-induced neuromuscular block. Anesthesiology 96:45, 2002.
96. Kopman AF, Zank LM, Ng J, et al: Antagonism of cisatracurium and rocuronium block at a tactile train-of-four count of 2: Should quantitative assessment of neuromuscular function be mandatory? Anesth Analg 98:102, 2004.
97. Pedersen T, Viby-Mogensen J, Bang U, et al: Does perioperative tactile evaluation of the train-of-four response influence the frequency of postoperative residual neuromuscular blockade? Anesthesiology 73:835, 1990.

Daniel I. Sessler

48 Temperature Regulation and Monitoring

Key Points

1. General anesthetics decrease the thresholds (triggering core temperatures) for vasoconstriction and shivering by 2°C to 3°C.
2. Anesthetic-induced impairment of thermoregulatory control, combined with a cool operating room environment, makes most patients hypothermic.
3. The major initial cause of hypothermia in most patients is core-to-peripheral redistribution of body heat.
4. Neuraxial anesthesia impairs both central and peripheral thermoregulatory control and is associated with substantial hypothermia.
5. Large randomized trials have proved that even mild hypothermia (i.e., 1.5°C to 2.0°C) causes adverse outcomes, including a threefold increase in morbid myocardial outcomes, a threefold increase in risk for wound infection, coagulopathy and need for allogeneic transfusion, prolonged recovery, and prolonged hospitalization.
6. Body temperature should be monitored in patients undergoing surgery lasting longer than 30 minutes, and core temperature should be maintained at 36°C or higher whenever possible. Forced-air warming currently offers the best combination of high efficacy, low cost, and remarkable safety.

Mammals and birds are homeothermic and require a nearly constant internal body temperature. When internal temperature deviates significantly from normal, metabolic functions usually deteriorate, and death may result. The thermoregulatory system generally maintains core body temperature within a few tenths of a degree centigrade of "normal," which is about 37°C in humans. Anesthetic-induced inhibition of thermoregulation combined with exposure to a cold operating room environment makes most unwarmed patients hypothermic. In recent years, major outcome studies have shown that mild hypothermia (≈1°C to 2°C): (1) triples the incidence of morbid cardiac outcomes, (2) triples the incidence of surgical wound infections, (3) increases surgical blood loss and the need for allogeneic transfusion by about 20%, and, (4) prolongs postanesthesia recovery and the duration of hospitalization. An understanding of normal and anesthetic-influenced thermoregulation will facilitate prevention and management of these and numerous other temperature-related complications.

Normal Thermoregulation

Thermoregulation is based on multiple, redundant signals from nearly every type of tissue. Processing of thermoregulatory information occurs in three phases: *afferent thermal sensing*, *central regulation*, and *efferent responses*.

Afferent Input

Information on temperature is obtained from thermally sensitive cells throughout the body. Cold-sensitive cells are anatomically and physiologically distinct from those that detect warmth. Warm receptors increase their firing rates when temperature increases, whereas cold receptors do so when temperature decreases. Cutaneous warm receptors rarely depolarize at normal skin temperatures and are probably important only during heat stress. The actual sensors appear to be a recently discovered class of transient receptor potential (TRP) protein receptors.[1]

Cold signals travel primarily via Aδ nerve fibers, and warm information, by unmyelinated C fibers, although there is some overlap.[2] C fibers also detect and convey pain sensation, which is why intense heat cannot be distinguished from sharp pain. Most ascending thermal information traverses the spinothalamic tracts in the anterior spinal cord, but no single spinal tract is critical for conveying thermal information. Consequently, the entire anterior cord must be destroyed to ablate thermoregulatory responses.

The hypothalamus, other parts of the brain, the spinal cord, deep abdominal and thoracic tissues, and the skin surface each contribute roughly 20% of total thermal input to the central regulatory system.[3]

Central Control

Temperature is regulated by central structures (primarily the hypothalamus) that compare integrated thermal input from the skin surface, neuraxis, and deep tissues with *threshold* temperatures for each thermoregulatory response. Although integrated by the hypothalamus, most thermal information is "preprocessed" in the spinal cord and other parts of the central nervous system. This hierarchic arrangement presumably developed when the evolving thermoregulatory control system co-opted previously existing mechanisms (e.g., shivering from muscles previously used for posture and locomotion). Some thermoregulatory responses can be mounted by the spinal cord alone.[4] For example, animals and patients with high spinal cord transection regulate temperature better than might be expected.

The slope of response intensity versus core temperature defines the *gain* of a thermoregulatory response. Response intensity no longer increasing with further deviation in core temperature identifies the *maximum intensity*. This system of thresholds and gains is a model for a thermoregulatory system that is further complicated by interactions between other regulatory responses (i.e., vascular volume control) and time-dependent effects.

How the body determines absolute threshold temperatures is unknown, but the mechanism appears to be mediated by norepinephrine, dopamine, 5-hydroxytryptamine, acetylcholine, prostaglandin E_1, and neuropeptides. The thresholds vary daily in both sexes (circadian rhythm) and monthly in women by approximately 0.5°C. Exercise, food intake, infection, hypothyroidism and hyperthyroidism, anesthetic and other drugs (including alcohol, sedatives, and nicotine), and cold and warm adaptation all alter threshold temperatures.

Control of autonomic responses is approximately 80% determined by thermal input from core structures (Fig. 48-1).[5] In contrast, a large fraction of the input controlling behavioral responses is derived from the skin surface. The *interthreshold range* (core temperatures *not* triggering autonomic thermoregulatory responses) is a few tenths of a degree centigrade.[6] This range is bounded by the sweating threshold at its upper end and by vasoconstriction at the lower end. Because energy cost and nutrients are conserved without excessive autonomic control within this range, some animals such as camels and desert rats use this strategy extensively and exhibit core temperature changes of up to 10°C each day. However, most mammals—including humans—normally regulate core temperature tightly.

Both sweating and vasoconstriction thresholds are 0.3°C to 0.5°C higher in women than in men, even during the follicular phase of the menstrual cycle (first 10 days).[7] These differences are even greater during the luteal phase.[8] Central thermoregulatory control is apparently intact even in somewhat premature infants.[9] In contrast, thermoregulatory control is sometimes impaired in the elderly.[10]

Efferent Responses

The body responds to thermal perturbations (body temperatures differing from the appropriate threshold) via effector mechanisms that increase metabolic heat production or alter environmental heat loss. Each thermoregulatory effector has its own threshold and gain, so there is an orderly progression of responses and response intensities in proportion to need. In general, energy-efficient effectors such as vasoconstriction are maximized before metabolically costly responses such as shivering are initiated. Figure 48-2 shows the normal values for the major autonomic response thresholds.

Effectors determine the ambient temperature range that the body will tolerate while maintaining a normal core temperature. When specific effector mechanisms are inhibited (e.g., when shivering is prevented by the administration of muscle relaxants), the

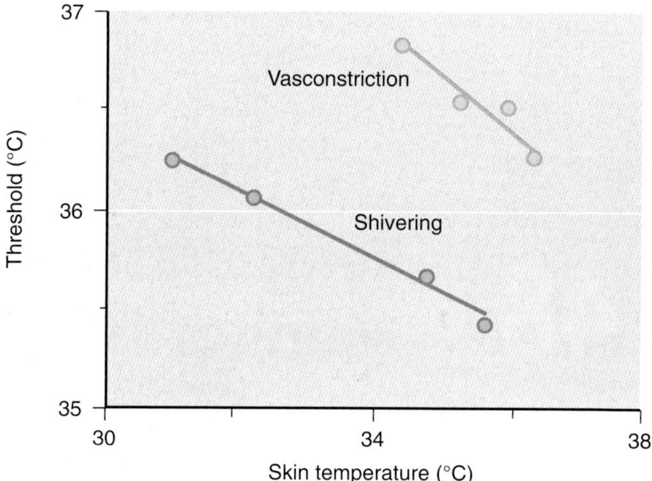

Figure 48-1 There is a linear relationship between mean skin temperature and the core temperature triggering vasoconstriction and shivering. Skin temperature contributes about 20% to control of each thermoregulatory defense. *(From Cheng C, Matsukawa T, Sessler DI, et al: Increasing mean skin temperature linearly reduces the core-temperature thresholds for vasoconstriction and shivering in humans. Anesthesiology 82:1160-1168, 1995.)*

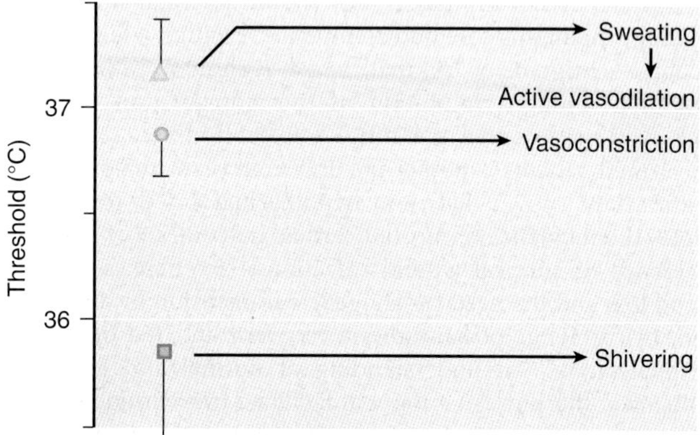

Figure 48-2 A core temperature below the threshold for response to cold provokes vasoconstriction, nonshivering thermogenesis, and shivering. A core temperature exceeding the hyperthermic threshold produces active vasodilation and sweating. No thermoregulatory responses are initiated when the core temperature is between these thresholds; these temperatures identify the interthreshold range, which in humans is usually only about 0.2°C. *(Threshold data from Lopez M, Sessler DI, Walter K, et al: Rate and gender dependence of the sweating, vasoconstriction, and shivering thresholds in humans. Anesthesiology 80:780-788, 1994.)*

tolerable range is decreased. Still, temperature will remain normal unless other effectors cannot compensate for the imposed stress. Quantitatively, *behavioral regulation* is the most important effector mechanism. Behavioral compensations include dressing appropriately, modifying environmental temperature, assuming positions that oppose skin surfaces, and voluntary movement.

Infants regulate their temperature remarkably well. In contrast, advanced age, infirmity, or medications can diminish the efficacy of thermoregulatory responses and increase the risk for hypothermia. For example, decreased muscle mass, neuromuscular diseases, and muscle relaxants all inhibit shivering, which increases the minimum tolerable ambient temperature. Similarly, anticholinergic drugs inhibit sweating, which decreases the maximum tolerable temperature.

Cutaneous vasoconstriction is the most consistently used autonomic effector mechanism. Metabolic heat is lost primarily via convection and radiation from the skin surface, and vasoconstriction reduces this loss. Total digital skin blood flow is divided into nutritional (mostly capillary) and thermoregulatory (mostly arteriovenous shunt) components.[11] The arteriovenous shunts are anatomically and functionally distinct from the capillaries supplying nutritional blood to the skin (thus vasoconstriction does not compromise the needs of peripheral tissues).

Control of blood flow through arteriovenous shunts tends to be "on" or "off." In other words, the gain of this response is high, with digital flow increasing from trivial to maximal levels after changes in core temperature of only a few tenths of a degree centigrade. Local α-adrenergic sympathetic nerves mediate constriction in the thermoregulatory arteriovenous shunts, and flow is minimally affected by *circulating* catecholamines. Roughly 10% of cardiac output traverses the arteriovenous shunts; consequently, shunt vasoconstriction increases mean arterial pressure approximately 15 mm Hg.[12]

Nonshivering thermogenesis increases metabolic heat production (measured as whole-body oxygen consumption) without producing mechanical work. It doubles heat production in infants[13] but increases it only slightly in adults.[14] The intensity of nonshivering thermogenesis increases in linear proportion to the difference between mean body temperature and its threshold. Skeletal muscle and brown fat tissue are the major sources of nonshivering heat in adults. The metabolic rate in both tissues is controlled primarily by norepinephrine released from adrenergic nerve terminals and is further mediated locally by an uncoupling protein.[15]

Sustained shivering augments metabolic heat production by 50% to 100% in adults. This increase is small in comparison to that produced by exercise (which can, at least briefly, increase metabolism by 500%) and thus is surprisingly ineffective. Shivering does not occur in newborn infants and probably is not fully effective until children are several years old. The rapid tremor (up to 250 Hz) and unsynchronized muscular activity of thermogenic shivering suggest no central oscillator. However, superimposed on the fast activity, there is usually a slow (4 to 8 cycles/min), synchronous "waxing-and-waning" pattern that presumably is centrally mediated.[16]

Sweating is mediated by postganglionic, cholinergic nerves.[17] It thus is an active process that is prevented by nerve block or administration of atropine.[18] Sweating is the only mechanism by which the body can dissipate heat in an environment exceeding core temperature. Fortunately, the process is remarkably effective, with 0.58 kcal dissipated per gram of evaporated sweat.

Active vasodilation is apparently mediated by nitric oxide.[19] Because active vasodilation requires intact sweat gland function, it is also largely inhibited by nerve blockade. The threshold for active vasodilation is usually similar to the sweating threshold, but the gain may be less. Consequently, maximum cutaneous vasodilation is generally delayed until core temperature is well above that provoking maximum sweating intensity.

Thermoregulation During General Anesthesia

Behavioral regulation is not relevant during general anesthesia because patients are unconscious and frequently paralyzed. All general anesthetics tested thus far markedly impair normal autonomic thermoregulatory control and cause slightly elevated warm-response thresholds, whereas cold-response thresholds are markedly reduced. Consequently, the interthreshold range is increased from its normal value near 0.3°C to about 2°C to 4°C.[20-24] The gain and maximum intensity of some responses remain normal,[7] whereas others are reduced by general anesthesia.[25,26]

Response Thresholds

Propofol,[20] alfentanil,[21] and dexmedetomidine[22] all produce a slight linear increase in the sweating threshold combined with a marked and linear decrease in the vasoconstriction and shivering thresholds. Isoflurane[24] and desflurane[23] also slightly increase the sweating threshold; however, they decrease the cold-response threshold nonlinearly. Consequently, the volatile anesthetics inhibit vasoconstriction and shivering less than propofol does at low concentrations but more than propofol does at typical anesthetic doses. In all cases (except during meperidine[27] and nefopam[28] administration), vasoconstriction and shivering decrease synchronously and thus maintain their normal approximate 1°C difference.

The dose-dependent response thresholds for four anesthetic drugs are shown in Figure 48-3. The combination of increased sweating thresholds and reduced vasoconstriction thresholds increases the interthreshold range about 20-fold, from its normal value near 0.2°C to approximately 2°C to 4°C. Temperatures within this range do *not* trigger thermoregulatory defenses, and patients are thus by definition poikilothermic within this temperature range.

Isoflurane,[24] desflurane,[23,25] enflurane,[29] halothane,[30] and the combination of nitrous oxide and fentanyl[31] decrease the vasoconstriction threshold 2°C to 4°C from its normal value near 37°C. The dose dependence is nonlinear; that is, greater concentrations produce disproportionate threshold reductions. The shivering thresholds decrease synchronously. In contrast, these drugs increase the sweating threshold only slightly.

Clonidine synchronously decreases cold-response thresholds[32] while slightly increasing the sweating threshold.[33] Nitrous oxide decreases the vasoconstriction[34] and shivering[35] thresholds less than equipotent concentrations of volatile anesthetics do. In

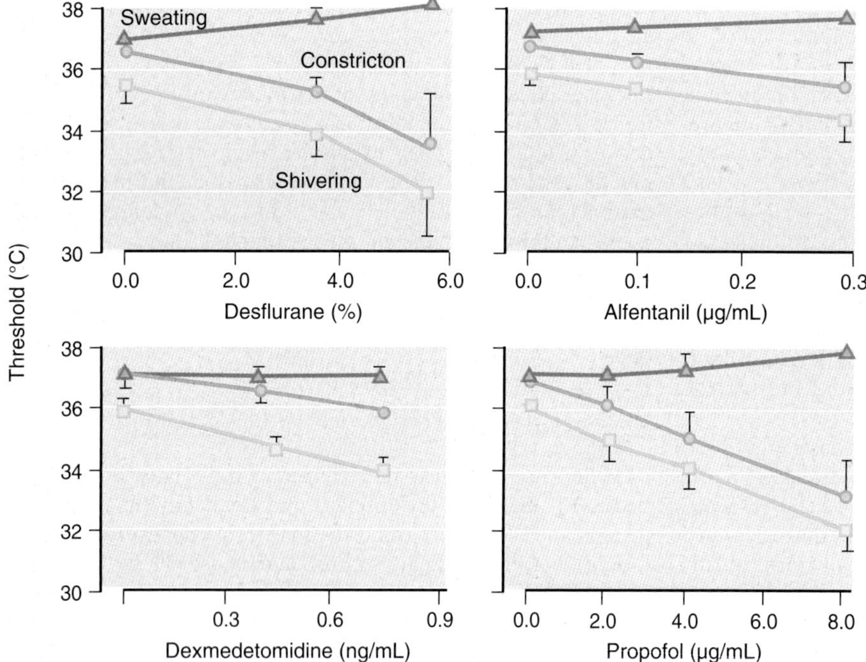

Figure 48-3 Major autonomic thermoregulatory response thresholds in volunteers given desflurane, alfentanil, dexmedetomidine, or propofol. All the anesthetics slightly increase the sweating threshold (triggering core temperature) while markedly and synchronously decreasing the vasoconstriction and shivering thresholds. Standard deviation bars smaller than the data markers have been deleted. *(From Annadata RS, Sessler DI, Tayefeh F, et al: Desflurane slightly increases the sweating threshold, but produces marked, non-linear decreases in the vasoconstriction and shivering thresholds. Anesthesiology 83:1205-1211, 1995; Kurz A, Go JC, Sessler DI, et al: Alfentanil slightly increases the sweating threshold and markedly reduces the vasoconstriction and shivering thresholds. Anesthesiology 83:293-299, 1995; Talke P, Tayefeh F, Sessler DI, et al: Dexmedetomidine does not alter the sweating threshold, but comparably and linearly reduces the vasoconstriction and shivering thresholds. Anesthesiology 87:835-841, 1997; and Matsukawa T, Kurz A, Sessler DI, et al: Propofol linearly reduces the vasoconstriction and shivering thresholds. Anesthesiology 82:1169-1180, 1995.)*

contrast, midazolam only slightly impairs thermoregulatory control.[36,37] Painful stimulation slightly increases the vasoconstriction thresholds[29]; consequently, thresholds will be somewhat lower when surgical pain is prevented by simultaneous local or regional anesthesia.

Responses in Infants and the Elderly

Thermoregulatory vasoconstriction is comparably impaired in infants, children, and adults given isoflurane[38] or halothane (Fig. 48-4).[39] In contrast, the vasoconstriction threshold is about 1°C less in patients aged 60 to 80 years than in those between 30 and 50 years (see Chapters 69, 71, 82, and 84).

Nonshivering thermogenesis does not occur in anesthetized adults,[40] but it is an important thermoregulatory response in animals and human infants. However, nonshivering thermogenesis in animals is inhibited by volatile anesthetics,[41] and it fails to increase the metabolic rate in infants anesthetized with propofol (Fig. 48-5).[42]

Gain and Maximum Response Intensity

Both the gain and maximum intensity of sweating remain normal during isoflurane[7] and enflurane anesthesia.[43] However, the gain of arteriovenous shunt vasoconstriction is reduced threefold during desflurane anesthesia (Fig. 48-6),[25] even though the maximum vasoconstriction intensity remains normal.[44]

Shivering is rare at surgical levels of general anesthesia, which is consistent with its threshold being roughly 1°C less than the vasoconstriction threshold.[20-24] (Vasoconstriction usually prevents additional hypothermia,[45] so even unwarmed patients rarely become cold enough to shiver.) Nonetheless, shivering can be induced by sufficient active cooling.

Gain and maximum shivering intensity remain normal during both meperidine and alfentanil administration.[46] Gain also remains nearly intact during nitrous oxide administration, although maximum intensity is reduced.[47] Isoflurane changes the macroscopic pattern of shivering to such an extent that it is no longer possible to easily determine gain. The drug does, however, reduce maximum shivering intensity.[26]

In summary, sweating is the best preserved major thermoregulatory defense during anesthesia. Not only is the

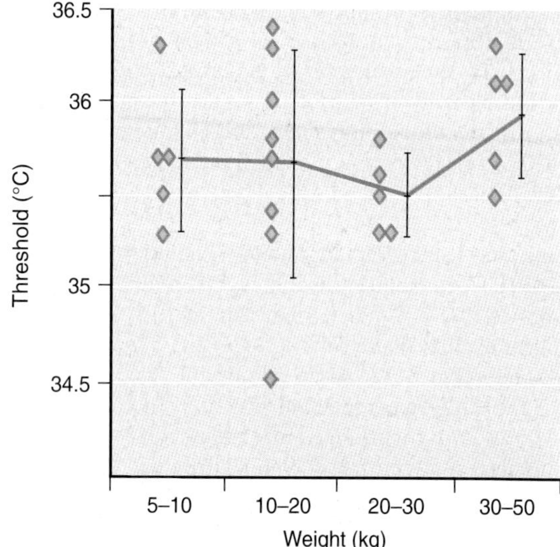

Figure 48-4 Core thermoregulatory threshold in 23 healthy children and infants undergoing abdominal surgery with halothane anesthesia. Differences among the groups are not statistically significant. Results are presented as means ± SD. *(From Bissonnette B, Sessler DI: Thermoregulatory thresholds for vasoconstriction in pediatric patients anesthetized with halothane or halothane and caudal bupivacaine. Anesthesiology 76:387-392, 1992.)*

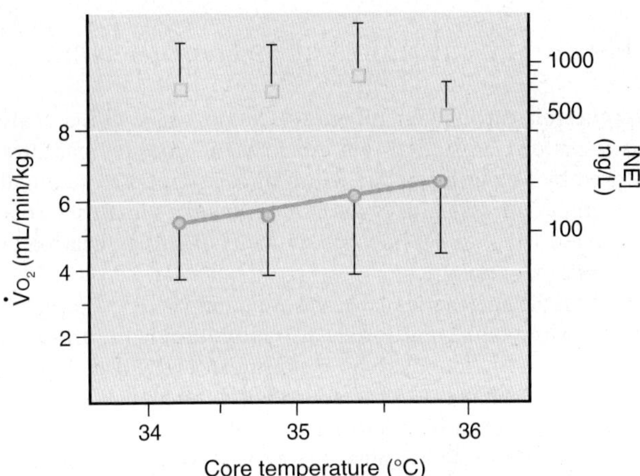

Figure 48-5 Progressive reduction in core temperature did not trigger an increase in oxygen consumption ($\dot{V}O_2$) that might indicate nonshivering thermogenesis. Instead, hypothermia decreased systemic oxygen consumption: $\dot{V}O_2 = 0.83$ (Core temperature) – 23.3 ; $r^2 = .92$. Intraoperative plasma norepinephrine concentrations ([NE]) were variable but did not change significantly as a function of core temperature. Data are presented as means ± SD. *(From Plattner O, Semsroth M, Sessler DI, et al: Lack of nonshivering thermogenesis in infants anesthetized with fentanyl and propofol. Anesthesiology 86:772-777, 1997.)*

threshold only slightly increased, but the gain and maximum intensity also remain normal. In contrast, the thresholds for vasoconstriction and shivering are markedly reduced, and furthermore, the efficacy of these responses is diminished even after being activated.

Development of Hypothermia During General Anesthesia

Inadvertent hypothermia is by far the most common perioperative thermal disturbance during anesthesia. Hypothermia results from a combination of anesthetic-impaired thermoregulation and exposure to a cold operating room environment. Of these two causes, impaired thermoregulation is much more important.

Heat Transfer

Heat can be transferred from a patient to the environment in four ways: radiation, conduction, convection, and evaporation. Among these mechanisms, radiation and convection contribute most to perioperative heat loss.

All surfaces with a temperature above absolute zero radiate heat; similarly, all surfaces absorb heat radiating from surrounding surfaces. Heat transfer via this mechanism is proportional to the difference of the fourth power of the absolute temperature difference between the surfaces. It is likely that radiation is the major type of heat loss in most surgical patients.[48]

Conductive heat loss is proportional to the temperature difference between two adjacent surfaces and the strength of the thermal insulation separating them. In general, conductive losses are negligible during surgery because patients usually only directly contact the foam pad (an excellent thermal insulator) covering most operating room tables.

Conductive loss of heat directly to air molecules is limited by the development of a layer of still air adjacent to the skin that serves as an insulator. When this layer is disturbed by air currents, the insulating properties diminish substantially, thereby increasing heat loss. This increase is termed convection and is proportional to the square root of the air speed; this is the basis of the familiar "wind chill" factor. Air speed in operating rooms—even those with high rates of air turnover—is typically only approximately 20 cm/sec, which only slightly increases loss when compared with still air. Nonetheless, convective loss is usually the second most important mechanism by which heat is transferred from patients to the environment. Presumably, convective loss increases substantially in operating rooms equipped to provide laminar flow. However, the actual augmentation has not been quantified and may be less than expected from the increase in air speed because surgical draping provides considerable thermal insulation.

Sweating increases cutaneous evaporative loss enormously but is rare during anesthesia. In the absence of sweating, evaporative loss from the skin surface is limited to less than 10% of metabolic heat production in adults. In contrast, infants lose a higher fraction of their metabolic heat from transpiration of water through thin skin. The problem becomes especially acute in

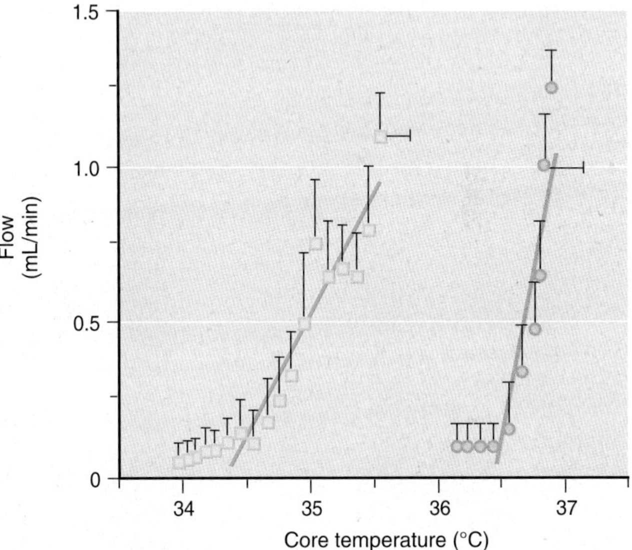

Figure 48-6 Finger blood flow without (*circles*) and with (*squares*) desflurane administration. Values were computed relative to the thresholds (finger flow = 1.0 mL/min) in each subject. Flows of exactly 1.0 mL/min are not shown because flows in each individual were averaged over 0.1°C or 0.05°C increments; each data point thus includes both higher and lower flows. The horizontal standard deviation bars indicate variability in the thresholds among the volunteers; although error bars are shown only at a flow near 1.0 mL/min, the same temperature variability applies to each data point. Slopes of the flow-versus–core temperature relationships (1.0 to ≈0.15 mL/min) were determined by linear regression. These slopes defined the gain of vasoconstriction with and without desflurane anesthesia. Gain was reduced by a factor of 3, from 2.4 to 0.8 mL/min/°C ($P < .01$). *(From Kurz A, Xiong J, Sessler DI, et al: Desflurane reduces the gain of thermoregulatory arterio-venous shunt vasoconstriction in humans. Anesthesiology 83:1212-1219, 1995.)*

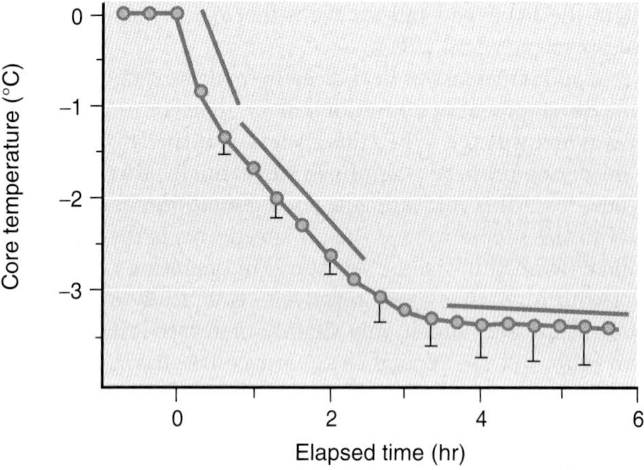

Figure 48-7 Hypothermia during general anesthesia develops with a characteristic pattern. An initial rapid decrease in core temperature results from a core-to-peripheral redistribution of body heat. This is followed by a slow, linear reduction in core temperature that results simply from heat loss exceeding heat production. Finally, core temperature stabilizes and subsequently remains virtually unchanged. This plateau phase may be a passive thermal steady state or result when sufficient hypothermia triggers thermoregulatory vasoconstriction. Results are presented as means ± SD.

premature infants, who may lose one fifth of their metabolic heat production via transcutaneous evaporation.[49] Simple thermodynamic calculations and clinical measurements indicate that only trivial amounts of heat are lost from the respiratory system.[50] Evaporation inside surgical wounds may contribute substantially to total heat loss[51] but has never been quantified in humans.

Patterns of Intraoperative Hypothermia

Hypothermia during general anesthesia develops with a characteristic pattern. An initial rapid decrease in core temperature is followed by a slow, linear reduction in core temperature. Finally, core temperature stabilizes and subsequently remains virtually unchanged (Fig. 48-7). Each component of this typical pattern has a different etiology.

Volatile anesthetics cause vasodilation via direct peripheral action.[52] More importantly, they also inhibit tonic thermoregulatory vasoconstriction, thereby resulting in arteriovenous shunt dilation.[20-24] Nonetheless, anesthetic-induced vasodilation increases cutaneous heat loss only slightly.[53] Anesthetics reduce the metabolic rate 20% to 30%.[54] However, even the combination of increased heat loss and reduced heat production is insufficient to explain the 0.5°C to 1.5°C decrease in core temperature generally observed during the first hour of anesthesia.

The key to understanding the initial decrease in core temperature is to appreciate that body heat is not normally distributed evenly. Core temperature represents only about half the body mass (mostly the trunk and head); the remaining mass is typically 2°C to 4°C cooler than the core. This core-to-peripheral tissue temperature gradient is normally maintained by tonic thermoregulatory vasoconstriction. Anesthetic-induced vasodilation, however, allows core heat to flow peripherally. This warms the arms and legs but does so at the expense of the core (Figs. 48-8 and 48-9).[55] The extent to which redistribution reduces core temperature depends on the core-to-peripheral tissue temperature gradient at the time of induction. This gradient, in turn, depends

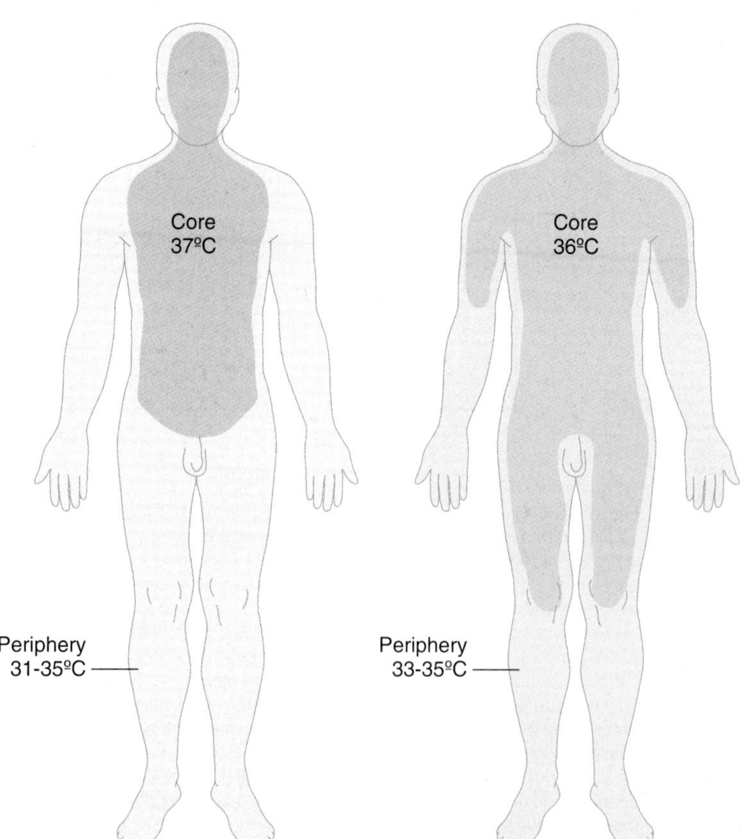

Figure 48-8 Drawing illustrating internal redistribution of body heat after induction of general anesthesia. Hypothermia after induction of spinal or epidural anesthesia results similarly, but redistribution is restricted to the legs.

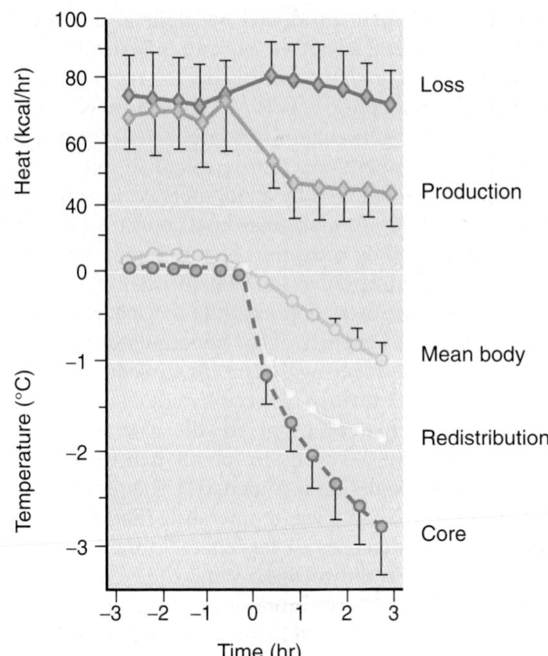

Figure 48-9 Changes in body heat content and distribution of heat within the body during induction of general anesthesia (at elapsed time zero). Subtraction of the change in mean body temperature from the change in core (tympanic membrane) temperature leaves the core hypothermia specifically resulting from redistribution. Redistribution hypothermia was thus not a measured value; instead, it is defined by the decrease in core temperature not explained by the relatively small decrease in systemic heat content. After 1 hour of anesthesia, core temperature had decreased 1.6 ± 0.3°C, with redistribution contributing 81% to the decrease. Even after 3 hours of anesthesia, redistribution contributed 65% to the entire 2.8 ± 0.5°C decrease in core temperature. Results are presented as means ± SD. *(Modified from Matsukawa T, Sessler DI, Sessler AM, et al: Heat flow and distribution during induction of general anesthesia. Anesthesiology 82:662-673, 1995.)*

on the patient's prior thermal environment and thermoregulatory status, both of which are difficult to determine clinically.

After initial redistribution hypothermia, core temperature usually decreases in a slow, linear fashion for 2 to 4 hours. This reduction results simply from heat loss exceeding metabolic heat production,[56] and the rate at which core temperature decreases depends on the difference and size of the patient. After 3 to 4 hours of anesthesia, core temperature usually reaches a plateau and remains virtually constant for the duration of surgery.[31] The core temperature plateau may simply represent a thermal steady state (heat production equaling heat loss) in patients remaining relatively warm. In others, however, the plateau phase is associated with peripheral thermoregulatory vasoconstriction triggered by core temperatures of 33°C to 35°C.

Thermoregulatory vasoconstriction during anesthesia decreases cutaneous heat loss,[44] but this decrease alone is usually insufficient to produce a thermal steady state. Furthermore, neither adults[40] nor infants[42] appear to be able to increase intraoperative heat production in response to hypothermia. An additional mechanism must therefore contribute to the core temperature plateau. Evidence suggests that a primary factor is constraint of metabolic heat to the core thermal compartment. In this scenario, distribution of metabolic heat (which is largely produced centrally) is restricted to the core compartment, thereby maintaining its temperature. Peripheral tissue temperature, in contrast, continues to decrease because it is no longer being supplied with sufficient heat from the core.[45] A core temperature plateau resulting from thermoregulatory vasoconstriction is thus not a thermal steady state, and body heat content continues to decrease even though core temperature remains nearly constant.

Neuraxial Anesthesia

Autonomic thermoregulation is impaired during regional anesthesia, and the result is typically intraoperative core hypothermia. Interestingly, this hypothermia is often not consciously perceived by patients but nonetheless triggers shivering. The result is frequently a potentially dangerous clinical paradox: a hypothermic patient who denies feeling cold (see Chapters 51, 52 and 87).

Thermoregulation

Epidural[57,58] and spinal[58,59] anesthesia each decrease the thresholds triggering vasoconstriction and shivering (above the level of the block) by about 0.6°C (Fig. 48-10). Presumably, this decrease does not result from recirculation of neuraxially administered local anesthetic because impairment is similar during epidural and spinal anesthesia,[57-59] although the amount and location of administered local anesthetic differ substantially. Furthermore, lidocaine administered intravenously in doses producing plasma concentrations similar to those occurring during epidural anesthesia has no thermoregulatory effect.[60] Finally, neuraxial administration of 2-choloprocaine, a local anesthetic with a plasma half-life of only about 20 seconds, also impairs thermoregulatory control.[61]

The vasoconstriction and shivering thresholds are comparably decreased during regional anesthesia,[59] suggesting an alteration in central, rather than peripheral control. The mechanism by

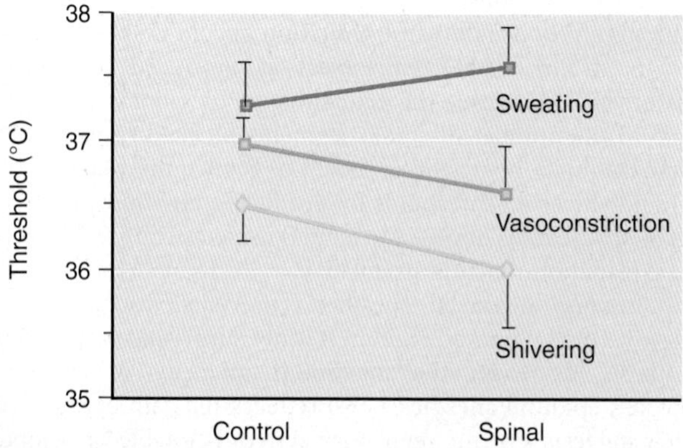

Figure 48-10 Spinal anesthesia increased the sweating threshold but reduced the thresholds for vasoconstriction and shivering. Consequently, the interthreshold range increased substantially. The vasoconstriction-to-shivering range, however, remained normal during spinal anesthesia. Results are presented as means ± SD. *(From Kurz A, Sessler DI, Schroeder M, Kurz M: Thermoregulatory response thresholds during spinal anesthesia. Anesth Analg 77:721-726, 1993.)*

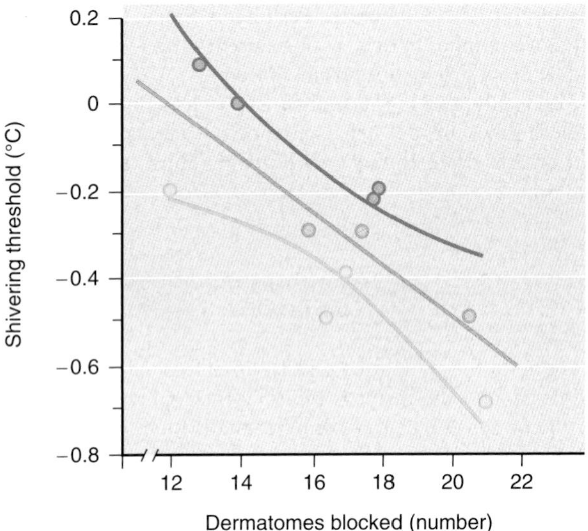

Figure 48-11 The number of dermatomes blocked (sacral segments = 5; lumbar segments = 5; thoracic segments = 12) versus reduction in the shivering threshold (difference between the control shivering threshold and the spinal shivering threshold). The shivering threshold was reduced more by extensive spinal blocks than by less extensive ones (Δ threshold = 0.74 – 0.06 [dermatomes blocked]; $r^2 = .58$, $P < .006$). The *curved lines* indicate 95% confidence intervals for the slope. *(From Leslie K, Sessler DI: Reduction in the shivering threshold is proportional to spinal block height. Anesthesiology 84:1327-1331, 1996.)*

which peripheral administration of local anesthesia impairs centrally mediated thermoregulation may involve alteration of afferent thermal input from the legs. The key factor here is that tonic cold signals dominate thermal input at leg skin temperatures in typical operating room environments.[2] Regional anesthesia blocks all thermal input from the blocked regions, which in the typical case is primarily cold information. The brain may then interpret decreased cold information as relative leg warming. This appears to be an unconscious process in that perceived temperature does not increase.[62] Because skin temperature is an important input to the thermoregulatory control system, leg warming proportionately reduces the vasoconstriction and shivering thresholds. Consistent with this theory, a leg skin temperature near 38°C is required to produce the same reduction in cold-response thresholds in an unanesthetized subject as produced by regional anesthesia.[63] Moreover, the reduction in thresholds is proportional to the number of spinal segments blocked (Fig. 48-11).[64] Major conduction anesthesia may thus reduce the vasoconstriction and shivering thresholds by producing an abnormal elevation in *apparent* (as opposed to actual) leg temperature. However, this explanation remains speculative.

Because neuraxial anesthesia prevents vasoconstriction and shivering in blocked regions, it is not surprising that epidural anesthesia decreases the maximum intensity of shivering. However, epidural anesthesia also reduces the gain of shivering, which suggests that the regulatory system is unable to compensate for lower body paralysis (Fig. 48-12).[26] Thermoregulatory defenses, once triggered, are thus less effective than usual during regional anesthesia.

Neuraxial anesthesia is frequently supplemented with sedative and analgesic medications that impair thermoregulatory control.[20,21,27] Such inhibition may be severe when combined with the intrinsic impairment produced by regional anesthesia and other factors, including advanced age and preexisting illness.

Interestingly, core hypothermia during regional anesthesia may not trigger a perception of cold.[57,65] The reason is that thermal perception (behavioral regulation) is largely determined by skin rather than core temperature. During regional anesthesia, core hypothermia is accompanied by a real increase in skin temperature. The result is typically a perception of continued or increased warmth accompanied by activation of autonomic thermoregulatory responses including shivering (Fig. 48-13).[57,65]

Taken together, these data indicate that neuraxial anesthesia inhibits numerous aspects of thermoregulatory control. The vasoconstriction and shivering thresholds are reduced by regional anesthesia[57-59,63,64] and further reduced by adjuvant drugs[21,36] and advanced age.[10] Even once triggered, the gain and maximum response intensity of shivering are about half-normal. Finally, behavioral thermoregulation is impaired.[65] The result is that cold defenses are triggered at a lower temperature than normal during regional anesthesia, defenses are less effective once triggered, and patients frequently do not recognize that they are hypothermic. Because core temperature monitoring remains rare during regional anesthesia, substantial hypothermia often goes undetected in these patients.[66]

Heat Balance

Hypothermia is common during regional anesthesia and may be nearly as severe as during general anesthesia.[67] Core temperature

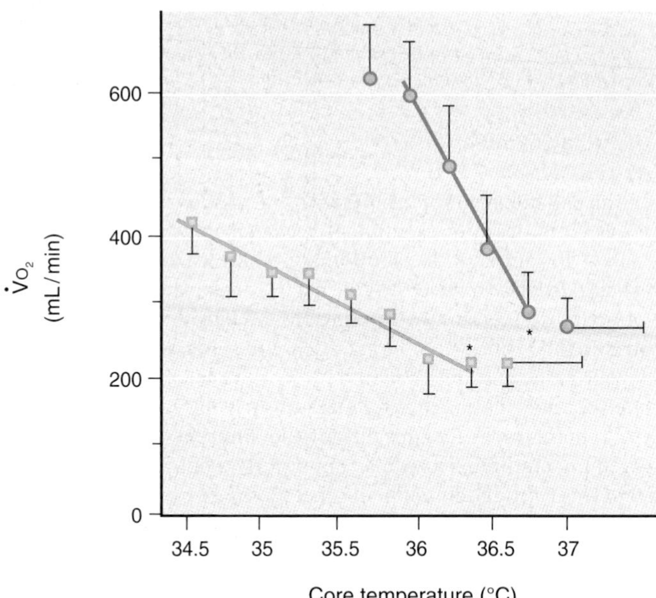

Figure 48-12 Systemic oxygen consumption without (*circles*) and with (*squares*) epidural anesthesia. The horizontal standard deviation bars indicate variability in the thresholds among the volunteers; although error bars are shown only once in each series, the same temperature variability applies to each data point. Slopes of the oxygen consumption–versus–core temperature relationships (*solid lines*) were determined by linear regression. These slopes defined the gain of shivering with and without epidural anesthesia. Gain was reduced 3.7-fold, from −412 mL/min/°C ($r^2 = .99$) to −112 mL/min/°C ($r^2 = .96$). *(From Kim J-S, Ikeda T, Sessler D, et al: Epidural anesthesia reduces the gain and maximum intensity of shivering. Anesthesiology 88:851-857, 1998.)*

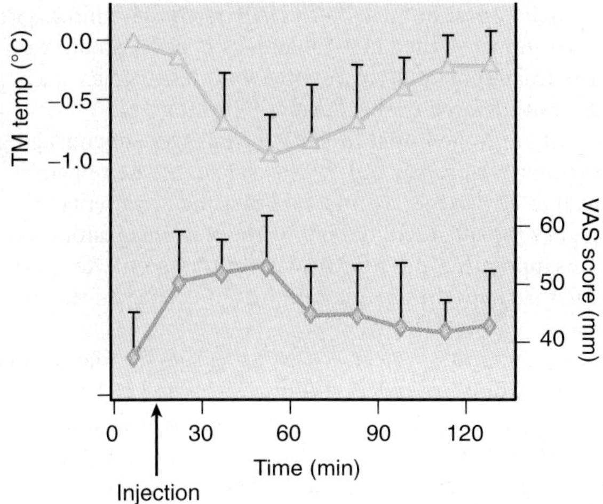

Figure 48-13 Induction of epidural anesthesia at an elapsed time of 15 minutes decreased core temperature and increased thermal comfort as determined by a 100-mm visual analog scale (VAS). Interesting, however, that maximal thermal comfort coincided with *minimum* core temperature. The results are presented as means ± SD. TM, tympanic membrane. *(Modified from Sessler DI, Ponte J: Shivering during epidural anesthesia. Anesthesiology 72:816-821, 1990.)*

typically decreases 0.5°C to 1.0°C shortly after induction of anesthesia. However, the vasodilation induced by regional anesthesia only slightly increases cutaneous heat loss. Furthermore, metabolic heat production remains constant or increases because of shivering thermogenesis. This rapid decrease in core temperature, similar to that seen after induction of general anesthesia, also results from an internal core-to-peripheral redistribution of body heat.[68] As during general anesthesia,[69,70] redistribution hypothermia during regional anesthesia can be minimized by cutaneous warming before induction.[71]

Subsequent hypothermia results simply from heat loss exceeding metabolic heat production. Unlike patients given general anesthesia, however, core temperature does not necessarily plateau after several hours of surgery. Not only is the vasoconstriction threshold centrally impaired by regional anesthesia,[58,59] but more importantly, vasoconstriction in the legs is also directly prevented by nerve block.[72] Because the legs constitute the bulk of the peripheral thermal compartment, an effective plateau cannot develop without vasoconstriction in the legs and the resulting decrease in cutaneous heat loss and constraint of metabolic heat to the core.

The importance of intraoperative leg vasoconstriction is illustrated during combined regional/general anesthesia. Consistent with the impairment of thermoregulatory responses with regional anesthesia alone,[58,59] vasoconstriction during combined regional/general anesthesia is triggered at a core temperature approximately 1°C lower than during general anesthesia alone. Moreover, once triggered, vasoconstriction produces a core temperature plateau during general anesthesia alone but not during combined regional/general anesthesia. The result is that core temperature during combined regional/general anesthesia continues to decrease throughout surgery.[73] Consequently, core temperature monitoring and thermal management are especially important in patients given simultaneous regional and general anesthesia.

Shivering

Shivering-like tremor in volunteers given neuraxial anesthesia is always preceded by core hypothermia and vasoconstriction (above the level of the block).[57] Furthermore, electromyographic analysis indicates that the tremor has the 4- to 8-cycle/min waxing-and-waning pattern that characterizes normal shivering.[61] The tremor is thus apparently normal thermoregulatory shivering, triggered when redistribution hypothermia decreases core temperature.

Spinal thermal receptors have been detected in every mammal and bird tested. Experimental stimulation of these receptors reliably produces shivering in animals. Stimulation of these putative receptors in humans by epidural anesthetic injection could theoretically initiate thermoregulatory responses, including shivering. However, epidural administration of large amounts of ice-cold saline does not trigger shivering in volunteers.[74] In addition, the incidence of shivering is comparable in volunteers[57] and patients[75] given warm or cold epidural anesthetic injections. These data indicate that the temperature of an injected local anesthetic does not influence the incidence of shivering during major conduction anesthesia.

The risk of shivering during neuraxial anesthesia is markedly diminished by maintaining strict normothermia.[57] However, there is a distinct incidence of low-intensity, shivering-like tremor that occurs in normothermic patients and is not thermoregulatory.[76] The cause of this muscular activity remains unknown, but it is associated with pain[77] and may thus result from activation of the sympathetic nervous system (Fig. 48-14).

Shivering during neuraxial anesthesia can sometimes be treated by warming sentient skin. This augments cutaneous

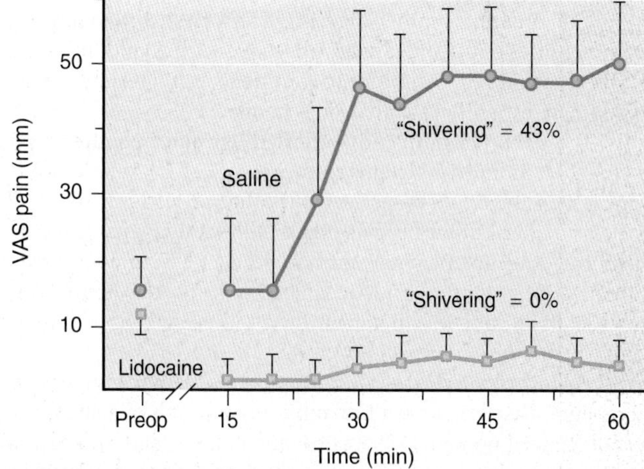

Figure 48-14 Visual analog pain scores (VAS) in normothermic patients given intra-articular lidocaine or saline after knee surgery. Pain was assessed postoperatively by an investigator blinded to the group assignment. Time zero indicates discontinuation of anesthesia. Data are presented as means ± SD. Patients receiving a local anesthetic block (lidocaine) had significantly less postoperative pain than those given saline; all values after 10 elapsed minutes differed significantly in the two groups. Shivering-like tremor was observed in 43% of the patients given saline versus 0% of those given lidocaine, thus indicating that the tremor is related to pain. *(From Horn E-P, Schroeder F, Wilhelm S, et al: Postoperative pain facilitates non-thermoregulatory tremor. Anesthesiology 91:979-984, 1999.)*

thermal input to the central regulatory system and thus increases the degree of core hypothermia tolerated. Because the entire skin surface contributes 20% to thermoregulatory control[5] and the lower body contributes about 10%,[63] sentient skin warming is likely to compensate for only small reductions in core temperature. The same drugs that are effective for postanesthetic tremor are also useful for shivering during regional anesthesia; such drugs include meperidine (25 mg intravenously [IV] or epidurally),[78] clonidine (75 µg IV),[79] dexmedetomine,[80] ketanserin (10 mg IV),[79] and magnesium sulfate (30 mg/kg IV).[81]

Consequences of Mild Intraoperative Hypothermia

Perianesthetic hypothermia produces potentially severe complications, as well as distinct benefits. Thermal management thus deserves the same thoughtful analysis of potential risks and benefits as other therapeutic decisions do.

Benefits

Substantial protection against cerebral ischemia and hypoxia is provided by hypothermia of just 1°C to 3°C in animals.[82,83] Protection was initially thought to result from the approximate 8%/°C linear reduction in tissue metabolic rate. However, the efficacy of mild hypothermia far exceeds that of treatments such as high-dose isoflurane or barbiturate coma, which comparably reduce the metabolic rate.[84] These data suggest that other actions (e.g., decreased release of excitatory amino acids) explain the protective action of hypothermia.[85] Accordingly, there is no reason to expect protection to augment linearly with temperature, and in animals it appears that much of the total benefit from moderate hypothermia takes place within the first couple of degrees.

Therapeutic hypothermia has twice been shown to improve outcomes after out-of-hospital cardiac arrest.[86,87] Rapid induction of hypothermia is thus becoming routine for patients after recovery from arrest and for asphyxiated neonates.[88-90]

The potential protection afforded by mild hypothermia is so great that reduced core temperature (i.e., ≈34°C) is increasingly being used during neurosurgery and other procedures in which tissue ischemia can be anticipated. The difficulty is that there are currently few outcome data substantiating an extrapolation from animal data to clinical practice. Furthermore, the appropriate target temperature for therapeutic hypothermia has yet to be established.

Hypothermia for brain trauma was initially claimed to be therapeutic based on a post hoc subgroup analysis of a study that overall showed no benefit.[91] A subsequent large randomized trial was unable to demonstrate any benefit overall or in subgroups—although interpretation of the study was limited by violations in the fluid administration protocol in some patients.[92] Most recently, hypothermia was shown to be beneficial in a nonrandomized study in which brain trauma patients with elevated intracranial pressure refractory to conventional treatment were assigned to therapeutic hypothermia. Despite being sicker than the comparison patients (who had low intracranial pressure), the hypothermic patients demonstrated improved outcomes.[93]

Small nonrandomized series suggested that mild hypothermia might improve the outcome after stroke.[94] A small feasibility trial for treatment of stroke with hypothermia has been published,[95] but no large trial is currently in progress.

Although the initial feasibility trials were encouraging,[95,96] a subsequent large outcome trial failed to demonstrate any improvement with therapeutic hypothermia in patients undergoing surgery for subarachnoid hemorrhage.[97] This result was especially disappointing because surgery is one of the few times in humans that hypothermia can be instituted before the onset of ischemia.

Hypothermic protection against ischemia may extend to other organs. For example, mild hypothermia markedly reduces infarct size in experimental acute myocardial infarction in human-sized pigs,[98] and a preliminary study in patients was encouraging.[99] However, a subsequent major outcome trial in humans failed to demonstrate convincing benefit (unpublished).

A limitation of most therapeutic hypothermia studies is that cooling began well after the ischemic insult and that patients typically took many hours to cool. It thus remains possible that benefit will yet be identified in future studies that initiate hypothermia earlier and use recently developed systems to cool patients faster. Table 48-1 lists selected major studies that have evaluated the potential benefits of mild perioperative hypothermia.

Complications

Coagulation is impaired by mild hypothermia. The most important factor is a cold-induced defect in platelet function.[107] Interestingly, the defect in platelet function is related to local temperature, not core temperature. Wound temperature, however, is largely determined by core temperature and will be distinctly higher in normothermic patients. Perhaps as important, hypothermia directly impairs enzymes of the coagulation cascade. This will not be apparent during routine coagulation screening because the tests are performed at 37°C. When these tests are performed at hypothermic temperatures, however, the defect becomes apparent.[108]

Consistent with these in vitro defects, nearly all randomized trials indicate that mild hypothermia increases blood loss during hip arthroplasty and increases allogeneic transfusion requirements.[109] Similarly, nearly all randomized trials report an increased transfusion requirement in hypothermic patients. Meta-analyses indicate that both blood loss and transfusion requirements are significantly increased by hypothermia.[106] The treatment effect is substantial, with just 1°C of core hypothermia increasing each by about 20%.

Wound infections are among the most common serious complications of anesthesia and surgery and probably cause more morbidity than all other anesthetic complications combined.[110] Hypothermia can contribute to wound infections both by directly impairing immune function[111] and by triggering thermoregulatory vasoconstriction, which in turn decreases oxygen delivery to wounds.[112] It is well established that fever is protective and that infections are aggravated when naturally occurring fever is prevented.[113] Similarly, mild hypothermia, maintained only during anesthesia, impairs subsequent resistance to both *Escherichia coli* and *Staphylococcus aureus* dermal infections in guinea pigs. As

Table 48-1 Major Complications of Mild Perioperative Hypothermia in Humans

Consequence	First Author	Year	N	ΔT_{core} (°C)	Normothermic	Hypothermic	P
Surgical wound infection	Kurz	1996	200	1.9	6%	19%	<.01
Duration of hospitalization	Kurz	1996	200	1.9	12.1 ± 4.4 days	14.7 ± 6.5 days	<.01
Duration of hospitalization	Frank	1997	300	1.3	8 (range, 5-13)	8 (5-11)	NS
Postoperative troponin I	Nesher[100]	2003	60	1.0	22 ± 9 ng/mL	8 ± 5 ng/mL	
Morbid cardiac events	Frank	1997	300	1.3	1%	6%	<.05
Myocardial damage	Nesher[100]	2003	60	1.0	8 ± 5 ng/ml	22 ± 9 ng/mL	<.01
Postoperative shivering	Just[101]	1992	14	2.3	141 ± 9 mL/min/m²	269 ± 60 mL/min/m²	<.001
Duration of postanesthetic recovery	Lenhardt[102]	1997	150	1.9	53 ± 36 min	94 ± 65 min	<.001
Adrenergic activation	Frank[103]	1995	74	1.5	330 ± 30 pg/mL	480 ± 70 pg/mL	<.05
Thermal discomfort	Kurz[104]	1995	74	2.6	50 ± 10 mm VAS	18 ± 9 mm VAS	<.001
Mortality after major trauma	Gentillo[105]	1997	57	≈1.5	2/29 (7%)	12/28 (43%)	<.05

Only prospective, randomized human trials are included; subjective responses were evaluated by observers blinded to the treatment group and core temperature. *N* = total number of subjects. ΔT_{core} = difference in core temperature between the treatment groups. Different outcomes of some studies are shown in separate rows. VAS is a 100-mm-long visual analog scale (0 mm = intense cold; 100 mm = intense heat). The study by Just and colleagues is but one of dozens of studies showing that hypothermia provokes shivering. The results are presented as means ± SD or median (interquartile range) unless otherwise specified. NS = not significant. For the effects of hypothermia on perioperative blood loss and transfusion requirement, see the meta-analysis by Rajagopalan and coworkers.[106]

might be expected from these in vitro and animal data, a prospective, randomized clinical trial indicated that mild intraoperative hypothermia triples the incidence of surgical wound infection in patients undergoing colon surgery. Furthermore, hypothermia delayed wound healing and prolonged the duration of hospitalization 20% even in patients without infection. Consistent with poor wound healing, urinary nitrogen excretion remains elevated for several postoperative days in patients allowed to become hypothermic during surgery.

Thermal comfort is markedly impaired by postoperative hypothermia, a feeling that persists for several hours in patients who are several degrees centigrade hypothermic at the beginning of recovery (Fig. 48-15).[104] Patients, asked years after surgery, often identify feeling cold in the immediate postoperative period as the worst part of their hospitalization—sometimes rating it worse than surgical pain. Postoperative thermal discomfort is also physiologically stressful in that it elevates blood pressure, heart rate, and plasma catecholamine concentrations.[103] These factors presumably contribute to what may be the most important consequence of mild perioperative hypothermia: a threefold increase in morbid myocardial outcomes. Given that myocardial ischemia is among the leading causes of unanticipated perioperative death, the results of this prospective, randomized trial must be taken extremely seriously. Drug metabolism is markedly decreased by perioperative hypothermia. For further information see Chapters 26 and 29. Table 48-2 lists the major studies that have evaluated complications caused by mild perioperative hypothermia.

Postanesthetic Shivering

The incidence of postoperative shivering-like tremor is reportedly about 40% but now appears to be less as more patients are kept normothermic and opioids are administered more frequently and in larger doses than in the past. It is a potentially serious complication that increases oxygen consumption roughly 100% in proportion to intraoperative heat loss.[116] Interestingly, though, myocardial ischemia is poorly correlated with shivering, suggesting that an increased metabolic rate is not the primary cause of this complication. In addition to increasing intraocular and

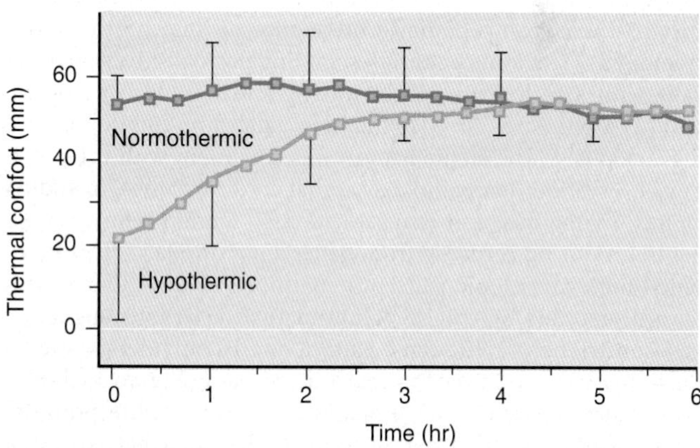

Figure 48-15 Patients who started recovery while about 2°C hypothermic reported feeling unpleasantly cold, and the sensation persisted longer than 2 hours. Only a few of the warmed patients shivered at any time during the recovery period. In contrast, most of the hypothermic patients demonstrated grade 2 or 3 tremor during the first postoperative hour. By the end of the first elapsed hour, however, shivering was rare, even in the hypothermic patients. Error bars indicate standard deviations. Thermal comfort is shown on a 100-mm visual analog scale, where 0 mm is the worst possible cold sensation, 50 mm is neutral, and 100 mm is extreme heat. *(From Kurz A, Sessler DI, Narzt E, et al: Postoperative hemodynamic and thermoregulatory consequences of intraoperative core hypothermia. J Clin Anesth 7:359-366, 1995.)*

Table 48-2 Potential Benefits of Mild Perioperative Hypothermia in Humans

Consequence	First author	Year	N	ΔT_{core} (°C)	Normothermic	Hypothermic	P
Mortality after brain trauma	Clifton[92]	2001	392	4.2	27%	28%	NS
Favorable Glasgow outcome score 3 months after brain trauma	Shiozaki[114]	2001	91	4	59%	47%	NS
Glasgow outcome score 12 months after brain trauma (1-3/4-5)	Marion[91]	1997	81	≈4	62%/38%	39%/61%	NS
Neurologic outcome after cardiac arrest (good)	Bernard[86]	2002	77	≈4	26%	49%	.01
Neurologic outcome 6 months after cardiac arrest (good recovery or moderate disability)	Hypothermia Group[87]	2002	273	≈4.5	55%	39%	.009
Mortality at 6 months	Hypothermia Group[87]	2002	273	≈4.5	55%	41%	.02
Neurologic outcome of neonatal hypoxia (death or moderate to severe disability)	Gluckman[88]	2005	218	≈2	66%	59%	.1
Neurologic outcome of neonatal hypoxia (death or moderate to severe disability)	Shankaran[89]	2005	208	3.8	62%	44%	.01
Good neurologic outcome after intracranial aneurysm surgery	Todd[97]	2005	1001	3.5	63	66	NS

Only prospective, randomized human trials are included; subjective responses were evaluated by observers blinded to the treatment group and core temperature. *N* = total number of subjects. ΔT_{core} = difference in core temperature between the treatment groups. Different outcomes of some studies are shown in separate rows. Results are presented as means ± SD or median (interquartile range) unless otherwise specified. NS = not significant. For the effects of mild hypothermia on neonatal asphyxia, see the Cochrane meta-analysis by Jacobs and coworkers.[115]

intracranial pressure, postoperative shivering possibly aggravates wound pain by stretching incisions. The most important determinants of shivering risk are young age and low core temperature.[117]

Unfortunately, the etiology of postanesthetic shivering-like tremor is unclear. Certainly, much postoperative tremor is simply normal shivering. As early as 1972, however, investigators recognized the existence of at least two distinct tremor patterns.[118] That perceptive observation was subsequently confirmed in a study that used electromyography to demonstrate that postoperative tremor has (1) a tonic pattern resembling normal shivering, typically with a 4- to 8-cycle/min waxing-and-waning component, and (2) a phasic, 5- to 7-Hz bursting pattern resembling pathologic clonus.[119] The clonic pattern was consistent with the previous observation that pathologic spinal cord responses, including clonus, nystagmus, and exaggerated deep tendon reflexes, were common during recovery from general anesthesia.[120] This combined tonic and clonic pattern is thermoregulatory; that is, it is always preceded by core hypothermia and arteriovenous shunt vasoconstriction.[121] The tonic pattern consistently demonstrated the 4- to 8-cycle/min waxing-and-waning pattern of normal shivering[16] and apparently is a simple thermoregulatory response to intraoperative hypothermia. In contrast, the clonic pattern is not a normal component of thermoregulatory shivering and appears to be specific to recovery from volatile anesthetics. Although the precise etiology of this tremor pattern remains unknown, it may result from anesthetic-induced disinhibition of normal descending control over spinal reflexes. Earlier data in surgical patients, however, belie the simple conclusion from a volunteer study[121] that all postanesthetic tremor is thermoregulatory. Instead, there appears to be a distinct incidence of non-thermoregulatory tremor in normothermic postoperative patients[122]; similar non-thermoregulatory tremor has been observed in women during labor.[76] The etiology of this tremor and why volunteers and patients should respond differently remain unknown, but surgical pain appears to be a key factor.[77]

Postanesthetic shivering can be treated by skin surface warming because the regulatory system tolerates more core hypothermia when cutaneous warm input is augmented. However, the skin surface contributes only 20% to control of shivering,[5] and available skin surface warmers increase mean skin temperature only a few degrees centigrade.[123] Consequently, cutaneous warming compensates for only small amounts of core hypothermia and will not usually prove effective in most patients with core temperatures much below 35°C.[124]

Postanesthetic shivering can also be treated with a variety of drugs, including clonidine (75 μg IV),[79] ketanserin (10 mg IV),[79] tramadol,[125] physostigmine (0.04 mg/kg IV),[126] nefopam (0.15 mg/kg),[127] dexmedetomidine, and magnesium sulfate (30 mg/kg IV).[81] The specific mechanisms by which ketanserin, tramadol, physostigmine, and magnesium sulfate stop shivering remain unknown. Similarly, how clonidine arrests shivering also remains unknown, but clonidine[32] and dexmedetomidine[22] comparably reduce the vasoconstriction and shivering thresholds, thus suggesting that they act on the central thermoregulatory system rather than preventing shivering peripherally. Postoperative shivering has been reviewed in detail[128] and treatment options have been subjected to a systematic review.[129]

Alfentanil, a pure μ-receptor agonist, significantly impairs thermoregulatory control.[21] However, meperidine is considerably more effective in treating shivering than equi-analgesic doses of other μ-agonists are.[130] Clinically, this efficacy is manifested as a shivering threshold that is reduced twice as much as the vasoconstriction threshold[27] without a decrease in the gain or maximum intensity of shivering.[46] The efficacy of meperidine is at least partially preserved during the administration of moderate doses of naloxone (0.5 μg/kg/min) but virtually obliterated by enormous doses (5.0 μg/kg/min).[131] These data suggest that the action of this drug is in part mediated by non–μ-opioid receptors. Meperidine possesses considerable κ activity[132] and also has central anticholinergic activity. However, neither mechanism appears to mediate meperidine's special antishivering activity.

Perioperative Thermal Manipulations

Intraoperative thermoregulatory vasoconstriction, once triggered, is remarkably effective in preventing further core hypothermia.[39,45] Nonetheless, most patients are poikilothermic during surgery because they do not become sufficiently hypothermic to trigger thermoregulatory responses.[20,21,23,24] Therefore, intraoperative hypothermia can be minimized by any technique that limits cutaneous heat loss to the environment, such as loss caused by cold operating rooms, evaporation from surgical incisions, or conductive cooling produced by the administration of cold intravenous fluids. The efficacy of various approaches differs enormously, however.

Mean body temperature will decrease when heat loss to the environment exceeds metabolic heat production. Heat production during anesthesia is approximately 0.8 kcal/kg/hr. Because the specific heat of the human body is about 0.83 kcal/kg,[133] body temperature decreases approximately 1°C/hr when heat lost to the environment exceeds metabolic production by a factor of 2. Normally, about 90% of metabolic heat is lost through the skin surface. During anesthesia, additional heat is also lost directly from surgical incisions and by the administration of cold intravenous fluids.

Effects of Vasomotor Tone on Heat Transfer

Thermoregulatory vasodilation causes the initial core-to-peripheral redistribution of body heat[55]; similarly, re-emergence of vasoconstriction in patients becoming sufficiently hypothermic produces a core temperature plateau.[45] It is thus evident that vasomotor tone alters intercompartmental heat transfer. In addition to thermoregulatory arteriovenous shunt status, arteriolar tone is directly modulated by anesthetics per se.[52] Both factors potentially influence the speed with which peripherally applied heat reaches the core thermal compartment.

Thermoregulatory vasoconstriction slightly impairs induction of therapeutic hypothermia during neurosurgery.[134] However, arteriovenous shunt tone has little effect on intraoperative cooling[135] or heating.[136] Intraoperative vasoconstriction thus only slightly impedes peripheral-to-core transfer of cutaneous heating and cooling. Little clinical effect presumably results because intraoperative thermoregulatory vasoconstriction is opposed by direct anesthetic-induced peripheral vasodilation.

During postanesthetic recovery, however, the situation differs markedly. Here, dissipation of anesthetic-induced peripheral dilation[52,137] leaves thermoregulatory vasoconstriction unopposed. As might be expected, this vasoconstriction then becomes an important factor and significantly impairs transfer of peripherally applied heat to the core thermal compartment. Patients with residual spinal anesthetic block thus warm considerably faster than those recovering from general anesthesia alone

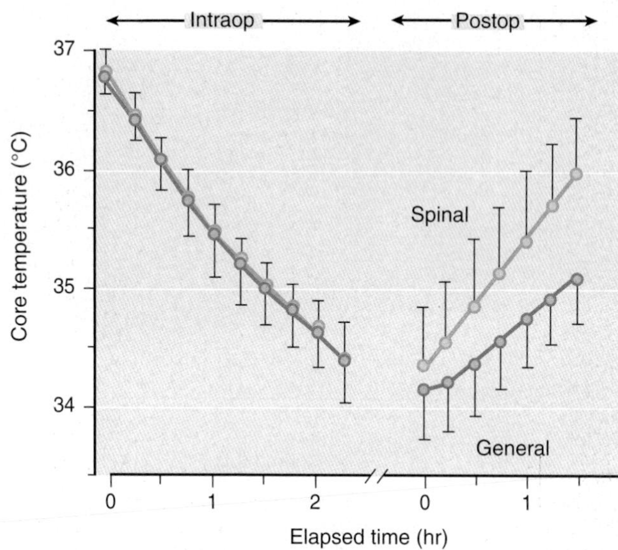

Figure 48-16 Intraoperative and postoperative core temperatures in patients assigned to general anesthesia (n = 20) and spinal anesthesia (n = 20). All patients were warmed with forced air during the postoperative period. Core temperature did not differ significantly during surgery but increased significantly faster postoperatively in patients given spinal anesthesia (1.2 ± 0.1°C/hr versus 0.7 ± 0.2°C/hr, means ± SD). *(From Szmuk P, Ezri T, Sessler DI, et al: Spinal anesthesia only minimally increases the efficacy of postoperative forced-air rewarming. Anesthesiology 87:1050-1054, 1997.)*

(Fig. 48-16).[138] Heat balance studies indicate that core warming is slowed because vasoconstriction constrains up to 30 kcal in peripheral tissues.[139]

Furthermore, it is easier to maintain intraoperative normothermia (when most patients are vasodilated) than rewarm patients postoperatively (when virtually all hypothermic patients are vasoconstricted). In addition to being more effective, intraoperative warming is more appropriate than postoperative treatment of hypothermia because it prevents the complications resulting from hypothermia.[109] Patients unavoidably becoming hypothermic during surgery should nonetheless be actively heated postoperatively to increase thermal comfort, decrease shivering, and hasten rewarming.

Preventing Redistribution Hypothermia

The initial 0.5°C to 1.5°C reduction in core temperature is difficult to prevent because it results from redistribution of heat from the central thermal compartment to cooler peripheral tissues.[55] Consequently, surface warming usually fails to prevent hypothermia during the first hour of anesthesia.[56] Lack of efficacy during this period results both because the central-to-peripheral flow of heat is massive and because transfer of applied cutaneous heat to the core requires nearly an hour, even in vasodilated patients.

Although redistribution is difficult to treat,[56] it can be prevented. Redistribution results when anesthetic-induced vasodilation allows heat to flow peripherally down the normal temperature gradient. Skin surface warming before induction of anesthesia does not significantly alter core temperature (which remains well regulated), but it does increase body heat content. Most of the increase is in the legs, the most important component of the

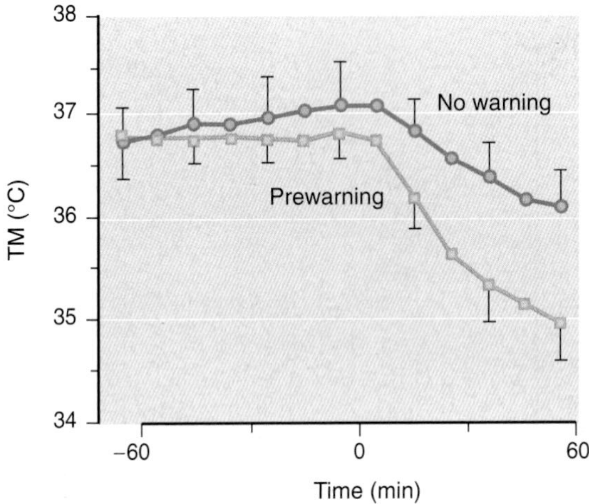

Figure 48-17 During the preinduction period (−120 to 0 minutes), volunteers were either actively warmed or passively cooled (no warming). At induction of anesthesia (time = 0 minutes), active warming was discontinued and volunteers were exposed to the ambient environment. Initial tympanic membrane (TM) temperatures were similar before each preinduction treatment. During the 60 minutes after induction of anesthesia, core temperature decreased less when volunteers were prewarmed. ($\Delta T = -1.1 \pm 0.3$°C) than when the same volunteers were not warmed ($\Delta T = -1.9 \pm 0.3$°C). Data are presented as means ± SD. *(From Hynson JM, Sessler DI, Moayeri A, et al: The effects of pre-induction warming on temperature and blood pressure during propofol/nitrous oxide anesthesia. Anesthesiology 79:219-228, 1993.)*

peripheral thermal compartment. When peripheral tissue temperature is sufficiently increased, subsequent inhibition of normal tonic thermoregulatory vasoconstriction produces little redistribution hypothermia because heat can flow only down a temperature gradient (Fig. 48-17).[69,70] Although substantial amounts of heat must be transferred across the skin surface, active prewarming for as little as 30 minutes probably prevents considerable redistribution.[140]

The "afterdrop" associated with discontinuation of cardiopulmonary bypass is a type of redistribution hypothermia that results from a substantial core-to-peripheral tissue temperature gradient. As might be expected, it is more impressive after bypass at 17°C[141] than at 27°C to 31°C.[142] Cutaneous warming during and after bypass reduces core temperature afterdrop by 60%. However, heat balance data indicate that this reduction results primarily because cutaneous warming prevents the typical decrease in body heat content after discontinuation of bypass rather than by reducing redistribution.[143]

Airway Heating and Humidification

Simple thermodynamic calculations indicate that less than 10% of metabolic heat production is lost via the respiratory tract. The loss results from both heating and humidifying inspiratory gases, but humidification requires two thirds of the heat.[50] Because little heat is lost via respiration, even active airway heating and humidification minimally influence core temperature.[56]

Because respiratory heat loss remains virtually constant during anesthesia, the fraction of total heat lost via the respiratory tract decreases dramatically during large operations in which substantial heat is lost from evaporation within surgical incisions.[51] Consequently, airway heating and humidification are even less effective than usual in patients most in need of effective warming.

Intravenous Fluids

Patients cannot be warmed by administering heated fluids because the fluids cannot (much) exceed body temperature. On the other hand, heat loss from cold intravenous fluids becomes substantial when large amounts of crystalloid solution or blood are administered. One unit of refrigerated blood or 1 L of crystalloid solution administered at room temperature each decreases mean body temperature approximately 0.25°C. (The blood is twice as cold, but only half the volume.) Fluid warmers minimize these losses and should be used when large amounts of intravenous fluid or blood are administered. In smaller cases, though, they contribute little.

For routine cases, there are no clinically important differences among the available fluid warmers. Although most warmers allow fluid to cool in the tubing between the heater and the patient, this cooling is of little consequence in adults: at high flow there is little cooling, and at low flow the amount of fluid given is trivial.[144] Special high-volume systems with powerful heaters and little resistance to flow facilitate care of trauma victims and are useful in other cases in which a large amount of fluid must be administered quickly.

Cutaneous Warming

Operating room temperature is the most critical factor influencing heat loss because it determines the rate at which metabolic heat is lost by radiation and convection from the skin and by evaporation from within surgical incisions. Consequently, increasing room temperature is one way to minimize heat loss. However, room temperatures exceeding 23°C are generally required to maintain normothermia in patients undergoing all but the smallest procedures[145]; most operating room personnel find such temperatures uncomfortably warm. Infants may require ambient temperatures exceeding 26°C to maintain normothermia. Such temperatures are sufficiently high to impair the performance of operating room personnel and decrease their vigilance.

The easiest method of decreasing cutaneous heat loss is to apply passive insulation to the skin surface. Insulators readily available in most operating rooms include cotton blankets, surgical drapes, plastic sheeting, and reflective composites ("space blankets"). A single layer of each reduces heat loss approximately 30%, and there are no clinically important differences among the types of insulation. The reduction in heat loss from all the commonly used passive insulators is similar because most of the insulation is provided by the layer of still air trapped beneath the covering. As a result, adding additional layers of insulation further reduces heat loss only slightly. For example, one cotton blanket reduces heat loss by about 30%, but three cotton blankets reduces heat loss only by 50%. Furthermore, warming the cotton blankets provides little benefit, and the benefit is short-lived.[146] These data indicate that simply adding additional layers of passive insulation or warming the insulation before application will usually be insufficient in patients becoming hypothermic while covered with a single layer of insulation.

Cutaneous heat loss is roughly proportional to surface area throughout the body.[147] (The popular perception that a large fraction of metabolic heat is lost from the head is false in adults. Loss from the head can be substantial in small infants,[148] but the loss is high mostly because the head represents a large fraction of the total surface area.) Consequently, the amount of skin covered is more important than which surfaces are insulated. It does not make sense, for example, to cover the head and leave the arms exposed because the arms have more surface area than the head and account for more heat loss.

Passive insulation alone is rarely sufficient to maintain normothermia in patients undergoing large operations; active warming will be required in such cases. Because about 90% of metabolic heat is lost via the skin surface, only cutaneous warming will transfer sufficient heat to prevent hypothermia. Consequently, for intraoperative use, circulating water and forced air are the two major systems requiring consideration.

Studies consistently report that circulating-water mattresses are nearly ineffective.[149] Presumably, they are unable to maintain normothermia because little heat is lost from the back into the 5 cm of foam insulation covering most operating room tables. Moreover, the combination of heat and decreased local perfusion (resulting when the patient's weight reduces capillary blood flow) increases the propensity for pressure/heat necrosis ("burns"). Such tissue injury can occur even when the water temperature does not exceed 40°C.[150] Circulating water is more effective—and safer—when placed *over* patients rather than *under* them and, in that position, can almost completely eliminate metabolic heat loss. Metabolic heat production will increase mean body temperature approximately 1°C/hr when cutaneous heat loss is eliminated. Recently developed circulating-water garments transfer large amounts of heat by increasing the warmed surface area or using materials that facilitate conduction.[151,152]

The most common perianesthetic warming system is forced air. The best forced-air systems completely eliminate heat loss from the skin surface.[123] Forced air usually maintains normothermia even during the largest operations[56] and is superior to circulating-water mattresses.[153] It is also remarkably safe, with few if any injuries reported with proper use.

Induction of Mild Therapeutic Hypothermia

There remains a paucity of evidence supporting the application of therapeutic hypothermia for indications other than out-of-hospital cardiac arrest and asphyxiated neonates. Nonetheless, hypothermia is occasionally used during neurosurgery or acute myocardial infarction. Typically, target core temperatures are 32°C to 34°C, and it is thought that reaching the target temperature quickly is important.

Passive cooling is far too slow for induction of therapeutic hypothermia. Immersion in cold water is the quickest noninvasive method of actively cooling patients. However, immersion is difficult under clinical conditions and poses a substantial electrical safety risk. Administration of refrigerated intravenous fluids is also effective and reduces mean body temperature 0.5°C/L.[154] However, this method may be impractical in neurosurgical patients, in whom fluids must be restricted.

Forced-air cooling is easy to implement but relatively slow in that it takes about 2.5 hours to cool neurosurgical patients to 33°C.[134] Conventional circulating-water mattresses are unlikely to be efficient because relatively little skin surface contacts the mattress and the patient's own body weight reduces blood-borne convection of heat to the back. Newer circulating-water systems include garment-like covers or "energy exchange pads" that cover far more skin surface and transfer large amounts of heat, and they are fairly effective.[155]

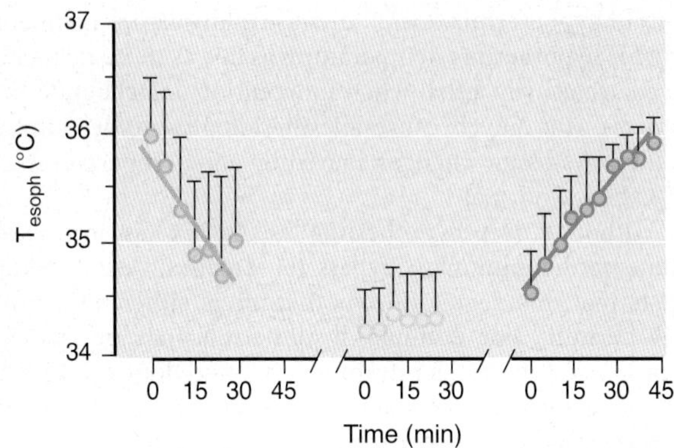

Figure 48-18 Average (±SD) intraoperative esophageal temperatures (T_{esoph}) during the cooling, temperature maintenance, and rewarming periods in eight neurosurgical patients who were cooled with endovascular heat-exchanging catheters in the vena cava. Time zero identified the beginning of each thermal management period; the duration of these periods differed in individual patients, depending on the duration of surgery and other factors. Regression lines are shown for the cooling and rewarming periods. *(From Doufas AG, Akça O, Barry A, et al: Initial experience with a novel heat-exchanging catheter in neurosurgical patients. Anesth Analg 95:1752-1756, 2002.)*

The best way to rapidly induce therapeutic hypothermia is probably endovascular cooling. These systems consist of a heat-exchanging catheter, usually inserted into the inferior vena cava via the femoral artery, and a servocontroller. They can decrease core temperatures at rates approaching 4°C/hr (Fig. 48-18).[156]

Inducing therapeutic hypothermia during surgery is relatively easy because anesthetics profoundly impair thermoregulatory responses. In contrast, unanesthetized patients—even those who have suffered a stroke—vigorously defend core temperature by vasoconstriction and shivering.[157] It is thus necessary to pharmacologically induce tolerance to hypothermia. The best method thus far identified is the combination of buspirone and meperidine, drugs that synergistically reduce the shivering threshold to around 34°C without provoking excessive sedation or respiratory toxicity.[158] The combination of dexmedetomidine and meperidine may also be helpful, although the interaction is simply additive in this case.[80] In contrast, ondansetron,[159] doxapram,[160] and magnesium sulfate[161] only slightly reduce the shivering threshold in humans. Although initially reported to be effective,[162] neither arm nor face warming reduces the shivering threshold by clinically important amounts.[163]

Deliberate Severe Intraoperative Hypothermia

Severe hypothermia may be induced deliberately to confer protection against tissue ischemia, specifically during cardiac surgery and, occasionally, neurosurgery. Drugs such as barbiturates and volatile anesthetics provide considerably less protection than even mild hypothermia does.[84] Because many organs compensate poorly for hypothermia, temperatures as low as those deliberately induced are usually lethal when unintentional. Deliberate hypothermia is safe only because anesthesiologists understand and treat the physiologic changes caused by core temperatures 10°C to 15°C below normal.

Although deep hypothermia (i.e., 28°C) has been used to facilitate cardiopulmonary bypass for decades, recent evidence suggests that this degree of hypothermia is either unhelpful or simply harmful. For example, hypothermia may be associated with prolonged ventricular dysfunction[164] and does not limit cognitive impairment after bypass.[165] Consequently, cardiac surgery is increasingly being performed at either "tepid" temperatures (i.e., 33°C) or normothermia. There is increasing evidence that outcomes after bypass surgery, whether on- or off-pump, are improved by maintaining normothermia or near-normothermia.[166,167] Deep hypothermia (i.e., 18°C) remains routine for intentional circulatory arrest cases.[141]

Organ Function

Hypothermia decreases the whole-body metabolic rate by approximately 8%/°C[40] to approximately one half the normal rate at 28°C.[168] Whole-body oxygen demand diminishes, and oxygen consumption in tissues that have higher than normal metabolic rates, such as the brain, is especially reduced. Brain oxygenation is thus improved by hypothermia.[169] Low metabolic rates allow aerobic metabolism to continue during periods of compromised oxygen supply; toxic waste production declines in proportion to the metabolic rate. Although a decreased metabolic rate certainly contributes to the observed protection against tissue ischemia, other effects of hypothermia, including "membrane stabilization" and decreased release of toxic metabolites and excitatory amino acids, appear to be most important.[85]

Cerebral blood flow also decreases in proportion to the metabolic rate during hypothermia because of an autoregulatory increase in cerebrovascular resistance.[85] The arteriovenous Po_2 difference thus remains constant, and the venous lactate concentration does not increase. Cerebral function is well maintained until core temperatures reach approximately 33°C, but consciousness is lost at temperatures below 28°C. Primitive reflexes such as the gag, pupillary constriction, and monosynaptic spinal reflexes remain intact until approximately 25°C. Nerve conduction decreases, but peripheral muscle tone increases and results in rigidity and myoclonus at temperatures near 26°C. Somatosensory and audio evoked potentials are temperature dependent, but not significantly modified at core temperatures of 33°C or higher.

Hypothermic effects on the heart include a decrease in heart rate, increased contractility, and well-maintained stroke volume.[170] Cardiac output and blood pressure both decrease. At temperatures below 28°C, sinoatrial pacing becomes erratic and ventricular irritability increases. Fibrillation usually occurs between 25°C and 30°C, and electrical defibrillation is generally ineffective at these temperatures. Because coronary artery blood flow decreases in proportion to cardiac work, hypothermia per se does not cause myocardial ischemia. However, even mild hypothermia decreases tissue damage in response to experimental cardiac ischemia.[98]

Hypothermia decreases blood flow to the kidneys by increasing renovascular resistance. Inhibition of tubular absorption maintains normal urinary volume. As temperature decreases, reabsorption of sodium and potassium is progressively inhibited and thereby results in an antidiuretic hormone–mediated "cold diuresis." Despite increased excretion of these ions, plasma electrolyte concentrations usually remain normal. Kidney functions return to normal when patients are rewarmed. Respiratory strength is diminished at core temperatures lower than 33°C, but the ventilatory CO_2 response is minimally affected. Hepatic blood flow and function also decrease and thus significantly inhibit the metabolism of some drugs.

Acid-Base Changes

The pH of neutral water ($[OH^-] = [H^+]$) increases 0.017 unit for each 1°C reduction in temperature[171]; the pH of blood in a closed system (e.g., test tube or artery) changes similarly (see Chapter 49). Cold-blooded animals allow pH to vary with body temperature as it would in vitro (i.e., blood becomes more alkalotic as temperature decreases); in contrast, homeotherms, which decrease body temperature during hibernation, maintain an arterial pH near 7.4, a process known as pH-stat management. Interpretation of arterial pH in hypothermic humans is difficult because it is unclear which strategy is optimal.[172]

To mimic the compensatory mechanisms used by hibernating homeotherms, blood pH (which is measured by electrodes at 37°C) has traditionally been "corrected" to the patient's actual body temperature. Without correction, tissue oxygen availability decreases because hemoglobin's affinity for oxygen increases about 1.7%/°C. This effect is small in comparison to the 5.7%/°C increase in oxyhemoglobin affinity caused by hypothermia itself. Fortunately, the combined increases in affinity are offset by the 8%/°C reduction in metabolic rate caused by hypothermia. Tissue hypoxia is thus unlikely, with or without correction, and has not been demonstrated experimentally.

Ectothermic strategy is also known as "alpha-stat" because the dissociation constant of the α-imidazole group in histidine changes in parallel with that of water. Maintaining constant imidazole ionization results in optimal enzyme function as temperature changes. In contrast, homeothermic dynamics significantly decreases metabolic function, and animals are essentially anesthetized by cold. Constant relative alkalinity also maintains a stable intracellular-to-extracellular gradient that promotes the removal of acidic products of intracellular metabolism, which might be salutary.[173]

Both alpha- and pH-stat management seem to work well, and physiologic differences between them appear to be subtle. However, there is increasing evidence that pH-stat management better preserves neurons in the context of ischemic stress.[174-176] Furthermore, clinical outcomes seem to be improved by pH-stat management[177]—or at least not worsened.[178] Nonetheless, alpha-stat management remains common, and there is no consensus that either strategy markedly influences the outcome of cardiac surgery.

Hyperthermia and Fever

Hypothermia is by far the most common perianesthetic thermal perturbation. However, hyperthermia is probably more dangerous than a comparable degree of hypothermia, and hyperthermia

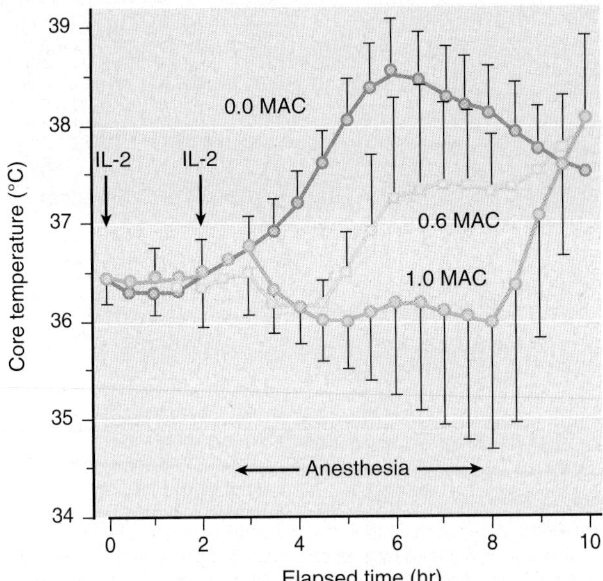

Figure 48-19 Change in core temperature after the administration of 50,000 IU/kg of interleukin-2 (IL-2), followed by a second dose of 100,000 IU/kg 2 hours later. The first dose of IL-2 defined elapsed time zero; anesthesia was started after 3 elapsed hours and continued for 5 hours. Data are presented as means ± SD. *(From Negishi C, Lenhardt R, Sessler DI, et al: Desflurane reduces the febrile response to interleukin-2 administration. Anesthesiology 88:1162-1169, 1998.)*

is certainly more dangerous when perturbations exceed a few degrees centigrade. Hyperthermia is a generic term simply indicating a core body temperature exceeding normal values. In contrast, fever is a regulated increase in the core temperature targeted by the thermoregulatory system. Hyperthermia can result from a variety of causes and usually indicates a problem of sufficient severity that physician intervention is required.

Passive Hyperthermia

Passive intraoperative hyperthermia results from excessive patient heating and is most common in infants and children. It is especially frequent when effective active warming is used without adequate core temperature monitoring. Passive hyperthermia, by definition, does not result from thermoregulatory intervention. Consequently, it can easily be treated by discontinuing active warming and removing excessive insulation.

For information on malignant hyperthermia, see Chapter 37.

Fever

Normal body temperature is neither set nor maintained by circulating factors. In contrast, fever results when endogenous pyrogens increase the thermoregulatory target temperature ("set point"). Endogenous pyrogens identified include interleukin-1, tumor necrosis factor, interferon-α, and macrophage inflammatory protein-1.[179] Although it was initially believed that these factors act directly on hypothalamic thermoregulatory centers,[180] there is increasing evidence of a more complicated system involving vagal afferents.[181] Most endogenous pyrogens have peripheral actions (e.g., activation of the immune system) in addition to their central generating capabilities.

Fever is relatively rare during general anesthesia even though febrile stimuli are frequently present. It is rare because volatile anesthetics per se inhibit expression of fever (Fig. 48-19),[182] as do opioids.[183] Infection is by far the most common cause of fever. However, perioperative fever also occurs in response to mismatched blood transfusions, blood in the fourth cerebral ventricle, and allergic reactions. Some degree of fever is also typical after surgery.[184] The causes of fever are sufficiently diverse—and potentially serious—that a search for a specific etiology is usually warranted.

Treatment of hyperthermia depends on the cause, with the critical distinction being between fever and other causes of hyperthermia. (In general, patients with fever and increasing core temperature will have constricted fingertips, whereas those with other types of hyperthermia will be vasodilated.) It is always appropriate to treat the underlying causes, but nonfebrile hyperthermia will also improve with cooling.

The first- and second-line treatments of fever are amelioration of the underlying cause and administration of antipyretic medications. The first treatment strategy often fails because the etiology of the fever remains unknown; alternatively, the source may be known but unresponsive. The second strategy also often fails or is only partially effective, perhaps because some fever is mediated by mechanisms that bypass conventional antipyretics.[179] It is in these patients that third-line treatment is most likely to be implemented: active cooling (Table 48-3). Active cooling of febrile

Table 48-3 Active Cutaneous Cooling as Treatment of Fever

	Control	Cooling	Warming
Integrated core temperature (°C/hr)	6.0 ± 1.6	5.7 ± 2.2	6.4 ± 1.2
Oxygen consumption (mL/min)	330 ± 50	430 ± 40*	310 ± 30
Duration of shivering (min)	33 ±11	229 ± 35	20 ± 0
Mean arterial pressure (mm Hg)	90 ± 4	98 ± 6*	86 ± 6†
Mean [norepinephrine] (nM)	1.0 ± 0.4	1.4 ± 0.7*	1.1 ± 0.5†
Baseline [epinephrine] (nM)	0.3 ± 0.1	0.3 ± 0.1	0.3 ± 0.1
Mean [epinephrine] during treatment (nM)	0.3 ± 0.1	0.5 ± 0.1*	0.4 ± 0.1
Severe cold sensation (% of time)	27	89*	11

Volunteers were given 30,000 IU/kg of interleukin-2 (IL-2), followed 2 hours later by an additional dose of 70,000 IU/kg. The first dose of IL-2 defined elapsed time zero; thermal management started after 3 elapsed hours and continued for 5 hours. Each volunteer participated on 3 separate days: no warming or cooling, active cooling, and active warming. Mean and integrated values are presented over the treatment period, from 3 to 8 elapsed hours. Times are presented in terms of hours elapsed since the first injection of IL-2. Data are presented as means ± SD.
*Statistically significant differences from control.
†Statistically significant differences from the cooling day.
From Lenhardt R, Negishi C, Sessler DI, et al: The effects of physical treatment on induced fever in humans. Am J Med 106:550-555, 1999.

patients is intuitive. However, it frequently fails to reduce core temperature—while simultaneously worsening the situation by triggering thermoregulatory defenses, including intense discomfort, shivering, and activation of the autonomic nervous system.[185] Active cooling of febrile patients should thus be instituted with considerable care to be sure that the putative benefits outweigh the stress induced by the activation of thermoregulatory defenses.

Hyperthermia During Epidural Analgesia

Hyperthermia frequently complicates epidural analgesia for labor and delivery[186] and in nonpregnant postoperative patients.[187] It is more likely during prolonged labor (i.e., >8 hours). A clinical consequence of this hyperthermia is that women given epidural analgesia are more often administered antibiotics than those treated conventionally are, and their offspring are more commonly treated for sepsis.[188]

Because passive hyperthermia and excessive heat production are unlikely causes, elevated body temperature in laboring and postoperative patients is presumably true fever (i.e., a regulated increase in core temperature) resulting from infection or inflammation.[189] For example, Dashe and coworkers concluded that "Epidural analgesia is associated with intrapartum fever, but only in the presence of placental inflammation. This suggests that the fever reported with epidural analgesia is due to infection rather than the analgesia itself."[189]

The conventional assumption is that hyperthermia is *caused* by the technique, although no convincing mechanism has been proposed. It is worth remembering, though, that pain in "control" patients is usually treated with opioids—which themselves attenuate fever.[178] Fever associated with infection or tissue injury might then be suppressed by the low doses of opioids that are usually given to the "control" patients while being expressed normally in patients given epidural analgesia (Fig. 48-20).[190] The extent to which this mechanism contributes remains to be determined and has been disputed,[191] but no convincing alternative explanation has been advanced.

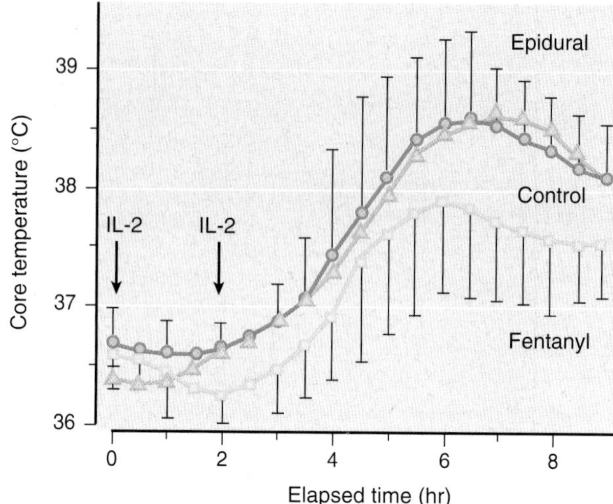

Figure 48-20 Core temperatures after the administration of 50 IU/g of interleukin-2 (IL-2), followed by a second dose of 100 IU/g 2 hours later. The first dose of IL-2 defined elapsed time zero. Data are presented as means ± SD. Error bars for the epidural days are omitted for clarity but were similar to those shown for control and intravenous fentanyl. *(From Negishi C, Lenhardt R, Ozaki M, et al: Opioids inhibit febrile responses in humans, whereas epidural analgesia does not: An explanation for hyperthermia during epidural analgesia. Anesthesiology 94:218-222, 2001.)*

Temperature Monitoring

Core temperature measurements (e.g., tympanic membrane measured with a thermocouple, pulmonary artery, distal part of the esophagus, and nasopharynx) are used to monitor intraoperative hypothermia, prevent overheating, and facilitate detection of malignant hyperthermia. Muscle or skin surface temperatures may be used to evaluate vasomotion[192] and ensure the validity of peripheral neuromuscular monitoring.[193]

Both core and skin surface temperature measurements are required to determine the thermoregulatory effects of different anesthetic drugs. The combination of core and mean skin temperature can be used to estimate mean body temperature—and therefore body heat content—with remarkable accuracy.[194] Temperatures are not uniform within the body; consequently, temperatures measured at each site have different physiologic and practical significance.

Thermometers

Mercury-in-glass thermometers are slow and cumbersome and thus have universally been replaced with electronic systems. The most common electronic thermometers are thermistors and thermocouples. Both devices are sufficiently accurate for clinical use and inexpensive enough to be disposable. Also sufficiently accurate for clinical use are "deep tissue" thermometers that are based on actively reducing the cutaneous heat flux to zero[195]; unfortunately, "deep tissue" thermometers are not currently available in Europe or the United States. Infrared monitors that extrapolate tympanic membrane temperature from outer ear temperature are unreliable,[196] as are infrared systems that scan forehead skin.[197]

Temperature-Monitoring Sites

The core thermal compartment is composed of highly perfused tissues whose temperature is uniform and high in comparison to the rest of the body. Temperature in this compartment can be evaluated in the pulmonary artery, distal part of the esophagus, tympanic membrane, or nasopharynx.[198,199] Temperature probes incorporated into esophageal stethoscopes must be positioned at the point of maximal heart sounds, or even more distally, to provide accurate readings. Even during rapid thermal perturbations such as cardiopulmonary bypass, these temperature-monitoring sites remain reliable. Core temperature can be estimated with reasonable accuracy by using oral, axillary, rectal, and bladder temperatures, except during extreme thermal perturbations.[198,199]

Skin surface temperatures are considerably lower than core temperature. Skin surface temperatures—when adjusted with an appropriate offset—nonetheless reflect core temperature reasonably well.[200] However, skin temperatures fail to reliably confirm

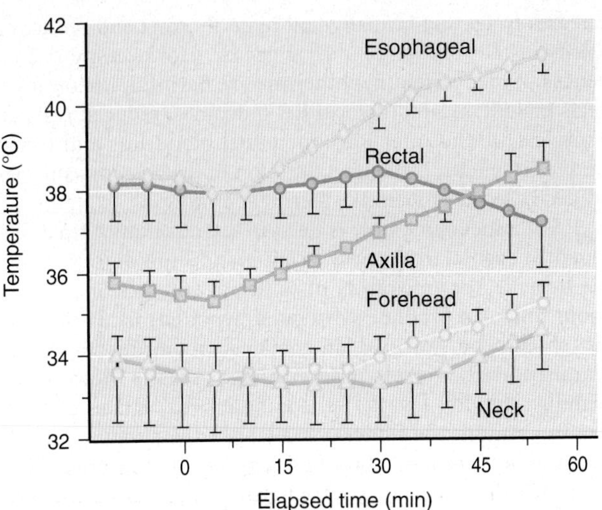

Figure 48-21 Axillary and esophageal temperatures correlated well during acute malignant hyperthermia in swine, but forehead and neck skin temperatures did not. Rectal temperature also failed to promptly identify the onset of malignant hyperthermia. Elapsed time zero indicates an end-tidal Pco_2 of 70 mm Hg. These data indicate that forehead and neck skin surface temperatures will not adequately confirm other clinical signs of malignant hyperthermia. Valid core temperature–monitoring sites include the distal part of the esophagus, pulmonary artery, nasopharynx, and tympanic membrane. Except during cardiopulmonary bypass, body temperature can also be measured in the mouth, axilla, and bladder. Data are presented as means ± SD. *(Modified from Iaizzo PA, Kehler CH, Zink RS, et al: Thermal response in acute porcine malignant hyperthermia. Anesth Analg 82:803-809, 1996.)*

the clinical signs of malignant hyperthermia (tachycardia and hypercapnia) in swine[201] and have not been evaluated for this purpose in humans (Fig. 48-21). Rectal temperature also normally correlates well with core temperature[198,199] but fails to increase appropriately during malignant hyperthermia crises[201] and under other documented situations.[202] Consequently, rectal and skin surface temperatures must be used with considerable caution.

Even during cardiopulmonary bypass, the core temperature–monitoring sites (e.g., tympanic membrane, nasopharynx, pulmonary artery, and esophagus) remain useful. In contrast, rectal temperatures lag behind those measured in core sites. Consequently, rectal temperature is considered an "intermediate" temperature in deliberately cooled patients. During cardiac surgery, bladder temperature is equal to rectal temperature (and therefore intermediate) when urine flow is low, but it is equal to pulmonary artery temperature (and thus core) when flow is high.[203] Because bladder temperature is strongly influenced by urine flow, it may be difficult to interpret in these patients. Adequacy of rewarming is best evaluated by considering both "core" and "intermediate" temperatures.

When Temperature Monitoring Is Required

Core hypothermia is as common during epidural and spinal anesthesia as during general anesthesia and can be nearly as severe.[66] Therefore, core temperature should be measured during regional anesthesia in patients likely to become hypothermic, which at the very least includes those undergoing body cavity surgery.

Core temperature monitoring is appropriate during most general anesthetics both to facilitate detection of malignant hyperthermia and to quantify hyperthermia and hypothermia. By far the most common perioperative thermal disturbance is inadvertent hypothermia. Core temperature usually decreases 0.5°C to 1.5°C in the first 30 minutes after induction of anesthesia. Hypothermia results from internal redistribution of heat and a variety of other factors whose importance in individual patients is hard to predict.[55,68] Core temperature perturbations during the first 30 minutes of anesthesia are thus difficult to interpret, and measurements are not usually required. Body temperature should, however, be monitored in patients undergoing general anesthesia exceeding 30 minutes in duration and in all patients whose surgery lasts longer than 1 hour.

Temperature-Monitoring and Thermal Management Guidelines

The objective of temperature monitoring and perioperative thermal management is to detect thermal disturbances and maintain appropriate body temperature during anesthesia. The data available suggest the following guidelines:

1. Core body temperature should be measured in most patients given general anesthesia for longer than 30 minutes.
2. Temperature should also be measured during regional anesthesia when changes in body temperature are intended, anticipated, or suspected.
3. Unless hypothermia is specifically indicated (e.g., for protection against ischemia), effort should be made to maintain intraoperative core temperature higher than 36°C.*

Various organizations have also proposed temperature-monitoring and thermal management strategies. The ASA standards requires only that "every patient receiving anesthesia shall have temperature monitored when clinically significant changes in body temperature are intended, anticipated or suspected." For office-based sedation, regional anesthesia, or general anesthesia, the ASA also requires that "the body temperature of pediatric patient shall be measured continuously."

The state of New Jersey has stronger requirements, specifically that the body temperature of each patient under general or regional anesthesia shall be continuously monitored. Italy probably has the strongest standards, which require, among other things, that (1) core temperature is measured in adults undergoing general anesthesia for longer than 30 minutes (and all children), (2) ambient operating room temperature exceeds 21°C, (3) patients are kept normothermic, and (4) patients who become hypothermic remain in the postanesthesia care unit until normothermia is restored.

In 2007, the American College of Cardiology and American Heart Association published guidelines for the care of patients undergoing noncardiac surgery. The guidelines include a class 1 recommendation that "maintenance of body temperature in a

*Opinions are the author's and not necessarily shared by the American Society of Anesthesiologists (ASA), but they should be.

normothermic range is recommended for most procedures other than during periods in which mild hypothermia is intended to provide organ protection (e.g., during high aortic cross-clamping)."[204] Based on overwhelming evidence of hypothermia-induced complications, maintaining perioperative normothermia is likely to be among the first anesthetic "pay-for-performance" measures.

Summary

Body temperature is normally controlled by a negative-feedback system in the hypothalamus that integrates thermal information from most tissues. Approximately 80% of this thermal input is derived from core body temperature, which can be measured with distal esophageal, nasopharyngeal, or tympanic membrane thermometer probes. The hypothalamus coordinates increases in heat production (nonshivering thermogenesis and shivering), increases in environmental heat loss (sweating), and decreases in heat loss (vasoconstriction) as needed to maintain normothermia.

Thermal steady state requires that heat loss to the environment equals metabolic heat production; hypothermia occurs when heat loss exceeds production. Mild core hypothermia is common during surgery and anesthesia and results initially from redistribution of body heat from the core to peripheral tissues and subsequently from heat loss exceeding metabolic heat production. Clinical doses of general anesthetics decrease the threshold for response to hypothermia from approximately 37°C (normal) to 33°C to 35°C. Anesthetized patients whose core temperatures exceed these values are usually poikilothermic and do not actively respond to thermal perturbations. Patients becoming sufficiently hypothermic do trigger thermoregulatory vasoconstriction, and the vasoconstriction is remarkably effective in minimizing further core hypothermia.

Mild intraoperative hypothermia provides significant protection against tissue ischemia and hypoxia in animals. Nonetheless, the only situations in which improved outcome has been demonstrated with therapeutic hypothermia in humans is out-of-hospital cardiac arrest and neonatal asphyxia. Hypothermia also decreases triggering of malignant hyperthermia and reduces the severity of the syndrome, once triggered. However, most consequences of inadvertent hypothermia are harmful. Major adverse effects include morbid myocardial outcomes, reduced resistance to surgical wound infections, increased blood loss and transfusion requirements, prolonged duration of drug action, shivering, and decreased postoperative thermal comfort.

Little metabolic heat is lost via the respiratory tract. Consequently, even active airway heating and humidification are of little benefit. Administration of sufficient volumes of cold intravenous fluid can produce substantial hypothermia. Fluids therefore should be warmed in patients requiring intravenous administration of more than several liters per hour; however, fluid warming should always be secondary to active cutaneous warming. Among the clinically available active systems, forced air offers the best combination of efficacy, safety, and price. Forced air can usually maintain normothermia even during the largest operations.

Regional anesthesia produces both peripheral and central inhibition of thermoregulatory control. Peripheral inhibition results when local anesthetics block nerves that are required for thermoregulatory defenses. Hypothermia during neuraxial anesthesia results initially from core-to-peripheral redistribution of body heat and subsequently from heat loss exceeding heat production. Hypothermia during major conduction anesthesia may be as severe as that during general anesthesia.

Increased core temperature can result from augmented thermogenesis (malignant hyperthermia), excessive heating (passive hyperthermia), or a specific increase in the thermoregulatory target temperature (fever). Because the causes of hyperthermia are varied and often serious, the etiology of observed increases in core temperature should be sought and appropriate treatments should be instituted.

A reasonable strategy for detecting and preventing thermal disturbances is to monitor core temperature in patients in whom general anesthesia will last longer than 30 minutes and in those undergoing major surgery with regional anesthesia. Unless hypothermia is specifically indicated (i.e., for protection against cerebral ischemia), core temperature should be maintained above 36°C.

References

1. Brauchi S, Orta G, Salazar M, et al: A hot-sensing cold receptor: C-terminal domain determines thermosensation in transient receptor potential channels. J Neurosci 26:4835-4840, 2006.
2. Poulos DA: Central processing of cutaneous temperature information. Fed Proc 40:2825-2829, 1981.
3. Jessen C, Feistkorn G: Some characteristics of core temperature signals in the conscious goat. Am J Physiol 247:R456-R464, 1984.
4. Simon E: Temperature regulation: The spinal cord as a site of extrahypothalamic thermoregulatory functions. Rev Physiol Biochem Pharmacol 71:1-76, 1974.
5. Cheng C, Matsukawa T, Sessler DI, et al: Increasing mean skin temperature linearly reduces the core-temperature thresholds for vasoconstriction and shivering in humans. Anesthesiology 82:1160-1168, 1995.
6. Lopez M, Sessler DI, Walter K, et al: Rate and gender dependence of the sweating, vasoconstriction, and shivering thresholds in humans. Anesthesiology 80:780-788, 1994.
7. Washington D, Sessler DI, Moayeri A, et al: Thermoregulatory responses to hyperthermia during isoflurane anesthesia in humans. J Appl Physiol 74:82-87, 1993.
8. Hessemer V, Brück K: Influence of menstrual cycle on thermoregulatory, metabolic, and heart rate responses to exercise at night. J Appl Physiol 59:1911-1917, 1985.
9. Mestyan J, Jarai I, Bata G, Fekete M: The significance of facial skin temperature in the chemical heat regulation of premature infants. Biol Neonate 7:243-254, 1964.
10. Vassilieff N, Rosencher N, Sessler DI, Conseiller C: The shivering threshold during spinal anesthesia is reduced in the elderly. Anesthesiology 83:1162-1166, 1995.
11. Hales JRS: Skin arteriovenous anastomoses, their control and role in thermoregulation. *In* Johansen K, Burggren W (eds): Cardiovascular Shunts: Phylogenetic, Ontogenetic and Clinical Aspects. Copenhagen, Munksgaard, 1985, pp 433-451.
12. Greif R, Laciny S, Rajek A, et al: Blood pressure response to thermoregulatory vasoconstriction during isoflurane and desflurane anesthesia. Acta Anaesthesiol Scand 47:847-852, 2003.
13. Dawkins MJR, Scopes JW: Non-shivering thermogenesis and brown adipose tissue in the human new-born infant. Nature 206:201-202, 1965.
14. Jessen K: An assessment of human regulatory non-shivering thermogenesis. Acta Anaesthesiol Scand 24:138-143, 1980.
15. Nedergaard J, Cannon B: The uncoupling protein thermogenin and mitochondrial thermogenesis. New Comp Biochem 23:385-420, 1992.

16. Israel DJ, Pozos RS: Synchronized slow-amplitude modulations in the electromyograms of shivering muscles. J Appl Physiol 66:2358-2363, 1989.
17. Hemingway A, Price WM: The autonomic nervous system and regulation of body temperature. Anesthesiology 29:693-701, 1968.
18. Boudet J, Qing W, Boyer-Chammard A, et al: Dose-response effects of atropine in human volunteers. Fundam Clin Pharmacol 5:635-640, 1991.
19. Kellogg DL Jr: In vivo mechanisms of cutaneous vasodilation and vasoconstriction in humans during thermoregulatory challenges. J Appl Physiol 100:1709-1718, 2006.
20. Matsukawa T, Kurz A, Sessler DI, et al: Propofol linearly reduces the vasoconstriction and shivering thresholds. Anesthesiology 82:1169-1180, 1995.
21. Kurz A, Go JC, Sessler DI, et al: Alfentanil slightly increases the sweating threshold and markedly reduces the vasoconstriction and shivering thresholds. Anesthesiology 83:293-299, 1995.
22. Talke P, Tayefeh F, Sessler DI, et al: Dexmedetomidine does not alter the sweating threshold, but comparably and linearly reduces the vasoconstriction and shivering thresholds. Anesthesiology 87:835-841, 1997.
23. Annadata RS, Sessler DI, Tayefeh F, et al: Desflurane slightly increases the sweating threshold, but produces marked, non-linear decreases in the vasoconstriction and shivering thresholds. Anesthesiology 83:1205-1211, 1995.
24. Xiong J, Kurz A, Sessler DI, et al: Isoflurane produces marked and non-linear decreases in the vasoconstriction and shivering thresholds. Anesthesiology 85:240-245, 1996.
25. Kurz A, Xiong J, Sessler DI, et al: Desflurane reduces the gain of thermoregulatory arterio-venous shunt vasoconstriction in humans. Anesthesiology 83:1212-1219, 1995.
26. Ikeda T, Kim J-S, Sessler DI, et al: Isoflurane alters shivering patterns and reduces maximum shivering intensity. Anesthesiology 88:866-873, 1998.
27. Kurz A, Ikeda T, Sessler DI, et al: Meperidine decreases the shivering threshold twice as much as the vasoconstriction threshold. Anesthesiology 86:1046-1054, 1997.
28. Alfonsi P, Adam F, Passard A, et al: Nefopam, a non-sedative benzoxazocine analgesic, selectively reduces the shivering threshold. Anesthesiology 100:37-43, 2004.
29. Washington DE, Sessler DI, McGuire J, et al: Painful stimulation minimally increases the thermoregulatory threshold for vasoconstriction during enflurane anesthesia in humans. Anesthesiology 77:286-290, 1992.
30. Sessler DI, Olofsson CI, Rubinstein EH, Beebe JJ: The thermoregulatory threshold in humans during halothane anesthesia. Anesthesiology 68:836-842, 1988.
31. Sessler DI, Olofsson CI, Rubinstein EH: The thermoregulatory threshold in humans during nitrous oxide–fentanyl anesthesia. Anesthesiology 69:357-364, 1988.
32. Delaunay L, Bonnet F, Liu N, et al: Clonidine comparably decreases the thermoregulatory thresholds for vasoconstriction and shivering in humans. Anesthesiology 79:470-474, 1993.
33. Delaunay L, Herail T, Sessler DI, et al: Clonidine increases the sweating threshold, but does not reduce the gain of sweating. Anesth Analg 83:844-848, 1996.
34. Ozaki M, Sessler DI, Suzuki H, et al: Nitrous oxide decreases the threshold for vasoconstriction less than sevoflurane or isoflurane. Anesth Analg 80:1212-1216, 1995.
35. Imamura M, Matsukawa T, Ozaki M, et al: Nitrous oxide decreases the shivering threshold less than isoflurane in rabbits. Br J Anaesth 90:88-90, 2003.
36. Kurz A, Sessler DI, Annadata R, et al: Midazolam minimally impairs thermoregulatory control. Anesth Analg 81:393-398, 1995.
37. Matsukawa T, Hanagata K, Ozaki M, et al: I.M. midazolam as premedication produces a concentration dependent decrease in core temperature in male volunteers. Br J Anaesth 78:396-399, 1997.
38. Bissonnette B, Sessler DI: The thermoregulatory threshold in infants and children anesthetized with isoflurane and caudal bupivacaine. Anesthesiology 73:1114-1118, 1990.
39. Bissonnette B, Sessler DI: Thermoregulatory thresholds for vasoconstriction in pediatric patients anesthetized with halothane or halothane and caudal bupivacaine. Anesthesiology 76:387-392, 1992.
40. Hynson JM, Sessler DI, Moayeri A, McGuire J: Absence of nonshivering thermogenesis in anesthetized humans. Anesthesiology 79:695-703, 1993.
41. Dicker A, Ohlson KB, Johnson L, et al: Halothane selectively inhibits nonshivering thermogenesis. Anesthesiology 82:491-501, 1995.
42. Plattner O, Semsroth M, Sessler DI, et al: Lack of nonshivering thermogenesis in infants anesthetized with fentanyl and propofol. Anesthesiology 86:772-777, 1997.
43. Lopez M, Ozaki M, Sessler DI, Valdes M: Physiological responses to hyperthermia during epidural anesthesia and combined epidural/enflurane anesthesia in women. Anesthesiology 78:1046-1054, 1993.
44. Sessler DI, Hynson J, McGuire J, et al: Thermoregulatory vasoconstriction during isoflurane anesthesia minimally decreases heat loss. Anesthesiology 76:670-675, 1992.
45. Kurz A, Sessler DI, Christensen R, Dechert M: Heat balance and distribution during the core-temperature plateau in anesthetized humans. Anesthesiology 83:491-499, 1995.
46. Ikeda T, Sessler DI, Tayefeh F, et al: Meperidine and alfentanil do not reduce the gain or maximum intensity of shivering. Anesthesiology 88:858-865, 1998.
47. Passias TC, Mekjavic IB, Eiken O: The effect of 30% nitrous oxide on thermoregulatory responses in humans during hypothermia. Anesthesiology 76:550-559, 1992.
48. Hardy JD, Milhorat AT, DuBois EF: Basal metabolism and heat loss of young women at temperatures from 22 degrees C to 35 degrees C. J Nutr 21:383-403, 1941.
49. Maurer A, Micheli JL, Schutz Y, et al: Transepidermal water loss and resting energy expenditure in preterm infants. Helv Paediatr Acta 39:405-418, 1984.
50. Bickler P, Sessler DI: Efficiency of airway heat and moisture exchangers in anesthetized humans. Anesth Analg 71:415-418, 1990.
51. Roe CF: Effect of bowel exposure on body temperature during surgical operations. Am J Surg 122:13-15, 1971.
52. Robinson BJ, Ebert TJ, O'Brien TJ, et al: Mechanisms whereby propofol mediates peripheral vasodilation in humans. Anesthesiology 86:64-72, 1997.
53. Sessler DI, McGuire J, Moayeri A, Hynson J: Isoflurane-induced vasodilation minimally increases cutaneous heat loss. Anesthesiology 74:226-232, 1991.
54. Stevens WC, Cromwell TH, Halsey MJ, et al: The cardiovascular effects of a new inhalation anesthetic, Forane, in human volunteers at constant arterial carbon dioxide tension. Anesthesiology 35:8-16, 1971.
55. Matsukawa T, Sessler DI, Sessler AM, et al: Heat flow and distribution during induction of general anesthesia. Anesthesiology 82:662-673, 1995.
56. Hynson J, Sessler DI: Intraoperative warming therapies: A comparison of three devices. J Clin Anesth 4:194-199, 1992.
57. Sessler DI, Ponte J: Shivering during epidural anesthesia. Anesthesiology 72:816-821, 1990.
58. Ozaki M, Kurz A, Sessler DI, et al: Thermoregulatory thresholds during spinal and epidural anesthesia. Anesthesiology 81:282-288, 1994.
59. Kurz A, Sessler DI, Schroeder M, Kurz M: Thermoregulatory response thresholds during spinal anesthesia. Anesth Analg 77:721-726, 1993.
60. Glosten B, Sessler DI, Ostman LG, et al: Intravenous lidocaine does not cause tremor or alter thermoregulation. Reg Anesth 16:218-222, 1991.
61. Hynson J, Sessler DI, Glosten B, McGuire J: Thermal balance and tremor patterns during epidural anesthesia. Anesthesiology 74:680-690, 1991.
62. Rajek A, Greif R, Sessler DI: Effects of epidural anesthesia on thermal sensation. Reg Anesth Pain Med 26:527-531, 2001.
63. Emerick TH, Ozaki M, Sessler DI, et al: Epidural anesthesia increases apparent leg temperature and decreases the shivering threshold. Anesthesiology 81:289-298, 1994.
64. Leslie K, Sessler DI: Reduction in the shivering threshold is proportional to spinal block height. Anesthesiology 84:1327-1331, 1996.
65. Glosten B, Sessler DI, Faure EAM, et al: Central temperature changes are not perceived during epidural anesthesia. Anesthesiology 77:10-16, 1992.
66. Arkilic CF, Akça O, Taguchi A, et al: Temperature monitoring and management during neuraxial anesthesia: An observational study. Anesth Analg 91:662-666, 2000.
67. Frank SM, Beattie C, Christopherson R, et al: Epidural versus general anesthesia, ambient operating room temperature, and patient age as predictors of inadvertent hypothermia. Anesthesiology 77:252-257, 1992.
68. Matsukawa T, Sessler DI, Christensen R, et al: Heat flow and distribution during epidural anesthesia. Anesthesiology 83:961-967, 1995.
69. Hynson JM, Sessler DI, Moayeri A, et al: The effects of pre-induction warming on temperature and blood pressure during propofol/nitrous oxide anesthesia. Anesthesiology 79:219-228, 1993.
70. Just B, Trévien V, Delva E, Lienhart A: Prevention of intraoperative hypothermia by preoperative skin-surface warming. Anesthesiology 79:214-218, 1993.
71. Glosten B, Hynson J, Sessler DI, McGuire J: Preanesthetic skin-surface warming reduces redistribution hypothermia caused by epidural block. Anesth Analg 77:488-493, 1993.
72. Valley MA, Bourke DL, Hamill MP, Srinivasa NR: Time course of sympathetic blockade during epidural anesthesia: Laser Doppler flowmetry studies of regional skin perfusion. Anesth Analg 76:289-294, 1993.
73. Joris H, Ozaki M, Sessler DI, et al: Epidural anesthesia impairs both central and peripheral thermoregulatory control during general anesthesia. Anesthesiology 80:268-277, 1994.
74. Ponte J, Sessler DI: Extradurals and shivering: Effects of cold and warm extradural saline injections in volunteers. Br J Anaesth 64:731-733, 1990.
75. Harris MM, Lawson D, Cooper CM, Ellis J: Treatment of shivering after epidural lidocaine. Reg Anesth 14:13-18, 1989.

76. Panzer O, Ghazanfari N, Sessler DI, et al: Shivering and shivering-like tremor during labor with and without epidural analgesia. Anesthesiology 90:1609-1616, 1999.
77. Horn E-P, Schroeder F, Wilhelm S, et al: Postoperative pain facilitates non-thermoregulatory tremor. Anesthesiology 91:979-984, 1999.
78. Brownbridge P: Shivering related to epidural blockade with bupivacaine in labour, and the influence of epidural pethidine. Anaesth Intensive Care 14:412-417, 1986.
79. Joris J, Banache M, Bonnet F, et al: Clonidine and ketanserin both are effective treatments for postanesthetic shivering. Anesthesiology 79:532-539, 1993.
80. Doufas AG, Lin CM, Suleman MI, et al: Dexmedetomidine and meperidine additively reduce the shivering threshold in humans. Stroke 34:1218-1223, 2003.
81. Kizilirmak S, Karakas SE, Akça O, et al: Magnesium sulphate stops postanesthetic shivering. Proc N Y Acad Sci 813:799-806, 1997.
82. Wass CT, Lanier WL, Hofer RE, et al: Temperature changes of 1°C alter functional neurologic outcome and histopathology in a canine model of a complete cerebral ischemia. Anesthesiology 83:325-335, 1995.
83. Kawai N, Okauchi M, Morisaki K, Nagao S: Effects of delayed intraischemic and postischemic hypothermia on a focal model of transient cerebral ischemia in rats. Stroke 31:1982-1989, discussion 1989, 2000.
84. Todd MM, Warner DS: A comfortable hypothesis reevaluated: Cerebral metabolic depression and brain protection during ischemia [editorial]. Anesthesiology 76:161-164, 1992.
85. Conroy BP, Lin CY, Jenkins LW, et al: Hypothermic modulation of cerebral ischemic injury during cardiopulmonary bypass in pigs. Anesthesiology 88:390-402, 1998.
86. Bernard SA, Gray TW, Buist MD, et al: Treatment of comatose survivors of out-of-hospital cardiac arrest with induced hypothermia. N Engl J Med 346:557-563, 2002.
87. Hypothermia after Cardiac Arrest Study Group: Mild therapeutic hypothermia to improve the neurologic outcome after cardiac arrest. N Engl J Med 346:549-556, 2002.
88. Gluckman PD, Wyatt JS, Azzopardi D, et al: Selective head cooling with mild systemic hypothermia after neonatal encephalopathy: Multicentre randomised trial. Lancet 365:663-670, 2005.
89. Shankaran S, Laptook AR, Ehrenkranz RA, et al: Whole-body hypothermia for neonates with hypoxic-ischemic encephalopathy. N Engl J Med 353:1574-1584, 2005.
90. Gunn AJ, Gluckman PD, Gunn TR: Selective head cooling in newborn infants after perinatal asphyxia: A safety study. Pediatrics 102:885-892, 1998.
91. Marion DW, Penrod LE, Kelsey SF, et al: Treatment of traumatic brain injury with moderate hypothermia. N Engl J Med 336:540-546, 1997.
92. Clifton GL, Miller ER, Choi SC, et al: Lack of effect of induction of hypothermia after acute brain injury. N Engl J Med 344:556-563, 2001.
93. Polderman KH, Joe RTT, Peerdeman SM, et al: Effects of therapeutic hypothermia on intracranial pressure and outcome in patients with severe head injury. Intensive Care Med 28:1563-1573, 2002.
94. Schwab S, Schwarz S, Spranger M, et al: Moderate hypothermia in the treatment of patients with severe middle cerebral artery infarction. Stroke 29:2461-2466, 1998.
95. Krieger DW, De Georgia MA, Abou-Chebl A, et al: Cooling for acute ischemic brain damage (cool aid): An open pilot study of induced hypothermia in acute ischemic stroke. Stroke 32:1847-1854, 2001.
96. Hindman BJ, Todd MM, Gelb AW, et al: Mild hypothermia as a protective therapy during intracranial aneurysm surgery: A randomized prospective pilot trial. Neurosurgery 44:23-32, 1999.
97. Todd MM, Hindman BJ, Clarke WR, Torner JC: Mild intraoperative hypothermia during surgery for intracranial aneurysm. N Engl J Med 352:135-145, 2005.
98. Dae MW, Gao DW, Sessler DI, et al: Effect of endovascular cooling on myocardial temperature, infarct size, and cardiac output in human-sized pigs. Am J Physiol Heart Circ Physiol 282:H1584-H1591, 2002.
99. Dixon SR, Whitbourn RJ, Dae MW, et al: Induction of mild systemic hypothermia with endovascular cooling during primary percutaneous coronary intervention for acute myocardial infarction. J Am Coll Cardiol 40:1928-1934, 2002.
100. Nesher N, Zisman E, Wolf T, et al: Strict thermoregulation attenuates myocardial injury during coronary artery bypass graft surgery as reflected by reduced levels of cardiac-specific troponin I. Anesth Analg 96:328-335, 2003.
101. Just B, Delva E, Camus Y, Lienhart A: Oxygen uptake during recovery following naloxone. Anesthesiology 76:60-64, 1992.
102. Lenhardt R, Marker E, Goll V, et al: Mild intraoperative hypothermia prolongs postoperative recovery. Anesthesiology 87:1318-1323, 1997.
103. Frank SM, Higgins MS, Breslow MJ, et al: The catecholamine, cortisol, and hemodynamic responses to mild perioperative hypothermia. Anesthesiology 82:83-93, 1995.
104. Kurz A, Sessler DI, Narzt E, et al: Postoperative hemodynamic and thermoregulatory consequences of intraoperative core hypothermia. J Clin Anesth 7:359-366, 1995.
105. Gentilello LM, Jurkovich GJ, Stark MS, et al: Is hypothermia in the victim of major trauma protective or harmful? A randomized, prospective study. Ann Surg 226:439-447, discussion 447-449, 1997.
106. Rajagopalan S, Mascha E, Na J, Sessler DI: The effects of mild perioperative hypothermia on blood loss and transfusion requirement: A meta-analysis. Anesthesiology 108:71-77, 2008.
107. Michelson AD, MacGregor H, Barnard MR, et al: Reversible inhibition of human platelet activation by hypothermia in vivo and in vitro. Thromb Haemost 71:633-640, 1994.
108. Staab DB, Sorensen VJ, Fath JJ, et al: Coagulation defects resulting from ambient temperature–induced hypothermia. J Trauma 36:634-638, 1994.
109. Schmied H, Kurz A, Sessler DI, et al: Mild intraoperative hypothermia increases blood loss and allogeneic transfusion requirements during total hip arthroplasty. Lancet 347:289-292, 1996.
110. Bremmelgaard A, Raahave D, Beir-Holgersen R, et al: Computer-aided surveillance of surgical infections and identification of risk factors. J Hosp Infect 13:1-18, 1989.
111. Van Oss CJ, Absolam DR, Moore LL, et al: Effect of temperature on the chemotaxis, phagocytic engulfment, digestion and O_2 consumption of human polymorphonuclear leukocytes. J Reticuloendothel Soc 27:561-565, 1980.
112. Sheffield CW, Sessler DI, Hopf HW, et al: Centrally and locally mediated thermoregulatory responses alter subcutaneous oxygen tension. Wound Rep Reg 4:339-345, 1997.
113. Kluger MJ: Is fever beneficial? Yale J Biol Med 59:89-95, 1986.
114. Shiozaki T, Hayakata T, Taneda M, et al: A multicenter prospective randomized controlled trial of the efficacy of mild hypothermia for severely head injured patients with low intracranial pressure. Mild Hypothermia Study Group in Japan. J Neurosurg 94:50-54, 2001.
115. Jacobs S, Hunt R, Tarnow-Mordi W, et al: Cooling for newborns with hypoxic ischaemic encephalopathy. Cochrane Database Syst Rev 4:CD003311, 2007.
116. Lienhart A, Fiez N, Deriaz H: Frisson postopératoire: Analyse des principaux facteurs associés. Ann Fr Anesth Reanim 11:488-495, 1992.
117. Eberhart LH, Doderlein F, Eisenhardt G, et al: Independent risk factors for postoperative shivering. Anesth Analg 101:1849-1857, 2005.
118. Soliman MG, Gillies DMM: Muscular hyperactivity after general anaesthesia. Can Anaesth Soc J 19:529-535, 1972.
119. Sessler DI, Israel D, Pozos RS, et al: Spontaneous post-anesthetic tremor does not resemble thermoregulatory shivering. Anesthesiology 68:843-850, 1988.
120. Rosenberg H, Clofine R, Bialik O: Neurologic changes during awakening from anesthesia. Anesthesiology 54:125-130, 1981.
121. Sessler DI, Rubinstein EH, Moayeri A: Physiological responses to mild perianesthetic hypothermia in humans. Anesthesiology 75:594-610, 1991.
122. Horn E-P, Sessler DI, Standl T, et al: Non-thermoregulatory shivering in patients recovering from isoflurane or desflurane anesthesia. Anesthesiology 89:878-886, 1998.
123. Giesbrecht GG, Ducharme MB, McGuire JP: Comparison of forced-air patient warming systems for perioperative use. Anesthesiology 80:671-679, 1994.
124. Alfonsi P, Nourredine KE, Adam F, et al: Effect of postoperative skin-surface warming on oxygen consumption and the shivering threshold. Anaesthesia 58:1228-1234, 2003.
125. De Witte J, Rietman GW, Vandenbroucke G, Deloof T: Post-operative effects of tramadol administered at wound closure. Eur J Anaesthesiol 15:190-195, 1998.
126. Horn E-P, Standl T, Sessler DI, et al: Physostigmine prevents postanesthetic shivering as does meperidine or clonidine. Anesthesiology 88:108-113, 1998.
127. Bilotta F, Pietropaoli P, Sanita R, et al: Nefopam and tramadol for the prevention of shivering during neuraxial anesthesia. Reg Anesth Pain Med 27:380-384, 2002.
128. De Witte J, Sessler DI: Perioperative shivering: Physiology and pharmacology. Anesthesiology 96:467-484, 2002.
129. Kranke P, Eberhart LH, Roewer N, Tramer MR: Pharmacological treatment of postoperative shivering: A quantitative systematic review of randomized controlled trials. Anesth Analg 94:453-460, 2002.
130. Guffin A, Girard D, Kaplan JA: Shivering following cardiac surgery: Hemodynamic changes and reversal. J Cardiothorac Vasc Anesth 1:24-28, 1987.
131. Kurz M, Belani K, Sessler DI, et al: Naloxone, meperidine, and shivering. Anesthesiology 79:1193-1201, 1993.
132. Magnan J, Paterson SJ, Tavani A, Kosterlitz HW: The binding spectrum of narcotic analgesic drugs with different agonist and antagonist properties. Naunyn Schmiedebergs Arch Pharmacol 319:197-205, 1982.
133. Burton AC: Human calorimetry: The average temperature of the tissues of the body. J Nutr 9:261-280, 1935.
134. Kurz A, Sessler DI, Birnbauer F, et al: Thermoregulatory vasoconstriction impairs active core cooling. Anesthesiology 82:870-876, 1995.

135. Plattner O, Xiong J, Sessler DI, et al: Rapid core-to-peripheral tissue heat transfer during cutaneous cooling. Anesth Analg 82:925-930, 1996.
136. Clough D, Kurz A, Sessler DI, et al: Thermoregulatory vasoconstriction does not impede core warming during cutaneous heating. Anesthesiology 85:281-288, 1996.
137. Weiskopf RB: Cardiovascular effects of desflurane in experimental animals and volunteers. Anaesthesia 50:S14-S27, 1995.
138. Szmuk P, Ezri T, Sessler DI, et al: Spinal anesthesia only minimally increases the efficacy of postoperative forced-air rewarming. Anesthesiology 87:1050-1054, 1997.
139. Plattner O, Ikeda T, Sessler DI, et al: Postanesthetic vasoconstriction slows postanesthetic peripheral-to-core transfer of cutaneous heat, thereby isolating the core thermal compartment. Anesth Analg 85:899-906, 1997.
140. Sessler DI, Schroeder M, Merrifield B, et al: Optimal duration and temperature of pre-warming. Anesthesiology 82:674-681, 1995.
141. Rajek A, Lenhardt R, Sessler DI, et al: Tissue heat content and distribution during and after cardiopulmonary bypass at 17°C. Anesth Analg 88:1220-1225, 1999.
142. Rajek A, Lenhardt R, Sessler DI, et al: Tissue heat content and distribution during and after cardiopulmonary bypass at 31°C and 27°C. Anesthesiology 88:1511-1518, 1998.
143. Rajek A, Lenhardt R, Sessler DI, et al: Efficacy of two methods for reducing post-bypass afterdrop. Anesthesiology 92:447-456, 2000.
144. Faries G, Johnston C, Pruitt KM, Plouff RT: Temperature relationship to distance and flow rate of warmed IV fluids. Ann Emerg Med 20:1198-1200, 1991.
145. Morris RH: Operating room temperature and the anesthetized, paralyzed patient. Surgery 102:95-97, 1971.
146. Sessler DI, Schroeder M: Heat loss in humans covered with cotton hospital blankets. Anesth Analg 77:73-77, 1993.
147. Sessler DI, Moayeri A, Støen R, et al: Thermoregulatory vasoconstriction decreases cutaneous heat loss. Anesthesiology 73:656-660, 1990.
148. Simbruner G, Weninger W, Popow C, Herholdt WJ: Regional heat loss in newborn infants: Part II. Heat loss in newborns with various diseases—a method of assessing local metabolism and perfusion. S Afr Med J 68:945-948, 1985.
149. Morris RH, Kumar A: The effect of warming blankets on maintenance of body temperature of the anesthetized, paralyzed adult patient. Anesthesiology 36:408-411, 1972.
150. Crino MH, Nagel EL: Thermal burns caused by warming blankets in the operating room. Anesthesiology 29:149-151, 1968.
151. Stanley TO, Grocott HP, Phillips-Bute B, et al: Preliminary evaluation of the Arctic Sun temperature controlling system during off pump coronary artery bypass surgery. Ann Thorac Surg 75:1140-1144, 2003.
152. Taguchi A, Ratnaraj J, Kabon B, et al: Effects of a circulating-water garment and forced-air warming on body heat content and core temperature. Anesthesiology 100:1058-1064, 2004.
153. Kurz A, Kurz M, Poeschl G, et al: Forced-air warming maintains intraoperative normothermia better than circulating-water mattresses. Anesth Analg 77:89-95, 1993.
154. Rajek A, Greif R, Sessler DI, et al: Core cooling by central-venous infusion of 4°C and 20°C fluid: Isolation of core and peripheral thermal compartments. Anesthesiology 93:629-637, 2000.
155. Mayer SA, Kowalski RG, Presciutti M, et al: Clinical trial of a novel surface cooling system for fever control in neurocritical care patients. Crit Care Med 32:2508-2515, 2004.
156. Doufas AG, Akça O, Barry A, et al: Initial experience with a novel heat-exchanging catheter in neurosurgical patients. Anesth Analg 95:1752-1756, 2002.
157. Zweifler RM, Sessler DI, Zivin JA: Thermoregulatory vasoconstriction and shivering impede therapeutic hypothermia in acute ischemic stroke victims. J Stroke Cerebrovasc Dis 6:100-104, 1997.
158. Mokhtarani M, Mahgob AN, Morioka N, et al: Buspirone and meperidine synergistically reduce the shivering threshold. Anesth Analg 93:1233-1239, 2001.
159. Komatsu R, Orhan-Sungur M, In J, et al: Ondansetron does not reduce the shivering threshold in healthy volunteers. Br J Anaesth 96:732-737, 2006.
160. Komatsu R, Sengupta P, Cherynak G, et al: Doxapram only slightly reduces the shivering threshold in healthy volunteers. Anesth Analg 101:1368-1373, 2005.
161. Wadhwa A, Sengupta P, Durrani J, et al: Magnesium sulphate only slightly reduces the shivering threshold in humans. Br J Anaesth 94:756-762, 2005.
162. Iaizzo PA, Jeon YM, Sigg DC: Facial warming increases the threshold for shivering. J Neurosurg Anesthesiol 11:231-239, 1999.
163. Doufas AG, Wadhwa A, Lin C-M, et al: Neither arm nor face warming reduces the shivering threshold in unanesthetized humans. Stroke 34:1736-1740, 2003.
164. Tveita T, Ytrehus K, Myhre ES, Hevroy O: Left ventricular dysfunction following rewarming from experimental hypothermia. J Appl Physiol 85:2135-2139, 1998.
165. Grigore AM, Mathew J, Grocott HP, et al: Prospective randomized trial of normothermic versus hypothermic cardiopulmonary bypass on cognitive function after coronary artery bypass graft surgery. Anesthesiology 95:1110-1119, 2001.
166. Warm Heart Investigators: Randomised trial of normothermic versus hypothermic coronary bypass surgery. Lancet 343:559-563, 1994.
167. Nesher N, Uretzky G, Insler S, et al: Thermo-wrap technology preserves normothermia better than routine thermal care in patients undergoing off-pump coronary artery bypass and is associated with lower immune response and lesser myocardial damage. J Thorac Cardiovasc Surg 129:1371-1378, 2005.
168. Suga H, Goto Y, Igarashi Y, et al: Cardiac cooling increases Emax without affecting relation between O_2 consumption and systolic pressure-volume area in dog left ventricle. Circ Res 63:61-71, 1988.
169. Okano N, Owada R, Fujita N, et al: Cerebral oxygenation is better during mild hypothermic than normothermic cardiopulmonary bypass. Can J Anaesth 47:131-136, 2000.
170. Weisser J, Martin J, Bisping E, et al: Influence of mild hypothermia on myocardial contractility and circulatory function. Basic Res Cardiol 96:198-205, 2001.
171. Satoh-Kuriwada S, Sasano T, Date H, et al: Centrally mediated reflex vasodilation in the gingiva induced by painful tooth-pulp stimulation in sympathectomized human subjects. J Periodont Res 38:218-222, 2003.
172. Mortola JP, Frappell PB: Ventilatory responses to changes in temperature in mammals and other vertebrates. Annu Rev Physiol 62:847-874, 2000.
173. Piccioni MA, Leirner AA, Auler JO Jr: Comparison of pH-stat versus alpha-stat during hypothermic cardiopulmonary bypass in the prevention and control of acidosis in cardiac surgery. Artif Organs 28:347-352, 2004.
174. Markowitz SD, Mendoza-Paredes A, Liu H, et al: Response of brain oxygenation and metabolism to deep hypothermic circulatory arrest in newborn piglets: Comparison of pH-stat and alpha-stat strategies. Ann Thorac Surg 84:170-176, 2007.
175. Kurth CD, O'Rourke MM, O'Hara IB: Comparison of pH-stat and alpha-stat cardiopulmonary bypass on cerebral oxygenation and blood flow in relation to hypothermic circulatory arrest in piglets. Anesthesiology 89:110-118, 1998.
176. Kurth CD, O'Rourke MM, O'Hara IB, Uher B: Brain cooling efficiency with pH-stat and alpha-stat cardiopulmonary bypass in newborn pigs. Circulation 96:II-358-II-363, 1997.
177. du Plessis AJ, Jonas RA, Wypij D, et al: Perioperative effects of alpha-stat versus pH-stat strategies for deep hypothermic cardiopulmonary bypass in infants. J Thorac Cardiovasc Surg 114:991-1000, discussion 1000-1001, 1997.
178. Bellinger DC, Wypij D, du Plessis AJ, et al: Developmental and neurologic effects of alpha-stat versus pH-stat strategies for deep hypothermic cardiopulmonary bypass in infants. J Thorac Cardiovasc Surg 121:374-383, 2001.
179. Davatelis G, Wolpe SD, Sherry B, et al: Macrophage inflammatory protein-1: A prostaglandin-independent endogenous pyrogen. Science 243: 1066-1068, 1989.
180. Blatteis C: Role of the OVLT in the febrile response to circulating pyrogens. Prog Brain Res 91:409-412, 1992.
181. Blatteis C, Sehic E: Fever: How may circulating pyrogens signal the brain? News Physiol Sci 12:1-9, 1997.
182. Negishi C, Lenhardt R, Sessler DI, et al: Desflurane reduces the febrile response to interleukin-2 administration. Anesthesiology 88:1162-1169, 1998.
183. Negishi C, Kim J-S, Lenhardt R, et al: Alfentanil reduces the febrile response to interleukin-2 in humans. Crit Care Med 28:1295-1300, 2000.
184. Frank SM, Kluger MJ, Kunkel SL: Elevated thermostatic setpoint in postoperative patients. Anesthesiology 93:1426-1431, 2000.
185. Lenhardt R, Negishi C, Sessler DI, et al: The effects of physical treatment on induced fever in humans. Am J Med 106:550-555, 1999.
186. Vinson DC, Thomas R, Kiser T: Association between epidural analgesia during labor and fever. J Fam Pract 36:617-622, 1993.
187. Bredtmann RD, Herden HN, Teichmann W, et al: Epidural analgesia in colonic surgery: Results of a randomized prospective study. Br J Surg 77:638-642, 1990.
188. Lieberman E, Cohen A, Lang J, et al: Maternal intrapartum temperature elevation as a risk factor for cesarean delivery and assisted vaginal delivery. Am J Public Health 89:506-510, 1999.
189. Dashe JS, Rogers BB, McIntire DD, Leveno KJ: Epidural analgesia and intrapartum fever: Placental findings. Obstet Gynecol 93:341-344, 1999.
190. Negishi C, Lenhardt R, Ozaki M, et al: Opioids inhibit febrile responses in humans, whereas epidural analgesia does not: An explanation for hyperthermia during epidural analgesia. Anesthesiology 94:218-222, 2001.
191. Gross JB, Cohen AP, Lang JM, et al: Differences in systemic opioid use do not explain increased fever incidence in parturients receiving epidural analgesia. Anesthesiology 97:157-161, 2002.
192. Rubinstein EH, Sessler DI: Skin-surface temperature gradients correlate with fingertip blood flow in humans. Anesthesiology 73:541-545, 1990.

193. Heier T, Caldwell JE, Sessler DI, et al: The relationship between adductor pollicis twitch tension and core, skin and muscle temperature during nitrous oxide–isoflurane anesthesia in humans. Anesthesiology 71:381-384, 1989.
194. Lenhardt R, Sessler DI: Estimation of mean body temperature from mean skin and core temperature. Anesthesiology 105:1117-1121, 2006.
195. Matsukawa T, Sessler DI, Ozaki M, Kumazawa T: Comparison of distal esophageal temperature to "deep sternal," "deep forehead," and tracheal temperatures. Can J Anaesth 44:433-438, 1997.
196. Imamura M, Matsukawa T, Ozaki M, et al: The accuracy and precision of four infrared aural canal thermometers during cardiac surgery. Acta Anaesthesiol Scand 42:1222-1226, 1998.
197. Suleman MI, Doufas AG, Akça O, et al: Insufficiency in a new temporal-artery thermometer for adult and pediatric patients. Anesth Analg 95:67-71, 2002.
198. Bissonnette B, Sessler DI, LaFlamme P: Intraoperative temperature monitoring sites in infants and children and the effect of inspired gas warming on esophageal temperature. Anesth Analg 69:192-196, 1989.
199. Cork RC, Vaughan RW, Humphrey LS: Precision and accuracy of intraoperative temperature monitoring. Anesth Analg 62:211-214, 1983.
200. Ikeda T, Sessler DI, Marder D, Xiong J: The influence of thermoregulatory vasomotion and ambient temperature variation on the accuracy of core-temperature estimates by cutaneous liquid-crystal thermometers. Anesthesiology 86:603-612, 1997.
201. Iaizzo PA, Kehler CH, Zink RS, et al: Thermal response in acute porcine malignant hyperthermia. Anesth Analg 82:803-809, 1996.
202. Ash CJ, Cook JR, McMurry TA, Auner CR: The use of rectal temperature to monitor heat stroke. Mo Med 89:283-288, 1992.
203. Horrow JC, Rosenberg H: Does urinary catheter temperature reflect core temperature during cardiac surgery? Anesthesiology 69:986-989, 1988.
204. Fleisher LA, Beckman JA, Brown KA, et al: ACC/AHA 2007 guidelines on perioperative cardiovascular evaluation and care for noncardiac surgery. J Am Coll Cardiol 50:1707-1732, 2007.

Index

Note: Page numbers followed by b, f, and t indicate boxes, figures, and tables, respectively.

J

K